KAPLAN & SADOCK'S

Synopsis of Psychiatry

Behavioral Sciences/Clinical Psychiatry

Ninth Edition

Drugs Used in Psychiatry

This guide contains color reproductions of some commonly prescribed psychotherapeutic drugs. This guide mainly illustrates tablets and capsules. A † symbol preceding the name of a drug indicates that other doses are available. Check directly with the manufacturer. (*Although the photos are intended as accurate reproductions of the drug, this guide should be used only as a quick identification aid.*)

†ADDERALL XR®

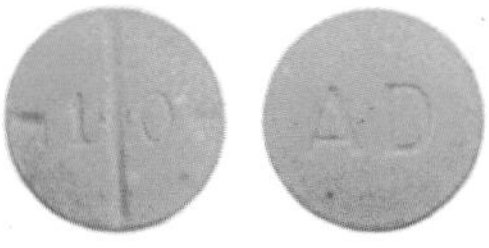

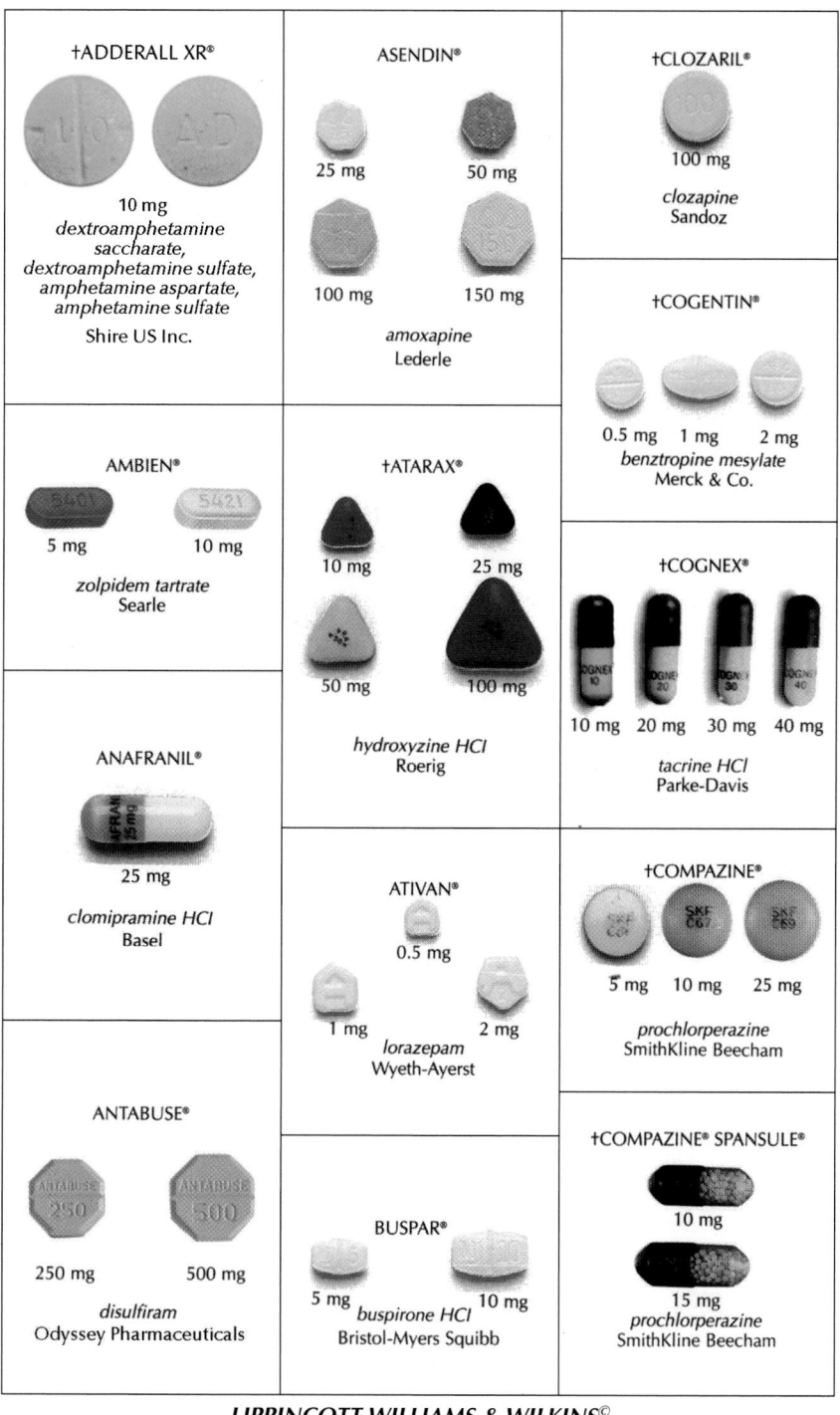

10 mg
dextroamphetamine saccharate, dextroamphetamine sulfate, amphetamine aspartate, amphetamine sulfate
Shire US Inc.

AMBIEN®

5 mg 10 mg
zolpidem tartrate
Searle

ANAFRANIL®

25 mg
clomipramine HCl
Basel

ANTABUSE®

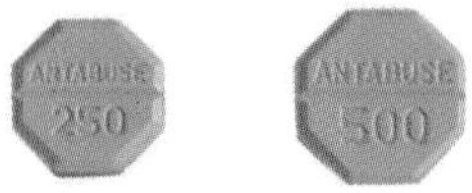

250 mg 500 mg
disulfiram
Odyssey Pharmaceuticals

ASENDIN®

25 mg 50 mg

100 mg 150 mg
amoxapine
Lederle

†ATARAX®

10 mg 25 mg

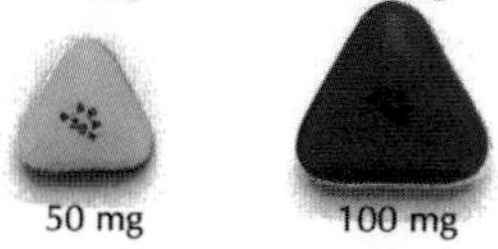

50 mg 100 mg
hydroxyzine HCl
Roerig

ATIVAN®

0.5 mg

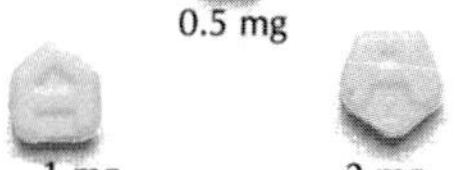

1 mg 2 mg
lorazepam
Wyeth-Ayerst

BUSPAR®

5 mg 10 mg
buspirone HCl
Bristol-Myers Squibb

†CLOZARIL®

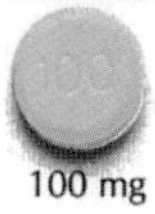

100 mg
clozapine
Sandoz

†COGENTIN®

0.5 mg 1 mg 2 mg
benztropine mesylate
Merck & Co.

†COGNEX®

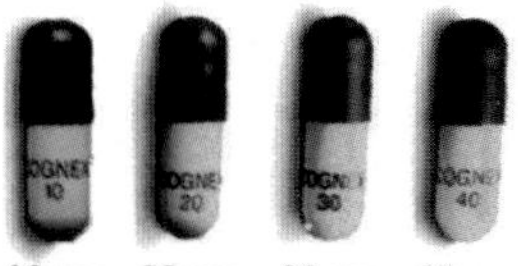

10 mg 20 mg 30 mg 40 mg
tacrine HCl
Parke-Davis

†COMPAZINE®

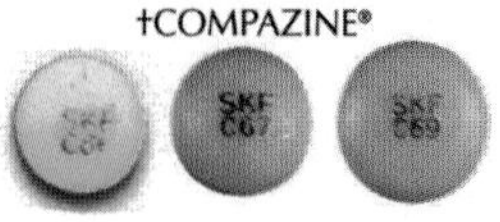

5 mg 10 mg 25 mg
prochlorperazine
SmithKline Beecham

†COMPAZINE® SPANSULE®

10 mg

15 mg
prochlorperazine
SmithKline Beecham

CYLERT®

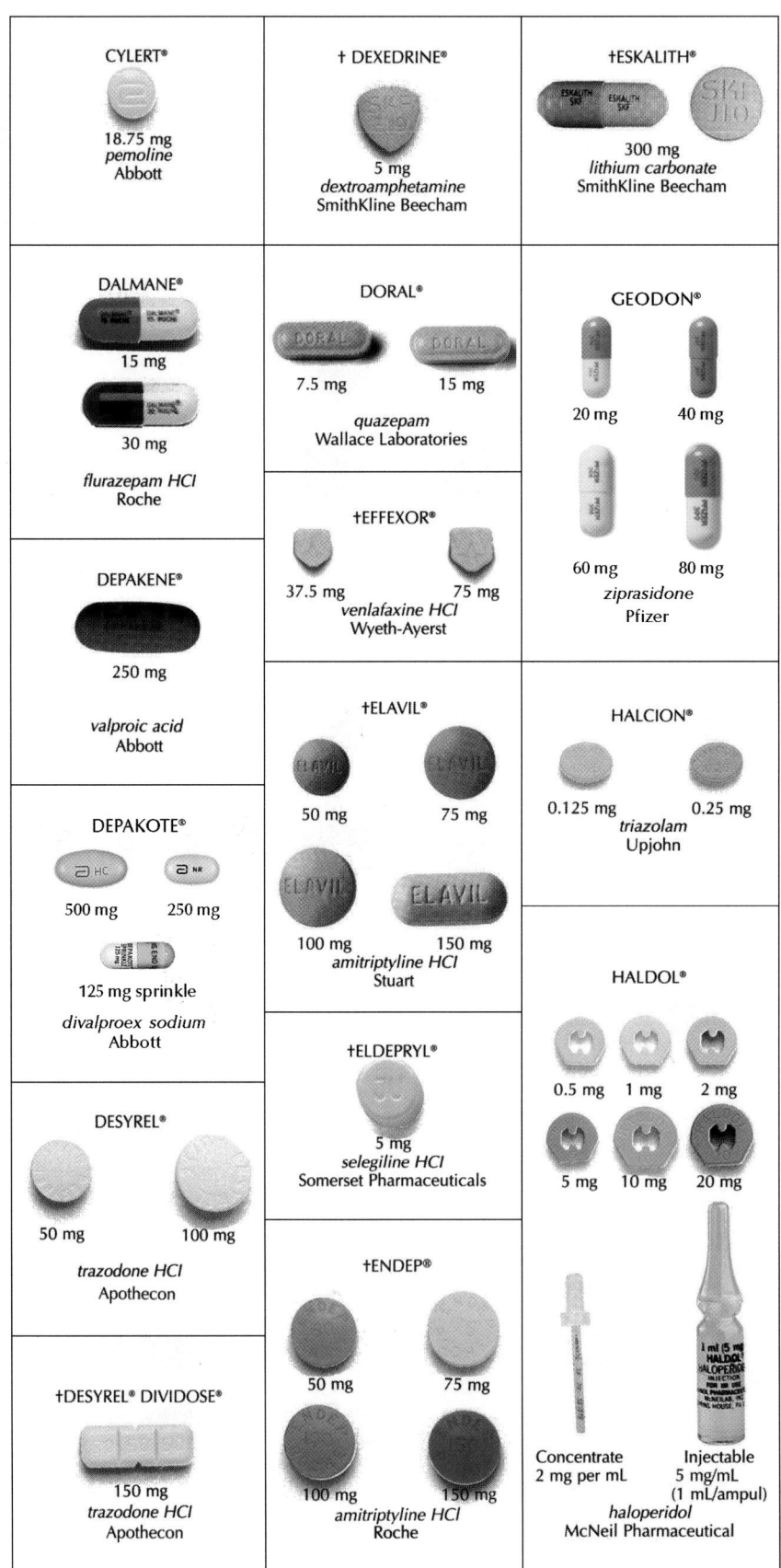

18.75 mg
pemoline
Abbott

DALMANE®

15 mg

30 mg

flurazepam HCl
Roche

DEPAKENE®

250 mg

valproic acid
Abbott

DEPAKOTE®

500 mg   250 mg

125 mg sprinkle

divalproex sodium
Abbott

DESYREL®

50 mg   100 mg

trazodone HCl
Apothecon

†DESYREL® DIVIDOSE®

150 mg
trazodone HCl
Apothecon

† DEXEDRINE®

5 mg
dextroamphetamine
SmithKline Beecham

DORAL®

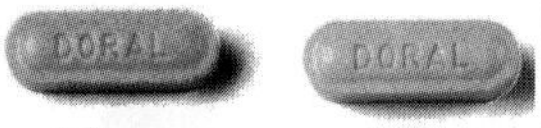

7.5 mg   15 mg

quazepam
Wallace Laboratories

†EFFEXOR®

37.5 mg   75 mg
venlafaxine HCl
Wyeth-Ayerst

†ELAVIL®

50 mg   75 mg

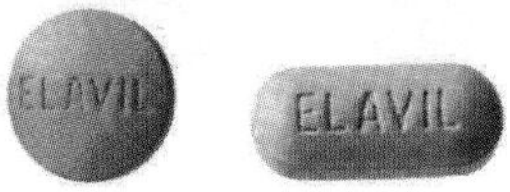

100 mg   150 mg
amitriptyline HCl
Stuart

†ELDEPRYL®

5 mg
selegiline HCl
Somerset Pharmaceuticals

†ENDEP®

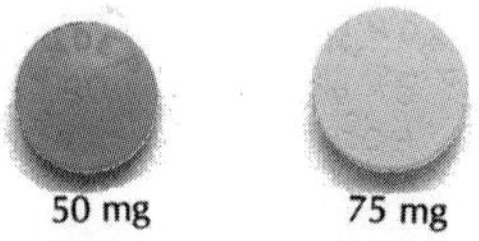

50 mg   75 mg

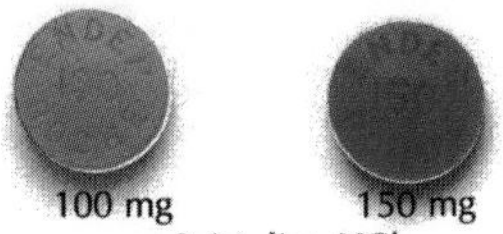

100 mg   150 mg
amitriptyline HCl
Roche

†ESKALITH®

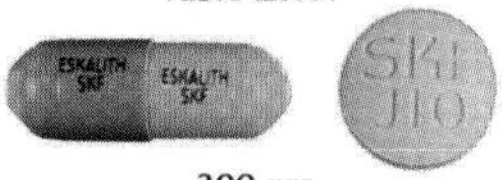

300 mg
lithium carbonate
SmithKline Beecham

GEODON®

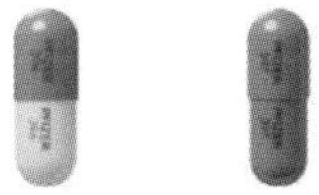

20 mg   40 mg

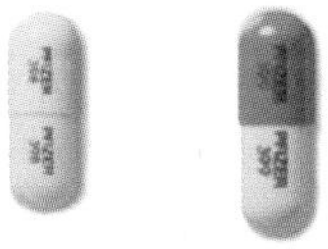

60 mg   80 mg
ziprasidone
Pfizer

HALCION®

0.125 mg   0.25 mg
triazolam
Upjohn

HALDOL®

0.5 mg   1 mg   2 mg

5 mg   10 mg   20 mg

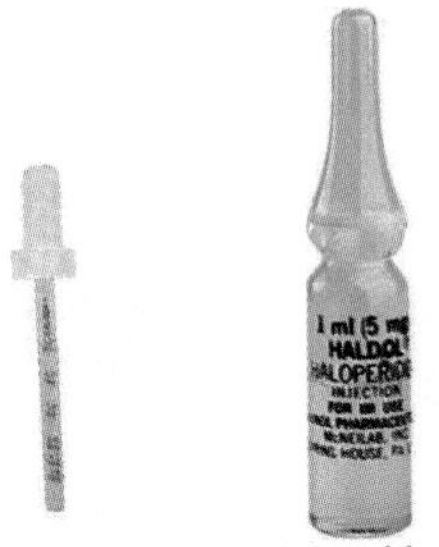

Concentrate
2 mg per mL

Injectable
5 mg/mL
(1 mL/ampul)

haloperidol
McNeil Pharmaceutical

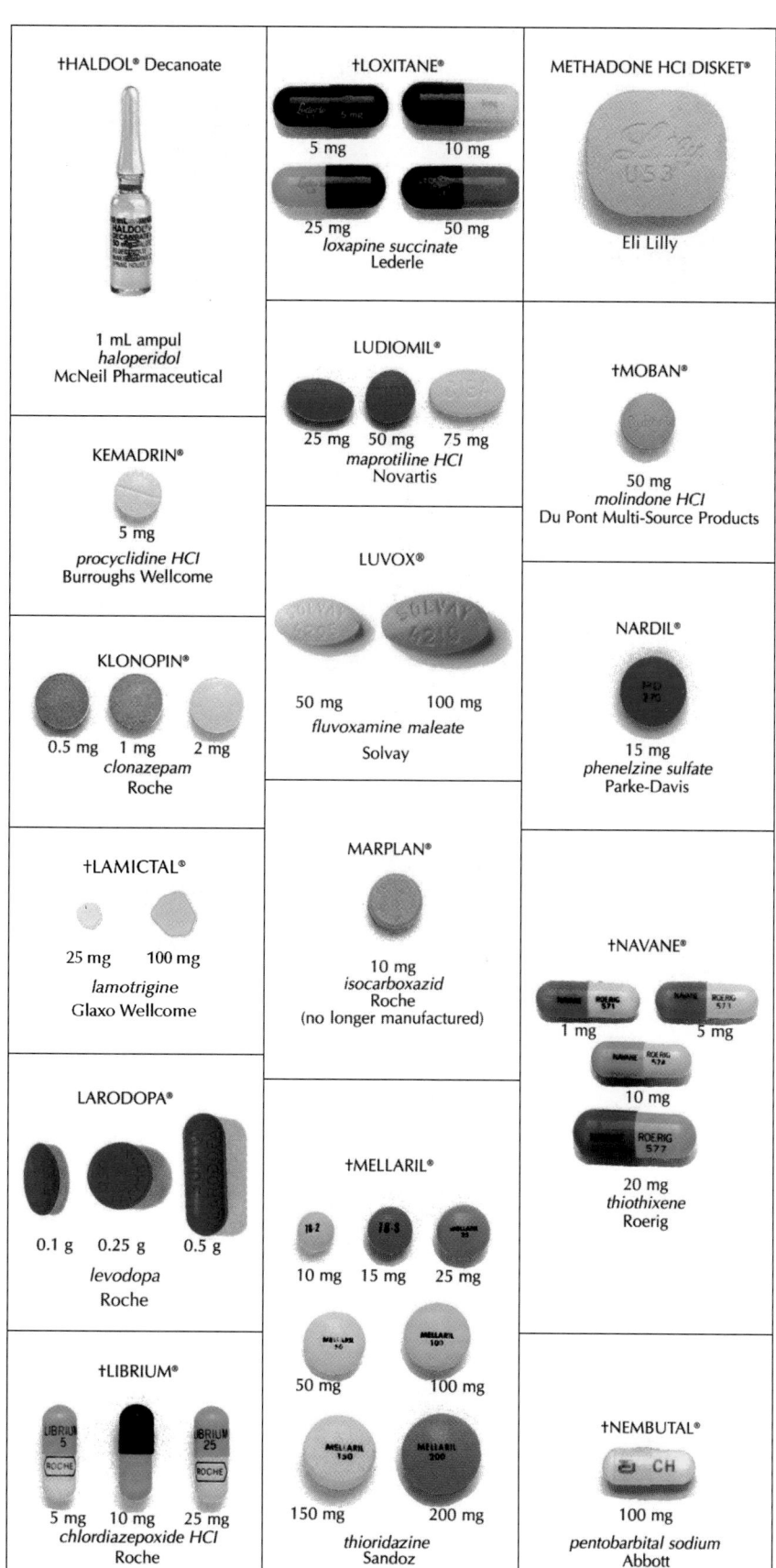

†HALDOL® Decanoate

1 mL ampul
haloperidol
McNeil Pharmaceutical

KEMADRIN®

5 mg
procyclidine HCl
Burroughs Wellcome

KLONOPIN®

0.5 mg 1 mg 2 mg
clonazepam
Roche

†LAMICTAL®

25 mg 100 mg
lamotrigine
Glaxo Wellcome

LARODOPA®

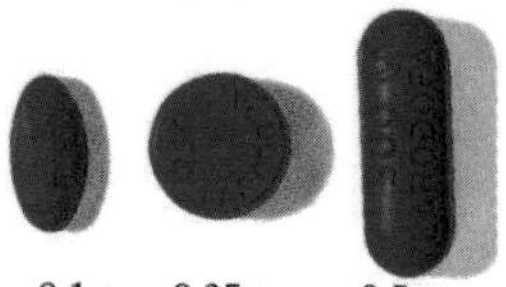

0.1 g 0.25 g 0.5 g
levodopa
Roche

†LIBRIUM®

5 mg 10 mg 25 mg
chlordiazepoxide HCl
Roche

†LOXITANE®

5 mg 10 mg

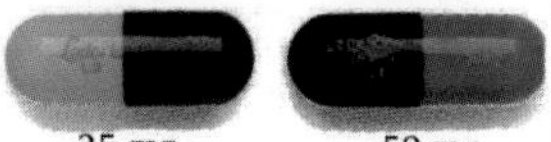

25 mg 50 mg
loxapine succinate
Lederle

LUDIOMIL®

25 mg 50 mg 75 mg
maprotiline HCl
Novartis

LUVOX®

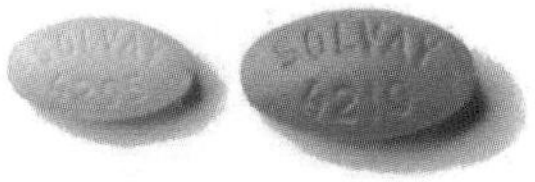

50 mg 100 mg
fluvoxamine maleate
Solvay

MARPLAN®

10 mg
isocarboxazid
Roche
(no longer manufactured)

†MELLARIL®

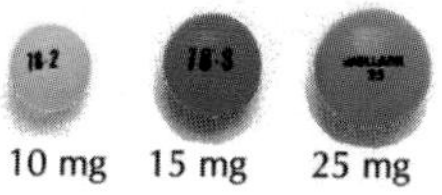

10 mg 15 mg 25 mg

50 mg 100 mg

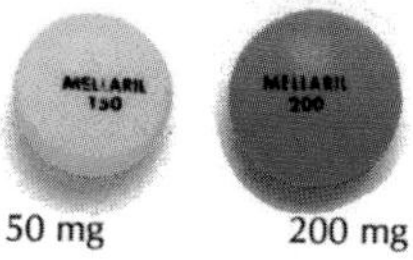

150 mg 200 mg
thioridazine
Sandoz

METHADONE HCl DISKET®

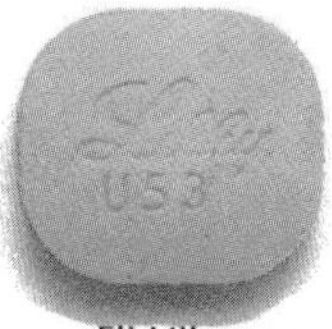

Eli Lilly

†MOBAN®

50 mg
molindone HCl
Du Pont Multi-Source Products

NARDIL®

15 mg
phenelzine sulfate
Parke-Davis

†NAVANE®

1 mg 5 mg

10 mg

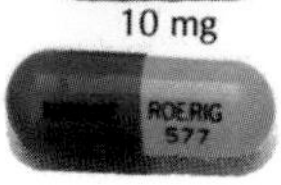

20 mg
thiothixene
Roerig

†NEMBUTAL®

100 mg
pentobarbital sodium
Abbott

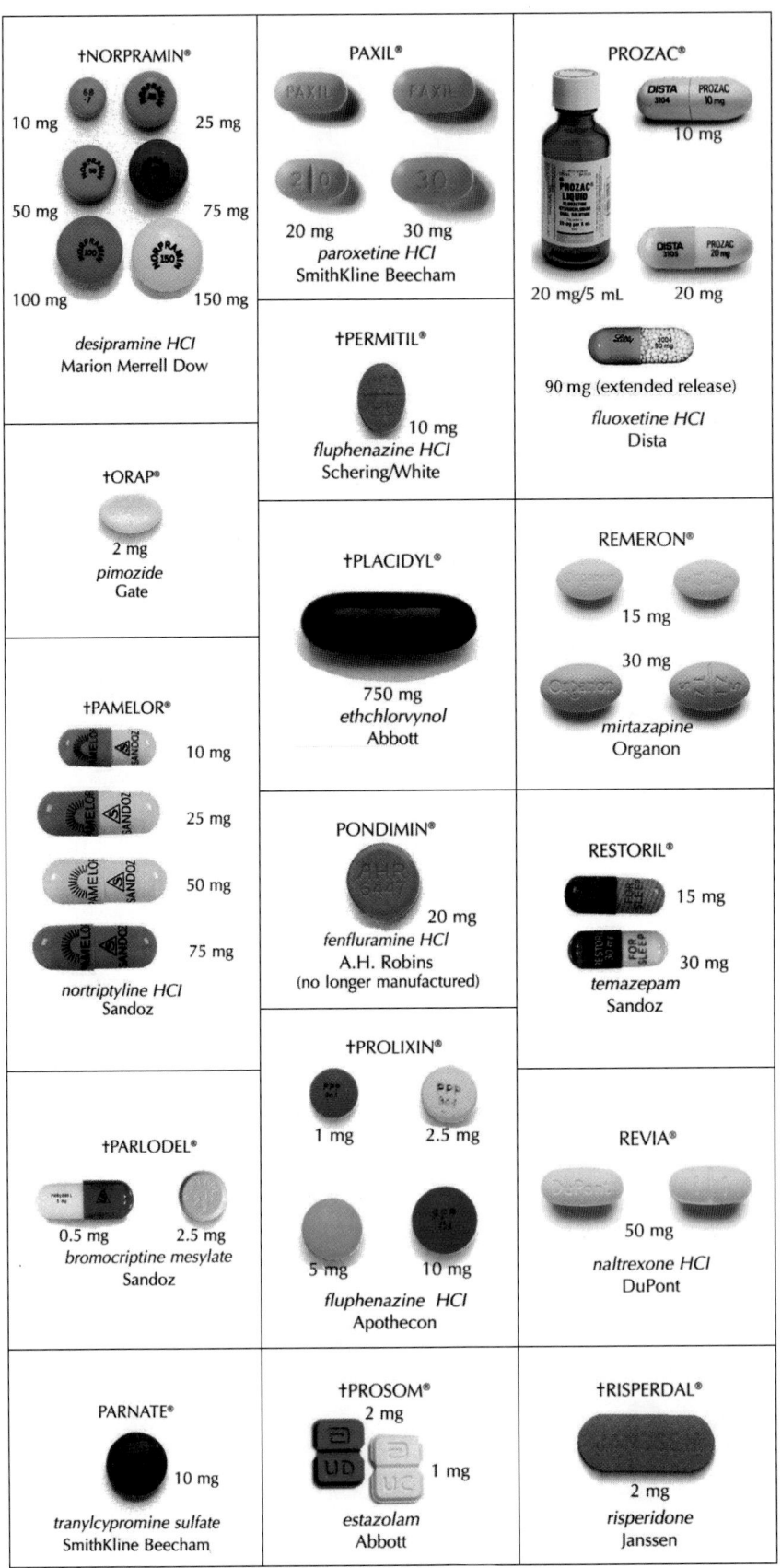

†NORPRAMIN®

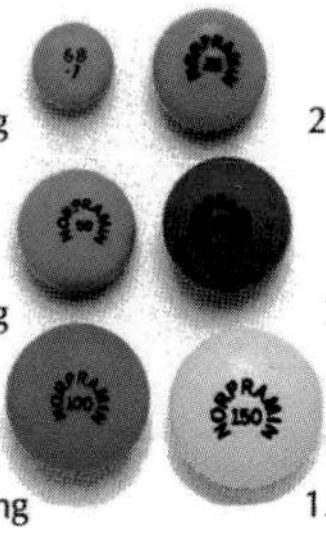

10 mg 25 mg

50 mg 75 mg

100 mg 150 mg

desipramine HCl
Marion Merrell Dow

†ORAP®

2 mg
pimozide
Gate

†PAMELOR®

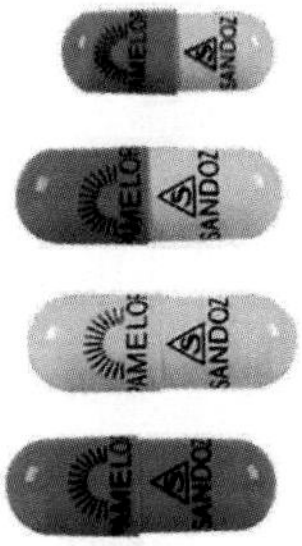

10 mg

25 mg

50 mg

75 mg

nortriptyline HCl
Sandoz

†PARLODEL®

0.5 mg 2.5 mg
bromocriptine mesylate
Sandoz

PARNATE®

10 mg

tranylcypromine sulfate
SmithKline Beecham

PAXIL®

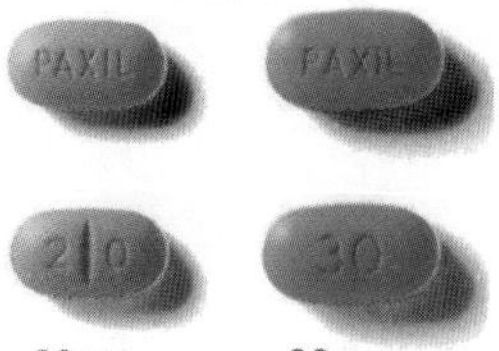

20 mg 30 mg
paroxetine HCl
SmithKline Beecham

†PERMITIL®

10 mg
fluphenazine HCl
Schering/White

†PLACIDYL®

750 mg
ethchlorvynol
Abbott

PONDIMIN®

20 mg
fenfluramine HCl
A.H. Robins
(no longer manufactured)

†PROLIXIN®

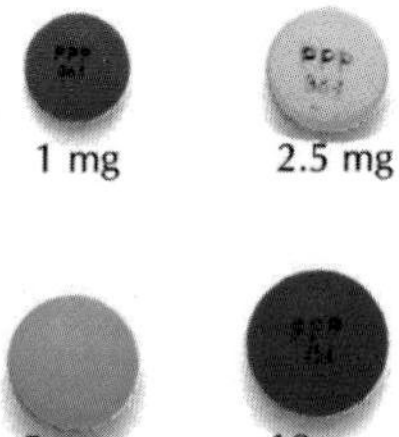

1 mg 2.5 mg

5 mg 10 mg

fluphenazine HCl
Apothecon

†PROSOM®

2 mg

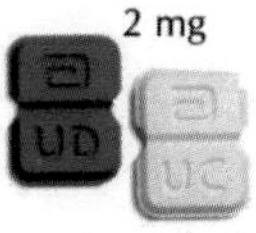

1 mg

estazolam
Abbott

PROZAC®

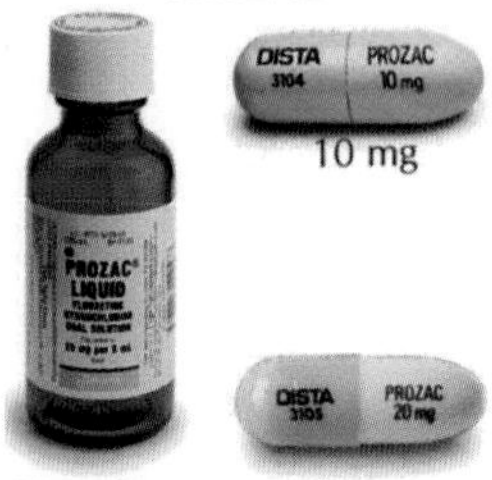

10 mg

20 mg/5 mL 20 mg

90 mg (extended release)

fluoxetine HCl
Dista

REMERON®

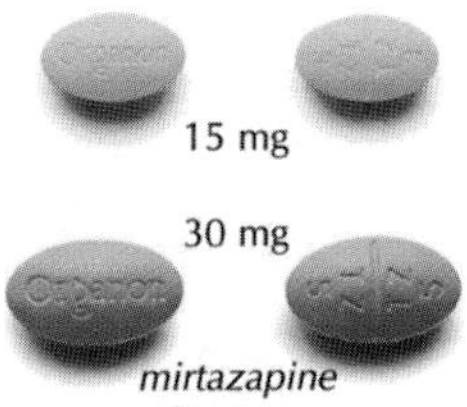

15 mg

30 mg

mirtazapine
Organon

RESTORIL®

15 mg

30 mg

temazepam
Sandoz

REVIA®

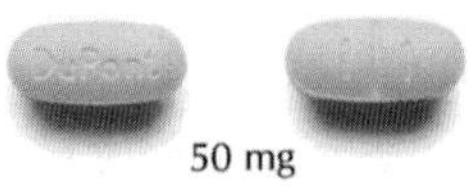

50 mg

naltrexone HCl
DuPont

†RISPERDAL®

2 mg
risperidone
Janssen

RITALIN®

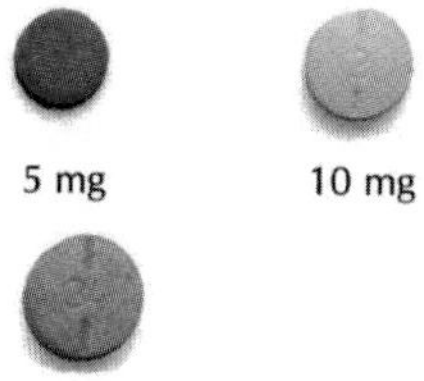

5 mg 10 mg 20 mg

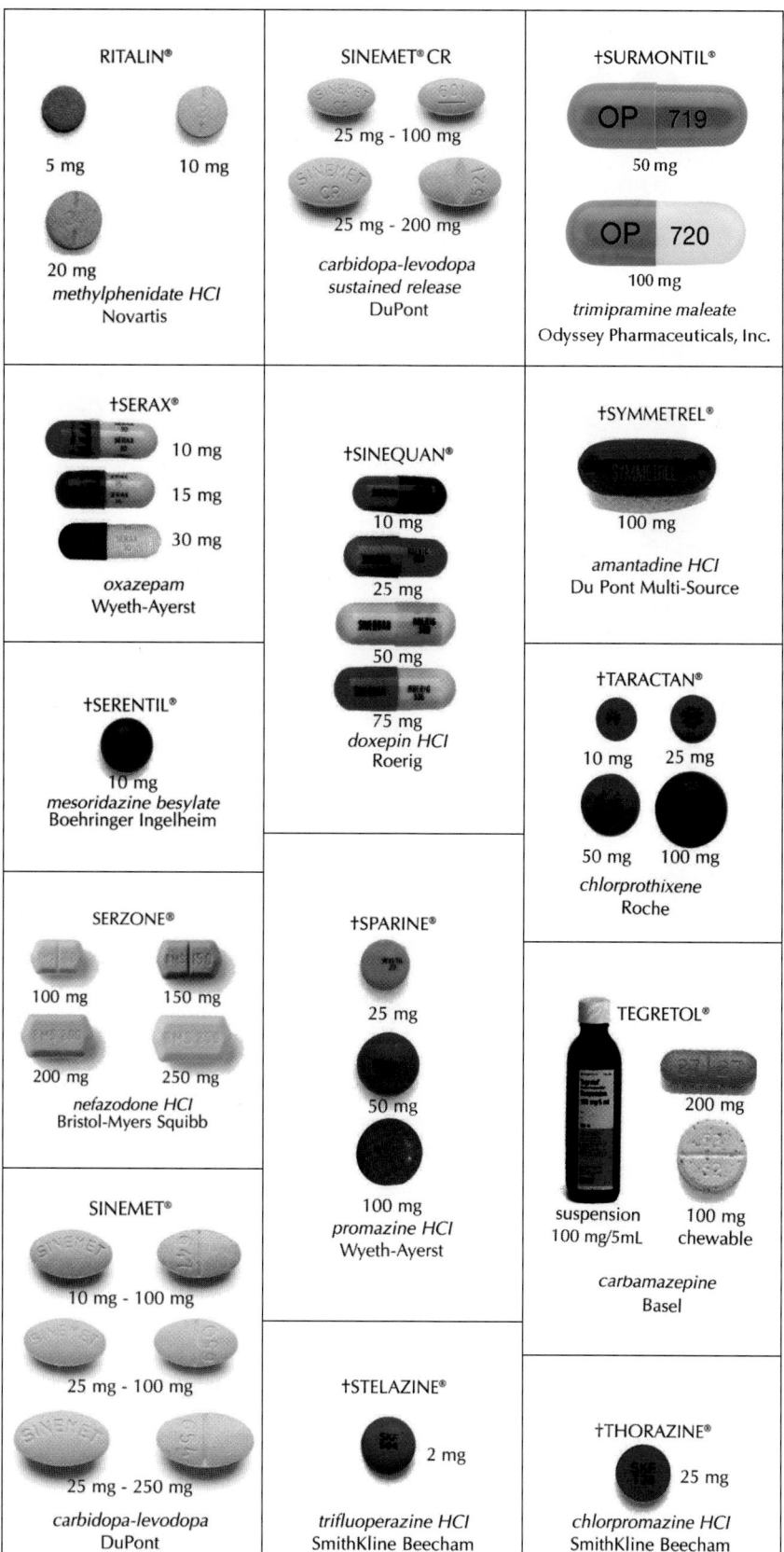

methylphenidate HCl
Novartis

†SERAX®

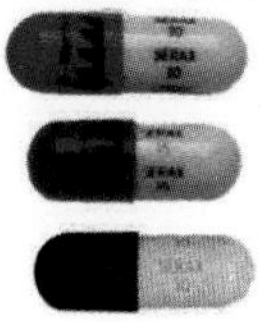

10 mg 15 mg 30 mg

oxazepam
Wyeth-Ayerst

†SERENTIL®

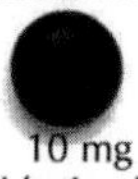

10 mg

mesoridazine besylate
Boehringer Ingelheim

SERZONE®

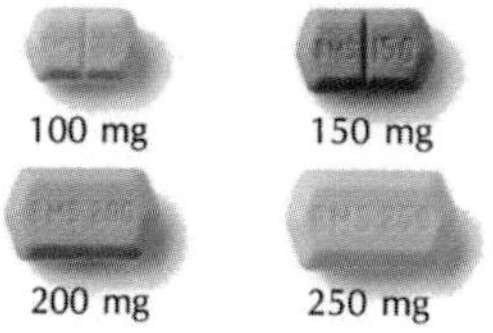

100 mg 150 mg 200 mg 250 mg

nefazodone HCl
Bristol-Myers Squibb

SINEMET®

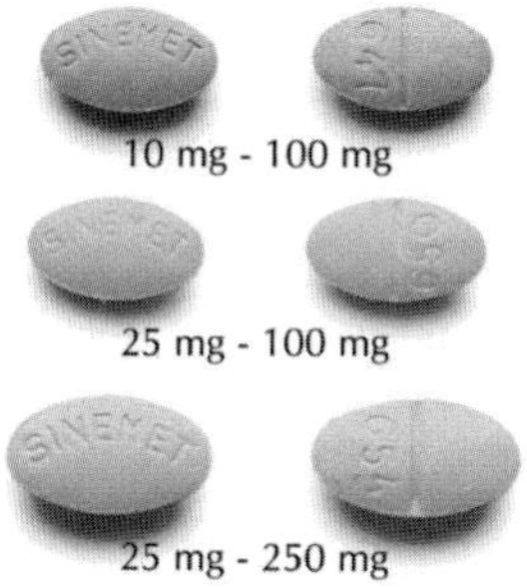

10 mg - 100 mg
25 mg - 100 mg
25 mg - 250 mg

carbidopa-levodopa
DuPont

SINEMET® CR

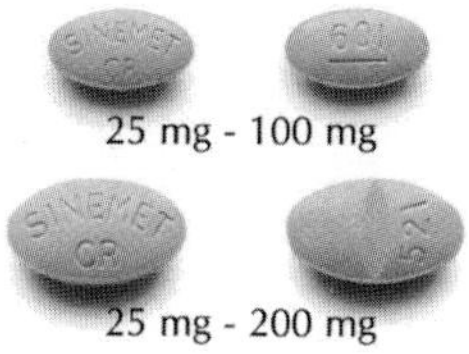

25 mg - 100 mg
25 mg - 200 mg

carbidopa-levodopa sustained release
DuPont

†SINEQUAN®

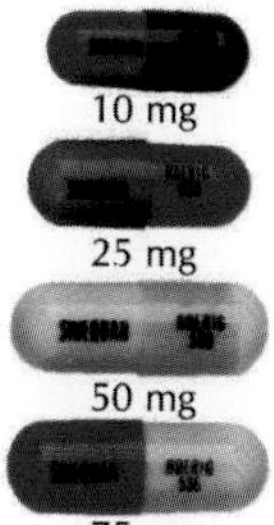

10 mg 25 mg 50 mg 75 mg

doxepin HCl
Roerig

†SPARINE®

25 mg 50 mg 100 mg

promazine HCl
Wyeth-Ayerst

†STELAZINE®

2 mg

trifluoperazine HCl
SmithKline Beecham

†SURMONTIL®

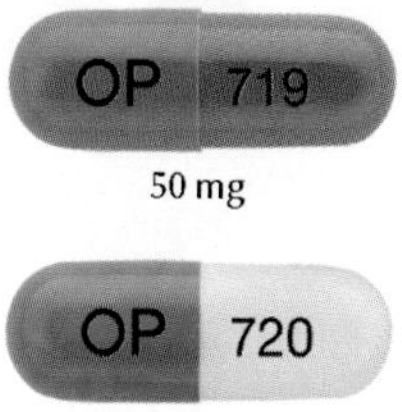

50 mg 100 mg

trimipramine maleate
Odyssey Pharmaceuticals, Inc.

†SYMMETREL®

100 mg

amantadine HCl
Du Pont Multi-Source

†TARACTAN®

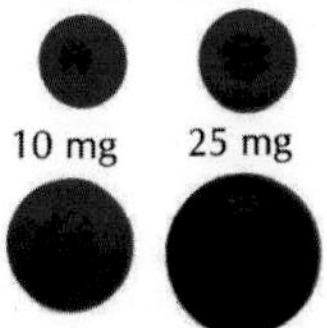

10 mg 25 mg 50 mg 100 mg

chlorprothixene
Roche

TEGRETOL®

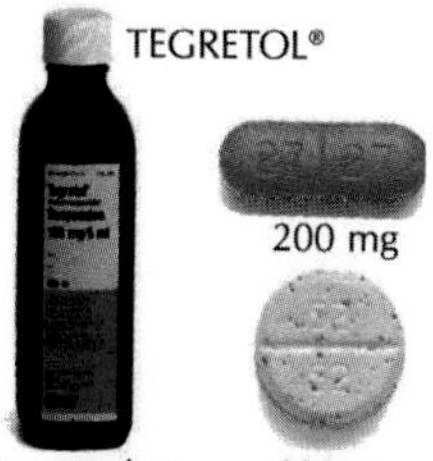

200 mg
suspension 100 mg/5mL
100 mg chewable

carbamazepine
Basel

†THORAZINE®

25 mg

chlorpromazine HCl
SmithKline Beecham

LIPPINCOTT WILLIAMS & WILKINS©

†TOFRANIL®

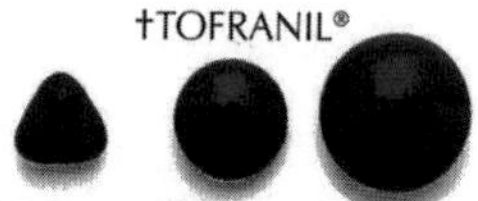

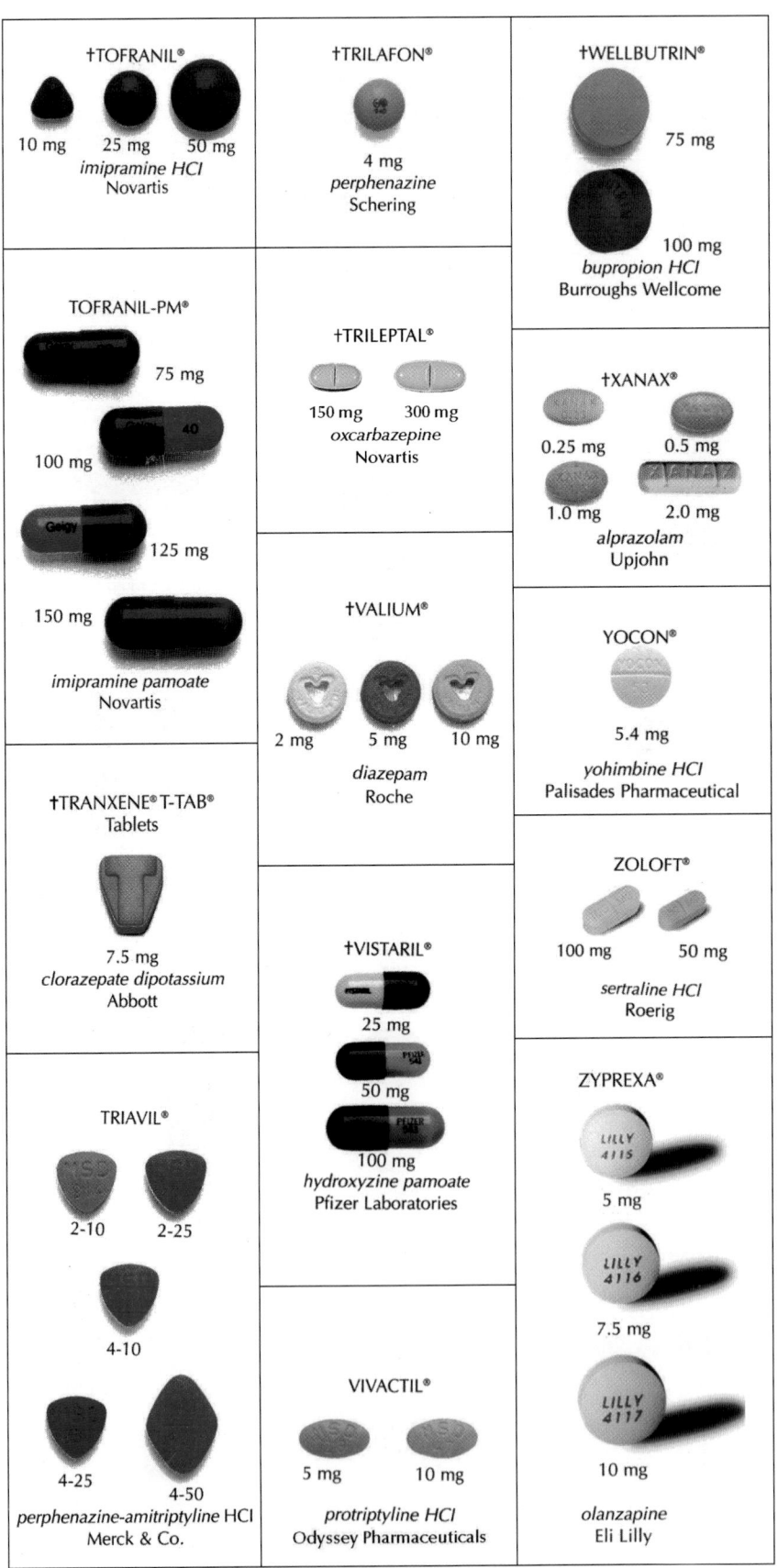

10 mg 25 mg 50 mg
imipramine HCl
Novartis

TOFRANIL-PM®

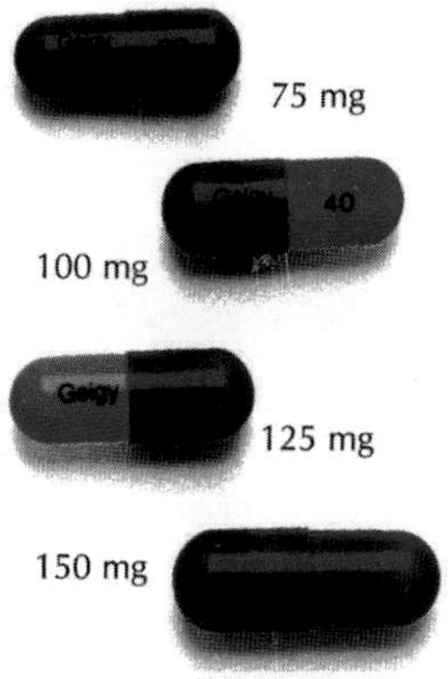

75 mg
100 mg
125 mg
150 mg
imipramine pamoate
Novartis

†TRANXENE® T-TAB®
Tablets

7.5 mg
clorazepate dipotassium
Abbott

TRIAVIL®

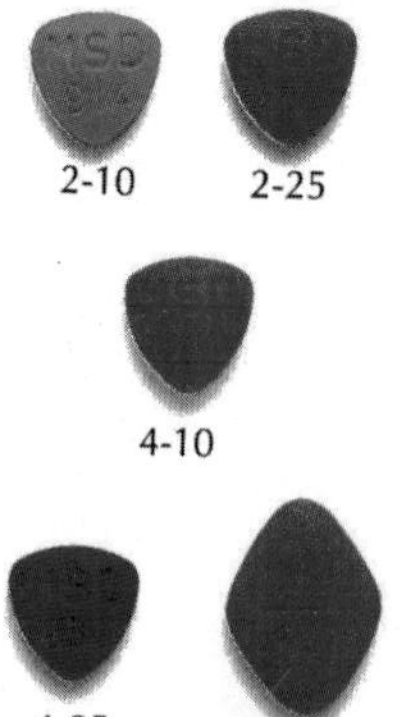

2-10 2-25
4-10
4-25 4-50
perphenazine-amitriptyline HCl
Merck & Co.

†TRILAFON®

4 mg
perphenazine
Schering

†TRILEPTAL®

150 mg 300 mg
oxcarbazepine
Novartis

†VALIUM®

2 mg 5 mg 10 mg
diazepam
Roche

†VISTARIL®

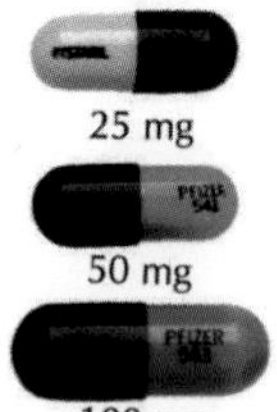

25 mg
50 mg
100 mg
hydroxyzine pamoate
Pfizer Laboratories

VIVACTIL®

5 mg 10 mg
protriptyline HCl
Odyssey Pharmaceuticals

†WELLBUTRIN®

75 mg
100 mg
bupropion HCl
Burroughs Wellcome

†XANAX®

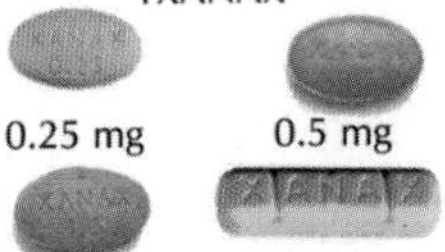

0.25 mg 0.5 mg
1.0 mg 2.0 mg
alprazolam
Upjohn

YOCON®

5.4 mg
yohimbine HCl
Palisades Pharmaceutical

ZOLOFT®

100 mg 50 mg
sertraline HCl
Roerig

ZYPREXA®

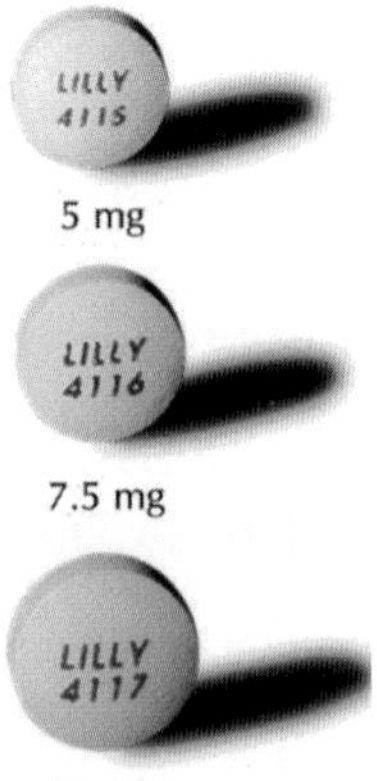

5 mg
7.5 mg
10 mg
olanzapine
Eli Lilly

KAPLAN & SADOCK'S

Synopsis of Psychiatry

Behavioral Sciences/Clinical Psychiatry

Ninth Edition

Senior Consulting Editor

Robert Cancro, M.D., Med.D.Sc.

Lucius N. Littauer Professor and Chairman, Department of Psychiatry, New York University School of Medicine; Director of Psychiatry, Tisch Hospital, The University Hospital of the New York University Medical Center, New York, New York; Director, Nathan S. Kline Institute for Psychiatric Research, Orangeburg, New York

Contributing Editors

James Edmondson, M.D., Ph.D.

Assistant Professor of Psychiatry, Department of Psychiatry, New York University School of Medicine, New York, New York

Glen O. Gabbard, M.D.

Professor of Psychiatry and Director, Menninger Baylor Psychiatry Clinic, Baylor College of Medicine, Houston, Texas

Jack A. Grebb, M.D.

Professor of Psychiatry, Department of Psychiatry, New York University School of Medicine, New York, New York

Myrl Manley, M.D.

Associate Professor of Psychiatry and Director of Medical Student Education in Psychiatry, New York University School of Medicine, New York, New York

Caroly S. Pataki, M.D.

Associate Clinical Professor of Psychiatry and Associate Director of Training and Education for Child and Adolescent Psychiatry, University of California at Los Angeles School of Medicine; Attending Psychiatrist, UCLA Neuropsychiatric Institute, Los Angeles, California

Norman Sussman, M.D.

Professor of Psychiatry, New York University School of Medicine; Director, Psychopharmacology Research and Consultation Service, Bellevue Hospital Center, New York, New York

KAPLAN & SADOCK'S

Synopsis of Psychiatry

Behavioral Sciences/Clinical Psychiatry

NINTH EDITION

Benjamin James Sadock, M.D.

Menas S. Gregory Professor of Psychiatry and Vice Chairman,
Department of Psychiatry, New York University School of Medicine;
Attending Psychiatrist, Tisch Hospital;
Attending Psychiatrist, Bellevue Hospital Center;
Consulting Psychiatrist, Lenox Hill Hospital,
New York, New York

Virginia Alcott Sadock, M.D.

Professor of Psychiatry, Department of Psychiatry,
New York University School of Medicine;
Attending Psychiatrist, Tisch Hospital;
Attending Psychiatrist, Bellevue Hospital Center,
New York, New York

LIPPINCOTT WILLIAMS & WILKINS
A **Wolters Kluwer** Company
Philadelphia • Baltimore • New York • London
Buenos Aires • Hong Kong • Sydney • Tokyo

Acquisitions Editor: Charles W. Mitchell
Developmental Editors: Joyce Murphy and Sarah Mercure
Supervising Editor: Melanie Bennitt
Production Editor: Alyson Langlois, Silverchair Science + Communications
Compositor: Silverchair Science + Communications
Printer: Quebecor Versailles

Printed in the USA

Previous Editions
First Edition 1972
Second Edition 1976
Third Edition 1981
Fourth Edition 1985
Fifth Edition 1988
Sixth Edition 1991
Seventh Edition 1994
Eighth Edition 1998

Library of Congress Cataloging-in-Publication Data
Sadock, Benjamin J.
Kaplan & Sadock's synopsis of psychiatry : behavioral sciences, clinical psychiatry.--
9th ed. / Benjamin James Sadock, Virginia Alcott Sadock.
p. ; cm.
Rev. ed. of: Kaplan and Sadock's synopsis of psychiatry / Harold I. Kaplan, Benjamin J.
Sadock. c1998.
Includes bibliographical references and index.
ISBN 0-7817-3183-6
1. Mental illness. 2. Psychiatry. I. Title: Kaplan and Sadock's synopsis of psychiatry.
II. Title: Synopsis of psychiatry. III. Kaplan, Harold I., 1927-1998, Kaplan and Sadock's
synopsis of psychiatry. IV. Sadock, Virginia A. V. Title.
[DNLM: 1. Mental Disorders. WM 140 S126k 2002]
RC454 .K35 2002
616.89--dc21

2002030009

---

10 9 8 7 6 5 4 3 2 1

Dedicated to all those persons who work with
and care for the mentally ill

Preface

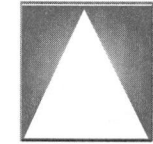

This is the ninth edition of *Synopsis of Psychiatry* to be published since the book first appeared over 30 years ago. It has been updated and revised continually to serve the needs of diverse professional groups—psychiatrists and nonpsychiatric physicians, medical students, psychologists, social workers, psychiatric nurses, and others who work with and care for the mentally ill. It has also been used by nonprofessionals as an authoritative guide to help them collaborate in the care of a family member or friend with mental illness. As authors and editors, we have been extremely gratified by its wide acceptance and use both in this country and around the world.

BACKGROUND

This textbook evolved from our experience editing the *Comprehensive Textbook of Psychiatry.* That book is nearly 3,500 double-column pages long, composed of over 400 contributions by outstanding psychiatrists and behavioral scientists. It serves the needs of those persons who require an exhaustive, detailed, and encyclopedic survey of the entire field. But the *Comprehensive Textbook of Psychiatry,* in an effort to be as comprehensive as possible, spans two volumes in covering the material suitably, clearly rendering it unwieldy for some groups, especially medical students, who need a brief and more condensed statement of the field of psychiatry. For that reason, the authors of *Synopsis* decided to abbreviate, condense, and modify the content of the *Comprehensive Textbook of Psychiatry.* To accomplish this, sections were deleted or condensed, new subjects were introduced, and all sections were brought up to date, especially certain key areas, such as psychopharmacology. We wish to acknowledge our great and obvious debt to the more than 1,500 contributors to the current and previous editions of the *Comprehensive Textbook of Psychiatry* who have allowed us to synopsize their work; at the same time, we must accept responsibility for the modifications and changes in the new work.

Synopsis of Psychiatry stands as a complementary volume to the *Comprehensive Textbook,* characterized by compactness, portability, and up-to-date coverage of the field. It has evolved over the years as a separate and independent textbook that has the reputation of being a consistent, accurate, objective, and reliable compendium of new events in the field of psychiatry.

DSM-IV-TR

A revision of the fourth edition of the *American Psychiatric Association Diagnostic and Statistical Manual of Mental Disorders* (DSM-IV), called DSM-IV-TR (TR stands for text revision), was published in 2000. It contains the official nomenclature used by psychiatrists and other mental health professionals in the United States; the psychiatric disorders discussed in the textbook are consistent with and follow that nosology. Every section dealing with clinical disorders has been updated thoroughly and completely to include the revisions contained in DSM-IV-TR.

DSM is a manual on nosology; it is not, nor has it ever claimed to be, a textbook. *Synopsis* covers the *entire* field of psychiatry and, unlike DSM, allows room for varying points of view, especially about diagnostic categories in which there is ambiguity or controversy. Some psychiatrists have reservations about DSM, and in several sections of *Synopsis* these objections are noted. Terms such as *psychogenic, neurosis,* and *psychosomatic,* among others, are used in this book even though these terms are not part of the official nosology.

ICD-10

Synopsis was the first U.S. textbook to include the definitions and diagnostic criteria of mental disorders used in the tenth revision of the World Health Organization's *International Statistical Classification of Diseases and Related Health Problems* (ICD-10). There are textual differences between DSM and ICD, but according to treaties between the United States and the World Health Organization, the diagnostic code numbers must be identical to ensure uniform reporting of national and international psychiatric statistics. Currently, both DSM and ICD diagnoses and numerical codes are accepted by Medicare, Medicaid, and private insurance companies for reimbursement purposes in the United States. Readers can find the DSM-IV-TR classification with the equivalent ICD-10 classification listed in Chapter 9.

Philosophy

Throughout the years, the goal of this book has been to foster professional competence and ensure the highest quality of care. An eclectic, multidisciplinary approach has been its hallmark,

and this edition maintains that tradition; thus, biological, psychological, and sociological factors are equitably presented as they affect the person in health and disease. The authors are committed to the philosophy of humanitarianism that stresses the dignity, worth, and capacity for self-realization in each individual. Unfortunately, prejudice toward mental illness still exists in many quarters—political policy makers, insurance companies, the general public, and, sadly, the medical profession itself. A principal aim of this textbook is to help eliminate such prejudice, which is largely responsible for the discrimination toward persons with emotional disorders.

Comprehensive Teaching System

The textbook forms one part of a comprehensive system developed by the authors to facilitate the teaching of psychiatry and the behavioral sciences. At the head of the system is the *Comprehensive Textbook of Psychiatry*, which is global in depth and scope; it is designed for and used by psychiatrists, behavioral scientists, and all workers in the mental health field. *Kaplan & Sadock's Synopsis of Psychiatry* is a relatively brief, highly modified, original, and current version useful for medical students, psychiatric residents, practicing psychiatrists, and mental health professionals. Another part of the system is *Study Guide and Self-Examination Review for Synopsis of Psychiatry*, which consists of multiple-choice questions and answers; it is designed for students of psychiatry and for clinical psychiatrists who require a review of the behavioral sciences and general psychiatry in preparation for a variety of examinations. The questions are modeled after and consistent with the format used by the National Board of Medical Examiners and the United States Medical Licensing Examination. Other parts of the system are the pocket handbooks *Pocket Handbook of Clinical Psychiatry, Pocket Handbook of Psychiatric Drug Treatment, Pocket Handbook of Emergency Psychiatric Medicine,* and *Pocket Handbook of Primary Care Psychiatry*. Those books cover the diagnosis and treatment of psychiatric disorders, psychopharmacology, psychiatric emergencies, and primary care psychiatry, respectively, and are designed and written to be carried in the pocket by clinical clerks and practicing physicians, whatever their specialty, to provide a quick reference. Finally, *Comprehensive Glossary of Psychiatry and Psychology* provides simply written definitions for psychiatrists and other physicians, psychologists, students, other mental health professionals, and the general public. Taken together, these books create a multiple approach to the teaching, study, and learning of psychiatry.

CHANGES IN THIS EDITION

Format

Synopsis was among the first textbooks to illustrate psychiatric subjects to enrich the learning experience and to avoid having the reader founder in a sea of type. New illustrations and colorplates have been added to many sections. Colorplates of all psychiatric drugs and their dosage forms, including all new drugs developed since the last edition was published, are also included, as in all *Kaplan & Sadock* books. Color cues differentiate DSM-IV-TR and ICD-10 diagnostic tables as a further aid to the reader.

Case Histories

Case histories make clinical disorders more vital for the student and are an integral part of *Synopsis*. All cases in this edition are new, derived from various sources: *ICD-10 Casebook, DSM-IV Casebook, DSM-IV Case Studies*, contributors to the *Comprehensive Textbook of Psychiatry*, and the authors' clinical experience at New York's Bellevue Hospital Center. We especially wish to thank the American Psychiatric Press and the World Health Organization for permission to use many of their cases. Cases appear in tinted type to help the reader find them easily.

New and Updated Sections

Chapter 3, "The Brain and Behavior," has been reorganized, revised, updated, and extensively rewritten. A new section, "Functional and Behavioral Neuroanatomy," was written to emphasize the influence of function rather than structure on behavior. Another new section, "Psychoneuroendocrinology and Psychoneuroimmunology," reflects the rapid advances in these fields. A newly written section, "Neurogenetics and Molecular Biology," details the complex interaction between nature and nurture in the etiology of psychiatric disorders.

Several chapters appear for the first time. "End-of-Life Care and Palliative Medicine" reflects our belief that psychiatrists have a unique role to play in the emerging clinical specialty of palliative care and pain control. Too little time—especially in medical school—is provided in training students to care for the dying patient with sensitivity and compassion. A new chapter, "Psychiatry and Reproductive Medicine," was written to keep pace with the rapid advances in women's health issues, including the controversial role of hormone replacement therapy in the treatment of mental and other disorders.

This edition continues the tradition of speaking out forcefully on sociopolitical issues that affect the delivery of health care. Practitioners have a special obligation to know about such issues that inform the physical and psychological well-being of their patients. Two new chapters, "Public and Hospital Psychiatry" and "Health Care Delivery in Psychiatry and Medicine," include discussions on many areas of controversy: the homeless mentally ill, deinstitutionalization, working conditions and number of hours medical housestaff are on duty, the role of managed care in medicine and psychiatry, the regulation of medicine by government agencies, and the need for parity between mental and physical illness. The chapter "Ethics in Psychiatry" was completely revised and updated and includes an extensive discussion of the role of euthanasia and physician-assisted suicide and their impact on the practice of medicine.

The section "Mental Disorders Due to a General Medical Condition" contains a new discussion of prion disorders and "mad cow disease." The section "Posttraumatic Stress Disorder and Acute Stress Disorder" includes a discussion of the psychological sequelae of the tragic events of September 11, 2001, involving the World Trade Center in New York and the Pentagon in Washington. The reader will also find a new discussion of the psychiatric aspects of torture and survivors of torture. A new section, "Anthropology and Cross-Cultural Psychiatry,"

reflects the global scope of psychiatry and the need for clinicians to understand disorders that appear around the world. The section "Medical Record" was added because of its relevance to issues of privacy and the interference of government and insurance companies with medical care.

Finally, every section on clinical psychiatry has been updated to include the latest information about diagnosing and treating mental disorders. The references are also completely up-to-date.

Psychopharmacology

Drugs used to treat mental disorders are classified according to their pharmacological activity and mechanism of action to replace such categories as antidepressants, antipsychotics, anxiolytics, and mood stabilizers, which are overly broad and do not reflect the clinical use of psychotropic medication. For example, many antidepressant drugs are used to treat anxiety disorders; some anxiolytics are used to treat depression and bipolar disorders; and drugs from all categories are used to treat other clinical disorders, such as eating disorders, panic disorders, and impulse-control disorders. There are also many drugs used to treat a variety of mental disorders that do not fit into any broad classification. Information about all pharmacological agents used in psychiatry, including pharmacodynamics, pharmacokinetics, dosages, adverse effects, and drug–drug interactions, was thoroughly updated and includes all drugs approved since the last edition was published.

Childhood Disorders

Two chapters, "Adolescent Substance Abuse" and "Forensic Issues in Child Psychiatry," were expanded for this edition to reflect the epidemic of illicit drug use among youth and the problems of violence and delinquency. New data about posttraumatic stress disorders in children have been added, including discussions of false memory syndrome and psychological sequelae in children who have been affected by terrorist activities. Every clinical disorder section was updated and revised, especially those that deal with the use of pharmacological agents in children, which is increasing rapidly.

Acknowledgments

We deeply appreciate the work of our contributing editors, who gave generously of their time and expertise. They include Glen Gabbard, M.D., on psychoanalysis and psychodynamics of clinical disorders; James Edmondson, M.D., on brain and behavior; Caroly Pataki, M.D., on childhood and adolescent disorders; Myrl Manley, M.D., on behavioral sciences; Norman Sussman, M.D., on psychopharmacology; and Jack Grebb, M.D., on biological psychiatry. Dorice Viera, Associate Curator of the Frederick L. Ehrman Medical Library at the New York University School of Medicine, provided valuable assistance. We thank her for her extraordinary help.

Justin Hollingsworth played a key and invaluable role as project editor, as he has in many of our previous books. He was ably assisted by Yande McMillan and Peggy Cuzzolino. Others who deserve thanks are Jay K. Kantor, Ph.D., Jonathan Tobkes, M.D., Henry York, M.D., Mercedes Blackstone, M.D., Tracy Farkas, M.D., Samoon Ahmad, M.D., Lillia de Bosch, M.D., Larry Maayan, M.D., Kathleen Rey, Pamela Miles, Marissa Kaminsky, and Nitza Jones. We also want to thank Anne Schwartz for her excellent editing of this textbook.

We especially wish to acknowledge the contributions of James Sadock, M.D., and Victoria Sadock, M.D., for help in their areas of expertise: emergency adult and emergency pediatric medicine, respectively.

The staff at Lippincott Williams & Wilkins was most efficient. We thank Joyce Murphy, Managing Editor, who worked with us on previous projects, and Charley Mitchell, Executive Editor, who helped us in countless ways.

Finally, we want to express our deepest thanks to Robert Cancro, M.D., Professor and Chairman of the Department of Psychiatry at New York University School of Medicine. Dr. Cancro's commitment to psychiatric education and psychiatric research is recognized throughout the world. He is a much valued and highly esteemed colleague and friend. Our collaboration and association with this outstanding American educator has been a source of great inspiration.

B.J.S.

V.A.S.

Contents

Preface vii

1 The Doctor–Patient Relationship and Interviewing Techniques 1

2 Human Development Throughout the Life Cycle 16

2.1 Normality, Mental Health, and Life Cycle Theory 16
2.2 Prenatal Period, Infancy, and Childhood 21
2.3 Adolescence 35
2.4 Adulthood 41
2.5 Late Adulthood (Old Age) 50
2.6 Death, Dying, and Bereavement 58

3 The Brain and Behavior 66

3.1 Functional and Behavioral Neuroanatomy 66
3.2 Neurophysiology and Neurochemistry 88
3.3 Neuroimaging 108
3.4 Neurogenetics and Molecular Biology 122
3.5 Psychoneuroendocrinology and Psychoneuroimmunology 128

4 Contributions of the Psychosocial Sciences 136

4.1 Jean Piaget 136
4.2 Attachment Theory 139
4.3 Learning Theory 143
4.4 Aggression 150
4.5 Ethology and Sociobiology 158
4.6 Anthropology and Cross-Cultural Psychiatry 166
4.7 Epidemiology and Biostatistics 170

5 Clinical Neuropsychological Testing 178

5.1 Clinical Neuropsychological Testing of Intelligence and Personality 178
5.2 Clinical Neuropsychological Assessment of Adults 185

6 Theories of Personality and Psychopathology 193

6.1 Sigmund Freud: Founder of Classic Psychoanalysis 193
6.2 Erik Erikson 211
6.3 Schools Derived from Psychoanalysis and Psychology 217

7 Clinical Examination of the Psychiatric Patient 229

7.1 Psychiatric History and Mental Status Examination 229
7.2 Medical Record 250
7.3 Physical Examination of the Psychiatric Patient 254
7.4 Laboratory Tests in Psychiatry 260

8 Signs and Symptoms in Psychiatry 275

9 **Classification in Psychiatry and Psychiatric Rating Scales** **288**

10 **Delirium, Dementia, and Amnestic and Other Cognitive Disorders and Mental Disorders Due to a General Medical Condition** **319**

10.1 Overview 319
10.2 Delirium 323
10.3 Dementia 329
10.4 Amnestic Disorders 345
10.5 Mental Disorders Due to a General Medical Condition 350

11 **Neuropsychiatric Aspects of HIV Infection and AIDS** **371**

12 **Substance-Related Disorders** **380**

12.1 Introduction and Overview 380
12.2 Alcohol-Related Disorders 395
12.3 Amphetamine (or Amphetaminelike)-Related Disorders 413
12.4 Caffeine-Related Disorders 419
12.5 Cannabis-Related Disorders 424
12.6 Cocaine-Related Disorders 428
12.7 Hallucinogen-Related Disorders 435
12.8 Inhalant-Related Disorders 440
12.9 Nicotine-Related Disorders 444
12.10 Opioid-Related Disorders 448
12.11 Phencyclidine (or Phencyclidinelike)-Related Disorders 456
12.12 Sedative-, Hypnotic-, or Anxiolytic-Related Disorders 460
12.13 Anabolic Steroid Abuse 466
12.14 Other Substance-Related Disorders 468

13 **Schizophrenia** **471**

14 **Other Psychotic Disorders** **505**

14.1 Schizophreniform Disorder 505
14.2 Schizoaffective Disorder 508
14.3 Delusional Disorder and Shared Psychotic Disorder 511
14.4 Brief Psychotic Disorder, Psychotic Disorder Not Otherwise Specified, and Secondary Psychotic Disorders 520
14.5 Culture-Bound Syndromes 529

15 **Mood Disorders** **534**

15.1 Major Depression and Bipolar Disorder 534
15.2 Dysthymia and Cyclothymia 572
15.3 Other Mood Disorders 578

16 **Anxiety Disorders** **591**

16.1 Overview 591
16.2 Panic Disorder and Agoraphobia 599
16.3 Specific Phobia and Social Phobia 609
16.4 Obsessive-Compulsive Disorder 616
16.5 Posttraumatic Stress Disorder and Acute Stress Disorder 623
16.6 Generalized Anxiety Disorder 632
16.7 Other Anxiety Disorders 636

17 **Somatoform Disorders** **643**

18 **Chronic Fatigue Syndrome and Neurasthenia** **661**

19 **Factitious Disorders** **668**

20 **Dissociative Disorders** **676**

21 **Human Sexuality** **692**

21.1 Normal Sexuality 692
21.2 Abnormal Sexuality and Sexual Dysfunctions 701
21.3 Sexual Disorder Not Otherwise Specified and Paraphilias 718

22 Gender Identity Disorders 730

23 Eating Disorders 739
23.1 Anorexia Nervosa 739
23.2 Bulimia Nervosa and Eating Disorder Not Otherwise Specified 746
23.3 Obesity 751

24 Normal Sleep and Sleep Disorders 756
24.1 Normal Sleep 756
24.2 Sleep Disorders 760

25 Impulse-Control Disorders Not Elsewhere Classified 782

26 Adjustment Disorders 795

27 Personality Disorders 800

28 Psychological Factors Affecting Medical Condition and Psychosomatic Medicine 822
28.1 Overview 822
28.2 Specific Disorders 826
28.3 Treatment of Psychosomatic Disorders 840
28.4 Consultation-Liaison Psychiatry 843

29 Complementary and Alternative Medicine in Psychiatry 851

30 Psychiatry and Reproductive Medicine 868

31 Relational Problems 879

32 Problems Related to Abuse or Neglect 883

33 Additional Conditions That May Be a Focus of Clinical Attention 894

34 Emergency Psychiatric Medicine 901
34.1 Psychiatric Emergencies 901
34.2 Suicide 913

35 Psychotherapies 923
35.1 Psychoanalysis and Psychoanalytic Psychotherapy 923
35.2 Brief Psychotherapy 930
35.3 Group Psychotherapy, Combined Individual and Group Psychotherapy, and Psychodrama 935
35.4 Family Therapy and Couples Therapy 941
35.5 Biofeedback 948
35.6 Behavior Therapy 950
35.7 Cognitive Therapy 956
35.8 Hypnosis 960
35.9 Psychosocial Treatment and Rehabilitation 964
35.10 Combined Psychotherapy and Pharmacotherapy 967

36 Biological Therapies 974
36.1 General Principles of Psychopharmacology 974
36.2 Drug Augmentation Therapy 989
36.3 Medication-Induced Movement Disorders 992
36.4 Psychotherapeutic Drugs 999
36.4.1 α_2-Adrenergic Receptor Agonists: Clonidine and Guanfacine 1005
36.4.2 β-Adrenergic Receptor Antagonists 1008
36.4.3 Amantadine 1011
36.4.4 Anticholinergics 1012
36.4.5 Antihistamines 1015

36.4.6 Barbiturates and Similarly Acting Drugs 1017
36.4.7 Benzodiazepines 1022
36.4.8 Bupropion 1029
36.4.9 Buspirone 1031
36.4.10 Calcium Channel Inhibitors 1033
36.4.11 Carbamazepine 1036
36.4.12 Chloral Hydrate 1040
36.4.13 Cholinesterase Inhibitors 1041
36.4.14 Dantrolene 1045
36.4.15 Disulfiram 1046
36.4.16 Dopamine Receptor Agonists and Precursors: Bromocriptine, Levodopa, Pergolide, Pramipexole, and Ropinirole 1047
36.4.17 Dopamine Receptor Antagonists: Typical Antipsychotics 1050
36.4.18 Lithium 1067
36.4.19 Mirtazapine 1074
36.4.20 Monoamine Oxidase Inhibitors 1076
36.4.21 Nefazodone 1080
36.4.22 Opioid Receptor Agonists: Methadone, Levomethadyl, and Buprenorphine 1082
36.4.23 Opioid Receptor Antagonists: Naltrexone and Nalmefene 1085
36.4.24 Other Anticonvulsants: Gabapentin, Lamotrigine, and Topiramate 1089
36.4.25 Reboxetine 1092
36.4.26 Selective Serotonin Reuptake Inhibitors 1093
36.4.27 Serotonin-Dopamine Antagonists: Atypical Antipsychotics 1104
36.4.28 Sibutramine 1113
36.4.29 Sildenafil 1114
36.4.30 Sympathomimetics and Related Drugs 1116
36.4.31 Thyroid Hormones 1122
36.4.32 Trazodone 1123
36.4.33 Tricyclics and Tetracyclics 1125
36.4.34 Valproate 1131
36.4.35 Venlafaxine 1135
36.4.36 Yohimbine 1137
36.5 Electroconvulsive Therapy 1138
36.6 Other Biological and Pharmacological Therapies 1144

37 Child Psychiatry: Assessment, Examination, and Psychological Testing 1151

38 Mental Retardation 1161

39 Learning Disorders 1180

40 Motor Skills Disorder: Developmental Coordination Disorder 1190

41 Communication Disorders 1194

42 Pervasive Developmental Disorders 1208

43 Attention-Deficit Disorders 1223

44 Disruptive Behavior Disorders 1232

45 Feeding and Eating Disorders of Infancy or Early Childhood 1241

46 Tic Disorders 1246

47 Elimination Disorders 1254

48 Other Disorders of Infancy, Childhood, and Adolescence 1259

48.1 Separation Anxiety Disorder 1259
48.2 Selective Mutism 1265
48.3 Reactive Attachment Disorder of Infancy or Early Childhood 1266

48.4 Stereotypic Movement Disorder and Disorder of Infancy, Childhood, or Adolescence Not Otherwise Specified 1271

49 Mood Disorders and Suicide in Children and Adolescents 1274

50 Early-Onset Schizophrenia 1282

51 Adolescent Substance Abuse 1286

52 Child Psychiatry: Additional Conditions That May Be a Focus of Clinical Attention 1290

53 Psychiatric Treatment of Children and Adolescents 1295

53.1 Individual Psychotherapy 1295
53.2 Group Psychotherapy 1300
53.3 Residential, Day, and Hospital Treatment 1302
53.4 Biological Therapies 1305
53.5 Psychiatric Treatment of Adolescents 1311

54 Forensic Issues in Child Psychiatry 1315

55 Geriatric Psychiatry 1318

56 End-of-Life Care and Palliative Medicine 1338

57 Forensic Psychiatry 1351

58 Ethics in Psychiatry 1365

59 Public and Hospital Psychiatry 1374

60 Health Care Delivery in Psychiatry and Medicine 1382

Index 1391

1

The Doctor–Patient Relationship and Interviewing Techniques

The doctor–patient relationship is at the core of the practice of medicine. It is of utmost concern to all physicians and should be evaluated in all cases. The patient expects a good relationship as much as a cure, and it is common experience that patients are most tolerant of the therapeutic limitations of medicine when there is mutual respect between both parties. Therefore, it is incumbent on all clinicians to consider the nature of the relationship, the factors in themselves and their patients that influence the relationship, and the manner in which good rapport can be achieved.

Rapport is the spontaneous, conscious feeling of harmonious responsiveness that promotes the development of a constructive therapeutic relationship. It implies an understanding and trust between the doctor and patient. With rapport, patients feel accepted with both their assets and liabilities. Frequently, the doctor is the only person to whom they can talk about things that they cannot tell anyone else. Most patients trust their doctors to keep secrets, and this confidence must not be betrayed. Patients who feel that someone knows them, understands them, and accepts them find that a source of strength. "The secret of the care of the patient is in caring for the patient," remarked Francis Peabody (1881–1927), who was a talented teacher, clinician, and researcher.

Whether or not patients feel satisfied with their visits to the doctor is influenced more by interpersonal factors—the perception that the doctor is concerned, caring, and understanding—than by technical competence. This holds true for patients whose purpose in visiting the doctor is to receive medication or undergo a procedure. Medicine is an intensely human and personal endeavor, and the doctor–patient relationship itself becomes part of the therapeutic process.

Self-reflection and understanding are necessary to keep the doctor–patient relationship a positive force. Doctors must empathize with patients, but not to the point of assuming their patients' burdens or fantasizing that they can be their patients' savior. They should be able to leave their patients' problems behind when away from the office or the hospital and should not use their patients as substitutes for intimacy or relationships that may be missing in their personal lives. Otherwise they are handicapped in their efforts to help sick people, who need sympathy and understanding, not sentimentality and overinvolvement.

Physicians are sometimes prone to some defensiveness, partly with good reason; many doctors have been sued, attacked, and even killed because they did not give particular patients the satisfaction they desired. Consequently, some physicians may assume a defensive attitude toward all patients. Although such rigidity may create the image of thoroughness and efficiency, it is frequently inappropriate. Flexibility is necessary to respond to the subtle interplay between doctor and patient and allows a certain tolerance for the uncertainty present in the clinical situation with any patient. Physicians must learn to accept that although they may wish to control everything in a patient's care, this wish can never be fully realized. In some situations a disease cannot be cured, and death cannot be prevented, no matter how conscientious, competent, or caring the physician is. Physicians must also avoid sidestepping issues that they find difficult to deal with because of their own sensitivities, prejudices, or peculiarities, especially when these issues are important to a patient.

THE BIOPSYCHOSOCIAL MODEL

In 1977, George Engel, at the University of Rochester, published a seminal paper that articulated the *biopsychosocial model* of disease, which stressed an integrated approach to human behavior and disease. The biological system refers to the anatomical, structural, and molecular substrates of disease and its effects on patients' biological functioning; the psychological system refers to the effects of psychodynamic factors, motivation, and personality on the experience of, and reaction to, illness; and the social system examines cultural, environmental, and familial influences on the expression and experience of illness. Engle postulates that each system affects and is affected by the others. The model does not treat medical illness as a direct result of a person's psychological or sociocultural makeup but, rather, promotes a more comprehensive understanding of disease and treatment.

A dramatic example of Engel's concept of the biopsychosocial model was a 1971 study of the relationship between sudden death and psychological factors. After investigating 170 sudden deaths over about 6 years, Engel observed that serious illness or even death might be associated with psychological stress or trauma. Among the potential triggering events he listed are the death of a close friend, grief, anniversary reactions, loss of self-esteem, personal danger or threat, the letdown after the threat has passed, and reunions or triumphs.

Beyond the Biopsychosocial Model

Since Engel's paper was first published, the importance of the biopsychosocial model has been recognized and repeated to the point of becoming a kind of catechism in medical education—endlessly repeated but increasingly distant from the way medicine is actually practiced in the real world. While psychological and social variables are unquestionably important in medicine, their proportional importance varies depending on the person and his or her medical circumstances. Chronic conditions such as hypertension or diabetes are affected by multiple aspects of personality and the social environment; however, the short-term treatment of an acute infection may not be. Because the biopsychosocial model offers no guidance on when and which psychosocial factors are important, physicians are often left with the impression that they must know everything about every patient—so obviously impossible that by default they fall back on a biomedical approach, focusing instead on physical pathology and the use of biological, physical interventions.

The biopsychosocial model provides a conceptual framework for dealing with disparate information and serves as a reminder that there may be important issues beyond the purely biological; however, it is not a template for practicing medicine or for treating individual patients. It cannot substitute for a relationship between the patient and doctor that reflects warmth, genuine concern, and mutual trust. For example, attempting to elicit a biopsychosocial understanding of disease outside a doctor–patient relationship that conveys understanding, acceptance, and trust can be destructive rather than helpful, as in the following case:

A 45-year-old professional man recently diagnosed with hepatitis C and mild-to-moderate cirrhosis was referred by his physician to the transplant service of a large teaching hospital for evaluation for a liver transplant. After waiting for over an hour, he was first interviewed by a financial coordinator who asked detailed questions about insurance and resources. He was then shown into a room where he sat across from three people he had never met before: a transplant physician, a nurse practitioner, and a psychiatric social worker. The physician proceeded to read from a series of written questions, seldom looking up from his clipboard to make eye contact. As the patient answered, the physician made notes. The questions were increasingly personal, ranging from "Are you married? Do you have any children? What is your occupation?" to "Do you drink? Did you ever drink? Do you use any intravenous drugs? What is your sexual orientation?" The patient became increasingly uncomfortable and defensive and subsequently registered with a different transplant center despite the original center's strong national reputation.

Spirituality

The role of spirituality and religion in sickness and health has gained ascendancy in recent years, with some suggesting that it become part of the biopsychosocial model. There is some evidence that strong religious beliefs, spiritual yearnings, prayer, and devotional acts have positive influences on a person's mental and physical health. These issues are better attended to by theologians than by physicians; however, doctors need to be aware of spirituality in their patients' lives and sensitive to their patients' religious beliefs. In some instances beliefs may impede medical care, such as the refusal of some religious groups to accept blood transfusions. In most cases, however, when treating patients with strong religious beliefs, the wise physician will welcome the collaboration of the pastoral counselor.

ILLNESS BEHAVIOR

The term *illness behavior* describes patients' reactions to the experience of being sick. Aspects of illness behavior have sometimes been termed the *sick role*, the role that society ascribes to people when they are ill. The sick role can include being excused from responsibilities and the expectation of wanting to obtain help to get well. Illness behavior and the sick role are affected by people's previous experiences with illness and by their cultural beliefs about disease. The influence of culture on reporting and manifestation of symptoms must be evaluated. For some disorders this varies little among cultures, whereas for others the way a person deals with the disorder may strongly shape the way the condition presents itself. The relation of illness to family processes, class status, and ethnic identity is also important. The attitudes of peoples and cultures about dependency and helplessness greatly influence whether and how a person asks for help, as do such psychological factors as personality type and the personal meaning the person attributes to being ill. People react to illness in different ways, which depend on their habitual modes of thinking, feeling, and behaving. Some people experience illness as overwhelming loss; others see in the same illness a challenge they must overcome or a punishment they deserve. Table 1–1 lists essential areas to be addressed in assessing illness behavior and helpful questions for making the assessment.

MODELS OF INTERACTION BETWEEN DOCTOR AND PATIENT

The interactions between a doctor and patient—the questions a patient asks, the way in which news is conveyed and treatment

Table 1–1
Assessment of Individual Illness Behavior

Prior illness episodes, especially illnesses of standard severity (childbirth, renal stones, surgery)
Cultural degree of stoicism
Cultural beliefs concerning the specific problem
Personal meaning of or beliefs about the specific problem
Particular questions to ask to elicit the patient's explanatory model:

1. What do you call your problem? What name does it have?
2. What do you think caused your problem?
3. Why do you think it started when it did?
4. What does your sickness do to you?
5. What do you fear most about your sickness?
6. What are the chief problems that your sickness has caused you?
7. What are the most important results you hope to receive from treatment?
8. What have you done so far to treat your illness?

Courtesy of Mack Lipkin, Jr., M.D.

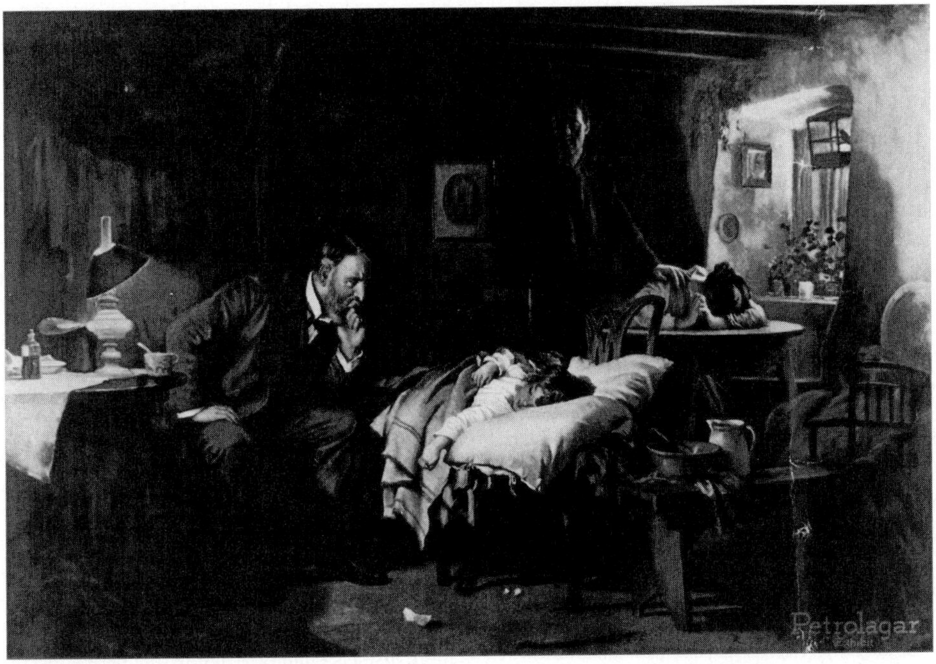

FIGURE 1–1
Painting by Sir Luke Fildes of a physician watching over a sick child. The worried father is standing in the background, and the mother is weeping with her head buried in her arm on the table. (By permission of The New York Academy of Medicine Library, New York, NY.)

recommendations are made—can take different shapes. It is helpful in thinking about the relationship to formulate "models" of interaction. However, these are fluid concepts. A talented, sensitive physician will have different approaches with different patients and indeed may have different approaches with the same patient as time and medical circumstances vary.

1. *The paternalistic model.* In a paternalistic relationship between the doctor and patient, it is assumed that the doctor knows best. He or she will prescribe treatment, and the patient is expected to comply without questioning. Moreover, the doctor may decide to withhold information when it is believed to be in the patient's best interests. In this model, also called the "autocratic model," the physician asks most of the questions and generally dominates the interview.

There are circumstances in which a paternalistic approach is desirable. In emergency situations the doctor needs to take control and make potentially life-saving decisions without long deliberation. In addition, some patients feel overwhelmed by their illness and are comforted by a doctor who can take charge. In general, however, the paternalistic approach risks a clash of values. A paternalistic obstetrician, for example, might insist on spinal anesthesia for delivery when the patient wants to experience natural childbirth.

2. *The informative model.* The doctor in this model dispenses information. All available data are freely given, but the choice is left wholly up to the patient. For example, doctors may quote 5-year survival statistics for various treatments of breast cancer and expect women to make up their own minds without suggestion or interference from them. This model may be appropriate for certain one-time consultations where no established relationship exists and the patient will be returning to the regular care of a known physician. At other times this purely informative approach is likely to be perceived by the patient as cold and uncaring, as it tends to see the patient as unrealistically autonomous.

3. *The interpretive model.* Doctors who have come to know their patients better and understand something of the circumstances of their lives, their families, their values, and their hopes and aspirations, are better able to make recommendations that take into account the unique characteristics of an individual patient. There will be a sense of shared decision making as the doctor presents and discusses alternatives, to find, with the patient's participation, the one that is best for that particular person. The doctor in this model does not abrogate the responsibility for making decisions, but is flexible, and is willing to consider criticism and alternative suggestions.

4. *The deliberative model.* The physician in this model acts as a friend or counselor to the patient, not just by presenting information, but in actively advocating a particular course of action. The deliberative approach is commonly used by doctors hoping to modify injurious behavior, for example, in trying to get their patients to stop smoking or lose weight.

These models are only guides for thinking about the doctor–patient relationship. One is not intrinsically superior to any other, and a physician may use approaches from all four in dealing with a patient during a single visit. Difficulties are most likely to arise not from the use of one or another of the models, but with the physician who is rigidly fixed in one approach and cannot switch strategies, even when indicated and desirable. The models do not, moreover, describe the presence or absence of interpersonal warmth. It is entirely possible for patients to see a paternalistic or autocratic physician as personable, caring, and concerned. In fact a common image of the small town or country doctor in the early part of the 20th century was a man (seldom a woman) totally committed to the welfare of his patients, who would come in the middle of the night and sit at the bedside holding the patient's hand, who would be invited to Sunday dinner, and who expected his instructions to be followed exactly and without question (Fig. 1–1).

TRANSFERENCE AND COUNTERTRANSFERENCE

Doctors and patients may have divergent, distorted, and unrealistic views about each other, about what happens during a clinical encounter, and about what the patient has a right to expect. *Transference* and *countertransference* are terms originating in psychoanalytic theory. They are purely hypothetical constructs, but they have proved extremely useful as organizing principles for explaining certain developments of the doctor–patient relationship that can be upsetting and that can interfere with good medical care.

Transference describes the process of patients unconsciously attributing to their doctors aspects of important past relationships, especially those with their parents. A patient may come to see the doctor as cold, harsh, critical, threatening, seductive, caring, or nurturing, not because of anything the physician says or does, but because that has been the patient's experience in the past. The residue of the experience leads the patient unwittingly to "transfer" the feeling from past relationships to the doctor. The transference can be positive or negative, and it can swing back and forth—sometimes abruptly—between the two. Many a physician has become unsettled when a pleasant, cooperative, and admiring patient suddenly and for no discernible reason becomes enraged and breaks off the relationship or threatens a lawsuit.

In many respects the role of the psychiatrist differs from that of a nonpsychiatric physician, and yet many patients expect the same from the psychiatrist as they do from other physicians. Transference reactions may be strongest with psychiatrists for a number of reasons. For example, as part of intensive, insight-oriented psychotherapy, the encouragement of transference feelings is an integral part of treatment. In some types of therapy, a psychiatrist is more or less neutral. The more neutral or less information the patient has about the psychiatrist, the more transferential fantasies and concerns are mobilized and projected onto the doctor. Once the fantasies are stimulated and projected, the psychiatrist can help patients gain insight into how these fantasies and concerns affect all the important relationships in their lives. Although a nonpsychiatrist does not use transference attitudes in this intensive way, a solid understanding of the power and manifestations of transference is necessary for optimal treatment results in any doctor–patient relationship.

The words and deeds of doctors have a power far beyond the commonplace because of their unique authority and the patients' dependence on them. How a particular physician behaves and interacts has a direct bearing on the emotional and even the physical reactions of the patient. One patient repeatedly had high blood pressure when examined by a physician he considered cold, aloof, and stern. He had normal blood pressure, however, when seen by a doctor he regarded as warm, understanding, and sympathetic.

Physicians themselves are not immune to distorted perceptions of the doctor–patient relationship. When doctors unconsciously ascribe motives or attributes to patients that come from the doctor's past relationships, the process is called *countertransference.* Countertransference may take the form of negative, disruptive feelings, but it may also encompass disproportionately positive, idealizing, or even eroticized reactions. Just as patients have expectations for physicians—for example, competence, objectivity, comfort, and relief—physicians often have unconscious or unspoken expectations of patients. Most commonly patients are thought of as "good" patients if their expressed severity of symptoms correlates with an overtly diagnosable biological disorder, if they are compliant and generally nonchallenging with treatment, if they are emotionally controlled, and if they are grateful. If these expectations are not met, even if this is a result of unconscious unrealistic needs on the part of the physician, the patient may be blamed and considered unlikable, untreatable, or "difficult."

A physician who actively dislikes a patient is apt to be ineffective in dealing with him or her. Emotion breeds counteremotion. For example, if the physician is hostile, the patient becomes more hostile; the physician then becomes even angrier, and the relationship deteriorates rapidly. If the physician can rise above such emotions and handle the resentful patient with equanimity, the interpersonal relationship may shift from mutual overt antagonism to at least increased acceptance and grudging respect. Rising above such emotions involves being able to step back from the intense countertransferential reactions and explore the nature of the relationship more dispassionately. After all, the patient needs the doctor, and hostility ensures that the needed help will not occur. If the doctor can understand that the patient's antagonism is in some way defensive or self-protective and most likely reflects transferential fears of disrespect, abuse, and disappointment, the doctor may be less angry and more empathic.

Patients' responses to their doctors are not invariably transferential and may be based on the real interaction between them. A woman who gets mad at her doctor for keeping her waiting, failing to keep appointments, and not remembering important parts of her medical history is reacting to the reality of her treatment and is not necessarily manifesting transference. Doctors need to be aware of the distorting and disruptive power of transference, but they must not use transference as an excuse for failing to consider the real relationship and the effects their actions have on patients.

INTERVIEWING EFFECTIVELY

One of a physician's most important tools is the ability to interview effectively. Through a skilled interview, physicians can gather the data necessary to understand and treat patients and, in the process, to increase patients' understanding of, and compliance with, the physicians' advice.

Many factors influence both the content and the process of interviews. Patients' personalities and character styles significantly influence reactions as well as the emotional context in which interviews unfold. Various clinical situations—including whether patients are seen on a general hospital ward, on a psychiatric ward, in an emergency room, or as outpatients—shape the questions asked and the recommendations offered. Technical factors such as telephone interruptions, the use of an interpreter, note taking, and the patient's illness itself—whether in an acute stage or in remission—influence the content and process of the interview. Interviewers' styles, experiences, and theoretical orientations also have a significant impact. Even the timing of interjections such as "uh huh" can influence when patients speak and what they do or do not say

Table 1–2
Three Functions of the Medical Interview

Functions	Objectives	Skills
I. Determining the nature of the problem	1. To enable the clinician to establish a diagnosis or recommend further diagnostic procedures, suggest a course of treatment, and predict the nature of the illness	1. Knowledge base of diseases, disorders, problems, and clinical hypotheses from multiple conceptual domains: biomedical, sociocultural, psychodynamic, and behavioral 2. Ability to elicit data for the above conceptual domains (encouraging the patient to tell his or her story; organizing the flow of the interview, the form of questions, the characterization of symptoms, the mental status examination) 3. Ability to perceive data from multiple sources (history, mental status examination, physician's subjective response to the patient, nonverbal cues, listening at multiple levels) 4. Hypothesis generation and testing 5. Developing a therapeutic relationship (function II)
II. Developing and maintaining a therapeutic relationship	1. The patient's willingness to provide diagnostic information 2. Relief of physical and psychological distress 3. Willingness to accept a treatment plan or a process of negotiation 4. Patient satisfaction 5. Physician satisfaction	1. Defining the nature of the relationship 2. Allowing the patient to tell his or her story 3. Hearing, bearing, and tolerating the patient's expression of painful feelings 4. Appropriate and genuine interest, empathy, support, and cognitive understanding 5. Attending to common patient concerns over embarrassment, shame, and humiliation 6. Eliciting the patient's perspective 7. Determining the nature of the problem 8. Communicating information and recommending treatment (function III)
III. Communicating information and implementing a treatment plan	1. Patient's understanding of the illness 2. Patient's understanding of the suggested diagnostic procedures 3. Patient's understanding of the treatment possibilities 4. Consensus between physician and patient about the above items 1 to 3 5. Informed consent 6. Improve coping mechanisms 7. Lifestyle changes	1. Determining the nature of the problem (function I) 2. Developing a therapeutic relationship (function II) 3. Establishing the differences in perspective between physician and patient 4. Educational strategies 5. Clinical negotiations for conflict resolution

Reprinted with permission from Lazare A, Bird J, Lipkin M Jr, Putnam S. Three functions of the medical interview: An integrative conceptual framework. In: Lipkin Jr M, Putnam S, Lazare A, eds. *The Medical Interview.* New York: Springer; 1989:103.

as they unconsciously try to follow the subtle leads and cues provided by the doctor.

Psychiatric versus Medical-Surgical Interviews

Mack Lipkin, Jr., described three functions of medical interviews: to assess the nature of the problem, to develop and maintain a therapeutic relationship, and to communicate information and implement a treatment plan (Table 1–2). These functions are exactly the same as those of psychiatric and surgical interviews. Also universal are the predominant coping mechanisms, both adaptive and maladaptive. These mechanisms include such reactions as anxiety, depression, regression, denial, anger, and dependency (Table 1–3). Physicians must anticipate, recognize, and address such reactions if any treatment and intervention are to be effective.

Psychiatric interviews have two major technical goals: (1) recognition of the psychological determinants of behavior and (2) symptom classification. These goals are reflected in two styles of interviewing: the insight-oriented, or psychodynamic, style and the symptom-oriented, or descriptive, style. *Insight-oriented* interviewing attempts to elicit unconscious conflicts, anxieties, and defenses. The *symptom-oriented* approach emphasizes the classification of patients' complaints and dysfunctions as defined by specific diagnostic categories. The approaches are not mutually exclusive and, in fact, can be compatible. A diagnosis can be described as precisely as possible by eliciting such details as symptoms, course of illness, and family history and by understanding a patient's personality, developmental history, and unconscious conflicts.

Psychiatric patients must often contend with stresses and pressures that differ from those suffered by patients who do not have a psychiatric disorder. These stresses include the stigma attached to being a psychiatric patient (it is more acceptable to have a medical or surgical problem than a mental problem); communication difficulty because of disorders of thinking, and oddities of behavior and impairments of insight and judgment that might make compliance with treatment difficult. Because psychiatric patients often find it difficult to describe fully what is going on, physicians must be prepared to obtain information from other sources. Family members, friends, and spouses can provide critical data such as past psychiatric history, responses to medication, and precipitating stresses that patients may not be able to describe themselves.

Table 1–3
Predictable Reactions to Illness

Intrapsychic	Clinical
Lowered self image → loss → grief	Anxiety or depression
Threat to homeostasis → fear	Denial or anxiety
Failure of (self) care → helplessness, hopelessness	Depression
	Bargaining and blaming
Sense of loss of control → shame (guilt)	Regression
	Isolation
	Dependency
	Anger
	Acceptance

Courtesy of Mack Lipkin, Jr., M.D.

Psychiatric patients may not be able to tolerate a traditional interview format, especially in the acute stages of a disorder. For instance, a patient suffering from increased agitation or depression may not be able to sit for 30 to 45 minutes of discussion or questioning. In such cases, physicians must be prepared to conduct multiple brief interactions over time, for as long as the patient is able, then stopping and returning when the patient appears able to tolerate more.

Physicians must be particularly prepared to use their powers of observation with psychiatric patients who cannot communicate well verbally. Their specific observations should include patients' general appearance, behavior, and body language and the ways in which these factors provide diagnostic clues. According to the American Psychiatric Association's "Practice Guidelines for Psychiatric Evaluation of Adults," the psychiatrists' assessment tool "is the face-to-face interview of the patient: evaluations based solely on review of records and interviews of persons close to the patient are inherently limited."

All physicians who treat psychiatric patients should be familiar with this guideline (Table 1–4) because many nonpsychiatric physicians see psychiatric patients. Studies show that about 60 percent of all patients with mental disorders visit a nonpsychiatric physician during any 6-month period and that patients with mental disorders are twice as likely to visit a primary care physician as are other patients. Nonpsychiatric physicians should be knowledgeable about the special problems of psychiatric patients and the specific techniques used to treat them.

Rapport

Establishing rapport is the first step of a psychiatric interview, and interviewers often use their own empathic responses to facilitate the development of rapport. Ekkehard and Sieglinde Othmer defined the development of rapport as encompassing six strategies: (1) putting patients and interviewers at ease; (2) finding patients' pain and expressing compassion; (3) evaluating patients' insight and becoming an ally; (4) showing expertise; (5) establishing authority as physicians and therapists; and (6) balancing the roles of empathic listener, expert, and authority. As part of a strategy for increasing rapport, Othmer and Othmer developed a checklist (Table 1–5) that enables interviewers to recognize problems and refine their skills in establishing rapport.

In one survey of 700 patients, patients substantially agreed that physicians do not have the time or inclination to listen and consider patients' feelings, that physicians do not have enough knowledge of the emotional problems and socioeconomic background of patients' families, and that physicians increase patients' fear by giving explanations in technical language.

Physicians' failure to establish good rapport with patients accounts for much of the ineffectiveness of care. Rapport implies understanding and trust between doctor and patient. Psychosocial and economic factors exert a profound influence on human relations, and physicians should have as much understanding as possible of patients' subcultures. Differences in social, intellectual, and educational status can interfere seriously with rapport.

Evaluating the social pressures in patients' early lives helps psychiatrists better understand patients. Emotional reactions, healthy or unhealthy, are the result of a constant interplay of biological, sociological, and psychological forces. Each stress leaves behind a trace of its influence and continues to manifest itself throughout life in proportion to the intensity of its effect and the susceptibility of the human being involved. Stresses and strains should be determined to the fullest extent possible. The

Table 1–4
Outline of the APA Practice Guidelines for Psychiatric Evaluation

I. Introduction
  A. General psychiatric evaluation
  B. Emergency evaluation
  C. Clinical consultation
  D. Other consultations
II. Site of the clinical evaluation
  A. Inpatient settings
  B. Outpatient settings
  C. General medical settings
  D. Other settings
III. Domains of the clinical evaluation
  A. Reason for the evaluation
  B. History of the present illness
  C. Past psychiatric history
  D. General medical history
  E. History of substance abuse
  F. Psychosocial developmental history (personal history)
  G. Social history
  H. Occupational history
  I. Family history
  J. Review of systems
  K. Physical examination
  L. Mental status examination
  M. Functional assessment
  N. Diagnostic test
  O. Information derived from the interview process
IV. Evaluation process
  A. Methods of obtaining information
  B. The process of assessment
V. Special considerations
  A. Interactions with third-party payers and their agents
  B. The process of the assessment
VI. Developmental process

Adapted from American Psychiatric Association. Practice guidelines for psychiatric evaluation of adults. *Am J Psychiatry.* 1995;152(11 suppl):66.

Table 1–5
Checklist for Clinicians

The following checklist allows clinicians to rate their skills in establishing and maintaining rapport. It helps them detect and eliminate weaknesses in interviews that failed in some significant way. Each item is rated "yes," "no," or "not applicable."

	Yes	No	N/A
1. I put the patient at ease.			
2. I recognized the patient's state of mind.			
3. I addressed the patient's distress.			
4. I helped the patient warm up.			
5. I helped the patient overcome suspiciousness.			
6. I curbed the patient's intrusiveness.			
7. I stimulated the patient's verbal production.			
8. I curbed the patient's rambling.			
9. I understood the patient's suffering.			
10. I expressed empathy for the patient's suffering.			
11. I tuned in on the patient's affect.			
12. I addressed the patient's affect.			
13. I became aware of the patient's level of insight.			
14. I assumed the patient's view of the disorder.			
15. I had a clear perception of the overt and the therapeutic goals of treatment.			
16. I stated the overt goal of treatment to the patient.			
17. I communicated to the patient that I am familiar with the illness.			
18. My questions convinced the patient that I am familiar with the symptoms of the disorder.			
19. I let the patient know that he or she is not alone with the illness.			
20. I expressed my intent to help the patient.			
21. The patient recognized my expertise.			
22. The patient respected my authority.			
23. The patient appeared fully cooperative.			
24. I recognized the patient's attitude toward the illness.			
25. The patient viewed the illness with distance.			
26. The patient presented as a sympathy-craving sufferer.			
27. The patient presented as a very important patient.			
28. The patient competed with me for authority.			
29. The patient was submissive.			
30. I adjusted my role to the patient's role.			
31. The patient thanked me and made another appointment.			

Reprinted with permission from Othmer E, Othmer SC. *The Clinical Interview Using DSM-IV.* Washington, DC: American Psychiatric Press; 1994.

significant point may not be a stress itself but a person's reaction to it.

Beginning the Interview

How a physician begins an interview provides a powerful first impression to patients, and the manner in which a doctor opens communication with a patient can affect the way the remainder of the interview proceeds. Patients are often anxious on first encounters with physicians and feel both vulnerable and intimidated. A physician who can establish rapport quickly, put the patient at ease, and show respect is well on the way to conducting a productive exchange of information. This exchange is critical to making a correct diagnosis and to establishing treatment goals.

All physicians should initially make sure that they know a patient's name and that the patient knows the physician's name. Physicians should introduce themselves to other people who have come with the patient and should find out if the patient wants another person present during the initial interview. The request for the presence of another person should be granted, but the physician should also attempt to speak with patients privately to determine if there is anything that they want the doctor to know but were reluctant to say in front of someone else.

Patients have a right to know the position and professional status of persons involved in their care. For example, medical students should introduce themselves as such and not as doctors, and physicians should make it clear whether they are consultants (called in by another physician to see the patient), are covering for another physician, or are involved in the interview to teach students rather than to treat the patient.

After the introductions and other initial assessments have been made, a useful and appropriate opening remark is "Can you tell me about the troubles that bring you in today?" or "Tell me about the problems you have been having." Following up with a second one such as "What other problems have you been experiencing?" often elicits information that patients were reluctant to give initially. It also indicates to the patient that the doctor is interested in hearing as much as a patient wants to say.

A less directive approach is to ask a patient "Where shall we start?" or "Where would you prefer to begin?" If a patient has

been referred by another doctor for consultation, the initial remarks can indicate that the consulting doctor already knows something about the patient. For instance, the consulting doctor may say, "Your doctor has told me something about what has been troubling you but I'd like to hear from you in your own words what you've been experiencing."

Most patients do not speak freely unless they have privacy and are sure that their conversations cannot be overheard. Physicians who make sure at the beginning of an interview that such factors as privacy, quiet, and a lack of interruptions are attended to convey to patients that what they say is important and worthy of serious consideration.

Sometimes a patient will appear frightened at the beginning of an interview and may not want to answer questions. If this seems to be the case, the physician may comment on this impression directly in a gentle and supportive way and encourage the patient to talk about his or her feelings about the interview itself. Acknowledging a patient's anxiety is the first step in understanding and reducing it. An example of what could be said is "I can't help but notice that you seem to be feeling anxious about talking with me. Is there anything I can do or any questions I can answer that will make it easier?" or "I know it can be frightening to talk to a doctor, especially one you've never met before, but I'd like to make it as comfortable for you as possible. Is there anything you can put your finger on that's making it tough for you to talk with me?"

Another important initial question is "Why now?" A physician should be clear about why a patient has chosen that particular time to ask for help. The reason may be as simple as that it was the first available appointment hour. Very often, however, people seek out doctors as the result of particular events that have increased stress. These stressful events may be thought of as precipitants, and they often contribute significantly to patients' current problems. Examples of stressful precipitants include real or symbolic losses such as deaths or separations, milestone events (e.g., birthdays or anniversaries), and physical changes such as the presence or intensification of symptoms. Physicians who are unaware of such stresses in people's lives may miss unspoken fears and questions that can compromise the patient's care and well-being.

The Interview Proper

In the interview proper, physicians discover in detail what is troubling patients. They must do so in a systematic way that facilitates the identification of relevant problems in the context of an ongoing empathic working alliance with patients.

The *content* of an interview is literally what is said between doctor and patient: the topics discussed, the subjects mentioned. The *process* of the interview is what occurs nonverbally between doctor and patient, that is, what is happening in the interview beneath the surface. Process involves feelings and reactions that are unacknowledged or unconscious. Patients may use body language to express feelings they cannot express verbally, for example, a clenched fist or nervous tearing at a tissue by a patient with an apparently calm outward demeanor. Patients may shift the interview away from an anxiety-provoking subject onto a neutral topic without realizing that they are doing so. Patients may return again and again to a particular topic, regardless of what direction the interview appears to be taking. Trivial remarks and apparently casual asides may reveal serious underlying concerns, for example, "Oh, by the way, a neighbor of mine tells me that he knows someone with the same symptoms as my son, and that person has cancer."

Table 1–6
Common Interview Techniques

1. Establish rapport as early in the interview as possible.
2. Determine the patient's chief complaint.
3. Use the chief complaint to develop a provisional differential diagnosis.
4. Rule the various diagnostic possibilities out or in by using focused and detailed questions.
5. Follow up on vague or obscure replies with enough persistence to accurately determine the answer to the question.
6. Let the patient talk freely enough to observe how tightly the thoughts are connected.
7. Use a mixture of open-ended and closed-ended questions.
8. Don't be afraid to ask about topics that you or the patient may find difficult or embarrassing.
9. Ask about suicidal thoughts.
10. Give the patient a chance to ask questions at the end of the interview.
11. Conclude the initial interview by conveying a sense of confidence and, if possible, of hope.

Reprinted with permission from Andreasen NC, Black DW. *Introductory Textbook of Psychiatry.* Washington, DC: American Psychiatric Association Press; 1991.

Specific Techniques. Table 1–6 lists some common interview techniques.

OPEN-ENDED VERSUS CLOSED-ENDED QUESTIONS. Interviewing any patient involves a fine balance between allowing the patient's story to unfold at will and obtaining the necessary data for diagnosis and treatment. Most experts on interviewing agree that in an ideal interview, an interviewer begins with broad, open-ended questioning, continues by becoming specific, and closes with detailed direct questioning.

The early part of the interview is generally the most open-ended, in that physicians allow patients to speak as much as possible in their own words. A closed-ended, or directive, question is one that asks for specific information and allows a patient few options in answering. Too many closed-ended questions, especially in the early part of the interview, can restrict patients' responses. Sometimes, directive questions are necessary to obtain important data, but when they are used too often, a patient may think that information is to be given only in response to direct questioning by the doctor. An example of an open-ended question is "Can you tell me more about that?" A closed-ended question would be "How long have you been taking the medication?"

Closed-ended questions can be effective in generating specific and quick responses about a clearly delineated topic. They are effective in eliciting information about the absence of certain symptoms (e.g., auditory hallucinations or suicidal thinking). Closed-ended questions have also been found effective in assessing such factors as the frequency, severity, and duration of symptoms. Table 1–7 summarizes some of the pros and cons of open- and closed-ended questions.

Table 1–7
Pros and Cons of Open-Ended and Closed-Ended Questions

Aspect	Broad, Open-Ended Questions	Narrow, Closed-Ended Questions
Genuineness	High They produce spontaneous formulations.	Low They lead the patient.
Reliability	Low They may lead to nonreproducible answers.	High Narrow focus, but they may suggest answers.
Precision	Low Intent of question is vague.	High Intent of question is clear.
Time efficiency	Low Circumstantial elaborations.	High May invite yes or no answers.
Completeness of diagnostic coverage	Low Patient selects topic.	High Interviewer selects topic.
Acceptance by patient	Varies Most patients prefer expressing themselves freely; others feel guarded and insecure.	Varies Some patients enjoy clear-cut checks; others hate to be pressed into a yes or no format.

Reprinted with permission from Othmer E, Othmer SC. *The Clinical Interview Using DSM-IV.* Washington, DC: American Psychiatric Press; 1994.

REFLECTION. In the technique of reflection, a doctor repeats to a patient, in a supportive manner, something that the patient has said. The goal of reflection is twofold: to assure the doctor that he or she has correctly understood what the patient is trying to say and to let the patient know that the doctor is perceiving what is being said. It is an empathic response meant to let the patient know that the doctor is both listening to the patient's concerns and understanding them. For example, if a patient is speaking about fears of dying and the effects of talking about these fears with his or her family, the doctor might say, "It seems that you are concerned with becoming a burden to your family." This reflection is not an exact repetition of what the patient has said, but rather a paraphrase that indicates the doctor has perceived the essential meaning.

FACILITATION. Doctors help patients continue in the interview by providing both verbal and nonverbal cues that encourage patients to keep talking. Nodding one's head, leaning forward in the chair, and saying "Yes, and then ...?" or "Uh-huh, go on," are all examples of facilitation.

SILENCE. Silence can be used in many ways in normal conversations, even to indicate disapproval or disinterest. In the doctor–patient relationship, however, silence may be constructive and in certain situations may allow patients to contemplate, to cry, or just to sit in an accepting, supportive environment in which the doctor makes it clear that not every moment must be filled with talk.

CONFRONTATION. The technique of confrontation is meant to point out to a patient something that the doctor thinks the patient is not paying attention to, is missing, or is in some way denying. Confrontation must be done skillfully so that patients are not forced to become hostile and defensive. The confrontation is meant to help patients face whatever needs to be faced in a direct but respectful way. For example, a patient who has just made a suicidal gesture but is telling the doctor that it was not serious may be confronted with the statement, "What you have done may not have killed you, but it's telling me that you are in serious trouble right now and that you need help so that you don't try suicide again."

CLARIFICATION. In clarification, doctors attempt to get details from patients about what they have already said. For example, a doctor may say, "You are feeling depressed. When do you feel most depressed?"

INTERPRETATION. The technique of interpretation is most often used when a doctor states something about a patient's behavior or thinking that the patient may not be aware of. The technique follows on the doctor's careful listening to the underlying themes and patterns in the patient's story. Interpretations usually help clarify interrelationships that the patient may not see. The technique is a sophisticated one and should generally be used only after the doctor has established some rapport with the patient and has a reasonably good idea of what some interrelationships are. For example, a doctor may say, "When you talk about how angry you are that your family has not been supportive, I think you're also telling me how worried you are that I won't be there for you either. What do you think?"

SUMMATION. Periodically during the interview, a doctor can take a moment and briefly summarize what a patient has said thus far. Doing so assures both the patient and doctor that the doctor has heard the same information that the patient has actually conveyed. For example, the doctor may say, "OK, I just want to make sure that I've got everything right up to this point."

EXPLANATION. Doctors explain treatment plans to patients in easily understandable language and allow patients to respond and ask questions. For example, a doctor may say, "It is essential that you come into the hospital now because of the seriousness of your condition. You will be admitted tonight through the emergency room, and I will be there to make all the arrangements. You will be given a small dose of medication that will make you sleepy. The medication is called lorazepam, and the dose you will be getting is 0.25 mg. I will see you again first thing in the morning, and we'll go over all the procedures that will be required before anything else happens. Now, what are your questions? I know you must have some."

TRANSITION. The technique of transition allows doctors to convey the idea that enough information has been obtained on one subject; the doctor's words encourage patients to continue on to another subject. For example, a doctor may say, "You've given me a good sense of that particular time in your life. Perhaps now you could tell me a bit more about an even earlier time in your life."

SELF-REVELATION. Limited, discreet self-disclosure by physicians may be useful in certain situations, and physicians should feel at ease and should communicate a sense of self-comfort. Conveying this sense may involve answering a patient's questions about whether a physician is married and where he or she comes from. A doctor who practices self-revelation excessively, however, is using a patient to gratify unfulfilled needs in his or her own life and is abusing the role of physician. If a doctor thinks that a piece of information will help a patient be more comfortable, the doctor can decide in each case whether to be self-revealing. The decision depends on whether the information will further a patient's care or if it will provide nothing useful. Even if the doctor decides that self-revelation is not warranted, he or she should be careful not to make the patient feel embarrassed for asking. For example, the doctor may say, "I will be happy to tell you whether or not I am married, but first let's talk a little about why it is important for you to know that. If we talk about it, I'll have a bit more information about who you are and what your concerns are regarding me and my involvement in your care." Do not take patients' questions at face value alone. Many questions, especially personal ones, convey not just natural curiosity but also hidden concerns about the doctor that should not be ignored.

POSITIVE REINFORCEMENT. The technique of positive reinforcement allows patients to feel comfortable telling a doctor anything, even about such things as noncompliance with treatment. Encouraging a patient to feel that the doctor is not upset by whatever the patient has to say facilitates an open exchange. For example, a doctor might say, "I appreciate your telling me that you have stopped taking your medication. Can you tell me what the problem was?"

An experienced psychiatrist, in response to patients who were afraid of revealing "shocking" material in the initial interview, would sometimes respond in the following manner: "After all these years in practice I don't think I have heard anything new that could shock me. As a matter of fact, it would be interesting to hear something that might." The implied acceptance of all things human usually puts patients at ease.

REASSURANCE. Truthful reassurance of a patient can lead to increased trust and compliance and can be experienced as an empathic response of a concerned physician. False reassurance, however, is essentially lying to a patient and can badly impair the patient's trust and compliance. False reassurance is often given from a desire to make a patient feel better, but once a patient knows that a doctor has not told the truth, the patient is unlikely to accept or believe truthful reassurance. In an example of false reassurance, a patient with a terminal illness asks, "Am I going to be all right, Doctor?" and the doctor responds, "Of course you're going to be all right. Everything's fine." An example of truthful reassurance is "I'm going to do everything possible to make you comfortable, and part of being comfortable is for you to know as much as I know about what is going on with you. We both know that what you have is serious. I'd like to know exactly what you think is happening to you and to clarify any questions you have." The patient may then be able to talk openly about his or her fear of dying.

ADVICE. In many situations it is not only acceptable but desirable for doctors to give patients advice. To be effective and to be perceived as empathic rather than inappropriate or intrusive, the advice should be given only after patients are allowed to talk freely about their problems so that physicians have an adequate information base from which to make suggestions. At times, after a doctor has listened carefully to a patient, it becomes clear that the patient does not, in fact, want advice as much as an objective, caring, nonjudgmental ear. Giving advice too quickly can lead a patient to feel that the doctor is not really listening but, rather, is responding, either out of anxiety or from the belief that the doctor inherently knows better than the patient what should be done in a particular situation. In an example of advice given too quickly, a patient says, "I can't take this medication. It's bothering me," and the physician responds, "Fine. I think you should stop taking it, and I'll prescribe something different." A more appropriate response is, "I'm sorry to hear that. Tell me what about the medication has been bothering you, and I'll have a better idea what we should do to make you more comfortable." In another example, the patient says, "I've really been feeling down lately," and the doctor replies, "Well in that case, I think it's important that you go out and do some things that are fun, such as going to a movie or taking a walk in the park." In this case, a more appropriate and helpful response could be, "Tell me more about what you mean by 'feeling down.'"

ENDING THE INTERVIEW. Physicians want patients to leave an interview feeling understood and respected and believing that all the pertinent and important information has been conveyed to an informed, empathic listener. To this end, doctors should give patients a chance to ask questions and should let patients know as much as possible about future plans. Doctors should thank patients for sharing the necessary information and let patients know that the information conveyed has been helpful in clarifying the next steps. Any prescription of medication should be spelled out clearly and simply, and doctors should ascertain whether patients understand the prescription and how to take it. Doctors should make another appointment or give a referral and some indication about how patients can reach help quickly if it is necessary before the next appointment.

COMPLIANCE

Compliance, also known as adherence, is the degree to which a patient carries out the clinical recommendations of a treating physician. Examples of compliance include keeping appointments, entering into and completing a treatment program, taking medications correctly, and following recommended changes in behavior or diet.

Compliance behavior depends on the specific clinical situation, the nature of the illness, and the treatment program. In general, about one third of all patients comply with treatment, one third sometimes comply with certain aspects of treatment, and one third never comply with treatment. An overall figure derived from a number of studies indicates that 54 percent of patients comply with treatment at any given time. One study found that up to 50 percent of patients with hypertension do not comply at all with treatment and that 50 percent of those who do leave treatment within 1 year.

In an attempt to understand why such a high percentage of patients fail to comply regularly, researchers have investigated several variables. For example, increased complexity of the reg-

Table 1–8
Common Reasons for Noncompliance with Medication

1. The instructions are poorly given or the patient incompletely understands them.

   Example: A 34-year-old woman suffering from a first episode of major depression is prescribed paroxetine 20 mg/day. She responds well with full resolution of all symptoms within four weeks. Two weeks later, feeling back to normal, she stops taking the medication. Three weeks later she suffers a relapse.

   Comment: The woman did not understand (perhaps it was not well explained) that it would be necessary to continue medication for several months after full recovery to minimize the risk of relapse.

2. The patient may find side effects intolerable.

   Example: A 20-year-old man is given a provisional diagnosis of schizophrenia when he begins to experience auditory hallucinations. He is treated with haloperidol 5 mg twice a day. The hallucinations resolve but he begins to experience erectile dysfunction and stops the medication without telling anyone.

   Comment: Common potential side effects and toxicities should always be reviewed with patients before they start medication. It is equally important to encourage the patient to discuss with the physician any adverse experiences, and to reassure the patient that it is not necessary to put up with intolerable side effects since there are alternative medications that can be tried.

3. Psychiatric symptoms interfere with treatment.

   Example: A 41-year-old woman with a diagnosis of paranoid schizophrenia is admitted to an inpatient service with the delusion that she is being poisoned by an alien force. She is treated with risperidone 2 mg/day and discharged after one week. She stops taking medication the day of her discharge, believing it also to be poison and part of the plot to hurt her.

   Comment: The clinician must be alert to the possibility that symptoms may interfere with treatment, establish as best as possible a trusting rapport, and inquire about the possibility ("Are you sometimes frightened that I might want to hurt you, too?"). If medications are prescribed, they must be in doses sufficient to provide benefit.

4. Patients like their symptoms and don't want them treated.

   Example: A 37-year-old man with bipolar disorder, well controlled with lithium for 2 years, begins to feel mildly euphoric, more energetic, and more gregarious than usual. He stops taking lithium because he feels it slows him down. Within two weeks he is in a full manic episode.

   Comment: Psychoeducation is part of the ongoing therapeutic process and may take time to be fully accomplished. Compliance is more easily achieved when a solid collaborative relationship has been established, when the physician is receptive to the patient's subjective experience of illness and treatment, and when the patient fully understands that mildly pleasant symptoms can become destructive and very unpleasant if inadequately treated.

5. The lives of some patients are so chaotic and disorganized that good compliance is difficult without close monitoring and follow-up.

   Example: A 47-year-old homeless woman with a diagnosis of chronic undifferentiated schizophrenia was treated in an emergency room, given a prescription for a month's supply of an antipsychotic, and told to come back to the outpatient clinic in a month. Following discharge, the woman lived in a series of shelters and church refuges. Her bags containing her Medicaid and Medicare cards, prescription and appointment card were stolen. She could not remember the date or place of follow-up and forgot about them.

   Comment: Failure to provide close, structured follow-up for this patient almost guarantees treatment failure. Individual case managers help, although sometimes the number of cases they are assigned to follow is overwhelming.

6. Patients stop taking medications because they can't afford them.

   Example: An elderly man living on a modest fixed income consulted his internist because of fatigue. She diagnosed depression and prescribed a relatively new SSRI. When the man went to fill the prescription at his pharmacy he was told a month's supply would cost $300. He did not fill the prescription and was embarrassed to tell his internist why.

   Comment: The cost of medications is too seldom factored into prescribing decisions. This is particularly important for patients relying on Medicare since Medicare currently has no outpatient prescription benefits. Generic drugs are always cheaper than brand name equivalents. However, when a drug is new and still under patent, there may be no low-cost alternatives.

imen, along with an increased number of required behavioral changes, appears to be associated with noncompliance. There is no clear association, however, between compliance and a patient's sex, marital status, race, religion, socioeconomic status, intelligence, or educational level. Psychiatric patients, however, exhibit a higher degree of noncompliant behavior than do medical patients. Compliance increases when physicians have such characteristics as enthusiasm and a nonpunitive attitude. Older doctors with experience, the amount of time spent talking to patients, a short waiting room time, and increased frequency of visits are also associated with high rates of compliance.

The doctor-patient relationship, or doctor-patient match, is one of the most important factors in compliance issues. When doctor and patient have different priorities and beliefs, different styles of communication (including a different understanding of medical advice), and different medical expectations, compliance decreases. Compliance can be increased when physicians explain to patients the value of a particular treatment outcome and emphasize that following the recommendation will produce this outcome. Compliance can also increase if patients know the names and effects of each drug they are taking.

A highly significant factor in compliance seems to be patients' subjective feelings of distress or illness, as opposed to doctors' often objective medical estimates of the disease and required therapy. Patients who believe they are ill tend toward compliance. Asymptomatic patients such as those with hypertension are at greater risk for noncompliance than are patients with symptoms.

When there are problems in communication, compliance decreases. When effective communication is coupled with close patient supervision and a patient's subjective sense of satisfaction that a doctor has met expectations, compliance increases. Studies have shown that noncompliance is associated with physicians who are perceived as rejecting and unfriendly. Noncompliance is also associated with asking a patient for information and then not giving feedback or with failing to explain a diagnosis or the cause of a patient's symptoms. Doctors who are aware of patients' belief systems, feelings, and habits and who enlist the patient in establishing a treatment regimen increase compliant behavior.

Noncompliance with medication has many causes. The physician must explore the reasons for noncompliance rather than dismiss the patient as uncooperative. Some common reasons for noncompliance are listed in Table 1–8. Other strate-

gies to improve compliance include asking patients to describe what they believe is wrong with them and what should be done, what they understand to be the reasons for the doctor's recommendations, and what they see as the risks and benefits of following the prescribed treatment. Common errors are patients not taking medications for as long as they should and not taking the proper amount each day. Patients are more likely to be noncompliant if they have to take more than three kinds of medications in one day or if they must take medications more than four times a day. Older people and others who have trouble seeing or hearing may misread or misunderstand medication instructions. In these instances, it is helpful to print the instructions on a piece of paper, ask the patient to read them back, ask whether the patient has any questions, and then ask the patient to explain specifically and in what amounts the medication is to be taken.

Sometimes instead of making errors, patients deliberately change the treatment regimen, for example, by not showing up for appointments or by taking medications in a manner different from that recommended. In these instances, which may involve competing pressures from family or work, the doctor needs to negotiate a compromise with the patient. The doctor and patient together specify what they can expect from each other. Implicit in this approach are the ideas that the contract can be renegotiated and the patient can be assured that suggestions can be made by either the doctor or the patient to improve compliance.

SPECIFIC ISSUES IN PSYCHIATRY

Fees

Before clinicians can establish an ongoing relationship with patients, they must address certain issues. For instance, they must openly discuss payment of fees. Discussing these issues and any other questions about fees from the beginning of the relationship can minimize misunderstanding later. Most patients have medical insurance through health maintenance organizations (HMOs) or Medicare. HMOs pay for doctors' visits in whole or in part, but only if the doctor is a member (or provider) in the patient's plan. Some plans (called point of service plans) offer partial payments even if the doctor is not a member (i.e., he or she is called "out-of-network"). That should be clarified; otherwise, the patient may have to pay out-of-pocket, which he or she may be unwilling or unable to do. (See Chapter 60 for a discussion of health care delivery systems.)

Confidentiality

Psychiatrists should discuss the extent and limitations of confidentiality with patients, so that patients are clear about what can and cannot remain confidential. As much as physicians must legally and ethically respect patients' confidentiality, it may be wholly or partially broken in some specific situations. For example, if a patient makes clear that he or she intends to harm someone, the doctor has a responsibility to notify the intended victim. Other issues related to confidentiality include who has access to the patient's medical record, information required by insurance companies (which may be extensive), and the degree to which the patient's case will be used for teaching purposes. In all such situations, the patient must give permission for the use of medical records. (See Chapter 58 for a discussion of confidentiality.)

Supervision

It is both commonplace and necessary for doctors in training to receive supervision from experienced physicians. This practice is the norm in large teaching hospitals, and most patients are aware of it. When young doctors are receiving supervision from senior physicians, patients should know from the beginning. Informing patients is particularly important in psychiatry, in which the supervision of individual psychotherapy cases is a routine and established practice and in which the psychiatric resident is required to present verbatim accounts of an entire therapy session (process notes) to a senior supervisor. If a patient is curious about the level of the treating doctor's experience, the doctor or medical student should respond honestly and not mislead the patient. If the doctor is less than truthful and the patient later discovers this, the relationship between doctor and patient may become untenable.

Missed Appointments and Length of Sessions

Patients need to be informed about a doctor's policies for missed appointments and length of sessions. Psychiatrists generally see patients in regularly scheduled blocks of time ranging from 15 to 45 minutes. At the end of this time, psychiatrists expect patients to accept the fact that the session is over. Nonpsychiatric physicians may schedule somewhat differently, by putting aside 30 minutes to an hour for an initial visit and then perhaps scheduling patient visits every 15 to 20 minutes for follow-up appointments. Psychiatrists who are treating psychotic inpatients may determine that a patient cannot tolerate a lengthy session and may decide to see the patient in a series of 10-minute sessions throughout the week. Whatever the policies, patients must be made aware of them to prevent misunderstandings.

The same can be said about policies for missed appointments. Some doctors ask patients to give 24 hours' notice to avoid being billed for a missed session. Others bill for missed sessions regardless of advance notification. Still others decide on a case-by-case basis or perhaps state a 24-hour rule but make exceptions when warranted. Some doctors state that if they receive advance notice and can fill the appointment time, they won't charge for missed sessions; others do not charge for missed appointments at all. The choice is up to the individual physician, but patients must know in advance to make an informed decision about whether to accept the doctor's policy or to choose another doctor.

Availability of Doctor

What are a doctor's obligations to be available between scheduled appointments? Is it incumbent on physicians to be available 24 hours a day? Once a patient enters into a contract to receive care from a particular physician, the doctor is responsible for having a mechanism in place for providing emergency service outside scheduled appointment times. Patients should be told what the mechanism is, whether it is an emergency phone number or a covering physician. If the physician is going

to be away for a period of time, coverage by another physician is necessary, and patients must be informed how to reach the covering doctor. They should know that their doctor will be available between appointments to answer pressing questions and that extra appointments can be scheduled if necessary.

Within these general parameters, however, physicians must make their own decisions about their availability to specific patients. In some cases, doctors may have to place firm limits on availability between sessions. For instance, patients who repeatedly call at all hours with concerns that are best addressed during scheduled appointments should be respectfully but firmly discouraged from calling unnecessarily. They can be reassured that all concerns will be addressed and that if there is not enough time during the regular appointment, another appointment can be made, but told that all nonemergency concerns will be postponed until the next session.

Follow-Up

Many events can disrupt the continuity of the doctor-patient relationship. Some of these events are routine (e.g., residents ending their training and moving on to another hospital); others are out of the ordinary and thus unpredictable (e.g., when physicians become ill and can no longer take care of their patients). Patients must be assured that regardless of what occurs in the course of a particular doctor-patient relationship, their care will be ongoing.

A complex situation arises when physicians become ill and are unable to continue caring for patients. When they know in advance that they will have to interrupt therapy, clear arrangements for referral to other doctors can be made. Although there are arguments both for and against physicians revealing their illnesses to patients, it seems best to err on the side of truth. The information should be conveyed in as calm and nonthreatening a way as possible. The reason for telling the truth is that patients will fantasize reasons about why the doctor has stopped seeing them and may fear that something about them has made the doctor leave. Untruthfulness in this situation also encourages the view that being ill is shameful or frightening and that doctors who cannot handle their own illness should not expect patients to be able to. It is not the role of patients, however, to take care of their doctors; informing patients should not carry with it any sense that a doctor's illness is a patient's burden.

Problem Patients and Special Interview Situations

Almost all physicians treat so-called problem patients who are difficult to work with not because of their medical illness but because they engage in power struggles, are demanding, or are uncooperative. It is a natural human quality to feel anger and resentment toward difficult patients, to try to limit the amount of time spent with them, and to secretly (or explicitly) hope that they move on to another physician. While these reactions are understandable, they are likely to make a bad situation worse and to interfere with the doctor's primary mission—providing the best possible medical care. Understanding some of the hidden fears and conflicts shaping the behavior of difficult patients helps the physician develop patience and greater compassion and makes it easier to provide interventions that are medically sound. In special situations, interview techniques need to be varied according to the personality reactions of the patient, the type and severity of illness, and the objective of the interview. Varying degrees of permissiveness and directiveness may be used. Different approaches to different patients are indicated, and the approach to the same patient should be changed when appropriate.

Histrionic Patients. Patients who are histrionic have a dramatic, emotional, and impressionistic style. They may be seductive with their physicians and others out of an unconscious need for reassurance and the fear that they will not be taken seriously unless they are sexually desirable. They often come across as overly emotional and flirtatious. The physician needs to be calm, reassuring, and accepting of such patients. Most do not really want to seduce their doctor, but they do not know other ways of getting the attention they need.

Dependent Patients. Some patients seem to need an inordinate amount of attention and yet never seem reassured. They are the patients likely to make repeated urgent calls between scheduled appointments and to demand special consideration. The doctor needs to be firm in establishing limits while reassuring the patient that his or her needs are taken seriously and treated professionally.

Demanding Patients. Some patients have a difficult time delaying gratification and demand that their discomfort be eliminated immediately. They are easily frustrated and can become petulant or even angry and hostile if they do not get what they want when they want it. They may impulsively do something self-destructive if they feel thwarted, and they appear manipulative and attention seeking. What they may be feeling underneath their surface behavior is the fear that they will never get what they need from others and thus must act in that inappropriately aggressive way. They can be particularly difficult for any doctor to treat. The doctor must be firm with these patients from the outset and clearly define acceptable and unacceptable behavior. These patients must be treated with respect and care, but must also be confronted with their behavior so they learn to be responsible for their actions.

Narcissistic Patients. Narcissistic patients act as though they are superior to everyone around them, including the doctor. They have a tremendous need to appear perfect and are contemptuous of others whom they perceive to be imperfect. They may be rude, abrupt, arrogant, and demanding. They may initially idealize the doctor out of a need to have their doctor be as perfect as they are, but the idealization can quickly turn to disdain when they discover the doctor is human after all. Underneath their surface arrogance, narcissistic patients feel desperately inadequate and fear that others will see through them.

Suspicious Patients. Some persons, usually those with a paranoid personality, have a chronic, deeply ingrained suspicion that other people want to cause them harm. They misinterpret neutral events as evidence of a conspiracy against them. They are critical and evasive, and they are sometimes called "grievance collectors" because they tend to blame other people for everything bad in their lives. They are extremely mistrustful

and may question everything the doctor says or does. The physician should try to maintain a respectful but somewhat formal and distant approach with these patients. Expressions of warmth often heighten the suspicions. The doctor should explain in detail every decision and planned procedure and should try to respond nondefensively to the patient's suspiciousness.

Isolated Patients. Isolated and solitary patients do not appear to need or want much contact with other people. Intimate contact with the doctor is viewed with distaste, and such patients would prefer to take care of themselves entirely without a doctor's help if it were possible. Some isolated patients would receive the psychiatric diagnosis of schizoid personality disorder. They are withdrawn, absorbed in a world of fantasy, and unable to talk about their feelings. The doctor should treat these patients with as much respect for their privacy as possible and should not expect them to respond to the doctor's concern in kind.

Obsessive Patients. Obsessive patients are orderly, punctual, and so concerned with detail that they often don't see the larger picture. They often appear unemotional, even aloof, especially when confronted with anything disturbing or frightening. They have a strong need to be in control of everything in their lives and may struggle with their doctor whenever they feel decisions are being imposed. Underneath, obsessive patients are often frightened of losing control and becoming helpless and dependent. Their physicians should try to include them in their own care and treatment as much as possible. Doctors should explain in detail what is going on and what is being planned, making sure the patient can make choices in his or her own behalf.

Help-Rejecting Complainer. Some patients appear to communicate only through a long litany of complaints and disappointments. They often covertly blame others for all their problems and make people feel guilty about not doing or caring enough. They may not be able to express angry feelings directly and thus express them indirectly or passively by being late for appointments or not making payments on time. They may see themselves as self-sacrificing. When help is offered they usually respond by saying, "Yes, but . . ." Doctors should take such patients' concerns seriously, but without encouraging the sick role. Firm limits must be set on the doctor's availability. At the same time physicians can offer the reassurance of frequent, regularly scheduled appointments. The doctor must often be involved with family members. The family is dealing with the patient's difficult style everyday and is likely to feel angry, frustrated, and guilty because of it.

Manipulative Patients. Manipulative patients are described in psychiatric terminology as having antisocial personality traits. They do not appear to experience appropriate guilt and, in fact, may not even be aware of what it is to feel guilty. On the surface they may be charming, intelligent, and socially adept, but these are poses they have perfected over years of practice. They often have histories of criminal acts, and they get by in the world through lying and manipulation. These patients frequently malinger—that is, they consciously pretend to be sick to gain some specific external objective such as an insurance settlement or access to narcotic analgesics. When they are truly sick, the doctor must treat them with respect, but with a heightened sense of vigilance. If they have violent histories, the doctor may feel threatened by such patients and should unashamedly seek assistance, not feel compelled to see them alone. Firm limits must be set on behavior (e.g., no drugs brought into the hospital), and the consequences of transgression clearly stated and adhered to. If inappropriate behavior is discovered, these patients must be confronted directly and held responsible for their actions. These patients often lie; however, believing a patient's lies is not a professional failure. Psychiatrists are trained to detect, understand, and treat psychopathology, not to function as lie detectors. While a certain level of suspicion is essential in the practice of psychiatry, clinicians determined never to be taken in by deceitful patients will approach them with such exaggerated suspiciousness that therapeutic work will be impossible.

Patients from Different Cultures and Backgrounds. Differences in race, nationality, and religion and other significant cultural differences between patient and doctor can impair communication and lead to misunderstanding. Such differences can affect the way people present themselves to physicians, the kinds of symptoms they complain of, and their understanding of the causes of illness and need for treatment. Cultural differences can also interfere with establishing rapport. The use of honorifics, the extent of direct eye contact considered appropriate, and whether it is appropriate for men and women to shake hands can all lead unwary physicians astray. The psychiatrist must proceed with humility and respect, especially when unfamiliar with the patient's background. Asking about differences is better than assuming. Patients will not be offended when the doctor asks, "Have I understood this in the way you meant it?"

Additional problems arise when doctor and patient speak different languages. If a translator is needed it is best to use a disinterested third party unknown to the patient. Using family or friends to translate will limit what the patient is comfortable saying and will inevitably invite distortions in what the patient is reported to have said. Translators must be instructed to translate verbatim what the patient says—a difficult task for even the most experienced professional translators. Many beginners will try to impose organization and meaning on a patient's disorganized and nonsensical statements. Some words and expressions are untranslatable.

STRESSES ON THE PHYSICIAN

In addition to the vast amount of knowledge and the skills required for the practice of medicine, an effective physician must also develop the capacity for balancing compassionate concern with dispassionate objectivity, the wish to relieve pain with the ability to make painful decisions, and the desire to cure and control with an acceptance of one's human limitations. Learning to balance these interrelated aspects of the physician's role is essential to allow the doctor to cope productively within daily work that involves illness, pain, sadness, suffering, and death. A lack of balance can lead a physician to feel overwhelmed and depressed. A sense of futility

Table 1–9
Character and Qualities of the Physician As Described by William S. Osler, M.D., in *Aequanimitas*

Imperturbability	The ability to maintain extreme calm and steadiness
Presence of mind	Self-control in an emergency or embarrassing situation so that one can say or do the right thing
Clear judgment	The ability to make an informed opinion that is intelligible and free of ambiguity
Ability to endure frustration	The capacity to remain firm and deal with insecurity and dissatisfaction
Infinite patience	The unlimited ability to bear pain or trial calmly
Charity toward others	To be generous and helpful, especially toward the needy and suffering
The search for absolute truth	To investigate facts and pursue reality
Composure	Calmness of mind, bearing, and appearance
Bravery	The capacity to face or endure events with courage
Tenacity	To be persistent in attaining a goal or adhering to something valued
Idealism	Forming standards and ideals and living under their influence
Equanimity	The ability to handle stressful situations with an undisturbed, even temper

and failure can begin to permeate a physician's attitude, setting the stage for frustration and anger with one's profession, patients, and self. Many people drawn to the field of medicine are perfectionistic, demanding of themselves, and attentive to details. These qualities can be adaptive—in fact are probably necessary—but need to be balanced with healthy doses of self-knowledge, humility, humor, and kindness. William Osler, physician and teacher, discussed the characteristics and quality of the physician in his book *Aequanimitas,* which are summarized in Table 1–9. They are ideals to be strived for, but they are rarely reached. Physicians (and other health care providers) must be tolerant about the limits on what they can realistically and honestly accomplish.

References

American Psychiatric Association. Practice guidelines for psychiatric evaluation of adults. *Am J Psychiatry.* 1995;152(11 suppl):66.

Bishop J. Guidelines for a nonsexist (gender-sensitive) doctor-patient relationship. *Can J Psychiatry.* 1992;37:62.

Bradley EH, Hallemeier AG, Fried TR, Johnson-Hurzeler R, Cherlin EJ, Kasl S, Horwitz SM. Documentation of discussions about prognosis with terminally ill patients. *Am J Med.* 2001;111:218.

Engel GL. The clinical application of the biopsychosocial model. *Am J Psychiatry.* 1980;137:535.

Freud S. Recommendations to physicians practicing psychoanalysis. In: *Standard Edition of the Complete Psychological Works of Sigmund Freud.* Vol 12. London: Hogarth; 1958:109.

Greengold NL, Ault M. Crossing the cultural doctor-patient barrier. *Acad Med.* 1995;71:112.

Jordan JV, Kim D, Silver MH. Shattered trust: Technical and moral lessons from an interrupted first visit. *Harv Rev Psychiatry.* 2002;10:37.

Mechanic D. Are patient's office visits with physicians getting shorter? *N Engl J Med.* 2001;344:1476.

O'Brien R. The doctor-patient relationship. *Ann N Y Acad Sci.* 1994;729:22.

Ong LM, de Haes JC, Hoos AM, Lammas FB. Doctor-patient communication: a review of the literature. *Soc Sci Med.* 1995;40:903.

Othmer E, Othmer SC. *The Clinical Interview Using DSM-IV.* Washington, DC: American Psychiatric Press; 1994.

Silver A, Weiss D. Paternalistic attitudes and moral reasoning among physicians at a large teaching hospital. *Acad Med.* 1992;67:62.

Verhulst J, Tucker G. Medical and narrative approaches in psychiatry. *Psychiatr Ser.* 1995;46:513.

West C. Reconceptualizing gender in physician-patient relationships. *Soc Sci Med.* 1993;36:57.

Wink P, Dillon M. Spiritual development across the adult life course: Findings from a longitudinal study. *Adult Development.* 2002;9:79.

2

Human Development Throughout the Life Cycle

▲ 2.1 Normality, Mental Health, and Life Cycle Theory

NORMALITY AND MENTAL HEALTH

Normality and mental health are central issues in psychiatric theory and practice but are difficult to define. For example, *normality* has been defined as patterns of behavior or personality traits that are typical or that conform to some standard of proper and acceptable ways of behaving and being. The use of terms such as *typical* or *acceptable,* however, has been criticized because they are ambiguous, involve value judgments, and vary from one culture to another. To overcome this objection psychiatrist and historian George Mora devised a system to describe behavioral manifestations that are normal in one context but not in another, depending on how the person is viewed by the society (Table 2.1–1). This paradigm, however, may give too much weight to peer group observations and judgments. The World Health Organization (WHO) defines *normality* as a state of complete physical mental, and social well-being; but again, this definition is limited, because it defines physical and mental health simply as the absence of physical or mental disease.

The text revision of the fourth edition of *Diagnostic and Statistical Manual of Mental Disorders* (DSM-IV-TR) offers no definition of normality or mental health; although a definition of *mental disorder* is presented. According to DSM-IV-TR, a mental disorder is conceptualized as a behavioral or psychological syndrome or pattern that is associated with distress (e.g., a painful symptom) or disability (i.e., impairment in one or more important areas of functioning). In addition, the syndrome or pattern must not be merely an expected and culturally sanctioned response to a particular event, such as the death of a loved one. DSM-IV-TR emphasizes that neither deviant behavior (e.g., political, religious, or sexual) nor conflicts that are primarily between the individual and society are mental disorders.

In *Mental Health: A Report of the Surgeon General,* mental health is defined as "the successful performance of mental functions, in terms of thought, mood, and behavior that results in productive activities, fulfilling relationships with others, and the ability to adapt to change and to cope with adversity."

Finally, a controversial view is held by the psychiatrist Thomas Szasz, who believes that the concept of mental illness should be abandoned entirely. In his book *The Myth of Mental Illness* Szasz states that normality can be measured only in terms of what persons do or do not do and that defining normality is beyond the realm of psychiatry.

Psychiatry has been criticized over the years by certain groups for its portrayal of normality. The psychology of women, for example, has been criticized as sexist because it was formulated initially by men; similar criticism comes from other groups who believe the portrayal of their psychological issues is biased by placing undue emphasis on psychopathology rather than healthy attributes. A much discussed issue is the change in psychiatry's view of homosexuality from abnormal to normal that took place 25 years ago, an evolution shaped by cultural norms, society's expectations and values, professional biases, individual differences, and the political climate of the time.

FUNCTIONAL PERSPECTIVES OF NORMALITY

The many theoretical and clinical concepts of normality seem to fall into four functional perspectives. Although each perspective is unique and has its own definition and description, the perspectives complement each other, and together they represent the totality of the behavioral science and social science approaches to the subject. The four perspectives of normality as described by Daniel Offer and Melvin Sabshin are (1) normality as health, (2) normality as utopia, (3) normality as average, and (4) normality as process.

Normality as Health

The first perspective is basically the traditional medical psychiatric approach to health and illness. Most physicians equate normality with health and view health as an almost universal phenomenon. As a result, behavior is assumed to be within normal limits when no manifest psychopathology is present. If all behavior were to be put on a scale, normality would encompass the major portion of the continuum, and abnormality would be the small remainder.

This definition of normality correlates with the traditional model of the doctor who attempts to free his patient from grossly observable signs and symptoms. To this physician, the lack of signs or symptoms indicates health. Health in this con-

Table 2.1–1
Normality in Context

Term	Concept
Autonormal	Person seen as normal by his or her own society
Autopathological	Person seen as abnormal by his or her own society
Heteronormal	Person seen as normal by members of another society observing him or her
Heteropathological	Person seen as unusual or pathological by members of another society observing him or her

Data from George Mora, M.D.

text refers to a *reasonable,* rather than an *optimal,* state of functioning. In its simplest form, this perspective described by John Romano views a healthy person as one who is reasonably free of undue pain, discomfort, and disability.

Normality as Utopia

The second perspective conceives of normality as that harmonious and optimal blending of the diverse elements of the mental apparatus that culminates in optimal functioning. Such a definition emerges when psychiatrists or psychoanalysts talk about the ideal person, when they grapple with a complex problem, or when they discuss their criteria for a successful treatment. This approach can be traced back to Sigmund Freud, who when discussing normality stated, "A normal ego is like normality in general, an ideal fiction."

Although this approach is characteristic of many psychoanalysts, it is by no means unique to them. It can also be found among other psychotherapists in the field of psychiatry and among psychologists of quite different persuasions.

Normality as Average

The third perspective is commonly used in normative studies of behavior and is based on a mathematical principle of the bell-shaped curve. This approach considers the middle range normal and both extremes deviant. The normative approach based on this statistical principal describes each individual in terms of general assessment and total score. Variability is described only within the context of groups, not within the context of the individual.

Although this approach is more commonly used in psychology than in psychiatry, psychiatrists have been relying on normative pencil-and-paper tests to a much larger extent than in the past. Not only do psychiatrists use instruments such as the Minnesota Multiple Personality Inventory (MMPI), they also construct their own tests and questionnaires. (Psychiatric rating scales are discussed in Chapter 9.)

Normality as Process

The fourth perspective stresses that normal behavior is the end result of interacting systems. Based on this definition, temporal changes are essential to a complete definition of normality. In other words, the normality-as-process perspective stresses changes or processes rather than a cross-sectional definition of normality.

Investigators who subscribe to this approach can be found in all the behavioral and social sciences. A typical example of the concepts in this perspective is Erik Erikson's conceptualization of the epigenesis of personality development and the seven development stages essential in the attainment of mature adult functioning. (Erikson's theories are discussed in Section 6.2.)

PSYCHOANALYTIC THEORIES OF NORMALITY

Some psychoanalysts base their concepts of normality on the absence of symptoms; but while the disappearance of symptoms is necessary for cure or improvement, the absence of symptoms alone does not suffice for a comprehensive definition of normality. Accordingly, most psychoanalysts view a capacity for work and enjoyment as indicating normality or, as Freud put it, the ability "to love and to work."

The psychoanalyst Heinz Hartmann conceptualized normality by describing the "autonomous functions of the ego." These are psychological capacities present at birth that are conflict free, that is, uninfluenced by the internal psychic world. They include perception, intuition, comprehension, thinking, language, certain aspects of motor development, learning, and intelligence. The concept of autonomous and conflict-free functions of the ego helps explain the mechanisms whereby some persons lead relatively normal lives in the presence of extraordinary external experiential traumas—the so-called invulnerable child, that is, a child who is invulnerable to the "slings and arrows of outrageous fortune" by virtue of autonomous ego strengths. A summary of some psychoanalytic views of normality is given in Table 2.1–2.

Karl Jaspers

Karl Jaspers (1883–1969), the German psychiatrist and philosopher, described a "personal world"—the way a person thinks or feels—that could be either normal or abnormal. According to Jaspers, the personal world is abnormal when it (1) springs from a condition that is recognized universally as abnormal, such as schizophrenia, (2) when it separates the person from others emotionally, and (3) when it does not provide the person with a sense of "spiritual and material" security.

Jaspers was a proponent of phenomenology, in which the clinician studies psychological signs and symptoms with the goal of understanding the internal experience of the patient. By listening carefully to the patient, the psychiatrist temporarily enters the mental life of the patient. Jaspers believed that to fully understand the signs and symptoms observed in the patient, the clinician must have no prior assumptions. A person who reports a hallucinatory experience, for example, must not be judged thereby as being abnormal or psychotic. To be used diagnostically, the phenomenon must occur repeatedly and be characteristic of a known disorder.

Some investigators are developing a research strategy that defines normality by examining a person's mental state at various times during the day in different life settings. What is abnormal in one setting or at one time of day may be normal in another.

Table 2.1–2
Psychoanalytic Concepts of Normality

Theorist	Concept
Sigmund Freud	Normality is an idealized fiction
Kurt Eissler	Absolute normality cannot be obtained because the normal person must be totally aware of his or her thoughts and feelings
Melanie Klein	Normality is characterized by strength of character, the capacity to deal with conflicting emotions, the ability to experience pleasure without conflict, and the ability to love
Erik Erikson	Normality is the ability to master the periods of life: trust vs. mistrust; autonomy vs. shame and doubt; initiative vs. guilt; industry vs. inferiority; identity vs. role confusion; intimacy vs. isolation; generativity vs. stagnation; and ego integrity vs. despair
Laurence Kubie	Normality is the ability to learn by experience, to be flexible, and to adapt to a changing environment
Heinz Hartman	Conflict-free ego functions represent the person's potential for normality; the degree the ego can adapt to reality and be autonomous is related to mental health
Karl Menninger	Normality is the ability to adjust to the external world with contentment and to master the task of acculturation
Alfred Adler	The person's capacity to develop social feeling and to be productive is related to mental health; the ability to work heightens self-esteem and makes one capable of adaptation
R. E. Money-Kryle	Normality is the ability to achieve insight into one's self, an ability that is never fully accomplished
Otto Rank	Normality is the capacity to live without fear, guilt, or anxiety and to take responsibility for one's own actions

Robert Campbell

Finally, there is the commonly accepted and widely used definition of mental health adapted from Campbell's *Psychiatric Dictionary*: Psychically normal persons are those who are in harmony with themselves and with their environment. They conform with the cultural requirements or injunctions of their community. They may possess medical deviation or disease, but as long as this does not impair their reasoning, judgment, intellectual capacity, and ability to make a harmonious personal and social adaptation, they may be regarded as psychically sound or normal.

NORMALITY IN ADOLESCENCE

In addition to studying adult normality Offer and Sabshin studied a group of adolescents throughout their high school years and identified three normal types of development: continuous growth, surgent growth, and tumultuous growth. Although persons of each type are different, they can be placed along a continuum of normality. They formulated an operational definition of normality that is not absolute but, rather, describes one type of middle-class adolescent population. Healthy teenagers are characterized by

1. Almost complete absence of gross psychopathology, severe physical defects, and severe physical illness
2. Mastery of previous development tasks without serious setbacks
3. Ability to experience emotional states flexibly and to resolve conflicts actively with reasonable success
4. Relatively good relationship with parents, siblings, and peers
5. Feeling part of a larger cultural environment and being aware of its norms and values

(Section 2.3 discusses adolescence in detail.)

LIFE CYCLE THEORY

The life cycle represents the stages through which all humans pass from birth to death. The fundamental assumption of all life cycle theories is that development occurs in successive, clearly defined stages. This sequence is invariant; that is, it occurs in a particular order in every person's life, whether or not all stages are completed. A second assumption of life cycle theory is the *epigenetic principle,* which maintains that each stage is characterized by events or crises that must be resolved satisfactorily for development to proceed smoothly. According to the epigenetic model, if resolution is not achieved within a given life period, all subsequent stages reflect that failure in the form of physical, cognitive, social, or emotional maladjustment. A third assumption is that each phase of the life cycle contains a dominant feature, complex of features, or a crisis point that distinguishes it from phases that either preceded or will follow it.

Charting of the life cycle lies within the study of developmental psychology and involves such diverse elements as biological maturity, psychological capacity, adaptive techniques, defense mechanisms, symptom complexes, role demands, social behavior, cognition, perception, language development, and interpersonal relationships. Various models of the life cycle describe the major developmental phases but emphasize different elements. Taken together however, they demonstrate that there is an order to human life, despite the fact that each person is unique.

Theodore Lidz, a major exponent of life cycle theory describes several factors that account for the phasic nature of the life cycle.

1. The acquisition of many abilities must wait for the physical maturation of the organism. For example, the infant cannot become a toddler until the pyramidal nerve tracts that permit voluntary discrete movements of the lower limbs become functional. Then, after such maturation occurs, it takes considerable practice to gain the skills needed to master a function, but the function becomes amenable to training and education. Adequate mastery of simple skills must precede their incorporation into more complex activities. In a somewhat different way, shifts in the physiological equilibrium can initiate a new phase in the life cycle, as when the new inner forces that come with puberty require changes in personality functioning, whatever the preparation in prior phases of childhood.

2. Cognitive development plays a significant role in creating phasic shifts. The ability to communicate needs and desires verbally and to understand what parents say is a major factor in ending the period of infancy, and children's ability to attend school depends to a great extent on their gaining the ability to

form concrete categories at the age of 5 or 6. Cognitive development does not progress at an even pace, because qualitatively different capacities emerge in rather discrete stages.

3. Society establishes roles and sets of expectations for persons of different ages and statuses. At 5 or 6, a child becomes a schoolchild with new demands and opportunities. As adults, interpersonal relationships such as marriage require that the person attend to the needs of the other.

4. Children attain many attributes and capacities for directing the self and controlling impulses by internalizing parental characteristics to gradually overcome the need for surrogate egos to direct their lives and provide security. Such internalizations take place in stages in relation to the child's physical, intellectual, and emotional development.

5. Finally, time itself is a determinant of phasic changes not only because of the need to move into age-appropriate roles but because changes in physical make-up at puberty and old age require changes in self-concepts and attitudes. Awareness of the passage of time also fosters entry into new stages of life, as when persons realize that more time lies behind than ahead of them as they enter late middle age.

Each phase of the life cycle presents a critical task to be surmounted to enable the person to cope with the tasks of the next phase. By mastering those crises, the person gains greater confidence, self-sufficiency, and integration. Many of the so-called traumas that initiate neuroses are simply the person's inability to cope with, or difficulty in coping with, the critical events that are inevitable aspects of the developmental process. Although each person meets each developmental crisis somewhat differently, there are similarities in the ways persons meet and seek to cope with similar developmental problems. The similarities in the developmental tasks, common problems in coping with them, and knowledge of the likely consequences of failure to master them provide major guidelines for psychotherapists in their attempt to help persons understand themselves better.

Developmental Approaches

Freud. A seminal work on the subject is the developmental scheme introduced in 1905 by Freud in his *Three Essays on the Theory of Sexuality.* Freud conceptualized a development scheme that he believed to be universal, which focused on the childhood period and his idea of libido. According to Freud, childhood phases of development correspond to successive shifts in the investment of sexual energy to areas of the body usually associated with eroticism: the mouth, the anus, and the genitalia. Freud's developmental stages were accordingly classified as the oral phase, birth to 1 year; the anal phase, ages 1 to 3 years; and the phallic phase, ages 3 to 5 years. Freud also described a fourth period, latency, which extends from ages 5 and 6 years until puberty. Latency is marked by a diminution of sexual interest, which is reactivated at puberty. Freud believed that successful resolution of these childhood phases was essential to normal adult functioning and that by comparison, adult experiences are of relatively little consequence. (Freud's theories are discussed extensively in Section 6.1.)

Carl Gustav Jung. Carl Gustav Jung viewed external factors as playing an important role in a person's normal growth and adaptation. He described the process of individuation as the growth and expansion of personality that occurs through the person's realizing and learning what he or she is intrinsically. According to Jung, libido is every possible manifestation of psychic energy; it is not limited to sexuality or to aggression but includes religious and spiritual urges and the drive to seek a clear, deep understanding of the meaning of life.

Harry Stack Sullivan. Harry Stack Sullivan conceived of human development as largely shaped by external events, specifically by social interaction. According to his influential model of the life cycle, each phase of development is marked by a need for interactions with certain persons, and the quality of these interactions influences human personality. Normality, for Sullivan, is the capacity to see oneself and the world as they really are.

Erik Erikson. Although Erikson accepted Freud's theory of infantile sexuality, he also thought that development potentials occurred at all stages of life. Erikson constructed a life cycle model consisting of eight stages that extend into adulthood and old age:

Stage 1. Trust versus mistrust
Stage 2. Autonomy versus shame and doubt
Stage 3. Initiative versus guilt
Stage 4. Industry versus inferiority
Stage 5. Ego identity versus role confusion
Stage 6. Intimacy versus isolation
Stage 7. Generativity versus stagnation
Stage 8. Ego integrity versus despair

Erikson ascribed five of these psychological stages to childhood: trust, autonomy, initiative, industry, and identity, which correlate with Freud's psychosexual stages. In addition, Erikson added three stages that extend beyond young adulthood into old age: intimacy, generativity, and integrity. For Erikson, normality implied the ability to be responsible for oneself and not to blame or fault others. His eight stages have both positive and negative aspects, have specific emotional crises, and are affected by the interaction of the person's biology, culture, and society. Each stage has two possible outcomes, one positive, or healthy, and the other negative, or unhealthy. Under ideal circumstances, the crisis is resolved when the person achieves a new, higher level of functioning after achieving a positive outcome at the end of the stage. According to Erikson, most persons do not achieve perfect positive polarity but fall more toward the positive pole than toward the negative pole. (Erikson's theories are discussed in depth in Section 6.2.)

Jean Piaget. By conducting intensive studies of the way children think and behave, Jean Piaget formulated a theory of cognition, which he divided into four stages: sensorimotor, preoperational thought, concrete operations, and formal operations. Infants grow by predetermined steps through various stages. Each stage has its own characteristics and needs and must be negotiated successfully before going to the next. The sequence of stages is not automatic but depends on both central nervous system growth and life experiences. Ample evidence indicates that an unfavorable environment can delay some of the developmental stages, but particularly favorable environ-

mental stimulators can accelerate progress through the stages. (Piaget's theories are discussed in depth in Section 4.1.)

Daniel Levinson. Daniel Levinson, at Yale University, focuses on personality development throughout the course of life. He suggests that the human life cycle is composed of four major eras, each lasting about 25 years, with some overlap, so that a new era is starting as the previous one is ending. Levinson identified a typical age of onset, that is, the age at which an era usually begins. The evolving sequence of eras and their age spans described by Levinson are childhood and adolescence, birth to 22 years; early adulthood, 17 to 45 years; middle adulthood, 40 to 65 years; and late adulthood, 65 years and beyond. Levinson also identified 4- to 5-year transitional periods between eras, which function as boundary zones during which a person terminates the outgoing era and initiates the incoming one.

Bernice Neugarten. Bernice Neugarten contributed to an understanding of normality in old age. Most studies of this period are deficit focused, that is, they emphasize what the elderly cannot do rather than what they can do. Neugarten observed that elders remain psychologically flexible and are able to adapt to the changing circumstances—both internal and external—of aging. She emphasized a normative approach to aging. In a normative framework researchers ask in effect, "How do old persons cope with the adaptational tasks of the 60s, 70s, and beyond?" These tasks include maintaining physical and intellectual functioning, sustaining flexibility and the capacity for change, and continuing interpersonal relationships. Aging and some disability are normal; whereas extreme disability is neither normal nor inevitable. Most older persons do not fear death but come to accept it as the normal end to the life cycle.

Neugarten and her group have been among the few workers to study the psychology of women. In particular, she has found that most women successfully adapt to the various crisis points of marriage, pregnancy, childbirth, and the menopause.

ADAPTIVE MENTAL MECHANISMS

George Vaillant and his group studied a cohort of men for almost 50 years, starting when they were freshmen at Harvard University. A happy childhood manifested by few oral-dependent traits, little psychopathology, the capacity to play, and good object relationships was found to correlate significantly with positive traits in middle life.

Vaillant noted that a hierarchy of ego mechanisms was constructed as the men advanced in age. Defenses were organized along a continuum that reflected two aspects of the personality: immaturity versus maturity and psychopathology versus objective adaptation to the external environment. Moreover, the defensive style shifted as a person matured. Vaillant concluded that adaptive styles mature over the years and that the maturation depends more on development from within than on changes in the interpersonal environment. He also corroborated Erikson's model of the life cycle.

Vaillant described a scheme for a positive psychology that focuses on the normal, or positive, aspects of thinking, feeling, and behavior rather than on its negative, or pathological, aspects. He identified a group of adaptive or mature defense mechanisms that enable a person to cope with the stresses of life. Persons who use them are likely to have a normal adjustment in life as measured by economic stability, joy in living, marital satisfaction, and both a subjective sense and objective evidence of physical health. The mature, adaptive defenses according to Vaillant are altruism, sublimation, anticipation, and humor. Some also consider asceticism and suppression mature defenses (Table 2.1–3).

Table 2.1–3
The Mature Defenses

Altruism. The vicarious but constructive and instinctually gratifying service to others. This must be distinguished from altruistic surrender, which involves a surrender of direct gratification or of instinctual needs in favor of fulfilling the needs of others to the detriment of the self, with vicarious satisfaction only being gained through introjection.

Anticipation. The realistic anticipation of, or planning for, future inner discomfort; implies overly concerned planning, worrying, and anticipation of dire and dreadful possible outcomes.

Asceticism. The elimination of directly pleasurable affects attributable to an experience. The moral element is implicit in setting values on specific pleasures. Asceticism is directed against all "base" pleasures perceived consciously, and gratification is derived from the renunciation.

Humor. The overt expression of feelings without personal discomfort or immobilization and without unpleasant effect on others. Humor allows one to bear, and yet focus on, what is too terrible to be borne, in contrast to wit, which always involves distraction or displacement away from the affective issue.

Sublimation. The gratification of an impulse whose goal is retained, but whose aim or object is changed from a socially objectionable one to a socially valued one. Libidinal sublimation involves desexualization of drive impulses and placing a value judgment that substitutes what is valued by the superego or society. Sublimation of aggressive impulses takes place through pleasurable games and sports. Unlike neurotic defenses, sublimation allows instincts to be channeled rather than to be dammed up or diverted. Thus, in sublimation, feelings are acknowledged, modified, and directed toward a relatively significant person or goal so that modest instinctual satisfaction results.

Suppression. The conscious or semiconscious decision to postpone attention to a conscious impulse or conflict.

Courtesy of William W. Meissner, M.D.

Adaptive defenses occur equally in men and women and are seen in all socioeconomic groups. Persons who used the most adaptive defenses were less likely to become depressed after stressful life events than those who did not. An incidental finding among men who had been in combat was that adaptive defenses were protective against posttraumatic stress disorders (PTSD).

Normal Child Development

Normal child development may be approached from a variety of perspectives. Melvin Lewis describes normal childhood behavior as that which conforms to the expectations of the majority in a given society at a given time. According to Lewis, disordered behavior in a child is behavior that most adults consider inappropriate in form, frequency, or intensity. Lewis points out that the criteria for such a judgment "are often nebulous," and different biases come into play that infuse the boundary between normal and abnormal.

As mentioned above, Freud described four psychosexual stages of child development—oral, anal, phallic, and latency—derived from the analysis of adults with various types of psy-

chopathology. On the basis of direct observations of children, other psychoanalysts elaborated on many of Freud's theories.

Anna Freud delineated aspects of normal growth and development in children and was interested in empirical research directed at helping to clarify how children cope with adaptive tasks. She described stages of development—such as dependence to independence, wetting to bladder control, self-involvement to companionship—that represent the movement from the immature infant to the complexity of the developed child.

Margaret Mahler studied early childhood object relations and made a significant contribution to the understanding of personality development. She described the separation-individuation process, resulting in a person's subjective sense of separateness from the world around him or her. The separation-individuation phase of development begins in the fourth or fifth month of life and is completed by age 3 years.

In view of the various models for conceptualizing the phases of development, it has become customary to organize developmental stages in chronological order as follows: infancy; toddler period; preschool period; school period or middle years; early, middle, and late adolescence; and early, middle, and late adulthood (old age). In the sections that follow these stages are discussed in greater detail.

References

Austrian SG, ed. *Developmental Theories through the Life Cycle.* New York: Columbia University Press; 2002.
Craig GJ. *Human Development.* 7th ed. Upper Saddle River, NJ: Prentice-Hall; 1996.
Cui X-J, Vaillant GE. Antecedents and consequences of negative life events in adulthood: a longitudinal study. *Am J Psychiatry.* 1996;153:21.
Dacey JS, Travers JF. *Human Development across the Lifespan.* 3rd ed. Madison, WI: Brown & Benchmark; 1996.
Erikson E. *Childhood and Society.* New York: WW Norton; 1950.
Ferraro KF, Farmer MM. Utility of health data from social surveys: is there a gold standard for measuring morbidity? *Am Sociol Rev.* 1999;64:303.
Freud A. *The Ego and the Mechanisms of Defense.* New York: International Universities Press; 1966.
Haw C. Psychological perspectives on women's vulnerability to mental illness. In: Kohen D, ed. *Women and Mental Health.* London: Routledge; 2000:65.
Lidz T. *The Person: His and Her Development throughout the Life Cycle.* New York: Basic Books; 1976.
Offer D, Sabshin M. *Normality and the Life Cycle.* New York: Basic Books; 1984.
Phelan JC, Link BG. The labeling theory of mental disorder (1): the role of social contingencies in the application of psychiatric labels. In: Horwitz AV, Scheid TL, eds. *A Handbook for the Study of Mental Health: Social Contexts, Theories, and Systems.* Cambridge: Cambridge University Press; 1999:139.
Robins LN, Rutter M, eds. *Straight and Devious Pathways from Childhood to Adulthood.* Cambridge: Cambridge University Press, 1989.
Strayer J. The dynamics of emotions and life cycle identity. *Identity.* 2002;2:47.
Vaillant GE, ed. *Empirical Studies of Ego Mechanism and Defense.* Washington, DC: American Psychiatric Association Press; 1986.

▲ 2.2 Prenatal Period, Infancy, and Childhood

The conventional stages of early development include the prenatal period, infancy (from birth to about 15 months), the toddler period (15 months to 2½ years), the preschool period (2½ to 6 years), and the middle years (6 to 12 years). These stages form a continuum along which development proceeds, and after birth there is rarely a clear-cut division between them.

Arnold Gesell described developmental schedules that are widely used in both pediatrics and child psychiatry. These schedules outline the qualitative sequence of children's motor, adaptive, and personal-social behavior from birth to 6 years (Table 2.2–1).

PRENATAL PERIOD

After implantation the egg begins to divide and is known as an *embryo.* Growth and development occur at a rapid pace; by the end of 8 weeks, the shape is recognizably human, and the embryo has become a *fetus.* Figure 2.2–1 illustrates a 12-week fetus in utero.

The fetus maintains an internal equilibrium that, with variable effects, interacts continuously with the intrauterine environment. In general, most disorders that occur are multifactorial—the result of a combination of effects, some of which may be additive. Damage at the fetal stage usually has a more global impact than damage after birth, because rapidly growing organs are the most vulnerable. Boys are more vulnerable to developmental damage than girls; geneticists recognize that in humans and animals, girls show a propensity for greater biological vigor than boys, possibly because of the girls' second X chromosome.

Fetal Life

A great deal of biological activity occurs in utero. A fetus is involved in a variety of behaviors that are necessary for adaptation outside the womb. For example, a fetus sucks on thumb and fingers; it folds and unfolds its body and eventually assumes a position in which its occiput is in an anterior vertex position, which is the position in which fetuses usually exit the uterus.

Behavior. Pregnant women are extraordinarily sensitive to prenatal movements. They describe their unborn babies as active or passive, as kicking vigorously or rolling around, as quiet when the mothers are active but as kicking as soon as the mothers try to rest.

Women usually detect fetal movements 16 to 20 weeks into the pregnancy; the fetus can be artificially set into total body motion by in utero stimulation of its ventral skin surfaces by the 14th week. The fetus may be able to hear by the 18th week, and it responds to loud noises with muscle contractions, movements, and an increased heart rate. Bright light flashed on the abdominal wall of the 20-week pregnant woman causes changes in fetal heart rate and position. The retinal structures begin to function at that time. Eyelids open at 7 months. Smell and taste are also developed at this time, and the fetus responds to substances that may be injected into the amniotic sac, such as contrast medium. Some reflexes present at birth exist in utero: the grasp reflex, which appears at 17 weeks; the Moro (startle) reflex, which appears at 25 weeks; and the sucking reflex, which appears at about 28 weeks.

Nervous System. The nervous system arises from the neural plate, which is a dorsal ectodermal thickening that appears on about the 16th day of gestation. By the sixth week, part of the neural tube becomes the cerebral vesicle, which later becomes the cerebral hemispheres (Fig. 2.2–2).

The cerebral cortex begins to develop by the 10th week, but layers do not appear until the sixth month of pregnancy; the sensory cortex and the motor cortex are formed before the association cortex. Some brain function has been detected in utero by

Table 2.2–1
Landmarks of Normal Behavioral Development

Age	Motor and Sensory Behavior	Adaptive Behavior	Personal and Social Behavior
Birth to 4 weeks	Hand-to-mouth reflex, grasping reflex Rooting reflex (puckering lips in response to perioral stimulation), Moro reflex (digital extension when startled), sucking reflex, Babinski reflex (toes spread when sole of foot is touched) Differentiates sounds (orients to human voice) and sweet and sour tastes Visual tracking Fixed focal distance of 8 inches Makes alternating crawling movements Moves head laterally when placed in prone position	Anticipatory feeding-approach behavior at 4 days Responds to sound of rattle and bell Regards moving objects momentarily	Responsiveness to mother's face, eyes, and voice within first few hours of life Endogenous smile Independent play (until 2 years) Quiets when picked up Impassive face
4 weeks	Tonic neck reflex positions predominate Hands fisted Head sags but can hold head erect for a few seconds Visual fixation, stereoscopic vision (12 weeks)	Follows moving objects to the midline Shows no interest and drops object immediately	Regards face and diminishes activity Responds to speech Smiles preferentially to mother
16 weeks	Symmetrical postures predominate Holds head balanced Head lifted 90° when prone on forearm Visual accommodation	Follows a slowly moving object well Arms activate on sight of dangling object	Spontaneous social smile (exogenous) Aware of strange situations
28 weeks	Sits steadily, leaning forward on hands Bounces actively when placed in standing position	One-hand approach and grasp of toy Bangs and shakes rattle Transfers toys	Takes feet to mouth Pats mirror image Starts to imitate mother's sounds and actions
40 weeks	Sits alone with good coordination Creeps Pulls self to standing position Points with index finger	Matches two objects at midline Attempts to imitate scribble	Separation anxiety manifest when taken away from mother Responds to social play, such as pat-a-cake and peekaboo Feeds self cracker and holds own bottle
52 weeks	Walks with one hand held Stands alone briefly	Seeks novelty	Cooperates in dressing
15 months	Toddles Creeps up stairs		Points or vocalizes wants Throws objects in play or refusal
18 months	Coordinated walking, seldom falls Hurls ball Walks up stairs with one hand held	Builds a tower of three or four cubes Scribbles spontaneously and imitates a writing stroke	Feeds self in part, spills Pulls toy on string Carries or hugs a special toy, such as a doll Imitates some behavioral patterns with slight delay
2 years	Runs well, no falling Kicks large ball Goes up and down stairs alone Fine motor skills increase	Builds a tower of six or seven cubes Aligns cubes, imitating train Imitates vertical and circular strokes Develops original behaviors	Pulls on simple garment Domestic mimicry Refers to self by name Says "no" to mother Separation anxiety begins to diminish Organized demonstrations of love and protest Parallel play (plays side by side but does not interact with other children)
3 years	Rides tricycle Jumps from bottom steps Alternates feet going up stairs	Builds tower of 9 or 10 cubes Imitates a three-cube bridge Copies a circle and a cross	Puts on shoes Unbuttons buttons Feeds self well Understands taking turns
4 years	Walks down stairs one step to a tread Stands on one foot for 5 to 8 seconds	Copies a cross Repeats four digits Counts three objects with correct pointing	Washes and dries own face Brushes teeth Associative or joint play (plays cooperatively with other children)
5 years	Skips, using feet alternately Usually has complete sphincter control Fine coordination improves	Copies a square Draws a recognizable person with a head, a body, and limbs Counts 10 objects accurately	Dresses and undresses self Prints a few letters Plays competitive exercise games
6 years	Rides two-wheel bicycle	Prints name Copies triangle	Ties shoelaces

Adapted from Arnold Gessell, M.D., and Stella Chess, M.D.

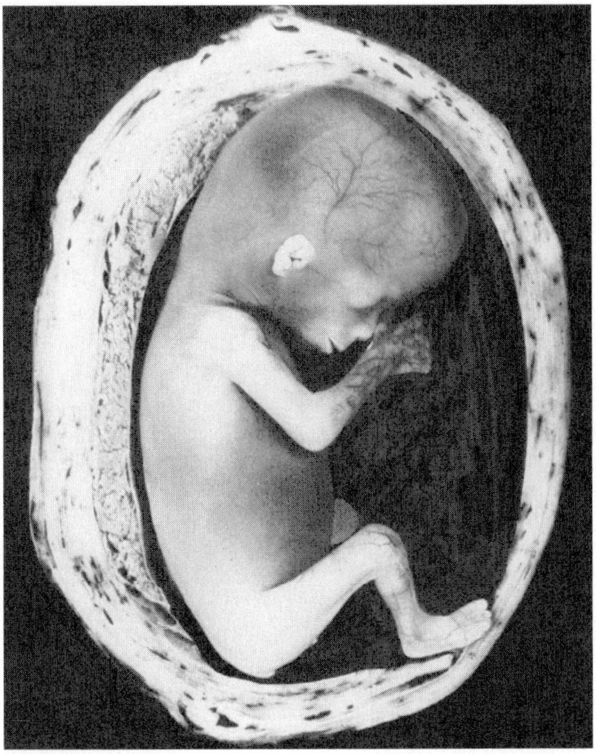

FIGURE 2.2–1
Photograph of a 12-week fetus in utero. Note the extremely thin skin and the underlying blood vessels. The face has all the human characteristics, but the ears are still primitive. Movements begin at this time but are usually not felt by the mother. (From Langman J. *Medical Embryology.* 8th ed. Baltimore: Williams & Wilkins; 2000:78, with permission.)

fetal encephalographic responses to sound. The human brain weighs about 350 g at birth and 1,450 g at full adult development, a fourfold increase, mainly in the neocortex. This increase is almost entirely due to growth in the number and branching of dendrites establishing new connections. After birth, the number of new neurons is negligible. Uterine contractions may contribute to fetal neural development by causing the developing neural network to receive and transmit sensory impulses.

Maternal Stress

Maternal stress correlates with high levels of stress hormones (epinephrine, norepinephrine, and adrenocorticotropic hormone) in the fetal bloodstream, which act directly on the fetal neuronal network to increase blood pressure, heart rate, and activity level. Mothers with high levels of anxiety are more likely to have babies who are hyperactive, irritable, and of low birthweight and who have problems feeding and sleeping than are mothers with low anxiety levels. A fever in the mother causes the fetus's temperature to rise.

Genetic Disorders

In many cases, genetic counseling depends on prenatal diagnosis. The diagnostic techniques used include amniocentesis (transabdominal aspiration of fluid from the amniotic sac), ultrasound examinations, X-rays, fetoscopy (direct visualization of the fetus), fetal blood and skin sampling, chorionic villus sampling, and α-fetoprotein screening. In about 2 percent of women tested, the results are positive for some abnormality, including X-linked disorders, neural tube defects (detected by high levels of α-fetoprotein), chromosomal disorders (e.g., trisomy 21), and various inborn errors of metabolism (e.g., Tay-Sachs disease and lipoidoses).

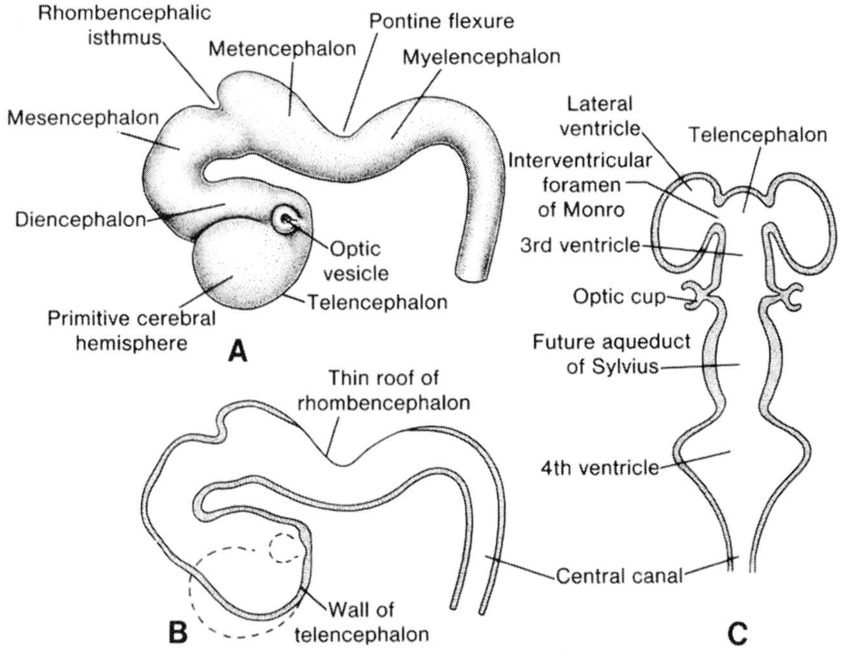

FIGURE 2.2–2
A. Lateral view of the brain vesicles of the human embryo in the beginning of the sixth week (modified after Hochstetter). **B.** Midline section through the brain vesicles and spinal cord of an embryo of the same age as shown in **A.** Note the thin roof of the rhombencephalon. **C.** Diagram to show the lumina of the spinal cord and brain vesicles. (From Langman J. *Medical Embryology.* 4th ed. Baltimore: Williams & Wilkins; 1981:322, with permission.)

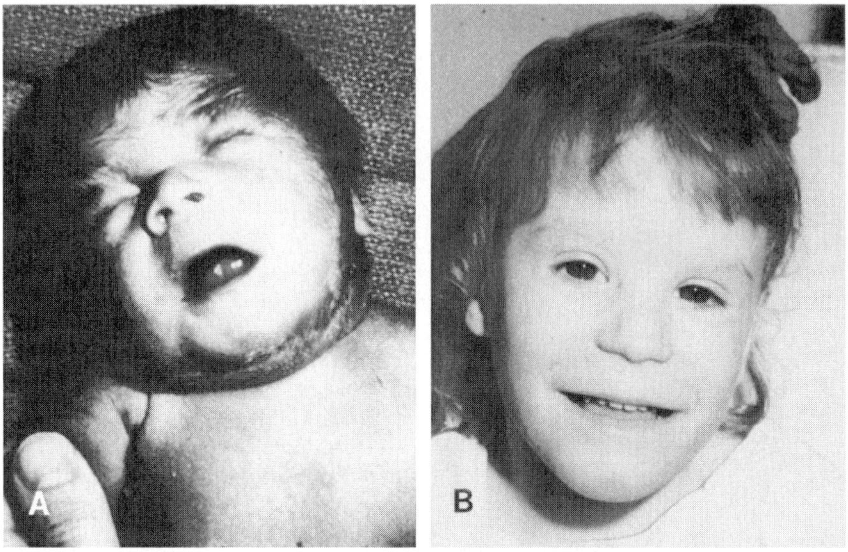

FIGURE 2.2–3
Photographs of children with "fetal-alcohol syndrome." **A.** Severe case. **B.** Slightly affected child. Note in both children the short palpebral fissures and hypoplasia of the maxilla. Usually the defect includes other craniofacial abnormalities. Cardiovascular defects and limb deformities are also common symptoms of the fetal alcohol syndrome. (From Langman J. *Medical Embryology.* 7th ed. Baltimore: Williams & Wilkins; 1995:108, with permission.)

Some diagnostic tests carry a risk; for instance, about 5 percent of women who undergo fetoscopy miscarry. Amniocentesis, which is usually performed between the 14th and 16th weeks of pregnancy, causes fetal damage or miscarriage in less than 1 percent of women tested. Fully 98 percent of all prenatal tests in pregnant women reveal no abnormality in the fetus. Prenatal testing is recommended for women over 35 and for those with a family history of a congenital defect.

Maternal Drug Use

Fetal alcohol syndrome (Fig. 2.2–3) affects about one third of all infants born to alcoholic women. The syndrome is characterized by growth retardation of prenatal origin (height, weight); minor anomalies, including microphthalmia (small eyeballs), short palpebral fissures, midface hypoplasia (underdevelopment), a smooth or short philtrum, and a thin upper lip; and central nervous system (CNS) manifestations, including microcephaly (head circumference below the third percentile), a history of delayed development, hyperactivity, attention deficits, learning disabilities, intellectual deficits, and seizures. The incidence of infants born with fetal alcohol syndrome is about 0.5 per 1,000 live births.

Smoking during pregnancy is associated with below-average infant birthweight. Infants born to mothers dependent on narcotics go through a withdrawal syndrome at birth. Crack cocaine use by women during pregnancy has been correlated with a number of behavioral abnormalities including increased irritability and crying and decreased desire for human contact. No direct causal relation has been established because of confounding variables including maternal use of other drugs.

Prenatal exposure to various medications can also result in abnormalities. Common drugs with teratogenic effects include antibiotics (tetracyclines), anticonvulsants (valproate [Depakene], carbamazepine [Tegretol], and phenytoin [Dilantin]), progesterone-estrogens, lithium (Eskalith), and warfarin (Coumadin).

When a woman is exposed to severe radiation during the first 20 weeks of her pregnancy, the baby will be born with gross deformities. Estimates are that 3 to 6 percent of all newborns have some sort of birth defect that is fatal at birth or that causes permanent disability. Table 2.2–2 lists malformations that occur during the first year of life.

Table 2.2–2
Causes of Human Malformations Observed During the First Year of Life

Suspected Cause	% of Total
Genetic	
Autosomal genetic disease	15–20
Cytogenic (chromosomal abnormalities)	5
Unknown	
Polygenic	
Multifactorial (genetic-environmental interactions)	
Spontaneous error of development	
Synergistic interactions of teratogens	
Environmental	
Maternal conditions: diabetes; endocrinopathies; nutritional deficiencies, starvation; drug and substance addictions	4
Maternal infections: rubella, toxoplasmosis, syphilis, herpes, cytomegalic inclusion disease, varicella, Venezuelan equine encephalitis, parvovirus B19	3
Mechanical problems (deformations): abnormal cord constrictions, disparity in uterine size and uterine contents	1–2
Chemicals, drugs, radiation, hyperthermia	<1
Preconception exposures (excluding mutagens and infectious agents)	<1

Reprinted with permission from Brent RL, Beckman DA. Environmental teratogens. *Bull N Y Acad Med.* 1990;66:125.

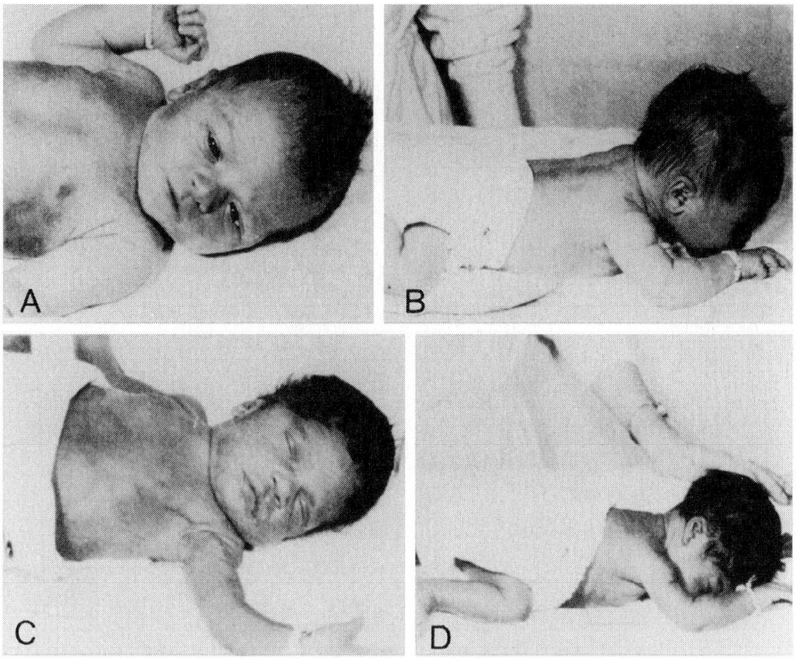

FIGURE 2.2–4
Contrast between full-term (**A** and **B**) and premature (**C** and **D**) infants. Note the limp sprawl of the baby in **C** and the difficulty in raising the head to clear nose and mouth in **D**. (Reprinted with permission from Stone LJ, Church J. *Childhood and Adolescence.* 4th ed. New York: Random House; 1979:7.)

INFANCY

The delivery of the fetus marks the start of infancy. The average newborn weighs about 3,400 g (7$^1/_2$ lb). *Small fetuses*, defined as those with a birthweight below the 10th percentile for their gestational age, occur in about 7 percent of all pregnancies. At the 26th to the 28th week of gestation, the prematurely born fetus has a good chance of survival.

Premature infants are defined as those with a gestation of less than 34 weeks or a birthweight under 2,500 g. Such infants are at increased risk for learning disabilities such as dyslexia, emotional and behavioral problems, mental retardation, and child abuse. With each 100-g increment of weight, beginning at about 1,000 g, infants have a progressively better chance of survival. A 36-week-old fetus has less chance of survival than a 3,000-g fetus born close to term. The difference between normal and preterm infants is shown in Figure 2.2–4.

Postmature infants are defined as infants born 2 weeks or more beyond the expected date of birth. Because pregnancy at term is calculated as extending 40 weeks from the last menstrual period and since the exact time of fertilization varies, the incidence of postmaturity is high if based on menstrual history alone. The postmature baby typically has long nails, scanty lanugo hair, more scalp hair than usual, and increased alertness.

Developmental Landmarks

Reflexes and Survival Systems at Birth. Reflexes are present at birth. They include the rooting reflex (puckering of the lips in response to perioral stimulation), the grasp reflex, the plantar (Babinski) reflex, the knee reflex, the abdominal reflexes, the startle (Moro) reflex (Fig. 2.2–5), and the tonic neck reflex. In normal children, the grasp reflex, the startle reflex, and the tonic neck reflex disappear by the fourth month. The Babinski reflex usually disappears by the 12th month.

Survival systems—breathing, sucking, swallowing, and circulatory and temperature homeostasis—are relatively functional at birth, but the sensory organs are incompletely developed. Further differentiation of neurophysiological functions depends on an active process of stimulatory reinforcement from the external environment, such as persons touching and stroking the infant. The newborn infant is awake for only a short period each day; rapid eye movement (REM) and non-REM sleep are present at birth. Other spontaneous behaviors include crying, smiling, and penile erection in males. One-day-old infants can detect the smell of their mother's milk, and 3-day-old infants distinguish their mother's voice.

Language and Cognitive Development. At birth, infants can make noises, such as crying, but they do not vocalize until about 8 weeks. At that time, guttural or babbling sounds occur spontaneously, especially in response to the mother. The persistence and further evolution of children's vocalizations depend on parental reinforcement. Language development occurs in well-delineated stages as outlined in Table 2.2–3.

By the end of infancy (about 2 years), infants have transformed reflexes into voluntary actions that are the building blocks of cognition. They begin to interact with the environment, to experience feedback from their own bodies, and to become intentional in their actions. By the end of the second year of life, children begin to use symbolic play and language.

Jean Piaget (1896–1980), a Swiss psychologist, observed the growing capacity of young children (including his own) to think and to reason. An outline of the main stages of his theory

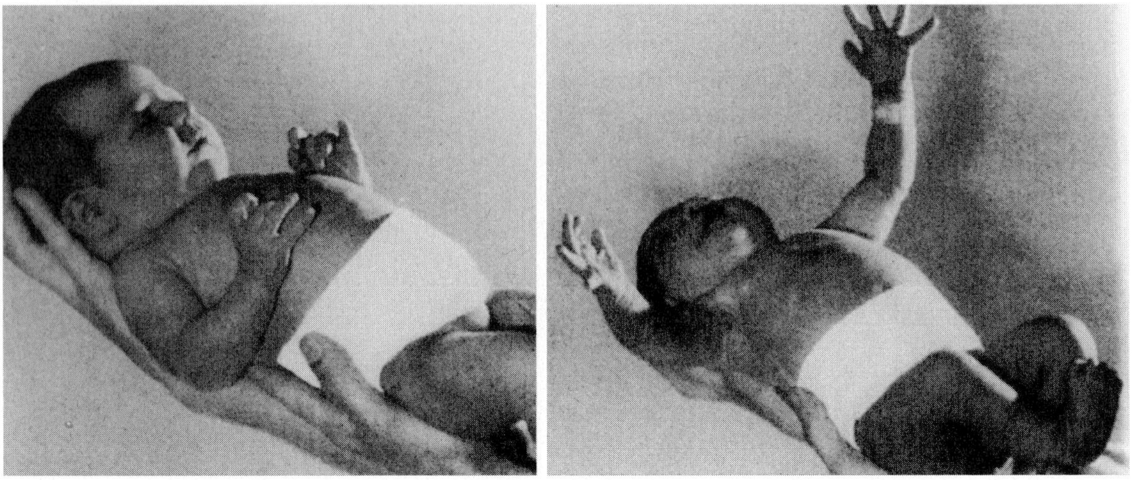

FIGURE 2.2–5
Moro reflex. (Reprinted with permission from Stone LJ, Church J. *Childhood and Adolescence.* 4th ed. New York: Random House; 1979:14.)

of cognitive development is presented in Table 2.2–4, and his work is discussed extensively in Section 4.1.

Emotional and Social Development. By the age of 3 weeks, infants imitate the facial movements of adult caregivers. They open their mouths and thrust out their tongues in response to adults who do the same. By the third and fourth months of life, these behaviors are easily elicited. These imitative behaviors are believed to be the precursors of infants' emotional life. The smiling response occurs in two phases: the first phase is endogenous smiling, which occurs spontaneously within the first 2 months and is unrelated to external stimulation; the second phase is exogenous smiling, which is stimulated from the outside, usually by the mother, and occurs by the 16th week.

The stages of emotional development parallel those of cognitive development. Indeed, the caregiving person provides the major stimulus for both aspects of mental growth. Human infants depend totally on adults for survival. Through regular and predictable interaction, an infant's behavioral repertoire expands as a consequence of caregivers' social responses (Table 2.2–5).

In the first year, infants' moods are highly variable and intimately related to internal states such as hunger. Toward the second two thirds of the first year, infants' moods grow increasingly related to external social cues; a parent can get even a hungry infant to smile. When the infant is internally comfortable, a sense of interest and pleasure in the world and in its primary caregivers should prevail. The development of infants' personal and social behavior is outlined in Table 2.2–1. Prolonged separation from the mother (or other primary caregiver) during the second 6 months of life can lead to depression that may persist into adulthood as part of an individual's character.

Temperamental Differences

There are strong suggestions of inborn differences and wide variability in autonomic reactivity and temperament among individual infants. Stella Chess and Alexander Thomas (husband and wife psychiatric collaborators) identified the following nine behavioral dimensions, in which reliable differences among infants can be observed.

1. Activity level—the motor component present in a given child's functioning
2. Rhythmicity—the predictability of such functions as hunger, feeding pattern, elimination, and the sleep-wake cycle
3. Approach or withdrawal—the response to a new stimulus, such as a food, toy, or person
4. Adaptability—the speed and ease with which a current behavior can be modified in response to altered environmental structuring
5. Intensity of reaction—the amount of energy used in mood expression
6. Threshold of responsiveness—the stimulation intensity required to evoke a discernable response to sensory stimuli, environmental objects, and social contacts
7. Quality of mood—pleasant, joyful, friendly behavior versus unpleasant, crying, unfriendly behavior
8. Distractibility—the effectiveness of extraneous environmental stimuli interfering with, or altering the direction of, ongoing behavior
9. Attention span and persistence—the length of time a particular activity is pursued (attention span) and the continuation of an activity in the face of obstacles (persistence)

The ratings of individual children showed considerable stability over a 25-year follow-up period, but some temperamental traits did not persist. This finding was attributed to genetic effects on personality; that is, some gene actions were discontinuous. There is a complex interplay among the initial characteristics of infants, the mode of parental management, children's subsequent behavior, and even the appearance of symptoms. These connections support the concept of the importance of both genetic endowment (nature) and environmental experience (nurture) in behavior.

Table 2.2–3
Language Development

Age and Stage of Development	Mastery of Comprehension	Mastery of Expression
0–6 months	Shows startle response to loud or sudden sounds Attempts to localize sounds, turning eyes or head Appears to listen to speakers, may respond with smile Recognizes warning, angry, and friendly voices Responds to hearing own name	Has vocalizations other than crying Has differential cries for hunger, pain Makes vocalizations to show pleasure Plays at making sounds Babbles (a repeated series of sounds)
7–11 months Attending-to-language stage	Shows listening selectivity (voluntary control over responses to sounds) Listens to music or singing with interest Recognizes "no," "hot," own name Looks at pictures being named for up to 1 minute Listens to speech without being distracted by other sounds	Responds to own name with vocalizations Imitates the melody of utterances Uses jargon (own language) Has gestures (shakes head for no) Has exclamation ("oh-oh") Plays language games (pat-a-cake, peekaboo)
12–18 months Single-word stage	Shows gross discriminations between dissimilar sounds (bells vs. dog vs. horn vs. mother's or father's voice) Understands basic body parts, names of common objects Acquires understanding of some new words each week Can identify simple objects (baby, ball, etc.) from a group of objects or pictures Understands up to 150 words by age 18 months	Uses single words (mean age of first word is 11 months; by age 18 months, child is using up to 20 words) "Talks" to toys, self, or others using long patterns of jargon and occasional words Approximately 25% of utterances are intelligible All vowels articulated correctly Initial and final consonants often omitted
12–24 months Two-word messages stage	Responds to simple directions ("Give me the ball") Responds to action commands ("Come here," "Sit down") Understands pronouns (me, him, her, you) Begins to understand complex sentences ("When we go to the store, I'll buy you some candy")	Uses two-word utterances ("Mommy sock," "all gone," "ball here") Imitates environmental sounds in play ("moo," "mmm, mmm," etc.) Refers to self by name, begins to use pronouns Echoes two or more last words of sentences Begins to use three-word telegraphic utterances ("all gone ball," "me go now") Utterances 26% to 50% intelligible Uses language to ask for needs
24–36 months Grammar formation stage	Understands small body parts (elbow, chin, eyebrow) Understands family name categories (grandma, baby) Understands size (little one, big one) Understands most adjectives Understands functions (why do we eat, why do we sleep)	Uses real sentences with grammatical function words (can, will, the, a) Usually announces intentions before acting "Conversations" with other children, usually just monologues Jargon and echolalia gradually drop from speech Increased vocabulary (up to 270 words at 2 years, 895 words at 3 years) Speech 50% to 80% intelligible *P, b, m* articulated correctly Speech may show rhythmic disturbances
36–54 months Grammar development stage	Understands prepositions (under, behind, between) Understands many words (up to 3,500 at 3 years, 5,500 at 4 years) Understands cause and effect (What do you do when you're hungry?, cold?) Understands analogies (Food is to eat, milk is to _____)	Correct articulation of *n, w, ng, h, t, d, k, g* Uses language to relate incidents from the past Uses wide range of grammatical forms: plurals, past tense, negatives, questions Plays with language: rhymes, exaggerates Speech 90% intelligible, occasional errors in the ordering of sounds within words Able to define words Egocentric use of language rare Can repeat a 12-syllable sentence correctly Some grammatical errors still occur
55 months on True communication stage	Understands concepts of number, speed, time, space Understands left and right Understands abstract terms Is able to categorize items into semantic classes	Uses language to tell stories, share ideas, and discuss alternatives Increasing use of varied grammar; spontaneous self-correction of grammatical errors Stabilizing of articulation *f, v, s, z, l, r, th*, and consonant clusters Speech 100% intelligible

Reprinted with permission from Rutter M, Hersov L, eds. *Child and Adolescent Psychiatry.* London: Blackwell; 1985.

Table 2.2–4
Stages of Cognitive Development Proposed by Piaget

1. Sensorimotor (birth to 2 years)
   From the outset, biology and experience blend to produce learned behavior. A stimulus is received, a response elicited, accompanied by awareness. As children become more mobile, these experiences build on one another.
   Critical achievements by the end of this period:
   a. Object permanence (objects have an existence independent of children's involvement with them)
   b. Symbolization, expressed in mental symbols and words
2. Preoperational thought (2 to 7 years)
   Children use symbols and language more extensively, but thinking and reasoning are intuitive. Children are unable to think logically or deductively.
   Characteristics:
   a. Sense of "immanent justice"—punishment for bad deeds is unavoidable
   b. Egocentrism—children see themselves as center of the universe, are unable to understand another's point of view
   c. "Phenomenalistic causality"—events that occur together are thought to cause one another
   d. "Animistic thinking"—physical events and objects are endowed with feelings and intentions
3. Concrete operations (7 to 11 years)
   Egocentric thought is replaced by "operational" thought, which involves attending to information outside; children are able to understand another's point of view. Children in this stage can serialize, order, and group things according to common characteristics.
   Critical achievements:
   a. Conservation—recognizing that a ball of clay rolled out into a tube contains the same amount of clay
   b. Reversibility—ice can change to water and back to ice again
4. Formal operations (11 years through the end of adolescence)
   Children can think abstractly, reason deductively, and define abstract concepts. Not all children enter this stage at the same time or to the same degree.

Attachment

Bonding is the term used to describe the intense emotional and psychological relationship a mother develops for her baby. *Attachment* is the relationship the baby develops with its caregivers. Infants in the first months after birth become attuned to social and interpersonal interaction. They show a rapidly increasing responsivity to the external environment and an ability to form a special relationship with significant primary caregivers—that is, to form an attachment.

Table 2.2–5
Emotional Development from Infancy Through Childhood

Age	Emotional Capacity and Expression
Birth	Pleasure, surprise, disgust, distress
6–8 weeks	Joy
3–4 months	Anger
8–9 months	Sadness, fear
12–18 months	Tender affection, shame (begins at 18 months)
24 months	Pride
3–4 years	Guilt, envy
5–6 years	Insecurity, humility, confidence

Data adapted from Joseph Campas at the University of Denver and other researchers.

Harry Harlow. Harry Harlow studied social learning and the effects of social isolation in monkeys. Harlow placed newborn rhesus monkeys with two types of surrogate mothers—one a wire-mesh surrogate with a feeding bottle and the other a wire-mesh surrogate covered with terry cloth. The monkeys preferred the terry-cloth surrogates, which provided contact and comfort, to the feeding surrogate. (When hungry, the infant monkeys would go to the feeding bottle but then would quickly return to the terry-cloth surrogate.) When frightened, monkeys raised with terry-cloth surrogates showed intense clinging behavior and appeared to be comforted, whereas those raised with wire-mesh surrogates gained no comfort and appeared to be disorganized. The results of Harlow's experiments were widely interpreted as indicating that infant attachment is not simply the result of feeding.

Both types of surrogate-reared monkeys were subsequently unable to adjust to life in a monkey colony and had extraordinary difficulty learning to mate. When impregnated, the females failed to mother their young. These behavioral peculiarities were attributed to the isolates' lack of mothering in infancy.

John Bowlby. John Bowlby studied the attachment of infants to mothers and concluded that early separation of infants from their mothers had severe negative effects on children's emotional and intellectual development. He described *attachment behavior,* which develops during the first year of life, as the maintenance of physical contact between the mother and child when the child is hungry, frightened, or in distress. (Section 4.2 discusses attachment theory.)

Mary Ainsworth. Mary Ainsworth expanded on Bowlby's observations and found that the interaction between mother and baby during the attachment period influences the baby's current and future behavior significantly. Many observers believe that patterns of infant attachment affect future adult emotional relationships. Patterns of attachment vary among babies; for example, some babies signal or cry less than others. Sensitive responsiveness to infant signals, such as cuddling the baby when it cries, causes infants to cry less in later months. Close bodily contact with the mother when the baby signals for her is also associated with the growth of self-reliance, rather than clinging dependence, as the baby grows older. Unresponsive mothers produce anxious babies.

Ainsworth also confirmed that attachment serves to reduce anxiety. What she called the *secured base effect* enables a child to move away from the attachment figure and explore the environment. Inanimate objects, such as a teddy bear or a blanket (called the *transitional object* by Donald Winnicott), also serve as a secure base, one that often accompanies children as they investigate the world. A growing body of literature derived from direct observation of mother-infant interactions and longitudinal studies has expanded on, and refined, Ainsworth's original descriptions. Maternal sensitivity and responsiveness are the main determinants of secure attachment. But when the attachment is insecure, the type of insecurity (avoidant, anxious, ambivalent) is determined by infant temperament. Overall, male infants are less likely to have secure attachments and are more vulnerable to changes in maternal sensitivity than are female infants.

The attachment of the firstborn child is decreased by the birth of a second; but it is decreased much more when the firstborn is 2 to 5 years of age when the younger sibling is born than when the firstborn is under 24 months. Not surprisingly, the extent of the decrease also depends on the mother's own sense of security, confidence, and mental health.

Social Deprivation Syndromes and Maternal Neglect. Investigators, especially René Spitz, have long documented the severe developmental retardation that accompanies maternal rejection and neglect. Infants in institutions characterized by low staff-to-infant ratios and frequent turnover of personnel tend to display marked developmental retardation, even with adequate physical care and freedom from infection. The same infants, placed in adequate foster or adoptive care, exhibit marked acceleration in development.

Fathers and Attachment. Babies become attached to fathers as well as to mothers, but the attachment is different. Generally, mothers hold babies for caregiving, and fathers hold babies for purposes of play. Given a choice of either parent after separation infants usually go to the mother, but if the mother is unavailable they turn to the father for comfort. Babies raised in extended families or with multiple caregivers are able to establish many attachments.

Stranger Anxiety. A fear of strangers is first noted in infants at about 26 weeks of age but is not fully developed until about 32 weeks (8 months). At the approach of a stranger infants cry and cling to their mothers. Babies exposed to only one caregiver are more likely to have stranger anxiety than are those exposed to a variety of caregivers. Stranger anxiety is believed to result from a baby's growing ability to distinguish caregivers from all other persons.

Separation anxiety, which occurs between 10 and 18 months of age, is related to stranger anxiety but is not identical to it. Separation from the person to whom the infant is attached precipitates separation anxiety. Stranger anxiety, however, occurs even when the infant is in the mother's arms. The infant learns to separate as it starts to crawl and move away from the mother, but the infant constantly looks back and frequently returns to the mother for reassurance.

Margaret Mahler (1897–1985) proposed a theory to describe how young children acquire a sense of identity separate from their mothers'. Her theory of separation-individuation was based on observations of the interactions of children and their mothers. This theory is outlined in Table 2.2–6.

Table 2.2–6
Stages of Separation-Individuation Proposed by Mahler

1. Normal autism (birth to 2 months)
   Periods of sleep outweigh periods of arousal in a state reminiscent of intrauterine life.
2. Symbiosis (2 to 5 months)
   Developing perceptual abilities gradually enable infants to distinguish the inner from the outer world; mother–infant is perceived as a single fused entity.
3. Differentiation (5 to 10 months)
   Progressive neurological development and increased alertness draw infants' attention away from self to the outer world. Physical and psychological distinctiveness from the mother is gradually appreciated.
4. Practicing (10 to 18 months)
   The ability to move autonomously increases children's exploration of the outer world.
5. Rapprochement (18 to 24 months)
   As children slowly realize their helplessness and dependence, the need for independence alternates with the need for closeness. Children move away from their mothers and come back for reassurance.
6. Object constancy (2 to 5 years)
   Children gradually comprehend and are reassured by the permanence of mother and other important people, even when not in their presence.

Infant Care

Clinicians are now beginning to view infants as important actors in the family drama, ones who partly determine its course. Infants' behavior controls mothers' behavior, just as mothers' behavior modulates infants' behavior. A calm, smiling, predictable infant is a powerful reward for tender maternal care. A jittery, irregular, irritable infant tries a mother's patience. When a mother's capacity for giving is marginal, such infant traits may cause her to turn away from her child and thus complicate the child's already-troubled beginnings.

Parental Fit. Parental fit describes how well the mother or father relates to the newborn or developing infant; the idea takes into account temperamental characteristics of both parent and child. Each newborn has innate psychophysiological characteristics, which are known collectively as temperament. Chess and Thomas identified a range of normal temperamental patterns, from the difficult child at one end of the spectrum to the easy child at the other end.

Difficult children, who make up 10 percent of all children, have a hyperalert physiological makeup. They react intensely to stimuli (cry easily at loud noises), sleep poorly, eat at unpredictable times, and are difficult to comfort. *Easy children,* who make up 40 percent of all children, are regular in eating, eliminating, and sleeping; are flexible; can adapt to change and new stimuli with a minimum of distress; and are easily comforted when they cry. The other 50 percent of children are mixtures of these two types. The difficult child is harder to raise and places greater demands on the parent than the easy child. Chess and Thomas used the term *goodness of fit* to characterize the harmonious and consonant interaction between a mother and a child in their motivations, capacities, and styles of behavior. Poorness of fit is likely to lead to distorted development and maladaptive functioning. A difficult child must be recognized, because parents of such infants often have feelings of inadequacy and believe that they are doing something wrong to account for the difficulty in sleeping and eating and the problems comforting the child. In addition, most difficult children have emotional disturbances later in life.

Good-Enough Mothering. Winnicott believed that infants begin life in a state of nonintegration, with unconnected and diffuse experiences, and that mothers provide the relationship that enables infants' incipient selves to emerge. Mothers supply a holding environment in which infants are contained and experienced. During the last trimester of pregnancy and for the first

few months of a baby's life, the mother is in a state of primary maternal preoccupation, absorbed in fantasies about, and experiences with, her baby. The mother need not be perfect, but she must provide good-enough mothering. She plays a vital role in bringing the world to the child and offering empathic anticipation of the infant's needs. If the mother can resonate with the infant's needs, the baby can become attuned to its own bodily functions and drives that are the basis for the gradually evolving sense of self.

TODDLER PERIOD

The second year of life is marked by accelerated motor and intellectual development. The ability to walk gives toddlers some control over their own actions; this mobility enables children to determine when to approach and when to withdraw. The acquisition of speech profoundly extends their horizons. Typically, children learn to say "no" before they learn to say "yes." Toddlers' negativism is vital to the development of independence, but if it persists, oppositional behavior connotes a problem.

Learning language is a crucial task in the toddler period. Vocalizations become distinct, and toddlers can name a few objects and make needs known in one or two words. Near the end of the second year and into the third year toddlers sometimes use short sentences. The pace of language development varies considerably from child to child, and although a small number of children are truly late developers, most child experts recommend a hearing test if the child is not making two-word sentences by age 2.

Developmental Landmarks

Language and Cognitive Development. Toddlers begin to listen to explanations that can help them tolerate delay. They create new behaviors from old ones (originality) and engage in symbolic activities (e.g., using words and playing with dolls when the dolls represent something, such as a feeding sequence). Toddlers have varied capacities for concentration and self-regulation.

Emotional and Social Development. In the second year, pleasure and displeasure become further differentiated. "Social referencing" is often apparent at this age; the child looks to parents and others for emotional cues about how to respond to novel events. Toddlers show exploratory excitement, assertive pleasure, and pleasure in discovery and in developing new behavior (e.g., new games), including teasing and surprising or fooling the parent (e.g., hiding). The toddler has capacities for an organized demonstration of love (e.g., running up and hugging, smiling, and kissing the parent at the same time) and of protest (e.g., turning away, crying, banging, biting, hitting, yelling, and kicking). Comfort with family and apprehension with strangers may increase. Anxiety appears to be related to disapproval and the loss of a loved caregiver and can be disorganizing. (Additional information appears in Table 2.2–1.)

Sexual Development. Sexual differentiation is evident from birth, when parents start dressing and treating infants differently because of the expectations evoked by sex typing. Through imitation, reward, and coercion, children assume the behaviors that their cultures define as appropriate for their sexual roles. Children exhibit curiosity about anatomical sex. When their curiosity is recognized as healthy and is met with honest, age-appropriate replies, children acquire a sense of the wonder of life and are comfortable with their own roles. If the subject of sex is taboo and children's questions are rebuffed, shame and discomfort may result.

Gender identity, the unshakeable conviction of being male or female, begins to manifest at 18 months of age and is often fixed by 24 to 30 months. It was once widely believed that gender identity was primarily a function of social learning. John Money reported on children with ambiguous or damaged external genitalia who were raised as the sex opposite to their chromosomal sex. Long-term follow-up of those individuals suggests that the major part of gender identity is innate and that rearing may not affect the genetic diathesis.

Gender role describes the behavior that society deems appropriate for one sex or another, and it is not surprising that significant cultural differences exist. There may be different expectations for boys and girls in what and whom they play with, their tone of voice, the expression of emotions, and how they dress. Nevertheless, some generalizations are possible. Boys are more likely than girls to engage in rough and tumble play. Mothers talk more to girls than to boys, and by the time the child is two, fathers generally pay more attention to boys. Many educated, middle-class parents determined to raise nonsexist children are startled to see their children's determined preference for sex-stereotyped toys: girls want to play with dolls, boys with guns.

Sphincter Control and Sleep. The second year of life is a period of increasing social demands on children. Toilet training serves as a paradigm of the family's general training practices; that is, the parent who is overly severe in the area of toilet training is likely to be punitive and restrictive in other areas also. Control of daytime urination is usually complete by the age of 2½, and control of nighttime urination is usually complete by the age of 4 years, when bowel control is usually accomplished. Since 1900, there have been pendulum swings between extremes of permissiveness and control in toilet training. The trend in the United States has been toward delayed training, but in the last few years this trend appears to be shifting back to early training.

Toddlers may have sleep difficulties related to fear of the dark, which can often be managed by using a nightlight. Most toddlers generally sleep about 12 hours a day, including a 2-hour nap. Parents must be aware that children of this age may need reassurance before going to bed and that the average 2-year-old takes about 30 minutes to fall asleep.

Parenting

Paralleling the changing tasks for children are changing tasks for parents. In infancy, the major responsibility for parents is to meet the infant's needs in a sensitive and consistent fashion. The parental task in the toddler stage requires firmness about the boundaries of acceptable behavior and encouragement of the child's progressive emancipation. Parents must be careful not to be too authoritarian at this stage; children must be allowed to operate for themselves and to learn from their mis-

takes and must be protected and assisted when challenges are beyond their abilities.

During the toddler period, children are likely to struggle for the exclusive affection and attention of their parents. This struggle includes rivalry both with siblings and with one or another parent for the star role in the family. Although children are beginning to be able to share, they do so reluctantly. When the demands for exclusive possession are not resolved effectively, the result is likely to be jealous competitiveness in relationships with peers and lovers. The fantasies aroused by the struggle lead to fear of retaliation and to displacement of fear onto external objects. In an equitable, loving family a child elaborates a moral system of ethical rights. Parents need to balance between punishment and permissiveness and set realistic limits on a toddler's behavior.

PRESCHOOL PERIOD

The preschool period is characterized by marked physical and emotional growth. Generally, between 2 and 3 years of age, children reach half their adult height. The 20 baby teeth are in place at the beginning of the stage, and by the end they begin to fall out. Children are ready to enter school by the time the stage ends at age 5 or 6. They have mastered the tasks of primary socialization—to control their bowels and urine, to dress and feed themselves, and to control their tears and temper outbursts, at least most of the time.

The term *preschool* for the age group of $2^{1}/_{2}$ to 6 years may be a misnomer; many children are already in schoollike settings, such as preschool nurseries and day care centers, where working mothers must often place their children. Preschool education can be valuable, but stressing academic advancement too far beyond a child's capabilities can be counterproductive.

Developmental Landmarks

Language and Cognitive Development. In the preschool period, children's use of language expands, and they use sentences. Individual words have regular and consistent meanings at the beginning of the period, and children begin to think symbolically. In general, however, their thinking is egocentric; they cannot place themselves in the position of another child and are incapable of empathy. Children think intuitively and prelogically and do not understand causal relations.

Emotional and Social Behavior. At the start of the preschool period, children can express such complex emotions as love, unhappiness, jealousy, and envy, both preverbally and verbally. Their emotions are still easily influenced by somatic events, such as tiredness and hunger. Although they still think mostly egocentrically, children's capacity for cooperation and sharing is emerging. Anxiety is related to loss of a person who was loved and depended on and to loss of approval and acceptance. Although still potentially disorganizing, anxiety can be tolerated better than in the past. Four-year-olds are learning to share and to have concern for others. Feelings of tenderness are sometimes expressed. Anxiety over bodily injury and the loss of a loved person's approval is sometimes disruptive.

By the end of the preschool period, children have many relatively stable emotions. Expansiveness, curiosity, pride, and gleeful excitement related to the self and the family are balanced with coyness, shyness, fearfulness, jealousy, and envy. Shame and humiliation are evident. Capacities for empathy and love are developed but fragile and easily lost if competitive or jealous strivings intervene. Anxiety and fears are related to bodily injury and loss of respect, love, and emerging self-esteem. Guilt feelings are possible. Additional information appears in Table 2.2–1.

Children between the ages of 3 and 6 years are aware of their bodies, of the genitalia, and of differences between the sexes. In their play, doctor-nurse games allow children to act out their sexual fantasies. Their awareness of their bodies extends beyond the genitalia; they show a preoccupation with illness or injury, so much so that the period has been called "the Band-Aid phase." Every injury must be examined and taken care of by a parent.

Children develop a division between what they want and what they are told to do. The division increases until a gap grows between their set of expanded desires, their exuberance at unlimited growth, and their parents' restrictions; they gradually turn parental values into self-obedience, self-guidance, and self-punishment.

At the end of the preschool stage, the child's conscience is established. The development of a conscience sets the tone for the moral sense of right and wrong. Until about 7 years of age, children experience rules as absolute and as existing for their own sake. They do not understand that there may be more than one point of view to a moral issue; a violation of the rules calls for absolute retribution—that is, children have the notion of immanent justice.

SIBLING RIVALRY. In the preschool period children relate to others in new ways. The birth of a sibling (a common occurrence during this time) tests a preschool child's capacity for further cooperation and sharing but may also evoke sibling rivalry, which is most likely to occur at this time. Sibling rivalry depends on child-rearing practice. Favoritism for any reason commonly aggravates such rivalry. Children who get special treatment because they are gifted, are defective in some way, or have a preferred gender are likely to receive angry feelings from their siblings. Experiences with siblings may influence growing children's relationships with peers and authority; for example, a problem may result if the needs of a new baby prevent the mother from attending to a firstborn child's needs. If not handled properly, the displacement of the firstborn can be a traumatic event.

PLAY. In the preschool years, children begin to distinguish reality from fantasy, and play reflects this growing awareness. Pretend games are popular and help test real-life situations in a playful manner. Dramatic play in which children act out a role, such as a housewife or a truck driver, is common. One-to-one play relationships advance to complicated patterns with rivalries, secrets, and two-against-one intrigues. Children's play behavior reflects their level of social development.

Between $2^{1}/_{2}$ and 3 years, children commonly engage in *parallel play,* solitary play alongside another child with no interaction between them. By age 3, play is often *associative,* that is, playing with the same toys in pairs or in small groups, but still with no real interaction among them. By age 4, children are usually able to share and engage in *cooperative play.* Real interactions and taking turns become possible.

Between 3 and 6 years of age, growth can be traced through drawings. A child's first drawing of a human being is a circular line with marks for the mouth, nose, and eyes; ears and hair are added later; arms

and sticklike fingers appear next; and then legs appear. Last to appear is a torso in proportion to the rest of the body. Intelligent children can deal with details in their art. Drawings express creativity throughout a child's development: They are representational and formal in early childhood, make use of perspective in middle childhood, and become abstract and affect laden in adolescence. Drawings also reflect children's body image concepts and sexual and aggressive impulses.

IMAGINARY COMPANIONS. Imaginary companions most often appear during preschool years, usually in children with above-average intelligence and usually in the form of persons. Imaginary companions may also be things, such as toys that are anthropomorphized. Some studies indicate that up to 50 percent of children between the ages of 3 and 10 years have imaginary companions at one time or another. Their significance is not clear, but these figures are usually friendly, relieve loneliness, and reduce anxiety. In most instances, imaginary companions disappear by age 12, but they may occasionally persist into adulthood.

TELEVISION. Most children in the United States grow up watching an extraordinary amount of television. Preschoolers watch, on average, 3 to 4 hours per day, most of it unsupervised. Recent studies have confirmed a correlation between children watching a lot of violence on television and exhibiting more aggressiveness. Heavy television watching also appears to interfere with a child's learning to read.

MIDDLE YEARS

The period between age 6 and puberty is often called the *middle years*. During this time, children enter elementary school. The formal demands for academic learning and accomplishment become major determinants of further personality development.

Developmental Landmarks

Language and Cognitive Development. In the middle years, language expresses complex ideas with relations among several elements. Logical exploration tends to dominate fantasy, and children show an increased interest in rules and orderliness and an increased capacity for self-regulation. During this period, children's conceptual skills develop, and thinking becomes organized and logical. The ability to concentrate is well established by age 9 or 10, and by the end of the period, children begin to think in abstract terms. Improved gross motor coordination and muscle strength enable children to write fluently and draw artistically. They are also capable of complex motor tasks and activities, such as tennis, gymnastics, golf, baseball, and skateboarding.

Recent evidence has shown that changes in thinking and reasoning during the middle years result from maturational changes in the brain. Children are now capable of increased independence, learning, and socialization. Theorists consider moral development a gradual, stepwise process spanning childhood, adolescence, and young adulthood.

In the middle years, both girls and boys make new identifications with other adults, such as teachers and counselors. These identifications may so influence girls that their goals of wanting to marry and have babies, as their mothers did, may be combined with a desire for a career or may be postponed or abandoned entirely.

Girls who cannot identify with their mothers or whose fathers are overly attached may become fixated at about a 6-year-old level; as a result, they may fear men or women or both or become seductively close to them. In either case, such girls may not be seen as normal during the school-age years. A similar situation may occur in boys who have been unable to identify successfully with fathers who were aloof, brutal, or absent. Perhaps his mother prevented a boy from identifying with his father by being overprotective or by binding the son too closely to herself. As a result, boys may enter this period with a variety of problems. They may be fearful of men, unsure of their sense of masculinity, or unwilling to leave their mothers (sometimes manifested by a school phobia); they may lack initiative and be unable to master school tasks, thus incurring academic problems.

The school-age period is a time when peer interaction assumes major importance. Interest in relationships outside the family takes precedence over those within the family. Nevertheless, a special relationship exists with the same-sex parent, with whom children identify and who is now an ideal and a role model.

Empathy and concern for others begin to emerge early in the middle years; by the time children are 9 or 10, they have well-developed capacities for love, compassion, and sharing. They have a capacity for long-term, stable relationships with family, peers, and friends, including best friends. Emotions about sexual differences begin to emerge as either excitement or shyness with the opposite sex. School-age children prefer to interact with children of the same sex. Although the middle years have sometimes been referred to as a "latency period"—a moratorium on psychosexual exploration and play until the eruption of sexual impulses with puberty—it is now recognized that a considerable amount of sexual interest continues through these years. Sex play and curiosity are common, especially among boys, but also among girls, Boys compare genitals and sometimes engage in group or mutual masturbation. An interest in anal humor and toilet jokes is often seen. Children this age often start using sexual and excretory words as expletives.

CHUM PERIOD. Harry Stack Sullivan postulated that a chum, or buddy, is an important phenomenon during the school years. By about 10 years of age, children develop a close same-sex relationship, which Sullivan believed is necessary for further healthy psychological growth. Moreover, Sullivan believed that the absence of a chum during the middle years of childhood is an early harbinger of schizophrenia.

SCHOOL REFUSAL. Some children refuse to go to school at this time, generally because of separation anxiety. A fearful mother may transmit her own fear of separation to a child, or a child who has not resolved dependence needs panics at the idea of separation. School refusal is usually not an isolated problem; children with the problem typically avoid many other social situations.

OTHER ISSUES IN CHILDHOOD

Sex Role Development

Persons' sex roles are similar to their gender identity; persons see themselves as male or female. The sex role also involves identification with culturally acceptable masculine or feminine ways of behaving; but changing expectations in society (particularly in the United States) of what constitutes masculine and feminine behavior can create ambiguity.

Parents react differently to their male and female children. Independence, physical play, and aggressiveness are encouraged in boys; dependence, verbalization, and physical intimacy are encouraged in girls. Nowadays, however, boys are encouraged to verbalize their feelings and to pursue interests traditionally associated with girls, while girls are encouraged to pursue careers traditionally dominated by men and to participate in competitive sports. As society grows more tolerant in its expectations of the sexes, roles become less rigid, and opportunities for boys and girls enlarge and broaden.

Biologically, boys are more physically aggressive than girls; and parental expectations, particularly the expectations of fathers, reinforce this trait. Differences also exist between boys and girls in the influence of persons outside the family. Girls tend to respond to the expectations and opinions of girls and of teachers of either sex but to ignore boys. Boys on the other hand tend to respond to other boys, but to ignore girls and teachers.

Dreams and Sleep

Children's dreams can have a profound effect on behavior. During the first year of life, when reality and fantasy are not yet fully differentiated, dreams may be experienced as if they were, or could be, true. At age 3, many children believe dreams are shared directly by more than one person, but most 4-year-olds understand that dreams are unique to each individual. Children view dreams either with pleasure or, as is most often reported, with fear. The dream content should be seen in connection with children's life experience, developmental stage, mechanisms used during dreaming, and sex.

Disturbing dreams peak when children are 3, 6, and 10 years old. Two-year-old children may dream about being bitten or chased; at the age of 4 they may have many animal dreams and also dream of persons who either protect or destroy. At age 5 or 6, dreams of being killed or injured, of flying and being in cars, and of ghosts become prominent; the role of conscience, moral values, and increasing conflicts are concerned with these themes. In early childhood, aggressive dreams rarely seem to occur; instead, dreamers are in danger, a state that perhaps reflects children's dependent position. By about the age of 5, children realize that their dreams are not real; before then they believe them to be real events. By age 7, children know that they create their dreams themselves.

Between the ages of 3 and 6 years, children normally want to keep their bedroom door open or to have a nightlight, so that they can either maintain contact with their parents or view the room in a realistic, nonfearful way. At times, children resist going to sleep to avoid dreaming. Disorders associated with falling asleep, therefore, are often connected with dreaming. Children often create rituals to protect them in the withdrawal from the world of reality into the world of sleep. Parasomnias such as sleep walking, sleep talking, enuresis (bed-wetting), and night terrors are common at this age. They usually occur during stage 4 sleep when dreaming is minimal, and they do not indicate emotional trouble or underlying psychopathology. Most children grow out of parasomnias by adolescence.

Periods of REM occur about 60 percent of the time during the first few weeks of life, a period when infants sleep two thirds of the time. Premature babies sleep even longer than full-term babies, and a greater proportion of their sleep is REM sleep. The sleep-wake cycle of newborns is about 3 hours long. Among adults, the dream-to-sleep ratio is stable: 20 percent of sleeping time is spent dreaming. Even newborns have brain activity similar to that of the dreaming state.

Spacing of Children

For women in the United States, 10 percent of conceptions that lead to live births are considered unwanted, and 20 percent are wanted but considered ill timed. The implications of these figures are that some couples may be poorly prepared or may feel guilty about not wanting to be parents. It is desirable to plan pregnancies and to have mutual agreement on the spacing of children. The typical number of children in a present-day family is two, half the typical number at the beginning of the century. Repeated childbearing prevents adequate recuperation from the birth process and places mothers at risk for complications and injury. New mothers require time to adapt; the period of adaptation may range from a few weeks to several months. The demands of other children at home can be taxing, and if these children are also young, the family may be stressed beyond its capacity.

Studies of children from large families (of four or five children) show that they are more likely to have conduct disorder and to have a slightly lower level of verbal intelligence than children from small families. Decreased parental interaction and discipline may account for these findings.

Birth Order

The effects of birth order vary. Firstborn children are often more highly valued than subsequent children, particularly if the firstborn is male, especially in non-Western cultures, but also sometimes in the United States. Firstborns have been found to have higher intelligence quotients (IQs) than their younger siblings, a finding that may reflect parents' having more time to interact with a firstborn child. Firstborn children appear to be more achievement oriented than subsequent children born to the same parents. As more children enter the family, parental time for each child diminishes; prenatal stress may also increase as more children have to be cared for.

Second and third children have the advantage of their parents' previous experience. Younger children also learn from their older siblings. For example, they may show more sophisticated use of pronouns at an earlier age than firstborns did. When children are spaced too closely, however, there may not be enough lap time for each child. The arrival of new children in the family affects not only the parents but also the siblings. Firstborn children may resent the birth of a new sibling, who threatens their sole claim on parental attention. In some cases, regressive behavior such as enuresis or thumb sucking occurs.

In general, the oldest children achieve the most and are the most authoritarian; middle children usually receive the least attention in the home and may develop strong peer relationships to compensate; and the youngest children may receive too much attention and be spoiled. According to Frank Sulloway, firstborn children tend to be conservative and conformists; by contrast, youngest children tend to be independent and rebellious in regard to family and cultural

norms. Sulloway found that a high proportion of prominent persons were lastborn children. He ascribes these differences to birth order and suggests that each child develops personality traits to fit an unfilled slot in the family. His findings need to be replicated.

Children and Divorce

Many children live in homes in which divorce has occurred. Approximately 30 percent of all children in the United States live in homes in which one parent (usually the mother) is the sole head of the household, and 61 percent of all children born in any given year can expect to live with only one parent before they reach the age of 18 years. A child's age at the time of the parents' divorce affects the child's reaction to the divorce. Immediately after a divorce, an increase in behavioral and emotional disorders appears in all age groups. Three- to 6-year-old children do not understand what is happening, and those who do understand often assume that they are somehow responsible for the divorce. If divorce occurs when a child is between 7 and 12 years, school performance generally declines. Older children, especially adolescents, comprehend the situation and believe that they could have prevented the divorce had they intervened in some way—had they, in effect, served as surrogate marriage therapists—but they are still hurt, angry, and critical of their parents' behavior.

Some children harbor the fantasy that their parents will be reunited in the future. Such children show animosity toward a parent's real or potential new mate because they are forced to recognize that no reconciliation is taking place. Recovery from, and adaptation to, the effects of divorce usually take 3 to 5 years, but about one third of all children from divorced homes have lasting psychological trauma. Among boys, physical aggression is a common sign of distress. Adolescents tend to spend more time away from the parental home after the divorce. Suicide attempts may occur as a direct result of the divorce; one of the predictors of suicide in adolescence is the recent divorce or separation of the parents. Children who adapt well to divorce do so if each parent makes an effort to continue to relate to the child in spite of the child's anger. To facilitate recovery, the divorced couple must avoid arguing with one another and must show consistent behavior toward the child. Despite childhood behavioral problems at the time of divorce, the prevalence of serious psychiatric problems such as depression or anxiety disorders in adulthood is not higher among children from divorced homes.

Stepparents. When remarriage occurs, children must learn to adapt to the stepparent and to the so-called reconstituted family. Such adaptation is usually difficult, especially when the stepparent is nonsupportive, resents the stepchild, or favors his or her own natural children. A natural child born to the new couple—a stepsibling—sometimes receives more attention than a stepchild and, as a result, is the object of sibling rivalry.

Adoption

Adoption is defined as the process by which a child is taken into a family by one or more adults who are not the biological parents but are recognized by law as the child's parents. About 2.5 million persons under 18 years of age are adopted each year. Fifty-two percent of children are adopted by persons not related to them by birth or marriage, and the remainder are adopted by relatives or stepparents. Most adopted children are born out of wedlock, and 40 percent of all such children are born to mothers between 15 and 19 years of age.

Adoptive parents most often tell their children of their status between the ages of 2 and 4 years. Informing children about their adoption reduces the possibility that the children learn of it from extrafamilial sources and then feel betrayed by their adoptive parents and abandoned by their biological parents.

Emotional and behavior disorders such as aggressive behavior, stealing, and learning disturbances have been reported to be higher among adopted than nonadopted children. The later the age of adoption, the higher the incidence and the more severe the behavior problems.

Throughout childhood and adolescence, children may be preoccupied with fantasies of two sets of parents. An adopted child may split the two sets of parents into good and bad parents. Adopted children usually have a strong desire to know their biological parents; some children pattern themselves after their fantasies of their absent biological parents and create a conflict with their adoptive parents. In most cases in which adopted children have sought out and met their biological parents (and vice versa), the experience has been generally positive, especially if the child is in late adolescence or early adulthood.

Family Factors in Child Development

Family Stability. Parents and children living under the same roof in harmonious interaction is the expected cultural norm in Western society. Within this framework, childhood development presumably proceeds most expeditiously. Deviations from the norm (e.g., divorced- and single-parent families) are associated with a broad range of problems in children, including low self-esteem, increased risk of child abuse, increased incidence of divorce when they eventually marry, and increased incidence of mental disorders, particularly depressive disorders and antisocial personality disorder as adults. Why some children from unstable homes are less affected than others (or even immune to these deleterious effects) is of great interest. Michael Rutter has postulated that vulnerability is influenced by sex (boys are more affected than girls), age (older children are less vulnerable than younger ones), and inborn personality characteristics. For example, children who have a placid temperament are less likely to be victims of abuse within a family than are hyperactive children; by virtue of their placidity, they may be less affected by the emotional turmoil surrounding them.

Other Family Factors. In childhood and adolescence the death of a parent is associated with adverse effects, such as an increase in later emotional problems, particularly a susceptibility to depression and divorce. This finding contrasts sharply to the results of separations caused by less traumatic events. For example, no evidence indicates that working mothers raise children who are less healthy than those brought up by mothers who stay at home. Home caregivers can act as surrogate moth-

ers, and in such cases the children do not become more attached to the caregiver than to the parent.

The role of day care centers for children is under continuous investigation. Some studies show that children placed in day care centers before the age of 5 years are less assertive and less effectively toilet trained than home-reared children. Other studies have shown that young children in day care are more advanced in social and cognitive development than young children who are not in day care. Such studies must take into account the quality of both the day care center and the homes from which children come. For example, a child from a disadvantaged home may be better off in a day care center than a child from an advantaged home. Similarly, a woman who wishes to leave the home to work for financial or other reasons and cannot do so may resent being forced to remain in the home in a child-rearing role, which may adversely affect the child.

Parenting Styles. The ways in which children are raised vary considerably between and within cultures. Rutter has clustered the diversity into four general styles. Subsequent research has confirmed that certain styles tend to correlate with certain behavior in the children, although the outcomes are by no means absolute. The *authoritarian* style, characterized by strict, inflexible rules, can lead to low self-esteem, unhappiness, and social withdrawal. The *indulgent-permissive* style, which includes little or no limit setting coupled with unpredictable parental harshness, can lead to low self-reliance, poor impulse control, and aggression. The *indulgent-neglectful* style, one of uninvolvement in the child's life and rearing, puts the child at risk for low self-esteem, impaired self-control and increased aggression. The *authoritative-reciprocal* style, marked by firm rules and shared decision making in a warm, loving environment, is believed to be the style most likely to result in self-reliance, self-esteem, and a sense of social responsibility.

REFERENCES

Bowlby J. *Attachment and Loss.* Vol 1: *Attachment.* New York: Basic Books; 1969.

Brodzinsky DM, Smith DW, Brodzinsky AB. *Children's Adjustment to Adoption: Developmental and Clinical Issues.* Thousand Oaks, CA: Sage; 1998.

Clulow C. Attachment theory and the therapeutic frame. In: Clulow C, ed. *Adult Attachment and Couple Psychotherapy: The 'Secure Base' in Practice and Research.* Philadelphia: Brunner-Routledge; 2001:85.

Crittenden PM, Claussen AH, eds. *The Organization of Attachment Relationships: Maturation, Culture, and Context.* New York: Cambridge University Press; 2000.

Diener ML, Goldstein LH, Mangelsdorf SC. The role of prenatal expectations in parents' reports of infant temperament. *Merrill-Palmer Q.* 1995;41:172.

Gordon MF. Normal child development. In: Sadock BJ, Sadock VA, eds. *Kaplan & Sadock's Comprehensive Textbook of Psychiatry.* 7th ed. Vol 2. Baltimore: Lippincott Williams & Wilkins; 2000:2534.

Kasen S, Cohen P, Brook JS, Hartmark C. A multiple-risk interaction model: effects of temperament and divorce on psychiatric disorders in children. *Abnorm Child Psychol.* 1996;24:121.

Levy TM, ed. *Handbook of Attachment Interventions.* San Diego: Academic Press; 2000.

Lidz T. *The Person: His and Her Development Throughout the Life Cycle.* New York: Basic Books; 1976.

Manassis K. Child-parent relations: attachment and anxiety disorders. In: Silverman WK, Treffers PDA, eds. *Cambridge Child and Adolescent Psychiatry.* New York: Cambridge University Press; 2001.

O'Brien M: Child-rearing difficulties reported by parents of infants and toddlers. *J Pediatr Psychol.* 1996;21:433.

Smotherman WP, Robinson SR. The development of behavior before birth. *Dev Psychol.* 1996;32:425.

Strauss B, ed. *Involuntary Childlessness: Psychological Assessment, Counseling, and Psychotherapy.* Kirkland, WA: Hogrefe & Huber Publishers; 2002.

Susman-Stillman A, Kalkose M, Egeland B, Waldman I. Infant temperament and maternal sensitivity as predictors of attachment security. *Infant Behav Dev.* 1996;19:33.

Woodcock J. Refugee children and their families: theoretical and clinical perspectives. In: Dwivedi KN, ed. *Post-traumatic Stress Disorder in Children and Adolescents.* London: Whurr Publishers; 2000:213.

▲ 2.3 Adolescence

Adolescence is characterized by profound biological, psychological, and social developmental changes. The biological onset of adolescence is signaled by rapid acceleration of skeletal growth and the beginnings of physical sexual development. The psychological onset is characterized by acceleration of cognitive development and consolidation of personality formation. Socially, adolescence is a period of intensified preparation for the coming role of young adulthood.

Many societies have marked the beginning of adolescence with puberty rites or rites of passage that celebrate adolescents' attainment of adult status, with its corresponding duties and responsibilities. The complexities of modern life have postponed attaining adult status; the onset of the teens is sometimes celebrated with religious rites, and adolescence remains an acknowledged stage of human development. As a stage, however, adolescence is variable—in age of onset, in length, in rate of growth, in sexual development, and in mental maturation. Jean Piaget, for example, proposed that formal operational thinking—which involves deductive logic—inevitably begins in adolescence, but later researchers have shown that the ability to solve complex problems depends on education and knowledge as well as an innate facility.

Adolescence is commonly divided into three periods: early (ages 11 to 14), middle (ages 14 to 17), and late (ages 17 to 20). These divisions are arbitrary; growth and development occur along a continuum that varies from person to person. Puberty, a physical process of change characterized by the development of secondary sex characteristics, differs from adolescence, largely a psychological process of change. Under ideal circumstances the processes are synchronous; when they do not occur simultaneously, as they often do not, adolescents must cope with the imbalance as an added stress. Adolescence terminates in adulthood.

PUBERTY

The onset of puberty, triggered by maturation of the hypothalamic-pituitary-adrenal-gonadal axes, is marked by the secretion of sex steroids. This hormonal activity produces the manifestations of puberty traditionally categorized as primary and secondary sex characteristics. The primary sex characteristics are those directly involved in coitus and reproduction, the reproductive organs and the external genitalia. The secondary sex characteristics include enlarged breasts and hips in girls and facial hair and lowered voices in boys. Height and weight increase earlier in girls than in boys; by age 12, girls are generally both taller and heavier than boys. Table 2.3–1 gives a summary of puberty changes.

Precocious or delayed growth, acne, obesity (about 15 percent of adolescents), and enlarged mammary glands in boys and small or overabundant breasts in girls are some deviations from the expected patterns of maturation. Although these conditions

Table 2.3–1
Pubertal Stages

	Characteristics		
Stage	**Genital Development in Boys**	**Pubic Hair Development**	**Breast Development in Girls**
1	Testes, scrotum, and penis are about the same size and shape as in early childhood.	The vellus over the pubis is not further developed than over the abdominal wall (i.e., no pubic hair).	There is elevation of the papillae only.
2	Scrotum and testes are slightly enlarged. The skin of the scrotum is reddened and changed in texture. There is little or no enlargement of the penis at this stage.	There is sparse growth of long, slightly pigmented, tawny hair, straight or slightly curled, chiefly at the base of the penis or along the labia.	Breast bud stage. There is elevation of the breasts and papillae as small mounds. Areolar diameter is enlarged over that of stage 1.
3	Penis is slightly enlarged, at first mainly in length. Testes and scrotum are larger than in stage 2.	The hair is considerably darker, coarser, and more curled. It spreads sparsely over the pubis.	Breasts and areolae are both enlarged and elevated more than in stage 2 but with no separation of their contours.
4	Penis is further enlarged, with growth in breadth and development of glans. Testes and scrotum are larger than in stage 3; scrotum skin is darker than in earlier stages.	Hair is now adult in type, but the area covered is still considerably smaller than in the adult. There is no spread to the medial surface of the thighs.	The areolae and papillae form secondary mounds projecting above the contours of the breasts.
5	Genitalia are adult in size and shape.	The hair is adult in quantity and type, with distribution of the horizontal (or classically feminine) pattern. Spread is to the medial surface of the thighs but not up the linea alba or elsewhere above the base of the inverse triangle.	Mature stage. The papillae only project, with the areolae recessed to the general contours of the breasts.

may not be medically significant, they often have psychological sequelae. Adolescents are sensitive to the opinions of their peers and constantly compare themselves with others. Any deviation, real or imagined, can lead to feelings of inferiority, low self-esteem, and loss of confidence. Girls are more sensitive to early physical manifestations of puberty than are boys. For example, tall girls feel more self-conscious about their height than do tall boys when they compare themselves with their peers.

Onset of Puberty

The onset of puberty varies, with girls entering puberty 12 to 18 months earlier than boys. The average age is 11 for girls (range, 8 to 13) and 13 for boys (range, 10 to 14). Twins of either sex tend to have onset of puberty later than nontwins. The age of onset of puberty has been steadily declining over the past 100 years. One of the consequences is a longer period of sexual maturity before the individual is culturally and socially considered an adult. In general, earlier-than-normal puberty is an advantage for boys and a disadvantage for girls.

Changes in Hormones

Sex hormone levels increase slowly throughout adolescence and correspond to bodily changes. Follicle-stimulating hormone (FSH) and luteinizing hormone (LH) levels also increase throughout adolescence, but between ages 17 and 18, the LH level is frequently above the adult value. LH levels characteristic of adult functioning begin in late adolescence.

From ages 16 and 17, a large increase seems to occur in average testosterone levels, which then decrease and stabilize at the adult level. Testosterone is the hormone responsible for masculinization of boys, and estradiol is the hormone responsible for feminization of girls. Both hormones also influence central nervous system functioning, including mood and behavior. Low estrogen levels may be associated with depressed mood (as happens in some women's premenstrual periods). High testosterone levels have been correlated with aggression and impulsivity in some men. Testosterone levels correlate with libido and are manifested by sex drive and masturbation in both sexes. In boys, androgens are produced by the testes and the adrenal gland; in girls, by the adrenal gland only. Levels are usually much higher in boys than in girls, and the effect of hormone changes on sexual behavior is usually more pronounced in boys than in girls. With the physical changes accompanying puberty, both boys and girls tend to become preoccupied with their appearance.

PSYCHOSEXUAL DEVELOPMENT

The sex drive is triggered by certain androgens, such as testosterone, which are at higher levels during adolescence than at any other time of life. According to William Masters and Virginia Johnson, the male sex drive peaks between 17 and 18 years of age. Early adolescents vent libidinal urges most often through masturbation, a safe way to satisfy sexual impulses.

Because girls enter puberty 2 years earlier than boys, they may begin dating and having sexual intercourse at an earlier age; but adolescent girls are less sexually active than boys of the same age. Boys are easily aroused by stimuli, and erections are frequent. For girls, the sexual impulse is associated with other feelings. Girls tend to view sex and love as related; boys find desire or lust and love to be separable.

Anna Freud described intellectualism and asceticism as two defense mechanisms commonly used by adolescents to deal

with sexual drives. Intellectualization is manifested by involvement in ideas and books; asceticism is manifested by a retreat into grand ideas and a renunciation of bodily pleasures. Most adolescents struggle with control of their libidinal drives. Early adolescents are still attached to their families and sometimes have resurgent oedipal feelings and even sexual fantasies about the same-sex or opposite-sex parent. These thoughts and feelings are generally repressed, and sexuality is directed outward; crushes, hero worship, and the idealization of movie and music stars are characteristic of this stage.

In middle adolescence, sexual behavior and experimentation with a variety of sexual roles are common. Masturbation occurs as a normal activity about equally in both sexes at this time, but a strict religious upbringing may engender strong feelings of guilt. Heterosexual crushes, often with an unattainable person of the same age or older, are common.

Homosexual experiences, usually transient, may also occur in middle adolescence. Many adolescents need reassurance about the normality of an isolated homosexual experience and confirmation that it does not indicate a permanent homosexual orientation. For others, a homosexual orientation is already determined by this time. These adolescents (estimated to be between 1 and 4 percent of all adolescent boys and 0.5 to 2 percent of all adolescent girls) may require counseling about dealing with their sexual orientation.

Although many adolescents experiment with sex at an early age, recent surveys indicate that the average age for the first sexual intercourse in both sexes is 16 years. The trend in U.S. society is toward greater, and more frequent, sexual activity at earlier ages than in the past. A decade ago, for example, the average age for first sexual intercourse was 18, and only 55 percent of women had had sexual intercourse by that time. Currently, 80 percent of men and 70 percent of women have engaged in coitus by age 19.

Menarche

The onset of the menstrual function, menarche, is one of the pubertal changes in girls. The current trend is toward an earlier menarche than in the past. During the1880s, the average age at menarche was 15 to 16 years. In the 1920s in the United States, the average age at menarche was 14.5 years; by the 1980s, it had dropped to 13 years. The time of menarche is determined by a complex interaction of biological and psychosocial factors. Good nutrition, fewer serious illnesses, and overall good physical health promote earlier menarche. The mother's age at menarche correlates loosely with her daughter's. Psychological or social distress has not been found to either delay or advance menarche. Cultural views of menarche vary from a curse at one extreme to a joyful affirmation of womanhood at the other. Most adolescent girls still do not receive information on the menses from their parents but rely on information from peers, schools, and the media.

Neurological Changes

During adolescence, the brain acquires the number of dendritic connections that will persist into adulthood. This is actually fewer than existed during the middle and early years of childhood, when a tremendous proliferation of connections was generated. Connections that are reinforced by environmental stimuli are retained. Those that are not are pruned back.

COGNITIVE AND PERSONALITY DEVELOPMENT

At the beginning of adolescence, thinking usually becomes abstract, conceptual, and future oriented. Many adolescents show remarkable creativity, which they express in writing, music, art, and poetry. Creativity is also expressed in sports and in adolescents' interests in the world of ideas—humanitarian issues, morals, ethics, and religion. Keeping a personal diary is a common creative outlet during this period.

A major task of adolescence is to achieve a secure sense of self. *Identity diffusion* is a failure to develop a cohesive self or self-awareness. Adolescent identity crisis is partly resolved by the move from dependency to independence. The initial struggles often revolve around the established concepts of sex roles and gender identification. Old techniques that a child earlier used to master separation may return.

Negativism

"No, I can do it myself. Don't tell me how long my hair can be. Don't tell me how short my skirt can be." This negativism is a renewed attempt to tell parents and the world that young persons have minds of their own. Negativism becomes an active, verbal way of expressing anger; adolescents may seize almost any issue to express their independence. Parents and adolescents may argue about the adolescents' choice of friends, peer groups, school plans and courses, and points of philosophy and etiquette. Members of each generation recall the clothes, hairstyles, and other external badges—the more shocking the better—used to define adolescents' differences from their parents.

Early psychoanalytic thinkers believed that a period of significant psychological upheaval, personality disorganization, and mood and behavior changes—called *adolescent turmoil*—was not only widespread, but desirable as a necessary part of the process of adolescents separating from their parents. It is now recognized that adolescent turmoil is neither common nor normal. Most teenagers can negotiate the demands of school and family life with little disruption. Serious mood and behavior disturbances during adolescence should be considered potential symptoms of psychopathology and be investigated.

Adolescents slowly blend values from many sources into their own belief systems, which must have the flexibility to change and grow to accommodate new life situations. As adolescents begin to feel independent of their families and as families support and encourage their emerging maturity, the questions "Who am I?" and "Where am I going?" begin to be answered.

PEER GROUP

The school experience accelerates and intensifies separation from the family. More and more, adolescents live in a world unfamiliar to parents. Home is a base; the real world is school, and the most important relationships, besides the adolescent's family, are with persons of similar ages and interests. Adolescents attempt to establish a personal identity separate from their parents but close enough to the family structure to be included.

Although adolescents tend to rely on peers for day-to-day support, the social support provided by parents has a stress-buffering effect in emergency situations. Adolescents often view themselves through the eyes of their peers, and any deviation in appearance, dress code, or behavior can result in diminished self-esteem. Parents must be aware of the sudden, frequent changes in friendships, personal appearance, and interests but must abrogate their authority.

PARENTING

The concept of the generation gap between parents and children has emerged from persons' experience being parents of adolescents. The gap represents the differences in experiences and perceptions of life events. In addition to having to deal with the turmoil that accompanies adolescent development, parents of adolescents are usually middle-aged and must also make adjustments to work, to marriage, and to their own parents. Many difficulties surround adolescents' need to assume increased independence from home, a move that can be threatening to parents who cannot let go and who want to maintain control of their children. Some parents may be unable to set limits on behavior; others act out their hidden or unconscious fantasies through the lives of their children. Superego lacunae (gaps or holes in the conscience) in parents may engender similar lacunae in children, and these gaps are then acted out. Moreover, the strong emerging sexuality of adolescents may trigger anxiety in parents. A few parents may be attracted to their opposite-sex or same-sex offspring and deal with the subsequent anxiety in maladaptive ways, such as getting angry (reaction formation).

In spite of these possibilities, parents of adolescents report few major altercations and get along with their children. For the most part, adolescents are receptive to parental approval and disapproval, and most adolescents and their parents can bridge the generation gap successfully. When they do not, the failure may arise from mental disorders in children, parents, or both. About 20 percent of adolescents have a diagnosable mental disorder. Among the most common diagnoses are adjustment disorders; anxiety disorders and depressive disorders are also common. These disorders are often associated with delinquent behavior, rebelliousness, and academic failure—all of which may contribute to family disharmony.

DEVELOPMENT OF MORALS

For most persons, developing a well-defined sense of morality is a major accomplishment of late adolescence and adulthood. *Morality* is defined as conformity to shared standards, rights, and duties. When two socially accepted standards conflict, a person learns to make judgments based on an individualized sense of conscience. Persons are morally obliged to abide by established norms but only to the degree that they serve human ends. The adolescent stage of development internalizes ethical principles and the control of conduct.

Piaget described morality as developing gradually, in conjunction with the stages of cognitive development. Preschool children simply follow rules set forth by the parents; in the middle years, children accept rules but show an inability to allow for exceptions; and during adolescence, young persons recognize rules in terms of what is good for the society at large.

Lawrence Kohlberg integrated Piaget's concepts and described three major levels of morality. The first level is pre–conventional morality, in which punishment and obedience to the parent are the determining factors. The second level is morality of conventional role-conformity, in which children try to conform to gain approval and to maintain good relationships with others. The third and highest level is morality of self-accepted moral principles, in which children voluntarily comply with rules on the basis of a concept of ethical principles and make exceptions to rules in certain circumstances.

CHOICE OF OCCUPATION

Occupational choice stems from the question, "Where am I going?" Both men and women need to feel independent, autonomous, and content with their vocational choices. Adolescents are beleaguered by peers, parents, teachers, and counselors, as well as by unconscious forces in attempting to decide on a vocation. Whether there are opportunities for further schooling plays a role in their decisions. Among college graduates, 30 percent go on to some type of graduate education. Those adolescents who are unable to continue schooling are severely hampered in establishing a satisfactory vocational identity. Many are fated for lives of economic and emotional depression.

The psychological basis for a sense of individual worth as an adult rests on the acquisition of competence during adolescence. A sense of competence is acquired by experiencing success in a task that today's society views as important. The sustained motivation necessary for mastering a difficult work role is possible only when adolescents have a likelihood of fulfilling this role in adult life and of gaining the respect of others.

RISK-TAKING BEHAVIOR

Risk-taking behavior in adolescence can involve alcohol, tobacco, and other substance use; promiscuous sexual activity, which is especially dangerous in view of the risk of acquired immune deficiency syndrome (AIDS); and accident-prone behavior, such as fast driving, skydiving, and hang gliding. Most mortality statistics for teenagers cite accidents as the leading cause of death, with vehicular accidents accounting for about 40 percent of all teenage deaths. The reasons for risk-taking behavior vary and relate to counterphobic dynamics, the fear of inadequacy, the need to affirm a sexual identity, and group dynamics such as peer pressure. The behavior may also reflect some adolescents' omnipotent fantasies, in which they view themselves as invulnerable to harm and injury. Information alone does not decrease risk: High levels of knowledge about human immunodeficiency virus (HIV) and AIDS do not correlate with decreased high-risk behaviors (about 6,000 teenagers are infected with HIV each year, most by sexual contact). Recently, a genetic predisposition to risk-taking behavior was identified; as adolescence proceeds, risk-taking behavior abates, and responsible decision-making activity occurs.

USE OF DRUGS

Although cocaine use is declining among U.S. teenagers, the use of other drugs of abuse has increased. This increase reverses a trend of declining drug use since the peak years in the 1970s. In

2000, a survey of high school students found that marijuana was the most popular illegal drug, and about 40 percent of high school seniors reported having used it. Alcohol use was reported by over 85 percent of seniors and binge drinking (defined as five or more drinks in a row on one or more occasions in 1 month) by 32 percent of high school students. About 3 percent of teenagers smoke cigarettes, with higher use by girls than by boys. White students smoke more than black students. Among youths 12 and 13 years old, 3 percent used illicit drugs in 2000.

PREGNANCY

Each year about 1 million teenage girls under the age of 19 become pregnant. Of this number, 600,000 give birth; the rest (400,000 [40 percent]) obtain abortions. The number of teenagers who engage in sexual intercourse is increasing. Boys generally have more sexual partners than do girls, and boys are less likely than girls to seek emotional attachments with their sexual partners. Pregnancy rates for girls 15 to19 years old are higher for blacks than for whites.

Contrary to earlier beliefs, sexual abuse during childhood does not increase teenage pregnancy rates. (Sexually abused girls are, however, more likely to exhibit socially deviant behaviors and to have older boyfriends.) Among pregnant teenagers, minimal prenatal care is a major contributing factor in maternal morbidity and mortality. Only one third of sexually active teenagers use contraceptives; most are uneducated about contraceptive use or are unwilling or unable to obtain contraceptives. Table 2.3–2 lists reasons for contraceptive misuse or rejection. In some subcultures, teenagers view pregnancy as a rite of passage into adulthood. An adolescent girl who is depressed, insecure about her attractiveness, or the child of a conflicted or divorced couple is more likely to become pregnant than an adolescent from a stable background.

The average adolescent mother cannot care for her child, who is either placed in foster care or raised by the teenager's already overburdened parents or other relatives. Few girls marry the fathers of their children; the fathers, usually teenagers, cannot care for themselves, much less the mothers of their children. If the two do marry, they usually divorce.

Table 2.3–2
Factors in the Misuse or Rejection of Contraceptives

Factors	Comments
Denial	Belief that pregnancy will not or cannot occur
Opportunism	Taking advantage of the opportunity (possibly unexpected) for coitus without regard for the consequences
Love	Coitus is driven by passionate enthusiasm with the expectation of marriage if pregnancy occurs
Guilt	Contraceptive use represents planned coitus, which engenders feelings of guilt
Embarrassment	Self-consciousness about using condom or inserting diaphragm in front of the partner
Entrapment	Desire to impregnate or to become pregnant to force the partner to become attached emotionally
Eroticism	Belief that contraceptive use decreases or interferes with erotic pleasure
Nihilism	Belief that contraceptives are ineffective or useless
Fear and anxiety	Coitus is associated with high levels of anxiety; fear of performance ability interferes with contraceptive use
Abortion	Belief that if one gets pregnant, an abortion can be obtained; therefore, a contraceptive is not needed
Education	Lack of education about effective contraceptive use from parents and school
Availability	Access to, or cost of, contraceptive prohibits its use

Abortion

Teenage girls often use abortion services. Almost all the girls are unwed mothers from low socioeconomic groups; their pregnancies result from sex with boys to whom they felt emotionally attached. Most teenagers elect to have abortions with their parents' consent, but laws of mandatory parental consent put two rights into competition: a girl's claim to privacy and a parent's need to know. Most adults believe that teenagers should have parental permission for an abortion; but when parents refuse to give their consent, most states prohibit parents from vetoing the teenager's decision.

The abortion rate in many European countries tends to be far lower than that in the United States. In the United States, the rate of abortion among girls between the ages of 15 and 19 is about 30 per 1,000 girls, according to the Centers for Disease Control and Prevention. In France, for instance, about 10.5 of every 1,000 girls under the age of 20 had an abortion in 2000, according to World Health Organization statistics. The rate of abortion in Germany was 6.8; in Italy, 6.3; and in Spain, 4.5. Britain has a higher rate, 18.5. Family planning experts believe that more sex education and availability of contraceptive devices help keep the number of abortions down. In Holland, where contraceptives are freely available in schools, the teenage pregnancy rate is among the lowest in the world.

PROSTITUTION

Teenagers constitute a large portion of all prostitutes, with estimates ranging up to 1 million teenagers involved in prostitution. Most adolescent prostitutes are girls, but boys are involved as homosexual prostitutes. Most teenagers who enter a life of prostitution come from broken homes or were abused as children. Many were victims of rape. Most teenagers ran away from home and were taken in by pimps and substance abusers; the adolescents themselves then became substance abusers. They are at high risk for AIDS, and many (up to 70 percent in some studies) are infected with HIV.

VIOLENCE

Although rates of violent crime have decreased throughout the United States in the past 5 years—for example, the homicide rate in New York City fell by almost 50 percent between 1998 and 2000—violent crimes by young offenders are on the increase. Homicides are the second leading cause of death among persons aged 15 to 25. (Accidents are first; suicides,

third.) Black male teenagers are far more likely to be murder victims than are boys from any other racial or ethnic group or girls of any race. The factor most strongly associated with violence among adolescent boys is growing up in a household without a father or father surrogate; this factor aside, race, socioeconomic status, and education show no effect on the propensity toward violence.

EVOLUTION OF ADULTHOOD

As opposed to the legal definition of adulthood, the end of adolescence occurs when persons begin to assume the actual tasks of young adulthood, which involve choosing an occupation and developing a sense of intimacy that leads, in most cases, to marriage and parenthood. Daniel Levinson described an early-adult transition between adolescence and adulthood in which a young person begins to leave home and live independently. This period sees a peaking of biological development, assumption of new social roles, socialization into these roles (which involves learning skills and attitudes required to perform the roles well), and eventual assumption of an adult self and life structure.

The rate of depression may be as high as 1 in 8 adolescents. Adolescents often refuse health care because they fear the doctors will disclose confidential information about sensitive issues to their parents. In many situations, however, adolescents can make their own health care decisions. Table 2.3–3 presents a

Table 2.3–3
Teenagers and the Law

Vignette	Response
Sarah asks her doctor for a confidential pregnancy test. Her friend calls later to find out the results for her. Can the doctor disclose the results to Sarah's friend?	Not without Sarah's permission. The information is confidential and cannot be disclosed to anyone but Sarah.
Dana is 17. She goes to her doctor to be treated for genital herpes. Does the doctor need her parents' permission before treating her?	No. A minor can consent to care for sexually transmitted diseases; parental consent is not required.
The public health officer tells Lisa that she may have an STD. Can the officer tell Lisa who transmitted it?	No. The officer can reveal only that Lisa is at risk. He or she cannot reveal the name of the contact.
Qiao-Ling is 15. She is severely depressed and wants mental health treatment, but her parents refuse to allow it. The physician believes that she needs to be treated. Can the doctor treat Qiao-Ling?	Yes—if Qiao-Ling consents to the treatment.
Can Rahim, who is 15, consent to his own admission for inpatient mental health treatment?	No. A minor must be 16 or over to consent to inpatient mental health treatment.
Jacob is 16. He is thinking about talking to a school counselor about his drinking problem, but is afraid that his parents will be notified. Can he receive counseling without parental consent?	Variable. Parental consent is not necessary for a minor to receive alcohol counseling, but in some states counselors may tell parents.
A 14-year-old girl, Carla, wants to get a prescription for the pill. Does she need parental consent?	No. Birth control pills, like all other forms of contraception, must be made available to minors without parental consent.
Can a pregnant 15-year-old decide whether to have a cesarean section or a vaginal delivery?	Yes. Physicians may strongly encourage a young woman to seek a supportive adult's assistance when making a difficult decision such as this, but a minor who understands the risks and benefits can make the decision for herself.
Kim is 15. She is from Iowa, but is staying in New York for the summer for a dance program. She has found out that she is pregnant and wants to terminate the pregnancy. Does she need parental consent?	No. While Kim is in New York, she will be treated according to New York law. She does not need parental consent.
Rebecca, a 15-year-old who lives with her mother, is HIV positive. She has never told her mother that she is HIV positive, and now she has developed an AIDS-related illness. She wants medical care but will avoid treatment if she is required to tell her mother. Can the physician treat her without parental consent?	Yes. The physician can treat Rebecca without consulting with either of Rebecca's parents, but the physician may wish to help Rebecca find a supportive adult in whom she can confide about her situation.
James is 14 years old. He is HIV positive and suffers from an AIDS-related illness. He will not agree to medical treatment if he must tell his parents. The physician determines that requesting parental consent would be detrimental to James' health and that James is capable of consenting to his own care. James receives treatment. Can the medical facility inform his parents that he has received treatment?	No. The facility is prohibited from releasing information to James' parents for two reasons. First, when a minor consents to his or her own AIDS treatment, the parent cannot be informed about the treatment. Second, when a physician finds that disclosing information would not be in the best interests of the minor, information cannot be disclosed to the parents.
Tom is 6 years old and needs a hepatitis B shot. His parents are out of town and he is staying with his aunt and uncle. Can they consent to the vaccination for him?	Yes. Even though they are only caring for him temporarily, they can consent to his vaccination.
Tanya is 15. She thinks she might have herpes, but she doesn't want to tell her parents. Can she obtain medical attention without telling them?	Yes. Whether it's a diagnosis, a prescription, or a surgical treatment, physicians may treat adolescents for STDs without parental consent.

Table derived from Faierman J, Lieberman D, Chu Y, eds. *Teenagers' Health Care and the Law: A Guide to the Law on Minors Rights in New York.* New York: New York Civil Liberties Union Reproductive Rights Project; 2000.

series of vignettes covering a wide range of problems common to adolescents, with the appropriate decisions to be made by clinicians. The law defines a minor as a person under the age of 18; at 18, for legal matters, a person is considered an adult.

References

Auerswald CL, Eyre SL. Youth homelessness in San Francisco: A life cycle approach. *Soc Sci Med.* 2002;54:1497.

Campbell BC, Udry JR. Stress and age at menarche of mothers and daughters. *J Biosoc Sci.* 1995;27:127.

Connolly J, Furman W, Konarski R. The role of peers in the emergence of heterosexual romantic relationships in adolescence. *Child Dev.* 2000;71:1395.

Cotton NS. Normal adolescence. In: Sadock BJ, Sadock VA, eds. *Kaplan & Sadock's Comprehensive Textbook of Psychiatry.* 7th ed. Vol 2. Baltimore: Lippincott Williams & Wilkins; 2000:2550.

Freud A. Adolescence. *Psychoanal Study Child.* 1958;13:255.

Frey CU, Rothlisberger C. Social support in healthy adolescents. *J Youth Adolesc.* 1996;25:17.

Garger JA, Brooks-Gunn J, Warren MP. The antecedents of menarcheal age: heredity, family environment, and stressful life events. *Child Dev.* 1995;66:346.

Jarvinen DW, Nicholls JG. Adolescents' social goals, belief about the causes of social success, and satisfaction in peer relationships. *Dev Psychol.* 1996;32:432.

Loevinger J. Ego development in adolescence. In: Muuss RE, Porton HD. *Adolescent Behavior and Society: A Book of Readings.* 5th ed. New York: McGraw-Hill; 2000:234.

Rainey DY, Stevens-Simon C, Kaplan DW. Are adolescents who report prior sexual abuse at a higher risk for pregnancy? *Child Abuse Negl.* 1995; 19:1283.

Shields G, Adams J. HIV/AIDS among youth: a community needs assessment study. *Child Adolesc Soc Work J.* 1995;12:361.

Skoe E, von der Lippe, eds. *Personality Development in Adolescence: A Cross National and Life Span Perspective.* New York: Routledge; 1998.

▲ 2.4 Adulthood

Early developmental psychologists and theorists focused primarily on childhood, especially the first 3 years of life. Adulthood was seen as the culmination of all developmental steps that had gone before; it is now recognized that development continues throughout the entire lifespan. Most adults are forced to confront and adapt to similar circumstances: establishing an independent identity, forming a marriage or other partnership, raising children, building and maintaining careers, and accepting the disability and death of one's parents. Persons meet these challenges in different ways and with different degrees of success. All can be stressful, and all can result in physical and psychiatric symptoms. Clearly, there is no single trajectory to a successful, fulfilling adulthood. Some persons assume responsibility for full-time jobs, marriage, and children right after high school. Others, especially those pursuing professional degrees, may have a period of extended adolescence into their late 20s before full adult independence. There is no fixed sequence of events (career can come before marriage and vice-versa), and many persons' lives include momentary regressions and resetting goals.

In modern Western societies, adulthood is the longest phase of human life. Although the exact age of consent varies from person to person, adulthood can be divided into three main parts: young or early adulthood (ages 20 to 40), middle adulthood (ages 40 to 65), and late adulthood or old age.

This section deals with early and middle adulthood, when the processes of marriage, child rearing, and work are most significant—a time of changes, dramatic and subtle but always continuous. Calvin Colarusso, one of the major proponents of adult development, outlined the transition to early adulthood as follows:

> As they leave childhood and adolescence behind and journey through young adulthood and midlife, men and women attempt to achieve the following:

1. Separate psychologically from the parents of childhood and achieve self-sufficiency in the adult world
2. Find a gratifying place in the world of work
3. Experience sexual and emotional intimacy within a committed relationship
4. Become a parent
5. Accept the aging process in the body
6. Integrate the growing awareness of time limitation and personal death
7. Maintain physical and emotional intimacy in the face of the powerful physical, psychological, and environmental pressures of midlife
8. Facilitate the emergence of childhood into adulthood
9. Develop and sustain friendships with individuals of different ages and backgrounds
10. Continue to play
11. Leave a legacy for future generations by facilitating the development of younger individuals

EARLY ADULTHOOD

Usually considered to begin at the end of adolescence (about age 20) and to end at age 40, early adulthood is characterized by peaking biological development, the assumption of major social roles, and the evolution of an adult self and life structure. The successful passage into adulthood depends on satisfactory resolution of childhood and adolescent crises.

During late adolescence, young persons generally leave home and begin to function independently. Sexual relationships become serious, and the quest for intimacy begins. The transition to early adulthood involves many important events: graduating from high school, starting a job or entering college, and living independently. The 20s are spent, for the most part, exploring options for occupation and marriage or alternative relationships, and making commitments in various areas.

Early adulthood requires choosing new roles (e.g., husband, father) and establishing an identity congruent with those new roles. It involves asking and answering the questions Who am I and Where am I going? The choices made during this time may be tentative; young adults may make several false starts.

Developmental Tasks

During early adulthood, options for occupation and marriage (or other intimate relationships) are explored. For most young adults, selecting a mate and starting a family are of paramount importance. At about age 30, young adults are likely to question their choices and may ask themselves whether the life they have is the one they really want. Daniel J. Levinson called this period of reappraisal the age 30 transition. Some young persons who think that their lives are going well reaffirm their commitments and experience a smooth transition. Others, however, may experience a major crisis, manifested by marital problems, job

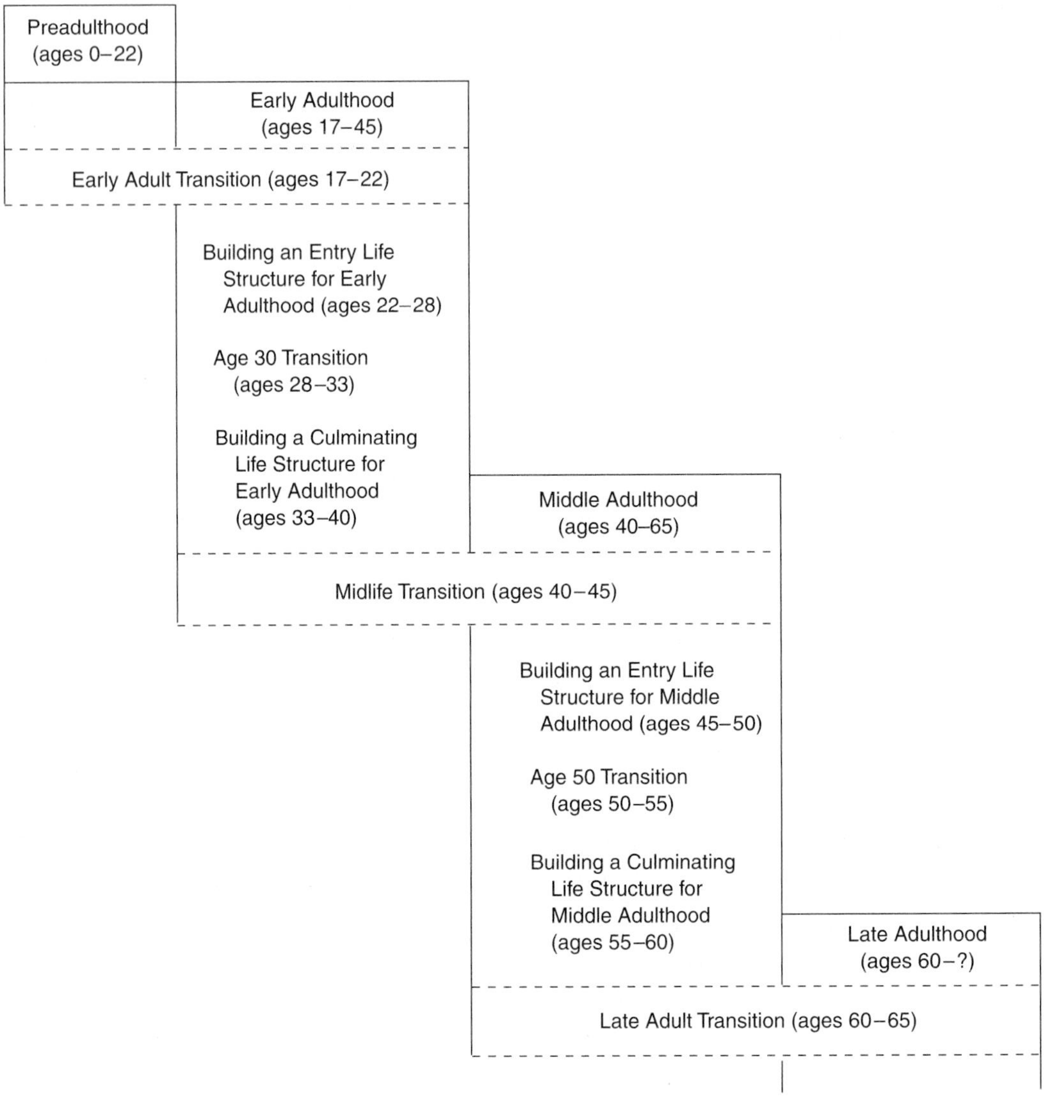

FIGURE 2.4–1
Developmental periods in the eras of early and middle adulthood. (Adapted from Levinson DJ, Darrow NC, Klein EB, Levinson MH, McKee B. *The Seasons of a Man's Life.* New York: Knopf; 1978.)

changes, and psychiatric symptoms such as anxiety and depression. Levinson described developmental periods through all phases of adulthood (Fig. 2.4–1).

A number of different models have been proposed for understanding adult development. They are all theoretical and somewhat idealized. They all use metaphors to describe complex social, psychological, and interpersonal interactions. The models are *heuristic:* they provide a conceptual framework for thinking about common important experiences. They are *descriptive* rather than *prescriptive;* that is, they provide a useful way of looking at what many persons do, not a formula for what all persons should do. Some of the terms and concepts commonly used are explained in Table 2.4–1. These periods involve individuation, that is, leaving the family of origin and becoming one's own man or woman, passing through midlife, and preparing in middle adulthood for the transition into late adulthood.

Colarusso outlined the developmental tasks of young adulthood as follows:

1. To develop a young-adult sense of self and others: the third individuation
2. To develop adult friendships
3. To develop the capacity for intimacy; to become a spouse
4. To become a biological and psychological parent
5. To develop a relationship of mutuality and equality with parents while facilitating their midlife development
6. To establish an adult work identity
7. To develop adult forms of play
8. To integrate new attitudes toward time

Roger Gould reported similar processes among persons in their late 20s and early 30s who discover talents, wishes, tendencies, and interests not previously appreciated or acknowledged. This awareness may produce either disillusionment and

Table 2.4–1
Psychological Development Concepts

Concept	Definition	Example
Transition	The bridge between two successive stages	Late adolescence
Normative crisis	A period of rapid change or turmoil that strains a person's adaptive capacities	Midlife crisis
Stage	Period of consolidation of skills and capacities	Mature adulthood
Plateau	Period of developmental stability	Adulthood up to midlife
Rite of passage	Social ritual that facilitates a transition	Graduation; marriage

Adapted from Wolman T, Thompson T. Adult and later-life development. In: Stoudemire A, ed. *Human Behavior.* Philadelphia: Lippincott-Raven; 1998.

depression or a new sense of self with a realistic appraisal of one's strengths and weaknesses.

As mentioned in Section 6.3, Erik Erikson is one of the major proponents of adult developmental theory. The specific *phase* that applies to young adulthood is the development of intimacy vs. isolation. This is the time that contacts with others are made, when intimate relationships develop, and when commitment to another person—the marriage partner, the significant other—develops. Not negotiating this developmental crisis (to use Erikson's term) can lead to a state of isolation. Persons may become withdrawn, and depression may be a psychopathological outcome.

Occupation. Socioeconomic group, gender, and race affect the pursuit and development of particular occupational choices. Blue-collar workers generally enter the work force directly after high school; white-collar workers and professionals usually enter the work force after college or professional school.

A healthy adaptation to work provides an outlet for creativity, satisfactory relationships with colleagues, pride in accomplishment, and increased self-esteem. Job satisfaction does not depend wholly on money. In contrast, maladaptation can lead to dissatisfaction with oneself and with the job, insecurity, decreased self-esteem, anger, and resentment at having to work. Symptoms of job dissatisfaction are a high rate of job changes, absenteeism, mistakes at work, accident proneness, and even sabotage. Members of minorities are frequently burdened with low socioeconomic status, which limits their opportunities for rewarding and satisfying work. They frequently begin their 20s with hopes of becoming successful but are often disappointed in this endeavor later in life.

WOMEN AND WORK. Since the 1970s, women have become a significant economic force in the United States. Women's wages have steadily increased relative to men's, although the typical hourly wage for women is still less than that for men. More women have been entering the workplace. The proportion of working-age women with jobs has increased from 35 percent in 1960 to over 70 percent in 2000. Even more impressive is the fact that women now own one third of all businesses. Undoubtedly some, but not all, married women work only because of financial necessity.

In general, families whose income is below $50,000 per year are more likely to include a working mother. Most nonworking mothers are found in families with an annual income over $100,000 per year (1999 data from the U.S. Bureau of the Census). In spite of this, however, the greatest increase in working wives has occurred toward the top of the income scale.

Women's increasing economic power has been accompanied by increasing political power (if not yet widespread representation on the national level). The political gender gap (men and women voting for different parties) has widened; women disproportionately favor Democrats. Political observers noted numerous instances in which presidential and other campaigns appeal specifically to women. The term *soccer moms* was coined to describe well-to-do, ethnically diverse suburban women balancing the demands of work and family. Soccer moms were supposedly hard-headed and pragmatic; their votes were up for grabs. One pundit wrote, "As the soccer mom votes, so goes the election."

UNEMPLOYMENT. The effects of unemployment transcend those of loss of income; the psychological and physical tolls are enormous. The incidence of alcohol dependence, homicide, violence, suicide, and mental illness rises with unemployment. One's core identity, which is often tied to occupation and work, is seriously damaged when a job is lost, whether through firing, attrition, or early or sometimes even regular retirement. Seventy percent of married women with children under the age of 6 have paid employment. For many of these women, work enhances their self-esteem in addition to providing needed income.

One must not underestimate the self-esteem that work offers, as the following vignette demonstrates.

A young-adult female patient had greatly enjoyed her 5 years in college and only reluctantly accepted a job with a large real estate firm. During college she had had limited interest in her appearance, and she began work in clothing borrowed from family and friends. She scoffed when her boss began to criticize her dress and gave her an advance to buy an upscale wardrobe; but she began to enjoy the fine clothing and the respect engendered by her appearance and position. As her income began to rise, work became a source of pleasure and self-esteem and the way to acquire some of the trappings of adulthood. (Courtesy of Calvin Colarusso, M.D.)

Marriage

Most persons in the United States marry for the first time in their mid- to late 20s. The median age of first marriage has been rising steadily since 1950 for both men and women, and the number of persons who never marry has been increasing. By 2000, the proportion of 30- to 34-year-olds who never married

almost tripled, and the proportion of never-married 35- to 39-year-olds doubled. The rate of divorce has also been declining. In 1998, it reached the lowest level in almost 20 years. However, since the marriage rate in the general population is declining faster than the divorce rate, the likelihood that marriage will end in divorce has increased. Currently there are about 55 million married couples in America, and half of them have children. Most divorced persons marry again—in most cases more successfully than the first time—an indication that the marital unit still provides a means for sustained intimacy, perpetuates the culture, and gratifies interpersonal needs.

The change in mores from the 1950s restrictive moral climate to the modern-day permissive moral climate is seen in the number of unmarried adults who live together (cohabitation). In the 1960s, only 8 percent of couples lived together before marrying; currently, more than 50 percent of first marriages are preceded by cohabitation. Domestic demographics in the United States are listed in Table 2.4–2.

INTERRACIAL MARRIAGE. Mixed-race marriages were banned in 19 states until a Supreme Court decision in 1967. In 1970, they accounted for only 2 percent of all marriages involving at least one black partner. The trend has been steadily upward. About 15 percent of all new black marriages involve a white partner. In more than two thirds of these mixed weddings, the groom was black and the bride was white.

Despite the trend toward more interracial marriages, they still remain a small proportion of all marriages. Most persons are more likely to marry someone from the same racial and ethnic background. Marriages between Hispanic whites and non-Hispanic whites and between Asians and whites are more common than those between blacks and whites.

Table 2.4–2
Domestic Demographics

	2000	Approximate Change Since 1970 (%)
Total family population†	70,000,000	+30
Annual births	4,000,000	+5
Marital births	3,000,000	–20
Nonmarital births	1,000,000	+200
Women aged 40–44 who have not married	10%	+80
Men aged 40–44 who have not married	16%	+110
All married couples	55,000,000	+20
Married with children	25,000,000	–1
Single-parent families	10,000,000	+200
Children living with unmarried couples	2,000,000	+660
Single mothers who have never married	40%	+350
Distribution of births		
White	60%	–20
Black	15%	–10
Hispanic	20%	+175
Asian & other	5%	+365
	100%	

†Family consists of married couples/male householder, no spouse present/female householder, no spouse present.
Data adapted from U.S. Bureau of the Census, Current population survey, 2000. Figures have been rounded.

MARITAL ADJUSTMENT. In the United States a high value is placed on marital stability, love, and happiness. Although most persons marry for love, it is not possible to predict who will marry whom and which marriages will be successful. Most persons marry within their own socioeconomic group to persons from their own neighborhoods. The decision to marry also hinges on group and family pressures. Most persons are expected to marry in their 20s.

David Reed, who studied emotional adjustment in marriage and the factors that account for marital happiness, wrote:

> Most studies concur that happiness in a marriage implies happiness in the general relationship. However, those who report very happy marriages tend to dwell on their relationship in surveys, and those who are unhappy tend to indicate external sources of stress. None of this research includes objective observation of actual behavior. In relations in which need satisfaction is measured, researchers are inconclusive as to how emotional adjustment is achieved. It has become popular to advocate communication and verbal confrontation as important ingredients in emotional adjustment in marriage. Advocates of this view proselytize that openness, more talking, increased sensitivity to feelings, personalizing of language symbols, and keeping the communication channels open all contribute to happiness. Some studies agree with this view . . . However, other studies report that communication can disturb a relationship, particularly when there is an emphasis on verbal overkill. Complete openness can be destructive. There may be a secret intolerance of weakness or an inability to perceive accurately the emotional strength of one's spouse. In such a relationship the verbally active partner becomes the better fighter who always wins. Thus, conflict is never well handled, and fights become a chronic source of despair . . .
>
> It is likely that there is a general correlation between happiness and stability . . . it is likely that in most relationships some form of success precedes general emotional fulfillment. By and large, this means that the husband needs to succeed in his role performance before there is an overwhelming concern with companionship. This is particularly true in disadvantaged families in which survival is an issue of far greater importance than pleasure. Moreover, satisfaction should not be confused with bliss, for satisfaction may include overt hostility more than peaceful companionship.

MARITAL PROBLEMS. Although marriage tends to be regarded as a permanent tie, unsuccessful unions may be terminated, as indeed they are in most societies. Nevertheless, many marriages that do not end in separation or divorce are disturbed. In considering marital problems, clinicians are concerned not only with the persons involved but also with the marital unit itself. How any marriage works out relates to the partners selected, the personality organization or disorganization of each, the interaction between them, and the original reasons for the union. Persons marry for a variety of reasons—emotional, social, economic,

and political, among others. One person may look to the spouse to meet unfulfilled childhood needs for good parenting. Another may see the spouse as someone to be saved from an otherwise unhappy life. Irrational expectations between spouses increase the risk of marital problems.

MARRIAGE AND COUPLES THERAPY. When families consist of grandparents, parents, children, and other relatives living under the same roof, assistance for marital problems can sometimes be obtained from a member of the extended family with whom one or both partners have rapport. With the contraction of the extended family in recent times, however, this source of informal help is no longer as accessible as it once was. Similarly, religion once played a more important role than now in the maintenance of family stability. Wise religious leaders are available to provide counseling, but they are not sought out to the extent that they once were, which reflects the decline in religious influence among large segments of the population. Formerly, both the extended family and religion not only provided guidance for couples in distress but also prevented dissolution of marriages by virtue of the social pressures that the extended family and religion exerted on couples to stay together. As family, religious, and societal pressures have relaxed, legal procedures for relatively easy separation and divorce have expanded. Concurrently, the need for formalized marriage counseling services has developed.

Marital therapy is a form of psychotherapy for married persons in conflict with each other. A trained person establishes a professional contract with the patient-couple and, through definite types of communication, attempts to alleviate the disturbance, to reverse or change maladaptive patterns of behavior, and to encourage personality growth and development.

In *marriage counseling,* only a particular conflict related to the immediate concerns of the family is discussed; marriage counseling is conducted much more superficially by persons with less psychotherapeutic training than is marital therapy. *Marriage therapy* places greater emphasis on restructuring the interaction between the couple—including, at times, exploration of the psychodynamics of each partner. Both therapy and counseling emphasize helping marital partners cope effectively with their problems.

Parenthood. By age 30, most have established families and must deal with parent–child problems. In addition to the economic burden of raising a child (estimated to be $250,000 for a middle-class family whose child goes to college), there are emotional costs. Children may reawaken conflicts that parents themselves had as children, or children may have chronic illnesses that challenge families' emotional resources. In general, men have been more concerned with their work and occupational advancement than with child rearing, and women have been more concerned about their role as mothers than with advancement in their occupation; but this emphasis is changing dramatically for both sexes. A small, but growing, number of couples are choosing to split a job (or work at two part-time jobs) and share child-rearing duties.

For persons in their 20s and 30s, parenting has been described as a continuing process of letting go. Children must be allowed to separate from parents and, in some cases, must be encouraged to do so. When parents are in their 20s, letting go involves separation from children who are starting school. School phobias and school refusal syndromes that are accompanied by extreme separation anxiety may have to be dealt with. Often, a parent who cannot let go of a child accounts for this situation; some parents want their children to remain tightly bound to them emotionally. Family therapy that explores these dynamics may be needed to resolve such problems.

As children get older and enter adolescence, the process of establishing identity assumes great importance. Peer relationships become crucial to a child's development, and overprotective parents who keep a child from developing friendships or having the freedom to experiment with friends that the parents disapprove of can interfere with the child's passage through adolescence. Parents need not try to refrain from exerting influence over their children; guidance and involvement are crucial. But they must recognize that adolescents, especially, need parental approval; although rebellious on the surface, adolescents are much more tractable than they appear, provided parents are not overbearing or generally punitive.

SINGLE-PARENT FAMILIES. There are more than 10 million single-parent families with one or more children under the age of 18; of these families, 20 percent are single-parent homes in which a woman is the sole head of the household. Although most of these children were left in the custody of their mothers by the courts in divorce proceedings, other children have been abandoned by their fathers. The increase in number of single-parent families has risen almost 200 percent since 1980.

The number of children born to unwed mothers has declined over the past 10 years, but in 1998 they still accounted for about one quarter of all births in the United States. Similarly, the birth rate for teenage women has been declining every year since 1991 when it peaked.

ALTERNATIVE LIFESTYLE PARENTING. Both single and married homosexual men and women are choosing to raise children. In most cases, such children are obtained through adoption. Some, however, may be born to a lesbian woman through artificial insemination or obtained from a willing mother surrogate. The number of such family units is increasing. The scant data about the development of children in these homes indicate that they are at no greater risk for emotional problems (or for a homosexual orientation) than children raised in conventional households.

ADOPTION. Adoption laws were enacted in the United States in about 1850, and since the turn of the century, adoption or foster placement has replaced institutional care as the preferred way to raise children who are neglected, unwanted, or abandoned. Many couples who are unable to conceive (and some couples who already have children) turn to adoption.

In addition to the full range of normal parent–child developmental issues, adoptive parents face special problems. They must decide how and when to tell the child about the adoption. They must deal with the child's possible desire for information about his or her biological parents. Recent high-profile cases in which children were removed from adoptive and psychological parents to be placed with biological parents may cast a shadow of uncertainty over the first few years of adoption. Whether these events have any impact on parent–child bonding or the child's subsequent emotional development has not been studied. Adopted children are more likely to develop conduct disorders, problems with drug abuse, and antisocial personality traits. It is unclear whether these problems result from the process of adoption or whether parents who give up children for adoption are more likely to pass along a genetic predisposition for these behaviors.

Table 2.4–3
Features Salient to Middle Life

Issues	Positive Features	Negative Features
Prime of life	Responsible use of power; maturity; productivity	Winner-loser view; competitiveness
Stock taking: what to do with the rest of one's life	Possibility; alternatives; organization of commitments; redirection	Closure; fatalism
Fidelity and commitments	Commitment to self, others, career, society; filial maturity	Hypocrisy; self-deception
Growth-death (to grow is to die); juvenescence and rejuvenation fantasies	Naturality regarding body, time	Obscene or frenetic efforts (e.g., to be youthful); hostility and envy of youth and progeny; longing
Communication and socialization	Matters understood; continuity; picking up where left off; large social network; rootedness of relationships, places, and ideas	Repetitiveness; boredom; impatience; isolation; conservatism; confusion; rigidity

Adapted from Robert N. Butler, M.D.

With widespread use of birth control and access to abortions, the number of infants available for adoption has declined steeply. Wealthy parents may prefer to arrange for private adoption rather than wait many uncertain years for an institutional adoption. (In private adoptions a biological mother is paid for her legal and medical expenses but not for the baby. Baby selling is a felony in all states.) International adoptions (especially from Bosnia, Latin America, Eastern Europe, and China) have also become more common. Questionable regulation in these countries has raised concern that some infants put up for adoption in poor countries may not be orphans but are being sold by destitute mothers.

Additional controversy has surrounded the adoption of black babies by white families. In 1972 the National Association of Black Social Workers issued a position paper condemning such adoptions in all circumstances. Several prospective studies have found that white parents can raise black children who have solid self-esteem and unambivalent racial identity.

MIDDLE ADULTHOOD

The ages that define middle adulthood vary among theorists, but the period typically spans the years from 40 to 65. Carl Jung referred to age 40 as "the noon of life." The transition from early adulthood involves a process of reviewing the past, considering how life has gone, and deciding what the future will be like. With regard to occupation, many persons begin to experience the gap between early aspirations and current achievements. They may wonder whether the lifestyle and the commitments they chose in early adulthood are worth continuing; they may feel that they would like to live their remaining years in a different, more satisfying way, without knowing exactly how. As children grow up and leave home, parental roles change, and persons redefine their roles as husbands and wives.

Important gender changes occur in middle adulthood. Many women who no longer need to nurture young children can release their energy into independent pursuits that require assertiveness and a competitive spirit, traits that were traditionally considered masculine. Alternatively, men in middle adulthood may develop qualities that enable them to express their emotions and recognize their dependency needs, traits that were traditionally considered feminine. With the new balance of the masculine and the feminine, a person may now be able to relate more effectively to someone of the other sex than in the past.

Developmental Tasks

Robert Butler described several underlying themes in middle adulthood that appear to be present regardless of marital and family status, gender, or economic level (Table 2.4–3). These themes include aging (as changes in bodily functions are noticed in middle adulthood); taking stock of accomplishments and setting goals for the future; reassessing commitments to family, work, and marriage; dealing with parental illness and death; and attending to all the developmental tasks without losing the capacity to experience pleasure or to engage in playful activity.

Erik Erikson. Erikson described middle adulthood as characterized either by generativity or by stagnation. Erikson defined *generativity* as the process by which persons guide the oncoming generation or improve society. This stage includes having and raising children, but wanting or having children does not ensure generativity. A childless person can be generative by helping others, by being creative, and by contributing to society. Parents must be secure in their own identities to raise children successfully: They cannot be preoccupied with themselves and act as if they were, or wished to be, the child in the family.

To be *stagnant* means that a person stops developing. For Erikson, stagnation was anathema, and he referred to adults without any impulses to guide the new generation or to those who produce children without caring for them as being "within a cocoon of self-concern and isolation." Such persons are in great danger. Because they are unable to negotiate the developmental tasks of middle adulthood, they are unprepared for the next stage of the life cycle, old age, which places more demands on the psychological and physical capacities than all the preceding stages.

George Vaillant. In his longitudinal study of 173 men who were interviewed at 5-year intervals after they graduated from Harvard, Vaillant found a strong correlation between physical and emotional health in middle age. In addition, those with the poorest psychological adjustment during college years had a high incidence of physical illness in middle age. No single factor in childhood accounted for adult mental health, but an overall sense

of stability in the parental home predicted a well-adjusted adulthood. A close sibling relationship during college years was correlated with emotional and physical well-being in middle age. In another study Vaillant found that childhood and adult work habits were correlated and that adult mental health and good interpersonal relationships were associated with the capacity to work in childhood. Vaillant's studies are ongoing and represent the longest continuous study of adulthood ever performed.

Sexuality

Sexuality is a major issue in midlife. Although William Masters and Virginia Johnson reported, as did Alfred Kinsey and others, that enjoyable sexual activity (including coitus) may continue well into old age, sexual functioning may decline. For some persons, however, the erroneous belief that vigorous sexual activity is the prerogative of youth suffices to interfere with their normal physiological sexual responses.

Fears and the reality of impotence are common problems in middle-aged men. The most common cause of impotence in the middle years is not aging but excessive alcohol intake, drugs (e.g., tranquilizers and antidepressants), and stress with fatigue and anxiety; most chronic impotence in middle adulthood is due to psychological rather than organic causes.

Middle-aged women may also experience a decline in sexual functioning related more to psychological, than to physical, causes. Women do not reach their sexual prime until their mid-30s; consequently, they have a greater capacity for orgasm in middle adulthood than in young adulthood. Women, however, are more vulnerable than men to narcissistic blows to their self-esteem as they lose their youthful appearance, which is overvalued in today's society. During middle adulthood they may feel less sexually desirable than in early adulthood and thus feel less entitled to an adequate sex life. An inability to deal with changes in body image prompts many women and men to undergo cosmetic surgery in an effort to maintain their youthful appearance.

Climacterium

Middle adulthood is the time of the male and female *climacterium,* the period in life characterized by decreased biological and physiological functioning. For women, the menopausal period is considered the climacterium, and it may start anywhere from the 40s to the early 50s. Bernice Neugarten studied this period and found that more than 50 percent of women described the menopause as an unpleasant experience, but a significant portion believed that their lives had not changed in any significant way, and many women experienced no adverse effects. Because they no longer had to worry about becoming pregnant, some women report feeling sexually freer after the menopause than before its onset. Generally, the female climacterium has been stereotyped as a sudden or radical psychophysiological experience; but it is more often a gradual experience as estrogen secretion decreases with changes in the flow, timing, and eventual cessation of the menses. Vasomotor instability (hot flashes) may occur, and the menopause may extend over several years. Some women experience anxiety and depression, but usually women who have a history of poor adaptation to stress are predisposed to the menopausal syndrome. (Chapter 30 on reproductive medicine provides further discussion of menopause and its management.)

For men, the climacterium has no clear demarcation; male hormones stay fairly constant through the 40s and 50s and then begin to decline. Nevertheless, men must adapt to a decline in biological functioning and overall physical vigor. About age 50 there is a slight decrease in healthy sperm and seminal fluid; not sufficient, however, to preclude insemination. Coincident with the decreased testosterone level, there may be fewer and less firm erections and decreased sexual activity generally. Some men experience a so-called midlife crisis during this period. The crisis can be mild or severe, characterized by a sudden drastic change in work or marital relationships, severe depression, increased use of alcohol or drugs, or a shift to an alternate lifestyle.

Midlife Crisis

The physical changes of middle age are accompanied by new emotional and psychological demands. Arguably the most profound is the ability to surrender the fantasy of unlimited possibilities. Adolescents and young adults can look to the future and imagine almost anything for themselves: successful careers, loving partners, adventure, recognition, and wealth. Such fantasies are often a helpful comfort in dealing with the sometimes discouraging realities of everyday life. As men and women reach middle age, and as the recognition of a finite lifespan becomes more real, persons begin to face the prospect that some of life's goals will be left unaccomplished and that the possibility of exciting new relationships, dramatic new adventures, or major career changes is increasingly less likely. It is a period of growing appreciation for what one does have and a gradual letting go of what might have been.

Some persons feel a sense of urgency in middle age to do and accomplish all they can before time runs out. This impulse can be adaptive and enriching, for example, when a person decides to learn French or to take a trip up the Amazon. Occasionally it becomes destructive. Persons may leave their families to have sexual affairs with younger partners or abandon careers to pursue interests of the moment. The term *midlife crisis* does not have fixed meaning and has been used by writers to describe a wide range of emotional struggles a person may face during this period. In general, however, it is reserved for serious maladaptive behavior that often occurs in the context of severe or unexpected life events such as the death of a spouse, the loss of a job, or serious illness. Men and women who are most prone to midlife crises tend to come from families characterized by one or more of the following during their adolescence: parental discord, withdrawal by the same-sex parent, anxious parents, or impulsive parents with a low sense of responsibility.

Dr. C., a prominent, 45-year-old surgeon, had been married for 22 years and was the father of three adolescent children. One Saturday he left home for the golf course and did not return. Although he had been somewhat bored by his wife for some time, he did not have any conscious plans to

leave her. As he reconstructed his thoughts, he was standing on the tenth tee, after making par on the ninth, when the thought occurred to him "I'm never going home again." After showering and lingering over a drink with his friends, he drove for several hours and checked into a motel. The next day was spent in thought "about my life, its meaning and purpose. I suddenly knew it wasn't right for me and I had to change it." On Monday morning he returned home, left his wife a note in the mailbox telling her, without any explanation, that he was leaving, and drove to his office. There he saw his patients, went to the bank and cashed in a $100,000 certificate of deposit from his pension plan, and got on a plane for a distant city. Upon arriving he left a message for one of his partners asking him to take over his practice. For the next 2 months he did nothing but exercise and think. Eventually he wrote his wife a letter informing her of his whereabouts and of his decision to remain away.

When he came for treatment 16 months later he was working in an emergency room and had begun a relationship with a 43-year-old divorcee with two teenage sons, "not so very different from the family I left," he said.

Therapeutic efforts to reconstruct the patient's thinking during the acute phase of the crisis were limited by his inability to remember. He just knew he had to change, now.

Therapeutic exploration of the probable dynamics behind the crisis—the recent death of his father, occasional impotence and dissatisfaction with his wife—were illuminating but did not change Dr. C.'s determination to avoid his former life. He refused to meet with his wife and eventually agreed through a lawyer to a divorce settlement that gave her almost all of their assets. He did agree to see his children when they sought him out but did not initiate contacts with them. All of his energies were directed toward "doing what I want to do, meeting new persons, and finding myself."

The therapy seemed to meet the patient's need to understand himself and build a new life. He eventually remarried and supported his new family by continuing to work in emergency rooms, making far less money than he had in his surgery practice. He even took up golf again. (Courtesy of Calvin Colarusso, M.D.)

Empty-Nest Syndrome. Another phenomenon described in middle adulthood has been called the *empty-nest syndrome,* a depression that occurs in men and women when their youngest child is about to leave home. Most parents, however, perceive the departure of the youngest child as a relief rather than a stress. If no compensating activities have been developed, particularly by the mother, some parents become depressed. This is especially true of women whose predominant role in life has been mothering or of couples who decided to stay in an otherwise unhappy marriage "for the sake of the children."

Other Tasks of Middle Adulthood

As persons approach the age of 50, they clearly define what they want from work, family, and leisure. Men who have reached their highest level of advancement in work may experience disillusionment or frustration when they realize that they can no longer anticipate new work challenges. For women who have invested themselves completely in mothering, this period leaves them with no suitable identity after the children leave home. Sometimes, social rules become rigidly established; lack of freedom in lifestyle and a sense of entrapment may lead to depression and a loss of confidence. There may also be unique financial burdens in middle age, produced by pressures to care for aged parents at one end of the spectrum and children at the other end.

Levinson described a transitional period between the ages of 50 and 55 during which a developmental crisis may occur when persons feel incapable of changing an intolerable life structure. Although no single event characterizes the transition, the physiological changes that begin to appear may have a dramatic effect on a person's sense of self. For example, a person may experience a decrease in cardiovascular efficiency that accompanies aging. Chronological age and physical infirmity are not linear, however; those who exercise regularly, who do not smoke, and who eat and drink in moderation can maintain their physical health and emotional well-being.

Middle adulthood is when persons frequently feel overwhelmed by too many obligations and duties, but it is also a time of great satisfaction for most persons. They have developed a wide array of acquaintances, friendships, and relationships, and the satisfaction they express about their network of friends predicts positive mental health. Some social ties, however, may be a source of stress when demands either cannot be met or assault a person's self-esteem. Power, leadership, wisdom, and understanding are most generally possessed by persons who are middle aged, and if their health and vitality remain intact, it is truly the prime of life.

DIVORCE

Divorce is a major crisis of life. Spouses often grow, develop, and change at different rates; one spouse may discover that the other is not the same as when they first married. In truth, both partners have changed and evolved, not necessarily in complementary directions. Frequently, one spouse blames a third person for alienation of affections and refuses to examine his or her own role in the marital problems. Certain aspects of marital deterioration and divorce seem to be related to specific qualities of middle life—need for change, weariness with acting responsibly, fear of facing up to oneself. The following cases reported by Colarusso are informative.

A 55-year-old patient, Mrs. A., sought treatment "in order to leave my marriage. We've been married for 35 years but I haven't loved my husband for the last 20. I've been so dependent on him all of my adult life that I don't know if I have the courage to leave." Twice-weekly psychotherapy that lasted 15 months helped her leave her husband, start a business, and begin a new relationship. "I have less money and I'm scared about the future, but I feel alive and in control of my life. I think Bill is happier, too."

Fifty-year-old Mrs. T. left her "wonderful" husband because "I've missed something. I just have to get out on my own." She married at age 18, "going from my parent's home to his home." She recognized that her rage at her husband for "not being all the other men I could have married, for closing off all the living I could have done" was irrational but uncontrollable. "I have to live on my own for awhile, to see if I can do it, before it's too late." Fully intending to return to her husband, she continued exploring the infantile and adult issues that precipitated the separation, leaving the future of the marriage in doubt.

A 43-year-old patient, Mr. S. was continually preoccupied with his marriage during his 4-year analysis. Sexually inhibited during adolescence, he "married the only girl in the world who knew less about sex than I did." Exploration of his sexual inhibitions led to a decision to stay in the marriage. "I've learned in this analysis that sex is not the rare, extraordinary thing I thought it was as a kid; billions of persons do it every day. I know I could go out and sleep with a lot of different women, but how different, or better, would it actually be? Jane and I have built a pretty good life together. She's changed a lot and so have I. I think we can make the next 20 years better than the last 20."

Types of Separation

Paul Bohannan, an anthropologist with expertise in marriage and divorce, described the types of separations that take place at the time of divorce.

Psychic Divorce. In psychic divorce the love object is given up, and a grief reaction about the death of the relationship occurs. Sometimes a period of anticipatory mourning sets in before the divorce. Separating from a spouse forces a person to become autonomous, to change from a position of dependence. The separation may be difficult to achieve, especially if both are used to being dependent on each other (as normally happens in marriage) or if one was so dependent as to be afraid or incapable of becoming independent. Most persons report such feelings as depression, ambivalence, and mood swings at the time of divorce. Studies indicate that recovery from divorce takes about 2 years; by then the ex-spouse may be viewed neutrally, and each spouse accepts his or her new identity as a single person.

Legal Divorce. Legal divorce involves going through the courts so that each of the parties is remarriageable. Seventy-five percent of divorced women and eighty percent of divorced men remarry within 3 years of divorce. No-fault divorce, in which neither person is judged to be the guilty party, has become the most widely used legal mechanism for divorce.

Economic Divorce. Major concerns are the division of the couple's property between them and economic support for the wife. Many men who are ordered by the courts to pay alimony or child support flout the law and create a major social problem.

Community Divorce. The social network of the divorced couple changes markedly. A few relatives and friends are retained from the community, and new ones are added. The task of meeting new friends is often difficult for divorced persons, who may realize how dependent they were on their spouses for social exchanges.

Coparental Divorce. Coparental divorce is the separation of a parent from the child's other parent. Being a single parent differs from being a married parent.

Custody

The parental right doctrine is a legal concept that awards custody to the more fit natural parent and attempts to ensure that the best interest of the child is served. In the past, mothers were almost always awarded custody, but custody is now given to fathers in about 15 percent of cases. Custodial fathers are likely to be white, married, older, and better educated than custodial mothers. Women who are granted custody have a better chance of being awarded child support and of actually receiving payment than do men who are granted custody. Nevertheless, women who receive payments still have lower incomes than men who receive payment.

The types of custody include joint custody, in which a child spends equal time with each parent, an increasingly common practice; split custody, in which siblings are separated and each parent has custody of one or more of the children; and single custody, in which the children live solely with one parent and the other parent has rights of visitation that may be limited in some way by the court. Child support payments are more likely to be made when parents have joint custody or when the noncustodial parent is given visitation rights.

Problems may surface in the parent–child relationship with the custodial or the noncustodial parent. The absence of the noncustodial parent in the home represents the reality of the divorce, and the custodial parent may become the target of the child's anger about the divorce. The parent under such stress may not be able to deal with the child's increased needs and emotional demands.

The noncustodial parent must cope with limits placed on time spent with the child. This parent loses the day-to-day gratification and the responsibilities involved with parenting. Emotional distress is common in parent and child. Joint custody offers a solution with some advantages, but it requires substantial maturity on the part of the parents and can present some problems. Parents must separate their child-rearing practices from their postdivorce resentments, and they must develop a spirit of cooperation about rearing the child. They must also be able to tolerate frequent communication with the ex-spouse.

Reasons for Divorce

Divorce tends to run in families and rates are highest in couples who marry as teenagers or come from different socioeconomic backgrounds. Every marriage is psychologically unique and so is each divorce. If a person's parents were divorced, he or she may choose to resolve a marital problem in the same way, through divorce. Expectations of the spouse may be unrealistic: One partner may expect the other to act as an all-giving mother or a magically protective father. The parenting experience places the greatest strain on a marriage. In surveys of couples with and without children, those without children reported getting more pleasure from the spouse than those with children. Illness in the child creates the

greatest strain of all, and more than 50 percent of marriages in which a child has died through illness or accident end in divorce.

Other causes of marital distress are problems about sex and money. Both areas may be used as a means of control, and withholding sex or money is a means of expressing aggression. There is also less social pressure now than in the past to remain married. As discussed above, the easing of divorce laws and the declining influence of religion and the extended family make divorce an acceptable course of action today.

Intercourse outside of Marriage. *Adultery* is defined as voluntary sexual intercourse between a married person and someone other than his or her spouse. A 1994 survey by the University of Chicago reported that 85 percent of married women and 75 percent of married men remain faithful to their spouses. These numbers are much higher than earlier researchers found. For men, the first extramarital affair is often associated with the wife's pregnancy, when coitus may be interdicted. Most of these incidents are kept secret from the spouse and, if known, rarely account for divorce. Nevertheless the infidelity may serve as the catalyst for basic dissatisfactions in the marriage to surface, and these problems may then lead to its dissolution. Adultery may decline, as potentially fatal sexually transmitted diseases such as acquired immune deficiency syndrome (AIDS) serve as sobering deterrents.

Adult Maturity

Success and happiness in adulthood are made possible by achieving a modicum of maturity—a mental state, not an age. However, the capacity for maturity is a direct outgrowth of the engagement and mastery of the developmental tasks of young and middle adulthood. From a developmental perspective, *maturity* may be defined as a mental state found in healthy adults that is characterized by detailed knowledge of the parameters of human existence, a sophisticated level of self-awareness based on an honest appraisal of one's own experience within those basic parameters, and the ability to use this intellectual and emotional knowledge and insight caringly in relation to one's self and others.

The achievement of maturity in midlife leads to emergence of the capacity for wisdom. Those who possess wisdom have learned from the past and are fully engaged in life in the present. Just as important, they anticipate the future and make the necessary decisions to enhance prospects for health and happiness. In other words, a philosophy of life has been developed that includes understanding and acceptance of the person's place in the order of human existence.

References

Brent DA, Johnson B, Bartle S, Bridge J. Personality disorders, tendency to impulsive violence, and survival behavior in adolescents. *J Am Acad Child Adolesc Psychiatry.* 1993;32:69.

Campbell BC, Udry JR. Stress and age at menarche of mothers and daughters. *J Biosoc Sci.* 1995;27:127.

Colarusso CA. Adulthood. In: Sadock BJ, Sadock VA, eds. *Kaplan & Sadock's Comprehensive Textbook of Psychiatry.* 7th ed. Vol 2. Baltimore: Lippincott Williams & Wilkins; 2000:2962.

Feeney A, Noller P, Wark C. Marital satisfaction and spousal interaction. In: Sternberg J, Hojjat A, et al., eds. *Satisfaction in Close Relationships.* New York: Guildford Press; 1997:160.

Flanagan CA, Eccles JS. Changes in parents' work status and adolescents' adjustment at school. *Child Dev.* 1993;64:246.

Freud A. Adolescence. *Psychoanal Study Child.* 1958;13:255.

Frey CU, Rothlisberger C. Social support in healthy adolescents. *J Youth Adolesc.* 1996;25:17.

Garber J, Weiss SB, Shanley N. Cognitions, depressive symptoms, and development in adolescents. *J Abnorm Psychol.* 1993;102:47.

Graber JA, Brooks-Gunn J, Warren MP. The antecedents of menarcheal age: heredity, family environment, and stressful life events. *Child Dev.* 1995;66:346.

Jarvinen DW, Nicholls JG. Adolescents' social goals, belief about the causes of social success, and satisfaction in peer relationships. *Dev Psychol.* 1996;32:432.

Murry VM. Incidence of first pregnancy among black adolescent females over three decades. *Youth Soc.* 1992;23:478.

Mussen PH, Conger JJ, Kagan J. Adolescence. In: *Essentials of Child Development and Personality.* New York: Harper & Row, 1984.

Newcomb MD. Life change events among adolescents. *J Nerv Ment Dis.* 1986;175:280.

Rainey DY, Stevens-Simon C, Kaplan DW. Are adolescents who report prior sexual abuse at a higher risk for pregnancy? *Child Abuse Negl.* 1995;19:1283.

Shields G, Adams J. HIV/AIDS among youth: a community needs assessment study. *Child Adolesc Soc Work J.* 1995;12:361.

Takanishi R. The opportunities of adolescence: research, interventions, and policy. *Am Psychol.* 1993;48:85.

Vaillant G. *Aging Well.* Boston: Little, Brown and Company; 2002.

Waughan VC, Litt IF. *Child and Adolescent Development.* Philadelphia: WB Saunders; 1990.

▲ 2.5 Late Adulthood (Old Age)

Late adulthood, or old age, usually refers to the stage of the life cycle that begins at age 65. Gerontologists—those who study the aging process—divide older adults into two groups: young-old, ages 65 to 74; and old-old, ages 75 and beyond. Some use the term *oldest old* to refer to those over 85. Older adults can also be described as well-old (persons who are healthy) and sick-old (persons who have an infirmity that interferes with functioning and requires medical or psychiatric attention). The health needs of older adults have grown enormously as the population ages, and geriatric physicians and psychiatrists play major roles in treating this population.

DEMOGRAPHICS

The number of individuals over age 65 is rapidly expanding. In 1900, for example, 4 percent of the U.S. population was older than 65 years. By 1990 it was 12.5 percent, and by 2030, it is projected to be 20 percent. That increase far exceeds the general population growth—10-fold compared with just over 3-fold between 1900 and 2000—and is projected to continue (e.g., 2½ times vs. just over 1½ times between 1990 and 2050) (Table 2.5–1).

The life expectancy for women at birth is projected to continue to exceed that for men by 7 years until the year 2050. By 2050, the composition of the U.S. population by age and sex is estimated to differ markedly from that today. Such changes are bound to influence income and marital statistics, the percentage of elderly persons living alone or in long-term care facilities, and other aspects of the social network.

The accuracy of the above projections, however, depends on the accuracy of other predications such as birth rates, immigration, and emigration—all of which are more difficult to gauge for the future than the remaining variables, death rates or life expectancies. Projections concerning life expectancy, for example, can change substantially within a single decade.

Table 2.5–1
Aging Population of the United States: 1900–2050

			Population, in Millions and as a Percentage of Total Population				
			All Ages	65 and Over		85 and Over	
Year	Median Age	Mean Age	(*N*)	(*N*)	(%)	(*N*)	(%)
1900			76.0	3.1	4.1%	0.1	0.1%
1950			150.1	12.3	8.2%	0.6	0.4%
1990			248.7	31.1	12.5%	3.0	1.2%
2000	35.7	36.5	276.2	35.3	12.8%	4.3	1.6%
2010	37.2	37.8	300.4	40.1	13.3%	6.0	2.0%
2030	38.5	39.9	350.0	70.2	20.1%	8.8	2.5%
2050	38.1	40.3	392.0	80.1	20.4%	18.9	4.8%

Population: U.S. Bureau of the Census. *Current Population Reports, Special Studies, P23–190, 65+ in the United States.* Washington, DC: U.S. Government Printing Office; 1996.
Mean/Median Age, 2000–2050: Day JC. Population projections of the United States by age, sex, race and Hispanic origin: 1995 to 2050. In *U.S. Bureau of the Census, Current Population Reports, P25–1130.* Washington, DC: U.S. Government Printing Office; 1996.

BIOLOGY OF AGING

The aging process, or senescence (from the Latin *senescere*, "to grow old"), is characterized by a gradual decline in the functioning of all the body's systems—cardiovascular, respiratory, genitourinary, endocrine, and immune, among others. But the belief that old age is invariably associated with profound intellectual and physical infirmity is a myth. Most older persons retain their cognitive abilities and physical capacities to a remarkable degree.

An overview of the biological changes that accompany old age is given in Table 2.5–2. The various decrements listed do not occur in a linear fashion in all systems. Not all organ systems deteriorate at the same rate, nor do they follow a similar pattern of decline for all persons. Each person is genetically endowed with one or more vulnerable systems, or a system may become vulnerable because of environmental stressors or intentional misuse (e.g., excessive ultraviolet exposure, smoking, alcohol). Moreover, not all organ systems deteriorate at the same time. Any one of a number of organ systems begins to deteriorate, and this deterioration then leads to illness or death.

Aging generally means the aging of cells. In the most commonly held theory, each cell has a genetically determined life span during which it can replicate itself a limited number of times before it dies. Structural changes occur in cells with age. In the central nervous system, for example, age-related cell changes occur in neurons, which show signs of degeneration. In senility (characterized by severe memory loss and a loss of intellectual functioning), signs of degeneration are much more severe. An example is the neurofibrillary degeneration seen most commonly in dementia of the Alzheimer's type.

Structural changes and mutations in deoxyribonucleic acid (DNA) and ribonucleic acid (RNA) are also found in aging cells; these have been attributed to genotypic programming, X-rays, chemicals, and food products, among others. There is probably no single cause of aging, and all areas of the body are affected to some degree. Genetic factors have been implicated in disorders that commonly occur in older persons, such as hypertension, coronary artery disease, arteriosclerosis, and neoplastic disease. Family studies indicate inheritance factors for breast and stomach cancer, colon polyps, and certain mental disorders of old age. Huntington's disease shows an autosomal dominant mode of inheritance with complete penetrance. The average age of onset is between 35 and 40, but cases have occurred as late as 70 years of age.

Longevity

Longevity has been studied since the beginning of recorded history and has always been a topic of great interest. The research about longevity reveals that a family history of longevity is the best indicator of a long life; almost half of fathers of persons who live past 80 also lived past 80. Nevertheless, many conditions leading to a shortened life can be prevented, ameliorated, or delayed with effective intervention. Heredity is but one factor—one beyond a person's control. Predictors of longevity that are within a person's control include regular medical checkups, minimal or no caffeine or alcohol consumption, work gratification, and a perceived sense of the self as being socially useful in an altruistic role, such as spouse, teacher, mentor, parent, or grandparent. Healthy eating and adequate exercise are also associated with health and longevity.

Life Expectancy

In the United States, the average life expectancy of both sexes has increased in every decade—from 48 years in 1900 to 73.5 years for men and 80.4 years for women in 2000. The projected life expectancy at birth and at age 65 is indicated in Table 2.5–3. Changes in morbidity and mortality have also occurred. Over the past 30 years, for example, there has been a 60 percent decline in mortality from cerebrovascular disease and a 30 percent decline in mortality from coronary artery disease. In contrast, mortality from cancer, which rises steeply with age, has increased, especially cancer of the lung, colon, stomach, skin, and prostate.

The oldest old, persons over 85 years of age, is the most rapidly growing segment of the older population. Over the last 25 years the population of all older persons increased by 100 percent, compared with 45 percent for the entire U.S. population,

Table 2.5–2
Biological Changes Associated with Aging

Cellular level	Change in cellular DNA and RNA structures: intracellular organelle degeneration
	Neuronal degeneration in central nervous system, primarily in superior temporal precentral and inferior temporal gyri; no loss in brainstem nuclei
	Receptor sites and sensitivity altered
	Decreased anabolism and catabolism of cellular transmitter substances
	Intercellular collagen and elastin increase
Immune system	Impaired T-cell response to antigen
	Increase in function of autoimmune bodies
	Increased susceptibility to infection and neoplasia
	Leukocytes unchanged, T lymphocytes reduced
	Increased erythrocyte sedimentation (nonspecific)
Musculoskeletal	Decrease in height because of shortening of spinal column (2-inch loss in both men and women from the second to the seventh decade)
	Reduction in lean muscle mass and muscle strength; deepening of thoracic cage
	Increase in body fat
	Elongation of nose and ears
	Loss of bone matrix, leading to osteoporosis
	Degeneration of joint surfaces may produce osteoarthritis
	Risk of hip fracture is 10–25% by age 90
	Continual closing of cranial sutures (parietomastoid suture does not attain complete closure until age 80)
	Men gain weight until about age 60, then lose; women gain weight until age 70, then lose
Integument	Graying of hair results from decreased melanin production in hair follicles (by age 50, 50% of all persons male and female are at least 50% gray; pubic hair is last to turn gray)
	General wrinkling of skin
	Less active sweat glands
	Decrease in melanin
	Loss of subcutaneous fat
	Nail growth slowed
Genitourinary and reproductive	Decreased glomerular filtration rate and renal blood flow
	Decreased hardness of erection, diminished ejaculatory spurt
	Decreased vaginal lubrication
	Enlargement of prostate
	Incontinence
Special senses	Thickening of optic lens, reduced peripheral vision
	Inability to accommodate (presbyopia)
	High-frequency sound hearing loss (presbyacusis)—25% show loss by age 60, 65% by age 80
	Yellowing of optic lens
	Reduced acuity of taste, smell, and touch
	Decreased light-dark adaption
Neuropsychiatric	Takes longer to learn new material, but complete learning still occurs
	Intelligence quotient (IQ) remains stable until age 80
	Verbal ability maintained with age
	Psychomotor speed declines
Memory	Tasks requiring shifting attentions performed with difficulty
	Encoding ability diminishes (transfer of short-term to long-term memory and vice versa)
	Recognition of right answer on multiple-choice tests remains intact
	Simple recall declines
Neurotransmitters	Norepinephrine decreases in central nervous system
	Increased monoamine oxidase and serotonin in brain
Brain	Decrease in gross brain weight, about 17% by age 80 in both sexes
	Widened sulci, smaller convolutions, gyral atrophy
	Ventricles enlarge
	Increased transport across blood–brain barrier
	Decreased cerebral blood flow and oxygenation
Cardiovascular	Increase in size and weight of heart (contains lipofuscin pigment derived from lipids)
	Decreased elasticity of heart valves
	Increased collagen in blood vessels
	Increased susceptibility to arrhythmias
	Altered homeostasis of blood pressure
	Cardiac output maintained in absence of coronary heart disease
Gastrointestinal (GI) system	At risk for atrophic gastritis, hiatal hernia, diverticulosis
	Decreased blood flow to gut, liver
	Diminished saliva flow
	Altered absorption from GI tract (at risk for malabsorption syndrome and avitaminosis)
	Constipation
Endocrine	Estrogen levels decrease in women
	Adrenal androgen decreases
	Testosterone production declines in men
	Increase in follicle-stimulating hormone (FSH) and luteinizing hormone (LH) in postmenopausal women
	Serum thyroxine (T_4) and thyroid-stimulating hormone (TSH) normal, triiodothyronine (T_3) reduced
	Glucose tolerance test result decreases
Respiratory	Decreased vital capacity
	Diminished cough reflex
	Decreased bronchial epithelium ciliary action

but the increase for the 85 and older group exceeded 275 percent. It is expected that by 2050, the oldest old will make up about 25 percent of the elderly population and 5 percent of the total population in the United States. Figure 2.5–1 gives projected percentages for the average annual growth rate of the elderly population to the year 2050.

The leading causes of death among older persons are heart disease, cancer, and stroke. Accidents are among the leading causes

Table 2.5–3
Projected Life Expectancy at Birth and Age 65, by Sex: 1990–2050 (in Years)

	At Birth			At Age 65		
Year	Men	Women	Difference	Men	Women	Difference
1990	72.1	79.0	6.9	15.0	19.4	4.4
2000	73.5	80.4	6.9	15.7	20.3	4.6
2010	74.4	81.3	6.9	16.2	21.0	4.8
2020	74.9	81.8	6.9	16.6	21.4	4.8
2030	75.4	82.3	6.9	17.0	21.8	4.8
2040	75.9	82.8	6.9	17.3	22.3	5.0
2050	76.4	83.3	6.9	17.7	22.7	5.0

Data from U.S. Bureau of the Census, Washington, DC.

of death of persons over 65. Most fatal accidents are caused by falls, pedestrian incidents, and burns. Falls are most commonly the result of cardiac arrhythmias and hypotensive episodes.

Some gerontologists consider death in very old persons (over 85) to result from an aging syndrome characterized by diminished elastic-mechanical properties of the heart, arteries, lungs, and other organs. Death results from trivial tissue injuries that would not be fatal to a younger person; accordingly, senescence is viewed as the cause of death.

Ethnicity and Race

The proportion of older persons in the black, Hispanic, and Asian populations is smaller than that in the white population, but it is increasing rapidly. By 2050, 20 percent of older persons will be nonwhite. The proportion of older persons who are Hispanic will increase from 4 to approximately 14 percent over the same period. According to the U.S. Census Bureau, *Hispanic* refers to persons "whose origins are Mexican, Puerto Rican, Cuban, Central or South American or other Hispanic/Latino, regardless of race."

Sex Ratios

On average, women live longer than men and are more likely than men to live alone. The number of men per 100 women decreases sharply from age 65 to 85 (Fig. 2.5–2).

Geographic Distribution

The most populous states have the largest number of older persons. California has the most (3.3 million), followed by New York, Pennsylvania, Texas, Michigan, Illinois, Florida, and Ohio, each with more than 1 million. States with high proportions of older persons include Pennsylvania, Florida, Nebraska, and North Dakota. The high proportion in Florida is due to those who move into the state for retirement; in the others it is due to young persons moving out.

Exercise, Diet, and Health

Diet and exercise play a role in preventing or ameliorating chronic diseases of older persons, such as arteriosclerosis and hypertension. Hyperlipidemia correlates with coronary artery disease and can be controlled by reducing body weight, decreasing the intake of saturated fat, and limiting the intake of cholesterol. Increasing the daily intake of dietary fiber can also help decrease serum lipoprotein levels. A daily intake of 1 ounce (about 30 mL) of alcohol has been correlated with longevity and elevated high-density lipoproteins (HDL). Studies have also clearly demonstrated that statin drugs that reduce cholesterol have a dramatic effect on reducing cardiovascular disease in persons with diet- or exercise-resistant hyperlipidemia.

Low salt intake (less than 3 g a day) is associated with a lowered risk of hypertension. Hypertensive geriatric patients can often correct their condition by moderate exercise and decreased salt intake without the addition of drugs.

A regimen of daily moderate exercise (walking for 30 minutes a day) has been associated with a reduction in cardiovascular disease, decreased incidence of osteoporosis, improved respiratory function, the maintenance of ideal weight, and a general sense of well-being. Exercise has been shown to improve strength and function even among the very old. In many cases a disease process has been reversed and even cured by diet and exercise, without additional medical or surgical intervention.

Table 2.5–4 lists the biological changes associated with diet and exercise. A comparison with Table 2.5–1 reveals that almost every biological change associated with aging is positively affected by diet and exercise.

Stage Theories of Personality Development

Early personality theorists proposed that development was completed by the end of childhood or adolescence. One of the first development theorists to propose that personality continues to develop and grow over the life span was Erik Erikson (Table 2.5–5). Erikson believed that development proceeded through a series of psychosocial stages, each with its own conflict that is resolved by the individual with greater or lesser success. Erikson termed the crisis of the last epoch of life *integrity versus despair* and believed that successful resolution of this crisis involved a process of life review and achieved a sense of peace and wisdom through coming to terms with how one's life was lived. For example, Erikson proposed that successful resolution of this crisis would be characterized by a sense of having lived one's life well, while a less successful resolution would be

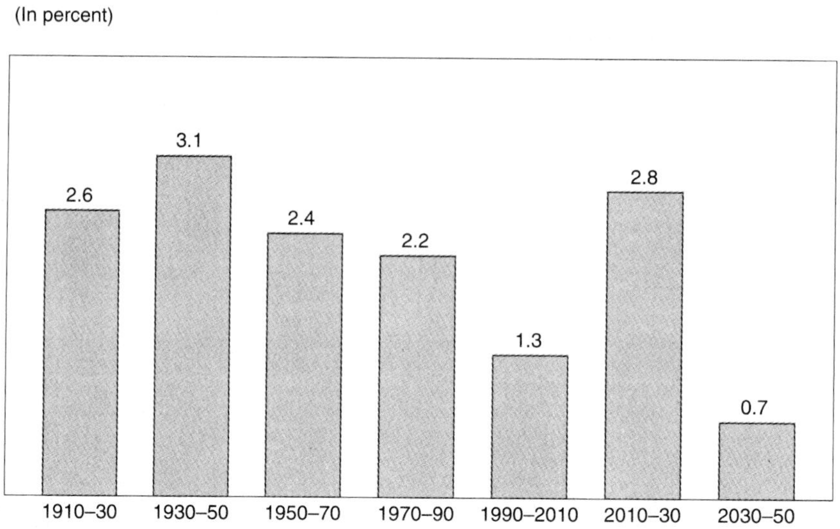

FIGURE 2.5–1
Average annual growth rate of the elderly population. (Data from U.S. Bureau of the Census.)

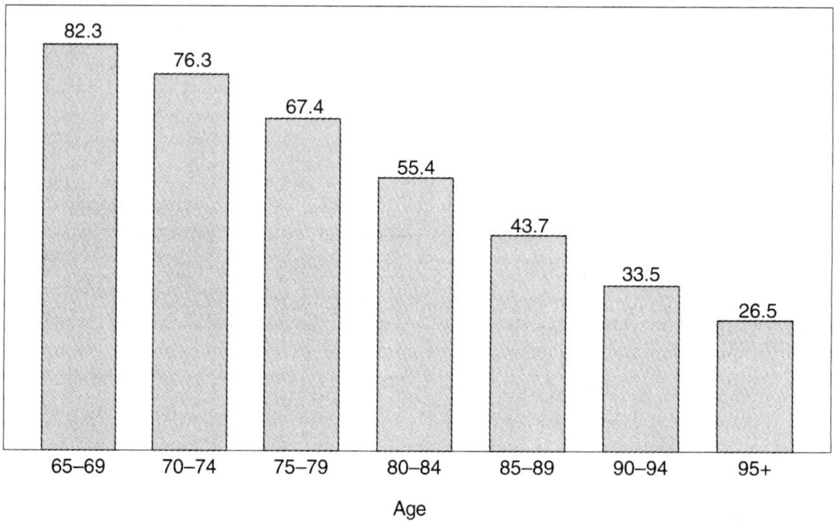

FIGURE 2.5–2
Number of men per 100 women by age. (Data from U.S. Bureau of the Census.)

characterized by feeling that life was too short, that one did not choose wisely, and bitterness that one will not have a chance to live life over.

Several studies have attempted to validate aspects of Erikson's theory. In one study, a sample of over 400 men was studied prospectively, and the highest eriksonian life stage each achieved was rated according to data gathered on the circumstances of his life. For example, if a man had achieved independence from his family of origin and was self-sufficient but was unable to develop an intimate relationship, the highest life stage achieved would be the identity stage, not the intimacy stage. This study found that eriksonian stages are passed through in sequential order, although often not at the same age for different individuals, and that the stages are surprisingly universal in populations that are ethnically and socioeconomically diverse.

A longitudinal study of approximately 500 subjects from two age cohorts found that the earlier age cohort scored significantly higher on integrity than the later age cohort, and scores for both age cohorts on integrity had declined significantly by the final time of testing. These data suggest that the conflict of integrity versus despair may have a more favorable outcome in earlier age cohorts than in later ones, raising the possibility that changing societal values have had a negative impact on the struggle for integrity. Another study found that *wisdom,* a construct related to integrity, bore a stronger relation to life satisfaction in elderly adults than other variables, including finances, health, and living situation.

Personality over the Life Span: Stability or Change? While Erikson and other stage theorists focused on unique developmental tasks and stages central to each

Table 2.5–4
Positive and Healthy Physiological Effects of Exercise and Nutrition

Increases
- Strength of bones, ligaments, and muscles
- Muscle mass and body density
- Articular cartilage thickness
- Skeletal muscle ATP, CRP, K+, and myoglobin
- Skeletal muscle oxidative enzyme content and mitochondria
- Skeletal muscle arterial collaterals and capillary density
- Heart volume and weight
- Blood volume and total circulating hemoglobin
- Cardiac stroke volume
- Myocardial contractility
- Maximal CO_2(A-V)
- Maximal blood lactate concentration
- Maximal pulmonary ventilation
- Maximal respiratory work
- Maximal oxygen diffusing capacity
- Maximal exercise capacity as measured by the maximal oxygen intake, exercise time, and distance
- Serum high-density lipoprotein concentration
- Anaerobic threshold
- Plasma insulin concentration with submaximal exercise

Decreases
- Heart rate at rest and during submaximal exercise
- Blood lactate concentration during submaximal exercise
- Pulmonary ventilation during submaximal work
- Respiratory quotient during submaximal work
- Serum triglyceride concentration
- Body fatness
- Serum low-density lipoprotein concentration
- Systolic blood pressure
- Core temperature threshold for initiation of sweating
- Sweat sodium and chloride content
- Plasma epinephrine and norepinephrine with submaximal exercise
- Plasma glucagon and growth hormone concentrations with submaximal exercise
- Relative hemoconcentration with submaximal exercise in the heat

Reprinted with permission from Buskirk ER. In: White PL, Monderka T, eds. *Diet and Exercise: Synergism in Health Maintenance.* Chicago: American Medical Association; 1982:133.

phase of life, other theorists have focused on defining core personality traits within the individual and determining their course over the life span. For example, do those who are gregarious or extraverted during early childhood and adolescence remain extraverted through midlife and old age? Several well-designed longitudinal studies that have followed individuals over periods ranging from 10 to 50 years have found strong evidence for stability in five basic personality traits: extraversion, neuroticism, agreeableness, openness to experience, and conscientiousness. Some studies found slight decreases in extraversion and slight increases in agreeableness as individuals move into the oldest-old category, which contrasts with early theories that proposed that personality rigidifies as individuals age.

Table 2.5–5
Old Age Developmental Theorists

Sigmund Freud	Increasing control of the ego and id with aging results in increased autonomy. Regression may permit primitive modes of functioning to reappear.
Erik Erikson	The central conflict in old age is between *integrity,* the sense of satisfaction people feel reflecting on a life lived productively, and *despair,* the sense that life has little purpose or meaning. Contentment in old age comes only with getting beyond narcissism and into intimacy and generativity.
Heinz Kohut	Old people must continually cope with narcissistic injury as they attempt to adapt to the biological, psychological, and social losses associated with the aging process. The maintenance of self-esteem is a major task of old age.
Bernice Neugarten	The major conflict of old age relates to giving up the position of authority and evaluating achievements and former competence. It is a time of reconciliation with others and resolution of grief over the death of others and the approaching death of self.
Daniel Levinson	Ages 60–65 is a transition period ("the late adult transition"). People who are narcissistic and too heavily invested in body appearance are liable to become preoccupied with death. Creative mental activity is a normal and healthy substitute for reduced physical activity.

Is the fact that personality appears to have considerable stability over time inconsistent with the basic tenets of stage theories? Perhaps not. It may be that while individuals are consistent over time in their basic personality structure, the themes and conflicts with which they struggle change considerably over the life span, from concerns about developing identity and a stable sense of self, to finding a life partner, to issues related to life review, as hypothesized by the stage theories. In addition, in developing theories about personality change, few studies have examined the impact of significant historical events on personality; thus the ways in which these events may result in personality change has not been studied systematically.

PSYCHOSOCIAL ASPECTS OF AGING

Social Activity

Healthy older persons usually maintain a level of social activity that is only slightly changed from that of earlier years. For many, old age is a period of continued intellectual, emotional, and psychological growth. In some cases, however, physical illness or the death of friends and relatives may preclude continued social interaction. Moreover, as persons experience an increased sense of isolation, they may become vulnerable to depression. Growing evidence indicates that maintaining social activities is valuable for physical and emotional well-being. Contact with younger persons is also important. Old persons can pass on cultural values and provide care services to the younger generation and thereby maintain a sense of usefulness that contributes to self-esteem.

Table 2.5–6
Top 10 Chronic Conditions for People 65+, by Age and Race (number per 1,000 people)

	Age				Race (65+)		
Condition	**65+**	**45 to 64**	**65 to 74**	**75+**	**White**	**Black**	**Black as % of White**
Arthritis	483.0	253.8	437.3	554.5	483.2	522.6	108
Hypertension	380.6	229.1	383.8	375.6	367.4	517.7	141
Hearing impairment	286.5	127.7	239.4	360.3	297.4	174.5	59
Heart disease	278.9	118.9	231.6	353.0	286.5	220.5	77
Cataracts	156.8	16.1	107.4	234.3	160.7	139.8	87
Deformity or orthopedic impairment	155.2	155.5	141.4	177.0	156.2	150.8	97
Chronic sinusitis	153.4	173.5	151.8	155.8	157.1	125.2	80
Diabetes	88.2	58.2	89.7	85.7	80.2	165.9	207
Visual impairment	81.9	45.1	69.3	101.7	81.1	77.0	95
Varicose veins	78.1	57.8	72.6	86.6	80.3	64.0	80

Data from National Center for Health Statistics, Washington, DC.

Ageism

Ageism, a term coined by Robert Butler, refers to discrimination toward old persons and to the negative stereotypes about old age that are held by younger adults. Old persons may themselves resent and fear other old persons and discriminate against them. In Butler's scheme, persons often associate old age with loneliness, poor health, senility, and general weakness or infirmity. The experience of older persons, however, does not consistently support this attitude. For example, although 50 percent of young adults expect poor health to be a problem for those over 65 years old, 75 percent of persons 65 to 74 years of age describe their health as good. Two thirds of persons 75 and older feel the same way. Health problems, when they do exist, more often involve chronic than acute conditions. More than four of five persons over the age of 65 have at least one chronic condition (Table 2.5–6).

Good health, however, is not the sole determinant of a good quality of life in old age. Surveys of old persons show that social contacts are at least as highly valued. In fact, the factors affecting good aging appear to be multidimensional. Aging "robustly" means considering aging in terms of productive involvement, affective status, functional status, and cognitive status. These four indicators are only minimally correlated. The most robustly aging individuals report greater social contact, better health and vision, and fewer significant life events in the past 3 years than their less robustly aging counterparts. There is a linear, age-related decrease in robustness, but it can still be found among the oldest old.

George Vaillant followed up a group of Harvard freshmen into old age and found the following about emotional health at age 65: Having been close to brothers and sisters during college correlated with emotional well-being; undergoing early traumatic life experiences, such as the death of a parent or parental divorce, did not correlate with poor adaptation in old age; being depressed at some point between ages 21 and 50 predicted emotional problems at age 65; and possessing the personality traits of pragmatism and dependability as a young adult was associated with a sense of well-being at age 65.

Countertransference

Physicians' feelings and attitudes toward older persons stem from a variety of sources: countertransference, societal attitudes, and patients' attitudes about being old. Countertransference feelings about aging are determined by a physician's needs and past experiences, and they function on both a conscious and an unconscious level. Physicians may have fears about their own old age or may have had conflicts about the aging or death of parents or grandparents. Physicians must be aware of these feelings, especially negative ones. Some older persons may act out the poor expectations held by their physicians; they may lose confidence in their abilities and appear to be less able than they are in fact.

Socioeconomics

The economics of old age is of paramount importance to older persons themselves and to society at large. The past 30 years has seen a dramatic decline in the proportion of the U.S. elderly population who are poor, primarily as a result of Medicare, Social Security, and private pensions. In 1959, 35.2 percent of persons over 65 lived below the poverty line, but by 1995 this figure had declined to 10.5 percent, the first time that the poverty rate for older persons dipped below that for persons of working age. Persons over age 65 make up 12 percent of the population, but they include only 9 percent of those living at low socioeconomic levels. Women are more likely than men to be poor. Income sources vary for persons age 65 and older. Despite overall economic gains, many older persons are so preoccupied by money worries that their enjoyment of life is lessened. Obtaining proper medical care may be especially difficult when personal funds are not available or are insufficient.

Medicare (Title 18) provides both hospital and medical insurance for those over age 65. About 150 million medical bills are reimbursed under the Medicare program each year; but only about 40 percent of all medical expenses incurred by older

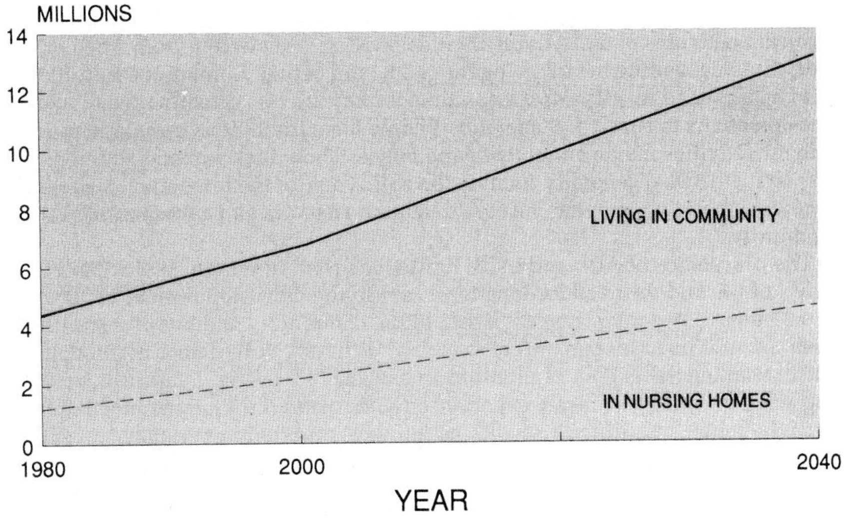

FIGURE 2.5–3

People age 65+ in need of long-term care: 1980–2040. (Reproduced with permission from Manton B, Soldo J. Dynamics of health changes in the oldest old: New perspectives and evidence. *Milbank Q.* 1985;63:12.)

persons is covered under Medicare. The rest is paid by private insurance, state insurance, or personal funds. Some services—such as outpatient psychiatric treatment, skilled nursing care, physical rehabilitation, and preventive physical examinations—are covered minimally or not at all.

In addition to Medicare, the Social Security program pays benefits to persons over age 65 (over age 66 in the year 2009 and age 67 in 2027) and pays benefits at reduced rates from age 62 on. To qualify for benefits, a person must have worked long enough to become insured: A worker must have worked for 10 years to be eligible for benefits. Benefits are also paid to widows, widowers, and dependent children if those receiving benefits or contributing to Social Security die (survivor benefits). Social Security is not a pension scheme but a pay-as-you-go income supplement to prevent mass destitution among older persons. Benefits are paid by those currently working to those retired. Serious difficulties for Social Security are forecast for the next 3 decades, when the number of baby boomers reaching old age will greatly exceed the number of younger workers paying into the plan.

Retirement

For many older persons, retirement is a time for the pursuit of leisure and for freedom from the responsibility of previous working commitments. For others, it is a time of stress, especially when retirement results in economic problems or a loss of self-esteem. Ideally, employment after age 65 should be a matter of choice. With the passage of the Age Discrimination in Employment Act of 1967 and its amendments, forced retirement at age 70 has been virtually eliminated in the private sector, and it is not legal in federal employment.

Most of those who retire voluntarily reenter the work force within 2 years, for a variety of reasons—negative reactions to being retired, feelings of being unproductive, economic hardship, and loneliness. The amount of time spent in retirement has increased as the life span has nearly doubled since 1900. Currently, the number of years spent in retirement is almost equal to the number of years spent working.

Sexual Activity

An estimated 70 percent of men and 20 percent of women over age 60 are sexually active; sexual activity is usually limited by the absence of an available partner. Longitudinal studies have found that the sex drive does not decrease as men and women age; in fact, some report an increased sex drive. William Masters and Virginia Johnson reported sexual functioning among those in their 80s. Expected physiological changes in men include a longer time for erection to occur, decreased penile turgidity, and ejaculatory seepage; in women, decreased vaginal lubrication and vaginal atrophy are associated with lowered estrogen levels. Medications can also adversely affect sexual behavior. A significant finding was that the more active a person's sex life was in early adulthood, the more likely it is to be active in old age.

Long-Term Care

Many older persons who are infirm require institutional care. Although only 5 percent are institutionalized in nursing homes at any one time, about 35 percent of older persons require care in a long-term facility at some time during their lives (Fig. 2.5–3). Older nursing home residents are mainly widowed women, and about 50 percent are over age 85.

Nursing home care costs are not covered by Medicare; they range from $20,000 to $50,000 a year. About 20,000 long-term nursing care institutions are available in the United States—not enough to meet the need. Those older persons who do not require skilled nursing care can be managed in other types of health-related facilities, such as centers they attend during the daytime hours, but the need for care far exceeds the availability of such centers.

Outside institutions, care for older persons is provided by their children (primarily their daughters and daughters-in-law),

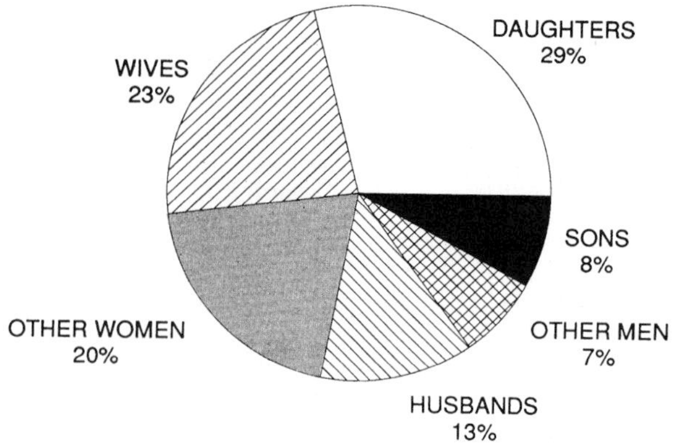

FIGURE 2.5–4
Caretakers and their relationship to the elderly care recipient. (Data from Select Committee on Aging, U.S. House of Representatives.)

their wives, and other women (Fig. 2.5–4). Over 50 percent of these women caregivers also work in jobs outside the home, and about 40 percent also care for their own children. In general, women end up as caregivers more often than men because of cultural and societal expectations. According to the American Association of Retired Persons, daughters with jobs spend an average of 12 hours a week providing care and currently spend about $150 a month for travel, telephone calls, special foods, and medication for older persons.

PSYCHIATRIC PROBLEMS OF OLDER PERSONS

Despite the ubiquity of loss in old age, the prevalence of major depressive disorder and dysthymia is actually less than in younger age groups. Several explanations for this phenomenon have been proposed: rarity of late-onset depression, higher mortality among persons with depression, and a general decrease in disorders caused by emotional upheavals or substance abuse in older persons. Depression in old persons is often accompanied by physical symptoms or cognitive changes that may mimic dementia.

The incidence of suicide among older persons is high (40 per 100,000 population) and is highest for older white men. The suicide of older persons is perceived differently by surviving friends and family members on the basis of gender: Men are thought to have been physically ill, and women are thought to have been mentally ill.

The relation between good mental and good physical health is clear in older persons. Adverse effects on the course of chronic medical illness are correlated with emotional problems. (An extensive discussion of psychiatric problems in older persons appears in Chapter 55.)

The reader is referred to Chapter 60 for an extensive discussion of health care delivery in psychiatry and medicine in which more socioeconomic and demographic data reflecting the entire life cycle can be found.

REFERENCES

Aging America: Trends and Projections. Washington, DC: US Government Printing Office; 1991.

Butler RN, Lewis MI. *Aging and Mental Health; Positive Psychosocial and Biomedical Approaches*. 3rd ed. St. Louis: CV Mosby; 1982.

Erikson EH, Erikson JM, Kivnick HG. *Vital Involvement in Old Age*. New York: WW Norton; 1986.

Ernst C, Angst J. Depression in old age. Is there a real decrease in prevalence? A review. *Eur Arch Psychiatry Clin Neurosci*. 1995;245:272.

Farquhar M. Elderly people's definitions of quality of life. *Soc Sci Med*. 1995;41:1439.

Garfein AJ, Herzog AR. Robust aging among the young-old, old-old, and oldest-old. *J Gerontol B Psychol Sci Soc Sci*. 1995;50:S77.

Gutmann D. *The Human Elder in Nature, Culture, and Society: Lives in Context*. Boulder, CO: Westview Press; 1997.

Jarvik LF. Geriatric psychiatry. In: Sadock BJ, Sadock VA, eds. *Kaplan & Sadock's Comprehensive Textbook of Psychiatry*. 7th ed. Vol 2. Baltimore: Lippincott Williams & Wilkins; 2000:2980.

Marris P. Holding onto meaning through the life cycle. In: Weiss RS, Bass SA, eds. *Challenges of the Third Age: Meaning and Purpose in Later Life*. London: Oxford University Press; 2002:13.

Pollock GH, Greenspan SI, eds. *The Course of Life*. Vol 7: *Completing the Journey*. Madison, CT: International Universities Press; 1998.

Pruchno R, Kleban MH. Caring for an institutionalized parent: the role of coping strategies. *Psychol Aging*. 1993;8:18.

Schiavi RC, Schreiner-Engel P, Mandeli J, Schanzer H, Cohen E. Healthy aging and male sexual function. *Am J Psychiatry*. 1990;147:766.

Stoller EP, Forster E, Portugal S. Self-care responses to symptoms by older people: a healthy diary study of illness behavior. *Med Care*. 1993;31:24.

West RL, Crook TH, Barron KL. Everyday memory performance across the life span: effects of age and noncognitive individual differences. *Psychol Aging*. 1992;7:72.

▲ 2.6 Death, Dying, and Bereavement

Death is a universal and unavoidable phenomenon. It arouses strong feelings of dread and fear in dying patients as well as in their families and health care providers. In clinical practice death is not the special province of any single discipline or the specialty of any one branch of medicine; rather, it is the universal reminder of life and its meanings. Physicians, mental health workers, and clergy are involved in terminal-care situations, and increasingly, persons die in hospital or hospice settings rather than at home. This brings the medical community to the forefront of decisions on when and how life should end. Similarly, the role of physicians in regard to their patients' suicidal impulses is becoming more complex. Rather than uniformly being on the side of preserving life and preventing suicide, physicians now are being urged in certain circumstances and in the name of compassion and dignity to help some patients carry out their suicidal wishes. This section covers *thanatology,* which is the study of the experience of death, dying, and bereavement. The reader will find an extensive discussion of related issues in Chapter 56 on end-of-life care and palliative medicine.

DEFINITIONS

The terms *death* and *dying* are not synonymous and have no unequivocal definitions. However, because medical, legal, and moral issues cluster around when and how death takes place, definitions are necessary. *Death* may be considered the absolute cessation of vital functions, while *dying* is the process of losing these functions. Dying may also be seen as a developmental concomitant of living, a part of the birth-to-death continuum. Living may entail numerous "minideaths": the end of growth and its potential; health-compromising illness; multiple losses;

decreasing vitality; growing dependency with aging; and finally, dying. Dying and persons' awareness of it imbues humans with values, passions, wishes, and the incentive to make the most of time.

Advances in technology have changed the focus of death definitions. Since the late 1960s the definition of death has shifted from a focus on respiratory and circulatory function to a focus on brain activity. Brain functioning and the resuscitation potential of mechanically maintained patients are a current focus. Heart transplant in the 1960s caused "brain death" to gain in prominence. Viable, intact donor organs are needed for transplants, but because organs lose viability with prolonged use of artificial respiration, physicians must be able to pinpoint when brain death occurs in potential donor patients.

Uniform Determination of Death Act

Responding to that need, the President's Commission for the Study of Ethical Problems in Medicine and Biomedical and Behavioral Research published its definition of death in 1981. The Uniform Determination of Death Act established that one who has sustained either (1) irretrievable cessation of circulatory and respiratory functions or (2) irretrievable cessation of all functions of the entire brain, including the brainstem, is dead. Determination of death must be in accordance with accepted medical standards. The guidelines recommended the use of a 24-hour observation period for patients, with confirmatory tests during that period (Table 2.6–1).

Table 2.6–1
Clinical Criteria for Brain Death in Adults and Children

Coma
Absence of motor responses
Absence of pupillary responses to light and pupils at midposition with respect to dilatation (4–6 mm)
Absence of corneal reflexes
Absence of caloric responses
Absence of gag reflex
Absence of coughing in response to tracheal suctioning
Absence of sucking and rooting reflexes
Absence of respiratory drive at a $PaCO_2$ that is 60 mm Hg or 20 mm Hg above normal base-line values[a]
Interval between two evaluations, according to patient's age
Term to 2 mo old, 48 hr
>2 mo to 1 yr old, 24 hr
>1 yr to <18 yr old, 12 hr
≥18 yr old, interval optional
Confirmatory tests
Term to 2 mo old, 2 confirmatory tests
>2 mo to 1 yr old, 1 confirmatory test
>1 yr to <18 yr old, optional
≥18 yr old, optional

[a]$PaCO_2$ denotes the partial pressure of arterial carbon dioxide.
From Wijdicks EFM. The diagnosis of brain death. *N Engl J Med.* 2001;344:1216.

REACTIONS TO DEATH

Persons react to death partly according to its context. For instance, persons may experience death as timely or untimely: timely when a person's expected survival and actual life span are approximately equal, and untimely when a person's death is unexpected or premature. Those left to grieve a timely death are usually not surprised or shocked by it, unlike those who grieve an untimely death, such as that of a young person, a person who dies suddenly, or a person whose catastrophic death is associated with violence, an accident, or utter meaninglessness.

Death can also be regarded as intentional (suicide), unintentional (trauma or disease), and subintentional (substance abuse, alcohol dependence, cigarette smoking). Death may have multiple psychological meanings, both for the person who is dying and for society in general. In Susan Sontag's formulation, death may even take on the power of metaphor. For example, some view death and certain terminal illnesses as deserved punishment for what are perceived as immoral or sinful lifestyles.

PSYCHOGENIC DEATH

Emotional factors alone may suffice to trigger sudden death in certain persons not otherwise at risk. For instance, ventricular fibrillation and myocardial infarction may follow sudden psychic stress. Voodoo death, or death secondary to a hex, occurs when a person believed to have the psychic power to cause death puts a curse on someone who believes in that person's power. In such cases, the hypothalamic-pituitary-adrenal axis and the autonomic nervous system probably become dysfunctional because of emotional stress, which causes the cessation of vital functions. Unless a healer removes the curse, a person under such a spell or hex may die.

Out-of-Body Experiences

Many persons believe in an afterlife, and afterlife phenomena have been reported throughout history. In recent years, large numbers of persons have claimed near-death or out-of-body experiences; as many as 40 percent of persons in the United States have described such events. The manner of the brush with death (illness, accident, or attempted suicide), the demographics (age, education, race, sex), and religious beliefs did not predispose one group over another to report such events.

Descriptions of near-death experience are often strikingly similar; they can involve an out-of-body experience of a person's viewing his or her own body and overhearing conversations; feelings of peace and quiet; hearing a distant noise; entering a dark tunnel; leaving the body behind; meeting dead loved ones; witnessing beings of light; returning to life to complete unfinished business; and a deep sadness if they recover and leave the new dimension. The experience is almost always described as peaceful and loving; it feels real to the participants, who distinguish it from dreams and hallucinations. Such experiences may provoke sweeping lifestyle changes. Because they have been widely reported in the popular press, patients may want to discuss such events with their physicians.

LEGAL ASPECTS OF DEATH

According to law, physicians must sign the death certificate, which attests to the cause of death (e.g., congestive heart fail-

ure or pneumonia). They must also attribute the death to natural, accidental, suicidal, homicidal, or unknown causes. A medical examiner, coroner, or pathologist must examine anyone who dies unattended by a physician and perform an autopsy to determine the cause of death. In some cases, a psychological autopsy is performed: A person's sociocultural and psychological background is examined retrospectively by interviewing friends, relatives, and doctors to determine whether a mental illness, such as a depressive disorder, was present. For example, a determination can be made that a person died because he or she was pushed (murder) or because he or she jumped (suicide) from a high building. Each situation has clear medical and legal implications.

IMPENDING DEATH

Elisabeth Kübler-Ross, a psychiatrist and thanatologist, made a comprehensive and useful organization of reactions to impending death. A dying patient seldom follows a regular series of responses that can be clearly identified; no established sequence is applicable to all patients. Nevertheless, the following five stages proposed by Kübler-Ross are widely encountered.

Stage 1—Shock and Denial

On being told that they are dying, persons initially react with shock. They may appear dazed at first and then may refuse to believe the diagnosis; they may deny that anything is wrong. Some persons never pass beyond this stage and may go from doctor to doctor until they find one who supports their position. The degree to which denial is adaptive or maladaptive appears to depend on whether a patient continues to obtain treatment even while denying the prognosis. In such cases, physicians must communicate to patients and their families, respectfully and directly, basic information about the illness, its prognosis, and the options for treatment. For effective communication, physicians must allow for patients' emotional responses and reassure them that they will not be abandoned.

Stage 2—Anger

Persons become frustrated, irritable, and angry at being ill. They commonly ask, "Why me?" They may become angry at God, their fate, a friend, or a family member; they may even blame themselves. They may displace their anger onto the hospital staff members and the doctor, whom they blame for the illness. Patients in the stage of anger are difficult to treat. Doctors who have difficulty understanding that anger is a predictable reaction and is really a displacement may withdraw from patients or transfer them to other doctors' care.

Physicians treating angry patients must realize that the anger being expressed cannot be taken personally. An empathic, nondefensive response can help defuse patients' anger and can help them refocus on their own deep feelings (e.g., grief, fear, loneliness) that underlie the anger. Physicians should also recognize that anger may represent patients' desire for control in a situation in which they feel completely out of control.

Stage 3—Bargaining

Patients may attempt to negotiate with physicians, friends, or even God; in return for a cure, they promise to fulfill one or many pledges, such as giving to charity and attending church regularly. Some patients believe that if they are good (compliant, nonquestioning, cheerful), the doctor will make them better. The treatment of such patients involves making it clear that they will be taken care of to the best of the doctor's abilities and that everything that can be done will be done, regardless of any action or behavior on the patients' part. Patients must also be encouraged to participate as partners in their treatment and to understand that being a good patient means being as honest and straightforward as possible.

Stage 4—Depression

In the fourth stage, patients show clinical signs of depression—withdrawal, psychomotor retardation, sleep disturbances, hopelessness, and, possibly, suicidal ideation. The depression may be a reaction to the effects of the illness on their lives (e.g., loss of a job, economic hardship, helplessness, hopelessness, and isolation from friends and family), or it may be in anticipation of the loss of life that will eventually occur. A major depressive disorder with vegetative signs and suicidal ideation may require treatment with antidepressant medication or electroconvulsive therapy (ECT). All persons feel some sadness at the prospect of their own death, and normal sadness does not require biological intervention. But major depressive disorder and active suicidal ideation can be alleviated and should not be accepted as normal reactions to impending death. A person who suffers from major depressive disorder may be unable to sustain hope, which can enhance the dignity and quality of life and even prolong longevity. Studies have shown that some terminally ill patients can delay their death until after a loved one's significant event (e.g., graduation of a grandson from college).

Stage 5—Acceptance

In the stage of acceptance, patients realize that death is inevitable, and they accept the universality of the experience. Their feelings may range from a neutral to a euphoric mood. Under ideal circumstances, patients resolve their feelings about the inevitability of death and can talk about facing the unknown. Those with strong religious beliefs and a conviction of life after death sometimes find comfort in the ecclesiastical maxim, "Fear not death; remember those who have gone before you and those who will come after."

ATTITUDES TOWARD DEATH ACROSS THE LIFE CYCLE

Children

The stages of children's emotional and cognitive development play a significant role in their perception, interpretation, and understanding of death. Children's ability to understand death reflects their ability to understand any abstract concept. Preschool children under the age of 5 years (Jean Piaget's preoperational phase) are animistic. They believe that everything, even

an inanimate object, is alive, and they are aware of death only in the sense that it is a separation similar to sleep. Between the ages of 5 and 10 years (concrete operations), children have a developing sense of inevitable human mortality; they fear that their parents will die and that they will be abandoned. About the age of 9 or 10, children conceptualize death as something that can happen to a child as well as to a parent. Usually by puberty, children conceptualize death as universal, irreversible, and inevitable, as do adults. Unlike parents in other parts of the world, middle-class parents in the United States tend to shield children from a knowledge of death. Rather than protecting children, the air of mystery surrounding death in such instances may create irrational fears in them.

Children with fatal illnesses create major emotional stresses for their caregivers, be they parents, relatives, hospital staff members, or physicians. A consistently present, trusted person is essential to provide optimal care for a dying child. The separation of a child from its mother is as traumatic an event for the hospitalized child as the illness itself, perhaps even more so. As John Bowlby pointed out, having the mother or an equally valued and familiar caregiver room with a hospitalized child can help alleviate the child's anxiety and can facilitate necessary medical care.

Adolescents

Capable of formal cognitive operations, adolescents understand that death is inevitable and final. Their major fears parallel those of all teenagers: loss of control, being imperfect, and being different. Concerns about body image, hair loss, or loss of bodily control may generate great resistance to continuing treatment. Alternating emotions of despair, rage, grief, bitterness, terror, and joy are common. An adolescent's cognitive capacity to understand death may not translate into an understanding that their own personal death is possible. The potential for withdrawal and isolation is great, because teenagers may deny their fear of abandonment by actually repulsing friendly gestures. Teenagers must be part of the decision-making process surrounding their death. Many are capable of great courage, grace, and dignity in facing death.

Adults

Unlike children and teenagers, older adults often readily accept that their time has come. Elderly patients may talk or joke openly about dying and sometimes welcome it. In their 70s or beyond, they no longer harbor illusions of indestructibility; most have already had several close calls, their parents have died, and they have gone to funerals for friends and relatives. Although they may not be happy to die, they can be reconciled to it.

According to Erik Erikson, the eighth and final stage in the life cycle brings either a sense of integrity or despair. As elderly adults enter the last phase of their lives, they reflect on their time and how it has been lived. When one has taken care of things and is relatively successful and adapted to the triumphs and disappointments of life, one can look back with satisfaction and only a few regrets; one experiences a sense of integrity about oneself, feeling that one has lived totally and well and that one's life has been meaningful. Integrity of the self allows an individual to accept inevitable disease and death without fear of succumbing helplessly. However, a person who looks back on life as a series of missed opportunities or as filled with personal misfortunes has a sense of bitter despair, a preoccupation with what might have been if only this or that had happened; then death is viewed with fear, because it symbolizes emptiness and failure.

BEREAVEMENT, GRIEF, AND MOURNING

Bereavement, grief, and *mourning* are terms that apply to the psychological reactions of those who survive a significant loss. *Grief* is the subjective feeling precipitated by the death of a loved one. The term is used synonymously with *mourning,* although, in the strictest sense, *mourning* is the process by which grief is resolved; it is the societal expression of postbereavement behavior and practices. *Bereavement* literally means the state of being deprived of someone by death and refers to being in the state of mourning. Regardless of the fine points that differentiate these terms, the experiences of grief and bereavement have enough similarities to warrant a syndrome that has signs, symptoms, a demonstrable course, and an expected resolution.

The expression of grief encompasses a wide range of emotions, depending on cultural norms and expectations (e.g., some cultures encourage or demand an intense display of emotions, whereas others expect just the opposite) and on the circumstances of the loss (e.g., a sudden unexpected death versus one that is clearly anticipated). Grief work is a complex psychological process of withdrawing attachment and working through the pain of bereavement. Figure 2.6–1 summarizes one concept of some recognizable and predictable manifestations of the phases of uncomplicated grief.

Normal Grief

Uncomplicated grief is a normal response, in view of the predictability of its symptoms and its course. Initial grief is often manifested as a state of shock that may be expressed as a feeling of numbness and a sense of bewilderment. This apparent inability to comprehend what has happened may be short-lived and is followed by such expressions of suffering and distress as sighing and crying, a feature of grief that is less common among men in Western cultures than among women. Feelings of weakness, decreased appetite, weight loss, and difficulty concentrating, breathing, and talking also appear. Sleep disturbances may include difficulty falling asleep, waking up during the night, and awakening early. Often, dreams of the deceased person occur, after which the dreamer awakens with a sense of disappointment in finding that the experience was only a dream.

Self-reproach is common, although it is less intense in normal, than in pathological, grief. Self-reproachful thoughts usually center on some relatively minor act of omission or commission toward the deceased. A phenomenon known as survivor guilt occurs in those who are relieved that someone other than them has died. Survivors sometimes believe that they should have been the person who died and may (if the guilt persists) have difficulty establishing new intimate relationships from fear of betraying the deceased person. Forms of denial occur throughout the period of bereavement; often, the bereaved person inadvertently denies the death or acts as if the loss had not occurred. Efforts to perpetuate the lost relationship

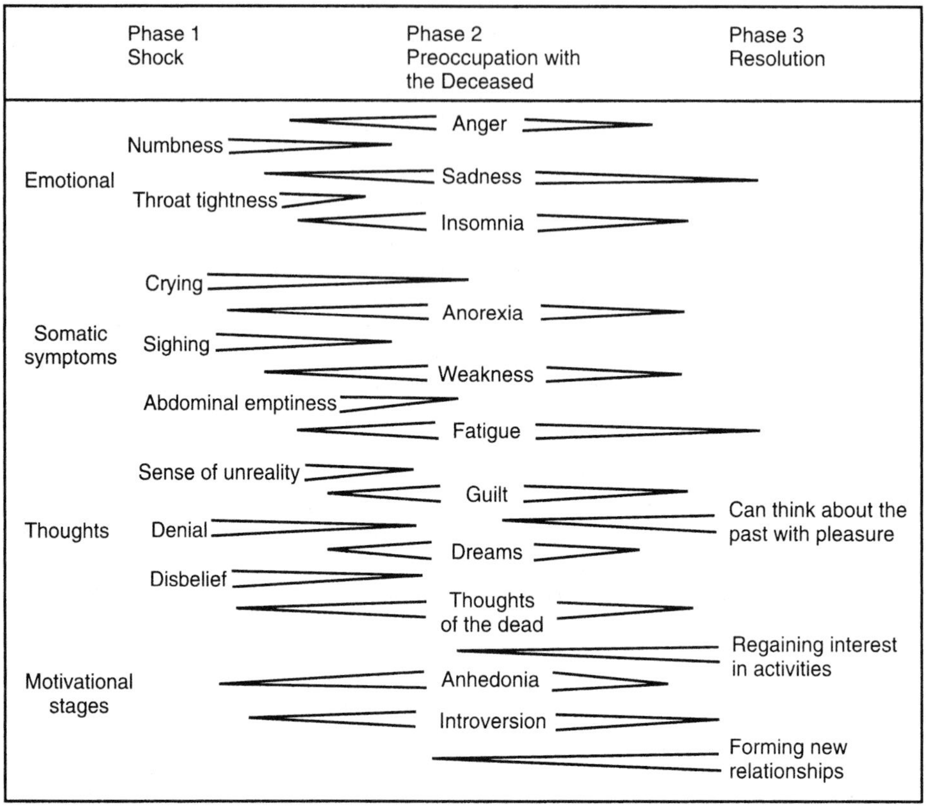

FIGURE 2.6–1
Phases of uncomplicated grief. (Reprinted with permission from Brown JT, Stoudemire A. Normal and pathological grief. *JAMA*. 1983;250:378.)

are evidenced by an investment in objects that were treasured by the deceased person or that remind the grief-stricken person of the one who has died (linkage objects).

A sense of the deceased person's presence may be so intense that it constitutes an illusion or a hallucination (e.g., hearing the deceased person's voice or feeling the person's presence). In normal grief, however, the survivor realizes that the perception is not real. As part of what has been labeled *identification phenomena,* a survivor may take on the qualities, mannerisms, or characteristics of the deceased person to perpetuate the person in some concrete way. This maneuver can reach potentially pathological expression with the development of physical symptoms similar to those experienced by the person who died or suggesting the illness from which the deceased person died.

Bowlby hypothesized four stages of bereavement. Stage 1 is an early phase of acute despair characterized by numbness and protest. Denial may be immediate, and outbursts of anger and distress are common. The stage may last moments to days and may be periodically revisited by the grieving person throughout the mourning process. Stage 2, a phase of intense yearning and searching for the person who has died, is characterized by physical restlessness and an all-consuming preoccupation with the deceased. The phase may last several months or even years in an attenuated form. In stage 3, which has been described as a phase of disorganization and despair, the reality of the loss begins to sink in. A sense of going through the motions of living is dominant, and the grieving person appears withdrawn, apathetic, and listless. Insomnia and weight loss often occur, as does a feeling that life has lost its meaning. The grieving person constantly relives memories of the deceased; an associated inevitable feeling of disappointment occurs when the bereaved person recognizes that the memories are just memories. Stage 4 is a phase of reorganization during which the acutely painful aspects of grief begin to recede and the grieving person begins to feel like returning to life. The deceased person is now remembered with a sense of joy as well as sadness, and the image of the lost person becomes internalized.

Grief Period

Because persons vary greatly in their expressions of grief, the signs, symptoms, and phases of mourning and bereavement are not as discrete as their characterizations might imply. Nevertheless, the manifestations of grief usually tend to subside over time. The length and intensity of grief, especially the acute phases, can be shaped by the suddenness of the death. If death occurs without warning, shock and disbelief may last for a long time; when death has been long anticipated, much of the mourning process may have already occurred by the time death intervenes. Traditionally, grief lasts about 6 months to 1 year, as the grieving person experiences the calendar year at least once without the lost person. Some signs and symptoms of grief may persist much longer than 1 or 2 years, and a survivor may have various grief-related feelings, symptoms, and behavior throughout life. Even-

tually, however, normal grief resolves, and persons return to a state of productivity and relative well-being. In general, the acute grief symptoms gradually lessen, and within 1 or 2 months the grieving person is able to eat, sleep, and return to functioning.

Anticipatory Grief

Anticipatory grief is expressed in advance of a loss perceived as inevitable, as distinguished from grief that occurs at or after the loss. By definition, anticipatory grief ends with the occurrence of the anticipated loss, regardless of what reactions follow. Unlike conventional grief, which diminishes in intensity with the passage of time, anticipatory grief may either increase or decrease in intensity as the expected loss becomes imminent. In some instances, particularly when the occurrence of the loss is delayed, anticipatory grief may be expended, and the bereaved person shows few manifestations of acute grief when the loss occurs. Once anticipatory grief has been expended, the bereaved person may find it difficult to reestablish a previous relationship; this phenomenon is experienced with the return of persons long gone (e.g., to war or confined to concentration camps) and of those thought to have been dead.

Anniversary Reactions. When the trigger for an acute grief reaction is a special occasion such as a holiday or birthday, the rekindled grief is called an *anniversary reaction.* It is not unusual for anniversary reactions to occur each year on the day the person died, or in some cases, when the bereaved individual becomes the same age the deceased was at the time of death. Although these anniversary reactions tend to become relatively mild and brief over time, they can be experienced as the reliving of one's original grief and may prevail for hours or days.

Complicated, Pathological, or Abnormal Grief

Some persons experience an abnormal course of grief and mourning. Pathological grief can take several forms, ranging from absent or delayed grief to excessively intense and prolonged grief to grief associated with suicidal ideation or frank psychotic symptoms. Persons at greatest risk for an abnormal grief reaction are those who suffer a loss suddenly or through horrific circumstances, those who are socially isolated, those who believe they are responsible (whether the responsibility is real or imagined) for the death, those with a history of traumatic losses, and those with an intensely ambivalent or dependent relationship to the person who died.

Some relationships between persons, regardless of their public appearances, are sufficiently negative that reduced or absent grief is a normal and appropriate reflection of their animosities. In these cases, the consequences of the death of the person, even if it is a spouse or a parent, may be decidedly positive for the survivor.

Other forms of abnormal grief occur when some aspects of normal grieving are distorted or intensified to psychotic proportions. Identifying with the deceased person, such as taking on certain admired traits or treasuring certain possessions, is normal; believing that one is the deceased person or is dying of exactly what the deceased person died of (if, in fact, this is untrue) is not normal. Hearing the fleeting, transient voice of a deceased person may be normal; persistent, intrusive, complex auditory hallucinations are not normal. Denial of certain aspects of the death is normal; denial that includes the belief that the dead person is still alive is not normal.

Grief versus Depression

Grief and depression share many features: sadness, tearfulness, loss of appetite, poor sleep, and diminished interest in the world. There are, however, enough differences that psychiatrists regard them as separate syndromes (Table 2.6–2).

The mood disturbance in depression is typically pervasive and unremitting; any mood fluctuations are relatively minor. Fluctuations in grief are common. Persons often describe grief coming in waves, washing over them, and then subsiding. Even in intense grief, moments of lightheartedness and happy reminiscence are possible. Shame and guilt are common in depression. When they occur in grief, they usually involve not having done enough for the deceased before his or her death; in depression they commonly arise from a fundamental belief that one is wicked or worthless. The realization that grief is time limited is very important. Many persons suffering from major depression lack hope; they cannot imagine ever feeling better. Persons who have experienced previous depression are at risk for becoming depressed at times of major loss, and a bereaved person's clinical history may be helpful in judging a current reaction. Depressed persons threaten suicide more often than grieving persons, who, except in unusual instances—for example, physically dependent and older persons—do not seriously wish to die, even if they claim that life is unbearable.

Physicians must determine when grief has become pathological and has evolved into major depressive disorder. Grief is

Table 2.6–2
Differentiating the Depressive Symptoms Associated with Bereavement from Major Depressive Disorder

Bereavement	Major Depressive Disorder
Symptoms may meet syndromal criteria for major depressive episode, but survivor rarely has morbid feelings of guilt and worthlessness, suicidal ideation, or psychomotor retardation	Any symptoms as defined by DSM-IV-TR
Dysphoria often triggered by thoughts or reminders of the deceased	Dysphoria often autonomous and independent of thoughts or reminders of the deceased
Onset within the first 2 months of bereavement	Onset at any time
Duration of depressive symptoms is less than 2 months	Depression often becomes chronic, intermittent, or episodic
Functional impairment is transient and mild	Clinically significant distress or impairment
No family or past personal history of major depressive disorder	Family or past personal history of major depressive disorder

Courtesy of Sidney Zisook, M.D., and Nancy S. Downs, M.D.

a normal, albeit intensely painful state that responds to support, empathy, and the passage of time. Major depressive disorder is potentially a medical emergency that requires immediate intervention to forestall a complication such as suicide.

The Grieving Child

Bowlby also studied the bereavement process in children, a process similar to that in adults, especially once a child can understand the irrevocability of death. The mourning process resembles the separation process in having three phases: protest, despair, and detachment. In the protest phase, a child has a strong desire for the mother or other caregiver who died and cries for her return; in the despair phase, a child begins to lose hope about the mother's return, crying is intermittent, and withdrawal and apathy set in. In the detachment phase, a child begins to relinquish some emotional attachment to the dead parent and exhibit a reawakened interest in the surroundings.

In dealing with a bereaved child, the clinician should recognize the child's need to find a person to substitute for the lost parent. Children may transfer their need for a parent to several adults rather than to one. If there is no consistently available person, severe psychological damage may result, so that the child no longer looks for, or expects, intimacy in any relationship. The importance of managing grief reactions in children is highlighted by the increased evidence that depressive disorders and suicide attempts occur more frequently in adults who experienced the death of a parent in early childhood.

The question of whether children should attend funerals is a common one, and no hard and fast rule exists. Most child experts agree that if a child expresses a desire to go, the wish should be respected; if a child is reluctant or refuses to go, this wish should also be respected. In most circumstances it is probably best to encourage a child to attend so that the ritual is not enveloped in a frightening and distorted fantasy or mystery.

Parental Grief

Parents react to a child's death or to the birth of a malformed infant in stages similar to those that Kübler-Ross described in terminal illness: shock, denial, anger, bargaining, depression, and acceptance. The death of a child is often a more intense emotional experience than the death of an adult. Parental feelings of guilt and helplessness may be overwhelming; parents may believe that somehow they did not protect their children and have unnaturally outlived them. Lost hopes, wishes, and fulfillments associated with a new generation cause additional pain. Manifestations of the grief may well last a lifetime.

A sudden death is often more traumatic than a prolonged death, because anticipatory grief can occur when death is expected. A parent may become overprotective of a dying child or shower the child with gifts that were previously denied. The stress of dealing with a child's death may cause a marriage that has had conflicts to disintegrate. One parent may blame the other for the child's fatal illness, especially if the child's disease had a hereditary basis. Physicians should be alert to these patterns of dissension. Some studies indicate that up to 50 percent of marriages in which a child dies or is born malformed end in divorce.

Psychodynamics

In 1917, Sigmund Freud wrote in *Mourning and Melancholia* that normal grief (mourning) results from the withdrawal of the libido from its attachment to the lost object. In normal mourning, the loss is clearly and unambivalently perceived, and the person who died is eventually, through the grief work, internalized as a loving and loved object. In abnormal grief (melancholia), the lost object is not given up but is incorporated in the survivor's psyche as an object infused with negative feelings. These negative feelings toward the deceased person are experienced as part of the self, and the survivor becomes depressed, has low self-esteem, feels worthless, and becomes self-accusatory, with possible delusional expectations of punishment. Freud's distinction between mourning and melancholia is still considered valid—that is, an exaggerated loss of self-esteem is not part of normal grieving.

Other psychoanalytic theorists have stressed the role of unconscious dynamics in grief reactions. The greater the role of unconscious and ambivalent factors (e.g., anger toward a person who died), the greater the likelihood of an abnormal grief reaction. Karl Abraham described the introjection of an ambivalently loved lost object and the subsequent direction of anger toward the introjected object.

Biology of Grief

Grief is both a physiological and an emotional response. During acute grief (as with other stressful events), persons may suffer disruption of biological rhythms. Grief is also accompanied by impaired immune functioning: decreased lymphocyte proliferation and impaired functioning of natural killer cells. Whether the immune changes are clinically significant has not been established, but the mortality rate for widows and widowers following the death of a spouse is higher than that in the general population. Widowers appear to be at risk longer than widows.

Phenomenology of Grief. Bereavement reactions involve alternations in feelings states, coping strategies, interpersonal relationships, biopsychosocial functioning, self-esteem, and world views that may last indefinitely. Manifestations of grief reflect the individual's personality, previous life experiences, past psychological history, the significance of the loss, the bereaved's relationship with the deceased, the existing social network, intercurrent life events, health, and other resources. Despite individual variations in the bereavement process, investigators have proposed grieving process models, which include at least three partially overlapping phases or states: (1) initial shock, disbelief, and denial; (2) an intermediate period of acute discomfort and social withdrawal; and (3) a culminating period of restitution and reorganization. Like Kübler-Ross's stages of dying, the stages of grief do not prescribe a correct course of grief; rather, they are general guidelines that describe an overlapping and fluid process that varies with the survivors (Table 2.6–3).

Grief Therapy

Persons in normal grief seldom seek psychiatric help because they accept their reactions and behavior as appropriate. Accord-

Table 2.6–3
Phases of Grief

Shock and denial (minutes, days, weeks)
Disbelief and numbness
Searching behaviors: pining, yearning, protest
Acute anguish (weeks, months)
Waves of somatic distress
Withdrawal
Preoccupation
Anger
Guilt
Lost patterns of conduct
Restless and agitated
Aimless and amotivational
Identification with the bereaved
Resolution (months, years)
Have grieved
Return to work
Resume old roles
Acquire new roles
Reexperience pleasure
Seek companionship and love of others

Courtesy of Sidney Zisook, M.D., and Nancy S. Downs, M.D.

ingly, an attending physician should not routinely recommend that a bereaved person see a psychiatrist or psychologist unless a markedly divergent reaction to the loss is noted. For example, under usual circumstances a bereaved person does not make a suicide attempt; if someone seriously contemplates suicide, psychiatric intervention is indicated.

When professional assistance is sought, it usually involves a request for sleeping medication from a family physician. A mild sedative to induce sleep may be useful in some situations, but antidepressant medication or antianxiety agents are rarely indicated in normal grief. Bereaved persons may have to go through the mourning process, however painful it is, for successful resolution to occur. Narcotizing patients with drugs interferes with the normal process that ultimately can lead to a favorable outcome.

Because grief reactions may develop into a depressive disorder or pathological mourning, specific counseling sessions for those bereaved are often valuable. Grief therapy is an increasingly important skill. In regularly scheduled sessions, grieving persons are encouraged to talk about feelings of loss and about the person who has died. Many bereaved persons have difficulty recognizing and expressing angry or ambivalent feelings toward a deceased person, and they must be reassured that these feelings are normal.

Grief therapy need not be conducted only on a one-to-one basis; group counseling is also effective. Self-help groups also have great value in certain cases. About 30 percent of widows and widowers report that they become isolated from friends, withdraw from social life, and thus experience feelings of isolation and loneliness. Self-help groups offer companionship, social contacts, and emotional support; they eventually enable their members to reenter society in a meaningful way. Bereavement care and grief therapy have been most effective with widows and widowers. The necessity for this therapy stems, in part, from the contraction of the family unit; extended family members were once able to provide the needed emotional support and guidance during the mourning period. In the World Trade Center disaster in 2001, such support groups were of great help in enabling New York City uniformed firefighters and police who lost over 500 of their colleagues to deal with the grieving process.

References

Aarli J. The immune system and the nervous system. *J Neurol.* 1983;229:137.

Baker JE, Sedney MA, Gross E. Psychological tasks for bereaved children. *Am J Orthopsychiatry.* 1992;62:105.

Conwell Y, Caine ED. Rational suicide and the right to die: reality and myth. *N Engl J Med.* 1991;325:1100.

Hendin H, Klerman G. Physician-assisted suicide: the dangers of legalization. *Am J Psychiatry.* 1993;150:143.

Hinohara S. Sir William Osler's philosophy on death. *Ann Intern Med.* 1993;118:639.

Horowitz MJ. Depression after the death of a spouse. *Am J Psychiatry.* 1992;149:579.

Jeret JS. Discussing dying: changing attitudes among patients, physicians, and medical students. *Pharos.* 1989;52:15.

Kübler-Ross E. *On Death and Dying.* New York: Macmillan; 1969.

Leming MR, Dickinson GE. *Understanding Dying, Death and Bereavement.* New York: Holt, Rinehart & Winston; 1985.

Lo B, Ruston D, Kates LW, Arnold RM. Discussing religious and spiritual issues at the end of life. *JAMA.* 2002;287:749.

Ness DE, Pfeffer CR. Sequelae of bereavement resulting from suicide. *Am J Psychiatry.* 1990;147:279.

Nuss WS, Zubenko GS. Correlates of persistent depressive symptoms in widows. *Am J Psychiatry.* 1992;149:346.

Parkes CM, Weiss RS. *Recovery from Bereavement.* New York: Basic Books; 1983.

Reisman AS. Death of a spouse: illusory basic assumptions and continuation of bonds. *Death Stud.* 2001;25:445.

Roberts G, Owen J. The near-death experience. *Br J Psychiatry.* 1988;153:607.

Schleifer SJ, Keller SE, Camerino M, et al. Suppression of lymphocyte stimulation following bereavement. *JAMA.* 1983;250:374.

Schulz J, Beach A, Lind B. Involvement in caregiving and adjustment to death of a spouse: findings from the Caregiver Health Effects Study. *JAMA.* 2001;285:3123.

Speece MW, Brent SB. The acquisition of a mature understanding of three components of the concept of death. *Death Stud.* 1992;16:211.

Tedeschi RG, Calhoun LG. Using the support group to respond to the isolation of bereavement. *J Ment Health Counsel.* 1993;15:47.

Weiss L, Frischer L, Richman J. Parental adjustment to intrapartum and delivery room loss: the role of hospital-based support program. *Clin Perinatol.* 1989;16:1009.

Wijdicks EFM. The diagnosis of brain death. *N Engl J Med.* 2001;344:1216.

3 The Brain and Behavior

▲ 3.1 Functional and Behavioral Neuroanatomy

FUNCTIONAL UNITS OF THE BRAIN

The *nervous system* may be considered as a set of functional units classified as sensory, motor, and association. By processing external stimuli into neuronal impulses, *sensory systems* create an internal representation of the external world. A separate map is formed for each sensory modality. *Motor systems* enable persons to manipulate their environment and to influence others' behavior through communication. In the brain, sensory input, representing the external world, is integrated with internal drivers and emotional stimuli in *association units,* which in turn drive the actions of motor units. Although psychiatry is primarily concerned with the brain's association function, an appreciation of the sensory and motor systems' information processing is essential for sorting logical thought from the distortions introduced by psychopathology.

SENSORY SYSTEMS

The external world offers an infinite amount of potentially relevant information. In this overwhelming volume of sensory information in the environment, the sensory systems must both detect and discriminate stimuli; they winnow relevant information from the mass of confounding input by applying filtration at all levels. Sensory systems first transform external stimuli into neural impulses and then filter out irrelevant information to create an internal image of the environment, which serves as a basis for reasoned thought. Feature extraction is the quintessential role of sensory systems. They achieve this goal with their hierarchical organizations, which first transform physical stimuli into neural activity in the primary sense organs and then refine and narrow the neural activity in a series of higher cortical processing areas. This neural processing eliminates irrelevant data from higher representations and reinforces crucial features. At the highest levels of sensory processing, neural images are transmitted to the association areas to be acted on in the light of emotions and drives.

The Five Primary Senses

Somatosensory System. The *somatosensory system,* an intricate array of parallel point-to-point connections from the body surface to the brain, was the first sensory system to be understood in anatomical detail. There are six somatosensory modalities: light touch, pressure, pain, temperature, vibration, and proprioception (position sense). The organization of nerve bundles and synaptic connections in the somatosensory system encodes spatial relationships at all levels, so that the organization is strictly *somatotopic* (Fig. 3.1–1). Within a given patch of skin, various receptor nerve terminals act in concert to mediate distinct modalities. The mechanical properties of the skin's mechanoreceptors and thermoreceptors generate neural impulses in response to dynamic variations in the environment while they suppress static input. Nerve endings are either fast or slow responders; their depth in the skin also determines their sensitivity to sharp or blunt stimuli. Thus, the representation of the external world is significantly refined at the level of the primary sensory organs.

The receptor organs generate coded neural impulses that travel proximally along the sensory nerve axons to the spinal cord. These far-flung routes are susceptible to varying systemic medical conditions and to pressure palsies. Pain, tingling, and numbness are the typical presenting symptoms of peripheral neuropathies.

After sensory fibers enter the spinal cord, they are sorted into one of three fiber tracts. Some fibers travel locally and synapse within one or two spinal segments; these local projections participate in further filtering of the sensory input by suppressing unwanted "noise" to allow sharper delineation of the signal. Second, fibers for conscious perception of touch, pain, and temperature decussate, or cross the midline, at the level of entry into the spinal cord and ascend to the brain in the spinothalamic tract. The perception of pain is divided into the lateral spinothalamic tract, which registers localized, discrete, acute pains, and the medial spinothalamic tract, which, along with the spinoreticulothalamic pathway, registers diffuse, chronic pains. Surgical interruption of these pathways may ablate pain perception but may also produce a central pain syndrome. Third, fibers for conscious perception of touch, vibration sense, and proprioception ascend, without immediate decussation, in the posterior columns. The somatotopic organization of the sensory projections is rigorously maintained in the spinal cord; input from the upper body is layered onto fibers from the legs and is segregated by modality. Facial sensation is mediated by the trigeminal nerve, whose fibers lie atop those of the arms and legs.

All somatosensory fibers project to, and synapse in, the thalamus. The thalamic neurons preserve the somatotopic representation by projecting fibers to the somatosensory cortex, located immediately posterior to the sylvian fissure in the parietal lobe (Fig. 3.1–2, Brodmann areas 1, 2, and 3). Despite considerable overlap, several bands of cortex roughly parallel to the sylvian fissure are segregated by somatosensory

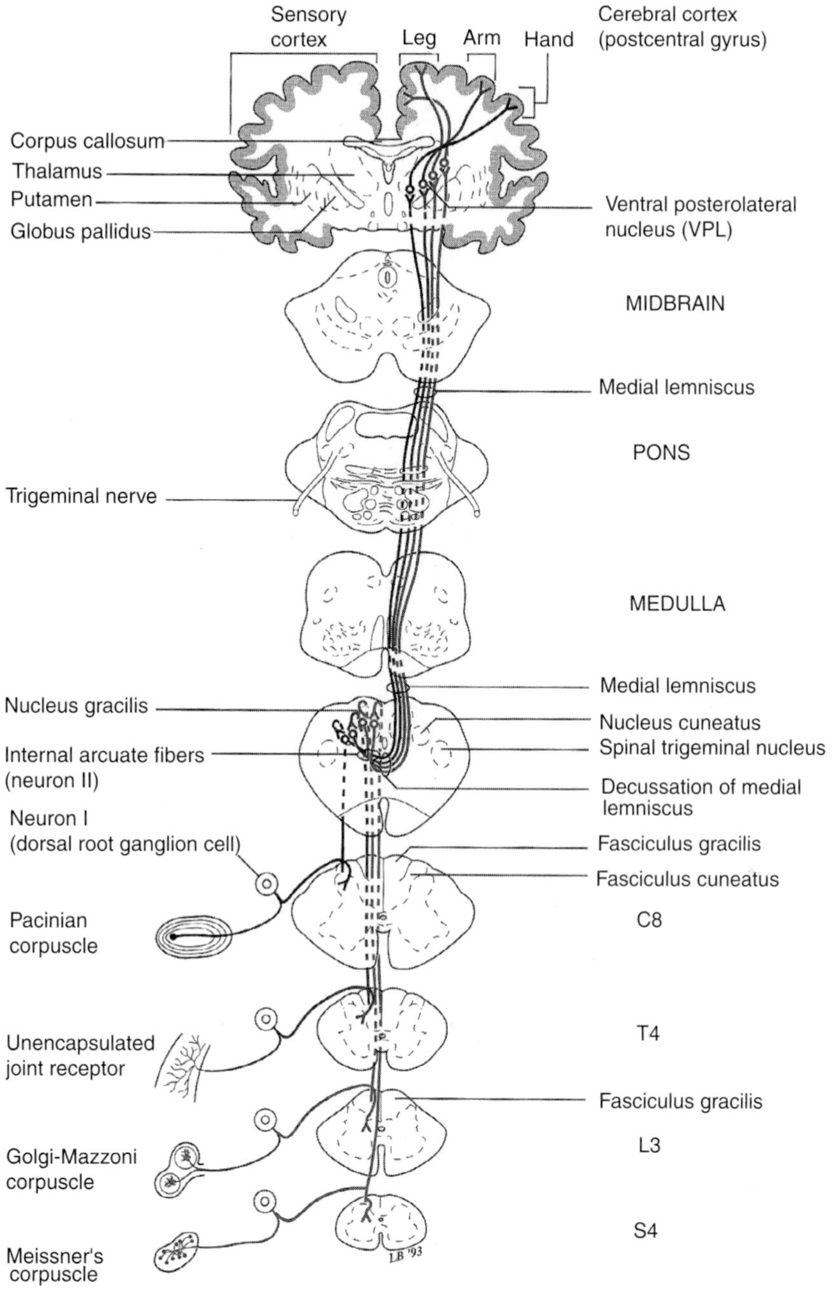

FIGURE 3.1–1
Somatotopic organization of the somatosensory system. Each somatosensory modality is carefully segregated from the other modalities, and the fibers of different spinal levels are segregated as they ascend to the somatosensory cortex. (From Parent A. *Carpenter's Human Neuroanatomy.* 9th ed. Baltimore: Williams & Wilkins; 1996:369, with permission.)

modality. Within each band is the sensory "homunculus" (Fig. 3.1–3), the culmination of the careful somatotopic segregation of the sensory fibers at the lower levels. The clinical syndrome of *tactile agnosia* (*astereognosis*) is defined by the inability to recognize objects based on touch, although the primary somatosensory modalities—light touch, pressure, pain, temperature, vibration, and proprioception—are intact. This syndrome, localized at the border of the somatosensory and association areas in the posterior parietal lobe, appears to represent an isolated failure of only the highest order of feature extraction, with preservation of the more basic levels of the somatosensory pathway.

Reciprocal connections are a key anatomical feature of crucial importance to conscious perception; as many fibers project down from the cortex to the thalamus as project up from the thalamus to the cortex. These reciprocal fibers play a critical role in filtering sensory input. In normal states, they facilitate the sharpening of internal representations, but in pathological states, they may generate false signals or inappropriately suppress sensation. Such cortical interference with sensory perception is thought to underlie many psychosomatic syndromes, such as the hemisensory loss that characterizes conversion disorder.

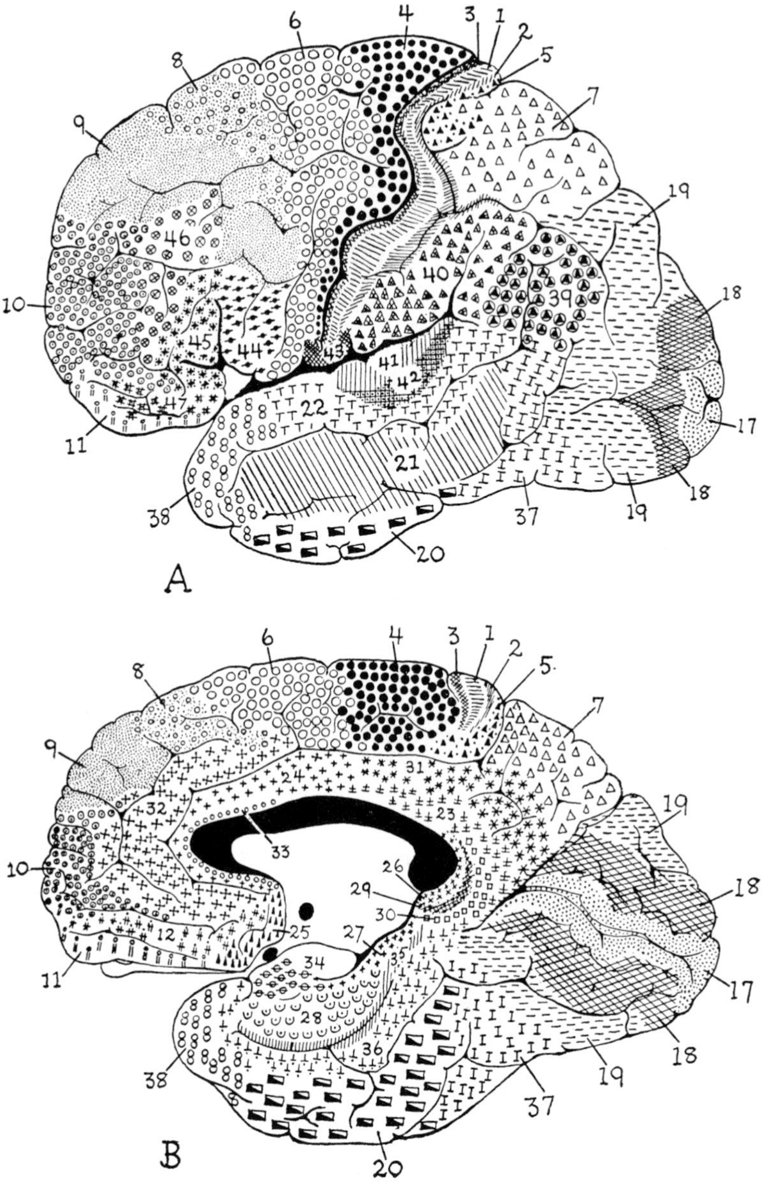

FIGURE 3.1–2

Cytoarchitectonic regions of the brain according to Brodmann. **A.** Lateral surface. **B.** Medial surface. (From Carpenter MB. *Core Text of Neuroanatomy.* 4th ed. Baltimore: Williams & Wilkins; 1991:399, with permission.)

The prenatal development of the strict point-to-point pattern that characterizes the somatosensory system remains an area of active study. Patterns of sensory innervation result from a combination of axonal guidance by particular molecular cues and pruning of exuberant synaptogenesis on the basis of an organism's experience. Leading hypotheses weigh contributions from a genetically determined molecular map, in which the arrangement of fiber projections is organized by fixed and diffusible chemical cues, against contributions from the modeling and remodeling of projections on the basis of coordinated neural activity. Thumbnail calculations suggest that the 30,000 to 40,000 genes in human DNA are far too few to encode completely the position of all the trillions of synapses in the brain. In fact, genetically determined positional cues probably steer growing fibers toward the general target, and the pattern of projections is fine-tuned by activity-dependent mechanisms. Recent data suggest that well-established adult thalamocortical sensory projections can be gradually remodeled as a result of a reorientation of coordinated sensory input or in response to loss of part of the somatosensory cortex, for instance, in stroke.

Visual System. Visual images are transduced into neural activity within the retina and are processed through a series of brain cells, which respond to increasingly complex features, from the eye to the higher visual cortex. The neurobiological basis of feature extraction is best understood in finest detail in the visual system. Beginning with classical work in the 1960s, research in the visual pathway has produced two main para-

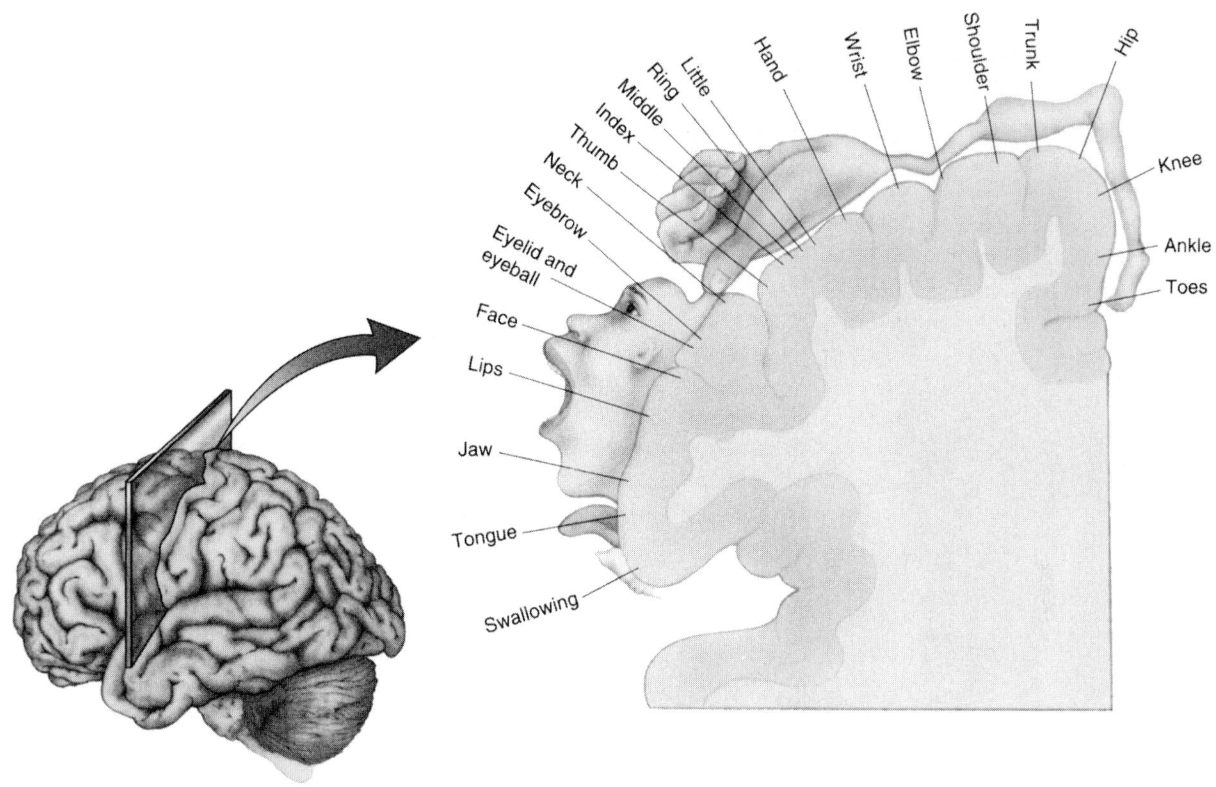

FIGURE 3.1–3
Somatotopic map of the human precentral gyrus. (From Bear MF, Connors BW, Paradiso MA. *Neuroscience: Exploring the Brain*. Baltimore: Williams & Wilkins; 1996:383, with permission.)

digms for all sensory systems. The first paradigm, mentioned above with respect to the somatosensory system, weighs the contributions of genetics and experience—or nature and nurture—to the formation of the final synaptic arrangement. Transplantation experiments, resulting in an accurate point-to-point pattern of connectivity even when the eye was surgically inverted, suggested an innate, genetically determined mechanism of synaptic pattern formation. The crucial role of early visual experience in establishing the adult pattern of visual connections, on the other hand, crystallized the hypothesis of activity-dependent formation of synaptic connectivity. The final adult pattern is the result of both factors.

The second main paradigm, most clearly revealed in the visual system, is that of highly specialized brain cells that respond exclusively to extremely specific stimuli. Recent work, for example, has defined cells in the inferior temporal cortex that respond only to faces viewed at a specific angle. Extrapolating this specialization to an extreme, researchers have postulated a "grandmother cell," a cell that would fire only when a subject was regarding his or her own grandmother. Such a cell, representing a fixed site for important memories, has not yet been identified, perhaps simply because scientists have not yet found it or, more significantly, perhaps because evoking the memory of a person's response to the presence of his or her grandmother requires the activity of large neural networks and may not be limited to a single neuron. Nevertheless, the cellular localization of specific feature extraction is of critical importance in defining the boundary between sensory and association systems, but only in the visual system has this significant question been posed experimentally.

In the visual pathway, light passes through the eye and stimulates the photoreceptor cells. In response to light, the receptor molecules change conformation and trigger an intracellular cascade that generates neural impulses. Feature extraction begins in the retina, where stimulating a point immediately suppresses the response of the circle of neighboring cells, termed a *center-surround response*. This response sharpens edges in the image. The retina consists of rods, which respond only to the intensity of light, and three types of cones, each of which is tuned to respond most strongly to one of the three primary colors. Perception of color ultimately emerges in the cortex, from comparisons of the ratio of intensities of signals from each of the three classes of cones. An exact point-to-point visuotopic projection, from the halves of each retina that respond to the same half of the visual field, travels to the lateral geniculate nucleus (LGN), where additional center-surround sharpening occurs. The optic tracts project from the LGN to the primary visual cortex at the posterior pole of the occipital lobe. In the visual cortex of each hemisphere, the input from each eye is segregated into ocular dominance columns: Radial columns of cortex that are activated by input from only one eye are adjacent to columns that respond only to the other eye (Fig. 3.1–4). This segregation may underlie the stereoscopic localization of objects in space.

In the primary visual cortex, columns of cells respond specifically to lines of a specific orientation. The cells of the primary visual cortex project to the secondary visual cortex, where cells respond specifically to particular movements of lines and to angles. In turn, these cells project to

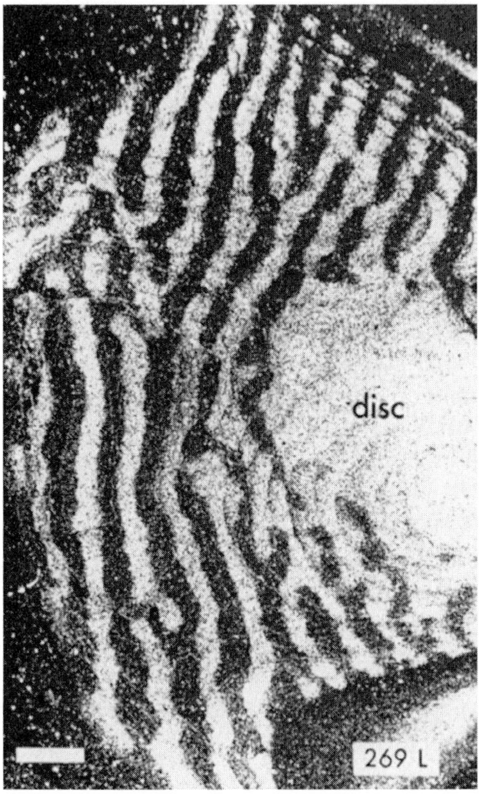

FIGURE 3.1–4

Ocular dominance columns. Projection of the retina onto the visual cortex in the occipital lobe. Axons from the left eye are labeled black; axons from the right eye are unlabeled. In the cortex, the retinal projections form a neatly ordered alternating pattern called the ocular dominance columns. These columns form as a result of postnatal visual activity and are thus determined through a combination of genetics and experience. (From Carpenter MB. *Core Text of Neuroanatomy.* 4th ed. Baltimore: Williams & Wilkins; 1991:412, with permission.)

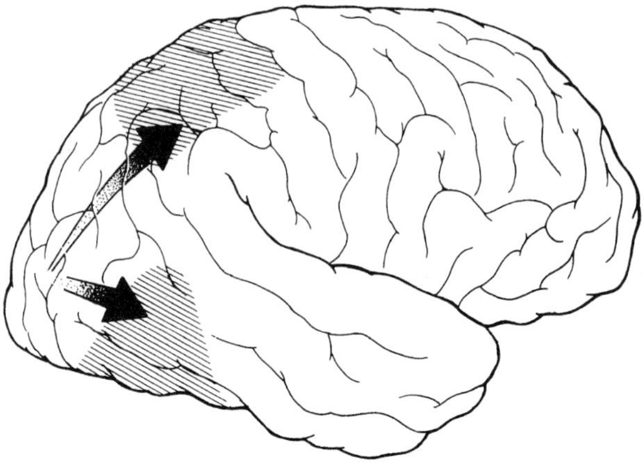

FIGURE 3.1–5

Visual association areas. At the far left pole of the cortex, impulses from the primary visual cortex spread both to the parietal lobe (*upper shaded area*), which tracks *where* the image is in space, and to the temporal lobe (*lower shaded area*), which determines *what* the image is. (From Filley CM. *Neurobehavioral Anatomy.* Niwot, CO: University Press of Colorado; 1995, with permission.)

two association areas, where additional features are extracted and conscious awareness of images forms (Fig. 3.1–5). The inferior temporal lobe detects the shape, form, and color of the object—the *what* questions; the posterior parietal lobe tracks the location, motion, and distance—the *where* questions. The posterior parietal lobe contains distinct sets of neurons that signal the intention either to look into a certain part of visual space or to reach for a particular object. In the inferior temporal cortices (ITCs), adjacent cortical columns respond to complex forms. Responses to facial features tend to occur in the left ITC, and responses to complex shapes tend to occur in the right ITC. The brain devotes specific cells to the recognition of facial expressions and to the aspect and position of faces of others with respect to the individual. Other body parts have a less complete representation among feature-specific cells, and inanimate objects occupy another set of cellular addresses.

The crucial connections between the feature-specific cells and the association areas involved in memory and conscious thought remain to be delineated. Much elucidation of feature recognition is based on invasive animal studies. In humans, the clinical syndrome of *prosopagnosia* describes the inability to recognize faces, in the presence of preserved recognition of other environmental objects. On the basis of pathological and radiological examination of individual patients, prosopagnosia is thought to result from disconnection of the left ITC from the visual association area in the left parietal lobe. Such lesional studies are useful in identifying necessary components of a mental pathway, but they may be inadequate to define the entire pathway. One noninvasive technique that is still being perfected and is beginning to reveal the full anatomical relation of the human visual system to conscious thought and memory is functional neuroimaging (Chapter 3, Section 3.3).

As is true for language, there appears to be a hemispheric asymmetry for certain components of visuospatial orientation. Although both hemispheres cooperate in perceiving and drawing complex images, the right hemisphere, especially the parietal lobe, contributes the overall contour, perspective, and right-left orientation, and the left hemisphere adds internal detail, embellishment, and complexity. The brain can be fooled in optical illusions (Fig. 3.1–6).

Neurological conditions such as strokes and other focal lesions have permitted the definition of several disorders of visual perception. *Apperceptive visual agnosia* is the inability to identify and draw items using visual cues, with preservation of other sensory modalities. It represents a failure of transmission of information from the higher visual sensory pathway to the association areas and is due to bilateral lesions in the visual association areas. *Associative visual agnosia* is the inability to name or use objects despite the ability to draw them. It is caused by bilateral medial occipitotemporal lesions and may occur along with other visual impairments. Color perception may be ablated in lesions of the dominant occipital lobe that include the splenium of the corpus callosum. *Color agnosia* is the inability to recognize a color despite being able to match it. *Color anomia* is the inability to name a color despite being able to point to it. *Central achromatopsia* is a complete inability to perceive color. *Anton's syndrome* is a failure to acknowledge blindness, possibly owing to interruption of fibers involved in self-assessment. It is seen with bilateral occipital lobe lesions. The most common causes are hypoxic injury, stroke, metabolic encephalopathy, migraine, herniation resulting from mass lesions, trauma, and leukodystrophy. *Balint's syndrome* consists of a triad of optic ataxia (the

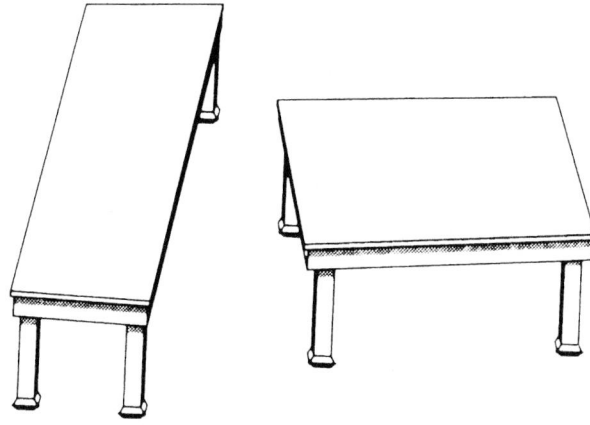

FIGURE 3.1–6

Optical illusion: perspective. Two tables are drawn in a perspective view. The left table appears to be long and narrow, while the right table appears to be short and wide. In fact, both tabletops are drawn exactly the same size on the page (the reader can measure them). Closest attention is paid to those feature recognition modules that identify items that can be used best. Unlike the brain's very familiar ideal of a table top, the two-dimensional shapes depicted by the actual printed lines on the paper are so unfamiliar that we find it almost impossible to see them as abstract drawings. This is because the ability to draw a perspectival image such as this one is evolutionarily extremely recent—at most a few thousand years—whereas the ability to recognize a "raised, flat surface on which to prepare food" is probably 100 million years old or older. (Modified from Gazzaniga MS. *The Mind's Past.* Berkeley: University of California Press; 1988:88, with permission.)

inability to direct optically guided movements), *oculomotor apraxia* (inability to direct gaze rapidly), and *simultanagnosia* (inability to integrate a visual scene to perceive it as a whole). Balint's syndrome is seen in bilateral parieto-occipital lesions. *Gerstmann syndrome* includes agraphia, calculation difficulties (acalculia), right-left disorientation, and finger agnosia. It has been attributed to lesions of the dominant parietal lobe.

Auditory System. Sounds are instantaneous, incremental changes in ambient air pressure. The pressure changes cause the ear's tympanic membrane to vibrate; the vibration is then transmitted to the ossicles (malleus, incus, and stapes) and thereby to the endolymph or fluid of the cochlear spiral. Vibrations of the endolymph move cilia on hair cells, which generate neural impulses. The hair cells respond to sounds of different frequency in a tonotopic manner within the cochlea, like a long, spiral piano keyboard. Neural impulses from the hair cells travel in a tonotopic arrangement to the brain in the fibers of the cochlear nerve. They enter the brainstem cochlear nuclei, are relayed through the lateral lemniscus to the inferior colliculi, and then to the medial geniculate nucleus (MGN) of the thalamus. MGN neurons project to the primary auditory cortex in the posterior temporal lobe. Dichotic listening tests, in which different stimuli are presented to each ear simultaneously, demonstrate that most of the input from one ear activates the contralateral auditory cortex and that the left hemisphere tends to be dominant for auditory processing.

In the auditory system, the temporal and tonotopic pattern of cortical projections to the primary auditory cortex encodes pitch and begins to localize sounds in space. Sound localization relative to the ears is achieved by subtle comparisons of sound intensity and phase between the two ears. This function occurs in a brain region that is spatially distinct from the primary auditory cortex and that has cells that respond specifically to movements of the sound source relative to the listener. There is evidence that this task is mediated by the right hemisphere. The helices of the pinna facilitate localization by producing characteristic echoes, depending on the angle at which the sound hits the ear.

Sonic features are extracted through a combination of mechanical and neural filters. The representation of sound is roughly tonotopic in the primary auditory cortex, whereas *lexical processing* (i.e., the extraction of vowels, consonants, and words from the auditory input) occurs in higher language association areas, especially in the left temporal lobe. The syndrome of *word deafness,* characterized by intact hearing for voices but an inability to recognize speech, may reflect damage to the left parietal cortex. This syndrome is thought to result from disconnection of the auditory cortex from Wernicke's area. A rare, complementary syndrome, *auditory sound agnosia,* is defined as the inability to recognize nonverbal sounds, such as a horn or a cat's meow, in the presence of intact hearing and speech recognition. Researchers consider this syndrome the right hemisphere correlate of pure word deafness. The evolution of vocalization innervation is shown in Figure 3.1–7.

Olfaction. Odorants, or volatile chemical cues, enter the nose, are solubilized in the nasal mucus, and bind to odorant receptors displayed on the surface of the sensory neurons of the olfactory epithelium. Each neuron in the epithelium displays a unique odorant receptor, and cells displaying a given receptor are randomly arranged within the olfactory epithelium. Humans possess several hundred distinct receptor molecules that bind the huge variety of environmental odorants; workers estimate that humans can discriminate 10,000 different odors. Odorant binding generates neural impulses, which travel along the axons of the sensory nerves through the cribriform plate to the olfactory bulb. Within the bulb, all axons corresponding to a given receptor converge onto only 1 or 2 of 3,000 processing units called *glomeruli.* Because each odorant activates several receptors that activate a characteristic pattern of glomeruli, the identity of external chemical molecules is represented internally by a spatial pattern of neural activity in the olfactory bulb.

Each glomerulus projects to a unique set of 20 to 50 separate columns in the olfactory cortex. In turn, each olfactory cortical column receives projections from a unique combination of glomeruli. The connectivity of the olfactory system is genetically determined. Because each odorant activates a unique set of several receptors and thus a unique set of olfactory bulb glomeruli, each olfactory cortical column is tuned to detect a different odorant of some evolutionary significance to the species. Unlike the signals of the somatosensory, visual, and auditory systems, olfactory signals do not pass through the thalamus but project directly to the frontal lobe and the limbic system, especially the pyriform cortex. The connections to the limbic system (amygdala, hippocampus, pyriform cortex) are significant. Olfactory cues stimulate strong emotional responses and may evoke powerful memories.

Olfaction, the most ancient sense in evolutionary terms, is tightly associated with sexual and reproductive responses. A related chemosensory structure, the vomeronasal organ, is thought to detect *pheromones,* chemical cues that trigger unconscious, stereotyped responses. In some animals, ablation of the vomeronasal organ in early

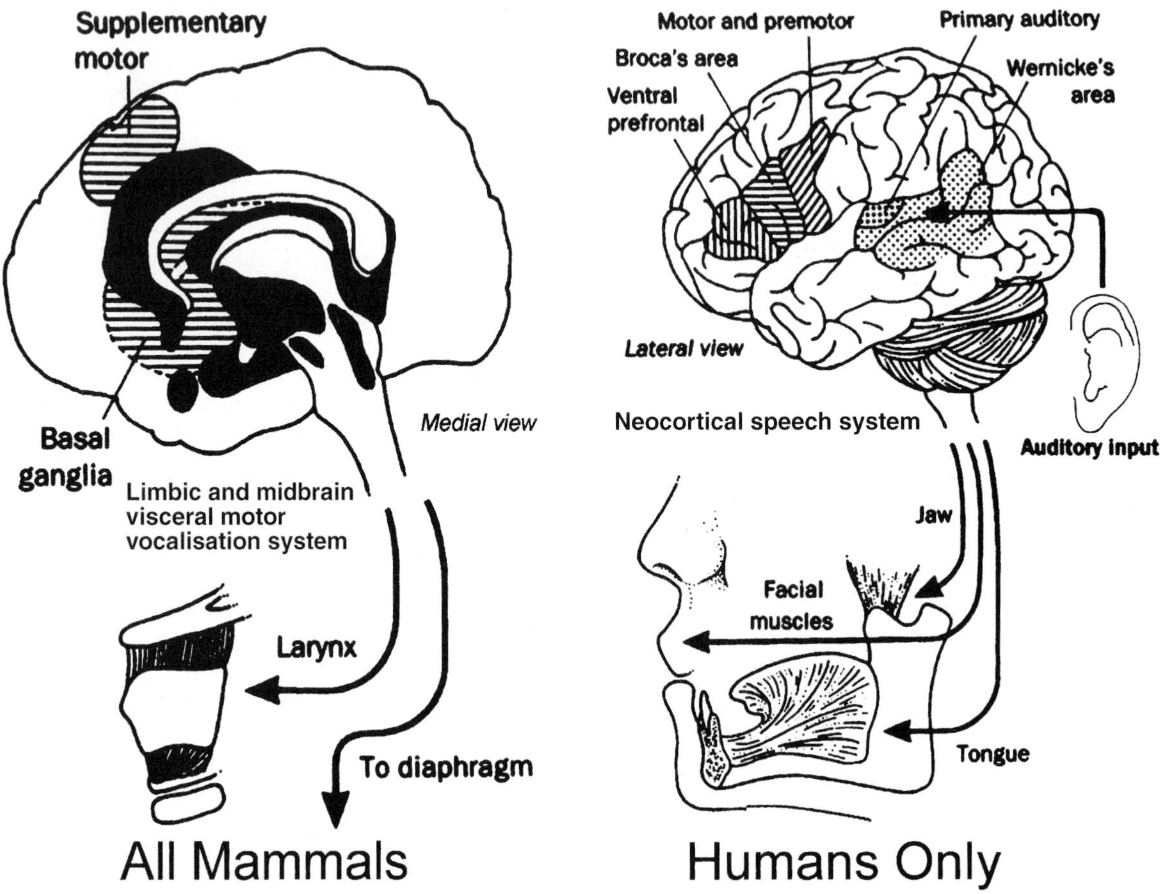

FIGURE 3.1–7

Evolution of vocalization innervation. Descending neural pathways controlling vocalization in all mammals (*left*) and those specific to human speech (*right*). The general mammalian pathways originate from subcortical limbic structures that are the source of emotional experience and expression. The subcortical call system produces automatic movements of the visceral muscles of the larynx and diaphragm. It is probably involved in human "innate calls," such as laughter and sobbing, and it may play a part in human speech intonation, tone, and rhythm. The human-specific pathways originate from neocortical areas controlling skilled behavior. The neocortical speech system produces skilled movements of the face and mouth muscles necessary for articulation of words. Although shown separately, the subcortical and neocortical vocal control pathways work together in humans and converge on the same output nuclei for the larynx, tongue, and facial muscles. In humans, the subcortical call system can interfere with speech at times of intense emotion. (Modified from Jones S, Martin R, Pilbeam D. *The Cambridge Encyclopedia of Human Evolution*. Cambridge, UK: Cambridge University Press; 1992:132, with permission.)

life may prevent the onset of puberty. Recent studies have suggested that humans also respond to pheromones in a manner that varies according to the menstrual cycle. The structures of higher olfactory processing in phylogenetically more primitive animals have evolved in humans into the limbic system, the center of the emotional brain and the gate through which experience is admitted into memory according to emotional significance. The elusive basic animal drives with which clinical psychiatry constantly grapples may therefore, in fact, originate from the ancient centers of higher olfactory processing.

Taste. Soluble chemical cues in the mouth bind to receptors in the tongue and stimulate the gustatory nerves, which project to the nucleus solitarius in the brainstem. The sense of taste is believed to discriminate only broad classes of stimuli: sweet, sour, bitter, and salty. Each modality is mediated through a unique set of cellular receptors and channels, of which several may be expressed in each taste neuron. The detection and the discrimination of foods, for example, involve a combination of the senses of taste, olfaction, touch, vision, and hearing. Taste fibers activate the medial temporal lobe, but the higher cortical localization of taste is only poorly understood.

Autonomic Sensory System (ANS)

The autonomic nervous system monitors the basic functions necessary for life. The activity of visceral organs, blood pressure, cardiac output, blood glucose levels, and body temperature are all transmitted to the brain by autonomic fibers. Most autonomic sensory information remains unconscious; if such information rises to conscious levels, it is only as a vague sensation, in contrast to the capacity of the primary senses to transmit sensations rapidly and exactly.

Development of Sensory Networks

Somatosensory System. A strict somatotopic representation exists at each level of the somatosensory system. During

development, neurons extend axons to connect to distant brain regions; after arriving at the destination, a set of axons must therefore sort itself to preserve the somatotopic organization. A classical experimental paradigm for this developmental process is the representation of a mouse's whiskers in the somatosensory cortex. The murine somatosensory cortex contains a barrel field of cortical columns, each of which corresponds to one whisker. When mice are inbred to produce fewer whiskers, fewer somatosensory cortex barrels appear. Each barrel is expanded in area, and the entire barrel field covers the same area of the somatosensory cortex as it does in normal animals. This experiment demonstrates that certain higher cortical structures may form in response to peripheral input and that different input complexities determine different patterns of synaptic connectivity. Although the mechanisms by which peripheral input molds cortical architecture are largely unknown, animal model paradigms are beginning to yield clues. For example, in a mutant mouse that lacks monoamine oxidase A and thus has extremely high cortical levels of serotonin, barrels fail to form in the somatosensory cortex. This result indirectly implicates serotonin in the mechanism of barrel field development.

In adults, the classic mapping studies of Wilder Penfield suggested the existence of a homunculus, an immutable cortical representation of the body surface. More recent experimental evidence from primate studies and from stroke patients, however, has promoted a more plastic conception than Penfield's. Minor variations exist in the cortical pattern of normal individuals, yet dramatic shifts in the map can occur in response to loss of cortex from stroke or injury. When a stroke ablates a significant fraction of the somatosensory homunculus, the homuncular representation begins to contract and shift proportionately to fill the remaining intact cortex.

Moreover, the cortical map can be rearranged solely in response to a change in the pattern of tactile stimulation of the fingers. The somatotopic representation of the proximal and distal segments of each finger normally forms a contiguous map, presumably because both segments contact surfaces simultaneously. But under experimental conditions in which the distal segments of all fingers are simultaneously stimulated while contact of the distal and proximal parts of each finger is separated, the cortical map gradually shifts 90 degrees to reflect the new sensory experience. In the revised map, the cortical representation of the proximal segment of each finger is no longer contiguous with that of the distal segment.

These data support the notion that the internal representation of the external world, while static in gross structure, may be continuously modified at the level of synaptic connectivity to reflect relevant sensory experiences. The cortical representation also tends to shift to fit entirely into the available amount of cortex.

These results also support the notion that cortical representations of sensory input or of memories may be holographic rather than spatially fixed: The pattern of activity, rather than the physical structure, may encode information. In sensory systems, this plasticity of cortical representation allows recovery from brain lesions; the phenomenon may also underlie learning. Figure 3.1–8 depicts localized functional areas of the brain.

Visual System. In humans, the initial projections from both eyes intermingle in the cortex. During the development of visual connections in the early postnatal period, there is a window of time during which binocular visual input is required for development of ocular dominance columns in the primary visual cortex. *Ocular dominance columns* are stripes of cortex that receive input from only one eye, separated by stripes innervated only by fibers from the other eye (Fig. 3.1–4). Occlusion of one eye during this critical period completely eliminates the persistence of its fibers in the cortex and allows the fibers of the active eye to innervate the entire visual cortex. In contrast, when normal binocular vision is allowed during the critical development window, the usual dominance columns form; occluding one eye after the completion of innervation of the cortex produces no subsequent alteration of the ocular dominance columns. This paradigm crystallizes the importance of early childhood experience on the formation of adult brain circuitry.

An interesting experimental twist occurs in frogs; namely, each visual cortex is normally innervated by only one eye. If a third eye is grafted onto the brain before development of the visual connections and if its fibers arrive at the cortex coincidentally with those of the native eyes, a pattern of ocular dominance columns forms where none is normally seen. This finding suggests that the neural mechanism by which competing inputs are organized and compartmentalized in the cortex is a property with high evolutionary conservation.

Auditory System. Certain children are unable to process auditory input clearly and therefore have impaired speech and comprehension of spoken language. Studies on some of these children have determined that they can in fact discriminate speech if the consonants and vowels—the phonemes—are slowed two- to fivefold by a computer. Based on this observation, a tutorial computer program was designed that initially asked questions in a slowed voice and, as subjects answered questions correctly, gradually increased the rate of phoneme presentation to approximate normal rates of speech. Subjects gained some ability to discriminate routine speech over a period of 2 to 6 weeks and appeared to retain these skills after the tutoring period was completed. This finding probably has therapeutic applicability to 5 to 8 percent of children with speech delay, but ongoing studies may expand the eligible group of students. This finding, moreover, suggests that neuronal circuits required for auditory processing can be recruited and be made more efficient long after language is normally learned, provided that the circuits are allowed to finish their task properly, even if this requires slowing the rate of input. Circuits thus functioning with high fidelity can then be trained to speed their processing.

A recent report has extended the age at which language acquisition may be acquired for the first time.

A boy who suffered from intractable epilepsy of one hemisphere was mute because the uncontrolled seizure activity precluded the development of organized language functions. At the age of 9 years he had the abnormal hemisphere removed to cure the epilepsy. Although he had not spoken to that point of his life, he initiated an accelerated acquisition of language milestones beginning at that age and ultimately gained language abilities only a few years delayed relative to his chronological age.

Researchers cannot place an absolute upper limit on the age at which language abilities may be learned, although acquisition at ages beyond the usual childhood period is usually incomplete. Anecdotal reports document acquisition of reading skills after the age of 80 years.

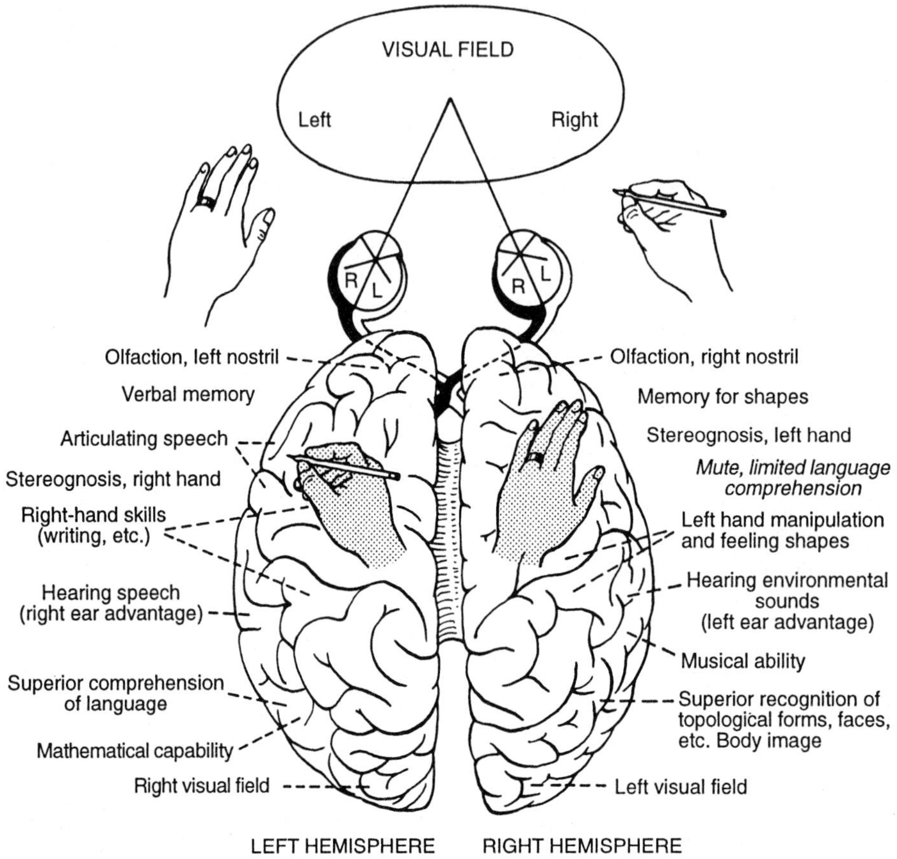

FIGURE 3.1–8

Drawing of the dorsal surface of the human brain showing the tendency for certain functions to be preferentially localized to one hemisphere. However, the intact brain may not be as lateralized as some studies (e.g., of patients with commissurotomies) suggest, the degree of lateralization differs across individuals, and in the intact brain it is rare that one hemisphere can mediate a function that the other hemisphere is completely unable to perform. (From Fuchs AF, Phillips JO. Association cortex. In: Patton HD, et al. *Textbook of Physiology.* 21st ed. Vol 1. Philadelphia: WB Saunders; 1989.)

Olfaction. During normal development, axons from the nasal olfactory epithelium project to the olfactory bulb and segregate into about 3,000 equivalent glomeruli. If in the early postnatal period an animal is exposed to a single dominant scent, then one glomerulus expands massively within the bulb at the expense of the surrounding glomeruli. Thus, as discussed above with reference to the barrel fields of the somatosensory cortex, the size of brain structures may reflect the environmental input.

Alteration of Conscious Sensory Perception through Hypnosis

Hypnosis is a state of heightened suggestibility attainable by a certain proportion of the population. Under a state of hypnosis, gross distortions of perception in any sensory modality can be achieved instantaneously. The anatomy of the sensory system does not change, yet the same specific stimuli may be perceived with diametrically opposed emotional value before and after induction of the hypnotic state. For example, under hypnosis a person may savor an onion as if it were a luscious chocolate truffle, only to reject the onion as abhorrently pungent seconds later, when the hypnotic suggestion is reversed. The localization of the hypnotic switch has not been determined, but it presumably involves both sensory and association areas of the brain. Experiments tracing neural pathways in human volunteers via functional neuroimaging have demonstrated that shifts in attention in an environmental setting determine changes in the regions of the brain that are activated, on an instantaneous time scale. Thus the organizing centers of the brain may route conscious and unconscious thoughts through different sequences of neural processing centers, depending on a person's ultimate goals and emotional state. These attention-mediated variations in synaptic utilization can occur instantaneously, much like the alteration in the routing of associational processing that may occur in hypnotic states.

MOTOR SYSTEMS

Layers of Evolutionary Sophistication

The movements of the body muscles are controlled by the lower motor neurons, which extend axons—some as long as 1 meter—to the muscle fibers. The firing of the lower motor neurons is regulated by the summation of upper motor neuron activity. In the brainstem, primitive systems produce gross coordinated movements of the entire body. Activation of the rubrospinal tract stimulates flexion of all limbs, whereas activation of the vestibu-

lospinal tract causes all limbs to extend. Newborn infants, for example, have all limbs tightly flexed, presumably through the dominance of the rubrospinal system. In fact, the movements of an anencephalic infant, who completely lacks a cerebral cortex, may be indistinguishable from the movements of a normal newborn. In the first few months of life, the flexor spasticity is gradually mitigated by the opposite actions of the vestibulospinal fibers, and more limb mobility occurs.

At the top of the motor hierarchy is the corticospinal tract, which controls fine movements and which eventually dominates the brainstem system during the first years of life. The upper motor neurons of the corticospinal tract reside in the posterior frontal lobe, in a section of cortex known as the *motor strip* (Fig. 3.1–2, Brodmann area 4). Planned movements are conceived in the association areas of the brain, and in consultation with the basal ganglia and cerebellum, the motor cortex directs their smooth execution. The importance of the corticospinal system becomes immediately evident in strokes, in which spasticity returns as the cortical influence is ablated and the actions of the brainstem motor systems are released from cortical modulation.

Basal Ganglia

The *basal ganglia,* a subcortical group of gray matter nuclei, appear to mediate postural tone. There are four functionally distinct ganglia: the striatum, the pallidum, the substantia nigra, and the subthalamic nucleus. Collectively known as the corpus striatum, the caudate and putamen harbor components of both motor and association systems. The caudate nucleus plays an important role in the modulation of motor acts. Anatomical and functional neuroimaging studies have correlated decreased activation of the caudate with obsessive-compulsive behavior. When functioning properly, the caudate nucleus acts as a gatekeeper to allow the motor system to perform only those acts that are goal directed. When it fails to perform its gatekeeper function, extraneous acts are performed as in obsessive-compulsive disorder or in the tic disorders, such as Tourette's disorder. Overactivity of the striatum owing to lack of dopaminergic inhibition (e.g., in parkinsonian conditions) results in *bradykinesia,* an inability to initiate movements. The caudate, in particular, shrinks dramatically in Huntington's disease. This disorder is characterized by rigidity, on which is gradually superimposed choreiform, or "dancing," movements. Psychosis may be a prominent feature of Huntington's disease, and suicide is not uncommon. The caudate is also thought to influence associative, or cognitive, processes. Figure 3.1–9 is a schematic drawing of the basal ganglia.

The globus pallidus contains two parts linked in series. In a cross section of the brain, the internal and external parts of the globus pallidus are nested within the concavity of the putamen. The globus pallidus receives input from the corpus striatum and projects fibers to the thalamus. This structure may be severely damaged in Wilson's disease and in carbon monoxide poisoning, which are characterized by dystonic posturing and flapping movements of the arms and legs.

The substantia nigra is named the black substance because the presence of melanin pigment causes it to appear black to the naked eye. It has two parts, one of which is functionally equivalent to the globus pallidus interna. The other part degenerates in Parkinson's disease. Parkinsonism is characterized by rigidity and tremor and is associated with depression in over 30 percent of cases.

Finally, lesions in the subthalamic nucleus yield ballistic movements, sudden limb jerks of such velocity that they are compared to projectile movement.

Together, the nuclei of the basal ganglia appear capable of initiating and maintaining the full range of useful movements. Workers have speculated that the nuclei serve to configure the activity of the overlying motor cortex to fit the purpose of the association areas. In addition, they appear to integrate proprioceptive feedback to maintain an intended movement.

Cerebellum

The cerebellum consists of a simple six-cell pattern of circuitry that is replicated roughly 10 million times. Simultaneous recordings of the cerebral cortex and the cerebellum have shown that the cerebellum is activated several milliseconds before a planned movement. Moreover, ablation of the cerebellum renders intentional movements coarse and tremulous. These data suggest that the cerebellum carefully modulates the tone of agonistic and antagonistic muscles by predicting the relative contraction needed for smooth motion. This prepared motor plan is used to ensure that exactly the right amount of flexor and extensor stimuli is sent to the muscles. Recent functional imaging data have shown that the cerebellum is active even during the mere imagination of motor acts, when no movements ultimately result from its calculations. The cerebellum harbors two, and possibly more, distinct "homunculi" or cortical representations of the body plan. Figure 3.1–10 depicts the cerebellar nuclei.

Motor Cortex

Penfield's groundbreaking work defined a motor homunculus in the precentral gyrus, Brodmann area 4 (Fig. 3.1–2), where a somatotopic map of the motor neurons is found. Individual cells within the motor strip cause contraction of single muscles. The brain region immediately anterior to the motor strip is called the *supplementary motor area,* Brodmann area 6. This region contains cells that when individually stimulated can trigger more complex movements, by influencing a firing sequence of motor strip cells. Recent studies have demonstrated wide representation of motor movements in the brain (see Color Plate 3.1–11 on p. 115).

The skillful use of the hands is called *praxis,* and deficits in skilled movements are termed *apraxias.* The three levels of apraxia are limb-kinetic, ideomotor, and ideational. *Limb-kinetic apraxia* is the inability to use the contralateral hand in the presence of preserved strength; it results from isolated lesions in the supplementary motor area, which contains neurons that stimulate functional sequences of neurons in the motor strip.

Ideomotor apraxia is the inability to perform an isolated motor act upon command, despite preserved comprehension, strength, and spontaneous performance of the same act. Ideomotor apraxia simultaneously affects both limbs and involves functions so specialized that they are localized to only one hemisphere. Conditions in two separate areas can produce this apraxia. Disconnection of the language comprehension area, Wernicke's area, from the motor regions causes an inability to

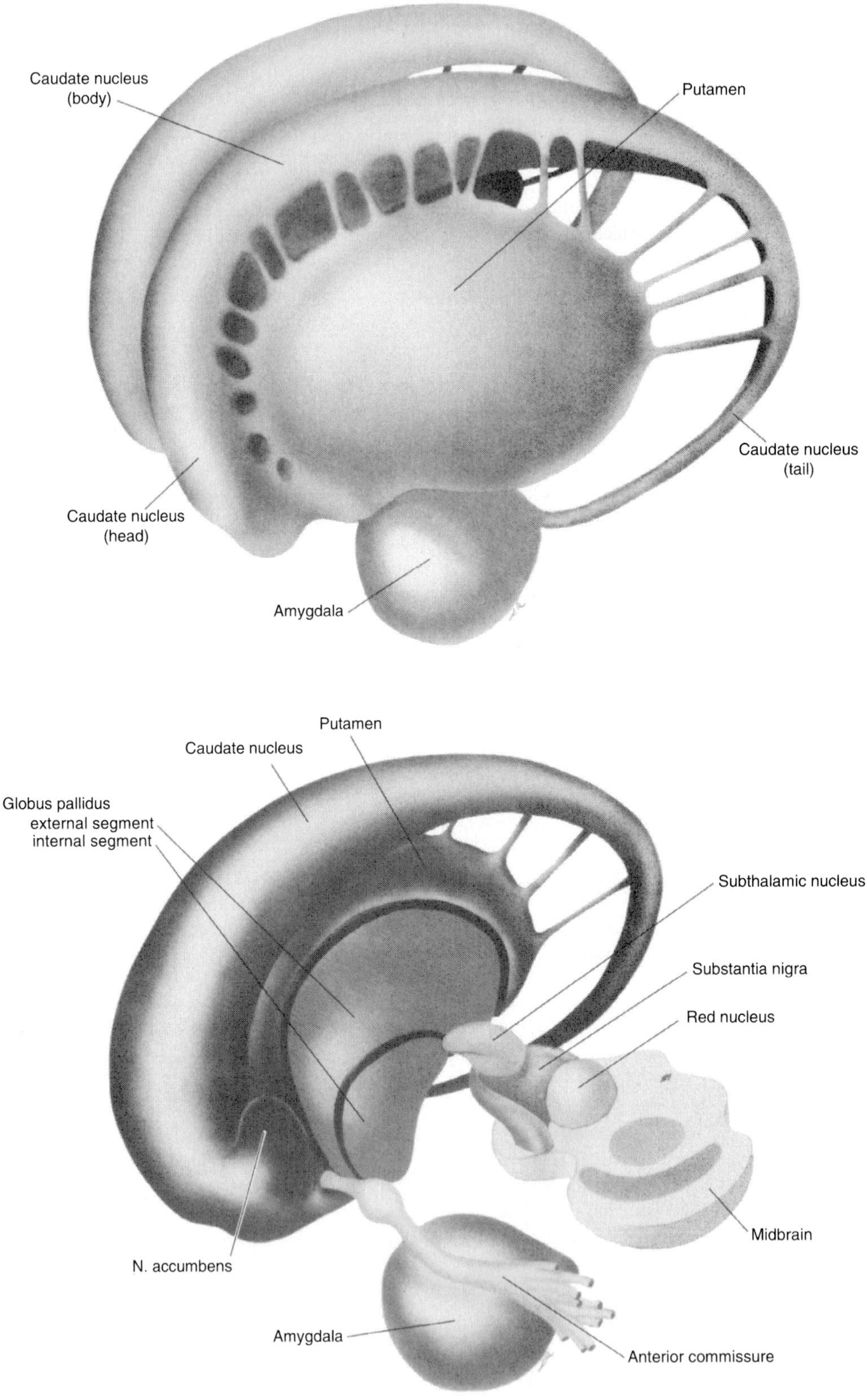

FIGURE 3.1–9

Schematic drawing of the isolated basal ganglia as seen from the dorsolateral perspective, so that the caudate nucleus is apparent bilaterally. In the *bottom panel*, the basal ganglia from the left hemisphere has been removed, exposing the medial surface of the right putamen and globus pallidus, as well as the subthalamic nucleus and substantia nigra. (Adapted from Hendelman WJ. *Student's Atlas of Neuroanatomy*. Philadelphia: WB Saunders; 1994.)

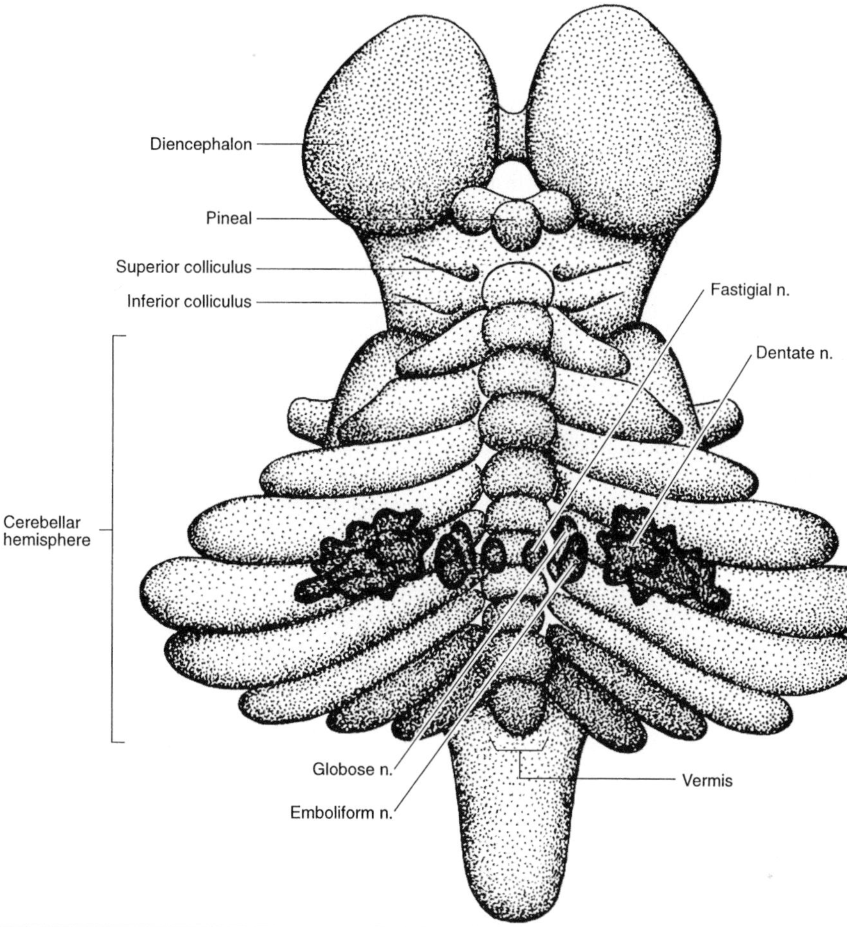

FIGURE 3.1–10
Schematic drawing of the dorsal view of the cerebellum showing the relative location and size of the cerebellar nuclei situated deep within the cerebellum. (Adapted from Hendelman WJ. *Student's Atlas of Neuroanatomy.* Philadelphia: WB Saunders; 1994.)

follow spoken commands, and lesions to the left premotor area may impair the actual motor program as it is generated by the higher-order motor neurons. This program is transmitted across the corpus callosum to the right premotor area, which directs the movements of the left hand. A lesion in this callosal projection may also cause an isolated ideomotor apraxia in the left hand. This syndrome implies the representation of specific motor acts within discrete sections of the left premotor cortex. Thus, just as some cells respond selectively to specific environmental features in the higher sensory cortices, some cells in the premotor cortex direct specific complex motor tasks.

Ideational apraxia occurs when the individual components of a sequence of skilled acts can be performed in isolation, but the entire series cannot be organized and executed as a whole. For example, the sequence of opening an envelope, removing the letter, unfolding it, and placing it on the table cannot be performed in order, even though the individual acts can be performed in isolation. The representation of the concept of a motor sequence may involve several areas, specifically the left parietal cortex, but it likely also relies on the sequencing and executive functions of the prefrontal cortex. This apraxia is a typical finding of diffuse cortical degeneration, such as Alzheimer's disease.

Autonomic Motor System

The *autonomic system* is divided into a sensory component (described above) and a motor component. The *autonomic motor system* is divided into two branches, the sympathetic and the parasympathetic. As a rule, organs are innervated by both types of fibers, which often serve antagonistic roles. The *parasympathetic system* slows the heart rate and begins the process of digestion. In contrast, the *sympathetic system* mediates the fight or flight response, with increased heart rate, shunting of blood away from the viscera, and increased respiration. The sympathetic system is highly activated by sympathomimetic drugs, such as amphetamine and cocaine, and may also be activated by withdrawal from sedating drugs such as alcohol, benzodiazepines, and opioids. Investigators who have found an increased risk of heart attacks in persons with high levels of hostility have suggested that chronic activation of the sympathetic fight or flight response, with elevated secretion of adrenaline, may underlie this association.

The brain center that drives the autonomic motor system is the *hypothalamus,* which houses a set of paired nuclei that appear to control appetite, rage, temperature, blood pressure, perspiration, and sexual drive. For example, lesions to the ventromedial nucleus, the satiety center, produce a voracious appetite and rage. In contrast, lesions to the upper region of the lateral nucleus, the hunger center, produce a profound loss of appetite. Numerous research groups are making intense efforts to define the biochemical regulation of appetite and obesity and frequently target the role of the hypothalamus.

In the regulation of sexual attraction, the role of the hypothalamus has also become an area of active research. In the 1990s, three groups independently reported neuroanatomical differences between certain of the hypothalamic nuclei of heterosexual and homosexual men. Researchers interpreted this finding to suggest that human sexual orientation has a neuroanatomical basis, and this result has stimulated several follow-up studies of the biological basis of sexual orientation. At present, however, these controversial findings are not accepted without question, and no clear consensus has emerged about whether the structure of the hypothalamus consistently correlates with sexual orientation. In animal studies, early nurturing and sexual experiences consistently alter the size of specific hypothalamic nuclei.

ASSOCIATION SYSTEMS

Primitive Reflex Circuit

Sensory pathways function as extractors of specific features from the overwhelming multitude of environmental stimuli, whereas motor pathways carry out the wishes of the organism. These pathways may be linked directly, for example, in the spinal cord, where a primitive reflex arc may mediate the brisk withdrawal of a limb from a painful stimulus, without immediate conscious awareness. In this loop, the peripheral stimulus activates the sensory nerve, the sensory neuron synapses on and directly activates the motor neuron, and the motor neuron drives the muscle to contract. This response is strictly local and all-or-none. Such primitive reflex arcs, however, rarely generate an organism's behaviors. In most behaviors, sensory systems project to association areas, where sensory information is interpreted in terms of internally determined memories, motivations, and drives. The exhibited behavior results from a plan of action determined by the association components and carried out by the motor systems.

Basic Organization of the Brain

Many theorists have subdivided the brain into functional systems. Korbinian Brodmann defined 47 areas on the basis of cytoarchitectonic distinctions, a cataloguing that has been remarkably durable as the functional anatomy of the brain has been elucidated (Fig. 3.1–2). A separate function, based on data from lesion studies and from functional neuroimaging, has been assigned to nearly all Brodmann areas. At the other extreme, certain experts have distinguished only three processing blocks: the brainstem and the thalamic reticular activating system provide arousal and set up attention; the posterior cortex integrates perceptions and generates language; and at the highest level, the frontal cortex generates programs and executes plans like an orchestra conductor.

Hemispheric lateralization of function is a key feature of higher cortical processing. The primary sensory cortices for touch, vision, hearing, smell, and taste are represented bilaterally, and the first level of abstraction for these modalities is also usually represented bilaterally. The highest levels of feature extraction, however, are generally unified in one brain hemisphere only. For example, recognition of familiar and unfamiliar faces seems localized to the left inferior temporal cortex, and cortical processing of olfaction occurs in the right frontal lobe. The clearest known example of hemispheric lateralization is the localization of language functions to the left hemisphere. Starting with the work of Pierre Broca and Karl Wernicke in the 19th century, researchers have drawn a detailed map of language comprehension and expression (Fig. 3.1–12). At least eight types of aphasias in which one or more components of the language pathway are injured have been defined (Table 3.1–1). *Prosody,* the emotional and affective components of language, or "body language," appears to be localized in a mirror set of brain units in the right hemisphere.

The *limbic system,* a circuit of phylogenetically ancient structures, is responsible for generating and modifying memories and for assigning emotional weight to sensory and recalled experience (Fig. 3.1–13). One nucleus in the limbic system, the *amygdala,* receives fibers from all sensory areas and appears to serve as a gate for the assignment of emotional significance to memories. The limbic structures in lower animals are devoted in large measure to processing olfactory input, a role superseded in humans by memory functions. The behavioral aspects of the limbic system are discussed below.

Hypotheses about the flow of thought in the brain are based on few experimental data, although this scarcity of findings has not impeded numerous theoreticians from speculating about functional neuroanat-

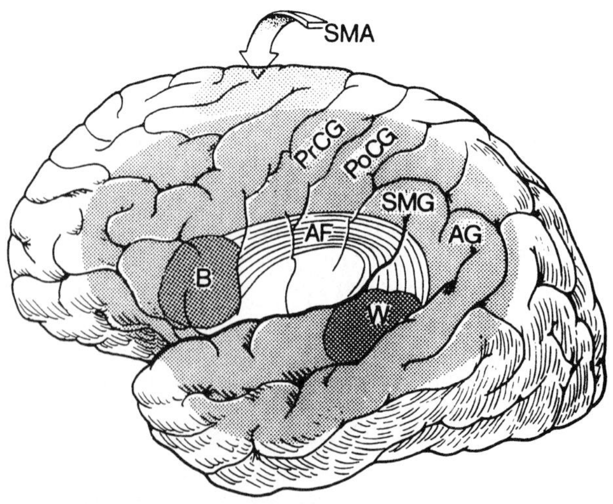

FIGURE 3.1–12

Language areas of the left hemisphere: *B,* Broca's area; *W,* Wernicke's area; *AF,* arcuate fasciculus; *SMA,* supplementary motor area; *PrCG,* precentral gyrus; *PoCG,* postcentral gyrus; *SMG,* supramarginal gyrus; and *AG,* angular gyrus. Language comprehension occurs in Wernicke's area, which is connected to Broca's area by the arcuate fasciculus. Generation of speech occurs in Broca's area. (From Filley CM. *Neurobehavioral Anatomy.* Niwot, CO: University of Colorado Press; 1995:76, with permission.)

Table 3.1–1
Localization of Aphasia Syndromes

Aphasia Type	Spontaneous Speech	Auditory Comprehension	Repetition	Naming	Localization (Left Hemisphere)
Broca's	Nonfluent	Good	Poor	Poor	Broca's area
Wernicke's	Fluent	Poor	Poor	Poor	Wernicke's area
Conduction	Fluent	Good	Poor	Poor	Arcuate fasciculus
Global	Nonfluent	Poor	Poor	Poor	Perisylvian region
Transcortical motor	Nonfluent	Good	Good	Poor	Anterior border zone
Transcortical sensory	Fluent	Poor	Good	Poor	Posterior border zone
Anomic	Fluent	Good	Good	Poor	Angular gyrus
Mixed transcortical	Nonfluent	Poor	Good	Poor	Anterior and posterior border zone

Reprinted with permission from Filley CM. *Neurobehavioral Anatomy.* Niwot, CO: University Press of Colorado; 1995:80.

omy. Several roles have been tentatively assigned to specific lobes of the brain, on the basis of the functional deficits resulting from localized injury. These data indicate that certain regions of cortex may be necessary for a specific function, but they do not define the complete set of structures that suffices for a complex task. Anecdotal evidence from surface electrocorticography for the study of epilepsy, for example, suggests that a right parietal seizure impulse may shoot immediately to the left frontal lobe and then to the right temporal lobe before spreading locally to the remainder of the parietal lobe. This evidence illustrates the limitations of naively assigning a mental function to a single brain region. Functional neuroimaging studies frequently reveal simultaneous activation of disparate brain regions during the performance of

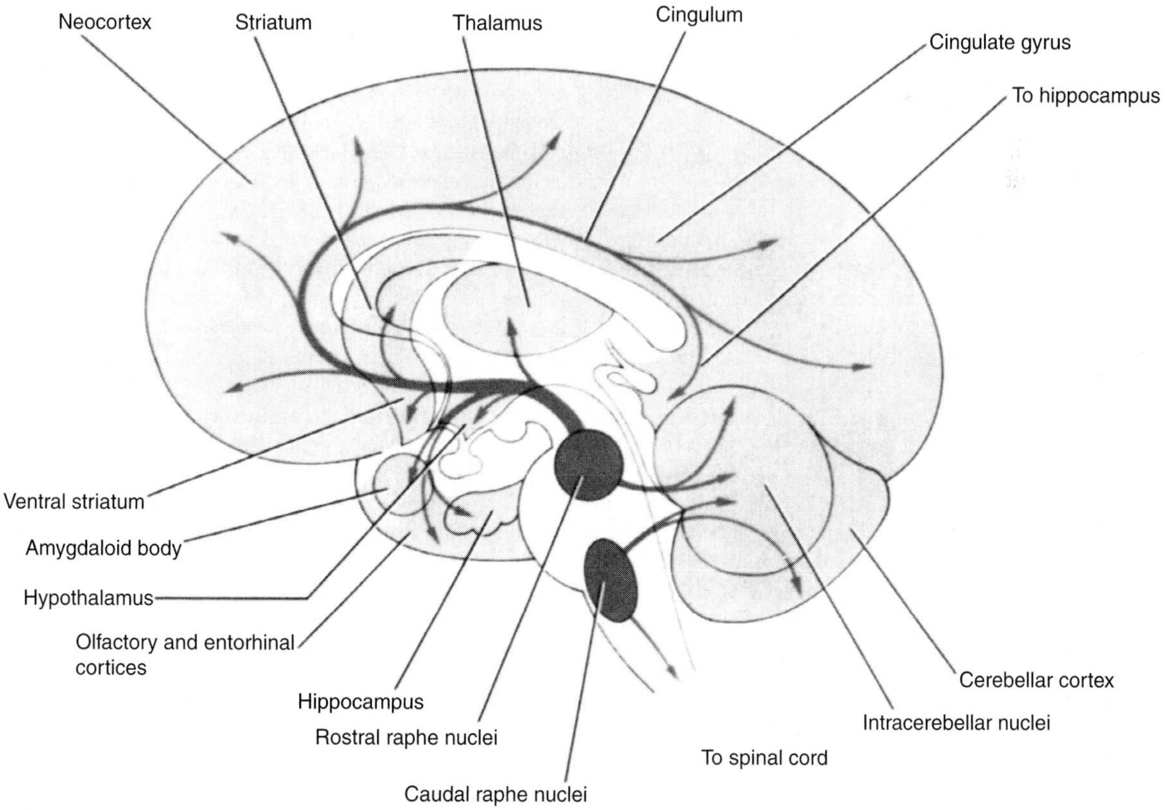

FIGURE 3.1–13

Serotonergic (5-HT) pathways. The raphe nuclei form a more or less continuous collection of cell groups close to the midline throughout the brainstem, but for the sake of simplicity, they have been subdivided into a rostral group and a caudal group in the drawing. The rostral raphe nuclei project to a large number of forebrain structures. The fibers that project laterally through the internal and external capsules to widespread areas of the neocortex are not indicated in this highly schematic drawing. (From Heimer L. *The Human Brain and Spinal Cord.* New York: Springer; 1983, with permission.)

Table 3.1–2
Regional Functions of the Human Brain

Frontal lobes	
	Voluntary movement
	Language production (left)
	Motor prosody (right)
	Comportment
	Executive function
	Motivation
Temporal lobes	
	Audition
	Language comprehension (left)
	Sensory prosody (right)
	Memory
	Emotion
Parietal lobes	
	Tactile sensation
	Visuospatial function (right)
	Reading (left)
	Calculation (left)
Occipital lobes	
	Vision
	Visual perception

Reprinted with permission from Filley CM. *Neurobehavioral Anatomy.* Niwot, CO: University Press of Colorado; 1995:6.

even a simple cognitive task. Nevertheless, particularly in the processing of vision and language, fairly well-defined lobar syndromes have been confirmed (Table 3.1–2).

Localization of Specific Brain Functions

Arousal and Attention. *Arousal,* or the establishment and maintenance of an awake state, appears to require at least three brain regions. Within the brainstem, the ascending reticular activating system (ARAS), a diffuse set of neurons, appears to set the level of consciousness. The ARAS projects to the intralaminar nuclei of the thalamus, and these nuclei in turn project widely throughout the cortex. Electrophysiological studies show that both the thalamus and the cortex fire rhythmical bursts of neuronal activity at the rates of 20 to 40 cycles per second. During sleep, these bursts are not synchronized. During wakefulness, the ARAS stimulates the thalamic intralaminar nuclei, which in turn coordinate the oscillations of different cortical regions. The greater the synchronization, the higher the level of wakefulness. The absence of arousal produces stupor and coma. In general, small discrete lesions of the ARAS may produce a stuporous state, whereas at the hemispheric level, large bilateral lesions are required to cause the same depression in alertness. One particularly unfortunate but instructive condition involving extensive, permanent, bilateral cortical dysfunction is the persistent vegetative state. Sleep–wake cycles may be preserved, and the eyes may appear to gaze; but the external world does not register and there is no evidence of conscious thought. This condition represents the expression of the isolated actions of the ARAS and the thalamus.

The maintenance of attention appears to require an intact right frontal lobe. For example, a widely used test of persistence requires scanning and identifying only the letter *A* from a long list of random letters. Normal persons can usually maintain performance of such a task for several minutes, but in patients with right frontal lobe dysfunction, this capacity is severely curtailed. Lesions of similar size in other regions of the cortex usually do not affect persistence tasks. In contrast, the more generally adaptive skill of maintaining a coherent line of thought is diffusely distributed throughout the cortex. Many medical conditions may affect this skill and may produce acute confusion or delirium (Table 3.1–3).

One widely diagnosed disorder of attention is attention-deficit/hyperactivity disorder. No pathological findings have been consistently associated with this disorder. Functional neuroimaging studies, however, have variously documented either frontal lobe or right hemisphere hypometabolism in patients with attention-deficit/hyperactivity disorder, compared with normal controls. These findings strengthen the notion that the frontal lobes—especially the right frontal lobe—are essential to the maintenance of attention.

Memory. The clinical assessment of memory should test three periods, which have distinct anatomical correlates. *Immediate memory* functions over a period of seconds; *recent memory* applies on the scale of minutes to days; and *remote memory* encompasses months to years. Immediate memory is implicit in the concept of attention and the ability to follow a train of thought. This ability has been divided into phonological and visuospatial components, and functional imaging has localized them to the left and right hemispheres, respectively. A related concept, incorporating immediate and recent memory, is *working memory,* which is the ability to store information for several seconds, while other, related cognitive operations take place on this information. Recent studies have shown that single neurons in the dorsolateral prefrontal cortex not only record features necessary for working memory, but also record the certainty with which the information is known and the degree of expectation assigned to the permanence of a particular environmental feature. Some neurons fire rapidly for an item that is eagerly awaited, but may cease firing if hopes are dashed unexpectedly. The encoding of the emotional value of an item contained in the working memory may be of great usefulness in determining goal-directed behavior. Some researchers localize working memory predominantly to the left frontal cortex. Clinically, however, bilateral prefrontal cortex lesions are required for severe impairment of working memory.

Three brain structures are critical to the formation of memories: the medial temporal lobe, certain diencephalic nuclei, and the basal forebrain. The *medial temporal lobe* houses the *hippocampus,* an elongated, highly repetitive network. The amygdala is adjacent to the anterior end of the hippocampus. The *amygdala* has been suggested to rate the emotional importance of an experience and to activate the level of hippocampal activity accordingly. Thus, an emotionally intense experience is indelibly etched in memory, but indifferent stimuli are quickly disregarded.

Animal studies have defined a hippocampal place code, a pattern of cellular activation in the hippocampus that corresponds to the animal's location in space. When the animal is introduced to a novel environment, the hippocampus is broadly activated. As the animal explores and roams, the firing of cer-

Table 3.1–3
Major Causes of Acute Confusion

Toxic
Prescription drugs
Nonprescription drugs
Drug withdrawal
Metabolic
Hypoxia
Hypoglycemia
Uremia
Hepatic disease
Thiamine deficiency
Electrolyte disturbances
Endocrinopathies
Infectious and inflammatory
Meningitis
Encephalitis
Vasculitis
Abscess
Epileptic
Postictal state
Complex partial status epilepticus
Absence status epilepticus
Vascular
Stroke
Subarachnoid hemorrhage
Traumatic
Concussion
Severe traumatic brain injury
Neoplastic
Deep midline tumors
Increased intracranial pressure
Postsurgical
Preoperative atropine
Hypoxia
Analgesics
Electrolyte imbalance
Fever

Reprinted with permission from Filley CM. *Neurobehavioral Anatomy.* Niwot, CO: University Press of Colorado; 1995:52.

tain hippocampal regions begins to correspond to specific locations in the environment. In about 1 hour, a highly detailed internal representation of the external space (a "cognitive map") appears in the form of specific firing patterns of the hippocampal cells. These patterns of neuronal firing may bear little spatial resemblance to the environment they represent; rather, they may seem randomly arranged in the hippocampus. If the animal is manually placed in a certain part of a familiar space, only the corresponding hippocampal regions show intense neural activity. When recording continues into sleep periods, firing sequences of hippocampal cells outlining a coherent path of navigation through the environment are registered, even though the animal is motionless. If the animal is removed from the environment for several days and then returned, the previously registered hippocampal place code is immediately reactivated. A series of animal experiments has dissociated the formation of the hippocampal place code from either visual, auditory, or olfactory cues, although each of these modalities may contribute to place code generation. Other factors may include internal calculations of distances based on counting footsteps or other proprioceptive information. Data from targeted genetic mutations in mice have implicated both the *N*-methyl-D-aspartate (NMDA) glutamate receptors and the calcium-calmodulin kinase II (CaMKII) in the proper formation of hippocampal place fields. These data suggest that the hippocampus is a significant site for formation and storage of immediate and recent memories. Although no data yet support the notion, it is conceivable that the hippocampal cognitive map is inappropriately reactivated during a *déjà vu* experience.

The most famous human subject in the study of memory is H. M., a man with intractable epilepsy, who had both his hippocampi and amygdalae surgically removed to alleviate his condition. The epilepsy was controlled, but he was left with a complete inability to form and recall memories of facts. H. M.'s learning and memory skills were relatively preserved, which led to the suggestion that declarative or factual memory may be separate within the brain from procedural or skill-related memory. A complementary deficit in procedural memory with preservation of declarative memory may be seen in persons with Parkinson's disease, in whom dopaminergic neurons of the nigrostriatal tract degenerate. Because this deficit in procedural memory can be ameliorated with treatment with levodopa (Larodopa), which is thought to potentiate dopaminergic neurotransmission in the nigrostriatal pathway, a role has been postulated for dopamine in procedural memory. Additional case reports have further implicated the amygdala and the afferent and efferent fiber tracts of the hippocampus as essential to the formation of memories. Lesional studies have also suggested a mild lateralization of hippocampal function in which the left hippocampus is more efficient at forming verbal memories and the right hippocampus tends to form nonverbal memories. After unilateral lesions in humans, however, the remaining hippocampus may compensate to a large extent. Medical causes of amnesia include alcoholism, seizures, migraine, drugs, vitamin deficiencies, trauma, strokes, tumors, infections, and degenerative diseases.

The motor system within the cortex receives directives from the association areas. The performance of a novel act requires constant feedback from the sensory and association areas for completion, and functional neuroimaging studies have demonstrated widespread activation of the cortex during unskilled acts. Memorized motor acts initially require activation of the medial temporal lobe. With practice, however, the performance of ever-larger segments of an act necessary to achieve a goal become encoded within discrete areas of the premotor and parietal cortices, particularly the left parietal cortex, with the result that a much more limited activation of the cortex is seen during highly skilled acts, and the medial temporal lobe is bypassed. This process is called the *corticalization of motor commands.* In lay terms, the process suggests a neuroanatomical basis for the adage "practice makes perfect."

Within the diencephalon, the dorsal medial nucleus of the thalamus and the mamillary bodies appear necessary for memory formation. These two structures are damaged in thiamine deficiency states usually seen in chronic alcoholics, and their inactivation is associated with Korsakoff's syndrome. This syndrome is characterized by severe inability to form new memories and a variable inability to recall remote memories.

The most common clinical disorder of memory is Alzheimer's disease. Alzheimer's disease is characterized pathologically by the degeneration of neurons and their replacement by senile plaques and neurofibrillary tangles. Clinicopathological studies have suggested that the cognitive decline is best correlated with the loss of synapses. Initially, the parietal and temporal lobes are affected, with relative sparing of the frontal lobes. This pattern of degeneration correlates with the early loss of memory, which is largely a temporal lobe function. Also, syntactical language comprehension and visuospatial organization, functions that rely heavily on the parietal lobe, are impaired early in the course of Alzheimer's disease. In contrast, personality changes, which reflect frontal lobe function, are relatively late consequences of Alzheimer's disease. Alzheimer's disease is discussed in Chapter 3, Section 3.4, and in Chapter 10. A rarer, complementary cortical degeneration syndrome, Pick's disease, first affects the frontal lobes while sparing the temporal and parietal lobes. In Pick's disease, disinhibition and impaired language expression, which are signs of frontal dysfunction, appear early, with relatively preserved language comprehension and memory.

Memory loss can also result from disorders of the subcortical gray matter structures, specifically the basal ganglia and the brainstem nuclei, from disease of the white matter, or from disorders that affect both gray and white matter.

Language. Because of the major role of verbal and written language in human communication, the neuroanatomical basis of language is the most completely understood association function. Language disorders, also called aphasias, are readily diagnosed in routine conversation, whereas perceptual disorders may escape notice except during detailed neuropsychological testing, although these disorders may be due to injury of an equal volume of cortex. Among the earliest models of cortical localization of function were Broca's 1865 description of a loss of fluent speech caused by a lesion in the left inferior frontal lobe and Wernicke's 1874 localization of language comprehension to the left superior temporal lobe. Subsequent analyses of patients rendered aphasic by strokes, trauma, or tumors have led to the definition of the entire language association pathway from sensory input through the motor output (Fig. 3.1–12).

Language most clearly demonstrates hemispheric localization of function. In most persons, the hemisphere dominant for language also directs the dominant hand. Ninety percent of the population is right-handed, and 99 percent of right-handers have left hemispheric dominance for language. Of the 10 percent who are left-handers, 67 percent also have left hemispheric language dominance; the other 33 percent have either mixed or right hemispheric language dominance. This innate tendency to lateralization of language in the left hemisphere is highly associated with an asymmetry of the planum temporale, a triangular cortical patch on the superior surface of the temporal lobe that appears to harbor Wernicke's area. Patients with mixed hemispheric dominance for language lack the expected asymmetry of the planum temporale. The fact that asymmetry has been observed in prenatal brains suggests a genetic determinant. Indeed, the absence of asymmetry runs in families, although both genetic and intrauterine influences probably contribute to the final pattern.

Language comprehension is processed at three levels. First, in *phonological processing,* individual sounds, such as vowels or consonants, are recognized in the inferior gyrus of the frontal lobes. Phonological processing improves if lip reading is allowed, if speech is slowed, or if contextual clues are provided. Second, *lexical processing* matches the phonological input with recognized words or sounds in the individual's memory. Lexical processing determines whether a sound is a word or not. Recent evidence has localized lexical processing to the left temporal lobe, where the representations of lexical data are organized according to semantic category. Third, *semantic processing* connects the words to their meaning. Persons with an isolated defect in semantic processing may retain the ability to repeat words in the absence of an ability to understand or spontaneously generate speech. Semantic processing activates the middle and superior gyri of the left temporal lobe, whereas the representation of the conceptual content of words is widely distributed in the cortex. Language production proceeds in the opposite direction, from the cortical semantic representations through the left temporal lexical nodes to either the oromotor phonological processing area (for speech) or the graphomotor system (for writing). Each of these areas may be independently or simultaneously damaged by stroke, trauma, infection, or tumor, resulting in a specific type of aphasia.

The garbled word salad or illogical utterances of an aphasic patient leave little uncertainty about the diagnosis of left-sided cortical injury, but the right hemisphere contributes a somewhat more subtle, but equally important, affective quality to language. For example, the phrase "I feel good" may be spoken with an infinite variety of shadings, each of which is understood differently. The perception of prosody and the appreciation of the associated gestures, or "body language," appear to require an intact right hemisphere. Behavioral neurologists have mapped an entire pathway for prosody association in the right hemisphere that mirrors the language pathway of the left hemisphere. Patients with right hemisphere lesions, who have impaired comprehension or expression of prosody, may find it difficult to function in society despite their intact language skills.

Developmental dyslexia is defined as an unexpected difficulty with learning in the context of adequate intelligence, motivation, and education. Whereas speech consists of the logical combination of 44 basic phonemes of sounds, reading requires a broader set of brain functions and is thus more prone to disruption. The awareness of specific phonemes develops about the age of 4 to 6 years and appears to be prerequisite to acquisition of reading skills. Inability to recognize distinct phonemes is the best predictor of a reading disability. Functional neuroimaging studies have localized the identification of letters to the occipital lobe adjacent to the primary visual cortex. Phonological processing occurs in the inferior frontal lobe, and semantic processing requires the superior and middle gyri of the left temporal lobe. A recent finding of uncertain significance is that phonological processing in men activates only the left inferior frontal gyrus, whereas phonological processing in women activates the inferior frontal gyrus bilaterally. Careful analysis of an individual's particular reading deficits can guide remedial tutoring efforts that can focus on weaknesses and thus

attempt to bring the reading skills up to the general level of intelligence and verbal skills.

In children, developmental nonverbal learning disorder is postulated to result from right hemisphere dysfunction. Nonverbal learning disorder is characterized by poor fine-motor control in the left hand, deficits in visuoperceptual organization, problems with mathematics, and incomplete or disturbed socialization.

Patients with nonfluent aphasia, who cannot complete a simple sentence, may be able to sing an entire song, apparently because many aspects of music production are localized to the right hemisphere. Music is represented predominantly in the right hemisphere, but the full complexity of musical ability seems to involve both hemispheres. Trained musicians appear to transfer many musical skills from the right hemisphere to the left as they gain proficiency in musical analysis and performance.

Emotion. Persons' emotional experiences occupy the attention of all mental health professionals. Emotion derives from basic drives, such as feeding, sex, reproduction, pleasure, pain, fear, and aggression, which all animals share. The neuroanatomical basis for these drives appears to be centered in the limbic system. Distinctly human emotions, such as affection, pride, guilt, pity, envy, and resentment, are largely learned and most likely are represented in the cortex. The regulation of drives appears to require an intact frontal cortex. The complex interplay of the emotions, however, is far beyond the understanding of functional neuroanatomists. Where, for example, are the representations of the id, the ego, and the superego? Through what pathway are ethical and moral judgments shepherded? What processes allow beauty to be in the eye of the beholder? These philosophical questions represent a true frontier of human discovery.

Within the cortex, several studies have suggested a hemispheric dichotomy of emotional representation. The left hemisphere houses the analytical mind but may have a limited emotional repertoire. For example, lesions to the right hemisphere, which cause profound functional deficits, may be noted with indifference by the intact left hemisphere. The denial of illness and of the inability to move the left hand in cases of right hemisphere injury is called *anosognosia.* In contrast, left hemisphere lesions, which cause profound aphasia, may trigger a catastrophic depression, as the intact right hemisphere struggles with the realization of the loss. The right hemisphere also appears dominant for affect, socialization, and body image.

Damage to the left hemisphere produces intellectual disorder and loss of the narrative aspect of dreams. Damage to the right hemisphere produces affective disorders, loss of the visual aspects of dreams, and a failure to respond to humor, shadings of metaphor, and connotations. In dichotic vision experiments, two scenes of varied emotional content were displayed simultaneously to each half of the visual field and were perceived separately by each hemisphere. A more intense emotional response attended the scenes displayed to the left visual field that were processed by the right hemisphere. Moreover, hemisensory changes representing conversion disorders have been repeatedly noted to involve the left half of the body more often than the right, an observation that suggests an origin in the right hemisphere.

Within the hemispheres, the temporal and frontal lobes play a prominent role in emotion. The temporal lobe exhibits a high frequency of epileptic foci, and temporal lobe epilepsy (TLE) presents an interesting model for the role of the temporal lobe in behavior. In studies of epilepsy, abnormal brain activation is analyzed, rather than the deficits in activity analyzed in classical lesional studies. TLE is of particular interest in psychiatry because patients with temporal lobe seizures may often manifest bizarre behavior without the classic grand mal shaking movements caused by seizures in the motor cortex. A proposed TLE personality is characterized by hyposexuality, emotional intensity, and a perseverative approach to interactions, termed *viscosity.* Patients with left TLE may generate references to personal destiny and philosophical themes and may display a humorless approach to life. In contrast, patients with right TLE may display excessive emotionality, ranging from elation to sadness. Although TLE patients may display excessive aggression between seizures, the seizure itself may evoke fear.

The inverse of a TLE personality appears in persons with bilateral injury to the temporal lobes after head trauma, cardiac arrest, herpes simplex encephalitis, or Pick's disease. This lesion resembles the one described in the Klüver-Bucy syndrome, an experimental model of temporal lobe ablation in monkeys. Behavior in this syndrome is characterized by hypersexuality, placidity, a tendency to explore the environment with the mouth, inability to recognize the emotional significance of visual stimuli, and constantly shifting attention, called *hypermetamorphosis.* In contrast to the aggression-fear spectrum sometimes seen in patients with TLE, complete experimental ablation of the temporal lobes appears to produce a uniform, bland reaction to the environment, possibly due to inability to access memories.

The prefrontal cortices influence mood in a complementary way. Whereas activation of the left prefrontal cortex appears to lift the mood, activation of the right prefrontal cortex causes depression. A lesion to the left prefrontal area, at either the cortical or the subcortical level, abolishes the normal mood-elevating influences and produces depression and uncontrollable crying. In contrast, a comparable lesion to the right prefrontal area may produce laughter, euphoria, and *witzelsucht,* a tendency to joke and make puns. Effects opposite to those caused by lesions appear during seizures, in which there is abnormal, excessive activation of either prefrontal cortex. A seizure focus within the left prefrontal cortex may cause gelastic seizures, for example, in which the ictal event is laughter. Functional neuroimaging has documented left prefrontal hypoperfusion during depressive states, which normalized after the depression was treated successfully.

Behavioral Aspects of the Limbic System

The limbic system was delineated by James Papez in 1937. The Papez circuit consists of the hippocampus, the fornix, the mamillary bodies, the anterior nucleus of the thalamus, and the cingulate gyrus (Fig. 3.1–13). The boundaries of the limbic system were subsequently expanded to include the amygdala, septum, basal forebrain, nucleus accumbens, and orbitofrontal cortex. Although this schema creates an anatomical loop for emotional processing, the specific contributions of the individual components other than the hippocampus or even whether a given train of neural impulses actually travels along the entire pathway is unknown.

The amygdala appears to be a critically important gate through which internal and external stimuli are integrated. Information from the primary senses is interwoven with internal drives, such as hunger and thirst, to assign emotional significance to sensory experiences. The amygdala may mediate learned fear responses, such as anxiety and panic, and may direct the expres-

sion of certain emotions by producing a particular affect. Neuroanatomical data suggest that the amygdala exerts a more powerful influence on the cortex, to stimulate or suppress cortical activity, than the cortex exerts on the amygdala. Pathways from the sensory thalamic relay stations separately send sensory data to the amygdala and the cortex, but the subsequent effect of the amygdala on the cortex is the more potent of the two reciprocal connections. In contrast, damage to the amygdala has been reported to ablate the ability to distinguish fear and anger in other persons' voices and facial expressions. Persons with such injuries may have a preserved ability to recognize happiness, sadness, or disgust. The limbic system appears to house the emotional association areas, which direct the hypothalamus to express the motor and endocrine components of the emotional state.

Fear and Aggression. Electrical stimulation of animals throughout the subcortical area involving the limbic system produces rage reactions (e.g., growling, spitting, arching of the back). Whether the animal flees or attacks depend on the intensity of the stimulation.

Feeding. Electrical stimulation of the lateral hypothalamus causes fully satiated animals to eat avidly. Bilateral lesions in the area produce aphagia and adipsia.

Sex. Lesions of the pyriform cortex produce hypersexuality in cats, who will attempt copulation almost continually with any object they can grasp.

Self-Stimulation. By training an animal to press a lever to obtain food and then arranging things so that each lever press also delivers stimuli to particular loci in the brain it is possible to determine whether the animal seeks, avoids, or is indifferent to stimulation in various neural systems. Such studies revealed that the overwhelming majority of points where stimulation was either sought or avoided lay within the limbic system. Findings show that for reasons that remain unclear, rats will stimulate the lateral hypothalamus rather than eat, sometimes leading to starvation.

Self-stimulation studies on human subjects have yielded interesting results. A few patients have apparently found that stimulation in septal areas relieves "anger and frustration." There seems little question but that such stimulation might have important therapeutic value if enough of its neurophysiology were understood. On the other hand, the conscious concomitants of self-stimulation in humans are often so vague or bizarre that they engender little hope of being able to comprehend the psychological effects on man or animals in any simple terms. Some of the effects are overtly sexual, and a "cool taste," a "high" feeling, a feeling of being "about to remember something interesting," and "almost reaching an orgasm" are some of the verbal reports of these effects that some self-stimulating patients give. Drastic changes of mood affirm the import of activity of the limbic system. Reliably specific therapeutic control of these powerful effects by means of localized stimulation will require great extension of present knowledge and techniques, but few areas of research hold greater promise than this for relief of human suffering.

Limbic System and Schizophrenia

The limbic system has been particularly implicated in neuropathological studies of schizophrenia. Eugen Bleuler's well-known four *A*s of schizophrenia—affect, associations, ambivalence, and autism—refer to brain functions served in part by limbic structures. Several clinicopathological studies have found a reduction in the brain weight of the gray matter but not of the white matter in persons with schizophrenia. In pathological as well as in magnetic resonance imaging (MRI) reports, persons with schizophrenia may have reduced volume of the hippocampus, amygdala, and parahippocampal gyrus. Schizophrenia may be a late sequela of a temporal epileptic focus, with some studies reporting an association in 7 percent of patients with TLE.

Functional neuroimaging studies have demonstrated decreased activation of the frontal lobes in a large number of patients with schizophrenia, particularly during tasks requiring willed action. A reciprocal increase in activation of the temporal lobe may occur during willed actions, such as finger movements or speaking, in persons with schizophrenia. Neuropathological studies have shown a decreased density of neuropil, the intertwined axons and dendrites of the neurons, in the frontal lobes of these patients. During development, the density of neuropil is highest around age 1 and then is reduced somewhat through synaptic pruning; the density plateaus throughout childhood and is further reduced to adult levels in adolescence. One hypothesis of the appearance of schizophrenia in the late teenage years is that excessive adolescent synaptic pruning occurs and results in too little frontolimbic activity. Some experts have suggested that hypometabolism and paucity of interneuronal connections in the prefrontal cortex may reflect inefficiencies in working memory, which permits the disjointed discourse and loosening of associations that characterize schizophrenia. At present, the molecular basis for the regulation of the density of synapses within the neuropil is unknown. Other lines of investigation aimed at understanding the biological basis of schizophrenia have documented inefficiencies in the formation of cortical synaptic connections in the middle of the second trimester of gestation, which may be due to a viral infection or malnutrition. Neurodevelopmental surveys administered during childhood have found an increased incidence of subtle neurological abnormalities prior to the appearance of the thought disorder in persons who subsequently exhibited signs of schizophrenia.

In one intriguing study, positron emission tomography (PET) scanning was used to identify the brain regions that are activated when a person hears spoken language. A consistent set of cortical and subcortical structures demonstrated increased metabolism when speech was processed. The researchers then studied a group of patients with schizophrenia who were experiencing active auditory hallucinations. During the hallucinations, the same cortical and subcortical structures were activated as were activated by the actual sounds, including the primary auditory cortex. At the same time, there was decreased activation of areas thought to monitor speech, including the left middle temporal gyrus and the supplementary motor area. This study raises the questions of what brain structure is activating the hallucinations and by what mechanism do neuroleptic drugs suppress the hallucinations. Clearly, functional imaging has much to tell about the neuroanatomical basis of schizophrenia.

Frontal Lobe Function

The *frontal lobes,* the region that determines how the brain acts on its knowledge, constitute a category unto themselves. In

comparative neuroanatomical studies, the massive size of the frontal lobes is the main feature that distinguishes the human brain from that of other primates and that lends it uniquely human qualities. There are four subdivisions of the frontal lobes. The first three—the motor strip, the supplemental motor area, and Broca's area—are mentioned above in the discussion of the motor system and language. The fourth, most anterior, division is the prefrontal cortex. The prefrontal cortex contains three regions in which lesions produce distinct syndromes: the *orbitofrontal,* the *dorsolateral,* and the *medial.* Dye-tracing studies have defined dense reciprocal connections between the prefrontal cortex and all other brain regions. Therefore, to the extent that anatomy can predict function, the prefrontal cortex is ideally connected to allow sequential use of the entire palette of brain functions in executing goal-directed activity. Indeed, frontal lobe injury usually impairs the executive functions: motivation, attention, and sequencing of actions.

Bilateral lesions of the frontal lobes are characterized by changes in personality—how persons interact with the world. The *frontal lobe syndrome,* which is most commonly produced by trauma, infarcts, tumors, lobotomy, multiple sclerosis, or Pick's disease, consists of slowed thinking, poor judgment, decreased curiosity, social withdrawal, and irritability. Patients typically display apathetic indifference to experience that can suddenly explode into impulsive disinhibition. Unilateral frontal lobe lesions may be largely unnoticed because the intact lobe can compensate with high efficiency.

Frontal lobe dysfunction may be difficult to detect by means of highly structured, formal neuropsychological tests. Intelligence, as reflected in the intelligence quotient (IQ), may be normal, and functional neuroimaging studies have shown that the IQ seems to require mostly parietal lobe activation. For example, during administration of the Wechsler Adult Intelligence Scale–Revised (WAIS-R), the highest levels of increased metabolic activity during verbal tasks occurred in the left parietal lobe, whereas the highest levels of increased metabolic activity during performance skills occurred in the right parietal lobe. In contrast, frontal lobe pathology may become apparent only under unstructured, stressful, real-life situations.

A famous case illustrating the result of frontal lobe damage involves Phineas Gage, a 25-year-old railroad worker. While he was working with explosives, an accident drove an iron rod through Gage's head. He survived, but both frontal lobes were severely damaged. After the accident his behavior changed dramatically. The case was written up by J. M. Harlow, M.D., in 1868, as follows:

> [George] is fitfull, irreverent, indulging at times in the grossest profanity (which was not previously his custom), manifesting but little deference for his fellows, impatient of restraint or advice when it conflicts with his desires . . . His mind was radically changed, so decidedly that his friends and acquaintances said he was "no longer Gage."

In one study of right-handed males, lesions of the right prefrontal cortex eliminated the tendency to use internal, associative memory cues and led to an extreme tendency to interpret the task at hand in terms of its immediate context. In contrast, right-handed males who had lesions of the left prefrontal cortex produced no context-dependent interpretations and interpreted the tasks entirely in terms of their own internal drives. A mirror image of the functional lateralization appeared in left-handed subjects. This test thus revealed the clearest known association of higher cortical functional lateralization with the subjects' dominant hand. Future experiments in this vein will attempt to reproduce these findings with functional neuroimaging. If corroborated, these studies suggest a remarkable complexity of functional localization within the prefrontal cortex and may also have implications for the understanding of psychiatric diseases in which prefrontal pathology has been postulated, such as schizophrenia and mood disorders.

The heavy innervation of the frontal lobes by dopamine-containing nerve fibers is of interest because of the action of antipsychotic medications. At the clinical level, antipsychotic medications may help to organize the rambling associations of a patient with schizophrenia. At the neurochemical level, most typical antipsychotic medications block the actions of dopamine at the dopamine D_2 receptors. Therefore, the frontal lobes may be a major therapeutic site of action for antipsychotic medications.

DEVELOPMENT

The nervous system is divided into the central and peripheral nervous systems (CNS and PNS). The CNS consists of the brain and spinal cord; the PNS refers to all the sensory, motor, and autonomic fibers and ganglia outside the CNS. During development, both divisions arise from a common precursor, the neural tube, which in turn is formed through folding of the neural plate, a specialization of the ectoderm, the outermost of the three layers of the primitive embryo. During embryonic development, the neural tube itself becomes the CNS, while the ectoderm immediately superficial to the neural tube becomes the neural crest, which gives rise to the PNS. The formation of these structures requires chemical communication between the neighboring tissues in the form of cell surface molecules and diffusible chemical signals. In many cases, an earlier-formed structure, such as the notochord, is said to *induce* the surrounding ectoderm to form a later structure, in this case the neural plate. Identification of the chemical mediators of tissue induction is an active area of research. Investigators have begun to examine whether failures of the interactions of these mediators and their receptors could underlie errors in brain development that cause psychopathology.

Neuronal Migration and Connections

The life cycle of a neuron consists of cell birth, migration to the adult position, extension of an axon, elaboration of dendrites, synaptogenesis, and, finally, the onset of chemical neurotransmission. Individual neurons are born in proliferative zones generally located along the inner surface of the neural tube. At the peak of neuronal proliferation in the middle of the second trimester, 250,000 neurons are born each minute. Postmitotic neurons migrate outward to their adult locations in the cortex, guided by radially oriented astrocytic glial fibers. Glial-guided neuronal migration in the cerebral cortex occupies much of the first 6

months of gestation. For some neurons in the prefrontal cortex, migration occurs over a distance 5,000 times the diameter of the neuronal cell body. Neuronal migration requires a complex set of cell–cell interactions and is susceptible to errors in which neurons fail to reach the cortex and instead reside in ectopic positions. A group of such incorrectly placed neurons is called a *heterotopia.* Neuronal heterotopias have been shown to cause epilepsy and are highly associated with mental retardation. In a neuropathological study of the planum temporale of four consecutive patients with dyslexia, heterotopias were a common finding. Recently, heterotopic neurons within the frontal lobe have been postulated to play a causal role in some cases of schizophrenia.

Many neurons lay an axon down as they migrate, while others do not initiate axon outgrowth until they have reached their cortical targets. Thalamic axons that project to the cortex initially synapse on a transient layer of neurons called the *subplate neurons.* In normal development, the axons subsequently detach from the subplate neurons and proceed superficially to synapse on the true cortical cells. The subplate neurons then degenerate. Some brains from persons with schizophrenia reveal an abnormal persistence of subplate neurons, suggesting a failure to complete axonal pathfinding in the brains of these persons. This finding does not correlate with the presence of schizophrenia in every case, however. A characteristic branched dendritic tree elaborates once the neuron has completed migration. Synaptogenesis occurs at a furious rate from the second trimester through the first 10 years or so of life. The peak of synaptogenesis occurs within the first 2 postnatal years, when as many as 30 million synapses form each second. Ensheathment of axons by myelin begins prenatally; it is largely complete in early childhood but does not reach its full extent until late in the third decade of life. Myelination of the brain is also sequential (Fig. 3.1–14).

Neuroscientists are tremendously interested in the effect of experience on the formation of brain circuitry in the first years of life. As noted above, there are many examples of the impact of early sensory experience on the wiring of cortical sensory processing areas. Similarly, early movement patterns are known to reinforce neural connections in the supplemental motor area that drive specific motor acts. Neurons rapidly form a fivefold excess of synaptic connections; then, through a darwinian process of elimination, only those synapses that serve a relevant function persist. This synaptic pruning appears to preserve input in which the presynaptic cell fires in synchrony with the postsynaptic cell, a process that reinforces repeatedly activated neural circuits. One molecular component that is thought to mediate synaptic reinforcement is the postsynaptic NMDA glutamate receptor. This receptor allows the influx of calcium ions only when activated by glutamate at the same time as the membrane in which it sits is depolarized. Thus, glutamate binding without membrane depolarization or membrane depolarization without glutamate binding fails to trigger calcium influx. NMDA receptors open in dendrites that are exposed to repeated activation, and their activation stimulates stabilization of the synapse. Calcium is a crucial intracellular messenger that initiates a cascade of events, including gene regulation and the release of trophic factors that strengthen particular synaptic connections. Although there is less experimental evidence for the role of experience in modulating synaptic connectivity of association areas than has been demonstrated in sensory and motor areas, neuroscientists assume that similar activity-dependent mechanisms may apply in all areas of the brain.

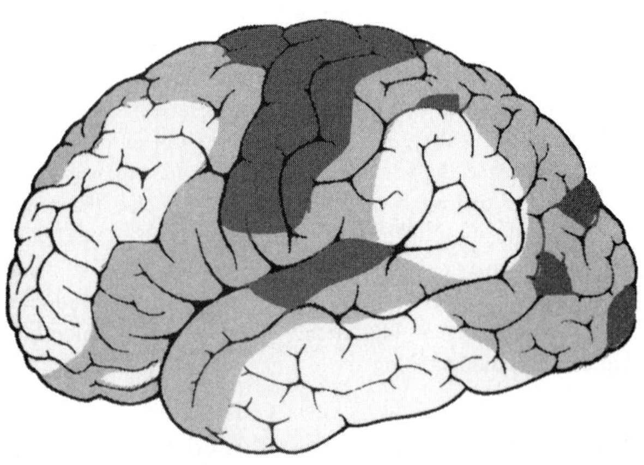

FIGURE 3.1–14

Sequence of myelination of the brain. Myelination occurs first in brain areas involved with leg movements, primitive vision, and primitive hearing, shown in *dark gray.* Next, shown in *light gray,* are the brain areas involved in arm movements, the supplementary motor areas, the higher visual and auditory areas, and the lower association areas. Finally, the frontal executive cortex, the parieto-occipital association area, and temporal object recognition areas, shown in *white,* do not complete their myelination until the time of puberty. (Modified from Spitzer M. *The Mind within the Net: Models of Learning, Thinking, and Acting.* Cambridge, MA: Bradford; 1991:179, with permission.)

Auditory Processing and Language

An emerging concept of great significance in both child and adult psychiatry is the existence of early windows of time during which the brain establishes the basic circuitry for language, emotion, logic, mathematics, movements, and music. These windows open within the first few months of life and may close in some cases by 1 year of age. For example, a "perceptual map" of *phonemes,* the building blocks of language, is formed in the higher auditory processing regions of Wernicke's area during the first 12 months of life.

Certain sounds used by non–English-speaking persons do not occur in English. Studies in the United States have shown that babies less than 6 months of age can be taught to discriminate these non-English sounds, but babies older than 6 months can no longer hear them. Moreover, the map for English differs, for instance, from that for Japanese in the location of neurons that respond to the sounds *ra* and *la.* In English, these neurons are located far apart within the somatosensory cortex, whereas in Japanese persons, who have difficulty distinguishing these sounds, the neurons are so closely intertwined as to be virtually overlapping. Thus, to a Japanese person, *la* and *ra* elicit nearly the same pattern of neural activity, a fact that may underlie the difficulties of Japanese speakers in discriminating these sounds. Within the English language, studies have shown that babies of mothers who spoke loquaciously to them acquired a larger vocabulary than babies of taciturn mothers. These findings suggest that very early experiences may establish the density and fidelity of neural circuits for specific brain functions, the consequences of which may affect persons for the rest of their lives. An interesting study of human laughter explained how some types are more natural than others, on the basis of neurobiological structure (Fig. 3.1–15).

Workers have recently studied a particular learning disorder, the auditory processing defect, with electroencephalography. Patients with

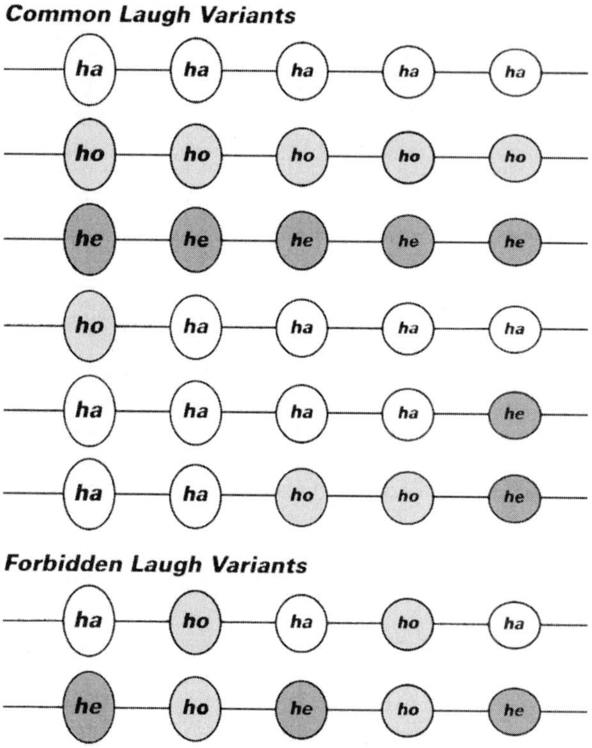

FIGURE 3.1–15
Variations of a five-note laugh. Laughter can be visualized as a series of beads on a string, with each "bead" having a duration of about $1/15$ second and repeating every $1/5$ second. Some laugh variants are common and easy to mimic, while "forbidden" types do not occur naturally and are difficult to produce; a sample of each type is shown. The gradual decrease in note amplitude is due to the loss of air needed to produce notes late in a sequence. (Modified from Provine RR. *Laughter: A Scientific Investigation*. New York: Viking Penguin; 2000:58, with permission.)

this defect may have difficulty discriminating the phonemes *da* and *ga*. When the string *da-da-da-ga* is played to normal subjects while an electroencephalogram is recorded, a change in the brain wave pattern accompanies the transition from *da* to *ga*. In contrast, the same stimulus fails to alter the brain waves of subjects with the auditory processing defect. Nevertheless, with proper training over the course of several weeks, many persons with the auditory processing defect acquired the ability to discriminate the two sounds. This finding shows that in some cases, with intensive modification of experience, neural circuits may be at least partially altered after the window of development has closed.

Neurological Basis of Development Theories

In the realm of emotion, early childhood experiences have been suspected to be at the root of psychopathology since the earliest theories of Sigmund Freud. Freud's psychoanalytic method aimed at tracing the threads of a patient's earliest childhood memories. Franz Alexander added the goal of allowing the patient to relive them in a less pathological environment, a process known as a "corrective emotional experience." Although neuroscientists have no data demonstrating that this method operates at the level of neurons and circuits, emerging results reveal a profound effect of early caregivers on an adult individual's emotional repertoire. For example, the concept of *attunement* is defined as the process by which caregivers "play back a child's inner feelings." If a baby's emotional expressions are reciprocated in a consistent and sensitive manner, certain emotional circuits are reinforced. These circuits likely include the limbic system, in particular, the amygdala, which serves as a gate to the hippocampal memory circuits for emotional stimuli. In one anecdote, for example, a baby whose mother repeatedly failed to mirror her level of excitement emerged from childhood an extremely passive girl, who was unable to experience a thrill or a feeling of joy.

The relative contributions of nature and nurture are perhaps nowhere more indistinct than in the maturation of emotional responses, partly because the localization of emotion within the adult brain is only poorly understood. It is reasonable to assume, however, that the reactions of caregivers during a child's first 2 years of life are eventually internalized as distinct neural circuits, which may be only incompletely subject to modification through subsequent experience. For example, axonal connections between the prefrontal cortex and the limbic system, which probably play a role in modulating basic drives, are established between the ages of 10 and 18 months. Recent work suggests that a pattern of terrifying experiences in infancy may flood the amygdala and drive memory circuits to be specifically alert to threatening stimuli, at the expense of circuits for language and other academic skills. Thus, infants raised in a chaotic and frightening home may be neurologically disadvantaged for the acquisition of complex cognitive skills in school.

An adult correlate to this cascade of detrimental overactivity of the fear response is found in posttraumatic stress disorder, in which persons exposed to an intense trauma involving death or injury may have feelings of fear and helplessness for years after the event. A PET scanning study of posttraumatic stress disorder patients revealed abnormally high activity in the right amygdala while the patients were reliving their traumatic memories. The researchers hypothesized that the stressful hormonal milieu present during the registration of the memories may have served to burn the memories into the brain and to prevent their erasure by the usual memory modulation circuits. As a result, the traumatic memories exerted a pervasive influence and led to a state of constant vigilance, even in safe, familiar settings.

Workers in the related realms of mathematics have produced results documenting the organizing effects of early experiences on internal representations of the external world. Since the time of Pythagoras, music has been considered a branch of mathematics. A series of recent studies has shown that groups of children who were given 8 months of intensive classical music lessons during preschool years later had significantly better spatial and mathematical reasoning in school than a control group. Nonmusical tasks such as navigating mazes, drawing geometric figures, and copying patterns of two-color blocks were performed significantly more skillfully by the musical children. Early exposure to music may thus be ideal preparation for later acquisition of complex mathematical and engineering skills.

These tantalizing observations suggest a neurological basis for the developmental theories of Jean Piaget, Erik Erikson, Margaret Mahler, John Bowlby, Freud, and others. Erikson's epigenetic theory states that normal adult behavior results

from the successful, sequential completion of each of several infantile and childhood stages (see Chapter 6, Section 6.3). According to the epigenetic model, failure to complete an early stage is reflected in subsequent physical, cognitive, social, or emotional maladjustment. By analogy, the experimental data just discussed suggest that early experience, particularly during the critical window of opportunity for establishing neural connections, primes the basic circuitry for language, emotions, and other advanced behaviors. Clearly, miswiring of an infant's brain may lead to severe handicaps later when the person attempts to relate to the world as an adult. These findings support the vital need for adequate public financing of Early Intervention and Head Start programs, programs that may be the most cost-effective means of improving persons' mental health.

References

Allen DN, Seaton BE, Goldstein G, et al. Neuroanatomic differences among cognitive and symptom subtypes of schizophrenia. *J Nerv Ment Dis*. 2000;188:381.

Altshuler LL, Bartzokis G, Grieder T, et al. An MRI study of temporal lobe structures in men with bipolar disorder or schizophrenia. *Biol Psychiatry*. 2000;48:147.

Austin MP, Mitchell P, Wilhelm K, et al. Cognitive function in depression: a distinct pattern of frontal impairment in melancholia? *Psychol Med*. 1999;29:73.

Bryant NL, Buchanan RW, Vladar K, Breier A, Rothman M. Gender differences in temporal lobe structures of patients with schizophrenia: a volumetric MRI study. *Am J Psychiatry*. 1999;156:603.

Chacko RC, Corbin MA, Harper RG. Acquired obsessive-compulsive disorder associated with basal ganglia lesions. *J Neuropsychiatry Clin Neurosci*. 2000;12:269.

Cowan WM, Harter DH, Kandel ER. The emergence of modern neuroscience: some implications for neurology and psychiatry. *Annu Rev Neurosci*. 2000;23:343.

Dougherty DD, Shin LM, Alpert NM, et al. Anger in healthy men: a PET study using script-driven imagery. *Biol Psychiatry*. 1999;46:466.

Flashman LA, McAllister TW, Andreasen NC, Saykin AJ. Smaller brain size associated with unawareness of illness in patients with schizophrenia. *Am J Psychiatry*. 2000;157:1167.

Giannakopoulos P, Gold G, Duc M, Michel JP, Hof PR, Bouras C. Neuroanatomic correlates of visual agnosia in Alzheimer's disease: a clinicopathologic study. *Neurology*. 1999;52:71.

Goodnick PJ, Rush AJ, George MS, Marangell LB, Sackeim HA. Vagus nerve stimulation in depression. *Expert Opin Pharmacother*. 2001;2:1061.

Gray TS. Functional and anatomical relationships among the amygdala, basal forebrain, ventral striatum, and cortex. An integrative discussion. *Ann N Y Acad Sci*. 1999;877:439.

Gur RE, Cowell PE, Latshaw A, et al. Reduced dorsal and orbital prefrontal gray matter volumes in schizophrenia. *Arch Gen Psychiatry*. 2000;57:761.

Gur RE, Turetsky BI, Cowell PE, et al. Temporolimbic volume reductions in schizophrenia. *Arch Gen Psychiatry*. 2000;57:769.

Joseph R. Frontal lobe psychopathology: mania, depression, confabulation, catatonia, perseveration, obsessive compulsions, and schizophrenia. *Psychiatry*. 1999;62:138.

Kim JS, Choi-Kwon S. Poststroke depression and emotional incontinence: correlation with lesion location. *Neurology*. 2000;54:1805.

Laakso MP, Vaurio O, Koivisto E, et al. Psychopathy and the posterior hippocampus. *Behav Brain Res*. 2001;118:187.

Menon V, Anagnoson RT, Mathalon DH, Glover GH, Pfefferbaum A. Functional neuroanatomy of auditory working memory in schizophrenia: relation to positive and negative symptoms. *Neuroimage*. 2001;13:433.

Narayan M, Bremner JD, Kumar A. Neuroanatomic substrates of late-life mental disorders. *J Geriatr Psychiatry Neurol*. 1999;12:95.

Nofzinger EA, Price JC, Meltzer CC, et al. Towards a neurobiology of dysfunctional arousal in depression: the relationship between beta EEG power and regional cerebral glucose metabolism during NREM sleep. *Psychiatry Res*. 2000;98:71.

Pearlson GD. New insights on the neuroanatomy of schizophrenia. *Curr Psychiatry Rep*. 1999;1:41.

Remschmidt H. Early-onset schizophrenia as a progressive-deteriorating developmental disorder: evidence from child psychiatry. *J Neural Transm Gen Sect*. 2002;109:101.

Simpson S, Baldwin RC, Jackson A, Burns A, Thomas P. Is the clinical expression of late-life depression influenced by brain changes? MRI subcortical neuroanatomical correlates of depressive symptoms. *Int Psychogeriatr*. 2000;12:425.

Stern E, Silbersweig DA, Chee KY, et al. A functional neuroanatomy of tics in Tourette syndrome. *Arch Gen Psychiatry*. 2000;57:741.

Sullivan GM, Coplan JD, Kent JM, Gorman JM. The noradrenergic system in pathological anxiety: a focus on panic with relevance to generalized anxiety and phobias. *Biol Psychiatry*. 1999;46:1205.

▲ 3.2 Neurophysiology and Neurochemistry

In the previous section, the gross structure of the brain is defined, and the various functional units of the brain are presented as being generally stable for the life of the organism. Indeed, the anatomical relations between neurons undoubtedly play a major role in determining personality traits and thought processes. At a finer level of analysis, however, an equally important determinant of the quality of thought is the efficiency of information processing by individual neurons. Single neurons communicate by interpreting their chemical environment, by instantly changing the chemical cues to electrical activity for transport down axons, and, finally, by efficiently translating the electrical data into finely modulated chemical emissions that can be secreted to influence other neuronal or nonneuronal cells. Thus electrical impulses facilitate instantaneous responses, and the chemical milieu is of paramount importance in maintaining the fidelity of the brain's image of the world.

History

The study of chemical interneuronal communication is called *neurochemistry*. With the acceptance in the late 19th century of the neuronal theory of Wilhelm His and Santiago Ramon y Cajal, which stated that the brain consists of individual cells rather than a syncytium of cytoplasm, a search was initiated for the mediators of intercellular communication. At the turn of the century, the effects of extracts of the adrenal gland on sympathetic nerve tissue was elucidated, and soon scientists discovered chemicals in the brain—neurotransmitters—with similar stimulatory actions. Postulating that cells also contained inhibitory and excitatory "receptive substances," Karl Lashley envisioned the entire basic apparatus of chemical neurotransmission: neurotransmitters and specific receptor molecules. In the first half of the 20th century, the major biogenic amine neurotransmitters were characterized; the more abundant amino acid neurotransmitters were not recognized as transmitters until much more recently. Recent years have seen a massive proliferation in known peptide neurotransmitters and receptors, and novel classes of neurotransmitters have been identified, including nucleotides, prostaglandins, and gases. Through advanced molecular cloning techniques, dozens of orphan receptor genes have been sequenced, for which no known ligand exists. Moreover, in addition to their role in modulating cellular electrical excitability, molecules identified initially as neurotransmitters (e.g., serotonin) have been found to influence gene expression and synapse formation. The field of neurochemistry has thus exploded into a massive complexity of molecules and gone beyond the study of the chemical mediation of nerve impulses into a broad discipline that overlaps with neuroanatomy, developmental neurobiology, and behavioral genetics.

In psychopharmacology, the major available therapeutic interventions center on modification of biogenic amine neurotransmission and, to a lesser extent, amino acid neurotransmission. While these systems are discussed in detail below, students of psychiatry must be aware of the entire range of neurochemistry, because many new classes of psychopharmacological agents that act on more recently defined neurotransmitter systems are likely to emerge in the near

future. Moreover, neuronal electrical activity is continuously modulated by excitatory and inhibitory neurotransmitters, by circulating hormones, by immune surveillance, by general medical homeostasis, and by chronobiological rhythms, each of which may be influenced with existing therapeutic methods. Neuronal electrical activity, along with the chemical factors, simultaneously modifies the abundance and phosphorylation status of cellular proteins, the level of expression of certain genes, and the connectivity of a neuron to thousands of neighboring neurons. Each of these avenues of therapeutic influence may open in the future.

BASIC ELECTROPHYSIOLOGY

Membranes and Charge

In the resting state, the intracellular compartment of a neuron is more negatively charged than the extracellular compartment. The charge gradient is maintained across the hydrophobic plasma membrane, which consists of a lipid bilayer containing embedded cholesterol molecules, which modify membrane rigidity, and numerous proteins including ion pumps, ion channels, and neurotransmitter receptors. Ion pumps and ion channels maintain a gradient of cations; potassium ions are 15 to 20 times more concentrated inside neurons, and sodium ions are 8 to 15 times less concentrated inside neurons than in the extracellular space. The principal ion pump is the energy-requiring sodium-potassium–adenosine triphosphatase (ATPase) exchange pump, which maintains an electrical gradient by pumping sodium out and potassium in. The principal ion channels are the sodium, potassium, calcium, and chloride ion channels. The membrane is described as *semipermeable* because it is selective regarding which ions can pass through it. The semipermeability of the membrane is the basis for its functional role, which is similar to the role of a capacitor. A capacitor stores an electrical charge by isolating positive and negative ions with an insulator. The hydrophobic neuronal membrane serves this insulator role. The charge can be released by bypassing the insulator, which occurs in neurons by opening channels that allow passage of ions through the membrane. The electrical potential of the membrane obeys *Ohm's law,* $E = IR$, where E is the transmembrane potential, I is the current, and R is the resistance.

Ion Channels

The rapid transmission of information along neuronal axons, which may exceed a velocity of 60 meters per second, is mediated by instantaneous changes in membrane potential called *action potentials.* These changes in membrane potential occur when the charge gradients maintained by the insulator function of the membrane are allowed to flow unimpeded through protein pores called *ion channels.* Ion channels are selective for specific ions, such as sodium channels that may not allow passage of potassium ions. In the resting state, ion channels are closed. Ion channels open in response to binding of ligands to receptors—*ligand-gated ion channels*—or in response to changes in membrane potential—*voltage-gated ion channels.* Among ligand-gated ion channels, certain ligands, called *excitatory neurotransmitters,* open cation channels that depolarize the membrane and increase the likelihood of the generation of an action potential. These ligands are said to elicit excitatory postsynaptic potentials (EPSPs). Other ligands, called *inhibitory neurotransmitters,* open chloride channels that hyperpolarize the membrane and decrease the likelihood of the generation of an action potential. These ligands are said to elicit inhibitory postsynaptic potentials (IPSPs). In the central nervous system (CNS), the binding of a single ligand to a ligand-gated ion channel may change the neuronal membrane potential by 1 mV. Therefore, the combined activation of several ligand-gated channels is needed to trigger an action potential. In clinical medicine, sodium channel blockers are used as local anesthetics and antiarrhythmics, and potassium channel blockers are used as antiarrhythmics. In psychiatry, blockers of CNS calcium channels are used to treat bipolar disorder. A blocker of calcium channels in skeletal muscle, dantrolene (Dantrium), is used to treat neuroleptic malignant syndrome.

The ion channels themselves are glycoproteins (proteins with sugar moieties) that span the neuronal membrane and contain a pore that can be opened and closed, through which specific ions can flow. The ligand-gated channels are particularly relevant in the study of psychiatry, since many psychotherapeutic and psychoactive drugs affect these channels directly (Table 3.2–1).

Action Potentials

In the resting state, the intracellular compartment of the neuron is negatively charged at a potential of –70 to –80 mV, but during an action potential this membrane potential reverses in a thin zone immediately adjacent to the membrane. For an action potential to be generated by a neuron, ligand-gated ion channels open, and sodium ions begin to enter the cell and gradually make the inner surface of the membrane less negatively charged relative to the outside. The point at which the negative charge on the interior of the membrane is low enough to open adjacent voltage-gated sodium channels is called the *spike threshold,* characteristically approximately –55 mV. The inward flow of sodium ions then rapidly depolarizes the membrane and initiates an action potential, which propagates itself along the membrane by sequentially triggering adjacent voltage-gated sodium channels. The action potential itself is a brief (0.1 to 2 msec) wave of reversal of membrane potential that moves along an axon (Fig. 3.2–1). During the action potential the interior of the membrane is positively charged with respect to the outside of the membrane. The initial ion channel involved in the action potential is the Na^+ channel, which, when opened, allows positively charged sodium ions to enter the neuron. The Ca^{2+} channels open next, allowing the positively charged calcium ions to enter the neuron and further contribute to the spike of the action potential. Not only does the entry of calcium ions affect the membrane potential, but also the calcium ion is an important second-messenger molecule that is involved in initiating protein-protein interactions and gene regulation. Entry of the calcium ion into the synaptic terminal is also critical for the release of neurotransmitter molecules, and calcium ion entry activates ion channels that carry an outflow of potassium ions that are involved in arresting the action potential. Activation of those K^+ channels results in after-

Table 3.2–1
Some Ligand-Gated Ion Channels

Neurotransmitter	Receptor Subtype	G Protein or Direct[a]	Ion Channel Activated	Physiological Response[b]
Acetylcholine	Nicotinic	D	Na^+/K^+	E
	Muscarinic	G	K^+	E
Dopamine	D_2	G	K^+	I
Norepinephrine	α_1	G	K^+	E
	α_2	G	K^+	I
	β	G	K^+	E
Serotonin	5-HT_{1A}	G	K^+	I
	5-$HT_{1C/2}$	G	K^+	E
	5-HT_3	D	Na^+/K^+	E
GABA	$GABA_A$	D	Cl^-	I
Glutamate	AMPA	D	Na^+/K^+	E
	Kainate	D	Na^+/K^+	E
	NMDA	D	Ca^{2+}	E
Opioid	μ, δ	G	K^+	I
Substance P	NK	G	K^+	E

[a]D, directly coupled; G, G protein coupled.
[b]E, excitatory; I, inhibitory.

hyperpolarization of the membrane after an action potential. During the afterhyperpolarization the inside of the membrane is even more negatively charged than it was at baseline. Afterhyperpolarization contributes to the refractory period of a neuron after an action potential; during this period, no other action potential can be generated.

The rate of local spread of an action potential determines the rate of conduction of the impulse along the nerve. A bare axon may conduct an action potential at a velocity of 1 meter per second. At this rate, for example, only about three new visual images could reach the visual cortex per second, and polysynaptic image processing would be considerably slower. However, the brain can distinguish up to 50 new images per second. The increased nerve conduction velocity that accounts for the rapid processing capabilities of the brain is due to the presence of myelin sheaths, which encircle larger axons. *Myelin* is a highly hydrophobic substance that completely prevents the passage of ions. It is laid down in segments along the axon, which are separated by gaps of bare axonal membrane called *nodes of Ranvier.* The local changes in membrane charge that constitute the action potential occur at the nodes of Ranvier, and they then jump over the myelin segment to the next node of Ranvier. The presence of myelin segments reduces the number of times the action potential must trigger neighboring voltage-gated ion channels to conduct an impulse along that length of the axon. The nerve conduction velocity may thus reach as high as 65 meters per second in large, myelinated fibers.

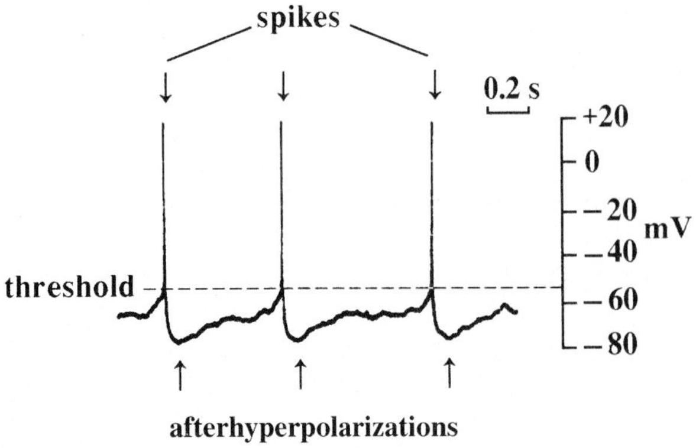

FIGURE 3.2–1
Action potentials. An oscilloscope trace shows a repetitively firing neuron recorded intracellularly *in vivo.* This example was taken from a serotonergic neuron in the dorsal raphe nucleus of the rat midbrain. As can be seen from the trace, when the membrane potential, in millivolts, reaches the spike threshold (–55 mV), an all-or-none spike occurs. After each spike, an afterhyperpolarization moves the cell away from the threshold into a more negative potential (near –80 mV). As the afterhyperpolarization decays, the cell again approaches the spike threshold. (Courtesy of George K. Aghajanian, M.D., and Meenakshi Alreja, Ph.D.)

Translation of the Action Potential into Chemical Neurotransmission

At the synaptic terminus of the axon, action potentials trigger the release of neurotransmitters (Fig. 3.2–2) into the synaptic cleft, where they may act on other neurons or muscles. The presynaptic nerve terminals contain voltage-gated calcium channels that locally raise the intracellular calcium concentration. This initiates a cascade of protein-protein and protein-lipid interactions in which neurotransmitter-containing synaptic vesicles fuse with the presynaptic membrane and release their contents into the synaptic cleft. In muscles, voltage-gated calcium channels that are opened by the arriving action potentials trigger the movement of myosin on actin fibers, a process called *excitation-contraction coupling.* In each of these instances, the electrical impulse causes changes in local calcium concentrations, which in turn rapidly trigger physical changes in the ultrastructure of the cell (Fig. 3.2–3). (Specific neurotransmitters are discussed below.)

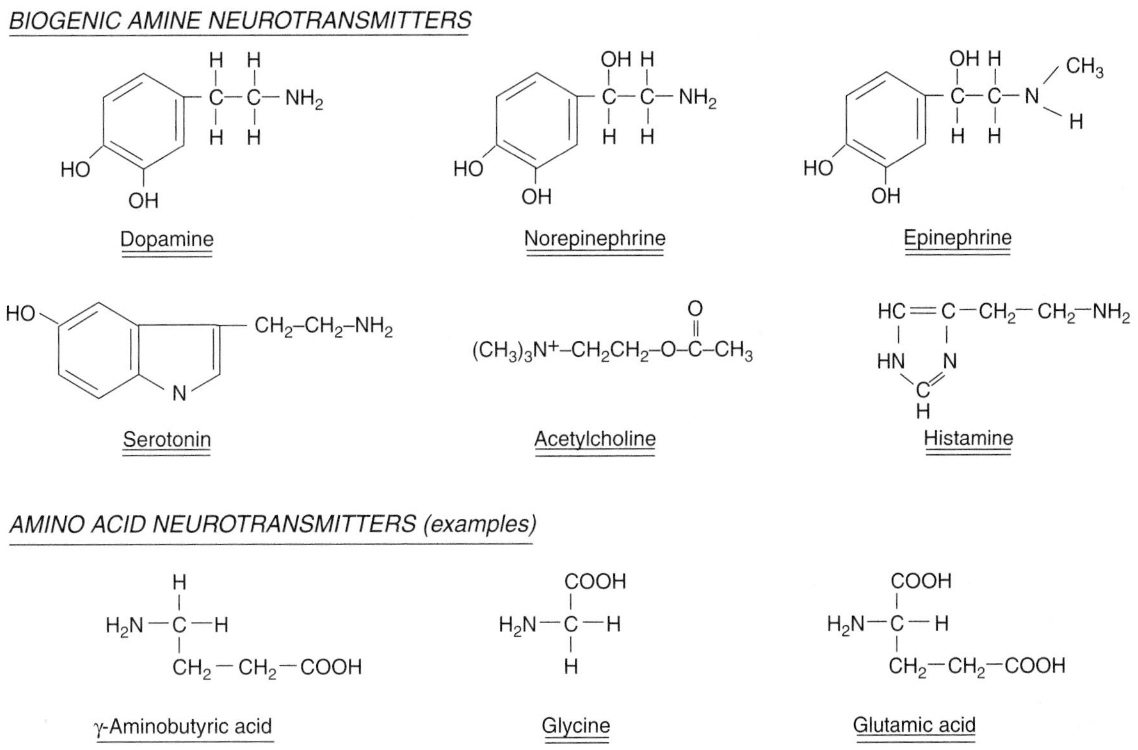

PEPTIDE NEUROTRANSMITTERS

NEUROTENSIN:

Glu – Leu – Tyr – Glu – Asn – Lys – Pro – Arg – Arg – Pro – Tyr – Ile – Leu

THYROTROPIN – RELEASING HORMONE (TRH):

Glu – His – Pro

CHOLECYSTOKININ OCTAPEPTIDE (CCK-8):

Asp – Tyr – Met – Gly – Trp – Met – Asp – Phe

FIGURE 3.2–2
Three classes of neurotransmitters.

SYNAPSES

The propagation of an action potential along an axon is described as an *all-or-none phenomenon;* that is, once an action potential has been triggered, it is propagated at full strength for the entire length of the axon. Subtleties of neuronal processing are thus generally not represented by modulation of the intensity of the action potential, although an exception to this rule may occur at axoaxonal synapses. In most neurons, however, the essence of neuronal processing occurs in the regulation of whether an action potential is generated. This determination is the summation of excitatory and inhibitory chemical influences that act on the *axon hillock,* which originates the action potential. The *synapse* is the site at which stimuli are given and received and where the finest shadings of neuronal activity are negotiated.

The components of the synapse are the axon terminal of the presynaptic neuron, the synaptic cleft, and the dendrite of the postsynaptic neuron. When an action potential develops in the presynaptic neuron, the action potential moves down the axon to the axon terminal or to other, functionally similar regions of the axons called *axonal varicosities.* The action potential causes the release of neurotransmitter molecules discussed below into the *synaptic cleft,* the small space between the presynaptic neuron and the postsynaptic neuron. The neurotransmitter molecules diffuse across the synaptic cleft and then bind to their specific receptors on the external membrane of the dendrite of the postsynaptic neuron. The most common type of synapse involves the termination of the presynaptic neuronal axon on the postsynaptic neuronal cell body, an axon, or a dendrite. These synapses are called *axosomatic, axoaxonic,* and *axodendritic,* respectively. In addition to the chemical synapses, electrical synapses, also called *gap junctions,* allow the direct transfer of ions between two neurons as a form of interneuronal neurochemical communication. *Conjoint synapses* are synapses that have both electrical and chemical characteristics.

During development, a severalfold excess of synapses forms, and only those synapses of functional relevance survive into adulthood. In

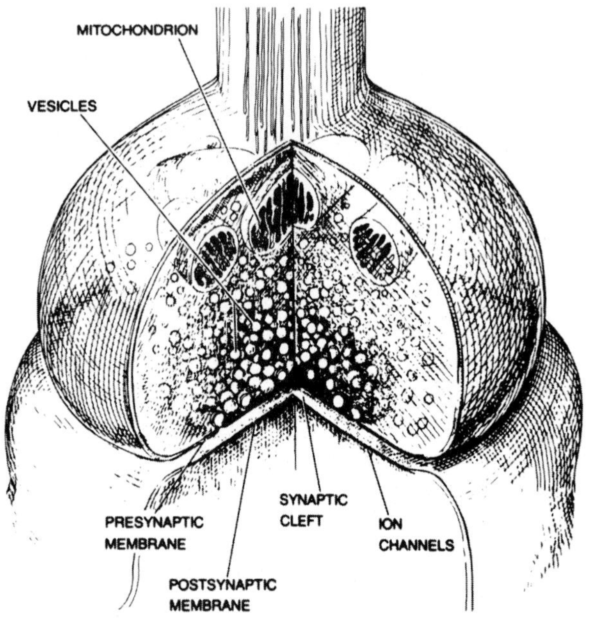

FIGURE 3.2–3

Synapse consists of two parts: the knoblike tip of an axon terminal and the receptor region on the surface of another neuron. The membranes are separated by a synaptic cleft some 20 to 30 nm across. Molecules of chemical transmitter, stored in vesicles in the axon terminal, are released into the cleft by arriving nerve impulses and change the electrical state of the receiving neuron, making it either more likely or less likely to fire an impulse. (From Stevens CF. The neuron. In: Llinás RL, ed. *The Biology of the Brain from Neurons to Networks.* New York: Freedman; 1988:3, with permission.)

the adult, synaptic relations are constantly remodeled through increases or decreases in the size and strength of individual synapses, as well as the formation of new synapses and the elimination of unnecessary synapses. The mechanical adhesive properties of synapses are mediated by various combinations of the calcium-dependent cadherin family of adhesion molecules. Changes in the structure of synapses are mediated by trophic substances known as *growth factors,* which act on specific receptors to regulate local protein-protein interactions and to modify levels of gene expression. Thus, not only neurotransmitters subtly modulate intercellular communication, trophic substances constantly remodel the synaptic channels through which chemical neurotransmission occurs. *N*-Methyl-D-aspartate (NMDA) glutamate receptors are particularly important to the process of synaptic remodeling. NMDA receptors are essential to certain forms of long-term potentiation (LTP) in which coordinated neuronal activity strengthens certain synapses. On the basis of a large amount of electrophysiological data, LTP has been proposed to be the cellular correlate of long-term memory, although molecular biological experiments suggest that other systems must also contribute.

Presynaptic Components

The presynaptic terminals contain the synthetic machinery responsible for the synthesis of all neurotransmitters except peptide neurotransmitters, which are synthesized in the cell body. Neurotransmitter synthesis may be stimulated by an influx of calcium ions, variations in levels of the second-messenger cyclic adenosine monophosphate (cAMP), or changes in levels of circulating hormones. Once synthesized, neurotransmitters are packaged into synaptic vesicles, which may store a mixture of amine and peptide neurotransmitters. Data indicate that all termini of a single neuron secrete the same combination of neurotransmitters. In practice, however, probably a minority of neurons has more than one axonal terminus, and newer techniques suggest a possible heterogeneity of neurotransmitter composition among different vesicles in a single neuron. Energy for the synthesis, storage, release, and degradation of neurotransmitters is provided by mitochondria. (The life cycle of specific neurotransmitters is discussed below.) The presynaptic membrane contains ion channels, neurotransmitter receptors, and neurotransmitter transporters. Voltage-gated calcium channels trigger vesicle release. Presynaptic neurotransmitter receptors mediate feedback inhibition of neurotransmitter synthesis and release. For example, many norepinephrine-releasing neurons have presynaptic α_2-adrenergic receptors that, when occupied by the released norepinephrine, cause the releasing neuron to decrease or stop the release of norepinephrine. Transporters take neurotransmitters up from the synaptic cleft for recycling or degradation. Additional transporters in the membranes of storage vesicles load the vesicles with neurotransmitters.

Neurotransmitter storage vesicles in the presynaptic terminal fuse with the presynaptic membrane and release their components into the synaptic cleft in a process called *exocytosis.* Many details of synaptic vesicle fusion have become known recently. Synaptotagmin and synaptobrevin, components of the vesicle membrane, and neurexins and syntaxins, components of the plasma membrane, mediate the fusion of the vesicle to the inner surface of the presynaptic membrane. Synaptophysin helps to create a pore in the presynaptic membrane.

Once a monoamine neurotransmitter such as norepinephrine, dopamine, or serotonin has been released into the synaptic cleft, it acts until it diffuses away or, more commonly, is removed by reuptake mechanisms. Specific presynaptic transmembrane transporter molecules return free monoamine neurotransmitters to the nerve terminal, where they are either repackaged into vesicles for release in response to subsequent action potentials or degraded by monoamine oxidases (MAOs). Transporters have gained increasing appreciation in psychopharmacology as the sites of the major mechanism of action of both therapeutic and illicit drugs. They form a family of integral membrane proteins with 12 transmembrane domains and several intracellular sites of potential phosphorylation. The tricyclic drugs, discovered almost 40 years ago, are thought to inhibit the norepinephrine and serotonin reuptake mechanisms. On the basis of this fact, several newer antidepressant medications have been identified in assays specifically designed to detect the inhibition of monoamine reuptake through transporters. The most widely used of these are the selective serotonin reuptake inhibitors (SSRIs); others, developed more recently, exhibit varying ratios of inhibitory activity on the dopamine, norepinephrine, and serotonin transporters. Cocaine appears to block all three monoamine transporters. A recent study found a correlation between a genetic variant serotonin transporter, which is present in lower amounts on the presynaptic membrane, and increased levels of anxiety and neuroticism. Decreased numbers of transporter molecules would be expected to reduce the rate of serotonin reuptake. Based on a relatively small patient sample, the genetic variant was calculated to account for 3 to 4 percent of the behavioral variation for anxiety in the population of normal subjects. This result appears to conflict with the fact that pharmacological block-

ers of serotonin transporters, such as fluoxetine (Prozac), which would be expected to have the same net effect as the mutation (specifically, lowering reuptake and hence increasing synaptic serotonin activity) nevertheless reduce, rather than increase, anxiety. Clearly, more research is needed to understand the role of serotonin in anxiety and mood disorders.

Degradation of recycled biogenic amine neurotransmitters is mediated principally by MAOs, which are attached to the outer mitochondrial membrane. MAO type A (MAO_A) metabolizes norepinephrine and serotonin, and its inhibition by MAO inhibitors is associated with an elevation in mood. MAO type B (MAO_B) metabolizes dopamine.

Synapse

Although it makes up less than 1 percent of the total volume of the brain, the *synaptic compartment*—the space between the presynaptic and postsynaptic membranes—contains the mixture of neurotransmitters with the greatest influence on thought and behavior. These molecules are available to act on specific receptors and to initiate or inhibit the generation of action potentials in the postsynaptic cell. The list of neurotransmitters runs into the hundreds of distinct molecules, including amino acids (glutamate, γ-aminobutyric acid [GABA], glycine, aspartate, homocystine), biogenic amines (norepinephrine, serotonin, dopamine, epinephrine, acetylcholine, histamine), neuropeptides (vasopressin, oxytocin, enkephalins, endorphins, substance P, neurotensin, and several hundred others), nucleotides (adenosine, cAMP), gases (nitric oxide [NO], carbon monoxide [CO], ammonia [NH_3]), and prostaglandins. The synaptic cleft of cholinergic synapses harbors acetylcholinesterase, which inactivates acetylcholine by cleaving it into acetate and choline. The concentrations of various neurotransmitters in the synaptic cleft are carefully regulated by feedback inhibition of transmitter release and by reuptake into the presynaptic terminal by transporter molecules. This regulation is critically important because the concentration of each neurotransmitter determines the degree to which it activates its specific receptors.

Postsynaptic Components

Receptors. Neurotransmitter receptors are the sites of action for many of the psychotherapeutic and psychoactive drugs used today. The techniques of molecular biology have led to the identification and sequencing of many new subtypes of receptors. The importance of those advances lies in the long-standing hypothesis that the ability to subtype receptors would refine both the hunt for pathology in disease states and the design of specifically acting drugs.

The principal function of postsynaptic neurotransmitter receptors is to alter the transmembrane electrical potential, to either increase or decrease the likelihood of triggering an action potential. Excitatory neurotransmitters cause depolarization of the postsynaptic membrane. Because binding a single neurotransmitter results in a change of only 1 mV, there is much room for subtle modulation of the postsynaptic response by the combined actions of several neurotransmitters before the membrane potential is raised from the resting potential of –70 to –80 mV to the threshold potential of –55 mV. The fine modulation of receptor activation results from changes in the synaptic concentration of neurotransmitters, in combination with variations in the efficiency of the translation of receptor binding to the opening of ion channels, which are due to chemical modulation of the intracellular segments of the receptor, the association of the receptor with other cellular proteins, the number of receptors, or levels of second messengers. Once the threshold potential is reached at the axon hillock, however, the all-or-none action potential is initiated by the opening of voltage-gated sodium channels, and there is virtually no further chance for modification of the impulse.

Two terms often used in conjunction with receptors are *supersensitivity* and *subsensitivity*. These terms refer, respectively, to a greater than usual response and a less than usual response of the receptor to a constant amount of neurotransmitter. The sensitivity of a receptor may be due to the number of receptors present, the affinity of the receptor for the neurotransmitter, and the efficiency with which binding of the neurotransmitter to the receptor is translated into an intraneuronal message. All these steps in receptor function are variable and subject to regulation.

Fundamentally, there are two types of neurotransmitter receptors: seven-transmembrane-domain receptors, which require G proteins to open channels, and ligand-gated ion channels, in which the channel is an integral part of the complex that binds the ligand. Many of the receptors located directly on ion channels are listed in Table 3.2–1. Many of the biogenic amine receptors, regardless of whether they are associated with G proteins or directly with ion channels, are listed in Table 3.2–2. The seven-transmembrane-domain receptors all have a characteristic structure in which the NH_2-terminal end of the protein is located extracellularly and the COOH-terminal end of the protein is located intracellularly. Moreover, the third intracytoplasmic loop of the receptor tends to be the largest loop. Occasionally, the second intracytoplasmic loop is also fairly large. The first intracytoplasmic loop seems invariably to be the smallest. The length of the COOH-terminal intracytoplasmic tail varies. The large intracytoplasmic loops and the COOH-tail contain identified or potential sites of phosphorylation, a feature that is involved in the regulation of receptor function. For example, when a β-adrenergic receptor is activated, it is rapidly inactivated by phosphorylation of the third intracytoplasmic loop by β-adrenergic receptor kinase, which then allows binding of an inhibitor protein called β-arrestin.

Another type of postsynaptic membrane receptor, which does not cause changes in membrane potential, is the family of tyrosine kinase receptors, which have an extracellular ligand-binding component, a single transmembrane domain, and an intracellular tyrosine kinase that phosphorylates both itself and other cytoplasmic proteins and so triggers a cascade of intracellular phosphorylations that ultimately lead to changes in gene expression. Tyrosine kinase receptors often associate as dimers, either homodimers or heterodimers. There is a vast diversity of tyrosine kinase receptors, much of which is due to various combinations of modular segments of the receptor genes that have arisen during evolution. Tyrosine kinase receptors bind growth factors and mediate the plasticity of synaptic associations. Two such factors are nerve growth factor (NGF) and brain-derived neurotropic factor (BDNF), which have opposite effects on the size of developing cortical somatosensory receptive fields and thus may collaborate in the remodeling of neuronal circuits that underlies synaptic plasticity during development and in adults.

Table 3.2–2
Receptor Subtypes for Biogenic Amine Neurotransmitters

Neurotransmitter	Receptor Subtype	G/I[a]	Effector Mechanism[b]
Acetylcholine	M_1	G	IP_3/DG, increase cGMP
	M_2	G	Decrease cAMP, increase K^+ conductance
	M_3	G	IP_3/DG, increase cGMP
	M_4	G	Decrease cAMP
	M_5	G	IP_3/DG
	Nicotinic	I	Na^+/K^+
Dopamine	D_1	G	Increase cAMP
	D_2	G	Decrease cAMP, increase K^+ conductance
	D_3	G	?Decrease cAMP
	D_4	G	?Decrease cAMP
	D_5	G	Increase cAMP
Epinephrine and norepinephrine	$\alpha_{1a, b, c, and d}$	G	IP_3/DG
	$\alpha_{2a, b, and c}$	G	Decrease cAMP, increase K^+ conductance
	$\beta_{1, 2, and 3}$	G	Increase cAMP
Histamine	H_1	G	IP_3/DG
	H_2	G	Increase cAMP
	H_3	?	?
Serotonin	5-HT_{1A}	G	Decrease cAMP, increase K^+ conductance
	5-HT_{1B}	G	Decrease cAMP
	5-HT_{1C}	G	IP_3/DG
	5-HT_{1D}	G	Increase cAMP
	5-HT_{1E}	G	Decrease cAMP
	5-HT_{1F}	G	Decrease cAMP
	5-HT_{2A}	G	IP_3/DG
	5-HT_{2B}	G	IP_3/DG
	5-HT_{2C}	G	IP_3/DG
	5-HT_3	I	Na^+/K^+
	5-HT_4	G	Increase cAMP
	5-HT_{5A}	G	?
	5-HT_{5B}	G	?
	5-HT_6	G	Increase cAMP
	5-HT_7	G	Increase cAMP

[a]G, G protein linked; I, directly linked to an ion channel.
[b]IP_3, stimulation of phosphoinositide turnover, resulting in an increase in the concentrations of inositol triphosphate and diacylglycerol.

Postsynaptic cells also are regulated by circulating hormones, such as thyroid hormone or steroids. These hormones diffuse through the membrane and bind to cytoplasmic receptors, which then are translocated into the nucleus, where they regulate gene expression.

G Proteins. G proteins are a family of guanosine triphosphate (GTP)-binding proteins with similar structures, which interact with members of the very large family of seven-transmembrane-domain receptors, of which the adrenergic receptor is a prototype. GTP is interconvertible with guanosine diphosphate (GDP). The G proteins themselves consist of three smaller proteins, called the α, β, and γ subunits. When an intact G protein (all three subunits, with GDP bound to the α subunit) binds to a receptor, the receptor assumes a state with a high affinity for the neurotransmitter molecule. When the neurotransmitter binds to this complex, it triggers the replacement of GDP with GTP on the α subunit, thereby destabilizing the associations among the neurotransmitter, the receptor, and the G protein. The G protein further dissociates into the GTP-binding α subunit and the βγ subunit, which contains both the β and γ subunits. The GTP-associated α subunit is the active fragment involved in activating or inhibiting a particular effector molecule (e.g., adenylyl cyclase or an ion channel). Because that α subunit itself has the ability to convert GTP to GDP, the activity of the GTP-associated α subunit is stopped when the GTP is converted to GDP. The conversion of GTP to GDP allows reassociation of the α subunit with a βγ subunit.

The family of G proteins is created by the diversity of subunit types that have been identified. The greatest diversity has been found for the α subunit, although an increasing number of reports describe diversity of the β and γ subunits. The classically described α subunits are α_s, α_i, and α_o. The α_s subunit has been associated with the stimulation of adenylyl cyclase activity; the α_i subunit has been associated with the inhibition of adenylyl cyclase activity; and the α_o subunit has been associated with the stimulation of the phosphoinositol second-messenger system. At least 10 other α subunit genes have been sequenced.

Second Messengers. The neurotransmitters themselves are conceptualized as the first messengers that bring a signal to a

neuron. For the neuron to act on the signal, the first-messenger signal must be translated into an intraneuronal signal via formation of second-messenger molecules. The most classic second messengers are the cyclic nucleotides (cAMP and cyclic guanosine monophosphate [cGMP]), the calcium ion (Ca^{2+}), and the phosphoinositol metabolites (inositol triphosphate [IP_3] and diacylglycerol [DAG]). Another increasingly appreciated class of second messengers is the eicosanoid metabolites. Gases, such as NO and CO, not only mediate interneuronal communication but also serve as intraneuronal second-messenger molecules.

CYCLIC NUCLEOTIDES. cAMP is produced from ATP by the enzyme adenylyl cyclase. Adenylyl cyclase is linked to receptors by G proteins. The G_s protein stimulates the activity of adenylyl cyclase, and the G_i protein inhibits the activity of adenylyl cyclase. Once formed, cAMP has its biological effects; then the cAMP activity is terminated by its conversion into 5'-AMP by phosphodiesterase. An exactly analogous pathway is involved in the formation of cGMP, where the involved enzyme is guanylyl cyclase. cAMP binds to a cAMP-responsive element binding protein (CREBP), which is a transcription factor that stimulates transcription from several genes, including the synthetic machinery for certain neurotransmitters. On the basis of studies with mutant "knockout" mice that lack CREBP, CREBP appears to mediate learning and memory, as well as opiate addiction, which may be viewed as an extreme form of associative learning.

CALCIUM. In the resting cell, the intracellular calcium concentration is maintained at a very low level (10^{-7} M) relative to the extracellular concentration (10^{-3} M). Calcium, as a second messenger, can come from two sources. First, calcium can enter the cell from the extracellular space through either voltage-gated or ligand-gated ion channels. Second, calcium can be released from intraneuronal storage vesicles by the action of a phosphoinositol metabolite, IP_3. Calcium can act either alone as a second messenger or in tandem with a variety of calcium-binding proteins (e.g., calmodulin). Calcium stimulates formation of NO and may trigger excitotoxic cellular damage under some circumstances. Very small increases in the intraneuronal calcium concentration can have profound biological effects. Recent data demonstrate that significant changes in intracellular calcium concentrations may be very localized—for example, to a single dendrite—without involving the entire cellular domain. This ability to sequester calcium may underlie local changes in synaptic efficiency and may provide a subcellular basis for learning and memory.

PHOSPHOINOSITOL METABOLITES. In a manner analogous to adenylyl cyclase activity, another receptor-activated enzyme, phospholipase C, converts a membrane lipid (phosphatidylinositol 4,5-bisphosphate) into two active metabolites (IP_3 and DAG). As mentioned above, the major effect of IP_3 is to cause the release of calcium from intraneuronal stores of calcium in the endoplasmic reticulum. The major activity of DAG is to activate a specific protein kinase.

EICOSANOIDS. In a manner analogous to phospholipase C activity, another receptor-activated enzyme, phospholipase A_2, converts membrane phospholipids into free arachidonic acid. Arachidonic acid can then be cleaved by cyclooxygenase and other enzymes to produce a wide array of second-messenger molecules, including several types of prostaglandins, cyclic endoperoxides (e.g., prostacyclins and thromboxanes), and leukotrienes. These three classes of molecules have a variety of second-messenger activities that are the subject of many ongoing basic science investigations.

GASES. NO is formed from L-arginine and molecular oxygen by the enzyme nitric oxide synthase, which has at least four recognized forms. NO was originally discovered because of its ability to relax vascular muscle, and it may mediate local increases in cerebral blood flow associated with neuronal activity. The action of NO to dilate blood vessels accounts for its use in the drug sildenafil (Viagra) to produce penile erections. NO diffuses readily within cells and between cells, and among its activities is the potent activation of guanylyl cyclase. NO synthase is stimulated by nitroprusside and inhibited by nitroarginine and methylarginine. CO also activates guanylyl cyclase and is formed in neurons by heme oxygenase.

JAK-STAT. The Janus kinase (Jak) is a receptor for cytokines. Upon activation by its ligand, Jak phosphorylates members of the signal transducers and activators of transcription (STAT) family of transcription factors, which then translocate directly into the nucleus, where they regulate gene expression. This system is unusual in not using one of the common second messengers but, rather, allowing specific communication between the cytokine ligand and the resulting regulation of gene transcription. This distinction raises one perplexing issue regarding the regulation of gene expression by the common transcription factors: how can a general increase in a small molecule elicit a specific change in gene expression? One suggestion has been that the response of a particular cell to a rise in second-messenger levels is determined by the state of differentiation of the cell, so that only a small number of genes may be regulated by a common second messenger at any one time. The Jak-STAT mechanism may represent an alternative pathway in which a variety of second messengers may be used independently, depending on the extracellular stimulus. In the brain, the Jak-STAT system has so far only been shown to mediate trophic signals that support neuronal survival. Researchers are actively investigating other possible roles for this novel second-messenger system.

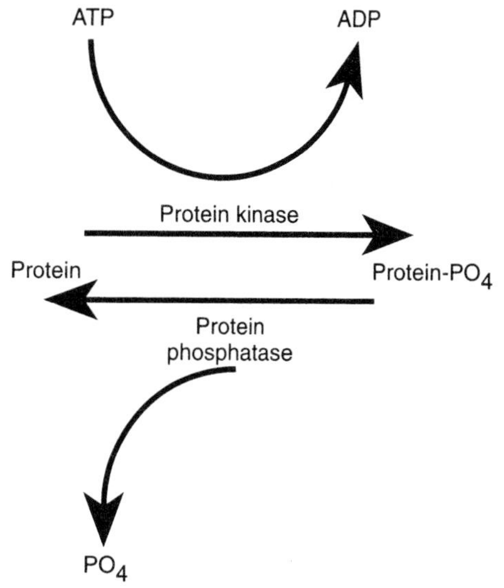

FIGURE 3.2–4

Regulation of protein function by phosphorylation. Numerous cellular proteins are activated or inactivated by the addition of a phosphate group (PO_4) from adenosine triphosphate (ATP). Addition of the phosphate is catalyzed by specific protein kinases, while removal of the phosphate is catalyzed by protein phosphatases. (Courtesy of Jack A. Grebb, M.D.)

Protein Kinases. One of the primary activities of the second-messenger molecules is to activate a class of molecules known as the protein kinases. *Protein kinases* catalyze the transfer of the terminal phosphate group of ATP onto protein molecules (Fig. 3.2–4). Each of the second-messenger molecules is associated with the activation of a specific protein kinase. Four protein kinases (cAMP-dependent protein kinase [PKA], cGMP-dependent protein kinase [PKG], calcium/calmodulin-dependent protein kinase [CaMK], and calcium/phosphatidylserine-dependent protein kinase, also known as protein kinase C [PKC]) phosphorylate serine or threonine residues in proteins. In contrast, the receptor tyrosine kinases phosphorylate tyrosine residues in proteins without involving a second messenger. Tyrosine kinases are activated by growth factors binding to specific transmembrane receptors.

Protein phosphorylation is the best-studied example of how reversible, posttranslational modification of a protein can change its function. Protein phosphorylation is reversible by the activities of another class of enzymes, the protein phosphatases, which remove the phosphate group from the protein (Fig. 3.2–4). The addition or the deletion of the negatively charged phosphate group changes the charge and can change the shape of the protein molecule. This change in charge and shape can affect the function of the protein and essentially serves as a molecular on-off switch for the function of the protein. Moreover, proteins are usually phosphorylated on multiple sites by different protein kinases; therefore, fine adjustment of the function of the protein is possible, in addition to simply turning the protein on or off. An example of regulation by phosphorylation is the β-receptor. The sensitivity of this receptor to its ligand is regulated by the state of the receptor's phosphorylation.

Protein phosphorylation has been traced through many metabolic pathways in which a cascade of phosphorylations regulates a chain of enzymatic reactions. The regulation of glucose metabolism and the citric acid cycle are two examples. Kinases also play an important role in the regulation of cellular proliferation—many oncogenes are kinases—and the regulation of numerous other genes. In psychiatry, lithium therapy has been shown to reduce the activity of protein kinase C in concert with its salutary effects on bipolar disorder. It is very likely that ongoing investigations will implicate kinases in the etiology of other psychiatric disorders.

NEUROTRANSMITTERS

A molecule must meet a number of criteria to be classified as a neurotransmitter (Table 3.2–3). These criteria must usually be met through a variety of basic science and clinical research studies. Substances that have only been shown to meet a few of the criteria are referred to as *putative neurotransmitters,* meaning they have not been shown experimentally to meet all of the criteria.

Table 3.2–3
Criteria for a Neurotransmitter

1. The molecule is synthesized in the neuron.
2. The molecule is present in the presynaptic neuron and is released on depolarization in physiologically significant amounts.
3. When administered exogenously as a drug, the exogenous molecule mimics the effects of the endogenous neurotransmitter.
4. A mechanism in the neurons or the synaptic cleft acts to remove or deactivate the neurotransmitter.

Chemical Neurotransmission

Chemical neurotransmission is the process involving the release of a neurotransmitter by one neuron and the binding of the neurotransmitter molecule to a receptor on another neuron. The process of chemical neurotransmission is affected by most drugs used in psychiatry. Older antipsychotics, but not the serotonin-dopamine antagonists, are believed to exert their effects mainly by blocking dopamine type 2 (D_2) receptors; virtually all antidepressants are believed to exert their effects by increasing the amount of serotonin or norepinephrine or both in the synaptic cleft; and almost all benzodiazepine anxiolytics are believed to exert their effects on the $GABA_A$ receptors that are linked to chloride ion channels.

Neuromodulators and Neurohormones. The word used most commonly to denote the chemical signals that flow between neurons is *neurotransmitter,* although the words *neuromodulators* and *neurohormones* are also used in some cases to emphasize specific characteristics. In contrast to the characteristically immediate and short-lived effects of a neurotransmitter, a neuromodulator, as the name implies, modulates the response of a neuron to a neurotransmitter. The modulatory effect may be present for a longer time than is usual for a neurotransmitter molecule to be present. Thus, a neuromodulating substance may have an effect on a neuron over a long period of time, and that effect may be more involved with fine tuning than with activating or directly inhibiting the generation of an action potential. A neurohormone is distinguished by the fact that it is released into the bloodstream rather than into the extraneuronal space in the brain. Once in the bloodstream, the neurohormone can then diffuse into the extraneuronal space and have its effects on neurons.

Classification. The three major types of neurotransmitters in the brain are the biogenic amines, the amino acids, and the peptides (Fig. 3.2–2). The biogenic amines are the best known and most understood neurotransmitters because they were the first to be discovered. However, they constitute the neurotransmitter substance in only a small percentage of neurons. The amino acid neurotransmitters were late to be discovered, principally because of the difficulty in differentiating amino acids present in most proteins from the same amino acids acting separately as neurotransmitters. The amino acid neurotransmitters are present in upward of 70 percent of neurons. The peptide neurotransmitters are intermediate in terms of the percentage of neurons that contain a neurotransmitter of that type, but they far surpass the other two categories in the sheer number (about 200 to 300) of neurotransmitters of that type that have been putatively identified. The full neurotransmitter criteria have been met for only a few of these peptides at this time (Table 3.2–3). Nevertheless, the evidence indicating that the putative peptide neurotransmitters are, in fact, neurotransmitters is generally robust. Recent data have led to the identification of at least four other classes of neurotransmitters—nucleotides, gases, eicosanoids, and anandamides—and have hinted at receptors for others, including so-called sigma (Σ) receptors.

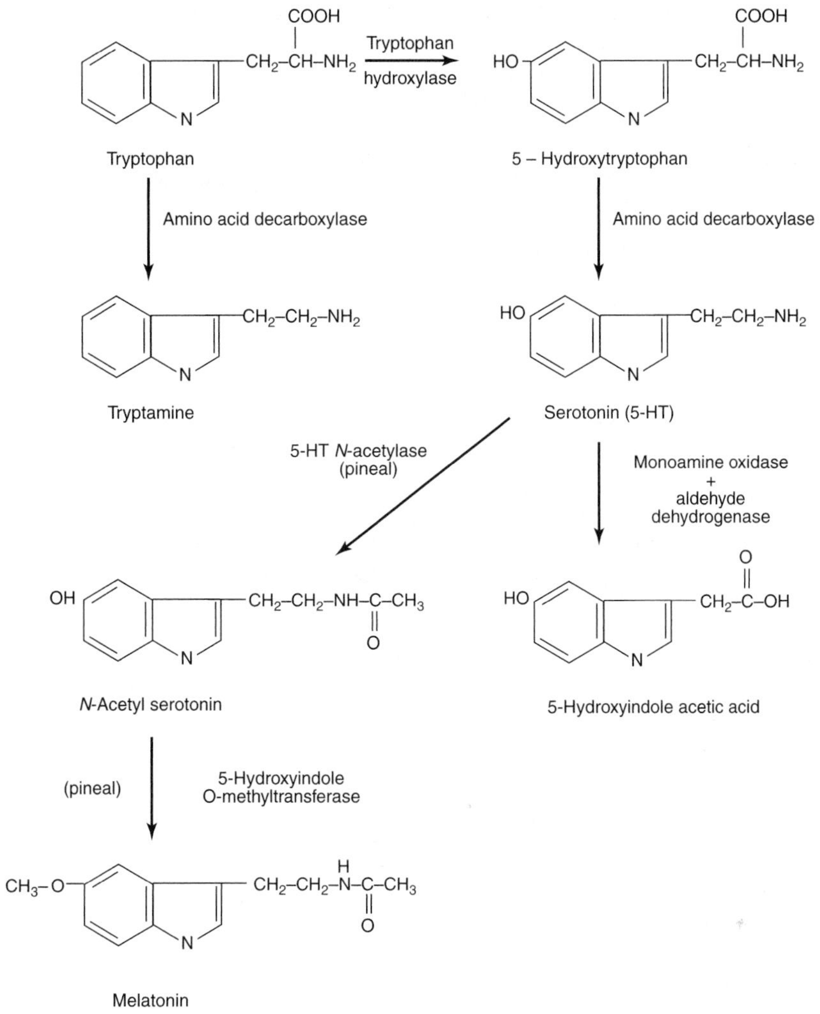

FIGURE 3.2–5
Synthetic and metabolic pathways of serotonin. (From Cooper JR, Bloom FE, Roth RH. *The Biochemical Basis of Neuropharmacology.* 7th ed. New York: Oxford University Press; 1996:355.)

Thus, the current psychopharmacological agents influence only a small fraction of the neurons in the brain. This may represent a fortunate coincidence, as drugs that influence amino acid neurotransmitters generally have adverse effects at low doses, and relatively few drugs have been found to act on peptide receptors, most notably the opiates. The small number of biogenic amine-containing neurons belies their significant functional importance, because they project widely throughout the brain and modulate activity in practically every brain region.

BIOGENIC AMINES

Each of these neurotransmitters is synthesized in a discrete nucleus of neurons from which axons project widely throughout the brain and spinal cord. They therefore exert a disproportionate influence on the activity of the brain, and they are of central importance to the pharmacological therapy of thought disorders, mood disorders, and anxiety disorders. Dopamine, norepinephrine, and epinephrine are products of the catecholamine synthetic pathway, whereas serotonin, acetylcholine, and histamine are derived from distinct precursors (Fig. 3.2–5). A full understanding of the role of these neurotransmitters in psychiatry includes knowledge of their anatomy, their life cycle (synthesis, secretion, reuptake, and degradation), receptors, and the drugs that modify their activity (Fig. 3.2–6).

Dopamine

CNS Dopaminergic Tracts. The three most important dopaminergic tracts for psychiatry are the nigrostriatal tract, the mesolimbic-mesocortical tract, and the tuberoinfundibular tract (Fig. 3.2–7). The nigrostriatal tract projects from its cell bodies in the substantia nigra to the corpus striatum. When the D_2 receptors at the end of this tract are blocked by classic antipsychotic drugs, parkinsonian side effects emerge. In Parkinson's disease the nigrostriatal tract degenerates, resulting in the motor symptoms of the disease. Because of the significant association between Parkinson's disease and depression, the nigrostriatal tract may somehow be involved with the control of mood, in addition to its classic role in motor control.

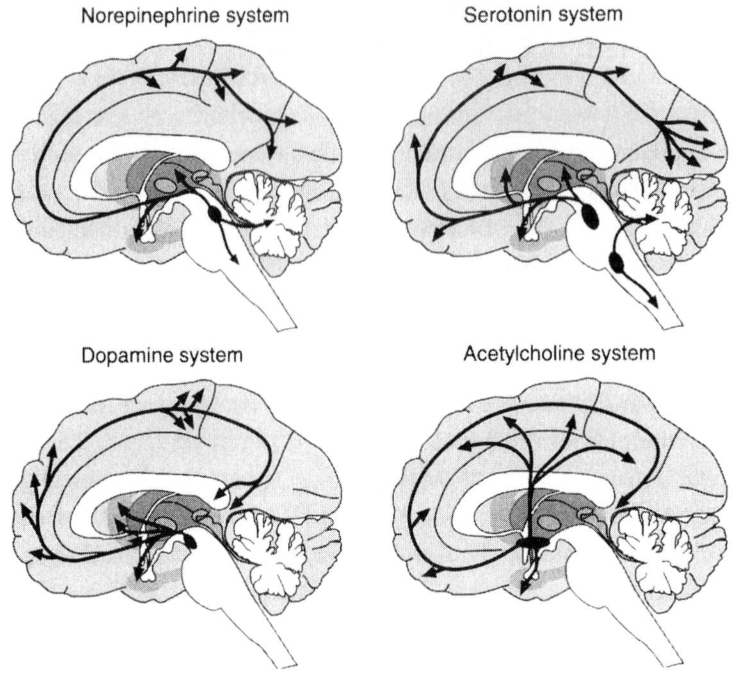

FIGURE 3.2–6

The four major biogenic amine neuromodulatory systems. Each biogenic amine neurotransmitter system originates in a subcortical nucleus (*black ovals*) and sends numerous projections diffusely throughout the higher brain regions (*black arrows*). Norepinephrine system: cell bodies reside in the locus ceruleus **(top left)**. Serotonin system: cell bodies reside in the rostral and caudal raphe nuclei **(top right)**. Dopamine system: cell bodies reside in the contiguous substantia nigra and ventral tegmental area **(bottom left)**. Acetylcholine system: cell bodies reside in the nucleus basalis of Meynert **(bottom right)**. (Modified from Spitzer M. *The Mind Within the Net: Models of Learning, Thinking, and Acting*. Cambridge, MA: Bradford; 1999:270, with permission.)

D_2 receptors in the caudate nucleus suppress the activity of the caudate nucleus. The caudate neurons regulate motor acts by gating which intended acts are actually carried out. The absence of D_2 receptor activity allows the caudate to dampen motor activity excessively, resulting in the bradykinesia that typifies parkinsonism. At the other extreme, excess dopamine activity in the caudate removes the gating control and may result in extraneous motor acts, such as tics. A recent study of obsessive-compulsive disorder patients, for example, correlated increased caudate dopamine analogue binding, which reflects increased numbers of the D_2 receptors, with more prominent clinical tics.

The mesolimbic-mesocortical tract projects from its cell bodies in the ventral tegmental area (VTA), which lies adjacent to the substantia nigra, to most areas of the cerebral cortex and the limbic system. Because the tract projects to the limbic system and the neocortex, the tract may be involved in mediating the antipsychotic effects of antipsychotic drugs.

The cell bodies of the tuberoinfundibular tract are in the arcuate nucleus and the periventricular area of the hypothalamus and project to the infundibulum and the anterior pituitary. Dopamine acts as a release-inhibiting factor in the tract by inhibiting the release of prolactin from the anterior pituitary. Patients who take dopamine receptor antagonists often have roughly threefold elevated prolactin levels because the blockade of dopamine receptors in the tract eliminates the inhibitory effect of dopamine.

Dopamine Life Cycle. The dopaminergic axon terminal is the site of synthesis for dopamine. Dopamine is one of the three catecholamine neurotransmitters that are synthesized starting with the amino acid tyrosine. The other two catecholamine neurotransmitters are norepinephrine and epinephrine (Fig. 3.2–8). The rate-limiting enzymatic step in the synthesis of any of the catecholamines is catalyzed by tyrosine hydroxylase. Therefore, dietary changes in tyrosine levels do not influence the synthesis of catecholamines. Tyrosine hydroxylase is a phosphoprotein that is subject to regulation by a range of protein kinases and protein phosphatases. Tyrosine hydroxylase transforms tyrosine into 3,4-dihydroxyphenylalanine (dopa). Because it is beyond the rate-limiting synthetic step, dopa may be administered orally to increase the rate of synthesis of its product, dopamine, and dopa is used for this purpose to treat Parkinson's disease. Once dopamine is produced, it is taken into synaptic vesicles by specific transporters and then released into the synaptic cleft on depolarization of the axon terminal.

The actions of dopamine are terminated by two general routes. First, dopamine can be taken back up into the presynaptic neuron and recycled as a neurotransmitter; this pathway is generally referred to as the *reuptake mechanism*. Reuptake occurs by the passage of the dopamine molecule from the synaptic space, through the presynaptic dopamine transporter, into the intracellular space, where it is packaged into vesicles. Second, dopamine can be metabolized. The two major enzymes involved in the metabolism of dopamine are MAO and, less importantly, catechol-*O*-methyltransferase (COMT). MAO is localized on the outer mitochondrial membrane, principally in the presynaptic terminal, where it acts on dopamine that has been taken up into the presynaptic terminal but not yet repackaged into vesicles. COMT is a soluble enzyme localized in the cytoplasm of the postsynaptic cell and of glial cells and, possibly also, extracellularly. When dopamine is metabolized extraneuronally by COMT, the resulting metabolites are then taken back into the neuron and further metabolized by MAO. As dis-

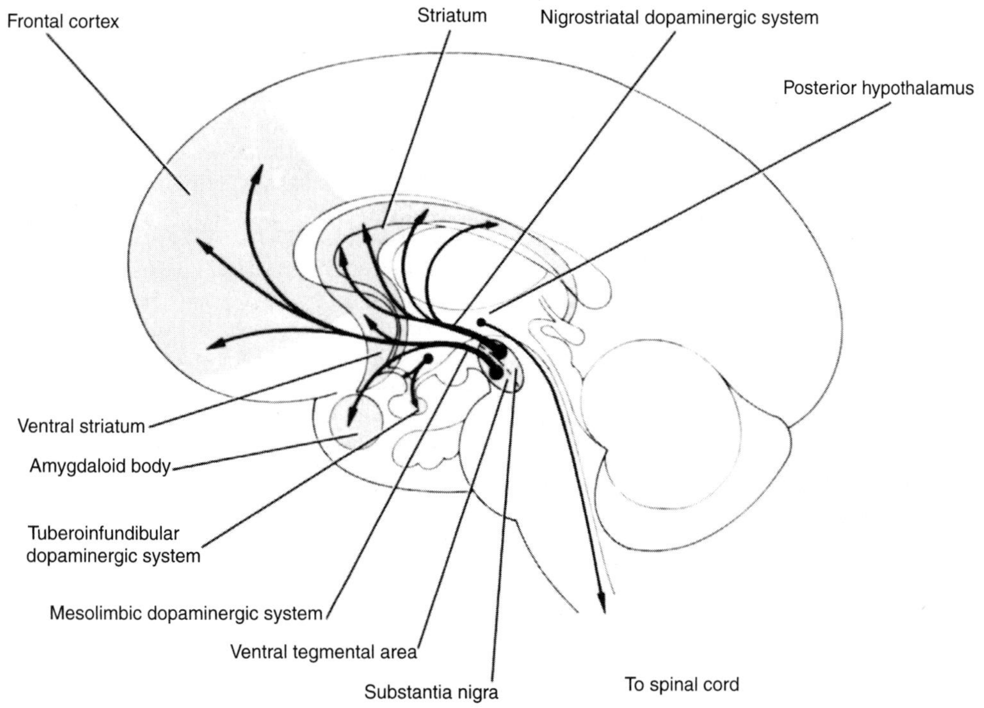

FIGURE 3.2–7

Dopaminergic (DA) pathways. The nigrostriatal DA system originates in the substantia nigra and terminates in the main dorsal part of the striatum. The ventral tegmental area gives rise to the mesolimbic DA system, which terminates in the ventral striatum, the amygdaloid body, the frontal lobe, and some other basal forebrain areas. The tuberoinfundibular system innervates the median eminence and the posterior and intermediate lobes of the pituitary, and dopamine neurons in the posterior hypothalamus project to the spinal cord. (Reprinted with permission from Heimer L. *The Human Brain and Spinal Cord.* New York: Springer; 1983.)

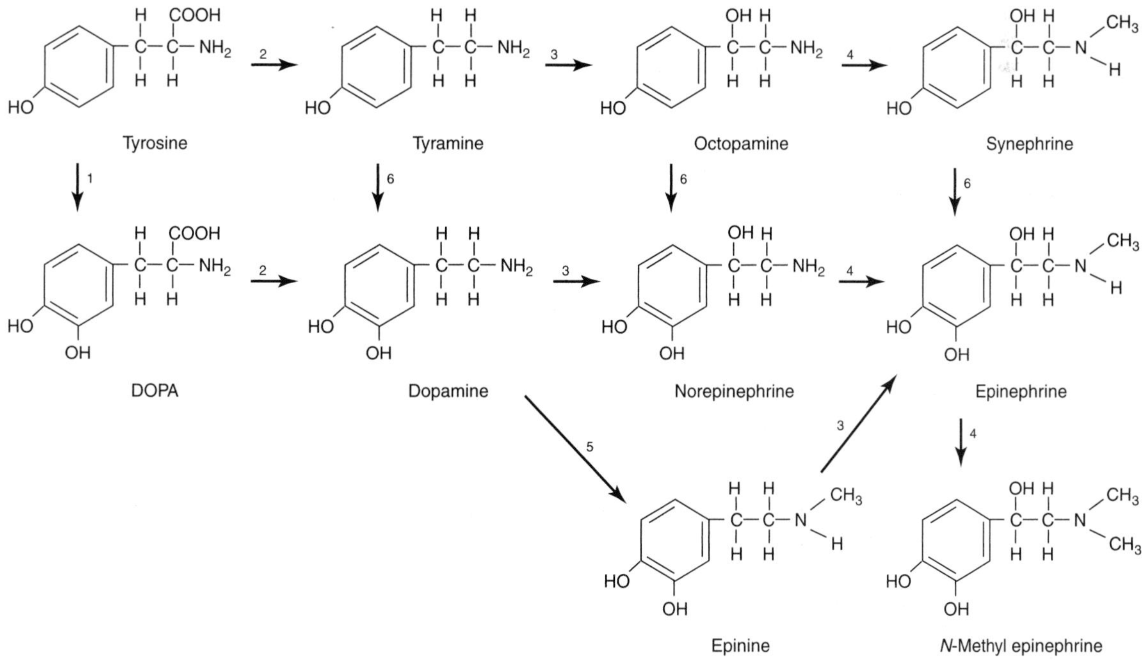

FIGURE 3.2–8

Primary and alternative pathways for the formation of catecholamines: (1) tyrosine hydroxylase; (2) aromatic amino acid decarboxylase; (3) dopamine-β-hydroxylase; (4) phenylethanolamine-*N*-methyltransferase; (5) nonspecific *N*-methyltransferase in lung and folate-dependent *N*-methyltransferase in brain; (6) catechol-forming enzyme. (Reprinted with permission from Cooper JR, Bloom FE, Roth RH. *The Biochemical Basis of Neuropharmacology.* 7th ed. New York: Oxford University Press; 1996:232.)

cussed above there are two types of MAOs; MAO_B selectively metabolizes dopamine. The primary metabolite of dopamine is homovanillic acid (HVA), and many research studies of cerebrospinal fluid, urine, and serum attempt to assess dopamine activity in the CNS by measuring concentrations of HVA.

Dopamine Receptors. The five subtypes of dopamine receptors (listed in Table 3.2–2) can be put into two groups. In the first group the D_1 and D_5 receptors stimulate the formulation of cAMP by activating the stimulatory G protein, G_s. The D_5 receptor has only recently been discovered, and less is known about it than about the D_1 receptor. One difference between these two receptors is that the D_5 receptor has a much higher affinity for dopamine than does the D_1 receptor. The second group of dopamine receptors is made up of the D_2, D_3, and D_4 receptors. The D_2 receptor inhibits the formation of cAMP by activating the inhibitory G protein, G_i, and some data indicate that the D_3 and D_4 receptors act similarly. One of the differences among the D_2, D_3, and D_4 receptors is their differential distribution. The D_2 receptor is prominent in the striatum (caudate nucleus and putamen), the D_3 receptor is especially concentrated in the nucleus accumbens, in addition to other regions, and the D_4 receptor is especially concentrated in the frontal cortex, in addition to other regions.

In a recent study, a scale of emotional detachment, with high values for aloofness and vindictiveness and low values for overly nurturing behavior and excessive exploitability, was used to rate 24 individuals, and then the density of D_2 receptors was determined in each person's putamen. A strong correlation was found between high levels of detachment and a low density of putaminal D_2 receptors, while low levels of detachment correlated strongly with high D_2 receptor density. This finding is in keeping with the clinical observation that D_2 receptor antagonists (i.e., typical antipsychotic drugs) reduce the positive symptoms of schizophrenia, such as hallucinations and delusions, but may worsen the negative symptoms, such as social ambivalence and catatonia. In another study, experts postulate that dopamine activity may act in the medial left prefrontal cortex to suppress signals of emotional distress. A recent report supporting this hypothesis correlated a genetic polymorphism in the D_4 receptor with differences in subjective reports of mood.

Dopamine and Drugs. In the past, the potency of antipsychotic compounds has been correlated with their affinity for the D_2 receptor. Since blockade of dopamine receptors, particularly the D_2 receptor, has been associated with the efficacy of antipsychotic drugs, long-term administration of dopamine receptor antagonists results in an upregulation in the number of dopamine receptors present. This upregulation may be involved in the development of tardive dyskinesia. The development of a new class of highly effective antipsychotic agents, called the serotonin-dopamine antagonists because they block predominantly the serotonin type $5\text{-}HT_2$ and, to a lesser extent, the D_2 receptors, has led to a reassessment of the D_2 receptor affinity hypothesis of antipsychotic potency. Serotonin-dopamine antagonists are associated with a greatly reduced risk of development of parkinsonian side effects and tardive dyskinesia, and not only do they treat the positive symptoms of schizophrenia, effectively treated by pure D_2 receptor antagonists (psychosis, hallucinations, agitation), they also improve the negative symptoms of schizophrenia (blunted affect, ambivalence, catatonia).

Other substances that affect the dopamine system are amphetamines and cocaine. Amphetamines cause the release of dopamine, and cocaine blocks the uptake of dopamine. Thus, the substances increase the amount of dopamine present in the synapse. Cocaine and methamphetamine (Desoxyn) are among the most addicting substances. Their use may permanently deplete the brain's stores of dopamine. The dopaminergic systems may be particularly involved in the brain's so-called reward or pleasure-seeking system, and this involvement may explain the high addiction potential of cocaine. Mutant "knockout mice," in which the dopamine transporter gene has been experimentally deleted, do not respond biochemically or behaviorally to cocaine. This suggests that the dopamine transporter is necessary for the pharmacological effects of cocaine. Studies in rats showed that D_2 receptor agonists increased cocaine self-administration, while D_1 receptor agonists lowered the desire for cocaine. Nicotine, the most psychoactive ingredient in cigarette smoke, stimulates the release of dopamine and glutamate. Epidemiological studies have found that smokers have a reduced risk of developing Parkinson's disease, Alzheimer's disease, and ulcerative colitis. A nicotine analogue that stimulates dopamine release is under study for treatment of Parkinson's disease, and the nicotine transdermal patch is being studied to counteract the cognitive impairment caused by treatment with haloperidol (Haldol). The nicotine-stained fingers of many schizophrenia patients may be a sign that they are medicating themselves unknowingly with their powerful neurotransmitter.

The dopamine transporter may be blocked by benztropine (Cogentin) and bupropion (Wellbutrin), though it is unlikely that sufficient CNS concentrations of these drugs are routinely obtained to have an appreciable effect on dopamine transport. The transporter is the portal of entry of the neurotoxin methylphenyltetrahydropyridine (MPTP), which may cause parkinsonism by killing the nigral dopaminergic neurons. Dopamine-containing storage vesicles are depleted irreversibly by reserpine (Serpasil) and reversibly by tetrabenazine.

Dopamine and Psychopathology. The *dopamine hypothesis of schizophrenia* grew from the observations that drugs that block dopamine receptors (e.g., haloperidol) have antipsychotic activity and drugs that stimulate dopamine activity (e.g., amphetamine) can induce psychotic symptoms in nonschizophrenic persons when given in high enough doses. The dopamine hypothesis remains the leading neurochemical hypothesis for schizophrenia, but room is being made for a role for serotonin, based on the therapeutic success of the serotonin-dopamine antagonists. A recent series of studies showed that plasma concentrations of HVA are, in fact, reduced in many schizophrenic patients who respond to antipsychotic drugs. A major problem with the hypothesis is that blockade of dopamine receptors reduces psychotic symptoms in virtually any disorder, such as psychosis associated with a brain tumor and psychosis associated with mania. Thus, some as yet unrecognized neurochemical abnormality in schizophrenia may be unique to the condition.

Dopamine may also be involved in the pathophysiology of mood disorders. Dopamine activity may be low in depression and high in mania. Amphetamines, which potentiate dopamine activity, are highly effective antidepressants. The observation that levodopa (Larodopa) can cause mania and psychosis in some parkinsonian patients also supports the hypothesis. Some studies have found low levels of dopamine metabolites in depressed patients.

Norepinephrine and Epinephrine

Although norepinephrine and epinephrine are discussed together, norepinephrine is the more important and more abun-

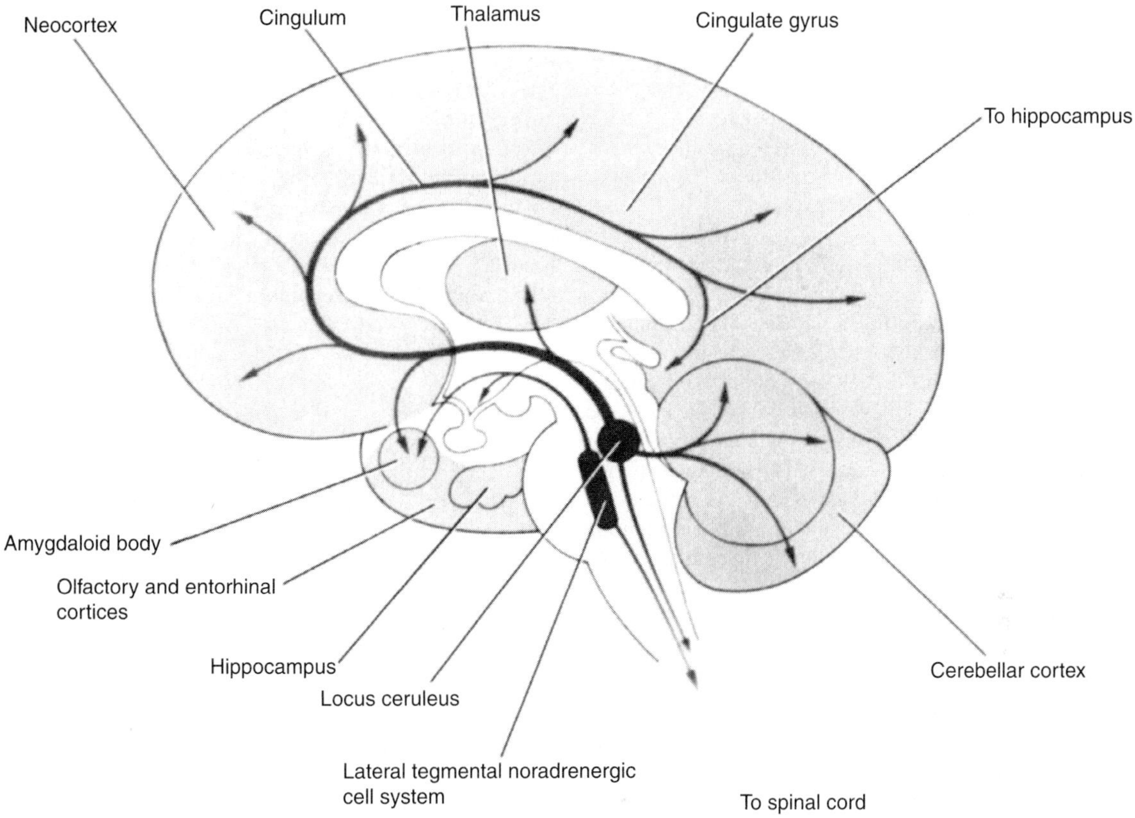

FIGURE 3.2–9

Noradrenergic pathways. The locus ceruleus, which is located immediately underneath the floor of the fourth ventricle in the rostrolateral part of the pons, is the most important noradrenergic nucleus in the brain. Its projections reach many areas in the forebrain, the cerebellum, and the spinal cord. Noradrenergic neurons in the lateral brainstem tegmentum innervate several structures in the basal forebrain, including the hypothalamus and the amygdaloid body. (Reprinted with permission from Heimer L. *The Human Brain and Spinal Cord.* New York: Springer; 1983.)

dant of the two related neurotransmitters in the brain, although adrenally derived epinephrine is more abundant than norepinephrine in the serum. The norepinephrine system and the epinephrine system are also referred to as the noradrenergic system and the adrenergic system, respectively. The receptors are referred to simply as adrenergic receptors, however, because they are receptors for both epinephrine and norepinephrine.

CNS Noradrenergic Tracts. The major concentration of noradrenergic (and adrenergic) cell bodies that project upward in the brain is in the compact locus ceruleus in the pons (Fig. 3.2–9). The axons of these neurons project through the medial forebrain bundle to the cerebral cortex, the limbic system, the thalamus, and the hypothalamus.

Norepinephrine and Epinephrine Life Cycle. Norepinephrine and epinephrine, along with dopamine, constitute the catecholamines. As discussed above, the catecholamines are synthesized from tyrosine, and the rate-limiting enzyme is tyrosine hydroxylase (Fig. 3.2–8). In neurons that release norepinephrine, the enzyme dopamine β-hydroxylase converts dopamine to norepinephrine; neurons that release dopamine lack this enzyme. In neurons that release epinephrine, the enzyme phenylethanolamine-*N*-methyltransferase (PNMT) converts norepinephrine into epinephrine. Neurons that release either dopamine or norepinephrine do not have PNMT.

Once norepinephrine or epinephrine is formed, it is taken through specific transporter proteins into synaptic vesicles, from which it is released on depolarization of the axonal terminal. As with dopamine, the two major routes of deactivation are uptake back into the presynaptic neuron and metabolism by MAO and COMT. The MAO_A subtype preferentially metabolizes norepinephrine and epinephrine, as well as serotonin.

Noradrenergic and Adrenergic Receptors. The two broad groups of adrenergic and noradrenergic receptors, often just referred to as adrenergic receptors, are the α-adrenergic receptors and the β-adrenergic receptors (Table 3.2–2). The advances of molecular biology have now subtyped these receptors into three types of α_1-receptors (α_{1a}, α_{1b}, and α_{1d}), three types of α_2-receptors (α_{2a}, α_{2c}, α_{2b}), one type of α_3-receptor, and three types of β-receptors (β_1, β_2, and β_3). Although the field is changing rapidly, all α_1-receptors seem to be linked to the phosphoinositol turnover system, α-receptors seem to inhibit the formation of cAMP, and β-receptors seem to stimulate the formation of cAMP. The surface availability and the efficiency of signal transduction of the adrenergic receptors are constantly regulated by phosphorylations and changes in pro-

tein-protein interactions. Significant data have long been available on the β_1- and β_2-receptors, which regulate the function of nearly every organ in the body, often in antagonism to the effects of the α receptors. The β_3-receptors have recently been found to regulate energy metabolism. They are expressed in adipocytes, and their activation by agonists reduces the amount of body fat. They are therefore a target for the development of antiobesity drugs.

Norepinephrine and Drugs. The psychiatric drugs that are most associated with norepinephrine are the classic antidepressant drugs, the tricyclic drugs and the MAO inhibitors (MAOIs), and, more recently, venlafaxine (Effexor), mirtazapine (Remeron), bupropion, and nefazodone (Serzone). The tricyclic drugs, venlafaxine, bupropion, and nefazodone block the reuptake of norepinephrine (and serotonin) into the presynaptic neuron, and the MAOIs block the catabolism of norepinephrine (and serotonin). Thus, the immediate effect of tricyclic drugs and MAOIs is to increase the concentrations of norepinephrine (and serotonin) in the synaptic cleft. Since antidepressants take 2 to 4 weeks to exert their therapeutic effects, it is obviously not the immediate effect alone that results in their beneficial effects. However, the immediate effects may eventually lead to a downregulation of the number of postsynaptic β-receptors, and this downregulation of postsynaptic β-receptors has been correlated with clinical improvement. Mirtazapine acts by blocking the presynaptic α_2-receptors and thus removing the feedback inhibition normally exerted on the release of norepinephrine. The net effect of mirtazapine is to increase norepinephrine secretion.

The α-adrenergic system is also involved in the production of some of the adverse events that can be seen with many psychotherapeutic drugs. Blockade of the α_1-receptors is commonly associated with sedation and postural hypotension. Another drug that affects the α-adrenergic system is clonidine (Catapres), which is an α-receptor agonist. The α_2-receptors are generally located on the presynaptic neuron in the CNS, and activation of these receptors downregulates the production and the release of norepinephrine. The sympatholytic actions of clonidine have been used for a variety of psychiatric disorders, including opioid withdrawal. The antihypertensive agent methyldopa (Aldomet) is a competitive inhibitor of L-aromatic amino acid decarboxylase, which transforms methyldopa to methyldopamine and eventually to methylnorepinephrine, which displaces norepinephrine from storage vesicles. Methylnorepinephrine acts as an α_2-receptor agonist to lower blood pressure. The α_2-receptor antagonist yohimbine (Yocon) is used to reverse the antisexual effects of antidepressants, especially those of the serotonergic class.

The β-adrenergic receptor antagonists, such as propranolol (Inderal), have also been used in psychiatry. In general, β-receptors are located postsynaptically, and inhibition of their activity results in a decrease in cAMP formation in the postsynaptic neuron. The β-adrenergic antagonists have been used to treat social phobia (e.g., performance anxiety), akathisia (a movement disorder associated with antipsychotic compounds), and lithium-induced tremor.

Norepinephrine and Psychopathology. The *biogenic amine hypothesis of mood disorders* was based on the observation that the tricyclic drugs and the MAOIs are effective in alleviating the symptoms of depression. What the relative roles of serotonin and norepinephrine are in the pathophysiology of depression is still unclear. Drugs that affect both neurotransmitters are effective, and drugs that affect primarily norepinephrine—for example, desipramine (Norpramin)—and drugs that affect primarily serotonin—for example, fluoxetine—are also effective. When noradrenergic neurons are destroyed in experimental animal models, however, drugs that affect serotonin do not have their usual effects; and when serotonergic neurons are destroyed, drugs that affect norepinephrine do not have their usual effects. These experimental results indicate that the interrelationships between serotonergic and noradrenergic neurons are incompletely understood.

Serotonin

CNS Serotonergic Tracts. The major site of serotonergic cell bodies is in the upper pons and the midbrain—specifically, the median and dorsal raphe nuclei and, to a lesser extent, the caudal locus ceruleus, the area postrema, and the interpeduncular area (Fig. 3.2–10). These neurons project to the basal ganglia, the limbic system, and the cerebral cortex.

Serotonin Life Cycle. As with the catecholamines, serotonin is synthesized in the axonal terminal (Fig. 3.2–5). The precursor amino acid is tryptophan. In contrast to the catecholamines, the availability of tryptophan is the rate-limiting function, and the enzyme tryptophan hydroxylase is not rate limiting. Therefore, dietary variations in tryptophan can measurably affect serotonin levels in the brain. For example, tryptophan depletion causes irritability and hunger, whereas tryptophan supplementation may induce sleep, relieve anxiety, and increase a sense of well-being. Once synthesized, serotonin is packaged into vesicles for release upon the arrival of an action potential. The synaptic action of serotonin is terminated by reuptake into the presynaptic terminal by the plasma membrane transporter. The promotor of the transporter gene contains a polymorphism that creates a twofold variation in the amount of transporter between different individuals, which in some way may account for 3 to 4 percent of the biological variation in levels of anxiety. The key enzyme involved in the metabolism of serotonin is MAO, preferentially MAO_A, and the primary metabolite is 5-hydroxyindoleacetic acid (5-HIAA) (Fig. 3.2–6).

Serotonergic Receptors. Seven types of serotonin receptors are now recognized—$5\text{-}HT_1$ through $5\text{-}HT_7$, with numerous subtypes, totaling 14 distinct receptors. The various functional effector mechanisms of some of these receptors are listed in Table 3.2–2. The diversity of serotonin receptors has initiated a significant effort to study the distribution of serotonin receptor subtypes in pathological states and to design subtype-specific drugs that may be of particular therapeutic benefit in specific conditions. For example, buspirone (BuSpar), a clinically effective anxiolytic, is a potent $5\text{-}HT_{1A}$ agonist, and other $5\text{-}HT_{1A}$ agonists are being developed for the treatment of anxiety and depression. Clozapine (Clozaril), the prototypical serotonin-dopamine antagonist antipsychotic agent, has significant activity as an antagonist of $5\text{-}HT_2$ receptors, and this observation has initiated a major effort to study the role of this seroto-

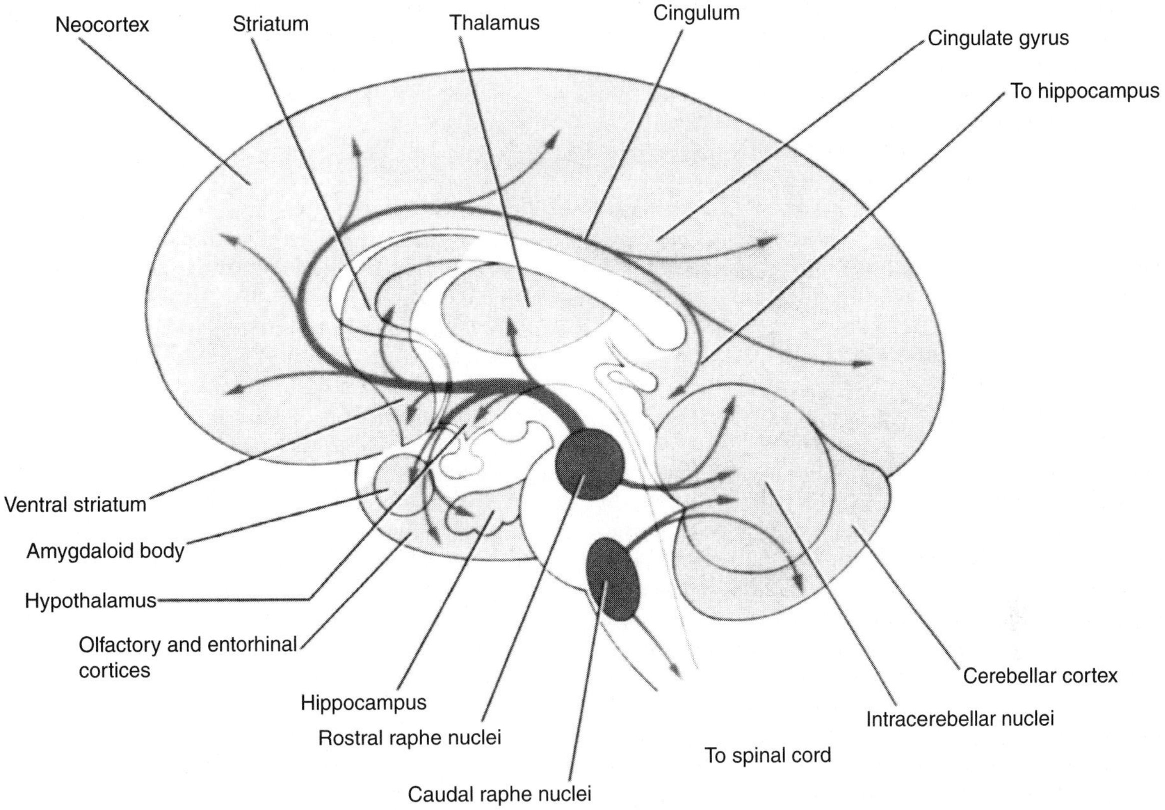

FIGURE 3.2–10

Serotonergic (5-HT) pathways. The raphe nuclei form a more or less continuous collection of cell groups close to the midline throughout the brainstem, but for the sake of simplicity, they have been subdivided into a rostral group and a caudal group in the drawing. The rostral raphe nuclei project to a large number of forebrain structures. The fibers that project laterally through the internal and external capsules to widespread areas of the neocortex are not indicated in this highly schematic drawing. (Reprinted with permission from Heimer L. *The Human Brain and Spinal Cord.* New York: Springer; 1983.)

nin receptor subtype and to develop drugs that are 5-HT_2 antagonists for the treatment of schizophrenia.

Antagonists of the 5-HT_3 receptor are also under study as potential antianxiety and antipsychotic compounds. The distributed serotonin receptors are sometimes responsible for the side effects of serotonergic drugs, many of which nonspecifically raise serotonin levels and thus indiscriminately increase receptor activation. Serotonin receptors in the basal ganglia may be responsible for akathisia and agitation; 5-HT_3 receptors in the brainstem vomiting center (area postrema) or the hypothalamus may cause nausea and vomiting; receptors in the limbic system may cause an initial increase in anxiety; receptors in various parts of the brainstem sleep centers may produce either insomnia or somnolence; spinal cord pathways may produce sexual dysfunction; receptors in the intestines (where 90 percent of the body's serotonin is found) may cause gastrointestinal upset and diarrhea; and receptors in the cranial blood vessel may cause headache. One cannot predict which adverse effects, if any, will occur in a particular patient.

Serotonin and Drugs. Some of the new relations between serotonin and drugs under development are discussed above; however, the historical association of serotonin and psychotropic drugs was first made with the tricyclic drugs and the MAOIs, as described for norepinephrine and epinephrine. The tricyclic drugs and the MAOIs, respectively, block the uptake and the metabolism of serotonin and norepinephrine, thus increasing the concentration of both neurotransmitters in the synaptic cleft. Fluoxetine is one of the SSRIs that are used in the treatment of depression. Other drugs in that class include paroxetine (Paxil), sertraline (Zoloft), fluvoxamine (Luvox), and citalopram (Celexa), all of which are usually associated with minimal adverse effects, especially in comparison with the tricyclic drugs and the MAOIs.

Venlafaxine blocks the reuptake of both serotonin and norepinephrine. With respect to serotonin, both trazodone (Desyrel) and nefazodone block the reuptake of serotonin and directly antagonize 5-HT_2 receptors, with the net effect stimulating 5-HT_1 receptors. Trazodone and nefazodone and the 5-HT_1 receptor agonist buspirone are the first of what will likely be a series of drugs that target subtypes of serotonin receptors.

Another serotonergic drug that has been used in psychiatry is L-tryptophan. Because the concentration of L-tryptophan is the rate-limiting function in the synthesis of serotonin, ingestion of L-tryptophan can increase the concentration of serotonin in the CNS. L-Tryptophan was withdrawn from the market in 1990 in the United States by the Food and Drug Administration (FDA) because a contaminant from the production process at one particular manufacturing site caused an eosinophilia-myal-

gia syndrome in some patients taking the drug. Recent data suggest that L-tryptophan itself may cause the eosinophilia-myalgia syndrome.

Serotonin is also involved in the mechanism of at least two major substances of abuse, lysergic acid diethylamide (LSD) and 3,4-methylenedioxymethamphetamine (MDMA), also known as "ecstasy." The serotonin system is the major site of action for LSD, but exactly how LSD exerts its effects remains unclear. MDMA has dual effects: blocking the uptake of serotonin and inducing the massive release of the serotonin contents of serotonergic neurons.

Serotonin and Psychopathology. The principal association of serotonin with a psychopathological condition is with depression, as suggested in the biogenic amine hypothesis of mood disorders. This hypothesis is simply that depression is associated with too little serotonin and that mania is associated with too much serotonin. As explained above for norepinephrine, that simplified view is undoubtedly not entirely accurate. The *permissive hypothesis* postulates that low levels of serotonin permit abnormal levels of norepinephrine to cause depression or mania. With the introduction of a variety of new drugs, serotonin is one of the most exciting areas for research in the anxiety disorders and schizophrenia, in addition to its role in depression. For example, early theories about the causes of anxiety focused on the GABA system because the first effective anxiolytics were the benzodiazepines, which potentiate GABAergic neurotransmission. With the recent success of SSRIs and buspirone, which are effective antianxiety agents, the theory of anxiety needed room for a role for serotonin. Similarly, schizophrenia was previously thought to result from an imbalance of dopamine, but since the therapeutic success of the serotonin-dopamine antagonists, schizophrenia is now thought to result from misregulation of both dopamine and serotonin function. It is likely that theories will need to be revised several times over in the near future as agents become available for modification of particular receptor subtypes.

PEPTIDE NEUROTRANSMITTERS

As many as 300 peptide neurotransmitters may be in the human brain. A peptide is a short protein consisting of fewer than 100 amino acids. Peptides are made in the neuronal cell body by the transcription and translation of a genetic message. Peptides are stored in synaptic vesicles and are released from the axon terminals. The activity of peptides is terminated by the action of enzymes, peptidases, which cleave the peptides between specific amino acid residues. In addition to the regulatory mechanisms shared with other neurotransmitters, neuroactive peptides are subject to additional refinements in regulation. Differential ribonucleic acid (RNA) processing of the RNA first transcribed from the deoxyribonucleic acid (DNA) (heterogeneous nuclear RNA [hnRNA]) can result in different messenger RNAs (mRNAs). Most of these initial mRNAs for peptide neurotransmitters actually code for much longer peptides, called preprohormones, which are cleaved in the cell body before they are packaged as prohormones into vesicles for transport to the axon terminals. During the transport phase, the prohormone is usually further cleaved to form the final form of the peptide, which can then be subject to additional posttranslational modifications. Peptide receptors are members of the seven-transmembrane-domain, G protein-linked receptor family. In addition, most if not all peptide neurotransmitters coexist in storage vesicles with other neurotransmitters.

Selected Peptide Neurotransmitters

Endogenous Opioids. The remarkable analgesic and psychological effects of opium have been recognized since biblical times. The isolation of the alkaloid morphine in 1806 led in this century to the development of extensive pharmacological assays for opiate agents and raised the question of whether there were endogenous opiatelike compounds. In the mid-1970s, peptides isolated from brain extracts were shown to interact with opioid receptors and were called *opioids.* The endogenous opioids act on three major receptors, μ, κ, and δ, and are believed to be involved in the regulation of stress, pain, and mood. Three classes of endogenous opioids were recognized, the enkephalins, endorphins, and dynorphins, and recently, the endomorphins, which at last rival morphine itself in potency, were discovered. These range in size from the 31-amino-acid β-endorphin down to the tetrapeptide endomorphins. These peptides bind to members of the opioid receptor family. Enkephalins bind strongly to δ-opioid receptors and with less affinity to μ-receptors. The β-endorphin binds with modest affinity to μ- and δ-receptors. Dynorphins bind strongly to κ- and μ-receptors. None of these binds as strongly as morphine or elicits as strong an analgesic response as the plant alkaloid, however, and for years many questioned whether they in fact represented the true endogenous opioids. Endomorphins 1 and 2, in contrast, equal the affinity of morphine for the μ-receptors and also the analgesic activity of morphine in animals. It is therefore postulated that endogenous ligands of high affinity for the δ- and κ-receptors remain to be discovered. The enkephalins, endorphins, and dynorphins are derived by processing of their respective precursor polypeptides, proopiomelanocortin (POMC), proenkephalin, and prodynorphin. Processing of POMC results in adrenocorticotrophic hormone (ACTH), melanocyte-stimulating hormones, and β-endorphin. Processing of proenkephalin produces metenkephalin and leuenkephalin, and processing of prodynorphin produces β-neoendorphin and dynorphin. The precursor molecule or molecules for endomorphins have not been found but are assumed also to be larger polypeptides. Although evidence of opioids as true neurotransmitters has been difficult to distinguish from their potentiating effects on glutamatergic or adrenergic neurotransmission, a true role for endogenous opioid neurotransmission has been established in the hippocampus, where associative learning may contribute to addiction. Endogenous opioid-containing neurons are found in several brain regions, including the medial hypothalamus, diencephalon, pons, hippocampus, and midbrain, and their axons project both locally and widely. Examination of enkephalins, endorphins, and dynorphins in models of addiction have failed to yield insight in the form of variations in levels of ligands. This may be because they are not the endogenous ligands of highest affinity and specificity. Emerging data on endomorphins and other, so far unknown ligands may yet unlock the mystery of addiction.

Substance P. Substance P is the primary neurotransmitter in most primary afferent sensory neurons and in the striatonigral pathway. They are most prominently associated with mediation of the perception of pain. Abnormalities affecting substance P have been hypothesized for Huntington's disease, dementia of the Alzheimer's type, and mood disorders.

Neurotensin. Neurotensin has been hypothesized to be involved in the pathophysiology of schizophrenia, mostly because of its coexistence with dopamine in some axon terminals. Some preliminary reports suggest that neurotensin-related peptides or drugs have beneficial effects for some psychotic symptoms.

Cholecystokinin. Like neurotensin and for the same reasons, cholecystokinin (CCK) has been hypothesized to be involved in the pathophysiology of schizophrenia. CCK has also been implicated in the pathophysiologies of eating disorders and movement disorders. CCK causes anxiety and triggers panic attacks in people with panic disorder. CCK antagonists are under study as possible anxiolytic agents.

Somatostatin. Somatostatin is also known as growth hormone-inhibiting factor. Postmortem studies have implicated somatostatin in Huntington's disease and dementia of the Alzheimer's type.

Vasopressin and Oxytocin. Vasopressin and oxytocin, two related peptides, have been postulated to be involved in the regulation of mood. They are both synthesized in the hypothalamus and are released in the posterior pituitary.

Neuropeptide Y. Neuropeptide Y has been shown to stimulate the appetite, and development of neuropeptide Y receptor antagonists is an active area of interest for obesity researchers.

AMINO ACID NEUROTRANSMITTERS

Amino acids are the building blocks of proteins. Because of their abundance, it was long assumed that they could not also serve as neurotransmitters. However, glutamate and aspartate are present in disproportionately high concentrations in the brain, and their roles as neurotransmitters have been broadly accepted. The two major amino acid neurotransmitters are GABA and glutamate. GABA is an inhibitory amino acid, and glutamate is an excitatory amino acid. It is occasionally suggested that a simplified way to look at the brain is as a balance between just those two neurotransmitters, with all the biogenic amine and peptide neurotransmitters simply involved in modulating that balance. Recent discoveries have further increased the importance of the study of amino acid neurotransmitters. These discoveries include the observations that the benzodiazepines, barbiturates, and several anticonvulsants act primarily through GABAergic mechanisms and that an important substance of abuse, phencyclidine (PCP), acts at glutamate receptors. One of the most active areas of recent neuroscience research is the role of NMDA glutamate receptors in learning and memory. These observations have led to an intensive study of these receptors with regard to major psychiatric disorders, such as anxiety disorders and schizophrenia.

Glycine. Glycine is synthesized primarily from serine by the actions of serine *trans*-hydroxymethylase and β-glycerate dehydrogenase, both of which are rate limiting. Glycine does double duty as a mandatory adjunctive neurotransmitter for glutamate activity and an independent inhibitory neurotransmitter at its own receptors. The excitatory amino acid–binding site for glycine on the NMDA glutamate receptor is referred to as the non–strychnine-sensitive glycine receptor, and it contrasts with the strychnine-sensitive glycine receptor, which is an inhibitory receptor. Improvement of NMDA receptor activity by occupancy of the glycine-binding site has been hypothesized to present an adjunctive mode for the treatment of schizophrenia. Some, but not all, clinical trials of this hypothesis have shown a reduction in the negative symptoms of schizophrenia by glycine or glycine as the omega (ω) receptors. The β-carbolines are a class of drugs that are inverse agonists of the benzodiazepine receptors; thus, their activity results in anxiety and convulsions.

Histamine

Neurons that release histamine as their neurotransmitter are located in the hypothalamus and project to the cerebral cortex, the limbic system, and the thalamus. There are three types of histamine receptors: H_1-receptor stimulation increases the production of IP_3 and DAG; H_2 stimulation increases the production of cAMP; and the H_3 receptor may regulate vascular tone. Blockade of H_1 receptors is the mechanism of action for allergy medications and is partly the mechanism for commonly observed side effects (e.g., sedation, weight gain, and hypotension) of some psychotropic drugs.

Acetylcholine

CNS Cholinergic Tracts. A group of cholinergic neurons in the nucleus basalis of Meynert projects to the cerebral cortex and the limbic system. Additional cholinergic neurons in the reticular system project to the cerebral cortex, the limbic system, the hypothalamus, and the thalamus. Some patients with dementia of the Alzheimer's type or Down syndrome appear to have specific degeneration of the neurons in the nucleus basalis of Meynert.

Acetylcholine Life Cycle. Acetylcholine is synthesized in the cholinergic axon terminal from acetylcoenzyme A (acetyl-CoA) and choline by the enzyme choline acetyltransferase. Once made, acetylcholine is packaged into storage vesicles for release when triggered by an action potential. Acetylcholine is metabolized in the synaptic cleft by acetylcholinesterase, and the resulting choline is taken back up into the presynaptic neuron and is recycled to make new acetylcholine molecules. Acetylcholinesterase is affected by the drugs currently in use for the treatment of Alzheimer's disease.

Cholinergic Receptors. The two major subtypes of cholinergic receptors are muscarinic and nicotinic (Table 3.2–2). There are five recognized types of muscarinic receptors with various effects on phosphoinositol turnover, cAMP and cGMP production, and potassium ion channel activity. Muscarinic receptors are antagonized by atropine and by the anticholinergic drugs. The nicotinic receptors are ligand-gated ion channels that have the receptor site directly on the ion channel itself. The nicotinic receptor is actually made up of four subunits (α, β, γ, and δ). Nicotinic receptors can vary in the number of each of those subunits; thus, there is a multitude of subtypes of nicotinic receptors, based on the specific configuration of the subunits.

Acetylcholine and Drugs. The most common use of anticholinergic drugs in psychiatry is in treatment of the motor

abnormalities caused by the use of classic antipsychotic drugs (e.g., haloperidol). The efficacy of the drugs for that indication is determined by the balance between acetylcholine activity and dopamine activity in the basal ganglia. In normal people, the activity of the nigrostriatal dopamine pathway is partially balanced by the activity of cholinergic pathways in the basal ganglia. Blockade of D_2 receptors in the striatum upsets this balance, but the balance may be partially restored, albeit at a lower set point, by antagonism of muscarinic receptors. Blockade of muscarinic cholinergic receptors is a common pharmacodynamic effect of many psychotropic drugs. Blockade of those receptors leads to the commonly seen adverse effects of blurred vision, dry mouth, constipation, and difficulty in initiating urination. Excessive blockade of CNS cholinergic receptors causes confusion and delirium. Drugs that increase cholinergic activity by blocking breakdown by acetylcholinesterase (e.g., donepezil [Aricept]) have been shown to be effective in the treatment of dementia of the Alzheimer's type.

When bound by nicotine, CNS presynaptic nicotinic receptors mediate a large influx of calcium and therefore cause neurotransmitter release in many types of neurons. Recent evidence has shown that nicotine increases the strength of synaptic connections in the hippocampus, the brain region that supports short-term memory. Several nicotinelike compounds that stimulate acetylcholine release are under study as cognitive enhancers for treatment of Alzheimer's disease.

Acetylcholine and Psychopathology. The most common association with acetylcholine is dementia of the Alzheimer's type and other dementias. Anticholinergic agents can impair learning and memory in normal people. With the recent identification of the protein structures of the various muscarinic and nicotinic receptors, many researchers are working on specific muscarinic and nicotinic agonists that may have some benefit in the treatment of dementia of the Alzheimer's type. Acetylcholine may also be involved in mood and sleep disorders.

γ-Aminobutyric Acid (GABA). SYNTHESIS, METABOLISM, AND PATHWAYS. GABA is found almost exclusively in the CNS, and it does not cross the blood–brain barrier. The highest concentrations are in the midbrain and diencephalon, with lower amounts in the cerebral hemispheres, the pons, and the medulla. GABA is synthesized from glutamate by the rate-limiting enzyme glutamic acid decarboxylase (GAD), which requires pyridoxine (vitamin B_6) as a cofactor. Once released into the synaptic cleft, GABA is taken up by a specific transporter into the presynaptic neuron and adjacent glia, where it is metabolized by mitochondria-associated GABA transaminase (GABA-T). GABA is the primary neurotransmitter in intrinsic neurons that function as local mediators for the inhibitory feedback loops. GABA commonly coexists with biogenic amine neurotransmitters, glycine, and peptide neurotransmitters, including somatostatin, NPY, CCK, substance P, and vasoactive intestinal peptide (VIP).

RECEPTORS AND DRUGS. There are three types of GABA receptors, $GABA_A$, $GABA_B$, and $GABA_C$, each with a discrete pattern of expression in the brain. The $GABA_B$ receptor is a G protein–associated receptor; $GABA_A$ and $GABA_C$ are directly acting, ligand-gated chloride ion channels that increase membrane polarization (Fig. 3.2–8). $GABA_A$ is the predominant species, consisting of five subunits in variable combinations. The $GABA_B$ receptor agonist baclofen is used to treat spasticity. The $GABA_A$ receptor antagonists bicuculline and picrotoxin strongly induce seizures. Because GABA is thought to suppress seizure activity, anxiety, and mania, considerable effort has been devoted to synthesizing drugs that potentiate GABA activity. One such drug, progabide, is a hydrophobic GABA receptor agonist with good brain penetration, which has anticonvulsant activity. Tiagabine (Gabitril), which inhibits the GABA transporter, and vigabatrin (Sabril), which inhibits GABA-T, raise the effective synaptic levels of GABA and exhibit anticonvulsant activity. The anticonvulsant topiramate (Topamax) potentiates $GABA_A$ receptor activity by unclear mechanisms. Gabapentin (Neurontin), a GABA derivative, is an effective anticonvulsant with good brain penetration; yet, curiously, it has no activity at GABA receptors or the GABA transporter. The $GABA_A$ receptor has binding sites for GABA, the benzodiazepines, and the barbiturates. The benzodiazepines increase the affinity of the $GABA_A$ receptor for GABA. The benzodiazepine receptors are sometimes referred to as the ω-receptors. As mentioned above, the β-carbolines are a class of drugs that are inverse agonists of the benzodiazepine receptors; thus, their activity results in anxiety and convulsions. Flumazenil (Romazicon) is a benzodiazepine antagonist that is currently being used in hospital emergency rooms as a treatment for benzodiazepine overdose.

GABA AND PSYCHOPATHOLOGY. Clinical research on the GABAergic system, because it is associated with benzodiazepines, has focused on its potential role in the pathophysiology of anxiety disorders. Many of the standard anticonvulsants also have their effects on the GABA system; therefore, researchers in epilepsy also are actively studying the GABA system. The success of the anticonvulsants carbamazepine (Tegretol) and valproic acid (Depakote) for the treatment of rapid cycling bipolar I disorder has stimulated trials of the GABAergic anticonvulsants listed above for this indication.

Glutamate. SYNTHESIS, METABOLISM, AND PATHWAYS. Glutamate is synthesized from glucose and glutamine in presynaptic neuron terminals and is stored in synaptic vesicles. Once released into the synaptic cleft, it acts on receptors, and its action is terminated by highly efficient uptake into the presynaptic neuron or adjacent glia. Glutamate is the primary neurotransmitter in cerebellar granule cells, the striatum, the cells of the hippocampal molecular layer and entorhinal cortex, the pyramidal cells of the cortex, and the thalamocortical and corticostriatal projections. Glutamate release is stimulated by nicotine.

RECEPTORS AND DRUGS. There are five major types of glutamate receptors. The NMDA receptor is the best understood and most complex of the receptors, because it may play an essential role in learning and memory, as well as psychopathology. The other four receptor types are therefore referred to as the non-NMDA glutamate receptors. The NMDA receptor allows the passage of sodium, potassium, and calcium. It opens only under conditions in which it is bound by two molecules of glutamate and a molecule of glycine at the same time as the potential of the membrane in which it sits rises above –65 mV, which allows the magnesium ion that normally blocks the ion pore to fall off. Since most cells that respond to glutamate display both NMDA and non-NMDA receptors, the initial depolarization response is mediated by the non-NMDA receptors until the membrane potential rises above –65 mV, at which time the NMDA receptors open. The NMDA receptor is also blocked by physiological concentrations of magnesium, PCP, and PCP-related substances (e.g., dizocilpine [MK-801]). The requirement of

simultaneous membrane depolarization and glutamate receptor occupancy for activation of NMDA-mediated calcium flux has piqued interest in the receptor as the essential feature of the cellular mechanism of memory. In this model, a prolonged set of temporally coordinated stimuli is required for NMDA receptor opening, which uniquely triggers a cascade of intracellular events leading to the expression of a certain set of genes, and this in turn reinforces and stabilizes the synapses responsible for the initial receptor activation. Thus, a physical change in the synaptic relationships results from a specific pattern of receptor stimulation. Although the details of this pathway remain to be completely elucidated, NMDA receptor antagonists have been shown to prevent the formation of memory.

Two of the other receptors are the α-amino-3-hydroxy-5-methyl-4-isoxazole propionic acid (AMPA) and the kainate receptors, which share depolarization as their principal effect with the NMDA receptor. The two remaining types of glutamate receptors are the AP4 (1-2-amino-4-phosphorobutyrate) and ACPD *trans*-1-aminocyclopentane-1-3-dicarboxylic acid) receptors. The AP4 receptor is thought to be an inhibitory autoreceptor. The ACPD receptor (also called the metabotropic receptor) is a seven-transmembrane-domain, G protein-linked receptor that exerts its effects through the phosphoinositol second-messenger system.

GLUTAMATE AND PSYCHOPATHOLOGY. The major pathophysiological conditions currently associated with the glutamate systems are excitotoxicity and schizophrenia. *Excitotoxicity* is the hypothesis that excessive stimulation of glutamate receptors leads to prolonged and excessive intraneuronal concentrations of calcium and NO. Such conditions activate many enzymes (especially proteases) that are destructive to neuronal integrity. The association with schizophrenia is partly due to the psychotomimetic effects observed with PCP. In this model, a reduction in NMDA receptor activity is thought to cause psychotic symptoms. Attempts to reduce excitotoxicity during strokes with the NMDA receptor blocker MK-801 were terminated because of precipitation of psychosis. It seems, therefore, that the glutamate neurotransmitter-receptor system is poorly suited to be a target for psychotherapeutic drugs; too much NMDA receptor activity kills neurons, and too little NMDA receptor activity induces psychosis. A few NMDA receptor inhibitors with a reassuring safety profile are under development, including remacemide. Some basic science studies show that dopamine and glutamate have opposing effects. Because of that association or because of the sensitivity of nigral dopamine-containing neurons to excitotoxicity, glutamate may be involved in the pathophysiology of Parkinson's disease.

Other Neurotransmitters.

NUCLEOTIDES. Of the four nucleotides in deoxyribonucleic acid (DNA), the purine adenosine and its high-energy phosphorylated form ATP have also been shown to be neurotransmitters. Receptors for purines have been found in the brain. P_1 receptors have a high affinity for adenosine, and P_2 receptors have a high affinity for ATP. Two subtypes of the P_1 receptor are the adenosine A_1 and A_2 receptors, both of which are G protein-linked receptors. Binding of adenosine to A_1 receptors results in cellular responses opposite to those of binding of adenosine to A_2 receptors in some systems. The P_1 receptors are blocked by xanthines, such as caffeine and theophylline. Adenosine is concentrated in specific cellular layers of discrete regions of the brain and appears to have the general effect of inhibiting the release of most other neurotransmitters. During a seizure, it is released from cells and appears to act to terminate the seizure. The actions of adenosine, which are opposite to those of caffeine, have led to various research efforts to study adenosine analogues for use as anticonvulsants or sedatives. In clinical use as a cardiac antiarrhythmic agent, intravenous adenosine has a half-life on the order of less than 5 minutes. ATP itself may also serve as a neurotransmitter. It is stored in synaptic vesicles along with catecholamines and is released when the catecholamines are released. It preferentially acts on P_2 receptors, and data show that at least one function of ATP is the opening of Na^+, K^+, and Ca^+ ion channels.

EICOSANOIDS. The metabolites of arachidonic acid, prostaglandins, prostacyclins, thromboxane, and leukotrienes, also called eicosanoids or prostanoids, are all present in the brain. To date, eight prostanoid receptors have been identified in various neural and nonneural tissues: the thromboxane A_2 receptor, prostacyclin receptor, prostaglandin F receptor, prostaglandin D receptor, and four subtypes of prostaglandin E receptors (EP_1R to EP_4R). They are coupled to different signal transduction systems. In addition, leukotriene-binding sites have been found in the brain. Although these substances have not yet fulfilled all the criteria for neurotransmitters, efforts are being made to explore this possible role.

ANANDAMIDES. A novel compound formed from arachidonic acid and ethanolamine, *N*-arachidonoylethanolamine (anadamide), and 2-arachnidonylglycerol are now recognized as weak and strong endogenous ligands, respectively, for the cannabinoid receptor family. Cannabinoids are the active ingredients in marijuana, and a lengthy search for an endogenous ligand for the cannabinoid receptor has recently ended. There are two types of cannabinoid receptors, central (CB_1) and peripheral (CB_2), each of which has several subtypes. These receptors are members of the seven-transmembrane-domain, G protein–linked family of receptors, and they bind tetrahydrocannabinol (THC), the active ingredient of marijuana. Anandamides generally exhibit pharmacological effects that are less potent, but similar to those of THC, including lowering intraocular pressure, decreasing activity level, and relieving pain. The colocalization of anandamides and cannabinoid receptors in the thalamus suggests that anandamides may act as neurotransmitters. Researchers are continuing to seek more potent endogenous ligands.

SIGMA RECEPTORS. The Σ-receptor site has been defined pharmacologically but has not yet been purified or cloned, and the endogenous ligand for the receptors has not been identified. Only recently has the site now known as the Σ receptor been distinguished from the PCP receptor. It is now clear that the principal site of action for PCP is the NMDA glutamate receptor, where PCP binding results in an indirect inhibition of calcium ion influx. The Σ site binds pentazocine (Talwin) and haloperidol, which belong to distinct drug classes. Although the study of the Σ-binding characteristic remains an area of active research, consistent results from efforts to purify the receptor have been elusive.

REFERENCES

Arranz MJ, Mancama D, Kerwin RW. Neurotransmitter receptor variants and their influence on antipsychotic treatment. *Int J Mol Med.* 2001;7:27.

Fernstrom JD, Fernstrom MH. Diet, monoamine neurotransmitters and appetite control. *Nestle Nutr Workshop Ser Clin Perform Programme.* 2001;117.

Hyde TM, Crook JM. Cholinergic systems and schizophrenia: primary pathology or epiphenomena? *J Chem Neuroanat.* 2001;22:53.

Kronfol Z, Remick DG. Cytokines and the brain: implications for clinical psychiatry. *Am J Psychiatry.* 2000;157:683.

Lesch KP. Variation of serotonergic gene expression: neurodevelopment and the complexity of response to psychopharmacologic drugs. *Eur Neuropsychopharmacol.* 2001;11:457.

Licht EA, Jacobsen RH, Fujikawa DG. Chronically impaired frontal lobe function from subclinical epileptiform discharges. *Epilepsy & Behavior.* 2002;3:96.
Martinez D, Broft A, Laruelle M. Imaging neurochemical endophenotypes: promises and pitfalls. *Pharmacogenomics.* 2001;2:223.
Mathew SJ, Coplan JD, Gorman JM. Neurobiological mechanisms of social anxiety disorder. *Am J Psychiatry.* 2001;158:1558.
Mignot E. A commentary on the neurobiology of the hypocretin/orexin system. *Neuropsychopharmacology.* 2001;25(5 suppl 1):S5.
Mortensen OV, Kristensen AS, Wiborg O. Species-scanning mutagenesis of the serotonin transporter reveals residues essential in selective, high-affinity recognition of antidepressants. *J Neurochem.* 2001;79:237.
Murai T, Muller U, Werheid K, et al. In vivo evidence for differential association of striatal dopamine and midbrain serotonin systems with neuropsychiatric symptoms in Parkinson's disease. *J Neuropsychiatry Clin Neurosci.* 2001; 13:222.
Pollmacher T, Haack M, Schuld A, Kraus T, Hinze-Selch D. Effects of antipsychotic drugs on cytokine networks. *J Psychiatr Res.* 2000;34:369.
Sakai K, Gao XM, Hashimoto T, Tamminga CA. Traditional and new antipsychotic drugs differentially alter neurotransmission markers in basal ganglia-thalamocortical neural pathways. *Synapse.* 2001;39:152.
Soudijn W, van Wijngaarden I. The GABA transporter and its inhibitors. *Curr Med Chem.* 2000;7:1063.
Sukonick DL, Pollock BG, Sweet RA, et al. The 5-HTTPR*S/*L polymorphism and aggressive behavior in Alzheimer disease. *Arch Neurol.* 2001;58:1425.

▲ 3.3 Neuroimaging

Neuroimaging has evolved tremendously, providing psychiatrists with unprecedented information about brain structure and function. Computer tomographic (CT) scanners, the first widely used neuroimaging devices, allowed assessment of structural brain lesions such as tumors or strokes. Magnetic resonance imaging (MRI) scans, developed next, distinguished gray and white matter better than CT scans did and allowed visualizations of smaller brain lesions as well as white matter abnormalities. In addition to structural neuroimaging with CT and MRI, a revolution in functional neuroimaging has enabled clinical scientists to obtain unprecedented insights into the diseased human brain. The foremost techniques for functional neuroimaging include positron emission tomography (PET) and single photon emission computer tomography (SPECT).

Primary observation of structural and functional brain imaging in neuropsychiatric disorders such as dementia, movement disorders, demyelinating disorders, and epilepsy has not only contributed to a greater understanding of the pathophysiology of neurological and psychiatric illnesses, but also can help practicing clinicians in difficult diagnostic situations.

USES OF NEUROIMAGING

Indications for Ordering Neuroimaging in Clinical Practice

Neurological Deficits. In a neurological examination, any change that can be localized to the brain or spinal cord requires neuroimaging. Neurological examination includes mental status, cranial nerves, motor system, coordination, sensory system, and reflex components. The mental status examination assesses arousal, attention, and motivation; memory; language; visuospatial function; complex cognition; and mood and affect. Consultant psychiatrists should consider a workup including neuroimaging for patients with new-onset psychosis and acute changes in mental status. The clinical examination always assumes priority, and neuroimaging is ordered on the basis of clinical suspicion of a central nervous system (CNS) disorder.

Dementia. Loss of memory and cognitive abilities affects more than 10 million persons in the United States and will affect an increasing number as the population ages. Reduced mortality from cancer and heart disease has increased life expectancy and has allowed persons to survive to the age of onset of degenerative brain disorders, which have proved more difficult to treat. Depression, anxiety, and psychosis are common in patients with dementia. The most common cause of dementia is Alzheimer's disease, which does not have a characteristic appearance on routine neuroimaging but, rather, is associated with diffuse loss of brain volume.

One treatable cause of dementia that requires neuroimaging for diagnosis is *normal pressure hydrocephalus,* a disorder of the drainage of cerebrospinal fluid. This condition does not progress to the point of acutely increased intracranial pressure but stabilizes at a pressure at the upper end of the normal range. The dilated ventricles, which may be readily visualized with CT or MRI, exert pressure on the frontal lobes. A gait disorder is almost uniformly present; dementia, which may be indistinguishable from that of Alzheimer's disease, appears less consistently. Relief of the increased cerebrospinal fluid pressure may completely restore gait and mental function.

Infarction of the cortical or subcortical areas, or stroke, may produce focal neurological deficits, including cognitive and emotional changes. Strokes are easily seen on MRI scans. Depression is common among stroke patients, either because of direct damage to the emotional centers of the brain or because of the patient's reaction to the disability. Depression, in turn, may cause pseudodementia. In addition to large strokes, extensive atherosclerosis in brain capillaries may cause countless tiny infarctions of brain tissue; patients with this phenomenon may develop dementia as fewer and fewer neural pathways participate in cognition. This state, called *vascular dementia,* is characterized on MRI scans by patches of increased signal in the white matter. Recent clinicopathological studies of brain tissue with typical Alzheimer's disease changes (senile plaques and neurofibrillary tangles) suggest that dementia results from these changes plus microscopic infarctions. Patients with Alzheimer's neuropathology but without strokes may not have dementia.

Certain degenerative disorders of basal ganglia structures, associated with dementia, may have a characteristic appearance on MRI scans. Huntington's disease typically produces atrophy of the caudate nucleus; thalamic degeneration may interrupt the neural links to the cortex (Fig. 3.3–1).

Space-occupying lesions can cause dementia. Chronic subdural hematomas and cerebral contusions, caused by head trauma, may produce focal neurological deficits or may only produce dementia. Brain tumors can affect cognition in several ways. Skull-based meningiomas can compress the underlying cortex and impair its processing. Infiltrative glial cell tumors, such as astrocytoma or glioblastoma multiforme, may cut off communication between brain centers by interrupting white matter tracts. Tumors located near the ventricular system can obstruct the flow of cerebrospinal fluid and gradually increase the intracranial pressure.

Chronic infections, including neurosyphilis, cryptococcosis, tuberculosis, and Lyme disease, may cause symptoms of

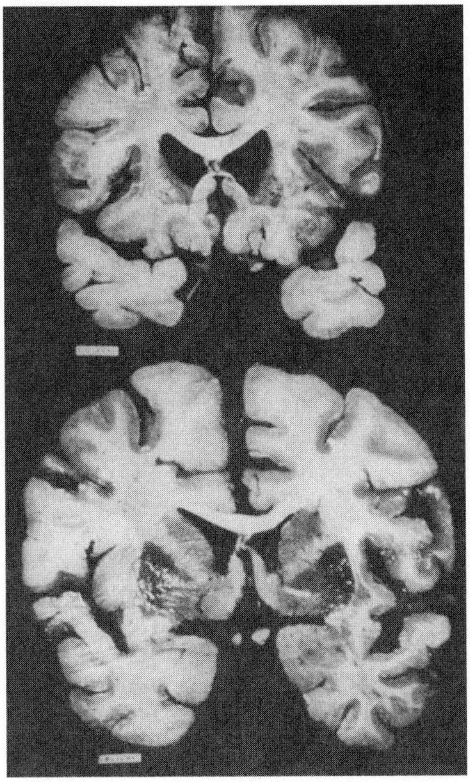

FIGURE 3.3–1

Brain slices. **Top**: Huntington disease. Atrophy of caudate nucleus and lentiform nuclei with dilatation of lateral ventricle. **Bottom**: Normal brain. (From Fahn S. Huntington Disease. In: Rowland LP, ed. *Merritt's Textbook of Neurology.* 10th ed. Philadelphia: Lippincott Williams & Wilkins; 2000:659.)

dementia and may produce a characteristic enhancement of the meninges, especially at the base of the brain. Serological studies are needed to complete the diagnosis. Human immunodeficiency virus (HIV) infection can cause dementia directly, in which case there is a diffuse loss of brain volume, or can allow the proliferation of the JC virus to yield progressive multifocal leukoencephalopathy, which affects white matter tracts and appears as increased white matter signal on MRI scans.

Chronic demyelinating diseases, such as multiple sclerosis, may affect cognition because of white matter disruption. Multiple sclerosis plaques are easily seen on MRI scans as periventricular patches of increased signal intensity.

Any evaluation of dementia should consider medication effects, metabolic derangements, infections, and nutritional causes that may not produce abnormalities on neuroimaging.

Indications for Neuroimaging in Clinical Research

Analysis of Clinically Defined Groups of Patients. Psychiatric research aims to categorize patients with psychiatric disorders to facilitate the discovery of neuroanatomical and neurochemical bases of mental illness. Researchers have used functional neuroimaging to study groups of patients with such psychiatric conditions as schizophrenia, affective disorders, and anxiety disorders, among others. In schizophrenia, for example, neuropathological volumetric analyses have suggested a loss of brain weight, specifically of gray matter. There appears to be a paucity of axons and dendrites in the cortex, and CT and MRI may show compensatory enlargement of the lateral and third ventricles. Specifically, the temporal lobes of persons with schizophrenia appear to suffer the most loss of volume relative to normal persons. Recent studies have found that the left temporal lobe is generally more affected than the right. The frontal lobe may also have abnormalities, not in the volume of the lobe, but in the level of activity detected by functional neuroimaging. Persons with schizophrenia consistently exhibit decreased metabolic activity in the frontal lobes, especially during tasks that require the prefrontal cortex. As a group, schizophrenia patients are also more likely to have an increase in ventricular size than are nonschizophrenic controls.

Disorders of mood and affect may also be associated with loss of brain volume and decreased metabolic activity in the frontal lobes. Inactivation of the left prefrontal cortex appears to depress mood; inactivation of the right prefrontal cortex elevates it. Among anxiety disorders, studies of obsessive-compulsive disorder with conventional CT and MRI have shown either no specific abnormalities or a smaller caudate nucleus. Functional PET and SPECT studies suggest abnormalities in the corticolimbic, basal ganglial, and thalamic structures in the disorder. When patients are experiencing obsessive-compulsive disorder symptoms, the orbital prefrontal cortex shows abnormal activity. A partial normalization of caudate glucose metabolism appears in patients taking medications such as fluoxetine (Prozac) or clomipramine (Anafranil) or undergoing behavior modification.

Functional neuroimaging studies of persons with attention-deficit/hyperactivity disorder (ADHD) either have shown no abnormalities or have shown decreased volume of the right prefrontal cortex and the right globus pallidus. In addition, whereas normally the right caudate nucleus is larger than the left caudate nucleus, persons with ADHD may have caudate nuclei of equal size. These findings suggest dysfunction of the right prefrontal-striatal pathway for control of attention.

Analysis of Brain Activity during Performance of Specific Tasks. Many original conceptions of different brain region functions emerged from observing deficits caused by local injuries, tumors, or strokes. Functional neuroimaging allows researchers to review and reassess classical teachings in the intact brain. Most work, to date, has been aimed at language and vision. Although many technical peculiarities and limitations of SPECT, PET, and functional MRI (fMRI) have been overcome, none of these techniques has demonstrated clear superiority. Studies require carefully controlled conditions, which subjects may find arduous. Nonetheless, functional neuroimaging has contributed major conceptual advances, and the methods are now limited mainly by the creativity of the investigative protocols.

Studies have been designed to reveal the functional neuroanatomy of all sensory modalities, gross and fine motor skills, language, memory, calculations, learning, and disorders of thought, mood, and anxiety. Unconscious sensations transmitted by the autonomic nervous system have been localized to specific brain regions. These analyses provide a basis for comparison with results of studies of clinically defined patient groups and may lead to improved therapies for mental illnesses.

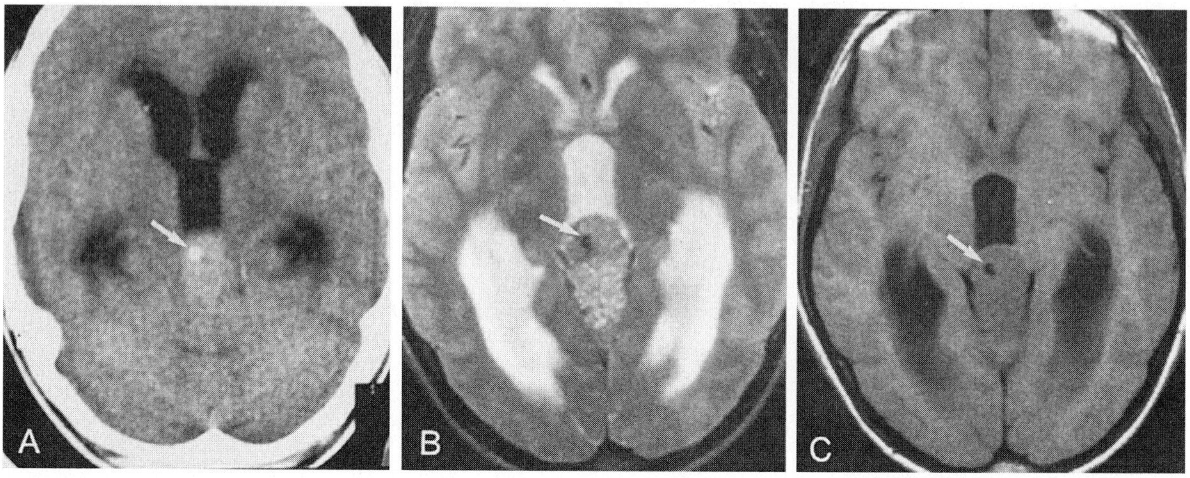

FIGURE 3.3–2

Comparison of CT and MRI. **A.** Computed tomography (CT) scan in the axial plane at the level of the third ventricle. The cerebrospinal fluid (CSF) within the ventricles appears black, the brain tissue appears gray, and the skull appears white. There is very poor discrimination between the gray and white matter of the brain. The *arrow* indicates a small calcified lesion in a tumor of the pineal gland. Detection of calcification is one role in which CT is superior to MRI. **B.** T2-weighted image of the same patient at roughly the same level. With T2, the CSF appears white, the gray matter appears gray, the white matter is clearly distinguished from the gray matter, and the skull and indicated calcification appear black. Much more detail of the brain is visible than with CT. **C.** T1-weighted image of the same patient at roughly the same level. With T1, the CSF appears dark, the brain appears more uniformly gray, and the skull and indicated calcification appear black. T1 MRI images are the most similar to CT images. (Reprinted with permission from Grossman CB. *Magnetic Resonance Imaging and Computed Tomography of the Head and Spine.* 2nd ed. Baltimore: Williams & Wilkins; 1996:101.)

SPECIFIC TECHNIQUES

Computed Tomography (CT) Scans

In 1972, CT scanning revolutionized diagnostic neuroradiology by permitting imaging of the brain tissue in live patients. CT scanners are currently the most widely available and convenient imaging tools available in clinical practice; practically every hospital emergency room has immediate access to a CT scanner at all times. CT scanners effectively take a series of head X-ray pictures from all vantage points, 360 degrees around a patient's head. The amount of radiation that passes through, or is not absorbed, from each angle is digitized and entered into a computer. The computer uses matrix algebra calculations to assign a specific density to each point within the head and displays these data as a set of two-dimensional images. When viewed in sequence, the images allow mental reconstruction of the shape of the brain.

The CT image is determined only by the degree to which tissues absorb X-irradiation. The bony structures absorb high amounts of irradiation and tend to obscure details of neighboring structures, an especially troublesome problem in the brainstem, which is surrounded by a thick skull base. Within the brain itself, there is relatively little difference in the attenuation of X-rays between gray matter and white matter. Although the gray-white border is usually distinguishable, details of the gyral pattern may be difficult to appreciate in CT scans. Certain tumors may be invisible on CT because they absorb as much irradiation as the surrounding normal brain.

Appreciation of tumors and areas of inflammation, which may cause changes in behavior, can be increased by intravenous infusion of iodine-containing contrast agents. Iodinated compounds, which absorb much more irradiation than the brain, appear white. The intact brain is separated from the bloodstream by the blood–brain barrier, which normally prevents the passage of the highly charged contrast agents. The blood–brain barrier, however, breaks down in the presence of inflammation or fails to form within tumors and thus allows accumulation of contrast agents. These sites appear whiter than the surrounding brain. Iodinated contrast agents must be used with caution in patients who are allergic to these agents or to shellfish.

With the introduction of MRI scanning, CT scans have been supplanted as the nonemergency neuroimaging study of choice. The increased resolution and delineation of detail afforded by MRI scanning is often required for diagnosis in psychiatry. In addition, performing the most detailed study available inspires the most confidence in the analysis. The only component of the brain better seen on CT scanning is calcification, which may be invisible on MRI (Fig. 3.3–2).

Magnetic Resonance Imaging (MRI) Scans

MRI scanning entered clinical practice in 1982 and soon became the test of choice for clinical psychiatrists and neurologists. The technique does not rely on the absorption of X-rays but is based on nuclear magnetic resonance (NMR). The principle of NMR is that the nuclei of all atoms are thought to spin about an axis, which is randomly oriented in space. When atoms are placed in a magnetic field, the axes of all odd-numbered nuclei align with the magnetic field. The axis of a nucleus deviates away from the magnetic field when exposed to a pulse of radiofrequency electromagnetic radiation oriented at 90 or 180 degrees to the magnetic field. When the pulse terminates, the axis of the spinning nucleus realigns itself with the magnetic field, and during this realignment, it emits its own radiofrequency signal. MRI scanners collect the emissions of individual, realigning nuclei and use computer analysis to generate a series of two-dimensional

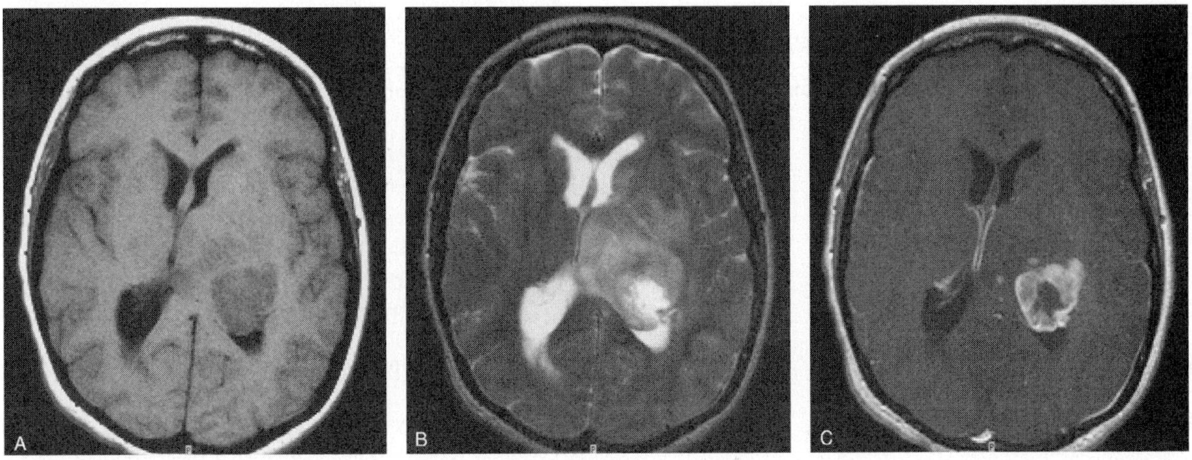

FIGURE 3.3–3
Three axial images from a 46-year-old woman who was hospitalized for the first time for depression and suicidality following the end of a long-standing relationship. A malignant neoplasm extending into the posterior aspect of the left lateral ventricle is clearly seen in all three images. Images **A** and **B** are T1- and T2-weighted, respectively. Image **C** demonstrates the effects of postcontrast enhancement. (Courtesy of Craig N. Carson, M.D., and Perry F. Renshaw, M.D.)

images that represent the brain. The images may be in the axial, coronal, or sagittal planes.

By far the most abundant odd-numbered nucleus in the brain belongs to hydrogen. The rate of realignment of the hydrogen axis is determined by its immediate environment, a combination of both the nature of the molecule of which it is a part and the degree to which it is surrounded by water. Hydrogen nuclei within fat realign rapidly, and hydrogen nuclei within water realign slowly. Hydrogen nuclei in proteins and carbohydrates realign at intermediate rates.

Routine MRI studies use three different radiofrequency pulse sequences. The two parameters that are varied are the duration of the radiofrequency excitation pulse and the length of the time that data are collected from the realigning nuclei. Because T1 pulses are brief and data collection is brief, hydrogen nuclei in hydrophobic environments are emphasized. Thus, fat is bright on T1, and cerebrospinal fluid is dark. The T1 image most closely resembles that of CT scans and is most useful for assessing overall brain structure. T1 is also the only sequence that allows contrast enhancement with the contrast agent gadolinium-diethylenetriamine pentaacetic acid (gadolinium-DTPA). Like the iodinated contrast agents used in CT scanning, gadolinium remains excluded from the brain by the blood-brain barrier, except in areas where this barrier breaks down, such as inflammation or tumor. On T1 images, gadolinium-enhanced structures appear white.

T2 pulses last four times as long as T1 pulses, and the collection times are also extended, to emphasize the signal from hydrogen nuclei surrounded by water. Thus, brain tissue is dark, and cerebrospinal fluid is white on T2 images. Areas within the brain tissue that have abnormally high water content, such as tumors, inflammation, or strokes, appear brighter on T2 images. T2 images reveal brain pathology most clearly. The third routine pulse sequence is the proton density, or balanced, sequence. In this sequence, a short radio pulse is followed by a prolonged period of data collection, which equalizes the density of the cerebrospinal fluid and the brain and allows distinction of tissue changes immediately adjacent to the ventricles.

An additional technique, sometimes used in clinical practice for specific indications, is fluid-attenuated inversion recovery (FLAIR). In this method, the T1 image is inverted and added to the T2 image to double the contrast between gray matter and white matter. Inversion recovery imaging is useful for detecting sclerosis of the hippocampus caused by temporal lobe epilepsy and for localizing areas of abnormal metabolism in degenerative neurological disorders.

MRI magnets are rated in teslas (T), units of magnetic field strength. MRI scanners in clinical use range from 0.3 to 2.0 T. Higher field-strength scanners produce images of markedly higher resolution. In research settings for humans, magnets as powerful as 4.7 T are used; for animals, magnets up to 12 T are used. Unlike the well-known hazards of X-irradiation, exposure to electromagnetic fields of the strength used in MRI machines has not been shown to damage biological tissues.

MRI scans may not be used for patients with pacemakers or implants of ferromagnetic metals. MRI involves enclosing a patient in a narrow tube, in which the patient must remain motionless for up to 20 minutes. The radiofrequency pulses create a loud banging noise that may be obscured by music played in headphones. A significant number of patients cannot tolerate the claustrophobic conditions of routine MRI scanners and may need an open MRI scanner, which has less power and thus produces images of lower resolution. The resolution of brain tissue of even the lowest-power MRI scan, however, exceeds that of CT scanning. Figure 3.3–3 reveals that a brain tumor is the cause of a patient's depression.

Magnetic Resonance Spectroscopy (MRS)

Whereas routine MRI detects hydrogen nuclei to determine brain structure, magnetic resonance spectroscopy (MRS) can detect several odd-numbered nuclei (Table 3.3–1). The ability of MRS to detect a wide range of biologically important nuclei permits the use of the technique to study many metabolic processes. Although the resolution and sensitivity of MRS machines are poor compared with those of currently available PET and SPECT devices, the use of stronger magnetic fields will improve this feature to some extent in the future.

MRS can image nuclei with an odd number of protons and neutrons (Table 3.3–1). The unpaired protons and neutrons (nucleons)

Table 3.3–1
Nuclei Available for In Vivo Magnetic Resonance Spectroscopy (MRS)[a]

Nucleus	Natural Abundance	Relative Sensitivity	Potential Clinical Uses
^{1}H	99.99	1.00	MRI Analysis of metabolism Identification of unusual metabolites Characterization of hypoxia
^{19}F	100.00	0.83	Measurement of pO_2 Analysis of glucose metabolism Measurement of pH Noninvasive pharmacokinetics
^{7}Li	92.58	0.27	Pharmacokinetics
^{23}Na	100.00	0.09	MRI
^{31}P	100.00	0.07	Analysis of bioenergetics Identification of unusual metabolites Characterization of hypoxia Measurement of pH
^{14}N	93.08	0.001	Measurement of glutamate, urea, ammonia
^{39}K	93.08	0.0005	?
^{13}C	1.11	0.0002	Analysis of metabolite turnover rate Pharmacokinetics of labeled drugs
^{17}O	0.04	0.00001	Measurement of metabolic rate
^{2}H	0.02	0.000002	Measurement of perfusion

[a]Natural abundance is given as percentage abundance of the isotope of interest. Nuclei are tabulated in order of decreasing relative sensitivity; relative sensitivity is calculated by multiplying the relative sensitivity for equal numbers of nuclei (at a given field strength) by the natural abundance of that nucleus. A considerable gain in relative sensitivity can be obtained by isotopic enrichment of the nucleus of choice or by the use of novel pulse sequences.

Reprinted with permission from Dager SR, Steen RG. Applications of magnetic resonance spectroscopy to the investigation of neuropsychiatric disorders. *Neuropsychopharmacology.* 1992;6:249.

appear naturally and are nonradioactive. As in MRI, the nuclei align themselves in the strong magnetic field produced by an MRS device. A radiofrequency pulse causes the nuclei of interest to absorb and then emit energy. The readout of an MRS device is usually in the form of a spectrum, such as those for phosphorus-31 and hydrogen-1 nuclei, although the spectrum can also be converted into a pictorial image of the brain. The multiple peaks for each nucleus reflect the fact that the same nucleus is exposed to different electron environments (electron clouds) in different molecules. The hydrogen-1 nuclei in a molecule of creatine, therefore, have a different chemical shift (position in the spectrum) than the hydrogen-1 nuclei in a choline molecule, for example. Thus, the position in the spectrum (the chemical shift) indicates the identity of the molecule in which the nuclei are present. The height of the peak with respect to a reference standard of the molecule indicates the amount of the molecule present.

MRS of the hydrogen-1 nuclei is best at measuring *N*-acetylaspartate (NAA), creatine, and choline-containing molecules; but MRS can also detect glutamate, glutamine, lactate, and *myo*-inositol. Although glutamate and γ-aminobutyric acid (GABA), the major amino acid neurotransmitters, can be detected by MRS, the biogenic amine neurotransmitters (e.g., dopamine) are present in concentrations too low to be detected with the technique. MRS of phosphorus-31 can be used to determine the pH of brain regions and the concentrations of phosphorus-containing compounds (e.g., adenosine triphosphate [ATP] and guanosine triphosphate [GTP]), which are important in the energy metabolism of the brain.

MRS has revealed decreased concentrations of NAA in the temporal lobes and increased concentrations of inositol in the occipital lobes of persons with dementia of the Alzheimer's type. In a series of subjects with schizophrenia, decreased NAA concentrations were found in the temporal and frontal lobes. MRS has been used to trace the levels of ethanol in various brain regions. In panic disorder, MRS was used to record the levels of lactate, whose intravenous infusion can precipitate panic episodes in about three fourths of patients with either panic disorder or major depression. Brain lactate concentrations were found to be elevated during panic attacks, even without provocative infusion.

Additional indications include the use of MRS to measure concentrations of psychotherapeutic drugs in the brain. One study used MRS to measure lithium concentrations in the brains of patients with bipolar disorder and found that lithium concentrations in the brain were half those in the plasma during depressed and euthymic periods but exceeded those in the plasma during manic episodes. Some compounds, such as fluoxetine and trifluoperazine (Stelazine), contain fluorine-19, which can also be detected in the brain and measured by MRS. For example, MRS has demonstrated that it takes 6 months of steady use for fluoxetine to reach maximum concentrations in the brain, which equilibrate at about 20 times the serum concentrations.

Functional Magnetic Resonance Imaging (fMRI)

Recent advances in data collection and computer data processing have reduced the acquisition time for an MRI image to less than 1 second. A new sequence of particular interest to psychiatrists is the T2*, or blood oxygen level–dependent (BOLD) sequence, which detects levels of oxygenated hemoglobin in the blood. Neuronal activity within the brain causes a local increase in blood flow, which in turn increases the local hemoglobin con-

centration. Although neuronal metabolism extracts more oxygen in active areas of the brain, the net effect of neuronal activity is to increase the local amount of oxygenated hemoglobin. This change can be detected essentially in real time with the T2* sequence, which thus detects the functionally active brain regions. This process is the basis for the technique of fMRI.

What fMRI detects is not brain activity per se, but blood flow. The volume of brain in which blood flow increases exceeds the volume of activated neurons by about 1 to 2 cm and limits the resolution of the technique. Sensitivity and resolution can be improved with the use of nontoxic, ultrasmall iron oxide particles. Thus, two tasks that activate clusters of neurons 5 mm apart, such as recognizing two different faces, yield overlapping signals on fMRI and so are usually indistinguishable by this technique. Functional MRI is useful to localize neuronal activity to a particular lobe or subcortical nucleus and has even been able to localize activity to a single gyrus. The method detects tissue perfusion, not neuronal metabolism. In contrast, PET scanning may give information specifically about neuronal metabolism.

No radioactive isotopes are administered in fMRI, a great advantage over PET and SPECT. A subject can perform a variety of tasks, both experimental and control, in the same imaging session. First, a routine T1 MRI image is obtained; then the T2* images are superimposed to allow more precise localization. Acquisition of enough images for study may require 20 minutes to 3 hours, during which time the subject's head must remain in exactly the same position. Several methods, including a frame around the head and a special mouthpiece, have been used. Although realignments of images can correct for some head movement, small changes in head position may lead to erroneous interpretations of brain activation.

fMRI has recently revealed unexpected details about the organization of language within the brain. Using a series of language tasks requiring semantic, phonemic, and rhyming discrimination, one study found that rhyming (but not other types of language processing) produced a different pattern of activation in men and women. Rhyming activated the inferior frontal gyrus bilaterally in women, but only on the left in men. In another study, fMRI revealed a previously suspected, but unproved, neural circuit for lexical categories, interpolated between the representations for concepts and those for phonemes. This novel circuit was located in the left anterior temporal lobe. Data from patients with dyslexia (reading disorder) doing simple rhyming tasks demonstrated a failure to activate Wernicke's area and the insula, which were active in normal subjects doing the same task (see Color Plate 3.3–4 on p. 116).

Sensory functions have also been mapped in detail with fMRI. The activation of the visual and auditory cortices has been visualized in real time. In a recent intriguing study, the areas that were activated while a subject with schizophrenia listened to speech were also activated during auditory hallucinations. These areas included the primary auditory cortex as well as higher-order auditory processing regions. fMRI is the imaging technique most widely used to study brain abnormality related to cognitive dysfunction.

Single Photon Emission Computed Tomography (SPECT) Scanning

SPECT uses manufactured radioactive compounds to study regional differences in cerebral blood flow within the brain. This high-resolution imaging technique records the pattern of photon emission from the bloodstream according to the level of perfusion in different regions of the brain. Like fMRI, it provides information on the cerebral blood flow, which is highly correlated with the rate of glucose metabolism, but does not measure neuronal metabolism directly.

SPECT uses compounds labeled with single photon-emitting isotopes: iodine-123, technetium-99m, and xenon-133. Xenon-133 is a noble gas that is inhaled directly. The xenon quickly enters the blood and is distributed to areas of the brain as a function of regional blood flow. Xenon-SPECT is thus referred to as the *regional cerebral blood flow (rCBF) technique*. For technical reasons, xenon-SPECT can measure blood flow only on the surface of the brain, which is an important limitation. Many mental tasks require communication between the cortex and subcortical structures, and this activity is poorly measured by xenon-SPECT.

Assessment of blood flow over the whole brain with SPECT requires the injectable tracers, technetium-99m–*d,l*-hexamethylpropyleneamine oxime (HMPAO [Ceretec]) or iodoamphetamine (Spectamine). These isotopes are attached to molecules that are highly lipophilic and rapidly cross the blood–brain barrier and enter cells. Once inside the cell, the ligands are enzymatically converted to charged ions, which remain trapped in the cell. Thus, over time, the tracers are concentrated in areas of relatively higher blood flow. Although blood flow is usually assumed to be the major variable tested in HMPAO SPECT, local variations in the permeability of the blood–brain barrier and in the enzymatic conversion of the ligands within cells also contribute to regional differences in signal levels.

In addition to these compounds used for measuring blood flow, iodine-123 (^{123}I)-labeled ligands for the muscarinic, dopaminergic, and serotonergic receptors, for example, can be used to study these receptors by SPECT technology. Once photon-emitting compounds reach the brain, detectors surrounding the patient's head pick up their light emissions. This information is relayed to a computer, which constructs a two-dimensional image of the isotope's distribution within a slice of the brain. A key difference between SPECT and PET is that in SPECT a single particle is emitted, whereas in PET two particles are emitted; the latter reaction gives a more precise location for the event and better resolution of the image. Increasingly, for both SPECT and PET studies, investigators are performing prestudy MRI or CT studies, then superimposing the SPECT or PET image on the MRI or CT image to obtain a more accurate anatomical location for the functional information (see Color Plate 3.3–5 on p. 116). SPECT is useful in diagnosing decreased or blocked cerebral blood flow in stroke victims. Some workers have described abnormal flow patterns in the early stage of Alzheimer's disease that may aid in early diagnosis.

Positron Emission Tomography (PET) Scanning

The isotopes used in PET decay by emitting positrons, antimatter particles that bind with and annihilate electrons, thereby giving off photons that travel in 180-degree opposite directions. Because detectors have twice as much signal from which to generate an image as SPECT scanners have, the resolution of the PET image is higher. A wide range of compounds can be used in PET studies, and the resolution of PET continues to be refined closer to its theoretical minimum of 3 mm, which is the distance positrons move before colliding with an electron. There are relatively few PET scanners because they require an on-site cyclotron to make the isotopes.

The most commonly used isotopes in PET are fluorine-18, nitrogen-13, and oxygen-15. These isotopes are usually linked to another molecule, except in the case of oxygen-15 (^{15}O). The most commonly reported ligand has been [^{18}F]fluorodeoxyglucose (FDG), an analogue of glucose that the brain cannot metabolize. Thus, the brain regions with the highest metabolic rate and the highest blood flow take up the most FDG but cannot metabolize and excrete the usual metabolic products. The concentration of ^{18}F builds up in these neurons and is detected by the PET camera. Water-15 ($H_2{}^{15}O$) and nitrogen-13 (^{13}N) are used to measure blood flow, and oxygen-15 (^{15}O) can be used to determine metabolic rate. Glucose is by far the predominant energy source available to brain cells, and its use is thus a highly sensitive indicator of the rate of brain metabolism. [^{18}F]-labeled 3,4-dihydroxyphenylalanine (dopa), the fluorinated precursor to dopamine, has been used to localize dopaminergic neurons.

PET has been used increasingly to study normal brain development and function as well as to study neuropsychiatric disorders. With regard to brain development, PET studies have found that glucose use is greatest in the sensorimotor cortex, thalamus, brainstem, and cerebellar vermis when an infant is 5 weeks of age or younger. By 3 months of age, most areas of the cortex show increased use except for the frontal and association cortices, which do not begin to exhibit an increase until the infant is 8 months old. An adult pattern of glucose metabolism is achieved by the age of 1 year, but use in the cortex continues to rise above adult levels until the child is about 9 years old, when use in the cortex begins to decrease and reaches its final adult level in the late teen years. In another study, subjects listened to a rapidly presented list of thematically related words. When asked to recall words in the thematic category that may or may not have been on the list, some subjects falsely recalled that they had heard words that were actually not on the list. By PET scanning, the hippocampus was active during both true and false recollections, whereas the auditory cortex was only active during recollection of words that were actually heard. When pressed to determine

COLOR PLATE 3.1–11

Wide distribution of brain activity during repeated movement of the right hand. Areas of increased neuronal activity, shown in red, are superimposed on a computer-reconstructed 3-dimensional MRI image of the human brain projected in six views: (*top left*) front coronal view, (*top right*) back coronal view, (*middle left*) right sagittal view, (*middle right*) left sagittal view, (*bottom left*) bottom axial view, and (*bottom right*) top axial view. The patterns of neuronal activity are defined using functional MRI neuroimaging. Activity is seen in widely distributed, discrete areas, most strongly in the left cerebral hemisphere and the right cerebellum. Most higher-order functional brain modules, such as that for hand movements, are widely distributed among local networks in the brain. (Modified from Lawler A. New brain institute struggles for traction. *Science.* 2001;293:1421, with permission.)

COLOR PLATE 3.3–4

Functional MRI during rhyming tasks in normal people and people with dyslexia. The left hemisphere is depicted in green. Normal (*top*) and dyslexic (*bottom*) subjects were shown two letters and asked to determine whether the letters rhymed (B-T) or not (B-K). To perform the task, the subjects had to translate the letters into sounds, or phonemes, (/bee/,/tee/), then compare only the rhyming part of the phonemes (/ee/). In normals, three contiguous areas were activated, including Broca's area, Wernicke's area, and the intervening insula. In those with dyslexia, only Broca's area was activated. Dyslexic patients required much more time to complete the task and were more prone to make errors. (Reprinted with permission from Frith C, Frith U. A biological marker for dyslexia. *Nature.* 1996;382:19.)

COLOR PLATE 3.3–5

Stages of the superimposition of a SPECT cerebral blood-flow image **(A)**, which has been redefined **(B)**, and an MRI T1-weighted image **(C)**, to produce a combination **(D)**. (Reprinted with permission from Besson JAO. Magnetic resonance imaging and its application in neuropsychiatry. *Br J Psychiatry.* 1990;25(9 Suppl):157.)

COLOR PLATE 3.3–6

PET scans with [^{18}F]fluorodeoxyglucose in a control (*top*) and six patients with neurological disorders. The three images from the control show transverse sections of the brain at a high level through the parietal lobes (*left*), an intermediate level through the basal ganglia and the thalamus (*center*), and a low level through the base of the frontal lobes, the temporal lobes, and the cerebellum (*right*). The level of each image corresponds approximately to the level of the scans below. The *bar* indicates the level of glucose metabolic activity in the images, with colors on the left indicating low levels of metabolism and colors on the right indicating high levels. The middle and bottom scans are from patients with multi-infarct dementia (*MID*) (also known as vascular dementia), Alzheimer's disease (*AD*), temporal lobe epilepsy, brain tumor (primitive neuroectodermal tumor), Huntington's disease (*HD*), and olivopontocerebellar atrophy (*OPCA*). A small region of absent glucose metabolism is seen in the patient with multi-infarct dementia (*arrow*); PET scans at other levels in the patient revealed a number of similar areas, which represent small focal infarctions. The scan in the patient with Alzheimer's disease shows hypometabolism in both parietal lobes (*arrows*). The image in the patient with epilepsy shows hypometabolism in the right temporal lobe (*arrow*), which is the site of origin of the seizure disorder. The scan in the patient with a tumor shows a region of hypermetabolism in the thalamus, which is the location of the tumor (*arrow*). The image in the patient with Huntington's disease shows hypometabolism in the caudate nuclei bilaterally (*arrows*). The scan in the patient with olivopontocerebellar atrophy shows hypometabolism in the cerebellum (*arrows*) and the brainstem. (Reprinted with permission from Gilman S. Advances in neurology. *N Engl J Med.* 1992;326:1610.)

COLOR PLATE 3.3–7

PET images showing radioactivity in a horizontal brain section through the striatal level after an intravenous injection of [^{11}C]raclopride, a dopamine receptor agonist, into a healthy volunteer. **A.** PET image before medication. Corresponding PET images at different time points after the administration of 4 mg haloperidol are shown after 3 hours **(B)**, after 6 hours **(C)**, and after 27 hours **(D)**. (Reprinted with permission from Nordström A-L, Farde L, Halldin D. Time course of D_2-dopamine receptor occupancy examined by PET after single oral doses of haloperidol. *Psychopharmacology.* 1992;106:436.)

COLOR PLATE 3.3–8

Three-dimensional PET FDG images demonstrate markedly lower glucose metabolism in the temporoparietal region in patient with Alzheimer's disease than in normal control. (From Sadock BJ, Sadock VA. *Kaplan and Sadock's Comprehensive Textbook of Psychiatry.* 7th ed. Vol 1. Baltimore: Lippincott Williams & Wilkins; 2000.)

COLOR PLATE 3.4–2

The human karyotype. The normal human genetic material contains two copies of the 3,000,000,000 DNA-base genomic sequence, packaged into 22 matched pairs of autosomes and X and Y sex chromosomes. Here the human karyotype has been stained using different colored chromosome-specific probes. Identical twins share identical copies of genomic DNA. (Adapted from Bentley D. *The Geography of Our Genome.* Supplement to *Nature,* 2001, with permission.)

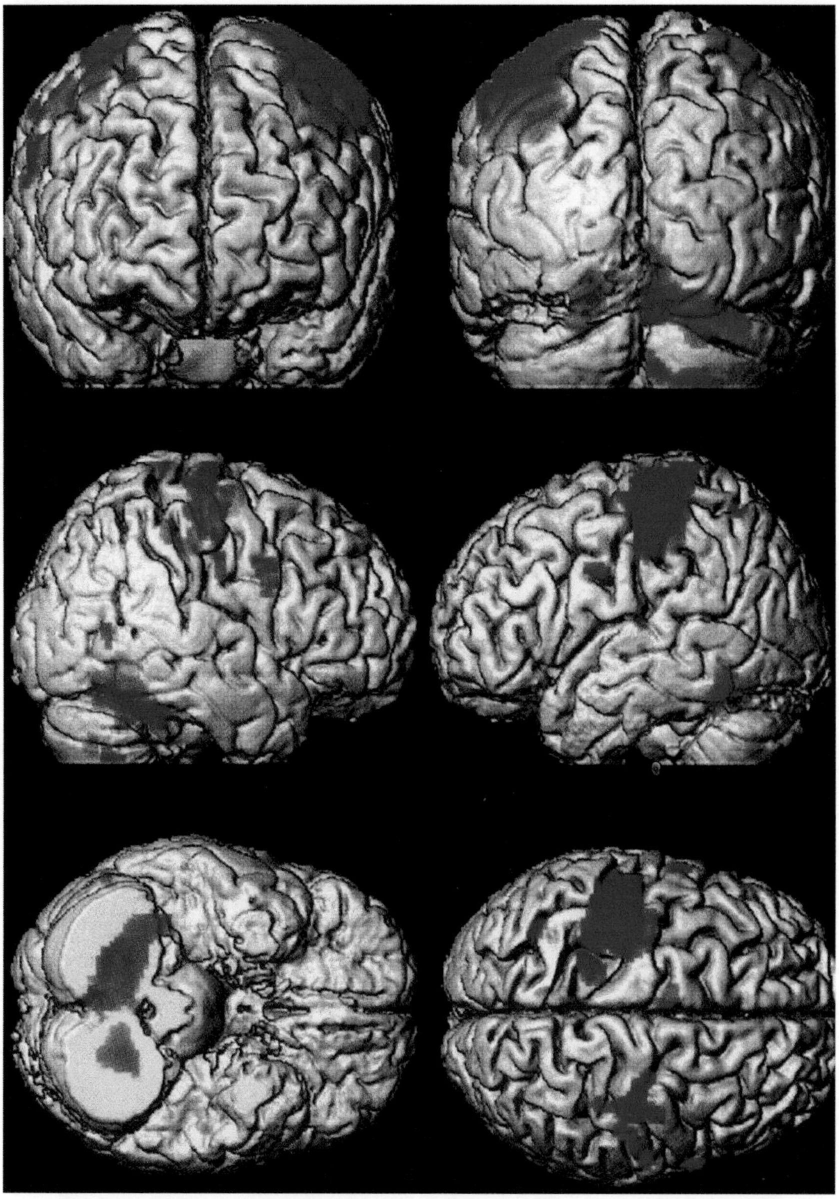

COLOR PLATE 3.1–11

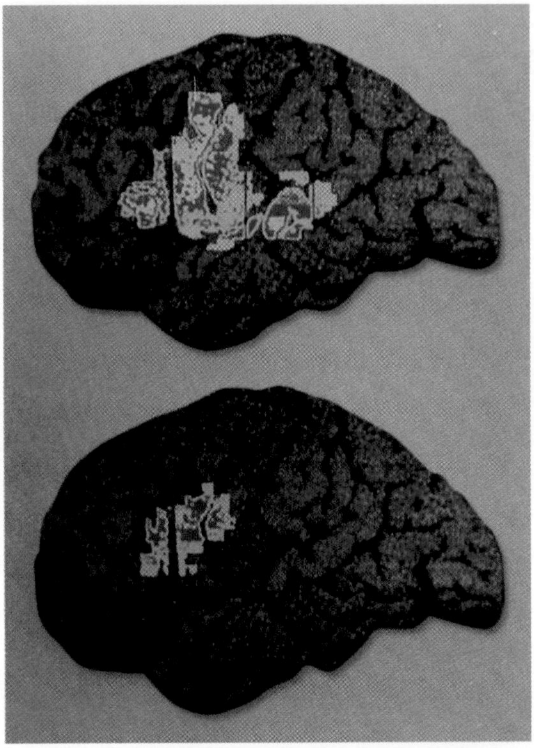

COLOR PLATE 3.3–4

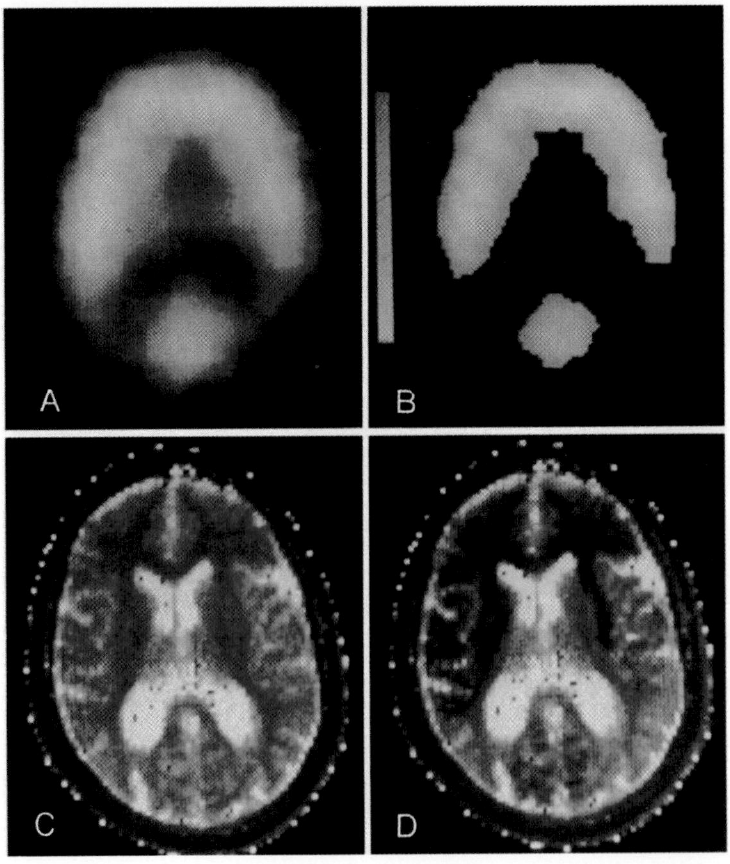

COLOR PLATE 3.3–5

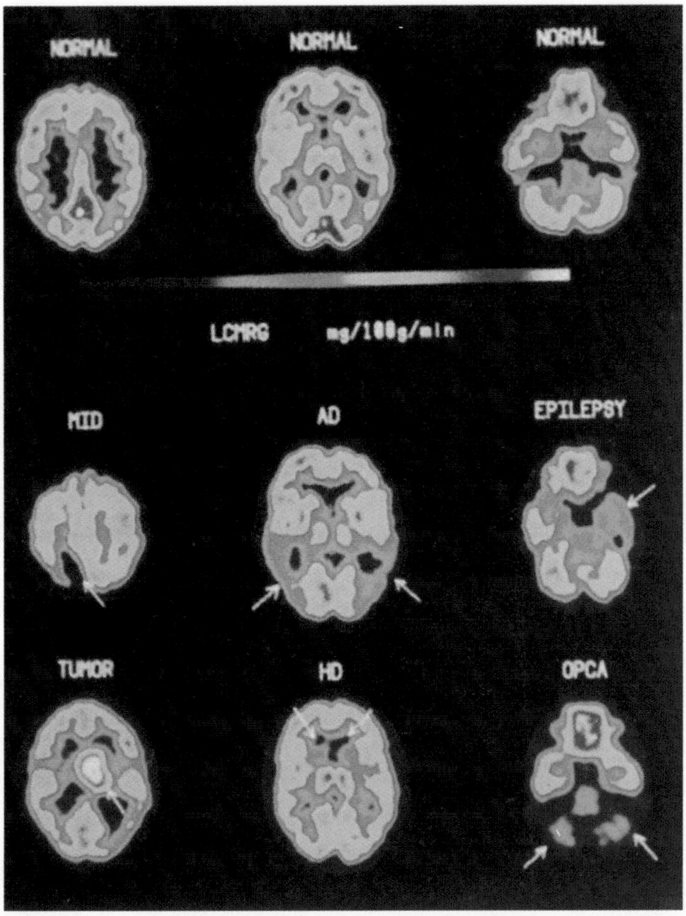

COLOR PLATE 3.3–6

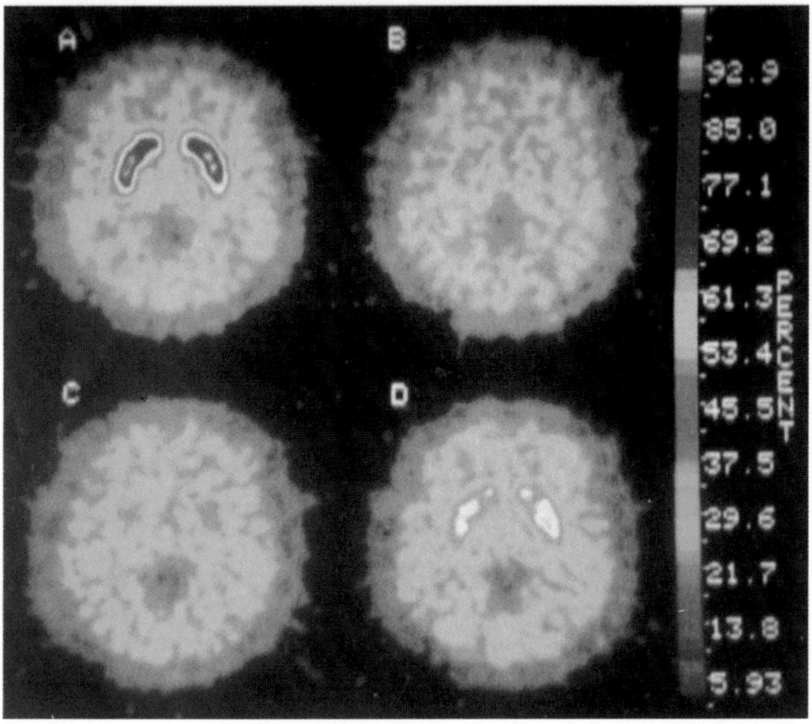

COLOR PLATE 3.3–7

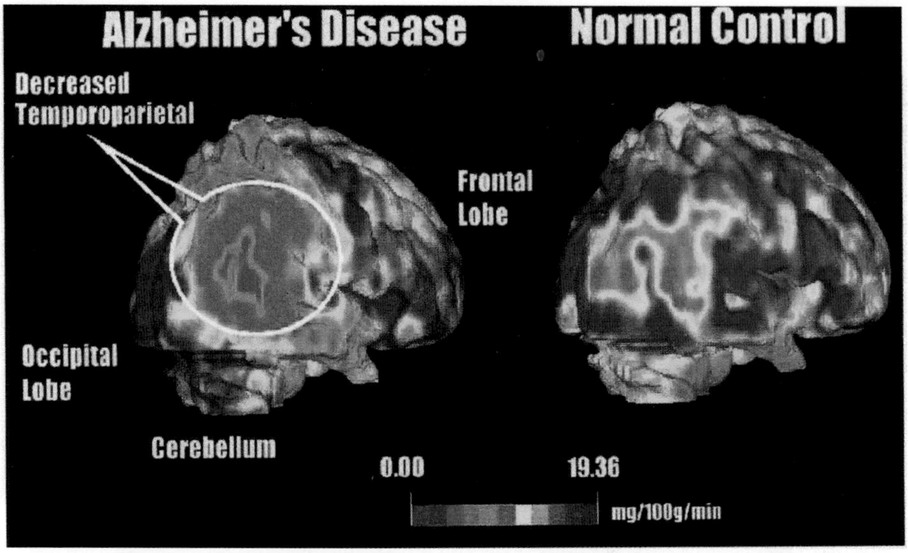

COLOR PLATE 3.3–8

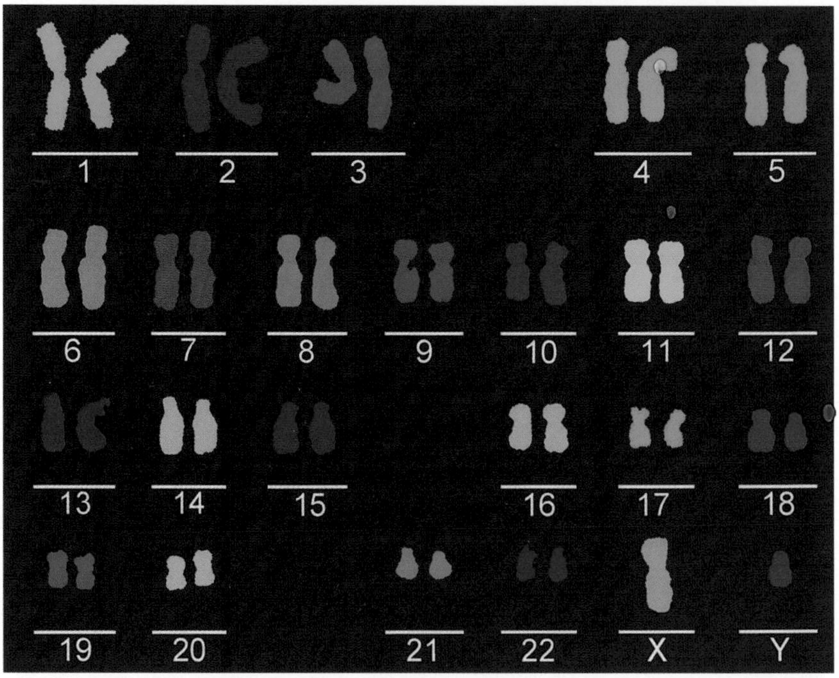

COLOR PLATE 3.4–2

whether memories were true or false, subjects activated the frontal lobes. FDG studies have also investigated pathology in neurological disorders and psychiatric disorders (see Color Plate 3.3–6 on p. 117). Two other types of studies use precursor molecules and receptor ligands. The dopamine precursor dopa has been used to visualize pathology in patients with Parkinson's disease, and radiolabeled ligands for receptors have been useful in determining the occupancy of receptors by specific psychotherapeutic drugs (see Color Plate 3.3–7 on p. 117).

For example, dopamine receptor antagonists such as haloperidol (Haldol) block almost 100 percent of D_2 receptors. The atypical antipsychotic drugs block serotonin 5-HT_2 receptors in addition to D_2 receptors; hence they are referred to as *serotonin-dopamine receptor antagonists*.

The following case illustrates the potential diagnostic value of three-dimensional PET imaging.

Patient A. is a 70-year-old man who had gotten more forgetful, to the point that his family was worried about him. The patient's family was interested in getting a diagnostic workup to evaluate the possible causes for his memory disorder. His PET scan showed that he had functional parietotemporal decrease (see Color Plate 3.3–8 on p. 118), which corroborated other neurological evaluations suggesting that he had Alzheimer's disease. The patient was treated with tacrine (Cognex) and benefited from some stabilization of his symptoms. (Courtesy of Joseph C. Wu, M.D., Daniel G. Amen, M.D., and H. Stefan Bracha, M.D.)

Pharmacological and Neuropsychological Probes

With both PET and SPECT and eventually with MRS, more studies and possibly more diagnostic procedures will use pharmacological and neuropsychological probes. The purpose of such probes is to stimulate particular regions of brain activity, so that, when compared with a baseline, workers can reach conclusions about the functional correspondence to particular brain regions. One example of the approach is the use of PET to detect regions of the brain involved in the processing of shape, color, and velocity in the visual system. Another example is the use of cognitive activation tasks (e.g., the Wisconsin Card Sorting Test) to study frontal blood flow in patients with schizophrenia. A key consideration in the evaluation of reports that measure blood flow is the establishment of a true baseline value in the study design. Typically, the reports use an awake, resting state, but there is variability in whether the patients have their eyes closed or their ears blocked; both conditions can affect brain function. There is also variability in such baseline brain function factors as gender, age, anxiety about the test, nonpsychiatric drug treatment, vasoactive medications, and time of day.

Electroencephalography

Neural electrical activity consists of patterned changes in electrical potential across cell membranes. Individual cells generate membrane potentials that can be detected only within a few micrometers of the cell, but assemblies of brain cells that fire synchronously may generate potentials on the order of microvolts, which can be detected through the skull and skin with an array of scalp electrodes. The regional variation in electrical potential across the scalp forms the basis of *electroencephalography,* which is the recording of the electrical activity of the brain. Electroencephalography is used in clinical psychiatry principally to evaluate the presence of seizures, particularly temporal lobe or frontal lobe seizures, which may produce complex behaviors.

Summation of the electrical potential changes in the cortex is thought to occur at the radially oriented large pyramidal cells of the cortex. When two scalp electrodes are placed far enough apart (at least several millimeters), they subsume enough pyramidal cell generators to detect changes in the electrical potential on the order of 2 to 200 microvolts. Although a random pattern of voltage changes might be expected, the normal human electroencephalogram (EEG), in fact, contains rhythmical activity at frequencies of 1 Hz (1 cycle per second) to 50 Hz. The most obvious rhythm in adults is the alpha rhythm of 9 to 10 Hz, present over the occipital lobe. On the basis of animal experiments in which stimulation or ablation of the thalamus stimulated or abolished rhythmical cortical activity, respectively, researchers concluded that rhythmical cortical activity detected by the EEG originates in thalamocortical circuits driven by thalamic pacemaker cells. The nuclei of the thalamus may project widely or to discrete regions of the cortex and may also project branches that stimulate thalamic inhibitory interneurons. Certain of these interneurons inhibit the thalamic projection for one tenth of a second, which according to one theory may be the basis of the 10-Hz alpha rhythm. In an alternative view, cortical-cortical interactions alone have cortical rhythmicity; this view is based on observations that cortical activity may be better synchronized to activity in other parts of the cortex than to the thalamus. Besides the thalamus and cortex, lesional studies have demonstrated that an intact brainstem ascending reticular activating system (ARAS) is necessary for cortical rhythms. Finally, cortical rhythms in humans may be abolished by arousal, heightened attention, drowsiness, or sleep.

The principal source of EEG activity is the electrical potential of the brain. Activity immediately below the scalp electrodes contributes most to the recording, but distant brain activity may modulate the tracing. The EEG must be recorded with the patient as motionless as possible, to eliminate the introduction of muscle artifact. Muscle contraction, of course, also involves electrical activity, and muscle twitching, especially of the face and scalp muscles, may generate electrical potentials high enough to obscure brain electrical activity completely. Other sources of muscle artifact include eye movements; eye movements are a normal component of the rapid eye movement (REM) stage of sleep and may clue an electroencephalographer to the presence of REM sleep. Since artifacts may also be introduced from a strong source of alternating current, an EEG is usually recorded in a shielded room.

The electrodes normally used to record the EEG are attached to the scalp with a conductive paste. Under special circumstances, needle electrodes may be placed into the nasopharynx or the masseter muscle to approximate the temporal lobes. With the realization that surgical removal of an epileptic focus

within the brain may cure epilepsy in a patient otherwise refractory to medical management, several epilepsy centers have refined the use of strips or arrays of electrodes applied directly to the surface of the brain at craniotomy, from which discharges are recorded for several days. To localize deeper epileptogenic foci, depth electrodes may be inserted into the brain. These invasive recording methods offer greatly improved spatial resolution of epileptiform activity. They may also be used to stimulate the brain to map out the sites of critical functions and to guide the hand of the neurosurgeon during the resection of diseased brain.

Routine electroencephalography uses the international 10–20 system of electrode placement to provide a uniform assessment of the entire scalp. Lines are drawn between bony landmarks and then divided into segments of either 10 or 20 percent of their length, making a grid that covers the scalp. The standard array consists of 21 electrodes, but extra electrodes may be interpolated on the grid for finer spatial resolution. Three montages are used to represent cortical activity. In the longitudinal bipolar montage, each channel registers positive or negative signals by comparing the potential of adjacent electrodes, which are oriented in anterior-posterior chains. In the transverse bipolar montage, the chains are connected from left to right across the head. The deflection of adjacent electrodes in opposite directions, called a *phase reversal,* localizes the site of a spike in electrical potential in the bipolar montage. *Bipolar montages* yield the best localization of cerebral activity. In contrast to the bipolar montage, the *referential montage* compares the electrical potential of each electrode to a common ground electrode, usually located at one ear. The advantage of the referential montage is that it may reveal potentials with a wider distribution across the brain.

The normal EEG consists of a mixture of frequencies, which are divided into four bandwidths. Delta waves oscillate below 4 Hz, and theta waves oscillate from 4 to 8 Hz; activity below 8 Hz is also called *slow wave activity.* Alpha waves, the frequency of the posterior dominant rhythm, are from 8 to 13 Hz. Beta waves (fast activity) are over 13 Hz. Normal activity contains a posterior alpha rhythm with the eyes closed; more anterior regions have random admixtures of theta, alpha, or beta activity. The appearance of delta activity is abnormal, except in sleep, and may reflect an underlying structural lesion. Upon alerting and eye opening, the posterior alpha is replaced by random activity.

Abnormal discharges suggesting a seizure focus consist of rapid changes in potential, or spikes, which may be organized in rhythmical patterns. The spikes may be followed by a broad slow wave, yielding a spike-wave pattern. If spike or spike-wave activity is localized to one area of the montage, the underlying brain is referred to as a *potentially epileptogenic focus.* Such a focus may originate a focal seizure, which is a series of spikes or spike-wave complexes that persists to the point of affecting a patient's movements or behavior. If the seizure focus recruits neighboring brain tissue and spreads throughout the cortex, it is said to *generalize;* generalized seizures are accompanied by loss of consciousness. Generalized seizures may not be preceded by focal cortical seizure activity but may appear throughout the EEG simultaneously. Such generalized-onset seizures are thought to originate in deep structures, such as the thalamus.

Routine surface electroencephalography is useful in evaluating epilepsy. In patients with epileptic seizures, a single EEG will be abnormal 70 percent of the time. After three routine EEGs, the sensitivity increases to 95 percent. Therefore, an abnormal EEG may strongly suggest epilepsy, but a normal EEG does not rule out the disorder. In patients with episodes of bizarre behavior who do not exhibit the classical tonic-clonic seizure movements, it may be difficult to diagnose seizure activity on the basis of history alone. When routine EEGs do not show epileptiform activity, one may have to record the EEG for a prolonged period, as much as several days, with closed-circuit television (CCTV) observation, to capture an actual seizure event. This method, called *24-hour CCTV electroencephalographic monitoring,* is performed in specified epilepsy monitoring units at major referral centers or on an ambulatory basis in the home.

In clinical psychiatry, electroencephalography is useful to distinguish temporal lobe seizures from pseudoseizures. Another indication for electroencephalography is in the differentiation of dementia from pseudodementia caused by depression. In dementia, the EEG reveals excessive slow wave activity, whereas in depression the recording is normal. For most psychiatric patients, however, electroencephalography is of little value; however, it has been used to explain abnormal behavior as in the following case:

A 37-year-old left-handed man with epilepsy presented with aggressive episodes. The seizures consisted of an olfactory aura followed by "spacing out," or alteration of consciousness, for approximately 1 minute. In addition to these complex partial seizures the patient had occasional secondary generalized tonic-clonic seizures with urinary incontinence and tongue-biting. During the postictal period, as he began to recover consciousness he experienced an overwhelming sense of threat or of having been harmed. These feelings became focused on any individual who was in his immediate environment. He believed that person had beaten or otherwise hurt him and was going to harm him further. The patient felt compelled to attack these individuals, often inflicting significant physical injury. Although his postictal confusion would clear in about 1 hour, his sense of being harmed or threatened diminished slowly over about 24 hours after a seizure. After the resolution of these feelings, he felt great remorse over the harm that he had done. Nevertheless, on several occasions he was charged with aggravated assault. Sleep-deprived EEGs confirmed the presence of left anterior temporal epileptiform activity. The patient's aggressive postictal episodes abated with control of his complex partial seizures with carbamazepine (Tegretol).

Electroencephalography is used during electroconvulsive therapy (ECT) to monitor the success of the stimulus in producing seizure activity. The EEG is an essential part of the polysomnogram, or sleep study, used in the evaluation of sleep disorders. The definition of sleep stages is based on the EEG patterns.

The EEG has been used in research settings to evaluate the registration of sensations by the cortex. If the responses to a

sufficient series of stimuli are summed, the subconscious registration of environmental events may be detected with an EEG. As a tool for establishing the function of different brain regions, the EEG provides excellent temporal resolution, but spatial resolution is poor. Because of the constant random brain activity seen over most parts of the brain, it has not been possible to use the EEG to localize the activation of specific brain regions during complex cognitive tasks as one can use fMRI, SPECT, or PET scanning.

In theory, a sufficiently detailed recording of the electrical activity of the brain should reveal a specific pattern of activity when a person thinks of a specific word or idea. In practice, however, this level of interpretive sophistication is many years away. Preliminary efforts have succeeded in interpreting EEG activity in terms of simple conscious thought. In an effort to harness the complexity of brain waves to direct computers and machines (e.g., as a communication tool for patients unable to speak because of severe spasticity), researchers have categorized the frequency and waveforms of the EEG during thoughts. Alpha waves (8 to 13 Hz) appear when the eyes close, and they attenuate when the eyes open or the person concentrates on vivid imagination. Beta waves (fast waves, usually 14 to 30 Hz) increase with heightened mental activity and may reach 50 Hz during intense thought. Theta waves (4 to 7 Hz) appear during emotional stress, especially frustration or disappointment. Delta waves (less than 4 Hz) occur during deep sleep.

A particular type of alpha-range waves, called mu waves, are recorded over the motor cortex, and they attenuate in amplitude with actual or imagined movements. In the past decade, researchers have trained individuals to regulate the amplitude of their mu waves by visualizing various motions, such as chewing, swallowing, or smiling. EEG electrodes placed over the motor strip and attached to an amplitude analyzer can determine the size of the mu waves with sufficient precision to guide a computer cursor and operate a program solely by means of thoughts. Other EEG-computer machines use the presence or absence of alpha waves, determined by unfocusing or focusing attention, to operate an electronic switch. With time and the application of increased computer-processing power, researchers may begin to decipher the electrical signature of complex cognition.

Magnetoencephalography (MEG) and Transcranial Magnetic Stimulation (TMS)

Physics teaches that every electrical field has a corresponding magnetic field oriented at right angles to it. This fact applies to the electrical activity of the brain and forms the basis for magnetoencephalography (MEG). Much of the previous discussion of electroencephalography can be translated for MEG. The changes in membrane potential of neurons during normal activity generate tiny magnetic fields. When the activities of the billions of neurons in the cortex are summed, the changes in magnetic field can be detected with special magnets placed on the scalp. But although electroencephalography uses simple wires and can be performed almost anywhere, MEG requires supercooled magnets, called *single superconducting quantum interference devices* (SQUIDs), which operate near absolute zero temperature. The technique is therefore limited to a handful of facilities.

MEG offers the best temporal and the lowest spatial resolution of any technique currently available. It also detects only tangentially flowing fields, complementing electroencephalography, which detects radially oriented fields. MEG is the superior technique for detection of activity deep within the brain because the fields are less attenuated by the skull and scalp tissues. In addition, since it is a true monopolar technique, it does not require a reference electrode and therefore can avoid certain artifacts. The fields registered by MEG are tiny; recordings need careful shielding and extensive computerized computational algorithms for maximum localization within the brain. MEG thus remains almost exclusively a research tool.

The major area in which the existence of magnetic fields in the brain provides a unique opportunity for study is the ability to alter the magnetic fields by transcranial magnetic stimulation (TMS). In theory, applying electrical fields to the brain is also possible, and this is the central therapeutic intervention in ECT. In practice, however, attenuation of the scalp and nonneural tissues, which generates heat and pain and may produce burns, limits the usefulness of electrical stimulation. TMS involves a strong electromagnet, in which the field is oscillated at 0.1 to 60 Hz. The frequency, pulse duration, and intensity of the magnetic field all contribute to the amount of neuronal stimulation caused by TMS. Low-frequency (0.1 to 5 Hz) pulses may in some cases reduce metabolism in the underlying cortex, whereas higher-frequency pulses (15 to 25 Hz) may increase local cerebral metabolism. Pulse rates above 25 Hz are associated with the induction of seizures and are avoided in human subjects. When applied accurately in a single pulse, TMS can inactivate neural activity. When given as a train of pulses, it can transiently inhibit discrete regions of the brain, which then rebound and exhibit prolonged increased activity, sometimes for as long as days to months. For example, a pulse aimed at a specific part of the basal ganglia can eliminate the tremor of Parkinson's disease.

In psychiatric research, the prevailing view that the left hemisphere generates positive emotions and the right hemisphere mediates negative emotions has been addressed with TMS. Pulses that inactivate brain regions suppress positive thoughts and elicit sadness when directed toward the left frontal lobe. When the right frontal lobe is suppressed by TMS, subjects feel happier and more energetic. In tests, these mood changes lasted a few hours. In another experimental paradigm, severely depressed patients, who might otherwise have been candidates for ECT, instead received TMS over the left frontal lobe for 20 minutes a day over 2 weeks. A significant number of patients reported an improved mood for a few days, whereas patients subjected to sham treatments showed no improvement. As a practical therapy for depression, TMS would have to be readministered frequently. Researchers are attempting to prolong the effects.

An interesting application of TMS and electroencephalography or MEG involves timing the flow of neural impulses through the brain. When one part of the brain is stimulated with TMS, the transmission of this information to distant brain regions can be registered to millisecond accuracy with electroencephalography, MEG, or both. This process may allow systematic functional mapping of intracortical circuits, to build on the scaffolding of cortical connections defined by classical neuroanatomical methods.

Evoked Potentials (EPs) and Event-Related Potentials (ERPs)

Sensory evoked potentials, reflecting the brain's electrical response to reproducible sensory stimuli, are extracted from the EEG by computer-assisted signal averaging. The recording of EPs uses electrode and recording arrangements similar to those

used in electroencephalography. Sensory EPs provide a measure of how the cortex responds to particular sensory stimuli. In evaluating demyelinating disorders, such as multiple sclerosis, well-established protocols exist for somatosensory evoked potentials (SEPs), brainstem auditory evoked potentials (BAEPs), and visual evoked potentials (VEPs). In EP testing, a stimulus from one sensory modality (e.g., a mild electric shock, a click, or a light flash) is presented multiple times while the resulting neural EPs are recorded at various levels over the sensory pathway, always including electrodes over the corresponding sensory cortex. Because of the inherent random and rhythmical brain activity recorded by scalp electrodes, one must average the cortical responses to 100 to 2000 identical repetitions of a particular sensory stimulus. The random activity tends to cancel itself out, whereas the sensory response adds up to a recognizable waveform. The result is a smooth curve (the EP) that includes peaks and valleys.

Positive waves are downward deflections, and negative waves are upward deflections. Particular waves are further identified by the number of milliseconds that occur after the stimulus. The P300 wave, therefore, is a downward (positive) deflection that occurs approximately 300 ms after the stimulus. The magnitude and the timing of EP waves constitute the basis of the clinical and research evaluation of an EP recording.

The EP waves have been classified into early (<50 ms after the stimulus), middle (50 to 250 ms), and late (>250 ms) components. The relay of sensory information as it passes from a sensory organ (e.g., the eyes) to the primary sensory cortex and to the association cortex is reflected in the early EP components. Increasingly complex cognitive and psychological processing of sensory information is reflected in the late EP components. EP recordings are especially subject to contamination by various artifacts in addition to those affecting EEG recordings. Attention, compliance, fatigue, coffee and cigarette consumption, the age of the person, and diurnal variations all reportedly affect the data from EP recordings.

In research settings, a dense (64-channel) EEG electrode array, recording brain activity in a time-locked fashion during cognitive tasks such as reading, is used to correlate late EP components with higher cognitive processing. In one study, when subjects read a passage and recording began at the arrival at a certain trigger word, the event-related potential (ERP) began at about 70 ms, with bilateral positive current sources over the occipitoparietal visual processing areas. A negative potential then followed at about 180 ms over the left temporal lobe, accompanied by an anterior positivity. A separate posterior positive pattern then emerged that seemed to repeat the topography of the initial positive current. Next, at about 350 ms, the ERP for the trigger word developed diffuse positivity over the superior surface of the head and several negativities over inferior regions. This superior source–inferior sink pattern, called the P300, or the late positive component (LPC), was greater over the left hemisphere. Under similar recording conditions, when the trigger word was replaced with a semantically unexpected word, the brain electrical activity showed no potential at 350 ms, but then developed an LPC at 400 ms, which remained relatively symmetrical over the two hemispheres.

In a further refinement of this approach, ERPs, which have relatively poor spatial resolution, nevertheless provide enough spatial discrimination to permit temporal ordering of the activation of several brain regions that are identified as essential to the performance of a task by fMRI or PET. In one example of this approach, functional brain imaging studies with PET identified blood flow changes in widely separated areas of the brain during the performance of word-related tasks. ERPs were then used to investigate the temporal relationships among cortical areas previously identified by PET to be differentially activated when performing a language task. ERPs showed strong task-related differences over left and middle inferior frontal and left parietotemporal regions. Frontal and left parietotemporal channels revealed these differences about 200 and 700 ms, respectively, after word presentation. These results provided the time course for parts of the anatomical circuit involved in generating the meaning of a word. Although labor intensive, studies combining functional neuroimaging and ERP hold great promise for understanding the neuroanatomical basis for normal and abnormal human cognition.

References

Bonne O, Brandes D, Gilboa A, et al. Longitudinal MRI study of hippocampal volume in trauma survivors with PTSD. *Am J Psychiatry.* 2001;158:1248.

Boutros NN, Struve F. Electrophysiological assessment of neuropsychiatric disorders. *Semin Clin Neuropsychiatry.* 2002;7:30.

Bressan RA, Jones HM, Ell PJ, Pilowsky LS. Dopamine D(2) receptor blockade in schizophrenia. *Am J Psychiatry.* 2001;158:971.

Camargo EE. Brain SPECT in neurology and psychiatry. *J Nucl Med.* 2001;42:611.

Carter CS, MacDonald AW 3rd, Ross LL, Stenger VA. Anterior cingulate cortex activity and impaired self-monitoring of performance in patients with schizophrenia: an event-related fMRI study. *Am J Psychiatry.* 2001;158:1423.

Danos P, Guich S, Abel L, Buchsbaum MS. EEG alpha rhythm and glucose metabolic rate in the thalamus in schizophrenia. *Neuropsychobiology.* 2001;43:265.

Drevets WC. Neuroimaging studies of mood disorders. In: Helzer JE, Hudziak JJ, eds. *Defining Psychopathology in the 21st Century: DSM-V and Beyond.* Washington, DC: American Psychiatric Publishing, Inc.; 2002:71.

Durston S, Hulshoff Pol HE, Casey BJ, Giedd JN, Buitelaar JK, van Engeland H. Anatomical MRI of the developing human brain: what have we learned? *J Am Acad Child Adolesc Psychiatry.* 2001;40:1012.

Halldin C, Gulyas B, Langer O, Farde L. Brain radioligands—state of the art and new trends. *Q J Nucl Med.* 2001;45:139.

Herpertz SC, Dietrich TM, Wenning B, et al. Evidence of abnormal amygdala functioning in borderline personality disorder: a functional MRI study. *Biol Psychiatry.* 2001;50:292.

Kircher TT, Bulimore ET, Brammer MJ, et al. Differential activation of temporal cortex during sentence completion in schizophrenic patients with and without formal thought disorder. *Schizophr Res.* 2001;50:27.

Maria Moresco R, Messa C, Lucignani G, et al. PET in psychopharmacology. *Pharmacol Res.* 2001;44:151.

Markianos M, Hatzimanolis J, Lykouras L. Neuroendocrine responsivities of the pituitary dopamine system in male schizophrenic patients during treatment with clozapine, olanzapine, risperidone, sulpiride, or haloperidol. *Eur Arch Psychiatry Clin Neurosci.* 2001;251:141.

Migneco O, Benoit M, Koulibaly PM, et al. Perfusion brain SPECT and statistical parametric mapping analysis indicate that apathy is a cingulate syndrome: a study in Alzheimer's disease and nondemented patients. *Neuroimage.* 2001;13:896.

Rauch SL, Whalen PJ, Curran T, et al. Probing striato-thalamic function in obsessive-compulsive disorder and Tourette syndrome using neuroimaging methods. *Adv Neurol.* 2001;85:207.

Sackeim HA. Functional brain circuits in major depression and remission. *Arch Gen Psychiatry.* 2001;58:649.

Shenton ME, Dickey CC, Frumin M, McCarley RW. A review of MRI findings in schizophrenia. *Schizophr Res.* 2001;49:1.

Strafella AP, Paus T, Barrett J, Dagher A. Repetitive transcranial magnetic stimulation of the human prefrontal cortex induces dopamine release in the caudate nucleus. *J Neurosci.* 2001;21:RC157.

Videbech P, Ravnkilde B, Pedersen AR, et al. The Danish PET/depression project: PET findings in patients with major depression. *Psychol Med.* 2001;31:1147.

▲ 3.4 Neurogenetics and Molecular Biology

The human genome consists of between 30,000 and 50,000 genes, of which over 20,000 have been identified. Over 5,000 genetic disorders, each transmitted through a single mutant gene, have been characterized. The application of more power-

ful quantitative methods of analysis, new molecular technologies, and more detailed maps of the human genome have permitted localization to chromosomal regions of over 400 of these disease genes, with precise identification of more than 80.

There are major public health implications to identifying genes that influence an individual's risk of developing the more common familiar mental disorders such as schizophrenia, bipolar I disorder, alcoholism (alcohol abuse or dependence) and obsessive-compulsive disorder. Such findings may ultimately have relevance for many affected individuals and their relatives, given the potential for developing a genetic test to identify individuals at risk, and equally important for providing the pharmaceutical industry with new drug therapy targets. Clinicians and researchers must understand the basic principles of genetics and genetic epidemiology so that they will be able to appreciate the relevance of new data derived from the genetic analysis of mental disorders.

BASIC MOLECULAR BIOLOGY

The central dogma of molecular biology is "DNA makes RNA makes protein." Deoxyribonucleic acid (DNA) is a genetic code consisting of a series of bases, adenine (A), cytosine (C), guanine (G), and thymine (T), which are covalently linked to form extremely long molecules (Fig. 3.4–1). *Genes* consist of strings of DNA code that specify a series of base triplets, called *codons,* that determine a specific sequence of *amino acids,* the building blocks of proteins. DNA resides in the nucleus, where it serves as a template for the formation of messenger ribonucleic acid (mRNA) molecules. Messenger RNA is assembled according to the DNA code by the stepwise addition of bases according to a complementation algorithm. Ribonucleic adenine (rA) is complementary to deoxyribonucleic thymine (T), rG to C, rC to G, and ribonucleic uracil (rU) to adenine (A). Thus, the DNA string ATGTCTTAG would encode the mRNA string UACAGAAUC. Messenger RNA has stretches of protein-coding sequences, called *exons,* which are interrupted by noncoding sequences, called *introns.* Soon after the mRNA is transcribed from the DNA, the exons are spliced together to form a continuous stretch of coding sequence. The mRNA moves into the cytoplasm and binds to ribosomes, which read the triplet codons and assemble a string of amino acids to form a specific protein. There are 20 common amino acids, each with a different atomic configuration. Depending on the primary amino acid sequence, the protein folds into a three-dimensional molecule that interacts specifically with other proteins, carbohydrates, nucleic acids, or lipids to carry out the functions of the cell.

The relative abundance of various proteins in the cell may be regulated by the rate of mRNA transcription, at the level of mRNA translation into protein, or at the level of the degradation of the protein molecules. mRNA transcriptional control is the most common type of specific gene regulation. Initiation of mRNA transcription involves general factors, called *transcription factors,* common to all genes, but it is regulated by specific transcription factors that bind only to certain genes and are themselves regulated by intracellular and extracellular signals. Thus, thyroid hormones diffuse into the cell and bind to the thyroid receptors, and the hormone-receptor complex, which acts as a transcription factor, enters the nucleus and activates certain genes by binding to specific DNA sequences immediately adjacent to these genes. There is much interest in psychiatry in gene regulation by neurotransmitters and in the regulation of the synaptic neurochemical milieu by variations in the levels of gene transcription.

The human genetic material consists of 3 billion bases of DNA, which are divided into units of roughly 60 million bases, called *chromosomes.* The normal cell nucleus contains 23 pairs of chromosomes—22 matched pairs of autosomes and the X and Y sex chromosomes (see Color Plate 3.4–2 on p. 118). A typical gene spans about 10,000 bases, and the longest known gene covers 2 million bases. Humans are estimated to have about 30,000 to 40,000 distinct genes. The site of the chromosomes where a gene is located is called a *locus.* About 1 percent of the total DNA encodes genes that may be translated into proteins; and the remaining 99 percent is noncoding, "junk," DNA. The functions of only a few thousand of the genes are known at this time. Some genes encode proteins that play housekeeping roles within the cell; that is, they are present in all cells and are essential to the survival of the cell. Other genes play specific regulatory roles and are cell-type specific. Among these latter genes are those of particular interest to psychiatrists. Intense research is under way to identify both those genes that, when altered, may cause psychiatric illness and those that may determine normal emotional behaviors and responses. At this time, these goals tax, and in most cases exceed, the data-processing capabilities of even the most sophisticated investigators, but major technical advances are appearing at a rapid rate. With the complete sequencing of the human genome, most gene experts now anticipate significant advances in the identification of the genetic basis of complex human behaviors early in the 21st century.

PREMISES OF NEUROGENETICS

Many major psychiatric disorders have been shown to have a strong hereditary predisposition. In the case of schizophrenia, for example, a first-degree relative of an affected patient has about a 10 percent chance of having the illness, far in excess of the 1 percent risk in the general population. Monozygotic twins display nearly 50 percent concordance for schizophrenia. Bipolar I disorder and major depressive disorder exhibit similar familial clustering, in that first-degree relatives are 8 to 18 times more likely to have a mood disorder than is the general population, and monozygotic twins show a 33 to 90 percent concordance rate. Tourette's disorder shows an even more convincing genetic association. Several family pedigrees have been constructed in which transmission of the disorder is consistent with an autosomal dominant mode with penetrance of 99 percent in males and 70 percent in females. Only 10 percent of patients with Tourette's disorder do not have an affected family member. These facts stimulate the expectation that a specific genetic basis will emerge for certain psychiatric diseases.

Medicine has provided many models of genetically determined pathology. There are thousands of examples of inherited human traits and disorders, many of which have been traced to a single aberrant gene. One classic model is sickle cell anemia. A mutation at a single point in the β-globin gene causes this disorder by producing a single amino acid substitution in the β-globin protein, which forms half of hemoglobin. The mutation promotes crystallization of hemoglobin red blood cells and causes them to assume the shape of a sickle. Clinically, this effect leads to sludging in cap-

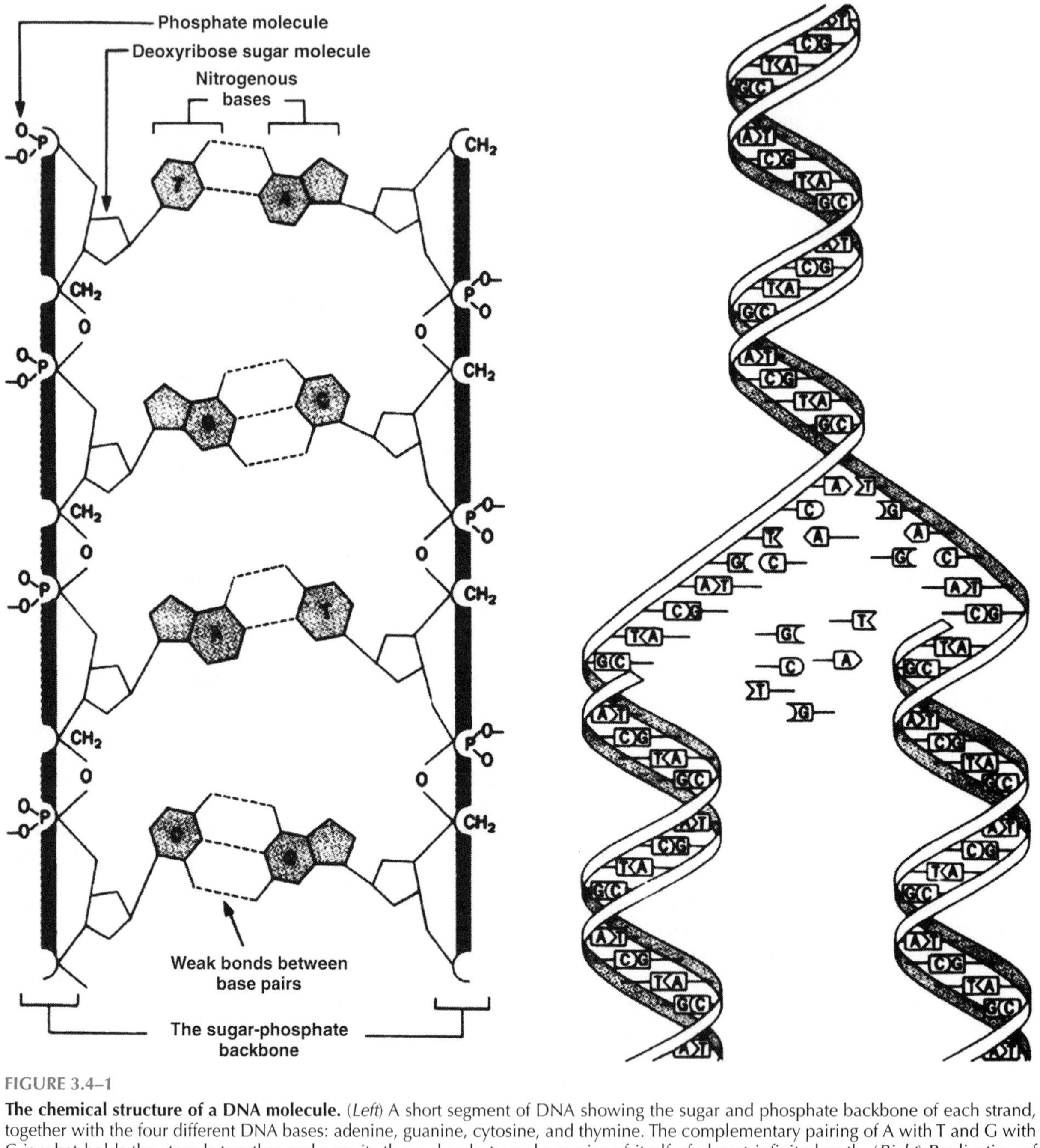

FIGURE 3.4–1

The chemical structure of a DNA molecule. (*Left*) A short segment of DNA showing the sugar and phosphate backbone of each strand, together with the four different DNA bases: adenine, guanine, cytosine, and thymine. The complementary pairing of A with T and G with C is what holds the strands together and permits the molecule to make copies of itself of almost infinite length. (*Right*) Replication of DNA, showing how the molecule unwinds and, by pairing of the complementary bases with each other, makes two identical copies of the original DNA sequence. (Modified from Jones S, Martin R, and Pilbeam D. *The Cambridge Encyclopedia of Human Evolution*. Cambridge, UK: Cambridge University Press, 1992:11.)

illaries and bone pain, as well as ischemic events such as strokes. The sickle cell anemia model is unusual among genetic diseases for the detail in which the molecular abnormality is known and for the simplicity with which the clinical syndrome can be traced to the biochemical mutation. Nevertheless, sickle cell anemia displays wide clinical variability, ranging from patients who are asymptomatic to severely impaired patients who die prematurely. This fact demonstrates the clinical variability introduced by *modifier genes,* which encode proteins that the aberrant protein interacts with. Two variants of sickle cell anemia, sickle-thalassemia and hemoglobin SC disease, have been traced to specific modifier genes, but most clinical variability is due to unknown factors. Thus, sickle cell anemia demonstrates the incompleteness of even the best understood genetic determination of human disease. This model tempers the optimism of researchers pursuing the genetic basis of behavior and emotion, which are considerably less well defined at a clinical level than sickle cell anemia.

Traits are clinically defined features, such as sickle crises or blue eyes. Some traits are determined by a single gene,

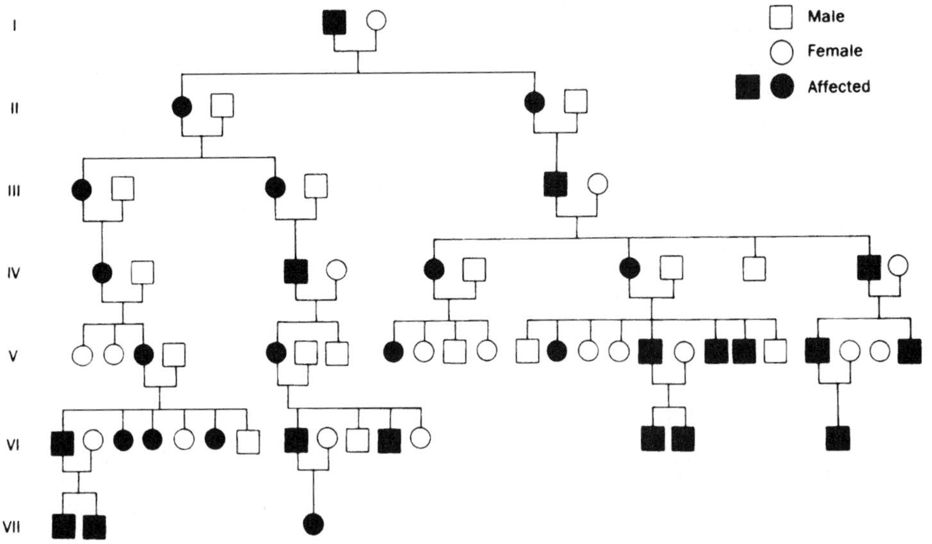

FIGURE 3.4–3

Transmission of traits through sexual reproduction. Sexual reproduction permits the propagation of novel advantageous mutations through a population. This pedigree shows seven generations in which a dominant trait (*dark circles and squares*) is transmitted from generation to generation. From a single trait-bearing individual in generation I, the trait is transmitted to roughly half of the offspring of seventeen unaffected individuals (*open circles and squares*): one in generation I, two in generation II, three in generation III, five in generation IV, four in generation V, and two in generation VI. (Modified from Jones S, Martin R, and Pilbeam D. *The Cambridge Encyclopedia of Human Evolution*. Cambridge, UK: Cambridge University Press; 1992:258.)

whereas others emerge from the interactions of the products of (in some cases) hundreds of genes. Behavior likely is the expression of the products of thousands of genes, although specific single-gene mutations may influence certain behaviors in consistent ways. Studies of animal behavior, especially that of the fruit fly and the laboratory mouse, have documented many behaviors inherited as single-gene traits. These heritable behaviors have often been traced to a specific gene, whereas others are only known to be heritable. Fortunately, the former category is rapidly expanding at the expense of the latter. Identifying a gene that determines a specific behavioral trait requires rigorous clinical definition of the trait and the largest possible pedigree or family tree in which the pattern of the trait's inheritance is unambiguously defined. Mapping genes essentially involves correlating the inheritance of the trait with the inheritance of molecular markers scattered throughout an animal's genetic material. This method is called *linkage analysis* or *positional cloning.*

For traits determined by single genes, three common inheritance patterns are recognized: autosomal dominant, autosomal recessive, and X-linked recessive transmission. In *autosomal dominant transmission* of disease only one of the two copies of the gene in the cell nucleus needs to mutate to produce the clinical trait. A parent with one copy of a dominant mutation has a 50 percent chance of passing the trait to a child. In *autosomal recessive transmission,* the trait can be passed on only when both copies are mutated. Thus a parent with an autosomal recessive trait can transmit it to a child only when the other parent also passes on the mutant gene. In *X-linked recessive transmission,* the gene is found on an unpaired X chromosome and is thus the only copy of the gene in the nucleus. An X-linked recessive trait therefore occurs in males, who have only one X chromosome; females are carriers, but they do not display the clinical traits because they have a second, normal X chromosome (Fig. 3.4–3).

In psychiatry, the largest hurdle in the process of assigning behavioral traits to specific genes is the rigorous clinical definition of psychiatric traits. The text revision of the fourth edition of *Diagnostic and Statistical Manual of Mental Disorders* (DSM-IV-TR), which provides exact categorization for most psychiatric disorders, nonetheless probably includes a genetically heterogeneous population of patients under each diagnostic category. The situation is further muddled by the lack of objective, quantifiable tests for psychiatric disorders. Moreover, because familial clustering of certain behavioral traits can be due to either genetics (nature) or upbringing (nurture), constructing accurate pedigrees strictly according to genetic criteria may be impossible. Finally, the multigenic determination of behavioral traits serves to increase the complexity of analysis exponentially. If all hurdles can be overcome, the process of screening chromosomes for linkage between a trait and a specific chromosome location is virtually automated.

At this time, pedigrees have been assembled for each of the main psychiatric disorders, and chromosomal linkage has been sought with the tools of molecular genetics. Even in the apparently straightforward case of Tourette's disorder, screening of almost all chromosomes has failed to identify a specific genetic locus always inherited with the clinical behavior. This finding suggests that Tourette's syndrome is a *multigenic trait,* that is, a disorder that may be due to the combined influences of several genes. Screening for mutations in genes that regulate the dopamine pathway in patients with Tourette's syndrome, as well as neurotransmitters in other disorders, is ongoing.

Genetic causes are being sought for other psychiatric disorders. Based on an analysis of 22 pedigrees, a locus that confers an increased risk of bipolar disorder has been identified on

chromosome 18. The correlation is not robust, which indicates a need for further investigation. For the personality trait of anxiety, a genetic variant of the serotonin transporter gene has been described that alters the number of transporter molecules in the presynaptic membrane of serotonergic neurons. This alternative version of the transporter has been calculated to account for less than 5 percent of the genetic variance for anxiety in the general population.

Persons with schizophrenia may have difficulty filtering auditory input to screen out extraneous sounds. A carefully performed positional cloning project has identified a locus on chromosome 15 that encodes the α_1 nicotinic acetylcholine receptor and appears to account for the abnormality in auditory processing in several pedigrees of patients with schizophrenia. Another study, examining the previously described negative association between schizophrenia and rheumatoid arthritis, found that the human lymphocyte antigen (HLA) *DRB1*04* allele was significantly associated with a reduced risk of rheumatoid arthritis in 94 unrelated patients with schizophrenia. A study of 265 Irish families with a high incidence of schizophrenia found two loci, one on chromosome 8 and the other on chromosome 6, each of which accounted for the vulnerability to schizophrenia in 10 to 30 percent of the families. These findings should be viewed as preliminary, and each will require further work.

Alzheimer's disease can be definitively diagnosed only by pathological examination of brain tissue, either at autopsy or from brain biopsy. Whereas shrinkage of neuronal volume without loss of neurons is a feature of normal aging, loss of neurons is typical of Alzheimer's disease. The two characteristic neuropathological features are senile plaques and neurofibrillary tangles. A recent clinicopathological study found that elderly nuns with senile plaques and neurofibrillary tangles do not always have dementia, but the risk is greatly increased (from 57 to 93 percent) if they also have suffered strokes. A separate study of nuns showed that writing style at age 20 years predicted the onset of dementia (presumably Alzheimer's) over the age of 70 years. Nuns with a simple writing style in their youth were more likely to develop dementia than nuns with a complex command of written language. These two studies illustrate that dementia of the Alzheimer's type likely results from a combination of genetically determined and acquired factors.

Four genetic loci have been associated with the risk of Alzheimer's disease. Ten percent of cases of Alzheimer's disease are hereditary, and the remaining 90 percent are sporadic. Of the hereditary cases, 70 to 80 percent are attributable to mutations in the presenilin 1 gene, located on chromosome 14, which causes onset of symptoms at age 40 to 50 years. Another 20 to 30 percent are attributable to mutations in a related gene, presenilin 2, located on chromosome 1, which causes onset of symptoms at age 50 years. A final 2 to 3 percent of the familial cases are attributable to mutations in the β-amyloid precursor protein (APP) gene, located on chromosome 21, which causes onset of symptoms at age 50 years. APP and a cytoskeletal protein called *tau* are prominent components of senile plaques and neurofibrillary tangles in both familial and sporadic cases of Alzheimer's disease. Tau protein appears to polymerize into the paired helical filaments that are the main components of neurofibrillary tangles if it is not protected from phosphorylation. This protection is afforded by apolipoprotein E (apo ε), encoded by a gene on chromosome 19 that has three alleles. The $\varepsilon 2$ allele protects tau, whereas the $\varepsilon 3$ and (especially) the $\varepsilon 4$ alleles do not associate as strongly with tau and leave it susceptible to phosphorylation and eventual polymerization. Presence of the $\varepsilon 3/\varepsilon 4$ or the $\varepsilon 4/\varepsilon 4$ alleles has been claimed to account for 10 to 50 percent of the risk of sporadic Alzheimer's disease with onset of symptoms about age 60 years. Such individuals seem to have a particular loss of acetylcholine-containing neurons and thus may be less likely to respond to acetylcholinesterase inhibitors, such as donepezil (Aricept). In summary, the known genetic risk factors for Alzheimer's disease so far account for less than 50 percent of cases (Fig. 3.4–4).

The process of correlating a specific gene to a clinical trait by linkage analysis is called *positional cloning*. Positional cloning may involve identifying a change in 1 base of the 3 billion bases of DNA in the human nucleus, potentially a highly tedious task. Presently, researchers do linkage analysis using 6,000 unique DNA markers that are scattered evenly across the chromosomes at an average interval of 500,000 bases. To establish linkage of a trait with one of these markers, each member of a pedigree is tested for the presence of the markers, and patterns of inheritance of the markers are correlated with presence or absence of the trait of interest. This task is now almost fully automated but still requires several months of work for even a small pedigree. Although positional cloning projects for human behavioral traits have been initiated several times, no psychiatric disorder has been completely analyzed.

In positional cloning, once a researcher identifies a marker that is inherited exactly as the trait is, the genetic mutation can be assumed to lie within 1 million bases of the marker. In this interval, several dozen genes may be identified in DNA databases. In each gene, each variant in the primary sequence could represent the critical mutation; therefore, each must be tested systematically in all members of the pedigree. If a mutation is determined likely to cause the trait, the mutation can be artificially produced in mice to see whether the clinical trait is reproduced, within the limitations of the behavioral repertoire of laboratory mice. The entire process resembles searching for a needle in a haystack, with clues obtained only at great effort and expense.

ANIMAL MODELS OF HUMAN BEHAVIOR

Researchers have customarily used small mammals and birds in screening and testing pharmacological agents. Animals share many neurotransmitter systems acted on by psychiatric drugs and are thus good models for pharmacokinetic studies. Numerous behavioral assays have been devised to test activity levels, aggression and passivity, exploration and withdrawal, and other basic behavioral tendencies. Nevertheless, animals are poor models for many complex human behavioral traits. This fact is explained partly by neuroanatomy; small mammals and birds lack a prefrontal cortex, a part of the human brain that is increasingly thought necessary for complex behaviors as well as for psychiatric abnormalities.

Animals can be bred for specific traits and may rapidly provide extensive pedigrees for positional cloning projects. Among the genes recently discovered in this manner are those that control obesity in mice. Breeding the *ob* mouse strain with a normal strain led to the discovery of *leptin*, a hormone made by fat cells, which acts on the brain to suppress eating behavior. Leptin is also found in humans, although its role in human obesity is still unclear, and it remains to be seen whether exogenous administration of leptin can reduce overeating in

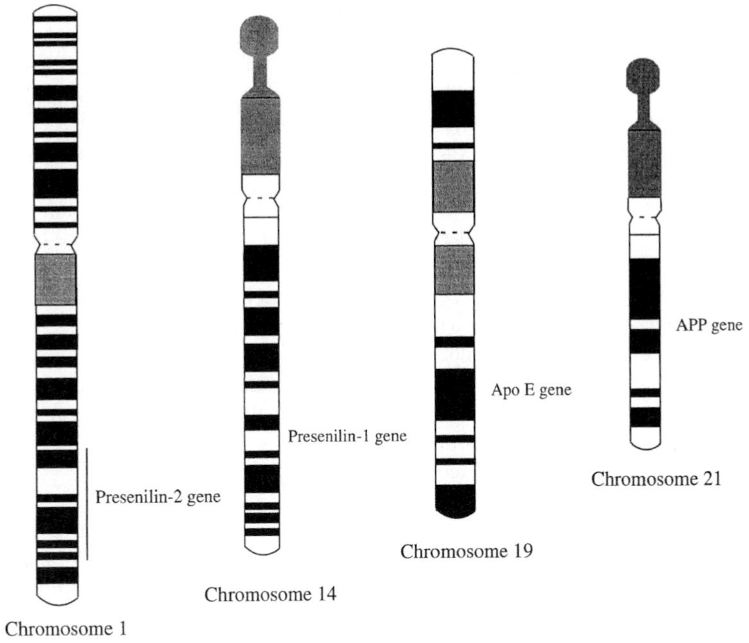

FIGURE 3.4–4
Chromosomal location of the genes implicated in Alzheimer's disease. Apo E, apolipoprotein E; APP, amyloid precursor protein. (Courtesy of Carol A. Matthews, M.D., and Nelson B. Freimer, M.D.)

humans. Hundreds of mutant mouse strains have been isolated on the basis of unusual behavior, and positional cloning projects are slowly identifying specific mutant genes that determine the behavioral variation. The techniques of positional cloning are becoming ever more powerful and efficient, and a proliferation of reports on genes that influence animal behavior can be expected in the next few years.

On the basis of pharmacological evidence, some genes have been assumed to encode proteins needed for behavior, such as neurotransmitter receptors. Methods of gene targeting, called *knockout technology,* can assess the contribution of specific candidate genes to mouse behavior. Gene targeting allows the creation of mice with deletions or modifications in a specific candidate gene. The resulting mutant mice have one of three phenotypes. Some have no detectable abnormalities, either because the gene is redundant or because the abnormality is too subtle to be detected. Some gene knockouts are lethal in the embryonic period and cannot be assayed in adulthood. Neither of these outcomes is particularly informative about behavior. Sometimes, however, the mutant animals display specific behavioral abnormalities against a background of otherwise normal behavior. In some cases, the abnormalities are predictable; in other cases they are unexpected.

Calcium-calmodulin kinase II (CaMKII) was considered a critical component of the intracellular signaling pathway during learning and memory, on the basis of biochemical data. CaMKII knockout mice, in which this protein is completely absent, cannot learn a maze easily mastered by normal mice. They also show an abnormal hippocampal "place code," which is an internal map representing the external environment that normally can be recalled for most of an animal's life span. This example of a successful predicted outcome is unfortunately a relatively rare result. In another example, based on the fact that cocaine blocks the serotonin transporter and raises synaptic levels of serotonin, a deletion was made in the serotonin 5- HT_{1B} receptor, and cocaine was administered. Normal mice become very active and aggressive when given a dose of cocaine, but the 5-HT_{1B}-receptor knockout mice failed to respond to injections of the same dose. This result confirms the role of the 5-HT_{1B} receptors in the response to cocaine. Mice that lack the dopamine transporter show excessive locomotor activity reminiscent of the behavior of mice given amphetamine, which stimulates dopamine release into the synapse.

Targeted deletion of another serotonin receptor, the 5-HT_{2C} receptor, yielded mice that were obese and aggressive. This result was interesting because it was not fully expected on the basis of pharmacological data. The deletion of monoamine oxidase type B (MAO_B), the enzyme that metabolizes serotonin and catecholamines, caused failure of formation of the barrel fields in the somatosensory cortex. This finding was associated with significantly elevated amounts of serotonin in the cortex, and the results suggest that careful modulation of serotonin levels may be necessary for the proper formation of certain cortical circuits during development. This result was quite unexpected. Another unexpected finding was that mice lacking the transcription factor *fosB* grew and developed apparently normally but failed to nurture their young. A defect in olfactory imprinting in mothers was considered responsible for this behavior.

Presently, hundreds of ongoing knockout projects are targeted to known candidate genes, and as more such genes are isolated, hundreds more knockout projects will undoubtedly begin. Because most mouse genes have a human counterpart, inferences can be made about the role of particular candidate genes in human behavior, on the basis of the mouse data. This approach is limited, however, by the fact that human genes cannot be manipulated; the assumptions must remain untested, unless a human mutation appears coincidentally.

NEW METHODS FOR ISOLATION OF HUMAN GENES RESPONSIBLE FOR BEHAVIORAL TRAITS

DNA microassays are powerful tools for the analysis of the organization and regulation of messenger RNA expression.

The advantages of microassay analyses include the ability to study the regulation of several genes or even the entire genome in a single experiment. This method can potentially link specific clinical manifestations of psychiatric disorders to the expression of particular alleles of a large array of behaviorally relevant genes. The new field of pharmacogenomics, which focuses on genetic determinants of drug response at the level of the entire human genome, is important for the development of safer and more effective drugs. Pharmacogenomics will aid in understanding how genetics influences disease development and drug response and facilitate the discovery of new treatments.

The major need in behavioral genetics is clinical research to better define the genetic subtypes of major disease categories. Breakthroughs in behavioral genetics can only arise with a more complete understanding of clinical phenotypes. Once clinical research can tease out inherited components from environmental influences and can construct reliable pedigrees, the mechanical task of finding a specific genetic mutation that is inherited with the behavioral trait is almost an afterthought.

To speculate on the uses of a specific genetic linkage, beyond the intellectual satisfaction of the discovery, researchers must consider drugs and gene therapy. Although pharmacologists have probably tested millions of known biochemical compounds to assess their clinical effectiveness, a specific genetic linkage may possibly suggest a novel class of drugs that has not yet been tried. With respect to gene therapy, this hypothetical method would use a gene delivery system, most likely a modified virus, to insert a functional copy of a mutant gene into the brain cells that require the gene for normal function. This prospect is unlikely to be realized for a long while.

References

Berrettini WH. The human genome: susceptibility loci. *Am J Psychiatry.* 2001;158:865.

Cardno AG, Holmans PA, Rees MI, et al. A genome-wide linkage study of age at onset in schizophrenia. *Am J Med Genet.* 2001;105:439.

Cravchik A, Goldman D. Neurochemical individuality: genetic diversity among human dopamine and serotonin receptors and transporters. *Arch Gen Psychiatry.* 2000;57:1105.

Eaden J, Mayberry MK, Sherr A, Mayberry JF. Screening: the legal view. *Public Health.* 2001;115:218.

Enoch MA, Goldman D. The genetics of alcoholism and alcohol abuse. *Curr Psychiatry Rep.* 2001;3:144.

Evans KL, Muir WJ, Blackwood DH, Porteous DJ. Nuts and bolts of psychiatric genetics: building on the Human Genome Project. *Trends Genet.* 2001;17:35.

Gratacos M, Nadal M, Martin-Santos R, et al. A polymorphic genomic duplication on human chromosome 15 is a susceptibility factor for panic and phobic disorders. *Cell.* 2001;106:367.

Hurko O. Genetics and genomics in neuropsychopharmacology: the impact on drug discovery and development. *Eur Neuropsychopharmacol.* 2001;11:491.

Johnston-Wilson NL, Bouton CM, Pevsner J, Breen JJ, Torrey EF, Yolken RH. Emerging technologies for large-scale screening of human tissues and fluids in the study of severe psychiatric disease. *Int J Neuropsychopharmacol.* 2001;4:83.

Mundo E, Richter MA, Sam F, Macciardi F, Kennedy JL. Is the 5-HT(1Dbeta) receptor gene implicated in the pathogenesis of obsessive-compulsive disorder? *Am J Psychiatry.* 2000;157:1160.

Mundo E, Walker M, Tims H, Macciardi F, Kennedy JL. Lack of linkage disequilibrium between serotonin transporter protein gene (SLC6A4) and bipolar disorder. *Am J Med Genet.* 2000;96:379.

Niculescu AB 3rd, Kelsoe JR. Convergent functional genomics: application to bipolar disorder. *Ann Med.* 2001;33:263.

Ohara K. Anticipation, imprinting, trinucleotide repeat expansions and psychoses. *Prog Neuropsychopharmacol Biol Psychiatry.* 2001;25:167.

Patenaude AF, Guttmacher AE, Collins FS. Genetic testing and psychology. *Am Psychol.* 2002;57:271.

Roubertoux PL, Le Roy-Duflos I. Quantitative trait locus mapping: fishing strategy or replicable results? *Behav Genet.* 2001;31:141.

Tamminga CA. The human genome sequence: the human genome II: sources of genetic variation. *Am J Psychiatry.* 2001;158:691.

▲ 3.5 Psychoneuroendocrinology and Psychoneuroimmunology

The term *psychoneuroendocrinology* refers to the structural and functional relations between the hormonal system and the central nervous system (CNS) and the behaviors that modulate and arise from both. Endocrine disorders are frequently associated with secondary psychiatric symptoms such as depressed mood and disturbances in thought, while a significant percentage of patients suffering from defined psychiatric syndromes display regular patterns of endocrine dysfunction.

Hormone Secretion

Hormones are divided into two general classes: (1) proteins, polypeptides, and glycoproteins and (2) steroids and steroidlike compounds (Table 3.5–1) that are secreted by an endocrine gland into the bloodstream and are transported to their sites of action. When a hormone is colocalized and cosecreted with a neurotransmitter (e.g., norepinephrine), it may be referred to as a *neuromodulator,* although some hormones or neuromodulators have been shown to meet criteria for neurotransmitters themselves.

Hormone secretion is stimulated by the action of a neurohormone, a neuronal secretory product of neuroendocrine transducer cells of the hypothalamus. Neurohormones (Table 3.5–2) include corticotropin-releasing hormone (CRH), which stimulates adrenocorticotropin (adrenocorticotropic hormone [ACTH]); thyrotropin-releasing hormone (TRH), which stimulates release of thyroid-stimulating hormone (TSH); gonadotropin-releasing hormone (GnRH), which stimulates release of luteinizing hormone (LH) and follicle-stimulating hormone (FSH); and somatostatin (somatotropin release-inhibiting factor [SRIF]) and growth-hormone-releasing hormone (GHRH), both of which stimulate growth hormone (GH) release. Chemical signals cause the release of these neurohormones from the median eminence of the hypothalamus into the portal hypophyseal bloodstream and coordinate their transport to the anterior pituitary to regulate the release of target hormones. Pituitary hormones in turn act directly on target cells (e.g., ACTH on the adrenal gland) or stimulate release of other hormones from peripheral endocrine organs. In addition, these hormones have feedback actions that regulate neurohormone secretion and effects in the brain itself, both directly and as modulators of neurotransmitter action (neuromodulation).

Developmental Psychoneuroendocrinology

Hormones can have both organizational and activational effects. Exposure to gonadal hormones during critical stages of neural development directs changes in brain morphology and function (e.g., sex-specific behavior in adulthood). Similarly, thyroid hormones are essential for the normal development of the CNS, and thyroid deficiency during critical stages of postnatal life will severely impair growth and development of the brain, resulting in behavioral disturbances that may be permanent if replacement therapy is not instituted.

Table 3.5–1
Classifications of Hormones

Structure	Examples	Storage	Lipid Soluble
Proteins, polypeptides, glycoproteins	ACTH, β-endorphin, TRH, LH, FSH	Vesicles	No
Steroids, steroid-like compounds	Cortisol, estrogen, thyroxine	Diffusion after synthesis	Yes
Functions			
Autocrine	Self-regulatory effects		
Paracrine	Local or adjacent cellular action		
Endocrine	Distant target site		

ACTH, adrenocorticotropin; TRH, thyrotropin-releasing hormone; LH, luteinizing hormone; FSH, follicle-stimulating hormone.
Courtesy of Victor I Reus, M.D., and Sydney Frederick-Osborne, Ph.D.

Hypothalamic-Pituitary-Adrenal Axis

Since the earliest conceptions of the stress response, by Hans Selye and others, investigation of hypothalamic-pituitary-adrenal function has occupied a central position in psychoendocrine research. CRH, ACTH, and cortisol levels all rise in response to a variety of physical and psychic stresses and serve as prime factors in maintaining homeostasis and developing adaptive responses to novel or challenging stimuli. The hormonal response depends not only on the characteristics of the stressor itself, but also on how the individual assesses and is able to cope with it. Aside from generalized effects on arousal, distinct effects on sensory processing, stimulus habituation and sensitization, pain, sleep, and memory storage and retrieval have been documented. In primates, social status can influence adrenocortical profiles and in turn be affected by exogenously induced changes in hormone concentration.

Pathological alterations in hypothalamic-pituitary-adrenal function have been associated primarily with mood disorders, posttraumatic stress disorder, and dementia of the Alzheimer's type, although recent animal evidence points toward a role of this system in substance use disorders as well; disturbances of mood are found in more than 50 percent of patients with Cushing's syndrome (characterized by elevated cortisol concentrations), with psychosis or suicidal thought apparent in more than 10 percent of patients studied. Cognitive impairments similar to those seen in major depressive disorder (principally in visual memory and higher cortical functions) are common and relate to the severity of the hypercortisolemia and possible reduction in hippocampal size. In general, reduced cortisol levels normalize mood and mental status. Conversely, in Addison's disease (characterized by adrenal insufficiency), apathy, social withdrawal, impaired sleep, and decreased concentration frequently accompany prominent fatigue. Replacement of glucocorticoid (but not of electrolyte) resolves behavioral symptomatology. Similarly, hypothalamic-pituitary-adrenal abnormalities are reversed in persons who are treated successfully with antidepressant medications, and these drugs have been found to stimulate corticosteroid receptor gene expression. Failure to normalize hypothalamic-pituitary-adrenal abnormalities is a poor prognostic sign. Alterations in hypothalamic-pituitary-adrenal function associated with depression include elevated cortisol concentrations, failure to suppress cortisol in response to dexamethasone, increased adrenal size and sensitivity to ACTH, a blunted ACTH response to CRH, and, possibly, elevated CRH concentrations in the brain.

Table 3.5–2
Neurohormones

Neurohormone	Hormone Stimulated
Corticotropin-releasing hormone (CRH)	Adrenocorticotropic hormone (ACTH)
Thyrotropin-releasing hormone (TRH)	Thyroid-stimulating hormone (TSH)
	Luteinizing hormone (LH)
Gonadotropin-releasing hormone (GnRH)	Follicle-stimulating hormone (FSH)
Somatostatin (SRIF)	Growth hormone (GH)
Growth-hormone-releasing hormone (GHRH)	GH
Oxytocin	Prolactin
Arginine vasopressin (AVP)	ACTH

Courtesy of Victor I Reus, M.D., and Sydney Frederick-Osborne, Ph.D.

Insulin. Increasing evidence indicates that insulin may be integrally involved in learning and memory. Insulin receptors occur in high density in the hippocampus and are thought to help neurons metabolize glucose. Patients with Alzheimer's disease have lower insulin concentrations in the cerebrospinal fluid (CSF) than controls, and both insulin and glucose dramatically improve verbal memory. Depression is frequent in patients with diabetes, as are indexes of impaired hormonal response to stress. It is not known whether these findings represent direct effects of the disease or are secondary, nonspecific effects. Some antipsychotics are known to dysregulate insulin metabolism.

Hypothalamic-Pituitary-Gonadal Axis

The gonadal hormones (progesterone, androstenedione, testosterone, estradiol, and others) are steroids that are secreted principally by the ovary and testes, but significant amounts of androgens arise from the adrenal cortex as well. The prostate gland and adipose tissue are also involved in the synthesis and storage of dihydrotestosterone and contribute to individual variance in sexual function and behavior.

The timing and presence of gonadal hormones play a critical role in the development of sexual dimorphisms in the brain.

Developmentally, these hormones direct the organization of many sexually dimorphic CNS structures and functions, such as the size of the hypothalamic nuclei and corpus callosum, neuronal density in the temporal cortex, the organization of language ability, and responsivity in Broca's area. Women with congenital adrenal hyperplasia, a deficiency of the enzyme 21-hydroxylase, which leads to high exposure to adrenal androgens in prenatal and postnatal life, have in some studies been found to be more aggressive and assertive and less interested in traditional female roles than control female subjects. Sexual dimorphisms may also reflect acute and reversible actions of relative steroid concentrations (e.g., higher estrogen levels transiently increase CNS sensitivity to serotonin).

Testosterone. Testosterone is the primary androgenic steroid, with both androgenic (i.e., facilitating linear body growth) and somatic growth functions. Testosterone is associated with increased violence and aggression in animals and in correlation studies in humans, but anecdotal reports of increased aggression with testosterone treatment have not been substantiated in investigations in humans. In hypogonadal men, testosterone improves mood and decreases irritability. Varying effects of anabolic-androgenic steroids on mood have been noted anecdotally. A prospective, placebo-controlled study of anabolic-androgenic steroid administration in normal subjects reported positive mood symptoms including euphoria, increased energy, and sexual arousal, in addition to increases in the negative mood symptoms of irritability, mood swings, violent feelings, anger, and hostility.

Testosterone is important for sexual desire in both men and women. In males, muscle mass and strength, sexual activity, desire, thoughts, and intensity of sexual feelings depend on normal testosterone levels, but these functions are not clearly augmented by supplemental testosterone in those with normal androgen levels. Adding small amounts of testosterone to normal hormonal replacement in postmenopausal women has, however, proved to be as beneficial as its use in hypogonadal men.

Dihydroepiandrosterone (DHEA), an adrenal androgen, is the most abundant circulating steroid. It has many physiological effects, but behavioral interest has centered on its steady decrement over the life span in humans, and its possible involvement in memory. Several controlled trials of DHEA administration point to improved well-being and functional status in both depressed and normal individuals. Its effects may result from its transformation into estrogen or testosterone or from its antiglucocorticoid activity.

Estrogen and Progesterone. Estrogens can influence neural activity in the hypothalamus and limbic system directly through modulation of neuronal excitability, and they have complex multiphasic effects on nigrostriatal dopamine receptor sensitivity. Accordingly, evidence indicates that the antipsychotic effect of psychiatric drugs may change over the menstrual cycle and that the risk of tardive dyskinesia depends partly on estrogen concentrations. Several studies have suggested that gonadal steroids modulate spatial cognition and verbal memory and are involved in impeding age-related neuronal degeneration. There is also increasing evidence that estrogen administration decreases the risk and severity of dementia of the Alzheimer's type in postmenopausal women. Estrogen has mood-enhancing properties and can also increase sensitivity to serotonin, possibly by inhibiting monoamine oxidase. In animal studies long-term estrogen treatment results in a decrease in serotonin 5-HT_1 receptors and an increase in 5-HT_2 receptors. In oophorectomized women, significant reductions in tritiated imipramine binding sites (which modulate presynaptic serotonin uptake) were restored with estrogen treatment.

The association of these hormones with serotonin is hypothetically relevant to mood change in premenstrual and postpartum mood disturbances. In premenstrual dysphoric disorder a constellation of symptoms resembling major depressive disorder occurs in most menstrual cycles, appearing in the luteal phase and disappearing within a few days of the onset of menses. No definitive abnormalities in estrogen or progesterone levels have been demonstrated in women with premenstrual dysphoric disorder, but decreased serotonin uptake with premenstrual reductions in steroid levels have been correlated with the severity of some symptoms.

Most psychological symptoms associated with the menopause are actually reported during perimenopause rather than after complete cessation of menses. Although studies suggest no increased incidence of major depressive disorder, reported symptoms include worry, fatigue, crying spells, mood swings, diminished ability to cope, and diminished libido or intensity of orgasm. Hormone replacement therapy (HRT) is effective in preventing osteoporosis and reinstating energy, a sense of well-being, and libido; however, its use is extremely controversial. A 2002 National Institutes of Health study found that combined estrogen-progestin drugs (e.g., Premarin) caused small increases in breast cancer, heart attack, strokes, and blood clots among menopausal women. Studies of the effects of estrogen alone in women who have had hysterectomies (since estrogen alone increases the risk for uterine cancer) are ongoing.

Prolactin. Prolactin is primarily involved in reproductive functions. During maturation, prolactin secretion participates in gonadal development. In adults, prolactin contributes to the regulation of the behavioral aspects of reproduction and infant care, including estrogen-dependent sexual receptivity and breast-feeding.

Although prolactin metabolism is not clearly altered in psychiatric disorders, hyperprolactinemic patients often complain of depression, decreased libido, stress intolerance, anxiety, and increased irritability. These behavioral symptoms usually resolve in parallel with decrements in serum prolactin with either surgical or pharmacological treatment. Serum prolactin concentrations also correlate positively with the severity of tardive dyskinesia, particularly in women who have been exposed to antipsychotic medication.

Hypothalamic-Pituitary-Thyroid Axis

Thyroid hormones are involved in the regulation of nearly every organ system, particularly those integral to the metabolism of food and the regulation of temperature, and are responsible for optimal development and function of all body tissues. In addition to its prime endocrine function, TRH has direct effects on neuronal excitability, behavior, and neurotransmitter regulation.

Thyroid disorders may induce virtually any psychiatric symptom or syndrome, although no consistent associations of specific syndromes and thyroid conditions are found. Hyperthyroidism is commonly associated with fatigue, irritability, insomnia, anxiety, restlessness, weight loss, and emotional lability; marked impairment in concentration and memory may also be evident. Such states can progress into delirium or mania or they can be episodic. On occasion, a true psychosis develops, with paranoia as a particularly common presenting feature. In some cases psychomotor retardation, apathy, and withdrawal are the presenting features rather than agitation and anxiety. Symptoms of mania have also been reported following rapid normalization

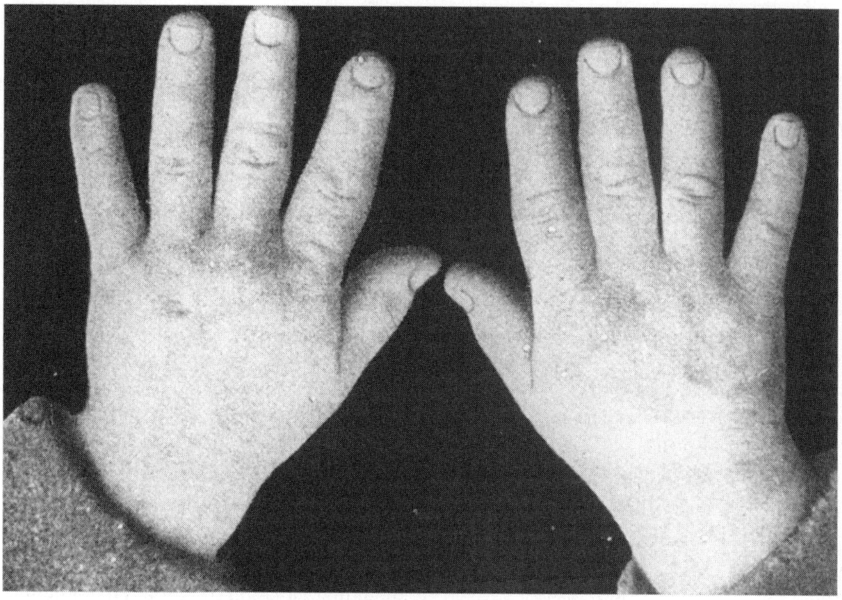

FIGURE 3.5–1
Hands of a patient suffering from hypothyroidism (myxedema), illustrating the swelling of the soft parts, the broadening of the fingers, and their consequent stumpy or pudgy appearance. (Reprinted from Waterfield RL. Anæmia. In: *French's Index of Differential Diagnosis.* 7th ed. AH Douthwaite, ed. Baltimore: Williams & Wilkins; 1954.)

of thyroid status in hypothyroid individuals and may covary with thyroid level in individuals with episodic endocrine dysfunction. In general, behavioral abnormalities resolve with normalization of thyroid function and respond symptomatically to traditional psychopharmacological regimens.

The psychiatric symptoms of chronic hypothyroidism are generally well recognized (Fig. 3.5–1). Classically, fatigue, decreased libido, memory impairment, and irritability are noted, but a true secondary psychotic disorder or dementialike state can also develop. Suicidal ideation is common, and the lethality of actual attempts is profound. In milder, subclinical states of hypothyroidism, the absence of gross signs accompanying endocrine dysfunction may result in its being overlooked as a possible cause of a mental disorder.

Growth Hormone

GH deficiencies interfere with growth and delay the onset of puberty. Low GH levels may result from a stressful experience. Administration of GH to individuals with GH deficiency benefits cognitive function in addition to its more obvious somatic effects, but evidence indicates poor psychosocial adaptation in adulthood for children who were treated for GH deficiency. A significant percentage of patients with major depressive disorder and dysthymic disorder may have a GH deficiency. Some prepubertal and adult patients with diagnoses of major depressive disorder exhibit hyposecretion of GHRH during an insulin tolerance test, a deficit that has been interpreted as reflecting alterations in both cholinergic and serotonergic mechanisms. A number of GH abnormalities have been noted in patients with anorexia nervosa. Secondary factors such as weight loss, however, in both major depressive disorder and eating disorders, may be responsible for alterations in endocrine release. Nonetheless, at least one study has reported that GHRH stimulates food consumption in patients with anorexia nervosa and lowers food consumption in patients with bulimia. Administration of GH to elderly men increases lean body mass and improves vigor. Growth hormone is released in pulses throughout the day, but the pulses are closer together during the first hours of sleep than at other times.

Endogenous Opioids

Since the discovery of endogenous opioid receptors and their endogenous ligands in the early 1970s, research into the possible behavioral roles of such compounds has flourished. The term *opioid* was initially introduced to differentiate endogenous opioid peptides from exogenous opiate drugs but is now used to refer to all drugs with opioid activity.

In animal models a number of stressors, including purely psychological ones, induce opiate-mediated effects such as analgesia and hypomotility that are reversed by the opiate antagonist naloxone (Narcan). Several studies have found that concentrations of plasma β-endorphin in humans are correlated with measures of stress elicited by surgery, exercise, parachuting, or pain. Opioids also affect eating behavior. Most commonly, short-term administration of opioid agonists increases eating, whereas antagonists reduce food intake by up to 30 percent, diminish intake of fats and highly palatable foods, and increase caloric expenditure. Recently, in double-blind trials naltrexone (ReVia) was found to be an effective adjunct in the treatment of alcohol dependence, reducing drinking, craving, the high derived from drinking alcohol, and the likelihood that sampling alcohol would precipitate a relapse; however, these results need to be replicated.

Melatonin

Melatonin is a pineal hormone that is derived from the serotonin molecule and controls photoperiodically mediated endo-

crine events (particularly those of the hypothalamic-pituitary-gonadal axis). It also modulates immune function, mood, and reproductive performance and is a potent antioxidant and free-radical scavenger. Melatonin has a depressive effect on CNS excitability, is an analgesic, and has seizure-inhibiting effects in animal studies. Melatonin can be a useful therapeutic agent in the treatment of circadian phase disorders such as jet lag. Intake of melatonin increases the speed of falling asleep, as well as its duration and quality.

Oxytocin

Oxytocin, also a posterior pituitary hormone, is involved in osmoregulation, the milk ejection reflex, food intake, and female maternal and sexual behaviors. Oxytocin is theorized to be released during orgasm, more so in females than in males, and is presumed to promote bonding between the sexes.

Substance P

Substance P, an 11-amino-acid peptide discovered in 1930, has neurotrophic effects and acts as an excitatory transmitter in primary afferent nerve terminals in mammalian spinal cord, helping to regulate sympathetic noradrenergic function. Depending on the pain paradigm used, administration of substance P can produce either hyperalgesia or analgesia. Substance P also has been found to have memory-promoting and reinforcing effects. Although substance P has been implicated in the pathogenesis of several neuropsychiatric disorders, evidence regarding any specific role is mixed.

Endocrine Assessment

Neuroendocrine function can be studied by assessing baseline measures and by measuring the response of the axis to some neurochemical or hormonal challenge. The first method has two approaches. One approach is to measure a single time point—for example, morning levels of growth hormone; this approach is subject to significant error because of the pulsatile nature of the release of most hormones. The second approach is to collect blood samples at multiple points or to collect 24-hour urine samples; these measurements are less prone to major errors. The best approach, however, is to do a neuroendocrine challenge test, in which the person is given a drug or a hormone that perturbs the endocrine axis in some standard way. Nondiseased persons show much less variation in their responses to such challenge studies than in their baseline measurements.

PSYCHONEUROIMMUNOLOGY

The nervous system and the immune system represent two networks within the body. Each contains a massive diversity of cell types and uses a large pharmacopoeia of chemical signals. Until about 20 years ago, these two systems were considered to act as parallel but independent entities. Since the 1980s, however, a small but growing number of elegant studies has revealed a set of direct interactions between the two systems and has spawned the field of psychoneuroimmunology.

Behavioral Conditioning

Demonstration that learning processes can influence immunological function is another example of interactions between the immune system and the nervous system. Several classical conditioning paradigms have been associated with suppression or enhancement of the immune response in various experimental designs.

In an effort to condition rats to avoid saccharine-flavored water, the flavored water was presented simultaneously with an injection of cyclophosphamide (Cytoxan), to induce nausea. While the method engendered an aversion to saccharine, the immunosuppressive effect of cyclophosphamide also became a conditioned response. Thus, conditioned rats, when given saccharine-flavored water, suppressed their T cells, contracted infectious diseases, and died unexpectedly.

Stress and the Immune Response

Experiments conducted on laboratory animals in the late 1950s and the early 1960s indicated that a wide variety of stressors—including isolation, rotation, crowding, exposure to a predator, and electric shock—increased morbidity and mortality in response to several types of tumors and infectious diseases caused by viruses and parasites. Evidence indicates that stressful life events can increase the susceptibility to infectious diseases in humans. For example, investigators have found that infection rates by five separate rhinoviruses administered intranasally are significantly higher in persons under high psychological stress than in those under low stress. Some studies have indicated a relation between depressive symptoms (presumably secondary to increased stress and inability to cope) and cancer development; others have been unable to replicate these findings. Once cancer has developed, however, data on women with metastatic breast cancer indicate that supportive group therapy may increase the time of survival and reduce pain episodes. Other studies report that quality of life rather than survival is improved, but even that is significant.

Studies on academic stress among medical students found less natural killer cell activity during the final examination period than during a preexamination baseline. Examination stress has also been associated with decreased numbers of T cells, mitogen responses, interferon production, and antibody responses to recombinant hepatitis B vaccine. In addition, increased antibody titers to latent herpes viruses, presumably secondary to impaired cellular immunity, have been observed. Investigators have also reported decreases in measures of immune function in persons exposed to chronic life stressors, such as divorce and taking care of patients with Alzheimer's disease. For example, caregivers to Alzheimer's disease patients showed alterations in lymphocyte subpopulations, increased antibody titers to herpes simplex virus, decreased proliferative response to mitogens, more days of illness from infectious disease, impaired antibody responses to an influenza virus vaccine, and longer latency for wound healing. Conjugal bereavement, one of the most stressful commonly occurring life events, has been associated with increased medical morbidity and mortality.

Finally, a great deal of attention has been directed to the notion that stress and depression may influence immunocompetence in human immunodeficiency virus (HIV)–seropositive persons, thereby serving as cofactors in the progression of HIV

infection to acquired immune deficiency syndrome (AIDS). Studies found that HIV-positive subjects who experienced severe stress had relevant changes in immune parameters, including lower CD8+ and lower natural killer cell counts. Ongoing studies are examining psychosocial variables and immunological and clinical endpoints in persons with HIV infection.

Psychiatric Disorders and Manifestations

The idea that altered CNS function results from a combination of the direct effects of an injurious event on various cell types and the effects of inflammatory mediators on neurons and supporting cells is a cornerstone of neuroimmunology. The idea that infectious agents can lead to psychiatric disorders is well established. Obvious examples include the mental retardation that may develop after congenital infection with rubella or cytomegalovirus, the delirium that accompanies acute meningoencephalitis after CNS infection by herpes simplex virus type I, dementias due to slow viruses (e.g., kuru and Creutzfeldt-Jakob disease), and the neuropsychiatric manifestations that occur during neurosyphilis.

Schizophrenia. Several lines of evidence suggest that virus infection during neural development may be involved in the pathogenesis of some cases of schizophrenia. The data include (1) an excess number of patient births in the late winter and early spring, suggesting possible exposure to viral infection in utero during the fall and winter peak of viral illnesses; (2) an association between exposure to viral epidemics in utero and later development of schizophrenia; (3) an increased likelihood for schizophrenic patients to have had older siblings in the household (a potential source of viral infections) compared with controls; and (4) geographical variation in prevalence, with schizophrenia being more common at greater distance from the equator. Investigators have also reported various alterations in immune markers in patients with schizophrenia, including increased levels of interferon, lower interleukin-2 (IL-2) production, and increased numbers of IL-2 receptors. Some studies have found an increase in immunoglobulin levels in the CSF.

Neural cells are the targets for autoantibodies in many syndromes. For example, autoantibodies to cytoplasmic proteins of Purkinje cells are associated with subacute cortical cerebellar degeneration, which is a rare complication of breast or ovarian cancers. Autoantibodies to γ-aminobutyric acid (GABA)-ergic neurons in the serum and the CSF appear to be the mechanism behind the stiff-man syndrome, a rare disorder characterized by progressive rigidity accompanied by recurrent painful muscle spasms. Antineuronal antibodies can also arise following infection with group A β-hemolytic streptococci, as exemplified by Sydenham's chorea. Considering that children with Sydenham's chorea frequently exhibit obsessive-compulsive symptoms, emotional lability, and hyperactivity, there may be a spectrum of pediatric autoimmune neuropsychiatric disorders associated with streptococcal infections (PANDAS). In particular, sudden onset of obsessive-compulsive disorder, tics, attention-deficit/hyperactivity disorder, and other psychiatric syndromes have been characterized in children following infection with group A β-hemolytic streptococci.

Major Depressive Disorder. There has been increasing interest in the possibility that immune activation may contribute to the pathophysiology of depression. For example, elevated serum concentrations of the proinflammatory cytokines IL-1 and IL-6 as well as increased acute-phase proteins including C-reactive protein, haptoglobin, and α_1-acid glycoprotein have been found in patients with major depressive disorder. In addition, cellular markers of immune activation have been described. The source of immune activation in major depressive disorder is unknown, although studies have shown that both stress and CRH can induce proinflammatory cytokines in the absence of a formal immune challenge. Administration of a variety of cytokines in clinical trials also has been associated with the development of depressive syndromes (sickness behavior).

Alzheimer's Disease. Although Alzheimer's disease is not considered primarily an inflammatory disease, emerging evidence indicates that the immune system may contribute to its pathogenesis. The discovery that amyloid plaques are associated with acute-phase proteins such as complement proteins and C-reactive protein suggests the possibility of an ongoing immune response. The idea that inflammatory processes are involved in Alzheimer's disease has been bolstered by recent studies showing that long-term use of nonsteroidal antiinflammatory drugs (NSAIDs) is negatively correlated with the development of Alzheimer's disease.

HIV Infection. Infection with HIV is an immunological disease associated with a variety of neurological manifestations including dementia. HIV encephalitis results in synaptic abnormalities and loss of neurons in the limbic system, basal ganglia, and neocortex. A thorough discussion of HIV is provided in Chapter 11.

Multiple Sclerosis. Multiple sclerosis is a demyelinating disease characterized by disseminated inflammatory lesions of white matter. Considerable progress has been made in elucidating the immunopathology of myelin destruction that occurs in multiple sclerosis and in the animal model for the disease, experimental allergic encephalomyelitis. Although the initial step in lesion formation has not been determined, disruption of the blood–brain barrier and infiltration of T cells, B cells, plasma cells, and macrophages appear to be associated with lesion formation.

Other Disorders. Finally, there are several disorders in which neural-immune interactions are suspected but not well documented. Chronic fatigue syndrome is an illness with a controversial etiology and pathogenesis. Besides persistent fatigue, symptoms frequently include depression and sleep disturbances. Tests of immune function have found indications of both immune activation and immunosuppression. Neuroendocrine assessments indicate that patients with chronic fatigue syndrome may be hypocortisolemic because of impaired activation of the hypothalamic-pituitary-adrenal axis. Although an acute viral infection frequently precedes the onset of chronic fatigue syndrome, no infectious agent has been causally associated with the disease. In contrast, Lyme disease, in which sleep disturbances and depression are also common, is clearly caused by infection with the tick-borne spirochete *Borrelia burgdorferi,* which can invade the CNS and cause encephalitis and neurological symptoms. Lyme disease is remarkable because it appears to produce a spectrum of neuropsychiatric disorders

including anxiety, irritability, obsessions, compulsions, hallucinations, and cognitive deficits. Immunopathology of the CNS may be involved, because symptoms can persist or reappear even after a lengthy course of antibiotic treatment, and the spirochete is frequently difficult to isolate from the brain. Gulf War syndrome is a controversial condition with inflammatory and neuropsychiatric features. The condition has been attributed variously to combat stress, chemical weapons (e.g., cholinesterase inhibitors), infections, and vaccines. Given the impact of stress on neurochemistry and immune responses, these pathogenic mechanisms are not mutually exclusive.

BIOLOGICAL RHYTHMS AND CHRONOBIOLOGY

Biological systems constantly oscillate between different states at different rates. The obvious physical cycles to which a person's biological rhythms conform include the day–night cycle, the lunar month, the solar year, and biophysical constraints, such as the rate of pulmonary gas diffusion that determines the respiratory rate and the cardiac contractile parameters that dictate the heart rate. Patterned mealtimes and the 9-to-5 workday are examples of other exogenous influences. The brain is filled with oscillations, some of which provide a constant drone over which others weave an elaborate melody. Theorists of higher perception and thought such as Rudolfo Llinas, are increasingly interested in how the brain may use rhythmical patterns of neuronal firing to encode information, in addition to using different spatial combinations of synaptic connections. Thus, biological rhythms range from the monthly menstrual cycle to brain oscillations occurring at the rate of 30 to 60 times per second.

Sleep is one of several biological rhythms within the body. Circadian biological rhythms are set by both internal and external forces, generally called *zeitgebers* (time givers, time clues, synchronizers), which constitute a widely distributed set of nuclei. The principal circadian influences emanate from the pontine reticular formation as well as the suprachiasmatic nuclei of the hypothalamus. Recent evidence has shown that the suprachiasmatic nucleus can entrain circadian rhythms even in the absence of physical synaptic connections with the remainder of the hypothalamus, suggesting that this zeitgeber may act through elaboration of diffusible substances. In the absence of exogenous clues, the period of human circadian rhythms is a bit longer than a day (24.5 hours).

The sleep–wake cycle, hormonal levels, body temperature, and the menstrual cycle are all examples of biological rhythms in the human body that can be measured. When a person is in a healthy state, all the rhythms have a natural relation, and they are said to be in phase. When the system is perturbed (e.g., by staying up all night), certain biological rhythms are thrown off (e.g., those for growth hormone and cortisol), and the rhythms are then considered out of phase. The state of having one's biological rhythms out of phase contributes to the ill effects experienced by the person. Some disorders have phase perturbations as part of their symptoms. When rhythms are disordered, a particular rhythm may have an *abnormal phase advance,* in which it begins earlier than usual, or a *phase delay,* in which it begins later than usual. Under experimental conditions a phase-responsive curve for a biological rhythm may show that a particular stimulus (e.g., light) can cause either a phase advance or a phase delay depending on when it is delivered in a cycle (e.g., the sleep–wake cycle). Lithium (Eskalith) and many of the tricyclic drugs and MAO inhibitors (MAOIs) delay rhythms in experimental animal models, supporting the hypothesis that at least some forms of depression represent phase-advance disorders.

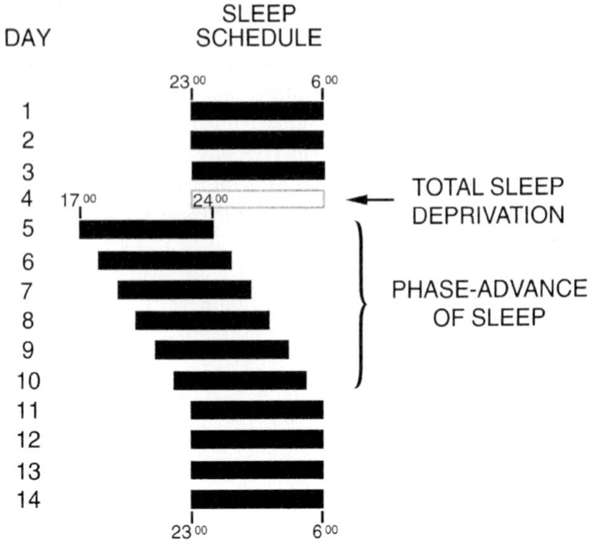

FIGURE 3.5–2

Treatment of depression by shifting the sleep–wake cycle earlier (phase advancing it), relative to other circadian rhythms, then gradually shifting it back to a normal schedule. The phase-advance treatment is based on experimental observations that sleep is depressant when it coincides with late night and early morning circadian phases but not when it coincides with late afternoon and early evening circadian phases. (See Wehr TA, Wirz-Justice A, Duncan WC, Gillin JC, Goodwin FK. Phase-advance of the circadian sleep-wake cycle as an antidepressant. *Science.* 1979;206:710; Berger M, Vollmann J, Hohagen F, et al. Sleep deprivation combined with consecutive sleep phase advance as a fast-acting therapy in depression: an open pilot trial in medicated and unmedicated patients. *Am J Psychiatr.* 1997;154:870.)

Sleep is an essential phase of human daily existence in which a great amount of mental activity occurs. While most of the period of sleep remains unconscious, dream states may engrave vivid and bizarre memories. Freud, in *The Interpretation of Dreams,* called dreams the "royal road to the unconscious." The sleep–wake cycle is synchronized with cyclic changes in the levels of several circulating hormones. Serum cortisol levels are lowest at the onset of sleep and highest in morning. TSH secretion is suppressed by the onset of sleep, while melatonin is secreted at night and terminates upon retinal stimulation by sunlight. GH levels surge during deep sleep, and this stimulus for growth gradually ceases by late adult life as deep sleep disappears. Prolactin and LH also reach their highest levels during sleep. Other hormones such as testosterone vary markedly throughout the day (thus a single reading does not measure testosterone accurately).

The necessity for sleep is demonstrated by experiments in which animals deprived of sleep die within a few weeks. Humans deprived of sleep for 60 to 200 hours begin to exhibit a breakdown in concentration, motor skills, self-care, attention, judgment, and eventually communication. Hallucinations and illusions may appear. However, a wide variation exists in the

requirement for sleep, which is determined by genetic factors, habits formed early in life, and particular physical and emotional states. The circadian (24-hour) rhythm appears in the first few months of life and remains intact until old age, when it may begin to fragment.

Depression is the psychiatric symptom that has been most associated with disruptions in biological rhythms. Early morning awakening, decreased latency of rapid eye movement (REM) sleep, and neuroendocrine perturbations seen in depression can all be conceptualized as reflecting a disorder of coordination of biological rhythms. One hypothesis is that depression occurs in some persons when the sleep-sensitive phase of the circadian system advances from the first hours of awakening to the last hours of sleep. Research indicates that alterations in the light–dark cycle (by exposing the patient to artificial light or by changing the patient's sleep–wake cycle) (Fig. 3.5–2) can relieve the symptoms.

References

Abbas AK, Lichtman AH, Pober JS. *Cellular and Molecular Immunology.* 2nd ed. Philadelphia: WB Saunders; 1994.

Arborelius L, Owens MJ, Plotsky PM, Nemeroff CB. The role of corticotropin-releasing factor in depression and anxiety disorders. *J Endocrinol.* 1999;160:1.

Besedovsky HO, Rey AD. Immune-neuro-endocrine interactions: facts and hypotheses. *Endocr Rev.* 1996;17:64.

Brzezinski A. Melatonin in humans. *N Engl J Med.* 1997;336:186.

Connor TJ, Leonard BE. Depression, stress and immunological activation: the role of cytokines in depressive disorders. *Proc Natl Sci Counc Repub China B.* 1998;62:583.

Coplan JD, Andrews MW, Rosenblum LA, et al. Persistent elevations of cerebrospinal fluid concentrations of corticotropin-releasing factor in adult nonhuman primates exposed to early-life stressors: implications for pathophysiology of mood and anxiety disorders. *Proc Natl Acad Sci U S A.* 1996;93:1619.

Goehler LE, Gaykema RPA, Nguyen KT, et al. Interleukin-1B in immune cells of the abdominal vagus nerve. A link between the immune and nervous systems? *J Neurosci.* 1999;19:2799.

Insel TR, O'Brien DJ, Leckman JF. Oxytocin, vasopressin, and autism: is there a connection? *Biol Psychiatry.* 1999;45:145.

Kawata M. Roles of steroid hormones and their receptors in structural organization in the nervous system. *Neurosci Res.* 1995;24:1.

Kunz D, Herrmann WM. Sleep-wake cycle, sleep-related disturbances, and sleep disorders: a chronobiological approach. *Compr Psychiatry.* 2000;41(2 suppl 1):104.

Lamberts SWJ, van den Beld AW, van der Lely A-J. The endocrinology of aging. *Science.* 1997;278:419.

Liu D, Diorio J, Tannenbaum B, et al. Maternal care, hippocampal glucocorticoid receptors, and hypothalamic-pituitary-adrenal responses to stress. *Science.* 1997;277:1659.

Lyons DM, Wang OJ, Lindley SE, Levin S. Kalin NH, Schatzberg A. Separation induced changes in squirrel monkey hypothalamic-pituitary-adrenal physiology resemble aspects of hypercortisolism in humans. *Psychoneuroendocrinology.* 1999;24:131.

Muller N, Riedel M, Gruber R, Ackenheil M, Schwarz MJ. The immune system and schizophrenia. an integrative view. *Ann N Y Acad Sci.* 2000;917:456.

Porter SS, Hopkins RO, Weaver LK, et al. Corpus callosum atrophy and neuropsychological outcome following carbon monoxide poisoning. *Arch Clin Neuropsychol.* 2002;17:195.

Stevens JR. Schizophrenia: reproductive hormones and the brain. *Am J Psychiatry.* 2002;159:713.

4 Contributions of the Psychosocial Sciences

▲ 4.1 Jean Piaget

Jean Piaget created a broad theoretical system for the development of cognitive abilities; in this sense, his work was similar to that of Sigmund Freud, but Piaget emphasized the ways that children think and acquire knowledge.

Piaget (1896–1980) was born in Neuchatel, Switzerland, where he studied at the university and received a doctorate in biology at the age of 22 (Fig. 4.1–1). Becoming interested in psychology, he studied and carried out research at several centers, including the Sorbonne in Paris, and worked with Eugen Bleuler at the Burghölztli Psychiatric Hospital.

Widely renowned as a child (or developmental) psychologist, Piaget referred to himself primarily as a *genetic epistemologist,* which he defined as the study of the development of abstract thought on the basis of a biological or innate substrate. That self-designation reveals that Piaget's central project was more than the articulation of a *developmental child psychology,* as this term is generally understood, but rather an account of the progressive development of human knowledge.

COGNITIVE DEVELOPMENT STAGES

Piaget described four major stages leading to the capacity for adult thought. Each stage is a prerequisite for the following one, but the rate at which different children move through different stages varies with their native endowment and environmental circumstances. Piaget's four stages are the sensorimotor stage, the stage of preoperational thought, the stage of concrete operations, and the stage of formal operations.

Sensorimotor Stage (Birth to 2 Years)

Piaget used the term *sensorimotor* to describe the first stage: Infants begin to learn through sensory observation, and they gain control of their motor functions through activity, exploration, and manipulation of the environment. Piaget divided this stage into six substages, listed in Table 4.1–1.

From the outset, biology and experience blend to produce learned behavior. For example, infants are born with a sucking reflex, but a type of learning occurs when infants discover the location of the nipple and alter the shape of their mouths. A stimulus is received, and a response results, accompanied by a sense of awareness that is the first schema, or elementary concept. As infants become more mobile, one schema is built on another, and new and more complex schemata are developed. Infants' spatial, visual, and tactile worlds expand during this period; children interact actively with the environment and use previously learned behavior patterns. For example, having learned to use a rattle, infants shake a new toy like the rattle they have already learned to use. Infants also use the rattle in new ways.

The critical achievement of this period is the development of *object permanence* or the *schema of the permanent object.* This phrase relates to a child's ability to understand that objects have an existence independent of the child's involvement with them. Infants learn to differentiate themselves from the world and are able to maintain a mental image of an object, even when it is not present and visible. When an object is dropped in front of infants, they look down to the ground to search for the object; that is, they behave for the first time as though the object has a reality outside themselves.

At about 18 months, infants begin to develop mental symbols and to use words, a process known as *symbolization.* Infants are able to create a visual image of a ball or a mental symbol of the word *ball* to stand for, or signify, the real object. Such mental representations allow children to operate on new conceptual levels. The attainment of object permanence marks the transition from the sensorimotor stage to the preoperational stage of development.

Stage of Preoperational Thought (2 to 7 years)

During the stage of preoperational thought, children use symbols and language more extensively than in the sensorimotor stage. Thinking and reasoning are intuitive; children learn without the use of reasoning. They are unable to think logically or deductively, and their concepts are primitive; they can name objects but not classes of objects. Preoperational thought is midway between socialized adult thought and the completely autistic freudian unconscious. Events are not linked by logic. Early in this stage, if children drop a glass that then breaks, they have no sense of cause and effect. They believe that the glass was ready to break, not that they broke the glass. Children in this stage also cannot grasp the sameness of an object in different circumstances: The same doll in a carriage, a crib, or a chair

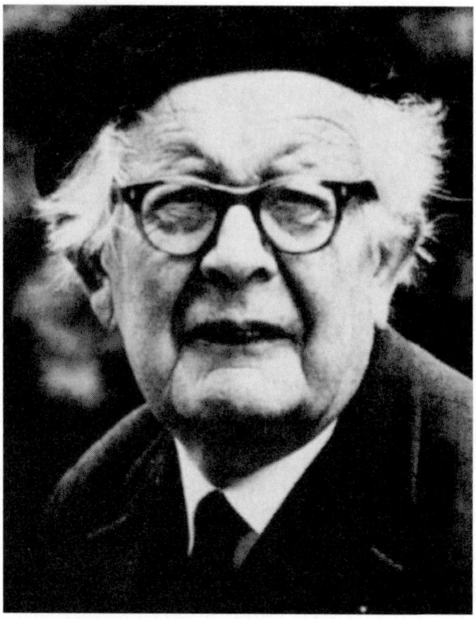

FIGURE 4.1–1
Jean Piaget. (Reprinted with permission from the Jean Piaget Society, Temple University, Philadelphia, PA.)

is perceived to be three different objects. During this time, things are represented in terms of their function. For example, a child defines a bike as "to ride" and a hole as "to dig."

In this stage, children begin to use language and drawings in more elaborate ways. From one-word utterances, two-word phrases, made up of either a noun and a verb or a noun and an objective, develop. A child may say, "Bobby eat," or "Bobby up."

Children in the preoperational stage cannot deal with moral dilemmas, although they have a sense of what is good and bad. For example, when asked, "Who is more guilty, the person who breaks one dish on purpose or the person who breaks 10 dishes by accident?" a young child usually answers that the person who breaks 10 dishes by accident is more guilty because more dishes are broken. Children in this stage have a sense of *immanent justice,* the belief that punishment for bad deeds is inevitable.

Children in this developmental stage are *egocentric*: They see themselves as the center of the universe; they have a limited point of view; and they are unable to take the role of another person. Children are unable to modify their behavior for someone else; for example, children are not being negativistic when they do not listen to a command to be quiet because their brother has to study. Instead, egocentric thinking prevents an understanding of their brother's point of view.

During this stage, children also use a type of magical thinking, called *phenomenalistic causality,* in which events that occur together are thought to cause one another (e.g., thunder causes lightning, and bad thoughts cause accidents). In addition, children use *animistic thinking,* which is the tendency to endow physical events and objects with lifelike psychological attributes, such as feelings and intentions.

Semiotic Function. The semiotic function emerges during the preoperational period. With this new ability, children can represent something—such as an object, an event, or a conceptual scheme—with a signifier, which serves a representative function (e.g., language, mental image, symbolic gesture). That is, children use a symbol or sign to stand for something else. Drawing is a semiotic function initially done as a playful exercise but eventually signifying something else in the real world.

Table 4.1–1
Piaget's Sensorimotor Period of Cognitive Development

Age	Characteristics
Birth–2 months	Uses inborn motor and sensory reflexes (sucking, grasping, looking) to interact and accommodate to the external world
2–5 months	Primary circular reaction—coordinates activities of own body and five senses (e.g., sucking thumb); reality remains subjective—does not seek stimuli outside of its visual field; displays curiosity
5–9 months	Secondary circular reaction—seeks out new stimuli in the environment; starts both to anticipate consequences of own behavior and to act purposefully to change the environment; beginning of intentional behavior
9 months–1 year	Shows preliminary signs of object permanence; has a vague concept that objects exist apart from itself; plays peekaboo; imitates novel behaviors
1 year–18 months	Tertiary circular reaction—seeks out new experiences; produces novel behaviors
18 months–2 years	Symbolic thought—uses symbolic representations of events and objects; shows signs of reasoning (e.g., uses one toy to reach for and get another); attains object permanence

Stage of Concrete Operations (7 to 11 Years)

The stage of concrete operations is so named because in this period children operate and act on the concrete, real, and perceivable world of objects and events. Egocentric thought is replaced by *operational thought,* which involves dealing with a wide array of information outside the child. Therefore, children can now see things from someone else's perspective.

Children in this stage begin to use limited logical thought processes and can serialize, order, and group things into classes on the basis of common characteristics. *Syllogistic reasoning,* in which a logical conclusion is formed from two premises, appears during this stage; for example, all horses are mammals (premise); all mammals are warm blooded (premise); therefore, all horses are warm blooded (conclusion). Children are able to reason and to follow rules and regulations. They can regulate themselves, and they begin to develop a moral sense and a code of values.

Children who become overly invested in rules may show obsessive-compulsive behavior; children who resist a code of values often seem willful and reactive. The most desirable developmental outcome in this stage is that a child attains a healthy respect for rules and understands that there are legitimate exceptions to rules.

Conservation is the ability to recognize that although the shape of objects may change, the objects still maintain or con-

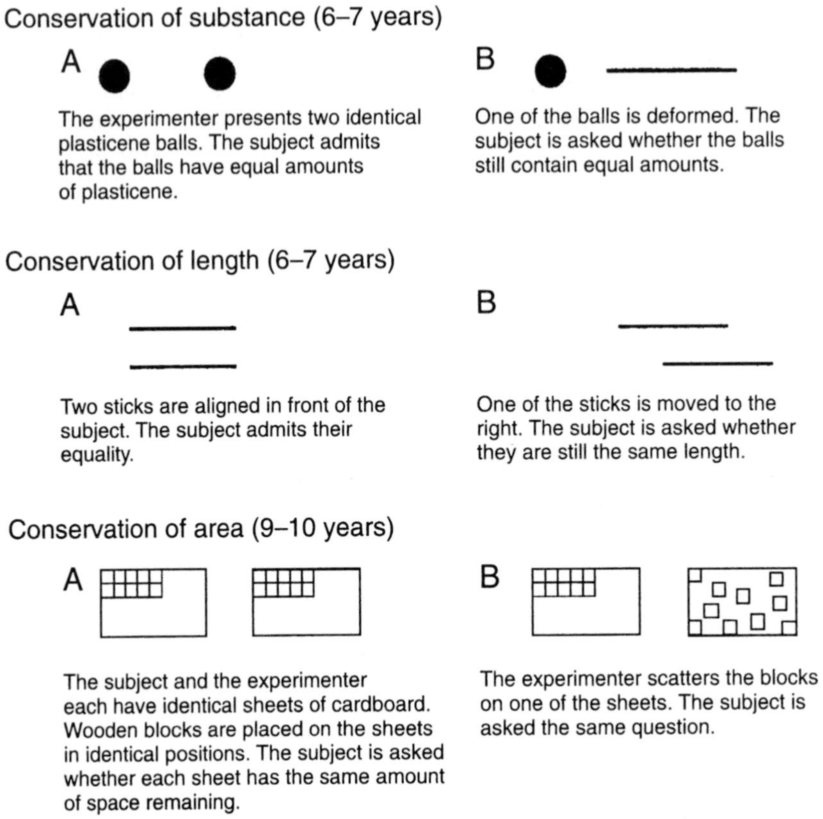
Conservation of substance (6–7 years)
A
B
The experimenter presents two identical plasticene balls. The subject admits that the balls have equal amounts of plasticene.
One of the balls is deformed. The subject is asked whether the balls still contain equal amounts.
Conservation of length (6–7 years)
A
B
Two sticks are aligned in front of the subject. The subject admits their equality.
One of the sticks is moved to the right. The subject is asked whether they are still the same length.
Conservation of area (9–10 years)
A
B
The subject and the experimenter each have identical sheets of cardboard. Wooden blocks are placed on the sheets in identical positions. The subject is asked whether each sheet has the same amount of space remaining.
The experimenter scatters the blocks on one of the sheets. The subject is asked the same question.

FIGURE 4.1–2
Some simple tests for conservation, with approximate ages of attainment. When the sense of conservation is achieved, the child answers that **B** contains the same quantity as **A.** (Modified from Lefrancois GR. *Of Children: An Introduction to Child Development.* Belmont, CA: Wadsworth; 1973:305, with permission.)

serve other characteristics that enable them to be recognized as the same. For example, if a ball of clay is rolled into a long, thin sausage shape, children recognize that each form contains the same amount of clay. An inability to conserve (which is characteristic of the preoperational stage) is observed when a child declares that there is more clay in the sausage-shaped piece because it is longer. *Reversibility* is the capacity to understand the relation between things, to realize that one thing can turn into another and back again—for example, ice and water.

The most important sign that children are still in the preoperational stage is that they have not achieved conservation or reversibility. The ability of children to understand concepts of quantity is one of Piaget's most important cognitive developmental theories. Measures of quantity include measures of substance, length, number, liquids, and area (Fig. 4.1–2).

The 7- to 11-year-old child must organize and order occurrences in the real world. Dealing with the future and its possibilities occurs in the formal operational stage.

Stage of Formal Operations (11 through the End of Adolescence)

The stage of formal operations is so named because young persons' thinking operates in a formal, highly logical, systematic, and symbolic manner. This stage is characterized by the ability to think abstractly, to reason deductively, and to define concepts and also by the emergence of skills for dealing with permutations and combinations; young persons can grasp the concept of probabilities. Adolescents attempt to deal with all possible relations and hypotheses to explain data and events during this stage; language use is complex, follows formal rules of logic, and is grammatically correct. Abstract thinking is shown by adolescents' interest in a variety of issues—philosophy, religion, ethics, and politics.

Hypotheticodeductive Thinking. Hypotheticodeductive thinking is the highest organization of cognition and enables persons to make a hypothesis or proposition and to test it against reality. *Deductive reasoning* moves from the general to the particular and is a more complicated process than *inductive reasoning,* which moves from the particular to the general.

Because young persons can reflect on their own and other persons' thinking, they are prone to self-conscious behavior. As adolescents attempt to master new cognitive tasks, they may return to egocentric thought, but on a higher level than in the past. For example, adolescents may think that they can accomplish everything or can change events by thought alone. Not all adolescents enter the stage of formal operations at the same time or to the same degree. Depending on individual capacity and intervening experience, some may not reach the stage of formal operational thought at all and may remain in the concrete operational mode throughout life.

PSYCHIATRIC APPLICATIONS

Piaget's theories have many psychiatric implications. Hospitalized children who are in the sensorimotor stage have not achieved object permanence and, therefore, suffer from separation anxiety. They are best off if their mothers are allowed to stay with them overnight. Children at the preoperational stage, who are unable to deal with concepts and abstractions, benefit more from role-playing proposed medical procedures and situations than by having them verbally described in detail. For example, a child who is to receive intravenous therapy is helped by acting out the procedure with a toy intravenous set and dolls.

Because children at the preoperational stage do not understand cause and effect, they may interpret physical illness as punishment for bad thoughts or deeds; and because they have not yet mastered the capacity to conserve and do not understand the concept of reversibility (which normally occurs during the concrete operational stage), they cannot understand that a broken bone mends or that blood lost in an accident is replaced.

Adolescents' thinking, during the stage of formal operations, may appear overly abstract when it is, in fact, a normal developmental stage. Adolescent turmoil may not herald a psychotic process but may well result from a normal adolescent's coming to grips with newly acquired abilities to deal with the unlimited possibilities of the surrounding world.

Adults under stress may regress cognitively as well as emotionally. Their thinking can become preoperational, egocentric, and sometimes animistic.

Implications for Psychotherapy

Piaget was not an applied psychologist and did not develop the implications of his cognitive model for psychotherapeutic intervention. Nevertheless, his work formed one of the foundations of the "cognitive revolution" in psychology. One aspect of this revolution was an increasing emphasis on the cognitive components of the therapeutic endeavor. In contrast to classical psychodynamic therapy, which focused primarily on drives and affects, and in contrast to behavior therapy, which focused on overt actions, cognitive approaches to therapy focused on thoughts, including automatic assumptions, beliefs, plans, and intentions.

Aaron Beck, for example, developed an entire school of cognitive therapy that focuses on the role of cognitions in causing or maintaining psychopathology. Cognitive therapy has been shown to be an effective treatment for problems as diverse as depression, anxiety disorders, and substance abuse.

A core idea in cognitive therapy is that the patient can be assisted to identify the negative automatic thoughts and underlying dysfunctional attitudes or beliefs that contribute to emotional distress or addictive behavior. The cognitive component of the therapy begins with identification of automatic thoughts, so designated because they are rapid, overlearned responses that instantaneously mediate between an event and an affective reaction. The key therapeutic process after identification of the maladaptive thoughts is to help the patient view these thoughts more objectively rather than accepting them unquestioningly as valid.

Developmentally Based Psychotherapy

Developmentally based psychotherapy, developed by Stanley Greenspan, M.D., integrates cognitive, affective, drive, and relationship-based approaches with new understanding of the stages of human development. The clinician first determines the level of the patient's ego or personality development and the presence or absence of deficits or constrictions. For example, can the person regulate activity and sensations, relate to others, read nonverbal affective symbols, represent experience, build bridges between representations, integrate emotional polarities, abstract feelings, and reflect on internal wishes and feelings?

From a developmental point of view, the integral parts of the therapeutic process include learning how to regulate experience; to engage more fully and deeply in relationships; to perceive, comprehend, and respond to complex behaviors, and interactive patterns; and to be able to engage in the ever-changing opportunities, tasks, and challenges during the course of life (e.g., adulthood and aging) and, throughout, to observe and reflect on one's own and others' experiences. These processes are the foundation of the ego, and more broadly, the personality. Their presence constitutes emotional health and their absence, emotional disorder. The developmental approach describes how to harness these core processes and so assist the patients in mobilizing their own growth.

REFERENCES

Chapman M. *Constructive Evolution: Origins and Development of Piaget's Thought.* Cambridge, UK: Cambridge University Press; 1988.

Elkind D. Piagetian psychology and the practice of child psychiatry. *J Am Acad Child Psychiatry.* 1982;21:435.

Ferreiro W. On the links between equilibration, causality and 'prise de conscience' in Piaget's theory. *Hum Dev.* 2001;44:220.

Flavell J. *The Developmental Psychology of Jean Piaget.* New York: Van Nostrand; 1963.

Greenspan SI. *Developmentally Based Psychotherapy.* Madison, CT: International Universities Press; 1997.

Greenspan SI, Curry JF. Extending Piaget's Approach to Intellectual Functioning. In: Sadock BJ, Sadock VA, eds. *Kaplan & Sadock's Comprehensive Textbook of Psychiatry.* 7th ed. Vol 1. Baltimore: Lippincott Williams & Wilkins; 2000:402.

Piaget J. *The Language and Thought of the Child.* London: Routledge & Kegan Paul; 1926.

Piaget J. *The Moral Judgement of the Child.* New York: Harcourt; 1932.

Piaget J. *Play, Dreams, and Imitation in Childhood.* New York: Norton; 1951.

Piaget J. *The Origins of Intelligence in Children.* New York: International Universities Press; 1952.

Piaget J. *Logic and Psychology.* New York: Basic Books; 1957.

Piaget J. *The Early Growth of Logic in the Child.* New York: WW Norton; 1969.

Piaget J. *Structuralism.* New York: Basic Books; 1970.

Piaget J. *Genetic Epistemology.* New York: Columbia University Press; 1973.

Piaget J. *The Grasp of Consciousness.* Cambridge, MA: Harvard University Press; 1976.

Piaget J, Inhelder B. *The Psychology of the Child.* New York: Basic Books; 1969.

Piaget J, Inhelder B. *Memory and Intelligence.* New York: Basic Books; 1973.

Piaget J, Inhelder B. *The Origin of the Idea of Chance in Children.* New York: WW Norton; 1975.

Pons F, Harris P. Piaget's conception of the development of consciousness: an examination of two hypotheses. *Hum Dev.* 2001;44:220.

▲ 4.2 Attachment Theory

ATTACHMENT AND DEVELOPMENT

John Bowlby, a British psychoanalyst (1907–1990), formulated the theory that normal attachment in infancy is crucial to a person's healthy development (Fig. 4.2–1). According to Bowlby, attachment occurs when there is a "warm, intimate and continu-

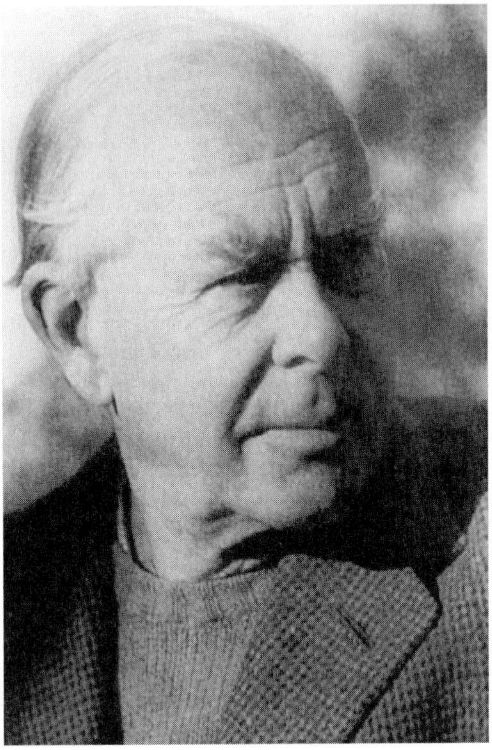

FIGURE 4.2–1
John Bowlby.

ous relationship with the mother in which both find satisfaction and enjoyment." Being monotropic, infants tend to attach to one person; but they may form attachments to several persons, such as the father or a surrogate. Attachment develops gradually; it results in an infant's wanting to be with a preferred person, who is perceived as stronger, wiser, and able to reduce anxiety or distress. Attachment thus gives infants feelings of security. The process is facilitated by interaction between mother and infant; the amount of time together is less important than the amount of activity between the two.

Attachment can be defined as the emotional tone between children and their caregivers and is evidenced by an infant's seeking and clinging to the caregiving person, usually the mother. By their first month, infants usually have begun to show such behavior, which is designed to promote proximity to the desired person.

The term *bonding* is sometimes used synonymously with attachment, but the two are different phenomena. *Bonding* concerns the mother's feelings for her infant and differs from attachment. Mothers do not normally rely on their infants as a source of security, as is the case in attachment behavior. Much research reveals that the bonding of mother to infant occurs when there is skin-to-skin contact between the two or when other types of contact, such as voice and eye contact, are made. Some workers have concluded that a mother who has skin-to-skin contact with her baby immediately after birth shows a stronger bonding pattern and may provide more attentive care than a mother who does not have this experience. Some researchers have even proposed a critical period immediately after birth, during which such skin-to-skin contact must occur if bonding is to take place. This concept is much disputed: Many mothers are clearly bonded to their infants and display excellent maternal care even though they did not have skin-to-skin contact immediately postpartum. Because human beings can develop representational models of their babies in utero and even before conception, this representational thinking may be as important to the bonding process as skin, voice, or eye contact.

Ethological Studies

Bowlby suggested a darwinian evolutionary basis for attachment behavior; namely, such behavior ensures that adults protect their young. Ethological studies show that nonhuman primates and other animals show attachment behavior patterns that are presumably instinctual and are governed by inborn tendencies. An example of an instinctual attachment system is *imprinting,* in which certain stimuli can elicit innate behavior patterns during the first few hours of an animal's behavioral development; thus, the animal offspring becomes attached to its mother at a critical period early in its development. A similar sensitive or critical period during which attachment occurs has been postulated for human infants. The presence of imprinting behavior in humans is highly controversial, but bonding and attachment behavior during the first year of life closely approximate the critical period; in humans, however, this period occurs over a span of years rather than hours.

Harry Harlow. Harry Harlow's work with monkeys is relevant to attachment theory. Harlow demonstrated the emotional and behavioral effects of isolating monkeys from birth and keeping them from forming attachments. The isolates were withdrawn, unable to relate to peers, unable to mate, and incapable of caring for their offspring. (Harlow's work is discussed further in Section 4.5.)

PHASES OF ATTACHMENT

In the first attachment phase, sometimes called the *preattachment stage* (birth to 8 or 12 weeks), babies orient to their mothers, follow them with their eyes over a 180-degree range, and turn toward and move rhythmically with their mother's voice. In the second phase, sometimes called *attachment in the making* (8 to 12 weeks to 6 months), infants become attached to one or more persons in the environment. In the third phase, sometimes called *clear-cut attachment* (6 through 24 months), infants cry and show other signs of distress when separated from the caretaker or mother; this phase may occur as early as 3 months in some infants. On being returned to the mother, the infant stops crying and clings, as if to gain further assurance of the mother's return. Sometimes, seeing the mother after a separation is sufficient for crying to stop. In the fourth phase (25 months and beyond), the mother figure is seen as independent, and a more complex relationship between the mother and the child develops. Table 4.2–1 summarizes the development of normal attachment from birth through 3 years.

Mary Ainsworth

Mary Ainsworth expanded on Bowlby's observations and found that the interaction between the mother and her baby during the

Table 4.2–1
Normal Attachment

Birth to 30 days
- Reflexes at birth
  - Rooting
  - Head turning
  - Sucking
  - Swallowing
  - Hand-mouth
  - Grasp
  - Digital extension
  - Crying—signal for particular kind of distress
  - Responsiveness and orientation to mother's face, eyes, and voice
- 4 days—anticipatory approach behavior at feeding
- 3 to 4 weeks—infant smiles preferentially to mother's voice

Age 30 days through 3 months
- Vocalization and gaze reciprocity further elaborated from 1 to 3 months; babbling at 2 months, more with the mother than with a stranger
- Social smile
- In strange situation, increased clinging response to mother

Age 4 through 6 months
- Briefly soothed and comforted by sound of mother's voice
- Spontaneous, voluntary reaching for mother
- Anticipatory posturing to be picked up
- Differential preference for mother intensifies
- Subtle integration of responses to mother

Age 7 through 9 months
- Attachment behaviors further differentiated and focused specifically on mother
- Separation distress, stranger distress, strange-place distress

Age 10 through 15 months
- Crawls or walks toward mother
- Subtle facial expressions (coyness, attentiveness)
- Responsive dialogue with mother clearly established
- Early imitation of mother (vocal inflections, facial expression)
- More fully developed separation distress and mother preference
- Pointing gesture
- Walking to and from mother
- Affectively positive reunion responses to mother after separation or, paradoxically, short-lived, active avoidance or delayed protest

Age 16 months through 2 years
- Involvement in imitative jargon with mother (12 to 14 months)
- Head-shaking "no" (15 to 16 months)
- Transitional object used during the absence of mother
- Separation anxiety diminishes
- Mastery of strange situations and persons when mother is near
- Evidence of delayed imitation
- Object permanence
- Microcosmic symbolic play

Age 25 months through 3 years
- Able to tolerate separations from mother without distress when familiar with surroundings and given reassurances about mother's return
- Two- and three-word speech
- Stranger anxiety much reduced
- Object consistency achieved—maintains composure and psychosocial functioning without regression in absence of mother
- Microcosmic play and social play; cooperation with others begins

Based on material by Justin Call, M.D.

Table 4.2–2
The Strange Situation

Episode[a]	Persons Present	Change
1	Parent, infant	Enter room
2	Parent, infant, stranger	Unfamiliar adult joins the dyad
3	Infant, stranger	Parent leaves
4	Parent, infant	Parent returns, stranger leaves
5	Infant	Parent leaves
6	Infant, stranger	Stranger returns
7	Parent, infant	Parent returns, stranger leaves

Reprinted with permission from Lamb ME, Nash A, Teti DM, Bornstein MH. Infancy. In Lewis M, ed. *Child and Adolescent Psychiatry: A Comprehensive Textbook*. 2nd ed. Baltimore: Williams & Wilkins; 1996:256.

[a]All episodes are usually 3 minutes long, but episodes 3, 5, and 6 can be curtailed if the infant becomes too distressed, and episodes 4 and 7 are sometimes extended.

attachment period significantly influences the baby's current and future behavior. Patterns of attachments vary among babies; for example, some babies signal or cry less than others. Sensitive responsiveness to infant signals, such as cuddling a crying baby, causes infants to cry less in later months, rather than reinforcing crying behavior. Close bodily contact with the mother when the baby signals for her is also associated with the growth of self-reliance, rather than a clinging dependence, as the baby grows older. Unresponsive mothers produce anxious babies; these mothers often have lower intelligence quotients (IQs) and are emotionally more immature and younger than responsive mothers.

Ainsworth also confirmed that attachment serves the purpose of reducing anxiety. What she called the *secure base effect* enables children to move away from attachment figures and to explore the environment. Inanimate objects, such as a teddy bear and a blanket (called the *transitional object* by Donald Winnicott), also serve as a secure base, one that often accompanies them as they investigate the world.

Strange Situation. Ainsworth developed *strange situation*, the research protocol for assessing the quality and security of an infant's attachment. In this procedure, the infant is exposed to escalating amounts of stress; for example, the infant and the parent enter an unfamiliar room, an unfamiliar adult then enters the room, and the parent leaves the room. The protocol has seven steps (Table 4.2–2). According to Ainsworth's studies, about 65 percent of infants are securely attached by the age of 24 months.

ANXIETY

Bowlby's theory of anxiety holds that a child's sense of distress during separation is perceived and experienced as anxiety and is the prototype of anxiety. Any stimuli that alarm children and cause fear (e.g., loud noises, falling, and cold blasts of air) mobilize signal indicators (e.g., crying) that cause the mother to respond in a caring way by cuddling and reassuring the child. The mother's ability to relieve the infant's anxiety or fear is fundamental to the growth of attachment in the infant. When

the mother is close to the child and the child experiences no fear, the child gains a sense of *security*, the opposite of anxiety. When the mother is unavailable to the infant because of physical absence (e.g., if the mother is in prison) or because of psychological impairment (e.g., severe depression), anxiety develops in the infant.

Expressed as tearfulness or irritability, *separation anxiety* is the response of a child who is isolated or separated from its mother or caretaker. It is most common at 10 to 18 months of age and disappears generally by the end of the third year. Somewhat earlier (at about 8 months) *stranger anxiety*, an anxiety response to someone other than the caregiver, appears.

Signal Indicators

Signal indicators are infants' signs of distress that prompt or elicit a behavioral response in the mother. The primary signal is crying. There are three types: hunger (the most common), anger, and pain. Some mothers can distinguish between them, but most mothers generalize the hunger cry to represent distress from pain, frustration, or anger. Other signal indicators that reinforce attachment are smiling, cooing, and looking. The sound of an adult human voice can prompt these indicators.

Losing Attachments

Persons' reactions to the death of a parent or a spouse can be traced to the nature of their past and present attachment to the lost figure. An absence of demonstrable grief may be due to real experiences of rejection and to the lack of closeness in the relationship. The person may even consciously offer an idealized picture of the deceased. Persons who show no grief usually try to present themselves as independent and as disinterested in closeness and attachment.

Sometimes, however, the severing of attachments is traumatic. The death of a parent or a spouse can precipitate a depressive disorder, and even suicide, in some persons. The death of a spouse increases the chance that the surviving spouse will experience a physical or mental disorder during the next year. The onset of depression and other dysphoric states often involves having been rejected by a significant figure in a person's life.

DISORDERS OF ATTACHMENT

Attachment disorders are characterized by biopsychosocial pathology that results from maternal deprivation, a lack of care by, and interaction with, the mother or caregiver. Failure-to-thrive syndromes, psychosocial dwarfism, separation anxiety disorder, avoidant personality disorder, depressive disorders, delinquency, academic problems, and borderline intelligence have been traced to negative attachment experiences. When maternal care is deficient because a mother is mentally ill, because a child is institutionalized for a long time, or because the primary object of attachment dies, children suffer emotional damage. Bowlby originally thought that the damage was permanent and invariable, but he revised his theories to take into account the time at which the separation occurred, the type and degree of separation, and the level of security that the child experienced before the separation.

Bowlby described a predictable set and sequence of behavior patterns in children who are separated from their mothers for long periods (more than 3 months): *protest*, in which the child protests the separation by crying, calling out, and searching for the lost person; *despair*, in which the child appears to lose hope that the mother will return; and *detachment*, in which the child emotionally separates himself or herself from the mother. Bowlby believed that this sequence involves ambivalent feelings toward the mother; the child both wants her and is angry with her for her desertion.

Children in the detachment stage respond in an indifferent manner when the mother returns; the mother has not been forgotten, but the child is angry at her for having gone away in the first place and fears that she will go away again. Some children have affectionless personalities characterized by emotional withdrawal, little or no feeling, and a limited ability to form affectionate relationships.

Anaclitic Depression. Anaclitic depression, also known as hospitalism, was first described by René Spitz in infants who had made normal attachments but were then suddenly separated from their mothers for varying times and placed in institutions or hospitals. The children became depressed, withdrawn, nonresponsive, and vulnerable to physical illness but recovered when their mothers returned or when surrogate mothering was available.

CHILD MALTREATMENT

Abused children often maintain their attachments to abusive parents. Studies of dogs have shown that severe punishment and maltreatment increase attachment behavior. When children are hungry, sick, or in pain, they too show clinging attachment behavior. Similarly, when children are rejected by their parents or are afraid of them, their attachment may increase; some children want to remain with an abusive parent. Nevertheless, when a choice must be made between a punishing and a nonpunishing figure, the nonpunishing person is the preferable choice, especially if the person is sensitive to the child's needs. (Child abuse is discussed at length in Chapter 32.)

PSYCHIATRIC APPLICATIONS

The applications of attachment theory in psychotherapy are numerous. When a patient is able to attach to a therapist, a secure base effect is seen. The patient may then be able to take risks, mask anxiety, and practice new patterns of behavior that otherwise might not have been attempted. Patients whose impairments can be traced to never having made an attachment in early life may do so for the first time in therapy, with salutary effects.

Patients whose pathology stems from exaggerated early attachments may attempt to replicate them in therapy. Therapists must enable such patients to recognize the ways their early experiences have interfered with their ability to achieve independence.

For patients who are children and whose attachment difficulties may be more apparent than those of adults, therapists represent consistent and trusted figures who can engender a sense of warmth and self-esteem in children, often for the first time.

Relationship Disorders

A person's psychological health and sense of well-being depend significantly upon the quality of his or her relationships and attachment to others, and a core issue in all close personal relationships is establishing and regulating that connection. In a typical attachment interaction, one person seeks more proximity and affection, and the other either reciprocates, rejects, or disqualifies the request. A pattern is shaped through repeated exchanges. Distinct attachment styles have been observed. Adults with an *anxious-ambivalent* attachment style tend to be obsessed with romantic partners, suffer from extreme jealousy, and have a high divorce rate. Persons with an *avoidant* attachment style are relatively uninvested in close relationships, though they often feel lonely. They seem afraid of intimacy and tend to withdraw when there is stress or conflict in the relationship. Break-up rates are high. Persons with a *secure* attachment style are highly invested in relationships and tend to behave without much possessiveness or fear of rejection.

References

Ainsworth MS. Attachments across the life span. *Bull N Y Acad Med.* 1985;61:792.

Bowlby J. *Maternal Care and Mental Health.* Geneva: World Health Organization; 1951.

Bowlby J. The nature of the child's tie to his mother. *Int J Psychoanal.* 1958;39:350.

Bowlby J. *Attachment and Loss.* Vols 1, 2, 3. New York: Basic Books; 1969, 1973, 1980.

Bus AG. Parent-child book reading through the lens of attachment theory. In: Verhoeven L, Snow C, eds. *Literacy and Motivation: Reading Engagement in Individuals and Groups.* Mahwah, NJ: Lawrence Erlbaum; 2001:39.

DeFrain JD, Jakub DK, Mendoza BL. The psychological effects of sudden infant death on grandmothers and grandfathers. *Omega J Death Dying.* 1992;24:165.

George C. A representational perspective of child abuse and prevention: internal working models of attachment and caregiving. *Child Abuse Negl.* 1996;20:411.

Gullestad SE. Attachment theory and psychoanalysis: controversial issues. *Scand Psychoanal Rev.* 2001;24:3.

Johnson S, Sims A. Attachment theory: a map for couples therapy. In: Levy TM, ed. *Handbook of Attachment Interventions.* San Diego, CA: Academic Press; 2000;169.

Klaus MH, Kennell JH. *Parent–Infant Bonding.* 2nd ed. St. Louis: Mosby; 1982.

MacDonald SG. The real and the researchable: a brief review of the contribution of John Bowlby (1907–1990). *Perspect Psychiatr Care.* 2001;37:60.

Routh CP, Hill JW, Steele H, Elliott CE, Dewey ME. Maternal attachment status, psychosocial stressors and problem behaviour: follow-up after parent training courses for conduct disorder. *J Child Psychol Psychiatry.* 1995;36:1179.

Ward MJ, Carlson EA. Associations among adult attachment representations, maternal sensitivity, and infant-mother attachment in a sample of adolescent mothers. *Child Dev.* 1995;66:69.

▲ 4.3 Learning Theory

Learning is defined as a change in behavior resulting from repeated practice, and both the environment and the behavior interact to produce the learned change. To assess learning one measures an aspect of performance such as the accuracy of a motor skill or the ability to recognize and repeat words. Learning and performance are related but should not be confused; when performance is adversely affected by insufficient motivation or by anxiety, learning that has occurred may not be demonstrable.

Learning may be state dependent, that is, it may occur when the person is in a special internal state (e.g., under the influence of a drug) or in a special environment. Such learning is best recalled when the person is in the same internal state or external environment in which the information was first acquired. For example, when a behavior is acquired under the influence of a pharmacological agent and tests for learning are carried out in the absence of the drug, there may be little or no evidence of acquisition. When the learning test is carried out under the influence of the drug, however, performance may change, and learning may then be demonstrated.

TYPES OF LEARNING

There are three types of learning: (1) In *classical conditioning,* learning is thought to take place as a result of the contiguity of environmental events; when events occur closely together in time, persons will probably come to associate the two. (2) In *operant conditioning,* learning is thought to result from the consequences of a person's actions. (3) *Social learning theory* incorporates both classical and operant models of learning but also considers a reciprocal interaction between the person and the environment. Cognitive processes are viewed as important factors in modulating a person's responses to environmental events.

Psychoanalytic theory and practice developed concurrently with learning theory, and attempts have been made over the past half century to integrate the two theoretical approaches. For example, in 1950 John Dollard and Neal Miller reformulated many psychoanalytic concepts in terms of learning theory. Such attempts, however, have had little lasting influence on psychoanalytic thought or therapy.

Classical Conditioning

Classical (also called *respondent*) *conditioning* results from the repeated pairing of a neutral (conditioned) stimulus with one that evokes a response (unconditioned stimulus), such that the neutral stimulus eventually comes to evoke the response. The time relation between the presentation of the conditioned and unconditioned stimuli is important and varies for optimal learning from a fraction of a second to several seconds.

The Russian physiologist and Nobel prize winner Ivan Petrovich Pavlov (1849–1936) (Fig. 4.3–1), observed in his work on gastric secretion that a dog salivated not only when food was placed in its mouth but also at the sound of the footsteps of the person coming to feed it, even though the dog could not see or smell the food. Pavlov analyzed these events and called the saliva flow that occurred with the sound of footsteps a *conditioned response* (CR)—a response elicited under certain conditions by a particular stimulus.

In a typical pavlovian experiment, a *stimulus* (S) that had no capacity to evoke a particular response before training did so after consistent association with another stimulus. For example, under normal circumstances, a dog does not salivate at the sound of a bell, but when the bell sound is always followed by the presentation of food, the dog ultimately pairs the bell and the food. Eventually, the bell sound alone elicits salivation (CR).

Because the food naturally produces salivation, it is referred to as an *unconditioned stimulus* (UCS). Salivation, a response that is reliably elicited by food (UCS), is referred to as an *unconditioned response* (UCR). The bell, which was originally unable to evoke salivation but came to do so when paired with

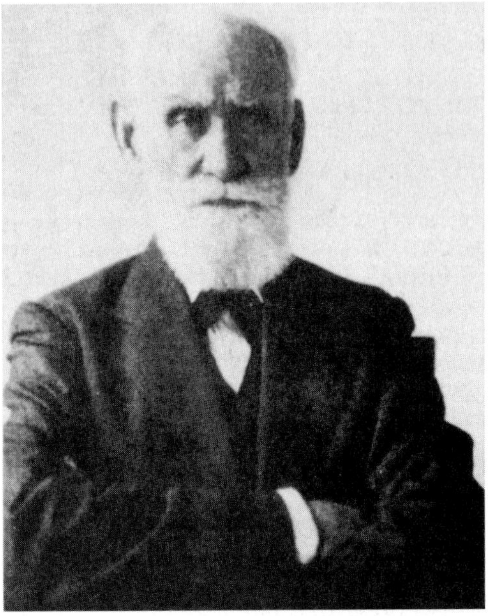

FIGURE 4.3–1
Ivan Pavlov.

food, is referred to as a *conditioned stimulus* (CS). Classical conditioning is most often applied to responses mediated by the autonomic nervous system.

Classical conditioning is diagramed as follows:

Before conditioning

Food (UCS) → Salivation (UCR)

Bell (CS) paired with food (UCS) → Salivation (UCR)

After conditioning

Bell (CS) → Salivation (CR)

Extinction. Extinction occurs when the conditioned stimulus is constantly repeated without the unconditioned stimulus until the response evoked by the conditioned stimulus gradually weakens and eventually disappears. In the previous example, extinction would occur if the bell (CS) is rung repeatedly without the food (UCS) being given. Eventually, salivation (CR) does not occur when the bell sounds, and extinction occurs. Extinction, however, does not completely destroy a conditioned response. If an animal is rested after extinction, the conditioned response returns, although less strong than originally, a phenomenon known as *partial recovery*.

The American psychologist John B. Watson (1878–1958) used Pavlov's theory of classical conditioning to explain certain aspects of human behavior. In 1920, Watson described producing a phobia in an 11-month-old boy called Little Albert. At the same time that the boy was shown a white rat that he initially did not fear, he was exposed to a loud, frightening noise. After several such pairings, Albert became fearful of the white rat, even when he heard no loud noise. Watson and his colleagues obtained the same results using a white rabbit and eventually managed to generalize the response to any furry object. Many theorists believe that this process accounts for the development of childhood phobias, which are considered learned responses based on classical conditioning.

Stimulus Generalization. *Stimulus generalization* describes a process whereby a conditioned response is transferred from one stimulus to another. Animals respond to stimuli similar to the original conditioned stimulus: A dog conditioned to respond to a bell also responds to the sound of a tuning fork. The theory of stimulus generalization is sometimes used to explain higher learning by showing how persons learn similarities. For example, a street sign is recognized whether it is on a pole, a building, or a curb, because there is sufficient stimulus similarity for generalization to occur.

Discrimination. *Discrimination* is the process of recognizing and responding to differences between similar stimuli. If the two stimuli are sufficiently different, an animal can learn to respond to one and not to the other; for example, an animal can learn to respond differentially to similar bells. A child learns to discriminate four-legged animals (the common stimulus) into dogs, cats, cows, and other quadrupeds.

When learning is viewed as a balance of generalization and discrimination, some disorders of thinking can be considered to stem from difficulties with these two processes. A person who had a traumatic childhood experience with a person who wore a moustache may transfer these negative feelings to all men with moustaches; this example shows both faulty discrimination and stimulus generalization.

Operant Conditioning

B. F. Skinner (1904–1990) developed a theory of learning and behavior known as *operant conditioning*. Whereas in classical conditioning an animal is passive or restrained and behavior is reinforced by the experimenter, in operant conditioning the animal is active and behaves in a way that produces a reward; thus learning occurs as a consequence of action. For example, a rat receives a reinforcing stimulus (food) only when it correctly responds by pressing a lever. Food, approval, praise, good grades, or any other response that satisfies a need in an animal or a person can serve as a reward.

Operant conditioning is related to trial-and-error learning, as described by the American psychologist Edward L. Thorndike (1874–1949). In trial-and-error learning, a person or animal attempts to solve a problem by trying different actions until one proves successful. A freely moving organism behaves in a way that is instrumental in producing a reward. For example, a cat in a Thorndike puzzle box must learn to lift a latch to escape from the box. For this reason, operant conditioning is sometimes called *instrumental conditioning*. Thorndike's law of effect states that certain responses are reinforced by reward, and the organism learns from these experiences. Four kinds of operant conditioning are described in Table 4.3–1: primary reward conditioning, escape conditioning, avoidance conditioning, and secondary reward conditioning.

Respondent and Operant Behavior. Skinner described two types of behavior: *respondent behavior*, which results from known stimuli (e.g., the knee jerk reflex to patellar stimulation

Table 4.3–1
Four Kinds of Operant or Instrumental Conditioning

Primary reward conditioning	The simplest kind of conditioning. The learned response is instrumental in obtaining a biologically significant reward, such as a pellet of food or a drink of water.
Escape conditioning	The organism learns a response that is instrumental in getting out of some place it prefers not to be.
Avoidance conditioning	The kind of learning in which a response to a cue is instrumental in avoiding a painful experience. A rat on a grid, for example, may avoid a shock if it quickly pushes a lever when a light signal goes on.
Secondary reward conditioning	The kind of learning in which instrumental behavior to get at a stimulus has no biological usefulness itself but has in the past been associated with a biologically significant stimulus. For example, chimpanzees learn to press a lever to obtain poker chips, which they insert into a slot to secure grapes. Later, they work to accumulate poker chips even when they are not interested in grapes.

or the pupillary constriction to light), and *operant behavior,* which is independent of a stimulus (e.g., the random movements of an infant or the aimless movements of a laboratory rat in a cage). Skinner took advantage of operant behavior by placing a rat in a Skinner box (named after him, its developer). The rat was deprived of food; in the course of moving around the box, it randomly pressed a bar. At some point in the experiment, food was released by the experimenter when the bar was pressed. The food reinforced the bar pressing, which increased or decreased in rate depending on the level of reinforcement given by the experimenter. A *reinforcer* is anything that maintains a response or increases its strength; the term is used synonymously with *reward.* Some workers, however, distinguish between the two and point out that responses are reinforced, whereas subjects are rewarded.

Reinforcement Schedule (Programming). Reinforcers are described as *primary* when they are independent of previous learning (e.g., the need for food or water) and *secondary* when they are based on previously rewarded learning (e.g., giving money to a child with good grades). In operant conditioning, one can vary the schedule of reward or reinforcement for a behavioral pattern in a process known as programming. The intervals between reinforcements may be *fixed* (e.g., every third response is rewarded) or *variable* (e.g., sometimes the third response is rewarded; at other times, the sixth response is rewarded).

A *continuous reinforcement* (also called *contingency reinforcement* or *management*) schedule, in which every response is reinforced, leads to the most rapid acquisition of a behavior, not the maintenance of behavior. Reinforcing a response only a fraction of the times the behavior occurs is called *partial reinforcement.* Partial, or intermittent, reinforcement is most effective in maintaining behavior that is resistant to extinction. For example, a person uses a gambling slot machine most frequently when the reward is partially reinforced—that is, when money is won at variable times. This procedure keeps the gambler guessing or trying to anticipate when a payoff will occur. The strength of operant learning is reflected in the frequency of responses: A high response frequency indicates strong operant learning, and a decrease in frequency indicates that extinction is occurring. Table 4.3–2 lists the effects of various reinforcement schedules on behavior.

In operant conditioning, *positive reinforcement* is the process by which certain consequences of a response increase the probability that the response will recur. Food, water, praise, and money are positive reinforcers. On the other hand, events aversive to some may be reinforcing for others. For example, the behavior of some children is reinforced by scolding, which, after all, is a form of attention. Many substances also appear to be positive reinforcers, including opium, cocaine, nicotine, and barbiturates.

Positive reinforcement is a useful therapeutic method for severely ill psychiatric patients, as in the following case.

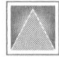

Table 4.3–2
Reinforcement Schedules in Operant Conditioning

Reinforcement Schedule	Example	Behavioral Effect
Fixed-ratio (FR) schedule	Reinforcement occurs after every 10 responses (10:1 ratio); 10 bar presses release a food pellet; workers are paid for every 10 items they make.	Rapid rate of response to obtain the greatest number of rewards. Animal knows that the next reinforcement depends on a certain number of responses being made.
Variable-ratio (VR) schedule	Variable reinforcement occurs (e.g., after the third, sixth, then second response, and so on).	Generates a fairly constant rate of response because the probability of reinforcement at any given time remains relatively stable.
Fixed-interval (FI) schedule	Reinforcement occurs at regular intervals (e.g., every 10 minutes or every third hour).	Animal keeps track of time. Rate of responding drops to near 0 after reinforcement and then increases at about the expected time of reward.
Variable-interval (VI) schedule	Reinforcement occurs after variable intervals (e.g., every 3, 6, and then 2 hours), similar to VR schedule.	Response rate does not change between reinforcements. Animal responds at a steady rate to get the reward when it is available; common in trout fishing, use of slot machines, checking mailbox.

The patient was a 21-year-old-man who was extremely withdrawn. He spent most of his time in his hospital room, rarely approaching others or initiating conversation. Skilled psychiatric nursing care had not altered his behavior. As a first step in increasing his conversational ability, reinforcement for approaching nurses was instituted. The patient was first carefully observed, and it was noted that he enjoyed listening to the radio and watching television. He was told that for every 2 minutes during which he talked with the nurses in three daily sessions he would earn a token that could be exchanged for 3 minutes of listening to the radio or watching television, and that talking was the only way in which he would earn the right to engage in those activities. The nurses, in turn, were instructed not to approach him during the sessions but to engage in conversation only if he initiated and maintained it, thus reinforcing a chain of behaviors: approaching nurses, initiating conversation, and maintaining conversational behavior. The nurses also timed the number of minutes of conversation, using a stopwatch.

The patient engaged in little conversation with the nurses during the baseline measurement period. When the token system was introduced, he began to speak with the nurses for increasing lengths of time. In the third phase of the treatment study, the patient was given a free supply of tokens equivalent to what he had earned in the previous phase; the tokens were no longer contingent on his behavior. Under those conditions the amount of conversation gradually declined, an example of extinction. When the original reinforcement conditions were reintroduced, the patient's conversational ability improved. Similar procedures were used to generalize his newfound conversational ability to other staff members, eventually allowing the patient to engage successfully in a rehabilitation program. (Courtesy of W. Stewart Agras, M.D., and G. Terence Wilson, Ph.D.)

Negative reinforcement is a process by which a response that leads to the removal of an aversive event is increased. For example, a teenager mows the lawn to avoid parental complaints, or an animal jumps off a grid to escape a painful shock. Any behavior that enables a person or animal to avoid or escape a punishing consequence is strengthened.

Negative reinforcement is not punishment. *Punishment* is an aversive stimulus (e.g., a slap) that is presented specifically to weaken or suppress an undesired response; punishment reduces the probability that a response will recur. The usual use of the term *punishment* must be distinguished from the technical use of the term. In learning theory, the punishing event delivered is always contingent on performance and demonstrably reduces the frequency of the behavior being punished. This meaning differs from the use of the term to denote imprisonment, for example, because the prison sentence follows long after the crime has been committed and may not affect future criminal behavior.

Aversive Control. In aversive control or conditioning, an organism changes its behavior to avoid a painful, noxious, or aversive stimulus. Electric shocks are common aversive stimuli used in laboratory experiments. Any behavior that avoids an aversive stimulus is reinforced as a result.

Escape Learning and Avoidance Learning. Negative reinforcement is related to two types of learning, escape learning and avoidance learning. In *escape learning,* an animal learns a response to get out of a place where it does not want to be (e.g., an animal jumps off an electric grid whenever the grid is charged). *Avoidance learning* requires an additional response. The rat on the grid learns to avoid a shock if it quickly pushes a lever when a light signal goes on. To move from escape learning to avoidance learning, an animal must make an *anticipatory response* to prevent the punishment. Escape learning and avoidance learning are two forms of aversive control; behavior that terminates the source of aversive stimuli is strengthened and maintained.

Shaping Behavior. Shaping involves changing behavior in a deliberate and predetermined way. By reinforcing those responses that are in the desired direction, an experimenter shapes an animal's behavior. An experimenter who wants to train a seal to ring a bell with its nose can give a food reinforcement as the animal's random behavior brings its nose near the bell. To teach a mute schizophrenic patient to talk, a therapist may first reward the patient for simply looking at the therapist; later the therapist reinforces any vocalizations and then simple speech. The closer the time of the reinforcement to the operant behavior, the better the learning. Shaping is also called *successive approximation.*

Adventitious Reinforcement. Responses accidentally reinforced by coincidental pairing of response and reinforcement are adventitious. Such events may have clinical implications in the development of phobias and other behavior.

Premack's Principle. A concept developed by David Premack states that a behavior engaged in with high frequency can be used to reinforce a low-frequency behavior. In one experiment, Premack observed that children spent more time playing with a pinball machine than eating candy when both were freely available. When he made playing with the pinball machine contingent on eating a certain amount of candy, the children increased the amount of candy they ate. In a therapeutic application of this principle, patients with schizophrenia were observed to spend more time in a rehabilitation center sitting down doing nothing than they did working at a simple task. When 5 minutes of sitting down was made contingent on a certain amount of work, the work output was considerably increased, as was skill acquisition. This principle is also known as Grandma's rule ("If you eat your spinach, you can have dessert").

SOCIAL LEARNING THEORY

Social learning theory relies on role modeling, identification, and human interactions. A person can learn by imitating the behavior of another person, but personal factors are involved. When a person dislikes a role model, imitative behavior is unlikely. Social learning theorists combine operant and classical conditioning theories. For example, although the observation of models may be a major factor in the learning process, imitation of the model must be reinforced or rewarded if the behaviors are to become part of the person's repertoire.

Albert Bandura is a major proponent of the social learning school. According to Bandura, behavior results from the interplay between cognitive and environmental factors, a concept known as *reciprocal determinism.* Persons learn by observing others, intentionally or accidentally; this process is described as modeling, or learning through imitation. A person's choice of model is influenced by a variety of factors, such as age, sex, status, and similarity. If a chosen model reflects healthy norms and values, the person develops *self-efficacy,* the capacity to adapt to normal, everyday life as well as to threatening situations. It is possible to eliminate negative behavior patterns by having a person learn alternative techniques from other role models. For example, fearful children become less fearful when they watch other children acting fearlessly in the same situation. Similarly, demonstrating a fearless approach to a phobic situation may be useful to motivate a patient's approach to the feared object or situation.

Modeling has also been used in weight reduction and smoking cessation programs. It is an important component of group treatment plans in which members of the group learn from one another.

COGNITIVE LEARNING

Cognition is the process of obtaining, organizing, and using intellectual knowledge. Persons perform mental operations and store bits of information in memory to be retrieved later. Cognitive learning theories focus on the role of understanding: Cognition implies understanding the connection between cause and effect, between action and the consequences of the action. *Cognitive strategies* are mental plans that persons use to understand themselves and the environment.

The cognitive strategy of patients with depression focuses on what is wrong rather than what is right. A form of cognitive therapy developed by Aaron Beck for the treatment of depression teaches patients to recognize and value their assets and alerts them to the cognitive pattern that causes their depression. Beck described the cognitive triad that exists in depression as consisting of a person's negative view of self, negative interpretation of experience, and negative expectation of the future.

Many theorists, such as Jean Piaget, have defined a series of stages in cognitive growth. Another approach toward cognition is *information processing,* a sequence of mental operations involving input, storage, and output of information. Cognition involves calling up and processing relevant information from stored memory.

Behavior can change through techniques in which persons learn by listening to or reading instructions. Therapeutic instructions modify both a person's outcome and efficacy expectations. For example, patients told that their blood pressure readings would drop if they followed certain relaxation procedures showed a decline in blood pressure. To learn new patterns of behavior persons can monitor their behavior by charting events, such as when they eat or smoke. Self-monitoring also reduces the rate of relapse. If a therapist helps patients define and set realistic and well-specified goals, they have a greater likelihood of achieving them than if goals are poorly defined or unrealistic. Goal attainment enhances self-efficacy, which in turn affects future performance positively.

Piaget was a major theorist of cognitive development. His work is discussed in Section 4.1.

Cognitive Dissonance

Cognitive dissonance means incongruity or disharmony among a person's beliefs, knowledge, and behavior. When dissonance becomes too great, persons change their ways of thinking or behaving to lessen the disharmony. An example of cognitive dissonance is a person's unwillingness to believe that a very expensive car or one that is considered a status symbol could have anything wrong with it or could be defective in any way. Another example is believing strongly in a decision after it has been made. Dissonance generally occurs when there is a palpable disparity between two experimental or behavioral elements. Cognitive dissonance apparently produces an uncomfortable tension state (like hunger) that persons are motivated to change.

Attribution Theory

Attribution theory is a cognitive approach concerned with how persons perceive the causes of behavior. According to attribution theory, persons are likely to attribute their own behavior to situational causes but are likely to attribute others' behavior to stable internal dispositions (personality traits); the particular cause that a person attributes to a given event influences subsequent feelings and behavior. In psychiatry, attribution theory may help explain why some persons attribute a change in behavior to an external event (situation) or to a change in internal state (disposition or ability). Similarly, behavioral change may be attributed to the effects of taking a drug or to interpersonal events. Research on drug effects by attribution theorists has shown that it may be unwise to describe a drug as very strong or as very effective because, if it does have the desired effect, patients may believe that is the only reason they got better.

NEUROPHYSIOLOGY OF LEARNING

One of the first theorists to explore the neurophysiological aspects of learning was Clark L. Hull (1884–1952), who developed a drive reduction theory of learning. Hull postulated that neurophysiological connections established in the central nervous system reduce the level of a drive (e.g., obtaining food reduces hunger). An external stimulus stimulates an efferent system and elicits a motor impulse. The critical connection is between the stimulus and the motor response, which is a neurophysiological reaction that leads to what Hull called a *habit.* Habits are strengthened when a response further reduces the drive associated with the aroused need.

By exploring the human brain, researchers such as Pierre Broca and Karl Wernicke identified specific areas of the brain involved in the development and retention of speech and language. Electrical stimulation of certain brain sites evoked vivid mental imagery in patients, and lesions of the amygdaloid nucleus in animals interfered with learning. Learning produces changes in the structure and function of nerve cells. In one study, monkeys that were trained to use a particular finger to obtain food showed hypertrophy of the area of the brain responsible for finger control.

Habituation and Sensitization

In the study of the snail *Aplysia,* Eric Kandel showed how simple forms of learning, such as habituation and sensitization, can occur. Kandel studied a defensive reflex involving the with-

drawal of the snail's siphon when the animal is tactually stimulated. If the snail is touched repeatedly, it is subject to habituation and learns not to withdraw its siphon and gill. Habituation causes the organism to stop responding reflexively as a result of the repeated stimulus.

Aplysia can also be sensitized; that is, a reflex response can be made more sensitive, so that a subthreshold stimulus elicits a response. If the snail receives a strong stimulus (e.g., an electric shock), it becomes sensitized; then, even a previously subthreshold stimulation causes the animal to withdraw its gill and siphon. Experimental work with *Aplysia* has also shown that habituation develops before sensitization. Kandel's research with simple organisms, such as *Aplysia,* revealed that learning avoidance behavior alters the chemical structure of cells in the nervous system. When the avoidance is unlearned, these chemical changes are reversed. Such research provides a foundation for understanding the neurochemistry of learning and for exploring reciprocal interactions between ongoing biological processes in the central nervous system and behavior changes resulting from environmental influences. Kandel received the Nobel prize for his work in 2000.

Memory Formation and Storage

The neurobiological basis of learning is located in the structures of the brain involved in forming and storing information, which include the hippocampus, the cortex, and the cerebellum. One hundred billion neurons in the brain are involved in forming memories, including a layer of 4.6 million cells in the hippocampus.

Learning begins with the senses taking in an environmental stimulus that is eventually transformed into a memory trace or memory link. An electrical or chemical impulse, passing through a neuron when the brain receives information, triggers the formation of connections between synapses. Animal experiments have shown an increase in synaptic connections when learning occurs.

Long-term memories have increased time to link with many locations in the cortex and thus are retained longer than short-term memories. The more connections, the better the chance of contacting a neural pathway leading to the memory; repeated reliving of a memory enhances its permanence.

Storage is the key to a good memory. Relating material to something that is already known creates more pathways and increases the storage power. Processing information at a semantic level involves more of the mind than does rote memorization. Semantic information decays at a slower rate than information superficially memorized, without meaning and comprehension.

Memory is divided into short-term and long-term types; long-term memory is also known as *recent memory, recent past memory, remote memory,* and *secondary memory.* Short-term memory—also called *immediate memory, working memory, primary memory,* and *buffer memory*—is adversely affected by chronic emotional stress, psychological exhaustion, or too much input. Short-term and long-term memory differ in the amount of information that can be stored. The capacity of short-term memory is limited (five to nine bits of information).

Smell and emotion may underlie long-term memories. Scent conveys information through the olfactory nerve to the hippocampus, which plays a role in the control of emotion. Learning and memory are affected by stress. The increase in adrenaline resulting from stress can enhance learning, but if stress is too great, learning is inhibited. A persons' mood affects learning and the recall of material; a person learning material in a happy mood enhances his or her memory and has better recall. Those childhood memories that survive are memories associated with the time the child learned to speak, between the ages of 3 and 5 years. Before then, only memories associated with traumatic events or with smell are likely to be remembered.

MOTIVATION

Motivation is a state of being that produces a tendency toward action. The state may be one of deprivation (e.g., hunger), a value system, or a strongly held belief (e.g., religion). In the mediation of learning and perception, biological mechanisms play an important role in motivating behavior. An organism tries to maintain homeostasis or internal balance against any disturbance of equilibrium (e.g., a thirsty animal is motivated to find water and drink). Social motives, such as the need for recognition and achievement, also account for behavioral patterns (e.g., studying hard to get good grades). But the intensity of motivation to master any task in a particular situation is determined by at least two factors: the achievement motive (desire to achieve) and the likelihood of success.

Persons show marked individual differences in the values placed on objects and goals. Some students strive for As; others depreciate the importance of grades and place higher value on intellectual satisfaction or on extracurricular activities. The expectancy factor refers to the subjective probability that by expending sufficient effort, the object may be acquired or the goal reached.

Psychiatric Applications

In 1950, Joseph Wolpe defined *anxious behavior* as persistent habits of learned or conditioned responses acquired in anxiety-generating situations. If a response inhibitory to anxiety can occur in the presence of anxiety-evoking stimuli, it weakens the connection between the stimuli and the anxiety response. Wolpe referred to this process as *reciprocal inhibition.* Relaxation, for instance, is considered incompatible with anxiety and, therefore, inhibits it. Wolpe was a pioneer in the development of behavior therapy.

Anxiety Hierarchy. In Wolpe's method of therapy, known as *systematic desensitization,* the goal is to eliminate maladaptive anxiety and behavior. To accomplish this goal, Wolpe asked his patients to imagine the least disturbing item on a list of potentially anxiety-evoking stimuli and then to proceed step by step up the list to the most disturbing stimulus. For example, a patient with a fear of heights ranked the sight of a tall building lower in the anxiety hierarchy than standing on a high ledge; being on the 10th floor of a building fell somewhere in between. In a relaxed state (usually induced by hypnosis but sometimes induced by drugs), the patient was instructed to visualize the least anxiety-producing situation; if this visualization did not produce anxiety, the person moved up the hierarchy. Eventually, the patient was desensitized to the source of anxiety.

Tension Reduction Theory. Dollard and Miller attempted to reconcile behavioral theory and freudian psychodynamics by stressing the commonalities between the two. Subscribing to

Table 4.3–3
Behavioral and Psychoanalytic Models

Behavioral Model	Psychoanalytic Model
Behavior is determined by current contingencies, reinforcement history, and genetic endowment	Behavior is determined by intrapsychic processes
Problem behavior is the focus of study and treatment	Behavior is but a symbol of intrapsychic processes and a symptom of unconscious conflict; the underlying conflict is the focus of treatment
Contemporary variables, such as contingencies of reinforcement, are the focus of the analysis	Historical variables, such as childhood experiences, are the focus of the analysis
Treatment entails the application of the principles of operant or classical conditioning	Treatment consists of bringing unconscious conflicts into consciousness
Objective observation, measurement, and experimentation are the methods used; the focus is on observable behavior and environmental events (antecedents and consequences)	Subjective methods of interpretation of behavior and inference regarding unobservable events (e.g., intrapsychic processes) are used
Theory is based on experimentation	Theory is predominantly based on case histories
Tenets can be formulated into testable hypotheses and evaluated through experimentation	Many tenets cannot be formulated into testable hypotheses to be evaluated through experimentation

Reprinted with permission from Dorsett PC. Behavioral and social learning psychology. In: Stoudemire A, ed. *Human Behavior: An Introduction for Medical Students.* Philadelphia: JB Lippincott; 1990:105.

Table 4.3–4
Common Terms Used in Learning Theory

Aversive conditioning: A procedure in which punishment or aversive stimulation is used to reduce the frequency of a target behavior.

Avoidance learning: A form of operant learning in which an organism learns to avoid certain responses or situations.

Classical conditioning: The association of a neutral stimulus with an unconditioned stimulus such that the neutral stimulus comes to bring about a response similar to that originally elicited by the unconditioned stimulus.

Conditioned response (CR): In classical conditioning the response elicited by the conditioned stimulus.

Conditioned stimulus (CS): In classical conditioning the originally neutral stimulus that comes to be associated with the unconditioned stimulus and eventually elicits a conditioned response.

Continuous reinforcement: A schedule of reinforcement in which a reward is administered every time a response is emitted.

Covert reinforcement: A method of increasing behavioral frequency by using the imagination of pleasant events as a reinforcement.

Covert sensitization: A method of reducing the frequency of behavior by associating it with the imagination of unpleasant consequences.

Discrimination learning: A process in which the tendency toward stimulus generalization is counteracted and responses are made only to specific stimuli.

Experimental neurosis: An abnormal behavior pattern produced in animals through the application of classical or operant conditioning techniques.

Extinction: The reduction of frequency of a learned response as a result of the cessation of reinforcement.

Fixed-interval schedule: A reinforcement schedule in which a reward is given after a specific amount of time has passed.

Fixed-ratio schedule: A reinforcement schedule in which a reward is given after a specific number of responses have been emitted.

Habituation: A simple form of learning in which the response to a repeated stimulus lessens over time.

Higher-order conditioning: In classical conditioning the establishment of a new conditioned stimulus through association with an established conditioned stimulus.

Instrumental learning: Operant conditioning.

Law of effect: The principle that behaviors followed by pleasant consequences are strengthened and those followed by negative consequences are weakened.

Modeling: Observational learning.

Negative practice: A method for reducing the frequency of a behavior by the intense repetition of the response.

Observational learning: Learning new behaviors by observing others responding and receiving some form of consequence; vicarious learning.

Operant conditioning: A form of learning in which behavioral frequency is altered through the application of positive and negative consequences.

Partial reinforcement: A schedule of reinforcement in which rewards are not given each time a response is made, rendering a learned response highly resistant to extinction.

Primary reinforcer: A stimulus affecting a biological process (e.g., food that increases the probability of behaviors it follows).

Reinforcer: A stimulus that increases the frequency of responses it follows.

Respondent learning: Classical conditioning.

Secondary reinforcers: Stimuli that gain the power to reinforce a behavior through association with primary reinforcers.

Shaping: An operant procedure in which a desirable behavior pattern is learned by the successive reinforcement of approximations to that behavior.

Spontaneous recovery: The increase in the strength of an extinguished behavior after the passage of a period of time.

Successive approximation: See *Shaping.*

Unconditioned response: In classical conditioning a response that occurs spontaneously to the unconditioned stimulus.

Unconditioned stimulus: A stimulus that, without any training, produces a specific response.

Variable-interval schedule: A reinforcement schedule in which a reward is given after varying periods of time have passed.

Variable-ratio schedule: A reinforcement schedule in which a reward is given after a varying number of responses have been emitted.

Table by Marshall P. Duke, Ph.D., and Stephen Nowicki, Jr., Ph.D.

the tension reduction theory of behavior, they considered behavior to be motivated by an organism's attempt to reduce tension produced by unsatisfied or unconscious drives. Similarly, Sigmund Freud's pleasure principle is a tension-reducing force and, consequently, a strong motivator. When a drive is repressed, anxiety occurs and acts as an acquired drive; a person's behavior may be motivated by an attempt to reduce that anxiety. Adults may avoid situations that are likely to stimulate anxiety, but they may be completely unaware of their avoidance patterns. Therapy, in part, is an unlearning process. The patient learns that certain behaviors can reduce anxiety, and avoidance patterns are replaced by approach patterns. (Table 4.3–3 gives a comparison of the behavioral and psychoanalytic models.)

Learned Helplessness Model of Depression. A laboratory animal may be classically conditioned to accept a painful stimulus when restrained. Such restraint eventually teaches the animal that it has no way to avoid the aversive stimulus. A condition known as *learned helplessness* develops when an organism learns that no behavioral pattern can influence the environment. The learned helplessness paradigm has been used to explain depression in humans who feel helpless, without options, and unable to control events.

Brain Stimulation and Reinforcement. When certain areas of the hypothalamus are electrically stimulated, intense pleasure is experienced by both humans and other animals. When nonhuman primates were provided with a way to stimulate pleasure centers in their brains, they preferred stimulating themselves to eating or drinking. In human beings, similar phenomena occur; in one case, a patient stimulated his brain 1,000 times in a 6-hour period until he was forced to stop.

Table 4.3–4 provides an overview of terms used in this section in addition to the common terms used in learning theory.

References

Agras WS, Wilson GT. Learning theory. In: Sadock BJ, Sadock VA, eds. *Kaplan & Sadock's Comprehensive Textbook of Psychiatry.* 7th ed. Vol 1. Baltimore: Lippincott Williams & Wilkins; 2000:413.

Byrnes JP. Categorizing and combining theories of cognitive development and learning. *Educ Psychol Rev.* 1992;4:309.

Case R, Griffin S, Kelly WM. Socioeconomic differences in children's early cognitive development and their readiness for schooling. In: Golbeck SL, ed. *Psychological Perspectives on Early Childhood Education: Reframing Dilemmas in Research and Practice.* The Rutgers invitational symposium on education series. Mahwah, NJ: Lawrence Erlbaum; 2001:37.

Cattell RB. *Psychotherapy by Structured Learning Theory.* New York: Springer; 1987.

Daum I, Schugens M. On the cerebellum and classical conditioning. *Curr Dir Psychol Sci.* 1996;5:58.

Hall G. Learning about associatively activated stimulus representations: implications for acquired equivalence and perceptual learning. *Anim Learn Behav.* 1996;24:233.

Lovibond PF. Animal learning theory and the future of human pavlovian conditioning. *Biol Psychol.* 1988;27:199.

Mowrer OH. *Learning Theory and Behavior.* New York: Wiley, 1960.

Nathan M, Robinson C. Considerations of learning and learning research: revisiting the "media effects" debate. *J Interact Learn Res.* 2001;12:69.

Pavlov IP. *Conditioned Reflexes.* London: Oxford University Press; 1927.

Rescorla RA, Holland PC. Behavioral studies of associative learning in animals. *Annu Rev Psychol.* 1982;33:265.

Skinner BF. *Science and Human Behavior.* New York: Macmillan; 1953.

Slangen JL, Early B, Jaffard R, Richelle M, Olton DS. Behavioral models of memory and amnesia. *Pharmacopsychiatry.* 1990;23:81.

Sudakov KV. The development of the scientific ideas of I. P. Pavlov on the goal reflex in studies of the mechanisms of biological motivation. *Neurosci Behav Physiol.* 2001;31:87.

Waelti P, Dickinson JA, Schultz W. Dopamine responses comply with basic assumptions of formal learning theory. *Nature.* 2001;412:43.

Walker S. *Learning Theory and Behavior Modification.* London: Methuen; 1984.

Watson JB, Rayner R. Conditioned emotional reactions. *J Exp Psychol.* 1920;3:1.

Windholz G. Pavlov's conceptualization of learning. *Am J Psychol.* 1992;105:459.

▲ 4.4 Aggression

Although many definitions of *aggression* have been put forth, the term is not easily defined. In humans, aggressive behavior assumes the form of violent actions against others, who may avoid such treatment or may fight back. Aggression implies the intent to harm or otherwise injure another person, an implication inferred from events preceding or following the act of aggression.

A classification system of aggression has been organized around behavior patterns; that is, behavior patterns similar in form are assigned to the same category. For example, one category of aggression behavior might include physical attacks against the self, and another, physical attacks against objects or others.

The term *aggression* is not specifically defined in the text revision of the fourth edition of the American Psychiatric Association's *Diagnostic and Statistical Manual of Mental Disorders* (DSM-IV-TR). The definition used in this section, which refers to behavior intended to cause physical injury to others, is descriptive by virtue of its short-term consequence, harm to others. Many behaviors are aggressive even though they do not involve physical injury. Verbal aggression is one example. There are others, such as coercion, intimidation, managerial styles that result in harmful psychological consequences to others, and premeditated social ostracism of others. The importance of these behaviors in day-to-day living should not be underestimated, nor should their effects on recipients' self-esteem, social status, and happiness.

FANTASIES VERSUS ACTS

Persons may have violent thoughts or fantasies, but unless they lose control, thoughts do not become acts. However, any set of conditions that produce increased aggressive impulses in the context of diminished control may produce violent acts. Situations with combinations of factors include toxic and organic states, developmental disabilities, florid psychosis, conduct disorder, and overwhelming psychological and environmental stress. Table 4.4–1 outlines some of the disorders listed in DSM-IV-TR that have been associated with violent and aggressive behavior.

Distinguishing fantasies from the threat of a real act is extremely important, because there are laws that require psychiatrists to warn both legal authorities and potential victims when they suspect one of their patients will actually commit foul play. Fantasies, however—even the most violent, murderous, or sadistic—are not subject to such reporting requirements. (Chapter 58 on forensic psychiatry discusses these issues further.)

PREDICTORS OF AGGRESSION

Most adults with and without mental disorders who commit aggressive acts are likely to do so against persons they know, usu-

Table 4.4–1
Some DSM-IV-TR Disorders Associated with Aggression

Mental retardation
Attention-deficit/hyperactivity disorder
Conduct disorder
Cognitive disorders
Delirium
Dementia
Psychotic disorders
Schizophrenia
Psychotic disorder not otherwise specified
Mood disorders
Mood disorder due to a general medical condition
Substance-induced mood disorder
Intermittent explosive disorder
Adjustment disorder with disturbance of conduct
Personality disorders
Paranoid personality disorder
Antisocial personality disorder
Borderline personality disorder
Narcissistic personality disorder
Axis V conditions
Childhood, adolescent, or adult antisocial behavior

ally family members. This fact indicates that aggression is not directed indiscriminately. A possible exception to the familiar-person generalization is reported among male adolescents, who often behave aggressively toward casual acquaintances or strangers.

Generally, the probability of aggressive behavior increases when persons become psychologically decompensated and perhaps also when the onset of a mental disorder is rapid. Otherwise, little is known about the relation between the course of illness and aggression. Episodic decompensation may occur in those who ingest large quantities of alcohol; more than 50 percent of persons who commit criminal homicides and who engage in assaultive behavior are reported to have imbibed significant amounts of alcohol immediately beforehand.

Researchers have recently turned their attention to sex differences in the predisposition to, and frequency of, aggression. For aggression classified as homicide, battery, assault with a weapon, or rape, the frequency among males clearly exceeds that among females. In domestic violence, when one marital partner acts to hurt another, the frequency among men and women is about equal. Studies of persons who are hospitalized in psychiatric facilities for long periods indicate that the prevalence of male and female aggression is about equal. Tables 4.4–2 and 4.4–3 summarize predictors of violence. Among all factors, the best predictor of violence is a history of violent behavior.

ETIOLOGY

Psychological Factors

Instinctive Behavior. FREUD'S VIEW. In his early writings, Sigmund Freud held that all human behavior stems either directly or indirectly from Eros—the life instinct—whose energy, or libido, is directed toward the enhancement or reproduction of life. In this framework, aggression was viewed simply as a reaction to the blocking or thwarting of libidinal impulses and was neither an automatic nor an inevitable part of life.

Table 4.4–2
Commonly Cited Predictors of Dangerousness to Others

High degree of intent to harm
Presence of a victim
Frequent and open threats
Concrete plan
Access to instruments of violence
History of loss of control
Chronic anger, hostility, or resentment
Enjoyment in watching or inflicting harm
Lack of compassion
Self-view as victim
Resentful of authority
Childhood brutality or deprivation
Decreased warmth and affection in home
Early loss of parent
Fire setting, bed-wetting, and cruelty to animals
Prior violent acts
Reckless driving

After the tragic events of World War I, Freud gradually came to adopt a gloomier position about the nature of human aggression. He proposed the existence of a second major instinct—Thanatos, the death force—whose energy is directed toward the destruction or termination of life. According to Freud, all human behavior stems from the complex interplay of Thanatos and Eros and the constant tension between them.

Because the death instinct, if unrestrained, soon results in self-destruction, Freud hypothesized that through mechanisms such as displacement, the energy of Thanatos is redirected outward and serves as the basis for aggression against others. Thus in Freud's latest view, aggression stems primarily from the redirection of the self-destructive death instinct away from the self and toward others.

LORENZ'S VIEW. According to Konrad Lorenz, aggression that causes physical harm to others springs from a fighting instinct that humans share with other organisms. The energy associated with this instinct is produced spontaneously in organisms at a more or less constant rate. The probability of aggression increases as a function of the amount of stored energy and the presence and strength of aggression-releasing stimuli. Aggression is inevitable, and, at times, spontaneous eruptions occur.

Learned Behavior. From another perspective, aggression is primarily a learned form of social behavior—one that is acquired and maintained in much the same manner as other forms of activity. According to Albert Bandura, neither innate urges toward violence nor aggressive drives aroused by frustration are the roots of human aggression. Rather, persons engage in assaults against others because they acquired aggressive responses through past experience; they receive or anticipate various forms of reward for performing such actions; or they are directly instigated to aggression by specific social or envi-

Table 4.4–3
Assessing the Risk of Committing a Homicide[a]

Clinical Characteristics	Low Risk	Medium Risk	High Risk
Hostility indicators (history)			
Family life	Wanted child, good loving family	Some family disruption, loss of a parent or one-parent family	Early violence, battered child, poor parent model
Significant others	Several reliable family members or friends available	Few or one available	None available
Daily functioning	Good in most activities	Moderately good in some activities	Not good in any activities
Lifestyle	Stable	Moderately stable	Unstable
Socioeconomic	Upper	Middle	Lower
Employment	Employed	Employment history fairly stable	Unemployed
Education	High school graduate or more (university or technical training)	High school dropout, can read and write	School dropout, semiliterate to illiterate
Housing	Lives in adequate housing, clean environment and space	Fair housing, some overcrowding	Poor housing, crowded, slums
Isolation or withdrawal	Able to relate well to others, outgoing	Mild, some withdrawal and feelings of hopelessness	Long history of being a loner, antisocial, withdrawn, hopeless and helpless feelings
Alcohol or other substance use	Nondrinker, occasional social use	Social drinker or user to occasional abuse	Chronic abuse
Psychological help	No history of need for or use of psychiatric hospitalization	Some outpatient psychiatric help, moderately satisfied with self	History of psychiatric hospitalization, negative view of help
Personal history	No history of violence or impulsive behavior	Occasional history of violence or impulsive behavior	Frequent history of violence or impulsive behavior
Perturbation (negative emotional states)			
Anxiety	Low, good emotional control	Occasional feelings of anxiety	Easily aroused to anxiety, high or panic state
Depression	Low	Occasional depression	Severe, chronically moody
Self-esteem	Good, has reinforcements from others	Usually good	Chronically poor self-image
Hostility	Low	Some	Marked, aggressive
Impulse control	Controlled	Some impulsive acting out not physically violent	Feels need for violence
Constriction (narrowing of vision)			
Coping strategies and devices being used	Able to cope with stress and outside irritating influences; well-developed defense mechanisms	Usually can cope under most pressures; sometimes becomes constrictive in thinking and acts out	Becomes constrictive under most stress; acts out in destructive, socially unacceptable ways
Disorientation and disorganization	None, is in good contact with what is happening	Little to moderate	Marked, losing contact with reality
Resources	Able to make good use of resources available	Some use of resources, aware of most resources	Unable either to use resources available or to recognize that help is available
Cessation (stop the person causing the problem)			
Previous arrests	None	Has been arrested, has not served time	Multiple arrest history, served time in prison, would murder to avoid going back to prison
Previous homicide	None	Has exhibited aggressive behavior; been in fights but no attempt to kill another	Yes, looks at the killing of another as a feasible act
Homicide plan	None	Has held fleeting thoughts of killing another, no definite plan	Frequent or constant thoughts with a specific plan
Weapon available	None that person thinks of	Yes, person aware of weapons in immediate environment but not seriously considering use	Yes, and planning on use (a loaded gun should be considered highly lethal)

[a]No one clinical characteristic predicts homicide. However, the greater the number of clinical characteristics in the medium-risk and high-risk categories, the greater is the risk.
Adapted from Allen N. *Homicide: Perspectives on Prevention.* New York: Human Sciences; 1979.

Table 4.4–4
Theoretical Perspectives on Aggression

Theory	Assumed Source of Aggression	Possibility of Preventing or Controlling Aggression
Instinct theory	Innate tendencies or instincts	Low: aggressive impulses are constantly generated and impossible to avoid
Drive theory	Externally elicited aggressive drive	Low: external sources of aggressive drive are common (e.g., frustration) and impossible to eliminate
Social learning theory	Present social or environmental conditions plus past social learning	Moderate to high: appropriate changes in current social and environmental conditions or in reinforcement contingencies can reduce or prevent overt aggressive actions

Courtesy of Robert A. Baron, Ph.D.

ronmental conditions. In contrast to instinct and drive theories (the psychological representation of a need that impels an organism to seek a goal), the social learning perspective does not attribute aggression to one or a few potential causes but suggests that the roots of such behavior are varied and involve an aggressor's past experience, learning, and a wide range of external situational factors. For example, soldiers receive medals for killing enemy troops during times of war, and professional athletes earn widespread admiration and large financial rewards by competing aggressively (Table 4.4–4).

Social Factors

Frustration. The single most potent means of inciting human beings to aggression is frustration. Widespread acceptance of this view stems mainly from John Dollard's frustration-aggression hypothesis. In its original form, the hypothesis indicated that frustration always leads to a form of aggression and that aggression always stems from frustration.

Frustrated persons, however, do not always respond with aggressive thoughts, words, or deeds. They may show a wide variety of reactions, ranging from resignation, depression, and despair to attempts to overcome the sources of their frustration. And not all aggression results from frustration. Persons (e.g., boxers and football players) act aggressively for many reasons and in response to many stimuli.

Examination of the evidence indicates that whether frustration increases or fails to enhance overt aggression depends largely on two factors. First, frustration appears to increase aggression only when the frustration is intense. When it is mild or moderate, aggression may not be enhanced. Second, frustration is likely to facilitate aggression when it is perceived as arbitrary or illegitimate, rather than when it is viewed as deserved or legitimate.

Direct Provocation. Evidence indicates that physical abuse and verbal taunts from others often elicit aggressive actions. Once aggression begins, it often shows an unsettling pattern of escalation; as a result, even mild verbal slurs or glancing blows may initiate a process in which stronger and stronger provocations are exchanged.

Television Violence. A link between aggression and exposure to televised violence has been noted. The more televised violence children watch, the greater is their level of aggression against others. The strength of the relation appears to increase over time; this finding points to the cumulative effects of media violence. The processes that account for the effects of filmed and televised violence on the behavior of viewers are outlined in Table 4.4–5. Similar concerns have been raised about computer games with violent themes. Some studies indicate that adolescents become desensitized to homicidal activities after repeated exposure, especially if the game involves their killing virtual opponents, which is common in many computer programs.

Environmental Factors

Air Pollution. Exposure to noxious odors, such as those produced by chemical plants and other industries, may increase personal irritability and, therefore, aggression, although this effect appears to be true only up to a point. If the odors in question are truly foul, aggression appears to decrease—perhaps because escaping from the unpleasant environment becomes a dominant goal for those involved.

Noise. Several studies have reported that persons exposed to loud, irritating noise direct stronger assaults against others than those not exposed to such environmental conditions.

Table 4.4–5
Mechanisms Underlying the Effects of Televised and Filmed Violence on the Behavior of Viewers

Mechanism	Effects
Observational learning	Viewers acquire new means of harming others not previously present in their behavior repertoires.
Disinhibition	Viewers' restraints or inhibitions against performing aggressive actions are weakened as a result of observing others engaging in such behavior.
Desensitization	Viewers' emotional responsivity to aggressive actions and their consequences—signs of suffering on the part of victims—is reduced. As a result, they show little, if any, emotional arousal in response to such stimuli.

Courtesy of Robert A. Baron, Ph.D.

Crowding. Some studies indicate that overcrowding may produce elevated levels of aggression, but other investigations have failed to obtain evidence of such a link. Crowding may enhance the likelihood of aggressive outbursts when typical reactions are negative (e.g., annoyance, irritation, and frustration). The crowding of airline passengers in coach class has been suggested as contributing to violent incidents among passengers.

Situational Factors

Heightened Physiological Arousal. Some research indicates that heightened arousal stemming from such diverse sources as participation in competitive activities, vigorous exercise, and exposure to provocative films enhances overt aggression.

Sexual Arousal. Recent investigations indicate that the effects of sexual arousal on aggression depend strongly on the erotic materials used to induce such reactions and on the precise nature of the reactions themselves. When the erotica viewed are mild, such as photos of attractive nudes, aggression is reduced. When they are explicit, such as films of couples engaged in various sex acts, aggression is enhanced.

Pain. Physical pain may arouse an aggressive drive—the motive to harm or injure others. This drive, in turn, may find expression against any available target, including those not in any way responsible for the aggressor's discomfort. This hypothesis may partly explain why persons exposed to aggression act aggressively toward others.

Biological Factors

Aggression has been linked in animals with testosterone, progesterone, luteinizing hormone, renin, β-endorphin, prolactin, melatonin, norepinephrine, dopamine, epinephrine, acetylcholine, serotonin, 5-hydroxyindoleacetic acid (5-HIAA), and phenylacetic acid, among others. Some studies have related the level of aggression to androgen levels. These studies point to the androgen insensitivity syndrome (in which there is defective binding of androgens to proteins, resulting in male offspring with a feminine appearance and a decreased propensity for rough-and-tumble play) and to the adrenogenital syndrome (in which the mother's adrenal cortex exposes the fetus to elevated adrenal androgens, resulting in masculinization, partly evidenced by increased rough-and-tumble play in masculinized girls).

In regard to drugs and substances of abuse, several generalizations appear to hold. Small doses of alcohol inhibit aggression, and large doses facilitate it. Barbiturate effects are similar to the effects of alcohol, as are the effects of aerosols and commercial solvents. Anxiolytics generally inhibit aggression, although paradoxical aggression is sometimes observed. Opioid dependence (but not opioid intoxication) is associated with increased aggression, as is the use of stimulants, cocaine, hallucinogens, and, in some cases, variable doses of marijuana.

Neuroanatomical Damage. Increasingly, several investigators are hypothesizing that the root of the aggressive behavior of certain chronically aggressive persons is organic brain damage. This perspective is an elaboration of the theory that aggression is a learned social behavior, in that persons who have been the victims of severe physical abuse may suffer neurological sequelae secondary to the abuse, and the sequelae biologically predispose them to violent behavior. In 1986, Dorothy Lewis reported that every death-row inmate studied by her team of researchers had a history of head injury, often inflicted by abusive parents. This study concluded that death-row inmates constitute an especially neuropsychiatrically impaired prison population. Researchers investigating the association between head injury and violent behavior have been careful to point out that the linkage of physical abuse, head injury, and violence is uncertain, although most studies do show an association between early physical abuse and later aggressive behavior. Some researchers speculate that the combination of brain injury and a history of undergoing and observing chronic severe abuse is particularly lethal.

Neurotransmitters. Generally, cholinergic and catecholaminergic mechanisms seem to be involved in the induction and enhancement of predatory aggression, whereas serotonergic systems and γ-aminobutyric acid (GABA) seem to inhibit such behavior. The catecholaminergic and serotonergic systems evidently modulate affective aggression. Dopamine seems to facilitate aggression, whereas norepinephrine and serotonin appear to inhibit it. Recently, serotonin has again gained attention as a potentially important mediating factor in aggression. Rapid declines in serotonin levels or function are associated with increased irritability and, in nonhuman primates, with increased aggression. Some human studies have indicated that 5-HIAA levels in cerebrospinal fluid inversely correlate with the frequency of aggression, particularly among persons who commit suicide.

Genetic Factors

Twin Studies. Research involving monozygotic twins indicates a hereditary component to aggressive behavior. Thus far, most studies have focused on nonpsychiatric populations, in which the concordance rates for monozygotic twins exceed the rates for dizygotic twins.

Pedigree Studies. Several studies show that persons with family histories of mental disorders are more prone to mental disorders and engage in more aggressive behavior than those without such histories. Those with low intelligence quotient (IQ) scores appear to have a higher frequency of delinquency and aggression than those with normal IQ scores. Observed correlations between aggressive behavior and other atypical behaviors indicate that genetic predispositions to atypical behavior, including behaviors associated with mental disorders, are associated with atypical physiological functions, one consequence of which is an increase in the probability of aggression.

Chromosomal Influences. Behavior research involving the influence of chromosomes has concentrated primarily on abnormalities in X and Y chromosomes, particularly the 47-chromosome XYY syndrome. Early studies indicated that persons with the syndrome could be characterized as tall, of below-average intelligence, and likely to be apprehended and in prison for engaging in criminal behavior. Subsequent studies indicated, however, that, at most, the XYY syndrome contributes to aggressive behavior in only a small percentage of

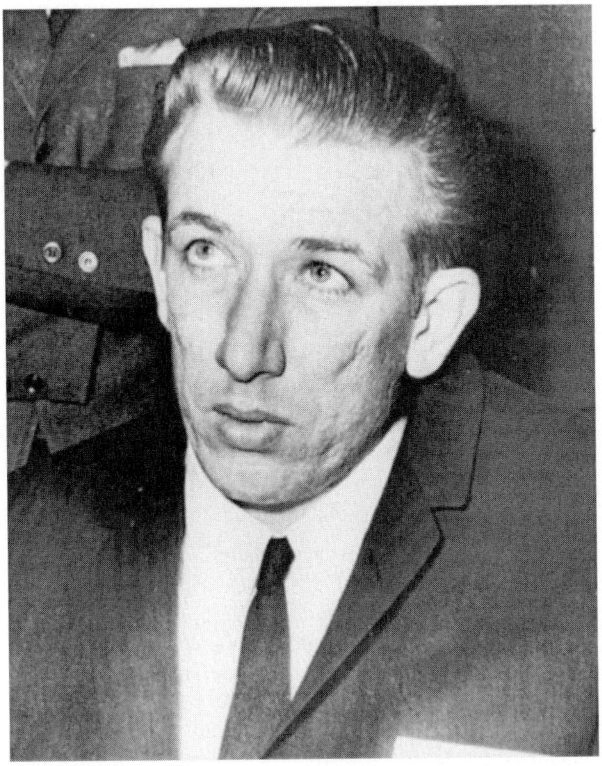

FIGURE 4.4–1
Richard Speck. He was convicted in 1966 of slaying eight nurses in Chicago by stabbing and strangulation. His legal defense was based on his genetic makeup, which was "XYY." Individuals with these genes have been reported to be tall, mentally retarded, have acne, and show aggressive behavior. A jury found him guilty, and he was sentenced to death in the electric chair. (Courtesy of Wide World Photos.)

cases. Studies of the androgen and gonadotropin characteristics of persons with XYY syndrome have been inconclusive. A famous case of an "XYY" insanity defense is illustrated in Figure 4.4–1.

EPIDEMIOLOGY

According to the Federal Bureau of Investigation (FBI) *Uniform Crime Reports,* there are about 1½ million violent crimes (murder, rape, forcible robbery, and aggravated assault) committed in the United States each year. Of this number, about 90,000 are rapes, and about 15,000 are homicides. These statistics have decreased by 25.5 percent since 1991. Violent crime rates are highest in large metropolitan areas and lowest in rural areas.

Violent acts are most often committed by persons who know or knew each other. Homicides are most prevalent among strangers (55 percent); more than 65 percent of homicides are committed with handguns. In the United States, homicide is the second leading cause of death among persons 15 to 24 years of age. Furthermore, a young black man is eight times more likely to be murdered than a white man of the same age. Much lower homicide rates have been reported in such countries as England, Sweden, Japan, and Canada, which all have strict handgun-control laws. Homicide is most prevalent in low socioeconomic groups and is more commonly committed by men than by women.

One national survey of high school students reported that 28 percent of the boys and 7 percent of the girls had been in a physical fight in the previous month. Nearly 35 percent of those surveyed reported having been in at least one physical fight that resulted in an injury requiring medical attention.

PREVENTION AND CONTROL

For physicians, the prevention of death and disability resulting from aggressive, violent, or homicidal behavior begins at the individual level. For instance, violence within a family (such as sexual and physical abuse of children, wife beating, and self-destructive behavior) is often revealed through sensitive questioning and a high index of suspicion on the clinician's part. Preventive interventions include psychiatric referral, notification of the proper legal or other authorities (mandatory in such cases as child abuse and specific threats of harm to persons), and skilled counseling by appropriately trained therapists. Many experts advocate limiting exposure to violence on television and in movies and computer games as way to decrease violence.

Punishment

Punishment is sometimes an effective deterrent to overt aggression. Research findings indicate that the frequency or intensity of such behavior can be reduced by even mild forms of punishment, such as social disapproval; but punishment may not always, or even usually, produce such effects.

The recipients of punishment often interpret it as an attack against them. To the extent that it is, aggressors may respond even more aggressively. Strong punishment is more likely to provoke desires for revenge or retribution than to instill lasting restraints against violence. Persons who administer punishment may serve as aggressive models for those on the receiving end of such discipline, and as noted above, exposure to such models may potentiate violent acts. Because of the conditions under which it is usually administered (a long time after the aggression is committed), punishment may only temporarily reduce the strength or frequency of aggressive behavior. Once the punishment is discontinued, the aggressive acts quickly reappear. For these reasons, certain punishments may backfire and actually encourage, rather than inhibit, the dangerous actions they are designed to prevent.

Catharsis

For many years workers have widely believed that providing angry persons with an opportunity to engage in expressive but noninjurious behaviors reduces their tension or arousal and weakens their tendency to engage in overt and potentially dangerous acts of aggression—the so-called catharsis hypothesis. Although Freud accepted the existence of such catharsis, he was relatively pessimistic about its usefulness in preventing overt aggression. At present, catharsis is thought to help some persons discharge aggression; other persons may become more aggressive as a result of the expressive behaviors.

Training in Social Skills

A major reason why many persons become involved in repeated aggressive encounters is their lack of basic social skills. These persons do not know how to communicate effectively, and thus they adopt an abrasive style of self-expression. Their ineptness in performing such basic tasks as making requests, engaging in negotiations, and lodging complaints often irritates friends, acquaintances, and strangers. Their severe social deficits seem to ensure that they experience repeated frustration and frequently anger those with whom they have direct contact. A technique for reducing the frequency of such behavior involves providing such persons with the social skills that they sorely lack. Social skills training has been applied to diverse groups, including highly aggressive teenagers, police, and even child-abusing parents. In many cases, dramatic changes in the targeted behaviors have been produced (e.g., enhanced interpersonal communication and improved ability to handle rejection and stress), and reduced aggressive behavior related to these shifts is frequently observed. The results are encouraging and indicate that training in appropriate social skills can offer a promising approach to the reduction of human violence.

Induction of Incompatible Responses

Empathy. When aggressors attack other persons in face-to-face confrontations, the aggressors may block out, ignore, or deny signs of pain and suffering on the part of their victims. If aggressors are exposed to such feedback, they may feel empathy and subsequently reduce further aggression. In several experiments, exposure to signs of pain or discomfort on the victim's part has inhibited further aggression.

Humor. Informal observation indicates that anger can often be reduced through exposure to humorous material, and some laboratory studies support this hypothesis. Several types of humor, presented in various formats, may induce reactions or emotions incompatible with aggression among the persons who observe the humor.

Other Factors. Many other reactions may also be incompatible with anger or overt aggression. As already noted, mild sexual arousal sometimes operates in this fashion. Similarly, feelings of guilt about the performance of aggressive actions often reduce such behavior. Participation in absorbing cognitive tasks, such as solving mathematics problems, may induce reactions incompatible with anger and aggressive actions. A summary of mechanisms of violence is given in Figure 4.4–2.

Pharmacotherapy

Several types of drugs and clinical monitoring—for example, blood pressure and electroencephalogram (EEG)—are essential for the optimal treatment of specific aggressive persons. Lithium (Eskalith) appears to be a drug of major promise for some violent patients, especially delinquent adolescent boys. Anticonvulsants occasionally reduce seizure-induced forms of aggression, and they may have the same effect on persons who do not have epilepsy. Antipsychotic medications seem to reduce aggression in both psychotic and nonpsychotic violent patients. Antidepressants may be effective in reducing violence in some depressed patients. Antianxiety agents appear to have a limited role in reducing aggression. Anticonvulsant agents such as gabapentin (Neurontin) have been of use in reducing aggressive outbursts. Antiandrogenic agents may be effective in the treatment of aggressive sex offenders. β-Adrenergic receptor antagonists (beta-blockers) and stimulants may be effective in aggressive children. And electroconvulsive therapy may be effective in a small group of selected patients. Table 4.4–6 outlines some possible psychopharmacological interventions for aggression.

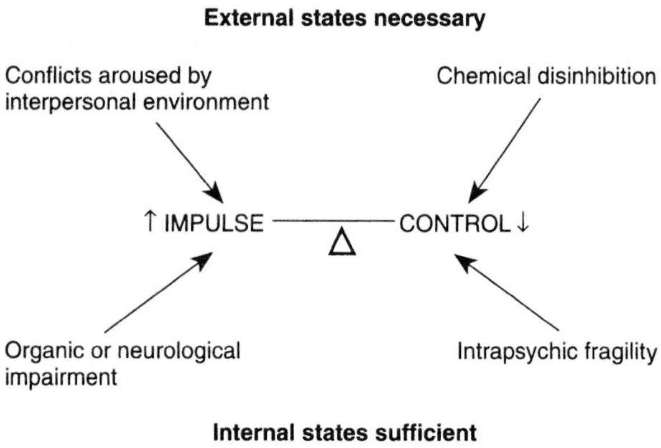

FIGURE 4.4–2
Mechanisms of violence.

VICTIMS

An estimated 18 million persons in the United States at some time have suffered psychiatric disturbance as a result of crime. At any given moment, up to 5 million persons in the United States may suffer from crime-related symptoms. The National Institute of Justice estimates that a 12-year-old American has an 80 percent chance of being the victim of a serious crime at some point in his or her life. Recent research indicates that many victims of violent crimes are at increased risk for major psychiatric problems. Long-term depressive disorders and phobias are two mental disorders reported to occur more frequently in victims of crime than in the general population. Many researchers believe that distinct, characteristic emotional effects are associated with being the victim of a crime and that these effects are related to the fact that victims are the targets of another person's intentional aggression. Table 4.4–7 lists the main emotional aftereffects of crime.

ACCIDENTS

An accident is an event that occurs by chance or unexpectedly, without conscious planning. Studies of accidents show that causes can sometimes be determined and possibly corrected, but they are often multiple and require a multifaceted approach to the problem. For instance, both behavioral and psychological characteristics can be related to the occurrence of accidents. These characteristics include anxiety, boredom, fatigue, and the ingestion of substances that alter concentration and motor coordination. In 2000, according to the National Safety Council, a total of about 97,000 deaths and more than 20 million disabling injuries resulted from accidents.

Table 4.4–6
Schematic Differential Diagnosis and the Pharmacological Treatment of Violence

Psychotic Dimension
Organic Dimension
Characterological Dimension

	Functional	Toxic-metabolic	Structural		Episodic dyscontrol	Other
	Schizophrenia Mania	Drug ETOH	OBS	Epilepsy	Intermittent explosive disorder	Antisocial personality disorder Emotionally unstable character
			Deliriums	Attention-deficit/hyperactivity disorder		
	Depressive disorders	Substance withdrawal	Dementias	Mental retardation		
Acute	Antipsychotics	Benzodiazepines Antihistamines Antipsychotics Physostigmine	Antipsychotics	Benzodiazepines		
Chronic	Antipsychotics Lithium Antidepressants	Benzodiazepines Disulfiram Antidepressants	Antipsychotics Cerebral vasodilators	Anticonvulsants Benzodiazepines Barbiturates Stimulants Antidepressants	Anticonvulsants Lithium Antipsychotics	

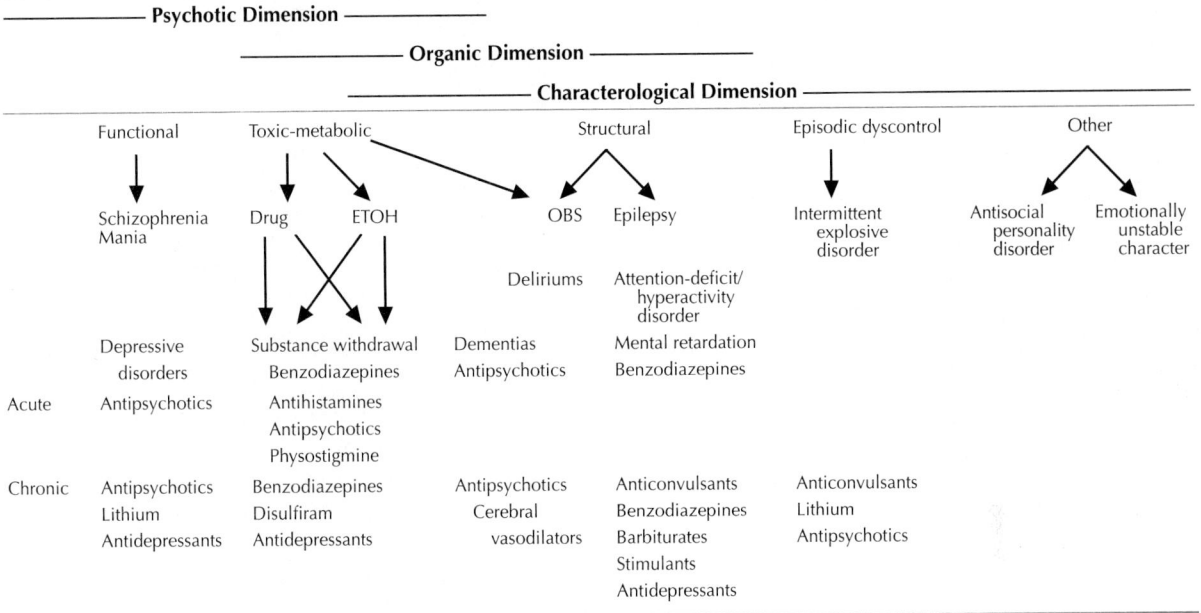

ETOH, ethanol; OBS, organic brain syndrome.
Adapted from Skodol A. Emergency management of potentially violent patients. In: Bassul E, Birk A, eds. *Emergency Psychiatry: Concepts, Methods and Practice.* New York: Plenum; 1984.

For persons 15 to 24 years of age, accidents are the most common cause of death in the United States. Accidents are the fifth most common cause of death overall in the United States. The most recent national data on the cost of injuries reported that for the noninstitutionalized population, accidents were the second leading cause of direct medical costs (second only to heart disease and exceeding cancer) and also accounted for major indirect costs, such as work loss and disability.

Vehicular accidents, industrial accidents, and home accidents were the most frequent types of injuries. One third of all injury deaths are secondary to automobile accidents, and one third are secondary to other accidents; the remaining one third are evenly divided between suicide and homicide. After motor vehicle accidents, the most common causes of accidental death are falls, followed by fire, drowning, and poisoning.

Table 4.4–7
Aftermath of Crime: Main Emotional Effects

Sense of helplessness: The world seems unsafe; victims lack confidence in their judgment and competence to deal with the world.

Rage at being a victim: Intense anger is usually expressed toward family members and those who try to help; conversely, sometimes the victim is unable to express any anger at anything.

Sense of being permanently damaged: Rape victims, for example, may feel that they will never be attractive again.

Inability to trust or to be intimate with others: The effect can include a loss of faith in institutions like the police and the courts.

Persistent preoccupation with the crime: Excessive concern with the crime and its details may reach the point of obsession.

Loss of belief that the world is just: The effect may include self-blame and a sense of having done something to deserve being a victim.

Courtesy of Stuart Kleinman, M.D.

Psychophysiological Considerations

Victims' psychophysiological states must be considered in all injuries and accidents. A physical condition such as fatigue may lead to either distraction or an inability to respond quickly enough to avoid an accident. Such toxic substances as barbiturates, antihistamines, marijuana, and particularly alcohol are important. About one half of reported automobile accidents occur in conjunction with alcohol intake. Persons with diabetes, epilepsy, cardiovascular disease, and mental disorders are involved in more than twice as many accidents per 1,000 miles of driving as those who do not have these illnesses. Age-related impairments, both motor and cerebral function deficits, may lead to potentially impaired judgment, which contributes to fatal accidents among persons 65 and older.

Motivations

From a motivational point of view, the first writings on the subject of an accident-prone personality date to Freud's *The Psychopathology of Everyday Life* (1904):

> Many apparently accidental injuries that happen to such patients are really instances of self-injuries. What happens is an impulse to self-punishment, which is constantly on the watch and which normally finds expression in self-reproach or contributes to the formation of a symptom, takes ingenious advantage of an external situation that chance happens to offer, or lends assistance to that situation until the desired injurious effect is brought about.

Many retrospective studies have explored the personality characteristics of persons who have had severe or frequent accidents. In these studies, workers have speculated that persons repeatedly involved in accidents may have an underlying self-destructive tendency suggesting the existence of

depression, poor control of hostility, a tendency to be more action oriented and less reflective than the general population, and a propensity for intrapsychic or interpersonal difficulties at least partially resolved by the occurrence of the accident. The concept of an unconscious sense of guilt and a need to atone or to be punished for such guilt feelings may provide the motivation for many accidents. Motivations other than an unconscious sense of guilt may be found by examining the life situations of persons involved in accidents. An unconscious wish to escape or to avoid something is often apparent. The desire to escape may be related to external situations in which an accident provides a convenient way of avoiding a possibly humiliating experience. One such example is the man who has an accident on his way to a job interview and thereby avoids the possible humiliation of not obtaining the position he was seeking. Accidents help a person avoid new responsibilities by providing a convenient and acceptable rationale for not entering into the new situation without losing self-esteem or the esteem of others.

REFERENCES

Cairns RB, Cairns BD. The natural history and developmental functions of aggression. In: Sameroff AJ, Lewis M, eds. *Handbook of Developmental Psychology.* 2nd ed. New York: Kluwer Academic/Plenum; 2000:403.

Council on Scientific Affairs. Assault weapons as a public health hazard in the United States. *JAMA.* 1992;267:3067.

Crusio WE. The neurobehavioral genetics of aggression. *Behav Genet.* 1996;26:459.

Cueva JE, Overall JE, Small AM, Armenteros JL, Perry R, Campbell M. Carbamazepine in aggressive children with conduct disorder: a double-blind and placebo-controlled study. *Child Adolesc Psychiatry.* 1996;35:480.

Elliott FA. Violence: the neurologic contribution: an overview. *Arch Neurol.* 1992;49:595.

Federal Bureau of Investigation. *Uniform Crime Reports.* Washington, DC: US Government Printing Office; 2000.

Fishbein DH, ed. The science, treatment, and prevention of antisocial behaviors: application to the criminal justice system. Kingston, NJ: Civic Research Institute; 2000:5.

Gentry J, Eron LD. American Psychological Association Commission on Violence and Youth. *Am Psychol.* 1993;48:89.

Kinzie JD, Boehnlein JK. Psychotherapy of the victims of massive violence: countertransference and ethical issues. *Am Psychother.* 1993;47:90.

National Center for Environmental Health and Injury Control. Physical fighting among high school students: United States, 1990. *MMWR Morb Mortal Wkly Rep.* 1992;41:91.

Pinard G-F, Pagani L, eds. *Clinical Assessment of Dangerousness: Empirical Contributions.* New York: Cambridge University Press; 2001:47.

Serbin LA, Peters PL, Schwartzman AE. Longitudinal study of early childhood injuries and acute illnesses in the offspring of adolescent mothers who were aggressive, withdrawn, or aggressive-withdrawn in childhood. *Abnorm Psychol.* 1996;105:500.

Tardiff K. Adult antisocial behavior and criminality. In: Sadock BJ, Sadock VA, eds. *Kaplan & Sadock's Comprehensive Textbook of Psychiatry.* 7th ed. Vol 2. Baltimore: Lippincott Williams & Wilkins; 2000:1908.

Tardiff K, Marzuk PM, Leon AC, Portera L, Weiner C. Violence by patients admitted to a private psychiatric hospital. *Am J Psychiatry.* 1997;154:88.

Verhoeven WMA, Tuinier S. Pharmacotherapy in aggressive and auto-aggressive behavior. In: Dosen A, Day K, eds. *Treating Mental Illness and Behavior Disorders in Children and Adults with Mental Retardation.* Washington, DC: American Psychiatric Press; 2001:283.

▲ 4.5 Ethology and Sociobiology

ETHOLOGY

Ethology is the systematic study of animal behavior. Its roots lie in the natural science of biology, in particular, in zoology. In 1973 the Nobel prize in psychiatry and medicine was awarded to three ethologists, Karl von Frisch, Konrad Lorenz, and Nikolaas Tinbergen. Those awards highlighted the special relevance of ethology not only for medicine but also for psychiatry.

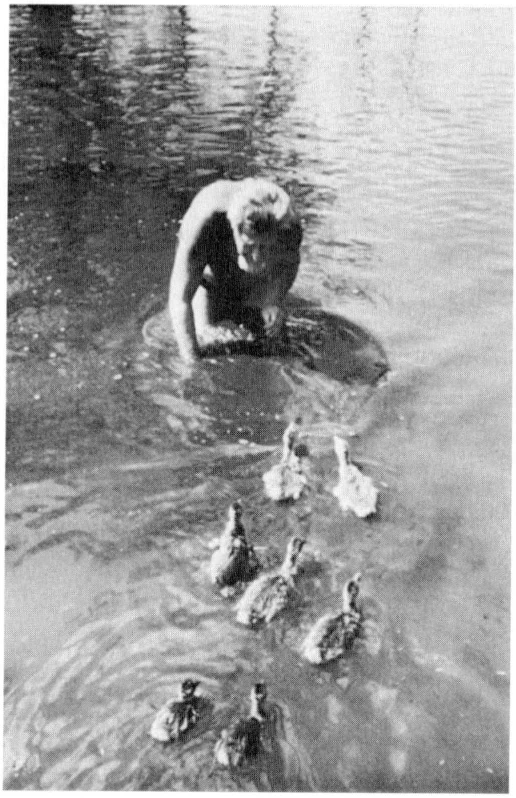

FIGURE 4.5–1

In a famous experiment, Konrad Lorenz demonstrated that goslings responded to him as if he were the natural mother. (Reprinted with permission from Hess EH. Imprinting: An effect of an early experience. *Science* 1959;130:133.)

KONRAD LORENZ

Born in Austria, Konrad Lorenz (1903–1988) is best known for his studies of imprinting. *Imprinting* implies that, during a certain short period of development, a young animal is highly sensitive to a certain stimulus that then, but not at other times, provokes a specific behavior pattern. Lorenz described newly hatched goslings that are programmed to follow a moving object and thereby become imprinted rapidly to follow it and, possibly, similar objects. Typically, the mother is the first moving object the gosling sees, but should it see something else first, the gosling follows it. For instance, a gosling imprinted by Lorenz followed him and refused to follow a goose (Fig. 4.5–1). Imprinting is an important concept for psychiatrists to understand in their effort to link early developmental experiences with later behaviors.

Lorenz also studied the behaviors that function as sign stimuli—that is, social releasers—in communications between individual animals of the same species. Many signals have the character of fixed motor patterns that appear automatically; the reaction of other members of the species to the signals is equally automatic.

Lorenz is also well known for his study of aggression. He wrote about the practical function of aggression, such as territorial defense by fish and birds. Aggression among members of the same species is common, but Lorenz pointed out that in normal conditions, it seldom leads

to killing or even to serious injury. Although animals attack one another, a certain balance appears between tendencies to fight and flight, with the tendency to fight being strongest in the center of the territory and the tendency to flight strongest at a distance from the center.

In many works, Lorenz tried to draw conclusions from his ethological studies of animals that could also be applied to human problems. The postulation of a primary need for aggression in humans, cultivated by the pressure for selection of the best territory, is a primary example. Such a need may have served a practical purpose at an early time, when human beings lived in small groups that had to defend themselves from other groups. Competition with neighboring groups could become an important factor in selection. Lorenz pointed out, however, that this need has survived the advent of weapons that can be used not merely to kill individuals but to wipe out all human beings.

NIKOLAAS TINBERGEN

Born in the Netherlands, Nikolaas Tinbergen (1907–1988), a British zoologist, conducted a series of experiments to analyze various aspects of animals' behavior. He was also successful in quantifying behavior and in measuring the power or strength of various stimuli in eliciting specific behavior. Tinbergen described displacement activities, which have been studied mainly in birds. For example, in a conflict situation, when the needs for fight and for flight are of roughly equal strength, birds sometimes do neither. Rather, they display behavior that appears to be irrelevant to the situation (e.g., a herring gull defending its territory can start to pick grass). Displacement activities of this kind vary according to the situation and the species concerned. Human beings can engage in displacement activities when under stress.

Lorenz and Tinbergen described *innate releasing mechanisms,* animals' responses triggered by releasers, which are specific environmental stimuli. Releasers (including shapes, colors, and sounds) evoke sexual, aggressive, or other responses. For example, big eyes in human infants evoke more caretaking behavior than do small eyes.

In his later work, Tinbergen, along with his wife, studied early childhood autistic disorder. They began by observing the behavior of autistic and normal children when they meet strangers, analogous to the techniques used in observing animal behavior. In particular, they observed in animals the conflict that arises between fear and the need for contact and noted that the conflict can lead to behavior similar to that of autistic children. They hypothesized that, in certain predisposed children, fear can greatly predominate and can also be provoked by stimuli that normally have a positive social value for most children. This innovative approach to studying infantile autistic disorder opened up new avenues of inquiry. Although their conclusions about preventive measures and treatment must be considered tentative, their method shows another way in which ethology and clinical psychiatry can relate to each other.

KARL VON FRISCH

Born in Austria, Karl von Frisch (1886–1982) conducted studies on changes of color in fish and demonstrated that fish could learn to distinguish among several colors and that their sense of color was fairly congruent with that of human beings. He later went on to study the color vision and behavior of bees and is most widely known for his analysis of how bees communicate with one another—that is, their language, or what is known as their dances. His description of the exceedingly complex behavior of bees prompted an investigation of communication systems in other animal species, including humans.

Characteristics of Human Communication. A human being's communicative operations are based on two fundamentally different symbolization systems: nonverbal communication rests on the analogue principle, and verbal codification rests on the digital principle. The inner experience of what is going on at any moment involves nonverbal images that in some way reflect the total situation. Bodily movements and spontaneous, immediate reactions require an analogical appreciation of events. Persons thus develop within themselves a small-scale model of the world based on the recognition of similarities or differences. This method is used for gaining a bird's-eye view of events and for implementing quick reactions necessary for survival. But when persons have time to analyze a situation they use words or numbers, which can detail aspects of events without recourse to analogies. In the digital-verbal system, numbers or letters are arbitrarily assigned to events, and a legend indicates what these symbols refer to. In complex human encounters, verbal and nonverbal communication is used together. The object-oriented parts of the message are expressed in words, and the subject- or participant-oriented parts are expressed nonverbally.

SUBHUMAN PRIMATE DEVELOPMENT

An area of animal research that has relevance to human behavior and psychopathology is the longitudinal study of nonhuman primates. Monkeys have been observed from birth to maturity, not only in their natural habitats and laboratory facsimiles but also in laboratory settings that involve various degrees of social deprivation early in life. Social deprivation has been produced through two predominant conditions: social isolation and separation. Socially isolated monkeys are raised in varying degrees of isolation and are not permitted to develop normal attachment bonds. Monkeys separated from their primary caretakers thereby experience disruption of an already developed bond. Social isolation techniques illustrate the effects of an infant's early social environment on subsequent development (Figs. 4.5–2 and 4.5–3), and

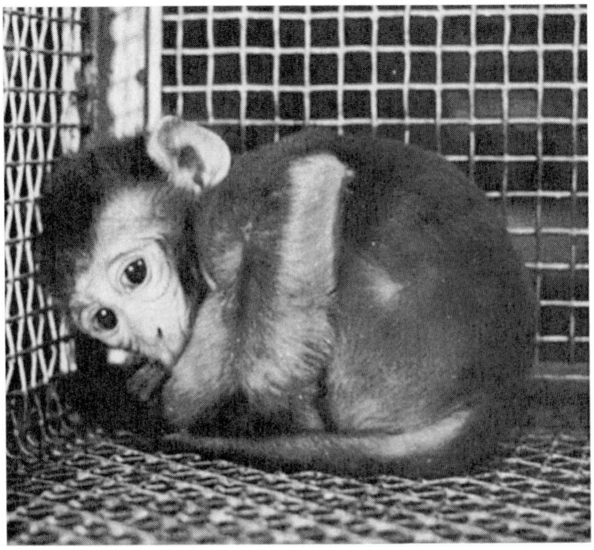

FIGURE 4.5–2
Social isolate after removal of isolation screen.

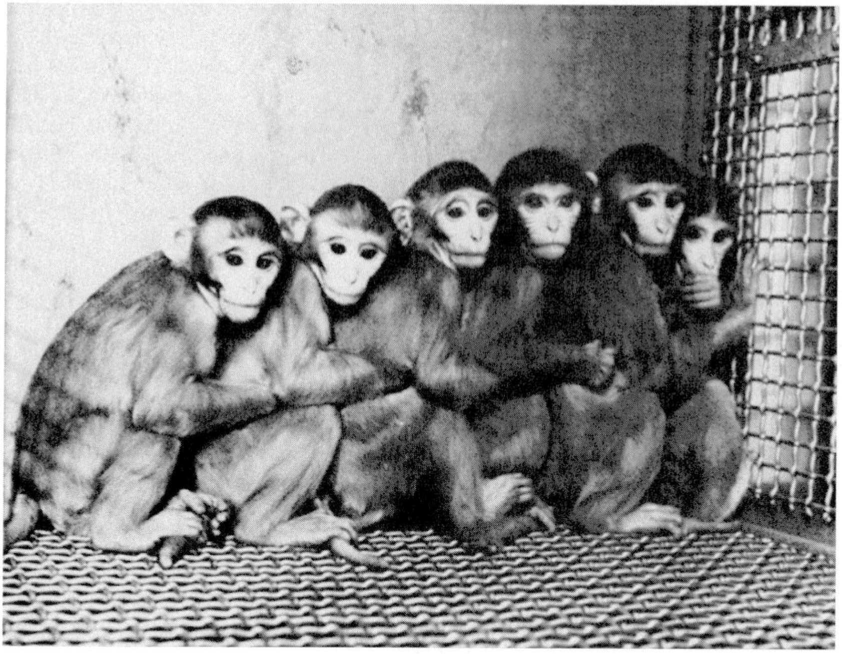

FIGURE 4.5–3
Choo-choo phenomenon in peer-only–reared infant rhesus monkeys.

separation techniques illustrate the effects of loss of a significant attachment figure. The name most associated with isolation and separation studies is Harry Harlow. A summary of Harlow's work is presented in Table 4.5–1.

In a series of experiments, Harlow separated rhesus monkeys from their mothers during their first weeks of life. During this time, the monkey infant depends on its mother for nourishment and protection, as well as for physical warmth and emotional security—*contact comfort*, as Harlow first termed it in 1958. Harlow substituted a surrogate mother made from wire or cloth for the real mother. The infants preferred the cloth-covered surrogate mother, which provided contact comfort, to the wire-covered surrogate, which provided food but no contact comfort (Fig. 4.5–4).

Table 4.5–1
Social Deprivation in Nonhuman Primates

Type of Social Deprivation	Effect
Total isolation (not allowed to develop caretaker or peer bond)	Self-orality, self-clasping, very fearful when placed with peers, unable to copulate. If impregnated, female is unable to nurture young (motherless mothers). If isolation goes beyond 6 months, no recovery is possible.
Mother-only reared	Fails to leave mother and explore. Terrified when finally exposed to peers. Unable to play or to copulate.
Peer-only reared	Engages in self-orality, grasps others in clinging manner, easily frightened, reluctant to explore, timid as adult, play is minimal.
Partial isolation (can see, hear, and smell other monkeys)	Stares vacantly into space, engages in self-mutilation, stereotyped behavior patterns.
Separation (taken from caretaker after bond has developed)	Initial protest stage changing to despair 48 hours after separation; refuses to play. Rapid reattachment when returned to mother.

Adapted from work of Harry Harlow, M.D.

Treatment of Abnormal Behavior

Stephen Suomi demonstrated that monkey isolates can be rehabilitated if they are exposed to monkeys that promote physical contact without threatening the isolates with aggression or overly complex play interactions. These monkeys were called *therapist monkeys*. To fill such a therapeutic role, Suomi chose young normal monkeys that would play gently with the isolates and approach and cling to them. Within 2 weeks, the isolates were reciprocating the social contact, and their incidence of abnormal self-directed behaviors began to decline significantly. By the end of the 6-month therapy period, the isolates were actively initiating play bouts with both the therapists and each other, and most of their self-directed behaviors had disappeared. The isolates were observed closely for the next 2 years, and their improved behavioral repertoires did not regress over time. The results of this and subsequent monkey-therapist studies underscored the potential reversibility of early cognitive and social deficits at the human level. The studies also served as a model for developing therapeutic treatments for socially retarded and withdrawn children.

Several investigators have argued that social separation manipulations with nonhuman primates provide a compelling basis for animal models of depression and anxiety. Some monkeys react to separations with behavioral and physiological symptoms similar to those seen in depressed human patients; both electroconvulsive therapy (ECT) and tricyclic drugs are

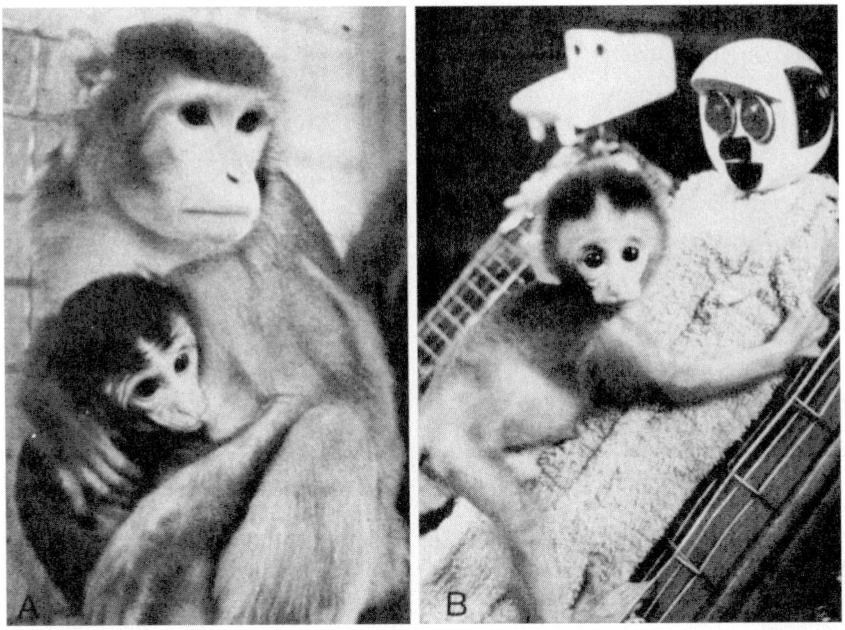

FIGURE 4.5–4
Monkey infant with mother (**A**) and with cloth-covered surrogate (**B**).

effective in reversing the symptoms in monkeys. Not all separations produce depressive reactions in monkeys, just as separation does not always precipitate depression in humans, young and old.

Individual Differences

Recent research has revealed that some rhesus monkey infants consistently display fearfulness and anxiety in situations in which similarly reared peers show normal exploratory behavior and play. These situations generally involve exposure to a novel object or situation. Once the object or situation has become familiar, any behavioral differences between the anxiety-prone, or timid, infants and their outgoing peers disappear, but the individual differences appear to be stable during development. Infant monkeys at 3 to 6 months of age that are at high risk for fearful or anxious reactions tend to remain at high risk for such reactions, at least until adolescence.

Long-term follow-up study of these monkeys has revealed some behavioral differences between fearful and nonfearful female monkeys when they become adults and have their first infants. Fearful female monkeys who grow up in socially benign and stable environments typically become fine mothers, but fearful female monkeys who have reacted with depression to frequent social separations during childhood are at high risk for maternal dysfunction; more than 80 percent of these mothers either neglect or abuse their first offspring. Yet nonfearful female monkeys that encounter the same number of social separations but do not react to any of these separations with depression turn out to be good mothers.

EXPERIMENTAL DISORDERS

Stress Syndromes. Several researchers, including Ivan Petrovich Pavlov in Russia and W. Horsley Gantt and Howard Scott Liddell in the United States, studied the effects of stressful environments on animals, such as dogs and sheep. Pavlov produced a phenomenon in dogs, which he labeled *experimental neurosis,* by the use of a conditioning technique that led to symptoms of extreme and persistent agitation. The technique involved teaching dogs to discriminate between a circle and an ellipse and then progressively diminishing the difference between the two. Gantt used the term *behavior disorders* to describe the reactions he elicited from dogs forced into similar conflictual learning situations. Liddell described the stress response he obtained in sheep, goats, and dogs as *experimental neurasthenia,* which was produced in some cases by merely doubling the number of daily test trials in an unscheduled manner.

Learned Helplessness. The learned helplessness model of depression, developed by Martin Seligman, is a good example of an experimental disorder. Dogs were exposed to electric shocks from which they could not escape. The dogs eventually gave up and made no attempt to escape new shocks. The apparent giving up generalized to other situations, and eventually the dogs always appeared to be helpless and apathetic. Because the cognitive, motivational, and affective deficits displayed by the dogs resembled symptoms common to human depressive disorders, learned helplessness, although controversial, was proposed as an animal model of human depression. In connection with learned helplessness and the expectation of inescapable punishment, research on subjects has revealed brain release of endogenous opiates, destructive effects on the immune system, and elevation of the pain threshold.

A social application of this concept involves school children who have learned that they fail in school no matter what they do; they view themselves as helpless losers, and this self-concept causes them to stop trying. Teaching them to persist may reverse the process, with excellent results in self-respect and school performance.

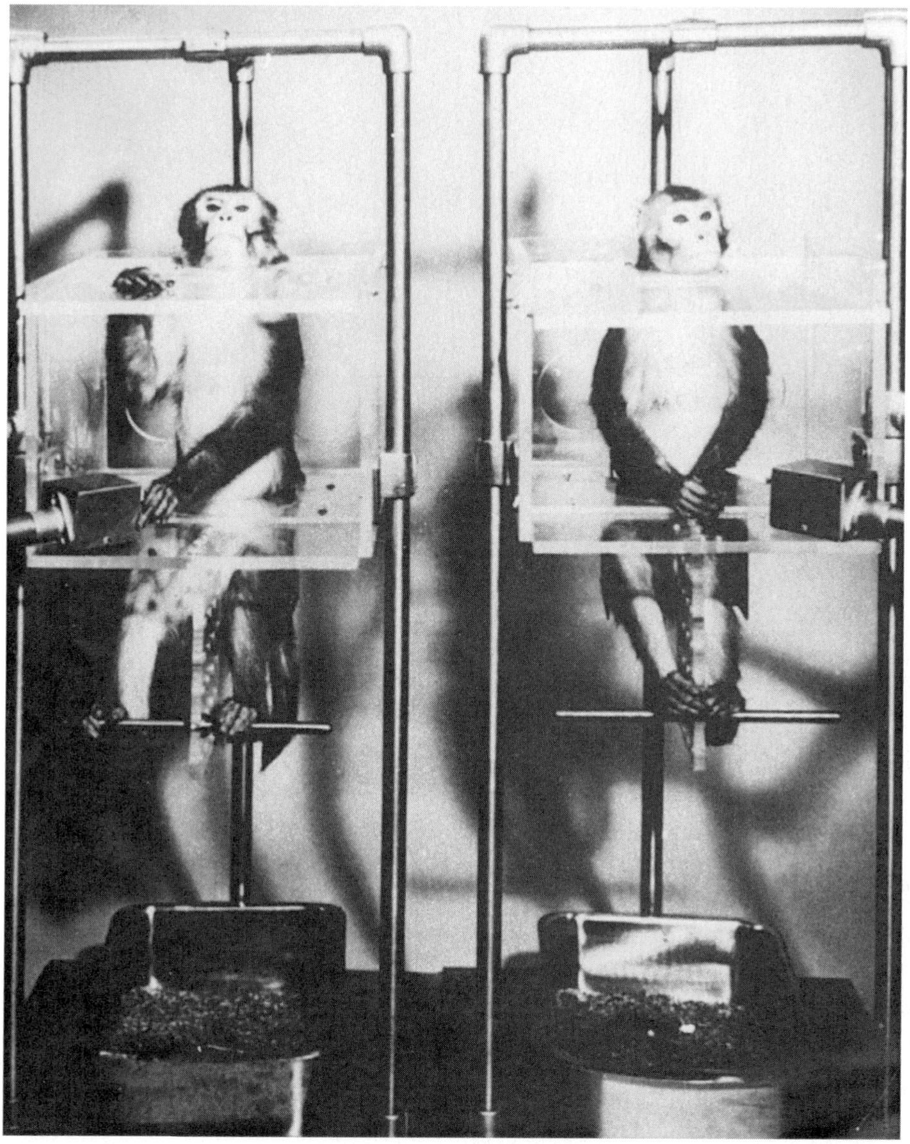

FIGURE 4.5–5
The monkey on the left, known as the executive monkey, controls whether or not both will receive an electric shock. The decision-making task produces a state of chronic tension. Note the more relaxed attitude of the monkey on the right. (From U.S. Army photographs.)

Unpredictable Stress. Rats subjected to chronic unpredictable stress (crowding, shocks, irregular feeding, and interrupted sleep time) show decreases in movement and exploratory behavior; this finding illustrates the roles of unpredictability and lack of environmental control in producing stress. These behavioral changes can be reversed by antidepressant medication. Animals under experimental stress (Fig. 4.5–5) become tense, restless, hyperirritable, or inhibited in certain conflict situations.

Dominance. Animals in a dominant position in a hierarchy have certain advantages (e.g., in mating and feeding). Being more dominant than peers is associated with elation, and a fall in position in the hierarchy is associated with depression. When persons lose jobs, are replaced in organizations, or otherwise have their dominance or hierarchical status changed, they can experience depression.

Temperament. Temperament mediated by genetics plays a role in behavior. For example, one group of pointer dogs was bred for fearfulness and a lack of friendliness toward persons, and another group was bred for the opposite characteristics. The phobic dogs were extremely timid and fearful and showed decreased exploratory capacity, increased startle response, and cardiac arrhythmias. Benzodiazepines diminished these fearful, anxious responses. Amphetamines and cocaine aggravated the responses of genetically nervous dogs to a greater extent than they did the responses of the stable dogs.

Brain Stimulation. Pleasurable sensations have been produced in both humans and animals through self-stimulation of certain brain areas, such as the medial forebrain bundle, the septal area, and the lateral hypothalamus. Rats have engaged in repeated self-stimulation (2,000 stimulations per hour) to gain

rewards. Catecholamine production increases with self-stimulation of the brain area, and drugs that decrease catecholamines decrease the process. The centers for sexual pleasure and opioid reception are closely related anatomically. Heroin addicts report that the so-called rush after intravenous injection of heroin is akin to an intense sexual orgasm.

Pharmacological Syndromes. With the emergence of biological psychiatry, many researchers have used pharmacological means to produce syndrome analogues in animal subjects. Two classic examples are the reserpine (Serpasil) model of depression and the amphetamine psychosis model of paranoid schizophrenia. In the depression studies, animals given the norepinephrine-depleting drug reserpine exhibited behavioral abnormalities analogous to those of major depressive disorder in humans. The behavioral abnormalities produced were generally reversed by antidepressant drugs. These studies tended to corroborate the theory that depression in humans is, in part, the result of diminished levels of norepinephrine. Similarly, animals given amphetamines acted in a stereotypical, inappropriately aggressive, and apparently frightened manner that resembled paranoid psychotic symptoms in humans. Both of these models are considered too simplistic in their concepts of cause, but they remain as early paradigms for this type of research.

Studies have also been done on the effects of catecholamine-depleting drugs on monkeys during separation and reunion periods. These studies showed that catecholamine depletion and social separation can interact in a highly synergistic fashion and can yield depressive symptoms in subjects for whom mere separation or low-dosage treatment by itself does not suffice to produce depression.

Reserpine has produced severe depression in humans and as a result is rarely used as either an antihypertensive (its original indication) or an antipsychotic. Similarly, amphetamine and its congeners (including cocaine) can induce psychotic behavior in persons who use it in overdose or over long periods of time.

SENSORY DEPRIVATION

The history of sensory deprivation and its potentially deleterious effects evolved from instances of aberrant mental behavior in explorers, shipwrecked sailors, and prisoners in solitary confinement. Toward the end of World War II, startling confessions, induced by brainwashing prisoners of war, caused a rise of interest in this psychological phenomenon brought about by the deliberate diminution of sensory input.

To test the hypothesis that an important element in brainwashing is prolonged exposure to sensory isolation, D. O. Hebb and his coworkers brought solitary confinement into the laboratory and demonstrated that volunteer subjects—under conditions of visual, auditory, and tactile deprivation for periods of up to 7 days—reacted with increased suggestibility. Some subjects also showed characteristic symptoms of the sensory deprivation state: anxiety, tension, inability to concentrate or organize thoughts, increased suggestibility, body illusions, somatic complaints, intense subjective emotional distress, and vivid sensory imagery—usually visual and sometimes reaching the proportions of hallucinations with a delusionary quality.

Psychological Theories

Anticipating psychological explanation, Sigmund Freud wrote: "It is interesting to speculate what could happen to ego function if the excitations or stimuli from the external world were either drastically diminished or repetitive. Would there be an alteration in the unconscious mental processes and an effect upon the conceptualization of time?"

Indeed, under conditions of sensory deprivation, the abrogation of such ego functions as perceptual contact with reality and logical thinking brings about confusion, irrationality, fantasy formation, hallucinatory activity, and wish-dominated mental reactions. In the sensory-deprivation situation, the subject becomes dependent on the experimenter and must trust the experimenter for the satisfaction of such basic needs as feeding, toileting, and physical safety. A patient undergoing psychoanalysis may be in a kind of sensory deprivation room (e.g., a soundproof room with dim lights and a couch) in which primary-process mental activity is encouraged through free association.

Cognitive. Cognitive theories stress the fact that the organism is an information-processing machine, whose purpose is optimal adaptation to the perceived environment. Lacking sufficient information, the machine cannot form a cognitive map against which current experience is matched. Disorganization and maladaptation then result. To monitor their own behavior and to attain optimal responsiveness, persons must receive continuous feedback; otherwise they are forced to project outward idiosyncratic themes that have little relation to reality. This situation is similar to that of many psychotic patients.

Physiological Theories

The maintenance of optimal conscious awareness and accurate reality testing depends on a necessary state of alertness. This alert state, in turn, depends on a constant stream of changing stimuli from the external world, mediated through the ascending reticular activating system in the brainstem. In the absence or impairment of such a stream, as occurs in sensory deprivation, alertness drops away, direct contact with the outside world diminishes, and impulses from the inner body and the central nervous system may gain prominence. For example, idioretinal phenomena, inner ear noise, and somatic illusions may take on a hallucinatory character.

SOCIOBIOLOGY

Sociobiology, also called *evolutionary psychology,* is the study of human behavior based upon the transmission and modification of genetically influenced behavioral traits. A major thinker in the field is E. O. Wilson, whose book *Sociobiology* emphasized the role of evolution in shaping behavior.

Evolution

Evolution is described as any change in the genetic makeup of a population. Evolution occurs through natural selection, as formulated by Charles Darwin, which is the reproduction of those genes produced by mutation that account for the most successful offspring. Lamarckian evolution, which occurs through the inheritance of acquired characteristics, describes the evolution of culture.

Competition. Animals vie with one another for resources and territory, the area that is defended for the exclusive use of the animal and that ensures access to food and reproduction. The ability of one animal to defend a disputed territory or resource is called *resource holding potential*, and the greater this potential, the more successful the animal.

Aggression. Aggression serves both to increase territory and to eliminate competitors. Defeated animals can emigrate, disperse, or remain in the social group as subordinate animals. A dominance hierarchy in which animals are associated with one another in subtle but well-defined ways is part of every social pattern.

Reproduction. Because behavior is influenced by heredity, those behaviors that promote reproduction and survival of the species are among the most important. Males usually compete for the females with other males, a process that produces fit offspring. Male-male competition can take various forms; for example, sperm can be thought of as competing for access to the ovum. Females compete with females but in more subtle ways, primarily in terms of dominance, nest-building ability, and breeding potential. *Sexual dimorphism,* or different behavioral patterns for males and females, evolves to ensure the maintenance of resources and reproduction.

Altruism. Behavior that is altruistic benefits others and appears to enhance others' success, with no benefit for the altruist. Sociobiologists explain altruism as a way of maintaining the gene pool at its highest level. In a sense, altruism is selfishness at the level of the gene rather than at the level of the individual animal. A classic case of altruism is the female worker classes of certain wasps, bees, and ants. These workers are sterile and do not reproduce but labor altruistically for the reproductive success of the queen.

Another possible mechanism for the evolution of altruism is group selection. If groups containing altruists are more successful than those composed entirely of selfish members, the altruistic groups succeed at the expense of the selfish ones, and altruism evolves. But within each group, altruists are at a severe disadvantage relative to selfish members, however well the group as a whole does.

Implications for Psychiatry. Evolutionary theory provides possible explanations for some disorders. Some may be manifestations of adaptive strategies. For example, cases of anorexia nervosa may be partially understood as a strategy ultimately caused to delay mate selection, reproduction, and maturation in situations where males are perceived as scarce. Persons who take risks may do so to obtain resources and gain social influence. An erotomanic delusion in a postmenopausal single woman may represent an attempt to compensate for the painful recognition of reproductive failure.

Studies of Identical Twins Reared Apart: Nature versus Nurture

Studies in sociobiology have stimulated one of the oldest debates in psychology. Does human behavior owe more to nature or to nurture? Curiously, humans readily accept the fact that genes determine most of the behaviors of nonhumans but tend to attribute their own behavior almost exclusively to nurture. In fact, however, recent data unequivocally identify our genetic endowment as an equally important, if not more important, factor.

The best "experiments of nature" permitting an assessment of the relative influences of nature and nurture are cases of genetically identical twins separated in infancy and raised in different social environments. If nurture is the most important determinant of behavior, they should behave differently. On the other hand, if nature dominates, each will closely resemble the other, despite their never having met. Several hundred pairs of twins separated in infancy, raised in separate environments, then reunited in adulthood have been rigorously analyzed. Nature has emerged as a key determinant of human behavior.

Jim L. and Jim S. were first reunited at age 39. They were genetically identical twins, reared apart since infancy by different adoptive families in Ohio and unaware of each other's existence. As children, each twin had had a dog named Toy. Each bit his fingernails and, since age 18, had suffered from mixed headache syndrome, a combined tension and migraine headache. Each had been married twice, first to a Linda and then to a Betty. One twin had named his son James Alan, and the other, James Allen. Each had put a circular bench around a tree in his garden. Each had worked at a gas station and later part-time in law enforcement as a sheriff. Each chain-smoked Salems and preferred an occasional Miller Lite beer. Each scattered love notes to his wife around the house. Every summer, unbeknownst to the other, each had driven his family in a light blue Chevrolet from Ohio to the Pas-Grille Beach in St. Petersburg, Florida, for their summer vacation. They had similar voices, hand gestures, and mannerisms.

Jerry L. and Mark N., identical twins separated in infancy, were first reunited at age 30. Each was nearly bald and had a bushy mustache. Each was a volunteer firefighter and made his living installing safety equipment. Each wore aviator glasses, big belt buckles, and big key rings. Each drank Budweiser with his pinky hooked on the bottom of the can and crushed the can when he was finished.

Jack Y. and Oskar S., identical twins born in Trinidad in 1933 and separated in infancy by their parents' divorce, were first reunited at age 46. Oskar was raised by his Catholic mother and grandmother in Nazi-occupied Sudetenland, Czechoslovakia. Jack was raised by his Orthodox Jewish father in Trinidad and spent time on an Israeli kibbutz. Each wore aviator glasses and a blue sport shirt with shoulder plackets, had a trim mustache, liked sweet liqueurs, stored rubber bands on his wrists, read books and magazines from back to

front, dipped buttered toast in his coffee, flushed the toilet before and after using it, enjoyed sneezing loudly in crowded elevators to frighten other passengers, and routinely fell asleep at night while watching television. Each was impatient, squeamish about germs, and gregarious.

Bessie and Jessie, identical twins separated at 8 months of age after their mother's death, were first reunited at age 18. Each had had a bout of tuberculosis, and they had similar voices, energy levels, administrative talents, and decision-making styles. Each had had her hair cut short in early adolescence. Jessie had a college-level education, while Bessie had had only 4 years of formal education; yet Bessie scored 156 on intelligence quotient testing, while Jessie scored 153. Each read avidly, which may have compensated for Bessie's sparse education; she created an environment compatible with her inherited potential.

Neuropsychological Testing Results

A dominant influence of genetics on behavior has been documented in several sets of identical twins on the Minnesota Multiphasic Personality Inventory (MMPI). Twins reared apart generally showed the same degree of genetic influence across the different scales as twins reared together. Two particularly fascinating identical twin pairs, despite being reared on different continents, in countries with different political systems and different languages, generated scores more closely correlated across 13 MMPI scales than the already tight correlation noted among all tested identical twin pairs, most of whom had shared similar rearing.

Reared-apart twin studies report a high correlation (r = 0.75) for intelligence quotient (IQ) similarity. In contrast, the IQ correlation for reared-apart nonidentical twin siblings is 0.38, and for sibling pairs in general, is in the 0.45 to 0.50 range. Strikingly, IQ similarities are not influenced by similarities in access to dictionaries, telescopes, and original artwork; in parental education and socioeconomic status; or in characteristic parenting practices. These data overall suggest that tested intelligence is determined roughly two thirds by genes and one third by environment.

Studies of reared-apart identical twins reveal a genetic influence on alcohol use, substance abuse, childhood antisocial behavior, adult antisocial behavior, risk aversion, and visuomotor skills, as well as on psychophysiological reactions to music, voices, sudden noises, and other stimulation, as revealed by brain wave patterns and skin conductance tests. Moreover, reared-apart identical twins show that genetic influence is pervasive, affecting virtually every measured behavioral trait. For example, many individual preferences previously assumed to be due to nurture (e.g., religious interests, social attitudes, vocational interests, job satisfaction, and work values) are strongly determined by nature.

A selected glossary of some terms used in this section and other ethological terms is given in Table 4.5–2.

Table 4.5–2
Selected Glossary of Ethological Terms

Action-specific energy	Energy associated with the innate releasing mechanism and specific to a particular behavior pattern, which builds up if the releasing stimulus is not present to activate the behavior pattern, and conversely is depleted by repetition.
Aggression	Intraspecific conflict manifested by physical attack or social signaling.
Appetitive behavior	Phase of behavior involving the active seeking of sign stimuli and thought to be driven by action-specific energy accumulating through inactivity of the specific behavior pattern.
Consummatory response	Phase of behavior whereby the energy driving the appetitive phase is released. Involves the perception of sign stimuli, the activation of the innate releasing mechanism (IRM), and the performance of the fixed action pattern (FAP).
Critical period	The time during which imprinting must occur, usually shortly after birth or early in life. Also, "sensitive period."
Displacement activity	A set of behavior patterns occurring alongside an unrelated set of behavior patterns. Originally, irrelevant movements from one behavioral system occurring in the presence of powerful but thwarted drive from another behavior system.
Ethology	The biological study of behavior. From the Greek *ethos,* meaning custom, usage, manner, habit. The modern usage is attributed to Oskar Heinroth, Konrad Lorenz's teacher.
Fixed action pattern (FAP)	A genetically determined behavior pattern that is initiated by stimuli particular to the pattern and that consists of species-specific stereotyped movements.
Imprinting	A specialized form of learning occurring early in life and often influencing behavior later in life. The exposure to the stimulus situation must occur during a particular period, the critical period, and the exposure can be of short duration and without obvious reward. The learning is particularly resistant to change.
Innate	Genetically determined behavior patterns, in theory not influenced by experience.
Innate releasing mechanism (IRM)	Sensory mechanism selectively responsive to specific external stimuli and responsible for triggering the stereotyped motor response.
Instinct	A developmental process resulting in species-typical behavior.
Redirection activity	The venting of one drive from two or more incompatible, but simultaneously activated, drives on some third animal or object.
Ritualization	Process of a behavior pattern being incorporated through evolution into a primary signaling function, frequently with exaggeration and embellishment of some of the movements.

Courtesy of William T. McKinney, Jr., M.D.

References

Ainsworth MS, Bowlby J. An ethological approach to personality development. *Am Psychol.* 1991;46:333.

Barash DP. *Sociobiology and Behavior.* 2nd ed. New York: Elsevier; 1982.

Barash DP. *Revolutionary Biology: The New Gene-Centered View of Life.* New Brunswick, NJ: Transaction Publishers; 2001.

Baron-Cohen S, ed. *The Maladapted Mind: Classic Readings in Evolutionary Psychopathology.* Hove, UK: Psychology Press; 1997.

Buss DM. *The Evolution of Desire.* New York: Basic Books; 1994.

Darwin C. *The Expression of the Emotions in Man and Animals.* Chicago: University of Chicago Press; 1965.

Flinn MV. Culture and the evolution of social learning. *Evol Hum Behav.* 1997;18:23.

Harlow HF. The nature of love. *Am Psychol.* 1958;13:673.

Kraemer GW, Ebert MH, Schmidt DE, McKinney WT. Strangers in a strange land: a psychobiological study of infant monkeys before and after separation from real or inanimate mothers. *Child Dev.* 1991;62:548.

McEwan KL, Costello CG, Taylor PJ. Adjustment to infertility. *J Abnorm Psychol.* 1987;96:108.

McGuire MT, Troisi A. Evolutionary biology and psychiatry. In: Sadock BJ, Sadock VA, eds. *Kaplan & Sadock's Comprehensive Textbook of Psychiatry.* 7th ed. Vol 1. Baltimore: Lippincott Williams & Wilkins; 2000:492.

McGuire MT, Troisi A, Raleigh M. Depression in evolutionary context. In: Baron-Cohen S, ed. *The Maladapted Mind: Classic Readings in Evolutionary Psychopathology.* Hove, UK: 1997.

Segal NL. *Entwined Lives: Twins and What They Tell Us About Human Behavior.* Plume: New York; 1999:116–151.

Trujillo M. Cultural psychiatry. In: Sadock BJ, Sadock VA, eds. *Kaplan & Sadock's Comprehensive Textbook of Psychiatry.* 7th ed. Vol 1. Baltimore: Lippincott Williams & Wilkins; 2000:492.

Wilson EO. *Sociobiology: The New Synthesis.* Cambridge, MA: Harvard University Press; 1975.

▲ 4.6 Anthropology and Cross-Cultural Psychiatry

Anthropology is the study of human beings. It is relevant to psychiatry in three critical areas. First, from a theoretical standpoint, the documentation of particular mental disorders in different sociocultural contexts provides evidence for their syndromal significance (e.g., schizophrenia is found in all cultures). Second, from a clinical standpoint, the explanatory models about patients from culturally and ethnically diverse backgrounds help in both formulating illness and responding to it in culturally appropriate ways. Finally, from a public health perspective, understanding the social production and social course of mental illness suggests means of improving outcome or even preventing illness.

Researchers in human behavior often turn to anthropology for examples of normal and maladaptive behavior in various cultures. Because psychiatric theorists have long predicted that cultural variables influence behavior, these variables may help further the understanding of the nature–nurture controversy; namely, which aspects of human beings are innate and biological, which aspects are shaped by the environment, and how the constant feedback between these two aspects affects human beings.

In psychiatry the increasingly acknowledged evidence of biological factors has altered the view of persons as largely determined by the outcome of relationships shaping children's earliest years. And although anthropological cross-cultural studies have focused on differences as well as similarities in human beings, some anthropologists have emphasized that people cannot be independent of their cultures and that even the attempt to study cross-cultural behavior is a culturally bound viewpoint.

PSYCHOANALYTICAL THEORY

Beginning with Sigmund Freud, psychoanalysts have applied their insights to cultural data. In his 1913 work *Totem and Taboo,* Freud described the earliest humans as a group of brothers who killed and devoured their violent primal father. This criminal act and the so-called totem meal made the brothers feel guilty. Consequently, they formulated rules to prevent similar acts from occurring, and these rules were the beginning of social organization. Carl Gustav Jung's writings include many anthropological references, especially to archaeology and mythology. In *Symbols and Transformations*, written in 1912, Jung traced patients' fantasies back to earliest human artifacts. Neither Freud nor Jung had field experience, but Erik Erikson did. Erikson is best known for his psychocultural biographies of Mohandas Gandhi and Martin Luther and for his 1950 book *Childhood and Society,* in which he attempted to integrate individual psychosexual development with cultural influences. Many of his conclusions were based on his experiences with the Pine Ridge Indians in the Dakotas and the Yurok Indians in Oregon.

George Devereux studied American Plains Native Americans and provided insights into the problems that arise in dealing with patients from diverse ethnic backgrounds. In the 1930s and the 1940s, Abraham Kardiner worked with the concept of national character and suggested that each culture is associated with a common (or at least widely shared) personality structure. Kardiner believed that the adult Russian personality, for example, is characterized by depressive and manic traits. Other such generalities about national character were set forth by various workers, but these descriptions were often used to foster political, ideological, or discriminatory attitudes and so have fallen out of favor. The current consensus is that a clinically meaningful prediction about personality cannot be made on the basis of nationality alone. But as Ruth Benedict wrote in *Patterns of Culture,* personality types may reflect a culture's configuration because people are malleable and they assume a society's expected behavior pattern.

Bronislaw Malinowski and Margaret Mead were among the anthropologists who examined the psychoanalytic concept that adult personality and mental functioning are largely determined during childhood. Malinowski examined childhood and adult sexuality in the Trobriand Islanders and claimed that he found no evidence of the Oedipus complex, which at the time was believed to be universal. Margaret Mead examined gender and sex-role behavior. She observed three tribes in New Guinea and found different patterns of sex-role behavior for men and women in each tribe. According to Mead, behavior is relative, and a society can create deviance by either condoning or condemning certain behavior patterns. Mead considered the Oedipus complex a useful concept in its widest meaning, which is that in all societies adults are involved in the growing child's sexual attitudes, especially those toward the parent of the opposite sex.

Margaret Mead

In her *Coming of Age in Samoa,* published in 1928, Mead (Fig. 4.6–1) described a society in the South Pacific in which adolescent turmoil—widely believed at the time to be universal—appeared not to exist. This was the result, she argued, of the unusual Samoan culture that nurtured open, nonpossessive sexual relationships among adolescents, encour-

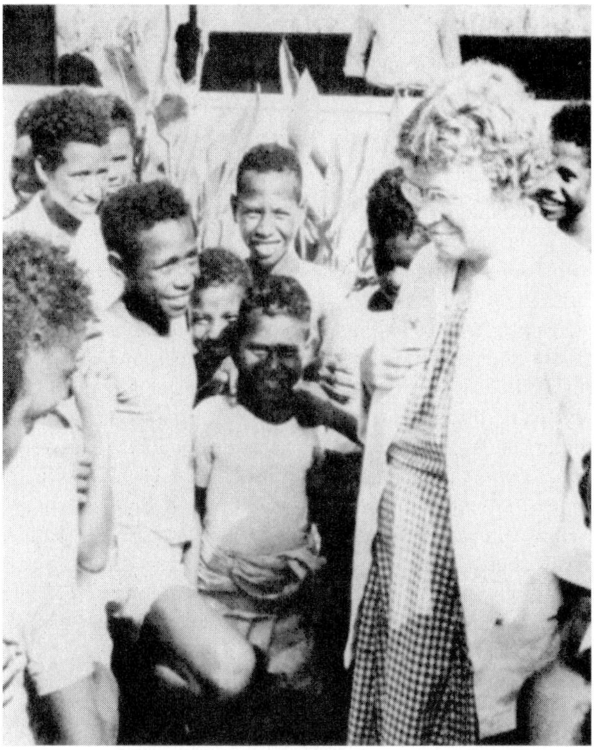

FIGURE 4.6–1

Margaret Mead (1901–1978), the world-famous anthropologist, spent years studying other societies and amassing cross-cultural data. Her *Coming of Age in Samoa* (published in 1928) gave a favorable picture of many aspects of life in a "primitive" society and was influential in establishing an attitude of cultural relativism among many scientists and thinkers. Here she is pictured meeting with schoolchildren in New Guinea. (From Carson RC, Butcher JN, Coleman JC. *Abnormal Psychology and Modern Life.* 8th ed. Boston: Scott, Foresman; 1988:83. © Institute for Cultural Studies, Inc.)

aged communal child rearing, and denigrated aggressiveness and competitiveness. Growing up was "so easy," she stated, because of "the general casualness of the whole society."

Widely publicized and discussed, Mead's observations helped to entrench a belief in cultural determinism that persisted for decades. Research has shown, however, that Mead's methodology was seriously flawed, and her conclusions were questionable. When Mead went to Samoa at the age of 23, she spoke no Samoan language, and her data were based, not on direct observation, but on the hearsay reports of adolescent and preadolescent girls from nearby villages.

Rather than an idyllic paradise of free love among gentle people, most observers, including Samoans themselves, describe a competitive society marked by interfamily and intervillage networks in which female virginity is highly prized at the time of marriage. Ample evidence (e.g., teenage delinquency and suicide rates) shows that during the 1920s, "adolescent turmoil" was not only present, but pronounced. One critic has described Mead's Samoan study as an example of how "as evidence is sought to substantiate a cherished doctrine, the deeply held beliefs of those involved may lead them unwillingly into error."

The absolute cultural determinism advocated by Mead arose in response to the absolute biological determinism of an earlier generation. Neither extreme is believed credible by behavioral researchers today.

Psychosocial Growth

The effects of early life experiences on adult mental health and the explanations for deviance or maladaptive behavior are still controversial issues. Psychodynamic psychiatrists and theorists rely on historical data about adverse experiences to explain later behavior; but new work shows that few experiences are irreversible. Some affection-deprived children described by John Bowlby were able to grow up capable of forming attachments if other experiences later in life were favorable. Similarly, many successful adults come from deprived or otherwise toxic homes and appear to be, or are, invulnerable to these stressors.

Freud postulated a universal sequence of emotional development. Beyond some very general elements (the existence of infantile sexuality, the formation of an attachment to a primary caretaker who is usually the mother, the ubiquity of conflicts and jealousies within the family), this allegedly universal sequence has never found empirical support in cross-cultural studies of human behavioral psychological development. Such studies have, however, produced extensive evidence supporting empirically grounded putative universals of psychosocial growth.

Among the well-established cross-cultural universals of psychosocial development, the best supported and most plausibly related to underlying neural or neuroendocrine maturational events are the emergence of sociality, as heralded by social smiling, during the first 4 months of life, in parallel with the maturation of basal ganglia and cortical motor circuits; the emergence of strong attachments, awareness of separation, and recognition of strangers, in the second half of the first year of life, in parallel with the maturation of the major fiber tracts of the limbic system; the emergence of language during the second year and after, in parallel with the maturation of the thalamic projection to the auditory cortex among other circuits; the emergence of a sex difference in physical aggressiveness in early and middle childhood, with male children on average more aggressive than female children, a consequence in part of prenatal androgenization of the hypothalamus; the emergence of adult sexual motivation and functioning in adolescence, in parallel with and following the maturation of the hypothalamic-pituitary-gonadal axis at puberty, against the background of the previously mentioned prenatal androgenization of the hypothalamus in males.

As for the effect of early life experiences on psychological development, recent work has established an extraordinary fact. In rigorous twin, adoption, and family studies, variance in personality as well as in mental ability can be statistically apportioned among various sources. The results routinely accord a large proportion of the variance to environmental influence (roughly half in numerous studies). The effect of family relationships on personality and mental ability, however, appears to be minimal.

The portion of the variance in outcome measures (e.g., behavior and questionnaire results) attributable to environment is composed almost entirely of within-family variance, such as sibling differences. Identical twins reared together are routinely found to be no more similar in personality than identical twins reared in separate families; sometimes, the separately reared twins are found to be more similar. (See the discussion in Section 4.5 on identical twins.) To the extent that children in different families differ in personality, the difference can be explained almost entirely by their genetic differences. Differences between nonidentical twin siblings, however, cannot be

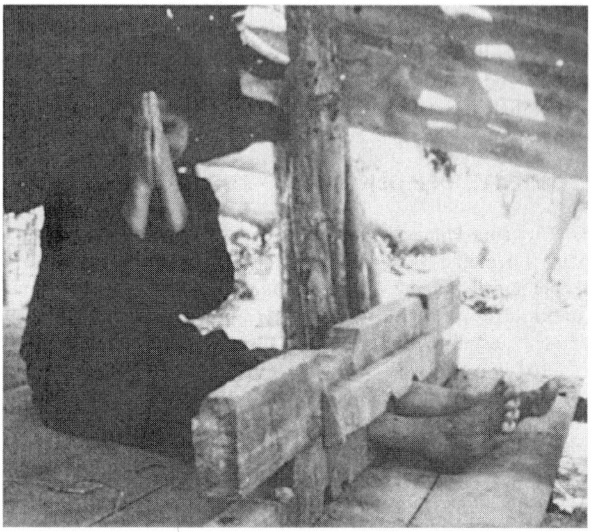

FIGURE 4.6–2
Psychotic woman in Laos. She was kept in stocks for several months to prevent her from running off into the forest, a well-known fatal outcome of psychosis in the area. (Courtesy of Joseph Westermeyer, M.D.)

explained by their genetic differences alone but require environmental explanations as well, such as birth order.

This conclusion seems to indicate that parents' attempts to treat their children similarly (rules, religion, schooling, toys, television) do not make their offspring more similar in personality, or more different from their counterparts in other families, than they would be on the basis of genes alone. No one understands the reason for this phenomenon. Whatever the explanation, the challenge posed by the extremely small measurable between-family variance poses a major challenge to the explanatory paradigms of child psychiatry, psychodynamic theory, and developmental psychology.

Although cultural anthropologists have described and analyzed cross-cultural variation, they have also studied the features of human behavior that do not vary. The concept of universals has several different meanings. Behaviors such as coordinated bipedal walking or smiling in social greeting are exhibited by all normal members of every known society. Behaviors are universal within an age or sex class, such as the Moro reflex in all normal neonates or the ejaculatory motor action pattern in all postpubertal males. Population characteristics apply to all populations but not to all individual members of the populations, such as the sex difference in physical aggressiveness. Universal features of culture rather than of behavior exist, such as the taboos against incest and homicide, or the highly variable but always present institution of marriage, or the social construction of illness and attempts at healing (Fig. 4.6–2). Characteristics, although unusual or even rare, are found at some low level in every population, such as homicidal violence, thought disorder, depression, suicide, and incest.

CROSS-CULTURAL PSYCHIATRY

Psychiatrists, particularly those who practice in urban settings, are increasingly called upon to evaluate and treat patients in the many cultural and linguistic groups that constitute today's multicultural society. In treating a patient who speaks a language other than English and holds beliefs at variance with mainstream culture, the clinician needs different attitudes, knowledge, and skills to provide technically correct and culturally competent services.

Cultural psychiatry draws on many basic and applied disciplines to build its essential constructs. Anthropology (both cultural and medical anthropology) supplies cultural psychiatry with essential insights into the behavior of people in their natural habitats, native views on health and illness, descriptions of indigenous healing systems, and the role of the healer and rituals of healing in different ethnic and cultural groups. Sociology elucidates the relation of basic psychological processes and psychiatric disorders to such human universals as age, gender, and social and occupational status. Epidemiology generates data about the differential incidence and prevalence of psychological distress and disorders in different cultural groups as well as comparative studies of the pathogenesis, onset, pathoplasty, course, and outcome of diagnostic entities across diverse cultural groups. Developmental psychology and psychopathology illuminate the impact of culture on normative personality development and its disorders. Cultural psychopathology investigates the various culture-bound or culture-specific syndromes, and finally, ethnic psychopharmacology studies the impact of race and ethnicity on use, metabolism, and differential effects of standard psychotropic medication and expands our knowledge of the biological and psychological effects of ancient systems of diets and curative herbs.

In the text revision of the fourth edition of *Diagnostic and Statistical Manual of Mental Disorders* (DSM-IV-TR), the American Psychiatric Association discusses the importance of culture and ethnicity on diagnosis and treatment of psychiatric disorders. Special efforts were made in its preparation to incorporate an awareness that the manual is used in culturally diverse populations in the United States and internationally. Clinicians are called on to evaluate individuals from numerous different ethnic groups and cultural backgrounds (including many who are recent immigrants). Diagnostic assessment can be especially challenging when a clinician from one ethnic or cultural group uses the DSM-IV-TR classification to evaluate an individual from a different ethnic or cultural group. A clinician who is unfamiliar with the nuances of an individual's cultural frame of reference may incorrectly judge as psychopathology those normal variations in behavior, belief, or experience that are particular to the individual's culture. For example, certain religious practices or beliefs (e.g., hearing or seeing a deceased relative during bereavement) may be misdiagnosed as manifestations of a psychotic disorder. Applying personality disorder criteria across cultural settings may be especially difficult because of the wide cultural variation in concepts of self, styles of communication, and coping mechanisms.

Definitions and Key Concepts

Culture. For its application to psychiatric practice, perhaps the best definition of culture is provided by the National Institute of Mental Health's Culture and Diagnosis Group: "Culture refers to meanings, values and behavioral norms that are learned and transmitted in the

dominant society and within its social groups. Culture powerfully influences cognition, feelings, and self-concept as well as the diagnostic process and treatment decisions."

Culture is thus best conceptualized as a totality, composed of a complex system of symbols possessing subjective dimensions such as values, feelings, and ideals and objective dimensions including beliefs, traditions, and behavioral prescriptions, articulated into laws and rituals. This unique capacity of culture to bind the objective world of perceived reality to the subjective world of the personal and intimate lends it its powerful role as expressor, mediator, and moderator of psychological processes and, ultimately, emotional disorders.

Scope of Culture. Though the manifestations of culture are broad enough to be considered almost infinite, the noted American anthropologist George P. Murdock described a long list of features considered to be universally present in the hundreds of societies studied by contemporary anthropologists. In alphabetical order, they are "age-grading, athletic sports, bodily adornment, calendar, cleanliness training, community organization, cooking, cooperative labor, cosmology, courtship, dancing, decorative art, divination, division of labor, dream interpretation, education, eschatology, ethics, ethnobotany, etiquette, faith healing, family feasting, fire-making, folklore, food taboos, funeral rites, games, gestures, gift-giving, government, greetings, hair styles, hospitality, housing, hygiene, incest taboos, inheritance rules, joking, kin groups, kinship nomenclature, language, law, luck, magic, marriage, mealtimes, medicine, obstetrics, penal sanction, personal names, population policy, postnatal care, pregnancy usages, property rights, propitiation of supernatural beings, puberty customs, religious ritual, residence rules, sexual restrictions, soul concepts, status differentiation, superstition, surgery, tool-making, trade, visiting, weather control and weaving." Obviously some of these dimensions are more central than others to the relation of culture to psychology and psychopathology. Among these are rules related to sexuality and reproduction (incest taboo and rules of marriage), community and social organizations (kinship, kin groups, power relations, and division of labor), and cosmological visions (magic, superstition, and creational myths).

Race and Ethnicity. Traditionally, *race* denotes human groupings that are biologically (and in theory genetically) determined. In fact other contemporary biologists consider race to be poorly correlated with any measurable biological or cultural phenomenon. Although some characteristics of a given "racial" group (e.g., skin color) may appear phenotypically compelling, the use of the *race* to aggregate individuals displaying that characteristic may convey a false sense of distinctiveness and may imply the existence of a biological basis for such classification systems. Such is not the case for any of the phenotypic characteristics used to establish race. On the other hand *ethnicity,* a term increasingly preferred by cross-cultural researchers, connotes groups of individuals sharing a sense of common identity, a common ancestry, and shared beliefs and history. A given patient's ethnicity can be assessed by focusing the clinical history taking on key ethnically shaped developmental experiences, such as special rituals and rites of passage, and adherence to ethnically prescribed family roles, religious observances, food preferences, and the like. Cultural identity denotes the internalized self-definition resulting from the person's selective, developmentally mediated incorporation of values, beliefs, history, and customs from those available in that person's native environment. Typically, it contains many dimensions of self-experience including age, gender, race, sexual orientation, ethnicity, language, class, and religious and spiritual beliefs.

CULTURE AND PSYCHOPATHOLOGY

Culture is an all-pervasive medium for humans. It is driven by the human brain's unique ability to create images and symbols and structure them into complex wholes that in turn can drive brain function to produce defined behaviors and modulate instinctually driven ones. The ability to mediate biological functions via symbolic (and image) representation and manipulation is dramatically expanded in humans by the function of awareness or consciousness leading to the notion of the self.

Humans structure symbols into progressively more complex sequences ranging from basic, simple ideas to complex holistic beliefs, values, and ideals. These in turn are codified by language, images, and other means and shared with others to constitute the building blocks of common culture. Culture thus becomes a hierarchical array of complex symbols that affect the individual's emotions and behaviors and, when communicated to others, affect social and group function.

All cultures develop both processes that facilitate adjustment and conflict resolution and pressures that foster conflict, deviance, and maladjustment. These pressures can act broadly on large social groups and selectively on specific cultural subgroups. All cultures define a spectrum of "normal behaviors" as well as thresholds of tolerance for diverse "abnormalities," imposing different social consequences on different patterns of deviance.

Each culture provides its own unique stresses as well as beliefs and rituals to reduce psychological tension. Ashley Montagu has indicated, for example, that cultures that provide adaptive channels for the expression of aggression and the satisfaction of dependency needs can significantly reduce personal and interpersonal conflict. In the modern era, cultures and subcultures change at increasing rates in response to the adaptive demands represented by a global world in increasing economic, political, and social competition. This progressive globalization imposes additional adaptive stresses on individuals and cultural groups.

Cultural Identity. DSM-IV-TR recommends that in assessing an individual's cultural identity, the clinician should "note the individual's ethnic or cultural reference group. For immigrants and ethnic minorities, they should assess the degree of involvement with both culture of origin and host culture." Frances G. Lu and coworkers summarized the essential components of cultural identity (Table 4.6–1).

Table 4.6–1
Aspects of Cultural Identity Development

Ethnicity	Gender
Race	Age
Country of origin	Sexual orientation
Language	Religious and spiritual beliefs
Acculturation	Socioeconomic class and education

From Lu FG, Russell FL, Mezzich JE. Issues in the assessment and diagnosis of culturally diverse individuals. In: Oldham J, Riba M, eds: *Annual Review of Psychiatry.* Vol 14. Washington, DC: American Psychiatric Press; 1995.

To these factors one must add migration history, which is commonly left out of the clinical evaluation of cross-cultural patients. Culturally uninformed clinicians often treat their immigrant patients as if their lives began when they arrived in the United States, and their clinical narratives often lack key data from the patients' preimmigration experience. Careful attention must be paid to the traumas and losses encountered by refugees in their country of origin, often including exposure (as witness or victims) to physical or emotional torture or both. The process of acculturation is once again key to understanding the psychological distress and psychopathology of immigrants. There are three major sources of stress in the migration experience: (1) entry into the host society, frequently at lower occupational and social levels; (2) disruption of interpersonal relationships; and (3) the acculturation process. The clinician can assess the degree of acculturation and the nature of the acculturation process through many indirect means. Age at immigration, number of years in the United States, occupational status, language proficiency, and participation in the host culture social networks give the clinician some idea of the rate and ease of acculturation for a given patient.

Families can also be classified by degree of acculturation. From this perspective immigrant families may be described along a continuum of acculturation as traditional, transitional bicultural, and Americanized. Each of these family structures presents different assets and vulnerabilities in relation to the immigration experience.

CULTURE-BOUND SYNDROMES

These syndromes are generally discussed as exotic disturbances of thought, mood, or behavior displaying dramatic presentation, occurring in the context of specific local cultures, and at least partially understood through the lens of the psychosocial forces—often conflictual—relevant to that particular culture. As psychiatry reaches out to all parts of the world, the significance of these syndromes is increasing. The reader is referred to Section 14.5 for an extensive discussion of culture-bound syndromes.

References

Al-Issa I, ed. *Handbook of Culture and Mental Illness: An International Perspective*. Madison, CT: International Universities Press; 1995.

Andrews GR. Cross cultural studies: an important development in aging research. *J Am Geriatr Soc*. 1989;37:483.

Armelagos GJ, Leatherman T, Ryan M, Sibley L. Biocultural synthesis in medical anthropology. *Med Anthropol*. 1992;14:35.

Bracken PJ. Post-empiricism and psychiatry: meaning and methodology in cross-cultural research. *Soc Sci Med*. 1993;36:265.

Erikson E. *Childhood and Society*. New York: WW Norton; 1950.

Fabrega H Jr. An ethnomedical perspective of Anglo-American psychiatry. *Am J Psychiatry*. 1989;146:588.

Fabrega H Jr. Culture and the psychosomatic tradition. *Psychosom Med*. 1992;54:561.

Freud S. *Totem and Taboo*. In: *Standard Edition of the Complete Psychological Works of Sigmund Freud*. Vol 13. London: Hogarth Press; 1955:1.

Fullilove MT. Psychiatric implications of displacement: contributions from the psychology of place. *Am J Psychiatry*. 1996;153:1516.

Jung C. *Symbols and Transformations*. 2nd ed. Princeton, NJ: Princeton University Press; 1967.

Kirmayer LJ. Cultural variations in the response to psychiatric disorders and emotional distress. *Soc Sci Med*. 1989;29:327.

Koegel P. Through a different lens: an anthropological perspective on the homeless mentally ill. *Cult Med Psychiatry*. 1992;16:1.

Landrine H, Klonoff EA. Culture and health-related schemas: a review and proposal for interdisciplinary integration. *Health Psychol*. 1992;11:267.

Mooij A. Towards an anthropological psychiatry. *Theoret Med*. 1995;16:73.

Murray SO, Darnell R. Margaret Mead and paradigm shifts within anthropology during the 1920s. *J Youth Adolesc*. 2000;29:557.

Parron DL. DSM-IV: making it culturally relevant. In: Friedman S, ed. *Anxiety Disorders in African Americans*. New York: Springer; 1994:15.

Rendon M. Toward a genealogy of culture. *Am J Psychoanal*. 2001;61:325.

Truijillo M. Cultural psychiatry. In: Sadock BJ, Sadock VA, eds. *Kaplan & Sadock's Comprehensive Textbook of Psychiatry*. 7th ed. Vol 1. Baltimore: Lippincott Williams & Wilkins; 2000:492.

▲ 4.7 Epidemiology and Biostatistics

EPIDEMIOLOGY

Psychiatric epidemiology has contributed to a broad range of clinical, research, and health policy fields. Recent findings provide data on the course and co-occurrence of psychiatric disorders, identify their possible risk factors, measure the functional impairment they cause, establish a basis for policy decisions on mental health, and set a starting point for analyzing access to care and use of mental health services.

Results from epidemiological studies are routinely included in the *Diagnostic and Statistical Manual of Mental Disorders* (DSM) to describe the frequency and correlates of mental disorders. In developing the diagnostic criteria themselves, secondary analyses of many epidemiological studies assessed the frequency with which discrete symptoms appeared together, to define syndromes in large community and clinical populations. Epidemiological studies that demonstrate the significance of depression as a risk factor for death in persons with cardiovascular disease have engendered new interest in pathophysiological mechanisms that might account for the relation between these disorders.

One of the most visible indicators of the policy use of epidemiological data is found in the joint publication by the World Bank and the World Health Organization (WHO) entitled *The Global Burden of Disease*. Based on data developed over the past two decades, mental disorders have been found to be among the leading causes of disability worldwide, with major depression currently the fourth leading cause of disability.

DEFINITION

Epidemiology is the study of the distribution, incidence, prevalence, and duration of disease. In psychiatry, epidemiological methods contribute to an understanding of the causes, treatment, and prevention of mental disorders. Such methods also help define and evaluate strategies to prevent and control disease and disability. In addition, epidemiological studies help in the overall planning and evaluating of mental health programs on both local and national levels.

Epidemiological surveys reveal that about one third of all Americans have had or will have a mental disorder at some time in their lives. The most common mental disorders are anxiety disorders, and the next most common are depressive disorders and alcohol or other substance abuse. In addition, surveys have found that about 15 percent—if not more—of all patients seen for a medical or surgical problem by nonpsychiatric physicians have an associated emotional disorder, most often depression or alcohol abuse or both.

Epidemiology advances psychiatric research by correlating clinical findings with such sociodemographic variables as age, gender, and socioeconomic status. For example, higher rates of almost every mental disorder are found in persons under age 45 than in those over 45. In general, women have significantly higher rates than men for all disorders, particularly depressive and anxiety disorders. Men, however, have significantly higher rates of substance-related disorders and antisocial personality disorder. Schizophrenia, which affects about 1 percent of the population, shows similar rates for men and women.

Epidemiological studies are also used to compare the incidence and the prevalence of diseases internationally and cross-culturally. In general, the prevalence of mental disorders appears to be fairly constant, regardless of nationality or cultural background; however, schizophrenia has a better prognosis and outcome in less developed third-world countries than it does in better developed societies such as the United States and the United Kingdom.

Types of Clinical and Epidemiological Studies

Clinical and epidemiological studies in psychiatry attempt to answer questions relating to the causes, treatment, course, prognosis, and prevention of various disorders. There are two main types: (1) *observational*, in which the natural course of an illness is followed without any intervention, and (2) *experimental*, in which some or all factors under study are controlled by the investigator. Most studies are experimental; however, because of the many variables involved in mental disorders; it is difficult to design well-controlled experimental studies. The most common types of experimental designs used in psychiatry are described below.

Cohort Study. A *cohort* is a group chosen from a well-defined population and studied over a long period of time. Cohort studies are also known as longitudinal studies. An example is the study by Stella Chess and Alexander Thomas of temperamental characteristics of the same group of infants at ages 3 months, 2 years, 5 years, and 20 years. The researchers detected a relation between the initial characteristics of the infant and a subgroup of children who eventually had clinical psychiatric problems. In that study the cohort was the group born and studied in the year the study began.

Cohort studies provide direct estimates of risk associated with a suspected causal factor. They are more time-consuming and expensive to perform than case history studies, which are usually quick and inexpensive. Cohort studies are usually conducted when ample evidence from case-history studies indicates that a relation exists between a risk factor and a disorder. For example, in the relation between lung cancer and smoking, many case-history studies had been published before the first cohort study was reported.

Retrospective and Prospective Studies. Prospective studies, also called longitudinal studies, are based on observing events as they occur. A major problem in psychiatric longitudinal studies is that some persons are lost to follow-up over time. Retrospective studies are based on past data or past events.

Cross-Sectional Study. Cross-sectional studies provide information about the prevalence of disease in a representative study population at a particular point in time. For that reason, they are also known as prevalence studies.

Case-History Study. A case-history study is a retrospective study that examines persons with a particular disease.

Case-Control Study. A case-control study is a retrospective study that examines persons without a particular disease.

Clinical Trial. In a clinical trial, specially selected patients receive a course of treatment, and another group does not. Eligible patients are randomly assigned to the treatment group or to the control group. The goal of the study is to determine the effects of a given treatment.

Double-Blind Study. A double-blind study helps eliminate bias because neither the patient nor the persons involved in the study know which, if any, treatment is being given to the patient. In drug studies, a control group of patients may receive a placebo (i.e., an inert substance prepared to resemble the active drug being tested in the experiment). A response to the placebo may represent the psychological effect of taking a pill, a response not due to any psychopharmacological property (so-called placebo effect). In addition, the investigators do not know the treatment given because drugs are identified by special codes unknown to them. The outcome may be assessed by persons other than those administering the treatment (so-called blind evaluators). Control subjects may receive an alternative comparison treatment, rather than just a placebo.

Crossover Study. A crossover study is a variation of the double-blind study. The treatment group and the control or placebo group change places at some point, so that the placebo group gets the treatment and the treatment group now receives the placebo. That procedure eliminates bias because, if the treatment group improves in both instances and the placebo group does not, one can conclude that the makeup of the two groups was truly random. Each group serves as the control for the other.

Psychiatric Case Register. A case register maintains a longitudinal record of psychiatric contacts for each person receiving care in a geographically defined community. Not all areas lend themselves to a register because persons may leave the area for treatment or the population may be highly mobile. A well-maintained register is of great value in determining accurate treated-incidence rates, lifetime- or period-treated prevalence rates, comparative rates for different time periods for the same population, and information regarding the use of services over time as well as in identifying high-risk groups for further study.

Major Epidemiological Studies

Major psychiatric epidemiological research studies have been conducted over the years. The goal of each study was to determine the prevalence of psychopathology in a defined community. Persons in a particular community were interviewed directly (usually using a structured interview protocol) to determine the presence or absence of psychological symptoms. The major studies are described below.

Chicago Study. A team under the direction of Robert E. L. Faris and Henry Warren Dunham examined about 35,000 admissions to mental hospitals in Chicago between 1922 and 1934. The survey found that first hospital admissions for schizophrenia were highest among persons from the central sections of Chicago, members of the city's lowest socioeconomic group. Rates of admission decreased as one moved away from the central areas and into more affluent communities. Faris and Dunham

developed a *drift hypothesis,* which holds that impaired persons slide down the social scale because of their illness. By contrast, a *segregation hypothesis* holds that instead of helplessly drifting downward, schizophrenic persons actively seek city areas where anonymity and isolation protect them from the demands that more organized societies make on them. That study helped conceptualize two additional hypotheses about mental illness: (1) the *social causation theory,* which holds that being a member of a low socioeconomic group is significant in causing illness, and (2) the *social selection theory,* which holds that having a mental disorder leads one to become a member of the low socioeconomic group as a secondary phenomenon. In other words, the disorder is caused by genetic or psychological factors, and the drift downward results.

Midtown Manhattan Study. In 1954 a team directed by Thomas Rennie and Leo Srole designed and conducted a survey involving 1,660 adults sampled from a specific section of New York City. The objective of the study was to determine the effects of demographic, social, and personal factors on mental health and illness by use of a structured interview conducted by nonpsychiatrists. Mental disorder was rated not present, mild, moderate, or marked. The main objective was to test the association between life stress and psychological symptoms, and some of the findings follow. The incidence of mental disorders rose as age increased; 81 percent of persons from 20 to 59 years of age had symptoms that were mild to severely incapacitating, and 23.4 percent of persons in that age group were substantially impaired. Socioeconomic status was the single most significant variable affecting mental illness, persons in the low socioeconomic group had six times as many symptoms as those in the high groups.

New Haven Study. In 1950 August De Belmont Hollingshead and Fredrick Carl Redlich studied the relation of social class to the prevalence of treated mental disorders in New Haven, Connecticut. Their studies included a census of psychiatric patients, a survey of the population at large, a study of psychiatrists, and a controlled-case study. Analysis of the data revealed a definite relation between social class and mental disorders. Neurosis was most prevalent among persons in the high socioeconomic groups; psychosis was most prevalent among persons in the low socioeconomic groups. The poor were more often seen in mental health clinics than by private psychiatrists. In addition, low socioeconomic status, occupational instability, and downward mobility were associated with the highest frequency of psychiatric disability. Hollingshead and Redlich devised a subgrouping of class structure in the county based on education, occupation, and income. Their class distinctions, described in Table 4.7–1, are used by sociologists and epidemiologists. Another New Haven study used a structured diagnostic interview to make specific diagnoses. A major finding of that study was that 15.1 percent of the adult population over age 26 showed evidence of a mental disorder, and a probable mental disorder was present in an additional 2.7 percent.

Stirling County Study. In 1952, Alexander H. Leighton conducted a psychiatric epidemiological study of Stirling County, a Nova Scotian county of 20,000 persons. Information was recorded by nonclinician interviewers using structured interviews. The information was later rated by a psychiatrist. Unlike the New Haven and Midtown Manhattan surveys, the subjects of the Stirling County study lived in rural areas—small villages, one small town, and many isolated farms. Male and female household heads were interviewed. The major findings were that 57 percent of the persons interviewed had experienced some mental disorder, 24 percent had a notable impairment, and 20 percent needed psychiatric attention. Women exhibited considerably more psychiatric disorders than men, and mental disorders were found to increase in number with age and degree of poverty.

Table 4.7–1
Class Status and Cultural Characteristics of Subjects in the New Haven Study

Class	Class Status and Cultural Characteristics
I	Class I, containing the community's business and professional leaders, has two segments: a long-established core group of interrelated families and a smaller, upwardly mobile group of new people. Members of the core group usually inherit money, along with group values that stress tradition, stability, and social responsibility. Those in the new group are highly educated, self-made, able, and aggressive. Their family relationships often are not cohesive or stable. Socially, they are rejected by the core group, to whom they are, however, a threat by the vigor of their leadership in community affairs.
II	Class II is marked by at least some education beyond high school and occupations as managers or in the lower-ranking professions. Four of five are upwardly mobile. They are joiners at all ages and tend to have stable families, but they have usually gone apart from parental families and often from their home communities. Tensions arise generally from striving for educational, economic, and social success.
III	Class III men for the most part are in salaried administrative and clerical jobs (51 percent) or own small businesses (24 percent); many of the women also have jobs. Typically, they are high school graduates. They usually have economic security but little opportunity for advancement. Families tend to be less stable than those in class II. Family members of all ages tend to join organizations and to be active in them. There is less satisfaction with present living conditions and less optimism than in class II.
IV	In class IV, 53 percent say they belong to the working class. Seven of 10 show no generational mobility. Most are content and make no sacrifices to get ahead. Most of the men are semiskilled (53 percent) or skilled (35 percent) manual employees. Practically all the women who are able to hold jobs do so. Education usually stops shortly after graduation from grammar school for both parents and children. Families are much different from those in class III. Families are larger, and they are more likely to include three generations. Households are more likely to include boarders and roomers. Homes are more likely to be broken.
V	Class V adults usually have not completed elementary school. Most are semiskilled factory workers or unskilled laborers. They are concentrated in tenement and cold-water-flat areas of New Haven or in suburban slums. There are generally brittle family ties. Very few participate in organized community institutions. Leisure activities in the household and on the street are informal and spontaneous. Adolescent boys frequently have contact with the law in their search for adventure. There is a struggle for existence. There is much resentment, expressed freely in primary groups, about how they are treated by those in authority. There is much acting out of hostility.

NIMH Epidemiologic Catchment Area (NIMH-ECA) Survey. The NIMH-ECA project evolved from the report of the 1977 President's Commission on Mental Health, which

highlighted the need to identify the mentally ill and indicate how they are treated and by whom. Darrel Regier and his associates at the Division of Biometry and Epidemiology of the National Institute of Mental Health (NIMH) sought to identify the percentage of the population with mental disorders. The objective was to determine the percentages of the population with mental disorders that were receiving treatment in mental health settings (such as psychiatric clinics), private psychiatrists' offices, and such nonpsychiatric settings as general medical treatment centers and internists' offices. Estimates indicated that at least 15 percent of the population of the United States is affected by mental disorders in one year, and only one fifth of those persons received care from mental health specialists. Three fifths of persons with identified mental disorders were treated by primary care physicians. Various sites around the country are being studied to assess mental disorder prevalence, incidence, and service use in geographically defined community populations of at least 200,000 residents. Random samples are drawn to obtain completed interviews on at least 20,000 community and institutional residents. The *Diagnostic Interview Schedule* (DIS)—which assesses the presence, duration, and severity of symptoms—is the major instrument that the trained lay interviewer uses to interview each subject. Compared with all previous studies, the NIMH-ECA study uses better diagnostic tools and more specific criteria to make a reliable diagnosis, including careful clinical descriptions and follow-up studies. Much larger samples are used than in the previously described studies. In general, findings of the ECA survey show the following: rates of depression are twice as high for females as for males, males are more likely than females to have alcohol dependence, and substance abuse is more common in persons under age 30 than in older persons. The epidemiological findings of 1-year and lifetime prevalence rates for specific mental disorders in the five ECA sites are listed in Table 4.7–2. More specific data about each disorder are found in the chapter that discusses the disorder in depth.

Table 4.7–2
Comparison of One-Year and Lifetime Prevalence Rates Limited to Common Age Range of 18–54 Years

Disorder	Prevalence (%)
Any 12-month disorder	29.8 (0.6)
Any lifetime disorder	46.9 (0.7)
Any substance use or dependence	
12 month	10.5 (0.4)
Lifetime	24.3 (0.6)
Alcohol dependence	
12 month	4.4 (0.2)
Lifetime	11.3 (0.4)
Drug dependence	
12 month	2.4 (0.2)
Lifetime	6.4 (0.3)
Any affective (mood) disorder	
12 month	10.1 (0.4)
Lifetime	14.9 (0.4)
Major depressive episode	
12 month	6.4 (0.3)
Lifetime	12.5 (0.4)
Dysthymia—lifetime	5.5 (0.3)
Any anxiety disorder	
12 month	11.8 (0.4)
Lifetime	19.2 (0.5)
Panic disorder	
12 month	1.5 (0.1)
Lifetime	2.8 (0.2)
Social phobia	
12 month	2.1 (0.2)
Lifetime	3.7 (0.3)
Schizophrenia	
12 month	0.9 (0.1)
Lifetime	1.5 (0.1)
Somatization	
12 month	0.1 (0.0)
Lifetime	0.1 (0.0)

Adapted from Regier DA, Kaelber CT, Rae DS, et al. Limitations of diagnostic criteria and assessment instruments for mental disorders: implications for research and policy. *Arch Gen Psychiatry.* 1998;55:109.

Assessment Instruments

The major obstacle to the identification of cases has been the lack of an explicit set of criteria for diagnostic classification. Over the years a variety of diagnostic procedures and assessment instruments have been developed. Information about a subject can be collected in several ways. Medical records are often used for patients in clinical settings. Records in central data banks called *case registers* can be used. In Scandinavian countries, particularly Sweden, control data banks are extensive. An important source of information about a subject is the *direct interview,* which is a person-to-person interaction. *Indirect surveys* using a structured self-report form may be used, but they lack the clinical judgment of an experienced practitioner that is necessary in some instances. The most common assessment approach is an interview format, which may be *structured* (the same questions asked of all subjects) or *unstructured* (interviewers use their own clinical judgment in choosing their questions. Several structured instruments with acceptable interrater reliability are outlined in Table 4.7–3. An effective assessment instrument must be reliable, valid, and free of bias. *Reliability* concerns whether or not the findings of the assessment instrument or diagnostic procedure are reproducible and can be replicated when the instrument is used by different examiners (*interrater reliability*) or on different occasions (*test-retest reliability*). *Validity* concerns whether the test measures what it is supposed to measure. Does the assessment instrument identify the cases it is designed to identify? Validity can be broken down further into the following categories: *criterion validity,* in which results from one test instrument are compared with the results of another test whose validity has already been established; *face validity,* which concerns whether the test makes sense to the investigator using it; *content validity,* which concerns whether the test covers specific types of information that can be interpreted or scored at a later date; *concurrent validity,* which concerns whether the results correspond to the results of another test with the same variable; and *construct validity,* which concerns whether the test instrument is in fact measuring what it was designed to measure. The two

Table 4.7–3
Commonly Used Assessment Instruments

Instrument	Condition	Interviewer	Comments
Present State Examination (PSE)	Psychotic disorders, schizophrenia	Psychiatrists	Limited to 1-month period before interview; can be used with computer program CATEGO
Schedule for Affective Disorders and Schizophrenia (SADS)	Schizophrenia and mood disorders	Psychiatrists or specially trained interviewer	Variations: SADS-C measures current disorder, and SADS-L measures lifetime disorders
General Health Questionnaire (GHQ)	Medical patients with psychiatric symptoms of anxiety or depression	Self-report	Does not identify specific mental disorders
Diagnostic Interview Schedule (DIS)	Covers more than 30 mental disorders, including schizophrenia, mood disorders, anxiety disorders, substance abuse, cognitive disorders	Self-report combined with specially trained interviewers	Correlates with range of DSM-III diagnostic classification; assesses symptoms over lifetime; used in the NIMH-ECA program
Iowa Structured Psychiatric Interview (ISPI)	Major mental disorders	Trained interviewer	Provides detailed psychosocial and family history; covers lifetime prevalence

properties of validity and reliability are extremely important in psychiatric epidemiology, especially if one is attempting to identify a specific disorder or syndrome. Analytic studies can also be flawed by *bias*, an error in construction that favors one outcome over another. Bias can occur if examiners know something about the status of the case that influences their judgment (e.g., they know that one group is receiving medication). These potential flaws can affect the validity of a study's findings. To eliminate this kind of bias, researchers developed the double-blind method. Bias is also diminished by randomizing the sample so that each member of the total group studied has an equal chance of being selected—for example, by assigning each person a number from a table of random numbers.

Assessment instruments must be *sensitive*; that is, they must be able to detect the thing being evaluated (e.g., to diagnose a disorder when it is present). If an instrument detects a disorder in a person who does not have the disorder, the result is called a *false positive*, rather than a *true positive*. Tests must also be *specific*; that is, they must not detect things not being evaluated. For example, tests must be able to determine the absence of a disorder in a person who does not have the disorder, which is called a *true-negative* result. A disorder reported to be absent in a person when it is present is a *false-negative result*. Assessment instruments should also have good *predictive value*, which is the proportion of true-positive or true-negative results. Predictive values indicate what percentage of test outcomes are expected to coincide with assigned diagnoses. Table 4.7–4 summarizes the interpretation of sensitivity, specificity, and predictive value.

BIOSTATISTICS

Biostatistics is the mathematical science of describing, organizing, and interpreting data related to medicine. Epidemiology relies on statistics to enable investigators to examine possible causes of disease and to evaluate treatment strategies. The principles of statistics are beyond the scope of this book, but a glossary of statistical terms used in most elementary textbooks of statistics is presented here. Knowledge of such terms is necessary not only for understanding epidemiological concepts but also for accurately assessing statistical methods that appear in scientific publications.

The two major types of statistics are descriptive and inferential. *Descriptive statistics* are numerical values that summarize, organize, and describe observations (e.g., the average number of symptoms associated with an anxiety disorder). Examples include mean, standard deviation, and variance. *Inferential statistics* are numerical values used to generalize about probabilities on the basis of a sample (e.g., comparing the effect of drug A with that of drug B in the treatment of a group of depressed patients). Examples include the analysis of variance, probability, and probability (P) value.

One derives data (factual information) from a population or a sample. A *population* is the entire collection of a set of objects, persons, or events in a particular context (e.g., all patients with schizophrenia in a particular hospital). A *sample* is a subset selected from this population (e.g., one half of the patients with schizophrenia in a particular hospital). Data can be *nominal* (organized into categories), *ordinal* (ranked in order), or *organized into interval ratios* (measured on a scale, graph, or table).

Glossary of Statistical Terms

Analysis of Variance (ANOVA). A set of statistical procedures designed to compare two or more groups of observations. It determines whether the differences between groups are due to experimental influence or to chance alone.

Chi-Square Test. A set of statistical procedures used to evaluate the relative frequency or proportion of events in a population that fall into well-defined categories.

Confidence Interval. An interval that is likely to capture the population mean with a specified level of confidence. For the 95 per-

Table 4.7–4
Definitions and Calculations for Interpreting Performance of Diagnostic Tests

Term	Definition	Calculation
True positive (TP)	Diseased person with abnormal test results	
True negative (TN)	Nondiseased person with normal test results	
False positive (FP)	Nondiseased person with abnormal test results	
False negative (FN)	Diseased person with normal test results	
Referent value	A value to which laboratory results can be referred and from which the probability of disease or predictive value can be calculated	
Sensitivity	True positive rate	$\frac{TP}{TP + FN} \times 100$
Specificity	True negative rate	$\frac{TN}{TN + FP} \times 100$
Predictive value of abnormal test results (PV +)	Proportion of abnormal test results that are true positive	$\frac{TP}{TP + FP} \times 100$
Predictive value of normal test results (PV –)	Proportion of normal test results that are true negative	$\frac{TN}{TN + FN} \times 100$
Efficiency	Percentage of all results that are true results, whether positive or negative	$\frac{TP + TN}{\text{Grand total}} \times 100$

Table by John F. Greden, M.D.

cent confidence interval, the chances are estimated to be 95 in 100 that the true mean falls within that interval.

Control Group. A group that does not receive treatment and is used as a standard of comparison.

Correlation Coefficient. A measurement of the direction and strength of the relation between two variables. Two of the most commonly used are the Spearman rank order coefficient for ordinal data and the Pearson correlation coefficient for nominal data. The Pearson correlation coefficient (r) takes any value between –1 and +1. A *positive correlation* means that as one variable increases (or decreases) the other moves in the same direction. A negative r indicates that the variables move in opposite directions. A correlation approaching –1 or +1 indicates a strong relationship; a correlation approaching 0 indicates a weak relationship. Correlation coefficients indicate only the degree of relationship; they say nothing about cause and effect.

Dependent Variable. The phenomenon of interest in a research study, often called the *outcome variable.*

Descriptive Statistics. Methods used to summarize, organize, and describe observations. Examples include the mean, standard deviation, and variance.

Discriminant Analysis. A multivariate method for finding the relation between a single discrete outcome and a linear combination of two or more predictors.

Distribution. A series or range of values that can be organized according to their frequency of occurrence (*frequency distribution*). A symmetrical, bell-shaped frequency distribution of scores is called a *normal distribution* (the bell curve). Distribution may be normal or skewed in a positive or negative direction (Fig. 4.7–1).

Incidence. The number of new cases occurring over a specified time. The most common period used is 1 year, which produces an annual incidence calculated as follows:

$$\text{Incidence} = \frac{\text{Number of new cases of a disease (over a 1-year period)}}{\text{Total number of persons in the population (over a 1-year period)}}$$

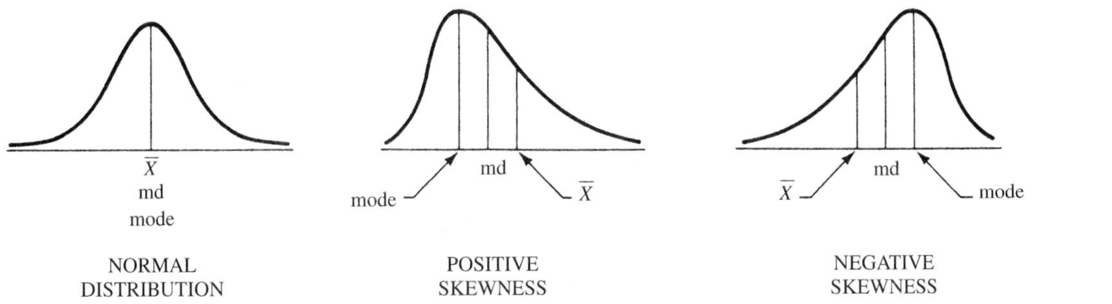

FIGURE 4.7–1
Examples of normal distribution, positive skewness, and negative skewness.

A study of incidence is more difficult to do than a study of prevalence cases because those who already have the disease must be excluded from the incidence numerator; they cannot be considered new cases. Since those who have had the disease are no longer at risk for it, they also must be excluded from the denominator. A broader concept of total incidence includes those with a new episode of illness, regardless of whether they have had previous episodes.

Lifetime Expectancy. The total probability of a person's having a disorder during his or her lifetime. Prevalence and incidence vary for sex and age; thus, sex-specific and age-specific rates are used to express the relative frequency of cases in each category.

Measure of Central Tendency. A central value in a distribution around which other values are distributed. Three measures of central tendency are the mean, the median, and the mode.

MEAN. A statistical measurement derived from adding a set of scores and then dividing by the number of scores. The mean is the average score.

Multivariate Analysis. Method of considering the relation of three or more variables. Multivariate methods include multiple regression, discriminant analysis, canonical correlation, and factor analysis.

Multivariate Analysis of Variance. A multivariate technique that uses an analysis of variance design but includes a dependent variable that is a linear combination of variables.

Null Hypothesis. The assumption that there is no significant difference between two random samples of a population. When the null hypothesis is rejected, observed differences between groups are deemed improbable by chance alone.

Percentile Rank. The percentage of scores in a distribution exceeded by any particular score. For example, a percentile rank of 80 for a given score means that this score exceeds 80 percent of all scores in the distribution.

Population. The entire collection of a set of objects or persons with the same definition.

Power Analysis. Analytical method for estimating the sample size required to detect statistical effects of defined size for variables with known variances.

Prevalence. The number of existing cases of a disorder. There are several types of prevalence.

POINT PREVALENCE. The number of persons who have a disorder at a specified point in time. The point can be a certain calendar day (e.g., April 1, 1993) or any day during a particular study (e.g., the fourth day of the study), regardless of the calendar day. It is calculated as follows:

$$\text{Point prevalence} = \frac{\text{Number of persons with a disorder at a specified point in time}}{\text{Total population at a specified point in time}}$$

PERIOD PREVALENCE. The number of persons who have a disorder at any time during a specified period (longer than a calendar day or a point in time). It is calculated as follows:

$$\text{Period prevalence} = \frac{\text{Number of persons with a disorder during a time period}}{\text{Total population during time period}}$$

The numerator includes any existing cases at the start of the period and any new cases that develop during the period. Period prevalence may be used to determine the number of persons with a disorder, the number of those in treatment, and the duration of an illness.

LIFETIME PREVALENCE. A measure at a point in time of the number of persons who had a disorder at some time during their lives. A potential problem with determining lifetime prevalence is that it is almost always based on subject recall, which can be inaccurate.

TREATED PREVALENCE. The number of persons being treated for a disorder, determined by counting all those in a defined geographic area who are receiving treatment. Treated point prevalence (e.g., the number of patients being treated for a disorder in a clinic on a certain day) or treated period prevalence (e.g., the number of patients being treated for a disorder at a clinic over the past year) can be measured.

Probability. A quantitative statement of the likelihood that an event will occur. A probability of 0 means that the event is certain not to occur; a probability of 1 means that the event will occur with certainty.

***P* Value.** The probability of obtaining a result by chance alone. A *P* value of .01 means that the probability of obtaining a result by chance alone is 1 in 100; a value of .05 means that the result will occur 5 times out of every 100 times by chance alone.

Randomization. The process allowing each patient in a clinical trial to have an equal chance to be assigned to a control or experimental treatment group. It protects against selection bias and guarantees the validity of statistical tests of significance.

Regression Analysis. A method for obtaining a prediction from observed data to predict the value of one variable (x) in relation to the value of another variable (y).

Risk Factor. A disorder-associated factor that may support a causal connection. A risk may be factor specific (e.g., it occurs in only one sex) or factor related (e.g., it is likely to occur in a certain environment). A causal connection between a risk factor and a disorder is shown by temporality, in which a factor precedes the disorder being studied; the repeated appearance of the same risk factor in multiple studies; specificity, in which a risk factor is associated with one disorder only; and a determination that the experimental intervention eliminating the risk factor also eliminates the disorder. Determining what factor or factors account for the increased risk of a disorder is one of the challenges of psychiatric epidemiology

RELATIVE RISK. The ratio of the incidence of the disease among persons exposed to the risk factor to the incidence among those not exposed. For example, the relative risk of lung cancer is much greater for heavy smokers than for nonsmokers.

ATTRIBUTABLE RISK. The absolute incidence of the disease in exposed persons that can be attributed to the exposure. The measure is derived by subtracting the incidence of the disease in question among unexposed persons from its total incidence among those exposed. For example, the lung cancer death rate for nonsmokers may be subtracted from the total community lung cancer death rate. The results are the attributable community risk for lung cancer. Attributable risk is a useful concept that shows what may be expected if the risk is removed. For example, on the basis of available data, the attributable risk for deaths from lung cancer could be avoided if smoking were eliminated.

Sample. A subset of observations selected from a population.

Sensitivity. The number of true-positive results divided by the sum of the number of true positives and false negatives. It is the proportion of patients with the condition in question that the test can detect.

Specificity. The number of true-negative results divided by the sum of the number of true negatives and false positives. It is the proportion of patients without the condition that the test finds to be negative.

Standard Deviation (SD). A measure of variation derived by squaring each deviation in a set of scores, taking the average of these squares, and then taking the square root of the result. The standard deviation is represented by the Greek letter sigma (σ). In a normal distribution, ±1 SD includes 68 percent of the population; ±2 SD includes 95 percent of the population; and ±3 SD includes 99 percent of the population.

Standardized or Z-Score. The deviation of a score from its group mean expressed in standard deviation units.

Survival Analysis. Method for evaluating the timing of events. These methods can be used to evaluate life expectancy, age of onset of psychological illness, time to relapse for those in treatment, or the timing of developmental milestones such as first word, age of initiation of smoking, or age at marriage or any other time-dependent variable.

***t*-Test.** A statistical procedure designed to compare two sets of observations.

Type I Error. The error that occurs when the null hypothesis is rejected when it should have been retained; the false claim of a true difference because the observed difference is due entirely to chance.

Type II Error. The error that occurs when the null hypothesis is retained when it should have been rejected; the false acceptance of the null hypothesis when, in fact, there is a true difference, but the difference is so small that it falls within the acceptance region of the null hypothesis.

Variable. A characteristic that can assume different values in different experimental situations. In research, independent variables are those qualities that the experimenter systematically varies (e.g., time, age, sex, type of drug) in the experiment. Dependent variables are those qualities that measure the influence of the independent variable or the outcome of the experiment (e.g., the measurement of a person's specific physiological reactions to a drug).

References

Bird HR. Epidemiology of childhood disorders in a cross-cultural context. *Child Psychol Psychiatry.* 1996;37:35.

Cooper B. Epidemiology and prevention in the mental health field. *Soc Psychiatry Psychiatr Epidemiol.*1990;25:9.

Doll B. Prevalence of psychiatric disorders in children and youth: an agenda for advocacy by school psychology. *School Psychol O.* 1996;11:20.

Fenton WS, Robinowitz CB, Leaf PJ. Male and female psychiatrists and their patients. *Am J Psychiatry.* 1987;144:358.

Ford DE, Cooper-Patrick L. Sleep disturbances and mood disorders: an epidemiologic perspective. *Depression Anxiety.* 2001;14:3.

Gurland B. Epidemiology of psychiatric disorders. In: Sadavoy J, Lazarus LW, Jarvik LF, Grossberg GT, eds. *Comprehensive Review of Geriatric Psychiatry-II.* 2nd ed. Washington, DC: American Psychiatric Press; 1196:3.

Henderson AS. The present state of psychiatric epidemiology. *Aust N Z J Psychiatry.* 1996;30:9.

Kaplan RM, Grant IG. Statistics and experimental design. In: Sadock BJ, Sadock VA, eds. *Kaplan & Sadock's Comprehensive Textbook of Psychiatry.* 7th ed. Vol 1. Baltimore: Lippincott Williams & Wilkins; 2000:522.

Klerman GI. Paradigm shifts in USA psychiatric epidemiology since World War II. *Soc Psychiatry Psychiatr Epidemiol.* 1990;25:27.

Regier DA, Burke JD. Epidemiology. In: Sadock BJ, Sadock VA, Eds. *Kaplan & Sadock's Comprehensive Textbook of Psychiatry.* 7th ed. Vol 1. Baltimore: Lippincott Williams & Wilkins; 2000:500.

Roger JL, Howard KI, Vesey JT. Using significance test to evaluate equivalence between two experimental groups. *Psychol Bull.* 1993;113:553.

Samuels JF, Nestadt G. Epidemiology: the distribution of mental disorders in the community. In: Breakey WK, ed. *Integrated Mental Health Services: Modern Community Psychiatry.* New York: Oxford University Press; 1996:71.

Toussaint LL, Williams DR, Musick MA, Everson SA. Forgiveness and health: age differences in a U.S. probability sample. *J Adult Develop.* 2001;8:249.

Visotsky HM. Courage, creativity, and cost-effectiveness: the challenge for a psychiatric program administration. *New Dir Ment Health Serv.* 1991;49:51.

5

Clinical Neuropsychological Testing

▲ 5.1 Clinical Neuropsychological Testing of Intelligence and Personality

Clinical neuropsychological testing of intelligence and personality plays a relatively minor role in establishing a psychiatric diagnosis, which is based primarily on observable signs and symptoms and clinical interviews. However, these tests, which are designed to measure specific aspects of a person's intelligence, thinking, or personality, are helpful in special situations. Intelligence testing is necessary to establish the degree of mental retardation, and neuropsychological tests (described in Section 5.2) help quantify and localize brain damage. Some tests may highlight areas of conflict or concern in a person's life that should be a focus of therapeutic attention, and certain tests may reveal severely disordered thinking not otherwise evident. The tests are usually administered by psychologists specifically trained in their use and interpretation.

Most commonly used assessment instruments are standardized against normal control subjects, who are required to respond to the same stimuli or set of questions. Their responses are tabulated into a normal distribution pattern against which new subjects are compared. With *standardization,* test administration and scoring are invariant across time and examiners. Related to the standardization of any test are the available data that presumably show whether the test is valid and reliable. *Reliability* assesses the reproducibility of results; *validity* assesses whether the test measures what it purports to measure (see Chapter 4, Section 4.7, which discusses biostatistics).

TYPES OF TESTS

Objective Tests

Objective tests are typically pencil-and-paper tests based on specific items and questions. They yield numerical scores and profiles easily subjected to mathematical or statistical analysis. An example is the Minnesota Multiphasic Personality Inventory (MMPI).

Projective Tests

Projective tests present stimuli whose meanings are not immediately obvious; some ambiguity forces persons to project their own needs into the test situation. Projective tests presumably have no right or wrong answers. Those being tested impute meanings to the stimulus, apparently based on psychological and emotional factors. Examples include the Thematic Apperception Test (TAT), the Draw-a-Person test, the Rorschach test, and the Sentence Completion Test.

INTELLIGENCE TESTING

Intelligence can be defined as the ability to assimilate factual knowledge, to recall either recent or remote events, to reason logically, to manipulate concepts (either numbers or words), to translate the abstract to the literal and the literal to the abstract, to analyze and synthesize forms, and to deal meaningfully and accurately with problems and priorities deemed important in a particular setting. Intelligence varies tremendously from person to person.

In 1905, Alfred Binet introduced the concept of the mental age (MA), which is the average intellectual level of a particular age. The intelligence quotient (IQ) is the ratio of MA to CA (chronological age), multiplied by 100 to eliminate the decimal point; it is represented by the following equation:

$$IQ = \frac{MA}{CA} \times 100$$

An IQ of 100, or average, results when chronological and mental ages are equal. Because it is impossible to measure age-associated changes in intellectual power after the age of 15 with available intelligence tests, the highest divisor in the IQ formula is 15. One way of expressing a person's relative standing within a group is by using percentile. The higher the percentile, the higher the rank within a group. An IQ of 100 corresponds to the 50th percentile in intellectual ability for the general population.

As measured by most intelligence tests, IQ is an interpretation or classification of a total test score in relation to norms established by a group. IQ is a measure of present functioning ability, not necessarily of future potential. Although under ordinary circumstances the IQ is stable throughout life, there is no absolute certainty about its predictive properties. A person's IQ must be examined in the light of past experiences and future opportunities.

The IQ itself does not indicate the origins of its reflected capacities—genetic (innate) or environmental. The most useful intelligence test must measure a variety of skills and abilities, including verbal and performance, early learned and recently learned, timed and untimed, culture free, and culture bound. No

intelligence test is totally culture free, although tests do differ significantly in degree.

Wechsler Adult Intelligence Scale (WAIS)

The Wechsler Adult Intelligence Scale (WAIS) is the best standardized and most widely used intelligence test in clinical practice today. It was constructed by David Wechsler at New York University Medical Center and Bellevue Psychiatric Hospital. Designed in 1939, the original WAIS has gone through several revisions. The latest revision, the WAIS-III, is designed for persons 16 to 89 years of age. A scale for children ages 5 through 15 years has been devised (Wechsler Intelligence Scale for Children-III [WISC-III]) and a scale for children ages 4 to 6½ years (Wechsler Preschool and Primary Scale of Intelligence-Revised [WPPSI-R]).

The WAIS comprises 11 subtests made up of six verbal subtests and five performance subtests, which yield a verbal IQ, a performance IQ, and a combined or full-scale IQ. Intelligence levels are based on the assumption that intellectual abilities are normally distributed (in a bell-shaped curve) throughout the population (Fig. 5.1–1). Verbal and performance IQs and the full-scale IQ are determined by the use of separate tables for each of the seven age groups (from 16 to 64 years) on which the test was standardized. Variability in functioning is revealed through discrepancies between verbal and performance IQs and by the scatter pattern between subtests.

Construction of the Test.

The following subtests are described in the order in which they are presented to the subject.

VERBAL SKILLS. *Information.* This subtest covers general information and knowledge and is subject to cultural variables. Persons from low socioeconomic groups with little schooling do not perform as well as those from high socioeconomic groups with more schooling.

Comprehension. This subtest measures subjects' knowledge of social conventions and common sense and examines qualities of a person's reasoning and thinking by posing questions about proverbs and how persons ought to behave under certain circumstances.

Arithmetic. The ability to do arithmetic and other simple calculations is reflected on this subtest, which is adversely influenced by anxiety and poor attention and concentration.

Similarities. This subtest is a sensitive indicator of intelligence. It covers the ability to abstract by asking subjects to explain the similarity between two things.

Digit Span. Immediate retention is measured in this subtest. Subjects are asked to learn a series of two to nine digits, which are immediately recalled both forward and backward. Anxiety, poor attention span, and brain dysfunction interfere with recall.

Vocabulary. Subjects are asked to define 35 vocabulary words of increasing difficulty. Intelligence has a high correlation with vocabulary, which is related to level of education. Idiosyncratic definitions of words may give clues to personality structure.

PERFORMANCE. *Picture Completion.* This subtest initiates the performance part of the WAIS and consists of completing a picture in which a part is missing. Visuoperceptive defects become evident when mistakes are made on this test.

Block Design. This subtest requires subjects to match colored blocks and visual designs. Brain dysfunction involving impairment of left-right dominance interferes with performance.

Picture Arrangement. Subjects are required to arrange a series of pictures in a sequence that tells a story (e.g., a person committing a crime). In addition to testing performance, this subtest provides data about a subject's cognitive style.

Object Assembly. Subjects must assemble objects, such as the figure of a woman or an animal, in the proper order and organization. Visuoperception, somatoperception, and manual dexterity are tested.

Digit Symbol. In this final subtest of the WAIS, subjects receive a code that pairs symbols with digits. The test consists of matching a series of digits to their corresponding symbols in as little time as possible.

Distribution of IQ Scores.

The average, or normal, range of IQ is 90 to 110; IQ scores of at least 120 are considered supe-

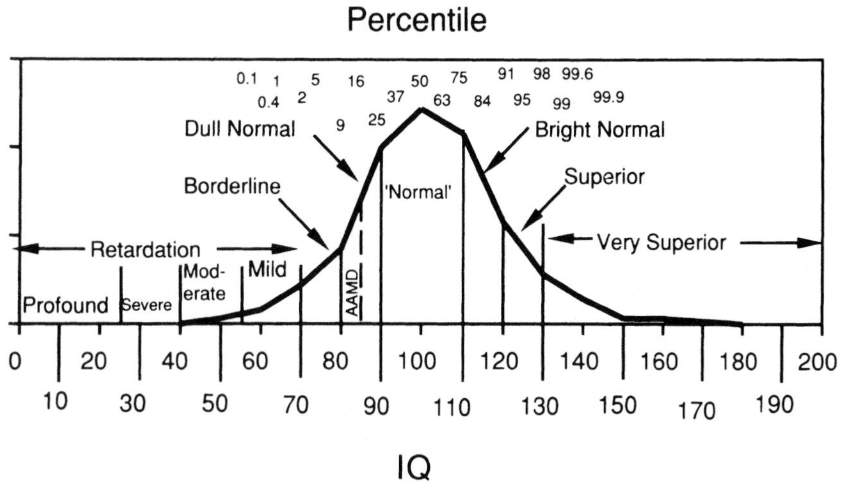

FIGURE 5.1–1
The distribution of Wechsler Adult Intelligence Scale IQ categories. (Adapted from Matarazzo JD. *Wechsler's Measurement and Appraisal of Adult Intelligence.* 5th ed. New York: Oxford University Press; 1972:124.)

Table 5.1–1
Classification of Intelligence by IQ Range

Classification	IQ Range
Profound mental retardation (MR)[a]	Below 20 or 25
Severe MR[a]	20–25 to 35–40
Moderate MR[a]	35–40 to 50–55
Mild MR[a]	50–55 to about 70
Borderline	70–79
Dull normal	80 to 90
Normal	90 to 110
Bright normal	110 to 120
Superior	120 to 130
Very superior	130 and above

[a]According to the text revision of the fourth edition of *Diagnostic and Statistical Manual of Mental Disorders* (DSM-IV-TR).

rior (Table 5.1–1). According to the American Association of Mental Deficiency (AAMD) and the text revision of the fourth edition of *Diagnostic and Statistical Manual of Mental Disorders* (DSM-IV-TR), mental retardation is defined as an IQ below 70, which corresponds to the lowest 2.2 percent of the population. Consequently, 2 of every 100 persons have IQ scores consistent with mental deficiency, which can range from mild to profound.

Reliability and Validity. The reliability of the WAIS is very high. Retesting of persons 18 years and older rarely reveals changes in IQ scores.

The verbal scale of the IQ measures the retention of previously acquired factual information, and the performance scale measures visuospatial capacity and visuomotor speed in problem-solving tasks. The performance scale is more sensitive to normal aging than the verbal scale, which is more sensitive to education. Arithmetic and memory for digits are adversely affected by anxiety. The validity of the WAIS is high in identifying mental retardation and in predicting future school performance. A disparity between the verbal test and the performance test (usually more than 15 points) may indicate psychopathology, such as attention-deficit/hyperactivity disorder, which requires further testing.

Lewis Terman at Stanford University devised the Stanford-Binet Test in 1916, and it is now in its fourth revision. It is a comprehensive intelligence test that is used in psychiatry and education, although less widely than the WAIS.

ADULT PERSONALITY ASSESSMENT

Objective Personality Assessment

The objective approach to personality assessment is characterized by the reliance on structured, standardized measurement devices, which typically have a self-report nature. *Structured* reflects the tendency to use straightforward test stimuli, such as direct questions about persons' opinions of themselves and unambiguous instructions about completing the test.

Response sets are attitudes or styles in responding to personality questionnaires. Some persons answer incorrectly to present themselves in a more favorable light or to please the examiner. Other persons attempt to look worse than they truly are. Well-designed tests, such as the MMPI, have built-in scales designed to detect such response sets and to adjust scores accordingly. A list of various objective personality measures is given in Table 5.1–2.

Minnesota Multiphasic Personality Inventory (MMPI). This self-report inventory is the most widely used and most thoroughly researched objective personality assessment instrument. The MMPI was developed in 1937 by Starke Hathaway, a psychologist, and J. Charnley McKinley, a psychiatrist. The test was eventually updated and is now called the MMPI-2. The test consists of more than 500 statements—such as, "I worry about sex matters"; "I sometimes tease animals"; "I believe I am being plotted against"—to which subjects must respond with "true," "false," or "cannot say." The test may be used in card or booklet form, and several computer programs exist to process responses.

The MMPI gives scores on 10 standard clinical scales, each of which was derived empirically (i.e., homogeneous criterion groups of psychiatric patients were used in developing the scales). The items for each scale were selected for their ability to separate medical and psychiatric patients from normal control subjects.

CLINICAL SCALES. The clinical scales are numbered and are often referred to by number rather than by name, particularly in coding abnormally high scores. A high score on a particular scale does not mean that a subject has the illness. For example, an elevated 8 (schizophrenia) score does not indicate that a patient necessarily has schizophrenia. The scales are listed in Table 5.1–3.

INTERPRETATION. Accurate interpretation requires great experience in administering the test and some understanding of the social, educational, and socioeconomic backgrounds of patients. Recent evidence indicates that religion and race are both potential variables in MMPI responses.

Although the MMPI was initially considered a diagnostic aid (i.e., a patient with major depressive disorder would score high on the depression scale), the advantages of a configural approach to interpretation quickly became apparent. The configural approach, which involves interpretation based on the patterning of the entire profile, has become the preferred method and has increased the effectiveness of the MMPI as a personality measurement device. Various researchers have identified numerous personality correlates of various MMPI scale configurations, frequently by using the two highest scales as the basis for interpretive statements.

Actuarial research of such nature has also served as the basis for computerized interpretative services. These services, although not a substitute for a comprehensive personality evaluation, can assist clinicians in hypothesis formulation. Computerized services are especially useful when the MMPI is to be interpreted by a person knowledgeable in all aspects of the MMPI and in the nature of the development of the computerized program. Blind use of these services by professionals not trained in the use of the MMPI, however, is clearly inappropriate and perhaps even unethical.

The fact that the MMPI and MMPI-2 are the most widely used and researched psychological personality measurement devices is undoubtedly one of their major strengths. Several hundred research papers on the MMPI appear in the literature each year, and it has been used extensively in cross-cultural clinical and research applications. The huge body of literature generated has resulted in a catalog of MMPI correlates on a wide variety of clinical cases, which provides descriptive, predictive, diagnostic, and prognostic information. Another strength of the MMPI is its atheoretical nature, a characteristic that probably increases its usefulness over a broad spectrum. The presence of validity scales designed to assess test-taking attitude, in addition to clinical and personality information, is a distinct advantage that the MMPI maintains over many personality

Table 5.1–2
Objective Measures of Personality in Adults

Name	Description	Strengths	Weaknesses
Minnesota Multiphasic Personality Inventory (MMPI)	566 items, true-false; self-report format; 17 primary scales (numerous special scales)	Provides wide range of data on numerous personality variables; strong research base	Tends to emphasize major psychopathology; needs revision with current normative data
Minnesota Multiphasic Personality Inventory-2 (MMPI-2)	567 items; true-false; self-report format; 20 primary scales	Current revision of MMPI with updated response booklet; revised scaling methods, and new validity scores; new normative data	Preliminary data indicate that the MMPI-2 and the MMPI can provide discrepant results; normative sample biased toward upper socioeconomic status; no normative data for adolescents
Million Clinical Multiaxial Inventory (MCMI)	175 items; true-false; self-report format; 20 primary scales	Brief administration time; corresponds well with DSM-III diagnostic classifications	Needs more validation research; no information on disorder severity; needs revision for DSM-IV
Million Clinical Multiaxial Inventory-II (MCMI-II)	175 items; true-false; self-report format; 25 primary scales	Brief administration time; corresponds well with DSM-III-R	High degree of item overlap in various scales; no information on disorder or trait severity
16 Personality Factor Questionnaire (16 PF)	True-false; self-report format; 16 personality dimensions	Sophisticated psychometric instrument with considerable research conducted on nonclinical populations	Limited usefulness with clinical populations
Personality Assessment Inventory (PAI)	344 items; Likert-type format; self-report; 22 scales	Includes measures of psychopathology, personality dimensions, validity scales, and specific concerns to psychotherapeutic treatment	Inventory is new and has not yet generated a supportive research base
California Personality Inventory (CPI)	True-false; self-report format; 17 scales	Well-accepted method of assessing patients who do not exhibit major psychopathology	Limited usefulness with clinical populations
Jackson Personality Inventory (JPI)	True-false; self-report format; 15 personality scales	Constructed in accord with sophisticated psychometric techniques; controls for response sets	Unproved usefulness in clinical settings
Edwards Personal Preference Schedule (EPPS)	Forced choice; self-report format	Follows Murray's theory of personology; accounts for social desirability	Not widely used clinically because restricted information obtained
Psychological Screening Inventory (PSI)	103 items; true-false; self-report format	Yields 4 scores that can be used as screening measures for the possibility of a need for psychological help	Scales are short and have correspondingly low reliability
Eysenck Personality Questionnaire (EPQ)	True-false; self-report format	Useful as a screening device; test has a theoretical basis with research support	Scales are short, and items are transparent as to purpose; not recommended for other than a screening device
Adjective Checklist (ACL)	True-false; self-report or informant report	Can be used for self-rating or other rating	Scores rarely correlate highly with conventional personality inventories
Comrey Personality Scales (CPS)	True-false; self-report format; 8 scales	Factor-analytical techniques used with a high degree of sophistication in test constructed	Not widely used; factor-analytical interpretation problems
Tennessee Self-Concept Scale (TSCS)	100 items; true-false; self-report format; 14 scales	Brief administration time yields considerable information	Brevity is also a disadvantage, lowering reliability and validity; useful as a screening device only

Courtesy of Robert W. Butler, Ph.D., and Paul Satz, Ph.D.

assessment tools. The MMPI has been restandardized on the basis of a contemporary sample of normal persons, and questions and language have been updated to reflect current cultural views.

Structured Clinical Diagnostic Assessments. Several structured and semistructured interviews based on DSM-IV-TR criteria have been designed to provide numerical scores on diagnostic scales. The scales are useful in establishing the severity of illness and in monitoring recovery. Although used clinically, their greatest use is as research instruments; they help to standardize a subject cohort and provide objective outcome measures for assessing treatment response. Among these instruments are the Hamilton Rating Scale for Depression, the Hamilton Anxiety Rating Scale, the Yale-Brown Obsessive-Compulsive Scale (YBOCS), and the Structural Clinical Interview for DSM-IV Dissociative Disorders (SCID-D).

Table 5.1–3
MMPI Validity and Clinical Scales

Validity

L: Lie Scale A nonempirically derived social desirability scale. Items tend to reflect behaviors that are considered socially desirable but rarely practiced. The score can suggest defensiveness, illiteracy, psychosis, or personality processes, depending on various factors.

F: Infrequency Scale Measures a tendency to endorse selected items that are statistically rare responses (less than 10 percent of the original normal sample). Useful in identifying illiteracy, malingering, panic, confusion, psychosis, and personality processes.

K: Suppressor Scale Used to adjust mathematically certain clinical scales to decrease false positives and false negatives. The scale is also useful in determining overall test-taking attitude and is an indication of personality variables.

Clinical

1: Hypochondriasis Reflects somatic concerns and preoccupation with bodily functioning. Interpretation needs to take into account such factors as age and actual health status. As with all MMPI scales, interpretation is furthered by looking at its relation to other scales.

2: Depression Tends to reflect depression as a mood disorder. The fact that the scale is sensitive to situational variables suggests that it may be a good index of state personality status.

3: Hysteria Involves the identification of classic histrionic symptoms, including the presence of physical symptoms coupled with indifference, denial, repression, and inhibition. The scale does not necessarily measure other popularly conceived traits, such as liability and melodramatic attitude.

4: Psychopathic Deviance Developed to assess the amorality and asociality aspects of psychopathy, rather than the criminal or antisocial. Its meaning depends on other scale configurations. The scale provides good information on the quality of interpersonal relationships.

5: Masculinity-Femininity Originally developed to identify homosexuality but rarely used for that purpose, although it does provide information on gender identity. The scale reflects a variety of personality and interest areas, such as dependence, sensitivity, intellectuality, and tendencies toward introspection.

6: Paranoia Developed by the empirical identification of classic paranoiacs, assesses vigilance, sensitivity, delusional thought, distrust, and suspicion. Except for the paranoid areas, the members of the original criterion group were considered functional in their lives.

7: Psychasthenia A diverse scale designed to measure anxiety and obsessive-compulsive traits. Endorsed items can reflect fear, obsessive-compulsive symptoms, interpersonal hostility, tension, specific phobias, and impaired concentration.

8: Schizophrenia Reflects the acute positive symptoms of psychotic breaks with reality, rather than the chronic negative symptoms. The scale also assesses alienation, impaired self-identity, and isolation.

9: Hypomania Measures the classic symptoms of mania, including elated and unstable mood, psychomotor excitement, and flight of ideas. It also appears to reflect narcissistic personality traits. In general, the scale provides information on the degree of drivenness of the person's personality characteristics. It has a strong age component.

10: Social Introversion Provides information on social withdrawal, shyness, leadership, talkativeness, levels of gregariousness, and, to a small degree, self-concept and neurotic tendencies. It is more two-dimensional and bipolar (introversion versus extroversion) than the other scales.

Special

A: Anxiety The first general factor extracted from factor analytic studies on the MMPI. It is thought to reflect generalized endorsement of psychopathology.

R: Repression The second factor that is found on factor analytic studies of the MMPI. It can be conceptualized as measuring the tendency to engage in denial.

ES: Ego Strength Provides an index of how functional the patient may be in terms of work and other social areas, regardless of level of psychopathology.

MAS: *McAndrews Alcoholism Scale* Estimates the person's degree of addiction proneness, especially with alcohol, opiates, and opioids. It is especially sensitive to daily substance abuse, rather than episodic abuse.

Courtesy of Robert W. Butler, Ph.D., and Paul Satz, Ph.D., with the assistance of Alex Caldwell, Ph.D.

Projective Personality Assessment

The projective approach to personality assessment is defined by the use of unstructured, often ambiguous test stimuli. A basic assumption is that when confronted with a vague stimulus and required to respond to it in some manner, persons cannot help but reveal information about themselves—not only in the way the ambiguity is confronted but also in the content of their responses.

The projective approach is essentially idiographic, and the tests most commonly are not interpreted by comparing a person's responses with a set of criterion-referenced normative data. Typically, interpretation is based on a theory of human behavior and personality; it is assumed that persons bring certain needs, characteristics, defenses, and other qualities that become apparent through the testing process.

Several semistructured situations and projective-type stimuli have been developed, including perceiving inkblots, drawing pictures, and telling stories on the basis of presented pictures. Various projective personality measures are listed in Table 5.1–4.

Rorschach Test. The Rorschach test was devised by Hermann Rorschach, a Swiss psychiatrist (Fig. 5.1–2), who in about 1910 began to experiment with ambiguous inkblots. A standard set of 10 inkblots serves as a stimulus for associations; one inkblot is shown in Figure 5.1–3. In the standard series, the blots are reproduced on cards 7 by 9½ inches and are numbered from I to X. Five of the blots are black and white; the other five include colors. The cards are shown to a patient in a particular order, and the psychologist keeps a record of the patient's verbatim responses, along with initial reaction times and total time spent on each card. After completion of what is called the free-association phase, the examiner conducts an inquiry phase to determine important aspects of each response that are crucial to its scoring. Table 5.1–5 contains examples of responses to Rorschach stimuli.

SCORING. The scoring of responses converts the important aspects of each response into a symbol system related to location areas, determinants, content areas, and popularity.

Table 5.1–4
Projective Measures of Personality

Name	Description	Strengths	Weaknesses
Rorschach test	10 stimulus cards of inkblots, some colored, others achromatic	Most widely used projective device and certainly the best researched; considerable interpretative data available	Some Rorschach interpretive systems have unproved validity
Thematic Apperception Test (TAT)	20 stimulus cards depicting a number of scenes of varying ambiguity	A widely used method that, in the hands of a well-trained person, provides valuable information	No generally accepted scoring system results in poor consistency in interpretation; time-consuming administration
Sentence completion test	A number of different devices available, all sharing the same format with more similarities than differences	Brief administration time; can be a useful adjunct to clinical interviews if supplied beforehand	Stimuli are obvious in intent and subject to easy falsification
Holtzman Inkblot Technique (HIT)	Two parallel forms of inkblot cards with 45 cards per form	Only one response is allowed per card, making research less troublesome	Not widely accepted and rarely used; not directly comparable to Rorschach interpretive strategies
Figure drawing	Typically human forms but can involve houses or other forms	Quick administration	Interpretive strategies have typically been unsupported by research
Make-a-Picture Story (MAPS)	Similar to TAT; however, stimuli can be manipulated by the patient	Provides idiographic personality information through thematic analysis	Minimal research support; not widely used

Courtesy of Robert W. Butler, Ph.D., and Paul Satz, Ph.D.

Location. Location is scored in terms of which portion of the blot was used as the basis for a response (e.g., the whole blot, a common detail of the blot, an unusual detail of the blot, or an area of white space). Attention to the whole blot with accurate form perception reflects good organizational ability and high intelligence. Overattention to detail is common in obsessive and paranoid subjects.

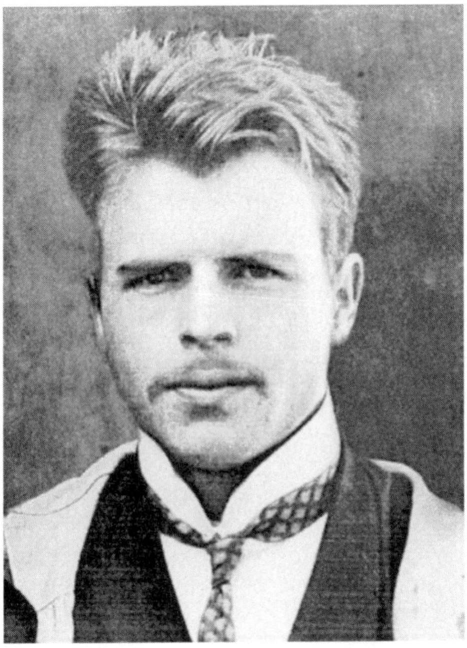

FIGURE 5.1–2
Herman Rorschach. (Courtesy of New York Academy of Medicine, New York, NY.)

Determinants. The determinants of each response reflect the features of the blot that make it look the way the patient thought it looked (e.g., form, shading, color, movement of either humans or animals, inanimate movements, or combinations of these determinants with varying emphasis). Overemphasis on form suggests rigidity and constriction of the personality. Color responses relate to the emotional reactions of the person to the environment and to the control of emotion.

Content. Responses are scored in terms of the content they reflect—human, animal, anatomy, sex, food, nature, and so on. In general, content areas reflect the subject's breadth and range of interests.

Popularity. Certain responses to the cards are more popular than others.

INTERPRETATION. The Rorschach test brings subjects' thinking and association patterns clearly into focus because the ambiguity of the stimulus provides relatively few cues about conventional, standard, or normal responses. Proper interpretation, however, requires a great deal of experience. There is a high reliability among experienced clinicians who administer

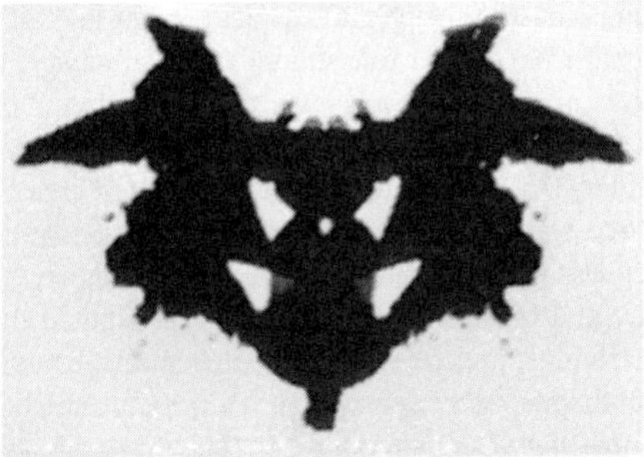

FIGURE 5.1–3
Plate 1 of the Rorschach test. (Reprinted with permission from Huber Medical Publisher, Bern.)

Table 5.1–5
Sample Rorschach Responses and Interpretation to Card I by Diagnostic Category

Diagnostic Category	Patient's Response Proper	Patient's Response on Inquiry	Interpretation
Nonpatient	Well the first impression is of a wolf's head, ears here and eyes.	"Overall the head, nose, eyes, ears, the whole thing."	Common response using the white space as the eyes, responding to the whole blot
Schizophrenic patient	I will say the first thing that comes to mind, it would be a predator on the movie, lost of ink, predator, have you seen that movie?	"The whole picture all the way, and I liked the movie and the reason why is because you said the first thing that comes to mind. I've seen the movie over and over again, 10 times. The whole picture, something that looks at me mean. (Looks at you mean?) Because it's a person that kills without any feeling, that's why I thought the movie was good."	The response shows difficulty staying focused on the task at hand, tangential thought process, some paranoia and distortion of the form of the card
Depression	Could be a leaf.	"Could be a leaf that has fallen off the tree and started to decay, leafs have jagged edges. (You said decayed?) Because if it was a perfect leaf all this would be part of the blot, and here parts of it that have fallen off. That would have been the stem. Also you have the main vein running down the middle, this is more prevalent because it's biggest, if it was on a tree it would get nutrients to the leaf like our blood system."	The response shows morbid content (decay) that indicates a poor view of self and the world; leaf responses also weigh on the isolation index
Anxiety	I don't know, I'd have to think about it. It could be trees.	"Like if you are in the forest, stalks you know, when trees blend together they are nondescript. I'm a real outdoor person, I like to go to the forest and spend time there. (Can you help me see the trees?) Just this little Christmas tree here and here, the outline."	The response shows discomfort in committing to a response, and discomfort in beginning the task; some anxiety is also seen in the rambling personalization used to justify the response

Courtesy of Dana Foley, Ph.D.

the test. In proper hands, the test is extremely useful, especially in eliciting psychodynamic formulations, defense mechanisms, and subtle disorders of thinking.

Thematic Apperception Test (TAT). This test was designed by Henry Murray and Christiana Morgan as part of a normal personality study conducted at the Harvard Psychological Clinic in 1943. The TAT consists of a series of 30 pictures and one blank card, but not all the pictures are used. The choice depends on what conflict area the examiner wishes to clarify with a patient. Examples of TAT pictures are a young woman seated on a couch looking up at an older man, a man standing beside a nude woman in a bed, a gray-haired man looking at a younger man, and an older woman standing behind a younger woman (Fig. 5.1–4).

Although most of the pictures depict persons and all are representational (making the test stimuli more structured than are the inkblots of the Rorschach test), there is ambiguity in each picture. Unlike the Rorschach blots to which patients are asked to associate, the TAT requires patients to construct or create a story.

As the test was originally conceived, an important aspect of each story was the figure (the hero) with whom subjects seemed to identify and to whom they presumably attributed their own wishes, strivings, and conflicts. The characteristics of persons other than the hero were considered to represent subjects' views of other persons in their environment. It is now assumed that all the figures in a TAT story are equally representative of subjects; the more accepted and conscious traits and motives are attributed to figures closest to the subject in age, sex, and appearance, and the more unacceptable and unconscious traits and motives are attributed to figures most unlike the subject.

The stories must be considered from the standpoint of unusualness of theme or plot. Whether subjects deal with a

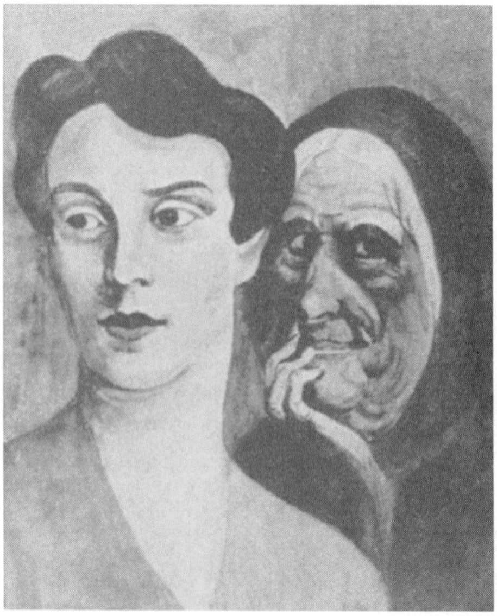

FIGURE 5.1–4
Card 12F of the Thematic Apperception Test. (Courtesy of Harvard University Press, Cambridge, MA.)

common or uncommon theme, their stories reflect their own idiosyncratic approaches to organization, sequence, vocabulary, style, preconceptions, assumptions, and outcome. TAT cards have varying stimulus values and can be assumed to elicit data pertaining to various areas of functioning. Generally, the TAT is more useful as a technique for inferring motivational aspects of behavior than as a basis for making a diagnosis.

Sentence Completion Test (SCT). This test is designed to tap patients' conscious associations to areas of functioning in which clinicians may be interested. The SCT is composed of a series of sentence stems (usually 75 to 100)—such as, "I like . . ."; "Sometimes I wish . . ."—that patients are asked to complete in their own words.

Time pressure is usually applied; patients are instructed to write down the first thing that comes to mind. In other instances, the test is administered orally by the examiner, as in the word-association technique. Sentence stems vary in their ambiguity; hence, some items serve as projective test stimuli ("Sometimes I . . ."). Others closely resemble direct-response questionnaires ("My greatest fear is . . .").

With the individual protocol, most clinicians use an inspection technique and note particularly those responses that express strong affects, that tend to be given repetitively, or that are unusual or particularly informative in any way. Areas in which denial operates are often revealed through omissions, bland expressions, or factual reports ("My mother is a woman"). Humor may also reflect an attempt to deny anxiety about a particular issue, person, or event. Important historical material is sometimes revealed directly ("I feel guilty about the way my sister was drowned").

Word-Association Technique. Carl Gustav Jung devised the word-association technique. Jung presented stimulus words to patients and had them respond with the first word that came to mind. After the initial administration of the list, some clinicians today repeat the list and ask the patient to respond with the same words that he or she used previously; discrepancies between the two administrations may reveal associational difficulties. Complex indicators include long reaction times, blocking difficulties in making responses, unusual responses, repetition of the stimulus word, apparent misunderstanding of the word, slang associations, perseveration of earlier responses, and ideas or unusual mannerisms or movements accompanying a response. Because it is easily quantified, the test continues to be used as a research instrument, although its popularity has diminished greatly over the years.

Draw-a-Person Test. This test was first used as a measure of intelligence in children. Detail was correlated with intelligence and developmental level. It has since become useful as an adult test. The Draw-a-Person test is easily administered, usually with the instructions, "I'd like you to draw a picture of a person; draw the best person you can." After completion of the first drawing, the patient is asked to draw a picture of a person of the sex opposite that of the figure in the drawing. Some clinicians use an interrogation procedure in which the patient is questioned about his or her drawings. ("What is he doing?" "What are her best qualities?") Modifications include asking for a drawing of a house and a tree (House-Tree-Person test), of the patient's family, and of an animal.

A general assumption is that the drawing of a person represents the expression of the self or of the body in the environment. Interpretive principles rest largely on the assumed functional significance of each body part. Most clinicians use drawings primarily as a screening technique, particularly for the detection of brain damage.

INTEGRATION OF TEST FINDINGS

The integration of test findings into a comprehensive, meaningful report is probably the most difficult aspect of psychological evaluation. Inferences from various tests must be related to one another in terms of clinicians' confidence in them and of a patient's presumed level of awareness that consciousness is being tapped.

Most clinicians follow some general outline in preparing a psychological report, such as test behavior, intellectual functioning, personality functioning (reality-testing ability, impulse control, manifest depression and guilt, manifestations of major dysfunction, major defenses, overt symptoms, interpersonal conflicts, self-concept, affects), inferred diagnosis, degree of present overt disturbance, prognosis for social recovery, motivation for personality change, primary assets and weaknesses, recommendations, and summary.

References

Adams RL, Culbertson JL. Personality assessment: adults and children. In: BJ Sadock, VA Sadock, eds. *Kaplan & Sadock's Comprehensive Textbook of Psychiatry.* 7th ed. Vol 1. Baltimore: Lippincott Williams & Wilkins; 2000:702.

Bremner J, Steinberg M, Southwick SM, Johnson DR, Charney DS. Use of the Structured Clinical Interview for DSM-IV Dissociative Disorders for systematic assessment of dissociative symptoms in posttraumatic stress disorder. *Am J Psychiatry.* 1993;150:1011.

Chick D, Sheaffer CI, Goggin WC, Sison GF. The relationship between MCMI personality scales and clinician-generated DSM-III-R personality disorder diagnoses. *J Pers Assess.* 1993;61:264.

Edwards DW, Morrison TL, Weissman HN. The MMPI and MMPI-2 in an outpatient sample: comparisons of code types, validity scales and clinical scales. *J Pers Assess.* 1993;61:1.

Fischer J, Corcoran K. *Measures for Clinical Practice: A Sourcebook.* 2nd ed. Vol 1: *Couples, Families and Children.* New York: Free Press; 1994.

Fischer J, Corcoran K. *Measures for Clinical Practice: A Sourcebook.* 2nd ed. Vol 2: *Adults.* New York: Free Press; 1994.

Goldstein G, Hersen M, eds. *Handbook of Psychological Assessment.* New York: Pergamon; 1990.

Graham JR. *Assessing Personality and Psychopathology.* New York: Oxford University Press; 1990.

Kardum I, Hudek-Knezevic J. The relationship between Eysenck's personality traits, coping styles and moods. *Pers Individ Diff.* 1996;20:341.

Lezak MD. *Neuropsychological Assessment.* 2nd ed. New York: Oxford University Press; 1983.

McCann JR. Convergent and discriminant validity of the MCMI-II and MMPI personality disorder scales. *Psych Assess.* 1991;3:9.

Rorschach H. *Psychodiagnostik.* Bern: Bircher; 1921.

Schnurr PP, Friedman MJ, Rosenberg SD. Preliminary MMPI scores as predictors of combat-related PTSD symptoms. *Am J Psychiatry.* 1993;150:479.

Smith LL. On the usefulness of item bias analysis to personality psychology. *J Pers Soc Psychol.* 2002;28:754.

Swanda RM, Haaland KY, LaRue A. Clinical neuropsychology and intellectual assessment of adults. In: Sadock BJ, Sadock VA, eds. *Kaplan & Sadock's Comprehensive Textbook of Psychiatry.* 7th ed. Vol 1. Baltimore: Lippincott Williams & Wilkins; 2000:689.

▲ 5.2 Clinical Neuropsychological Assessment of Adults

Clinical neuropsychology is a specialty in psychology that examines the relationship between behavior and brain functioning in the realms of cognitive, motor, sensory, and emotional functioning. In general, the clinical neuropsychologist inte-

grates the medical and psychosocial history with the reported complaints and the pattern of performance on neuropsychological procedures to determine whether results are consistent with a particular area of brain damage or a particular diagnosis.

The aim of neuropsychological tests is to achieve quantifiable and reproducible results that can be compared with the test scores of normal persons of comparable age and demographic background. Standardized techniques for assessing adult functioning include psychological tests, scales that rate behavior, and controlled interviews.

Neuropsychological assessment is indicated to identify cognitive defects, to differentiate incipient depression from dementia, to determine the course of an illness, to assess neurotoxic effects (such as memory impairment by substance abuse), to evaluate the effects of treatment (e.g., surgery for epilepsy, pharmacotherapy), and to evaluate learning disorders.

REASONING, CONCEPT FORMATION, AND PROBLEM SOLVING

Patients with cerebral disease are likely to lose the capacity to reason abstractly and to lack flexibility in problem solving or adapting to changed situations. Frontal lobe disease is often associated with impaired abstract reasoning, although other areas of the brain may also be involved. Workers can use many tests to assess the capacity for concept formation.

Wisconsin Card Sorting Test (WCST)

The Wisconsin Card Sorting Test (WCST) assesses abstract reasoning and flexibility in problem solving. Stimulus cards of different color, form, and number are presented to patients to sort into groups according to a principle established by the examiner but unknown to the patient (e.g., to sort by color, ignoring form and number). As the patient sorts the cards, he or she is told whether the responses are correct or incorrect, and the number of trials required to achieve 10 consecutive correct responses is recorded. When (or if) the patient has mastered the task, the examiner changes the principle of sorting, and the number of trials required to achieve correct sorting is recorded. The procedure, repeated several times, measures the capacity for abstract thinking (i.e., the number of trials required to achieve a solution) and flexibility (perseverative errors on successive sorting trials). Persons with damage to the frontal lobes or to the caudate and some persons with schizophrenia give abnormal responses.

MEMORY

Impairment of various types of memory, most notably short-term and recent memory, is a prominent behavioral deficit in patients with brain damage. In addition, it is often the first sign of cerebral disease and of aging. *Memory* is a comprehensive term that covers the retention of all types of material over various times and involves diverse forms of response. Consequently, a neuropsychological examiner is more inclined to give specific memory tests and evaluate them separately than to use an omnibus battery that provides a brief assessment of a large variety of performances and yields a single score.

Types of Memory

Immediate (or *short-term*) *memory* may be defined as the reproduction, recognition, or recall of perceived material within a period up to 30 seconds after presentation. It is most often assessed by digit repetition and reversal (auditory) and memory-for-designs (visual) tests. Both an auditory-verbal task, such as digit span or memory for words or sentences, and a nonverbal visual task, such as memory for designs or for objects or faces, should be given to assess a patient's immediate memory. Patients can also be asked to listen to a standardized story and then repeat it as accurately as possible. Patients with lesions of the right hemisphere are likely to show more severe defects on visual nonverbal tasks than on auditory verbal tasks. Conversely, patients with left hemisphere disease, including those who are not aphasic, are likely to show severe deficits on the auditory verbal tests, with variable performance on the visual nonverbal tasks.

Recent memory concerns events over the past few hours or days and can be tested by asking patients what they had for breakfast and who visited with them in the hospital.

Recent past memory concerns the retention of information over the past few months. Patients can be asked questions about current events.

Remote memory is the ability to remember events in the distant past. It is commonly believed that remote memory is well preserved in patients who show pronounced defects in recent memory, but the remote memory of senile and amnestic patients is usually significantly inferior to that of normal persons of comparable age and education. Even patients who appear to be able to recount their past fairly accurately show gaps and inconsistencies in their recitals on close examination.

Memory theorists have described three other types of memories: episodic, for specific events (e.g., a telephone message); semantic, for knowledge and facts (e.g., the first president of the United States); and implicit, for automatic skills (e.g., speaking grammatically or driving a car). Semantic and implicit memory do not decline with age, and persons continue to accumulate information over a lifetime. A minimal decline in episodic memory with aging may relate to impaired frontal lobe functioning.

Testing Memory

Wechsler Memory Scale. The Wechsler Memory Scale-Revised (WMS-R) is the most widely used memory test battery for adults. It is a composite of verbal paired associate and paragraph retention, visual memory for designs, orientation, digit span, rote recall of the alphabet, and counting backward. The scale yields a memory quotient (MQ), which is corrected for age and generally approximates the Wechsler Adult Intelligence Scale intelligence quotient (WAIS IQ); amnestic conditions, such as Korsakoff's syndrome, are characterized by a disproportionately low MQ but a relatively preserved IQ.

Benton Visual Retention Test. The Benton Visual Retention Test is sensitive to short-term memory loss (Fig. 5.2–1).

ORIENTATION

Orientation for person or place is rarely disturbed in brain-damaged patients who are not psychotic or severely demented, although defects in temporal orientation, which can reflect the integrity of recent memory, are common. Clinical examiners often miss these defects because of the tendency to regard as inconsequential slight inaccuracies in giving the day of the week or the date of the month. About 25 percent of nonpsy-

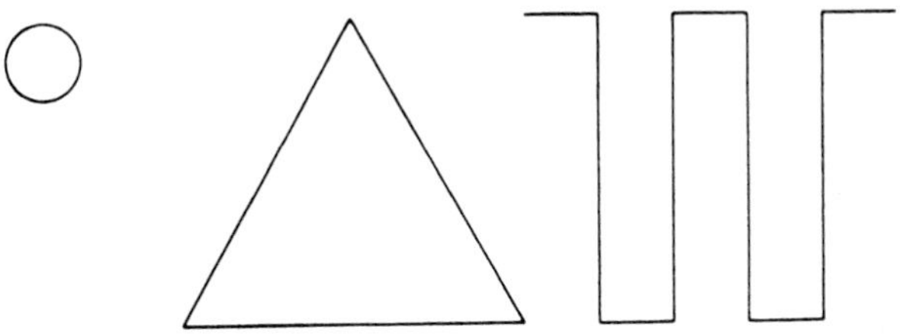

FIGURE 5.2–1
Test item from the Benton Visual Retention Test. The most frequently used testing condition involves the presentation of each geometric figure for 10 seconds, after which the patient attempts to draw the figure from memory. (Reprinted with permission from Benton AL. *The Revised Visual Retention Test: Clinical and Experimental Applications.* 4th ed. New York: Psychological Corporation; 1974:32.)

chotic patients with hemispheric cerebral disease, however, are likely to show significantly decreased performance with respect to the precision of temporal orientation. A simple test for orientation is outlined in Table 5.2–1.

PERCEPTUAL AND PERCEPTUOMOTOR PERFORMANCE

Many patients with brain disease show an impaired ability to analyze complex stimulus constellations or an inability to translate their perception into appropriate motor action. Unless the impairment is gross (e.g., as in visual object agnosia or dressing apraxia) or it interferes with a specific occupation skill, these deficits are not likely to be the subject of spontaneous complaint. Appropriate testing, however, discloses a remarkably high incidence of impaired performance on visuoanalytic, visuospatial, and visuoconstructive tasks in brain-damaged patients, particularly in persons with disease involving the right hemisphere. This type of impairment also extends to tactile and auditory perceptual task performances.

Visuoperceptive and visuoconstructive capacity and somatoperceptual defects can be assessed by tests. Double simultaneous stimulation is tested by lightly touching one of the patient's cheeks with one hand and simultaneously touching the back of one of the patient's hands with the other. A patient with brain dysfunction is unable to recognize one or both of the stimuli. The double simultaneous stimulation is a general test of defective capacity for perceptual integration.

Perceptuomotor tests often help localize cerebral lesions. A significant portion of patients with lesions of the right hemisphere who do not show obvious impairment in language functions perform poorly on perceptual tests (Fig. 5.2–2).

HEMISPHERIC DOMINANCE AND INTRAHEMISPHERIC LOCALIZATION

Many functions are mediated by both the right and left cerebral hemispheres. However, important qualitative differences between the two hemispheres can be demonstrated in the presence of lateralized brain injury. Various cognitive skills that have been linked to the left or right hemisphere in right-handed people are listed in Table 5.2–2. Although language is the most obvious area that is largely controlled by the left hemisphere, the left hemisphere is also generally considered to be dominant for limb praxis (i.e., performing complex movements, such as brushing teeth, to command or imitation) and has been associated with the cluster of deficits identified as Gerstmann syndrome (i.e., finger agnosia, dyscalculia, dysgraphia, and right-left disorientation). In contrast, the right hemisphere is thought to play a more important role in controlling visuospatial abilities and hemispatial attention, which are associated with the clinical presentations of constructional apraxia and neglect, respectively.

Although lateralized deficits such as these are typically characterized in terms of damage to the right or left hemisphere, the patient's performance can also be characterized in terms of preserved brain functions. In other words, it is the remaining intact brain tissue that drives many behavioral responses following injury to the brain—not only the absence of critical brain tissue.

Table 5.2–1
Temporal Orientation Schedule

Administration

What is today's date? (The patient is required to give month, day, and year)

What day of the week is it?

What time is it now? (Examiner makes sure that the patient cannot look at a watch or clock)

Scoring

Day of week: 1 error point for each day removed from the correct day to a maximum of 3 points

Day of month: 1 error point for each day removed from the correct day to a maximum of 15 points

Month: 5 error points for each month removed from the correct month with the qualification that, if the stated date is within 15 days of the correct date, no points are scored for the incorrect month (for example, May 29 for June 2 = 4 points off)

Year: 10 error points for each year removed from the correct year to a maximum of 60 points with the qualification that, if the stated date is within 15 days of the correct date, no points are scored for the incorrect year (for example, December 26, 1982, for January 2, 1983 = 7 points off)

Time of day: 1 error point for each 30 minutes removed from the correct time to a maximum of 5 points

Courtesy of Arthur L. Benton, Ph.D.

Bender Visual Motor Gestalt Test

This test of visuomotor coordination is useful for both children and adults. It was designed in 1938 by Lauretta Bender of New York University Medical Center and Bellevue Psychiatric Hospital, who used it to evaluate maturational levels in children. Developmentally, a child younger than 3 years of age is generally unable to reproduce any of the test's designs meaningfully. About 4 years of age, a child may be able to copy several designs but does so poorly. At about age 6, a child should produce some recognizable, although still uneven, representations of all the designs. By age 10 and certainly by age 12, a child's copies should be reasonably accurate and well organized. Bender also presented studies of adults with cognitive disorders, mental retardation, aphasias, psychoses, neuroses, and malingering.

The test material consists of nine separate designs, adapted from those used by Max Wertheimer in his studies in gestalt psychology. Each design is printed against a white background on a separate card (Fig. 5.2–3). Presented with unlined paper, patients are asked to copy each design with the card in

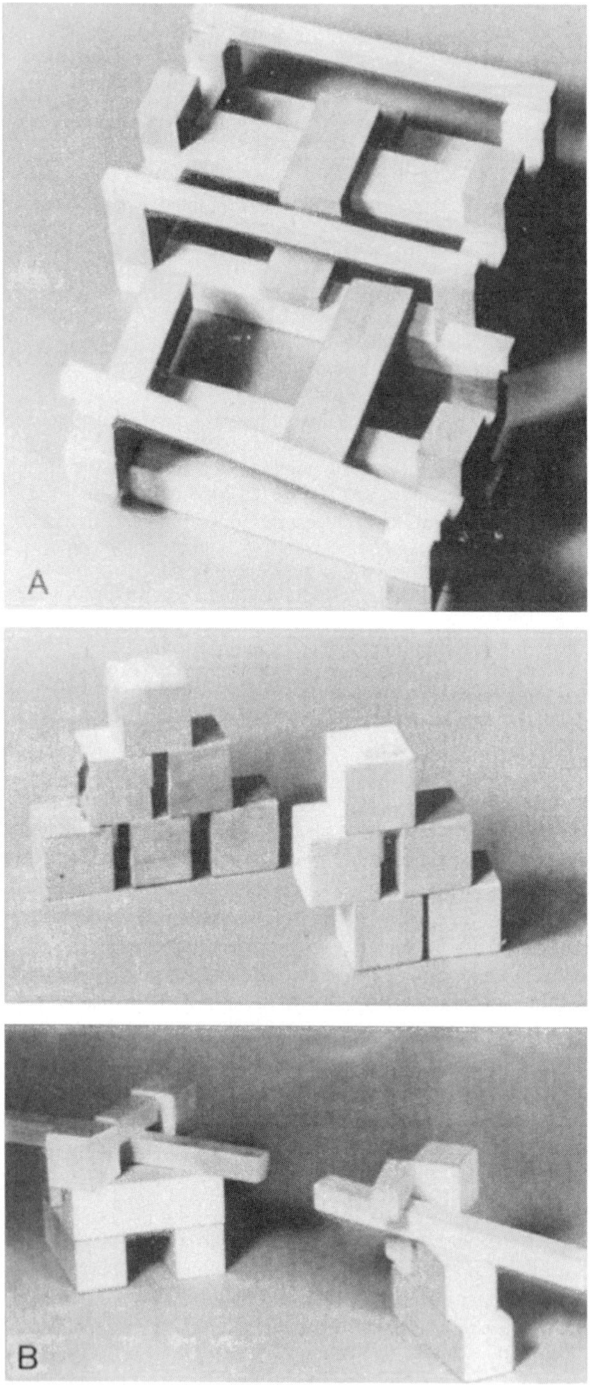

FIGURE 5.2–2

Examples of "closing-in" error **(A)** and neglect of left side **(B)** on the three-dimensional constructional praxis test. (Reprinted with permission from Benton AL, Sivan AB, Hamsher K deS, Varney NR, Spreen O. *Contributions to Neuropsychological Assessment.* 2nd ed. New York: Oxford University Press; 1983:121.)

Table 5.2–2
Selected Neuropsychological Deficits Associated with Left or Right Hemisphere Damage

Left Hemisphere	Right Hemisphere
Aphasia	Visuospatial deficits
Right-left disorientation	Impaired visual perception
Finger agnosia	Neglect
Dysgraphia (aphasic)	Dysgraphia (spatial, neglect)
Dyscalculia (number alexia)	Dyscalculia (spatial)
Constructional apraxia (details)	Constructional apraxia (Gestalt)
Limb apraxia	Dressing apraxia
	Anosognosia

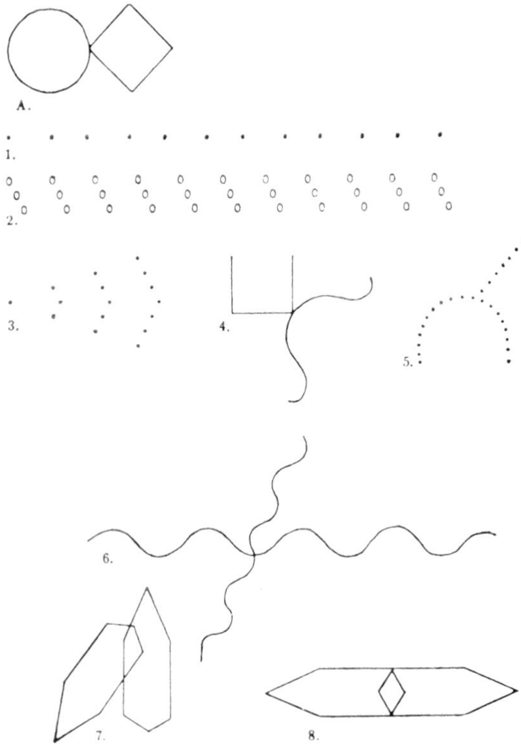

FIGURE 5.2–3

Text figures from the Bender Visual Motor Gestalt test, adapted from Max Wertheimer. (From Bender L. *A Visual Motor Gestalt Test and Its Clinical Use.* New York: American Orthopsychiatric Association; 1938:33.)

front of them. There is no time limit. This phase of the test is highly structured and does not investigate memory function, because the cards remain in front of patients while they copy them. Many clinicians include a subsequent recall phase, in which (after an interval of 45 to 60 seconds) patients are asked to reproduce as many of the designs as they can from memory. This phase not only investigates visual memory, but also presents a less structured situation, in which patients must rely essentially on their own resources. It is often particularly helpful to compare the patient's functioning under the two conditions.

The Bender Gestalt Test is probably used most frequently with adults as a screening device for signs of organic dysfunction. Evaluation of the protocol depends on the form of the reproduced figures and on their relation to one another and to the whole spatial background (Figs. 5.2–4 and 5.2–5).

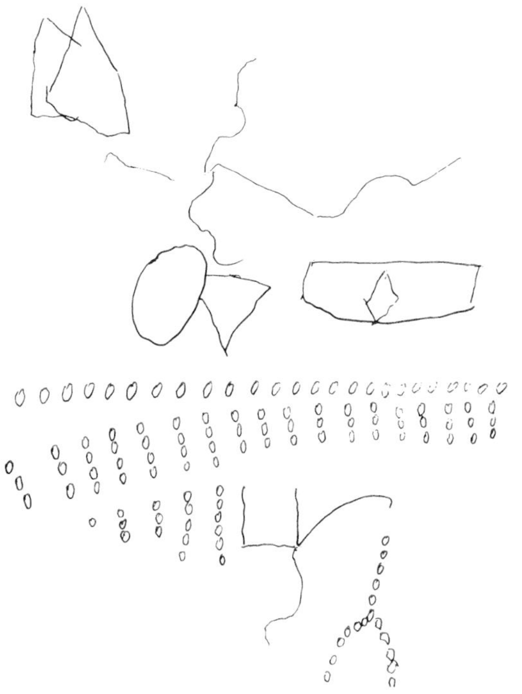

FIGURE 5.2–4
Bender gestalt drawing of a 57-year-old, brain-damaged female patient.

Complex Visual Discrimination

Although the inability to recognize familiar faces (prosopagnosia) is an uncommon disorder, defective discrimination of unfamiliar faces is a common finding in patients with right-hemisphere or bilateral lesions. The Facial Recognition Test, in which a patient is required to identify a photograph of a face originally presented in a front view when it is included in various displays (e.g., side view and a front view with shadows), produces a high frequency of failure in patients with posterior right hemisphere lesions. Performance is generally intact in patients with left hemisphere lesions (provided that receptive language is not seriously limited) and in patients with schizophrenia.

The Judgment of Line Orientation Test has been found to demonstrate failing performance in an impressive proportion of patients with right hemisphere disease. The test requires matching the slope of visually presented lines or pairs of lines. As depicted in Figure 5.2–6, the patient points to or verbally identifies the lines of the display that correspond to the angular orientation of each pair of lines. As with facial recognition, patients with right hemisphere lesions are frequently defective in visuospatial tests, whereas patients with left hemisphere disease perform within the normal range.

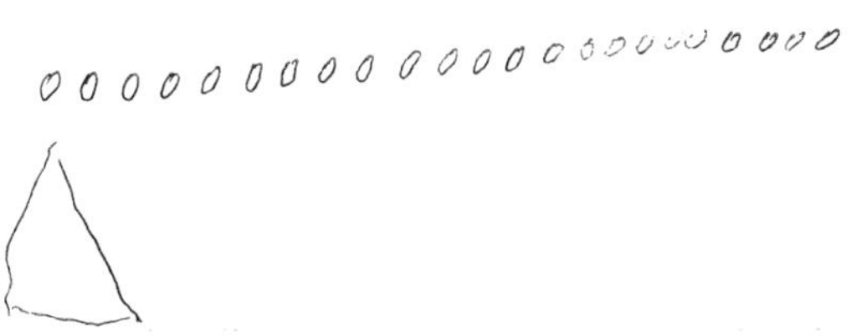

FIGURE 5.2–5
Bender gestalt recall of the 57-year-old, brain-damaged female patient in Figure 5.2–4.

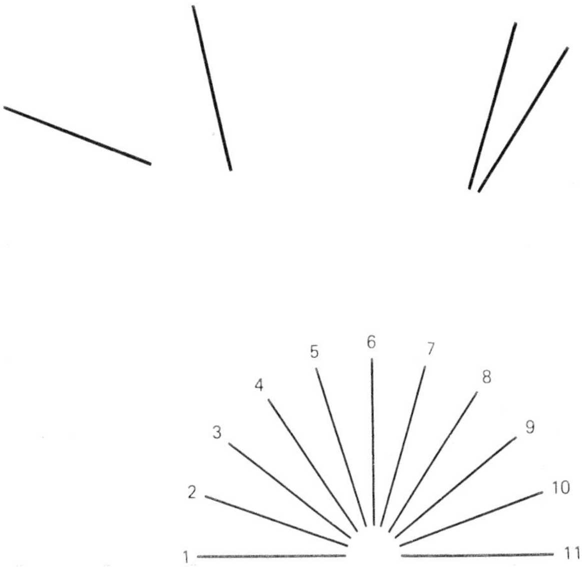

FIGURE 5.2–6
Double-line stimuli that are matched to the multiple choice card below on the Judgment of Line Orientation Test. (Reprinted with permission from Benton AL, Sivan AB, Hamsher K deS, Varney NR, Spreen O. *Contributions to Neuropsychological Assessment. A Clinical Manual.* 2nd ed. New York: Oxford University Press; 1994.)

LANGUAGE

Relatively minor defects in the use of language may be valid indicators of the presence of brain disease. The dominant hemisphere controls language function. The affective part of speech that conveys mood is called *prosody* and is controlled by the nondominant hemisphere. Fluency is tested by asking patients to give all the words they can think of beginning with a given letter of the alphabet. Aphasic patients with left hemisphere disease fail this task. Variables influencing language tests are educational background, sex, and age. Reading and writing are also associated with the dominant hemisphere and are tested by asking patients to read aloud from prepared material and to write their names or a brief passage. Dyslexia and dysgraphia are suspected if patients have difficulties in performing these tasks.

The Boston Diagnostic Aphasia Examination includes a speech rating scale that is useful for comparing with test scores and a brief schedule of items for assessing ideomotor praxis—that is, symbolic buccofacial and limb movements to exhibit gestures and to demonstrate the use of imagined or real objects.

ATTENTION AND CONCENTRATION

The capacity to sustain a maximal level of attention over a period is sometimes impaired in brain-damaged patients, and this impairment is reflected in an oscillation in performance level for a continuous or repeated activity. Some evidence indicates that the instability in performance is related to an electro-

encephalographic abnormality and that an inexplicable decline in performance is related temporally to the occurrence of certain types of abnormal electrical activity. Simple reaction time provides a convenient measure of the variability and speed of simple responses.

The reaction time needed to respond to a stimulus is impaired in 40 to 45 percent of brain-damaged patients and is a sensitive indicator of overall cerebral integrity. Comparison of the reaction times of the right and left hands often provides an indication of the site of the lesion in a patient and of unilateral cerebral disease.

COMPREHENSIVE TESTING

Several test batteries have been developed to help in neuropsychological and neuropsychiatric evaluation. Among them are the Luria-Nebraska and the Halstead-Reitan neuropsychological test batteries.

Luria-Nebraska Neuropsychological Battery

Based on the work of the Russian neuropsychologist Alexander Luria, the Luria-Nebraska Neuropsychological Battery was developed at the University of Nebraska. The test assesses a wide range of cognitive functions: memory; motor functions; rhythm; tactile, auditory, and visual functions; receptive and expressive speech; writing; spelling; reading; and arithmetic. The test is designed for persons who are at least 15 years of age, and a children's version can be used with 8- to 12-year-olds. The test is extremely sensitive for identifying specific types of problems (e.g., dyslexia and dyscalculia), rather than being limited to global impressions of brain dysfunction. It also helps localize the various cortical zones that are involved in a particular function and is useful in establishing left or right cerebral dominance.

Halstead-Reitan Battery of Neuropsychological Tests

In the early 1940s, Ward Halstead and his student Ralph Reitan developed a battery of tests that was used to determine the location and the effects of specific brain lesions. The battery is composed of 10 tests.

1. Category test: Patients must discover the common element in a set of pictures; the test measures concept function, abstraction, and visual acuity.
2. Tactual performance test: Patients place shapes in a form board while blindfolded and then must recall the arrangement of the board; the performance tests dexterity, spatial memory, and tactual discrimination.
3. Rhythm test: Patients identify 30 pairs of rhythmic beats as either the same or different to test auditory perception, attention, and concentration.
4. Finger-oscillation test: Patients tap the index finger of each hand in a measured 10-second period; the test measures dexterity and motor speed.
5. Speech-sounds perception test: Patients match 60 nonsense syllables that they hear with several printed alternatives; the test measures auditory discrimination and phonetic skills.
6. Trail-making test: Patients first connect 25 numbered circles in order and then connect 25 lettered and numbered circles in order, alternating between numbered and alphabetical circles; the procedure tests visuomotor perception and motor speed.
7. Critical flicker frequency: Patients note when a flickering light becomes steady for a test of visual perception.
8. Time sense test: Patients judge, without looking, the time it takes for the second hand of a watch to make several revolutions as a test of memory and spatial perception.
9. Aphasia screening test: Patients must name objects, read, write, calculate, draw shapes, identify body parts, perform acts, and differentiate between left and right as a means of testing a wide range of verbal and nonverbal brain functions.
10. Sensory-perceptual tests: Patients perform several tasks with eyes closed—such as identifying where they are touched simultaneously on the hand and the face (simultaneous sensory stimulation test), which finger is touched (finger localization), what coins are placed in the hand (stereognosis), and what numbers are written on the skin (tactile perception).

The Halstead-Reitan Battery has the advantage of providing a uniform profile of scores that must be weighed against the considerable time required for administration. The test can differentiate those who are brain damaged from neurologically intact persons. Persons with schizophrenia tend to perform above the level of subacutely brain-damaged patients but not differently from those with chronic brain damage. Moreover, the pattern of deficits on the Halstead-Reitan Battery is similar in patients with brain damage and with schizophrenia.

RELIABILITY AND VALIDITY

The reliability and validity of neuropsychological tests may be affected by many factors. Mood states, especially anxiety and depression, may change scores from one test administration to the next. Reliability is also affected by motivation, effort, and cooperation, and changes in clinical status can alter test-retest performance.

Results may be confounded by medication effects. Anticonvulsants typically decrease performance in all areas. Antipsychotics, however, have either negligible or mildly positive effects in patients with schizophrenia.

THERAPEUTIC DISCUSSION OF RESULTS

A key component of the neuropsychological examination process is the opportunity to discuss results of the examination with the patient and family or other caregivers. This meeting can be a powerful therapeutic opportunity to educate them and clarify individual and relationship issues that can affect the patient's functioning. If the patient's active cooperation in the initial examination was enlisted appropriately, the patient will be optimally prepared to invest value and confidence in the findings of the examination. At the time of the results discussion, it is useful to review the goals of the examination with the patient and supportive family or caregivers and to clarify the expectations of those who are present. Typically, these sessions include information about the patient's diagnosis,

Table 5.2–3
Selected Neuropsychological Tests and Function Assessed by Cognitive Domain

Executive functioning	
Category Test	Concept generation, mental shifting
Wisconsin Card Sorting Test	Concept generation, mental shifting
Tower of Hanoi	Planning, organization
Verbal Fluency	Word generation to phonemes
Raven's Progressive Matrices Test	Nonverbal reasoning
Trail Making Test	Simple mental shifting
Mazes (WISC-III)	Planning, visuomotor organization

Attention, concentration, orientation, vigilance	
Continuous Performance Test	Target stimulus selection
Cancellation Tests	Target search amid competing arrays
Stroop Color Word Test	Suppression of distracting visual stimuli
Paced Auditory Serial Addition Task	Sustained attention and mental tracking
WISC-III Symbol Search	Target stimulus search
Symbol Digit Modalities Test	Written and oral coding

Receptive and expressive language	
Peabody Picture Vocabulary Test-III	One-word receptive and expressive vocabulary
Gardner Expressive One Word Picture Vocabulary Test—Revised	Single-word expressive language
Gardner Receptive One Word Picture Vocabulary Test—Revised	Single-word receptive language
Auditory Analysis Test	Sort, order, synthesize auditory perceptual elements
Token Test	Comprehend verbal instructions, grammatical complexity, attention
Boston Naming Test	Visual confrontation naming
Verbal Fluency	Word retrieval to letter cue
Aphasia Screening Test	Receptive and expressive language screen
Comprehensive Evaluation of Language Functions—Revised	Receptive and expressive language
Test of Language Development—2	Receptive and expressive language
Automatic Language Sequences	Alphabet and number sequencing

Sensory-perceptual examination	
Reitan-Klove Sensory-Perceptual Examination	Tactile, auditory, and visual stimulation screen

Motor examination	
Reitan-Klove Lateral Dominance Examination	Knowledge of right and left, body parts
Benton Right-Left Orientation Test	Knowledge of right and left
Finger Tapping Test	Fine-motor speed
Grip Strength (Dynamometer) Test	Comparative strength
Grooved Pegboard Test	Fine-motor dexterity and speed
Purdue Pegboard Test	Fine-motor dexterity and speed
Luria Motor Sequences	Organization of motor sequences
Rapid Alternating Movements	Cerebellar screen

Visuospatial analysis and constructional skills	
Developmental Test of Visual-Motor Integration	Design copying
Benton Judgment of Line Orientation	Perception, matching of visuospatial orientation
Benton Facial Recognition Test	Face discrimination
Hooper Visual Organization Test Drawings	Mental organization of visual percept free drawing

Learning and retrieval	
Selective Reminding Test	Word list learning and retrieval
California Verbal Learning Test	Word list learning and retrieval
Rey-Osterrieth Complex Figure	Design copying, immediate recall, delayed retrieval
Benton Visual Recognition Test	Design copying, immediate retrieval
Story recall	Retrieval of contextual verbal information
Sentence memory	Auditory and verbal retrieval
Composite memory batteries	
Wide range assessment of memory and language	
Test of memory and learning	
Children's Memory Scale	

Courtesy of Ida Sue Baron, Ph.D., and Eileen B. Fennell, Ph.D.

with emphasis upon the natural course and prognosis as well as compensation and coping strategies for the patient and family. If findings show evidence of chronic or progressive neurological disease, these issues must be explicitly discussed, including rehabilitative sources. It is equally important to relate the impact of the results to the patient's current living circumstances, future goals, and course of adjustment. Strong emotions and underlying tensions within family relationships frequently come to light in the context of honest discussion, and so the results discussion can be an important therapeutic opportunity to model effective communication and problem-solving techniques.

A list of selected neuropsychological tests used by psychologists is provided in Table 5.2–3.

References

Axelrod BN, Goldman RS, Henry RR. Sensitivity of the Mini-Mental State Examination to frontal lobe dysfunction in normal aging. *J Clin Psychol.* 1992;48:68.

Bryson GJ, Silverstein ML, Nathan A, Stephen L. Differential rate of neuropsychological dysfunction in psychiatric disorders: comparison between the Halstead-Reitan and Luria-Nebraska batteries. *Percept Mot Skills.* 1993;76:305.

Chouinard MJ, Braun CM-J. A meta analysis of the relative sensitivity of neuropsychological screening tests. *J Clin Exp Neuropsychol.* 1993;15:591.

Cohen RJ, Swerdlik ME. *Psychological Testing and Assessment: An Introduction to Tests and Measurement.* 5th ed. New York: McGraw-Hill; 2002.

Crossen JR, Wiens AN. Comparison of the Auditory-Verbal Learning Test (AVLT) and California Verbal Learning Test (CVLT) in a sample of normal subjects. *J Clin Exp Neuropsychol.* 1995;16:190.

Csepe V, Osman-Sagi J, Molnar M, Gosy M. Impaired speech perception in aphasic patients: event-related potential and neuropsychological assessment. *Neuropsychologia.* 2001;39:1194.

Goldberg TE, Hyde TM, Kleinman JE, Weinberger DR. Course of schizophrenia:

neuropsychological evidence for a static encephalopathy. *Schizophr Bull.* 1993;19:797.

Grant I, Adams KM. *Neuropsychological Assessment of Neuropsychiatric Disorders.* 2nd ed. New York: Oxford University Press; 1996.

Hanson SL, Tucker DM. *Neuropsychological Assessment.* Philadelphia: Hanley & Belfus; 1992.

Heilman KM, Valenstein E, eds. *Clinical Neuropsychology.* 3rd ed. New York: Oxford University Press; 1993.

Kempen JM, Kritchevsky M, Feldman ST. Effect of visual impairment on neuropsychological test performance. *J Clin Exp Neuropsychol.* 1994;16:223.

Lemsky CM. Neuropsychological assessment and treatment planning. In: Groth-Marnat G, ed. *Neuropsychological Assessment in Clinical Practice: A Guide to Test Interpretation and Integration.* New York: John Wiley & Sons; 2000:535.

Lezak MD. *Neuropsychological Assessment.* 3rd ed. New York: Oxford University Press; 1995.

Mittenberg W, Azrin R, Millsaps C, Heilbronner R. Identification of malingered head injury on the Wechsler Memory Scale–Revised. *Psychol Assess.* 1993;5:34.

Nadolne MJ, Stringer AY. Ecologic validity in neuropsychological assessment: prediction of wayfinding. *J Int Neuropsychol Soc.* 2001;7:675.

Reitan RM, Wolfson D. Conventional intelligence measurements and neuropsychological concepts of adaptive abilities. *J Clin Psychol.* 1992;48:521.

Swanda RM, Haaland KY, LaRue A. Clinical neuropsychology and intellectual assessment of adults. In: Sadock BJ, Sadock VA, eds. *Kaplan & Sadock's Comprehensive Textbook of Psychiatry.* 7th ed. Vol 1. Baltimore: Lippincott Williams & Wilkins; 2000:689.

6 Theories of Personality and Psychopathology

▲ 6.1 Sigmund Freud: Founder of Classic Psychoanalysis

Psychoanalysis both as a theory and a treatment has evolved immeasurably since Sigmund Freud created the discipline in the waning years of the 19th century. Some of Freud's ideas have been revised as a result of systematic research from experimental psychology and neuroscience. Freud always predicted that such revisions would occur as knowledge about brain mechanisms increased. Nevertheless, certain basic tenets of Freud's thinking have remained central to psychiatric and psychotherapeutic practice. Among these are the notion of psychic determination, unconscious mental activity, and the role of childhood experience in shaping the adult personality.

The role of meaning was also central to Freud's vision of psychoanalysis. In his view, symptoms, thoughts, feelings, and behavior could all be viewed as the final common pathways of meaningful psychological processes, many of which were unconscious. Even when biological factors influence the pathogenesis of a disorder, the symptoms nevertheless have psychological meaning to the person. For example, in auditory hallucinations, biological mechanisms may produce the symptom, but the content of that symptom and its meaning to the patient relate to specific psychological characteristics unique to that patient. The role of unconscious factors in determining the shape of symptoms and their meaning is crucial to a psychoanalytic point of view.

In addition, as William Wordsworth noted, "The child is father of the man." In other words, childhood experiences are repeated throughout life and are critical in determining one's adult relationships. We now know that childhood experience is pivotal in creating neural networks that shape the personality and persons' expectations of how others will respond to them.

Certain principles of technique, such as resistance, transference, and countertransference, are also at the core of psychoanalysis as a treatment. Freud recognized that patients often *resist* the physician's efforts to heal. For example, when he asked patients to say whatever came to mind, a technique known as *free association*, some patients either became silent or were unable to follow his suggestion. Freud ultimately had the insight that patients are often unconsciously ambivalent about getting better, so they oppose the efforts of the physician to help them. Freud developed the idea while working with psychoanalytic patients, but the contemporary psychiatrist will see resistance with most patients in everyday practice. Mundane behaviors such as forgetting medication, missing a scheduled appointment, and neglecting to fill a prescription may all reflect unconscious resistance to getting better.

The other cornerstones of technique in psychoanalysis involve transference and countertransference. *Transference* is the patient's displacement onto the analyst of early wishes and feelings toward persons from the past. Some resistances may emerge because patients experience the psychiatrist as a parental figure from the past, and they seek to defy the perceived parental control. A contemporary view of transference would acknowledge that the analyst or physician's real characteristics always influence the transference. In other words, one could describe transference as an admixture of figures from the patient's past and the *real relationship* with the clinician in the present. *Countertransference* is the flip side of transference—the clinician's feelings toward the patient, based on a mixture of the real characteristics of the patient and qualities associated with figures from the clinician's past.

Freud was convinced that the unconscious could be directly observed in the psychoanalyst's consulting room. Slips of the tongue, which he called *parapraxes*, often reveal unconscious intent that is outside the individual's awareness. One woman who was asked about her religion responded, "Prostitute, I mean, Protestant." Her guilt feelings about her sexuality had overridden her conscious intent to identify her religious views. Unconscious mental activity is also seen in dreams and many nonverbal behaviors. As more and more knowledge about implicit and explicit memory has accumulated in neuroscience investigations, the fact that much of mental life is unconscious is no longer controversial.

Psychoanalysis today is recognized as having three crucial aspects: it is a therapeutic technique, a body of scientific and theoretical knowledge, and a method of investigation. This section focuses on psychoanalysis as both a theory and a treatment, but the basic tenets elaborated here have wide applications to nonpsychoanalytic settings in clinical psychiatry.

LIFE OF FREUD

Freud was born on May 6, 1856, in Freiburg, a small town in Moravia, which is now part of the Czech Republic. When Freud

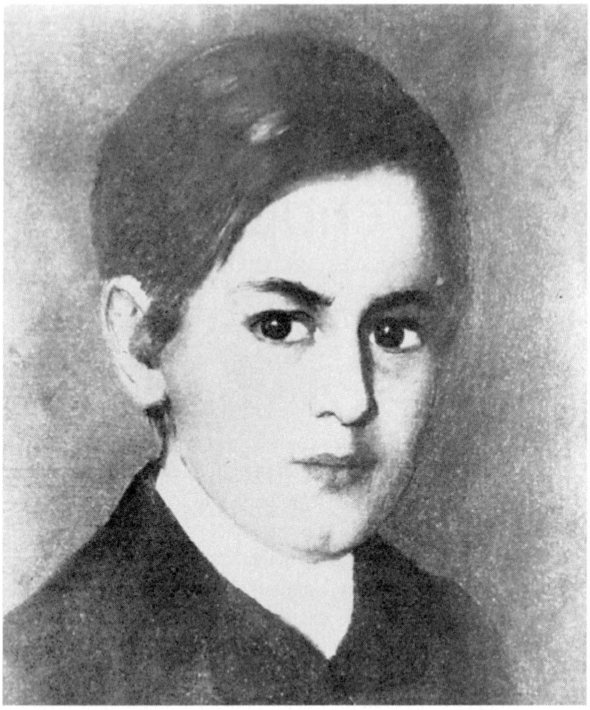

FIGURE 6.1–1
Sigmund Freud as a boy in 1870. (Courtesy of Menninger Foundation Archives, Topeka, KS.)

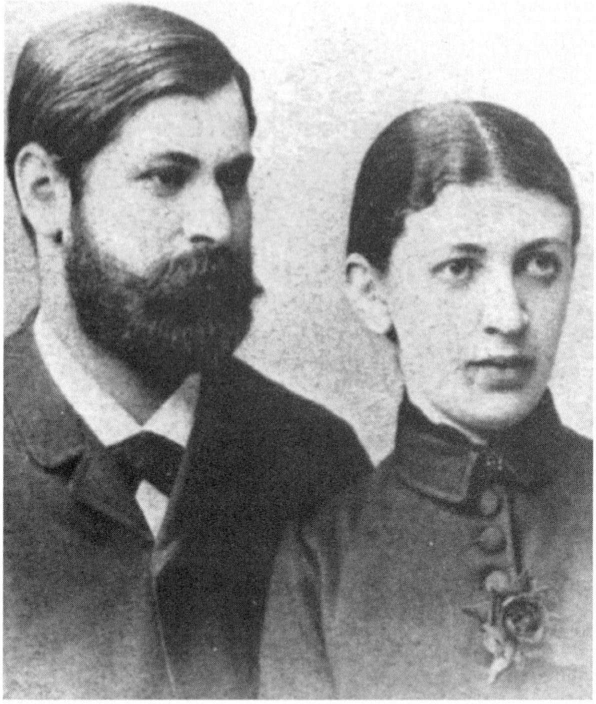

FIGURE 6.1–2
Sigmund Freud and his bride, Martha Bernays, in 1886. (Courtesy of Menninger Foundation Archives, Topeka, KS.)

was 4 years old, his father, a Jewish wool merchant, moved the family to Vienna, where Freud spent most of his life. Following medical school, he specialized in neurology and studied for a year in Paris with Jean-Martin Charcot. He was also influenced by Ambroise-August Liebault and Hippolyte-Marie Bernheim, both of whom taught him hypnosis while he was in France. After his education in France, he returned to Vienna and began clinical work with hysterical patients. Between 1887 and 1897, his work with these patients led him to develop psychoanalysis. Figures 6.1–1 through 6.1–9 trace the highlights of Freud's life. He died in London in 1939.

BEGINNINGS OF PSYCHOANALYSIS

Freud's early career as a neurologist inevitably led him to wonder about the interface between mind and body. In conjunction with his colleague Joseph Breuer (Fig. 6.1–10), he treated a series of female patients suffering from hysterical symptoms that defied neurological explanation. One particular patient, Bertha Pappenheim, who was treated by Breuer as Anna O., intrigued Freud and led him to investigate the use of hypnosis as a routine part of his clinical practice. In 1889, Freud turned to the cathartic method, which he used in conjunction with hypnosis. Using this approach, Freud attempted to remove symptoms through a process of recovering and verbalizing suppressed feelings with which the symptoms were associated. This method came to be known as *abreaction.*

Through his experiments with abreaction and catharsis, Freud learned that his patients were often unable or unwilling

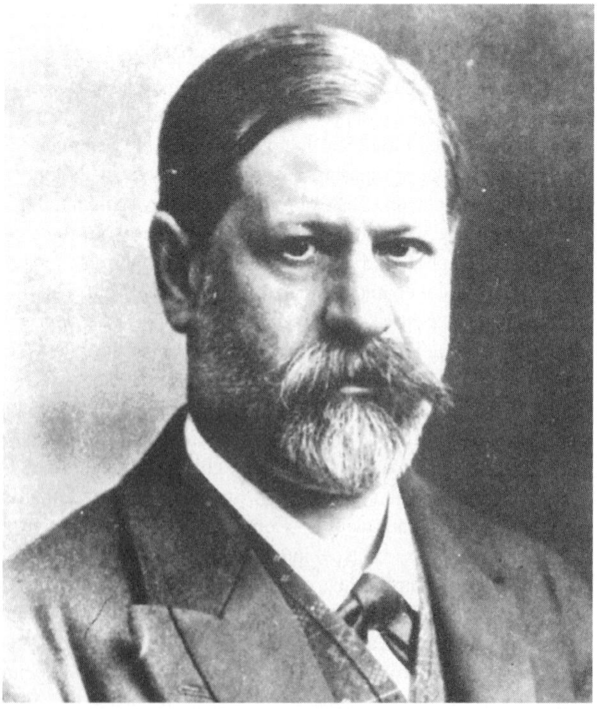

FIGURE 6.1–3
Sigmund Freud in 1903. (Courtesy of Menninger Foundation Archives, Topeka, KS.)

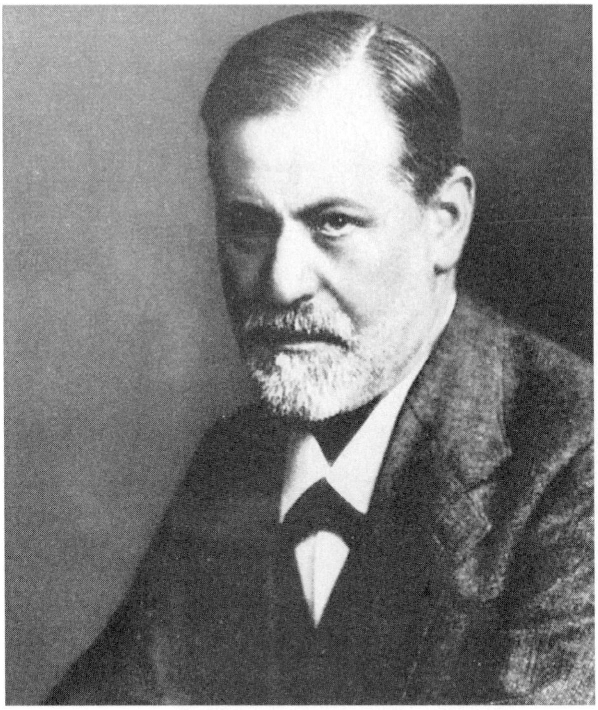

FIGURE 6.1–4
Sigmund Freud in 1911. (Courtesy of Menninger Foundation Archives, Topeka, KS.)

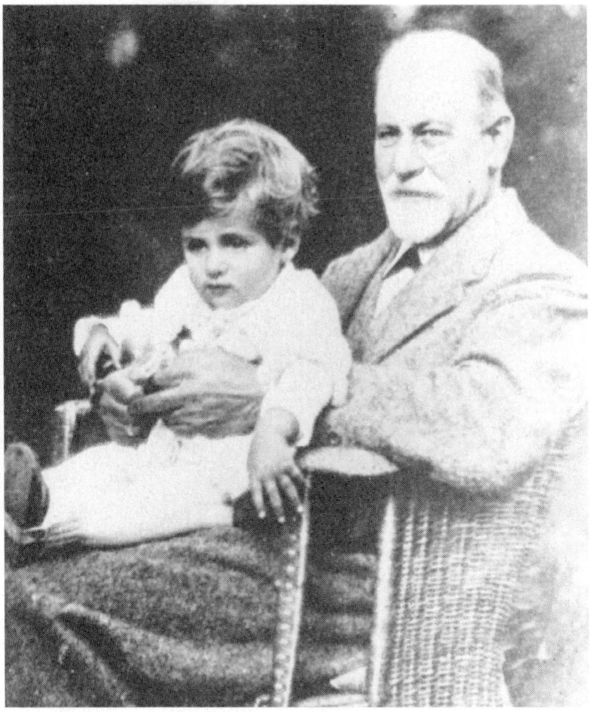

FIGURE 6.1–5
Sigmund Freud with his grandson in 1922. (Courtesy of Menninger Foundation Archives, Topeka, KS.)

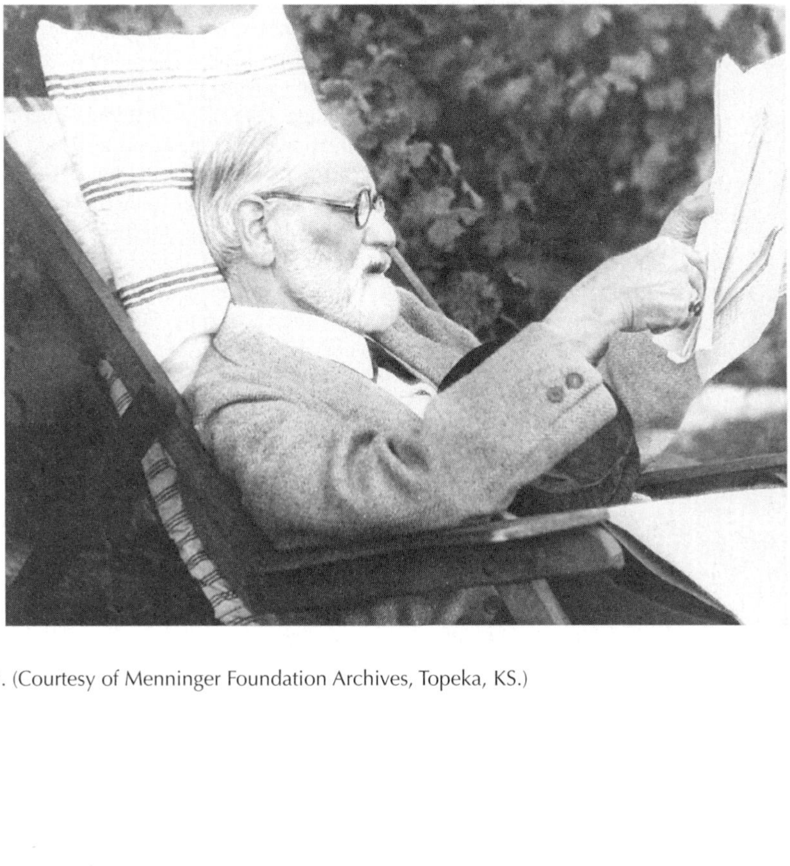

FIGURE 6.1–6
Sigmund Freud in 1935. (Courtesy of Menninger Foundation Archives, Topeka, KS.)

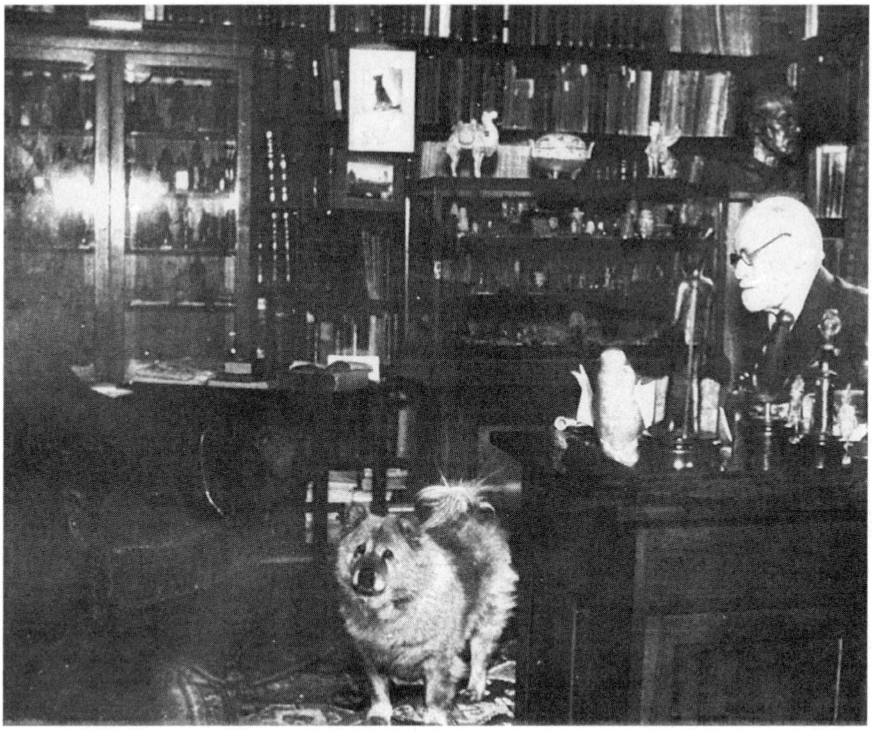

FIGURE 6.1–7
Sigmund Freud, with his chow dog, at work in his office in 1936. (Courtesy of Menninger Foundation Archives, Topeka, KS.)

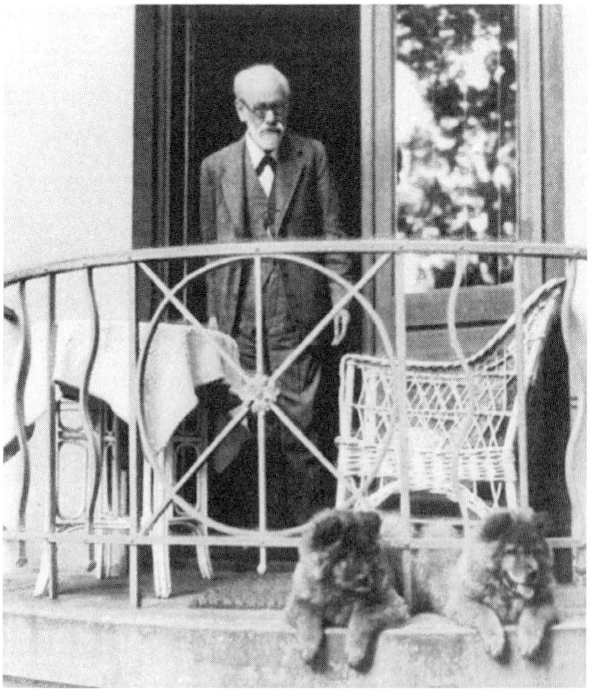

FIGURE 6.1–8
Sigmund Freud with two pet chows in 1938. (Courtesy of Menninger Foundation Archives, Topeka, KS.)

to recount memories that subsequently proved very significant. Freud referred to this reluctance as *resistance,* and later determined that resistance was caused by largely unconscious, active forces in patients' minds. Freud described this active process of excluding distressing material from conscious awareness as *repression,* which he came to regard as essential to symptom formation. Because of the forces of repression and resistance, Freud abandoned his cathartic method and switched to *free association*—inviting his patients to say whatever came into their minds without censoring their thoughts.

Freud's treatment of patients with hysteria during the early 1890s convinced him that childhood sexual seduction played a major role in causing the neuroses. Many of his patients reported such seductions by nursemaids, fathers, and caretakers, and Freud believed that repressed memories of actual sexual trauma created neurotic symptoms.

In the later 1890s, however, he began to reconsider these views; ultimately, he shifted his thinking. The idea that sexual seduction by parental figures was a fantasy began to displace his theory that actual seduction was a pivotal pathogenic factor in neuroses. This shift seemed to be influenced by Freud's own self-analysis, in which he became convinced of childhood sexual fantasies in himself as well as in his patients. Moreover, some patients' reports of abuse sounded so fantastic that it became difficult for Freud to distinguish truth from fiction in such accounts. Contrary to recent reports by Freud's critics, however, he never actually abandoned his belief that real incest

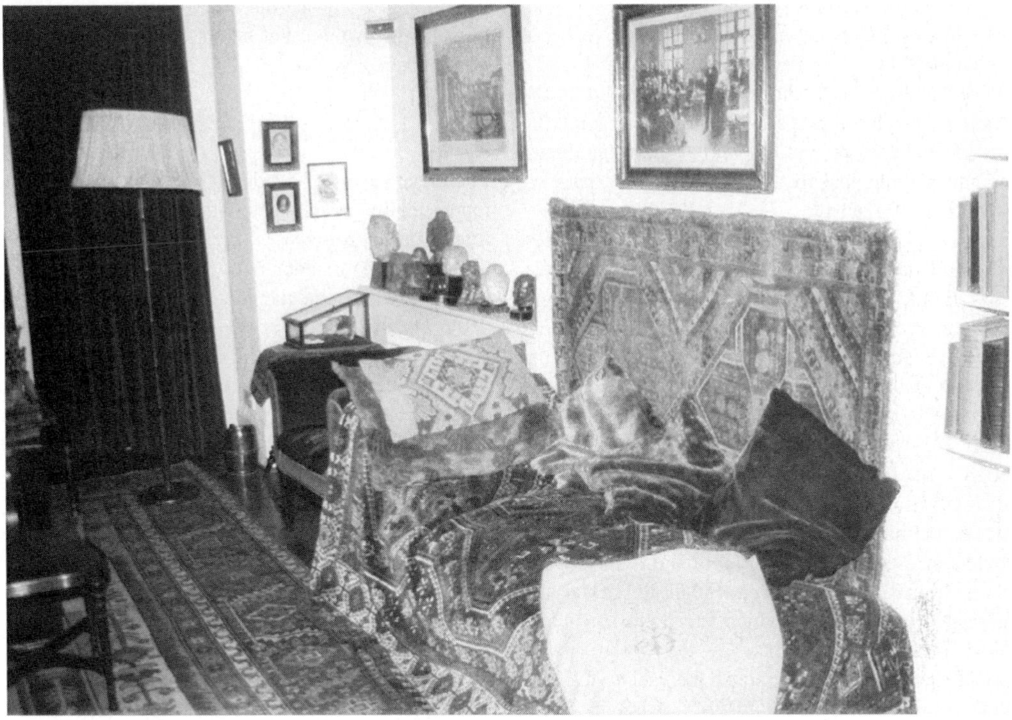

FIGURE 6.1–9
Sigmund Freud's couch in Freud Museum. (Courtesy of Menninger Foundation Archives, Topeka, KS.)

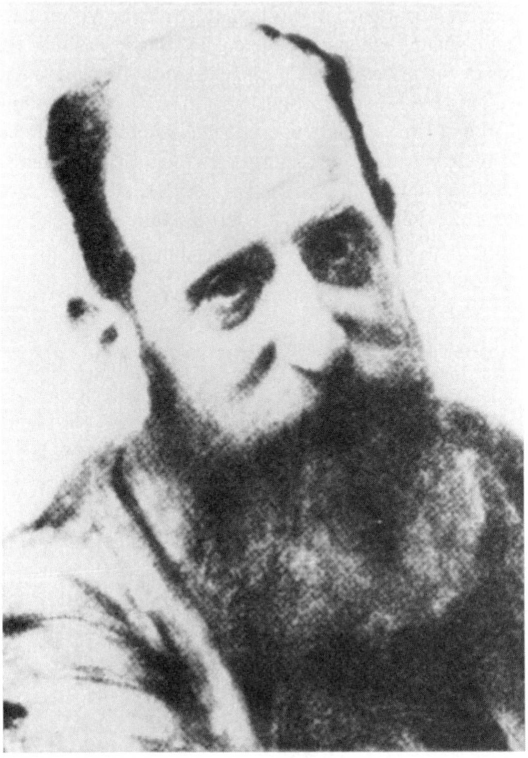

FIGURE 6.1–10
Joseph Breuer (1842–1925). (From Carson RC, Butcher JN, Coleman JC. *Abnormal Psychology and Modern Life.* 8th ed. Boston: Scott, Foresman; 1988:61. Copyright Culver Pictures.)

was a factor contributing to psychopathology in adults, and throughout his career he reasserted that he was convinced of actual sexual seductions of children by parents. Nevertheless, he placed much greater emphasis on childhood sexual fantasies as the core of neuroses. Freud's self-analysis also was instrumental in his deciphering of dreams and led to the appearance in 1900 of perhaps his most monumental work, *The Interpretation of Dreams.*

THE INTERPRETATION OF DREAMS

Freud became aware of the significance of dreams when he noted that patients frequently reported their dreams in the process of free association. Through their further associations to the dream content, he learned that dreams were definitely meaningful, even though meanings were often hidden or disguised. Most of all, Freud was struck by the intimate connection between dream content and unconscious memories or fantasies that were long repressed. This observation led Freud to declare that the interpretation of dreams was the royal road to understanding the unconscious.

In *The Interpretation of Dreams,* Freud asserted that a dream is the disguised fulfillment of an unconscious childhood wish that is not readily accessible to conscious awareness in waking life. In attempting to characterize the psychology of dreaming, Freud laid the foundations for ego psychology. He suggested that unconscious childhood wishes can be transformed into disguised conscious manifestations only if a censor exists in the mind. The censor, acting in the service of the ego, functions to preserve sleep. By disguising

disturbing thoughts and feelings, the censor makes sure that the dreamer's sleep is not disturbed. Moreover, early forms of defense mechanisms in the ego were delineated by Freud's investigation of the different methods of disguise used by the ego—for example, displacement, condensation, and symbolic representation. Freud drew beginning parallels between dream mechanisms and pathological thoughts of psychotic patients in the waking state.

The analysis of dreams elicits material that has been repressed. These unconscious thoughts and wishes include nocturnal sensory stimuli (sensory impressions such as pain, hunger, thirst, urinary urgency), the day residue (thoughts and ideas that are connected with the activities and preoccupations of the dreamer's current waking life), and repressed unacceptable impulses. Because motility is blocked by the sleep state, the dream enables partial but limited gratification of the repressed impulse that gives rise to the dream.

Freud distinguished between two layers of dream content. The *manifest* content refers to what is recalled by the dreamer; the *latent* content involves the unconscious thoughts and wishes that threaten to awaken the dreamer. Freud described the unconscious mental operations by which latent dream content is transformed into manifest dream as the *dream work.* Repressed wishes and impulses must attach themselves to innocent or neutral images to pass the scrutiny of the dream censor. This process involves selection of apparently meaningless or trivial images from the dreamer's current experience, images that are dynamically associated with the latent images that they resemble in some respect.

Condensation

In condensation, several unconscious impulses, wishes, or feelings can be combined and attached to one manifest dream image. For example, a composite character may appear in the dream with a name like one person in the dreamer's life, a beard like another person, and a musical instrument that reflects a third person.

Displacement

In displacement, the energy or intensity associated with one object is diverted to a substitute object that is associatively related but more acceptable to the dreamer's ego. Murderous wishes toward the dreamer's mother, for example, may be redirected toward a neutral or insignificant person in life. Thus, the dream censor displaces affective energy in such a way that the dreamer's sleep can continue undisturbed. Projection, a special instance of displacement, involves the attribution of the dreamer's own unacceptable impulses or wishes to another character in the dream.

Symbolic Representation

Freud noted that the dreamer would often represent highly charged ideas or objects by using innocent images that were in some way connected with the idea or object being represented. In this manner, an abstract concept or a complex set of feelings toward a person could be symbolized by a simple, concrete, or sensory image. Freud noted that symbols have unconscious meanings that can be discerned through the patient's associations to the symbol, but he also believed that certain symbols have universal meanings.

Secondary Revision

The mechanisms of condensation, displacement, and symbolic representation are characteristic of a type of thinking that Freud referred to as *primary process.* This primitive mode of cognitive activity is characterized by illogical, bizarre, and absurd images that seem incoherent. Freud believed that a more mature and reasonable aspect of the ego works during dreams to organize primitive aspects of dreams into a more coherent form. *Secondary revision* is Freud's name for this process, in which dreams become somewhat more rational. The process is related to mature activity characteristic of waking life, which Freud termed *secondary process.*

Affects in Dreams

Secondary emotions may not appear in the dream at all, or they may be experienced in somewhat altered form. For example, repressed rage toward a person's father may take the form of mild annoyance. Feelings may also appear as their opposites.

Anxiety Dreams

Freud's dream theory preceded his development of a comprehensive theory of the ego. Hence, his understanding of dreams stresses the importance of discharging drives or wishes through the hallucinatory contents of the dream. He viewed such mechanisms as condensation, displacement, symbolic representation, projection, and secondary revision primarily as facilitating the discharge of latent impulses, rather than as protecting dreamers from anxiety and pain. Freud understood anxiety dreams as reflecting a failure in the protective function of the dream-work mechanisms. In other words, the repressed impulses succeed in working their way into the manifest content in a more or less recognizable manner.

Punishment Dreams

Dreams in which dreamers experience punishment represented a special challenge for Freud because they appear to represent an exception to his wish fulfillment theory of dreams. He came to understand such dreams as reflecting a compromise between the repressed wish and the repressing agency or conscience. In a punishment dream, the ego anticipates condemnation on the part of the dreamer's conscience if the latent unacceptable impulses are allowed direct expression in the manifest dream content. Hence, the wish for punishment on the part of the patient's conscience is satisfied by giving expression to punishment fantasies.

TOPOGRAPHICAL MODEL OF THE MIND

The publication of *The Interpretation of Dreams* in 1900 heralded the arrival of Freud's topographical model of the mind, in which he divided the mind into three regions: the conscious

system, the preconscious system, and the unconscious system. Each system has its own unique characteristics.

The Conscious

The conscious system in Freud's topographical model is the part of the mind in which perceptions coming from the outside world or from within the body or mind are brought into awareness. Consciousness is a subjective phenomenon whose content can be communicated only by means of language or behavior. Freud assumed that consciousness used a form of neutralized psychic energy that he referred to as *attention cathexis.* In other words, persons were aware of a particular idea or feeling as a result of investing a discrete amount of psychic energy in the idea or feeling.

The Preconscious

The preconscious system comprises those mental events, processes, and contents that can be brought into conscious awareness by the act of focusing attention. Although most persons are not consciously aware of the appearance of their first-grade teacher, they ordinarily can bring this image to mind by deliberately focusing attention on the memory. Conceptually, the preconscious interfaces with both unconscious and conscious regions of the mind. To reach conscious awareness, contents of the unconscious must become linked with words and thus become preconscious. The preconscious also serves to maintain the repressive barrier and to censor unacceptable wishes and desires.

The Unconscious

The unconscious system is dynamic. Its mental contents and processes are kept from conscious awareness through the force of censorship or repression. The unconscious is closely related to instinctual drives. At this point in Freud's theory of development, instincts were thought to consist of sexual and self-preservative drives, and the unconscious was thought to contain primarily the mental representations and derivatives of the sexual instinct.

The content of the unconscious is limited to wishes seeking fulfillment. These wishes provide the motivation for dream and neurotic symptom formation. This view is now considered reductionist.

The unconscious system is characterized by *primary process thinking,* which is principally aimed at facilitating wish fulfillment and instinctual discharge. It is governed by the pleasure principle and therefore disregards logical connections, has no concept of time, represents wishes as fulfillments, permits contradictions to exist simultaneously, and denies the existence of negatives. The primary process is also characterized by extreme mobility of drive cathexis; the investment of psychic energy can shift from object to object without opposition. Memories in the unconscious have been divorced from their connection with verbal symbols. Hence, when words are reapplied to forgotten memory traits, as in psychoanalytic treatment, the verbal recathexis allows the memories to reach consciousness again.

The contents of the unconscious can become conscious only by passing through the preconscious. When censors are overpowered, the elements can enter consciousness.

Limitations of the Topographical Theory

Freud soon realized that two main deficiencies in the topographical theory limited its usefulness. First, many patients' defense mechanisms that guard against distressing wishes, feelings, or thoughts were themselves not initially accessible to consciousness. Thus, repression cannot be identical with the preconscious, because by definition this region of the mind is accessible to consciousness. Second, Freud's patients frequently demonstrated an unconscious need for punishment. This clinical observation made it unlikely that the moral agency making the demand for punishment could be allied with anti-instinctual forces that were available to conscious awareness in the preconscious. These difficulties led Freud to discard the topographical theory, but certain concepts derived from the theory continue to be useful, particularly, primary and secondary thought processes, the fundamental importance of wish fulfillment, the existence of a dynamic unconscious, and a tendency toward regression under frustrating conditions.

INSTINCT OR DRIVE THEORY

After the development of the topographical model, Freud turned his attention to the complexities of instinct theory. Freud was determined to anchor his psychological theory in biology. His choice led to terminological and conceptual difficulties when he used terms derived from biology to denote psychological constructs. *Instinct,* for example, refers to a pattern of species-specific behavior that is genetically derived and therefore is more or less independent of learning. Modern research demonstrating that instinctual patterns are modified through experiential learning, however, has made Freud's instinctual theory problematic. Further confusion has stemmed from the ambiguity inherent in a concept on the borderland between the biological and the psychological: Should the mental representation aspect of the term and the physiological component be integrated or separated? Although *drive* may have been closer than *instinct* to Freud's meaning, in contemporary usage, the two terms are often used interchangeably.

In Freud's view, an instinct has four principal characteristics: source, impetus, aim, and object. The *source* refers to the part of the body from which the instinct arises. The *impetus* is the amount of force or intensity associated with the instinct. The *aim* refers to any action directed toward tension discharge or satisfaction, and the *object* is the target (often a person) for this action.

Instincts

Libido. Freud defined *libido* as "that force by which the sexual instinct is represented in the mind." The association of libido with sexuality is somewhat misleading. Freud's intent was to encompass the general notion of pleasure as well as sexuality and to include both the physiological underpinnings and the mental representations. The linkage of genital sexuality with libido was viewed as the end result of a course of development in which libidinal expression took a variety of forms.

Ego Instincts. From 1905 on, Freud maintained a dual instinct theory, subsuming sexual instincts and ego instincts

connected with self-preservation. Until 1914, with the publication of *On Narcissism,* Freud had paid little attention to ego instincts; in this communication, however, Freud invested ego instinct with libido for the first time by postulating an ego libido and an object libido. Freud thus viewed narcissistic investment as an essentially libidinal instinct and called the remaining nonsexual components the *ego instincts.*

Aggression. When psychoanalysts today discuss the dual instinct theory, they are generally referring to libido and aggression. Freud, however, originally conceptualized aggression as a component of the sexual instincts in the form of sadism. As he became aware that sadism had nonsexual aspects to it, he made finer gradations, which enabled him to categorize aggression and hate as part of the ego instincts and the libidinal aspects of sadism as components of the sexual instincts. Finally, in 1923, to account for the clinical data he was observing, he was compelled to conceive of aggression as a separate instinct in its own right. The source of this instinct, according to Freud, was largely in skeletal muscles, and the aim of the aggressive instincts was destruction.

Life and Death Instincts. Before designating aggression as a separate instinct, Freud, in 1920, subsumed the ego instincts under a broader category of life instincts. These were juxtaposed with death instincts and were referred to as *Eros* and *Thanatos* in *Beyond the Pleasure Principle.* The life and death instincts were regarded as forces underlying the sexual and aggressive instincts. Although Freud could not provide clinical data that directly verified the death instinct, he thought the instinct could be inferred by observing *repetition compulsion,* a person's tendency to repeat past traumatic behavior. Freud thought that the dominant force in biological organisms had to be the death instinct. In contrast to the death instinct, Eros (the life instinct) refers to the tendency of particles to reunite or bind to one another, as in sexual reproduction. The prevalent view today is that the dual instincts of sexuality and aggression suffice to explain most clinical phenomena without recourse to a death instinct.

Pleasure and Reality Principles

In 1911, Freud described two basic tenets of mental functioning, the pleasure principle and the reality principle. He essentially recast the primary process and secondary process dichotomy into the pleasure and reality principles and thus took an important step toward solidifying the notion of the ego. Both principles, in Freud's view, are aspects of ego functioning. The *pleasure principle* is defined as an inborn tendency of the organism to avoid pain and to seek pleasure through the discharge of tension. The *reality principle,* on the other hand, is considered to be a learned function closely related to the maturation of the ego; this principle modifies the pleasure principle and requires delay or postponement of immediate gratification.

Infantile Sexuality

Freud set forth the three major tenets of psychoanalytic theory when he published *Three Essays on the Theory of Sexuality.* First, he broadened the definition of sexuality to include forms of pleasure that transcend genital sexuality. Second, he established a developmental theory of childhood sexuality that delineated the vicissitudes of erotic activity from birth through puberty. Third, he forged a conceptual linkage between neuroses and perversions.

Freud's notion that children are influenced by sexual drives has made some persons reluctant to accept psychoanalysis. Freud noted that infants are capable of erotic activity from birth, but the earliest manifestations of infantile sexuality are basically nonsexual and are associated with such bodily functions as feeding and bowel-bladder control. As libidinal energy shifts from the oral zone to the anal zone to the phallic zone, each stage of development is thought to build on and to subsume the accomplishments of the preceding stage. The *oral stage* occupies the first 12 to 18 months of life, centers on the mouth and lips, and is manifested in chewing, biting, and sucking. The dominant erotic activity of the *anal stage,* from 18 to 36 months of age, involves bowel function and control. The *phallic stage,* from 3 to 5 years of life, initially focuses on urination as the source of erotic activity. Freud suggested that phallic erotic activity in boys is a preliminary stage leading to adult genital activity. Whereas the penis remains the principal sexual organ throughout male psychosexual development, Freud postulated that females have two principal erotogenic zones, the vagina and the clitoris. He thought that the clitoris was the chief erotogenic focus during the infantile genital period but that erotic primacy shifted to the vagina after puberty. Studies of human sexuality have subsequently questioned the validity of this distinction.

Freud discovered that in the psychoneuroses, only a limited number of the sexual impulses that had undergone repression and were responsible for creating and maintaining the neurotic symptoms were normal. For the most part, these were the same impulses that were given overt expression in the perversions. The neuroses, then, were the negative of perversions.

Object Relationships in Instinct Theory

Freud suggested that the choice of a love object in adult life, the love relationship itself, and the nature of all other object relationships depend primarily on the nature and quality of children's relationships during the early years of life. In describing the libidinal phases of psychosexual development, Freud repeatedly referred to the significance of a child's relationships with parents and other significant persons in the environment.

The awareness of the external world of objects develops gradually in infants. Soon after birth, they are primarily aware of physical sensations, such as hunger, cold, and pain, which give rise to tension, and caregivers are regarded primarily as persons who relieve their tension or remove painful stimuli. Recent infant research, however, suggests that awareness of others begins much sooner than Freud originally thought. Table 6.1–1 provides a summary of the stages of psychosexual development and the object relationships associated with each stage. Although the table goes only as far as young adulthood, development is now recognized as continuing throughout adult life.

Table 6.1–1
Stages of Psychosexual Development

Oral Stage			
Definition	The earliest stage of development in which the infant's needs, perceptions, and modes of expression are primarily centered in the mouth, lips, tongue, and other organs related to the oral zone.	Objectives	To establish a trusting dependence on nursing and sustaining objects, to establish comfortable expression and gratification of oral libidinal needs without excessive conflict or ambivalence from oral sadistic wishes.
Description	The oral zone maintains its dominant role in the organization of the psyche through approximately the first 18 months of life. Oral sensations include thirst, hunger, pleasurable tactile stimulations evoked by the nipple or its substitute, sensations related to swallowing, and satiation. Oral drives consist of two separate components: libidinal and aggressive. States of oral tension lead to a seeking for oral gratification, typified by quiescence at the end of nursing. The oral triad consists of the wish to eat, to sleep, and to reach that relaxation that occurs at the end of sucking just before the onset of sleep. Libidinal needs (oral erotism) are thought to predominate in the early parts of the oral phase, whereas they are mixed with more aggressive components later (oral sadism). Oral aggression may express itself in biting, chewing, spitting, or crying. Oral aggression is connected with primitive wishes and fantasies of biting, devouring, and destroying.	Pathological traits	Excessive oral gratifications or deprivation can result in libidinal fixations that contribute to pathological traits. Such traits can include excessive optimism, narcissism, pessimism (often seen in depressive states), and demandingness. Oral characters are often excessively dependent and require others to give to them and to look after them. Such persons want to be fed but may be exceptionally giving to elicit a return of being given to. Oral characters are often extremely dependent on objects for the maintenance of their self-esteem. Envy and jealousy are often associated with oral traits.
		Character traits	Successful resolution of the oral phase provides a basis in character structure for capacities to give to and receive from others without excessive dependence or envy and a capacity to rely on others with a sense of trust, as well as with a sense of self-reliance and self-trust.
Anal Stage			
Definition	The stage of psychosexual development that is prompted by maturation of neuromuscular control over sphincters, particularly the anal sphincters, thus permitting more voluntary control over retention or expulsion of feces.	Objectives	The anal period is essentially a period of striving for independence and separation from the dependence on and control by the parent. The objectives of sphincter control without overcontrol (fecal retention) or loss of control (messing) are matched by the child's attempts to achieve autonomy and independence without excessive shame or self-doubt from loss of control.
Description	This period, which extends roughly from 1 to 3 years of age, is marked by a recognizable intensification of aggressive drives mixed with libidinal components and in sadistic impulses. Acquisition of voluntary sphincter control is associated with an increasing shift from passivity to activity. The conflicts over anal control and the struggle with the parent over retaining or expelling feces in toilet training give rise to increased ambivalence, together with a struggle over separation, individuation, and independence. Anal erotism refers to the sexual pleasure in anal functioning, both in retaining the precious feces and in presenting them as a precious gift to the parent. Anal sadism refers to the expression of aggressive wishes connected with discharging feces as powerful and destructive weapons. These wishes are often displayed in such children's fantasies as bombing and explosions.	Pathological traits	Maladaptive character traits, often apparently inconsistent, are derived from anal erotism and the defenses against it. Orderliness, obstinacy, stubbornness, willfulness, frugality, and parsimony are features of the anal character derived from a fixation on anal functions. When defenses against anal traits are less effective, the anal character reveals traits of heightened ambivalence, lack of tidiness, messiness, defiance, rage, and sadomasochistic tendencies. Anal characteristics and defenses are most typically seen in obsessive-compulsive neuroses.
		Character traits	Successful resolution of the anal phase provides the basis for the development of personal autonomy, a capacity for independence and personal initiative without guilt, a capacity for self-determining behavior without a sense of shame or self-doubt, a lack of ambivalence and a capacity for willing cooperation without either excessive willfulness or sense of self-diminution or defeat.

(*continued*)

Table 6.1–1 (*continued*)

		Urethral Stage	
Definition	This stage was not explicitly treated by Freud but is envisioned as a transitional stage between the anal and the phallic stages of development. It shares some of the characteristics of the preceding anal stage and some from the subsequent phallic stage.	Objectives	Issues of control and urethral performance and loss of control. It is not clear whether or to what extent the objectives of urethral functioning differ from those of the anal period.
Description	The characteristics of the urethral stage are often subsumed under those of the phallic stage. Urethral erotism, however, is used to refer to the pleasure in urination, as well as the pleasure in urethral retention analogous to anal retention. Similar issues of performance and control are related to urethral functioning. Urethral functioning may also be invested with a sadistic quality, often reflecting the persistence of anal sadistic urges. Loss of urethral control, as in enuresis, may frequently have regressive significance that reactivates anal conflicts.	Pathological traits	The predominant urethral trait is that of competitiveness and ambition, probably related to the compensation for shame due to loss of urethral control. In control this may be the start for the development of penis envy, related to the feminine sense of shame and inadequacy in being unable to match the male urethral performance. This is also related to issues of control and shaming.
		Character traits	Besides the healthy effects analogous to those from the anal period, urethral competence provides a sense of pride and self-competence derived from performance. Urethral performance is an area in which the small boy can imitate and match his father's more adult performance. The resolution of urethral conflicts sets the stage for budding gender identity and subsequent identifications.
		Phallic Stage	
Definition	The phallic stage of sexual development begins sometime during the third year of life and continues until approximately the end of the fifth year.	Pathological traits	The derivation of pathological traits from the phallic-oedipal involvement is sufficiently complex and subject to such a variety of modifications that it encompasses nearly the whole of neurotic development. The issues, however, focus on castration in males and on penis envy in females. The other important focus of developmental distortions in this period derives from the patterns of identification that are developed out of the resolution of the oedipal complex. The influence of castration anxiety and penis envy, the defenses against both, and the patterns of identification that emerge from the phallic phase are the primary determinants of the development of human character. They also subsume and integrate the residues of previous psychosexual stages, so that fixations or conflicts that derive from any of the preceding stages can contaminate and modify the oedipal resolution.
Description	The phallic phase is characterized by a primary focus of sexual interests, stimulation, and excitement in the genital area. The penis becomes the organ of principal interest to children of both sexes, with the lack of a penis in the female being considered evidence of castration. The phallic phase is associated with an increase in genital masturbation accompanied by predominantly unconscious fantasies of sexual involvement with the opposite-sex parent. The threat of castration and its related castration anxiety arise in connection with guilt over masturbation and oedipal wishes. During this phase the oedipal involvement and conflict are established and consolidated.		
Objectives	The objective of this phase is to focus erotic interest in the genital area and genital functions. This focusing lays the foundation for gender identity and serves to integrate the residues of previous stages of psychosexual development into a predominantly genital-sexual orientation. The establishing of the oedipal situation is essential for the furtherance of subsequent identifications that will serve as the basis for important and enduring dimensions of character organization.	Character traits	The phallic stage provides the foundations for an emerging sense of sexual identity, a sense of curiosity without embarrassment, initiative without guilt, as well as a sense of mastery not only over objects and persons in the environment but also over internal processes and impulses. The resolution of the oedipal conflict at the end of the phallic period gives rise to powerful internal resources for regulation of drive impulses and their direction to constructive ends. This internal source of regulation is the superego, and it is based on identifications derived primarily from parental figures.

(*co.ntinued*)

Table 6.1–1 (*continued*)

Latency Stage			
Definition	The stage of relative quiescence or inactivity of the sexual drive during the period from the resolution of the Oedipus complex until pubescence (from about 5–6 years until about 11–13 years).	Pathological traits	The danger in the latency period can arise from either a lack of development of inner controls or an excess of them. The lack of control can lead to a failure of the child to sufficiently sublimate energies in the interests of learning and development of skills; an excess of inner control, however, can lead to premature closure of personality development and the precocious elaboration of obsessive character traits.
Description	The institution of the superego at the close of the oedipal period and the further maturation of ego functions allow considerably greater control of instinctual impulses. Sexual interests during this period are generally thought to be quiescent. This is a period of primarily homosexual affiliations for both boys and girls, as well as a sublimation of libidinal and aggressive energies into energetic learning and play activities, exploring the environment, and becoming more proficient in dealing with the world of things and persons around them. It is a period for the development of important skills. The relative strength of regulatory elements often gives rise to patterns of behavior that are somewhat obsessive and hypercontrolling.	Character traits	The latency period has frequently been regarded as a period of relatively unimportant inactivity in the developmental scheme. Recently, great respect has been gained for the developmental processes that take place in this period. Important consolidations and additions are made to the basic postoedipal identifications. It is a period of integrating and consolidating previous attainments in psychosexual development and establishing decisive patterns of adaptive functioning. The child can develop a sense of industry and a capacity for mastery of objects and concepts that allows autonomous function with a sense of initiative without running the risk of failure or defeat or a sense of inferiority. These important attainments need to be further integrated, ultimately as the essential basis for a mature adult life of satisfaction in work and love.
Objectives	The primary objective in this period is the further integration of oedipal identifications and a consolidation of sex-role identity and sex roles. The relative quiescence and control of instinctual impulses allow for the development of ego apparatuses and mastery skills. Further identificatory components may be added to the oedipal ones on the basis of broadening contacts with other significant figures outside the family, such as teachers, coaches, and other adults.		
Genital Stage			
Definition	The genital or adolescent phase of psychosexual development extends from the onset of puberty from ages 11–13 until the person reaches young adulthood. In current thinking, there is a tendency to subdivide this stage into preadolescent, early adolescent, middle adolescent, late adolescent, and even postadolescent periods.	Pathological traits	The pathological deviations due to a failure to achieve successful resolution of this stage of development are multiple and complex. Defects can arise from the whole spectrum of psychosexual residues, since the developmental task of the adolescent period is in a sense a partial reopening and reworking and reintegrating of all those aspects of development. Previous unsuccessful resolutions and fixations in various phases or aspects of psychosexual development will produce pathological defects in the emerging adult personality. A more specific defect from a failure to resolve adolescent issues has been described by Erikson as identity diffusion.
Description	The physiological maturation of systems of genital (sexual) functioning and attendant hormonal systems leads to an intensification of drives, particularly libidinal drives. This produces a regression in personality organization, which reopens conflicts of previous stages of psychosexual development and provides the opportunity for a reresolution of these conflicts in the context of achieving a mature sexual and adult identity.	Character traits	The successful resolution and reintegration of previous psychosexual stages in the adolescent, fully genital phase sets the stage normally for a fully mature personality with a capacity for full and satisfying genital potency and a self-integrated and consistent sense of identity. Such a person has reached a satisfying capacity for self-realization and meaningful participation in the areas of work and love and in the creative and productive application to satisfying and meaningful goals and values. Only in the last few years has the presumed relationship between psychosexual genitality and maturity of personality functioning been put in question.
Objectives	The primary objectives of this period are the ultimate separation from dependence on and attachment to the parents and the establishment of mature, nonincestuous object relations. Related to this are the achievement of a mature sense of personal identity and acceptance and the integration of a set of adult roles and functions that permit new adaptive integrations with social expectations and cultural values.		

Adapted by Glen O. Gabbard, M.D., from Meissner WW. Theories of personality and psychopathology. In: Kaplan HI, Sadock BJ, eds. *Comprehensive Textbook of Psychiatry.* 4th ed. Vol. 1. Baltimore: Williams & Wilkins; 1985:360.

Concept of Narcissism

According to Greek myth, Narcissus, a beautiful youth, fell in love with his reflection in the water of a pool and drowned in his attempt to embrace his beloved image. Freud used the term *narcissism* to describe situations in which an individual's libido was invested in the ego itself rather than in other persons. This concept of narcissism presented him with vexing problems for his instinct theory and essentially violated his distinction between libidinal instincts and ego or self-preservative instincts. Freud's understanding of narcissism led him to use the term to describe a wide array of psychiatric disorders, very much in contrast to the term's contemporary use to describe a specific personality disorder. Freud lumped several disorders together as the narcissistic neuroses, in which a person's libido is withdrawn from objects and turned inward. He believed that this withdrawal of libidinal attachment to objects accounted for the loss of reality testing in psychotic patients; grandiosity and omnipotence in such patients reflected excessive libidinal investment in the ego.

Freud did not limit his use of narcissism to psychoses. In states of physical illness and hypochondriasis, he observed that libidinal investment was frequently withdrawn from external objects and from outside activities and interests. Similarly, he suggested that in normal sleep, libido was also withdrawn and reinvested in a sleeper's own body. Freud regarded homosexuality as an instance of a narcissistic form of object choice, in which persons fall in love with an idealized version of themselves projected onto another person. He also found narcissistic manifestations in the beliefs and myths of primitive people, especially those involving the ability to influence external events through the magical omnipotence of thought processes. In the course of normal development, children also exhibit this belief in their own omnipotence.

Freud postulated a state of primary narcissism at birth in which the libido is stored in the ego. He viewed the neonate as completely narcissistic, with the entire libidinal investment in physiological needs and their satisfaction. He referred to this self-investment as *ego libido*. The infantile state of self-absorption changes only gradually, according to Freud, with the dawning awareness that a separate person—the mothering figure—is responsible for gratifying an infant's needs. This realization leads to the gradual withdrawal of the libido from the self and its redirection toward the external object. Hence, the development of object relations in infants parallels the shift from primary narcissism to object attachment. The libidinal investment in the object is referred to as *object libido*. If a developing child suffers rebuffs or trauma from the caretaking figure, object libido may be withdrawn and reinvested in the ego. Freud called this regressive posture *secondary narcissism*.

Freud used the term *narcissism* to describe many different dimensions of human experience. At times, he used it to describe a perversion in which persons used their own bodies or body parts as objects of sexual arousal. At other times, he used the term to describe a developmental phase, as in the state of primary narcissism. In still other instances, the term referred to a particular object choice. Freud distinguished love objects who are chosen "according to the narcissistic type," in which case the object resembles the subject's idealized or fantasied self-image, from objects chosen according to the "anaclitic," in which the love object resembles a caretaker from early in life. Finally, Freud also used the word *narcissism* interchangeably and synonymously with *self-esteem*.

EGO PSYCHOLOGY

Although Freud had used the construct of the ego throughout the evolution of psychoanalytic theory, ego psychology as it is known today really began with the publication in 1923 of *The Ego and the Id*. This landmark publication also represented a transition in Freud's thinking from the topographical model of the mind to the tripartite structural model of ego, id, and superego. He had observed repeatedly that not all unconscious processes can be relegated to a person's instinctual life. Elements of the conscience, as well as functions of the ego, are clearly also unconscious.

Structural Theory of the Mind

The structural model of the psychic apparatus is the cornerstone of ego psychology. The three provinces—id, ego, and superego—are distinguished by their different functions (Fig. 6.1–11).

Id. Freud used the term *id* to refer to a reservoir of unorganized instinctual drives. Operating under the domination of the primary process, the id lacks the capacity to delay or modify the instinctual drives with which an infant is born. The id should not, however, be viewed as synonymous with the unconscious, because both the ego and the superego have unconscious components.

Ego. The ego spans all three topographical dimensions of conscious, preconscious, and unconscious. Logical and abstract thinking and verbal expression are associated with conscious and preconscious functions of the ego. Defense mechanisms reside in the unconscious domain of the ego. The ego is the executive organ of the psyche and controls motility, perception, contact with reality, and, through the mechanisms of defense available to it, the delay and modulation of drive expression.

Freud believed that the id is modified as a result of the impact of the external world on the drives. The pressures of external reality enable the ego to appropriate the energies of the id to do its work. As the ego brings influences from the external

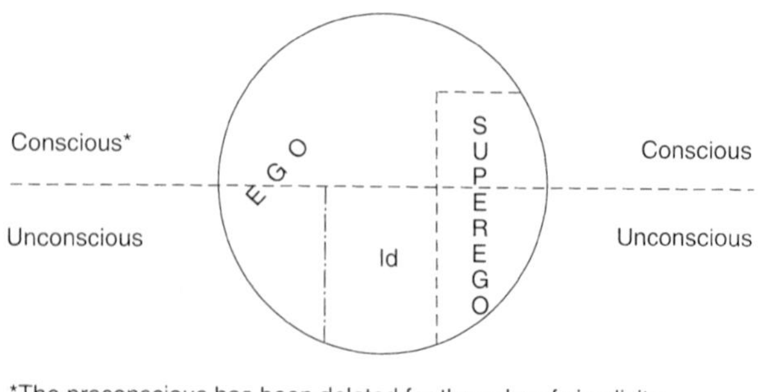

*The preconscious has been deleted for the sake of simplicity.

FIGURE 6.1–11

Freud's structural model. (Reprinted with permission from Gabbard GO. *Psychodynamic Psychiatry in Clinical Practice: The DSM-IV Edition*. Washington, DC: American Psychiatric Press; 1994:31.)

world to bear on the id, it simultaneously substitutes the reality principle for the pleasure principle. Freud emphasized the role of conflict within the structural model and observed that conflict occurs initially between the id and the outside world, only to be transformed later to conflict between the id and the ego.

The third component of the tripartite structural model is the superego. The superego establishes and maintains an individual's moral conscience on the basis of a complex system of ideals and values internalized from parents. Freud viewed the superego as the heir to the Oedipus complex. Children internalize parental values and standards at about the age of 5 or 6 years. The superego then serves as an agency that provides ongoing scrutiny of a person's behavior, thoughts, and feelings; makes comparisons with expected standards of behavior; and offers approval or disapproval. These activities occur largely unconsciously.

The ego ideal is often regarded as a component of the superego. It is an agency that prescribes what a person should do according to internalized standards and values. The superego, by contrast, is an agency of moral conscience that *proscribes*—that is, dictates what a person should *not* do. Throughout the latency period and thereafter, persons continue to build on early identifications through their contact with admired figures who contribute to the formation of moral standards, aspirations, and ideals.

Functions of the Ego

Modern ego psychologists have identified a set of basic ego functions that characterize the operations of the ego. These descriptions reflect the ego activities that are generally regarded as fundamental.

Control and Regulation of Instinctual Drives. The development of the capacity to delay or postpone drive discharge, like the capacity to test reality, is closely related to the early childhood progression from the pleasure principle to the reality principle. This capacity is also an essential aspect of the ego's role as mediator between the id and the outside world. Part of infants' socialization to the external world is the acquisition of language and secondary process or logical thinking.

Judgment. A closely related ego function is judgment, which involves the ability to anticipate the consequences of actions. As with control and regulation of instinctual drives, judgment develops in parallel with the growth of *secondary process thinking.* The ability to think logically allows assessment of how contemplated behavior may affect others.

Relation to Reality. The mediation between the internal world and external reality is a crucial function of the ego. Relations with the outside world can be divided into three aspects: the sense of reality, reality testing, and adaptation to reality. The *sense of reality* develops in concert with an infant's dawning awareness of bodily sensations. The ability to distinguish what is outside the body from what is inside is an essential aspect of the sense of reality, and disturbances of body boundaries, such as depersonalization, reflect impairment in this ego function. *Reality testing,* an ego function of paramount importance, refers to the capacity to distinguish internal fantasy from external reality. This function differentiates psychotic from nonpsychotic persons. *Adaptation to reality* involves persons' ability to use their resources to develop effective responses to changing circumstances on the basis of previous experience with reality.

Object Relationships. The capacity to form mutually satisfying relationships is related in part to patterns of internalization stemming from early interactions with parents and other significant figures. This ability is also a fundamental function of the ego, in that satisfying relatedness depends on the ability to integrate positive and negative aspects of others and self and to maintain an internal sense of others even in their absence. Similarly, mastery of drive derivatives is also crucial to the achievement of satisfying relationships. Although Freud did not develop an extensive object relations theory, British psychoanalysts, such as Ronald Fairbairn (1889–1964) and Michael Balint (1886–1970), elaborated greatly on the early stages in infants' relationships with need-satisfying objects and on the gradual development of a sense of separateness from the mother. Another of their British colleagues, Donald W. Winnicott (1897–1971), described the *transitional object* (e.g., a blanket, teddy bear, or pacifier) as the link between developing children and their mothers. A child can separate from the mother because a transitional object provides feelings of security in her absence. The stages of human development and object relations theory are summarized in Figure 6.1–12.

Synthetic Function of the Ego. First described by Herman Nunberg in 1931, the *synthetic function* refers to the ego's capacity to integrate diverse elements into an overall unity. Different aspects of self and others, for example, are synthesized into a consistent representation that endures over time. The function also involves organizing, coordinating, and generalizing or simplifying large amounts of data.

Primary Autonomous Ego Functions. Heinz Hartmann described the so-called primary autonomous functions of the ego as rudimentary apparatuses present at birth that develop independently of intrapsychic conflict between drives and defenses. These functions include perception, learning, intelligence, intuition, language, thinking, comprehension, and motility. In the course of development, some of these conflict-free aspects of the ego may eventually become involved in conflict. They will develop normally if the infant is raised in what Hartmann referred to as an *average expectable environment.*

Secondary Autonomous Ego Functions. Once the sphere where primary autononomous function develops becomes involved with conflict, so-called *secondary autonomous ego functions* arise in the defense against drives. For example, a child may develop caretaking functions as a reaction formation against murderous wishes during the first few years of life. Later, the defensive functions may be neutralized or deinstinctualized when the child grows up to be a social worker and cares for homeless persons.

Defense Mechanisms

At each phase of libidinal development, specific drive components evoke characteristic ego defenses. The anal phase, for example, is associated with reaction formation, as manifested

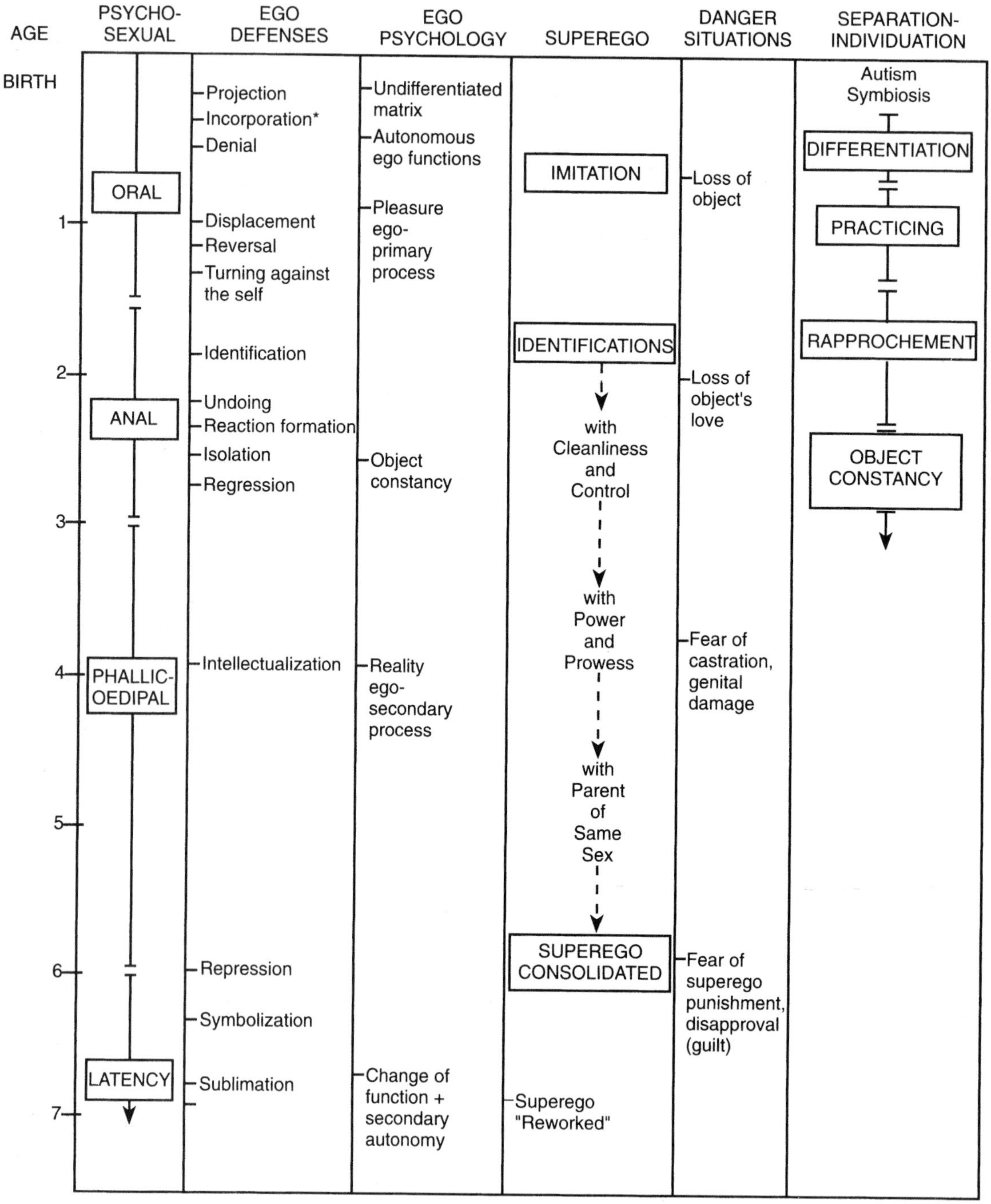

FIGURE 6.1–12

Parallel lines of human development. Asterisk indicates also introjection. (Reprinted with permission from Inderbitzin LB, Luke CM, James ME..Psychoanalytic psychotherapy. In: Stoudemire A, ed. *Human Behavior: An Introduction for Medical Students.* Philadelphia: JB Lippincott; 1990:74.)

by the development of shame and disgust in relation to anal impulses and pleasures.

Defenses can be grouped hierarchically according to the relative degree of maturity associated with them. Narcissistic defenses are the most primitive and appear in children and persons who are psychotically disturbed. Immature defenses are seen in adolescents and some nonpsychotic patients. Neurotic defenses are encountered in obsessive-compulsive and hysterical patients as well as in adults under stress. Table 6.1–2 lists the defense mechanisms according to George Vaillant's classification of the four types.

Theory of Anxiety

Freud initially conceptualized anxiety as "dammed up libido." In other words, a physiological increase in sexual tension leads

Table 6.1–2
Classification of Defense Mechanisms

Narcissistic Defenses[a]			
Denial	Avoiding the awareness of some painful aspect of reality by negating sensory data. Although repression defends against affects and drive derivatives, denial abolishes external reality. Denial may be used in both normal and pathological states.	Projection	Perceiving and reacting to unacceptable inner impulses and their derivatives as though they were outside the self. On a psychotic level, this defense mechanism takes the form of frank delusions about external reality (usually persecutory) and includes both perception of one's own feelings in another and subsequent acting on the perception (psychotic paranoid delusions). The impulses may derive from the id or the superego (hallucinated recriminations) but may undergo transformation in the process. Thus, according to Freud's analysis of paranoid projections, homosexual libidinal impulses are transformed into hatred and then projected onto the object of the unacceptable homosexual impulse.
Distortion	Grossly reshaping external reality to suit inner needs (including unrealistic megalomania beliefs, hallucinations, wish-fulfilling delusions) and using sustained feelings of delusional superiority or entitlement.		
Immature Defenses			
Acting out	Expressing an unconscious wish or impulse through action to avoid being conscious of an accompanying affect. The unconscious fantasy is lived out impulsively in behavior, thereby gratifying the impulse, rather than the prohibition against it. Acting out involves chronically giving in to an impulse to avoid the tension that would result from the postponement of expression.	Passive-aggressive behavior	Expressing aggression toward others indirectly through passivity, masochism, and turning against the self. Manifestations of passive-aggressive behavior include failure, procrastination, and illnesses that affect others more than oneself.
Blocking	Temporarily or transiently inhibiting thinking. Affects and impulses may also be involved. Blocking closely resembles repression but differs in that tension arises when the impulse, affect, or thought is inhibited.	Regression	Attempting to return to an earlier libidinal phase of functioning to avoid the tension and conflict evoked at the present level of development. It reflects the basic tendency to gain instinctual gratification at a less-developed period. Regression is a normal phenomenon as well, as a certain amount of regression is essential for relaxation, sleep, and orgasm in sexual intercourse. Regression is also considered an essential concomitant of the creative process.
Hypochondriasis	Exaggerating or overemphasizing an illness for the purpose of evasion and regression. Reproach arising from bereavement, loneliness, or unacceptable aggressive impulses toward others is transformed into self-reproach and complaints of pain, somatic illness, and neurasthenia. In hypochondriasis, responsibility can be avoided, guilt may be circumvented, and instinctual impulses are warded off. Because hypochondriacal introjects are ego-alien, the afflicted person experiences dysphoria and a sense of affliction.	Schizoid fantasy	Indulging in autistic retreat to resolve conflict and to obtain gratification. Interpersonal intimacy is avoided, and eccentricity serves to repel others. The person does not fully believe in the fantasies and does not insist on acting them out.
Introjection	Internalizing the qualities of an object. Although vital to development, introjection also serves specific defensive functions. When used as a defense, it can obliterate the distinction between the subject and the object. Through the introjection of a loved object, the painful awareness of separateness or the threat of loss may be avoided. Introjection of a feared object serves to avoid anxiety when the aggressive characteristics of the object are internalized, thus placing the aggression under one's own control. A classic example is identification with the aggressor. An identification with the victim may also take place, whereby the self-punitive qualities of the objects are taken over and established within one's self as a symptom or character trait.	Somatization	Converting psychic derivatives into bodily symptoms and tending to react with somatic manifestations, rather than psychic manifestations. In desomatization, infantile somatic responses are replaced by thought and affect; in resomatization, the person regresses to earlier somatic forms in the face of unresolved conflicts.

(continued)

Table 6.1–2 (*continued*)

Neurotic Defenses	
Controlling	Attempting to manage or regulate events or objects in the environment to minimize anxiety and to resolve inner conflicts.
Displacement	Shifting an emotion or drive cathexis from one idea or object to another that resembles the original in some aspect or quality. Displacement permits the symbolic representation of the original idea or object by one that is less highly cathected or evokes less distress.
Externalization	Tending to perceive in the external world and in external objects elements of one's own personality, including instinctual impulses, conflicts, moods, attitudes, and styles of thinking. Externalization is a more general term than projection.
Inhibition	Consciously limiting or renouncing some ego functions, alone or in combination, to evade anxiety arising out of conflict with instinctual impulses, the superego, or environmental forces or figures.
Intellectualization	Excessively using intellectual processes to avoid affective expression or experience. Undue emphasis is focused on the inanimate to avoid intimacy with people, attention is paid to external reality to avoid the expression of inner feelings, and stress is excessively placed on irrelevant details to avoid perceiving the whole. Intellectualization is closely allied to rationalization.
Isolation	Splitting or separating an idea from the affect that accompanies it but is repressed. Social isolation refers to the absence of object relationships.
Rationalization	Offering rational explanations in an attempt to justify attitudes, beliefs, or behavior that may otherwise be unacceptable. Such underlying motives are usually instinctually determined.
Dissociation	Temporarily but drastically modifying a person's character or one's sense of personal identity to avoid emotional distress. Fugue states and hysterical conversion reactions are common manifestations of dissociation. Dissociation may also be found in counterphobic behavior, dissociative identity disorder, the use of pharmacological highs or religious joy.
Reaction formation	Transforming an unacceptable impulse into its opposite. Reaction formation is characteristic of obsessional neurosis, but it may occur in other forms of neuroses as well. If this mechanism is frequently used at any early stage of ego development, it can become a permanent character trait, as in an obsessional character.
Repression	Expelling or withholding from consciousness an idea or feeling. Primary repression refers to the curbing of ideas and feelings before they have attained consciousness: secondary repression excludes from awareness what was once experienced at a conscious level. The repressed is not really forgotten in that symbolic behavior may be present. This defense differs from suppression by effecting conscious inhibition of impulses to the point of losing and not just postponing cherished goals. Conscious perception of instincts and feelings is blocked in repression.
Sexualization	Endowing an object or function with sexual significance that it did not previously have or possessed to a smaller degree to ward off anxieties associated with prohibited impulses or their derivatives.
Mature Defenses	
Altruism	Using constructive and instinctually gratifying service to others to undergo a vicarious experience. It includes benign and constructive reaction formation. Altruism is distinguished from altruistic surrender, in which a surrender of direct gratification or of instinctual needs takes place in favor of fulfilling the needs of others to the detriment of the self, and the satisfaction can only be enjoyed vicariously through introjection.
Anticipation	Realistically anticipating or planning for future inner discomfort. The mechanism is goal-directed and implies careful planning or worrying and premature but realistic affective anticipation of dire and potentially dreadful outcomes.
Asceticism	Eliminating the pleasurable effects of experiences. There is a moral element in assigning values to specific pleasures. Gratification is derived from renunciation, and asceticism is directed against all base pleasures perceived consciously.
Humor	Using comedy to overtly express feelings and thoughts without personal discomfort or immobilization and without producing an unpleasant effect on others. It allows the person to tolerate and yet focus on what is too terrible to be borne; it is different from wit, a form of displacement that involves distraction from the affective issue.
Sublimation	Achieving impulse gratification and the retention of goals but altering a socially objectionable aim or object to a socially acceptable one. Sublimation allows instincts to be channeled, rather than blocked or diverted. Feelings are acknowledged, modified, and directed toward a significant object or goal, and modest instinctual satisfaction occurs.
Suppression	Consciously or semiconsciously postponing attention to a conscious impulse or conflict. Issues may be deliberately cut off, but they are not avoided. Discomfort is acknowledged but minimized.

[a]The categorization of these defenses as narcissistic is controversial. Many psychoanalysts would subsume them under "Immature Defenses."

Adapted by Glen O. Gabbard, M.D., from Vaillant GE. *Adaptation to Life.* Boston: Little, Brown; 1977; Semrad E. The operation of ego defenses in object loss. In: Moriarily DM, ed. *The Loss of Loved Ones.* Springfield, IL: Charles C Thomas; 1967; and Bibring GL, Dwyer TF, Huntington DS, Valenstein AA. A study of the psychological process in pregnancy and of the earliest mother-child relationship: methodological considerations. *Psychoanal Stud Child.* 1961;16:25.

to a corresponding increase in libido, the mental representation of the physiological event. (See Chapter 18 for a discussion of neurasthenia.) The *actual neuroses* are caused by this buildup. Later, with the development of the structural model, Freud developed a new theory of a second type of anxiety that he referred to as *signal anxiety.* In this model, anxiety operates at an unconscious level and serves to mobilize the ego's resources to avert danger. Either external or internal sources of danger may produce a signal that leads the ego to marshal specific defense mechanisms to guard against, or reduce, instinctual excitation.

Freud's later theory of anxiety explains neurotic symptoms as the ego's partial failure to cope with distressing stimuli. The drive derivatives associated with danger may not have been adequately contained by the defense mechanisms used by the ego. In phobias, for example, Freud explained that fear of an external threat (e.g., dogs or snakes) is an externalization of an internal danger.

Danger situations can also be linked to developmental stages and thus can create a developmental hierarchy of anxiety. The earliest danger situation is a fear of disintegration or annihilation, often associated with concerns about fusion with an external object. As infants mature and recognize the mothering figure as a separate person, separation anxiety, or fear of the loss of an object, becomes more prominent. During the oedipal psychosexual stage, girls are most concerned about losing the love of the most important figure in their lives, their mother. Boys are primarily anxious about bodily injury or castration. After resolution of the oedipal conflict, a more mature form of anxiety occurs, often termed *superego anxiety.* This latency-age concern involves the fear that internalized parental representations, contained in the superego, will cease to love, or will angrily punish, the child.

Character

In 1913, Freud distinguished between neurotic symptoms and personality or character traits. *Neurotic symptoms* develop as a result of the failure of repression; *character traits* owe their existence to the success of repression, that is, to the defense system that achieves its aim through a persistent pattern of reaction formation and sublimation. In 1923, Freud also observed that the ego can only give up important objects by identifying with them or introjecting them. This accumulated pattern of identifications and introjections also contributes to character formation. Freud specifically emphasized the importance of superego formation in the construction of character.

Contemporary psychoanalysts regard character as a person's habitual or typical pattern of adaptation to internal drive forces and to external environmental forces. *Character* and *personality* are used interchangeably and are distinguished from the ego in that they largely refer to styles of defense and of directly observable behavior rather than to feeling and thinking.

Character is also influenced by constitutional temperament; the interaction of drive forces with early ego defenses and with environmental influences; and various identifications with, and internalizations of, other persons throughout life. The extent to which the ego has developed a capacity to tolerate the delay of impulse discharge and to neutralize instinctual energy determines the degree to which such character traits emerge in later life. Exaggerated development of certain character traits at the expense of others may lead to personality disorders or produce a vulnerability or predisposition to psychosis.

CLASSIC PSYCHOANALYTIC THEORY OF NEUROSES

The classic view of the genesis of neuroses regards conflict as essential. The conflict may arise between instinctual drives and external reality or between internal agencies, such as the id and the superego or the id and the ego. Moreover, because the conflict has not been worked through to a realistic solution, the drives or wishes that seek discharge have been expelled from consciousness through repression or another defense mechanism. Their expulsion from conscious awareness, however, does not make the drives any less powerful or influential. As a result, the unconscious tendencies (e.g., the disguised neurotic symptoms) fight their way back into consciousness. This theory of the development of neurosis assumes that a rudimentary neurosis based on the same type of conflict existed in early childhood.

Deprivation during the first few months of life because of absent or impaired caretaking figures may adversely affect ego development. This impairment, in turn, may result in failure to make appropriate identifications. The resulting ego difficulties create problems in mediating between the drives and the environment. Lack of capacity for constructive expression of drives, especially aggression, may lead some children to turn their aggression on themselves and become overtly self-destructive. Parents who are inconsistent, excessively harsh, or overly indulgent may influence children to develop disordered superego functioning. Severe conflict that cannot be managed through symptom formation may lead to extreme restrictions in ego functioning and fundamentally impair the capacity to learn and develop new skills.

Traumatic events that seem to threaten survival may break through defenses when the ego has been weakened. More libidinal energy is then required to master the excitation that results. The libido thus mobilized, however, is withdrawn from the supply that is normally applied to external objects. This withdrawal further diminishes the strength of the ego and produces a sense of inadequacy. Frustrations or disappointments in adults may revive infantile longings that are then dealt with through symptom formation or further regression.

In his classic studies, Freud described four different types of childhood neuroses, three of which had later neurotic developments in adult life. This well-known series of cases shown in tabulated form in Table 6.1–3 exemplifies some of Freud's important conclusions: (1) neurotic reactions in the adult are associated frequently with neurotic reactions in childhood; (2) the connection is sometimes continuous but more often separated by a latent period of nonneurosis; and (3) infantile sexuality, both fantasized and real, occupies a memorable place in the early history of the patient.

Certain differences are worth noting in the four cases shown in Table 6.1–3. First, the phobic reactions tend to start at about 4 or 5 years of age, the obsessional reactions between 6 and 7, and the conversion reactions at 8. The amount of background disturbance is greatest in the conversion reaction and the mixed neurosis, and it seems only slight in the phobic and

Table 6.1–3
Classic Psychoneurotic Reactions of Childhood

	Conversion Reaction (Dora)	Phobic Reaction (Hans)	Obsessive-Compulsive Reaction (Rat Man)	Mixed Neurotic Reaction (Wolf Man)
Family history	Striking family history of psychiatric and physical illness	Both parents treated for neurotic conflict but not severe	No family history of mental illness	Striking family history of psychiatric and physical illness
Symptoms	Enuresis and masturbation, 6–8 yr; onset of neurosis at 8; migraine, nervous cough, and hoarseness at 12; aphonia at 16; "appendicitis" at 16; convulsions at 16; facial neuralgia at 19; change of personality at 8 from "wild creature" to quiet child	Compulsive questions at 3–3 1/2 yr in regard to sex difference; jealous reaction to sibling birth at 3 1/2; overt castration threat; overt masturbation at 3 1/2; overeating and constipation at 4–5; phobic reaction at 4–5; attack of flu at 5 worsens phobia; tonsillectomy at 5 worsens phobia	Naughty period at 3–4 yr; marked timidity after beating by father at 4; recognizing people by their smells as a child (*Renifleur*); precocious ego development; onset of obsessive ideas at 6–7	Tractable and quiet up to 3 1/4 yr; "naughty" period at 3 1/4–4 yr; phobias at 4–5 with nightmares; obsessional reaction at 6–7 (pious ceremonials). Disappearance of neuroses at 8
Causes	Seduction by older man; father's illness; father's affair	Seductive care by mother; sibling birth at 3 1/2	Seduction by governess at 4; death of sibling at 4; beating by father at 4	Seduction by older sister at 3 1/4; mother's illness; conflict between maid and governess

Courtesy of E. James Anthony, M.D.

obsessional reactions. The course of the phobic reaction seems little influenced by severe traumatic factors, whereas traumatic factors, such as sexual seductions, play an important role in the three other subgroups. It was during this period that Freud elaborated his seduction hypothesis for the cause of the neuroses, in terms of which the obsessive-compulsive and hysterical reactions were alleged to originate in active and passive sexual experiences.

TREATMENT AND TECHNIQUE

The cornerstone of psychoanalytic technique is *free association,* in which patients say whatever comes to mind. Free association does more than provide content for the analysis: It also induces the necessary regression and dependency connected with establishing and working through the transference neurosis. When this development occurs, all the original wishes, drives, and defenses associated with the infantile neurosis are transferred to the person of the analyst.

As patients attempt to free associate, they soon learn that they have difficulty saying whatever comes to mind, without censoring certain thoughts. They develop conflicts about their wishes and feelings toward the analyst that reflect childhood conflicts. The *transference* that develops toward the analyst may also serve as resistance to the process of free association. Freud discovered that *resistance* was not simply a stoppage of a patient's associations, but also an important revelation of the patient's internal object relations as they were externalized and manifested in the transference relationship with the analyst. The systematic analysis of transference and resistance is the essence of psychoanalysis. Freud was also aware that the analyst might have transferences to the patient, which he called *countertransference.* Countertransference, in Freud's view, was an obstacle that the analyst needed to understand so that it did not interfere with treatment. In this spirit, he recognized the need for all analysts to have been analyzed themselves.

Analysts after Freud began to recognize that countertransference was not only an obstacle, but also a source of useful information about the patient. In other words, the analyst's feelings in response to the patient reflect how other persons respond to the patient and provide some indication of the patient's own internal object relations. By understanding the intense feelings that occur in the analytic relationship, the analyst can help the patient broaden understanding of past and current relationships outside the analysis. The development of insight into neurotic conflicts also expands the ego and provides an increased sense of mastery. (Psychoanalysis and other techniques derived from it are discussed in greater detail in Chapter 35, Section 35.1.)

REFERENCES

Brenner C. *The Mind in Conflict.* New York: International Universities Press; 1982.

Fenichel O. *The Psychoanalytic Theory of Neurosis.* New York: WW Norton; 1945.

Freud A. *The Ego and the Mechanisms of Defense* (1936). In: *The Writings of Anna Freud.* Vol 2. Rev ed. New York: International Universities Press; 1966.

Freud S. *The Standard Edition of the Complete Psychological Works of Sigmund Freud.* Vols 1–24. London: Hogarth; 1953–1966.

Freud S. *The Ego and the Id.* New York: WW Norton; 1960.

Freud S. *Beyond the Pleasure Principle.* New York: WW Norton; 1961.

Freud S. *An Outline of Psycho-Analysis.* New York: WW Norton; 1969.

Gabbard GO. Psychoanalysis. In: *Kaplan & Sadock's Comprehensive Textbook of Psychiatry.* 7th ed. Vol 1. Sadock BJ, Sadock VA, eds. Baltimore: Lippincott Williams & Wilkins; 2000:563.

Gabbard GO. *Psychodynamic Psychiatry in Clinical Practice: The Third Edition.* Washington, DC: American Psychiatric Press; 2000.

Holt RR. *Freud Reappraised: A Fresh Look at Psychoanalytic Theory.* New York: Guilford; 1989.

Katz AJ. The implications of revising Freud's empiricism for drive theory. *Psychoanal Contemp Thought.* 2001;24:253.

Winer JA, Anderson JW, eds. *The Annual of Psychoanalysis.* Vol XXIX: *Sigmund Freud and his impact on the modern world.* Hillsdale, NJ: Analytic Press; 2001:145.

Winnicott DW. *Playing and Reality.* New York: Basic Books; 1971.

▲ 6.2 Erik Erikson

Erik Homburger Erikson (Fig. 6.2–1) was born on June 15, 1902, in Karlsruhe, Germany. He died in 1994. His father, a Danish Protestant, and his mother, a Danish Jew, separated before he was born, and he grew up in the home of his mother and German-Jewish stepfather, Theodore Homburger, a pediatrician. Erikson was never able to learn the identity of his biological father; his mother withheld that information from him all her life.

Erikson immigrated to the United States in 1933. He worked at the Austen Riggs Center in Stockbridge, Massachusetts, and conducted research at Harvard, Yale, and the University of California at Berkeley. He became interested in the influence of culture on child development, and as a result of his studies in the 1930s and the 1940s, including anthropological work with the Sioux in South Dakota and the Yurok in northern California, his book *Childhood and Society* was published in 1950. In this publication, he presented a psychosocial theory of development that describes crucial steps in persons' relationships with the social world, based on the interplay between biology and society.

Erikson drew on much of freudian psychology, but he added to Sigmund Freud's theory of infantile sexuality by concentrating on children's development beyond puberty. Erikson concluded that human personality is determined not only by childhood experiences, but also by those of adulthood. Erikson stated: "If everything goes back into childhood, then everything is somebody else's fault and taking responsibility for oneself is undermined." Most important, Erikson formulated a theory of human development that covers the entire span of the life cycle, from infancy and childhood through old age and senescence.

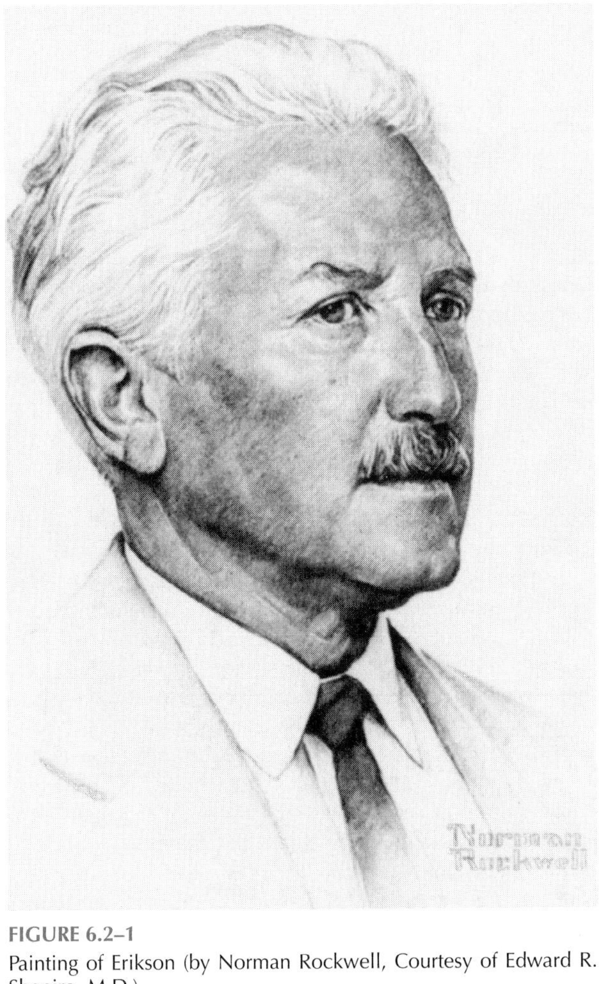

FIGURE 6.2–1
Painting of Erikson (by Norman Rockwell, Courtesy of Edward R. Shapiro, M.D.).

EPIGENETIC PRINCIPLE

Erikson's formulations were based on the concept of epigenesis, a term borrowed from embryology. His *epigenetic principle* holds that development occurs in sequential, clearly defined stages, and that each stage must be satisfactorily resolved for development to proceed smoothly. According to the epigenetic model, if successful resolution of a particular stage does not occur, all subsequent stages reflect the failure in the form of physical, cognitive, social, or emotional maladjustment.

Relation to Freudian Theory

Erikson accepted Freud's concepts of instinctual development and infantile sexuality. For each of Freud's psychosexual stages (e.g., oral, anal, and phallic), Erikson described a corresponding zone with a specific pattern or mode of behavior. Thus, the oral zone is associated with sucking or taking-in behavior; the anal zone is associated with holding on and letting go. Erikson emphasized that the development of the ego is more than the result of intrapsychic wants or inner psychic energies. It is also a matter of mutual regulation between growing children and a society's culture and traditions.

Eight Stages of the Life Cycle

Erikson's conception of the eight stages of ego development across the life cycle is the centerpiece of his life's work, and he elaborated the conception throughout his subsequent writings (Table 6.2–1). The eight stages represent points along a continuum of development in which physical, cognitive, instinctual, and sexual changes combine to trigger an internal crisis whose resolution results in either psychosocial regression or growth and the development of specific *virtues*. In *Insight and Responsibility* Erikson defined virtue as "inherent strength," as in the active quality of a medicine or liquor. He wrote in *Identity: Youth and Crisis* that "crisis" refers not to a "threat of catastrophe, but to a turning point, a crucial period of increased vulnerability and heightened potential, and therefore, the ontogenetic source of generational strength and maladjustment."

Stage 1: Trust versus Mistrust (Birth to about 18 Months). In *Identity: Youth and Crisis*, Erikson noted that the infant "lives through and loves with" its mouth. Indeed, the mouth forms the basis of its first mode or pattern of behavior, that of incorporation. The infant is taking the world in through the mouth, eyes, ears, and sense of touch. The baby is learning a cultural modality that Erikson termed *to get*, that is, to receive what is offered and elicit what is desired. As the infant's teeth develop and it discovers the pleasure of biting, it enters the second oral stage, the active-incorporative mode. The infant is no

Table 6.2–1
Erikson's Psychosocial Stages

Psychosocial Stage	Associated Virtue	Related Forms of Psychopathology	Positive and Negative Forerunners of Identity Formation	Enduring Aspects of Identity Formation
Trust vs. mistrust (birth—)	Hope	Psychosis Addictions Depression	Mutual recognition vs. autistic isolation	Temporal perspective vs. time confusion
Autonomy vs. shame and doubt (~18 months—)	Will	Paranoia Obsessions Compulsions Impulsivity	Will to be oneself vs. self-doubt	Self-certainty vs. self-consciousness
Initiative vs. guilt (~3 years—)	Purpose	Conversion disorder Phobia Psychosomatic disorder Inhibition	Anticipation of roles vs. role inhibition	Role experimentation vs. role fixation
Industry vs. inferiority (~5 years—)	Competence	Creative inhibition Inertia	Task identification vs. sense of futility	Apprenticeship vs. work paralysis
Identity vs. role confusion (~13 years—)	Fidelity	Delinquent behavior Gender-related identity disorders Borderline psychotic episodes		Identity vs. identity confusion
Intimacy vs. isolation (~20s—)	Love	Schizoid personality disorder Distantiation		Sexual polarization vs. bisexual confusion
Generativity vs. stagnation (~40s—)	Care	Mid-life crisis Premature invalidism		Leadership and followership vs. abdication of responsibility
Integrity vs. despair (~60s—)	Wisdom	Extreme alienation Despair		Ideological commitment vs. confusion of values

Adapted from Erikson E. *Insight and Responsibility*. New York: WW Norton; 1964; Erikson E. *Identity: Youth and Crisis*. New York: WW Norton; 1968.

longer passively receptive to stimuli; it reaches out for sensation and grasps at its surroundings. The social modality shifts to that of *taking and holding on* to things.

The infant's development of basic trust in the world stems from its earliest experiences with its mother or primary caretaker. In *Childhood and Society* Erikson asserts that trust depends not on "absolute quantities of food or demonstrations of love, but rather on the quality of maternal relationship." A baby whose mother can anticipate and respond to its needs in a consistent and timely manner despite its oral aggression will learn to tolerate the inevitable moments of frustration and deprivation. The defense mechanisms of introjection and projection will provide the infant with the means to internalize pleasure and externalize pain such that "consistency, continuity, and sameness of experience provide a rudimentary sense of ego identity." Trust will predominate over mistrust, and hope will crystallize. For Erikson, the element of society corresponding to this stage of ego identity is religion, as both are founded upon "trust born of care."

In keeping with his emphasis on the epigenetic character of psychosocial change, Erikson conceived of many forms of psychopathology as examples of what he termed *aggravated development crisis,* development that, having gone awry at one point, affects subsequent psychosocial change. A person who, as a result of severe disturbances in the earliest dyadic relationships, fails to develop a basic sense of trust or the virtue of hope may be predisposed as an adult to the profound withdrawal and regression characteristic of schizophrenia. Erikson hypothesized that the depressed patient's experience of being empty and of being no good is an outgrowth of a developmental derailment that causes oral pessimism to predominate. Addictions may also be traced to the mode of oral incorporation.

Stage 2: Autonomy versus Shame and Doubt (about 18 Months to about 3 Years). In the development of speech and sphincter and muscular control, the toddler practices the social modalities of *holding on and letting go,* and experiences the first stirrings of the virtue that Erikson termed *will.* Much depends on the amount and type of control exercised by adults over the child. Control that is exerted too rigidly or too early defeats the toddler's attempts to develop its own internal controls, and regression or false progression results. Parental control that fails to protect the toddler from the consequences of his or her own lack of self-control or judgment can be equally disastrous to the child's development of a healthy sense of autonomy. In *Identity: Youth and Crisis,* Erikson asserted: "This stage, therefore, becomes decisive for the ratio between loving good will and hateful self-insistence, between cooperation and willfulness, and between self-expression and compulsive self-restraint or meek compliance."

Where that ratio is favorable, the child will develop an appropriate sense of autonomy and the capacity to "have and to hold"; where it is unfavorable, doubt and shame will undermine free will. According to Erikson, the principle of law and order has at its roots this early preoccupation with the protection and regulation of will. In *Childhood and Society*, he concluded, "The sense of autonomy fostered in the child and modified as life progresses, serves (and is served by) the preservation in economic and political life of a sense of justice."

A person who becomes fixated at the transition between the development of hope and autonomous will, with its residue of mistrust and doubt, may develop paranoiac fears of persecution. When psychosocial development is derailed in the second stage, other forms of pathology may emerge. The perfectionism, inflexibility, and stinginess of the person with an obsessive-compulsive personality disorder may stem from conflicting tendencies to hold on and to let go. The ruminative and ritualistic behavior of the person who suffers from an obsessive-compulsive disorder may be an outcome of the triumph of doubt over autonomy and the subsequent development of a primitively harsh conscience.

Stage 3: Initiative versus Guilt (about 3 Years to about 5 Years). The child's increasing mastery of locomotor and language skills expands its participation in the outside world and stimulates omnipotent fantasies of wider exploration and conquest. Here the youngster's mode of participation is active and intrusive; its social modality is that of *being on the make*. The intrusiveness is manifested in the child's fervent curiosity and genital preoccupations, competitiveness, and physical aggression. The Oedipus complex is in ascendance as the child competes with the same-sex parent for the fantasized possession of the other parent. In *Identity: Youth and Crisis*, Erikson wrote that "jealousy and rivalry now come to a climax in a final contest for a favored position with one of the parents: the inevitable and necessary failure leads to guilt and anxiety."

Guilt over the drive for conquest and anxiety over the anticipated punishment are both assuaged in the child through repression of the forbidden wishes and development of a superego to regulate its initiative. This conscience, the faculty of self-observation, self-regulation, and self-punishment, is an internalized version of parental and societal authority. Initially the conscience is harsh and uncompromising; however, it constitutes the foundation for the subsequent development of morality. Having renounced oedipal ambitions, the child begins to look outside the family for arenas in which it can compete with less conflict and guilt. This is the stage that highlights the child's expanding initiative and forms the basis for the subsequent development of realistic ambition and the virtue of *purpose*. As Erikson noted in *Childhood and Society*, "The 'oedipal' stage sets the direction toward the possible and the tangible which permits the dreams of early childhood to be attached to the goals of an active adult life." Toward this end, social institutions provide the youngster with an economic ethos in the form of adult heroes who begin to take the place of their storybook counterparts.

When there has been an inadequate resolution of the conflict between initiative and guilt, the person may ultimately develop a conversion disorder, inhibition, or phobia. Those who overcompensate for the conflict by driving themselves too hard may experience enough stress to produce psychosomatic symptoms.

Stage 4: Industry versus Inferiority (about 5 Years to about 13 Years). With the onset of latency, the child discovers the pleasures of production. He or she develops industry by learning new skills and takes pride in the things made. Erikson wrote in *Childhood and Society* that the child's "ego boundaries include his tools and skills: the work principle teaches him the pleasure of work completion by steady attention and persevering diligence." Across cultures, this is a time when the child receives systematic instruction and learns the fundamentals of technology as they pertain to the use of basic utensils and tools. As children work they identify with their teachers and imagine themselves in various occupational roles.

A child who is unprepared for this stage of psychosocial development, either through insufficient resolution of previous stages or by current interference, may develop a sense of inferiority and inadequacy. In the form of teachers and other role models, society becomes crucially important in the child's ability to overcome that sense of inferiority and to achieve the virtue known as competence. In *Identity: Youth and Crisis*, Erikson noted: "This is socially a most decisive stage. Since industry involves doing things beside and with others, a first sense of division of labor and of differential opportunity, that is, a sense of the technological ethos of a culture, develops at this time."

The pathological outcome of a poorly navigated stage of industry versus inferiority is less well defined than in previous stages, but it may concern the emergence of a conformist immersion into the world of production in which creativity is stifled and identity is subsumed under the worker's role.

Stage 5: Identity versus Role Confusion (about 13 Years to about 21 Years). With the onset of puberty and its myriad social and physiological changes, the adolescent becomes preoccupied with the question of identity. Erikson noted in *Childhood and Society* that youth are now "primarily concerned with what they appear to be in the eyes of others as compared to what they feel they are, and with the question of how to connect the roles and skills cultivated earlier with the occupational prototypes of the day." Childhood roles and fantasies are no longer appropriate, yet the adolescent is far from equipped to become an adult. In *Childhood and Society* Erikson writes that the integration that occurs in the formation of ego identity encompasses far more than the summation of childhood identifications. "It is the accrued experience of the ego's ability to integrate these identifications with the vicissitudes of the libido, with the aptitudes developed out of endowment, and with the opportunities offered in social roles."

The formation of cliques and an identity crisis occur at the end of adolescence. Erikson calls the crisis normative because it is a normal event. Failure to negotiate this stage leaves adolescents without a solid identity; they suffer from identity diffusion or role confusion, characterized by not having a sense of self and by confusion about their place in the world. Role confusion may manifest in such behavioral abnormalities as running away, criminality, and overt psychosis. Problems in gender

identity and sexual role may manifest at this time. Adolescents may defend against role diffusion by joining cliques or cults or by identifying with folk heroes. Intolerance of individual differences is a way in which the young person attempts to ward off a sense of identity loss. Falling in love, a process by which the adolescent may clarify a sense of identity by projecting a diffused self-image onto the partner and seeing it gradually assume a more distinctive shape, and an overidentification with idealized figures are means by which the adolescent seeks self-definition. With the attainment of a more sharply focused identity, the youth develops the virtue of *fidelity*—faithfulness not only to the nascent self-definition but also to an ideology that provides a version of self-in-world. As Erikson, Joan Erikson, and Helen Kivnick wrote in *Vital Involvement in Old Age,* "Fidelity is the ability to sustain loyalties freely pledged in spite of the inevitable contradictions of value systems. It is the cornerstone of identity and receives inspiration from confirming ideologies and affirming companionships." Role confusion ensues when the youth is unable to formulate a sense of identity and belonging. Erikson held that delinquency, gender-related identity disorders, and borderline psychotic episodes can result from such confusion.

Stage 6: Intimacy versus Isolation (about 21 Years to about 40 Years). Freud's famous response to the question of what a normal person should be able to do well, "Lieben und arbeiten" (to love and to work), is one that Erikson often cited in his discussion of this psychosocial stage, and it emphasizes the importance he placed on the virtue of *love* within a balanced identity. Erikson asserted in *Identity: Youth and Crisis* that Freud's use of the term *love* referred to "the generosity of intimacy as well as genital love; when he said love and work, he meant a general work productiveness which would not preoccupy the individual to the extent that he might lose his right or capacity to be a sexual and a loving being."

Intimacy in the young adult is closely tied to fidelity; it is the ability to make and honor commitments to concrete affiliations and partnerships even when that requires sacrifice and compromise. The person who cannot tolerate the fear of ego loss arising out of experiences of self-abandonment (e.g., sexual orgasm, moments of intensity in friendships, aggression, inspiration, and intuition) is apt to become deeply isolated and self-absorbed. *Distantiation*, an awkward term coined by Erikson to mean "the readiness to repudiate, isolate, and, if necessary, destroy those forces and persons whose essence seems dangerous to one's own," is the pathological outcome of conflicts surrounding intimacy and, in the absence of an ethical sense where intimate, competitive, and combative relationships are differentiated, forms the basis for various forms of prejudice, persecution, and psychopathology.

Erikson's separation of the psychosocial task of achieving identity from that of achieving intimacy, and his assertion that substantial progress on the former task must precede development on the latter have engendered much criticism and debate. Critics have argued that Erikson's emphasis on separation and occupationally based identity formation fails to take into account the importance for women of continued attachment and the formation of an identity based on relationships.

Stage 7: Generativity versus Stagnation (about 40 Years to about 60 Years). Erikson asserted in *Identity: Youth and Crisis* that "generativity is primarily the concern for establishing and guiding the next generation." The term *generativity* applies not so much to rearing and teaching one's offspring as to a protective concern for all the generations and for social institutions. It encompasses productivity and creativity as well. Having previously achieved the capacity to form intimate relationships, the person now broadens the investment of ego and libidinal energy to include groups, organizations, and society. *Care* is the virtue that coalesces at this stage. In *Childhood and Society* Erikson emphasized the importance to the mature person of feeling needed. "Maturity needs guidance as well as encouragement from what has been produced and must be taken care of." Through generative behavior the individual can pass on knowledge and skills while obtaining a measure of satisfaction in having achieved a role with senior authority and responsibility in the tribe.

When persons cannot develop true generativity, they may settle for pseudoengagement in occupation. Often such persons restrict their focus to the technical aspects of their roles, at which they may now have become highly skilled, eschewing larger responsibility for the organization or profession. This failure of generativity can lead to profound personal stagnation, masked by a variety of escapisms, such as alcohol and drug abuse, and sexual and other infidelities. Mid-life crisis or premature invalidism (physical and psychological) may occur. In this case, pathology appears not only in middle-aged persons but also in the organizations that depend upon them for leadership. Thus, the failure to develop at mid-life can lead to sick, withered, or destructive organizations that spread the effects of failed generativity throughout society; examples of such failures have become so common that they constitute a defining feature of modernity.

Stage 8: Integrity versus Despair (about 60 Years to Death). In *Identity: Youth and Crisis*, Erikson defined integrity as "the acceptance of one's one and only life cycle and of the persons who have become significant to it as something that had to be and that, by necessity, permitted of no substitutions." From the vantage point of this stage of psychosocial development, the individual relinquishes the wish that important persons in his life had been different and is able to love in a more meaningful way—one that reflects accepting responsibility for one's own life. The individual in possession of the virtue of *wisdom* and a sense of integrity has room to tolerate the proximity of death and to achieve what Erikson termed in *Identity: Youth and Crisis* a "detached yet active concern with life."

Erikson underlined the social context for this final stage of growth. In *Childhood and Society*, he wrote, "The style of integrity developed by his culture or civilization thus becomes the 'patrimony' of his soul. . . .In such final consolidation, death loses its sting."

When the attempt to attain integrity has failed, the individual may become deeply disgusted with the external world and contemptuous of persons as well as institutions. Erikson wrote in *Childhood and Society* that such disgust masks a fear of death and a sense of despair that "time is now short, too short for the attempt to start another life and to try out alternate roads to integrity." Looking back on the eight ages of man, he noted

the relation between adult integrity and infantile trust, "Healthy children will not fear life if their elders have integrity enough not to fear death."

PSYCHOPATHOLOGY

Each stage of the life cycle has its own psychopathological outcome if it is not mastered successfully.

Basic Trust

An impairment of basic trust leads to basic mistrust. In infants, social trust is characterized by ease of feeding, depth of sleep, smiling, and general physiological homeostasis. Prolonged separation during infancy can lead to hospitalism or anaclitic depression (see Chapter 4, Section 4.2). In later life, this lack of trust may be manifested by dysthymic disorder, a depressive disorder, or a sense of hopelessness. Persons who develop and rely on the defense of projection—in which, according to Erikson, "we endow significant persons with the evil which actually is in us"—experienced a sense of social mistrust in the first years of life and are likely to develop paranoid or delusional disorders. Basic mistrust is a major contribution to the development of schizoid personality disorder and, in most severe cases, to the development of schizophrenia. Substance-related disorders can also be traced to social mistrust; substance-dependent personalities have strong oral-dependency needs and use chemical substances to satisfy themselves because of their belief that human beings are unreliable and, at worst, dangerous. If not nurtured properly, infants may feel empty, starved not just for food but also for sensual and visual stimulation. They may become, as adults, seekers after stimulating thrills that do not involve intimacy and that help ward off feelings of depression.

Autonomy

The stage in which children attempt to develop into autonomous beings is often called the *terrible twos*, referring to toddlers' willfulness at this period of development. If shame and doubt dominate over autonomy, compulsive doubting may occur. The inflexibility of the obsessive personality also results from an overabundance of doubt. Too rigorous toilet training, commonplace in today's society, which requires a clean, punctual, and deodorized body, can produce an overly compulsive personality that is stingy, meticulous, and selfish. Known as anal personalities, such persons are parsimonious, punctual, and perfectionistic (the three Ps).

Too much shaming causes children to feel evil or dirty and may pave the way for delinquent behavior. In effect, children say, "If that's what they think of me, that's the way I'll behave." Paranoid personalities feel that others are trying to control them, a feeling that may have its origin during the stage of autonomy versus shame and doubt. When coupled with mistrust, the seeds are planted for persecutory delusions. Impulsive disorder may be explained as a person's refusing to be inhibited or controlled.

Initiative

Erikson stated: "In pathology, the conflict over initiative is expressed either in hysterical denial, which causes the repression of the wish or the abrogation of its executive organ by paralysis or impotence; or in overcompensatory showing off, in which the scared individual, so eager to 'duck,' instead 'sticks his neck out.'" In the past, hysteria was the usual form of pathological regression in this area, but a plunge into psychosomatic disease is now common.

Excessive guilt may lead to a variety of conditions, such as generalized anxiety disorder and phobias. Patients feel guilty because of normal impulses, and they repress these impulses, with resulting symptom formation. Punishment or severe prohibitions during the stage of initiative versus guilt can produce sexual inhibitions. Conversion disorder or specific phobia may result when the oedipal conflict is not resolved. As sexual fantasies are accepted as unrealizable, children may punish themselves for these fantasies by fearing harm to their genitals. Under the brutal assault of the developing superego, they may repress their wishes and begin to deny them. If this pattern is carried forward, paralysis, inhibition, or impotence can result. Sometimes, in fear of not being able to live up to what others expect, children may turn to psychosomatic disease.

Industry

Erikson described industry as a "sense of being able to make things and make them well and even perfectly." When children's efforts are thwarted, they are made to feel that personal goals cannot be accomplished or are not worthwhile, and a sense of inferiority develops. In adults, this sense of inferiority can result in severe work inhibitions and a character structure marked by feelings of inadequacy. For some persons, the feelings may result in a compensatory drive for money, power, and prestige. Work can become the main focus of life, at the expense of intimacy.

Identity

Many disorders of adolescence can be traced to identity confusion. The danger is role diffusion. Erikson stated:

> Where this is based on a strong previous doubt as to one's sexual identity, delinquent and outright psychotic incidents are not uncommon. If diagnosed and treated correctly, those incidents do not have the same fatal significance that they have at other ages. It is primarily the inability to settle on an occupational identity that disturbs young persons. Keeping themselves together, they temporarily overidentify, to the point of apparent complete loss of identity, with the heroes of cliques and crowds.

Other disorders during the stage of identity versus role diffusion include conduct disorder, disruptive behavior disorder, gender identity disorder, schizophreniform disorder, and other psychotic disorders. The ability to leave home and live independently is an important task during this period. An inability to separate from the parent and prolonged dependence may occur.

Intimacy

The successful formation of a stable marriage and family depends on the capacity to become intimate. The years of early adulthood are crucial for deciding whether to get married and to whom. Gender identity determines object choice, either heterosexual or homosexual, but making an intimate connection with another person is a major task. Persons with schizoid personal-

ity disorder remain isolated from others because of fear, suspicion, the inability to take risks, or the lack of a capacity to love.

Generativity

From about 40 to 65 years, the period of middle adulthood, specific disorders are less clearly defined than in the other stages described by Erikson. Persons who are middle aged show a higher incidence of depression than younger adults, which may be related to middle-aged persons' disappointments and failed expectations as they review the past, consider their lives, and contemplate the future. The increased use of alcohol and other psychoactive substances also occurs during this time.

Integrity

Anxiety disorders often develop in older persons. In Erikson's formulation, this development may be related to persons' looking back on their lives with a sense of panic. Time has run out, and chances are used up. The decline in physical functions can contribute to psychosomatic illness, hypochondriasis, and depression. The suicide rate is highest over the age of 65. Persons facing dying and death may find it intolerable not to have been generative or able to make significant attachments in life. Integrity, for Erikson, is characterized by an acceptance of life. Without acceptance, persons feel despair and hopelessness that can result in severe depressive disorders.

TREATMENT

Although no independent eriksonian psychoanalytic school exists in the same way that freudian and jungian schools do, Erikson made many important contributions to the therapeutic process. Among his most important contributions is his belief that establishing a state of trust between doctor and patient is the basic requirement for successful therapy. When psychopathology stems from basic mistrust (e.g., depression), a patient must reestablish trust with the therapist, whose task, like that of the good mother, is to be sensitive to the patient's needs. The therapist must have a sense of personal trustworthiness that can be transmitted to the patient.

Techniques

For Erikson, a psychoanalyst is not a blank slate in the therapeutic process, as he or she commonly is in freudian psychoanalysis. To the contrary, effective therapy requires that therapists actively convey to patients the belief that they are understood. This is done not only through empathetic listening but also by verbal assurances, which enable a positive transference built on mutual trust to develop.

Beginning as an analyst for children, Erikson tried to provide this mutuality and trust while he observed children recreating their own worlds by structuring dolls, blocks, vehicles, and miniature furniture into the dramatic situations that were bothering them. Then Erikson correlated his observations with statements by the children and their family members. He began treatment of a child only after eating an evening meal with the entire family, and his therapy was usually conducted with much cooperation from the family. After each regressive episode in the treatment of a schizophrenic child, for instance, Erikson discussed with every member of the family what had been going on with them before the episode. Only when he was thoroughly satisfied that he had identified the problem did treatment begin. Erikson sometimes provided corrective information to the child—for instance, telling a boy who could not release his feces and had made himself ill from constipation that food is not an unborn infant.

Erikson often turned to play, which, along with specific recommendations to parents, proved fruitful as a treatment modality. Play, for Erikson, is diagnostically revealing and thus helpful for a therapist who seeks to promote a cure, but it is also curative in its own right. Play is a function of the ego and gives children a chance to synchronize social and bodily processes with the self. Children playing with blocks or adults playing out an imagined dramatic situation can manipulate the environment and develop the sense of control that the ego needs. Play therapy is not the same for children and adults, however. Children create models in an effort to gain control of reality; they look ahead to new areas of mastery. Adults use play to correct the past and to redeem their failures.

Mutuality, which is important in Erikson's system of health, is also vital to a cure. Erikson applauded Freud for the moral choice of abandoning hypnosis, as hypnosis heightens the demarcation between the healer and the sick and heightens the inequality that Erikson compares to the inequality of child and adult. Erikson urged that the relationship of the healer to the sick person be one of equals "in which the observer who has learned to observe himself teaches the observed to become self-observant."

Dreams and Free Association

Like Freud, Erikson worked with the patient's associations to the dream as the "best leads" to understanding its meaning. He valued the first association to the dream, which he believed to be powerful and important. Ultimately, Erikson listened for "a central theme which, once found, gives added meaning to all the associated material."

Erikson believed that interpretation was the primary therapeutic agent, sought as much by the patient as by the therapist. He emphasized free-floating attention as the method that enabled discovery to occur. Erikson once described this attentional stance by commenting that in clinical work, "You need a history and you need a theory, and then you must forget them both and let each hour stand for itself." This frees both parties from counterproductive pressures to advance in the therapy and allows them both to notice the gaps in the patient's narrative that signal the unconscious.

Goals

Erikson discussed four dimensions of the psychoanalyst's job. The patient's desire to be cured and the analyst's desire to cure is the first dimension. There is mutuality in that patient and therapist are motivated by cure, and there is a division of labor. The goal is always to help the patient's ego get stronger and cure itself. The second dimension Erikson called objectivity-participation. Therapists must keep their

minds open. "Neuroses change," wrote Erikson. New generalizations must be made and arranged in new configurations. The third dimension runs along the axis of knowledge-participation. The therapist "applies selected insights to more strictly experimental approaches." The fourth dimension is tolerance-indignation. Erikson stated: "Identities based on Talmudic argument, on messianic zeal, on punitive orthodoxy, on faddist sensationalism, on professional and social ambition" are harmful and tend to control patients. Control widens the gap of inequality between the doctor and the patient and makes realization of the recurrent idea in Erikson's thought—mutuality—difficult.

According to Erikson, therapists have the opportunity to work through past unresolved conflicts in the therapeutic relationship. Erikson encouraged therapists not to shy away from guiding patients; he believes that therapists must offer patients both prohibitions and permissions. Nor should therapists be so engrossed in patients' past life experiences that current conflicts are overlooked.

The goal of therapy is to recognize how patients have passed through the various stages of the life cycle and how the various crises in each stage have or have not been mastered. Equally important, future stages and crises must be anticipated, so that they can be negotiated and mastered appropriately. Unlike Freud, Erikson does not believe that the personality is so inflexible that change cannot occur in middle and late adulthood. For Erikson, psychological growth and development occur throughout the entire span of the life cycle.

The Austen Riggs Center in Stockbridge, Massachusetts, is a repository of Erikson's work and many of his theories are put into practice there. Erik's wife, Joan, developed an activities program at the Austen Riggs Center as an "interpretation-free zone" where patients could take up work roles or function as students with artists and craftspersons, without the burden of the patient role. This workspace encouraged the play and creativity required for the patients' work development to parallel the process of their therapy.

References

Coles R. *Erik H. Erikson: The Growth of His Work.* Boston: Little, Brown; 1970.
Erikson E. Observations on Sioux education. *J Psychol.* 1939;7:101.
Erikson E. Hitler's imagery and German youth. *Psychiatry.* 1942;5:475.
Erikson E. *Childhood and Society.* New York: WW Norton; 1950.
Erikson E. The dream specimen of psychoanalysis. *J Am Psychoanal Assoc.* 1954;2:5.
Erikson E. Freud's "The Origins of Psychoanalysis." *Int J Psychoanal.* 1955;36:1.
Erikson E. The first psychoanalyst. *Yale Rev.* 1956;46:40.
Erikson E. The problem of ego identity. *Psychol Issues.* 1959;1:379.
Erikson E. *Young Man Luther.* New York: WW Norton; 1962.
Erikson E. *Insight and Responsibility.* New York: WW Norton; 1964.
Erikson E. *Identity: Youth and Crisis.* New York: WW Norton; 1968.
Erikson E. *Gandhi's Truth.* New York: WW Norton; 1969.
Erikson E. *Life History and the Historical Moment.* New York: WW Norton; 1975.
Erikson E. *Identity and the Life Cycle.* New York: WW Norton; 1980.
Erikson E, Erikson J, Kivnick H. *Vital Involvement in Old Age.* New York: WW Norton; 1986.
Evans R. *Dialogue with Erik Erikson.* New York: Harper & Row; 1967.
Friedman L. *Identity's Architect: A Biography of Erik Erikson.* New York: Scribner; 1999.
Ginsburg HJ. Childhood injuries and Erikson's psychosocial stages. *Soc Behav Pers.* 1992;20:95.
Schein S, ed. *Erik Erikson: A Way of Looking at Things.* New York: WW Norton; 1987.
Shapiro ER, Fromm MG. Eriksonian clinical theory and psychiatric treatment. In: Sadock BJ, Sadock VA, eds. *Kaplan & Sadock's Comprehensive Textbook of Psychiatry.* 7th ed. Vol 2. Baltimore: Lippincott Williams & Wilkins; 2000:2200.

▲ 6.3 Schools Derived from Psychoanalysis and Psychology

Many theories have been proposed to explain the basis of normal and abnormal behavior. Essentially, these theoretical models are designed to facilitate the understanding, prediction, and eventual therapeutic control of human behavior. Different theories of personality and psychopathology generally deal with the same basic issues and operate on comparable levels of description. However, they tend to vary in emphasis; they use different theoretical constructs and are often based on different underlying hypotheses. At the present time, no one theory can explain and predict normal human behavior in an entirely satisfactory manner; nor has any single theory been able to account adequately for the many forms of abnormal behavior encountered in clinical practice. Nevertheless, many theories of personality and psychopathology have contributed valuable concepts and methods of treatment.

Brief synopses of the theories that exert the greatest influence on current psychiatric thought are listed below in alphabetical order of their proponent. Each of these theories contains insights that merit consideration because they enhance our understanding of the complexities of human behavior. They also illustrate the diversity of theoretical orientation that characterizes psychiatry today.

KARL ABRAHAM (1877–1925)

Karl Abraham, one of Sigmund Freud's earliest disciples, was the first psychoanalyst in Germany. He is best known for his explication of depression from a psychoanalytic perspective and for his elaboration of Freud's stages of psychosexual development. Abraham divided the oral stage into a biting phase and a sucking phase; the anal stage into a destructive-expulsive (anal-sadistic) phase and a mastering-retentive (anal-erotic) phase; and the phallic stage into an early phase of partial genital love (true phallic phase) and a later mature genital phase. Abraham also linked the psychosexual stages to specific syndromes. For example, he postulated that obsessional neurosis resulted from fixation at the anal-sadistic phase, and depression from fixation at the oral stage.

ALFRED ADLER (1870–1937)

Alfred Adler (Fig. 6.3–1) was one of Freud's prized pupils, but theoretical differences led to their eventual estrangement. Adler thought that Freud had overemphasized the sexual theory of neurosis and that aggression was far more important, specifically in its manifestation as a striving for power, which he believed to be a masculine trait. He introduced the term *masculine protest* to describe the tendency to move from a passive, feminine role to a masculine, active role. Adler's theories are collectively known as *individual psychology.*

Adler coined the term *inferiority complex* to refer to a sense of inadequacy and weakness that is universal and inborn. A developing child's self-esteem is compromised by a physical defect, and Adler referred to

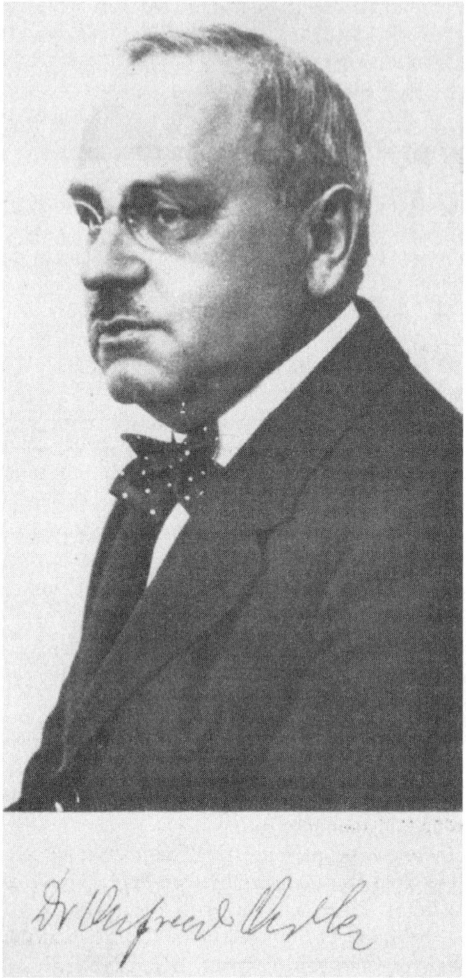

FIGURE 6.3–1
Alfred Adler (print includes signature). (Courtesy of Alexandra Adler.)

this phenomenon as *organ inferiority.* He also thought that a basic inferiority tied to children's oedipal longings could never be gratified.

Adler was one of the first developmental theorists to recognize the importance of children's birth order in their families of origin. The first-born child reacts with anger to the birth of siblings and struggles against giving up the powerful position of only child. The second-born child must constantly strive to compete with the firstborn. Adler thought that a child's sibling position results in lifelong influences on character and lifestyle.

The primary therapeutic approach in adlerian therapy is encouragement, through which Adler believed his patients could overcome feelings of inferiority. Consistent human relatedness, in his view, leads to greater hope, less isolation, and greater affiliation with society. He believed that patients needed to develop a greater sense of their own dignity and worth and renewed appreciation of their abilities and strengths.

FRANZ ALEXANDER (1891–1964)

Franz Alexander (Fig. 6.3–2) emigrated from his native Germany to the United States, where he settled in Chicago and founded the Chicago Institute for Psychoanalysis. He wrote extensively about the association between specific personality traits and certain psychosomatic ailments, a point of view that came to be known as the

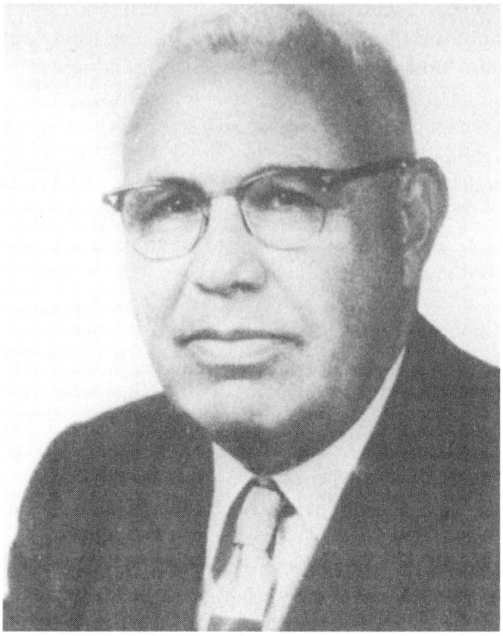

FIGURE 6.3–2
Franz Alexander. (Courtesy of Franz Alexander.)

specificity hypothesis. Alexander fell out of favor with classic analysts for advocating the *corrective emotional experience* as part of analytic technique. In this approach, Alexander suggested that an analyst must deliberately adopt a particular mode of relatedness with a patient to counteract noxious childhood influences from the patient's parents. He believed that the trusting, supportive relationship between patient and analyst enabled the patient to master childhood traumas and to grow from the experience.

GORDON ALLPORT (1896–1967)

Gordon Allport, a psychologist in the United States, is known as the founder of the humanistic school of psychology, which holds that each person has an inherent potential for autonomous function and growth. At Harvard University, he taught the first course in the psychology of personality offered at a college in the United States.

Allport believed that a person's only real guarantee of personal existence is a sense of self. Selfhood develops through a series of stages, from awareness of the body to self-identity. Allport used the term *propriem* to describe strivings related to maintenance of self-identity and self-esteem. He used the term *traits* to refer to the chief units of personality structure. *Personal dispositions* are individual traits that represent the essence of an individual's unique personality. *Maturity* is characterized by a capacity to relate to others with warmth and intimacy and an expanded sense of self. In Allport's view, mature persons have security, humor, insight, enthusiasm, and zest. Psychotherapy is geared to helping patients realize these characteristics.

MICHAEL BALINT (1896–1970)

Michael Balint was considered a member of the independent or middle group of object relations theorists in the United Kingdom. Balint believed that the urge for the primary love object underlies

virtually all psychological phenomena. Infants wish to be loved totally and unconditionally, and when a mother is not forthcoming with appropriate nurturance, a child devotes his or her life to a search for the love missed in childhood. According to Balint, the *basic fault* is the feeling of many patients that something is missing. Like Ronald Fairbairn and Donald W. Winnicott, Balint understood this deficit in internal structure to result from maternal failures. He viewed all psychological motivations as stemming from the failure to receive adequate maternal love.

Unlike Fairbairn, however, Balint did not entirely abandon drive theory. He suggested that libido, for example, is both pleasure seeking and object seeking. He also worked with seriously disturbed patients, and like Winnicott, he thought that certain aspects of psychoanalytic treatment occur at a more profound level than that of the ordinary verbal explanatory interpretations. Although some material involving genital psychosexual stages of development can be interpreted from the perspective of intrapsychic conflict, Balint believed that certain preverbal phenomena are reexperienced in analysis and that the relationship itself is decisive in dealing with this realm of early experience.

ERIC BERNE (1910–1970)

Eric Berne (Fig. 6.3–3) began his professional life as a training and supervising analyst in classic psychoanalytic theory and technique, but ultimately developed his own school, known as transactional analysis. A *transaction* is a stimulus presented by one person that evokes a corresponding response in another. Berne defined psychological *games* as stereotyped and predictable transactions that persons learn in childhood and continue to play throughout their lives. *Strokes,* the basic motivating factors of human behavior, consist of specific rewards, such as approval and love. All persons have three ego states that exist within them: the *Child,* which represents primitive elements that become fixed in early childhood; the *Adult,* which is the part of the personality capable of objective appraisals of reality; and the *Parent,* which is an introject of the values of a person's actual parents. The therapeutic process is geared toward helping patients understand whether they are functioning in the child, adult, or parent mode in their interactions with others. As patients learn to recognize characteristic games played again and again throughout life, they can ultimately function in the adult mode as much as possible in interpersonal relationships.

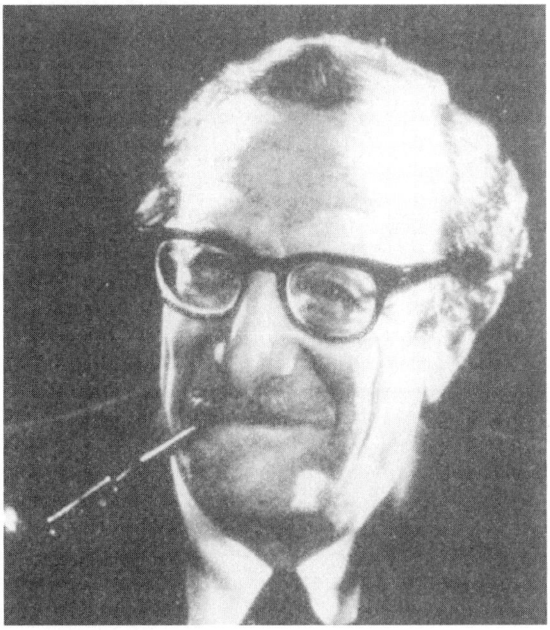

FIGURE 6.3–3
Eric Berne. (Courtesy of Grove Press.)

WILFRED BION (1897–1979)

Wilfred Bion expanded Melanie Klein's concept of *projective identification* to include an interpersonal process in which a therapist feels coerced by a patient into playing a particular role in the patient's internal world. He also developed the notion that the therapist must contain what the patient has projected so that it is processed and returned to the patient in modified form. Bion believed that a similar process occurs between mother and infant. He also observed that "psychotic" and "nonpsychotic" aspects of the mind function simultaneously as suborganizations. Bion is probably best known for his application of psychoanalytic ideas to groups. Whenever a group gets derailed from its task, it deteriorates into one of three *basic states*: dependency, pairing, or fight–flight.

JOHN BOWLBY (1907–1990)

John Bowlby is generally considered the founder of attachment theory. He formed his ideas about attachment in the 1950s while he was consulting with the World Health Organization on the problems of homelessness in children. He stressed that the essence of attachment is *proximity* (i.e., the tendency of a child to stay close to the mother or caregiver). His theory of the mother–infant bond was firmly rooted in biology and drew extensively from ethology and evolutionary theory. A basic sense of security and safety is derived from a continuous and close relationship with a caregiver, according to Bowlby. This readiness for attachment is biologically driven, and Bowlby stressed that attachment is reciprocal. Maternal bonding and caregiving is always intertwined with the child's attachment behavior. Bowlby felt that without this early proximity to the mother or caregiver, the child does not develop a *secure base*, which he considered a launching pad for independence. In the absence of a secure base, the child feels frightened or threatened, and development is severely compromised. Bowlby and attachment theory are discussed in detail in Chapter 4, Section 4.2.

RAYMOND CATTELL (1905–1998)

Raymond Cattell obtained his Ph.D. in England before moving to the United States. He introduced the use of *multivariate analysis* and *factor analysis*—statistical procedures that simultaneously examine the relations among multiple variables and factors—to the study of personality. By examining a person's life record objectively, using personal interviewing and questionnaire data, Cattell described a variety of traits that represent the building blocks of personality.

Traits are both biologically based and environmentally determined or learned. Biological traits include sex, gregariousness, aggression, and

parental protectiveness. Environmentally learned traits include cultural ideas, such as work, religion, intimacy, romance, and identity. An important concept is the *law of coercion to the biosocial mean,* which holds that society exerts pressure on genetically different persons to conform to social norms. For example, a person with a strong genetic tendency toward dominance is likely to receive social encouragement for restraint, whereas the naturally submissive person will be encouraged toward self-assertion.

RONALD FAIRBAIRN (1889–1964)

Ronald Fairbairn, a Scottish analyst who worked most of his life in relative isolation, was one of the major psychoanalytic theorists in the British school of object relations. He suggested that infants are not primarily motivated by the drives of libido and aggression but by an object-seeking instinct. Fairbairn replaced the freudian ideas of energy, ego, and id with the notion of *dynamic structures.* When an infant encounters frustration, a portion of the ego is defensively split off in the course of development and functions as an entity in relation to internal objects and to other subdivisions of the ego. He also stressed that not only an object but also an object *relationship* is internalized during development, so that a self is always in relationship to an object, and the two are connected with an affect.

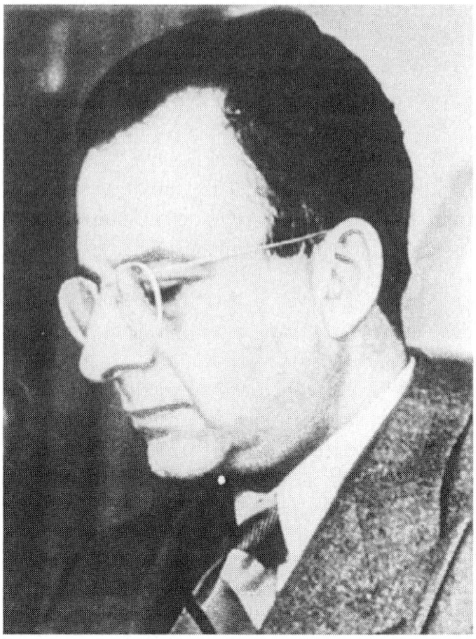

FIGURE 6.3–4
Erich Fromm. (Courtesy of Erich Fromm.)

SÁNDOR FERENCZI (1873–1933)

Although Sándor Ferenczi, a Hungarian analyst, had been analyzed by Freud and was influenced by him, he later discarded Freud's techniques and introduced his own method of analysis. He understood the symptoms of his patients as related to sexual and physical abuse in childhood and proposed that analysts need to love their patients in a way that compensates them for the love they did not receive as children. He developed a procedure known as *active therapy,* in which he encouraged patients to develop an awareness of reality through active confrontation by the therapist. He also experimented with *mutual analysis,* in which he would analyze his patient for a session and then allow the patient to analyze him for a session.

ERICH FROMM (1900–1980)

Erich Fromm (Fig. 6.3–4) came to the United States in 1933 from Germany, where he had received his Ph.D. He was instrumental in founding the William Alanson White Institute for Psychiatry in New York. Fromm identified five character types that are common to, and determined by, Western culture; each person may possess qualities from one or more types. The types are (1) the *receptive personality,* who is passive; (2) the *exploitative personality,* who is manipulative; (3) the *marketing personality,* who is opportunistic and changeable; (4) the *hoarding personality,* who saves and stores; and (5) the *productive personality,* who is mature and enjoys love and work. The therapeutic process involves strengthening the person's sense of ethical behavior toward others and developing productive love, which is characterized by care, responsibility, and respect for other persons.

ANNA FREUD (1895–1982)

Anna Freud (Fig. 6.3–5), the daughter of Sigmund Freud, ultimately made her own set of unique contributions to psychoanalysis. While her father focused primarily on repression as the central defense mechanism, Anna Freud greatly elaborated on individual defense mechanisms, including reaction formation, regression, undoing, introjection, identification, projection, turning against the self, reversal, and sublimation. She was also a key

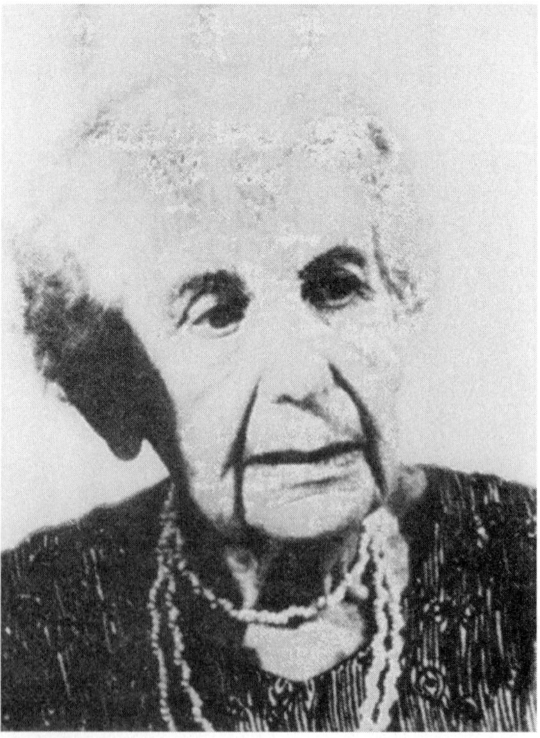

FIGURE 6.3–5
Anna Freud (1895–1982). (From Carson RC, Butcher JN, Coleman JC. *Abnormal Psychology and Modern Life.* 8th ed. Boston: Scott, Foresman; 1988:66. Copyright UPI/Bettman Newsphotos.)

figure in the development of modern ego psychology in that she emphasized that there was "depth in the surface." In other words, the defenses marshaled by the ego to avoid unacceptable wishes from the id were in and of themselves complex and worthy of attention. Up to that point the primary focus had been on uncovering unconscious sexual and aggressive wishes. She also made seminal contributions to the field of child psychoanalysis and studied the function of the ego in personality development. She founded the Hampstead child therapy course and clinic in London in 1947 and served as its director.

MERTON M. GILL (1914–1994)

Merton M. Gill began his career at the Menninger Clinic in the 1940s, working with David Rappaport on the elaboration of ego psychology. As his career evolved, he became a leader in what is now termed the *social constructivist* view. Gill suggested that the facts within the psychoanalytic process are not objectively or authoritatively observed by the analyst but, rather, are a matter of agreement between analyst and analysand. Gill advocated two major elements of the social constructivist perspective: A patient's transference perception of the analyst is to some degree based on the analyst's *real* behavior, and the analyst's ongoing personal participation in the analytic process has a continuous effect on the patient and on how the analyst understands the patient.

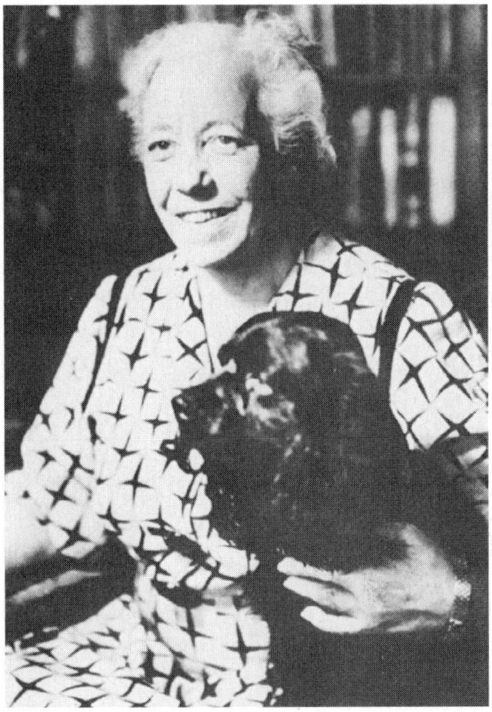

FIGURE 6.3–6
Karen Horney. (Courtesy of the Association for the Advancement of Psychoanalysis, New York.)

KURT GOLDSTEIN (1878–1965)

Kurt Goldstein was born in Germany and received his M.D. from the University of Breslau. He was influenced by existentialism and Gestalt psychology—every organism has dynamic properties, which are energy supplies that are relatively constant and evenly distributed. When states of tension-disequilibrium occur, an organism automatically attempts to return to its normal state. What happens in one part of the organism affects every other part, a phenomenon known as *holocoenosis.*

Self-actualization was a concept Goldstein used to describe persons' creative powers to fulfill their potentialities. Because each person has a different set of innate potentialities, persons strive for self-actualization along different paths. Sickness severely disrupts self-actualization. Responses to disruption of an organism's integrity may be rigid and compulsive; regression to more primitive modes of behavior is characteristic. One of Goldstein's major contributions was his identification of the *catastrophic reaction* to brain damage, in which a person becomes fearful and agitated and refuses to perform simple tasks because of the fear of possible failure.

KAREN HORNEY (1885–1952)

Born and educated in Germany, Karen Horney (Fig. 6.3–6) taught at the Institute of Psychoanalysis in Berlin before immigrating to the United States. Horney believed that a person's current personality attributes result from the interaction between the person and the environment and are not solely based on infantile libidinal strivings carried over from childhood. Her theory, known as *holistic psychology,* maintains that a person needs to be seen as a unitary whole who influences, and is influenced by, the environment. She thought that the Oedipus complex was overvalued in terms of its contribution to adult psychopathology, but she also believed that rigid parental attitudes about sexuality led to excessive concern with the genitals.

She proposed three separate concepts of the self: the *actual self,* the sum total of a person's experience; the *real self,* the harmonious, healthy person; and the *idealized self,* the neurotic expectation or glorified image that a person feels he or she should be. A person's *pride system* alienates him or her from the real self by overemphasizing prestige, intellect, power, strength, appearance, sexual prowess, and other qualities that can lead to self-effacement and self-hatred. Horney also established the concepts of *basic anxiety* and *basic trust.* The therapeutic process, in her view, aims for *self-realization* by exploring distorting influences that prevent the personality from growing.

EDITH JACOBSON (1897–1978)

Edith Jacobson, a psychiatrist in the United States, believed that the structural model and an emphasis on object relations are not fundamentally incompatible. She thought that the ego, self-images, and object images exert reciprocal influences on each other's development. She also stressed that the infant's disappointment with the maternal object is not necessarily related to the mother's actual failure. In Jacobson's view, disappointment is related to a specific, drive-determined demand, rather than to a global striving for contact or engagement. She viewed an infant's experience of pleasure or "unpleasure" as the core of the early mother–infant relationship. Satisfactory experiences lead to the formation of good or gratifying images, whereas unsatisfactory experiences create bad or frustrating images. Normal and pathological development is based on the evolution of these self-images and object images. Jacobson believed that

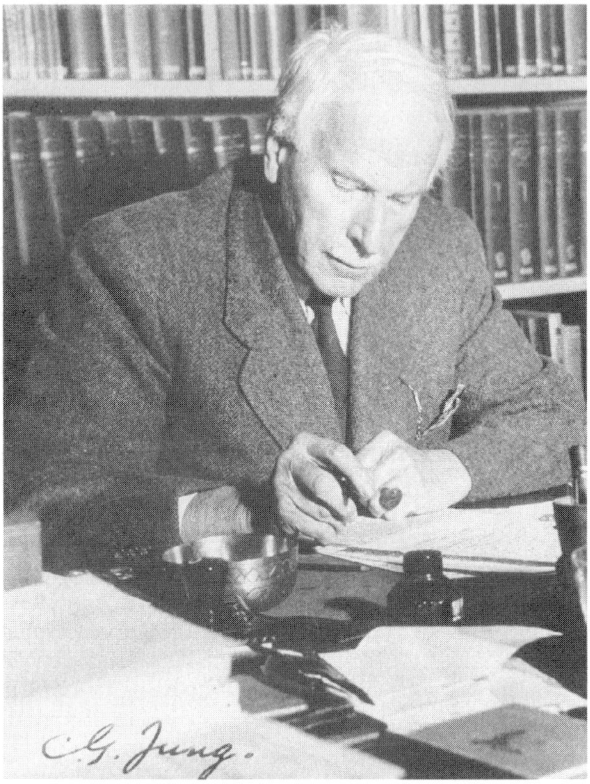

FIGURE 6.3–7
Carl Gustave Jung (print includes signature). (Courtesy of National Library of Medicine, Bethesda, MD.)

the concept of *fixation* refers to modes of object relatedness, rather than to modes of gratification.

CARL GUSTAV JUNG (1875–1961)

Carl Gustav Jung (Fig. 6.3–7), a Swiss psychiatrist, formed a psychoanalytic school known as analytic psychology, which includes basic ideas related to, but going beyond, Freud's theories. After initially being Freud's disciple, Jung broke with Freud over the latter's emphasis on infantile sexuality. He expanded on Freud's concept of the unconscious by describing the *collective unconscious* as consisting of all humankind's common, shared mythological and symbolic past. The collective unconscious includes *archetypes*—representational images and configurations with universal symbolic meanings. Archetypal figures exist for the mother, father, child, and hero, among others. Archetypes contribute to *complexes,* feeling-toned ideas that develop as a result of personal experience interacting with archetypal imagery. Thus, a mother complex is determined not only by the mother–child interaction but also by the conflict between archetypal expectation and actual experience with the real woman who functions in a motherly role.

Jung noted that there are two types of personality organizations: introversion and extroversion. *Introverts* focus on their inner world of thoughts, intuitions, emotions, and sensations; *extroverts* are more oriented toward the outer world, other persons, and material goods. Each person has a mixture of both components. The *persona,* the mask covering the personality, is the face a person presents to the outside world. The persona may become fixed, and the real person hidden from himself or herself. *Anima* and *animus* are unconscious traits possessed by men and women, respectively, and are contrasted with the persona. *Anima* refers to a man's undeveloped femininity, whereas *animus* refers to a woman's undeveloped masculinity.

The aim of jungian treatment is to bring about an adequate adaptation to reality, which involves a person's fulfilling his or her creative potentialities. The ultimate goal is to achieve *individuation,* a process continuing throughout life whereby persons develop a unique sense of their own identity. This developmental process may lead them down new paths away from their previous directions in life.

OTTO KERNBERG (B. 1928)

Otto Kernberg is perhaps the most influential object relations theorist in the United States. Influenced by both Klein and Jacobson, much of his theory is derived from his clinical work with patients who have borderline personality disorder. Kernberg places great emphasis on the splitting of the ego and the elaboration of good and bad self-configurations and object configurations. Although he has continued to use the structural model, he views the id as composed of self-images, object images, and their associated affects. Drives appear to manifest themselves only in the context of internalized interpersonal experience. Good and bad self-representations and object relations become associated, respectively, with libido and aggression. Object relations not only constitute the building blocks of structure, but also the building blocks of drives. Goodness and badness in relational experiences precede drive cathexis. In other words, the dual instincts of libido and aggression arise from object-directed affective states of love and hate.

Kernberg proposed the term *borderline personality organization* for a broad spectrum of patients characterized by a lack of an integrated sense of identity, ego weakness, absence of superego integration, reliance on primitive defense mechanisms such as splitting and projective identification, and a tendency to shift into primary process thinking. He suggested a specific type of psychoanalytic psychotherapy for such patients in which transference issues are interpreted early in the process.

MELANIE KLEIN (1882–1960)

Melanie Klein (Fig. 6.3–8) was born in Vienna, worked with Abraham and Ferenczi, and later moved to London. Klein evolved a theory of internal object relations that was intimately linked to drives. Her unique perspective grew largely from her psychoanalytic work with children, in which she became impressed with the role of unconscious intrapsychic fantasy. She postulated that the ego undergoes a splitting process to deal with the terror of annihilation. She also thought that Freud's concept of the death instinct was central to understanding aggression, hatred, sadism, and other forms of "badness," all of which she viewed as derivatives of the death instinct.

Klein viewed projection and introjection as the primary defensive operations in the first months of life. Infants project derivatives of the death instinct into the mother and then fear attack from the "bad mother," a phenomenon that Klein referred to as *persecutory anxiety.* This anxiety is intimately associated with the *paranoid-schizoid position,* infants' mode of organizing experience in which all aspects of infant and mother are split into good and bad elements. As the disparate views are integrated, infants become concerned that they may have

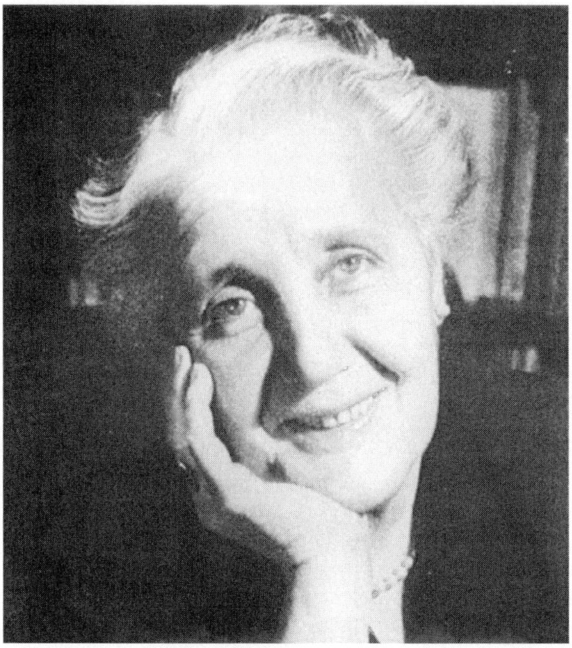

FIGURE 6.3–8
Melanie Klein. (Courtesy of Melanie Klein and Douglas Glass.)

harmed or destroyed the mother through the hostile and sadistic fantasies directed toward her. At this developmental point, children have arrived at the *depressive position,* in which the mother is viewed ambivalently as having both positive and negative aspects and as the target of a mixture of loving and hateful feelings. Klein was also instrumental in the development of child analysis, which evolved from an analytic play technique in which children used toys and played in a symbolic fashion that allowed analysts to interpret the play.

HEINZ KOHUT (1913–1981)

Heinz Kohut is best known for his writings on narcissism and the development of self psychology. He viewed the development and maintenance of self-esteem and self-cohesion as more important than sexuality or aggression. Kohut described Freud's concept of narcissism as judgmental, in that development was supposed to proceed toward object relatedness and away from narcissism. He conceived of two separate lines of development, one moving in the direction of object relatedness and the other in the direction of greater enhancement of the self.

In infancy, children fear losing the protection of the early mother–infant bliss and resort to one of three pathways to save the lost perfection: the grandiose self, the alter ego or twinship, and the idealized parental image. These three poles of the self manifest themselves in psychoanalytic treatment in terms of characteristic transferences, known as *self-object transferences.* The *grandiose self* leads to a *mirror transference,* in which patients attempt to capture the gleam in the analyst's eye through exhibitionistic self-display. The *alter ego* leads to the *twinship transference,* in which patients perceive the analyst as a twin. The *idealized parental image* leads to an *idealizing transference,* in which patients feel enhanced self-esteem by being in the presence of the exalted figure of the analyst.

Kohut suggested that empathic failures in the mother lead to a developmental arrest at a particular stage when children need to use others to perform self-object functions. Although Kohut originally applied this formulation to narcissistic personality disorder, he later expanded it to apply to all psychopathology.

JACQUES LACAN (1901–1981)

Born in Paris and trained as a psychiatrist, Jacques Lacan founded his own institute, the Freudian School of Paris. He attempted to integrate the intrapsychic concepts of Freud with concepts related to linguistics and semiotics (the study of language and symbols). Whereas Freud saw the unconscious as a seething cauldron of needs, wishes, and instincts, Lacan saw it as a sort of language that helps to structure the world. Two of his principal concepts are that the unconscious is structured like a language and that the unconscious is a discourse. Primary process thoughts are actually uncontrolled free-flowing sequences of meaning. Symptoms are signs or symbols of underlying processes. The role of the therapist is to interpret the semiotic text of the personality structure. Lacan's most basic phase is the mirror stage; it is here that infants learn to recognize themselves by taking the perspective of others. In that sense, the ego is not part of the self but, rather, is something outside of, and viewed by, the self. The ego comes to represent parents and society more than it represents the actual self of the person.

Lacan's therapeutic approach involves the need to become less alienated from the self and more involved with others. Relationships are often fantasized, which distorts reality and which must be corrected. Among his most controversial beliefs was that the resistance to understanding the real relationship can be reduced by shortening the length of the therapy session and that psychoanalytic sessions need to be standardized not to time but, rather, to content and process.

KURT LEWIN (1890–1947)

Kurt Lewin received his Ph.D. in Berlin, came to the United States in the 1930s, and taught at Cornell, Harvard, and the Massachusetts Institute of Technology. He adapted the field approach of physics to a concept called *field theory.* A *field* is the totality of coexisting, mutually interdependent parts. Behavior becomes a function of persons and their environment, which together make up the *life space.* The life space represents a field in constant flux, with *valences* or needs that require satisfaction. A hungry person is more aware of restaurants than someone who has just eaten, and a person who wants to mail a letter is aware of mailboxes.

Lewin applied field theory to groups. *Group dynamics* refers to the interaction among members of a group, each of whom depends on the others. The group can exert pressure on a person to change behavior, but the person also influences the group when change occurs.

ABRAHAM MASLOW (1908–1970)

Abraham Maslow (Fig. 6.3–9) was born in Brooklyn, New York, and completed both his undergraduate and graduate work at the University of Wisconsin. Along with Goldstein, Maslow believed in *self-actualization theory*—the need to understand the totality of a person. A leader in humanistic psychology, Maslow described a hierarchical organization of needs present in everyone. As the more primitive needs such as hunger and

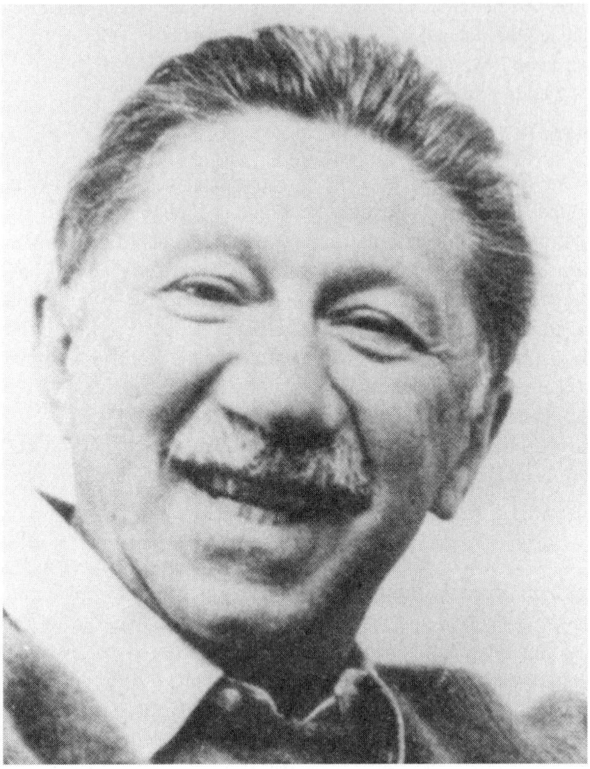

FIGURE 6.3–9

Abraham H. Maslow (1908–1970). (From Carson RC, Butcher JN, Coleman JC. *Abnormal Psychology and Modern Life,* 8th ed. Boston: Scott, Foresman; 1988:74. Copyright The Bettman Archive.)

thirst are satisfied, more advanced psychological needs such as affection and self-esteem become the primary motivators. Self-actualization is the highest need.

A *peak experience,* frequently occurring in self-actualizers, is an episodic, brief occurrence in which a person suddenly experiences a powerful transcendental state of consciousness—a sense of heightened understanding, an intense euphoria, an integrated nature, unity with the universe, and an altered perception of time and space. This powerful experience tends to occur most often in the psychologically healthy and may produce long-lasting beneficial effects.

KARL A. MENNINGER (1893–1990)

Karl A. Menninger was one of the first physicians in the United States to receive psychiatric training. With his brother, Will, he pioneered the concept of a psychiatric hospital based on psychoanalytic principles and founded the Menninger Clinic in Topeka, Kansas. He also was a prolific writer; *The Human Mind,* one of his most popular books, brought psychoanalytic understanding to the lay public. He made a compelling case for the validity of Freud's death instinct in *Man Against Himself. The Vital Balance* was his magnum opus, in which he formulated a unique theory of psychopathology. Menninger maintained a lifelong interest in the criminal justice system and argued in *The Crime of Punishment* that many convicted criminals needed treatment rather than punishment. Finally, his volume entitled *Theory of Psychoanalytic Technique* was one of the few books to examine the theoretical underpinnings of psychoanalysts' interventions.

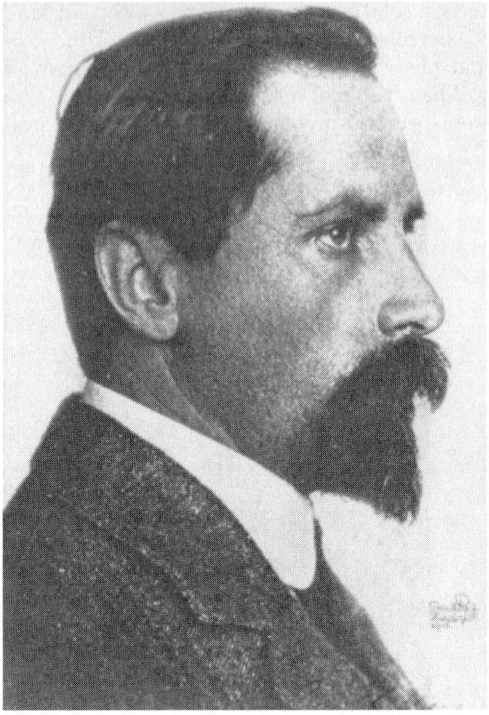

FIGURE 6.3–10

Adolf Meyer, 1866–1950. (From the National Library of Medicine, Bethesda, MD.)

ADOLPH MEYER (1866–1950)

Adolph Meyer (Fig. 6.3–10) came to the United States from Switzerland in 1892 and eventually became director of the psychiatric Henry Phipps Clinic of the Johns Hopkins Medical School. Although he did not entirely reject Freud's theoretical emphasis of mental functioning, Meyer preferred to examine the verifiable and objective aspects of a person's life. His theory of psychobiology explained disordered behavior as reactions to genetic, physical, psychological, environmental, and social stresses. Meyer introduced the concept of *common sense psychiatry,* and focused on ways in which a patient's current life situation could be realistically improved. He coined the concept of *ergasia,* the action of the total organism. His goal in therapy was to aid patients' adjustment by helping them modify unhealthy adaptations. One of Meyer's tools was an autobiographical life chart constructed by the patient during therapy.

GARDNER MURPHY (1895–1979)

Gardner Murphy was born in Ohio and received his Ph.D. from Columbia University. He was among the first to publish a comprehensive history of psychology and made major contributions to social, general, and educational psychology. According to Murphy, three essential stages of personality development are the stage of undifferentiated wholeness, the stage of differentiation, and the stage of integration. This development is frequently

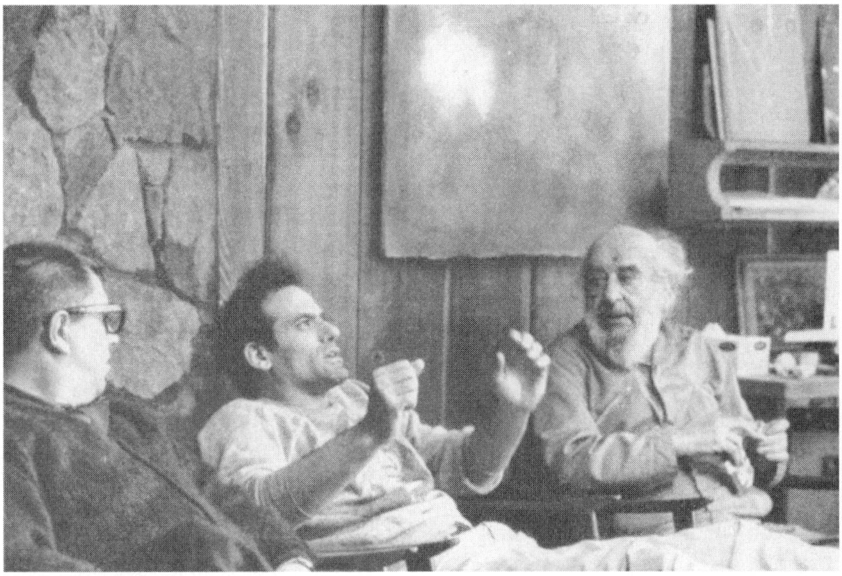

FIGURE 6.3–11
Fritz Perls, at right, conducting a group session. (Courtesy of Michael Alexander.)

uneven, with both regression and progression occurring along the way. There are four inborn human needs: visceral, motor, sensory, and emergency-related. These needs become increasingly specific in time as they are molded by a person's experiences in various social and environmental contexts. *Canalization* brings about these changes by establishing a connection between a need and a specific way of satisfying the need.

Murphy was interested in parapsychology. States such as sleep, drowsiness, certain drug and toxic conditions, hypnosis, and delirium tend to be favorable to paranormal experiences. Impediments to paranormal awareness include various intrapsychic barriers, conditions in the general social environment, and a heavy investment in ordinary sensory experiences.

HENRY MURRAY (1893–1988)

Henry Murray was born in New York City, attended medical school there, and was a founder of the Boston Psychoanalytic Institute. He proposed the term *personology* to describe the study of human behavior. He focused on *motivation,* a need that is aroused by internal or external stimulation; once aroused, motivation produces continued activity until the need is reduced or satisfied. He developed the *Thematic Apperception Test* (TAT), a projective technique used to reveal both unconscious and conscious mental processes and problem areas.

FREDERICK S. PERLS (1893–1970)

Gestalt theory developed in Germany under the influence of several men: Max Wertheimer (1880–1943), Wolfgang Köhler (1887–1967), and Lewin. Frederick "Fritz" Perls (Fig. 6.3–11) applied Gestalt theory to a therapy that emphasizes the current experiences of the patient in the here and now, as contrasted to the there and then of psychoanalytic schools. In terms of motivation, patients learn to recognize their needs at any given time and the ways that the drive to satisfy these needs may influence their current behavior. According to the Gestalt point of view, behavior represents more than the sum of its parts. A *gestalt,* or a whole, both includes, and goes beyond, the sum of smaller, independent events; it deals with essential characteristics of actual experience, such as value, meaning, and form.

SANDOR RADO (1890–1972)

Sandor Rado (Fig. 6.3–12) came to the United States from Hungary in 1945 and founded the Columbia Psychoanalytic Institute in New

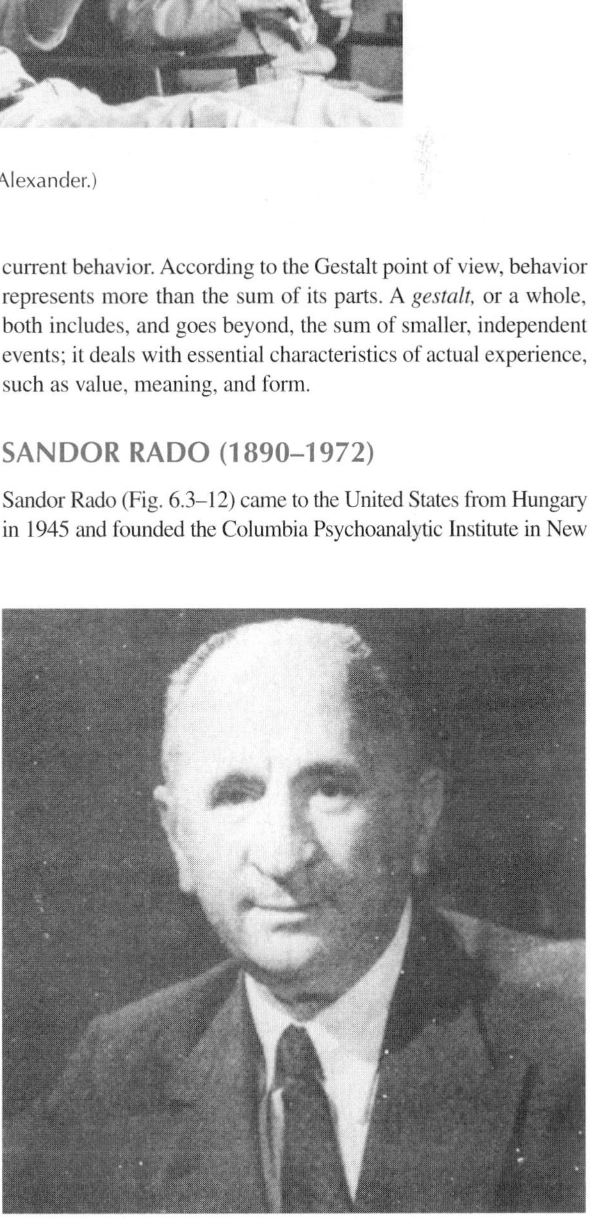

FIGURE 6.3–12
Sandor Rado. (Courtesy of New York Academy of Medicine, New York.)

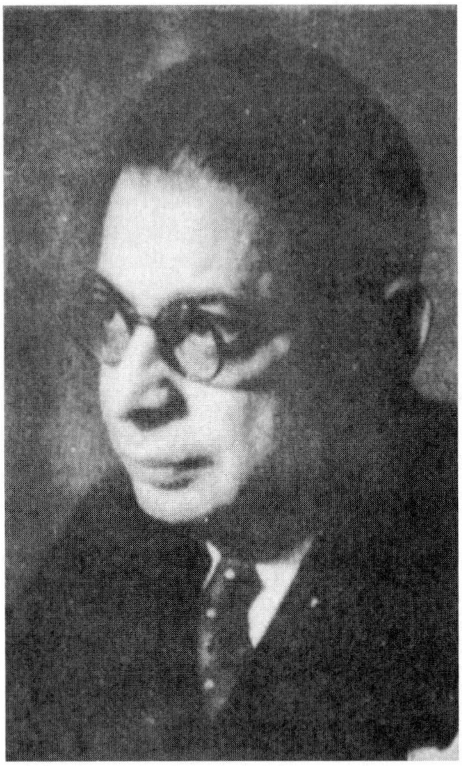

FIGURE 6.3–13
Otto Rank. (Courtesy of New York Academy of Medicine, New York.)

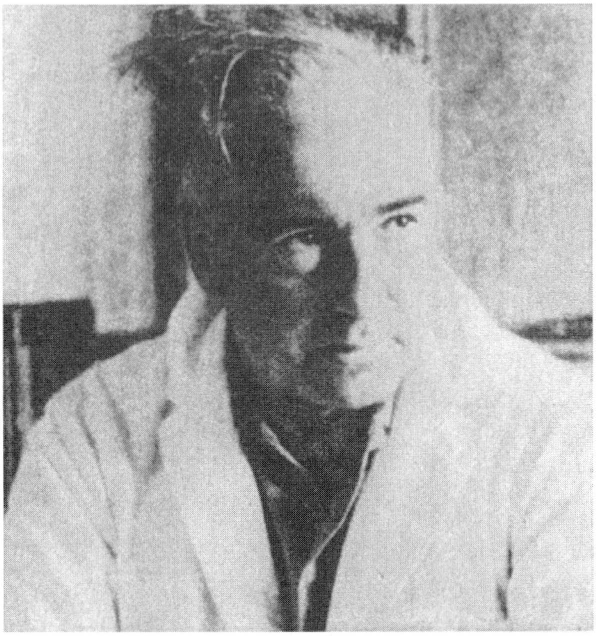

FIGURE 6.3–14
Wilhelm Reich. (Courtesy of New York Academy of Medicine, New York.)

York. His theories of *adaptational dynamics* hold that the organism is a biological system operating under hedonic control, which is somewhat similar to Freud's pleasure principle. Cultural factors often cause excessive hedonic control and disordered behavior by interfering with the organism's ability for *self-regulation*. In therapy, the patient needs to relearn how to experience pleasurable feelings.

OTTO RANK (1884–1939)

An Austrian psychologist and a protégé of Sigmund Freud, Otto Rank (Fig. 6.3–13) broke with Freud in his 1924 publication, *The Trauma of the Birth,* and developed a new theory, which he called *birth trauma*. Anxiety is correlated with separation from the mother—specifically, with separation from the womb, the source of effortless gratification. This painful experience results in primal anxiety. Sleep and dreams symbolize the return to the womb.

The personality is divided into impulses, emotions, and will. Children's impulses seek immediate discharge and gratification. As impulses are mastered, as in toilet training, children begin the process of will development. If will is carried too far, pathological traits (e.g., stubbornness, disobedience, and inhibitions) may develop.

WILHELM REICH (1897–1957)

Wilhelm Reich (Fig. 6.3–14), an Austrian psychoanalyst, made major contributions to psychoanalysis in the area of character formation and character types. The term *character armor* refers to the personality's defenses that serve as resistance to self-understanding and change. There are four major character types: the *hysterical character* is sexually seductive, anxious, and fixated at the phallic phase of libido development; the *compulsive character* is controlled, distrustful, indecisive, and fixated at the anal phase; the *narcissistic character* is fixated at the phallic state of development, and if the person is male, there is contempt for women; and the *masochistic character* is long-suffering, complaining, and self-deprecatory, with an excessive demand for love.

The therapeutic process, called *will therapy,* emphasizes the relationship between patient and therapist; the goal of treatment is to help patients accept their separateness. A definite termination date for therapy is used to protect against excessive dependence on the therapist.

CARL ROGERS (1902–1987)

Carl Rogers (Fig. 6.3–15) received his Ph.D. in psychology from Columbia University. After attending Union Theological Seminary in New York, Rogers studied for the ministry. His name is most clearly associated with the *person-centered theory* of personality and psychotherapy, in which the major concepts are self-actualization and self-direction. Specifically, persons are born with a capacity to direct themselves in the healthiest way, toward a level of completeness called self-actualization. From his person-centered approach, Rogers viewed personality not as a static entity composed of traits and patterns but as a dynamic phenomenon involving ever-changing communications, relationships, and self-concepts.

Rogers developed a treatment program called *client-centered psychotherapy*. Therapists attempt to produce an atmosphere in which clients can reconstruct their strivings for self-actualization. Therapists hold clients in *unconditional positive regard,* which is the total nonjudgmental acceptance of clients as they are. Other therapeutic prac-

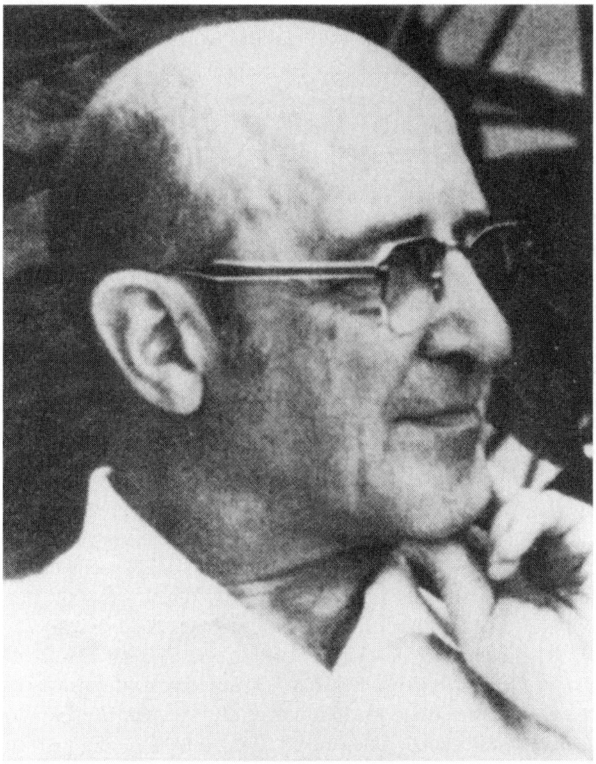

FIGURE 6.3–15
Carl Rogers (b. 1902). (From Carson RC, Butcher JN, Coleman JC. *Abnormal Psychology and Modern Life.* 8th ed. Boston: Scott, Foresman; 1988:75. Copyright Hugh L. Wilkerson.)

tices include attention to the present, focus on clients' feelings, emphasis on process, trust in the potential and self-responsibility of clients, and a philosophy grounded in a positive attitude toward them, rather than a preconceived structure of treatment.

JEAN-PAUL SARTRE (1905–1980)

Born in Paris, Jean-Paul Sartre wrote plays and novels before turning to psychology. He was a German prisoner of war from 1940 to 1941 during World War II. Influenced by the ideas of Martin Heidegger, he developed what he called existential psychoanalysis. The reflective self was a key concept in Sartre's psychology. He recognized that humans alone could reflect on themselves as objects, so that the experience of "Being" in humans is unique in the natural world. This capacity to reflect leads humans to impose a meaning on existence. For Sartre, this meaning allows a human being to create his or her own essence.

Sartre denied the realm of the unconscious; he thought that human beings were condemned to be free and to face the fundamental existential dilemma—their aloneness without a god to provide meaning. As a result, each individual creates values and meanings. Neurosis is an escape from freedom, which is the key to maintaining psychological health. Sartre made no distinction between philosophy and psychology. Psychologists, like philosophers, search for the truth about the world. Part of this truth, in Sartre's view, was the dialectic between consciousness and Being. Consciousness introduces nothingness and is a negation of being-in-itself. Ideals are revealed in actions, not in professed beliefs.

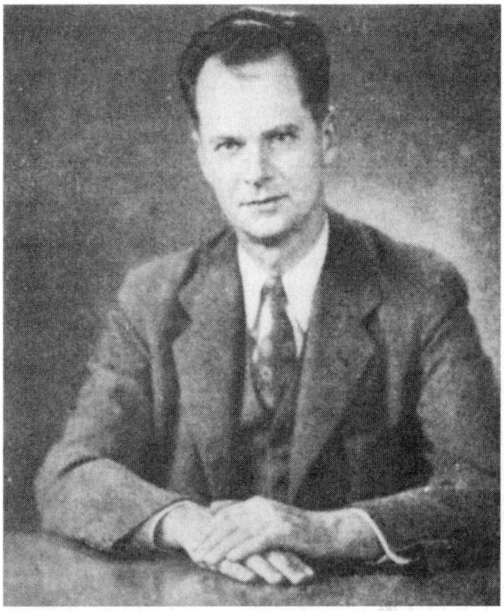

FIGURE 6.3–16
B. F. Skinner.

B. F. SKINNER (1904–1990)

Burrhus Frederic Skinner (Fig. 6.3–16), commonly known as B. F. Skinner, received his Ph.D. in psychology from Harvard University, where he taught for many years. Skinner's seminal work in operant learning laid much of the groundwork for many current methods of behavior modification, programmed instruction, and general education. His global beliefs about the nature of behavior have been applied more widely, it can be argued, than those of any other theorist except, perhaps, Freud. His impact has been impressive in scope and magnitude.

Skinner's approach to personality was derived more from his basic beliefs about behavior than from a specific theory of personality per se. To Skinner, personality did not differ from other behaviors or sets of behaviors; it is acquired, maintained, and strengthened or weakened according to the same rules of reward and punishment that alter any other form of behavior. *Behaviorism,* as Skinner's basic theory is most commonly known, is concerned only with observable, measurable behavior that can be operationalized. Many abstract and mentalistic hallmarks of other dominant personality theories have little place in Skinner's framework. Concepts such as self, ideas, and ego are considered unnecessary for understanding behavior and are shunned. Through the process of operant conditioning and the application of basic principles of learning, persons are believed to develop sets of behavior that characterize their responses to the world of stimuli that they face in their lives. Such a set of responses is called *personality.*

HARRY STACK SULLIVAN (1892–1949)

Harry Stack Sullivan (Fig. 6.3–17) received his training in psychiatry in the United States in the 1920s and 1930s, during the early years of Freud's profound influence on American psychiatry. Like Meyer, under whom he studied, however, Sullivan insisted on formulating his concepts on observable data.

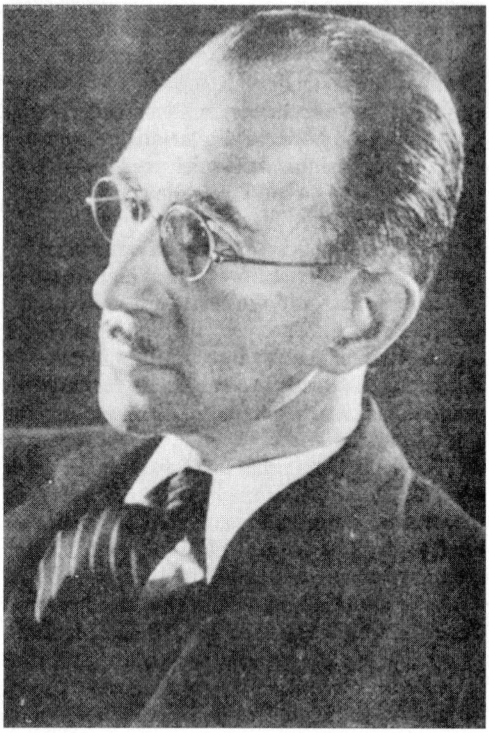

FIGURE 6.3–17
Harry Stack Sullivan. (Courtesy of New York Academy of Medicine, New York.)

Sullivan described three modes of experiencing and thinking about the world. The *prototaxic mode* is undifferentiated thought that cannot separate the whole into parts or use symbols. It occurs normally in infancy and also appears in patients with schizophrenia. In the *parataxic mode,* events are causally related because of temporal or serial connections. Logical relationships, however, are not perceived. The *syntaxic mode* is the logical, rational, and most mature type of cognitive functioning of which a person is capable. These three types of thinking and experiencing occur side by side in all persons; it is the rare person who functions exclusively in the syntaxic mode.

The total configuration of personality traits is known as the *self-system,* which develops in various stages and is the outgrowth of interpersonal experiences, rather than an unfolding of intrapsychic forces. During infancy, anxiety occurs for the first time when infants' primary needs are not satisfied. During childhood, from 2 to 5 years, a child's main tasks are to learn the requirements of the culture and how to deal with powerful adults. As a juvenile, from 5 to 8 years, a child has a need for peers and must learn how to deal with them. In preadolescence, from 8 to 12 years, the capacity for love and for collaboration with another person of the same sex develops. This so-called chum period is the prototype for a sense of intimacy. In the history of patients with schizophrenia, this experience of chums is often missing. During adolescence, major tasks include the separation from the family, the development of standards and values, and the transition to heterosexuality.

The therapy process requires the active participation of the therapist, who is known as a *participant observer.* Modes of experience, particularly the parataxic, need to be clarified, and new patterns of behavior need to be implemented. Ultimately, persons need to see themselves as they really are, instead of as they think they are or as they want others to think they are.

Sullivan is best known for his creative psychotherapeutic work with severely disturbed patients. He believed that even the most psychotic patients with schizophrenia could be reached through the human relationship of psychotherapy.

DONALD W. WINNICOTT (1897–1971)

Donald W. Winnicott was one of the central figures in the British school of object relations theory. His theory of *multiple self-organizations* included a *true self,* which develops in the context of a responsive *holding environment* provided by a *good-enough mother.* When infants experience a traumatic disruption of their developing sense of self, however, a false self emerges and monitors and adapts to the conscious and unconscious needs of the mother; it thus provides a protected exterior behind which the true self is afforded a privacy that it requires to maintain its integrity.

Winnicott also developed the notion of the *transitional object.* Ordinarily a pacifier, blanket, or teddy bear, this object serves as a substitute for the mother during infants' efforts to separate and become independent. It provides a soothing sense of security in the absence of the mother. Winnicott viewed the transitional space in which the transitional object functions as the source of art, creativity, and religion.

References

Ansbacher HL, Ansbacher RR, eds. *The Individual Psychology of Alfred Adler: A Systematic Presentation in Selections from His Writings.* New York: Basic Books; 1956.

Baker HS, Baker MN. Heinz Kohut's self psychology: an overview. *Am J Psychiatry.* 1987;144:1.

Bowlby J. *A Secure Base: Parent–Child Attachment and Healthy Human Development.* New York: Basic Books; 1988.

Chessick R. *What Constitutes the Patient in Psychotherapy: Alternative Approaches to Understanding.* Northvale, NJ: Jason Aronson; 1992.

Edgcumbe R. *Anna Freud: A View of Development, Disturbance and Therapeutic Techniques.* London: Routledge; 2000.

Gabbard GO. Psychoanalysis. In: Kaplan BJ, Sadock V, eds. *Kaplan & Sadock's Comprehensive Textbook of Psychiatry.* 7th ed. Vol 1. Baltimore: Lippincott Williams & Wilkins; 2000:431.

Gabbard GO. *Psychodynamic Psychiatry in Clinical Practice: The Third Edition.* Washington, DC: American Psychiatric Press; 2000.

Gill MM. *Psychoanalysis in Transition: A Personal View.* Hillsdale, NJ: Analytic Press; 1994.

Greenberg JR, Mitchell SA. *Object Relations in Psychoanalytic Theory.* Cambridge, MA: Harvard University Press; 1983.

Groskurth P. *Melanie Klein: Her World and Her Work.* New York: AA Knopf; 1986.

Horney K. *The Neurotic Personality of Our Time.* New York: WW Norton; 1937.

Jung CG. *Memories, Dreams, Reflections.* New York: Random House; 1961.

Menninger KA. *The Vital Balance: The Life Process in Mental Health and Illness.* New York: Viking; 1963.

Monroe RL. *Schools of Psychoanalytic Thought.* New York: Dryden Press; 1955.

Perry HS. *Psychiatrist of America: The Life of Harry Stack Sullivan.* Cambridge, MA: Belknap Press, Harvard University Press; 1982.

Rayner E. *The Independent Mind in British Psychoanalysis.* Northvale, NJ: Jason Aronson; 1991.

Schultz DP, Schultz SE. *Theories of Personality.* 7th ed. Belmont, CA: Wadsworth/Thomson Learning; 2001.

Segal H. *Melanie Klein.* New York: Viking; 1980.

Smith S. *Ideas of the Great Psychologists.* Philadelphia: Harper & Row; 1983.

7 Clinical Examination of the Psychiatric Patient

7.1 Psychiatric History and Mental Status Examination

The diagnosis of psychiatric patients differs in several important ways from the diagnosis of patients with physical disease. Despite impressive advances in such fields as neuroimaging, molecular biology, and genetics, our knowledge of the causes of most psychiatric disorders remains primitive and incomplete. Diagnosis based on etiology is therefore not likely. Moreover, in the absence of etiological certainty, there have grown up over the past several decades a variety of sometimes competing theoretical schools, which attempt to explain the origins of symptoms on the basis of theories of general behavior. For example, psychoanalytic theory, drawing on the work of Sigmund Freud and subsequent generations of analysts, suggests that psychiatric symptoms result from unconscious intrapsychic conflict—that is, conflict within a person's own thinking; a wish to do something may coexist with a fear that the thing will be done. Behavioral theory, on the other hand, explains symptoms as conditioned by a complex interplay of rewards and punishments. For a diagnosis to be widely useable, it cannot be tied to one theoretical school to the exclusion of the other.

Another difference between diagnosis in psychiatry and that in physical medicine is that psychiatry has no external validating criteria. Few independent markers such as laboratory tests exist to confirm or refute an initial diagnosis. Consequently, a psychiatric diagnosis is only as good as the knowledge and skill of the clinician who is making it. As might be expected, this has led over the years to a serious problem of diagnostic reliability—different psychiatrists examining the same patient come up with different diagnoses.

These difficulties were addressed in the various editions of *Diagnostic and Statistical Manual of Mental Disorders* (DSM) of the American Psychiatric Association. The DSM diagnostic criteria are based on descriptive phenomenology. Phenomenology describes what is known through the senses—what is directly seen or heard, for example—as opposed to what is interpreted or inferred. Observed data are always more reliable than inferred data, and the move away from interpretive, intuitive, and impressionistic diagnoses to a phenomenological descriptive system has improved psychiatric diagnostic reliability. It has also strengthened the medical model. DSM is currently in its fourth edition, and its evolution is one of the major recent advances in psychiatric diagnosis. A text revision of the fourth edition of DSM (DSM-IV-TR) was published in 2000.

The psychiatric evaluation comprises two sections. The first, a section of histories (e.g., psychiatric, medical, family), includes the patient's description of how symptoms of the current episode have evolved, a review of past episodes and treatments, a description of current and past medical conditions, a summary of family members' psychiatric problems and treatments, and the patient's personal history, which reveals interpersonal and adaptive functioning over time. Information for the history will come from the patient but may be supplemented by collateral information from family members, social referral agencies, previous treating physicians, and old hospital records. The second section of the psychiatric evaluation, the mental status examination, systematically reviews the patient's emotional and cognitive functioning at the time the interview is conducted.

PSYCHIATRIC HISTORY

The psychiatric history is the record of the patient's life; it allows a psychiatrist to understand who the patient is, where the patient has come from, and where the patient is likely to go in the future. The history is the patient's life story told to the psychiatrist in the patient's own words from his or her own point of view. Many times, the history also includes information about the patient obtained from other sources, such as a parent or spouse. Obtaining a comprehensive history from a patient and, if necessary, from informed sources is essential to making a correct diagnosis and formulating a specific and effective treatment plan. As mentioned above, a psychiatric history differs slightly from histories taken in medicine or surgery. In addition to gathering the concrete and factual data related to the chronology of symptom formation and to the psychiatric and medical history, a psychiatrist strives to derive from the history the elusive picture of a patient's individual personality characteristics, including both strengths and weaknesses. The psychiatric history provides insight into the nature of relationships with those closest to the patient and includes all the important persons in his or her life. One can usually elicit a reasonably comprehensive picture of the patient's development from the earliest formative years until the present.

Table 7.1–1
Outline of Psychiatric History

I. Identifying data
II. Chief complaint
III. History of present illness
  A. Onset
  B. Precipitating factors
IV. Past illnesses
  A. Psychiatric
  B. Medical
  C. Alcohol and other substance history
V. Family history
VI. Personal history (anamnesis)
  A. Prenatal and perinatal
  B. Early childhood (through age 3)
  C. Middle childhood (ages 3–11)
  D. Late childhood (puberty through adolescence)
  E. Adulthood
    1. Occupational history
    2. Marital and relationship history
    3. Military history
    4. Educational history
    5. Religion
    6. Social activity
    7. Current living situation
    8. Legal history
  F. Sexual history
  G. Fantasies and dreams
  H. Values

The most important technique for obtaining a psychiatric history is to allow patients to tell their stories in their own words in the order that they consider most important. As patients relate their stories, skillful interviewers recognize the points at which they can introduce relevant questions about the areas described in the outline of the history and mental status examination.

The structure of the history and mental status examination presented in this section is not intended to be a rigid plan for interviewing a patient; it is meant to be a guide for organizing the patient's history when it is written up. Several acceptable and standard formats for a psychiatric history are available; one such format is presented in Table 7.1–1. Examples of questions to ask the patient when obtaining the psychiatric history are listed in Table 7.1–2.

Identifying Data

The identifying data provide a succinct demographic summary of the patient by name, age, marital status, sex, occupation, language (if other than English), ethnic background, and religion, insofar as they are pertinent, and current circumstances of living. The information can also include the place or situation in which the current interview took place, the source(s) of the information, the reliability of the source(s), and whether the current disorder is the first episode for the patient. The psychiatrist should indicate whether the patient came in on his or her own, was referred by someone else, or was brought in by someone else. The identifying data are meant to provide a thumbnail sketch of potentially important patient characteristics that may

Table 7.1–2
Common Questions for the Psychiatric History and Mental Status

Topic	Questions	Comments and Helpful Hints
Identifying data: Name, age, sex, marital status, religion, education, address, phone number, occupation, source of referral	Be direct in obtaining identifying data. Request specific answers.	If patient cannot cooperate get information from family member or friend; if referred by a physician, obtain medical record.
Chief complaint (CC): Brief statement in patient's own words of why patient is in the hospital or is being seen in consultation	Why are you going to see a psychiatrist? What brought you to the hospital? What seems to be the problem?	Record answers verbatim; a bizarre complaint points to psychotic process.
History of present illness (HPI): Development of symptoms from time of onset to present; relation of life events, conflicts, stressors; drugs; change from previous level of functioning	When did you first notice something happening to you? Were you upset about anything when symptoms began? Did they begin suddenly or gradually?	Record in patient's own words as much as possible. Get history of previous hospitalizations and treatment. Sudden onset of symptoms may indicate drug-induced disorder.
Previous psychiatric and medical disorders: Psychiatric disorders; psychosomatic, medical, neurological illnesses (e.g., craniocerebral trauma, convulsions)	Did you ever lose consciousness? Have a seizure?	Ascertain extent of illness, treatment, medications, outcomes, hospitals, doctors. Determine whether illness serves some additional purpose (secondary gain).
Personal history: Birth and infancy: To the extent known by the patient, ascertain mother's pregnancy and delivery, planned or unwanted pregnancy, developmental landmarks—standing, walking, talking, temperament	Do you know anything about your birth? If so, from whom? How old was your mother when you were born? Your father?	Older mothers (>35) have high risk for Down syndrome baby; older father (>45) may contribute damaged sperm producing deficits including schizophrenia.

(*continued*)

Table 7.1–2 (*continued*)

Topic	Questions	Comments and Helpful Hints
Childhood: Feeding habits, toilet training, personality (shy, outgoing), general conduct and behavior, relationship with parents or caregivers, peers. Separations, nightmares, bed-wetting, fears	Toilet training? Bedwetting? Sex play with peers? What is your first childhood memory?	Separation anxiety and school phobia associated with adult depression; enuresis associated with fire setting. Childhood memories before the age of 3 are usually imagined, not real.
Adolescence: Peer and authority relationships, school history, grades, emotional problems, drug use, age of puberty	Adolescents may refuse to answer questions; but they should be asked. Adults may distort memories of emotionally charged adolescent experience. Sexual molestation?	Poor school performance is a sensitive indicator of emotional disorder. Schizophrenia begins in late adolescence.
Adulthood: Work history, choice of career, marital history, children, education, finances, military history, religion	Open-ended questions are preferable. Tell me about your marriage. Be nonjudgmental: What role does religion play in your life, if any? What is your sexual preference in a partner?	Depending on chief complaint some areas require more detailed inquiry. Manic patients frequently go into debt or are promiscuous. Overvalued religious ideas associated with paranoid personality disorder.
Sexual history: Sexual development, masturbation, anorgasmia, erectile disorder, premature ejaculation, paraphilia, sexual orientation, general attitudes and feelings	Are there or have there been any problems or concerns about your sex life? How did you learn about sex? Has there been any change in your sex drive?	Be nonjudgmental. Asking *when* masturbation began is a better approach than asking *do you* or *did you ever* masturbate.
Family history: Psychiatric, medical, and genetic illness in mother, father, siblings; age of parents and occupations; if deceased, date and cause; feelings about each family member, finances	Have any members in your family been depressed? Alcoholic? In a mental hospital? In jail? Describe your living conditions. Did you have your own room?	Genetic loading in anxiety, depression, schizophrenia. Get medication history of family (medications effective in family members for similar disorders may be effective in patient).
	Mental Status	
General appearance: Note appearance, gait, dress, grooming (neat or unkempt), posture, gestures, facial expressions. Does patient appear older or younger than stated age?	Introduce yourself and direct patient to take a seat. In the hospital, bring your chair to bedside; do not sit on the bed.	Unkempt and disheveled in cognitive disorder; pinpoint pupils in narcotic addiction; withdrawal and stooped posture in depression.
Motoric behavior: Level of activity: psychomotor agitation or psychomotor retardation—tics, tremors, automatisms, mannerisms, grimacing, stereotypes, negativism, apraxia, echopraxia, waxy flexibility; emotional appearance—anxious, tense, panicky, bewildered, sad, unhappy; voice—faint, loud, hoarse; eye contact	Have you been more active than usual? Less active? You may ask about obvious mannerisms, e.g., "I notice that your hand still shakes, can you tell me about that?" Stay aware of smells, e.g., alcoholism/ketoacidosis.	Fixed posturing, odd behavior in schizophrenia. Hyperactive with stimulant (cocaine) abuse and in mania. Psychomotor retardation in depression; tremors with anxiety or medication side effect (lithium). Eye contact is normally made approximately half the time during the interview. Minimal eye contact in schizophrenia. Scanning of environment in paranoid states.
Attitude during interview: How patient relates to examiner—irritable, aggressive, seductive, guarded, defensive, indifferent, apathetic, cooperative, sarcastic	You may comment about attitude. You seem irritated about something; is that an accurate observation?	Suspiciousness in paranoia; seductive in hysteria; apathetic in conversion disorder (*la belle indifference*); punning (*witzlesucht*) in frontal lobe syndromes.
Mood: Steady or sustained emotional state—gloomy, tense, hopeless, ecstatic, resentful, happy, bashful, sad, exultant, elated, euphoric, depressed, apathetic, anhedonic, fearful, suicidal, grandiose, nihilistic	How do you feel? How are your spirits? Do you have thoughts that life is not worth living or that you want to harm yourself? Do you have plans to take your own life? Do you want to die? Has there been a change in your sleep habits?	Suicidal ideas in 25% of depressives; elation in mania. Early morning awakening in depression; decreased need for sleep in mania.
Affect: Feeling tone associated with idea—labile, blunt, appropriate to content, inappropriate, flat	Observe nonverbal signs of emotion, body movements, facies, rhythm of voice (prosody). Laughing when talking about sad subjects, e.g., death, is inappropriate.	Changes in affect usual with schizophrenia: loss of prosody in cognitive disorder, catatonia. Do not confuse medication adverse effect with flat affect.
Speech: Slow, fast, pressured, garrulous, spontaneous, taciturn, stammering, stuttering, slurring, staccato. Pitch, articulation, aphasia, coprolalia, echolalia, incoherent, logorrhea, mute, paucity, stilted	Ask patient to say "Methodist Episcopalian" to test for dysarthria.	Manic patients show pressured speech; paucity of speech in depression; uneven or slurred speech in cognitive disorders.

(*continued*)

Table 7.1–2 (*continued*)

Topic	Questions	Comments and Helpful Hints
Perceptual disorders: Hallucinations—olfactory, auditory, haptic (tactile), gustatory, visual; illusions; hypnopompic or hypnagogic experiences; feeling of unreality, *déjà vu, déjà entendu,* macropsia	Do you ever see things or hear voices? Do you have strange experiences as you fall asleep or upon awakening? Has the world changed in any way? Do you have strange smells?	Visual hallucinations suggest schizophrenia. Tactile hallucinations suggest cocainism, delirium tremens (DTs). Olfactory hallucinations common in temporal lobe epilepsy.
Thought content: Delusions—persecutory (paranoid), grandiose, infidelity, somatic, sensory, thought broadcasting, thought insertion, ideas of reference, ideas of unreality, phobias, obsessions, compulsions, ambivalence, autism, dereism, blocking, suicidal or homicidal preoccupation, conflicts, nihilistic ideas, hypochondriasis, depersonalization, derealization, flight of ideas, *idée fixe,* magical thinking, neologisms	Do you feel people want to harm you? Do you have special powers? Is anyone trying to influence you? Do you have strange body sensations? Are there thoughts that you can't get out of your mind? Do you think about the end of the world? Can people read your mind? Do you ever feel the TV is talking to you? Ask about fantasies and dreams.	Are delusions congruent with mood (grandiose delusions with elated mood) or incongruent? Mood incongruent delusions point to schizophrenia. Illusions are common in delirium. Thought insertion is characteristic of schizophrenia.
Thought process: Goal-directed ideas, loosened associations, illogical, tangential, relevant, circumstantial, rambling, ability to abstract, flight of ideas, clang associations, perseveration	Ask meaning of proverbs to test abstraction, e.g., "People in glass houses should not throw stones." Concrete answer is, "Glass breaks." Abstract answers deal with universal themes or moral issues. Ask similarity between bird and butterfly (both alive), bread and cake (both food).	Loose associations point to schizophrenia; flight of ideas, to mania; inability to abstract, to schizophrenia, brain damage.
Sensorium: Level of consciousness—alert, clear, confused, clouded, comatose, stuporous; orientation to time, place, person; cognition	What place is this? What is today's date? Do you know who I am? Do you know who you are?	Delirium or dementia shows clouded or wandering sensorium. Orientation to person remains intact longer than orientation to time or place.
Memory: Remote memory (long-term memory): Past several days, months, years	Where were you born? Where did you go to school? Date of marriage? Birthdays of children? What were last week's newspaper headlines?	Patients with dementia of the Alzheimer's type retain remote memory longer than recent memory. Gaps in memory may be localized or filled in with confabulatory details. Hypermnesia is seen in paranoid personality.
Recent memory (short-term): Recall of events in past day or two	Where were you yesterday? What did you eat at your last meal?	In brain disease, recent memory loss (amnesia) usually occurs before remote memory loss.
Immediate memory (very short-term memory): Laying down of immediate information with ability to quickly recall data	Ask patient to repeat six digits forward, then backward (normal responses). Ask patient to try to remember three nonrelated items; test patient after 5 minutes.	Loss of memory occurs with cognitive, dissociative, or conversion disorder. Anxiety can impair immediate retention and recent memory. Anterograde memory loss (amnesia) occurs after taking certain drugs, e.g., benzodiazepines. Retrograde memory loss occurs after head trauma.
Concentration and calculation: Ability to pay attention; distractibility; ability to do simple math	Ask patient to count from 1 to 20 rapidly; do simple calculations (2 × 3, 4 × 9); do serial 7 test, i.e., subtract 7 from 100 and keep subtracting 7. How many nickels in $1.35?	Rule out medical cause for any defects versus anxiety or depression (pseudodementia). Make tests congruent with educational level of patient.
Information and intelligence: Use of vocabulary; level of education; fund of knowledge	Distance from New York City to Los Angeles. Name some vegetables. What is the largest river in the United States?	Check educational level to judge results. Rule out mental retardation, borderline intellectual functioning.
Judgment: Ability to understand relations between facts and to draw conclusions; responses in social situations	What is the thing to do if you find an envelope in the street that is sealed, stamped, and addressed?	Impaired in brain disease, schizophrenia, borderline intellectual functioning, intoxication.
Insight level: Realizing that there are physical or mental problems; denial of illness, ascribing blame to outside factors; recognizing need for treatment	Do you think you have a problem? Do you need treatment? What are your plans for the future?	Impaired in delirium, dementia, frontal lobe syndrome, psychosis, borderline intellectual functioning.

affect diagnosis, prognosis, treatment, and compliance. An example of the written report of the identifying data follows.

Mr. J. Jones is a 25-year-old white, single, Catholic man, currently unemployed and homeless, living in public shelters and on the street. The current interview occurred in the emergency room (ER), with the patient in four-point restraints in the presence of two clinical staff members and one police officer. It was the 10th such visit to the ER for Mr. Jones in the past year. The sources of information on Mr. Jones included the patient himself and the police officer who brought him to the ER. The police officer had witnessed the patient on the street and knew him from previous episodes.

Chief Complaint

The chief complaint, in the patient's own words, states why he or she has come or been brought in for help. It should be recorded even if the patient is unable to speak, and the patient's explanation, regardless of how bizarre or irrelevant it is, should be recorded verbatim in the section on the chief complaint. The other individuals present as sources of information can then give their versions of the presenting events in the section on the history of the present illness.

Examples of chief complaints follow:

"I was feeling very depressed and thinking about killing myself."
"Every car outside my house has a license plate number that is sending me hidden messages concerning a plot to kill the president."
"There's nothing wrong with me; it's her that's crazy."
"The patient was mute."

History of Present Illness

The history of present illness provides a comprehensive and chronological picture of the events leading up to the current moment in the patient's life. This part of the psychiatric history is probably the most helpful in making a diagnosis: When was the onset of the current episode, and what were the immediate precipitating events or triggers? An understanding of the history of the present illness helps answer the question Why now? Why did the patient come to the doctor at this time? What were the patient's life circumstances at the onset of the symptoms or behavioral changes, and how did they affect the patient so that the presenting disorder became manifest? Knowing the previously well patient's personality also helps give perspective on the currently ill patient.

The evolution of the patient's symptoms should be determined and summarized in an organized and systematic way. Symptoms not present should also be delineated. The more detailed the history of the present illness, the more likely the clinician is to make an accurate diagnosis. What past precipitating events were part of the chain leading up to the immediate events? In what ways has the patient's illness affected his or her life activities (e.g., work, important relationships)? What is the nature of the dysfunction (e.g., details about changes in such factors as personality, memory, speech)? Are there psychophysiological symptoms? If so, they should be described in terms of location, intensity, and fluctuation. Any relation between physical and psychological symptoms should be noted. A description of the patient's current anxieties, whether they are generalized and nonspecific (free floating) or are specifically related to particular situations, is helpful. How does the patient handle these anxieties? Frequently, a relatively open-ended question such as "How did this all begin?" leads to an adequate unfolding of the history of the present illness. A well-organized patient is generally able to present a chronological account of the history, but a disorganized patient is difficult to interview, as the chronology of events is confused. In this case, contacting other informants, such as family members and friends, can be a valuable aid in clarifying the patient's story.

Past Illnesses

The past illnesses section of the psychiatric history is a transition between the story of the present illness and the patient's personal history (also called the *anamnesis*). Past episodes of both psychiatric and medical illnesses are described. Ideally, a detailed account of the patient's preexisting and underlying psychological and biological substrates is given at this point, and important clues to, and evidence of, vulnerable areas in the patient's functioning are provided. The patient's symptoms, extent of incapacity, type of treatment received, names of hospitals, length of each illness, effects of previous treatments, and degree of compliance should all be explored and recorded chronologically. Particular attention should be paid to the first episodes that signaled the onset of illness, because first episodes can often provide crucial data about precipitating events, diagnostic possibilities, and coping capabilities.

With regard to medical history, the psychiatrist should obtain a medical review of symptoms and note any major medical or surgical illnesses and major traumas, particularly those requiring hospitalization. Episodes of craniocerebral trauma, neurological illness, tumors, and seizure disorders are especially relevant to psychiatric histories, as is a history of testing positive for the human immunodeficiency virus (HIV) or having acquired immune deficiency syndrome (AIDS). Specific questions need to be asked about the presence of a seizure disorder, episodes of loss of consciousness, changes in usual headache patterns, changes in vision, and episodes of confusion and disorientation. A history of infection with syphilis is critical and relevant.

Causes, complications, and treatment of any illness and the effects of the illness on the patient should be noted. Specific questions about psychosomatic disorders should be asked and the answers noted. Included in this category are hay fever, rheumatoid arthritis, ulcerative colitis, asthma, hyperthyroidism, gastrointestinal upsets, recurrent colds, and skin conditions. All patients must be asked about alcohol and other substances used, including details about the quantity and frequency of use. It is often advisable to frame questions in the form of an assumption of use, such as, "How much alcohol would you say you drink in a day?" rather than "Do you drink?" The latter question may put the patient on the defensive, concerned about what the physician will think if the answer is yes. If the physician assumes that drinking is a fact, the patient is likely to feel comfortable admitting use.

The importance of a thorough, accurate medical history is difficult to overstate. Many medical conditions and their treatments cause psychiatric symptoms that without an attentive medical history may be mistaken for a primary psychiatric disorder. Endocrinopathies such as hypothyroidism or Addison's disease may manifest with depression. Treatment with corticosteroids may precipitate manic and psychotic symptoms. In addition, the coexistence of physical disease may result in secondary psychiatric symptoms. A middle-aged man in the aftermath of a heart attack may suffer from anxiety and depression. A patient's medical status will also guide psychiatric treatment decisions. A depressed patient with cardiac conduction abnormalities will not be treated (at least initially) with a tricyclic antidepressant. A bipolar disorder patient with kidney disease will receive an anticonvulsant mood stabilizer rather than lithium. The names and dosing schedules for all currently prescribed nonpsychiatric drugs should be obtained to avoid adverse interactions with prescribed psychiatric medication.

Family History

A brief statement about any psychiatric illness, hospitalization, and treatment of the patient's immediate family members should be placed in the family history part of the report. Is there a family history of alcohol and other substance abuse or of antisocial behavior? In addition, the family history should provide a description of the personalities and intelligence of the various persons living in the patient's home from childhood to the present as well as a description of the various households in which the patient lived. The psychiatrist should also define the role each person played in the patient's upbringing and this person's current relationship with the patient. What were and are the family ethnic, national, and religious traditions? Informants other than the patient may be available to contribute to the family history, and the source should be cited in the written record. Various members of the family often give different descriptions of the same persons and events. The psychiatrist should determine the family's attitude toward, and insight into, the patient's illness. Does the patient feel that the family members are supportive, indifferent, or destructive? What is the role of illness in the family?

Other questions that provide useful information in this section include the following: What is the patient's attitude toward his or her parents and siblings? The psychiatrist should ask the patient to describe each family member. Who is mentioned first? Who is left out? What does each parent do for a living? What do the siblings do? How do the siblings' occupations compare with the patient's work, and how does the patient feel about it? Who does the patient feel most similar to in the family and why?

Table 7.1–3
Outline of a Developmental History

A. Prenatal and perinatal
  1. Full-term pregnancy or premature
  2. Vaginal delivery or caesarian
  3. Drugs taken by mother during pregnancy (prescription and recreational)
  4. Birth complications
  5. Defects at birth
B. Infancy and early childhood
  1. Infant–mother relationship
  2. Problems with feeding and sleep
  3. Significant milestones
    a. Standing/walking
    b. First words/two-word sentences
    c. Bowel and bladder control
  4. Other caregivers
  5. Unusual behaviors, e.g., head banging
C. Middle childhood
  1. Preschool and school experiences
  2. Separations from caregivers
  3. Friendships/play
  4. Methods of discipline
  5. Illness, surgery, or trauma
D. Adolescence
  1. Onset of puberty
  2. Academic achievement
  3. Organized activities (sports, clubs)
  4. Areas of special interest
  5. Romantic involvements and sexual experience
  6. Work experience
  7. Drug/alcohol use
  8. Symptoms (moodiness, irregularity of sleeping or eating, fights and arguments)
E. Young adulthood
  1. Meaningful long-term relationship
  2. Academic and career decisions
  3. Military experience
  4. Work history
  5. Prison experience
  6. Intellectual pursuits and leisure activities
F. Middle adulthood and old age
  1. Changing family constellation
  2. Social activities
  3. Work and career changes
  4. Aspirations
  5. Major losses
  6. Retirement and aging

Personal History (Anamnesis)

In addition to studying the patient's present illness and current life situation, the psychiatrist needs a thorough understanding of the patient's past and its relation to the present emotional problem. The anamnesis, or personal history, is usually divided into early childhood, late childhood, and adulthood (Table 7.1–3). The predominant emotions associated with the different life periods (e.g., painful, stressful, conflictual) should be noted. Depending on time and situation, the psychiatrist may go into detail with regard to each of the following.

Prenatal and Perinatal History. The psychiatrist considers the home situation into which the patient was born and whether the patient was planned and wanted. Were there any problems with the mother's pregnancy and delivery? What was the mother's emotional and physical state at the time of the patient's birth? Were there any maternal health problems during

CURRENT LIVING SITUATION. Ask the patient to describe where he or she lives in terms of the neighborhood and the residence as well as the number of rooms, the number of family members living in the home, and the sleeping arrangements. Inquire how issues of privacy are handled, with particular emphasis on parental and sibling nudity and bathroom arrangements. Also ask about the sources of family income and any financial hardships. If applicable, inquire about public assistance and the patient's feelings about it. If the patient has been hospitalized, have provisions been made so that he or she will not lose a job or an apartment? Ask who is caring for the children at home, who visits the patient in the hospital, and how frequently.

LEGAL HISTORY. Has the patient ever been arrested and, if so, for what? How many times? Was the patient ever in jail? For how long? Is the patient on probation, or are charges pending? Is the patient mandated to be in treatment as part of a stipulation of probation? Does the patient have a history of assault or violence? Against whom? Were weapons used? What is the patient's attitude toward the arrests or prison terms? An extensive legal history, as well as the patient's attitude toward it, may indicate antisocial trends or a litigious personality. An extensive history of violence may alert the psychiatrist to the potential for violence in the future.

Sexual History.

Much of the history of infantile sexuality is not recoverable, although many patients can recall curiosities and sexual games played from the ages of 3 to 6 years. The psychiatrist should ask how the patient learned about sex and what he or she felt were parents' attitudes about sexual development. Also inquire whether the patient was sexually abused in childhood. Some material discussed in this section may also be covered in the section on adolescent sexuality. It is not important where in the history it is covered, as long as it is included.

The onset of puberty and the patient's feelings about this milestone are important. Adolescent masturbatory history, including the nature of the patient's fantasies and feelings about them, is of significance. Attitudes toward sex should be described in detail. Is the patient shy, timid, aggressive? Does the patient need to impress others and boast of sexual conquests? Did the patient experience anxiety in the sexual setting? Was there promiscuity? What is the patient's sexual orientation?

The sexual history (Table 7.1–4) should include any sexual symptoms, such as anorgasmia, vaginismus, erectile disorder (impotence), premature or retarded ejaculation, lack of sexual desire, and paraphilias (e.g., sexual sadism, fetishism, voyeurism). Attitudes toward fellatio, cunnilingus, and coital techniques may be discussed. The topic of sexual adjustment should include a description of how sexual activity is usually initiated, the frequency of sexual relations, and sexual preferences, variations, and techniques. It is usually appropriate to inquire whether the patient has engaged in extramarital relationships and, if so, under what circumstances and whether the spouse knew of the affair. If the spouse did learn of the affair, the psychiatrist should ask the patient to describe what happened. The reasons underlying an extramarital affair are just as important as understanding its effect on the marriage. Attitudes toward contraception and family planning are important. What form of contraception does the patient use? The psychiatrist, however, should not assume that the patient uses birth control. If an interviewer asks a lesbian patient to describe what type of birth control she uses (on the assumption that she is heterosexual), the patient may surmise that the interviewer will not understand or accept her sexual orientation. A more helpful question is "Do you need to use birth control?" or "Is contraception something that is part of your sexuality?"

The psychiatrist should ask whether the patient wants to mention other areas of sexual functioning and sexuality. Is the patient aware of the issues involved in safe sex? Does the patient have a sexually transmitted disease, such as herpes or AIDS? Does the patient worry about being HIV positive?

Table 7.1–4
Sexual History

1. Screening questions
   a. Are you sexually active?
   b. Have you noticed any changes or problems with sex recently?
2. Developmental
   a. Acquisition of sexual knowledge
   b. Onset of puberty/menarche
   c. Development of sexual identity and orientation
   d. First sexual experiences
   e. Sex in romantic relationship
   f. Changing experiences or preferences over time
   g. Sex and advancing age
3. Clarification of sexual problems
   a. Desire phase
      Presence of sexual thoughts or fantasies
      When do they occur and what is their object?
      Who initiates sex and how?
   b. Excitement phase
      Difficulty in sexual arousal (achieving or maintaining erections, lubrication), during foreplay and preceding orgasm
   c. Orgasm phase
      Does orgasm occur?
      Does it occur too soon or too late?
      How often and under what circumstances does orgasm occur?
      If orgasm doesn't occur is it because of not being excited or lack of orgasm despite being aroused?
   d. Resolution phase
      What happens after sex is over? (e.g., contentment, frustration, continued arousal)

Fantasies and Dreams.

Freud stated that dreams are the royal road to the unconscious. Repetitive dreams have particular value. If the patient has nightmares, what are their repetitive themes? Some of the most common dream themes are food, examinations, sex, helplessness, and feelings of impotence. Can the patient describe a recent dream and discuss its possible meanings? Fantasies and daydreams are another valuable source of unconscious material. As with dreams, the psychiatrist can explore and record details of the fantasy and attendant feelings.

What are the patient's fantasies about the future? If the patient could make any change in his or her life, what would it be? What are the patient's most common or favorite current fantasies? Does the patient experience daydreams? Are the patient's fantasies grounded in reality, or is the patient unable to tell the difference between fantasy and reality?

Values. The psychiatrist may inquire about the patient's system of values—both social and moral—including values about work, money, play, children, parents, friends, sex, community concerns, and cultural issues. For instance, are children a burden or a joy? Is work a necessary evil, an unavoidable chore, or an opportunity? What is the patient's concept of right and wrong?

MENTAL STATUS EXAMINATION

The mental status examination is the part of the clinical assessment that describes the sum total of the examiner's observations and impressions of the psychiatric patient at the time of the interview. Whereas the patient's history remains stable, the patient's mental status can change from day to day or hour to hour. The mental status examination is the description of the patient's appearance, speech, actions, and thoughts during the interview. Even when a patient is mute, is incoherent, or refuses to answer questions, the clinician can obtain a wealth of information through careful observation. Although practitioners' organizational formats for writing up the mental status examination vary slightly, the format must contain certain categories of information. One such format is outlined in Table 7.1–5.

General Description

Appearance. In this category, the psychiatrist describes the patient's appearance and overall physical impression, as reflected by posture, poise, clothing, and grooming. If the patient appears particularly bizarre, the clinician may ask, "Has anyone ever commented on how you look?" "How would you describe how you look?" "Can you help me understand some of the choices you make in how you look?"

Examples of items in the appearance category include body type, posture, poise, clothes, grooming, hair, and nails. Common terms used to describe appearance are healthy, sickly, ill at ease, poised, old looking, young looking, disheveled, childlike, and bizarre. Signs of anxiety are noted: moist hands, perspiring forehead, tense posture, wide eyes.

Table 7.1–5
Outline for the Mental Status Examination

1. Appearance
2. Speech
3. Mood
   a. Subjective
   b. Objective
4. Thinking
   a. Form
   b. Content
5. Perceptions
6. Sensorium
   a. Alertness
   b. Orientation (person, place, time)
   c. Concentration
   d. Memory (immediate, recent, long term)
   e. Calculations
   f. Fund of knowledge
   g. Abstract reasoning
7. Insight
8. Judgment

Overt Behavior and Psychomotor Activity. This category refers to both the quantitative and qualitative aspects of the patient's motor behavior. Included are mannerisms, tics, gestures, twitches, stereotyped behavior, echopraxia, hyperactivity, agitation, combativeness, flexibility, rigidity, gait, and agility. Describe restlessness, wringing of hands, pacing, and other physical manifestations. Note psychomotor retardation or generalized slowing of body movements. Describe any aimless, purposeless activity.

Attitude toward Examiner. The patient's attitude toward the examiner can be described as cooperative, friendly, attentive, interested, frank, seductive, defensive, contemptuous, perplexed, apathetic, hostile, playful, ingratiating, evasive, or guarded; any number of other adjectives can be used. Record the level of rapport established.

Mood and Affect

Mood. *Mood* is defined as a pervasive and sustained emotion that colors the person's perception of the world. The psychiatrist is interested in whether the patient remarks voluntarily about feelings or whether it is necessary to ask the patient how he or she feels. Statements about the patient's mood should include depth, intensity, duration, and fluctuations. Common adjectives used to describe mood include depressed, despairing, irritable, anxious, angry, expansive, euphoric, empty, guilty, hopeless, futile, self-contemptuous, frightened, and perplexed. Mood may be labile, fluctuating or alternating rapidly between extremes (e.g., laughing loudly and expansively one moment, tearful and despairing the next).

Affect. *Affect* may be defined as the patient's present emotional responsiveness, inferred from the patient's facial expression, including the amount and the range of expressive behavior. Affect may or may not be congruent with mood. Affect can be described as within normal range, constricted, blunted, or flat. In the normal range of affect, there is variation in facial expression, tone of voice, use of hands, and body movements. When affect is constricted, the range and intensity of expression are reduced. In blunted affect, emotional expression is further reduced. To diagnose flat affect, there should be virtually no signs of affective expression; the patient's voice should be monotonous, and the face should be immobile. Note the patient's difficulty in initiating, sustaining, or terminating an emotional response.

Appropriateness of Affect. The psychiatrist can consider the appropriateness of the patient's emotional responses in the context of the subject the patient is discussing. Delusional patients who are describing a delusion of persecution should be angry or frightened about the experiences they believe are happening to them. Anger or fear in this context is an appropriate expression. Psychiatrists use the term *inappropriate affect* for a quality of response found in some schizophrenic patients, in which the patient's affect is incongruent

with what the patient is saying (e.g., flattened affect when speaking about murderous impulses).

Speech Characteristics

This part of the report describes the physical characteristics of speech. Speech can be described in terms of its quantity, rate of production, and quality. The patient may be described as talkative, garrulous, voluble, taciturn, unspontaneous, or normally responsive to cues from the interviewer. Speech may be rapid or slow, pressured, hesitant, emotional, dramatic, monotonous, loud, whispered, slurred, staccato, or mumbled. Speech impairments, such as stuttering, are included in this section. Any unusual rhythms (termed *dysprosody*) or accent should be noted. The patient's speech may be spontaneous.

Perception

Perceptual disturbances, such as hallucinations and illusions, may be experienced in reference to the self or the environment. The sensory system involved (e.g., auditory, visual, taste, olfactory, or tactile) and the content of the illusion or the hallucinatory experience should be described. The circumstances of the occurrence of any hallucinatory experience are important; hypnagogic hallucinations (occurring as a person falls asleep) and hypnopompic hallucinations (occurring as a person awakens) have much less serious significance than other types of hallucinations. Hallucinations may also occur in particular times of stress for individual patients. Feelings of depersonalization and derealization (extreme feelings of detachment from the self or the environment) are other examples of perceptual disturbance. Formication, the feeling of bugs crawling on or under the skin, is seen in cocainism.

Examples of questions used to elicit the experience of hallucinations include the following: Have you ever heard voices or other sounds that no one else could hear or when no one else was around? Have you experienced any strange sensations in your body that others do not seem to see?

A young man with schizophrenia heard an insistent voice repeatedly telling him to stop his antipsychotic medication. After resisting the command for many weeks, the patient felt that he could no longer fight the voice, and he discontinued treatment. Two months later, he was hospitalized involuntarily and near cardiovascular collapse. He later said that once he stopped the medication, the voice further insisted that he should stop eating and drinking to purify himself.

A terrified 37-year-old man in acute delirium tremens glanced agitatedly about the room. He pointed out the window and said: "My God, the Spanish armada is on the lawn. They're about to attack." He experienced the hallucination as real, and it persisted intermittently for 3 days before abating. Subsequently, the patient had no memory of the experience.

Table 7.1–6
Formal Thought Disorders

Circumstantiality. Overinclusion of trivial or irrelevant details that impede the sense of getting to the point.

Clang associations. Thoughts are associated by the sound of words rather than by their meaning, e.g., through rhyming or assonance.

Derailment. (Synonymous with loose associations) A breakdown in both the logical connection between ideas and the overall sense of goal-directedness. The words make sentences, but the sentences don't make sense.

Flight of ideas. A succession of multiple associations so that thoughts seem to move abruptly from idea to idea; often (but not invariably) expressed through rapid, pressured speech.

Neologism. The invention of new words or phrases or the use of conventional words in idiosyncratic ways.

Perseveration. Repetition out of context of words, phrases, or ideas.

Tangentiality. In response to a question, the patient gives a reply that is appropriate to the general topic without actually answering the question. Example:

Doctor: "Have you had any trouble sleeping lately?"

Patient: "I usually sleep in my bed, but now I'm sleeping on the sofa."

Thought blocking. A sudden disruption of thought or a break in the flow of ideas.

Thought Content and Mental Trends. Thought can be divided into process (or form) and content. *Process* refers to the way in which a person puts together ideas and associations, the form in which a person thinks. Process or form of thought may be logical and coherent or completely illogical and even incomprehensible. *Content* refers to what a person is actually thinking about: ideas, beliefs, preoccupations, obsessions. Table 7.1–6 lists common thought disorders.

Thought Process (Form of Thinking). The patient may have either an overabundance or a poverty of ideas. There may be rapid thinking, which, if carried to the extreme, is called a *flight of ideas*. A patient may exhibit slow or hesitant thinking.

Thought may be vague or empty. Do the patient's replies really answer the questions asked, and does the patient have the capacity for goal-directed thinking? Are the responses relevant or irrelevant? Is there a clear cause-and-effect relation in the patient's explanations? Does the patient have *loose associations* (e.g., do the ideas expressed seem unrelated and idiosyncratically connected)? Disturbances of the continuity of thought include statements that are tangential, circumstantial, rambling, evasive, or perseverative.

Blocking is interruption of the train of thought before an idea has been completed; the patient may indicate an inability to recall what was being said or intended to be said. *Circumstantiality* indicates the loss of capacity for goal-directed thinking; in the process of explaining an idea, the patient brings in many irrelevant details and parenthetical comments but eventually does get back to the original point. *Tangentiality* is a disturbance in which the patient loses the thread of the conversation, pursues divergent thoughts stimulated by various external or internal irrelevant stimuli, and never returns to the original point. Thought process impairments may be reflected by incoherent or incomprehensible connections of thoughts (*word salad*), *clang associations* (association by rhyming), *punning* (association by

double meaning), and *neologisms* (new words created by the patient by combining or condensing other words).

Thought Content. Disturbances in content of thought include delusions, preoccupations (which may involve the patient's illness), obsessions ("Do you have ideas that are intrusive and repetitive?"), compulsions ("Are there things you do over and over, in a repetitive manner?" "Are there things you must do in a particular way or order?" "If you do not do them that way, must you repeat them?" "Do you know why you do things that way?"), phobias, plans, intentions, recurrent ideas about suicide or homicide, hypochondriacal symptoms, and specific antisocial urges.

> A 32-year-old woman with a mild viral syndrome picked up a carton of milk in the supermarket and then returned it to its shelf, after deciding not to buy it. Over the next few days, she spent increasing amounts of time thinking about the act. She could not stop herself from thinking that the mother of a young child picked up the same container, contracted the patient's virus, and gave it to her child, who may then have become ill and died as a result of a fulminant infection. Despite knowing that this sequence of events was extremely unlikely, the woman could not stop replaying the scenario in her mind.

Does the patient have thoughts of doing self-harm? Is there a plan? A major category of disturbances of thought content involves delusions. Delusions—fixed, false beliefs out of keeping with the patient's cultural background—may be mood congruent (thoughts that are in keeping with a depressed or elated mood, e.g., a depressed patient thinks he is dying or an elated patient thinks she is the Virgin Mary) or mood incongruent (e.g., an elated patient thinks he has a brain tumor). The psychiatrist should describe the content of any delusional system and attempt to evaluate its organization and the patient's conviction about its validity. The manner in which it affects the patient's life is appropriately described in the history of the present illness. Delusions may be bizarre and may involve beliefs about external control. Delusions may have themes that are persecutory or paranoid, grandiose, jealous, somatic, guilty, nihilistic, or erotic. The clinician should describe ideas of reference and of influence. Examples of *ideas of reference* include a person's belief that the television or radio is speaking to or about him or her. Examples of *ideas of influence* are beliefs about another person or force controlling some aspect of one's behavior.

> A young man with schizophrenia, a college dropout who could work only part-time at low-level jobs and who lived with his high-achieving family, believed he was the Messiah. He was fully convinced that his struggles and lack of occupational success were merely God's tests until the patient's true identity would be revealed. As he improved, he would, if asked, say that he was God's chosen but, when questioned further, would admit the slight possibility that he was wrong. On reaching his best clinical state, he would muse on the possibility that he was the Messiah but state that he was not sure.

Sensorium and Cognition

The sensorium and cognition portion of the mental status examination seeks to assess brain function, including intelligence, capacity for abstract thought, and level of insight and judgment. The Mini-Mental State Examination (MMSE) is a brief instrument designed to grossly assess cognitive functioning. It assesses orientation, memory, calculations, reading and writing capacity, visuospatial ability, and language. The patient is measured quantitatively on these functions; a perfect score is 30 points. The MMSE is widely used as a simple, quick assessment of possible cognitive deficits. (See Table 10.1–4 in Section 10.1 for an example of the MMSE.) Questions that test cognitive function are listed in Table 7.1–7.

Consciousness. Disturbances of consciousness usually indicate organic brain impairment. Clouding of consciousness is an overall reduced awareness of the environment. A patient may be unable to sustain attention to environmental stimuli or to maintain goal-directed thinking or behavior. Clouding or obtunding of consciousness is frequently not a fixed mental state. A patient typically exhibits fluctuations in the level of awareness of

Table 7.1–7
Questions Used to Test Cognitive Functions in the Sensorium Section of the MSE

1. Alertness	(Observation)
2. Orientation	What is your name? Who am I?
	What place is this? Where is it located?
	What city are we in?
3. Concentration	Starting at 100, count backward by 7 (or 3)
	Say the letters of the alphabet backward starting with Z
	Name the months of the year backward starting with December
4. Memory	
Immediate	Repeat these numbers after me: 1, 4, 9, 2, 5.
Recent	What did you have for breakfast?
	What were you doing before we started talking this morning?
	I want you to remember these three things: a yellow pencil, a cocker spaniel, and Cincinnati. After a few minutes I'll ask you to repeat them.
Long term	What was your address when you were in the third grade?
	Who was your teacher?
	What did you do during the summer between high school and college?
5. Calculations	If you buy something that costs $3.75 and you pay with a $5 bill, how much change should you get?
	What is the cost of 3 oranges if a dozen oranges cost $4.00?
6. Fund of knowledge	What is the distance between New York and Los Angeles? What body of water lies between South America and Africa?
7. Abstract reasoning	Which one doesn't belong in this group: a pair of scissors, a canary, and a spider? Why?
	How are an apple and an orange alike?

the surrounding environment. The patient who has an altered state of consciousness often shows some impairment of orientation as well, although the reverse is not necessarily true. Some terms used to describe the patient's level of consciousness are *clouding*, *somnolence*, *stupor*, *coma*, *lethargy*, or *alert*.

Orientation and Memory. Disorders of orientation are traditionally separated according to time, place, and person. Any impairment usually appears in this order (i.e., sense of time is impaired before sense of place); similarly, as the patient improves, the impairment clears in the reverse order. The psychiatrist must determine whether a patient can give the approximate date and time of day. In addition, if hospitalized, does the patient know how long he or she has been there? Does the patient seem to be oriented to the present? In questions about orientation to place, patients should be able to state the name and the location of the hospital correctly and to behave as though they know where they are. In assessing orientation for person, the psychiatrist asks patients whether they know the names of the people around them and whether they understand their roles in relationship to them. Do they know who the examiner is? Only in the most severe instances do patients not know who they themselves are.

A 42-year-old alcoholic man in delirium tremens, examined in a California hospital in 1995, was asked the date and where he was. He replied: "I'm standing on a street corner in Kansas City in 1966 minding my own business. Why don't you mind yours?"

Memory functions have traditionally been divided into four areas: remote memory, recent past memory, recent memory, and immediate retention and recall. Recent memory may be checked by asking patients about their appetite and then about what they had for breakfast or for dinner the previous evening. Patients may be asked at this point if they recall the interviewer's name. Asking patients to repeat six digits forward and then backward is a test of immediate retention. Remote memory can be tested by asking patients for information about their childhood that can be later verified. Asking patients to recall important news events from the past few months checks recent past memory. Often in cognitive disorders, recent or short-term memory is impaired first, and remote or long-term memory is impaired later. If there is impairment, what efforts are made to cope with it or to conceal it? Is denial, confabulation, or circumstantiality used to conceal a deficit? Reactions to the loss of memory can give important clues to underlying disorders and coping mechanisms. For instance, a patient who appears to have memory impairment but, in fact, is depressed is more likely to be concerned about memory loss than is someone with memory loss secondary to dementia. The clinician must also determine whether a catastrophic reaction is present (anxious crying when unable to remember).

A 40-year-old chronically alcoholic man, whose memory on the mental status examination was markedly impaired, frantically demanded to be released from the hospital, saying that his wife had just been in an automobile accident and that he had to rush to another hospital to see her. He said it with sincere conviction and appropriate fearful concern; for the patient, at least, the story was real. In fact, his wife had been dead for 15 years. The patient told the same story over and over again, always with evident conviction, in spite of the fact that staff members confronted him with the reality that his wife had been dead for years. The patient was never influenced by their assertions, because he could not register new memories. Although his past memory was patchy at best, he could repeatedly recall the story of his wife's emergency.

Table 7.1–8
Summary of Memory Tests

Try to assess whether the process of registration, retention, or recollection of material is involved.

Remote memory: Childhood data, important events known to have occurred when the patient was younger or free of illness, personal matters, neutral material

Recent past memory: The past few months

Recent memory: The past few days, what the patient did yesterday, the day before, what the patient had for breakfast, lunch, dinner

Immediate retention and recall: Digit-span measures; ability to repeat six figures after examiner dictates them—first forward, then backward (patients with unimpaired memory can usually repeat six digits backward); ability to repeat three words immediately and 3 to 5 minutes later

Confabulation (unconsciously making up false answers when memory is impaired) is most closely associated with cognitive disorders. Table 7.1–8 gives a summary of memory tests.

Concentration and Attention. A patient's concentration may be impaired for many reasons. A cognitive disorder, anxiety, depression, and internal stimuli, such as auditory hallucinations, all may contribute to impaired concentration. Subtracting serial 7s from 100 is a simple task that requires intact concentration and cognitive capacities. Could the patient subtract 7 from 100 and keep subtracting 7s? If the patient could not subtract 7s, could 3s be subtracted? Were easier tasks accomplished—4 × 9, 5 × 4? The examiner must always assess whether anxiety, some disturbance of mood or consciousness, or a learning deficit (dyscalculia) is responsible for the difficulty.

Attention is assessed by calculations or by asking the patient to spell the word *world* (or others) backward. The patient can also be asked to name five things that start with a particular letter.

During his most recent manic episode, a 48-year-old man with bipolar disorder had intense, grandiose, psychotic ideas. He was convinced that he could control the traffic in Los Angeles by driving on certain freeways at specified times and willing others to leave the road. After the manic episode ended and during the depressive episode that immediately followed, he could recall virtually no details of his

previous thought content while he was manic. Later, when euthymic, he remembered only a few hazy images. A year later, the beginning of a new hypomanic period was heralded by the patient's spontaneously remembering and describing in great detail the psychotic plans of the previous episode.

Reading and Writing. The psychiatrist should ask the patient to read a sentence (e.g., "Close your eyes") and then to do what the sentence says. The patient should also be asked to write a simple but complete sentence.

Visuospatial Ability. The patient should be asked to copy a figure, such as a clock face or interlocking pentagons.

Abstract Thought. Abstract thinking is the ability to deal with concepts. Patients may have disturbances in the manner in which they conceptualize or handle ideas. Can the patient explain similarities, such as those between an apple and a pear or between truth and beauty? Are the meanings of simple proverbs, such as "A rolling stone gathers no moss," understood? Answers may be concrete (giving specific examples to illustrate the meaning) or overly abstract (giving too generalized an explanation). The appropriateness of answers and the manner in which they are given should be noted. In a catastrophic reaction, brain-damaged patients become extremely emotional and cannot think abstractly.

Information and Intelligence. If a possible cognitive impairment is suspected, does the patient have trouble with mental tasks, such as counting the change from $10 after a purchase of $6.37? If this task is too difficult, are easy problems (such as how many nickels are in $1.35) solved? The patient's intelligence is related to vocabulary and general fund of knowledge (e.g., the distance from New York to Paris, presidents of the United States). The patient's educational level (both formal and self-education) and socioeconomic status must be taken into account. Handling difficult or sophisticated concepts can reflect intelligence, even in the absence of formal education or an extensive fund of information. Ultimately, the psychiatrist estimates the patient's intellectual capability and capacity to function at the level of basic endowment.

Impulsivity

Is the patient capable of controlling sexual, aggressive, and other impulses? An assessment of impulse control is critical in ascertaining the patient's awareness of socially appropriate behavior and is a measure of the patient's potential danger to self and others. Patients may be unable to control impulses secondary to cognitive and psychotic disorders or because of chronic characterological defects, as observed in the personality disorders. Impulse control can be estimated from information in the patient's recent history and from behavior observed during the interview.

Judgment and Insight

Judgment. During the course of history taking, the psychiatrist should be able to assess many aspects of the patient's capability for social judgment. Does the patient understand the likely outcome of his or her behavior, and is he or she influenced by this understanding? Can the patient predict what he or she would do in imaginary situations (e.g., smelling smoke in a crowded movie theater)?

Insight. Insight is a patient's degree of awareness and understanding about being ill. Patients may exhibit complete denial of their illness or may show some awareness that they are ill but place the blame on others, on external factors, or even on organic factors. They may acknowledge that they have an illness but ascribe it to something unknown or mysterious in themselves.

An 18-year-old man went to an emergency room with the belief that he was controlled by a computer on an *Enterprise*-like starship, an elaboration from the television series *Star Trek*. He was convinced that all his thoughts, actions, and feelings were being programmed on board the starship, which was located light years away and, therefore, could never be detected by anyone else.

Intellectual insight is present when patients can admit that they are ill and acknowledge that their failures to adapt are, in part, due to their own irrational feelings. Patients' inability to apply their knowledge to alter future experiences, however, is the major limitation to intellectual insight. True emotional insight is present when patients' awareness of their own motives and deep feelings leads to a change in their personality or behavior patterns.

A summary of 6 levels of insight follows:

1. Complete denial of illness
2. Slight awareness of being sick and needing help but denying it at the same time
3. Awareness of being sick but blaming it on others, on external factors, or on organic factors
4. Awareness that illness is due to something unknown in the patient
5. Intellectual insight: admission that the patient is ill and that symptoms or failures in social adjustment are due to the patient's own particular irrational feelings or disturbances without applying this knowledge to future experiences
6. True emotional insight: emotional awareness of the motives and feelings within the patient and the important persons in his or her life, which can lead to basic changes in behavior

Reliability

The mental status part of the report concludes with the psychiatrist's impressions of the patient's reliability and capacity to report his or her situation accurately. It includes an estimate of the psychiatrist's impression of the patient's truthfulness or veracity. For instance, if the patient is open about significant active substance abuse or about circumstances that the patient knows may reflect badly (e.g., trouble with the

law), the psychiatrist may estimate the patient's reliability to be good.

PSYCHIATRIC REPORT

The psychiatric report is a written document that details the findings obtained from the psychiatric history and mental status examination. It may also be formatted in other ways, provided that all the pertinent data are recorded. It includes a final summary of both positive and negative findings and an interpretation of the data. It has more than descriptive value; it has meaning that helps provide an understanding of the case. The examiner addresses critical questions in the report: Are future diagnostic studies needed and if so which ones? Is a consultant needed? Is a comprehensive neurological workup needed including an electroencephalogram or computerized tomography scan? Are psychological tests indicated? Are psychodynamic factors relevant? The report includes a diagnosis made according to the DSM-IV-TR, which uses a multiaxial classification scheme consisting of five axes, each of which should be covered (see Table 9.1–6 in Section 9.1). A prognosis is also discussed in the report, with both good and bad prognostic factors listed. Finally, a treatment plan discusses, and makes firm recommendations about, management issues. A detailed outline of the psychiatric report is found in Table 7.1–9.

Table 7.1–9
Psychiatric Report

I. Psychiatric history
  A. Identification: Name, age, marital status, sex, occupation, language if other than English, race, nationality, and religion if pertinent; previous admissions to a hospital for the same or a different condition; with whom the patient lives
  B. Chief complaint: Exactly why the patient came to the psychiatrist, preferably in the patient's own words; if that information does not come from the patient, note who supplied it
  C. History of present illness: Chronological background and development of the symptoms or behavioral changes that culminated in the patient's seeking assistance; patient's life circumstances at the time of onset; personality when well; how illness has affected life activities and personal relations—changes in personality, interests, mood, attitudes toward others, dress, habits, level of tenseness, irritability, activity, attention, concentration, memory, speech; psychophysiological symptoms—nature and details of dysfunction; pain—location, intensity, fluctuation; level of anxiety—generalized and nonspecific (free floating) or specifically related to particular situations, activities, or objects; how anxieties are handled—avoidance, repetition of feared situation, use of drugs or other activities for alleviation
  D. Past psychiatric and medical history: (1) Emotional or mental disturbances—extent of incapacity, type of treatment, names of hospitals, length of illness, effect of treatment; (2) psychosomatic disorders: hay fever, arthritis, colitis, rheumatoid arthritis, recurrent colds, skin conditions; (3) medical conditions: follow customary review of systems—sexually transmitted diseases, alcohol or other substance abuse, at risk for AIDS; (4) neurological disorders: headache, craniocerebral trauma, loss of consciousness, seizures or tumors
  E. Family history: Elicited from patient and from someone else, since quite different descriptions may be given of the same persons and events; ethnic, national, and religious traditions; other persons in the home, descriptions of them—personality and intelligence—and what has become of them since patient's childhood; descriptions of different households lived in; present relationships between patient and those who were in family; role of illness in the family; family history of mental illness; where does patient live—neighborhood and particular residence of the patient; is home crowded; privacy of family members from each other and from other families; sources of family income and difficulties in obtaining it; public assistance (if any) and attitude about it; will patient lose job or apartment by remaining in the hospital; who is caring for children
  F. Personal history (anamnesis): History of the patient's life from infancy to the present to the extent it can be recalled; gaps in history as spontaneously related by the patient; emotions associated with different life periods (painful, stressful, conflictual) or with phases of life cycle
    1. Early childhood (through age 3)
      a. Prenatal history and mother's pregnancy and delivery: Length of pregnancy, spontaneity and normality of delivery, birth trauma, whether patient was planned and wanted, birth defects
      b. Feeding habits: Breast-fed or bottle-fed, eating problems
      c. Early development: Maternal deprivation, language development, motor development, signs of unmet needs, sleep pattern, object constancy, stranger anxiety, separation anxiety
      d. Toilet training: Age, attitude of parents, feelings about it
      e. Symptoms of behavior problems: Thumb sucking, temper tantrums, tics, head bumping, rocking, night terrors, fears, bedwetting or bed soiling, nail biting, masturbation
      f. Personality and temperament as a child: Shy, restless, overactive, withdrawn, studious, outgoing, timid, athletic, friendly patterns of play, reactions to siblings
    2. Middle childhood (ages 3 to 11): Early school history—feelings about going to school, early adjustment, gender identification, conscience development, punishment; social relationships, attitudes toward siblings and playmates
    3. Later childhood (prepuberty through adolescence)
      a. Peer relationships: Number and closeness of friends, leader or follower, social popularity, participation in group or gang activities, idealized figures; patterns of aggression, passivity, anxiety, antisocial behavior
      b. School history: How far the patient went, adjustment to school, relationships with teachers—teacher's pet or rebellious—favorite studies or interests, particular abilities or assets, extracurricular activities, sports, hobbies, relationships of problems or symptoms to any school period

(continued)

Table 7.1–9 (*continued*)

c. Cognitive and motor development: Learning to read and other intellectual and motor skills, minimal cerebral dysfunction, learning disabilities—their management and effects on the child
d. Particular adolescent emotional or physical problems: Nightmares, phobias, masturbation, bed-wetting, running away, delinquency, smoking, drug or alcohol use, weight problems, feeling of inferiority
e. Psychosexual history
   i. Early curiosity, infantile masturbation, sex play
   ii. Acquiring of sexual knowledge, attitude of parents toward sex, sexual abuse
   iii. Onset of puberty, feelings about it, kind of preparation, feelings about menstruation, development of secondary sexual characteristics
   iv. Adolescent sexual activity: Crushes, parties, dating, petting, masturbation, wet dreams and attitudes toward them
   v. Attitudes toward same and opposite sex: Timid, shy, aggressive, need to impress, seductive, sexual conquests, anxiety
   vi. Sexual practices: Sexual problems, homosexual and heterosexual experiences, paraphilias, promiscuity
f. Religious background: Strict, liberal, mixed (possible conflicts), relation of background to current religious practices

4. Adulthood
   a. Occupational history: Choice of occupation, training, ambitions, conflicts; relations with authority, peers, and subordinates; number of jobs and duration; changes in job status; current job and feelings about it
   b. Social activity: Whether patient has friends or not; is patient withdrawn or socializing well; social, intellectual, and physical interests; relationships with same sex and opposite sex; depth, duration, and quality of human relations
   c. Adult sexuality
      i. Premarital sexual relationships, age of first coitus, sexual orientation
      ii. Marital history: Common-law marriages, legal marriages, description of courtship and role played by each partner, age at marriage, family planning and contraception, names and ages of children, attitudes toward raising children, problems of any family members, housing difficulties if important to the marriage, sexual adjustment, extramarital affairs, areas of agreement and disagreement, management of money, role of in-laws
      iii. Sexual symptoms: Anorgasmia, impotence, premature ejaculation, lack of desire
      iv. Attitudes toward pregnancy and having children; contraceptive practices and feelings about them
      v. Sexual practices: Paraphilias such as sadism, fetishes, voyeurism; attitude toward fellation, cunnilingus; coital techniques, frequency
   d. Military history: General adjustment, combat, injuries, referral to psychiatrists, type of discharge, veteran status
   e. Value systems: Whether children are seen as a burden or a joy; whether work is seen as a necessary evil, an avoidable chore, or an opportunity; current attitude about religion; belief in heaven and hell

Summation of the examiner's observations and impressions derived from the initial interview

II. Mental status
   A. Appearance
      1. Personal identification: May include a brief nontechnical description of the patient's appearance and behavior as a novelist might write it; attitude toward examiner can be described here—cooperative, attentive, interested, frank, seductive, defensive, hostile, playful, ingratiating, evasive, guarded
      2. Behavior and psychomotor activity: Gait, mannerisms, tics, gestures, twitches, stereotypes, picking, touching examiner, echopraxia, clumsy, agile, limp, rigid, retarded, hyperactive, agitated, combative, waxy
      3. General description: Posture, bearing, clothes, grooming, hair, nails; healthy, sickly, angry, frightened, apathetic, perplexed, contemptuous, ill at ease, poised, old looking, young looking, effeminate, masculine; signs of anxiety—moist hands, perspiring forehead, restlessness, tense posture, strained voice, wide eyes; shifts in level of anxiety during interview or with particular topic
   B. Speech: Rapid, slow, pressured, hesitant, emotional, monotonous, loud, whispered, slurred, mumbled, stuttering, echolalia, intensity, pitch, ease, spontaneity, productivity, manner, reaction time, vocabulary, prosody
   C. Mood and affect
      1. Mood (a pervasive and sustained emotion that colors the person's perception of the world): How does patient say he or she feels; depth, intensity, duration, and fluctuations of mood—depressed, despairing, irritable, anxious, terrified, angry, expansive, euphoric, empty, guilty, awed, futile, self-contemptuous, anhedonic, alexithymic
      2. Affect (the outward expression of the patient's inner experiences): How examiner evaluates patient's affects—broad, restricted, blunted or flat, shallow, amount and range of expression; difficulty in initiating, sustaining, or terminating an emotional response; is the emotional expression appropriate to the thought content, culture, and setting of the examination; give examples if emotional expression is not appropriate
   D. Thinking and perception
      1. Form of thinking
         a. Productivity: Overabundance of ideas, paucity of ideas, flight of ideas, rapid thinking, slow thinking, hesitant thinking; does patient speak spontaneously or only when questions are asked, stream of thought, quotations from patient
         b. Continuity of thought: Whether patient's replies really answer questions and are goal directed, relevant, or irrelevant; loose associations; lack of causal relations in patient's explanations; illogical, tangential, circumstantial, rambling, evasive, perseverative statements, blocking or distractibility

(*continued*)

Table 7.1–9 (*continued*)

c. Language impairments: Impairments that reflect disordered mentation, such as incoherent or incomprehensible speech (word salad), clang associations, neologisms

2. Content of thinking
   a. Preoccupations: About the illness, environmental problems; obsessions, compulsions, phobias; obsessions or plans about suicide, homicide; hypochondriacal symptoms, specific antisocial urges or impulses
3. Thought disturbances
   a. Delusions: Content of any delusional system, its organization, the patient's convictions as to its validity, how it affects his or her life: persecutory delusions—isolated or associated with pervasive suspiciousness; mood-congruent or mood-incongruent
   b. Ideas of reference and ideas of influence: How ideas began, their content, and the meaning the patient attributes to them
4. Perceptual disturbances
   a. Hallucinations and illusions: Whether patient hears voices or sees visions; content, sensory system involvement, circumstances of the occurrence; hypnagogic or hypnopompic hallucinations; thought broadcasting
   b. Depersonalization and derealization: Extreme feelings of detachment from self or from the environment
5. Dreams and fantasies
   a. Dreams: Prominent ones, if patient will tell them; nightmares
   b. Fantasies: Recurrent, favorite, or unshakable daydreams

E. Sensorium
1. Alertness: Awareness of environment, attention span, clouding of consciousness, fluctuations in levels of awareness, somnolence, stupor, lethargy, fugue state, coma
2. Orientation
   a. Time: Whether patient identifies the day correctly; or approximate date, time of day; if in a hospital, knows how long he or she has been there; behaves as though oriented to the present
   b. Place: Whether patient knows where he or she is
   c. Person: Whether patient knows who the examiner is and the roles or names of the persons with whom in contact
3. Concentration and calculation: Subtracting 7 from 100 and keep subtracting 7s; if patient cannot subtract 7s, can easier tasks be accomplished—4 × 9; 5 × 4; how many nickels are in $1.35; whether anxiety or some disturbance of mood or concentration seems to be responsible for difficulty
4. Memory: Impairment, efforts made to cope with impairment—denial, confabulation, catastrophic reaction, circumstantiality used to conceal deficit; whether the process of registration, retention, or recollection of material is involved
   a. Remote memory: Childhood data, important events known to have occurred when the patient was younger or free of illness, personal matters, neutral material
   b. Recent past memory: Past few months
   c. Recent memory: Past few days, what did patient do yesterday, the day before, have for breakfast, lunch, dinner
   d. Immediate retention and recall: Ability to repeat six figures after examiner dictates them—first forward, then backward, then after a few minutes' interruption; other test questions; did same questions, if repeated, call forth different answers at different times
   e. Effect of defect on patient: Mechanisms patient has developed to cope with defect
5. Fund of knowledge: Level of formal education and self-education; estimate of the patient's intellectual capability and whether capable of functioning at the level of his or her basic endowment; counting, calculation, general knowledge; questions should have relevance to the patient's educational and cultural background
6. Abstract thinking: Disturbances in concept formation; manner in which the patient conceptualizes or handles his or her ideas; similarities (e.g., between apples and pears), differences, absurdities; meanings of simple proverbs, e.g., "A rolling stone gathers no moss"; answers may be concrete (giving specific examples to illustrate the meaning) or overly abstract (giving generalized explanation); appropriateness of answers

F. Insight: Degree of personal awareness and understanding of illness
1. Complete denial of illness
2. Slight awareness of being sick and needing help but denying it at the same time
3. Awareness of being sick but blaming it on others, on external factors, on medical or unknown organic factors
4. Intellectual insight: Admission of illness and recognition that symptoms or failures in social adjustment are due to irrational feelings or disturbances, without applying that knowledge to future experiences
5. True emotional insight: Emotional awareness of the motives and feelings within, of the underlying meaning of symptoms; does the awareness lead to changes in personality and future behavior; openness to new ideas and concepts about self and the important persons in his or her life

G. Judgment
1. Social judgment: Subtle manifestations of behavior that are harmful to the patient and contrary to acceptable behavior in the culture; does the patient understand the likely outcome of personal behavior and is patient influenced by that understanding; examples of impairment
2. Test judgment: Patient's prediction of what he or she would do in imaginary situations; e.g., what patient would do with a stamped, addressed letter found in the street

(*continued*)

Table 7.1–9 (*continued*)

III. Further diagnostic studies
   A. Physical examination
   B. Neurological examination
   C. Additional psychiatric diagnostic
   D. Interviews with family members, friends, or neighbors by a social worker
   E. Psychological, neurological, or laboratory tests as indicated: Electroencephalogram, computed tomography scan, magnetic resonance imaging, tests of other medical conditions, reading comprehension and writing tests, test for aphasia, projective or objective psychological tests, dexamethasone-suppression test, 24-hour urine test for heavy metal intoxication, urine screen for drugs of abuse

IV. Summary of findings

Summarize mental symptoms, medical and laboratory findings, and psychological and neurological test results, if available; include medications patient has been taking, dosage, duration. Clarity of thinking is reflected in clarity of writing. When summarizing the mental status, e.g., the phrase "Patient denies hallucinations and delusions" is not as precise as "Patient denies hearing voices or thinking that he is being followed." The latter indicates the specific question asked and the specific response given. Similarly, in the conclusion of the report one would write "Hallucinations and delusions were not elicited."

V. Diagnosis

Diagnostic classification is made according to DSM-IV-TR, which uses a multiaxial classification scheme consisting of five axes, each of which should be covered in the diagnosis

Axis I: Clinical syndromes (e.g., mood disorders, schizophrenia, generalized anxiety disorder) and other conditions that may be a focus of clinical attention

Axis II: Personality disorders, mental retardation, and defense mechanisms

Axis III: Any general medical conditions (e.g., epilepsy, cardiovascular disease, endocrine disorders)

Axis IV: Psychosocial and environmental problems (e.g., divorce, injury, death of a loved one) relevant to the illness

Axis V: Global assessment of functioning exhibited by the patient during the interview (e.g., social, occupational, and psychological functioning); a rating scale with a continuum from 100 (superior functioning) to 1 (grossly impaired functioning) is used

VI. Prognosis

Opinion about the probable future course, extent, and outcome of the disorder; good and bad prognostic factors; specific goals of therapy

VII. Psychodynamic formulation

Causes of the patient's psychodynamic breakdown—influences in the patient's life that contributed to present disorder; environmental, genetic, and personality factors relevant to determining patient's symptoms; primary and secondary gains; outline of the major defense mechanism used by the patient

VIII. Comprehensive treatment plan

Modalities of treatment recommended, role of medication, inpatient or outpatient treatment, frequency of sessions, probable duration of therapy; type of psychotherapy; individual, group, or family therapy; symptoms or problems to be treated. Initially, treatment must be directed toward any life-threatening situations such as suicidal risk or risk of danger to others that require psychiatric hospitalization. Danger to self or others is an acceptable reason (both legally and medically) for involuntary hospitalization. In the absence of the need for confinement, a variety of outpatient treatment alternatives are available: day hospitals, supervised residences, outpatient psychotherapy or pharmacotherapy, among others. In some cases, treatment planning must attend to vocational and psychosocial skills training and even legal or forensic issues.

Comprehensive treatment planning requires a therapeutic team approach using the skills of psychologists, social workers, nurses, activity and occupational therapists, and a variety of other mental health professionals, with referral to self-help groups (e.g., Alcoholics Anonymous [AA]) if needed. If either the patient or family members are unwilling to accept the recommendations of treatment and the clinician thinks that the refusal of the recommendations may have serious consequences, the patient, parent, or guardian should sign a statement to the effect that the recommended treatment was refused.

PRACTICAL ASPECTS OF THE PSYCHIATRIC INTERVIEW

Session Length

The initial consultation lasts for 30 minutes to 1 hour, depending on the circumstances. Interviews with patients who are psychotic or medically ill are brief because patients may find the interview stressful. Similarly, emergency room interviews vary in length. Initial interviews to evaluate patients for pharmacotherapy or psychotherapy tend to be longer; second visits and ongoing therapeutic interviews vary in length. The American Board of Psychiatry and Neurology, in its clinical oral examination in psychiatry, allows 30 minutes for candidates to conduct a psychiatric examination.

Patients' management of appointment times reveals important aspects of personality and coping. Most often, patients arrive a few minutes before their appointments. An anxious patient may arrive as much as 30 minutes early. When a patient arrives very early, the clinician may want to explore the reasons. The patient who arrives significantly late for an appointment also poses potential questions. The first time a patient is late, the clinician may listen to the explanation offered and respond sympathetically if the lateness is due to circumstances

beyond the patient's control. A patient who states, "I forgot all about the appointment," however, is offering a clue that something about going to the doctor makes the patient anxious or uncomfortable. This reaction needs to be explored further. The psychiatrist may ask, "Did you feel reluctant to come in today?" If the answer is, "Yes," the psychiatrist can begin to explore the possible reasons for the patient's reluctance. If the answer is, "No," it is probably best to drop the direct questioning about the lateness and just listen to the patient. By listening carefully, the psychiatrist can usually detect themes that the patient may not recognize. These themes can then be explored by both the patient and the psychiatrist in an attempt to understand better what the patient is experiencing.

A psychiatrist's handling of time is also an important factor in the interview. Carelessness about time indicates a lack of concern for the patient. If a psychiatrist is unavoidably detained for an interview, it is appropriate to express regret at having kept the patient waiting.

Seating and Arrangement of Office

The arrangement of chairs in the psychiatrist's office affects the interview. Both chairs should be of approximately equal height, so that neither person looks down on the other. Most psychiatrists think that it is desirable to place the chairs without any furniture between the clinician and the patient. If the room contains several chairs, the psychiatrist indicates his or her own chair and then allows the patient to choose the chair in which he or she will feel most comfortable.

The evaluation should be conducted in a comfortable room with pleasant lighting. Better rapport can be established and fuller observations made if the psychiatrist is not sitting behind a desk. While there is no reason to make the room impersonal, dramatic paintings, spectacular, panoramic views, or expensive antiques may distract the patient. A comfortable waiting area should be provided for patients who arrive early.

A psychiatrist can never remain entirely unknown to patients, and the office can tell patients a good deal about the doctor's personality. The colors in the office, paintings and diplomas on the wall, the furniture, plants, books, and personal photographs—all describe the psychiatrist in ways that are not directly verbalized. Patients often have reactions to their doctors' offices that may or may not be distortions, and carefully listening to any comments can help a psychiatrist understand the patient. Studies have shown that patients respond more positively to male physicians who wear jackets and ties than to those who do not. No studies have been done on the dress of female physicians, but, by extrapolation, professional attire would probably elicit a positive response.

Table 7.1–10
Supportive and Obstructive Interventions

Supportive

Acknowledging emotion

Doctor: "Even after all these years, talking about your mother brings tears to your eyes."

Encouragement

Patient: "I've never been very good at putting things into words."

Doctor: "I think you've described the situation well—in a way that helps me understand what you've been going through."

Reassurance

Doctor: "The hopelessness you feel right now seems overwhelming. I think it is very likely with the proper treatment you can get back to feeling yourself."

Nonverbal

Facial expression and body posture that convey interest, concern, and attentiveness.

Obstructive

Compound questions

Doctor: "Do you take a vacation every year, and are you able to relax?"

Trapping the patient in his or her own words

Doctor: "When I asked you before, you said nothing had gone well over the last year, and now you're telling me you got a raise and have been exercising more."

Why questions

Doctor: "Why do you keep waking up so early in the morning?"

Dismissal or minimization

Patient: "Over the last month I've had trouble with sex."

Doctor: "That happens from time to time."

Premature advice

Patient: "Ever since my girlfriend and I split up last year, I can't seem to meet anyone new."

Doctor: "Why not try spending time in bookstores and coffee houses? There are usually lots of single people in those places."

Not following the patient's lead

Doctor: "How long have you been feeling so sad?"

Patient: "Over 6 months. Nothing is getting better. I'm starting to wonder if it's worth it."

Doctor: "Do you have trouble sleeping through the night?"

Judgmental

Doctor: "Have you been using any drugs?"

Patient: "Well besides drinking, I smoke a little grass on weekends."

Doctor: "Don't you know that marijuana can cause serious problems with motivation over the long term?"

Nonverbal

Facial expression, body posture, and behavior that indicate lack of interest or inattentiveness such as yawning, or checking one's watch. The doctor who shows no emotional reaction to what a patient is saying usually conveys a sense of not listening or being uninterested.

Types of Interventions

Psychiatrists do much more during an interview than ask questions. They provide feedback and information, offer reassurances, and respond emotionally to what the patient is saying. The psychiatrist's facial expression and body posture also convey information to the patient. Interventions are described as "supportive" or "obstructive," depending on the extent to which they increase the flow of information and enhance or diminish rapport. Table 7.1–10 contains examples of both.

The concept of supportive and obstructive interventions has broad, general use, but it cannot be applied rigidly. The psychiatric interview is a complex, multifaceted task that is shaped by the personalities and circumstances of the interview. Above all it is a human endeavor. The personality of the interviewer is an inevitable and desirable component of the interview and it need not to be veiled behind a mask of austerity or indifference. The concept of "neutrality" as proposed in psychoanalytic psychia-

try means that the psychiatrist does not take sides in the patient's intrapsychic conflicts. It does not mean the clinician is a nonresponding robot.

Ending the Interview

At the end of the evaluation the psychiatrist must give the patient his or her impressions and suggestions, even if they are preliminary. Patients seeing a psychiatrist for the first time are often apprehensive. They wonder if they are "crazy," if their problems can be understood, if they will be judged, and most importantly whether they can be helped. Although patients may experience significant relief just in talking with another person about their concerns, these fears should be explicitly addressed and realistic reassurance offered about available treatments. The concluding moments of the initial interview prepare the patient for follow-up, and handling them well increases the likelihood of helping the patient. It is especially important to give persons who have become emotionally distraught a few minutes to collect themselves before they are asked to leave the office. For example, a psychiatrist might say to a patient who is sobbing heavily near the end of the interview, "It's clear these things are still very painful to talk about. We have to finish in a few minutes, but let me take a moment to give you my impressions and tell you what I think is best to do next."

Note Taking

For legal and medical reasons, an adequate written record of each patient's treatment must be maintained. The patient's record also aids the psychiatrist's memory. Each clinician must establish a system of record keeping and decide which information to record. Many psychiatrists make complete notes during the first few sessions while eliciting historical data. Afterward, most psychiatrists record only new historical information, important events in the patient's life, medications prescribed, dreams, and general comments about the patient's progress. Some psychiatrists maintain detailed process notes (verbatim record of a session) for specific patients by writing out immediately after a session as much of the session as they can remember. Process notes make it much easier to determine trends in the treatment (with regard to transference and countertransference issues) and to go back over the session to pick up ideas that may have been missed. Process notes are also helpful if a psychiatrist is working with a supervisor or a consultant who needs an accurate presentation of a particular session.

Most psychiatrists do not recommend taking extensive notes during a session; writing can cut down on the ability to listen. Some patients, however, may express resentment if a psychiatrist does not write notes during an interview; they may fear that their comments were not important enough to record or that the psychiatrist was not interested in them. As not taking notes during a session presumably has no relation to the psychiatrist's listening, this feeling on a patient's part can be further explored to understand the fear of not being taken seriously.

An increasing number of psychiatrists are communicating with patients through e-mail. E-mail has the advantages of being quick, usually brief, and often less disruptive than telephone calls. As a result, e-mail communication often feels more spontaneous and casual than a telephone call or letter. However, for all their apparent casualness, e-mail messages constitute a formal part of the treatment record and are subject to review in court proceedings.

Stress Interview

A stress interview has its advocates and has a minor place in the armamentarium of interview techniques. Most patients feel some anxiety or other emotion when talking to a psychiatrist. Through his or her manner or a word of reassurance or praise the psychiatrist can often decrease this emotion so that the patient can continue to tell his or her story. However, certain patients are monotonously repetitious or show insufficient emotion for motivation. Apathy, indifference, and emotional blunting are not conducive to discussion of personality problems. In patients with such reactions, stimulation of emotions can be constructive. These patients may require probing, challenging, or confrontation to arouse feelings that will promote progress in furthering understanding. For example, the *la belle indifférence* of the hysteric may be converted into anxiety so that the patient can experience enough discomfort to talk about his or her conflicts.

Follow-Up Interviews

Interviews after the initial one allow patients to correct any misinformation provided in the first meeting. It is often helpful to start the second interview by asking a patient whether he or she has thought about the first interview and what his or her reactions to the experience were. Another variation is to say: "Frequently, people think of additional things they wanted to discuss after they leave. What thoughts have you had?"

Psychiatrists often learn something of value when they ask patients whether they have discussed the interview with anyone else. If the patient has done so, the details of the conversation and the person with whom the patient spoke are enlightening. There are no set rules about which topics are best deferred until the second interview. In general, as patients' comfort and familiarity with the psychiatrist increase, they become increasingly able to reveal the intimate details of their lives.

INTERVIEWING SPECIAL TYPES OF PSYCHIATRIC PATIENTS

Psychotic Patients

Patients with psychotic symptoms have difficulty thinking clearly and reasoning logically. Their ability to concentrate may be impaired, and they may be distracted by delusions, beliefs, and hallucinations. Psychotic patients are often frightened and may be quite guarded. Often the evaluation of a psychotic patient needs to be more focused and structured than that of other patients. Open-ended questions and long periods of silence tend to be disorganizing. Short questions are easier than long ones. Questions calling for abstract responses or hypothetical conjecture may be unanswerable.

Patients with hallucinations should be asked to describe the phenomenology of the sensory misperception as fully as possible. Patients with auditory hallucinations should be asked about content, context, volume, clarity, and their response. The evaluation needs to distinguish between true hallucination on the one

hand and illusions, hypnagogic, hypnopompic, and vivid imagining on the other.

Delusions are by definition fixed false beliefs. Attempting to reason a person away from a delusional belief will not succeed and will be counterproductive. Delusional patients often come to a psychiatric evaluation having had their beliefs dismissed or belittled by friends and family, and they will be on guard for similar reactions from the examiner. It is possible to discuss delusions without conveying belief or disbelief. Careless use of psychiatric jargon must be avoided. Words such as *grandiose*, *paranoid*, and indeed the word *delusion* itself will seem harsh and judgmental and are unlikely to be helpful in eliciting information.

Persons with paranoid delusions or with high levels of nondelusional suspiciousness are best evaluated with respectful, but somewhat distant, formality. Efforts to reassure or ingratiate will increase suspicion. The psychiatrist must keep in mind the possibility of being incorporated into a delusional belief and may need to ask about it directly. "Are you concerned that I might try to hurt you, too?"

Disorders of thought form can seriously impair communication. Their presence usually requires very short, focused questions and considerable structure. The psychiatrist needs to provide an organization for thinking that the patient cannot provide.

Depressed and Potentially Suicidal Patients

Severely depressed patients may also have difficulty concentrating, thinking clearly, and speaking spontaneously. The intensity of mood disturbances can seem all-consuming and may well lead to distortions in thinking and perception. Some depressed patients will need the doctor to be more forceful and directive than usual. It will sometimes seem that the examiner must provide all the emotional and intellectual energy for doctor and patient. Long silences are seldom helpful, and the examiner may need to repeat questions. Ruminative patients will need to be interrupted and redirected.

All patients must be asked about suicidal thoughts, and depressed patients may need to be questioned more fully. A thorough assessment of suicidal potential addresses intent, plans, means, and perceived consequences as well as "Do you ever think of hurting yourself?" or "Does it ever seem that life isn't worth living?" The psychiatrist must be comfortable asking simple, direct questions. Asking about suicide does not increase the risk. On the contrary, most patients are relieved to be able to discuss openly such painful thoughts that they have been struggling with in private.

Agitated and Potentially Violent Patients

The risk for violence and aggression is inherent in working with psychiatric patients; the coexistence of diminished judgment, increased impulsivity, and paranoid thinking greatly increases the risk. Some conditions in which the potential for violence is high include alcohol and central nervous system (CNS) stimulant intoxication, delirium, paranoid psychoses, and manic states. When faced with a potentially violent patient, the psychiatrist's task is twofold: to contain the behavior and limit the potential for harm but also to conduct an evaluation and provide treatment. In the case of a patient with delirium, the need for evaluation may be a medical emergency.

Most unpremeditated violence is preceded by a prodrome of accelerating psychomotor agitation. The patient may begin pacing and pounding his fist in his hand. (Most—but not all—violent psychiatric patients are men.) His speech becomes loud, abusive, obscene, and threatening. His temporal arteries begin to throb. The prodrome commonly lasts from 30 to 60 minutes before erupting into physical violence, thus offering a window of opportunity to intervene before violence occurs.

Several steps can be taken to minimize the potential risk. The interview should be conducted in a quiet, nonstimulating environment. Both doctor and patient should have enough space to be comfortable, and neither should have any physical barrier to leaving the room. During the interview, the psychiatrist must try not to behave in any manner that could be construed as threatening by the patient such as standing over him, staring, or touching without permission. The psychiatrist must ask the questions essential for evaluation. Bargaining, threatening or bullying is counterproductive. Above all, the psychiatrist must feel safe enough to perform a professional evaluation; a fearful psychiatrist cannot do an adequate job. There will be times when the threat is sufficient to require terminating the interview. In the emergency room and on inpatient services, physical and chemical restraints are occasionally necessary to protect both the medical staff and the patient.

Patients Who Lie

Psychiatrists recognize that what patients report may not be the literal truth. The unreliability of memory and the vagaries of psychopathology through which a patient's narrative is processed will distort and falsify. The examiner knows that what is historically untrue may still be emotionally true and, therefore, a meaningful part of the diagnostic assessment.

At times patients lie consciously with the explicit intent of deceiving the therapist. The purpose may be secondary gain such as exemption from jury duty, financial gain, or a supply of addictive drugs. Such patients are falsifying symptoms. (Malingering is not listed as a mental disorder in DSM-IV-TR.)

Patients also lie to gain whatever benefit there is in assuming the sick role and not for any obvious external advantage. The diagnosis of factitious disorder is used for most persons who pretend to be sick for unclear, internal emotional reasons. Because psychiatrists do not have available biological markers to define pathology, they have to accept the patient's report as an honest statement of his or her experience. There is no way of knowing whether a patient is or is not experiencing auditory hallucinations other than through self-report. Nevertheless, an experienced interviewer can detect subtle discrepancies, internal inconsistencies, or suspiciously atypical symptoms; these can be questioned without assuming the patient is lying.

Being lied to angers most people, certainly no less psychiatrists who depend on trust to perform their work. However, believing a patient's lies is not a professional failure. Psychiatrists are trained to detect, understand, and treat psychopathology, not to serve as lie detectors. While a certain level of suspicion is essential in the practice of psychiatry, the clinician who is determined never to be taken in will approach patients with such exaggerated suspiciousness that therapeutic work will be impossible.

The reader is referred to Chapter 1 on the doctor–patient relationship for a discussion of other types of difficult patients (e.g., the seductive patient).

Empathy

A diagnostic interview often gives patients considerable relief. Puzzling and sometimes frightening symptoms are frames in the context of medical understanding. Bizarre experiences can be understood rationally and organized intelligently in meaningful ways that allow us to make informed predictions about treatment response and recovery. Equally important to an intellectual understanding is an emotional understanding of what patients have been going through. Empathy is a human capacity, essential for psychiatry. The expression of empathy is a skill that grows more refined with experience.

While empathic statements can be extremely important in strengthening the relationship between doctor and patient, they can also be disruptive. Since empathic observations derive from intuition as much as observation, care must be taken to make sure they are not just projections of the psychiatrist's own feelings. Guarded patients may find such observations intrusive and threatening, especially when they are stated categorically ("You're feeling hurt") rather than conditionally ("It sounds as though your feelings were hurt"). Empathic statements made prematurely, while a patient is still strongly defended against an unpleasant feeling, are not likely to be helpful. For the most part, patients are not looking for someone who feels the way they feel, but for a person who will try to understand what they are feeling.

References

Bjorkly S. Clinical assessment of dangerousness in psychotic patients: some risk indicators and pitfalls. *Aggression Violent Behav.* 1997;2:167.

Corty E, Lehman AF, Myers CP. Influence of psychoactive substance use on the reliability of psychiatric diagnosis. *J Consult Clin Psychol.* 1993;61:165.

Janca A, Hiller W. ICD-10 checklists—a tool for clinician's use of the ICD-10 classification of mental and behavioral disorders. *Compr Psychiatry.* 1996;37:180.

Kosten TA, Rounsaville BJ. Sensitivity of psychiatric diagnosis based on the best estimate procedure. *Am J Psychiatry.* 1992;149:1225.

Lewis NDC. *Outlines for Psychiatric Examinations.* 3rd ed. Albany: New York State Department of Mental Hygiene; 1943.

MacKinnon RA, Yudofsky SC. *The Psychiatric Interview in Clinical Practice.* Philadelphia: JB Lippincott; 1986.

Manley MRS. The psychiatric interview, history, and mental status examination. In: Sadock BJ, Sadock VA, eds. *Kaplan & Sadock's Comprehensive Textbook of Psychiatry.* 7th ed. Vol 1. Baltimore: Lippincott Williams & Wilkins; 2000:6520.

Shaffer D, Gould MS, Fisher P, et al. Psychiatric diagnosis in child and adolescent suicide. *Arch Gen Psychiatry.* 1996;53:339.

Tangalos EG, Smith GE, Ivnik RJ, et al. The Mini-Mental State Examination in general medical practice: clinical utility and acceptance. *Mayo Clin Proc.* 1996;71:829.

Wiley SD. Deception and detection in psychiatric diagnosis. *Psychiatr Clin North Am.* 1998;21:869.

Williams JW Jr, Noel PH, Cordes JA, et al. Is this patient clinically depressed? *JAMA.* 2002;287:1160.

Zarin DA, Earls F. Diagnostic decision making in psychiatry. *Am J Psychiatry.* 1993;150:197.

▲ 7.2 Medical Record

The medical record includes the psychiatric report but contains much more information than that. It is a narrative that documents all events that occur during the course of treatment, most often referring to the patient's stay in the hospital. However, it applies equally to outpatients treated in doctors' offices. Progress notes record every interaction between doctor and patient (including psychotherapy sessions), reports of all special studies including laboratory tests, and prescriptions and orders for all medications. In the hospital, nurses' notes are an important part of the medical record. They help describe the patient's course: Is the patient beginning to respond to treatment? Are there times during the day or night when symptoms get worse or remit? Are there adverse effects or complaints by the patient about prescribed medication? Are there signs of agitation, violence, or mention of suicide? If the patient requires restraints or seclusion are the proper supervisory procedures being followed? Taken as a whole, the medical record tells what happened to the patient since first making contact with the health care system. It concludes with a discharge summary that provides a concise overview of the patient's course, with recommendations for future treatment, if necessary. Evidence of contact with a referral agency should be documented in the medical record to establish continuity of care if further intervention is necessary.

USE OF THE RECORD

The medical record is used not only by physicians but also by regulatory agencies and managed care companies to determine length of stay, quality of care, and reimbursement to doctors and hospitals. In theory, the inpatient medical record is accessible to authorized persons only and is safeguarded for confidentiality. In practice, however, absolute confidentiality cannot be guaranteed. Guidelines for what material needs to be incorporated into the medical record are given in Table 7.2–1.

Table 7.2–1
Medical Record

There shall be an individual record for each person admitted to the psychiatric inpatient unit. Patient records shall be safeguarded for confidentiality and be accessible only to authorized persons. Each case record shall include

1. Legal admission documents
2. Identifying information on the individual and family
3. Source of referral, date of commencing service, and name of staff member carrying overall responsibility for treatment and care
4. Initial, intercurrent, and final diagnoses, including psychiatric or mental retardation diagnoses in official terminology
5. Reports of all diagnostic examinations and evaluations, including findings and conclusions
6. Reports of all special studies performed, including X-rays, clinical laboratory tests, clinical psychological testing, electroencephalograms, psychometric tests
7. The individual written plan of care, treatment, and rehabilitation
8. Progress notes written and signed by all staff members having significant participation in the program of treatment and care
9. Summaries of case conferences and special consultations
10. Dated and signed prescriptions or orders for all medications, with notation of termination dates
11. A closing summary of the course of treatment and care
12. Documentation of any referrals to another agency

Adapted from the 1995 guidelines of the New York State Office of Mental Health.

The medical record is also crucial in malpractice litigation. Robert I. Simon summarized the liability issues as follows:

> Properly kept medical records can be the psychiatrist's best ally in malpractice litigation. If no record is kept, numerous questions will be raised regarding the psychiatrist's competence and credibility. This failure to keep medical records may also violate state statutes or licensing provisions. Failure to keep medical records may arise out of the psychiatrist's concern that patient treatment information be totally protected. Although this is an admirable ideal, in real life the psychiatrist may be legally compelled under certain circumstances to testify about confidential treatment matters.

Outpatient records are also subject to scrutiny by third parties under certain circumstances, and psychiatrists in private practices are under the same obligation to maintain a record of the patient in treatment as hospital psychiatrists. Table 7.2–2 lists documentation issues of concern to third-party payers.

Records need not be kept indefinitely by the doctor; the length of time varies according to state laws. In general, records of children are kept for longer periods than those for adults.

Table 7.2–2
Documentation Issues[a]

1. Are patient's areas of dysfunction described? From the biological, psychological, and social points of view?
2. Is alcohol or substance abuse addressed?
3. Do clinical activities happen at the expected time? If too late or never—why?
4. Are issues identified in the treatment plan and followed in progress notes?
5. When there is a variance in the patient's outcome: Is there a note in the progress notes to that effect? Is there also a note in the progress notes reflecting the clinical strategies recommended to overcome the impediments to the patient's improvement?
6. If new clinical strategies are implemented, how is their impact evaluated? When?
7. Is there a sense of multidisciplinary input and coordination of treatment in the progress notes?
8. Do progress notes indicate the patient's functioning in the therapeutic community and its relationship to their discharge criteria?
9. Can one extrapolate from the patients' behavior in the therapeutic community how they will function in the community at large?
10. Are there notes depicting the patients' understanding of their discharge planning? Family participation in discharge planning must be entered in the progress notes with their reaction to the plan.
11. Do attending progress notes bridge the differences in thinking of other disciplines?
12. Are the patient's needs addressed in the treatment plan?
13. Are the patient's family needs evaluated and implemented?
14. Is patient and family satisfaction evaluated in any way?
15. Is alcohol and substance abuse addressed as a possible contributor to readmission?
16. If the patient was readmitted, are there indications that previous records were reviewed, and if the patient is on medication other than that prescribed on discharge is there a rationale for this change?
17. Do the progress notes identify the type of medication used and the rationale for increase, decrease, discontinuation, or augmentation of medication.
18. Are medication effects documented, including dosages, response, and adverse or other side effects?

[a]Documentation issues are of concern to third-party payers such as insurance companies and HMOs who examine patients' charts to see if the areas listed above are covered. In many cases, however, the review is conducted by persons with little or no background in psychiatry or psychology who do not recognize the complexities of psychiatric diagnosis and treatment. Payments to hospitals, doctors, and patients are often denied because of what such reviewers consider "inadequate documentation."

Personal Notes and Observations

According to laws relating to access to medical records, some jurisdictions have a provision that applies to a physician's personal notes and observations (e.g., that in the Public Health Law of New York State). Personal notes are defined as "a practitioner's speculations, impressions (other than tentative or actual diagnosis)." The data are maintained only by the clinician and cannot be disclosed to any other person. Psychiatrists concerned about material that may prove damaging or otherwise hurtful to the patient if released to a third party may consider using this provision to maintain doctor–patient confidentiality.

Patient Access to Records

Patients have a legal right to access their medical records. This right represents society's belief that the responsibility for medical care has become a collaborative process between doctor and patient. Patients see many different physicians, and they can be more effective historians and coordinators of their own care with such information.

Psychiatrists must be careful in releasing their records to the patient if, in their judgment, the patient can be harmed emotionally as a result. Under these circumstances, the psychiatrist may choose to prepare a summary of the patient's course of treatment, holding back material that might be hurtful—especially if it were to get into the hands of third parties. In malpractice cases, however, it may not be possible to do so.

Requests by Third Parties

As mentioned above, outpatient records may be sought by third parties such as attorneys and insurance carriers. Patients usually give insurance companies the right to access their records when they sign member contracts, but many persons are unaware of that particular clause. Because of that, it is prudent to obtain the patient's authorization separately before giving out any information. If served with a legal request to release patient records, legal advice should be obtained before acceding to that request. A subpoena does not necessarily invalidate physician–patient confidentiality. Similarly, one doctor may request a medical record from another doctor. This generally facilitates patient care and is good practice; however, a separate authorization should be obtained from the patient before doing so.

Problem-Oriented Medical Record

In 1969 Lawrence L. Weed published *Medical Records, Medical Education and Patient Care,* in which he described the problem-oriented medical record. The problem-oriented medical record lists all health problems discovered in the initial workup. Problem areas are added to and corrected over time. Active problems are listed in one column, and as they are

resolved, they are transferred to an inactive column. Progress notes are dated, titled, and numbered according to the problem list. As a final check, the record is audited for thoroughness, reliability, efficiency, and standards of treatment and outcome.

Problem-Oriented Record in Medical Education

Many medical schools are using educational techniques based upon the problem-oriented medical record. Teaching and testing organizations such as the United States Medical Licensing Examination (USMLE) are relying on the ability of a student to deal with a problem-oriented medical record as an evaluation tool. In such exercises, students are provided with general patient information, which may include a summary of the physical examination and positive elements in the psychiatric report. Students must delineate the problem areas that need attention, determine preventive or treatment options for each problem, and understand the patient from biological, social, and psychological points of view.

Although the problem-oriented medical record is not the standard format used by psychiatrists, it has influenced how patients are viewed. For example, in DSM-IV-TR specific psychosocial and environmental problems that may affect diagnosis of mental disorders are recorded on Axis IV. The problems are divided into nine categories that can each affect the person adversely: (1) problems with the primary support group (e.g., death of a family member), (2) problems related to the social environment (e.g., absence of friends), (3) educational problems (e.g., discord with teachers or classmates), (4) occupational problems (e.g., stress at work), (5) housing problems (e.g., unsafe neighborhood), (6) economic problems (e.g., excess debt), (7) problems with access to health care services (e.g., no health insurance), (8) problems with the legal system (e.g., litigation), and (9) other problems (e.g., floods, earthquakes).

A 55-year-old married man complains of being fearful that he will be forced to resign from an administrative job because his company is being downsized. He complains of anxiety, insomnia, and irritability and gives no history of previous dysphoric states. After a thorough evaluation it becomes apparent that the proximate cause of his symptoms is the probability of losing his job. Symptom removal is relatively simple with the aid of anxiolytic or hypnotic drugs; however, a more comprehensive approach is required. The therapist has to attend to the occupational problem that might include having the patient confront his superiors, applying for reassignment to another area within the company, seeking other employment, evaluating his assets for early retirement, job retraining, or other approaches directed toward the vocational crisis.

E-Mail

E-mail is increasingly being used by physicians as a quick and efficient way to communicate not only with patients but with other doctors about their patients; however, it is a public document and should be treated as such. The dictum of not diagnosing or prescribing medication over the telephone to a patient one has not examined should also apply to e-mail. It is not only dangerous, but also unethical. All e-mail messages should be printed out for the paper chart unless electronic archives are regularly backed up and secure.

ETHICAL ISSUES

Psychiatrists continually make judgments about what is not appropriate material to include in the psychiatric report, the medical record, the case report, and other written communications about the patient. Such judgments often involve ethical issues. In a case report, for example, the patient should not be identifiable, a position made clear in the American Psychiatric Association's *Principles of Medical Ethics with Annotations Especially Applicable to Psychiatry,* which states that published case reports must be suitably disguised to safeguard patient confidentiality without altering material to provide a less-than-complete portrayal of the patient's actual condition. In some instances obtaining a written release from the patient that allows the psychiatrist to publish the case may also be advisable, even if the patient is appropriately disguised.

Psychiatrists sometimes include material in the medical record that is specifically directed toward warding off future culpability if liability issues are ever raised. The following vignette illustrates one such instance.

A psychiatrist noted in the chart that he discussed with the patient the important adverse effects of a particular medication he was about to prescribe. In fact, he only discussed the two adverse effects most commonly observed. He chose not to discuss others because he was concerned that the patient (who was highly suggestible) would develop them, and he wrote that in the chart. When the patient developed an adverse effect (even though minor and not life threatening), he sued the psychiatrist for not advising him of that possibility. The case was settled in the psychiatrist's favor on the basis of the note in the medical records.

Military Psychiatry. Psychiatrists in the military face unique ethical problems because confidentiality does not exist under the military code of conduct.

A 19-year-old single, white male, new to military service, presented with a history of periodic episodes of anxiety when taking showers in groups with other men. He identified himself as gay and recognized that his anxiety was related to his fear of acting out his sexual impulses, thus risking court-martial and dishonorable discharge should he ever be discovered. The psychiatrist was on the horns of a dilemma: whether to report the soldier to his commanding officer (as he was obliged to do under the military code) or to protect the soldier from acting on his impulses that would place him in danger (in keeping with the medical ethic to do no harm). After discussing various options, he and the patient agreed on the latter option. A diagnosis of anxiety disorder was made that allowed the patient to receive an honorable discharge on medical grounds, based on a recognized psychiatric disorder. No record of his homosexual orientation was made.

Managed Care. With the advent of managed care and the need to send periodic progress reports and documentation of signs and symptoms to third-party reviewers to pay for treatment, some psychiatrists may diminish or exaggerate symptomatology. The following case report and discussion illustrates the ethical difficulties psychiatrists face in dealing with managed care.

Mrs. P. admitted herself to the hospital because she was afraid she might kill herself. She was suffering from a major depressive episode, but she improved markedly during the first weeks on Dr. A.'s ward. Although Dr. A. believed that Mrs. P. was no longer suicidal, he thought she would benefit greatly from continued hospitalization. Because he knew that Mrs. P. could not afford to pay for hospitalization and that the insurance company would pay only if the patient was suicidally depressed, he decided not to document Mrs. P.'s improvement. He noted in the chart "the patient continues to have a risk of suicide."

This case illustrates one of the difficulties posed by cost constraints and managed care. Dr. A. responds to this difficulty by tailoring the chart. Does he engage in a form of deception? Yes, he intentionally misleads by what he writes and what he omits writing in the chart. Although what he writes is true in some literal sense, his statement is misleading in the context of treatment. Mrs. P. is not suicidally depressed in the way she was.

What Dr. A. omits from the chart is also deceptive. Whether a particular omission is deceptive depends, in part, on the roles and expectations of the people involved. Not telling your colleague that you dislike his tie is not a deception. It is simply tact, unless your role or relationship involves the expectation that you will offer your candid opinion. Dr. A.'s case is different. His professional role is to document the patient's course, and the expectation is that he will note any significant improvement. Thus his failure to document Mrs. P.'s progress accurately is a kind of deception.

The second and more difficult question is whether deception is justified in this instance. The answer to that question depends on the reasons for the deception, the reasons against it, and the alternatives available.

The reasons for this deception are obvious. Dr. A.'s aim and primary obligation is to help the patient. He believes that Mrs. P. would benefit greatly from continued hospitalization that she cannot afford. He may also believe that it is unfair for the insurance company to refuse to pay for inpatient treatment of nonsuicidal depression and that his deception rectifies that unfair practice.

There are also important reasons against this deception. The first reason concerns honesty and social trust. It is a good thing if a person can rely on what others say and write. Without some honesty and trust, many social exchanges and practices would be impossible. Deception, even for beneficent purposes, has real potential to damage social trust. A risk exists that deception may damage a person's trust in the profession of psychiatry and even patients' trust in their psychiatrists. Damage to trust may, in turn, compromise treatment.

The second reason concerns future medical treatment. If Mrs. P. seeks medical treatment in the future, the physicians who attend her will read the misleading notes. If they believe that the notes are an accurate account of the previous treatment, they may suggest an inappropriate treatment for the present problem. Even if they have doubts about the accuracy of the notes in her chart, they are deprived of an accurate history and report. In either case, the prior deception can hinder treatment.

The third reason concerns obligations and coverage policies. Dr. A. seems to ignore the obligation he has to the population that is covered by the insurance policy. He shifts a burden onto this population by forcing the insurance company to pay for treatment it did not agree to cover. Perhaps the insurance company should pay for inpatient treatment in cases like Mrs. P.'s; perhaps its policies are unreasonable and unfair. But Dr. A.'s deception does not challenge the insurance company and pressure it to change its policy; nor does his deception encourage patients and their families to contest the company's policies. The use of deception is simply an ad hoc circumvention of a policy that should be challenged and discussed.

Dr. A. also seems to ignore his obligation to future patients. By introducing an inaccuracy into the chart, he compromises the value of medical records research. In a small way, his deception deprives future patients of the benefit of research that relies on medical records.

Whether the deception is justified depends not only on the weight of the reasons for and against the deception but also on the available alternatives. One alternative is to tailor the chart. Another alternative is to describe Mrs. P.'s response accurately and discharge her to outpatient care. But a third alternative exists. Dr. A. can accurately document the patient's course and recommend continued hospitalization. He can petition the insurance company for coverage. If the insurance company decides not to approve further inpatient care for the patient, Dr. A. can appeal that decision. This alternative is more time consuming, and there is no guarantee it will succeed, but it avoids all the problems associated with the use of deception. (Courtesy of J. Dwyer and A. Shih.)

The issues of documentation and access to medical records will receive much more study in future years. Legislative patient privacy bills are before Congress as of this writing to protect and limit third-party access to medical records. In spite of this, however, the trend toward less patient privacy continues. Proposed legislation would give each person in America a unique medical identifier that could encode on a microchip one's medical record from the cradle to the grave. Should this or similar legislation be enacted into law, medical privacy will continue to erode.

Finally, critics of current documentation processes claim that filling out forms developed by governmental agencies—more necessary for fiscal than for medical needs—takes time away from direct patient care. In the future, society will have to determine how far the process of documentation must proceed

before the need to archive material unrelated to direct patient care interferes with the care of the patient.

References

Baur C. Limiting factors on the transformative powers of e-mail in patient-physician relationships: a critical analysis. *Health Commun.* 2000;12:239.

Botkin JR. Protecting the privacy of family members in survey and pedigree research. *JAMA.* 2001;285:207.

Dunivin DL, Foust MJ Jr. A case study from the Department of Defense Psychopharmacology Demonstration Project: mania and neurosyphilis. *Profess Psychol Res Pract.* 1999;30:346.

Gostin LO. National health information privacy: regulations under the Health Insurance Portability and Accountability Act. *JAMA.* 2001;285:3015.

Lowrance WW. *Privacy and Health Research: A Report to the US Secretary of Health and Human Services.* Washington, DC: Dept of Health and Human Services; 1997.

Mitchell AC, McCabe EM, Brown KW. Psychiatrists' attitudes to physical examination of new out-patients with a major depressive disorder. *Psychiatr Bull.* 1998;22:82.

National Research Council. *For the Record: Protecting Electronic Health Information.* Washington, DC: National Academy Press; 1997.

Sadock BJ. Psychiatric report and medical record. In: Sadock BJ, Sadock VA, eds. *Kaplan & Sadock's Comprehensive Textbook of Psychiatry.* 7th ed. Vol 1. Baltimore: Lippincott Williams & Wilkins; 2000:665.

▲ 7.3 Physical Examination of the Psychiatric Patient

Although psychiatrists do not perform routine physical examinations on their patients, a knowledge and understanding of physical signs and symptoms is part of their training, which enables them to recognize signs and symptoms that may indicate possible medical or surgical illness. For example, palpitations may be associated with mitral valve prolapse, which is diagnosed by cardiac auscultation. Psychiatrists are also able to recognize and treat the adverse effects of psychotropic medication, which are used by an increasing number of patients seen by psychiatrists and nonpsychiatric physicians.

Some psychiatrists insist that every patient have a complete medical workup; others may not. Whatever their policy, psychiatrists should consider patients' medical status at the outset of a psychiatric evaluation. Psychiatrists must often decide whether a patient needs a medical examination and, if so, what it should include—most commonly, a thorough medical history, including a review of systems, a physical examination, and relevant diagnostic laboratory studies. A recent study of 1,000 medical patients found that in 75 percent of cases no cause of symptoms (i.e., subjective complaints) could be found, and a psychological basis was assumed in 10 percent of those cases.

HISTORY OF MEDICAL ILLNESS

In the course of conducting a psychiatric evaluation, information should be gathered about known bodily diseases or dysfunctions, hospitalizations and operative procedures, medications taken recently or at present, personal habits and occupational history, family history of illnesses, and specific physical complaints. Information about medical illnesses should be gathered from the patient, the referring physician, and the family if necessary.

Information about previous episodes of illness may provide valuable clues about the nature of the present disorder. For example, a distinctly delusional disorder in a patient with a history of several similar episodes that responded promptly to diverse forms of treatment strongly suggests the possibility of substance-induced psychotic disorder. To pursue this lead, the psychiatrist should order a drug screen. The history of a surgical procedure may also be useful; for instance, a thyroidectomy suggests hypothyroidism as the cause of depression.

Depression is an adverse effect of several medications prescribed for hypertension. Medication taken in a therapeutic dosage occasionally reaches high concentrations in the blood. Digitalis intoxication, for example, may occur under such circumstances and result in impaired mental functioning. Proprietary drugs may cause or contribute to an anticholinergic delirium. Therefore, the psychiatrist must inquire about over-the-counter remedies as well as prescribed medications. A history of herbal intake and alternative therapy is essential in view of their increased use.

An occupational history may also provide essential information. Exposure to mercury may result in complaints suggesting a psychosis, and exposure to lead, as in smelting, may produce a cognitive disorder. The latter clinical picture can also result from imbibing moonshine whiskey with a high lead content.

In eliciting information about specific symptoms, the psychiatrist brings medical and psychological knowledge into full play. For example, the psychiatrist should elicit sufficient information from the patient complaining of headache to predict whether the pain results from intracranial disease that requires neurological testing. Also, the psychiatrist should be able to recognize that the pain in the right shoulder of a hypochondriacal patient with abdominal discomfort may be the classic referred pain of gallbladder disease.

REVIEW OF SYSTEMS

An inventory by systems should follow the open-ended inquiry. The review may be organized according to organ systems (e.g., liver, pancreas), functional systems (e.g., gastrointestinal), or a combination of the two, as in the following outline. In all cases, the review should be comprehensive and thorough. Even if a psychiatric component is suspected, a complete workup is still indicated.

Head

Many patients give a history of headache; its duration, frequency, character, location, and severity should be ascertained. Headaches often result from substance abuse, including alcohol, nicotine, and caffeine. Vascular (migraine) headaches are precipitated by stress. Temporal arteritis causes unilateral throbbing headaches and may lead to blindness. Brain tumors are associated with headaches as a result of increased intracranial pressure. A history of head injury may result in subdural hematoma and in boxers can cause progressive dementia with extrapyramidal symptoms. The headache of subarachnoid hemorrhage is sudden, severe, and associated with changes in the sensorium. Normal pressure hydrocephalus may follow a head injury or encephalitis and may be associated with dementia, shuffling gait, and urinary incontinence. Dizziness occurs in up

Table 7.3–1
Approach to the Differentiation of Dizziness Subtypes

Dizziness Subtype	Type of Sensation	Temporal Characteristics	Other Specifications
Vertigo	A feeling that one or one's surroundings are moving (typically, spinning)	Episodic vertigo occurs in attacks that last seconds to days Continuous vertigo is present all or most of the time for at least a week	Descriptions of episodic vertigo should include the characteristics, duration, and date of the first episode; length of episodes; and exacerbating factors
Presyncope	A lightheaded, faint feeling, as though one were about to pass out	Typically occurs in episodes lasting seconds to hours	The following questions should be answered: (1) Has syncope ever occurred during an episode? (2) Do episodes occur only when the patient is upright, or do they occur in other positions? (3) Are episodes associated with palpitations, medication, meals, bathing, dyspnea, or chest discomfort?
Disequilibrium	A sense of unsteadiness that is (1) primarily felt in the lower extremities, (2) most prominent when standing or walking, and (3) relieved by sitting or lying down	Usually present, although it may fluctuate in intensity	Identify whether symptom occurs in isolation or accompanies another dizziness subtype; describe exacerbating factors
Other dizziness: anxiety-related, ocular, tilting environment, other	A feeling not covered by the above definitions. May include swimming or floating sensations, vague lightheadedness, or feelings of dissociation. May be difficult for the patient to describe	Usually present all or most of the time for days or weeks, sometimes years	The following questions should be answered: (1) Is dizziness associated with anxiety or hyperventilation? (2) Was change in vision connected with dizziness onset? (3) Is dizziness a sensation that the environment is tilting sideways (suggests an otolith problem)?

From Sloane PD, Coeytaux RR, Beck RS, Dallara J. Dizziness. State of the science. *Ann Intern Med.* 2001;134:825.

to 30 percent of persons and determining its cause is challenging (Table 7.3–1) and often difficult. A change in the size or shape of the head may be indicative of Paget's disease.

Eye, Ear, Nose, and Throat

Visual acuity, diplopia, hearing problems, tinnitus, glossitis, and bad taste are covered in this area. A patient taking antipsychotics who gives a history of twitching about the mouth or disturbing movements of the tongue may be in the early and potentially reversible stage of tardive dyskinesia. Impaired vision may occur with thioridazine (Mellaril) in high dosages (over 800 mg a day). A history of glaucoma contraindicates drugs with anticholinergic effects. Aphonia may be hysterical in nature. The late stage of cocaine abuse can result in perforations of the nasal septum and difficulty breathing. A transitory episode of diplopia may herald multiple sclerosis. Delusional disorder is more common in hearing-impaired persons than in those with normal hearing. Complaints of bad odors may be a symptom of temporal lobe epilepsy rather than schizophrenia.

Respiratory System

Cough, asthma, pleurisy, hemoptysis, dyspnea, and orthopnea are considered in this section. Hyperventilation is suggested if the patient's symptoms include all or a few of the following: onset at rest, sighing respirations, apprehension, anxiety, depersonalization, palpitations, inability to swallow, numbness of the feet and hands, and carpopedal spasm. Dyspnea and breathlessness may occur in depression. In pulmonary or obstructive airway disease, the onset of symptoms is usually insidious, whereas in depression, it is sudden. In depression, breathlessness is experienced at rest, shows little change with exertion, and may fluctuate within a matter of minutes; the onset of breathlessness coincides with the onset of a mood disorder and is often accompanied by attacks of dizziness, sweating, palpitations, and paresthesias.

In obstructive airway disease, patients with the most-advanced respiratory incapacity experience breathlessness at rest. Most striking and of greatest assistance in making a differential diagnosis is the emphasis placed on the difficulty in inspiration experienced by patients with depression and on the difficulty in expiration experienced by patients with pulmonary disease. Bronchial asthma has sometimes been associated with a childhood history of extreme dependence on the mother. Patients with bronchospasm should not receive propranolol (Inderal) because it may block catecholamine-induced bronchodilation; propranolol is specifically contraindicated for patients with bronchial asthma because epinephrine given to such patients in an emergency will not be effective. Patients taking angiotensin-converting enzyme (ACE) inhibitors may develop a dry cough as an adverse effect of the drug.

Cardiovascular System

Tachycardia, palpitations, and cardiac arrhythmia are among the most common signs of anxiety about which the patient may complain. Pheochromocytoma usually produces symptoms that

mimic anxiety disorders, such as rapid heartbeat, tremors, and pallor. Increased urinary catecholamines are diagnostic of pheochromocytoma. Patients taking guanethidine (Ismelin) for hypertension should not receive tricyclic drugs, which reduce or eliminate the antihypertensive effect of guanethidine. A history of hypertension may preclude the use of monoamine oxidase inhibitors (MAOIs) because of the risk of a hypertensive crisis if such hypertensive patients inadvertently ingest foods high in tyramine. Patients with a suspected cardiac disease should have an electrocardiogram before tricyclics or lithium (Eskalith) is prescribed. A history of substernal pain should be evaluated, and the clinician should keep in mind that psychological stress can precipitate angina-type chest pain in the presence of normal coronary arteries. Patients taking opioids should never receive MAOIs; the combination can cause cardiovascular collapse.

Gastrointestinal System

This area covers such topics as appetite, distress before or after meals, food preferences, diarrhea, vomiting, constipation, laxative use, and abdominal pain. A history of weight loss is common in depressive disorders, but depression may accompany the weight loss caused by ulcerative colitis, regional enteritis, and cancer. Anorexia nervosa is accompanied by severe weight loss in the presence of normal appetite. Avoidance of certain foods may be a phobic phenomenon or part of an obsessive ritual. Laxative abuse and induced vomiting are common in bulimia nervosa. Constipation can be caused by opioid dependence and by psychotropic drugs with anticholinergic side effects. Cocaine or amphetamine abuse causes a loss of appetite and weight loss. Weight gain can occur under stress or in association with atypical depression. Polyphagia, polyuria, and polydipsia are the triad of diabetes mellitus. Polyuria, polydipsia, and diarrhea are signs of lithium toxicity.

Genitourinary System

Urinary frequency, nocturia, pain or burning on urination, and changes in the size and the force of the stream are some of the signs and symptoms in this area. Anticholinergic adverse effects associated with antipsychotics and tricyclic drugs may cause urinary retention in men with prostate hypertrophy. Erectile difficulty and retarded ejaculation are also common adverse effects of these drugs, and retrograde ejaculation occurs with thioridazine. A baseline level of sexual responsiveness before using pharmacological agents should be obtained. A history of sexually transmitted diseases—for example, gonorrheal discharge, chancre, herpes, and pubic lice—may indicate sexual promiscuity or unsafe sexual practices. In some cases, the first symptom of acquired immune deficiency syndrome (AIDS) is the gradual onset of mental confusion leading to dementia. Incontinence should be evaluated carefully, and if it persists, further investigation for more extensive disease should include a workup for human immunodeficiency virus (HIV) infection. Drugs with anticholinergic adverse effects should be avoided in men with prostatism.

Menstrual History

A menstrual history should include the age of the onset of menarche and menopause; the interval, regularity, duration, and amount of flow of periods; irregular bleeding; dysmenorrhea; and abortions. Amenorrhea is characteristic of anorexia nervosa and also occurs in women who are psychologically stressed. Women who are afraid of becoming pregnant or who have a wish to be pregnant may have delayed periods. *Pseudocyesis* is false pregnancy with complete cessation of the menses. Perimenstrual mood changes (e.g., irritability, depression, and dysphoria) should be noted. Painful menstruation can result from uterine disease (e.g., myomata), from psychological conflicts about the menses, or from a combination of the two. Some women report a premenstrual increase in sexual desire. The emotional reaction associated with abortion should be explored, since it can be mild or severe.

GENERAL OBSERVATION

An important part of the medical examination is subsumed under the broad heading of general observation—visual, auditory, and olfactory. Such nonverbal clues as posture, facial expression, and mannerisms should also be noted.

Vision

Scrutiny of the patient begins at the first encounter. When the patient goes from the waiting room to the interview room, the psychiatrist should observe the patient's gait. Is the patient unsteady? Ataxia suggests diffuse brain disease, alcohol or other substance intoxication, chorea, spinocerebellar degeneration, weakness based on a debilitating process, and an underlying disorder, such as myotonic dystrophy. Does the patient walk without the usual associated arm movements and turn in a rigid fashion, like a toy soldier, as is seen in early Parkinson's disease? Does the patient have asymmetry of gait, such as turning one foot outward, dragging a leg, or not swinging one arm, suggesting a focal brain lesion?

As soon as the patient is seated, the psychiatrist should direct attention to grooming. Is the patient's hair combed, are the nails clean, and are the teeth brushed? Has clothing been chosen with care, and is it appropriate? Although inattention to dress and hygiene is common in mental disorders—in particular, depressive disorders—it is also a hallmark of cognitive disorders. Lapses—such as mismatching socks, stockings, or shoes—may suggest a cognitive disorder.

The patient's posture and automatic movements or the lack of them should be noted. A stooped, flexed posture with a paucity of automatic movements may be due to Parkinson's disease or diffuse cerebral hemispheric disease or be an adverse effect of antipsychotics. An unusual tilt of the head may be adopted to avoid eye contact, but it can also result from diplopia, a visual field defect, or focal cerebellar dysfunction. Frequent quick, purposeless movements are characteristic of anxiety disorders, but they are equally characteristic of chorea and hyperthyroidism. Tremors, although commonly seen in anxiety disorders, may point to Parkinson's disease, essential tremor, or adverse effects of psychotropic medication. Patients with essential tremor sometimes seek psychiatric treatment because they believe the tremor must be due to unrecognized fear or anxiety, as others often suggest. Unilateral paucity or excess of movement suggests focal brain disease.

The patient's appearance is then scrutinized to assess general health. Does the patient appear to be robust, or is there a

sense of ill health? Does looseness of clothing indicate recent weight loss? Is the patient short of breath or coughing? Does the patient's general physiognomy suggest a specific disease? Men with Klinefelter's syndrome have a feminine fat distribution and lack the development of secondary male sex characteristics. Acromegaly is usually immediately recognizable by the large head and jaw.

What is the patient's nutritional status? Recent weight loss, although often seen in depressive disorders and schizophrenia, may be due to gastrointestinal disease, diffuse carcinomatosis, Addison's disease, hyperthyroidism, and many other somatic disorders. Obesity may result from either emotional distress or organic disease. Moon facies, truncal obesity, and buffalo hump are striking findings in Cushing's syndrome. The puffy, bloated appearance seen in hypothyroidism and the massive obesity and periodic respiration seen in Pickwickian syndrome are easily recognized in patients referred for psychiatric help. Hyperthyroidism is indicated by exophthalmos.

The skin frequently provides valuable information. The yellow discoloration of hepatic dysfunction and the pallor of anemia are reasonably distinctive. Intense reddening may be due to carbon monoxide poisoning or to photosensitivity resulting from porphyria or phenothiazines. Eruptions may be manifestations of such disorders as systemic lupus erythematosus (e.g., the butterfly on the face), tuberous sclerosis with adenoma sebaceum, and sensitivity to drugs. A dusky purplish cast to the face, plus telangiectasia, is almost pathognomonic of alcohol abuse.

A young woman, complaining of depression and listlessness, mentioned in an off-hand manner that she had a rash. An on-the-spot examination of her skin revealed petechial hemorrhages on both arms and both legs. Further inquiry disclosed information about bleeding from several sites. Her blood platelet count was 4,000/mm^3. The diagnosis was thrombocytopenia.

Careful observation may reveal clues that lead to the correct diagnosis in patients who create their own skin lesions. For example, the location and shape of the lesions and the time of their appearance may be characteristic of dermatitis factitia.

The patient's face and head should be scanned for evidence of disease. Premature whitening of the hair occurs in pernicious anemia, and thinning and coarseness of the hair occur in myxedema. In alopecia areata patches of hair are lost, leaving bald spots; trichotillomania presents a similar picture. Pupillary changes are produced by various drugs—constriction by opioids and dilation by anticholinergic agents and hallucinogens. The combination of dilated and fixed pupils and dry skin and mucous membranes should immediately suggest the likelihood of atropine use or atropinelike toxicity. Diffusion of the conjunctiva suggests alcohol abuse, cannabis abuse, or obstruction of the superior vena cava. Flattening of the nasolabial fold on one side or weakness of one side of the face—as manifested in speaking, smiling, and grimacing—may be the result of focal dysfunction of the contralateral cerebral hemisphere or of Bell's palsy.

The patient's state of alertness and responsiveness should be evaluated carefully. Drowsiness and inattentiveness may be due to a psychological problem, but they are more likely to result from organic brain dysfunction, whether secondary to an intrinsic brain disease or to an exogenous factor, such as substance intoxication.

Hearing

Listening intently is just as important as looking intently for evidence of somatic disorders. Slowed speech is characteristic not only of depression but also of diffuse brain dysfunction and subcortical dysfunction; unusually rapid speech is characteristic not only of manic episodes and anxiety disorders but also of hyperthyroidism. A weak voice with monotonous tone may be a clue to Parkinson's disease in patients who complain mainly of depression. A slow, low-pitched, hoarse voice should suggest the possibility of hypothyroidism; this voice quality has been described as sounding like a drowsy, slightly intoxicated person with a bad cold and a plum in the mouth.

Difficulty initiating speech may be due to anxiety or stuttering or may indicate Parkinson's disease or aphasia. Easy fatigability of speech is sometimes a manifestation of an emotional problem, but it is also characteristic of myasthenia gravis. Patients with these complaints are likely to be seen by a psychiatrist before the correct diagnosis is made.

Word production, as well as the quality of speech, is important. When words are mispronounced or incorrect words are used, there is a possibility of aphasia caused by a lesion of the dominant hemisphere. The same possibility exists when the patient perseverates, has trouble finding a name or a word, or describes an object or an event in an indirect fashion (paraphasia). When not consonant with patients' socioeconomic and educational levels, coarseness, profanity, or inappropriate disclosures may indicate loss of inhibition caused by dementia.

Smell

Much less is learned through the sense of smell than through the senses of sight and hearing, but smell occasionally provides useful information. The unpleasant odor of a patient who fails to bathe suggests a cognitive disorder or a depressive disorder. The odor of alcohol or of substances used to hide it is revealing in a patient who attempts to conceal a drinking problem. Occasionally, a uriniferous odor calls attention to bladder dysfunction secondary to a nervous system disease. Characteristic odors are also noted in patients with diabetic acidosis, uremia, and hepatic coma. Precocious puberty can be associated with the smell of adult sweat produced by mature apocrine glands.

PHYSICAL EXAMINATION

Patient Selection

The nature of the patient's complaints is critical to determine whether a complete physical examination is required. Complaints fall into the three categories of body, mind, and social interactions. Bodily symptoms (e.g., headaches and palpitations) call for a thorough medical examination to determine what part, if any, somatic processes play in causing the distress. The same can be said for mental symptoms such as depression, anxiety, hallucinations, and persecutory delusions, which can be expres-

sions of somatic processes. If the problem is clearly limited to the social sphere (e.g., long-standing difficulties in interactions with teachers, employers, parents, or a spouse), there may be no special indication for a physical examination. Personality changes, however, may result from a medical disorder (e.g., early Alzheimer's disease) and cause interpersonal conflicts.

Psychological Factors

Even a routine physical examination may evoke adverse reactions; instruments, procedures, and the examining room may be frightening. A simple running account of what is being done can prevent much needless anxiety. Moreover, if the patient is consistently forewarned of what will be done, the dread of being suddenly and painfully surprised recedes. Comments such as "There's nothing to this" and "You don't have to be afraid because this won't hurt" leave the patient in the dark and are much less reassuring than a few words about what actually will be done.

Although the physical examination is likely to engender or intensify a reaction of anxiety, it can also stir up sexual feelings. Some women with fears or fantasies of being seduced may misinterpret an ordinary movement in the physical examination as a sexual advance. Similarly, a delusional man with homosexual fears may perceive a rectal examination as a sexual attack. Lingering over the examination of a particular organ because an unusual but normal variation has aroused the physician's scientific curiosity is likely to raise concern in the patient that a serious pathological process has been discovered. Such a reaction may be profound in an anxious or hypochondriacal patient.

The physical examination occasionally serves a psychotherapeutic function. Anxious patients may be relieved to learn that, in spite of troublesome symptoms, there is no evidence of the serious illness that they fear. The young person who complains of chest pain and is certain that the pain heralds a heart attack can usually be reassured by the report of normal findings after a physical examination and electrocardiogram. The reassurance relieves only the worry occasioned by the immediate episode, however. Unless psychiatric treatment succeeds in dealing with the determinants of the reaction, recurrent episodes are likely.

Sending a patient who has a deeply rooted fear of malignancy for still another test that is intended to be reassuring is usually unrewarding. Some patients may have a false fixed belief that a disorder is present.

> In spite of repeated examinations, a patient who was a physician was convinced that he had carcinoma of the pharynx. A colleague, in an effort to produce positive proof, performed a biopsy of the area of complaint. When the patient was shown a microscopic section of normal tissue, he immediately declared that the normal section had been substituted for one showing malignant cells.

During the performance of the physical examination, an observant physician may note indications of emotional distress. For instance, during genital examinations, a patient's behavior may reveal information about sexual attitudes and problems, and these reactions may be used later to open this area for exploration.

Timing of the Physical Examination

Circumstances occasionally make it desirable or necessary to defer a complete medical assessment. For example, a delusional or manic patient may be combative or resistive or both. In this instance, a medical history should be elicited from a family member if possible, but unless there is a pressing reason to proceed with the examination, it should be deferred until the patient is tractable.

For psychological reasons, it may be ill advised to recommend a medical assessment at the time of an initial office visit. In view of today's increased sensitivity and openness about sexual matters and a tendency to turn quickly to psychiatric help, young men may complain about their failure to consummate their first coital attempt. After taking a detailed history, the psychiatrist may conclude that the failure was due to situational anxiety. If so, neither a physical examination nor psychotherapy should be recommended; they would have the undesirable effect of reinforcing the notion of pathology. Should the problem be recurrent, further evaluation would be warranted.

Neurological Examination

If the psychiatrist suspects that the patient has an underlying somatic disorder, such as diabetes mellitus or Cushing's syndrome, referral is usually made to a medical physician for diagnosis and treatment. The situation is different when a cognitive disorder is suspected. The psychiatrist often chooses to assume responsibility in these cases. At some point, however, a thorough neurological evaluation may be indicated.

During the history-taking process in such cases, the patient's level of awareness, attentiveness to the details of the examination, understanding, facial expression, speech, posture, and gait are noted. It is also assumed that a thorough mental status examination will be performed. The neurological examination is carried out with two objectives in mind: to elicit signs pointing to focal, circumscribed cerebral dysfunction and to elicit signs suggesting diffuse, bilateral cerebral disease. The first objective is met by the routine neurological examination, which is designed primarily to reveal asymmetries in the motor, perceptual, and reflex functions of the two sides of the body, caused by focal hemispheric disease. The second objective is met by seeking to elicit signs that have been attributed to diffuse brain dysfunction and to frontal lobe disease. These signs include the sucking, snout, palmomental, and grasp reflexes and the persistence of the glabella tap response. Regrettably, with the exception of the grasp reflex, such signs do not correlate strongly with the presence of underlying brain pathology.

Other Findings

Psychiatrists should be able to evaluate the significance of findings uncovered by consultants. With a patient who complains of a lump in the throat (globus hystericus) and who is found on examination to have hypertrophied lymphoid tissue, it is tempting to wonder about a causal relation. How can a clinician be sure that the finding is not incidental? Has the patient been

known to have hypertrophied lymphoid tissue at a time when no complaint was made? Do many persons with hypertrophied lymphoid tissue never experience the sensation of a lump in the throat?

With a patient with multiple sclerosis who complains of an inability to walk but, on neurological examination, has only mild spasticity and a unilateral Babinski sign, it is tempting to ascribe the symptom to the neurological disorder; but the complaint may be aggravated by emotional distress. The same holds true for a patient with profound dementia in whom a small frontal meningioma is seen on a computed tomography (CT) scan. Dementia is not always correlated with the findings. Significant brain atrophy could cause very mild dementia, and minimal brain atrophy could cause significant dementia.

A lesion is often found that can account for a symptom, but the psychiatrist should make every effort to separate an incidental finding from a causative one and to distinguish a lesion merely found in the area of the symptom from a lesion producing the symptom.

PATIENTS UNDERGOING PSYCHIATRIC TREATMENT

While patients are being treated for psychiatric disorders, psychiatrists should be alert to the possibility of intercurrent illnesses that call for diagnostic studies. Patients in psychotherapy, particularly those in psychoanalysis, may be all too willing to ascribe their new symptoms to emotional causes. Attention should be given to the possible use of denial, especially if the symptoms seem to be unrelated to the conflicts currently in focus.

At a time of increased psychological stress, a patient had urinary frequency, which she ascribed to her current situation. Only after much urging did she agree to see a urologist, who diagnosed and treated her cystitis.

Not only may patients in psychotherapy be prone to attribute new symptoms to emotional causes, but sometimes their therapists do so as well. The danger of providing psychodynamic explanations for physical symptoms is ever present.

A disturbed young woman in a psychiatric unit, who would curl up in a clothes basket and remain there for long periods, was described as regressing and assuming the fetal position. Later, when the diagnosis of meningoencephalitis was confirmed, it seemed that a better explanation for her behavior was the need to relieve pressure on nerve roots.

Symptoms such as drowsiness and dizziness and signs such as a skin eruption and a gait disturbance, common adverse effects of psychotropic medication, call for a medical reevaluation if the patient fails to respond in a reasonable time to changes in the dosage or the kind of medication prescribed. If patients who are receiving tricyclic or antipsychotic drugs complain of blurred vision (usually an anticholinergic adverse effect) and the condition does not recede with a reduction in dosage or a change in medication, they should be evaluated to rule out other causes. In one case, the diagnosis proved to be *Toxoplasma* chorioretinitis. The absence of other anticholinergic adverse effects, such as a dry mouth and constipation, is an additional clue alerting the psychiatrist to the possibility of a concomitant medical illness.

Early in an illness, there may be few if any positive physical or laboratory results. In such instances, especially if the evidence of psychic trauma or emotional conflicts is glaring, all symptoms are likely to be regarded as psychosocial in origin, and new symptoms also seen in this light. Indications for repeating portions of the medical workup may be missed unless the psychiatrist is alert to clues suggesting that some symptoms do not fit the original diagnosis and point, instead, to a medical illness. Occasionally, a patient with an acute illness, such as encephalitis, is hospitalized with the diagnosis of schizophrenia, or a patient with a subacute illness, such as carcinoma of the pancreas, is treated in a private office or clinic with the diagnosis of a depressive disorder. Although it may not be possible to make the correct diagnosis at the time of the initial psychiatric evaluation, continued surveillance and attention to clinical details usually provide clues leading to the recognition of the cause.

The likelihood of intercurrent illness is greater with some psychiatric disorders than with others. Substance abusers, for example, because of their life patterns, are susceptible to infection and are likely to suffer from the adverse effects of trauma, dietary deficiencies, and poor hygiene. Depression decreases the immune response.

When somatic and psychological dysfunctions are known to coexist, the psychiatrist should be thoroughly conversant with the patient's medical status. In cases of cardiac decompensation, peripheral neuropathy, and other disabling disorders, the nature and degree of impairment that can be attributed to the physical disorder should be assessed. It is important to answer the question: Does the patient exploit a disability, or is it ignored or denied with resultant overexertion? To answer this question, the psychiatrist must assess the patient's capabilities and limitations, rather than make sweeping judgments based on a diagnostic label.

Special vigilance about medical status is required for some patients in treatment for somatoform and eating disorders. Such is the case for patients with ulcerative colitis who are bleeding profusely and for patients with anorexia nervosa who are losing appreciable weight. These disorders can become life threatening.

Importance of Medical Illness

Numerous articles have called attention to the need for thorough medical screening of patients seen in psychiatric inpatient services and clinics. (A similar need has been demonstrated for the psychiatric evaluation of patients seen in medical inpatient services and clinics.) The concept of *medical clearance* remains ambiguous and has meaning in the context of psychiatric admission or clearance for transfers from different settings or institutions. It implies that no medical condition exists to account for the patient's condition.

Among identified psychiatric patients, anywhere from 24 to 60 percent have been shown to suffer from associated physical disorders. In a survey of 2,090 psychiatric clinic patients, 43

percent were found to have associated physical disorders; of these, almost half the physical disorders had not been diagnosed by the referring sources. (In this study, 69 patients were found to have diabetes mellitus, but only 12 of these patients had been diagnosed before referral.)

Expecting all psychiatrists to be experts in internal medicine is unrealistic, but expecting them to recognize or have high suspicion of physical disorders that are present is realistic. Moreover, they should make appropriate referrals and collaborate in treating patients who have both physical and mental disorders.

Psychiatric symptoms are nonspecific; they can herald medical as well as psychiatric illness. They often precede the appearance of definitive medical symptoms. Some psychiatric symptoms (e.g., visual hallucinations, distortions, and illusions) should evoke a high level of suspicion of a medical toxicity.

The medical literature abounds with case reports of patients whose disorders were initially considered emotional but ultimately proved to be secondary to medical conditions. The data in most of the reports revealed features pointing toward organicity. Diagnostic errors arose because such features were accorded too little weight.

References

Aronowitz RA. When do symptoms become a disease? *Ann Intern Med.* 2001;134:803.

Ellenhorn MJ, Barceloux DG. *Medical Toxicology: Diagnosis and Treatment of Human Poisoning.* New York: Elsevier; 1988.

Kaaya S, Goldberg D, Gask L. Management of somatic presentations of psychiatric illness in general medical settings: evaluation of a new training course for general practitioners. *Med Educ.* 1992;26:138.

Kroenke K. Studying symptoms: sampling and measurement issues. *Ann Intern Med.* 2001;134:844.

Kroenke K, Harris L. Symptoms research: a fertile field. *Ann Intern Med.* 2001;134:801.

Mitchell AC, McCabe EM, Brown KW. Psychiatrists' attitudes to physical examination of new out-patients with a major depressive disorder. *Psychiatr Bull.* 1998;22:82.

Osterloh JD, Becker CE. Chemical dependency and drug testing in the workplace. *West J Med.* 1990;152:506.

Rosse RB, Deutsch LH, Deutsch SI. Medical assessment and laboratory testing in psychiatry. In: Sadock BJ, Sadock VA, eds. *Kaplan & Sadock's Comprehensive Textbook of Psychiatry.* 7th ed. Vol 1. Baltimore: Lippincott Williams & Wilkins; 2000:732.

Waddington D. GP monitoring of lithium levels. *Br J Psychiatry.* 1996;168:383.

Weinberger DR. Brain disease and psychiatric illness: when should a psychiatrist order a CT scan? *Am J Psychiatry.* 1984;141:1521.

Wessely S. Chronic fatigue: symptom and syndrome. *Ann Intern Med.* 2001;134:838.

Winston AP. Physical assessment of the eating disordered patient. *Eur Eating Disord Rev.* 2000;8:188.

▲ 7.4 Laboratory Tests in Psychiatry

Laboratory testing is an integral part of psychiatric assessment and treatment. Compared with other medical specialists, however, psychiatrists depend more on clinical examinations and patients' signs and symptoms than on laboratory tests. For example, no test can establish or rule out a diagnosis of schizophrenia, bipolar I disorder, or major depressive disorder. Nevertheless, advances in neuropsychiatry and biological psychiatry have made laboratory tests more and more useful to psychiatrists as well as to biological researchers.

MEDICAL HISTORY

Psychiatrists must be sensitive to the possibility of comorbid medical illness in their patients, particularly in elderly, chronically mentally ill, indigent, and substance-abusing populations. The possibility of occult medical illness must always be considered when patients present with psychiatric syndromes. Thyroid and adrenal disease may manifest as a psychotic or mood disorder, and cancer may manifest as depression. Table 7.4–1 lists medical conditions that can manifest psychiatric symptoms. Each of these diagnoses can argue for a different set of laboratory or diagnostic tests. Laboratory testing is also used to monitor dosing, compliance, and toxic effects of various psychotropic medications (e.g., lithium [Eskalith] and other mood stabilizers).

The initial evaluation must always include a thorough assessment of the prescribed and over-the-counter medications that the patient is taking. Many psychiatric syndromes can be of iatrogenic origin, caused by medications (e.g., depression by antihypertensives, delirium by anticholinergics, and psychosis by steroids). Often, if clinically possible, a washout of medications may aid the diagnosis. Screening tests for medical illnesses are given in Table 7.4–2.

NEUROENDOCRINE TESTS

Thyroid Function Tests

Several thyroid function tests are available, including tests for thyroxine (T_4) by competitive protein binding (T_4D) and by radioimmunoassay (T_4RIA) involving a specific antigen-antibody reaction. Table 7.4–3 lists some common thyroid function tests. More than 90 percent of T_4 is bound to serum protein and is responsible for thyroid-stimulating hormone (TSH) secretion and cellular metabolism. Other thyroid measures include the free T_4 index (FT_4I), triiodothyronine uptake, and total serum triiodothyronine measured by radioimmunoassay (T_3RIA). These tests are used to rule out hypothyroidism, which can appear with symptoms of depression. In some studies, up to 10 percent of patients complaining of depression and associated fatigue had incipient hypothyroid disease. Other associated signs and symptoms common to both depression and hypothyroidism include weakness, stiffness, poor appetite, constipation, menstrual irregularities, slowed speech, apathy, impaired memory, and even hallucinations and delusions. Lithium can cause hypothyroidism and, more rarely, hyperthyroidism. Table 7.4–4 outlines the suggested monitoring of thyroid function for patients taking lithium. Neonatal hypothyroidism results in mental retardation and is preventable if the diagnosis is made at birth. Table 7.4–5 lists the thyroid function test changes associated with hypothyroidism.

The thyrotropin-releasing hormone (TRH) stimulation test is indicated for patients whose marginally abnormal thyroid test results suggest subclinical hypothyroidism, which may account for clinical depression. The test is also used for patients with possible lithium-induced hypothyroidism. The procedure entails an intravenous (IV) injection of 500 μg of TRH, which produces a sharp rise in serum TSH when measured at 15, 30, 60, and 90 minutes. Table 7.4–6 summarizes one suggested TRH test protocol. An increase in serum TSH from 5 to 25 IU/

Table 7.4–1
Some Medical Conditions That May Manifest with Neuropsychiatric Symptoms

Neurological
- Cerebrovascular disorders (hemorrhage, infarction)
- Head trauma (concussion, posttraumatic hematoma)
- Epilepsy (especially complex partial seizures)
- Narcolepsy
- Brain neoplasms (primary or metastatic)
- Normal-pressure hydrocephalus
- Parkinson's disease
- Multiple sclerosis
- Huntington's disease
- Dementia of the Alzheimer's type
- Metachromatic leukodystrophy
- Migraine

Endocrine
- Hypothyroidism
- Hyperthyroidism
- Hypoadrenalism
- Hyperadrenalism
- Hypoparathyroidism
- Hyperparathyroidism
- Hypoglycemia
- Hyperglycemia
- Diabetes mellitus
- Panhypopituitarism
- Pheochromocytoma
- Gonadotropic hormonal disturbances
- Pregnancy

Metabolic and systemic
- Fluid and electrolyte disturbances (e.g., syndrome of inappropriate antidiuretic hormone secretion [SIADH])
- Hepatic encephalopathy
- Uremia
- Porphyria
- Hepatolenticular degeneration (Wilson's disease)
- Hypoxemia (chronic pulmonary disease)
- Hypotension
- Hypertensive encephalopathy

Toxic
- Intoxication or withdrawal associated with drug or alcohol abuse
- Adverse effects of prescribed and over-the-counter medications
- Environmental toxins (volatile hydrocarbons, heavy metals, carbon monoxide, organophosphates)

Nutritional
- Vitamin B_{12} deficiency (pernicious anemia)
- Nicotinic acid deficiency (pellagra)
- Folate deficiency (megaloblastic anemia)
- Thiamine deficiency (Wernicke-Korsakoff syndrome)
- Trace metal deficiency (zinc, magnesium)
- Nonspecific malnutrition and dehydration

Infectious
- AIDS
- Neurosyphilis
- Viral meningitides and encephalitides (e.g., herpes simplex)
- Brain abscess
- Viral hepatitis
- Infectious mononucleosis
- Tuberculosis
- Systemic bacterial infections (especially pneumonia) and viremia
- Streptococcal infections
- Pediatric infection-triggered, autoimmune neuropsychiatric disorders

Autoimmune
- Systemic lupus erythematosus

Neoplastic
- CNS primary and metastatic tumors
- Endocrine tumors
- Pancreatic carcinoma
- Paraneoplastic syndromes

Table adapted from Darrell G. Kirch, M.D.

mL above baseline is normal. An increase of less than 7 IU/mL is considered a blunted response, which may correlate with a diagnosis of a depressive disorder. Eight percent of all patients with depressive disorders have some thyroid illness.

Table 7.4–2
Screening Tests for Medical Illness

1. CBC count with differential
2. Complete blood chemistries (including measurements of electrolytes, glucose, calcium, and magnesium and tests of hepatic and renal function)
3. Thyroid function tests
4. Rapid plasma reagent (RPR) or VDRL test
5. Urinalysis
6. Urine toxicology screen
7. ECG
8. Chest roentgenography (for patients over age 35)
9. Plasma levels of any drugs being taken, if appropriate

Dexamethasone-Suppression Test

Dexamethasone is a long-acting synthetic glucocorticoid with a long half-life. About 1 mg of dexamethasone is equivalent to 25 mg of cortisol. The dexamethasone suppression test (DST) is used to help confirm a diagnostic impression of major depressive disorder.

Procedure. The patient is given 1 mg of dexamethasone by mouth at 11 PM, and the plasma cortisol level is measured at 8 AM, 4 PM, and 11 PM. Plasma cortisol concentrations above 5 µg/dL (known as nonsuppression) are considered abnormal (i.e., a positive result). Suppression of cortisol indicates that the hypothalamic-adrenal-pituitary axis is functioning properly. Since the 1930s, dysfunction of this axis has been known to be associated with stress.

The DST can be used to follow a depressed person's response to treatment. Normalization of the DST result, however, is not an indication to stop antidepressant treatment, because the DST result may normalize before the depression resolves.

Table 7.4–3
Common Thyroid Function Tests

Type of Test[a]	Normal Values	Cost ($)	Interference
In vitro (serum tests)			
T_4	4.5–13 μg/100 mL 58–167 nmol/L	7–22	Changes in TBG, drugs, etc.
Resin T_3 uptake	25–35%	3–10	Changes in TBG, drugs, etc.
T_7 and ETR	Combinations of values for T_4 and resin T_3 uptake		
TSH	0–10 μIU/mL 2–7 μIU/mL	39	Pituitary disease
T_3RIA	80–200 ng/100 mL 1.2–3.1 nmol/L	41	Changes in TBG, drugs, etc.
Autoantibodies	Absent	30–60	
In vivo tests			
Radioiodine uptake (^{131}I, ^{123}I)	10–25%/24 hours	60–95	Never use in pregnancy: iodides T_3 and T_4 therapy, antithyroid drugs, thyroiditis
Thyroid scan radioiodine	Both lobes homogeneous	80	Iodides T_3, T_4: never use in pregnancy
TRH injection	TSH increase to 2× control	115	
TSH stimulation	No effect or increased uptake	115	
T_4 suppression	Uptake reduced to half of original value	115	Heart disease or other contraindication of T_4 therapy
Histology (biopsy)			
Fine-needle aspiration biopsy	Normal cytology	28	Inadequate sample
Cutting-needle biopsy	Normal cytology	[b]	Significant danger of hemorrhage

[a]Tests are listed in order of decreasing frequency of practical application. Adapted from Halsted JA, Halsted CH, eds. *The Laboratory in Clinical Medicine: Interpretation and Application.* 2nd ed. Philadelphia: WB Saunders; 1981.
[b]Cost varies from laboratory to laboratory.
Reprinted with permission from MacKinnon RA, Yudofsky SC. *Principles of the Psychiatric Evaluation.* Philadelphia: JB Lippincott; 1991:96.

Table 7.4–4
Thyroid Monitoring for Patients Taking Lithium

Evaluation	Before Treatment	Repeat at 6 Months	Repeat Yearly
Medical			
1. Careful medical and family history to detect family history of thyroid disease	x		
2. Review of symptoms of hyperthyroidism and hypothyroidism	x	x	x
3. Physical examination, including palpation of thyroid	x		x
Laboratory			
T_3RU	x		x
T_4RIA	x		x
T_2I (free thyroxine index)	x		x
TSH	x	x	x
Antithyroid antibodies	x		x

Reprinted with permission from MacKinnon RA, Yudofsky SC. *Principles of the Psychiatric Evaluation.* Philadelphia: JB Lippincott; 1991:104.

Reliability. The problems associated with the DST include varying reports of sensitivity and specificity. False-positive and false-negative results are common and are listed in Table 7.4–7. The sensitivity of the DST is considered to be 45 percent in major depressive disorders and 70 percent in major depressive episodes with psychotic features. The specificity is 90 percent compared with controls and 77 percent compared with other psychiatric diagnoses. Figure 7.4–1 illustrates the suppression

Table 7.4–5
Thyroid Function Test Changes in Patients with Hypothyroidism

1. Serum T_4 concentration is decreased.
2. Serum-free thyroxine is decreased.
3. Serum T_3 concentration is decreased.
4. Serum T_3 uptake is decreased.
5. Serum PBI is decreased.
6. Serum thyroxine-binding globulin is normal.
7. Serum T_3–T_4 ratio is increased.
8. Serum TSH is increased.

Reprinted with permission from MacKinnon RA, Yudofsky SC. *Principles of the Psychiatric Evaluation.* Philadelphia: JB Lippincott; 1991:97.

Table 7.4–6
TRH Test Protocol

1. Patient takes nothing by mouth after midnight and is at rest in bed at 8:30 AM.
2. Indwelling venous catheter is placed, and a normal saline drip is started to keep the line open.
3. At 8:59 AM, blood is taken through a three-way stopcock for determination of T_3RU, T_3RIA, T_4, and TSH levels (reverse T_3 is optional).
4. At 9 AM, intravenous TRH (protirelin) 500 μg is given slowly over 30 seconds. Side effects from the infusions may include a transient sensation of warmth, desire to urinate, nausea, metallic taste, headache, dry mouth, chest tightness, or a pleasant genital sensation. Those effects are generally short-lived and mild.
5. Blood samples are taken through the stopcock before the TRH is administered and at 15, 30, 60, and 90 minutes after infusion to measure changes in TSH.

Reprinted with permission from MacKinnon RA, Yudofsky SC. *Principles of the Psychiatric Evaluation.* Philadelphia: JB Lippincott; 1991:94.

Table 7.4–7
Medical Conditions and Pharmacological Agents That May Interfere with Results of the Dexamethasone-Suppression Test

False-positive results are associated with
- Phenytoin
- Barbiturates
- Meprobamate
- Glutethimide
- Carbamazepine
- Cardiac failure
- Hypertension
- Renal failure
- Disseminated cancer and serious infections
- Recent major trauma or surgery
- Fever
- Nausea
- Dehydration
- Temporal lobe disease
- High-dosage estrogen treatment
- Pregnancy
- Cushing's disease
- Unstable diabetes mellitus
- Extreme weight loss (malnutrition, anorexia nervosa)
- Alcohol abuse
- Benzodiazepine withdrawal
- Tricyclic drug withdrawal
- Dementia
- Bulimia nervosa
- Acute psychotic disorder
- Advanced age

False-negative results are associated with
- Hypopituitarism
- Addison's disease
- Long-term synthetic steroid therapy
- Indomethacin
- High-dosage cyproheptadine treatment
- High-dosage benzodiazepine treatment

Reprinted with permission from Young M, Stanford J. The dexamethasone suppression test for the detection, diagnosis, and management of depression. *Arch Intern Med.* 1984;100:309.

of plasma cortisol in a patient with major depressive disorder before and 6 weeks after the initiation of treatment with a tricyclic drug. Some evidence indicates that patients with a positive DST result (especially 10 μg/dL) will have a good response to somatic treatment, such as electroconvulsive therapy (ECT) or cyclic antidepressant therapy.

Other Endocrine Tests

Many other hormones affect behavior. Exogenous hormonal administration has been shown to affect behavior, and known endocrine diseases have associated mental disorders. In addition to thyroid hormones, these hormones include the anterior pituitary hormone prolactin, growth hormone, somatostatin, gonadotrophin-releasing hormone (GnRH), the sex steroids, luteinizing hormone (LH), follicle-stimulating hormone (FSH), testosterone, and estrogen. Melatonin from the pineal gland has been implicated in seasonal affective disorder (called mood disorder with seasonal pattern in the text revision of the fourth edition of *Diagnostic and Statistical Manual of Mental Disorders* [DSM-IV-TR]). Symptoms of anxiety or depression in some patients may be explained on the basis of unspecified changes in endocrine function or homeostasis.

Catecholamines

The level of serotonin metabolite 5-hydroxyindoleacetic acid (5-HIAA) is elevated in the urine of patients with carcinoid tumors. Elevated levels are noted at times in patients who take phenothiazine medication and in those who eat foods high in serotonin (e.g., walnuts, bananas, and avocados). The concentration of 5-HIAA in cerebrospinal fluid is low in some persons who are in a suicidal depression and in postmortem studies of those who have committed suicide in particularly violent ways. Low 5-HIAA levels in cerebrospinal fluid are associated with violence in general. Norepinephrine and its metabolic products—metanephrine, normetanephrine, and vanillylmandelic acid (VMA)—can be measured in urine, blood, and plasma. Plasma catecholamine levels are markedly elevated in pheochromocytoma, which is associated with anxiety, agitation, and hypertension. Some patients with chronic anxiety may exhibit elevated blood norepinephrine and epinephrine levels. Some depressed patients have a low urinary norepinephrine-to-epinephrine ratio (NE:E).

High levels of urinary norepinephrine and epinephrine have been found in some patients with posttraumatic stress disorder. The norepinephrine metabolite 3-methoxy-4-hydroxyphenylglycol (MHPG) concentration is decreased in patients with severe depressive disorders, especially those patients who attempt suicide.

Kidney Function Tests

Creatinine clearance detects early kidney damage and can be serially monitored to follow the course of renal disease. Blood urea nitrogen (BUN) is also elevated in renal disease and is excreted via the kidneys; serum BUN and creatinine levels are monitored in patients taking lithium. If the serum BUN or creatinine level is abnormal, the patient's 2-hour creatinine clearance and ultimately the 24-hour creatinine clearance are tested.

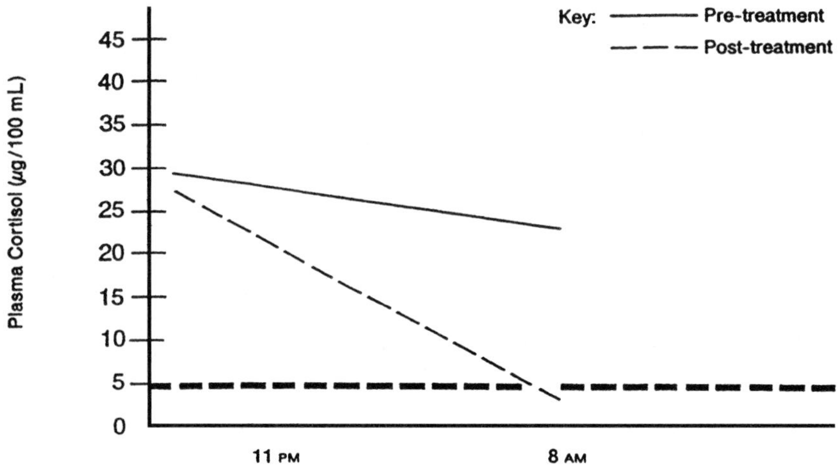

FIGURE 7.4–1
Dexamethasone-suppression test results for a patient with major depressive disorder. (Reprinted with permission from MacKinnon A, Yudofsky SC. *Principles of the Psychiatric Evaluation.* Philadelphia: JB Lippincott; 1991.)

Table 7.4–8 outlines a suggested protocol for monitoring renal function in patients taking lithium. Table 7.4–9 summarizes other laboratory testing for patients taking lithium.

Liver Function Tests

Total bilirubin and direct bilirubin values are elevated in hepatocellular injury and intrahepatic bile stasis, which can occur with phenothiazine or tricyclic medication and with alcohol and other substance abuse. Certain drugs (e.g., phenobarbital [Solfoton, Luminal]) may lower the serum bilirubin concentration. Liver damage or disease, which is reflected by abnormal findings in liver function tests (LFTs), may manifest with signs and symptoms of a cognitive disorder, including disorientation and delirium. Impaired hepatic function may increase the elimination half-lives of certain drugs, including some benzodiazepines, so that the drug may stay in a patient's system longer than it would under normal circumstances. LFTs must be monitored routinely when using certain drugs, such as carbamazepine (Tegretol) and valproate (Depakene).

Table 7.4–8
Renal Monitoring for Patients Taking Lithium

Evaluation	Before Treatment	Repeat at 6 Months	Repeat Yearly
Medical			
1. Careful medical and family history to detect presence of familial kidney disease or predisposition to kidney disease (diabetes, hypertension)	x		
2. Specific comprehensive review of genitourinary system symptoms	x	x	x
3. Physical examination	x		x
Laboratory			
BUN	x		x
Creatinine	x	x	x
Creatinine clearance (24-hour urine) urinalysis	x		x
24-hour urine volume	x		x
12-hour fluid deprivation test	x		

Reprinted with permission from MacKinnon RA, Yudofsky SC. *Principles of the Psychiatric Evaluation.* Philadelphia: JB Lippincott; 1991:103.

BLOOD TEST FOR SEXUALLY TRANSMITTED DISEASES

The Venereal Disease Research Laboratory (VDRL) test is used as a screening test for syphilis. If positive, the result is confirmed by using the specific fluorescent treponemal antibody-absorption test (FTA-ABS test), in which the spirochete *Treponema pallidum* is used as the antigen. A central nervous system (CNS) VDRL test is performed in patients with suspected neurosyphilis. A positive HIV test result indicates that a

Table 7.4–9
Other Laboratory Testing for Patients Taking Lithium

Test	Frequency
1. Complete blood count	Before treatment and yearly
2. Serum electrolytes	Before treatment and yearly
3. Fasting blood glucose	Before treatment and yearly
4. Electrocardiogram	Before treatment and yearly
5. Pregnancy testing for women of childbearing age[a]	Before treatment

[a]Test more frequently when compliance with treatment plan is uncertain.
Reprinted with permission from MacKinnon RA, Yudofsky SC. *Principles of the Psychiatric Evaluation.* Philadelphia: JB Lippincott; 1991:106.

person has been exposed to infection with the virus that causes acquired immune deficiency syndrome (AIDS).

TESTS RELATED TO PSYCHOTROPIC DRUGS

In caring for patients receiving psychotropic medication, the trend is to measure the concentration of the prescribed drug in plasma regularly. For some drugs, such as lithium, the monitoring is essential; for other drugs, such as antipsychotics, it is mainly of academic or research interest. A clinician need not practice defensive medicine by insisting that all patients receiving psychotropic drugs have blood levels determined for medicolegal purposes. The current status of psychopharmacological treatment is such that a psychiatrist's clinical judgment and experience, except in rare instances, are better indications of a drug's therapeutic efficacy than determining its level in plasma. Moreover, the reliance on plasma levels cannot replace clinical skills and the need to maintain the humanitarian aspects of patient care. The major classes of drugs and the suggested guidelines are outlined below.

Benzodiazepines

No special tests are needed for patients taking benzodiazepines. Among the benzodiazepines metabolized in the liver by oxidation, impaired hepatic function increases the half-life. Baseline LFTs are indicated for patients with suspected liver damage. Urine is tested routinely for benzodiazepines in patients with substance abuse.

Antipsychotics

No special tests are needed for patients taking antipsychotics, although it is a good idea to obtain baseline values for liver function and a complete blood cell count. Antipsychotics are metabolized primarily in the liver, with metabolites excreted primarily in urine. Many metabolites are active. Peak plasma concentration usually is reached 2 to 3 hours after an oral dose. Elimination half-life is 12 to 30 hours but may be much longer. Steady state requires at least 1 week at a constant dose (months at a constant dose of depot antipsychotics). With the exception of clozapine (Clozaril), all antipsychotics cause a short-term elevation in serum prolactin concentration (secondary to tuberoinfundibular activity). A normal prolactin level often indicates either noncompliance or nonabsorption. Adverse effects include leukocytosis, leukopenia, impaired platelet function, mild anemia (both aplastic and hemolytic), and agranulocytosis. Bone marrow and blood element adverse effects can occur abruptly, even when the dosage has remained constant. Low-potency antipsychotics are most likely to cause agranulocytosis, which is the most common bone marrow adverse effect. These agents may cause hepatocellular injury and intrahepatic biliary stasis (indicated by elevated total and direct bilirubin and elevated transaminases). They also can cause electrocardiographic changes (not as frequently as with tricyclic antidepressants), including a prolonged QT interval; flattened, inverted, or bifid T waves; and U waves. The relation of dose to plasma concentration differs widely among patients.

Clozapine. Because of the risk of agranulocytosis (1 to 2 percent), patients who are being treated with clozapine must have a baseline white blood cell (WBC) and differential count before the initiation of treatment, a WBC count every week throughout treatment, and a weekly WBC count for 4 weeks after discontinuation of clozapine treatment. Physicians and pharmacists who provide clozapine must be registered through the Clozaril National Registry (1-800-448-5938). Table 7.4–10 summarizes the clinical management of reduced WBC, leukopenia, and agranulocytosis in patients treated with clozapine.

Tricyclic and Tetracyclic Drugs

An electrocardiogram (ECG) should be taken before starting a regimen of cyclic drugs to assess for conduction delays, which may lead to heart block at therapeutic levels. Some clinicians believe that all patients receiving prolonged cyclic drug therapy should have an annual ECG. At therapeutic levels, the drugs suppress arrhythmias through a quinidinelike effect.

Blood levels should be determined routinely when using imipramine (Tofranil), desipramine (Norpramin), or nortriptyline (Pamelor) in the treatment of depressive disorders. Blood level determinations may also be useful for patients with a poor response at normal dosage ranges and with high-risk patients for whom there is an urgent need to know whether a therapeutic or toxic plasma level of the drug has been reached. Blood level determinations should also include the measurement of active metabolites (e.g., imipramine is converted to desipramine, amitriptyline [Elavil] to nortriptyline). Some characteristics of tricyclic drug plasma levels are described as follows.

Imipramine. The percentage of favorable responses correlates with plasma levels in a linear manner between 200 and 250 ng/mL, but some patients may respond at a lower level. Levels above 250 ng/mL yield no improved favorable response, and adverse effects increase.

Nortriptyline. The therapeutic window (the range within which a drug is most effective) is between 50 and 150 ng/mL. The response rate decreases at levels above 150 ng/mL.

Desipramine. Levels above 125 ng/mL correlate with a higher percentage of favorable responses.

Amitriptyline. Different studies have produced conflicting results with regard to blood levels, but they range from 75 to 175 ng/mL.

Procedure for Determining Blood Concentrations. The blood specimen should be drawn 10 to 14 hours after the last dose, usually in the morning after a bedtime dose. Patients must have received a stable daily dose for at least 5 days for the test to be valid. Some patients who metabolize cyclic drugs unusually poorly may have levels as high as 2,000 ng/mL while taking normal dosages and before showing a favorable clinical response. Such patients must be monitored closely for cardiac adverse effects. Patients with levels above 1,000 ng/mL are generally at risk for cardiotoxicity.

Monoamine Oxidase Inhibitors

Patients taking monoamine oxidase inhibitors (MAOIs) are instructed to avoid tyramine-containing foods because of the

Table 7.4–10
Clinical Management of Reduced White Blood Cell Count, Leukopenia, and Agranulocytosis

Problem Phase	WBC Findings	Clinical Findings	Treatment Plan
Reduced WBC count	WBC count reveals a significant drop (even if WBC count is still in normal range). "Significant drop" is (1) drop of more than 3,000 cells from prior test or (2) three or more consecutive drops in WBC counts	No symptoms of infection	1. Monitor patient closely 2. Institute twice-weekly CBC tests with differentials if deemed appropriate by attending physician 3. Clozapine therapy may continue
Mild leukopenia	WBC = 3,000–3,500	Patient may or may not show clinical symptoms, such as lethargy, fever, sore throat, weakness	1. Monitor patient closely 2. Institute a minimum of twice-weekly CBC tests with differentials 3. Clozapine therapy may continue
Leukopenia or granulocytopenia	WBC = 2,000–3,000 or granulocytes = 1,000–1,500	Patient may or may not show clinical symptoms, such as fever, sore throat, lethargy, weakness	1. Interrupt clozapine at once 2. Institute daily CBC tests with differentials 3. Increase surveillance, consider hospitalization 4. Clozapine therapy may be reinstituted after normalization of WBC
Agranulocytosis (uncomplicated)	WBC count less than 2,000 or granulocytes less than 1,000	The patient may or may not show clinical symptoms, such as fever, sore throat, lethargy, weakness	1. Discontinue clozapine at once 2. Place patient in protective isolation in a medical unit with modern facilities 3. Consider a bone marrow specimen to determine if progenitor cells are being suppressed 4. Monitor patient every 2 days until WBC and differential counts return to normal (about 2 weeks) 5. Avoid use of concomitant medications with bone marrow–suppressing potential
Agranulocytosis (with complications)	WBC count less than 2,000 or granulocytes less than 1,000	Definite evidence of infection, such as fever, sore throat, lethargy, weakness, malaise, skin ulcerations, etc.	1. Consult with hematologist or other specialist to determine appropriate antibiotic regimen 2. Start appropriate therapy; monitor closely
Recovery	WBC count more than 4,000 and granulocytes more than 2,000	No symptoms of infection	1. Once-weekly CBC with differential counts for 4 consecutive normal values 2. Clozapine must not be restarted

Reprinted with permission from Sandoz Pharmaceuticals Corporation and MacKinnon RA, Yudofsky SC. *Principles of the Psychiatric Evaluation.* Philadelphia: JB Lippincott; 1991:118.

danger of a hypertensive crisis. A baseline normal blood pressure (BP) must be recorded, and the BP must be monitored during treatment. MAOIs may also cause orthostatic hypotension as a direct drug adverse effect unrelated to diet. Other than their potential for elevating BP when taken with certain foods, MAOIs are relatively free of other adverse effects. A test used both in a research setting and in current clinical practice involves correlating the therapeutic response with the degree of platelet MAO inhibition.

Lithium

Patients receiving lithium should have baseline thyroid function tests, electrolyte monitoring, a WBC, renal function tests (specific gravity, BUN, and creatinine), and a baseline ECG. The rationale for these tests is that lithium can cause renal concentrating defects, hypothyroidism, and leukocytosis; sodium depletion can cause toxic lithium levels; and about 95 percent of lithium is excreted in the urine. Lithium has also been shown to cause ECG changes, including various conduction defects.

Lithium is most clearly indicated in the prophylactic treatment of manic episodes (its direct antimanic effect may take up to 2 weeks), and it is commonly coupled with antipsychotics for the treatment of acute manic episodes. Lithium itself may also have antipsychotic activity. The maintenance level is 0.6 to 1.2 mEq/L, although acutely manic patients can tolerate up to 1.5 to 1.8 mEq/L. Some patients may respond at lower levels; others may require higher levels. A response below 0.4 mEq/L is probably a placebo effect. Toxic reactions may occur with levels above 2.0 mEq/L. Regular lithium monitoring is essential; there is a narrow therapeutic range beyond which cardiac problems and CNS effects can occur.

Table 7.4–11
Laboratory Monitoring of Patients Taking Carbamazepine

Test	Frequency
1. Complete blood count	Before treatment and every 2 weeks for the first 2 months of treatment; thereafter, once every 3 months
2. Platelet count and reticulocyte count	Before treatment and yearly
3. Serum electrolytes	Before treatment and yearly
4. Electrocardiogram	Before treatment and yearly
5. SGOT, SGPT, LDH alkaline phosphatase	Before treatment and every month for the first 2 months of treatment; thereafter, every 3 months
6. Pregnancy test for women of childbearing age	Before treatment and as frequently as monthly in noncompliant patients

Reprinted with permission from MacKinnon RA, Yudofsky SC. *Principles of the Psychiatric Evaluation.* Philadelphia: JB Lippincott; 1991:108.

Blood for lithium level determination is drawn 8 to 12 hours after the last dose, usually in the morning after the bedtime dose. The level should be measured at least twice a week while stabilizing the patient and may be determined monthly thereafter.

Carbamazepine

A pretreatment complete blood cell (CBC) count including a platelet count should be done. Reticulocyte count and serum iron tests are also desirable. These tests should be repeated weekly during the first 3 months of treatment and monthly thereafter. Carbamazepine can cause aplastic anemia, agranulocytosis, thrombocytopenia, and leukopenia. Because of the minor risk of hepatotoxicity, LFTs should be done every 3 to 6 months. The medication should be discontinued if the patient shows any signs of bone marrow suppression as measured with periodic CBC counts. The therapeutic level of carbamazepine is 8 to 12 ng/mL, with toxicity most often reached at levels of 15 ng/mL. Most clinicians report that levels as high as 12 ng/mL are hard to achieve. Table 7.4–11 summarizes one suggested protocol for laboratory monitoring of patients taking carbamazepine.

Valproate

Serum levels of valproic acid and divalproex (Depakote) are therapeutic in the range of 45 to 50 ng/mL. Above 125 ng/mL, adverse effects occur, including thrombocytopenia. Serum levels should be determined periodically, and LFTs should be run every 6 to 12 months.

Tacrine

Tacrine (Cognex) may cause liver damage. A baseline of liver function should be established, and follow-up serum transaminase levels should be determined every other week for about 5 months. Patients who develop jaundice or who have bilirubin levels above 3 mg/dL must be withdrawn from the drug.

PROVOCATION OF PANIC ATTACKS WITH SODIUM LACTATE

Up to 72 percent of patients with panic disorder have a panic attack when administered IV injection of sodium lactate. Therefore, lactate provocation is used to confirm a diagnosis of panic disorder. Lactate provocation has also been used to trigger flashbacks in patients with posttraumatic stress disorder. Hyperventilation, another known trigger of panic attacks in predisposed persons, is not as sensitive as lactate provocation in inducing panic attacks. Carbon dioxide (CO_2) inhalation also precipitates panic attacks in those so predisposed. Panic attacks triggered by sodium lactate are not inhibited by peripherally acting β-adrenergic receptor antagonists (beta-blockers) but are inhibited by alprazolam (Xanax) and tricyclic drugs.

DRUG-ASSISTED INTERVIEW

Interviews with amobarbital (Amytal) have both diagnostic and therapeutic indications. Diagnostically, the interviews are helpful in differentiating nonorganic and organic conditions, particularly in patients with symptoms of catatonia, stupor, and muteness. Organic conditions tend to worsen with infusions of amobarbital, but nonorganic or psychogenic conditions tend to get better because of disinhibition, decreased anxiety, or increased relaxation. Therapeutically, amobarbital interviews are useful in disorders of repression and dissociation—for example, in the recovery of memory in psychogenic amnestic disorders and fugue, in the recovery of function in conversion disorder, and in facilitation of emotional expression in posttraumatic stress disorder. Benzodiazepines can be substituted for amobarbital in the infusion. The procedure is outlined in Table 7.4–12.

Table 7.4–12
Drug-Assisted Interview Procedure

1. Have patient recline in an environment in which cardiopulmonary resuscitation is readily available should hypotension or respiratory depression develop.
2. Explain to patient that medication should help him or her relax and feel like talking.
3. Insert a narrow-bore needle into a peripheral vein.
4. Inject a 5% solution of sodium amobarbital (500 mg dissolved in 10 mL of sterile water) at a rate no faster than 1 mL/min (50 mg/min).
5. Begin interview by discussing neutral topics: often, it is helpful to prompt the patient with known facts about his or her life.
6. Continue infusion until either sustained lateral nystagmus or drowsiness is noted.
7. To maintain the level of narcosis, continue infusion at a rate of 0.5 to 1.0 mL/5 min (25 to 50 mg/5 min).
8. Have the patient recline for at least 15 minutes after the interview is terminated, until the patient can walk without supervision.
9. Use the same method every time to avoid dosage errors.

Table 7.4–13
Substances of Abuse That Can Be Tested in Urine

Substance	Length of Time Detected in Urine
Alcohol	7–12 hours
Amphetamine	48 hours
Barbiturate	24 hours (short-acting)
	3 weeks (long-acting)
Benzodiazepine	3 days
Cannabis	3 days to 4 weeks (depending on use)
Cocaine	6–8 hours (metabolites 2–4 days)
Codeine	48 hours
Heroin	36–72 hours
Methadone	3 days
Methaqualone	7 days
Morphine	48–72 hours
Phencyclidine (PCP)	8 days
Propoxyphene	6–48 hours

LUMBAR PUNCTURE

Lumbar puncture is useful in patients who have a sudden manifestation of new psychiatric symptoms, especially changes in cognition. The clinician should be especially vigilant if there is fever or neurological symptoms such as seizures. Lumbar puncture is of use in diagnosing CNS infection (e.g., meningitis).

URINE TESTING FOR SUBSTANCE ABUSE

A number of substances may be detected in a patient's urine if the urine is tested within a specific (and variable) period after ingestion of the substance. Knowledge of urine substance testing is becoming crucial for practicing physicians in view of the controversial issue of mandatory or random substance testing. Table 7.4–13 provides a summary of substances of abuse that can be detected in urine.

Laboratory tests are also used in the detection of substances that may be contributing to cognitive disorders. Table 7.4–14 is an outline of therapeutic, toxic, and lethal levels of substances most commonly implicated in cognitive disorders.

Table 7.4–14
Blood Level Data for Clinical Assessment

		Blood Levels	
Substance	Therapeutic or Normal (%)	Toxic (%)	Lethal (%)
Acetaminophen (Tylenol)	1.0–2.0 mg	15.0 mg	150.0 mg
Acetylsalicylic acid (salicylate)	10–30.0 mg	>39.0 mg	50.0 mg
Aminophylline (theophylline)	1.0–2.0 mg	3.0–4.0 mg	21.0–25.0 mg
Amitriptyline (Elavil)	5.0–20.0 μg	>50.0 μg	1.0–2.0 mg
Amphetamines	2.0–3.0 μg	50.0 μg	200.0 μg
Arsenic	0.0–2.0 μg	0.10 mg	1.5 mg
Barbiturates			
Short-acting	0.1 mg	0.7 mg	1.0 mg
Intermediate-acting	0.1–0.5 mg	1.0–3.0 mg	>3.0 mg
Phenobarbital	1.5–3.9 mg	4.0–6.0 mg	8.0–>15 mg
Barbital	1.0 mg	6.0–8.0 mg	>10.0 mg
Bromide	5.0–30 mg	50–150 mg	200 mg
Carbamazepine (Tegretol)	0.8–1.2 mg	>1.5 mg	—
Chloral hydrate	0.2–1.0 mg	10.0 mg	25.0 mg
Chlordiazepoxide (Librium)	0.1–0.3 mg	0.55 mg	2.0 mg
Chlorpromazine (Thorazine)	0.05 mg	0.1–0.2 mg	0.3–1.2 mg
Cocaine	5.0–15.0 μg	90.0 μg	0.1–2.0 mg
Codeine	2.5–12.0 μg	—	20.0–60.0 μg
Desipramine (Norpramin)	15.0–30.0 μg	>50.0 μg	1.0–2.0 mg
Diazepam (Valium)	0.05–0.25 mg	0.5–2.0 mg	>2.0 mg
Digoxin	0.06–0.20 μg	0.21–0.90 μg	1.5 μg
Diphenhydramine (Benadryl)	1.0–10.0 μg	0.5 mg	>1.0 mg
Doxepin (Sinequan)	10.0–25.0 μg	50.0–200.0 μg	>1.0 mg
Ethanol	—	100.0 mg (legal intoxication)	350.0 mg
Glutethimide (Doriden)	0.02–0.08 mg	1.0–8.0 mg	3.0–10.0 mg
Haloperidol (Haldol)	0.05–0.9 μg	1.0–4.0 mg	—
Imipramine (Tofranil)	15.0–25.0 μg	50.0–150.0 μg	0.2 mg
Lead	0.0–30.0 μg	130 μg	110.0–350.0 μg
Lithium	0.42–0.83 mg (0.6–1.2 mEq/L)	1.39 mg (2.0 mEq/L)	>3.47 mg (>4.0 mEq/L)
LSD	—	0.1–0.4 μg	—
Meperidine (Demerol)	0.03–0.10 mg	0.5 mg	3.0 mg
Meprobamate	0.8–2.4 mg	6.0–10.0 mg	14.0–35.0 mg

(*continued*)

Table 7.4–14 (*continued*)

Substance	Therapeutic or Normal (%)	Blood Levels Toxic (%)	Lethal (%)
Mercury	0.0–8 μg	100 μg	600.0 μg
Methadone (Dolophine)	30.0–110.0 μg	0.2 mg	>0.4 mg
Methamphetamine	0.02–0.06 mg	0.06–0.5 mg	1.0–4.0 mg
Methanol	—	20.0 mg	>89.0 mg
Methaqualone (Quaalude)	0.3–0.6 mg	1.0–3.0 mg	>3.0 mg
Methylphenidate (Ritalin)	1.0–6.0 μg	80.0 μg	230.0 μg
Morphine	10.0 μg	—	5.0–400 μg (free morphine from heroin)
Nortriptyline (Pamelor)	12.0–16.0 μg	0.05 mg	1.3 mg
Oxycodone (Percodan)	1.7–3.6 μg	20.0–500.0 μg	—
Paraldehyde	2.0–11.0 mg	20.0–40.0 mg	>50.0 mg
Pentazocine (Talwin)	0.01–0.06 mg	0.2–0.5 mg	1.0–2.0 mg
Perphenazine (Trilafon)	0.5 μg	100.0 μg	—
Phencyclidine (PCP)	—	0.7–24.0 μg	100.0–500.0 μg
Phenytoin (Dilantin)	1.0–2.0 mg	2.0–5.0 mg	>10 mg
Primidone (Mysoline)	0.5–1.2 mg	5.0–8.0 mg	10.0 mg
Propoxyphene (Darvon)	5.0–20.0 μg	30.0–60.0 μg	80.0–200.0 μg
Propranolol (Inderal)	2.5–20.0 μg	—	0.8–1.2 mg
Quinidine	0.03–0.6 mg	1.0 mg	3.0–5.0 mg
Quinine	0.18 mg	—	1.2 mg
Thioridazine (Mellaril)	0.10–0.15 mg	1.0 mg	2.0–8.0 mg
Trifluoperazine (Stelazine)	0.08 mg	0.12–0.3 mg	0.3–0.8 mg

Reprinted with permission from Winek L. *Drug and Chemical Blood-Level Data*. Pittsburgh: Fisher Scientific; 1985.

OTHER LABORATORY TESTS

Laboratory tests not already discussed are covered in Table 7.4–15 in terms of their indications and significance in medical conditions that affect behavior. See Chapter 11 for information about testing for HIV.

BIOCHEMICAL MARKERS

Many potential biochemical markers, including neurotransmitters and their metabolites, may help in the diagnosis and treatment of psychiatric disorders. Research in this area is still evolving. Table 7.4–16 summarizes some new developments.

Table 7.4–15
Other Laboratory Tests

Test	Major Psychiatric Indications	Comments
Acid phosphatase	Organic workup for cognitive disorders	Increased in prostate cancer, benign prostatic hypertrophy, excessive platelet destruction, bone disease
Adrenocorticotropic hormone (ACTH)	Organic workup	Increased in steroid abuse; may be increased in seizures, psychotic disorders, Cushing's disease, and in response to stress Decreased in Addison's disease
Alanine aminotransferase (ALT) (formerly called serum glutamic-pyruvic transaminase [SGPT])	Organic workup	Increased in hepatitis, cirrhosis, liver metastases Decreased in pyridoxine (vitamin B_6) deficiency
Albumin	Organic workup	Increased in dehydration Decreased in malnutrition, hepatic failure, burns, multiple myeloma, carcinomas
Aldolase	Eating disorders Schizophrenia	Increased in patients who abuse ipecac (e.g., bulimic patients), schizophrenia (60–80%)
Alkaline phosphatase	Organic workup Use of psychotropic medications	Increased in Paget's disease, hyperparathyroidism, hepatic disease, hepatic metastases, heart failure, phenothiazine use Decreased in pernicious anemia (vitamin B_{12} deficiency)
Ammonia, serum	Organic workup	Increased in hepatic encephalopathy

(*continued*)

Table 7.4–15 (*continued*)

Test	Major Psychiatric Indications	Comments
Amylase, serum	Eating disorders	May be increased in bulimia nervosa
Antinuclear antibodies	Organic workup	Found in systemic lupus erythematosus (SLE) and drug-induced lupus (e.g., secondary to phenothiazines, anticonvulsants); SLE can be associated with delirium, psychotic disorders, mood disorders
Aspartate aminotransferase (AST) (formerly SGOT)	Organic workup	Increased in heart failure, hepatic disease, pancreatitis, eclampsia, cerebral damage, alcohol dependence
		Decreased in pyridoxine (vitamin B_6) deficiency, terminal stages of liver disease
Bicarbonate, serum	Panic disorder	Decreased in hyperventilation syndrome, panic disorder, anabolic steroid abuse
	Eating disorders	May be elevated in patients with bulimia nervosa, in laxative abuse, in psychogenic vomiting
Bilirubin	Organic workup	Increased in hepatic disease
Blood urea nitrogen (BUN)	Delirium	Elevated in renal disease, dehydration
	Use of psychotropic medications	Elevations associated with lethargy, delirium
		If elevated, can increase toxic potential of psychiatric medications, especially lithium and amantadine (Symmetrel)
Bromide, serum	Dementia	Bromide intoxication can cause psychosis, hallucinations, delirium
	Psychosis	Part of dementia workup, especially when serum chloride is elevated
Caffeine level, serum	Anxiety	Evaluation of patients with suspected caffeinism
Calcium (Ca), serum	Organic workup	Increased in hyperparathyroidism, bone metastases
	Mood disorders	Increase associated with delirium, depression, psychosis
	Psychosis	Decreased in hypoparathyroidism, renal failure
	Eating disorders	Decrease associated with depression, irritability, delirium, long-term laxative abuse
Carotid ultrasound	Dementia	Occasionally included in dementia workup, especially to rule out multi-infarct dementia
		Primary value is in search for possible infarct causes
Catecholamines, urinary and plasma	Panic attacks	Elevated in pheochromocytoma
	Anxiety disorders	
Cerebrospinal fluid (CSF)	Organic workup	Increased protein and cells in infection, positive VDRL result in neurosyphilis, bloody CSF in hemorrhagic conditions
Ceruloplasmin, serum; copper, serum	Organic workup	Low in Wilson's disease (hepatolenticular disease)
Chloride (Cl), serum	Eating disorders	Decreased in patients with bulimia nervosa and psychogenic vomiting
	Panic disorder	Mild elevation in hyperventilation syndrome, panic disorder
Cholecystokinin (CCK)	Eating disorders	Compared with controls, blunted in bulimic patients after eating meal (may normalize after treatment with antidepressants)
CO_2 inhalation; sodium bicarbonate infusion	Anxiety	Panic attacks produced in subgroup of patients
Coombs test, direct and indirect	Hemolytic anemias secondary to psychotropic medications	Evaluation of drug-induced hemolytic anemias, such as those secondary to chlorpromazine, phenytoin, levodopa, and methyldopa
Copper, urine	Organic workup	Elevated in Wilson's disease
Cortisol (hydrocortisone)	Organic workup Mood disorders	Excessive level may indicate Cushing's disease associated with anxiety, depression, and a variety of other conditions
Creatine phosphokinase (CPK)	Use of antipsychotics Use of restraints Substance abuse	Increased in neuroleptic malignant syndrome, intramuscular injection, rhabdomyolysis (secondary to substance abuse), patients in restraints, patients experiencing dystonic reactions; asymptomatic elevations seen with use of antipsychotics
Creatinine, serum	Organic workup	Elevated in renal disease
Dopamine (DA) (L-dopa stimulation of dopamine)	Depression	Inhibits prolactin
		Test used to assess functional integrity of dopaminergic system, which is impaired in Parkinson's disease, depression
Doppler ultrasound	Impotence Organic workup	Carotid occlusion, transient ischemic attack (TIA), reduced penile blood flow in impotence

(*continued*)

Table 7.4–15 (*continued*)

Test	Major Psychiatric Indications	Comments
Echocardiogram	Panic disorder	10–40% of patients with panic disorder show mitral valve prolapse
Electroencephalogram (EEG)	Organic workup	Seizures, brain death, lesions; shortened REM latency in depression High-voltage activity in stupor; low-voltage fast activity in excitement; in functional nonorganic cases (e.g., dissociative disorders), alpha activity is present in the background, which responds to auditory and visual stimuli Biphasic or triphasic slow bursts seen in dementia of Creutzfeldt-Jakob disease
Epstein-Barr virus (EBV); cytomegalovirus (CMV)	Organic workup Chronic fatigue Mood disorders	Part of herpesvirus group EBV is causative agent for infectious mononucleosis, which can manifest with depression and personality change CMV can produce anxiety, confusion, mood disorders EBV associated with chronic mononucleosislike syndrome associated with chronic depression and fatigue; may be association between EBV and major depressive disorder
Erythrocyte sedimentation rate (ESR)	Organic workup	An increase in ESR represents a nonspecific test of infectious, inflammatory, autoimmune, or malignant disease; sometimes recommended in the evaluation of anorexia nervosa
Estrogen	Mood disorder	Decreased in menopausal depression and premenstrual syndrome; variable changes in anxiety
Ferritin, serum	Organic workup	Most sensitive test for iron deficiency
Folate (folic acid), serum	Alcohol abuse Use of specific medications	Usually measured with vitamin B_{12} deficiencies associated with psychotic disorders, paranoia, fatigue, agitation, dementia, delirium Associated with alcohol dependence, use of phenytoin, oral contraceptives, estrogen
Follicle-stimulating hormone (FSH)	Depression	High normal in anorexia nervosa, higher values in postmenopausal women; low levels in patients with panhypopituitarism
Glucose, fasting blood (FBS)	Panic attacks Anxiety Delirium Depression	Very high FBS associated with delirium Very low FBS associated with delirium, agitation, panic attacks, anxiety, depression
Glutamyl transaminase, serum	Alcohol abuse Organic workup	Increased in alcohol abuse, cirrhosis, liver disease
Gonadotropin-releasing hormone (GnRH)	Depression Anxiety Schizophrenia	Decreased in schizophrenia; increased in anorexia nervosa; variable in depression, anxiety
Growth hormone (GH)	Depression Schizophrenia	Blunted GH responses to insulin-induced hypoglycemia in depressed patients; increased GH responses to dopamine agonist challenge in schizophrenic patients; increased in some patients with anorexia nervosa
Hematocrit (Hct); hemoglobin (Hb)	Organic workup	Assessment of anemia (anemia may be associated with depressive and psychotic disorders)
Hepatitis A viral antigen (HAAg)	Mood disorders Organic workup	Less severe, better prognosis than hepatitis B; may present with anorexia nervosa, depression
Hepatitis B surface antigen (HBsAg); hepatitis Bc antigen (HBcAg)	Mood disorders Organic workup	Active hepatitis B infection indicates greater infectivity and progression to chronic liver disease May present with depression
Holter monitor	Panic disorder	Evaluation of panic-disordered patients with palpitations and other cardiac symptoms
Human immunodeficiency virus (HIV)	Organic workup	CNS involvement: AIDS dementia, personality change due to a general medical condition, mood disorder due to a general medical condition, acute psychotic disorders
17-Hydroxycorticosteroid	Depression	Deviations detect hyperadrenocorticalism, which can be associated with major depressive disorder Increased in steroid abuse
5-Hydroxyindoleacetic acid (5-HIAA)	Depression Suicide Violence	Decreased in CSF in aggressive or violent patients with suicidal or homicidal impulses May indicate decreased impulse control and predict suicide

(*continued*)

Table 7.4–15 (*continued*)

Test	Major Psychiatric Indications	Comments
Iron, serum	Organic workup	Iron-deficiency anemia
Lactate dehydrogenase (LDH)	Organic workup	Increased in myocardial infarction, pulmonary infarction, hepatic disease, renal infarction, seizures, cerebral damage, megaloblastic (pernicious) anemia, factitious elevations secondary to rough handling of blood specimen tube
Lupus anticoagulant (LA)	Use of phenothiazines	An antiphospholipid antibody, which has been described in some patients using phenothiazines, especially chlorpromazine
Lupus erythematosus (LE) test	Depression Psychosis Delirium Dementia	Positive test result associated with SLE, which may manifest with various psychiatric disturbances, such as psychotic disorders, depressive disorders, delirium, dementia; also tested for with antinuclear antibody (ANA) and anti-DNA antibody tests
Luteinizing hormone (LH)	Depression	Low in patients with panhypopituitarism; decrease associated with depression
Magnesium, serum	Alcohol abuse Organic workup	Decreased in alcohol dependence; low levels associated with agitation, delirium, seizures
MAO, platelet	Depression	Low in depression
MCV (mean corpuscular volume) (average volume of a red blood cell)	Alcohol abuse	Elevated in alcohol dependence, vitamin B_{12}, folate deficiency
Melatonin	Mood disorder with seasonal pattern	Produced by light and pineal gland and decreased in mood disorder with seasonal pattern
Metal (heavy) intoxication (serum or urinary)	Organic workup	Lead—apathy, irritability, anorexia nervosa, confusion Mercury—psychosis, fatigue, apathy, decreased memory, emotional lability, "mad hatter" Manganese—manganese madness, Parkinsonlike syndrome Aluminum—dementia Arsenic—fatigue, blackouts, hair loss
3-Methoxy-4-hydroxyphenylglycol (MHPG)	Depression Anxiety	Most useful in research; decreases in urine may indicate decreases centrally
Myoglobin, urine	Phenothiazine use Substance abuse Use of restraints	Increased in neuroleptic malignant syndrome; in PCP, cocaine, or lysergic acid diethylamide (LSD) intoxication; in patients in restraints
Nicotine	Anxiety Nicotine addiction	Anxiety, smoking
Nocturnal penile tumescence	Impotence	Quantification of penile circumference changes, penile rigidity, frequency of penile tumescence Evaluation of erectile function during sleep Erections associated with rapid eye movement (REM) sleep Helpful in differentiation between organic and functional causes of impotence
Parathyroid (parathormone) hormone	Anxiety Organic workup	Low level causes hypocalcemia and anxiety Dysregulation associated with wide variety of cognitive disorders
Phosphorus, serum	Organic workup Panic disorder	Increased in renal failure, diabetic acidosis, hypoparathyroidism, hypervitamin D Decreased in cirrhosis, hypokalemia, hyperparathyroidism, panic attack, hyperventilation syndrome
Platelet count	Use of psychotropic medications	Decreased by certain psychotropic medications (carbamazepine, clozapine, phenothiazines)
Porphobilinogen (PBG)	Organic workup	Increased in acute porphyria
Porphyria-synthesizing enzyme	Psychosis Organic workup	Acute panic attack or a cognitive disorder can occur in acute porphyria attack, which may be precipitated by barbiturates, imipramine
Potassium (K), serum	Organic workup Eating disorders	Increased in hyperkalemic acidosis; increase is associated with anxiety in cardiac arrhythmia Decreased in cirrhosis, metabolic alkalosis, laxative abuse, diuretic abuse; decrease is common in bulimic patients and in psychogenic vomiting, anabolic steroid abuse

(*continued*)

Table 7.4–15 (*continued*)

Test	Major Psychiatric Indications	Comments
Prolactin, serum	Use of antipsychotic medications Cocaine use Pseudoseizures	Antipsychotics, by decreasing dopamine, increase prolactin synthesis and release, especially in women Elevated prolactin levels may be seen secondary to cocaine withdrawal Lack of prolactin rise after seizure suggests pseudoseizure
Protein, total serum	Organic workup Use of psychotropic medications	Increased in multiple myeloma, myxedema, lupus Decreased in cirrhosis, malnutrition, overhydration Low serum protein can result in greater sensitivity to conventional doses of protein-bound medications (lithium is not protein bound)
Prothrombin time (PT)	Organic workup	Elevated in significant liver damage (cirrhosis), patients with lupus anticoagulant, which can be found in certain patients receiving antipsychotic medications, especially chlorpromazine
Reticulocyte count (estimate of red blood cell production in bone marrow)	Organic workup Use of carbamazepine	Low in megaloblastic or iron deficiency anemia and anemia of chronic disease Must be monitored in patient taking carbamazepine
Salicylate, serum	Psychotic disorder due to a general medical condition with hallucinations Suicide attempts	Toxic levels may be seen in suicide attempts and may cause psychotic disorder due to a general medical condition with hallucinations
Sodium (Na), serum	Organic workup	Decreased with water intoxication; SIADH Increased with excessive salt intake; diabetes Decreased in hypoadrenalism, myxedema, congestive heart failure, diarrhea, polydipsia, use of carbamazepine, anabolic steroids Low levels associated with greater sensitivity to conventional dose of lithium
Testosterone, serum	Impotence Hypoactive sexual desire disorder	Increased in anabolic steroid abuse Follow-up of sex offenders treated with medroxyprogesterone May be decreased in organic workup of impotence Decrease may be seen in hypoactive sexual desire disorder Decreased with medroxyprogesterone treatment
Thyroid function tests	Organic workup Depression	Detection of hypothyroidism or hyperthyroidism Abnormalities can be associated with depression, anxiety, psychosis, dementia, delirium
Urinalysis	Organic workup Pretreatment workup of lithium Drug screening	Provides clues to cause of various cognitive disorders (assessing general appearance, pH, specific gravity, bilirubin, glucose, blood, ketones, protein, etc.); specific gravity may be affected by lithium
Urinary creatinine	Organic workup Substance abuse Lithium use	Increased in renal failure, dehydration Part of pretreatment workup for lithium
Venereal Disease Research Laboratory (VDRL)	Syphilis	Positive (high titers) in secondary syphilis (may be positive or negative in primary syphilis) Low titers (or negative) in tertiary syphilis
Vitamin A, serum	Depression Delirium	Hypervitaminosis A is associated with a variety of mental status changes
Vitamin B_{12}, serum	Organic workup Dementia	Part of workup of megaloblastic anemia and dementia B_{12} deficiency associated with psychosis, paranoia, fatigue, agitation, dementia, delirium Often associated with chronic alcohol abuse
White blood cell (WBC)	Use of psychotropic medications	Leukopenia and agranulocytosis associated with certain psychotropic medications, such as phenothiazines, carbamazepine, clozapine Leukocytosis associated with lithium and neuroleptic malignant syndrome

Table 7.4–16
Biochemical Markers in Psychiatry

A. Monoamines
   1. Plasma homovanillic acid (pHVA), a major dopamine metabolite, may have value in identifying schizophrenic patients who respond to antipsychotics
   2. 3-Methoxy-4-hydroxyphenylglycol (MHPG) is a norepinephrine metabolite
   3. 5-Hydroxyindoleacetic acid (5-HIAA) is associated with suicidal behavior, aggression, poor impulse control, and depression; elevated levels may be associated with anxious, obsessional, and inhibited behaviors

B. Alzheimer's disease
   1. Apolipoprotein E allele—associated with increased risk for Alzheimer's disease; some asymptomatic middle-aged persons exhibit reduced glucose metabolism on positron emission tomography (PET), similar to findings in Alzheimer's patients
   2. Neural thread protein—reported to be increased in patients with Alzheimer's disease; CSF neural thread protein is marketed as a diagnostic test
   3. Other potential CSF tests include CSF tau (increased), CSF amyloid (decreased), ratio of CSF albumin to serum albumin (normal in Alzheimer's disease, elevated in vascular dementia), and inflammatory markers (e.g., CSF acute-phase reactive proteins); the gene for the amyloid precursor protein is considered to have possible etiological significance, but further research is needed

References

Anfinson TJ, Kathol RG. Screening laboratory evaluation in psychiatric patients: a review. *Gen Hosp Psychiatry.* 1992;14(suppl 4):248.

Belkin B, Miller NS. Agreement among laboratory tests, self-reports, and collateral reports of alcohol and drug use. *Ann Clin Psychiatry.* 1992;4:33.

Bowden CL, Janicak PG, Orsulak P, et al. Relation of serum valproate concentration to response in mania. *Am J Psychiatry.* 1996;153:765.

Brower KJ, Catlin DH, Blow FC, Eliopulos GA, Beresford TP. Clinical assessment and urine testing for anabolic-androgenic steroid abuse and dependence. *Am J Drug Alcohol Abuse.* 1991;17:161.

Davidson M, Kahn RS, Knott P, et al. Effects of neuroleptic treatment on symptoms of schizophrenia and plasma homovanillic acid concentrations. *Arch Gen Psychiatry.* 1991;48:910.

Dunivin DL, Foust MJ Jr. A case study from the Department of Defense Psychopharmacology Demonstration Project: mania and neurosyphilis. *Profess Psychol Res Pract.* 1999;30:346.

Heuser I, Yassouridis A, Holsboer F. The combined dexamethasone/CRH test: a refined laboratory test for psychiatric disorders. *J Psychiatr Res.* 1994;28:341.

Hughes JR. A review of the usefulness of the standard EEG in psychiatry. *Clin Electroencephalogr.* 1996;27:35.

Mookhoek EJ, Sterrenburg CM. Annual laboratory screening for chronic hospitalized elderly psychiatric patients: habit or necessity? *Int J Geriatr Psychiatry.* 1996;11:477.

Rosse RB, Deutsch LH, Deutsch SI. Medical assessment and laboratory testing in psychiatry. In: Sadock BJ, Sadock VA, eds. *Kaplan & Sadock's Comprehensive Textbook of Psychiatry.* 7th ed. Vol 2. Baltimore: Lippincott Williams & Wilkins; 2000:2329.

8

Signs and Symptoms in Psychiatry

The reader will find over 350 terms in this section used to describe the signs and symptoms of psychiatric illness. Experienced psychiatrists have encountered most of them; however, it is the rare psychiatrist who has encountered them all. As John Nemiah wrote: "Psychiatry is a science of inexhaustible complexity. It is as infinite as the range of human emotion and behavior. One cannot possibly learn it all."

The language of psychiatry is precise, which allows clinicians to articulate their observations reliably. This facilitates accurate diagnosis, which informs effective treatment. Accuracy in language enables psychiatrists and other clinicians to communicate fruitfully not only with one another but also with their patients. *Signs* are observations and objective findings elicited by the clinician, such as a patient's constricted affect or psychomotor retardation. *Symptoms* are the subjective experiences described by the patient, often expressed as the chief complaints, such as depressed mood or lack of energy. A *syndrome* is a group of signs and symptoms that together make up a recognizable condition, which can be more equivocal than a specific disorder or disease.

Many of the signs and symptoms listed below can be understood as various points on a spectrum of behavior ranging from normal to abnormal. It is extremely rare to have a pathognomonic sign or symptom in psychiatry. In internal medicine, by contrast, one is more likely to find signs indicating a specific disorder (e.g., the Kayser-Fleischer ring of Wilson's disease).

PHENOMENOLOGY

Phenomenology is a school of philosophy and psychiatry developed by Edmund Husserl (1859–1938) and the psychiatrist and philosopher Karl Jaspers (1883–1969) that focuses on the sign or symptom as an event that can be described and experienced. Phenomenologists try not to judge whether or not a phenomenon, such as a hallucination, is abnormal. Rather they attempt to understand it through intuition and experience it through empathy. By listening carefully, the psychiatrist temporarily lives the mental life of the patient.

Jaspers described a "personal world"—the way a person thinks or feels—that could be either normal or abnormal. According to Jaspers, the personal world is abnormal when it (1) springs from a condition that is recognized universally as abnormal, such as schizophrenia, (2) separates the person from others emotionally, and (3) does not provide the person with a sense of "spiritual and material" security. Jaspers believed that for a full understanding of the signs and symptoms observed in the patient, the clinician must have no prior assumptions. A person who reports a hallucination must not be judged thereby as being abnormal or psychotic. To be used diagnostically the phenomenon must occur repeatedly, and be characteristic of a known disorder.

DESCRIPTIVE TERMS

Descriptions of signs and symptoms in psychiatry have remained fairly constant over the years; however, some terms fall in and out of favor. In the various editions of the *Diagnostic and Statistical Manual of Mental Disorders* (DSM), for example, some terms have been retained and others omitted, and some terms are not common to DSM and the *International Classification of Diseases* (ICD).

The fourth edition of DSM (DSM-IV) eliminated the diagnosis of organic mental disorder in an attempt to indicate that all mental disorders may have a biological basis, or medical cause. Thus, the diagnosis of organic mental disorder is now called "delirium, dementia, and amnestic and other cognitive disorders." The 10th revision of the *International Statistical Classification of Diseases and Related Health Problems* (ICD-10), however, retains the diagnostic category organic mental disorders to refer to these conditions.

In a further effort to emphasize the biological aspects of mental illness, DSM-IV and the text revision of DSM-IV (DSM-IV-TR) eschew the term *psychogenic*. Nevertheless, it still appears in ICD-10 to refer to the fact that life events or difficulties play an important role in the genesis of many psychiatric disorders. Similarly, DSM has eliminated the term *neurosis,* which is also used in ICD-10. Both terms—*organic* and *neurosis*—remain in common parlance among health professionals, however.

Neurosis

A neurosis is a chronic or recurrent nonpsychotic disorder characterized mainly by anxiety, which is experienced or expressed directly or is altered through defense mechanisms; it appears as a symptom, such as an obsession, a compulsion, a phobia, or a sexual dysfunction. In the third edition of DSM (DSM-III), a neurotic disorder was defined as follows:

> A mental disorder in which the predominant disturbance is a symptom or group of symptoms that is distressing to the individual and is recognized by him or her as unacceptable and alien (ego-dystonic); reality testing is grossly intact. Behavior does not actively violate gross social norms (though it may be quite disabling). The disturbance is relatively enduring or recurrent without treatment, and is not limited to a transitory reaction to stressors. There is no demonstrable organic etiology or factor.

The term *neuroses* encompasses a broad range of disorders of various signs and symptoms. As such, it has lost precision, except to signify that the person's gross reality testing and personality organization are intact. However, a neurosis can be, and usually is, sufficient to impair the person's functioning in a number of areas. It remains a useful term, especially when compared to the term *psychosis,* described below, still used in DSM-IV-TR.

Psychosis

The traditional meaning of the term *psychotic* emphasized loss of reality testing and impairment of mental functioning—manifested by delusions, hallucinations, confusion, and impaired memory. In the most common psychiatric use of the term, *psychotic* became synonymous with severe impairment of social and personal functioning characterized by social withdrawal and inability to perform the usual household and occupational roles. Another use of the term—based upon psychoanalytic concepts—specifies the degree of ego regression as the criterion for psychotic illness. As a consequence of those multiple meanings, the term has lost its precision in current clinical and research practice.

According to the *American Psychiatric Glossary* of the American Psychiatric Association, the term *psychotic* means grossly impaired reality testing. The term may be used to describe the behavior of a person at a given time or a mental disorder in which at some time during its course all persons with the disorder have grossly impaired reality testing. With gross impairment in reality testing, persons incorrectly evaluate the accuracy of their perceptions and thoughts and make incorrect inferences about external reality, even in the face of contrary evidence. The term *psychotic* does not apply to minor distortions of reality that involve matters of relative judgment. For example, depressed persons who underestimate their achievements are not described as psychotic; those who believe that they have caused natural catastrophes are so described.

Classification

Patients are more than a collection of signs and symptoms. The trend toward collecting symptoms and its possible dehumanizing effects was described by Karl Menninger over 35 years ago. As if anticipating the mathematical device currently in use in DSM-IV-TR, he wrote: "If the patient has, let us say, five symptoms, one can look up each of these symptoms and find which disease is so characterized under all five headings. Then, *voilà!* The diagnosis!" Menninger suggested that the trend toward tabulating disease states was antithetical to understanding the person experiencing the illness and deemphasized the compassionate approach toward the patient that is the hallmark of psychiatry. The algorithms and decision trees used in DSM-IV-TR and in the various computer programs that record signs and symptoms to provide a diagnosis are useful; however, Menninger's cautionary note must not be forgotten. A description of signs and symptoms is the science of psychiatry; the skill of the observers and their creative imaginations and ability to empathize is the art of psychiatry.

The outline that follows is a comprehensive list of signs and symptoms, each of which has a definition or description. As mentioned above, most psychiatric signs and symptoms are rooted in normal behavior and can be understood as various points on a spectrum of behavior ranging from normal to pathological. Table 8–1 presents an alphabetical list of the mental phenomena and the signs and symptoms of psychiatric illness outlined in this chapter. The numbers and letters in the right-hand column refer to the place in the chapter where each item is defined.

Table 8–1
Index to Signs and Symptoms of Psychiatric Illness (This table lists in alphabetical order the mental phenomena and the signs and symptoms of psychiatric illness discussed in this chapter. The numbers and letters in the right-hand column refer to the place in the chapter where each item is defined.)

Abreaction	II, C, 9	Akinesia	III, 2g
Abstract thinking	IV	Akinetic mutism	I, A, 6
Abulia	III, 15	Alexia	VIII, B, 3
Acalculia	VIII, B, 1	Alexithymia	II, B, 12
Acathexis	II, C, 14	Algophobia	IV, C, 11e
Acrophobia	IV, C, 11c	Alogia	V, B, 7
Acting out	III, 14	Ambivalence	II, C, 8
Aculalia	V, A, 11	Amimia	III, 27
Adiadochokinesia	VI, B, 9	Amnesia	VII, A, 1
Adynamic	II, D, 12	Amnestic aphasia	V, B, 3
Affect	II, A	Anergia	III, 16
Aggression	III, 13	Anhedonia	II, B, 10
Agitation	II, C, 4	Anomia	V, B, 3
Agnosia	VI, B, 1	Anorexia	II, D, 1
Agoraphobia	IV, C, 11d	Anosognosia	VI, B, 2
Agraphia	VIII, B, 2	Anterograde amnesia	VII, A, 1a
Ailurophobia	IV, C, 11f	Anxiety	II, C, 1
Akathisia	III, 10e	Apathy	II, C, 7

(continued)

Table 8–1 (*continued*)

Aphasic disturbances	V, B	Constricted affect	II, A, 4
Apperception	I	Conversion phenomena	VI, C
Appropriate affect	II, A, 1	Convulsion	III, 24
Apraxia	VI, B, 7	Coprolalia	IV, C, 10
Astasia abasia	III, 17	Coprophrasia	V, B, 8
Astereognosis	VI, B, 4	Coprophagia	III, 18
Ataxia	III, 10g	Cryptolalia	IV, B, 16
Attention	I, B	Decathexis	II, C, 15
Auditory hallucination	VI, A, 1c	*Déjà entendu*	VII, A, 2e
Aura	VI, B, 10	*Déjà pensé*	VII, A, 2f
Autistic thinking	IV, A, 7	*Déjà vu*	VII, A, 2d
Automatic judgment	X, B	Delirium	I, A, 4
Automatic obedience	III, 8	Delirium tremens	VI, A, 1l
Automatism	III, 7	Delusion	IV, C, 3
Autotopagnosia	VI, B, 2	Delusion of control	IV, C, 3j
Bereavement	II, B, 11	Delusion of grandeur	IV, C, 3h, ii
Bizarre delusion	IV, C, 3a	Delusion of infidelity	IV, C, 3k
Blackout	VII, A, 8	Delusion of persecution	IV, C, 3h, i
Blocking	IV, B, 15	Delusion of poverty	IV, C, 3f
Blood injection phobia	IV, C, 11l	Delusion of reference	IV, C, 3h, iii
Blunted affect	II, A, 3	Delusion of self-accusation	IV, C, 3i
Bradykinesia	III, 22	Delusional jealousy	IV, C, 3k
Bradylalia	V, A, 12	Dementia	VIII, B
Broca's aphasia	V, B, 1	Dementia syndrome of depression	VIII, C
Bulimia	II, D, 11	Depersonalization	VI, C, 4
Catalepsy	III, 2a	Depression	II, B, 9
Cataplexy	III, 4	Derailment	IV, B, 12
Catatonia	III, 2	Derealization	VI, C, 5
Catatonic excitement	III, 2b	Dereism	IV, A, 6
Catatonic posturing	III, 2e	Diminished libido	II, D, 6
Catatonic rigidity	III, 2d	Dipsomania	III, 10f, i
Catatonic stupor	III, 2c	Disinhibition	I, B, 5
Cathexis	II, C, 14	Disorientation	I, A, 1
Cenesthesic hallucination	VI, A, 1h	Dissociation	VI, C, 8
Cerea flexibilitas (waxy flexibility)	III, 21	Dissociative identity disorder	VI, C, 7
Chorea	III, 23	Distractibility	I, B, 1
Circumstantiality	IV, B, 3	Disturbances associated with cognitive disorder	VI, B
Clang association	IV, B, 14	Disturbances associated with conversion and dissociative phenomena	VI, C
Claustrophobia	IV, C, 11i		
Clérambault-Kandinsky complex	IV, C, 3l	Disturbances in content of thought	IV, C
Clonic convulsion	III, 24a	Disturbances in form of thinking	IV, A
Clouding of consciousness	I, A, 2	Disturbances in speech	V, A
Cluttering	V, A, 10	Disturbances in suggestibility	I, C
Coma	I, A, 5	Disturbances of attention	I, B
Coma vigil	I, A, 6	Disturbances of consciousness	I, A
Command automatism	III, 8	Disturbances of memory	VII, A
Command hallucination	VI, A, 1o	Diurnal variation	II, D, 5
Complex partial seizure	III, 25, c	Dreamlike state	I, A, 8
Compulsion	IV, C, 9; III, 10f	Drowsiness	I, A, 10
Conation	III	Dysarthria	V, A, 7
Concrete thinking	VIII, D	Dyscalculia	VIII, B, 1
Condensation	IV, B, 9	Dysgraphia	VIII, B, 2
Confabulation	VII, A, 2c	Dyskinesia	III, 19
Confusion	I, A, 10	Dysphoria	V, A, 13
Consciousness	I	Dysphoric mood	II, B, 1
Constipation	II, D, 7	Dysprosody	V, A, 6

(*continued*)

Table 8–1 (*continued*)

Dystonia	III, 26	Immediate memory	VII, B, 1
Echolalia	IV, B, 8	Impaired insight	IX, C
Echopraxia	III, 1	Impaired judgment	X, C
Ecstasy	II, B, 8	Impulse control	II, C, 12
Egomania	IV, C, 5	Inappropriate affect	II, A, 2
Eidetic image	VII, A, 4	Incoherence	IV, B, 5
Elation	II, B, 14	Increased libido	II, D, 6
Elevated mood	II, B, 6	Ineffability	II, C, 13
Emotion	II	Initial insomnia	II, D, 3a
Emotional insight	IV, A, 10	Insight	IX
Erotomania	IV, C, 31	Insomnia	II, D, 3
Erythrophobia	IV, C, 11g	Intellectual insight	IX, A
Euphoria	II, B, 7	Intelligence	VIII
Euthymic mood	II, B, 2	Irrelevant answer	IV, B, 10
Excessively loud or soft speech	V, A, 8	Irritability	II, C, 4
Expansive mood	II, B, 3	Irritable mood	II, B, 4
Expressive aphasia	V, B, 1	*Jamais vu*	VII, A, 2g
False memory	VII, A, 2h	Jargon aphasia	V, B, 5
Fatigue	II, D, 8	Kleptomania	III, 10f, ii
Fausse reconnaissance	VII, A, 2a	*La belle indifférence*	II, B, 18
Fear	II, C, 3	Labile affect	II, A, 6
Flat affect	II, A, 5	Labile mood	II, B, 5
Flight of ideas	IV, B, 13	Lethologica	VII, A, 7
Floccillation	III, 10j	Lilliputian hallucination	VI, A, 1i
Fluent aphasia	V, B, 2	Logorrhea	V, A, 2
Folie à deux (*folie à trois*)	I, C, 1	Loosening of associations	IV, B, 11
Formal thought disorder	IV, A, 4	Macropsia	VI, C, 2
Formication	VI, A, 1g	Magical thinking	IV, A, 8
Free-floating anxiety	II, C, 2	Mania	II, B, 16
Freudian slip	IV	Mannerism	III, 6
Fugue	VI, C, 6	Melancholia	II, C, 13
Generalized tonic-clonic seizure	III, 25, a	Memory	VII
Global aphasia	V, B, 6	Mental disorder	IV, A, 1
Glossolalia	IV, B, 16	Mental retardation	VIII, A
Grief	II, B, 11	Micropsia	VI, C, 3
Guilt	II, C, 11	Middle insomnia	II, D, 3b
Gustatory hallucination	VI, A, 1f	Mimicry	III, 12
Hallucination	VI, A, 1	Monomania	IV, C, 6
Hallucinosis	VI, A, 1l	Mood	II, B
Haptic hallucination	VI, A, 1g	Mood-congruent delusion	IV, C, 3c
Hyperactivity (hyperkinesis)	III, 10b	Mood-congruent hallucination	VI, A, 1j
Hypermnesia	VII, A, 3	Mood-incongruent delusion	IV, C, 3d
Hyperphagia	II, D, 2	Mood-incongruent hallucination	VI, A, 1k
Hyperpragia	I, B, 3	Mood swings	II, B, 5
Hypersomnia	II, D, 4	Motor aphasia	V, B, 1
Hypervigilance	I, B, 3	Motor behavior (conation)	III
Hypnagogic hallucination	VI, A, 1a	Mourning	II, B, 11
Hypnopompic hallucination	VI, A, 1b	Multiple personality	VI, C, 7
Hypnosis	I, C, 2	Munchausen syndrome	IV, C, 3m
Hypoactivity (hypokinesis)	III, 11	Muscle rigidity	III, 20
Hypochondria	IV, C, 7	Mutism	III, 9
Hypomania	II, B, 15	Needle phobia	IV, C, 111
Hysterical anesthesia	VI, C, 1	Negativism	III, 3
Idea of reference	IV, C, 3h, iii	Neologism	IV, B, 1
Illogical thinking	IV, A, 5	Nihilistic delusion	IV, C, 3e
Illusion	VI, A, 2	Noesis	IV, C, 12

(*continued*)

Table 8–1 (*continued*)

Nominal aphasia	V, B, 3	Shame	II, C, 10
Nonfluent aphasia	V, B, 1	Simple partial seizure	III, 25b
Nymphomania	III, 10f, iii	Simultagnosia	VI, B, 8
Obsession	IV, C, 8	Sleepwalking	III, 10d
Olfactory hallucination	VI, A, 1e	Social phobia	IV, C, 11b
Orientation	VII	Somatic delusion	IV, C, 3g
Overactivity	III, 10	Somatic hallucination	VI, A, 1h
Overvalued idea	IV, C, 2	Somatopagnosia	VI, B, 3
Panic	II, C, 6	Somnambulism	III, 10d
Panphobia	IV, C, 11h	Somnolence	I, A, 9
Paramnesia	VII, A, 2	Speaking in tongues	IV, B, 16
Paranoid delusions	IV, C, 3h	Specific disturbances in form of thought	IV, B
Paranoid ideation	IV, C, 3h	Specific phobia	IV, C, 11a
Parapraxis	IV	Stereotypy	III, 5
Pathological jealousy	IV, C, 3k	Stupor	I, A, 3; III, 2c
Perception	VI	Stuttering	V, A, 9
Persecutory delusion	IV, C, 3h, i	Suicidal ideation	II, B, 13
Perseveration	IV, B, 6	Sundowning	I, A, 12
Phantom limb	VI, A, 1g	Synesthesia	VI, A, 1m
Phobia	IV, C, 11	Syntactical aphasia	V, B, 4
Physiological disturbances associated with mood	II, D	Systematized delusion	IV, C, 3b
Pica	II, D, 9	Tactile (haptic) hallucination	VI, A, 1g
Polyphagia	III, 10h	Tangentiality	IV, B, 4
Posturing	III, 2e	Tension	II, C, 5
Poverty of content of speech	V, A, 5	Terminal insomnia	II, D, 3c
Poverty of speech	V, A, 3	Thinking	IV
Preoccupation of thought	IV, C, 4	Thought broadcasting	IV, C, 3j, iii
Pressure of speech	V, A, 1	Thought control	IV, C, 3j, iv
Primary process thinking	IV, A, 9	Thought deprivation	IV, B, 15
Prosopagnosia	VI, B, 6	Thought insertion	IV, C, 3j, ii
Pseudocyesis	II, D, 10	Thought withdrawal	IV, C, 3j, i
Pseudodementia	VIII, C	Tic	III, 10c
Pseudologia phantastica	IV, C, 3m	Tonic convulsion	III, 24, b
Psychomotor agitation	III, 10a	Trailing phenomenon	VI, A, 1n
Psychosis	IV, A, 2	Trance	I, B, 4
Reality testing	IV, A, 3	Tremor	III, 10i
Recent memory	VII, B, 2	Trend of thought	IV, C, 4
Recent past memory	VII, B, 3	Trichotillomania	III, 10f, v
Receptive aphasia	V, B, 2	True insight	IX, B
Remote memory	VII, B, 4	Twilight state	I, A, 7
Repression	VII, A, 6	Twirling	III, 21
Restricted affect	II, A, 4	*Unio mystica*	IV, C, 13
Retrograde amnesia	VII, A, 1b	Vegetative signs	II, D
Retrospective falsification	VII, A, 2b	Verbigeration	IV, B, 7
Rigidity	III, 2d	Visual agnosia	VI, B, 4
Ritual	III, 10f, vi	Visual hallucination	VI, A, 1d
Rumination	IV, C, 8	Volubility	V, A, 2
Satyriasis	III, 10f, iv	Waxy flexibility	III, 2f
Screen memory	VII, A, 5	Wernicke's aphasia	V, B, 2
Seizure	III, 25	Word salad	IV, B, 2
Selective inattention	I, B, 2	Xenophobia	IV, C, 11j
Sensorium	I	Zoophobia	IV, C, 11k
Sensory aphasia	V, B, 2		

I. Consciousness: state of awareness.

A. Disturbances of consciousness: *apperception* is perception modified by a person's own emotions and thoughts; *sensorium* is the state of cognitive functioning of the special senses (sometimes used as a synonym for *consciousness*); disturbances of consciousness are most often associated with brain pathology.

1. Disorientation: disturbance of orientation in time, place, or person.
2. Clouding of consciousness: incomplete clear-mindedness with disturbances in perception and attitudes.
3. Stupor: lack of reaction to, and unawareness of, surroundings.
4. Delirium: bewildered, restless, confused, disoriented reaction associated with fear and hallucinations.
5. Coma: profound unconsciousness.
6. Coma vigil: coma in which a patient appears to be awake with eyes open but cannot be aroused (also known as *akinetic mutism*).
7. Twilight state: disturbed consciousness with hallucinations.
8. Dreamlike state: often used as a synonym for *complex partial seizure* or *psychomotor epilepsy.*
9. Somnolence: abnormal drowsiness.
10. Confusion: disturbance of consciousness in which reactions to environmental stimuli are inappropriate; manifested by disordered orientation in relation to time, place, or person.
11. Drowsiness: a state of impaired awareness associated with a desire or inclination to sleep.
12. Sundowning: syndrome in older persons that usually occurs at night and is characterized by drowsiness, confusion, ataxia, and falling as the result of being overly sedated with medications; also called *sundowner's syndrome.*

B. Disturbances of attention: *attention* is the amount of effort exerted in focusing on certain portions of an experience; ability to sustain a focus on one activity; ability to concentrate.

1. Distractibility: inability to concentrate attention; state in which attention is drawn to unimportant or irrelevant external stimuli.
2. Selective inattention: blocking out only those things that generate anxiety.
3. Hypervigilance: excessive attention and focus on all internal and external stimuli, usually secondary to delusional or paranoid states; similar to hyperpragia, excessive thinking and mental activity.
4. Trance: focused attention and altered consciousness, usually seen in hypnosis, dissociative disorders, and ecstatic religious experiences.
5. Disinhibition: removal of an inhibitory effect that permits persons to lose control of impulses as occurs in alcohol intoxication.

C. Disturbances in suggestibility: compliant and uncritical response to an idea or influence.

1. *Folie à deux* (or *folie à trois*): communicated emotional illness between two (or three) persons.
2. Hypnosis: artificially induced modification of consciousness characterized by heightened suggestibility.

II. Emotion: complex feeling state with psychic, somatic, and behavioral components that is related to affect and mood.

A. Affect: observed expression of emotion, possibly inconsistent with patient's description of emotion.

1. Appropriate affect: condition in which the emotional tone is in harmony with the accompanying idea, thought, or speech; also further described as broad or full affect in which a full range of emotions is appropriately expressed.
2. Inappropriate affect: disharmony between the emotional feeling tone and the idea, thought, or speech accompanying it.
3. Blunted affect: disturbance in affect manifested by severe reduction in the intensity of externalized feeling tone.
4. Restricted or constricted affect: reduction in intensity of feeling tone, less severe than blunted affect but clearly reduced.
5. Flat affect: absence or near absence of any signs of affective expression; voice monotonous, face immobile.
6. Labile affect: rapid and abrupt changes in emotional feeling tone, unrelated to external stimuli.

B. Mood: pervasive and sustained emotion subjectively experienced and reported by a patient and observed by others; examples include depression, elation, and anger.

1. Dysphoric mood: an unpleasant mood.
2. Euthymic mood: normal range of mood, implying absence of depressed or elevated mood.
3. Expansive mood: a person's expression of feelings without restraint, frequently with overestimation of their significance or importance.
4. Irritable mood: state in which a person is easily annoyed and provoked to anger.
5. Mood swings (labile mood): oscillations between euphoria and depression or anxiety.
6. Elevated mood: air of confidence and enjoyment; mood more cheerful than usual.
7. Euphoria: intense elation with feelings of grandeur.
8. Ecstasy: feeling of intense rapture.
9. Depression: psychopathological feeling of sadness.
10. Anhedonia: loss of interest in, and withdrawal from, all regular and pleasurable activities, often associated with depression.
11. Grief or mourning: sadness appropriate to a real loss; also called *bereavement.*
12. Alexithymia: a person's inability to, or difficulty in, describing or being aware of emotions or mood.
13. Suicidal ideation: thoughts or act of taking one's own life.
14. Elation: feelings of joy, euphoria, triumph, intense self-satisfaction, or optimism.
15. Hypomania: mood abnormality with the qualitative characteristics of mania but somewhat less intense.

16. Mania: mood state characterized by elation, agitation, hyperactivity, hypersexuality, and accelerated thinking and speaking.
17. Melancholia: severe depressive state; used in the term *involutional melancholia* both descriptively and also in reference to a distinct diagnostic entity.
18. *La belle indifférence*: inappropriate attitude of calm or lack of concern about one's disability.

C. Other emotions

1. Anxiety: feeling of apprehension caused by anticipation of danger, which may be internal or external.
2. Free-floating anxiety: pervasive, unfocused fear not attached to any idea.
3. Fear: anxiety caused by consciously recognized and realistic danger.
4. Agitation: severe anxiety associated with motor restlessness; similar to irritability characterized by excessive excitability with easily triggered anger or annoyance.
5. Tension: increased and unpleasant motor and psychological activity.
6. Panic: acute, episodic, intense attack of anxiety associated with overwhelming feelings of dread and autonomic discharge.
7. Apathy: dulled emotional tone associated with detachment or indifference.
8. Ambivalence: coexistence of two opposing impulses toward the same thing in the same person at the same time.
9. Abreaction: emotional release or discharge after recalling a painful experience.
10. Shame: failure to live up to self-expectations.
11. Guilt: emotion secondary to doing what is perceived as wrong.
12. Impulse control: ability to resist an impulse, drive, or temptation to perform an action.
13. Ineffability: ecstatic state in which person states it is indescribable, inexpressible, and impossible to convey to another person.
14. Acathexis: lack of feeling associated with an ordinarily emotionally charged subject; in *cathexis,* the feeling is connected.
15. Decathexis: detaching emotions from thoughts, ideas, or persons.

D. Physiological disturbances associated with mood: signs of somatic (usually autonomic) dysfunction, most often associated with depression (also called *vegetative signs*).

1. Anorexia: loss of, or decrease in, appetite.
2. Hyperphagia: increase in intake of food.
3. Insomnia: lack of, or diminished, ability to sleep.
   a. Initial: difficulty falling asleep.
   b. Middle: difficulty sleeping through the night without waking up and difficulty going back to sleep.
   c. Terminal: early morning awakening.
4. Hypersomnia: excessive sleeping.
5. Diurnal variation: mood is regularly worst in the morning, immediately after awakening, and improves as the day progresses.
6. Diminished libido: decreased sexual interest, drive, and performance (increased libido is often associated with manic states).
7. Constipation: inability to defecate or difficulty defecating.
8. Fatigue: a feeling of weariness, sleepiness, or irritability following a period of mental or bodily activity.
9. Pica: craving and eating nonfood substances, such as paint and clay.
10. Pseudocyesis: rare condition in which a patient has the signs and symptoms of pregnancy, such as abdominal distention, breast enlargement, pigmentation, cessation of menses, and morning sickness.
11. Bulimia: insatiable hunger and voracious eating; seen in bulimia nervosa and atypical depression.
12. Adynamia: weakness and fatigability.

III. Motor behavior (conation): aspect of the psyche that includes impulses, motivations, wishes, drives, instincts, and cravings, as expressed by a person's behavior or motor activity.

1. Echopraxia: pathological imitation of movements of one person by another.
2. Catatonia and postural abnormalities: seen in catatonic schizophrenia and some patients with brain diseases, such as encephalitis.
   a. Catalepsy: general term for an immobile position that is constantly maintained.
   b. Catatonic excitement: agitated, purposeless motor activity, uninfluenced by external stimuli.
   c. Catatonic stupor: markedly slowed motor activity, often to the point of immobility and seeming unawareness of surroundings.
   d. Catatonic rigidity: voluntary assumption of a rigid posture, held against all efforts to be moved.
   e. Catatonic posturing: voluntary assumption of an inappropriate or bizarre posture, generally maintained for long periods.
   f. *Cerea flexibilitas* (waxy flexibility): condition in which a person can be molded into a position that is then maintained; when an examiner moves the person's limb, the limb feels as if it were made of wax.
   g. Akinesia: lack of physical movement, as in the extreme immobility of catatonic schizophrenia; may also occur as an extrapyramidal adverse effect of antipsychotic medication.
3. Negativism: motiveless resistance to all attempts to be moved or to all instructions.
4. Cataplexy: temporary loss of muscle tone and weakness precipitated by a variety of emotional states.
5. Stereotypy: repetitive fixed pattern of physical action or speech.
6. Mannerism: ingrained, habitual involuntary movement.
7. Automatism: automatic performance of an act or acts generally representing unconscious symbolic activity.

8. Command automatism: automatic following of suggestions (also automatic obedience).
9. Mutism: voicelessness without structural abnormalities.
10. Overactivity.
    a. Psychomotor agitation: excessive motor and cognitive activity, usually nonproductive and in response to inner tension.
    b. Hyperactivity (hyperkinesis): restless, aggressive, destructive activity, often associated with some underlying brain pathology.
    c. Tic: involuntary, spasmodic motor movement.
    d. Sleepwalking (somnambulism): motor activity during sleep.
    e. Akathisia: subjective feeling of muscular tension secondary to antipsychotic or other medication, which can cause restlessness, pacing, repeated sitting and standing; can be mistaken for psychotic agitation.
    f. Compulsion: uncontrollable impulse to perform an act repetitively.
        i. Dipsomania: compulsion to drink alcohol.
        ii. Kleptomania: compulsion to steal.
        iii. Nymphomania: excessive and compulsive need for coitus in a woman.
        iv. Satyriasis: excessive and compulsive need for coitus in a man; in women called *nymphomania*.
        v. Trichotillomania: compulsion to pull out hair.
        vi. Ritual: automatic compulsive activity, anxiety reducing in origin.
    g. Ataxia: failure of muscle coordination; irregularity of muscle action.
    h. Polyphagia: pathological overeating.
    i. Tremor: rhythmical alteration in movement, which is usually faster than one beat a second; typically, tremors decrease during periods of relaxation and sleep and increase during periods of anger and increased tension.
    j. Floccillation: aimless picking usually at clothing or bedclothes, commonly seen in delirium.
11. Hypoactivity (hypokinesis): decreased motor and cognitive activity, as in psychomotor retardation; visible slowing of thought, speech, and movements.
12. Mimicry: simple, imitative motor activity of childhood.
13. Aggression: forceful, goal-directed action that may be verbal or physical; the motor counterpart of the affect of rage, anger, or hostility.
14. Acting out: direct expression of an unconscious wish or impulse in action; living out unconscious fantasy impulsively in behavior.
15. Abulia: reduced impulse to act and think, associated with indifference about consequences of action; a result of neurological deficit.
16. Anergia: lack of energy (anergy).
17. Astasia abasia: inability to stand or walk in a normal manner, even though normal leg movements can be performed in a sitting or lying down position. The gait is bizarre and does not suggest a specific organic lesion; seen in conversion disorder.
18. Coprophagia: eating of filth or feces.
19. Dyskinesia: difficulty performing voluntary movements, as in extrapyramidal disorders.
20. Muscle rigidity: state in which the muscles remain immovable; seen in schizophrenia.
21. Twirling: a sign present in autistic children who continually rotate in the direction in which their head is turned.
22. Bradykinesia: slow motor activity with decreased normal, spontaneous movement.
23. Chorea: random and involuntary quick, jerky, purposeless movements.
24. Convulsion: involuntary, violent muscular contraction or spasm.
    a. Clonic convulsion: convulsion in which the muscles alternately contract and relax.
    b. Tonic convulsion: convulsion in which the muscle contraction is sustained.
25. Seizure: an attack or sudden onset of certain symptoms, such as convulsions, loss of consciousness, and psychic or sensory disturbances; seen in epilepsy and can be substance induced.
    a. Generalized tonic-clonic seizure: generalized onset of tonic-clonic movements of the limbs, tongue biting, and incontinence followed by slow, gradual recovery of consciousness and cognition; also called *grand mal seizure* and *psychomotor seizure*.
    b. Simple partial seizure: localized ictal onset of seizure without altered consciousness.
    c. Complex partial seizure: localized ictal onset of seizure with altered consciousness.
26. Dystonia: slow, sustained contractions of the trunk or limbs; seen in medication-induced dystonia.
27. Amimia: inability to make gestures or to comprehend those made by others.

IV. Thinking: goal-directed flow of ideas, symbols, and associations initiated by a problem or task and leading toward a reality-oriented conclusion; when a logical sequence occurs, thinking is normal; *parapraxis* (unconsciously motivated lapse from logic, also called a *freudian slip*) is considered part of normal thinking. *Abstract thinking* is the ability to grasp the essentials of a whole, to break a whole into its parts, and to discern common properties.

A. General disturbances in form or process of thinking

1. Mental disorder: clinically significant behavior or psychological syndrome associated with distress or disability, not just an expected response to a particular event or limited to relations between a person and society.
2. Psychosis: inability to distinguish reality from fantasy; impaired reality testing, with the creation of a new reality (as opposed to *neurosis:* mental disorder in which reality testing is intact; behavior may not violate gross social norms, but is relatively enduring or recurrent without treatment).

3. Reality testing: objective evaluation and judgment of the world outside the self.
4. Formal thought disorder: disturbance in the form of thought rather than the content of thought; thinking characterized by loosened associations, neologisms, and illogical constructs; thought process is disordered, and the person is defined as psychotic.
5. Illogical thinking: thinking containing erroneous conclusions or internal contradictions; psychopathological only when it is marked and when not caused by cultural values or intellectual deficit.
6. Dereism: mental activity not concordant with logic or experience.
7. Autistic thinking: preoccupation with inner, private world; term used somewhat synonymously with *dereism*.
8. Magical thinking: a form of dereistic thought; thinking similar to that of the preoperational phase in children (Jean Piaget), in which thoughts, words, or actions assume power (e.g., to cause or prevent events).
9. Primary process thinking: general term for thinking that is dereistic, illogical, magical; normally found in dreams, abnormally in psychosis.
10. Emotional insight: deep level of understanding or awareness that is likely to lead to positive changes in personality and behavior.

B. Specific disturbances in form of thought

1. Neologism: new word created by a patient, often by combining syllables of other words, for idiosyncratic psychological reasons.
2. Word salad: incoherent mixture of words and phrases.
3. Circumstantiality: indirect speech that is delayed in reaching the point but eventually gets from original point to desired goal; characterized by overinclusion of details and parenthetical remarks.
4. Tangentiality: inability to have goal-directed associations of thought; speaker never gets from point to desired goal.
5. Incoherence: thought that generally is not understandable; running together of thoughts or words with no logical or grammatical connection, resulting in disorganization.
6. Perseveration: persisting response to a previous stimulus after a new stimulus has been presented; often associated with cognitive disorders.
7. Verbigeration: meaningless repetition of specific words or phrases.
8. Echolalia: psychopathological repeating of words or phrases of one person by another; tends to be repetitive and persistent; may be spoken with mocking or staccato intonation.
9. Condensation: fusion of various concepts into one.
10. Irrelevant answer: answer that is not in harmony with question asked (person appears to ignore or not attend to question).
11. Loosening of associations: flow of thought in which ideas shift from one subject to another in a completely unrelated way; when severe, speech may be incoherent.
12. Derailment: gradual or sudden deviation in train of thought without blocking; sometimes used synonymously with *loosening of associations*.
13. Flight of ideas: rapid, continuous verbalizations or plays on words produce constant shifting from one idea to another; ideas tend to be connected, and in the less severe form a listener may be able to follow them.
14. Clang association: association of words similar in sound but not in meaning; words have no logical connection; may include rhyming and punning.
15. Blocking: abrupt interruption in train of thought before a thought or idea is finished; after a brief pause, person indicates no recall of what was being said or was going to be said (also known as *thought deprivation*).
16. Glossolalia: expression of a revelatory message through unintelligible words (also known as *speaking in tongues*); not considered a disturbance in thought if associated with practices of specific Pentecostal religions; also known as *cryptolalia,* a private spoken language.

C. Specific disturbances in content of thought

1. Poverty of content: thought that gives little information because of vagueness, empty repetitions, or obscure phrases.
2. Overvalued idea: unreasonable, sustained false belief maintained less firmly than a delusion.
3. Delusion: false belief, based on incorrect inference about external reality, not consistent with patient's intelligence and cultural background; cannot be corrected by reasoning.
   a. Bizarre delusion: an absurd, totally implausible, strange false belief (e.g., invaders from space have implanted electrodes in a person's brain).
   b. Systematized delusion: false belief or beliefs united by a single event or theme (e.g., a person is being persecuted by the CIA, the FBI, or the Mafia).
   c. Mood-congruent delusion: delusion with mood-appropriate content (e.g., a depressed patient believes that he or she is responsible for the destruction of the world).
   d. Mood-incongruent delusion: delusion with content that has no association to mood or is mood neutral (e.g., a depressed patient has delusions of thought control or thought broadcasting).
   e. Nihilistic delusion: false feeling that self, others, or the world is nonexistent or coming to an end.
   f. Delusion of poverty: a person's false belief that he or she is bereft or will be deprived of all material possessions.

g. Somatic delusion: false belief involving functioning of the body (e.g., belief that the brain is rotting or melting).
h. Paranoid delusions: include persecutory delusions and delusions of reference, control, and grandeur (distinguished from *paranoid ideation,* which is suspiciousness of less than delusional proportions).
   i. Delusion of persecution: a person's false belief that he or she is being harassed, cheated, or persecuted; often found in litigious patients who have a pathological tendency to take legal action because of imagined mistreatment.
   ii. Delusion of grandeur: a person's exaggerated conception of his or her importance, power, or identity.
   iii. Delusion of reference: a person's false belief that the behavior of others refers to himself or herself; that events, objects, or other persons have a particular and unusual significance, usually of a negative nature; derived from idea of reference, in which a person falsely feels that others are talking about him or her (e.g., belief that persons on television or radio are talking to, or about, the person).
i. Delusion of self-accusation: false feeling of remorse and guilt.
j. Delusion of control: false feeling that a person's will, thoughts, or feelings are being controlled by external forces.
   i. Thought withdrawal: delusion that thoughts are being removed from a person's mind by other persons or forces.
   ii. Thought insertion: delusion that thoughts are being implanted in a person's mind by other persons or forces.
   iii. Thought broadcasting: delusion that a person's thoughts can be heard by others, as though they were being broadcast over the air.
   iv. Thought control: delusion that a person's thoughts are being controlled by other persons or forces.
k. Delusion of infidelity (delusional jealousy): false belief derived from pathological jealousy about a person's lover being unfaithful.
l. Erotomania: delusional belief, more common in women than in men, that someone is deeply in love with them (also known as *Clérambault-Kandinsky complex*).
m. Pseudologia phantastica: a type of lying in which a person appears to believe in the reality of his or her fantasies and acts on them; associated with Munchausen syndrome, repeated feigning of illness.

4. Trend or preoccupation of thought: centering of thought content on a particular idea, associated with a strong affective tone, such as a paranoid trend or a suicidal or homicidal preoccupation.
5. Egomania: pathological self-preoccupation.
6. Monomania: preoccupation with a single object.
7. Hypochondria: exaggerated concern about health that is based not on real organic pathology but, rather, on unrealistic interpretations of physical signs or sensations as abnormal.
8. Obsession: pathological persistence of an irresistible thought or feeling that cannot be eliminated from consciousness by logical effort; associated with anxiety.
9. Compulsion: pathological need to act on an impulse that, if resisted, produces anxiety; repetitive behavior in response to an obsession or performed according to certain rules, with no true end in itself other than to prevent something from occurring in the future.
10. Coprolalia: compulsive utterance of obscene words.
11. Phobia: persistent, irrational, exaggerated, and invariably pathological dread of a specific stimulus or situation; results in a compelling desire to avoid the feared stimulus.
    a. Specific phobia: circumscribed dread of a discrete object or situation (e.g., dread of spiders or snakes).
    b. Social phobia: dread of public humiliation, as in fear of public speaking, performing, or eating in public.
    c. Acrophobia: dread of high places.
    d. Agoraphobia: dread of open places.
    e. Algophobia: dread of pain.
    f. Ailurophobia: dread of cats.
    g. Erythrophobia: dread of red (refers to a fear of blushing).
    h. Panphobia: dread of everything.
    i. Claustrophobia: dread of closed places.
    j. Xenophobia: dread of strangers.
    k. Zoophobia: dread of animals.
    l. Needle phobia: the persistent, intense, pathological fear of receiving an injection; also called *blood injection phobia.*
12. Noesis: a revelation in which immense illumination occurs in association with a sense that a person has been chosen to lead and command.
13. *Unio mystica*: an oceanic feeling of mystic unity with an infinite power; not considered a disturbance in thought content if congruent with person's religious or cultural milieu.

V. Speech: ideas, thoughts, feelings as expressed through language; communication through the use of words and language.

A. Disturbances in speech

1. Pressure of speech: rapid speech that is increased in amount and difficult to interrupt.
2. Volubility (logorrhea): copious, coherent, logical speech.
3. Poverty of speech: restriction in the amount of speech used; replies may be monosyllabic.
4. Nonspontaneous speech: verbal responses given only when asked or spoken to directly; no self-initiation of speech.

5. Poverty of content of speech: speech that is adequate in amount but conveys little information because of vagueness, emptiness, or stereotyped phrases.
6. Dysprosody: loss of normal speech melody (called *prosody*).
7. Dysarthria: difficulty in articulation, not in word finding or in grammar.
8. Excessively loud or soft speech: loss of modulation of normal speech volume; may reflect a variety of pathological conditions ranging from psychosis to depression to deafness.
9. Stuttering: frequent repetition or prolongation of a sound or syllable, leading to markedly impaired speech fluency.
10. Cluttering: erratic and dysrhythmic speech, consisting of rapid and jerky spurts.
11. Aculalia: nonsense speech associated with markedly impaired comprehension.
12. Bradylalia: Abnormally slow speech.
13. Dysphonia: difficulty or pain in speaking.

B. Aphasic disturbances: disturbances in language output.

1. Motor aphasia: disturbance of speech caused by a cognitive disorder in which understanding remains but ability to speak is grossly impaired; halting, laborious, and inaccurate speech (also known as *Broca's, nonfluent, and expressive aphasia*).
2. Sensory aphasia: organic loss of ability to comprehend the meaning of words; fluid and spontaneous but incoherent and nonsensical speech (also known as *Wernicke's, fluent, and receptive aphasia*).
3. Nominal aphasia: difficulty finding correct name for an object (also termed *anomia* and *amnestic aphasia*).
4. Syntactical aphasia: inability to arrange words in proper sequence.
5. Jargon aphasia: words produced are totally neologistic; nonsense words repeated with various intonations and inflections.
6. Global aphasia: combination of a grossly nonfluent aphasia and a severe fluent aphasia.
7. Alogia: inability to speak because of mental deficiency or an episode of dementia.
8. Coprophrasia: involuntary use of vulgar or obscene language; seen in Tourette's disorder and some patients with schizophrenia.

VI. Perception: process of transferring physical stimulation into psychological information; mental process by which sensory stimuli are brought to awareness.

A. Disturbances of perception

1. Hallucination: false sensory perception not associated with real external stimuli; there may or may not be a delusional interpretation of the hallucinatory experience.
   a. Hypnagogic hallucination: false sensory perception occurring while falling asleep; generally considered nonpathological.
   b. Hypnopompic hallucination: false perception occurring while awakening from sleep; generally considered nonpathological.
   c. Auditory hallucination: false perception of sound, usually voices but also other noises, such as music; most common hallucination in psychiatric disorders.
   d. Visual hallucination: false perception involving sight consisting of both formed images (e.g., persons) and unformed images (e.g., flashes of light); most common in medically determined disorders.
   e. Olfactory hallucination: false perception of smell; most common in medical disorders.
   f. Gustatory hallucination: false perception of taste, such as unpleasant taste, caused by an uncinate seizure; most common in medical disorders.
   g. Tactile (haptic) hallucination: false perception of touch or surface sensation, as from an amputated limb (*phantom limb*); crawling sensation on or under the skin (*formication*).
   h. Somatic hallucination: false sensation of things occurring in or to the body, most often of visceral origin (also known as *cenesthesic hallucination*).
   i. Lilliputian hallucination: false perception in which objects are seen as reduced in size (also termed *micropsia*).
   j. Mood-congruent hallucination: hallucination in which the content is consistent with either a depressed or a manic mood (e.g., a depressed patient hears voices saying that the patient is a bad person; a manic patient hears voices saying that the patient is of inflated worth, power, and knowledge).
   k. Mood-incongruent hallucination: hallucination in which the content is not consistent with either depressed or manic mood (e.g., in depression, hallucinations not involving such themes as guilt, deserved punishment, or inadequacy; in mania, hallucinations not involving such themes as inflated worth or power).
   l. Hallucinosis: hallucinations, most often auditory, that are associated with chronic alcohol abuse and that occur within a clear sensorium, as opposed to delirium tremens (DTs), hallucinations that occur in the context of a clouded sensorium.
   m. Synesthesia: sensation or hallucination caused by another sensation (e.g., an auditory sensation accompanied by, or triggering, a visual sensation; a sound experienced as being seen or a visual experience experienced as heard).
   n. Trailing phenomenon: perceptual abnormality associated with hallucinogenic drugs in which moving objects are seen as a series of discrete and discontinuous images.
   o. Command hallucination: false perception of orders that a person may feel obliged to obey or unable to resist.
2. Illusion; misperception or misinterpretation of real external sensory stimuli.

B. Disturbances associated with cognitive disorder and medical conditions

1. Agnosia: an inability to recognize and interpret the significance of sensory impressions.
2. Anosognosia (ignorance of illness): a person's inability to recognize a neurological deficit as occurring to himself or herself.
3. Somatopagnosia (ignorance of the body): a person's inability to recognize a body part as his or her own (also called *autotopagnosia*).
4. Visual agnosia: inability to recognize objects or persons.
5. Astereognosis: inability to recognize objects by touch.
6. Prosopagnosia: inability to recognize faces.
7. Apraxia: inability to carry out specific tasks.
8. Simultagnosia: inability to comprehend more than one element of a visual scene at a time or to integrate the parts into a whole.
9. Adiadochokinesia: inability to perform rapid alternating movements.
10. Aura: warning sensations such as automatisms, fullness in the stomach, blushing, and changes in respiration, cognitive sensations, and affective states usually experienced before a seizure; a sensory prodrome that precedes a classic migraine headache.

C. Disturbances associated with conversion and dissociative phenomena: somatization of repressed material or the development of physical symptoms and distortions involving the voluntary muscles or special sense organs; not under voluntary control and not explained by any physical disorder.

1. Hysterical anesthesia: loss of sensory modalities resulting from emotional conflicts.
2. Macropsia: state in which objects seem larger than they are.
3. Micropsia: state in which objects seem smaller than they are (both macropsia and micropsia can also be associated with clear organic conditions, such as complex partial seizures).
4. Depersonalization: a person's subjective sense of being unreal, strange, or unfamiliar.
5. Derealization: a subjective sense that the environment is strange or unreal; a feeling of changed reality.
6. Fugue: taking on a new identity with amnesia for the old identity; often involves travel or wandering to new environments.
7. Multiple personality: one person who appears at different times to be two or more entirely different personalities and characters (called *dissociative identity disorder* in DSM-IV).
8. Dissociation: unconscious defense mechanism involving the segregation of any group of mental or behavioral processes from the rest of the person's psychic activity; may entail separation of an idea from its accompanying emotional tone, as seen in dissociative and conversion disorders.

VII. Memory: function by which information stored in the brain is later recalled to consciousness. *Orientation* is the normal state of oneself and one's surroundings in terms of time, place, and person.

A. Disturbances of memory

1. Amnesia: partial or total inability to recall past experiences; may be of organic or emotional origin.
   a. Anterograde: amnesia for events occurring after a point in time.
   b. Retrograde: amnesia for events occurring before a point in time.
2. Paramnesia: falsification of memory by distortion of recall.
   a. *Fausse reconnaissance:* false recognition.
   b. Retrospective falsification: memory becomes unintentionally (unconsciously) distorted by being filtered through a person's present emotional, cognitive, and experiential state.
   c. Confabulation: unconscious filling of gaps in memory by imagined or untrue experiences that a person believes but that have no basis in fact; most often associated with organic pathology.
   d. *Déjà vu*: illusion of visual recognition in which a new situation is incorrectly regarded as a repetition of a previous memory.
   e. *Déjà entendu*: illusion of auditory recognition.
   f. *Déjà pensé*: illusion that a new thought is recognized as a thought previously felt or expressed.
   g. *Jamais vu*: false feeling of unfamiliarity with a real situation that a person has experienced.
   h. False memory: a patient's recollection of, and belief in, an event that did not actually occur.
3. Hypermnesia: exaggerated degree of retention and recall.
4. Eidetic image: visual memory of almost hallucinatory vividness.
5. Screen memory: a consciously tolerable memory covering for a painful memory.
6. Repression: a defense mechanism characterized by unconscious forgetting of unacceptable ideas or impulses.
7. Lethologica: temporary inability to remember a name or a proper noun.
8. Blackout: amnesia experienced by alcoholics about behavior during drinking bouts; usually indicates that reversible brain damage has occurred.

B. Levels of memory

1. Immediate: reproduction or recall of perceived material within seconds to minutes.
2. Recent: recall of events over past few days.
3. Recent past: recall of events over past few months.
4. Remote: recall of events in distant past.

VIII. Intelligence: ability to understand, recall, mobilize, and constructively integrate previous learning in meeting new situations.

A. Mental retardation: sufficient lack of intelligence to interfere with social and vocational performance: mild (IQ of 50 or 55 to approximately 70), moderate (IQ of 35 or 40 to 50 or 55), severe (IQ of 20 or 25 to 35 or 40), or profound (IQ below 20 or 25); obsolete terms are *idiot* (mental age less than 3 years), *imbecile* (mental age of 3 to 7 years), and *moron* (mental age of about 8).

B. Dementia: organic and global deterioration of intellectual functioning without clouding of consciousness.

1. Dyscalculia (acalculia): loss of ability to do calculations; not caused by anxiety or impairment in concentration.
2. Dysgraphia (agraphia): loss of ability to write in cursive style; loss of word structure.
3. Alexia: loss of a previously possessed reading facility; not explained by defective visual acuity.

C. Pseudodementia: clinical features resembling a dementia not caused by an organic condition; most often caused by depression (dementia syndrome of depression).

D. Concrete thinking: literal thinking; limited use of metaphor without understanding nuances of meaning; one-dimensional thought.

E. Abstract thinking: ability to appreciate nuances of meaning; multidimensional thinking with ability to use metaphors and hypotheses appropriately.

IX. Insight: ability to understand the true cause and meaning of a situation (such as a set of symptoms).

A. Intellectual insight: understanding of the objective reality of a set of circumstances without the ability to apply the understanding in any useful way to master the situation.

B. True insight: understanding of the objective reality of a situation, coupled with the motivation and the emotional impetus to master the situation.

C. Impaired insight: diminished ability to understand the objective reality of a situation.

X. Judgment: ability to assess a situation correctly and to act appropriately in the situation.

A. Critical judgment: ability to assess, discern, and choose among various options in a situation.

B. Automatic judgment: reflex performance of an action.

C. Impaired judgment: diminished ability to understand a situation correctly and to act appropriately.

References

American Psychiatric Association. *Diagnostic and Statistical Manual of Mental Disorders*. 4th ed. Text revision. Washington, DC: American Psychiatric Association; 2000.

Andreasen NC. The clinical assessment of thought, language, and communication disorders: I. The definition of terms and evaluation of their reliability. *Arch Gen Psychiatry*. 1979;36:1315.

Campbell RJ. *Psychiatric Dictionary*. 7th ed. New York: Oxford University Press; 1996.

Cassano GB, Perugi G, Musetti L, Akiskal HS. The nature of depression presenting concomitantly with panic disorder. *Compr Psychiatry*. 1989;30:473.

Coleman M, Gillberg C. *The Schizophrenias; A Biological Approach to the Schizophrenia Spectrum Disorders*. New York: Springer; 1996.

Geschwind N. Aphasia. *N Engl J Med*. 1971;284:654.

McConville M. Let the straw man speak: Husserl's phenomenology in contest. *Gestalt Rev*. 2001;5:195.

Rapaport MH, Judd LL, Schettler PJ, et al. A descriptive analysis of minor depression. *Am J Psychiatry*. 2002;159:637.

Sadler JZ, Hulgus UF. Clinical problem solving and the biopsychosocial model. *Am J Psychiatry*. 1992;149:1315.

Sadock BJ. Signs and symptoms in psychiatry. In: Sadock BJ, Sadock VA, eds. *Kaplan & Sadock's Comprehensive Textbook of Psychiatry*. 7th ed. Vol 1. Baltimore: Lippincott Williams & Wilkins; 2000.

Sadock BJ, Sadock VA. *Kaplan & Sadock's Pocket Handbook of Clinical Psychiatry*. 3rd ed. Baltimore: Lippincott Williams & Wilkins; 2001.

Spitzer RL, Gibbon M, Skodol AE, Williams JBW, First MB. *DSM-IV Casebook: A Learning Companion to the Diagnostic and Statistical Manual of Mental Disorders*. 4th ed. Washington, DC: American Psychiatric Press; 1994.

9

Classification in Psychiatry and Psychiatric Rating Scales

Advances in scientific psychiatry are to a great extent shaped by its system of classification. Systems of classification are fundamental to all sciences, containing the concepts upon which theory is based and influencing what can and cannot be seen. The classification of illnesses (*nosology*) has always been an integral part of the theory and practice of medicine.

Systems of classification for psychiatric diagnoses have several purposes: to distinguish one psychiatric diagnosis from another, so that clinicians can offer the most effective treatment; to provide a common language among health care professionals; and to explore the still unknown causes of many mental disorders. The two most important psychiatric classifications are the *Diagnostic and Statistical Manual of Mental Disorders* (DSM) developed by the American Psychiatric Association in collaboration with other groups of mental health professionals, and the *International Classification of Diseases* (ICD), developed by the World Health Organization.

DSM-IV-TR's Relation to ICD-10

The text revision of the fourth edition of DSM (DSM-IV-TR) was designed to correspond to the 10th revision of the *International Statistical Classification of Diseases and Related Health Problems* (ICD-10), developed in 1992. There was a strong consensus that diagnostic systems used in the United States must be compatible with the ICD to ensure uniform reporting of national and international health statistics. In addition, Medicare requires that billing codes for reimbursement follow ICD.

ICD-10 is the official classification system used in Europe and many other parts of the world. All categories used in DSM-IV-TR are found in ICD-10, but not all ICD-10 categories are in DSM-IV-TR. The code numbers for disorders in DSM are fully compatible with ICD and are listed in an appendix.

History

The various classification systems used in psychiatry date back to Hippocrates, who introduced the terms *mania* and *hysteria* as forms of mental illness in the fifth century BC. Since then, each era has introduced its own psychiatric classification. The first U.S. classification was introduced in 1869 at the annual meeting of the American Medico-Psychological Association, which later became the American Psychiatric Association.

In 1952, the American Psychiatric Association's Committee on Nomenclature and Statistics published the first edition of DSM (DSM-I). Five editions have been published since then: DSM-II (1968); DSM-III (1980); a revised DSM-III, DSM-III-R (1987), DSM-IV (1994), and DSM-IV-TR (2000).

DSM-IV-TR

DSM-IV-TR is the official psychiatric coding system used in the United States. Although some psychiatrists have been critical of the many versions of DSM that have appeared since 1952, DSM-IV-TR is the official U.S. nomenclature. All terminology used in this textbook conforms to DSM-IV-TR nomenclature.

Basic Features

Descriptive Approach. The approach to DSM-IV-TR is atheoretical with regard to causes. Thus, DSM-IV-TR attempts to describe the manifestations of the mental disorders and only rarely attempts to account for how the disturbances come about. The definitions of the disorders usually consist of descriptions of clinical features.

Diagnostic Criteria. Specified diagnostic criteria are provided for each specific mental disorder. These criteria include a list of features that must be present for the diagnosis to be made. Such criteria increase the reliability of the process of diagnosis.

Systematic Description. DSM-IV-TR also systematically describes each disorder in terms of its associated features: specific age-, culture-, and gender-related features; prevalence, incidence, and risk; course; complications; predisposing factors; familial pattern; and differential diagnosis. In some instances, when many specific disorders share common features, this information is included in the introduction to the entire section. Laboratory findings and associated physical examination signs and symptoms are described when relevant. DSM-IV-TR is not, and does not purport to be, a textbook: No mention is made of theories of causes, management, or treatment, and the controversial issues surrounding a particular diagnostic category are not discussed.

Table 9–1
DSM-IV-TR Axis I: Clinical Disorders and Other Disorders That May Be a Focus of Clinical Attention

Disorders usually first diagnosed in infancy, childhood, or adolescence (excluding mental retardation)
Delirium, dementia, and amnestic and other cognitive disorders
Mental disorders due to a general medical condition not elsewhere classified
Substance-related disorders
Schizophrenia and other psychotic disorders
Mood disorders
Anxiety disorders
Somatoform disorders
Factitious disorders
Dissociative disorders
Sexual and gender identity disorders
Eating disorders
Sleep disorders
Impulse-control disorders not elsewhere classified
Adjustment disorders
Other conditions that may be a focus of clinical attention

From American Psychiatric Association. *Diagnostic and Statistical Manual of Mental Disorders.* 4th ed. Text rev. Washington, DC: American Psychiatric Association; copyright 2000, with permission.

Diagnostic Uncertainties. DSM-IV-TR provides explicit rules to be used when the information is insufficient (diagnosis to be deferred or provisional) or the patient's clinical presentation and history do not meet the full criteria of a prototypical category (an atypical, residual, or not otherwise specified type within the general category).

Multiaxial Evaluation

DSM-IV-TR is a multiaxial system that evaluates patients along several variables and contains five axes. Axis I and Axis II make up the entire classification of mental disorder: 17 major classifications (Tables 9–1 and 9–2) and more than 300 specific disorders. In many instances, patients have a disorder on both axes. For example, a patient may have major depressive disorder noted on Axis I and obsessive-compulsive personality disorder on Axis II.

Axis I. Axis I consists of clinical disorders and other conditions that may be a focus of clinical attention (Table 9–1).

Axis II. Axis II consists of personality disorders and mental retardation (Table 9–2). The habitual use of a particular defense mechanism can be indicated on Axis II.

Axis III. Axis III lists any physical disorder or general medical condition that is present in addition to the mental disorder. The physical condition may be causative (e.g., kidney failure causing delirium), the result of a mental disorder (e.g., alcohol gastritis secondary to alcohol dependence), or unrelated to the mental disorder. When a medical condition is causative or causally related to a mental disorder, a mental disorder due to a general condition is listed on Axis I, and the general medical condition is listed on both Axis I and Axis III. In DSM-IV-TR's example—a case in which hypothyroidism is a direct cause of major depressive disorder—the designation on Axis I is mood disorder due to hypothyroidism with depressive features, and hypothyroidism is listed again on Axis III (Table 9–3).

Table 9–2
DSM-IV-TR Axis II: Personality Disorders and Mental Retardation

Paranoid personality disorder
Schizoid personality disorder
Schizotypal personality disorder
Antisocial personality disorder
Borderline personality disorder
Histrionic personality disorder
Narcissistic personality disorder
Avoidant personality disorder
Dependent personality disorder
Obsessive-compulsive personality disorder
Personality disorder not otherwise specified
Mental retardation

From American Psychiatric Association. *Diagnostic and Statistical Manual of Mental Disorders.* 4th ed. Text rev. Washington, DC: American Psychiatric Association; copyright 2000, with permission.

Axis IV. Axis IV is used to code the psychosocial and environmental problems that contribute significantly to the development or exacerbation of the current disorder (Table 9–4). The evaluation of stressors is based on a clinicians' assessment of the stress that an average person with similar sociocultural values and circumstances

Table 9–3
DSM-IV-TR Axis III: ICD-9-CM General Medical Conditions

Infectious and parasitic diseases (001–139)
Neoplasms (140–239)
Endocrine, nutritional, and metabolic diseases and immunity disorders (240–279)
Diseases of the blood and blood-forming organs (280–289)
Diseases of the nervous system and sense organs (320–389)
Diseases of the circulatory system (390–459)
Diseases of the respiratory system (460–519)
Diseases of the digestive system (520–579)
Diseases of the genitourinary system (580–629)
Complications of pregnancy, childbirth, and the puerperium (630–676)
Diseases of the skin and subcutaneous tissue (680–709)
Diseases of the musculoskeletal system and connective tissue (710–739)
Congenital anomalies (740–759)
Certain conditions originating in the perinatal period (760–779)
Symptoms, signs, and ill-defined conditions (780–799)
Injury and poisoning (800–999)

From American Psychiatric Association. *Diagnostic and Statistical Manual of Mental Disorders.* 4th ed. Text rev. Washington, DC: American Psychiatric Association; copyright 2000, with permission.

Table 9–4
DSM-IV-TR Axis IV: Psychosocial and Environmental Problems

Problems with primary support group
Problems related to the social environment
Educational problems
Occupational problems
Housing problems
Economic problems
Problems with access to health care services
Problems related to interaction with the legal system/crime
Other psychosocial and environmental problems

From American Psychiatric Association. *Diagnostic and Statistical Manual of Mental Disorders.* 4th ed. Text rev. Washington, DC: American Psychiatric Association; copyright 2000, with permission.

would experience from the psychosocial stressors. This judgment is based on the amount of change that the stressor causes in the person's life, the degree to which the event is desired and under the person's control, and the number of stressors. Stressors may be positive (such as a job promotion) or negative (such as the loss of a loved one). Information about stressors may be important in formulating a treatment plan that includes attempts to remove the psychosocial stressors or to help the patient cope with them.

Axis V. Axis V is a global assessment of functioning (GAF) scale in which clinicians judge patients' overall levels of functioning during a particular time (e.g., at the time of the evaluation or the patient's highest level of functioning for at least a few months during the past year). Functioning is considered a composite of three major areas: social functioning, occupational functioning, and psychological functioning. The GAF scale, based on a continuum of mental health and mental illness, is a 100-point scale, 100 representing the highest level of functioning in all areas (Table 9–5). Per-

Table 9–5
Global Assessment of Functioning (GAF) Scale

Consider psychological, social, and occupational functioning on a hypothetical continuum of mental health–illness. Do not include impairment in functioning due to physical (or environmental) limitations.

Code	(**Note:** Use intermediate codes when appropriate, e.g., 45, 68, 72.)
100–91	Superior functioning in a wide range of activities, life's problems never seem to get out of hand, is sought out by others because of his or her many positive qualities. No symptoms.
90–81	Absent or minimal symptoms (e.g., mild anxiety before an exam), good functioning in all areas, interested and involved in a wide range of activities, socially effective, generally satisfied with life, no more than everyday problems or concerns (e.g., an occasional argument with family members).
80–71	If symptoms are present, they are transient and expectable reactions to psychosocial stressors (e.g., difficulty concentrating after family argument): no more than slight impairment in social, occupational, or school functioning (e.g., temporarily falling behind in schoolwork).
70–61	Some mild symptoms (e.g., depressed mood and mild insomnia) OR some difficulty in social, occupational, or school functioning (e.g., occasional truancy, or theft within the household), but generally functioning pretty well, has some meaningful interpersonal relationships.
60–51	Moderate symptoms (e.g., flat affect and circumstantial speech, occasional panic attacks) OR moderate difficulty in social, occupational, or school functioning (e.g., few friends, conflicts with peers or coworkers).
50–41	Serious symptoms (e.g., suicidal ideation, severe obsessional rituals, frequent shoplifting) OR any serious impairment in social, occupational, or school functioning (e.g., no friends, unable to keep a job).
40–31	Some impairment in reality testing or communication (e.g., speech is at times illogical, obscure, or irrelevant) OR major impairment in several areas, such as work or school, family relations, judgment, thinking, or mood (e.g., depressed man avoids friends, neglects family, and is unable to work; child frequently beats up younger children, is defiant at home, and is failing at school).
30–21	Behavior is considerably influenced by delusions or hallucinations OR serious impairment in communication or judgment (e.g., sometimes incoherent, acts grossly inappropriately, suicidal preoccupation) OR inability to function in almost all areas (e.g., stays in bed all day; no job, home, or friends).
20–11	Some danger of hurting self or others (e.g., suicide attempts without clear expectation of death, frequently violent, manic excitement) OR occasionally fails to maintain minimal personal hygiene (e.g., smears feces) OR gross impairment in communication (e.g., largely incoherent or mute).
10–1	Persistent danger of severely hurting self or others (e.g., recurrent violence) OR persistent inability to maintain minimal personal hygiene OR serious suicidal act with clear expectation of death.
0	Inadequate information.

The GAF Scale is a revision of the GAS (Endicott J, Spitzer RL, Fleiss JL, Cohen I. The Global Assessment Scale: a procedure for measuring overall severity of psychiatric disturbance. *Arch Gen Psychiatry.* 1976;33:766) and CGAS (Shaffer D, Gould MS, Brasio J, et al. Children's Global Assessment Scale (CGAS). *Arch Gen Psychiatry.* 1983;40:1228). They are revisions of the Global Scale of the Health-Sickness Rating Scale (Luborsky I. Clinicians' judgments of mental health. *Arch Gen Psychiatry.* 1962;7:407).

From American Psychiatric Association. *Diagnostic and Statistical Manual of Mental Disorders.* 4th ed. Text rev. Washington, DC: American Psychiatric Association; copyright 2000, with permission.

Table 9–6
DSM-IV-TR Multiaxial Evaluation Report Form

The following form is offered as one possibility for reporting multiaxial evaluations. In some settings, this form may be used exactly as is; in other settings, the form may be adapted to satisfy special needs.

AXIS I: Clinical Disorders
Other Conditions That May Be a Focus of Clinical Attention

Diagnostic code ___ ___ ___ . ___ ___ DSM-IV name ____________
___ ___ ___ . ___ ___ ____________
___ ___ ___ . ___ ___ ____________

AXIS II: Personality Disorders
Mental Retardation

Diagnostic code ___ ___ ___ . ___ ___ DSM-IV name ____________
___ ___ ___ . ___ ___ ____________

AXIS III: General Medical Conditions

ICD-9-CM code ___ ___ ___ . ___ ___ ICD-9-CM name ____________
___ ___ ___ . ___ ___ ____________
___ ___ ___ . ___ ___ ____________

AXIS IV: Psychosocial and Environmental Problems

Check:

- ❑ Problems with primary support group *Specify:* ____________
- ❑ Problems related to the social environment *Specify:* ____________
- ❑ Educational problems *Specify:* ____________
- ❑ Occupational problems *Specify:* ____________
- ❑ Housing problems *Specify:* ____________
- ❑ Economic problems *Specify:* ____________
- ❑ Problems with access to health care services *Specify:* ____________
- ❑ Problems related to interaction with the legal system/crime *Specify:* ____________
- ❑ Other psychosocial and environmental problems *Specify:* ____________

AXIS V: Global Assessment of Functioning Scale

Score: ____________
Time Frame: ____________

From American Psychiatric Association. *Diagnostic and Statistical Manual of Mental Disorders.* 4th ed. Text rev. Washington, DC: American Psychiatric Association; copyright 2000, with permission.

Table 9–7
DSM-IV Examples of How to Record the Results of a DSM-IV Multiaxial Evaluation

Example 1:		
Axis I	296.23	Major depressive disorder, single episode, severe without psychotic features
	305.00	Alcohol abuse
Axis II	301.6	Dependent personality disorder
		Frequent use of denial
Axis III		None
Axis IV		Threat of job loss
Axis V	GAF = 35	(current)
Example 2:		
Axis I	300.4	Dysthymic disorder
	315.00	Reading disorder
Axis II	V71.09	No diagnosis
Axis III	382.9	Otitis media, recurrent
Axis IV		Victim of child neglect
Axis V	GAF = 53	(current)
Example 3:		
Axis I	293.83	Mood disorder due to hypothyroidism, with depressive features
Axis II	V71.09	No diagnosis, histrionic personality features
Axis III	244.9	Hypothyroidism
	365.23	Chronic angle-closure glaucoma
Axis IV		None
Axis V	GAF = 45	(on admission)
	GAF = 65	(at discharge)
Example 4:		
Axis I	V61.1	Partner relational problem
Axis II	V71.09	No diagnosis
Axis III		None
Axis IV		Unemployment
Axis V	GAF = 83	(highest level past year)

From American Psychiatric Association. *Diagnostic and Statistical Manual of Mental Disorders.* 4th ed. Text rev. Washington, DC: American Psychiatric Association; copyright 2000, with permission.

sons who had a high level of functioning before an episode of illness generally have a better prognosis than do those who had a low level of functioning.

Multiaxial Evaluation Report Form. Table 9–6 shows the DSM-IV-TR Multiaxial Evaluation Report form. Examples of how to record the results of a DSM-IV-TR multiaxial evaluation are given in Table 9–7.

Nonaxial Format

DSM-IV-TR also allows clinicians who do not wish to use the multiaxial format to list the diagnoses serially, with the principal diagnosis listed first (Table 9–8).

Severity of Disorder

Depending on the clinical picture and the presence or absence of signs and symptoms and their intensity, the severity of a disorder may be mild, moderate, or severe, and the disorder may be in partial or full remission. The following guidelines are used by DSM-IV-TR.

Mild. Few, if any, symptoms in excess of those required to make the diagnosis are present, and symptoms result in no more than minor impairment in social or occupational functioning.

Moderate. Symptoms or functional impairment between "mild" and "severe" are present.

Table 9–8
DSM-IV-TR Nonaxial Format

Clinicians who do not wish to use the multiaxial format may simply list the appropriate diagnoses. Those choosing this option should follow the general rule of recording as many coexisting mental disorders, general medical conditions, and other factors that are relevant to the care and treatment of the individual. The principal diagnosis or the reason for visit should be listed first.

The examples below illustrate the reporting of diagnoses in a format that does not use the multiaxial system.

Example 1:	
296.23	Major depressive disorder, single episode, severe without psychotic features
305.00	Alcohol abuse
301.6	Dependent personality disorder
	Frequent use of denial
Example 2:	
300.4	Dysthymic disorder
315.00	Reading disorder
382.9	Otitis media, recurrent
Example 3:	
293.83	Mood disorder due to hypothyroidism with depressive features
244.9	Hypothyroidism
365.23	Chronic angle-closure glaucoma
	Histrionic personality features
Example 4:	
V61.1	Partner relational problem

From American Psychiatric Association. *Diagnostic and Statistical Manual of Mental Disorders.* 4th ed. Text rev. Washington, DC: American Psychiatric Association; copyright 2000, with permission.

Severe. Many symptoms in excess of those required to make the diagnosis, or several symptoms that are particularly severe are present, or the symptoms result in marked impairment in social or occupational functioning.

In Partial Remission. The full criteria for the disorder were previously met, but currently only some of the symptoms or signs of the disorder remain.

In Full Remission. There are no longer any symptoms or signs of the disorder, but it is still clinically relevant to note the disorder. The differentiation of In Full Remission from recovered requires consideration of many factors, including the characteristic course of the disorder, the length of time since the last period of disturbance, the total duration of the disturbance, and the need for continued evaluation or prophylactic treatment.

Other Criteria

Multiple Diagnoses. When a person has more than one Axis I disorder, the principal diagnosis is indicated by listing it first. According to DSM-IV-TR, the *principal diagnosis* is the condition chiefly responsible for the signs and symptoms of the individual. It may be difficult in situations of "dual diagnosis" (a substance-related diagnosis such as amphetamine dependence accompanied by a non–substance-related diagnosis such as schizophrenia), which is the principal diagnosis. DSM-IV-TR states: "For example, it may be unclear which diagnosis should be considered 'principal' for an individual hospitalized with both Schizophrenia and Amphetamine Intoxication, because each condition may have contributed equally to the need for admission and treatment."

Provisional Diagnosis. If there is diagnostic uncertainty, the clinician can write "(Provisional)" following the diagnosis. A person may appear to have major depressive disorder but be unable to give an adequate history to establish that the full criteria are met. The differential diagnosis depends on the duration of illness. For example, DSM-IV-TR states, "a diagnosis of Schizophreniform Disorder requires a duration of less than 6 months and can only be given provisionally if assigned before remission has occurred."

Prior History. For some purposes, noting a prior history of a disorder may be useful. DSM states that a past diagnosis of mental disorder can "be indicated by using the specifier Prior History (e.g., Separation Anxiety Disorder, Prior History, for an individual with a history of Separation Anxiety Disorder who has no current disorder or who currently meets criteria for Panic Disorder)."

Not Otherwise Specified Categories

Each diagnosis has a "not otherwise specified" (NOS) category. According to DSM-IV-TR, an NOS diagnosis may be appropriate (1) either when the symptoms are below the diagnostic threshold for one of the specific disorders or when there is an atypical or mixed presentation, (2) the symptom pattern has not been included in the DSM-IV-TR classification but it causes clinically significant distress or impairment (research criteria for some of these symptom patterns have been included in an appendix), or (3) the cause is uncertain (i.e., whether it is primary or secondary).

Frequently Used Criteria

Criteria Used to Exclude Other Diagnoses and to Suggest Differential Diagnoses. Most criteria sets used in DSM-IV-TR include exclusion criteria to establish boundaries between disorders and to clarify differential diagnoses. The wording of the exclusion criteria reflects the various types of relations between disorders:

- **"Criteria have never been met for . . ."** This exclusion criterion is used to define a lifetime hierarchy between disorders. For example, a diagnosis of Major Depressive Disorder can no longer be given once a Manic Episode has occurred and must be changed to a diagnosis of Bipolar I Disorder.
- **"Criteria are not met for . . ."** This exclusion criterion is used to establish a hierarchy between disorders (or subtypes) defined cross-sectionally. For example, the specifier With Melancholic Features takes precedence over With Atypical Features for describing the current Major Depressive Episode.
- **"Does not occur exclusively during the course of . . ."** This exclusion criterion prevents a disorder from being diagnosed when its symptom presentation occurs only during the course of another dis-

order. For example, dementia is not diagnosed separately if it occurs only during delirium; Conversion Disorder is not diagnosed separately if it occurs only during Somatization Disorder; Bulimia Nervosa is not diagnosed separately if it occurs only during Anorexia Nervosa. This exclusion criterion is typically used in situations in which the symptoms of one disorder are associated features or a subset of the symptoms of the preempting disorder. The clinician should consider periods of partial remission as part of the "course of another disorder." It should be noted that the excluded diagnosis can be given at times when it occurs independently (e.g., when the excluding disorder is in full remission).

- **"Not due to the direct physiological effects of a substance (e.g., a drug of abuse, a medication) or a general medical condition."** This exclusion criterion is used to indicate that a substance-induced and general medical etiology must be considered and ruled out before the disorder can be diagnosed (e.g., Major Depressive Disorder can be diagnosed only after etiologies based on substance use and a general medical condition have been ruled out).
- **"Not better accounted for by . . ."** This exclusion criterion is used to indicate that the disorders mentioned in the criterion must be considered in the differential diagnosis of the presenting psychopathology and that, in boundary cases, clinical judgment will be necessary to determine which disorder provides the most appropriate diagnosis. In such cases, the "Differential Diagnosis" section of the text for the disorders should be consulted for guidance.

The general convention in DSM-IV is to allow multiple diagnoses to be assigned for those presentations that meet criteria for more than one DSM-IV disorder. In three situations, the previous exclusion criteria help to establish a diagnostic hierarchy (and thus prevent multiple diagnoses) or to highlight differential diagnostic considerations (and thus discourage multiple diagnoses):

When a Mental Disorder Due to a General Medical Condition or a Substance-Induced Disorder is responsible for the symptoms, it preempts the diagnosis for the corresponding primary disorder with the same symptoms (e.g., Cocaine-Induced Mood Disorder preempts Major Depressive Disorder). In such cases, an exclusion criterion containing the phrase "not due to the direct effects of . . ." is included in the criteria set for the primary disorder.

When a more pervasive disorder (e.g., Schizophrenia) has among its defining symptoms (or associated symptoms) what are the defining symptoms of a less pervasive disorder (e.g., Dysthymic Disorder), one of the following three exclusion criteria appears in the criteria set of the less pervasive disorder, indicating that only the more pervasive disorder is diagnosed: "Criteria have never been met for . . . ," "Criteria are not met for . . .," "does not occur exclusively during the course of. . . ".

When there are particularly difficult differential diagnostic boundaries, the phrase "not better accounted for by . . ." is included to indicate that clinical judgment is necessary to determine which diagnosis is most appropriate. For example, Panic Disorder With Agoraphobia includes the criterion "not better accounted for by Social Phobia" and Social Phobia includes the criterion "not better accounted for by Panic Disorder With Agoraphobia" in recognition of the fact that this is a particularly difficult boundary to draw. In some cases, both diagnoses might be appropriate.

Criteria for Substance-Induced Disorders. It is often difficult to determine whether presenting symptomatology is substance induced, that is, the direct physiological consequence of Substance Intoxication or Withdrawal, medication use, or toxin exposure. In an effort to provide some assistance in making this determination, two criteria have been added to each of the Substance-Induced Disorders. These criteria are intended to provide general guidelines, but at the same time allow for clinical judgment in determining whether or not the presenting symptoms are best accounted for by the direct physiological effects of the substance:

There is evidence from the history, physical examination, or laboratory findings of either or:

1. The symptoms developed during, or within a month of, Substance Intoxication or Withdrawal.
2. Medication use is etiologically related to the disturbance.

> The disturbance is not better accounted for by a disorder that is not substance induced. Evidence that the symptoms are better accounted for by a disorder that is not substance induced might include the following: symptoms precede the onset of the substance use (or medication use); symptoms persist for a substantial period of time (about 1 month) after the cessation of acute withdrawal or severe intoxication or are substantially in excess of what would be expected given the type, duration, or amount of the substance used; or other evidence suggests the existence of an independent non–substance-induced disorder (a history of recurrent non–substance-related episodes).

Criteria for a Mental Disorder Due to a General Medical Condition. The following criterion is necessary to establish the etiological requirements for each of the mental disorders due to a general medical condition (such as mood disorder due to hypothyroidism): "There is evidence from the history, physical examination, or laboratory findings that the disturbance is the direct physiological consequence of a general medical condition."

DSM-IV-TR Classification of Mental Disorders

The DSM-IV-TR classification of mental disorders (Axis I and Axis II) is provided near the end of this chapter.

Definition of Mental Disorder. According to DSM-IV-TR:

> [E]ach of the mental disorders is conceptualized as a clinically significant behavioral or psychological syndrome or pattern that occurs in an individual and that is associated with present distress (e.g., a painful symptom) or disability (i.e., impairment in one or more important areas of functioning) or with a significantly increased risk of suffering death, pain, disability, or an important loss of freedom. In addition, this syndrome or pattern must not be merely an expectable and culturally sanctioned response to a particular event, for example, the death of a loved one. Whatever its original cause, it must currently be considered a manifestation of a behavioral, psychological, or biological dysfunction in the individual. Neither deviant behavior (e.g., political, religious, or sexual) nor conflicts that are primarily between the individual and society are mental disorders unless the deviance or conflict is a symptom of a dysfunction in the individual, as described above . . . .

Distinction Between *Mental Disorder* and *General Medical Condition.*

> The terms *mental disorder* and *general medical condition* are used throughout this manual. The term *mental disorder* is explained above. The term *general medical condition* is used merely as a convenient shorthand to refer to conditions and disorders that are listed outside the "Mental and Behavioral Disorders" chapter of ICD. It should be recognized that these are merely terms of convenience and should not be taken to imply that there is any fundamental distinction between mental disorders and general medical conditions, that mental disorders are unrelated to physical or biological factors or processes, or that general medical conditions are unrelated to behavioral or psychosocial factors or processes.

Organization. The DSM-IV-TR organizational plan is described as follows:

> The first section is devoted to "Disorders Usually First Diagnosed in Infancy, Childhood, or Adolescence." This division of the Classification according to age at presentation is for convenience only and is not absolute. Although disorders in this section are usually first evident in childhood and adolescence, some individuals diagnosed with disorders located in this section (e.g., Attention-Deficit/Hyperactivity Disorder) may not present for clinical attention until adulthood. In addition, it is not uncommon for the age at onset for many disorders placed in other sections to be during childhood or adolescence (e.g., Major Depressive Disorder, Schizophrenia, Generalized Anxiety Disorder). Clinicians who work primarily with children and adolescents should therefore be familiar with the entire manual, and those who work primarily with adults should also be familiar with this section.
>
> The next three sections—"Delirium, Dementia, and Amnestic and Other Cognitive Disorders"; "Mental Disorders Due to a General Medical Condition"; and "Substance-Related Disorders"—were grouped together in DSM-III-R under the single heading of "Organic Mental Syndromes and Disorders." . . . As in DSM-III-R, these sections are placed before the remaining disorders in the manual because of their priority in differential diagnosis (e.g., substance-related causes of depressed mood must be ruled out before making a diagnosis of Major Depressive Disorder). To facilitate differential diagnosis, complete lists of Mental Disorders Due to a General Medical Condition and Substance-Related Disorders appear in these sections, whereas the text and criteria for these disorders are placed in the diagnostic sections with disorders with which they share phenomenology. For example, the text and criteria for Substance-Induced Mood Disorder and Mood Disorder Due to a General Medical Condition are included in the Mood Disorders section.
>
> The organizing principle for all the remaining sections (except for Adjustment Disorders) is to group disorders based on their shared phenomenological features in order to facilitate differential diagnosis. The "Adjustment Disorders" section is organized differently in that these disorders are grouped based on their common etiology (e.g., maladaptive reaction to a stressor). Therefore, the Adjustment Disorders include a variety of heterogeneous clinical presentations (e.g., Adjustment Disorder With Depressed Mood, Adjustment Disorder With Anxiety, Adjustment Disorder With Disturbance of Conduct).
>
> Finally, DSM-IV-TR includes a section for Other Conditions That May Be a Focus of Clinical Attention.

ICD-10. In ICD-10, a class called *neurotic, stress-related, and somatoform disorders* encompasses the following: phobic anxiety disorders, other anxiety disorders (including panic disorder, generalized anxiety disorder, and mixed anxiety and depressive disorder), obsessive-compulsive disorder, adjustment disorders, dissociative (conversion) disorders, and somatoform disorders. In addition, ICD-10 includes neurasthenia as a neurotic disorder, characterized by mental and physical fatigability, a sense of general instability, irritability, anhedonia, and sleep disturbances. Many of the cases so diagnosed outside the United States fit the descriptions of anxiety disorders and depressive disorders and are diagnosed as such by U.S. psychiatrists.

An appendix was added to DSM-IV to reflect the influence of culture and ethnicity on psychiatric assessment and diagnosis. This appendix describes culturally specific symptom patterns, preferred idioms for describing distress, and prevalence when such information is available. It also provides clinicians with guidance on how clinical presentations may be influenced by patients' cultural settings.

New and Controversial Categories

Proposed new categories that were considered controversial or for which there was insufficient information to warrant inclusion in DSM-IV-TR were placed in Appendix B, "Criteria Sets and Axes Provided for Further Study." Not all psychiatrists agree that these categories are discrete psychological disorders, and they do not agree on the essential diagnostic features. Each category requires systematic research to determine whether it will eventually be included in the official nomenclature. Nevertheless, clinicians should be familiar with the conditions, some of which are already included in ICD-10. These conditions are described briefly below.

Postconcussional Disorder. Postconcussional disorder is discussed in Chapter 10, Section 10.5. In ICD-10, it is referred to as *postconcussional syndrome,* which occurs after head trauma that usually is severe enough to result in loss of consciousness. Symptoms include headache, dizziness (usually lacking the features of true vertigo), fatigue, irritability, difficulty concentrating and performing mental tasks, memory impairment, insomnia, and reduced tolerance for stress, emotional excitement, and alcohol abuse.

Mild Neurocognitive Disorder. This condition is discussed in Chapter 10, Section 10.1.

Caffeine Withdrawal. This disorder is covered in Chapter 12, Section 12.4.

Postpsychotic Depressive Disorder of Schizophrenia. This disorder is discussed in Chapter 15, Section 15.3. In ICD-10, postschizophrenic depression is described as follows:

A depressive episode, which may be prolonged, arising in the aftermath of a schizophrenic illness. Some schizophrenic symptoms must still be present but no longer dominate the clinical picture. These persisting schizophrenic symptoms may be "positive" or "negative," though the latter are more common. It is uncertain, and immaterial to the diagnosis, to what extent the depressive symptoms have merely been uncovered by the resolution of earlier psychotic symptoms (rather than being a new development) or are an intrinsic part of schizophrenia rather than a psychological reaction to it. They are rarely sufficiently severe or extensive to meet criteria for a severe depressive episode, and it is often difficult to decide which of the patient's symptoms are due to depression and which to neuroleptic medication or to the impaired volition and affective flattening of schizophrenia itself. This depressive disorder is associated with an increased risk of suicide.

Simple Deteriorative Disorder. This disorder is covered in Chapter 13 and Chapter 14, Section 14.4. In ICD-10, it is described as an uncommon disorder characterized by oddities of conduct, inability to meet the demands of society, blunting of affect, loss of volition, and social impoverishment. Delusions and hallucinations are not evident.

Minor Depressive Disorder, Recurrent Brief Depressive Disorder, and Premenstrual Dysphoric Disorder. These disorders are covered in Chapter 15, Section 15.3. Minor depressive disorder is associated with comparatively mild symptoms, such as worry and overconcern with minor autonomic symptoms (e.g., tremor and palpitations). Most cases never come to medical or psychiatric attention. In ICD-10, recurrent brief depressive disorder is characterized by recurrent episodes of depression, each of which lasts less than 2 weeks (typically 2 to 3 days) and ends with complete recovery.

Mixed Anxiety-Depressive Disorder. This disorder is covered in Chapter 16, Section 16.7. Mixed anxiety and depressive disorder is listed in ICD-10, where it is described as encompassing symptoms of both anxiety and depression, neither of which predominates.

Factitious Disorder by Proxy. This disorder, also known as Munchausen syndrome by proxy, is discussed in Chapter 19. In the disorder, parents feign illness in their children.

Dissociative Trance Disorder. The dissociative disorders are discussed in Chapter 20. ICD-10 lists trance and possession disorders, in which a patient experiences temporary loss of both the sense of personal identity and full awareness of the surroundings. The disorders are involuntary or unwanted. In some cases, patients act as if taken over by another personality, spirit, or force.

Binge-Eating Disorder. This disorder is a variant of bulimia nervosa, which is discussed in Chapter 23, Section 23.2. It consists of recurrent episodes of binge eating without compensatory behavior, such as self-induced vomiting and laxative abuse.

Depressive Personality Disorder and Passive-Aggressive Personality Disorder. These personality disorders are classified in the NOS category of personality disorders. Each is described in Chapter 27.

Medication-Induced Movement Disorders. These disorders are caused by the adverse effects of medication. They include parkinsonism, neuroleptic malignant syndrome, acute dystonia, acute akathisia, tardive dyskinesia, postural tremor, and NOS movement disorder. These disorders are discussed in Chapter 36, Section 36.3.

Culture-Bound Syndromes

An appendix of culturally related syndromes includes the name of each condition, the culture in which it was first described, a brief description of its psychopathology, and a list of possibly related DSM-IV-TR categories. Chapter 14, Section 14.5 includes a discussion of culture-bound syndromes.

The implication of culture and its relation to diagnosis is set forth in DSM-IV-TR as follows:

> Diagnostic assessment can be especially challenging when a clinician from one ethnic or cultural group uses the DSM-IV Classification to evaluate an individual from a different ethnic or cultural group. A clinician who is unfamiliar with the nuances of an individual's cultural frame of reference may incorrectly judge as psychopathology those normal variations in behavior, belief, or experience that are particular to the individual's culture. For example, certain religious practices or beliefs (e.g., hearing or seeing a deceased relative during bereavement) may be misdiagnosed as manifestations of a Psychotic Disorder. Applying Personality Disorder criteria across cultural settings may be especially difficult because of the wide cultural variation in concepts of self, styles of communication, and coping mechanisms.

Guidelines

Cautionary Statement. The American Psychiatric Association has issued a cautionary statement about the proper use and interpretation of the diagnostic categories in DSM-IV. It reads as follows:

> These diagnostic criteria and the DSM-IV Classification of mental disorders reflect a consensus of current formulations of evolving knowledge in our field. They do not encompass, however, all the conditions for which people may be treated or appropriate topics for research efforts.

Caveats. DSM-IV-TR describes specific caveats regarding its use:

> LIMITATIONS OF THE CATEGORICAL APPROACH. There is no assumption that each category of mental disorder is a completely discrete entity with absolute boundaries dividing it from other mental disorders or from no mental disorder. There is also no assumption that all individuals described as having the same mental disorder are alike in all important ways. The clinician using the DSM-IV should

therefore consider that individuals sharing a diagnosis are likely to be heterogeneous even in regard to the defining features of the diagnosis and that boundary cases will be difficult to diagnose in any but a probabilistic fashion.

USE OF CLINICAL JUDGMENT. The specific diagnostic criteria included in DSM-IV are meant to serve as guidelines to be informed by clinical judgment and are not meant to be used in a cookbook fashion. For example, the exercise of clinical judgment may justify giving a certain diagnosis to an individual even though the clinical presentation falls just short of meeting the full criteria for the diagnosis as long as the symptoms that are present are persistent and severe.

USE OF DSM-IV IN FORENSIC SETTINGS. In most situations, the clinical diagnosis of a DSM-IV mental disorder is not sufficient to establish the existence for legal purposes of a "mental disorder," "mental disability," "mental disease," or "mental defect." In determining whether an individual meets a specified legal standard (e.g., for competence, criminal responsibility, or disability), additional information is usually required beyond that contained in the DSM-IV diagnosis.

Decision Trees. Decision trees, also known as algorithms, are diagrammatic tracks that organize a clinician's thinking so that all differential diagnoses are considered and ruled in or out, resulting in a presumptive diagnosis. Beginning with specific signs or symptoms, the psychiatrist follows the positive or negative track down the tree (by answering yes or no) until a point in the tree with no outgoing branches (known as a leaf) is found. This point is the final diagnosis. Figure 9–1 is an example of a decision tree for psychotic disorders. DSM-IV-TR includes an appendix of diagnostic decision trees.

PSYCHIATRIC RATING SCALES

Psychiatric rating scales, also called *rating instruments,* provide a way to quantify aspects of a patient's psyche, behavior, and relationships with individuals and society. The measurement of pathology in these areas of a person's life may initially seem less straightforward than the measurement of pathology—hypertension, for example—by other medical specialists. Nevertheless, many psychiatric rating scales can measure carefully chosen features of well-formulated concepts. Moreover, psychiatrists who do not use these rating scales are left with only their clinical impressions, which are difficult to record in a manner that allows reliable future comparison and communication. Without psychiatric rating scales, quantitative data in psychiatry are crude (e.g., length of hospitalization or other treatment, discharge and readmission to hospital, length of relationships or employment, and presence of legal troubles). Table 9–9 lists a variety of rating scales and the initial reference source for each. Some commonly used instruments are found in Tables 9–10 through 9–15.

Characteristics of Rating Scales

Rating scales can be specific or comprehensive, and they can measure both internally experienced variables (e.g., mood) and externally observable variables (e.g., behavior). Specific scales measure discrete thoughts, moods, or behaviors, such as obsessive thoughts and temper tantrums; comprehensive scales measure broad abstractions, such as depression and anxiety.

Signs and Symptoms. Classic items from the mental status examination are the most frequently assessed items on rating scales. These items include thought disorders, mood disturbances, and gross behaviors. Rating scales also cover the assessment of adverse effects from psychotherapeutic drugs. Social adjustments (e.g., occupational success and quality of relationships) and psychoanalytic concepts (e.g., ego strength and defense mechanisms) are also measured by some rating scales, although the reliability and the validity of such scales are lowered by the absence of agreed-on norms, the high level of inference required on some items, and the lack of independence between measures.

Other Characteristics. Other characteristics of rating scales include the time covered, the level of judgment required, and the method of recording answers. The time covered by a rating scale must be specified, and the rate must adhere to this period. For example, a particular rating scale may rate a 5-minute observation period, a week-long period, or a patient's entire life.

The most reliable rating scales require a limited amount of judgment or inference on the part of the rater. Whatever the level of judgment required, clear definitions of the answer scale, preferably with clinical examples, should be provided by the developer of the scale and should be read by the rater.

The actual answer given may be recorded as either a dichotomous variable (e.g., true or false, present or absent) or a continuous variable. Continuous items may ask the rater to choose a term to describe severity (absent, slight, mild, moderate, severe, or extreme) or frequency (never, rarely, occasionally, often, very often, or always). Although many psychiatric symptoms are thought of as existing in dichotomous states—for example, the presence or absence of delusions—most experienced clinicians know that the world is not so simple.

Rating Scales Used in DSM-IV-TR

Rating scales form an integral part of DSM-IV-TR. The rating scales used are broad and measure the overall severity of a patient's illness.

GAF Scale. Axis V in DSM-IV uses the GAF scale (Table 9–5). This axis is used to report a clinician's judgment of a patient's overall level of functioning. The information is used to decide on a treatment plan and later to measure the plan's effect.

Social and Occupational Functioning Assessment Scale. This scale can be used to track a patient's progress in social and occupational areas (Table 9–16). It is independent of the psychiatric diagnosis and the severity of the patient's psychological symptoms.

Other Scales. Two other scales that may be useful are the Global Assessment of Relational Functioning (GARF) Scale (Table 9–17) and the Defensive Functioning Scale (Table 9–18).

DSM-IV-TR and ICD-10 Classifications and Codes

Table 9–19 lists the DSM-IV-TR classification with ICD-9-CM codes. Table 9–20 lists the ICD-10 classification of mental disorders and ICD-10 codes.

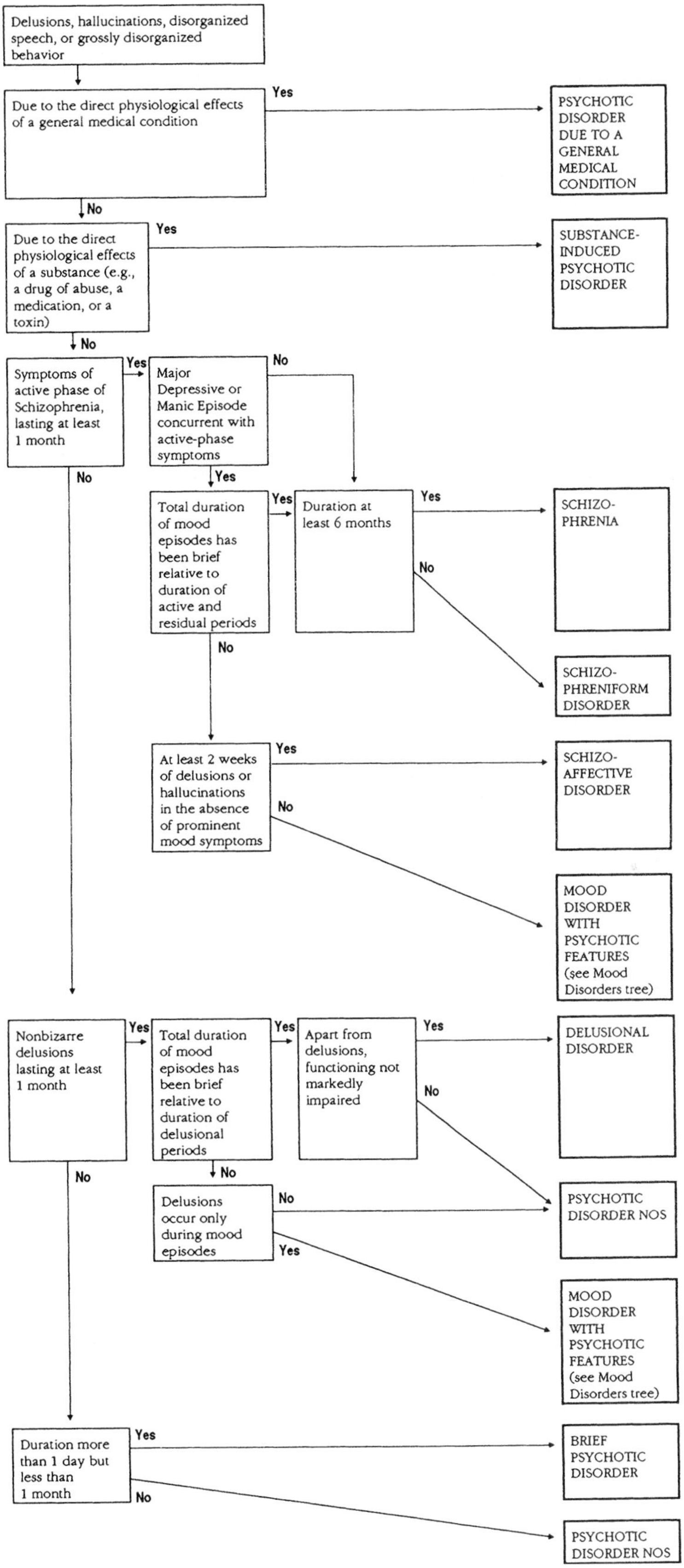

FIGURE 9–1

Differential diagnosis of psychotic disorders. (Reprinted with permission from American Psychiatric Association: *Diagnostic and Statistical Manual of Mental Disorders,* 4th ed. Washington, DC: American Psychiatric Association; 2000.)

Table 9–9
Psychiatric Rating Scales

Scale	Source
Rating scales used for schizophrenia and psychosis	
Brief Psychiatric Rating Scale	*Psychological Reports* 1962;10:799.
Schedule for Affective Disorders and Schizophrenia (SADS)	*Archives of General Psychiatry* 1978;35:837.
Scale for the Assessment of Negative Symptoms (SANS)	University of Iowa Press, 1983.
Scale for the Assessment of Thought, Language, and Communication (TLC)	University of Iowa Press, 1978.
Thought Disorder Index (TDI)	*Archives of General Psychiatry* 1983;40:1281.
Quality of Life Scale (QLS)	*Schizophrenia Bulletin* 1984;10:383.
Chestnut Lodge Prognostic Scale for Chronic Schizophrenia	*Schizophrenia Bulletin* 1987;13:277.
Rating scales used for mood disorders	
Beck Depression Inventory	*Archives of General Psychiatry* 1961;4:561.
Standard Assessment of Depressive Disorders (SADD)	*Psychological Medicine* 1979;10:743.
Zung Self-Rating Scale for Depression	*Archives of General Psychiatry* 1965;12:63.
Carroll Rating Scale for Depression	*British Journal of Psychiatry* 1981;138:194.
Montgomery-Asberg Scale	*British Journal of Psychiatry* 1979;134:382.
Raskin Depression Rating Scale	*Journal of Nervous and Mental Disease* 1969;148:87.
Inventory to Diagnose Depression	*Archives of General Psychiatry* 1986;43:1976.
Mania Rating Scale	*Journal of Clinical Psychiatry* 1983;44:98.
Manic State Rating Scale	*Archives of General Psychiatry* 1971;25:256.
Rating scales used for anxiety disorders	
Brief Outpatient Psychopathology Scale	*Journal of Clinical Pharmacology* 1969;9:187.
Physicians Questionnaire	*Psychopharmacologia* 1970;17:338.
Covi Anxiety Scale	*Psychopharmacology Bulletin* 1982;18:69.
Anxiety States Inventory	*Psychosomatics* 1971;12:371.
Fear Questionnaire	*Behavioral Research and Therapeutics* 1979;17:263.
Mobility Inventory for Agoraphobia	*Behavioral Research and Therapeutics* 1985;23:35.
Social Avoidance and Distress Scale	*Journal of Consulting and Clinical Psychology* 1969;33:448.
Acute Panic Inventory	*Archives of General Psychiatry* 1984;41:764.
Leyton Obsessional Inventory	*Psychological Medicine* 1970;1:48.
Maudsley Obsessional-Compulsive Inventory	*Behavioral Research and Therapeutics* 1977;15:389.
Fear Thermometer	*Journal of Consulting and Clinical Psychiatry* 1983;15:488.
Impact of Events Scale	*Psychosomatic Medicine* 1979;41:209.
Other rating scales	
Child and adolescent patients	
General reference for adult scales that have been modified for children	*Psychopharmacology Bulletin* 1985;21:737.
Adverse effects of drugs	
Systematic Assessment for Treatment of Emergent Events (SAFTEE): General Inquiry (GI) Systematic Inquiry (SI)	*Psychopharmacology Bulletin* 1986;22:343.
Quality of life	
Patterns of Individual Change Scale (PICS)	*Archives of General Psychiatry* 1985;42:703.
Dissociative disorders	
Structured Clinical Interview for DSM-IV Dissociative Disorders (SCID-IV)	*American Journal of Psychiatry* 1993;150:1011.

Table 9–10
Brief Psychiatric Rating Scale

DIRECTIONS: Place an X in the appropriate box to represent the level of severity of each symptom.

PATIENT______________________________

RATER______________________________

NO.______________________________

DATE______________________________

	Not present = 0	**Very mild = 1**	**Mild = 2**	**Moderate = 3**	**Mod. severe = 4**	**Severe = 5**	**Extremely severe = 6**
	0	**1**	**2**	**3**	**4**	**5**	**6**
1. Somatic concern—preoccupation with physical health, fear of physical illness, hypochondriases	❑	❑	❑	❑	❑	❑	❑
2. Anxiety—worry, fear, overconcern for present or future	❑	❑	❑	❑	❑	❑	❑
3. Emotional withdrawal—lack of spontaneous interaction, isolation, deficiency in relating to others	❑	❑	❑	❑	❑	❑	❑
4. Conceptual disorganization—thought processes confused, disconnected, disorganized, disrupted	❑	❑	❑	❑	❑	❑	❑
5. Guilt feelings—self-blame, shame, remorse for past behavior	❑	❑	❑	❑	❑	❑	❑
6. Tension—physical and motor manifestations or nervousness, overactivation, tension	❑	❑	❑	❑	❑	❑	❑
7. Mannerisms and posturing—peculiar, bizarre, unnatural motor behavior (not including tic)	❑	❑	❑	❑	❑	❑	❑
8. Grandiosity—exaggerated self-opinion, arrogance, conviction of unusual power or abilities	❑	❑	❑	❑	❑	❑	❑
9. Depressive mood—sorrow, sadness, despondency, pessimism	❑	❑	❑	❑	❑	❑	❑
10. Hostility—animosity, contempt, belligerence, disdain for others	❑	❑	❑	❑	❑	❑	❑
11. Suspiciousness—mistrust, belief that others harbor malicious or discriminatory intent	❑	❑	❑	❑	❑	❑	❑
12. Hallucinatory behavior—perceptions without normal external stimulus correspondence	❑	❑	❑	❑	❑	❑	❑
13. Motor retardation—slowed, weakened movements or speech, reduced body tone	❑	❑	❑	❑	❑	❑	❑
14. Uncooperativeness—resistance, guardedness, rejection of authority	❑	❑	❑	❑	❑	❑	❑
15. Unusual thought content—unusual, odd, strange, bizarre thought content	❑	❑	❑	❑	❑	❑	❑
16. Blunted affect—reduced emotional tone, reduction in normal intensity of feelings, flatness	❑	❑	❑	❑	❑	❑	❑
17. Excitement—heightened emotional tone, agitation, increased reactivity	❑	❑	❑	❑	❑	❑	❑
18. Disorientation—confusion or lack of proper association for person, place, or time	❑	❑	❑	❑	❑	❑	❑

Courtesy of John E. Overall, Ph.D.

Table 9–11
Hamilton Anxiety Rating Scale

Instructions: This checklist is to assist the physician or psychiatrist in evaluating each patient as to his degree of anxiety and pathological condition. Please fill in the appropriate rating:

NONE = 0 MILD = 1 MODERATE = 2 SEVERE = 3 SEVERE, GROSSLY DISABLING = 4

Item		**Rating**	**Item**		**Rating**
Anxious	Worries, anticipation of the worst, fearful anticipation, irritability	______	Somatic (sensory)	Tinnitus, blurring of vision, hot and cold flushes, feelings of weakness, picking sensation	______
Tension	Feelings of tension, fatigability, startle response, moved to tears easily, trembling, feelings of restlessness, inability to relax	______	Cardiovascular symptoms	Tachycardia, palpitations, pain in chest, throbbing of vessels, fainting feelings, missing beat	______
Fears	Of dark, of strangers, of being left alone, of animals, of traffic, of crowds	______	Respiratory symptoms	Pressure or constriction in chest, choking feelings, sighing, dyspnea	______
Insomnia	Difficulty in falling asleep, broken sleep, unsatisfying sleep and fatigue on waking, dreams, nightmares, night-terrors	______	Gastrointestinal symptoms	Difficulty in swallowing, wind, abdominal pain, burning sensations, abdominal fullness, nausea, vomiting, borborygmi, looseness of bowels, loss of weight, constipation	______
Intellectual (cognitive)	Difficulty in concentration, poor memory	______	Genitourinary symptoms	Frequency of micturition, urgency of micturition, amenorrhea, menorrhagia, development of frigidity, premature ejaculation, loss of libido, impotence	______
Depressed mood	Loss of interest, lack of pleasure in hobbies, depression, early waking, diurnal swing	______	Autonomic symptoms	Dry mouth, flushing, pallor, tendency to sweat, giddiness, tension headache, raising of hair	______
Somatic (muscular)	Pains and aches, twitching, stiffness, myoclonic jerks, grinding of teeth, unsteady voice, increased muscular tone	______	Behavior at interview	Fidgeting, restlessness or pacing, tremor of hands, furrowed brow, strained face, sighing or rapid respiration, facial pallor, swallowing, belching, brisk tendon jerks, dilated pupils, exophthalmos	______

ADDITIONAL COMMENTS

Investigator's signature:

Reprinted with permission from Hamilton M. The assessment of anxiety states by rating. *Br J Psychiatry.* 1959;32:50.

Table 9–12
Hamilton Rating Scale for Depression

For each item select the "cue" which best characterizes the patient.

1: Depressed mood (Sadness, hopeless, helpless, worthless)
- 0 Absent
- 1 These feeling states indicated only on questioning
- 2 These feeling states spontaneously reported verbally
- 3 Communicates feeling states nonverbally—i.e., through facial expression, posture, voice, and tendency to weep
- 4 Patient reports VIRTUALLY ONLY these feeling states in his spontaneous verbal and nonverbal communication

2: Feelings of guilt
- 0 Absent
- 1 Self-reproach, feels he has let people down
- 2 Ideas of guilt or rumination over past errors or sinful deeds
- 3 Present illness is a punishment. Delusions of guilt
- 4 Hears accusatory or denunciatory voices and/or experiences threatening visual hallucinations

3: Suicide
- 0 Absent
- 1 Feels life is not worth living
- 2 Wishes he were dead or any thoughts of possible death to self
- 3 Suicide ideas or gesture
- 4 Attempts at suicide (any serious attempt rates 4)

4: Insomnia early
- 0 No difficulty falling asleep
- 1 Complains of occasional difficulty falling asleep—i.e., more than 1/4 hour
- 2 Complains of nightly difficulty falling asleep

5: Insomnia middle
- 0 No difficulty
- 1 Patient complains of being restless and disturbed during the night
- 2 Waking during the night—any getting out of bed rates 2 (except for purpose of voiding)

(*continued*)

Table 9–12 (*continued*)

6: Insomnia late
- 0 No difficulty
- 1 Waking in early hours of the morning but goes back to sleep
- 2 Unable to fall asleep again if gets out of bed

7: Work and activities
- 0 No difficulty
- 1 Thoughts and feelings of incapacity, fatigue, or weakness related to activities, work, or hobbies
- 2 Loss of interest in activity, hobbies, or work—either directly reported by patient, or indirect in listlessness, indecision, and vacillation (feels he has to push self to work or activities)
- 3 Decrease in actual time spent in activities or decrease in productivity. In hospital, rate 3 if patient does not spend at least three hours a day in activities (hospital job or hobbies) exclusive of ward chores
- 4 Stopped working because of present illness. In hospital, rate 4 if patient engages in no activities except ward chores, or if patient fails to perform ward chores unassisted

8: Retardation (Slowness of thought and speech; impaired ability to concentrate; decreased motor activity)
- 0 Normal speech and thought
- 1 Slight retardation at interview
- 2 Obvious retardation at interview
- 3 Interview difficult
- 4 Complete stupor

9: Agitation
- 0 None
- 1 "Playing with" hands, hair, etc.
- 2 Hand-wringing, nail biting, hair pulling, biting of lips

10: Anxiety psychic
- 0 No difficulty
- 1 Subjective tension and irritability
- 2 Worrying about minor matters
- 3 Apprehensive attitude apparent in face or speech
- 4 Fears expressed without questioning

11: Anxiety somatic

0 Absent	Physiological concomitants of anxiety, such as:
1 Mild	Gastrointestinal—dry mouth, wind, indigestion, diarrhea, cramps, belching
2 Moderate	Cardiovascular—palpitations, headaches
3 Severe	Respiratory—hyperventilation, sighing
4 Incapacitating	Urinary frequency
	Sweating

12: Somatic symptoms gastrointestinal
- 0 None
- 1 Loss of appetite but eating without staff encouragement. Heavy feelings in abdomen
- 2 Difficulty eating without staff urging; requests or requires laxatives or medication for bowels or medication for G.I. symptoms

13: Somatic symptoms general
- 0 None
- 1 Heaviness in limbs, back or head. Backaches, headache, muscle aches. Loss of energy and fatigability
- 2 Any clear-cut symptom rates 2

14: Genital symptoms

0 Absent	Symptoms such as:
1 Mild	Loss of libido
2 Severe	Menstrual disturbances

15: Hypochondriasis
- 0 Not present
- 1 Self-absorption (bodily)
- 2 Preoccupation with health
- 3 Frequent complaints, requests for help, etc.
- 4 Hypochondriacal delusions

16: Loss of weight
- A: When rating by history
  - 0 No weight loss
  - 1 Probable weight loss associated with present illness
  - 2 Definite (according to patient) weight loss
- B: On weekly ratings by ward psychiatrist, when actual weight changes are measured
  - 0 Less than 1 lb weight loss in week
  - 1 Greater than 1 lb weight loss in week
  - 2 Greater than 2 lb weight loss in week

17: Insight
- 0 Acknowledges being depressed and ill
- 1 Acknowledges illness but attributes cause to bad food, climate, overwork, virus, need for rest, etc.
- 2 Denies being ill at all

18: Diurnal variation

AM	PM		
0	0	Absent	If symptoms are worse in the morning or evening, note which it is and rate severity of variation
1	1	Mild	
2	2	Severe	

19: Depersonalization and derealization

0 Absent	
1 Mild	Such as:
2 Moderate	Feeling of unreality
3 Severe	Nihilistic ideas
4 Incapacitating	

20: Paranoid symptoms
- 0 None
- 1, 2 Suspiciousness
- 3 Ideas of reference
- 4 Delusions of reference and persecution

21: Obsessional and compulsive symptoms
- 0 Absent
- 1 Mild
- 2 Severe

22: Helplessness
- 0 Not present
- 1 Subjective feelings which are elicited only by inquiry
- 2 Patient volunteers his helpless feelings
- 3 Requires urging, guidance, and reassurance to accomplish ward chores or personal hygiene
- 4 Requires physical assistance for dress, grooming, eating, bedside tasks, or personal hygiene

23: Hopelessness
- 0 Not present
- 1 Intermittently doubts that "things will improve" but can be reassured
- 2 Consistently feels "hopeless" but accepts reassurances
- 3 Expresses feelings of discouragement, despair, pessimism about future, which cannot be dispelled
- 4 Spontaneously and inappropriately perseverates: "I'll never get well" or its equivalent

24: Worthlessness (Ranges from mild loss of esteem, feelings of inferiority, self-deprecation to delusional notions of worthlessness)
- 0 Not present
- 1 Indicates feelings of worthlessness (loss of self-esteem) only on questioning
- 2 Spontaneously indicates feelings of worthlessness (loss of self-esteem)
- 3 Different from 2 by degree. Patient volunteers that he is "no good," "inferior," etc.
- 4 Delusional notions of worthlessness—i.e., "I am a heap of garbage" or its equivalent

Reprinted with permission from Hamilton M. A rating scale for depression. *J Neurol Neurosurg Psychiatry.* 1960;23:56.

Table 9–13
Yale-Brown Obsessive-Compulsive Scale

For each item circle the number identifying the response which best characterizes the patient.

1. Time occupied by obsessive thoughts
   How much of your time is occupied by obsessive thoughts?
   How frequently do the obsessive thoughts occur?
   0 None
   1 Mild (less than 1 hr/day) or occasional (intrusion occurring no more than 8 times a day)
   2 Moderate (1 to 3 hr/day) or frequent (intrusion occurring more than 8 times a day, but most of the hours of the day are free of obsessions)
   3 Severe (greater than 3 and up to 8 hr/day) or very frequent (intrusion occurring more than 8 times a day and occurring during most of the hours of the day)
   4 Extreme (greater than 8 hr/day) or near consistent intrusion (too numerous to count and an hour rarely passes without several obsessions occurring)
2. Interference due to obsessive thoughts
   How much do your obsessive thoughts interfere with your social or work (or role) functioning? Is there anything that you don't do because of them?
   0 None
   1 Mild, slight interference with social or occupational activities, but overall performance not impaired
   2 Moderate, definite interference with social or occupational performance but still manageable
   3 Severe, causes substantial impairment in social or occupational performance
   4 Extreme, incapacitating
3. Distress associated with obsessive thoughts
   How much distress do your obsessive thoughts cause you?
   0 None
   1 Mild, infrequent, and not too disturbing
   2 Moderate, frequent, and disturbing but still manageable
   3 Severe, very frequent, and very disturbing
   4 Extreme, near constant, and disabling distress
4. Resistance against obsessions
   How much of an effort do you make to resist the obsessive thoughts?
   How often do you try to disregard or turn your attention away from these thoughts as they enter your mind?
   0 Makes an effort to always resist, or symptoms so minimal doesn't need to actively resist
   1 Tries to resist most of the time
   2 Makes some effort to resist
   3 Yields to all obsessions without attempting to control them, but does so with some reluctance
   4 Completely and willingly yields to all obsessions
5. Degree of control over obsessive thoughts
   How much control do you have over your obsessive thoughts?
   How successful are you in stopping or diverting your obsessive thinking?
   0 Complete control
   1 Much control, usually able to stop or divert obsessions with some effort and concentration
   2 Moderate control, sometimes able to stop or divert obsessions
   3 Little control, rarely successful in stopping obsessions
   4 No control, experienced as completely involuntary, rarely able to even momentarily divert thinking
6. Time spent performing compulsive behaviors
   How much time do you spend performing compulsive behaviors? How frequently do you perform compulsions?
   0 None
   1 Mild (less than 1 hr/day performing compulsions) or occasional (performance of compulsions occurring no more than 8 times a day)
   2 Moderate (1 to 3 hr/day performing compulsions) or frequent (performance of compulsions occurring more than 8 times a day, but most of the hours of the day are free of compulsive behaviors)
   3 Severe (greater than 3 and up to 8 hr/day performing compulsions) or very frequent (performance of compulsions occurring more than 8 times a day and occurring during most of the hours of the day)
   4 Extreme (greater than 8 hr/day performing compulsions) or near consistent performance of compulsions (too numerous to count and an hour rarely passes without several compulsions being performed)
7. Interference due to compulsive behaviors
   How much do your compulsive behaviors interfere with your social or work (or role) functioning? Is there anything that you don't do because of the compulsions?
   0 None
   1 Mild, slight interference with social or occupational activities, but overall performance not impaired
   2 Moderate, definite interference with social or occupational performance but still manageable
   3 Severe, causes substantial impairment in social or occupational performance
   4 Extreme, incapacitating
8. Distress associated with compulsive behavior
   How would you feel if prevented from performing your compulsions?
   How anxious would you become? How anxious do you get while performing compulsions until you are satisfied they are completed?
   0 None
   1 Mild, only slightly anxious if compulsions prevented or only slightly anxious during performance of compulsions
   2 Moderate, reports that anxiety would mount but remain manageable if compulsions prevented or that anxiety increases but remains manageable during performance of compulsions
   3 Severe, prominent, and very disturbing increase in anxiety if compulsions interrupted or prominent and very disturbing increases in anxiety during performance of compulsions
   4 Extreme, incapacitating anxiety from any intervention aimed at modifying activity or incapacitating anxiety develops during performance of compulsions
9. Resistance against compulsions
   How much of an effort do you make to resist the compulsions?
   0 Makes an effort to always resist, or symptoms so minimal doesn't need to actively resist
   1 Tries to resist most of the time
   2 Makes some effort to resist
   3 Yields to all compulsions without attempting to control them but does so with some reluctance
   4 Completely and willingly yields to all compulsions
10. Degree of control over compulsive behavior
   0 Complete control
   1 Much control, experiences pressure to perform the behavior but usually able to exercise voluntary control over it
   2 Moderate control, strong pressure to perform behavior, can control it only with difficulty
   3 Little control, very strong drive to perform behavior, must be carried to completion, can only delay with difficulty
   4 No control, drive to perform behavior experienced as completely involuntary

Reprinted with permission from Goodman WK, Price LH, Rasmussen SA, et al. The Yale-Brown Obsessive-Compulsive Scale, I: Development, use, and reliability. *Arch Gen Psychiatry.* 1989;46:1006.

Table 9–14
Scale for the Assessment of Negative Symptoms (SANS)

0 = None 1 = Questionable 2 = Mild 3 = Moderate 4 = Marked 5 = Severe

Affective flattening or blunting	
1 *Unchanging facial expression* The patient's face appears wooden, changes less than expected as emotional content of discourse changes.	0 1 2 3 4 5
2 *Decreased spontaneous movements* The patient shows few or no spontaneous movements, does not shift position, move extremities, etc.	0 1 2 3 4 5
3 *Paucity of expressive gestures* The patient does not use hand gestures, body position, etc., as an aid to expressing his ideas.	0 1 2 3 4 5
4 *Poor eye contact* The patient avoids eye contact or "stares through" interviewer even when speaking.	0 1 2 3 4 5
5 *Affective nonresponsivity* The patient fails to smile or laugh when prompted.	0 1 2 3 4 5
6 *Lack of vocal inflections* The patient fails to show normal vocal emphasis patterns, is often monotonic.	0 1 2 3 4 5
7 *Global rating of affective flattening* This rating should focus on overall severity of symptoms, especially unresponsiveness, eye contact, facial expression, and vocal inflections.	0 1 2 3 4 5
Alogia	
8 *Poverty of speech* The patient's replies to questions are restricted in *amount,* tend to be brief, concrete, and unelaborated.	0 1 2 3 4 5
9 *Poverty of content of speech* The patient's replies are adequate in amount but tend to be vague, overconcrete, or overgeneralized, and convey little information.	0 1 2 3 4 5
10 *Blocking* The patient indicates, either spontaneously or with prompting, that his [her] train of thought was interrupted.	0 1 2 3 4 5
11 *Increased latency of response* The patient takes a long time to reply to questions; prompting indicates the patient is aware of the question.	0 1 2 3 4 5
12 *Global rating of alogia* The core features of alogia are poverty of speech and poverty of content.	0 1 2 3 4 5
Avolition-apathy	
13 *Grooming and hygiene* The patient's clothes may be sloppy or soiled, and he [she] may have greasy hair, body odor, etc.	0 1 2 3 4 5
14 *Impersistence at work or school* The patient has difficulty seeking or maintaining employment, completing school work, keeping house, etc. If an inpatient, cannot persist at ward activities, such as occupational therapy, playing cards, etc.	0 1 2 3 4 5
15 *Physical anergia* The patient tends to be physically inert. He [she] may sit for hours and does not initiate spontaneous activity.	0 1 2 3 4 5
16 *Global rating of avolition-apathy* Strong weight may be given to one or two prominent symptoms if particularly striking.	0 1 2 3 4 5
Anhedonia-asociality	
17 *Recreational interests and activities* The patient may have few or no interests. Both the quality and quantity of interests should be taken into account.	0 1 2 3 4 5
18 *Sexual activity* The patient may show a decrease in sexual interest and activity, or enjoyment when active.	0 1 2 3 4 5
19 *Ability to feel intimacy and closeness* The patient may display an inability to form close or intimate relationships, especially with the opposite sex and family.	0 1 2 3 4 5
20 *Relationships with friends and peers* The patient may have few or no friends and may prefer to spend all of his [her] time isolated.	0 1 2 3 4 5
21 *Global rating of anhedonia-asociality* This rating should reflect overall severity, taking into account the patient's age, family status, etc.	0 1 2 3 4 5
Attention	
22 *Social inattentiveness* The patient appears uninvolved or unengaged. He [she] may seem spacey.	0 1 2 3 4 5
23 *Inattentiveness during mental status testing* Tests of "serial 7s" (at least five subtractions) and spelling *world* backwards: Score: 2 = 1 error; 3 = 2 errors; 4 = 3 errors.	0 1 2 3 4 5
24 *Global rating of attention* This rating should assess the patient's overall concentration, clinically and on tests.	0 1 2 3 4 5

Bracketed words are our addition.

Table 9–15
Scale for the Assessment of Positive Symptoms (SAPS)

0 = None 1 = Questionable 2 = Mild 3 = Moderate 4 = Marked 5 = Severe

Hallucinations	
1 *Auditory hallucinations* The patient reports voices, noises, or other sounds that no one else hears.	0 1 2 3 4 5
2 *Voices commenting* The patient reports a voice which makes a running commentary on his [her] behavior or thoughts.	0 1 2 3 4 5
3 *Voices conversing* The patient reports hearing two or more voices conversing.	0 1 2 3 4 5
4 *Somatic or tactile hallucinations* The patient reports experiencing peculiar physical sensations in the body.	0 1 2 3 4 5
5 *Olfactory hallucinations* The patient reports experiencing unusual smells which no one else notices.	0 1 2 3 4 5
6 *Visual hallucinations* The patient sees shapes or people that are not actually present.	0 1 2 3 4 5
7 *Global rating of hallucinations* This rating should be based on the duration and severity of the hallucinations and their effects on the patient's life.	0 1 2 3 4 5
Delusions	
8 *Persecutory delusions* The patient believes he [she] is being conspired against or persecuted in some way.	0 1 2 3 4 5
9 *Delusions of jealousy* The patient believes his [her] spouse is having an affair with someone.	0 1 2 3 4 5
10 *Delusions of guilt or sin* The patient believes that he [she] has committed some terrible sin or done something unforgivable.	0 1 2 3 4 5
11 *Grandiose delusions* The patient believes he [she] has special powers or abilities.	0 1 2 3 4 5
12 *Religious delusions* The patient is preoccupied with false beliefs of a religious nature.	0 1 2 3 4 5
13 *Somatic delusions* The patient believes that somehow his [her] body is diseased, abnormal, or changed.	0 1 2 3 4 5
14 *Delusions of reference* The patient believes that insignificant remarks or events refer to him [her] or have some special meaning.	0 1 2 3 4 5
15 *Delusions of being controlled* The patient feels that his [her] feelings or actions are controlled by some outside force.	0 1 2 3 4 5
16 *Delusions of mind reading* The patient feels that people can read his [her] mind or know his [her] thoughts.	0 1 2 3 4 5
17 *Thought broadcasting* The patient believes that his [her] thoughts are broadcast so that he himself [she herself] or others can hear them.	0 1 2 3 4 5
18 *Thought insertion* The patient believes that thoughts that are not his [her] own have been inserted into his [her] mind.	0 1 2 3 4 5
19 *Thought withdrawal* The patient believes that thoughts have been taken away from his [her] mind.	0 1 2 3 4 5
20 *Global rating of delusions* This rating should be based on the duration and persistence of the delusions and their effect on the patient's life.	0 1 2 3 4 5
Bizarre behavior	
21 *Clothing and appearance* The patient dresses in an unusual manner or does other strange things to alter his [her] appearance.	0 1 2 3 4 5
22 *Social and sexual behavior* The patient may do things considered inappropriate according to usual social norms (e.g., masturbating in public).	0 1 2 3 4 5
23 *Aggressive and agitated behavior* The patient may behave in an aggressive, agitated manner, often unpredictably.	0 1 2 3 4 5
24 *Repetitive or stereotyped behavior* The patient develops a set of repetitive actions or rituals that he [she] must perform over and over.	0 1 2 3 4 5
25 *Global rating of bizarre behavior* This rating should reflect the type of behavior and the extent to which it deviates from social norms.	0 1 2 3 4 5
Positive formal thought disorder	
26 *Derailment* A pattern of speech in which ideas slip off track onto ideas obliquely related or unrelated.	0 1 2 3 4 5
27 *Tangentiality* Replying to a question in an oblique or irrelevant manner.	0 1 2 3 4 5
28 *Incoherence* A pattern of speech which is essentially incomprehensible at times.	0 1 2 3 4 5
29 *Illogicality* A pattern of speech in which conclusions are reached which do not follow logically.	0 1 2 3 4 5
30 *Circumstantiality* A pattern of speech which is very indirect and delayed in reaching its goal idea.	0 1 2 3 4 5
31 *Pressure of speech* The patient's speech is rapid and difficult to interrupt; the amount of speech produced is greater than that considered normal.	0 1 2 3 4 5
32 *Distractible speech* The patient is distracted by nearby stimuli which interrupt his [her] flow of speech.	0 1 2 3 4 5
33 *Clanging* A pattern of speech in which sounds rather than meaningful relationships govern word choice.	0 1 2 3 4 5
34 *Global rating of positive formal thought disorder* This rating should reflect the frequency of abnormality and degree to which it affects the patient's ability to communicate.	0 1 2 3 4 5
Inappropriate affect	
35 *Inappropriate affect* The patient's affect is inappropriate or incongruous, not simply flat or blunted.	0 1 2 3 4 5

Bracketed words are our addition.

Table 9–16
Social and Occupational Functioning Assessment Scale (SOFAS)

Consider social and occupational functioning on a continuum from excellent functioning to grossly impaired functioning. Include impairments in functioning due to physical limitations, as well as those due to mental impairments. To be counted, impairment must be a direct consequence of mental and physical health problems; the effects of lack of opportunity and other environmental limitations are not to be considered.

Code	(**Note:** Use intermediate codes when appropriate, e.g., 45, 68, 72.)
100–91	Superior functioning in a wide range of activities.
90–81	Good functioning in all areas, occupationally and socially effective.
80–71	No more than a slight impairment in social, occupational, or school functioning (e.g., infrequent interpersonal conflict, temporarily falling behind in schoolwork).
70–61	Some difficulty in social, occupational, or school functioning, but generally functioning well, has some meaningful interpersonal relationships.
60–51	Moderate difficulty in social, occupational, or school functioning (e.g., few friends, conflicts with peers or coworkers).
50–41	Serious impairment in social, occupational, or school functioning (e.g., no friends, unable to keep a job).
40–31	Major impairment in several areas, such as work or school, family relations (e.g., depressed man avoids friends, neglects family, and is unable to work; child frequently beats up younger children, is defiant at home, and is failing at school).
30–21	Inability to function in almost all areas (e.g., stays in bed all day; no job, home, or friends).
20–11	Occasionally fails to maintain minimal personal hygiene; unable to function independently.
10–1	Persistent inability to maintain minimal personal hygiene. Unable to function without harming self or others or without considerable external support (e.g., nursing care and supervision).
0	Inadequate information.

Note: The rating of overall psychological functioning on a scale of 0–100 was operationalized by Luborsky in the Health-Sickness Rating Scale.
Luborsky L. Clinicians' judgments of mental health. *Arch Gen Psychiatry.* 1962;7:407. Spitzer and colleagues developed a revision of the Health-Sickness Rating Scale called the Global Assessment Scale (GAS) (Endicott J, Spitzer RL, Fleiss JL, et al. The Global Assessment Scale: a procedure for measuring overall severity of psychiatric disturbance. *Arch Gen Psychiatry.* 1976;33:766). The SOFAS is derived from the GAS and its development is described in Goldman HH, Skodol AE, Lave TR. Revising Axis V for DSM-IV: a review of measures of social functioning. *Am J Psychiatry.* 1992;149:1148.

Table 9–17
Global Assessment of Relational Functioning (GARF)

INSTRUCTIONS: The GARF Scale can be used to indicate an overall judgment of the functioning of a family or other ongoing relationship on a hypothetical continuum ranging from competent, optimal relational functioning to a disrupted, dysfunctional relationship. It is analogous to Axis V (Global Assessment of Functioning Scale) provided for individuals in DSM-IV. The GARF Scale permits the clinician to rate the degree to which a family or other ongoing relational unit meets the affective and/or instrumental needs of its members in the following areas:

A. *Problem solving*—skills in negotiating goals, rules, and routines; adaptability to stress; communication skills; ability to resolve conflict.

B. *Organization*—maintenance of interpersonal roles and subsystem boundaries; hierarchical functioning, coalitions and distribution of power, control and responsibility.

C. *Emotional climate*—tone and range of feelings; quality of caring, empathy, involvement and attachment/commitment; sharing of values; mutual affective responsiveness, respect, and regard; quality of sexual functioning.

In most instances, the GARF Scale should be used to rate functioning during the current period (i.e., the level of relational functioning at the time of the evaluation). In some settings, the GARF Scale may also be used to rate functioning for other time periods (i.e., the highest level of relational functioning for at least a few months during the past year). **Note:** Use specific, intermediate codes when possible, for example, 45, 68, 72. If detailed information is not adequate to make specific ratings, use midpoints of the five ranges, that is, 90, 70, 50, 30, or 10.

(81–100) Overall: Relational unit is functioning satisfactorily from self-report of participants and from perspectives of observers.

Agreed-on patterns or routines exist that help meet the usual needs of each family/couple member; there is flexibility for change in response to unusual demands or events; occasional conflicts and stressful transitions are resolved through problem-solving communication and negotiation.

There is a shared understanding and agreement about roles and appropriate tasks; decision making is established for each functional area, and there is recognition of the unique characteristics and merit of each subsystem (e.g., parents/spouses, siblings, and individuals).

There is a situationally appropriate, optimistic atmosphere in the family; a wide range of feelings is freely expressed and managed within the family; there is a general atmosphere of warmth, caring, and sharing of values among all family members. Sexual relations of adult members are satisfactory.

(61–80) Overall: Functioning of relational unit is somewhat unsatisfactory. Over a period of time, many but not all difficulties are resolved without complaints.

Daily routines are present but there is some pain and difficulty in responding to the unusual. Some conflicts remain unresolved, but do not disrupt family functioning.

(*continued*)

Table 9–17 (*continued*)

Decision making is usually competent, but efforts at control of one another quite often are greater than necessary or are ineffective. Individuals and relationships are clearly demarcated but sometimes a specific subsystem is depreciated or scapegoated.

A range of feeling is expressed, but instances of emotional blocking or tension are evident. Warmth and caring are present but are marred by a family member's irritability and frustrations. Sexual activity of adult members may be reduced or problematic.

(41–60) Overall: Relational unit has occasional times of satisfying and competent functioning together, but clearly dysfunctional, unsatisfying relationships tend to predominate.

Communication is frequently inhibited by unresolved conflicts that often interfere with daily routines; there is significant difficulty in adapting to family stress and transitional change.

Decision making is only intermittently competent and effective; either excessive rigidity or significant lack of structure is evident at these times. Individual needs are quite often submerged by a partner or coalition.

Pain or ineffective anger or emotional deadness interferes with family enjoyment. Although there is some warmth and support for members, it is usually unequally distributed. Troublesome sexual difficulties between adults are often present.

(21–40) Overall: Relational unit is obviously and seriously dysfunctional; forms and time periods of satisfactory relating are rare.

Family/couple routines do not meet the needs of members; they are grimly adhered to or blithely ignored. Life cycle changes, such as departures or entries into the relational unit, generate painful conflict and obviously frustrating failures of problem solving.

Decision making is tyrannical or quite ineffective. The unique characteristics of individuals are unappreciated or ignored by either rigid or confusingly fluid coalitions.

There are infrequent periods of enjoyment of life together; frequent distancing or open hostility reflect significant conflicts that remain unresolved and quite painful. Sexual dysfunction among adult members is commonplace.

(1–20) Overall: Relational unit has become too dysfunctional to retain continuity of contact and attachment.

Family/couple routines are negligible (e.g., no mealtime, sleeping, or waking schedule); family members often do not know where others are or when they will be in or out; there is little effective communication among family members.

Family/couple members are not organized in such a way that personal or generational responsibilities are recognized. Boundaries of relational unit as a whole and subsystems cannot be identified or agreed upon. Family members are physically endangered or injured or sexually attacked.

Despair and cynicism are pervasive; there is little attention to the emotional needs of others; there is almost no sense of attachment, commitment, or concern about one another's welfare.

0 Inadequate information.

From American Psychiatric Association. *Diagnostic and Statistical Manual of Mental Disorders.* 4th ed. Text rev. Washington, DC: American Psychiatric Association; copyright 2000, with permission.

Table 9–18
Defensive Functioning Scale

High adaptive level. This level of defensive functioning results in optimal adaptation in the handling of stressors. These defenses usually maximize gratification and allow the conscious awareness of feelings, ideas, and their consequences. They also promote an optimum balance among conflicting motives. Examples of defenses characteristically at this level are

- anticipation
- affiliation
- altruism
- humor
- self-assertion
- self-observation
- sublimation
- suppression

Mental inhibitions (compromise formation) level. Defensive functioning at this level keeps potentially threatening ideas, feelings, memories, wishes, or fears out of awareness. Examples are

- displacement
- dissociation
- intellectualization
- isolation of affect
- reaction formation
- repression
- undoing

Minor image-distorting level. This level is characterized by distortions in the image of the self, body, or others that may be employed to regulate self-esteem. Examples are

- devaluation
- idealization
- omnipotence

Disavowal level. This level is characterized by keeping unpleasant or unacceptable stressors, impulses, ideas, affect, or responsibility out of awareness with or without a misattribution of these to external causes. Examples are

- denial
- projection
- rationalization

Major image-distorting level. This level is characterized by gross distortion or misattribution of the image of self or others. Examples are

- autistic fantasy
- projective identification
- splitting of self-image or image of others

Action level. This level is characterized by defensive functioning that deals with internal or external stressors by action or withdrawal. Examples are

- acting out
- apathetic withdrawal
- help-rejecting complaining
- passive aggression

Level of defensive dysregulation. This level is characterized by failure of defensive regulation to contain the individual's reaction to stressors, leading to a pronounced break with objective reality. Examples are

- delusional projection
- psychotic denial
- psychotic distortion

From American Psychiatric Association. *Diagnostic and Statistical Manual of Mental Disorders.* 4th ed. Text rev. Washington, DC: American Psychiatric Association; copyright 2000, with permission.

Table 9–19
DSM-IV-TR Classification (with ICD-9-CM Numerical Codes)

NOS, not otherwise specified.

An *x* appearing in a diagnostic code indicates that a specific code number is required.

An ellipsis (. . .) is used in the names of certain disorders to indicate that the name of a specific mental disorder or general medical condition should be inserted for the name when recording (e.g., 293.0 Delirium due to hypothyroidism).

If criteria are currently met, one of the following severity specifiers may be noted after the diagnosis:
- Mild
- Moderate
- Severe

If criteria are no longer met, one of the following specifiers may be noted:
- In partial remission
- In full remission
- Prior history

Disorders Usually First Diagnosed in Infancy, Childhood, or Adolescence

MENTAL RETARDATION

Note: *These are coded on Axis II.*

317	Mild mental retardation
318.0	Moderate mental retardation
318.1	Severe mental retardation
318.2	Profound mental retardation
319	Mental retardation, severity unspecified

LEARNING DISORDERS

315.00	Reading disorder
315.1	Mathematics disorder
315.2	Disorder of written expression
315.9	Learning disorder NOS

MOTOR SKILLS DISORDER

315.4	Developmental coordination disorder

COMMUNICATION DISORDERS

315.31	Expressive language disorder
315.32	Mixed receptive-expressive language disorder
315.39	Phonological disorder
307.0	Stuttering
307.9	Communication disorder NOS

PERVASIVE DEVELOPMENTAL DISORDERS

299.00	Autistic disorder
299.80	Rett's disorder
299.10	Childhood disintegrative disorder
299.80	Asperger's disorder
299.80	Pervasive developmental disorder NOS

ATTENTION-DEFICIT AND DISRUPTIVE BEHAVIOR DISORDERS

314.xx	Attention-deficit/hyperactivity disorder
.01	Combined type
.00	Predominantly inattentive type
.01	Predominantly hyperactive-impulsive type
314.9	Attention-deficit/hyperactivity disorder NOS
312.xx	Conduct disorder
.81	Childhood-onset type
.82	Adolescent-onset type
.89	Unspecified onset
313.81	Oppositional defiant disorder
312.9	Disruptive behavior disorder NOS

FEEDING AND EATING DISORDERS OF INFANCY OR EARLY CHILDHOOD

307.52	Pica
307.53	Rumination disorder
307.59	Feeding disorder of infancy or early childhood

TIC DISORDERS

307.23	Tourette's disorder
307.22	Chronic motor or vocal tic disorder
307.21	Transient tic disorder (115)
	Specify if: single episode/recurrent
307.20	Tic disorder NOS

ELIMINATION DISORDERS

___.__	Encopresis
787.6	With constipation and overflow incontinence
307.7	Without constipation and overflow incontinence
307.6	Enuresis (not due to a general medical condition)
	Specify type: nocturnal only/diurnal only/nocturnal and diurnal

OTHER DISORDERS OF INFANCY, CHILDHOOD, OR ADOLESCENCE

309.21	Separation anxiety disorder
	Specify if: early onset
313.23	Selective mutism
313.89	Reactive attachment disorder of infancy or early childhood
	Specify type: inhibited type/disinhibited type
307.3	Stereotypic movement disorder
	Specify if: with self-injurious behavior
313.9	Disorder of infancy, childhood, or adolescence NOS

Delirium, Dementia, and Amnestic and Other Cognitive Disorders

DELIRIUM

293.0	Delirium due to ... *[indicate the general medical condition]*
___.__	Substance intoxication delirium *(refer to Substance-Related Disorders for substance-specific codes)*
___.__	Substance withdrawal delirium *(refer to Substance-Related Disorders for substance-specific codes)*
___.__	Delirium due to multiple etiologies *(code each of the specific etiologies)*
780.09	Delirium NOS

DEMENTIA

294.xx	Dementia of the Alzheimer's type, with early onset *(also code 331.0 Alzheimer's disease on Axis III)*
.10	Without behavioral disturbance
.11	With behavioral disturbance

(continued)

Table 9–19 (*continued*)

294.xx	Dementia of the Alzheimer's type, with late onset *(also code 331.0 Alzheimer's disease on Axis III)*
.10	Without behavioral disturbance
.11	With behavioral disturbance
290.xx	Vascular dementia
.40	Uncomplicated
.41	With delirium
.42	With delusions
.43	With depressed mood
	Specify if: with behavioral disturbance
Code presence or absence of a behavioral disturbance in the fifth digit for dementia due to a general medical condition:	
	0 = Without behavioral disturbance
	1 = With behavioral disturbance
294.1x	Dementia due to HIV disease *(also code 042 HIV on Axis III)*
294.1x	Dementia due to head trauma *(also code 854.00 head injury on Axis III)*
294.1x	Dementia due to Parkinson's disease *(also code 332.0 Parkinson's disease on Axis III)*
294.1x	Dementia due to Huntington's disease *(also code 333.4 Huntington's disease on Axis III)*
294.1x	Dementia due to Pick's disease *(also code 331.1 Pick's disease on Axis III)*
294.1x	Dementia due to Creutzfeldt-Jakob disease *(also code 046.1 Creutzfeldt-Jakob disease on Axis III)*
294.1x	Dementia due to ... *[indicate the general medical condition not listed above] (also code the general medical condition on Axis III)*
___.__	Substance-induced persisting dementia *(refer to Substance-Related Disorders for substance-specific codes)*
___.__	Dementia due to multiple etiologies *(code each of the specific etiologies)*
294.8	Dementia NOS
AMNESTIC DISORDERS	
294.0	Amnestic disorder due to ... *[indicate the general medical condition]*
	Specify if: transient/chronic
___.__	Substance-induced persisting amnestic disorder *(refer to Substance-Related Disorders for substance-specific codes)*
294.8	Amnestic disorder NOS
OTHER COGNITIVE DISORDERS	
294.9	Cognitive disorder NOS
Mental Disorders Due to a General Medical Condition Not Elsewhere Classified	
293.89	Catatonic disorder due to ... *[indicate the general medical condition]*
310.1	Personality change due to ... *[indicate the general medical condition]*
	Specify type: labile type/disinhibited type/aggressive type/apathetic type/paranoid type/other type/combined type/unspecified type
293.9	Mental disorder NOS due to ... *[indicate the general medical condition]*

Substance-Related Disorders

The following specifiers apply to substance dependence as noted:

[a]With physiological dependence/without physiological dependence

[b]Early full remission/early partial remission/sustained full remission/sustained partial remission

[c]In a controlled environment

[d]On agonist therapy

The following specifiers apply to substance-induced disorders as noted:

[I]With onset during intoxication/[W]With onset during withdrawal

ALCOHOL-RELATED DISORDERS	
Alcohol Use Disorders	
303.90	Alcohol dependence[a,b,c]
305.00	Alcohol abuse
Alcohol-Induced Disorders	
303.00	Alcohol intoxication
291.81	Alcohol withdrawal
	Specify if: with perceptual disturbances
291.0	Alcohol intoxication delirium
291.0	Alcohol withdrawal delirium
291.2	Alcohol-induced persisting dementia
291.1	Alcohol-induced persisting amnestic disorder
291.x	Alcohol-induced psychotic disorder
.5	With delusions[I,W]
.3	With hallucinations[I,W]
291.89	Alcohol-induced mood disorder[I,W]
291.89	Alcohol-induced anxiety disorder[I,W]
291.89	Alcohol-induced sexual dysfunction[I]
291.89	Alcohol-induced sleep disorder[I,W]
291.9	Alcohol-related disorder NOS
AMPHETAMINE- (OR AMPHETAMINE-LIKE) RELATED DISORDERS	
Amphetamine Use Disorders	
304.40	Amphetamine dependence[a,b,c]
305.70	Amphetamine abuse
Amphetamine-Induced Disorders	
292.89	Amphetamine intoxication
	Specify if: with perceptual disturbances
292.0	Amphetamine withdrawal
292.81	Amphetamine intoxication delirium
292.xx	Amphetamine-induced psychotic disorder
.11	With delusions[I]
.12	With hallucinations[I]
292.84	Amphetamine-induced mood disorder[I,W]
292.89	Amphetamine-induced anxiety disorder[I]
292.89	Amphetamine-induced sexual dysfunction[I]
292.89	Amphetamine-induced sleep disorder[I,W]
292.9	Amphetamine-related disorder NOS
CAFFEINE-RELATED DISORDERS	
Caffeine-Induced Disorders	
305.90	Caffeine intoxication
292.89	Caffeine-induced anxiety disorder[I]
292.89	Caffeine-induced sleep disorder[I]
292.9	Caffeine-related disorder NOS

(*continued*)

Table 9–19 (*continued*)

CANNABIS-RELATED DISORDERS	
Cannabis Use Disorders	
304.30	Cannabis dependence[a,b,c]
305.20	Cannabis abuse
Cannabis-Induced Disorders	
292.89	Cannabis intoxication
	Specify if: with perceptual disturbances
292.81	Cannabis intoxication delirium
292.xx	Cannabis-induced psychotic disorder
.11	With delusions[I]
.12	With hallucinations[I]
292.89	Cannabis-induced anxiety disorder
292.9	Cannabis-related disorder NOS
COCAINE-RELATED DISORDERS	
Cocaine Use Disorders	
304.20	Cocaine dependence[a,b,c]
305.60	Cocaine abuse
Cocaine-Induced Disorders	
292.89	Cocaine intoxication
	Specify if: with perceptual disturbances
292.0	Cocaine withdrawal
292.81	Cocaine intoxication delirium
292.xx	Cocaine-induced psychotic disorder
.11	With delusions[I]
.12	With hallucinations[I]
292.84	Cocaine-induced mood disorder[I,W]
292.89	Cocaine-induced anxiety disorder[I,W]
292.89	Cocaine-induced sexual dysfunction[I]
292.89	Cocaine-induced sleep disorder[I,W]
292.9	Cocaine-related disorder NOS
HALLUCINOGEN-RELATED DISORDERS	
Hallucinogen Use Disorders	
304.50	Hallucinogen dependence[b,c]
305.30	Hallucinogen abuse
Hallucinogen-Induced Disorders	
292.89	Hallucinogen intoxication
292.89	Hallucinogen persisting perception disorder (flashbacks)
292.81	Hallucinogen intoxication delirium
292.xx	Hallucinogen-induced psychotic disorder
.11	With delusions[I]
.12	With hallucinations[I]
292.84	Hallucinogen-induced mood disorder[I]
292.89	Hallucinogen-induced anxiety disorder[I]
292.9	Hallucinogen-related disorder NOS
INHALANT-RELATED DISORDERS	
Inhalant Use Disorders	
304.60	Inhalant dependence[b,c]
305.90	Inhalant abuse
Inhalant-Induced Disorders	
292.89	Inhalant intoxication
292.81	Inhalant intoxication delirium
292.82	Inhalant-induced persisting dementia
292.xx	Inhalant-induced psychotic disorder
.11	With delusions[I]
.12	With hallucinations[I]
292.84	Inhalant-induced mood disorder[I]
292.89	Inhalant-induced anxiety disorder[I]
292.9	Inhalant-related disorder NOS
NICOTINE-RELATED DISORDERS	
Nicotine Use Disorder	
305.1	Nicotine dependence[a,b]
Nicotine-Induced Disorder	
292.0	Nicotine withdrawal
292.9	Nicotine-related disorder NOS
OPIOID-RELATED DISORDERS	
Opioid Use Disorders	
304.00	Opioid dependence[a,b,c,d]
305.50	Opioid abuse
Opioid-Induced Disorders	
292.89	Opioid intoxication
	Specify if: with perceptual disturbances
292.0	Opioid withdrawal
292.81	Opioid intoxication delirium
292.xx	Opioid-induced psychotic disorder
.11	With delusions[I]
.12	With hallucinations[I]
292.84	Opioid-induced mood disorder[I]
292.89	Opioid-induced sexual dysfunction[I]
292.89	Opioid-induced sleep disorder[I,W]
292.9	Opioid-related disorder NOS
PHENCYCLIDINE- (OR PHENCYCLIDINE-LIKE) RELATED DISORDERS	
Phencyclidine Use Disorders	
304.60	Phencyclidine dependence[b,c]
305.90	Phencyclidine abuse
Phencyclidine-Induced Disorders	
292.89	Phencyclidine intoxication
	Specify if: with perceptual disturbances
292.81	Phencyclidine intoxication delirium
292.xx	Phencyclidine-induced psychotic disorder
.11	With delusions[I]
.12	With hallucinations[I]
292.84	Phencyclidine-induced mood disorder[I]
292.89	Phencyclidine-induced anxiety disorder[I]
292.9	Phencyclidine-related disorder NOS
SEDATIVE-, HYPNOTIC-, OR ANXIOLYTIC-RELATED DISORDERS	
Sedative, Hypnotic, or Anxiolytic Use Disorders	
304.10	Sedative, hypnotic, or anxiolytic dependence[a,b,c]
305.40	Sedative, hypnotic, or anxiolytic abuse
Sedative-, Hypnotic-, or Anxiolytic-Induced Disorders	
292.89	Sedative, hypnotic, or anxiolytic intoxication
292.0	Sedative, hypnotic, or anxiolytic withdrawal
	Specify if: with perceptual disturbances
292.81	Sedative, hypnotic, or anxiolytic intoxication delirium
292.81	Sedative, hypnotic, or anxiolytic withdrawal delirium
292.82	Sedative-, hypnotic-, or anxiolytic-induced persisting dementia
292.83	Sedative-, hypnotic-, or anxiolytic-induced persisting amnestic disorder
292.xx	Sedative-, hypnotic-, or anxiolytic-induced psychotic disorder

(*continued*)

Table 9–19 (*continued*)

Code	Disorder
.11	With delusions[l,W]
.12	With hallucinations[l,W]
292.84	Sedative-, hypnotic-, or anxiolytic-induced mood disorder[l,W]
292.89	Sedative-, hypnotic-, or anxiolytic-induced anxiety disorder[W]
292.89	Sedative-, hypnotic-, or anxiolytic-induced sexual dysfunction[l]
292.89	Sedative-, hypnotic-, or anxiolytic-induced sleep disorder[l,W]
292.9	Sedative-, hypnotic-, or anxiolytic-related disorder NOS
POLYSUBSTANCE-RELATED DISORDER	
304.80	Polysubstance dependence[a,b,c,d]
OTHER (OR UNKNOWN) SUBSTANCE-RELATED DISORDERS	
Other (or Unknown) Substance Use Disorders	
304.90	Other (or unknown) substance dependence[a,b,c,d]
305.90	Other (or unknown) substance abuse
Other (or Unknown) Substance-Induced Disorders	
292.89	Other (or unknown) substance intoxication
	Specify if: with perceptual disturbances
292.0	Other (or unknown) substance withdrawal
	Specify if: with perceptual disturbances
292.81	Other (or unknown) substance-induced delirium
292.82	Other (or unknown) substance-induced persisting dementia
292.83	Other (or unknown) substance-induced persisting amnestic disorder
292.xx	Other (or unknown) substance-induced psychotic disorder
.11	With delusions[l,W]
.12	With hallucinations[l,W]
292.84	Other (or unknown) substance-induced mood disorder[l,W]
292.89	Other (or unknown) substance-induced anxiety disorder[l,W]
292.89	Other (or unknown) substance-induced sexual dysfunction[l]
292.89	Other (or unknown) substance-induced sleep disorder[l,W]
292.9	Other (or unknown) substance-related disorder NOS
Schizophrenia and Other Psychotic Disorders	
295.xx	Schizophrenia
The following classification of longitudinal course applies to all subtypes of schizophrenia:	
Episodic with interepisode residual symptoms (*specify* if: with prominent negative symptoms)/episodic with no interepisode residual symptoms	
Continuous (*specify* if: with prominent negative symptoms)	
Single episode in partial remission (*specify* if: with prominent negative symptoms)/single episode in full remission	
Other or unspecified pattern	
.30	Paranoid type
.10	Disorganized type
.20	Catatonic type
.90	Undifferentiated type
.60	Residual type
295.40	Schizophreniform disorder
	Specify if: without good prognostic features/with good prognostic features
295.70	Schizoaffective disorder
	Specify if: bipolar type/depressive type
297.1	Delusional disorder
	Specify if: erotomanic type/grandiose type/jealous type/persecutory type/somatic type/mixed type/unspecified type
298.8	Brief psychotic disorder
	Specify if: with marked stressor(s)/without marked stressor(s)/with postpartum onset
297.3	Shared psychotic disorder
293.xx	Psychotic disorder due to ... *[indicate the general medical condition]*
.81	With delusions
.82	With hallucinations
___.___	Substance-induced psychotic disorder (*refer to Substance-Related Disorders for substance-specific codes*)
	Specify if: with onset during intoxication/with onset during withdrawal
298.9	Psychotic Disorder NOS
Mood Disorders	
Code current state of major depressive disorder or bipolar I disorder in fifth digit:	
1 = Mild	
2 = Moderate	
3 = Severe without psychotic features	
4 = Severe with psychotic features	
Specify: mood-congruent psychotic features/mood-incongruent psychotic features	
5 = In partial remission	
6 = In full remission	
0 = Unspecified	
The following specifiers apply (for current or most recent episode) to mood disorders as noted:	
[a]Severity/psychotic/remission specifiers/[b]Chronic/[c]With catatonic features/[d]With melancholic features/[e]With atypical features/[f]With postpartum onset	
The following specifiers apply to mood disorders as noted:	
[g]With or without full interepisode recovery/[h]With seasonal pattern/[i]With rapid cycling	
DEPRESSIVE DISORDERS	
296.xx	Major depressive disorder
.2x	Single episode[a,b,c,d,e,f]
.3x	Recurrent[a,b,c,d,e,f,g,h]
300.4	Dysthymic disorder
	Specify if: early onset/late onset
	Specify if: with atypical features
311	Depressive disorder NOS

(*continued*)

Table 9–19 (*continued*)

BIPOLAR DISORDERS	
296.xx	Bipolar I disorder
.0x	Single manic episode[a,c,f]
	Specify if: mixed
.40	Most recent episode hypomanic[g,h,i]
.4x	Most recent episode manic[a,c,f,g,h,i]
.6x	Most recent episode mixed[a,c,f,g,h,i]
.5x	Most recent episode depressed[a,b,c,d,e,f,g,h,i]
.7	Most recent episode unspecified[g,h,i]
296.89	Bipolar II disorder[a,b,c,d,e,f,g,h,i]
	Specify (current or most recent episode): hypomanic/depressed
301.13	Cyclothymic disorder
296.80	Bipolar disorder NOS
293.83	Mood disorder due to ... *[indicate the general medical condition]*
	Specify type: with depressive features/with major depressive-like episode/with manic features/ with mixed features
___.__	Substance-induced mood disorder *(refer to Substance-Related Disorders for substance-specific codes)*
	Specify type: with depressive features/with manic features/with mixed features
	Specify if: with onset during intoxication/with onset during withdrawal
296.90	Mood disorder NOS
Anxiety Disorders	
300.01	Panic disorder without agoraphobia
300.21	Panic disorder with agoraphobia
300.22	Agoraphobia without history of panic disorder
300.29	Specific phobia
	Specify type: animal type/natural environment type/blood-injection-injury type/situational type/other type
300.23	Social phobia
	Specify if: generalized
300.3	Obsessive-compulsive disorder
	Specify if: with poor insight
309.81	Posttraumatic stress disorder
	Specify if: acute/chronic
	Specify if: with delayed onset
308.3	Acute stress disorder
300.02	Generalized anxiety disorder
293.84	Anxiety disorder due to ... *[indicate the general medical condition]*
	Specify if: with generalized anxiety/with panic attacks/with obsessive-compulsive symptoms
___.__	Substance-induced anxiety disorder *(refer to Substance-Related Disorders for substance-specific codes)*
	Specify if: with generalized anxiety/with panic attacks/with obsessive-compulsive symptoms/ with phobic symptoms
	Specify if: with onset during intoxication/with onset during withdrawal
300.00	Anxiety disorder NOS
Somatoform Disorders	
300.81	Somatization disorder
300.82	Undifferentiated somatoform disorder
300.11	Conversion disorder
	Specify type: with motor symptom or deficit/with sensory symptom or deficit/with seizures or convulsions/with mixed presentation
307.xx	Pain disorder
.80	Associated with psychological factors
.89	Associated with both psychological factors and a general medical condition
	Specify if: acute/chronic
300.7	Hypochondriasis
	Specify if: with poor insight
300.7	Body dysmorphic disorder
300.82	Somatoform disorder NOS
Factitious Disorders	
300.xx	Factitious disorder
.16	With predominantly psychological signs and symptoms
.19	With predominantly physical signs and symptoms
.19	With combined psychological and physical signs and symptoms
300.19	Factitious disorder NOS
Dissociative Disorders	
300.12	Dissociative amnesia
300.13	Dissociative fugue
300.14	Dissociative identity disorder
300.6	Depersonalization disorder
300.15	Dissociative disorder NOS
Sexual and Gender Identity Disorders	
SEXUAL DYSFUNCTIONS	
The following specifiers apply to all primary sexual dysfunctions:	
Lifelong type/acquired type	
Generalized type/situational type	
Due to psychological factors/due to combined factors	
Sexual Desire Disorders	
302.71	Hypoactive sexual desire disorder
302.79	Sexual aversion disorder
Sexual Arousal Disorders	
302.72	Female sexual arousal disorder
302.72	Male erectile disorder
Orgasmic Disorders	
302.73	Female orgasmic disorder
302.74	Male orgasmic disorder
302.75	Premature ejaculation
Sexual Pain Disorders	
302.76	Dyspareunia (not due to a general medical condition)
306.51	Vaginismus (not due to a general medical condition)
Sexual Dysfunction Due to a General Medical Condition	
625.8	Female hypoactive sexual desire disorder due to ... *[indicate the general medical condition]*
608.89	Male hypoactive sexual desire disorder due to ... *[indicate the general medical condition]*

(*continued*)

Table 9–19 (*continued*)

607.84	Male erectile disorder due to ... *[indicate the general medical condition]*
625.0	Female dyspareunia due to ... *[indicate the general medical condition]*
608.89	Male dyspareunia due to ... *[indicate the general medical condition]*
625.8	Other female sexual dysfunction due to ... *[indicate the general medical condition]*
608.89	Other male sexual dysfunction due to ... *[indicate the general medical condition]*
___.__	Substance-induced sexual dysfunction *(refer to Substance-Related Disorders for substance-specific codes)*
	Specify if: with impaired desire/with impaired arousal/with impaired orgasm/with sexual pain
	Specify if: with onset during intoxication
302.70	Sexual dysfunction NOS
PARAPHILIAS	
302.4	Exhibitionism
302.81	Fetishism
302.89	Frotteurism
302.2	Pedophilia
	Specify if: sexually attracted to males/sexually attracted to females/sexually attracted to both
	Specify if: limited to incest
	Specify type: exclusive type/nonexclusive type
302.83	Sexual masochism
302.84	Sexual sadism
302.3	Transvestic fetishism
	Specify if: with gender dysphoria
302.82	Voyeurism
302.9	Paraphilia NOS
GENDER IDENTITY DISORDERS	
302.xx	Gender identity disorder
.6	in children
.85	in adolescents or adults
	Specify if: sexually attracted to males/sexually attracted to females/sexually attracted to both/sexually attracted to neither
302.6	Gender identity disorder NOS
302.9	Sexual disorder NOS
Eating Disorders	
307.1	Anorexia nervosa
	Specify type: restricting type; binge-eating/purging type
307.51	Bulimia nervosa
	Specify type: Purging type/nonpurging type
307.50	Eating disorder NOS
Sleep Disorders	
PRIMARY SLEEP DISORDERS	
Dyssomnias	
307.42	Primary insomnia
307.44	Primary hypersomnia
	Specify if: recurrent
347.0	Narcolepsy
780.59	Breathing-related sleep disorder
307.45	Circadian rhythm sleep disorder
	Specify if: delayed sleep phase type/jet lag type/shift work type/unspecified type
307.47	Dyssomnia NOS
Parasomnias	
307.47	Nightmare disorder
307.46	Sleep terror disorder
307.46	Sleepwalking disorder
307.47	Parasomnia NOS
SLEEP DISORDERS RELATED TO ANOTHER MENTAL DISORDER	
307.42	Insomnia related to ... *[indicate the Axis I or Axis II disorder]*
307.44	Hypersomnia related to ... *[indicate the Axis I or Axis II disorder]*
OTHER SLEEP DISORDERS	
780.xx	Sleep disorder due to ... *[indicate the general medical condition]*
.52	Insomnia type
.54	Hypersomnia type
.59	Parasomnia type
.59	Mixed type
___.__	Substance-induced sleep disorder *(refer to Substance-Related Disorders for substance-specific codes)*
	Specify type: insomnia type/hypersomnia type/parasomnia type/mixed type
	Specify if: with onset during intoxication/with onset during withdrawal
Impulse-Control Disorders Not Elsewhere Classified	
312.34	Intermittent explosive disorder
312.32	Kleptomania
312.33	Pyromania
312.31	Pathological gambling
312.39	Trichotillomania
312.30	Impulse-control disorder NOS
Adjustment Disorders	
309.xx	Adjustment disorder
.0	With depressed mood
.24	With anxiety
.28	With mixed anxiety and depressed mood
.3	With disturbance of conduct
.4	With mixed disturbance of emotions and conduct
.9	Unspecified
	Specify if: acute/chronic
Personality Disorders	
Note: *These are coded on Axis II.*	
301.0	Paranoid personality disorder
301.20	Schizoid personality disorder
301.22	Schizotypal personality disorder
301.7	Antisocial personality disorder
301.83	Borderline personality disorder
301.50	Histrionic personality disorder
301.81	Narcissistic personality disorder

(*continued*)

Table 9–19 (*continued*)

301.82	Avoidant personality disorder
301.6	Dependent personality disorder
301.4	Obsessive-compulsive personality disorder
301.9	Personality disorder NOS
Other Conditions That May Be a Focus of Clinical Attention	
PSYCHOLOGICAL FACTORS AFFECTING MEDICAL CONDITION	
316.0	... *[specified psychological factor] affecting ... [indicate the general medical condition]*
	Choose name based on nature of factors:
	Mental disorder affecting medical condition
	Psychological symptoms affecting medical condition
	Personality traits or coping style affecting medical condition
	Maladaptive health behaviors affecting medical condition
	Stress-related physiologic response affecting medical condition
	Other or unspecified psychological factors affecting medical condition
MEDICATION-INDUCED MOVEMENT DISORDERS	
332.1	Neuroleptic-induced parkinsonism
333.92	Neuroleptic malignant syndrome
333.7	Neuroleptic-induced acute dystonia
333.99	Neuroleptic-induced acute akathisia
333.82	Neuroleptic-induced tardive dyskinesia
333.1	Medication-induced postural tremor
333.90	Medication-induced movement disorder NOS
OTHER MEDICATION-INDUCED DISORDER	
995.2	Adverse effects of medication NOS
RELATIONAL PROBLEMS	
V61.9	Relational problem related to a mental disorder or general medical condition
V61.20	Parent–child relational problem
V61.10	Partner relational problem
V61.8	Sibling relational problem
V62.81	Relational problem NOS
PROBLEMS RELATED TO ABUSE OR NEGLECT	
V61.21	Physical abuse of child *(code 995.54 if focus of attention is on victim)*
V61.21	Sexual abuse of child *(code 995.53 if focus of attention is on victim)*
V61.21	Neglect of child *(code 995.52 if focus of attention is on victim)*
___.__	Physical abuse of adult
V61.12	(if by partner)
V62.83	(if by person other than partner) *(code 995.81 if focus of attention is on victim)*
___.__	Sexual abuse of adult
V61.12	(if by partner)
V62.83	(if by person other than partner) *(code 995.83 if focus of attention is on victim)*
ADDITIONAL CONDITIONS THAT MAY BE A FOCUS OF CLINICAL ATTENTION	
V15.81	Noncompliance with treatment
V65.2	Malingering
V71.01	Adult antisocial behavior
V71.02	Child or adolescent antisocial behavior
V62.89	Borderline intellectual functioning **Note:** *This is coded on Axis II.*
780.9	Age-related cognitive decline
V62.82	Bereavement
V62.3	Academic problem
V62.2	Occupational problem
313.82	Identity problem
V62.89	Religious or spiritual problem
V62.4	Acculturation problem
V62.89	Phase-of-life problem
Additional Codes	
300.9	Unspecified mental disorder (nonpsychotic)
V71.09	No diagnosis or condition on Axis I
799.9	Diagnosis or condition deferred on Axis II
V71.09	No diagnosis an Axis II
799.9	Diagnosis deferred on Axis II
Multiaxial System	
Axis I	Clinical disorders Other conditions that may be a focus of clinical attention
Axis II	Personality disorders, mental retardation
Axis III	General medical conditions
Axis IV	Psychosocial and environmental problems
Axis V	Global assessment of functioning

From American Psychiatric Association. *Diagnostic and Statistical Manual of Mental Disorders.* 4th ed. Text rev. Washington, DC: American Psychiatric Association; copyright 2000, with permission.

Table 9–20
ICD-10 Classification of Mental Disorders

F00–F09
Organic, including symptomatic, mental disorders

F00 Dementia in Alzheimer's disease
- F00.0 Dementia in Alzheimer's disease with early onset
- F00.1 Dementia in Alzheimer's disease with late onset
- F00.2 Dementia in Alzheimer's disease, atypical or mixed type
- F00.9 Dementia in Alzheimer's disease, unspecified

F01 Vascular dementia
- F01.0 Vascular dementia of acute onset
- F01.1 Multi-infarct dementia
- F01.2 Subcortical vascular dementia
- F01.3 Mixed cortical and subcortical vascular dementia
- F01.8 Other vascular dementia
- F01.9 Vascular dementia, unspecified

F02 Dementia in other diseases classified elsewhere
- F02.0 Dementia in Pick's disease
- F02.1 Dementia in Creutzfeldt-Jakob disease
- F02.2 Dementia in Huntington's disease
- F02.3 Dementia in Parkinson's disease
- F02.4 Dementia in human immunodeficiency virus [HIV] disease
- F02.8 Dementia in other specified diseases classified elsewhere

F03 Unspecified dementia

A fifth character may be added to specify dementia in F00–F03, as follows:
- .x 0 Without additional symptoms
- .x 1 Other symptoms, predominantly delusional
- .x 2 Other symptoms, predominantly hallucinatory
- .x 3 Other symptoms, predominantly depressive
- .x 4 Other mixed symptoms

F04 Organic amnestic syndrome, not induced by alcohol and other psychoactive substances

F05 Delirium, not induced by alcohol and other psychoactive substances
- F05.0 Delirium, not superimposed on dementia, so described
- F05.1 Delirium, superimposed on dementia
- F05.8 Other delirium
- F05.9 Delirium, unspecified

F06 Other mental disorders due to brain damage and dysfunction and to physical disease
- F06.0 Organic hallucinosis
- F06.1 Organic catatonic disorder
- F06.2 Organic delusional [schizophrenialike] disorder
- F06.3 Organic mood [affective] disorders
  - .30 Organic manic disorder
  - .31 Organic bipolar disorder
  - .32 Organic depressive disorder
  - .33 Organic mixed affective disorder
- F06.4 Organic anxiety disorder
- F06.5 Organic dissociative disorder
- F06.6 Organic emotionally labile [asthenic] disorder
- F06.7 Mild cognitive disorder
- F06.8 Other specified mental disorders due to brain damage and dysfunction and to physical disease
- F06.9 Unspecified mental disorder due to brain damage and dysfunction and to physical disease

F07 Personality and behavioral disorders due to brain disease, damage, and dysfunction
- F07.0 Organic personality disorder
- F07.1 Postencephalitic syndrome
- F07.2 Postconcussional syndrome
- F07.8 Other organic personality and behavioral disorders due to brain disease, damage, and dysfunction
- F07.9 Unspecified organic personality and behavioral disorder due to brain disease, damage, and dysfunction

F09 Unspecified organic or symptomatic mental disorder

F10–F19
Mental and behavioral disorders due to psychoactive substance use

F10—Mental and behavioral disorders due to use of alcohol

F11—Mental and behavioral disorders due to use of opioids

F12—Mental and behavioral disorders due to use of cannabinoids

F13—Mental and behavioral disorders due to use of sedatives or hypnotics

F14—Mental and behavioral disorders due to use of cocaine

F15—Mental and behavioral disorders due to use of other stimulants, including caffeine

F16—Mental and behavioral disorders due to use of hallucinogens

F17—Mental and behavioral disorders due to use of tobacco

F18—Mental and behavioral disorders due to use of volatile solvents

F19—Mental and behavioral disorders due to multiple drug use and use of other psychoactive substances

Four- and five-character categories may be used to specify the clinical conditions, as follows:
- F1x.0 Acute intoxication
  - .00 Uncomplicated
  - .01 With trauma or other bodily injury
  - .02 With other medical complications
  - .03 With delirium
  - .04 With perceptual distortions
  - .05 With coma
  - .06 With convulsions
  - .07 Pathological intoxication
- F1x.1 Harmful use
- F1x.2 Dependence syndrome
  - .20 Currently abstinent
  - .21 Currently abstinent, but in a protected environment
  - .22 Currently on a clinically supervised maintenance or replacement regime [controlled dependence]
  - .23 Currently abstinent, but receiving treatment with aversive or blocking drugs
  - .24 Currently using the substance [active dependence]
  - .25 Continuous use
  - .26 Episodic use [dipsomania]
- F1x.3 Withdrawal state
  - .30 Uncomplicated
  - .31 Convulsions
- F1x.4 Withdrawal state with delirium
  - .40 Without convulsions
  - .41 With convulsions
- F1x.5 Psychotic disorder
  - .50 Schizophrenialike
  - .51 Predominantly delusional
  - .52 Predominantly hallucinatory
  - .53 Predominantly polymorphic
  - .54 Predominantly depressive symptoms
  - .55 Predominantly manic symptoms
  - .56 Mixed
- F1x.6 Amnestic syndrome
- F1x.7 Residual and late-onset psychotic disorder
  - .70 Flashbacks
  - .71 Personality or behavior disorder
  - .72 Residual affective disorder
  - .73 Dementia
  - .74 Other persisting cognitive impairment
  - .75 Late-onset psychotic disorder
- F1x.8 Other mental and behavioral disorders
- F1x.9 Unspecified mental and behavioral disorder

(*continued*)

Table 9–20 (*continued*)

F20–F29
Schizophrenia, schizotypal and delusional disorders

F20 Schizophrenia
F20.0 Paranoid schizophrenia
F20.1 Hebephrenic schizophrenia
F20.2 Catatonic schizophrenia
F20.3 Undifferentiated schizophrenia
F20.4 Postschizophrenic depression
F20.5 Residual schizophrenia
F20.6 Simple schizophrenia
F20.8 Other schizophrenia
F20.9 Schizophrenia, unspecified
A fifth character may be used to classify course:
.x 0 Continuous
.x 1 Episodic with progressive deficit
.x 2 Episodic with stable deficit
.x 3 Episodic remittent
.x 4 Incomplete remission
.x 5 Complete remission
.x 8 Other
.x 9 Period of observation less than one year

F21 Schizotypal disorders
F22 Persistent delusional disorders
F22.0 Delusional disorder
F22.8 Other persistent delusional disorders
F22.9 Persistent delusional disorder, unspecified

F23 Acute and transient psychotic disorders
F23.0 Acute polymorphic psychotic disorder without symptoms of schizophrenia
F23.1 Acute polymorphic psychotic disorder with symptoms of schizophrenia
F23.2 Acute schizophrenialike psychotic disorder
F23.3 Other acute predominantly delusional psychotic disorders
F23.8 Other acute transient psychotic disorders
F23.9 Acute and transient psychotic disorders unspecified
A fifth character may be used to identify the presence or absence of associated acute stress:
.x 0 Without associated acute stress
.x 1 With associated acute stress

F24 Induced delusional disorder

F25 Schizoaffective disorders
F25.0 Schizoaffective disorder, manic type
F25.1 Schizoaffective disorder, depressive type
F25.2 Schizoaffective disorder, mixed type
F25.8 Other schizoaffective disorders
F25.9 Schizoaffective disorder, unspecified

F28 Other nonorganic psychotic disorders

F29 Unspecified nonorganic psychosis

F30–F39
Mood [affective] disorders

F30 Manic episode
F30.0 Hypomania
F30.1 Mania without psychotic symptoms
F30.2 Mania with psychotic symptoms
F30.8 Other manic episodes
F30.9 Manic episode, unspecified

F31 Bipolar affective disorder
F31.0 Bipolar affective disorder, current episode hypomanic
F31.1 Bipolar affective disorder, current episode manic without psychotic symptoms
31.2 Bipolar affective disorder, current episode manic with psychotic symptoms
F31.3 Bipolar affective disorder, current episode mild or moderate depression
.30 Without somatic symptoms
.31 With somatic symptoms
F31.4 Bipolar affective disorder, current episode severe depression without psychotic symptoms
F31.5 Bipolar affective disorder, current episode severe depression with psychotic symptoms
F31.6 Bipolar affective disorder, current episode mixed
F31.7 Bipolar affective disorder, currently in remission
F31.8 Other bipolar affective disorders
F31.9 Bipolar affective disorder, unspecified

F32 Depressive episode
F32.0 Mild depressive episode
.00 Without somatic symptoms
.01 With somatic symptoms
F32.1 Moderate depressive episode
.10 Without somatic symptoms
.11 With somatic symptoms
F32.2 Severe depressive episode without psychotic symptoms
F32.3 Severe depressive episode with psychotic symptoms
F32.8 Other depressive episodes
F32.9 Depressive episode, unspecified

F33 Recurrent depressive disorder
F33.0 Recurrent depressive disorder, current episode mild
.00 Without somatic symptoms
.01 With somatic symptoms
F33.1 Recurrent depressive disorder, current episode moderate
.00 Without somatic symptoms
.01 With somatic symptoms
F33.2 Recurrent depressive disorder, current episode severe without psychotic symptoms
F33.3 Recurrent depressive disorder, current episode severe with psychotic symptoms
F33.4 Recurrent depressive disorder, currently in remission
F33.8 Other recurrent depressive disorders
F33.9 Recurrent depressive disorder, unspecified

F34 Persistent mood [affective] disorders
F34.0 Cyclothymia
F34.1 Dysthymia
F34.8 Other persistent mood [affective] disorders
F34.9 Persistent mood [affective] disorder, unspecified

F38 Other mood [affective] disorders
F38.0 Other single mood [affective] disorders
.00 Mixed affective episode
F38.1 Other recurrent mood [affective] disorders
.10 Recurrent brief depressive disorder
F38.8 Other specified mood [affective] disorders

F39 Unspecified mood [affective] disorder

F40–F48
Neurotic stress-related and somatoform disorders

F40 Phobic anxiety disorders
F40.0 Agoraphobia
.00 Without panic disorder
.01 With panic disorder
F40.1 Social phobias
F40.2 Specific (isolated) phobias
F40.8 Other phobic anxiety disorders
F40.9 Phobic anxiety disorder, unspecified

F41 Other anxiety disorders
F41.0 Panic disorder [episodic paroxysmal anxiety]
F41.1 Generalized anxiety disorder
F41.2 Mixed anxiety and depressive disorder
F41.3 Other mixed anxiety disorders
F41.8 Other specified anxiety disorders
F41.9 Anxiety disorder, unspecified

(*continued*)

Table 9–20 (*continued*)

F42 Obsessive-compulsive disorder
- F42.0 Predominantly obsessional thoughts or ruminations
- F42.1 Predominantly compulsive acts [obsessional rituals]
- F42.2 Mixed obsessional thoughts and acts
- F42.8 Other obsessive-compulsive disorders
- F42.9 Obsessive-compulsive disorder, unspecified

F43 Reaction to severe stress, and adjustment disorders
- F43.0 Acute stress reaction
- F43.1 Posttraumatic stress disorder
- F43.2 Adjustment disorders
  - .20 Brief depressive reaction
  - .21 Prolonged depressive reaction
  - .22 Mixed anxiety and depressive reaction
  - .23 With predominant disturbance of other emotions
  - .24 With predominant disturbance of conduct
  - .25 With mixed disturbance of emotions and conduct
  - .28 With other specified predominant symptoms
- F43.8 Other reactions to severe stress
- F43.9 Reaction to severe stress, unspecified

F44 Dissociative [conversion] disorders
- F44.0 Dissociative amnesia
- F44.1 Dissociative fugue
- F44.2 Dissociative stupor
- F44.3 Trance and possession disorders
- F44.4 Dissociative motor disorders
- F44.5 Dissociative convulsions
- F44.6 Dissociative anesthesia and sensory loss
- F44.7 Mixed dissociative [conversion] disorders
- F44.8 Other dissociative [conversion] disorders
  - .80 Ganser's syndrome
  - .81 Multiple personality disorder
  - .82 Transient dissociative [conversion] disorders occurring in childhood and adolescence
  - .88 Other specified dissociative [conversion] disorders
- F44.9 Dissociative [conversion] disorder, unspecified

F45 Somatoform disorders
- F45.0 Somatization disorder
- F45.1 Undifferentiated somatoform disorder
- F45.2 Hypochondriacal disorder
- F45.3 Somatoform autonomic dysfunction
  - .30 Heart and cardiovascular system
  - .31 Upper gastrointestinal tract
  - .32 Lower gastrointestinal tract
  - .33 Respiratory system
  - .34 Genitourinary system
  - .38 Other organ or system
- F45.4 Persistent somatoform pain disorder
- F45.8 Other somatoform disorders
- F45.9 Somatoform disorder, unspecified

F48 Other neurotic disorders
- F48.0 Neurasthenia
- F48.1 Depersonalization-derealization syndrome
- F48.8 Other specified neurotic disorders
- F48. 9 Neurotic disorder, unspecified

F50–F59

Behavioral syndromes associated with physiological disturbances and physical factors

F50 Eating disorders
- F50.0 Anorexia nervosa
- F50.1 Atypical anorexia nervosa
- F50.2 Bulimia nervosa
- F50.3 Atypical bulimia nervosa
- F50.4 Overeating associated with other psychological disturbances
- F50.5 Vomiting associated with other psychological disturbances
- F50.8 Other eating disorders
- F50.9 Eating disorder, unspecified

F51 Nonorganic sleep disorders
- F51.0 Nonorganic insomnia
- F51.1 Nonorganic hypersomnia
- F51.2 Nonorganic disorder of the sleep-wake schedule
- F51.3 Sleepwalking [somnambulism]
- F51.4 Sleep terrors [night terrors]
- F51.5 Nightmares
- F51.8 Other nonorganic sleep disorders
- F51.9 Nonorganic sleep disorder, unspecified

F52 Sexual dysfunction, not caused by organic disorder or disease
- F52.0 Lack or loss of sexual desire
- F52.1 Sexual aversion and lack of sexual enjoyment
  - .10 Sexual aversion
  - .11 Lack of sexual enjoyment
- F52.2 Failure of genital response
- F52.3 Orgasmic dysfunction
- F52.4 Premature ejaculation
- F52.5 Nonorganic vaginismus
- F52.6 Nonorganic dyspareunia
- F52.7 Excessive sexual drive
- F52.8 Other sexual dysfunction, not caused by organic disorders or disease
- F52.9 Unspecified sexual dysfunction, not caused by organic disorder or disease

F53 Mental and behavioral disorders associated with the puerperium, not elsewhere classified
- F53.0 Mild and behavioral disorders associated with the puerperium, not elsewhere classified
- F53.1 Severe mental and behavioral disorders associated with the puerperium, not elsewhere classified
- F53.8 Other mental and behavioral disorders associated with the puerperium, not elsewhere classified
- F53.9 Puerperal mental disorder, unspecified

F54 Psychological and behavioral factors associated with disorders or disease classified elsewhere

F55 Abuse of non-dependence-producing substances
- F55.0 Antidepressants
- F55.1 Laxatives
- F55.2 Analgesics
- F55.3 Antacids
- F55.4 Vitamins
- F55.5 Steroids or hormones
- F55.6 Specific herbal or folk remedies
- F55.8 Other substances that do not produce dependence
- F55.9 Unspecified

F59 Unspecified behavioral syndromes associated with physiological disturbances and physical factors

F60–69

Disorders of adult personality and behavior

F60 Specific personality disorders
- F60.0 Paranoid personality disorder
- F60.1 Schizoid personality disorder
- F60.2 Dissocial personality disorder
- F60.3 Emotionally unstable personality disorder
  - .30 Impulsive type
  - .31 Borderline type
- F60.4 Histrionic personality disorder
- F60.5 Anankastic personality disorder
- F60.6 Anxious [avoidant] personality disorder
- F60.7 Dependent personality disorder
- F60.8 Other specific personality disorders
- F60.9 Personality disorder, unspecified

F61 Mixed and other personality disorders
- F61.0 Mixed personality disorders
- F61.1 Troublesome personality changes

(*continued*)

Table 9–20 (*continued*)

F62 Enduring personality changes, not attributable to brain damage and disease
- F62.0 Enduring personality change after catastrophic experience
- F62.1 Enduring personality change after psychiatric illness
- F62.8 Other enduring personality changes
- F62.9 Enduring personality change, unspecified

F63 Habit and impulse disorders
- F63.0 Pathological gambling
- F63.1 Pathological fire-setting [pyromania]
- F63.2 Pathological stealing [kleptomania]
- F63.3 Trichotillomania
- F63.8 Other habit and impulse disorders
- F63.9 Habit and impulse disorder, unspecified

F64 Gender identity disorders
- F64.0 Transsexualism
- F64.1 Dual-role transvestism
- F64.2 Gender identity disorder of childhood
- F64.8 Other gender identity disorders
- F64.9 Gender identity disorder, unspecified

F65 Disorders of sexual preference
- F65.0 Fetishism
- F65.1 Fetishistic transvestism
- F65.2 Exhibitionism
- F65.3 Voyeurism
- F65.4 Pedophilia
- F65.5 Sadomasochism
- F65.6 Multiple disorders of sexual preference
- F65.8 Other disorders of sexual preference
- F65.9 Disorder of sexual preference, unspecified

F66 Psychological and behavioral disorders associated with sexual development and orientation
- F66.0 Sexual maturation disorder
- F66.1 Egodystonic sexual orientation
- F66.2 Sexual relationship disorder
- F66.8 Other psychosexual development disorders
- F66.9 Psychosexual development disorder, unspecified

A fifth character may be used to indicate association with:
- .x 0 Heterosexuality
- .x 1 Homosexuality
- .x 2 Bisexuality
- .x 3 Other, including prepubertal

F68 Other disorders of adult personality and behavior
- F68.0 Elaboration of physical symptoms for psychological reasons
- F68.1 Intentional production or feigning of symptoms or disabilities, either physical or psychological [factitious disorder]
- F68.8 Other specified disorders of adult personality and behavior

F69 Unspecified disorder of adult personality and behavior

F70–F79
Mental retardation

F70 Mild mental retardation

F71 Moderate mental retardation

F72 Severe mental retardation

F73 Profound mental retardation

F78 Other mental retardation

F79 Unspecified mental retardation

A fourth character may be used to specify the extent of associated behavioral impairment:
- F7x.0 No, or minimal, impairment of behavior
- F7x.1 Significant impairment of behavior requiring attention or treatment
- F7x.8 Other impairments of behavior
- F7x.9 Without mention of impairment of behavior

F80–F89
Disorders of psychological development

F80 Specific developmental disorders of speech and language
- F80.0 Specific speech articulation disorder
- F80.1 Expressive language disorder
- F80.2 Receptive language disorder
- F80.3 Acquired aphasia with epilepsy [Landau-Kleffner syndrome]
- F80.8 Other developmental disorders of speech and language
- F80.9 Developmental disorder of speech and language, unspecified

F81 Specific developmental disorders of scholastic skills
- F81.0 Specific reading disorder
- F81.1 Specific spelling disorder
- F81.2 Specific disorder of arithmetical skills
- F81.3 Mixed disorder of scholastic skills
- F81.8 Other developmental disorders of scholastic skills
- F81.9 Developmental disorder of scholastic skills, unspecified

F82 Specific developmental disorder of motor function

F83 Mixed specific developmental disorders

F84 Pervasive developmental disorders
- F84.0 Childhood autism
- F84.1 Atypical autism
- F84.2 Rett's syndrome
- F84.3 Other childhood disintegrative disorder
- F84.4 Overactive disorder associated with mental retardation and stereotyped movements
- F84.5 Asperger's syndrome
- F84.8 Other pervasive developmental disorders
- F84.9 Pervasive developmental disorder, unspecified

F88 Other disorders of psychological development

F89 Unspecified disorder of psychological development

F90–F98
Behavioral and emotional disorders with onset usually occurring in childhood and adolescence

F90 Hyperkinetic disorders
- F90.0 Disturbance of activity and attention
- F90.1 Hyperkinetic conduct disorder
- F90.8 Other hyperkinetic disorders
- F90.9 Hyperkinetic disorder, unspecified

F91 Conduct disorders
- F91.0 Conduct disorder confined to the family context
- F91.1 Unsocialized conduct disorder
- F91.2 Socialized conduct disorder
- F91.3 Oppositional defiant disorder
- F91.8 Other conduct disorders
- F91.9 Conduct disorder, unspecified

F92 Mixed disorders of conduct and emotions
- F92.0 Depressive conduct disorder
- F92.8 Other mixed disorders of conduct and emotions
- F92.9 Mixed disorder of conduct and emotions, unspecified

F93 Emotional disorders with onset specific to childhood
- F93.0 Separation anxiety disorder of childhood
- F93.1 Phobic anxiety disorder of childhood
- F93.3 Sibling rivalry disorder
- F93.8 Other childhood emotional disorders
- F93.9 Childhood emotional disorder, unspecified

F94 Disorders of social functioning with onset specific to childhood and adolescence
- F94.0 Elective mutism
- F94.1 Reactive attachment disorder of childhood
- F94.2 Disinhibited attachment disorder of childhood
- F94.8 Other childhood disorders of social functioning
- F94.9 Childhood disorders of social functioning, unspecified

(*continued*)

Table 9–20 (*continued*)

F95 Tic disorders
- F95.0 Transient tic disorder
- F95.1 Chronic motor or vocal tic disorder
- F95.2 Combined vocal and multiple motor tic disorder [de la Tourette's syndrome]
- F95.8 Other tic disorders
- F95.9 Tic disorder, unspecified

F98 Other behavioral and emotional disorders with onset usually occurring in childhood and adolescence
- F98.0 Nonorganic enuresis
- F98.1 Nonorganic encopresis
- F98.2 Feeding disorder of infancy and childhood
- F98.3 Pica of infancy and childhood
- F98.4 Stereotyped movement disorders
- F98.5 Stuttering [stammering]
- F98.6 Cluttering
- F98.8 Other specified behavioral and emotional disorders with onset usually occurring in childhood and adolescence
- F98.9 Unspecified behavioral and emotional disorders with onset usually occurring in childhood and adolescence

F99 Mental disorder, not otherwise specified

Reprinted with permission from World Health Organization. *The ICD-10 Classification of Mental and Behavioral Disorders: Clinical Descriptions and Diagnostic Guidelines*. Geneva: World Health Organization; 1992.

References

American Psychiatric Association. *Diagnostic and Statistical Manual of Mental Disorders*. 4th ed. Text revision. Washington, DC: American Psychiatric Association; 2000.

Berrios GE, Hauser R. The early development of Kraepelin's ideas on classification: a conceptual history. *Psychol Med*. 1988;18:813.

Bryan KJ, Rounsaville B, Spitzer RL, Williams JB. Reliability of dual diagnosis: substance dependence and psychiatric disorders. *J Nerv Ment Dis*. 1992;180:251.

Burros OK, ed. *Personality Tests and Reviews*. Highland Park, NJ: Gryphon; 1970.

Frances A. An introduction of DSM-IV. *Hosp Community Psychiatry*. 1990;41:49.

Janca A, Hiller W. ICD-10 checklists—a tool for clinician's use of the ICD-10 classification of mental and behavioral disorders. *Compr Psychiatry*. 1996;37:180.

Liddle PF, Ngan ET, Duffield G, et al. Signs and Symptoms of Psychotic Illness (SSPI): a rating scale. *Br J Psychiatry*. 2002;180:45.

Lyerly SB. *Handbook of Psychiatric Rating Scales*. 2nd ed. Bethesda, MD: National Institute of Mental Health; 1973.

Ventureyra VAG, Yao S-N, Cottraux J, et al. The validation of the Posttraumatic Stress Disorder Checklist Scale in posttraumatic stress disorder and nonclinical subjects. *Psychother Psychosom*. 2002;71:47.

Wilson M. DSM-III and the transformation of American psychiatry. A history. *Am J Psychiatry*. 1993;150:399.

World Health Organization. *The ICD-10 Classification of Mental and Behavioural Disorders: Clinical Descriptions and Diagnostic Guidelines*. Geneva: World Health Organization; 1992.

World Health Organization. *The ICD-10 Classification of Mental and Behavioural Disorders: Diagnostic Criteria for Research*. Geneva: World Health Organization; 1992.

Zarin DA, Earls F. Diagnostic decision making in psychiatry. *Am J Psychiatry*. 1993;150:197.

Zimmerman M. Is DSM-IV needed at all? *Am J Psychiatry*. 1990;147:974.

Zimmerman M, Coryell W, Black D. Variability in the application of contemporary diagnostic criteria: endogenous depression as an example. *Am J Psychiatry*. 1990;147:1173.

10

Delirium, Dementia, and Amnestic and Other Cognitive Disorders and Mental Disorders Due to a General Medical Condition

▲ 10.1 Overview

In the text revision of the fourth edition of *Diagnostic Statistical Manual of Mental Disorders* (DSM-IV-TR) three groups of disorders–delirium, dementia, and the amnestic disorders—are characterized by the primary symptom common to all the disorders, which is an impairment in cognition (as in memory, language, or attention). Although DSM-IV-TR acknowledges that other psychiatric disorders can exhibit some cognitive impairment as a symptom, cognitive impairment is the cardinal symptom in delirium, dementia, and the amnestic disorders. Within each of these diagnostic categories, DSM-IV-TR delimits specific types (Table 10.1–1).

In the past, these conditions were classified under the heading "organic mental" or "organic brain disorders." Traditionally, those disorders were defined as disorders that had an identifiable pathological condition such as brain tumor, cerebrovascular disease, or drug intoxication. Those brain disorders with no generally accepted organic basis (such as depression) were called functional disorders.

This century-old distinction between organic and functional disorders is outdated and has been deleted from the nomenclature. The only unbiased conclusion to be made from evaluation of the available data is that every psychiatric disorder has an organic (that is, biological or chemical) component. Because of this reassessment of the data, the concept of functional disorders has been determined to be misleading, and the term *functional* and its historical opposite, *organic,* are not used in that context in DSM-IV-TR.

A further indication that the dichotomy is no longer valid is the revival of the term *neuropsychiatry.* As defined in the seventh edition of *Campbell's Psychiatric Dictionary, neuropsychiatry* emphasizes the somatic substructure on which mental operations and emotions are based; it is concerned with the psychopathological accompaniments of brain dysfunction as observed in seizure disorders, for example. Neuropsychiatry focuses on the psychiatric aspects of neurological disorders and the role of brain dysfunction in psychiatric disorders.

CLASSIFICATION

For each of the three major groups—delirium, dementia, and amnestic disorders—there are subcategories based on etiology. They are defined and summarized as follows:

Delirium

Delirium is marked by short-term confusion and changes in cognition. There are four subcategories based upon several causes: (1) general medical condition, e.g., infection; (2) substance induced, e.g., cocaine, opioids, phencyclidine (PCP); (3) multiple causes, e.g., head trauma and kidney disease; and (4) delirium not otherwise specified, e.g., sleep deprivation.

Dementia

Dementia is marked by severe impairment in memory, judgment, orientation, and cognition. There are six subcategories: (1) dementia of the Alzheimer's type, which usually occurs in persons over 65 and is manifested by progressive intellectual disorientation and dementia, delusions, or depression; (2) vascular dementia, caused by vessel thrombosis or hemorrhage; (3) other medical conditions, e.g., human immunodeficiency virus (HIV) disease, head trauma, Pick's disease, Creutzfeldt-Jakob disease (caused by a slow-growing transmittable virus); (4) substance induced, caused by toxin or medication, e.g., gasoline fumes, atropine; (5) multiple etiologies; and (6) not otherwise specified (if cause is unknown).

Amnestic Disorder

Amnestic disorder is marked by memory impairment and forgetfulness. There are three subcategories: (1) caused by medical condition (hypoxia); (2) caused by toxin or medication, e.g., marijuana, diazepam; and (3) not otherwise specified.

Table 10.1–1
DSM-IV Cognitive Disorders

Delirium
- Delirium due to a general medical condition
- Substance-induced delirium
- Delirium due to multiple etiologies
- Delirium not otherwise specified

Dementia
- Dementia of the Alzheimer's type
- Vascular dementia
- Dementia due to other general medical conditions
  - Dementia due to HIV disease
  - Dementia due to head trauma
  - Dementia due to Parkinson's disease
  - Dementia due to Huntington's disease
  - Dementia due to Pick's disease
  - Dementia due to Creutzfeldt-Jakob disease
  - Dementia due to other general medical conditions
- Substance-induced persisting dementia
- Dementia due to multiple etiologies
- Dementia not otherwise specified

Amnestic disorders
- Amnestic disorder due to a general medical condition
- Substance-induced persisting amnestic disorder
- Amnestic disorder not otherwise specified
- Cognitive disorder not otherwise specified

Cognitive Disorder Not Otherwise Specified

Cognitive disorder not otherwise specified is a DSM-IV-TR category that allows for the diagnosis of a cognitive disorder that does not meet the criteria for delirium, dementia, or amnestic disorders (Table 10.1–2). The cause of these syndromes is presumed to involve a specific general medical condition, a pharmacologically active agent, or possibly both.

Table 10.1–2
DSM-IV-TR Diagnostic Criteria for Cognitive Disorder Not Otherwise Specified

This category is for disorders that are characterized by cognitive dysfunction presumed to be due to the direct physiological effect of a general medical condition that do not meet criteria for any of the specific deliriums, dementias, or amnestic disorders listed in this section and that are not better classified as delirium not otherwise specified, dementia not otherwise specified, or amnestic disorder not otherwise specified. For cognitive dysfunction due to a specific or unknown substance, the specific substance-related disorder not otherwise specified category should be used.

Examples include

1. Mild neurocognitive disorder: impairment in cognitive functioning as evidenced by neuropsychological testing or quantified clinical assessment, accompanied by objective evidence of a systemic general medical condition or central nervous system dysfunction
2. Postconcussional disorder: following a head trauma, impairment in memory or attention with associated symptoms

From American Psychiatric Association. *Diagnostic and Statistical Manual of Mental Disorders.* 4th ed. Text rev. Washington, DC: American Psychiatric Association; copyright 2000, with permission.

CLINICAL EVALUATION

Psychiatric History

During the history taking, the clinician seeks to elicit the development of the illness. Subtle cognitive disorders, fluctuating symptoms, and progressing disease processes may be tracked effectively. The clinician should obtain a detailed rendition of changes in the patient's daily routine involving such factors as self-care, job responsibilities, and work habits; meal preparation; shopping and personal support; interactions with friends; hobbies and sports; reading interests; religious, social, and recreational activities; and ability to maintain personal finances. Understanding the past life of each patient provides an invaluable source of baseline data regarding changes in function such as attention and concentration, intellectual abilities, personality, motor skills, and mood and perception. The examiner seeks to find the particular pursuits that the patient considers most important, or central, to his or her lifestyle and attempts to discern how those pursuits have been affected by the emerging clinical condition. Such a method provides the opportunity to appraise both the impact of the illness and the patient-specific baseline for monitoring the effects of future therapies.

Mental Status Examination

Following a thorough history, the clinician's primary tool is the assessment of the mental status. Like the physical examination, the mental status examination is a means of surveying functions and abilities, to allow a definition of personal strengths and weakness. It is a repeatable, structured assessment of symptoms and signs that promotes effective communication between clinicians. It also establishes the basis for future comparison, essential for documenting therapeutic effectiveness, and it allows comparisons between different patients, with a generalization of findings from one patient to another. Table 10.1–3 lists the components of a comprehensive neuropsychiatric mental status examination.

Cognition

When testing cognitive functions the clinician should evaluate memory; visuospatial and constructional abilities; and reading, writing, and mathematical abilities. Assessment of abstraction ability is also valuable, but although a patient's performance on tasks such as proverb interpretation may be a useful bedside projective test in some patients, the specific interpretation may result from a variety of factors, such as poor education, low intelligence, and failure to understand the concept of proverbs, as well as from a broad array of primary and secondary psychopathological disturbances.

Although formal evaluation of cognitive impairment requires time-consuming consultation with an expert in psychological testing, one practical and clinically useful test for practitioners is the Mini-Mental State Examination (MMSE) (Table 10.1–4). MMSE is a screening test that can be used during a patient's clinical examination. It is also a practical test to track the changes in a patient's cognitive state. Of a possible 30

Table 10.1–3
Neuropsychiatric Mental Status Examination

A. General Description

1. General appearance, dress, sensory aids (glasses, hearing aid)
2. Level of consciousness and arousal
3. Attention to environment
4. Posture (standing and seated)
5. Gait
6. Movements of limbs, trunk, and face (spontaneous, resting, and after instruction)
7. General demeanor (including evidence of responses to internal stimuli)
8. Response to examiner (eye contact, cooperation, ability to focus on interview process)
9. Native or primary language

B. Language and Speech

1. Comprehension (words, sentences, simple and complex commands, and concepts)
2. Output (spontaneity, rate, fluency, melody or prosody, volume, coherence, vocabulary, paraphasic errors, complexity of usage)
3. Repetition
4. Other aspects
   a. Object naming
   b. Color naming
   c. Body part identification
   d. Ideomotor praxis to command

C. Thought

1. Form (coherence and connectedness)
2. Content
   a. Ideational (preoccupations, overvalued ideas, delusions)
   b. Perceptual (hallucinations)

D. Mood and Affect

1. Internal mood state (spontaneous and elicited; sense of humor)
2. Future outlook
3. Suicidal ideas and plans
4. Demonstrated emotional status (congruence with mood)

E. Insight and Judgment

1. Insight
   a. Self-appraisal and self-esteem
   b. Understanding of current circumstances
   c. Ability to describe personal psychological and physical status
2. Judgment
   a. Appraisal of major social relationships
   b. Understanding of personal roles and responsibilities

F. Cognition

1. Memory
   a. Spontaneous (as evidenced during interview)
   b. Tested (incidental, immediate repetition, delayed recall, cued recall, recognition; verbal, nonverbal; explicit, implicit)
2. Visuospatial skills
3. Constructional ability
4. Mathematics
5. Reading
6. Writing
7. Fine sensory function (stereognosis, graphesthesia, two-point discrimination)
8. Finger gnosis
9. Right-left orientation
10. "Executive functions"
11. Abstraction

Courtesy of Eric D. Caine, M.D., and Jeffrey M. Lyness, M.D.

Table 10.1–4
Mini-Mental State Examination (MMSE) Questionnaire

Orientation (score 1 if correct)	
Name this hospital or building.	____
What city are you in now?	____
What year is it?	____
What month is it?	____
What is the date today?	____
What state are you in?	____
What county is this?	____
What floor of the building are you on?	____
What day of the week is it?	____
What season of the year is it?	____
Registration (score 1 for each object correctly repeated)	
Name three objects and have the patient repeat them. Score number repeated by the patient. Name the three objects several more times if needed for the patient to repeat correctly (record trials____).	____
Attention and calculation	
Subtract 7 from 100 in serial fashion to 65. Maximum score = 5	____
Recall (score 1 for each object recalled)	
Do you recall the three objects named before?	____
Language tests	
Confrontation naming: watch, pen = 2	____
Repetition: "No ifs, ands, or buts" = 1	____
Comprehension: Pick up the paper in your right hand, fold it in half, and set it on the floor = 3	____
Read and perform the command "close your eyes" = 1	____
Write any sentence (subject, verb, object) = 1	____
Construction	
Copy the design below = 1	____

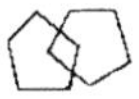

Total MMSE questionnaire score (maximum = 30)	____

Adapted from Folstein MF, Folstein S, McHugh PR. Mini-mental state: a practical method for grading the cognitive state of patients for the clinician. *J Psychiatr Res.* 1975;12:189.

points, a score below 25 suggests possible impairment, and a score below 20 indicates definite impairment.

PATHOLOGY AND LABORATORY EXAMINATION

Like all medical tests, psychiatric evaluations such as the mental status examination must be interpreted in the overall context of thorough clinical and laboratory assessment. Psychiatric and neuropsychiatric patients require careful physical examination (Table 10.1–5), especially when there are issues involving etiologically related or comorbid medical conditions. When consulting internists and other medical specialists, the clinician must ask specific questions to focus the differential diagnostic process and use the consultation most effectively. In particular, most systemic medical or primary cerebral diseases that lead to psychopathological disturbances also manifest with a variety of peripheral or central abnormalities.

Table 10.1–5
Comprehensive Workup of Dementia and Other Cognitive Disorders

Physical examination including thorough neurological examination
Vital signs
Mental status examination
Mini-Mental State Examination (MMSE)
Review of medications and drug levels
Blood and urine screens for alcohol, drugs, and heavy metals[a]
Physiological workup
Serum electrolytes/glucose/Ca^{2+}, Mg^{2+}
Liver, renal function tests
SMA-12 or equivalent serum chemistry profile
Urinalysis
Complete blood cell count with differential cell type count
Thyroid function tests (including TSH level)
RPR (serum screen)
FTA-ABS (if CNS disease is suspected)
Serum B_{12}
Folate levels
Urine corticosteroids[a]
Erythrocyte sedimentation rate (Westergren)
Antinuclear antibody[a] (ANA), C_3C_4, anti-DS DNA[a]
Arterial blood gases[a]
HIV screen[a,b]
Urine porphobilinogens[a]
Chest radiograph
Electrocardiogram
Neurological workup
CT or MRI scan of head[a]
SPECT[b,c]
Lumbar puncture[a]
EEG[a]
Neuropsychological testing[d]

[a]All indicated by history and physical examination.
[b]Requires special consent and counseling.
[c]May detect cerebral blood flow perfusion deficits.
[d]May be useful in differentiating dementia from other neuropsychiatric syndromes if it cannot be done clinically.
Adapted with permission from Stoudemire A, Thompson TL. Recognizing and treating dementia. *Geriatrics.* 1981;36:112.

A screening laboratory evaluation is sought initially and may be followed by a variety of ancillary tests to increase the diagnostic specificity. Table 10.1–6 lists such procedures, some of which are described below.

Table 10.1–6
Screening Laboratory Tests

General Tests
Complete blood cell count
Erythrocyte sedimentation rate
Electrolytes
Glucose
Blood urea nitrogen and serum creatinine
Liver function tests
Serum calcium and phosphorus
Thyroid function tests
Serum protein
Levels of all drugs
Urinalysis
Pregnancy test for women of childbearing age
Electrocardiography
Ancillary Laboratory Tests
Blood
Blood cultures
Rapid plasma reagin test
HIV testing (ELISA and Western blot)
Serum heavy metals
Serum copper
Ceruloplasmin
Serum B_{12}, RBC folate levels
Urine
Culture
Toxicology
Heavy metal screen
Electrography
Electroencephalography
Evoked potentials
Polysomnography
Nocturnal penile tumescence
Cerebrospinal fluid
Glucose, protein
Cell count
Cultures (bacterial, viral, fungal)
Cryptococcal antigen
Venereal Disease Research Laboratory test
Radiography
Computed tomography
Magnetic resonance imaging
Positron emission tomography
Single photon emission computed tomography

Courtesy of Eric D. Caine, M.D., and Jeffrey M. Lyness, M.D.

ELECTROENCEPHALOGRAPHY

Electroencephalography (EEG) is an easily accessible, noninvasive test of brain dysfunction that has high sensitivity in many disorders but relatively low specificity. Beyond its recognized uses in epilepsy, EEG's greatest utility is in detecting altered electrical rhythms associated with mild delirium, space-occupying lesions, and continuing complex partial seizures (in which the patient remains conscious although behaviorally impaired). EEG is also sensitive to metabolic and toxic states, often showing a diffuse slowing of brain activity. Focal slowing may indicate a variety of causes such as space-occupying lesions (tumors, cerebral abscesses) or subdural hematomas. However, a superficial EEG (one that is recorded through the skull) is often insufficient for source localization and may prove insensitive to a variety of abnormal processes. Nasopharyngeal recordings may better define abnormalities generated by the temporal lobes. Direct cortical (surface) recordings are also used to localize seizure foci. EEG findings change with aging, with a general reduction in alpha wave activity, and with increases in the relative amounts of theta and delta wave activity. Early in the course of disorders such as Alzheimer's disease the standard EEG finding usually remains normal and therefore is often unrevealing. As part of sleep polysomnography, recent studies have suggested that EEG may aid in the future in distinguishing between elderly subjects with major depressive disorder associated with cognitive impairment and those with a primary neurodegenerative process underlying their dementia.

COMPUTED TOMOGRAPHY AND MAGNETIC RESONANCE IMAGING

Computed tomography (CT) and magnetic resonance imaging (MRI) have proved to be powerful neuropsychiatric research tools. Recent developments in MRI allow the direct measurement of structures such as the thalamus, basal ganglia, hippocampus, and amygdala, as well as temporal and apical areas of the brain and the structures of the posterior fossa. MRI has largely replaced CT as the most utilitarian and cost-effective method of imaging in neuropsychiatry. Patients with acute cerebral hemorrhages or hematomas must continue to be assessed using CT, but these patients present infrequently in psychiatric settings. MRI better discriminates the interface between gray and white matter and is useful in detecting a variety of white matter lesions in the periventricular and subcortical regions. The pathophysiological significance of such findings remains to be defined. White matter abnormalities are detected in younger patients with multiple sclerosis or HIV infection and in older patients with hypertension, vascular dementia, or dementia of the Alzheimer's type. However, their prevalence is also increased in healthy, aging individuals who have no defined disease process. Like CT, the greatest utility of MRI in the evaluation of patients with dementia arises from what it may exclude (tumors, vascular disease) rather than what it can demonstrate specifically.

POSITRON EMISSION TOMOGRAPHY, SINGLE PHOTON EMISSION COMPUTED TOMOGRAPHY, AND FUNCTIONAL MAGNETIC RESONANCE IMAGING

Physiologically based techniques for imaging the brain, such as positron emission tomography (PET) and single photon emission computed tomography (SPECT), involve the injection of radioactively labeled, naturally occurring compounds or a radiopharmaceutical, with subsequent demonstration of cerebral blood flow or the incorporation of the labeled compounds into specific metabolic pathways. Such imaging methods have shown promise in studying the neurochemical and physiological bases of a variety of neuropsychiatric disorders. However, the cost of PET currently precludes its use as a routine diagnostic procedure, and insufficient data exist to project its ultimate utility for routine clinical evaluation. SPECT can be performed more readily and more cheaply, but whether it will have specific diagnostic utility in general psychiatry remains to be determined. Functional MRI (fMRI) holds great promise as a research tool to explore the physiological bases of complex behavioral processes. However, its potential utility as a clinical diagnostic tool remains to be defined.

NEUROPSYCHOLOGICAL TESTING

Neuropsychological testing provides a standardized, quantitative, reproducible evaluation of a patient's cognitive abilities. Such procedures may be useful for initial evaluation and periodic assessment. Tests are available that assess abilities across the broad array of cognitive domains, and many offer comparative normative groups or adjusted scores based on normative samples. The clinician seeking neuropsychological consultation should understand enough about the strengths and weaknesses of selected procedures to benefit fully from the results obtained. (Chapter 5 includes a complete survey of neuropsychological tests.)

ICD-10

Unlike in DSM-IV-TR, organic (including symptomatic) mental disorders are organized in the 10th revision of the *International Statistical Classification of Disease and Related Health Problems* (ICD-10) on the basis of "their common, demonstrable etiology in cerebral disease, brain injury, or other insult leading to cerebral dysfunction." In the ICD-10, rather than being deleted, the term *organic* implies only that "the syndrome . . . can be attributed to an independently diagnosable cerebral or systemic disease or disorder." Primary dysfunction affects the brain directly; secondary dysfunctions occur as a result of diseases or disorders attacking several organs or body systems *including* the brain. According to ICD-10, all the disorders can be divided into two groups: one in which the invariable and most prominent features are disturbances of cognitive functions or of the sensorium and one in which the most conspicuous manifestations are in the areas of perception, thought contents, or mood and emotion or in the overall pattern of personality and behavior.

Consequently, categories included as organic mental disorders, including symptomatic ones, in ICD-10 are dementia in Alzheimer's disease; vascular dementia; dementia in other diseases classified elsewhere (such as dementia in Pick's disease); unspecified dementia; organic amnesia syndrome, not induced by alcohol and other psychoactive substances; delirium, not induced by alcohol and other psychoactive substances; other mental disorders due to brain damage and dysfunction and due to physical disease (such as organic mood disorders due to brain disease, damage, and dysfunction); and unspecified organic or symptomatic mental disorder. Alcohol- and drug-caused brain disorders are discussed in a separate section.

References

Caine ED. Should age-associated cognitive decline be included in DSM-IV? *J Neuropsychiatry Clin Neurosci.* 1993;5:1.

Caine ED, Lyness JM. Delirium, dementia, and amnestic and other cognitive disorders. In: Sadock BJ, Sadock VA, eds. *Kaplan & Sadock's Comprehensive Textbook of Psychiatry.* 7th ed. Vol 1. Baltimore: Lippincott Williams & Wilkins; 2000:854.

Janicki MP, Dalton AJ, eds. *Dementia, Aging and Intellectual Disabilities: A Handbook.* Philadelphia: Brunner/Mazel; 1999.

Kawas CH, Brookmeyer R. Aging and the public health effects of dementia. *N Engl J Med.* 2001;344:1160.

Newman MF. Coronary-artery bypass surgery and the brain. *N Engl J Med.* 2001;344:451.

Reynolds EH. Structure and function in neurology and psychiatry. *Br J Psychiatry.* 1990;157:481.

Rowland LP. *Merritt's Neurology.* 10th ed. Philadelphia: Lippincott Williams & Wilkins; 2000.

▲ 10.2 Delirium

Delirium is a syndrome, not a disease, and it has many causes, all of which result in a similar pattern of signs and symptoms relating to the patient's level of consciousness and cognitive impairment. Delirium remains an underrecognized and underdiagnosed clinical disorder. Part of the problem is that the syndrome has a variety of other names, for example, acute confusional state, acute brain syndrome, metabolic encephalopathy, toxic psychosis, and acute brain failure. The intent of the text revision of the fourth edition of the *Diagnostic and Statistical Manual of Mental Disorders* (DSM-IV-TR) was to help consolidate the myriad of terms into a single diagnostic label.

In DSM-IV-TR, delirium is "characterized by a disturbance of consciousness and a change in cognition that develop over a

short . . . time." The hallmark symptom of delirium is an impairment of consciousness, usually occurring in association with global impairments of cognitive functions. Abnormalities of mood, perception, and behavior are common psychiatric symptoms; tremor, asterixis, nystagmus, incoordination, and urinary incontinence are common neurological symptoms. Classically, delirium has a sudden onset (hours or days), a brief and fluctuating course, and rapid improvement when the causative factor is identified and eliminated, but each of these characteristic features can vary in individual patients. Physicians must recognize delirium to identify and treat the underlying cause and to avert the development of delirium-related complications such as accidental injury because of the patient's clouded consciousness.

EPIDEMIOLOGY

Delirium is a common disorder. According to DSM-IV-TR, the point prevalence of delirium in the general population is 0.4 percent for people 18 and older and 1.1 percent for people 55 and older. Approximately 10 to 30 percent of medically ill patients who are hospitalized exhibit delirium. Approximately 30 percent of patients in surgical intensive care units and cardiac intensive care units and 40 to 50 percent of patients who are recovering from surgery for hip fractures have an episode of delirium. The highest rate of delirium is found in postcardiotomy patients, more than 90 percent in some studies. An estimated 20 percent of patients with severe burns and 30 to 40 percent of patients with acquired immune deficiency syndrome (AIDS) have episodes of delirium while they are hospitalized. Delirium develops in 80 percent of terminally ill patients. The causes of postoperative delirium include the stress of surgery, postoperative pain, insomnia, pain medication, electrolyte imbalances, infection, fever, and blood loss.

Advanced age is a major risk factor for the development of delirium. Approximately 30 to 40 percent of hospitalized patients older than age 65 have an episode of delirium, and another 10 to 15 percent of elderly persons exhibit delirium on admission to the hospital. Of nursing home residents over age 75, 60 percent have repeated episodes of delirium. Other predisposing factors for the development of delirium are preexisting brain damage (such as dementia, cerebrovascular disease, tumor), a history of delirium, alcohol dependence, diabetes, cancer, sensory impairment (such as blindness), and malnutrition. Male gender is an independent risk factor for delirium according to DSM-IV-TR.

Delirium is a poor prognostic sign. Rates of institutionalization are increased threefold for patients 65 years and older who exhibit delirium while in the hospital. The 3-month mortality rate of patients who have an episode of delirium is estimated to be 23 to 33 percent. The 1-year mortality rate for patients who have an episode of delirium may be as high as 50 percent. Elderly patients who experience delirium while hospitalized have a 20 to 75 percent mortality rate during that hospitalization. After discharge, up to 15 percent of these persons die within a 1-month period, and 25 percent die within 6 months.

ETIOLOGY

The major causes of delirium are central nervous system disease (such as epilepsy), systemic disease (such as cardiac failure), and either intoxication or withdrawal from pharmacological or toxic agents (Table 10.2–1). When evaluating patients with delirium,

Table 10.2–1
Causes of Delirium

- Intracranial causes
  - Epilepsy and postictal states
  - Brain trauma (especially concussion)
  - Infections
    - Meningitis
    - Encephalitis
  - Neoplasms
  - Vascular disorders
- Extracranial causes
  - Drugs (ingestion or withdrawal) and poisons
    - Anticholinergic agents
    - Anticonvulsants
    - Antihypertensive agents
    - Antiparkinsonian agents
    - Antipsychotic drugs
    - Cardiac glycosides
    - Cimetidine
    - Clonidine
    - Disulfiram
    - Insulin
    - Opiates
    - Phencyclidine
    - Phenytoin
    - Ranitidine
    - Salicylates
    - Sedatives (including alcohol) and hypnotics
    - Steroids
  - Poisons
    - Carbon monoxide
    - Heavy metals and other industrial poisons
  - Endocrine dysfunction (hypofunction or hyperfunction)
    - Pituitary
    - Pancreas
    - Adrenal
    - Parathyroid
    - Thyroid
  - Diseases of nonendocrine organs
    - Liver
      - Hepatic encephalopathy
    - Kidney and urinary tract
      - Uremic encephalopathy
    - Lung
      - Carbon dioxide narcosis
      - Hypoxia
    - Cardiovascular system
      - Cardiac failure
      - Arrhythmias
      - Hypotension
  - Deficiency diseases
    - Thiamine, nicotinic acid, B_{12}, or folic acid deficiencies
  - Systemic infections with fever and sepsis
  - Electrolyte imbalance of any cause
  - Postoperative states
  - Trauma (head or general body)

Adapted from Charles E. Wells, M.D.

clinicians should assume that any drug that a patient has taken may be etiologically relevant to the delirium.

DIAGNOSIS AND CLINICAL FEATURES

The syndrome of delirium is almost always caused by one or more systemic or cerebral derangements that affect brain function.

A 74-year-old African-American woman, Ms. Richardson, was brought to a city hospital emergency room by the police. She is unkempt, dirty, and foul smelling. She does not look at the interviewer and is apparently confused and unresponsive to most of his questions. She knows her name and address, but not the day or the month. She is unable to describe the events that led to her admission.

The police reported that they were called by neighbors because Ms. Richardson had been wandering around the neighborhood and not taking care of herself. The medical center mobile crisis unit went to her house twice, but could not get in and presumed she was not home. Finally, the police came and broke into the apartment, where they were met by a snarling German shepherd. They shot the dog with a tranquilizing gun, and then found Ms. Richardson hiding in the corner, wearing nothing but a bra. The apartment was filthy, the floor was littered with dog feces. The police found a gun, which they took into custody.

The following day, while Ms. Richardson was awaiting transfer to a medical unit for treatment of her out-of-control diabetes, the supervising psychiatrist attempted to interview her. Her facial expression was still mostly unresponsive, and she still didn't know the month and couldn't say what hospital she was in. She reported that the neighbors had called the police because she was "sick," and indeed she had felt sick and weak, with pains in her shoulder; in addition, she had not eaten for 3 days. She remembered that the dog was not in "the shop" and would be returned to her when she got home. She refused to give the name of a neighbor who was a friend, saying, "He's got enough troubles of his own." She denied ever being in a psychiatric hospital or hearing voices, but acknowledged that she had at one point seen a psychiatrist "near Lincoln Center" because she couldn't sleep. He had prescribed medication that was too strong, so she didn't take it. She didn't remember the name so the interviewer asked if it was Thorazine. She said no, it was "allal." "Haldol?" asked the interviewer. She nodded. The interviewer was convinced that was the drug, but other observers thought she might have said yes to anything that sounded remotely like it, such as "Elavil." When asked about the gun, she denied, with some annoyance, that it was real and said it was a toy gun that had been brought to the house by her brother, who had died 8 years ago. She was still feeling weak and sick, complained of pain in her shoulder, and apparently had trouble swallowing. She did manage to smile as the team left her bedside. (Reprinted with permission from *DSM-IV Casebook*.)

DSM-IV-TR gives separate diagnostic criteria for each type of delirium: (1) delirium due to a general medical condition (Table 10.2–2), (2) substance intoxication delirium (Table 10.2–3),

Table 10.2–2
DSM-IV-TR Diagnostic Criteria for 293.0 Delirium Due to General Medical Condition

A. Disturbance of consciousness (i.e., reduced clarity of awareness of the environment) with reduced ability to focus, sustain, or shift attention.

B. A change in cognition (such as memory deficit, disorientation, language disturbance) or the development of a perceptual disturbance that is not better accounted for by a preexisting, established, or evolving dementia.

C. The disturbance develops over a short period of time (usually hours to days) and tends to fluctuate during the course of the day.

D. There is evidence from the history, physical examination, or laboratory findings that the disturbance is caused by the direct physiological consequences of a general medical condition.

Coding note: If delirium is superimposed on a preexisting vascular dementia, indicate the delirium by coding vascular dementia, with delirium.

Coding note: Include the name of the general medical condition on Axis I, e.g., Delirium due to hepatic encephalopathy; also code the general medical condition on Axis III.

From American Psychiatric Association. *Diagnostic and Statistical Manual of Mental Disorders.* 4th ed. Text rev. Washington, DC: American Psychiatric Association; copyright 2000, with permission.

Table 10.2–3
DSM-IV-TR Diagnostic Criteria for Substance Intoxication Delirium

A. Disturbance of consciousness (i.e., reduced clarity of awareness of the environment) with reduced ability to focus, sustain, or shift attention.

B. A change in cognition (such as memory deficit, disorientation, language disturbance) or the development of a perceptual disturbance that is not better accounted for by a preexisting, established, or evolving dementia.

C. The disturbance develops over a short period of time (usually hours to days) and tends to fluctuate during the course of the day.

D. There is evidence from the history, physical examination, or laboratory findings of either (1) or (2):

(1) the symptoms in Criteria A and B developed during substance intoxication

(2) medication use is etiologically related to the disturbance*

Note: This diagnosis should be made instead of a diagnosis of substance intoxication only when the cognitive symptoms are in excess of those usually associated with the intoxication syndrome and when the symptoms are sufficiently severe to warrant independent clinical attention.

***Note:** The diagnosis should be recorded as substance-induced delirium if related to medication use.

Code (Specific substance) intoxication delirium:

(Alcohol; Amphetamine [or amphetaminelike substance]; Cannabis; Cocaine; Hallucinogen; Inhalant; Opioid; Phencyclidine [or phencyclidinelike substance]; Sedative, hypnotic, or anxiolytic; Other [or unknown] substance [e.g., cimetidine, digitalis, benztropine])

From American Psychiatric Association. *Diagnostic and Statistical Manual of Mental Disorders.* 4th ed. Text rev. Washington, DC: American Psychiatric Association; copyright 2000, with permission.

Table 10.2–4
DSM-IV-TR Diagnostic Criteria for Substance Withdrawal Delirium

A. Disturbance of consciousness (i.e., reduced clarity of awareness of the environment) with reduced ability to focus, sustain, or shift attention.
B. A change in cognition (such as memory deficit, disorientation, language disturbance) or the development of a perceptual disturbance that is not better accounted for by a preexisting, established, or evolving dementia.
C. The disturbance develops over a short period of time (usually hours to days) and tends to fluctuate during the course of the day.
D. There is evidence from the history, physical examination, or laboratory findings that the symptoms in Criteria A and B developed during, or shortly after, a withdrawal syndrome.

Note: This diagnosis should be made instead of a diagnosis of substance withdrawal only when the cognitive symptoms are in excess of those usually associated with the withdrawal syndrome and when the symptoms are sufficiently severe to warrant independent clinical attention.

Code (Specific substance) withdrawal delirium:

(Alcohol; Sedative, hypnotic, or anxiolytic; Other [or unknown] substance)

From American Psychiatric Association. *Diagnostic and Statistical Manual of Mental Disorders.* 4th ed. Text rev. Washington, DC: American Psychiatric Association; copyright 2000, with permission.

Table 10.2–6
DSM-IV-TR Diagnostic Criteria for Delirium Not Otherwise Specified

This category should be used to diagnose a delirium that does not meet criteria for any of the specific types of delirium described in this section.

Examples include

1. A clinical presentation of delirium that is suspected to be due to a general medical condition or substance use but for which there is insufficient evidence to establish a specific etiology
2. Delirium due to causes not listed in this section (e.g., sensory deprivation)

From American Psychiatric Association. *Diagnostic and Statistical Manual of Mental Disorders.* 4th ed. Text rev. Washington, DC: American Psychiatric Association; copyright 2000, with permission.

(3) substance withdrawal delirium (Table 10.2–4), (4) delirium due to multiple etiologies (Table 10.2–5), and (5) delirium not otherwise specified (Table 10.2–6) for a delirium of unknown cause or due to causes not listed, such as sensory deprivation. However, the syndrome is the same, regardless of cause.

The core features of delirium include altered consciousness, such as decreased level of consciousness; altered attention, which may include diminished ability to focus, sustain, or shift attention; impairment in other realms of cognitive function, which may manifest as disorientation (especially to time and space) and decreased memory; relatively rapid onset (usually hours to days); brief duration (usually days to weeks); and often marked, unpredictable fluctuations in severity and other clinical manifestations during the course of the day, sometimes worse at night (sundowning), which may range from periods of lucidity to quite severe cognitive impairment and disorganization.

Table 10.2–5
DSM-IV-TR Diagnostic Criteria for Delirium Due to Multiple Etiologies

A. Disturbance of consciousness (i.e., reduced clarity of awareness of the environment) with reduced ability to focus, sustain, or shift attention.
B. A change in cognition (such as memory deficit, disorientation, language disturbance) or the development of a perceptual disturbance that is not better accounted for by a preexisting, established, or evolving dementia.
C. The disturbance develops over a short period of time (usually hours to days) and tends to fluctuate during the course of the day.
D. There is evidence from the history, physical examination, or laboratory findings that the delirium has more than one etiology (e.g., more than one etiological general medical condition, a general medical condition plus substance intoxication or medication side effect).

Coding note: Use multiple codes reflecting specific delirium and specific etiologies, e.g., Delirium due to viral encephalitis; Alcohol withdrawal delirium.

From American Psychiatric Association. *Diagnostic and Statistical Manual of Mental Disorders.* 4th ed. Text rev. Washington, DC: American Psychiatric Association; copyright 2000, with permission.

Associated clinical features are often present and may be prominent. They may include disorganization of thought processes (ranging from mild tangentiality to frank incoherence), perceptual disturbances such as illusions and hallucinations, psychomotor hyperactivity and hypoactivity, disruption of the sleep–wake cycle (often manifested as fragmented sleep at night, with or without daytime drowsiness), mood alterations (from subtle irritability to obvious dysphoria, anxiety, or even euphoria), and other manifestations of altered neurological function (e.g., autonomic hyperactivity or instability, myoclonic jerking, and dysarthria). The electroencephalogram (EEG) usually shows diffuse slowing of background activity, although patients with delirium due to alcohol or sedative-hypnotic withdrawal have low-voltage fast activity.

The major neurotransmitter hypothesized to be involved in delirium is acetylcholine, and the major neuroanatomical area is the reticular formation. The reticular formation of the brainstem is the principal area regulating attention and arousal; the major pathway implicated in delirium is the dorsal tegmental pathway, which projects from the mesencephalic reticular formation to the tectum and thalamus. Several studies have reported that a variety of delirium-inducing factors result in decreased acetylcholine activity in the brain. One of the most common causes of delirium is toxicity from too many prescribed medications with anticholinergic activity. In addition to the anticholinergic drugs themselves, many of the most common drugs used in psychiatry have similar effects, e.g., atropine, amitriptyline (Elavil), doxepin (Sinequan), nortriptyline (Aventyl), imipramine (Tofranil), thioridazine (Mellaril), and chlorpromazine (Thorazine). Researchers have suggested other pathophysiological mechanisms for delirium. In particular, the delirium associated with alcohol withdrawal has been associated with hyperactivity of the locus ceruleus and its noradrenergic neurons. Other neurotransmitters that have been implicated are serotonin and glutamate.

Table 10.2–7
Physical Examination of the Delirious Patient

Parameter	Finding	Clinical Implication
1. Pulse	Bradycardia	Hypothyroidism Stokes-Adams syndrome Increased intracranial pressure
	Tachycardia	Hyperthyroidism Infection Heart failure
2. Temperature	Fever	Sepsis Thyroid storm Vasculitis
3. Blood pressure	Hypotension	Shock Hypothyroidism Addison's disease
	Hypertension	Encephalopathy Intracranial mass
4. Respiration	Tachypnea	Diabetes Pneumonia Cardiac failure Fever Acidosis (metabolic)
	Shallow	Alcohol or other substance intoxication
5. Carotid vessels	Bruits or decreased pulse	Transient cerebral ischemia
6. Scalp and face	Evidence of trauma	
7. Neck	Evidence of nuchal rigidity	Meningitis Subarachnoid hemorrhage
8. Eyes	Papilledema	Tumor Hypertensive encephalopathy
	Pupillary dilatation	Anxiety Autonomic overactivity (e.g., delirium tremens)
9. Mouth	Tongue or cheek lacerations	Evidence of generalized tonic-clonic seizures
10. Thyroid	Enlarged	Hyperthyroidism
11. Heart	Arrhythmia	Inadequate cardiac output, possibility of emboli
	Cardiomegaly	Heart failure Hypertensive disease
12. Lungs	Congestion	Primary pulmonary failure Pulmonary edema Pneumonia
13. Breath	Alcohol Ketones	 Diabetes
14. Liver	Enlargement	Cirrhosis Liver failure
15. Nervous system		
a. Reflexes—muscle stretch	Asymmetry with Babinski's signs	Mass lesion Cerebrovascular disease Preexisting dementia
	Snout	Frontal mass Bilateral posterior cerebral artery occlusion
b. Abducent nerve (sixth cranial nerve)	Weakness in lateral gaze	Increased intracranial pressure
c. Limb strength	Asymmetrical	Mass lesion Cerebrovascular disease
d. Autonomic	Hyperactivity	Anxiety Delirium

Reprinted with permission from Strub RL, Black FW. *Neurobehavioral Disorders: A Clinical Approach.* Philadelphia: FA Davis; 1981:120.

Table 10.2–8
Laboratory Workup of the Patient with Delirium

Standard studies
- Blood chemistries (including electrolytes, renal and hepatic indexes, and glucose)
- Complete blood count with white cell differential
- Thyroid function tests
- Serologic tests for syphilis
- Human immunodeficiency virus (HIV) antibody test
- Urinalysis
- Electrocardiogram
- Electroencephalogram
- Chest radiograph
- Blood and urine drug screens

Additional tests when indicated
- Blood, urine, and cerebrospinal fluid (CSF) cultures
- B_{12}, folic acid concentrations
- Computed tomography or magnetic resonance imaging brain scan
- Lumbar puncture and CSF examination

PHYSICAL AND LABORATORY EXAMINATIONS

Delirium is usually diagnosed at the bedside and is characterized by the sudden onset of symptoms. A bedside mental status examination—such as the Mini-Mental State Examination (see Table 10.1–4), the mental status examination, or neurologic signs—can be used to document the cognitive impairment and to provide a baseline from which to measure the patient's clinical course. The physical examination often reveals clues to the cause of the delirium (Table 10.2–7). The presence of a known physical illness or a history of head trauma or alcohol or other substance dependence increases the likelihood of the diagnosis.

The laboratory workup of a patient with delirium should include standard tests and additional studies indicated by the clinical situation (Table 10.2–8). In delirium, the EEG characteristically shows a generalized slowing of activity and may be useful in differentiating delirium from depression or psychosis. The EEG of a delirious patient sometimes shows focal areas of hyperactivity. In rare cases, it may be difficult to differentiate delirium related to epilepsy from delirium related to other causes.

DIFFERENTIAL DIAGNOSIS

Delirium versus Dementia

A number of clinical features help distinguish delirium from dementia (Table 10.2–9). In contrast to the sudden onset of delirium, the onset of dementia is usually insidious. Although both conditions include cognitive impairment, the changes in dementia are more stable over time and, for example, usually do not fluctuate over the course of a day. A patient with dementia is usually alert; a patient with delirium has episodes of decreased consciousness. Occasionally, delirium occurs in a patient with dementia, a condition known as beclouded dementia. A dual diagnosis of delirium can be made when there is a definite history of preexisting dementia.

Table 10.2–9
Frequency of Clinical Features of Delirium Contrasted with Dementia

Feature	Delirium	Dementia
Impaired memory	+++	+++
Impaired thinking	+++	+++
Impaired judgment	+++	+++
Clouding of consciousness	+++	–
Major attention deficits	+++	+[a]
Fluctuation over course of a day	+++	+
Disorientation	+++	++[a]
Vivid perceptual disturbances	++	+
Incoherent speech	++	+[a]
Disrupted sleep–wake cycle	++	+[a]
Nocturnal exacerbation	++	+[a]
Insight	++[b]	+[b]
Acute or subacute onset	++	–[c]

+++, always present; ++, usually present; +, occasionally present; –, usually absent.
[a]More frequent in advanced stages of dementia.
[b]Present during lucid intervals or on recovery from delirium; present during early stages of dementia.
[c]Onset may be acute or subacute in some dementias, e.g., multi-infarction, hypoxemia, certain reversible dementias.
Reprinted with permission from Liston EH. Diagnosis and management of delirium in the elderly patient. *Psychiatr Ann.* 1984;14:117.

Delirium versus Schizophrenia or Depression

Delirium must also be differentiated from schizophrenia and depressive disorder. Some patients with psychotic disorders, usually schizophrenia or manic episodes, may have periods of extremely disorganized behavior difficult to distinguish from delirium. In general, however, the hallucinations and delusions of patients with schizophrenia are more constant and better organized than those of patients with delirium. Patients with schizophrenia usually experience no change in their level of consciousness or in their orientation. Patients with hypoactive symptoms of delirium may appear somewhat similar to severely depressed patients, but they can be distinguished on the basis of an EEG. Other psychiatric diagnoses to consider in the differential diagnosis of delirium are brief psychotic disorder, schizophreniform disorder, and dissociative disorders. Patients with factitious disorders may attempt to simulate the symptoms of delirium but usually reveal the factitious nature of their symptoms by inconsistencies on their mental status examinations, and an EEG can easily separate the two diagnoses.

COURSE AND PROGNOSIS

Although the onset of delirium is usually sudden, prodromal symptoms (such as restlessness and fearfulness) may occur in the days preceding the onset of florid symptoms. The symptoms of delirium usually persist as long as the causally relevant factors are present, although delirium generally lasts less than a week. After identification and removal of the causative factors, the symptoms of delirium usually recede over a 3- to 7-day period, although some symptoms may take up to 2 weeks to resolve completely. The older a patient and the longer the patient has been delirious, the longer the delirium takes to resolve. Recall of what transpired during a delirium, once it is over, is characteristically spotty; a patient may refer to the episode as a bad dream or a nightmare only vaguely remembered. As stated in the discussion on epidemiology, the occurrence of delirium is associated with a high mortality rate in the ensuing year, primarily because of the serious nature of the associated medical conditions that lead to delirium.

Whether delirium progresses to dementia has not been demonstrated in carefully controlled studies, although many clinicians believe that they have seen such a progression. A clinical observation that has been validated by some studies, however, is that periods of delirium are sometimes followed by depression or posttraumatic stress disorder.

TREATMENT

In treating delirium, the primary goal is to treat the underlying cause. When the underlying condition is anticholinergic toxicity, the use of physostigmine salicylate (Antilirium), 1 to 2 mg intravenously or intramuscularly, with repeated doses in 15 to 30 minutes may be indicated. The other important goal of treatment is to provide physical, sensory, and environmental support. Physical support is necessary so that delirious patients do not get into situations in which they may have accidents. Patients with delirium should be neither sensory deprived nor overly stimulated by the environment. They are usually helped by having a friend or relative in the room or by the presence of a regular sitter. Familiar pictures and decorations, the presence of a clock or a calendar, and regular orientations to person, place, and time help make patients with delirium comfortable. Delirium can sometimes occur in older patients wearing eye patches after cataract surgery ("black-patch delirium"). Such patients can be helped by placing pinholes in the patches to let in some stimuli or by occasionally removing one patch at a time during recovery.

Pharmacotherapy

The two major symptoms of delirium that may require pharmacological treatment are psychosis and insomnia. A commonly used drug for psychosis is haloperidol (Haldol), a butyrophenone antipsychotic drug. Depending on a patient's age, weight, and physical condition, the initial dose may range from 2 to 10 mg intramuscularly, repeated in an hour if the patient remains agitated. As soon as the patient is calm, oral medication in liquid concentrate or tablet form should begin. Two daily oral doses should suffice, with two thirds of the dose being given at bedtime. To achieve the same therapeutic effect, the oral dose should be approximately 1.5 times the parenteral dose. The effective total daily dose of haloperidol may range from 5 to 50 mg for most patients with delirium. Droperidol (Inapsine) is a butyrophenone available as an alternative intravenous formulation, although careful monitoring of the electrocardiogram may be prudent with this treatment. Phenothiazines should be avoided in delirious patients because these drugs are associated with significant anticholinergic activity.

Insomnia is best treated with benzodiazepines with short or intermediate half-lives, e.g., lorazepam (Ativan) 1 to 2 mg at bedtime. Benzodiazepines with long half-lives and barbiturates

Table 10.2–10
ICD-10 Diagnostic Criteria for Delirium, Not Induced by Alcohol and Other Psychoactive Substances

A. There is clouding of consciousness, i.e., reduced clarity of awareness of the environment, with reduced ability to focus, sustain, or shift attention.
B. Disturbance of cognition is manifest by both:
  (1) impairment of immediate recall and recent memory, with relatively intact remote memory;
  (2) disorientation in time, place, or person.
C. At least one of the following psychomotor disturbances is present:
  (1) rapid, unpredictable shifts from hypoactivity to hyperactivity;
  (2) increased reaction time;
  (3) increased or decreased flow of speech;
  (4) enhanced startle reaction.
D. There is disturbance of sleep or of the sleep–wake cycle, manifest by at least one of the following:
  (1) insomnia, which in severe cases may involve total sleep loss, with or without daytime drowsiness, or reversal of the sleep–wake cycle;
  (2) nocturnal worsening of symptoms;
  (3) disturbing dreams and nightmares, which may continue as hallucinations or illusions after awakening.
E. Symptoms have rapid onset and show fluctuations over the course of the day.
F. There is objective evidence from history, physical and neurological examination, or laboratory tests of an underlying cerebral or systemic disease (other than psychoactive substance-related) that can be presumed to be responsible for the clinical manifestations in Criteria A–D.

Comments

Emotional disturbances such as depression, anxiety or fear, irritability, euphoria, apathy, or wondering perplexity, disturbances of perception (illusions or hallucinations, often visual), and transient delusions are typical but are not specific indications for the diagnosis. A fourth character may be used to indicate whether or not the delirium is superimposed on dementia:

Delirium, not superimposed on dementia
Delirium, superimposed on dementia
Other delirium
Delirium, unspecified

should be avoided unless they are being used as part of the treatment for the underlying disorder (such as alcohol withdrawal). There have been case reports of improvement in or remission of delirious states due to intractable medical illnesses with electroconvulsive therapy (ECT); however, routine consideration of ECT for delirium is not advised. If delirium is due to severe pain or dyspnea, a physician should not hesitate to prescribe opioids for both their analgesic and sedative effects.

ICD-10

The 10th revision of *International Statistical Classification of Diseases and Related Health Problems* (ICD-10) criteria for delirium, not induced by alcohol and other psychoactive substances, are presented in Table 10.2–10. Delirium associated with the use of a substance are listed in Table 12.1–8 in section 12.1.

References

Breitbart W, Gibson C, Tremblay A. The delirium experience: delirium recall and delirium-related distress in hospitalized patients with cancer, their spouses/caregivers, and their nurses. *Psychosomatics.* 2002;43:183.

Caine ED, Lyness JM. Delirium, dementia, and amnestic and other cognitive disorders. In: Sadock BJ, Sadock VA, eds. *Kaplan & Sadock's Comprehensive Textbook of Psychiatry.* 7th ed. Vol 1. Baltimore: Lippincott Williams & Wilkins; 2000:854.

Flacker JM, Lipsitz LA. Neural mechanisms of delirium: current hypotheses and evolving concepts. *J Gerontol A Biol Sci Med Sci.* 1999;54:B239-246.

Fleminger S. Remembering delirium. *Br J Psychiatry.* 2002;180:4.

Francis J, Kapoor WN. Delirium in hospitalized elderly. *J Gen Intern Med.* 1990;5:65.

Liptzin B, Levkoff SE, Cleary PD, Pilgrim DM, Reilly CH, Albert M, Wetle TT. An empirical study of diagnostic criteria for delirium. *Am J Psychiatry.* 1991;148:454.

Meagher DJ. Delirium: Optimising management. *BMJ.* 2001;322:144–149.

Parikh SS, Chung F. Postoperative delirium in the elderly. *Anesth Analg.* 1995;80:1223.

Pompei P. Delirium in hospitalized elderly patients. *Hosp Pract Off Ed.* 1993;28:69.

Rockwood K. Educational interventions in delirium. *Demential & Geriatric Cognitive Disorders.* 1999;10:426–429.

Rummans TA, Evans JM, Krahn LE, Fleming KC. Delirium in elderly patients: evaluation and management. *Mayo Clin Proc.* 1995;70:989.

Shapira J, Roper J, Schulzinger J. Managing delirious patients. *Nursing.* 1993;23:78.

Taylor D, Lewis S. Delirium. *J Neurol Neurosurg Psychiatry.* 1993;56:742.

Trzepacz PT. The delirium rating scale: its use in consultation-liaison research. *Psychosomatics.* 1999;40:193–204.

▲ 10.3 Dementia

Dementia is a diminution in cognition in the setting of a stable level of consciousness. The persistent and stable nature of the impairment distinguishes dementia from the altered consciousness and fluctuating deficits of delirium. In the text revision of the fourth edition of *Diagnostic and Statistical Manual of Mental Disorders* (DSM-IV-TR), dementia is "characterized by multiple cognitive defects that include impairment in memory," without impairment in consciousness. The cognitive functions that can be affected in dementia include general intelligence, learning and memory, language, problem solving, orientation, perception, attention and concentration, judgment, and social abilities. A person's personality is also affected. A diagnosis of dementia, according to DSM-IV-TR, requires that the symptoms result in significant impairment in social or occupational functioning and that they represent a significant decline from a previous level of functioning.

The critical clinical points of dementia are the identification of the syndrome and the clinical workup of its cause. The disorder may be progressive or static, permanent or reversible. An underlying cause is always assumed, although in rare cases it is impossible to determine a specific cause. The potential reversibility of dementia is related to the underlying pathological condition and to the availability and application of effective treatment. Approximately 15 percent of people with dementia have reversible illnesses if treatment is initiated before irreversible damage takes place.

EPIDEMIOLOGY

Dementia is essentially a disease of older people. In the United States the prevalence rate is 1.5 percent for persons over 65

years old and rises to between 16 and 25 percent for those over 85. Approximately 5 percent of persons older than age 65 have severe dementia, and 15 percent have mild dementia. Of those older than age 80, approximately 20 percent have severe dementia. Of all patients with dementia, 50 to 60 percent have the most common type of dementia, dementia of the Alzheimer's type (Alzheimer's disease). Dementia of the Alzheimer's type increases in prevalence with increasing age. For persons aged 65 years old, males have a prevalence rate of 0.6 percent and females of 0.8 percent. At age 90, rates are 21 percent. For all these figures, 40 to 60 percent of cases are moderate to severe. The rates of prevalence (males to females) are 11 and 14 percent at age 85, 21 and 25 percent at age 90, and 36 and 41 percent at age 95. Patients with dementia of the Alzheimer's type occupy more than 50 percent of nursing home beds. Over 2 million persons with dementia are cared for in these homes. The risk factors for development of Alzheimer's disease include being female, having a first-degree relative with the disorder, and having a history of head injury. Down syndrome is also characteristically associated with the development of dementia of the Alzheimer's type.

According to the 2000 American Psychiatric Association (APA) *Practice Guideline for the Treatment of Patients with Alzheimer's Disease and Other Dementias of Late Life*, the onset of the disease generally occurs in late life, most commonly in the 60s, 70s, and 80s and beyond, but in rare instances the disorder appears in the 40s and 50s (known as early-onset dementia). The incidence of Alzheimer's disease also increases with age, and it is estimated to be 0.5 percent per year from age 65 to 69, 1 percent per year from age 70 to 74, 2 percent per year from age 75 to 79, 3 percent per year from 80 to 84, and 8 percent per year from age 85 onward. The disease has a gradual but steadily downward progression. Previous estimates of time of death after onset of symptoms ranged from 5 to 9 years; however, in a 2001 study of patients with Alzheimer's disease, the median survival was only 3 years after onset of symptoms.

The second most common type of dementia is vascular dementia, which is causally related to cerebrovascular diseases. Hypertension predisposes a person to the disease. Vascular dementias account for 15 to 30 percent of all dementia cases. Vascular dementia is most common in persons between the ages of 60 and 70 and is more common in men than in women. Approximately 10 to 15 percent of patients have coexisting vascular dementia and dementia of the Alzheimer's type.

Other common causes of dementia, each representing 1 to 5 percent of all cases, include head trauma, alcohol-related dementias, and various movement disorder–related dementias such as Huntington's disease and Parkinson's disease (Table 10.3–1). Because dementia is a fairly general syndrome, it has many causes, and clinicians must embark on a careful clinical workup of a patient with dementia to establish its cause.

Table 10.3–1
Disorders That May Produce Dementia

Alzheimer's disease[a]
Vascular dementia[b]
  Varieties: Multiple infarcts (called multi-infarct dementia)
    Lacunae
    Binswanger's disease
    Cortical microinfarction
Drugs and toxins (including chronic alcoholic dementia)[c]
Intracranial masses: tumors, subdural masses, brain abscesses[c]
Anoxia
Trauma
  Head injury[c]
  Dementia pugilistica (punch-drunk syndrome)
Normal-pressure hydrocephalus[c]
Neurodegenerative disorders
  Parkinson's disease[d]
  Huntington's disease[d]
  Progressive supranuclear palsy[d]
  Pick's disease[d]
  Amyotrophic lateral sclerosis
  Spinocerebellar degenerations
  Olivopontocerebellar degeneration
  Ophthalmoplegia plus
  Metachromatic leukodystrophy (adult form)
  Hallervorden-Spatz disease
  Wilson's disease
Infections
  Creutzfeldt-Jakob disease
  AIDS[d]
  Viral encephalitis
  Progressive multifocal leukoencephalopathy
  Behçet's syndrome
  Neurosyphilis
  Chronic bacterial meningitis
  Cryptococcal meningitis
  Other fungal meningitides
Nutritional disorders
  Wernicke-Korsakoff syndrome (thiamine deficiency)[c]
  Vitamin B_{12} deficiency
  Folate deficiency
  Pellagra
  Marchiafava-Bignami disease
  ?Zinc deficiency
Metabolic disorders
  Metachromatic leukodystrophy
  Adrenal leukodystrophy
  Dialysis dementia
  Hypothyroidism and hyperthyroidism
  Renal insufficiency, severe
  Cushing's syndrome
  Hepatic insufficiency
  Parathyroid disease
Chronic inflammatory disorders[d]
  Lupus and other collagen-vascular[d] disorders with intracerebral vasculitis
  Multiple sclerosis
  Whipple's disease

[a]Accounts for 50 to 60 percent of cases.
[b]Accounts for 10 to 20 percent of cases.
[c]Accounts for 1 to 5 percent of cases.
[d]Accounts for about 1 percent of cases.
No symbol: less than 1 percent of cases.
Reprinted with permission from Bosser M. Dementia. In: Asbury AK, McKhann GM, McDonald WI, eds. *Diseases of the Nervous System: Clinical Neurobiology.* 2nd ed. Philadelphia: WB Saunders; 1992:789.

ETIOLOGY

Dementia has many causes (see Table 10.3–1), but dementia of the Alzheimer's type and vascular dementia together represent up to 75 percent of all cases. Other causes of dementia specified in DSM-IV-TR are Pick's disease, Creutzfeldt-Jakob disease,

Huntington's disease, Parkinson's disease, human immunodeficiency virus (HIV), and head trauma.

Dementia of the Alzheimer's Type

In 1907, Alois Alzheimer first described the condition that later assumed his name. He described a 51-year-old woman with a 4½-year course of progressive dementia. The final diagnosis of Alzheimer's disease requires a neuropathological examination of the brain; nevertheless, dementia of the Alzheimer's type is commonly diagnosed in the clinical setting after other causes of dementia have been excluded from diagnostic consideration.

Genetic Factors. Although the cause of dementia of the Alzheimer's type remains unknown, progress has been made in understanding the molecular basis of the amyloid deposits that are a hallmark of the disorder's neuropathology. Some studies have indicated that as many as 40 percent of patients have a family history of dementia of the Alzheimer's type; thus, genetic factors are presumed to play a part in the development of the disorder, at least in some cases. Additional support for a genetic influence is the concordance rate for monozygotic twins, which is higher than the rate for dizygotic twins (43 percent versus 8 percent, respectively). In several well-documented cases, the disorder has been transmitted in families through an autosomal dominant gene, although such transmission is rare. Alzheimer's type dementia has shown linkage to chromosomes 1, 14, and 21.

AMYLOID PRECURSOR PROTEIN

The gene for amyloid precursor protein is on the long arm of chromosome 21. The process of differential splicing yields four forms of amyloid precursor protein. The β/A4 protein, the major constituent of senile plaques, is a 42–amino acid peptide that is a breakdown product of amyloid precursor protein. In Down syndrome (trisomy 21), there are three copies of the amyloid precursor protein gene, and in a disease in which there is a mutation at codon 717 in the amyloid precursor protein gene, a pathological process results in the excessive deposition of β/A4 protein. Whether the processing of abnormal amyloid precursor protein is of primary causative significance in Alzheimer's disease is unknown, but many research groups are studying both the normal metabolic processing of amyloid precursor protein and its processing in patients with dementia of the Alzheimer's type in an attempt to answer this question.

MULTIPLE E4 GENES

One study implicated gene E4 in the origin of Alzheimer's disease. People with one copy of the gene have Alzheimer's disease three times more frequently than do those with no E4 gene, and people with two E4 genes have the disease eight times more frequently than do those with no E4 gene. Diagnostic testing for this gene is not currently recommended because it is found in persons without dementia and not found in all cases of dementia.

Neuropathology. The classic gross neuroanatomical observation of a brain from a patient with Alzheimer's disease is diffuse atrophy (Fig. 10.3–1) with flattened cortical sulci and enlarged cerebral ventricles. The classic and pathognomonic microscopic findings are senile plaques, neurofibrillary tangles, neuronal loss (particularly in the cortex and the hippocampus), synaptic loss (perhaps as much as 50 percent in the cortex), and granulovascular degeneration of the neurons. Neurofibrillary tangles (Fig. 10.3–2) are composed of cytoskeletal elements, primarily phosphorylated tau protein, although other cytoskeletal proteins are also present. Neurofibrillary tangles are not unique to Alzheimer's disease, but also occur in Down syndrome, dementia pugilistica (punch-drunk syndrome), Parkinson–

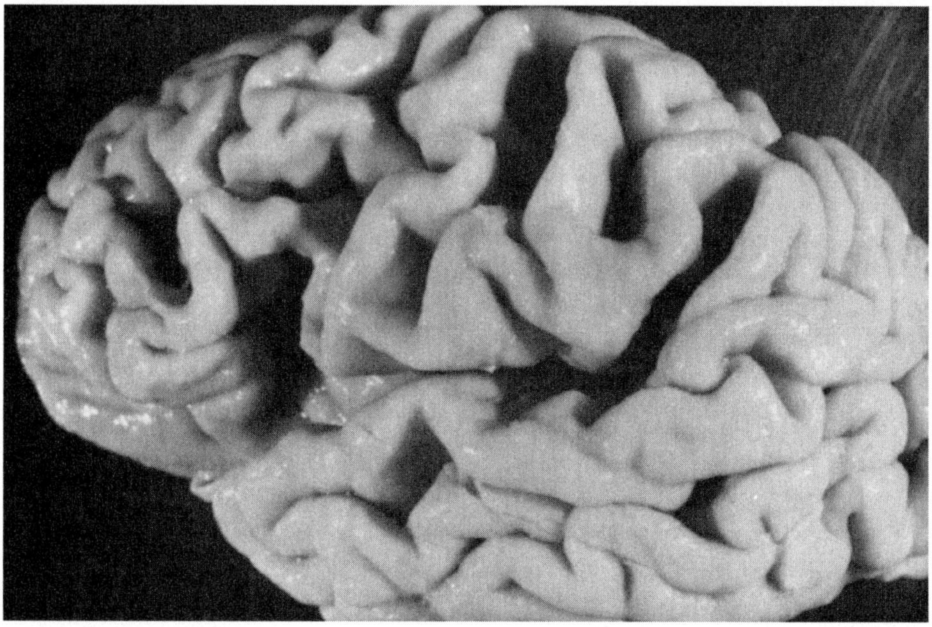

FIGURE 10.3–1
Gross external appearance of the brain of a patient who had dementia of the Alzheimer's type, with late onset. The leptomeninges have been removed so that the generalized atrophy may be fully appreciated. (Courtesy of Daniel P. Perl, M.D.)

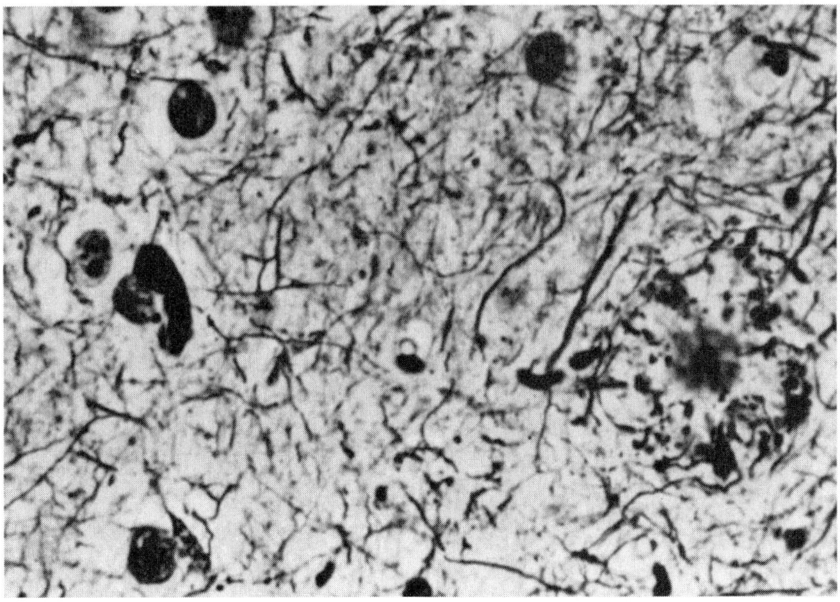

FIGURE 10.3–2
Alzheimer's disease. Prominent senile plaques on left. Several neurons with neurofibrillary tangles on right. Note also disruption of cortical organization. (Reprinted from Mayeux R, Chun MR. Acquired and hereditary dementias. In: Rowland LP, ed. *Merritt's Textbook of Neurology.* 10th ed. Philadelphia: Lippincott Williams & Wilkins; 2000:636.)

dementia complex of Guam, Hallervorden-Spatz disease, and the brains of normal people as they age. Neurofibrillary tangles are commonly found in the cortex, the hippocampus, the substantia nigra, and the locus ceruleus.

Senile plaques, also referred to as amyloid plaques, more strongly indicate Alzheimer's disease, although they are also seen in Down syndrome and, to some extent, in normal aging. Senile plaques are composed of a particular protein, β/A4, and astrocytes, dystrophic neuronal processes, and microglia. The number and the density of senile plaques present in postmortem brains have been correlated with the severity of the disease that affected the persons.

Neurotransmitters. The neurotransmitters that are most often implicated in the pathophysiological condition of Alzheimer's disease are acetylcholine and norepinephrine, both of which are hypothesized to be hypoactive in Alzheimer's disease. Several studies have reported data consistent with the hypothesis that specific degeneration of cholinergic neurons is present in the nucleus basalis of Meynert in persons with Alzheimer's disease. Other data supporting a cholinergic deficit in Alzheimer's disease demonstrate decreased acetylcholine and choline acetyltransferase concentrations in the brain. Choline acetyltransferase is the key enzyme for the synthesis of acetylcholine, and a reduction in choline acetyltransferase concentration suggests a decrease in the number of cholinergic neurons present. Additional support for the cholinergic deficit hypothesis comes from the observation that cholinergic antagonists, such as scopolamine and atropine, impair cognitive abilities, whereas cholinergic agonists, such as physostigmine and arecoline, enhance cognitive abilities. Decreased norepinephrine activity in Alzheimer's disease is suggested by the decrease in norepinephrine-containing neurons in the locus ceruleus found in some pathological examinations of brains from persons with Alzheimer's disease. Two other neurotransmitters implicated in the pathophysiological condition of Alzheimer's disease are the neuroactive peptides somatostatin and corticotropin; decreased concentrations of both have been reported in persons with Alzheimer's disease.

Other Causes. Another theory to explain the development of Alzheimer's disease is that an abnormality in the regulation of membrane phospholipid metabolism results in membranes that are less fluid—that is, more rigid—than normal. Several investigators are using molecular resonance spectroscopic imaging to assess this hypothesis directly in patients with dementia of the Alzheimer's type. Aluminum toxicity has also been hypothesized to be a causative factor, because high levels of aluminum have been found in the brains of some patients with Alzheimer's disease; but this is no longer considered a significant etiological factor. Excessive stimulation by the transmitter glutamate that may damage neurons is another theory of causation.

Familial Multiple System Taupathy with Presenile Dementia. A recently discovered type of dementia, familial multiple system taupathy, shares some brain abnormalities found in people with Alzheimer's disease. The gene that causes the disorder is thought to be carried on chromosome 17. The symptoms of the disorder include short-term memory problems and difficulty maintaining balance and walking. The onset of disease occurs in the 40s and 50s, and persons with the disease live an average of 11 years after the onset of symptoms.

As in Alzheimer's disease patients, tau protein builds up in neurons and glial cells of persons with familial multiple system taupathy. Eventually, the protein buildup kills brain cells. The

disorder is not associated with the senile plaques associated with Alzheimer's disease.

Vascular Dementia

The primary cause of vascular dementia, formerly referred to as multi-infarct dementia, is presumed to be multiple cerebral vascular disease, resulting in a symptom pattern of dementia. Vascular dementia is most common in men, especially those with preexisting hypertension or other cardiovascular risk factors. The disorder affects primarily small- and medium-sized cerebral vessels, which undergo infarction and produce multiple parenchymal lesions spread over wide areas of the brain (Fig. 10.3–3). The causes of the infarctions may include occlusion of the vessels by arteriosclerotic plaques or thromboemboli from distant origins (such as heart valves). An examination of a patient may reveal carotid bruits, funduscopic abnormalities, or enlarged cardiac chambers.

Binswanger's Disease. Binswanger's disease, also known as subcortical arteriosclerotic encephalopathy, is characterized by the presence of many small infarctions of the white matter that spare the cortical regions. Although Binswanger's disease was previously considered a rare condition, the advent of sophisticated and powerful imaging techniques, such as magnetic resonance imaging (MRI), has revealed that the condition is more common than previously thought.

Pick's Disease

In contrast to the parietal-temporal distribution of pathological findings in Alzheimer's disease, Pick's disease is characterized by a preponderance of atrophy in the frontotemporal regions. These regions also have neuronal loss, gliosis, and neuronal Pick's bodies, which are masses of cytoskeletal elements. Pick's bodies are seen in some postmortem specimens but are not necessary for the diagnosis. The cause of Pick's disease is unknown, but the disease constitutes approximately 5 percent of all irreversible dementias. It is most common in men, especially those who have a first-degree relative with the condition. Pick's disease is difficult to distinguish from dementia of the Alzheimer's type, although the early stages of Pick's disease are more often characterized by personality and behavioral changes, with relative preservation of other cognitive functions. Features of Klüver-Bucy syndrome (such as hypersexuality, placidity, and hyperorality) are much more common in Pick's disease than in Alzheimer's disease.

Lewy Body Disease

Lewy body disease is a dementia clinically similar to Alzheimer's disease and often characterized by hallucinations, parkinsonian features, and extrapyramidal signs. Lewy inclusion bodies are found in the cerebral cortex. The exact incidence is unknown. These patients show marked adverse effects when given antipsychotic medications.

Huntington's Disease

Huntington's disease is classically associated with the development of dementia. The dementia seen in this disease is the subcortical type of dementia, characterized by more motor abnormalities and fewer language abnormalities than in the cortical type of dementia (Table 10.3–2). The dementia of Huntington's disease exhibits psychomotor slowing and difficulty with complex tasks, but memory, language, and insight remain relatively intact in the early and middle stages of the illness. As the disease progresses, however, the dementia becomes complete; the features distinguishing it from dementia of the Alzheimer's type are the high incidence of depres-

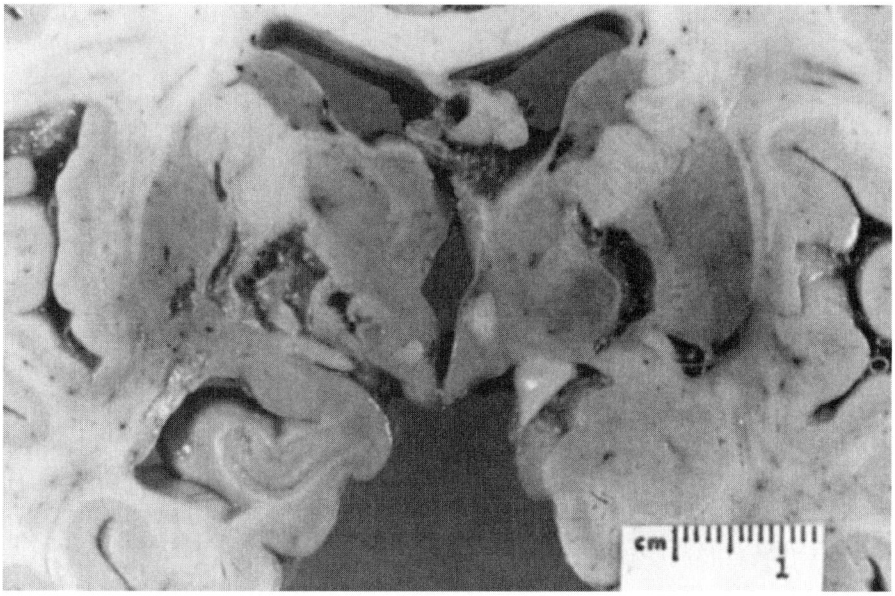

FIGURE 10.3–3

Gross appearance of the cerebral cortex on coronal section from a case of vascular dementia. The multiple bilateral lacunar infarcts involve the thalamus, the internal capsule, and the globus pallidus. (Courtesy of Daniel P. Perl, M.D.)

Table 10.3–2
Distinguishing Features of Subcortical and Cortical Dementias

Characteristic	Subcortical Dementia	Cortical Dementia	Recommended Tests
Language	No aphasia (anomia, if severe)	Aphasia early	FAS test Boston Naming test WAIS-R vocabulary test
Memory	Impaired recall (retrieval) > recognition (encoding)	Recall and recognition impaired	Wechsler memory scale; Symbol Digit Paired Associate Learning (Brandt)
Attention and immediate recall	Impaired	Impaired	WAIS-R digit span
Visuospatial skills	Impaired	Impaired	Picture arrangement, object assembly and block design; WAIS subtests
Calculation	Preserved until late	Involved early	Mini-Mental State
Frontal system abilities (executive function)	Disproportionately affected	Degree of impairment consistent with other involvement	Wisconsin Card Sorting Test; Odd Man Out test; Picture Absurdities
Speed of cognitive processing	Slowed early	Normal until late in disease	Trail making A and B: Paced Auditory Serial Addition Test (PASAT)
Personality	Apathetic, inert	Unconcerned	MMPI
Mood	Depressed	Euthymic	Beck and Hamilton depression scales
Speech	Dysarthric	Articulate until late	Verbal fluency (Rosen, 1980)
Posture	Bowed or extended	Upright	
Coordination	Impaired	Normal until late	
Motor speed and control	Slowed	Normal	Finger-tap; grooved pegboard
Adventitious movements	Chorea, tremor tics, dystonia	Absent (Alzheimer's dementia—some myoclonus)	
Abstraction	Impaired	Impaired	Category test (Halstead Battery)

Reprinted with permission from Pajeau AK, Román GC. HIV encephalopathy and dementia. In: J Biller, RG Kathol, eds. *The Psychiatric Clinics of North America: The Interface of Psychiatry and Neurology.* Vol. 15. Philadelphia: WB Saunders; 1992:457.

sion and psychosis, in addition to the classic choreoathetoid movement disorder.

Parkinson's Disease

Like Huntington's disease, parkinsonism is a disease of the basal ganglia, commonly associated with dementia and depression. An estimated 20 to 30 percent of patients with Parkinson's disease have dementia, and an additional 30 to 40 percent have measurable impairment in cognitive abilities. The slow movements of persons with Parkinson's disease are paralleled in the slow thinking of some affected patients, a feature that clinicians may refer to as bradyphrenia.

HIV-Related Dementia

Infection with HIV commonly leads to dementia and other psychiatric symptoms. Patients infected with HIV experience dementia at an annual rate of approximately 14 percent. An estimated 75 percent of patients with acquired immune deficiency syndrome (AIDS) have involvement of the central nervous system (CNS) at the time of autopsy. The development of dementia in people infected with HIV is often paralleled by the appearance of parenchymal abnormalities in MRI scans. Other infectious dementias are caused by *Cryptococcus* and *Treponema pallidum.*

Head Trauma–Related Dementia

Dementia can be a sequela of head trauma. The so-called punch-drunk syndrome (dementia pugilistica) occurs in boxers after repeated head trauma over many years. It is characterized by emotional lability, dysarthria, and impulsivity.

DIAGNOSIS AND CLINICAL FEATURES

The dementia diagnoses in DSM-IV-TR are dementia of the Alzheimer's type (Table 10.3–3), vascular dementia (Table 10.3–4), dementia due to other general medical conditions (Table 10.3–5), substance-induced persisting dementia (Table 10.3–6), dementia due to multiple etiologies (Table 10.3–7), and dementia not otherwise specified (Table 10.3–8).

The diagnosis of dementia is based on the clinical examination, including a mental status examination, and on information from the patient's family, friends, and employers. Complaints of a personality change in a patient older than age 40 suggest that a diagnosis of dementia should be carefully considered.

Clinicians should note patients' complaints about intellectual impairment and forgetfulness as well as evidence of patients' evasion, denial, or rationalization aimed at concealing cognitive deficits. Excessive orderliness, social withdrawal, or a tendency to relate events in minute detail can be characteristic, and sudden outbursts of anger or sarcasm may occur. Patients' appearance and behavior should be observed. Lability of emotions, sloppy grooming, uninhibited remarks, silly jokes, or a dull, apathetic, or vacuous facial expression and manner suggest the presence of dementia, especially when coupled with memory impairment.

Memory impairment is typically an early and prominent feature in dementia, especially in dementias involving the cortex, such as dementia of the Alzheimer's type. Early in the

Table 10.3–3
DSM-IV-TR Diagnostic Criteria for Dementia of the Alzheimer's Type

A. The development of multiple cognitive deficits manifested by both
   (1) memory impairment (impaired ability to learn new information or to recall previously learned information)
   (2) one (or more) of the following cognitive disturbances:
      (a) aphasia (language disturbance)
      (b) apraxia (impaired ability to carry out motor activities despite intact motor function)
      (c) agnosia (failure to recognize or identify objects despite intact sensory function)
      (d) disturbance in executive functioning (i.e., planning, organizing, sequencing, abstracting)

B. The cognitive deficits in Criteria A1 and A2 each cause significant impairment in social or occupational functioning and represent a significant decline from a previous level of functioning.

C. The course is characterized by gradual onset and continuing cognitive decline.

D. The cognitive deficits in Criteria A1 and A2 are not due to any of the following:
   (1) other central nervous system conditions that cause progressive deficits in memory and cognition (e.g., cerebrovascular disease, Parkinson's disease, Huntington's disease, subdural hematoma, normal-pressure hydrocephalus, brain tumor)
   (2) systemic conditions that are known to cause dementia (e.g., hypothyroidism, vitamin B_{12} or folic acid deficiency, niacin deficiency, hypercalcemia, neurosyphilis, HIV infection)
   (3) substance-induced conditions

E. The deficits do not occur exclusively during the course of a delirium.

F. The disturbance is not better accounted for by another Axis I disorder (e.g., major depressive disorder, schizophrenia).

Code based on presence or absence of a clinically significant behavioral disturbance:

Without behavioral disturbance: if the cognitive disturbance is not accompanied by any clinically significant behavioral disturbance.

With behavioral disturbance: if the cognitive disturbance is accompanied by a clinically significant behavioral disturbance (e.g., wandering, agitation).

Specify subtype:

With early onset: if onset is at age 65 years or below

With late onset: if onset is after age 65 years

Coding note: Also code Alzheimer's disease on Axis III. Indicate other prominent clinical features related to the Alzheimer's disease on Axis I (e.g., Mood disorder due to Alzheimer's disease, with depressive features, and Personality change due to Alzheimer's disease, aggressive type).

From American Psychiatric Association. *Diagnostic and Statistical Manual of Mental Disorders.* 4th ed. Text rev. Washington, DC: American Psychiatric Association; copyright 2000, with permission.

Table 10.3–4
DSM-IV-TR Diagnostic Criteria for Vascular Dementia

A. The development of multiple cognitive deficits manifested by both
   (1) memory impairment (impaired ability to learn new information or to recall previously learned information)
   (2) one (or more) of the following cognitive disturbances:
      (a) aphasia (language disturbance)
      (b) apraxia (impaired ability to carry out motor activities despite intact motor function)
      (c) agnosia (failure to recognize or identify objects despite intact sensory function)
      (d) disturbance in executive functioning (i.e., planning, organizing, sequencing, abstracting)

B. The cognitive deficits in Criteria A1 and A2 each cause significant impairment in social or occupational functioning and represent a significant decline from a previous level of functioning.

C. Focal neurological signs and symptoms (e.g., exaggeration of deep tendon reflexes, extensor plantar response, pseudobulbar palsy, gait abnormalities, weakness of an extremity) or laboratory evidence indicative of cerebrovascular disease (e.g., multiple infarctions involving cortex and underlying white matter) that are judged to be etiologically related to the disturbance.

D. The deficits do not occur exclusively during the course of a delirium.

Code based on predominant features:

With delirium: if delirium is superimposed on the dementia

With delusions: if delusions are the predominant feature

With depressed mood: if depressed mood (including presentations that meet full symptom criteria for a major depressive episode) is the predominant feature. A separate diagnosis of mood disorder due to a general medical condition is not given.

Uncomplicated: if none of the above predominates in the current clinical presentation

Specify if:

With behavioral disturbance

Coding note: Also code cerebrovascular condition on Axis III.

From American Psychiatric Association. *Diagnostic and Statistical Manual of Mental Disorders.* 4th ed. Text rev. Washington, DC: American Psychiatric Association; copyright 2000, with permission.

course of dementia, memory impairment is mild and usually most marked for recent events; people forget telephone numbers, conversations, and events of the day. As the course of dementia progresses, memory impairment becomes severe, and only the earliest learned information (such as a person's place of birth) is retained.

Inasmuch as memory is important for orientation to person, place, and time, orientation can be progressively affected during the course of a dementing illness. For example, patients with dementia may forget how to get back to their rooms after going to the bathroom. No matter how severe the disorientation seems, however, patients show no impairment in their level of consciousness.

Dementing processes that affect the cortex, primarily dementia of the Alzheimer's type and vascular dementia, can affect patients' language abilities. DSM-IV-TR includes aphasia as one of the diagnostic criteria. The language difficulty may be characterized by a vague, stereotyped, imprecise, or circumstantial locution, and patients may also have difficulty naming objects.

Table 10.3–5
DSM-IV-TR Diagnostic Criteria for Dementia Due to Other General Medical Conditions

A. The development of multiple cognitive deficits manifested by both
  (1) memory impairment (impaired ability to learn new information or to recall previously learned information)
  (2) one (or more) of the following cognitive disturbances:
    (a) aphasia (language disturbance)
    (b) apraxia (impaired ability to carry out motor activities despite intact motor function)
    (c) agnosia (failure to recognize or identify objects despite intact sensory function)
    (d) disturbance in executive functioning (i.e., planning, organizing, sequencing, abstracting)

B. The cognitive deficits in Criteria A1 and A2 each cause significant impairment in social or occupational functioning and represent a significant decline from a previous level of functioning.

C. There is evidence from the history, physical examination, or laboratory findings that the disturbance is the direct physiological consequence of a general medical condition other than Alzheimer's disease or cerebrovascular disease (e.g., HIV infection, traumatic brain injury, Parkinson's disease, Huntington's disease, Pick's disease, Creutzfeldt-Jakob disease, normal-pressure hydrocephalus, hypothyroidism, brain tumor, or vitamin B_{12} deficiency).

D. The deficits do not occur exclusively during the course of a delirium.

Code based on presence or absence of a clinically significant behavioral disturbance:

Without behavioral disturbance: if the cognitive disturbance is not accompanied by any clinically significant behavioral disturbance.

With behavioral disturbance: if the cognitive disturbance is accompanied by a clinically significant behavioral disturbance (e.g., wandering, agitation).

Coding note: Also code the general medical condition on Axis III (e.g., HIV infection, head injury, Parkinson's disease, Huntington's disease, Pick's disease, Creutzfeldt-Jakob disease).

From American Psychiatric Association. *Diagnostic and Statistical Manual of Mental Disorders.* 4th ed. Text rev. Washington, DC: American Psychiatric Association; copyright 2000, with permission.

Table 10.3–6
DSM-IV-TR Diagnostic Criteria for Substance-Induced Persisting Dementia

A. The development of multiple cognitive deficits manifested by both
  (1) memory impairment (impaired ability to learn new information or to recall previously learned information)
  (2) one (or more) of the following cognitive disturbances:
    (a) aphasia (language disturbance)
    (b) apraxia (impaired ability to carry out motor activities despite intact motor function)
    (c) agnosia (failure to recognize or identify objects despite intact sensory function)
    (d) disturbance in executive functioning (i.e., planning, organizing, sequencing, abstracting)

B. The cognitive deficits in Criteria A1 and A2 each cause significant impairment in social or occupational functioning and represent a significant decline from a previous level of functioning.

C. The deficits do not occur exclusively during the course of a delirium and persist beyond the usual duration of substance intoxication or withdrawal.

D. There is evidence from the history, physical examination, or laboratory findings that the deficits are etiologically related to the persisting effects of substance use (e.g., a drug of abuse, a medication).

Code (Specific substance)-induced persisting dementia:

(Alcohol; Inhalant; Sedative, hypnotic, or anxiolytic; Other [or unknown] substance)

From American Psychiatric Association. *Diagnostic and Statistical Manual of Mental Disorders.* 4th ed. Text rev. Washington, DC: American Psychiatric Association; copyright 2000, with permission.

Table 10.3–7
DSM-IV-TR Diagnostic Criteria for Dementia Due to Multiple Etiologies

A. The development of multiple cognitive deficits manifested by both
  (1) memory impairment (impaired ability to learn new information or to recall previously learned information)
  (2) one (or more) of the following cognitive disturbances:
    (a) aphasia (language disturbance)
    (b) apraxia (impaired ability to carry out motor activities despite intact motor function)
    (c) agnosia (failure to recognize or identify objects despite intact sensory function)
    (d) disturbance in executive functioning (i.e., planning, organizing, sequencing, abstracting)

B. The cognitive deficits in Criteria A1 and A2 each cause significant impairment in social or occupational functioning and represent a significant decline from a previous level of functioning.

C. There is evidence from the history, physical examination, or laboratory findings that the disturbance has more than one etiology (e.g., head trauma plus chronic alcohol use, dementia of the Alzheimer's type with the subsequent development of vascular dementia).

D. The deficits do not occur exclusively during the course of a delirium.

Coding note: Use multiple codes based on specific dementias and specific etiologies, e.g., Dementia of the Alzheimer's type, with late onset, without behavioral disturbance; Vascular dementia, uncomplicated.

From American Psychiatric Association. *Diagnostic and Statistical Manual of Mental Disorders.* 4th ed. Text rev. Washington, DC: American Psychiatric Association; copyright 2000, with permission.

Psychiatric and Neurological Changes

Personality. Changes in the personality of a person with dementia are especially disturbing for the families of affected patients. Preexisting personality traits may be accentuated during the development of a dementia. Patients with dementia may also become introverted and may seem to be less concerned than they previously were about the effects of their behavior on others. Persons with dementia who have paranoid delusions are generally hostile to family members and caretakers. Patients with frontal and temporal involvement are likely to have marked personality changes and may be irritable and explosive.

Hallucinations and Delusions. An estimated 20 to 30 percent of patients with dementia (primarily patients with dementia of the Alzheimer's type) have hallucinations, and 30 to 40 percent have delusions, primarily of a paranoid or persecutory and unsystematized nature, although complex, sustained, and

Table 10.3–8
DSM-IV-TR Diagnostic Criteria for Dementia Not Otherwise Specified

This category should be used to diagnose a dementia that does not meet criteria for any of the specific types described in this section.

An example is a clinical presentation of dementia for which there is insufficient evidence to establish a specific etiology.

From American Psychiatric Association. *Diagnostic and Statistical Manual of Mental Disorders.* 4th ed. Text rev. Washington, DC: American Psychiatric Association; copyright 2000, with permission.

well-systematized delusions are also reported by these patients. Physical aggression and other forms of violence are common in demented patients who also have psychotic symptoms.

Mood. In addition to psychosis and personality changes, depression and anxiety are major symptoms in an estimated 40 to 50 percent of patients with dementia, although the full syndrome of depressive disorder may be present in only 10 to 20 percent. Patients with dementia may also exhibit pathological laughter or crying—that is, extremes of emotions—with no apparent provocation.

Cognitive Change. In addition to the aphasias in patients with dementia, apraxias and agnosias are common, and they are included as potential diagnostic criteria in DSM-IV-TR. Other neurological signs that can be associated with dementia are seizures, seen in approximately 10 percent of patients with dementia of the Alzheimer's type and in 20 percent of patients with vascular dementia, and atypical neurological presentations, such as nondominant parietal lobe syndromes. Primitive reflexes—such as the grasp, snout, suck, tonic-foot, and palmomental reflexes—may be present on neurological examination, and myoclonic jerks are present in 5 to 10 percent of patients.

Patients with vascular dementia may have additional neurological symptoms, such as headaches, dizziness, faintness, weakness, focal neurological signs, and sleep disturbances, possibly attributable to the location of the cerebrovascular disease. Pseudobulbar palsy, dysarthria, and dysphagia are also more common in vascular dementia than in other dementing conditions.

Catastrophic Reaction. Patients with dementia also exhibit a reduced ability to apply what Kurt Goldstein called the "abstract attitude." Patients have difficulty generalizing from a single instance, forming concepts, and grasping similarities and differences among concepts. Furthermore, the ability to solve problems, to reason logically, and to make sound judgments is compromised. Goldstein also described a catastrophic reaction marked by agitation secondary to the subjective awareness of intellectual deficits under stressful circumstances. Persons usually attempt to compensate for defects by using strategies to avoid demonstrating failures in intellectual performance; they may change the subject, make jokes, or otherwise divert the interviewer. Lack of judgment and poor impulse control appear commonly, particularly in dementias that primarily affect the frontal lobes. Examples of these impairments include coarse language, inappropriate jokes, neglect of personal appearance and hygiene, and a general disregard for the conventional rules of social conduct.

Sundowner Syndrome. Sundowner syndrome is characterized by drowsiness, confusion, ataxia, and accidental falls. It occurs in older people who are overly sedated and in patients with dementia who react adversely to even a small dose of a psychoactive drug. The syndrome also occurs in demented patients when external stimuli, such as light and interpersonal orienting cues, are diminished.

Dementia of the Alzheimer's Type

The DSM-IV-TR diagnostic criteria for dementia of the Alzheimer's type emphasize the presence of memory impairment and the associated presence of at least one other symptom of cognitive decline (aphasia, apraxia, agnosia, or abnormal executive functioning). The diagnostic criteria also require a continuing and gradual decline in functioning, impairment in social or occupational functioning, and the exclusion of other causes of dementia. According to DSM-IV-TR, the age of onset can be characterized as early (at age 65 or younger) or late (after age 65) and any predominant behavioral symptom should be coded with the diagnosis, if appropriate.

Mr. E. is a 68-year-old married man with two children who has been followed by a multidisciplinary team at a Department of Veterans Affairs (VA) geriatric research and clinical center for the past 6 years. The occasion for this evaluation is Mrs. E.'s request for residential placement for her husband.

Mr. E. was first evaluated 9 years ago when his wife observed changes in his memory and behavior and suggested that they seek medical advice. At that time, Mr. E. was still employed as a security guard. During the couple's initial visit to a physician, Mr. E. acknowledged that he had been aware of increasing memory problems for at least the past 2 years. He said that he frequently forgot his keys or would go into the house to get something and then forget what he wanted. Mrs. E. noted that he had changed from an outgoing, pleasant person to one who avoided conversation. She said that he also seemed hostile at times for no apparent reason. Mr. E. was in good general health and was not taking any medications. His alcohol consumption was limited to two to three beers a day. He had no significant medical or psychiatric history and no significant family history for either cognitive or psychiatric disorders.

Three years later, Mrs. E. contacted the VA center for treatment of her husband's cognitive and behavior symptoms. The neurological examination demonstrated an absence of focal abnormalities, but glabellar, snout, and palmomental responses were present. Mr. E. was hesitant and had difficulty with sustained attention, which made determination of visual fields difficult. There was no evidence of any disturbance of mood. On examination of his sensorium, Mr. E. was disoriented about place and date; he missed the actual date by 2 years and 1 month. However, he seemed to comprehend most of the questions and was aware that he was experiencing cognitive difficulties.

On neuropsychological testing, Mr. E. showed moderate to severe impairment in memory, attention, visual spatial reasoning, set shifting, and judgment and planning abilities. Results of laboratory screening tests were unremarkable. An electroencephalogram (EEG) was mildly abnormal, showing nonspecific theta waves and sharp discharge bilaterally. A computed tomographic (CT) head scan showed slight enlargement of the lateral ventricles and the third ventricle, which was consistent with mild atrophy.

Mr. E. was started on 1 mg of haloperidol at bedtime. Shortly after this, his wife became concerned that the medication was actually increasing his agitated behavior because he had begun to lock himself in the bedroom and would not allow her to clean him up after he was incontinent of stool in his clothing. The haloperidol dosage was then reduced to 0.5 mg a day. Mr. E.'s behavior did not improve after 4 months of medication, so the drug was discontinued at Mrs. E.'s request.

A year and a half after Mr. E.'s initial visit to the geriatric center (and 6 years after he began experiencing cognitive and behavioral symptoms), Mrs. E. first began discussing long-term placement for Mr. E. with the treatment team. By this time, the dementia was severe; Mr. E. paced most of the night, experienced frequent crying spells, and had become physically threatening to his wife. On one occasion, Mrs. E. had gotten up during the night to find that her husband had turned up the thermostat to the maximum temperature, turned on all the burners on the stove, and turned the oven on at 500°.

However, after exploring family support options with the team, Mrs. E. decided to continue to care for her husband in their home. A selective serotonin reuptake inhibitor (SSRI) was prescribed for him, after which Mrs. E. noted an initial decrease in Mr. E.'s crying, an improvement in his sleep, and an increased willingness to help with some of the household chores. However, Mrs. E. soon felt that the medication was making Mr. E. more confused and unmanageable, and after 4 months it was discontinued.

About 7 months later, Mrs. E. brings her husband in for this evaluation to seriously investigate residential placement for him. She says she is at the end of her rope because Mr. E. constantly wanders off when she isn't watching him and has nearly been run over on several occasions. Although she describes feeling terribly guilty about "abandoning" him, she does not think she can cope any longer with the responsibility of ensuring his safety. She doesn't see any alternative but to arrange for his placement in a residential facility. Mr. E. is therefore transferred from the geriatric center to a VA long-term-care center 120 miles away.

DSM-IV-TR DIAGNOSIS

Axis I: Dementia of Alzheimer's type, with early onset, uncomplicated
Axis II: No diagnosis
Axis III: Alzheimer's disease
Axis IV: Financial difficulties
Axis V: GAF = 15 (current); 20 (highest level in the past year)

(From *DSM-IV Case Studies.*)

Vascular Dementia

The general symptoms of vascular dementia are the same as those for dementia of the Alzheimer's type, but the diagnosis of vascular dementia requires either clinical or laboratory evidence in support of a vascular cause of the dementia. Vascular dementia is more likely to show a decremental, stepwise deterioration than is Alzheimer's disease.

Dementia Due to Other General Medical Conditions

DSM-IV-TR lists six specific causes of dementia that can be coded directly: HIV disease, head trauma, Parkinson's disease, Huntington's disease, Pick's disease, and Creutzfeldt-Jakob disease. A seventh category allows clinicians to specify other nonpsychiatric medical conditions associated with dementia.

Substance-Induced Persisting Dementia

To facilitate the clinician's thinking about differential diagnosis, substance-induced persisting dementia is listed in two places in the DSM-IV-TR, with the dementias and with the substance-related disorders. The specific substances that DSM-IV-TR cross-references are alcohol; inhalant; sedatives, hypnotics, or anxiolytics; and other or unknown substances.

PATHOLOGY, PHYSICAL FINDINGS, AND LABORATORY EXAMINATION

A comprehensive laboratory workup must be performed when one is evaluating a patient with dementia. The purposes of the workup are to detect reversible causes of dementia and to provide the patient and family with a definitive diagnosis. The range of possible causes of dementia mandates selective use of laboratory tests. The evaluation should follow informed clinical suspicion, based on the history and physical and mental status examination results. Table 10.1–6 in Section 10.1 lists a number of laboratory tests that are useful in evaluating specific diseases presenting as dementia. The continued improvements in brain imaging techniques, particularly MRI, have, in some cases, made differentiation between dementia of the Alzheimer's type and vascular dementia somewhat more straightforward than in the past. An active area of research is the use of single photon emission computed tomography (SPECT) to detect patterns of brain metabolism in various types of dementias; the use of SPECT images may soon help in the clinical differential diagnosis of dementing illnesses.

A general physical examination is a routine component of the workup for dementia. It may reveal evidence of systemic disease causing brain dysfunction, such as an enlarged liver and hepatic encephalopathy, or it may demonstrate systemic disease related to particular CNS processes. The detection of Kaposi's sarcoma, for example, should alert the clinician to the probable presence of AIDS and the associated possibility of AIDS dementia complex. Focal neurological findings, such as asymmetrical hyperreflexia or weakness, are seen more often in vascular than in degenerative disease. Frontal lobe signs and

primitive reflexes occur in many disorders and often point to greater progression.

DIFFERENTIAL DIAGNOSIS

Dementia of the Alzheimer's Type versus Vascular Dementia

Classically, vascular dementia has been distinguished from dementia of the Alzheimer's type by the decremental deterioration that may accompany cerebrovascular disease over time. Although the discrete, stepwise deterioration may not be apparent in all cases, focal neurological symptoms are more common in vascular dementia than in dementia of the Alzheimer's type, as are the standard risk factors for cerebrovascular disease.

Vascular Dementia versus Transient Ischemic Attacks

Transient ischemic attacks (TIAs) are brief episodes of focal neurological dysfunction lasting less than 24 hours (usually 5 to 15 minutes). Although a variety of mechanisms may be responsible, the episodes are frequently the result of microembolization from a proximal intracranial arterial lesion that produces transient brain ischemia, and the episodes usually resolve without significant pathological alteration of the parenchymal tissue. Approximately one third of persons whose TIAs were untreated experience a brain infarction later; therefore, recognition of TIAs is an important clinical strategy to prevent brain infarction.

Clinicians should distinguish episodes involving the vertebrobasilar system from those involving the carotid arterial system. In general, symptoms of vertebrobasilar disease reflect a transient functional disturbance in either the brainstem or the occipital lobe; carotid distribution symptoms reflect unilateral retinal or hemispheric abnormality. Anticoagulant therapy, antiplatelet agglutinating drugs such as aspirin, and extracranial and intracranial reconstructive vascular surgery are effective in reducing the risk of infarction in patients with transient ischemic attacks.

Delirium

Differentiating between delirium and dementia can be more difficult than the DSM-IV classification indicates. In general, delirium is distinguished by rapid onset, brief duration, fluctuation of cognitive impairment during the course of the day, nocturnal exacerbation of symptoms, marked disturbance of the sleep–wake cycle, and prominent disturbances in attention and perception.

Depression

Some patients with depression have symptoms of cognitive impairment difficult to distinguish from symptoms of dementia. The clinical picture is sometimes referred to as *pseudodementia*, although the term *depression-related cognitive dysfunction* is preferable and more descriptive (Table 10.3–9). Patients with depression-related cognitive dysfunction generally have prominent depressive symptoms, have more insight into their symptoms than do demented patients, and often have a past history of depressive episodes.

Factitious Disorder

Persons who attempt to simulate memory loss, as in factitious disorder, do so in an erratic and inconsistent manner. In true dementia, memory for time and place is lost before memory for person, and recent memory is lost before remote memory.

Schizophrenia

Although schizophrenia may be associated with some acquired intellectual impairment, its symptoms are much less severe than are the related symptoms of psychosis and thought disorder seen in dementia.

Normal Aging

Aging is not necessarily associated with any significant cognitive decline, but minor memory problems can occur as a normal part of aging. These normal occurrences are sometimes referred to as benign senescent forgetfulness or age-associated memory impairment. They are distinguished from dementia by their minor severity and by the fact that they do not interfere significantly with a person's social or occupational behavior.

Other Disorders

Mental retardation does not include memory impairment and occurs in childhood. Amnestic disorder is characterized by circumscribed loss of memory and no deterioration. Major depression in which there is impaired memory responds to antidepressant medication. Malingering and pituitary disorder must be ruled out but are unlikely.

COURSE AND PROGNOSIS

The classic course of dementia is an onset in the patient's 50s or 60s, with gradual deterioration over 5 to 10 years, leading eventually to death. The age of onset and the rapidity of deterioration vary among different types of dementia and within individual diagnostic categories. The average survival expectation for patients with dementia of the Alzheimer's type is approximately 8 years, with a range of 1 to 20 years. Data suggest that persons with an early onset of dementia or with a family history of dementia are likely to have a rapid course. In a recent study of 821 persons with Alzheimer's disease, the median survival time was 3.5 years. Once dementia is diagnosed, patients must undergo a complete medical and neurological workup, because 10 to 15 percent of all patients with dementia have a potentially reversible condition if treatment is initiated before permanent brain damage occurs.

The most common course of dementia begins with a number of subtle signs that may, at first, be ignored by both the patient and the people closest to the patient. A gradual onset of symptoms is most commonly associated with dementia of the Alzheimer's type, vascular dementia, endocrinopathies, brain tumors, and metabolic disorders. Conversely, the onset

Table 10.3–9
Major Clinical Features Differentiating Pseudodementia from Dementia

Pseudodementia	Dementia
Clinical course and history	
Family always aware of dysfunction and its severity	Family often unaware of dysfunction and its severity
Onset can be dated with some precision	Onset can be dated only within broad limits
Symptoms of short duration before medical help is sought	Symptoms usually of long duration before medical help is sought
Rapid progression of symptoms after onset	Slow progression of symptoms throughout course
History of previous psychiatric dysfunction common	History of previous psychiatric dysfunction unusual
Complaints and clinical behavior	
Patients usually complain much of cognitive loss	Patients usually complain little of cognitive loss
Patients' complaints of cognitive dysfunction usually detailed	Patients' complaints of cognitive dysfunction usually vague
Patients emphasize disability	Patients conceal disability
Patients highlight failures	Patients delight in accomplishments, however trivial
Patients make little effort to perform even simple tasks	Patients struggle to perform tasks
	Patients rely on notes, calendars, etc., to keep up
Patients usually communicate strong sense of distress	Patients often appear unconcerned
Affective change often pervasive	Affect labile and shallow
Loss of social skills often early and prominent	Social skills often retained
Behavior often incongruent with severity of cognitive dysfunction	Behavior usually compatible with severity of cognitive dysfunction
Nocturnal accentuation of dysfunction uncommon	Nocturnal accentuation of dysfunction common
Clinical features related to memory, cognitive, and intellectual dysfunctions	
Attention and concentration often well preserved	Attention and concentration usually faulty
"Don't know" answers typical	Near-miss answers frequent
On tests of orientation, patients often give "don't know" answers	On tests of orientation, patients often mistake unusual for usual
Memory loss for recent and remote events usually severe	Memory loss for recent events usually more severe than for remote events
Memory gaps for specific periods or events common	Memory gaps for specific periods unusual[a]
Marked variability in performance on tasks of similar difficulty	Consistently poor performance on tasks of similar difficulty

[a]Except when caused by delirium, trauma, seizures, etc.
Reprinted with permission from Wells CE. Pseudodementia. *Am J Psychiatry.* 1979;36:898.

of dementia resulting from head trauma, cardiac arrest with cerebral hypoxia, or encephalitis may be sudden. Although the symptoms of the early phase of dementia are subtle, the symptoms become conspicuous as the dementia progresses, and family members may then bring a patient to a physician's attention. People with dementia may be sensitive to the use of benzodiazepines or alcohol, which can precipitate agitated, aggressive, or psychotic behavior. In the terminal stages of dementia, patients become empty shells of their former selves—profoundly disoriented, incoherent, amnestic, and incontinent of urine and feces.

With psychosocial and pharmacological treatment and possibly because of self-healing properties of the brain, the symptoms of dementia may progress slowly for a time or may even recede somewhat. The regression of symptoms is certainly a possibility in reversible dementias (dementias caused by hypothyroidism, normal pressure hydrocephalus, and brain tumors) once treatment is initiated. The course of the dementia varies from a steady progression (commonly seen with dementia of the Alzheimer's type) to an incrementally worsening dementia (commonly seen with vascular dementia) to a stable dementia (as may be seen in dementia related to head trauma).

Psychosocial Determinants

The severity and course of dementia can be affected by psychosocial factors. The greater a person's premorbid intelligence and education, the better the ability to compensate for intellectual deficits. People who have a rapid onset of dementia use fewer defenses than do those who experience an insidious onset. Anxiety and depression may intensify and aggravate the symptoms. Pseudodementia occurs in depressed people who complain of impaired memory but are, in fact, suffering from a depressive disorder. When the depression is treated, the cognitive defects disappear.

TREATMENT

The first step in the treatment of dementia is verification of the diagnosis. Accurate diagnosis is imperative, for the progression may be halted or even reversed if appropriate therapy is provided. Preventive measures are important, particularly in vascular dementia. Such measures might include changes in diet, exercise, and control of diabetes and hypertension. Pharmacological agents might include antihypertensive, anticoagulant, or antiplatelet agents. Blood pressure control should aim for the

higher end of the normal range, as that has been demonstrated to improve cognitive function in patients with vascular dementia. Blood pressure below the normal range has been demonstrated to further impair cognitive function in the patient with dementia. The choice of antihypertensive agent can be significant in that β-adrenergic receptor antagonists have been associated with exaggeration of cognitive impairment. Angiotensin-converting enzyme (ACE) inhibitors and diuretics have not been linked to exaggeration of cognitive impairment and are thought to lower blood pressure without affecting cerebral blood flow, which is presumed to be correlated with cognitive function. Surgical removal of carotid plaques may prevent subsequent vascular events in carefully selected patients. The general treatment approach to patients with dementia is to provide supportive medical care, emotional support for the patients and their families, and pharmacological treatment for specific symptoms, including disruptive behavior.

Psychosocial Therapies

The deterioration of mental faculties has significant psychological meaning for patients with dementia. The experience of a sense of continuity over time depends on memory. Recent memory is lost before remote memory in most cases of dementia, and many patients are highly distressed by clearly recalling how they used to function while observing their obvious deterioration. At the most fundamental level, the self is a product of brain functioning. Patients' identities begin to fade as the illness progresses, and they can recall less and less of their past. Emotional reactions ranging from depression to severe anxiety to catastrophic terror can stem from the realization that the sense of self is disappearing.

Patients often benefit from a supportive and educational psychotherapy in which the nature and course of their illness are clearly explained. They may also benefit from assistance in grieving and accepting the extent of their disability and from attention to self-esteem issues. Any areas of intact functioning should be maximized by helping patients identify activities in which successful functioning is possible. A psychodynamic assessment of defective ego functions and cognitive limitations can also be useful. Clinicians can help patients find ways to deal with the defective ego functions, such as keeping calendars for orientation problems, making schedules to help structure activities, and taking notes for memory problems.

Psychodynamic interventions with family members of patients with dementia may be of great assistance. Those who take care of a patient struggle with feelings of guilt, grief, anger, and exhaustion as they watch a family member gradually deteriorate. A common problem that develops among caregivers involves their self-sacrifice in caring for a patient. The gradually developing resentment from this self-sacrifice is often suppressed because of the guilt feelings it produces. Clinicians can help caregivers understand the complex mixture of feelings associated with seeing a loved one decline and can provide understanding as well as permission to express these feelings. Clinicians must also be aware of the caregivers' tendencies to blame themselves or others for patients' illnesses and must appreciate the role that patients with dementia play in the lives of family members.

Pharmacotherapy

Clinicians may prescribe benzodiazepines for insomnia and anxiety, antidepressants for depression, and antipsychotic drugs for delusions and hallucinations, but they should be aware of possible idiosyncratic drug effects in older people (such as paradoxical excitement, confusion, and increased sedation). In general, drugs with high anticholinergic activity should be avoided.

Donepezil (Aricept), rivastigmine (Exelon), galantamine (Remiryl), and tacrine (Cognex) are cholinesterase inhibitors used for the treatment of mild to moderate cognitive impairment in Alzheimer's disease. They reduce the inactivation of the neurotransmitter acetylcholine and thus potentiate the cholinergic neurotransmitter, which in turn produces a modest improvement in memory and goal-directed thought. These drugs are most useful for persons with mild to moderate memory loss who have enough preservation of their basal forebrain cholinergic neurons to benefit from augmentation of cholinergic neurotransmission.

Donepezil is well tolerated and widely used. Tacrine is rarely used, because of its potential for hepatotoxicity. There are fewer clinical data available for rivastigmine and galantamine, which appear more likely to cause gastrointestinal (GI) and neuropsychiatric adverse effects than is donepezil. None of these medications prevents the progressive neuronal degeneration of the disorder. Prescribing information for anticholinesterase inhibitors can be found in Section 36.4.13.

Other Treatment Approaches. Other drugs that are being tested for cognitive-enhancing activity include general cerebral metabolic enhancers, calcium channel inhibitors, and serotonergic agents. Some studies have shown that selegiline (Eldepryl), a selective type B monoamine oxidase (MAO_B) inhibitor, may slow the advance of this disease.

Memantine (Akatinol) protects neurons from excessive amounts of glutamate, which may be neurotoxic. The drug is used in Europe. Ondansetron (Zofran), a 5-HT_3 receptor antagonist, is under investigation.

Estrogen replacement therapy may reduce the risk of cognitive decline in postmenopausal women; however, more studies are needed to confirm this effect. Complementary and alternative medicine studies are examining ginkgo biloba and other phytomedicinals to see if they have a positive effect on cognition. Reports of patients using nonsteroidal antiinflammatory agents having a lower risk of developing Alzheimer's disease have appeared.

ICD-10

Except for dementia due to head trauma, all the dementias included in DSM-IV-TR are also in the 10th revision of *International Statistical Classification of Diseases and Related Health Problems* (ICD-10). ICD-10 also includes general criteria for dementia (Table 10.3–10). Dementia in Alzheimer's disease is divided into four types (Table 10.3–11). ICD-10 divides vascular dementia into nine types based on the nature of the vascular disease (Table 10.3–12). ICD-10 includes two residual categories—dementia in other diseases classified elsewhere (such as dementia in Pick's disease) (Table 10.3–13) and unspecified dementia (dementia with an unknown cause).

Table 10.3–10
ICD-10 Diagnostic Criteria for Dementia

G1. There is evidence of each of the following:

(1) A decline in memory, which is most evident in the learning of new information, although, in more severe cases, the recall of previously learned information may also be affected. The impairment applies to both verbal and nonverbal material. The decline should be objectively verified by obtaining a reliable history from an informant, supplemented, if possible, by neuropsychological tests or quantified cognitive assessments. The severity of the decline, with mild impairment as the threshold for diagnosis, should be assessed as follows:

Mild. The degree of memory loss is sufficient to interfere with everyday activities, though not so severe as to be incompatible with independent living. The main function affected is the learning of new material. For example, the individual has difficulty in registering, storing, and recalling elements involved in daily living, such as where belongings have been put, social arrangements, or information recently imparted by family members.

Moderate. The degree of memory loss represents a serious handicap to independent living. Only highly learned or very familiar material is retained. New information is retained only occasionally and very briefly. Individuals are unable to recall basic information about their own local geography, what they have recently been doing, or the names of familiar people.

Severe. The degree of memory loss is characterized by the complete inability to retain new information. Only fragments of previously learned information remain. The individual fails to recognize even close relatives.

(2) A decline in other cognitive abilities characterized by deterioration in judgment and thinking, such as planning and organizing, and in the general processing of information. Evidence for this should ideally be obtained from an informant and supplemented, if possible, by neuropsychological tests or quantified objective assessments. Deterioration from a previously higher level of performance should be established. The severity of the decline, with mild impairment as the threshold for diagnosis, should be assessed as follows:

Mild. The decline in cognitive abilities causes impaired performance in daily living, but not to a degree that makes the individual dependent on others. Complicated daily tasks or recreational activities cannot be undertaken.

Moderate. The decline in cognitive abilities makes the individual unable to function without the assistance of another in daily living, including shopping and handling money. Within the home, only simple chores can be performed. Activities are increasingly restricted and poorly sustained.

Severe. The decline is characterized by an absence, or virtual absence, of intelligible ideation.

The overall severity of the dementia is best expressed as the level of decline in memory *or* other cognitive abilities, whichever is the more severe (e.g., mild decline in memory *and* moderate decline in cognitive abilities indicate a dementia of moderate severity).

G2. Awareness of the environment (i.e., absence of clouding of consciousness [as defined in delirium, not induced by alcohol and other psychoactive substances, Criterion A]) is preserved during a period sufficiently long to allow the unequivocal demonstration of the symptoms in Criterion G1. When there are superimposed episodes of delirium, the diagnosis of dementia should be deferred.

G3. There is a decline in emotional control or motivation, or a change in social behavior manifest as at least one of the following:

(1) emotional lability
(2) irritability
(3) apathy
(4) coarsening of social behavior

G4. For a confident clinical diagnosis, the symptoms in criterion G1 should have been present for at least 6 months; if the period since the manifest onset is shorter, the diagnosis can be only tentative.

Comments

The diagnosis is further supported by evidence of damage to other higher cortical functions, such as aphasia, agnosia, apraxia.

Judgment about independent living or the development of dependence (upon others) should take account of the cultural expectation and context.

Dementia is specified here as having a minimum duration of 6 months to avoid confusion with reversible states with identical behavioral syndromes, such as traumatic subdural hemorrhage, normal pressure hydrocephalus, and diffuse or focal brain injury.

A fifth character may be used to indicate the presence of additional symptoms: Dementia in Alzheimer's disease, vascular dementia, dementia in diseases classified elsewhere, unspecified dementia, as follows:

Without additional symptoms
With other symptoms, predominantly delusional
With other symptoms, predominantly hallucinatory
With other symptoms, predominantly depressive
With other mixed symptoms

A sixth character may be used to indicate the severity of the dementia:

Mild
Moderate
Severe

As mentioned above, the overall severity of the dementia depends on the level of memory *or* intellectual impairment, whichever is the more severe.

Table 10.3–11
ICD-10 Diagnostic Criteria for Dementia in Alzheimer's Disease

A. The general criteria for dementia G1–G4 must be met.

B. There is no evidence from the history, physical examination, or special investigations for any other possible cause of dementia (e.g., cerebrovascular disease, HIV disease, Parkinson's disease, Huntington's disease, normal pressure hydrocephalus), a systemic disorder (e.g., hypothyroidism, vitamin B_{12} or folic acid deficiency, hypercalcemia), or alcohol or drug abuse.

Comments

The diagnosis is confirmed by postmortem evidence of neurofibrillary tangles and neuritic plaques in excess of those found in normal aging of the brain.

The following features support the diagnosis, but are not necessary elements: involvement of cortical functions as evidenced by aphasia, agnosia, or apraxia; decrease of motivation and drive, leading to apathy and lack of spontaneity; irritability and disinhibition of social behavior; evidence from special investigations that there is cerebral atrophy, particularly if this can be shown to be increasing over time. In severe cases there may be Parkinson-like extrapyramidal changes, logoclonia, and epileptic fits.

Specification of features for possible subtypes

Because of the possibility that subtypes exist, it is recommended that the following characteristics be ascertained as a basis for a further classification: age at onset; rate of progression; configuration of the clinical features, particularly the relative prominence (or lack) of temporal, parietal, or frontal lobe signs; any neuropathological or neurochemical abnormalities, and their pattern.

The division of Alzheimer's disease into subtypes can at present be accomplished in two ways: first by taking only the age of onset and labeling the disease as either early or late, with an approximate cutoff point at 65 years; or second, by assessing how well the individual conforms to one of the two putative syndromes, early- or late-onset type.

It should be noted that a sharp distinction between early- and late-onset types is unlikely. Early-onset type may occur in late life, just as late-onset type may occasionally have an onset before the age of 65. The following criteria may be used to differentiate dementia in Alzheimer's disease with early and late onset, but it should be remembered that the status of this subdivision is still controversial.

Dementia in Alzheimer's disease with early onset

1. The criteria for dementia in Alzheimer's disease must be met, and the age at onset must be below 65 years.
2. In addition, at least one of the following requirements must be met:
   (a) evidence of a relatively rapid onset and progression;
   (b) in addition to memory impairment, there must be aphasia (amnesic or sensory), agraphia, alexia, acalculia, or apraxia (indicating the presence of temporal, parietal, and/or frontal lobe involvement).

Dementia in Alzheimer's disease with late onset

1. The criteria for dementia in Alzheimer's disease must be met and the age at onset must be 65 years or more.
2. In addition, at least one of the following requirements must be met:
   (a) evidence of a very slow, gradual onset and progression (the rate of the latter may be known only retrospectively after a course of 3 years or more);
   (b) predominance of memory impairment G1(1), over intellectual impairment G1(2) (see general criteria for dementia).

Dementia in Alzheimer's disease, atypical or mixed type

This term and code should be used for dementias that have important atypical features or that fulfill criteria for both early- and late-onset types of Alzheimer's disease. Mixed Alzheimer's and vascular dementia are also included here.

Dementia in Alzheimer's disease, unspecified

Table 10.3–12
ICD-10 Diagnostic Criteria for Vascular Dementia

G1. The general criteria for dementia (G1–G4) must be met.

G2. Deficits in higher cognitive functions are unevenly distributed, with some functions affected and others relatively spared. Thus, memory may be markedly affected while thinking, reasoning, and information processing may show only mild decline.

G3. There is clinical evidence of focal brain damage, manifest as at least one of the following:
   (1) unilateral spastic weakness of the limbs;
   (2) unilaterally increased tendon reflexes;
   (3) extensor plantar response;
   (4) pseudobulbar palsy.

G4. There is evidence from the history, examination, or tests of a significant cerebrovascular disease, which may reasonably be judged to be etiologically related to the dementia (e.g., a history of stroke, evidence of cerebral infarction).

The following criteria may be used to differentiate subtypes of vascular dementia, but it should be remembered that the usefulness of this subdivision may not be generally accepted.

Vascular dementia of acute onset

A. The general criteria for vascular dementia must be met.

B. The dementia develops rapidly (i.e., usually within 1 month, but within no longer than 3 months) after a succession of strokes or (rarely) after a single large infarction.

Multi-infarct dementia

A. The general criteria for vascular dementia must be met.

B. The onset of the dementia is gradual (i.e., within 3–6 months), following a number of minor ischemic episodes.

Comments

It is presumed that there is an accumulation of infarcts in the cerebral parenchyma. Between the ischemic episodes there may be periods of actual clinical improvement.

Subcortical vascular dementia

A. The general criteria for vascular dementia must be met.

B. There is a history of hypertension.

C. There is evidence from clinical examination and special investigations of vascular disease located in the deep white matter of the cerebral hemispheres, with preservation of the cerebral cortex.

Mixed cortical and subcortical vascular dementia

Mixed cortical and subcortical components of the vascular dementia may be suspected from the clinical features, the results of investigations (including autopsy), or both.

Other vascular dementia

Vascular dementia, unspecified

Table 10.3–13
ICD-10 Diagnostic Criteria for Dementia in Other Diseases

Classified elsewhere

Dementia in Pick's disease

A. The general criteria for dementia (G1–G4) must be met.

B. Onset is slow with steady deterioration.

C. Predominance of frontal lobe involvement is evidenced by two or more of the following:
(1) emotional blunting;
(2) coarsening of social behavior;
(3) disinhibition;
(4) apathy or restlessness;
(5) aphasia.

D. In the early stages, memory and parietal lobe functions are relatively preserved.

Dementia in Creutzfeldt-Jakob disease

A. The general criteria for dementia (G1–G4) must be met.

B. There is very rapid progression of the dementia, with disintegration of virtually all higher cerebral functions.

C. One or more of the following types of neurological symptoms and signs emerge, usually after or simultaneously with the dementia:
(1) pyramidal symptoms;
(2) extrapyramidal symptoms;
(3) cerebellar symptoms;
(4) aphasia;
(5) visual impairment.

Comments

An akinetic and mute state is the typical terminal stage. An amyotrophic variant may be seen, where the neurological signs precede the onset of the dementia. A characteristic electroencephalogram (periodic spikes against a slow and low-voltage background), if present in association with the above clinical signs, increases the probability of the diagnosis. However, the diagnosis can be confirmed only by neuropathological examination (neuronal loss, astrocytosis, and spongiform changes). Because of the risk of infection, this should be carried out only under special protective conditions.

Dementia in Huntington's disease

A. The general criteria for dementia (G1–G4) must be met.

B. Subcortical functions are affected first and dominate the picture of dementia throughout; subcortical involvement is manifested by slowness of thinking or movement and personality alteration with apathy or depression.

C. There are involuntary choreiform movements, typically of the face, hands, or shoulders, or in the gait. The patient may attempt to conceal them by converting them into a voluntary action.

D. There is a history of Huntington's disease in one parent or a sibling, or a family history that suggests the disorder.

E. There are no clinical features that otherwise account for the abnormal movements.

Comments

In addition to involuntary choreiform movements, there may be development of extrapyramidal rigidity or of spasticity with pyramidal signs.

Dementia in Parkinson's disease

A. The general criteria for dementia (G1–G4) must be met.

B. A diagnosis of Parkinson's disease has been established.

C. None of the cognitive impairment is attributable to antiparkinsonian medication.

D. There is no evidence from the history, physical examination, or special investigations for any other possible cause of dementia, including other forms of brain disease, damage, or dysfunction (e.g., cerebrovascular disease, HIV disease, Huntington's disease, normal pressure hydrocephalus), a systemic disorder (e.g., hypothyroidism, vitamin B_{12} or folic acid deficiency, hypercalcemia), or alcohol or drug abuse.

If criteria are also fulfilled for dementia in Alzheimer's disease with late onset, that category should be used in combination with Parkinson's disease.

Dementia in human immunodeficiency virus (HIV) disease

A. The general criteria for dementia (G1–G4) must be met.

B. A diagnosis of HIV infection has been established.

C. There is no evidence from the history, physical examination, or special investigations for any other possible cause of dementia, including other forms of brain disease, damage, or dysfunction (e.g., Alzheimer's disease, cerebrovascular disease, Parkinson's disease, Huntington's disease, normal pressure hydrocephalus), a systemic disorder (e.g., hypothyroidism, vitamin B_{12} or folic acid deficiency, hypercalcemia), or alcohol or drug abuse.

Dementia in other specified diseases classified elsewhere

Dementia can occur as a manifestation or consequence of a variety of cerebral and somatic conditions. To specify the etiology, the ICD-10 code for the underlying condition should be added.

Reprinted with permission from World Health Organization. *The ICD-10 Classification of Mental and Behavioural Disorders: Diagnostic Criteria for Research.* Copyright, World Health Organization, Geneva, 1993.

References

Almkvist O, Bäckman L. Detection and staging of early clinical dementia. *Acta Neurol Scand.* 1993;88:10.

Bookheimer SY. Patterns of brain activation in people at risk for Alzheimer's disease. *N Engl J Med.* 2001;345:450.

Caine ED, Lyness JM. Delirium, dementia, and amnestic and other cognitive disorders. In: Sadock BJ, Sadock VA, eds. *Kaplan & Sadock's Comprehensive Textbook of Psychiatry.* 7th ed. Vol 1. Baltimore: Lippincott Williams & Wilkins; 2000:854.

Corder EH, Saunders AM, Strittmatter WJ, et al. Gene dose of apolipoprotein E type 4 allele and the risk of Alzheimer's disease in late onset families. *Science.* 1993;261:921.

Davis RE, Emmerling MR, Jaen JC, Moos WH, Spiegel K. Therapeutic intervention in dementia. *Crit Rev Neurobiol.* 1993;7:41.

Ghetti B. Familial multiple system taupath with presenile dementia. *Proc Natl Acad Sci U S A.* 1997;94:4113.

Gold G, Bouras C, Canuto A, et al. Clinicopathological validation study of four sets of clinical criteria for vascular dementia. *Am J Psychiatry.* 2002;159:82.

Kawas CH, Brookmeyer R. Aging and the public health effects of dementia. *N Engl J Med.* 2001;344:1160.

Krasuski J, Alexander G, Horwitz B, et al. Relation of medial temporal lobe volumes to age and memory function in nondemented adults with down's syndrome: implications for the prodromal phase of Alzheimer's disease. *Am J Psychiatry.* 2002;159:74.

Luchins DJ, Cohen D, Hanrahan P, et al. Are there clinical differences between familial and non familial Alzheimer's disease? *Am J Psychiatry.* 1992; 149:1023.

Moulignier A, Allo S, Zittoun R, Gout O. Recombinant interferon-alpha-induced chorea and frontal subcortical dementia. *Neurology.* 2002;58:328.

Pajeau AK, Roman GC. HIV encephalopathy and dementia. *Psychiatr Clin North Am.* 1992;15:455.

Sano M, Ernesto C, Thomas RG, et al., for the Alzheimer's Disease Cooperative Study. A controlled trial of selegiline, alpha-tocopherol, or both as treatment for Alzheimer's disease. *N Engl J Med.* 1997;336:1216.

Serby M, Samuels SC. Diagnostic criteria for dementia with Lewy bodies reconsidered. *Am J Geriatr Psychiatry.* 2001;9:212.

Will RG, Ironside JW, Zeidler M, et al. A new variant of Creutzfeldt-Jakob disease in the UK. *Lancet.* 1996;347:921.

Wolfson C, Wolfson DB. A reevaluation of the duration of survival after the onset of dementia. *N Engl J Med.* 2001;344:1111.

World Health Organization consultation on public health issues related to bovine spongiform encephalopathy and the emergence of a new variant of Creutzfeldt-Jakob disease. *MMWR Morb Mortal Wkly Rep*. 1996;45:295.

▲ 10.4 Amnestic Disorders

The essential feature of amnestic disorders is the acquired impaired ability to learn and recall new information, or the inability to recall previously learned knowledge or past events. The impairment must be sufficiently severe to compromise personal, social, or occupational functioning. The diagnosis is not made if the memory impairment exists in the context of reduced ability to maintain and shift attention, as encountered in delirium, or in association with significant functional problems due to the compromise of multiple intellectual abilities, as seen in dementia. Amnestic disorders are secondary syndromes caused by systemic medical or primary cerebral disease, substance use disorders, or medication adverse effects, as evidenced by findings from clinical history, physical examination, or laboratory examination.

Table 10.4–1
Major Causes of Amnestic Disorders

Systemic medical conditions
Thiamine deficiency (Korsakoff's syndrome)
Hypoglycemia
Primary brain conditions
Seizures
Head trauma (closed and penetrating)
Cerebral tumors (especially thalamic and temporal lobe)
Cerebrovascular diseases (especially thalamic and temporal lobe)
Surgical procedures on the brain
Encephalitis due to herpes simplex
Hypoxia (including nonfatal hanging attempts and carbon monoxide poisoning)
Transient global amnesia
Electroconvulsive therapy
Multiple sclerosis
Substance-related causes
Alcohol use disorders
Neurotoxins
Benzodiazepines (and other sedative-hypnotics)
Many over-the-counter preparations

EPIDEMIOLOGY

No adequate studies have reported on the incidence or prevalence of amnestic disorders. Amnesia is most commonly found in alcohol use disorders and in head injury. In general practice and hospital settings, the frequency of amnesia related to chronic alcohol abuse has decreased, and the frequency of amnesia related to head trauma has increased.

ETIOLOGY

The major neuroanatomical structures involved in memory and in the development of an amnestic disorder are particular diencephalic structures such as the dorsomedial and midline nuclei of the thalamus and midtemporal lobe structures such as the hippocampus, the mamillary bodies, and the amygdala. Although amnesia is usually the result of bilateral damage to these structures, some cases of unilateral damage result in an amnestic disorder, and evidence indicates that the left hemisphere may be more critical than the right hemisphere in the development of memory disorders. Many studies of memory and amnesia in animals have suggested that other brain areas may also be involved in the symptoms accompanying amnesia. Frontal lobe involvement may result in such symptoms as confabulation and apathy, which can be seen in patients with amnestic disorders.

Amnestic disorders have many potential causes (Table 10.4–1). Thiamine deficiency, hypoglycemia, hypoxia (including carbon monoxide poisoning), and herpes simplex encephalitis all have a predilection to damage the temporal lobes, particularly the hippocampi, and thus can be associated with the development of amnestic disorders. Similarly, when tumors, cerebrovascular diseases, surgical procedures, or multiple sclerosis plaques involve the diencephalic or temporal regions of the brain, the symptoms of an amnestic disorder may develop. General insults to the brain such as seizures, electroconvulsive therapy (ECT), and head trauma may also result in memory impairment. Transient global amnesia is presumed to be a cerebrovascular disorder involving transient impairment in blood flow through the vertebrobasilar arteries.

Many drugs have been associated with the development of amnesia, and clinicians should review all drugs taken, including nonprescription drugs, in the diagnostic workup of a patient with amnesia. The benzodiazepines are the most commonly used prescription drugs associated with amnesia. All benzodiazepines can be associated with amnesia, especially if combined with alcohol. When triazolam (Halcion) is used in doses of 0.25 mg or less, which are generally equivalent to standard doses of other benzodiazepines, amnesia is no more often associated with triazolam than with other benzodiazepines. With alcohol and higher doses, anterograde amnesia has been reported.

DIAGNOSIS

For the diagnosis of amnestic disorder, the text revision of the fourth edition of *Diagnostic and Statistical Manual of Mental Disorders* (DSM-IV-TR) requires the "development of memory impairment as manifested by impairment in the ability to learn new information or the inability to recall previously learned information," and the "memory disturbance [must cause] . . . significant impairment in social or occupational functioning." A diagnosis of amnestic disorder due to a general medical condition (Table 10.4–2) is made when there is evidence of a causatively relevant specific medical condition (including physical trauma). DSM-IV-TR further categorizes the diagnosis as transient or chronic. A diagnosis of substance-induced persisting amnestic disorder is made when there is evidence that the symptoms are caus-

Table 10.4–2
DSM-IV-TR Diagnostic Criteria for Amnestic Disorder Due to a General Medical Condition

A. The development of memory impairment as manifested by impairment in the ability to learn new information or the inability to recall previously learned information.

B. The memory disturbance causes significant impairment in social or occupational functioning and represents a significant decline from a previous level of functioning.

C. The memory disturbance does not occur exclusively during the course of a delirium or a dementia.

D. There is evidence from the history, physical examination, or laboratory findings that the disturbance is the direct physiological consequence of a general medical condition (including physical trauma).

Specify if:

Transient: if memory impairment lasts for 1 month or less

Chronic: if memory impairment lasts for more than 1 month

Coding note: Include the name of the general medical condition on Axis I, e.g., Amnestic disorder due to head trauma; also code the general medical condition on Axis III.

atively related to the use of a substance (Table 10.4–3). DSM-IV-TR refers clinicians to specific diagnoses within substance-related disorders: alcohol-induced persisting amnestic disorder; sedative, hypnotic, or anxiolytic-induced persisting amnestic disorder; and other (or unknown) substance-induced persisting amnestic disorder. DSM-IV-TR also provides the diagnosis of amnestic disorder not otherwise specified (Table 10.4–4).

Table 10.4–3
DSM-IV-TR Diagnostic Criteria for Substance-Induced Persisting Amnestic Disorder

A. The development of memory impairment as manifested by impairment in the ability to learn new information or the inability to recall previously learned information.

B. The memory disturbance causes significant impairment in social or occupational functioning and represents a significant decline from a previous level of functioning.

C. The memory disturbance does not occur exclusively during the course of a delirium or a dementia and persists beyond the usual duration of substance intoxication or withdrawal.

D. There is evidence from the history, physical examination, or laboratory findings that the memory disturbance is etiologically related to the persisting effects of substance use (e.g., a drug of abuse, a medication).

Code (Specific substance)-induced persisting amnestic disorder:

(Alcohol; Sedative, hypnotic, or anxiolytic; Other [or unknown] substance)

Table 10.4–4
DSM-IV-TR Diagnostic Criteria for Amnestic Disorder Not Otherwise Specified

This category should be used to diagnose an amnestic disorder that does not meet criteria for any of the specific types described in this section.

An example is a clinical presentation of amnesia for which there is insufficient evidence to establish a specific etiology (i.e., dissociative, substance induced, or due to a general medical condition).

CLINICAL FEATURES AND SUBTYPES

The central symptom of amnestic disorders is the development of a memory disorder characterized by impairment in the ability to learn new information (anterograde amnesia) and the inability to recall previously remembered knowledge (retrograde amnesia). The symptom must result in significant problems for patients in their social or occupational functioning. The time in which a patient is amnestic may begin directly at the point of trauma or may include a period before the trauma. Memory for the time during the physical insult (e.g., during a cerebrovascular event) may also be lost.

Short-term and recent memory are usually impaired. Patients cannot remember what they had for breakfast or lunch, the name of the hospital, or their doctors. In some patients, the amnesia is so profound that they cannot orient themselves to city and time, although orientation to person is seldom lost in amnestic disorders. Memory for overlearned information or events from the remote past, such as childhood experiences, is good; but memory for events from the less remote past (over the past decade) is impaired. Immediate memory (tested, for example, by asking a patient to repeat six numbers) remains intact. With improvement, patients may experience a gradual shrinking of the time for which memory has been lost, although some patients experience a gradual improvement in memory for the entire period.

The onset of symptoms may be sudden, as in trauma, cerebrovascular events, and neurotoxic chemical assaults, or gradual, as in nutritional deficiency and cerebral tumors. The amnesia can be of short duration (specified by DSM-IV-TR as transient if lasting 1 month or less) or of long duration (specified by DSM-IV-TR as persistent if lasting more than 1 month).

A variety of other symptoms can be associated with amnestic disorders. For patients with other cognitive impairments, a diagnosis of dementia or delirium is more appropriate than a diagnosis of an amnestic disorder. Both subtle and gross changes in personality can accompany the symptoms of memory impairment in amnestic disorders. Patients may be apathetic, lack initiative, have unprovoked episodes of agitation, or appear to be overly friendly or agreeable. Patients with amnestic disorders may also appear bewildered and confused and may attempt to cover their confusion with confabulatory answers to questions. Characteristically, patients with amnestic disorders do not have good insight into their neuropsychiatric conditions.

Ms. R. is a 48-year-old woman who is divorced and has three teenage children. Until 3 years earlier, Ms. R. worked as a buyer for a department store. At that time, she experienced fatigue, forgetfulness, a sense of apathy, and headaches, which she attributed to a preexisting migraine condition. She visited a psychiatrist who prescribed an antidepressant to which she did not respond. The headaches worsened, and Ms. R. visited a neurologist who found nothing on neurological examination but recommended a CT scan as a precautionary measure. The CT scan revealed a large, grade II of IV right frontal glioma. This was resected surgically followed by 7,500 rads of radiotherapy focused on the right frontal quadrant. Ms. R. recovered well from the surgery and radiation, with no focal neurological deficits. She had a surprisingly benign course and was able to return to work. The only medication she was taking was carbamazepine as a prophylactic against seizures, which she has never had.

Three years after her surgery, the patient and her family began to notice a problem in her short-term memory, which began with forgetting appointments and losing objects. On one occasion, she was unable to find her car in the airport parking lot because she forgot its make and where she had parked it. With time, this forgetfulness progressed and became severe enough to interfere with her work. For example, she would forget she had placed orders and would repeat them. At first, Ms. R. became irritable about these incidents and often blamed others for her problems (e.g., her secretary for losing her papers, her children for misplacing things at home). Ms. R.'s memory problems were especially distressing to her because she had always prided herself on her memory and had been the one to find things for others in the household. With time, however, she developed insight and accepted that this memory problem was a result of the radiation she had received. Her long-term memory is intact as are her other cognitive abilities, except for some reduced ability to plan ahead, but because this had been very well developed before, the patient can still function better than average. Ms. R. eventually began to make so many mistakes at work that it was obvious she could no longer continue in her job. She is able to function reasonably well at home, however, with the assistance of "things to do" lists and cuing bulletin boards in many rooms of the house.

DSM-IV-TR DIAGNOSIS

Axis I: Amnestic disorder due to central nervous system radiation, chronic
Axis II: No diagnosis
Axis III: Postradiation for brain tumor
Axis IV: Inability to work causing financial stress
Axis V: GAF = 55

Cerebrovascular Diseases

Cerebrovascular diseases affecting the hippocampus involve the posterior cerebral and basilar arteries and their branches. Infarctions are rarely limited to the hippocampus; they often involve the occipital or parietal lobes. Thus, common accompanying symptoms of cerebrovascular diseases in this region are focal neurological signs involving vision or sensory modalities. Cerebrovascular diseases affecting the bilateral medial thalamus, particularly the anterior portions, are often associated with symptoms of amnestic disorders. A few case studies report amnestic disorders from rupture of an aneurysm of the anterior communicating artery, resulting in infarction of the basal forebrain region.

Multiple Sclerosis

The pathophysiological process of multiple sclerosis involves the seemingly random formation of plaques within the brain parenchyma. When the plaques occur in the temporal lobe and the diencephalic regions, symptoms of memory impairment can occur. In fact, the most common cognitive complaints in patients with multiple sclerosis involve impaired memory, which occurs in 40 to 60 percent of patients. Characteristically, digit span memory is normal, but immediate recall and delayed recall of information are impaired. The memory impairment can affect both verbal and nonverbal material.

Korsakoff's Syndrome

Korsakoff's syndrome is an amnestic syndrome caused by thiamine deficiency, most commonly associated with the poor nutritional habits of people with chronic alcohol abuse. Other causes of poor nutrition (such as starvation), gastric carcinoma, hemodialysis, hyperemesis gravidarum, prolonged intravenous hyperalimentation, and gastric plication may also result in thiamine deficiency. Korsakoff's syndrome is often associated with Wernicke's encephalopathy, which is the associated syndrome of confusion, ataxia, and ophthalmoplegia. In patients with these thiamine deficiency–related symptoms, the neuropathological findings include hyperplasia of the small blood vessels with occasional hemorrhages, hypertrophy of astrocytes, and subtle changes in neuronal axons. Although the delirium clears up within a month or so, the amnestic syndrome either accompanies or follows untreated Wernicke's encephalopathy in approximately 85 percent of all cases.

The onset of Korsakoff's syndrome may be gradual. Recent memory tends to be affected more than is remote memory, but this feature is variable. Confabulation, apathy, and passivity are often prominent symptoms in the syndrome. With treatment, patients may remain amnestic for up to 3 months and then gradually improve over the ensuing year. Administration of thiamine may prevent the development of additional amnestic symptoms, but the treatment can seldom reverse severe amnestic symptoms once they are present. Approximately one third to one fourth of all patients recover completely, and approximately one fourth of all patients have no improvement of their symptoms.

Alcoholic Blackouts

Some persons with severe alcohol abuse may exhibit the syndrome commonly referred to as an alcoholic blackout. Characteristically, these persons awake in the morning with a conscious awareness of being unable to remember a period the night before during which they were intoxicated. Sometimes, specific behaviors (hiding money in a secret place and provoking fights) are associated with the blackouts.

Electroconvulsive Therapy

ECT treatments are usually associated with retrograde amnesia for a period of several minutes before the treatment and anterograde amnesia after the treatment. The anterograde amnesia usually resolves within 5

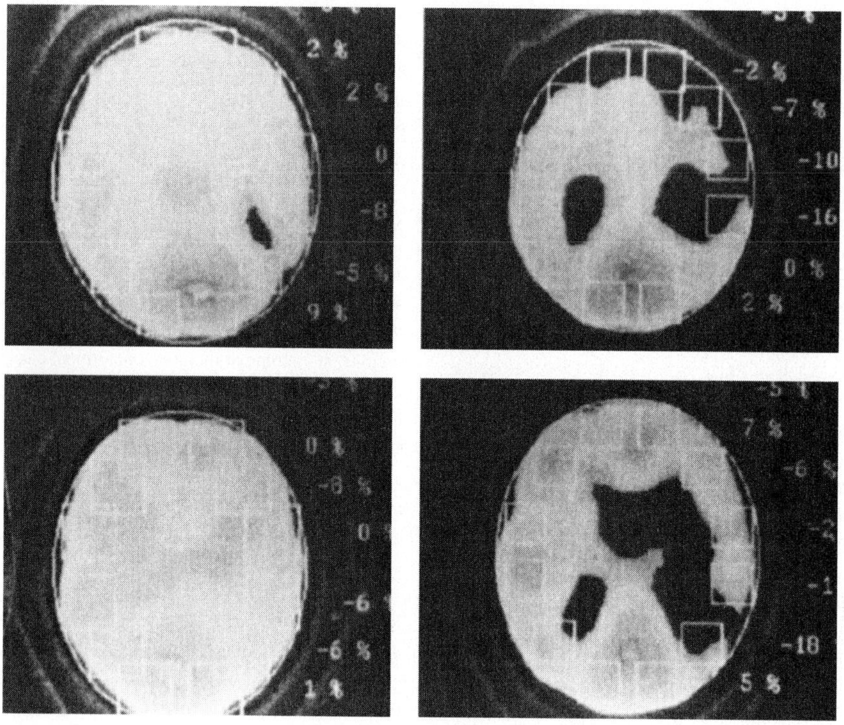

FIGURE 10.4–1

Technetium-99m HP-PAO single photon emission computed tomography scans. Left-sided temporal hypoperfusion is seen in **patients 2** (*top left*), **3** (*top right*), **4** (*bottom left*), and **5** (*bottom right*), 18 months, 4 days, 1 day, and 4 days, respectively, after the transient global amnestic attack. The right side of the patient is at the left side of the figure. (Reprinted with permission from Laloux P, Brichant C, Cauwe F, Decoster P. Technetium-99m HM-PAO single photon emission computed tomography imaging in transient global amnesia. *Arch Neurol.* 1992;49:545.)

hours. Mild memory deficits may remain for 1 to 2 months after a course of ECT treatments, but the symptoms are completely resolved 6 to 9 months after treatment.

Head Injury

Head injuries (both closed and penetrating) can result in a wide range of neuropsychiatric symptoms, including dementia, depression, personality changes, and amnestic disorders. Amnestic disorders caused by head injuries are commonly associated with a period of retrograde amnesia leading up to the traumatic incident and amnesia for the traumatic incident itself. The severity of the brain injury correlates somewhat with the duration and severity of the amnestic syndrome, but the best correlate of eventual improvement is the degree of clinical improvement in the amnesia during the first week after the patient regains consciousness.

Transient Global Amnesia

Transient global amnesia is characterized by the abrupt loss of the ability to recall recent events or to remember new information. The syndrome is often characterized by mild confusion and a lack of insight into the problem, a clear sensorium, and, occasionally, the inability to perform some well-learned complex tasks. Episodes last from 6 to 24 hours. Studies suggest that transient global amnesia occurs in 5 to 10 cases per 100,000 persons per year; although, for patients older than age 50, the rate may be as high as 30 cases per 100,000 persons per year. The pathophysiology is unknown, but it is likely to involve ischemia of the temporal lobe and the diencephalic brain regions. Several studies of patients with single photon emission computed tomography (SPECT) have shown decreased blood flow in the temporal and parietotemporal regions, particularly in the left hemisphere (Fig. 10.4–1). Patients with transient global amnesia almost universally experience complete improvement, although one study found that approximately 20 percent of patients may have recurrence of the episode, and another study found that approximately 7 percent of patients may have epilepsy. Patients with transient global amnesia have been differentiated from patients with transient ischemic attacks in that fewer patients have diabetes, hypercholesterolemia, and hypertriglyceridemia but more have hypertension and migrainous episodes.

PATHOLOGY AND LABORATORY EXAMINATION

Laboratory findings diagnostic of the disorder may be obtained using quantitative neuropsychological testing. Standardized tests also are available to assess recall of well-known historical events or public figures, to characterize an individual's inability to remember previously learned information. Performance on such tests varies among individuals with amnestic disorder. Subtle deficits in other cognitive functions may be noted in individuals with amnestic disorder. However, memory deficits constitute the predominant feature of the mental status examination and account largely for any functional deficits. No specific or diagnostic features are detectable on imaging studies such as magnetic resonance imagery (MRI) or computed

tomography (CT). However, damage of midtemporal lobe structures is common and may be reflected in enlargement of third ventricle or temporal horns or in structural atrophy detected by MRI.

DIFFERENTIAL DIAGNOSIS

Table 10.4–1 lists the major causes of amnestic disorders. To make the diagnosis, clinicians must obtain a patient's history, conduct a complete physical examination, and order all appropriate laboratory tests. Other diagnoses, however, can be confused with the amnestic disorders.

Dementia and Delirium

Clinicians must differentiate amnestic disorders from dementia and delirium. Memory impairment is commonly present in dementia but is accompanied by other cognitive deficits. Memory impairment is also commonly present in delirium but occurs in the setting of impaired attention and consciousness.

Normal Aging

Some minor impairment in memory may accompany normal aging, but the DSM-IV requirement that the memory impairment cause significant impairment in social or occupational functioning should exclude normal aging from the diagnosis.

Dissociative Disorders

The dissociative disorders can sometimes be difficult to differentiate from the amnestic disorders. Patients with dissociative disorders, however, are more likely to have lost their orientation to self and may have more selective memory deficits than do patients with amnestic disorders. For example, patients with dissociative disorders may not know their names or home addresses but still be able to learn new information and remember selected past memories. Dissociative disorders are also often associated with emotionally stressful life events involving money, the legal system, or troubled relationships.

Factitious Disorders

Patients with factitious disorders who are mimicking an amnestic disorder often have inconsistent results on memory tests and have no evidence of an identifiable cause. These findings, coupled with evidence of primary or secondary gain for a patient, should suggest a factitious disorder.

COURSE AND PROGNOSIS

The specific cause of the amnestic disorder determines the course and the prognosis for a patient. The onset may be sudden or gradual, the symptoms may be transient or persistent, and the outcome can range from no improvement to complete recovery. Transient amnestic disorder with full recovery is common in temporal lobe epilepsy, ECT, the intake of such drugs as benzodiazepines and barbiturates, and resuscitation from cardiac arrest. Permanent amnestic syndromes may follow head trauma, carbon monoxide poisoning, a cerebral infarction, a subarachnoid hemorrhage, and herpes simplex encephalitis.

TREATMENT

The primary approach to treating amnestic disorders is to treat the underlying cause. Although a patient is amnestic, supportive prompts about the date, the time, and the patient's location can be helpful and can reduce the patient's anxiety. After resolution of the amnestic episode, psychotherapy of some type (cognitive, psychodynamic, or supportive) may help patients incorporate the amnestic experience into their lives.

Psychotherapy

Psychodynamic interventions may be of considerable value for patients suffering from amnestic disorders that result from insults to the brain. Understanding the course of recovery in such patients helps clinicians to be sensitive to the narcissistic injury inherent in damage to the central nervous system.

The first phase of recovery, in which patients are incapable of processing what happened because the ego defenses are overwhelmed, requires clinicians to serve as a supportive auxiliary ego who explains to a patient what is happening and provides missing ego functions. In the second phase of recovery, as the realization of the injury sets in, patients may become angry and feel victimized by the malevolent hand of fate. They may view others, including the clinician, as bad or destructive, and clinicians must contain these projections without becoming punitive or retaliatory. Clinicians can build a therapeutic alliance with patients by explaining slowly and clearly what happened and by offering an explanation for a patient's internal experience. The third phase of recovery is integrative. As a patient accepts what happened, a clinician can help the patient form a new identity by connecting current experiences of the self with past experiences. Grieving over the lost faculties may be an important feature of the third phase.

Most patients who are amnestic because of brain injury engage in denial. Clinicians must respect and empathize with the patient's need to deny the reality of what has happened. Insensitive and blunt confrontations destroy any developing therapeutic alliance and may cause patients to feel attacked. In a sensitive approach, clinicians help patients accept their cognitive limitations by exposing them to these deficits bit by bit over time. When patients fully accept what has happened, they may need assistance in forgiving themselves and any others involved, so that they can get on with their lives. Clinicians must also be wary of being seduced into thinking that all of the patient's symptoms are directly related to the brain insult. An evaluation of preexisting personality disorders, such as borderline, antisocial, and narcissistic personality disorders, must be part of the overall assessment; many patients with personality disorders place themselves in situations that predispose them to injuries. These personality features may become a crucial part of the psychodynamic psychotherapy.

Recently, centers for cognitive rehabilitation have been established whose rehabilitation-oriented therapeutic milieu is intended to promote recovery from brain injury, especially that from traumatic causes. Despite the high cost of extended care at these sites, which provide both long-term institutional and day-

Table 10.4–5
ICD-10 Diagnostic Criteria for Organic Amnesic Syndrome, Not Induced by Alcohol and Other Psychoactive Substances

A. There is memory impairment, manifest in both
 1. A defect of recent memory (impaired learning of new material) to a degree sufficient to interfere with daily living
 2. A reduced ability to recall past experiences
B. There is no
 1. Defect in immediate recall (as tested, for example, by the digit span)
 2. Clouding of consciousness and disturbance of attention. Delirium, not induced by alcohol and other psychoactive substances
 3. Global intellectual decline (dementia)
C. There is objective evidence (from physical and neurological examination, laboratory tests) and/or history of an insult to, or a disease of, the brain (especially involving bilaterally the diencephalic and medial temporal structures but other than alcohol encephalopathy) that can reasonably be presumed to be responsible for the clinical manifestations

Comments

Associated features, including confabulations, emotional changes (apathy, lack of initiative), and lack of insight are useful additional pointers to the diagnosis but are not invariably present.

Adapted with permission from World Health Organization. *The ICD-10 Classification of Mental and Behavioural Disorders: Diagnostic Criteria for Research.* Copyright, World Health Organization, Geneva, 1993.

time services, no data have been developed to define therapeutic effectiveness for the heterogeneous groups of patients who participate in such tasks as memory retaining.

ICD-10

The criteria for organic amnesic syndrome, not induced by alcohol and other psychoactive substances, in the 10th revision of *International Statistical Classification of Diseases and Related Health Problems* (ICD-10) are presented in Table 10.4–5. In ICD-10, deliriums associated with the use of a substance are classified under the category of mental and behavioral disorders due to psychoactive substance use as a withdrawal state with delirium, as a subtype of acute intoxication (e.g., acute intoxication due to the use of alcohol with delirium), and as an additional specifier to alcohol withdrawal state and sedative or hypnotic withdrawal state.

References

Ahmed S, Bierley R, Sheikh JI, et al. Post-traumatic amnesia after closed head injury. A review of the literature and some suggestions for further research. *Brain Inj.* 2000;14:765–780.

Caine ED, Lyness JM. Delirium, dementia, and amnestic and other cognitive disorders. In: Sadock BJ, Sadock VA, eds. *Kaplan & Sadock's Comprehensive Textbook of Psychiatry.* 7th ed. Vol 1. Baltimore: Lippincott Williams & Wilkins; 2000:854.

Erickson KR. Amnestic disorders: pathophysiology and patterns of memory dysfunction. *West J Med.* 1990;152:159.

Farah MJ, Feinberg TE. *Patient-Based Approaches to Cognitive Neuroscience. Issues in Clinical and Cognitive Neuropsychology.* Cambridge: The MIT Press; 2000:291–299.

Feinstein A, Hershkop S, Ouchterlony D, et al. Posttraumatic amnesia and recall of a traumatic event following traumatic brain surgery. *J Neuropsychiatry Clin Neurosci.* 2002;14:25.

Gasquonine PG. Learning in post-traumatic amnesia following extremely severe closed head injury. *Brain Inj.* 1991;5:169.

Hodges JR, McCarthy RA. Loss of remote memory: a cognitive neuropsychological perspective. *Curr Opin Neurobiol.* 1995;5:178.

Hodges JR, Warlow CP. The aetiology of transient global amnesia: a case-control study of 114 cases with prospective follow-up. *Brain.* 1990;113:639.

Kin JJ, Fanselow MS. Modality-specific retrograde amnesia of fear. *Science.* 1992;256:675.

Kopelman MD. Focal retrograde amnesia and the attribution of causality: an exceptionally critical review. *Cognitive Neuropsychology.* 2000;17:585–621.

Laloux P, Brichant C, Cauwe F, Decoster P. Technetium-99m HM-PAO single photon emission computed tomography imaging in transient global amnesia. *Arch Neurol.* 1992;49:543.

Paul RH, Graber JR, Bowlby DC, et al. Remote memory in neurodegenerative disease. In: Troester AI, ed. *Memory in Neurodegenerative Disease: Biological, Cognitive, and Clinical Perspectives.* New York: Cambridge University Press; 1998:184–196.

Squire LR, Zola-Morgan S. The medical temporal lobe memory system. *Science.* 1991;253:1380.

▲ 10.5 Mental Disorders Due to a General Medical Condition

As a general rule, the differential diagnosis for a mental syndrome in a patient should always include consideration of any general medical condition that a patient may have and consideration of any prescription, nonprescription, or illegal substances that a patient may be taking. Although some specific medical conditions have classically been associated with mental syndromes, a much larger number of general medical conditions have been associated with mental syndromes in case reports and small studies.

In the text revision of the fourth edition of *Diagnostic and Statistical Manual of Mental Disorders* (DSM-IV-TR), each mental disorder due to a general medical condition is classified within the category that most resembles the symptoms (Table 10.5–1). For example, the diagnosis of psychotic disorder due to general medical condition is found in the DSM-IV-TR section on schizophrenia and other psychotic disorders. A clinician evaluating a patient with depression can refer to the DSM-IV-TR section on mood disorders and find mood disorder due to a general medical condition as one of the diagnoses.

MOOD DISORDER DUE TO A GENERAL MEDICAL CONDITION

Also known as secondary mood disorders, these conditions are characterized by a prominent mood alteration thought to be the direct physiological effect of a specific medical illness or agent. These disorders are often difficult to define and have not been extensively researched; however, the key feature is prominent, persistent, distressing, or functionally impairing depressed mood (anhedonia) or elevated, expansive, or irritable mood, judged to be caused either by medical or surgical illness or by substance intoxication or withdrawal. Cognitive impairment is not the predominant clinical feature; otherwise, the mood disturbance would be viewed as part of delirium, dementia, or other cognitive deficit disorder. The diagnostician is asked to specify if the mood syndrome is manic, depressed, or mixed and if criteria for a fully symptomatic major depressive or manic syndromic are fulfilled.

Table 10.5–1
Mental Disorders Due to a General Medical Condition

DSM-IV-TR Category	Mental Disorders Due to a General Medical Condition	Section
Delirium, dementia, amnestic and other cognitive disorders	Delirium due to a general medical condition	10.2
	Dementia due to other general medical conditions	10.3
	Amnestic disorder due to a general medical condition	10.4
Schizophrenia and other psychotic disorders	Psychotic disorder due to a general medical condition	14.1
Mood disorders	Mood disorder due to a general medical condition	15.1
Anxiety disorders	Anxiety disorder due to a general medical condition	16.1
Sexual disorders	Sexual dysfunction due to a general medical condition	21.2
Sleep disorders	Sleep disorder due to a general medical condition	24.2
Mental disorders due to a general medical condition not elsewhere classified	Catatonic disorder due to a general medical condition	10.5
	Personality change due to a general medical condition	10.5
	Mental disorder not otherwise specified due to a general medical condition	10.5

Epidemiology

The incidence and prevalence of secondary mood disorders are unknown. Depression in the medically ill appears to be equally prevalent by sex or, possibly, slightly higher in men than in women. Major and minor depressive episodes are common after certain illnesses such as strokes, Parkinson's disease, Huntington's disease, human immunodeficiency virus (HIV) infection, and multiple sclerosis. Secondary mania is less prevalent in neurological disease than is depression; however, many experienced clinicians report a high rate of euphoria in patients with multiple sclerosis.

Etiology

The list of potential causes for both depressive and manic syndromes is long. Table 10.5–2 lists some of the causes most commonly considered.

Diagnosis and Clinical Features

The depressive or manic symptoms found in secondary mood disorders are phenomenologically similar to those found in primary (idiopathic) mood disorders. It is not known if certain symptoms occur more commonly in the secondary disorders; presumably the prevalence may vary depending on the specific etiology of the secondary disorder. For example, anxiety has been described as prominent in major depressive syndromes seen in patients with Parkinson's disease; however, no studies have compared depressed patients with Parkinson's disease with similarly aged patients experiencing idiopathic major depressive disorder.

Differential Diagnosis

There are two broad domains of differential diagnosis to consider when establishing the presence of a secondary mood disorder. The first is symptom related: Does the patient have clinically significant manic or depressive symptoms in the absence of evidence of a predominant cognitive deficit? That assessment requires attention to symptoms and function in the history and mental status examination. As part of the process,

Table 10.5–2
Causes of Secondary Mood Disorders

Drug intoxication
Alcohol or sedative-hypnotics
Antipsychotics
Antidepressants
Metoclopramide, H_2-receptor blockers
Antihypertensives (especially centrally acting agents, e.g., methyldopa, clonidine, reserpine)
Sex steroids (e.g., oral contraceptives, anabolic steroids)
Glucocorticoids
Levodopa
Bromocriptine
Drug withdrawal
Nicotine, caffeine, alcohol or sedative-hypnotics, cocaine, amphetamines
Tumor
Primary cerebral
Systemic neoplasm
Trauma
Cerebral contusion
Subdural hematoma
Infection
Cerebral (e.g., meningitis, encephalitis, HIV, syphilis)
Systemic (e.g., sepsis, urinary tract infection, pneumonia)
Cardiac and vascular
Cerebrovascular (e.g., infarcts, hemorrhage, vasculitis)
Cardiovascular (e.g., low-output states, congestive heart failure, shock)
Physiological or metabolic
Hypoxemia, electrolyte disturbances, renal or hepatic failure, hypo- or hyperglycemia, postictal states
Endocrine
Thyroid or glucocorticoid disturbances
Nutritional
Vitamin B_{12}, folate deficiency
Demyelinating
Multiple sclerosis
Neurodegenerative
Parkinson's disease, Huntington's disease

Courtesy of Eric D. Caine, M.D., and Jeffrey M. Lyness, M.D.

the clinician is also establishing whether there is a clearly defined mood syndrome sufficient to warrant an empirical treatment trial with antidepressant medications.

The second domain is etiological: Does the patient have an Axis III condition or a state of substance intoxication or withdrawal that is causing the mood disturbance? Establishing the presence of the relevant condition depends on standard psychiatric and medical-neurological assessments; establishing the causal relation to the mood disorder may be difficult.

Course and Prognosis

Depressive conditions that are comorbid with general medical illnesses or substance-related disorders have poorer prognoses than those that have no demonstrated associations. Secondary depressive illness is most often a chronic disease that is sometimes characterized by periods of remission followed by recurrences and sometimes by continuous illness. The prognosis varies, depending on the etiological disease state; depression secondary to a readily treatable disease (e.g., hypothyroidism) has a better outcome than depression associated with a terminal, essentially untreatable condition (e.g., metastatic pancreatic carcinoma).

Treatment

Standard antidepressant medications, including tricyclic drugs, monoamine oxidase inhibitors (MAOIs), selective serotonin reuptake inhibitors (SSRIs), and psychostimulants, are effective in many depressed patients with medical and neurological illnesses or substance use disorders. Electroconvulsive therapy (ECT) may be useful in patients who do not respond to medication.

The clinician treating a patient with a secondary mood disorder should treat the underlying medical cause as effectively as possible. Standard treatment approaches for the corresponding primary mood disorder should be used, although the risk of toxic effects from psychotropic drugs may require more gradual dosage increases. At a minimum, psychotherapy should focus on psychoeducational issues. The concept of a behavioral disturbance secondary to medical illness may be new or difficult for many patients and families to understand. Specific intrapsychic, interpersonal, and family issues are addressed as indicated in psychotherapy.

PSYCHOTIC DISORDER DUE TO A GENERAL MEDICAL CONDITION

To establish the diagnosis of psychotic disorder due to a general medical condition, the clinician first must exclude syndromes in which psychotic symptoms may be present in association with cognitive impairment (e.g., delirium and dementia of the Alzheimer's type). Disorders in this category are not associated usually with changes in the sensorium.

Epidemiology

The incidence and prevalence of secondary psychotic disorders in the general population are unknown. The prevalence of psychotic symptoms is increased in selected clinical populations, such as nursing home residents, but it is unclear how to extrapolate these findings to other patient groups.

Etiology

Virtually any cerebral or systemic disease that affects brain function can produce psychotic symptoms. Table 10.3–1 in Section 10.3 lists examples within each of the broad categories of diseases that can produce dementia; each of those diseases can also produce psychotic symptoms, both in the presence and in the absence of cognitive impairment. Degenerative disorders, such as Alzheimer's disease or Huntington's disease, may present initially with new-onset psychosis, with minimal evidence of cognitive impairment at the earliest stages.

Diagnosis and Clinical Features

To establish the diagnosis of a secondary psychotic syndrome, the clinician first determines that the patient is not delirious, as evidenced by a stable level of consciousness. A careful mental status assessment is conducted to exclude significant cognitive impairments, such as those encountered in dementia or amnestic disorder. The next step is to search for systemic or cerebral diseases that might be causally related to the psychosis. Psychotic symptomatology per se is not helpful in distinguishing a secondary from a primary (idiopathic) cause.

A systematic physical and neurological examination should be performed. The examiner should bear in mind, however, that nonlocalizing, soft neurological signs and a variety of dyskinesias can be present in schizophrenia. An evaluation with magnetic resonance imaging (MRI) for any new-onset psychosis is recommended, irrespective of patient age. The detection of a systemic or cerebral abnormality such as a brain tumor may lead to the determination of secondary psychosis; however, establishing a diagnosis of secondary psychotic syndrome requires thoughtful clinical reasoning. Table 10.5–3 lists a number of specific psychotic symptoms that have been consistently associated with disease in particular brain regions.

Course and Prognosis

The course and prognosis of secondary psychotic syndromes depend on their etiology. Vivid psychotic symptoms arising from head trauma may improve dramatically during recovery. Delusions associated with degenerative diseases may diminish as the disease worsens, for the capacity to generate those more complex cognitions is gradually lost. Some secondary psychotic disorders improve with treatment of the underlying disorder, such as the interictal psychosis of epilepsy, which often improves with the pharmacological or surgical control of seizures. Psychotic disorders secondary to infectious disease may not improve, despite eradication of the infectious organism, because of irreversible tissue damage sustained during the acute infection.

Treatment

The principles of treatment for a secondary psychotic disorder are similar to those for any secondary neuropsychiatric disorder, namely, rapid identification of the etiological agent and

Table 10.5–3
Psychotic Symptoms Associated with Abnormality of Specific Brain Regions

Symptoms	Site	Laterality
First-rank symptoms	Temporal lobe	Dominant hemisphere
Thoughts spoken aloud		
Voices commenting		
Third-person voices arguing		
Made actions		
Made feelings		
Thought withdrawal		
Thought diffusion		
Delusional perception		
Complex delusions	Subcortical or limbic	
Anton syndrome	Occipital lobe, optic tract	Bilateral
Anosognosia	Parietal lobe	Nondominant hemisphere
Misidentification syndromes	Parietal, temporal, frontal lobes	Nondominant hemisphere, bilateral
Capgras syndrome		
Reduplicative paramnesia		
Fregoli syndrome		
Intermetamorphosis syndrome		

Courtesy of Eric D. Caine, M.D., and Jeffrey M. Lyness, M.D.

treatment of the underlying cause. Antipsychotic medication may provide symptomatic relief.

ANXIETY DISORDER DUE TO A GENERAL MEDICAL CONDITION

Definition

The key feature of anxiety disorder due to a general medical condition is the presence of prominent anxiety symptoms, which may include generalized anxiety, panic attacks, obsessions, compulsions, or phobias and which are caused either by a medical or surgical (Axis III) condition or by substance intoxication or withdrawal.

Epidemiology

The prevalence of anxiety symptoms is high in general medical patients and in patients with many of the specific medical illnesses that are putative potential causes for secondary anxiety syndromes.

Etiology

Causes most commonly described in anxiety syndromes include substance-related states (intoxication with caffeine, cocaine, amphetamines, and other sympathomimetic agents; withdrawal from nicotine, sedative-hypnotics, and alcohol), endocrinopathies (especially pheochromocytoma, hyperthyroidism, hypercortisolemic states, and hyperparathyroidism), metabolic derangements (e.g., hypoxemia, hypercalcemia, and hypoglycemia), and neurological disorders (including vascular, trauma, and degenerative types). Many of these conditions are either inherently transient or easily remediable. Whether that reflects the pathophysiology of secondary anxiety or is an artifact of reporting (e.g., anxiety with subacute onset and complete resolution after removal of a pheochromocytoma is more likely to be reported as an example of anxiety due to a medical illness than is chronic anxiety in the context of chronic obstructive pulmonary disease) is not known. Much attention has been paid to the association of panic attacks and mitral valve prolapse. The nature of that association is unknown, and therefore the diagnosis of panic attacks secondary to mitral valve prolapse currently is premature. Interestingly, several recent reports have sought to tie obsessive-compulsive symptoms to the development of pathology in the basal ganglia.

Diagnosis and Clinical Features

The symptoms of secondary anxiety disorders are by definition phenomenologically similar to those found in the corresponding primary anxiety disorder (e.g., panic attacks and obsessions).

Course and Prognosis

The outcome presumably depends on the specific cause; thus, anxiety due to hyperthyroidism may well remit with treatment of the hyperthyroid state, whereas anxiety due to cardiomyopathy with a low-output state may run a more chronic course.

Treatment

Aside from treating the underlying causes, clinicians have found benzodiazepines helpful in decreasing anxiety symptoms; supportive psychotherapy (including psychoeducational issues focusing on the diagnosis and prognosis) may also be useful. The efficacy of other, more specific therapies in secondary syndromes (e.g., antidepressant medications for panic attacks, SSRIs for obsessive-compulsive symptoms, behavior therapy for simple phobias) is unknown; but they may be of use.

SLEEP DISORDER DUE TO A GENERAL MEDICAL CONDITION

Diagnosis

Sleep disorders can manifest in four ways: by an excess of sleep (hypersomnia), by a deficiency of sleep (insomnia), by abnormal behavior or activity during sleep (parasomnia), and by a disturbance in the timing of sleep (circadian rhythm sleep disorders). Primary sleep disorders occur unrelated to any other medical or psychiatric illness.

Etiology and Differential Diagnosis

Table 10.5–4 lists a number of conditions in which a sleep disturbance has been frequently described.

Table 10.5–4
Medical Conditions Commonly Associated with a Secondary Sleep Disorder

Condition	Sleep Symptoms
Parkinsonism	Frequent awakenings, disturbance of circadian rhythms
Dementia	Sundowning, frequent awakenings
Epilepsy	Difficulty initiating sleep, frequent awakenings, parasomnias
Cerebrovascular disease	Difficulty initiating sleep, frequent awakenings
Huntington's disease	Frequent awakening
Kleine-Levin syndrome	Hypersomnia
Uremia	Restless legs, nocturnal myoclonus

Courtesy of Eric D. Caine, M.D., and Jeffrey M. Lyness, M.D.

Treatment

The diagnosis of a secondary sleep disorder hinges on the identification of an active disease process known to exert the observed effect on sleep. Treatment first addresses the underlying neurological or medical disease. Symptomatic treatments focus on behavior modification, such as improvement of sleep hygiene. Pharmacological options may also be used, such as benzodiazepines for restless legs syndrome or nocturnal myoclonus, stimulants for hypersomnia, and tricyclic antidepressant medications for manipulation of REM sleep.

SEXUAL DYSFUNCTION DUE TO A GENERAL MEDICAL CONDITION

Specific syndromes characterized by sexual dysfunction thought to be physiologically caused by a general medical condition are female or male hypoactive sexual desire disorder, male erectile disorder, dyspareunia, and other male or female sexual dysfunction.

Epidemiology

Although surveys have repeatedly demonstrated a high prevalence of sexual dysfunction in the general population, valid data on secondary dysfunctions are lacking. Similarly, certain medications may be associated with specific rates of sexual symptoms, but the percentage of patients with true secondary syndromes is not known.

Etiology

Potential causes of sexual dysfunctions are listed in Table 10.5–5. The type of sexual dysfunction is affected by the cause, but specificity is rare; that is, a given cause may manifest as one (or more than one) of several syndromes. General categories include medications and drugs of abuse, local disease processes that affect the primary or secondary sexual organs, and systemic illnesses that affect sexual organs via neurological, vascular, or endocrinological routes.

Table 10.5–5
Causes of Secondary Sexual Dysfunctions

Medications
- Cardiac drugs, antihypertensives (e.g., reserpine, β-adrenergic receptor antagonists, clonidine, α-methyldopa, diuretics)
- H_2-receptor blockers
- Carbonic anhydrase inhibitors
- Anticholinergics
- Anticonvulsants (e.g., carbamazepine, phenytoin, primidone)
- Antipsychotics
- Antidepressants (e.g., tricyclic drugs, MAO oxidase inhibitors, trazodone, SSRIs)
- Sedative-hypnotics

Substances of abuse
- Alcohol
- Opioids
- Stimulants
- Cannabis
- Sedative-hypnotics

Local disease processes that affect primary or secondary sexual organs
- Congenital anomalies or malformations
- Trauma
- Tumor
- Infection
- Postsurgical or postirradiation local neurological and vascular pathology

Systemic disease processes
- Neurological
  - Central nervous system (e.g., strokes, multiple sclerosis)
  - Peripheral nervous system (e.g., peripheral neuropathy)
- Vascular
  - Atherosclerosis, vasculitis (as examples)
- Endocrine
  - Diabetes mellitus, alterations in function of thyroid, adrenal cortex, gonadotropins, gonadal hormones (as examples)

Courtesy of Eric D. Caine, M.D., and Jeffrey M. Lyness, M.D.

Course and Prognosis

The course and prognosis of secondary sexual dysfunctions vary widely, depending on the cause. Drug-induced syndromes generally remit with discontinuation (or dosage reduction) of the offending agent. Endocrine-based dysfunctions also generally improve with restoration of normal physiology. By contrast, dysfunctions due to neurological disease may run protracted, even progressive, courses.

Treatment

The treatment approach varies widely, depending on the etiology. When reversal of the underlying cause is not possible, supportive and behaviorally oriented psychotherapy with the patient (and perhaps the partner) may minimize distress and increase sexual satisfaction (e.g., by developing sexual interactions that are not limited by the specific dysfunction). Support groups for people with specific types of dysfunctions are avail-

Table 10.5–6
DSM-IV-TR Diagnostic Criteria for Catatonic Disorder Due to General Medical Condition

A. The presence of catatonia as manifested by motoric immobility, excessive motor activity (that is apparently purposeless and not influenced by external stimuli), extreme negativism or mutism, peculiarities of voluntary movement, or echolalia or echopraxia.
B. There is evidence from the history, physical examination, or laboratory findings that the disturbance is the direct physiological consequence of a general medical condition.
C. The disturbance is not better accounted for by another mental disorder (e.g., a manic episode).
D. The disturbance does not occur exclusively during the course of a delirium.

Coding note: Include the name of the general medical condition on Axis I, e.g., Catatonic disorder due to hepatic encephalopathy; also code the general medical condition on Axis III.

From American Psychiatric Association. *Diagnostic and Statistical Manual of Mental Disorders.* 4th ed. Text rev. Washington, DC: American Psychiatric Association; copyright 2000, with permission.

able. Other symptom-based treatments may be used in certain conditions; for example, sildenafil (Viagra) administration or surgical implantation of a penile prosthesis may be used in the treatment of male erectile dysfunction.

MENTAL DISORDERS DUE TO A GENERAL MEDICAL CONDITION NOT ELSEWHERE CLASSIFIED

DSM-IV-TR has three additional diagnostic categories for clinical presentations of mental disorders due to a general medical condition that do not meet the diagnostic criteria for specific diagnoses. The first of the diagnoses is catatonic disorder due to a general medical condition (Table 10.5–6). The second is personality change due to a general medical condition. The third diagnosis is mental disorder not otherwise specified due to a general medical condition (Table 10.5–7).

Table 10.5–7
DSM-IV-TR Diagnostic Criteria for Mental Disorder Not Otherwise Specified Due to a General Medical Condition

This residual category should be used for situations in which it has been established that the disturbance is caused by the direct physiological effects of a general medical condition, but the criteria are not met for a specific mental disorder due to a general medical condition (e.g., dissociative symptoms due to complex partial seizures).

Coding note: Include the name of the general medical condition on Axis I, e.g., Mental disorder not otherwise specified due to HIV disease; also code the general medical condition on Axis III.

From American Psychiatric Association. *Diagnostic and Statistical Manual of Mental Disorders.* 4th ed. Text rev. Washington, DC: American Psychiatric Association; copyright 2000, with permission.

Catatonia Due to a Medical Condition

Catatonia may be caused by a variety of medical or surgical conditions. It is characterized usually by fixed posture and waxy flexibility. Mutism, negativism, and echolalia may be associated features.

Epidemiology. The incidence of catatonia due to a general medical condition is unknown. Catatonic symptoms are more likely to be associated with schizophrenia than with other disorders.

Diagnosis and Clinical Features. Peculiarities of movement are the most characteristic feature, usually rigidity. Hyperactivity and psychomotor agitation may also occur (Table 10.5–7). A thorough medical workup is necessary to confirm the diagnosis.

Course and Prognosis. The course and prognosis are intimately related to the cause. Neoplasms, encephalitis, head trauma, diabetes, and other metabolic disorders may manifest with catatonic features. If the underlying disorder is treatable, the catatonic syndrome will resolve.

Treatment. Treatment must be directed to the underlying cause. Antipsychotic medications may improve postural abnormalities even though they have no effect on the underlying disorder. Schizophrenia must always be ruled out in patients who present with catatonic symptoms.

Personality Change Due to a General Medical Condition

Personality change means that the person's fundamental means of interacting and behaving have been altered. When a true personality change occurs in adulthood, the clinician should always suspect brain injury. Almost every medical disorder can be accompanied by personality change, however.

Epidemiology. No reliable epidemiological data exist on personality trait changes in medical conditions. Specific personality trait changes for particular brain diseases—for example, passive and self-centered behaviors in patients with dementia of the Alzheimer's type—have been reported. Similarly, apathy has been described in patients with frontal lobe lesions.

Etiology. Diseases that preferentially affect the frontal lobes or subcortical structures are more likely to manifest with prominent personality change. Head trauma is a common cause. Frontal lobe tumors, such as meningiomas and gliomas, can grow to considerable size before coming to medical attention, as they may be neurologically silent (i.e., without focal signs). Progressive dementia syndromes, especially those with a subcortical pattern of degeneration, such as acquired immune deficiency syndrome (AIDS) dementia complex, Huntington's disease, or progressive supranuclear palsy, often cause significant personality disturbance. Multiple sclerosis can impinge on the personality, reflecting subcortical white matter degeneration. Exposure to toxins with a predilection for white matter, such as irradiation, may also produce significant personality change disproportionate to the cognitive or motor impairment.

Table 10.5–8
DSM-IV-TR Diagnostic Criteria for Personality Change Due to General Medical Condition

A. A persistent personality disturbance that represents a change from the individual's previous characteristic personality pattern. (In children, the disturbance involves a marked deviation from normal development or a significant change in the child's usual behavior patterns lasting at least 1 year.)
B. There is evidence from the history, physical examination, or laboratory findings that the disturbance is the direct physiological consequence of a general medical condition.
C. The disturbance is not better accounted for by another mental disorder (including other mental disorders due to a general medical condition).
D. The disturbance does not occur exclusively during the course of a delirium.
E. The disturbance causes clinically significant distress or impairment in social, occupational, or other important areas of functioning.

Specify type:

Labile type: if the predominant feature is affective lability
Disinhibited type: if the predominant feature is poor impulse control as evidenced by sexual indiscretions, etc.
Aggressive type: if the predominant feature is aggressive behavior
Apathetic type: if the predominant feature is marked apathy and indifference
Paranoid type: if the predominant feature is suspiciousness or paranoid ideation
Other type: if the presentation is not characterized by any of the above subtypes
Combined type: if more than one feature predominates in the clinical picture
Unspecified type

Coding note: Include the name of the general medical condition on Axis I, e.g., Personality change due to temporal lobe epilepsy; also code the general medical condition on Axis III.

From American Psychiatric Association. *Diagnostic and Statistical Manual of Mental Disorders.* 4th ed. Text rev. Washington, DC: American Psychiatric Association; copyright 2000, with permission.

Diagnosis and Clinical Features. The DSM-IV-TR diagnostic criteria for personality change due to a general medical condition are listed in Table 10.5–8.

Course and Prognosis. Personality change secondary to mass lesions or hydrocephalus can improve dramatically with surgery, chemotherapy, or radiation therapy. Personality change secondary to head trauma may improve slowly and gradually over the course of months or years, although residual disturbances may remain. Personality change due to degenerative processes can be disruptive early in the disease process; however, management of such patients may ease as the disease progresses and the personality evolves into greater apathy, unresponsiveness, and akinesia. Personality change associated with epilepsy can improve dramatically with seizure control by pharmacotherapy or surgery.

Treatment. Treatment of secondary personality syndromes is first directed toward correcting the underlying cause. Lithium carbonate (Eskalith), carbamazepine (Tegretol), and valproic acid (Depakote) have been used for the control of affective lability and impulsivity. Aggression or explosiveness may be treated with lithium, anticonvulsant medications, or a combination of lithium and an anticonvulsant agent. Centrally active β-adrenergic receptor antagonists, such as propranolol (Inderal), have some efficacy as well. Apathy and inertia have occasionally improved with psychostimulant agents. Because cognition and verbal skills may be preserved in patients with secondary personality changes, they may be candidates for psychotherapy. Families should be involved in the therapy process, with a focus on education and understanding the origins of the patient's inappropriate behaviors. Issues such as competency, disability, and advocacy are frequently of clinical concern with these patients in light of the unpredictable and pervasive behavior change.

SPECIFIC DISORDERS

Epilepsy

Epilepsy is the most common chronic neurological disease in the general population and affects approximately 1 percent of the population in the United States. For psychiatrists, the major concerns about epilepsy are consideration of an epileptic diagnosis in psychiatric patients, the psychosocial ramifications of a diagnosis of epilepsy for a patient, and the psychological and cognitive effects of commonly used anticonvulsant drugs. With regard to the first of these concerns, 30 to 50 percent of all persons with epilepsy have psychiatric difficulties sometime during the course of their illness. The most common behavioral symptom of epilepsy is a change in personality. Psychosis and violence occur much less commonly than was previously believed.

Definitions. A seizure is a transient paroxysmal pathophysiological disturbance of cerebral function caused by a spontaneous, excessive discharge of neurons. Patients are said to have epilepsy if they have a chronic condition characterized by recurrent seizure. The ictus, or ictal event, is the seizure itself. The nonictal periods are categorized as preictal, postictal, and interictal. The symptoms during the ictal event are determined primarily by the site of origin in the brain for the seizure and by the pattern of the spread of seizure activity through the brain. Interictal symptoms are influenced by the ictal event and other neuropsychiatric and psychosocial factors, such as coexisting psychiatric or neurological disorders, the presence of psychosocial stressors, and premorbid personality traits.

Classification. The two major categories of seizures are partial and generalized. Partial seizures involve epileptiform activity in localized brain regions. Generalized seizures involve the entire brain (Fig. 10.5–1). A classification system for seizures is outlined in Table 10.5–9.

GENERALIZED SEIZURES. Generalized tonic-clonic seizures exhibit the classic symptoms of loss of consciousness, generalized tonic-clonic movements of the limbs, tongue biting, and incontinence. Although the diagnosis of the ictal events of the seizure is relatively straightforward, the postictal state, characterized by a slow, gradual recovery of consciousness

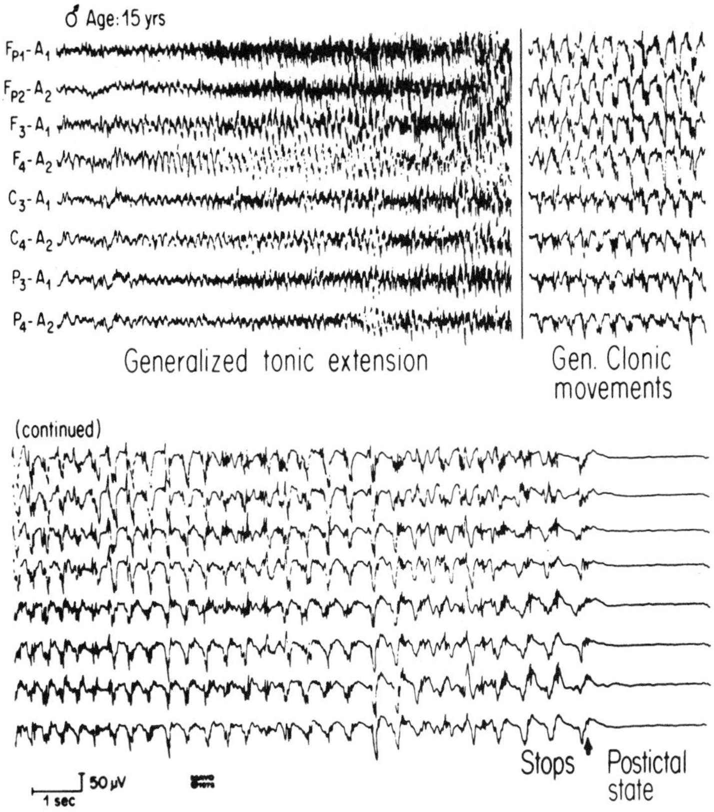

FIGURE 10.5–1

Electroencephalographic recording during generalized tonic-clonic seizure, showing rhythmic sharp waves and muscle artifact during tonic phase, spike and wave discharges during clonic phase, and attenuation of activity during postictal state. (Courtesy of Barbara F. Westmoreland, M.D.)

and cognition, occasionally presents a diagnostic dilemma for a psychiatrist in an emergency room. The period of recovery from a generalized tonic-clonic seizure ranges for a few minutes to many hours, and the clinical picture is that of a gradually clearing delirium. The most common psychiatric problems associated with generalized seizures involve helping patients adjust to a chronic neurological disorder and assessing the cognitive or behavioral effects of anticonvulsant drugs.

Absence Seizure (Petit Mal). A difficult type of generalized seizure for a psychiatrist to diagnose is an absence, or petit mal, seizure. The epileptic nature of the episodes may go unrecognized, because the characteristic motor or sensory manifestations of epilepsy may be absent or so slight that they do not arouse suspicion. Petit mal epilepsy usually begins in childhood between the ages of 5 and 7 years and ceases by puberty. Brief disruptions of consciousness, during which the patient suddenly loses contact with the environment, are characteristic of petit mal epilepsy, but the patient has no true loss of consciousness and no convulsive movements during the episodes. The electroencephalogram (EEG) produces a characteristic pattern of three-per-second spike-and-wave activity (Fig. 10.5–2). In rare instances, petit mal epilepsy begins in adulthood. Adult-onset petit mal epilepsy can be characterized by sudden, recurrent psychotic episodes or deliriums that appear and disappear abruptly. The symptoms may be accompanied by a history of falling or fainting spells.

PARTIAL SEIZURES. Partial seizures are classified as either simple (without alterations in consciousness) or complex (with an alteration in consciousness). Somewhat more than half of all patients with partial seizures have complex partial seizures. Other terms used for complex partial seizures are temporal lobe epilepsy, psychomotor seizures, and limbic epilepsy; these terms, however, are not accurate descriptions of the clinical situation. Complex partial epilepsy, the most common form of epilepsy in adults, affects approximately 3 in 1,000 persons. About 30 percent of patients with complex partial seizures have major mental illness such as depression.

Symptoms. **PREICTAL SYMPTOMS.** Preictal events (auras) in complex partial epilepsy include autonomic sensations (e.g., fullness in the stomach, blushing, and changes in respiration), cognitive sensations (e.g., *déjà vu*, *jamais vu*, forced thinking, and dreamy states), affective states (e.g., fear, panic, depression, and elation), and, classically, automatisms (e.g., lip smacking, rubbing, and chewing).

ICTAL SYMPTOMS. Brief, disorganized, and uninhibited behavior characterizes the ictal event. Although some defense attorneys may claim otherwise, rarely does a person exhibit organized, directed violent behavior during an epileptic episode. The cognitive symptoms include amnesia for the time during the seizure and a period of resolving delirium after the

Table 10.5–9
International Classification of Epileptic Seizures

I. Partial seizures (seizures beginning locally)
  A. Partial seizures with elementary symptoms (generally without impairment of consciousness)
    1. With motor symptoms
    2. With sensory symptoms
    3. With autonomic symptoms
    4. Compound forms
  B. Partial seizures with complex symptoms (generally with impairment of consciousness; temporal lobe or psychomotor seizures)
    1. With impairment of consciousness only
    2. With cognitive symptoms
    3. With affective symptoms
    4. With psychosensory symptoms
    5. With psychosensory symptoms (automatisms)
    6. Compound forms
  C. Partial seizures secondarily generalized
II. Generalized seizures (bilaterally symmetrical and without local onset)
  A. Absences (petit mal)
  B. Myoclonus
  C. Infantile spasms
  D. Clonic seizures
  E. Tonic seizures
  F. Tonic-clonic seizures (grand mal)
  G. Atonic seizures
  H. Akinetic seizures
III. Unilateral seizures
IV. Unclassified seizures (because of incomplete data)

Adapted from Gastaut H. Clinical and electroencephalographical classification of epileptic seizures. *Epilepsia.* 1970;11:102.

seizure. A seizure focus can be found on an EEG in 25 to 50 percent of all patients with complex partial epilepsy (Fig. 10.5–3). The use of sphenoidal or anterior temporal electrodes and sleep-deprived EEGs may increase the likelihood of finding an EEG abnormality. Multiple normal EEGs are often obtained for a patient with complex partial epilepsy; therefore, normal EEGs cannot be used to exclude a diagnosis of complex partial epilepsy. The use of long-term EEG recordings (usually 24 to 72 hours) can help clinicians detect a seizure focus in some patients. Most studies show that the use of nasopharyngeal leads does not add much to the sensitivity of an EEG, but they do add to the discomfort of the procedure for the patient.

INTERICTAL SYMPTOMS. *Personality Disturbances.* The most frequent psychiatric abnormalities reported in epileptic patients are personality disorders, and they are especially likely to occur in patients with epilepsy of temporal lobe origin. The most common features are religiosity, a heightened experience of emotions—a quality usually called viscosity of personality—and changes in sexual behavior. The syndrome in its complete form is relatively rare, even in those with complex partial seizures of temporal lobe origin. Many patients are not affected by personality disturbances; others suffer from a variety of disturbances that differ strikingly from the classic syndrome.

A striking religiosity may be manifested not only by increased participation in overtly religious activities but also by unusual concern for moral and ethical issues, preoccupation with right and wrong, and heightened interest in global and philosophical concerns. The hyperreligious features can sometimes seem like the prodromal symptoms of schizophrenia and can result in a diagnostic problem in an adolescent or a young adult.

The symptom of viscosity of personality is usually most noticeable in a patient's conversation, which is likely to be slow, serious, ponderous, pedantic, overly replete with nonessential details, and often circumstantial. The listener may grow bored but be unable to find a

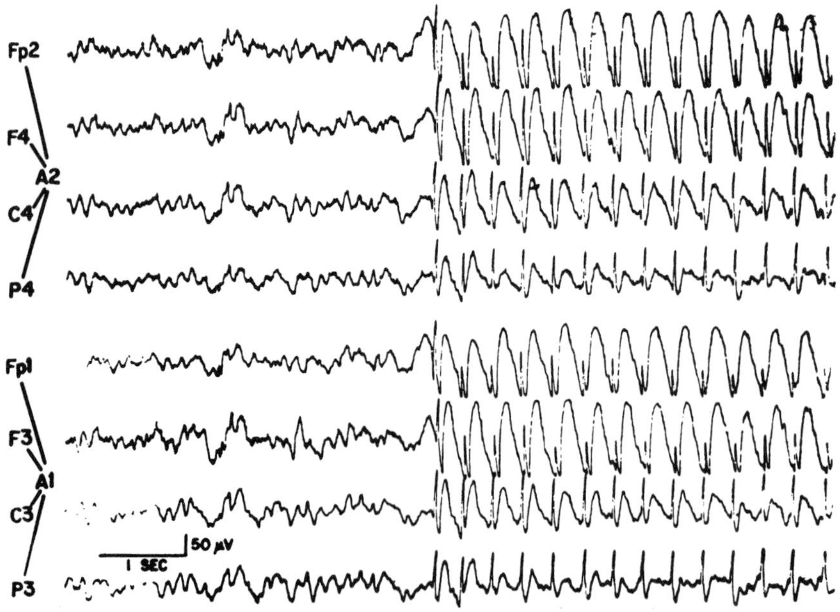

FIGURE 10.5–2
Petit mal epilepsy characterized by bilaterally synchronous 3-Hz spike and slow-wave activity.

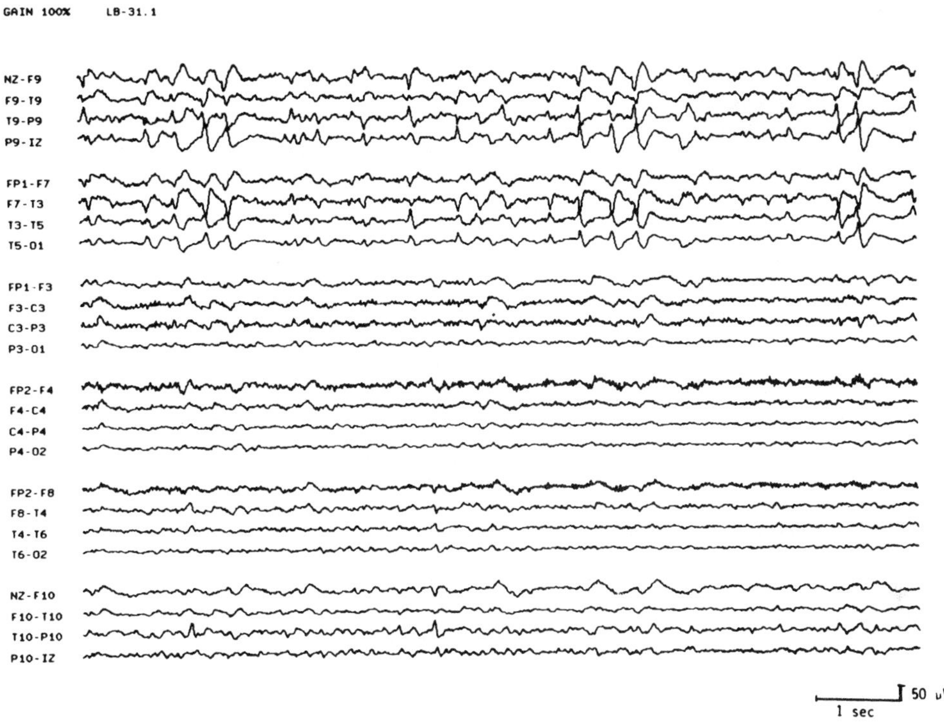

FIGURE 10.5–3
An interictal encephalograph in a patient with complex partial seizures reveals frequent left-temporal spike discharges and rare, independent right-temporal sharp-wave activity. (Reprinted with permission from Cascino GD. Complex partial seizures: clinical features and differential diagnosis. *Psychiatr Clin North Am.* 1992;15:377.)

courteous and successful way to disengage from the conversation. The speech tendencies, often mirrored in the patient's writing, result in a symptom known as hypergraphia, which some clinicians consider virtually pathognomonic for complex partial epilepsy.

Changes in sexual behavior may be manifested by hypersexuality; deviations in sexual interest, such as fetishism and transvestism; and, most commonly, hyposexuality. The hyposexuality is characterized both by a lack of interest in sexual matters and by reduced sexual arousal. Some patients with the onset of complex partial epilepsy before puberty may fail to reach a normal level of sexual interest after puberty, although this characteristic may not disturb the patient. For patients with the onset of complex partial epilepsy after puberty, the change in sexual interest may be bothersome and worrisome.

Psychotic Symptoms. Interictal psychotic states are more common than ictal psychoses. Schizophrenia-like interictal episodes can occur in patients with epilepsy, particularly those with temporal lobe origins. An estimated 10 percent of all patients with complex partial epilepsy have psychotic symptoms. Risk factors for the symptoms include female gender, left-handedness, the onset of seizures during puberty, and a left-sided lesion.

The onset of psychotic symptoms in epilepsy is variable. Classically, psychotic symptoms appear in patients who have had epilepsy for a long time, and the onset of psychotic symptoms is preceded by the development of personality changes related to the epileptic brain activity. The most characteristic symptoms of the psychoses are hallucinations and paranoid delusions. Patients usually remain warm and appropriate in affect, in contrast to the abnormalities of affect commonly seen in patients with schizophrenia. The thought disorder symptoms in patients with psychotic epilepsy are most commonly those involving conceptualization and circumstantiality, rather than the classic schizophrenic symptoms of blocking and looseness.

Violence. Episodic violence has been a problem in some patients with epilepsy, especially epilepsy of temporal and frontal lobe origin. Whether the violence is a manifestation of the seizure itself or is of interictal psychopathological origin is uncertain. Most evidence points to the extreme rarity of violence as an ictal phenomenon. Only in rare cases should an epileptic patient's violence be attributed to the seizure itself.

Mood Disorder Symptoms. Mood disorder symptoms, such as depression and mania, are seen less often in epilepsy than are schizophrenialike symptoms. The mood disorder symptoms that do occur tend to be episodic and appear most often when the epileptic foci affect the temporal lobe of the nondominant cerebral hemisphere. The importance of mood disorder symptoms may be attested to by the increased incidence of attempted suicide in people with epilepsy.

Diagnosis. A correct diagnosis of epilepsy can be particularly difficult when the ictal and interictal symptoms of epilepsy are severe manifestations of psychiatric symptoms in the absence of significant changes in consciousness and cognitive abilities. Therefore, psychiatrists must maintain a high level of suspicion during the evaluation of a new patient and must consider the possibility of an epileptic disorder, even in the absence of the classic signs and symptoms. Another differential diagnosis to consider is pseudoseizure, in which a patient has some conscious control over mimicking the symptoms of a seizure (Table 10.5–10).

Table 10.5–10
Differentiating Features of Pseudoseizures and Epileptic Seizures

Feature	Epileptic Seizures	Pseudoseizure
Clinical features		
Nocturnal seizure	Common	Uncommon
Stereotyped aura	Usually	None
Cyanotic skin changes during seizures	Common	None
Self-injury	Common	Rare
Incontinence	Common	Rare
Postictal confusion	Present	None
Body movements	Tonic or clonic or both	Nonstereotyped and asynchronous
Affected by suggestion	No	Yes
EEG features		
Spike and waveforms	Present	Absent
Postictal slowing	Present	Absent
Interictal abnormalities	Variable	Variable

Reprinted with permission from Stevenson JM, King JH. Neuropsychiatric aspects of epilepsy and epileptic seizures. In: Hales RE, Yodofsky SC, eds. *American Psychiatric Press Textbook of Neuropsychiatry.* Washington, DC: American Psychiatric Press; 1987:220.

For patients who have previously received a diagnosis of epilepsy, the appearance of new psychiatric symptoms should be considered as possibly representing an evolution in their epileptic symptoms. The appearance of psychotic symptoms, mood disorder symptoms, personality changes, or symptoms of anxiety (e.g., panic attacks) should cause a clinician to evaluate the control of the patient's epilepsy and to assess the patient for the presence of an independent mental disorder. In such circumstances, the clinician should evaluate the patient's compliance with the anticonvulsant drug regimen and should consider whether the psychiatric symptoms could be adverse effects from the antiepileptic drugs themselves. When psychiatric symptoms appear in a patient who has had epilepsy diagnosed or considered as a diagnosis in the past, the clinician should obtain results of one or more EEG examinations.

In patients who have not previously received a diagnosis of epilepsy, four characteristics should cause a clinician to be suspicious of the possibility: the abrupt onset of psychosis in a person previously regarded as psychologically healthy, the abrupt onset of delirium without a recognized cause, a history of similar episodes with abrupt onset and spontaneous recovery, and a history of previous unexplained falling or fainting spells.

Treatment. First-line drugs for generalized tonic-clonic seizures are valproate and phenytoin (Dilantin). First-line drugs for partial seizures include carbamazepine, oxcarbazepine (Trileptal), and phenytoin. Ethosuximide (Zarontin) and valproate are first-line drugs for absence (petit mal) seizures. The drugs used for various types of seizures are listed in Table 10.5–11. Carbamazepine and valproic acid may be helpful in controlling the symptoms of irritability and outbursts of aggression, as are the typical antipsychotic drugs. Psychotherapy, family counseling, and group therapy may be useful in addressing the psychosocial issues associated with epilepsy. In addition, clinicians should be aware that many antiepileptic drugs cause mild to moderate cognitive impairment, and an adjustment of the dosage or a change in medications should be considered if symptoms of cognitive impairment are a problem in a patient.

Brain Tumors

Brain tumors and cerebrovascular diseases can cause virtually any psychiatric symptom or syndrome, but cerebrovascular diseases, by the nature of their onset and symptom pattern, are rarely misdiagnosed as mental disorders. In general, tumors are associated with fewer psychopathological signs and symptoms than are cerebrovascular diseases affecting a similar volume of brain tissue. The two key approaches to the diagnosis of either

Table 10.5–11
Commonly Used Anticonvulsant Drugs

Drug	Use	Maintenance Dosage (mg/day)
Carbamazepine (Tegretol, Carbatrol)	Generalized tonic-clonic, partial	600–1,200
Clonazepam (Klonopin)	Absence, atypical myoclonic	2–12
Ethosuximide (Zarontin)	Absence	1,000–2,000
Gabapentin (Neurontin)	Complex partial seizures (augmentation)	900–3,600
Lamotrigine (Lamictal)	Complex partial seizures, generalized (augmentation)	300–500
Oxcarbazepine (Trileptal)	Partial	600–2,400
Phenobarbital	Generalized tonic-clonic	100–200
Phenytoin (Dilantin)	Generalized tonic-clonic, partial, status epilepticus	300–500
Primidone (Mysoline)	Partial	750–1,000
Tiagabine (Gabitril)	Generalized	32–56
Topiramate (Topamax)	Complex partial seizures (augmentation)	200–400
Valproate	Absence, myoclonic generalized tonic-clonic akinetic, partial seizures	750–1,000
Zonisamide (Zonegran)	Generalized	400–600

condition are a comprehensive clinical history and a complete neurological examination. Performance of the appropriate brain imaging technique is usually the final diagnostic procedure; the imaging should confirm the clinical diagnosis.

Clinical Features, Course, and Prognosis. Mental symptoms are experienced at some time during the course of illness in approximately 50 percent of patients with brain tumors. In approximately 80 percent of these patients with mental symptoms, the tumors are located in frontal or limbic brain regions rather than in parietal or temporal regions. Meningiomas are likely to cause focal symptoms by compressing a limited region of the cortex, whereas gliomas are likely to cause diffuse symptoms. Delirium is most often a component of rapidly growing, large, or metastatic tumors. If a patient's history and a physical examination reveal bowel or bladder incontinence, a frontal lobe tumor should be suspected; if the history and examination reveal abnormalities in memory and speech, a temporal lobe tumor should be suspected.

COGNITION. Impaired intellectual functioning often accompanies the presence of a brain tumor, regardless of its type or location.

LANGUAGE SKILLS. Disorders of language function may be severe, particularly if tumor growth is rapid. In fact, defects of language function often obscure all other mental symptoms.

MEMORY. Loss of memory is a frequent symptom of brain tumors. Patients with brain tumors exhibit Korsakoff's syndrome and retain no memory of events that occurred since the illness began. Events of the immediate past, even painful ones, are lost. Patients, however, retain old memories and are unaware of their loss of recent memory.

PERCEPTION. Prominent perceptual defects are often associated with behavioral disorders, especially because patients must integrate tactile, auditory, and visual perceptions to function normally.

AWARENESS. Alterations of consciousness are common late symptoms of increased intracranial pressure caused by a brain tumor. Tumors arising in the upper part of the brainstem may produce a unique symptom called akinetic mutism, or vigilant coma. The patient is immobile and mute, yet alert.

Table 10.5–12
DSM-IV-TR Research Criteria for Postconcussional Disorder

A. A history of head trauma that has caused significant cerebral concussion.
Note: The manifestations of concussion include loss of consciousness, posttraumatic amnesia, and, less commonly, posttraumatic onset of seizures. The specific method of defining this criterion needs to be established by further research.

B. Evidence from neuropsychological testing or quantified cognitive assessment of difficulty in attention (concentrating, shifting focus of attention, performing simultaneous cognitive tasks) or memory (learning or recalling information).

C. Three (or more) of the following occur shortly after the trauma and last at least 3 months:
(1) becoming fatigued easily
(2) disordered sleep
(3) headache
(4) vertigo or dizziness
(5) irritability or aggression on little or no provocation
(6) anxiety, depression, or affective lability
(7) changes in personality (e.g., social or sexual inappropriateness)
(8) apathy or lack of spontaneity

D. The symptoms in Criteria B and C have their onset following head trauma or else represent a substantial worsening of preexisting symptoms.

E. The disturbance causes significant impairment in social or occupational functioning and represents a significant decline from a previous level of functioning. In school-age children, the impairment may be manifested by a significant worsening in school or academic performance dating from the trauma.

F. The symptoms do not meet criteria for dementia due to head trauma and are not better accounted for by another mental disorder (e.g., amnestic disorder due to head trauma, personality change due to head trauma).

From American Psychiatric Association. *Diagnostic and Statistical Manual of Mental Disorders.* 4th ed. Text rev. Washington, DC: American Psychiatric Association; copyright 2000, with permission.

Colloid Cysts. Although they are not brain tumors, colloid cysts located in the third ventricle can exert physical pressure on structures within the diencephalon and produce such mental symptoms as depression, emotional lability, psychotic symptoms, and personality changes. The classic associated neurological symptoms are position-dependent intermittent headaches.

Head Trauma

Head trauma can result in an array of mental symptoms and can lead to a diagnosis of dementia due to head trauma or to mental disorder not otherwise specified due to a general medical condition (such as postconcussional disorder). The postconcussive syndrome remains controversial, because it focuses on the wide range of psychiatric symptoms, some serious, that can follow what seems to be minor head trauma. DSM-IV-TR includes a set of research criteria for postconcussional disorder in an appendix (Table 10.5–12).

Pathophysiology. Head trauma is a common clinical situation; an estimated 2 million incidents involve head trauma each year. Head trauma most commonly occurs in people 15 to 25 years of age and has a male-to-female predominance of approximately 3 to 1. Gross estimates based on the severity of the head trauma suggest that virtually all patients with serious head trauma, more than half of patients with moderate head trauma, and about 10 percent of patients with mild head trauma have ongoing neuropsychiatric sequelae resulting from the head trauma. Head trauma can be divided grossly into penetrating head trauma (such as trauma produced by a bullet) and blunt trauma, in which there is no physical penetration of the skull. Blunt trauma is far more common than penetrating head trauma. Motor vehicle accidents account for more than half of all the incidents of blunt central nervous system (CNS) trauma; falls, violence, and sports-related head trauma account for most of the remaining cases (Fig. 10.5–4).

Whereas brain injury from penetrating wounds is usually localized to the areas directly affected by the missile, brain

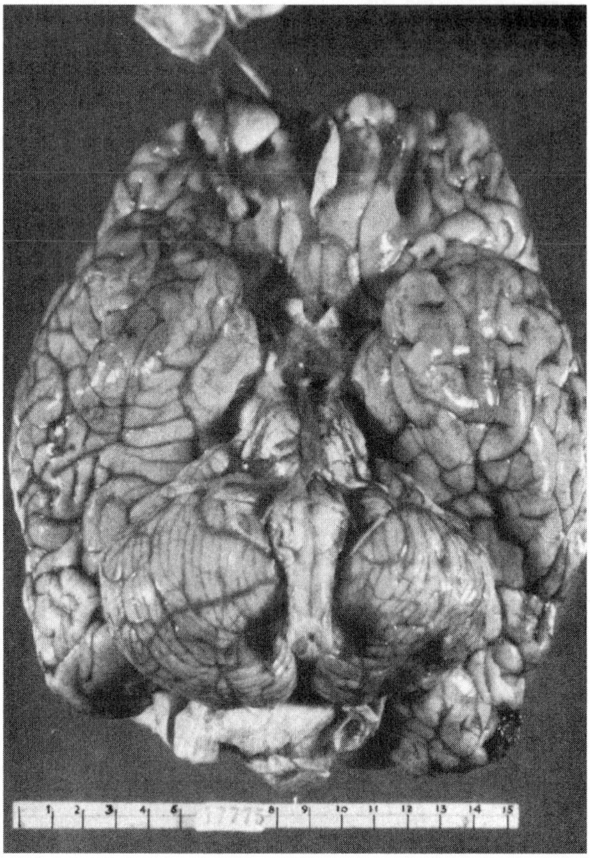

FIGURE 10.5–4
Severe contusion of the frontal poles has resulted in their atrophy and distortion. (Courtesy of Dr. H. M. Zimmerman.)

injury from blunt trauma involves several mechanisms. During the actual head trauma, the head usually moves back and forth violently, so that the brain hits repeatedly against the skull as it and the skull are mismatched in their rapid deceleration and acceleration. This crashing results in focal contusions, and the stretching of the brain parenchyma produces diffuse axonal injury. Later-developing processes, such as edema and hemorrhaging, may result in further damage to the brain.

Symptoms. The two major clusters of symptoms related to head trauma are those of cognitive impairment and of behavioral sequelae. After a period of posttraumatic amnesia, there is usually a 6- to 12-month period of recovery, after which the remaining symptoms are likely to be permanent. The most common cognitive problems are decreased speed in information processing, decreased attention, increased distractibility, deficits in problem solving and in the ability to sustain effort, and problems with memory and learning new information. A variety of language disabilities may also occur.

Behaviorally, the major symptoms involve depression, increased impulsivity, increased aggression, and changes in personality. These symptoms may be further exacerbated by the use of alcohol, which is often involved in the head trauma event itself. A debate has ensued about how preexisting character and personality traits affect the development of behavioral symptoms after head trauma. The critical studies needed to answer the question definitively have not yet been done, but the weight of opinion is leaning toward a biologically and neuroanatomically based association between the head trauma and the behavioral sequelae.

Treatment. The treatment of the cognitive and behavioral disorders in head trauma patients is basically similar to the treatment approaches used in other patients with these symptoms. One difference is that head trauma patients may be particularly susceptible to the side effects associated with psychotropic drugs; therefore, treatment with these agents should be initiated in lower dosages than usual, and they should be titrated upward more slowly than usual. Standard antidepressants can be used to treat depression, and either anticonvulsants or antipsychotics can be used to treat aggression and impulsivity. Other approaches to the symptoms include lithium, calcium channel blockers, and β-adrenergic receptor antagonists.

Clinicians must support patients through individual or group psychotherapy and should support the major caretakers through couples and family therapy. Patients with minor and moderate head trauma often rejoin their families and restart their jobs; therefore, all involved parties need help to adjust to any changes in the patient's personality and mental abilities.

Demyelinating Disorders

Multiple sclerosis (MS) is the major demyelinating disorder. Other demyelinating disorders include amyotrophic lateral sclerosis (ALS), metachromatic leukodystrophy, adrenoleukodystrophy, gangliosidoses, subacute sclerosing panencephalitis, and Kufs' disease. All these disorders can be associated with neurological, cognitive, and behavioral symptoms.

Multiple Sclerosis. MS is characterized by multiple episodes of symptoms, pathophysiologically related to multifocal lesions in the white matter of the CNS (Fig. 10.5–5). The cause remains unknown, but studies have focused on slow viral infections and disturbances in the immune system. The estimated prevalence of multiple sclerosis in the Western Hemisphere is 50 per 100,000 people. The disease is much more frequent in cold and temperate climates than in the tropics and subtropics and more common in women than in men; it is predominantly a disease of young adults. In most patients, the onset occurs between the ages of 20 and 40 years.

The neuropsychiatric symptoms of MS can be divided into cognitive and behavioral types. Research reports have found that 30 to 50 percent of patients with MS have mild cognitive impairment and that 20 to 30 percent of MS patients have serious cognitive impairments. Although evidence indicates that MS patients experience a decline in their general intelligence, memory is the most commonly affected cognitive function. The severity of the memory impairment does not seem to be correlated with the severity of the neurological symptoms or the duration of the illness.

The behavioral symptoms associated with MS are varied and may include euphoria, depression, and personality changes. Psychosis is a rare complication. Approximately 25 percent of

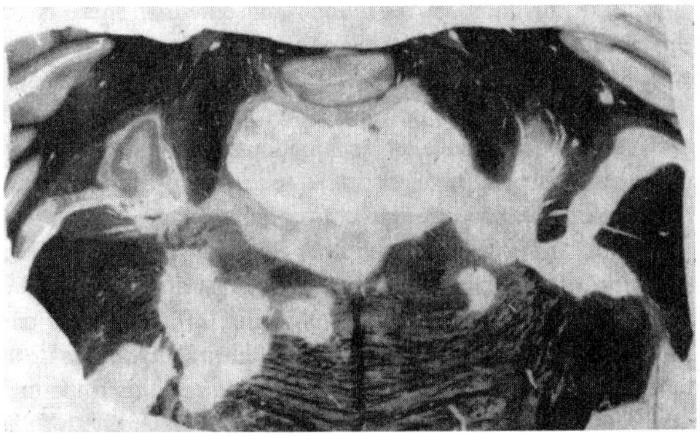

FIGURE 10.5–5
Multiple sclerosis. Irregular, seemingly punched out zones of demyelination are evident in this section through the level of the fourth ventricle. Myelin stain. 2.6×. (Courtesy of Dr. H. M. Zimmerman.)

persons with MS exhibit a euphoric mood that is not hypomanic, but somewhat more cheerful than their situation warrants and not necessarily in character with their disposition before the onset of MS. Only 10 percent of MS patients have a sustained and elevated mood, although it is still not truly hypomanic. Depression, however, is common; it affects 25 to 50 percent of patients with MS and results in a higher rate of suicide than is seen in the general population. Risk factors for suicide in MS patients are male sex, onset of MS before age 30, and a relatively recent diagnosis of the disorder. Personality changes are also common in MS patients; they affect 20 to 40 percent of patients and are often characterized by increased irritability or apathy.

Amyotrophic Lateral Sclerosis. ALS is a progressive, noninherited disease of asymmetrical muscle atrophy. It begins in adult life and progresses over months or years to involve all the striated muscles except the cardiac and ocular muscles. In addition to muscle atrophy, patients have signs of pyramidal tract involvement. The illness is rare and occurs in approximately 1.6 persons per 100,000 annually. A few patients have concomitant dementia. The disease progresses rapidly, and death generally occurs within 4 years of onset.

Infectious Diseases

Herpes Simplex Encephalitis. Herpes simplex encephalitis is the most common type of focal encephalitis and most commonly affects the frontal and temporal lobes. The symptoms often include anosmia, olfactory and gustatory hallucinations, and personality changes and can also involve bizarre or psychotic behaviors. Complex partial epilepsy may also develop in patients with herpes simplex encephalitis. Although the mortality rate for the infection has decreased, many patients exhibit personality changes, symptoms of memory loss, and psychotic symptoms.

Rabies Encephalitis. The incubation period for rabies ranges from 10 days to 1 year, after which symptoms of restlessness, overactivity, and agitation can develop. Hydrophobia, present in up to 50 percent of patients, is characterized by an intense fear of drinking water. The fear develops from the severe laryngeal and diaphragmatic spasms that the patients experience when they drink water. Once rabies encephalitis develops, the disease is fatal within days or weeks.

Neurosyphilis. Neurosyphilis (also known as general paresis) appears 10 to 15 years after the primary *Treponema* infection. Since the advent of penicillin, neurosyphilis has become a rare disorder, although AIDS is associated with reintroducing neurosyphilis into medical practice in some urban settings. Neurosyphilis generally affects the frontal lobes and results in personality changes, development of poor judgment, irritability, and decreased care for self. Delusions of grandeur develop in 10 to 20 percent of affected patients. The disease progresses with the development of dementia and tremor, until patients are paretic. The neurological symptoms include Argyll-Robertson pupils, which are small, irregular, and unequal and have light–near reflex dissociation, tremor, dysarthria, and hyperreflexia. Cerebrospinal fluid (CSF) examination shows lymphocytosis, increased protein, and a positive result on a Venereal Disease Research Laboratory (VDRL) test.

Chronic Meningitis. Chronic meningitis is now seen more often than in the recent past because of the immunocompromised condition of people with AIDS. The usual causative agents are *Mycobacterium tuberculosis, Cryptococcus,* and *Coccidioides.* The usual symptoms are headache, memory impairment, confusion, and fever.

Subacute Sclerosing Panencephalitis. Subacute sclerosing panencephalitis is a disease of childhood and early adolescence, with a 3-to-1 male-to-female ratio. The onset usually follows either an infection with measles or a vaccination for measles. The initial symptoms may be behavioral change, temper tantrums, sleepiness, and hallucinations, but the classic symptoms of myoclonus, ataxia, seizures, and intellectual deterioration eventually develop. The disease progresses relentlessly to coma and death in 1 to 2 years.

Lyme Disease. Lyme disease is caused by infection with the spirochete *Borrelia burgdorferi* transmitted through the bite of the deer tick (*Ixodes scapularis*), which feed on infected deer and mice. About 16,000 cases are reported annually in the United States.

A characteristic bull's-eye rash (Fig. 10.5–6) is found at the site of the tick bite, followed shortly thereafter by flulike symptoms. Impaired cognitive functioning and mood changes are associated with the illness and may be the presenting complaint. These include memory lapses, difficulty concentrating, irritability, and depression.

There is no clear-cut diagnostic test available. About 50 percent of patients become seropositive to *B. burgdorferi.* Prophylaxis vaccine is not always effective and is controversial. Treatment consists of a 14- to 21-day course of doxycycline (Vibramycin), which results in a 90 percent cure rate. Specific psychotropic drugs can be targeted to treat the psychiatric sign or symptom (e.g., diazepam [Valium] for anxiety). Left untreated, about 60 percent of persons develop a

Table 11–1
AIDS Safe-Sex Guidelines

Remember: Any activity that allows for the exchange of body fluids of one person through the mouth, anus, vagina, bloodstream, cuts, or sores of another person is considered unsafe at this time.

Safe-sex practices
- Massage, hugging, body-to-body rubbing
- Dry social kissing
- Masturbation
- Acting out sexual fantasies (that do not include any unsafe-sex practices)
- Using vibrators or other instruments (provided they are not shared)

Low-risk sex practices

These activities are not considered completely safe:
- French (wet) kissing (without mouth sores)
- Mutual masturbation
- Vaginal and anal intercourse while using a condom
- Oral sex, male (fellatio), while using a condom
- Oral sex, female (cunnilingus), while using a barrier
- External contact with semen or urine, provided there are no breaks in the skin

Unsafe-sex practices
- Vaginal or anal intercourse without a condom
- Semen, urine, or feces in the mouth or the vagina
- Unprotected oral sex (fellatio or cunnilingus)
- Blood contact of any kind
- Sharing sex instruments or needles

Reprinted with permission from Moffatt B, Spiegel J, Parrish S, Helquist M. *AIDS: A Self-Care Manual.* Santa Monica, CA: IBS Press; 1987:125.

Table 11–2
Centers for Disease Control and Prevention (CDC) Guidelines for the Prevention of HIV Transmission from Infected to Uninfected Persons

Infected persons should be counseled to prevent the further transmission of HIV by:

1. Informing prospective sex partners of their infection with HIV, so they can take appropriate precautions. Abstention from sexual activity with another person is one option that would eliminate any risk of sexually transmitted HIV infection.
2. Protecting a partner during any sexual activity by taking appropriate precautions to prevent that person's coming into contact with the infected person's blood, semen, urine, feces, saliva cervical secretions, or vaginal secretions. Although the efficacy of using condoms to prevent infections with HIV is still under study, the consistent use of condoms should reduce the transmission of HIV by preventing exposure to semen and infected lymphocytes.
3. Informing previous sex partners and any persons with whom needles were shared of their potential exposure to HIV and encouraging them to seek counseling and testing.
4. For IV drug abusers, enrolling or continuing in programs to eliminate the abuse of IV substances. Needles, other apparatus and drugs must never be shared.
5. Never sharing toothbrushes, razors, or other items that could become contaminated with blood.
6. Refraining from donating blood, plasma, body organs, other tissue, or semen.
7. Avoiding pregnancy until more is known about the risks of transmitting HIV from the mother to the fetus or newborn.
8. Cleaning and disinfecting surfaces on which blood or other body fluids have spilled, in accordance with previous recommendations.
9. Informing physicians, dentists, and other appropriate health professionals of antibody status when seeking medical care, so that the patient can be appropriately evaluated.

Reprinted from *MMWR Morb Mortal Wkly Rep.* 1986;35:152.

out proper sterilization techniques. Transmission of HIV through blood transfusions, organ transplantation, and artificial insemination is no longer a problem now that donors are tested for HIV infection. Tragically, many hemophilia patients received transfusions of HIV-infected blood products before HIV was identified as the causative agent. The risk of infection of health care workers after a needlestick is rare, about 1 in 300 incidents.

Children can be infected in utero or through breast-feeding when their mothers are infected with HIV. Zidovudine (Retrovir) and protease inhibitors taken by the HIV-infected pregnant woman prevent perinatal transmission in over 95 percent of cases. Health workers are theoretically at risk because of potential contact with bodily fluids from HIV-infected patients. In practice, however, the incidence of such transmission is very low, and almost all reported cases have been traced to accidental needle punctures with contaminated hypodermic needles. No evidence has been found that HIV can be contracted through casual contact, such as by sharing a living space or a classroom with a person who is infected, although direct and indirect contact with an infected person's bodily fluids, such as blood and semen, should be avoided (Table 11–2).

After infection with HIV, AIDS is estimated to develop in 8 to 11 years, although this time is gradually increasing because of early treatment. Once a person is infected with HIV, the virus primarily targets T4 (helper) lymphocytes, also called CD4+ lymphocytes, to which the virus binds because a glycoprotein (gp-120) on the viral surface has a high affinity for the CD4 receptor on T4 lymphocytes. After binding, the virus can inject its RNA into the infected lymphocyte, where the RNA is transcribed into deoxyribonucleic acid (DNA) by the action of reverse transcriptase. The resultant DNA can then be incorporated into the host cell's genome and translated and eventually transcribed, once the lymphocyte is stimulated to divide. After viral proteins have been produced by lymphocytes, the various components of the virus assemble, and new mature viruses bud off from the host cell. Although the process of budding may cause lysis of the lymphocyte, other HIV pathophysiological mechanisms can gradually disable a patient's entire complement of T4 lymphocytes.

Diagnosis

Serum Testing. Two assay techniques are now widely available to detect the presence of anti-HIV antibodies in human serum. Both health care workers and their patients must understand that the presence of HIV antibodies indicates infection, not immunity to infection. Those with a positive finding on an HIV test have been exposed to the virus, have the virus within their

11

Neuropsychiatric Aspects of HIV Infection and AIDS

Acquired immune deficiency syndrome (AIDS) is a lethal neuromedical disorder associated with infection by viruses of the *Retroviridae* family known as human immunodeficiency viruses (HIV). Although the central feature of HIV infection involves gradual collapse of the body's ability to mount an appropriate cell-mediated immune response with attendant medical complications, neuropsychiatric phenomena can also be prominent.

The first case of AIDS was reported in 1981. Analysis of specimens retained from persons who died before 1981, however, has shown that HIV infections were present as early as 1959. This suggests that in the 1960s and 1970s, HIV-related disorders and AIDS were increasingly common but unrecognized, particularly in Africa and North America. According to the Centers for Disease Control and Prevention (CDC), in 2001 an estimated 500,000 to 600,000 Americans were infected with HIV infection and another 320,000 persons have full-blown AIDS. New infections, which peaked at over 150,000 annually in the mid-1980s were reduced to an estimated 40,000 a year in the early 1990s. The World Health Organization (WHO) estimates that, worldwide, 2.5 million adults and 1 million children have AIDS and about 30 million persons are infected with HIV.

AIDS and HIV-related disorders have profoundly altered health care throughout the world. Mental health clinicians have played an important part in efforts to cope with these disorders in three areas. First, workers have reported pathological involvement of the brain in 75 to 90 percent of autopsies performed on those who had had AIDS. At least 50 percent of patients have neuropsychiatric complications, such as HIV encephalopathy; in about 10 percent of patients such complications are the first sign of the disorder. Second, because classic psychiatric syndromes such as anxiety and depressive disorders and psychotic disorders are commonly associated with HIV-related disorders, mental health clinicians must assess and treat these syndromes both pharmacologically and psychotherapeutically. Third, everyone in the mental health field is involved in helping society deal with this modern plague. Mental health organizations and professionals have worked to educate persons about the societal effects of the disorders and the necessity to change private behaviors, such as sexual and substance-using actions.

HIV AND ITS TRANSMISSION

HIV is a retrovirus related to the human T-cell leukemia viruses (HTLV) and to retroviruses that infect animals, including nonhuman primates. At least two types of HIV have been identified, HIV-1 and HIV-2. HIV-1 is the causative agent for most HIV-related diseases; HIV-2, however, seems to be causing an increasing number of infections in Africa. There may be other subtypes of HIV, which are now classified as HIV-O. HIV is present in blood, semen, cervical and vaginal secretions, and, to a lesser extent, in saliva, tears, breast milk, and the cerebrospinal fluid of those who are infected. HIV is most often transmitted through sexual intercourse or the transfer of contaminated blood from one person to another. Unprotected anal or vaginal sex are the sexual activities most likely to transmit the virus. Oral sex has also been implicated, but rarely. Health providers should be aware of the guidelines for safe sexual practices and should advise their patients to practice safe sex (Table 11–1).

The chance of becoming infected after a single exposure to an HIV-infected person is relatively low: 0.8 to 3.2 percent for unprotected receptive anal intercourse, 0.05 to 0.15 percent with unprotected vaginal sex, 0.32 percent after puncture with an HIV-contaminated needle, and 0.67 percent after using a contaminated needle to inject drugs. However, the probability of transmission could be higher, depending on the viral load of the contact person (which tends to be higher at the beginning and end of the course of the illness) or other factors, such as sexually transmitted diseases. The presence of sexually transmitted diseases, such as herpes or syphilis, or other lesions that compromise the integrity of skin or mucosa, further increases the risk of transmission. Transmission also occurs through exposure to contaminated needles, thus accounting for the high incidence of HIV infection among drug users. HIV is also transmitted by infusions of whole blood, plasma, and clotting factors but not immune serum globulin or hepatitis B vaccine.

Although male-to-male transmission has been the most common route of sexual transmission in North America, male-to-female and female-to-male transmissions are increasing, and they represent most transmission worldwide. Some studies have shown that about 50 percent of the regular sex partners of persons with HIV infection become infected themselves, a statistic suggesting that some persons do not yet understand immunity or resistance to HIV infection.

Transmission by contaminated blood most often occurs when those abusing a substance intravenously (IV) share hypodermic needles with-

Table 11–1
AIDS Safe-Sex Guidelines

Remember: Any activity that allows for the exchange of body fluids of one person through the mouth, anus, vagina, bloodstream, cuts, or sores of another person is considered unsafe at this time.

Safe-sex practices
- Massage, hugging, body-to-body rubbing
- Dry social kissing
- Masturbation
- Acting out sexual fantasies (that do not include any unsafe-sex practices)
- Using vibrators or other instruments (provided they are not shared)

Low-risk sex practices

These activities are not considered completely safe:
- French (wet) kissing (without mouth sores)
- Mutual masturbation
- Vaginal and anal intercourse while using a condom
- Oral sex, male (fellatio), while using a condom
- Oral sex, female (cunnilingus), while using a barrier
- External contact with semen or urine, provided there are no breaks in the skin

Unsafe-sex practices
- Vaginal or anal intercourse without a condom
- Semen, urine, or feces in the mouth or the vagina
- Unprotected oral sex (fellatio or cunnilingus)
- Blood contact of any kind
- Sharing sex instruments or needles

Reprinted with permission from Moffatt B, Spiegel J, Parrish S, Helquist M. *AIDS: A Self-Care Manual.* Santa Monica, CA: IBS Press; 1987:125.

Table 11–2
Centers for Disease Control and Prevention (CDC) Guidelines for the Prevention of HIV Transmission from Infected to Uninfected Persons

Infected persons should be counseled to prevent the further transmission of HIV by:

1. Informing prospective sex partners of their infection with HIV, so they can take appropriate precautions. Abstention from sexual activity with another person is one option that would eliminate any risk of sexually transmitted HIV infection.
2. Protecting a partner during any sexual activity by taking appropriate precautions to prevent that person's coming into contact with the infected person's blood, semen, urine, feces, saliva cervical secretions, or vaginal secretions. Although the efficacy of using condoms to prevent infections with HIV is still under study, the consistent use of condoms should reduce the transmission of HIV by preventing exposure to semen and infected lymphocytes.
3. Informing previous sex partners and any persons with whom needles were shared of their potential exposure to HIV and encouraging them to seek counseling and testing.
4. For IV drug abusers, enrolling or continuing in programs to eliminate the abuse of IV substances. Needles, other apparatus and drugs must never be shared.
5. Never sharing toothbrushes, razors, or other items that could become contaminated with blood.
6. Refraining from donating blood, plasma, body organs, other tissue, or semen.
7. Avoiding pregnancy until more is known about the risks of transmitting HIV from the mother to the fetus or newborn.
8. Cleaning and disinfecting surfaces on which blood or other body fluids have spilled, in accordance with previous recommendations.
9. Informing physicians, dentists, and other appropriate health professionals of antibody status when seeking medical care, so that the patient can be appropriately evaluated.

Reprinted from *MMWR Morb Mortal Wkly Rep.* 1986;35:152.

out proper sterilization techniques. Transmission of HIV through blood transfusions, organ transplantation, and artificial insemination is no longer a problem now that donors are tested for HIV infection. Tragically, many hemophilia patients received transfusions of HIV-infected blood products before HIV was identified as the causative agent. The risk of infection of health care workers after a needlestick is rare, about 1 in 300 incidents.

Children can be infected in utero or through breast-feeding when their mothers are infected with HIV. Zidovudine (Retrovir) and protease inhibitors taken by the HIV-infected pregnant woman prevent perinatal transmission in over 95 percent of cases. Health workers are theoretically at risk because of potential contact with bodily fluids from HIV-infected patients. In practice, however, the incidence of such transmission is very low, and almost all reported cases have been traced to accidental needle punctures with contaminated hypodermic needles. No evidence has been found that HIV can be contracted through casual contact, such as by sharing a living space or a classroom with a person who is infected, although direct and indirect contact with an infected person's bodily fluids, such as blood and semen, should be avoided (Table 11–2).

After infection with HIV, AIDS is estimated to develop in 8 to 11 years, although this time is gradually increasing because of early treatment. Once a person is infected with HIV, the virus primarily targets T4 (helper) lymphocytes, also called CD4+ lymphocytes, to which the virus binds because a glycoprotein (gp-120) on the viral surface has a high affinity for the CD4 receptor on T4 lymphocytes. After binding, the virus can inject its RNA into the infected lymphocyte, where the RNA is transcribed into deoxyribonucleic acid (DNA) by the action of reverse transcriptase. The resultant DNA can then be incorporated into the host cell's genome and translated and eventually transcribed, once the lymphocyte is stimulated to divide. After viral proteins have been produced by lymphocytes, the various components of the virus assemble, and new mature viruses bud off from the host cell. Although the process of budding may cause lysis of the lymphocyte, other HIV pathophysiological mechanisms can gradually disable a patient's entire complement of T4 lymphocytes.

Diagnosis

Serum Testing. Two assay techniques are now widely available to detect the presence of anti-HIV antibodies in human serum. Both health care workers and their patients must understand that the presence of HIV antibodies indicates infection, not immunity to infection. Those with a positive finding on an HIV test have been exposed to the virus, have the virus within their

Table 10.5–14 (*continued*)

B. There is a disorder in cognitive function for most of the time over a period of at least 2 weeks, as reported by the individual or a reliable informant. The disorder is exemplified by difficulties in any of the following areas: (1) memory (particularly recall) or new learning; (2) attention or concentration; (3) thinking (e.g., slowing in problem solving or abstraction); (4) language (e.g., comprehension, word finding); (5) visual-spatial functioning. C. There is an abnormality or decline in performance in quantified cognitive assessments (e.g., neuropsychological tests or mental status examination). D. None of the difficulties listed in criterion B(1)–(5) is such that a diagnosis made of dementia, organic amnesic syndrome, delirium, postencephalitic syndrome, postconcussional syndrome, or other persisting cognitive impairment due to psychoactive substance use.	**Comments** If criterion G1 for other mental disorders due to brain damage and dysfunction and to physical disease is fulfilled by the presence of central nervous system dysfunction, it is usually presumed that this is the cause of the mild cognitive disorder. If criterion G1 is fulfilled by the presence of a systemic physical disorder, it is often unjustified to assume that there is a direct causative relationship. Nevertheless, it may be useful in such instances to record the presence of the systemic physical disorder as "associated," without implying a necessary causation. An additional fifth character may be used for this: **Not associated with a systemic physical disorder** **Associated with a systemic physical disorder** The systemic physical disorder should be recorded separately by its appropriate ICD-10 code. **Other specified mental disorders due to brain damage and dysfunction and to physical disease** Examples of this category are transient or mild abnormal mood states occurring during treatment with steroids or antidepressants which do not meet the criteria for organic mood disorder. **Unspecified mental disorder due to brain damage and dysfunction and to physical disease**

References

Biller J, Kathol RH. The interface of psychiatry and neurology. *Psychiatr Clin North Am.* 1992;15(2):283.

Caine ED, Lyness JM. Delirium, dementia, and amnestic and other cognitive disorders. In: Sadock BJ, Sadock VA, eds. *Kaplan & Sadock's Comprehensive Textbook of Psychiatry.* 7th ed. Vol 1. Baltimore: Lippincott Williams & Wilkins; 2000:854.

Chiu HF. Psychiatric aspects of progressive supranuclear palsy. *Gen Hosp Psychiatry.* 1995;17:135.

Currier MB, Murray GB, Elch CC. Electroconvulsive therapy for poststroke depressed geriatric patients. *J Neuropsychiatry Clin Neurosci.* 1992;4:140.

Fedoroff JP, Startstein SE, Forrester AW, et al. Depression in patients with acute traumatic brain injury. *Am J Psychiatry.* 1992;149:918.

Fornazzari L, Farcnik K, Smith I, Heasman GA, Ichise M. Violent visual hallucinations and aggression in frontal lobe dysfunction: clinical manifestations of deep orbitofrontal foci. *J Neuropsychiatry Clin Neurosci.* 1992;4:42.

Hajet T. Higher prevalence of antibiodies to *Borrelia Burgdorferi* in psychiatric patients than in healthy subjects. *Am J Psych.* 2002;159:297.

Herman BP, Seidenberg M, Haltiner A, Wyler AR. Mood state in unilateral temporal lobe epilepsy. *Biol Psychiatry.* 1991;30:1205.

Iverson GL. Psychopathology associated with systemic lupus erythematosus: a methodological review. *Semin Arthritis Rheum.* 1993;22:242.

Jorge RE, Robinson RG, Starkstein SE, Arndt SV. Depression and anxiety following traumatic brain injury. *J Neuropsychiatry.* 1993;5:369.

Kanemoto K, Kim Y, Miyamoto T, Kawasaki J. Presurgical postictal and acute interictal psychoses are differentially associated with postoperative mood and psychotic disorders. *J Neuropsychiatry Clin Neurosci.* 2001;13:243.

Lendvai I, Sarvay SM, Steinberg MD. Creutzfeldt-Jakob disease presenting as secondary mania. *Psychosomatics.* 1999;40:524.

Masand P, Murray GB, Pickett P. Psychostimulants in post-stroke depression. *J Neuropsychiatry Clin Neurosci.* 1991;3:23.

Steere AC. Medical progress: Lyme disease. *N Engl J Med.* 2001;345:115.

Stenager EN, Stenager E, Kock-Henriksen N, et al. Suicide and multiple sclerosis: an epidemiological investigation. *J Neurol Neurosurg Psychiatry.* 1992;55:542.

Table 10.5–14
ICD-10 Diagnostic Criteria for Other Mental Disorders Due to Brain Damage and Dysfunction and Due to Physical Disease

G1. There is objective evidence (from physical and neurological examination and laboratory tests) and/or history of cerebral disease, damage, or dysfunction, or of systemic physical disorder known to cause cerebral dysfunction, including hormonal disturbances (other than alcohol- or other psychoactive substance–related) and nonpsychoactive drug effects.

G2. There is a presumed relationship between the development (or marked exacerbation) of the underlying disease, damage, or dysfunction, and the mental disorder, the symptoms of which may have immediate onset or may be delayed.

G3. There is recovery from or significant improvement in the mental disorder following removal or improvement of the underlying presumed cause.

G4. There is insufficient evidence for an alternative causation of the mental disorder, e.g., a strong family history of a clinically similar or related disorder.

If criteria G1, G2, and G4 are met, a provisional diagnosis is justified; if, in addition, there is evidence of G3, the diagnosis can be regarded as certain.

Organic hallucinosis

A. The general criteria for other mental disorders due to brain damage and dysfunction and to physical disease must be met.

B. The clinical picture is dominated by persistent or recurrent hallucinations (usually visual or auditory).

C. Hallucinations occur in clear consciousness.

Comments

Delusional elaboration of the hallucinations, as well as full or partial insight, may or may not be present: these features are not essential for the diagnosis.

Organic catatonic disorder

A. The general criteria for other mental disorders due to brain damage and dysfunction and to physical disease must be met.

B. One of the following must be present:

(1) stupor, i.e., profound diminution or absence of voluntary movements and speech, and of normal responsiveness to light, noise, and touch, but with normal muscle tone, static posture, and breathing maintained (and often limited coordinated eye movements);

(2) negativism (positive resistance to passive movement of limbs or body or rigid posturing).

C. There is catatonic excitement (gross hypermotility of a chaotic quality, with or without a tendency to assaultiveness).

D. There is rapid and unpredictable alternation of stupor and excitement.

Comments

Confidence in the diagnosis is increased if additional catatonic phenomena are present, e.g., stereotypies, waxy flexibility, and impulsive acts. Care should be taken to exclude delirium; however, it is not known whether an organic catatonic state always occurs in clear consciousness, or whether it represents an atypical manifestation of a delirium in which criteria A, B, and D are only marginally met, whereas criterion C is prominent.

Organic delusional (schizophrenialike) disorder

A. The general criteria for other mental disorders due to brain damage and dysfunction and to physical disease must be met.

B. The clinical picture is dominated by delusions (of persecution, bodily change, disease, death, jealousy), which may exhibit a varying degree of systematization.

C. Consciousness is clear and memory is intact.

Comments

Further features that complete the clinical picture but that are not invariably present include: hallucinations (in any modality); schizophrenic-type thought disorder; isolated catatonic phenomena such as stereotypies, negativism, or impulsive acts. The clinical picture may meet the symptomatic criteria for schizophrenia, persistent delusional disorder, or acute and transient psychotic disorders. However, if the state also meets the general criteria for a presumptive organic etiology laid down in the introduction to other mental disorders due to brain damage and dysfunction and to physical disease, it should be classified here. Marginal or nonspecific findings such as enlarged cerebral ventricles or "soft" neurological signs do not qualify as evidence for criterion G1 of other mental disorders due to brain damage and dysfunction and to physical disease.

Organic mood (affective) disorder

A. The general criteria for other medical disorders due to brain damage and dysfunction and to physical disease must be met.

B. The condition must meet the criteria for one of the affective disorders.

The diagnosis of the affective disorder may be specified by using a fifth character:

Organic manic disorder

Organic bipolar disorder

Organic depressive disorder

Organic mixed affective disorder

Organic anxiety disorder

A. The general criteria for other medical disorders due to brain damage and dysfunction and to physical disease must be met.

B. The condition must meet the criteria for either panic disorder or generalized anxiety disorder.

Organic dissociative disorder

A. The general criteria for other mental disorders due to brain damage and dysfunction and to physical disease must be met.

B. The condition must meet the criteria for one of the dissociative (conversion) disorders categories.

Organic emotionally labile (asthenic) disorder

A. The general criteria for other mental disorders due to brain damage and dysfunction and to physical disease must be met.

B. The clinical picture is dominated by emotional lability (uncontrolled, unstable, and fluctuating expression of emotions).

C. There is a variety of unpleasant physical sensations such as dizziness or pains and aches.

Comments

Fatigability and listlessness (asthenia) are often present but are not essential for the diagnosis.

Mild cognitive disorder

Note: The status of this construct is being examined. Specific research criteria must be viewed as tentative. One of the principal reasons for its inclusion is to obtain further evidence, allowing its differentiation from disorders such as dementia, organic amnesic syndrome, delirium, and several disorders in personality and behavioral disorders due to brain disease, damage, and dysfunction.

A. The general criteria for other mental disorders due to brain damage and dysfunction and to physical disease must be met.

(*continued*)

Table 10.5–13
ICD-10 Diagnostic Criteria for Personality and Behavioral Disorders Due to Brain Disease, Damage, and Dysfunction

G1. There must be objective evidence (from physical and neurological examination and laboratory tests) and/or history of cerebral disease, damage, or dysfunction.

G2. There is no clouding of consciousness or significant memory deficit.

G3. There is insufficient evidence for an alternative causation of the personality or behavior disorder that would justify its placement in disorders of adult personality and behavior category.

Organic personality disorder

A. The general criteria for personality and behavioral disorders due to brain disease, damage, and dysfunction must be met.

B. At least three of the following features must be present over a period of 6 months or more:

(1) consistently reduced ability to persevere with goal-directed activities, especially those involving relatively long periods and postponed gratification;

(2) one or more of the following emotional changes:

(a) emotional lability (uncontrolled, unstable, and fluctuating expression of emotions);

(b) euphoria and shallow, inappropriate jocularity, unwarranted by the circumstances;

(c) irritability and/or outbursts of anger and aggression;

(d) apathy;

(3) disinhibited expression of needs or impulses without consideration of consequences or of social conventions (the individual may engage in dissocial acts such as stealing, inappropriate sexual advances, or voracious eating, or exhibit extreme disregard for personal hygiene);

(4) cognitive disturbances, typically in the form of:

(a) excessive suspiciousness and paranoid ideas;

(b) excessive preoccupation with a single theme such as religion, or rigid categorization of other people's behavior in terms of "right" and "wrong";

(5) marked alteration of the rate and flow of language production, with features such as circumstantiality, overinclusiveness, viscosity, and hypergraphia;

(6) altered sexual behavior (hyposexuality or change in sexual preference).

Specification of features for possible subtypes

Option 1. A marked predominance of the symptoms in criteria (1) and (2)(d) is thought to define a pseudoretarded or apathetic type; a predominance of (1), (2)(c), and (3) is considered a pseudopsychopathic type; and a combination of (4), (5), and (6) is regarded as characteristic of the limbic epilepsy personality syndrome. None of these entities has yet been sufficiently validated to warrant a separate description.

Option 2. If desired, the following types may be specified: labile type, disinhibited type, aggressive type, apathetic type, paranoid type, mixed type, and other.

Postencephalitic syndrome

A. The general criteria for personality and behavioral disorders due to brain disease, damage, and dysfunction must be met.

B. At least one of the following residual neurological dysfunctions must be present:

(1) paralysis;

(2) deafness;

(3) aphasia;

(4) constructional apraxia;

(5) acalculia.

C. The syndrome is reversible, and its duration rarely exceeds 24 months.

Comments

Criterion C constitutes the main difference between this disorder and organic personality disorder.

Residual symptoms and behavioral change following either viral or bacterial encephalitis are nonspecific and do not provide a sufficient basis for a clinical diagnosis. They may include: general malaise, apathy, or irritability; some lowering of cognitive functioning (learning difficulties); disturbances in the sleep–wake pattern; or altered sexual behavior.

Postconcussional syndrome

Note: The nosological status of this syndrome is uncertain, and criterion G1 of the introduction to this rubric is not always ascertainable. However, for those undertaking research into this condition, the following criteria are recommended:

A. The general criteria of personality and behavioral disorders due to brain disease, damage, and dysfunction must be met.

B. There must be a history of head trauma with loss of consciousness, preceding the onset of symptoms by a period of up to 4 weeks. (Objective EEG, brain imaging, or oculonystagmographic evidence for brain damage may be lacking.)

C. At least three of the following features must be present:

(1) complaints of unpleasant sensations and pains, such as headache, dizziness (usually lacking the features of true vertigo), general malaise, and excessive fatigue, or noise intolerance;

(2) emotional changes, such as irritability, emotional lability (both easily provoked or exacerbated by emotional excitement or stress), or some degree of depression and/or anxiety;

(3) subjective complaints of difficulty in concentration and in performing mental tasks, and of memory problems (without clear objective evidence, e.g., psychological tests, of marked impairment);

(4) insomnia;

(5) reduced tolerance to alcohol;

(6) preoccupation with the above symptoms and fear of permanent brain damage, to the extent of hypochondriacal, overvalued ideas and adoption of a sick role.

Other organic personality and behavioral disorders due to brain disease, damage, and dysfunction

Brain disease, damage, or dysfunction may produce a variety of cognitive, emotional, personality, and behavioral disorders, some of which may not be classifiable under organic personality disorder, postencephalitic syndrome, postconcussional syndrome. However, since the nosological status of the tentative syndromes in this area is uncertain, they should be coded as "other." A fifth character may be added, if necessary, to identify presumptive individual entities.

Unspecified organic personality and behavioral disorder due to brain disease, damage, and dysfunction

insomnia, depression, and delirium; the medical symptoms include dermatitis, peripheral neuropathies, and diarrhea. The course of pellagra has traditionally been described as "five Ds": dermatitis, diarrhea, delirium, dementia, and death. The response to treatment with nicotinic acid is rapid, but dementia from prolonged illness may improve only slowly and incompletely.

Thiamine Deficiency. Thiamine (vitamin B_1) deficiency leads to beriberi, characterized chiefly by cardiovascular and neurological changes, and to Wernicke-Korsakoff syndrome, which is most often associated with chronic alcohol abuse. Beriberi occurs primarily in Asia and in areas of famine and poverty. The psychiatric symptoms include apathy, depression, irritability, nervousness, and poor concentration; severe memory disorders can develop with prolonged deficiencies.

Cobalamin Deficiency. Deficiencies in cobalamin (vitamin B_{12}) arise because of the failure of the gastric mucosal cells to secrete a specific substance, intrinsic factor, required for the normal absorption of vitamin B_{12} in the ileum. The deficiency state is characterized by the development of a chronic macrocytic megaloblastic anemia (pernicious anemia) and by neurological manifestations resulting from degenerative changes in the peripheral nerves, the spinal cord, and the brain. Neurological changes are seen in approximately 80 percent of all patients. These changes are commonly associated with megaloblastic anemia, but they occasionally precede the onset of hematological abnormalities.

Mental changes such as apathy, depression, irritability, and moodiness are common. In a few patients, encephalopathy and its associated delirium, delusions, hallucinations, dementia, and, sometimes, paranoid features are prominent and are sometimes called megaloblastic madness. The neurological manifestations of vitamin B_{12} deficiency can be rapidly and completely arrested by early and continued administration of parenteral vitamin therapy.

Toxins

Environmental toxins are becoming an increasingly serious threat to physical and mental health in contemporary society.

Mercury. Mercury poisoning can be caused by either inorganic or organic mercury. Inorganic mercury poisoning results in the "mad hatter" syndrome (previously seen in workers in the hat industry who softened felt by putting it in their mouths), with depression, irritability, and psychosis. Associated neurological symptoms are headache, tremor, and weakness. Organic mercury poisoning can be caused by contaminated fish or grain and can result in depression, irritability, and cognitive impairment. Associated symptoms are sensory neuropathies, cerebellar ataxia, dysarthria, paresthesias, and visual field defects. Mercury poisoning in pregnant women causes abnormal fetal development. No specific therapy is available, although chelation therapy with dimercaprol has been used in acute poisoning.

Lead. Lead poisoning occurs when the amount of lead ingested exceeds the body's ability to eliminate it. It takes several months for toxic symptoms to appear.

The signs and symptoms of lead poisoning depend on the level of lead in the blood. When lead reaches levels above 200 mg/mL, symptoms of severe lead encephalopathy occur, with dizziness, clumsiness, ataxia, irritability, restlessness, headache, and insomnia. Later, an excited delirium occurs, with associated vomiting and visual disturbances, and progresses to convulsions, lethargy, and coma.

Treatment of lead encephalopathy should be instituted as rapidly as possible, even without laboratory confirmation, because of the high mortality. The treatment of choice to facilitate lead excretion is intravenous administration of calcium disodium edetate (calcium disodium versenate) daily for 5 days.

Manganese. Early manganese poisoning (sometimes called manganese madness) causes symptoms of headache, irritability, joint pains, and somnolence. An eventual picture appears of emotional lability, pathological laughter, nightmares, hallucinations, and compulsive and impulsive acts associated with periods of confusion and aggressiveness. Lesions involving the basal ganglia and pyramidal system result in gait impairment, rigidity, monotonous or whispering speech, tremors of the extremities and tongue, masked facies (manganese mask), micrographia, dystonia, dysarthria, and loss of equilibrium. The psychological effects tend to clear 3 or 4 months after the patient's removal from the site of exposure, but neurological symptoms tend to remain stationary or to progress. There is no specific treatment for manganese poisoning, other than removal from the source of poisoning. The disorder is found in persons working in refining ore, brick workers, and those making steel casings.

Arsenic. Chronic arsenic poisoning most commonly results from prolonged exposure to herbicides containing arsenic or from drinking water contaminated with arsenic. Arsenic is also used in the manufacture of silicon-based computer chips. Early signs of toxicity are skin pigmentation, gastrointestinal complaints, renal and hepatic dysfunction, hair loss, and a characteristic garlic odor to the breath. Encephalopathy eventually occurs, with generalized sensory and motor loss. Chelation therapy with dimercaprol has been used successfully to treat arsenic poisoning.

ICD-10

In the 10th revision of *International Statistical Classification of Disease and Related Health Problems* (ICD-10), mental disorders related to medical conditions are covered by two categories: personality and behavioral disorders due to brain disease, damage, and dysfunction (Table 10.5–13) and other mental disorders due to brain damage and dysfunction and to physical disease (Table 10.5–14).

ical symptoms include weight gain, a deep voice, thin and dry hair, loss of the lateral eyebrow, facial puffiness, cold intolerance, and impaired hearing. Approximately 10 percent of all patients have residual neuropsychiatric symptoms after hormone replacement therapy.

Parathyroid Disorders. Dysfunction of the parathyroid gland results in the abnormal regulation of calcium metabolism. Excessive secretion of parathyroid hormone causes hypercalcemia, which can result in delirium, personality changes, and apathy in 50 to 60 percent of patients and cognitive impairments in approximately 25 percent of patients. Neuromuscular excitability, which depends on proper calcium ion concentration, is reduced, and muscle weakness may appear.

Hypocalcemia can occur with hypoparathyroid disorders and can result in neuropsychiatric symptoms of delirium and personality changes. If the calcium level decreases gradually, clinicians may see the psychiatric symptoms without the characteristic tetany of hypocalcemia. Other symptoms of hypocalcemia are cataract formation, seizures, extrapyramidal symptoms, and increased intracranial pressure.

Adrenal Disorders. Adrenal disorders disturb the normal secretion of hormones from the adrenal cortex and produce significant neurological and psychological changes. Patients with chronic adrenocortical insufficiency (Addison's disease), which is most frequently the result of adrenocortical atrophy or granulomatous invasion caused by tuberculous or fungal infection, exhibit mild mental symptoms, such as apathy, easy fatigability, irritability, and depression. Occasionally, confusion or psychotic reactions develop. Cortisone or one of its synthetic derivatives is effective in correcting such abnormalities.

Excessive quantities of cortisol produced endogenously by an adrenocortical tumor or hyperplasia (Cushing's syndrome) lead to a secondary mood disorder, a syndrome of agitated depression, and often suicide. Decreased concentration and memory deficits may also be present. Psychotic reactions, with schizophrenialike symptoms, are seen in a small number of patients. The administration of high doses of exogenous corticosteroids typically leads to a secondary mood disorder similar to mania. Severe depression may follow the termination of steroid therapy.

Pituitary Disorders. Patients with total pituitary failure can exhibit psychiatric symptoms, particularly postpartum women who have hemorrhaged into the pituitary, a condition known as Sheehan's syndrome. Patients have a combination of symptoms, especially of thyroid and adrenal disorders, and can show virtually any psychiatric symptom.

Metabolic Disorders

A common cause of organic brain dysfunction, metabolic encephalopathy can produce alterations in mental processes, behavior, and neurological functions. The diagnosis should be considered whenever recent and rapid changes in behavior, thinking, and consciousness have occurred. The earliest signals are likely to be impairment of memory, particularly recent memory, and impairment of orientation. Some patients become agitated, anxious, and hyperactive; others become quiet, withdrawn, and inactive. As metabolic encephalopathies progress, confusion or delirium gives way to decreased responsiveness, to stupor, and, eventually, to death.

Hepatic Encephalopathy. Severe hepatic failure can result in hepatic encephalopathy, characterized by asterixis, hyperventilation, EEG abnormalities, and alterations in consciousness. The alterations in consciousness can range from apathy to drowsiness to coma. Associated psychiatric symptoms are changes in memory, general intellectual skills, and personality.

Uremic Encephalopathy. Renal failure is associated with alterations in memory, orientation, and consciousness. Restlessness, crawling sensations on the limbs, muscle twitching, and persistent hiccups are associated symptoms. In young people with brief episodes of uremia, the neuropsychiatric symptoms tend to be reversible; in elderly people with long episodes of uremia, the neuropsychiatric symptoms can be irreversible.

Hypoglycemic Encephalopathy. Hypoglycemic encephalopathy can be caused either by excessive endogenous production of insulin or by excessive exogenous insulin administration. The premonitory symptoms, which do not occur in every patient, include nausea, sweating, tachycardia, and feelings of hunger, apprehension, and restlessness. As the disorder progresses, disorientation, confusion, and hallucinations, as well as other neurological and medical symptoms, can develop. Stupor and coma may occur, and a residual and persistent dementia can sometimes be a serious neuropsychiatric sequela of the disorder.

Diabetic Ketoacidosis. Diabetic ketoacidosis begins with feelings of weakness, easy fatigability, and listlessness and increasing polyuria and polydipsia. Headache and sometimes nausea and vomiting appear. Patients with diabetes mellitus have an increased likelihood of chronic dementia with general arteriosclerosis.

Acute Intermittent Porphyria. The porphyrias are disorders of heme biosynthesis that result in excessive accumulation of porphyrins. The triad of symptoms is acute, colicky abdominal pain, motor polyneuropathy, and psychosis. Acute intermittent porphyria is an autosomal dominant disorder that affects more women than men and has its onset between ages 20 and 50. The psychiatric symptoms include anxiety, insomnia, lability of mood, depression, and psychosis. Some studies have found that between 0.2 and 0.5 percent of chronic psychiatric patients may have undiagnosed porphyrias. Barbiturates precipitate or aggravate the attacks of acute porphyria, and the use of barbiturates for any reason is absolutely contraindicated in a person with acute intermittent porphyria and in anyone who has a relative with the disease.

Nutritional Disorders

Niacin Deficiency. Dietary insufficiency of niacin (nicotinic acid) and its precursor tryptophan is associated with pellagra, a globally occurring nutritional deficiency disease seen in association with alcohol abuse, vegetarian diets, and extreme poverty and starvation. The neuropsychiatric symptoms of pellagra include apathy, irritability,

were young (under 40), and none had risk factors of CJD. At autopsy, prion disease was found. The disease was attributed to the transmission in the United Kingdom of BSE between cattle and from cattle to humans in the 1980s. BSE appears to have originated from sheep scrapie–contaminated feed given to cattle. Scrapie is a spongiform encephalopathy found in sheep and goats that has not been shown to cause human disease; however, it is transmissible to other animal species.

By the end of 2001, about 100 cases had been reported, with a mean age of onset of 29 years. Clinicians must be alert to the diagnosis in young people with behavioral and psychiatric abnormalities in association with cerebellar signs such as ataxia or myoclonus. The psychiatric presentation of vCJD is not specific. Most patients reported depression, withdrawal, anxiety, and sleep disturbance. Paranoid delusions have occurred. Neuropathological changes are similar to those in vCJD, with the addition of amyloid plaques.

Epidemiological data are still being gathered. The incubation period for vCJD and the amount of infected meat product required to cause infection are unknown. One patient was reported to have been a vegetarian for 5 years before his disease was diagnosed. vCJD can be diagnosed antemortem by examining the tonsils with Western blot immunostains to detect PrP^{Sc} in lymphoid tissue. Diagnosis relies on the development of progressive neurodegenerative features in persons who have ingested contaminated meat or brains. There is no cure, and death usually occurs within 2 to 3 years after diagnosis.

KURU. Kuru is an epidemic prion disease found in New Guinea that is caused by cannibalistic funeral rituals in which the brains of the deceased are eaten. Women are more affected by the disorder than men, presumably because they participate in the ceremony to a greater extent. Death usually occurs within 2 years after symptoms develop. Neuropsychiatric signs and symptoms consist of ataxia, chorea, strabismus, delirium, and dementia. Pathological changes are similar to those with other prion disease: neuronal loss, spongiform lesions, and astrocytic proliferation. The cerebellum is most affected. Iatrogenic transmission of kuru has occurred when cadaveric material such as dura mater and cornea was transplanted into normal recipients. Since the cessation of cannibalism in New Guinea, the incidence of the disease has decreased drastically.

GERSTMANN-STRAUSSLER-SCHEINKER DISEASE. First described in 1928, this disorder is a neurodegenerative syndrome characterized by ataxia, chorea, and cognitive decline leading to dementia. It is caused by a mutation in the PrP gene that is fully penetrant and autosomal dominant; thus the disease is inherited, and affected families have been identified over several generations. Genetic testing can confirm the presence of the abnormal genes before onset. Pathological changes characteristic of prion disease are present: spongiform lesions, neuronal loss, and astrocyte proliferation. Amyloid plaques have been found in the cerebellum. Onset of the disease occurs between 30 and 40 years of age. The disease is fatal within 5 years of onset.

FATAL FAMILIAL INSOMNIA. FFI is an inherited prion disease that primarily affects the thalamus. A syndrome of insomnia and autonomic nervous system dysfunction consisting of fever, sweating, labile blood pressure, and tachycardia occurs that is debilitating. Onset is in middle adulthood, and death usually occurs in 1 year. There is no treatment.

FUTURE DIRECTIONS. Determining how prions mutate to produce disease phenotypes and determining how prions are transmitted between different mammalian species are major areas of research. Public health measures to prevent transmission of animal disease to humans is ongoing and must be relentless, especially since these disorders are invariably fatal within a few years of onset. Developing genetic interventions that prevent or repair damage to the normal prion gene offers the best hope of cure. Psychiatrists are faced with having to manage patients who actually have the disease and those with hypochondriacal fears of having contracted the disease. In some patients such fears can reach delusional proportions. Treatment is symptomatic and involves anxiolytics, antidepressants, and psychostimulants, depending on symptoms. Supportive psychotherapy may be of use in early stages to help patients and family cope with the illness.

Preventing unintentional human-to-human or animal-to-human transmission of prions remains the best way to limit the scope of these diseases. However, sporadic cases of CJD will still appear because of the rare spontaneous mutation of the normal prion protein into the abnormal form. At present, there is little to offer patients with prion disease other than supportive treatment and emotional support.

Immune Disorders

The major immune disorder in contemporary society is AIDS, but other immune disorders can also present diagnostic and treatment challenges to mental health clinicians.

Systemic Lupus Erythematosus. Systemic lupus erythematosus (SLE) is an autoimmune disease that involves inflammation of multiple organ systems. The officially accepted diagnosis of SLE requires a patient to have 4 of 11 criteria that have been defined by the American Rheumatism Association. Between 5 and 50 percent of SLE patients have mental symptoms at the initial presentation, and approximately 50 percent of patients eventually show neuropsychiatric manifestations. The major symptoms are depression, insomnia, emotional lability, nervousness, and confusion. Treatment with steroids commonly induces further psychiatric complications, including mania and psychosis.

Endocrine Disorders

Thyroid Disorders. Hyperthyroidism is characterized by confusion, anxiety, and an agitated, depressive syndrome. Patients may also complain of being easily fatigued and of feeling generally weak. Insomnia, weight loss despite increased appetite, tremulousness, palpitations, and increased perspiration are also common symptoms. Serious psychiatric symptoms include impairments in memory, orientation, and judgment; manic excitement; delusions; and hallucinations.

In 1949, Irvin Asher named hypothyroidism "myxedema madness." In its most severe form, hypothyroidism is characterized by paranoia, depression, hypomania, and hallucinations. Slowed thinking and delirium can also be symptoms. The phys-

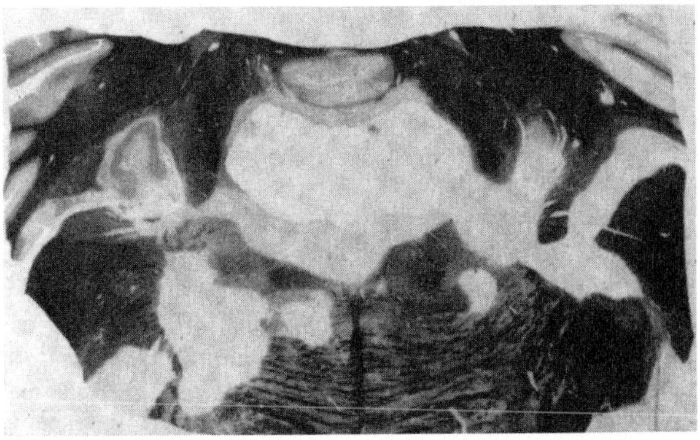

FIGURE 10.5–5
Multiple sclerosis. Irregular, seemingly punched out zones of demyelination are evident in this section through the level of the fourth ventricle. Myelin stain. 2.6×. (Courtesy of Dr. H. M. Zimmerman.)

persons with MS exhibit a euphoric mood that is not hypomanic, but somewhat more cheerful than their situation warrants and not necessarily in character with their disposition before the onset of MS. Only 10 percent of MS patients have a sustained and elevated mood, although it is still not truly hypomanic. Depression, however, is common; it affects 25 to 50 percent of patients with MS and results in a higher rate of suicide than is seen in the general population. Risk factors for suicide in MS patients are male sex, onset of MS before age 30, and a relatively recent diagnosis of the disorder. Personality changes are also common in MS patients; they affect 20 to 40 percent of patients and are often characterized by increased irritability or apathy.

Amyotrophic Lateral Sclerosis. ALS is a progressive, noninherited disease of asymmetrical muscle atrophy. It begins in adult life and progresses over months or years to involve all the striated muscles except the cardiac and ocular muscles. In addition to muscle atrophy, patients have signs of pyramidal tract involvement. The illness is rare and occurs in approximately 1.6 persons per 100,000 annually. A few patients have concomitant dementia. The disease progresses rapidly, and death generally occurs within 4 years of onset.

Infectious Diseases

Herpes Simplex Encephalitis. Herpes simplex encephalitis is the most common type of focal encephalitis and most commonly affects the frontal and temporal lobes. The symptoms often include anosmia, olfactory and gustatory hallucinations, and personality changes and can also involve bizarre or psychotic behaviors. Complex partial epilepsy may also develop in patients with herpes simplex encephalitis. Although the mortality rate for the infection has decreased, many patients exhibit personality changes, symptoms of memory loss, and psychotic symptoms.

Rabies Encephalitis. The incubation period for rabies ranges from 10 days to 1 year, after which symptoms of restlessness, overactivity, and agitation can develop. Hydrophobia, present in up to 50 percent of patients, is characterized by an intense fear of drinking water. The fear develops from the severe laryngeal and diaphragmatic spasms that the patients experience when they drink water. Once rabies encephalitis develops, the disease is fatal within days or weeks.

Neurosyphilis. Neurosyphilis (also known as general paresis) appears 10 to 15 years after the primary *Treponema* infection. Since the advent of penicillin, neurosyphilis has become a rare disorder, although AIDS is associated with reintroducing neurosyphilis into medical practice in some urban settings. Neurosyphilis generally affects the frontal lobes and results in personality changes, development of poor judgment, irritability, and decreased care for self. Delusions of grandeur develop in 10 to 20 percent of affected patients. The disease progresses with the development of dementia and tremor, until patients are paretic. The neurological symptoms include Argyll-Robertson pupils, which are small, irregular, and unequal and have light–near reflex dissociation, tremor, dysarthria, and hyperreflexia. Cerebrospinal fluid (CSF) examination shows lymphocytosis, increased protein, and a positive result on a Venereal Disease Research Laboratory (VDRL) test.

Chronic Meningitis. Chronic meningitis is now seen more often than in the recent past because of the immunocompromised condition of people with AIDS. The usual causative agents are *Mycobacterium tuberculosis, Cryptococcus,* and *Coccidioides*. The usual symptoms are headache, memory impairment, confusion, and fever.

Subacute Sclerosing Panencephalitis. Subacute sclerosing panencephalitis is a disease of childhood and early adolescence, with a 3-to-1 male-to-female ratio. The onset usually follows either an infection with measles or a vaccination for measles. The initial symptoms may be behavioral change, temper tantrums, sleepiness, and hallucinations, but the classic symptoms of myoclonus, ataxia, seizures, and intellectual deterioration eventually develop. The disease progresses relentlessly to coma and death in 1 to 2 years.

Lyme Disease. Lyme disease is caused by infection with the spirochete *Borrelia burgdorferi* transmitted through the bite of the deer tick (*Ixodes scapularis*), which feed on infected deer and mice. About 16,000 cases are reported annually in the United States.

A characteristic bull's-eye rash (Fig. 10.5–6) is found at the site of the tick bite, followed shortly thereafter by flulike symptoms. Impaired cognitive functioning and mood changes are associated with the illness and may be the presenting complaint. These include memory lapses, difficulty concentrating, irritability, and depression.

There is no clear-cut diagnostic test available. About 50 percent of patients become seropositive to *B. burgdorferi.* Prophylaxis vaccine is not always effective and is controversial. Treatment consists of a 14- to 21-day course of doxycycline (Vibramycin), which results in a 90 percent cure rate. Specific psychotropic drugs can be targeted to treat the psychiatric sign or symptom (e.g., diazepam [Valium] for anxiety). Left untreated, about 60 percent of persons develop a

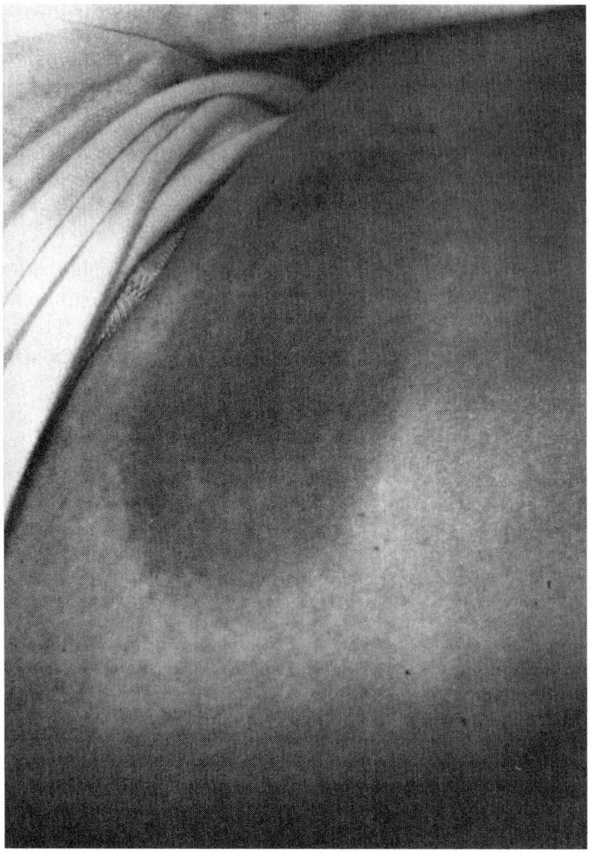

FIGURE 10.5–6
Erythema migrans ("bull's-eye" rash) on the thigh. (From Barbour R. Lyme disease. In: Hoeprich PD, Jordan MC, Ronald AR, eds. *Infectious Diseases: A Treatise of Infectious Processes.* Philadelphia: JB Lippincott; 1994:1329.)

chronic condition. Such patients may be given an erroneous diagnosis of a primary depression rather than one secondary to the medical condition. Support groups for patients with chronic Lyme disease are important. Group members provide each other with emotional support that helps improve their quality of life.

Prion Disease. Prion disease is a group of related disorders caused by a transmissible infectious protein known as a prion. Included in this group are Creutzfeldt-Jakob disease (CJD), Gerstmann-Straussler syndrome (GSS), fatal familial insomnia (FFI), and kuru. A variant of CJD (vCJD), also called "mad cow disease," appeared in 1995 in the United Kingdom and is attributed to the transmission of bovine spongiform encephalopathy (BSE) from cattle to humans. Collectively, these disorders are also known as subacute spongiform encephalopathy because of shared neuropathological changes that consist of (1) spongiform vacuolization, (2) neuronal loss, and (3) astrocyte proliferation in the cerebral cortex. Amyloid plaques may or may not be present.

ETIOLOGY. Prions are transmissible agents but differ from viruses in that they lack nucleic acid. Prions are mutated proteins generated from the human prion protein gene (PrP), which is located on the short arm of chromosome 20. There is no direct link between prion disease and Alzheimer's disease, which has been traced to chromosome 21.

PrP mutates into a disease-related isoform PrP–Super–C (PrP^{Sc}) that can replicate and is infectious. The neuropathological changes that occur in prion disease are presumed to be caused by direct neurotoxic effects of PrP^{Sc}.

The specific prion disease that develops depends on the mutation of PrP that occurs. Mutations at PrP 178N/129V cause CJD; mutations at 178N/129M cause FFI; and mutations at 102L/129M cause GSS and kuru. Other mutations of PrP have been described, and research continues in this important area of genomic identification. Some mutations are both fully penetrant and autosomal dominant and account for inherited forms of prion disease. For example, both GSS and FFI are inherited disorders, and about 10 percent of cases of CJD are also inherited. Prenatal testing for the abnormal PrP gene is available; whether or not such testing should be routinely done is open to question at this time.

CREUTZFELDT-JAKOB DISEASE. First described in 1920, this is an invariably fatal, rapidly progressive disorder that occurs mainly in middle-aged or older adults. It manifests initially with fatigue, flulike symptoms, and cognitive impairment. As the disease progresses, focal neurological findings such as aphasia and apraxia occur. Psychiatric manifestations are protean and include emotional lability, anxiety, euphoria, depression, delusions, hallucinations, or marked personality changes. The disease progresses over months, leading to dementia, akinetic mutism, coma, and death.

The rates of Creutzfeldt-Jakob disease range from 1 to 2 cases per million persons a year, worldwide. The infectious agent self-replicates and can be transmitted to humans by inoculation with infected tissue and sometimes by ingestion of contaminated food. Iatrogenic transmission has been reported via transplantation of contaminated cornea or dura mater or to children via contaminated supplies of human growth hormone derived from infected persons. Neurosurgical transmission has also been reported. Household contacts are not at greater risk for developing the disease than the general population, unless there is direct inoculation.

Diagnosis requires pathological examination of the cortex, which reveals the classic triad of spongiform vacuolation, loss of neurons, and astrocyte cell proliferation. The cortex and basal ganglia are most affected. An immunoassay test for Creutzfeldt-Jakob disease in the CSF shows promise in supporting the diagnosis; however, this needs to be tested more extensively. Although not specific for Creutzfeldt-Jakob disease, EEG abnormalities are present in nearly all patients, consisting of a slow and irregular background rhythm with periodic complex discharges. Computed tomography (CT) and MRI studies may reveal cortical atrophy later in the course of disease. Single photon emission computed tomography (SPECT) and positron emission tomography (PET) reveal heterogeneously decreased uptake throughout the cortex.

There is no known treatment for Creutzfeldt-Jakob disease. Death usually occurs within 6 months after diagnosis.

VARIANT CJD. In 1995 a variant of CJD (vCJP) appeared in the United Kingdom. The patients affected all died; they

bodies, have the potential to transmit the virus to another person, and will almost certainly eventually develop AIDS. Those with a negative HIV test result have either not been exposed to the HIV virus and are not infected or were exposed to the HIV virus but have not yet developed antibodies, a possibility if the exposure occurred less than a year before the testing.

The two assay techniques used are the enzyme-linked immunosorbent assay (ELISA) and the Western blot assay. The ELISA is used as an initial screening test because it is less expensive than the Western blot assay and better suited for large-scale screening. The ELISA is sensitive and reasonably specific; it is unlikely to report a false-negative result, but it may indicate a false-positive one. For this reason, positive results from an ELISA are confirmed by using the more expensive and cumbersome Western blot assay, which is sensitive and specific.

Seroconversion is the change, after infection with HIV, from a negative HIV antibody test result to a positive one. Seroconversion most commonly occurs 6 to 12 weeks after infection, although in rare cases seroconversion can take 6 to 12 months.

Counseling. The major issues in counseling persons about HIV serum testing are who should be tested; why a particular person should or should not be tested; what the test results signify; and what the implications are. Although specific groups of persons are at high risk for contracting HIV and should be tested (Table 11–3), any person who wants to be tested should probably be tested. The reasons for requesting a test should be ascertained to detect unspoken concerns and motivations that may merit psychotherapeutic intervention. Counseling both before and after testing should be done in person, not over the telephone, and should cover both the significance of the test results and their implications for behavioral changes. It is good practice to repeat the meaning of the test results and their implications several times at both pretest and posttest interviews; many persons are so anxious at these sessions that they may miss something told to them only once.

During pretest counseling, counselors should review past practices that may have put the testee at risk for HIV infection and should discuss safe sexual practices (Table 11–4). During posttest counseling (Table 11–5), counselors should explain that a negative test finding implies that safe sexual behavior and the avoidance of shared hypodermic needles are recommended for the person to remain free of HIV infection. A positive test result indicates that the person is infected with HIV and can spread the disease. Those with positive results must receive counseling about safe practices and potential treatment options. They may need additional psychotherapeutic interventions if anxiety or depressive disorders develop after they discover that they are infected. Common issues and concerns are fear of disclosure, relationships with friends and family, employment and financial security, medical condition, and such psychological issues as self-esteem and self-blame. A person may react to a positive HIV test finding with a syndrome similar to posttraumatic stress disorder. Concern about minor physical symptoms, insomnia, and dependence on health care workers commonly arise. Adjustment disorder with anxiety or depressed mood may develop in as many as 25 percent of those informed of a positive HIV test result. Clinical interactions with patients should emphasize the meaning of a positive test result and should encourage reestablishment of emotional and functional stability.

Couples who are considering taking the HIV antibody test must decide who will be tested and whether to go alone or together. The therapist should ask why they are considering taking the test; partners often for the first time discuss issues of commitment, honesty, and trust, such as sexual contacts outside the relationship. They need to be prepared for the possibility that one or both are infected and must discuss what effect this will have on their relationship.

Table 11–3
Possible Indications for HIV Testing

1. Patients who belong to a high-risk group: (1) men who have had sex with another man since 1977; (2) intravenous drug abusers since 1977; (3) hemophiliacs and other patients who have received since 1977 blood or blood product transfusions not screened for HIV; (4) sexual partners of people from any of those groups; (5) sexual partners of people with known HIV exposure—people with cuts, wounds, sores, or needlesticks whose lesions have had direct contact with HIV-infected blood.
2. Patients who request testing. Not all patients admit to the presence of risk factors (e.g., because of shame, fear).
3. Patients with symptoms or AIDS.
4. Women belonging to a high-risk group who are planning pregnancy or who are pregnant.
5. Blood, semen, or organ donors.

Adapted with permission from Rosse RB, Giese AA, Deutsch S, Morihisa JM. *Laboratory and Diagnostic Testing in Psychiatry.* Washington, DC: American Psychiatric Press; 1989:54.

Table 11–4
Pretest HIV Counseling

1. Discuss meaning of a positive result and clarify distortions (e.g., the test detects exposure to the AIDS virus; it is not a test for AIDS).
2. Discuss the meaning of a negative result (e.g., seroconversion requires time, recent high-risk behavior may require follow-up testing).
3. Be available to discuss the patient's fears and concerns (unrealistic fears may require appropriate psychological intervention).
4. Discuss why the test is necessary. (Not all patients will admit to high-risk behaviors.)
5. Explore the patient's potential reactions to a positive result (e.g. "I'll kill myself if I'm positive"). Take appropriate necessary steps to intervene in a potentially catastrophic reaction.
6. Explore past reactions to severe stresses.
7. Discuss the confidentiality issues relevant to the testing situation (e.g., is it an anonymous or nonanonymous setting?). Inform the patient of other possible testing options where the counseling and testing can be done completely anonymously (e.g., where the result is not made a permanent part of a hospital chart). Discuss who has access to the test results.
8. Discuss with the patient how being seropositive can potentially affect social status (e.g., health and life insurance coverage, employment, housing).
9. Explore high-risk behaviors and recommend risk-reducing interventions.
10. Document discussions in chart.
11. Allow the patient time to ask questions.

Reprinted with permission from Rosse RB, Giese AA, Deutsch SI, Morihisa JM. *Laboratory and Diagnostic Testing in Psychiatry.* Washington, DC: American Psychiatric Press; 1989:55.

Table 11–5
Posttest HIV Counseling

1. Interpretation of test result:
   Clarify distortion (e.g., "a negative test still means you could contract the virus at a future time; it does not mean you are immune from AIDS").
   Ask questions about the patient's understanding and emotional reaction to the test result.
2. Recommendations for prevention of transmission (careful discussion of high-risk behaviors and guidelines for prevention of transmission).
3. Recommendations on the follow-up of sexual partners and needle contacts.
4. If test result is positive, recommendations against donating blood, sperm, or organs and against sharing razors, toothbrushes, and anything else that may have blood on it.
5. Referral for appropriate psychological support: HIV-positive patients often need access to a mental health team (assess need for inpatient versus outpatient care; consider individual or group supportive therapy). Common themes include the shock of the diagnosis, the fear of death, and social consequences, grief over potential losses, and dashed hopes for good news.
   Also look for depression, hopelessness, anger, frustration, guilt, and obsessional themes. Activate supports available to patient (e.g., family, friends, community services).

Reprinted with permission from Rosse RB, Giese AA, Deutsch SI, Morihisa JM. *Laboratory and Diagnostic Testing in Psychiatry.* Washington, DC: American Psychiatric Press; 1989:58.

Confidentiality. Confidentiality is a key issue in serum testing. No one should be given an HIV test without previous knowledge and consent, although various jurisdictions and organizations, such as the military, now require HIV testing for all inhabitants or members. The results of an HIV test can be shared with other members of a medical team, although the information should be provided to no one else except in the special circumstances discussed below. The patient should be advised against disclosing the results of HIV testing too readily to employers, friends, and family members; the information could result in discrimination in employment, housing, and insurance.

The major exception to restriction of disclosure is the need to notify potential and past sexual or IV substance partners. Most HIV-positive patients act responsibly. If, however, a treating physician knows that an HIV-infected patient is putting another person at risk of becoming infected, the physician may try either to hospitalize the infected person involuntarily (to prevent danger to others) or to notify the potential victim. Clinicians should be aware of the laws about such issues, which vary among the states. These guidelines also apply to inpatient psychiatric wards when an HIV-infected patient is believed to be sexually active with other patients.

CLINICAL FEATURES

Nonneurological Factors

About 30 percent of persons infected with HIV experience a flulike syndrome 3 to 6 weeks after becoming infected; most never notice any symptoms immediately or shortly after their infection. When symptoms do appear, the flulike syndrome includes fever, myalgia, headaches, fatigue, gastrointestinal symptoms, and sometimes a rash. The syndrome may be accompanied by splenomegaly and lymphadenopathy. Rarely, acute aseptic meningitis develops shortly after infection, as does encephalopathy or Guillain-Barré syndrome.

In the United States, the median duration of the asymptomatic stages is 10 years, although nonspecific symptoms—lymphadenopathy, chronic diarrhea, weight loss, malaise, fatigue, fevers, night sweats—may variably appear. During the asymptomatic period, however, the T4 cell count almost always declines from normal values (>1,000/mm^3) to grossly abnormal values (<200/mm^3).

The most common infection in HIV-infected persons who have AIDS is *Pneumocystis carinii* pneumonia, which is characterized by a chronic, nonproductive cough and dyspnea, sometimes severe enough to result in hypoxemia and its resultant cognitive effects. Diagnosis is made with fiberoptic bronchoscopy and alveolar lavage. The pneumonia is usually treatable with trimethoprim and sulfamethoxazole (Bactrim, Septra) or pentamidine isethionate (Pentam), which can also be used for prophylaxis against the pneumonia. The other disease that was initially associated with the development of AIDS is Kaposi's sarcoma, a previously rare, blue-purple–tinted skin lesion. For unknown reasons, Kaposi's sarcoma is less commonly associated with cases of recently diagnosed AIDS.

Although *Pneumocystis carinii* pneumonia and Kaposi's sarcoma are the two classic AIDS-related infectious and neoplastic disorders, the severely disabled cellular immune system of HIV-infected patients permits the development of a staggering array of infections and neoplasms. The most common infections are from protozoa such as *Toxoplasma gondii,* fungi such as *Cryptococcus neoformans* and *Candida albicans,* bacteria such as *Mycobacterium avium-intracellulare,* and viruses such as cytomegalovirus and herpes simplex virus.

For psychiatrists, the importance of these nonneurological, nonpsychiatric complications lies in their biological effects on patients' brain functions (e.g., hypoxia with *Pneumocystis carinii* pneumonia) and their psychological effects on patients' moods and anxiety states. Further, because each of the conditions is usually treated by an additional drug, psychiatrists need to be aware of the adverse CNS effects of many medications.

Neurological Factors

An extensive array of disease processes can affect the brain of a patient infected with HIV (Table 11–6). The most important diseases for mental health workers to be aware of are *HIV mild neurocognitive disorder* and *HIV-associated dementia*. The latter is a cortical or subcortical type of dementia that may affect 50 percent of HIV-infected patients to some degree. Other diseases and complications of treatment must also be considered in the differential diagnosis of an HIV-infected patient with neuropsychiatric symptoms. Symptoms such as photophobia, headache, stiff neck, motor weakness, sensory loss, and changes in level of consciousness should alert a mental health worker that the patient should be examined for possible development of a CNS opportunistic infection or a CNS neoplasm. HIV infection can also result in a variety of peripheral neuropathies that should prompt mental health clinicians to reconsider the extent of CNS involvement.

Psychiatric Syndromes

HIV-Associated Dementia. The text revision of the fourth edition of the *Diagnostic and Statistical Manual of Men-*

Table 11–6
Conditions Associated with HIV Infection

Bacterial infections, multiple or recurrent[a]
Candidiasis of bronchi, trachea, or lungs
Candidiasis, esophageal
Cervical cancer, invasive[b]
Coccidioidomycosis, disseminated or extrapulmonary
Cryptococcosis, extrapulmonary
Cryptosporidiosis, chronic intestinal (>1 month's duration)
Cytomegalovirus disease (other than liver, spleen, or nodes)
Cytomegalovirus retinitis (with loss of vision)
Encephalopathy, HIV-related
Herpes simplex, chronic ulcers (>1 month's duration); or bronchitis, pulmonitis, or esophagitis
Histoplasmosis, disseminated or extrapulmonary
Isosporiasis, chronic intestinal (>1 month's duration)
Kaposi's sarcoma
Lymphoid interstitial pneumonia and/or pulmonary lymphoid hyperplasia[a]
Lymphoma, Burkitt's (or equivalent term)
Lymphoma, immunoblastic (or equivalent term)
Lymphoma, primary, of brain
Mycobacterium avium complex or *M. kansasii*, disseminated or extrapulmonary
Mycobacterium tuberculosis, any site (pulmonary[b] or extrapulmonary)
Mycobacterium, other species or unidentified species, disseminated or extrapulmonary
Pneumocystis carinii pneumonia
Pneumonia, recurrent[b]
Progressive multifocal leukoencephalopathy
Salmonella septicemia, recurrent
Toxoplasmosis of brain
Wasting syndrome due to HIV

[a]Children <13 years old.
[b]Added in the 1993 expansion of the AIDS surveillance case definition for adolescents and adults.
Adapted from 1993 revised classification system for HIV infection and expanded surveillance, case definition for AIDS among adolescents and adults. *MMWR Morb Mortal Wkly Rep*. 1992:41.

tal Disorders (DSM-IV-TR) allows the diagnosis of dementia due to HIV disease when there is "the presence of a dementia that is judged to be the direct pathophysiological consequence of human immunodeficiency virus (HIV) disease." (See Table 10.3–5 in Chapter 10.)

Although HIV-associated dementia is found in a large proportion of patients infected with HIV, other causes of dementia in these patients must be considered. These causes include CNS infections, CNS neoplasms, CNS abnormalities caused by systemic disorders and endocrinopathies, and adverse CNS responses to drugs. The development of dementia is generally a poor prognostic sign, and 50 to 75 percent of patients with dementia die within 6 months.

Mild Neurocognitive Disorder. A less severe form of brain involvement is called *HIV-associated neurocognitive disorder*, also known as *HIV encephalopathy*. It is characterized by impaired cognitive functioning and reduced mental activity that interferes with work, homemaking, or social functioning. There are no laboratory findings specific to the disorder, and it occurs independently of depression and anxiety. Progression to HIV-associated dementia usually occurs but may be prevented by early treatment.

ICD-10. In the 10th revision of the *International Statistical Classification of Diseases and Related Health Problems* (ICD-10), dementia in HIV disease is briefly covered under organic, including symptomatic, mental disorders (see Chapter 10). Here the dementia is defined as "a disorder characterized by cognitive deficits meeting the clinical diagnostic criteria for dementia, in the absence of concurrent illness or condition other than HIV infection that could explain the findings." AIDS–dementia complex and HIV encephalopathy or subacute encephalitis are also included in this dementia.

Delirium. Delirium can result from the same causes that lead to dementia in patients infected with HIV (Table 11–6). Clinicians have classified delirious states characterized by both increased and decreased activity. Delirium in HIV-infected patients is probably underdiagnosed, but it should always precipitate a medical workup of an HIV-infected patient to determine whether a new CNS-related process has begun.

Anxiety Disorders. Patients with HIV infection may have any of the anxiety disorders, but generalized anxiety disorder, posttraumatic stress disorder, and obsessive-compulsive disorder are particularly common.

Adjustment Disorder. Adjustment disorder with anxiety or depressed mood has been reported to occur in 5 to 20 percent of patients infected with HIV. The incidence of adjustment disorder in persons infected with HIV is higher than usual in some special populations, such as military recruits and prison inmates.

Depressive Disorders. A range of 4 to 40 percent of HIV-infected patients have been reported to meet the diagnostic criteria for depressive disorders. The pre-HIV infection prevalence of depressive disorders may be higher than usual in some groups who are at risk for contracting HIV. Another reason for the reported variation in prevalence rates is the variable application of the diagnostic criteria; some of the criteria for depressive disorders (poor sleep and weight loss) can also be caused by the HIV infection itself. Depression is higher in women than in men.

Mania. Mood disorder with manic features, with or without hallucinations, delusions, or a disorder of thought process can complicate any stage of HIV infection, but most commonly occurs in late-stage disease complicated by neurocognitive impairment.

Substance Abuse. Substance abuse is a problem not only for IV substance abusers who contract HIV-related diseases but also for other patients with HIV, who may have used illegal substances only occasionally in the past but may now be tempted to use them regularly to deal with depression or anxiety.

Suicide. Suicidal ideation and suicide attempts may increase in patients with HIV infection and AIDS. The risk factors for suicide among persons infected with HIV are having

friends who died from AIDS, recent notification of HIV seropositivity, relapses, difficult social issues relating to homosexuality, inadequate social and financial support, and the presence of dementia or delirium.

Psychotic Disorder. Psychotic symptoms are usually later-stage complications of HIV infection. They require immediate medical and neurological evaluation and often require management with antipsychotic medications.

Worried Well. The so-called worried well are those in high-risk groups who, although they are seronegative and disease free, are anxious about contracting the virus. Some are reassured by repeated negative serum test results, but others cannot be reassured. Their worried well status can progress to generalized anxiety, panic attacks, obsessive-compulsive disorder, and hypochondriasis.

TREATMENT

Prevention is the primary approach to HIV infection. Primary prevention involves protecting persons from getting the disease; secondary prevention involves modification of the disease's course. All persons with any risk of HIV infection should be informed about safe-sex practices and about the necessity to avoid sharing contaminated hypodermic needles. Preventive strategies, however, are complicated by the complex societal values surrounding sexual acts, sexual orientation, birth control, and substance abuse. Many public health officials have advocated condom distribution in schools and the distribution of clean needles to drug addicts. These issues remain controversial, although condom use has been shown to be a fairly (although not completely) safe and effective preventive strategy against HIV infection. Those who are conservative and religious argue that the educational message should be sexual abstinence. Many university laboratories and pharmaceutical companies are attempting to develop a vaccine to protect persons from infection by HIV. The development of such a vaccine, however, is probably at least a decade away.

The assessment of patients infected with HIV should include a complete sexual and substance-abuse history, a psychiatric history, and an evaluation of the support systems available to them. Clinicians must understand a patient's history with regard to sexual orientation and substance abuse, and the patient must feel that the therapist is not judging past or present behaviors. A therapist can often encourage a sense of trust and empathy in the patient by asking specific, well-informed, straightforward questions about the homosexual or substance-using culture. The therapist must also determine the patient's knowledge about HIV and AIDS.

The homosexual community has provided a significant support system for those infected with HIV, particularly for persons who are gay and bisexual. Public education campaigns within this community have resulted in significant (more than 50 percent) reductions in the highest-risk sexual practices, although some gay men still practice high-risk sex. Homosexual men are likely to practice safe sex if they know the safe-sex guidelines, have access to a support group, are in a steady relationship, and have a close relationship with a person with AIDS. Partly because of the many biases against them, IV substance users with AIDS have received little support, and there has been little progress in educating these persons who are a major reservoir for spread of the virus to women, heterosexual men, and children.

PHARMACOTHERAPY

A growing list of agents that act at different points in viral replication has raised for the first time the hope that HIV might be permanently suppressed or actually eradicated from the body. At the time of this writing, the active agents were in two general classes: reverse transcriptase inhibitors and protease inhibitors. The reverse transcriptase inhibitors are further subdivided into the nucleoside reverse transcriptase inhibitor group and the nonnucleoside reverse transcriptase inhibitors. Table 11–7 lists available agents in each of these three categories.

Currently recommendations are that treatment should be initiated with triple therapy, that is, a combination of two reverse transcriptase inhibitors plus one protease inhibitor. Three agents are recommended because an individual with a plasma viral load of 20,000 copies per milliliter is likely to harbor all possible resistant genotypes of HIV that can result from one or two point mutations. Thus, even the use of two agents leaves the distinct possibility that a few resistant strains will escape, leading to treatment failure. The likelihood that an infected person will harbor HIV genotypes with three independent mutations is very low; thus, triple therapy should be initiated where possible.

In choosing specific drug combinations, clinicians take into account both the mode of action of specific agents and their drug–drug interactions. For example, zidovudine and lamivudine (Epivir) are both reverse transcriptase inhibitors; however, zidovudine appears to work best in actively replicating cells whereas lamivudine is most active in resting infected cells. Furthermore, zidovudine penetrates into the CNS, while the penetration of lamivudine is low.

Triple therapy may be used for persons who have had an unexpected sexual encounter with a potentially infected partner. It is also used in

Table 11–7
Antiretroviral Agents

Generic Name	Trade Name	Usual Abbreviation
Nucleoside reverse transcriptase inhibitors		
Zidovudine	Retrovir	AZT or ZDV
Didanosine	Videx	ddI
Zalcitabine	Hivid	ddC
Stavudine	Zerit	d4T
Lamivudine	Epivir	3TC
Abacavir	Ziagen	
Nonnucleoside reverse transcriptase inhibitors		
Nevirapine	Viramune	
Delavirdine	Rescriptor	
Efavirenz	Sustiva	
Protease inhibitors		
Saquinavir	Invirase	
Ritonavir	Norvir	
Indinavir	Crixivan	
Nelfinavir	Viracept	

health care workers who have been pricked by a needle from an infected patient. In both instances, triple therapy is started immediately after the event and is usually continued for 3 months.

The antiretroviral agents have many adverse effects too numerous to describe. Of importance to psychiatrists is that protease inhibitors are metabolized by the hepatic cytochrome P450 oxidase system and can therefore increase levels of certain psychotropic drugs that are similarly metabolized. These include bupropion (Wellbutrin), meperidine (Demerol), various benzodiazepines, and selective serotonin reuptake inhibitors (SSRIs). Therefore, one must exercise caution in prescribing psychotropic drugs to persons taking protease inhibitors.

In addition to the new nucleoside reverse transcriptase inhibitors, nonnucleoside reverse transcriptase inhibitors, and protease inhibitors that may soon become available, other classes of drugs are under investigation. These include agents that interfere with HIV cell binding and fusion, the action of HIV integrase, and certain HIV genes such as *gag,* among others.

Beyond treatment directed specifically against HIV, many interventions are available to prevent and treat various complications of immunodeficiency caused by opportunistic viral, bacterial, fungal, and protozoan infections. Both survival and quality of life have improved substantially because of early diagnosis and treatment of these opportunistic conditions.

The use of combination antiretroviral regimens in conjunction with more specific treatments of complications has prolonged the survival of both asymptomatic and symptomatic HIV-infected persons. However, despite progress in maintaining patients longer and in better states of health, the ultimate outcome is still uncertain; that is, it is unclear at present whether any HIV-infected person can expect to escape developing AIDS and ultimately dying. HIV-infected persons are keenly aware of this prognosis, and their concern sometimes takes the form of psychiatric disturbances. These phenomena and the primary and secondary neurocognitive complications related to HIV infection are discussed below.

The introduction of potent antiretroviral drug combinations and the development of sensitive quantitative assays of HIV RNA concentrations have begun to revolutionize the treatment of HIV cognitive disorders as they have done for systemic disease. There is hope that measuring the viral load in CSF will be a window into brain infection and a guide for monitoring response to therapy.

High concentrations of HIV RNA in CSF are associated with neurocognitive impairment in AIDS. High-dosage zidovudine monotherapy can ameliorate HIV-associated neurocognitive impairment, perhaps in part because it penetrates the blood–brain barrier well. Since the introduction of protease inhibitors and combination antiretroviral therapy, zidovudine monotherapy is no longer an option for treatment; nevertheless, it remains an important component of combination regimens. Protease inhibitors cannot cross the blood–brain barrier in therapeutic amounts and thus might not be expected to be effective in treating neurocognitive disorders. Nevertheless, combination of these drugs with other first-generation agents such as zidovudine appears to prevent or even reverse the progression of these disorders. Clinical improvement, both in terms of enhanced performance on standardized neuropsychological testing and of the pattern and severity of white matter signal abnormalities on magnetic resonance imagery (MRI), can be seen within 2 to 3 months of beginning therapy. Perhaps one of every three affected patients will show clinically significant improvement in neurocognitive function. It is not clear how protease inhibitors could arrest or even reverse HIV-associated neurocognitive impairment. It may be that a markedly reduced viral load no longer triggers the production of neurotoxic cytokines, excitatory neurotransmitters, and inflammatory agents by the immune system.

Novel treatments may also be useful. Neuronal excitotoxicity, mediated through the activation of glutamatergic receptors by the HIV envelope protein gp120, is a potentially important mechanism by which brain dysfunction might occur in HIV infection. Memantine is an open-channel antagonist of *N*-methyl-D-aspartate (NMDA)–type glutamate receptors that is generally well tolerated. It is currently being used as a treatment for dementia of the Alzheimer's type in Europe. On the assumption that an agent that could dislodge gp120 from neural receptor sites might be useful, an octapeptide called *d*-ala-peptide-t-amide (peptide t) has been used in phase II clinical trials. Compared with placebo, peptide t was associated with neuropsychological improvement in cognitively impaired individuals (with CD4 counts <200) and a reduced likelihood of progression of impairment on 6-month follow-up. Calcium channel inhibitors, which theoretically seemed potentially useful, have not proven successful.

The remaining forms of treatment are principally supportive. The most important step is to exclude other potentially treatable conditions, such as secondary infections or neoplasia, metabolic abnormalities with low-grade delirium, or other psychiatric disorders (e.g., major depressive disorder). Once the diagnosis is clear, then the usual supportive measures for neurocognitively impaired persons should be used. These include identifying areas of cognitive strength and deficit, reducing emphasis on areas that are now impaired (e.g., divided attention, speeded processing), emphasizing efforts to maintain good orientation and reality testing, and avoiding medications that might further compromise cognitive function, in particular, benzodiazepine drugs. If they must be used, such medications should be given at lower-than-usual doses. Antidepressant and antipsychotic agents, if indicated, may also have to be prescribed in much lower dosages (e.g., 25 percent of the usual recommended dosage).

INTERACTIONS OF PSYCHOTROPIC DRUGS AND ANTIRETROVIRAL DRUGS

Manufacturers of the protease inhibitors have as a first step listed many psychotropic drugs as relatively or absolutely contraindicated in combination with protease inhibitors, which may be an overstatement. Because these presumptive drug interactions have not been studied systematically, it would be unfortunate to deny patients entire classes of potentially safe and beneficial psychotropic drug interventions. For now the most sensible policy is to be aware of the likely major drug–drug interactions and to monitor patients for treatment-emergent adverse effects and, when possible, for psychotropic drug concentrations in plasma. The most likely interactions are as follows. All protease inhibitors will increase psychotropic drug concentrations if the major route of metabolism of the psychotropic agent involves the 3A

isoenzyme of the cytochrome P450 (CYP) CYP 3A system. If the CYP 2D6 system is the primary route of metabolism (e.g., tricyclic medications, SSRIs), ritonavir (Norvir) will specifically inhibit their metabolism. Thus the protease inhibitors may inhibit the metabolism of many antidepressants and antipsychotic agents as well as benzodiazepines. For example, plasma concentrations of alprazolam (Xanax), midazolam (Versed), triazolam (Halcion), and zolpidem (Ambien) may be increased, and dosage reduction and careful monitoring may be required to prevent oversedation or other toxic effects. Protease inhibitors have been reported to increase concentrations of bupropion, nefazodone (Serzone), and fluoxetine (Prozac) to toxic levels and to increase the concentration of desipramine (Norpramin) in plasma by 100 to 150 percent. Drug interactions with antipsychotic agents are less well studied, but ritonavir particularly may increase concentrations. Concentrations of methadone (Dolophine) and meperidine are also reported to be elevated. Additionally, concentrations of some drugs of abuse such as methylenedioxymethamphetamine (MDMA) may be increased. In turn, protease inhibitors may induce the metabolism of valproate (Depakene) and lorazepam (Ativan) and lead to lower concentrations in plasma.

Some psychotropic medications may induce metabolism of protease inhibitors. Carbamazepine (Tegretol) and phenobarbital (Luminal, Solfoton) may reduce the concentration of protease inhibitors in serum. The clinical relevance of this potential interaction is not clear, but use of an alternate mood stabilizer may be indicated. No interactions with lithium (Eskalith) and gabapentin (Neurontin) have been reported.

Finally, psychotropic drugs may reduce the metabolism of some protease inhibitors, with an increase in protease inhibitor adverse effects. This has been reported with nefazodone and fluoxetine.

PSYCHOTHERAPY

Approaches. Major psychodynamic themes for HIV-infected patients involve self-blame, self-esteem, and issues regarding death. The psychiatrist can help patients deal with feelings of guilt regarding behaviors that contributed to infection or AIDS. Some HIV and AIDS patients feel that they are being punished. Difficult health care decisions, such as whether to initiate or continue taking antiretroviral medication and terminal care and life-support systems, should be explored, and here denial of illness may be evident. Major practical themes involve employment, medical benefits, life insurance, career plans, dating and sex, and relationships with families and friends. The entire range of psychotherapeutic approaches may be appropriate for patients with HIV-related disorders. Both individual therapy and group therapy can be effective. Individual therapy may be either short-term or long-term and may be supportive, cognitive, behavioral, or psychodynamic. Group therapy techniques can range from psychodynamic to completely supportive in nature.

At the time of testing positive, the HIV-infected person is almost immediately faced with questions about disclosing his or her serostatus. Most counselors suggest that recently infected individuals withhold disclosure to others until they feel well-enough informed about HIV and its treatment and are ready to answer questions that may arise. Others may ask questions that relate to their own safety, differences between HIV and AIDS, stage of disease, and life span. A patient's readiness to accept the emotional consequences of disclosure—such as another's fury and rejection—must also be anticipated. In brief the HIV-infected person must assess not only his or her readiness, but also the readiness of others to hear the announcement of seropositivity.

Among the fears that must be confronted is the concern that once the individual's serostatus has been revealed, he or she has lost control of who next learns of the seroconversion. In deciding whether or not to tell others, the patient must also address their sense of betrayal if they are not told. The same issues apply to the person's work environment. As a practical matter the individual may need to decide whether to tell a trusted colleague in case of a job-related accident that might put others at risk of infection. Similarly, parents must decide when or whether to tell their children. Some parents want to tell very young children as soon as possible, while other parents prefer to withhold this information until their child's teenage years, for fear of "taking away their childhood." The question of custody of children after the parent's death must be considered. The same question of timing will arise about when to tell children that they are seropositive. The parent must balance fears that telling the child's school will lead to discrimination while guarding their child's and others' safety in case of an accident.

The psychiatrist may have a special role regarding HIV treatment. The advent of protease inhibitors and the promise of additional increasingly effective therapies has brought hopes of a "cure" to patients and physicians alike. Even patients who have failed one or more rounds of combination therapies may find that family, friends, and physicians continue to be optimistic. The psychiatrist may be the only "safe" person to whom the patient can express discouragement, weariness, fear of treatment failure, and fury or guilt for not being able to tolerate successful therapy or for not responding to regimens that have benefited others. The psychiatrist also may be the only one confronting unrealistic expectations of cure or the assumption that safe sex practices are no longer relevant. Paradoxically, the therapeutic task also may be to examine the patient's reaction to a reprieve from certain death—the so-called second-life agenda.

Direct counseling regarding substance use and its potential adverse effects on the HIV-infected patient's health is indicated. Specific treatments for particular substance-related disorders should be initiated if necessary for the total well-being of the patient.

Therapist-Related Issues. Countertransference issues and burnout of therapists who treat many HIV-infected patients must be evaluated regularly. Therapists must acknowledge to themselves their predetermined attitudes toward sexual orientation and substance use so that those attitudes do not interfere with the treatment of the patient. Issues regarding the therapist's own sexual identity, past behaviors, and eventual death may also give rise to countertransference issues. Psychotherapists who have practices with many HIV-infected patients can begin to have their effectiveness impaired by professional burnout. Some studies have found that seeing many HIV-infected patients in a short time seems to be more stressful to therapists than seeing a smaller number of HIV-infected patients over a longer period.

Involvement of Significant Others. The patient's family, lover, and close friends are often important allies in treatment. The patient's spouse or lover may have guilt feelings about possibly having infected the patient or may experience

anger at the patient for possibly infecting him or her. The involvement of members of the patient's support group can help the therapist assess the patient's cognitive function and can also aid in planning financial and living arrangements for the patient. The patient's significant others may themselves benefit from the attention of the therapist in helping them cope with the illness and the impending loss of a friend or family member.

References

Angrist B, d'Hollosy M, Sanfilipo M, et al. Central nervous system stimulants as symptomatic treatments for AIDS-related neuropsychiatric impairments. *J Clin Psychopharmacol.* 1992;12:268.

Castellon SA, Hinkin CH, Myers HF. Neuropsychiatric disturbance is associated with executive dysfunction in HIV-1 infection. *J Int Neuropsychol Soc.* 2000;6:336.

Graham NMH, Zeger SL, Park LP, et al. The effects on survival of early treatment of human immunodeficiency virus infection. *N Engl J Med.* 1992;326:1037.

Grant I, Atkinson JH Jr. Neuropsychiatric aspects of HIV infection and AIDS. In: Sadock BJ, Sadock VA, eds. *Kaplan & Sadock's Comprehensive Textbook of Psychiatry.* 7th ed. Vol II. Baltimore: Lippincott Williams & Wilkins; 2000:308.

Handelsman L, Aronson M, Maurer G, et al. Neuropsychological and neurological manifestations of HIV-1 dementia in drug users. *J Neuropsychiatry Clin Neurosci.* 1992;4:21.

Harris MJ, Jests DV, Gleghorn A, Sewell DD. New-onset psychosis in HIV-infected patients. *J Clin Psychiatry.* 1991;52:369.

Hirsch MS, D'Aquilla RT. Therapy for human immunodeficiency virus infection. *N Engl J Med.* 1993;328:1686.

Jansen RS, St Louis ME, Satten GA, et al. HIV infection among patients in US acute care hospitals. The Hospital HIV Surveillance Group. *N Engl J Med.* 1992;327:445.

Katz MH, Gerberding JL. Postexposure treatment of people exposed to the human immunodeficiency virus through sexual contact or injection-drug use. *N Engl J Med.* 1997;336:1097.

Kieburtz K, Zettelmaier AE, Ketonen L, Tuite M, Caine ED. Manic syndrome in AIDS. *Am J Psychiatry.* 1991;148:1068.

Levy JK, Fernandez F, Lachar BL, et al. Neuropsychiatry of human immunodeficiency virus infection. In: Ovsiew F, ed. *Neuropsychiatry and Mental Health Services.* Washington, DC: American Psychiatric Press; 1999:221.

LoPiccolo CJ, Goodkin K. The role of precise conceptualization in the treatment of a complicated HIV-1 infected neuropsychiatric patient. *J Neuropsychiatry Clin Neurosci.* 1999;11:234.

Maldonado JL, Fernandez F, Levy JK. Acquired immunodeficiency syndrome. In: Lauterbach EC, ed. *Psychiatric Management in Neurological Disease.* Washington, DC: American Psychiatric Press; 2000:271.

Mapou RL, Law WA, Martin A, Kampen D, Salazar AM, Rundell JR. Neuropsychological performance, mood, and complaints of cognitive and motor difficulties in individuals infected with the human immunodeficiency virus. *J Neuropsychiatry Clin Neurosci.* 1993;5:86.

Martin L, Tummala R, Fernandez F. Psychiatric management of HIV infection and AIDS. *Psychiatr Ann.* 2002;32:133.

Morrison MF, Petitto JM, Have TT, et al. Depressive anxiety disorders in women with HIV infection. *Am J Psychiatry.* 2002;159:789.

Norton J. The neuropsychiatric symptoms of AIDS. *Am J Psychiatry.* 2000;157:2059.

Pajeau AK, Roma Román GC. HIV encephalopathy and dementia. *Psychiatr Clin North Am.* 1992;15:455.

Ricart F, Cohen M, Alfonso CA, et al. Understanding the psychodynamics of non-adherence to medical treatment in persons with HIV infection. *Gen Hosp Psychiatry.* 2002;24:176.

Rourke SB, Halman MH, Bassel C. Neuropsychiatric correlates of memory-metamemory dissociations in HIV-infection. *J Clin Exp Neuropsychol.* 1999;21:757.

Ruiz P. Living and dying with HIV/AIDS: a psychosocial perspective. *Am J Psychiatry.* 2000;157:1101.

Sacks M, Dermatis H, Looser-Ott S, Burton W, Perry S. Undetected HIV infection among acutely ill psychiatric inpatients. *Am J Psychiatry.* 1992; 149:544.

Sepkowitz KA. AIDS—the first 20 years. *N Engl J Med.* 2001;344:1764.

Silverman DC. Psychosocial impact of HIV-related caregiving on health providers: a review and recommendations for the role of psychiatry. *Am J Psychiatry.* 1993;150:705.

Steinbrook R. Drazen JM. AIDS—will the next 20 years be different? *N Engl J Med.* 2001;344:1781.

Van Gorp EG, Mandlekern MA, Gee M, et al. Cerebral metabolic dysfunction in AIDS: findings in a sample with and without dementia. *J Neuropsychiatry Clin Neurosci.* 1992;4:280.

12 Substance-Related Disorders

▲ 12.1 Introduction and Overview

Whether a society views substance use primarily as a moral or a legal problem, when it creates difficulties for the user or ceases to be entirely volitional it becomes the concern of all the helping professions, including psychiatry. This chapter on substance-related disorders is made up of separate sections organized around the syndromes engendered by the use of each of the major groups of pharmacological agents that are commonly misused (abused).

Aside from the percentage of the population who report using one or more illicit substances in their lifetimes (almost 40 percent) and the staggering cost to society (over $200 billion per year), the phenomenon of substance abuse has many implications for brain research and for clinical psychiatry. Some substances can affect both internally perceived mental states, such as mood, and externally observable activities, such as behavior. Substances can cause neuropsychiatric symptoms indistinguishable from those of common psychiatric disorders with no known causes (e.g., schizophrenia and mood disorders), and thus primary psychiatric disorders and disorders involving the use of substances are possibly related. If the depressive symptoms seen in some persons who have not taken a brain-altering substance are indistinguishable from the depressive symptoms in a person who has taken a brain-altering substance, there may be a brain-based commonality between substance-taking behavior and depression. The very existence of brain-altering substances is a fundamental clue to the ways in which the brain works in both normal and abnormal states.

There is a perennial debate in the United States about the most effective way to handle drug problems. In the past few years, a small but growing number of government officials, commentators, and academics have argued that the present policy of aggressively prosecuting drug sellers and users should be reconsidered. They have compared the current drug policy with the prohibition of alcohol from 1920 to 1934 and have argued that abolishing drug laws would eliminate the profit motive, the gangs, and the drug dealers. Although she stopped short of endorsing such a radical reversal of the nation's drug policy, the former U.S. Surgeon General Joycelyn Elders, M.D., recommended that the government study the possibility of legalizing drugs of abuse and suggested that doing so might reduce the incidence of violent crimes.

TERMINOLOGY

The complexity of the subject of illicit substance use is reflected in the associated terminology, which seems to change regularly as various professional and governmental committees convene to discuss the problem. One question is what to call the brain-altering substances. The text revision of the fourth edition of *Diagnostic and Statistical Manual of Mental Disorders* (DSM-IV-TR) refers to brain-altering substances as *substances* and to the related disorders as *substance-related disorders*. In DSM-IV-TR, the concept of *psychoactive substance* does not include chemicals with brain-altering properties such as organic solvents, which may be ingested either on purpose or by accident. Legal substances cannot be separated from illegal substances; many legal substances, such as morphine, are often obtained by illegal means and used for nonprescribed purposes. The word *substance* is generally preferable to the word *drug,* because *drug* implies a manufactured chemical, whereas many substances associated with abuse patterns occur naturally (e.g., opium) or are not meant for human consumption (e.g., airplane glue). Thus, in DSM-IV-TR, the topic is described by the general heading of substance-related disorders.

The substance-related disorders are cross-referenced in the DSM-IV-TR categories that cover these particular symptoms or syndromes (Table 12.1–1). For example, a patient with depression related to cocaine withdrawal receives a diagnosis of cocaine-induced mood disorder with depressive features, with onset during withdrawal. This diagnosis is also cross-referenced within the DSM-IV-TR section on mood disorders. The cross-referencing emphasizes the differential diagnosis of mood disorder symptoms while emphasizing that a single substance of abuse can result in many neuropsychiatric symptoms and syndromes.

Although all substances considered by DSM-IV-TR in the substance-related disorders category are associated with a pathological intoxication state, the substances vary as to whether the pathological state is associated with withdrawal or persists after the elimination of the substance from the body (Table 12.1–2). Within the DSM-IV-TR system, patients who are experiencing substance intoxication or withdrawal accompanied by psychiatric symptoms but who do not meet the criteria for a specific syndromal pattern of symptoms (e.g., depression) receive the diagnosis of substance intoxication (Table 12.1–3) or substance withdrawal (Table 12.1–4), possibly along with dependence or abuse.

Table 12.1–1
DSM-IV-TR Substance-Induced Disorders Outside of Substance-Related Disorders Category

Diagnosis	DSM-IV Category	Synopsis Section
Substance intoxication delirium	Delirium, dementia, and amnestic and other cognitive disorders	10.2
Substance withdrawal delirium	Delirium, dementia, and amnestic and other cognitive disorders	10.2
Substance-induced persisting dementia	Delirium, dementia, and amnestic and other cognitive disorders	10.3
Substance-induced persisting amnestic disorder	Delirium, dementia, and amnestic and other cognitive disorders	10.4
Substance-induced psychotic disorder	Schizophrenia and other psychotic disorders	14
Substance-induced mood disorder	Mood disorders	15.3
Substance-induced anxiety disorder	Anxiety disorders	16.7
Substance-induced sexual dysfunction	Sexual and gender identity disorders	21.2
Substance-induced sleep disorder	Sleep disorders	24.2

Substance Dependence and Abuse

In 1964, the World Health Organization concluded that the term *addiction* is no longer a scientific term and recommended substituting the term *drug dependence*. The concept of substance dependence has had many officially recognized and commonly used meanings over the decades. Two concepts have been used to define aspects of dependence: behavioral and physical. In behavioral dependence, substance-seeking activities and related evidence of pathological use patterns are emphasized, whereas physical dependence refers to the physical (physiological) effects of multiple episodes of substance use. In definitions stressing physical dependence, ideas of tolerance or withdrawal appear in the classification criteria.

Somewhat related to *dependence* are the related words *addiction* and *addict*. The word *addict* has acquired a distinctive, unseemly, and pejorative connotation that ignores the concept of substance abuse as a medical disorder. *Addiction* has also been trivialized in popular usage, as in the phrases *TV addiction* and *money addiction*. Although these connotations have helped the officially sanctioned nomenclature to avoid use of the word *addiction*, there may be common neurochemical and neuroanatomical substrates among all the addictions, whether to substances or to gambling, sex, stealing, or eating. These various addictions may have similar effects on the activities of specific reward areas of the brain, such as the ventral tegmental area, the locus ceruleus, and the nucleus accumbens.

DSM-IV-TR allows clinicians to specify whether symptoms of physiological abuse dependence are present (Table 12.1–5 or Table 12.1–6). The presence or absence of physiological dependence need not be distinguished from physical and psychological dependence, respectively. Such a distinction parallels the flawed organic-functional distinction; psychological or behavioral dependence undoubtedly reflects physiological changes in the behavioral centers of the brain. DSM-IV-TR also allows clinicians to assess the current state of the substance dependence by providing a list of course modifiers (Table 12.1–7). *Psychological dependence,* also referred to as *habituation,* is characterized by a continuous or intermittent craving for the substance to avoid a dysphoric state. DSM-IV-TR defines substance abuse as characterized by the presence of at least one specific symptom indicating that substance use has interfered with the person's life (Table 12.1–5). Persons cannot meet the diagnosis of substance abuse for a particular substance if they have ever met the criteria for dependence on the same substance.

Codependence

The terms *coaddiction, coalcoholism,* and, more commonly, *codependency* or *codependence* are used to designate the behavioral patterns of family members who have been significantly affected by another family member's substance use or addiction. The terms have been used in various ways, and there are no established criteria for codependence.

Enabling. Enabling was one of the first, and more agreed upon, characteristics of codependence or coaddiction. Sometimes family members feel that they have little or no control over the enabling acts. Either because of the social pressures for protecting and supporting family members or because of pathological interdependencies, or both, enabling behavior often resists modification. Other characteristics of codependence include unwillingness to accept the notion of addiction as a disease. The family members continue to behave as if the substance-using behavior were voluntary and willful (if not actually spiteful) and the user cares more for alcohol and drugs than for the members of the family. This results in feelings of anger, rejection, and failure. In addition to those feelings, family members may feel guilty and depressed because addicts, in an effort to deny loss of control over drugs and to shift the focus of concern away from their use, often try to place the responsibility for such use on other family members, who often seem willing to accept some or all of it.

Denial. Family members, like the substance users themselves, often behave as if the substance use that is causing obvious problems were not really a problem; that is, they engage in denial. The reasons for the unwillingness to accept the obvious vary. Sometimes denial is self-protecting, in that the family members believe that if there is a drug or alcohol problem, then they are responsible.

Like the addicts themselves, codependent family members seem unwilling to accept the notion that outside intervention is needed and, despite repeated failures, continue to believe that greater willpower and greater efforts at control can restore tran-

Table 12.1–2
Diagnoses Associated with Class of Substances

	Dependence	Abuse	Intoxication	Withdrawal	Intoxication Delirium	Withdrawal Delirium	Dementia	Amnestic Disorder	Psychotic Disorders	Mood Disorders	Anxiety Disorders	Sexual Dysfunctions	Sleep Disorders
Alcohol	X	X	X	X	I	W	P	P	I/W	I/W	I/W	I	I/W
Amphetamines	X	X	X	X	I				I	I/W	I	I	I/W
Caffeine			X								I		I
Cannabis	X	X	X		I				I		I		
Cocaine	X	X	X	X	I				I	I/W	I/W	I	I/W
Hallucinogens	X	X	X		I				I[a]	I	I		
Inhalants	X	X	X		I		P		I	I	I		
Nicotine	X			X									
Opioids	X	X	X	X	I				I	I		I	I/W
Phencyclidine	X	X	X		I				I	I	I		
Sedatives, hypnotics, or anxiolytics	X	X	X	X	I	W	P	P	I/W	I/W	W	I	I/W
Polysubstance	X												
Other	X	X	X	X	I	W	P	P	I/W	I/W	I/W	I	I/W

Note: X, I, W, I/W, or P indicates that the category is recognized in DSM-IV. In addition, *I* indicates that the specifier With Onset During Intoxication may be noted for the category (except for Intoxication Delirium); *W* indicates that the specifier With Onset During Withdrawal may be noted for the category (except for Withdrawal Delirium); and *I/W* indicates that either With Onset During Intoxication or With Onset During Withdrawal may be noted for the category. *P* indicates that the disorder is Persisting.

[a]Also hallucinogen persisting perception disorder (flashbacks).

From American Psychiatric Association. *Diagnostic and Statistical Manual of Mental Disorders.* 4th ed. Text rev. Washington, DC: American Psychiatric Association; copyright 2000, with permission.

Table 12.1–3
DSM-IV-TR Criteria for Substance Intoxication

A. The development of a reversible substance-specific syndrome due to recent ingestion of (or exposure to) a substance. **Note:** Different substances may produce similar or identical syndromes.
B. Clinically significant maladaptive behavioral or psychological changes that are due to the effect of the substance on the central nervous system (e.g., belligerence, mood lability, cognitive impairment, impaired judgment, impaired social or occupational functioning) and develop during or shortly after use of the substance.
C. The symptoms are not due to a general medical condition and are not better accounted for by another mental disorder.

From American Psychiatric Association. *Diagnostic and Statistical Manual of Mental Disorders.* 4th ed. Text rev. Washington, DC: American Psychiatric Association; copyright 2000, with permission.

Table 12.1–4
DSM-IV-TR Criteria for Substance Withdrawal

A. The development of a substance-specific syndrome due to the cessation of (or reduction in) substance use that has been heavy and prolonged.
B. The substance-specific syndrome causes clinically significant distress or impairment in social, occupational, or other important areas of functioning.
C. The symptoms are not due to a general medical condition and are not better accounted for by another mental disorder.

From American Psychiatric Association. *Diagnostic and Statistical Manual of Mental Disorders.* 4th ed. Text rev. Washington, DC: American Psychiatric Association; copyright 2000, with permission.

Table 12.1–5
DSM-IV-TR Criteria for Substance Abuse

A. A maladaptive pattern of substance use leading to clinically significant impairment or distress, as manifested by one (or more) of the following, occurring within a 12-month period:
   (1) recurrent substance use resulting in a failure to fulfill major role obligations at work, school, or home (e.g., repeated absences or poor work performance related to substance use; substance-related absences, suspensions, or expulsions from school; neglect of children or household)
   (2) recurrent substance use in situations in which it is physically hazardous (e.g., driving an automobile or operating a machine when impaired by substance use)
   (3) recurrent substance-related legal problems (e.g., arrests for substance-related disorderly conduct)
   (4) continued substance use despite having persistent or recurrent social or interpersonal problems caused or exacerbated by the effects of the substance (e.g., arguments with spouse about consequences of intoxication, physical fights)
B. The symptoms have never met the criteria for Substance Dependence for this class of substance.

From American Psychiatric Association. *Diagnostic and Statistical Manual of Mental Disorders.* 4th ed. Text rev. Washington, DC: American Psychiatric Association; copyright 2000, with permission.

Table 12.1–6
DSM-IV-TR Diagnostic Criteria for Substance Dependence

A maladaptive pattern of substance use, leading to clinically significant impairment or distress, as manifested by three (or more) of the following, occurring at any time in the same 12-month period:

(1) tolerance, as defined by either of the following:
   (a) a need for markedly increased amounts of the substance to achieve intoxication or desired effect
   (b) markedly diminished effect with continued use of the same amount of the substance
(2) withdrawal, as manifested by either of the following:
   (a) the characteristic withdrawal syndrome for the substance (refer to Criteria A and B of the criteria sets for Withdrawal from the specific substances)
   (b) the same (or a closely related) substance is taken to relieve or avoid withdrawal symptoms
(3) the substance is often taken in larger amounts or over a longer period than was intended
(4) there is a persistent desire or unsuccessful efforts to cut down or control substance use
(5) a great deal of time is spent in activities necessary to obtain the substance (e.g., visiting multiple doctors or driving long distances), use the substance (e.g., chain-smoking), or recover from its effects
(6) important social, occupational, or recreational activities are given up or reduced because of substance use
(7) the substance use is continued despite knowledge of having a persistent or recurrent physical or psychological problem that is likely to have been caused or exacerbated by the substance (e.g., current cocaine use despite recognition of cocaine-induced depression, or continued drinking despite recognition that an ulcer was made worse by alcohol consumption)

Specify if:

With Physiological Dependence: evidence of tolerance or withdrawal (i.e., either Item 1 or 2 is present)

Without Physiological Dependence: no evidence of tolerance or withdrawal (i.e., neither Item 1 nor 2 is present)

Course specifiers (see Table 12.1–7 for definitions):

Early Full Remission
Early Partial Remission
Sustained Full Remission
Sustained Partial Remission
On Agonist Therapy
In a Controlled Environment

From American Psychiatric Association. *Diagnostic and Statistical Manual of Mental Disorders.* 4th ed. Text rev. Washington, DC: American Psychiatric Association; copyright 2000, with permission.

quility. When additional efforts at control fail, they often attribute the failure to themselves rather than to the addict or the disease process, and along with failure come feelings of anger, lowered self-esteem, and depression.

EPIDEMIOLOGY

The National Institute of Drug Abuse (NIDA) and other agencies conduct periodic surveys of the use of illicit drugs in the United States. In general, about 40 percent of the population

Table 12.1–7
DSM-IV Course Modifiers for Substance Dependence

Six course specifiers are available for substance dependence. The four remission specifiers can be applied only after none of the criteria for substance dependence or substance abuse has been present for at least 1 month. The definition of these four types of remission is based on the interval of time that has elapsed since the cessation of dependence (early versus sustained remission) and whether there is continued presence of one or more of the items included in the criteria sets for dependence or abuse (partial versus full remission). Because the first 12 months following dependence is a time of particularly high risk for relapse, this period is designated early remission. After 12 months of early remission have passed without relapse to dependence, the person enters into sustained remission. For both early remission and sustained remission, a further designation of full is given if no criteria for dependence or abuse have been met during the period of remission; a designation of partial is given if at least one of the criteria for dependence or abuse has been met, intermittently or continuously, during the period of remission. The differentiation of sustained full remission from recovered (no current substance use disorder) requires consideration of the length of time since the last period of disturbance, the total duration of the disturbance, and the need for continued evaluation. If, after a period of remission or recovery, the individual again becomes dependent, the application of the early remission specifier requires that there again be at least 1 month in which no criteria for dependence or abuse are met. Two additional specifiers have been provided: on agonist therapy and in a controlled environment. For an individual to qualify for early remission after cessation of agonist therapy or release from a controlled environment, there must be a 1-month period in which none of the criteria for dependence or abuse is met.

The following remission specifiers can be applied only after no criteria for dependence or abuse have been met for at least 1 month. Note that these specifiers do not apply if the individual is on agonist therapy or in a controlled environment (see below).

Early full remission. This specifier is used if, for at least 1 month, but for less than 12 months, no criteria for dependence or abuse have been met.

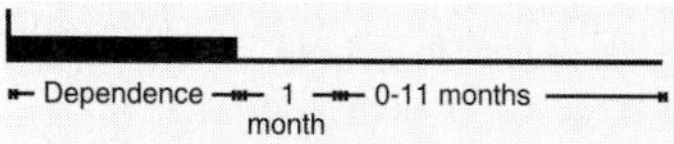

Early partial remission. This specifier is used if, for at least 1 month, but less than 12 months, one or more criteria for dependence or abuse have been met (but the full criteria for dependence have not been met).

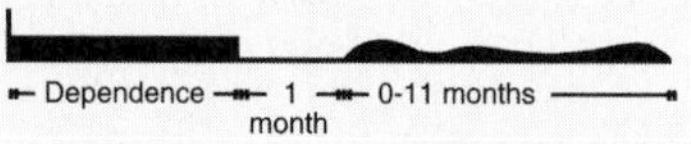

Sustained full remission. This specifier is used if none of the criteria for dependence or abuse has been met at any time during a period of 12 months or longer.

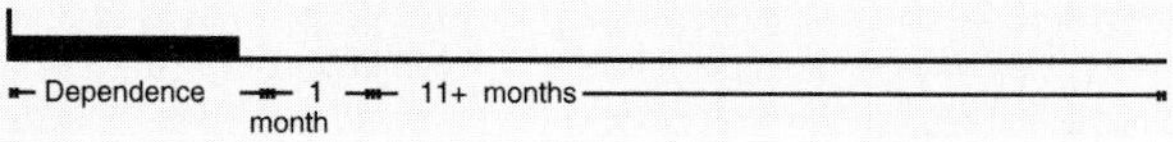

Sustained partial remission. This specifier is used if full criteria for dependence have not been met for a period of 12 months or longer; however, one or more criteria for dependence or abuse have been met.

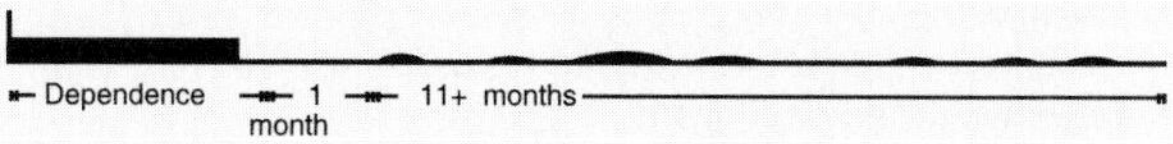

The following specifiers apply if the individual is on agonist therapy or in a controlled environment:

On agonist therapy. This specifier is used if the individual is on a prescribed agonist medication, and no criteria for dependence or abuse have been met for the class of medication for at least the past month (except tolerance to, or withdrawal from, the agonist). This category also applies to those being treated for dependence using a partial agonist or an agonist/antagonist.

In a controlled environment. This specifier is used if the individual is in an environment where access to alcohol and controlled substances is restricted, and no criteria for dependence or abuse have been met for at least the past month. Examples of these environments are closely supervised and substance-free jails, therapeutic communities, or locked hospital units.

From American Psychiatric Association. *Diagnostic and Statistical Manual of Mental Disorders.* 4th ed. Text rev. Washington, DC: American Psychiatric Association; copyright 2000, with permission.

reports using one or more illicit substances in their lifetime, and about 15 percent have used illicit substances in the past year. The lifetime prevalence of substance abuse is about 20 percent.

Lower educational and lower income levels predict a lifetime history of dependence (odds ratios greater than 2), but race, ethnicity, or living in an urban environment do not. Differences also exist in the likelihood that users of a particular drug will become dependent on it. For example, for heroin, the lifetime dependence rate for opioids is about 23 percent; for tobacco, the lifetime dependence rate is 32 percent; for cocaine, 17 percent; and for alcohol, 17 percent, but for psychedelics, only 5 percent. Men who used alcohol were more likely to become dependent (21.4 percent) than women (9.2 percent), possibly because they drink more than women, but genetics may also play a role.

Table 12.1–8 shows data from the 1998 National Household Survey on Drug Abuse (NHSDA) on the percentage of respondents who reported using various drugs. The data are shown for four age groups. Persons aged 18 to 25 years reported the highest level of use of illicit drugs during the 30 days preceding the interview; those ages 26 to 34 had the next highest rate and reported a higher lifetime experience with cocaine. Illicit drug use during the 30 days preceding the interview is far more prevalent among young adults (ages 18 to 34, particularly those 18 to 25 years old) than among those above age 35 or below age 18. Also, whereas recent use is more common in large metropolitan areas than in rural areas, regional, racial, and ethnic differences vary with the age group considered. With the exception of tobacco dependence, all forms of substance abuse or dependence are more common among men than among women. However, recent data indicate that when adjustment is made for differences in rates of use and experimentation with illicit drugs, women are about as likely as men to become

Table 12.1–8
Use of Illicit Drugs, Alcohol, and Tobacco in the U.S. Population by Age Groups

	Lifetime Use (%)				Past-Year Use (%)				Past-Month Use (%)			
Drug	12 to 17	18 to 25	26 to 34	>35	12 to 17	18 to 25	26 to 34	>35	12 to 17	18 to 25	26 to 34	>35
Any illicit drug[a]	23.7	48.0	53.1	29.0	16.7	26.8	14.6	5.3	9.0	15.6	8.4	2.9
Marijuana and hashish	16.8	44.0	50.5	27.0	13.0	23.8	11.3	3.8	7.1	13.2	6.3	2.0
Cocaine	1.9	10.2	20.9	8.9	1.4	4.7	3.5	0.9	0.6	2.0	1.5	0.4
Crack	0.7	3.0	4.4	1.6	0.4	1.3	1.1	0.4	0.2	0.6	0.5	0.2
Inhalants	5.9	10.8	8.3	3.6	4.0	3.0	0.7	0.3	1.7	1.0	0.3	0.1
Hallucinogens	5.6	16.3	15.4	7.3	4.3	6.9	1.1	0.2	2.0	2.3	0.2	0.1
PCP	1.2	2.3	4.2	3.4	0.7	0.5	0.0	0.1	0.2	0.1	*b*	0.0
LSD	4.3	13.9	11.7	5.8	2.8	4.6	0.5	*b*	0.8	0.9	0.1	*b*
Heroin	0.5	1.3	1.3	1.2	0.3	0.9	0.2	0.0	0.2	0.4	0.1	0.0
Nonmedical use of any psychotherapeutic[c]	6.8	12.7	13.4	8.3	4.7	6.7	4.2	1.8	1.9	2.9	1.9	0.9
Stimulants	2.2	4.3	6.5	4.7	1.5	2.0	1.3	0.4	0.5	0.6	0.4	0.3
Sedatives	1.1	1.3	2.9	2.5	0.4	0.7	0.5	0.2	0.2	0.3	0.2	0.0
Tranquilizers	1.7	5.0	5.8	3.1	1.0	2.6	1.6	0.7	0.2	0.9	0.5	0.4
Analgesics	5.5	8.9	7.5	4.2	3.7	4.9	2.5	1.1	1.5	2.0	1.1	0.5
Any illicit drug other than marijuana[d]	13.0	26.6	30.2	15.1	9.3	12.7	7.2	2.7	4.6	6.3	3.6	1.4
Alcohol	38.8	83.8	90.3	87.8	32.7	75.3	77.2	64.9	18.8	60.0	61.6	51.7
"Binge" alcohol use[e]	*f*								7.2	32.0	22.8	11.3
Heavy alcohol use[c]									2.9	12.9	7.1	3.8
Cigarettes	36.3	68.5	73.8	77.8	24.2	44.7	39.2	29.1	18.3	38.3	35.0	27.0
Smokeless tobacco	10.0	23.4	24.4	14.8	4.6	9.7	7.2	2.9	1.9	6.1	4.9	2.3

[a]Use at least once of marijuana or hashish, cocaine (including crack), inhalants, hallucinogens (including PCP and LSD), heroin, or any prescription-type psychotherapeutic used nonmedically.
[b]Low precision; no estimate reported.
[c]Nonmedical use of any prescription-type stimulant, sedative, tranquilizer, or analgesic, does not include over-the-counter drugs.
[d]Use at least once of any of these listed drugs, regardless of marijuana use, marijuana users who also have used any of the other listed drugs are included.
[e]Drinking five or more drinks on the same occasion on at least 1 day in the past 30 days. "Occasion" means at the same time or within a couple hours of each other. Heavy alcohol use is defined as drinking five or more drinks on the same occasion on each of five or more days in the past 30 days; all heavy alcohol users are also "binge" alcohol users.
[f]Not available.
From National Household Survey on Drug Abuse, Substance Abuse and Mental Health Services Administration (SAMHSA) Office of Applied Studies, Department of Health and Human Services, preliminary data, June 1997.

dependent. Current illicit drug use (past 30 days) was more common among male (8.1 percent) than female (4.2 percent) respondents, was more common among the unemployed, and was slightly more common among blacks and in the western states. The DSM-IV-TR epidemiological data are included in the sections on specific substances.

Trends

The 2000 NHSDA found that rates of illicit drug use in the U.S. population remained largely unchanged from those in 1999. A slight decrease in drug use was noted among the youngest teenagers. The survey also showed that current cigarette use declined among youths 12 to 17 years old and young adults aged 18 to 25.

An estimated 14 million Americans, or 6.3 percent of the population 12 years old and older, reported that they had used an illicit drug at least once during the 30 days before the 2000 survey interview. Among 12- to 17-year-olds, 9.7 percent were illicit drug users in 2000, compared with 9.8 percent in 1999.

A leading indicator of drug use—the rate of use in the youngest age group—suggests that rates may decline in the future. Among youths 12 and 13 years old, a key target audience of the National Youth Anti-Drug Media Campaign, the rate of past-month illicit drug use declined from 3.9 percent in 1999 to 3 percent in 2000.

Patterns of drug use showed substantial variation by age. Among youths, rates increased with age, peaking in the 18- to 20-year age group at 19.6 percent. After age 20, the rates generally declined with age, except among adults aged 40 to 44 years, whose drug use rates were higher than those in the 35- to 39-year-old group. Persons in their early 40s in 2000 were teenagers during the 1970s, a period when the incidence and prevalence of drug use were rising dramatically.

About 15.4 percent of unemployed adults were current illicit drug users in 2000, compared with 6.3 percent of full-time employed adults and 7.8 percent of part-time employed adults. Of the 11.8 million adult illicit drug users in 2000, 9.1 million (77 percent) were employed either full-time or part-time.

Marijuana is the most commonly used illicit drug. In 2000 it was used by 76 percent of current illicit drug users. Approximately 59 percent of illicit drug users consumed only marijuana, 17 percent used

marijuana and another illicit drug, and the remaining 24 percent reported use of an illicit drug other than marijuana.

An estimated 65.5 million Americans aged 12 and older—29.3 percent—reported current use of a tobacco product in 2000. Of these, 55.7 million (24.9 percent) smoked cigarettes, 10.7 million (4.8 percent) smoked cigars, 7.6 million (3.4 percent) used smokeless tobacco, and 2.1 million (1.0 percent) smoked pipes.

For youths aged 12 to 17, the rate of cigarette use declined from 14.9 percent in 1999 to 13.4 percent in 2000. This decrease was primarily a result of a decline among boys. Among youths, the rate of smoking was higher in 2000 for females than for males—14.1 percent and 12.8 percent, respectively. Rates of cigarette use among young adults declined from 39.7 percent in 1999 to 38.3 percent in 2000.

The rates of alcohol use among youths aged 12 to 20 and the general population have remained relatively flat for the past several years. In 2000, almost half of Americans 12 years old and older—46.6 percent, or 104 million persons—reported being current drinkers. The prevalence of current alcohol use increased with age, from 2.4 percent at age 12 to a peak of 65.2 percent for 21-year-olds. About 9.7 million persons in the 12- to 20-year age group, or 27.5 percent, reported drinking alcohol in the past month. Of these, 6.6 million, or 18.7 percent, were binge drinkers, and 2.1 million, or 6 percent, were heavy drinkers.

The percentage of persons who reported driving under the influence of alcohol during the past year declined from 10.9 percent in 1999 to 10 percent in 2000. The percentage driving under the influence of drugs also declined—from 3.4 percent in 1999 to 3.1 percent in 2000.

The survey report notes that the use of one substance often goes hand in hand with the use of others. For example, 4.6 percent of nonsmokers aged 12 to 17 in 2000 used illicit drugs, whereas 42.7 percent of youths who used cigarettes also reported current illicit drug use.

The survey is based on a representative sample of the U.S. population aged 12 and older, including persons living in households and in some group quarters, such as dormitories and homeless shelters. In 2000, interviews were conducted with more than 71,000 individuals. Complete findings of the survey are available at www.samhsa.gov. (The reader is also referred to Chapter 60, Health Care Delivery in Psychiatry and Medicine.)

ETIOLOGY

At one level, substance abuse and substance dependence result from a person's taking a particular substance in an abusive pattern, but such simplification does not answer questions about why only some persons have substance abuse or substance dependence. As with all psychiatric disorders, the initial causative theories grew from psychodynamic models; subsequent models invoked behavioral, genetic, or neurochemical explanations. Most recent causative models for substance abuse invoke the entire range of theories (Fig. 12.1–1).

Psychodynamic Factors

The range of psychodynamic theories about substance abuse reflects the various popular theories during the past 100 years. According to classic theories, substance abuse is a masturbatory equivalent (i.e., the need for orgasm), a defense against anxious impulses, or a manifestation of oral regression (i.e., dependency). Recent psychodynamic formulations relate substance use to depression or treat substance use as a reflection of disturbed ego functions (i.e., the inability to deal with reality).

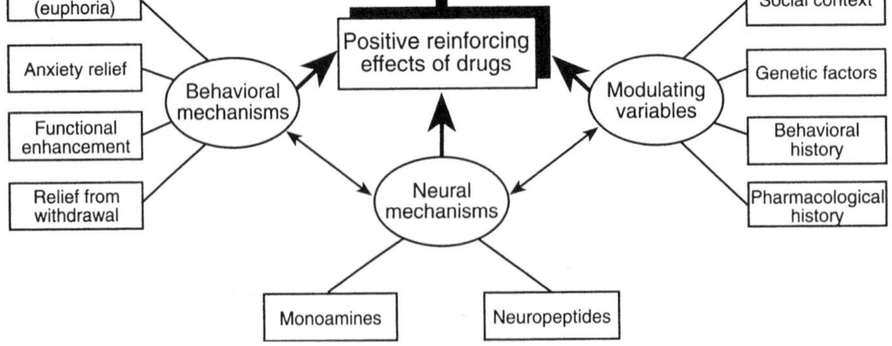

FIGURE 12.1–1

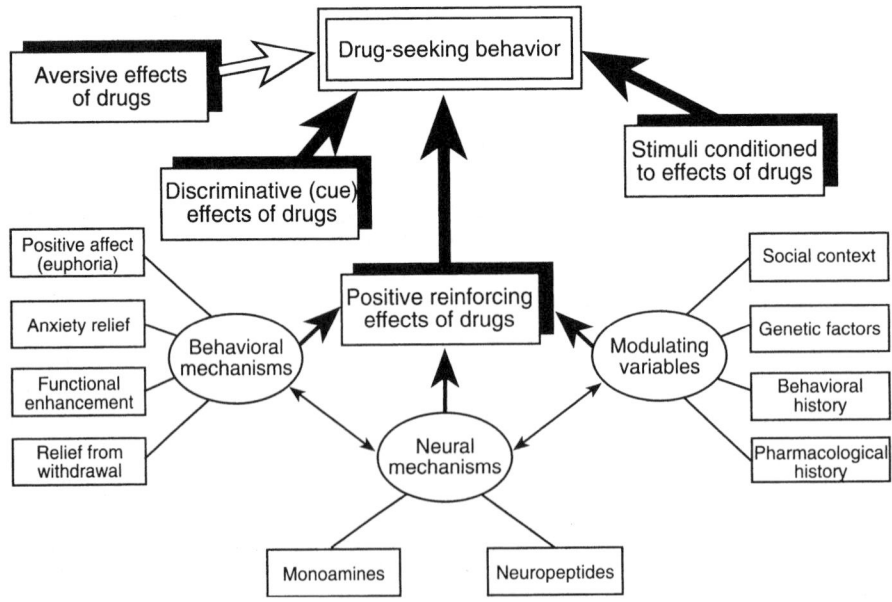

A psychopharmacological model of dependence as substance-seeking behavior controlled by four main processes: positive reinforcing and discriminative effects of substances and of stimuli associated with them (which facilitate substance seeking) and aversive effects of substances (which weaken the behavior). The four processes are common to substances of many classes. A detailed framework for analyzing positive reinforcing effects is shown (similar analyses could be made for discriminative and aversive effects); at this level the relative importance of the factors shown in the diagram varies considerably between classes of substances. (Reprinted with permission from Stolerman I. Drugs of abuse: Behavior principles, methods, and terms. *Trends Pharmacol Sci.* 1992;13:171.)

Psychodynamic approaches to persons with substance abuse are more widely valued and accepted than they are in the treatment of patients with alcohol abuse. In contrast to alcoholic patients, individuals with polysubstance abuse are more likely to have had unstable childhoods, more likely to self-medicate with substances, and more likely to benefit from psychotherapy. Considerable research links personality disorders with the development of substance dependence.

Other psychosocial theories invoke relationships with the family and with society in general, and there are many reasons to suspect a societal role in the development of patterns of substance abuse and substance dependence. Urban newspapers are filled with gripping stories about the drug culture permeating areas of urban poverty. Such articles often describe children brought into this culture at early ages. Yet even under these social pressures, not every child receives a diagnosis of substance abuse or substance dependence, a fact that suggests the involvement of other causal factors.

Behavioral Theories

Some behavioral models of substance abuse have focused on substance-seeking behavior rather than on the symptoms of physical dependence (Fig. 12.1–1). For a behavioral model to have relevance to all substances, the model must not depend on the presence of withdrawal symptoms or of tolerance; many substances of abuse are not associated with development of physiological dependence. Some researchers hypothesize that four major behavioral principles work to induce substance-seeking behavior. The first two principles are the positive reinforcing qualities and the adverse effects of some substances. Most substances of abuse produce a positive experience after their first use, and thus the substance acts as a positive reinforcer for substance-seeking behavior. Many substances also result in adverse effects, which act to reduce substance-seeking behavior. According to principles three and four, a person must be able to discriminate the substance of abuse from other substances, and almost all substance-seeking behavior is associated with cues that become connected with the substance-taking experience.

Genetic Factors

Strong evidence from studies of twins, adoptees, and siblings brought up separately indicates that the cause of alcohol abuse has a genetic component. Many less conclusive data show that other types of substance abuse or substance dependence have a genetic pattern in their development. Researchers recently have used restriction fragment length polymorphism (RFLP) in the study of substance abuse and substance dependence, and a few reports of RFLP associations have been published.

Neurochemical Factors

Receptors and Receptor Systems. With the exception of alcohol, researchers have identified particular neurotransmitters or neurotransmitter receptors involved with most substances of abuse. Some researchers base their studies on such hypotheses. The opioids, for example, act on opioid receptors. A person with too little endogenous opioid activity (e.g., low concentrations of endorphins) or with too much activity of an endogenous opioid antagonist may be at risk for developing opioid dependence. Even in a person with completely normal endogenous receptor function and neurotransmitter concentration, the long-term use of a particular substance of abuse may eventually modulate receptor systems in the brain so that the presence of the exogenous substance is needed to maintain homeostasis. Such a receptor-level process may be the mechanism for developing tolerance within the central nervous system (CNS). Demonstrating modulation of neurotransmitter release and neurotransmitter receptor function has proved difficult, however, and recent research focuses on the effects of substances on the second-messenger system and on gene regulation.

Pathways and Neurotransmitters. The major neurotransmitters possibly involved in developing substance abuse and substance dependence are the opioid, catecholamine (particularly dopamine), and γ-aminobutyric acid (GABA) systems (Fig. 12.1–2). The dopaminergic neurons in the ventral tegmental area are particularly important. These neurons project to the cortical and limbic regions, especially the nucleus accumbens. This pathway is probably involved in the sensation of reward and may be the major mediator of the effects of such substances as amphetamine and cocaine. The locus ceruleus, the largest group of adrenergic neurons, probably mediates the effects of the opiates and the opioids. These pathways have collectively been called the *brain-reward circuitry.*

COMORBIDITY

Comorbidity is the cooccurrence of two or more psychiatric disorders in a single patient. A high prevalence of additional psychiatric disorders is found among persons seeking treatment for alcohol, cocaine, or opioid dependence. Although opioid, cocaine, and alcohol abusers with current psychiatric problems are more likely to seek treatment, those who do not seek treatment are not necessarily free of comorbid psychiatric problems; such persons may have social supports that enable them to deny the impact that drug use is having on their lives. Two large epidemiological studies have shown that even among representative samples of the population, those who meet the criteria for alcohol or drug abuse and dependence (excluding tobacco dependence) are far more likely to meet the criteria for other psychiatric disorders also.

Antisocial Personality Disorder

In various studies, a range of 35 to 60 percent of patients with substance abuse or substance dependence also meet the diagnostic criteria for antisocial personality disorder. The range is even higher when investigators include persons who meet all the antisocial personality disorder diagnostic criteria except the requirement that the symptoms started at an early age. That is, a high percentage of patients with substance abuse or substance dependence diagnoses have a pattern of antisocial behavior, whether it was present before the substance use started or developed during the course of the substance use. Patients with substance abuse or substance dependence diagnoses who have antisocial personality disorder are likely to use more illegal substances; to have more

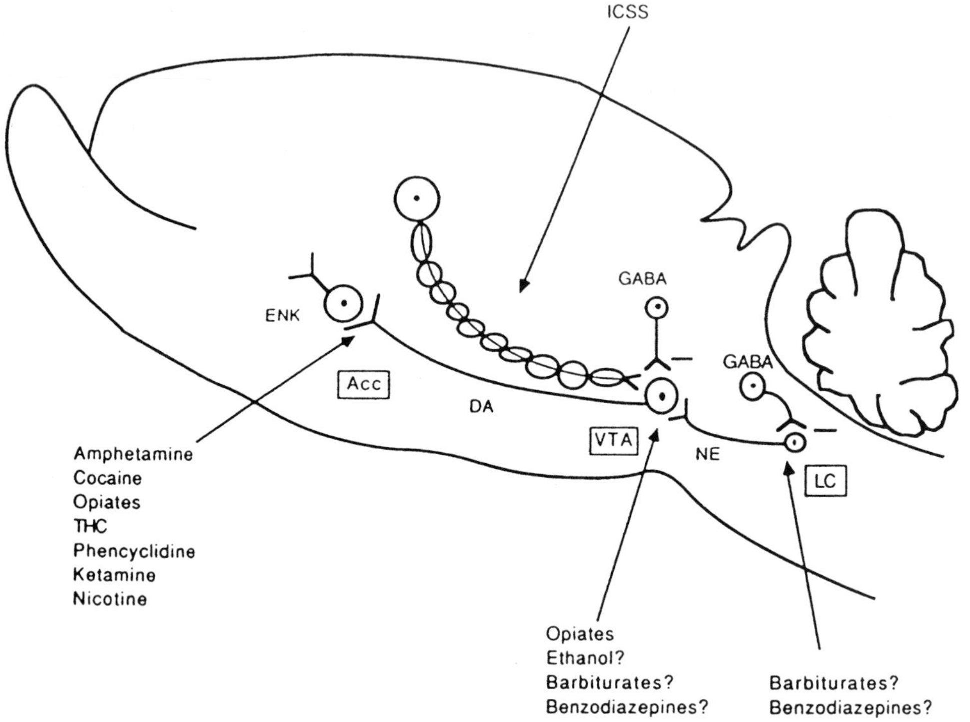

FIGURE 12.1–2

The brain-reward circuitry of the mammalian (laboratory rat) brain, with sites at which various abusable substances appear to act to enhance brain reward and thus to induce substance-using behavior and possibly craving. *ICSS*, the descending, myelinated, moderately fast-conducting component of the brain-reward circuitry that is preferentially activated by electrical intracranial self-stimulation; *DA*, the subcomponent of the ascending mesolimbic dopaminergic system that appears to be preferentially activated by abusable substances; *LC*, locus ceruleus; *VTA*, central tegmental area; *Acc*, nucleus accumbens; *ENK*, enkephalins; *NE*, noradrenergic fibers, which originate in the locus ceruleus and synapse into the general vicinity of the ventral mesencephalic DA cell fields; *GABA*, the GABAergic inhibitory fiber systems synapsing on both the locus ceruleus noradrenergic fibers and the ventral mesencephalic DA cell fields. (Reprinted with permission from Gardner E. Brain reward mechanism. In: Lowinson JH, Ruiz P, Millman RB, eds. *Substance Abuse: A Comprehensive Textbook*. 2nd ed. Baltimore: Williams & Wilkins; 1992:87.)

psychopathology; to be less satisfied with their lives; and to be more impulsive, isolated, and depressed than patients with antisocial personality disorders alone.

Depression and Suicide

Depressive symptoms are common among persons diagnosed with substance abuse or substance dependence. About one third to one half of all those with opioid abuse or opioid dependence and about 40 percent of those with alcohol abuse or alcohol dependence meet the criteria for major depressive disorder sometime during their lives. Substance use is also a major precipitating factor for suicide. Persons who abuse substances are about 20 times more likely to die by suicide than the general population. About 15 percent of persons with alcohol abuse or alcohol dependence have been reported to commit suicide. This frequency of suicide is second only to the frequency in patients with major depressive disorder.

TREATMENT AND REHABILITATION

Some persons who develop substance-related problems recover without formal treatment, especially as they age. For those patients with less severe disorders, such as nicotine addiction, relatively brief interventions are often as effective as more intensive treatments. Since these brief interventions do not change the environment, alter drug-induced brain changes, or provide new skills, a change in the patient's motivation (cognitive change) probably best explains their impact on the drug-using behavior. For those individuals who do not respond or whose dependence is more severe, a variety of interventions appear to be effective.

It is useful to distinguish among specific procedures or techniques (e.g., individual therapy, family therapy, group therapy, relapse prevention, and pharmacotherapy) and treatment programs. Most programs use a number of specific procedures and involve several professional disciplines as well as nonprofessionals who have special skills or personal experience with the substance problem being treated. The best treatment programs combine specific procedures and disciplines to meet the needs of the individual patient after a careful assessment.

There is no generally accepted classification either for the specific procedures used in treatment or for programs using various combinations of procedures. This lack of standardized terminology for categorizing procedures and programs presents a problem, even when the field of interest is narrowed from substance problems in general to treatment for a single substance, such as alcohol, tobacco, or cocaine. Except in carefully monitored research projects, even the definitions of specific procedures (e.g., individual counseling, group therapy, and methadone

maintenance) tend to be so imprecise that one usually cannot infer just what transactions are supposed to occur. Nevertheless, for descriptive purposes, programs are often broadly grouped on the basis of one or more of their salient characteristics: whether the program is aimed at merely controlling acute withdrawal and consequences of recent drug use (detoxification) or is focused on longer-term behavioral change; whether the program makes extensive use of pharmacological interventions; and the degree to which the program is based on individual psychotherapy, Alcoholics Anonymous (AA) or other 12-step principles, or therapeutic community principles. For example, government agencies recently categorized publicly funded treatment programs for drug dependence as either methadone maintenance (mostly outpatient), outpatient drug-free programs, therapeutic communities, or short-term inpatient programs.

Selecting a Treatment

Not all interventions are applicable to all varieties of substance use or dependence, and some of the more coercive interventions used for illicit drugs are not applicable to substances that are legally available, such as tobacco. Addictive behaviors do not change abruptly, but through a series of stages. Five stages in this gradual process have been proposed: precontemplation, contemplation, preparation, action, and maintenance. For some types of addictions the therapeutic alliance is enhanced when the treatment approach is tailored to the patient's stage of readiness to change. Interventions for some drug use disorders may have a specific pharmacological agent as an important component; for example, disulfiram, naltrexone (ReVia), or acamprosate for alcoholism; methadone (Dolophine), levomethadyl acetate (ORLAAM), or buprenorphine (Buprenex) for heroin addiction; and nicotine delivery devices or bupropion (Zyban) for tobacco dependence. Not all interventions are likely to be useful to health care professionals. For example, many youthful offenders with histories of drug use or dependence are now remanded to special facilities (boot camps); other programs for offenders (and sometimes for employees) rely almost exclusively on the deterrent effect of frequent urine testing; and a third group are built around religious conversion or rededication in a specific religious sect or denomination. In contrast to the numerous studies suggesting some value for brief interventions for smoking and for problem drinking, there are few controlled studies of brief interventions for those seeking treatment for dependence on illicit drugs.

In general, brief interventions (such as a few weeks of detoxification, whether in or out of a hospital) used for persons who are severely dependent on illicit opioids have limited effect on outcome measured a few months later. Substantial reductions in illicit drug use, antisocial behaviors, and psychiatric distress among patients dependent on cocaine or heroin are much more likely following treatment lasting at least 3 months. Such a time-in-treatment effect is seen across very different modalities, from residential therapeutic communities to ambulatory methadone maintenance programs. Although some patients appear to benefit from a few days or weeks of treatment, a substantial percentage of users of illicit drugs drop out (or are dropped) from treatment before they have achieved significant benefits.

Some of the variance in treatment outcomes can be attributed to differences in the characteristics of patients entering treatment and by events and conditions following treatment. However, programs based on similar philosophical principles and using what seem to be similar therapeutic procedures vary greatly in effectiveness. Some of the differences among programs that seem to be similar reflect the range and intensity of services offered. Programs with professionally trained staffs that provide more comprehensive services to patients with more severe psychiatric difficulties are more likely to be able to retain those patients in treatment and help them make positive changes. Differences in the skills of individual counselors and professionals can strongly affect outcomes.

Such generalizations concerning programs serving illicit drug users may not hold for programs dealing with those seeking treatment for alcohol, tobacco, or even cannabis problems uncomplicated by heavy use of illicit drugs. In such cases, relatively brief periods of individual or group counseling can produce long-lasting reductions in drug use. The outcomes usually considered in programs dealing with illicit drugs have typically included measures of social functioning, employment, and criminal activity, as well as decreased drug-using behavior.

Treatment of Comorbidity—Integrated versus Concurrent

The treatment of the severely mentally ill (primarily those with schizophrenia and schizoaffective disorders) who are also drug dependent continues to pose problems for clinicians. Although some special facilities have been developed that use both antipsychotic drugs and therapeutic community principles, for the most part, specialized addiction agencies have difficulty treating these patients. Generally, integrated treatment in which the same staff can treat both the psychiatric disorder and the addiction is more effective than either parallel treatment (a mental health and a specialty addiction program providing care concurrently) or sequential treatment (treating either the addiction or the psychiatric disorder first and then dealing with the comorbid condition).

Services and Outcome

The extension of managed care into the public sector has produced a major reduction in the use of hospital-based detoxification and virtual disappearance of residential rehabilitation programs for alcoholics. Unfortunately, managed-care organizations tend to assume that the relatively brief courses of outpatient counseling that are effective with private-sector alcoholic patients are also effective with patients who are dependent on illicit drugs and who have minimal social supports. For the present, the trend is to provide the care that costs least over the short term and to ignore studies showing that more services can produce better long-term outcomes.

Treatment is often a worthwhile social expenditure. For example, treatment of antisocial illicit drug users in outpatient settings can decrease antisocial behavior and reduce rates of HIV seroconversion that more than offset the treatment cost. Treatment in a prison setting can decrease postrelease costs associated with drug use and rearrests. Despite such evidence there are problems maintaining public support for treatment of substance dependence in both the public and private sectors. This lack of support suggests that these problems con-

tinue to be viewed, at least in part, as moral failings rather than as medical disorders.

ICD-10

The approach used in the 10th revision of *International Statistical Classification of Diseases and Related Health Problems* (ICD-10) differs somewhat from that in DSM-IV-TR. In the section titled "Mental and Behavioral Disorders Due to Psychoactive Substance Use," the term *psychoactive substance* refers to alcohol, opioids, cannabinoids, sedatives and hypnotics, cocaine, other stimulants such as caffeine, hallucinogens, tobacco, volatile solvents, multiple drugs, and other psychoactive substances (Table 12.1–9). Thus, solvents are considered psychoactive, although their accidental ingestion is not mentioned. ICD-10 does not distinguish between legal and illegal substances but stipulates that the substances may or may not have been medically prescribed.

The disorders related to psychoactive substance use are described as mental and behavioral, with diagnostic guidelines provided for identifying the substance and for determining the specific nature of the disorder. When appropriate, references to other categories are given. For instance, under *psychotic disorder* in the substance use section, ICD-10 mentions schizophrenia, mood disorder, and paranoid or schizoid personality disorder as possible diagnoses for mental disorders "aggravated or precipitated by psychoactive substance use." In addition, ICD-10 includes a separate category for non–dependence-producing substances (Table 12.1–10), including antidepressants, laxatives, analgesics, and vitamins, among others. DSM-IV-TR does not contain a similar category.

Table 12.1–9
ICD-10 Diagnostic Criteria for Mental and Behavioral Disorders Due to Psychoactive Substance Use

Mental and behavioral disorders due to use of alcohol
Mental and behavioral disorders due to use of opioids
Mental and behavioral disorders due to use of cannabinoids
Mental and behavioral disorders due to use of sedatives or hypnotics
Mental and behavioral disorders due to use of cocaine
Mental and behavioral disorders due to use of other stimulants, including caffeine
Mental and behavioral disorders due to use of hallucinogens
Mental and behavioral disorders due to use of tobacco
Mental and behavioral disorders due to use of volatile solvents
Mental and behavioral disorders due to multiple drug use and use of other psychoactive substances

Acute intoxication

G1. There must be clear evidence of recent use of a psychoactive substance (or substances) at sufficiently high dose levels to be consistent with intoxication.

G2. There must be symptoms or signs of intoxication compatible with the known actions of the particular substance (or substances), as specified below, and of sufficient severity to produce disturbances in the level of consciousness cognition, perception, affect, or behavior that are of clinical importance.

G3. The symptoms or signs present cannot be accounted for by a medical disorder unrelated to substance use, and are not better accounted for by another mental or behavioral disorder.

Acute intoxication frequently occurs in persons who have more persistent alcohol- or drug-related problems in addition. Where there are such problems, e.g., harmful use, dependence syndrome, or psychotic disorder, they should also be recorded.

The following may be used to indicate whether the acute intoxication was associated with any complications:

Uncomplicated
Symptoms are of varying severity, usually dose dependent
With trauma or other bodily injury
With other medical complications
Examples are hematemesis, inhalation of vomit
With delirium
With perceptual distortions
With coma
With convulsions
Pathological intoxication

Applies only to alcohol

Acute intoxication due to use of alcohol

A. The general criteria for acute intoxication must be met.

B. There must be dysfunctional behavior, as evidenced by at least one of the following:
   (1) disinhibition
   (2) argumentativeness
   (3) aggression
   (4) lability of mood
   (5) impaired attention
   (6) impaired judgment
   (7) interference with personal functioning

C. At least one of the following signs must be present:
   (1) unsteady gait
   (2) difficulty in standing
   (3) slurred speech
   (4) nystagmus
   (5) decreased level of consciousness (e.g., stupor, coma)
   (6) flushed face
   (7) conjunctival injection

Comment

When severe, acute alcohol intoxication may be accompanied by hypotension, hypothermia, and depression of the gag reflex. If desired, the blood alcohol level may be specified.

Pathological alcohol intoxication

Note. The status of this condition is being examined. These research criteria must be regarded as tentative.

A. The general criteria for acute intoxication must be met, with the exception that pathological intoxication occurs after drinking amounts of alcohol insufficient to cause intoxication in most people.

B. There is verbally aggressive or physically violent behavior that is not typical of the person when sober.

C. The intoxication occurs very soon (usually a few minutes) after consumption of alcohol.

D. There is no evidence of organic cerebral disorder or other mental disorders.

Comment

This is an uncommon condition. The blood alcohol levels found in this disorder are lower than those that would cause acute intoxication in most people, i.e., below 40 mg/100 mL.

(*continued*)

Table 12.1–9 (*continued*)

Acute intoxication due to use of opioids

A. The general criteria for acute intoxication must be met.

B. There must be dysfunctional behavior, as evidenced by at least one of the following:

(1) apathy and sedation
(2) disinhibition
(3) psychomotor retardation
(4) impaired attention
(5) impaired judgment
(6) interference with personal functioning

C. At least one of the following signs must be present:

(1) drowsiness
(2) slurred speech
(3) pupillary constriction (except in anoxia from severe overdose, when pupillary dilatation occurs)
(4) decreased level of consciousness (e.g., stupor, coma)

Comment

When severe, acute opioid intoxication may be accompanied by respiratory depression (and hypoxia), hypotension, and hypothermia.

Acute intoxication due to use of cannabinoids

A. The general criteria for acute intoxication must be met.

B. There must be dysfunctional behavior or perceptual abnormalities, including at least one of the following:

(1) euphoria and disinhibition
(2) anxiety or agitation
(3) suspiciousness or paranoid ideation
(4) temporal slowing (a sense that time is passing very slowly, and/or the person is experiencing a rapid flow of ideas)
(5) impaired judgment
(6) impaired attention
(7) impaired reaction time
(8) auditory, visual, or tactile illusions
(9) hallucinations with preserved orientation
(10) depersonalization
(11) derealization
(12) interference with personal functioning

C. At least one of the following signs must be present:

(1) increased appetite
(2) dry mouth
(3) conjunctival injection
(4) tachycardia

Acute intoxication due to use of sedatives or hypnotics

A. The general criteria for acute intoxication must be met.

B. There is dysfunctional behavior, as evidenced by at least one of the following:

(1) euphoria and disinhibition
(2) apathy and sedation
(3) abusiveness or aggression
(4) lability of mood
(5) impaired attention
(6) anterograde amnesia
(7) impaired psychomotor performance
(8) interference with personal functioning

C. At least one of the following signs must be present:

(1) unsteady gait
(2) difficulty in standing
(3) slurred speech
(4) nystagmus
(5) decreased level of consciousness (e.g., stupor, coma)
(6) erythematous skin lesions or blisters

Comment

When severe, acute intoxication from sedative or hypnotic drugs may be accompanied by hypotension, hypothermia, and depression of the gag reflex.

Acute intoxication due to use of cocaine

A. The general criteria for acute intoxication must be met.

B. There must be dysfunctional behavior or perceptual abnormalities, as evidenced by at least one of the following:

(1) euphoria and sensation of increased energy
(2) hypervigilance
(3) grandiose beliefs or actions
(4) abusiveness or aggression
(5) argumentativeness
(6) lability of mood
(7) repetitive stereotyped behaviors
(8) auditory, visual, or tactile illusions
(9) hallucinations, usually with intact orientation
(10) paranoid ideation
(11) interference with personal functioning

C. At least two of the following signs must be present:

(1) tachycardia (sometimes bradycardia)
(2) cardiac arrhythmias
(3) hypertension (sometimes hypotension)
(4) sweating and chills
(5) nausea or vomiting
(6) evidence of weight loss
(7) pupillary dilatation
(8) psychomotor agitation (sometimes retardation)
(9) muscular weakness
(10) chest pain
(11) convulsions

Comment

Interference with personal functioning is most readily apparent from the social interactions of cocaine users, which range from extreme gregariousness to social withdrawal.

Acute intoxication due to use of other stimulants, including caffeine

A. The general criteria for acute intoxication must be met.

B. There must be dysfunctional behavior or perceptual abnormalities, as evidenced by at least one of the following:

(1) euphoria and sensation of increased energy
(2) hypervigilance
(3) grandiose beliefs or actions
(4) abusiveness or aggression
(5) argumentativeness
(6) lability of mood
(7) repetitive stereotyped behaviors
(8) auditory, visual, or tactile illusions
(9) hallucinations, usually with intact orientation
(10) paranoid ideation
(11) interference with personal functioning

(*continued*)

Table 12.1–9 (*continued*)

C. At least two of the following signs must be present:
  (1) tachycardia (sometimes bradycardia)
  (2) cardiac arrhythmias
  (3) hypertension (sometimes hypotension)
  (4) sweating and chills
  (5) nausea or vomiting
  (6) evidence of weight loss
  (7) pupillary dilatation
  (8) psychomotor agitation (sometimes retardation)
  (9) muscular weakness
  (10) chest pain
  (11) convulsions

Comment

Interference with personal functioning is most readily apparent from the social interactions of the substance users, which range from extreme gregariousness to social withdrawal.

Acute intoxication due to use of hallucinogens

A. The general criteria for acute intoxication must be met.
B. There must be dysfunctional behavior or perceptual abnormalities, as evidenced by at least one of the following:
  (1) anxiety and fearfulness
  (2) auditory, visual, or tactile illusions or hallucinations occurring in a state of full wakefulness and alertness
  (3) depersonalization
  (4) derealization
  (5) paranoid ideation
  (6) ideas of reference
  (7) lability of mood
  (8) hyperactivity
  (9) impulsive acts
  (10) impaired attention
  (11) interference with personal functioning
C. At least two of the following signs must be present:
  (1) tachycardia
  (2) palpitations
  (3) sweating and chills
  (4) tremor
  (5) blurring of vision
  (6) pupillary dilatation
  (7) incoordination

Acute intoxication due to use of tobacco [acute nicotine intoxication]

A. The general criteria for acute intoxication must be met.
B. There must be dysfunctional behavior or perceptual abnormalities, as evidenced by at least one of the following:
  (1) insomnia
  (2) bizarre dreams
  (3) lability of mood
  (4) derealization
  (5) interference with personal functioning
C. At least one of the following signs must be present:
  (1) nausea or vomiting
  (2) sweating
  (3) tachycardia
  (4) cardiac arrhythmias

Acute intoxication due to use of volatile solvents

A. The general criteria for acute intoxication must be met.
B. There must be dysfunctional behavior, evidenced by at least one of the following:
  (1) apathy and lethargy
  (2) argumentativeness
  (3) abusiveness or aggression
  (4) lability of mood
  (5) impaired judgment
  (6) impaired attention and memory
  (7) psychomotor retardation
  (8) interference with personal functioning
C. At least one of the following signs must be present:
  (1) unsteady gait
  (2) difficulty in standing
  (3) slurred speech
  (4) nystagmus
  (5) decreased level of consciousness (e.g., stupor, coma)
  (6) muscle weakness
  (7) blurred vision or diplopia

Comment

Acute intoxication from inhalation of substances other than solvents should also be coded here.

When severe, acute intoxication from volatile solvents may be accompanied by hypotension, hypothermia, and depression of the gag reflex.

Acute intoxication due to multiple drug use and use of other psychoactive substances

This category should be used when there is evidence of intoxication caused by recent use of other psychoactive substances (e.g., phencyclidine) or of multiple psychoactive substances where it is uncertain which substance has predominated.

Harmful use

A. There must be clear evidence that the substance use was responsible for (or substantially contributed to) physical or psychological harm, including impaired judgment or dysfunctional behavior, which may lead to disability or have adverse consequences for interpersonal relationships.
B. The nature of the harm should be clearly identifiable (and specified).
C. The pattern of use has persisted for at least 1 month or has occurred repeatedly within a 12-month period.
D. The disorder does not meet the criteria for any other mental or behavioral disorder related to the same drug in the same time period (except for acute intoxication).

Dependence syndrome

A. Three or more of the following manifestations should have occurred together for at least 1 month or, if persisting for periods of less than 1 month, should have occurred together repeatedly within a 12-month period:
  (1) a strong desire or sense of compulsion to take the substance
  (2) impaired capacity to control substance-taking behavior in terms of its onset, termination, or levels of use, as evidenced by: the substance being often taken in larger amounts or over a longer period than intended; or by a persistent desire or unsuccessful efforts to reduce or control substance use

(*continued*)

Table 12.1–9 (*continued*)

(3) a physiological withdrawal state when substance use is reduced or ceased, as evidenced by the characteristic withdrawal syndrome for the substance, or by use of the same (or closely related) substance with the intention of relieving or avoiding withdrawal symptoms

(4) evidence of tolerance to the effects of the substance, such that there is a need for significantly increased amounts of the substance to achieve intoxication or the desired effect, or a marked diminished effect with continued use of the same amount of the substance

(5) preoccupation with substance use, as manifested by important alternative pleasures or interests being given up or reduced because of substance use; or a great deal of time being spent in activities necessary to obtain, take, or recover from the effects of the substance

(6) persistent substance use despite clear evidence of harmful consequences, as evidenced by continued use when the individual is actually aware, or may be expected to be aware, of the nature and extent of harm

Diagnosis of the dependence syndrome may be further specified by the following:

Currently abstinent

Early remission

Partial remission

Full remission

Currently abstinent but in a protected environment (e.g., in a hospital, in a therapeutic community, in prison, etc.)

Currently on a clinically supervised maintenance or replacement regime (controlled dependence) (e.g., with methadone; nicotine gum or nicotine patch)

Currently abstinent, but receiving treatment with aversive or blocking drugs (e.g., naltrexone or disulfiram)

Currently using the substance (active dependence)

Without physical features

With physical features

The course of the dependence may be further specified, if desired, as follows:

Continuous use

Episodic use (dipsomania)

Withdrawal state

G1. There must be clear evidence of recent cessation or reduction of substance use after repeated, and usually prolonged and/or high-dose, use of that substance.

G2. Symptoms and signs are compatible with the known features of a withdrawal state from the particular substance or substances (see below).

G3. Symptoms and signs are not accounted for by a medical disorder unrelated to substance use, and not better accounted for by another mental or behavioral disorder.

The diagnosis of withdrawal state may be further specified by using the following:

Uncomplicated

With convulsions

Alcohol withdrawal state

A. The general criteria for withdrawal state must be met.

B. Any three of the following signs must be present:

(1) tremor of the tongue, eyelids, or outstretched hands

(2) sweating

(3) nausea, retching, or vomiting

(4) tachycardia or hypertension

(5) psychomotor agitation

(6) headache

(7) insomnia

(8) malaise or weakness

(9) transient visual, tactile, or auditory hallucinations or illusions

(10) grand mal convulsions

Comment

If delirium is present, the diagnosis should be alcohol withdrawal state with delirium (delirium tremens).

A. The general criteria for withdrawal state must be met. (Note that an opioid withdrawal state may also be induced by administration of an opioid antagonist after a brief period of opioid use.)

B. Any three of the following signs must be present:

(1) craving for an opioid drug

(2) rhinorrhea or sneezing

(3) lacrimation

(4) muscle aches or cramps

(5) abdominal cramps

(6) nausea or vomiting

(7) diarrhea

(8) pupillary dilatation

(9) piloerection, or recurrent chills

(10) tachycardia or hypertension

(11) yawning

(12) restless sleep

Cannabinoid withdrawal state

Note. This is an ill-defined syndrome for which definitive diagnostic criteria cannot be established at the present time. It occurs following cessation of prolonged high-dose use of cannabis. It has been reported variously as lasting from several hours to up to 7 days.

Symptoms and signs include anxiety, irritability, tremor of the outstretched hands, sweating, and muscle aches.

Sedative or hypnotic withdrawal state

A. The general criteria for withdrawal state must be met.

B. Any three of the following signs must be present:

(1) tremor of the tongue, eyelids, or outstretched hands

(2) nausea or vomiting

(3) tachycardia

(4) postural hypotension

(5) psychomotor agitation

(6) headache

(7) insomnia

(8) malaise or weakness

(9) transient visual, tactile, or auditory hallucinations or illusions

(10) paranoid ideation

(11) grand mal convulsions

Comment

If delirium is present, the diagnosis should be sedative or hypnotic withdrawal state with delirium.

(*continued*)

Table 12.1–9 (*continued*)

Cocaine withdrawal state

A. The general criteria for withdrawal state must be met.

B. There is dysphoric mood (e.g., sadness or anhedonia).

C. Any two of the following signs must be present:

(1) lethargy and fatigue
(2) psychomotor retardation or agitation
(3) craving for cocaine
(4) increased appetite
(5) insomnia or hypersomnia
(6) bizarre or unpleasant dreams

Withdrawal state from other stimulants, including caffeine

A. The general criteria for withdrawal state must be met.

B. There is dysphoric mood (e.g., sadness or anhedonia).

C. Any two of the following signs must be present:

(1) lethargy and fatigue
(2) psychomotor retardation or agitation
(3) craving for stimulant drugs
(4) increased appetite
(5) insomnia or hypersomnia
(6) bizarre or unpleasant dreams

Hallucinogen withdrawal state

Note: There is no recognized hallucinogen withdrawal state.

Tobacco withdrawal state

A. The general criteria for withdrawal state must be met.

B. Any two of the following signs must be present:

(1) craving for tobacco (or other nicotine-containing products)
(2) malaise or weakness
(3) anxiety
(4) dysphoric mood
(5) irritability or restlessness
(6) insomnia
(7) increased appetite
(8) increased cough
(9) mouth ulceration
(10) difficulty in concentrating

Volatile solvents withdrawal state

Note: There is inadequate information on withdrawal states from volatile solvents for research to be formulated.

Multiple drug withdrawal state

Withdrawal state with delirium

A. The general criteria for withdrawal state must be met.

B. The criteria for delirium must be met.

The diagnosis of withdrawal state with delirium may be further specified by using the following:

Without convulsions

With convulsions

Psychotic disorder

A. Onset of psychotic symptoms must occur during or within 2 weeks of substance use.

B. The psychotic symptoms must persist for more than 48 hours.

C. Duration of the disorder must not exceed 6 months.

The diagnosis of psychotic disorder may be further specified by using the following:

Schizophrenialike

Predominantly delusional

Predominantly hallucinatory

Predominantly polymorphic

Predominantly depressive symptoms

Predominantly manic symptoms

Mixed

For research purposes it is recommended that change of the disorder from a nonpsychotic to a clearly psychotic state be further specified as either abrupt (onset within 48 hours) or acute (onset in more than 48 hours but less than 2 weeks).

Amnesic syndrome

A. Memory impairment is manifest in both:

(1) a defect of recent memory (impaired learning of new material) to a degree sufficient to interfere with daily living
(2) a reduced ability to recall past experiences

B. All of the following are absent (or relatively absent):

(1) defect in immediate recall (as tested, for example, by the digit span)
(2) clouding of consciousness and disturbance of attention, as defined in delirium, not induced by alcohol and other psychoactive substances, Criterion A
(3) global intellectual decline (dementia).

C. There is no objective evidence from physical and neurological examination, laboratory tests, or history of a disorder or disease of the brain (especially involving bilaterally the diencephalic and medial temporal structures), other than that related to substance use, that can reasonably be presumed to be responsible for the clinical manifestations described under Criterion A.

Residual and late-onset psychotic disorder

A. Conditions and disorders meeting the criteria for the individual syndromes listed below should be clearly related to substance use. Where onset of the condition or disorder occurs subsequent to use of psychoactive substances, strong evidence should be provided to demonstrate a link.

Comments

In view of the considerable variation in this category, the characteristics of such residual states or conditions should be clearly documented in terms of their type, severity, and duration. For research purposes full descriptive details should be specified.

If required, use as follows:

Flashbacks

Personality or behavior disorder

B. The general criteria for personality and behavioral disorder due to brain disease, damage and dysfunction must be met.

Residual affective disorder

B. The criteria for organic mood (affective) disorder must be met.

Dementia

B. The general criteria for dementia must be met.

Other persisting cognitive impairment

B. The criteria for mild cognitive disorder must be met, except for the exclusion of psychoactive substance use in Criterion D.

Late-onset psychotic disorder

B. The general criteria for psychotic disorder must be met, except with regard to the onset of the disorder, which is more than 2 weeks but not more than 6 weeks after substance use.

Other mental and behavioral disorders

Unspecified mental and behavioral disorder

Table 12.1–10
ICD-10 Diagnostic Criteria for Abuse of Non–Dependence-Producing Substances

A wide variety of medicaments and folk remedies may be involved, but the particularly important groups are: psychotropic drugs that do not produce dependence, such as antidepressants; laxatives; and analgesics that may be purchased without medical prescription, such as aspirin and paracetamol. Although the medication may have been medically prescribed or recommended in the first instance, prolonged, unnecessary, and often excessive dosage develops, which is facilitated by the availability of the substances without medical prescription.

Persistent and unjustified use of these substances is usually associated with unnecessary expense, often involves unnecessary contacts with medical professionals or supporting staff, and is sometimes marked by the harmful physical effects of the substances. Attempts to discourage or forbid the use of the substance are often met with resistance; for laxatives and analgesics this may be in spite of warnings about (or even the development of) physical harm such as renal dysfunction or electrolyte disturbances. Although it is usually clear that the patient has a strong motivation to take the substance, no dependence or withdrawal symptoms develop as in the case of the psychoactive substances specified in mental and behavioral disorders due to psychoactive substance use.

Identify the type of substance involved:

Antidepressants
(such as tricyclic and tetracyclic antidepressants and monoamine oxidase inhibitors)

Laxatives

Analgesics
(such as aspirin, paracetamol, phenacetin, not specified as psychoactive mental and behavioral disorders due to psychoactive substance use)

Antacids

Vitamins

Steroids or hormones

Specific herbal or folk remedies

Other substances that do not produce dependence
(such as diuretics)

Unspecified

Reprinted with permission from World Health Organization. *The ICD-10 Classification of Mental and Behavioural Disorders: Diagnostic Criteria for Research.* Copyright, World Health Organization, Geneva, 1993.

The sections that follow deal with substances of abuse according to the particular drug (e.g., alcohol, caffeine) and discuss their diagnosis, etiology, pharmacology, and treatment in depth.

References

Akil H, Owens C, Gutstein H, Taylor L, Curran E, Watson S. Endogenous opioids: overview and current issues. *Drug Alcohol Depend.* 1998;51:127.

Anglin MD, Hser Y-I, Grella CE. Drug addiction and treatment careers among clients in the Drug Abuse Treatment Outcome Study (DATOS). *Psychol Addict Behav.* 1997;11:308.

Baumohl J, Jaffe JH. History of alcohol and drug abuse treatment in the United States. In Jaffe JH, ed. *Encyclopedia of Drugs and Alcohol.* Vol 3. New York: Macmillan; 1995:432.

Beirut LJ, Dinwiddie SH, Begleiter H, et al. Familial transmission of substance dependence: alcohol, marijuana, cocaine, and habitual smoking. *Arch Gen Psychiatry.* 1998;55:982.

Gerstein DR, Harwood HJ, eds. *Treating Drug Problems.* Vol 1. Committee for the Substance Abuse Coverage Study, Division of Health Care Services, Institute of Medicine. Washington, DC: National Academy Press; 1990.

Goldman D, Bergen A. General and specific inheritance of substance abuse and alcoholism. *Arch Gen Psychiatry.* 1998;55:964.

Harrison PA, Fulkerson JA, Beebe TJ. DSM-IV substance use disorder criteria for adolescents: a critical examination based on a statewide school survey. *Am J Psychiatry.* 1998;155:486.

Institute of Medicine. *Broadening the Base of Treatment for Alcohol Problems.* Washington, DC: National Academy Press; 1990.

Institute of Medicine. *Pathways of Addiction.* Washington, DC: National Academy Press; 1996.

Inturrisi CE. Preclinical evidence for a role of glutamatergic systems in opioid tolerance and dependence. *Semin Neurosci.* 1997;9:110.

Jaffe JH. Substance-related disorders: introduction and overview. In: Sadock BJ, Sadock VA, eds. *Kaplan & Sadock's Comprehensive Textbook of Psychiatry.* 7th ed. Vol 1. Baltimore: Lippincott Williams & Wilkins; 2000:924.

Jaffe JH, Knapp CM, Ciraulo DA. Opiates: clinical aspects. In: Lowinson JH, Ruiz P, Millman RB, Langrod JG, eds. *Substance Abuse: A Comprehensive Textbook.* 3rd ed. Baltimore: Williams & Wilkins; 1997.

Johnston LD, O'Malley PM, Bachman JG. *National Survey Results on Drug Use from the Monitoring the Future Study. College Students and Young Adults.* Rockville, MD: National Institute on Drug Abuse; 1999.

Prescott CA, Kendler KS. Genetic and environmental contributions to alcohol abuse and dependence in a population-based sample of male twins. *Am J Psychiatry.* 1999;156:34.

Project MATCH Research Group. Matching alcoholism treatment to client heterogeneity: Project MATCH posttreatment drinking outcomes. *J Stud Alcohol.* 1997;58:2.

Simkin DR. Adolescent substance abuse disorders and comorbidity. *Pediatr Clin North Am.* 2002;49:463.

Staines GL, Magura S, Foote J, Deluca A, Kosanke N. Polysubstance use among alcoholics. *J Addict Dis.* 2001;20:53.

Substance Abuse and Mental Health Services Administration Office of Applied Studies. Preliminary Results from the 1996 National Household Survey on Drug Abuse. National Household Survey on Drug Abuse series: H-3. DHHS publ no. (SMA) 97–3149. Rockville, MD: SAMHSA, Office of Applied Studies; 1997.

Tucker, JA, Vuchinich RE, Murphy G. Substance use disorders. In: Antony MM, Barlow DH, ed. *Handbook of Assessment and Treatment Planning for Psychological Disorders.* New York: Guilford Press; 2002:415.

Uhl GR. Molecular genetics of substance abuse vulnerability: a current approach. *Neuropsychopharmacology.* 1999;20:1.

Wise RA. Drug-activation of brain reward pathways. *Drug Alcohol Depend.* 1998;51:13.

▲ 12.2 Alcohol-Related Disorders

An understanding of the effects of alcohol and the clinical importance of alcohol-related disorders is essential for the practice of psychiatry. Alcohol intoxication can cause irritability, violent behavior, feelings of depression, and, in rare instances, hallucinations and delusions. Longer-term, escalating levels of alcohol consumption can produce tolerance as well as such intense adaptation of the body that cessation of use can precipitate a withdrawal syndrome usually marked by insomnia, evidence of hyperactivity of the autonomic nervous system, and feelings of anxiety. Thus, in an adequate evaluation of life problems and psychiatric symptoms in a patient the clinician must consider the possibility that the clinical situation reflects the effects of alcohol.

Although alcohol abuse and dependency are commonly called *alcoholism,* the text revision of the fourth edition of the *Diagnostic and Statistical Manual of Mental Disorders* (DSM-IV-TR) does not use the term because it lacks a precise definition. Table 12.2–1 lists various categories and definitions of alcohol use.

EPIDEMIOLOGY

Drinking alcohol-containing beverages is generally considered an acceptable and common habit in the United States. About 90

Table 12.2–1
Categories and Definitions for Patterns of Alcohol Use

Category	Definition	Organization
Moderate drinking	Men, ≤2 drinks/d Women, ≤1 drink/d Persons >65 years of age, ≤1 drink/d	NIAAA
At-risk drinking	Men, >14 drinks/wk or >4 drinks per occasion Women, >7 drinks/wk or >3 drinks per occasion	NIAAA
Hazardous drinking	At risk for adverse consequences from alcohol	WHO
Harmful drinking	Alcohol causing physical or psychological harm	WHO
Alcohol abuse	≤1 of the following events in a year: recurrent use resulting in failure to fulfill major role obligations, recurrent use in hazardous situations, recurrent alcohol-related legal problems (e.g., citations for driving under the influence), continued use despite social or interpersonal problems caused or exacerbated by alcohol	APA
Alcohol dependence	≤3 of the following events in a year: tolerance; increased amounts to achieve effect; diminished effects from same amount; withdrawal; a great deal of time spent obtaining alcohol, using it, or recovering from its effects; important activities given up or reduced because of alcohol; drinking more or longer than intended; persistent desire or unsuccessful efforts to cut down or control alcohol use; continued use despite knowledge of a psychological problem caused or exacerbated by alcohol	APA

From Fiellin DA, Reid C, O'Connor PG. Outpatient management of patients with alcohol problems. *Ann Intern Med.* 2000;133:815.

percent of all U.S. residents have had an alcohol-containing drink at least once in their lives, and about 51 percent of all U.S. adults are current users of alcohol. After heart disease and cancer, alcohol-related disorders constitute the third largest health problem in the United States today; beer accounts for about one half of all alcohol consumption, liquor for about one third, and wine for about one sixth. About 30 to 45 percent of all adults in the United States have had at least one transient episode of an alcohol-related problem, usually an alcohol-induced amnestic episode like a blackout, driving a motor vehicle while intoxicated, or missing school or work because of excessive drinking. About 10 percent of women and 20 percent of men have met the diagnostic criteria for alcohol abuse during their lifetimes, and 3 to 5 percent of women and 10 percent of men have met the diagnostic criteria for the more serious diagnosis of alcohol dependence during their lifetimes. About 200,000 deaths each year are directly related to alcohol abuse. The common causes of death among persons with the alcohol-related disorders are suicide, cancer, heart disease, and hepatic disease. Although persons involved in automotive fatalities do not always meet the diagnostic criteria for an alcohol-related disorder, drunken drivers are involved in about 50 percent of all automotive fatalities, and this percentage increases to about 75 percent when only accidents occurring in the late evening are considered. Alcohol use and alcohol-related disorders are also associated with about 50 percent of all homicides and 25 percent of all suicides. Alcohol abuse reduces life expectancy by about 10 years, and alcohol leads all other substance in substance-related deaths.

Race and Ethnicity

Compared with other groups, whites have the highest rate of alcohol use, 56 percent. Rates for Hispanics and blacks are similar. The rate of binge use is lower among blacks than among whites and Hispanics. Heavy use shows no statistically significant differences by race or ethnicity (5.7 percent for whites, 6.3 percent for Hispanics, and 4.6 percent for blacks).

Gender

Sixty percent of men are past-month alcohol users, compared with 45 percent of women. Men are much more likely than women to be binge drinkers (23.8 and 8.5 percent, respectively) and heavy drinkers (9.4 and 2.0 percent, respectively).

Region and Urbanicity

The rate of current alcohol use was 59 percent in the North Central region, 54 percent in the Northeast region, 53 percent in the West, and 47 percent in the South in 1995. Rates of binge use were 20 percent in the North Central region, 16 percent in the West, and 14 percent in the South and Northeast. Heavy alcohol use rates were 7.0 percent in the North Central region, 5.6 percent in the West, 4.9 percent in the Northeast, and 4.8 percent in the South. The rate of past month alcohol use was 56 percent in large metropolitan areas, 52 percent in small metropolitan areas, and 46 percent in nonmetropolitan areas. There was little variation in binge and heavy alcohol use rates by population density.

Education

In contrast to the pattern for illicit drugs, the higher the educational attainment, the more likely is the current use of alcohol. About 70 percent of adults with college degrees are current drinkers, compared with only 40 percent of those with less than a high school education. Binge alcohol use rates are similar across different levels of education. The rate of heavy alcohol use, however, is 4 percent among adults who had completed college and 7 percent among adults who had not completed high school.

Socioeconomic Class

Alcohol-related disorders appear among persons of all socioeconomic classes. In fact, persons who are stereotypical skid-row alcoholics constitute less than 5 percent of those with alcohol-related disorders

in the United States. Moreover, these disorders are particularly frequent in persons with advanced academic degrees and upper socioeconomic standing.

Among high school students, alcohol-related problems are correlated with a history of school difficulties. High school dropouts and persons with a record of frequent truancy and delinquency appear to be at particularly high risk for alcohol abuse. These epidemiological data are consistent with the high comorbidity between alcohol-related disorders and antisocial personality disorder.

COMORBIDITY

The psychiatric diagnoses most commonly associated with the alcohol-related disorders are other substance-related disorders, antisocial personality disorder, mood disorders, and anxiety disorders. Although the data are somewhat controversial, most suggest that persons with alcohol-related disorders have a markedly higher suicide rate than the general population.

Antisocial Personality Disorder

A relation between antisocial personality disorder and alcohol-related disorders has frequently been reported. Some studies have suggested that antisocial personality disorder is particularly common in men with an alcohol-related disorder and can precede the development of the alcohol-related disorder. Other studies, however, have suggested that antisocial personality disorder and alcohol-related disorders are completely distinct entities that are not causally related.

Mood Disorders

About 30 to 40 percent of persons with an alcohol-related disorder meet the diagnostic criteria for major depressive disorder sometime during their lifetimes. Depression is more common in women than in men with these disorders. Several studies reported that depression is likely to occur in patients with alcohol-related disorders who have a high daily consumption of alcohol and a family history of alcohol abuse. Persons with alcohol-related disorders and major depressive disorder are at great risk for attempting suicide and are likely to have other substance-related disorder diagnoses. Some clinicians recommend that depressive symptoms that remain after 2 to 3 weeks of sobriety be treated with antidepressant drugs. Patients with bipolar I disorder are thought to be at risk for developing an alcohol-related disorder; they may use alcohol to self-medicate their manic episodes. Some studies have shown that persons with both alcohol-related disorder and depressive disorder diagnoses have concentrations of dopamine metabolites (homovanillic acid) and γ-aminobutyric acid (GABA) in their cerebrospinal fluid (CSF).

Anxiety Disorders

Many persons use alcohol for its efficacy in alleviating anxiety. Although the comorbidity between alcohol-related disorders and mood disorders is fairly widely recognized, it is less well known that perhaps 25 to 50 percent of all persons with alcohol-related disorders also meet the diagnostic criteria for an anxiety disorder. Phobias and panic disorder are particularly frequent comorbid diagnoses in these patients. Some data indicate that alcohol may be used in an attempt to self-medicate symptoms of agoraphobia or social phobia, but an alcohol-related disorder is likely to precede the development of panic disorder or generalized anxiety disorder.

Suicide

Most estimates of the prevalence of suicide among persons with alcohol-related disorders range from 10 to 15 percent, although alcohol use itself may be involved in a much higher percentage of suicides. Some investigators have questioned whether the suicide rate among persons with alcohol-related disorders is as high as the numbers suggest. Factors that have been associated with suicide among persons with alcohol-related disorders include the presence of a major depressive episode, weak psychosocial support systems, a serious coexisting medical condition, unemployment, and living alone.

ETIOLOGY

Alcohol-related disorders, like virtually all other psychiatric conditions, probably represent a heterogeneous group of disease processes. In any individual case, psychosocial, genetic, or behavioral factors may be more important than other factors. Within any single set of factors, such as biological factors, one element, such as a neurotransmitter receptor gene, may be more critically involved than another element, such as a neurotransmitter uptake pump. Except for research purposes, it is not necessary to identify the single causative factor; treating alcohol-related disorders requires taking whatever approaches are effective, regardless of theory.

Childhood History

Researchers have identified several factors in the childhood histories of persons with later alcohol-related disorders and in children at high risk for having an alcohol-related disorder because one or both of their parents are affected. In experimental studies, children at high risk for alcohol-related disorders have been found to possess, on average, a range of deficits on neurocognitive testing, low amplitude of the P300 wave on evoked potential testing, and a variety of abnormalities on electroencephalogram (EEG) recordings. Studies of high-risk offspring in their 20s have also shown a generally blunted effect of alcohol compared that seen in persons whose parents have not been diagnosed with alcohol-related disorder. These findings suggest that a heritable biological brain function may predispose a person to an alcohol-related disorder. A childhood history of attention-deficit/hyperactivity disorder or conduct disorder or both increases a child's risk for an alcohol-related disorder as an adult. Personality disorders, especially antisocial personality disorder, as noted above, also predispose a person to an alcohol-related disorder.

Psychodynamic Theories

Psychodynamic theories of alcohol-related disorders have centered on hypotheses about overly punitive superegos and fixation at the oral stage of psychosexual development. According to psychoanalytic theory, persons with harsh superegos who are self-punitive turn to alcohol as a way of diminishing unconscious stress. Anxiety in persons fixated at the oral stage may be reduced by taking substances, such as alcohol, by mouth.

Some psychodynamic psychiatrists describe the general personality of a person with an alcohol-related disorder as shy, isolated, impatient, irritable, anxious, hypersensitive, and sexually repressed. According to a common psychoanalytic aphorism, the superego is soluble in alcohol. On a less theoretical level, alcohol may be abused by some persons to reduce tension, anxiety, and psychic pain. Alcohol consumption can also lead to a sense of power and increased self-worth.

Sociocultural Theories

Some social settings commonly lead to excessive drinking. College dormitories and military bases are two such examples; in these settings, excessive and frequent drinking is often completely normal and socially expected. Colleges and universities have recently tried to educate students about the health risks of drinking large quantities of alcohol. Some cultural and ethnic groups are more restrained than others about alcohol consumption. For example, Asians and conservative Protestants use alcohol less frequently than do liberal Protestants and Catholics.

Behavioral and Learning Factors

Just as cultural factors can affect drinking habits, so can the habits within a family, specifically, parental drinking habits. Some evidence indicates, however, that familial drinking habits that affect children's drinking habits are less directly linked to development of alcohol-related disorders than was previously thought. From a behavioral viewpoint, the positive reinforcing aspects of alcohol can induce feelings of well-being and euphoria and can reduce fear and anxiety, which may further encourage drinking.

Genetic Theories

The best supported biological theory of alcoholism centers on genetics (Table 12.2–2). One finding supporting the genetic conclusion is the three- to fourfold higher risk for severe alcohol problems in close relatives of alcoholic persons. The rate of alcohol problems increases with the number of alcoholic relatives, the severity of their illness, and the closeness of their genetic relationship to the person under study. Family investigations do little to separate the importance of genetics and environment, but twin studies take the data a step further. The rate of similarity, or concordance, for severe alcohol-related problems is significantly higher in identical twins of alcoholic individuals than in fraternal twins in most studies. Adoption-type studies have all revealed a significantly enhanced risk for alcoholism in the offspring of alcoholic parents, even when the children were separated from their biological parents close to birth and raised without any knowledge of the problems within the biological family. The risk for severe alcohol-related difficulties is not further enhanced by being raised by an alcoholic adoptive family.

These data not only support the importance of genetic factors in alcoholism, but also highlight the complexity of the phenomenon. The absence of evidence of a single major locus indicates the possibility that a limited number of genes operate with incomplete penetrance or that a combination of genes is required before the disorder expresses itself (a polygenic mode of inheritance). Making matters even more complex is the likelihood that the disorder is solely an expression of environmental events in some families and that different genetic factors operate in different families to produce a picture of genetic heterogeneity.

Some evidence indicates that the brains of children with parents who have alcohol-related disorders exhibit unusual qualities in terms of electrophysiological measures—for example, evoked potentials and EEGs—and response to alcohol infusions. Neurotransmitter receptors such as the dopamine type 2 (D_2) receptors may be factors in the inheritance of alcohol-related disorders. Some studies have found abnormal concentrations of neurotransmitters and neurotransmitter metabolites in the CSF of patients with alcohol-related disorders. Results of many of these studies demonstrated low concentrations of serotonin, dopamine, and GABA or their metabolites.

Table 12.2–2
Data Supporting Genetic Influences in Alcoholism

Close family members have a fourfold increased risk.
The identical twin of an alcoholic person is at higher risk than a fraternal twin.
Adopted-away children of alcoholic persons have a fourfold higher risk.

EFFECTS OF ALCOHOL

The term *alcohol* refers to a large group of organic molecules that have a hydroxyl group (–OH) attached to a saturated carbon atom. Ethyl alcohol, also called *ethanol,* is the common form of alcohol; sometimes referred to as *beverage alcohol,* ethyl alcohol is used for drinking. The chemical formula for ethanol is $CH_3–CH_2–OH$.

The characteristic tastes and flavors of alcohol-containing beverages result from their methods of production, which produce various congeners in the final product, including methanol, butanol, aldehydes, phenols, tannins, and trace amounts of various metals. Although the congeners may confer some differential psychoactive effects on the various alcohol-containing beverages, these differences are minimal compared with the effects of ethanol itself. A single drink is usually considered to contain about 12 g of ethanol, which is the content of 12 ounces of beer (7.2 proof, 3.6 percent ethanol in the United States), one 4-ounce glass of nonfortified wine, or 1 to 1.5 ounces of an 80-proof (40 percent ethanol) liquor (e.g., whiskey or gin). In calculating patients' alcohol intake, however, clinicians should be aware that beers vary in their alcohol content, that beers are available in small and large cans and mugs, that glasses of wine range from 2 to 6 ounces, and that mixed drinks at some bars and in most homes contain 2 to 3 ounces of liquor. Nonetheless, using the moderate sizes of drinks, clinicians can estimate that a single drink increases the blood alcohol level of a 150-pound man by 15 to 20 mg/dL, which is about the concentration of alcohol that an average person can metabolize in 1 hour.

The possible beneficial effects of alcohol have been publicized, especially by the makers and the distributors of alcohol. Most attention has been focused on some epidemiological data that suggest that one or two glasses of red wine each day lower the incidence of cardiovascular disease; these findings, however, are highly controversial.

Absorption

About 10 percent of consumed alcohol is absorbed from the stomach, the remainder from the small intestine. Peak blood concentration of alcohol is reached in 30 to 90 minutes and usually in 45 to 60 minutes, depending on whether the alcohol was taken on an empty stomach (which enhances absorption) or with food (which delays absorption). The time to peak blood concentration also depends on the time during which the alcohol was consumed; rapid drinking reduces the time to peak concentration, slower drinking increases it. Absorption is most rapid with beverages containing 15 to 30 percent alcohol (30 to 60 proof). There is some dispute about whether carbonation (e.g., in champagne and in drinks mixed with seltzer) enhances the absorption of alcohol.

The body has protective devices against inundation by alcohol. For example, if the concentration of alcohol in the stomach becomes too high, mucus is secreted, and the pyloric valve closes. These actions slow the absorption and keep the alcohol from passing into the small intestine, where there are no significant restraints to absorption. Thus, a large amount of alcohol can remain unabsorbed in the stomach for hours. Furthermore, pylorospasm often results in nausea and vomiting.

Once alcohol is absorbed into the bloodstream, it is distributed to all body tissues. Because alcohol is uniformly dissolved in the body's water, tissues containing a high proportion of water receive a high concentration of alcohol. The intoxicating effects are greater when the blood alcohol concentration is rising than when it is falling (the Mellanby effects). For this reason, the rate of absorption bears directly on the intoxication response.

Metabolism

About 90 percent of absorbed alcohol is metabolized through oxidation in the liver; the remaining 10 percent is excreted unchanged by the kidneys and lungs. The rate of oxidation by the liver is constant and independent of the body's energy requirements. The body can metabolize about 15 mg/dL per hour, with a range of 10 to 34 mg/dL per hour. Stated another way, the average person oxidizes three fourths of an ounce of 40 percent (80 proof) alcohol in an hour. In persons with a history of excessive alcohol consumption, upregulation of the necessary enzymes results in rapid alcohol metabolism.

Alcohol is metabolized by two enzymes: alcohol dehydrogenase (ADH) and aldehyde dehydrogenase. ADH catalyzes the conversion of alcohol into acetaldehyde, which is a toxic compound; aldehyde dehydrogenase catalyzes the conversion of acetaldehyde into acetic acid. Aldehyde dehydrogenase is inhibited by disulfiram (Antabuse), often used in the treatment of alcohol-related disorders. Some studies have shown that women have a lower ADH blood content than men; this fact may account for women's tendency to become more intoxicated than men after drinking the same amount of alcohol. The decreased function of alcohol-metabolizing enzymes in some Asian persons can also lead to easy intoxication and toxic symptoms.

Effects on the Brain

Biochemistry. In contrast to most other substances of abuse with identified receptor targets—such as the *N*-methyl-D-aspartate (NMDA) receptor of phencyclidine (PCP)—no single molecular target has been identified as the mediator for the effects of alcohol. The long-standing theory about the biochemical effects of alcohol concerns its effects on the membranes of neurons. Data support the hypothesis that alcohol produces its effects by intercalating itself into membranes and thus increasing fluidity of the membranes with short-term use. With long-term use, however, the theory hypothesizes that the membranes become rigid or stiff. The fluidity of the membranes is critical to normal functioning of receptors, ion channels, and other membrane-bound functional proteins. In recent studies, researchers have attempted to identify specific molecular targets for the effects of alcohol. Most attention has been focused on the effects of alcohol at ion channels. Specifically, studies have found that alcohol ion channel activities associated with the nicotinic acetylcholine, serotonin 5-HT_3, and GABA type A ($GABA_A$) receptors are enhanced by alcohol, whereas ion channel activities associated with glutamate receptors and voltage-gated calcium channels are inhibited.

Behavioral Effects. As the net result of the molecular activities, alcohol functions as a depressant much like the barbiturates and the benzodiazepines, with which alcohol has some cross-tolerance and cross-dependence. At a level of 0.05 percent alcohol in the blood, thought, judgment, and restraint are loosened and sometimes disrupted. At a concentration of 0.1 percent, voluntary motor actions usually become perceptibly clumsy. In most states, legal intoxication ranges from 0.1 to 0.15 percent blood alcohol level. At 0.2 percent, the function of the entire motor area of the brain is measurably depressed, and the parts of the brain that control emotional behavior are also affected. At 0.3 percent, a person is commonly confused or may become stuporous; at 0.4 to 0.5 percent, the person falls into a coma. At higher levels, the primitive centers of the brain that control breathing and heart rate are affected, and death ensues secondary to direct respiratory depression or the aspiration of vomitus. Persons with long-term histories of alcohol abuse, however, can tolerate much higher concentrations of alcohol than can alcohol-naive persons; their alcohol tolerance may cause them to falsely appear less intoxicated than they really are. Table 12.2–3 provides information on the relation of alcohol blood concentration and its effect on driving. Practitioners may find these charts useful educational tools to give to their patients.

Sleep Effects. Although alcohol consumed in the evening usually increases the ease of falling asleep (decreased sleep latency), alcohol also has adverse effects on sleep architecture. Specifically, alcohol use is associated with a decrease in rapid eye movement sleep (REM or dream sleep) and deep sleep (stage 4) and more sleep fragmentation, with more and longer episodes of awakening. Therefore, the idea that drinking alcohol helps persons fall asleep is a myth.

Other Physiological Effects

Liver. The major adverse effects of alcohol use are related to liver damage. Alcohol use, even as short as week-long episodes of increased drinking, can result in an accumulation of fats and proteins, which produce the appearance of a fatty liver, sometimes found on physical examination as an enlarged liver. The association between fatty infiltration of the liver and serious liver damage remains unclear. Alcohol use, however, is associated with the development of alcoholic hepatitis and hepatic cirrhosis.

Table 12.2–3
Alcohol Impairment Charts

NEVER DRINK AND DRIVE

Drinks	For Males: Approximate Blood Alcohol Percentage — Body Weight in Pounds								
	100	120	140	160	180	200	220	240	
0	.00	.00	.00	.00	.00	.00	.00	.00	Only safe driving limit
1	.04	.03	.03	.02	.02	.02	.02	.02	Impairment begins
2	.08	.06	.05	.05	.04	.04	.03	.03	
3	.11	.09	.08	.07	.06	.06	.05	.05	Driving skills significantly affected
4	.15	.12	.11	.09	.08	.08	.07	.06	
5	.19	.16	.13	.12	.11	.09	.09	.08	Possible criminal penalties
6	.23	.19	.16	.14	.13	.11	.10	.09	
7	.26	.22	.19	.16	.15	.13	.12	.11	
8	.30	.25	.21	.19	.17	.15	.14	.13	Legally intoxicated
9	.34	.28	.24	.21	.19	.17	.15	.14	Criminal penalties
10	.38	.31	.27	.23	.21	.19	.17	.16	

Your body can get rid of one drink per hour. Each 1½ oz. of 80-proof liquor, 12 oz. of beer, or 5 oz. of table wine = 1 drink.

NEVER DRINK AND DRIVE

Drinks	For Females: Approximate Blood Alcohol Percentage — Body Weight in Pounds									
	90	100	120	140	160	180	200	220	240	
0	.00	.00	.00	.00	.00	.00	.00	.00	.00	Only safe driving limit
1	.05	.05	.04	.03	.03	.03	.02	.02	.02	Impairment begins
2	.10	.09	.08	.07	.06	.05	.05	.04	.04	Driving skills significantly affected
3	.15	.14	.11	.10	.09	.08	.07	.06	.06	
4	.20	.18	.15	.13	.11	.10	.09	.08	.08	Possible criminal penalties
5	.25	.23	.19	.16	.14	.13	.11	.10	.09	
6	.30	.27	.23	.19	.17	.15	.14	.12	.11	
7	.35	.32	.27	.23	.20	.18	.16	.14	.13	Legally intoxicated
8	.40	.36	.30	.26	.23	.20	.18	.17	.15	Criminal penalties
9	.45	.41	.34	.29	.26	.23	.20	.19	.17	
10	.51	.45	.38	.32	.28	.25	.23	.21	.19	

Your body can get rid of one drink per hour. Each 1½ oz. of 80-proof liquor, 12 oz. of beer, or 5 oz. of table wine = 1 drink.

Note: Separate charts for men and women are included because a woman drinking an equal amount of alcohol in the same period of time as a man of equivalent weight may have a higher blood alcohol level than that man.
This chart is intended as a guide, not a guarantee.
Alcohol affects individuals differently. Your blood alcohol level may be affected by your age, gender, physical condition, amount of food consumed, and any drugs or medication. In addition, different drinks may contain different amounts of alcohol, so it is important to know how much and the concentration of alcohol you consume. For purposes of this guide, "one drink" is equal to 1½ oz. of 80-proof liquor, 12 oz. of regular beer, or 5 oz. of table wine.
In Pennsylvania, a blood alcohol concentration (BAC) level of .10% or greater is all that is necessary to be convicted of driving under the influence (DUI). You may be convicted of DUI at .05% and above if there is supporting evidence of driving impairment. Some states have set .08% BAC as the legal limit. For commercial drivers, a BAC of .04% can result in a DUI conviction nationwide.
Impairment begins with your first drink. For safety's sake, never drive after drinking!
From The Pennsylvania Liquor Control Board (reprinted by permission).

Gastrointestinal System. Long-term heavy drinking is associated with developing esophagitis, gastritis, achlorhydria, and gastric ulcers. The development of esophageal varices can accompany particularly heavy alcohol abuse; the rupture of the varices is a medical emergency often resulting in death by exsanguination. Disorders of the small intestine occasionally occur, and pancreatitis, pancreatic insufficiency, and pancreatic cancer are also associated with heavy alcohol use. Heavy alcohol intake may interfere with the normal processes of food digestion and absorption; as a result, consumed food is inadequately digested. Alcohol abuse also appears to inhibit the intestine's capacity to absorb various nutrients, such as vitamins and amino acids. This effect, coupled with the often poor dietary habits of those with alcohol-related disorders, can cause serious vitamin deficiencies, particularly of the B vitamins.

Other Bodily Systems. Significant intake of alcohol has been associated with increased blood pressure, dysregulation of lipoprotein and triglyceride metabolism, and increased risk for myocardial infarctions and cerebrovascular diseases. Alcohol has been shown to affect the hearts of nonalcoholic persons who do not usually drink, increasing the resting cardiac output, the heart rate, and the myocardial oxygen consumption. Evidence indicates that alcohol intake can adversely affect the hematopoietic system and can increase the incidence of cancer, particularly head, neck, esophageal, stomach, hepatic, colonic, and

lung cancer. Acute intoxication may also be associated with hypoglycemia, which, when unrecognized, may be responsible for some of the sudden deaths of persons who are intoxicated. Muscle weakness is another side effect of alcoholism. Recent evidence shows that alcohol intake raises the blood concentration of estradiol in women. The increase in estradiol correlates with the blood alcohol level.

Laboratory Tests. The adverse effects of alcohol appear in common laboratory tests, which can be useful diagnostic aids in identifying persons with alcohol-related disorders. The γ-glutamyl transpeptidase levels are high in about 80 percent of those with alcohol-related disorders, and the mean corpuscular volume (MCV) is high in about 60 percent, more so in women than in men. Other laboratory test values that may be high in association with alcohol abuse are those of uric acid, triglycerides, aspartate aminotransferase (AST), and alanine aminotransferase (ALT).

Drug Interactions

The interaction between alcohol and other substances can be dangerous, even fatal. Certain substances such as alcohol and phenobarbital (Luminal) are metabolized by the liver, and their prolonged use may lead to acceleration of their metabolism. When persons with alcohol-related disorders are sober, this accelerated metabolism makes them unusually tolerant to many drugs such as sedatives and hypnotics; when they are intoxicated, however, these drugs compete with the alcohol for the same detoxification mechanisms, and potentially toxic concentrations of all involved substances can accumulate in the blood.

The effects of alcohol and other central nervous system (CNS) depressants are usually synergistic. Sedatives, hypnotics, and drugs that relieve pain, motion sickness, head colds, and allergy symptoms must be used with caution by persons with alcohol-related disorders. Narcotics depress the sensory areas of the cerebral cortex and can produce pain relief, sedation, apathy, drowsiness, and sleep; high doses can result in respiratory failure and death. Increasing the dosages of sedative-hypnotic drugs such as chloral hydrate (Noctec) and benzodiazepines, especially when they are combined with alcohol, produces a range of effects from sedation to motor and intellectual impairment to stupor, coma, and death. Because sedatives and other psychotropic drugs can potentiate the effects of alcohol, patients should be instructed about the dangers of combining CNS depressants and alcohol, particularly when they are driving or operating machinery.

Table 12.2–4
DSM-IV-TR Alcohol-Related Disorders

Alcohol use disorders
Alcohol dependence
Alcohol abuse
Alcohol-induced disorders
Alcohol intoxication
Alcohol withdrawal
  Specify if:
    With perceptual disturbances
Alcohol intoxication delirium
Alcohol withdrawal delirium
Alcohol-induced persisting dementia
Alcohol-induced persisting amnestic disorder
Alcohol-induced psychotic disorder, with delusions
  Specify if:
    With onset during intoxication
    With onset during withdrawal
Alcohol-induced psychotic disorder, with hallucinations
  Specify if:
    With onset during intoxication
    With onset during withdrawal
Alcohol-induced mood disorder
  Specify if:
    With onset during intoxication
    With onset during withdrawal
Alcohol-induced anxiety disorder
  Specify if:
    With onset during intoxication
    With onset during withdrawal
Alcohol-induced sexual dysfunction
  Specify if:
    With onset during intoxication
Alcohol-induced sleep disorder
  Specify if:
    With onset during intoxication
    With onset during withdrawal
Alcohol disorder not otherwise specified

From American Psychiatric Association. *Diagnostic and Statistical Manual of Mental Disorders.* 4th ed. Text rev. Washington, DC: American Psychiatric Association; copyright 2000, with permission.

DISORDERS

DSM-IV-TR lists the alcohol-related disorders (Table 12.2–4) and specifies the diagnostic criteria for alcohol intoxication (Table 12.2–5) and alcohol withdrawal (Table 12.2–6). The diagnostic criteria for the other alcohol-related disorders are listed in DSM-IV-TR under the major symptom. For example, the diagnostic criteria for alcohol-induced anxiety disorder are found in the anxiety disorders category, under the heading "Substance-Induced Anxiety Disorder."

Alcohol Dependence and Alcohol Abuse

Diagnosis and Clinical Features. In DSM-IV-TR, all substance-related disorders use the same criteria for dependence and abuse (see Tables 12.1–5 and 12.1–6). A need for daily use of large amounts of alcohol for adequate functioning, a regular pattern of heavy drinking limited to weekends, and long periods of sobriety interspersed with binges of heavy alcohol intake lasting for weeks or months strongly suggest alcohol dependence and alcohol abuse. The drinking patterns are often associated with certain behaviors: the inability to cut down or stop drinking; repeated efforts to control or reduce excessive drinking by "going on the wagon" (periods of temporary abstinence) or by restricting drinking to certain times of the day; binges (remaining intoxicated throughout the day for at least 2 days); occasional consumption of a fifth of spirits (or its equivalent in wine or beer); amnestic periods for events occurring while intoxicated (blackouts); the continuation of drinking despite a serious physical disorder that the

Table 12.2–5
DSM-IV-TR Diagnostic Criteria for Alcohol Intoxication

A. Recent ingestion of alcohol.
B. Clinically significant maladaptive behavioral or psychological changes (e.g., inappropriate sexual or aggressive behavior, mood lability, impaired judgment, impaired social or occupational functioning) that developed during, or shortly after, alcohol ingestion.
C. One (or more) of the following signs, developing during, or shortly after, alcohol use:
  (1) slurred speech
  (2) incoordination
  (3) unsteady gait
  (4) nystagmus
  (5) impairment in attention or memory
  (6) stupor or coma
D. The symptoms are not due to a general medical condition and are not better accounted for by another mental disorder.

From American Psychiatric Association. *Diagnostic and Statistical Manual of Mental Disorders.* 4th ed. Text rev. Washington, DC: American Psychiatric Association; copyright 2000, with permission.

person knows is exacerbated by alcohol use; and drinking nonbeverage alcohol, such as fuel and commercial products containing alcohol. In addition, persons with alcohol dependence and alcohol abuse show impaired social or occupational functioning because of alcohol use (e.g., violence while intoxicated, absence from work, job loss), legal difficulties (e.g., arrest for intoxicated behavior and traffic accidents while intoxicated), and arguments or difficulties with family members or friends about excessive alcohol consumption. According to DSM-IV-TR, the current rate of alcohol dependence is 5 percent.

Table 12.2–6
DSM-IV-TR Diagnostic Criteria for Alcohol Withdrawal

A. Cessation of (or reduction in) alcohol use that has been heavy and prolonged.
B. Two (or more) of the following, developing within several hours to a few days after Criterion A:
  (1) autonomic hyperactivity (e.g., sweating or pulse rate greater than 100)
  (2) increased hand tremor
  (3) insomnia
  (4) nausea or vomiting
  (5) transient visual, tactile, or auditory hallucinations or illusions
  (6) psychomotor agitation
  (7) anxiety
  (8) grand mal seizures
C. The symptoms in Criterion B cause clinically significant distress or impairment in social, occupational, or other important areas of functioning.
D. The symptoms are not due to a general medical condition and are not better accounted for by another mental disorder.

Specify if:
  With perceptual disturbances

From American Psychiatric Association. *Diagnostic and Statistical Manual of Mental Disorders.* 4th ed. Text rev. Washington, DC: American Psychiatric Association; copyright 2000, with permission.

A 25-year-old graduate student in physics was referred for evaluation by her adviser, who was concerned about tardiness at work and recent problems with a lack of clarity of thinking. As he discussed these difficulties with her, the student admitted being concerned about her drinking, which had been dramatically emphasized to her in a recent intervention carried out by her father and mother. She related that for the last 5 years or so she has regularly consumed 1.5 to 2 or 3 bottles of wine each evening (approximately 9 to 18 drinks). In the last 2 years she has noted a marked increase in the amount of alcohol needed to get the same effects and reported giving up activities with her family to drink, spending a great deal of her time drinking, and driving long distances to obtain alcohol. She has repeatedly tried to cut down, often setting a limit of two drinks in an evening, but regularly going on to nine or more standard drinks before stopping. Despite her high general level of functioning, her active participation in a graduate education program, and close interpersonal relationships, this history of alcohol dependency is fairly typical among alcohol-dependent individuals. (Courtesy of Marc A. Schuckit, M.D.)

Subtypes of Alcohol Dependence. Various researchers have attempted to divide alcohol dependence into subtypes based primarily on phenomenological characteristics. One recent classification notes that type A alcohol dependence is characterized by late onset, few childhood risk factors, relatively mild dependence, few alcohol-related problems, and little psychopathology. Type B alcohol dependence is characterized by many childhood risk factors, severe dependence, an early onset of alcohol-related problems, much psychopathology, a strong family history of alcohol abuse, frequent polysubstance abuse, a long history of alcohol treatment, and a high number of severe life stresses. Some researchers have found that type A persons who are alcohol dependent may respond to interactional psychotherapies, whereas type B persons who are alcohol dependent may respond to training in coping skills.

Other subtyping schemes of alcohol dependence have received fairly wide recognition in the literature. One group of investigators proposed three subtypes: *early-stage problem drinkers,* who do not yet have complete alcohol dependence syndromes; *affiliative drinkers,* who tend to drink daily in moderate amounts in social settings; and *schizoid-isolated drinkers,* who have severe dependence and tend to drink in binges and often alone.

Another investigator described gamma alcohol dependence, which is thought to be common in the United States and represents the alcohol dependence seen in those who are active in Alcoholics Anonymous (AA). This variant concerns control problems in which persons are unable to stop drinking once they start. When drinking is terminated as a result of ill health or lack of money, these persons can abstain for varying periods. In delta alcohol dependence, perhaps more common in Europe than in the United States, persons who are alcohol dependent

must drink a certain amount each day but are unaware of a lack of control. The alcohol use disorder may not be discovered until a person who must stop drinking for some reason exhibits withdrawal symptoms.

Another researcher has suggested a *type I, male-limited* variety of alcohol dependence, characterized by late onset, more evidence of psychological than of physical dependence, and the presence of guilt feelings. *Type II, male-limited* alcohol dependence is characterized by onset at an early age, spontaneous seeking of alcohol for consumption, and a socially disruptive set of behaviors when intoxicated.

Four subtypes of alcoholism were postulated by still another investigator. The first is *antisocial alcoholism,* typically with a predominance in men, a poor prognosis, early onset of alcohol-related problems, and a close association with antisocial personality disorder. The second is *developmentally cumulative alcoholism,* with a primary tendency for alcohol abuse that is exacerbated with time as cultural expectations foster increased opportunities to drink. The third is *negative-affect alcoholism,* which is more common in women than in men; according to this hypothesis, women are likely to use alcohol for mood regulation and to help ease social relationships. The fourth is *developmentally limited alcoholism,* with frequent bouts of consuming large amounts of alcohol; the bouts become less frequent as persons age and respond to the increased expectations of society about their jobs and families.

Alcohol Intoxication

DSM-IV-TR establishes formal criteria for diagnosing alcohol intoxication (Table 12.2–5): sufficient alcohol consumption, specific maladaptive behavioral changes, signs of neurological impairment, and the absence of other confounding diagnoses or conditions. Alcohol intoxication is not a trivial condition and, in extreme cases, can lead to coma, respiratory depression, and death from respiratory arrest or because of aspiration of vomitus. Treatment for severe alcohol intoxication requires mechanical ventilatory support in an intensive care unit, with attention to the patient's acid–base balance, electrolytes, and temperature. Some studies of cerebral blood flow (CBF) during alcohol intoxication have found a modest increase in CBF after the ingestion of small amounts of alcohol, but CBF decreases with continued drinking.

The severity of alcohol intoxication symptoms correlates roughly with the blood concentration of alcohol, which reflects the alcohol concentration in the brain. With the onset of intoxication, some persons become talkative and gregarious; others become withdrawn and sullen or belligerent. Some patients show lability of mood with intermittent episodes of laughing and crying. The person may show a short-term tolerance to alcohol and seem to be less intoxicated after many hours of drinking than after only a few hours.

The medical complications of intoxication include those that result from falls such as subdural hematomas and fractures. Telltale signs of frequent bouts of intoxication are facial hematomas, particularly about the eyes, the result of falls or fights while drunk. In cold climates, hypothermia and death may occur when a person is exposed to the elements. A person with alcohol intoxication may also be predisposed to infections secondary to a suppressed immune system.

Alcohol Withdrawal

Alcohol withdrawal, even without delirium, can be serious and can include seizures and autonomic hyperactivity. Conditions that may predispose to, or aggravate, withdrawal symptoms include fatigue, malnutrition, physical illness, and depression. The DSM-IV-TR criteria for alcohol withdrawal (Table 12.2–6) require the cessation or reduction of alcohol use that was heavy and prolonged as well as the presence of specific physical or neuropsychiatric symptoms. The diagnosis also allows for the specification "with perceptual disturbances." One recent positron emission tomographic (PET) study of blood flow during alcohol withdrawal in otherwise healthy persons with alcohol dependence reported a globally low rate of metabolic activity (Fig. 12.2–1), although, with further inspection of the data, the authors concluded that activity was especially low in the left parietal and right frontal areas.

The classic sign of alcohol withdrawal is tremulousness, although the spectrum of symptoms can expand to include psychotic and perceptual symptoms (e.g., delusions and hallucinations), seizures, and the symptoms of delirium tremens (DTs), called *alcohol withdrawal delirium* in DSM-IV-TR. Tremulousness (commonly called the "shakes" or the "jitters") develops 6 to 8 hours after the cessation of drinking, the psychotic and perceptual symptoms begin in 8 to 12 hours, seizures in 12 to 24 hours, and DTs during 72 hours, although physicians should watch for the development of DTs for the first week of withdrawal. The syndrome of withdrawal sometimes skips the usual progression and, for example, goes directly to DTs.

The tremor of alcohol withdrawal can be similar to either physiological tremor, with a continuous tremor of great amplitude and of more than 8 Hz, or familial tremor, with bursts of tremor activity slower than 8 Hz. Other symptoms of withdrawal include general irritability, gastrointestinal symptoms (e.g., nausea and vomiting), and sympathetic autonomic hyperactivity, including anxiety, arousal, sweating, facial flushing, mydriasis, tachycardia, and mild hypertension. Patients experiencing alcohol withdrawal are generally alert but may startle easily.

A 23-year-old computer consultant with alcohol dependence was unable to establish even 24 hours of sobriety as an outpatient. Therefore, reflecting his continued drinking, he was referred for inpatient care. Following approximately 10 hours of abstinence and with a documented blood alcohol concentration of 0 mg/dL, he was noted to be mildly diaphoretic, with a respiratory rate of 25 breaths per minute, blood pressure of 130/90, a mild bilateral tremor of the hands, and a pulse rate of 85 beats per minute. He had a history of jogging 2 to 5 miles a day, and these figures represented moderate elevation of his usual vital signs. Treated with multiple vitamins, good nutrition, oral fluids, and benzodiazepines, the symptoms rapidly improved, and his vital signs were close to normal by day 4 of abstinence. (Courtesy of Marc A. Schuckit, M.D.)

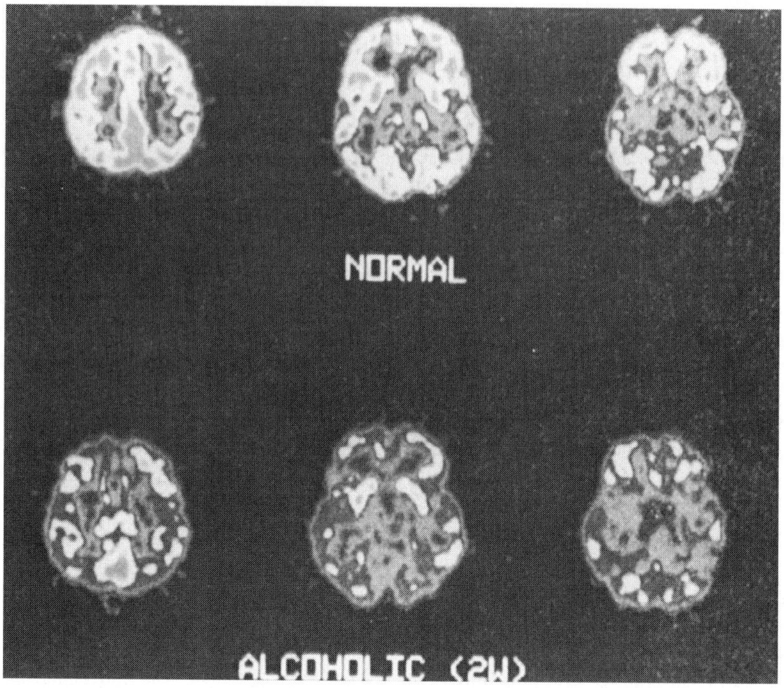

FIGURE 12.2–1

Brain PET metabolic images in a normal control subject and an alcoholic subject tested 2 weeks after the last use of alcohol. Notice the decreased cortical metabolic activity in the alcoholic person. (Reprinted with permission from Volkow ND, Hitzemann R, Wang G-J, et al. Decreased brain metabolism in neurologically intact healthy alcoholics. *Am J Psychiatry.* 1992;149:1019.)

Withdrawal Seizures. Seizures associated with alcohol withdrawal are stereotyped, generalized, and tonic-clonic in character. Patients often have more than one seizure 3 to 6 hours after the first seizure. Status epilepticus is relatively rare and occurs in less than 3 percent of patients. Although anticonvulsant medications are not required in the management of alcohol withdrawal seizures, the cause of the seizures is difficult to establish when a patient is first assessed in the emergency room; thus, many patients with withdrawal seizures receive anticonvulsant medications, which are then discontinued once the cause of the seizures is recognized. Seizure activity in patients with known alcohol abuse histories should still prompt clinicians to consider other causative factors, such as head injuries, CNS infections, CNS neoplasms, and other cerebrovascular diseases; long-term severe alcohol abuse can result in hypoglycemia, hyponatremia, and hypomagnesemia—all of which can also be associated with seizures.

Treatment. The primary medications for the control of alcohol withdrawal symptoms are the benzodiazepines (Table 12.2–7). Many studies have found that benzodiazepines help control seizure activity, delirium, anxiety, tachycardia, hypertension, diaphoresis, and tremor associated with alcohol withdrawal. Benzodiazepines can be given either orally or

Table 12.2–7
Drug Therapy for Alcohol Intoxication and Withdrawal

Clinical Problem	Drug	Route	Dosage	Comment
Tremulousness and mild to moderate agitation	Chlordiazepoxide	Oral	25–100 mg every 4–6 h	Initial dose can be repeated every 2 h until patient is calm; subsequent doses must be individualized and titrated
	Diazepam	Oral	5–20 mg every 4–6 h	
Hallucinosis	Lorazepam	Oral	2–10 mg every 4–6 h	
Extreme agitation	Chlordiazepoxide	Intravenous	0.5 mg/kg at 12.5 mg/min	Give until patient is calm; subsequent doses must be individualized and titrated
Withdrawal seizures	Diazepam	Intravenous	0.15 mg/kg at 2.5 mg/min	
Delirium tremens	Lorazepam	Intravenous	0.1 mg/kg at 2.0 mg/min	

Adapted from Koch-Weser J, Sellers EM, Kalant J. Alcohol intoxication and withdrawal. *N Engl J Med.* 1976;294:757.

parenterally; neither diazepam (Valium) nor chlordiazepoxide (Librium), however, should be given intramuscularly (IM) because of their erratic absorption by this route. Clinicians must titrate the dosage of the benzodiazepine, starting with a high dosage and lowering the dosage as the patient recovers. Enough benzodiazepines should be given to keep patients calm and sedated but not so sedated that they cannot be aroused for clinicians to perform appropriate procedures, including neurological examinations.

Although benzodiazepines are the standard treatment for alcohol withdrawal, studies have shown that carbamazepine (Tegretol) in daily doses of 800 mg is as effective as benzodiazepines and has the added benefit of minimal abuse liability. Carbamazepine use is gradually becoming common in the United States and Europe. The β-adrenergic receptor antagonists and clonidine (Catapres) have also been used to block the symptoms of sympathetic hyperactivity, but neither drug is an effective treatment for seizures or delirium.

Delirium

Diagnosis and Clinical Features. DSM-IV-TR contains the diagnostic criteria for alcohol intoxication delirium in the category of substance intoxication delirium and the diagnostic criteria for alcohol withdrawal delirium in the category of substance withdrawal delirium (see Tables 10.2–3 and 10.2–4 in Chapter 10, Section 10.2). Patients with recognized alcohol withdrawal symptoms should be carefully monitored to prevent progression to alcohol withdrawal delirium, the most severe form of the withdrawal syndrome, also known as DTs. Alcohol withdrawal delirium is a medical emergency that can result in significant morbidity and mortality. Patients with delirium are a danger to themselves and to others. Because of the unpredictability of their behavior, patients with delirium may be assaultive or suicidal or may act on hallucinations or delusional thoughts as if they were genuine dangers. Untreated, DTs has a mortality rate of 20 percent, usually as a result of an intercurrent medical illness such as pneumonia, renal disease, hepatic insufficiency, or heart failure. Although withdrawal seizures commonly precede the development of alcohol withdrawal delirium, delirium can also appear unheralded. The essential feature of the syndrome is delirium occurring within 1 week after a person stops drinking or reduces the intake of alcohol. In addition to the symptoms of delirium, the features of alcohol intoxication delirium include autonomic hyperactivity such as tachycardia, diaphoresis, fever, anxiety, insomnia, and hypertension; perceptual distortions, most frequently visual or tactile hallucinations; and fluctuating levels of psychomotor activity, ranging from hyperexcitability to lethargy.

About 5 percent of persons with alcohol-related disorders who are hospitalized have DTs. Because the syndrome usually develops on the third hospital day, a patient admitted for an unrelated condition may unexpectedly have an episode of delirium, the first sign of a previously undiagnosed alcohol-related disorder. Episodes of DTs usually begin in a patient's 30s or 40s after 5 to 15 years of heavy drinking, typically of the binge type. Physical illness (e.g., hepatitis or pancreatitis) predisposes to the syndrome; a person in good physical health rarely has DTs during alcohol withdrawal.

Mr. T. is a 35-year-old French factory worker. He is married and has three children, ages 7, 9, and 11.

PROBLEM

After falling downstairs and breaking his leg one evening, Mr. T. was admitted to the orthopedic department of a general hospital. On the third day of his stay, he grew increasingly nervous and started to tremble. He was asked about his drinking habits but denied having an alcohol problem. He told the physicians that he only occasionally had a glass of beer. During the night he could not sleep, and the nurses became concerned because he was talking incoherently and was obviously very anxious.

HISTORY

According to his wife, Mr. T. had drunk large quantities of beer for more than 3 years. During the preceding year, he had missed work several times and had been threatened with dismissal. Each day he started drinking when he came home from work in the evening and did not stop until he fell asleep. On the evening when he was admitted to the hospital, Mr. T. came home as usual but slipped on the stairs and broke his leg before he could start drinking. Consequently he had not had a drink prior to admission. Mrs. T. felt ashamed of her husband's alcohol problem and did not have the courage to tell the orthopedist about it when her husband went into the hospital. Three days later, when the doctors asked her directly, she told them the full story.

Mrs. T. said her husband had eaten very little during the previous few weeks. She had noticed that on several occasions he could not remember even important events that had happened the day before. He had a car accident when drunk 2 years earlier but without any major injury. Mr. T. had no other major health problems in the past. The relationship with his wife, however, had become extremely difficult since he started drinking, and Mrs. T. was seriously considering a divorce. The relationship with his children had been tense. He had often argued with them, but recently they had tried to avoid their father as much as possible.

According to Mrs. T., her husband's father had been a chronic alcoholic and died from liver cirrhosis when her husband was 24 years old.

DISCUSSION

Mr. T. has a long history of heavy alcohol use and developed severe withdrawal symptoms when he could not get alcohol. He presented with the characteristic symptoms of delirium: clouding of consciousness, global disturbance of cognition, psychomotor agitation, disturbances of the sleep–wake cycle (insomnia), rapid onset, and fluctuation of the symptoms.

The presence of a withdrawal state, associated with a delirium, shortly after cessation of heavy alcohol consumption indicates alcohol withdrawal state with delirium. Because the patient did not also have convulsions, the diagnosis according to ICD-10 is alcohol withdrawal state with delirium, without convulsions.

Mr. T.'s drinking problem has lasted for at least 3 years, and the information provided by his wife gives evidence that

points to an additional diagnosis of alcohol dependence syndrome. The memory problems observed by his wife make it possible that Mr. T. has, in addition, an amnesic syndrome caused by the use of alcohol. The description, however, does not provide us with enough information to make a reliable additional diagnosis of amnesic syndrome due to use of alcohol. This should be tested after the delirium and other withdrawal symptoms have subsided, as memory impairment is also a prominent feature in delirium.

Treatment. The best treatment for DTs is prevention. Patients withdrawing from alcohol who exhibit withdrawal phenomena should receive a benzodiazepine, such as 25 to 50 mg of chlordiazepoxide every 2 to 4 hours until they seem to be out of danger. Once the delirium appears, however, 50 to 100 mg of chlordiazepoxide should be given every 4 hours orally, or lorazepam (Ativan) should be given intravenously (IV) if oral medication is not possible (Table 12.2–7). Antipsychotic medications that may reduce the seizure threshold in patients should be avoided. A high-calorie, high-carbohydrate diet supplemented by multivitamins is also important.

Physically restraining patients with the DTs is risky; they may fight against the restraints to a dangerous level of exhaustion. When patients are disorderly and uncontrollable, a seclusion room can be used. Dehydration, often exacerbated by diaphoresis and fever, can be corrected with fluids given by mouth or IV. Anorexia, vomiting, and diarrhea often occur during withdrawal. Antipsychotic medications should be avoided because they may reduce the seizure threshold in the patient. The emergence of focal neurological symptoms, lateralizing seizures, increased intracranial pressure, or evidence of skull fractures or other indications of CNS pathology should prompt clinicians to examine a patient for additional neurological disease. Nonbenzodiazepine anticonvulsant medication is not useful in preventing or treating alcohol withdrawal convulsions, although benzodiazepines are generally effective.

Warm, supportive psychotherapy in the treatment of DTs is essential. Patients are often bewildered, frightened, and anxious because of their tumultuous symptoms, and skillful verbal support is imperative.

Alcohol-Induced Persisting Dementia

The legitimacy of the concept of alcohol-induced persisting dementia remains controversial; some clinicians and researchers believe that it is difficult to separate the toxic effects of alcohol abuse from the CNS damage done by poor nutrition and multiple trauma and that following the malfunctioning of other bodily organs such as the liver, the pancreas, and the kidneys. Although several studies have found enlarged ventricles and cortical atrophy in persons with dementia and a history of alcohol dependence, the studies do not help clarify the cause of the dementia. Nonetheless, DSM-IV-TR includes the diagnosis of alcohol-induced persisting dementia (Table 10.3–6). The controversy about the diagnosis should encourage clinicians to complete a diagnostic assessment of the dementia before concluding that it was caused by alcohol.

Alcohol-Induced Persisting Amnestic Disorder

Diagnosis and Clinical Features. The diagnostic criteria of alcohol-induced persisting amnestic disorder are contained in the DSM-IV category of substance-induced persisting amnestic disorder (Table 10.4–3). The essential feature of alcohol-induced persisting amnestic disorder is a disturbance in short-term memory caused by prolonged heavy use of alcohol. Because the disorder usually occurs in persons who have been drinking heavily for many years, the disorder is rare in persons younger than age 35.

Wernicke-Korsakoff Syndrome. The classic names for alcohol-induced persisting amnestic disorder are Wernicke's encephalopathy (a set of acute symptoms) and Korsakoff's syndrome (a chronic condition). Whereas Wernicke's encephalopathy is completely reversible with treatment, only about 20 percent of patients with Korsakoff's syndrome recover. The pathophysiological connection between the two syndromes is thiamine deficiency, caused either by poor nutritional habits or by malabsorption problems. Thiamine is a cofactor for several important enzymes and may also be involved in conduction of the axon potential along the axon and in synaptic transmission. The neuropathological lesions are symmetrical and paraventricular, involving the mammillary bodies, the thalamus, the hypothalamus, the midbrain, the pons, the medulla, the fornix, and the cerebellum.

Wernicke's encephalopathy, also called *alcoholic encephalopathy,* is an acute neurological disorder characterized by ataxia (affecting primarily the gait), vestibular dysfunction, confusion, and a variety of ocular motility abnormalities, including horizontal nystagmus, lateral orbital palsy, and gaze palsy. These eye signs are usually bilateral but not necessarily symmetrical. Other eye signs may include a sluggish reaction to light and anisocoria. Wernicke's encephalopathy may clear spontaneously in a few days or weeks or may progress into Korsakoff's syndrome.

Treatment. In the early stages, Wernicke's encephalopathy responds rapidly to large doses of parenteral thiamine, which is believed to be effective in preventing the progression into Korsakoff's syndrome. The dosage of thiamine is usually initiated at 100 mg by mouth two to three times daily and is continued for 1 to 2 weeks. In patients with alcohol-related disorders who are receiving IV administration of glucose solution, it is good practice to include 100 mg of thiamine in each liter of the glucose solution.

Korsakoff's syndrome is the chronic amnestic syndrome that can follow Wernicke's encephalopathy, and the two syndromes are believed to be pathophysiologically related. The cardinal features of Korsakoff's syndrome are impaired mental syndrome (especially recent memory) and anterograde amnesia in an alert and responsive patient. The patient may or may not have the symptom of confabulation. Treatment of Korsakoff's syndrome is also thiamine given 100 mg by mouth two to three times daily; the treatment regimen should continue for 3 to 12 months. Few patients who progress to Korsakoff's syndrome ever fully recover, although a substantial proportion have some improvement in their cognitive abilities with thiamine and nutritional support.

Blackouts. Alcohol-related blackouts are not included in DSM-IV-TR's diagnostic classification, although the symptom of alcohol intoxication is common. Blackouts are similar to episodes of transient global amnesia (see Chapter 10, Section 10.4) in that they are discrete episodes of anterograde amnesia that occur in association with alcohol intoxication. The periods of amnesia can be particularly distressing when persons fear that they have unknowingly harmed someone or behaved imprudently while intoxicated. During a blackout, persons have relatively intact remote memory but experience a specific short-term memory deficit in which they are unable to recall events that happened in the previous 5 or 10 minutes. Because their other intellectual faculties are well preserved, they can perform complicated tasks and appear normal to casual observers. The neurobiological mechanisms for alcoholic blackouts are now known at the molecular level; alcohol blocks the consolidation of new memories into old memories, a process that is thought to involve the hippocampus and related temporal lobe structures.

Alcohol-Induced Psychotic Disorder

Diagnosis and Clinical Features. The diagnostic criteria for alcohol-induced psychotic disorders, such as delusions and hallucinations, are found in the DSM-IV-TR category of substance-induced psychotic disorder (see Table 14.4–7). DSM-IV-TR further allows the specification of onset (during intoxication or withdrawal) and whether hallucinations or delusions are present. The most common hallucinations are auditory, usually voices, but they are often unstructured. The voices are characteristically maligning, reproachful, or threatening, although some patients report that the voices are pleasant and nondisruptive. The hallucinations usually last less than a week, but during that week impaired reality testing is common. After the episode, most patients realize the hallucinatory nature of the symptoms.

Hallucinations after alcohol withdrawal are considered rare, and the syndrome is distinct from alcohol withdrawal delirium. The hallucinations can occur at any age but usually appear in persons abusing alcohol for a long time. Although the hallucinations usually resolve within a week, some may linger; in these cases, clinicians must consider other psychotic disorders in the differential diagnosis. Alcohol withdrawal-related hallucinations are differentiated from the hallucinations of schizophrenia by the temporal association with alcohol withdrawal, the absence of a classic history of schizophrenia, and their usually short-lived duration. Alcohol withdrawal-related hallucinations are differentiated from the DTs by the presence of a clear sensorium in patients.

A 39-year-old male letter carrier was brought to an emergency room by the police after he behaved in an unusual fashion at home and complained that his neighbors were trying to kill him. The history obtained from the patient and his wife revealed that his psychotic thinking developed slowly over the preceding 3 weeks; he began with feelings that persons were looking at him at work, progressed to vague feelings that persons were against him, and went on to frank auditory hallucinations that persons at work and in the neighboring houses were talking about their plans to kill him. He had no insight into those paranoid delusions and auditory hallucinations. The relatively abrupt onset of the syndrome—he was in his late 30s—pointed to a potential organic cause, and further probing documented that he had been drinking between 6 and 18 beers daily for at least the preceding 10 weeks. A diagnosis of alcohol-induced psychotic disorder with onset during intoxication was made, and both hallucinations and delusions disappeared after 3 weeks of abstinence. After alcohol treatment, the man stayed sober for the next 8 months. Unfortunately, he later resumed heavy drinking and had a recurrence of both hallucinations and delusions. (Courtesy of Marc A. Schuckit, M.D.)

Treatment. The treatment of alcohol withdrawal–related hallucinations is much like the treatment of DTs—benzodiazepines, adequate nutrition, and fluids if necessary. If this regimen fails or for long-term cases, antipsychotics may be used.

Alcohol-Induced Mood Disorder

DSM-IV-TR allows for the diagnosis of alcohol-induced mood disorder with manic, depressive, or mixed features (see Table 15.3–10 in Chapter 15, Section 15.3) and also for the specification of onset during either intoxication or withdrawal. As with all the secondary and substance-induced disorders, clinicians must consider whether the abused substance and the symptoms have a causal relation.

A consultation was requested on a 42-year-old woman with alcohol dependence who complained of persisting severe depressive symptoms despite 5 days of abstinence. In the initial stage of the interview she noted that she had "always been depressed" and felt that she "drank to cope with the depressive symptoms." Her current complaint included a prominent sadness that had persisted for several weeks, difficulties concentrating, initial and terminal insomnia, and a feeling of hopelessness and guilt. In an effort to distinguish between an alcohol-induced mood disorder and an independent major depressive episode, a time-line–based history was obtained. This focused on the age of onset of alcohol dependence, periods of abstinence that extended for several months or more since the onset of dependence, and the ages of occurrence of clear major depressive episodes lasting several weeks or more at a time. Despite this patient's original complaints, it became clear that there had been no major depressive episodes prior to her mid-20s when alcohol dependence began, and that during a 1-year period of abstinence related to the gestation and neonatal period of her son, her mood had significantly improved. A provisional diagnosis of an alcohol-induced mood disorder was made. The patient was offered education, reassurance, and cognitive therapy to help her to deal with the depressive symptoms, but no antidepressant medications were prescribed. The depressive symptoms remained at their original intensity for several additional days and then began to improve. By

approximately 3 weeks abstinent the patient no longer met criteria for a major depressive episode, although she demonstrated mood swings similar to dysphemia for several additional weeks. This case is a fairly typical example of an alcohol-induced mood disorder in an individual with alcohol dependence. (Courtesy of Marc A. Shuckit, M.D.)

Alcohol-Induced Anxiety Disorder

DSM-IV-TR allows for the diagnosis of alcohol-induced anxiety disorder (see Table 16.7–3 in Section 16.7 of Chapter 16) and suggests that the diagnosis specify whether the symptoms are those of generalized anxiety, panic attacks, obsessive-compulsive symptoms, or phobic symptoms and whether the onset was during intoxication or during withdrawal. The association between alcohol use and anxiety symptoms is discussed above; deciding whether the anxiety symptoms are primary or secondary can be difficult.

A 52-year-old African American male lawyer entered treatment for alcohol dependence with the chief complaint of "panic attacks" as well as alcohol problems. In light of evidence of concomitant panic disorder and alcohol dependence, a time-line history was established. This individual first met criteria for panic disorder by approximately age 18, and occasional panic attacks intensified as he went off to college. After several visits to an emergency room during his freshman year, the diagnosis of panic disorder was made, and the current retrospective history revealed no evidence of dependence on alcohol or any other substance at that time. His panic disorder was treated with behavioral therapy and antidepressant medication and was under good control when, at approximately age 33, he intensified his alcohol intake and developed associated problems. He appears to have fulfilled criteria for alcohol dependence. During the course of his alcoholism, his panic disorder symptoms increased and decreased in intensity over time, with obvious exacerbations whenever he attempted to cut back on his alcohol intake. The diagnosis was alcohol dependence along with an independent panic disorder. Treatment focused on continuation of cognitive-behavioral therapy, antidepressant medications (when needed) for the panic disorder, and alcohol rehabilitation. (Courtesy of Marc A. Schuckit, M.D.)

Alcohol-Induced Sexual Dysfunction

In DSM-IV-TR, the formal diagnosis of symptoms of sexual dysfunction associated with alcohol intoxication is alcohol-induced sexual dysfunction (see Table 21.2–17 in Section 21.2 of Chapter 21).

Alcohol-Induced Sleep Disorder

In DSM-IV-TR, the diagnostic criteria for alcohol-induced sleep disorders with an onset during either alcohol intoxication or alcohol withdrawal are found in the sleep disorders section (see Table 24.2–21 in Section 24.2 of Chapter 24).

Table 12.2–8
DSM-IV-TR Diagnostic Criteria for Alcohol-Related Disorder Not Otherwise Specified

The alcohol-related disorder not otherwise specified category is for disorders associated with the use of alcohol that are not classifiable as alcohol dependence, alcohol abuse, alcohol intoxication, alcohol withdrawal, alcohol intoxication delirium, alcohol withdrawal delirium, alcohol-induced persisting dementia, alcohol-induced persisting amnestic disorder, alcohol-induced psychotic disorder, alcohol-induced mood disorder, alcohol-induced anxiety disorder, alcohol-induced sexual dysfunction, or alcohol-induced sleep disorder.

From American Psychiatric Association. *Diagnostic and Statistical Manual of Mental Disorders.* 4th ed. Text rev. Washington, DC: American Psychiatric Association; copyright 2000, with permission.

Alcohol-Related Use Disorder Not Otherwise Specified

DSM-IV-TR allows for the diagnosis of alcohol-related disorder not otherwise specified for alcohol-related disorders that do not meet the diagnostic criteria for any of the other diagnoses (Table 12.2–8).

Idiosyncratic Alcohol Intoxication. Whether there is such a diagnostic entity as idiosyncratic alcohol intoxication is under debate; DSM-IV-TR does not recognize this category as an official diagnosis. Several well-controlled studies of persons who supposedly have the disorder have raised questions about the validity of the designation. The condition has been variously called *pathologic, complicated, atypical,* and *paranoid alcohol intoxication;* all these terms indicate that a severe behavioral syndrome develops rapidly after a person consumes a small amount of alcohol that would have minimal behavioral effects on most persons. The diagnosis is important in the forensic arena because alcohol intoxication is not generally accepted as a reason for judging persons not responsible for their activities. Idiosyncratic alcohol intoxication, however, can be used in a person's defense if a defense lawyer can argue successfully that the defendant has an unexpected, idiosyncratic, pathological reaction to a minimal amount of alcohol.

In anecdotal reports, persons with idiosyncratic alcohol intoxication have been described as confused and disoriented and as experiencing illusions, transitory delusions, and visual hallucinations. Persons may display greatly increased psychomotor activity and impulsive, aggressive behavior. They may be dangerous to others and may also exhibit suicidal ideation and make suicide attempts. The disorder, usually described as lasting for a few hours, terminates in prolonged sleep, and those affected cannot recall the episodes on awakening. The cause of the condition is unknown, but it is reported to be most common in persons with high levels of anxiety. According to one hypothesis, alcohol causes sufficient disorganization and loss of control to release aggressive impulses. Another suggestion is that brain damage, particularly encephalitic or traumatic dam-

age, predisposes some persons to an intolerance for alcohol and thus to abnormal behavior after they ingest only small amounts. Other predisposing factors may include advancing age, using sedative-hypnotic drugs, and feeling fatigued. A person's behavior while intoxicated tends to be atypical; after one weak drink, a quiet, shy person becomes belligerent and aggressive.

In treating idiosyncratic alcohol intoxication, clinicians must help protect patients from harming themselves and others. Physical restraint may be necessary but is difficult because of the abrupt onset of the condition. Once a patient has been restrained, injection of an antipsychotic drug, such as haloperidol (Haldol), is useful for controlling assaultiveness. This condition must be differentiated from other causes of abrupt behavioral change, such as complex partial epilepsy. Some persons with the disorder reportedly showed temporal lobe spiking on an EEG after ingesting small amounts of alcohol.

Other Alcohol-Related Neurological Disorders

Only the major neuropsychiatric syndromes associated with alcohol use have been discussed here. The complete list of neurological syndromes is lengthy (Table 12.2–9). *Alcoholic pellagra encephalopathy* is one diagnosis of potential interest to psychiatrists presented with a patient who appears to be afflicted with Wernicke-Korsakoff syndrome but does not respond to thiamine treatment. The symptoms of alcoholic pellagra encephalopathy include confusion, clouding of consciousness, myoclonus, oppositional hypertonias, fatigue, apathy, irritability, anorexia, insomnia, and sometimes delirium. Patients suffer from a deficiency of niacin (nicotinic acid), and the specific treatment is 50 mg of niacin by mouth four times daily or 25 mg parenterally two to three times daily.

Fetal Alcohol Syndrome

Data indicate that women who are pregnant or are breast-feeding should not drink alcohol. Fetal alcohol syndrome, the leading cause of mental retardation in the United States, occurs when mothers drinking alcohol expose fetuses to alcohol in utero. The alcohol inhibits intrauterine growth and postnatal development. Microcephaly, craniofacial malformations, and limb and heart defects are common in affected infants. Short adult stature and development of a range of adult maladaptive behaviors have also been associated with fetal alcohol syndrome.

Table 12.2–9
Neurological and Medical Complications of Alcohol Use

- Alcohol intoxication
  - Acute intoxication
  - Pathological intoxication (atypical, complicated, unusual)
  - Blackouts
- Alcohol withdrawal syndromes
  - Tremulousness (the shakes or the jitters)
  - Alcoholic hallucinosis (horrors)
  - Withdrawal seizures (rum fits)
  - Delirium tremens (shakes)
- Nutritional diseases of the nervous system secondary to alcohol abuse
  - Wernicke-Korsakoff syndrome
  - Cerebellar degeneration
  - Peripheral neuropathy
  - Optic neuropathy (tobacco-alcohol amblyopia)
  - Pellagra
- Alcoholic diseases of uncertain pathogenesis
  - Central pontine myelinolysis
  - Marchiafava-Bignami disease
  - Fetal alcohol syndrome
  - Myopathy
  - Alcoholic dementia (?)
  - Alcoholic cerebral atrophy
- Systemic diseases due to alcohol with secondary neurological complications
  - Liver disease
    - Hepatic encephalopathy
    - Acquired (non-Wilsonian) chronic hepatocerebral degeneration
  - Gastrointestinal diseases
    - Malabsorption syndromes
    - Postgastrectomy syndromes
    - Possible pancreatic encephalopathy
  - Cardiovascular diseases
    - Cardiomyopathy with potential cardiogenic emboli and cerebrovascular disease
    - Arrhythmias and abnormal blood pressure leading to cerebrovascular disease
  - Hematological disorders
    - Anemia, leukopenia, thrombocytopenia (could possibly lead to hemorrhagic cerebrovascular disease)
  - Infectious disease, especially meningitis (especially pneumococcal and meningococcal)
  - Hypothermia and hyperthermia
  - Hypotension and hypertension
  - Respiratory depression and associated hypoxia
  - Toxic encephalopathies, including alcohol and other substances
  - Electrolyte imbalances leading to acute confusional states and, rarely, focal neurological signs and symptoms
    - Hypoglycemia
    - Hyperglycemia
    - Hyponatremia
    - Hypercalcemia
    - Hypomagnesemia
    - Hypophosphatemia
- Increased incidence of trauma
  - Epidural, subdural, and intracerebral hematoma
  - Spinal cord injury
  - Posttraumatic seizure disorders
  - Compressive neuropathies and brachial plexus injuries (Saturday night palsies)
  - Posttraumatic symptomatic hydrocephalus (normal pressure hydrocephalus)
  - Muscle crush injuries and compartmental syndromes

Reprinted with permission from Rubino FA. Neurologic complications of alcoholism. *Psychiatr Clin North Am.* 1992;15:361.

Women with alcohol-related disorders have a 35 percent risk of having a child with defects. Although the precise mechanism of the damage to the fetus is unknown, the damage seems to result from exposure in utero to ethanol or to its metabolites; alcohol may also cause hormone imbalances that increase the risk of abnormalities.

Prognosis

Between 10 and 40 percent of alcoholic persons enter some kind of formal treatment program during the course of their alcohol problems. A number of prognostic signs are favorable. First is the absence of preexisting antisocial personality disorder or a diagnosis of other substance abuse or dependence. Second, evidence of general life stability with a job, continuing close family contacts, and the absence of severe legal problems also bodes well for the patient. Third, if the patient stays for the full course of the initial rehabilitation (perhaps 2 to 4 weeks), the chances of maintaining abstinence are good. The combination of these three attributes predicts at least a 60 percent chance for 1 or more years of abstinence. Few studies have documented the long-term course, but researchers agree that 1 year of abstinence is associated with a good chance for continued abstinence over an extended period. However, alcoholic persons with severe drug problems (especially IV drug use or cocaine or amphetamine dependence) and those who are homeless may have only a 10 to 15 percent or so chance of achieving 1 year of abstinence.

Accurately predicting whether any specific person will achieve or maintain abstinence is impossible, but the prognostic factors listed above are associated with an increased likelihood of abstinence. However, the factors reflecting life stability probably explain only 20 percent or less of the course of alcohol use disorders. Many forces that are difficult to measure affect the clinical course significantly; they are likely to include such intangibles as motivational level and the quality of the patient's social support system.

In general, alcoholic persons with preexisting independent major psychiatric disorders—such as antisocial personality disorder, schizophrenia, and bipolar I disorder—are likely to run the course of their independent psychiatric illness. Thus, for example, clinicians must treat the patient with bipolar I disorder who has secondary alcoholism with appropriate psychotherapy and lithium (Eskalith), use relevant psychological and behavioral techniques for the patient with antisocial personality disorder, and offer appropriate antipsychotic medications on a long-term basis to the patient with schizophrenia. The goal is to minimize the symptoms of the independent psychiatric disorder in the hope that greater life stability will be associated with a better prognosis for the patient's alcohol problems.

TREATMENT AND REHABILITATION

Three general steps are involved in treating the alcoholic person after the disorder has been diagnosed—intervention, detoxification, and rehabilitation. These approaches assume that all possible efforts have been made to optimize medical functioning and to address psychiatric emergencies. Thus, for example, an alcoholic person with symptoms of depression severe enough to be suicidal requires inpatient hospitalization for at least several days until the suicidal ideation disappears. Similarly, a person presenting with cardiomyopathy, liver difficulties, or gastrointestinal bleeding first needs adequate treatment of the medical emergency.

The patient with alcohol abuse or dependence must then be brought face-to-face with the reality of the disorder (intervention), be detoxified if needed, and begin rehabilitation. The essentials of these three steps for an alcoholic person with independent psychiatric syndromes closely resemble the approaches used for the primary alcoholic person without independent psychiatric syndromes. However, in the former case the treatments are applied after the psychiatric disorder has been stabilized as much as possible.

Intervention

The goal in this step, which has also been called *confrontation,* is to break through feelings of denial and help the patient recognize the adverse consequences likely to occur if the disorder is not treated. Intervention is a process aimed at maximizing the motivation for treatment and continued abstinence.

This step often involves convincing patients that they are responsible for their own actions while reminding them of how alcohol has created significant life impairments. The psychiatrist often finds it useful to take advantage of the person's chief presenting complaint, whether it is insomnia, difficulties with sexual performance, an inability to cope with life stresses, depression, anxiety, or psychotic symptoms. The psychiatrist can then explain how alcohol has either created or contributed to these problems and can reassure the patient that abstinence can be achieved with a minimum of discomfort.

A physician was consulted by a 43-year-old businessman who was concerned about his wife. He had recently been confronted by their 21-year-old daughter, who felt that her mother was an alcoholic. The daughter noted her mother's slurred speech on several recent occasions when she had called home, noted times during the day when the mother was apparently home but did not answer the telephone, and observed high levels of alcohol consumption. A more detailed history revealed that the husband had been concerned about the wife's drinking pattern for at least 5 years; he related her practice of staying up after he went to bed and retiring later with alcohol on her breath. He also noted her consumption of 10 to 12 drinks at parties, with the resulting tendency to isolate herself from the remaining guests, her paniclike behavior regarding the need to pack liquor when they went on trips where alcohol might not be readily available, and what he observed to be a tremor of her hands some mornings during breakfast. The husband was given several potential courses of action, including the possibility of referring his wife for treatment with the physician. He was advised to share his concern with his wife when she was not actively intoxicated, emphasizing specific times and events when her impairment with alcohol was noted. He was also asked to consider whether a close friend of many years and the adult daughter might be included in this intervention, and it was suggested that a tentative appointment might be made with the clinician (or with an alcohol and drug treatment program) so that a next step could be established if the intervention was successful.

A physician intervening with a patient can use the same nonjudgmental but persistent approach each time an alcohol-related impairment is identified. It is the persistence rather than exceptional interpersonal skills that usually gets results. A single intervention is rarely enough. Most alcoholic persons need a series of reminders of how alcohol contributed to each developing crisis before they seriously consider abstinence as a long-term option.

Family

The family can be of great help in the intervention. Family members must learn not to protect the patient from the problems caused by alcohol; otherwise, the patient may not be able to gather the energy and the motivation necessary to stop drinking. During the intervention stage, the family can also suggest that the patient meet with persons who are recovering from alcoholism, perhaps through AA, and they can meet with groups, such as Al-Anon, that reach out to family members. Those support groups for families meet many times a week and help family members and friends see that they are not alone in their fears, worry, and feelings of guilt. Members share coping strategies and help each other find community resources. The groups can be most useful in helping family members rebuild their lives, even if the alcoholic person refuses to seek help.

Detoxification

Most persons with alcohol dependence have relatively mild symptoms when they stop drinking. If the patient is in relatively good health, is adequately nourished, and has a good social support system, the depressant withdrawal syndrome usually resembles a mild case of the flu. Even intense withdrawal syndromes rarely approach the severity of symptoms described by some early textbooks in the field.

The essential first step in detoxification is a thorough physical examination. In the absence of a serious medical disorder or combined drug abuse, severe alcohol withdrawal is unlikely. The second step is to offer rest, adequate nutrition, and multiple vitamins, especially those containing thiamine.

Mild or Moderate Withdrawal

Withdrawal develops because the brain has physically adapted to the presence of a brain depressant and cannot function adequately in the absence of the drug. Giving enough brain depressant on the first day to diminish symptoms and then weaning the patient off the drug over the next 5 days offers most patients optimal relief and minimizes the possibility that severe withdrawal will develop. Any depressant—including alcohol, barbiturates, or any of the benzodiazepines—can work, but most clinicians choose a benzodiazepine for its relative safety. Adequate treatment can be given with either short-acting drugs (e.g., lorazepam), or long-acting substances (e.g., chlordiazepoxide and diazepam).

An example of treatment is the administration of 25 mg of chlordiazepoxide by mouth three or four times a day on the first day, with a notation to skip a dose if the patient is asleep or feeling sleepy. An additional one or two 25-mg doses can be given during the first 24 hours if the patient is jittery or shows signs of increasing tremor or autonomic dysfunction. Whatever benzodiazepine dosage is required on the first day can be decreased by 20 percent each subsequent day, with a resulting need for no further medication after 4 or 5 days. When giving a long-acting agent, such as chlordiazepoxide, the clinician must avoid producing excessive sleepiness through overmedication; if the patient is sleepy, the next scheduled dose should be omitted. When taking a short-acting drug, such as lorazepam, the patient must not miss any dose because rapid changes in benzodiazepine concentrations in the blood may precipitate severe withdrawal.

A social model program of detoxification saves money by avoiding medications while using social supports. This less expensive regimen can be helpful for mild or moderate withdrawal syndromes. Some clinicians have also recommended β-adrenergic receptor antagonists (e.g., propranolol [Inderal]) or α-adrenergic receptor agonists (e.g., clonidine), although these medications do not appear to be superior to the benzodiazepines. Unlike the brain depressants, these other agents do little to decrease the risk of seizures or delirium.

Severe Withdrawal

For the approximately 1 to 3 percent of alcoholic patients with extreme autonomic dysfunction, agitation, and confusion—that is, those with alcoholic withdrawal delirium, or DTs—no optimal treatment has yet been developed. The first step is to ask why such a severe and relatively uncommon withdrawal syndrome has occurred; the answer often relates to a severe concomitant medical problem that needs immediate treatment. The withdrawal symptoms can then be minimized through the use of either benzodiazepines (in which case high doses are sometimes required) or antipsychotic agents, such as haloperidol. Once again, on the first or second day doses are used to control behavior, and the patient can be weaned off the medication by about the fifth day.

Another 1 to 3 percent of patients may have a single grand mal convulsion; the rare person has multiple fits, with the peak incidence on the second day of withdrawal. Such patients require neurological evaluation, but in the absence of evidence of a seizure disorder, they do not benefit from anticonvulsant drugs.

Rehabilitation

For most patients, rehabilitation includes three major components: (1) continued efforts to increase and maintain high levels of motivation for abstinence, (2) work to help the patient readjust to a lifestyle free of alcohol, and (3) relapse prevention. Because these steps are carried out in the context of acute and protracted withdrawal syndromes and life crises, treatment requires repeated presentations of similar materials that remind the patient how important abstinence is and that help the patient develop new day-to-day support systems and coping styles.

No single major life event, traumatic life period, or identifiable psychiatric disorder is known to be a unique cause of alcoholism. In addition, the effects of any causes of alcoholism are likely to have been diluted by the effects of alcohol on the brain and the years of an altered lifestyle, so that the alcoholism has developed a life of its own. This is true even though many alcoholic persons believe that the cause was depression, anxiety, life stress, or pain syndromes. Research, data from records, and resource persons usually reveal that alcohol contributed to the mood disorder, accident, or life stress, not vice versa.

The same general treatment approach is used in inpatient and outpatient settings. Selection of the more expensive and intensive inpatient mode often depends on evidence of additional severe medical or psychiatric syndromes, the absence of

appropriate nearby outpatient groups and facilities, and the patient's history of having failed in outpatient care. The treatment process in either setting involves intervention, optimizing physical and psychological functioning, enhancing motivation, reaching out to family, and using the first 2 to 4 weeks of care as an intensive period of help. Those efforts must be followed by at least 3 to 6 months of less frequent outpatient care. Outpatient care uses a combination of individual and group counseling, judicious avoidance of psychotropic medications unless needed for independent disorders, and involvement in such self-help groups as AA.

Counseling

Counseling efforts in the first several months should focus on day-to-day life issues to help patients maintain a high level of motivation for abstinence and to enhance their functioning. Psychotherapy techniques that provoke anxiety or that require deep insights have not been shown to be of benefit during the early months of recovery and, at least theoretically, may actually impair efforts at maintaining abstinence. Thus, this discussion focuses on the efforts likely to characterize the first 3 to 6 months of care.

Counseling or therapy can be carried out in an individual or group setting; few data indicate that either approach is superior. The technique used is not likely to matter greatly and usually boils down to simple day-to-day counseling or almost any behavioral or psychotherapeutic approach focusing on the here and now. To optimize motivation, treatment sessions should explore the consequences of drinking, the likely future course of alcohol-related life problems, and the marked improvement that can be expected with abstinence. Whether in an inpatient or an outpatient setting, individual or group counseling is usually offered a minimum of three times a week for the first 2 to 4 weeks, followed by less intense efforts, perhaps once a week, for the subsequent 3 to 6 months.

Much time in counseling deals with how to build a lifestyle free of alcohol. Discussions cover the need for a sober peer group, a plan for social and recreational events without drinking, and approaches for reestablishing communication with family members and friends.

The third major component, relapse prevention, first identifies situations in which the risk for relapse is high. The counselor must help the patient develop modes of coping to be used when the craving for alcohol increases or when any event or emotional state makes a return to drinking likely. An important part of relapse prevention is reminding the patient about the appropriate attitude toward slips. Short-term experiences with alcohol can never be used as an excuse for returning to regular drinking. The efforts to achieve and maintain a sober lifestyle are not a game in which all benefits are lost with that first sip. Rather, recovery is a process of trial and error; patients use slips that occur to identify high-risk situations and to develop more appropriate coping techniques.

Most treatment efforts recognize the effects that alcoholism has on the significant persons in the patient's life, and an important aspect of recovery involves helping family members and close friends understand alcoholism and realize that rehabilitation is an ongoing process that lasts for 6 to 12 or more months. Couples and family counseling and support groups for relatives and friends help the persons involved to rebuild relationships, to learn how to avoid protecting the patient from the consequences of any drinking in the future, and to be as supportive as possible of the alcoholic patient's recovery program.

Medications

If detoxification has been completed and the patient is not one of the 10 to 15 percent of alcoholic persons who have an independent mood disorder, schizophrenia, or anxiety disorder, little evidence favors prescribing psychotropic medications for the treatment of alcoholism. Lingering levels of anxiety and insomnia as part of a reaction to life stresses and protracted abstinence should be treated with behavior modification approaches and reassurance. Medications for these symptoms (including benzodiazepines) are likely to lose their effectiveness much faster than the insomnia disappears; thus, the patient may increase the dose and have subsequent problems. Similarly, sadness and mood swings can linger at low levels for several months. However, controlled clinical trials indicate no benefit in prescribing antidepressant medications or lithium to treat the average alcoholic person who has no independent or long-lasting psychiatric disorder. The mood disorder will clear before the medications can take effect, and patients who resume drinking while on the medications face significant potential dangers. With little or no evidence that the medications are effective, the dangers significantly outweigh any potential benefits from their routine use.

One possible exception to the proscription against the use of medications is the alcohol-sensitizing agent disulfiram. Disulfiram is given in daily doses of 250 mg before the patient is discharged from the intensive first phase of outpatient rehabilitation or from inpatient care. The goal is to place the patient in a condition in which drinking alcohol precipitates an uncomfortable physical reaction, including nausea, vomiting, and a burning sensation in the face and stomach. Unfortunately, few data prove that disulfiram is more effective than a placebo, probably because most persons stop taking the disulfiram when they resume drinking. Many clinicians have stopped routinely prescribing the agent, partly in recognition of the dangers associated with the drug itself: mood swings, rare instances of psychosis, the possibility of increased peripheral neuropathies, the relatively rare occurrence of other significant neuropathies, and potentially fatal hepatitis. Moreover, patients with preexisting heart disease, cerebral thrombosis, diabetes, and a number of other conditions cannot be given disulfiram because an alcohol reaction to the disulfiram could be fatal.

Two additional promising pharmacological interventions have recently been studied. The first involves the opioid antagonist naltrexone (ReVia), which is at least theoretically believed to possibly decrease the craving for alcohol or blunt the rewarding effects of drinking. In any event, two relatively small (approximately 90 patients on the active drug across the studies) and short-term (3 months of active treatment) investigations using 50 mg per day of this drug had potentially promising results. However, evaluating the full impact of this medication will require longer-term studies of relatively large groups of more diverse patients.

The second medication of interest, acamprosate (Campral), has been tested in over 5,000 alcohol-dependent patients in

Europe. This drug is not yet available in the United States. Used in dosages of approximately 2,000 mg per day, this medication was associated with approximately 10 to 20 percent more positive outcomes than placebo when used in the context of the usual psychological and behavioral treatment regimens for alcoholism. The mechanism of action of acamprosate is not known, but it may act directly or indirectly at GABA receptors or at NMDA sites, the effects of which alter the development of tolerance or physical dependence upon alcohol.

Another medication with potential promise in the treatment of alcoholism is the nonbenzodiazepine antianxiety drug buspirone (BuSpar), although the effect of this drug on alcohol rehabilitation is inconsistent between studies. However, no evidence exists that antidepressant medications such as the selective serotonin reuptake inhibitors (SSRIs), lithium, or antipsychotic medications are significantly effective in the treatment of alcoholism.

Self-Help Groups

Clinicians must recognize the potential importance of self-help groups like AA. Members of AA have help available 24 hours a day, associate with a sober peer group, learn that it is possible to participate in social functions without drinking, and are given a model of recovery by observing the accomplishments of sober members of the group. Learning about AA usually begins during inpatient or outpatient rehabilitation. The clinician can play a major role in helping patients understand the differences between specific groups. Some groups are composed of only men or only women; others are mixed. Some meetings are mostly for blue-collar men and women; others are mostly for professionals. Some groups place great emphasis on religion; others are eclectic. Patients with coexisting psychiatric disorders may need some additional education about AA. The clinician should remind them that some members of AA may not understand their special need for medications and should arm the patients with ways of coping when group members suggest inappropriately that the required medications be stopped.

References

Bierut LJ, Dinwiddie SH, Begleiter H, et al. Familial transmission of substance dependence: alcohol, marijuana, cocaine, and habitual smoking: a report from the Collaborative Study on the Genetics of Alcoholism. *Arch Gen Psychiatry.* 1998;55:982.

Blane HT, Leonard KE, eds. *Psychological Theories of Drinking and Alcoholism.* 2nd ed. New York: Guilford Press; 1999.

Heather N, Peters TJ, eds. *International Handbook of Alcohol Dependence and Problems.* New York: John Wiley & Sons; 2001:497.

Helander A, Carlsson AV, Borg S. Longitudinal comparison of carbohydrate-deficient transferrin and gamma-glutamyl transferase: complementary markers of excessive alcohol consumption. *Alcohol Alcohol.* 1996;31:101.

Kabel DI, Petty F. A placebo-controlled, double-blind study of fluoxetine in severe alcohol dependence: adjunctive pharmacotherapy during and after inpatient treatment. *Alcohol Clin Exp Res.* 1996;20:780.

Koob GF, Roberts AJ. Brain reward circuits in alcoholism. *CNS Spectrums.* 1999;4:23.

Kranzler HR, Burleson JA, Del Boca FK, et al. Buspirone treatment of anxious alcoholics: a placebo-controlled trial. *Arch Gen Psychiatry.* 1994;51:720.

Pfefferbaum A, Lim KO, Desmond JE, Sullivan EV. Thinning of the corpus callosum in older alcoholic men: a magnetic resonance imaging study. *Alcohol Clin Exp Res.* 1996;20:752.

Prescott CA, Kendler KS. Genetic and environmental contributions to alcohol abuse and dependence in a population-based sample of male twins. *Am J Psychiatry.* 1999;156:34.

Project MATCH Research Group. Matching alcoholism treatments to client heterogeneity. Project MATCH posttreatment drinking outcomes. *J Stud Alcohol.* 1997;58:7.

Roberts LJ, Linney KD. Alcohol problems and couples: drinking in an intimate relational context. In: Schmaling KB, Sher TG, eds. *The Psychology of Couples and Illness: Theory, Research, & Practice.* Washington, DC: American Psychological Association; 2000:269.

Schuckit MA. Alcohol-related disorders. In: Sadock, BJ, Sadock VA, editors. *Kaplan & Sadock's Comprehensive Textbook of Psychiatry.* 7th ed. Vol 1. Baltimore: Lippincott Williams &Wilkins; 2000:953.

Schuckit MA, Daeppen J-B, Tipp JE, Hesselbock M, Bucholz KK. The clinical course of alcohol-related problems in alcohol dependent and nonalcohol dependent drinking women and men. *J Stud Alcohol.* 1998;59:81.

Schuckit MA, Smith TL, Daeppen J-B, et al. Clinical relevance of the distinction between alcohol dependence with and without a physiological component. *Am J Psychiatry.* 1998;155:733.

Schuckit MA, Tipp JE, Bergman M, Reich W, Hesselbrock VM, Smith TL. Comparison of induced and independent major depressive disorders in 2945 alcoholics. *Am J Psychiatry.* 1997;154:948.

Schuckit MA, Tipp JE, Bucholz KK, et al. The lifetime rates of three major mood disorders and four major anxiety disorders in alcoholics and controls. *Addiction.* 1997;92:1289.

Thun MJ, Peto R, Lopez AD, et al. Alcohol consumption and mortality among middle-aged and elderly U.S. adults. *N Engl J Med.* 1997;337:1705.

Tsai G, Gastfriend DR, Coyle JT. The glutamatergic basis of human alcoholism. *Am J Psychiatry.* 1995;152:332.

Vaillant GE. A long-term follow-up of male alcohol abuse. *Arch Gen Psychiatry.* 1996;53:243.

Yeastedt J, La Grange L, Anton RF. Female alcoholic outpatients and female college students: a correlational study of self-reported alcohol consumption and carbohydrate-deficient transferrin levels. *J Stud Alcohol.* 1998;59:555.

Zernig G, Saria A, eds. *Handbook of Alcoholism. Pharmacology and Toxicology.* Boca Raton, FL: CRC Press; 2000:363.

▲ 12.3 Amphetamine (or Amphetaminelike)-Related Disorders

Amphetamines are the most widely used illicit drugs, second only to cannabis, in Great Britain, Australia, and several countries of Western Europe. In the United States, lifetime and current cocaine use still exceeds the nonmedical use of amphetamines; some studies report up to 600,000 abusers. In addition, methamphetamine (a congener of amphetamine) has also become a major drug of abuse.

The racemate amphetamine sulfate (Benzedrine) was first synthesized in 1887 and was introduced to clinical practice in 1932 as an over-the-counter inhaler for the treatment of nasal congestion and asthma. In 1937, amphetamine sulfate tablets were introduced for the treatment of narcolepsy, postencephalitic parkinsonism, depression, and lethargy. In the 1970s, a variety of social and regulatory factors began to curb widespread amphetamine distribution. The current U.S. Food and Drug Administration (FDA)–approved indications for amphetamine are limited to attention-deficit/hyperactivity disorder and narcolepsy. Amphetamines are also used in the treatment of obesity, depression, dysthymia, chronic fatigue syndrome, acquired immune deficiency syndrome (AIDS), and neurasthenia and as adjunctive therapy for depression resistant to drug treatment.

PREPARATIONS

The major amphetamines currently available and used in the United States are dextroamphetamine (Dexedrine), methamphetamine (Desoxyn), a mixed dextroamphetamine–amphetamine salt (Adderall), and methylphenidate (Ritalin). These drugs go by such street names as ice, crystal, crystal meth, and

speed. As a general class, the amphetamines are also referred to as analeptics, sympathomimetics, stimulants, and psychostimulants. The typical amphetamines are used to increase performance and to induce a euphoric feeling, for example, by students studying for examinations, by long-distance truck drivers on trips, by businesspeople with important deadlines, and by athletes in competition. Although not as addictive as cocaine, amphetamines are nonetheless addictive drugs.

Other amphetaminelike substances are ephedrine and pseudoephedrine, which are available over the counter in the United States as nasal decongestants. Phenylpropanolamine (PPA) is a psychostimulant, which, although less potent than the classic amphetamines, ephedrine, and PPA, is subject to abuse, partly because of its easy availability and low price. These drugs, PPA in particular, can dangerously exacerbate hypertension, precipitate a toxic psychosis, or result in death. The safety margin for PPA is particularly narrow, and three to four times the normal dose can result in life-threatening hypertension.

Methamphetamine

Methamphetamine (also called "ice") is a pure form that abusers of the substance inhale, smoke, or inject intravenously. Its psychological effects last for hours and are described as particularly powerful. Unlike crack cocaine (see Section 12.6), which must be imported, methamphetamine is a synthetic drug that can be manufactured domestically in illicit laboratories.

Amphetaminelike Substances

The classic amphetamine drugs (i.e., dextroamphetamine, methamphetamine, and methylphenidate) exert their major effects through the dopaminergic system. Substituted, so-called designer amphetamines (discussed below) have neurochemical effects on both the serotonergic and the dopaminergic systems and have behavioral effects that reflect a combination of amphetaminelike and hallucinogenlike activities. Some psychopharmacologists classify the substituted amphetamines as hallucinogens; in this textbook, however, they are classified with the amphetamines to which they are closely related structurally. Examples of the substituted amphetamines include 3,4-methylenedioxyamphetamine (MDMA), also referred to as "ecstasy," "XTC," and "Adam"; *N*-ethyl-3,4-methylenedioxyamphetamine (MDEA), also referred to as "Eve"; 5-methoxy-3,4-methylenedioxyamphetamine (MMDA); and 2,5-dimethoxy-4-methylamphetamine (DOM), also referred to as "STP." Of these drugs, MDMA has been studied most closely and is perhaps the most widely available. These drugs are discussed in greater detail below.

EPIDEMIOLOGY

In 2000, about 4 percent of the U.S. population used psychostimulants. The 18- to 25-year-old age group reported the highest level of use, followed by the 12- to 17-year-old group. Amphetamine use occurs in all socioeconomic groups, and amphetamine use is increasing among white professionals. Because amphetamines are available by prescription for specific indications, prescribing physicians must be aware of the risk of amphetamine abuse by others, including friends and family members of the patient receiving the amphetamine. No reliable data are available on the epidemiology of designer amphetamine use, but they are greatly abused. According to the text revision of the fourth edition of *Diagnostic and Statistical Manual of Mental Disorders* (DSM-IV-TR), the lifetime prevalence of amphetamine dependence and abuse is 1.5 percent, and the male to female ratio is 1.

NEUROPHARMACOLOGY

All the amphetamines are rapidly absorbed orally and have a rapid onset of action, usually within 1 hour when taken orally. The classic amphetamines are also taken intravenously and have an almost immediate effect by this route. Nonprescribed amphetamines and designer amphetamines are also inhaled ("snorting"). Tolerance develops with both classic and designer amphetamines, although amphetamine users often overcome the tolerance by taking more of the drug. Amphetamine is less addictive than cocaine, as evidenced by experiments on rats in which not all animals spontaneously self-administered low doses of amphetamine.

The classic amphetamines (i.e., dextroamphetamine, methamphetamine, and methylphenidate) produce their primary effects by causing the release of catecholamines, particularly dopamine, from presynaptic terminals. The effects are particularly potent for the dopaminergic neurons projecting from the ventral tegmental area to the cerebral cortex and the limbic areas. This pathway has been termed the *reward circuit pathway,* and its activation is probably the major addicting mechanism for the amphetamines.

The designer amphetamines (e.g., MDMA, MDEA, MMDA, and DOM) cause the release of catecholamines (dopamine and norepinephrine) and of serotonin, the neurotransmitter implicated as the major neurochemical pathway for hallucinogens. Therefore, the clinical effects of designer amphetamines are a blend of the effects of classic amphetamines and those of hallucinogens. The pharmacology of MDMA is the best understood of this group. MDMA is taken up in serotonergic neurons by the serotonin transporter responsible for serotonin reuptake. Once in the neuron, MDMA causes rapid release of a bolus of serotonin and inhibits the activity of serotonin-producing enzymes.

DIAGNOSIS

DSM-IV-TR lists many amphetamine (or amphetaminelike)-related disorders (Table 12.3–1) but specifies diagnostic criteria only for amphetamine intoxication (Table 12.3–2), amphetamine withdrawal (Table 12.3–3), and amphetamine-related disorder not otherwise specified (Table 12.3–4) in the section on amphetamine (or amphetaminelike)-related disorders. The diagnostic criteria for the other amphetamine (or amphetaminelike)-related disorders are contained in the DSM-IV-TR sections dealing with the primary phenomenological symptom (e.g., psychosis).

Amphetamine Dependence and Amphetamine Abuse

The DSM-IV-TR criteria for dependence and abuse are applied to amphetamine and its related substances (see Tables 12.1–5, 12.1–6, and 12.1–7 in Section 12.1). Amphetamine dependence

Table 12.3–1
DSM-IV-TR Amphetamine (or Amphetaminelike)-Related Disorders

Amphetamine use disorders
Amphetamine dependence
Amphetamine abuse
Amphetamine-induced disorders
Amphetamine intoxication
Specify if:
With perceptual disturbances
Amphetamine withdrawal
Amphetamine intoxication delirium
Amphetamine-induced psychotic disorder, with delusions
Specify if:
With onset during intoxication
Amphetamine-induced psychotic disorder, with hallucinations
Specify if:
With onset during intoxication
Amphetamine-induced mood disorder
Specify if:
With onset during intoxication
With onset during withdrawal
Amphetamine-induced anxiety disorder
Specify if:
With onset during intoxication
Amphetamine-induced sexual dysfunction
Specify if:
With onset during intoxication
Amphetamine-induced sleep disorder
Specify if:
With onset during intoxication
With onset during withdrawal
Amphetamine-related disorder not otherwise specified

From American Psychiatric Association. *Diagnostic and Statistical Manual of Mental Disorders.* 4th ed. Text rev. Washington, DC: American Psychiatric Association; copyright 2000, with permission.

can result in a rapid downward spiral of a person's abilities to cope with work- and family-related obligations and stresses. A person who abuses amphetamines requires increasingly high doses of amphetamine to obtain the usual high, and physical signs of amphetamine abuse (e.g., decreased weight and paranoid ideas) almost always develop with continued abuse.

Amphetamine Intoxication

The intoxication syndromes of cocaine (which blocks dopamine reuptake) and amphetamines (which cause the release of dopamine) are similar. Because more rigorous, in-depth research has been done on cocaine abuse and intoxication than on amphetamines, the clinical literature on amphetamines has been strongly influenced by the clinical findings of cocaine abuse. In DSM-IV-TR, the diagnostic criteria for amphetamine intoxication (Table 12.3–2) and cocaine intoxication (see Table 12.6–2 in Section 12.6) are separated but are virtually the same. DSM-IV-TR specifies perceptual disturbances as a symptom of amphetamine intoxication. If intact reality testing is absent, a diagnosis of amphetamine-induced psychotic disorder with onset during intoxication is indicated. The symptoms of amphetamine intoxication are mostly resolved after 24 hours and are generally completely resolved after 48 hours.

Table 12.3–2
DSM-IV-TR Diagnostic Criteria for Amphetamine Intoxication

A. Recent use of amphetamine or a related substance (e.g., methylphenidate).
B. Clinically significant maladaptive behavioral or psychological changes (e.g., euphoria or affective blunting; changes in sociability; hypervigilance; interpersonal sensitivity; anxiety, tension, or anger; stereotyped behaviors; impaired judgment; or impaired social or occupational functioning) that developed during, or shortly after, use of amphetamine or a related substance.
C. Two (or more) of the following, developing during, or shortly after, use of amphetamine or a related substance:
(1) tachycardia or bradycardia
(2) pupillary dilation
(3) elevated or lowered blood pressure
(4) perspiration or chills
(5) nausea or vomiting
(6) evidence of weight loss
(7) psychomotor agitation or retardation
(8) muscular weakness, respiratory depression, chest pain, or cardiac arrhythmias
(9) confusion, seizures, dyskinesias, dystonias, or coma
D. The symptoms are not due to a general medical condition and are not better accounted for by another mental disorder.

Specify if:
With perceptual disturbances

From American Psychiatric Association. *Diagnostic and Statistical Manual of Mental Disorders.* 4th ed. Text rev. Washington, DC: American Psychiatric Association; copyright 2000, with permission.

Table 12.3–3
DSM-IV-TR Diagnostic Criteria for Amphetamine Withdrawal

A. Cessation of (or reduction in) amphetamine (or a related substance) use that has been heavy and prolonged.
B. Dysphoric mood and two (or more) of the following physiological changes, developing within a few hours to several days after Criterion A:
(1) fatigue
(2) vivid, unpleasant dreams
(3) insomnia or hypersomnia
(4) increased appetite
(5) psychomotor retardation or agitation
C. The symptoms in Criterion B cause clinically significant distress or impairment in social, occupational, or other important areas of functioning.
D. The symptoms are not due to a general medical condition and are not better accounted for by another mental disorder.

From American Psychiatric Association. *Diagnostic and Statistical Manual of Mental Disorders.* 4th ed. Text rev. Washington, DC: American Psychiatric Association; copyright 2000, with permission.

Table 12.3–4
DSM-IV-TR Diagnostic Criteria for Amphetamine-Related Disorder Not Otherwise Specified

The amphetamine-related disorder not otherwise specified category is for disorders associated with the use of amphetamine (or a related substance) that are not classifiable as amphetamine dependence, amphetamine abuse, amphetamine intoxication, amphetamine withdrawal, amphetamine intoxication delirium, amphetamine-induced psychotic disorder, amphetamine-induced mood disorder, amphetamine-induced anxiety disorder, amphetamine-induced sexual dysfunction, or amphetamine-induced sleep disorder.

From American Psychiatric Association. *Diagnostic and Statistical Manual of Mental Disorders.* 4th ed. Text rev. Washington, DC: American Psychiatric Association; copyright 2000, with permission.

Amphetamine Withdrawal

After amphetamine intoxication, a crash occurs with symptoms of anxiety, tremulousness, dysphoric mood, lethargy, fatigue, nightmares (accompanied by rebound rapid eye movement [REM] sleep), headache, profuse sweating, muscle cramps, stomach cramps, and insatiable hunger. The withdrawal symptoms generally peak in 2 to 4 days and are resolved in 1 week. The most serious withdrawal symptom is depression, which can be particularly severe after the sustained use of high doses of amphetamine and which can be associated with suicidal ideation or behavior. The DSM-IV-TR diagnostic criteria for amphetamine withdrawal (Table 12.3–3) specify that a dysphoric mood and physiological changes are necessary for the diagnosis.

Amphetamine Intoxication Delirium

Under substance-related disorder, DSM-IV-TR includes a diagnosis of amphetamine intoxication delirium (see Table 10.2–3). Delirium associated with amphetamine use generally results from high doses of amphetamine or from sustained use, and so sleep deprivation affects the clinical presentation. The combination of amphetamines with other substances and the use of amphetamines by a person with preexisting brain damage can also cause development of delirium. It is not uncommon for university students using amphetamines to cram for examinations to exhibit this type of delirium.

Amphetamine-Induced Psychotic Disorder

The clinical similarity of amphetamine-induced psychosis to paranoid schizophrenia has prompted extensive study of the neurochemistry of amphetamine-induced psychosis to elucidate the pathophysiology of paranoid schizophrenia. The hallmark of amphetamine-induced psychotic disorder is the presence of paranoia. Amphetamine-induced psychotic disorder can be distinguished from paranoid schizophrenia by several differentiating characteristics associated with the former, including a predominance of visual hallucinations, generally appropriate affects, hyperactivity, hypersexuality, confusion and incoherence, and little evidence of disordered thinking (such as looseness of associations). In several studies, investigators also noted that although the positive symptoms of amphetamine-induced psychotic disorder and schizophrenia are similar, amphetamine-induced psychotic disorder generally lacks the affective flattening and alogia of schizophrenia. Clinically, however, acute amphetamine-induced psychotic disorder can be completely indistinguishable from schizophrenia, and only the resolution of the symptoms in a few days or a positive finding in a urine drug screen test eventually reveals the correct diagnosis.

The treatment of choice for amphetamine-induced psychotic disorder is the short-term use of an antipsychotic medication such as haloperidol (Haldol). DSM-IV-TR lists the diagnostic criteria for amphetamine-induced psychotic disorder with the other psychotic disorders (see Table 14.4–7) and allows clinicians to specify whether delusions or hallucinations are the predominant symptoms.

This agitated 42-year-old businessman was admitted to the psychiatric service after a 2½-month period in which he found himself becoming increasingly distrustful of others and suspicious of his business associates. He was taking their statements out of context, "twisting" their words, and making inappropriately hostile and accusatory comments; he had, in fact, lost several business deals that had been "virtually sealed." Finally, the patient fired a shotgun into his backyard late one night when he heard noises that convinced him that intruders were about to break into his house and kill him.

One and one-half years previously, the patient had been diagnosed as having Narcolepsy because of daily irresistible sleep attacks and episodes of sudden loss of muscle tone when he became emotionally excited, and had been placed on an amphetaminelike stimulant, methylphenidate. He became asymptomatic and was able to work quite effectively as the sales manager of a small office-machine company and to participate in an active social life with his family and a small circle of friends.

In the 4 months before admission, the patient had been using increasingly large doses of methylphenidate to maintain alertness late at night because of an increasing amount of work that could not be handled during the day. He reported that during this time he often could feel his heart race and had trouble sitting still.

DISCUSSION

The primary symptoms are palpitations, psychomotor agitation, hypervigilance, paranoid ideation about his coworkers, and delusions of reference (the patient acted on his belief that noises indicated the presence of intruders who were about to kill him). The presence of psychotic symptoms during these periods of drug-induced intoxication and the absence of preexisting psychotic disorder indicate Methylphenidate-Induced Psychotic Disorder. Because the clinical picture is dominated by delusions rather than hallucinations, With Delusions is noted. Had there not been any psychotic symptoms and the patient had sought help for the other symptoms; such as hypervigilance and psychomotor agitation, the diagnosis would have the residual category Methylphenidate Intoxication.

Narcolepsy, although traditionally considered a neurologic disorder, is a sleep disorder in DSM-IV, and is noted on Axis I. (From *DSM-IV Casebook.*)

Amphetamine-Induced Mood Disorder

According to DSM-IV-TR, the onset of amphetamine-induced mood disorder can occur during intoxication or withdrawal (see Table 15.3–10). In general, intoxication is associated with manic or mixed mood features, whereas withdrawal is associated with depressive mood features.

Amphetamine-Induced Anxiety Disorder

In DSM-IV-TR, the onset of amphetamine-induced anxiety disorder can also occur during intoxication or withdrawal (see Table 16.7–3). Amphetamine, like cocaine, can induce symptoms similar to those seen in obsessive-compulsive disorder, panic disorder, and phobic disorders, in particular.

Amphetamine-Induced Sexual Dysfunction

Amphetamine is often used to enhance sexual experiences; however, high doses and long-term use are associated with erectile disorder and other sexual dysfunctions. These dysfunctions are classified in DSM-IV-TR as amphetamine-induced sexual dysfunction with onset during intoxication (see Table 21.2–17).

Amphetamine-Induced Sleep Disorder

The diagnostic criteria for amphetamine-induced sleep disorder with onset during intoxication or withdrawal are found in the DSM-IV-TR section on sleep disorders (see Table 24.2–21). Amphetamine intoxication can produce insomnia and sleep deprivation, whereas persons undergoing amphetamine withdrawal can experience hypersomnolence and nightmares.

Disorder Not Otherwise Specified

If an amphetamine (or amphetaminelike)-related disorder does not meet the criteria of one or more of the categories discussed above, it can be diagnosed as an amphetamine-related disorder not otherwise specified (Table 12.3–4).

CLINICAL FEATURES

In persons who have not previously used amphetamines, a single 5-mg dose increases the sense of well-being and induces elation, euphoria, and friendliness. Small doses generally improve attention and increase performance on written, oral, and performance tasks. There is also an associated decrease in fatigue, induction of anorexia, and heightening of the pain threshold. Undesirable effects result from the use of high doses for long periods.

Adverse Effects

Amphetamines. PHYSICAL. Amphetamine abuse can produce adverse effects, the most serious of which include cerebrovascular, cardiac, and gastrointestinal effects. Among the specific life-threatening conditions are myocardial infarction, severe hypertension, cerebrovascular disease, and ischemic colitis. A continuum of neurological symptoms, from twitching to tetany to seizures to coma and death, is associated with increasingly high amphetamine doses. Intravenous use of amphetamines can transmit human immunodeficiency virus (HIV) and hepatitis and further the development of lung abscesses, endocarditis, and necrotizing angiitis. Several studies have shown that abusers of amphetamines knew little—or did not care—about safe-sex practices and the use of condoms. The non–life-threatening adverse effects of amphetamine abuse include flushing, pallor, cyanosis, fever, headache, tachycardia, palpitations, nausea, vomiting, bruxism (teeth grinding), shortness of breath, tremor, and ataxia. Pregnant women who use amphetamines often have babies with low birth weight, small head circumference, early gestational age, and growth retardation.

PSYCHOLOGICAL. The adverse psychological effects associated with amphetamine use include restlessness, dysphoria, insomnia, irritability, hostility, and confusion. Amphetamine use can also induce symptoms of anxiety disorders such as generalized anxiety disorder and panic disorder as well as ideas of reference, paranoid delusions, and hallucinations.

Other Agents

Substituted Amphetamines. MDMA is one of a series of substituted amphetamines that also includes MDEA, 3,4-methylenedioxyamphetamine (MDA), 2,5-dimethoxy-4-bromo-amphetamine (DOB), paramethoxyamphetamine (PMA), and others. These drugs produce subjective effects resembling those of amphetamine and lysergic acid diethylamide (LSD), and in that sense, MDMA and similar analogues may represent a distinct category of drugs.

A methamphetamine derivative that came into use in the 1980s, MDMA was not technically subject to legal regulation at the time. Although it has been labeled a "designer drug" in the belief that it was deliberately synthesized to evade legal regulation, it was actually synthesized and patented in 1914. Several psychiatrists used it as an adjunct to psychotherapy and concluded that it had value. At one time it was advertised as legal and was used in psychotherapy for its subjective effects. However, it was never approved by the FDA. Its use raised questions of both safety and legality, since the related amphetamine derivatives MDA, DOB, and PMA had caused a number of overdose deaths, and MDA was known to cause extensive destruction of serotonergic nerve terminals in the central nervous system (CNS). Using emergency scheduling authority, the Drug Enforcement Agency made MDMA a Schedule I drug under the CSA, along with LSD, heroin, and marijuana. Despite its illegal status, MDMA continues to be manufactured, distributed, and used in the United States, Europe, and Australia. Its use is common in Australia and Great Britain at extended dances ("raves") popular with adolescents and young adults.

MECHANISMS OF ACTION. The unusual properties of the drugs may be a consequence of the different actions of the optical isomers: the *R*(−) isomers produce LSD-like effects and the amphetaminelike properties are linked to *S*(+) isomers. The LSD-like actions, in turn, may be linked to the capacity to release serotonin. The various derivatives may exhibit significant differences in subjective effects and toxicity. Animals in laboratory experiments will self-administer the drugs, suggesting prominent amphetaminelike effects.

SUBJECTIVE EFFECTS. After taking usual doses (100 to 150 mg), MDMA users experience elevated mood and, according to various

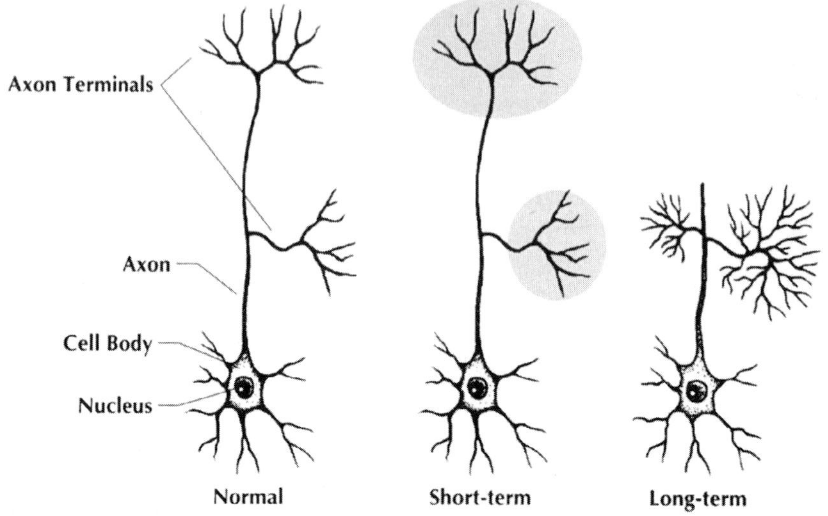

FIGURE 12.3–1

Neurotoxic effects of MDMA. Studies have found that MDMA damages serotonin-producing neurons in the brains of nonhuman primates. The *illustration* on the *left* shows a normal neuron. The *shaded area* in the *middle illustration* shows the axon terminals of the neuron that are damaged by MDMA. The *illustration* on the *right* shows how, 12 to 18 months after being damaged by MDMA, serotonin-producing nerve fibers have regrown excessively in some areas and not at all in others. (Reprinted from Mathias R. Like methamphetamine, "ecstasy" may cause long-term brain damage. *NIDA Notes.* 1996;11:7.)

reports, increased self-confidence and sensory sensitivity; peaceful feelings coupled with insight, empathy, and closeness to persons; and decreased appetite. Difficulty concentrating and an increased capacity to focus have both been reported. Dysphoric reactions, psychotomimetic effects, and psychosis have also been reported. Higher doses seem more likely to produce psychotomimetic effects. Sympathomimetic effects of tachycardia, palpitation, increased blood pressure, sweating, and bruxism are common. The subjective effects are reported to be prominent for about 4 to 8 hours, but they may not last as long or may last longer, depending on the dose and route of administration. The drug is usually taken orally but is also snorted and injected. Both tachyphylaxis and some tolerance are reported by users.

TOXICITY. Although it is not as toxic as MDA, various somatic toxicities have been attributed to MDMA use as well as fatal overdoses. It does not appear to be neurotoxic when injected into the brains of animals, but it is metabolized to MDA in both animals and humans. In animals, MDMA produces selective, long-lasting damage to serotonergic nerve terminals. It is not certain if the levels of the MDA metabolite reached in humans after the usual doses of MDMA suffice to produce lasting damage. Nonhuman primates are more sensitive than rodents to MDMA's toxic effects and show more prolonged or permanent neurotoxicity at doses not much higher than those used by humans (Fig. 12.3–1). Users of MDMA show differences in neuroendocrine responses to serotonergic probes, and studies of former MDMA users show global and regional decreases in serotonin transporter binding, as measured by positron emission tomography.

There are currently no established clinical uses for MDMA, although before its regulation, there were several reports of its beneficial effects as an adjunct to psychotherapy.

Khat. The fresh leaves of *Catha edulis,* a bush native to East Africa, have been used as a stimulant in the Middle East, Africa, and the Arabian Peninsula for at least 1,000 years. Khat is still widely used in Ethiopia, Kenya, Somalia, and Yemen. The amphetaminelike effects of khat have long been recognized, and although efforts to isolate the active ingredient were first undertaken in the 19th century, only since the 1970s has cathinone (*S*[–] α-aminopropiophenone or *S*[–]2-amino-1-phenyl-1-propanone) been identified as the substance responsible. Cathinone is a precursor moiety that is normally enzymatically converted in the plant to the less active entities norephedrine and cathine (norpseudoephedrine), which explains why only the fresh leaves of the plant are valued for their stimulant effects. Cathinone has most of the CNS and peripheral actions of amphetamine and appears to have the same mechanism of action. In humans it elevates mood, decreases hunger, and alleviates fatigue. At high doses it can induce an amphetaminelike psychosis in humans. Because it is typically absorbed buccally after chewing the leaf and because the alkaloid is metabolized relatively rapidly, high toxic blood levels are rarely reached. Concern about khat use is linked to its dependence-producing properties rather than to its acute toxicity. It is estimated that five million doses are consumed each day, despite prohibition of its use in a number of African and Arab countries.

In the 1990s, several clandestine laboratories began synthesizing methcathinone, a drug with actions quite similar to those of cathinone. Known by a number of street names (e.g., "CAT," "goob," and "crank"), its popularity is due primarily to its ease of synthesis from ephedrine or pseudoephedrine, which were readily available until placed under special controls. Methcathinone has been moved to Schedule (Control Level) I of the CSA. The patterns of use, adverse effects, and complications closely resemble those reported for amphetamine.

TREATMENT AND REHABILITATION

The treatment of amphetamine (or amphetaminelike)-related disorders shares with cocaine-related disorders the difficulty of helping patients remain abstinent from the drug, which is pow-

erfully reinforcing and induces craving. An inpatient setting and the use of multiple therapeutic methods (individual, family, and group psychotherapy) are usually necessary to achieve lasting abstinence. The treatment of specific amphetamine-induced disorders (e.g., amphetamine-induced psychotic disorder and amphetamine-induced anxiety disorder) with specific drugs (e.g., antipsychotic and anxiolytics) may be necessary on a short-term basis. Antipsychotics may be prescribed for the first few days. In the absence of psychosis, diazepam (Valium) is useful to treat patients' agitation and hyperactivity.

Physicians should establish a therapeutic alliance with patients to deal with the underlying depression or personality disorder or both. Because many patients are heavily dependent on the drug, however, psychotherapy may be especially difficult.

Comorbid conditions such as depression may respond to antidepressant medication. Bupropion (Wellbutrin) may be of use after patients have withdrawn from amphetamine. It has the effect of producing feelings of well-being as these patients cope with the dysphoria that may accompany abstinence.

References

Ail SF, ed. Neurobiological mechanisms of drugs of abuse: cocaine, ibogaine, and substituted amphetamines. *Ann Acad Sci.* 2000;914:1.

Anthony JC, Warner LA, Kessler RC. Comparative epidemiology of dependence on tobacco, alcohol, controlled substances, and inhalants: basic findings from the National Comorbidity Survey. *Exp Clin Psychopharmacol.* 1994;2:244.

Battaglia G, Napier TC. The effects of cocaine and the amphetamines on brain and behavior: a conference report. *Drug Alcohol Depend.* 1998;52:41.

Castner SA, Goldman-Rakic PS. Long-lasting psychotomimetic consequences of repeated low-dose amphetamine exposure in rhesus monkeys. *Neuropsychopharmacology.* 1999;20:10.

Center for Substance Abuse Treatment. *Proceedings of the National Consensus Meeting on the Use, Abuse and Sequelae of Abuse of Methamphetamine with Implications for Prevention, Treatment and Research.* DHHS publ. no. SMA 96–8013. Rockville, MD: Substance Abuse and Mental Health Services Administration; 1997.

Curran HV, Travill RA. Mood and cognitive effects of +/–3,4-methylenedioxymethamphetamine (MDMA, "ecstasy"): weekend "high" followed by mid-week low. *Addiction.* 1997;92:821.

Gawin FH, Ellinwood EH. Cocaine and other stimulants. *N Engl J Med.* 1988;318:1173.

Gorelick DA. Pharmacologic therapies for cocaine and other stimulant addiction. In: Graham AW, Schultz TK, eds. *Principles of Addiction Medicine.* 2nd ed. Chevy Chase, MD: American Society of Addiction Medicine; 1998.

Hall W, Hando J. Patterns of amphetamine use in Australia. In: Klee H, ed. *Amphetamine Misuse. International Perspectives on Current Trends.* Reading, Australia: Harwood Academic; 1997.

Hyman SE, Nestler EJ. Initiation and adaptation: a paradigm for understanding psychotropic drug action. *Am J Psychiatry.* 1996;153:151.

Jaffe JH. Amphetamine (or amphetamine-like)-related disorders. In: Sadock BJ, Sadock VA, eds. *Kaplan & Sadock's Comprehensive Textbook of Psychiatry.* 7th ed. Vol 1. Baltimore: Lippincott Williams & Wilkins; 2000:924.

Jaffe JH. Drug addiction and drug abuse. In: Gilman AG, Rall TW, Nies AS, Taylor P, eds. *Goodman and Gilman's The Pharmacological Basis of Therapeutics.* 8th ed. New York: Pergamon; 1990.

Jansen KLR. Ecstasy (MDMA) dependence. *Drug Alcohol Depend.* 1999;53:121.

McCann UD, Szabo Z, Scheffel U, Dannals RF, Ricaurte GA. Positron emission tomographic evidence of toxic effects of MDMA ("ecstasy") on brain serotonin neurons in human beings. *Lancet.* 1998;352:1433.

Meng Y, Dukat M, Bridgen DT, Martin BR, Lichtman AH. Pharmacological effects of methamphetamine and other stimulants via inhalation exposure. *Drug Alcohol Depend.* 1999;53:111.

Office of Applied Studies. *Preliminary Results from the 1997 National Household Survey on Drug Abuse.* National Household Survey on Drug Abuse Series: H6, DHHS publ. no. SMA 98–3251. Rockville, MD: Substance Abuse and Mental Health Services Administration; 1998.

Pope HG Jr, Kouri EM, Hudson JI. The effects of supraphysiologic doses of testosterone on mood and aggression in normal men: a randomized controlled trial. *Arch Gen Psychiatry.* 2000;57:133.

Self DW, Nestler EJ. Relapse to drug-seeking: neural and molecular mechanisms. *Drug Alcohol Depend.* 1998;51:49.

Strang J, Sheridan J. Prescribing amphetamines to drug misusers: data from the 1995 national survey of community pharmacies in England and Wales. *Addiction.* 1997;92:833.

Volkow ND, Wang G-J, Fowler JS, et al. Dopamine transporter occupancies in the human brain induced by therapeutic doses of oral methylphenidate. *Am J Psychiatry.* 1998;155:10.

▲ 12.4 Caffeine-Related Disorders

The most widely consumed psychoactive substance in the world is caffeine. It is estimated that over 80 percent of adults in the United States consume caffeine regularly, and throughout the world, caffeine consumption is well integrated into daily cultural practices (e.g., the coffee break in the United States, tea time in the United Kingdom, and kola nut chewing in Nigeria). Because caffeine use is so pervasive and widely accepted, disorders associated with caffeine use may be overlooked. However, one must recognize that caffeine is a psychoactive compound that can produce a wide variety of syndromes, and the text revision of the fourth edition of the American Psychiatric Association's *Diagnostic and Statistical Manual of Mental Disorders* (DSM-IV-TR) recognizes several caffeine-related disorders (e.g., caffeine intoxication, caffeine-induced anxiety disorder, and caffeine-induced sleep disorder). Other caffeine-related disorders, such as caffeine withdrawal and caffeine dependence, are not official diagnoses in DSM-IV-TR, but can also be of clinical interest.

EPIDEMIOLOGY

Caffeine is contained in drinks, foods, prescription medicines, and over-the-counter medicines (Table 12.4–1). An adult in the United States consumes about 200 mg of caffeine per day on average, although 20 to 30 percent of all adults consume more than 500 mg per day. The per capita use of coffee in the United States is 10.2 pounds per year. A cup of coffee generally contains 100 to 150 mg of caffeine; tea contains about one third as much. Many over-the-counter medications contain one third to one half as much caffeine as a cup of coffee, and some migraine medications and over-the-counter stimulants contain more caffeine than a cup of coffee. Cocoa, chocolate, and soft drinks contain significant amounts of caffeine, enough to cause some symptoms of caffeine intoxication in small children when they ingest a candy bar and a 12-ounce cola drink.

Caffeine consumption also varies by age. Figure 12.4–1 shows estimates of per capita caffeine consumption, by those who consume caffeine, for different age groups in the United States. These estimates demonstrate the wide variability in caffeine consumption for different ages. The figure shows that the average daily caffeine consumption of caffeine consumers of all ages is 2.79 mg/kg of body weight in the United States. There is substantial caffeine consumption even by young children (i.e., over 1 mg/kg for children between the ages of 1 and 5 years). Worldwide, estimates place the average daily per capita caffeine consumption at about 70 mg. According to DSM-IV-TR, the actual prevalence of caffeine-related disorders is unknown; but up to 85 percent of adults consume caffeine in any given year.

Table 12.4–1
Common Sources of Caffeine and Representative Decaffeinated Products

Source	Caffeine per Unit (mg)
Beverages and foods (5–6 oz)	
Fresh drip coffee, brewed coffee	90–140
Instant coffee	66–100
Tea (leaf or bagged)	30–100
Cocoa	5–50
Decaffeinated coffee	2–4
Chocolate bar or ounce of baking chocolate	25–35
Soft drinks (8–12 oz)	
Pepsi, Coke, Tab, Royal Crown, Dr. Pepper, Mountain Dew	25–50
Canada Dry Ginger Ale, Caffeine-Free Coke, Caffeine-Free Pepsi, 7-Up, Sprite, Squirt, Caffeine-Free Tab	0
Prescription medications (1 tablet or capsule)	
Cafergot, Migralam	100
Anoquan, Aspir-code, BAC, Darvon, Fiorinal	32–50
Over-the-counter analgesics and cold preparations (1 tablet or capsule)	
Excedrin	60
Aspirin compound, Anacin, B-C powder, Capron, Cope, Dolor, Midol, Nilain, Norgesic, PAC, Trigesic, Vanquish	~30
Advil, aspirin, Empirin, Midol 200, Nuprin, Pamprin	0
Over-the-counter stimulants and appetite suppressants (1 tablet or capsule)	
Caffin-TD, Caffedrine	250
Vivarin, Ver	200
Quick-Pep	140–150
Amostat, Anorexin, Appedrine, Nodoz, Wakoz	100

Adapted from table by Jerome H. Jaffe, M.D.

COMORBIDITY

Persons with caffeine-related disorders are more likely to have additional substance-related disorders than are those without diagnoses of caffeine-related disorders. About two thirds of those who consume large amounts of caffeine daily also use sedative and hypnotic drugs.

NEUROPHARMACOLOGY

Caffeine, a methylxanthine, is more potent than another commonly used methylxanthine, theophylline (Primatene). The half-life of caffeine in the human body is 3 to 10 hours, and the time of peak concentration is 30 to 60 minutes. Caffeine readily crosses the blood–brain barrier. Caffeine acts primarily as an antagonist of the adenosine receptors. Adenosine receptors activate an inhibitory G protein (Gi) and thus inhibit the formation of the second-messenger cyclic adenosine monophosphate (cAMP). Caffeine intake, therefore, results in an increase in intraneuronal cAMP concentrations in neurons with adenosine receptors. Three cups of coffee are estimated to deliver so much caffeine to the brain that about 50 percent of the adenosine receptors are occupied by caffeine. Several experiments indicate that caffeine, especially at high doses or concentrations, can affect dopamine and noradrenergic neurons. Specifically, dopamine activity may be enhanced by caffeine, a hypothesis that could explain clinical reports associating caffeine intake with an exacerbation of psychotic symptoms in patients with schizophrenia. Activation of noradrenergic neurons has been hypothesized to be involved in the mediation of some symptoms of caffeine withdrawal.

Genetics and Caffeine Use

Several investigations comparing coffee use in monozygotic and dizygotic twins have shown higher concordance rates for monozy-

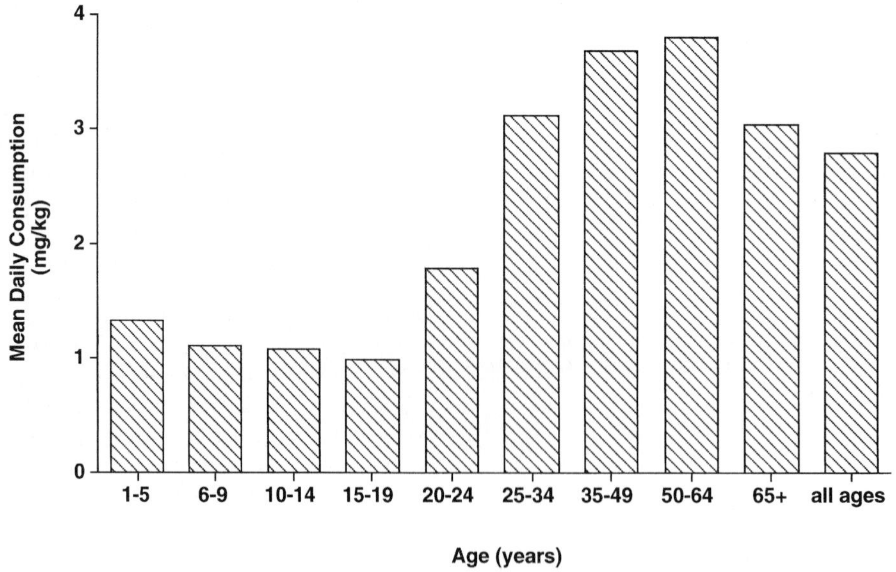

FIGURE 12.4–1

Mean daily caffeine consumption (mg/kg) for different age groups and all ages, in the United States of America. (Adapted from Barone JJ, Roberts HR. Caffeine consumption. *Food Chem Toxicol.* 1996;34:119.)

gotic twins, suggesting that there may be some genetic predisposition to continued coffee use following exposure to coffee.

Caffeine as a Substance of Abuse

Caffeine evidences all the traits associated with commonly accepted substances of abuse. First, caffeine can act as a positive reinforcer, particularly at low doses. Caffeine doses of about 100 mg induce a mild euphoria in humans and repeated substance-seeking behavior effects in other animals. Caffeine doses of 300 mg, however, do not act as positive reinforcers and can produce increased anxiety and mild dysphoria. Second, studies in animals and humans have reported that caffeine can be discriminated from a placebo in blind experimental conditions. Third, both animal and human studies have shown that physical tolerance develops to some effects of caffeine and that withdrawal symptoms occur.

Effects on Cerebral Blood Flow

Most studies have found that caffeine results in global cerebral vasoconstriction, with a resultant decrease in cerebral blood flow (CBF), although this effect may not occur in persons over 65 years of age. According to one recent study, tolerance does not develop to these vasoconstrictive effects, and the CBF shows a rebound increase after withdrawal from caffeine. Some clinicians believe that caffeine use can cause a similar constriction in the coronary arteries.

Table 12.4–3
DSM-IV-TR Diagnostic Criteria for Caffeine Intoxication

A. Recent consumption of caffeine, usually in excess of 250 mg (e.g., more than 2–3 cups of brewed coffee).

B. Five (or more) of the following signs, developing during, or shortly after, caffeine use:
  (1) restlessness
  (2) nervousness
  (3) excitement
  (4) insomnia
  (5) flushed face
  (6) diuresis
  (7) gastrointestinal disturbance
  (8) muscle twitching
  (9) rambling flow of thought and speech
  (10) tachycardia or cardiac arrhythmia
  (11) periods of inexhaustibility
  (12) psychomotor agitation

C. The symptoms in Criterion B cause clinically significant distress or impairment in social, occupational, or other important areas of functioning.

D. The symptoms are not due to a general medical condition and are not better accounted for by another mental disorder (e.g., an Anxiety Disorder).

From American Psychiatric Association. *Diagnostic and Statistical Manual of Mental Disorders.* 4th ed. Text rev. Washington, DC: American Psychiatric Association; copyright 2000, with permission.

DIAGNOSIS

The diagnosis of caffeine intoxication or other caffeine-related disorders depends primarily on a comprehensive history of a patient's intake of caffeine-containing products. The history should cover whether a patient has experienced any symptoms of caffeine withdrawal during periods when caffeine consumption was either stopped or severely reduced. The differential diagnosis for caffeine-related disorders should include the following psychiatric diagnoses: generalized anxiety disorder, panic disorder with or without agoraphobia, bipolar II disorder, attention-deficit/hyperactivity disorder, and sleep disorders. The differential diagnosis should include the abuse of caffeine-containing over-the-counter medications, anabolic steroids, and other stimulants, such as amphetamines and cocaine. A urine sample may be needed to screen for these substances. The differential diagnosis should also include hyperthyroidism and pheochromocytoma.

DSM-IV-TR lists the caffeine-related disorders (Table 12.4–2) and provides diagnostic criteria for caffeine intoxication (Table 12.4–3) but does not formally recognize a diagnosis of caffeine withdrawal, which is classified as a caffeine-related disorder not otherwise specified (Table 12.4–4). The diagnostic criteria for other caffeine-related disorders are contained in the sections specific for the principal symptom (e.g., as a substance-induced anxiety disorder for caffeine-induced anxiety disorder).

Table 12.4–2
DSM-IV-TR Caffeine-Related Disorders

Caffeine-induced disorders
  Caffeine intoxication
  Caffeine-induced anxiety disorder
    Specify if:
      With onset during intoxication
  Caffeine-induced sleep disorder
    Specify if:
      With onset during intoxication
  Caffeine-related disorder not otherwise specified

From American Psychiatric Association. *Diagnostic and Statistical Manual of Mental Disorders.* 4th ed. Text rev. Washington, DC: American Psychiatric Association; copyright 2000, with permission.

Table 12.4–4
DSM-IV-TR Diagnostic Criteria for Caffeine-Related Disorder Not Otherwise Specified

The caffeine-related disorder not otherwise specified category is for disorders associated with the use of caffeine that are not classifiable as caffeine intoxication, caffeine-induced anxiety disorder, or caffeine-induced sleep disorder. An example is caffeine withdrawal.

From American Psychiatric Association. *Diagnostic and Statistical Manual of Mental Disorders.* 4th ed. Text rev. Washington, DC: American Psychiatric Association; copyright 2000, with permission.

Caffeine Intoxication

DSM-IV-TR specifies the diagnostic criteria for caffeine intoxication (Table 12.4–3), including the recent consumption of caffeine, usually in excess of 250 mg. The annual incidence of caffeine intoxication is an estimated 10 percent, although some clinicians and investigators suspect that the actual incidence is much higher. The common symptoms associated with caffeine intoxication include anxiety, psychomotor agitation, restlessness, irritability, and psychophysiological complaints such as muscle twitching, flushed face, nausea, diuresis, gastrointestinal distress, excessive perspiration, tingling in the fingers and toes, and insomnia. Consumption of more than 1 g of caffeine can produce rambling speech, confused thinking, cardiac arrhythmias, inexhaustibleness, marked agitation, tinnitus, and mild visual hallucinations (light flashes). Consumption of more than 10 g of caffeine can cause generalized tonic-clonic seizures, respiratory failure, and death.

Caffeine Withdrawal

In spite of the fact that DSM-IV-TR does not include a diagnosis of caffeine withdrawal, several well-controlled studies indicate that caffeine withdrawal is a real phenomenon, and DSM-IV-TR gives research criteria for caffeine withdrawal (Table 12.4–5). The appearance of withdrawal symptoms reflects the tolerance and physiological dependence that develop with continued caffeine use. Several epidemiological studies have reported symptoms of caffeine withdrawal in 50 to 75 percent of all caffeine users studied. The most common symptoms are headache and fatigue; other symptoms include anxiety, irritability, mild depressive symptoms, impaired psychomotor performance, nausea, vomiting, craving for caffeine, and muscle pain and stiffness. The number and severity of the withdrawal symptoms are correlated with the amount of caffeine ingested and the abruptness of the withdrawal. Caffeine withdrawal symptoms have their onset 12 to 24 hours after the last dose; the symptoms peak in 24 to 48 hours and resolve within 1 week.

Table 12.4–5
DSM-IV-TR Research Criteria for Caffeine Withdrawal

A. Prolonged daily use of caffeine.

B. Abrupt cessation of caffeine use, or reduction in the amount of caffeine used, closely followed by headache and one (or more) of the following symptoms:
   (1) marked fatigue or drowsiness
   (2) marked anxiety or depression
   (3) nausea or vomiting

C. The symptoms in criterion B cause clinically significant distress or impairment in social, occupational, or other important areas of functioning.

D. The symptoms are not due to the direct physiological effects of a general medical condition (e.g., migraine, viral illness) and are not better accounted for by another mental disorder.

From American Psychiatric Association. *Diagnostic and Statistical Manual of Mental Disorders.* 4th ed. Text rev. Washington, DC: American Psychiatric Association; copyright 2000, with permission.

The induction of caffeine withdrawal can sometimes be iatrogenic. Physicians often ask their patients to discontinue caffeine intake before certain medical procedures, such as endoscopy, colonoscopy, and cardiac catheterization. Physicians also often recommend that patients with anxiety symptoms, cardiac arrhythmias, esophagitis, hiatal hernias, fibrocystic disease of the breast, and insomnia stop caffeine intake. Some persons simply decide that it would be good for them to stop using caffeine-containing products. In all these situations, caffeine users should taper the use of caffeine-containing products over a 7- to 14-day period rather than stop abruptly.

Ms. E. was a 32-year-old single white woman employed full-time at a local factory. She occasionally used nonsteroidal antiinflammatory drugs, but was taking no regular prescription medications. She had a history of alcohol dependence, in remission for 9 years, and was otherwise in good health.

She first began consuming caffeine when she started college, and her current beverage of choice was coffee. She typically drank 4 to 5 mugs of coffee each day and preferred to drink it without cream, milk, or sugar. She estimated that 5 minutes elapsed between the time she got up in the morning and the time she had her first cup of coffee; her roommate made a pot before Ms. E. got up, and Ms. E. immediately poured a mug when she got out of bed. She spaced her mugs over the course of the day, with her last mug either after lunch or with dinner.

Physicians had recommended that she cut down or stop her coffee use because of complaints of mild indigestion, but she had been unable to do so. Her roommate had also complained about her coffee use at times. Ms. E. routinely drank hot coffee in her car, and had spilled it and burned herself on one occasion.

When she stopped caffeine abruptly, Ms. E. experienced marked irritability; poor concentration; and a severe, generalized headache. When asked to rate the severity of the headache, she replied that "on a scale of 1 to 10 it's a 12." She also had muscle aches, low energy, lethargy, and a craving to drink a mug of coffee. On the day she had stopped coffee use abruptly, she left work 2 hours early because of problems concentrating on the job and went to bed several hours earlier than usual. She then returned to her usual pattern of coffee use. (Courtesy of Eric C. Strain, M.D., and Roland R. Griffiths, Ph.D.)

Caffeine-Induced Anxiety Disorder

Caffeine-induced anxiety disorder, which can occur during caffeine intoxication, is a DSM-IV-TR diagnosis (see Table 16.7–3 in Section 16.7 of Chapter 16). The anxiety related to caffeine use can resemble that of generalized anxiety disorder. Patients with the disorder may be perceived as "wired," overly talkative, and irritable; they may complain of not sleeping well and of having energy to burn. Caffeine may induce and exacerbate panic attacks in persons with a panic disorder, and although a causative association between caffeine and a panic disorder has not yet been demonstrated, patients with panic disorder should avoid caffeine.

Mr. B. was a 28-year-old single African American male graduate student who was in good health and had no history of previous psychiatric evaluation or treatment. He took no medications, did not smoke or consume alcohol, and had no current or past history of illicit drug use.

His chief complaint was that he had begun feeling mounting "anxiety" when working in the laboratory where he was pursuing his graduate studies. His work had been progressing well, he felt his relationship with his advisor was good and supportive, and he could not identify any problems with staff or peers that might explain his anxiety. He had been working long hours, but found the work interesting and had recently had his first paper accepted for publication.

Despite these successes, he reported feeling a "crescendoing anxiety" as his day progressed. He noted that by afternoon he would be experiencing palpitations, bursts of heart racing, tremors in his hands, and an overall feeling of "being on the edge." He also noted a nervous energy in the afternoons. These experiences were occurring daily and seemed confined to the laboratory (although he admitted he was in the laboratory every day of the week).

A review of Mr. B.'s caffeine intake revealed that he was consuming excessive amounts of coffee. Staff made a large urn of caffeinated coffee each morning, and Mr. B. routinely started with a large mug of coffee. Over the course of the morning he would consume three to four mugs of coffee (the equivalent of about six to eight 5-ounce cups of coffee), and he continued this level of use throughout the afternoon. He occasionally had a single can of caffeinated soda and used no other forms of caffeine on a regular basis. Mr. B. estimated he drank a total of six to eight or more mugs of coffee per day (which was estimated to be at least 1,200 mg of caffeine per day). Once pointed out to him, he realized this level of caffeine consumption was considerably higher than that at any other time in his life. He admitted he liked the taste of coffee and felt a burst of energy in the morning when he drank coffee, which helped him start his day. Mr. B. and his physician developed a plan to decrease his caffeine use by tapering off caffeine. Details of such a tapering schedule can be found in the section on treatment of caffeine dependence. Mr. B. successfully decreased his caffeine use and his anxiety symptoms resolved after his daily caffeine use had been markedly decreased. (Courtesy of Eric Strain, M.D.)

Caffeine-Induced Sleep Disorder

Caffeine-induced sleep disorder, which can occur during caffeine intoxication, is a DSM-IV-TR diagnosis (see Table 24.2–21). Caffeine is associated with delay in falling asleep, inability to remain asleep, and early morning awakening.

Caffeine-Related Disorder Not Otherwise Specified

DSM-IV-TR contains a residual category for caffeine-related disorders that do not meet the criteria for caffeine intoxication, caffeine-induced anxiety disorder, or caffeine-induced sleep disorder (Table 12.4–4).

CLINICAL FEATURES

Signs and Symptoms

After the ingestion of 50 to 100 mg of caffeine, common symptoms include increased alertness, a mild sense of well-being, and a sense of improved verbal and motor performance. Caffeine ingestion is also associated with diuresis, cardiac muscle stimulation, increased intestinal peristalsis, increased gastric acid secretion, and (usually mildly) increased blood pressure.

Adverse Effects

Although caffeine is not associated with cardiac-related risks in healthy persons, those with preexisting cardiac disease are often advised to limit their caffeine intake because of a possible association between cardiac arrhythmias and caffeine. Caffeine is clearly associated with increased gastric acid secretion, and clinicians usually advise patients with gastric ulcers not to ingest any caffeine-containing products. Limited data suggest that caffeine is associated with fibrocystic disease of the breasts in women. Although the question of whether caffeine is associated with birth defects remains controversial, women who are pregnant or breast-feeding should probably avoid caffeine-containing products. No solid data link caffeine intake with cancer.

TREATMENT

Analgesics, such as aspirin, almost always suffice to control the headaches and muscle aches that may accompany caffeine withdrawal. Rarely do patients require benzodiazepines to relieve withdrawal symptoms. If benzodiazepines are used for this purpose, they should be used in small dosages for a brief time, about 7 to 10 days at the longest.

The first step in reducing or eliminating caffeine use is to have patients determine their daily consumption of caffeine. This can best be accomplished by having the patient keep a daily food diary. The patient must recognize all sources of caffeine in the diet, including forms of caffeine (e.g., beverages, medications), and accurately record the amount consumed. After several days of keeping such a diary, the clinician can meet with the patient, review the diary, and determine the average daily caffeine dose in milligrams.

The patient and clinical should then decide upon a fading schedule for caffeine consumption. Such a schedule could involve a decrease in increments of 10 percent every few days. Since caffeine is typically consumed in beverage form, the patient can use a substitution procedure in which decaffeinated beverage is gradually used in place of caffeinated beverage. The diary should be maintained during this time, so that the patient's progress can be monitored. The fading should be individualized for each patient so that the rate of decrease in caffeine consumption minimizes withdrawal symptoms. One should probably avoid stopping all caffeine use abruptly, because withdrawal symptoms are likely to develop with sudden discontinuation of all caffeine use.

References

Dager SR, Layton ME, Strauss W, et al. Human brain metabolic response to caffeine and the effects of tolerance. *Am J Psychiatry.* 1999;156:229.

Evans SM, Griffiths RR. Dose-related caffeine discrimination in normal volun-

teers: individual differences in subjective effects and self-reported cues. *Behav Pharmacol.* 1991;2:345.

Griffiths RR, Mumford GK. Caffeine—a drug of abuse? In: Bloom FE, Kupfer DJ, eds. *Psychopharmacology: The Fourth Generation of Progress.* New York: Raven; 1995.

Griffiths RR, Woodson PP. Caffeine physical dependence: a review of human and laboratory animal studies. *Psychopharmacology.* 1988;94:437.

Hughes JR, Oliveto AH, Helzer JE, Higgins ST, Bickel WK. Should caffeine abuse, dependence, or withdrawal be added to DSM-IV and ICD-10? *Am J Psychiatry.* 1992;149:33.

James JE. *Understanding Caffeine: A Biobehavioral Analysis.* Thousand Oaks, CA: Sage; 1997.

Nehlig A. Are we dependent upon coffee and caffeine? A review on human and animal data. *Neurosci Biobehav Rev.* 1999;23:563.

Schuh KJ, Griffiths RR. Caffeine reinforcement: the role of withdrawal. *Psychopharmacology.* 1997;130:320.

Stanton CK, Gray RH. Effects of caffeine consumption on delayed conception. *Am J Epidemiol.* 1995;142:1322.

Strain EC, Griffiths RR. In: Sadock BJ, Sadock VA, eds. Kaplan & Sadock's *Comprehensive Textbook of Psychiatry.* 7th ed. Vol 2. Baltimore: Lippincott Williams & Wilkins; 2000:982.

Strain EC, Mumford GK, Silverman K, Griffiths RR. Caffeine dependence syndrome: evidence from case histories and experimental evaluations. *JAMA.* 1994;272:1043.

Tanda G, Golden SR. Alteration of the behavioral effects of nicotine by chronic caffeine exposure. *Pharmacol Biochem Behav.* 2000;66:47.

Weber JG, Ereth MH, Danielson DR. Perioperative ingestion of caffeine and postoperative headache. *Mayo Clin Proc.* 1993;68:842.

▲ 12.5 Cannabis-Related Disorders

Known in central Asia and China for at least 4,000 years, the Indian hemp plant *Cannabis sativa* is a hardy, aromatic annual herb (Fig. 12.5–1). The bioactive substances derived from it are collectively referred to as *cannabis.* By most estimates, cannabis remains the world's most commonly used illicit drug.

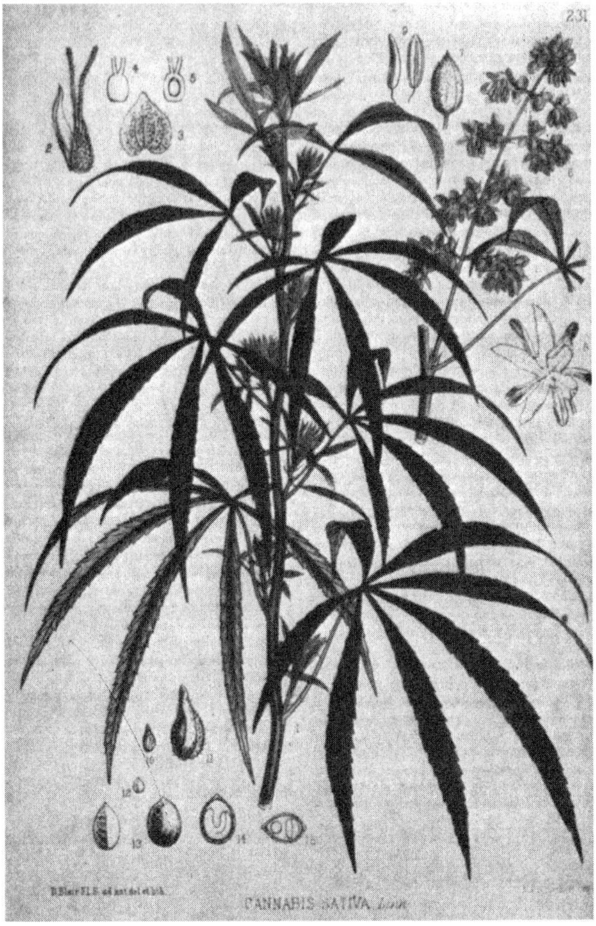

FIGURE 12.5–1
Marijuana (*Cannabis sativa*).

All parts of *Cannabis sativa* contain psychoactive cannabinoids, of which (–)-Δ9-tetrahydrocannabinol (Δ9-THC) is most abundant. The most potent forms of cannabis come from the flowering tops of the plants or from the dried, black-brown, resinous exudate from the leaves, which is referred to as *hashish* or *hash.* The cannabis plant is usually cut, dried, chopped, and rolled into cigarettes (commonly called "joints"), which are then smoked. The common names for cannabis are marijuana, grass, pot, weed, tea, and Mary Jane. Other names, which describe cannabis types of various strengths, are hemp, chasra, bhang, ganja, dagga, and sinsemilla.

EPIDEMIOLOGY

Prevalence and Recent Trends

The *Monitoring the Future* survey of adolescents in school indicates recent increases in lifetime, annual, current (within the past 30 days), and daily use of marijuana by eighth and tenth graders, continuing a trend that began in the early 1990s. In 1996, 23.1 percent of eighth graders and 39.8 percent of tenth graders reported lifetime marijuana use.

Another measure of the prevalence of marijuana use comes from the National Household Survey on Drug Abuse, a population-based random sample of households throughout the United States. Marijuana was the most commonly used illicit drug in the study. Lifetime prevalence of marijuana use increased with each age group until age 34 years, then decreased gradually. Those aged 18 to 21 were the most likely to have used marijuana in the past year (25 percent) or the past month (14 percent), and use was lowest among those aged 50 or older, where it was 1 percent or less. According to the text revision of the fourth edition of *Diagnostic and Statistical Manual of Mental Disorders* (DSM-IV-TR) there is a 5 percent lifetime rate of cannabis abuse or dependence.

Demographic Correlates

The rate of past year and current marijuana use by males was almost twice the rate for females overall among those aged 26 and older. This gap between the sexes narrows with younger users; at ages 12 to 17, there are no significant differences.

Race and ethnicity were also related to marijuana use, but the relationships varied by age group. Among those ages 12 to 17, whites had higher rates of lifetime and past-year marijuana use than blacks. Among 17- to 34-year-old adults, whites reported higher levels of lifetime use than blacks and Hispanics. But among those 35 and older, whites and blacks reported the same levels of use. The lifetime rates for black adults were significantly higher than those for Hispanics.

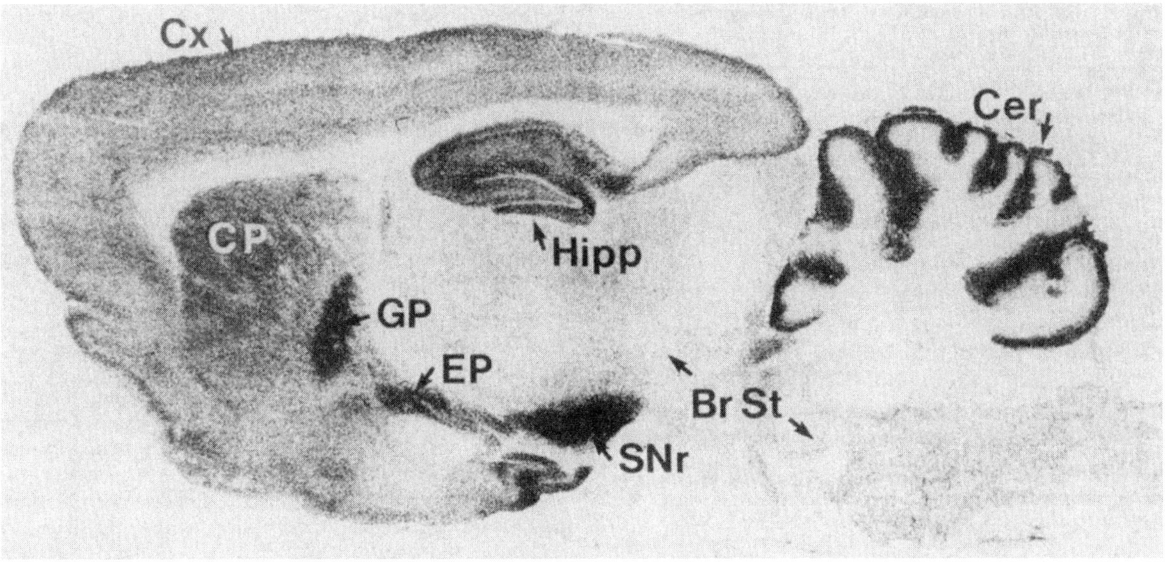

FIGURE 12.5–2

Autoradiography of cannabinoid receptor distribution in a sagittal section of rat brain. Binding of tritiated ligand is dense in the hippocampus (*Hipp*), the globus pallidus (*GP*), the entopeduncular nucleus (*EP*), the substantia nigra pars reticulata (*SNr*), and the cerebellum (*Cer*). Binding is moderate in the cerebral cortex (*Cx*) and the caudate putamen (*CP*) and sparse in the brainstem (*Br St*) and spinal cord. (Reprinted with permission from Howlett AC, Bidaut-Russell M, Devane WA, et al. The cannabinoid receptor: biochemical anatomical, and behavioral characterization. *Trends Neurosci.* 1990;13:422.)

NEUROPHARMACOLOGY

As stated above, the principal component of cannabis is Δ9-THC; however, the cannabis plant contains more than 400 chemicals, of which about 60 are chemically related to Δ9-THC. In humans, Δ9-THC is rapidly converted into 11-hydroxy-Δ9-THC, the metabolite that is active in the central nervous system (CNS).

A specific receptor for the cannabinols has been identified, cloned, and characterized. The cannabinoid receptor, a member of the G protein-linked family of receptors, is linked to the inhibitory G protein (Gi), which is linked to adenylyl cyclase in an inhibitory fashion. The cannabinoid receptor is found in highest concentrations in the basal ganglia, the hippocampus, and the cerebellum, with lower concentrations in the cerebral cortex (Fig. 12.5–2). It is not found in the brainstem, a fact consistent with cannabis's minimal effects on respiratory and cardiac functions. Studies in animals have shown that the cannabinoids affect the monoamine and γ-aminobutyric acid (GABA) neurons.

According to most studies, animals do not self-administer cannabinoids as they do most other substances of abuse. Moreover, there is some debate about whether the cannabinoids stimulate the so-called reward centers of the brain, such as the dopaminergic neurons of the ventral tegmental area. Tolerance to cannabis does develop, however, and psychological dependence has been found, although the evidence for physiological dependence is not strong. Withdrawal symptoms in humans are limited to modest increases in irritability, restlessness, insomnia, and anorexia and mild nausea; all these symptoms appear only when a person abruptly stops taking high doses of cannabis.

When cannabis is smoked, the euphoric effects appear within minutes, peak in about 30 minutes, and last 2 to 4 hours. Some motor and cognitive effects last 5 to 12 hours. Cannabis can also be taken orally when it is prepared in food, such as brownies and cakes. About two to three times as much cannabis must be taken orally to be as potent as cannabis taken by inhaling its smoke. Many variables affect the psychoactive properties of cannabis, including the potency of the cannabis used, the route of administration, the smoking technique, the effects of pyrolysis on the cannabinoid content, the dose, the setting, the user's past experience, the user's expectations, and the user's unique biological vulnerability to the effects of cannabinoids.

DIAGNOSIS AND CLINICAL FEATURES

The most common physical effects of cannabis are dilation of the conjunctival blood vessels (red eye) and mild tachycardia. At high doses, orthostatic hypotension may appear. Increased appetite—often referred to as "the munchies"—and dry mouth are common effects of cannabis intoxication. The fact that there has never been a clearly documented case of death caused by cannabis intoxication alone reflects the substance's lack of effect on the respiratory rate. The most serious potential adverse effects of cannabis use are those caused by inhaling the same carcinogenic hydrocarbons present in conventional tobacco, and some data indicate that heavy cannabis users are at risk for chronic respiratory disease and lung cancer. The practice of smoking cannabis-containing cigarettes to their very ends, so-called roaches, further increases the intake of tar (particulate matter). Many reports indicate that long-term cannabis use is associated with cerebral atrophy, seizure susceptibility, chromosomal damage, birth defects, impaired immune reactivity, alterations in testosterone concentrations, and dysregulation of menstrual cycles; these reports, however, have not been conclusively replicated, and the association between these findings and cannabis use is uncertain.

Table 12.5–1
DSM-IV-TR Cannabis-Related Disorders

Cannabis use disorders
Cannabis dependence
Cannabis abuse
Cannabis-induced disorders
Cannabis intoxication
Specify if:
With perceptual disturbances
Cannabis intoxication delirium
Cannabis-induced psychotic disorder, with delusions
Specify if:
With onset during intoxication
Cannabis-induced psychotic disorder, with hallucinations
Specify if:
With onset during intoxication
Cannabis-induced anxiety disorder
Specify if:
With onset during intoxication
Cannabis-related disorder not otherwise specified

From American Psychiatric Association. *Diagnostic and Statistical Manual of Mental Disorders.* 4th ed. Text rev. Washington, DC: American Psychiatric Association; copyright 2000, with permission.

DSM-IV-TR lists the cannabis-related disorders (Table 12.5–1) but has specific criteria within the cannabis-related disorders section only for cannabis intoxication (Table 12.5–2). The diagnostic criteria for the other cannabis-related disorders are contained in those DSM-IV-TR sections that focus on the major phenomenological symptom—for example, cannabis-induced psychotic disorder, with delusions, in the DSM-IV-TR section on substance-induced psychotic disorder (see Table 14.1–1 in Section 14.1 of Chapter 14).

Table 12.5–2
DSM-IV-TR Diagnostic Criteria for Cannabis Intoxication

A. Recent use of cannabis.
B. Clinically significant maladaptive behavioral or psychological changes (e.g., impaired motor coordination, euphoria, anxiety, sensation of slowed time, impaired judgment, social withdrawal) that developed during, or shortly after, cannabis use.
C. Two (or more) of the following signs, developing within 2 hours of cannabis use:
(1) conjunctival injection
(2) increased appetite
(3) dry mouth
(4) tachycardia
D. The symptoms are not due to a general medical condition and are not better accounted for by another mental disorder.

Specify if:
With perceptual disturbances

From American Psychiatric Association. *Diagnostic and Statistical Manual of Mental Disorders.* 4th ed. Text rev. Washington, DC: American Psychiatric Association; copyright 2000, with permission.

Cannabis Dependence and Cannabis Abuse

DSM-IV-TR includes the diagnoses of cannabis dependence and cannabis abuse (see Tables 12.1–7, 12.1–8, and 12.1–9). The experimental data clearly show tolerance to many of the effects of cannabis, but the data are less supportive of the existence of physical dependence. Psychological dependence on cannabis use does develop in long-term users.

Cannabis Intoxication

DSM-IV-TR formalizes the diagnostic criteria for cannabis intoxication (Table 12.5–2). These criteria state that the diagnosis can be augmented with the phrase "with perceptual disturbances." If intact reality testing is not present, the diagnosis is cannabis-induced psychotic disorder.

Cannabis intoxication commonly heightens users' sensitivities to external stimuli, reveals new details, makes colors seem brighter and richer than in the past, and subjectively slows the appreciation of time. In high doses, users may experience depersonalization and derealization. Motor skills are impaired by cannabis use, and the impairment in motor skills remains after the subjective, euphoriant effects have resolved. For 8 to 12 hours after using cannabis, users' impaired motor skills interfere with the operation of motor vehicles and other heavy machinery. Moreover, these effects are additive to those of alcohol, which is commonly used in combination with cannabis.

Cannabis Intoxication Delirium

Cannabis intoxication delirium is a DSM-IV-TR diagnosis (see Table 10.2–3). The delirium associated with cannabis intoxication is characterized by marked impairment on cognition and performance tasks. Even modest doses of cannabis impair memory, reaction time, perception, motor coordination, and attention. High doses that also impair users' levels of consciousness have marked effects on cognitive measures.

Cannabis-Induced Psychotic Disorder

Cannabis-induced psychotic disorder (see Table 14.1–2) is diagnosed in the presence of a cannabis-induced psychosis. Cannabis-induced psychotic disorder is rare; transient paranoid ideation is more common. Florid psychosis is somewhat common in countries in which some persons have long-term access to cannabis of particularly high potency. The psychotic episodes are sometimes referred to as "hemp insanity." Cannabis use rarely causes a "bad-trip" experience, which is often associated with hallucinogen intoxication. When cannabis-induced psychotic disorder does occur, it may be correlated with a preexisting personality disorder in the affected person.

Cannabis-Induced Anxiety Disorder

Cannabis-induced anxiety disorder (see Table 16.1–5) is a common diagnosis for acute cannabis intoxication, which in many persons induces short-lived anxiety states often provoked by paranoid thoughts. In such circumstances, panic attacks may be induced, based on ill-defined and disorganized fears. The appearance of anxiety symptoms is correlated with the dose and

Table 12.5–3
DSM-IV-TR Diagnostic Criteria for Cannabis-Related Disorder Not Otherwise Specified

The cannabis-related disorder not otherwise specified category is for disorders associated with the use of cannabis that are not classifiable as cannabis dependence, cannabis abuse, cannabis intoxication, cannabis intoxication delirium, cannabis-induced psychotic disorder, or cannabis-induced anxiety disorder.

From American Psychiatric Association. *Diagnostic and Statistical Manual of Mental Disorders.* 4th ed. Text rev. Washington, DC: American Psychiatric Association; copyright 2000, with permission.

is the most frequent adverse reaction to the moderate use of smoked cannabis. Inexperienced users are much more likely to experience anxiety symptoms than are experienced users.

Cannabis-Related Disorder Not Otherwise Specified

DSM-IV-TR does not formally recognize cannabis-induced mood disorders; therefore, such disorders are classified as cannabis-related disorders not otherwise specified (Table 12.5–3). Cannabis intoxication can be associated with depressive symptoms, although such symptoms may suggest long-term cannabis use. Hypomania, however, is a common symptom in cannabis intoxication.

DSM-IV-TR also does not formally recognize cannabis-induced sleep disorders or cannabis-induced sexual dysfunction; therefore, both are classified as cannabis-related disorders not otherwise specified. When either sleep disorder or sexual dysfunction symptoms are related to cannabis use, they almost always resolve within days or a week after cessation of cannabis use.

Flashbacks. Persisting perceptual abnormalities after cannabis use are not formally classified in DSM-IV-TR, although there are case reports of persons who have experienced—at times significantly—sensations related to cannabis intoxication after the short-term effects of the substance have disappeared. Continued debate concerns whether flashbacks are related to cannabis use alone or to the concomitant use of hallucinogens or of cannabis tainted with phencyclidine (PCP).

Amotivational Syndrome. Another controversial cannabis-related syndrome is amotivational syndrome. Whether the syndrome is related to cannabis use or reflects characterological traits in a subgroup of persons regardless of cannabis use is under debate. Traditionally, the amotivational syndrome has been associated with long-term heavy use and has been characterized by a person's unwillingness to persist in a task—be it at school, at work, or in any setting that requires prolonged attention or tenacity. Persons are described as becoming apathetic and anergic, usually gaining weight, and appearing slothful.

TREATMENT AND REHABILITATION

Treatment of cannabis use rests on the same principles as treatment of other substances of abuse—abstinence and support. Abstinence can be achieved through direct interventions, such as hospitalization, or through careful monitoring on an outpatient basis by the use of urine drug screens, which can detect cannabis for up to 4 weeks after use. Support can be achieved through the use of individual, family, and group psychotherapies. Education should be a cornerstone for both abstinence and support programs. A patient who does not understand the intellectual reasons for addressing a substance-abuse problem has little motivation to stop. For some patients, an antianxiety drug may be useful for short-term relief of withdrawal symptoms. For other patients, cannabis use may be related to an underlying depressive disorder that may respond to specific antidepressant treatment.

Medical Use of Marijuana

Marijuana has been used as a medicinal herb for centuries, and cannabis was listed in the U.S. pharmacopeia until the end of the 19th century as a remedy for anxiety, depression, and gastrointestinal disorders, among others. Currently, cannabis is a controlled substance with a high potential for abuse and no medical use recognized by the Drug Enforcement Agency (DEA); however, it is used to treat various disorders such as the nausea secondary to chemotherapy, multiple sclerosis, chronic pain, acquired immune deficiency syndrome (AIDS), and glaucoma. In 1996, California residents approved the California Compensation Use Act that allowed state residents to grow and use marijuana for these disorders, but in 2001 the U.S. Supreme Court ruled 8 to 0 that the manufacture and distribution of marijuana are illegal under any circumstances. It is unclear how that ruling will affect California. Dronabinol, a synthetic form of THC, has been approved by the U.S. Food and Drug Administration (FDA); however, taken orally, it is not considered as effective as smoking the entire plant product.

In 1996 an expert report by the Institute of Medicine suggested that marijuana be converted to a Schedule II drug with established controls on medical use. This would allow more controlled scientific drug trials to determine if there is unequivocal therapeutic efficacy in different conditions. The opposition to this is based on the illicit recreational use of marijuana, which obscures its legitimate medical use.

In addition to the Supreme Court ruling, President Clinton's Secretary of Health, Donna Shalala, and former Attorney General Janet Reno announced that any doctors who prescribed the drug would be prosecuted for a federal crime and could lose their license or be jailed. In a strongly worded editorial, the *New England Journal of Medicine* urged that "Federal authorities should rescind their prohibition of the medical use of marijuana for seriously ill patients and allow physicians to decide which patients to treat." They concluded the editorial by commenting on the role of the physician:

> Some physicians will have the courage to challenge the continued proscription of marijuana for the sick. Eventually, their actions will force the courts to adjudicate between the rights of those at death's door and the absolute power of bureaucrats whose decisions are based more on reflexive ideology and political correctness than on compassion.

For a further discussion of the federal government's intrusion into medical practice, the reader is referred to Chapter 56, End-of-Life Care and Palliative Medicine.

References

Bailey SL, Flewelling RL, Rachal JV. Predicting continued use of marijuana among adolescents: the relative influence of drug-specific and social context factors. *J Health Soc Behav.* 1992;33:51.
Chait LD, Zacny JP. Reinforcing and subjective effects of oral delta 9-THC and smoked marijuana in humans. *Psychopharmacology.* 1992;107:255.
Friedman H, Klein TW, Newton C, Daaka Y. Marijuana, receptors and immunomodulation. *Adv Exp Med Biol.* 1995;373:103.
Gardner EL, Lowinson JH. Marijuana's interaction with brain reward systems: update 1991. *Pharmacol Biochem Behav.* 1991;40:571.
Kassirer JP. Federal foolishness and marijuana [editorial]. *N Engl J Med.* 1997;5:336.
MacFadden W, Woody GE. Cannabis-related disorders. In: Sadock BJ, Sadock VA, eds. *Kaplan & Sadock's Comprehensive Textbook of Psychiatry.* 7th ed. Vol 1. Baltimore: Lippincott Williams & Wilkins; 2000:990.
Munro S, Thomas KL, Abu-Shaar M. Molecular characterization of a peripheral receptor for cannabinoids. *Nature.* 1993;365:61.
National Institute on Drug Abuse. *National Household Survey on Drug Abuse: Highlights, 1991.* Washington, DC: US Government Printing Office, 1991.
Stacy AW, Newcomb MD, Bentler PM. Cognitive motivation and drug use: a 9-year longitudinal study. *J Abnorm Psychol.* 1991;100:502.
Stenbacka M, Allebeck P, Romelsjo A. Do cannabis drug abusers differ from intravenous drug abusers? The role of social and behavioral risk factors. *Br J Addict.* 1992;87:259.
Tashkin DP, Gliederer F, Rose J, et al. Tar, CO and delta 9 THC delivery from the 1st to 2nd halves of a marijuana cigarette. *Pharmacol Biochem Behav.* 1991;40:657.
Vulcano BA, Barnes GE, Langstaff P. Predicting marijuana use among adolescents. *Int J Addict.* 1990;25:531.
Woody GE, MacFadden W. Cannabis-related disorders. In: Kaplan HI, Sadock BJ, eds. *Comprehensive Textbook of Psychiatry.* 6th ed. Vol 1. Baltimore: Williams & Wilkins; 1995:810.

▲ 12.6 Cocaine-Related Disorders

Cocaine is an alkaloid derived from the shrub *Erythroxylon coca,* which is indigenous to South America, where the leaves of the shrub are chewed by local inhabitants to obtain the stimulating effects (Fig. 12.6–1). The cocaine alkaloid was first isolated in 1860 and first used as a local anesthetic in 1880. It is still used as a local anesthetic, especially for eye, nose, and throat surgery, for which its vasoconstrictive and analgesic effects are helpful. In 1884, Sigmund Freud made a study of cocaine's general pharmacological effects and, for a period of time, according to his biographers, was addicted to the drug. In the 1880s and 1890s, cocaine was widely touted as a cure for many ills and was listed in the 1899 *Merck Manual.* In 1914, however, once its addictive and adverse effects had been recognized, cocaine was classified as a narcotic, along with morphine and heroin.

More than 25 million persons in the United States used cocaine at least once in the 1990s. For many of those persons, use progressed to abuse and dependence. In the early 1990s it was more common to have a lifetime history of cocaine dependence than of bipolar disorder (2.7 percent versus 1.6 percent). While the 20th-century epidemic appears to have passed its peak, cocaine use is still prevalent, and persons with cocaine abuse and dependence continue to come for treatment. A wealth of information now exists on the effects of cocaine on the brain and behavior and on cocaine toxicity, cocaine dependence, and the efficacy of treatment.

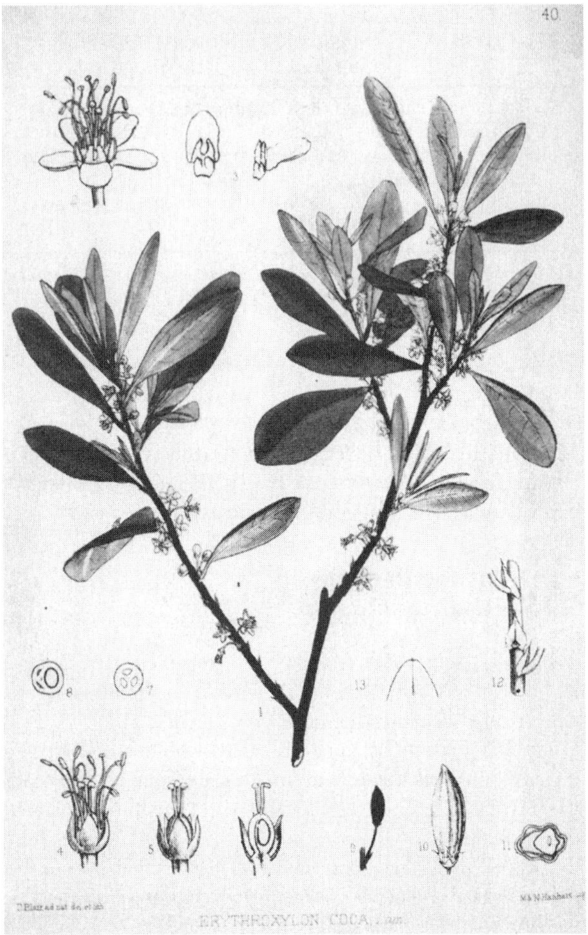

FIGURE 12.6–1
Cocaine is an alkaloid obtained from coca leaves.

DEFINITIONS

Substance use may be associated with a number of distinct disorders of which dependence and abuse are but two; the text revision of the fourth edition of *Diagnostic and Statistical Manual of Mental Disorders* (DSM-IV-TR) describes 10 others for cocaine. Cocaine dependence is defined in DSM-IV-TR as a cluster of physiological, behavioral, and cognitive symptoms that, taken together, indicate that the person continues to use cocaine despite significant problems related to such use. It is defined in the 10th revision of *International Statistical Classification of Diseases and Related Health Problems* (ICD-10) as a cluster of physiological, behavioral, and cognitive phenomena in which a person gives much higher priority to cocaine use than to other behaviors that once had a greater value. Central to these definitions is the emphasis placed on the drug-using behavior, its maladaptive nature, and how over time the voluntary choice to engage in that behavior shifts and becomes constrained as a result of interactions with the drug.

ICD-10 and DSM-IV-TR differ in their classification of what is called *substance abuse* in DSM-IV-TR. ICD-10 does not use the term *abuse* and includes instead the category of harmful use, which differs substantially from the concept of abuse used in DSM-IV-TR. However, the concept of harm is limited to physical and mental health (e.g., hepatitis, cardiac damage, episodes of depression, or toxic psychosis). It specifically excludes social impairments, as follows:

> Harmful patterns of use are often criticized by others and frequently associated with adverse social consequences

of various kinds. The fact that a pattern of use of a particular substance is disapproved of by another person or by the culture, or may have led to socially negative consequences such as arrest or marital arguments, is not in itself evidence of harmful use.

EPIDEMIOLOGY

According to DSM-IV-TR, about 10 percent of the U.S. population has tried cocaine, with 2 percent reporting use in the last year, 0.8 percent reporting use in the past month, and a lifetime rate of cocaine abuse or dependence of about 2 percent. Cocaine use is highest among persons ages 18 to 25 years (1.3 percent) and ages 26 to 34 (1.2 percent). Current cocaine use, however, is on the decline, primarily because of increased awareness of cocaine's risks as well as a comprehensive public campaign about cocaine and its effects. The societal effects of the decrease in cocaine use, however, have been somewhat offset by the frequent use over the past years of crack, a highly potent form of cocaine. Crack use is most common in persons ages 18 to 25, who are particularly attracted to the low street price of a single 50- to 100-mg dose. Males are twice as likely to be cocaine abusers as females, and all races and socioeconomic groups are equally affected.

COMORBIDITY

Like other substance-related disorders, cocaine-related disorders are often accompanied by additional psychiatric disorders. The development of mood disorders and alcohol-related disorders usually follows the onset of cocaine-related disorders, whereas anxiety disorders, antisocial personality disorder, and attention-deficit/hyperactivity disorder are thought to precede the development of cocaine-related disorders. Most studies of comorbidity in patients with cocaine-related disorders have shown that major depressive disorder, bipolar II disorder, cyclothymic disorder, anxiety disorders, and antisocial personality disorder are the most commonly associated psychiatric diagnoses. The percentages of comorbidity in cocaine users are presented in Table 12.6–1.

Table 12.6–1
Additional Psychiatric Diagnoses among Cocaine Users Seeking Treatment (New Haven Cocaine Diagnostic Study Results, Percentages)

Psychiatric Diagnosis	Current Disorder	Lifetime Disorder
Major depression	4.7	30.5
Cyclothymia/hyperthymia	19.9	19.9
Mania	0.0	3.7
Hypomania	2.0	7.4
Panic disorder	0.3	1.7
Generalized anxiety disorder	3.7	7.0
Phobia	11.7	13.4
Schizophrenia	0.0	0.3
Schizoaffective disorder	0.3	1.0
Alcoholism	28.9	61.7
Antisocial personality disorder—RDC	7.7	7.7
Antisocial personality disorder—DSM-III	32.9	32.9
Attention-deficit disorder		34.9

Adapted from Rounsaville BJ, Anton SI, Caroll K, et al. Psychiatric diagnoses of treatment-seeking cocaine abusers. *Arch Gen Psychiatry.* 1991;48:43.

ETIOLOGY

Genetic Factors

Laboratory animal strains differ greatly in their willingness to self-administer psychoactive drugs, including cocaine, and strains can be developed that differ even more markedly. The most convincing evidence to date of a genetic influence on cocaine dependence comes from studies of twins. Monozygotic twins have higher concordance rates for stimulant dependence (cocaine, amphetamines, and amphetaminelike drugs) than dizygotic twins. The analyses indicate that genetic factors and unique (unshared) environmental factors contribute about equally to the development of stimulant dependence.

Sociocultural Factors

Social, cultural, and economic factors are powerful determinants of initial use, continuing use, and relapse. Excessive use is far more likely in countries where cocaine is readily available. Different economic opportunities may influence certain groups more than others to engage in selling illicit drugs, and selling is more likely to be carried out in familiar communities than in those where the seller runs a high risk of arrest.

Learning and Conditioning

Learning and conditioning are also considered important in perpetuating cocaine use. Each inhalation or injection of cocaine yields a "rush" and a euphoric experience that reinforce the antecedent drug-taking behavior. In addition, the environmental cues associated with substance use become associated with the euphoric state so that long after a period of cessation, such cues (e.g., white powder and paraphernalia) can elicit memories of the euphoric state and reawaken craving for cocaine.

In cocaine abusers (but not in normal controls), cocaine-related stimuli activate brain regions subserving episodic and working memory and produce electroencephalographic (EEG) arousal (desynchronization). Increased metabolic activity in the limbic-related regions such as the amygdala, parahippocampal gyrus, and dorsolateral prefrontal cortex reportedly correlate with reports of craving for cocaine, but the degree of EEG arousal does not.

Pharmacological Factors

As a result of actions in the central nervous system (CNS), cocaine can produce a sense of alertness, euphoria, and well-being. There may be decreased hunger and less need for sleep. Performance impaired by fatigue is usually improved. Some users believe that cocaine enhances sexual performance.

NEUROPHARMACOLOGY

Cocaine's primary pharmacodynamic action related to its behavioral effects is competitive blockade of dopamine reuptake by the dopamine

transporter. This blockade increases the concentration of dopamine in the synaptic cleft and results in increased activation of both dopamine type 1 (D_1) and type 2 (D_2) receptors. The effects of cocaine on the activity mediated by D_3, D_4, and D_5 receptors are not yet well understood, but at least one preclinical study has implicated the D_3 receptor. Although the behavioral effects are attributed primarily to the blockade of dopamine reuptake, cocaine also blocks the reuptake of the other major catecholamine, norepinephrine, and that of serotonin. The behavioral effects related to these activities are receiving increased attention in the scientific literature. The effects of cocaine on cerebral blood flow and cerebral glucose use have also been studied. Results in most studies generally showed that cocaine is associated with decreased cerebral blood flow and possibly with the development of patchy areas of decreased glucose use.

The behavioral effects of cocaine are felt almost immediately and last for a relatively brief time (30 to 60 minutes); thus, users require repeated doses of the drug to maintain the feelings of intoxication. Despite the short-lived behavioral effects, metabolites of cocaine may be present in the blood and urine for up to 10 days.

Cocaine has powerful addictive qualities. Because of its potency as a positive reinforcer of behavior, psychological dependence on cocaine can develop after a single use. With repeated administration, both tolerance and sensitivity to various effects of cocaine can arise, although the development of tolerance or sensitivity is apparently due to many factors and is not easily predicted. Physiological dependence on cocaine does occur, although cocaine withdrawal is mild compared with withdrawal from opiates and opioids.

Researchers recently reported that positron emission tomography (PET) scans of the brains of patients being treated for cocaine addiction show high activation in the mesolimbic dopamine system when addicts profoundly crave a drug. Researchers exposed patients to cues that had previously caused them to crave cocaine, and patients described feelings of intense cravings for the drug while PET scans showed activation in areas from the amygdala and the anterior cingulate to the tip of both temporal lobes. Some researchers claim that the mesolimbic dopamine system is also active in patients with nicotine addiction, and the same system has been linked to cravings for heroin, morphine, amphetamines, marijuana, and alcohol.

D_2 receptors in the mesolimbic dopamine system have been held responsible for the heightened activity during periods of craving. PET scans of patients recovering from cocaine addiction are reported to show a drop in neuronal activity consistent with a lessened ability to receive dopamine, and the reduction in this ability, although it decreases over time, is apparent as long as a year and a half after withdrawal. The pattern of reduced brain activity reflects the course of the craving; between the third and fourth weeks of withdrawal, the activity is at its lowest level, and the risk of patient relapse is highest. After about 1 year, the brains of former addicts are almost back to normal, although whether the dopamine cells ever return to a completely normal state is debatable.

METHODS OF USE

Because drug dealers often dilute cocaine powder with sugar or procaine, street cocaine varies greatly in purity. Cocaine is sometimes cut with amphetamine. The most common method of using cocaine is inhaling the finely chopped powder into the nose, a practice referred to as "snorting" or "tooting." Other methods of ingesting cocaine are subcutaneous or intravenous (IV) injection and smoking (freebasing). Freebasing involves mixing street cocaine with chemically extracted pure cocaine alkaloid (the freebase) to get an increased effect. Smoking is also the method used for ingesting crack cocaine. Inhaling is the least dangerous method of cocaine use; IV injection and smoking are the most dangerous. The most direct methods of ingestion are often associated with cerebrovascular diseases, cardiac abnormalities, and death. Although cocaine can be taken orally, it is rarely ingested via this, the least effective, route.

Crack

Crack, a freebase form of cocaine, is extremely potent. It is sold in small, ready-to-smoke amounts, often called "rocks." Crack cocaine is highly addictive; even one or two experiences with the drug can cause intense craving for more. Users have been known to resort to extremes of behavior to obtain the money to buy more crack. Reports from urban emergency rooms have also associated extremes of violence with crack abuse.

DIAGNOSIS AND CLINICAL FEATURES

DSM-IV-TR lists many cocaine-related disorders (Table 12.6–2) but only specifies the diagnostic criteria for cocaine intoxica-

Table 12.6–2
DSM-IV-TR Cocaine-Related Disorders

Cocaine use disorders
Cocaine dependence
Cocaine abuse
Cocaine-induced disorders
Cocaine intoxication
Specify if:
With perceptual disturbances
Cocaine withdrawal
Cocaine intoxication delirium
Cocaine-induced psychotic disorder, with delusions
Specify if:
With onset during intoxication
Cocaine-induced psychotic disorder, with hallucinations
Specify if:
With onset during intoxication
Cocaine-induced mood disorder
Specify if:
With onset during intoxication
With onset during withdrawal
Cocaine-induced anxiety disorder
Specify if:
With onset during intoxication
With onset during withdrawal
Cocaine-induced sexual dysfunction
Specify if:
With onset during intoxication
Cocaine-induced sleep disorder
Specify if:
With onset during intoxication
With onset during withdrawal
Cocaine-related disorder not otherwise specified

From American Psychiatric Association. *Diagnostic and Statistical Manual of Mental Disorders.* 4th ed. Text rev. Washington, DC: American Psychiatric Association; copyright 2000, with permission.

Table 12.6–3
DSM-IV-TR Diagnostic Criteria for Cocaine Intoxication

A. Recent use of cocaine.

B. Clinically significant maladaptive behavioral or psychological changes (e.g., euphoria or affective blunting; changes in sociability; hypervigilance; interpersonal sensitivity; anxiety, tension, or anger; stereotyped behaviors; impaired judgment; or impaired social or occupational functioning) that developed during, or shortly after, use of cocaine.

C. Two (or more) of the following, developing during, or shortly after, cocaine use:

(1) tachycardia or bradycardia
(2) pupillary dilation
(3) elevated or lowered blood pressure
(4) perspiration or chills
(5) nausea or vomiting
(6) evidence of weight loss
(7) psychomotor agitation or retardation
(8) muscular weakness, respiratory depression, chest pain, or cardiac arrhythmias
(9) confusion, seizures, dyskinesias, dystonias, or coma

D. The symptoms are not due to a general medical condition and are not better accounted for by another mental disorder.

Specify if:

With perceptual disturbances

From American Psychiatric Association. *Diagnostic and Statistical Manual of Mental Disorders.* 4th ed. Text rev. Washington, DC: American Psychiatric Association; copyright 2000, with permission.

tion (Table 12.6–3) and cocaine withdrawal (Table 12.6–4) within the cocaine-related disorders section. The diagnostic criteria for the other cocaine-related disorders are in the DSM-IV-TR sections that focus on the principal symptom—for example, cocaine-induced mood disorder in the mood disorders section (see Table 15.3–10 in Section 15.3 of Chapter 15).

Table 12.6–4
DSM-IV-TR Diagnostic Criteria for Cocaine Withdrawal

A. Cessation of (or reduction in) cocaine use that has been heavy and prolonged.

B. Dysphoric mood and two (or more) of the following physiological changes, developing within a few hours to several days after Criterion A:

(1) fatigue
(2) vivid, unpleasant dreams
(3) insomnia or hypersomnia
(4) increased appetite
(5) psychomotor retardation or agitation

C. The symptoms in Criterion B cause clinically significant distress or impairment in social, occupational, or other important areas of functioning.

D. The symptoms are not due to a general medical condition and are not better accounted for by another mental disorder.

From American Psychiatric Association. *Diagnostic and Statistical Manual of Mental Disorders.* 4th ed. Text rev. Washington, DC: American Psychiatric Association; copyright 2000, with permission.

Cocaine Dependence and Abuse

DSM-IV-TR uses the general guidelines for substance dependence and substance abuse to diagnose cocaine dependence and cocaine abuse (see Tables 12.1–5, 12.1–6, and 12.1–7). Clinically and practically, cocaine dependence or cocaine abuse can be suspected in patients who evidence unexplained changes in personality. Common changes associated with cocaine use are irritability, impaired ability to concentrate, compulsive behavior, severe insomnia, and weight loss. Colleagues at work and family members may notice a person's general and increasing inability to perform the expected tasks associated with work and family life. The patient may show new evidence of increased debt or inability to pay bills on time because of the large sums used to buy cocaine. Cocaine abusers often excuse themselves from work or social situations every 30 to 60 minutes to find a secluded place to inhale more cocaine. Because of the vasoconstricting effects of cocaine, users almost always develop nasal congestion, which they may attempt to self-medicate with decongestant sprays.

Al S., a 39-year-old restaurant owner, is referred by a marriage counselor to a private outpatient substance abuse treatment program for evaluation and treatment of a possible "cocaine problem." According to the counselor, attempts to deal with the couple's marital problems have failed to produce any signs of progress over the past 6 or 7 months. The couple continues to have frequent, explosive arguments, some of which have led to physical violence. Fortunately, neither spouse has been seriously injured, but the continuing chaos in their relationship has led to a great deal of tension at home and appears to be contributing to the acting-out behavior and school problems of their two children, ages 9 and 13.

Several days ago the patient admitted to the counselor and to his wife that he had been using cocaine "occasionally" for at least the past year. The wife became angry and tearful, stating that if her husband failed to obtain treatment for his drug problem, she would separate from him and inform his parents of the problem. He reluctantly agreed to seek professional help, insisting that his cocaine use was "not a problem" and that he felt capable of stopping his drug use without entering a treatment program.

During the initial evaluation interview, Al reports that he is currently using cocaine, intranasally, 3 to 5 days a week, and that this pattern has been continuing for at least the past 2 years. On average, he consumes a total of 1 to 2 grams of cocaine weekly, for which he pays $80 per gram. Most of his cocaine use occurs at work, in his private office, or in the bathroom. He usually begins thinking about "coke" while driving to work in the morning. When he arrives at work, he finds it nearly impossible to avoid thinking of the cocaine vial in his desk drawer. Although he tries to distract himself and postpone using it as long as possible, he usually snorts his first "line" within an hour of arriving at work. On some days he may snort another two or three lines over the course

of the day. On other days, especially if he feels stressed or frustrated at work, he may snort a line or two every hour from morning through late afternoon. His cocaine use is sometimes fueled by offers of the drug from his business partner, whom the patient describes as a more controlled, infrequent user of the drug.

Al rarely uses cocaine at home and never in the presence of his wife or children. Occasionally he snorts a line or two on weekday evenings or weekends at home when everyone else is out of the house. Al denies current use of any other illicit drug but reports taking 10 to 20 mg of an antianxiety drug, diazepam (prescribed by a physician friend), at bedtime on days when cocaine leaves him feeling restless, irritable, and unable to fall asleep. When diazepam is unavailable, he drinks two or three beers instead.

He first tried cocaine 5 years ago at a friend's party. He enjoyed the energetic, euphoric feeling and the absence of any unpleasant side effects, except for a slightly uncomfortable "racing" feeling in his chest. For nearly 3 years thereafter, he used cocaine only when it was offered by others and never purchased his own supplies or found himself thinking about the drug between episodes of use. He rarely snorted more than four or five lines on any single occasion of use. During the past 2 years his cocaine use escalated to its current level, coincident with a number of significant changes in his life. His restaurant business became financially successful; he bought a large home in the suburbs; he had access to large sums of cash; and the pressures of a growing business made him feel entitled to the relief and pleasures offered by cocaine.

He denies any history of alcohol or drug abuse problems. The only other drug he has ever used is marijuana, which he smoked infrequently in college but never really liked. He also denies any history of other emotional problems and, except for marriage counseling, reports that he has never needed help from a mental health professional.

During the interview, Al remarks several times that although he thinks that his cocaine use "might be a problem," he does not consider himself to be "addicted" to it and is still not sure that he really requires treatment. In support of this view, he lists the following evidence: (1) His current level of cocaine use is not causing him any financial problems or affecting his standard of living. (2) He is experiencing no significant drug-related health problems that he is aware of, with the possible exception of feeling lethargic the next day following a day of heavy use. (3) On many occasions he has been able to stop using cocaine on his own, for several days at a time. (4) When he stops using the drug, he experiences no withdrawal syndrome and no continuous drug cravings. On the other hand, he does admit the following: (1) He often uses much more cocaine than intended on certain days. (2) The drug use is impairing his functioning at work because of negative effects on his memory, attention span, and attitude toward employees and customers. (3) Even when he is not actively intoxicated with cocaine, the aftereffects of the drug cause him to be short-tempered, irritable, and argumentative with his wife and children, leading to numerous family problems, including a possible breakup of his marriage. (4) Although he seems able to stop using cocaine for a few days at a time, somehow he always goes back to it. (5) As soon as he starts to use cocaine again, the craving and the preoccupation with the drug are immediately as intense as before he stopped using it.

At the end of the interview, Al agrees that although he came for the evaluation largely under pressure from his wife, he can see the potential benefits of trying to stop using cocaine on a more permanent basis. With a saddened expression, he explains how troubled and frightened he feels about the problems with his wife and children. He says that although marital problems existed before he started snorting cocaine, his continuing drug use has made them worse, and he now fears that his wife might leave him. He also feels extremely guilty about not being a "good father." He spends very little time with his children and often is distracted and irritable with them because of his cocaine use.

DISCUSSION

Al, like many people with a serious drug problem, does not like to think of himself as "addicted." However, Al's use of cocaine illustrates the core concept of psychoactive substance dependence: a cluster of cognitive, behavioral, and physiologic symptoms indicating that the person has impaired control of psychoactive substance despite adverse consequences. Al cannot stop himself from taking the first hit of cocaine in the morning; he uses it more often than he plans to; he keeps returning to it after stopping for a few days; he experiences withdrawal symptoms (lethargy); and he has reduced important social activities with his family because of mood changes caused by his taking cocaine. Therefore, the diagnosis is Cocaine Dependence, With Physiological Dependence.

FOLLOW-UP

Al entered the outpatient treatment program. His treatment included individual, group, and marital counseling combined with supervised urine screening and participation in a self-help group (Cocaine Anonymous). He initially had difficulty in fully acknowledging and accepting the seriousness of his drug dependency problem. He harbored fantasies about returning to "controlled" cocaine use and distrusted the program's requirement of total abstinence from all mood-altering substances, arguing that because he had never experienced problems with alcohol, he saw no reason to deny himself an occasional drink with dinner or at social gatherings. During the first 3 months of treatment he had two short "slips" back to taking cocaine, one of which was precipitated by drinking a glass of wine, which led to an intense craving for cocaine.

Subsequently, Al remained completely abstinent for the duration of the program (12 months) and became increasingly committed to maintaining a drug-free lifestyle. His relationship with his wife and children improved considerably. The violent arguments had stopped immediately with the cessation of cocaine use, and spending more time with his children became much easier without the negative influence of cocaine on his mood and mental state.

Three years later Al was still abstinent. He was no longer in treatment but continued to attend Cocaine Anonymous meetings at least two to three times every week. If he were diagnosed at this time, the Cocaine Dependence would be specified as Sustained Full Remission because of the absence of any of the signs or symptoms of Cocaine Dependence for over 12 months. (From *DSM-IV Casebook.*)

Cocaine Intoxication

DSM-IV-TR specifies the diagnostic criteria for cocaine intoxication (Table 12.6–3), which emphasizes the behavioral and physical signs and symptoms of cocaine use. The DSM-IV-TR diagnostic criteria allow for specification of the presence of perceptual disturbances. If hallucinations are present in the absence of intact reality testing, the appropriate diagnosis is cocaine-induced psychotic disorder, with hallucinations.

Persons use cocaine for its characteristic effects of elation, euphoria, heightened self-esteem, and perceived improvement on mental and physical tasks. Some studies have indicated that low doses of cocaine can actually be associated with improved performance on some cognitive tasks. With high doses, however, the symptoms of intoxication include agitation, irritability, impaired judgment, impulsive and potentially dangerous sexual behavior, aggression, a generalized increase in psychomotor activity, and, potentially, symptoms of mania. The major associated physical symptoms are tachycardia, hypertension, and mydriasis.

Cocaine Withdrawal

After cessation of cocaine use or after acute intoxication, postintoxication depression ("crash") may be associated with symptoms of dysphoria, anhedonia, anxiety, irritability, fatigue, hypersomnolence, and sometimes agitation. With mild to moderate cocaine use, these withdrawal symptoms end within 18 hours. With heavy use, as in cocaine dependence, withdrawal symptoms can last up to a week but usually peak in 2 to 4 days. Some patients and some anecdotal reports have described cocaine withdrawal syndromes that have lasted for weeks or months. The withdrawal symptoms can also be associated with suicidal ideation in affected persons. A person in the state of withdrawal can experience powerful and intense cravings for cocaine, especially because taking cocaine can eliminate the unpleasant withdrawal symptoms. Persons experiencing cocaine withdrawal often attempt to self-medicate with alcohol, sedatives, hypnotics, or antianxiety agents such as diazepam (Valium). The DSM-IV-TR diagnostic criteria for cocaine withdrawal are listed Table 12.6–4.

Cocaine Intoxication Delirium

DSM-IV-TR has specified a diagnosis for cocaine intoxication delirium (see Table 10.2–3). Cocaine intoxication delirium is most common when high doses of cocaine are used; when cocaine has been used over a short time, so that cocaine blood concentrations rapidly increase; or when cocaine is mixed with other psychoactive substances (e.g., amphetamine, opiates, opioids, and alcohol). Persons with preexisting brain damage (often resulting from previous episodes of cocaine intoxication) are also at increased risk for cocaine intoxication delirium.

Cocaine-Induced Psychotic Disorder

Paranoid delusions and hallucinations may occur in up to 50 percent of all persons who use cocaine. The occurrence of these psychotic symptoms depends on the dose, the duration of use, and the individual user's sensitivity to the substance. Cocaine-induced psychotic disorders are most common with IV users and crack users. Men are much more likely to have psychotic symptoms than are women. Paranoid delusions are the most frequent psychotic symptoms. Auditory hallucinations are also common, but visual and tactile hallucinations may be less common than paranoid delusions. The sensation of bugs crawling just beneath the skin (formication) has been reported to be associated with cocaine use. Psychotic disorders can develop with grossly inappropriate sexual and generally bizarre behavior and homicidal or other violent actions related to the content of the paranoid delusions or hallucinations. The DSM-IV-TR diagnostic criteria of cocaine-induced psychotic disorders are listed in Table 14.4–7. Clinicians can further specify whether delusions or hallucinations are the predominant symptom.

Cocaine-Induced Mood Disorder

DSM-IV-TR allows for the diagnosis of cocaine-induced mood disorder (see Table 15.3–10), which can begin during either intoxication or withdrawal. Classically, the mood disorder symptoms associated with intoxication are hypomanic or manic; the mood disorder symptoms associated with withdrawal are characteristic of depression.

Cocaine-Induced Anxiety Disorder

DSM-IV-TR also allows for the diagnosis of cocaine-induced anxiety disorder (see Table 16.7–3). Common anxiety disorder symptoms associated with cocaine intoxication or withdrawal are those of obsessive-compulsive disorder, panic disorders, and phobias.

Cocaine-Induced Sexual Dysfunction

DSM-IV-TR allows for the diagnosis of cocaine-induced sexual dysfunction (see Table 21.2–17), which can begin when a person is intoxicated with cocaine. Although cocaine is used as an aphrodisiac and as a way to delay orgasm, its repeated use can result in impotence.

Cocaine-Induced Sleep Disorder

Cocaine-induced sleep disorder, which can begin during either intoxication or withdrawal, is described under substance-induced sleep disorders (see Table 24.2–21). Cocaine intoxication is associated with the inability to sleep; cocaine withdrawal is associated with disrupted sleep or hypersomnolence.

Cocaine-Related Disorder Not Otherwise Specified

DSM-IV-TR provides a diagnosis of cocaine-related disorder not otherwise specified for cocaine-related disorders that can-

Table 12.6–5
DSM-IV-TR Diagnostic Criteria for Cocaine-Related Disorder Not Otherwise Specified

The cocaine-related disorder not otherwise specified category is for disorders associated with the use of cocaine that are not classifiable as cocaine dependence, cocaine abuse, cocaine intoxication, cocaine withdrawal, cocaine intoxication delirium, cocaine-induced psychotic disorder, cocaine-induced mood disorder, cocaine-induced anxiety disorder, cocaine-induced sexual dysfunction, or cocaine-induced sleep disorder.

From American Psychiatric Association. *Diagnostic and Statistical Manual of Mental Disorders.* 4th ed. Text rev. Washington, DC: American Psychiatric Association; copyright 2000, with permission.

not be classified into one of the previously discussed diagnoses (Table 12.6–5).

Adverse Effects

A common adverse effect associated with cocaine use is nasal congestion; serious inflammation, swelling, bleeding, and ulceration of the nasal mucosa can also occur. Long-term use of cocaine can also lead to perforation of the nasal septa. Freebasing and smoking crack can damage the bronchial passages and the lungs. The IV use of cocaine can result in infection, embolisms, and the transmission of human immunodeficiency virus (HIV). Minor neurological complications with cocaine use include the development of acute dystonia, tics, and migraine-like headaches. The major complications of cocaine use, however, are cerebrovascular, epileptic, and cardiac. About two thirds of these acute toxic effects occur within 1 hour of intoxication; about one fifth occur in 1 to 3 hours, and the remainder occur up to several days later.

Cerebrovascular Effects. The most common cerebrovascular diseases associated with cocaine use are nonhemorrhagic cerebral infarctions. When hemorrhagic infarctions do occur, they can include subarachnoid, intraparenchymal, and intraventricular hemorrhages. Transient ischemic attacks have also been associated with cocaine use. Although these vascular disorders usually affect the brain, spinal cord hemorrhages have also been reported. The obvious pathophysiological mechanism for these vascular disorders is vasoconstriction, but other pathophysiological mechanisms have also been proposed.

Seizures. Seizures have been reported to account for 3 to 8 percent of cocaine-related emergency room visits. Cocaine is the substance of abuse most commonly associated with seizures; the second most common substance is amphetamine. Cocaine-induced seizures are usually single events, although multiple seizures and status epilepticus are also possible. A rare and easily misdiagnosed complication of cocaine use is partial complex status epilepticus, which should be considered as a diagnosis in a patient who seems to have cocaine-induced psychotic disorder with an unusually fluctuating course. The risk of having cocaine-induced seizures is highest in patients with a history of epilepsy who use high doses of cocaine as well as crack.

Cardiac Effects. Myocardial infarctions and arrhythmias are perhaps the most common cocaine-induced cardiac abnormalities. Cardiomyopathies can develop with long-term use of cocaine, and cardioembolic cerebral infarctions can be a further complication of cocaine-induced myocardial dysfunction.

Death. High doses of cocaine are associated with seizures, respiratory depression, cerebrovascular diseases, and myocardial infarctions—all of which can lead to death in persons who use cocaine. Users may experience warning signs of syncope or chest pain but may ignore these signs because of the irrepressible desire to take more cocaine. Deaths have also been reported with the ingestion of "speedballs," which are combinations of opioids and cocaine.

TREATMENT AND REHABILITATION

Most cocaine users do not come to treatment voluntarily. Their experience with the substance is too positive, and the negative effects are perceived as too minimal, to warrant seeking treatment. Those who do not seek treatment often have polysubstance-related disorder, fewer negative consequences associated with cocaine use, fewer work-related or family-related obligations, and increased contact with the legal system and with illegal activities.

The major hurdle to overcome in the treatment of cocaine-related disorders is the user's intense craving for the drug. Although animal studies have shown that cocaine is a powerful inducer of self-administration, these studies have also shown that animals limit their use of cocaine when negative reinforcers are experimentally linked to the cocaine intake. In humans, negative reinforcers may take the form of work and family-related problems brought on by cocaine use. Therefore, clinicians must take a broad treatment approach and include social, psychological, and perhaps biological strategies in the treatment program.

Attaining abstinence from cocaine in their patients may require complete or partial hospitalization to remove patients from the usual social settings in which they had obtained or used cocaine. Frequent, unscheduled urine testing is almost always necessary to monitor patients' continued abstinence, especially in the first weeks and months of treatment. Relapse prevention therapy (RPT) is a therapy that relies on cognitive and behavioral techniques in addition to hospitalization and outpatient therapy to achieve the goal of abstinence.

Psychological intervention usually involves individual, group, and family modalities. In individual therapy, therapists should focus on the dynamics leading to cocaine use, the perceived positive effects of the cocaine, and other ways to achieve these effects. Group therapy and support groups, such as Narcotics Anonymous, often focus on discussions with other persons who use cocaine and on sharing past experiences and effective coping methods. Family therapy is often an essential component of the treatment strategy. Common issues discussed in family therapy are the ways the patient's past behavior has harmed the family and the responses of family members to these behaviors. Therapy should also focus, however, on the future and on changes in the family's activities that may help the patient stay off the drug and direct energies in different directions. This approach can be used on an outpatient basis.

Pharmacological Adjuncts

Presently, no pharmacological treatments produce decreases in cocaine use comparable to the decreases in opioid use seen when heroin users are treated with methadone, levomethadyl acetate (ORLAAM) (commonly called L-α-acetylmethadol [LAAM]) or buprenorphine (Buprenex). However, a variety of pharmacological agents, most of which are approved for other uses, have been, and are being, tested clinically for the treatment of cocaine dependence and relapse.

Cocaine users presumed to have preexisting attention-deficit/hyperactivity disorder or mood disorders have been treated with methylphenidate (Ritalin) and lithium (Eskalith), respectively. Those drugs are of little or no benefit in patients without the disorders, and clinicians should adhere strictly to maximal diagnostic criteria before using either of them in the treatment of cocaine dependence. In patients with attention-deficit/hyperactivity disorder, slow-release forms of methylphenidate may be less likely to trigger cocaine craving, but the impact of such pharmacotherapy on cocaine use remains to be demonstrated.

Many pharmacological agents have been explored on the premise that chronic cocaine use alters the function of multiple neurotransmitter systems, especially the dopaminergic and serotonergic transmitters regulating hedonic tone, and that cocaine induces a state of relative dopaminergic deficiency. Although the evidence for such alterations in dopaminergic function has been growing, it has been difficult to demonstrate that agents theoretically capable of modifying dopamine function can alter the course of treatment, even when studies in animal models and open-label studies suggested that they would be successful. In well-designed, controlled trials that obtained objective evidence of drug use, the following agents are among those that have not been found to reduce cocaine use: neurotransmitter precursors (e.g., dopa; tyrosine); dopaminergic agonists (e.g., bromocriptine [Parlodel]; lisuride [Dopergin]; pergolide [Permax]); and antiparkinson drugs that may also affect the dopaminergic system (amantadine [Symmetrel]).

Tricyclic antidepressant drugs such as desipramine (Norpramin) and imipramine (Tofranil) have also been tried. Although some double-blind studies that relied heavily on self-reports of drug use yielded some positive results, other studies did not find them significantly beneficial in inducing abstinence or preventing relapse. Used early in treatment, however, they may have some transient benefit for patients who are not severely dependent.

Also tried but not confirmed effective in controlled studies are other antidepressants, such as bupropion (Wellbutrin), monoamine oxidase (MAO) inhibitors (selegiline [Eldepryl]); selective serotonin uptake inhibitors (SSRIs; e.g., fluoxetine [Prozac]); mazindol (Sanorex); pemoline (Cylert); antipsychotics (e.g., flupenthixol [Depixol]); lithium; several different calcium channel inhibitors, anticonvulsants (e.g., carbamazepine [Tegretol] and valproic acid [Depakene]). One study found that 300 mg a day of phenytoin (Dilantin) reduced cocaine use; this study requires further replication.

Several agents are being developed that have not been tried in human studies. These include agents that would selectively block or stimulate dopamine receptor subtypes (e.g., selective D_1 agonists) and drugs that can selectively block the access of cocaine to the dopamine transporters but still permit the transporters to remove cocaine from the synapse. Another approach is aimed at preventing cocaine from reaching the brain by using antibodies to bind cocaine in the bloodstream (a so-called cocaine vaccine). Such cocaine-binding antibodies do reduce the reinforcing effects of cocaine in animal models. Also under study are catalytic antibodies that accelerate the hydrolysis of cocaine; and butyrylcholinesterase (pseudocholinesterase), which appears to hydrolyze cocaine selectively and is normally present in the body.

Detoxification

The cocaine withdrawal syndrome is distinct from that of opioids, alcohol, or sedative-hypnotic agents, since there are no physiological disturbances that necessitate inpatient or residential drug withdrawal. Thus it is generally possible to engage in a therapeutic trial of outpatient withdrawal before deciding whether a more intensive or controlled setting is required for patients unable to stop without help in limiting their access to cocaine. Patients withdrawing from cocaine typically experience fatigue, dysphoria, disturbed sleep, and some craving; some may experience depression. No pharmacological agents reliably reduce the intensity of withdrawal, but recovery over a week or two is generally uneventful. It may take longer, however, for sleep, mood, and cognitive function to recover fully.

References

Annas GJ. Testing poor pregnant patients for cocaine. *N Engl J Med.* 2001;344:152.

Ashton CH. Pharmacology and effects of cannabis: a brief review. *Br J Psychiatry.* 2001;178:10.

Crosby RD, Pearson VL, Eller C, Winegarden T, Graves NL. Phenytoin in the treatment of cocaine abuse: a double-blind study. *Clin Pharmacol Ther.* 1996;59:458.

Gallanter M, Egelko S, De Leon G, Rohrs C, Franco H. Crack-cocaine abusers in the general hospital: assessment and initiation of care. *Am J Psychiatry.* 1992;149:810.

Higgins ST, Budney AJ, Bickel WK, Hughes JR, Foerg F, Badger G. Achieving cocaine abstinence with a behavioral approach. *Am J Psychiatry.* 1993;150:763.

Jaffe JH. Cocaine-related disorders. In: Sadock BJ, Sadock VA, eds. *Kaplan & Sadock's Comprehensive Textbook of Psychiatry.* 7th ed. Vol 1. Baltimore: Lippincott Williams & Wilkins; 2000:999.

Self DW. Cocaine abuse takes a shot. *Nature.* 1995;378:666.

Silverman K, Higgins ST, Brooder RK, et al. Sustained cocaine abstinence in methadone maintenance patients through voucher-based reinforcement therapy. *Arch Gen Psychiatry.* 1996;53:409.

Strung J, Johns A, Can W. Cocaine in the UK—1991. *Br J Psychiatry.* 1993;162:1.

Substance Abuse and Mental Health Services Administration Office of Applied Studies. *Preliminary Estimates from the 1995 National Household Survey on Drug Abuse.* Washington, DC: US Government Printing Office; 1995.

Tims FM, Leukefeld CG, ed. *Relapse and Recovery in Addictions.* New Haven: Yale University Press; 2001:355.

Withers NW, Pulvirenti L, Koob GF, Gillin JC. Cocaine abuse and dependence. *J Clin Psychopharmacol.* 1995;15:63.

▲ 12.7 Hallucinogen-Related Disorders

Hallucinogens are natural and synthetic substances that are variously called *psychedelics* or *psychotomimetics* because, besides inducing hallucinations, they produce a loss of contact with reality and an experience of expanded and heightened consciousness. The hallucinogens are classified as Schedule I drugs; the U.S. Food and Drug Administration (FDA) has decreed that they have no medical use and a high abuse potential.

The classic, naturally occurring hallucinogens are *psilocybin* (from some mushrooms) and *mescaline* (from peyote cactus); others are harmine, harmaline, ibogaine, and *dimethyltryptamine* (DMT). The classic synthetic hallucinogen is *lysergic acid dieth-*

Table 12.7–1
Overview of Representative Hallucinogens

Agent	Locale	Chemical Classification	Biological Sources	Common Route	Typical Dose	Duration of Effects	Adverse Reactions
Lysergic acid diethylamide	Globally distributed, semisynthetic	Indolealkylamine	Fungus in rye yields lysergic acid	Oral	100 μg	6–12 h	Extensive, including pandemic 1965–1975
Mescaline	Southwestern U.S.	Phenethylamine	Peyote cactus, *L. williamsii*	Oral	200–400 mg or 4–6 cactus buttons	10–12 h	Little or none verified
Methylenedioxyamphetamine (MDA)	U.S., synthetic	Phenethylamine	Synthetic	Oral	80–160 mg	8–12 h	Documented
Methylenedioxymethamphetamine (MDMA)	U.S., synthetic	Phenethylamine	Synthetic	Oral	80–150 mg	4–6 h	Documented
Psilocybin	Southern U.S., Mexico, South America	Phosphorylated hydroxylated DMT	Psilocybin mushrooms	Oral	4–6 mg or 5–10 g of dried mushroom	4–6 h	Psychosis
Ibogaine	West Central Africa	Indolealkylamine	Tabernanthe iboga	Eating powdered root	200–400 mg	8–48 h	CNS excitation, death?
Ayahuasca	S. American tropics	Harmine, other β-carbolines	Bark or leaves of *Banisteriopsis caapi*	As a tea	300–400 mg	4–8 h	None reported
Dimethyltryptamine	S. America, synthetic	Substituted tryptamine	Leaves of *Virola calophylla*	As a snuff, IV	0.2 mg/kg I.V.	30 min	None reported
Morning glory	American tropics and warm zones	D-Lysergic acid alkaloids	Seeds of *I. violacea, T. corymbosa*	Orally as infusion	7–13 seeds	3 h	Toxic delirium
Nutmeg and mace	Warm zones of Europe, Africa, Asia	Myristicin and aromatic ethers	Fruit of *M. fragrans,* commercial spices	Orally or as a snuff	1 teaspoon, 5–15 g	Unknown	Similar to atropinism, with seizures, death
Yopo/Cohoba	Northern South America, Argentina	β-carbolines and tryptamines	Beans of *Anadenanthera peregrina*	Smoked or as a snuff	Unknown	Unknown	Ataxia, hallucinations, seizures?
Bufotenin	Northern South America, Argentina	5-OH-dimethyltryptamine	Skin glands of toads; seeds of *A. peregrina*	As a snuff or IV	Unknown	15 min	None reported

Courtesy of Henry David Abraham, M.D.

ylamide (LSD), synthesized in 1938 by Albert Hoffman, who later accidentally ingested some of the drug and experienced the first LSD-induced hallucinogenic episode. Some researchers classify the substituted or so-called designer amphetamines, such as 3,4-*methylenedioxyamphetamine* (MDMA), as hallucinogens. However, because these drugs are structurally related to amphetamines, this textbook classifies them as amphetaminelike substances, and they are covered in Section 12.3. Table 12.7–1 lists some representative hallucinogens.

EPIDEMIOLOGY

According to the text revision of the fourth edition of *Diagnostic and Statistical Manual of Mental Disorders* (DSM-IV-TR), 10 percent of persons in the United States had used a hallucinogen at least once. Hallucinogen use is most common among young (15 to 35 years of age) white men. The ratio of whites to blacks who have used a hallucinogen is 2 to 1, the white to Hispanic ratio is about 1.5 to 1. Men represent 62 percent of those who have used a hallucinogen at some time and 75 percent of those who have used a hallucinogen in the preceding month. Persons 26 to 34 years of age show the highest use of hallucinogens, with 15.5 percent having used a hallucinogen at least once. Persons 18 to 25 years of age have the highest recent use of a hallucinogen.

Cultural factors influence the use of hallucinogens; their use in the western United States is significantly higher than in the southern United States. Hallucinogen use is associated with less morbidity and less mortality than that of some other substances. For

example, one study found that only 1 percent of substance-related emergency room visits were related to hallucinogens, compared with 40 percent for cocaine-related problems. Of persons visiting the emergency room for hallucinogen-related reasons, however, more than 50 percent were younger than 20 years of age. A resurgence in the popularity of hallucinogens has been reported. According to DSM-IV-TR, the lifetime rate of hallucinogen abuse is about 0.6 percent, with a 12-month prevalence of about 0.1%.

NEUROPHARMACOLOGY

Although most hallucinogenic substances vary in their pharmacological effects, LSD can serve as a hallucinogenic prototype. The pharmacodynamic effect of LSD remains controversial, although it is generally agreed that the drug acts on the serotonergic system, whether as an antagonist or as an agonist. Data at this time suggest that LSD acts as a partial agonist at postsynaptic serotonin receptors.

Most hallucinogens are well absorbed after oral ingestion, although some are ingested by inhalation, smoking, or intravenous injection. Tolerance for LSD and other hallucinogens develops rapidly and is virtually complete after 3 or 4 days of continuous use. Tolerance also reverses quickly, usually in 4 to 7 days. Neither physical dependence nor withdrawal symptoms occur with hallucinogens, but a user can develop a psychological dependence on the insight-inducing experiences of episodes of hallucinogen use.

DIAGNOSIS

DSM-IV-TR lists a number of hallucinogen-related disorders (Table 12.7–2) but contains specific diagnostic criteria only for hallucinogen intoxication (Table 12.7–3) and hallucinogen persisting perception disorder (flashbacks) (Table 12.7–4). The diagnostic criteria for the other hallucinogen use disorders are contained in the DSM-IV-TR sections that are specific to each symptom—for example, hallucinogen-induced mood disorder (see Table 15.3–10 in Section 15.3 of Chapter 15).

Table 12.7–2
DSM-IV-TR Hallucinogen-Related Disorders

Hallucinogen use disorders
Hallucinogen dependence
Hallucinogen abuse
Hallucinogen-induced disorders
Hallucinogen intoxication
Hallucinogen persisting perception disorder (flashbacks)
Hallucinogen intoxication delirium
Hallucinogen-induced psychotic disorder, with delusions
Specify if:
With onset during intoxication
Hallucinogen-induced psychotic disorder, with hallucinations
Specify if:
With onset during intoxication
Hallucinogen-induced mood disorder
Specify if:
With onset during intoxication
Hallucinogen-induced anxiety disorder
Specify if:
With onset during intoxication
Hallucinogen-related disorder not otherwise specified

From American Psychiatric Association. *Diagnostic and Statistical Manual of Mental Disorders.* 4th ed. Text rev. Washington, DC: American Psychiatric Association; copyright 2000, with permission.

Table 12.7–3
DSM-IV-TR Diagnostic Criteria for Hallucinogen Intoxication

A. Recent use of a hallucinogen.
B. Clinically significant maladaptive behavioral or psychological changes (e.g., marked anxiety or depression, ideas of reference, fear of losing one's mind, paranoid ideation, impaired judgment, or impaired social or occupational functioning) that developed during, or shortly after, hallucinogen use.
C. Perceptual changes occurring in a state of full wakefulness and alertness (e.g., subjective intensification of perceptions, depersonalization, derealization, illusions, hallucinations, synesthesias) that developed during, or shortly after, hallucinogen use.
D. Two (or more) of the following signs, developing during, or shortly after, hallucinogen use:
(1) pupillary dilation
(2) tachycardia
(3) sweating
(4) palpitations
(5) blurring of vision
(6) tremors
(7) incoordination
E. The symptoms are not due to a general medical condition and are not better accounted for by another mental disorder.

From American Psychiatric Association. *Diagnostic and Statistical Manual of Mental Disorders.* 4th ed. Text rev. Washington, DC: American Psychiatric Association; copyright 2000, with permission.

Table 12.7–4
DSM-IV-TR Diagnostic Criteria for Hallucinogen Persisting Perception Disorder (Flashbacks)

A. The reexperiencing, following cessation of use of a hallucinogen, of one or more of the perceptual symptoms that were experienced while intoxicated with the hallucinogen (e.g., geometric hallucinations, false perceptions of movement in the peripheral visual fields, flashes of color, intensified colors, trails of images of moving objects, positive afterimages, halos around objects, macropsia, and micropsia).
B. The symptoms in Criterion A cause clinically significant distress or impairment in social, occupational, or other important areas of functioning.
C. The symptoms are not due to a general medical condition (e.g., anatomical lesions and infections of the brain, visual epilepsies) and are not better accounted for by another mental disorder (e.g., delirium, dementia, schizophrenia) or hypnopompic hallucinations.

From American Psychiatric Association. *Diagnostic and Statistical Manual of Mental Disorders.* 4th ed. Text rev. Washington, DC: American Psychiatric Association; copyright 2000, with permission.

Hallucinogen Dependence and Hallucinogen Abuse

Long-term hallucinogen use is not common. As stated above, there is no physical addiction. Although psychological dependence occurs, it is rare, in part because each LSD experience is different and in part because there is no reliable euphoria. Nonetheless, hallucinogen dependence and hallucinogen abuse are genuine syndromes, defined by DSM-IV-TR criteria (see Tables 12.1–5, 12.1–6, and 12.1–7 in Section 12.1).

Hallucinogen Intoxication

Intoxication with hallucinogens is defined in DSM-IV-TR as characterized by maladaptive behavioral and perceptual changes and by certain physiological signs (Table 12.7–3). The differential diagnosis for hallucinogen intoxication includes anticholinergic and amphetamine intoxication and alcohol withdrawal. The preferred treatment for hallucinogen intoxication is talking down the patient; during this process, guides can reassure patients that the symptoms are drug induced, that they are not going crazy, and that the symptoms will resolve shortly. In the most severe cases, dopaminergic antagonists—for example, haloperidol (Haldol)—or benzodiazepines—for example, diazepam (Valium)—can be used for a limited time. Hallucinogen intoxication usually lacks a withdrawal syndrome.

Hallucinogen Persisting Perception Disorder

Long after ingesting a hallucinogen, a person can experience a flashback of hallucinogenic symptoms. This syndrome is diagnosed as hallucinogen persisting perception disorder (Table 12.7–4) in DSM-IV-TR. According to studies, from 15 to 80 percent of users of hallucinogens report having experienced flashbacks. The differential diagnosis for flashbacks includes migraine, seizures, visual system abnormalities, and posttraumatic stress disorder. The following can trigger a flashback: emotional stress; sensory deprivation, such as monotonous driving; or use of another psychoactive substance, such as alcohol or marijuana.

Flashbacks are spontaneous, transitory recurrences of the substance-induced experience. Most flashbacks are episodes of visual distortion, geometric hallucinations, hallucinations of sounds or voices, false perceptions of movement in peripheral fields, flashes of color, trails of images from moving objects, positive afterimages and halos, macropsia, micropsia, time expansion, physical symptoms, or relived intense emotion. The episodes usually last a few seconds to a few minutes but can sometimes last longer. Most often, even in the presence of distinct perceptual disturbances, the person has insight into the pathological nature of the disturbance. Suicidal behavior, major depressive disorder, and panic disorders are potential complications.

Hallucinogen Intoxication Delirium

DSM-IV-TR allows for the diagnosis of hallucinogen intoxication delirium (see Table 10.2–3), a relatively rare disorder beginning during intoxication in those who have ingested pure hallucinogens. Hallucinogens are often mixed with other substances, however, and the other components or their interactions with the hallucinogens can produce clinical delirium.

Hallucinogen-Induced Psychotic Disorders

If psychotic symptoms are present in the absence of retained reality testing, a diagnosis of hallucinogen-induced psychotic disorder may be warranted (see Table 14.4–7 in Section 14.4). DSM-IV-TR also allows clinicians to specify whether hallucinations or delusions are the prominent symptoms. The most common adverse effect of LSD and related substances is a "bad trip," an experience resembling the acute panic reaction to cannabis but sometimes more severe; a bad trip can occasionally produce true psychotic symptoms. The bad trip generally ends when the immediate effects of the hallucinogen wear off, but its course is variable. Occasionally, a protracted psychotic episode is difficult to distinguish from a nonorganic psychotic disorder. Whether a chronic psychosis after drug ingestion is the result of the drug ingestion, is unrelated to the drug ingestion, or is a combination of both the drug ingestion and predisposing factors is currently unanswerable.

Occasionally, the psychotic disorder is prolonged, a reaction thought to be most common in persons with preexisting schizoid personality disorder and prepsychotic personalities, an unstable ego balance, or much anxiety. Such persons cannot cope with the perceptual changes, body-image distortions, and symbolic unconscious material stimulated by the hallucinogen. The rate of previous mental instability in persons hospitalized for LSD reactions is high. Adverse reactions occurred in the late 1960s when LSD was being promoted as a self-prescribed psychotherapy for emotional crises in the lives of seriously disturbed persons. Now that this practice is less frequent, prolonged adverse reactions are less common.

A 22-year-old female photography student presented to the hospital with inappropriate mood and bizarre thinking. She had no prior psychiatric history. Nine days prior to admission she ingested one or two psilocybin mushrooms. Following the immediate ingestion, the patient began to giggle. She then described euphoria, which progressed to auditory hallucinations and belief in the ability to broadcast her thoughts on the media. Two days later she repeated the ingestion, and continued to exhibit psychotic symptoms to the day of admission. When examined she heard voices telling her she could be president, and reported the sounds of "lambs crying." She continued to giggle inappropriately, bizarrely turning her head from side to side ritualistically. She continued to describe euphoria, but with an intermittent sense of hopelessness in a context of thought blocking. Her self-description was "feeling lucky." She was given haloperidol, 10 mg twice a day, along with benztropine (Cogentin) 1 mg three times a day and lithium carbonate (Eskalith) 300 mg twice a day. On this regimen her psychosis abated after 5 days.

Hallucinogen-Induced Mood Disorder

DSM-IV-TR provides a diagnostic category for hallucinogen-induced mood disorder (see Table 15.3–10 in Section 15.3). Unlike cocaine-induced mood disorder and amphetamine-

induced mood disorder, in which the symptoms are somewhat predictable, mood disorder symptoms accompanying hallucinogen abuse can vary. Abusers may experience maniclike symptoms with grandiose delusions or depressionlike feelings and ideas or mixed symptoms. As with the hallucinogen-induced psychotic disorder symptoms, the symptoms of hallucinogen-induced mood disorder usually resolve once the drug has been eliminated from the person's body.

Hallucinogen-Induced Anxiety Disorder

Hallucinogen-induced anxiety disorder (see Table 16.7–3) also varies in its symptom pattern, but few data about symptom patterns are available. Anecdotally, emergency room physicians who treat patients with hallucinogen-related disorders frequently report panic disorder with agoraphobia.

A 20-year-old man had a 7-year history of polysubstance abuse, including having used LSD an estimated 400 times. While driving with his girlfriend he ingested an unknown quantity of LSD and became intoxicated; he reported using no other drugs at this time. Within minutes after ingestion, he began to experience visual hallucinations that intensified as he drove. When he attempted to speak to his girlfriend, he saw that she had become a giant lizard. He became terrified and attempted to kill her by crashing the car, injuring himself and his passenger. By the time of discharge from the hospital 3 days later, his panic had resolved.

Hallucinogen-Related Disorder Not Otherwise Specified

When a patient with a hallucinogen-related disorder does not meet the diagnostic criteria for any of the standard hallucinogen-related disorders, the patient may be classified as having hallucinogen-related disorder not otherwise specified (Table 12.7–5). DSM-IV-TR does not have a diagnostic category of hallucinogen withdrawal, but some clinicians anecdotally report a syndrome with depression and anxiety after cessation of frequent hallucinogen use. Such a syndrome may best fit the diagnosis of hallucinogen-related disorder not otherwise specified.

Table 12.7–5
DSM-IV-TR Diagnostic Criteria for Hallucinogen-Related Disorder Not Otherwise Specified

The hallucinogen-related disorder not otherwise specified category is for disorders associated with the use of hallucinogens that are not classifiable as hallucinogen dependence, hallucinogen abuse, hallucinogen intoxication, hallucinogen persisting perception disorder, hallucinogen intoxication delirium, hallucinogen-induced psychotic disorder, hallucinogen-induced mood disorder, or hallucinogen-induced anxiety disorder.

From American Psychiatric Association. *Diagnostic and Statistical Manual of Mental Disorders.* 4th ed. Text rev. Washington, DC: American Psychiatric Association; copyright 2000, with permission.

CLINICAL FEATURES

The onset of action of LSD occurs within an hour, peaks in 2 to 4 hours, and lasts 8 to 12 hours. The sympathomimetic effects of LSD include tremors, tachycardia, hypertension, hyperthermia, sweating, blurring of vision, and mydriasis. Death caused by cardiac or cerebrovascular pathology related to hypertension or hyperthermia can occur with hallucinogenic use. A syndrome similar to neuroleptic malignant syndrome has reportedly been associated with LSD. Death can also be caused by a physical injury when LSD use impairs judgment about, for example, traffic or a person's ability to fly. The psychological effects are usually well tolerated, but when persons cannot recall experiences or appreciate that the experiences are substance induced, they may fear the onset of insanity.

With hallucinogen use, perceptions become unusually brilliant and intense. Colors and textures seem to be richer than in the past, contours sharpened, music more emotionally profound, and smells and tastes heightened. Synesthesia is common; colors may be heard or sounds seen. Changes in body image and alterations of time and space perception also occur. Hallucinations are usually visual, often of geometric forms and figures, but auditory and tactile hallucinations are sometimes experienced. Emotions become unusually intense and may change abruptly and often; two seemingly incompatible feelings may be experienced at the same time. Suggestibility is greatly heightened, and sensitivity or detachment from other persons may arise. Other common features are a seeming awareness of internal organs, the recovery of lost early memories, the release of unconscious material in symbolic form, and regression and the apparent reliving of past events, including birth. Introspective reflection and feelings of religious and philosophical insight are common. The sense of self is greatly changed, sometimes to the point of depersonalization, merging with the external world, separation of self from body, or total dissolution of the ego in mystical ecstasy.

There is no clear evidence of drastic personality change or chronic psychosis produced by long-term LSD use by moderate users not otherwise predisposed to these conditions. Some heavy users of hallucinogens, however, may experience chronic anxiety or depression and may benefit from a psychological or pharmacological approach that addresses the underlying problem.

Many persons maintain that a single experience with LSD has given them increased creative capacity, new psychological insight, relief from neurotic or psychosomatic symptoms, or a desirable change in personality. In the 1950s and 1960s, psychiatrists showed great interest in LSD and related substances, both as potential models for functional psychosis and as possible pharmacotherapeutic agents. The availability of these compounds to researchers in the basic neurosciences has led to many scientific advances.

TREATMENT

Hallucinogen Intoxication

Persons have historically been treated for hallucinogen intoxication by psychological support for the remainder of the trip, so-called talking down. This is a time-consuming and potentially hazardous undertaking given the lability of a patient with

hallucinogen-related delusions. Accordingly, treatment of hallucinogen intoxication is the oral administration of 20 mg of diazepam. This medication brings the LSD experience and any associated panic to a halt within 20 minutes and should be considered superior to "talking down" the patient over a period of hours or to administering antipsychotic agents. The marketing of lower doses of LSD and a more sophisticated approach to treatment of casualties by drug users themselves have combined to reduce the appearance of this once-common disorder in psychiatric treatment facilities.

Hallucinogen Persisting Disorder

Treatment for hallucinogen persisting perception disorder is palliative. The first step in the process is correct identification of the disorder; it is not uncommon for the patient to consult a number of specialists before the diagnosis is made. Pharmacological approaches include long-lasting benzodiazepines such as clonazepam (Klonopin) and, to a lesser extent, anticonvulsants including valproic acid (Depakene) and carbamazepine (Tegretol). Currently, no drug is completely effective in ablating symptoms. Antipsychotic agents should only be used in the treatment of hallucinogen-induced psychoses, because they may have a paradoxical effect and exacerbate symptoms. A second dimension of treatment is behavioral. The patient must be instructed to avoid gratuitous stimulation in the form of over-the-counter drugs, caffeine, alcohol, and avoidable physical and emotional stressors. Marijuana smoke is a particularly strong intensifier of the disorder, even when passively inhaled. Finally, three comorbid conditions are associated with hallucinogen persisting perception disorder—panic disorder, major depression, and alcohol dependence. All these conditions require primary prevention and early intervention.

Hallucinogen-Induced Psychosis

Treatment of hallucinogen-induced psychosis does not differ from conventional treatment for other psychoses. However, in addition to antipsychotic medications, a number of agents are reportedly effective including lithium carbonate, carbamazepine, and electroconvulsive therapy. Antidepressant drugs, benzodiazepines, and anticonvulsant agents may each have a role in treatment as well. One hallmark of this disorder is that as opposed to schizophrenia, in which negative symptoms and poor interpersonal relatedness may commonly be found, patients with hallucinogen-induced psychosis exhibit the positive symptoms of hallucinations and delusions while retaining the ability to relate to the psychiatrist. Medical therapies are best applied in a context of supportive, educational, and family therapies. The goals of treatment are the control of symptoms, a minimal use of hospitals, daily work, the development and preservation of social relationships, and the management of comorbid illnesses such as alcohol dependence.

References

Abraham HD. Hallucinogen-related disorders. In: Sadock BJ, Sadock VA, eds. *Kaplan & Sadock's Comprehensive Textbook of Psychiatry.* 7th ed. Vol 1. Baltimore: Lippincott Williams & Wilkins; 2000:1015.

Behan WM, Bakheit AM, Behan PO, More IA. The muscle findings in the neuroleptic malignant syndrome associated with lysergic acid diethylamide. *J Neurol Neurosurg Psychiatry.* 1991;54:741.

Cousineau D, Savard M, Allard D. Illicit drug use among adolescent students. A peer phenomenon? *Can Fam Physician Med Fam Can.* 1993;39:523.

Dinges MM, Oetting ER. Similarity in drug use patterns between adolescents and their friends. *Adolescence.* 1993;28:253.

Glennon RA. Do classical hallucinogens act as 5-HT2 agonists or antagonists? *Neuropsychopharmacology.* 1990;3:509.

Johnston LD, O'Malley PM, Bachman JG. *Drug Abuse among American High School Seniors, College Students, and Young Adults, 1975–1990.* Washington, DC: Department of Health and Human Services; 1991.

Kulig K. LSD. *Emerg Med Clin North Am.* 1990;8:551.

Lerner AG, Skladman I, Kodesh A, Sigal M, Shufman E. LSD-induced hallucinogen persisting perception disorder treated with clonazepam: two case reports. *Isr J Psychiatry Relat Sci.* 2001;38:133.

National Institute on Drug Abuse. *National Household Survey on Drug Abuse: Highlights, 1991.* Washington, DC: US Government Printing Office, 1991.

Pierce PA, Peroutka SJ. Antagonist properties of *d*-LSD at 5-hydroxytryptamine 2 receptors. *Neuropsychopharmacology.* 1990;3:503.

Popik P, Layer RT, Skolnick P. 100 years of ibogaine: neurochemical and pharmacological actions of a putative anti-addictive drug. *Pharmacol Rev.* 1995;47:235.

Schwartz RH. LSD: its rise, fall, and renewed popularity among high school students. *Pediatr Clin North Am.* 1995;42:403.

Spoerke DG, Hall AH. Plants and mushrooms of abuse. *Emerg Med Clin North Am.* 1990;8:579.

Stephens RS. Cannabis and hallucinogens. In: McCrady BS, Epstein EE, eds. *Addictions: A Comprehensive Guidebook.* New York: Oxford University Press; 1999:121.

Substance Abuse and Mental Health Services Administration Office of Applied Studies. *Preliminary Estimates from the 1995 National Household Survey on Drug Abuse.* Washington, DC: US Government Printing Office; 1995.

Ulrich RF, Patten BM. The rise, decline, and fall of LSD. *Perspect Biol Med.* 1991;34:561.

▲ 12.8 Inhalant-Related Disorders

The category of inhalant-related disorders includes the psychiatric syndromes resulting from the use of solvents, glues, adhesives, aerosol propellants, paint thinners, and fuels. Among specific examples of these substances are gasoline, varnish remover, lighter fluid, airplane glue, rubber cement, cleaning fluid, spray paint, shoe conditioner, and typewriter correction fluid. A resurgence of inhalants' popularity among young persons has been reported. The active compounds in these inhalants include toluene, acetone, benzene, trichloroethane, perchloroethylene, trichloroethylene, 1,2-dichloropropane, and halogenated hydrocarbons.

The text revision of the fourth edition of *Diagnostic and Statistical Manual of Mental Disorders* (DSM-IV-TR) specifically excludes anesthetic gases (e.g., nitrous oxide and ether) and short-acting vasodilators (e.g., amyl nitrite) from the inhalant-related disorders, which are classified as other (or unknown) substance-related disorders and are discussed in Section 12.14.

EPIDEMIOLOGY

Inhalant substances are easily available, legal, and inexpensive. These three factors contribute to the high use of inhalants among poor persons and young persons. According to DSM-IV-TR, about 6 percent of persons in the United States had used inhalants at least once, and about 1 percent were current users. Among young adults 18 to 25 years old, 11 percent had used inhalants at least once, and 2 percent were current users. Among adolescents 12 to 17 years old, 7 percent had used

Table 12.8–1
DSM-IV-TR Inhalant-Related Disorders

Inhalant use disorders
- **Inhalant dependence**
- **Inhalant abuse**

Inhalant-induced disorders
- **Inhalant intoxication**
- **Inhalant intoxication delirium**
- **Inhalant-induced persisting dementia**
- **Inhalant-induced psychotic disorder, with delusions**
  - *Specify* if:
    - With onset during intoxication
- **Inhalant-induced psychotic disorder, with hallucinations**
  - *Specify* if:
    - With onset during intoxication
- **Inhalant-induced mood disorder**
  - *Specify* if:
    - With onset during intoxication
- **Inhalant-induced anxiety disorder**
  - *Specify* if:
    - With onset during intoxication
- **Inhalant-related disorder not otherwise specified**

From American Psychiatric Association. *Diagnostic and Statistical Manual of Mental Disorders.* 4th ed. Text rev. Washington, DC: American Psychiatric Association; copyright 2000, with permission.

inhalants at least once, and 2 percent were current users. In one study of high school seniors, 18 percent reported having used inhalants at least once, and 2.7 percent reported having used inhalants within the preceding month. White users of inhalants are more common than either black or Hispanic users. Most users (up to 80 percent) are male. Some data suggest that inhalant use may be more common in suburban communities in the United States than in urban communities.

Inhalant use accounts for 1 percent of all substance-related deaths and fewer than 0.5 percent of all substance-related emergency room visits. About 20 percent of the emergency room visits for inhalant use involve persons younger than 18 years of age. Inhalant use among adolescents may be most common in those whose parents or older siblings use illegal substances. Inhalant use among adolescents is also associated with an increased likelihood of conduct disorder or antisocial personality disorder.

NEUROPHARMACOLOGY

Persons usually use inhalants with a tube, a can, a plastic bag, or an inhalant-soaked rag, through or from which a user can sniff the inhalant through the nose or "huff" it through the mouth. Inhalants generally act as a central nervous system (CNS) depressant. Tolerance for inhalants can develop, although withdrawal symptoms are usually fairly mild and are not classified as a disorder in DSM-IV-TR.

Inhalants are rapidly absorbed through the lungs and rapidly delivered to the brain. The effects appear within 5 minutes and may last for 30 minutes to several hours, depending on the inhalant substance and the dose. For example, 15 to 20 breaths of a 1 percent solution of gasoline may result in a high of several hours. The concentrations of many inhalant substances in blood are increased when used in combination with alcohol, perhaps because of competition for hepatic enzymes. Although about one fifth of an inhalant substance is excreted unchanged by the lungs, the remainder is metabolized by the liver. Inhalants are detectable in the blood for 4 to 10 hours after use, and blood samples should be taken in the emergency room when inhalant use is suspected.

Much like alcohol, inhalants have specific pharmacodynamic effects that are not well understood. Because their effects are generally similar and additive to the effects of other CNS depressants (e.g., ethanol, barbiturates, and benzodiazepines), some investigators have suggested that inhalants operate by enhancing the γ-aminobutyric acid (GABA) system. Other investigators have suggested that inhalants work through membrane fluidization, which has also been hypothesized to be a pharmacodynamic effect of ethanol.

DIAGNOSIS

DSM-IV-TR lists a number of inhalant-related disorders (Table 12.8–1) but contains specific diagnostic criteria only for inhalant intoxication (Table 12.8–2) within the inhalant-related disorders section. The diagnostic criteria of other inhalant-related disorders are specified in the DSM-IV-TR sections that specifically address

Table 12.8–2
DSM-IV-TR Diagnostic Criteria for Inhalant Intoxication

A. Recent intentional use or short-term, high-dose exposure to volatile inhalants (excluding anesthetic gases and short-acting vasodilators).
B. Clinically significant maladaptive behavioral or psychological changes (e.g., belligerence, assaultiveness, apathy, impaired judgment, impaired social or occupational functioning) that developed during, or shortly after, use of or exposure to volatile inhalants.
C. Two (or more) of the following signs, developing during, or shortly after, inhalant use or exposure:
   (1) dizziness
   (2) nystagmus
   (3) incoordination
   (4) slurred speech
   (5) unsteady gait
   (6) lethargy
   (7) depressed reflexes
   (8) psychomotor retardation
   (9) tremor
   (10) generalized muscle weakness
   (11) blurred vision or diplopia
   (12) stupor or coma
   (13) euphoria
D. The symptoms are not due to a general medical condition and are not better accounted for by another mental disorder.

From American Psychiatric Association. *Diagnostic and Statistical Manual of Mental Disorders.* 4th ed. Text rev. Washington, DC: American Psychiatric Association; copyright 2000, with permission.

the major symptoms—for example, inhalant-induced psychotic disorders (see Table 14.4–7 in Section 14.4 of Chapter 14).

Inhalant Dependence and Inhalant Abuse

Most persons probably use inhalants for a short time without developing a pattern of long-term use resulting in dependence and abuse. Nonetheless, dependence and abuse of inhalants occur and are diagnosed according to the standard DSM-IV-TR criteria for those syndromes (see Tables 12.1–5, 12.1–6, and 12.1–7 in Section 12.1).

Inhalant Intoxication

The DSM-IV-TR diagnostic criteria for inhalant intoxication (Table 12.8–2) specify the presence of maladaptive behavioral changes and at least two physical symptoms. The intoxicated state is often characterized by apathy, diminished social and occupational functioning, impaired judgment, and impulsive or aggressive behavior, and it can be accompanied by nausea, anorexia, nystagmus, depressed reflexes, and diplopia. With high doses and long exposures, a user's neurological status can progress to stupor and unconsciousness, and a person may later be amnestic for the period of intoxication. Clinicians can sometimes identify a recent user of inhalants by rashes around the patient's nose and mouth; unusual breath odors; the residue of the inhalant substances on the patient's face, hands, or clothing; and irritation of the patient's eyes, throat, lungs, and nose.

A group home referred a 16-year-old single Hispanic female to a university substance-treatment program for evaluation and recommendations regarding inhalant problems. The patient had been ordered to the group home for auto theft, menacing with a weapon, and being out of control by her family. By age 15 she had regularly been using inhalants and drinking alcohol heavily. She had tried typewriter-erasing fluid, bleach, tile cleaner, hairspray, nail polish, glue, and gasoline, but preferred spray paint. She had huffed paint many times each day for about 6 months at age 15, using a maximum of eight paint cans per day. The patient said, "It blacks out everything." Sometimes she had lost consciousness, and she believed that the paint had impaired her memory and made her "dumb."

The patient reported sexual abuse by an older, nonparental male relative beginning at age 3 and continuing for many years. By fifth grade she had begun showing extensive conduct problems, eventually including fighting, truancy, multiple runaways, gang involvement, and bringing weapons to school. Her family reportedly permitted gang meetings in their home. The patient reported stabbing one person with a screwdriver, another with a knife, and beating another unconscious with a bat. She said that her violence was greatest when she was intoxicated. The patient listed her strengths and abilities as drawing, cooking, staying clean, fighting, and giving good tattoos. In formal testing her thinking seemed slow, and she had some difficulty understanding questions. Her intelligence quotient (IQ) scores were Verbal, 72; Performance, 87; and Full Scale, 77. She met diagnostic criteria for inhalant dependence, alcohol abuse, and conduct disorder.

The evaluating program recommended (1) individual and group substance treatment, emphasizing the adverse cognitive and health effects of huffing; (2) urine monitoring; (3) further neurological and neuropsychological assessment; (4) family evaluation and treatment addressing the patient's anger about sexual abuse and her rebelliousness; (5) specific attention in treatment to the patient's anger and aggression; (6) psychoeducation concerning contraception and protection from sexually transmitted diseases; and (7) active support for continued schooling, with consideration of placement in special education. The patient returned to the group home for several months, and it is unclear which of these recommendations were implemented. She then rejoined her parents in a distant community. One year after the evaluation the patient and two others died when their speeding car hit a tree. An investigating officer said, "it appears that all of them had been sniffing or huffing paint." (Courtesy of Thomas J. Crowley, M.D.)

Inhalant Intoxication Delirium

DSM-IV-TR provides a diagnostic category for inhalant intoxication delirium (see Table 10.2–3 in Section 10.2). Delirium can be induced by the effects of the inhalants themselves, by pharmacodynamic interactions with other substances, and by the hypoxia that may be associated with either the inhalant or its method of inhalation. If the delirium results in severe behavioral disturbances, short-term treatment with a dopamine receptor antagonist, such as haloperidol (Haldol), may be necessary. Benzodiazepines should be avoided because of the possibility of increasing the patient's respiratory depression.

Inhalant-Induced Persisting Dementia

Inhalant-induced persisting dementia (see Table 10.3–6 in Section 10.3), like delirium, may be due to the neurotoxic effects of the inhalants themselves; the neurotoxic effects of the metals (e.g., lead) commonly used in inhalants; or the effects of frequent and prolonged periods of hypoxia. The dementia caused by inhalants is likely to be irreversible in all but the mildest cases.

Inhalant-Induced Psychotic Disorder

Inhalant-induced psychotic disorder is a DSM-IV-TR diagnosis (see Table 14.4–7 in Section 14.4). Clinicians can specify hallucinations or delusions as the predominant symptoms. Paranoid states are probably the most common psychotic syndromes during inhalant intoxication.

Inhalant-Induced Mood Disorder and Inhalant-Induced Anxiety Disorder

Inhalant-induced mood disorder (see Table 15.3–10 in Section 15.3) and inhalant-induced anxiety disorder (see Table 16.7–3 in Section 16.7) are DSM-IV-TR diagnoses that allow the classification of inhalant-related disorders characterized by prominent mood and anxiety symptoms. Depressive disorders are the most common mood disorders associated with inhalant use, and

Table 12.8–3
DSM-IV-TR Diagnostic Criteria for Inhalant-Related Disorder Not Otherwise Specified

The inhalant-related disorder not otherwise specified category is for disorders associated with the use of inhalants that are not classifiable as inhalant dependence, inhalant abuse, inhalant intoxication, inhalant intoxication delirium, inhalant-induced persisting dementia, inhalant-induced psychotic disorder, inhalant-induced mood disorder, or inhalant-induced anxiety disorder.

From American Psychiatric Association. *Diagnostic and Statistical Manual of Mental Disorders.* 4th ed. Text rev. Washington, DC: American Psychiatric Association; copyright 2000, with permission.

panic disorders and generalized anxiety disorder are the most common anxiety disorders.

Inhalant-Related Disorder Not Otherwise Specified

Inhalant-related disorder not otherwise specified is the recommended DSM-IV-TR diagnosis for inhalant-related disorders that do not fit into one of the diagnostic categories discussed above (Table 12.8–3).

CLINICAL FEATURES

In small initial doses, inhalants may be disinhibiting and may produce feelings of euphoria and excitement and pleasant floating sensations, the effects for which persons presumably use the drugs. High doses of inhalants can cause psychological symptoms of fearfulness, sensory illusions, auditory and visual hallucinations, and distortions of body size. The neurological symptoms can include slurred speech, decreased speed of talking, and ataxia. Long-term use can be associated with irritability, emotional lability, and impaired memory.

Tolerance for the inhalants does develop; although not recognized by DSM-IV-TR, a withdrawal syndrome can accompany the cessation of inhalant use. The withdrawal syndrome does not occur frequently; when it does, it can be characterized by sleep disturbances, irritability, jitteriness, sweating, nausea, vomiting, tachycardia, and (sometimes) delusions and hallucinations.

Adverse Effects

Inhalants are associated with many potentially serious adverse effects. Death can result from respiratory depression, cardiac arrhythmias, asphyxiation, aspiration of vomitus, or accident or injury (e.g., driving while intoxicated with inhalants). Other serious adverse effects of long-term inhalant use include irreversible hepatic or renal damage and permanent muscle damage associated with rhabdomyolysis. The combination of organic solvents and high concentrations of copper, zinc, and heavy metals has been associated with the development of brain atrophy, temporal lobe epilepsy, decreased IQ, and electroencephalogram (EEG) changes. Several studies of house painters and factory workers who have been exposed to solvents for long periods have shown evidence of brain atrophy on computed tomography (CT) scans and of decreases in cerebral blood flow. Additional adverse effects include cardiovascular and pulmonary symptoms (e.g., chest pain and bronchospasm), gastrointestinal symptoms (e.g., pain, nausea, vomiting, and hematemesis), and other neurological signs and symptoms (e.g., peripheral neuritis, headache, paresthesia, cerebellar signs, and lead encephalopathy). There are reports of brain atrophy, renal tubular acidosis, and long-term motor impairment in toluene users. Several reports concern serious adverse effects on fetal development when a pregnant woman uses or is exposed to inhalant substances.

TREATMENT

Inhalant intoxication, like alcohol intoxication, usually requires no medical attention and resolves spontaneously. However, effects of the intoxication, such as coma, bronchospasm, laryngospasm, cardiac arrhythmias, trauma, or burns, need treatment. Otherwise, care primarily involves reassurance, quiet support, and attention to vital signs and level of consciousness.

No established treatment exists for the cognitive and memory problems of inhalant-induced persisting dementia. Street outreach and extensive social service support have been offered to severely deteriorated, inhalant-dependent, homeless adults. Patients may require extensive support within their families or in foster or domiciliary care.

The course and treatment of inhalant-induced psychotic disorder are like those of inhalant intoxication. The disorder is brief, lasting a few hours to (at most) a very few weeks beyond the intoxication. Vigorous treatment of such life-threatening complications as respiratory or cardiac arrest, together with conservative management of the intoxication itself, is appropriate. Confusion, panic, and psychosis mandate special attention to patient safety. Severe agitation may require cautious control with haloperidol (5 mg intramuscularly per 70 kg body weight). Sedative drugs should be avoided as they may aggravate the psychosis. Inhalant-induced anxiety and mood disorders may precipitate suicidal ideation, and patients should be carefully evaluated for that possibility. Antianxiety and antidepressants are not useful in the acute phase of the disorder; they may be of use if there is a coexisting anxiety or depressive illness.

References

Brouette T, Anton R. Clinical review of inhalants. *Am J Addict.* 2001;10:79.
Crowley TJ. Inhalant-related disorders. In: Sadock BJ, Sadock VA, eds. *Kaplan & Sadock's Comprehensive Textbook of Psychiatry.* 7th ed. Vol 1. Baltimore: Lippincott Williams & Wilkins; 2000:982.
Dinwiddie SH, Reich T, Cloninger CR. The relationship of solvent use to other substance use. *Am J Drug Alcohol Abuse.* 1991;17:173.
Donnelly N, Oldenburg B, Quine S, et al. Changes in reported drug prevalence among New South Wales secondary school students, 1983–1989. *Aust J Public Health.* 1992;16:50.
Espeland K. Identifying the manifestations of inhalant abuse. *Nurs Pract.* 1995;20:49.
Espeland K. Inhalant abuse: assessment guidelines. *J Psychosoc Nurs Ment Health Serv.* 1993;31:11.
Keriotis AA, Upadhyaya HP. Inhalant dependence and withdrawal symptoms. *J Am Acad Child Adolesc Psychiatry.* 2000;39:679.
Lindren CH. Volatile substances of abuse. *Emerg Med Clin North Am.* 1990;8:559.
Miller NS, Gold MS. Organic solvent and aerosol abuse. *Am Fam Physician.* 1991;44:183.
Pollard TG. Relative addiction potential of major centrally-active drugs and drug classes: inhalants and anesthetics. *Adv Alcohol Subst Abuse.* 1990;9:149.
Substance Abuse and Mental Health Services Administration Office of Applied Studies. *Preliminary Estimates from the 1995 National Household Survey on Drug Abuse.* Washington, DC: US Government Printing Office; 1995.

Tenenbein M, Pillay N. Sensory evoked potentials in inhalant (volatile solvent) abuse. *J Pediatr Child Health*. 1993;29:206.

▲ 12.9 Nicotine-Related Disorders

The landmark 1988 publication called *The Surgeon General's Report on the Health Consequences of Smoking: Nicotine Addiction* increased the awareness of the hazards of smoking to the American public. But the fact that about 30 percent continue to smoke despite the mountain of data showing how dangerous the habit is to their health is testament to the powerfully addictive properties of nicotine. The ill effects of cigarette and cigar smoking are reflected in the estimate that 60 percent of the direct health care costs in the United States go to treat tobacco-related illnesses and amount to an estimated $1 billion a day.

EPIDEMIOLOGY

The World Health Organization (WHO) estimates there are 1 billion smokers worldwide, and they smoke 6 trillion cigarettes a year. The WHO also estimates that tobacco kills more than 3 million persons each year. Although the number of persons in the United States who smoke is decreasing, the number of persons smoking in developing countries is increasing. The rate of quitting smoking has been highest among well-educated white men and lowest among women, blacks, teenagers, and those with low levels of education.

Tobacco is the most common form of nicotine. It is smoked in cigarettes, cigars, and pipes and used as snuff and chewing tobacco (also called smokeless tobacco), both of which are increasingly popular in the United States. About 3 percent of all persons in the United States currently use snuff or chewing tobacco, but about 6 percent of young adults ages 18 to 25 use those forms of tobacco.

Currently, about 25 percent of Americans smoke, 25 percent are former smokers, and 50 percent have never smoked cigarettes. The prevalence of pipe, cigar, and smokeless tobacco use is less than 2 percent. The prevalence of smoking in the United States was decreasing about 1 percent a year, but it has not changed in the last 4 years. The mean age of onset of smoking is 16, and few persons start after 20. Dependence features appear to develop quickly. Classroom and other programs to prevent initiation are only mildly effective, but increased taxation does decrease initiation.

Over 75 percent of smokers have tried to quit, and about 40 percent try to quit each year. On a given attempt, only 30 percent remain abstinent for even 2 days, and only 5 to 10 percent stop permanently. However, most smokers make 5 to 10 attempts, so eventually 50 percent of "ever smokers" quit. In the past, 90 percent of successful attempts to quit involved no treatment. However, with the advent of over-the-counter (OTC) and nonnicotine medications in 1998, about one third of all attempts involved the use of medication.

In terms of the diagnosis of nicotine dependence per se, about 20 percent of the population develops nicotine dependence at some point, making it the most prevalent psychiatric disorder. According to the text revision of the fourth edition of *Diagnostic and Statistical Manual of Mental Disorders* (DSM-IV-TR), approximately 85 percent of current daily smokers are nicotine dependent. Nicotine withdrawal occurs in about 50 percent of smokers who try to quit.

Smoking is now as common in women as in men. Smoking is more prevalent in those with lower education and income and in most minority ethnic groups. According to the CDC, there are regional differences in smoking throughout the United States. The cigarette smoking prevalence by region varied by about a factor of two. The 12 areas with the highest prevalence of current smoking (Kentucky, Nevada, Missouri, Indiana, Ohio, West Virginia, North Carolina, Tennessee, New Hampshire, Alabama, Arkansas, and Alaska) differed significantly from the 12 areas with lowest prevalence (Utah, Puerto Rico, California, Arizona, Montana, Hawaii, Minnesota, Connecticut, Massachusetts, Colorado, Maryland, and Washington). The median smoking prevalence among men was 24.4 percent (range, 14.5 to 33.3 percent) and among women, 21.2 percent (range, 9.9 to 29.5 percent). Utah had the lowest prevalence for men (14.5 percent), and Puerto Rico had the lowest for women (9.9 percent).

Education

Level of education attainment correlated with tobacco usage. Thirty-seven percent of adults who had not completed high school smoked cigarettes, whereas only 17 percent of college graduates smoked.

Psychiatric Patients

Psychiatrists must be particularly concerned and knowledgeable about nicotine dependence because of the high proportion of psychiatric patients who smoke. Approximately 50 percent of all psychiatric outpatients, 70 percent of outpatients with bipolar I disorder, almost 90 percent of outpatients with schizophrenia, and 70 percent of substance use disorder patients smoke. Moreover, data indicate that patients with depressive disorders or anxiety disorders are less successful in their attempts to quit smoking than other persons; thus, a holistic health approach for these patients probably includes helping them address their smoking habits in addition to the primary mental disorder. The high percentage of schizophrenic patients who smoke has been attributed to the ability of nicotine to reduce their extraordinary sensitivity to outside sensory stimuli and to increase their concentration.

Death

Death is the primary adverse effect of cigarette smoking. Tobacco use is associated with approximately 400,000 premature deaths each year in the United States—25 percent of all deaths. The causes of death include chronic bronchitis and emphysema (51,000 deaths), bronchogenic cancer (106,000 deaths), 35 percent of fatal myocardial infarctions (115,000 deaths), cerebrovascular disease, cardiovascular disease, and almost all cases of chronic obstructive pulmonary disease and lung cancer. The increased use of chewing tobacco and snuff (smokeless tobacco) has been associated with the development of oropharyngeal cancer, and the resurgence of cigar smoking is likely to lead to an increase in the occurrence of this type of cancer.

Researchers have found that 30 percent of U.S. cancer deaths are caused by tobacco smoke, the single most lethal carcinogen in the United States. Smoking (mainly cigarette smoking) causes cancer of the lung, upper respiratory tract, esophagus, bladder, and pancreas and probably of the stomach, liver, and kidney. Smokers are eight times more likely than nonsmokers to develop lung cancer, and lung cancer has surpassed breast cancer as the leading cause of cancer-related deaths in women. Even second-hand smoke (discussed below) causes a few thousand cancer deaths each year in the United States, about the same number as are caused by radon exposure. Despite these staggering statistics, smokers can dramatically lower their chances of developing smoke-related cancers simply by quitting.

NEUROPHARMACOLOGY

The psychoactive component of tobacco is nicotine, which affects the central nervous system (CNS) by acting as an agonist at the nicotinic subtype of acetylcholine receptors. About 25 percent of the nicotine inhaled during smoking reaches the bloodstream, through which nicotine reaches the brain within 15 seconds. The half-life of nicotine is about 2 hours. Nicotine is believed to produce its positive reinforcing and addictive properties by activating the dopaminergic pathway projecting from the ventral tegmental area to the cerebral cortex and the limbic system. In addition to activating this dopamine reward system, nicotine causes an increase in the concentrations of circulating norepinephrine and epinephrine and an increase in the release of vasopressin, β-endorphin, adrenocorticotropic hormone (ACTH), and cortisol. These hormones are thought to contribute to the basic stimulatory effects of nicotine on the CNS.

DIAGNOSIS

DSM-IV-TR lists three nicotine-related disorders (Table 12.9–1) but contains specific diagnostic criteria for only nicotine withdrawal (Table 12.9–2) in the nicotine-related disorders section. The other nicotine-related disorders recognized by DSM-IV-TR are nicotine dependence and nicotine-related disorder not otherwise specified.

Nicotine Dependence

DSM-IV-TR allows for the diagnosis of nicotine dependence (see Tables 12.1–6 and 12.1–7 in Section 12.1 of this chapter) but not nicotine abuse. Dependence on nicotine develops quickly, probably because nicotine activates the ventral tegmental area dopaminergic system, the same system affected by cocaine and amphetamine. The development of dependence is enhanced by strong social factors that encourage smoking in some settings and by the powerful effects of tobacco company advertising. Persons are likely to smoke if their parents or siblings smoke and serve as role models. Several recent studies have also suggested a genetic diathesis toward nicotine dependence. Most persons who smoke want to quit and have tried many times to quit but have been unsuccessful.

Table 12.9–1
DSM-IV-TR Nicotine-Related Disorders

Nicotine use disorder
Nicotine dependence
Nicotine-induced disorder
Nicotine withdrawal
Nicotine-related disorder not otherwise specified

From American Psychiatric Association. *Diagnostic and Statistical Manual of Mental Disorders.* 4th ed. Text rev. Washington, DC: American Psychiatric Association; copyright 2000, with permission.

Table 12.9–2
DSM-IV-TR Diagnostic Criteria for Nicotine Withdrawal

A. Daily use of nicotine for at least several weeks.
B. Abrupt cessation of nicotine use, or reduction in the amount of nicotine used, followed within 24 hours by four (or more) of the following signs:
 (1) dysphoric or depressed mood
 (2) insomnia
 (3) irritability, frustration, or anger
 (4) anxiety
 (5) difficulty concentrating
 (6) restlessness
 (7) decreased heart rate
 (8) increased appetite or weight gain
C. The symptoms in Criterion B cause clinically significant distress or impairment in social, occupational, or other important areas of functioning.
D. The symptoms are not due to a general medical condition and are not better accounted for by another mental disorder.

From American Psychiatric Association. *Diagnostic and Statistical Manual of Mental Disorders.* 4th ed. Text rev. Washington, DC: American Psychiatric Association; copyright 2000, with permission.

Nicotine Withdrawal

DSM-IV-TR does not have a diagnostic category for nicotine intoxication but does have a diagnostic category for nicotine withdrawal (Table 12.9–2). Withdrawal symptoms can develop within 2 hours of smoking the last cigarette, generally peak in the first 24 to 48 hours, and can last for weeks or months. The common symptoms include an intense craving for nicotine, tension, irritability, difficulty concentrating, drowsiness and paradoxical trouble sleeping, decreased heart rate and blood pressure, increased appetite and weight gain, decreased motor performance, and increased muscle tension. A mild syndrome of nicotine withdrawal can appear when a smoker switches from regular to low-nicotine cigarettes.

Nicotine-Related Disorder Not Otherwise Specified

Nicotine-related disorder not otherwise specified is a diagnostic category for nicotine-related disorders that do not fit into one of the categories discussed above (Table 12.9–3). Such diagnoses may include nicotine intoxication, nicotine abuse, and mood disorders and anxiety disorders associated with nicotine use.

Table 12.9–3
DSM-IV-TR Diagnostic Criteria for Nicotine-Related Disorder Not Otherwise Specified

The nicotine-related disorder not otherwise specified category is for disorders associated with the use of nicotine that are not classifiable as nicotine dependence or nicotine withdrawal.

Table 12.9–4
Typical Quit Rates of Common Therapies

Therapy	Rate (%)
Self-quit	5
Self-help books	10
Physician advice	10
Over-the-counter patch or gum	15
Medication plus advice	20
Behavior therapy alone	20
Medication plus group therapy	30

CLINICAL FEATURES

Behaviorally, the stimulatory effects of nicotine produce improved attention, learning, reaction time, and problem-solving ability. Tobacco users also report that cigarette smoking lifts their mood, decreases tension, and lessens depressive feelings. Results of studies of the effects of nicotine on cerebral blood flow (CBF) suggest that short-term nicotine exposure increases CBF without changing cerebral oxygen metabolism, but long-term nicotine exposure decreases CBF. In contrast to its stimulatory CNS effects, nicotine acts as a skeletal muscle relaxant.

Adverse Effects

Nicotine is a highly toxic alkaloid. Doses of 60 mg in an adult are fatal secondary to respiratory paralysis; doses of 0.5 mg are delivered by smoking an average cigarette. In low doses the signs and symptoms of nicotine toxicity include nausea, vomiting, salivation, pallor (caused by peripheral vasoconstriction), weakness, abdominal pain (caused by increased peristalsis), diarrhea, dizziness, headache, increased blood pressure, tachycardia, tremor, and cold sweats. Toxicity is also associated with an inability to concentrate, confusion, and sensory disturbances. Nicotine is further associated with a decrease in the user's amount of rapid eye movement (REM) sleep. Tobacco use during pregnancy has been associated with an increased incidence of low-birth-weight babies and an increased incidence of newborns with persistent pulmonary hypertension.

Health Benefits of Smoking Cessation

Smoking cessation has major and immediate health benefits for persons of all ages and provides benefits for persons with and without smoking-related diseases. Former smokers live longer than those who continue to smoke. Smoking cessation decreases the risk for lung cancer and other cancers, myocardial infarction, cerebrovascular diseases, and chronic lung diseases. Women who stop smoking before pregnancy or during the first 3 to 4 months of pregnancy reduce their risk for having low-birth-weight infants to that of women who never smoked. The health benefits of smoking cessation substantially exceed any risks from the average 5-pound (2.3 kg) weight gain or any adverse psychological effects after quitting.

TREATMENT

Psychiatrists should advise all patients who are not in crisis to quit smoking. For patients who are ready to stop smoking, it is best to set a "quit date." Most clinicians and smokers prefer abrupt cessation, but because there are no good data to indicate that abrupt cessation is better than gradual cessation, patient preference for gradual cessation should be respected. Brief advice should focus on the need for medication or group therapy, weight gain concerns, high-risk situations, making cigarettes unavailable, and so forth. Because relapse is often rapid, the first follow-up phone call or visit should be 2 to 3 days after the quit date. These strategies have been shown to double self-initiated quit rates (Table 12.9–4).

Ms. H. was a 55-year-old patient with schizophrenia who smoked 35 cigarettes a day and smoked each cigarette intensely. She began her cigarette use at about the age of 20, during the prodromal stages of her first psychotic break. Over the next 35 years she had several psychotic breaks and was treated with conventional antipsychotic agents. During the first 30 years of treatment, no psychiatrist or physician advised her to stop smoking, largely because they believed she could not stop.

At age 53 she was diagnosed with diabetes and early ischemic heart disease. At that time her primary care physician recommended smoking cessation. The patient attempted to stop on her own but lasted only 48 hours, partly because her housemates and friends smoked. After a second failure on her own, she became discouraged and concluded that she could not stop smoking. During a routine medication check, her psychiatrist recommended that she stop smoking and the patient described her prior attempts. The psychiatrist and the patient discussed ways to avoid smokers and had the patient announce her intent to quit and request that her friends try not to smoke around her and offer encouragement for her attempt to quit. The psychiatrist also noted that she had become irritable, slightly depressed, and restless and suffered insomnia during prior cessation attempts and thus recommended medications, using the American Psychiatric Association (APA) brochure *Treatment Works* to help the patient decide which medication was best for her. She chose a nicotine patch.

The psychiatrist had the patient call 2 days after her attempt to quit. At this point the patient stated that the patch and gum were helping, but she still felt left out when her friends smoked and talked. One week later the patient returned after having relapsed back to smoking. The psychiatrist praised

the patient for not smoking for 4 days. He suggested that she contact him again if she wished to try to stop again. Seven months later, during another medication check the psychiatrist again asked the patient to consider cessation, but she was reluctant.

Two months later the patient called and said she wished to try again. She met with the psychiatrist and this time they listed several activities she could do to avoid being around friends who smoked, phoned the patient's boyfriend to ask him to assist her in stopping, asked the nurses on the inpatient ward to call the patient to encourage her, and decided to enroll her in a support group for the next 4 weeks. The nicotine patch was used again, but this time, the nonnicotine medication bupropion (Zyban) was added. The patient was followed with 15-minute visits for each of the first 3 weeks and two phone calls thereafter. She had two slips when she became angry with her boyfriend but did not go back to smoking and remained an exsmoker. An unexpected result of her successful cessation was an improved therapeutic alliance between the patient and her psychiatrist.

DISCUSSION

Most psychiatrists fail to diagnose and treat nicotine dependence. Unfortunately, sometimes psychiatrists find that although they have adequately treated the disorder that brought the patient into treatment, the patient has such morbidity or mortality from smoking that he or she cannot reap the benefits of psychiatric treatment. Ms. H.'s psychiatrist was correct in using pragmatic plans to help the patient overcome specific problems, in following the patient with short visits or phone calls, and in recommending nicotine replacement. The total amount of time spent with the patient on smoking was about 3 hours. Although this was not reimbursed, the psychiatrist knew that his intervention was an important contribution to the patient's health and was unlikely to be given by other care providers.

Psychosocial Therapies

Behavior therapy is the most widely accepted and well-proved psychological therapy for smoking. Behavior therapy consists of several techniques, three of which are supported by good evidence. Skills training and relapse prevention identify high-risk situations and plan and practice behavioral or cognitive coping skills for these situations. Stimulus control involves eliminating cues for smoking in the environment. Rapid smoking has smokers smoke repeatedly to the point of nausea in sessions to associate smoking with unpleasant, rather than pleasant, sensations. This last therapy appears to be effective but requires a good therapeutic alliance and patient compliance.

Psychopharmacological Therapies

Nicotine Replacement Therapies. All nicotine replacement therapies double cessation rates, presumably because they reduce nicotine withdrawal. These therapies can also be used to reduce withdrawal in patients on smoke-free wards. Replacement therapies use a short period of maintenance (6 to 12 weeks) often followed by a gradual reduction period (6 to 12 weeks).

Nicotine gum (Nicorette) is an OTC product that releases nicotine via chewing and buccal absorption. A 2-mg variety for those who smoke fewer than 25 cigarettes a day and a 4-mg variety for those who smoke more than 25 cigarettes a day are available. Smokers are to use one to two pieces of gum per hour after abrupt cessation. Venous blood concentrations from the gum are one third to one half the between-cigarette levels. Acidic beverages (coffee, tea, soda, and juice) should not be used before, during, or after gum use because they decrease absorption. Compliance with the gum has often been a problem. Adverse effects are minor and include bad taste and sore jaws. About 20 percent of those who quit use the gum for long periods, but 2 percent use gum for longer than a year; long-term use does not appear to be harmful. The major advantage of nicotine gum is its ability to provide relief in high-risk situations.

Nicotine patches, also sold OTC are available in a 16-hour no-taper preparation (Habitrol) and a 24- or 16-hour tapering preparation (Nicoderm CQ). Patches are administered each morning and produce blood concentrations about half those of smoking. Compliance is high, and the only major adverse effects are rashes and, with 24-hour wear, insomnia. Long-term use does not occur. Using gum and patches in high-risk situations increases quit rates by another 5 to 10 percent. No studies have been done to determine the relative efficacies of 24- or 16-hour patches or of taper and no-taper patches.

Nicotine nasal spray (Nicotrol), available only by prescription, produces nicotine concentrations in the blood that are more similar to those from smoking a cigarette, and it appears to be especially helpful for heavily dependent smokers. However, the spray causes rhinitis, watering eyes, and coughing in over 70 percent of patients. Although initial data suggested abuse liability, further trials have not found this.

The nicotine inhaler, a prescription product, was designed to deliver nicotine to the lungs, but the nicotine is actually absorbed in the upper throat. Resultant nicotine levels are low. The major asset of the inhaler is that it provides a behavioral substitute for smoking. The inhaler also doubles quit rates. These devices require frequent puffing, which can cause minor adverse effects.

Nonnicotine Medications. Nonnicotine therapy may help smokers who object philosophically to the notion of replacement therapy and smokers who fail replacement therapy. Bupropion (Zyban) (marketed as Wellbutrin for depression) is an antidepressant medication that has both dopaminergic and adrenergic actions. Daily dosages of 300 mg reliably double quit rates in smokers with and without a history of depression. In one study, combined bupropion and nicotine patch had higher quit rates than either alone. Adverse effects include insomnia and nausea, but these are rarely significant. Seizures have not occurred in smoking trials. Interestingly, nortriptyline (Pamelor) appears to be effective for smoking cessation.

Clonidine (Catapres) decreases sympathetic activity from the locus ceruleus and thus is thought to abate withdrawal symptoms. Whether given as a patch or orally, 0.2 to 0.4 mg a day of clonidine appears to double quit rates; however, the scientific database for the efficacy of clonidine is neither as extensive nor as reliable as that for nicotine replacement; also,

clonidine can cause drowsiness and hypotension. Some patients benefit from benzodiazepine therapy (10 to 30 mg per day) for the first 2 to 3 weeks of abstinence.

A nicotine vaccine that produces nicotine-specific antibodies in the brain is under investigation at the National Institute on Drug Abuse (NIDA).

Combined Psychosocial and Pharmacological Therapy

Several studies have shown that combining nicotine replacement and behavior therapy increases quit rates over either therapy alone (Table 12.12–4).

Smoke-Free Environment

Secondhand smoke may contribute to lung cancer death and coronary heart disease in adult nonsmokers. Each year, an estimated 3,000 lung cancer deaths and 62,000 deaths from coronary heart disease in adult nonsmokers are attributed to secondhand smoke. Among children, secondhand smoke is implicated in sudden infant death syndrome, low birth weight, chronic middle ear infections, and respiratory illnesses (e.g., asthma, bronchitis, and pneumonia). Two national health objectives for 2010 are to reduce cigarette smoking among adults to 12 percent and the proportion of nonsmokers exposed to environment tobacco smoke to 45 percent.

Involuntary exposure to secondhand smoke remains a common public health hazard that is preventable by appropriate regulatory policies. Bans on smoking in public places reduce exposure to secondhand smoke and the number of cigarettes smoked by smokers. There is nearly universal support for bans in schools and day-care centers and strong support for bans in indoor work areas and restaurants. Clean indoor air policies are one way to change social norms about smoking and reduce tobacco consumption.

References

Bolliger CT, Zellweger J-P, Danielsson T, et al. Smoking reduction with oral nicotine inhalers: double blind, randomised clinical trial of efficacy and safety. *BMJ.* 2000;321:329.

Brautbar N. Direct effects of nicotine on the brain: evidence for chemical addiction. *Arch Environ Health.* 1995;50:263.

Centers for Disease Control and Prevention. Prevalence of current cigarette smoking. *JAMA.* 2002;287:309.

Fiore MC. Trends in cigarette smoking in the United States: the epidemiology of tobacco use. *Med Clin North Am.* 1992;76:289.

Ginsberg D, Hall SM, Rosinski M. Partner support, psychological treatment, and nicotine gum in smoking treatment: an incremental study. *Int J Addict.* 1992;27:503.

Hughes JR. Nicotine-related disorders. In: Sadock BJ, Sadock VA, eds. *Kaplan & Sadock's Comprehensive Textbook of Psychiatry.* 7th ed. Vol 1. Baltimore: Lippincott Williams & Wilkins; 2000:1033.

Kessler DA. Nicotine addiction in young people. *N Engl J Med.* 1995;333:186.

Miller GH, Golish JA, Cox CE. A physician's guide to smoking cessation. *J Fam Pract.* 1992;34:759.

Newhouse PA, Hughes JR. The role of nicotine and nicotinic mechanisms in neuropsychiatric disease. *Br J Addict.* 1991;86:521.

Pettegrew JW, Panchalingam K, McClure RJ, Levine J. Brain metabolic effects of acute nicotine. *Neurochem Res.* 2001;26:181.

Rigotti NA. Treatment of tobacco use and dependence. *N Engl J Med.* 2002;346:506.

Russell MA, Stapleton JA, Feyerabend C, et al. Targeting heavy smokers in general practice: randomised controlled trial of transdermal nicotine patches. *Br Med J.* 1993;306:1308.

Schelling TC. Addictive drugs: the cigarette experience. *Science.* 1992;255:430.

Srivastava ED, Russell MA, Feyerabend C, Masterson JG, Rhodes J. Sensitivity and tolerance to nicotine in smokers and nonsmokers. *Psychopharmacology.* 1991;105:63.

Stolerman IP, Shoaib M. The neurobiology of tobacco addiction. *Trends Pharmacol Sci.* 1991;12:467.

Substance Abuse and Mental Health Services Administration Office of Applied Studies. *Preliminary Estimates from the 1995 National Household Survey on Drug Abuse.* Washington, DC: US Government Printing Office; 1995.

Vaughan DA. Frontiers in pharmacologic treatment of alcohol, cocaine, and nicotine dependence. *Psychiatr Ann.* 1990;20:695.

▲ 12.10 Opioid-Related Disorders

Opioids have been used for at least 3,500 years, mostly in the form of crude opium or in alcoholic solutions of opium. Morphine was first isolated in 1806 and codeine in 1832. Over the next century, pure morphine and codeine gradually replaced crude opium for medicinal purposes, although nonmedical use of opium (as for smoking) still persists in some parts of the world.

Throughout the world, more than 20 chemically distinct opioid drugs are in clinical use. In the developed countries, the opioid drug most frequently associated with abuse and dependence is heroin—a drug that is not used for therapeutic purposes in the United States. (Table 12.10–1) lists various opioids.

The text revision of the fourth edition of *Diagnostic and Statistical Manual of Mental Disorders* (DSM-IV-TR) divides opioid-related disorders into opioid use disorders (opioid abuse and opioid dependence) and nine other opioid-induced disorders (e.g., intoxication, withdrawal).

Opioid dependence is a cluster of physiological, behavioral, and cognitive symptoms, which taken together indicates repeated and continuing use of opioid drugs despite significant problems related to such use. Drug dependence in general has also been defined by the World Health Organization (WHO) as

Table 12.10–1
Opioids

Proprietary Name	Trade Name
Morphine	
Heroin (diacetylmorphine)	
Hydromorphone (dihydromorphinone)	Dilaudid
Oxymorphone (dihydrohydroxymorphinone)	Numorphan
Levorphanol	Levo-Dromoran
Methadone	Dolophine
Meperidine (pethidine)	Demerol, Pethadol
Fentanyl	Sublimaze
Codeine	
Hydrocodone (dihydrocodeinone)	Hycodan, others
Drocode (dihydrocodeine)	Synalgos-DC, Compal
Oxycodone (dihydrohydroxycodeinone)	Roxicodone, OxyContin, Percodan, Percocet
Propoxyphene	Darvon, others
Buprenorphine	Buprenex
Pentazocine	Talwin
Nalbuphine	Nubain
Butorphanol	Stadol

a syndrome in which the use of a drug or class of drugs takes on a much higher priority for a given person than other behaviors that once had a higher value. These brief definitions each have as their central features an emphasis on the drug-using behavior itself, its maladaptive nature, and how the choice to engage in that behavior shifts and becomes constrained as a result of interaction with the drug over time.

Opioid abuse is a term used to designate a pattern of maladaptive use of an opioid drug leading to clinically significant impairment or distress and occurring within a 12-month period, but one in which the symptoms have never met the criteria for opioid dependence.

The *opioid-induced disorders* as defined by DSM-IV-TR include such common phenomena as opioid intoxication, opioid withdrawal, opioid-induced sleep disorder, and opioid-induced sexual dysfunction. Opioid intoxication delirium is occasionally seen in hospitalized patients. Opioid-induced psychotic disorder, opioid-induced mood disorder, and opioid-induced anxiety disorder, by contrast, are quite uncommon with μ-agonist opioids but have been seen with certain mixed agonist-antagonist opioids acting at other receptors. DSM-IV-TR also includes *opioid-related disorder not otherwise specified* for situations that do not meet the criteria for any of the other opioid-related disorders.

In addition to the morbidity and mortality associated directly with the opioid-related disorders, the association between the transmission of the human immunodeficiency virus (HIV) and intravenous opioid and opiate use is now recognized as a leading national health concern. The words *opiate* and *opioid* come from the word *opium,* the juice of the opium poppy, *Papaver somniferum,* which contains approximately 20 opium alkaloids, including morphine.

Many synthetic opioids have been manufactured, including meperidine (Demerol), methadone (Dolophine), pentazocine (Talwin), and propoxyphene (Darvon). Methadone is the current gold standard in the treatment of opioid dependence. Opioid antagonists have been synthesized to treat opioid overdose and opioid dependence. This class of drugs includes naloxone (Narcan), naltrexone (ReVia), nalorphine, levallorphan, and apomorphine. Compounds with mixed agonist and antagonist activity at opioid receptors have been synthesized and include pentazocine, butorphanol (Stadol), and buprenorphine (Buprenex). Studies have found buprenorphine to be an effective treatment for opioid dependence.

EPIDEMIOLOGY

As stated above, persons with opioid dependence use heroin most widely. According to DSM-IV-TR the lifetime prevalence for heroin use is about 1 percent, with 0.2 percent having taken the drug during the prior year. The number of current heroin users has been questionably estimated to be between 600,000 and 800,000. The number of persons estimated to have used heroin at any time in their lives ("lifetime users") is approximately 2 million. The male-to-female ratio of persons with heroin dependence is about 3 to 1. Users of opioids typically started to use substances in their teens and early 20s; currently, most persons with opioid dependence are in their 30s and 40s. According to DSM-IV-TR, the tendency for dependence to remit generally begins after age 40 years and has been called "maturing out." However, many persons have remained opioid dependent for 50 years or longer. In the United States, persons tend to experience their first opioid-induced experience in their early teens or even as young as 10 years old. Early induction into the drug culture is likely in communities in which substance abuse is rampant and in families in which the parents are substance abusers. A heroin habit can cost a person hundreds of dollars a day; thus, a person with opioid dependence needs to obtain money through criminal activities and prostitution. The involvement of persons with opioid dependence in prostitution accounts for much of the spread of HIV.

NEUROPHARMACOLOGY

The primary effects of the opioids are mediated through the opioid receptors, which were discovered in the second half of the 1970s. The μ-opioid receptors are involved in the regulation and mediation of analgesia, respiratory depression, constipation, and dependence; the κ-opioid receptors, with analgesia, diuresis, and sedation; and the δ-opioid receptors, possibly with analgesia.

In 1974, enkephalin, an endogenous pentapeptide with opioidlike actions, was identified. This discovery led to the identification of three classes of endogenous opioids within the brain, including the endorphins and the enkephalins. Endorphins are involved in neural transmission and pain suppression. They are released naturally in the body when a person is physically hurt and account in part for the absence of pain during acute injuries.

The opioids also have significant effects on the dopaminergic and noradrenergic neurotransmitter systems. Several types of data indicate that the addictive rewarding properties of opioids are mediated through activation of the ventral tegmental area dopaminergic neurons that project to the cerebral cortex and the limbic system (Fig. 12.10–1).

Heroin is the most commonly abused opioid and is more potent and lipid soluble than morphine. Because of those properties, heroin crosses the blood–brain barrier faster and has a more rapid onset than morphine. Heroin was first introduced as a treatment for morphine addiction, but heroin, in fact, is more dependence producing than morphine. Codeine, which occurs naturally as about 0.5 percent of the opiate alkaloids in opium, is absorbed easily through the gastrointestinal tract and is subsequently transformed into morphine in the body. Results of at least one study using positron emission tomography (PET) have suggested that one effect of all opioids is decreased cerebral blood flow in selected brain regions in persons with opioid dependence.

Tolerance and Dependence

Tolerance does not develop uniformly to all actions of opioid drugs. Tolerance to some actions of opioids can be so high that a hundredfold increase in dose is required to produce the original effect. For example, terminally ill cancer patients may need 200 to 300 mg a day of morphine, whereas a dose of 60 mg can easily be fatal to an opioid-naive person. The symptoms of opioid withdrawal do not appear unless a person has been using opioids for a long time or when cessation is particularly abrupt, as occurs functionally when an opioid antagonist is given. The long-term use of opioids results in changes in the number and sensitivity of opioid receptors, which mediate at

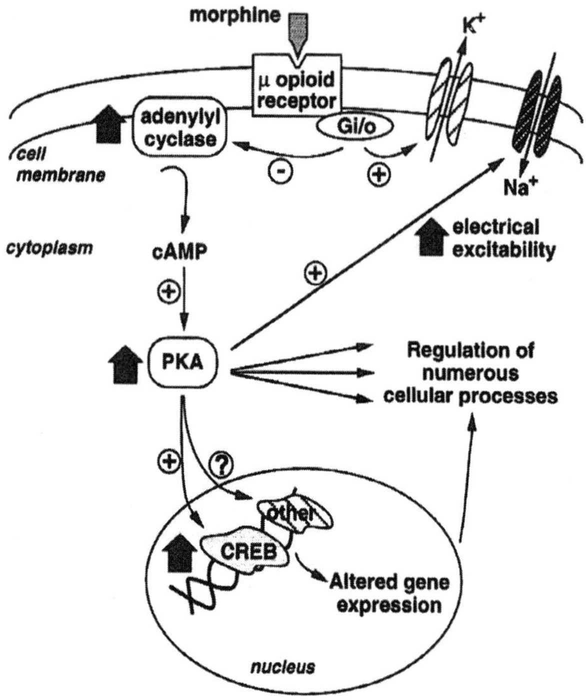

FIGURE 12.10–1

Scheme illustrating opioid actions in the locus ceruleus (LC). Opioids acutely inhibit LC neurons by increasing the conductance of a K^+ channel (*light cross-hatch*) via coupling with subtypes of G_i and/or G_0 and by decreasing an Na^+-dependent inward current (*dark cross-hatch*) via coupling with $G_{i/o}$ and the consequent inhibition if adenylyl cyclase. Reduced levels of cAMP decrease PKA and the phosphorylation of the responsible channel or pump. Inhibition of the cAMP pathway also decreases phosphorylation of numerous other proteins and thereby affects many additional processes in the neuron. For example, it reduces the phosphorylation state of CREB, which may initiate some of the longer-term changes in LC function. Upper bold arrows summarize effects of repeated morphine administration in the LC. Repeated morphine administration increases levels of adenylyl cyclase, PKA, and several phosphoproteins, including CREB. These changes contribute to the altered phenotype of the drug-addicted state. For example, the intrinsic excitability of LC neurons is increased via enhanced activity of the cAMP pathway and Na^+-dependent inward current, which contributes to the tolerance, dependence, and withdrawal exhibited by these neurons. This altered phenotypic state appears to be maintained in part by upregulation of CREB expression. (Reprinted with permission from Nestler EJ. Molecular mechanisms underlying opiate addiction: implications for medications development. *Semin Neurosci.*1997;0:84.)

least some of the effects of tolerance and withdrawal. Although long-term use is associated with increased sensitivity of the dopaminergic, cholinergic, and serotonergic neurons, the effect of opioids on the noradrenergic neurons is probably the primary mediator of the symptoms of opioid withdrawal. Short-term use of opioids apparently decreases the activity of the noradrenergic neurons in the locus ceruleus, long-term use activates a compensatory homeostatic mechanism within the neurons, and opioid withdrawal results in a rebound hyperactivity. This hypothesis also provides an explanation for why clonidine (Catapres), an α_2-adrenergic receptor agonist that decreases the release of norepinephrine, is useful in the treatment of opioid withdrawal symptoms.

Table 12.10–2
Non–Substance-Related Axis I Psychiatric Disorders in Opioid Users

	Lifetime Rates % (Current Rates %)		
Diagnostic Category[a]	**Men (*N* = 378)**	**Women (*N* = 338)**	**Total**
Any Axis I disorder	15.6 (5.0)	33.4 (11.2)	24.0 (8.0)
Mood disorder	11.4 (2.1)	27.5 (5.3)	19.0 (3.6)
Major depressive disorder	8.7 (1.3)	23.7 (5.3)	15.8 (3.2)
Dysthymic disorder	2.4 (2.4)	4.4 (4.4)	3.4 (3.4)
Bipolar I disorder	0.8 (0.8)	0.0 (0.0)	0.4 (0.4)
Anxiety disorder	6.1 (3.4)	10.7 (6.8)	8.2 (5.0)
Simple phobia	1.9 (1.9)	5.3 (3.6)	3.5 (2.7)
Social phobia	1.9 (0.8)	3.6 (2.7)	2.7 (1.7)
Panic disorder	2.1 (0.3)	1.8 (0.9)	2.0 (0.6)
Agoraphobia	0.0 (0.0)	0.6 (0.3)	0.3 (0.1)
Obsessive-compulsive disorder	0.5 (0.5)	0.0 (0.0)	0.3 (0.3)
General anxiety disorder	0.8 (0.8)	0.0 (0.0)	0.1 (0.1)
Eating disorders	0.0 (0.0)	1.5 (0.0)	0.7 (0.0)
Bulimia nervosa	0.0 (0.0)	0.9 (0.0)	0.4 (0.0)
Anorexia nervosa	0.0 (0.0)	0.6 (0.0)	0.3 (0.0)
Schizophrenia	0.0 (0.0)	0.3 (0.3)	0.1 (0.1)

[a]Multiple disorders possible.
Adapted from Brooner RK, King VL, Kidorf M, Schmidt CW, Bigelow GE. Psychiatric and substance use comorbidity among treatment-seeking opioid abusers. *Arch Gen Psychiatry.* 1997;54:71.

COMORBIDITY

About 90 percent of persons with opioid dependence have an additional psychiatric disorder. The most common comorbid psychiatric diagnoses are major depressive disorder, alcohol use disorders, antisocial personality disorder, and anxiety disorders. About 15 percent of persons with opioid dependence attempt to commit suicide at least once. The high prevalence of comorbidity with other psychiatric diagnoses highlights the need to develop a broad-based treatment program that also addresses patients' associated psychiatric disorders (Table 12.10–2).

ETIOLOGY

Psychosocial Factors

Opioid dependence is not limited to low socioeconomic classes, although the incidence of opioid dependence is greater in these groups than in higher socioeconomic classes. Social factors associated with urban poverty probably contribute to opioid dependence. About 50 percent of urban heroin users are children of single parents or divorced parents and are from families in which at least one other member has a substance-related disorder. Children from such settings are at high risk for opioid dependence, especially if they also evidence behavioral problems in school or other signs of conduct disorder.

Some consistent behavior patterns seem to be especially pronounced in adolescents with opioid dependence. These patterns have been called the *heroin behavior syndrome:* underly-

ing depression, often of an agitated type and frequently accompanied by anxiety symptoms; impulsiveness expressed by a passive-aggressive orientation; fear of failure; use of heroin as an antianxiety agent to mask feelings of low self-esteem, hopelessness, and aggression; limited coping strategies and low frustration tolerance, accompanied by the need for immediate gratification; sensitivity to drug contingencies, with a keen awareness of the relation between good feelings and the act of drug taking; feelings of behavioral impotence counteracted by momentary control over the life situation by means of substances; disturbances in social and interpersonal relationships with peers maintained by mutual substance experiences.

Biological and Genetic Factors

There is now evidence for common and drug-specific, genetically transmitted vulnerability factors that increase the likelihood of developing drug dependence. Individuals who abuse a substance from any category are more likely to abuse substances from other categories. Monozygotic twins are more likely than dizygotic twins to be concordant for opioid dependence. Multivariate modeling techniques indicated that not only was the genetic contribution high for heroin abuse in this group, but also a higher proportion of the variance due to genetic factors was not shared with the common vulnerability factor—that is, it was specific for opioids.

A person with an opioid-related disorder may have had genetically determined hypoactivity of the opiate system. Researchers are investigating the possibility that such hypoactivity may be caused by too few or less sensitive opioid receptors, by release of too little endogenous opioid, or by overly high concentrations of a hypothesized endogenous opioid antagonist. A biological predisposition to an opioid-related disorder may also be associated with abnormal functioning in either the dopaminergic or the noradrenergic neurotransmitter system.

Psychodynamic Theory

In psychoanalytic literature, the behavior of persons addicted to narcotics has been described in terms of libidinal fixation, with regression to pregenital, oral, or even more archaic levels of psychosexual development. The need to explain the relation of drug abuse, defense mechanisms, impulse control, affective disturbances, and adaptive mechanisms led to the shift from psychosexual formulations to formulations emphasizing ego psychology. Serious ego pathology is often thought to be associated with substance abuse and is considered to indicate profound developmental disturbances. Problems of the relation between the ego and affects emerge as a key area of difficulty.

DIAGNOSIS

DSM-IV-TR lists several opioid-related disorders (Table 12.10–3) but contains specific diagnostic criteria only for opioid intoxication (Table 12.10–4) and opioid withdrawal (Table 12.10–5) within the section on opioid-related disorders. The diagnostic criteria for the other opioid-related disorders are contained within the DSM-IV-TR sections that deal specifically with the

Table 12.10–3
DSM-IV-TR Opioid-Related Disorders

Opioid use disorders
Opioid dependence
Opioid abuse
Opioid-induced disorders
Opioid intoxication
  Specify if:
    With perceptual disturbances
Opioid withdrawal
Opioid intoxication delirium
Opioid-induced psychotic disorder, with delusions
  Specify if:
    With onset during intoxication
Opioid-induced psychotic disorder, with hallucinations
  Specify if:
    With onset during intoxication
Opioid-induced mood disorder
  Specify if:
    With onset during intoxication
Opioid-induced sexual dysfunction
  Specify if:
    With onset during intoxication
Opioid-induced sleep disorder
  Specify if:
    With onset during intoxication
    With onset during withdrawal
Opioid-related disorder not otherwise specified

From American Psychiatric Association. *Diagnostic and Statistical Manual of Mental Disorders.* 4th ed. Text rev. Washington, DC: American Psychiatric Association; copyright 2000, with permission.

Table 12.10–4
DSM-IV-TR Diagnostic Criteria for Opioid Intoxication

A. Recent use of an opioid.
B. Clinically significant maladaptive behavioral or psychological changes (e.g., initial euphoria followed by apathy, dysphoria, psychomotor agitation or retardation, impaired judgment, or impaired social or occupational functioning) that developed during, or shortly after, opioid use.
C. Pupillary constriction (or pupillary dilation due to anoxia from severe overdose) and one (or more) of the following signs, developing during, or shortly after, opioid use:
   (1) drowsiness or coma
   (2) slurred speech
   (3) impairment in attention or memory
D. The symptoms are not due to a general medical condition and are not better accounted for by another mental disorder.

Specify if:
  With perceptual disturbances

From American Psychiatric Association. *Diagnostic and Statistical Manual of Mental Disorders.* 4th ed. Text rev. Washington, DC: American Psychiatric Association; copyright 2000, with permission.

Table 12.10–5
DSM-IV-TR Diagnostic Criteria for Opioid Withdrawal

A. Either of the following:
  (1) cessation of (or reduction in) opioid use that has been heavy and prolonged (several weeks or longer)
  (2) administration of an opioid antagonist after a period of opioid use
B. Three (or more) of the following, developing within minutes to several days after Criterion A:
  (1) dysphoric mood
  (2) nausea or vomiting
  (3) muscle aches
  (4) lacrimation or rhinorrhea
  (5) pupillary dilation, piloerection, or sweating
  (6) diarrhea
  (7) yawning
  (8) fever
  (9) insomnia
C. The symptoms in Criterion B cause clinically significant distress or impairment in social, occupational, or other important areas of functioning.
D. The symptoms are not due to a general medical condition and are not better accounted for by another mental disorder.

From American Psychiatric Association. *Diagnostic and Statistical Manual of Mental Disorders.* 4th ed. Text rev. Washington, DC: American Psychiatric Association; copyright 2000, with permission.

predominant symptom—for example, opioid-induced mood disorder (see Table 15.3–10 in Section 15.3 of Chapter 15).

Opioid Dependence and Opioid Abuse

Opioid dependence and opioid abuse are defined in DSM-IV-TR according to the general criteria for these disorders (see Tables 12.1–6, 12.1–7, and 12.1–8).

Opioid Intoxication

DSM-IV-TR defines opioid intoxication as including maladaptive behavioral changes and some specific physical symptoms of opioid use (Table 12.10–4). In general, altered mood, psychomotor retardation, drowsiness, slurred speech, and impaired memory and attention in the presence of other indicators of recent opioid use strongly suggest a diagnosis of opioid intoxication. DSM-IV-TR allows for the specification of "with perceptual disturbances."

Opioid Withdrawal

The general rule about the onset and duration of withdrawal symptoms is that substances with short durations of action tend to produce short, intense withdrawal syndromes and substances with long durations of action produce prolonged but mild withdrawal syndromes. An exception to the rule, narcotic antagonist-precipitated withdrawal after long-acting opioid dependence can be severe.

An abstinence syndrome can be precipitated by administration of an opioid antagonist. The symptoms may begin within seconds of such an intravenous injection and may peak in about 1 hour. Opioid craving rarely occurs in the context of analgesic administration for pain from physical disorders or surgery. The full withdrawal syndrome, including intense craving for opioids, usually occurs only secondary to abrupt cessation of use in persons with opioid dependence.

Morphine and Heroin. The morphine and heroin withdrawal syndrome begins 6 to 8 hours after the last dose, usually after a 1- to 2-week period of continuous use or after the administration of a narcotic antagonist. The withdrawal syndrome reaches its peak intensity during the second or third day and subsides during the next 7 to 10 days, but some symptoms may persist for 6 months or longer.

Rafiq is a 43-year-old Egyptian fruit seller. He is married and has three children.

PROBLEM

Rafiq came to the outpatient clinic asking to be admitted for treatment of his heroin dependence. He was first introduced to heroin at the age of 27, when a friend offered him some of the substance to sniff. Rafiq liked the effect and for a while he would sniff one eighth of a gram every few days. When he tried to stop using it for fear he might become dependent on it, he experienced withdrawal symptoms. Afraid to tell anyone, he took some more heroin. In time he found he needed to increase the amount he took to get the same effect. During the ensuing years, he tried to abstain several times. He was admitted to the hospital for detoxification when he was 31, 32, 33, and again when he was 34 years old. His longest period of abstinence after discharge was 6 months. On his latest visit to the clinic, Rafiq said he could no longer live with the idea of being dependent on the drug. His dependence was disrupting his relationship with his wife, he said, and he despised himself for not being a better model for his children, who had already begun to suspect that their father was drug dependent. Before coming to the hospital, he had reached a dosage of 4 grams of heroin per day.

HISTORY

Rafiq had a history of normal development. His childhood and adolescence were rather miserable because of a very aggressive father. The father caused problems with the teachers at Rafiq's school, and the teachers took it out on the boy. He left school after only 3 years of education and spent his time at home doing nothing until the age of 14, when his father bought him some fruit to sell in the market. During his military service, Rafiq ran away once and was brought back to serve an extra 6 months as punishment. After finishing the military service, he met an elderly man who was looking for someone to help him in his fruit shop. Rafiq worked for him for a few years, and when the man died, he left the shop to Rafiq. Rafiq had always been an introvert who preferred being on his own. He got married when he was 26 years old and had three children who were all healthy and at different stages in their schooling.

FINDINGS

Rafiq came to the clinic by himself. He was appropriately dressed but looked exhausted. He showed withdrawal symptoms in the form of lacrimation, sneezing, vomiting, diarrhea, abdominal cramps, body aches, palpitations, shivering, and severe anxiety. His mood was dysphoric, and he had guilt feelings toward his family, especially his children. He felt ashamed and distressed. He repeatedly interrupted the interview to ask the staff to sedate him so he could avoid the withdrawal pains. He showed no evidence of thought or perceptual disturbances. He was oriented in time, place, and person, and his memory for recent and remote events was intact.

DISCUSSION

Rafiq was clearly in a state of heroin withdrawal without complications. The withdrawal state is one of the indicators of a dependence syndrome. The withdrawal symptoms in the case of Rafiq were mainly physical: rhinorrhea, diarrhea, lacrimation, and generalized body aches. The dependence is further evidenced by his long-standing need for heroin, the development of tolerance, and his lack of capacity to control the intake. (From *ICD-10 Casebook.*)

Meperidine. The withdrawal syndrome from meperidine begins quickly, reaches a peak in 8 to 12 hours, and ends in 4 to 5 days.

Methadone. Methadone withdrawal usually begins 1 to 3 days after the last dose and ends in 10 to 14 days.

Symptoms. Opioid withdrawal (Table 12.10–5) consists of severe muscle cramps and bone aches, profuse diarrhea, abdominal cramps, rhinorrhea, lacrimation, piloerection or gooseflesh (from which comes the term *cold turkey* for the abstinence syndrome), yawning, fever, pupillary dilation, hypertension, tachycardia, and temperature dysregulation, including hypothermia and hyperthermia. Persons with opioid dependence seldom die from opioid withdrawal, unless they have a severe preexisting physical illness such as cardiac disease. Residual symptoms—such as insomnia, bradycardia, temperature dysregulation, and a craving for opioids—may persist for months after withdrawal. Associated features of opioid withdrawal include restlessness, irritability, depression, tremor, weakness, nausea, and vomiting. At any time during the abstinence syndrome, a single injection of morphine or heroin eliminates all the symptoms.

Opioid Intoxication Delirium

Opioid intoxication delirium (Table 10.2–3) is most likely to happen when opioids are used in high doses, are mixed with other psychoactive compounds, or are used by a person with preexisting brain damage or a central nervous system (CNS) disorder (e.g., epilepsy).

Opioid-Induced Psychotic Disorder

Opioid-induced psychotic disorder can begin during opioid intoxication. The DSM-IV-TR diagnostic criteria are contained in the section on schizophrenia and other psychotic disorders (see Table 14.4–7 in Section 14.4). Clinicians can specify whether hallucinations or delusions are the predominant symptoms.

Table 12.10–6
DSM-IV-TR Diagnostic Criteria for Opioid-Related Disorder Not Otherwise Specified

The opioid-related disorder not otherwise specified category is for disorders associated with the use of opioids that are not classifiable as opioid dependence, opioid abuse, opioid intoxication, opioid withdrawal, opioid intoxication delirium, opioid-induced psychotic disorder, opioid-induced mood disorder, opioid-induced sexual dysfunction, or opioid-induced sleep disorder.

From American Psychiatric Association. *Diagnostic and Statistical Manual of Mental Disorders.* 4th ed. Text rev. Washington, DC: American Psychiatric Association; copyright 2000, with permission.

Opioid-Induced Mood Disorder

Opioid-induced mood disorder can begin during opioid intoxication (see Table 15.3–10). Opioid-induced mood disorder symptoms may have a manic, depressed, or mixed nature, depending on a person's response to opioids. A person coming to psychiatric attention with opioid-induced mood disorder usually has mixed symptoms, combining irritability, expansiveness, and depression.

Opioid-Induced Sleep Disorder and Opioid-Induced Sexual Dysfunction

Opioid-induced sleep disorder (see Table 24.2–20) and opioid-induced sexual dysfunction (see Table 21.2–12) are diagnostic categories in DSM-IV-TR. Hypersomnia is likely to be more common with opioids than insomnia. The most common sexual dysfunction is likely to be impotence.

Opioid-Related Disorder Not Otherwise Specified

DSM-IV-TR includes diagnoses for opioid-related disorders with symptoms of delirium, abnormal mood, psychosis, abnormal sleep, and sexual dysfunction. Clinical situations that do not fit into these categories exemplify appropriate cases for the use of the DSM-IV-TR diagnosis of opioid-related disorder not otherwise specified (Table 12.10–6).

CLINICAL FEATURES

Opioids can be taken orally, snorted intranasally, and injected intravenously (IV) (Fig. 12.10–2) or subcutaneously (Fig. 12.10–3). Opioids are subjectively addictive because of the euphoric high (the rush) that users experience, especially those who take the substances IV. The associated symptoms include a feeling of warmth, heaviness of the extremities, dry mouth, itchy face (especially the nose), and facial flushing. The initial euphoria is followed by a period of sedation, known in street

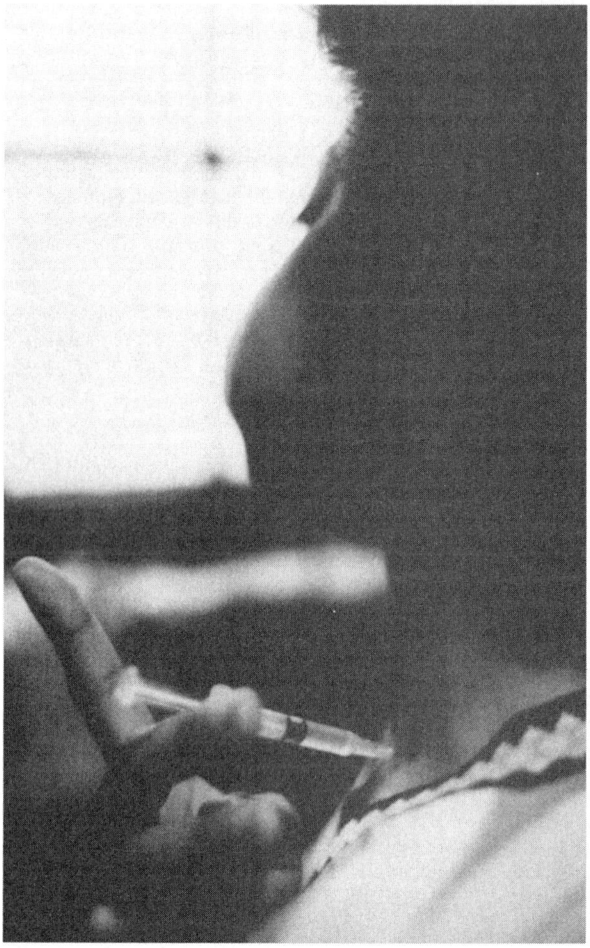

FIGURE 12.10–2
A heroin user puffs her cheeks to force blood into the jugular vein. (Courtesy of Steve Raymer, copyright, National Geographic Society, 1985.)

parlance as "nodding off." Opioid use can induce dysphoria, nausea, and vomiting in opioid-naive persons.

The physical effects of opioids include respiratory depression, pupillary constriction, smooth muscle contraction (including the ureters and the bile ducts), constipation, and changes in blood pressure, heart rate, and body temperature. The respiratory depressant effects are mediated at the level of the brainstem.

Adverse Effects

The most common and most serious adverse effect associated with the opioid-related disorders is the potential transmission of hepatitis and HIV through the use of contaminated needles by more than one person. Persons can experience idiosyncratic allergic reactions to opioids, which result in anaphylactic shock, pulmonary edema, and death if they do not receive prompt and adequate treatment. Another serious adverse effect is an idiosyncratic drug interaction between meperidine and monoamine oxidase inhibitors (MAOIs), which can produce gross autonomic instability, severe behavioral agitation, coma, seizures, and death. Opioids and MAOIs should not be given together for this reason.

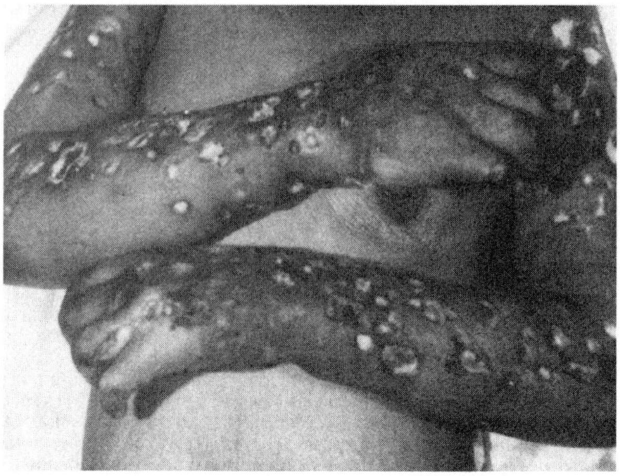

FIGURE 12.10–3
Skin popper. Circular depressed scars, often with underlying chronic abscesses, can result from skin popping. (Courtesy of Michael Baden, M.D.)

Opioid Overdose

Death from an overdose of an opioid is usually attributable to respiratory arrest from the respiratory depressant effect of the drug. The symptoms of overdose include marked unresponsiveness, coma, slow respiration, hypothermia, hypotension, and bradycardia. When presented with the clinical triad of coma, pinpoint pupils, and respiratory depression, clinicians should consider opioid overdose as a primary diagnosis. They can also inspect the patient's body for needle tracks in the arms, legs, ankles, groin, and even the dorsal vein of the penis.

MPTP-Induced Parkinsonism

In 1976, after ingesting an opioid contaminated with *N*-methyl-4-phenyl-1,2,3,6-tetrahydropyridine (MPTP), several persons developed a syndrome of irreversible parkinsonism. The mechanism for the neurotoxic effect is as follows: MPTP is converted into 1-methyl-4-phenylpyridinium (MPP+) by the enzyme monoamine oxidase and is then taken up by dopaminergic neurons. Because MPP+ binds to melanin in substantia nigra neurons, MPP+ is concentrated in these neurons and eventually kills the cells. PET studies of persons who ingested MPTP but remained asymptomatic have shown a decreased number of dopamine-binding sites in the substantia nigra. This decrease reflects a loss in the number of dopaminergic neurons in that region.

TREATMENT AND REHABILITATION

Overdose Treatment

The first task is to ensure an adequate airway. Tracheopharyngeal secretions should be aspirated; an airway may be inserted. The patient should be ventilated mechanically until naloxone, a specific opioid antagonist, can be given. Naloxone is administered IV at a slow rate—initially about 0.8 mg per 70 kg of body weight. Signs of improvement (increased respiratory rate

and pupillary dilation) should occur promptly. In opioid-dependent patients, too much naloxone may produce signs of withdrawal as well as reversal of overdosage. If there is no response to the initial dosage, naloxone administration may be repeated after intervals of a few minutes. In the past it was thought that if no response was observed after 4 to 5 mg the CNS depression was probably not due solely to opioids. The duration of action of naloxone is short compared with that of many opioids, such as methadone and levomethadyl acetate, and repeated administration may be required to prevent recurrence of opioid toxicity.

Withdrawal and Detoxification

Methadone. Methadone is a synthetic narcotic (an opioid) that substitutes for heroin and can be taken orally. When given to addicts to replace their usual substance of abuse, the drug suppresses withdrawal symptoms. A daily dosage of 20 to 80 mg suffices to stabilize a patient, although daily doses of up to 120 mg have been used. Methadone has a duration of action exceeding 24 hours; thus, once-daily dosing is adequate. Methadone maintenance is continued until the patient can be withdrawn from methadone, which itself causes dependence. An abstinence syndrome occurs with methadone withdrawal, but patients are detoxified from methadone more easily than from heroin. Clonidine (0.1 to 0.3 mg three to four times a day) is usually given during the detoxification period.

Methadone maintenance has several advantages. First, it frees persons with opioid dependence from using injectable heroin and thus reduces the chance of spreading HIV through contaminated needles. Second, methadone produces minimal euphoria and rarely causes drowsiness or depression when taken for a long time. Third, methadone allows patients to engage in gainful employment instead of criminal activity. The major disadvantage of methadone use is that patients remain dependent on a narcotic.

Other Opioid Substitutes. Levomethadyl (ORLAAM), also called L-α-acetylmethadol (LAMM), a longer-acting opioid than methadone, is also used to treat persons with opioid dependence. In contrast to the daily methadone treatment, LAMM can be administered in dosages of 30 to 80 mg three times a week; because of this less frequent dosing regimen, an increasing number of programs are using LAMM.

Buprenorphine is an opioid partial agonist and is an analgesic with opioid antagonist activity approved only for treatment of moderate to severe pain. Buprenorphine in a daily dose of 8 to 10 mg appears to reduce heroin use. Buprenorphine also is effective in thrice-weekly dosing because of its slow dissociation from opioid receptors.

Opioid Antagonists. Opioid antagonists block or antagonize the effects of opioids. Unlike methadone, they do not exert narcotic effects and do not cause dependence. Opioid antagonists include naloxone, which is used in the treatment of opioid overdose because it reverses the effects of narcotics, and naltrexone, the longest-acting (72 hours) antagonist. The theory for using an antagonist for opioid-related disorders is that blocking opioid agonist effects, particularly euphoria, discourages persons with opioid dependence from substance-seeking behavior and thus deconditions this behavior. The major weakness of the antagonist treatment model is the lack of any mechanism that compels a person to continue to take the antagonist.

Pregnant Women with Opioid Dependence

Neonatal addiction is a significant problem. About three fourths of all infants born to addicted mothers experience the withdrawal syndrome.

Neonatal Withdrawal. Although opioid withdrawal rarely is fatal for the otherwise healthy adult, it is hazardous to the fetus and can lead to miscarriage or fetal death. Maintaining a pregnant woman with opioid dependence on a low dosage of methadone (10 to 40 mg daily) may be the least hazardous course to follow. At this dosage, neonatal withdrawal is usually mild and can be managed with low doses of paregoric. If pregnancy begins while a woman is taking high doses of methadone, the dosage should be reduced slowly (e.g., 1 mg every 3 days), and fetal movements should be monitored. If withdrawal is necessary or desired, it is least hazardous during the second trimester.

Fetal AIDS Transmission. Acquired immune deficiency syndrome (AIDS) is the other major risk to the fetus of a woman with opioid dependence. Pregnant women can pass HIV, the causative agent of AIDS, to the fetus through the placental circulation. An HIV-infected mother can also pass HIV to the infant through breast-feeding. The use of zidovudine (Retrovir) alone or in combination with other anti-HIV medication in infected women can decrease the incidence of HIV in newborns.

Psychotherapy

The entire range of psychotherapeutic modalities is appropriate for treating opioid-related disorders. Individual psychotherapy, behavioral therapy, cognitive-behavioral therapy, family therapy, support groups (e.g., Narcotics Anonymous [NA]), and social skills training may all prove effective for specific patients. Social skills training should be particularly emphasized for patients with few social skills. Family therapy is usually indicated when the patient lives with family members.

Therapeutic Communities

Therapeutic communities are residences in which all members have a problem of substance abuse. Abstinence is the rule; to be admitted to such a community, a person must show a high level of motivation. The goals are to effect a complete change of lifestyle, including abstinence from substances; to develop personal honesty, responsibility, and useful social skills; and to eliminate antisocial attitudes and criminal behavior.

The staff members of most therapeutic communities are persons with former substance dependence who often put prospective candidates through a rigorous screening process to test their motivation. Self-help through the use of confronta-

tional groups and isolation from the outside world and from friends associated with the drug life are emphasized. The prototypical community for persons with substance dependence is Phoenix House, where the residents live for long periods (usually 12 to 18 months) while receiving treatment. They are allowed to return to their old environments only when they have demonstrated their ability to handle increased responsibility within the therapeutic community. Therapeutic communities can be effective but require large staffs and extensive facilities. Moreover, dropout rates are high; up to 75 percent of those who enter therapeutic communities leave within the first month.

Self-Help

NA is a self-help group of abstinent drug addicts modeled on the 12-step principles of Alcoholics Anonymous (AA). Such groups now exist in most large cities and can provide useful group support. The outcome for patients treated in 12-step programs is generally good, but the anonymity that is at the core of the 12-step model has made detailed evaluation of its efficacy in treating opioid dependence difficult.

Education and Needle Exchange

Although the essential treatment of opioid use disorders is encouraging persons to abstain from opioids, education about the transmission of HIV must receive equal attention. Persons with opioid dependence who use IV or subcutaneous routes of administration must be taught available safe-sex practices. Free needle-exchange programs are often subject to intense political and societal pressures but, where allowed, should be made available to persons with opioid dependence. Several studies have indicated that unsafe needle sharing is common when it is difficult to obtain enough clean needles and is also common in persons with legal difficulties, severe substance problems, and psychiatric symptoms. These are just the persons most likely to be involved in transmitting HIV.

References

Darke S, Wodak A, Hall W, Heather N, Ward J. Prevalence and predictors of psychopathology among opioid users. *Br J Addict.* 1992;87:771.

Di Chiara G, North RA. Neurobiology of opiate abuse. *Trends Pharmacol Sci.* 1992;13:185.

Gintzler AR. Relevance of opioid bimodality to tolerance/dependence formation: from transmitter release to second messenger formation. *Adv Exp Med Biol.* 1995;373:73.

Hurt PH, Ritchie EC. A case of ketamine dependence. *Am J Psychiatry.* 1994;151:779.

Jaffe JH. Opioid-related disorders. In: Sadock BJ, Sadock VA, eds. *Kaplan & Sadock's Comprehensive Textbook of Psychiatry.* 7th ed. Vol 1. Baltimore: Lippincott Williams & Wilkins; 2000:1038.

Koob GF, Maldonado R, Stinus L. Neural substrates of opiate withdrawal. *Trends Neurosci.* 1992;15:186.

Kosten TA, Bianchi MS, Kosten TR. The predictive validity of the dependence syndrome in opiate abusers. *Am J Drug Alcohol Abuse.* 1992;18:145.

Kreek MJ. Rationale for maintenance pharmacotherapy of opiate dependence. *Res Publ Assoc Res Nerv Ment Dis.* 1992;70:2.

Luthar SS, Anton SF, Merikangas KR, Rounsaville BJ. Vulnerability to substance abuse and psychopathology among siblings of opioid abusers. *J Nerv Ment Dis.* 1992;180:153.

Neslter EJ. Molecular mechanisms of drug addiction. *J Neurosci.* 1992;12:2439.

Robinson RC, Gatchel RJ, Polatin P, Deschner M, Noe C, Gajraj N. Screening for problematic prescription opioid use. *Clin J Pain.* 2001;17:220.

Substance Abuse and Mental Health Services Administration Office of Applied Studies. *Preliminary Estimates from the 1995 National Household Survey on Drug Abuse.* Washington, DC: US Government Printing Office; 1995.

▲ 12.11 Phencyclidine (or Phencyclidinelike)-Related Disorders

Phencyclidine (1,1[phenylcyclohexyl]piperidine; PCP), also known as "angel dust," was developed and is classified as a dissociative anesthetic. Its use as an anesthetic in humans, however, was associated with disorientation, agitation, delirium, and unpleasant hallucinations on awakening. Therefore, PCP is no longer used as an anesthetic in humans, although it is used in some countries as an anesthetic in veterinary medicine. Although PCP has a long duration of action and is very potent by any route of administration, PCP use carries a high risk of behavioral, physiological, and neurological toxicity, and it is highly reinforcing. A related compound, ketamine (Ketalar), also referred to as "special K," is still used as a human anesthetic in the United States; it has not been associated with the same adverse effects and is also subject to abuse.

PCP was first used illicitly in San Francisco in the late 1960s. Since then, about 30 chemical analogues have been produced and are intermittently available on the streets of major U.S. cities. The effects of PCP are similar to those of such hallucinogens as lysergic acid diethylamide (LSD). Because of differing pharmacology and some difference in clinical effects, however, the text revision of the fourth edition of *Diagnostic and Statistical Manual of Mental Disorders* (DSM-IV-TR) classifies the arylcyclohexylamines as a separate category. PCP has also been of interest to schizophrenia researchers, who have used PCP-induced chemical and behavioral changes in animals as a possible model of schizophrenia.

EPIDEMIOLOGY

PCP and some related substances are relatively easy to synthesize in illegal laboratories and relatively inexpensive to buy on the streets. The variable quality of the laboratories, however, results in a range of potency and purity. PCP use varies most markedly with geography. Some areas of some cities have a 10-fold higher usage rate of PCP than other areas. The highest PCP use in the United States is in Washington, D.C., where PCP accounts for 18 percent of all substance-related deaths. In Los Angeles, Chicago, and Baltimore, the comparable figure is 6 percent. Most users of PCP also use other substances, particularly alcohol, but also opiates, opioids, marijuana, amphetamines, and cocaine. PCP is frequently added to marijuana, with severe untoward effects on users. According to DSM-IV-TR, the actual rate of PCP dependence and abuse is not known, but PCP is associated with 3 percent of substance abuse deaths and 32 percent of substance-related emergency room visits nationally.

NEUROPHARMACOLOGY

PCP and its related compounds are variously sold as a crystalline powder, paste, liquid, or drug-soaked paper (blotter). PCP is most commonly used as an additive to a cannabis- or parsley-containing cigarette. Experienced users report that the effects of 2 to 3 mg of smoked PCP occur in about 5 minutes and pla-

Table 12.11–1
DSM-IV-TR Phencyclidine-Related Disorders

Phencyclidine use disorders
Phencyclidine dependence
Phencyclidine abuse
Phencyclidine-induced disorders
Phencyclidine intoxication
Specify if:
With perceptual disturbances
Phencyclidine intoxication delirium
Phencyclidine-induced psychotic disorder, with delusions
Specify if:
With onset during intoxication
Phencyclidine-induced psychotic disorder, with hallucination
Specify if:
With onset during intoxication
Phencyclidine-induced mood disorder
Specify if:
With onset during intoxication
Phencyclidine-induced anxiety disorder
Specify if:
With onset during intoxication
Phencyclidine-related disorder not otherwise specified

From American Psychiatric Association. *Diagnostic and Statistical Manual of Mental Disorders.* 4th ed. Text rev. Washington, DC: American Psychiatric Association; copyright 2000, with permission.

teau in 30 minutes. The bioavailability of PCP is about 75 percent when taken by intravenous administration and about 30 percent when smoked. The half-life of PCP in humans is about 20 hours, and the half-life of ketamine in humans is about 2 hours.

The primary pharmacodynamic effect of PCP and ketamine is as an antagonist at the *N*-methyl-D-aspartate (NMDA) subtype of glutamate receptors. PCP binds to a site within the NMDA-associated calcium channel and prevents the influx of calcium ions. PCP also activates the dopaminergic neurons of the ventral tegmental area, which project to the cerebral cortex and the limbic system. Activation of these neurons is usually involved in mediating the reinforcing qualities of PCP.

Tolerance for the effects of PCP occurs in humans, although physical dependence generally does not occur. In animals that are administered more PCP per pound for longer times than virtually any humans, however, PCP does induce physical dependence, with marked withdrawal symptoms of lethargy, depression, and craving. Physical symptoms of withdrawal in humans are rare, probably as a function of dose and duration of use. Although physical dependence on PCP is rare in humans, psychological dependence on PCP, as well as ketamine, is common, and some users become psychologically dependent on the PCP-induced psychological state.

The fact that PCP is made in illicit laboratories contributes to the increased likelihood of impurities in the final product. One such contaminant is 1-piperidenocyclohexane carbonitrite, which releases hydrogen cyanide in small quantities when ingested. Another contaminant is piperidine, which can be recognized by its strong, fishy odor.

DIAGNOSIS

DSM-IV-TR lists a number of PCP (or PCP-like)-related disorders (Table 12.11–1) but outlines the specific diagnostic criteria for only PCP intoxication (Table 12.11–2) within the PCP (or PCP-like)-related disorders section. Their diagnostic criteria for other PCP (or PCP-like)-related disorders are listed in the sections that deal with specific symptoms—for example, PCP-induced anxiety disorder is in the anxiety disorders section (see Table 16.7–3 in Section 16.7 of Chapter 16).

PCP Dependence and PCP Abuse

DSM-IV-TR uses the general criteria for PCP dependence and PCP abuse (see Tables 12.1–5, 12.1–6, and 12.1–7 in Section 12.1 of this chapter). Some long-term users of PCP are said to be "crystallized," a syndrome characterized by dulled thinking, decreased reflexes, loss of memory, loss of impulse control, depression, lethargy, and impaired concentration.

According to DSM-IV-TR, in the United States, more than 3 percent of those age 12 and older acknowledged ever using PCP, with 0.2 percent reporting use in the prior year. The highest lifetime prevalence was in those aged 26 to 34 years (4 percent), while the highest proportion using PCP in the prior year (0.7 percent) was in those aged 12 to 17 years.

PCP Intoxication

Short-term PCP intoxication can have potentially severe complications and must often be considered a psychiatric emergency. DSM-IV-TR gives specific criteria for PCP (Table 12.11–2). Clinicians can specify the presence of perceptual disturbances.

Table 12.11–2
DSM-IV-TR Diagnostic Criteria for Phencyclidine Intoxication

A. Recent use of phencyclidine (or a related substance).
B. Clinically significant maladaptive behavioral changes (e.g., belligerence, assaultiveness, impulsiveness, unpredictability, psychomotor agitation, impaired judgment, or impaired social or occupational functioning) that developed during, or shortly after, phencyclidine use.
C. Within an hour (less when smoked, "snorted," or used intravenously), two (or more) of the following signs:
(1) vertical or horizontal nystagmus
(2) hypertension or tachycardia
(3) numbness or diminished responsiveness to pain
(4) ataxia
(5) dysarthria
(6) muscle rigidity
(7) seizures or coma
(8) hyperacusis
D. The symptoms are not due to a general medical condition and are not better accounted for by another mental disorder.

Specify if:
With perceptual disturbances

From American Psychiatric Association. *Diagnostic and Statistical Manual of Mental Disorders.* 4th ed. Text rev. Washington, DC: American Psychiatric Association; copyright 2000, with permission.

Some patients may be brought to psychiatric attention within hours of ingesting PCP, but often 2 to 3 days elapse before psychiatric help is sought. The long interval between drug ingestion and the appearance of the patient in a clinic usually reflects the attempts of friends to deal with the psychosis by "talking down." Persons who lose consciousness are brought for help earlier than those who remain conscious. Most patients recover completely within a day or two, but some remain psychotic for as long as 2 weeks. Patients who are first seen in a coma often exhibit disorientation, hallucinations, confusion, and difficulty communicating on regaining consciousness. These symptoms may also be seen in noncomatose patients, but their symptoms appear to be less severe than those of comatose patients. Behavioral disturbances sometimes are severe; they may include public masturbation, stripping off clothes, violence, urinary incontinence, crying, and inappropriate laughing. Patients frequently have amnesia for the entire period of the psychosis.

A 17-year-old male was brought to the emergency room by the police, after being found, disoriented, on the street. As the police attempted to question him, he became increasingly agitated; when they attempted to restrain him, he became assaultive. Attempts to question or examine him in the emergency room evoked increased agitation. Initially it was impossible to determine vital signs or to draw blood. Based upon the observation of horizontal, vertical, and rotatory nystagmus, a diagnosis of PCP intoxication was entertained. Within a few minutes of being placed in a darkened examination room, his agitation decreased markedly.

His blood pressure was 170/100; other vital signs were within normal limits. Blood was drawn for toxicological examination. The patient agreed to take 20 mg of diazepam (Valium) orally. Thirty minutes later, he was less agitated and could be interviewed, although he responded to questions in a fragmented fashion and was slightly dysarthric. He stated that he must have inadvertently taken a larger-than-usual dose of "dust," which he reported having used once or twice a week for several years. He denied use of any other substance and any history of mental disorder. He was disoriented to time and place. The qualitative toxicology screen revealed PCP and no other drugs. Results of neurological examination were within normal limits but very brisk deep tendon reflexes were noted.

Some 90 minutes after arrival his temperature, initially normal, was 38°C, his blood pressure had increased to 182/110, and he responded poorly to stimulation. He was admitted to a medical bed. His blood pressure and level of consciousness continued to fluctuate over the ensuing 18 hours. Results of hematological and biochemical analyses of blood, as well as urinalyses, remained within normal limits. A history obtained from his family revealed that he had had multiple emergency-room visits for complications from PCP use during the previous several years. He had completed a 30-day residential treatment program and had participated in several outpatient programs but had consistently relapsed. The patient was discharged after vital signs and level of consciousness had been within normal limits for 8 hours. At discharge, nystagmus and dysarthria were no longer present. A referral to an outpatient treatment program was made. (Courtesy of Steven R. Zukin, M.D.)

PCP Intoxication Delirium

PCP intoxication delirium is included as a diagnostic category in DSM-IV-TR (see Table 10.2–3 in Section 10.2). An estimated 25 percent of all PCP-related emergency room patients may meet the criteria for the disorder, which can be characterized by agitated, violent, and bizarre behavior.

PCP-Induced Psychotic Disorder

PCP-induced psychotic disorder is included as a diagnostic category in DSM-IV-TR (see Table 14.4–7 in Section 14.4). Clinicians can further specify whether the predominant symptoms are delusions or hallucinations. An estimated 6 percent of PCP-related emergency room patients may meet the criteria for the disorder. About 40 percent of these patients have physical signs of hypertension and nystagmus, and 10 percent have been injured accidentally during the psychosis. The psychosis can last from 1 to 30 days, with an average of 4 to 5 days.

PCP-Induced Mood Disorder

PCP-induced mood disorder is included as a diagnostic category in DSM-IV-TR (see Table 15.3–10 in Section 15.3). An estimated 3 percent of PCP-related emergency room patients meet the criteria for the disorder, with most fitting the criteria for a maniclike episode. About 40 to 50 percent have been accidentally injured during the course of their manic symptoms.

PCP-Induced Anxiety Disorder

PCP-induced anxiety disorder is included as a diagnostic category in DSM-IV-TR (see Table 16.7–3 in Section 16.7). Anxiety is probably the most common symptom causing a PCP-intoxicated person to seek help in an emergency room.

PCP-Related Disorder Not Otherwise Specified

The diagnosis of PCP-related disorder not otherwise specified is the appropriate diagnosis for a patient who does not fit into any of the previously described diagnoses (Table 12.11–3).

Table 12.11–3
DSM-IV-TR Diagnostic Criteria for Phencyclidine-Related Disorder Not Otherwise Specified

The phencyclidine-related disorder not otherwise specified category is for disorders associated with the use of phencyclidine that are not classifiable as phencyclidine dependence, phencyclidine abuse, phencyclidine intoxication, phencyclidine intoxication delirium, phencyclidine-induced psychotic disorder, phencyclidine-induced mood disorder, or phencyclidine-induced anxiety disorder.

From American Psychiatric Association. *Diagnostic and Statistical Manual of Mental Disorders.* 4th ed. Text rev. Washington, DC: American Psychiatric Association; copyright 2000, with permission.

CLINICAL FEATURES

The amount of PCP varies greatly from PCP-laced cigarette to cigarette; 1 g may be used to make as few as four or as many as several dozen cigarettes. Less than 5 mg of PCP is considered a low dose, and doses above 10 mg are considered high. The variability of dose makes it difficult to predict the effect, although smoking PCP is the easiest and most reliable way for users to titrate the dose.

Persons who have just taken PCP are frequently uncommunicative, appear to be oblivious, and report active fantasy production. They experience speedy feelings, euphoria, bodily warmth, tingling, peaceful floating sensations, and, occasionally, feelings of depersonalization, isolation, and estrangement. Sometimes, they have auditory and visual hallucinations. They often have striking alterations of body image, distortions of space and time perception, and delusions. They may experience intensified dependence feelings, confusion, and disorganization of thought. Users may be sympathetic, sociable, and talkative at one moment but hostile and negative at another. Anxiety is sometimes reported; it is often the most prominent presenting symptom during an adverse reaction. Nystagmus, hypertension, and hyperthermia are common effects of PCP. Head-rolling movements, stroking, grimacing, muscle rigidity on stimulation, repeated episodes of vomiting, and repetitive chanting speech are sometimes observed.

The short-term effects last 3 to 6 hours and sometimes give way to a mild depression in which the user becomes irritable, somewhat paranoid, and occasionally belligerent, irrationally assaultive, suicidal, or homicidal. The effects can last for several days. Users sometimes find that it takes 1 to 2 days to recover completely; laboratory tests show that PCP may remain in the patient's blood and urine for more than a week.

DIFFERENTIAL DIAGNOSIS

Depending on a patient's status at the time of admission, the differential diagnosis may include sedative or narcotic overdose, psychotic disorder as a consequence of the use of psychedelic drugs, and brief psychotic disorder. Laboratory analysis may help to establish the diagnosis, particularly in the many cases in which the substance history is unreliable or unattainable.

TREATMENT AND REHABILITATION

The treatment for each of the PCP (or PCP-like)-related disorders is symptomatic. Talking down, which may work after hallucinogen use, is generally not useful for PCP intoxication. Benzodiazepines and dopamine receptor antagonists are the drugs of choice for controlling behavior pharmacologically. Physicians must monitor the patient's level of consciousness, blood pressure, temperature, and muscle activity and must be ready to treat severe medical abnormalities as necessary.

Clinicians must carefully monitor unconscious patients, particularly those who have toxic reactions to PCP; excessive secretions may interfere with already compromised respiration. In an alert patient who has recently taken PCP, gastric lavage presents a risk of inducing laryngeal spasm and aspiration of emesis. Muscle spasms and seizures are best treated with diazepam. The environment should afford minimal sensory stimulation. Ideally, one person stays with the patient in a quiet, dark room. Four-point restraint is dangerous because it may lead to rhabdomyolysis; total body immobilization may occasionally be necessary. A benzodiazepine is often effective in reducing agitation, but a patient with severe behavioral disturbances may require short-term treatment with a dopamine receptor antagonist—for example, haloperidol (Haldol). For patients with severe hypertension, a hypotensive-inducing drug such as phentolamine (Regitine) may be needed. Ammonium chloride in the early stage and ascorbic acid or cranberry juice later on are used to acidify the patient's urine and to promote the elimination of the substance, although the efficacy of the procedure is controversial.

If the symptoms are not severe and if the clinician can be certain that enough time has elapsed for all the PCP to have been absorbed, the patient may be monitored in the outpatient department and, if the symptoms improve, released to family or friends. Even at low doses, however, symptoms may worsen, and the person should be hospitalized to prevent violence and suicide.

In most cases, once any acute medical complications are successfully treated, both peripheral and central nervous system (CNS) complications, including psychosis, resolve completely within 24 to 72 hours. In the case of prolonged PCP-induced psychotic disorder, the rule is complete recovery within 4 to 6 weeks, regardless of whether antipsychotics have been administered. However, the rate of subsequent relapse to PCP use is very high. Persistence of a psychotic disorder beyond 8 weeks indicates the possible presence of an underlying psychotic disorder exacerbated, but not caused, by PCP.

Ketamine

Ketamine is a dissociative anesthetic agent, originally derived from PCP, that is available for use in human and veterinary medicine. It has become a drug of abuse, with sources exclusively from stolen supplies, and is available as a powder or in solution for intranasal, oral, inhalational, or (rarely) intravenous use. Ketamine functions by working at the NMDA receptor and, like PCP, can cause hallucinations and a dissociated state in which the patient has an altered sense of the body and reality and little concern for the environment.

Ketamine causes cardiovascular stimulation and no respiratory depression. On physical examination the patient may be hypertensive and tachycardic, have increased salivation, and have bidirectional and/or rotary nystagmus. The onset of action is within seconds when used intravenously, and analgesia lasting 40 minutes and dissociative effects lasting for hours have been described. Cardiovascular status should be monitored and supportive care administered. A dystonic reaction has been described, as have flashbacks, but a more common complication is related to a lack of concern for the environment or personal safety.

REFERENCES

Baldridge EB, Bessen HA. Phencyclidine. *Emerg Med Clin North Am.* 1990;8:541.

Gorelick DA, Wilkins JN. Inpatient treatment of PCP abusers and users. *Am J Drug Alcohol Abuse.* 1989;15:1.

Gorelick DA, Wilkins JN, Wong C. Outpatient treatment of PCP abusers. *Am J Drug Alcohol Abuse.* 1989;15:367.

Jansen KL. Ketamine: can chronic use impair memory? *Int J Addict.* 1990;25:133.

Javitt DC, Zukin SR. Recent advances in the phencyclidine model of schizophrenia. *Am J Psychiatry.* 1991;148:1301.
National Institute on Drug Abuse. *National Household Survey on Drug Abuse: Highlights, 1991.* Washington, DC: US Government Printing Office; 1991.
Polkis A, Graham M, Maginn D, Branch CA, Gantner GE. Phencyclidine and violent deaths in St. Louis, Missouri: a survey of medical examiners' cases from 1977 through 1986. *Am J Drug Alcohol Abuse.* 1990;16:265.
Rahbar F, Fomufod A, White D, Westney LS. Impact of intrauterine exposure to phencyclidine (PCP) and cocaine on neonates. *J Natl Med Assoc.* 1993;85:349.
Tabor BL, Smith-Wallace T, Yonekura ML. Perinatal outcome associated with PCP versus cocaine use. *Am J Drug Alcohol Abuse.* 1990;16:337.
Ubogu EE. Amaurosis fugax associated with phencyclidine inhalation. *Eur Neurol.* 2001;46:98.
Zukin SR. Phencyclidine (or phencyclidine-like)-related disorders. In: Sadock BJ, Sadock VA, eds. *Kaplan & Sadock's Comprehensive Textbook of Psychiatry.* 7th ed. Vol 1. Baltimore: Lippincott Williams & Wilkins; 2000:1063.

▲ 12.12 Sedative-, Hypnotic-, or Anxiolytic-Related Disorders

The drugs associated with this class of substance-related disorders are the benzodiazepines (e.g., diazepam [Valium], flunitrazepam [Rohypnol]), barbiturates (e.g., secobarbital [Seconal]), and the barbituratelike substances, which include methaqualone (formerly known as Quaalude) and meprobamate (Equanil). The major nonpsychiatric indications for these drugs are as antiepileptics, muscle relaxants, anesthetics, and anesthetic adjuvants. Alcohol and all drugs of this class are cross-tolerant, and their effects are additive. Physical and psychological dependence develop to all the drugs, and all are associated with withdrawal symptoms.

Sedatives are drugs that reduce subjective tension and induce mental calmness. The term *sedative* is virtually synonymous with the term *anxiolytic,* a drug that reduces anxiety. *Hypnotics* are drugs used to induce sleep. The differentiation between anxiolytics and sedatives as daytime drugs and hypnotics as nighttime drugs is not accurate. When sedatives and anxiolytics are given in high doses, they can induce sleep just as the hypnotics do. Conversely, when hypnotics are given in low doses, they can induce daytime sedation just as the sedatives and anxiolytics do. In some literature, especially older literature, the sedatives, anxiolytics, and hypnotics are grouped together as the *minor tranquilizers.* This term is poorly defined and subject to ambiguous meanings and, therefore, is best avoided.

SUBSTANCES

Benzodiazepines

Many benzodiazepines, differing primarily in their half-lives, are available in the United States. Examples of benzodiazepines are diazepam, flurazepam (Dalmane), oxazepam (Serax), and chlordiazepoxide (Librium). Benzodiazepines are used primarily as anxiolytics, hypnotics, antiepileptics, and anesthetics, as well as for alcohol withdrawal. After their introduction in the United States in the 1960s, benzodiazepines rapidly became the most prescribed drugs; about 15 percent of all persons in this country have had a benzodiazepine prescribed by a physician. Increasing awareness of the risks for dependence on benzodiazepines and increased regulatory requirements, however, have decreased the number of benzodiazepine prescriptions. The Drug Enforcement Agency (DEA) classifies all benzodiazepines as Schedule IV controlled substances.

Flunitrazepam, a benzodiazepine used in Mexico, South America, and Europe but not available in the United States, has become a drug of abuse. When taken with alcohol, it has been associated with promiscuous sexual behavior and rape. It is illegal to bring flunitrazepam into the United States. Although misused in the United States, it remains a standard anxiolytic in many countries.

Barbiturates

Before the introduction of benzodiazepines, barbiturates were frequently prescribed, but because of their high abuse potential, their use is much rarer today than in the past. Secobarbital (popularly known as "reds," "red devils," "seggies," and "downers"), pentobarbital (Nembutal) (known as "yellow jackets," "yellows," and "nembies"), and a secobarbital-amobarbital combination (known as "reds and blues," "rainbows," "double-trouble," and "tooies") are easily available on the street from drug dealers. Pentobarbital, secobarbital, and amobarbital (Amytal) are now under the same federal legal controls as morphine.

The first barbiturate, barbital (Veronal), was introduced in the United States in 1903. Barbital and phenobarbital (Solfoton, Luminal), which was introduced shortly thereafter, are long-acting drugs with half-lives of 12 to 24 hours. Amobarbital is an intermediate-acting barbiturate with a half-life of 6 to 12 hours. Pentobarbital and secobarbital are short-acting barbiturates with half-lives of 3 to 6 hours.

Barbituratelike Substances

The most commonly abused barbituratelike substance is methaqualone, which is no longer manufactured in the United States. It is often used by young persons who believe that the substance heightens the pleasure of sexual activity. Abusers of methaqualone commonly take one or two standard tablets (usually 300 mg per tablet) to obtain the desired effects. The street names for methaqualone include "mandrakes" (from the U.K. preparation Mandrax) and "soapers" (from the brand name Sopor). "Luding out" (from the brand name Quaalude) means getting high on methaqualone, which is often combined with excessive alcohol intake.

EPIDEMIOLOGY

According to DSM-IV-TR, about 6 percent of individuals have used either sedatives or tranquilizers illicitly, including 0.3 percent who reported illicit use of sedatives in the prior year and 0.1 percent who reported use of sedatives in the prior month. The age group with the highest lifetime prevalence of sedative (3 percent) or tranquilizer (6 percent) use was 26- to 34-year-olds, while those ages 18 to 25 were most likely to have used them in the prior year. About one quarter to one third of all substance-related emergency room visits involve substances of this class. The patients have a female-to-male ratio of 3 to 1 and a white-to-black ratio of 2 to 1. Some persons use benzodiazepines alone, but persons who use cocaine often use benzodiaz-

Table 12.12–1
DSM-IV-TR Sedative-, Hypnotic-, or Anxiolytic-Related Disorders

Sedative, hypnotic, or anxiolytic use disorders
Sedative, hypnotic, or anxiolytic dependence
Sedative, hypnotic, or anxiolytic abuse
Sedative-, hypnotic-, or anxiolytic-induced disorders
Sedative, hypnotic, or anxiolytic intoxication
Sedative, hypnotic, or anxiolytic withdrawal
Specify if:
With perceptual disturbances
Sedative, hypnotic, or anxiolytic intoxication delirium
Sedative, hypnotic, or anxiolytic withdrawal delirium
Sedative-, hypnotic-, or anxiolytic-induced persisting dementia
Sedative-, hypnotic-, or anxiolytic-induced psychotic disorder, with delusions
Specify if:
With onset during intoxication
With onset during withdrawal
Sedative-, hypnotic-, or anxiolytic-induced psychotic disorder, with hallucinations
Specify if:
With onset during intoxication
With onset during withdrawal
Sedative-, hypnotic-, or anxiolytic-induced mood disorder
Specify if:
With onset during intoxication
With onset during withdrawal
Sedative-, hypnotic-, or anxiolytic-induced anxiety disorder
Specify if:
With onset during withdrawal
Sedative-, hypnotic-, or anxiolytic-induced sexual dysfunction
Specify if:
With onset during intoxication
Sedative-, hypnotic-, or anxiolytic-induced sleep disorder
Specify if:
With onset during intoxication
With onset during withdrawal
Sedative-, hypnotic-, or anxiolytic-related disorder not otherwise specified

From American Psychiatric Association. *Diagnostic and Statistical Manual of Mental Disorders.* 4th ed. Text rev. Washington, DC: American Psychiatric Association; copyright 2000, with permission.

epines to reduce withdrawal symptoms, and opioid abusers use them to enhance the euphoric effects of opioids. Because they are easily obtained, benzodiazepines are also used by abusers of stimulants, hallucinogens, and phencyclidine (PCP) to help reduce the anxiety that can be caused by those substances.

Whereas barbiturate abuse is common among mature adults who have long histories of abuse of these substances, benzodiazepines are abused by a younger age group, usually under 40 years of age. This group may have a slight male predominance and has a white-to-black ratio of about 2 to 1. Benzodiazepines are probably not abused as frequently as other substances for the purpose of getting "high," or inducing a euphoric feeling. Rather, they are used when a person wishes to experience a general relaxed feeling.

NEUROPHARMACOLOGY

The benzodiazepines, barbiturates, and barbituratelike substances all have their primary effects on the γ-aminobutyric acid (GABA) type A ($GABA_A$) receptor complex, which contains a chloride ion channel, a binding site for GABA, and a well-defined binding site for benzodiazepines. The barbiturates and barbituratelike substances are also believed to bind somewhere on the $GABA_A$ receptor complex. When a benzodiazepine, barbiturate, or barbituratelike substance does bind to the complex, the effect is to increase the affinity of the receptor for its endogenous neurotransmitter, GABA, and to increase the flow of chloride ions through the channel into the neuron. The influx of negatively charged chloride ions into the neuron is inhibitory, and hyperpolarizes the neuron relative to the extracellular space.

Although all the substances in this class induce tolerance and physical dependence, the mechanisms behind these effects are best understood for the benzodiazepines. After long-term benzodiazepine use, the receptor effects caused by the agonist are attenuated. Specifically, GABA stimulation of the $GABA_A$ receptors results in less chloride influx than was caused by GABA stimulation before the benzodiazepine administration. This downregulation of receptor response is not due to a decrease in receptor number or to decreased affinity of the receptor for GABA. The basis for the downregulation seems to be in the coupling between the GABA binding site and the activation of the chloride ion channel. This decreased efficiency in coupling may be regulated within the $GABA_A$ receptor complex itself or by other neuronal mechanisms.

DIAGNOSIS

The text revision of the fourth edition of *Diagnostic and Statistical Manual of Mental Disorders* (DSM-IV-TR) lists a number of sedative-, hypnotic-, or anxiolytic-related disorders (Table 12.12–1), but includes specific diagnostic criteria only for sedative, hypnotic, or anxiolytic intoxication (Table 12.12–2) and

Table 12.12–2
DSM-IV-TR Diagnostic Criteria for Sedative, Hypnotic, or Anxiolytic Intoxication

A. Recent use of a sedative, hypnotic, or anxiolytic.
B. Clinically significant maladaptive behavioral or psychological changes (e.g., inappropriate sexual or aggressive behavior, mood lability, impaired judgment, impaired social or occupational functioning) that developed during, or shortly after, sedative, hypnotic, or anxiolytic use.
C. One (or more) of the following signs, developing during, or shortly after, sedative, hypnotic, or anxiolytic use:
(1) slurred speech
(2) incoordination
(3) unsteady gait
(4) nystagmus
(5) impairment in attention or memory
(6) stupor or coma
D. The symptoms are not due to a general medical condition and are not better accounted for by another mental disorder.

From American Psychiatric Association. *Diagnostic and Statistical Manual of Mental Disorders.* 4th ed. Text rev. Washington, DC: American Psychiatric Association; copyright 2000, with permission.

Table 12.12–3
DSM-IV-TR Diagnostic Criteria for Sedative, Hypnotic, or Anxiolytic Withdrawal

A. Cessation of (or reduction in) sedative, hypnotic, or anxiolytic use that has been heavy and prolonged.
B. Two (or more) of the following, developing within several hours to a few days after criterion A:
   (1) autonomic hyperactivity (e.g., sweating or pulse rate greater than 100)
   (2) increased hand tremor
   (3) insomnia
   (4) nausea or vomiting
   (5) transient visual, tactile, or auditory hallucinations or illusions
   (6) psychomotor agitation
   (7) anxiety
   (8) grand mal seizures
C. The symptoms in criterion B cause clinically significant distress or impairment in social, occupational, or other important areas of functioning.
D. The symptoms are not due to a general medical condition and are not better accounted for by another mental disorder.

Specify if:
With perceptual disturbances

From American Psychiatric Association. *Diagnostic and Statistical Manual of Mental Disorders.* 4th ed. Text rev. Washington, DC: American Psychiatric Association; copyright 2000, with permission.

sedative, hypnotic, or anxiolytic withdrawal (Table 12.12–3). The diagnostic criteria for other sedative-, hypnotic-, or anxiolytic-related disorders are outlined in the DSM-IV-TR sections that are specific for the major symptom—for example, sedative-, hypnotic-, or anxiolytic-induced psychotic disorder (see Table 14.4–7 in Section 14.4 of Chapter 14).

Dependence and Abuse

Sedative, hypnotic, or anxiolytic dependence and sedative, hypnotic, or anxiolytic abuse are diagnosed according to the general criteria in DSM-IV-TR for substance dependence and substance abuse (see Tables 12.1–5, 12.1–6, and 12.1–7).

Intoxication

DSM-IV-TR contains a single set of diagnostic criteria for intoxication by any sedative, hypnotic, or anxiolytic substance (Table 12.12–2). Although the intoxication syndromes induced by all these drugs are similar, subtle clinical differences are observable, especially with intoxications that involve low doses. The diagnosis of intoxication by one of this class of substances is best confirmed by obtaining a blood sample for substance screening.

Benzodiazepines. Benzodiazepine intoxication can be associated with behavioral disinhibition, potentially resulting in hostile or aggressive behavior in some persons. The effect is perhaps most common when benzodiazepines are taken in combination with alcohol. Benzodiazepine intoxication is associated with less euphoria than is intoxication by other drugs in this class. This characteristic is the basis for the lower abuse and dependence potential of benzodiazepines than of barbiturates.

Barbiturates and Barbituratelike Substances. When barbiturates and barbituratelike substances are taken in relatively low doses, the clinical syndrome of intoxication is indistinguishable from that associated with alcohol intoxication. The symptoms include sluggishness, incoordination, difficulty thinking, poor memory, slow speech and comprehension, faulty judgment, disinhibited sexual aggressive impulses, narrowed range of attention, emotional lability, and exaggerated basic personality traits. The sluggishness usually resolves after a few hours, but depending primarily on the half-life of the abused substance, impaired judgment, distorted mood, and impaired motor skills may remain for 12 to 24 hours. Other potential symptoms are hostility, argumentativeness, moroseness, and, occasionally, paranoid and suicidal ideation. The neurological effects include nystagmus, diplopia, strabismus, ataxic gait, positive Romberg's sign, hypotonia, and decreased superficial reflexes.

Withdrawal

DSM-IV-TR contains a single set of diagnostic criteria for withdrawal from any sedative, hypnotic, or anxiolytic substance (Table 12.12–3). Clinicians can specify "with perceptual disturbances" if illusions, altered perceptions, or hallucinations are present but accompanied by intact reality testing. Remember that benzodiazepines are associated with a withdrawal syndrome and that withdrawal from barbiturates can be life threatening. Withdrawal from benzodiazepines can also result in serious medical complications, such as seizures.

Benzodiazepines. The severity of the withdrawal syndrome associated with the benzodiazepines varies significantly depending on the average dose and the duration of use, but a mild withdrawal syndrome can follow even short-term use of relatively low doses of benzodiazepines. A significant withdrawal syndrome is likely to occur at cessation of dosages in the 40-mg-a-day range for diazepam, for example, although 10 to 20 mg a day, taken for a month, can also result in a withdrawal syndrome when drug administration is stopped. The onset of withdrawal symptoms usually occurs 2 to 3 days after the cessation of use, but with long-acting drugs, such as diazepam, the latency before onset may be 5 or 6 days. The symptoms include anxiety, dysphoria, intolerance for bright lights and loud noises, nausea, sweating, muscle twitching, and sometimes seizures (generally at dosages of 50 mg a day or more of diazepam).

Barbiturates and Barbituratelike Substances. The withdrawal syndrome for barbiturate and barbituratelike substances ranges from mild symptoms (e.g., anxiety, weakness, sweating, and insomnia) to severe symptoms (e.g., seizures, delirium, cardiovascular collapse, and death). Persons who have been abusing phenobarbital in the range of 400 mg a day may experience mild withdrawal symptoms; those who have been abusing the substance in the range of 800 mg a day experience orthostatic hypotension, weakness, tremor, and severe anxiety. About 75 percent of these persons have withdrawal-related seizures. Users of dosages higher than 800 mg a day may experience anorexia, delirium, hallucinations, and repeated seizures.

Most symptoms appear in the first 3 days of abstinence, and seizures generally occur on the second or third day, when the symptoms are worst. If seizures do occur, they always precede the development of delirium. The symptoms rarely occur more than a week after stopping the substance. A psychotic disorder, if it develops, starts on the third to eighth day. The various associated symptoms generally run their course within 2 to 3 days but may last as long as 2 weeks. The first episode of the syndrome usually occurs after 5 to 15 years of heavy substance use.

Delirium

DSM-IV-TR allows for the diagnosis of sedative, hypnotic, or anxiolytic intoxication delirium and sedative, hypnotic, or anxiolytic withdrawal delirium (see Tables 10.2–3 and 10.2–4 in Section 10.2). Delirium that is indistinguishable from delirium tremens associated with alcohol withdrawal is seen more commonly with barbiturate withdrawal than with benzodiazepine withdrawal. Delirium associated with intoxication can be seen with either barbiturates or benzodiazepines if the dosages are high enough.

Persisting Dementia

DSM-IV-TR allows for the diagnosis of sedative-, hypnotic-, or anxiolytic-induced persisting dementia (see Table 10.3–5). The existence of the disorder is controversial, since there is uncertainty whether a persisting dementia is due to the substance use itself or to associated features of the substance use. One must evaluate the diagnosis further by using DSM-IV-TR criteria to ascertain validity.

Persisting Amnestic Disorder

DSM-IV-TR allows for the diagnosis of sedative-, hypnotic-, or anxiolytic-induced persisting amnestic disorder (see Table 10.4–3 in Section 10.4). Amnestic disorders associated with sedatives, hypnotics, and anxiolytics may be underdiagnosed. One exception is the increased number of reports of amnestic episodes associated with short-term use of benzodiazepines with short half-lives (e.g., triazolam [Halcion]).

Psychotic Disorders

The psychotic symptoms of barbiturate withdrawal can be indistinguishable from those of alcohol-associated delirium tremens. Agitation, delusions, and hallucinations are usually visual, but sometimes tactile or auditory features develop after about 1 week of abstinence. Psychotic symptoms associated with intoxication or withdrawal are more common with barbiturates than with benzodiazepines and are diagnosed as sedative-, hypnotic-, or anxiolytic-induced psychotic disorders (see Table 14.4–7). Clinicians can further specify whether delusions or hallucinations are the predominant symptoms.

Other Disorders

Sedative, hypnotic, and anxiolytic use has also been associated with mood disorders (see Table 15.3–10 in Section 15.3), anxiety disorders (see Table 16.7–3 in Section 16.7), sleep disorders (see Table 24.2–20 in Section 24.2), and sexual dysfunctions (see Table 21.2–12 in Section 21.2). When none of the previously discussed diagnostic categories is appropriate for a person with a sedative, hypnotic, or anxiolytic use disorder, the appropriate diagnosis is sedative-, hypnotic-, or anxiolytic-related disorder not otherwise specified (Table 12.12–4).

Table 12.12–4
DSM-IV-TR Diagnostic Criteria for Sedative-, Hypnotic-, or Anxiolytic-Related Disorder Not Otherwise Specified

The sedative-, hypnotic-, or anxiolytic-related disorder not otherwise specified category is for disorders associated with the use of sedatives, hypnotics, or anxiolytics that are not classifiable as sedative, hypnotic, or anxiolytic dependence; sedative, hypnotic, or anxiolytic abuse; sedative, hypnotic, or anxiolytic intoxication; sedative, hypnotic, or anxiolytic withdrawal; sedative, hypnotic, or anxiolytic intoxication delirium; sedative, hypnotic, or anxiolytic withdrawal delirium; sedative-, hypnotic-, or anxiolytic-induced persisting dementia; sedative-, hypnotic-, or anxiolytic-induced persisting amnestic disorder; sedative-, hypnotic-, or anxiolytic-induced psychotic disorder; sedative-, hypnotic-, or anxiolytic-induced mood disorder; sedative-, hypnotic-, or anxiolytic-induced anxiety disorder; sedative-, hypnotic-, or anxiolytic-induced sexual dysfunction; or sedative-, hypnotic-, or anxiolytic-induced sleep disorder.

From American Psychiatric Association. *Diagnostic and Statistical Manual of Mental Disorders.* 4th ed. Text rev. Washington, DC: American Psychiatric Association; copyright 2000, with permission.

CLINICAL FEATURES

Patterns of Abuse

Oral Use. Sedatives, hypnotics, and anxiolytics can all be taken orally, either occasionally to achieve a time-limited specific effect or regularly to obtain a constant, usually mild, intoxication state. The occasional use pattern is associated with young persons who take the substance to achieve specific effects—relaxation for an evening, intensification of sexual activities, and a short-lived period of mild euphoria. The user's personality and expectations about the substance's effects and the setting in which the substance is taken also affect the substance-induced experience. The regular use pattern is associated with middle-aged, middle-class persons who usually obtain the substance from a family physician as a prescription for insomnia or anxiety. Abusers of this type may have prescriptions from several physicians, and the pattern of abuse may go undetected until obvious signs of abuse or dependence are noticed by the person's family, coworkers, or physicians.

Intravenous Use. A severe form of abuse involves the intravenous use of this class of substances. The users are mainly young adults intimately involved with illegal substances. Intravenous barbiturate use is associated with a pleasant, warm, drowsy feeling, and users may be inclined to use barbiturates more than opioids because barbiturates are less costly. The physical dangers of injection include transmission of the human immunodeficiency virus (HIV), cellulitis, vascular complications from accidental injection into an artery, infec-

Table 12.12–5
Approximate Therapeutic Equivalent Doses of Benzodiazepines

Generic Name	Trade Name	Dose (mg)
Alprazolam	Xanax	1
Chlordiazepoxide	Librium	25
Clonazepam	Klonopin	0.5–1
Clorazepate	Tranxene	15
Diazepam	Valium	10
Estazolam	ProSom	1
Flurazepam	Dalmane	30
Lorazepam	Ativan	2
Oxazepam	Serax	30
Prazepam	Paxipam	80
Temazepam	Restoril	20
Triazolam	Halcion	0.25
Quazepam	Doral	15
Zolpidem[a]	Ambien	10

[a]An imidazopyridine benzodiazepine agonist.

tions, and allergic reactions to contaminants. Intravenous use is associated with rapid and profound tolerance and dependence and a severe withdrawal syndrome.

Overdose

Benzodiazepines. In contrast to the barbiturates and the barbituratelike substances, the benzodiazepines have a large margin of safety when taken in overdoses, a feature that contributed significantly to their rapid acceptance. The ratio of lethal dose to effective dose is about 200 to 1 or higher, because of the minimal degree of respiratory depression associated with the benzodiazepines. A list of equivalent therapeutic doses of benzodiazepines is given in Table 12.12–5. Even when grossly excessive amounts (more than 2 g) are taken in suicide attempts, the symptoms include only drowsiness, lethargy, ataxia, some confusion, and mild depression of the user's vital signs. A much more serious condition prevails when benzodiazepines are taken in overdose in combination with other sedative-hypnotic substances, such as alcohol. In such cases, small doses of benzodiazepines can cause death. The availability of flumazenil (Romazicon), a specific benzodiazepine antagonist, has reduced the lethality of the benzodiazepines. Flumazenil can be used in emergency rooms to reverse the effects of the benzodiazepines.

Barbiturates. Barbiturates are lethal when taken in overdose because they induce respiratory depression. In addition to intentional suicide attempts, accidental or unintentional overdoses are common. Barbiturates in home medicine cabinets are a common cause of fatal drug overdoses in children. As with benzodiazepines, the lethal effects of the barbiturates are additive to those of other sedatives or hypnotics, including alcohol and benzodiazepines. Barbiturate overdose is characterized by the induction of coma, respiratory arrest, cardiovascular failure, and death.

The lethal dose varies with the route of administration and the degree of tolerance for the substance after a history of long-term abuse. For the most commonly abused barbiturates, the ratio of lethal dose to effective dose ranges between 3 to 1 and 30 to 1. Dependent users often take an average daily dose of 1.5 g of a short-acting barbiturate, and some have been reported to take as much as 2.5 g a day for months.

The lethal dose is not much greater for the long-term abuser than for the neophyte. Tolerance develops quickly to the point at which withdrawal in a hospital becomes necessary to prevent accidental death from overdose.

Barbituratelike Substances. The barbituratelike substances vary in their lethality and are usually intermediate between the relative safety of the benzodiazepines and the high lethality of the barbiturates. An overdose of methaqualone, for example, may result in restlessness, delirium, hypertonia, muscle spasms, convulsions, and, in very high doses, death. Unlike barbiturates, methaqualone rarely causes severe cardiovascular or respiratory depression, and most fatalities result from combining methaqualone with alcohol.

TREATMENT AND REHABILITATION

Withdrawal

Benzodiazepines. Because some benzodiazepines are eliminated from the body slowly, symptoms of withdrawal may continue to develop for several weeks. To prevent seizures and other withdrawal symptoms, clinicians should gradually reduce the dosage. Several reports indicate that carbamazepine (Tegretol) may be useful in the treatment of benzodiazepine withdrawal. Table 12.12–6 lists guidelines for treating benzodiazepine withdrawal.

Barbiturates. To avoid sudden death during barbiturate withdrawal, clinicians must follow conservative clinical guidelines. Clinicians should not give barbiturates to a comatose or grossly intoxicated patient. A clinician should attempt to determine a patient's usual daily dose of barbiturates and then verify the dosage clinically. For example, a clinician can give a test dose of 200 mg of pentobarbital every hour until a mild intoxication occurs but withdrawal symptoms are absent (Table 12.12–7). The clinician can then taper the total daily dose at a rate of about 10 percent of the total daily dose. Once the correct dosage is determined, a long-acting barbiturate can be used for the detoxification period. During this process, the patient may begin to experience withdrawal symptoms, in which case the clinician should halve the daily decrement.

In the withdrawal procedure, phenobarbital may be substituted for the more commonly abused short-acting barbiturates. The effects of phenobarbital last longer, and because there is less fluctuation of barbiturate blood levels, phenobarbital does not cause observable toxic signs or a serious overdose. An adequate dose is 30 mg of phenobarbital for every 100 mg of the short-acting substance. The user should be maintained for at least 2 days at that level before the dosage is reduced further. The regimen is analogous to the substitution of methadone for heroin.

After withdrawal is complete, the patient must overcome the desire to start taking the substance again. Although substitution of nonbarbiturate sedatives or hypnotics for barbiturates has been suggested as a preventive therapeutic measure, this often

Table 12.12–6
Guidelines for Treatment of Benzodiazepine Withdrawal

1. Evaluate and treat concomitant medical and psychiatric conditions
2. Obtain drug history and urine and blood sample for drug and ethanol assay
3. Determine required dose of benzodiazepine or barbiturate for stabilization, guided by history, clinical presentation, drug-ethanol assay, and (in some cases) challenge dose
4. Detoxification from supratherapeutic dosages:
   a. Hospitalize if there are medical or psychiatric indications, poor social supports, or polysubstance dependence or the patient is unreliable
   b. Some clinicians recommend switching to longer-acting benzodiazepine for withdrawal (e.g., diazepam, clonazepam); others recommend stabilizing on the drug that patient was taking or on phenobarbital
   c. After stabilization reduce dosage by 30 percent on the second or third day and evaluate the response, keeping in mind that symptoms that occur after decreases in benzodiazepines with short elimination half-lives (e.g., lorazepam) appear sooner than with those with longer elimination half-lives (e.g., diazepam)
   d. Reduce dosage further by 10 to 25 percent every few days if tolerated
   e. Use adjunctive medications if necessary—carbamazepine, β-adrenergic receptor antagonists, valproate, clonidine, and sedative antidepressants have been used but their efficacy in the treatment of the benzodiazepine abstinence syndrome has not been established)
5. Detoxification from therapeutic dosages:
   a. Initiate 10 to 25 percent dose reduction and evaluate response
   b. Dose, duration of therapy, and severity of anxiety influence the rate of taper and need for adjunctive medications
   c. Most patients taking therapeutic doses have uncomplicated discontinuation
6. Psychological interventions may assist patients in detoxification from benzodiazepines and in the long-term management of anxiety

Courtesy of Domenic A. Ciraulo, M.D., and Ofra Sarid-Segal, M.D.

Table 12.12–7
Pentobarbital Test Dose Procedure for Barbiturate Withdrawal

Symptoms after Test Dose of 200 mg Oral Pentobarbital	Estimated 24-Hour Oral Pentobarbital Dose (mg)	Estimated 24-Hour Oral Phenobarbital Dose (mg)
Level I: Asleep but arousable; withdrawal symptoms not likely	0	0
Level II: Mild sedation; patient may have slurred speech, ataxia, nystagmus	500–600	150–200
Level III: Patient is comfortable: no evidence of sedation; may have nystagmus	800	250
Level IV: No drug effect	1,000–1,200	300–600

Modified from Ciraulo DA, Shader RI, eds. *Clinical Manual of Chemical Dependence.* Washington, DC: American Psychiatric Press; 1991. From data in Ewing JA, Bakewell WE. Diagnosis and management of depressant drug dependence. *Am J Psychiatry* 1967;123:909.

results in replacing one substance dependence with another. If a user is to remain substance free, follow-up treatment, usually with psychiatric help and community support, is vital. Otherwise, a patient will almost certainly return to barbiturates or a substance with similar hazards.

Overdose

The treatment of overdose of this class of substances involves gastric lavage, activated charcoal, and careful monitoring of vital signs and central nervous system (CNS) activity. Overdose patients who come to medical attention while awake should be kept from slipping into unconsciousness. Vomiting should be induced, and activated charcoal should be administered to delay gastric absorption. If a patient is comatose, the clinician must establish an intravenous fluid line, monitor the patient's vital signs, insert an endotracheal tube to maintain a patent airway, and provide mechanical ventilation if necessary. Hospitalization of a comatose patient in an intensive care unit is usually required during the early stages of recovery from such overdoses.

LEGAL ISSUES

State and federal agencies have attempted to restrict the distribution of benzodiazepines by requiring special reporting forms. For example, through the use of New York State official prescription forms (formerly called *triplicate forms*), the names of doctors and patients are kept on file in a data bank. Governments have taken such measures to stem the tide of abuse. But most abuse results from the illicit manufacture, sale, and diversion of substances, particularly to cocaine and opioid addicts, not from physicians' prescriptions or legitimate pharmaceutical companies. The attempt to curtail the use of substances with unquestionable, invaluable therapeutic benefits exemplifies increasing government interference in the practice of medicine and in the confidential relationship between doctor and patient. Such restrictions do little to curb cocaine, opioid, or benzodiazepine abuse.

The number of benzodiazepine prescriptions decreased in New York State after the use of government forms was legislated. Whether or not this decrease was due to improved medical prescribing standards of practice or to the intimidation of physicians—or both—remains open to question. New York is now among 18 states that regulate Schedule II controlled substances with state-issued forms. In 1991, a symposium sponsored by the Medical Society of the State of New York concluded that triplicate prescriptions jeopardize patient care. The disadvantages of New York's program were summarized after conducting a survey of 1,513 physicians (Table 12.12–8).

Recent surveys of psychiatric patients (except those diagnosed as substance abusers) have demonstrated high rates of benzodiazepine prescription use but almost uniformly low abuse; thus physicians should not withhold benzodiazepines from their patients with emotional problems for fear of abuse.

Table 12.12–8
Disadvantages of New York's Triplicate Prescription Program

	%[a]
Inappropriately allows legislators to dictate practice of medicine	75
Consumes too much physician time	74
Violates physician–patient confidentiality	64
Imposes unnecessary physician monitoring	56
Increases cost burden to patients	49
Poses benzodiazepine withdrawal concerns	29
Other disadvantages	20
Increases possibility of robbery and assault	
Requires physician to practice defensive or reactive medicine	
Increases expense to physician	
Has not been proven to eliminate drug abuse	
Increases possibility of malpractice liability	
Forces prescribing of less efficacious, more hazardous medications	
Sets precedent for further government controls	
Coerces patient to seek alternative sources of drugs	

[a]Percentages reflect proportion of those ($N = 1,185$) who thought that the triplicate prescription program had any advantages.
Reprinted with permission from highlights of the symposium, "Triplicate Prescription: Issues and Answers," sponsored by the Medical Society of the State of New York, February 28, 1991.

References

American Psychiatric Association. *Benzodiazepine Dependence, Toxicity, and Abuse*. Washington, DC: American Psychiatric Association; 1990.

Ciraulo, DA, Sarid-Segal O. Sedative-, hypnotic-, or anxiolytic-related disorders. In: Sadock BJ, Sadock VA, eds. *Kaplan & Sadock's Comprehensive Textbook of Psychiatry*. 7th ed. Vol 1. Baltimore: Lippincott Williams & Wilkins; 2000:1071.

Cole JO, Chaiarello RJ. The benzodiazepines as drugs of abuse. *J Psychiatr Res*. 1990;24(3 suppl 2):135.

Juergens SM. Benzodiazepines and addiction. *Psychiatr Clin North Am*. 1993;16:75.

Klein RL, Whiting PJ, Harris RA. Benzodiazepine treatment causes uncoupling of recombinant GABA-A receptors expressed in stably transfected cells. *J Neurochem*. 1994;63:2349.

Lader M, Farr I, Morton S. A comparison of alpidem and placebo in relieving benzodiazepine withdrawal symptoms. *Int Clin Psychopharmacol*. 1993; 8:31.

Nutt DJ. Pharmacological mechanisms of benzodiazepine withdrawal. *J Psychiatr Res*. 1990;24(3 suppl 2):105.

Pandit SA, Argyropoulos S, Nutt DJ. Current status of anxiolytic drugs. *Prim Care Psychiatry*. 2001;7:1.

Patterson JF. Withdrawal from alprazolam dependency using clonazepam: clinical observations. *J Clin Psychiatry*. 1990;51(9 suppl):47.

Piper A Jr. Addiction to benzodiazepines—how common? *Arch Fam Med*. 1995;4:964.

Rickels K, Schweizer E, Case WG, Greenblatt DJ. Long-term therapeutic use of benzodiazepines: I. Effects of abrupt discontinuation. *Arch Gen Psychiatry*. 1990;47:899.

Romach M, Busto U, Somer G, Kaplan HL, Sellers E. Clinical aspects of chronic use of alprazolam and lorazepam. *Am J Psychiatry*. 1995;152:1161.

Schweizer E, Rickels K, Case WG, Greenblatt DJ. Long-term therapeutic use of benzodiazepines: II. Effects of gradual taper. *Arch Gen Psychiatry*. 1990;47:908.

Schweizer E, Rickels K, Case WG, Greenblatt DJ. Carbamazepine treatment in patients discontinuing long-term benzodiazepine therapy: effects on withdrawal severity and outcome. *Arch Gen Psychiatry*. 1991;48:448.

Seiverwright N, Dougal W. Withdrawal symptoms from high dose benzodiazepines in poly drug users. *Drug Alcohol Depend*. 1993;32:15.

Staley KJ, Soldo BL, Proctor WR. Ionic mechanisms of neuronal excitation by inhibitory GABAA receptors. *Science*. 1995;269:977.

▲ 12.13 Anabolic Steroid Abuse

The anabolic steroids are a family of drugs that includes the natural male hormone testosterone and a group of many synthetic analogues of testosterone synthesized since the 1940s (Table 12.13–1). All these drugs possess various degrees of *anabolic* (muscle-building) and *androgenic* (masculinizing) effects.

Many synthetic anabolic steroids, such as Dianabol, Anavar, and Winstrol-V, are now available in oral, transdermal, and intramuscular formulations. Anabolic steroids are Schedule III drugs and therefore are subject to the same regulatory dispensing requirements as narcotics. Although anabolic steroids have legitimate medical uses, they are used illegally to enhance physical performance and appearance and to increase muscle bulk.

EPIDEMIOLOGY

An estimated 1 million persons in the United States have used illegal steroids at least once. Users are primarily middle class and white. Male users of anabolic steroids greatly outnumber female users by approximately 6 to 1; about half the users started before the age of 16. In one survey, 1.5 percent of persons surveyed reported a lifetime nonmedical use of these drugs. The highest use was among 18- to 25-year-olds, and 26- to 34-year-olds had the next highest rate of use. Estimates for the rate of use in body builders have ranged up to 50 to 80 percent.

Table 12.13–1
Examples of Commonly Used Anabolic Steroids[a]

Compounds usually administered orally
Fluoxymesterone (Halotestin, Android-F, Ultandren)
Methandienone (formerly called methandrostenolone) (Dianabol)
Methyltestosterone (Android, Testred, Virilon)
Mibolerone (Cheque Drops[b])
Oxandrolone (Anavar)
Oxymetholone (Anadrol, Hemogenin)
Mesterolone (Mestoranum, Proviron)
Stanozolol (Winstrol)
Compounds usually administered intramuscularly
Nandrolone decanoate (Deca-Durabolin)
Nandrolone phenpropionate (Durabolin)
Methenolone enanthate (Primobolan depot)
Boldenone undecylenate (Equipoise[b])
Stanozolol (Winstrol-V[b])
Testosterone esters blends (Sustanon, Sten)
Testosterone cypionate
Testosterone enanthate (Delatestryl)
Testosterone propionate (Testoviron, Androlan)
Testosterone undecanoate (Andriol, Restandol)
Trenbolone acetate (Finajet, Finaplix[b])
Trenbolone hexahydrobencylcarbonate (Parabolan)

[a]Many of the brand names listed above are foreign, but are included because of the widespread illicit use of foreign steroid preparations in the United States.
[b]Veterinary compound.

NEUROPHARMACOLOGY

After oral administration of testosterone, only small amounts of the drug reach systemic circulation unchanged. The low bioavailability of orally administered testosterone results from metabolism of the drug in the gastrointestinal mucosa during first pass through the liver. The synthetic androgens (e.g., fluoxymesterone and methyltestosterone) are also less extensively metabolized following oral administration. In plasma, testosterone is 98 percent bound to a specific testosterone-estradiol-binding globulin. The plasma half-life of testosterone reportedly ranges from 10 to 100 minutes. Testosterone is metabolized principally in the liver to various 17-ketosteroids.

ETIOLOGY

Persons who use these drugs are usually involved in activities that require strength and endurance. These users include athletes involved in track and field, weight lifters, and others who desire extraordinary performance, usually in competitive sports settings. Use is reinforced if the drug-taking behavior results in a desired result, such as increased muscle mass or prolonged endurance. Psychodynamic vulnerability to anabolic steroid misuse includes low self-esteem and disturbances in the image and appearance of the body. Adolescent users—both heterosexual and homosexual—equate an Adonis-like body with the ability to attract sexual partners. These drugs may also be used to deny perceived narcissistic deficiencies.

DIAGNOSIS AND CLINICAL FEATURES

Because of their psychiatric effects, anabolic steroids have come to the attention of psychiatrists. Steroids may initially induce euphoria and hyperactivity. After relatively short periods, however, their use can become associated with increased anger, arousal, irritability, hostility, anxiety, somatization, and depression (especially during times when steroids are not used). Several studies have demonstrated that 2 to 15 percent of anabolic steroid abusers experience hypomanic or manic episodes, and a smaller percentage may have clearly psychotic symptoms. Also disturbing is a correlation between steroid abuse and violence ("roid rage" in the parlance of users). Steroid abusers with no record of antisocial behavior or violence have committed murders and other violent crimes.

Steroids are addictive substances. When abusers stop taking steroids, they can become depressed, anxious, and concerned about their bodies' physical state. Some similarities have been noted between athletes' views of their muscles and the views of patients with anorexia nervosa about their bodies; to an observer, both groups seem to distort realistic assessment of the body.

Iatrogenic addiction is a consideration in view of the increasing number of geriatric patients who are receiving testosterone from their physicians in an attempt to increase libido and reverse some aspects of aging.

Adverse Effects

Anabolic Steroids. Anabolic steroid use has obvious physical effects. Steroid use causes rapid development and enhancement of muscle bulk, definition, and power. Men who abuse steroids may have acne, premature balding, yellowing of the skin and the eyes, gynecomastia, and decreased size of the testicles and the prostate. Young boys abusing steroids can have painful enlargement of the genitalia. The use of steroids in young adolescents can also lead to stunted growth by causing premature closure of the bone plates. In women who abuse steroids, the voice may deepen, the breasts shrink, the clitoris enlarges, and the menstrual cycle becomes irregular.

Anabolic steroid use can also produce abnormal liver function test results, decrease high-density lipoprotein blood levels, and increase low-density lipoprotein blood levels. Decreased spermatogenesis has been reported, as has an association between anabolic steroid abuse and myocardial infarction and cerebrovascular diseases.

Adverse effects in women include clitoral enlargement (which may be irreversible), menstrual problems, alopecia or hirsutism, deepened voice (also irreversible), and acne.

Dehydroepiandrosterone (DHEA) and Androstenedione. DHEA and androstenedione are adrenal androgens marketed as food supplements and sold over the counter in health food stores. They are not approved or regulated by the Food and Drug Administration. They are steroid precursors of both androgens and estrogens; persons taking these substances report increased physical and psychological well-being. The adverse effects of the drugs in high doses are similar to those of anabolic steroids and include voice change, acne, hirsutism, and prostatic cancer. Because DHEA is available in U.S. health food stores and may have addictive potential, increased reports of misuse and adverse effects should be expected.

Mr. A. is a 26-year-old single white man. He is 69 inches tall and presently weights 204 pounds with a body fat of 11 percent. He reports that he began lifting weights at age 17, at which time he weighed 155 pounds. Within a year of beginning his weightlifting he began taking anabolic steroids after obtaining them through a friend at his gymnasium. His first cycle of steroids, lasting for 9 weeks, involved methandienone, 30 mg orally a day, and testosterone cypionate, 600 mg intramuscularly a week. During these 9 weeks he gained 20 pounds of muscle mass. He was so pleased with these results that he took five further cycles of anabolic steroids over the next 6 years. During his most ambitious cycle, approximately 1 year ago, he used testosterone cypionate, 600 mg per week; nandrolone decanoate (Deca-Durabolin), 400 mg a week; stanozolol (Winstrol), 12 mg a day; and oxandrolone (Anavar), 10 mg a day.

During each of the cycles Mr. A. has noted euphoria, irritability, and grandiose feelings. These symptoms were most prominent during his most recent cycle, when he felt invincible. During this cycle he also noted a decreased need for sleep, racing thoughts, and a tendency to spend excessive amounts of money. For example, he impulsively purchased a $2,700 stereo system when he realistically could not afford to spend more than $500. He also became uncharacteristically irritable with his girlfriend, and on one occasion put his fist through the side window of her car during an argument—an act inconsistent with his normally mild-mannered

personality. After this cycle of steroids ended, he became moderately depressed for about 2 months, with hypersomnia, anorexia, markedly decreased libido, and occasional suicidal ideation.

Mr. A. smoked marijuana almost daily during his last 2 years of high school and continues to smoke at least twice a week. He has experimented briefly with hallucinogens, cocaine, opiates, and stimulants, but has rarely used them in the last 5 years. However, he has used a number of drugs to lose weight in preparation for bodybuilding contests. These include ephedrine, amphetamine, triiodothyronine, and thyroxin. Recently, he has also begun to use the opioid agonist-antagonist nalbuphine (Nubain) intravenously to treat muscle aches from weightlifting. He reports that intravenous nalbuphine use is widespread among other anabolic steroid users of his acquaintance.

Mr. A. exhibits characteristic features of muscle dysmorphia. He checks his appearance dozens of times a day in mirrors, or when he sees his reflection in a store window or even in the back of a spoon. He becomes anxious if he misses even one day of working out at the gym, and acknowledges that his preoccupation with weightlifting has cost him both social and occupational opportunities. Although he has a 48-inch chest and 19-inch biceps, he has frequently declined invitations to go to the beach or a swimming pool for fear that he would look too small when seen in a bathing suit. He is anxious because he has lost some weight since the end of his previous cycle of steroids and is eager to resume another cycle of anabolic steroids in the near future. (Courtesy of Harrison G. Pope, Jr., M.D., and Kirk J. Brower, M.D.)

References

Abromowitz M. Dehydroepiandrosterone (DHEA). *Med Lett Drug Ther.* 1996;38:91.

Brower KJ. Anabolic steroids: a mind-body problem. *Psychiatry Ann.* 1992;22:2.

Clancy GP, Yates WR. Anabolic steroid use among substance abusers in treatment. *J Clin Psychiatry.* 1992;53:97.

DuRant RH, Rickert VI, Ashworth CS, et al. Use of multiple drugs among adolescents who use anabolic steroids. *N Engl J Med.* 1993;328:922.

Gonzalez A, McLachlan S, Keaney F. Anabolic steroid misuse: how much should we know? *Int J Psychiatry Clin Pract.* 2001;5:159.

Gruber AJ, Pope HG Jr. Psychiatric and medical effects of anabolic-androgenic steroid use in women. *Psychother Psychosom.* 2000;16:195.

Pope HG, Brower KJ. Anabolic-androgenic steroid abuse. In: Sadock BJ, Sadock VA, eds. *Kaplan & Sadock's Comprehensive Textbook of Psychiatry.* 7th ed. Vol 1. Baltimore: Lippincott Williams & Wilkins; 2000:1985.

▲ 12.14 Other Substance-Related Disorders

Substances that can be categorized according to some schema are described in the sections above. This section deals with a diverse group of drugs not covered above that cannot be easily grouped together. The text revision of the fourth edition of *Diagnostic and Statistical Manual of Mental Disorders* (DSM-IV-TR) includes a diagnostic category for these substances called other (or unknown) substance-related disorders (Table 12.14–1). Some of these substances are discussed below.

GAMMA HYDROXYBUTYRATE (GHB)

GHB is a naturally occurring transmitter in the brain that is related to sleep regulation. GHB increases dopamine levels in the brain. In general, GHB is a central nervous system (CNS) depressant with effects through the endogenous opioid system. It is used to induce anesthesia and long-term sedation, but its unpredictable duration of action limits its use. It has recently been studied for the treatment of alcohol and opioid withdrawal and narcolepsy.

Until 1990, GHB was sold in U.S. health food stores, and body builders used it as a steroid alternative. Reports indicate, however, that GHB is abused for its intoxicating effects and consciousness-altering properties. It is variously referred to as "GBH" and "liquid ecstasy" and is sold illicitly in various forms (e.g., powder and liquid). Similar chemicals, which the body converts to GBH, include gamma butyrolactone (GBL) and 1,4-butanediol. Adverse effects include nausea, vomiting, respiratory problems, seizures, coma, and death. In some reports, GHB abuse has been linked to Wernicke-Korsakoff–like syndrome.

NITRITE INHALANTS

The nitrite inhalants include amyl, butyl, and isobutyl nitrites, all of which are called "poppers" in popular jargon. The intoxication syndromes seen with nitrites can differ markedly from the syndromes seen with the standard inhalant substances, such as lighter fluid and airplane glue. Nitrite inhalants are used by persons seeking the associated mild euphoria, altered sense of time, feeling of fullness in the head, and, possibly, increased sexual feelings. The nitrite compounds are used by some gay men and users of other drugs to heighten sexual stimulation during orgasm and, in some cases, to relax the anal sphincter for penile penetration. Under such circumstances, a person may use the substance for a few or a dozen times within several hours.

Adverse reactions include a toxic syndrome characterized by nausea, vomiting, headache, hypotension, drowsiness, and irritation of the respiratory tract. Some evidence indicates that nitrite inhalants may adversely affect immune function. Because sildenafil (Viagra) is lethal when combined with nitrite compounds, persons at risk should be cautioned never to use the two together.

NITROUS OXIDE

Nitrous oxide, commonly known as "laughing gas," is a widely available anesthetic agent that is subject to abuse because of its ability to produce feelings of lightheadedness and of floating, sometimes experienced as pleasurable or specifically as sexual. With long-term abuse patterns, nitrous oxide use has been associated with delirium and paranoia. Female dental assistants exposed to high levels of nitrous oxide have reportedly experienced reduced fertility.

A 35-year-old male dentist with no history of other substance problems complained of problems with nitrous oxide abuse for 10 years. This had begun as experimentation with what he had considered a harmless substance. However, his rate of use increased over several years, eventually becoming almost daily for months at a time. He felt a craving before

Table 12.14–1
DSM-IV-TR Criteria for Other (or Unknown) Substance-Related Disorders

The other (or unknown) substance-related disorders category is for classifying substance-related disorders associated with substances not listed above. Examples of these substances, which are described in more detail below, include anabolic steroids, nitrite inhalants ("poppers"), nitrous oxide, over-the-counter and prescription medications not otherwise covered by the 11 categories (e.g., cortisol, antihistamines, benztropine), and other substances that have psychoactive effects. In addition, this category may be used when the specific substance is unknown (e.g., an intoxication after taking a bottle of unlabeled pills).

Anabolic steroids sometimes produce an initial sense of enhanced well-being (or even euphoria), which is replaced after repeated use by lack of energy, irritability, and other forms of dysphoria. Continued use of these substances may lead to more severe symptoms (e.g., depressive symptomatology) and general medical conditions (liver disease).

Nitrite inhalants ("poppers" forms of amyl, butyl, and isobutyl nitrite) produce an intoxication that is characterized by a feeling of fullness in the head, mild euphoria, a change in the perception of time, relaxation of smooth muscles, and a possible increase in sexual feelings. In addition to possible compulsive use, these substances carry dangers of potential impairment of immune functioning, irritation of the respiratory system, a decrease in the oxygen-carrying capacity of the blood, and a toxic reaction that can include vomiting, severe headache, hypotension, and dizziness.

Nitrous oxide ("laughing gas") causes rapid onset of an intoxication that is characterized by lightheadedness and a floating sensation that clears in a matter of minutes after administration is stopped. There are reports of temporary but clinically relevant confusion and reversible paranoid states when nitrous oxide is used regularly.

Other substances that are capable of producing mild intoxication include **catnip,** which can produce states similar to those observed with marijuana and which in high doses is reported to result in LSD-type perceptions; **betel nut,** which is chewed in many cultures to produce a mild euphoria and floating sensation; and **kava** (a substance derived from the South Pacific pepper plant), which produces sedation, incoordination, weight loss, mild forms of hepatitis, and lung abnormalities. In addition, individuals can develop dependence and impairment through repeated self-administration of **over-the-counter** and **prescription drugs,** including **cortisol, antiparkinsonian agents** that have anticholinergic properties, and **antihistamines.**

Texts and criteria sets have already been provided to define the generic aspects of substance dependence, substance abuse, substance intoxication, and substance withdrawal that are applicable across classes of substances. The other (or unknown) substance-induced disorders are described in the sections of the manual with disorders with which they share phenomenology (e.g., other for unknown) substance-induced mood disorder is included in the mood disorders section). Listed below are the other (or unknown) substance use disorders and the other (or unknown) substance-induced disorders.

Other (or unknown) substance use disorders

Other (or unknown) substance use dependence

Other (or unknown) substance abuse

Other (or unknown) substance-induced disorders

Other (or unknown) substance intoxication

Specify if:

With perceptual disturbances

Other (or unknown) substance withdrawal

Specify if:

With perceptual disturbances

Other (or unknown) substance-induced delirium

Other (or unknown) substance-induced persisting dementia

Other (or unknown) substance-induced persisting amnestic disorder

Other (or unknown) substance psychotic disorder, with delusions

Specify if:

With onset during intoxication

With onset during withdrawal

Other (or unknown) substance-induced psychotic disorder, with hallucinations

Specify if:

With onset during intoxication

With onset during withdrawal

Other (or unknown) substance-induced mood disorder

Specify if:

With onset during intoxication

With onset during withdrawal

Other (or unknown) substance-induced anxiety disorder

Specify if:

With onset during intoxication

With onset during withdrawal

Other (or unknown) substance-induced sexual dysfunction

Specify if:

With onset during intoxication

Other (or unknown) substance-induced sleep disorder

Specify if:

With onset during intoxication

Other (or unknown) substance-related disorder not otherwise specified

From American Psychiatric Association. *Diagnostic and Statistical Manual of Mental Disorders.* 4th ed. Text rev. Washington, DC: American Psychiatric Association; copyright 2000, with permission.

sessions of use. Then, using the gas while alone in his office, he immediately felt numbness, a change in his temperature and heart rate, and alleviation of depressed feelings. "Things would go through my mind. Time was erased." He sometimes fell asleep. Sessions might last a few minutes or up to 8 hours. They ended when the craving and euphoria ended. He had often tried to stop or cut down, sometimes consulting a professional about the problem.

OTHER SUBSTANCES

The spice nutmeg can be ingested in a number of preparations. When nutmeg is taken in sufficiently high doses, it can induce depersonalization, derealization, and a feeling of heaviness in the limbs. In high enough doses, morning glory seeds can produce a syndrome resembling that seen with lysergic acid diethylamide (LSD), characterized by altered sensory perceptions and mild visual hallucinations. Catnip can produce cannabis-like intoxication in low doses and LSD-like intoxication in high

doses. Betel nuts, when chewed, can produce a mild euphoria and a feeling of floating in space. Kava, derived from a pepper plant native to the South Pacific, produces sedation and incoordination and is associated with hepatitis, lung abnormalities, and weight loss. Some persons abuse over-the-counter and prescription medications such as cortisol, antiparkinsonian agents, and antihistamines. Ephedra, a natural substance found in herbal tea, acts like epinephrine and, when abused, produces cardiac arrhythmia and fatalities.

CHOCOLATE

A controversial possible substance of abuse is chocolate derived from the cacao bean. Anandamide, an ingredient in chocolate, stimulates the same receptors as marijuana. Other compounds in chocolate include tryptophan, the precursor of serotonin, and phenylalanine, an amphetamine-like substance, both of which improve mood. So-called chocoholics may be self-medicating because of a depressive diathesis.

POLYSUBSTANCE-RELATED DISORDER

Substance users often abuse more than one substance. In DSM-IV-TR, a diagnosis of polysubstance dependence is appropriate if, for a period of at least 12 months, a person has repeatedly used substances from at least three categories (not including nicotine and caffeine), even if the diagnostic criteria for a substance-related disorder are not met for any single substance, as long as, during this period, the criteria for substance dependence have been met for the substances considered as a group (Table 12.14–2).

Table 12.14–2
DSM-IV-TR Criteria for Polysubstance Dependence

This diagnosis is reserved for behavior during the same 12-month period in which the person was repeatedly using at least three groups of substances (not including caffeine and nicotine), but no single substance has predominated. Further, during this period, the dependence criteria were met for substances as a group but not for any specific substance.

From American Psychiatric Association. *Diagnostic and Statistical Manual of Mental Disorders.* 4th ed. Text rev. Washington, DC: American Psychiatric Association; copyright 2000, with permission.

TREATMENT AND REHABILITATION

Treatment approaches for the substances covered in this section vary according to substances, patterns of abuse, availability of psychosocial support systems, and patients' individual features. Two major treatment goals for substance abuse have been determined: the first is abstinence from the substance, and the second is the physical, psychiatric, and psychosocial well-being of the patient. Significant damage has often been done to a patient's support systems during prolonged periods of substance abuse. For a patient to stop a pattern of substance abuse successfully, adequate psychosocial supports must be in place to foster the difficult change in behavior.

In some rare cases, it may be necessary to initiate treatment on an inpatient unit. Although an outpatient setting is more desirable than an inpatient setting, the temptations available to an outpatient for repeated use may present too high a hurdle for the initiation of treatment. Inpatient treatment is also indicated in the case of severe medical or psychiatric symptoms, a history of failed outpatient treatments, a lack of psychosocial supports, or a particularly severe or long-term history of substance abuse. After an initial period of detoxification, patients need a sustained period of rehabilitation. Throughout treatment, individual, family, and group therapies can be effective. Education about substance abuse and support for patients' efforts are essential factors in treatment.

References

Brouette T, Anton R. Clinical review of inhalants. *Am J Addict.* 2001;10:79.
Jaffe JH. Substance-related disorders: introduction and overview. In: Sadock BJ, Sadock VA, eds. *Kaplan & Sadock's Comprehensive Textbook of Psychiatry.* 7th ed. Vol 1. Baltimore: Lippincott Williams & Wilkins; 2000:924.
Zvosec DL. Abuse of GHB-related compounds. *N Engl J Med.* 2001;344:87.

13 Schizophrenia

Schizophrenia, which afflicts approximately 1 percent of the population, usually begins before age 25, persists throughout life, and affects persons of all social classes. Both patients and their families often suffer from poor care and social ostracism because of widespread ignorance about the disorder. Although schizophrenia is discussed as if it is a single disease, it probably comprises a group of disorders with heterogeneous etiologies, and it includes patients whose clinical presentations, treatment response, and courses of illness vary. Clinicians should appreciate that the diagnosis of schizophrenia is based entirely on the psychiatric history and mental status examination. There is no laboratory test for schizophrenia.

Important advances in the understanding of schizophrenia have occurred in three major areas. First, advances in neuroimaging techniques, especially magnetic resonance imaging (MRI), and refinements in neuropathological techniques have focused much interest on certain brain areas as central to the pathophysiology of schizophrenia. The particular brain areas of interest are the frontal lobe, amygdala, hippocampus, parahippocampal gyrus, and cerebellum. The focus on these brain regions can generate hypotheses to expand the knowledge base regarding schizophrenia. Second, since the introduction of clozapine (Clozaril), an atypical antipsychotic with minimal neurological adverse effects, there has been a significant amount of research regarding other drugs effective in reducing the negative symptoms of schizophrenia with a low incidence of neurological adverse effects. Third, as drug treatments improve and the solid biological basis for schizophrenia is recognized, there is increased interest in the psychosocial factors affecting schizophrenia, including those that influence treatment approaches, including psychotherapy.

HISTORY

The magnitude of the clinical problem of schizophrenia has consistently attracted the attention of major figures in psychiatry and neurology throughout the history of the disorder. Two of these persons were Emil Kraepelin (1856–1926) and Eugen Bleuler (1857–1939). Earlier, Benedict Morel (1809–1873), a French psychiatrist, had used the term *démence précoce* for deteriorated patients whose illness began in adolescence; Karl Ludwig Kahlbaum (1828–1899) had described the symptoms of catatonia; and Ewold Hacker (1843–1909) had written about the bizarre behavior of patients with hebephrenia.

Emil Kraepelin

Kraepelin (Fig. 13–1) translated Morel's *démence précoce* into *dementia precox,* a term that emphasized the distinct cognitive process (*dementia*) and early onset (*precox*) of the disorder. Patients with dementia precox were described as having a long-term deteriorating course and the common clinical symptoms of hallucinations and delusions. Kraepelin distinguished these patients from those classified as having manic-depressive psychosis, who underwent distinct episodes of illness alternating with periods of normal functioning. The major symptoms of patients with paranoia were persistent persecutory delusions, and these patients were described as lacking the deteriorating course of dementia precox and the intermittent symptoms of manic-depressive psychosis. Although Kraepelin had acknowledged that about 4 percent of his patients recovered completely and 13 percent had significant remissions, later researchers sometimes mistakenly stated that he had considered dementia precox to have an inevitable deteriorating course.

Eugen Bleuler

Bleuler (Fig. 13–2) coined the term *schizophrenia,* which replaced *dementia precox* in the literature. He chose the term to express the presence of schisms between thought, emotion, and behavior in patients with the disorder. Bleuler stressed that, unlike Kraepelin's concept of dementia precox, schizophrenia need not have a deteriorating course. Before the publication of the third edition of *Diagnostic and Statistical Manual of Mental Disorders* (DSM-III), the incidence of schizophrenia increased in the United States (where psychiatrists followed Bleuler's principles) to perhaps as much as twice the incidence in Europe (where psychiatrists followed Kraepelin's principles). After the publication of DSM-III, the diagnosis of schizophrenia in the United States moved toward Kraepelin's concept. Bleuler's term *schizophrenia,* however, has become the internationally accepted label for the disorder. This term is often misconstrued, especially by lay people, to mean split personality. Split personality, now called *dissociative identity disorder,* is categorized in the text revision of the fourth edition of DSM (DSM-IV-TR) as a dissociative disorder and thus differs completely from schizophrenia.

The Four *A*s. Bleuler identified specific *fundamental* (*or primary*) *symptoms* of schizophrenia to develop his theory about the internal mental schisms of patients. These symptoms included associational disturbances, especially looseness, affective disturbances, autism, and ambivalence, summarized as the four *A*s: *a*ssociations, *a*ffect, *a*utism, and *a*mbivalence. Bleuler also identified *accessory* (*secondary*) *symp-*

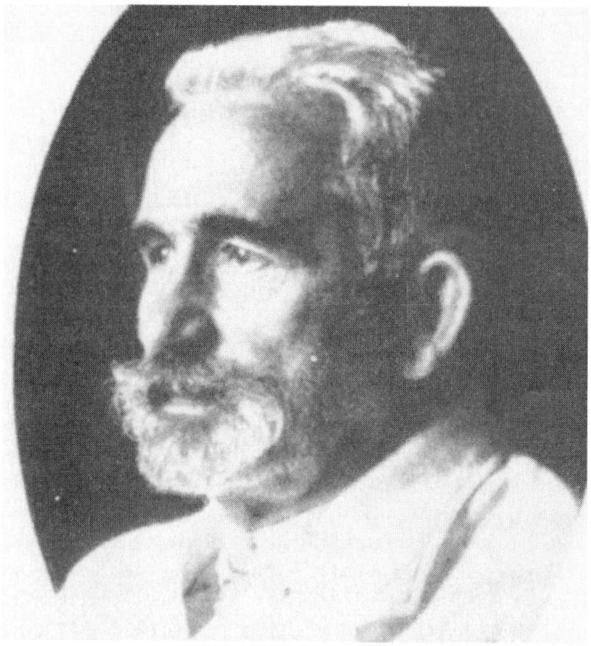

FIGURE 13–1
Emil Kraepelin. (Reprinted with permission from Davison GC, Neale JM. *Abnormal Psychology: An Experimental Clinical Approach.* New York, Wiley; 1974.)

toms, which included those symptoms that Kraepelin saw as major indicators of dementia precox: hallucinations and delusions.

Other Theorists. Adolf Meyer, Harry Stack Sullivan, Ernst Kretschmer, Gabriel Langfeldt, Kurt Schneider, and Karl Jaspers added much to the understanding of schizophrenia. Meyer, the founder of psychobiology, saw schizophrenia and other mental disorders as reactions to life stresses and called the syndrome a schizophrenic reaction. Sullivan, who founded the interpersonal psychoanalytic school, emphasized social isolation as a cause and a symptom of schizophrenia.

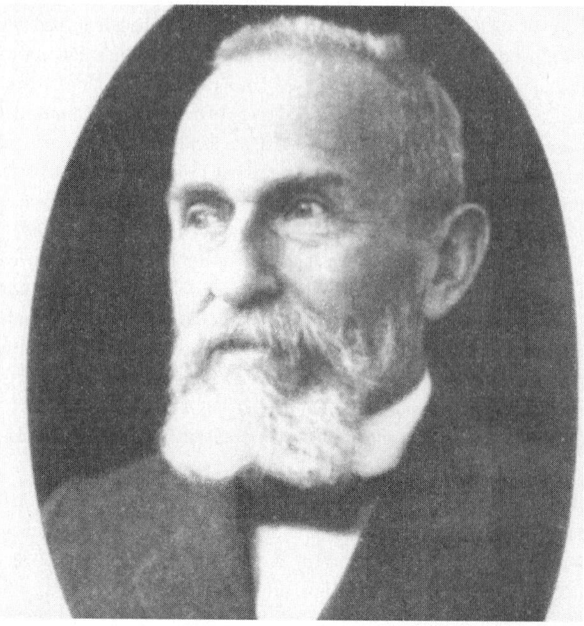

FIGURE 13–2
Eugen Bleuler. (Reprinted with permission from Davison GC, Neale JM. *Abnormal Psychology: An Experimental Clinical Approach.* New York, Wiley; 1974.)

Kretschmer compiled data to support the idea that schizophrenia occurred more often among persons with asthenic (i.e., slender, lightly muscled physiques), athletic, or dysplastic body types rather than among persons with pyknic (i.e., short, stocky physiques) body types. He thought the latter were more likely to incur bipolar disorders. His observations may seem strange, but they are not inconsistent with a superficial impression of the body types in many persons with schizophrenia.

Langfeldt classified patients with major psychotic symptoms into two groups, those with true schizophrenia and those with a schizophrenialike psychosis. In his description of *true schizophrenia,* Langfeldt stressed several factors: insidious onset, feelings of derealization and depersonalization, autism, and emotional blunting (Table 13–1). Researchers after Langfeldt gave *true schizophrenia* other names: nuclear schizophrenia, process schizophrenia, and nonremitting schizophrenia.

Schneider contributed a description of first-rank symptoms, which, he stressed, were not specific for schizophrenia and were not to be rigidly applied but were useful for making diagnoses (Table 13–1). He emphasized that in patients who showed no first-rank symptoms, the disorder could be diagnosed exclusively on the basis of second-rank symptoms and an otherwise typical clinical appearance. Clinicians frequently ignore his warnings and sometimes see the absence of first-rank symptoms during a single interview as evidence that a person does not have schizophrenia.

Jaspers, a psychiatrist and philosopher, played a major role in developing existential psychoanalysis. He was interested in the phenomenology of mental illness and the subjective feelings of patients with mental illness. His work paved the way toward trying to understand the psychological meaning of schizophrenic signs and symptoms such as delusions and hallucinations.

EPIDEMIOLOGY

In the United States, the lifetime prevalence of schizophrenia is about 1 percent, which means that about 1 person in 100 will develop schizophrenia during their lifetime. The Epidemiologic Catchment Area (ECA) study sponsored by the National Institute of Mental Health reported a lifetime prevalence of 0.6 to 1.9 percent. According to DSM-IV-TR, the annual incidence of schizophrenia ranges from 0.5 to 5.0 per 10,000, with some geographic variation (e.g., the incidence is higher for persons born in urban areas of industrialized nations). Schizophrenia is found in all societies and geographical areas, and incidence and prevalence rates are roughly equal worldwide. In the United States about 0.05 percent of the total population is treated for schizophrenia in any single year, and only about half of all patients with schizophrenia obtain treatment, in spite of the severity of the disorder.

Gender and Age

Schizophrenia is equally prevalent in men and women. The two sexes differ, however, in the onset and course of illness. Onset is earlier in men than in women. More than half of all male schizophrenia patients but only a third of all female schizophrenia patients are first admitted to a psychiatric hospital before age 25.

Table 13–1
Essential Features of Various Diagnostic Criteria for Schizophrenia

Kurt Schneider Criteria

1. First-rank symptoms
   a. Audible thoughts
   b. Voices arguing or discussing or both
   c. Voices commenting
   d. Somatic passivity experiences
   e. Thought withdrawal and other experiences of influenced thought
   f. Thought broadcasting
   g. Delusional perceptions
   h. All other experiences involving volition, made affects, and made impulses
2. Second-rank symptoms
   a. Other disorders of perception
   b. Sudden delusional ideas
   c. Perplexity
   d. Depressive and euphoric mood changes
   e. Feelings of emotional impoverishment
   f. ". . . and several others as well"

Gabriel Langfeldt Criteria

1. Symptom criteria
   Significant clues to a diagnosis of schizophrenia are (if no sign of cognitive impairment, infection, or intoxication can be demonstrated)
   a. Changes in personality, which manifest themselves as a special type of emotional blunting followed by lack of initiative, and altered, frequently peculiar behavior. (In hebephrenia, especially, the changes are characteristic and are a principal clue to the diagnosis.)
   b. In catatonic types, the history and the typical signs in periods of restlessness and stupor (with negativism, oily facies, catalepsy, special vegetative symptoms, etc.)
   c. In paranoid psychoses, essential symptoms of split personality (or depersonalization symptoms) and a loss of reality feeling (derealization symptoms) or primary delusions
   d. Chronic hallucinations
2. Course criterion
   A final decision about diagnosis cannot be made before a follow-up period of at least 5 years has shown a long-term course of disease

New Haven Schizophrenia Index

1. a. Delusions: not specified or other-than-depressive	2 points
b. Auditory hallucinations c. Visual hallucinations d. Other hallucinations	any one: 2 points
2. a. Bizarre thoughts b. Autism or grossly unrealistic private thoughts c. Looseness of associations, illogical thinking, overinclusion	any one: 2 points
d. Blocking e. Concreteness	either: 2 points
f. Derealization g. Depersonalization	each: 1 point
3. Inappropriate affect	1 point
4. Confusion	1 point
5. Paranoid ideation (self-referential thinking, suspiciousness)	1 point
6. Catatonic behavior a. Excitement b. Stupor c. Waxy flexibility d. Negativism e. Mutism f. Echolalia g. Stereotyped motor activity	any one: 1 point

Scoring: To be considered part of the schizophrenic group, the patient must score on Item 1 or Item 2a, 2b, or 2c and must receive a total score of at least 4 points.

(*continued*)

Table 13–1 (*continued*)

Flexible System

Minimum number of symptoms required can be four to eight, depending on investigator's choice:

1. Restricted affect
2. Poor insight
3. Thoughts aloud
4. Poor rapport
5. Widespread delusions
6. Incoherent speech
7. Unreliable information
8. Bizarre delusions
9. Nihilistic delusions
10. Absence of early awakening (1 to 3 hours)
11. Absence of depressed facies
12. Absence of elation

Research Diagnostic Criteria

Criteria 1 through 3 required for diagnosis:

1. At least two of the following for definite illness and one for probable (not counting those occurring during period of drug or alcohol abuse or withdrawal):
    a. Thought broadcasting, insertion, or withdrawal
    b. Delusions of being controlled or influenced, other bizarre delusions, or multiple delusions
    c. Delusions other than persecution or jealousy lasting at least 1 month
    d. Delusions of any type if accompanied by hallucinations of any type for at least 1 week
    e. Auditory hallucinations in which either a voice keeps up a running commentary on subject's behaviors or thoughts as they occur or two or more voices converse with each other
    f. Nonaffective verbal hallucinations spoken to subject
    g. Hallucinations of any type throughout day for several days or intermittently for at least 1 month
    h. Definite instances of marked formal thought disorders accompanied by blunted or inappropriate affect, delusions, or hallucinations of any type or grossly disorganized behavior
2. One of the following:
    a. Current period of illness lasted at least 2 weeks from onset of noticeable change in subject's usual condition
    b. Subject has had previous period of illness lasting at least 2 weeks, during which he or she met criteria, and residual signs of illness have remained (e.g., extreme social withdrawal, blunted or inappropriate affect, formal thought disorder, or unusual thoughts or perceptual experiences)
3. At no time during active period of illness being considered did subject meet criteria for probable or definite manic or depressive syndrome to the degree that it was a prominent part of illness.

St. Louis Criteria

1. Both necessary:
    a. Chronic illness with at least 6 months of symptoms before index evaluation without return to premorbid level of psychosocial adjustment
    b. Absence of period of depressive or manic symptoms sufficient to qualify for mood disorder or probable mood disorder
2. At least one of the following:
    a. Delusions or hallucinations without significant perplexity or disorientation
    b. Verbal production that makes communication difficult owing to lack of logical or understandable organization (in presence of muteness, diagnostic decision must be deferred)
3. At least three for definite, two for probable, illness:
    a. Never married
    b. Poor premorbid social adjustment or work history
    c. Family history of schizophrenia
    d. Absence of alcohol or other substance abuse within one year of onset
    e. Onset before age 40

(*continued*)

Table 13–1 (*continued*)

Present State Examination

The following 12 items from the Present State Examination correspond to a 12-point diagnostic system for schizophrenia, with varying levels of certainty of diagnosis based on the cutoff score determined by the examiner. Nine of the symptoms are scored 1 point each when present (+), and three are scored 1 point each when absent (–).

1. Restricted affect (+)
2. Poor insight (+)
3. Thoughts aloud (+)
4. Awaking early (–)
5. Poor rapport (+)
6. Depressed facies (–)
7. Elation (–)
8. Widespread delusions (+)
9. Incoherent speech (+)
10. Unreliable information (+)
11. Bizarre delusions (+)
12. Nihilistic delusions (+)

Tsuang and Winokur Criteria

I. Hebephrenic (A through D must be present):
   A. Age of onset and sociofamilial data (one of the following):
      1. Age of onset before 25 years
      2. Unmarried or unemployed
      3. Family history of schizophrenia
   B. Disorganized thought
   C. Affect changes (either 1 or 2):
      1. Inappropriate affect
      2. Flat affect
   D. Behavioral symptoms (either 1 or 2):
      1. Bizarre behavior
      2. Motor symptoms (either a or b):
         a. Hebephrenic traits
         b. Catatonic traits (if present, subtype may be modified to hebephrenia with catatonic traits)

II. Paranoid (A through C must be present):
   A. Age of onset and sociofamilial data (one of the following):
      1. Age of onset after 25 years
      2. Married or employed
      3. Absence of family history of schizophrenia
   B. Exclusion criteria:
      1. Disorganized thoughts must be absent or of mild degree, such that speech is intelligible
      2. Affective and behavioral symptoms, as described in hebephrenia, must be absent or of mild degree
   C. Preoccupation with extensive, well-organized delusions or hallucinations

The criteria of Schneider and Langfeld are reprinted with permission from World Psychiatric Association. *Diagnostic Criteria for Schizophrenic and Affective Psychoses.* Washington, DC: American Psychiatric Press; 1983. The criteria of St. Louis, Research Diagnostic Criteria, New Haven Schizophrenia Index and Flexible, are reprinted with permission from Endicott J, Nee J, Fleiss L, Cohen J, Williams JBW, Simon R. Diagnostic criteria for schizophrenia. *Arch Gen Psychiatry.* 1982;39:884. The criteria for Tsuang and Winokur are reprinted with permission from Tsuang MT, Winokur C. Criteria for hebephrenic and paranoid schizophrenia. *Arch Gen Psychiatry.* 1974;31:43.

The peak ages of onset are 10 to 25 years for men and 25 to 35 years for women. Unlike men, women display a bimodal age distribution, with a second peak occurring in middle age. Approximately 3 to 10 percent of women present with disease onset after age 40. About 90 percent of patients in treatment for schizophrenia are between 15 and 55 years old. Onset of schizophrenia before age 10 or after age 60 is extremely rare. Some studies have indicated that men are more likely to be impaired by negative symptoms (described below) than are women and that women are more likely to have better social functioning than are men prior to disease onset. In general, the outcome for female schizophrenia patients is better than that for male schizophrenia patients. When onset occurs after age 45, the disorder is characterized as late-onset schizophrenia.

Infection and Birth Season

A robust finding in schizophrenia research is that persons who develop schizophrenia are more likely to have been born in the winter and early spring and less likely to have been born in late spring and summer. In the Northern Hemisphere, including the United States, persons with schizophrenia are more often born in the months from January to April. In the Southern Hemisphere, persons with schizophrenia are more often born in the months

from July to September. One hypothesis is that a season-specific risk factor, such as a virus or a seasonal change in diet, may be operative. Viral hypotheses include slow viruses, retroviruses, and virally activated autoimmune reactions. Some studies show that the frequency of schizophrenia is increased following exposure to influenza—which occurs in the winter—during the second trimester of pregnancy. Another hypothesis is that persons with a genetic predisposition for schizophrenia have a decreased biological advantage to survive season-specific insults.

Geographical Distribution

Schizophrenia is not evenly distributed throughout the United States or the world. Historically, the prevalence of schizophrenia in the northeastern and western United States was greater than that in other areas, although this unequal distribution has eroded. Some geographical regions of the world such as Ireland have an unusually high prevalence of schizophrenia, and researchers have interpreted these geographical pockets of schizophrenia as possible support for an infective (e.g., viral) cause of schizophrenia.

Reproductive Factors

The use of psychotherapeutic drugs, the open-door policies in hospitals, the deinstitutionalization in state hospitals, the emphasis on rehabilitation, and community-based care for patients with schizophrenia have all led to an increase in the marriage and fertility rates among persons with schizophrenia. Because of these factors, the number of children born to parents with schizophrenia is continually increasing. The fertility rate for persons with schizophrenia is close to that for the general population. First-degree biological relatives of persons with schizophrenia have a 10 times greater risk for developing the disease than the general population.

Medical Illness

Persons with schizophrenia have a higher mortality rate from accidents and natural causes than the general population. Institution-related or treatment-related variables do not explain the increased mortality rate, but the higher rate may be related to the fact that the diagnosis and treatment of medical and surgical conditions in schizophrenia patients can be clinical challenges. Several studies have shown that up to 80 percent of all schizophrenia patients have significant concurrent medical illnesses and that up to 50 percent of these conditions may be undiagnosed.

Suicide Risk

Suicide is a leading cause of mortality in persons suffering from schizophrenia. Estimates vary, but as many as 15 percent of persons with schizophrenia may die because of a suicide attempt. Although the risk for suicide is greater in persons with schizophrenia than in the general population, some risk factors—such as being male, white, and socially isolated—are similar in both groups. Factors such as depressive illness, a history of suicide attempts, unemployment, and recent rejection also increase the risk for suicide in both populations. A postdischarge course involving high levels of psychopathology and functional impairment increases the risk for suicide. In addition, persons who have a realistic awareness of the deteriorative effects of the illness and a nondelusional assessment of their future mental deterioration, hopelessness, excessive dependence on treatment, or loss of faith in treatment have an increased risk of suicide. The risk of mortality is especially high in the young, during the early postdischarge period, and early in the course of illness, although the risk persists across the person's life span. Risk factors identified in previous studies may be helpful in assessing acute suicidal risk in a specific individual. Further research is needed to elucidate what risk factors best predict future suicide in persons with schizophrenia and what interventions are most helpful in preventing suicide.

Substance Use

Cigarette Smoking. Most surveys have reported that more than three fourths of all schizophrenia patients smoke cigarettes, compared with less than half of psychiatric patients as a whole. In addition to the well-known health risks associated with smoking, cigarette smoking affects other aspects of a schizophrenia patient's care. Several studies have reported that cigarette smoking is associated with the use of high dosages of antipsychotic drugs, possibly because cigarette smoking increases the metabolism of these drugs. On the other hand, cigarette smoking is associated with a decrease in antipsychotic drug–related parkinsonism, possibly because of nicotine-dependent activation of dopamine neurons. Recent studies have demonstrated that nicotine may decrease positive symptoms such as hallucinations in schizophrenia patients by its effect on nicotine receptors in the brain that reduce the perception of outside stimuli, especially noise. In that sense, smoking is a form of self-medication.

Other Substances. Comorbidity of schizophrenia and other substance-related disorders is common, although the implications of substance abuse in schizophrenia patients are unclear. About 30 to 50 percent of persons with schizophrenia may meet the diagnostic criteria for alcohol abuse or alcohol dependence; the two most commonly used other substances are cannabis (about 15 to 25 percent) and cocaine (about 5 to 10 percent). Patients report that they use these substances to obtain pleasure and to reduce their depression and anxiety. In schizophrenia patients, most studies have associated the comorbidity of substance-related disorders with a poor prognosis.

Population Factors

The prevalence of schizophrenia has been correlated with local population density in cities with populations of more than 1 million people. The correlation is weaker in cities of 100,000 to 500,000 people and is absent in cities with fewer than 10,000 people. The effect of population density is consistent with the observation that the incidence of schizophrenia in children of either one or two parents with schizophrenia is twice as high in cities as in rural communities. These observations suggest that social stressors in urban settings affect the development of schizophrenia in persons at risk.

Socioeconomic and Cultural Factors

Schizophrenia has been described in all cultures and socioeconomic status groups. In industrialized nations, a disproportionate

number of schizophrenia patients are in the low socioeconomic groups, an observation explained by two alternative hypotheses. The *downward drift hypothesis* suggests that affected persons move into, or fail to rise out of, a low socioeconomic group because of this illness. The *social causation hypothesis* proposes that stresses experienced by members of low socioeconomic groups contribute to the development of schizophrenia.

Some investigators have presented data indicating that in addition to the stress of industrialization as a cause of schizophrenia, the stress of immigration can lead to a schizophrenialike condition. Some studies report a high prevalence of schizophrenia among recent immigrants, a finding implicating abrupt cultural change as a stressor involved in the cause of schizophrenia. Perhaps consistent with both hypotheses is the observation that the prevalence of schizophrenia increases among Third World populations as contact with technologically advanced cultures increases.

Theorists advocating a social cause for schizophrenia argue that cultures may be more or less schizophrenogenic, depending on the perceptions of mental illness in the culture, the patient's role, the system of social and family supports, and the complexity of social communication. Schizophrenia has been reported to be prognostically more benign in developing countries where patients are reintegrated into their communities and families more completely than they are in highly developed Western societies.

Economics. The financial cost of schizophrenia in the United States is estimated to exceed that of all cancers combined. Factors contributing to this enormous financial demand include the following: the disease begins early in life; it causes significant and long-lasting impairments; it makes heavy demands for hospital care; and it requires ongoing clinical care, rehabilitation, and support services. About 1 percent of the national income goes toward the treatment of mental illness (excluding substance-related disorders). Schizophrenia accounts for 2.5 percent of all health care expenditures. Costs of treatment and indirect costs to society (e.g., lost production and mortality) amount to almost $50 billion annually. About 75 percent of persons with severe schizophrenia cannot work and are unemployed.

Hospitalization. The development of effective antipsychotic drugs and changes in political and popular attitudes toward the treatment and the rights of persons who are mentally ill have dramatically changed the patterns of hospitalization for schizophrenia patients over the past 50 years. Even with antipsychotic medication, however, the probability of readmission within 2 years after discharge from the first hospitalization is about 40 to 60 percent. Patients with schizophrenia occupy about 50 percent of all mental-hospital beds and account for about 16 percent of all psychiatric patients who receive any treatment.

Homelessness. The problem of persons who are homeless in large cities seems related to the deinstitutionalization of schizophrenia patients who were not adequately followed up. Although the exact percentage of homeless persons who have schizophrenia is difficult to obtain, an estimated one third to two thirds of homeless persons are probably afflicted with schizophrenia.

ETIOLOGY

Schizophrenia is discussed as if it is a single disease, but the diagnostic category includes a group of disorders, probably with heterogeneous causes, but with somewhat similar behavioral symptoms. Patients with schizophrenia show differing clinical presentations, treatment responses, and courses of illness.

Stress–Diathesis Model

According to the stress–diathesis model for the integration of biological, psychosocial, and environmental factors, a person may have a specific vulnerability (diathesis) that, when acted on by a stressful influence, allows the symptoms of schizophrenia to develop. In the most general stress–diathesis model, the diathesis or the stress can be biological, environmental, or both. The environmental component can be either biological (e.g., an infection) or psychological (e.g., a stressful family situation or the death of a close relative). The biological basis of a diathesis can be further shaped by epigenetic influences such as substance abuse, psychosocial stress, and trauma.

Neurobiology

The cause of schizophrenia is unknown. In the past decade, however, an increasing amount of research has indicated a pathophysiological role for certain areas of the brain, including the limbic system, the frontal cortex, cerebellum, and the basal ganglia. These four areas are interconnected, so that dysfunction in one area may involve a primary pathological process in another. Brain imaging of living persons and neuropathological examination of postmortem brain tissue have implicated the limbic system as a potential site for the primary pathological process in at least some, perhaps even most, schizophrenia patients.

Two areas of active research are the time that a neuropathological lesion appears in the brain and the interaction of the lesion with environmental and social stressors. The basis for the appearance of the brain abnormality may lie in abnormal development (e.g., abnormal migration of neurons along the radial glial cells during development) or in degeneration of neurons after development (e.g., abnormally early preprogrammed cell death, as appears to occur in Huntington's disease). The fact that monozygotic twins have a 50 percent discordance rate, however, implies a little-understood interaction between the environment and the development of schizophrenia. On the other hand, the factors regulating gene expression are just beginning to be understood. Although monozygotic twins have the same genetic information, differential gene regulation during their lives perhaps allows one monozygotic twin to have schizophrenia, whereas the other does not.

Dopamine Hypothesis. The simplest formulation of the *dopamine hypothesis of schizophrenia* posits that schizophrenia results from too much dopaminergic activity. The theory evolved from two observations. First, the efficacy and the potency of most antipsychotic drugs (i.e., the dopamine receptor antagonists) are correlated with their ability to act as antagonists of the dopamine D_2 receptor. Second, drugs that increase dopaminergic activity, notably amphetamine, are psychotomimetic. The basic theory does not elaborate on whether the dopaminergic hyperactivity is

due to too much release of dopamine, too many dopamine receptors, hypersensitivity of the dopamine receptors to dopamine, or a combination of these mechanisms. Which dopamine tracts in the brain are involved is also not specified in the theory, although the mesocortical and mesolimbic tracts are most often implicated. The dopaminergic neurons in these tracts project from their cell bodies in the midbrain to dopaminoceptive neurons in the limbic system and the cerebral cortex.

A significant role for dopamine in the pathophysiology of schizophrenia is consistent with studies that have measured plasma concentrations of the major dopamine metabolite, homovanillic acid. Several preliminary studies have indicated that under carefully controlled experimental conditions, plasma homovanillic acid concentrations can reflect central nervous system (CNS) concentrations of homovanillic acid. These studies have reported a positive correlation between high pretreatment concentrations of homovanillic acid and two factors: the severity of the psychotic symptoms and the treatment response to antipsychotic drugs. Studies of plasma homovanillic acid have also reported that with treatment, plasma homovanillic acid concentrations decline steadily. This decline is correlated with symptom improvement in at least some patients. The dopamine hypothesis of schizophrenia continues to be refined and expanded, and new dopamine receptors continue to be identified. One study has reported an increase in D_4 receptors in postmortem brain samples from schizophrenia patients.

Other Neurotransmitters. Although the neurotransmitter dopamine has received the most attention in schizophrenia research, increasing attention is being paid to other neurotransmitters for at least two reasons. First, because schizophrenia is likely to be a heterogeneous disorder, it is possible that abnormalities in different neurotransmitters lead to the same behavioral syndrome. For instance, hallucinogenic substances that affect serotonin, such as lysergic acid diethylamide (LSD), and high doses of substances that affect dopamine, such as amphetamine, can both cause psychotic symptoms that are difficult to distinguish from schizophrenia. Second, neuroscience research has shown that a single neuron may contain more than one neurotransmitter and may have neurotransmitter receptors for a half dozen more neurotransmitters. Thus the various neurotransmitters in the brain are involved in complex interactional relations, and abnormal functioning may result from changes in any single neurotransmitter.

SEROTONIN. Serotonin has received much attention in schizophrenia research since the observation was made that the serotonin-dopamine antagonists (SDAs) (e.g., clozapine, risperidone [Risperdal], sertindole [Serlect]) have potent serotonin-related activities. Specifically, antagonism at the serotonin 5-HT_2 receptor has been emphasized as important in reducing psychotic symptoms and in mitigating the development of D_2-antagonism–related movement disorders. Examination of the receptor affinity profiles for each of the SDAs reveals no uniform pattern or ratio of activities other than their relatively higher affinity for 5-HT_2 receptors than for D_2 receptors. Clozapine has its greatest affinity for histamine receptors, whereas quetiapine (Seroquel) binds most tightly to α_1-adrenergic receptors, and ziprasidone (Geodon) is the only member of the group to interact strongly with 5-HT_1 receptors. The affinity for 5-HT_2 and D_2 receptors varies over more than a 100-fold range within this class of drugs. Yet each is a more effective antipsychotic agent than hundreds of related compounds that differ only slightly in their affinities. It appears, therefore, that multiple neurotransmitter systems interact in a particular balance of activity levels to regulate the signs and symptoms of schizophrenia and, moreover, that antipsychotic drugs can modulate these circuits by subtly perturbing any of several neurotransmitter systems. As suggested in the research on mood disorders, serotonin activity has been implicated in suicidal and impulsive behavior that can also be seen in schizophrenia patients.

NOREPINEPHRINE. Several investigators have reported that long-term antipsychotic drug administration decreases the activity of noradrenergic neurons in the locus ceruleus and that the therapeutic effects of some antipsychotic drugs may involve their activities at α_1- and α_2-receptors. Although the relation between dopaminergic and noradrenergic activity remains unclear, an increasing amount of data suggest that the noradrenergic system modulates the dopaminergic system in such a way that abnormalities of the noradrenergic system predispose a patient to relapse frequently.

GABA. The inhibitory amino acid neurotransmitter γ-aminobutyric acid (GABA) has also been implicated in the pathophysiology of schizophrenia. The available data are consistent with the hypothesis that some patients with schizophrenia have a loss of GABAergic neurons in the hippocampus. The loss of inhibitory GABAergic neurons could theoretically lead to the hyperactivity of dopaminergic and noradrenergic neurons.

GLUTAMATE. The hypotheses proposed about glutamate include those of hyperactivity, hypoactivity, and glutamate-induced neurotoxicity. Glutamate has been implicated because ingestion of phencyclidine (PCP), a glutamate antagonist, produces an acute syndrome similar to schizophrenia.

NEUROPEPTIDES. Two neuropeptides, cholecystokinin and neurotensin, are found in a number of brain regions implicated in schizophrenia. Their concentrations are altered in psychotic states.

Neuropathology. In the 19th century, neuropathologists failed to find a neuropathological basis for schizophrenia, and thus they classified schizophrenia as a functional disorder. By the end of the 20th century, however, researchers had made significant strides in revealing a potential neuropathological basis for schizophrenia, primarily in the limbic system and the basal ganglia, including neuropathological or neurochemical abnormalities in the cerebral cortex, the thalamus, and the brainstem. The loss of brain volume widely reported in schizophrenic brains appears to result from reduced density of the axons, dendrites, and synapses that mediate associative functions of the brain. Synaptic density is highest at age 1, then is pared down to adult values in early adolescence. One theory, based in part on the observation that patients often develop schizophrenic symptoms during adolescence, holds that schizophrenia results from excessive pruning of synapses during this phase of development.

LIMBIC SYSTEM. Because of its role in controlling emotions, the limbic system has been hypothesized to be involved in the pathophysiological basis of schizophrenia. In fact, this area of the brain has proved to be the most fertile for neuropathological studies of

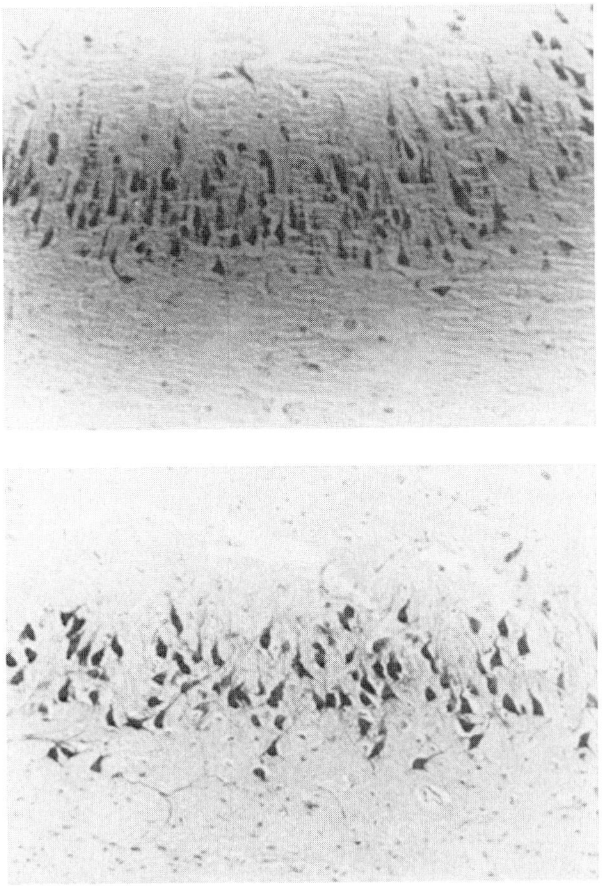

FIGURE 13–3

Comparison of cell orientation patterns of hippocampal pyramids at the CA1 to CA2 interface between nonschizophrenic control subjects **(top)** and schizophrenia patients **(bottom)** (Cresylecht violet stain, original magnification ×250). Positives were overexposed to enhance contrast. (Reprinted with permission from Conrad AJ, Abebe T, Austin R, Forsythe S, Scheibel AB. Hippocampal pyramidal cell disarray in schizophrenia as a bilateral phenomenon. *Arch Gen Psychiatry.* 1991;48:415.)

schizophrenia. Many well-controlled studies of postmortem brain samples from schizophrenia patients have shown a decrease in the size of the region including the amygdala, the hippocampus, and the parahippocampal gyrus. This neuropathological finding agrees with the observations made by MRI study of patients with schizophrenia. Disorganization of the neurons within the hippocampus of schizophrenia patients has also been reported (Fig. 13–3).

BASAL GANGLIA AND CEREBELLUM. The basal ganglia and cerebellum have been of theoretical interest in schizophrenia for at least two reasons. First, many patients with schizophrenia show odd movements, even in the absence of medication-induced movement disorders (e.g., tardive dyskinesia). The odd movements can include an awkward gait, facial grimacing, and stereotypies. Since the basal ganglia and cerebellum are involved in the control of movement, disease in these areas is implicated in the pathophysiology of schizophrenia. Second, of all the neurological disorders that can have psychosis as an associated symptom, the movement disorders involving the basal ganglia (e.g., Huntington's disease) are the ones most commonly associated with psychosis in affected patients. Furthermore, the basal ganglia and cerebellum are reciprocally connected to the frontal lobes, and the abnormalities in frontal lobe function seen in some brain-imaging studies may be due to disease in either area rather than in the frontal lobes themselves.

Neuropathological studies of the basal ganglia have produced variable and inconclusive reports about cell loss or the reduction of volume of the globus pallidus and the substantia nigra. In contrast, many studies have shown an increase in the number of D_2 receptors in the caudate, the putamen, and the nucleus accumbens. The question remains, however, whether the increase is secondary to the patients' having received antipsychotic medications. Some investigators have begun to study the serotonergic system in the basal ganglia; a role for serotonin in psychotic disorders is suggested by the clinical usefulness of antipsychotic drugs with serotonergic activity (e.g., clozapine, risperidone).

Neuroimaging. Before the advent of brain-imaging technologies, the study of schizophrenia depended on the distant measurement of brain activity—for example, the measurement of neurotransmitters in cerebrospinal fluid, plasma, or urine—in living patients or the direct measurement of the brain in deceased persons. Brain-imaging techniques now allow researchers to make specific measurements of neurochemicals or brain function in living patients. Calculations of the data derived from the brain-imaging machines are constructed from many assumptions, however, and differences in these mathematical models among research groups can potentially lead to different conclusions about the same data. To protect against this possibility, researchers constantly exchange their ideas about appropriate mathematical models.

COMPUTED TOMOGRAPHY. The initial studies using computed tomography (CT) in schizophrenic populations may have produced the earliest and most convincing data that schizophrenia is a bona fide brain disease. These studies have consistently shown that the brains of patients with schizophrenia have lateral and third ventricular enlargement and some reduction in cortical volume. These findings can be interpreted as consistent with a decrease in the usual amount of brain tissue in affected patients; whether this decrease is due to abnormal development or to degeneration is unknown.

Other CT studies have reported abnormal cerebral asymmetry, reduced cerebellar volume, and brain density changes in patients with schizophrenia. Many CT studies have correlated the presence of CT scan abnormalities with the presence of negative or deficit symptoms, neuropsychiatric impairment, increased neurological signs, frequent extrapyramidal symptoms from antipsychotic drugs, and poor premorbid adjustment. Although not all CT studies have confirmed these associations, it makes sense to conclude that the greater the evidence of neuropathological disease, the more serious the symptoms. The abnormalities reported in CT studies of patients with schizophrenia, however, have also been reported in other neuropsychiatric conditions, including mood disorders, alcohol-related disorders, and dementias. Thus, these changes are unlikely to be specific for the pathophysiological processes underlying schizophrenia.

Several investigators have attempted to determine whether the abnormalities detected by CT are progressive or static. Some studies have concluded that the lesions observed on CT scan are present at the onset of the illness and do not progress. Other studies, however, have concluded that the pathological process visualized on CT scan continues to progress during the illness. Thus, whether an active pathological process is continuing to evolve in schizophrenia patients is still uncertain.

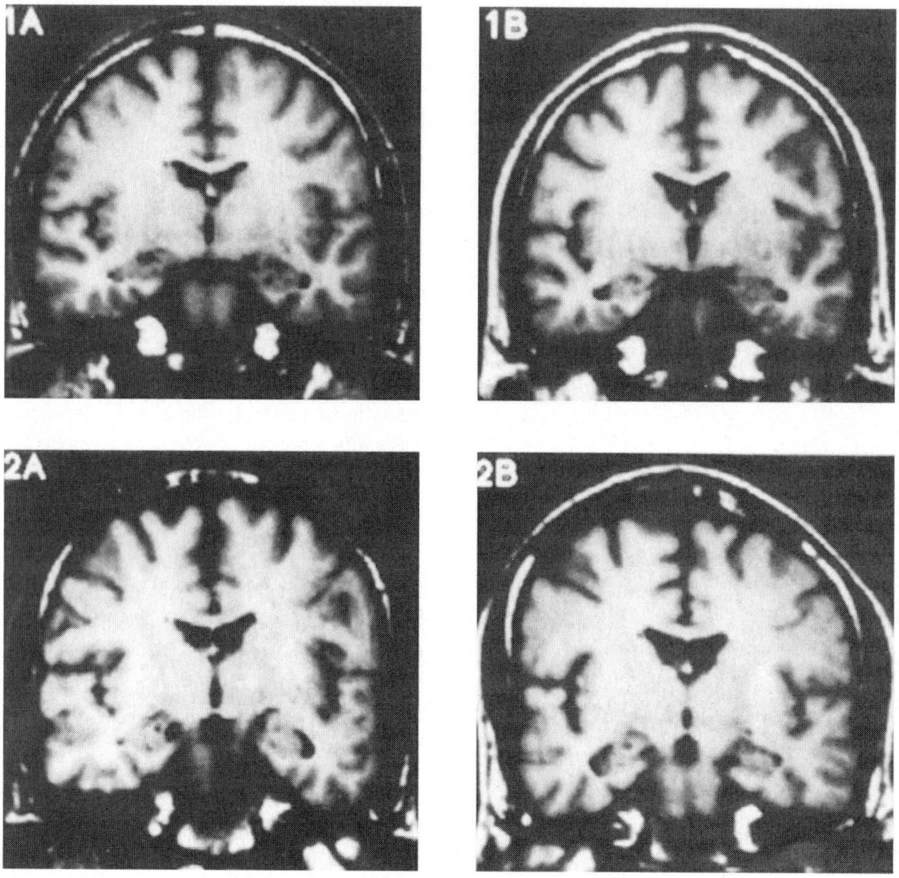

FIGURE 13–4

MRI coronal views from two sets of monozygotic twins discordant for schizophrenia show subtle enlargement of the lateral ventricles in the affected twins **(panels 1B** and **2B)** compared with the unaffected twins **(panels 1A** and **2A)**, even when the affected twin had small ventricles. (Reprinted with permission from Suddath RL, Christison GW, Torrey EF, Casanova MF, Weinberger DR. Anatomical abnormalities in the brains of monozygotic twins discordant for schizophrenia. *N Engl J Med.* 1990;322:789.)

Although the enlarged ventricles in schizophrenia patients are apparent when groups of patients and controls are used, the difference between affected and unaffected persons varies and is usually small. Therefore, the use of CT in the diagnosis of schizophrenia is limited. Some data indicate, however, that ventricles are more enlarged in patients with tardive dyskinesia than in patients without it, and some data show that ventricular enlargement is more frequent in male patients than in female patients.

MAGNETIC RESONANCE IMAGING. MRI was initially used to verify the findings of the CT studies but has subsequently served to expand the knowledge about the pathophysiology of schizophrenia. One of the most important MRI studies examined monozygotic twins who were discordant for schizophrenia (Fig. 13–4). The study found that virtually all the affected twins had larger cerebral ventricles than their nonaffected twins, although the cerebral ventricles of most affected twins fell within a normal range.

Investigators have used MRI in schizophrenia research because its resolution is superior to that with CT and for the qualitative information obtainable by using various signal sequences to get T1- or T2-weighted images, for example. As a result of the superior resolution of MRI, several reports have shown that the volumes of the hippocampus–amygdala complex and the parahippocampal gyrus are reduced in patients with schizophrenia. One study found a reduction of these brain areas in the left hemisphere (Fig. 13–5) and not in the right, although other studies have found bilateral reductions in volume. Some studies have correlated the reduction in limbic system volume with the degree of psychopathology or other measures of severity of illness.

FUNCTIONAL MRI (fMRI). fMRI is an ultrafast scanning technique that allows regional brain activity to be measured in vivo without ionizing radiation or invasive procedures. Several studies have shown differences in sensorimotor cortex activation between patients with schizophrenia and normal control subjects, as well as decreased blood flow to the occipital lobes. Regional brain activation is associated with changes in blood flow and blood volume. fMRI correlates well with positron emission tomography (PET) images of glucose uptake and with single photon emission computed tomography (SPECT) images of cerebral blood flow.

MAGNETIC RESONANCE SPECTROSCOPY (MRS). MRS is a technique that allows the measurement of the concentrations of specific molecules—for example, adenosine triphosphate (ATP)—in the brain. One study that used MRS imaging of the dorsolateral prefrontal cortex found that patients with schizophrenia had lower levels of phosphomonoesters and inorganic phosphate and higher levels of phosphodiesters and ATP than a control group. These data about the metabolism of phosphate-containing compounds were consistent with hypoactivity of that brain region and supported the findings of other brain-imaging

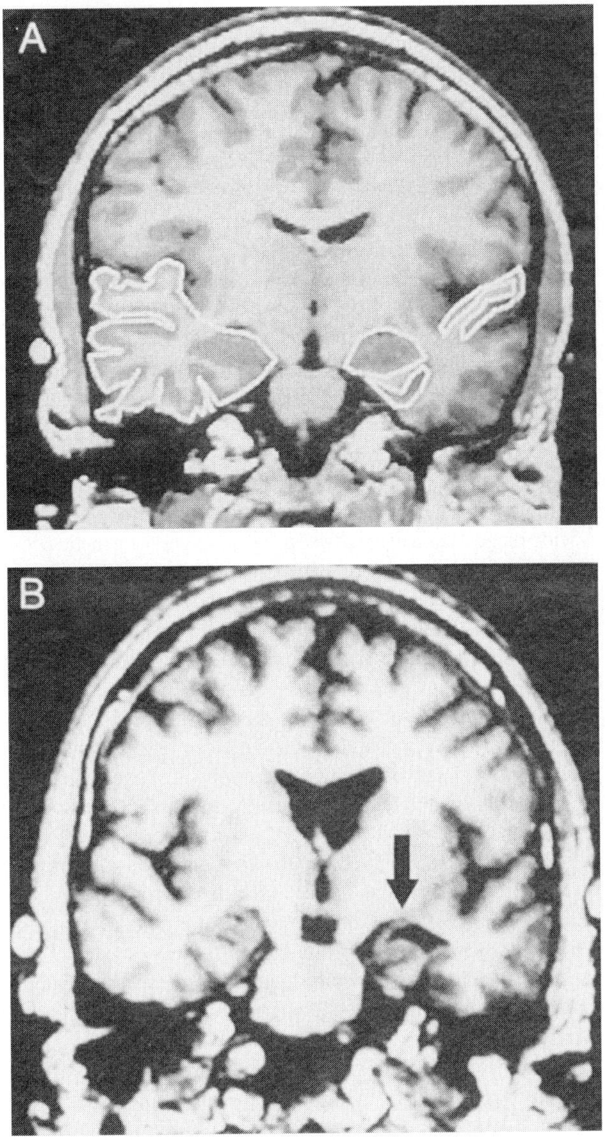

FIGURE 13–5

Coronal slice (1.5 mm) of the temporal lobe of a control subject **(A)** and a patient with schizophrenia **(B)**. In **A**, the regions of interest used to evaluate the temporal lobe have been outlined; the neocortical gray matter of the superior temporal gyrus is on the subject's left (viewer's right); more medially, the amygdala–hippocampal complex is shown as an almondlike shape, with the parahippocampal gyrus underneath. The temporal lobe is outlined on the subject's right. In **B**, the amount of cerebrospinal fluid (*black area*) surrounding the left superior temporal gyrus (sylvian fissure) is greater than the amount in the control. Tissue is lost in the parahippocampal gyrus, and the temporal horn surrounding the amygdala–hippocampal complex (*arrow*) is larger. (Reprinted with permission from Shenton ME, Kikinis R, Jolesz FA, et al. Abnormalities of the left temporal lobe and thought disorder in schizophrenia. *N Engl J Med.* 1992;327:606.)

studies (e.g., those of PET). Further, concentrations of *N*-acetyl aspartate (NAA), a marker of neurons, were lower in the hippocampus and frontal lobes of patients with schizophrenia and in the temporal lobes of persons with a first episode of psychosis.

POSITRON EMISSION TOMOGRAPHY. Although many studies using PET to study schizophrenia have been reported, few clear conclusions can be drawn at this time. Most PET studies have measured either glucose use or cerebral blood flow, and the positive findings have included hypoactivity of the frontal lobes, impaired activation of certain brain areas after psychological test stimulation, and hyperactivity of the basal ganglia relative to the cerebral cortex. Other studies, however, have failed to replicate these findings, although the abnormal-activation results seem to be robust. In these studies a person's blood flow is assayed by using PET, SPECT, or regional cerebral blood flow (rCBF) brain-imaging systems. While the cerebral blood flow is being measured, the patient performs a psychological task that presumably activates a particular part of the cerebral cortex in normal control subjects. One of the best-controlled studies of this design found that patients with schizophrenia, in contrast to the control group, failed to increase blood flow to the dorsolateral prefrontal cortex while performing the Wisconsin Card Sorting Test. One study found that a sample of patients with schizophrenia had reduced metabolic activity in the anterior left portion of the thalamus as measured by [^{18}F]luorodeoxyglucose PET and also had reduced volume in the same area as measured by MRI scan. Altered thalamic architecture and activity may play a role in schizophrenia.

A second type of PET study has used radioactive ligands to estimate the number of D_2 receptors present. The two most discussed studies disagree. One group reported an increased number of D_2 receptors in the basal ganglia, and the other group reported no change in the number of D_2 receptors in the basal ganglia. The difference between the two studies may involve the use of different ligands, different types of patients with schizophrenia, or other differences in method or data analysis. The controversy remains unresolved. The technique will, however, continue to be used in the study of schizophrenia, and subsequent research reports will use ligands for other neurotransmitter systems, such as the noradrenergic and glutamate systems.

Applied Electrophysiology. Electroencephalographic studies indicate that many schizophrenia patients have abnormal records, increased sensitivity to activation procedures (e.g., frequent spike activity after sleep deprivation), decreased alpha activity, increased theta and delta activity, possibly more epileptiform activity than usual, and possibly more left-sided abnormalities than usual. Schizophrenia patients also exhibit an inability to filter out irrelevant sounds and are extremely sensitive to background noise. The flooding of sound that results makes concentration difficult and may be a factor in the production of auditory hallucinations. This sound sensitivity may be associated with a genetic defect.

COMPLEX PARTIAL EPILEPSY. Schizophrenialike psychoses have been reported to occur more frequently than expected in patients with complex partial seizures, especially seizures involving the temporal lobes. Factors associated with the development of psychosis in these patients include a left-sided seizure focus, medial temporal location of the lesion, and early onset of seizures. The first-rank symptoms described by Schneider may be similar to symptoms of patients with complex partial epilepsy and may reflect the presence of a temporal lobe disorder when seen in patients with schizophrenia.

EVOKED POTENTIALS. A large number of abnormalities in evoked potential among patients with schizophrenia have been described. The P300 has been most studied and is defined as a large, positive evoked-potential wave that occurs about 300 ms after a sensory stimulus is detected. The major source of the P300 wave may be located in the limbic system structures of the

medial temporal lobes. In patients with schizophrenia, the P300 has been reported to be statistically smaller and later than that in comparison groups. Abnormalities in the P300 wave have also been reported to be more common in children who, because they have affected parents, are at high risk for schizophrenia. Whether the characteristics of the P300 represent a state or a trait phenomenon remains controversial. Other evoked potentials reported to be abnormal in patients with schizophrenia are the N100 and the contingent negative variation. The N100 is a negative wave that occurs about 100 ms after a stimulus, and the contingent negative variation is a slowly developing, negative-voltage shift following the presentation of a sensory stimulus that is a warning for an upcoming stimulus. The evoked-potential data have been interpreted as indicating that although patients with schizophrenia are unusually sensitive to a sensory stimulus (larger early evoked potentials), they compensate for the increased sensitivity by blunting the processing of information at higher cortical levels (indicated by smaller late evoked potentials).

Eye Movement Dysfunction. The inability to follow a moving visual target accurately is the defining basis for the disorders of smooth visual pursuit and disinhibition of saccadic eye movements seen in patients with schizophrenia. Eye movement dysfunction may be a trait marker for schizophrenia; it is independent of drug treatment and clinical state and is also seen in first-degree relatives of probands with schizophrenia. Various studies have reported abnormal eye movements in 50 to 85 percent of patients with schizophrenia, compared with about 25 percent in psychiatric patients without schizophrenia and less than 10 percent in non–psychiatrically ill control subjects. Because eye movement is partly controlled by centers in the frontal lobes, a disorder in eye movement is consistent with theories that implicate a frontal lobe pathological process in schizophrenia.

Psychoneuroimmunology. Several immunological abnormalities have been associated with patients who have schizophrenia. The abnormalities include decreased T-cell interleukin-2 production, reduced number and responsiveness of peripheral lymphocytes, abnormal cellular and humoral reactivity to neurons, and the presence of brain-directed (antibrain) antibodies. The data can be interpreted variously as representing the effects of a neurotoxic virus or of an endogenous autoimmune disorder. Most carefully conducted investigations that have searched for evidence of neurotoxic viral infections in schizophrenia have had negative results, although epidemiological data show a high incidence of schizophrenia after prenatal exposure to influenza during several epidemics of the disease. Other data supporting a viral hypothesis are an increased number of physical anomalies at birth, an increased rate of pregnancy and birth complications, seasonality of birth consistent with viral infection, geographical clusters of adult cases, and seasonality of hospitalizations. Nonetheless, the inability to detect genetic evidence of viral infection reduces the significance of all circumstantial data. The possibility of autoimmune brain antibodies has some data to support it; the pathophysiological process, if it exists, however, probably explains only a subset of the population with schizophrenia.

Psychoneuroendocrinology. Many reports describe neuroendocrine differences between groups of patients with schizophrenia and groups of control subjects. For example, results of the dexamethasone-suppression test have been reported to be abnormal in various subgroups of patients with schizophrenia, although the practical or predictive value of the test in schizophrenia has been questioned. One carefully done report, however, has correlated persistent nonsuppression on the dexamethasone-suppression test in schizophrenia with a poor long-term outcome.

Some data suggest decreased concentrations of luteinizing hormone–follicle-stimulating hormone (LH/FSH), perhaps correlated with age of onset and length of illness. Two additional reported abnormalities may be correlated with the presence of negative symptoms: a blunted release of prolactin and growth hormone on gonadotropin-releasing hormone (GnRH) or thyrotropin-releasing hormone (TRH) stimulation and a blunted release of growth hormone on apomorphine stimulation.

Genetic Factors

A wide range of genetic studies strongly suggests a genetic component to the inheritance of schizophrenia. In the 1930s, classic studies of the genetics of schizophrenia showed that a person is likely to have schizophrenia when other members of the family have the disorder and that the likelihood of the person's having schizophrenia is correlated with the closeness of the relationship (e.g., first-degree or second-degree relative; Table 13–2). Monozygotic twins have the highest concordance rate. In studies of adopted monozygotic twins, twins reared by adoptive parents are seen to have schizophrenia at the same rate as their twin siblings brought up by their biological parents. This finding suggests that the genetic influence outweighs the environmental influence, a finding corroborated by the observation that the more severe the schizophrenia, the more likely the twins are to be concordant for the disorder. One study supports the stress–diathesis model and shows that adopted monozygotic twins who later had schizophrenia were likely to have been adopted by psychologically disordered families.

Many associations between chromosomal sites and schizophrenia have been reported since the application of the techniques of molecular biology became widespread. More than half of all chromosomes have been associated with schizophrenia in various reports, but the long arms of chromosomes 5, 11, and 18, the short arm of chromosome 19, and the X chromosome have been implicated most commonly. Loci on chromosomes 6, 8, and 22 have also been implicated. The literature is best summarized as indicating a potentially heterogeneous genetic basis for schizophrenia.

Table 13–2
Prevalence of Schizophrenia in Specific Populations

Population	Prevalence (%)
General population	1.0
Nontwin sibling of a schizophrenia patient	8.0
Child with one parent with schizophrenia	12.0
Dizygotic twin of a schizophrenia patient	12.0
Child of two parents with schizophrenia	40.0
Monozygotic twin of a schizophrenia patient	47.0

Psychosocial Factors

If schizophrenia is a disease of the brain, it is likely to parallel diseases of other organs (e.g., myocardial infarctions and diabetes) whose courses are affected by psychosocial stress. Also, as with other chronic diseases (e.g., chronic congestive pulmonary disease), drug therapy alone rarely suffices to obtain maximal clinical improvement. Thus, clinicians should consider the psychosocial factors affecting schizophrenia. Although, historically, theorists have attributed the development of schizophrenia to psychosocial factors, contemporary clinicians can benefit from using the relevant theories and guidelines of these past observations and hypotheses.

Regardless of the controversies over the causes of schizophrenia, the disorder affects individual patients, each of whom has a unique psychological makeup. Although many psychodynamic theories about the pathogenesis of schizophrenia seem out of date, perceptive clinical observations can help contemporary clinicians understand how the disease may affect a patient's psyche.

PSYCHOANALYTIC THEORIES. Sigmund Freud postulated that schizophrenia resulted from developmental fixations that occurred earlier than those culminating in the development of neuroses. Freud also postulated that an ego defect contributed to the symptoms of schizophrenia. Ego disintegration in schizophrenia represents a return to the time when the ego was not yet, or had just begun to be, established. Thus, intrapsychic conflict arising from the early fixations and the ego defect, which may have resulted from poor early object relations, fuel the psychotic symptoms.

Central to Freud's theories of schizophrenia were a decathexis of objects and a regression in response to frustration and conflict with others. Many of Freud's ideas about schizophrenia were colored by his lack of intensive involvement with schizophrenia patients.

In the classic psychoanalytic view of schizophrenia, the ego defect affects the interpretation of reality and the control of inner drives, such as sex and aggression. The disturbances result from distortions in the reciprocal relationship between the infant and the mother. As described by Margaret Mahler, the child is unable to separate from, and progress beyond, the closeness and complete dependence that characterize the mother–child relationship in the oral phase of development. A person with schizophrenia never achieves object constancy, which is characterized by a sense of secure identity and which results from a close attachment to the mother during infancy. Paul Federn concluded that the fundamental disturbance in schizophrenia is the patient's early inability to achieve self–object differentiation. Some psychoanalysts hypothesize that the defect in rudimentary ego functions permits intense hostility and aggression to distort the mother–infant relationship and leads to a personality organization vulnerable to stress. The onset of symptoms during adolescence occurs when teenagers need a strong ego to function independently, to separate from the parents, to identify tasks, to control increased internal drives, and to cope with intense external stimulation.

Harry Stack Sullivan viewed schizophrenia as a disturbance in interpersonal relatedness. The patient's massive anxiety creates a sense of unrelatedness that is transformed into distortions called *parataxic distortions*, which are persecutory. To Sullivan schizophrenia is an adaptive method to avoid panic, terror, and disintegration of the sense of self. The source of pathological anxiety results from cumulative experimental traumas during development.

Psychoanalytic theory also postulates that the various symptoms of schizophrenia have symbolic meaning for individual patients. For example, fantasies of the world coming to an end may indicate a perception that a person's internal world has broken down. Feelings of grandeur may reflect reactivated narcissism, in which persons believe that they are omnipotent. Hallucinations may be substitutes for patients' inability to deal with objective reality and may represent their inner wishes or fears. Delusions, like hallucinations, are regressive, restitutive attempts to create a new reality or to express hidden fears or impulses (Fig. 13–6).

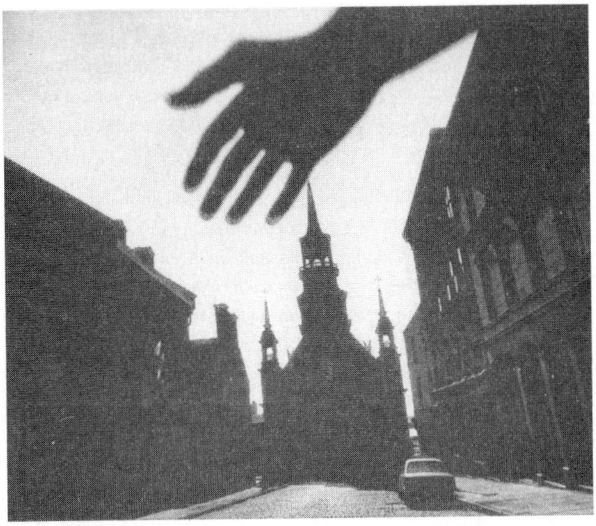

FIGURE 13–6
In schizophrenia, irrational and idiosyncratic ideas create a fearful world that is difficult for others to experience or understand, as symbolized above. (Courtesy of Arthur Tress.)

Regardless of the theoretical model, all psychodynamic approaches are founded on the premise that psychotic symptoms have meaning in schizophrenia. Patients, for example, may become grandiose after an injury to their self-esteem. Similarly, all theories recognize that human relatedness may be terrifying for persons with schizophrenia. Although research on the efficacy of psychotherapy with schizophrenia shows mixed results, concerned persons who offer compassion and a sanctuary in a confusing world must be a cornerstone of any overall treatment plan. Long-term follow-up studies show that some patients who bury psychotic episodes probably do not benefit from exploratory psychotherapy, but those who are able to integrate the psychotic experience into their lives may benefit from some insight-oriented approaches. There is renewed interest in the use of long-term individual psychotherapy in the treatment of schizophrenia, especially when combined with medication.

LEARNING THEORIES. According to learning theorists, children who later have schizophrenia learn irrational reactions and ways of thinking by imitating parents who have their own significant emotional problems. In learning theory, the poor interpersonal relationships of persons with schizophrenia develop because of poor models for learning during childhood.

Family Dynamics. No well-controlled evidence indicates that a specific family pattern plays a causative role in the development of schizophrenia. Clinicians must understand this important point—many parents of children with schizophrenia harbor anger against the psychiatric community for formerly correlating dysfunctional families with the development of schizophrenia. Advocacy organizations such as the National Alliance for the Mentally Ill (NAMI) have done much to edu-

cate parents not to blame themselves if schizophrenia develops in a child of theirs. Some patients with schizophrenia do come from dysfunctional families, just as many non–psychiatrically ill persons do. It is also clinically relevant, however, not to overlook pathological family behavior that can significantly increase the emotional stress with which a vulnerable patient with schizophrenia must cope.

DOUBLE BIND. The double-bind concept was formulated by Gregory Bateson and Donald Jackson to describe a hypothetical family in which children receive conflicting parental messages about their behavior, attitudes, and feelings. In Bateson's hypothesis, children withdraw into a psychotic state to escape the unsolvable confusion of the double bind. Unfortunately, the family studies that were conducted to validate the theory were seriously flawed methodologically. The theory has value only as a descriptive pattern, not as a causal explanation of schizophrenia. An example of a double bind is the parent who tells the child to provide cookies for his or her friends and then chastises the child for giving away too many cookies to playmates.

SCHISMS AND SKEWED FAMILIES. Theodore Lidz described two abnormal patterns of family behavior. In one family type, with a prominent schism between the parents, one parent is overly close to a child of the opposite sex. In the other family type, a skewed relationship between a child and one parent involves a power struggle between the parents and the resulting dominance of one parent. These dynamics stress the tenuous adaptive capacity of the schizophrenic person.

PSEUDOMUTUAL AND PSEUDOHOSTILE FAMILIES. As described by Lyman Wynne, some families suppress emotional expression by consistently using pseudomutual or pseudohostile verbal communication. In such families, a unique verbal communication develops, and when a child leaves home and must relate to other persons, problems may arise. The child's verbal communication may be incomprehensible to outsiders.

EXPRESSED EMOTION. Parents or other caretakers may behave with overt criticism, hostility, and overinvolvement toward a person with schizophrenia. Many studies have indicated that in families with high levels of expressed emotion (often abbreviated EE), the relapse rate for schizophrenia is high. The assessment of expressed emotion involves analyzing both what is said and the manner in which it is said.

Social Theories. Some researchers have suggested that industrialization and urbanization are involved in the causes of schizophrenia. Although some data support such theories, these stresses are now thought to have their major effects on the timing of onset and the severity of the illness.

DIAGNOSIS

The DSM-IV-TR diagnostic criteria are listed in Table 13–3. The criteria of other diagnostic systems appear in Table 13–1.

The DSM-IV-TR diagnostic criteria include course specifiers (i.e., prognosis) that offer clinicians several options and describe actual clinical situations (Table 13–3). The presence of hallucinations or delusions is not necessary for a diagnosis of schizophrenia; a patient's disorder is diagnosed as schizophrenia when the patient exhibits two of the symptoms listed as symptoms 3 through 5 in criterion A (discussed below). Criterion B requires that impaired functioning, although not deteriorations, be present during the active phase of the illness.

Table 13–3
DSM-IV-TR Diagnostic Criteria for Schizophrenia

A. *Characteristic symptoms:* Two (or more) of the following, each present for a significant portion of time during a 1-month period (or less if successfully treated):
(1) delusions
(2) hallucinations
(3) disorganized speech (e.g., frequent derailment or incoherence)
(4) grossly disorganized or catatonic behavior
(5) negative symptoms, i.e., affective flattening, alogia, or avolition

Note: Only one Criterion A symptom is required if delusions are bizarre or hallucinations consist of a voice keeping up a running commentary on the person's behavior or thoughts, or two or more voices conversing with each other.

B. *Social/occupational dysfunction:* For a significant portion of the time since the onset of the disturbance, one or more major areas of functioning such as work, interpersonal relations, or self-care are markedly below the level achieved prior to the onset (or when the onset is in childhood or adolescence, failure to achieve expected level of interpersonal, academic, or occupational achievement).

C. *Duration:* Continuous signs of the disturbance persist for at least 6 months. This 6-month period must include at least 1 month of symptoms (or less if successfully treated) that meet Criterion A (i.e., active-phase symptoms) and may include periods of prodromal or residual symptoms. During these prodromal or residual periods, the signs of the disturbance may be manifested by only negative symptoms or two or more symptoms listed in Criterion A present in an attenuated form (e.g., odd beliefs, unusual perceptual experiences).

D. *Schizoaffective and mood disorder exclusion:* Schizoaffective disorder and mood disorder with psychotic features have been ruled out because either (1) no major depressive, manic, or mixed episodes have occurred concurrently with the active-phase symptoms; or (2) if mood episodes have occurred during active-phase symptoms, their total duration has been brief relative to the duration of the active and residual periods.

E. *Substance/general medical condition exclusion:* The disturbance is not due to the direct physiological effects of a substance (e.g., a drug of abuse, a medication) or a general medical condition.

F. *Relationship to a pervasive developmental disorder:* If there is a history of autistic disorder or another pervasive developmental disorder, the additional diagnosis of schizophrenia is made only if prominent delusions or hallucinations are also present for at least a month (or less if successfully treated).

Classification of longitudinal course (can be applied only after at least 1 year has elapsed since the initial onset of active-phase symptoms):

Episodic with interepisode residual symptoms (episodes are defined by the reemergence of prominent psychotic symptoms); also *specify* if: **with prominent negative symptoms**

Episodic with no interepisode residual symptoms

Continuous (prominent psychotic symptoms are present throughout the period of observation); also *specify* if: **with prominent negative symptoms**

Single episode in partial remission: also *specify* if: **with prominent negative symptoms**

Single episode in full remission

Other or unspecified pattern

From American Psychiatric Association, *Diagnostic and Statistical Manual of Mental Disorders.* 4th ed. Text rev. Washington, DC: American Psychiatric Association; copyright 2000, with permission.

Table 13–4
DSM-IV-TR Diagnostic Criteria for Schizophrenia Subtypes

Paranoid type

A type of schizophrenia in which the following criteria are met:

A. Preoccupation with one or more delusions or frequent auditory hallucinations.

B. None of the following is prominent: disorganized speech, disorganized or catatonic behavior, or flat or inappropriate affect.

Disorganized type

A type of schizophrenia in which the following criteria are met:

A. All of the following are prominent:
(1) disorganized speech
(2) disorganized behavior
(3) flat or inappropriate affect

B. The criteria are not met for catatonic type.

Catatonic type

A type of schizophrenia in which the clinical picture is dominated by at least two of the following:

(1) motoric immobility as evidenced by catalepsy (including waxy flexibility) or stupor
(2) excessive motor activity (that is apparently purposeless and not influenced by external stimuli)
(3) extreme negativism (an apparently motiveless resistance to all instructions or maintenance of a rigid posture against attempts to be moved) or mutism
(4) peculiarities of voluntary movement as evidenced by posturing (voluntary assumption of inappropriate or bizarre postures), stereotyped movements, prominent mannerisms, or prominent grimacing
(5) echolalia or echopraxia

Undifferentiated type

A type of schizophrenia in which symptoms that meet Criterion A are present, but the criteria are not met for the paranoid, disorganized, or catatonic type.

Residual type

A type of schizophrenia in which the following criteria are met:

A. Absence of prominent delusions, hallucinations, disorganized speech, and grossly disorganized or catatonic behavior.

B. There is continuing evidence of the disturbance, as indicated by the presence of negative symptoms or two or more symptoms listed in Criterion A for schizophrenia, present in an attenuated form (e.g., odd beliefs, unusual perceptual experiences).

From American Psychiatric Association. *Diagnostic and Statistical Manual of Mental Disorders.* 4th ed. Text rev. Washington, DC: American Psychiatric Association; copyright 2000, with permission.

Symptoms must persist for at least 6 months, and a diagnosis of schizoaffective disorder or mood disorder must be absent.

Subtypes

DSM-IV-TR classifies the subtypes of schizophrenia as paranoid, disorganized, catatonic, undifferentiated, and residual (Table 13–4), based predominantly on clinical presentation. These subtypes are not closely correlated with different prognoses; for such differentiation, specific predictors of prognosis are best consulted (Table 13–5). The 10th revision of *International Statistical Classification of Diseases and Related Health Problems* (ICD-10), by contrast, uses nine subtypes: paranoid schizophrenia, hebephrenia, catatonic schizophrenia, undifferentiated schizophrenia, postschizophrenic depression, residual schizophrenia, simple schizophrenia, other schizophrenia, and schizophrenia, unspecified, with eight possibilities for classifying the course of the disorder, ranging from continuous to complete remission.

Table 13–5
Features Weighting toward Good to Poor Prognosis in Schizophrenia

Good Prognosis	Poor Prognosis
Late onset	Young onset
Obvious precipitating factors	No precipitating factors
Acute onset	Insidious onset
Good premorbid social, sexual, and work histories	Poor premorbid social, sexual, and work histories
Mood disorder symptoms (especially depressive disorders)	Withdrawn, autistic behavior
Married	Single, divorced, or widowed
Family history of mood disorders	Family history of schizophrenia
Good support systems	Poor support systems
Positive symptoms	Negative symptoms
	Neurological signs and symptoms
	History of perinatal trauma
	No remissions in 3 years
	Many relapses
	History of assaultiveness

Paranoid Type. The paranoid type of schizophrenia is characterized by preoccupation with one or more delusions or frequent auditory hallucinations. Classically, the paranoid type of schizophrenia is characterized mainly by the presence of delusions of persecution or grandeur. Patients with paranoid schizophrenia usually have their first episode of illness at an older age than do patients with catatonic or disorganized schizophrenia. Patients in whom schizophrenia occurs in the late 20s or 30s have usually established a social life that may help them through their illness, and the ego resources of paranoid patients tend to be greater than those of patients with catatonic and disorganized schizophrenia. Patients with the paranoid type of schizophrenia show less regression of their mental faculties, emotional responses, and behavior than do patients with other types of schizophrenia.

Patients with paranoid schizophrenia are typically tense, suspicious, guarded, reserved, and sometimes hostile or aggressive, but they can occasionally conduct themselves adequately in social situations. Their intelligence in areas not invaded by their psychosis tends to remain intact.

A 44-year-old single, unemployed man was brought into an emergency room by the police for striking an elderly woman in his apartment building. He complained that the woman he struck was a bitch and that she and "the others" deserved more than that for what they put him through.

The patient had been continually ill since the age of 22. During his first year of law school, he gradually became more and more convinced that his classmates were making fun of him. He noticed that they would snort and sneeze whenever he entered the classroom. When a girl he was dating broke off the relationship with him, he believed that she had been replaced by a look-alike. He called the police and asked for their help in solving the "kidnapping." His academic performance in school declined dramatically, and he was asked to leave and seek psychiatric care.

The patient got a job as an investment counselor at a bank, which he held for 7 months. However, he was getting an increasing number of distracting "signals" from coworkers, and he became more and more suspicious and withdrawn. At that time he first reported hearing voices. He was eventually fired and soon thereafter was hospitalized for the first time, at age 24. He has not worked since.

The patient has been hospitalized 12 times; the longest stay was for 8 months. However, in the past 5 years he was hospitalized only once, for 3 weeks. During the hospitalizations he received various antipsychotic drugs. Although outpatient medication had been prescribed, he usually stopped taking it shortly after leaving the hospital. Aside from twice-yearly lunch meetings with his uncle and his contact with mental health workers, he was totally isolated socially. He lived on his own and managed his own financial affairs, including a modest inheritance. He read the *Wall Street Journal* daily. He cooked and cleaned for himself.

The patient maintained that his apartment was the center of a large communication system that involved all three major television networks, his neighborhood, and apparently hundreds of "actors" in his neighborhood. There were secret cameras in his apartment that carefully monitored all his activities. When he was watching television, many of his minor actions (e.g., getting up to go to the bathroom) were soon directly commented on by the announcer. Whenever he went outside, the "actors" had all been warned to keep him under surveillance; everyone on the street watched him. His neighbors operated two "machines"; one was responsible for all his voices except the "joker." He was not certain who controlled that voice, which visited him only occasionally and was very funny. The other voices, which he heard many times each day, were generated by that machine, which he sometimes thought was directly run by the neighbor whom he attacked. For example, when he was going over his investments, those "harassing" voices constantly told him which stocks to buy. The other machine he called "the dream machine." That machine put erotic dreams into his head, usually of black women.

The patient described other unusual experiences. For example, he recently went to a shoe store 30 miles from his home in the hope of getting some shoes that would not be "altered." However, he soon found out that like the rest of the shoes he bought, special nails had been put into the bottoms of the shoe to annoy him. He was amazed that his decision about which shoe store to go to must have been known to his "harasser" before he himself knew it, so that they had time to get the altered shoes made up especially for him. He realized that great effort and "millions of dollars'" were involved in keeping him under surveillance. He sometimes thought that was all part of a large experiment to discover the secret of his superior intelligence.

At the interview, the patient was well groomed, and his speech was coherent and goal directed. His affect was, at most, only mildly blunted. He was initially angry at police. After several weeks of treatment with an antipsychotic that failed to control his psychotic symptoms, he was transferred to a long-stay facility with the plan to arrange a structured living situation for him.

DISCUSSION

The patient's long illness apparently began with delusions of reference (his classmates making fun of him by snorting and sneezing when he entered the classroom). Over the years his delusions had become increasingly complex and bizarre (his neighbors were actually actors; his thoughts were monitored; a machine put erotic dreams into his head). In addition, he had prominent hallucinations of voices that harassed him.

Bizarre delusions and prominent hallucinations are the characteristic psychotic symptoms of schizophrenia. The diagnosis was confirmed by the marked disturbance in his work and social functioning and the absence of a sustained mood disturbance and of any known organic factor that could account for the disturbance.

All the patient's delusions and hallucinations seemed to involve the single theme of a conspiracy to harass him. That systematized persecutory delusion—the absence of incoherence, marked loosening of associations, flat or grossly inappropriate affect or catatonic or grossly disorganized behavior—indicates the paranoid type. Schizophrenia, paranoid type, is further specified as continuous if, as in this case, all past and present active phases of the illness have been of the paranoid type. The prognosis for the continuous paranoid type is better than the prognosis for the disorganized and undifferentiated types. The patient did, in fact, do remarkably well in spite of a chronic psychotic illness; over the past 5 years he had been able to take care of himself.

Disorganized Type. The disorganized (formerly called hebephrenic) type of schizophrenia is characterized by a marked regression to primitive, disinhibited, and unorganized behavior and by the absence of symptoms that meet the criteria for the catatonic type. The onset of this subtype is generally early, before age 25. Disorganized patients are usually active but in an aimless, nonconstructive manner. Their thought disorder is pronounced, and their contact with reality is poor. Their personal appearance is dilapidated and then social behavior and their emotional responses are inappropriate, and they often burst into laughter without any apparent reason. Incongruous grinning and grimacing are common in these patients, whose behavior is best described as silly or fatuous.

Emilio is a 40-year-old man who looks 10 years younger. He is brought to the hospital, his 12th hospitalization, by his mother because she is afraid of him. He is dressed in a ragged overcoat, bedroom slippers, and a baseball cap and wears several medals around his neck. His affect ranges from anger at his mother ("She feeds me shit . . . what comes out of other people's rectums") to a giggling, obsequious seductiveness toward the interviewer. His speech and manner have a childlike quality, and he walks with a mincing step and exaggerated hip movements. His mother reports that he stopped taking his medication about a month ago, and has since begun to hear voices and to look and act more bizarre. When asked what he has been doing, he said, "Easting wired and lighting fires." His spontaneous speech is often incoherent and marked by frequent rhyming and clang associations (speech in which sounds, rather than meaningful relationships, govern word choice).

Emilio's first hospitalization occurred after he dropped out of school at age 16, and since that time he has never been able to attend school or hold a job. He has been treated with neuroleptics during his hospitalizations but doesn't continue to take medication when he leaves, so he quickly becomes disorganized again. He lives with his elderly mother but sometimes disappears for several months at a time and is eventually picked up by the police as he wanders in the streets. There is no known history of drug or alcohol abuse.

DISCUSSION

The combination of chronic illness with marked incoherence, inappropriate affect, auditory hallucinations, and grossly disorganized behavior leaves little doubt that the diagnosis is chronic schizophrenia. The course would be noted as continuous because Emilio apparently never has prolonged remissions of his psychosis. The prominence of his disorganized speech and behavior, grossly inappropriate affect, and the absence of prominent catatonic symptoms indicate the disorganized type.

FOLLOW-UP

Emilio has been hospitalized five more times in the 10 years following this admission to the hospital. During each of his hospitalizations, he was treated with high doses of antipsychotic drugs and within a few weeks began to behave appropriately and to be able to ignore the voices of his auditory hallucinations. During the first hospitalization, he was able to establish a relationship with a therapist and talk thoughtfully and with a full range of appropriate affect about his unhappy life, his inability to do any work because "nobody wants me," and his desire to be taken care of. However, soon after leaving the hospital Emilio stopped taking his medication, failed to keep clinic appointments, and within a few months was again grossly disorganized and psychotic.

Emilio's last psychiatric hospitalization was 2 years ago, when he was 48. His mother was now too feeble to care for him, and arrangements were made for him to live in an adult home after he left the hospital—supported by welfare, and with medication managed by the staff of the institution. In that setting he does fairly well. (From *DSM-IV Casebook*, with permission.)

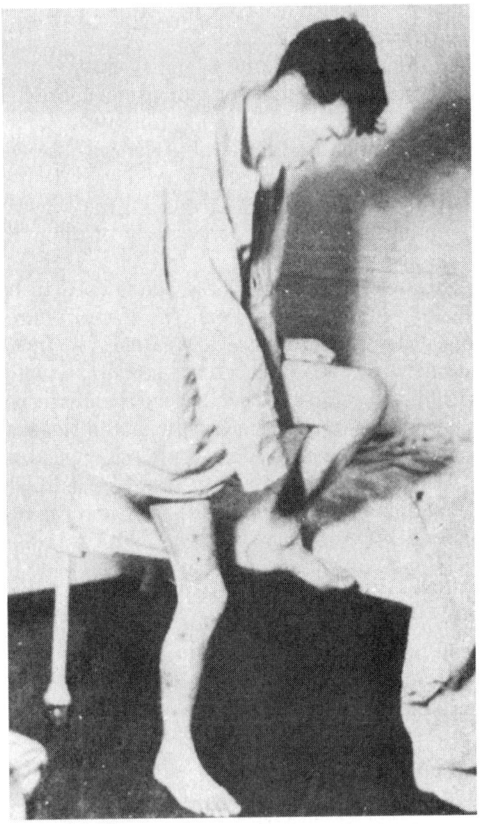

FIGURE 13–7
A chronic schizophrenia patient stands in a cataleptic position. He maintained this uncomfortable position for hours. (Courtesy of New York Academy of Medicine, New York, NY.)

Catatonic Type. The catatonic type of schizophrenia, which was common several decades ago, has become rare in Europe and North America. The classic feature of the catatonic type is a marked disturbance in motor function; this disturbance may involve stupor, negativism, rigidity, excitement, or posturing (Fig. 13–7). Sometimes, the patient shows rapid alteration between extremes of excitement and stupor. Associated features include stereotypies, mannerisms, and waxy flexibility. Mutism is particularly common. During catatonic stupor or excitement, patients need careful supervision to prevent them from hurting themselves or others. Medical care may be needed because of malnutrition, exhaustion, hyperpyrexia, or self-inflicted injury.

A young, unmarried woman, age 20, was admitted to a psychiatric hospital because she had become violent toward her parents, had been observed gazing into space with a rapt expression, and had been talking to invisible persons. She had been seen to strike odd postures. Her speech had become incoherent.

She had been a good student in high school, then went to business school and, a year before admission to the hospital, started to work in an office as a stenographer. She had always been shy, and although she was quite attractive, she had not been dating much. Another girl, who worked in the same office,

told the patient about boys and petting and began to exert a great deal of influence over her. The second girl would communicate with her from across the room. Even when they went home at night, the patient would get voice messages telling her to do certain things. Then pictures began to appear on the wall, most of them ugly and sneering. Those pictures had names—one was named shyness, another distress, another envy. Her office friend sent her messages to knock on the wall, to hit the pictures.

The patient was agitated, noisy, and uncooperative in the hospital for several weeks after she arrived, and required sedation. She received several courses of electroconvulsive treatment, which failed to influence the schizophrenic process to any significant degree. Ten years later, when antipsychotic drugs became available, she received pharmacotherapy.

Despite all those therapeutic efforts, her condition throughout her many years of stay in a mental hospital has remained one of chronic catatonic stupor. She is mute and practically devoid of any spontaneity, but she responds to simple requests. She stays in the same position for hours or sits curled up in a chair. Her facial expression is fixed and stony. (Courtesy of Robert Cancro, M.D., Med.D.Sc., and Heinz E. Lehmann, M.D.)

Undifferentiated Type. Frequently, patients who are clearly schizophrenic cannot be easily fitted into one or another type. DSM-IV-TR classifies these patients as having schizophrenia of the undifferentiated type.

Mr. D. is a 24-year-old, single, unemployed college dropout who was admitted to the hospital 3 weeks after he painted everything in sight black or white, including his room, his furniture, his clothes, and finally, even himself. He was responding to a persistent male voice that told him that his behavior would somehow solve the race problem in America and bring peace to his family.

Mr. D. has been hospitalized on at least five previous occasions during the past 5 years, each time for 4 to 6 weeks. Each hospitalization was due to an exacerbation of his illness with some combination of command hallucinations, strange behavior, and persecutory delusions. He has always responded fairly well to treatment with neuroleptics but hates to take the medication because it makes him feel "even deader than dead." Between hospitalizations, he is likely to take medication irregularly or not all and to miss more outpatient appointments than he keeps.

Mr. D. is the fourth of five children in an extremely close-knit, guilt-provoking, and argumentative family. His mother has been hospitalized twice for hallucinations and persecutory delusions but now functions reasonably well without medication. She believes that she knows better than the doctors what is best for her son. Her other children have left the family apartment, and Ms. D. has become increasingly attached to, and dependent on, "the only kid I have left." Mr. D. responds to his mother's ministrations with annoyance and avoidance but, when they are not forthcoming, also becomes annoyed.

Mr. D. spends most of his time in the apartment doing yoga and reading about jungian archetypes and social oppression. He sleeps all day and stays up most of every night and, except when hospitalized, rarely talks to anyone outside his immediate family circle. He is afraid to go outside, especially during the day, because he believes that strangers on the street are talking to each other about him and are able to control his thoughts and actions. He is convinced that the transmission of thought commands requires solar energy and that he is safer at night. He also believes that a "right-wing, neo-Nazi" group is attempting to ruin his reputation by spreading rumors that he is one-eighth Jewish.

As usual, Mr. D. responds well to neuroleptic medication during this hospitalization. He remains convinced of his delusions, but in a low-key way, and can to some extent be argued out of them. He is also able to talk to staff with less suspicion and greater coherence than when he was admitted, and his behavior is no longer overtly bizarre. He seems ready for discharge.

Mr. D.'s mother has had his room repainted and is eager to have him back. Mr. D.'s therapist focused attention on Mr. D.'s resistance to taking medication and the detrimental impact that this has on his treatment and his life. Mr. D. seems somewhat more insightful about this behavior than he has in the past. Efforts to enlist his mother's cooperation have not been conspicuously successful.

DIAGNOSIS

Axis 1: Schizophrenia, undifferentiated type episodic with interepisode residual symptoms
Axis II: No diagnosis
Axis III: None
Axis IV: GAF = 25 (current); (highest level past year)

(From *DSM-IV Case Studies*)

Residual Type. According to DSM-IV-TR, the residual type of schizophrenia is characterized by continuing evidence of the schizophrenic disturbance in the absence of a complete set of active symptoms or of sufficient symptoms to meet the diagnosis of another type of schizophrenia. Emotional blunting, social withdrawal, eccentric behavior, illogical thinking, and mild loosening of associations commonly appear in the residual type. When delusions or hallucinations occur, they are neither prominent nor accompanied by strong affect.

Other Subtypes

The subtyping of schizophrenia has had a long history; other subtyping schemes appear in the literature, especially literature from countries other than the United States.

***Bouffée Délirante* (Acute Delusional Psychosis).** This French diagnostic concept differs from a diagnosis of schizophrenia primarily on the basis of a symptom duration of less than 3 months. The diagnosis is similar to the DSM-IV-TR diagnosis of schizophreniform disorder. French clinicians report that about 40 percent of patients with a diagnosis of *bouffée*

délirante progress in their illness and are eventually classified as having schizophrenia.

Latent. The concept of latent schizophrenia was developed during a time when theorists conceived of the disorder in broad diagnostic terms. Currently, patients must be very mentally ill to warrant a diagnosis of schizophrenia, but with a broad diagnostic concept of schizophrenia, the condition of patients who would not currently be thought of as severely ill could have received a diagnosis of schizophrenia. Latent schizophrenia, for example, was often the diagnosis used for what are now called borderline schizoid and schizotypal personality disorders. These patients may occasionally show peculiar behaviors or thought disorders but do not consistently manifest psychotic symptoms. In the past, the syndrome was also termed *borderline schizophrenia.*

Oneiroid. The oneiroid state refers to a dreamlike state in which patients may be deeply perplexed and not fully oriented in time and place. The term *oneiroid schizophrenic* has been used for patients who are deeply engaged in their hallucinatory experiences to the exclusion of involvement in the real world. When an oneiroid state is present, clinicians should be particularly careful to examine patients for medical or neurological causes of the symptoms.

Paraphrenia. The term *paraphrenia* is sometimes used as a synonym for *paranoid schizophrenia* or for either a progressively deteriorating course of illness or the presence of a well-systemized delusional system. The multiple meanings of the term render it ineffectual in communicating information.

Pseudoneurotic Schizophrenia. Occasionally, patients who initially have such symptoms as anxiety, phobias, obsessions, and compulsions later reveal symptoms of thought disorder and psychosis. These patients are characterized by symptoms of pananxiety, panphobia, panambivalence, and sometimes chaotic sexuality. Unlike persons with anxiety disorders, pseudoneurotic patients have free-floating anxiety that rarely subsides. In clinical descriptions, the patients seldom become overtly and severely psychotic. This condition is currently diagnosed in DSM-IV-TR as borderline personality disorder.

Simple Deteriorative Disorder (Simple Schizophrenia). Simple deteriorative disorder is characterized by a gradual, insidious loss of drive and ambition. Patients with the disorder are usually not overtly psychotic and do not experience persistent hallucinations or delusions. Their primary symptom is withdrawal from social and work-related situations. The syndrome must be differentiated from depression, a phobia, a dementia, or an exacerbation of personality traits. Clinicians should be sure that patients truly meet the diagnostic criteria for schizophrenia before making the diagnosis. Simple deteriorative disorder appears as a diagnostic category in an appendix of DSM-IV-TR (Table 13–6).

Postpsychotic Depressive Disorder of Schizophrenia. Following an acute schizophrenia episode some patients become depressed (see Table 15.3–5). The symptoms of postpsychotic depressive disorder of schizophrenia can closely resemble the symptoms of the residual phase of schizophrenia as well as the adverse effects of commonly used antipsychotic medications. The diagnosis should not be made if they are substance induced or part of a mood disorder due to a general medical condition. ICD-10 describes a category called postschizophrenia depression arising in the aftermath of a schizophrenic illness. These depressive states occur in up to 25 percent of patients with schizophrenia and are associated with an increased risk of suicide. (Further discussion of the disorder can be found in Section 15.3.)

Table 13–6
DSM-IV-TR Research Criteria for Simple Deteriorative Disorder (Simple Schizophrenia)

A. Progressive development over a period of at least a year of all of the following:
  (1) marked decline in occupational or academic functioning
  (2) gradual appearance and deepening of negative symptoms such as affective flattening, alogia, and avolition
  (3) poor interpersonal rapport, social isolation, or social withdrawal

B. Criterion A for schizophrenia has never been met.

C. The symptoms are not better accounted for by schizotypal or schizoid personality disorder, a psychotic disorder, a mood disorder, an anxiety disorder, a dementia, or mental retardation and are not due to the direct physiological effects of a substance or a general medical condition.

From American Psychiatric Association. *Diagnostic and Statistical Manual of Mental Disorders.* 4th ed. Text rev. Washington, DC: American Psychiatric Association; copyright 2000, with permission.

Early-Onset Schizophrenia. A small minority of patients manifest schizophrenia in childhood. Such children may at first present diagnostic problems, particularly with differentiation from mental retardation and autistic disorder. Recent studies have established that the diagnosis of childhood schizophrenia may be based on the same symptoms used for adult schizophrenia. Its onset is usually insidious, its course tends to be chronic, and the prognosis is mostly unfavorable. (Chapter 50 contains further discussion of early-onset schizophrenia.)

Late-Onset Schizophrenia. Late-onset schizophrenia is clinically indistinguishable from schizophrenia but has an onset after age 45. This condition tends to appear more frequently in women and also tends to be characterized by a predominance of paranoid symptoms. The prognosis is favorable, and these patients usually do well on antipsychotic medication.

Other Diagnostic Criteria

A variety of research clinicians constructed their own criteria to describe the essential features of schizophrenia. Table 13–1 lists some of these schema, many of which are still in active use. The Present State Examination is among those extensively used by researchers.

Psychological Testing

Patients with schizophrenia generally perform poorly on a wide range of neuropsychological tests. Vigilance, memory, and concept formation are most affected and consistent with pathological involvement in the frontotemporal cortex.

Objective measures of neuropsychological performance, such as the Halstead-Reitan battery and the Luria-Nebraska battery, often give abnormal findings, such as bilateral frontal and temporal lobe dysfunction, including impairments in attention, retention time, and problem-solving ability. Motor ability is also impaired, possibly related to brain asymmetry.

Intelligence Tests. When groups of patients with schizophrenia are compared with groups of psychiatric patients without schizophrenia or with the general population, the schizophrenia patients tend to score lower on intelligence tests. Statistically, the evidence suggests that low intelligence is often present at the onset, and intelligence may continue to deteriorate with the progression of the disorder.

Projective and Personality Tests. Projective tests, such as the Rorschach test and the Thematic Apperception Test (TAT), may indicate bizarre ideation. Personality inventories, such as the Minnesota Multiphasic Personality Inventory (MMPI), often give abnormal results in schizophrenia, but the contribution to diagnosis and treatment planning is minimal.

CLINICAL FEATURES

A discussion of the clinical signs and symptoms of schizophrenia raises three key issues. First, no clinical sign or symptom is pathognomonic for schizophrenia; every sign or symptom seen in schizophrenia occurs in other psychiatric and neurological disorders. This observation is contrary to the often-heard clinical opinion that certain signs and symptoms are diagnostic of schizophrenia. Therefore, a patient's history is essential for the diagnosis of schizophrenia; clinicians cannot diagnose schizophrenia simply by results of a mental status examination, which may vary. Second, a patient's symptoms change with time. For example, a patient may have intermittent hallucinations and a varying ability to perform adequately in social situations, or significant symptoms of a mood disorder may come and go during the course of schizophrenia. Third, clinicians must take into account the patient's educational level, intellectual ability, and cultural and subcultural membership. An impaired ability to understand abstract concepts, for example, may reflect either the patient's education or his or her intelligence. Religious organizations and cults may have customs that seem strange to outsiders but are normal to those within the cultural setting.

Premorbid Signs and Symptoms

In theoretical formulations of the course of schizophrenia, premorbid signs and symptoms appear before the prodromal phase of the illness. The differentiation implies that premorbid signs and symptoms exist before the disease process evidences itself and that the prodromal signs and symptoms are parts of the evolving disorder. In the typical, but not invariable, premorbid history of schizophrenia, patients had schizoid or schizotypal personalities characterized as quiet, passive, and introverted; as children they had few friends. Preschizophrenic adolescents may have no close friends and no dates and may avoid team sports. They may enjoy watching movies and television or listening to music or playing computer games to the exclusion of social activities. Some adolescent patients may show a sudden onset of obsessive-compulsive behavior as part of the prodromal picture.

The validity of the prodromal signs and symptoms, almost invariably recognized after the diagnosis of schizophrenia has been made, is uncertain; once schizophrenia is diagnosed, the retrospective remembrance of early signs and symptoms is affected. Nevertheless, although the first hospitalization is often thought to mark the beginning of the disorder, signs and symptoms have often been present for months or even years. The signs may have started with complaints about somatic symptoms, such as headache, back and muscle pain, weakness, and digestive problems. The initial diagnosis may be malingering, chronic fatigue syndrome, or somatization disorder. Family and friends may eventually notice that the person has changed and is no longer functioning well in occupational, social, and personal activities. During this stage, a patient may begin to develop an interest in abstract ideas, philosophy, the occult, or religious questions. Additional prodromal signs and symptoms can include markedly peculiar behavior, abnormal affect, unusual speech, bizarre ideas, and strange perceptual experiences.

Positive and Negative Symptoms

In 1980, T. J. Crow proposed a classification of schizophrenia patients into types I and II, on the basis of the presence or absence of positive (or productive) and negative (or deficit) symptoms. Although the system was not accepted as part of the DSM-IV classification, the clinical distinction of the two types has significantly influenced psychiatric research. The *positive symptoms* include delusions and hallucinations. The *negative symptoms* include affective flattening or blunting, poverty of speech (alogia) or speech content, blocking, poor grooming, lack of motivation, anhedonia, and social withdrawal. Type I patients tend to have mostly positive symptoms, normal brain structures on CT scans, and relatively good response to treatment. Type II patients tend to have mostly negative symptoms, structural brain abnormalities on CT scans, and poor response to treatments. A third category, disorganized, includes disorganized speech (thought disorder), disorganized behavior, cognitive defects, and attention deficits. Nancy Andreason has studied positive and negative symptoms extensively (Table 13–7).

Mental Status Examination

General Description. The appearance of a patient with schizophrenia can range from that of a completely disheveled, screaming, agitated person to an obsessively groomed, completely silent, and immobile person. Between these two poles, patients may be talkative and may exhibit bizarre postures. Their behavior may become agitated or violent, apparently in an unprovoked manner but usually in response to hallucinations. By contrast, in catatonic stupor, often referred to as *catatonia,* patients seem completely lifeless and may exhibit such signs as muteness, negativism, and automatic obedience. Waxy flexibility, once a common sign in catatonia, has become rare, as has manneristic behavior (Fig. 13–8). A person with a less extreme subtype of catatonia may show marked social withdrawal and egocentricity, lack of spontaneous speech or movement, and an absence of goal-directed behavior (Fig. 13–9). Patients with catatonia may sit immobile and speechless in their chairs, respond to questions with only short answers, and move only when directed to. Other

Table 13–7
Percentage of Patients with Negative and Positive Symptoms (111 Consecutively Admitted Schizophrenic Patients)

Symptoms	Mild or Moderate	Severe or Extreme
Negative symptoms		
Affective flattening		
Unchanging facial expression	54	33
Decreased spontaneous movements	37	14
Paucity of expressive gestures	34	24
Poor eye contact	39	16
Affective nonresponsivity	18	18
Inappropriate affect	29	22
Lack of vocal inflections	40	9
Alogia		
Poverty of speech	20	20
Poverty of content of speech	33	6
Blocking	12	3
Increased response latency	17	6
Avolition–apathy		
Grooming and hygiene	33	41
Impersistence at work or school	13	74
Physical anergia	36	31
Anhedonia–asociality		
Recreational interests, activities	38	41
Sexual interest, activity	11	23
Intimacy, closeness	24	35
Relationship with friends, peers	25	63
Attention		
Social inattentiveness	25	32
Inattentiveness during testing	33	19
Positive symptoms		
Hallucinations		
Auditory	19	51
Voices commenting	22	12
Voices conversing	27	12
Somatic-tactile	10	6
Olfactory	5	1
Visual	16	15
Delusions		
Persecutory	19	47
Jealousy	2	1
Guilt, sin	16	2
Grandiose	15	15
Religious	12	11
Somatic	11	11
Delusions of reference	13	21
Delusions of being controlled	25	12
Delusions of mind reading	19	14
Thought broadcasting	11	2
Thought insertion	15	4
Thought withdrawal	11	6
Bizarre behavior		
Clothing, appearance	8	4
Social, sexual behavior	17	7
Aggressive/agitated behavior	14	6
Repetitive/stereotyped behavior	7	4
Positive formal thought disorder		
Derailment	30	4
Tangentiality	28	4
Incoherence	9	1
Illogicality	10	1
Circumstantiality	14	0
Pressure of speech	14	0
Distractible speech	12	1
Clanging	1	0

Adapted from Andreasen NC. The diagnosis of schizophrenia. *Schizophr Bull.* 1987;13:9.

obvious behavior may include odd clumsiness or stiffness in body movements, signs now seen as possibly indicating a disease process in the basal ganglia. Patients with schizophrenia often are poorly groomed, fail to bathe, and dress much too warmly for the prevailing temperatures. Other odd behaviors include tics, stereotypes, mannerisms, and, occasionally, *echopraxia,* in which patients imitate the posture or the behaviors of the examiner.

PRECOX FEELING. Some experienced clinicians report a precox feeling, an intuitive experience of their inability to establish an emotional rapport with a patient. Although the experience is common, no data indicate that it is a valid or reliable criterion in the diagnosis of schizophrenia.

Mood, Feelings, and Affect. Two common affective symptoms in schizophrenia are reduced emotional responsiveness, sometimes severe enough to warrant the label of anhedonia, and overly active and inappropriate emotions such as extremes of rage, happiness, and anxiety. A flat or blunted affect can be a symptom of the illness itself, of the parkinsonian adverse effects of antipsychotic medications, or of depression, and differentiating these symptoms can be a clinical challenge. Overly emotional patients may describe exultant feelings of omnipotence, religious ecstasy, terror at the disintegration of their souls, or paralyzing anxiety about the destruction of the universe. Other feeling tones include perplexity, a sense of isolation, overwhelming ambivalence, and depression.

Perceptual Disturbances. HALLUCINATIONS. Any of the five senses may be affected by hallucinatory experiences in patients with schizophrenia. The most common hallucinations, however, are auditory, with voices that are often threatening,

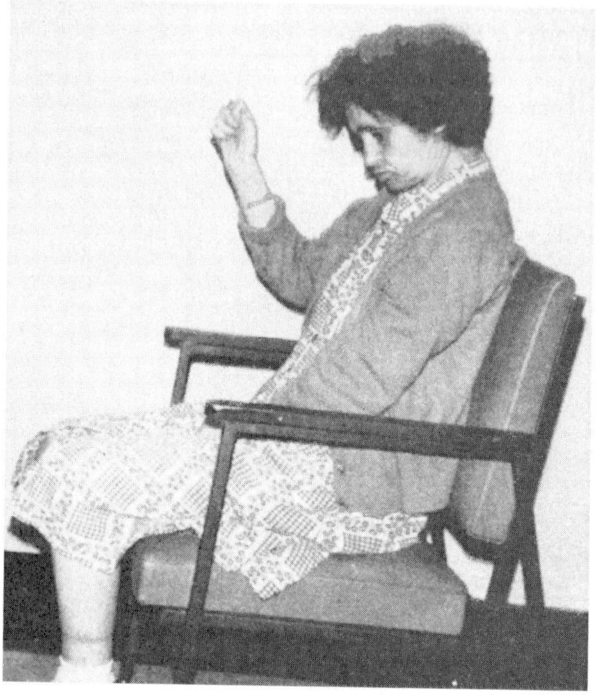

FIGURE 13–8
Long-term catatonic patient. This patient is immobile, demonstrating waxy flexibility. Her arm is in an uncomfortable position, elevated without support, and her stony facial expression has a *Schnauzkrampf,* or frozen snout. (Courtesy of Heinz E. Lehmann, M.D.)

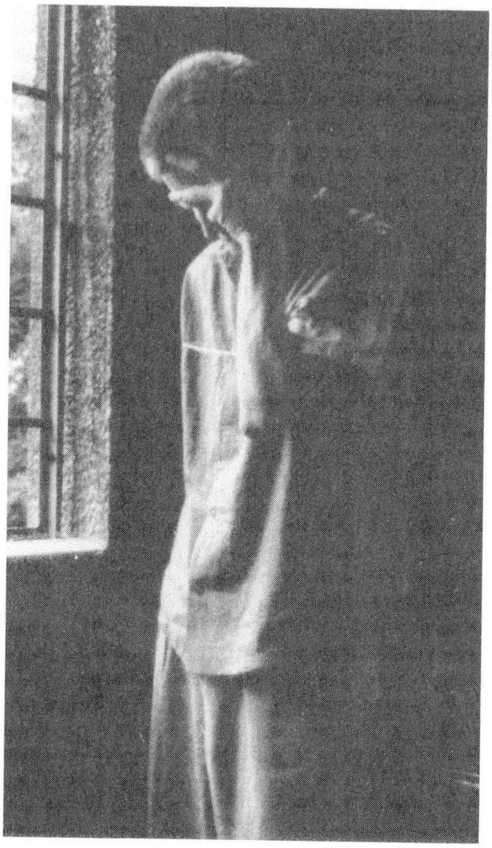

FIGURE 13–9
"Schizophrenic withdrawal." (Courtesy of Sid Bernstein, Research Facility, Orangeburg, NY.)

obscene, accusatory, or insulting. Two or more voices may converse among themselves, or a voice may comment on the patient's life or behavior. Visual hallucinations are common, but tactile, olfactory, and gustatory hallucinations are unusual; their presence should prompt the clinician to consider the possibility of an underlying medical or neurological disorder that is causing the entire syndrome.

Cenesthetic Hallucinations. Cenesthetic hallucinations are unfounded sensations of altered states in bodily organs. Examples of cenesthetic hallucinations include a burning sensation in the brain, a pushing sensation in the blood vessels, and a cutting sensation in the bone marrow. Bodily distortions may also occur (Fig. 13–10).

ILLUSIONS. As differentiated from hallucinations, *illusions* are distortions of real images or sensations, whereas *hallucinations* are *not* based on real images or sensations. Illusions can occur in schizophrenia patients during active phases, but they can also occur during the prodromal phases and during periods of remission. Whenever illusions or hallucinations occur, clinicians should consider the possibility of a substance-related cause for the symptoms, even when patients have already received a diagnosis of schizophrenia.

Thought. Disorders of thought are the most difficult symptoms for many clinicians and students to understand, but they may be the core symptoms of schizophrenia. Dividing the disorders of thought into disorders of thought content, form of thought, and thought process is one way to clarify them.

THOUGHT CONTENT. Disorders of thought content reflect the patient's ideas, beliefs, and interpretations of stimuli. Delusions, the most obvious example of a disorder of thought content, are varied in schizophrenia and may assume persecutory, grandiose, religious, or somatic forms.

Patients may believe that an outside entity controls their thoughts or behavior or, conversely, that they control outside events in an extraordinary fashion (e.g., by causing the sun to rise and set or by preventing earthquakes). Patients may have an intense and consuming preoccupation with esoteric, abstract, symbolic, psychological, or philosophical ideas. Patients may also worry about allegedly life-threatening but bizarre and implausible somatic conditions, such as the presence of aliens inside the patient's testicles affecting his ability to father children.

The phrase *loss of ego boundaries* describes the lack of a clear sense of where the patient's own body, mind, and influence end and where those of other animate and inanimate objects begin. For example, patients may think that other persons, the television, or the newspapers are referring to them (*ideas of reference*). Other symptoms of the loss of ego boundaries include the sense that the patient has physically fused with an outside object (e.g., a tree or another person) or that the patient has disintegrated and fused with the entire universe (*cosmic identity*). With such a state of mind, some patients with schizophrenia doubt their sex or their sexual orientation. These symptoms

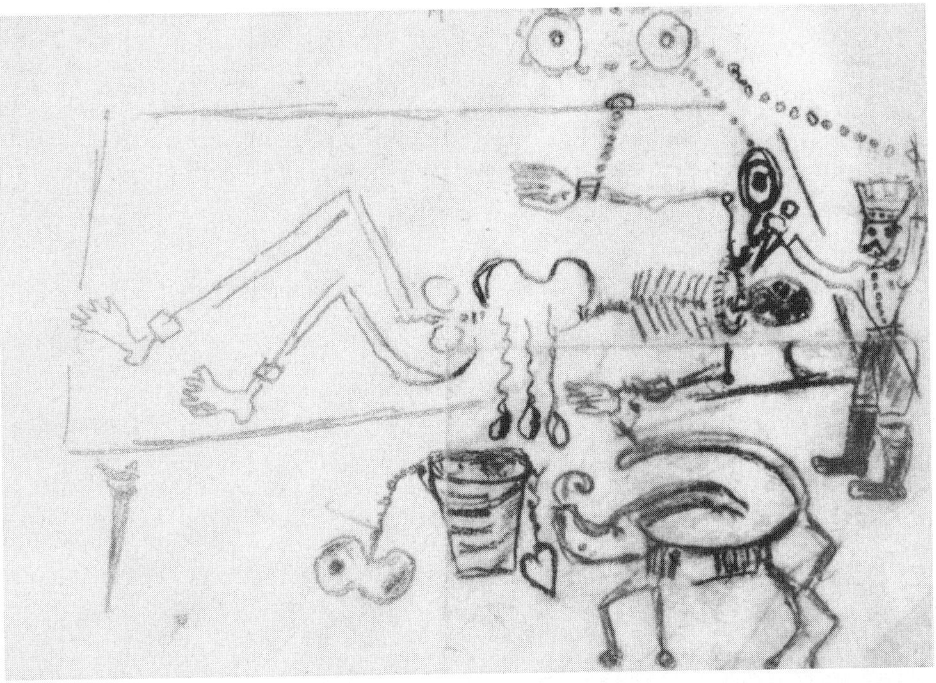

FIGURE 13–10
A 40-year-old schizophrenic man drew this picture, illustrating his elaborate fantasies of bodily torture and depicting a peculiar mixture of realistic and surrealistic details.

should not be confused with transvestism, transsexuality, or other gender identity problems.

FORM OF THOUGHT. Disorders of the form of thought are objectively observable in patients' spoken and written language (Fig. 13–11). The disorders include looseness of associations, derailment, incoherence, tangentiality, circumstantiality, neologisms (Fig. 13–12), echolalia, verbigeration, word salad, and mutism. Although looseness of associations was once described as pathognomonic for schizophrenia, the symptom is frequently seen in mania. Distinguishing between looseness of associations and tangentiality can be difficult for even the most experienced clinicians.

THOUGHT PROCESS. Disorders in thought process concern the way ideas and language are formulated. The examiner infers a disorder from what and how the patient speaks, writes, or draws. The examiner may also assess the patient's thought process by observing his or her behavior, especially in carrying out discrete tasks (e.g., in occupational therapy). Disorders of thought process include flight of ideas, thought blocking, impaired attention, poverty of thought content, poor abstraction abilities, perseveration, idiosyncratic associations (e.g., identical predicates and clang associations), overinclusion, and circumstantiality. *Thought control,* in which outside forces are controlling what the patient thinks or feels, is common as is *thought broadcasting,* in which patients think others can read their minds or that their thoughts are broadcast through television sets or radios.

Impulsiveness, Violence, Suicide, and Homicide.

Patients with schizophrenia may be agitated and have little impulse control when ill. They may also have decreased social sensitivity and appear to be impulsive when, for example, they grab another patient's cigarettes, change television channels abruptly, or throw food on the floor. Some apparently impulsive behavior, including suicide and homicide attempts, may be in response to hallucinations commanding the patient to act.

VIOLENCE. Violent behavior (excluding homicide) is common among untreated schizophrenia patients. Delusions of a persecutory nature, previous episodes of violence, and neurological deficits are risk factors for violent or impulsive behavior. Management includes appropriate antipsychotic medication. Emergency treatment consists of restraints and seclusion. Acute

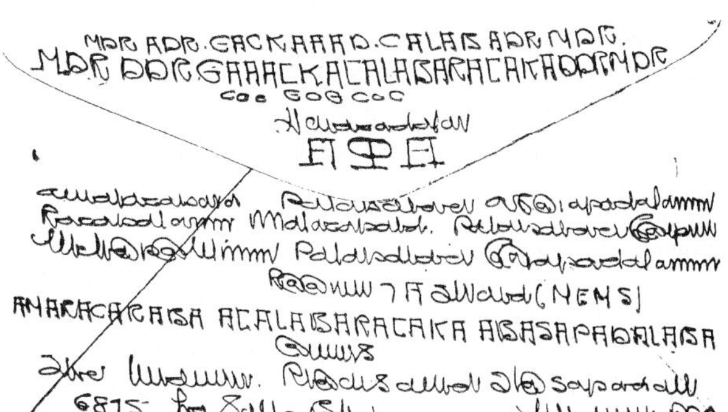

FIGURE 13–11
Sample of a chronic schizophrenic's noncommunicative writing. This addressed envelope illustrates manneristic writing, verbigeration, and possibly neologisms. Although the script appears to be exotic, note the recognizable Arabic numerals and English street names. (Courtesy of Heniz E. Lehmann.)

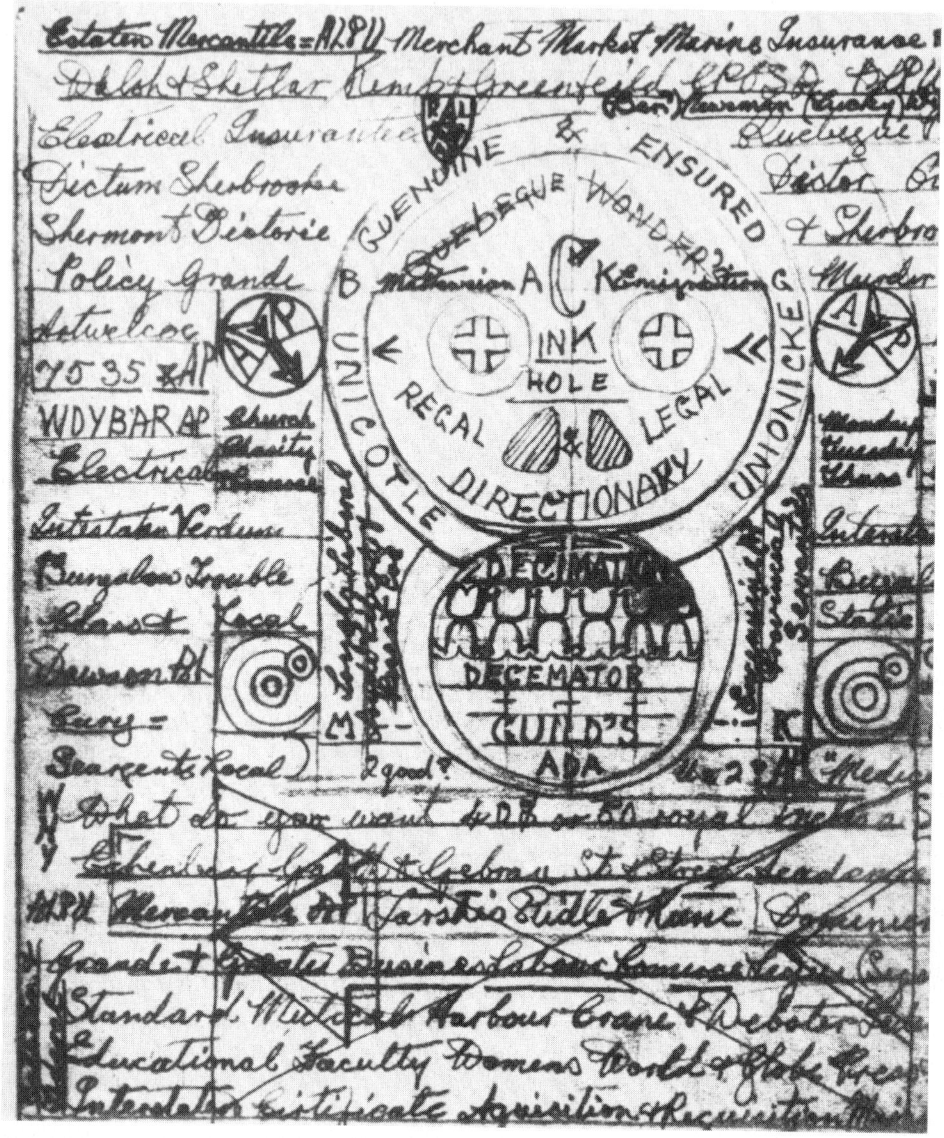

FIGURE 13–12
A schizophrenic woman expresses her incoherent thinking, combined with neologisms, in this drawing. (Courtesy of Heniz E. Lehmann.)

sedation with lorazepam (Ativan), 1 to 2 mg intramuscularly, repeated every hour as needed, may be necessary to prevent the patient from harming others. If a clinician feels fearful in the presence of a schizophrenia patient, that should be taken as an internal clue that the patient may be on the verge of acting out violently. In such cases, the interview should be terminated or be conducted with an attendant at the ready.

SUICIDE. As mentioned above, suicide is a risk. About 50 percent of all schizophrenia patients attempt suicide, and 10 to 15 percent of patients with schizophrenia die by suicide. Perhaps the most underappreciated factor involved in the suicide of these patients is depression that has been misdiagnosed as flat affect or as a medication adverse effect. Other precipitants of suicide include feelings of absolute emptiness, a need to escape from mental torture, or auditory hallucinations that command patients to kill themselves. The risk factors for suicide are the patient's awareness of the illness, male sex, college education, young age, a change in the course of the disease, an improvement after a relapse, dependence on the hospital, overly high ambitions, previous suicide attempts early in the course of the illness, and living alone. In the hospital, patients should be monitored closely if they are suicidal.

HOMICIDE. In spite of the sensational attention that the news media provide when a patient with schizophrenia murders someone, the available data indicate that these patients are no more likely to commit homicide than is a member of the general population. When a patient with schizophrenia does commit homicide, it may be for unpredictable or bizarre reasons based on hallucinations or delusions. Possible predictors of homicidal activity are a history of previous violence, dangerous behavior while hospitalized, and hallucinations or delusions involving such violence.

Sensorium and Cognition

Orientation. Patients with schizophrenia are usually oriented to person, time, and place. The lack of such orientation should prompt clinicians to investigate the possibility of a medical or neurological brain disorder. Some patients with schizophrenia may give incorrect or bizarre answers to questions about orientation, for example, "I am Christ; this is heaven; and it is AD 35."

Memory. Memory, as tested in the mental status examination, is usually intact, but there can be minor cognitive deficiencies. It may be impossible, however, to get a patient to attend closely enough to the memory tests for the ability to be assessed adequately.

Judgment and Insight. Classically, patients with schizophrenia are described as having poor insight into the nature and the severity of their disorder. The so-called lack of insight is associated with poor compliance with treatment. When examining schizophrenia patients, clinicians should carefully define various aspects of insight, such as awareness of symptoms, trouble getting along with people, and the reasons for these problems. Such information can be clinically useful in tailoring a treatment strategy and theoretically useful in postulating what areas of the brain contribute to the observed lack of insight (e.g., the parietal lobes).

Reliability. A patient with schizophrenia is no less reliable than any other psychiatric patient. The nature of the disorder, however, requires the examiner to verify important information through additional sources.

Neurological Findings

Localizing and nonlocalizing neurological signs (also known as hard and soft signs, respectively) have been reported to be more common in patients with schizophrenia than in other psychiatric patients. Nonlocalizing signs include dysdiadochokinesia, astereognosis, primitive reflexes, and diminished dexterity. The presence of neurological signs and symptoms correlates with increased severity of illness, affective blunting, and a poor prognosis. Other abnormal neurological signs include tics, stereotypies, grimacing, impaired fine motor skills, abnormal motor tone, and abnormal movements. One study has found that only about 25 percent of patients with schizophrenia are aware of their own abnormal involuntary movements and that the lack of awareness is correlated with lack of insight about the primary psychiatric disorder and the duration of illness.

Eye Examination. In addition to the disorder of smooth ocular pursuit (saccadic movement) patients with schizophrenia have an elevated blink rate. The elevated blink rate is thought to reflect hyperdopaminergic activity. In primates, blinking can be increased by dopamine agonists and reduced by dopamine antagonists.

Speech. Although the disorders of speech in schizophrenia (e.g., looseness of associations) are classically considered to indicate a thought disorder, they may also indicate a *forme fruste* of aphasia, perhaps implicating the dominant parietal lobe. The inability of schizophrenia patients to perceive the prosody of speech or to inflect their own speech can be seen as a neurological symptom of a disorder in the nondominant parietal lobe. Other parietal lobe–like symptoms in schizophrenia include the inability to carry out tasks (i.e., *apraxia*), right-left disorientation, and lack of concern about the disorder.

Other Physical Findings

An increased incidence of minor physical anomalies is associated with the diagnosis of schizophrenia. Such anomalies, most likely associated with early stages of embryonic and fetal growth, usually during the first trimester, have been reported in 30 to 75 percent of patients with schizophrenia, compared with 0 to 13 percent of the general population. Some current studies suggest that the anomalies are more common in men than in women and are probably associated with genetic factors, although obstetric complications cannot be ruled out as causative factors. Compulsive water drinking may occur in some patients who can consume up to 10 L a day and develop hyponatremia.

DIFFERENTIAL DIAGNOSIS

Secondary Psychotic Disorders

A wide range of nonpsychiatric medical conditions and a variety of substances can induce symptoms of psychosis and catatonia (Table 13–8). The most appropriate diagnosis for such psychosis or catatonia is psychotic disorder due to a general medical condition, catatonic disorder due to a general medical condition, or substance-induced psychotic disorder. The psychiatric manifestations of many nonpsychiatric medical conditions can come early in the course of the illness, often before the development of other symptoms. Therefore, clinicians must consider a wide range of nonpsychiatric medical conditions in the differential diagnosis of psychosis, even in the absence of obvious physical symptoms. Patients with neurological disorders generally have more insight into their illnesses and more distress from their psychiatric symptoms than do patients with schizophrenia. This fact can help clinicians distinguish the two groups of patients.

When evaluating a patient with psychotic symptoms, clinicians should follow the general guidelines for assessing nonpsychiatric conditions. First, clinicians should aggressively pursue an undiagnosed nonpsychiatric medical condition when a patient exhibits any unusual or rare symptoms or any variation in the level of consciousness. Second, clinicians should attempt to obtain a complete family history, including a history of medical, neurological, and psychiatric disorders. Third, clinicians should consider the possibility of a nonpsychiatric medical condition, even in patients with previous diagnoses of schizophrenia. A patient with schizophrenia is just as likely to have a brain tumor that produces psychotic symptoms as is a patient without schizophrenia.

Malingering and Factitious Disorders

For a patient who imitates the symptoms of schizophrenia but does not actually have the disorder, either malingering or a factitious disorder may be an appropriate diagnosis. Persons have faked schizophrenic symptoms and have been admitted into, and treated at, psychiatric hospitals. The condition of patients who are completely in control of their symptom production may qualify for a diagnosis of malingering; such patients usually have

Table 13–8
Differential Diagnosis of Schizophrenialike Symptoms

Medical and Neurological
Substance-induced—amphetamine, hallucinogens, belladonna alkaloids, alcohol hallucinosis, barbiturate withdrawal, cocaine, phencyclidine (PCP)
Epilepsy—especially temporal lobe epilepsy
Neoplasm, cerebrovascular disease, or trauma—especially frontal or limbic
Other conditions
Acquired immune deficiency syndrome
Acute intermittent porphyria
B_{12} deficiency
Carbon monoxide poisoning
Cerebral lipoidosis
Creutzfeldt-Jakob disease
Fabry's disease
Fahr's disease
Hallervorden-Spatz disease
Heavy metal poisoning
Herpes encephalitis
Homocystinuria
Huntington's disease
Metachromatic leukodystrophy
Neurosyphilis
Normal pressure hydrocephalus
Pellagra
Systemic lupus erythematosus
Wernicke-Korsakoff syndrome
Wilson's disease
Psychiatric
Atypical psychosis
Autistic disorder
Brief psychotic disorder
Delusional disorder
Factitious disorder with predominantly psychological signs and symptoms
Malingering
Mood disorders
Normal adolescence
Obsessive-compulsive disorder
Personality disorders—schizotypal, schizoid, borderline, paranoid
Schizoaffective disorder
Schizophrenia
Schizophreniform disorder

some obvious financial or legal reason to be considered mentally ill. The condition of patients who are less in control of their falsification of psychotic symptoms may qualify for a diagnosis of a factitious disorder. Some patients with schizophrenia, however, may falsely complain of an exacerbation of psychotic symptoms to obtain increased assistance benefits or to gain admission to a hospital. (Factitious disorders are the subject of Chapter 19.)

Other Psychotic Disorders

The psychotic symptoms of schizophrenia can be identical with those of schizophreniform disorder, brief psychotic disorder, schizoaffective disorder, and delusional disorders. *Schizophreniform disorder* differs from schizophrenia in that the symptoms have a duration of at least 1 month but less than 6 months. *Brief psychotic disorder* is the appropriate diagnosis when the symptoms have lasted at least 1 day but less than 1 month and when the patient has not returned to the premorbid state of functioning within that time. There may also be a precipitating traumatic event. When a manic or depressive syndrome develops concurrently with the major symptoms of schizophrenia, *schizoaffective disorder* is the appropriate diagnosis. Nonbizarre delusions present for at least 1 month without other symptoms of schizophrenia or a mood disorder warrant the diagnosis of *delusional disorder.*

Mood Disorders

The differential diagnosis of schizophrenia and mood disorders can be difficult but must be made because of the availability of specific and effective treatments for mania and depression. Compared with the duration of the primary symptoms, affective or mood symptoms in schizophrenia should be brief. Before making a premature diagnosis of schizophrenia and without more information than that gleaned from a single mental status examination, clinicians should delay a final diagnosis or should assume the presence of mood disorder. After remission of a schizophrenic episode, some patients experience a postpsychotic or secondary depression. Treatment with a serotonin-specific reuptake inhibitor or a tricyclic drug is indicated in that situation.

Personality Disorders

Various personality disorders may have some features of schizophrenia. Schizotypal, schizoid, and borderline personality disorders are the personality disorders with the most similar symptoms. Severe obsessive-compulsive personality disorder may mask an underlying schizophrenic process. Personality disorders, unlike schizophrenia, have mild symptoms and a history of occurring throughout a patient's life; they also lack an identifiable date of onset.

COURSE AND PROGNOSIS

Course

A premorbid pattern of symptoms may be the first evidence of illness, although the import of the symptoms is usually recognized only retrospectively. Characteristically, the symptoms begin in adolescence and are followed by the development of prodromal symptoms in days to a few months. Social or environmental changes, such as going away to college, using a substance, or a relative's death, may precipitate the disturbing symptoms, and the prodromal syndrome may last a year or more before the onset of overt psychotic symptoms.

The classic course of schizophrenia is one of exacerbations and remissions. After the first psychotic episode, a patient gradually recovers and may then function relatively normally for a long time. Patients usually relapse, however, and the pattern of illness during the first 5 years after the diagnosis generally indicates the patient's course. Further deterioration in the patient's

baseline functioning follows each relapse of the psychosis. This failure to return to baseline functioning after each relapse is the major distinction between schizophrenia and the mood disorders. Sometimes, a clinically observable postpsychotic depression follows a psychotic episode, and the schizophrenia patient's vulnerability to stress is usually lifelong. Positive symptoms tend to become less severe with time, but the socially debilitating negative or deficit symptoms may increase in severity. Although about one third of all schizophrenia patients have some marginal or integrated social existence, most have lives characterized by aimlessness, inactivity, frequent hospitalizations, and, in urban settings, homelessness and poverty.

Prognosis

Several studies have shown that over the 5- to 10-year period after the first psychiatric hospitalization for schizophrenia, only about 10 to 20 percent of patients can be described as having a good outcome. More than 50 percent of patients can be described as having a poor outcome, with repeated hospitalizations, exacerbations of symptoms, episodes of major mood disorders, and suicide attempts. In spite of these glum figures, schizophrenia does not always run a deteriorating course, and several factors have been associated with a good prognosis (see Table 13–5).

Reported remission rates range from 10 to 60 percent, and a reasonable estimate is that 20 to 30 percent of all schizophrenia patients are able to lead somewhat normal lives. About 20 to 30 percent of patients continue to experience moderate symptoms, and 40 to 60 percent of patients remain significantly impaired by their disorder for their entire lives. Patients with schizophrenia do much less well than patients with mood disorders, although 20 to 25 percent of mood disorder patients are also severely disturbed at long-term follow-up.

TREATMENT

Three observations about schizophrenia warrant attention when clinicians consider the treatment of the disorder. First, regardless of cause, schizophrenia occurs in a person with a unique individual, familial, and social psychological profile. Two factors—how the patient has been affected by the disorder and how the patient will be helped by the treatment—must shape the treatment approach. Second, many investigators consider that a 50 percent concordance rate for schizophrenia among monozygotic twins suggests that unknown, but probably specific, environmental and psychological factors have contributed to the development of the disorder. Thus, just as pharmacological agents are used to treat presumed chemical imbalances, nonpharmacological strategies must treat nonbiological issues. Third, the complexity of schizophrenia usually renders any single therapeutic approach inadequate to deal with the multifaceted disorder.

Although antipsychotic medications are the mainstay of the treatment for schizophrenia, research has found that psychosocial interventions, including psychotherapy; can augment the clinical improvement. Psychosocial modalities should be carefully integrated into the drug treatment regimen and should support it. Most patients with schizophrenia benefit more from the combined use of antipsychotic drugs and psychosocial treatment than from either treatment used alone.

Hospitalization

Hospitalization is indicated primarily for diagnostic purposes, for stabilization of medications, for patients' safety because of suicidal or homicidal ideation, and for grossly disorganized or inappropriate behavior, including the inability to take care of basic needs such as food, clothing, and shelter. Establishing an effective association between patients and community support systems is a primary goal of hospitalization. Other aspects of clinical management flow logically from medical models of the disorder. Because physicians are concerned with a patient's rehabilitation and adjustment, they must consider the patient's specific disabilities when planning treatment strategies. Physicians must also educate patients and their families and caretakers about schizophrenia.

Hospitalization decreases patients' stress and helps them structure their daily activities. The severity of a patient's illness and the availability of outpatient treatment facilities determine the length of the hospital stay. Research has shown that short stays of 4 to 6 weeks are just as effective as long-term hospitalizations and that hospital settings with active behavioral approaches produce better results than do custodial institutions.

Hospital treatment plans should be oriented toward practical issues of self-care, quality of life, employment, and social relationships. During hospitalization, patients should be coordinated with aftercare facilities including their family homes, foster families, board-and-care homes, and halfway houses. Day-care centers and home visits by counselors can sometimes help patients to remain out of the hospital for long periods and can improve the quality of their daily lives.

Biological Therapies

Pharmacotherapy. Antipsychotic medications, introduced in the early 1950s, have revolutionized the treatment of schizophrenia. About 2 to 4 times as many patients relapse when treated with a placebo as do those treated with antipsychotic drugs. These medications, however, treat the symptoms of the disorder and do not cure schizophrenia.

The antipsychotic drugs include two major classes: dopamine receptor antagonists (e.g., chlorpromazine [Thorazine], haloperidol [Haldol]), and SDAs (e.g., risperidone and clozapine).

DOPAMINE RECEPTOR ANTAGONISTS. The dopamine receptor antagonists are effective in the treatment of schizophrenia, particularly of the positive symptoms (e.g., delusions); however, the drugs have two major shortcomings. First, only a small percentage of patients (perhaps 25 percent) are helped enough to recover a reasonable amount of normal mental functioning. As noted above, even with treatment, about 50 percent of patients with schizophrenia lead severely debilitated lives. Second, the dopamine receptor antagonists are associated with both annoying and serious adverse effects. The most common annoying effects are akathisia and parkinsonianlike symptoms of rigidity and tremor. The potential serious effects include tardive dyskinesia and neuroleptic malignant syndrome.

SEROTONIN-DOPAMINE ANTAGONISTS. The SDAs produce minimal or no extrapyramidal symptoms, interact with different subtypes of dopamine receptors than do the standard antipsychotics, and affect both serotonin and glutamate receptors. They also pro-

duce fewer neurological and endocrinological adverse effects and are effective in treating negative symptoms of schizophrenia (e.g., withdrawal). Also called atypical antipsychotics, they appear to be effective for a broader range of patients with schizophrenia than the typical dopamine receptor antagonist antipsychotic agents. They are at least as effective as haloperidol for positive symptoms of schizophrenia, are uniquely effective for the negative symptoms, and cause few, if any, extrapyramidal symptoms. Approved SDAs include clozapine, risperidone, olanzapine (Zyprexa), sertindole, quetiapine, and ziprasidone. These drugs have replaced the dopamine receptor antagonists as the drugs of first choice for treatment of schizophrenia.

Risperidone. Risperidone is an effective antipsychotic medication with a mild profile of adverse effects. At doses commonly used, it is not associated with extrapyramidal symptoms. It causes less sedation and fewer anticholinergic effects than do dopamine receptor antagonists. A growing body of evidence supports its role as a first-line agent for first-break, mildly to moderately ill patients and for severely ill, treatment-refractory patients.

Clozapine. Clozapine, is probably the most effective for severely ill patients, but its use is complicated by the risk of significant adverse effects, which are not found in other SDAs. Clozapine is associated with potentially life-threatening agranulocytosis in 1 to 2 percent of patients, which requires weekly monitoring of the neutrophil count. It also presents a high risk for seizures and has significant anticholinergic effects. Clozapine remains useful for patients refractory to any other antipsychotic drug and for patients with tardive dyskinesia. Clozapine has little antagonist activity at the D_2 receptor and appears to reduce the symptoms of tardive dyskinesia without worsening the condition.

Olanzapine. Olanzapine is an effective medication for treatment of schizophrenia, with a mild, but somewhat different, profile of adverse effects than risperidone. It is less likely to produce extrapyramidal effects but is more likely to produce sedation, weight gain, orthostatic hypotension, and constipation. It is a useful first-line agent, in that patients who do not respond to one SDA may respond to another.

Sertindole. Sertindole is an effective agent, with a favorable profile of adverse effects, most of which are transient. It must be slowly titrated upward to avoid orthostatic hypotension. It may also cause sinus tachycardia, nasal congestion, and decreased ejaculatory volume. It causes little weight gain and does not cause anticholinergic symptoms. Its half-life of 3 days makes it ideal for poorly compliant patients.

Quetiapine. Quetiapine is an effective antipsychotic drug associated with no increased risk of extrapyramidal symptoms. The main adverse effects include sedation, tachycardia, weight gain, and agitation. The initial doses must be titrated upward over 4 days to avoid orthostatic hypotension and syncope.

Ziprasidone. Ziprasidone is an effective drug for treatment of schizophrenia. It has potential additional benefits for patients with affective symptoms, because it blocks reuptake of serotonin and norepinephrine, and for patients with anxiety, because it is an agonist for 5-HT_{1A} receptors. Adverse effects include sedation, nausea, dizziness, and lightheadedness, but not weight gain.

THERAPEUTIC PRINCIPLES. The use of antipsychotic medications in schizophrenia should follow five major principles. (1) Clinicians should carefully define the target symptoms to be treated. (2) An antipsychotic that has worked well in the past for a patient should be used again. In the absence of such information, the choice of an antipsychotic is usually based on the adverse effect profile. Currently available data indicate that SDAs may offer a superior adverse effect profile and the possibility of superior efficacy. (3) The minimum length of an antipsychotic trial is 4 to 6 weeks at adequate dosages. If the trial is unsuccessful, a different antipsychotic drug, usually from a different class, can be tried. An unpleasant reaction by the patient to the first dose of an antipsychotic drug, however, correlates strongly with future poor response and noncompliance. Negative experiences can include a peculiar subjective negative feeling, oversedation, or an acute dystonic reaction. When a severe negative initial reaction is observed, clinicians may consider switching to a different antipsychotic drug in less than 4 weeks. (4) In general, the use of more than one antipsychotic medication at a time is rarely, if ever, indicated. In especially treatment-resistant patients, however, combinations of antipsychotics with other drugs—for example, carbamazepine (Tegretol)—may be indicated. (5) Patients should be maintained on the lowest possible effective dosage of medication. The maintenance dosage is often lower than that used to achieve symptom control during the psychotic episode. A decision tree for the use of antipsychotic medication is given in Figure 13–13.

INITIAL WORKUP. In spite of the annoyance of the neurological effects and the looming possibility of tardive dyskinesia, antipsychotic drugs are remarkably safe, especially when given for a relatively short period. Thus, in emergency situations, clinicians can administer the drugs, with the exception of clozapine, without conducting a physical or laboratory examination of the patient. In the usual assessment, however, clinicians should obtain a complete blood count (CBC) with white blood cell indexes, liver function tests, and an electrocardiogram (ECG), especially in women older than 40 and men older than 30. The major contraindications to antipsychotic drugs are (1) a history of serious allergic response, (2) the possibility that a patient has ingested a substance that will interact with the antipsychotic to induce CNS depression (e.g., alcohol, opioids, opiates, barbiturates, benzodiazepines) or anticholinergic delirium (e.g., drugs containing atropine, scopolamine, and possibly PCP), (3) the presence of a severe cardiac abnormality, (4) a high risk for seizures from organic or idiopathic causes, and (5) the presence of narrow-angle glaucoma if an antipsychotic drug with significant anticholinergic activity is to be used.

TREATMENT OF REFRACTORY ILLNESS. In the acute state, virtually all patients eventually respond to repeated doses of an antipsychotic drug—every 1 to 2 hours by intramuscular (IM) administration or every 2 to 3 hours by mouth. A benzodiazepine is sometimes needed to sedate the patient further. The failure of a patient to respond in the acute state should cause clinicians to consider the possibility of an organic lesion.

Noncompliance with antipsychotic drugs is a major reason for relapse and for failure of a drug trial. Another major reason for a failed drug trial is insufficient time for the trial. It is generally a mistake to increase the dosage or to change antipsychotic medications in the first 2 weeks of treatment. If a patient is improving on the current regimen at the end of 2 weeks, continued treatment with the same regimen will probably result in steady clinical improvement. If, however, a patient has shown lit-

If a patient has a specific contraindication to any medication, remove that medication from the possibilities for that patient.

At each point in the algorithm, medications are chosen on the basis of

- Past response
- Side effects
- Patient preference
- Planned route of administration

GROUP 1: Conventional antipsychotic medications
GROUP 2: Risperidone
GROUP 3: Clozapine
GROUP 4: New antipsychotic medications—olanzapine, sertindole, quetiapine

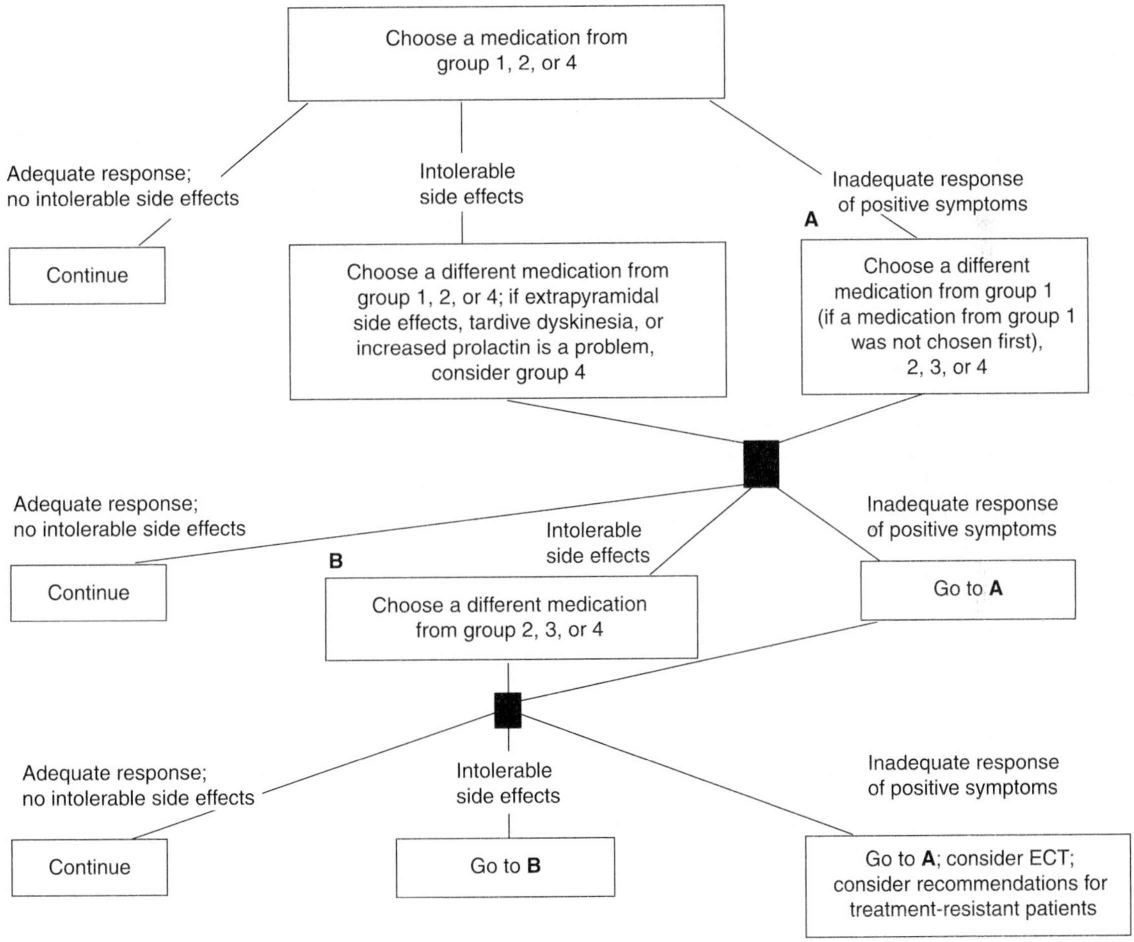

FIGURE 13–13
Pharmacological treatment of schizophrenia. (Reprinted with permission from American Psychiatric Association. Practice guideline for the treatment of patients with schizophrenia. *Am J Psychiatry.* 1997;154[suppl 4]:1.)

tle or no improvement in 2 weeks, the possible reasons for a drug failure, including noncompliance, should be considered. In a noncompliant patient, the use of a liquid preparation or depot forms of fluphenazine (Prolixin) or haloperidol may be indicated. Because of the diversity in the metabolism of drugs, clinicians should obtain plasma levels when the laboratory capability is available. Plasma levels of antipsychotic drugs provide only a gross measure of compliance, absorption, and metabolism. There are no clearly defined therapeutic blood level ranges for antipsychotic drugs similar to those for some antidepressants. Because neurological adverse effects are a common reason for noncompliance in patients with schizophrenia and a major cause of relapse, the more favorable adverse effect profiles of atypical agents may yield improved compliance and better outcome.

Having eliminated other possible reasons for the therapeutic failure of an antipsychotic drug, clinicians may try a second antipsychotic drug whose chemical structure differs from that of the first one. The use of so-called megadose antipsychotic therapy (e.g., 100 to 200 mg of haloperidol) is rarely indicated because almost no data support the practice.

Other Drugs. If adequate trials with one antipsychotic agent are unsuccessful, another may be tried. Combination therapy with one of these drugs and an adjuvant medication may also be tried. The adjuvant medications with the most supportive data are lithium, two anticonvulsants (carbamazepine and valproate), and the benzodiazepines.

LITHIUM. Lithium may be effective in further reducing psychotic symptoms in up to 50 percent of patients with schizophrenia. It is usually added with an antipsychotic drug that the patient is already taking. Lithium may also be a reasonable drug to try in patients who are unable to take any of the antipsychotic medications. It is also effective in schizophrenia patients with mood swings.

ANTICONVULSANTS. Carbamazepine or valproate is usually not used alone but is used in combination with lithium or an antipsychotic. Although neither of the anticonvulsants has been shown to be effective in reducing psychotic symptoms in schizophrenia when used alone, data suggest that the anticonvulsants reduce episodes of violence in some schizophrenia patients. Because of their effects on hepatic enzymes, anticonvulsants decrease blood levels of antipsychotics.

BENZODIAZEPINES. Data support the practice of coadministering alprazolam (Xanax) with antipsychotic drugs to patients who have not responded to antipsychotic administration alone. There are also reports of schizophrenia patients' responding to high dosages of diazepam (Valium) alone. The severity of the psychosis may, however, be exacerbated after the withdrawal of a benzodiazepine. Lorazepam may be preferable to diazepam because it is shorter acting and has less abuse potential.

Other Biological Therapies. Although much less effective than antipsychotic drugs, electroconvulsive therapy (ECT) may be indicated for catatonic patients and for patients who for some reason cannot take antipsychotic drugs. Patients who have been ill for less than 1 year are most likely to respond. Maintenance ECT may be of value in patients nonresponsive to pharmacological therapies.

In the past, psychosurgery, particularly frontal lobotomy, was used for the treatment of schizophrenia, with variable outcomes. Although sophisticated approaches to psychosurgery for schizophrenia may eventually be developed, psychosurgery is no longer considered an appropriate treatment. It is, however, practiced on a limited experimental basis for severe, intractable cases.

Psychosocial Therapies

Psychosocial therapies include a variety of methods to increase social abilities, self-sufficiency, practical skills, and interpersonal communication in schizophrenia patients. The goal is to enable persons who are severely ill to develop social and vocational skills for independent living. Such treatment is carried out at many sites: hospitals, outpatient clinics, mental health centers, day hospitals, and home or social clubs.

Social Skills Training. Social skills training is sometimes referred to as behavioral skills therapy (Table 13–9). The therapy can be directly supportive and useful to the patient along with pharmacological therapy. In addition to the symptoms seen in patients with schizophrenia, some of the most noticeable symptoms involve the person's relationships with others, including poor eye contact, unusual delays in response, odd facial expressions, lack of spontaneity in social situations, and inaccurate perceptions or lack of perception of emotions in other people. Behavioral skills training addresses these behaviors through the use of videotapes of others and of the patient, role playing in therapy, and homework assignments for the specific skills being practiced. Social skills training has been shown to reduce relapse rates as measured by the need for hospitalization.

Family-Oriented Therapies. Because patients with schizophrenia are often discharged in an only partially remitted state, a family to which a patient returns can often benefit from a brief but intensive (as often as daily) course of family therapy. The

Table 13–9
Goals and Targeted Behaviors for Social Skills Therapy

Phase	Goals	Targeted Behaviors
Stabilization and assessment	Establish therapeutic alliance	Empathy and rapport
	Assess social performance and perception skills	Verbal and nonverbal communication
	Assess behaviors that provoke expressed emotion	
Social performance within family	Express positive feelings within family	Compliments, appreciation, interest in others
	Teach effective strategies for coping with conflict	Avoidance response to criticism, stating preferences and refusals
Social perception in the family	Correctly identify content, context, and meaning of messages	Reading a message
		Labeling an idea
		Summarizing other's intent
Extrafamilial relationships	Enhance socialization skills	Conversational skills
	Enhance prevocational and vocational skills	Dating
		Recreational activities
		Job interviewing, work habits
Maintenance	Generalize skills to new situations	

Adapted with permission from Hogarty GE, Anderson CM, Reiss DJ, et al. Family psychoeducation, social skills training and maintenance chemotherapy: I. One-year effects of a controlled study on relapse and expressed emotion. *Arch Gen Psychiatry.* 1986;43:633.

therapy should focus on the immediate situation and should include identifying and avoiding potentially troublesome situations. When problems do emerge with the patient in the family, the aim of the therapy should be to resolve the problem quickly.

In wanting to help, family members too often encourage a relative with schizophrenia to resume regular activities too quickly, both from ignorance about the disorder and from denial of its severity. Without being overly discouraging, therapists must help the family and the patient understand and learn about schizophrenia and must encourage discussion of the psychotic episode and the events leading up to it. Ignoring the psychotic episode, a common occurrence, often increases the shame associated with the event and does not exploit the freshness of the episode to understand it better. Psychotic symptoms often frighten family members, and talking openly with the psychiatrist and with the relative with schizophrenia often eases all parties. Therapists can direct later family therapy toward long-range application of stress-reducing and coping strategies and toward the patient's gradual reintegration into everyday life.

Therapists must control the emotional intensity of family sessions with patients with schizophrenia. The excessive expression of emotion during a session can damage a patient's recovery process and can undermine potentially successful future family therapy. Several studies have shown that family therapy is especially effective in reducing relapses.

NATIONAL ALLIANCE FOR THE MENTALLY ILL. NAMI and similar organizations are support groups for family members and friends of patients who are mentally ill and for patients themselves. These organizations offer emotional and practical advice about obtaining care in the sometimes-complex health care delivery system and are useful sources to which to refer family members. NAMI has also waged a campaign to destigmatize mental illness and to increase government awareness of the needs and rights of persons who are mentally ill and their families.

Case Management. Because a variety of professionals with specialized skills, such as psychiatrists, social workers, and occupational therapists, among others, are involved in a treatment program, it is helpful to have one person aware of all the forces acting on the patient. The case manager ensures that their efforts are coordinated and that the patient keeps appointments and complies with treatment plans; the case manager may make home visits and even accompany the patient to work. The success of the program depends on the educational background, training, and competence of the individual case manager, which varies. Case managers often have too many cases to manage effectively. The ultimate benefits of the program have yet to be demonstrated.

Assertive Community Treatment (ACT). The Assertive Community Treatment (ACT) program was originally developed by researchers in Madison, Wisconsin, in the 1970s, for the delivery of services for persons with chronic mental illness. Patients are assigned to one multidisciplinary team (case manager, psychiatrist, nurse, general physicians, etc.). The team has a fixed caseload of patients and delivers all services when and where needed by the patient, 24 hours a day, 7 days a week. This is mobile and intensive intervention that provides treatment, rehabilitation, and support activities. These include home delivery of medications, monitoring of mental and physical health, in vivo social skills, and frequent contact with family members. There is a high staff-to-patient ratio (1:12). ACT programs can effectively decrease the risk of rehospitalization for persons with schizophrenia, but they are labor-intensive and expensive programs to administer.

Group Therapy. Group therapy for persons with schizophrenia generally focuses on real-life plans, problems, and relationships. Groups may be behaviorally oriented, psychodynamically or insight oriented, or supportive. Some investigators doubt that dynamic interpretation and insight therapy are valuable for typical patients with schizophrenia. But group therapy is effective in reducing social isolation, increasing the sense of cohesiveness, and improving reality testing for patients with schizophrenia. Groups led in a supportive manner appear to be most helpful for schizophrenia patients.

Cognitive Behavioral Therapy. Cognitive behavioral therapy has been used in schizophrenia patients to improve cognitive distortions, reduce distractibility, and correct errors in judgment. There are reports of ameliorating delusions and hallucinations in some patients using this method. Patients who might benefit generally have some insight into their illness.

Individual Psychotherapy. Studies of the effects of individual psychotherapy in the treatment of schizophrenia have provided data that the therapy is helpful and that the effects are additive to those of pharmacological treatment. In psychotherapy with a schizophrenia patient, developing a therapeutic relationship that the patient experiences as safe is critical. The therapist's reliability, the emotional distance between the therapist and the patient, and the genuineness of the therapist as interpreted by the patient all affect the therapeutic experience. Psychotherapy for a schizophrenia patient should be thought of in terms of decades, rather than sessions, months, or even years.

Some clinicians and researchers have emphasized that the ability of a patient with schizophrenia to form a therapeutic alliance with a therapist is predictive of the outcome. Schizophrenia patients who are able to form a good therapeutic alliance are likely to remain in psychotherapy, to remain compliant with their medications, and to have good outcomes at 2-year follow-up evaluations.

The relationship between clinicians and patients differs from that encountered in the treatment of nonpsychotic patients. Establishing a relationship is often difficult. Persons with schizophrenia are desperately lonely, yet defend against closeness and trust; they are likely to become suspicious, anxious, or hostile or to regress when someone attempts to draw close. Therapists should scrupulously respect a patient's distance and privacy and should demonstrate simple directness, patience, sincerity, and sensitivity to social conventions in preference to premature informality and the condescending use of first names. The patient is likely to perceive exaggerated warmth or professions of friendship as attempts at bribery, manipulation, or exploitation.

In the context of a professional relationship, however, flexibility is essential in establishing a working alliance with the patient. A therapist may have meals with the patient, sit on the floor, go for a walk, eat at a restaurant, accept and give gifts, play table tennis, remember the patient's birthday, or just sit

silently with the patient. The major aim is to convey the idea that the therapist is trustworthy, wants to understand the patient and tries to do so, and has faith in the patient's potential as a human being, no matter how disturbed, hostile, or bizarre the patient may be at the moment.

A flexible type of psychotherapy called personal therapy is a recently developed form of individual treatment for schizophrenia patients. Its objective is to enhance personal and social adjustment and to forestall relapse. It is a select method using social skills and relaxation exercises, psychoeducation, self-reflection, self-awareness, and exploration of individual vulnerability to stress. The therapist provides a setting that stresses acceptance and empathy. Patients receiving personal therapy show improvement in social adjustment (a composite measure that includes work performance, leisure and interpersonal relationships) and have a lower relapse rate after 3 years than patients not receiving personal therapy.

Vocational Therapy

A variety of methods and settings are used to help patients regain old skills or develop new ones. These include sheltered workshops, job clubs, and part-time or transitional employment programs. Enabling patients to become gainfully employed is both a means toward, and a sign of, recovery. Many schizophrenia patients are capable of performing high-quality work in spite of their illness. Others may exhibit exceptional skill or even brilliance in a limited field as a result of some idiosyncratic aspect of their disorder.

ICD-10

According to ICD-10, nine groups of symptoms are important for diagnosing schizophrenia: (1) thought echo, insertion, withdrawal, and broadcasting; (2) delusions of control, influence, or passivity; (3) hallucinatory voices; (4) other persistent delusions that are culturally inappropriate and impossible; (5) persistent hallucinations; (6) breaks or interpolation in thinking; (7) catatonic behavior; (8) "negative" symptoms resulting in social withdrawal and poor social performance but not caused by depression or medication; and (9) consistent, overall change in behavior. Unlike requirements in DSM-IV-TR for a diagnosis of schizophrenia, ICD-10 requires one clear symptom or two less clear symptoms from any one of groups 1 through 4 or symptoms from at least two of groups 5 through 8 to be present for most of the time during 1 month or more. Similar conditions lasting less than a month should be diagnosed as schizophrenialike disorders. DSM-IV-TR defines schizophrenia as a disturbance of at least 6 months' duration, with two or more symptoms active for at least a month. A disorder diagnosed as schizophrenia under ICD-10 standards may be diagnosed as schizophreniform disorder under DSM-IV-TR standards. The latter disorder is, according to DSM-IV-TR, equivalent to schizophrenia except for its duration, which is 1 to 6 months, and the absence of functional decline.

The ICD-10 general criteria for schizophrenia apply to all ICD-10 subtypes except simple schizophrenia. The ICD-10 diagnostic criteria for the schizophrenia subtypes are presented in Table 13–10, and ICD-10 includes two residual categories: other schizophrenia (e.g., cenesthopathic schizophrenia [a disorder in which patients complain about or have delusions of a general sense of bodily existence]) and unspecified schizophrenia.

Table 13–10
ICD-10 Diagnostic Criteria for Schizophrenia

This overall category includes the common varieties of schizophrenia, together with some less common varieties and closely related disorders.

General criteria for paranoid, hebephrenic, catatonic, and undifferentiated schizophrenia

G1. Either *at least one* of the syndromes, symptoms, and signs listed under (1) below, *or* at least two of the symptoms and signs listed under (2) should be present for most of the time during an episode of psychotic illness lasting for at least 1 month (or at some time during most of the days).

(1) At least one of the following must be present:

(a) thought echo, thought insertion or withdrawal, or thought broadcasting;

(b) delusions of control, influence, or passivity, clearly referred to body or limb movements or specific thoughts, actions, or sensations; delusional perception;

(c) hallucinatory voices giving a running commentary on the patient's behavior, or discussing the patient among themselves, or other types of hallucinatory voices coming from some part of the body;

(d) persistent delusions of other kinds that are culturally inappropriate and completely impossible (e.g., being able to control the weather, or being in communication with aliens from another world).

(2) *Or* at least two of the following:

(a) persistent hallucinations in any modality, when occurring every day for at least 1 month, when accompanied by delusions (which may be fleeting or half-formed) without clear affective content, or when accompanied by persistent overvalued ideas;

(b) neologisms, breaks, or interpolations in the train of thought, resulting in incoherence or irrelevant speech;

(c) catatonic behavior, such as excitement, posturing or waxy flexibility, negativism, mutism, and stupor;

(d) "negative" symptoms, such as marked apathy, paucity of speech, and blunting or incongruity of emotional responses (it must be clear that these are not due to depression or to neuroleptic medication).

G2. *Most commonly used exclusion clauses*

(1) If the patient also meets criteria for manic episode or depressive episode, the criteria listed under G1(1) and G1(2) above must have been met *before* the disturbance of mood developed.

(2) The disorder is not attributable to organic brain disease or to alcohol- or drug-related intoxication, dependence, or withdrawal.

(continued)

Table 13–10 (*continued*)

Comments

In evaluating the presence of these abnormal subjective experiences and behavior, special care should be taken to avoid false-positive assessments, especially where culturally or subculturally influenced modes of expression and behavior or a subnormal level of intelligence are involved.

Pattern of course

In view of the considerable variation of the course of schizophrenic disorders it may be desirable (especially for research) to specify the *pattern of course* by using a fifth character. Course should not usually be coded unless there has been a period of observation of at least 1 year.

Continuous

No remission of psychotic symptoms throughout the period of observation.

Episodic with progressive deficit

Progressive development of "negative" symptoms in the intervals between psychotic episodes.

Episodic with stable deficit

Persistent but nonprogressive "negative" symptoms in the intervals between psychotic episodes.

Episodic remittent

Complete or virtually complete remissions between psychotic episodes.

Incomplete remission

Complete remission

Other

Course uncertain, period of observation too short

Paranoid schizophrenia

A. The general criteria for schizophrenia must be met.

B. Delusions or hallucinations must be prominent (such as delusions of persecution, reference, exalted birth, special mission, bodily change, or jealousy; threatening or commanding voices, hallucinations of smell or taste, sexual or other bodily sensations.)

C. Flattening or incongruity of affect, catatonic symptoms, or incoherent speech must not dominate the clinical picture, although they may be present to a mild degree.

Hebephrenic schizophrenia

A. The general criteria for schizophrenia must be met.

B. Either of the following must be present:
 (1) definite and sustained flattening or shallowness of affect;
 (2) definite and sustained incongruity or inappropriateness of affect.

C. Either of the following must be present:
 (1) behavior that is aimless and disjointed rather than goal-directed;
 (2) definite thought disorder, manifesting as speech that is disjointed, rambling, or incoherent.

D. Hallucinations or delusions must not dominate the clinical picture, although they may be present to a mild degree.

Catatonic schizophrenia

A. The general criteria for schizophrenia must eventually be met, although this may not be possible initially if the patient is uncommunicative.

B. For a period of at least 2 weeks one or more of the following catatonic behaviors must be prominent:
 (1) stupor (marked decrease in reactivity to the environment and reduction of spontaneous movements and activity) or mutism;
 (2) excitement (apparently purposeless motor activity, not influenced by external stimuli);
 (3) posturing (voluntary assumption and maintenance of inappropriate or bizarre postures);
 (4) negativism (an apparently motiveless resistance to all instructions or attempts to be moved, or movement in the opposite direction);
 (5) rigidity (maintenance of a rigid posture against efforts to be moved);
 (6) waxy flexibility (maintenance of limbs and body in externally imposed positions);
 (7) command automatism (automatic compliance with instruction).

Undifferentiated schizophrenia

A. The general criteria for schizophrenia must be met.

Either of the following must apply:
 (1) insufficient symptoms to meet the criteria for any of the subtypes
 (2) so many symptoms that the criteria for more than one of the subtypes listed above are met.

Postschizophrenic depression

A. The general criteria for schizophrenia must have been met within the past 12 months but are not met at the present time.

B. One of the conditions in Criterion G1(2) a, b, c, or d for general schizophrenia must still be present.

C. The depressive symptoms must be sufficiently prolonged, severe, and extensive to meet criteria for at least a mild depressive episode.

Residual schizophrenia

A. The general criteria for schizophrenia must have been met at some time in the past but are not met at the present time.

B. At least four of the following "negative" symptoms have been present throughout the previous 12 months:
 (1) psychomotor slowing or underactivity;
 (2) definite blunting of affect;
 (3) passivity and lack of initiative;
 (4) poverty of either the quantity or the content of speech;
 (5) poor nonverbal communication by facial expression, eye contact, voice modulation, or posture;
 (6) poor social performance or self-care.

Simple schizophrenia

A. There is slow but progressive development, over a period of at least 1 year, of all three of the following:
 (1) a significant and consistent change in the overall quality of some aspects of personal behavior, manifest as loss of drive and interests, aimlessness, idleness, a self-absorbed attitude, and social withdrawal;
 (2) gradual appearance and deepening of "negative" symptoms such as marked apathy, paucity of speech, underactivity, blunting of affect, passivity and lack of initiative, and poor nonverbal communication (by facial expression, eye contact, voice modulation, and posture);
 (3) marked decline in social, scholastic, or occupational performance.

B. At no time are there any of the symptoms referred to in criterion G1 for general schizophrenia, nor are there hallucinations or well-formed delusions of any kind; i.e., the individual must never have met the criteria for any other type of schizophrenia or for any other psychotic disorder.

C. There is no evidence of dementia or any other organic mental disorder.

Other schizophrenia

Schizophrenia, unspecified

From World Health Organization. *The ICD-10 Classification of Mental and Behavioural Disorders: Diagnostic Criteria for Research.* Copyright, World Health Organization, Geneva, 1993.

References

Addington DE, Addington JM. Attempted suicide and depression in schizophrenia. *Acta Psychiatr Scand.* 1992;85:288.

American Psychiatric Association. Practice guidelines for the treatment of patients with schizophrenia. In: *Practice Guidelines for the Treatment of Psychiatric Disorders: Compendium 2000.* Washington, DC: American Psychiatric Association; 2000.

American Psychiatric Association. *Tardive Dyskinesia: A Task Force Report of the American Psychiatric Association.* Washington, DC: American Psychiatric Association; 1992.

Bogerst B, Lieberman JA, Ashtari M, et al. Hippocampus–amygdala volumes and psychopathology in chronic schizophrenia. *Biol Psychiatry.* 1993;33:236.

Breier A, Schreiber JL, Dyer J, Pickar D. National Institute of Mental Health longitudinal study of chronic schizophrenia: prognosis and predictors of outcome. *Arch Gen Psychiatry.* 1991;48:239.

Cancro R, Lehman HE. Schizophrenia: clinical features. In: Sadock BJ, Sadock VA, eds. *Comprehensive Textbook of Psychiatry.* 7th ed. Baltimore: Lippincott Williams & Wilkins; 2000.

Carone BJ, Harrow M, Westermeyer JF. Posthospital course and outcome in schizophrenia. *Arch Gen Psychiatry.* 1991;48:247.

Carpenter WT. The deficit syndrome. *Am J Psychiatry.* 1994;151:327.

Dalman C, Thomas HV, David AS, Gentz J, Lewis G, Alleback P. Signs of asphyxia at birth and risk of schizophrenia: population-based case-control study. *Br J Psychiatry.* 2001;179:403.

Gabbard GO. *Psychodynamic Psychiatry in Clinical Practice: The DSM-IV Edition.* Washington, DC: American Psychiatric Press; 1994.

Gaertner I, Gaertner, HJ, Vonthein R, Dietz K. Therapeutic drug monitoring of clozapine in relapse prevention. *J Clin Pharmacol.* 2001;305:21.

George TP, Potenza MN, Degan K. Acute tryptophan depletion in schizophrenic patients treated with clozapine. *Arch Gen Psychiatry.* 2002;291:59.

Goff DC, Henderson DC, Amico E. Cigarette smoking in schizophrenia: relationships to psychopathology and medication side effects. *Am J Psychiatry.* 1992;149:1189.

Harrison G, Gunnell D, Glazebrook C, Page K, Kwiecinski R. Association between schizophrenia and social inequality at birth: case-control study. *Br J Psychiatry.* 2001;179:346.

Harrison PJ. On the neuropathology of schizophrenia and its dementia: neurodevelopmental, neurodegenerative, or both? *Neurodegeneration.* 1995;4:1.

Harvey PD. Vulnerability to schizophrenia in adulthood. In: Ingram RE, Price JM, eds. *Vulnerability to Psychopathology: Risk across the Lifespan.* New York: Guilford Press; 2001;355.

Kane JM. Schizophrenia. *N Engl J Med.* 1996;334:34.

Kapur S, Remington G. Serotonin–dopamine interaction and its relevance to schizophrenia. *Am J Psychiatry.* 1996;153:466.

Kendler KS, Diehl SR. The genetics of schizophrenia: a current, genetic-epidemiologic perspective. *Schizophr Bull.* 1993;19:261.

Kinon BJ, Lieberman JA. Mechanisms of action of atypical antipsychotic drugs: a critical analysis. *Psychopharmacology.* 1996;124:2.

Kurumaji A, Okubo Y. D1 dopamine receptors, schizophrenia, and antipsychotic medications. In: Lidow MS, ed. *Neurotransmitter Receptors in Actions of Antipsychotic Medications. Pharmacology and Toxicology.* Boca Raton, FL: CRC Press; 2000:65.

Limpert C, Amador XF. Negative symptoms and the experience of emotion. In: Keefe RSE, McEvoy JP, eds. *Negative Symptom and Cognitive Deficit Treatment Response in Schizophrenia.* Washington, DC: American Psychiatric Press; 2001:111.

Lysaker PH, Bryson GJ, Bell MD. Insight and work performance in schizophrenia. *J Nerv Ment Dis.* 2002;190:142.

McClellan J, Werry J. Practice parameters for the assessment and treatment of children and adolescents with schizophrenia. *J Am Acad Child Adolesc Psychiatry.* 1994;33:616.

McGlashan TH, Fenton WS. Subtype progression and pathophysiologic deterioration in early schizophrenia. *Schizophr Bull.* 1993;19:17.

Moldin SO. Gender and schizophrenia: an overview. In: Frank E, ed. *Gender and Its Effects on Psychopathology.* Washington, DC: American Psychiatric Press; 2000:169.

Penn DL, Ritchie MF, Francis JC, Martin J. Social perception in schizophrenia: the role of context. *Psychiatry Res.* 2002;109:149.

Prikhojan A, Davis KL. Dementia in schizophrenia. In: Breier A, Tran PV, eds. *Current Issues in the Psychopharmacology of Schizophrenia.* Philadelphia: Lippincott Williams & Wilkins; 2001:513.

Sweeney JA, Haas G, Nimgaonkar V. Schizophrenia: etiology. In: Hersen M, Bellack AS. *Psychopathology in Adulthood.* Needham Heights, MA: Allyn & Bacon; 2000:278.

Yui K, Ikemoto S, Ishiguro T, Goto K. Studies of amphetamine or methamphetamine psychosis in Japan: relation of methamphetamine psychosis to schizophrenia. *Ann N Y Acad Sci.* 2000;914:1. Theme issue.

14 Other Psychotic Disorders

▲ 14.1 Schizophreniform Disorder

Schizophreniform disorder is similar to schizophrenia except that its symptoms last at least 1 month but less than 6 months. Patients with schizophreniform disorder return to their baseline level of functioning once the disorder has resolved. In contrast, for a patient to meet the diagnostic criteria for schizophrenia, the symptoms must have been present for at least 6 months. Gabriel Langfeldt first used the term *schizophreniform* in 1939, at the University Psychiatric Clinic in Oslo, Norway, to describe a disorder characterized by a brief, self-contained psychotic episode.

EPIDEMIOLOGY

Little is known about the incidence, prevalence, and sex ratio of schizophreniform disorder. The disorder is most common in adolescents and young adults and is less than half as common as schizophrenia. A lifetime prevalence rate of 0.2 percent and a 1-year prevalence rate of 0.1 percent have been reported.

Several studies have shown that the relatives of patients with schizophreniform disorder are at high risk of having other psychiatric disorders, but the distribution of the disorders differs from the distribution seen in the relatives of patients with schizophrenia and bipolar disorders. Specifically, the relatives of patients with schizophreniform disorders are more likely to have mood disorders than are the relatives of patients with schizophrenia. In addition, the relatives of patients with schizophreniform disorder are more likely to have a diagnosis of a psychotic mood disorder than are the relatives of patients with bipolar disorders.

ETIOLOGY

The cause of schizophreniform disorder is not known. As Langfeldt noted in 1939, the group of patients with this diagnostic label are likely to be heterogeneous. In general, some patients have a disorder similar to schizophrenia, whereas others have a disorder similar to a mood disorder. Because of the generally good outcome, the disorder probably has similarities to the episodic nature of mood disorders. Some data, however, indicate a close relation to schizophrenia.

In support of the relation to mood disorders, several studies have shown that patients with schizophreniform disorder, as a group, have more affective symptoms (especially mania) and a better outcome than patients with schizophrenia. Also, the increased occurrence of mood disorders in the relatives of patients with schizophreniform disorder indicates a relation to mood disorders. Thus, the biological and epidemiological data are most consistent with the hypothesis that the current diagnostic category defines a group of patients, some of whom have a disorder similar to schizophrenia, while others have a disorder resembling a mood disorder.

Brain Imaging

A relative activation deficit in the inferior prefrontal region of the brain while the patient is performing a region-specific psychological task (the Wisconsin Card Sorting Test), as reported for schizophrenia patients, has been reported in patients with schizophreniform disorder (Fig. 14.1–1). One study showed the deficit to be limited to the left hemisphere and also found impaired striatal activity suppression limited to the left hemisphere during the activation procedure. The data can be interpreted to indicate a physiological similarity between the psychosis of schizophrenia and the psychosis of schizophreniform disorder. Additional central nervous system (CNS) factors, as yet unidentified, may lead to either the long-term course of schizophrenia or the foreshortened course of schizophreniform disorder.

Although some data indicate that patients with schizophreniform disorder may have enlarged cerebral ventricles, as determined by computed tomography and magnetic resonance imaging, other data indicate that unlike the enlargement seen in schizophrenia, the ventricular enlargement in schizophreniform disorder is not correlated with outcome measures or other biological measures.

Other Biological Measures

Although brain imaging studies point to a similarity between schizophreniform disorder and schizophrenia, at least one study of electrodermal activity indicated a difference. Patients with schizophrenia born during the winter and spring months (a period of high risk for the birth of these patients) had hyporesponsive skin conductances, but this association was absent in patients with schizophreniform disorder. The significance and the meaning of this single study are difficult to interpret, but the

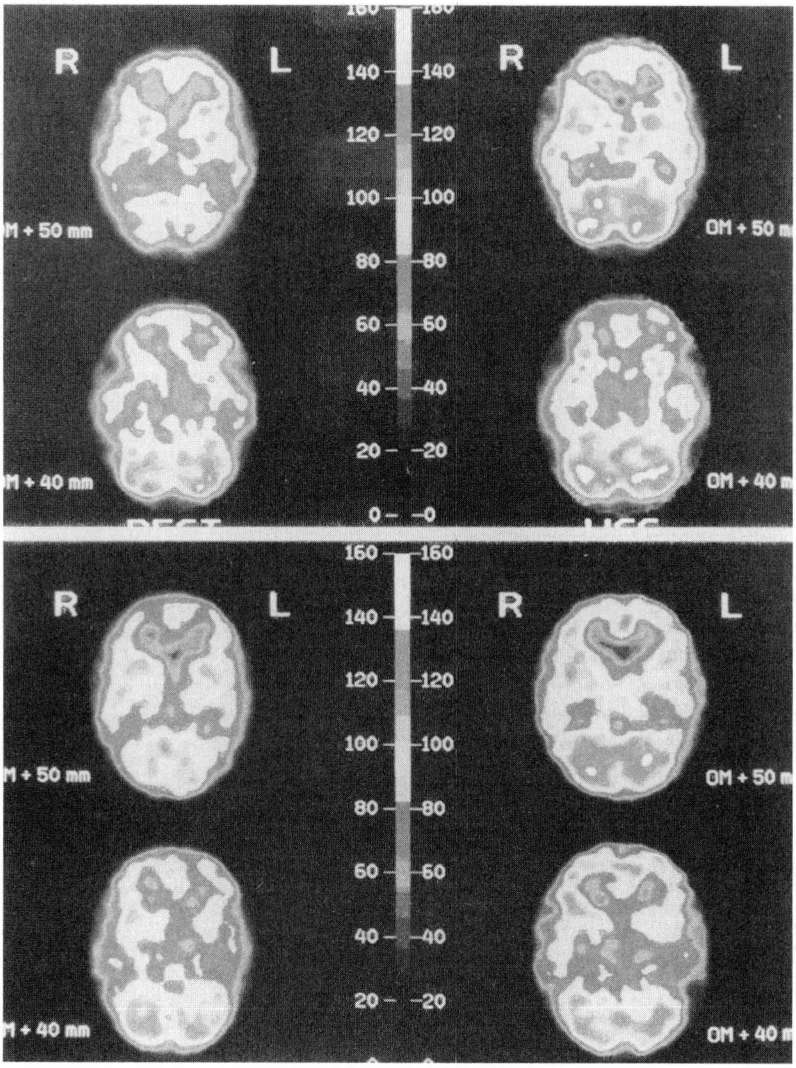

FIGURE 14.1–1

Regional cerebral blood flow distribution at rest **(left)** and during cerebral activation with the Wisconsin Card sorting Test **(right)** in a patient with schizophreniform disorder **(top)** and a healthy volunteer **(bottom)**. *OM* indicates orbitomeatal line. (Reprinted from Rubin P, Holm S, Friberg L, et al. Altered modulation of prefrontal and subcortical brain activity in newly diagnosed schizophrenia and schizophreniform disorder. *Arch Gen Psychiatry.* 1991;48:992, with permission.)

results do suggest caution in assuming similarity between patients with schizophrenia and those with schizophreniform disorder. Data from at least one study of eye tracking in the two groups also indicate that they may differ in some biological measures.

DIAGNOSTIC AND CLINICAL FEATURES

The text revision of the fourth edition of *Diagnostic and Statistical Manual of Mental Disorders* (DSM-IV-TR) criteria for schizophreniform disorder are listed in Table 14.1–1. Schizophreniform disorder in its typical presentation is a rapid-onset psychotic disorder without a significant prodrome. Hallucinations, delusions, or both will be present; negative symptoms of alogia and avolition may be present. Affect may be flattened, which is seen as a poor prognostic sign. Speech may be grossly disorganized and confused, and behavior may be disorganized or catatonic. The symptoms of psychosis, the negative symptoms, and those affecting speech and behavior will last at least 1 month but may last longer. The patient's degree of perplexity about what is happening should be assessed, as this is a differentiating prognostic sign.

Although the above is the typical presentation, a picture exactly resembling that of schizophrenia may also occur. In that case, the onset may be insidious, premorbid functioning may have been poor, and affect is quite blunted. The only differentiation from schizophrenia for this type of presentation is the duration of the total episode of illness. When it has lasted 6 months, the diagnosis becomes schizophrenia. In making the diagnosis in the case with insidious onset, the "attenuated symptoms" of the acute episode may have lasted for some time. If they have been present for at least 5 months and then the acute episode lasts 1 month, the diagnosis of schizophrenia is appropriate, without a prior diagnosis of schizophreniform disorder.

Table 14.1–1
DSM-IV-TR Diagnostic Criteria for Schizophreniform Disorder

A. Criteria A, D, and E of schizophrenia are met.
B. An episode of the disorder (including prodromal, active, and residual phases) lasts at least 1 month but less than 6 months. (When the diagnosis must be made without waiting for recovery, it should be qualified as "provisional.")
Specify if:
Without good prognostic features
With good prognostic features: as evidenced by two (or more) of the following:
(1) onset of prominent psychotic symptoms within 4 weeks of the first noticeable change in usual behavior or functioning
(2) confusion or perplexity at the height of the psychotic episode
(3) good premorbid social and occupational functioning
(4) absence of blunted or flat affect

From American Psychiatric Association. *Diagnostic and Statistical Manual of Mental Disorders.* 4th ed. Text rev. Washington, DC: American Psychiatric Association; copyright 2000, with permission.

In the typical form of the disorder, the patient returns to baseline functioning by the end of 6 months. Theoretically, repeated episodes of schizophreniform illness are possible, each lasting less than 6 months, but rarely is functioning not lost with repeated episodes of this severe illness, and schizophrenia is a more likely consideration.

Ms. L.J. was a 29-year-old Hispanic second daughter of an intact and stable family. She completed high school without problems and was described as outgoing and friendly. She considered college but opted to work. She spent several years as a factory worker and had decided to go back to school and become a teacher. Five months ago she had a sudden "awareness" that God was present and filling the souls of people around her. She became acutely distressed when she realized God was not going to "touch her." Her family was quite surprised and alarmed by her sudden change in behavior. She was brought to the local emergency room. While she occasionally drank alcohol and had smoked marijuana in the past, the family did not suspect a substance abuse problem.

Toxicology screening in the emergency room was negative for substances. She was admitted to the hospital for evaluation. She told the psychiatrist that she felt she had done something wrong and that was why God had abandoned her. She also reported that she felt people on the ward were reading her mind. She was particularly concerned that her critical thoughts about others could be heard and then these angry people would attack her. L.J. was stabilized on haloperidol (Haldol) and then switched to risperidone (Risperdal) because of adverse effects.

A family meeting was held to discuss her problems. At that time, the psychiatrist recommended a wait-and-see approach. The psychiatrist told the patient (and family) to follow up with an outpatient doctor and to continue taking the medication if the outpatient psychiatrist recommended it. Two months after her admission she no longer was distressed by her religious concerns. However, she still felt that people could read her mind. Three months after her admission she no longer felt that people could read her mind, and she had returned to her community college. A month later, she stopped taking her antipsychotic agent because she felt she didn't need it. Two weeks ago her family brought her to the emergency room because she was again talking about God and "hiding" from people who could read her thoughts. She initially refused medications but resumed taking them, with some improvement of her psychosis. A family meeting was held to discuss the return of her psychosis and the fact that she may eventually be diagnosed with schizophrenia. (Courtesy of John Lauriello, M.D., Brenda R. Erickson, M.D., and Samuel J. Keith, M.D.)

DIFFERENTIAL DIAGNOSIS

Although the major differential diagnoses are with brief psychotic disorder and schizophrenia, the rapid onset of acute psychosis may be the most important diagnostic point in a patient's course of illness. The clinician should focus on the prior 6 months, taking a detailed history of occupational and social functioning, the pattern of onset, the presence or absence of mood changes, alcohol and substance abuse, and other illness and prescriptive medication. Of special interest is any family history of psychiatric illness, mood disorders, or schizophrenia-like illnesses in particular. A recent study showed a high prevalence of personality disorders after recovery from the psychosis. One could hypothesize that the personality disorder predisposes one to psychosis especially when under stress.

A complete physical examination is always indicated with the presentation of a psychotic illness. Suggestions of endocrinological involvement, such as thyroid functioning, should be followed up with laboratory studies. Suspicion of substance abuse, no matter how remote a possibility, mandates a toxicology screening test. Changes in sensorium and a rapid onset of symptoms should raise clinical suspicion of substance toxicity. Alcohol may be involved in a number of ways. Certainly, alcohol withdrawal and the onset of delirium may be associated with psychotic symptoms. Further, alcohol abuse leads to unreliable medication taking, even of prescribed medications, which can lead to psychotic features.

Distinguishing mood disorders with psychotic features from a rapid-onset schizophreniform disorder may be difficult and tests the clinician's skills. Negative symptoms such as alogia, avolition, and blunted affect may be difficult to distinguish from the loss of interest and pleasure seen with major depressive episodes. Appetite, sleep, and other neurovegetative symptoms may also occur with both. The presence of the psychotic features of the illness, in the absence of these mood features, will help the to make the diagnosis of schizophreniform disorder, but this may take time to evolve.

A time cutoff has been established to differentiate schizophreniform disorder from brief psychotic disorder—more than 1 day but less than 1 month. During this period, the diagnosis

must be brief psychotic disorder. In diagnostic systems prior to DSM-IV-TR, the presence or absence of a stressor was used to differentiate these two conditions further, but it is no longer used in the nosology, except as a descriptor or modifier. Differentiation is based solely on the time line.

COURSE AND PROGNOSIS

The course of schizophreniform disorder is for the most part defined in the criteria. It is a psychotic illness lasting more than 1 month and less than 6 months. The real issue is what happens to persons with this illness over time. Most estimates of progression to schizophrenia range between 60 and 80 percent. What happens to the other 20 to 40 percent is currently not known. Some will have a second or third episode during which they will deteriorate into a more chronic condition of schizophrenia. A few, however, may have only this single episode and then continue on with their lives. While this is clearly the outcome desired by all clinicians and family members, it is probably a rare occurrence and should not be held out as likely.

TREATMENT

Hospitalization is often necessary in treating patients with schizophreniform disorder and allows effective assessment, treatment, and supervision of a patient's behavior. The psychotic symptoms can usually be treated by a 3- to 6-month course of antipsychotic drugs (e.g., risperidone). Several studies have shown that patients with schizophreniform disorder respond to antipsychotic treatment much more rapidly than patients with schizophrenia. In one study, about 75 percent of patients with schizophreniform disorder and only 20 percent of the patients with schizophrenia responded to antipsychotic medications within 8 days. A trial of lithium (Eskalith), carbamazepine (Tegretol), or valproate (Depakene) may be warranted for treatment and prophylaxis if a patient has a recurrent episode. Psychotherapy is usually necessary to help patients integrate the psychotic experience into their understanding of their minds, brains, and lives. Electroconvulsive therapy may be indicated for some patients, especially those with marked catatonic or depressed features.

Finally, most patients with schizophreniform disorder progress to full-blown schizophrenia despite treatment. In those cases, a course of management consistent with a chronic illness must be formulated.

REFERENCES

Cannon M, Caspi A, Moffitt TE, et al. Evidence for early-childhood pan-developmental impairment specific to schizophreniform disorder: results from a longitudinal birth cohort. *Arch Gen Psychiatry.* 2002;59:449.

Lauriello J, Erickson BR, Keith SJ. Schizoaffective disorder, schizophreniform disorder, and brief psychotic disorder. In: Sadock BJ, Sadock VA, eds. *Kaplan & Sadock's Comprehensive Textbook of Psychiatry.* 7th ed. Vol 1. Baltimore: Lippincott Williams & Wilkins; 2000:1232.

Marengo JT, Harrow M, Westermeyer JF. Early longitudinal course of acute-chronic and paranoid-undifferentiated schizophrenia subtypes and schizophreniform disorder. *J Abnorm Psychol.* 1991;100:600.

Poulton R, Caspi A, Moffitt TE, Cannon M, Murray R, Harrington H. Children's self-reported psychotic symptoms and adult schizophreniform disorder: a 15-year longitudinal study. *Arch Gen Psychiatry.* 2000;57:1053.

Pulver AE, Brown CH, Wolyniec PS, McGrath JA, Tam D. Psychiatric morbidity in the relatives of patients with DSM-III schizophreniform disorder: comparisons with the relatives of schizophrenic and bipolar disorder patients. *J Psychiatr Res.* 1991;25:19.

Rao ML, Gross G, Halaris A, et al. Hyperdopaminergia in schizophreniform psychosis: a chronobiological study. *Psychiatry Res.* 1993;47:187.

▲ 14.2 Schizoaffective Disorder

As the term implies, *schizoaffective disorder* has features of both schizophrenia and affective disorders (now called mood disorders). The diagnostic criteria for schizoaffective disorder have changed over time, mostly to reflect changes in the diagnostic criteria for schizophrenia and the mood disorders; however, it remains the best diagnosis for patients who present with mixtures of both.

George H. Kirby, in 1913, and August Hoch, in 1921, both described patients with mixed features of schizophrenia and affective (mood) disorders. Because their patients did not have the deteriorating course of dementia precox, Kirby and Hoch classified them in Emil Kraepelin's manic-depressive psychosis group.

In 1933, Jacob Kasanin introduced the term *schizoaffective disorder* to refer to a disorder with symptoms of both schizophrenia and mood disorders. In patients with the disorder, the onset of symptoms was sudden and often occurred in adolescence. Patients tended to have a good premorbid level of functioning, and often a specific stressor preceded the onset of symptoms. The family histories of the patients often included a mood disorder. Because Eugen Bleuler's broad concept of schizophrenia had eclipsed Kraepelin's narrow concept, Kasanin believed that the patients had a type of schizophrenia. From 1933 to about 1970, patients whose symptoms were similar to those of Kasanin's patients were variously classified as having schizoaffective disorder, atypical schizophrenia, good-prognosis schizophrenia, remitting schizophrenia, and cycloid psychosis—terms that emphasized a relation to schizophrenia.

Around 1970, two sets of data shifted the view of schizoaffective disorder from a schizophrenic illness to a mood disorder. First, lithium carbonate (Eskalith) was shown to be an effective and specific treatment for both bipolar disorders and some cases of schizoaffective disorder. Second, the United States–United Kingdom study published in 1968 by John Cooper and his colleagues showed that the variation in the number of patients classified as schizophrenic in the United States and in the United Kingdom resulted from an overemphasis in the United States on the presence of psychotic symptoms as a diagnostic criterion for schizophrenia.

EPIDEMIOLOGY

The lifetime prevalence of schizoaffective disorder is less than 1 percent, possibly in the range of 0.5 to 0.8 percent. These figures, however, are estimates; various studies of schizoaffective disorder have used varying diagnostic criteria. In clinical practice, a preliminary diagnosis of schizoaffective disorder is frequently used when a clinician is uncertain of the diagnosis.

Gender and Age Differences

The literature describing gender and age differences among patients with schizoaffective disorder is limited. The depressive type of schizoaffective disorder may be more common in older persons than in younger persons, and the bipolar type may be more common in young adults than in older adults.

The prevalence of the disorder has been reported to be lower in men than in women, particularly married women; the age of onset for women is later than that for men, as in schizophrenia. Men with schizoaffective disorder are likely to exhibit antisocial behavior and to have a markedly flat or inappropriate affect.

ETIOLOGY

The cause of schizoaffective disorder is unknown. The disorder may be a type of schizophrenia, a type of mood disorder, or the simultaneous expression of each. Schizoaffective disorder may also be a distinct third type of psychosis, one that is unrelated to either schizophrenia or a mood disorder. The most likely possibility is that schizoaffective disorder is a heterogeneous group of disorders encompassing all of these possibilities.

Studies designed to explore the etiology have examined family histories, biological markers, short-term treatment responses, and long-term outcomes. Most studies have considered patients with schizoaffective disorder to be a homogeneous group, but recent studies have examined the bipolar and depressive types of schizoaffective disorder separately, and the text revision of the fourth edition of *Diagnostic and Statistical Manual of Mental Disorders* (DSM-IV-TR) has a classification for each type.

Although much of the family and genetic research in schizoaffective disorder is based on the premise that schizophrenia and the mood disorders are completely separate entities, some data indicate that they may be genetically related. Studies of the relatives of patients with schizoaffective disorder have reported inconsistent results; however, according to DSM-IV-TR, there is an increased risk of schizophrenia among the relatives of probands with schizoaffective disorder.

As a group, patients with schizoaffective disorder have a better prognosis than patients with schizophrenia and a worse prognosis than patients with mood disorders. Also, as a group, patients with schizoaffective disorder tend to have a nondeteriorating course and respond better to lithium than patients with schizophrenia.

Consolidation of Data

A reasonable conclusion from the available data is that patients with schizoaffective disorder are a heterogeneous group: some have schizophrenia with prominent affective symptoms, others have a mood disorder with prominent schizophrenic symptoms, and still others have a distinct clinical syndrome. The hypothesis that schizoaffective disorder patients have both schizophrenia and a mood disorder is untenable, because the calculated co-occurrence of the two disorders is much lower than the incidence of schizoaffective disorder.

Diagnosis and Clinical Features

DSM-IV-TR diagnostic criteria are provided in Table 14.2–1. These criteria are a product of several revisions that sought to clarify several diagnoses, including schizophrenia, bipolar disorder, and major depressive disorder. The hope was that improving these diagnoses would make schizoaffective disorder begin to stand apart from them. However, the diagnostic criteria still leave much to interpretation. The diagnostician must accurately diagnose the affective illness, making sure it meets the criteria of either a manic or a depressive episode but also determining the exact length of each episode (not always easy or even possible).

Table 14.2–1
DSM-IV-TR Diagnostic Criteria for Schizoaffective Disorder

A. An uninterrupted period of illness during which, at some time, there is either a major depressive episode, a manic episode, or a mixed episode concurrent with symptoms that meet criterion A for schizophrenia.

Note: The major depressive episode must include Criterion A1: depressed mood.

B. During the same period of illness, there have been delusions or hallucinations for at least 2 weeks in the absence of prominent mood symptoms.

C. Symptoms that meet criteria for a mood episode are present for a substantial portion of the total duration of the active and residual periods of the illness.

D. The disturbance is not due to the direct physiological effects of a substance (e.g., a drug of abuse, a medication) or a general medical condition.

Specify type:

Bipolar type: if the disturbance includes a manic or a mixed episode (or a manic or a mixed episode and major depressive episodes)

Depressive type: if the disturbance only includes major depressive episodes

From American Psychiatric Association. *Diagnostic and Statistical Manual of Mental Disorders.* 4th ed. Text rev. Washington, DC: American Psychiatric Association; copyright 2000, with permission.

The length of each episode is critical for two reasons. First, to meet the B criterion (psychotic symptoms in the absence of the mood syndrome) one must know when the affective episode ends and the psychosis continues. Second, to meet criterion C, the length of all mood episodes must be combined and compared with the total length of the illness. If the mood component is present for a substantial portion of the total illness, then that criterion is met. Calculating the total length of the episodes can be difficult, and the term "substantial portion" is not defined. In practice, most clinicians look for the mood component to be 15 to 20 percent of the total illness. Patients who have one full manic episode lasting 2 months but who have suffered from symptoms of schizophrenia for 10 years do not meet the criteria for schizoaffective disorder. Instead, the diagnosis would be a mood episode superimposed on schizophrenia. Whether the bipolar or depressive type specifiers are helpful is unclear, but they may direct treatment options. These subtypes are often confused with earlier subtypes (schizophrenic versus affective type) thought to have implications in course and prognosis. Like most psychiatric diagnoses, schizoaffective disorder should not be used if the symptoms are caused by substance abuse or a secondary medical condition.

The 10th revision of *International Statistical Classification of Diseases and Related Health Problems* (ICD-10) diagnostic criteria for schizoaffective disorder are listed in Table 14.2–2.

Table 14.2–2
ICD-10 Diagnostic Criteria for Schizoaffective Disorders

Note: This diagnosis depends upon an approximate "balance" between the number, severity, and duration of the schizophrenic and affective symptoms.

G1. The disorder meets the criteria for one of the affective disorders of moderate or severe degree, as specified for each category.

G2. Symptoms from at least one of the groups listed below must be clearly present for most of the time during a period of at least 2 weeks (these groups are almost the same as for schizophrenia):
- (1) thought echo, thought insertion or withdrawal, thought broadcasting (Criterion G1(1)a for paranoid, hebephrenic, or catatonic schizophrenia);
- (2) delusions of control, influence, or passivity, clearly referred to body or limb movements or specific thoughts, actions, or sensations (Criterion G1(1)b for paranoid, hebephrenic, or catatonic schizophrenia);
- (3) hallucinatory voices giving a running commentary on the patient's behavior or discussing the patient among themselves, or other types of hallucinatory voices coming from some part of the body (Criterion G1(1)c for paranoid, hebephrenic, or catatonic schizophrenia);
- (4) persistent delusions of other kinds that are culturally inappropriate and completely impossible, but not merely grandiose or persecutory (Criterion G1(1)d for paranoid, hebephrenic, or catatonic schizophrenia), e.g., has visited other worlds; can control the clouds by breathing in and out; can communicate with plants or animals without speaking;
- (5) grossly irrelevant or incoherent speech, or frequent use of neologisms (a marked form of Criterion G1(2)b for paranoid, hebephrenic, or catatonic schizophrenia);
- (6) intermittent but frequent appearance of some forms of catatonic behavior, such as posturing, waxy flexibility, and negativism (Criterion G1(2)c for paranoid, hebephrenic, or catatonic schizophrenia).

G3. Criteria G1 and G2 above must be met within the same episode of the disorder, and concurrently for at least part of the episode. Symptoms from both G1 and G2 must be prominent in the clinical picture.

G4. *Most commonly used exclusion clause.* The disorder is not attributable to organic mental disorder, or to psychoactive substance-related intoxication, dependence, or withdrawal.

Schizoaffective disorder, manic type

A. The general criteria for schizoaffective disorder must be met.

B. Criteria for a manic disorder must be met.

Other schizoaffective disorders

Schizoaffective disorder, unspecified

Comments

If desired, further subtypes of schizoaffective disorder may be specified, according to the longitudinal development of the disorder, as follows:

Concurrent affective and schizophrenic symptoms only

Symptoms as defined in Criterion G2 for schizoaffective disorders

Concurrent affective and schizophrenic symptoms beyond the duration of affective symptoms

Reprinted with permission from World Health Organization. *The ICD-10 Classification of Mental and Behavioural Disorders: Diagnostic Criteria for Research.* Copyright, World Health Organization, Geneva, 1993.

Ms. A.D. was a 29-year-old unmarried white woman, with a 10-year history of schizoaffective disorder bipolar type. She was first hospitalized after child protection took her son away for alleged child abuse. When the patient was interviewed at that time, she was described as "dressed like a gypsy," with heavy makeup and pressured speech. She told the treatment team that her son had been abused by his father, a well-known rock star. During this time she was stabilized on lithium and haloperidol (Haldol). Ms. A.D.'s manic symptoms resolved, but her belief that she was a rock star's girlfriend remained. Since that first hospitalization she has lost custody of her son. She remains delusional about the child's famous father, and in addition, she believes that people are out to get her. She has had three distinct episodes of mania during which she needs little sleep and has racing thoughts and pressured speech. She has been intermittently compliant with medications and is currently receiving haloperidol in a long-acting form. In the 10 years of her illness she has never been free of her delusions. She has not been able to work and receives federal disability assistance. (Courtesy of John Lauriello, M.D., Brenda R. Erickson, M.D., and Samuel J. Keith, M.D.)

DIFFERENTIAL DIAGNOSIS

The psychiatric differential diagnosis includes all the possibilities usually considered for mood disorders and for schizophrenia. In any differential diagnosis of psychotic disorders a complete medical workup should be performed to rule out organic causes for the symptoms. A history of substance use (with or without positive results on a toxicology screening test) may indicate a substance-induced disorder. Preexisting medical conditions, their treatment, or both may cause psychotic and mood disorders. Any suspicion of a neurological abnormality warrants consideration of a brain scan to rule out anatomical pathology and an electroencephalogram (EEG) to determine any possible seizure disorders (e.g., temporal lobe epilepsy). Psychotic disorder due to seizure disorder is more common than that seen in the general population. It tends to be characterized by paranoia, hallucinations, and ideas of reference. Epileptic patients with psychosis are believed to have a better level of function than patients with schizophrenic spectrum disorders. Better control of the seizures can reduce the psychosis.

COURSE AND PROGNOSIS

Considering the uncertainty and evolving diagnosis of schizoaffective disorder, determining the long-term course and prognosis is difficult. Given the definition of the diagnosis, one might expect patients with schizoaffective disorder to have either a course similar to an episodic mood disorder, a chronic schizophrenic course, or some intermediate outcome. It has been presumed that an increasing presence of schizophrenic symptoms predicted worse prognosis. After 1 year, patients with schizoaffective disorder had different outcomes depending on whether their predominant symptoms were affective (better prognosis) or schizophrenic (worse prognosis). One study that followed patients diagnosed with schizoaffective disorder for 8 years

found that the outcomes of these patients more closely resembled schizophrenia than a mood disorder with psychotic features.

TREATMENT

Mood stabilizers are a mainstay of treatment for bipolar disorders and would be expected to be important in the treatment of patients with schizoaffective disorder. A recent study that compared lithium with carbamazepine (Tegretol) found that carbamazepine was superior for schizoaffective disorder, depressive type, but found no difference in the two agents for the bipolar type. In practice, however, these medications are used extensively alone, in combination with each other, or with an antipsychotic agent. In manic episodes, schizoaffective patients should be treated aggressively with dosages of a mood stabilizer in the middle to high therapeutic blood concentration range. As the patient enters maintenance phase, the dosage can be reduced to low to middle range to avoid adverse effects and potential effects on organ systems (e.g., thyroid and kidney) and to improve ease of use and compliance. Laboratory monitoring of plasma drug concentrations and periodic screening of thyroid, kidney, and hematological functioning should be performed.

By definition many schizoaffective patients suffer from major depressive episodes. Treatment with antidepressants mirrors treatment of bipolar depression. One should be careful not to precipitate a cycle of rapid switches from depression to mania with the antidepressant. The choice of antidepressant should take into account previous antidepressant successes or failures. Selective serotonin reuptake inhibitors (e.g., fluoxetine [Prozac] and sertraline [Zoloft]) are often used as first-line agents because they have less effect on cardiac status and have a favorable overdose profile. However, agitated or insomniac patients may benefit from a tricyclic drug. As in all cases of intractable mania, the use of electroconvulsive therapy (ECT) should be considered. As mentioned above, antipsychotic agents are important in the treatment of the psychotic symptoms of schizoaffective disorder.

Psychosocial Treatment

Patients benefit from a combination of family therapy, social skills training, and cognitive rehabilitation. Because the psychiatric field has had difficulty deciding on the exact diagnosis and prognosis of schizoaffective disorder, this uncertainty must be explained to the patient. The range of symptoms can be quite large as patients contend with both ongoing psychosis and varying mood states. It can be very difficult for family members to keep up with the changing nature and needs of these patients. Medication regimens can be complicated, with multiple medications from all classes of drugs.

REFERENCES

Goldstein JM, Faraone SV, Chen WJ, Tsuang MT. The role of gender in understanding the familial transmission of schizoaffective disorder. *Br J Psychiatry.* 1993;163:763.

Greil W, Ludwig-Mayerhofer W, Erazo N, et al. Lithium vs. carbamazepine in the maintenance treatment of schizoaffective disorder: a randomized study. *Eur Arch Psychiatry Clin Neurosci.* 1997;247:42.

Hummel B, Dittmann S, Forsthoff A, et al. Clozapine as add-on medication in the maintenance treatment of bipolar and schizoaffective disorders. *Neuropsychobiology.* 2002;45:37.

Keck PE, McElroy SL, Strakowski SM. New developments in the pharmacological treatment of schizoaffective disorder. *J Clin Psychiatry.* 1996;57:41.

Keck PE, McElroy SL, Strakowski SM, West SA. Pharmacological treatment of schizoaffective disorder. *Psychopharmacology.* 1994;114:529.

Lapensee MA. A review of schizoaffective disorder, I. Current concepts. *Can J Psychiatry.* 1992;37:335.

Lapensee MA. A review of schizoaffective disorder, II. Somatic treatment. *Can J Psychiatry.* 1992;37:347.

Lauriello J, Erickson BR, Keith SJ. Schizoaffective disorder, schizophreniform disorder, and brief psychotic disorder. In: Sadock BJ, Sadock VA, eds. *Kaplan & Sadock's Comprehensive Textbook of Psychiatry.* 7th ed. Vol 1. Baltimore: Lippincott Williams & Wilkins; 2000:1232.

Levitt JJ, Tsuang MT. The heterogeneity of schizoaffective disorder: implication for treatment. *Am J Psychiatry.* 1988;145:20.

Madhusoodanan S, Brenner R, Cohen CI. Risperidone for elderly patients with schizophrenia or schizoaffective disorder. *Psychiatr Ann.* 2000;30:175.

Susser E, Wanderling J. Epidemiology of nonaffective acute remitting psychosis vs. schizophrenia. *Arch Gen Psychiatry.* 1994;51:20.

Taylor MA, Amir N. Are schizophrenia and affective disorder related? The problem of schizoaffective disorder and the discrimination of the psychoses by signs and symptoms. *Compr Psychiatry.* 1994;35:420.

▲ 14.3 Delusional Disorder and Shared Psychotic Disorder

According to the text revision of the fourth edition of *Diagnostic and Statistical Manual of Mental Disorders* (DSM-IV-TR), the diagnosis of delusional disorder is made when a person exhibits nonbizarre delusions of at least 1 month's duration that cannot be attributed to other psychiatric disorders. Definitions of the term *delusion* and types relevant to delusional disorders are presented in Table 14.3–1. *Nonbizarre* means that the delusions must be about situations that can occur in real life, such as being followed, infected, loved at a distance, and so on; that is, they usually have to do with phenomena that, although not real, are nonetheless possible. There are several types of delusions, and the predominant type is specified when the diagnosis is made.

EPIDEMIOLOGY

An accurate assessment of the epidemiology of delusional disorder is hampered by the relative rareness of the disorder, as well as by its changing definitions in recent history. Moreover, delusional disorder may be underreported because delusional patients rarely seek psychiatric help unless forced to do so by their families or by the courts. Even with these limitations, however, the literature does support the contention that delusional disorder, although uncommon, has a relatively steady rate.

The prevalence of delusional disorder in the United States is currently estimated to be 0.025 to 0.03 percent. Thus, delusional disorder is much rarer than schizophrenia, which has a prevalence of about 1 percent, and the mood disorders, which have a prevalence of about 5 percent. The annual incidence of delusional disorder is 1 to 3 new cases per 100,000 persons. According to DSM-IV-TR, delusional disorders account for only 1 to 2 percent of all admissions to inpatient mental health facilities. The mean age of onset is about 40 years, but the range for age of onset runs from 18 to the 90s. There is a slight preponderance of female patients. Men are more likely to develop paranoid delusions than women, who are more likely to develop delusions of erotomania. Many patients are married and employed, but there may be some association with recent immigration and low socioeconomic status.

Table 14.3–1
DSM-IV-TR Definition of Delusion and Certain Common Types Associated with Delusional Disorders

Delusion A false belief based on incorrect inference about external reality that is firmly sustained despite what almost everyone else believes and despite what constitutes incontrovertible and obvious proof of evidence to the contrary. The belief is not one ordinarily accepted by other members of the person's culture or subculture (e.g., it is not an article of religious faith). When a false belief involves a value judgment, it is regarded as a delusion only when the judgment is so extreme as to defy credibility. Delusional conviction occurs on a continuum and can sometimes be inferred from an individual's behavior. It is often difficult to distinguish between a delusion and an overvalued idea (in which case the individual has an unreasonable belief or idea but does not hold it as firmly as is the case with a delusion). Delusions are subdivided according to their content. Some of the more common types are listed below:

Bizarre—A delusion that involves a phenomenon that the person's culture would regard as totally implausible.

Delusional jealousy—The delusion that one's sexual partner is unfaithful.

Erotomanic—A delusion that another person, usually of higher status, is in love with the individual.

Grandiose—A delusion of inflated worth, power, knowledge, identity, or special relationship to a deity or famous person.

Mood-congruent—See mood-congruent psychotic features.

Mood-incongruent—See mood-incongruent psychotic features.

Of being controlled—A delusion in which feelings, impulses, thoughts, or actions are experienced as being under the control of some external force rather than being under one's own control.

Of reference—A delusion whose theme is that events, objects, or other persons in one's immediate environment have a particular and unusual significance. These delusions are usually of a negative or pejorative nature, but also may be grandiose in content. This differs from an idea of reference, in which the false belief is not as firmly held nor as fully organized into a true belief.

Persecutory—A delusion in which the central theme is that one (or someone to whom one is close) is being attacked, harassed, cheated, persecuted, or conspired against.

Somatic—A delusion whose main content pertains to the appearance or functioning of one's body.

Thought broadcasting—The delusion that one's thoughts are being broadcast out loud so that they can be perceived by others.

Thought insertion—The delusion that certain of one's thought are not one's own, but rather are inserted into one's mind.

Mood-congruent psychotic features—Delusions or hallucinations whose content is entirely consistent with the typical themes of a depressed or manic mood. If the mood is depressed, the content of the delusions or hallucinations would involve themes of personal inadequacy, guilt, disease, death, nihilism, or deserved punishment. The content of the delusion may include themes of persecution if these are based on self-derogatory concepts such as deserved punishment. If the mood is manic, the content of the delusions or hallucinations would involve themes of inflated worth, power, knowledge, or identity, or a special relationship to a deity or a famous person. The content of the delusion may include themes of persecution if these are based on concepts such as inflated worth or deserved punishment.

Mood-incongruent psychotic features—Delusions or hallucinations whose content is not consistent with the typical themes of a depressed or manic mood. In the case of depression, the delusions or hallucinations would not involve themes of personal inadequacy, guilt, disease, death, nihilism, or deserved punishment. In the case of mania, the delusions or hallucinations would not involve themes of inflated worth, power, knowledge, or identity, or a special relationship to a deity or a famous person. Examples of mood-incongruent psychotic features include persecutory delusions (without self-derogatory or grandiose content), thought insertion, thought broadcasting, and delusions of being controlled whose content has no apparent relationship to any of the themes listed above.

From American Psychiatric Association. *Diagnostic and Statistical Manual of Mental Disorders.* 4th ed. Text rev. Washington, DC: American Psychiatric Association; copyright 2000, with permission.

ETIOLOGY

As with all major psychiatric disorders, the cause of delusional disorder is unknown. Moreover, patients currently classified as having delusional disorder probably have a heterogeneous group of conditions with delusions as the predominant symptom. The central concept about the cause of delusional disorder is its distinctness from schizophrenia and the mood disorders. Delusional disorder is much rarer than either schizophrenia or mood disorders, with a later onset than schizophrenia and a much less pronounced female predominance than the mood disorders. The most convincing data come from family studies that report an increased prevalence of delusional disorder and related personality traits (e.g., suspiciousness, jealousy, and secretiveness) in the relatives of delusional disorder probands. Family studies have reported neither an increased incidence of schizophrenia and mood disorders in the families of delusional disorder probands nor an increased incidence of delusional disorder in the families of probands with schizophrenia. Long-term follow-up of patients with delusional disorder indicates that the diagnosis of delusional disorder is relatively stable, with less than one fourth of the patients eventually being reclassified as having schizophrenia and less than 10 percent of patients eventually being reclassified as having a mood disorder. These data indicate that delusional disorder is not simply an early stage in the development of one or both of these two more common disorders.

Biological Factors

A wide range of nonpsychiatric medical conditions and substances, including clear-cut biological factors, can cause delusions, but not everyone with a brain tumor, for example, has delusions. Unique, and not yet understood, factors in a patient's brain and personality are likely to be relevant to the specific pathophysiology of delusional disorder.

The neurological conditions most commonly associated with delusions affect the limbic system and the basal ganglia. Patients whose

delusions are caused by neurological diseases and who show no intellectual impairment tend to have complex delusions similar to those in patients with delusional disorder. Conversely, patients with neurological disorder with intellectual impairments often have simple delusions unlike those in patients with delusional disorder. Thus, delusional disorder may involve the limbic system or basal ganglia in patients who have intact cerebral cortical functioning.

Delusional disorder may arise as a normal response to abnormal experiences in the environment, the peripheral nervous system, or the central nervous system. Thus, if patients have erroneous sensory experiences of being followed (e.g., hearing footsteps), they may come to believe that they are actually being followed. This hypothesis hinges on the presence of hallucinatorylike experiences that need to be explained. The presence of such hallucinatory experiences in delusional disorder has not been proved.

Psychodynamic Factors

Practitioners have a strong clinical impression that many patients with delusional disorder are socially isolated and have attained less than expected levels of achievement. Specific psychodynamic theories about the cause and the evolution of delusional symptoms involve suppositions regarding hypersensitive persons and specific ego mechanisms: reaction formation, projection, and denial.

Freud's Contributions. Sigmund Freud believed that delusions, rather than being symptoms of the disorder, are part of a healing process. In 1896, he described projection as the main defense mechanism in paranoia. Later, Freud read *Memories of My Nervous Illness,* an autobiographical account by Daniel Paul Schreber. Although he never met Schreber, Freud theorized from his review of the autobiography that unconscious homosexual tendencies are defended against by denial and projection. According to classic psychodynamic theory, the dynamics underlying the formation of delusions for a female patient are the same as for a male patient. Careful studies of patients with delusions have been unable to corroborate Freud's theories, although they may be relevant in individual cases. Overall, there is no higher incidence of homosexual ideation or activity in patients with delusions than in other groups. Freud's major contribution, however, was to demonstrate the role of projection in the formation of delusional thought.

Paranoid Pseudocommunity. Norman Cameron described seven situations that favor the development of delusional disorders: an increased expectation of receiving sadistic treatment, situations that increase distrust and suspicion, social isolation, situations that increase envy and jealousy, situations that lower self-esteem, situations that cause persons to see their own defects in others, and situations that increase the potential for rumination over probable meanings and motivations. When frustration from any combination of these conditions exceeds the tolerable limit, persons become withdrawn and anxious; they realize that something is wrong, seek an explanation for the problem, and crystallize a delusional system as a solution. Elaboration of the delusion to include imagined persons and attribution of malevolent motivations to both real and imagined persons result in the organization of the *pseudocommunity*—a perceived community of plotters. This delusional entity hypothetically binds together projected fears and wishes to justify the patient's aggression and to provide a tangible target for the patient's hostilities.

Other Psychodynamic Factors. Clinical observations indicate that many, if not all, paranoid patients experience a lack of trust in relationships. A hypothesis relates this distrust to a consistently hostile family environment, often with an overcontrolling mother and a distant or sadistic father. Erik Erikson's concept of trust versus mistrust in early development is a useful model to explain the suspiciousness of the paranoid who never went through the healthy experience of having his or her needs satisfied by what Erikson termed the "outer-providers." Thus, they have a general distrust of their environment.

Table 14.3–2
Risk Factors Associated with Delusional Disorder

Advanced age
Sensory impairment/isolation
Family history
Social isolation
Personality features (e.g., unusual interpersonal sensitivity)
Recent immigration

Defense Mechanisms. Patients with delusional disorder use primarily the defense mechanisms of reaction formation, denial, and projection. They use reaction formation as a defense against aggression, dependence needs, and feelings of affection and transform the need for dependence into staunch independence. Patients use denial to avoid awareness of painful reality. Consumed with anger and hostility and unable to face responsibility for the rage, they project their resentment and anger onto others and use projection to protect themselves from recognizing unacceptable impulses in themselves.

Other Relevant Factors. Delusions have been linked to a variety of additional factors such as social and sensory isolation, socioeconomic deprivation, and personality disturbance. The deaf, the visually impaired, and possibly immigrants with limited ability in a new language may be more vulnerable to delusion formation than the normal population. Vulnerability is heightened with advanced age. Delusional disturbance and other paranoid features are common in the elderly. In short, multiple factors are associated with the formation of delusions, and the source and pathogenesis of delusional disorders per se have yet to be specified (Table 14.3–2).

DIAGNOSIS AND CLINICAL FEATURES

The DSM-IV-TR diagnostic criteria for delusional disorder are listed in Table 14.3–3.

Mental Status

General Description. Patients are usually well groomed and well dressed, without evidence of gross disintegration of personality or of daily activities, yet they may seem eccentric, odd, suspicious, or hostile. They are sometimes litigious and may make this inclination clear to the examiner. The most remarkable feature of patients with delusional disorder is that the mental status examination shows them to be quite normal except for a markedly abnormal delusional system. Patients may attempt to engage clinicians as allies in their delusions, but a clinician should not pretend to accept the delusion; this collusion further confounds reality and sets the stage for eventual distrust between the patient and the therapist.

Table 14.3–3
DSM-IV-TR Diagnostic Criteria for Delusional Disorder

A. Nonbizarre delusions (i.e., involving situations that occur in real life, such as being followed, poisoned, infected, loved at a distance, or deceived by spouse or lover, or having a disease) of at least 1 month's duration.
B. Criterion A for schizophrenia has never been met. **Note:** Tactile and olfactory hallucinations may be present in delusional disorder if they are related to the delusional theme.
C. Apart from the impact of the delusion(s) or its ramifications, functioning is not markedly impaired and behavior is not obviously odd or bizarre.
D. If mood episodes have occurred concurrently with delusions, their total duration has been brief relative to the duration of the delusional periods.
E. The disturbance is not due to the direct physiological effects of a substance (e.g., a drug of abuse, a medication) or a general medical condition.

Specify type (the following types are assigned based on the predominant delusional theme):

Erotomanic type: delusions that another person, usually of higher status, is in love with the individual
Grandiose type: delusions of inflated worth, power, knowledge, identity, or special relationship to a deity or famous person
Jealous type: delusions that the individual's sexual partner is unfaithful
Persecutory type: delusions that the person (or someone to whom the person is close) is being malevolently treated in some way
Somatic type: delusions that the person has some physical defect or general medical condition
Mixed type: delusions characteristic of more than one of the above types but no one theme predominates
Unspecified type

From American Psychiatric Association. *Diagnostic and Statistical Manual of Mental Disorders.* 4th ed. Text rev. Washington, DC: American Psychiatric Association; copyright 2000, with permission.

Mood, Feelings, and Affect. Patients' moods are consistent with the content of their delusions. A patient with grandiose delusions is euphoric; one with persecutory delusions is suspicious. Whatever the nature of the delusional system, the examiner may sense some mild depressive qualities.

Perceptual Disturbances. By definition, patients with delusional disorder do not have prominent or sustained hallucinations. According to DSM-IV-TR, tactile or olfactory hallucinations may be present if they are consistent with the delusion (e.g., somatic delusion of body odor). A few delusional patients have other hallucinatory experiences—virtually always auditory rather than visual.

Thought. Disorder of thought content, in the form of delusions, is the key symptom of the disorder. The delusions are usually systematized and are characterized as being possible, for example, delusions of being persecuted, having an unfaithful spouse, being infected with a virus, or being loved by a famous person. These examples of delusional content contrast with the bizarre and impossible delusional content in some schizophrenia patients. The delusional system itself may be complex or simple. Patients lack other signs of thought disorder, although some may be verbose, circumstantial, or idiosyncratic in their speech when they talk about their delusions. Clinicians should not assume that all unlikely scenarios are delusional; the veracity of a patient's beliefs should be checked before deeming their content to be delusional. Table 14.3–4 lists the 10th revision of *International Statistical Classification of Diseases and Related Health Problems* (ICD-10) diagnostic criteria for delusional disorder.

Sensorium and Cognition. ORIENTATION. Patients with delusional disorder usually have no abnormality in orientation unless they have a specific delusion about a person, place, or time.

MEMORY. Memory and other cognitive processes are intact in patients with delusional disorder.

Table 14.3–4
ICD-10 Diagnostic Criteria for Delusional Disorders

Delusional disorder

A. A delusion or a set of related delusions, other than those listed as typically schizophrenic in Criterion G1(1)b or d for paranoid, hebephrenic, or catatonic schizophrenia (i.e., other than completely impossible or culturally inappropriate), must be present. The commonest examples are persecutory, grandiose, hypochondriacal, jealous (zelotypic), or erotic delusions.
B. The delusion(s) in Criterion A must be present for at least 3 months.
C. The general criteria for schizophrenia are not fulfilled.
D. There must be no persistent hallucinations in any modality (but there may be transitory or occasional auditory hallucinations that are not in the third person or giving a running commentary).
E. Depressive symptoms (or even a depressive episode) may be present intermittently, provided that the delusions persist at times when there is no disturbance of mood.
F. *Most commonly used exclusion clause.* There must be no evidence of primary or secondary organic mental disorder as listed under organic, including symptomatic, mental disorders, or of a psychotic disorder due to psychoactive substance use.

Specification for possible subtypes

The following types may be specified if desired: persecutory; litigious; self-referential; grandiose; hypochondriacal (somatic); jealous; erotomanic.

Other persistent delusional disorders

This is a residual category for persistent delusional disorders that do not meet the criteria for delusional disorder. Disorders in which delusions are accompanied by persistent hallucinatory voices or by schizophrenic symptoms that are insufficient to meet criteria for schizophrenia should be coded here. Delusional disorders that have lasted for less than 3 months should, however, be coded, at least temporarily, under acute and transient psychotic disorders.

Persistent delusional disorder, unspecified

Reprinted with permission from World Health Organization. *The ICD-10 Classification of Mental and Behavioural Disorders: Diagnostic Criteria for Research.* Copyright, World Health Organization, Geneva, 1993.

Impulse Control. Clinicians must evaluate patients with delusional disorder for ideation or plans to act on their delusional material by suicide, homicide, or other violence. Although the incidence of these behaviors is not known, therapists should not hesitate to ask patients about their suicidal, homicidal, or other violent plans. Destructive aggression is most common in patients with a history of violence; if aggressive feelings existed in the past, therapists should ask patients how they managed those feelings. If patients cannot control their impulses, hospitalization is probably necessary. Therapists can sometimes help foster a therapeutic alliance by openly discussing how hospitalization can help patients gain additional control of their impulses.

Judgment and Insight. Patients with delusional disorder have virtually no insight into their condition and are almost always brought to the hospital by the police, family members, or employers. Judgment can best be assessed by evaluating the patient's past, present, and planned behavior.

Reliability. Patients with delusional disorder are usually reliable in their information, except when it impinges on their delusional system.

Types

Persecutory Type. The delusion of persecution is a classic symptom of delusional disorder; persecutory-type and jealousy-type delusions are probably the forms seen most frequently by psychiatrists. In contrast to persecutory delusions in schizophrenia, the clarity, logic, and systematic elaboration of the persecutory theme in delusional disorder leave a remarkable stamp on this condition. The absence of other psychopathology, of deterioration in personality, or of deterioration in most areas of functioning also contrasts with the typical manifestations of schizophrenia.

A 56-year-old female X-ray technician who had emigrated as an adult from Europe and married late in life presented to the emergency room. Her complaints were that her husband's business partner of many years intended to get her husband to resign from the business and to destroy their home. Over a number of months she had become gradually aware that a variety of apparently inconsequential incidents (such as unusual cars parked on her isolated residential street, seeing individuals she knew at restaurants, and feeling as if she were being followed each time she drove her car) pointed to a conspiracy to disrupt and ultimately destroy their lives. Her delusion of persecution was remarkably systematized and detailed; her mood in describing this was tense and irritable. There was no evidence of hallucinations, confusion, thought disorder, or mood disorder. Cognition was intact. The patient was quite intelligent and saw the clinical consultation as a means of helping her husband deal with the distress of being targeted in such a manner. (The husband had accompanied his wife on these consultations. He also had experienced some delusional thinking in accord with hers.)

The patient showed no evidence that suggested suicidality or potential for violence toward others. She initially refused all medication but gradually, over several months of therapy and parallel frequent legal consultations, agreed reluctantly to take risperidone (Risperdal) and later, for postpsychotic depression, paroxetine (Paxil). She responded within weeks to 0.5 to 1 mg of risperidone administered daily or on alternate days; she refused to take the medication continuously. Within a year, she began to focus on other issues, and the emotional intensity of the delusional concerns diminished, although they could be aroused with modest stimulation in conversation or from happenings in her home or neighborhood. (Courtesy of Theo C. Manschreck, M.P.H., M.D.)

Jealous Type. Delusional disorder with delusions of infidelity has been called *conjugal paranoia* when it is limited to the delusion that a spouse has been unfaithful. The eponym *Othello syndrome* has been used to describe morbid jealousy that can arise from multiple concerns. The delusion usually afflicts men, often those with no prior psychiatric illness. It may appear suddenly and serve to explain a host of present and past events involving the spouse's behavior. The condition is difficult to treat and may diminish only on separation, divorce, or death of the spouse.

Marked jealousy (usually termed *pathological* or *morbid jealousy*) is thus a symptom of many disorders—including schizophrenia (in which female patients more commonly display this feature), epilepsy, mood disorders, drug abuse, and alcoholism—for which treatment is directed at the primary disorder. Jealousy is a powerful emotion; when it occurs in delusional disorder or as part of another condition it can be potentially dangerous and has been associated with violence, notably both suicide and homicide. The forensic aspects of the symptom have been noted repeatedly, especially its role as a motive for murder. However, physical and verbal abuse occur more frequently than extreme actions among individuals with this symptom. Caution and care in deciding how to deal with such presentations are essential not only for diagnosis, but also from the point of view of safety.

A 47-year-old carpenter was brought for psychiatric examination following complaints by neighbors about his loud yelling and verbal abuse of his girlfriend. The patient resented the psychiatric referral but was willing to give an account of his concerns. His girlfriend, he complained, was having an affair with someone, but he was not sure who the interloper was. On his own, however, he had begun gathering evidence: strands of hair found in the apartment, photographs of soiled sheets, and suspicious items from the trash—all of which he claimed proved that an affair was ongoing. He revealed plans to tape-record, possibly videotape, his girlfriend's activities while he was on the job. Upon disclosing that he had told his girlfriend that he would kill her if the affair persisted, he was admitted to the hospital. He was treated with a serotonin-dopamine antagonist in low

dosages and responded with a reduction in the intensity of his rage and preoccupation. Eventually, he left the hospital, but only after his girlfriend had moved away. He still harbored suspicions but accepted the termination of the relationship without voluble opposition.

Erotomanic Type. Patients with erotomania have delusions of secret lovers. Most frequently the patient is a woman, but men are also susceptible to the delusion. The patient believes that a suitor, usually more socially prominent than herself, is in love with her. The delusion becomes the central focus of the patient's existence, and the onset can be sudden. Erotomania, the *psychose passionelle,* is also referred to as *de Clérambault's syndrome* to emphasize its occurrence in different disorders. Besides being the key symptom in some cases of delusional disorder, it is known to occur in schizophrenia, mood disorder, and other organic disorders.

Patients with erotomania frequently show certain characteristics: They are generally unattractive women in low-level jobs who lead withdrawn, lonely lives, are single, and have few sexual contacts. They select secret lovers who differ substantially from them. They exhibit what has been called *paradoxical conduct,* the delusional phenomenon of interpreting all denials of love, no matter how clear, as secret affirmations of love. The course may be chronic, recurrent, or brief. Separation from the love object may be the only satisfactory intervention. Although men are less commonly afflicted by this condition than women, they may be more aggressive and possibly violent in their pursuit of love. Hence, in forensic populations, men with this condition predominate. The object of aggression may not be the loved individual but companions or protectors of the love object who are viewed as trying to come between the lovers. The tendency toward violence among men with erotomania may lead initially to police, rather than psychiatric, contact. In certain cases resentment and rage in response to an absence of reaction from all forms of love communication may escalate enough to put the love object in danger. So-called stalkers, who continually follow their perceived lovers, frequently have delusions. While most stalkers are men, women also stalk and both groups have a high potential for violence.

A 29-year-old male financial analyst, while having lunch in a downtown restaurant, observed the arrival of a well-known local media personality, an attractive woman about his age. He experienced several moments of eye contact with the woman and became convinced that she had fallen in love with him. There ensued a barrage of flowers, letters, phone calls, and even several attempts to meet with her at her workplace. The woman rebuffed all such efforts and eventually called the police. The man was arrested on a stalking charge after he was observed following the woman to her residence. He was angry and threatening to the police, finally admitting that he had purchased a handgun but refusing to give a reason for the purchase. He was remanded to a forensic psychiatric unit, treated with pimozide (Orap), and eventually discharged on court-supervised probation.

Somatic Type. Delusional disorder with somatic delusions has been called *monosymptomatic hypochondriacal psychosis.* The condition differs from other conditions with hypochondriacal symptoms in the degree of reality impairment. In delusional disorder the delusion is fixed, unarguable, and presented intensely, because the patient is totally convinced of the physical nature of the disorder. In contrast, persons with hypochondriasis often admit that their fear of illness is largely groundless. The content of the somatic delusion may vary widely from case to case. There are three main types: (1) delusions of infestation (including parasitosis); (2) delusions of dysmorphophobia, such as of misshapenness, personal ugliness, or exaggerated size of body parts (this category seems closest to that of body dysmorphic disorder); and (3) delusions of foul body odors or halitosis. This third category, sometimes referred to as *olfactory reference syndrome,* appears somewhat different from the category of delusions of infestation in that patients with the former have an earlier age of onset (mean 25 years), male predominance, single status, and absence of past psychiatric treatment. Otherwise, the three groups, although individually low in prevalence, appear to overlap.

The frequency of these conditions is low, but they may be underdiagnosed because patients present to dermatologists, plastic surgeons, and infectious disease specialists more often than to psychiatrists in the unremitting search for curative treatment.

Patients with this condition have a poor prognosis without treatment. It affects both sexes roughly equally. A previous history or family history of psychotic disorder is uncommon. Younger patients frequently have a history of substance abuse or head injury. Although anger and hostility are common, shame, depression, and avoidant behavior are even more characteristic. Suicide, apparently motivated by anguish, is not uncommon.

A 40-year-old single unemployed man is referred by his primary care physician because of repeated consultations related to his complaint of hair loss. A dermatologist evaluated the patient, found no pathology, and told him that the minimal hair loss was normal. The patient refused to accept this judgment and demanded a further consultation. Because of managed-care restrictions, the patient consulted two additional specialists with his own (meager) funds with similar results. He had quit his job because of embarrassment about the hair loss and had become increasingly indebted financially. The psychiatric consultation infuriated him, but he cooperated because he thought that the hair loss had begun with some "pills" he had been prescribed several years previously for anxiety and insomnia and that a psychiatrist might help him to understand his case and prescribe an antidote that might relieve the hair loss. Treatment with an antidepressant agent proved unsatisfactory, and the patient was given an atypical antipsychotic drug with modest success. He complained less frequently about the hair loss and eventually began to express concern about his loneliness and his fear of being a burden to his aging parents, whom he lived with for financial reasons. His insight, however, remained limited, and he intermittently voiced his concerns about his appearance and hair loss to his psychiatrist.

Grandiose Type. Delusions of grandeur (megalomania) have been noted for years. They were described in Kraepelin's paranoia and have been associated with conditions fitting the description of delusional disorder.

A 51-year-old man was arrested for disturbing the peace. Police had been called to a local park to stop him from carving his initials and those of a recently formed religious cult into various trees surrounding a pond in the park. When confronted, he had scornfully argued that having been chosen to begin a new townwide religious revival, it was necessary for him to publicize his intent in a permanent fashion. The police were unsuccessful in preventing the man from cutting another tree and arrested him. Psychiatric examination was ordered at the state hospital, and the patient was observed there for several weeks. He denied any emotional difficulty and had never received psychiatric treatment. There was no history of euphoria or mood swings. The patient was angry about being hospitalized and only gradually permitted the doctor to interview him. In a few days, however, he was busy preaching to his fellow patients and letting them know that he had been given a special mandate from God to bring in new converts through his ability to heal. Eventually, his preoccupation with special powers diminished, and no other evidence of psychopathology was observed. The patient was discharged, having received no medication at all. Two months later he was arrested at a local theater, this time for disrupting the showing of a film that depicted subjects he believed to be satanic.

Mixed Type. The category mixed type applies to patients with two or more delusional themes. This diagnosis should be reserved for cases in which no single delusional type predominates.

Unspecified Type. The category unspecified type is reserved for cases in which the predominant delusion cannot be subtyped within the previous categories. A possible example is certain delusions of misidentification, for example, Capgras's syndrome, named for the French psychiatrist who described the *illusion des sosies,* or the illusion of doubles. The delusion in Capgras's syndrome is the belief that a familiar person has been replaced by an impostor. Others have described variants of the Capgras's syndrome, namely, the delusion that persecutors or familiar persons can assume the guise of strangers (*Frégoli's phenomenon*) and the very rare delusion that familiar persons can change themselves into other persons at will (*intermetamorphosis*). Each disorder is not only rare but may be associated with schizophrenia, dementia, epilepsy, and other organic disorders. Reported cases have been predominantly in women, have had associated paranoid features, and have included feelings of depersonalization or derealization. The delusion may be short-lived, recurrent, or persistent. It is unclear whether delusional disorder can appear with such a delusion. Certainly, the Frégoli and intermetamorphosis delusions have bizarre content and are unlikely, but the delusion in Capgras's syndrome is a possible candidate for delusional disorder. The role of hallucination or perceptual disturbance in this condition needs to be explicated. Cases have appeared after sudden brain damage.

In the 19th century, the French psychiatrist Jules Cotard described several patients who suffered from a syndrome called *délire de négation,* sometimes referred to as *nihilistic delusional disorder* or *Cotard syndrome.* Patients with the syndrome complain of having lost not only possessions, status, and strength but also their heart, blood, and intestines. The world beyond them is reduced to nothingness. This relatively rare syndrome is usually considered a precursor to a schizophrenic or depressive episode. With the common use today of antipsychotic drugs, the syndrome is seen even less frequently than in the past.

Shared Psychotic Disorder

Shared psychotic disorder (also referred to over the years as *shared paranoid disorder, induced psychotic disorder, folie à deux, folie impose,* and *double insanity*) was first described by Lasegue and Falret in 1877. It is probably rare, but incidence and prevalence figures are lacking, and the literature consists almost entirely of case reports.

The disorder is characterized by the transfer of delusions from one person to another. Both persons are closely associated for a long time and typically live together in relative social isolation. In its most common form (which is covered by the DSM-IV-TR criteria in Table 14.3–5), the individual who first has the delusion (the primary case) is often chronically ill and typically is the influential member of a close relationship with a more suggestible person (the secondary case) who also develops the delusion. The secondary case is frequently less intelligent, more gullible, more passive, or more lacking in self-esteem than the primary case. If the pair separates, the secondary case may abandon the delusion, but this outcome is not seen uniformly. The occurrence of the delusion is attributed to the strong influence of the more dominant member. Old age, low intelligence, sensory impairment, cerebrovascular disease, and alcohol abuse are among the factors associated with this peculiar form of psychotic disorder. A genetic predisposition to idiopathic psychoses has also been suggested as a possible risk factor. The ICD-10 criteria for induced delusional disorder are given in Table 14.3–6.

Table 14.3–5
DSM-IV-TR Diagnostic Criteria for Shared Psychotic Disorder

A. A delusion develops in an individual in the context of a close relationship with another person(s), who has an already-established delusion.

B. The delusion is similar in content to that of the person who already has the established delusion.

C. The disturbance is not better accounted for by another psychotic disorder (e.g., schizophrenia) or a mood disorder with psychotic features and is not due to the direct physiological effects of a substance (e.g., a drug of abuse, a medication) or a general medical condition.

From American Psychiatric Association. *Diagnostic and Statistical Manual of Mental Disorders.* 4th ed. Text rev. Washington, DC: American Psychiatric Association; copyright 2000, with permission.

Table 14.3–6
ICD-10 Diagnostic Criteria for Induced Delusional Disorder

A. The individual(s) must develop a delusion or delusional system originally held by someone else with a disorder classified in schizophrenia, schizotypal disorder, persistent delusional disorder, or acute and transient psychotic disorders.

B. The people concerned must have an unusually close relationship with one another, and be relatively isolated from other people.

C. The individual(s) must not have held the belief in question before contact with the other person, and must not have suffered from any other disorder classified in schizophrenia, schizotypal disorder, persistent delusional disorder, or acute and transient psychotic disorders in the past.

Other special forms have been reported, such as *folie simultanée,* in which two persons become psychotic simultaneously and share the same delusion. Occasionally, more than two individuals are involved (e.g., *folie à trois, quatre, cinq;* also *folie à famille*), but such cases are especially rare. The most common relationships in *folie à deux* are sister–sister, husband–wife, and mother–child, but other combinations have also been described. Almost all cases involve members of a single family.

A 40-year-old woman consulted physicians to help cure her problem of disagreeable body odor. The physicians failed to satisfy the woman's hopes of diagnosis and treatment, because they found nothing wrong with her. They did occasionally recommend psychiatric consultation, which she refused. Her husband, a quiet, retiring man of 35, accompanied his wife to all medical specialist consultations. When questioned, he shared his wife's concerns about body odor and provided many examples of how distressing this problem had become. When he was told that there really was nothing wrong with his wife, he objected repeatedly and proclaimed that the doctors were incompetent. A psychiatrist was called to the clinic to see the couple and found consistent stories from both. The woman accepted a recommendation for hospitalization on the psychiatry-medical unit, and the husband returned home. After weeks of evaluation and treatment, the woman was discharged. The husband had stopped visiting her, and when informed that his wife would be coming home, he said that he thought she had been cured of her problem. However, 3 months later the couple was once again visiting different specialists.

DIFFERENTIAL DIAGNOSIS

Delirium, Dementia, and Substance-Related Disorders

Delirium and dementia should be considered in the differential diagnosis of a patient with delusions. Delirium can be differentiated by the presence of a fluctuating level of consciousness or impaired cognitive abilities. Delusions early in the course of a dementing illness, as in dementia of the Alzheimer's type, may give the appearance of a delusional disorder; however, neuropsychological testing usually detects cognitive impairment. Although alcohol abuse is an associated feature for patients with delusional disorder, delusional disorder should be distinguished from alcohol-induced psychotic disorder with hallucinations. Intoxication with sympathomimetics (including amphetamine), marijuana, or L-dopa is likely to result in delusional symptoms.

Other Disorders

The psychiatric differential diagnosis for delusional disorder includes malingering and factitious disorder with predominantly psychological signs and symptoms. The nonfactitious disorders in the differential diagnosis are schizophrenia, mood disorders, obsessive-compulsive disorder, somatoform disorders, and paranoid personality disorder. Delusional disorder is distinguished from schizophrenia by the absence of other schizophrenic symptoms and by the nonbizarre quality of the delusions; patients with delusional disorder also lack the impaired functioning seen in schizophrenia. The somatic type of delusional disorder may resemble a depressive disorder or a somatoform disorder. The somatic type of delusional disorder is differentiated from depressive disorders by the absence of other signs of depression and the lack of a pervasive quality to the depression. Delusional disorder can be differentiated from somatoform disorders by the degree to which the somatic belief is held by the patient. Patients with somatoform disorders allow for the possibility that their disorder does not exist, whereas patients with delusional disorder do not doubt its reality. Separating paranoid personality disorder from delusional disorder requires the sometimes difficult clinical distinction between extreme suspiciousness and frank delusion. In general, if clinicians doubt that a symptom is a delusion, the diagnosis of delusional disorder should not be made.

COURSE AND PROGNOSIS

Some clinicians and some research data indicate that an identifiable psychosocial stressor often accompanies the onset of the disorder. The nature of the stressor may in fact warrant some suspicion or concern. Examples of such stressors are recent immigration, social conflict with family members or friends, and social isolation. A sudden onset is generally thought to be more common than an insidious onset. Some clinicians believe that a person with delusional disorder is likely to have below-average intelligence and that the premorbid personality of such a person is likely to be extroverted, dominant, and hypersensitive. The person's initial suspicions or concerns gradually become elaborate, consume much of the person's attention, and finally become delusional. Persons may begin quarreling with coworkers, may seek protection from the FBI or the police, or may begin visiting many medical or surgical physicians to seek consultations, lawyers about suits, or police about delusional suspicions.

As mentioned above, delusional disorder is considered a fairly stable diagnosis. About 50 percent of patients have recovered at long-term follow-up, 20 percent show decreased symp-

toms, and 30 percent exhibit no change. The following factors correlate with a good prognosis: high levels of occupational, social, and functional adjustments; female sex; onset before age 30; sudden onset; short duration of illness; and the presence of precipitating factors. Although reliable data are limited, patients with persecutory, somatic, and erotic delusions are thought to have a better prognosis than patients with grandiose and jealous delusions.

TREATMENT

Delusional Disorder. Delusional disorder was generally regarded as resistant to treatment, and interventions often focused on managing the morbidity of the disorder by reducing the impact of the delusion on the patient's (and family's) life. However, in recent years the outlook has become less pessimistic or restricted in planning effective treatment. The goals of treatment are to establish the diagnosis, to decide on appropriate interventions, and to manage complications (Table 14.3–7). The success of these goals depends on an effective and therapeutic doctor–patient relationship, which is far from easy to establish. The patients do not complain about psychiatric symptoms and often enter treatment against their will; even the psychiatrist may be drawn into their delusional nets.

In shared psychiatric disorder, the patients must be separated. If hospitalization is indicated they should be placed on different units and have no contact. In general, the healthier of the two will give up the delusional belief (sometimes without any other therapeutic intervention). The sicker of the two will maintain the false fixed belief.

Psychotherapy

The essential element in effective psychotherapy is to establish a relationship in which patients begin to trust a therapist. Individual therapy seems to be more effective than group therapy; insight-oriented, supportive, cognitive, and behavioral therapies are often effective. A therapist should initially neither agree with nor challenge a patient's delusions. Although therapists must ask about a delusion to establish its extent, persistent questioning about it should probably be avoided. Physicians may stimulate the motivation to receive help by emphasizing a willingness to help patients with their anxiety or irritability, without suggesting that the delusions be treated, but therapists should not actively support the notion that the delusions are real.

The unwavering reliability of therapists is essential in psychotherapy. Therapists should be on time and make appointments as regularly as possible, with the goal of developing a solid and trusting relationship with a patient. Overgratification may actually increase patients' hostility and suspiciousness because ultimately they must realize that not all demands can be met. Therapists can avoid overgratification by not extending the designated appointment period, by not giving extra appointments unless absolutely necessary, and by not being lenient about the fee.

Therapists should avoid making disparaging remarks about a patient's delusions or ideas but can sympathetically indicate to patients that their preoccupation with their delusions is both distressing to themselves and interferes with a constructive life. When patients begin to waver in their delusional beliefs, therapists may increase reality testing by asking the patients to clarify their concerns.

A useful approach in building a therapeutic alliance is to empathize with the patient's internal experience of being overwhelmed by persecution. It may be helpful to make such comments as "You must be exhausted, considering what you've been through." Without agreeing with every delusional misperception, a therapist can acknowledge that from the patient's perspective, such perceptions create much distress. The ultimate goal is to help patients entertain the possibility of doubt about their perceptions. As they become less rigid, feelings of weakness and inferiority, associated with some depression, may surface. When a patient allows feelings of vulnerability to enter into the therapy, a positive therapeutic alliance has been established, and constructive therapy becomes possible.

When family members are available, clinicians may decide to involve them in the treatment plan. Without being delusionally seen as siding with the enemy, a clinician should attempt to enlist the family as allies in the treatment process. Consequently, both the patient and the family members need to understand that the therapist maintains physician–patient confidentiality and that communications from relatives are discussed with the patient. The family may benefit from the therapist's support and may thus support the patient.

A good therapeutic outcome depends on a psychiatrist's ability to respond to the patient's mistrust of others and the resulting interpersonal conflicts, frustrations, and failures. The mark of successful treatment may be a satisfactory social adjustment rather than abatement of the patient's delusions.

Hospitalization

Patients with delusional disorder can generally undergo treatment as outpatients, but clinicians should consider hospitalization for several reasons. First, patients may need a complete medical and neurological evaluation to determine whether a nonpsychiatric medical condition is causing the delusional symptoms. Second, patients need an assessment of their ability

Table 14.3–7
Diagnosis and Management of Delusional Disorder

Rule out other causes of paranoid features
Confirm the absence of other psychopathology
Assess consequences of delusion-related behavior
– Demoralization
– Despondency
– Anger, fear
– Depression
– Impact of search for "medical diagnosis," "legal solution," "proof of infidelity," etc. (i.e., financial, legal, personal, occupational, etc.)
Assess anxiety and agitation
Assess potential for violence, suicide
Assess need for hospitalization
Institute pharmacological and psychological therapies
Maintain connection through recovery

to control violent impulses (e.g., to commit suicide or homicide) that may be related to the delusional material. Third, patients' behavior about the delusions may have significantly affected their ability to function within their family or occupational settings; they may require professional intervention to stabilize social or occupational relationships.

If a physician is convinced that a patient would receive the best treatment in a hospital, then the physician should attempt to persuade the patient to accept hospitalization; failing that, legal commitment may be indicated. If a physician convinces a patient that hospitalization is inevitable, the patient often voluntarily enters a hospital to avoid legal commitment.

Pharmacotherapy

In an emergency, severely agitated patients should be given an antipsychotic drug intramuscularly. Although no adequately conducted clinical trials with large numbers of patients have been conducted, most clinicians consider antipsychotic drugs the treatment of choice for delusional disorder. Patients are likely to refuse medication because they can easily incorporate the administration of drugs into their delusional systems; physicians should not insist on medication immediately after hospitalization but, rather, should spend a few days establishing rapport with patients. Physicians should explain potential adverse effects to patients, so that they do not later suspect that the physician lied.

A patient's history of medication response is the best guide to choosing a drug. A physician should often start with low doses (e.g., 2 mg of haloperidol [Haldol]) and increase the dose slowly. If a patient fails to respond to the drug at a reasonable dosage in a 6-week trial, antipsychotic drugs from other classes should be tried. Some investigators have indicated that pimozide may be particularly effective in delusional disorder, especially in patients with somatic delusions. A common cause of drug failure is noncompliance, which should also be evaluated. Concurrent psychotherapy facilitates compliance with drug treatment.

If the patient receives no benefit from antipsychotic medication, use of the drug should be discontinued. In patients who do respond to antipsychotic drugs, some data indicate that maintenance doses can be low. Although essentially no studies evaluate the use of antidepressants, lithium (Eskalith), or anticonvulsants (e.g., carbamazepine [Tegretol] and valproate [Depakene]) in the treatment of delusional disorder, trials with these drugs may be warranted in patients who do not respond to antipsychotic drugs. Trials of these drugs should also be considered when a patient has either the features of a mood disorder or a family history of mood disorders.

References

Bentall RP, Kaney S, Dewey ME. Paranoia and social reasoning: an attribution theory analysis. *Br J Clin Psychol.* 1991;30:12.

Block B, Pristach CA. Diagnosis and management of the paranoid patient. *Am Fam Physician.* 1992;45:2634.

Conway CR, Bollini AM, Graham BG, et al. Sensory acuity and reasoning in delusional disorder. *Compr Psychiatry.* 2002;43:175.

Gabbard GO. *Psychodynamic Psychiatry in General Practice: The DSM-IV Edition.* Washington, DC: American Psychiatric Press; 1994.

Gambini O, Colombo C, Cavallaro R, Scarone S. Smooth pursuit eye movements and saccadic eye movements in patients with delusional disorder. *Am J Psychiatry.* 1993;150:1411.

Garfield D, Havens L. Paranoid phenomena and pathological narcissism. *Am J Psychother.* 1991;45:160.

Kennedy HG, Kemp LI, Dyer DE. Fear and anger delusional (paranoid) disorder: the association with violence. *Br J Psychiatry.* 1992;160:488.

Kennedy N, McDonough M, Kelly B, Berrios GE. Erotomania revisited: clinical course and treatment. *Compr Psychiatry.* 2002;43:1.

Manschreck TC. Delusional disorder and shared psychotic disorder. In: Sadock BJ, Sadock VA, eds. *Kaplan & Sadock's Comprehensive Textbook of Psychiatry.* 7th ed. Vol 1. Baltimore: Lippincott Williams & Wilkins; 2000:1243.

Marino C, Nobile M, Bellodi L, Smeraldi E. Delusional disorder and mood disorder: can they coexist? *Psychopathology.* 1993;26:53.

Opjordsmoen S, Retterstol N. Delusional disorder: the predictive validity of the concept. *Acta Psychiatr Scand.* 1991;84:250.

Opjordsmoen S, Retterstol N. Outcome in delusional disorder in different periods of time: possible implications for treatment with neuroleptics. *Psychopathology.* 1993;26:90.

Retterstol N, Opjordsmoen S. Fatherhood, impending or newly established, precipitating delusional disorders: long-term course and outcome. *Psychopathology.* 1991;24:232.

Rippon G. Paranoid-nonparanoid differences: psychophysiological parallels. *Int J Psychophysiol.* 1992;13:79.

Schanda H. Paranoia and dysphoria: historical developments, current concepts. *Psychopathology.* 2000;33:204.

Statel SL, Southwick SM, Gawin FH. Clinical features of cocaine-induced paranoia. *Am J Psychiatry.* 1991;148:495.

▲ 14.4 Brief Psychotic Disorder, Psychotic Disorder Not Otherwise Specified, and Secondary Psychotic Disorders

BRIEF PSYCHOTIC DISORDER

Brief psychotic disorder is an acute and transient psychotic syndrome. According to the text revision of the fourth edition of *Diagnostic and Statistical Manual of Mental Disorders* (DSM-IV-TR) the disorder lasts from 1 day to 1 month, and the symptoms may resemble those of schizophrenia (e.g., delusions and hallucinations). In addition, the disorder may develop in response to a severe psychosocial stressor or group of stressors. Because of the variable and unstable nature of the disorder, it is sometimes a difficult diagnosis to make in clinical practice.

History

Brief psychotic disorder has been poorly studied in psychiatry in the United States, partly because of the frequent changes in diagnostic criteria during the past 15 years. The diagnosis has been better appreciated and more completely studied in Scandinavia and other Western European countries than in the United States. Patients with disorders similar to brief psychotic disorder were previously classified as having reactive, hysterical, stress, and psychogenic psychoses.

Reactive psychosis was often used as a synonym for good-prognosis schizophrenia, but the DSM-IV-TR diagnosis of brief psychotic disorder is not meant to imply a relation with schizophrenia. In 1913, Karl Jaspers described several essential features for the diagnosis of reactive psychosis, including an identifiable and extremely traumatic stressor, a close temporal relation between the stressor and the development of the psychosis, and a generally benign course for the psychotic episode. Jaspers also stated that the content of the psychosis often reflected the nature of the traumatic experience and that the

development of the psychosis seemed to serve a purpose for the patient, often as an escape from a traumatic condition.

Epidemiology

The exact incidence and prevalence of brief psychotic disorder is not known, but it is generally considered uncommon. The disorder occurs more often among younger patients (20s and 30s) than older patients. Reliable data on sex and sociocultural determinants are limited, although some findings suggest a higher incidence in women and persons in developing countries. Such epidemiological patterns are sharply distinct from those of schizophrenia. Some clinicians indicate that the disorder may be seen most frequently in patients from low socioeconomic classes and in those who have experienced disasters or major cultural changes (such as immigrants). Persons who have gone through major psychosocial stressors may be at greater risk for subsequent brief psychotic disorder.

Comorbidity

The disorder is often seen in patients with personality disorders (most commonly, histrionic, narcissistic, paranoid, schizotypal, and borderline personality disorders).

Etiology

The cause of brief psychotic disorder is unknown. Patients who have a personality disorder may have a biological or psychological vulnerability for the development of psychotic symptoms, particularly those with borderline, schizoid, schizotypal, or paranoid qualities. Some patients with brief psychotic disorder have a history of schizophrenia or mood disorders in their families; but this is nonconclusive. Psychodynamic formulations have emphasized the presence of inadequate coping mechanisms and the possibility of secondary gain for patients with psychotic symptoms. Additional psychodynamic theories suggest that the psychotic symptoms are a defense against a prohibited fantasy, the fulfillment of an unattained wish, or an escape from a stressful psychosocial situation.

Diagnosis

DSM-IV-TR describes a continuum of diagnoses for psychotic disorders, based primarily on the duration of the symptoms. For psychotic symptoms that last at least 1 day but less than 1 month and that are not associated with a mood disorder, a substance-related disorder, or a psychotic disorder due to a general medical condition, a diagnosis of brief psychotic disorder is likely to be appropriate (Table 14.4–1).

Table 14.4–1
DSM-IV-TR Diagnostic Criteria for Brief Psychotic Disorder

A. Presence of one (or more) of the following symptoms:
  (1) delusions
  (2) hallucinations
  (3) disorganized speech (e.g., frequent derailment or incoherence)
  (4) grossly disorganized or catatonic behavior
  Note: Do not include a symptom if it is a culturally sanctioned response pattern.
B. Duration of an episode of the disturbance is at least 1 day but less than 1 month, with eventual full return to premorbid level of functioning.
C. The disturbance is not better accounted for by a mood disorder with psychotic features, schizoaffective disorder, or schizophrenia and is not due to the direct physiological effects of a substance (e.g., a drug of abuse, a medication) or a general medical condition.

Specify if:
  With marked stressor(s) (brief reactive psychosis): if symptoms occur shortly after and apparently in response to events that, singly or together, would be markedly stressful to almost anyone in similar circumstances in the person's culture
  Without marked stressor(s): if psychotic symptoms do *not* occur shortly after, or are not apparently in response to events that, singly or together, would be markedly stressful to almost anyone in similar circumstances in the person's culture
  With postpartum onset: if onset within 4 weeks postpartum

From American Psychiatric Association. *Diagnostic and Statistical Manual of Mental Disorders.* 4th ed. Text rev. Washington, DC: American Psychiatric Association; copyright 2000, with permission.

By contrast, in the 10th revision of the *International Statistical Classification of Diseases and Related Disorders* (ICD-10), acute and transient psychotic disorders are diagnosed by setting up a "diagnostic sequence that reflects the order of priority given to selected key features," including sudden (within 48 hours) or abrupt (more than 48 hours but within 2 weeks) onset, typical syndromes, and associated acute distress. For psychotic symptoms that last more than 1 month, the appropriate diagnoses to consider are delusional disorder (if delusions are the primary psychotic symptoms), schizophreniform disorder (if the symptoms have lasted less than 6 months), and schizophrenia (if the symptoms have lasted more than 6 months). Table 14.4–2 lists the ICD-IV diagnostic criteria for acute and transient psychiatric disorder.

DSM-IV-TR describes three subtypes: (1) the presence of stressors, (2) the absence of stressors, and (3) a postpartum onset (discussed below).

As with other acutely ill psychiatric patients, the history necessary to make the diagnosis may not be obtainable solely from the patient. Although psychotic symptoms may be obvious, information about prodromal symptoms, previous episodes of a mood disorder, and a recent history of ingestion of a psychotomimetic substance may not be available from the clinical interview alone. In addition, clinicians may not be able to obtain accurate information about the presence or absence of precipitating stressors. Such information is usually best and most accurately obtained from a relative or a friend.

Clinical Features

The symptoms of brief psychotic disorder always include at least one major symptom of psychosis, usually with an abrupt onset, but do not always include the entire symptom pattern

Table 14.4–2
ICD-10 Diagnostic Criteria for Acute and Transient Psychotic Disorders

G1. There is acute onset of delusions, hallucinations, incomprehensible or incoherent speech, or any combination of these. The time interval between the first appearance of any psychotic symptoms and the presentation of the fully developed disorder should not exceed 2 weeks.

G2. If transient states of perplexity, misidentification, or impairment of attention and concentration are present, they do not fulfill the criteria for organically caused clouding of consciousness as specified for delirium, not induced by alcohol and other psychoactive substances, criterion A.

G3. The disorder does not meet the symptomatic criteria for manic episode, depressive episode, or recurrent depressive disorder.

G4. There is insufficient evidence of recent psychoactive substance use to fulfill the criteria for intoxication, harmful use, dependence, or withdrawal states. The continued moderate and largely unchanged use of alcohol or drugs in amounts or with the frequency to which the individual is accustomed does not necessarily rule out the use of acute and transient psychotic disorders; this must be decided by clinical judgment and the requirements of the research project in question.

G5. *Most commonly used exclusion clause.* There must be no organic mental disorder or serious metabolic disturbances affecting the central nervous system (this does not include childbirth).

A fifth character should be used to specify whether the acute onset of the disorder is associated with acute stress (occurring 2 weeks or less before evidence of first psychotic symptoms):

Without associated acute stress

With associated acute stress

For research purposes, it is recommended that change of the disorder from a nonpsychotic to a clearly psychotic state is further specified as either abrupt (onset within 48 hours) or acute (onset in more than 48 hours but less than 2 weeks).

Acute polymorphic psychotic disorder without symptoms of schizophrenia

A. The general criteria for acute and transient psychotic disorders must be met.

B. Symptoms change rapidly in both type and intensity from day to day or within the same day.

C. Any type of either hallucinations or delusions occurs, for at least several hours, at any time from the onset of the disorder.

D. Symptoms from at least two of the following categories occur at the same time:
(1) emotional turmoil, characterized by intense feelings of happiness or ecstasy, or overwhelming anxiety or marked irritability;
(2) perplexity, or misidentification of people or places;
(3) increased or decreased motility, to a marked degree.

E. If any of the symptoms listed for schizophrenia, criterion G(1) and (2), are present, they are present only for a minority of the time from the onset; i.e., criterion B of acute polymorphic psychotic disorder with symptoms of schizophrenia is not fulfilled.

F. The total duration of the disorder does not exceed 3 months.

Acute polymorphic psychotic disorder with symptoms of schizophrenia

A. Criteria A, B, C, and D of acute polymorphic psychotic disorder must be met.

B. Some of the symptoms for schizophrenia must have been present for the majority of the time since the onset of the disorder, although the full criteria need not be met, i.e., at least one of the symptoms in criteria G1(1)a to G1(2)c.

C. The symptoms of schizophrenia in criterion B above do not persist for more than 1 month.

Acute schizophrenialike psychotic disorder

A. The general criteria for acute and transient psychotic disorders must be met.

B. The criteria for schizophrenia are met, with the exception of the criterion for duration.

C. The disorder does not meet criteria B, C, and D for acute polymorphic psychotic disorder.

D. The total duration of the disorder does not exceed 1 month.

Other acute predominantly delusional psychotic disorders

A. The general criteria for acute and transient psychotic disorders must be met.

B. Relatively stable delusions and/or hallucinations are present but do not fulfill the symptomatic criteria for schizophrenia.

C. The disorder does not meet the criteria for acute polymorphic psychotic disorder.

D. The total duration of the disorder does not exceed 3 months.

Other acute and transient psychotic disorders

Any other acute psychotic disorders that are not classifiable under any other category in acute and transient psychotic disorders (such as acute psychotic states in which definite delusions or hallucinations occur but persist for only small proportions of the time) should be coded here. States of undifferentiated excitement should also be coded here if more detailed information about the patient's mental state is not available, provided that there is no evidence of an organic cause.

Acute and transient psychotic disorder, unspecified

seen in schizophrenia. Some clinicians have observed that labile mood, confusion, and impaired attention may be more common at the onset of brief psychotic disorder than at the onset of eventually chronic psychotic disorders. Characteristic symptoms in brief psychotic disorder include emotional volatility, strange or bizarre behavior, screaming or muteness, and impaired memory for recent events. Some of the symptoms suggest a diagnosis of delirium and warrant a medical workup, especially to rule out adverse reactions to drugs.

Scandinavian and other European literature describes several characteristic symptom patterns in brief psychotic disorder, although these may differ somewhat in Europe and America. The symptom patterns include acute paranoid reactions, reactive confusion, reactive excitation, and reactive depression. Some data suggest that in the United States paranoia is often the predominant symptom in the disorder. In French psychiatry, *bouffée délirante* is similar to brief psychotic disorder. The following case from ICD-10 is an excellent example of the disorder:

Mrs. C. is a 25-year-old Frenchwoman.

PROBLEM

Mrs. C. was brought by ambulance to a hospital emergency department in the city where she lived. Her husband reported that she had been perfectly normal until the previous evening, when she had come home from work complaining that "strange things were going on" at her office. She had noticed that her colleagues were talking about her, that they had been quite different all of a sudden, and that they had started behaving as if they were acting a part. Mrs. C. was convinced that she had been put under surveillance and that someone was listening in on her telephone conversations. All day she had been feeling as if she were in a dream. When she looked in the mirror, she had seemed unreal to herself. She had become increasingly anxious, incoherent, and agitated during the course of the day and had not been able to sleep at all during the night. She had spent most of the night looking out of the window. Several times she pointed at the crows in a nearby tree and told her husband, "The birds are coming."

In the morning, Mr. C. found his wife on her knees as if she were praying. She knocked her head repeatedly against the floor and talked in a rambling way, declaring that she had been entrusted with a special mission, that her boss was a criminal, there were spies everywhere, and something terrible would happen soon. All of a sudden she calmed down, smiled at her husband, and told him that she had decided to convert from Catholicism to Islam. At that stage she became quite elated, started laughing and shouting, and declared that she and her husband could pray to the same god from then on. Shortly afterward she was terrified again and accused her husband of trying to poison her.

FINDINGS

On admission Mrs. C. was frightened and bewildered but was oriented in time, place, and person. She was restless and constantly changed position, standing and sitting, moving about the room, shouting and screaming, weeping and laughing. She talked in a rambling way, shifting from one subject to another without any transition. Something criminal was going on at her office, she said, and she had discovered a secret plot. There were microphones hidden everywhere, she added, and "the birds are coming." She wondered whether the physician was a real physician or "a spy in disguise." She went on to speak about "my mission," declared that Jesus had been a false prophet, that Muhammad was the real prophet, and that she would convince the world of what was right and wrong. She then began to explain that the truth was to be found in numbers. The digit "3" signifies good, she said, and the digit "8" represents evil. Suddenly she started to weep, explaining that her parents had died and that she wished to join them in heaven.

During the first days of hospitalization, Mrs. C. continued presenting a rapidly changing symptomatology. Her mood frequently shifted from sadness to elation, and the content of her delusions changed from persecution to mysticism. On several occasions she came out of her room and complained that she had heard people speaking about her, even when there was no one in the vicinity. When asked to describe what she was hearing, she spoke of voices coming from the corridor. She firmly denied that the voices might emanate from within her own body.

The physical examination did not reveal any abnormality. Results of blood tests, including thyroid function, were within normal limits, as were all other special investigations such as an electroencephalogram and brain scan.

COURSE

Mrs. C. was treated with 30 mg of haloperidol (Haldol) during the first week, and with half this dose for the following week. After 2 weeks all of her symptoms had disappeared, and she was discharged on medication. She was seen once a week in the outpatient department for another month, during which the medication was progressively reduced and then stopped completely. Two months after the onset of the delusional episode, the patient continued to be free of symptoms.

DISCUSSION

The significant features of Mrs. C.'s disorder were acute polymorphous delusions, rapidly changing mood disturbances, perplexity, depersonalization, and derealization without clouding of consciousness, and occasional auditory hallucinations. The disorder developed to its peak in 24 hours and was resolved in a few weeks, with complete recovery within 6 weeks. The patient had no psychiatric history.

The psychiatrist who dealt with this case made a diagnosis of *bouffée délirante*. This concept goes back to the French psychiatrist Valentin Magnan, whose pupil Paul Legrain proposed the following diagnostic criteria: an acute onset of the disorder "like a bolt from the blue" in the absence of a psychosocial stressor; the presence of unsystematized and rapidly changing "polymorphic" delusions; the presence of emotional turmoil with intense and changing feelings of anxiety, happiness, or sadness; the presence of perplexity, depersonalization, or derealization without clouding of consciousness; and resolution of the disorder with complete recovery within 2 months.

In ICD-10, the subtyping of acute and transient psychotic disorders rests on the acuteness of onset, the presence of typical syndromes, and the presence of associated stress. In the case of Mrs. C., the onset was abrupt (i.e., the symptoms appeared within less than 48 hours), the syndrome was polymorphic, there were no typically schizophrenic symptoms, and the onset of the disorder was not associated with acute stress. Therefore, Mrs. C.'s disorder must be coded as acute polymorphic psychotic disorder, without symptoms of schizophrenia, and without associated acute stress. (Reprinted with permission from *ICD-10 Casebook*.)

Precipitating Stressors. The clearest examples of precipitating stressors are major life events that would cause any person significant emotional upset. Such events include the loss of a close family member or a severe automobile accident. Some

clinicians argue that the severity of the event must be considered in relation to the patient's life. This view, although reasonable, may broaden the definition of precipitating stressor to include events unrelated to the psychotic episode. Others have argued that the stressor may be a series of modestly stressful events rather than a single markedly stressful event, but evaluating the amount of stress caused by a sequence of events calls for an almost impossibly high degree of clinical judgment.

R.S. was a 44-year-old Haitian male admitted for observation at the local emergency room. He was agitated and combative, requiring restraints and several intramuscular doses of droperidol (Inapsine) and lorazepam (Ativan). The psychiatrist could not interview him under these acute circumstances. His mother arrived soon after and was able to give corroborative history. According to his mother the patient had just learned that his wife and two children had died in a natural disaster in Haiti. Several hours after his first evaluation, the patient was calmer. He told staff that he was hearing his wife talking to him and he wished to "join her." He also believed the Haitian secret police were coming to arrest him. He was admitted to the inpatient ward and began a course of antipsychotic agent. By the third day of his hospitalization there was no evidence of the previous psychosis. He was discharged from the hospital and given a follow-up appointment in 1 month. When he returned the next month he had been medication free for that time. He was grieving the loss of his family but was not psychotic. He was referred to a grief group, which he attended for the next 6 months. In that time he remained sad, but there were no other episodes of paranoia or hallucinations. (Courtesy of John Lauriello, M.D., Brenda R. Erickson, M.D., and Samuel J. Keith, M.D.)

Differential Diagnosis

Clinicians must not assume that the correct diagnosis for a briefly psychotic patient is brief psychotic disorder, even when a clear precipitating psychosocial factor is identified. Such a factor may be merely coincidental. If psychotic symptoms are present longer than 1 month, the diagnoses of schizophreniform disorder, schizoaffective disorder, schizophrenia, mood disorders with psychotic features, delusional disorder, and psychotic disorder not otherwise specified must be entertained. However, if psychotic symptoms of sudden onset are present for less than a month in response to an obvious stressor, the diagnosis of brief psychotic disorder is strongly suggested. Other diagnoses to consider in the differential diagnosis include factitious disorder with predominantly psychological signs and symptoms, malingering, psychotic disorder caused by a general medical condition, and substance-induced psychotic disorder. In factitious disorder, symptoms are intentionally produced; in malingering there is a specific goal involved in appearing psychotic (e.g., to gain admission to the hospital); and when associated with a medical condition or drugs, the cause becomes apparent with proper medical or drug workups. If the patient admits to using illicit substances the clinician can make the assessment of substance intoxication or substance withdrawal without the use of laboratory testing. Patients with epilepsy or delirium can also show psychotic symptoms that resemble those seen in brief psychotic disorder. Additional psychiatric disorders to be considered in the differential diagnosis include dissociative identity disorder and psychotic episodes associated with borderline and schizotypal personality disorders.

Course and Prognosis

By definition, the course of brief psychotic disorder is less than 1 month. Nonetheless, the development of such a significant psychiatric disorder may signify a patient's mental vulnerability. Approximately half of patients who are first classified as having brief psychotic disorder later display chronic psychiatric syndromes such as schizophrenia and mood disorders. Patients with brief psychotic disorder, however, generally have good prognoses, and European studies have indicated that 50 to 80 percent of all patients have no further major psychiatric problems.

The length of the acute and residual symptoms is often just a few days. Occasionally, depressive symptoms follow the resolution of the psychotic symptoms. Suicide is a concern during both the psychotic phase and the postpsychotic depressive phase. Several indicators have been associated with a good prognosis (Table 14.4–3). Patients with these features are unlikely to have subsequent episodes, and schizophrenia or a mood disorder is unlikely to develop later.

Treatment

Hospitalization. An acutely psychotic patient may need brief hospitalization for both evaluation and protection. Evaluation requires close monitoring of symptoms and assessment of the patient's level of danger to self and others. In addition, the quiet, structured setting of a hospital may help patients regain their sense of reality. While clinicians wait for the setting or the drugs to have their effects, seclusion, physical restraints, or one-to-one monitoring of the patient may be necessary.

Pharmacotherapy. The two major classes of drugs to be considered in the treatment of brief psychotic disorder are the antipsychotic drugs and the benzodiazepines. When an antipsychotic drug is chosen, a high-potency antipsychotic drug such as haloperidol may be used. In patients who are at high risk for the

Table 14.4–3
Good Prognostic Features for Brief Psychotic Disorder

Good premorbid adjustment
Few premorbid schizoid traits
Severe precipitating stressor
Sudden onset of symptoms
Affective symptoms
Confusion and perplexity during psychosis
Little affective blunting
Short duration of symptoms
Absence of schizophrenic relatives

development of extrapyramidal adverse effects (e.g., young men), a serotonin-dopamine antagonist drug should be administered as prophylaxis against medication-induced movement disorder symptoms. Alternatively, benzodiazepines can be used in the short-term treatment of psychosis. Although benzodiazepines have limited or no usefulness in the long-term treatment of psychotic disorders, they can be effective for a short time and are associated with fewer adverse effects than the antipsychotic drugs. In rare cases, the benzodiazepines are associated with increased agitation and, more rarely still, with withdrawal seizures, which usually occur only with the sustained use of high dosages. The use of other drugs in the treatment of brief psychotic disorder, although reported in case studies, has not been supported in any large-scale studies. Anxiolytic medications, however, are often useful during the first 2 to 3 weeks after the resolution of the psychotic episode. Clinicians should avoid long-term use of any medication in the treatment of the disorder. If maintenance medication is necessary, a clinician may have to reconsider the diagnosis.

Psychotherapy. Although hospitalization and pharmacotherapy are likely to control short-term situations, the difficult part of treatment is the psychological integration of the experience (and possibly the precipitating trauma, if one was present) into the lives of the patients and their families. Psychotherapy is of use in providing an opportunity to discuss the stressors and the psychotic episode. Exploration and development of coping strategies are the major topics in psychotherapy. Associated issues include helping patients deal with the loss of self-esteem and to regain self-confidence. An individualized treatment strategy based on increasing problem-solving skills while strengthening the ego structure through psychotherapy appears to be the most efficacious. Involvement of the family in the treatment process may be crucial to a successful outcome.

PSYCHOTIC DISORDER NOT OTHERWISE SPECIFIED

The psychotic disorder not otherwise specified category is used for patients who have psychotic symptoms (e.g., delusions, hallucinations, and disorganized speech and behavior) but who do not meet the diagnostic criteria for other specifically defined psychotic disorders. In some cases the diagnosis of psychotic disorder not otherwise specified may be used when not enough information is available to make a specific diagnosis. DSM-IV-TR has listed some examples of the diagnosis to help guide clinicians (Table 14.4–4). ICD-10 criteria are listed in Table 14.4–5.

Table 14.4–4
DSM-IV-TR Diagnostic Criteria for Psychotic Disorder Not Otherwise Specified

This category includes psychotic symptomatology (i.e., delusions, hallucinations, disorganized speech, grossly disorganized or catatonic behavior) about which there is inadequate information to make a specific diagnosis or about which there is contradictory information, or disorders with psychotic symptoms that do not meet the criteria for any specific psychotic disorder.

Examples include

1. Postpartum psychosis that does not meet criteria for mood disorder with psychotic features, brief psychotic disorder, psychotic disorder due to a general medical condition, or substance-induced psychotic disorder
2. Psychotic symptoms that have lasted for less than 1 month but that have not yet remitted, so that the criteria for brief psychotic disorder are not met
3. Persistent auditory hallucinations in the absence of any other features
4. Persistent nonbizarre delusions with periods of overlapping mood episodes that have been present for a substantial portion of the delusional disturbance
5. Situations in which the clinician has concluded that a psychotic disorder is present, but is unable to determine whether it is primary, due to a general medical condition, or substance induced

From American Psychiatric Association. *Diagnostic and Statistical Manual of Mental Disorders.* 4th ed. Text rev. Washington, DC: American Psychiatric Association; copyright 2000, with permission.

Autoscopic Psychosis

The characteristic symptom of autoscopic psychosis is a visual hallucination of all or part of the person's own body. The hallucinatory perception, which is called a *phantom,* is usually colorless and transparent, and because the phantom imitates the person's movements, it is perceived as though appearing in a mirror. The phantom tends to appear suddenly and without warning.

Epidemiology. Autoscopy is a rare phenomenon. Some persons have an autoscopic experience only once or a few times; others have the experience more often. Although the data are limited, sex, age, heredity, and intelligence do not seem to be related to the occurrence of the syndrome.

Etiology. The cause of the autoscopic phenomenon is unknown. A biological hypothesis is that abnormal, episodic activity in areas of the temporoparietal lobes is involved with the sense of self, perhaps combined with abnormal activity in parts of the visual cortex. Psychological theories have associated the syndrome with personalities characterized by imagination, visual sensitivity, and, possibly, narcissistic personality disorder traits. Such persons may be likely to experience autoscopic phenomena during periods of stress.

Table 14.4–5
ICD-10 Diagnostic Criteria for Other Nonorganic Psychotic Disorders

Psychotic disorders that do not meet the criteria for schizophrenia or for psychotic types of mood (affective) disorders, and psychotic disorders that do not meet the symptomatic criteria for persistent delusional disorder should be coded here (persistent hallucinatory disorder is an example). Combinations of symptoms not covered by the previous categories, such as delusions other than those listed as typically schizophrenic under criterion G1(1)b or d for schizophrenia (i.e., other than completely impossible or culturally inappropriate) plus catatonia, should also be included here.

Reprinted with permission from World Health Organization. *The ICD-10 Classification of Mental and Behavioural Disorders: Diagnostic Criteria for Research.* Copyright, World Health Organization, Geneva, 1993.

Course and Prognosis. The classic descriptions of the phenomenon indicate that in most cases the syndrome is neither progressive nor incapacitating. Affected persons usually maintain some emotional distance from the phenomenon, an observation that suggests a specific neuroanatomical lesion. Rarely do the symptoms reflect the onset of schizophrenia or other psychotic disorders.

Postpartum Psychosis

Postpartum psychosis (sometimes called puerperal psychosis) is an example of psychotic disorder not otherwise specified that occurs in women who have recently delivered a baby; the syndrome is most often characterized by the mother's depression, delusions, and thoughts of harming either her infant or herself. Such ideation of suicide or infanticide must be carefully monitored; some mothers have acted on these ideas. Most available data suggest a close relation between postpartum psychosis and the mood disorders, particularly bipolar disorders and major depressive disorder.

Epidemiology. The incidence of postpartum psychosis is about 1 per 1,000 childbirths, although some reports have indicated that the incidence may be as high as 2 per 1,000. About 50 to 60 percent of affected women have just had their first child, and about 50 percent of cases involve deliveries associated with nonpsychiatric perinatal complications. About 50 percent of the affected women have a family history of mood disorders. Although postpartum psychosis is fundamentally a disorder of women, some rare cases affect fathers. In these instances, a husband may feel displaced by the child and may compete for the mother's love and attention. Such men, however, probably have a coexisting major mental disorder that has been exacerbated by the stress of fatherhood.

Etiology. The most robust data indicate that an episode of postpartum psychosis is essentially an episode of a mood disorder, usually a bipolar disorder but possibly a depressive disorder. Relatives of those with postpartum psychosis have an incidence of mood disorders that is similar to the incidence in relatives of persons with mood disorders. Schizoaffective disorder and delusional disorder are rarely appropriate diagnoses. The validity of diagnoses of mood disorders is usually verified in the year after the birth, when as many as two thirds of the patients have a second episode of the underlying disorder. The delivery process may best be seen as a nonspecific stress that causes the development of an episode of a major mood disorder, perhaps through a major hormonal mechanism.

A few instances of postpartum psychosis result from a general medical condition associated with perinatal events, such as infection, drug intoxication from, for example, scopolamine (Donnagel) and meperidine (Demerol), toxemia, and blood loss. The sudden decrease in estrogen and progesterone concentrations immediately after delivery may also contribute to the disorder, but treatment with these hormones has not been effective.

Some investigators have claimed that a purely psychosocial causal mechanism is suggested by the preponderance of primiparous mothers and by the association between postpartum psychosis and recent stressful events. Psychodynamic studies of postpartum mental illness have also suggested the presence of conflicted feelings in the mother about her mothering experience. Some women may not have wanted to become pregnant; others may feel trapped in unhappy marriages by motherhood. Marital discord during pregnancy has been associated with an increased incidence of illness, although the discord may be related to the slow development of mood disorder symptoms in the mother.

Diagnosis. Specific diagnostic criteria are not included in DSM-IV-TR. The diagnosis can be made when psychosis occurs in close temporal association with childbirth, although a DSM-IV-TR diagnosis of a mood disorder should be considered in the differential diagnosis. Characteristic symptoms include delusions, cognitive deficits, motility disturbances, mood abnormalities, and occasional hallucinations. The content of the psychotic material revolves around mothering and pregnancy. DSM-IV-TR also allows for the diagnoses of brief psychotic disorder and mood disorders with postpartum onset (see Table 15.1–24 in Section 15.1 of Chapter 15).

Clinical Features. The symptoms of postpartum psychosis can often begin within days of the delivery, although the mean time to onset is 2 to 3 weeks and almost always within 8 weeks of delivery. Characteristically, patients begin to complain of fatigue, insomnia, and restlessness and may have episodes of tearfulness and emotional lability. Later, suspiciousness, confusion, incoherence, irrational statements, and obsessive concerns about the baby's health and welfare may be present. Delusions may be present in 50 percent of patients and hallucinations in about 25 percent. Complaints regarding the inability to move, stand, or walk are also common.

Patients may have feelings of not wanting to care for the baby, of not loving the baby, and, in some cases, of wanting to do harm to the baby or to themselves or both. Delusional material may involve the idea that the baby is dead or defective. Patients may deny the birth and express thoughts of being unmarried, virginal, persecuted, influenced, or perverse. Hallucinations with similar content may involve voices telling the patient to kill the baby.

Differential Diagnosis. As with any psychotic disorder, clinicians should consider the possibility of either a psychotic disorder due to a general medical condition or a substance-induced psychotic disorder. Potential general medical conditions include hypothyroidism and Cushing's syndrome. Substance-induced psychotic disorder may be associated with the use of pain medications such as pentazocine (Talwin) or of antihypertensive drugs during pregnancy. Other potential medical causes include infections, toxemia, and neoplasms.

Women with a history of a mood disorder should be classified as having a recurrence of the disorder. Postpartum psychosis should not be confused with the so-called postpartum blues, a normal condition that occurs in up to 50 percent of women after childbirth. Postpartum blues is self-limited, lasts only a few days, and is characterized by tearfulness, fatigue, anxiety, and irritability that begin shortly after childbirth and lessen in severity over the course of a week. Postpartum nonpsychotic depression lacks delusional or hallucinatory activity. It is more severe than transient postpartum blues, occurs in 10 to 20 percent of women and is characterized by despondent mood, feelings of inadequacy as a parent, and sleep disturbances. There may be ruminative or obsessional thoughts of harming the

baby, but they lack delusional conviction. These patients should be observed carefully because it is sometimes difficult to differentiate between delusions and obsession and especially difficult to predict whether or not the patient will act on her fear of harming, or wish to harm, her baby.

Course and Prognosis. The onset of florid psychotic symptoms is usually preceded by prodromal signs such as insomnia, restlessness, agitation, lability of mood, and mild cognitive deficits. Once the psychosis occurs, the patient may be a danger to herself or to her newborn, depending on the content of her delusional system and her degree of agitation. In one study, 5 percent of patients committed suicide and 4 percent committed infanticide. A favorable outcome is associated with a good premorbid adjustment and a supportive family network.

The course of postpartum psychosis may be similar to that seen in patients with mood disorders. Specifically, mood disorders are usually episodic disorders, and patients with postpartum psychosis often experience another episode of symptoms within a year or two of the birth. Subsequent pregnancies are associated with an increased risk of another episode, sometimes as high as 50 percent.

Treatment. Postpartum psychosis is a psychiatric emergency. Antidepressants and lithium (Eskalith), sometimes in combination with an antipsychotic, are the treatments of choice. No pharmacological agents should be prescribed to a woman who is breast-feeding. Suicidal patients may require transfer to a psychiatric unit to help prevent a suicide attempt.

The mother is usually helped by contact with her baby if she so desires, but the visits must be closely supervised, especially if the mother is preoccupied with harming the infant. Psychotherapy is indicated after the period of acute psychosis, and therapy is usually directed at the conflictual areas that have become evident during the evaluation. Therapy may involve helping the patient accept and be at ease with the mothering role. Changes in environmental factors may also be indicated. Increased support from the husband and others in the environment may help reduce the woman's stress. Most studies report high rates of recovery from the acute illness.

Further information on postpartum conditions can be found in Chapter 30, Psychiatry and Reproductive Medicine.

PSYCHOTIC DISORDERS DUE TO A GENERAL MEDICAL CONDITION AND SUBSTANCE-INDUCED PSYCHOTIC DISORDER

The evaluation of a psychotic patient requires consideration of the possibility that the psychotic symptoms result from a general medical condition such as a brain tumor or the ingestion of a substance such as phencyclidine (PCP).

Epidemiology

Relevant epidemiological data about psychotic disorder due to a general medical condition and substance-induced psychotic disorder are lacking. The disorders are most often encountered in patients who abuse alcohol or other substances on a long-term basis. The delusional syndrome that may accompany complex partial seizures is more common in women than in men.

Etiology

Physical conditions such as cerebral neoplasms, particularly of the occipital or temporal areas, can cause hallucinations. Sensory deprivation, as in people who are blind or deaf, can also result in hallucinatory or delusional experiences. Lesions involving the temporal lobe and other cerebral regions, especially the right hemisphere and the parietal lobe, are associated with delusions.

Psychoactive substances are common causes of psychotic syndromes. The most commonly involved substances are alcohol, indole hallucinogens such as lysergic acid diethylamide (LSD), amphetamine, cocaine, mescaline, PCP, and ketamine. Many other substances, including steroids and thyroxine, can produce hallucinations. (See Table 13–8 for a list of general medical conditions and substances that can be associated with psychotic symptoms.)

Diagnosis

Psychotic Disorder Due to a General Medical Condition. The diagnosis of psychotic disorder due to a general medical condition (Table 14.4–6) is defined in DSM-IV-TR by specifying the predominant symptoms. When the diagnosis is used, the medical condition, along with the predominant symptoms pattern, should be included in the diagnosis, for example, psychotic disorder due to a brain tumor, with delusions. The DSM-IV-TR criteria further specify that the disorder does not occur exclusively while a patient is delirious or demented and that the symptoms are not better accounted for by another mental disorder.

Substance-Induced Psychotic Disorder

The diagnostic category of substance-induced psychotic disorder in DSM-IV-TR (Table 14.4–7) is reserved for those with sub-

Table 14.4–6
DSM-IV-TR Diagnostic Criteria for Psychotic Disorder Due to a General Medical Condition

A. Prominent hallucinations or delusions.

B. There is evidence from the history, physical examination, or laboratory findings that the disturbance is the direct physiological consequence of a general medical condition.

C. The disturbance is not better accounted for by another mental disorder.

D. The disturbance does not occur exclusively during the course of a delirium.

Code based on predominant symptom:

With delusions: if delusions are the predominant symptom

With hallucinations: if hallucinations are the predominant symptom

Coding note: Include the name of the general medical condition on Axis I, e.g., psychotic disorder due to malignant lung neoplasm, with delusions; also code the general medical condition on Axis III.

Coding note: If delusions are part of vascular dementia, indicate the delusions by coding the appropriate subtype, e.g., vascular dementia, with delusions.

From American Psychiatric Association. *Diagnostic and Statistical Manual of Mental Disorders.* 4th ed. Text rev. Washington, DC: American Psychiatric Association; copyright 2000, with permission.

Table 14.4–7
DSM-IV-TR Diagnostic Criteria for Substance-Induced Psychotic Disorder

A. Prominent hallucinations or delusions. **Note:** Do not include hallucinations if the person has insight that they are substance induced.

B. There is evidence from the history, physical examination, or laboratory findings of either (1) or (2):

(1) the symptoms in Criterion A developed during, or within a month of, substance intoxication or withdrawal

(2) medication use is etiologically related to the disturbance

C. The disturbance is not better accounted for by a psychotic disorder that is not substance induced. Evidence that the symptoms are better accounted for by a psychotic disorder that is not substance induced might include the following: the symptoms precede the onset of the substance use (or medication use); the symptoms persist for a substantial period of time (e.g., about a month) after the cessation of acute withdrawal or severe intoxication, or are substantially in excess of what would be expected given the type or amount of the substance used or the duration of use; or there is other evidence that suggests the existence of an independent non-substance-induced psychotic disorder (e.g., a history of recurrent non-substance-related episodes).

D. The disturbance does not occur exclusively during the course of a delirium.

Note: This diagnosis should be made instead of a diagnosis of substance intoxication or substance withdrawal only when the symptoms are in excess of those usually associated with the intoxication or withdrawal syndrome and when the symptoms are sufficiently severe to warrant independent clinical attention.

Code [Specific substance]-induced psychotic disorder:

(Alcohol, with delusions; alcohol, with hallucinations; amphetamine [or amphetaminelike substance], with delusions; amphetamine [or amphetaminelike substance], with hallucinations; cannabis, with delusions; cannabis, with hallucinations; cocaine, with delusions; cocaine, with hallucinations; hallucinogen, with delusions; hallucinogen, with hallucinations; inhalant, with delusions; inhalant, with hallucinations; opioid, with delusions; opioid, with hallucinations; phencyclidine [or phencyclidinelike substance], with delusions; phencyclidine [or phencyclidinelike substance], with hallucinations; sedative, hypnotic, or anxiolytic, with delusions; sedative, hypnotic, or anxiolytic, with hallucinations; other [or unknown] substance, with delusions; other [or unknown] substance, with hallucinations)

Specify if:

With onset during intoxication: if criteria are met for intoxication with the substance and the symptoms develop during the intoxication syndrome

With onset during withdrawal: if criteria are met for withdrawal from the substance and the symptoms develop during, or shortly after, a withdrawal syndrome

From American Psychiatric Association. *Diagnostic and Statistical Manual of Mental Disorders.* 4th ed. Text rev. Washington, DC: American Psychiatric Association; copyright 2000, with permission.

stance-induced psychotic symptoms and impaired reality testing. People with substance-induced psychotic symptoms (e.g., hallucinations) but with intact reality testing should be classified as having a substance-related disorder (e.g., PCP intoxication with perceptual disturbances). The diagnosis of substance-induced psychotic disorder is included with the other psychotic disorder diagnoses in DSM-IV-TR to prompt clinicians to consider the possibility that a substance is causally involved in the production of psychotic symptoms. The full diagnosis of substance-induced psychotic disorder should include the type of substance involved, the stage of substance use when the disorder began (e.g., during intoxication or withdrawal), and the clinical phenomena (e.g., hallucinations or delusions).

Clinical Features

Hallucinations. Hallucinations may occur in one or more sensory modalities. Tactile hallucinations (such as the sensation of bugs crawling on the skin) are characteristic of cocaine use. Auditory hallucinations are usually associated with psychoactive substance abuse; auditory hallucinations may also occur in persons who are deaf. Olfactory hallucinations can result from temporal lobe epilepsy; visual hallucinations may occur in persons who are blind because of cataracts. Hallucinations are either recurrent or persistent and are experienced in a state of full wakefulness and alertness; a hallucinating patient shows no significant changes in cognitive functions. Visual hallucinations often take the form of scenes involving diminutive (lilliputian) human figures or small animals. Rare musical hallucinations typically feature religious songs. Patients with psychotic disorder due to a general medical condition and substance-induced psychotic disorder may act on their hallucinations. In alcohol-related hallucinations, threatening, critical, or insulting third-person voices speak about the patients and may tell them to harm either themselves or others. Such patients are dangerous and are at significant risk for suicide or homicide. Patients may or may not believe that the hallucinations are real.

Delusions. Secondary and substance-induced delusions are usually present in a state of full wakefulness. Patients experience no change in the level of consciousness, although mild cognitive impairment may be observed. Patients may appear confused, disheveled, or eccentric, with tangential or even incoherent speech. Hyperactivity and apathy may be present, and an associated dysphoric mood is thought to be common. The delusions may be systematized or fragmentary, with varying content, but persecutory delusions are the most common.

Differential Diagnosis

Psychotic disorder due to a general medical condition and substance-induced psychotic disorder must be distinguished from delirium (in which patients have a clouded sensorium), from dementia (in which patients have major intellectual deficits), and from schizophrenia (in which patients have other symptoms of thought disorder and impaired functioning). Psychotic disorder due to a general medical condition and substance-induced psychotic disorder must also be differentiated from psychotic mood disorders (in which other affective symptoms are pronounced).

Treatment

Treatment involves identifying the general medical condition or the particular substance involved. At this point, treatment is directed toward the underlying condition and the patient's immediate behavioral control. Hospitalization may be neces-

sary to evaluate patients completely and to ensure their safety. Antipsychotic agents (e.g., olanzapine [Zyprexa] or haloperidol) may be necessary for immediate and short-term control of psychotic or aggressive behavior, although benzodiazepines may also be useful for controlling agitation and anxiety.

REFERENCES

Beighley PS, Brown GR, Thompson JW. DSM-III-R brief reactive psychosis among Air Force recruits. *J Clin Psychiatry.* 1992;53:283.

Jablensky A, Sartorius N, Ernberg G, et al. Schizophrenia: manifestations, incidence and course in different cultures; a World Health Organization ten-country study. *Psychol Med.* 1992:20(suppl).

Johnson FA. African perspectives on mental disorder. In: Mezzich JE, Honda Y, Kastrup MC, eds. *Psychiatric Diagnosis: A World Perspective.* New York: Springer-Verlag; 1994.

Karno M, Jenkins JH. Cultural considerations in the diagnosis of schizophrenia and related disorders and psychotic disorders not otherwise classified. In: Widiger TA, Frances A, Pincus HA, First MB, Ross R, Davis W, eds. *DSM-IV Source Book.* Washington, DC: American Psychiatric Press; 1994.

Kulhara P, Chakrabarti S. Culture and schizophrenia and other psychotic disorders. *Psychiatr Clin North Am.* 2001;24:449.

Lauriello J, Erickson BR, Keith SJ. Schizoaffective disorders, schizophreniform disorder, and brief psychotic disorder. In: Sadock BJ, Sadock VA, eds. *Kaplan & Sadock's Comprehensive Textbook of Psychiatry.* 7th ed. Vol 1. Baltimore: Lippincott Williams & Wilkins; 2000:1232.

Lin K-M. Cultural influences on the diagnosis of psychotic and organic disorders. In: Mezzich JE, Kleinman A, Fabrega H, Parron DL, eds. *Culture and Psychiatric Diagnosis.* Washington, DC: American Psychiatric Press; 1995.

Miller LJ. Postpartum depression. *JAMA.* 2002;287:762.

Nomacs R, Cohen LS. Postpartum psychiatric syndromes. In: Sadock BJ, Sadock VA, eds. *Kaplan & Sadock's Comprehensive Textbook of Psychiatry.* 7th ed. Vol 1. Baltimore: Lippincott Williams & Wilkins; 2000:1276.

Pull CB, Chaillet G. The nosological views of French-speaking psychiatry. In: Mezzich JE, Honda Y, Kastrup MC, eds. *Psychiatric Diagnosis: A World Perspective.* New York: Springer-Verlag; 1994.

Rosen JL, Woods SW, Miller TJ, McGlashan TH. Prospective observations of emerging psychosis. *J Nerv Ment Dis.* 2002;190:133.

Susser E, Fennig S, Jandorf L, Amador A, Bromet E. Epidemiology, diagnosis and course of brief psychoses. *Am J Psychiatry.* 1995;152:20.

Susser E, Wanderling E. Epidemiology of non-affective acute remitting psychosis vs schizophrenia. *Arch Gen Psychiatry.* 1994;51:294.

Thweatt R. European interest in transient psychotic episodes. *Am J Psychiatry.* 1986;143:557.

Vanderhart O, Witztum E, Friedman B. From hysterical psychosis to reactive dissociative psychosis. *J Trauma Stress.* 1993;6:43.

▲ 14.5 Culture-Bound Syndromes

While all psychiatric diagnoses are influenced by their cultural context, the most dramatic example of the difficulty in applying Western-based nosological concepts can be found in the so-called culture-bound syndromes. (See Chapter 1 for a further discussion of normality.) The term evolved to denote recurrent, locality-specific patterns of aberrant behavior and troubling experiences that appear to fall outside conventional Western psychiatric categories. The descriptive phrases formerly used to refer to such phenomena include "cultural and ethnic psychoses and neuroses" and "atypical and exotic psychotic syndromes." The *culture-bound syndrome* is now generally accepted to refer to culturally based signs and symptoms of mental distress or maladaptive behavior that are prominent in folk belief and practice. Such patterns are informed by native cultural assumptions, sorcery, breach of taboo, intrusion of a disease object, intrusion of a disease-causing spirit, or loss of soul.

Assessment of culture-bound syndromes must start with recognition that each human society has an indigenous body of beliefs and practices directed at explaining and treating disease and disorder and that patients internalize that world-view during the process of enculturation. They share their experiences and deal with distress through commonly understood symbols and meanings. In that light, the diagnostic encounter itself can be used as a point of entry into the patient's world. One cannot become an anthropological expert about each and every possible cultural group but one can try to learn by asking patients to share the cultural norms as they understand them.

REPRESENTATIVE SYNDROMES

Table 14.5–1 lists representative culture-bound syndromes from around the world with some of their clinical features. Two cases of cross-cultural syndromes compiled by Melvin Konner are reported below.

Marjorie Shostak's *Nisa: The Life and Words of a !Kung Woman* describes the life history of an essentially normal woman among hunter-gatherers in northwestern Botswana. The outlines of the culture and child-rearing pattern fit the model described for hunter-gatherers in general. Nisa was the third child (a second died in infancy) of a then stably married couple living traditionally. She remembered her life as idyllic until weaning, shortly before the birth of her younger brother, which she attended and whom she claimed to have saved from infanticide by her mother. She described intense sibling rivalry with her brother (e.g., continuing attempts to nurse) and attributed her small stature and other problems to allegedly early weaning. Her father fought violently with her mother but they remained together until Nisa was in adolescence. She was married several times premenarcheally and (despite a culturally typical pattern of sex play throughout childhood) had a stormy introduction to adult sexuality, but her parents tolerated her flight from her husbands.

She remained with her fourth husband, Tashy, and eventually had four children; two of them died in infancy and early childhood, one died of illness in his youth, and a fourth was killed by her own husband shortly after marriage. Those losses, along with Tashy's death shortly after the birth of her fourth child in her late 20s, shaped her adulthood. She had occasional contacts with lovers both before and after his death, a habit she had not given up by the time she was interviewed at ages 50 and 55, despite two further marriages, her then-current one being quite stable. Her menopause near age 50 caused a period of sadness and self-assessment, but at 55 she had accepted her childlessness and was bringing up her younger brother's two children. She was vibrant, mildly eccentric with a bawdy sense of humor, eloquent on both her own life and the culture, open to new relationships, including the interview relationship with its probing self-exploration, and proud of having surmounted difficulty and tragedy with a willingness to go forward and a continuing joy in life.

Table 14.5–1
Examples of Culture-Bound Syndromes

amok A dissociative episode characterized by a period of brooding followed by an outburst of violent, aggressive, or homicidal behavior directed at persons and objects. The episode tends to be precipitated by a perceived slight or insult and seems to be prevalent only among men. The episode is often accompanied by persecutory idea; automatism, amnesia, exhaustion, and a return to premorbid state following the episode. Some instances of amok may occur during a brief psychotic episode or constitute the onset or an exacerbation of a chronic psychotic process. The original reports that used this term were from Malaysia. A similar behavior pattern is found in Laos, Philippines, Polynesia (*cafard* or *cathard*), Papua New Guinea, and Puerto Rico (*mal de pelea*) and among the Navajo (*iich'aa*).

ataque de nervios An idiom of distress principally reported among Latinos from the Caribbean, but recognized among many Latin American and Latin Mediterranean groups. Commonly reported symptoms include uncontrollable shouting, attacks of crying, trembling, heat in the chest rising into the head, and verbal or physical aggression. Dissociative experiences, seizurelike or fainting episodes, and suicidal gestures are prominent in some attacks but absent in others. A general feature of an *ataque de nervios* is a sense of being out of control. *Ataques de nervios* frequently occur as a direct result of a stressful event relating to the family (e.g., death of a close relative, separation or divorce from a spouse, conflicts with a spouse or children, or witnessing an accident involving a family member). Persons may experience amnesia for what occurred during the *ataque de nervios,* but they otherwise return rapidly to their usual level of functioning. Although descriptions of some *ataques de nervios* most closely fit the DSM-IV description of panic attacks, the association of most *ataques* with a precipitating event and the frequent absence of the hallmark symptoms of acute fear or apprehension distinguish them from panic disorder. *Ataques* span the range from normal expressions of distress not associated with a mental disorder to symptom presentations associated with anxiety, mood, dissociative, or somatoform disorders.

bilis and colera (also referred to as *muina*) The underlying cause is thought to be strongly experienced anger or rage. Anger is viewed among many Latino groups as a particularly powerful emotion that can have direct effects on the body and exacerbate existing symptoms. The major effect of anger is to disturb core body balances (which are understood as a balance between hot and cold valences in the body and between the material and spiritual aspects of the body). Symptoms can include acute nervous tension, headache, trembling, screaming, stomach disturbances, and, in more severe cases, loss of consciousness. Chronic fatigue may result from an acute episode.

bouffée délirante A syndrome observed in West Africa and Haiti. The French term refers to a sudden outburst of agitated and aggressive behavior, marked confusion, and psychomotor excitement. It may sometimes be accompanied by visual and auditory hallucinations or paranoid ideation. The episodes may resemble an episode of brief psychotic disorder.

brain fag A term initially used in West Africa to refer to a condition experienced by high school or university students in response to the challenges of schooling. Symptoms include difficulties in concentrating, remembering, and thinking. Students often state that their brains are "fatigued." Additional somatic symptoms are usually centered around the head and neck and include pain, pressure or tightness, blurring of vision, heat, or burning. "Brain tiredness" or fatigue from "too much thinking" is an idiom of distress in many cultures, and resulting syndromes can resemble certain anxiety, depressive, and somatoform disorders.

dhat A folk diagnostic term used in India to refer to severe anxiety and hypochondriacal concerns associated with the discharge of semen, whitish discoloration of the urine, and feelings of weakness and exhaustion. Similar to *jiryan* (India), *sukra prameha* (Sri Lanka), and *shen-k'uei* (China).

falling-out or blackout Episodes that occur primarily in southern United States and Caribbean groups. They are characterized by a sudden collapse, which sometimes occurs without warning but is sometimes preceded by feelings of dizziness or "swimming" in the head. The person's eyes are usually open, but the person claims an inability to see. Those affected usually hear and understand what is occurring around them but feel powerless to move. This may correspond to a diagnosis of conversion disorder or a dissociative disorder.

ghost sickness A preoccupation with death and the deceased (sometimes associated with witchcraft), frequently observed among members of many American Indian tribes. Various symptoms can be attributed to ghost sickness, including bad dreams, weakness, feeling of danger, loss of appetite, fainting, dizziness, fear, anxiety, hallucinations, loss of consciousness, confusion, feelings of futility, and a sense of suffocation.

hwa-byung (also known as *wool-hwa-byung*) A Korean folk syndrome literally translated into English as "anger syndrome" and attributed to the suppression of anger. The symptoms include insomnia, fatigue, panic, fear of impending death, dysphoric affect indigestion, anorexia, dyspnea, palpitations, generalized aches and pains, and a feeling of a mass in the epigastrium.

koro A term probably of Malaysian origin, that refers to an episode of sudden and intense anxiety that the penis (or, in women, the vulva and nipples) will recede into the body and possibly cause death. The syndrome is reported in South and East Asia, where it is known by a variety of local terms, such as *shuk yang, shook yong,* and *suo yang* (Chinese); *jinjinia bemar* (Assam); or *rok-joo* (Thailand). It is occasionally found in the West. *Koro* at times occurs in localized epidemic form in East Asian areas. The diagnosis is included in the second edition of *Chinese Classification of Mental Disorders* (*CCMD-2*).

latah Hypersensitivity to sudden fright, often with echopraxia, echolalia, command obedience, and dissociative or trancelike behavior. The term *latah* is of Malaysian or Indonesian origin, but the syndrome has been found in many parts of the world. Other terms for the condition are *amurakh, irkunil, ikota, olan, myriachit,* and *menkeiti* (Siberian groups); *bah tschi, bah-tsi, baah-ji* (Thailand); *imu* (Ainu, Sakhalin, Japan); and *mali-mali* and *silok* (Philippines). In Malaysia it is more frequent in middle-aged women.

locura A term used by Latinos in the United States and Latin America to refer to a severe form of chronic psychosis. The condition is attributed to an inherited vulnerability, to the effect of multiple life difficulties, or to a combination of both factors. Symptoms exhibited by persons with *locura* include incoherence, agitation, auditory and visual hallucinations, inability to follow rules of social interaction, unpredictability, and possibly violence.

mal de ojo A concept widely found in Mediterranean cultures and elsewhere in the world. *Mal de ojo* is a Spanish phrase translated into English as "evil eye." Children are especially at risk. Symptoms include fitful sleep, crying without apparent cause, diarrhea, vomiting, and fever in a child or infant. Sometimes adults (especially women) have the condition.

nervios A common idiom of distress among Latinos in the United States and Latin America. A number of other ethnic groups have related, though often somewhat distinctive, ideas of nerves (such as *nerva* among Greeks in North America). *Nervios* refers both to a general state of vulnerability to stressful life experiences and to a syndrome brought on by difficult life circumstances. The term *nervios* includes a wide range of symptoms of emotional distress, somatic disturbance, and inability to function. Common symptoms include headaches and brain aches, irritability, stomach disturbances, sleep difficulties, nervousness, easy tearfulness, inability to concentrate, trembling, tingling sensations, and *mareos* (dizziness with occasional vertigolike exacerbations). *Nervios* tends to be an ongoing problem, although variable in the degree of disability that is manifest. *Nervios* is a very broad syndrome that spans the range from patients free of a mental disorder to presentations resembling adjustment, anxiety, depressive, dissociative, somatoform, or psychotic disorders. Differential diagnosis depends on the constellation of symptoms experienced, the kinds of social events that are associated with the onset and progress of *nervios,* and the level of disability experienced.

(*continued*)

Table 14.5–1 (*continued*)

piblokto An abrupt dissociative episode accompanied by extreme excitement of up to 30 minutes' duration and frequently followed by convulsive seizures and coma lasting up to 12 hours. It is observed primarily in Arctic and subarctic Eskimo communities, although regional variations in name exist. The person may be withdrawn or mildly irritable for a period of hours or days before the attack and typically reports complete amnesia for the attack. During the attack persons may tear off their clothing, break furniture, shout obscenities, eat feces, flee from protective shelters, or perform other irrational or dangerous acts.

***qi-gong* psychotic reactions** Acute, time-limited episodes characterized by dissociative, paranoid, or other psychotic or nonpsychotic symptoms that may occur after participation in the Chinese folk health-enhancing practice of *qi-gong* (exercise of vital energy). Especially vulnerable are persons who become overly involved in the practice. This diagnosis is included in CCMD-2.

rootwork A set of cultural interpretations that ascribe illness to hexing, witchcraft, sorcery, or evil influence of another person. Symptoms may include generalized anxiety and gastrointestinal complaints (e.g., nausea, vomiting, diarrhea), weakness, dizziness, the fear of being poisoned, and sometimes fear of being killed (voodoo death). Roots, spells, or hexes can be put or placed on other person, causing a variety of emotional and psychological problems. The hexed person may even fear death until the root has been taken off (eliminated), usually through the work of a root doctor (a healer in this tradition), who can also be called on to bewitched an enemy. Rootwork is found in the southern United States among both African-American and European-American populations and in Caribbean societies. It is also known as *mal puesto* or *brujeria* in Latino societies.

sangue dormido ("sleeping blood") A syndrome found among Portuguese Cape Verde Islanders (and immigrants from there to the United States). It includes pain, numbness, tremor, paralysis, convulsions, stroke, blindness, heart attack, infection, and miscarriages.

Shenjing shuariuo ("neurasthenia") In China a condition characterized by physical and mental fatigue, dizziness, headaches, other pains, concentration difficulties, sleep disturbance, and memory loss. Other symptoms include gastrointestinal problems, sexual dysfunction, irritability, excitability, and various signs suggesting disturbance of the autonomic nervous system. In many cases the symptoms would meet the criteria for a DSM-IV mood or anxiety disorder. The diagnosis is included in CCMD-2.

shen-k'uei (Taiwan); *shenkui* (China) A Chinese folk label describing marked anxiety or panic symptoms with accompanying somatic complaints for which no physical cause can be demonstrated. Symptoms include dizziness, backache, fatigability, general weakness, insomnia, frequent dreams, and complaints of sexual dysfunction, such as premature ejaculation and impotence. Symptoms are attributed to excessive semen loss from frequent intercourse, masturbation, nocturnal emission, or passing of white turbid urine believed to contain semen. Excessive semen loss is feared because of the belief that it represents the loss of one's vital essence and can therefore be life threatening.

shin-byung A Korean folk label for a syndrome in which initial phases are characterized by anxiety and somatic complaints (general weakness, dizziness, fear, anorexia, insomnia, gastrointestinal problems), with subsequent dissociation and possession by ancestral spirits.

spell A trance state in which persons "communicate" with deceased relatives or spirits. At times the state is associated with brief periods of personality change. The culture-specific syndrome is seen among African-Americans and European-Americans from the southern United States. Spells are not considered to be medical events in the folk tradition but may be misconstrued as psychotic episodes in clinical settings.

susto (*frigh* or "soul loss") A folk illness prevalent among some Latinos in the United States and among people in Mexico, Central America, and South America. *Susto* is also referred to as *espanto, pasmo, tripa ida, perdida del alma,* or *chibih. Susto* is an illness attributed to a frightening event that causes the soul to leave the body and results in unhappiness and sickness. Persons with *susto* also experience significant strains in key social roles. Symptoms may appear any time from days to years after the fright is experienced. It is believed that in extreme cases, *susto* may result in death. Typical symptoms include appetite disturbances, inadequate or excessive sleep, troubled sleep or dreams, feelings of sadness, lack of motivation to do anything, and feelings of low self-worth or dirtiness. Somatic symptoms accompanying *susto* include muscle aches and pains, headache, stomachache, and diarrhea. Ritual healings are focused on calling the soul back to the body and cleansing the person to restore bodily and spiritual balance. Different experience of *susto* may be related to major depressive disorder, posttraumatic stress disorders, and somatoform disorders. Similar etiological beliefs and symptom configurations are found in many parts of the world.

taijin kyofu sho A culturally distinctive phobia in Japan, in some ways resembling social phobia in DSM-IV. The syndrome refers to an intense fear that one's body, its parts or its functions, displease, embarrass, or are offensive to other people in appearance, odor, facial expressions, or movements. The syndrome is included in the official Japanese diagnostic system for mental disorders.

zar A general term applied in Ethiopia, Somalia, Egypt, Sudan, Iran, and other North African and Middle Eastern societies to the experience of spirits possessing a person. Persons possessed by a spirit may experience dissociative episodes that may include shouting, laughing, hitting the head against a wall, singing, or weeping. They may show apathy and withdrawal, refusing to eat or carry out daily tasks or may develop a long-term relationship with the possessing spirit. Such behavior is not considered pathological locally.

From American Psychiatric Association. *Diagnostic and Statistical Manual of Mental Disorders.* 4th ed. Text rev. Washington, DC: American Psychiatric Association; copyright 2000, with permission.

Gilbert Herdt's book *Guardians of the Flutes* is the best known of a series of ethnographies on cultures in a region of New Guinea (the semen belt) where male homosexuality is a universal aspect of adolescent development, and the symbolic framework involves the belief that semen must be absorbed, usually through fellatio, although also in some cultures through anal intercourse, for a boy to become a man. Among the Sambia studied by Herdt, boys engage in homosexual activity exclusively beginning at age 7 to 10 and continuing until they are married in their late teens or early 20s. They must suck the penises of postpubertal boys as often as possible until they go through puberty, after which

they are fellated very frequently by younger boys. It all proceeds in an atmosphere of extreme misogyny and of hypermasculine preparations for warriorhood and hunting. At the end of the period they marry and become exclusively heterosexual husbands and fathers in almost every case—a challenge to several theories of homosexuality and an answer to the obvious darwinian objections to such an apparently maladapative pattern.

The psychoanalyst Robert Stoller and Herdt published an aberrant case, Kalutwo, who had married four times by his mid-30s—marriages that were infertile and perhaps unconsummated. He was the illegitimate son of an older widow and a man married to someone else, who could have taken the widow as his second wife. Stigmatized, Kalutwo was raised by his mother, who was bitter about men and had no contact with his father. He showed an unusually keen enjoyment of fellatio, had unusually strong homoerotic feelings and attachments, and committed the serious indiscretion of continuing to fellate younger boys even after he reached puberty. Although he acted tough he never displayed what were considered masculine achievements, such as suffering war injuries or undertaking acts of courage. Stoller and Herdt argue for a classic psychoanalytic provenance of homosexuality in his case, but regardless of its cause, they argue that Kalutwo would be a homosexual anywhere, independent of the culture.

COURSE AND PROGNOSIS

Limited data on the longitudinal course of patients with culture-bound syndromes suggest that some of them eventually develop clinical features compatible with a diagnosis of schizophrenia, bipolar disorder, cognitive disorder, or other psychotic disorders. Thus, gathering information from all possible sources is crucial. Since clinical pictures evolve over time, thorough reevaluations should be conducted periodically to refine the diagnosis and improve clinical care.

TREATMENT

Treatment of a culture-bound syndrome poses several diagnostic challenges, the first of which is determining whether the symptomatology represents a culturally appropriate adaptive response to a situation. Clinicians are well advised to (1) know or search out the demographics of the local population or catchment area being served; (2) recognize that there is always a local pattern of conceptualization, naming, vocabulary, explanation, and treatment of patterns of distress that afflict a community, including mental disorders; and (3) talk with the family and learn about local customs or search out other modes of documentation. Persons within the culture will almost always recognize that one of their own is acting in a deviant manner, and their input can be extremely valuable in making an assessment of mental disorder.

When taking the history, patients should be asked what they think could have caused the problem and how they explain it to themselves. Some useful questions are (1) What do you think has caused your problem? (2) Why do you think it started when it did? (3) What do you think your sickness does to you? How does it work? (4) How severe is your sickness? Will it have a short or long course? (5) What kind of treatment do you think you should receive?

Insight into the dynamics of the patient's world facilitates the clinician's efforts to adapt his or her techniques (e.g., general activity level, mode of verbal intervention, content of remarks, tone of voice) to the patient's cultural background. It implies acceptance of, and respect for, the patient's cultural frame of reference and opens the possibility of direct intervention in the lives of patients, who may be willing to cooperate when they feel understood.

Indigenous Healers. One promising avenue is collaboration with indigenous healers. Several researchers have reported on their success in the use of indigenous and traditional healers in the treatment of psychiatric patients, especially those whose psychotic conditions are substantially connected to culture-specific beliefs (e.g., fear of voodoo death). Decisions about involving indigenous healers should be individualized and planned thoughtfully, taking into consideration the setting, the thoughtfulness and flexibility of the available healers, the type of psychopathology, and the patient's characteristics. The World Health Organization (WHO) has long advocated implementation at the local level of a policy of close collaboration between the conventional health system and traditional medicine, particularly between individual health professionals and traditional practitioners.

CULTURE AND PSYCHOPHARMACOLOGY

The relation between culture and psychopharmacology is as fascinating as it is complex. A web of incompletely understood relations links purely biological factors such as genes to factors deemed more socially generated, such as customary diets, nutrients, and herbs. To complete the picture, the clinician and researcher must consider additional factors such as the patient's culturally based expectations of optimum psychiatric treatment (pharmacotherapy or psychotherapy), expected rate of recovery (fast or slow), target symptoms, and threshold and tolerance for adverse effects. If a Hispanic patient has the culturally shared expectation that psychological disorders are somatically based and best treated by an authoritative physician with medication, alternative treatment recommendations will be met with resistance and reduced compliance, unless extensive psychoeducational efforts are deployed. Alternatively, middle-class, educated, urban professionals may reject psychopharmacological prescriptions for their anxiety or depressive syndromes as simplistic, because they had expected psychotherapy or psychoanalysis.

Thus, the therapeutic relationship across the language or cultural barrier should be initiated by carefully eliciting the patient's explanatory framework of illness, anticipated path to recovery, and expectations for treatment. Clinicians must spend time and effort in an educational dialogue with patients and their significant others and explain the reasons for an alternative to the patient's preferred course of treatment. Slow onset of action and the frequency of adverse effects interfere with the therapeutic cooperation of some Hispanic and Asian patients who expect rapid relief, fear toxicity, or are concerned with the addictive potential of medications to be taken long term. To obtain adequate compliance across the cultural barrier the clinician must make tactful efforts to learn the patient's (and the immediate family's) latent,

culturally shaped beliefs about the illness and its normative treatment, to provide therapeutic options compatible with the patient's culturally prescribed explanatory models, and to avoid having hidden miscommunication hinder the necessary compliance.

Pharmacogenetics. The field of pharmacogenetics grew out of observations of significant ethnic differences in response to drugs, in differential development, and in adverse-effect profiles, leading to the discovery of defects or deficiencies in the genetically controlled activity of enzyme systems responsible for the metabolism of psychotropic medications and toxins such as alcohol.

Acetylation Status. Observations of ethnic differences in the adverse-effects profile of the antituberculosis drug isoniazid (Nydrazid, Rifamate) led to the classification of persons as slow or rapid acetylators, which, among other biological effects, determines their metabolism of psychotropic medications such as clonazepam (Klonopin) and phenelzine (Nardil).

Alcohol Metabolism. P.H. Wolf, while studying racial differences in alcohol sensitivity, observed that about 80 percent of Asians and 50 percent of native Americans exhibited the flushing response to alcohol (compared with 10 percent of whites) and concluded that these differences had a genetic basis. They have been proved to be related to genetic polymorphism of isoenzymes of alcohol dehydrogenase (ADH) and aldehyde dehydrogenase (ALDH), enzymes critical for complete metabolism of alcohol and other neurotransmitters and which play a role in development of alcoholism or its avoidance. For example, Asians who are either homozygous or heterozygous for the atypical Asian-type *ALDH2* gene are alcohol sensitive and have a low risk for alcoholism and alcoholic liver disease.

Native Americans have a high frequency of both alcohol flushing and alcohol-related problems. Akira Yoshida's research team reported in 1993 that they had practically no detectable Asian type *ADH2* and *ALDH2* genes, a major alcohol-rejecting genetic factor.

Cytochrome P450 Isoenzymes. The cytochrome P450 enzyme system is key in the metabolism of psychotropic and nonpsychotropic drugs as well as a great variety of environmental toxins that find their way into the diets of animals and humans. The genetic defects that render these enzymes less effective and make humans poor metabolizers are unequally distributed among ethnic populations. This is particularly the case for two cytochrome P450 (CYP) isoenzymes: CYP 2D6 (debrisoquin hydroxylase), and CYP 2Cmp (mephenytoin hydroxylase). The percentage of CYP 2D6-poor metabolizers is lower for Asians (0.5 to 2.4 percent), and higher for whites (2.9 to 10 percent). Similar interethnic variance exists in the frequency of poor metabolizers of CYP 2Cmp, low among whites (3 percent), intermediate for African Americans (18 percent), and higher (up to 20 percent) in Asian and Japanese populations.

These interethnic differences in the P450 isoenzymes are of great importance in psychiatry and psychopharmacology because of their role in the metabolism of antipsychotics, antidepressants, sedatives such as barbiturates and benzodiazepines, and β-adrenergic receptor antagonists (beta-blockers) such as propranolol (Inderal).

Environmental Factors. In addition to being genetically regulated, enzymes that participate in the metabolism of psychotropic medications respond to environmental variables such as diet, alcohol, smoking status, and caffeine intake. All of these factors can accelerate or slow the metabolism of drugs through enzyme induction or inhibition.

Herbal Medicines. In parallel with available Western medicine-oriented psychiatric services, immigrants often retain their loyalty to ethnically based folk-medicine systems. Accounts by Vivian Garrison and Allan Hardwood document extensive use of folk healers by Puerto Ricans in New York City. Other investigators have reported that Mexican Americans are willing to accept prescribed medications from psychiatrists and herbs from a community healer, just as mainstream young urban professionals use natural serotonin-enhancing herbs such as St. John's wort in addition to, or instead of, the more conventional psychotropics prescribed by their psychiatrists. Culturally competent psychopharmacologists need to inquire about their patients' use of the traditional herbal medicines of Asians, African Americans, Hispanics, and other immigrants living in the United States. Many of these herbs possess high levels of psychoactive activity, such as anticholinergics (*Swertia japonica* used by Japanese patients or *Datura candida* used by Cubans), stimulants (the caffeine-loaded *Ibexguazusa* of Latin America), sedatives (*Schumanniophyton problematicans* of the Nigerians). Others, such as ginseng and glycyrrhiza, may stimulate or inhibit cytochrome P450.

References

Collins PY, Wig NN, Day R, et al. Psychosocial and biological aspects of acute brief psychoses in three developing country sites. *Psychiatr Q*. 1996;67:177.

Elmsley RA, Roberts MC, Rataemane S. Ethnicity and treatment response in schizophrenia: a comparison of 3 ethnic groups. *J Clin Psychiatry*. 2002;63:9.

Hughes CC. Culture in clinical psychiatry. In: Gaw A, ed. *Culture, Ethnicity, and Mental Illness*. Washington, DC: American Psychiatric Press; 1993.

Hughes CC. The culture-bound syndromes and psychiatric diagnosis. In: Mezzich JE, Kleinman A, Fabrega H, Parron DL, eds. *Culture and Psychiatry Diagnosis*. Washington, DC: American Psychiatric Press; 1996.

Jorge MR, Mezzich JE. Latin American contribution to psychiatric nosology and classification. In: Mezzich JE, Honda Y, Kastrup MC, eds. *Psychiatric Diagnosis: A World Perspective*. Berlin: Springer-Verlag; 1994.

Lin K-M. Cultural influences on the diagnosis of psychotic and organic disorders. In: Mezzich JE, Kleinman A, Fabrega H, Parron DL, eds. *Culture and Psychiatry Diagnosis*. Washington, DC: American Psychiatric Press; 1996.

Manschreck TC, Petri M. The atypical psychoses. *Cult Med Psychiatry*. 1978;2:233.

Mezzich JE, Kleinman A, Fabrega H, Parron DL. *Culture and Psychiatric Diagnosis*. Washington, DC: American Psychiatric Press; 1996.

Mezzich JE, Lin K-M, Hughes CC. Acute and transient psychotic disorders and culture-bound syndromes. In: Sadock BJ, Sadock VA, eds. *Kaplan & Sadock's Comprehensive Textbook of Psychiatry*. 7th ed. Vol 1. Baltimore: Lippincott Williams & Wilkins; 2000:1264.

Sartorius N, DeGirolano G, Andrews G, German GA, Eisenberg L. *Treatment of Mental Disorder: A Review of Effectiveness*. Washington, DC: World Health Organization and American Psychiatric Press; 1993.

Shen YC. On the second edition of the *Chinese Classification of Mental Disorder*. In: Mezzich JE, Honda Y, Kastrup MC, eds. *Psychiatric Diagnosis: A World Perspective*. Berlin: Springer-Verlag; 1994.

Truijillo M. Cultural psychiatry. In: Sadock BJ, Sadock VA, eds. *Kaplan & Sadock's Comprehensive Textbook of Psychiatry*. 7th ed. Vol 1. Baltimore: Lippincott Williams & Wilkins; 2000:492.

15 Mood Disorders

▲ 15.1 Major Depression and Bipolar Disorder

Mood disorders encompass a large group of disorders in which pathological mood and related disturbances dominate the clinical picture. Known in some previous editions of *Diagnostic and Statistical Manual of Mental Disorders* (DSM) as affective disorders, the term *mood disorders* is preferred because it refers to sustained emotional states, not merely to the external (affective) expression of a transitory emotional state. Mood disorders are best considered syndromes (rather than discrete diseases) consisting of a cluster of signs and symptoms sustained over weeks to months, which represent a marked departure from a person's habitual functioning and tend to recur, often in periodic or cyclical fashion. Mood may be normal, elevated, or depressed. Normal persons experience a wide range of moods and have an equally large repertoire of affective expressions; they feel in control, more or less, of their moods and affects. In mood disorders the sense of control is lost, and there is a subjective experience of great distress.

Patients with an elevated mood demonstrate expansiveness, flight of ideas, decreased sleep, heightened self-esteem, and grandiose ideas. Patients with depressed mood show loss of energy and interest, feelings of guilt, difficulty concentrating, loss of appetite, and thoughts of death or suicide. Other signs and symptoms include changes in activity level, cognitive abilities, speech, and vegetative functions (e.g., sleep, sexual activity, and other biological rhythms). These disorders virtually always result in impaired interpersonal, social, and occupational functioning.

Patients who are afflicted only with major depressive episodes are said to have major depressive disorder or unipolar depression. Patients with both manic and depressive episodes or patients with manic episodes alone are said to have bipolar disorder. The terms *unipolar mania, pure mania*, or *euphoric mania* are sometimes used for bipolar patients who do not have depressive episodes. *Hypomania* is an episode of manic symptoms that does not meet all the DSM-IV-TR criteria for a manic episode.

The field of psychiatry has considered major depression and bipolar disorder to be two separate disorders, particularly in the last 20 years. However, the possibility that bipolar disorder is actually a more severe expression of major depression has been reconsidered recently. Many patients given a diagnosis of major depressive disorder reveal, on careful examination, past episodes of manic or hypomanic behavior that have gone undetected.

HISTORY

People have recorded instances of depression since antiquity. Descriptions of what are now called mood disorders appear in many ancient documents. The Old Testament story of King Saul describes a depressive syndrome, as does the story of Ajax's suicide in Homer's *Iliad*. About 400 BC, Hippocrates used the terms *mania* and *melancholia* to describe mental disturbances. Around AD 30, the Roman physician Celsus described melancholia (from Greek *melan* ["black"] and *chole* ["bile"]) in his work *De re medicina* as a depression caused by black bile.

In 1854, Jules Falret described a condition called *folie circulaire,* in which patients experience alternating moods of depression and mania. In 1882, the German psychiatrist Karl Kahlbaum, using the term *cyclothymia,* described mania and depression as stages of the same illness. In 1899, Emil Kraepelin, building on the knowledge of previous French and German psychiatrists, described manic-depressive psychosis using most of the criteria that psychiatrists now use to establish a diagnosis of bipolar I disorder. According to Kraepelin, the absence of a dementing and deteriorating course in manic-depressive psychosis differentiated it from dementia precox (as schizophrenia was then called). Kraepelin also described a depression that came to be known as involutional melancholia, which has since come to be viewed as a form of mood disorder that begins in late adulthood (Fig. 15.1–1).

DSM-IV-TR CLASSIFICATION OF MOOD DISORDERS

According to the text revision of the fourth edition of DSM (DSM-IV-TR), a major depressive disorder (also known as unipolar depression) occurs without a history of a manic, mixed, or hypomanic episode. A major depressive episode must last at least 2 weeks, and typically a person with a diagnosis of a major depressive episode also experiences at least four symptoms from a list that includes changes in appetite and weight, changes in sleep and activity, lack of energy, feelings of guilt, problems thinking and making decisions, and recurring thoughts of death or suicide.

A manic episode is a distinct period of an abnormally and persistently elevated, expansive, or irritable mood lasting for at least 1 week, or less if a patient must be hospitalized. A hypomanic episode lasts at least 4 days and is similar to a manic episode except that it is not severe enough to cause impairment in social or occupational functioning, and no psy-

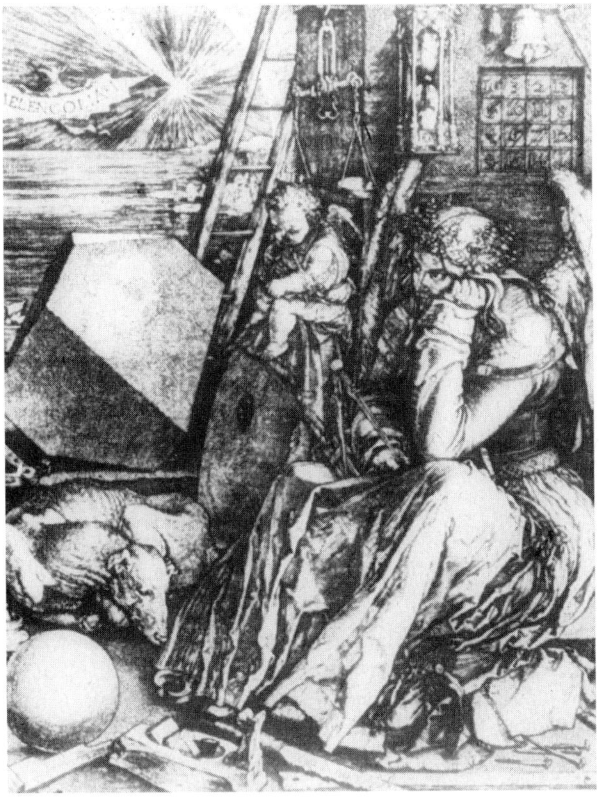

FIGURE 15.1–1
Melancholia (1514) by Albrecht Dürer.

chotic features are present. Both mania and hypomania are associated with inflated self-esteem, decreased need for sleep, distractibility, great physical and mental activity, and overinvolvement in pleasurable behavior. According to DSM-IV-TR, bipolar I disorder is defined as having a clinical course of one or more manic episodes and, sometimes, major depressive episodes. A mixed episode is a period of at least 1 week in which both a manic episode and a major depressive episode occur almost daily. A variant of bipolar disorder characterized by episodes of major depression and hypomania rather than mania is known as bipolar II disorder.

Two additional mood disorders, dysthymic disorder and cyclothymic disorder (discussed fully in Section 15.2), have also been appreciated clinically for some time. Dysthymic disorder and cyclothymic disorder are characterized by the presence of symptoms that are less severe than those of major depressive disorder and bipolar I disorder, respectively. DSM-IV-TR defines dysthymic disorder as characterized by at least 2 years of depressed mood that is not severe enough to fit the diagnosis of major depressive episode. Cyclothymic disorder is characterized by at least 2 years of frequently occurring hypomanic symptoms that cannot fit the diagnosis of manic episode and of depressive symptoms that cannot fit the diagnosis of major depressive episode.

DSM-IV-TR includes three mood disorder research categories (minor depressive disorder, recurrent brief depressive disorder, and premenstrual dysphoric disorder). Other DSM-IV-TR diagnoses are mood disorder due to a general medical condition and substance-induced mood disorder. These categories are designed to broaden the recognition of mood disorder diagnoses, to describe mood disorder symptoms more specifically than in the past, and to facilitate the differential diagnosis of mood disorders. Finally, DSM-IV-TR includes three residual disorders—bipolar disorder not otherwise specified, depressive disorder not otherwise specified, and mood disorder not otherwise specified (see Section 15.3).

EPIDEMIOLOGY

Incidence and Prevalence

Major depressive disorder is a common disorder, with a lifetime prevalence of about 15 percent, perhaps as high as 25 percent for women. The incidence of major depressive disorder is 10 percent in primary care patients and 15 percent in medical inpatients. Bipolar I disorder is less common than major depressive disorder, with a lifetime prevalence of about 1 percent, similar to the figure for schizophrenia. Table 15.1–1 lists the lifetime prevalence of mood disorders.

Sex

An almost universal observation, independent of country or culture, is the twofold greater prevalence of major depressive disorder in women than in men. The reasons for the difference have been hypothesized to involve hormonal differences, the effects of childbirth, differing psychosocial stressors for women and for men, and behavioral models of learned helplessness. In contrast to major depressive disorder, bipolar I disorder has an equal prevalence among men and women. Manic episodes are more common in men, and depressive episodes are more com-

Table 15.1–1
Lifetime Prevalence of Some DSM-IV-TR Mood Disorders

Mood Disorder	Lifetime Prevalence
Depressive disorders	
Major depressive disorder (MDD)	10–25% for women; 5–12% for men
Recurrent, with full interepisode recovery, superimposed on dysthymic disorder	Approximately 3% of persons with MDD
Recurrent, without full interepisode recovery, superimposed on dysthymic disorder (double depression)	Approximately 20–25% of persons with MDD
Dysthymic disorder	Approximately 6%
Bipolar disorders	
Bipolar I disorder	0.4–1.6%
Bipolar II disorder	Approximately 0.5%
Bipolar I disorder or bipolar II disorder, with rapid cycling	5–15% of persons with bipolar disorder
Cyclothymic disorder	0.4–1.0%

Data are from American Psychiatric Association. *Diagnostic and Statistical Manual of Mental Disorders.* 4th ed. Text rev. Washington, DC: American Psychiatric Association; copyright 2000, with permission.

mon in women. When manic episodes occur in women, they are more likely than men to present a mixed picture (e.g., mania and depression). Women also have a higher rate of being rapid cyclers, defined as having four or more manic episodes in a 1-year period.

Age

The onset of bipolar I disorder is earlier than that of major depressive disorder. The age of onset for bipolar I disorder ranges from childhood (as early as age 5 or 6) to 50 years or even older in rare cases, with a mean age of 30. The mean age of onset for major depressive disorder is about 40 years, with 50 percent of all patients having an onset between the ages of 20 and 50. Major depressive disorder can also begin in childhood or in old age. Recent epidemiological data suggest that the incidence of major depressive disorder may be increasing among people less than 20 years old. This may be related to the increased use of alcohol and drugs of abuse in this age group.

Marital Status

Major depressive disorder occurs most often in persons without close interpersonal relationships or in those who are divorced or separated. Bipolar I disorder is more common in divorced and single persons than among married persons, but this difference may reflect the early onset and the resulting marital discord characteristic of the disorder.

Socioeconomic and Cultural Factors

No correlation has been found between socioeconomic status and major depressive disorder. A higher than average incidence of bipolar I disorder is found among the upper socioeconomic groups. Depression is more common in rural areas than in urban areas. Bipolar I disorder is more common in persons who did not graduate from college than in college graduates, which may also reflect the relatively early age of onset for the disorder. The prevalence of mood disorder does not differ among races. There is a tendency, however, for examiners to underdiagnosis mood disorder and overdiagnosis schizophrenia in patients whose racial or cultural background differs from theirs.

ETIOLOGY

Biological Factors

Many studies have reported abnormalities in biogenic amine metabolites—such as 5-hydroxyindoleacetic acid (5-HIAA), homovanillic acid (HVA), and 3-methoxy-4-hydroxyphenylglycol (MHPG)—in blood, urine, and cerebrospinal fluid (CSF) of patients with mood disorders (Table 15.1–2). The data reported are most consistent with the hypothesis that mood disorders are associated with heterogeneous dysregulations of the biogenic amines.

Biogenic Amines. Of the biogenic amines, norepinephrine and serotonin are the two neurotransmitters most implicated in the pathophysiology of mood disorders (Table 15.1–3).

NOREPINEPHRINE. The correlation suggested by basic science studies between the downregulation of β-adrenergic receptors and clinical antidepressant responses is probably the single most compelling piece of data indicating a direct role for the noradrenergic system in depression. Other evidence has also implicated the presynaptic β_2-receptors in depression, as activation of these receptors results in a decrease of the amount of norepinephrine released. Presynaptic β_2-receptors are also located on serotonergic neurons and regulate the amount of serotonin released. The clinical effectiveness of antidepressant drugs with noradrenergic effects—for example, venlafaxine (Effexor)—further supports a role for norepinephrine in the pathophysiology of at least some of the symptoms of depression.

SEROTONIN. With the huge effect that the selective serotonin reuptake inhibitors (SSRIs)—for example, fluoxetine (Prozac)—have made on the treatment of depression, serotonin has become

Table 15.1–2
Frequently Reported Neurotransmitter and Metabolite Changes in Some Depressed Patients (Compared with Normal Controls)

	NE	MHPG	NM	VMA	Epi	MET	DA	HVA	5-HT	5-HIAA	GABA	GAD	CRH	Endorphins
CSF	nd	↓ ↑ ↔	nd	nd	nd	nd	nd	↓ ↑ psychotic dep.	nd	↓ ↔	↓	nd	↑	↑ mania ↔ dep.
Plasma	nd	nd	nd	nd	nd	nd	nd	nd	↓	nd	↓	nd	nd	↑ ↔
Uptake into platelets	nd	nd	nd	nd	nd	nd	nd	nd	↓	nd	nd	nd	nd	nd
Urine	↑ ↔	↓	↑ ↔	↑ ↔	↑ ↔	↑ ↔	↑ mania	nd	nd	nd	nd	nd	nd	nd
Brain tissue	nd	nd	nd	nd	nd	nd	nd	nd	↓	↓	nd	↓ ↔	nd	nd

nd, no data in this review; ↑, levels higher than control levels; ↓, lower than control levels; ↔, no change from control levels; NE, norepinephrine; MHPG, 3-methoxy-4-hydroxyphenethyleneglycol; NM, normetanephrine; VMA, 3-methoxy-4-hydroxymandelic acid; Epi, epinephrine; MET, metanephrine; DA, dopamine; HVA, homovanillic acid; 5-HT, serotonin; 5-HIAA, 5-hydroxyindoleacetic acid; GABA, γ-aminobutyric acid; GAD, glutamic acid decarboxylase; CRH, corticotropin-releasing hormone.

Reprinted with permission from Caldecott-Hazard S, Morgan DG, DeLeon-Jones F, Overstreet DH, Janowsky D. Clinical and biochemical aspects of depressive disorders. II. Transmitter/receptor theories. *Synapse.* 1991;9:253.

Table 15.1–3
Antidepressant-Induced Changes in Neurotransmitters, Metabolites, and Their Receptors in Humans and Animals

	Drugs					
What Was Measured	**Tricyclics**	**MAOIs**	**SUBs**	**Iprindole**	**LI**	**ECT**
Concentrations in brain tissue						
MHPG	↑	nd	nd	nd	nd	nd
Enkephalins	↑	nd	nd	↑	nd	↑
Concentrations in CSF						
MHPG	↓	↓	↓	nd	nd	nd
HVA	nd	↓	nd	nd	nd	nd
5-HIAA	↓	↓	↓	nd	nd	nd
β-Endorphin	nd	nd	nd	nd	nd	↑
Concentrations in urine						
MHPG	↓↑↔	nd	nd	nd	nd	nd
Effects on uptake of						
NE	↓	nd	↔	↔	nd	nd
5-HT	↓	nd	↓	↔	nd	nd
GABA	↓	nd	nd	nd	nd	nd
Number of receptors						
Brain α-2	↓↑↔	nd	nd	nd	nd	nd
Platelet α-2	nd	nd	nd	nd	↓	nd
Brain α-1	↑↔	nd	nd	nd	↑	nd
Brain β	↓	↓	↓↔	↓	nd	↓
Brain 5-HT-2	↓	↓	↓	↓	nd	↑
Brain 5-HT-1	↓↑↔	↓	↓↔	nd	nd	nd
Brain mACh	↑	nd	nd	nd	↑↔	nd
Brain dopamine-1	↓	nd	nd	nd	nd	↓
Brain $GABA_{\beta}$	↑↔	↑	↑	nd	nd	↑
Brain μ and Δ opioid	nd	nd	nd	nd	nd	↑↓
Sensitivity of somatodendritic DA receptors	↓↔	↓	nd	nd	nd	↓
Effect on stimulation of cAMP by NE	↓	↓	↓	↓	nd	↓
Effect on stimulation of PI by muscarinic agonists	nd	nd	nd	nd	↓↔	nd
Amount of glucocorticoid mRNA on receptor sites in brain	↑↓	nd	nd	nd	nd	nd

nd, no data in this review; ↑, higher; ↓, lower; ↔, no change. Arrows represent the most frequently observed (not necessarily all) effects of the drugs in each group. MAOI, monoamine oxidase inhibitor; SUB, serotonin uptake blocker; Li, lithium; ECT, electroconvulsive therapy; CSF, cerebrospinal fluid; MHPG, 3-methoxy-4-hydroxyphenethyleneglycol; HVA, homovanillic acid; 5-HIAA, 5-hydroxyindoleacetic acid; 5-HT, serotonin; NE, norepinephrine; DA, dopamine; GABA, γ-aminobutyric acid; mACh, muscarinic cholinergic; cAMP, cyclic adenosine monophosphate; PI, phosphoinositide; mRNA, messenger ribonucleic acid.

Reprinted with permission from Caldecott-Hazard S, Morgan DG, DeLeon-Jones F, Overstreet DH, Janowsky D. Clinical and biochemical aspects of depressive disorders. II. Transmitter/receptor theories. *Synapse.* 1991;9:254.

the biogenic amine neurotransmitter most commonly associated with depression. The identification of multiple serotonin receptor subtypes has also increased the excitement within the research community about the development of even more specific treatments for depression. Besides the fact that SSRIs and other serotonergic antidepressants are effective in the treatment of depression, other data indicate that serotonin is involved in the pathophysiology of depression. Depletion of serotonin may precipitate depression, and some patients with suicidal impulses have low CSF concentrations of serotonin metabolites and low concentrations of serotonin uptake sites on platelets.

DOPAMINE. Although norepinephrine and serotonin are the biogenic amines most often associated with the pathophysiology of depression, dopamine has also been theorized to play a role. The data suggest that dopamine activity may be reduced in depression and increased in mania. The discovery of new subtypes of the dopamine receptors and increased understanding of the presynaptic and postsynaptic regulation of dopamine function have further enriched research into the relation between dopamine and mood disorders. Drugs that reduce dopamine concentrations—for example, reserpine (Serpasil)—and diseases that reduce dopamine concentrations (e.g., Parkinson's disease) are associated with depressive symptoms. In contrast, drugs that increase dopamine concentrations, such as tyrosine, amphetamine, and bupropion (Wellbutrin), reduce the symptoms of depression. Two recent theories about dopamine and depression are that the mesolimbic dopamine pathway may be dysfunctional in depression and that the dopamine D_1 receptor may be hypoactive in depression.

Other Neurochemical Factors.

Although the data are not yet conclusive, amino acid neurotransmitters (particularly γ-aminobutyric acid [GABA]) and neuroactive peptides (partic-

ularly vasopressin and the endogenous opiates) have been implicated in the pathophysiology of mood disorders. Some investigators have suggested that second-messenger systems—such as adenylate cyclase, phosphatidylinositol, and calcium regulation—may also be causally relevant. The amino acids glutamate and glycine appear to be the major excitatory neurotransmitters in the central nervous system. Glutamate and glycine bind to sites associated with the *N*-methyl-D-aspartate (NMDA) receptor and, in excess, can have neurotoxic effects. The hippocampus has a high concentration of NMDA receptors; thus it is possible that glutamate in conjunction with hypercortisolemia mediate the neurocognitive effects of chronic stress. There is emerging evidence that drugs that antagonize NMDA receptors have antidepressants effects.

Neuroendocrine Regulation. The hypothalamus is central to the regulation of the neuroendocrine axes and itself receives many neuronal inputs that use biogenic amine neurotransmitters. Various neuroendocrine dysregulations have been reported in patients with mood disorders, and thus the abnormal regulation of neuroendocrine axes may result from abnormal functioning of biogenic amine–containing neurons. Although it is theoretically possible for a particular dysregulation of a neuroendocrine axis to be involved in the cause of a mood disorder, the dysregulations more likely reflect a fundamental underlying brain disorder. The major neuroendocrine axes of interest in mood disorders are the adrenal, thyroid, and growth hormone axes. Other neuroendocrine abnormalities that have been described in patients with mood disorders include decreased nocturnal secretion of melatonin, decreased prolactin release in response to tryptophan administration, decreased basal levels of follicle-stimulating hormone (FSH) and luteinizing hormone (LH), and decreased testosterone levels in men.

ADRENAL AXIS. *Role of Cortisol.* A correlation between the hypersecretion of cortisol and depression is one of the oldest observations in biological psychiatry. Basic and clinical research on this relation has produced an understanding of how cortisol release is regulated in persons with and without depression. About 50 percent of depressed patients have elevated cortical levels. Neurons in the paraventricular nucleus (PVN) release corticotropin-releasing hormone (CRH), which stimulates the release of adrenocorticotropic hormone (ACTH) from the anterior pituitary. ACTH is coreleased with β-endorphin and β-lipotropin, two peptides synthesized from the same precursor protein from which ACTH is synthesized. ACTH, in turn, stimulates the release of cortisol from the adrenal cortex. The cortisol feedback on the loop works through at least two mechanisms. A fast feedback mechanism, sensitive to the rate of cortisol concentration increase, operates through cortisol receptors on the hippocampus and decreases release of ACTH. A slow feedback mechanism, sensitive to the steady-state cortisol concentration, is thought to operate through pituitary and adrenal receptors.

Dexamethasone-Suppression Test. Dexamethasone (Decadron) is a synthetic analogue of cortisol. Many researchers have noted that a significant proportion, perhaps 50 percent, of depressed patients fail to have the normal cortisol suppression response to a single dose of dexamethasone. Although the dexamethasone-suppression test (DST) was initially thought to be of diagnostic usefulness, many patients with other psychiatric disorders also show a positive result (nonsuppression of cortisol); thus the test is not entirely valid for indicating mood disorders. New data indicate that DST results may, however, correlate with the likelihood of a relapse: Depressed patients whose DST results do not normalize with clinical response to treatment are more likely to relapse than are those whose DST results do normalize.

A recent advance in the assessment of the hypothalamic-pituitary-adrenal (HPA) axis in depression involved infusions of cortisol in persons who were and were not depressed. Cortisol, the naturally occurring hormone, is a better test substance than dexamethasone, which does not reach or activate all the relevant receptors. In one study, depressed patients had impaired function of the fast feedback loop; thus, for at least some of them, the functioning of cortisol receptors in the hippocampus may have been abnormal. Other researchers have found that hypercortisolemia can damage hippocampal neurons; thus a cycle involving stress, stimulation of cortisol release, and inability to stop cortisol release may result in increasing damage to an already impaired hippocampus.

THYROID AXIS. Thyroid disorders are often found in about 5 to 10 percent of persons with depression. One direct clinical implication of the association is the critical importance of determining the thyroid status of all affectively ill patients. About one third of all patients with major depressive disorder who have an otherwise normal thyroid axis have been found to have a blunted release of thyrotropin, the thyroid-stimulating hormone (TSH), to an infusion of the thyrotropin-releasing hormone (TRH) protirelin. This same abnormality has been reported in a wide range of other psychiatric diagnoses, however, so the diagnostic usefulness of the test is limited. Moreover, attempts to subtype depressed patients on the basis of their TRH test results have been contradictory.

Recent research has focused on the possibility that a subset of depressed persons have an unrecognized autoimmune disorder that affects their thyroid glands. Several studies have reported that about 10 percent of patients with mood disorders, perhaps particularly bipolar I disorder patients, have detectable concentrations of antithyroid antibodies. Whether the antibodies are in fact associated pathophysiologically with depression has not yet been determined. Another potential association exists between hypothyroidism and the development of a rapidly cycling course in patients with bipolar I disorder. Available research data indicate that the association is independent of the effects of lithium (Eskalith) treatment, which can cause hypothyroidism. Some depressed patients benefit from liothyronine (Cytomel).

GROWTH HORMONE. Several studies have shown a statistical difference between depressed patients and others in the regulation of growth hormone release. Depressed patients have a blunted sleep-induced stimulation of growth hormone release. Inasmuch as sleep abnormalities are common symptoms of depression, a neuroendocrine marker related to sleep is an avenue for research. Studies have also found that depressed patients have a blunted response to clonidine (Catapres)-induced increases in growth hormone secretion.

Somatostatin. In addition to inhibition of growth hormone and release of CRH, somatostatin inhibits GABA, ACTH, and TSH. Somatostatin levels are lower in the CSF of persons with

depression than in those with schizophrenia or normal controls, and increased levels have been observed in mania.

Prolactin. Prolactin release from the pituitary is stimulated by serotonin and inhibited by dopamine. Most studies have found no significant abnormalities of basal or circadian prolactin secretion in depression.

Sleep Abnormalities. Problems with sleeping—initial and terminal insomnia, multiple awakenings, hypersomnia—are common and classic symptoms of depression, and a perceived decreased need for sleep is a classic symptom of mania. Researchers have long recognized that the sleep electroencephalograms (EEGs) of many depressed persons show abnormalities. Common abnormalities are delayed sleep onset, shortened rapid eye movement (REM) latency (the time between falling asleep and the first REM period), a longer first REM period, and abnormal delta sleep. Some investigators have attempted to use the sleep EEG in the diagnostic assessment of patients with mood disorders.

Circadian Rhythms. The abnormalities of sleep architecture in depression and the transient clinical improvement associated with sleep deprivation have led to theories that depression reflects abnormal regulation of circadian rhythms. Some experimental studies with animals indicate that many of the standard antidepressant treatments are effective in changing the setting of internal biological clocks (endogenous *zeitgebers*).

Kindling. Kindling is the electrophysiological process in which repeated subthreshold stimulation of a neuron eventually generates an action potential. At the organ level, repeated subthreshold stimulation of an area of the brain results in a seizure. The clinical observation that anticonvulsants—for example, carbamazepine (Tegretol) and valproic acid (Depakene)—are useful in the treatment of mood disorders, particularly bipolar I disorder, has given rise to the theory that the pathophysiology of mood disorders may involve kindling in the temporal lobes. Although kindling has been found in laboratory animals, it has never been demonstrated convincingly in humans, and the salutary effects of anticonvulsants in bipolar disorder may also be due to electrochemical alterations unrelated to epilepsy.

Neuroimmune Regulation. Researchers have reported immunological abnormalities in depressed persons and in those grieving the loss of a relative, spouse, or close friend. The dysregulation of the cortisol axis may affect the immune status; there may be abnormal hypothalamic regulation of the immune system. A less likely possibility is that in some patients, a primary pathophysiological process involving the immune system leads to the psychiatric symptoms of mood disorders.

Brain Imaging. Brain imaging studies of patients with mood disorders have provided several inconclusive clues about abnormal brain function in these disorders. No brain imaging data about mood disorders have been replicated as consistently as the increased ventricular size in patients with schizophrenia. Nevertheless, structural brain imaging studies with computed tomography (CT) and magnetic resonance imaging (MRI) have produced interesting data. Although the studies have not reported consistent findings, the data indicate the following: A significant set of bipolar I disorder patients, predominantly men, have enlarged cerebral ventricles; ventricular enlargement is less common in patients with major depressive disorder than in those with bipolar I disorder, except that patients with major depressive disorder with psychotic features do tend to have enlarged cerebral ventricles. MRI studies have also indicated that patients with major depressive disorder have smaller caudate nuclei and smaller frontal lobes than control subjects; the depressed patients also have abnormal hippocampal T1 relaxation times, compared with control subjects. At least one MRI study reported that patients with bipolar I disorder have significantly more deep white matter lesions than control subjects.

Many reports in the literature concern cerebral blood flow in mood disorders, usually measured by using single photon emission computed tomography (SPECT) or positron emission tomography (PET). A slight majority of the studies have shown decreased blood flow affecting the cerebral cortex in general and the frontal cortical areas in particular. In contrast, investigators in one study found increased cerebral blood flow in patients with major depressive disorder. They found state-dependent increases in the cortex, the basal ganglia, and the medial thalamus, with the suggestion of a trait-dependent increase in the amygdala. Further studies are needed.

Another brain imaging technique that is being applied to a broad range of mental disorders is magnetic resonance spectroscopy (MRS). MRS studies of patients with bipolar I disorder have produced data consistent with the hypothesis that the pathophysiology of the disorder may involve an abnormal regulation of membrane phospholipid metabolism. ^{7}Li MRS is also used to study brain and plasma concentrations of lithium in patients with bipolar I disorder.

Neuroanatomical Considerations. Both the symptoms of mood disorders and biological research findings support the hypothesis that mood disorders involve pathology of the limbic system, the basal ganglia, and the hypothalamus (Fig. 15.1–2). Persons with neurological disorders of the basal ganglia and the limbic system (especially excitatory lesions of the nondominant hemisphere) are likely to show depressive symptoms. The limbic system and the basal ganglia are intimately connected, and the limbic system may well play a major role in the production of emotions. Depressed patients' alterations in sleep, appetite, and sexual behavior and biological changes in endocrine, immunological, and chronobiological measures suggest dysfunction of the hypothalamus. Depressed patients' stooped posture, motor slowness, and minor cognitive impairment are similar to the signs of disorders of the basal ganglia, such as Parkinson's disease and other subcortical dementias.

Genetic Factors

Genetic data strongly indicate that a significant genetic factor is involved in the development of a mood disorder, but the pattern of genetic inheritance is complex. Not only is it impossible to exclude psychosocial effects, but also, nongenetic factors probably have causative roles in the development of mood disorders in at least some persons. A genetic component plays a more significant role in transmitting bipolar I disorder than major depressive disorder.

Family Studies. Family studies have repeatedly found that first-degree relatives of bipolar I disorder probands (the first ill

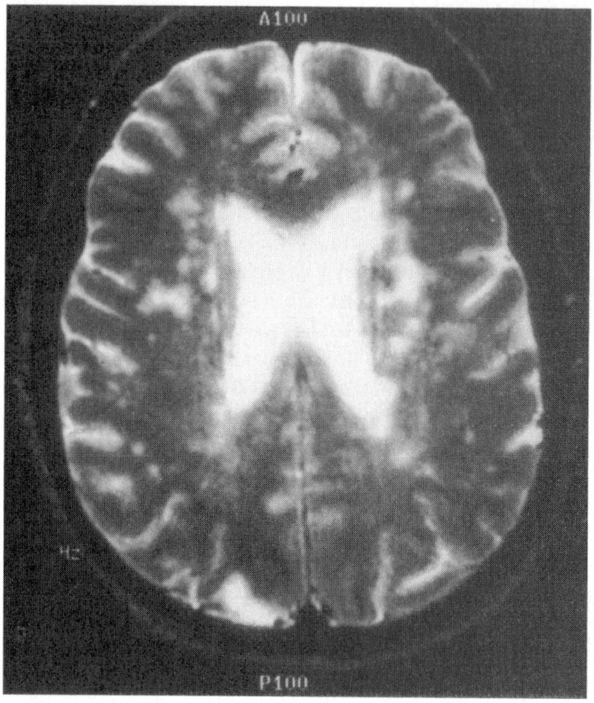

FIGURE 15.1–2

This magnetic resonance imaging (MRI) scan of a patient with late-onset major depressive disorder illustrates extensive periventricular hyperintensities associated with diffuse cerebrovascular disease.

subject identified in a family) are 8 to 18 times more likely than are the first-degree relatives of control subjects to have bipolar I disorder and 2 to 10 times more likely to have major depressive disorder. Family studies have also found that the first-degree relatives of major depressive disorder probands are 1.5 to 2.5 times more likely to have bipolar I disorder than are the first-degree relatives of normal control subjects and 2 to 3 times more likely to have major depressive disorder. The likelihood of having a mood disorder decreases as the degree of relationship widens. For example, a second-degree relative, such as a cousin, is less likely to be affected than is a first-degree relative, like a brother. The inheritability of bipolar I disorder is also apparent in the fact that about 50 percent of all bipolar I disorder patients have at least one parent with a mood disorder, most often major depressive disorder. If one parent has bipolar I disorder, there is a 25 percent chance that any child will have a mood disorder; if both parents have bipolar I disorder, there is a 50 to 75 percent chance that their child will have a mood disorder.

Adoption Studies. Adoption studies have also produced data supporting the genetic basis for the inheritance of mood disorders. Two of three adoption studies have found a strong genetic component for the inheritance of major depressive disorder; the only adoption study for bipolar I disorder also indicated a genetic basis. These adoption studies have shown that the biological children of affected parents remain at increased risk of a mood disorder, even if they are reared in nonaffected adoptive families. The prevalence of mood disorders in the adoptive parents is similar to the baseline prevalence in the general population.

Twin Studies. Twin studies have found a concordance rate for bipolar I disorder in monozygotic twins of 33 to 90 percent, depending on the particular study; for major depressive disorder, the concordance rate in monozygotic twins is about 50 percent. By contrast, the concordance rates in dizygotic twins are about 5 to 25 percent for bipolar I disorder and 10 to 25 percent for major depressive disorder.

Linkage Studies. The availability of modern techniques of molecular biology, including restriction fragment length polymorphisms (RFLPs), has led to many studies that have reported, replicated, or failed to replicate various associations between specific genes or gene markers and a mood disorders. At this time, no genetic association has been consistently replicated. The most reasonable interpretation of the study results is that the particular genes identified in the positive results may be involved with the genetic inheritance of the mood disorder in the families studied but may not be involved in the genetic inheritance of the mood disorder in other families. Associations between the mood disorders, particularly bipolar I disorder, and genetic markers have been reported for chromosomes 5, 11, 18, and X. The D_2 receptor gene is located on chromosome 5. The gene for tyrosine hydroxylase, the rate-limiting enzyme for catecholamine synthesis, is located on chromosome 11. In one study, markers on chromosome 18 were found in 28 nuclear families with bipolar disorder.

CHROMOSOME 11 AND BIPOLAR I DISORDER. In 1987, a study reported an association between bipolar I disorder among members of an Old Order Amish family and genetic markers on the short arm of chromosome 11. With subsequent extension of the pedigree and the development of bipolar I disorder in previously unaffected family members, the statistical association ceased to apply. That turn of events effectively illustrated the caution that must be used in carrying out and interpreting genetic linkage studies involving mental disorders.

X CHROMOSOME AND BIPOLAR I DISORDER. Linkage has long been suggested between bipolar I disorder and a region on the X chromosome that contains genes for color blindness and glucose-6-phosphate dehydrogenase deficiency. As with most linkage studies in psychiatry, the application of molecular genetic techniques has produced contradictory results; some studies find a linkage and others do not. The most conservative interpretation is the possibility that an X-linked gene is a factor in the development of bipolar I disorder in some patients and families.

Psychosocial Factors

Life Events and Environmental Stress. There is a long-standing clinical observation that stressful life events more often precede first, rather than subsequent, episodes of mood disorders. This association has been reported for both patients with major depressive disorder and patients with bipolar I disorder. One theory proposed to explain this observation is that the stress accompanying the first episode results in long-lasting changes in the brain's biology. These long-lasting changes may alter the functional states of various neurotransmitter and intraneuronal signaling systems, changes that may even include the loss of neurons and an excessive reduction in synaptic contacts. As a result, a person has a high risk of undergoing subsequent episodes of a mood disorder, even without an external stressor.

Some clinicians believe that life events play the primary or principal role in depression; others suggest that life events have only a limited role in the onset and timing of depression. The most compelling data indicate that the life event most often associated with development of depression is losing a parent before age 11. The environmental stressor most often associated with the onset of an episode of depression is the loss of a spouse. Another risk factor is unemployment—persons out of work are three times more likely to report symptoms of an episode of major depression than those who are employed.

Personality Factors. No single personality trait or type uniquely predisposes a person to depression; all humans, of whatever personality pattern, can and do become depressed under appropriate circumstances. Persons with certain personality disorders—obsessive-compulsive, histrionic, and borderline—may be at greater risk for depression than persons with antisocial or paranoid personality disorder. The latter can use projection and other externalizing defense mechanisms to protect themselves from their inner rage. No evidence indicates that any particular personality disorder is associated with later development of bipolar I disorder; however, patients with dysthymic disorder and cyclothymic disorder are at risk of later developing major depression or bipolar I disorder.

Recent stressful events are the most powerful predictors of the onset of a depressive episode. From a psychodynamic perspective, the clinician is always interested in the meaning of the stressor. Research has demonstrated that stressors that the patient experiences as reflecting more negatively on his or her self-esteem are more likely to produce depression. Moreover, what may seem to be a relatively mild stressor to outsiders may be devastating to the patient because of particular idiosyncratic meanings attached to the event.

Psychodynamic Factors in Depression. The psychodynamic understanding of depression defined by Sigmund Freud and expanded by Karl Abraham is known as the classical view of depression. That theory involves four key points: (1) disturbances in the infant–mother relationship during the oral phase (the first 10 to 18 months of life) predispose to subsequent vulnerability to depression; (2) depression can be linked to real or imagined object loss; (3) introjection of the departed objects is a defense mechanism invoked to deal with the distress connected with the object's loss; and (4) because the lost object is regarded with a mixture of love and hate, feelings of anger are directed inward at the self.

Melanie Klein understood depression as involving the expression of aggression toward loved ones, much as Freud did. Edward Bibring regarded depression as a phenomenon that sets in when a person becomes aware of the discrepancy between extraordinarily high ideals and the inability to meet those goals. Edith Jacobson saw the state of depression as similar to a powerless, helpless child victimized by a tormenting parent. Silvano Arieti observed that many depressed people have lived their lives for someone else rather than for themselves. He referred to this person for whom depressed patients live as the dominant other, which may be a principle, an ideal, or an institution, as well as an individual. Depression sets in when patients realize that the person or ideal for whom they have been living is never going to respond in a manner that will meet their expectations. Heinz Kohut's conceptualization of depression, derived from his self-psychological theory, rests on the assumption that the developing self has specific needs that must be met by parents to give the child a positive sense of self-esteem and self-cohesion. When others do not meet these needs, there is a massive loss of self-esteem that presents as depression. John Bowlby believed that damaged early attachments and traumatic separation in childhood predispose to depression. Adult losses are said to revive the traumatic childhood loss and so precipitate adult depressive episodes.

Psychodynamic Factors in Mania. Most theories of mania view manic episodes as a defense against underlying depression. Karl Abraham, for example, believed that the manic episodes may reflect an inability to tolerate a developmental tragedy, such as the loss of a parent. The manic state may also result from a tyrannical superego, which produces intolerable self-criticism that is then replaced by euphoric self-satisfaction. Bertram Lewin regarded the manic patient's ego as overwhelmed by pleasurable impulses such as sex or by feared impulses such as aggression. Klein also viewed mania as a defensive reaction to depression, using manic defenses such as omnipotence, in which the person develops delusions of grandeur.

Other Formulations of Depression

Cognitive Theory. According to cognitive theory, depression results from specific cognitive distortions present in persons prone to depression. Those distortions, referred to as depressogenic schemata, are cognitive templates that perceive both internal and external data in ways that are altered by early experiences. Aaron Beck postulated a cognitive triad of depression that consists of (1) views about the self—a negative self-precept, (2) about the environment—a tendency to experience the world as hostile and demanding, and (3) about the future—the expectation of suffering and failure. Therapy consists of modifying these distortions. The elements of cognitive theory are summarized in Table 15.1–4.

Table 15.1–4
Elements of Cognitive Theory

Element	Definition
Cognitive triad	Beliefs about oneself, the world, the future
Schemas	Ways of organizing and interpreting experiences
Cognitive distortions	
Arbitrary inference	Drawing a specific conclusion without sufficient evidence
Specific abstraction	Focus on a single detail while ignoring other, more important aspects of an experience
Overgeneralization	Forming conclusions based on too little and too narrow experience
Magnification and minimization	Over- or undervaluing the significance of a particular event
Personalization	Tendency to self-reference external events without basis
Absolutist, dichotomous thinking	Tendency to place experience into all-or-none categories

Courtesy of Robert M.A. Hirschfeld, M.D., and M. Tracie Shea, Ph.D.

Table 15.1–5
DSM-IV-TR Criteria for Major Depressive Episode

A. Five (or more) of the following symptoms have been present during the same 2-week period and represent a change from previous functioning; at least one of the symptoms is either (1) depressed mood or (2) loss of interest or pleasure.
Note: Do not include symptoms that are clearly due to a general medical condition, or mood-incongruent delusions or hallucinations.
(1) depressed mood most of the day, nearly every day, as indicated by either subjective report (e.g., feels sad or empty) or observation made by others (e.g., appears tearful). **Note:** In children and adolescents, can be irritable mood
(2) markedly diminished interest or pleasure in all, or almost all, activities most of the day, nearly every day (as indicated by either subjective account or observation made by others)
(3) significant weight loss when not dieting or weight gain (e.g., a change of more than 5% of body weight in a month), or decrease or increase in appetite nearly every day. **Note:** In children, consider failure to make expected weight gains.
(4) insomnia or hypersomnia nearly every day
(5) psychomotor agitation or retardation nearly every day (observable by others, not merely subjective feelings of restlessness or being slowed down)
(6) fatigue or loss of energy nearly every day
(7) feelings of worthlessness or excessive or inappropriate guilt (which may be delusional) nearly every day (not merely self-reproach or guilt about being sick)
(8) diminished ability to think or concentrate, or indecisiveness, nearly every day (either by subjective account or as observed by others)
(9) recurrent thoughts of death (not just fear of dying), recurrent suicidal ideation without a specific plan, or a suicide attempt or a specific plan for committing suicide

B. The symptoms do not meet criteria for a mixed episode.
C. The symptoms cause clinically significant distress or impairment in social, occupational, or other important areas of functioning.
D. The symptoms are not due to the direct physiological effects of a substance (e.g., a drug of abuse, a medication) or a general medical condition (e.g., hypothyroidism).
E. The symptoms are not better accounted for by bereavement, i.e., after the loss of a loved one, the symptoms persist for longer than 2 months or are characterized by marked functional impairment, morbid preoccupation with worthlessness, suicidal ideation, psychotic symptoms, or psychomotor retardation.

From American Psychiatric Association. *Diagnostic and Statistical Manual of Mental Disorders.* 4th ed. Text rev. Washington, DC: American Psychiatric Association; copyright 2000, with permission.

Table 15.1–6
DSM-IV-TR Criteria for Manic Episode

A. A distinct period of abnormally and persistently elevated, expansive, or irritable mood, lasting at least 1 week (or any duration if hospitalization is necessary).
B. During the period of mood disturbance, three (or more) of the following symptoms have persisted (four if the mood is only irritable) and have been present to a significant degree:
(1) inflated self-esteem or grandiosity
(2) decreased need for sleep (e.g., feels rested after only 3 hours of sleep)
(3) more talkative than usual or pressure to keep talking
(4) flight of ideas or subjective experience that thoughts are racing
(5) distractibility (i.e., attention too easily drawn to unimportant or irrelevant external stimuli)
(6) increase in goal-directed activity (either socially, at work or school, or sexually) or psychomotor agitation
(7) excessive involvement in pleasurable activities that have a high potential for painful consequences (e.g., engaging in unrestrained buying sprees, sexual indiscretions, or foolish business investments)

C. The symptoms do not meet criteria for a mixed episode.
D. The mood disturbance is sufficiently severe to cause marked impairment in occupational functioning or in usual social activities or relationships with others, or to necessitate hospitalization to prevent harm to self or others, or there are psychotic features.
E. The symptoms are not due to the direct physiological effects of a substance (e.g., a drug of abuse, a medication, or other treatment) or a general medical condition (e.g., hyperthyroidism).
Note: Maniclike episodes that are clearly caused by somatic antidepressant treatment (e.g., medication, electroconvulsive therapy, light therapy) should not count toward a diagnosis of bipolar I disorder.

From American Psychiatric Association. *Diagnostic and Statistical Manual of Mental Disorders.* 4th ed. Text rev. Washington, DC: American Psychiatric Association; copyright 2000, with permission.

Learned Helplessness. The learned helplessness theory of depression connects depressive phenomena to the experience of uncontrollable events. For example, when dogs in a laboratory were exposed to electrical shocks from which they could not escape, they showed behaviors that differentiated them from dogs who had not been exposed to such uncontrollable events. The dogs exposed to the shocks would not cross a barrier to stop the flow of electric shock when put in a new learning situation. They remained passive and did not move. According to the learned helplessness theory, the shocked dogs learned that outcomes were independent of responses, so they had both cognitive motivational deficit (i.e., they would not attempt to escape the shock) and emotional deficit (indicating decreased reactivity to the shock). In the reformulated view of learned helplessness as applied to human depression, internal causal explanations are thought to produce a loss of self-esteem after adverse external events. Behaviorists who subscribe to the theory stress that improvement of depression is contingent on the patient's learning a sense of control and mastery of the environment.

DIAGNOSIS

In addition to the diagnostic criteria for major depressive disorder and bipolar disorders, DSM-IV-TR includes specific criteria for mood episodes (Tables 15.1–5 through 15.1–8) and criteria such as severity (Tables 15.1–9 through 15.1–11) to qualify the most recent episode.

Table 15.1–7
DSM-IV-TR Criteria for Hypomanic Episode

A. A distinct period of persistently elevated, expansive, or irritable mood, lasting throughout at least 4 days, that is clearly different from the usual nondepressed mood.

B. During the period of mood disturbance, three (or more) of the following symptoms have persisted (four if the mood is only irritable) and have been present to a significant degree:
 (1) inflated self-esteem or grandiosity
 (2) decreased need for sleep (e.g., feels rested after only 3 hours of sleep)
 (3) more talkative than usual or pressure to keep talking
 (4) flight of ideas or subjective experience that thoughts are racing
 (5) distractibility (i.e., attention too easily drawn to unimportant or irrelevant external stimuli)
 (6) increase in goal-directed activity (either socially, at work or school, or sexually) or psychomotor agitation
 (7) excessive involvement in pleasurable activities that have a high potential for painful consequences (e.g., the person engages in unrestrained buying sprees, sexual indiscretions, or foolish business investments)

C. The episode is associated with an unequivocal change in functioning that is uncharacteristic of the person when not symptomatic.

D. The disturbance in mood and the change in functioning are observable by others.

E. The episode is not severe enough to cause marked impairment in social or occupational functioning, or to necessitate hospitalization, and there are no psychotic features.

F. The symptoms are not due to the direct physiological effects of a substance (e.g., a drug of abuse, a medication, or other treatment) or a general medical condition (e.g., hyperthyroidism).

Note: Hypomaniclike episodes that are clearly caused by somatic antidepressant treatment (e.g., medication, electroconvulsive therapy, light therapy) should not count toward a diagnosis of bipolar II disorder.

From American Psychiatric Association. *Diagnostic and Statistical Manual of Mental Disorders.* 4th ed. Text rev. Washington, DC: American Psychiatric Association; copyright 2000, with permission.

Table 15.1–8
DSM-IV-TR Criteria for Mixed Episode

A. The criteria are met both for a manic episode and for a major depressive episode (except for duration) nearly every day during at least a 1-week period.

B. The mood disturbance is sufficiently severe to cause marked impairment in occupational functioning or in usual social activities or relationships with others, or to necessitate hospitalization to prevent harm to self or others, or there are psychotic features.

C. The symptoms are not due to the direct physiological effects of a substance (e.g., a drug of abuse, a medication, or other treatment) or a general medical condition (e.g., hyperthyroidism).

Note: Mixedlike episodes that are clearly caused by somatic antidepressant treatment (e.g., medication, electroconvulsive therapy, light therapy) should not count toward a diagnosis of bipolar I disorder.

From American Psychiatric Association. *Diagnostic and Statistical Manual of Mental Disorders.* 4th ed. Text rev. Washington, DC: American Psychiatric Association; copyright 2000, with permission.

Table 15.1–9
DSM-IV-TR Criteria for Severity/Psychotic/Remission Specifiers for Current (or Most Recent) Major Depressive Episode

Note: Code in fifth digit. Mild, moderate, severe without psychotic features, and severe with psychotic features can be applied only if the criteria are currently met for a major depressive episode. In partial remission and in full remission can be applied to the most recent major depressive episode in major depressive disorder and to a major depressive episode in bipolar I or II disorder only if it is the most recent type of mood episode.

Mild: Few, if any, symptoms in excess of those required to make the diagnosis and symptoms result in only minor impairment in occupational functioning or in usual social activities or relationships with others.

Moderate: Symptoms or functional impairment between "mild" and "severe."

Severe without psychotic features: Several symptoms in excess of those required to make the diagnosis, **and** symptoms markedly interfere with occupational functioning or with usual social activities or relationships with others.

Severe with psychotic features: Delusions or hallucinations. If possible, specify whether the psychotic features are mood-congruent or mood-incongruent:

 Mood-congruent psychotic features: Delusions or hallucinations whose content is entirely consistent with the typical depressive themes of personal inadequacy, guilt, disease, death, nihilism, or deserved punishment.

 Mood-incongruent psychotic features: Delusions or hallucinations whose content does not involve typical depressive themes of personal inadequacy, guilt, disease, death, nihilism, or deserved punishment. Included are such symptoms as persecutory delusions (not directly related to depressive themes), thought insertion, thought broadcasting, and delusions of control.

In partial remission: Symptoms of a major depressive episode are present but full criteria are not met, or there is a period without any significant symptoms of a major depressive episode lasting less than 2 months following the end of the major depressive episode. (If the major depressive episode was superimposed on dysthymic disorder, the diagnosis of dysthymic disorder alone is given once the full criteria for a major depressive episode are no longer met.)

In full remission: During the past 2 months, no significant signs or symptoms of the disturbance were present.

Unspecified.

From American Psychiatric Association. *Diagnostic and Statistical Manual of Mental Disorders.* 4th ed. Text rev. Washington, DC: American Psychiatric Association; copyright 2000, with permission.

Major Depressive Disorder

DSM-IV-TR lists the criteria for a major depressive episode separately from the diagnostic criteria for depression-related diagnoses (Table 15.1–5) and also lists severity descriptors for a major depressive episode (Table 15.1–9).

Major Depressive Disorder, Single Episode. DSM-IV-TR specifies the diagnostic criteria for the first episode of major depressive disorder (Table 15.1–12). Differentiation between these patients and those who have two or more episodes of major depressive disorder is justified because of the uncertain course of the former patients' disorder. Several studies have

Table 15.1–10
DSM-IV-TR Criteria for Severity/Psychotic/Remission Specifiers for Current (or Most Recent) Manic Episode

Note: Code in fifth digit. Mild, moderate, severe without psychotic features, and severe with psychotic features can be applied only if the criteria are currently met for a manic episode. In partial remission and in full remission can be applied to a manic episode in bipolar I disorder only if it is the most recent type of mood episode.

Mild: Minimum symptom criteria are met for a manic episode.

Moderate: Extreme increase in activity or impairment in judgment.

Severe without psychotic features: Almost continual supervision required to prevent physical harm to self or others.

Severe with psychotic features: Delusions or hallucinations. If possible, specify whether the psychotic features are mood-congruent or mood-incongruent:

- **Mood-congruent psychotic features:** Delusions or hallucinations whose content is entirely consistent with the typical manic themes of inflated worth, power, knowledge, identity, or special relationship to a deity or famous person.
- **Mood-incongruent psychotic features:** Delusions or hallucinations whose content does not involve typical manic themes of inflated worth, power, knowledge, identity, or special relationship to a deity or famous person. Included are such symptoms as persecutory delusions (not directly related to grandiose ideas or themes), thought insertion, and delusions of being controlled.

In partial remission: Symptoms of a manic episode are present but full criteria are not met, or there is a period without any significant symptoms of a manic episode lasting less than 2 months following the end of the manic episode.

In full remission: During the past 2 months no significant signs or symptoms of the disturbance were present.

Unspecified.

From American Psychiatric Association. *Diagnostic and Statistical Manual of Mental Disorders.* 4th ed. Text rev. Washington, DC: American Psychiatric Association; copyright 2000, with permission.

Table 15.1–11
DSM-IV-TR Criteria for Severity/Psychotic/Remission Specifiers for Current (or Most Recent) Mixed Episode

Note: Code in fifth digit. Mild, moderate, severe without psychotic features, and severe with psychotic features can be applied only if the criteria are currently met for a mixed episode. In partial remission and in full remission can be applied to a mixed episode in bipolar I disorder only if it is the most recent type of mood episode.

Mild: No more than minimum symptom criteria are met for both a manic episode and a major depressive episode.

Moderate: Symptoms or functional impairment between "mild" and "severe."

Severe without psychotic features: Almost continual supervision required to prevent physical harm to self or others.

Severe with psychotic features: Delusions or hallucinations. If possible, specify whether the psychotic features are mood-congruent or mood-incongruent:

- **Mood-congruent psychotic features:** Delusions or hallucinations whose content is entirely consistent with the typical manic or depressive themes.
- **Mood-incongruent psychotic features:** Delusions or hallucinations whose content does not involve typical manic or depressive themes. Included are such symptoms as persecutory delusions (not directly related to grandiose or depressive themes), thought insertion, and delusions of being controlled.

In partial remission: Symptoms of a mixed episode are present but full criteria are not met, or there is a period without any significant symptoms of a mixed episode lasting less than 2 months following the end of the mixed episode.

In full remission: During the past 2 months, no significant signs or symptoms of the disturbance were present.

Unspecified.

From American Psychiatric Association. *Diagnostic and Statistical Manual of Mental Disorders.* 4th ed. Text rev. Washington, DC: American Psychiatric Association; copyright 2000, with permission.

reported data consistent with the notion that major depression covers a heterogeneous population of disorders. One type of study assessed the stability of a diagnosis of major depression in a patient over time. The studies found that 25 to 50 percent of the patients were later reclassified as having a different psychiatric condition or a nonpsychiatric medical condition with psychiatric symptoms. A second type of study evaluated first-degree relatives of affectively ill patients to determine the presence and types of psychiatric diagnoses for these relatives over time. Both types of studies found that depressed patients with more depressive symptoms are more likely to have stable diagnoses over time and are more likely to have affectively ill relatives than are depressed patients with fewer depressive symptoms. Also, patients with bipolar I disorder and those with bipolar II disorder (recurrent major depressive episodes with hypomania) are likely to have stable diagnoses over time.

Major Depressive Disorder, Recurrent. Patients who are experiencing at least a second episode of depression are classified in DSM-IV-TR as having major depressive disorder, recurrent (Table 15.1–13). The major problem with diagnosing recurrent episodes of major depressive disorder is choosing the criteria to designate the resolution of each period. Two variables are the degree of resolution of the symptoms and the length of the resolution. DSM-IV-TR requires that distinct episodes of depression be separated by at least 2 months during which a patient has no significant symptoms of depression.

Bipolar I Disorder

DSM-IV-TR contains a separate list of criteria for a manic episode (Table 15.1–6). DSM-IV-TR requires the presence of a distinct period of abnormal mood lasting at least 1 week and includes separate bipolar I disorder diagnoses for a single manic episode and a specific type of recurrent episode, based on the symptoms of the most recent episode.

The designation bipolar I disorder is synonymous with what was formerly known as bipolar disorder—a syndrome in which a complete set of mania symptoms occurs during the course of the disorder. DSM-IV-TR has formalized the diagnostic criteria for bipolar II disorder; it is characterized by depressive episodes and hypomanic episodes (see Table 15.1–7) during the course of the disorder, but the episodes of maniclike symptoms do not quite meet the diagnostic criteria for a full manic syndrome.

Table 15.1–12
DSM-IV-TR Diagnostic Criteria for Major Depressive Disorder, Single Episode

A. Presence of a single major depressive episode.
B. The major depressive episode is not better accounted for by schizoaffective disorder and is not superimposed on schizophrenia, schizophreniform disorder, delusional disorder, or psychotic disorder not otherwise specified.
C. There has never been a manic episode, a mixed episode, or a hypomanic episode. **Note:** This exclusion does not apply if all of the maniclike, mixedlike, or hypomaniclike episodes are substance or treatment induced or are due to the direct physiological effects of a general medical condition.

If the full criteria are currently met for a major depressive episode, *specify* its current clinical status and/or features:

Mild, moderate, severe without psychotic features/severe with psychotic features
Chronic
With catatonic features
With melancholic features
With atypical features
With postpartum onset

If the full criteria are not currently met for a major depressive episode, *specify* the current clinical status of the major depressive disorder or features of the most recent episode:

In partial remission, in full remission
Chronic
With catatonic features
With melancholic features
With atypical features
With postpartum onset

From American Psychiatric Association. *Diagnostic and Statistical Manual of Mental Disorders.* 4th ed. Text rev. Washington, DC: American Psychiatric Association; copyright 2000, with permission.

Table 15.1–13
DSM-IV-TR Diagnostic Criteria for Major Depressive Disorder, Recurrent

A. Presence of two or more major depressive episodes.
Note: To be considered separate episodes, there must be an interval of at least 2 consecutive months in which criteria are not met for a major depressive episode.
B. The major depressive episodes are not better accounted for by schizoaffective disorder and are not superimposed on schizophrenia, schizophreniform disorder, delusional disorder, or psychotic disorder not otherwise specified.
C. There has never been a manic episode, a mixed episode, or a hypomanic episode. **Note:** This exclusion does not apply if all of the maniclike, mixedlike, or hypomaniclike episodes are substance or treatment induced or are due to the direct physiological effects of a general medical condition.

If the full criteria are currently met for a major depressive episode, *specify* its current clinical status and/or features:

Mild, moderate, severe without psychotic features/severe with psychotic features
Chronic
With catatonic features
With melancholic features
With atypical features
With postpartum onset

If the full criteria are not currently met for a major depressive episode, *specify* the current clinical status of the major depressive disorder or features of the most recent episode:

In partial remission, in full remission
Chronic
With catatonic features
With melancholic features
With atypical features
With postpartum onset

Specify:

Longitudinal course specifiers (with and without interepisode recovery)
With seasonal pattern

From American Psychiatric Association. *Diagnostic and Statistical Manual of Mental Disorders.* 4th ed. Text rev. Washington, DC: American Psychiatric Association; copyright 2000, with permission.

DSM-IV-TR specifically states that manic episodes clearly precipitated by antidepressant treatment (e.g., pharmacotherapy, electroconvulsive therapy [ECT]) do not indicate bipolar I disorder.

Bipolar I Disorder, Single Manic Episode. According to DSM-IV-TR, patients must be experiencing their first manic episode to meet the diagnostic criteria for bipolar I disorder, single manic episode (Table 15.1–14). This requirement rests on the fact that patients who are having their first episode of bipolar I disorder depression cannot be distinguished from patients with major depressive disorder.

Bipolar I Disorder, Recurrent. The issues about defining the end of an episode of depression also apply to defining the end of an episode of mania. In DSM-IV-TR, episodes are considered distinct when they are separated by at least 2 months without significant symptoms of mania or hypomania. DSM-IV-TR specifies diagnostic criteria for recurrent bipolar I disorder on the basis of the symptoms of the most recent episode: bipolar I disorder, most recent episode manic (Table 15.1–15); bipolar I disorder, most recent episode hypomanic (Table 15.1–16); bipolar I disorder, most recent episode depressed (Table 15.1–17); bipolar I disorder, most recent episode mixed (Table 15.1–18); and bipolar I disorder, most recent episode unspecified (Table 15.1–19).

Bipolar II Disorder

The diagnostic criteria for bipolar II disorder specify a particular severity, frequency, and duration of the hypomanic symptoms. The diagnostic criteria for a hypomanic episode (Table 15.1–7) are listed separately from the criteria for bipolar II disorder (Table 15.1–20). The criteria have been established to decrease overdiagnosis of hypomanic episodes and the incorrect classification of patients with major depressive disorder as patients with bipolar II disorder. Clinically, psychiatrists may find it difficult to distinguish euthymia from hypomania in a patient who has been chronically depressed for many months or years. As with bipolar I disorder, antidepressant-induced hypomanic episodes are not diagnostic of bipolar II disorder.

Table 15.1–14
DSM-IV-TR Diagnostic Criteria for Bipolar I Disorder, Single Manic Episode

A. Presence of only one manic episode and no past major depressive episodes.
   Note: Recurrence is defined as either a change in polarity from depression or an interval of at least 2 months without manic symptoms.

B. The manic episode is not better accounted for by schizoaffective disorder and is not superimposed on schizophrenia, schizophreniform disorder, delusional disorder, or psychotic disorder not otherwise specified.

Specify if:
   Mixed: if symptoms meet criteria for a mixed episode

If the full criteria are currently met for a manic, mixed, or major depressive episode, *specify* its current clinical status and/or features:
   Mild, moderate, severe without psychotic features/severe with psychotic features
   With catatonic features
   With postpartum onset

If the full criteria are not currently met for a manic, mixed, or major depressive episode, *specify* the current clinical status of the bipolar I disorder or features of the most recent episode:
   In partial remission, in full remission
   With catatonic features
   With postpartum onset

From American Psychiatric Association. *Diagnostic and Statistical Manual of Mental Disorders.* 4th ed. Text rev. Washington, DC: American Psychiatric Association; copyright 2000, with permission.

Table 15.1–15
DSM-IV-TR Diagnostic Criteria for Bipolar I Disorder, Most Recent Episode Manic

A. Currently (or most recently) in a manic episode.

B. There has previously been at least one major depressive episode, manic episode, or mixed episode.

C. The mood episodes in Criteria A and B are not better accounted for by schizoaffective disorder and are not superimposed on schizophrenia, schizophreniform disorder, delusional disorder, or psychotic disorder not otherwise specified.

If the full criteria are currently met for a manic episode, *specify* its current clinical status and/or features:
   Mild, moderate, severe without psychotic features/severe with psychotic features
   With catatonic features
   With postpartum onset

If the full criteria are not currently met for a manic episode, *specify* the current clinical status of the bipolar I disorder and/or features of the most recent manic episode:
   In partial remission, in full remission
   With catatonic features
   With postpartum onset

Specify:
   Longitudinal course specifiers (with and without interepisode recovery)
   With seasonal pattern (applies only to the pattern of major depressive episodes)
   With rapid cycling

From American Psychiatric Association. *Diagnostic and Statistical Manual of Mental Disorders.* 4th ed. Text rev. Washington, DC: American Psychiatric Association; copyright 2000, with permission.

Specifiers Describing Most Recent Episode

In addition to the severity/psychotic/remission specifiers (Tables 15.1–9 through 15.1–11), DSM-IV-TR defines additional symptom features that can be used to describe patients with various mood disorders. Two of the cross-sectional features (melancholic and atypical) are limited to describing depressive episodes. Two others (catatonic features and with postpartum onset) can be applied to depressive and manic episodes.

With Psychotic Features. The presence of psychotic features (Table 15.1–9) in major depressive disorder reflects severe disease and is a poor prognostic indicator. A review of the literature comparing psychotic with nonpsychotic major depressive disorder indicates that the two conditions may be distinct in their pathogenesis. One difference is that bipolar I disorder is more common in the families of probands with psychotic depression than in the families of probands with nonpsychotic depression.

The psychotic symptoms themselves are often categorized as either mood congruent, that is, in harmony with the mood disorder ("I deserve to be punished because I am so bad"), or mood incongruent, not in harmony with the mood disorder. Mood disorder patients with mood-congruent psychoses have a psychotic type of mood disorder; however, mood disorder patients with mood-incongruent psychotic symptoms may have schizoaffective disorder or schizophrenia.

The following factors have been associated with a poor prognosis for patients with mood disorders: long duration of episodes, temporal dissociation between the mood disorder

Table 15.1–16
DSM-IV-TR Diagnostic Criteria for Bipolar I Disorder, Most Recent Episode Hypomanic

A. Currently (or most recently) in a hypomanic episode.

B. There has previously been at least one manic episode or mixed episode.

C. The mood symptoms cause clinically significant distress or impairment in social, occupational, or other important areas of functioning.

D. The mood episodes in Criteria A and B are not better accounted for by schizoaffective disorder and are not superimposed on schizophrenia, schizophreniform disorder, delusional disorder, or psychotic disorder not otherwise specified.

Specify:
   Longitudinal course specifiers (with and without interepisode recovery)
   With seasonal pattern (applies only to the pattern of major depressive episodes)
   With rapid cycling

From American Psychiatric Association. *Diagnostic and Statistical Manual of Mental Disorders.* 4th ed. Text rev. Washington, DC: American Psychiatric Association; copyright 2000, with permission.

Table 15.1–17
DSM-IV-TR Diagnostic Criteria for Bipolar I Disorder, Most Recent Episode Depressed

A. Currently (or most recently) in a major depressive episode.
B. There has previously been at least one manic episode or mixed episode.
C. The mood episodes in Criteria A and B are not better accounted for by schizoaffective disorder and are not superimposed on schizophrenia, schizophreniform disorder, delusional disorder, or psychotic disorder not otherwise specified.

If the full criteria are currently met for a major depressive episode, *specify* its current clinical status and/or features:

Mild, moderate, severe without psychotic features/severe with psychotic features
Chronic
With catatonic features
With melancholic features
With atypical features
With postpartum onset

If the full criteria are not currently met for a major depressive episode, *specify* the current clinical status of the bipolar I disorder and/or features of the most recent major depressive episode:

In partial remission, in full remission
Chronic
With catatonic features
With melancholic features
With atypical features
With postpartum onset

Specify:

Longitudinal course specifiers (with and without interepisode recovery)
With seasonal pattern (applies only to the pattern of major depressive episodes)
With rapid cycling

From American Psychiatric Association. *Diagnostic and Statistical Manual of Mental Disorders.* 4th ed. Text rev. Washington, DC: American Psychiatric Association; copyright 2000, with permission.

and the psychotic symptoms, and a poor premorbid history of social adjustment. The presence of psychotic features also has significant treatment implications. These patients typically require antipsychotic drugs in addition to antidepressants or mood stabilizers and may need ECT to obtain clinical improvement.

With Melancholic Features. *Melancholia* is one of the oldest terms used in psychiatry, dating back to Hippocrates in the 4th century to describe the dark mood of depression. It is still used to refer to a depression characterized by severe anhedonia, early morning awakening, weight loss, and profound feelings of guilt (often over trivial events). It is not uncommon for melancholic patients to have suicidal ideation. Melancholia is associated with change in the autonomic nervous system and in endocrine functions. For that reason melancholia is sometimes referred to as "endogenous depression" or depression that arises in the absence of external life stressors or precipitants. The DSM-IV-TR melancholic features can be applied to major depressive episodes in major

Table 15.1–18
DSM-IV-TR Diagnostic Criteria for Bipolar I Disorder, Most Recent Episode Mixed

A. Currently (or most recently) in a mixed episode.
B. There has previously been at least one major depressive episode, manic episode, or mixed episode.
C. The mood episodes in Criteria A and B are not better accounted for by schizoaffective disorder and are not superimposed on schizophrenia, schizophreniform disorder, delusional disorder, or psychotic disorder not otherwise specified.

If the full criteria are currently met for a mixed episode, *specify* its current clinical status and/or features:

Mild, moderate, severe without psychotic features/severe with psychotic features
With catatonic features
With postpartum onset

If the full criteria are not currently met for a mixed episode, *specify* the current clinical status of the bipolar I disorder and/or features of the most recent mixed episode:

In partial remission, in full remission
With catatonic features
With postpartum onset

Specify:

Longitudinal course specifiers (with and without interepisode recovery)
With seasonal pattern (applies only to the pattern of major depressive episodes)
With rapid cycling

From American Psychiatric Association. *Diagnostic and Statistical Manual of Mental Disorders.* 4th ed. Text rev. Washington, DC: American Psychiatric Association; copyright 2000, with permission.

Table 15.1–19
DSM-IV-TR Diagnostic Criteria for Bipolar I Disorder, Most Recent Episode Unspecified

A. Criteria, except for duration, are currently (or most recently) met for a manic, a hypomanic, a mixed, or a major depressive episode.
B. There has previously been at least one manic episode or mixed episode.
C. The mood symptoms cause clinically significant distress or impairment in social, occupational, or other important areas of functioning.
D. The mood symptoms in Criteria A and B are not better accounted for by schizoaffective disorder and are not superimposed on schizophrenia, schizophreniform disorder, delusional disorder, or psychotic disorder not otherwise specified.
E. The mood symptoms in Criteria A and B are not due to the direct physiological effects of a substance (e.g., a drug of abuse, a medication, or other treatment) or a general medical condition (e.g., hyperthyroidism).

Specify:

Longitudinal course specifiers (with and without interepisode recovery)
With seasonal pattern (applies only to the pattern of major depressive episodes)
With rapid cycling

From American Psychiatric Association. *Diagnostic and Statistical Manual of Mental Disorders.* 4th ed. Text rev. Washington, DC: American Psychiatric Association; copyright 2000, with permission.

Table 15.1–20
DSM-IV-TR Diagnostic Criteria for Bipolar II Disorder

A. Presence (or history) of one or more major depressive episodes.
B. Presence (or history) of at least one hypomanic episode.
C. There has never been a manic episode or a mixed episode.
D. The mood symptoms in Criteria A and B are not better accounted for by schizoaffective disorder and are not superimposed on schizophrenia, schizophreniform disorder, delusional disorder, or psychotic disorder not otherwise specified.
E. The symptoms cause clinically significant distress or impairment in social, occupational, or other important areas of functioning.

Specify current or most recent episode:

Hypomanic: if currently (or most recently) in a hypomanic episode

Depressed: if currently (or most recently) in a major depressive episode

If the full criteria are currently met for a major depressive episode, *specify* its current clinical status and/or features:

Mild, moderate, severe without psychotic features/severe with psychotic features. Note: Fifth-digit codes cannot be used here because the code for bipolar II disorder already uses the fifth digit.

Chronic

With catatonic features

With melancholic features

With atypical features

With postpartum onset

If the full criteria are not currently met for a hypomanic or major depressive episode, *specify* the clinical status of the bipolar II disorder and/or features of the most recent major depressive episode (only if it is the most recent type of mood episode):

In partial remission, in full remission. Note: Fifth-digit codes cannot be used here because the code for bipolar II disorder already uses the fifth digit.

Chronic

With catatonic features

With melancholic features

With atypical features

With postpartum onset

Specify:

Longitudinal course specifiers (with and without interepisode recovery)

With seasonal pattern (applies only to the pattern of major depressive episodes)

With rapid cycling

From American Psychiatric Association. *Diagnostic and Statistical Manual of Mental Disorders.* 4th ed. Text rev. Washington, DC: American Psychiatric Association; copyright 2000, with permission.

depressive disorder, bipolar I disorder, or bipolar II disorder (Table 15.1–21).

Table 15.1–21
DSM-IV-TR Criteria for Melancholic Features Specifier

Specify if:

With melancholic features (can be applied to the current or most recent major depressive episode in major depressive disorder and to a major depressive episode in bipolar I or bipolar II disorder only if it is the most recent type of mood episode)

A. Either of the following, occurring during the most severe period of the current episode:
   (1) loss of pleasure in all, or almost all, activities
   (2) lack of reactivity to usually pleasurable stimuli (does not feel much better, even temporarily, when something good happens)
B. Three (or more) of the following:
   (1) distinct quality of depressed mood (i.e., the depressed mood is experienced as distinctly different from the kind of feeling experienced after the death of a loved one)
   (2) depression regularly worse in the morning
   (3) early morning awakening (at least 2 hours before usual time of awakening)
   (4) marked psychomotor retardation or agitation
   (5) significant anorexia or weight loss
   (6) excessive or inappropriate guilt

From American Psychiatric Association. *Diagnostic and Statistical Manual of Mental Disorders.* 4th ed. Text rev. Washington, DC: American Psychiatric Association; copyright 2000, with permission.

With Atypical Features. The introduction of a formally defined depression with atypical features is a response to research and clinical data indicating that patients with atypical features have specific, predictable characteristics: overeating and oversleeping. These symptoms have sometimes been referred to as reversed vegetative symptoms, and the symptom pattern has sometimes been referred to as hysteroid dysphoria. When patients with major depressive disorder with these features are compared with patients without the features, the patients with atypical features are found to have a younger age of onset, more severe psychomotor slowing, and more frequent coexisting diagnoses of panic disorder, substance abuse or dependence, and somatization disorder. The high incidence and severity of anxiety symptoms in patients with atypical features have been correlated in some research with the likelihood of their being misclassified as having an anxiety disorder rather than a mood disorder. Patients with atypical features may also be likely to have a long-term course, a diagnosis of bipolar I disorder, or a seasonal pattern to their disorder. The major treatment implication of patients with atypical features is that they are more likely to respond to monoamine oxidase inhibitors (MAOIs) than to tricyclic drugs.

Yet the significance of atypical features remains controversial, as does the preferential treatment response to MAOIs. Moreover, the absence of specific diagnostic criteria has limited researchers' ability to assess the criteria's validity and the disorder's prevalence and to ascertain the existence of any other biological or psychological factors that may differentiate it from other symptom patterns.

The DSM-IV-TR atypical features can be applied to the most recent major depressive episode in major depressive disorder, bipolar I disorder, bipolar II disorder, or dysthymic disorder (Table 15.1–22).

Table 15.1–22
DSM-IV-TR Criteria for Atypical Features Specifier

Specify if:

With atypical features (can be applied when these features predominate during the most recent 2 weeks of a current major depressive episode in major depressive disorder or in bipolar I or bipolar II disorder when a current major depressive episode is the most recent type of mood episode, or when these features predominate during the most recent 2 years of dysthymic disorder; if the major depressive episode is not current, it applies if the feature predominates during any 2-week period)

A. Mood reactivity (i.e., mood brightens in response to actual or potential positive events)

B. Two (or more) of the following features:

(1) significant weight gain or increase in appetite
(2) hypersomnia
(3) leaden paralysis (i.e., heavy, leaden feelings in arms or legs)
(4) long-standing pattern of interpersonal rejection sensitivity (not limited to episodes of mood disturbance) that results in significant social or occupational impairment

C. Criteria are not met for with melancholic features or with catatonic features during the same episode.

From American Psychiatric Association. *Diagnostic and Statistical Manual of Mental Disorders.* 4th ed. Text rev. Washington, DC: American Psychiatric Association; copyright 2000, with permission.

Ms. G. is a 17-year-old high school senior who is referred for evaluation after she attempted suicide with an overdose of pills. Earlier on the night of the suicide attempt, she had a fight with her mother over a request to order pizza. The patient remembers her mother saying that she was a "spoiled brat" and asking whether she would be happier living elsewhere. The patient, feeling rejected and despondent, went to her room and wrote a note saying that she was having a mental breakdown and that she loved her parents but could not communicate with them. She added a request that her favorite glass animals be given to a particular friend. The parents, who had gone out to a movie, returned home later that evening to find their daughter comatose and immediately rushed her to the hospital emergency room.

During the last couple of months, Ms. G. has been crying frequently and has lost interest in her friends, school, and social activities. She has been eating more and more and has recently begun to gain weight, which her mother is very unhappy about. Ms. G. says that her mother is always harping about "taking care of herself," and in fact, the argument on the night of her suicide attempt was about Ms. G.'s desire to order a pizza that her mother did not think she needed. Ms. G.'s mother reports that all her daughter seems to want to do is sleep and that she never wants to go out with her friends or help around the house. When questioned about changes in her sleep habits, Ms. G. admits that she has been feeling very tired lately and that she often feels as if there is nothing to make it worth getting out of bed. She does mention that she is excited about an upcoming visit from her boyfriend, who attends a college a considerable distance away and has not been home for several months.

Upon evaluation, it is apparent that this teenager, the third of three children of upper-middle-class and very intelligent parents, is struggling with a view of herself as less bright, clever, and attractive than her two siblings. She feels ignored and essentially rejected by her seemingly omnipresent mother. The daughter is having difficulty developing a sense of separation from her mother and an image of her individual identity. She experienced her mother's directives as interference with her efforts to express autonomy and independence. (From *DSM-IV Case Studies.*)

With Catatonic Features. The decision to include a specific classification for catatonic features (Table 15.1–23) in the mood disorders category was motivated by two factors. First, because the authors intended DSM-IV-TR to serve as a guide in the differential diagnosis of mental disorders, the inclusion of a specifically catatonic type of mood disorder helps balance the presence of a catatonic type of schizophrenia. As a symptom, catatonia can be present in several mental disorders, most commonly, schizophrenia and the mood disorders. Second, although as yet incompletely studied, the presence of catatonic features in patients with mood disorders will probably be shown to have prognostic and treatment significance.

The hallmark symptoms of catatonia—stuporousness, blunted affect, extreme withdrawal, negativism, and marked psychomotor retardation—can be seen in both catatonic and noncatatonic schizophrenia, major depressive disorder (often with psychotic features), and medical and neurological disorders, but catatonic symptoms are probably most commonly associated with bipolar I disorder. Clinicians often do not asso-

Table 15.1–23
DSM-IV-TR Criteria for Catatonic Features Specifier

Specify if:

With catatonic features (can be applied to the current or most recent major depressive episode, manic episode, or mixed episode in major depressive disorder, bipolar I disorder, or bipolar II disorder)

The clinical picture is dominated by at least two of the following:

(1) motoric immobility as evidenced by catalepsy (including waxy flexibility) or stupor
(2) excessive motor activity (that is apparently purposeless and not influenced by external stimuli)
(3) extreme negativism (an apparently motiveless resistance to all instructions or maintenance of a rigid posture against attempts to be moved) or mutism
(4) peculiarities of voluntary movement as evidenced by posturing (voluntary assumption of inappropriate or bizarre postures), stereotyped movements, prominent mannerisms, or prominent grimacing
(5) echolalia or echopraxia

From American Psychiatric Association. *Diagnostic and Statistical Manual of Mental Disorders.* 4th ed. Text rev. Washington, DC: American Psychiatric Association; copyright 2000, with permission.

Table 15.1–24
DSM-IV-TR Criteria for Postpartum Onset Specifier

Specify if:

With postpartum onset (can be applied to the current or most recent major depressive, manic, or mixed episode in major depressive disorder, bipolar I disorder, or bipolar II disorder; or to brief psychotic disorder)

Onset of episode within 4 weeks postpartum

From American Psychiatric Association. *Diagnostic and Statistical Manual of Mental Disorders.* 4th ed. Text rev. Washington, DC: American Psychiatric Association; copyright 2000, with permission.

ciate catatonic symptoms with this disorder because of the marked contrast between the symptoms of stuporous catatonia and the classic symptoms of mania. Because catatonic symptoms are a behavioral syndrome appearing in several medical and psychiatric conditions, catatonic symptoms do not imply a single diagnosis. In DSM-IV-TR, catatonic features can be applied to the most recent manic episode or major depressive episode in major depressive disorder, bipolar I disorder, or bipolar II disorder.

Postpartum Onset. DSM-IV-TR allows the specification of a postpartum mood disturbance if the onset of symptoms is within 4 weeks postpartum (Table 15.1–24). Postpartum mental disorders commonly include psychotic symptoms. (Postpartum psychosis is discussed in Section 14.4.)

Chronic. DSM-IV-TR allows the specification of chronic to describe major depressive episodes that occur as a part of major depressive disorder, bipolar I disorder, and bipolar II disorder (Table 15.1–25).

Describing Course of Recurrent Episodes

DSM-IV-TR includes criteria for three distinct course specifiers for mood disorders. One of the course specifiers, with rapid cycling (Table 15.1–26), is restricted to bipolar I disorder and bipolar II disorder. Two other course specifiers, with seasonal pattern (Table 15.1–27) and with or without full interepisode recovery (Table 15.1–28), can be applied to bipolar I disorder, bipolar II disorder, and major depressive disorder, recurrent.

Table 15.1–25
DSM-IV-TR Criteria for Chronic Specifier

Specify if:

Chronic (can be applied to the current or most recent major depressive episode in major depressive disorder and to a major depressive episode in bipolar I or II disorder only if it is the most recent type of mood episode)

Full criteria for a major depressive episode have been met continuously for at least the past 2 years.

From American Psychiatric Association. *Diagnostic and Statistical Manual of Mental Disorders.* 4th ed. Text rev. Washington, DC: American Psychiatric Association; copyright 2000, with permission.

Table 15.1–26
DSM-IV-TR Criteria for Rapid-Cycling Specifier

Specify if:

With rapid cycling (can be applied to bipolar I disorder or bipolar II disorder)

At least four episodes of a mood disturbance in the previous 12 months that meet criteria for a major depressive, manic, mixed, or hypomanic episode.

Note: Episodes are demarcated either by partial or full remission for at least 2 months or a switch to an episode of opposite polarity (e.g., major depressive episode to manic episode).

From American Psychiatric Association. *Diagnostic and Statistical Manual of Mental Disorders.* 4th ed. Text rev. Washington, DC: American Psychiatric Association; copyright 2000, with permission.

The course specifier with postpartum onset can be applied to major depressive or manic episodes in bipolar I disorder, bipolar II disorder, major depressive disorder, and brief psychotic disorder.

Rapid Cycling. Patients with rapid cycling bipolar I disorder are likely to be female and to have had depressive and hypomanic episodes. No data indicate that rapid cycling has a familial pattern of inheritance, and thus an external factor such as stress or drug treatment may be involved in the pathogenesis of rapid cycling. The DSM-IV-TR criteria specify that the patient must have at least four episodes within a 12-month period (Table 15.1–26).

Table 15.1–27
DSM-IV-TR Criteria for Seasonal Pattern Specifier

Specify if:

With seasonal pattern (can be applied to the pattern of major depressive episodes in bipolar I disorder, bipolar II disorder, or major depressive disorder, recurrent)

A. There has been a regular temporal relationship between the onset of major depressive episodes in bipolar I or bipolar II disorder or major depressive disorder, recurrent, and a particular time of the year (e.g., regular appearance of the major depressive episode in the fall or winter).

Note: Do not include cases in which there is an obvious effect of seasonal-related psychosocial stressors (e.g., regularly being unemployed every winter).

B. Full remissions (or a change from depression to mania or hypomania) also occur at a characteristic time of the year (e.g., depression disappears in the spring).

C. In the last 2 years, two major depressive episodes have occurred that demonstrate the temporal seasonal relationships defined in Criteria A and B, and no nonseasonal major depressive episodes have occurred during that same period.

D. Seasonal major depressive episodes (as described above) substantially outnumber the nonseasonal major depressive episodes that may have occurred over the individual's lifetime.

From American Psychiatric Association. *Diagnostic and Statistical Manual of Mental Disorders.* 4th ed. Text rev. Washington, DC: American Psychiatric Association; copyright 2000, with permission.

Table 15.1–28
DSM-IV-TR Criteria for Longitudinal Course Specifiers

Specify if (can be applied to recurrent major depressive disorder or bipolar I or II disorder):

With full interepisode recovery: if full remission is attained between the two most recent mood episodes

Without full interepisode recovery: if full remission is not attained between the two most recent mood episodes

From American Psychiatric Association. *Diagnostic and Statistical Manual of Mental Disorders.* 4th ed. Text rev. Washington, DC: American Psychiatric Association; copyright 2000, with permission.

When Mr. E.'s desperate wife finally got him to agree to a comprehensive inpatient evaluation, he was 37, was unemployed, and had been essentially nonfunctional for several years. After a week during which he was partying all night and shopping all day, Mrs. E. said that she would leave him if he did not check into a psychiatric hospital. The admitting psychiatrist found him to be a fast-talking, jovial, seductive man with no evidence of delusions or hallucinations.

Mr. E.'s troubles began 7 years before when he was working as an insurance adjuster and had a few months of mild, intermittent, depressive symptoms, anxiety, fatigue, insomnia, and loss of appetite. At the time, he attributed these symptoms to stress at work, and within a few months was back to his usual self.

A few years later an asymptomatic thyroid mass was noted during a routine physical examination. One month after removal of the mass, a papillary cyst, Mr. E. noted dramatic mood changes. Twenty-five days of remarkable energy, hyperactivity, and euphoria were followed by 5 days of depression during which he slept a lot and felt that he could hardly move. This pattern of alternating periods of elation and depression, apparently with few "normal" days, repeated itself continuously over the following years.

During his energetic periods, Mr. E. was optimistic and self-confident, but short tempered and easily irritated. His judgment at work was erratic. He spent large sums of money on unnecessary and, for him, uncharacteristic purchases, such as a high-priced stereo system and several Doberman pinschers. He also had several impulsive sexual flings.

During his depressed periods, he often stayed in bed all day because of fatigue, lack of motivation, and depressed mood. He felt guilty about the irresponsibilities and excesses of the previous several weeks. He stopped eating, bathing, and shaving. After several days of this withdrawal, Mr. E. would rise from bed one morning feeling better and, within 2 days, be back at work, often working feverishly, though ineffectively, to catch up on work he had let slide during his depressed periods.

Although both he and his wife denied any drug use, other than drinking binges during his hyperactive periods, Mr. E. had been dismissed from his job 5 years previously because his supervisor was convinced that his overactivity must be due to drug use. His wife had supported him since then.

When he finally agreed to a psychiatric evaluation 2 years ago, Mr. E. was minimally cooperative and noncompliant with several medications that were prescribed, including lithium, neuroleptics, and antidepressants. His mood swings had continued with few interruptions up to the current hospitalization.

In the hospital results of his physical examination, blood chemistry, blood counts, computed tomography scan, and cognitive testing were unremarkable. Thyroid function testing revealed some laboratory evidence of thyroid hypofunction, but he was without clinical signs of thyroid disease. After a week he switched to his characteristic depressive state.

DISCUSSION

The diagnosis of bipolar I disorder, most recent episode manic, is not difficult to make in this case. In his energetic periods, Mr. E. had the characteristic symptoms of a manic episode: decreased need for sleep, overactivity, overtalkativeness, and excessive involvement in pleasurable activities without thinking of the consequences. In his depressed periods, he met the symptom, but not the duration, criteria for major depressive episode. Because he had had more than four episodes of mania in a 1-year period, separated by periods of depression, the bipolar I disorder is further qualified as rapid cycling.

Unlike Mr. E., not all persons with rapid cycling experience predictable shifts from mania to depression without intervening periods of euthymia. Rapid cycling usually involves one or more manic or hypomanic episodes, as in this case, but is also diagnosed if all of the episodes are depressed, manic, or hypomanic as long as they are separated by periods of remission (or switches to the opposite pole).

As noted previously, Mr. E.'s unusual behavior was attributed by his employers to drug use. It is not uncommon for such an erratic mood pattern to be mistakenly identified as evidence of drug abuse, which should also be part of the differential diagnosis when rapid cycling is being considered. Mr. E. is somewhat atypical among persons with rapid cycling in that the condition is much more common in women. The onset of his symptoms closely followed partial thyroidectomy, and he was found to have evidence of mild thyroid hypofunction. Thyroid disease has been reported in some studies to be a risk factor for rapid cycling. An additional risk factor, of unclear significance in this case, is the use of antidepressant medication. Because of high rates of nonresponse to lithium, rapid cycling is often treated with anticonvulsants.

FOLLOW-UP

After 3 weeks in the hospital, Mr. E.'s mood was stable on lithium and thyroxine, the latter being added for mood stabilization rather than to treat the laboratory evidence of thyroid hypofunction. He left the hospital, very quickly found a new job, and did well for the following year. Feeling well, he decided that he didn't need the medication and stopped taking the lithium. Within weeks he became extremely manic and had to be hospitalized again. (From *DSM-IV Casebook.*)

Seasonal Pattern. Patients with a seasonal pattern to their mood disorders tend to experience depressive episodes during a particular season, most commonly winter. The pattern has become known as seasonal affective disorder (SAD), although this term is not used in DSM-IV-TR (Table 15.1–27). Two types of evidence indicate that the seasonal pattern may represent a separate diagnostic entity. First, the patients are likely to respond to treatment with light therapy, although no adequate studies to evaluate light therapy in non–seasonally depressed patients have been conducted. Second, one PET study showed that patients show decreased metabolic activity in the orbital frontal cortex and in the left inferior parietal lobule. Future studies will probably focus on differentiating depressed persons with seasonal pattern from other depressed persons.

Longitudinal Course Specifiers. DSM-IV-TR includes specific descriptions of longitudinal courses for major depressive disorder, bipolar I disorder, and bipolar II disorder (Table 15.1–28). These longitudinal course specifiers allow clinicians and researchers to prospectively identify any treatment or prognostic significance in various longitudinal courses. Although preliminary studies of the DSM-IV-TR longitudinal course specifiers indicate that clinicians can assess the longitudinal course, more and larger studies are needed to develop a solid appreciation of the assessment and implications of variations in the longitudinal course.

Non–DSM-IV-TR Types. Other systems that identify types of patients with mood disorders usually separate patients with good and poor prognoses or patients who may respond to one treatment or another. They also differentiate endogenous-reactive and primary-secondary schemes.

The endogenous-reactive continuum is a controversial division. It implies that endogenous depressions are biological and that reactive depressions are psychological, primarily on the basis of the presence or absence of an identifiable precipitating stress. Other symptoms of endogenous depression have been described as diurnal variation, delusions, psychomotor retardation, early morning awakening, and feelings of guilt; thus, endogenous depression is similar to the DSM-IV-TR diagnosis of major depressive disorder with psychotic features or melancholic features or both. Symptoms of reactive depression have been described as including initial insomnia, anxiety, emotional lability, and multiple somatic complaints.

Primary depressions are what DSM-IV-TR refers to as mood disorders, except for the diagnoses of mood disorder caused by a general medical condition and substance-induced mood disorder, which are considered secondary depressions. Double depression is the condition in which major depressive disorder is superimposed on dysthymic disorder. A depressive equivalent is a symptom or syndrome that may be a *forme fruste* of a depressive episode. For example, a triad of truancy, alcohol abuse, and sexual promiscuity in a formerly well-behaved adolescent may constitute a depressive equivalent.

CLINICAL FEATURES

The two basic symptom patterns in mood disorders are depression and mania. Depressive episodes can occur in both major depressive disorder and bipolar I disorder. In many studies, researchers have attempted to find reliable differences between bipolar I disorder depressive episodes and episodes of major depressive disorder, but the differences are elusive. In a clinical situation, only the patient's history, family history, and future course can help differentiate the two conditions. Some patients with bipolar I disorder have mixed states with both manic and depressive features, and some seem to experience brief—minutes to a few hours—episodes of depression during manic episodes.

Depressive Episodes

A depressed mood and a loss of interest or pleasure are the key symptoms of depression. Patients may say that they feel blue, hopeless, in the dumps, or worthless. For a patient, the depressed mood often has a distinct quality that differentiates it from the normal emotion of sadness or grief. Patients often describe the symptom of depression as one of agonizing emotional pain and sometimes complain about being unable to cry, a symptom that resolves as they improve.

About two thirds of all depressed patients contemplate suicide, and 10 to 15 percent commit suicide. Those recently hospitalized with a suicide attempt or suicidal ideation have a higher lifetime risk of successful suicide than those never hospitalized. Some depressed patients sometimes seem unaware of their depression and do not complain of a mood disturbance, even though they exhibit withdrawal from family, friends, and activities that previously interested them. Almost all depressed patients (97 percent) complain about reduced energy; they have difficulty finishing tasks, are impaired at school and work, and have less motivation to undertake new projects. About 80 percent of patients complain of trouble sleeping, especially early morning awakening (i.e., terminal insomnia) and multiple awakenings at night, during which they ruminate about their problems. Many patients have decreased appetite and weight loss, but others experience increased appetite and weight gain and sleep longer than usual. These patients are classified in DSM-IV-TR as having atypical features.

Anxiety is a common symptom of depression and affects as many as 90 percent of all depressed patients. The various changes in food intake and rest can aggravate coexisting medical illnesses such as diabetes, hypertension, chronic obstructive lung disease, and heart disease. Other vegetative symptoms include abnormal menses and decreased interest and performance in sexual activities. Sexual problems can sometimes lead to inappropriate referrals, such as to marital counseling and sex therapy, when clinicians fail to recognize the underlying depressive disorder. Anxiety (including panic attacks), alcohol abuse, and somatic complaints (e.g., constipation and headaches) often complicate the treatment of depression. About 50 percent of all patients describe a diurnal variation in their symptoms, with increased severity in the morning and lessening of symptoms by evening. Cognitive symptoms include subjective reports of an inability to concentrate (84 percent of patients in one study) and impairments in thinking (67 percent of patients in another study).

Depression in Children and Adolescents. School phobia and excessive clinging to parents may be symptoms of depression in children. Poor academic performance, substance abuse, antisocial behavior, sexual promiscuity, truancy, and

running away may be symptoms of depression in adolescents. (This subject is further discussed in Chapter 49.)

Depression in Older People. Depression is more common in older persons than it is in the general population. Various studies have reported prevalence rates ranging from 25 to almost 50 percent, although the percentage of these cases that are caused by major depressive disorder is uncertain. Several studies have reported data indicating that depression in older persons may be correlated with low socioeconomic status, the loss of a spouse, a concurrent physical illness, and social isolation. Other studies have indicated that depression in older persons is underdiagnosed and undertreated, perhaps particularly by general practitioners. The underrecognition of depression in older persons may occur because the disorder appears more often with somatic complaints in older, than in younger, age groups. Further, ageism may influence and cause clinicians to accept depressive symptoms as normal in older patients.

Manic Episodes

An elevated, expansive, or irritable mood is the hallmark of a manic episode. The elevated mood is euphoric and often infectious and can even cause a countertransferential denial of illness by an inexperienced clinician. Although uninvolved persons may not recognize the unusual nature of a patient's mood, those who know the patient recognize it as abnormal. Alternatively, the mood may be irritable, especially when a patient's overtly ambitious plans are thwarted. Patients often exhibit a change of predominant mood from euphoria early in the course of the illness to later irritability.

The treatment of manic patients in an inpatient ward can be complicated by their testing of the limits of ward rules, their tendency to shift responsibility for their acts onto others, their exploitation of the weaknesses of others, and their propensity to create conflicts among staff members. Outside the hospital, manic patients often drink alcohol excessively, perhaps in an attempt to self-medicate. Their disinhibited nature is reflected in excessive use of the telephone, especially in making long-distance calls during the early morning hours.

Pathological gambling, a tendency to disrobe in public places, wearing clothing and jewelry of bright colors in unusual or outlandish combinations, and inattention to small details (e.g., forgetting to hang up the telephone) are also symptomatic of the disorder. Patients act impulsively and at the same time with a sense of conviction and purpose. They are often preoccupied by religious, political, financial, sexual, or persecutory ideas that can evolve into complex delusional systems. Occasionally, manic patients become regressed and play with their urine and feces.

Mania in Adolescents. Mania in adolescents is often misdiagnosed as antisocial personality disorder or schizophrenia. Symptoms of mania in adolescents may include psychosis, alcohol or other substance abuse, suicide attempts, academic problems, philosophical brooding, obsessive-compulsive disorder symptoms, multiple somatic complaints, marked irritability resulting in fights, and other antisocial behaviors. Although many of these symptoms are seen in normal adolescents, severe or persistent symptoms should cause clinicians to consider bipolar I disorder in the differential diagnosis.

Bipolar II Disorder

The clinical features of bipolar II disorder are those of major depressive disorder combined with those of a hypomanic episode. Although the data are limited, a few studies indicate that bipolar II disorder is associated with more marital disruption and with onset at an earlier age than bipolar I disorder. Evidence also indicates that patients with bipolar II disorder are at greater risk of both attempting and completing suicide than patients with bipolar I disorder and major depressive disorder.

Coexisting Disorders

Anxiety. In the anxiety disorders, DSM-IV-TR notes the existence of mixed anxiety-depressive disorder. Significant symptoms of anxiety can and often do coexist with significant symptoms of depression. Whether patients who exhibit significant symptoms of both anxiety and depression are affected by two distinct disease processes or by a single disease process that produces both sets of symptoms is not yet resolved. Patients of both types may constitute the group of patients with mixed anxiety-depressive disorder.

Alcohol Dependence. Alcohol dependence frequently coexists with mood disorders. Both patients with major depressive disorder and those with bipolar I disorder are likely to meet the diagnostic criteria for an alcohol use disorder. The available data indicate that alcohol dependence is more strongly associated with a coexisting diagnosis of depression in women than in men. In contrast, the genetic and family data about men who have both a mood disorder and alcohol dependence indicate that they are likely to be suffering from two genetically distinct disease processes.

Other Substance-Related Disorders. Substance-related disorders other than alcohol dependence are also commonly associated with mood disorders. The abuse of substances may be involved in precipitating an episode of illness or, conversely, may represent patients' attempts to treat their own illnesses. Although manic patients seldom use sedatives to dampen their euphoria, depressed patients often use stimulants, such as cocaine and amphetamines, to relieve their depression.

Medical Conditions. Depression commonly coexists with medical conditions, especially in older persons. When depression and medical conditions coexist, clinicians must try to determine whether the underlying medical condition is pathophysiologically related to the depression or whether any drugs that the patient is taking for the medical condition are causing the depression. Many studies indicate that treatment of a coexisting major depressive disorder can improve the course of the underlying medical disorder, including cancer.

MENTAL STATUS EXAMINATION

Depressive Episodes

General Description. Generalized psychomotor retardation is the most common symptom, although psychomotor agitation is also seen, especially in older patients. Hand wringing and hair pulling are the most common symptoms of agitation. Classically, a depressed patient has a stooped posture, no spon-

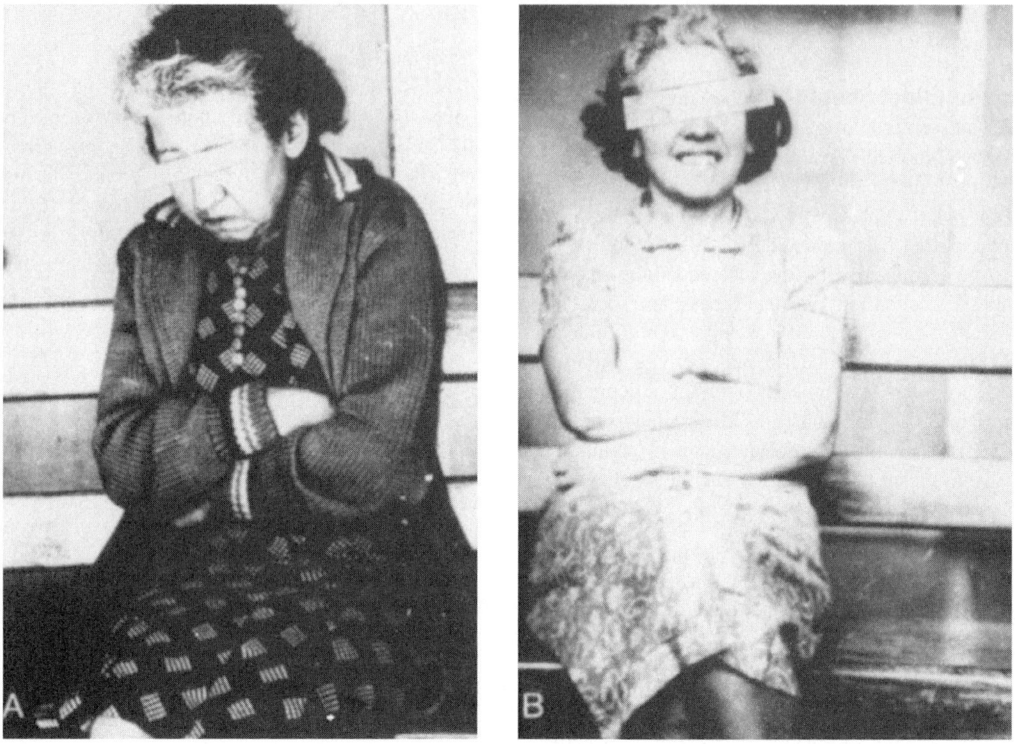

FIGURE 15.1–3
A 38-year-old woman during a state of deep retarded depression (**A**) and 2 months later, after recovery (**B**). The turned-down corners of her mouth, her stooped posture, her drab clothing, and her hairdo during the depressed episode are noteworthy. (Courtesy of Heinz E. Lehmann, M.D.)

taneous movements, and a downcast, averted gaze (Figs. 15.1–3 and 15.1–4). On clinical examination, depressed patients exhibiting gross symptoms of psychomotor retardation may appear identical to patients with catatonic schizophrenia. This fact is recognized in DSM-IV-TR by the inclusion of the symptom qualifier "with catatonic features" for some mood disorders.

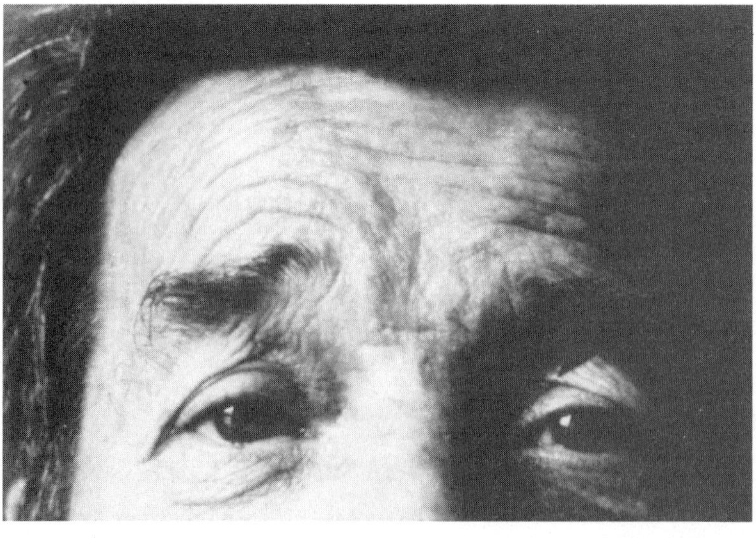

FIGURE 15.1–4
The Swiss neuropsychiatrist Otto Veraguth described a peculiar triangle-shaped fold in the nasal corner of the upper eyelid. The fold is often associated with depression and referred to as Veraguth's fold. The photograph illustrates this physiognomic feature in a 50-year-old man during a major depressive episode. Veraguth's fold may also be seen in persons who are not clinically depressed, usually while they are harboring a mild depressive affect. Distinct changes in the tone of the corrugator and zygomatic facial muscles accompany depression, as shown on electromyograms. (Courtesy of Heinz E. Lehmann, M.D.)

Mood, Affect, and Feelings. Depression is the key symptom, although about 50 percent of patients deny depressive feelings and do not appear to be particularly depressed. Family members or employers often bring or send these patients for treatment because of social withdrawal and generally decreased activity.

Speech. Many depressed patients evidence a decreased rate and volume of speech; they respond to questions with single words and exhibit delayed responses to questions. The examiner may literally have to wait 2 or 3 minutes for a response to a question.

Perceptual Disturbances. Depressed patients with delusions or hallucinations are said to have a major depressive episode with psychotic features. Even in the absence of delusions or hallucinations, some clinicians use the term *psychotic depression* for grossly regressed depressed patients—mute, not bathing, soiling. Such patients are probably better described as having catatonic features.

Delusions and hallucinations that are consistent with a depressed mood are said to be mood congruent. Mood-congruent delusions in a depressed person include those of guilt, sinfulness, worthlessness, poverty, failure, persecution, and terminal somatic illnesses (such as cancer and "rotting" brain). The content of mood-incongruent delusions or hallucinations is not consistent with a depressed mood. Mood-incongruent delusions in a depressed person involve grandiose themes of exaggerated power, knowledge, and worth—for example, the belief that a person is being persecuted because he or she is the Messiah. Although relatively rare, hallucinations can also occur in major depressive episodes with psychotic features.

Thought. Depressed patients customarily have negative views of the world and of themselves. Their thought content often includes nondelusional ruminations about loss, guilt, suicide, and death. About 10 percent of all depressed patients have marked symptoms of a thought disorder, usually thought blocking and profound poverty of content.

Sensorium and Cognition. ORIENTATION. Most depressed patients are oriented to person, place, and time, although some may not have enough energy or interest to answer questions about these subjects during an interview.

MEMORY. About 50 to 75 percent of all depressed patients have a cognitive impairment, sometimes referred to as depressive pseudodementia. Such patients commonly complain of impaired concentration and forgetfulness.

Impulse Control. About 10 to 15 percent of all depressed patients commit suicide, and about two thirds have suicidal ideation. Depressed patients with psychotic features occasionally consider killing a person as a result of their delusional systems, but the most severely depressed patients often lack the motivation or the energy to act in an impulsive or violent way. Patients with depressive disorders are at increased risk of suicide as they begin to improve and regain the energy needed to plan and carry out a suicide (paradoxical suicide). It is usually clinically unwise to give a depressed patient a large prescription for antidepressants, especially tricyclic drugs, at the time of their discharge from the hospital.

Judgment and Insight. Patients' judgment is best assessed by reviewing their actions in the recent past and their behavior during the interview. Depressed patients' insight into their disorder is often excessive; they overemphasize their symptoms, their disorder, and their life problems. It is difficult to convince such patients that improvement is possible.

Reliability. In interviews and conversations, depressed patients overemphasize the bad and minimize the good. A common clinical mistake is unquestioningly believing a depressed patient who states that a previous trial of antidepressant medications did not work. Such statements may be false, and they require confirmation from another source. Psychiatrists should not view patients' misinformation as an intentional fabrication; the admission of any hopeful information may be impossible for a person in a depressed state of mind.

Objective Rating Scales for Depression. Objective rating scales for depression can be useful in clinical practice for documenting the depressed patient's clinical state.

ZUNG. The Zung Self-Rating Depression Scale is a 20-item report scale. A normal score is 34 or less; a depressed score is 50 or more. The scale provides a global index of the intensity of a patient's depressive symptoms, including the affective expression of depression.

RASKIN. The Raskin Depression Scale is a clinician-rated scale that measures the severity of a patient's depression, as reported by the patient and as observed by the physician, on a five-point scale of three dimensions: verbal report, displayed behavior, and secondary symptoms. The scale has a range of 3 to 13; a normal score is 3, and a depressed score is 7 or more.

HAMILTON. The Hamilton Rating Scale for Depression (HAM-D) is a widely used depression scale with up to 24 items, each of which is rated 0 to 4 or 0 to 2, with a total score of 0 to 76. The clinician evaluates the patient's answers to questions about feelings of guilt, thoughts of suicide, sleep habits, and other symptoms of depression, and the ratings are derived from the clinical interview.

Manic Episodes

General Description. Manic patients are excited, talkative, sometimes amusing, and frequently hyperactive. At times, they are grossly psychotic and disorganized and require physical restraints and the intramuscular injection of sedating drugs.

Mood, Affect, and Feelings. Manic patients classically are euphoric, but they can also be irritable, especially when mania has been present for some time. They also have a low frustration tolerance, which may lead to feelings of anger and hostility. Manic patients may be emotionally labile, switching from laughter to irritability to depression in minutes or hours.

Speech. Manic patients cannot be interrupted while they are speaking, and they are often intrusive nuisances to those around them. Their speech is often disturbed. As the mania gets more intense, speech becomes louder, more rapid, and difficult to interpret and then is filled with puns, jokes, rhymes, plays on

words, and irrelevancies as the activated state increases. At a still greater activity level, associations become loosened, the ability to concentrate fades, and flight of ideas, word salad, and neologisms appear. In acute manic excitement, speech may be totally incoherent and indistinguishable from that of a person with schizophrenia.

Perceptual Disturbances. Delusions occur in 75 percent of all manic patients. Mood-congruent manic delusions are often concerned with great wealth, extraordinary abilities, or power. Bizarre and mood-incongruent delusions and hallucinations also appear in mania.

Thought. Manic patients' thought content includes themes of self-confidence and self-aggrandizement. Manic patients are often easily distracted, and cognitive functioning in the manic state is characterized by an unrestrained and accelerated flow of ideas.

Sensorium and Cognition. Although the cognitive deficits of patients with schizophrenia have been much discussed, less has been written about similar deficits in patients with bipolar I disorder, who may have similar minor cognitive deficits. The reported cognitive deficits can be interpreted as reflecting diffuse cortical dysfunction; subsequent work may localize the abnormal areas. Grossly, orientation and memory are intact, although some manic patients may be so euphoric that they answer incorrectly. Emil Kraepelin called the symptom "delirious mania."

Impulse Control. About 75 percent of all manic patients are assaultive or threatening. Manic patients do attempt suicide and homicide, but the incidence of these behaviors is unknown. Patients who threaten important people (such as the president of the United States) more often have bipolar I disorder than schizophrenia.

Judgment and Insight. Impaired judgment is a hallmark of manic patients. They may break laws about credit cards, sexual activities, and finances and sometimes involve their families in financial ruin. Manic patients also have little insight into their disorder.

Reliability. Manic patients are notoriously unreliable in their information. Because lying and deceit are common in mania, inexperienced clinicians may treat manic patients with inappropriate disdain.

DIFFERENTIAL DIAGNOSIS

Major Depressive Disorder

Medical Disorders. The DSM-IV-TR diagnosis of mood disorder due to a general medical condition describes a mood disorder caused by a nonpsychiatric medical condition. The DSM-IV-TR diagnosis of substance-induced mood disorder describes a mood disorder caused by a substance. Both these diagnostic categories are discussed in Section 15.3.

Failure to obtain a good clinical history or to consider the context of a patient's current life situation may lead to diagnostic errors. Clinicians should have depressed adolescents tested for mononucleosis, and patients who are markedly overweight or underweight should be tested for adrenal and thyroid dysfunctions. Homosexuals, bisexual men, and persons who abuse a substance intravenously should be tested for acquired immune deficiency syndrome (AIDS). Older patients should be evaluated for viral pneumonia and other medical conditions.

Many neurological and medical disorders and pharmacological agents can produce symptoms of depression (see Table 15.3–8 in Section 15.3). Patients with depressive disorders often first visit their general practitioners with somatic complaints. Most medical causes of depressive disorders can be detected with a comprehensive medical history, a complete physical and neurological examination, and routine blood and urine tests. The workup should include tests for thyroid and adrenal functions, because disorders of both of these endocrine systems can appear as depressive disorders. In substance-induced mood disorder, a reasonable rule of thumb is that any drug a depressed patient is taking should be considered a potential factor in the mood disorder. Cardiac drugs, antihypertensives, sedatives, hypnotics, antipsychotics, antiepileptics, antiparkinsonian drugs, analgesics, antibacterials, and antineoplastics are all commonly associated with depressive symptoms.

NEUROLOGICAL CONDITIONS. The most common neurological problems that manifest depressive symptoms are Parkinson's disease, dementing illnesses (including dementia of the Alzheimer's type), epilepsy, cerebrovascular diseases, and tumors. About 50 to 75 percent of all patients with Parkinson's disease have marked symptoms of depressive disorder that do not correlate with the patient's physical disability, age, or duration of illness but do correlate with the presence of abnormalities found on neuropsychological tests. The symptoms of depressive disorder may be masked by the almost identical motor symptoms of Parkinson's disease. Depressive symptoms often respond to antidepressant drugs or ECT. The interictal changes associated with temporal lobe epilepsy can mimic a depressive disorder, especially if the epileptic focus is on the right side. Depression is a common complicating feature of cerebrovascular diseases, particularly in the 2 years after the episode. Depression is more common in anterior brain lesions than in posterior brain lesions and in both cases often responds to antidepressant medications. Tumors of the diencephalic and temporal regions are particularly likely to be associated with depressive disorder symptoms.

PSEUDODEMENTIA. Clinicians can usually differentiate the pseudodementia of major depressive disorder from the dementia of a disease, such as dementia of the Alzheimer's type, on clinical grounds. The cognitive symptoms in major depressive disorder have a sudden onset, and other symptoms of the disorder, such as self-reproach, are also present. A diurnal variation in the cognitive problems, which is not seen in primary dementias, may occur. Depressed patients with cognitive difficulties often do not try to answer questions ("I don't know"), whereas patients with dementia may confabulate. In depressed patients, recent memory is affected more than remote memory. And, during an interview, depressed patients can sometimes be coached and encouraged into remembering, an ability that demented patients lack.

Mental Disorders. Depression can be a feature of virtually any mental disorder listed in DSM-IV-TR, but the mental disorders listed in Table 15.1–29 should be particularly considered in the differential diagnosis.

Table 15.1–29
Mental Disorders That Commonly Have Depressive Features

Adjustment disorder with depressed mood
Alcohol use disorders
Anxiety disorders
Generalized anxiety disorder
Mixed anxiety-depressive disorder
Panic disorder
Posttraumatic stress disorder
Obsessive-compulsive disorder
Eating disorders
Anorexia nervosa
Bulimia nervosa
Mood disorders
Bipolar I disorder
Bipolar II disorder
Cyclothymic disorder
Dysthymic disorder
Major depressive disorder
Minor depressive disorder
Mood disorder due to a general medical condition
Recurrent brief depressive disorder
Substance-induced mood disorder
Schizophrenia
Schizophreniform disorder
Somatoform disorders (especially somatization disorder)

OTHER MOOD DISORDERS. Clinicians must consider the range of DSM-IV-TR diagnosis categories available before arriving at a final diagnosis. First, they must rule out mood disorder caused by a general medical condition and substance-induced mood disorder. Next, clinicians must determine whether a patient has had episodes of manialike symptoms, indicating bipolar I disorder (complete manic and depressive syndromes), bipolar II disorder (recurrent major depressive episodes with hypomania), or cyclothymic disorder (incomplete depressive and manic syndromes). If a patient's symptoms are limited to those of depression, clinicians must assess the severity and duration of the symptoms to differentiate among major depressive disorder (complete depressive syndrome for 2 weeks), minor depressive disorder (incomplete but episodic depressive syndrome), recurrent brief depressive disorder (complete depressive syndrome but for less than 2 weeks per episode), and dysthymic disorder (incomplete depressive syndrome without clear episodes).

OTHER MENTAL DISORDERS. Substance-related disorders, psychotic disorders, eating disorders, adjustment disorders, somatoform disorders, and anxiety disorders are all commonly associated with depressive symptoms and must be considered in the differential diagnosis of a patient with depressive symptoms. Perhaps the most difficult differential is that between anxiety disorders with depression and depressive disorders with marked anxiety. The difficulty of distinguishing these is reflected in the inclusion of the diagnosis of mixed anxiety-depressive disorder in DSM-IV-TR. An abnormal result on the dexamethasone-suppression test, the presence of shortened REM latency on a sleep EEG, and a negative lactate infusion test result support a diagnosis of major depressive disorder in particularly ambiguous cases.

UNCOMPLICATED BEREAVEMENT. Uncomplicated bereavement is not considered a mental disorder, even though about one third of all bereaved spouses for a time meet the diagnostic criteria for major depressive disorder. Some patients with uncomplicated bereavement do develop major depressive disorder, but the diagnosis is not made unless no resolution of the grief occurs. The differentiation is based on the symptoms' severity and length. In major depressive disorder, common symptoms that evolve from unresolved bereavement are a morbid preoccupation with worthlessness, suicidal ideation, feelings that the person has committed an act (not just an omission) that caused the spouse's death, mummification (keeping the deceased's belongings exactly as they were), and a particularly severe anniversary reaction, which sometimes includes a suicide attempt.

Bipolar I Disorder

When a patient with bipolar I disorder has a depressive episode, the differential diagnosis is the same as that for a patient being considered for a diagnosis of major depressive disorder. When a patient is manic, however, the differential diagnosis includes bipolar I disorder, bipolar II disorder, cyclothymic disorder, mood disorder caused by a general medical condition, and substance-induced mood disorder. For manic symptoms, borderline, narcissistic, histrionic, and antisocial personality disorders need special consideration.

Schizophrenia. A great deal has been published about the clinical difficulty of distinguishing a manic episode from schizophrenia. Although difficult, a differential diagnosis is possible with a few clinical guidelines. Merriment, elation, and infectiousness of mood are much more common in manic episodes than in schizophrenia. The combination of a manic mood, rapid or pressured speech, and hyperactivity weights heavily toward a diagnosis of a manic episode. The onset in a manic episode is often rapid and is perceived as a marked change from a patient's previous behavior. Half of all patients with bipolar I disorder have a family history of mood disorder. Catatonic features may be a depressive phase of bipolar I disorder. When evaluating patients with catatonia, clinicians should look carefully for a past history of manic or depressive episodes and for a family history of mood disorders. Manic symptoms in persons from minority groups (particularly blacks and Hispanics) are often misdiagnosed as schizophrenic symptoms.

Medical Conditions. In contrast to depressive symptoms, which are present in almost all psychiatric disorders, manic symptoms are more distinctive, although they can be caused by a wide range of medical and neurological conditions and substances (see Table 15.1–8). Antidepressant treatment can also be associated with the precipitation of mania in some patients.

Bipolar II Disorder

The differential diagnosis of patients being evaluated for a mood disorder should include the other mood disorders, psychotic disorders, and borderline disorder. The differentiation

between major depressive disorder and bipolar I disorder on one hand and bipolar II disorder on the other hand rests on the clinical evaluation of the manialike episodes. Clinicians should not mistake euthymia in a chronically depressed patient for a hypomanic or manic episode. Patients with borderline personality disorder often have a severely disrupted life, similar to that of patients with bipolar II disorder, because of the multiple episodes of significant mood disorder symptoms.

COURSE AND PROGNOSIS

The many studies of the course and prognosis of mood disorders have generally concluded that mood disorders tend to have long courses and that patients tend to have relapses. Although mood disorders are often considered benign in contrast to schizophrenia, they exact a profound toll on affected patients. Another common conclusion from studies is that life stressors precede the first episode of mood disorders more frequently than subsequent episodes (Table 15.1–30). This finding has been interpreted to indicate that psychosocial stress may play a role in the initial cause of mood disorders and that even though the initial episode may resolve, a long-lasting change in the biology of the brain puts a patient at great risk for subsequent episodes.

Major Depressive Disorder

Course. ONSET. About 50 percent of patients undergoing their first episode of major depressive disorder exhibited significant depressive symptoms before the first identified episode. This observation implies that early identification and treatment of early symptoms may prevent the development of a full depressive episode. Although symptoms may have been present, patients with major depressive disorder usually have not had a premorbid personality disorder. The first depressive episode occurs before age 40 in about 50 percent of patients. A later onset is associated with the absence of a family history of mood disorders, antisocial personality disorder, and alcohol abuse.

DURATION. An untreated depressive episode lasts 6 to 13 months; most treated episodes last about 3 months. The withdrawal of antidepressants before 3 months has elapsed almost always results in the return of the symptoms. As the course of the disorder progresses, patients tend to have more frequent episodes that last longer. Over a 20-year period, the mean number of episodes is five or six.

DEVELOPMENT OF MANIC EPISODES. About 5 to 10 percent of patients with an initial diagnosis of major depressive disorder have a manic episode 6 to 10 years after the first depressive episode. The mean age for this switch is 32 years, and it often occurs after two to four depressive episodes. Although the data are inconsistent and controversial, some clinicians report that the depression of patients who are later classified as having bipolar I disorder is often characterized by hypersomnia, psychomotor retardation, psychotic symptoms, a history of postpartum episodes, a family history of bipolar I disorder, and a history of antidepressant-induced hypomania.

Prognosis. Major depressive disorder is not a benign disorder. It tends to be chronic, and patients tend to relapse. Patients who have been hospitalized for a first episode of major depressive disorder have about a 50 percent chance of recovering in the first year. The percentage of patients recovering after repeated hospitalization decreases with passing time. Many unrecovered patients remain affected with dysthymic disorder. Recurrences of major depressive episodes are also common. About 25 percent of patients experience a recurrence in the first 6 months after release from a hospital, about 30 to 50 percent in the first 2 years, and about 50 to 75 percent in 5 years. The incidence of relapse is lower than these figures in patients who continue prophylactic psychopharmacological treatment and in patients who have had only one or two depressive episodes. Generally, as a patient experiences more and more depressive episodes, the time between the episodes decreases, and the severity of each episode increases.

PROGNOSTIC INDICATORS. Many studies have focused on identifying both good and bad prognostic indicators in the course of major depressive disorder. Mild episodes, the absence of psychotic symptoms, and a short hospital stay are good prognostic indicators. Psychosocial indicators of a good course include a history of solid friendships during adolescence, stable family functioning, and generally sound social functioning for the 5 years preceding the illness. Additional good prognostic signs are the absence of a comorbid psychiatric disorder and of a personality disorder, no more than one previous hospitalization for major depressive disorder, and an advanced age of onset. The possibility of a poor prognosis is increased by coexisting dysthymic disorder, abuse of alcohol and other substances, anxiety disorder symptoms, and a history of more than one previous depressive episode. Men are more likely than women to experience a chronically impaired course.

Bipolar I Disorder

Course. The natural history of bipolar I disorder is such that it is often useful to make a graph of a patient's disorder and to keep it up-to-date as treatment progresses (Fig. 15.1–5). Although cyclothymic disorder is sometimes diagnosed retrospectively in patients with bipolar I disorder, no identified personality traits are specifically associated with bipolar I disorder.

Bipolar I disorder most often starts with depression (75 percent of the time in women, 67 percent in men) and is a recurring disorder. Most patients experience both depressive and manic episodes, although 10 to 20 percent experience only manic episodes. The manic episodes typically have a rapid onset (hours or days) but may evolve over a few weeks. An untreated manic episode lasts about 3 months; therefore, clinicians should not discontinue giving drugs before that time. Ninety percent of persons who have a single manic episode are likely to have another. As the disorder progresses, the time between episodes often decreases. After about five episodes, however, the interepisode interval often stabilizes at 6 to 9 months. Five to 15 percent of persons with bipolar disorder have four or more episodes per year and can be classified as rapid cyclers.

BIPOLAR I DISORDER IN CHILDREN AND OLDER PERSONS. Bipolar I disorder can affect both the very young and older persons. The incidence of bipolar I disorder in children and adolescents is about 1 percent, and the onset can be as early as age 8. Common misdiagnoses are schizophrenia and oppositional defiant disorder.

Table 15.1–30
Studies of Association between Life Events and First versus Subsequent Episodes of Mood Disorders

				Percentage of Patients for Whom Major Life Event Preceded Episode			
Author	Disorder	Number of Episodes	*N*	First Episode	Later Episode	*p*	Assessment
Matussek et al.	Depression	1	242	44		—	Stressors (138 psychological; 58 somatic) had to clearly precede onset of episode
		2	135		34	—	
		3	82		24	—	
		4	119		19	—	
Angst	Depression	1	103	60		—	No inventory
		≥4			38	—	
Okuma and Shimoyama	Bipolar	1	134	45		—	Any event (3 months prior)
		2	134		26	—	
		3	134		13	—	
Glassner et al.	Bipolar	1	25	75		—	Event rated stressful by patient and on Holmes and Rahe Scale (1 year prior; usually 2–24 days); role loss critical in patients and comparison subjects
		>1[a]			56		
Ambelas[b]	Mania	1	14	50		<.01	Paykel Life Events Scale (4 weeks prior); one third of cases followed bereavement
		≥2	67		28		
Gutierrez et al.	Depression	1	43	55.8		<.05	Social and somatic stressors; patients with late onset had more events than did those with early onset
		2	35		40.0		
		3	18		38.8		
		≥4	47		29.7		
Perris	Depression	1	37	62	50[c]	<.02	Semistructured interview; 56-item inventory (3 months prior)
		≥2	112	43	19[d]	<.001	
Dolan et al.	Depression	1	21	62		<.05	Bedford College-Life Events and Difficulties Schedule (6 months prior) (Brown, Harris, 1978)
		≥2	57		29		
Ezquiaga et al.	Depression	<3	52	50		<.01	Semistructured interview (Brown, Harris); no effect of chronic stress
		≥3	45		16		
Ambelas	Mania	1	50	66		<.001	Paykel Life Events Scale (4 weeks prior)
		≥2	40		20		
Ghaziuddin et al.	Depression	1	33	91		<.05	Paykel Life Events Scale (6 months prior)
		≥2	40		50		
Cassano et al.	Depression	1	94	66.0		<.05	Paykel Life Events Scale
		≥2	173		49.4		

[a]For this group, the most recent hospitalization was preceded by a life event resulting in role loss.
[b]Of surgical comparison subjects, 6.6% had experienced recent major life events.
[c]Percentage for negative or undesirable events.
[d]Percentage for events involving psychological conflict.
Reprinted with permission from Post RM. Transduction of psychosocial stress into the neurobiology of recurrent affective disorder. *Am J Psychiatry.* 1992;149:1000.

Bipolar I disorder with such an early onset is associated with a poor prognosis. Manic symptoms are common in older persons, although the range of causes is broad and includes nonpsychiatric medical conditions, dementia, delirium, and bipolar I disorder. Currently available data indicate that the onset of true bipolar I disorder in older persons is relatively uncommon.

Prognosis. Patients with bipolar I disorder have a poorer prognosis than do patients with major depressive disorder. About 40 to 50 percent of bipolar I disorder patients may have a second manic episode within 2 years of the first episode. Although lithium prophylaxis improves the course and prognosis of bipolar I disorder, probably only 50 to 60 percent of patients achieve significant control of their symptoms with lithium. One 4-year follow-up study of patients with bipolar I disorder found that a premorbid poor occupational status, alcohol dependence, psychotic features, depressive features, interepisode depressive features, and male gender were all factors that weighted toward a poor prognosis. Short duration of manic episodes, advanced age of onset, few suicidal thoughts, and few coexisting psychiatric or medical problems weight toward a good prognosis.

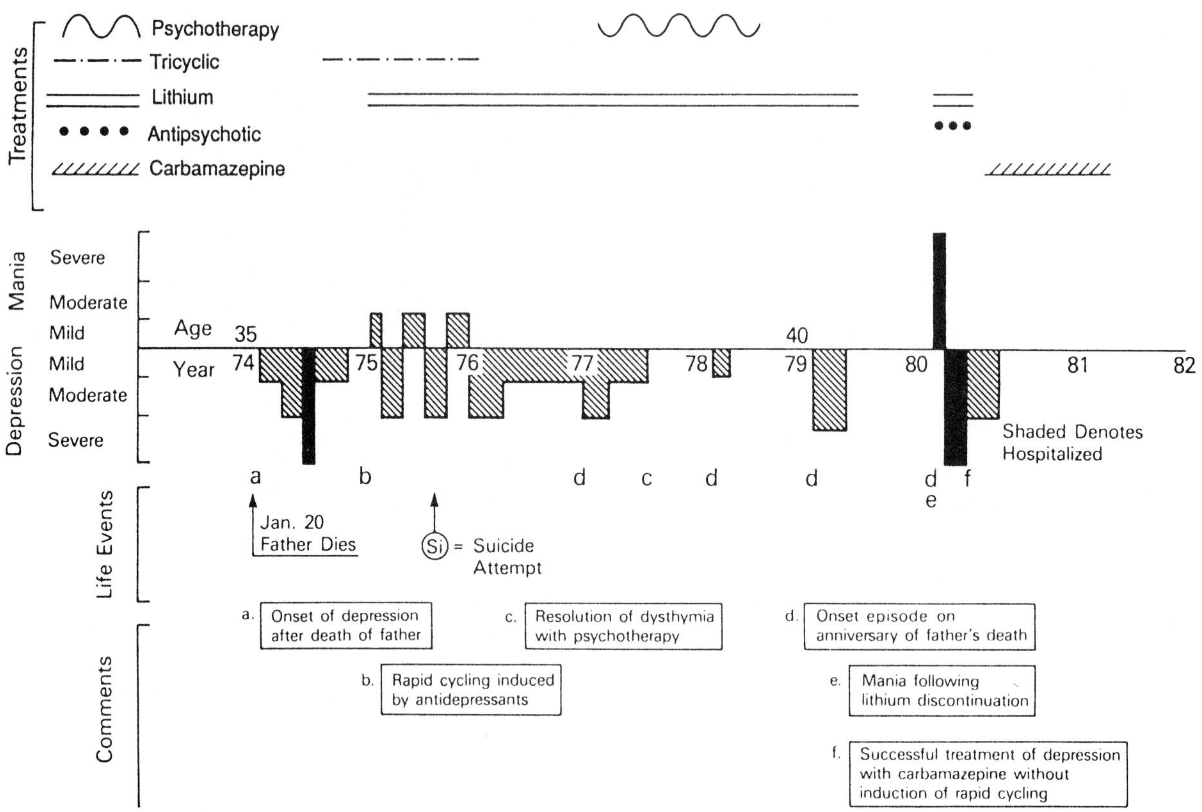

FIGURE 15.1–5
Graphing the course of a mood disorder. Prototype of a life chart. (Courtesy of Robert M. Post, M.D.)

About 7 percent of all patients with bipolar I disorder do not have a recurrence of symptoms; 45 percent have more than one episode, and 40 percent have a chronic disorder. Patients may have from 2 to 30 manic episodes, although the mean number is about 9. About 40 percent of all patients have more than 10 episodes. On long-term follow-up, 15 percent of all patients with bipolar I disorder are well, 45 percent are well but have multiple relapses, 30 percent are in partial remission, and 10 percent are chronically ill. One third of all patients with bipolar I disorder have chronic symptoms and evidence of significant social decline.

Bipolar II Disorder

The course and prognosis of bipolar II disorder have just begun to be studied. Preliminary data indicate, however, that the diagnosis is stable, as shown by the high likelihood that patients with bipolar II disorder will have the same diagnosis up to 5 years later. The data thus show that bipolar II disorder is a chronic disease that warrants long-term treatment strategies.

TREATMENT

The treatment of patients with mood disorders must be directed toward several goals. First, the patient's safety must be guaranteed. Second, a complete diagnostic evaluation of the patient must be carried out. Third, a treatment plan that addresses not only the immediate symptoms but also the patient's prospective well-being must be initiated. Although current treatment emphasizes pharmacotherapy and psychotherapy addressed to the individual patient, stressful life events are also associated with increases in relapse rates among patients with mood disorders. Thus, treatment must reduce the number and severity of stressors in patients' lives.

Overall, the treatment of mood disorders is rewarding for psychiatrists. Specific treatments are now available for both manic and depressive episodes, and data indicate that prophylactic treatment is also effective. Because the prognosis for each episode is good, optimism is always warranted and is welcomed by both the patient and the patient's family, even if initial treatment results are not promising. Mood disorders are chronic, however, and the psychiatrist must advise the patient and the family about future treatment strategies.

Hospitalization

The first and most critical decision a physician must make is whether to hospitalize a patient or attempt outpatient treatment. Clear indications for hospitalization are the need for diagnostic procedures, the risk of suicide or homicide, and a patient's grossly reduced ability to get food and shelter. A history of rapidly progressing symptoms and the rupture of a patient's usual support systems are also indications for hospitalization.

A physician may safely treat mild depression or hypomania in the office if he or she evaluates the patient frequently. Clinical signs of impaired judgment, weight loss, or insomnia should be minimal. The patient's support system should be strong, nei-

ther overinvolved nor withdrawing from the patient. Any adverse changes in the patient's symptoms or behavior or the attitude of the patient's support system may suffice to warrant hospitalization.

Patients with mood disorders are often unwilling to enter a hospital voluntarily, and may have to be involuntarily committed. These patients often cannot make decisions because of their slowed thinking, negative Weltanschauung (world view), and hopelessness. Manic patients often have such a complete lack of insight into their disorder that hospitalization seems absolutely absurd to them.

Psychosocial Therapy

Although most studies indicate—and most clinicians and researchers believe—that a combination of psychotherapy and pharmacotherapy is the most effective treatment for major depressive disorder, some data suggest another view: Either pharmacotherapy or psychotherapy alone is effective, at least in patients with mild major depressive episodes, and the regular use of combined therapy adds to the cost of treatment and exposes patients to unnecessary adverse effects.

Three types of short-term psychotherapies—cognitive therapy, interpersonal therapy, and behavior therapy—have been studied to determine their efficacy in the treatment of major depressive disorder. Although its efficacy in treating major depressive disorder is not as well researched as these three therapies, psychoanalytically oriented psychotherapy has long been used for depressive disorders, and many clinicians use the technique as their primary method. What differentiates the three short-term psychotherapy methods from the psychoanalytically oriented approach are the active and directive roles of the therapist, the directly recognizable goals, and the end points for short-term therapy.

Although less research has been conducted on the psychodynamic theory of depression than on some other forms of psychotherapy, the accumulating evidence is encouraging about the efficacy of dynamic therapy. In a randomized controlled trial comparing psychodynamic therapy with cognitive behavior therapy, the outcomes of the depressed patients in the study showed no differences between the two treatments.

Table 15.1–31 summarizes the features of the psychodynamic, cognitive, and interpersonal approaches; Table 15.1–32 summarizes some nonselective and selective patient variables for psychotherapy; Table 15.1–33 summarizes the advantages and limitations of the three approaches; and Tables 15.1–34 and 15.1–35 summarize features that may affect the choice of pharmacotherapy or psychotherapy or combined therapy. The National Institute of Mental Health (NIMH) Treatment of Depression Collaborative Research Program found the following predictors of response to various treatments: low social dysfunction suggested a good response

Table 15.1–31
Major Features of Three Psychotherapeutic Approaches to Depression

Feature	Psychodynamic Approach	Cognitive Approach	Interpersonal Approach
Major theorists	Freud, Abraham, Jacobson, Kohut	Plato, Adler, Beck, Rush	Meyer, Sullivan, Klerman, Weissman
Concepts of pathology and cause	Ego regression: damaged self-esteem and unresolved conflict due to childhood object loss and disappointment	Distorted thinking: dysphoria due to learned negative views of self, others, and the world	Impaired interpersonal relations: absent or unsatisfactory significant social bonds
Major goals and mechanisms of change	To promote personality change through understanding of past conflicts; to achieve insight into defenses, ego distortions, and superego defects; to provide a role model; to permit cathartic release of aggression	To provide symptomatic relief through alteration of target thoughts; to identify self-destructive cognitions; to modify specific erroneous assumptions; to promote self-control over thinking patterns	To provide symptomatic relief through solution of current interpersonal problems; to reduce stress involving family or work; to improve interpersonal communication skills
Primary techniques and practices	Expressive-empathic: fully or partially analyzing transference and resistance; confronting defenses; clarifying ego and superego distortions	Behavioral-cognitive: recording and monitoring cognitions; correcting distorted themes with logic and experimental testing; providing alternative thought content; homework	Communicative-environmental: clarifying and managing maladaptive relationships and learning new ones through communication and social skills training; providing information on illness
Therapist role–therapeutic relationship	Interpreter-reflector: establishment and exploration of transference; therapeutic alliance for benign dependence and empathic understanding	Educator-shaper: positive relationship instead of transference; collaborative empiricism as basis for joint scientific (logical) task	Explorer-prescriber: positive relationship-transference without interpretation; active therapist role for influence and advocacy
Marital-family role	Full individual confidentiality; exclusion of significant others except in life-threatening situations	Use of spouse as objective reporter; couples therapy for disturbed cognitions sustained in marital relationship	Integral role of spouse in treatment; examination of spouse's role in patient's predisposition to depression and effects of illness on marriage

Reprinted with permission from Karasu TB. Toward a clinical model of psychotherapy for depression. I. Systematic comparison of three psychotherapies. *Am J Psychiatry.* 1990;147:141.

Table 15.1–32
Nonselective and Selective Patient Variables for Psychotherapy for Depression

	Selective Patient Variables		
Nonselective Patient Variables	**Psychodynamic Therapy**	**Cognitive Therapy**	**Interpersonal Therapy**
Feelings of hopelessness and helplessness Apathy, decreased enjoyment, diminished desire or gratification Too high ego ideals and expectations Oversleeping, morbid dreams or nightmares Feelings of restlessness or being slowed down Lack of motivation or will Low self-esteem, inappropriate or excessive guilt and self-reproach Distractibility, sluggish thinking or decision making Wish or intention to be dead Social withdrawal, fear of rejection or failure Psychosomatic complaints, hypochondriasis	Long-term sense of emptiness and underestimation of self-worth Loss or long separation in childhood Conflicts in past relationships (e.g., with parent, sexual partner) Capacity for insight Ability to modulate regression Access to dreams and fantasy Little need for direction and guidance Stable environment	Obvious distorted thoughts about self, world, and future Pragmatic (logical) thinking Real inadequacies (including poor response to other psychotherapies) Moderate to high need for direction and guidance Responsiveness to behavioral training and self-help (high degree of self-control)	Recent, focused dispute with spouse or significant other Social or communication problems Recent role transition or life change Abnormal grief reaction Modest to moderate need for direction and guidance Responsiveness to environmental manipulation (available support network)

Reprinted with permission from Karasu TB. Toward a clinical model of psychotherapy for depression. II. An integrative and selective treatment approach. *Am J Psychiatry.* 1990;147:275.

Table 15.1–33
Advantages and Limitations of Three Psychotherapeutic Approaches to Depression

Feature	Psychodynamic Approach	Cognitive Approach	Interpersonal Approach
Theory			
Advantages	Individual depth approach encourages patient to look inward for solutions, rather than depending on external sources	Cognitive-behavioral orientation is tangible and objective	Interpersonal orientation addresses broader (e.g., social, family) context, useful in focusing on man–woman relations
Limitations	Focus on intrapsychic phenomena may obscure other (e.g., interpersonal, environmental) factors; aggression-depression theory can be overgeneralized and lead to overreliance on catharsis	Cognitive-behavioral emphasis may neglect whole person, especially affective component; symptom-oriented perspective overlooks past history, complex problem areas, and hidden conflicts	Emphasis on four designated interpersonal problems can bias toward preconceived themes; interpersonal orientation may stress marital/family factors while underplaying intrapsychic forces
Goals			
Advantages	Enduring structural change transcends symptomatic relief; strengthened adaptive capacities can be useful beyond specific depressive pathology	Primary goal of symptom relief is expedient in itself and is first stage in changing cognitive style	Improvement of interpersonal relations is expedient in itself and may also result in relief of symptoms
Limitations	Personality alteration can be too ambitious and may be unnecessary or excessive for most depression diagnoses	Symptom reduction may be insufficient, superficial, or temporary; focus on current problems can preclude enduring modification of personality or prophylactic function of treatment	Symptom relief may be fragile and temporary if it is highly dependent on external factors
Structure			
Advantages	Indefinite duration allows long-term or flexible goals[a]	Brief or fixed duration is cost-effective and can foster results in short period, may heighten expectation of rapid change and encourage optimism	Predetermined duration is cost-effective; approach reengages family and may have preventive effect
Limitations	Long-term or open-ended treatment is uneconomical and difficult to evaluate[a]	Short or predetermined duration may be insufficient or inflexible	Time limitation predetermines the extent of personal growth and independence

(continued)

Table 15.1–33 (*continued*)

Feature	Psychodynamic Approach	Cognitive Approach	Interpersonal Approach
Therapist role			
Advantages	Neutral, accepting stance ensures nonjudgmental attitude and objectivity; receptive listening encourages transference formation and ensuing analytic process	Active therapist can directly intervene to interrupt depressive schemata and suggest alternatives to faulty thinking	Therapist position between activity and reactivity can reassure patient and provide supportive person for patient to relate to
Limitations	Transference regression can produce overidealization of therapist and underestimation of patient self-worth; therapist silence may be misconstrued as rejection, which can perpetuate depression and cause premature termination	Active suggestion and direction can undermine patient responsibility and self-esteem by imposing therapist point of view or values	Supportive interpersonal role may encourage dependence and rage at withdrawal of therapist
Techniques			
Advantages	Free association provides verbal catharsis; interpretations provide new understanding of depressogenic conflicts and historical events	Specific approach is directly tailored to depressed population and aims at particular target symptoms; identification of depressogenic assumptions and homework to test new thinking foster cognitive modification	Specific approach is directly tailored to depressed population and can address particular current interpersonal maladaptions
Limitations	No specific techniques developed; focus on past events and spontaneous associations may encourage repetitive litany of depressive complaints at the expense of present therapeutic tasks	Emphasis on specific cognitive schemata may bias toward certain preconceived themes; overt simplicity of techniques may lead to underestimation of technical skill required	Identification of specific interpersonal problem areas may be overly restrictive, yet techniques are relatively nonspecific; legitimation of patient sick role may encourage passivity
Research status			
Advantages	Longitudinal case study approach useful for detailed examination and follow-up of individual patients	Operational manual allows for replication of treatment and training and empirical establishment of efficacy	Same as for cognitive approach
Limitations	Idiographic approach or anecdotal case history is not amenable to controlled or comparative research	Research-oriented operationalized approach may become oversimplified formula for complex clinical phenomena	Same as for cognitive approach
Relation to other modalities			
Advantages	Integrity of transference is maintained through elimination of outside influences	Competition with pharmacotherapy encourages research on relative efficacy, especially instances when cognitive therapy alone is most effective	Approach designed to be used alone or with drugs; it is especially amenable to combination with marital therapy
Limitations	Need for neutrality may limit use of other helpful treatment approaches (e.g., family therapy, drug treatment)	Competition with pharmacotherapy fosters polarization of approaches and partisan resistance to integration with drug treatment	Amenability to additive or eclectic modalities requires integrative theoretical model, clinical expertise in more than one modality, and ability to collaborate with other disciplines, which may lead to role diffusion and insufficient knowledge or training
Patient population			
Advantages	Special patient requisites (e.g., verbal orientation, psychological-mindedness) ensure maximal insight	Logical thinking ensures maximal potential to deal with and change depressogenic assumptions and thought patterns	Orientation toward interpersonal relations, especially marital interaction, can address gender issues in marriage, especially important given high prevalence of women among depressed patients
Limitations	Special patient requisites may limit usefulness to verbal, psychological-minded population	Cognitively impaired population may not benefit; sophisticated, introspective patients may find approach too simple-minded or superficial	Interpersonal orientation may overemphasize marriage; primarily female population may bias toward women; conjoint focus may bias against unmarried population

[a]Advantages and limitations of short-term psychodynamic therapy are similar to those for the cognitive and interpersonal approaches.
Reprinted with permission from Karasu TB. Toward a clinical model of psychotherapy for depression. I. Systematic comparison of three psychotherapies. *Am J Psychiatry.* 1990;147:142.

Table 15.1–34
Indications for Psychotherapy and Pharmacotherapy in the Treatment of Depression

Variable	Indication for Treatment[a]	
	Pharmacotherapy	Psychotherapy
Symptom criteria for major depressive episode		
Depressed mood	Marked vegetative signs; extreme or uncontrolled mood	Mild to moderate situational or characterological depressed mood
Diminished interest or pleasure	Anhedonia; loss of libido; impaired sexual function or performance	Apathy, decreased enjoyment; diminished sexual desire or gratification
Weight loss or gain	Significant weight loss	Insignificant weight gain
Insomnia or hypersomnia	Early morning wakening	Oversleeping, morbid dreams or nightmares
Psychomotor agitation	Hyperactivity or motor retardation	Restlessness or feelings of being slowed down
Fatigue or loss of energy (anergia)	Depressive stupor	Lack of motivation or will
Feelings of worthlessness or excessive guilt	Nihilistic or self-deprecatory delusions, self-berating auditory hallucinations	Low self-esteem, inappropriate guilt feelings, self-reproach
Diminished ability to think or concentrate, indecisiveness	Loss of control over thinking, obsessive rumination, inability to focus or act	Distractibility, sluggish thinking or decision making; negative cognitions
Recurrent thoughts of death or suicide	Acute, episodic, and uncontrolled suicidal acts or plans[b]	Chronic feelings of hopelessness or helplessness[c]
Associated features	Panic (anxiety) attacks or phobias; persecutory delusions; pseudodementia; physical symptoms or somatic delusions	Social withdrawal or fears of rejection or failure; psychosomatic complaints or hypochondriasis
Family history	Genetic loading (bipolar disorder or depressive disorder)	No genetic loading (dysthymic disorder)
Predisposing factors	Other mental disorders, e.g., schizophrenia, alcohol dependence, anorexia nervosa	Psychosocial stressors, e.g., loss of significant other, change in status or role
Personality disorders	Borderline, histrionic, obsessive-compulsive	Dependent, inadequate, masochistic

[a]These are not mutually exclusive categories.
[b]Hospitalization may be required.
[c]Medication may also be useful.
Reprinted with permission from Karasu TB. Toward a clinical model of psychotherapy for depression. II. An integrative and selective treatment approach. *Am J Psychiatry.* 1990;147:274.

to interpersonal therapy; low cognitive dysfunction suggested a good response to cognitive-behavioral therapy and pharmacotherapy; high work dysfunction suggested a good response to pharmacotherapy; and high depression severity suggested a good response to interpersonal therapy and pharmacotherapy.

Cognitive Therapy. Cognitive therapy, developed originally by Aaron Beck, focuses on the cognitive distortions postulated to be present in major depressive disorder. Such distortions include selective attention to the negative aspects of circumstances and unrealistically morbid inferences about con-

Table 15.1–35
Approach to Pharmacotherapy of Three Psychotherapies for Depression

Feature of Combined Treatment	Psychodynamic Therapy	Cognitive Therapy	Interpersonal Therapy
Basic stance	Medication is avoided except in life-threatening situation, used judiciously for severe vegetative signs	Pharmacotherapy and cognitive therapy alone are in ongoing competition, but drugs are used in case of poor response to cognitive therapy and for breaking psychotherapeutic impasses in severe depression when symptomatic relief is required	Interpersonal therapy and pharmacotherapy are considered having different effects and response timetables (early drug effects on vegetative symptoms, later psychotherapy effects on suicidal ideation, work, and interests)
Techniques	Personal (unconscious and conscious) meanings are explored and interpreted within therapy session	Information and rationale for use is provided; special tasks are assigned to increase adherence, e.g., postsession homework (lists of side effects); phone contact with therapist is encouraged	Information and rationale for use is provided, in line with medical model; time is set aside in each session to discuss pharmacological issues

Reprinted with permission from Karasu TB. Toward a clinical model of psychotherapy for depression. II. An integrative and selective treatment approach. *Am J Psychiatry.* 1990;147:272.

sequences. For example, apathy and low energy result from a patient's expectation of failure in all areas. The goal of cognitive therapy is to alleviate depressive episodes and prevent their recurrence by helping patients identify and test negative cognitions; develop alternative, flexible, and positive ways of thinking; and rehearse new cognitive and behavioral responses.

Studies have shown that cognitive therapy is effective in the treatment of major depressive disorder. Most of the studies found that cognitive therapy is equal in efficacy to pharmacotherapy and is associated with fewer adverse effects and better follow-up than pharmacotherapy. Some of the best controlled studies have indicated that the combination of cognitive therapy and pharmacotherapy is more efficacious than either therapy alone, although other studies have not found that additive effect. At least one study, the NIMH Treatment of Depression Collaborative Research Program, found that pharmacotherapy, either alone or with psychotherapy, may be the treatment of choice for patients with severe major depressive episodes.

Interpersonal Therapy. Interpersonal therapy, developed by Gerald Klerman, focuses on one or two of a patient's current interpersonal problems. This therapy is based on two assumptions. First, current interpersonal problems are likely to have their roots in early dysfunctional relationships. Second, current interpersonal problems are likely to be involved in precipitating or perpetuating the current depressive symptoms. Several controlled trials have compared interpersonal therapy, cognitive therapy, pharmacotherapy, and the combination of pharmacotherapy with psychotherapy. These trials indicated that interpersonal therapy is effective in the treatment of major depressive disorder and may, not surprisingly, be specifically helpful in addressing interpersonal problems. The data about the efficacy of interpersonal therapy in the treatment of severe major depressive episodes are less reliable, although some information indicates that interpersonal therapy may be the most effective method for severe major depressive episodes when the treatment choice is psychotherapy alone.

The interpersonal therapy program usually consists of 12 to 16 weekly sessions and is characterized by an active therapeutic approach. Intrapsychic phenomena, such as defense mechanisms and internal conflicts, are not addressed. Discrete behaviors—such as lack of assertiveness, impaired social skills, and distorted thinking—may be addressed but only in the context of their meaning in, or their effect on, interpersonal relationships.

Behavior Therapy. Behavior therapy is based on the hypothesis that maladaptive behavioral patterns result in a person's receiving little positive feedback and perhaps outright rejection from society. By addressing maladaptive behaviors in therapy, patients learn to function in the world in such a way that they receive positive reinforcement. Although individual and group therapies have been studied, behavior therapy for major depressive disorder has not yet been the subject of many controlled studies. The data to date indicate that behavior therapy is an effective treatment for major depressive disorder.

Psychoanalytically Oriented Therapy. The psychoanalytic approach to mood disorders is based on psychoanalytic theories about depression and mania. The goal of psychoanalytic psychotherapy is to effect a change in a patient's personality structure or character, not simply to alleviate symptoms. Improvements in interpersonal trust, intimacy, coping mechanisms, the capacity to grieve, and the ability to experience a wide range of emotions are some of the aims of psychoanalytic therapy. Treatment often requires the patient to experience periods of heightened anxiety and distress during the course of therapy, which may continue for several years.

Family Therapy. Family therapy is not generally viewed as a primary therapy for the treatment of major depressive disorder, but increasing evidence indicates that helping a patient with a mood disorder to reduce and cope with stress can lessen the chance of a relapse. Family therapy is indicated if the disorder jeopardizes a patient's marriage or family functioning or if the mood disorder is promoted or maintained by the family situation. Family therapy examines the role of the mood-disordered member in the overall psychological well-being of the whole family; it also examines the role of the entire family in the maintenance of the patient's symptoms. Patients with mood disorders have a high rate of divorce, and about 50 percent of all spouses report that they would not have married or had children if they had known that the patient was going to develop a mood disorder.

Pharmacotherapy

Although the specific, short-term psychotherapies such as interpersonal therapy and cognitive therapy have influenced the treatment approaches to major depressive disorder, the pharmacotherapeutic approach to mood disorders has revolutionized their treatment and has dramatically affected the courses of mood disorders and reduced their inherent costs to society. Physicians must integrate pharmacotherapy with psychotherapeutic interventions. If physicians view mood disorders as fundamentally evolving from psychodynamic issues, their ambivalence about the use of drugs may result in a poor response, noncompliance, and probably inadequate dosages for too short a treatment period. Alternatively, if physicians ignore the psychosocial needs of a patient, the outcome of pharmacotherapy may be compromised.

Major Depressive Disorder. Effective and specific treatments, such as tricyclic drugs, for major depressive disorder have been available for 40 years. The use of specific pharmacotherapy approximately doubles the chance that a depressed patient will recover in 1 month. Nevertheless, problems remain in the treatment of major depressive disorder: Some patients do not respond to the first treatment; all currently available antidepressants may take up to 3 to 4 weeks to exert significant therapeutic effects, although they may begin to show their effects earlier; and, until relatively recently, all available antidepressants have been toxic in overdoses and have had adverse effects. The introduction of the SSRIs, such as fluoxetine, paroxetine (Paxil), and sertraline (Zoloft), as well as bupropion, venlafaxine, nefazodone (Serzone), and mirtazapine (Remeron), offers clinicians drugs that are equally effective but safer and better tolerated than previous drugs. Recent indications (e.g., eating disorders and anxiety disorders) for antidepressant medications make the grouping of these drugs under the single label of antidepressants somewhat confusing.

The principal indication for antidepressants is a major depressive episode. The first symptoms to improve are often poor sleep and appetite patterns. Agitation, anxiety, depressive episodes, and hopelessness are the next symptoms to improve. Other target symptoms include low energy, poor concentration, helplessness, and decreased libido.

PATIENT EDUCATION. Adequate patient education about the use of antidepressants is as critical to treatment success as is choosing the most appropriate drug and dosage. When introducing the topic of a drug trial to a patient, physicians should emphasize that major depressive disorder is a combination of biological and psychological factors, both of which benefit from drug therapy. Physicians should also stress that the patient will not become addicted to antidepressants, because these drugs do not give immediate gratification. Further, it will probably take 3 to 4 weeks for the effects of the antidepressant to be felt, and even if the patient shows no improvement by that time, other medications are available. Some clinicians say that the appearance of side effects shows that the drug is working, but the expected side effects should be explained in detail. For example, some patients taking SSRIs may experience agitation, gastrointestinal upset, or nausea before any reduction in depression. The adverse effects pass with time. With tricyclic drugs and MAOIs, physicians may find it useful to tell the patient that sleep and appetite will improve first, followed by a sense of returned energy, and that the feeling of depression, unfortunately, will be the last symptom to change.

Physicians must always consider the risk of suicide in patients with mood disorder. Most antidepressants are lethal if taken in large amounts. It is unwise to give large prescriptions to most patients with mood disorder when they are discharged from the hospital unless another person monitors the drug's administration.

ALTERNATIVES TO DRUG TREATMENT. Two organic therapies that are alternatives to pharmacotherapy are ECT and phototherapy. ECT is generally used when a patient is unresponsive to pharmacotherapy or cannot tolerate pharmacotherapy or the clinical situation is so severe that the rapid improvement seen with ECT is needed. Although the use of ECT is often limited to these three situations, it is an effective antidepressant treatment and can be reasonably considered the treatment of choice in some patients, such as older depressed persons. Phototherapy is a novel treatment that has been used with patients with a seasonal pattern to their mood disorder. It can be used alone in mild cases of mood disorder with a seasonal pattern. For severely affected patients, it can be used in combination with pharmacotherapy, although studies of the efficacy of this combination have not yet produced definitive results.

AVAILABLE DRUGS. The SSRIs are the most widely used antidepressant drugs in the United States. They are the agents of choice because of their effectiveness, ease of use, and relative lack of adverse effects, even at high dosages. Because they are well tolerated, they have been prescribed by clinicians in a wide range of specialties. Of the other newer agents, bupropion, venlafaxine, and nefazodone have gained widespread use among psychiatrists. Each of these agents is safer than the tricyclic and tetracyclic drugs and MAOIs, and each has been shown to be as effective for depression in clinical trials. The tricyclic and tetracyclic drugs, trazodone (Desyrel), alprazolam (Xanax), and mirtazapine, may cause sedation. The MAOIs require dietary restrictions. Sympathomimetic drugs, such as dextroamphetamine (Dexedrine) and methylphenidate (Ritalin), may produce a rapid improvement of mood (within 1 week) and are indicated in closely monitored situations.

PHARMACOLOGICAL ACTIONS. In patients who tolerate full therapeutic dosages of the various available antidepressants, no one agent has shown an obvious superiority. There are marked differences, however, in adverse effect profiles, and individual patients may respond to one antidepressant and not to another. Most antidepressants interact with either serotonergic or noradrenergic neurotransmission or with both. Moreover, potentiation of either of these neurotransmitter systems has been shown to stimulate the other system, which makes the details of the pharmacodynamics of each drug difficult to translate into a prediction of efficacy. There is a fairly good correlation between in vitro evidence of interaction with a particular neurotransmitter and clinical evidence of particular adverse effects, which is outlined in Table 15.1–36.

The MAOIs are less frequently chosen because they may cause a hypertensive crisis if patients ingest foods with a high content of tyramine, which requires strict adherence to a simple set of dietary guidelines. Alprazolam, a benzodiazepine, is Food and Drug Administration (FDA) approved for treatment of depression, but it is rarely used because of concerns about sedation and because it may be addictive and may be very difficult to discontinue. Sympathomimetics, while among the most effective antidepressants, are rarely used because of concerns about abuse, even though this is unlikely at the low dosages usually necessary for treatment of depression.

ADVERSE EFFECTS. One of the most serious concerns about antidepressants is their lethality when taken in overdoses. Tricyclic and tetracyclic drugs are, by far, the most lethal of the antidepressants; the SSRIs, bupropion, trazodone, nefazodone, mirtazapine, venlafaxine, and the MAOIs are safer, although even these drugs can be lethal when taken in overdose in combination with alcohol or other drugs. Another concern about antidepressants is their cardiac safety. Again, tricyclic and tetracyclic drugs are generally the least safe. Hypotension is a potentially serious adverse effect of many antidepressants, particularly in older persons. Among the conventional antidepressants, amoxapine (Asendin), maprotiline (Ludiomil), nortriptyline (Aventyl), and trazodone are associated with little hypotension, and bupropion and the SSRIs are associated with the least hypotension. Many clinicians inappropriately ignore the sexual adverse effects of antidepressants. Almost all the antidepressants, except nefazodone and mirtazapine, have been associated with decreased libido, erectile dysfunction, or anorgasmia. The serotonergic drugs are probably more closely associated with sexual adverse effects than are the noradrenergic compounds. Table 15.1–37 lists adverse effects of many antidepressant drugs.

DRUG–DRUG INTERACTIONS. Another increasing concern among clinicians prescribing drugs for depressive disorders and conditions are possible drug–drug interactions, especially in regard to the hepatic cytochrome P450 enzyme. The cytochrome P450 isoenzyme system is involved in the metabolism of most drugs, but some people are genetically at risk for developing high

Table 15.1–36
Antidepressant Effects on CNS Neurotransmitters

	Serotonin	Norepinephrine	Dopamine	MAO Activity	Serotonin Type 2 Blockade
Amitriptyline	+++	++++	0	0	++
Amoxapine	+++	+++	–	0	+++
Bupropion	0	+	++	0	0
Clomipramine	++++	+++	+	0	++
Desipramine[a]	+	++++	0/+	0	+
Doxepin	+++	+	0	0	+
All SSRIs	+++++ (or more)	0/+	0/+	0	0/+
Imipramine	+++	++	0/+	0	++
Lithium	0/++[b]	–	–	0	0
Maprotiline	0	++++	0	0	NA
Moclobemide	0	0	0	Reversible type A	0
Nefazodone	+++[a]	0	0	0	++++
Nortriptyline[a]	++	+++	0	0	+
Phenelzine/tranylcypromine	0	0	0	Irreversible type A/B	0
Protriptyline	+	++++	0	0	NA
Trazodone	++	0	0	0	+++
Trimipramine	++	++	0	0	++
Venlafaxine	++++	+++	0/+	0	0

[a]Tertiary amine is demethylated to secondary amine.
[b]Acutely increases; chronically stabilizes.

Table 15.1–37
Adverse Effects of Antidepressants

	Anticholinergic Effects	Arrhythmias	Sedation	Seizures[a]	Orthostasis	GI	Sexual Dysfunction	Toxicity in Overdose
Amitriptyline	5	5	5	2	4	2	3	4
Amoxapine	2	1	3	3	1	1	3	5
Bupropion	0	0	0	4	0	1	0/1	3
Clomipramine	5	5	4	4	4	3	4	5
Desipramine	2	4	2	2	3	1	3	4
Doxepin	3	3	4	2	3	1	3	4
Fluoxetine	0	0	0/1	0	0	4	4	1
Fluvoxamine	1	0	0/1	0	0	5	4	1
Imipramine	3	5	3	2	4	2	3	5
Lithium	0	1	1	1	0	3	1	5
Maprotiline	3	3	3	3	2	1	3	5
Moclobemide	1	0	0	0	2	1	2	2
Nefazodone	1	0	3	0	1	3	1	1
Nortriptyline	3	4	2	2	1	2	3	5
Paroxetine	2	0	1/2	0	0	4	4	1
Protriptyline	3	3	0	2	2	1	3	4
Sertraline	0	0	0/1	0	0	4	4	1
Trazodone	0	1	4	1	3	1	2[b]	2
Trimipramine	4	5	5	2	3	2	4	5
Venlafaxine	1	0	0/1	0	0/1[c]	5	2/3	1

[a]Although ranked 1–4, "high risk" for seizures is still under 1%.
[b]Priapism.
[c]Slight increase in blood pressure also reported; dose related.
0, none; 1, minimal; 2, low; 3, moderate; 4, high; 5, very high.

Table 15.1–38
Drug Interactions and Cytochrome P450 Isoenzyme Systems

	Illustrative Antidepressant Risk Potential (In Vitro and In Vivo)			
Relative Ranking	**CYP 1A2**	**CYP 2C**	**CYP 2D6**	**CYP 3A3/4**
High	Fluvoxamine	Fluvoxamine Fluoxetine	Paroxetine Fluoxetine	Fluvoxamine Nefazodone TCAs
Moderate to minimal	Tertiary TCAs Fluoxetine	Tertiary TCAs	Secondary TCAs Sertraline	Sertraline Fluoxetine
Low to minimal	Paroxetine		Nefazodone Fluvoxamine Venlafaxine (in vitro)	Venlafaxine (in vitro)
	Unknown Risk			
	Nefazodone Sertraline Venlafaxine	Most antidepressants		Paroxetine

Illustrative Drugs That Might Interact with an Antidepressant			
CYP 1A2	**CYP 2C**	**CYP 2D6**	**CYP 3A3/4**
Theophylline	Mephenytoin	Desipramine, secondary TCAs	Terfenadine
Imipramine (minor)	Diazepam	Flecainide/ecainide	Astemizole
Caffeine	Hexobarbital	Risperidone	Ketoconazole
Phenacetin	Imipramine	Phenothiazines	Alprazolam
Acetaminophen	Phenacetin	Haloperidol (minor)	Triazolam
Warfarin (minor)	Warfarin	Reduced haloperidol	Erythromycin
Phenothiazines	Propranolol	Codeine	Nifedipine
	Tertiary TCAs	Propranolol (minor)	Cyclosporine
		Quinidine[a]	Corticosteroids

[a]Inhibitor at 2D6, not a substrate. Drug can be substrate and/or inhibitor at a given enzyme system.

blood concentrations of drugs that are metabolized by one of the cytochrome P450 isoenzymes, such as CYP 2D6 (Table 15.1–38).

TYPE-SPECIFIC TREATMENTS. Some clinical types of major depressive episodes may have varying responses to particular antidepressants. For example, patients with major depressive disorder with atypical features (sometimes called hysteroid dysphoria) may preferentially respond to treatment with MAOIs. Two other specific groups are patients with depressed bipolar I disorder and those with major depressive episodes with psychotic features.

Lithium is a potential first-line pharmacological agent for treating depression in patients with bipolar I disorder and some patients with major depressive disorder with a marked periodicity to their disorder. Patients with bipolar I disorder who are being treated with conventional antidepressants must be observed carefully for the emergence of manic symptoms.

Antidepressants alone are not likely to be effective in the treatment of major depressive episodes with psychotic features. One exception may be amoxapine, an antidepressant closely related to loxapine (Loxitane), an antipsychotic. Clinicians usually, however, use a combination of an antidepressant and an antipsychotic. Several studies have also shown that ECT is effective for this indication—perhaps more effective than pharmacotherapy.

GENERAL CLINICAL GUIDELINES. The most common clinical mistake leading to an unsuccessful trial of an antidepressant drug is the use of too low a dosage for too short a time. Table 15.1–39 lists the dosage ranges and indications for a range of drugs. Unless adverse events prevent it, the dosage of an antidepressant should be raised to the maximum recommended level and maintained at that level for at least 4 or 5 weeks before a drug trial is considered unsuccessful. Alternatively, if a patient is improving clinically on a low dosage of the drug, this dosage should not be raised unless clinical improvement stops before the maximal benefit is obtained. When a patient does not begin to respond to appropriate dosages of a drug after 2 or 3 weeks, clinicians may decide to obtain a plasma concentration of the drug if the test is available for the particular drug being used. The test may indicate either noncompliance or particularly unusual pharmacokinetic disposition of the drug and may thereby suggest an alternative dosage.

DURATION AND PROPHYLAXIS. Antidepressant treatment should be maintained for at least 6 months or the length of a previous episode, whichever is greater. Several studies show that prophylactic treatment with antidepressants is effective in reducing the number and severity of recurrences. One study concluded that when episodes are less than 2½ years apart, prophylactic treatment for 5 years is probably indicated. Another factor suggest-

Table 15.1–39
Selected Drugs Used to Treat Depression

Drug	Starting Dose (mg)	Dosage[a] (mg/d)	Therapeutic Plasma Concentration (ng/mL)
Amitriptyline (Elavil, Endep)	25 hs to 25 tid	50–300	60–200[b]
Amoxapine (Asendin)	50 bid[b]–50 tid	100–600	180–600[b]
Bupropion (Wellbutrin)	50–75 bid	150–450	50–100[b]
	SR:150[d]	150–400	50–100[b]
Citalopram (Celexa)	10–20	20–80	—
Clomipramine (Anafranil)	25 tid	100–250	200–300[b]
Desipramine (Norpramin, Pertofrane)	25 hs to 25 tid	50–300	125–250[c]
Doxepin (Adapin, Sinequan)	25 hs to 25 bid	75–300	110–250
Fluoxetine (Prozac)	20 qam	10–80	—
Fluvoxamine (Luvox)	50–100 qam	100–300	—
Imipramine (Janimine, Tofranil)	25 hs to 25 tid	50–300	>180[b,c]
Maprotiline (Ludiomil)	25 hs to 25 tid	50–225	200–400[b]
Mirtazapine (Remeron)	15	15–45	—
Nefazodone (Serzone)	100 mg tid	100–600	—
Nortriptyline (Aventyl, Pamelor)	25 hs to 25 tid	50–200	50–150[c]
Paroxetine (Paxil)	20 qam	10–50	—
Phenelzine (Nardil)	15 qam	15–90	80% inhibition of platelet MAO activity
Protriptyline (Vivactil)	10 qam	15–60	100–200
Sertraline (Zoloft)	50 qam	50–200	—
Trazodone (Desyrel)	50 tid	50–600	800–1600
Trimipramine (Surmontil)	25 hs to 25 tid	75–300	—
Tranylcypromine (Parnate)	10 qam	10–60	80% inhibition of platelet MAO activity
Venlafaxine (Effexor)	37.5 bid	75–375	—
	XR:37.5 qd[e]	75–225	—

[a]In geriatric patients, the appropriate dose is widely variable but in general is one half the young adult dosage range for tricyclic antidepressants and for those compounds with significant cardiovascular toxicity.
[b]Parent and metabolite.
[c]Therapeutic drug monitoring well established.
[d]Sustained-release formulation.
[e]Extended-release formulation.

ing prophylactic treatment is the seriousness of previous depressive episodes. Episodes that have involved significant suicidal ideation or impairment of psychosocial functioning may indicate that clinicians should consider prophylactic treatment. When antidepressant treatment is stopped, the drug dose should be tapered gradually over 1 to 2 weeks, depending on the half-life of the particular compound. Several studies indicate that maintenance antidepressant medication appears to be safe and effective for the treatment of chronic depression.

FAILURE OF DRUG TRIAL. When the first antidepressant drug has been used for an adequate trial and, if appropriate, clinicians are sure that adequate plasma concentrations were obtained, there are two options if symptoms have not improved satisfactorily: to augment the drug with lithium, liothyronine (the levorotatory isomer of triiodothyronine [T3]), or L-tryptophan, or to switch to an alternative primary agent. A now rarely used strategy is to combine a tricyclic or tetracyclic drug with an MAOI. When switching agents, clinicians should switch a patient who has been taking a tricyclic or tetracyclic drug to an SSRI (or possibly an MAOI) and should switch a patient who has been taking an SSRI to bupropion, venlafaxine, nefazodone, a tricyclic or tetracyclic drug, mirtazapine, trazodone, or possibly an MAOI. At least 2 weeks should elapse between the use of an SSRI and the use of an MAOI, and the two drugs should never be used concurrently, because a serotonin syndrome might develop.

Lithium. Lithium (900 to 1,200 mg a day, serum level between 0.6 and 0.8 mEq/L) can be added to the antidepressant dosage for 7 to 14 days. This approach converts a significant number of antidepressant nonresponders to responders. The mechanism of action is unknown, although the lithium may potentiate the serotonergic neuronal system. Some data indicate that pretreatment with the antidepressant alone is necessary for this effect and that beginning treatment with the two drugs simultaneously is not as effective as starting with an antidepressant and then adding lithium.

Liothyronine. The addition of 25 to 50 mg a day of liothyronine to an antidepressant regimen for 7 to 14 days may convert antidepressant nonresponders to responders. The adverse effects of liothyronine are minor but may include headaches and feelings of warmth. The mechanism of action for liothyronine augmentation is not known, although the modulation of β-receptors and the presence of undetectable thyroid axis abnormalities in major depressive disorder have been suggested. If liothyronine augmentation is successful, the liothyro-

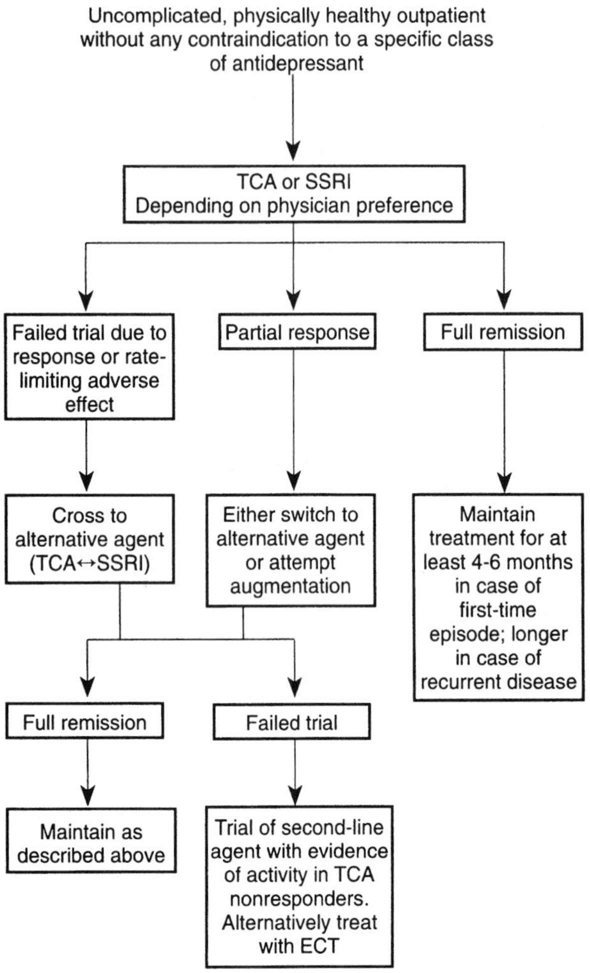

FIGURE 15.1–6

Algorithm for treating patient with major depressive disorder. *ECT,* electroconvulsive therapy; *SSRI,* serotonin-specific reuptake inhibitor; *TCA,* tricyclic antidepressant. (Reprinted with permission from Preskorn, SH, Burke M. Somatic therapy for major depressive disorder: selection of an antidepressant. *J Clin Psychiatry.* 1992;53[suppl 9]10.)

nine use should be continued for 2 months and then tapered at the rate of 12.5 mg a day every 3 to 7 days.

L-Tryptophan. L-Tryptophan, the amino acid precursor to serotonin, has been used as an adjuvant both to antidepressant drugs in major depressive disorder and to lithium in bipolar I disorder. L-Tryptophan has also been used alone as an antidepressant and a hypnotic. L-Tryptophan–containing products have been recalled in the United States because of an outbreak of eosinophilia-myalgia syndrome associated with the use of L-tryptophan. The symptoms of the syndrome include fatigue, myalgia, shortness of breath, rashes, and swelling of the extremities. Congestive heart failure and death can also occur. Several studies have shown that L-tryptophan is an effective adjuvant in the treatment of mood disorders; however, the drug should not be used for any purpose until the problem with the syndrome is completely resolved. The syndrome is probably related to a contaminant in a single manufacturing plant, but caution should still be used.

Tricyclic or Tetracyclic Drug and MAOI Combinations. The combination of a tricyclic or tetracyclic drug and an MAOI is sometimes used for patients who have not responded to several other pharmacological treatments. With the availability of a broad range of antidepressants, however, this combination therapy is rarely used. Because of the high incidence of adverse effects, it is not a treatment of choice. When this combination is used, clinicians should initiate treatment with the two drugs simultaneously at low dosages for each and should then raise the dosages slowly. Imipramine (Tofranil) or trimipramine (Surmontil) and an MAOI should not be used in combination because of their high incidence of toxic effects, including restlessness, dizziness, tremulousness, muscle twitching, sweating, convulsions, hyperpyrexia, and sometimes death.

When a patient has been taking a tricyclic or tetracyclic drug, physicians should quarter the dosage of the drug for 5 to 7 days and then slowly add the MAOI to the regimen. When the patient has been taking an MAOI, physicians should stop giving the drug for 2 weeks and then start giving the two drugs simultaneously. The reason for this strategy is that it takes about 2 weeks for normal MAO activity levels to be achieved after the use of MAOIs. Fig. 15.1–6 provides a useful treatment algorithm.

Bipolar I Disorder. Lithium, divalproex (Depakote), and olanzapine (Zyprexa) are standard treatments for the manic phase of bipolar disorder, but carbamazepine is also a well-established treatment. Gabapentin (Neurontin) and lamotrigine (Lamictal) are promising treatments for refractory or treatment-intolerant patients. The efficacy of the latter two agents is not well established, but their clinical use is expanding. Topiramate (Topamax) is another anticonvulsant showing benefit in bipolar patients. ECT is highly effective in all phases of bipolar disorder. Carbamazepine, divalproex, and valproic acid appear to be more effective than lithium in the treatment of mixed or dysphoric mania, rapid cycling, and psychotic mania and in the treatment of patients with a history of multiple manic episodes or comorbid substance abuse.

Treatment of acute manic episodes often requires adjunctive use of potent sedative drugs. Drugs commonly used at the start of treatment include clonazepam (Klonopin) (1 mg every 4 to 6 hours) and lorazepam (Ativan) (2 mg every 4 to 6 hours). Haloperidol (Haldol) (2 to 10 mg a day), olanzapine (2.6 to 10 mg a day), and risperidone (Risperdal) (0.5 to 6 mg a day) are also of use. Bipolar patients may be particularly sensitive to the side effects of typical antipsychotics. The atypical antipsychotics (e.g., olanzapine [10 to 15 mg a day]) are often used as monotherapy for short-term control and may have intrinsic antimanic properties. Physicians should attempt to taper dosages of these adjunctive agents when the patient stabilizes.

Patients who do not respond adequately to a mood stabilizer may do well with combination treatment. Lithium and valproic acid are commonly used together. Increased neurotoxicity is a risk, but the combination is safe. Other combinations include lithium plus carbamazepine plus valproic acid (which requires laboratory monitoring for drug interactions and hepatic toxicity) and combinations with the newer anticonvulsants.

LITHIUM. Lithium is still a standard treatment for bipolar I disorder. The adverse effects that may limit the use of lithium and cause clinicians to consider using either carbamazepine or valproate include renal effects (thirst, polyuria), nervous system effects (tremor, memory loss), metabolic effects (weight gain), gastrointestinal effects (diarrhea), dermatological effects (acne, psoriasis), and thyroid effects (goiter, myxedema). Of potentially serious concern with lithium treatment are its effects on the kidneys, which can include moderate and occasionally severe impairment of tubular function; uncommon, moderate, and unspecific morphological changes; and rarely, a nephrotic syndrome. These many adverse effects require careful monitoring of patients' renal and thyroid status.

Compliance with lithium treatment is increased with early initiation of treatment, adequate treatment of concomitant illness, treatment of coexisting substance abuse, early detection and prevention of adverse effects, and patient participation in individual and group psychotherapy. Responsiveness to lithium treatment is improved when adequate lithium levels are maintained, adjunctive medication is used as indicated, and laboratory and clinical monitoring is carried out. Nonresponsiveness to lithium treatment is most likely with severe illness, the presence of schizoaffective disorder symptoms, mixed manic and depressive symptoms, somatic symptoms, alcohol and other substance abuse, rapid cycling, and the absence of a family history of bipolar I disorder. A blood level of 0.8 to 1.2 mEq/L is the effective range.

VALPROATE. The efficacy data for valproate now suffice to warrant its use as a first-line drug. A significant number of patients seem to tolerate valproate better than they tolerate lithium and carbamazepine. Valproic acid and divalproex have a broad therapeutic index and appear to be effective at levels of 50 to 125 μg/mL. Pretreatment workup includes a complete blood cell count and liver function tests. A pregnancy test is needed because this drug can cause neural tube defects in developing fetuses. It can cause thrombocytopenia and increase transaminase levels, both of which are usually benign and self-limited but require increased blood monitoring. Fatal hepatic toxicity has been reported only in children under 10 who received multiple anticonvulsants. Typical adverse effects include hair loss (which can be treated with zinc and selenium), tremor, weight gain, and sedation. Gastrointestinal upset is common but can be minimized by using enteric-coated tablets (Depakote) and titrating gradually. Valproic acid can be loaded for short-term symptom control by administering at 20 mg/kg in divided doses. This strategy also produces a therapeutic level and may improve symptoms within 7 days. For outpatients, more physically brittle patients, or less severely ill patients, medication dosage can be started at 250 to 750 mg a day and gradually titrated to a therapeutic level. Blood level can be checked after 3 days at a particular dosage.

Carbamazepine. Carbamazepine is usually titrated to response rather than blood level, although many clinicians titrate to reach levels of 4 to 12 μg/mL. Pretreatment evaluation should include liver function tests and a complete blood cell count as well as an electrocardiogram (ECG), electrolyte levels, reticulocyte count, and pregnancy test. Adverse effects include nausea, sedation, and ataxia. Hepatic toxicity, hyponatremia, or bone marrow suppression may rarely occur. Rash occurs in 10% of patients. Exfoliative rashes (Stevens-Johnson syndrome) are rare but potentially fatal. Drug dosage can be started at 200 to 600 mg a day, with adjustments every 5 days based on clinical response. Improvement may be seen 7 to 14 days after a therapeutic dose has been achieved. Drug interactions complicate carbamazepine use and probably relegate it to second-line status. It is a potent enzyme inducer and can lower levels of other psychotropic drugs, such as haloperidol. Carbamazepine induces its own metabolism (autoinduction), and the dosage often needs to be increased during the first few months of treatment to maintain a therapeutic level and clinical response.

OTHER ANTICONVULSANTS. Lamotrigine and gabapentin are anticonvulsants that may have antidepressant, antimanic, and mood-stabilizing properties. They do not require blood monitoring. Gabapentin is excreted exclusively by the kidneys. It has a benign adverse effect profile that can include sedation, dizziness, and fatigue. It does not interact with other drugs. Dose reduction is required in patients with renal insufficiency. Gabapentin can be titrated aggressively, and therapeutic response has been reported at dosages of 300 to 3,600 mg a day. It has a short half-life, and dosing to three times a day is required. Lamotrigine requires gradual titration to decrease the risk for rash, which occurs in 10% of patients. Stevens-Johnson syndrome occurs in 0.1% of patients treated with lamotrigine. Other adverse effects include nausea, sedation, ataxia, and insomnia. Dosage can be initiated at 25 to 50 mg a day for 2 weeks and then increased slowly to 150 to 250 mg twice daily. Valproate raises lamotrigine levels. In the presence of valproate, lamotrigine titration should be slower and dosages lower (e.g., 25 mg orally four times daily for 2 weeks, with 25-mg increases every 2 weeks to a maximum of 150 mg a day).

Topiramate has shown efficacy in bipolar disorders. Its adverse effects include fatigue and cognitive dulling. This drug has the unique property of causing weight loss. One series of overweight patients with bipolar disorder lost an average of 5% of their body weight while taking topiramate as an adjunct to other medications. The starting dosage is usually 25 to 50 mg a day to a maximum of 400 mg a day.

Other Agents. Other agents used in bipolar disorder include verapamil (Isoptin, Calan), nimodipine (Nimotop), clonidine, clonazepam, and levothyroxine (Levoxyl, Levothroid, Synthroid). Clozapine (Clozaril) has been shown to have potent antimanic and mood-stabilizing properties in treatment-refractory patients. ECT may be considered in particularly severe or drug-resistant cases as another alternative treatment of bipolar I disorder.

RAPID CYCLING. The development of rapid cycling in patients with bipolar I disorder has been associated with the use of conventional antidepressants, especially tricyclic drugs, and with the presence of hypothyroidism. In addition to the use of thyroid treatments, that is, levothyroxine 0.3 to 0.5 mg a day, some researchers and clinicians have reported positive results with the use of other psychopharmacological agents, including SDAs, bupropion, and nimodipine.

MAINTENANCE. The decision to maintain a patient on lithium (or other drug) prophylaxis is based on the severity of the

patient's disorder, the risk of adverse effects from the particular drug, and the quality of the patient's support systems. Maintenance treatment is generally indicated for the prophylaxis of bipolar I disorder in any patient who has had more than one episode. The rationale for this practice is the relative safety of the available drugs, their demonstrated efficacy, and the significant potential for psychosocial problems if another bipolar I disorder episode occurs. During long-term treatment, laboratory monitoring is required for lithium, valproic acid, and carbamazepine.

Bipolar II Disorder. The treatment of bipolar II disorder must be approached cautiously; treatment for depressive episodes with antidepressants can frequently precipitate a manic episode. Whether typical bipolar I disorder medication strategies (e.g., lithium and anticonvulsants) are effective in the treatment of patients with bipolar II disorder is still under investigation. A trial of such agents seems warranted, especially when treatment with antidepressants alone has not been successful.

References

Akiskal HS, section ed. Mood disorders. In: Sadock BJ, Sadock VA, eds. *Kaplan & Sadock's Comprehensive Textbook of Psychiatry.* 7th ed. Vol I. Baltimore: Lippincott Williams & Wilkins; 2000:1284.

Baldessarini RJ, Tondo L. Does lithium treatment still work? Evidence of stable responses over three decades. *Arch Gen Psychiatry.* 2000;57:187.

Coryell W, Endicott J, Keller M. Major depression in a nonclinical sample: demographic and clinical risk factors for first onset. *Arch Gen Psychiatry.* 1992;49:117.

Coryell W, Endicott J, Keller M. Rapid cycling affective disorder: demographics, diagnosis, family history, and course. *Arch Gen Psychiatry.* 1992;49:126.

Gallagher-Thompson D, Steffen AM. Comparative effects of cognitive-behavioral and brief psychodynamic psychotherapies for depressed family caregivers. *J Consult Clin Psychol.* 1994;62:543.

Gotlib IH, Nolan SA. Depressive disorders. In: Hersen M, Bellack AS, ed. *Psychopathology in Adulthood.* 2nd ed. Needham Heights, MA: Allyn & Bacon; 2000:252.

Hammen C. Vulnerability to depression in adulthood. In: Ingram RE, Price JM, eds. *Vulnerability to Psychopathology: Risk across the Lifespan.* New York: Guilford Press; 2001:226.

Hammen C, Gitlin M. Stress reactivity in bipolar patients and its relation to prior history of disorder. *Am J Psychiatry.* 1997;154:856.

Johnson SL, Hayes AM, et al., eds. *Stress, Coping, and Depression.* Mahwah, NJ: Lawrence Erlbaum Associates; 2000:35.

Keck PE Jr, Nabulsi AA, Taylor JL, et al. A pharmacoeconomic model of divalproex vs. lithium in the acute and prophylactic treatment of bipolar I disorder. *J Clin Psychiatry.* 1996;57:213.

Keitner GI, Ryan CE, Miller IW, Norman WH. Recovery and major depression: factors associated with twelve-month outcome. *Am J Psychiatry.* 1992;149:93.

Kendler KS, Kessler RC, Walters EE, et al. Stressful life events, genetics liability, and onset of an episode of major depression in women. *Am J Psychiatry.* 1995;152:883.

MacKinnon DF, Zandi PP, Cooper J, et al. Comorbid bipolar disorder and panic disorder in families with a high prevalence of bipolar disorder. *Am J Psychiatry.* 2002;159:30.

Palmer KJ, ed. *Controversies in Depression Management.* Kwai Chung, Hong Kong: Adis International Publications; 2000:49.

Post RM, Ketter TA, Denicoff K, Pazzaglia PJ. The place of anticonvulsant therapy in bipolar illness. *Psychopharmacology.* 1996;128:115.

Power AC, Cowen PJ. Neuroendocrine challenge tests: assessment of 5-HT function in anxiety and depression. *Mol Aspects Med.* 1992;13:205.

Rice JP, Rochberg N, Endicott J, Lavori PW, Miller C. Stability of psychiatric diagnoses: an application to the affective disorder. *Arch Gen Psychiatry.* 1992;49:824.

Sachs GS, Thase ME. Bipolar disorder therapeutics: maintenance treatment. *Biol Psychiatry.* 2000;48:573.

Sands JR, Harrow M. Bipolar disorder: psychopathology, biology, and diagnosis. In: Hersen M, Bellack AS, ed. *Psychopathology in Adulthood.* 2nd ed. Needham Heights, MA: Allyn & Bacon; 2000:326.

▲ 15.2 Dysthymia and Cyclothymia

DYSTHYMIC DISORDER

Dysthymic disorder is a chronic disorder characterized by the presence of a depressed mood that lasts most of the day and is present almost continuously. According to the text revision of the fourth edition of *Diagnostic and Statistical Manual of Mental Disorders* (DSM-IV-TR), the most typical features of the disorder are feelings of inadequacy, guilt, irritability, and anger; withdrawal from society; loss of interest; and inactivity and lack of productivity. The term *dysthymia*, which means "ill humored," was introduced in 1980. Before that time, most patients now classified as having dysthymic disorder were classified as having depressive neurosis (also called neurotic depression).

Dysthymic disorder is distinguished from major depressive disorder by the fact that patients complain that they have always been depressed. Thus, most cases are of early onset, beginning in childhood or adolescence and certainly by the time patients reach their 20s. A late-onset subtype, much less prevalent and not well characterized clinically, has been identified among middle-aged and geriatric populations, largely through epidemiological studies in the community.

Although the dysthymia can occur as a secondary complication of other psychiatric disorders, the core concept of dysthymic disorder refers to a subaffective or subclinical depressive disorder with (1) low-grade chronicity for at least 2 years; (2) insidious onset, with origin often in childhood or adolescence; and (3) persistent or intermittent course. The family history of patients with dysthymia is typically replete with both depressive and bipolar disorders, which is one of the more robust findings supporting its link to primary mood disorder.

Epidemiology

Dysthymic disorder is common among the general population and affects 5 to 6 percent of all persons. It is seen among patients in general psychiatric clinics, where it affects between one half and one third of all patients. There are no gender differences for incidence rates. The disorder is more common in women younger than 64 years of age than in men of any age and is more common among unmarried and young persons and in those with low incomes. Dysthymic disorder frequently coexists with other mental disorders, particularly major depressive disorder and in persons with major depressive disorder there is less likelihood of full remission between episodes. The patients may also have coexisting anxiety disorders (especially panic disorder), substance abuse, and, borderline personality disorder. The disorder is more common among those with first-degree relatives with major depressive disorder. Patients with dysthymic disorder are likely to be taking a wide range of psychiatric medications, including antidepressants, antimanic agents such as lithium (Eskalith) and carbamazepine (Tegretol), and sedative-hypnotics.

Etiology

Biological Factors. Some studies of biological measures in dysthymic disorder support its classification with the mood disorders; other studies question this association. One hypothesis drawn from the data is that the biological basis for the symptoms of dysthymic disorder and major depressive disorder are similar, but the biological bases for the underlying pathophysiology in the two disorders differ.

SLEEP STUDIES. Decreased rapid eye movement (REM) latency and increased REM density are two state markers of depression in major depressive disorder that also occur in a significant proportion of patients with dysthymic disorder. Some investigators have reported preliminary data indicating that the presence of these sleep abnormalities in patients with dysthymic disorder predicts a response to antidepressant drugs.

NEUROENDOCRINE STUDIES. The two most studied neuroendocrine axes in major depressive disorder and dysthymic disorder are the adrenal axis and the thyroid axis, which have been tested by using the dexamethasone-suppression test (DST) and the thyrotropin-releasing hormone (TRH)–stimulation test, respectively. Although the results of studies are not absolutely consistent, most studies indicate that patients with dysthymic disorder are less likely to have abnormal results on a DST than are patients with major depressive disorder. Fewer studies of the TRH-stimulation test have been conducted, but they have produced preliminary data indicating that abnormalities in the thyroid axis may be a trait variably associated with chronic illness. A higher percentage of patients with dysthymic disorder have thyroid axis abnormalities than do normal control subjects.

Psychosocial Factors. Psychodynamic theories about the development of dysthymic disorder posit that the disorder results from personality and ego development and culminates in difficulty adapting to adolescence and young adulthood. Karl Abraham, for example, thought that the conflicts of depression center on oral- and anal-sadistic traits. Anal traits include excessive orderliness, guilt, and concern for others; they are postulated to be a defense against preoccupation with anal matter and with disorganization, hostility, and self-preoccupation. A major defense mechanism used is reaction formation. Low self-esteem, anhedonia, and introversion are often associated with the depressive character.

FREUD. In "Mourning and Melancholia," Sigmund Freud asserted that an interpersonal disappointment early in life can cause a vulnerability to depression that leads to ambivalent love relationships as an adult; real or threatened losses in adult life then trigger depression. Persons prone to depression are orally dependent and require constant narcissistic gratification. When deprived of love, affection, and care, they become clinically depressed; when they experience a real loss, they internalize or introject the lost object and turn their anger on it and, thus, on themselves.

COGNITIVE THEORY. The cognitive theory of depression also applies to dysthymic disorder. It holds that a disparity between actual and fantasized situations leads to diminished self-esteem and a sense of helplessness. The success of cognitive therapy in the treatment of some patients with dysthymic disorder may provide some support for the theoretical model.

Table 15.2–1
DSM-IV-TR Diagnostic Criteria for Dysthymic Disorder

A. Depressed mood for most of the day, for more days than not, as indicated either by subjective account or observation by others, for at least 2 years. **Note:** In children and adolescents, mood can be irritable and duration must be at least 1 year.

B. Presence, while depressed, of two (or more) of the following:
  (1) poor appetite or overeating
  (2) insomnia or hypersomnia
  (3) low energy or fatigue
  (4) low self-esteem
  (5) poor concentration or difficulty making decisions
  (6) feelings of hopelessness

C. During the 2-year period (1 year for children or adolescents) of the disturbance, the person has never been without the symptoms in Criteria A and B for more than 2 months at a time.

D. No major depressive episode has been present during the first 2 years of the disturbance (1 year for children and adolescents); i.e., the disturbance is not better accounted for by chronic major depressive disorder, or major depressive disorder, in partial remission.

  Note: There may have been a previous major depressive episode provided there was a full remission (no significant signs or symptoms for 2 months) before development of the dysthymic disorder. In addition, after the initial 2 years (1 year in children or adolescents) of dysthymic disorder, there may be superimposed episodes of major depressive disorder, in which case both diagnoses may be given when the criteria are met for a major depressive episode.

E. There has never been a manic episode, a mixed episode, or a hypomanic episode, and criteria have never been met for cyclothymic disorder.

F. The disturbance does not occur exclusively during the course of a chronic psychotic disorder, such as schizophrenia or delusional disorder.

G. The symptoms are not due to the direct physiological effects of a substance (e.g., a drug of abuse, a medication) or a general medical condition (e.g., hypothyroidism).

H. The symptoms cause clinically significant distress or impairment in social, occupational, or other important areas of functioning.

Specify if:
  Early onset: if onset is before age 21 years
  Late onset: if onset is age 21 years or older

Specify (for most recent 2 years of dysthymic disorder):
  With atypical features

From American Psychiatric Association. *Diagnostic and Statistical Manual of Mental Disorders.* 4th ed. Text rev. Washington, DC: American Psychiatric Association; copyright 2000, with permission.

Diagnosis and Clinical Features

The DSM-IV-TR diagnosis criteria for dysthymic disorder (Table 15.2–1) stipulate the presence of a depressed mood most of the time for at least 2 years (or 1 year for children and adolescents). To meet the diagnostic criteria, a patient should not have symptoms that are better accounted for as major depres-

Table 15.2–2
DSM-IV-TR Alternative Research Criterion B for Dysthymic Disorder

B. Presence, while depressed, of three (or more) of the following:
(1) low self-esteem or self-confidence, or feelings of inadequacy
(2) feelings of pessimism, despair, or hopelessness
(3) generalized loss of interest or pleasure
(4) social withdrawal
(5) chronic fatigue or tiredness
(6) feelings of guilt, brooding about the past
(7) subjective feelings of irritability or excessive anger
(8) decreased activity, effectiveness, or productivity
(9) difficulty in thinking, reflected by poor concentration, poor memory, or indecisiveness

From American Psychiatric Association. *Diagnostic and Statistical Manual of Mental Disorders.* 4th ed. Text rev. Washington, DC: American Psychiatric Association; copyright 2000, with permission.

Table 15.2–3
Attributes, Assets, and Liabilities of Depressive and Hyperthymic Temperaments

Depressive	Hyperthymic
Gloomy, incapable of fun, complaining	Cheerful and exuberant
Humorless	Articulate and jocular
Pessimistic and given to brooding	Overoptimistic and carefree
Guilt-prone, low self-esteem, and preoccupied with inadequacy or failure	Overconfident, self-assured, boastful, and grandiose
Introverted with restricted social life	Extroverted and people seeking
Sluggish, living a life out of action	High energy level, full of plans
Few but constant interests	Versatile with broad interests
Passive	Overinvolved and meddlesome
Reliable, dependable, and devoted	Uninhibited and stimulus seeking

Courtesy of Hagop S. Akiskal, M.D.

sive disorder and should never have had a manic or hypomanic episode. DSM-IV-TR allows clinicians to specify whether the onset was early (before age 21) or late (age 21 or older). DSM-IV-TR also allows specification of atypical features in dysthymic disorder.

The profile of dysthymic disorder overlaps with that of major depressive disorder but differs from it in that symptoms tend to outnumber signs (more subjective than objective depression). This means that disturbances in appetite and libido are uncharacteristic, and psychomotor agitation or retardation is not observed. This all translates into a depression with attenuated symptomatology. However, subtle endogenous features are observed: inertia, lethargy, and anhedonia that are characteristically worse in the morning. Because patients presenting clinically often fluctuate in and out of a major depression, the core DSM-IV-TR criteria for dysthymic disorder tend to emphasize vegetative dysfunction, whereas the alternative criterion B for dysthymic disorder (Table 15.2–2) in a DSM-IV appendix lists cognitive symptoms.

Dysthymic disorder is quite heterogeneous. Anxiety is not a necessary part of its clinical picture, yet dysthymic disorder is often diagnosed in patients with anxiety and neurotic disorders. That clinical situation is perhaps to be regarded as a secondary or "anxious dysthymia" or, in the framework of Peter Tyrer, as part of a "general neurotic syndrome." For greater operational clarity it is best to restrict dysthymic disorder to a primary disorder, one that cannot be explained by another psychiatric disorder. The essential features of such primary dysthymic disorder include habitual gloom, brooding, lack of joy in life, and preoccupation with inadequacy. Dysthymic disorder then is best characterized as long-standing, fluctuating, low-grade depression, experienced as part of the habitual self and representing an accentuation of traits observed in the depressive temperament (Table 15.2–3). The clinical picture of dysthymic disorder is quite varied, with some patients proceeding to major depression, while others manifest the pathology largely at the personality level.

A 27-year-old male grade-school teacher presented with the chief complaint that life was a painful duty that had always lacked luster for him. He said he felt enveloped by a sense of gloom that was nearly always with him. Although he was respected by his peers, he felt "like a grotesque failure, a self-concept I have had since childhood." He stated that he merely performed his responsibilities as a teacher and that he had never derived any pleasure from anything he had done in life. He said he had never had any romantic feelings; sexual activity, in which he had engaged with two different women, had involved pleasureless orgasm. He said he felt empty, going through life without any sense of direction, ambition, or passion, a realization that itself was tormenting. (Courtesy of Hagop S. Akiskal, M.D.)

Dysthymic Variants. Dysthymia is not uncommon in patients with chronically disabling physical disorders, particularly among elderly adults. Dysthymialike, clinically significant, subthreshold depression lasting 6 or more months has also been described in neurological conditions, including stroke. According to a recent World Health Organization (WHO) conference, this condition aggravates the prognosis of the underlying neurological disease and, therefore, deserves pharmacotherapy.

Prospective studies on children have revealed an episodic course of dysthymia with remissions, exacerbations, and eventual complications by major depressive episodes, 15 to 20 percent of which might even progress to hypomanic, manic, or mixed episodes postpuberty. Persons with dysthymic disorder presenting clinically as adults tend to pursue a chronic unipolar course that may or may not be complicated by major depression. They rarely develop spontaneous hypomania or mania. However, when treated with antidepressants, some of them may develop brief hypomanic switches that typically disappear when the antidepressant dose is decreased.

Differential Diagnosis

The differential diagnosis for dysthymic disorder is essentially identical to that for major depressive disorder. Many substances and medical illnesses can cause chronic depressive symptoms. Two disorders are particularly important to consider in the differential diagnosis of dysthymic disorder—minor depressive disorder and recurrent brief depressive disorder.

Minor Depressive Disorder. Minor depressive disorder (discussed in Section 15.3) is characterized by episodes of depressive symptoms that are less severe than those seen in major depressive disorder. The difference between dysthymic disorder and minor depressive disorder is primarily the episodic nature of the symptoms in the latter. Between episodes, patients with minor depressive disorder have a euthymic mood, whereas patients with dysthymic disorder have virtually no euthymic periods.

Recurrent Brief Depressive Disorder. Recurrent brief depressive disorder (discussed in Section 15.3) is characterized by brief periods (less than 2 weeks) during which depressive episodes are present. Patients with the disorder would meet the diagnostic criteria for major depressive disorder if their episodes lasted longer. Patients with recurrent brief depressive disorder differ from patients with dysthymic disorder on two counts: They have an episodic disorder, and their symptoms are more severe.

Double Depression. An estimated 40 percent of patients with major depressive disorder also meet the criteria for dysthymic disorder, a combination often referred to as double depression. Available data support the conclusion that patients with double depression have a poorer prognosis than patients with only major depressive disorder. The treatment of patients with double depression should be directed toward both disorders, as the resolution of the symptoms of major depressive episode still leaves these patients with significant psychiatric impairment.

Alcohol and Substance Abuse. Patients with dysthymic disorder commonly meet the diagnostic criteria for a substance-related disorder. This comorbidity can be logical; patients with dysthymic disorder tend to develop coping methods for their chronically depressed state. Therefore, they are likely to use alcohol, stimulants such as cocaine, or marijuana, the choice perhaps depending primarily on a patient's social context. The presence of a comorbid diagnosis of substance abuse presents a diagnostic dilemma for clinicians; the long-term use of many substances can result in a symptom picture indistinguishable from that of dysthymic disorder.

Course and Prognosis

About 50 percent of patients with dysthymic disorder experience an insidious onset of symptoms before age 25. Despite the early onset, patients often suffer with the symptoms for a decade before seeking psychiatric help and may consider early-onset dysthymic disorder simply part of life. Patients with an early onset of symptoms are at risk for either major depressive disorder or bipolar I disorder in the course of their disorder. Studies of patients with the diagnosis of dysthymic disorder indicated that about 20 percent progressed to major depressive disorder, 15 percent to bipolar II disorder, and less than 5 percent to bipolar I disorder.

The prognosis for patients with dysthymic disorder varies. Antidepressive agents (e.g., fluoxetine [Prozac] and bupropion [Wellbutrin]) and specific types of psychotherapies (e.g., cognitive and behavior therapies) have positive effects on the course and prognosis of dysthymic disorder. The available data about previously available treatments indicate that only 10 to 15 percent of patients are in remission 1 year after the initial diagnosis. About 25 percent of all patients with dysthymic disorder never attain a complete recovery. Overall, however, the prognosis is good with treatment.

Treatment

Historically, patients with dysthymic disorder either received no treatment or were seen as candidates for long-term, insight-oriented psychotherapy. Contemporary data offer the most objective support for cognitive therapy, behavior therapy, and pharmacotherapy. The combination of pharmacotherapy and either cognitive or behavior therapy may be the most effective treatment for the disorder.

Cognitive Therapy. Cognitive therapy is a technique in which patients are taught new ways of thinking and behaving to replace faulty negative attitudes about themselves, the world, and the future. It is a short-term therapy program oriented toward current problems and their resolution.

Behavior Therapy. Behavior therapy for depressive disorders is based on the theory that depression is caused by a loss of positive reinforcement as a result of separation, death, or sudden environmental change. The various treatment methods focus on specific goals to increase activity, to provide pleasant experiences, and to teach patients how to relax. Altering personal behavior in depressed patients is believed to be the most effective way to change the associated depressed thoughts and feelings. Behavior therapy is often used to treat the learned helplessness of some patients who seem to meet every life challenge with a sense of impotence.

Insight-Oriented (Psychoanalytic) Psychotherapy. Individual insight-oriented psychotherapy is the most common treatment method for dysthymic disorder, and many clinicians consider it the treatment of choice. The psychotherapeutic approach attempts to relate the development and maintenance of depressive symptoms and maladaptive personality features to unresolved conflicts from early childhood. Insight into depressive equivalents (such as substance abuse) or into childhood disappointments as antecedents to adult depression can be gained through treatment. Ambivalent current relationships with parents, friends, and others in the patient's current life are examined. Patients' understanding of how they try to gratify an excessive need for outside approval to counter low self-esteem and a harsh superego is an important goal in this therapy.

Dysthymic disorder involves a chronic state of depression that becomes a way of life for certain persons. These persons

consciously experience themselves at the mercy of a tormenting internal object that is unrelenting in its persecution. Usually conceptualized as a harsh superego, the internal agency criticizes them, punishes them for not measuring up to expectations, and generally contributes to their feelings of misery and unhappiness. This pattern may be associated with self-defeating tendencies, because patients do not feel that they deserve to be successful. They may also have a long-standing sense of despair about ever getting their emotional needs met by important persons in their lives. The patients' bleak outlook on life and their pessimism about relationships result in a self-fulfilling prophecy—many persons avoid them because their company is unpleasant.

Interpersonal Therapy. In interpersonal therapy for depressive disorders, a patient's current interpersonal experiences and ways of coping with stress are examined to reduce depressive symptoms and to improve self-esteem. Interpersonal therapy lasts for about 12 to 16 weekly sessions and can be combined with antidepressant medication.

Family and Group Therapies. Family therapy may help both the patient and the patient's family deal with the symptoms of the disorder, especially when a biologically based subaffective syndrome seems to be present. Group therapy may help withdrawn patients learn new ways to overcome their interpersonal problems in social situations.

Pharmacotherapy. Because of long-standing and commonly held theoretical beliefs that dysthymic disorder is primarily a psychologically determined disorder, many clinicians avoid prescribing antidepressants for patients; however, many studies have shown therapeutic success with antidepressants. The data generally indicate that selective serotonin reuptake inhibitors (SSRIs) are of use for patients with dysthymic disorder. Similarly, bupropion may also be an effective treatment for patients with dysthymic disorder. Monoamine oxidase inhibitors (MAOIs) are effective in a subgroup of dysthymic patients, a group who may also respond to the judicious use of amphetamines.

FAILURE OF THERAPEUTIC TRIAL. A therapeutic trial of an antidepressant in the treatment of dysthymic disorder should include maximal tolerated dosages for a minimum of 8 weeks before clinicians conclude that the trial was not effective. When a drug trial is unsuccessful, clinicians should reconsider the diagnosis, particularly the possibility of an underlying medical disorder (especially a thyroid disorder) or adult attention-deficit disorder. When reconsideration of the differential diagnosis still suggests that dysthymic disorder is the most likely diagnosis, clinicians may follow the same therapeutic strategy as for major depressive disorder and may attempt to augment the first antidepressant by adding lithium or liothyronine (Cytomel), although augmentation strategies for dysthymic disorder have not been studied. As an alternative, clinicians may decide to switch to an antidepressant from a completely different class of drugs. For example, if a trial with an SSRI is unsuccessful, a clinician may switch to bupropion, an MAOI, or a tricyclic drug. There are some reports of augmentation with testosterone in men who are treatment resistant.

Hospitalization. Hospitalization is usually not indicated for patients with dysthymic disorder, but particularly severe symptoms, marked social or professional incapacitation, the need for extensive diagnostic procedures, and suicidal ideation are all indications for hospitalization.

CYCLOTHYMIC DISORDER

Cyclothymic disorder is symptomatically a mild form of bipolar II disorder, characterized by episodes of hypomania and mild depression. In DSM-IV-TR, cyclothymic disorder is defined as a "chronic, fluctuating disturbance" with many periods of hypomania and of depression. The disorder is differentiated from bipolar II disorder, which is characterized by the presence of major (not minor) depressive and hypomanic episodes. As with dysthymic disorder, the inclusion of cyclothymic disorder with the mood disorders implies a relation, probably biological, to bipolar I disorder. Some psychiatrists, however, consider cyclothymic disorder to have no biological component and to result from chaotic object relations early in life.

Contemporary understanding of cyclothymic disorder is based to some extent on the observations of Emil Kraepelin and Kurt Schneider that one third to two thirds of patients with mood disorders exhibit personality disorders. Kraepelin described four types of personality disorders: depressive (gloomy), manic (cheerful and uninhibited), irritable (labile and explosive), and cyclothymic. He described the irritable personality as simultaneously depressive and manic and the cyclothymic personality as the alternation of the depressive and manic personalities.

Epidemiology

Patients with cyclothymic disorder may constitute from 3 to 5 percent of all psychiatric outpatients, perhaps particularly those with significant complaints about marital and interpersonal difficulties. In the general population, the lifetime prevalence of cyclothymic disorder is estimated to be about 1 percent. This figure is probably lower than the actual prevalence, because, as with patients with bipolar I disorder, the patients may not be aware that they have a psychiatric problem. Cyclothymic disorder, like dysthymic disorder, frequently coexists with borderline personality disorder. An estimated 10 percent of outpatients and 20 percent of inpatients with borderline personality disorder have a coexisting diagnosis of cyclothymic disorder. The female-to-male ratio in cyclothymic disorder is about 3 to 2, and 50 to 75 percent of all patients have an onset between ages 15 and 25. Families of persons with cyclothymic disorder often contain members with substance-related disorder.

Etiology

As with dysthymic disorder, there is controversy about whether cyclothymic disorder is related to the mood disorders, either biologically or psychologically. Some researchers have postulated that cyclothymic disorder has a closer relation to borderline personality disorder than to the mood disorders. In spite of these controversies, the preponderance of biological and

genetic data favors the idea of cyclothymic disorder as a bona fide mood disorder.

Biological Factors. The strongest evidence for the hypothesis that cyclothymic disorder is a mood disorder is the genetic data. About 30 percent of all patients with cyclothymic disorder have positive family histories for bipolar I disorder; this rate is similar to the rate for patients with bipolar I disorder. Moreover, the pedigrees of families with bipolar I disorder often contain generations of patients with bipolar I disorder linked by a generation with cyclothymic disorder. Conversely, the prevalence of cyclothymic disorder in the relatives of patients with bipolar I disorder is much higher than the prevalence of cyclothymic disorder either in the relatives of patients with other mental disorders or in persons who are mentally healthy. The observations that about one third of patients with cyclothymic disorder subsequently have major mood disorders, that they are particularly sensitive to antidepressant-induced hypomania, and that about 60 percent respond to lithium add further support to the idea of cyclothymic disorder as a mild or attenuated form of bipolar II disorder.

Psychosocial Factors. Most psychodynamic theories postulate that the development of cyclothymic disorder lies in traumas and fixations during the oral stage of infant development. Freud hypothesized that the cyclothymic state is the ego's attempt to overcome a harsh and punitive superego. Hypomania is explained psychodynamically as the lack of self-criticism and an absence of inhibitions occurring when a depressed person throws off the burden of an overly harsh superego. The major defense mechanism in hypomania is denial, by which the patient avoids external problems and internal feelings of depression.

Patients with cyclothymic disorder are characterized by periods of depression alternating with periods of hypomania. Psychoanalytic exploration reveals that such patients defend themselves against underlying depressive themes with their euphoric or hypomanic periods. Hypomania is frequently triggered by a profound interpersonal loss. The false euphoria generated in such instances is a patient's way to deny dependence on love objects while simultaneously disavowing any aggression or destructiveness that may have contributed to the loss of the loved person. Hypomania may also be associated with an unconscious fantasy that the lost object has been restored. This denial is generally short-lived, and the patient soon resumes the preoccupation with suffering and misery characteristic of dysthymic disorder.

Diagnosis and Clinical Features

Although many patients seek psychiatric help for depression, their problems are often related to the chaos that their manic episodes have caused. Clinicians must consider a diagnosis of cyclothymic disorder when a patient appears with what may seem to be sociopathic behavioral problems. Marital difficulties and instability in relationships are common complaints because patients with cyclothymic disorder are often promiscuous and irritable while in manic and mixed states. Although there are anecdotal reports of increased productivity and creativity when patients are hypomanic, most clinicians report that their patients become disorganized and ineffective in work and school during these periods.

Table 15.2–4
DSM-IV-TR Diagnostic Criteria for Cyclothymic Disorder

A. For at least 2 years, the presence of numerous periods with hypomanic symptoms and numerous periods with depressive symptoms that do not meet criteria for a major depressive episode. **Note:** In children and adolescents, the duration must be at least 1 year.

B. During the above 2-year period (1 year in children and adolescents), the person has not been without the symptoms in Criterion A for more than 2 months at a time.

C. No major depressive episode, manic episode, or mixed episode has been present during the first 2 years of the disturbance.

Note: After the initial 2 years (1 year in children and adolescents) of cyclothymic disorder, there may be superimposed manic or mixed episodes (in which case both bipolar I disorder and cyclothymic disorder may be diagnosed) or major depressive episodes (in which case both bipolar II disorder and cyclothymic disorder may be diagnosed).

D. The symptoms in Criterion A are not better accounted for by schizoaffective disorder and are not superimposed on schizophrenia, schizophreniform disorder, delusional disorder, or psychotic disorder not otherwise specified.

E. The symptoms are not due to the direct physiological effects of a substance (e.g., a drug of abuse, a medication) or a general medical condition (e.g., hyperthyroidism).

F. The symptoms cause clinically significant distress or impairment in social, occupational, or other important areas of functioning.

From American Psychiatric Association. *Diagnostic and Statistical Manual of Mental Disorders.* 4th ed. Text rev. Washington, DC: American Psychiatric Association; copyright 2000, with permission.

The DSM-IV-TR diagnostic criteria for cyclothymic disorder (Table 15.2–4) stipulate that a patient has never met the criteria for a major depressive episode and did not meet the criteria for a manic episode during the first 2 years of the disturbance. The criteria also require the more or less constant presence of symptoms for 2 years (or 1 year for children and adolescents).

Signs and Symptoms. The symptoms of cyclothymic disorder are identical to the symptoms of bipolar II disorder, except that they are generally less severe. On occasion, however, the symptoms may be equal in severity but of shorter duration than those seen in bipolar II disorder. About half of all patients with cyclothymic disorder have depression as their major symptom, and these patients are most likely to seek psychiatric help while depressed. Some patients with cyclothymic disorder have primarily hypomanic symptoms and are less likely to consult a psychiatrist than are primarily depressed patients. Almost all patients with cyclothymic disorder have periods of mixed symptoms with marked irritability.

Most patients with cyclothymic disorder seen by psychiatrists have not succeeded in their professional and social lives as a result of their disorder, but a few have become high achievers who have worked especially long hours and have required little sleep. Some persons' ability to control the symptoms of

the disorder successfully depends on multiple individual, social, and cultural attributes.

The lives of most patients with cyclothymic disorder are difficult. The cycles of the disorder tend to be much shorter than those in bipolar I disorder. In cyclothymic disorder, the changes in mood are irregular and abrupt and sometimes occur within hours. The unpredictable nature of the mood changes produces great stress. Patients often feel that their moods are out of control. In irritable, mixed periods, they may become involved in unprovoked disagreements with friends, family, and coworkers.

Substance Abuse. Alcohol abuse and other substance abuse are common in cyclothymic disorder patients, who use substances either to self-medicate (with alcohol, benzodiazepines, and marijuana) or to achieve even further stimulation (with cocaine, amphetamines, and hallucinogens) when they are manic. About 5 to 10 percent of all patients with cyclothymic disorder have substance dependence. Persons with this disorder often have a history of multiple geographical moves, involvements in religious cults, and dilettantism.

Differential Diagnosis

When a diagnosis of cyclothymic disorder is under consideration, all the possible medical and substance-related causes of depression and mania such as seizures and particular substances (cocaine, amphetamine, and steroids) must be considered. Borderline, antisocial, histrionic, and narcissistic personality disorders should also be considered in the differential diagnosis. Attention-deficit/hyperactivity disorder can be difficult to differentiate from cyclothymic disorder in children and adolescents. A trial of stimulants helps most patients with attention-deficit/hyperactivity disorder and exacerbates the symptoms of most patients with cyclothymic disorder. The diagnostic category of bipolar II disorder (discussed in Section 15.1) is characterized by the combination of major depressive and hypomanic episodes.

Course and Prognosis

Some patients with cyclothymic disorder are characterized as having been sensitive, hyperactive, or moody as young children. The onset of frank symptoms of cyclothymic disorder often occurs insidiously in the teens or early 20s. The emergence of symptoms at that time hinders a person's performance in school and the ability to establish friendships with peers. The reactions of patients to such a disorder vary; patients with adaptive coping strategies or ego defenses have better outcomes than patients with poor coping strategies. About one third of all patients with cyclothymic disorder develop a major mood disorder, most often bipolar II disorder.

Treatment

Biological Therapy. The mood stabilizers and antimanic drugs are the first line of treatment for patients with cyclothymic disorder. Although the experimental data are limited to studies with lithium, other antimanic agents—for example, carbamazepine and valproate (Depakene)—are reported to be effective. Dosages and plasma concentrations of these agents should be the same as those in bipolar I disorder. Antidepressant treatment of depressed patients with cyclothymic disorder should be done with caution, because these patients have increased susceptibility to antidepressant-induced hypomanic or manic episodes. About 40 to 50 percent of all patients with cyclothymic disorder who are treated with antidepressants experience such episodes. Anticonvulsants such as gabapentin (Neurontin) have been of use in some patients. Clonazepam (Klonopin) has been useful to control cyclothymic patients who are agitated periodically.

Psychosocial Therapy. Psychotherapy for patients with cyclothymic disorder is best directed toward increasing patients' awareness of their condition and helping them develop coping mechanisms for their mood swings. Therapists usually need to help patients repair any damage, both work and family related, done during episodes of hypomania. Because of the long-term nature of cyclothymic disorder, patients often require lifelong treatment. Family and group therapies may be supportive, educational, and therapeutic for patients and for those involved in their lives. The psychiatrist conducting psychotherapy is able to evaluate the degree of cyclothymia and so provide an early-warning system to prevent full-blown manic attacks before they occur.

References

Akiskal HS. Mood disorder: clinical features. In: Sadock BJ, Sadock VA, eds. *Kaplan & Sadock's Comprehensive Textbook of Psychiatry.* 7th ed. Vol 1. Baltimore: Lippincott Williams & Wilkins; 2000:1338.

Akiskal HS. Dysthymia and cyclothymia in psychiatric practice a century after Kraepelin. *J Affective Disorders.* 2001;62(1–2):17.

Baldwin DS. Dysthymia: options in pharmacotherapy. In: Palmer KJ, ed. *Managing Depressive Disorders.* Kwai Chung, Hong Kong: Adis International Publications; 2000:157.

Brunello N, Akiskal H, Boyer P, et al. Dysthymia: clinical picture, extent of overlap with chronic fatigue syndrome, neuropharmacological considerations, and new therapeutic vistas. *J Affective Disorders.* 1999;52(1–3):275.

De Lima MS, Hotoph M, Wessely S. The efficacy of drug treatments for dysthymia: a systematic review and meta-analysis. *Psychol Med.* 1999;29(6):1273.

Huprich SK. The overlap of depressive personality disorder and dysthymia, reconsidered. *Harvard Rev Psychiatry.* 2001;9(4):158.

Kocsis JH, Zisook S, Davidson J, et al. Double-blind comparison of sertraline, imipramine, and placebo in the treatment of dysthymia: psychosocial outcomes. *Am J Psychiatry.* 1997;154:390.

Shaffer D, Waslick BD. The many faces of depression in children and adolescents. *Rev Psychiatry.* 2002;21:105.

Verthoeven WMA, Tuinier S. Cyclothymia or unstable mood disorder? A systematic treatment evaluation with valproic acid. *J Appl Res Intellect Disabil.* 2001;14(2):147.

▲ 15.3 Other Mood Disorders

DEPRESSIVE DISORDER NOT OTHERWISE SPECIFIED

If a patient exhibits depressive symptoms as the major feature and does not meet the diagnostic criteria for any other mood disorder, the most appropriate diagnosis is a depressive disorder not otherwise specified (Table 15.3–1). Examples are minor depressive disorder, recurrent brief depressive disorder, and premenstrual dysphoric disorder.

Table 15.3–1
DSM-IV-TR Diagnostic Criteria for Depressive Disorder Not Otherwise Specified

The depressive disorder not otherwise specified category includes disorders with depressive features that do not meet the criteria for major depressive disorder, dysthymic disorder, adjustment disorder with depressed mood, or adjustment disorder with mixed anxiety and depressed mood. Sometimes depressive symptoms can present as part of an anxiety disorder not otherwise specified. Examples of depressive disorder not otherwise specified include

1. Premenstrual dysphoric disorder: in most menstrual cycles during the past year, symptoms (e.g., markedly depressed mood, marked anxiety, marked affective lability, decreased interest in activities) regularly occurred during the last week of the luteal phase (and remitted within a few days of the onset of menses). These symptoms must be severe enough to markedly interfere with work, school, or usual activities and be entirely absent for at least 1 week postmenses.
2. Minor depressive disorder: episodes of at least 2 weeks of depressive symptoms but with fewer than the five items required for major depressive disorder.
3. Recurrent brief depressive disorder: depressive episodes lasting from 2 days up to 2 weeks, occurring at least once a month for 12 months (not associated with the menstrual cycle).
4. Postpsychotic depressive disorder of schizophrenia: a major depressive episode that occurs during the residual phase of schizophrenia.
5. A major depressive episode superimposed on delusional disorder, psychotic disorder not otherwise specified, or the active phase of schizophrenia.
6. Situations in which the clinician has concluded that a depressive disorder is present but is unable to determine whether it is primary, due to a general medical condition, or substance induced.

From American Psychiatric Association. *Diagnostic and Statistical Manual of Mental Disorders.* 4th ed. Text rev. Washington, DC: American Psychiatric Association; copyright 2000, with permission.

Minor Depressive Disorder

The literature in the United States on minor depressive disorder is limited, in part because the term *minor depression* is used to describe a wide range of disorders, including what is called dysthymic disorder in the text revision of the fourth edition of *Diagnostic and Statistical Manual of Mental Disorders* (DSM-IV-TR). The European literature on minor depressive disorder is also limited, but it is more extensive than that in the United States. The information about this disorder is contained in an appendix of DSM-IV-TR that includes specific diagnostic guidelines. The disorder requires future study.

Epidemiology. The epidemiology of minor depressive disorder is unknown, but preliminary data indicate that it may be as common as major depressive disorder—that is, about 5 percent prevalence in the general population. Preliminary data also indicate that the disorder is more common in women than in men. Minor depressive disorder probably affects people of virtually any age, from childhood onward.

Etiology. The cause of minor depressive disorder is unknown. The same causative considerations given major depressive disorder should be considered. Specifically, the biological theories involve the activities of noradrenergic and serotonergic biogenic amine systems and the thyroid and adrenal neuroendocrine axes. The psychological theories center on issues of loss, guilt, and punitive superegos.

Diagnosis and Clinical Features. The DSM-IV-TR research criteria for minor depressive disorder include symptoms equal in duration to those of major depressive disorder but less severe (Table 15.3–2). The category allows a specific diagnosis for patients whose lives are affected by depressive symptoms but whose symptoms are not severe enough for a diagnosis of major depressive disorder.

Except that they are less severe, the clinical features of minor depressive disorder are virtually identical to those of major depressive disorder. The central symptom of both disorders is the same—a depressed mood.

Differential Diagnosis. The differential diagnosis for minor depressive disorder is the same as that for major depressive disorder. Of special importance for the differential diagnosis of minor depressive disorder are dysthymic disorder and recurrent brief depressive disorder. Dysthymic disorder is characterized by the presence of chronic depressive symptoms, whereas recurrent brief depressive disorder is characterized by multiple brief episodes of severe depressive symptoms.

Course and Prognosis. No definitive data on the course and the prognosis of minor depressive disorder are available, but minor depressive disorder, probably like major depressive disorder, has a long-term course that may require long-term treatment. A significant proportion of patients with minor depressive disorder are probably at risk for other mood disorders, including dysthymic disorder, bipolar I disorder, bipolar II disorder, and major depressive disorder.

Treatment. The treatment of minor depressive disorder can include psychotherapy, pharmacotherapy, or both. Insight-oriented psychotherapy, cognitive therapy, interpersonal therapy, and behavior therapy are the psychotherapeutic treatments for major depressive disorder and, by implication, for minor depressive disorder. Although the experimental data are limited, patients with minor depressive disorder are probably responsive to pharmacotherapy, particularly selective serotonin reuptake inhibitors (SSRIs) and bupropion (Wellbutrin).

Recurrent Brief Depressive Disorder

Recurrent brief depressive disorder is characterized by multiple, relatively brief episodes (of less than 2 weeks) of depressive symptoms that, except for their brief duration, meet the diagnostic criteria for major depressive disorder. Recurrent brief depressive disorder has been written about mostly in the European literature, but with its introduction as a research category in an appendix of DSM-IV-TR, the diagnosis is likely to gain rapid acceptance in the United States. This acceptance will likely be further facilitated by clinicians' increasing awareness that recurrent brief depressive disorder is relatively common and associated with significant morbidity.

Table 15.3–2
DSM-IV-TR Research Criteria for Minor Depressive Disorder

A. A mood disturbance, defined as follows:
   (1) at least two (but less than five) of the following symptoms have been present during the same 2-week period and represent a change from previous functioning; at least one of the symptoms is either (a) or (b):
      (a) depressed mood most of the day, nearly every day, as indicated by either subjective report (e.g., feels sad or empty) or observation made by others (e.g., appears tearful). **Note:** In children and adolescents, can be irritable mood.
      (b) markedly diminished interest or pleasure in all, or almost all, activities most of the day, nearly every day (as indicated by either subjective account or observation made by others)
      (c) significant weight loss when not dieting or weight gain (e.g., a change of more than 5% of body weight in a month), or decrease or increase in appetite nearly every day. **Note:** In children, consider failure to make expected weight gains.
      (d) insomnia or hypersomnia nearly every day
      (e) psychomotor agitation or retardation nearly every day (observable by others, not merely subjective feelings of restlessness or being slowed down)
      (f) fatigue or loss of energy nearly every day
      (g) feelings of worthlessness or excessive or inappropriate guilt (which may be delusional) nearly every day (not merely self-reproach or guilt about being sick)
      (h) diminished ability to think or concentrate, or indecisiveness, nearly every day (either by subjective account or as observed by others)
      (i) recurrent thoughts of death (not just fear of dying), recurrent suicidal ideation without a specific plan, or a suicide attempt or a specific plan for committing suicide
   (2) the symptoms cause clinically significant distress or impairment in social, occupational, or other important areas of functioning
   (3) the symptoms are not due to the direct physiological effects of a substance (e.g., a drug of abuse, a medication) or a general medical condition (e.g., hypothyroidism)
   (4) the symptoms are not better accounted for by bereavement (i.e., a normal reaction to the death of a loved one)

B. There has never been a major depressive episode, and criteria are not met for dysthymic disorder.

C. There has never been a manic episode, a mixed episode, or a hypomanic episode, and criteria are not met for cyclothymic disorder. **Note:** This exclusion does not apply if all of the manic-, mixed-, or hypomaniclike episodes are substance or treatment induced.

D. The mood disturbance does not occur exclusively during schizophrenia, schizophreniform disorder, schizoaffective disorder, delusional disorder, or psychotic disorder not otherwise specified.

From American Psychiatric Association. *Diagnostic and Statistical Manual of Mental Disorders.* 4th ed. Text rev. Washington, DC: American Psychiatric Association; copyright 2000, with permission.

Epidemiology

No extensive studies of the epidemiology of recurrent brief depressive disorder have been conducted in the United States. Using available data, the 10-year prevalence rate for the disorder is estimated to be 10 percent for people in their 20s; the 1-year prevalence rate for the general population is estimated to be 5 percent. These numbers indicate that recurrent brief depressive disorder is most common among young adults, but many more studies are needed to refine the data.

Etiology. One study showed that patients with recurrent brief depressive disorder share several biological abnormalities with patients with major depressive disorder, compared with control subjects who are mentally healthy. The variables include nonsuppression on the dexamethasone-suppression test (DST), a blunt response to thyrotropin-releasing hormone (TRH), and a shortening of rapid eye movement (REM) sleep latency. The data are consistent with the idea that recurrent brief depressive disorder is closely related to major depressive disorder in its cause and pathophysiology. The available data also suggest a close relation between the two disorders and indicate that family histories of patients with mood disorders are similar for recurrent brief depressive disorder and major depressive disorder.

Diagnosis and Clinical Features. The DSM-IV-TR research criteria for recurrent brief depressive disorder specify that the symptom duration for each episode is less than 2 weeks (Table 15.3–3). Otherwise, the diagnostic criteria for recurrent brief depressive disorder and major depressive disorder are essentially identical.

The clinical features of recurrent brief depressive disorder are almost identical to those of major depressive disorder. One subtle difference is that the frequent changes in their moods may make the lives of patients with recurrent brief depressive disorder seem more disrupted or chaotic than those of patients with major depressive disorder, whose depressive episodes occur at a measured pace. In one study, the mean length of time between depressive disorder episodes in recurrent brief depressive disorder was calculated to be 18 days. Results of another study showed that episodes of sleep disturbances closely coincide with the episodes of depression, thus helping clinicians establish the periodicity of the depressive episodes.

Differential Diagnosis. The differential diagnosis for recurrent brief depressive disorder is the same as that for major depressive disorder. Clinicians should consider bipolar disorders and major depressive disorder with seasonal pattern in the differential diagnosis. Research into recurrent brief depressive disorder may find an association with the rapid cycling type of bipolar disorder. Clinicians should also determine whether there is a seasonal pattern to the recurrence of depressive episodes in a patient being evaluated for a diagnosis of recurrent brief depressive disorder. At least one researcher has proposed that patients with recurrent brief depressive disorder be subtyped according to the relative frequencies of their depressive episodes. This differentiation is not included in DSM-IV-TR, although it may yet prove to have prognostic or treatment implications.

Course and Prognosis. The course and the prognosis for patients with recurrent brief depressive disorder are not well known. On the basis of available data, their course, including age of onset, and their prognosis are similar to those of patients with major depressive disorder.

Table 15.3–3
DSM-IV-TR Research Criteria for Recurrent Brief Depressive Disorder

A. Criteria, except for duration, are met for a major depressive episode.
B. The depressive periods in Criterion A last at least 2 days but less than 2 weeks.
C. The depressive periods occur at least once a month for 12 consecutive months and are not associated with the menstrual cycle.
D. The periods of depressed mood cause clinically significant distress or impairment in social, occupational, or other important areas of functioning.
E. The symptoms are not due to the direct physiological effects of a substance (e.g., a drug of abuse, a medication) or a general medical condition (e.g., hypothyroidism).
F. There has never been a major depressive episode, and criteria are not met for dysthymic disorder.
G. There has never been a manic episode, a mixed episode, or a hypomanic episode, and criteria are not met for cyclothymic disorder. **Note:** This exclusion does not apply if all of the manic-, mixed-, or hypomaniclike episodes are substance or treatment induced.
H. The mood disturbance does not occur exclusively during schizophrenia, schizophreniform disorder, schizoaffective disorder, delusional disorder, or psychotic disorder not otherwise specified.

From American Psychiatric Association. *Diagnostic and Statistical Manual of Mental Disorders.* 4th ed. Text rev. Washington, DC: American Psychiatric Association; copyright 2000, with permission.

Treatment. The treatment of patients with recurrent brief depressive disorder should be similar to the treatment of patients with major depressive disorder. The main treatments are psychotherapy (insight-oriented psychotherapy, cognitive therapy, interpersonal therapy, or behavioral therapy) and pharmacotherapy with the standard antidepressant drugs. Some of the treatments for bipolar I disorder—lithium (Eskalith) and anticonvulsants—may be of therapeutic value.

Premenstrual Dysphoric Disorder

In an appendix, DSM-IV-TR includes suggested diagnostic criteria for premenstrual dysphoric disorder to help researchers and clinicians evaluate the validity of the diagnosis. Premenstrual dysphoric disorder has also been referred to as late luteal phase dysphoric disorder. Whether the syndrome warrants an official diagnosis remains controversial. Nevertheless, the generally recognized syndrome involves mood symptoms (e.g., lability), behavior symptoms (e.g., changes in eating patterns), and physical symptoms (e.g., breast tenderness, edema, and headaches). This pattern of symptoms occurs at a specific time during the menstrual cycle, and the symptoms resolve for some period of time between menstrual cycles.

Epidemiology. Because of the absence of generally agreed-on diagnostic criteria, the epidemiology of premenstrual dysphoric disorder is not known with certainty. One study reported that about 40 percent of women have at least mild premenstrual symptoms and that 2 to 10 percent meet the full diagnostic criteria for the disorder.

Etiology. On the one hand, the cause of premenstrual dysphoric disorder is unknown. On the other hand, because the symptoms are timed to the menstrual cycle, the hormonal changes occurring during the menstrual cycle are probably involved in producing symptoms. A common theory among many proposed theories characterizes the disorder as the result of an abnormally high estrogen-to-progesterone ratio in affected women. Other hypotheses suggest that the biogenic amine neurons of affected women are abnormally affected by changes in the hormones, that the disorder is an example of a chronobiological phase disorder, and that it is the result of abnormal prostaglandin activity. In addition to the biological theories, societal and personal issues about menstruation and womanhood may affect the symptoms of individual patients.

Diagnosis and Clinical Features. An appendix of DSM-IV-TR contains suggested diagnostic criteria for premenstrual dysphoric disorder (Table 15.3–4). The criteria include symptoms about abnormal mood, abnormal behavior, and somatic complaints.

The most common mood and cognitive symptoms are lability of mood, irritability, anxiety, decreased interest in activities, increased fatigability, and difficulty concentrating. Behavioral symptoms often include changes in appetite and sleep patterns. The most common somatic complaints are headache, breast tenderness, and edema. In affected women, the symptoms appear during most (if not all) menstrual cycles, although they usually remit before the end of the blood flow. Affected women are symptom free for at least 1 week during each menstrual cycle.

Differential Diagnosis. If symptoms are present throughout the menstrual cycle, with no intercycle symptom relief, clinicians should consider one of the non–menstrual cycle–related mood disorders and anxiety disorders. The presence of especially severe symptoms, even if cyclical, should prompt clinicians to consider other mood disorders and anxiety disorder. A thorough medical workup is necessary to rule out medical or surgical conditions to account for symptoms (e.g., endometriosis).

Course and Prognosis. The course and the prognosis of premenstrual dysphoric disorder have not been studied enough to reach any reasonable conclusions. Anecdotally, the symptoms tend to be chronic unless effective treatment is initiated.

Treatment. Treatment of premenstrual dysphoric disorder includes support for the patient about the presence and recognition of the symptoms. SSRIs, for example, fluoxetine (Prozac, Sarafem) and alprazolam (Xanax), have all been reported to be effective, although no treatment has been conclusively demonstrated to be effective in multiple, well-controlled trials. Premenstrual dysphoric disorder is also covered in Chapter 30.

Table 15.3–4
DSM-IV-TR Research Criteria for Premenstrual Dysphoric Disorder

A. In most menstrual cycles during the past year, five (or more) of the following symptoms were present for most of the time during the last week of the luteal phase, began to remit within a few days after the onset of the follicular phase, and were absent in the week postmenses, with at least one of the symptoms being either (1), (2), (3), or (4):
  (1) markedly depressed mood, feelings of hopelessness, or self-deprecating thoughts
  (2) marked anxiety, tension, feelings of being "keyed up," or "on edge"
  (3) marked affective lability (e.g., feeling suddenly sad or tearful or increased sensitivity to rejection)
  (4) persistent and marked anger or irritability or increased interpersonal conflicts
  (5) decreased interest in usual activities (e.g., work, school, friends, hobbies)
  (6) subjective sense of difficulty in concentrating
  (7) lethargy, easy fatigability, or marked lack of energy
  (8) marked change in appetite, overeating, or specific food cravings
  (9) hypersomnia or insomnia
  (10) a subjective sense of being overwhelmed or out of control
  (11) other physical symptoms, such as breast tenderness or swelling, headaches, joint or muscle pain, a sensation of "bloating," weight gain

  Note: In menstruating females, the luteal phase corresponds to the period between ovulation and the onset of menses, and the follicular phase begins with menses. In nonmenstruating females (e.g., those who have had a hysterectomy), the timing of luteal and follicular phases may require measurement of circulating reproductive hormones.

B. The disturbance markedly interferes with work or school or with usual social activities and relationships with others (e.g., avoidance of social activities, decreased productivity and efficiency at work or school).

C. The disturbance is not merely an exacerbation of the symptoms of another disorder, such as major depressive disorder, panic disorder, dysthymic disorder, or a personality disorder (although it may be superimposed on any of these disorders).

D. Criteria A, B, and C must be confirmed by prospective daily ratings during at least two consecutive symptomatic cycles. (The diagnosis may be made provisionally prior to this confirmation.)

From American Psychiatric Association. *Diagnostic and Statistical Manual of Mental Disorders.* 4th ed. Text rev. Washington, DC: American Psychiatric Association; copyright 2000, with permission.

Table 15.3–5
DSM-IV-TR Research Criteria for Postpsychotic Depressive Disorder of Schizophrenia

A. Criteria are met for a major depressive episode.
  Note: The major depressive episode must include Criterion A1: depressed mood. Do not include symptoms that are better accounted for as medication side effects or negative symptoms of schizophrenia.

B. The major depressive episode is superimposed on and occurs only during the residual phase of schizophrenia.

C. The major depressive episode is not due to the direct physiological effects of a substance or a general medical condition.

From American Psychiatric Association. *Diagnostic and Statistical Manual of Mental Disorders.* 4th ed. Text rev. Washington, DC: American Psychiatric Association; copyright 2000, with permission.

Postpsychotic Depressive Disorder of Schizophrenia

Postpsychotic depressive disorder in schizophrenic patients is categorized in an appendix in DSM-IV-TR.

Epidemiology. In the absence of specific diagnostic criteria, the reported incidence of postpsychotic depression of schizophrenia varies widely, from less than 10 percent to more than 70 percent. A reasonable estimate based on large studies is about 25 percent, although a definitive incidence figure must wait for controlled studies using the DSM-IV-TR criteria.

Prognostic Significance. The prognostic significance of the DSM-IV-TR diagnosis is uncertain, because no studies using the official diagnostic category have been conducted. Nonetheless, data from other studies indicate that patients with postpsychotic depressive disorder of schizophrenia are likely to have had poor premorbid adjustment, marked schizoid personality disorder traits, and an insidious onset of their psychotic symptoms. They are also likely to have first-degree relatives with mood disorders. Although the findings have not been consistent, postpsychotic depressive disorder of schizophrenia has been associated with a less favorable prognosis, a higher likelihood of relapse, and a higher incidence of suicide than is seen in schizophrenia patients without postpsychotic depressive disorder. Some data indicate that schizophrenia patients with and without postpsychotic depressive disorder may differ in several biological variables such as DST and TRH test results.

Diagnosis and Differential Diagnosis. The clinical boundaries of the diagnosis are hard to define operationally. The symptoms of postpsychotic depressive disorder of schizophrenia can closely resemble the symptoms of the residual phase of schizophrenia as well as the adverse effects of commonly used antipsychotic medications. Distinguishing the diagnosis from schizoaffective disorder, depressive type, is also difficult. The DSM-IV-TR criteria for a major depressive episode must be met and the symptoms must occur only during the residual phase of schizophrenia (Table 15.3–5). The symptoms cannot be substance induced or part of a mood disorder due to a general medical condition.

The disorder may be almost entirely caused by antipsychotic medications, but several types of data indicate that antipsychotic medications cannot explain the entire extent of the symptoms. First, depressive symptoms are often present during the psychotic episode itself and, generally, decrease in severity with successful antipsychotic treatment. Second, the severity of depressive symptoms in patients with postpsychotic depressive disorder of schizophrenia has not been correlated with the use of antipsychotic medication. Third, depressive symptoms have been frequently reported in nonmedicated schizophrenia patients recovering from psychotic episodes. Nonetheless, clinicians should not confuse the antipsychotic-induced adverse

effects of akathisia and akinesia with symptoms of postpsychotic depressive disorder of schizophrenia.

Treatment. The use of antidepressants (e.g., fluoxetine [Prozac]) in the treatment of postpsychotic depressive disorder of schizophrenia has been reported in several studies. About half the studies reported positive effects, and the other half reported no effect in relieving depressive symptoms. Antidepressant medications probably relieve depressive symptoms in some patients, but the mixed results of the studies reflect the current inability to distinguish patients who will respond from those who will not.

BIPOLAR DISORDER NOT OTHERWISE SPECIFIED

If patients exhibit depressive and manic symptoms as the major features of their disorder and do not meet the diagnostic criteria for any other mood disorder or other DSM-IV-TR mental disorder, the most appropriate diagnosis is bipolar disorder not otherwise specified (Table 15.3–6).

Mixed Anxiety-Depressive Disorder

The inclusion of a mixed anxious depressive state in the DSM-IV-TR appendix acknowledges the simultaneous occurrence of anxious and depressive cognition in a person confronted with a major aversive life situation. The admixture implies that the psychopathology progresses from anxiety to depression and that the patient's mental state is still in flux. Patients with mixed pictures are reportedly most prevalent in general medical settings because they have many somatic complaints about which they are anxious, one of the most prominent being chronic fatigue. The criteria from the 10th revision of *International Statistical Classification of Diseases and Related Health Problems* (ICD-10) criteria would give many of these patients a diagnosis of neurasthenia. Some patients with chronic fatigue syndrome also have mixed anxiety and depressive symptomatology. This disorder is also discussed more fully in Chapter 18, which covers neurasthenia and chronic fatigue syndrome.

Table 15.3–6
DSM-IV-TR Diagnostic Criteria for Bipolar Disorder Not Otherwise Specified

The bipolar disorder not otherwise specified category includes disorders with bipolar features that do not meet criteria for any specific bipolar disorder. Examples include

1. Very rapid alternation (over days) between manic symptoms and depressive symptoms that meet symptom threshold criteria but not minimal duration criteria for manic, hypomanic, or major depressive episodes
2. Recurrent hypomanic episodes without intercurrent depressive symptoms
3. A manic or mixed episode superimposed on delusional disorder, residual schizophrenia, or psychotic disorder not otherwise specified
4. Hypomanic episodes, along with chronic depressive symptoms, that are too infrequent to qualify for a diagnosis of cyclothymic disorder
5. Situations in which the clinician has concluded that a bipolar disorder is present but is unable to determine whether it is primary, due to a general medical condition, or substance induced

From American Psychiatric Association. *Diagnostic and Statistical Manual of Mental Disorders.* 4th ed. Text rev. Washington, DC: American Psychiatric Association; copyright 2000, with permission.

Atypical Depression

A delimited version of atypical depression was incorporated into DSM-IV-TR as "atypical features" (see Table 15.1–22). Atypical depression refers to fatigue superimposed on a history of somatic anxiety and phobias, together with reverse vegetative signs (mood worse in the evening, insomnia, tendency to oversleep and overeat), so that weight gain occurs rather than weight loss. Sleep is disturbed in the first half of the night in many persons with atypical depressive disorder, so irritability, hypersomnolence, and daytime fatigue would be expected. The temperaments of these patients are characterized by extreme sensitivity. SSRIs may be of help; however, the monoamine oxidase inhibitors (MAOIs) seem to show some specificity for such patients. Others are helped by psychostimulants such as amphetamine.

OTHER DISORDERS NOT INCLUDED IN DSM-IV-TR

Atypical Cycloid Psychoses

Atypical cycloid psychoses show some features of bipolar I disorder but generally do not meet the complete diagnostic criteria for that category. Some patients with atypical cycloid psychoses may be classified as having bipolar disorder not otherwise specified.

Hysteroid Dysphoria

The category hysteroid dysphoria combines reverse vegetative signs with the following characteristics: (1) giddy responses to romantic opportunities and an avalanche of dysphoria (angry-depressive, even suicidal responses) upon romantic disappointment; (2) impaired anticipatory pleasure, yet the capability to respond with pleasure when such is provided by others (i.e., preservation of consummatory reward); (3) craving for chocolate and sweets, which contain phenylethylamine compounds and sugars believed to facilitate cellular and neuronal intake of the amino acid L-tryptophan, hypothetically leading to synthesis of endogenous antidepressants in the brain. The word "hysteroid" was used to imply that the apparent character pathology was secondary to biological disturbances. Patients are treated symptomatically. Some respond to SSRIs, others to MAOIs and mood stabilizers such as carbamazepine (Tegretol). This is not an "official" DSM-IV-TR diagnosis; it can be considered an atypical variant of depression.

Motility Psychosis

The two forms of motility psychosis are akinetic and hyperkinetic. The akinetic form of motility psychosis has a clinical presentation similar to that of catatonic stupor. In contrast to the catatonic type of schizophrenia, however, akinetic motility psychosis has a rapidly resolving and favorable course that does not lead to personality deterioration. In its hyperkinetic form, motility psychosis may resemble manic or catatonic

excitement. Like the akinetic form, the hyperkinetic form usually has a rapidly resolving and favorable course. Patients may switch from the akinetic to hyperkinetic form rapidly and may represent a danger to others during the excited phase. Mood is extremely labile in these patients.

Confusional Psychosis

As described originally, excited confusional psychosis is similar to mania but was differentiated from mania by several characteristics: more anxiety, less distractibility, and a degree of speech incoherence out of proportion to the severity of the flight of ideas. Confusional psychosis is probably a clinical variation of the mania seen in bipolar I disorder. Patients may switch rapidly from the akinetic to the hyperkinetic form and may represent a danger to others during the excited phase.

Anxiety-Blissfulness Psychosis

Anxiety-blissfulness psychosis may resemble agitated depression but may also be characterized by so much inhibition that a patient can hardly move. Periodic states of overwhelming anxiety and paranoid ideas of reference are characteristic of the condition, but self-accusation, hypochondriacal preoccupation, other depressive symptoms, and hallucinations may also accompany it. The blissful phase manifests most frequently in expansive behavior and grandiose ideas, which are concerned less with self-aggrandizement than with the mission of making others happy and saving the world.

SECONDARY MOOD DISORDERS

Secondary mood disorders consist of two broad categories that must be considered in the differential diagnosis of any patient with mood disorder symptoms. They are (1) mood disorder due to a general medical condition and (2) substance-induced mood disorder.

Mood Disorders Due to a General Medical Condition

When depressive or manic symptoms are present in a patient with a general medical condition, attributing the depressive symptoms either to the general medical condition or to a mood disorder can be difficult. Many general medical conditions present depressive symptoms, such as poor sleep, decreased appetite, and fatigue. This category is discussed extensively in Section 10.5. Table 15.3–7 lists the DSM-IV-TR criteria for the disorder

Table 15.3–7
DSM-IV-TR Diagnostic Criteria for Mood Disorder Due to a General Medical Condition

A. A prominent and persistent disturbance in mood predominates in the clinical picture and is characterized by either (or both) of the following:
   (1) depressed mood or markedly diminished interest or pleasure in all, or almost all, activities
   (2) elevated, expansive, or irritable mood

B. There is evidence from the history, physical examination, or laboratory findings that the disturbance is the direct physiological consequence of a general medical condition.

C. The disturbance is not better accounted for by another mental disorder (e.g., adjustment disorder with depressed mood in response to the stress of having a general medical condition).

D. The disturbance does not occur exclusively during the course of a delirium.

E. The symptoms cause clinically significant distress or impairment in social, occupational, or other important areas of functioning.

Specify type:

With depressive features: if the predominant mood is depressed but the full criteria are not met for a major depressive episode

With major depressivelike episode: if the full criteria are met (except Criterion D) for a major depressive episode

With manic features: if the predominant mood is elevated, euphoric, or irritable

With mixed features: if the symptoms of both mania and depression are present but neither predominates

Coding note: Include the name of the general medical condition on Axis I, e.g., mood disorder due to hypothyroidism, with depressive features; also code the general medical condition on Axis III.

Coding note: If depressive symptoms occur as part of a preexisting vascular dementia, indicate the depressive symptoms by coding the appropriate subtype, i.e., vascular dementia, with depressed mood.

From American Psychiatric Association. *Diagnostic and Statistical Manual of Mental Disorders.* 4th ed. Text rev. Washington, DC: American Psychiatric Association; copyright 2000, with permission.

Substance-Induced Mood Disorder

Substance-induced mood disorder must always be considered in the differential diagnosis of mood disorder symptoms. Clinicians should consider three possibilities. First, a patient may be taking drugs for the treatment of nonpsychiatric medical problems. Second, a patient may have been accidentally, and perhaps unknowingly, exposed to neurotoxic chemicals. Third, the patient may have taken a substance for recreational purposes or may be dependent on such a substance.

Epidemiology. The epidemiology of substance-induced mood disorder is unknown. The prevalence is probably high, however, given the widespread use of so-called recreational drugs, the many prescription drugs that can cause depression and mania, and the toxic chemicals that abound in the environment and the workplace.

Etiology. Medications, especially antihypertensives, are probably the most frequent cause of substance-induced mood disorder, although a wide range of drugs can produce depression (Table 15.3–8) and mania (see Table 15.3–9). Drugs such as reserpine (Serpasil) and methyldopa (Aldomet), both antihypertensive agents, can precipitate a depressive disorder, presumably by depleting serotonin, which happens in more than 10 percent of all persons who take the drugs.

Diagnosis and Clinical Features. The DSM-IV-TR diagnostic criteria for substance-induced mood disorder allow the specification of the substance involved, the time of onset (during intoxication or withdrawal), and the nature of the symptoms (e.g., manic or depressed) (Table 15.3–10). A maximum of 1 month between the use of the substance and the appearance of

Table 15.3–8
Pharmacological Causes of Depression

Cardiac and antihypertensive drugs	
Bethanidine	Digitalis
Clonidine	Prazosin
Guanethidine	Procainamide
Hydralazine	Veratrum
Methyldopa	Lidocaine
Propranolol	Oxprenolol
Reserpine	Methoserpidine
Sedatives and hypnotics	
Barbiturates	Benzodiazepines
Chloral hydrate	Chlormethiazole
Ethanol	Chlorazepate
Steroids and hormones	
Corticosteroids	Triamcinolone
Oral contraceptives	Norethisterone
Prednisone	Danazol
Stimulants and appetite suppressants	
Amphetamine	Diethylpropion
Fenfluramine	Phenmetrazine
Psychotropic drugs	
Butyrophenones	Phenothiazines
Neurological agents	
Amantadine	Baclofen
Bromocriptine	Carbamazepine
Levodopa	Methsuximide
Tetrabenazine	Phenytoin
Analgesics and antiinflammatory drugs	
Fenoprofen	Phenacetin
Ibuprofen	Phenylbutazone
Indomethacin	Pentazocine
Opiates	Benzydamine
Antibacterial and antifungal drugs	
Ampicillin	Griseofulvin
Sulfamethoxazole	Metronidazole
Clotrimazole	Nitrofurantoin
Cycloserine	Nalidixic acid
Dapsone	Sulfonamides
Ethionamide	Streptomycin
Tetracycline	Thiocarbanilide
Antineoplastic drugs	
C-Asparaginase	Bleomycin
Mithramycin	Trimethoprim
Vincristine	Zidovudine
6-Azauridine	
Miscellaneous drugs	
Acetazolamide	Methysergide
Choline	Meclizine
Cyproheptadine	Pizotifen
Disulfiram	
Anticholinesterases	
Cimetidine	Mebeverine
Diphenoxylate	Metoclopramide
Lysergide	Salbutamol

Adapted from Cummings JL. *Clinical Neuropsychiatry.* Orlando, FL: Grune & Stratton; 1985:187.

the symptoms is allowed in DSM-IV-TR, although the usual time frame is probably shorter. In some cases, the diagnosis may be warranted after more than 1 month.

Substance-induced manic and depressive features can be identical to those of bipolar I disorder and major depressive disorder. Substance-induced mood disorder, however, may show

Table 15.3–9
Pharmacological Causes of Mania

Amphetamines
Baclofen
Bromide
Bromocriptine
Captopril
Cimetidine
Cocaine
Corticosteroids (including ACTH)
Cyclosporine
Disulfiram
Hallucinogens (intoxication and flashbacks)
Hydralazine
Isoniazid
Levodopa
Methylphenidate
Metrizamide (following myelography)
Opiates and opioids
Phencyclidine (PCP)
Procarbazine
Procyclidine
Yohimbine

Adapted from Cummings JL. *Clinical Neuropsychiatry.* Orlando, FL: Grune & Stratton; 1985:187.

more waxing and waning of symptoms and a fluctuation in patients' level of consciousness.

Differential Diagnosis. A history of mood disorders in the patient or the patient's family weighs toward the diagnosis of a primary mood disorder, although such a history does not rule out the possibility of substance-induced mood disorder. Substances may also trigger an underlying mood disorder in a patient who is biologically vulnerable to mood disorders.

Course and Prognosis. The course and prognosis of substance-induced mood disorder vary. Shortly after the substance has been cleared from the body, a normal mood usually returns. Sometimes, however, the substance exposure seems to precipitate a long-lasting mood disorder that may take weeks or months to resolve completely.

Treatment. The primary treatment of substance-induced mood disorder is the identification of the causally involved substance. Stopping the intake of the substance usually suffices to cause the mood disorder symptoms to abate. If the symptoms linger, treatment with appropriate psychiatric drugs may be necessary.

Mood Disorder Not Otherwise Specified

If patients exhibit mood symptoms that are difficult to distinguish between depression and mania and do not meet the diagnostic criteria for any other mood disorder or other DSM-IV-TR mental disorder, the most appropriate diagnosis is mood disorder not otherwise specified (Table 15.3–11).

Table 15.3–10
DSM-IV-TR Diagnostic Criteria for Substance-Induced Mood Disorder

A. A prominent and persistent disturbance in mood predominates in the clinical picture and is characterized by either (or both) of the following:
  (1) depressed mood or markedly diminished interest or pleasure in all, or almost all, activities
  (2) elevated, expansive, or irritable mood

B. There is evidence from the history, physical examination, or laboratory findings of either (1) or (2):
  (1) the symptoms in Criterion A developed during, or within a month of, substance intoxication or withdrawal
  (2) medication use is etiologically related to the disturbance

C. The disturbance is not better accounted for by a mood disorder that is not substance induced. Evidence that the symptoms are better accounted for by a mood disorder that is not substance induced might include the following: the symptoms precede the onset of the substance use (or medication use); the symptoms persist for a substantial period of time (e.g., about a month) after the cessation of acute withdrawal or severe intoxication or are substantially in excess of what would be expected given the type or amount of the substance used or the duration of use; or there is other evidence that suggests the existence of an independent non–substance-induced mood disorder (e.g., a history of recurrent major depressive episodes).

D. The disturbance does not occur exclusively during the course of a delirium.

E. The symptoms cause clinically significant distress or impairment in social, occupational, or other important areas of functioning.

Note: This diagnosis should be made instead of a diagnosis of substance intoxication or substance withdrawal only when the mood symptoms are in excess of those usually associated with the intoxication or withdrawal syndrome and when the symptoms are sufficiently severe to warrant independent clinical attention.

Code [Specific substance]-induced mood disorder:

Alcohol; amphetamine [or amphetaminelike substance]; cocaine; hallucinogen; inhalant; opioid; phencyclidine [or phencyclidinelike substance]; sedative, hypnotic, or anxiolytic; other [or unknown] substance

Specify type:

With depressive features: if the predominant mood is depressed

With manic features: if the predominant mood is elevated, euphoric, or irritable

With mixed features: if symptoms of both mania and depression are present and neither predominates

Specify if:

With onset during intoxication: if the criteria are met for intoxication with the substance and the symptoms develop during the intoxication syndrome

With onset during withdrawal: if criteria are met for withdrawal from the substance and the symptoms develop during, or shortly after, a withdrawal syndrome

From American Psychiatric Association. *Diagnostic and Statistical Manual of Mental Disorders.* 4th ed. Text rev. Washington, DC: American Psychiatric Association; copyright 2000, with permission.

Table 15.3–11
DSM-IV-TR Diagnostic Criteria for Mood Disorder Not Otherwise Specified

This category includes disorders with mood symptoms that do not meet the criteria for any specific mood disorder and in which it is difficult to choose between depressive disorder not otherwise specified and bipolar disorder not otherwise specified (e.g., acute agitation).

From American Psychiatric Association. *Diagnostic and Statistical Manual of Mental Disorders.* 4th ed. Text rev. Washington, DC: American Psychiatric Association; copyright 2000, with permission.

ICD-10

ICD-10 describes mood (affective) disorders as characterized by "a change in mood or affect, usually to depression (with or without associated anxiety) or to elation." A change in activity level accompanies the mood change, and "most other symptoms are either secondary to, or easily understood in the context of, such changes." These disorders are recurrent, and the onset of the episodes may be related to "stressful events or situations." The mood disorders also include those occurring in children. Table 15.3–12 lists the ICD-10 criteria for mood disorders.

Table 15.3–12
ICD-10 Diagnostic Criteria for Mood [Affective] Disorders

Manic episode

Hypomania

A. The mood is elevated or irritable to a degree that is definitely abnormal for the individual concerned and sustained for at least 4 consecutive days.

B. At least three of the following signs must be present, leading to some interference with personal functioning in daily living:
  (1) increased activity or physical restlessness;
  (2) increased talkativeness;
  (3) distractibility or difficulty in concentration;
  (4) decreased need for sleep;
  (5) increased sexual energy;
  (6) mild overspending, or other types of reckless or irresponsible behavior;
  (7) increased sociability or overfamiliarity.

C. The episode does not meet the criteria for mania, bipolar affective disorder, depressive episode, cyclothymia, or anorexia nervosa.

(continued)

Table 15.3–12 (*continued*)

D. *Most commonly used exclusion clause.* The episode is not attributable to psychoactive substance use or to any organic mental disorder.

Mania without psychotic symptoms

A. Mood must be predominantly elevated, expansive, or irritable, and definitely abnormal for the individual concerned. The mood change must be prominent and sustained for at least 1 week (unless it is severe enough to require hospital admission).

B. At least three of the following signs must be present (four if the mood is merely irritable), leading to severe interference with personal functioning in daily living:
   (1) increased activity or physical restlessness;
   (2) increased talkativeness ("pressure of speech");
   (3) flight of ideas or the subjective experience of thoughts racing;
   (4) loss of normal social inhibitions, resulting in behavior that is inappropriate to the circumstances;
   (5) decreased need for sleep;
   (6) inflated self-esteem or grandiosity;
   (7) distractibility or constant changes in activity or plans;
   (8) behavior that is foolhardy or reckless and whose risks the individual does not recognize, e.g., spending sprees, foolish enterprises, reckless driving;
   (9) marked sexual energy or sexual indiscretions.

C. There are no hallucinations or delusions, although perceptual disorders may occur (e.g., subjective hyperacusis, appreciation of colors as especially vivid).

D. *Most commonly used exclusion clause.* The episode is not attributable to psychoactive substance use or to any organic mental disorder.

Mania with psychotic symptoms

A. The episode meets the criteria for mania without psychotic symptoms with the exception of Criterion C.

B. The episode does not simultaneously meet the criteria for schizophrenia or schizoaffective disorder, manic type.

C. Delusions or hallucinations are present, other than those listed as typically schizophrenic in Criterion G1(1)b, c, and d for schizophrenia (i.e., delusions other than those that are completely impossible or culturally inappropriate, and hallucinations that are not in the third person or giving a running commentary). The commonest examples are those with grandiose, self-referential, erotic, or persecutory content.

D. *Most commonly used exclusion clause.* The episode is not attributable to psychoactive substance use or to any organic mental disorder.

Specify whether the hallucinations or delusions are congruent or incongruent with the mood:

With mood-congruent psychotic symptoms (such as grandiose delusions or voices telling the individual that he or she has superhuman powers)

With mood-incongruent psychotic symptoms (such as voices speaking to the individual about affectively neutral topics, or delusions of reference or persecution)

Other manic episodes

Manic episode, unspecified

Bipolar affective disorder

Note. Episodes are demarcated by a switch to an episode of opposite mixed polarity or by a remission.

Bipolar affective disorder, current episode hypomanic

A. The current episode meets the criteria for hypomania.

B. There has been at least one other affective episode in the past, meeting the criteria for hypomanic or manic episode, depressive episode, or mixed affective episode.

Bipolar affective disorder, current episode manic without psychotic symptoms

A. The current episode meets the criteria for mania without psychotic symptoms.

B. There has been at least one other affective episode in the past, meeting the criteria for hypomanic or manic episode, depressive episode, or mixed affective episode.

Bipolar affective disorder, current episode manic without psychotic symptoms

A. The current episode meets the criteria for mania without psychotic symptoms.

B. There has been at least one other affective episode in the past, meeting the criteria for hypomanic or manic episode, depressive episode, or mixed affective episode.

Specify whether the psychotic symptoms are congruent or incongruent with the mood:

With mood-congruent psychotic symptoms

With mood-incongruent psychotic symptoms

Bipolar affective disorder, current episode moderate or mild depression

A. The current episode meets the criteria for a depressive episode of either mild or moderate severity.

B. There has been at least one other affective episode in the past, meeting the criteria for hypomanic or manic episode, depressive episode, or mixed affective episode.

Specify the presence of the "somatic syndrome" in the current episode of depression:

Without somatic syndrome

With somatic syndrome

Bipolar affective disorder, current episode severe depression without psychotic symptoms

A. The current episode meets the criteria for a severe depressive episode without psychotic symptoms.

B. There has been at least one well-authenticated hypomanic or manic episode or mixed affective episode in the past.

Bipolar affective disorder, current episode severe depression with psychotic symptoms

A. The current episode meets the criteria for a severe depressive episode without psychotic symptoms.

B. There has been at least one well-authenticated hypomanic or manic episode or mixed affective episode in the past.

Specify whether the psychotic symptoms are congruent or incongruent with the mood:

With mood-congruent psychotic symptoms

With mood-incongruent psychotic symptoms

Bipolar affective disorder, current episode mixed

A. The current episode is characterized by either a mixture or a rapid alternation (i.e., within a few hours) of hypomanic, manic, and depressive symptoms.

B. Both manic and depressive symptoms must be prominent most of the time during a period of at least 2 weeks.

C. There has been at least one well-authenticated hypomanic or manic episode, depressive episode, or mixed affective episode in the past.

(*continued*)

Table 15.3–12 (*continued*)

Bipolar affective disorder, currently in remission

A. The current state does not meet the criteria for depressive or manic episode of any severity or for any other mood [affective] disorder (possibly because of treatment to reduce the risk of future episodes).

B. There has been at least one well-authenticated hypomanic or manic episode in the past and in addition at least one other affective episode (hypomanic or manic, depressive, or mixed).

Other bipolar affective disorders

Bipolar affective disorder, unspecified

Depressive episode

G1. The depressive episode should last for at least 2 weeks.

G2. There have been no hypomanic or manic symptoms sufficient to meet the criteria for hypomanic or manic episode at any time in the individual's life.

G3. *Most commonly used exclusion clause.* The episode is not attributable to psychoactive substance use or to any organic mental disorder.

Somatic syndrome

Some depressive symptoms are widely regarded as having special clinical significance and are here called "somatic." (Terms such as biological, vital, melancholic, or endogenomorphic are used for this syndrome in other classifications.)

A fifth character may be used to specify the presence or absence of the somatic syndrome. To qualify for the somatic syndrome, *four* of the following symptoms should be present:

(1) marked loss of interest or pleasure in activities that are normally pleasurable;

(2) lack of emotional reactions to events or activities that normally produce an emotional response;

(3) waking in the morning 2 hours or more before the usual time;

(4) depression worse in the morning;

(5) objective evidence of marked psychomotor retardation or agitation (remarked on or reported by other people);

(6) marked loss of appetite;

(7) weight loss (5% or more of body weight in the past month);

(8) marked loss of libido.

In *The ICD-10 Classification of Mental and Behavioural Disorders: Clinical Descriptions and Diagnostic Guidelines,* the presence or absence of the somatic syndrome is not specified for severe depressive episode, since it is presumed to be present in most cases. For research purposes, however, it may be advisable to allow for the coding of the absence of the somatic syndrome in severe depressive episode.

Mild depressive episode

A. The general criteria for depressive episode must be met.

B. At least two of the following three symptoms must be present:

(1) depressed mood to a degree that is definitely abnormal for the individual, present for most of the day and almost every day, largely uninfluenced by circumstances, and sustained for at least 2 weeks;

(2) loss of interest or pleasure in activities that are normally pleasurable;

(3) decreased energy or increased fatigability.

C. An additional symptom or symptoms from the following list should be present, to give a total of at least *four:*

(1) loss of confidence or self-esteem;

(2) unreasonable feelings of self-reproach or excessive and inappropriate guilt;

(3) recurrent thoughts of death or suicide, or any suicidal behavior;

(4) complaints or evidence of diminished ability to think or concentrate, such as indecisiveness or vacillation;

(5) change in psychomotor activity, with agitation or retardation (either subjective or objective);

(6) sleep disturbance of any type;

(7) change in appetite (decrease or increase) with corresponding weight change.

A fifth character may be used to specify the presence or absence of the "somatic syndrome":

Without somatic syndrome

With somatic syndrome

Moderate depressive episode

A. The general criteria for depressive episode must be met.

B. At least two of the three symptoms listed for Criterion B above must be present.

C. Additional symptoms from depressive episode, Criterion C, must be present, to give a total of at least *six*.

A fifth character may be used to specify the presence or absence of the "somatic syndrome":

Without somatic syndrome

With somatic syndrome

Severe depressive episode without psychotic symptoms

Note: If important symptoms such as agitation or retardation are marked, the patient may be unwilling or unable to describe many symptoms in detail. An overall grading of severe episode may still be justified in such a case.

A. The general criteria for depressive episode must be met.

B. All three of the symptoms in Criterion B, depressive episode, must be present.

C. Additional symptoms from depressive episode, Criterion C, must be present, to give a total of at least *eight.*

D. There must be no hallucinations, delusions, or depressive stupor.

Severe depressive episode with psychotic symptoms

A. The general criteria for depressive episode must be met.

B. The criteria for severe depressive episode without psychotic symptoms must be met with the exception of Criterion D.

C. The criteria for schizophrenia or schizoaffective disorder, depressive type, are not met.

D. Either of the following must be present:

(1) delusions or hallucinations, other than those listed as typically schizophrenic in Criterion G1(1)b, c, and d for general criteria for paranoid, hebephrenic, catatonic, and undifferentiated schizophrenia (i.e., delusions other than those that are completely impossible or culturally inappropriate and hallucinations that are not in the third person or giving a running commentary), the commonest examples are those with depressive, guilty, hypochondriacal, nihilistic, self-referential, or persecutory content

(2) depressive stupor

A fifth character may be used to specify whether the psychotic symptoms are congruent or incongruent with mood:

With mood-congruent psychotic symptoms (i.e., delusions of guilt, worthlessness, bodily disease, or impending disaster, derisive or condemnatory auditory hallucinations)

With mood-incongruent psychotic symptoms (i.e., persecutory or self-referential delusions and hallucinations without an affective content)

(*continued*)

Table 15.3–12 (*continued*)

Other depressive episodes

Episodes should be included here which do not fit the descriptions given for depressive episodes, but for which the overall diagnostic impression indicates that they are depressive in nature. Examples include fluctuating mixtures of depressive symptoms (particularly those of the somatic syndrome) with nondiagnostic symptoms such as tension, worry, and distress, and mixtures of somatic depressive symptoms with persistent pain or fatigue not due to organic causes (as sometimes seen in general hospital services).

Depressive episode, unspecified

Recurrent depressive disorder

G1. There has been at least one previous episode, mild, moderate, or severe, lasting a minimum of 2 weeks and separated from the current episode by at least 2 months free from any significant mood symptoms.

G2. At no time in the past has there been an episode meeting the criteria for hypomanic or manic episode.

G3. *Most commonly used exclusion clause.* The episode is not attributable to psychoactive substance use or to any organic mental disorder.

It is recommended that the predominant type of previous episodes is specified (mild, moderate, severe, uncertain).

Recurrent depressive disorder, current episode mild

A. The general criteria for recurrent depressive disorder are met.

B. The current episode meets the criteria for mild depressive episode.

A fifth character may be used to specify the presence or absence of the "somatic syndrome," in the current episode:

Without somatic syndrome

With somatic syndrome

Recurrent depressive disorder, current episode moderate

A. The general criteria for recurrent depressive disorder are met.

B. The current episode meets the criteria for moderate depressive episode.

A fifth character may be used to specify the presence or absence of the "somatic syndrome," in the current episode:

Without somatic syndrome

With somatic syndrome

Recurrent depressive disorder, current episode without psychotic symptoms

A. The general criteria for recurrent depressive disorder are met.

B. The current episode meets the criteria for severe depressive episode without psychotic symptoms.

Recurrent depressive disorder, current episode severe with psychotic symptoms

A. The general criteria for recurrent depressive disorder are met.

B. The current episode meets the criteria for severe depressive episode with psychotic symptoms.

A fifth character may be used to specify whether the psychotic symptoms are congruent or incongruent with the mood:

With mood-congruent psychotic symptoms

With mood-incongruent psychotic symptoms

Recurrent depressive disorder, currently in remission

A. The general criteria for recurrent depressive disorder have been met in the past.

B. The current state does not meet the criteria for a depressive episode of any severity or for any other disorder in mood [affective] disorders.

Comment

This category can still be used if the patient receives treatment to reduce the risk of further episodes.

Other recurrent depressive disorders

Recurrent depressive disorder, unspecified

Persistent mood [affective] disorders

Cyclothymia

A. There must have been a period of at least 2 years of instability of mood involving several periods of both depression and hypomania, with or without intervening periods of normal mood.

B. None of the manifestations of depression or hypomania during such a 2-year period should be sufficiently severe or long-lasting to meet criteria for manic episode or depressive episode (moderate or severe); however, manic or depressive episode(s) may have occurred before, or may develop after, such a period of persistent mood instability.

C. During at least some of the periods of depression at least three of the following should be present:

(1) reduced energy or activity;
(2) insomnia;
(3) loss of self-confidence or feelings of inadequacy;
(4) difficulty in concentrating;
(5) social withdrawal;
(6) loss of interest in or enjoyment of sex and other pleasurable activities;
(7) reduced talkativeness;
(8) pessimism about the future or brooding over the past.

D. During at least some of the periods of mood elevation at least three of the following should be present:

(1) increased energy or activity;
(2) decreased need for sleep;
(3) inflated self-esteem;
(4) sharpened or unusually creative thinking;
(5) increased gregariousness;
(6) increased talkativeness or wittiness;
(7) increased interest and involvement in sexual and other pleasurable activities;
(8) overoptimism or exaggeration of past achievements.

Note. If desired, time of onset may be specified as early (in late teenage or the 20s) or late (usually between age 30 and 50 years, following an affective episode).

Dysthymia

A. There must be a period of at least 2 years of constant or constantly recurring depressed mood. Intervening periods of normal mood rarely last for longer than a few weeks, and there are no episodes of hypomania.

B. None, or very few, of the individual episodes of depression within such a 2-year period should be sufficiently severe or long-lasting to meet the criteria for recurrent mild depressive disorder.

C. During at least some of the periods of depression at least three of the following should be present:

(1) reduced energy or activity;
(2) insomnia;
(3) loss of self-confidence or feelings of inadequacy;
(4) difficulty in concentrating;
(5) frequent tearfulness;
(6) loss of interest in or enjoyment of sex and other pleasurable activities;
(7) feeling of hopelessness or despair;
(8) a perceived inability to cope with the routine responsibilities of everyday life;
(9) pessimism about the future or brooding over the past;
(10) social withdrawal;
(11) reduced talkativeness.

(*continued*)

Table 15.3–12 (*continued*)

Note. If desired, time of onset may be specified as early (in late teenage or the 20s) or late (usually between age 30 and 50 years, following an affective episode).

Other persistent mood [affective] disorders

This is a residual category for persistent affective disorders that are not sufficiently severe or long-lasting to fulfill the criteria for cyclothymia or dysthymia but that are nevertheless clinically significant. Some types of depression previously called "neurotic" are included here, provided that they do not meet the criteria for either cyclothymia or dysthymia or for depressive episode of mild or moderate severity.

Persistent mood [affective] disorder, unspecified

Other mood [affective] disorders

There are so many possible disorders that could be listed that no attempt has been made to specify criteria, except for mixed affective episode and recurrent brief depressive disorder. Investigators requiring criteria more exact than those available in *Clinical Descriptions and Diagnostic Guidelines* should construct them according to the requirements of their studies.

Other single mood [affective] disorders

Mixed affective episode

A. The episode is characterized by either a mixture or a rapid alternation (i.e., within a few hours) of hypomanic, manic, and depressive symptoms.

B. Both manic and depressive symptoms must be prominent most of the time during a period of at least 2 weeks.

C. There is no history of previous hypomanic, depressive, or mixed episodes.

Other recurrent mood [affective] disorders

Recurrent brief depressive disorder

A. The disorder meets the symptomatic criteria for mild, moderate, or severe depressive episode.

B. The depressive episodes have occurred about once a month over the past year.

C. The individual episodes last less than 2 weeks (typically 2–3 days).

D. The episodes do not occur solely in relation to the menstrual cycle.

Other specified mood [affective] disorders

This is a residual category for affective disorders that do not meet the criteria for any other categories above.

References

Akiskal HS, section ed. Mood disorders. In: Sadock BJ, Sadock VA, eds. *Kaplan & Sadock's Comprehensive Textbook of Psychiatry.* 7th ed. Vol 1. Baltimore: Lippincott Williams & Wilkins; 2000:1284.

Angst J, Dobler-Mikola A. The Zurich study: a prospective epidemiological study of depressive, neurotic and psychosomatic syndromes. IV. Recurrent and nonrecurrent brief depression. *Eur Arch Psychiatry Neurol Sci.* 1995;234:408.

Caine ED, Lyness JM. Delirium, dementia, and amnestic and other cognitive disorders. In: Sadock BJ, Sadock VA, eds. *Kaplan & Sadock's Comprehensive Textbook of Psychiatry.* 7th ed. Vol 1. Baltimore: Lippincott Williams & Wilkins; 2000:854.

Covinsky KE, Fortinsky RH, Palmer RM, Kresevic DM, Landefeld CS. Relation between symptoms of depression and health status outcomes in acutely ill hospitalized older persons. *Ann Intern Med.* 1997;126:417.

Larazue AA. The multimodal approach to the treatment of minor depression. *Am J Psychother.* 1992;46:50.

Tremblay LK, Naranjo CA, Cardenas L, Herrmann N, Busto UE. Probing brain reward system function in major depressive disorder: altered response to dextroamphetamine. *Arch Gen Psychiatry.* 2002;59:409.

Williamson GM, Shaffer DR, et al., eds. *Physical Illness and Depression in Older Adults: A Handbook of Theory, Research, and Practice.* The Plenum Series in Social/Clinical Psychology. New York: Kluwer Academic/Plenum Publishers; 2000:31.

16 Anxiety Disorders

▲ 16.1 Overview

Anxiety disorders are among the most prevalent psychiatric conditions in the United States and in most other populations studied. Further, studies have persistently shown that they produce inordinate morbidity, use of health care services, and functional impairment. Recent studies also suggest that chronic anxiety disorder may increase the rate of cardiovascular-related mortality. Hence, clinicians in psychiatry and other specialities must make the proper anxiety disorder diagnosis rapidly and initiate treatment.

From a neurobiological perspective, study of anxiety disorders is compelling. Understanding the neuroanatomy and molecular biology of anxiety promises new insights into etiology and more specific (and thus more effective) treatments in the future. Currently, the treatments available for anxiety disorders are among the most effective in psychiatric medicine. Pharmacological, cognitive-behavioral, and psychodynamic approaches have all proved useful in combating anxiety disorder. For many conditions (e.g., panic disorder), most patients should expect substantial relief from their symptoms in a relatively brief period.

Another fascinating aspect of anxiety disorders is the exquisite interplay of genetic and experiential factors. While there is little doubt that abnormal genes predispose to pathological anxiety states, evidence clearly indicates that traumatic life events and stress are also etiologically important. Study of the anxiety disorders thus presents a unique opportunity to understand the relation between nature and nurture. This arena should show little regard for purely biological versus psychological explanations about pathogenesis or therapeutics. Rather, anxiety disorder research aims at presenting a view of human function under pathological conditions that integrates multiple sources of theory and information.

HISTORY

Nearly a century ago, Sigmund Freud coined the term *anxiety neurosis,* which he believed resulted from dammed-up libido: A physiological increase in sexual tension leads to a corresponding increase in libido, the mental representation of the physiological event. The normal outlet for such tension is, in Freud's view, sexual intercourse, but sexual practices such as abstinence and coitus interruptus prevent tension release and produce neuroses. The conditions of heightened anxiety related to libidinal blockage include neurasthenia, hypochondriasis, and anxiety neuroses, all of which Freud regarded as having a biological basis.

NORMAL ANXIETY

Everyone experiences anxiety—a diffuse, unpleasant, vague sense of apprehension, often accompanied by autonomic symptoms (Table 16.1–1) such as headache, perspiration, palpitations, tightness in the chest, mild stomach discomfort, and restlessness, indicated by an inability to sit or stand still for long. The particular constellation of symptoms present during anxiety tends to vary among persons.

The Distinction between Fear and Anxiety

Anxiety is an alerting signal; it warns of impending danger and enables a person to take measures to deal with a threat. Fear is a similar alerting signal but should be differentiated from anxiety. Fear is a response to a known, external, definite, or nonconflictual threat; anxiety is a response to a threat that is unknown, internal, vague, or conflictual.

This distinction between fear and anxiety arose accidentally. When Freud's early translator mistranslated *angst,* the German word for "fear," as anxiety, Freud himself generally ignored the distinction that associates anxiety with a repressed, unconscious object and fear with a known, external object. The distinction may be difficult to make because fear may also be due to an unconscious, repressed, internal object displaced to another object in the external world. For example, a boy may fear barking dogs because he actually fears his father and unconsciously associates his father with barking dogs.

Nevertheless, according to postfreudian psychoanalytic formulations, the separation of fear and anxiety is psychologically justifiable. The emotion caused by a rapidly approaching car as a person crosses the street differs from the vague discomfort a person may experience when meeting new persons in a strange setting. The main psychological difference between the two emotional responses is the suddenness of fear and the insidiousness of anxiety.

Charles Darwin pointed out that the word *fear* is derived from words meaning "sudden" and "dangerous." Duration also seems to be vital in the neurophysiological phenomena of anxiety and fear. In 1896 Darwin gave the following psychophysiological description of acute fear merging into terror:

Table 16.1–1
Peripheral Manifestations of Anxiety

Diarrhea
Dizziness, light-headedness
Hyperhidrosis
Hyperreflexia
Hypertension
Palpitations
Pupillary mydriasis
Restlessness (e.g., pacing)
Syncope
Tachycardia
Tingling in the extremities
Tremors
Upset stomach ("butterflies")
Urinary frequency, hesitancy, urgency

> Fear is often preceded by astonishment, and is so far akin to it, that both lead to the senses of sight and learning being instantly aroused. In both cases the eyes and mouth are widely opened, and the eyebrows raised. The frightened man at first stands like a statue motionless and breathless, or crouches down as if instinctively to escape observation. The heart beats quickly and violently, so that it palpitates or knocks against the ribs; but it is very doubtful whether it then works more efficiently than usual, so as to send a greater supply of blood to all parts of the body; for the skin instantly becomes pale, as during incipient faintness. This paleness of the surface, however, is probably in large part, or exclusively, due to the vasomotor center being affected in such a manner as to cause the contraction of the small arteries of the skin. That the skin is much affected under the sense of great fear, we see in the marvelous and inexplicable manner in which perspiration immediately exudes from it. This exudation is all the more remarkable, as the surface is then cold, and hence the term a cold sweat; whereas, the sudorific glands are properly excited into action when the surface is heated. The hairs also on the skin stand erect; and the superficial muscles shiver. In connection with the disturbed action of the heart, the breathing is hurried. The salivary glands act imperfectly; the mouth becomes dry, and is often opened and shut. I have also noticed that under slight fear there is a strong tendency to yawn. One of the best-marked symptoms is the trembling of all the muscles of the body; and this is often first seen in the lips. From this cause, and from the dryness of the mouth, the voice becomes husky or indistinct, or may altogether fail. . . .
>
> As fear increases into an agony of terror, we behold, as under all violent emotions, diversified results. The heart beats wildly or may fail to act and faintness ensues; there is a deathlike pallor; the breathing is labored; the wings of the nostrils are widely dilated; there is a gasping and convulsive motion on the lips, a tremor on the hollow cheek, a gulping and catching of the throat; the uncovered and protruding eyeballs are fixed on the object of terror; or they may roll restlessly from side to side. The pupils are said to be enormously dilated. All the muscles of the body may become rigid, or may be thrown into convulsive movements. The hands are alternately clenched and opened, often with a twitching movement. The arms may be protruded, as if to avert some dreadful danger, or may be thrown wildly over the head. . . . In other cases there is a sudden and uncontrollable tendency to headlong flight; and so strong is this, that the boldest soldiers may be seized with a sudden panic.

Is Anxiety Adaptive?

When considered simply as an alerting signal, anxiety seems basically the same emotion as fear. As a warning of an external or internal threat, anxiety is adaptive and has lifesaving qualities. At a lower level, anxiety warns of threats of bodily damage, pain, helplessness, possible punishment, or the frustration of social or bodily needs; of separation from loved ones; of a menace to one's success or status; and ultimately of threats to unity or wholeness. It prompts a person to take the necessary steps to prevent the threat or to lessen its consequences. Examples of a person warding off threats in daily life include getting down to the hard work of preparing for an examination, dodging a ball thrown at the head, sneaking into the dormitory after curfew to prevent punishment, and running to catch the last commuter train. Thus, anxiety prevents damage by alerting the person to carry out certain acts that forestall the danger.

Stress and Anxiety

Whether an event is perceived as stressful depends on the nature of the event and on the person's resources, psychological defenses, and coping mechanisms. All involve the ego, a collective abstraction for the process by which a person perceives, thinks, and acts on external events or internal drives. A person whose ego is functioning properly is in adaptive balance with both external and internal worlds; if the ego is not functioning properly and the resulting imbalance continues long enough, the person experiences chronic anxiety.

Whether the imbalance is external, between the pressures of the outside world and the person's ego, or internal, between the person's impulses (e.g., aggressive, sexual, and dependent impulses) and conscience, the imbalance produces a conflict. Externally caused conflicts are usually interpersonal, whereas those that are internally caused are intrapsychic or intrapersonal. A combination of the two is possible, as in the case of employees whose excessively demanding and critical boss provokes impulses that they must control for fear of losing their jobs. Interpersonal and intrapsychic conflicts are, in fact, usually intertwined. Because human beings are social, their main conflicts are usually with other persons.

Symptoms of Anxiety

The experience of anxiety has two components: the awareness of the physiological sensations (such as palpitations and sweating) and the awareness of being nervous or frightened. A feeling of shame may increase anxiety—"Others will recognize that I am frightened." Many persons are astonished to find out that others are not aware of their anxiety or, if they are, do not appreciate its intensity.

In addition to motor and visceral effects (Table 16.1–1), anxiety affects thinking, perception, and learning. It tends to produce confusion and distortions of perception, not only of time and space but also of persons and the meanings of events.

These distortions can interfere with learning by lowering concentration, reducing recall, and impairing the ability to relate one item to another—that is, to make associations.

An important aspect of emotions is their effect on the selectivity of attention. Anxious persons are apt to select certain things in their environment and overlook others in their effort to prove that they are justified in considering the situation frightening. If they falsely justify their fear, they augment their anxieties by the selective response and set up a vicious circle of anxiety, distorted perception, and increased anxiety. If, alternatively, they falsely reassure themselves by selective thinking, appropriate anxiety may be reduced, and they may fail to take necessary precautions.

PATHOLOGICAL ANXIETY

Epidemiology

The anxiety disorders make up one of the most common groups of psychiatric disorders. The National Comorbidity Study reported that one in four persons met the diagnostic criteria for at least one anxiety disorder and that there is a 12-month prevalence rate of 17.7 percent. Women (30.5 percent lifetime prevalence) are more likely to have an anxiety disorder than are men (19.2 percent lifetime prevalence). Finally, the prevalence of anxiety disorders decreases with higher socioeconomic status.

Contributions of Psychological Sciences

Three major schools of psychological theory—psychoanalytic, behavioral, and existential—have contributed theories about the causes of anxiety. Each theory has both conceptual and practical usefulness in treating anxiety disorders.

Psychoanalytic Theories. Although Freud originally believed that anxiety stemmed from a physiological buildup of libido, he ultimately redefined anxiety as a signal of the presence of danger in the unconscious. Anxiety was viewed as the result of psychic conflict between unconscious sexual or aggressive wishes and corresponding threats from the superego or external reality. In response to this signal, the ego mobilized defense mechanisms to prevent unacceptable thoughts and feelings from emerging into conscious awareness. In his classic paper "Inhibitions, Symptoms, and Anxiety," Freud states that "it was anxiety which produced repression and not, as I formerly believed, repression which produced anxiety." Today, many neurobiologists continue to substantiate many of Freud's original ideas and theories. One example is the role of the amygdala, which subserves the fear response without any reference to conscious memory and substantiates Freud's concept of an unconscious memory system for anxiety responses. One of the unfortunate consequences of regarding the symptom of anxiety as a *disorder* rather than a *signal* is that the underlying sources of the anxiety may be ignored. From a psychodynamic perspective, the goal of therapy is not necessary to eliminate all anxiety but to increase anxiety tolerance, that is, the capacity to experience anxiety and use it as a signal to investigate the underlying conflict that has created it. Anxiety appears in response to various situations during the life cycle, and an attempt to eradicate it by psychopharmacological means may do nothing to address the life situation or its internal correlates that have induced the state of anxiety.

A 27-year-old woman entered the hospital complaining of multiple fears. She was too frightened to get on streetcars or buses, to go to the movies, and to go out to supper. She was also afraid that she would not live up to the expectations of her mother, was dubious about her own capabilities, and indicated that her marriage was in difficult straits and that she had previously been separated from her husband for 18 months. She stated that their only son was a bed wetter. In addition, she presented the symptoms of acute anxiety with palpitation, perspiration, dizziness, and shortness of breath.

Brief questioning elicited the information that her mother had been a nagging, sadistic person, who unmercifully hit the patient and her brother whenever they failed to obey her command. The father, a mild, subservient individual, had seldom been at home. The patient was a quiet and obedient, though fearful, child, usually timid and retiring, who felt that she must always acquiesce to the wishes of others or be subject to their criticism and withdrawal of affection.

The diagnosis in this case was anxiety disorder, associated with many phobias. The anxiety attacks occurred regularly in situations in which the patient's husband, mother, or even the doctor did or said something to arouse in her a fear of separation associated with a wish to retaliate angrily. She could not allow herself to express further criticism and rejections. Her anxiety attacks were relieved after several months of psychiatric treatment in which she was able to recognize her anger and how to assert herself appropriately. (Adapted from Kolb LC. *Modern Clinical Psychiatry.* 9th ed. Philadelphia: WB Saunders; 1977:507.)

To fully understand a particular patient's anxiety, it is often useful to think in terms of a developmental hierarchy that links the source of the anxiety to developmental issues. At the earliest level, disintegration anxiety may be present. This anxiety may derive either from the fear of losing the sense of self through merger with an object or from concern that the self will fragment because others are not responding with needed affirmation and validation. At a somewhat more advanced level, persecutory or paranoid anxiety may be connected with the perception that a person is at risk of being invaded and annihilated by an outside malevolent force. Another source of anxiety involves the child who fears losing the love or approval of a parent or loved object. Castration anxiety, linked to the oedipal phase of development in boys, concerns the fear of a retaliatory parental figure, usually the father, damaging the little boy's genitals or otherwise causing bodily harm. At the most mature level, superego anxiety is understood as related to guilt feelings about not living up to internalized standards of moral behavior derived from the parents. Often a psychodynamic interview can elucidate the principal level of anxiety with which a patient is dealing. Some anxiety is obviously related to multiple conflicts at various developmental levels.

Behavioral Theories. The behavioral or learning theories of anxiety have spawned some of the most effective treatments for anxiety disorders. According to these theories, anxiety is a

conditioned response to specific environmental stimuli. In a model of classic conditioning, persons without food allergies may become sick after eating contaminated shellfish in a restaurant. Subsequent exposures to shellfish may cause these persons to feel sick. Through generalization, they may come to distrust all food prepared by others. As an alternative causal possibility, they may learn to have an internal response of anxiety by imitating the anxiety responses of their parents (social learning theory). In either case, treatment is usually a form of desensitization by repeated exposure to the anxiogenic stimulus, coupled with cognitive psychotherapeutic approaches.

In recent years, proponents of behavioral theories have shown increasing interest in cognitive approaches to conceptualizing and treating anxiety disorders, and cognitive theorists have proposed alternatives to traditional learning theory causal models of anxiety. According to conceptualizations of nonphobic anxiety states, faulty, distorted, or counterproductive thinking patterns accompany or precede maladaptive behaviors and emotional disorders. According to one model, patients with anxiety disorders tend to overestimate the danger and the probability of harm in a given situation and tend to underestimate their abilities to cope with perceived threats to their physical or psychological well-being. This model asserts that patients with panic disorder often have thoughts of loss of control and fears of dying that follow inexplicable physiological sensations (such as palpitations, tachycardia, and light-headedness) but that precede and then accompany panic attacks. Cognitive-behavioral therapy is an effective way to treat anxiety disorders, and some studies suggest that psychotherapy may alter abnormal patterns of brain activation, but much more work is required in this area.

Existential Theories. Existential theories of anxiety provide models for generalized anxiety disorder, in which there is no specifically identifiable stimulus for a chronically anxious feeling. The central concept of existential theory is that persons become aware of feelings of profound nothingness in their lives, feelings that may be even more discomforting than an acceptance of their inevitable death. Anxiety is their response to the vast void in existence and meaning. Such existential concerns may have increased since the development of nuclear weapons and bioterrorism.

Contributions of Biological Sciences

Biological theories of anxiety have developed from preclinical studies with animal models of anxiety, the study of patients in whom biological factors were ascertained, the growing knowledge about basic neuroscience, and the actions of psychotherapeutic drugs. One pole of thought posits that measurable biological changes in patients with anxiety disorders reflect the results of psychological conflicts; the opposite pole posits that the biological events precede the psychological conflicts. Both situations may exist in specific persons, and a range of biologically based sensitivities may exist among persons with the symptoms of anxiety disorders.

Autonomic Nervous System. Stimulation of the autonomic nervous system causes certain symptoms—cardiovascular (e.g., tachycardia), muscular (e.g., headache), gastrointestinal (e.g., diarrhea), and respiratory (e.g., tachypnea). These peripheral manifestations of anxiety are neither peculiar to anxiety disorders nor necessarily correlated with the subjective experience of anxiety. In the first third of the 20th century, Walter Cannon demonstrated that cats exposed to barking dogs exhibit behavioral and physiological signs of fear that are associated with the adrenal release of epinephrine. The James-Lange theory states that subjective anxiety is a response to peripheral phenomena. It is currently generally thought that central nervous system anxiety precedes the peripheral manifestations of anxiety, except when a specific peripheral cause is present, such as when a patient has a pheochromocytoma. The autonomic nervous systems of some patients with anxiety disorder, especially those with panic disorder, exhibit increased sympathetic tone, adapt slowly to repeated stimuli, and respond excessively to moderate stimuli.

Neurotransmitters. The three major neurotransmitters associated with anxiety on the bases of animal studies and responses to drug treatment are norepinephrine, serotonin, and γ-aminobutyric acid (GABA). Much of the basic neuroscience information about anxiety comes from animal experiments involving behavioral paradigms and psychoactive agents. One such animal model of anxiety is the conflict test, in which the animal is simultaneously presented with stimuli that are positive (e.g., food) and negative (e.g., electric shock). Anxiolytic drugs (e.g., benzodiazepines) tend to facilitate the adaptation of the animal to this situation, whereas other drugs (e.g., amphetamines) further disrupt the animal's behavioral responses.

NOREPINEPHRINE. The general theory about the role of norepinephrine in anxiety disorders is that affected patients may have a poorly regulated noradrenergic system with occasional bursts of activity. The cell bodies of the noradrenergic system are primarily localized to the locus ceruleus in the rostral pons, and they project their axons to the cerebral cortex, the limbic system, the brainstem, and the spinal cord. Experiments in primates have demonstrated that stimulation of the locus ceruleus produces a fear response in the animals and that ablation of the same area inhibits or completely blocks the ability of the animals to form a fear response.

Human studies have found that in patients with panic disorder, β-adrenergic receptor agonists (e.g., isoproterenol [Isuprel]) and α_2-adrenergic receptor antagonists (e.g., yohimbine [Yocon]) can provoke frequent and severe panic attacks. Conversely, clonidine (Catapres), an α_2-receptor agonist, reduces anxiety symptoms in some experimental and therapeutic situations. A less consistent finding is that patients with anxiety disorders, particularly panic disorder, have elevated cerebrospinal fluid (CSF) or urinary levels of the noradrenergic metabolite 3-methoxy-4-hydroxyphenylglycol (MHPG).

SEROTONIN. The identification of many serotonin receptor types has stimulated the search for the role of serotonin in the pathogenesis of anxiety disorders. The interest in this relation was initially motivated by the observation that serotonergic antidepressants have therapeutic effects in some anxiety disorders—for example, clomipramine (Anafranil) in obsessive-compulsive disorder. The effectiveness of buspirone (BuSpar), a serotonin 5-HT_{1A} receptor agonist, in the treatment of anxiety disorders also suggests the possibility of an association between serotonin and anxiety. The cell bodies of most serotonergic neurons are located in the raphe nuclei in the rostral brainstem and project to the cerebral cortex, the limbic system (especially the amygdala and the hippocampus), and the hypothalamus. Although the administration of serotonergic agents to animals results in behavior suggesting anxiety, the data on similar effects in humans are less robust. Several reports indicate that *m*-chlorophenylpiperazine (mCPP), a drug with multiple serotonergic and nonserotonergic effects, and fenfluramine (Pondimin), which causes the release of serotonin, do

cause increased anxiety in patients with anxiety disorders; and many anecdotal reports indicate that serotonergic hallucinogens and stimulants—for example, lysergic acid diethylamide (LSD) and 3,4-methylenedioxymethamphetamine (MDMA)—are associated with the development of both acute and chronic anxiety disorders in persons who use these drugs.

GABA. A role of GABA in anxiety disorders is most strongly supported by the undisputed efficacy of benzodiazepines, which enhance the activity of GABA at the $GABA_A$ receptor, in the treatment of some types of anxiety disorders. Although low-potency benzodiazepines are most effective for the symptoms of generalized anxiety disorder, high-potency benzodiazepines, such as alprazolam (Xanax), are effective in the treatment of panic disorder. Studies in primates have found that autonomic nervous system symptoms of anxiety disorders are induced when a benzodiazepine inverse agonist, β-carboline-3-carboxylic acid (BCCE), is administered. BCCE also causes anxiety in normal control volunteers. A benzodiazepine antagonist, flumazenil (Romazicon), causes frequent severe panic attacks in patients with panic disorder. These data have led researchers to hypothesize that some patients with anxiety disorders have abnormal functioning of their $GABA_A$ receptors, although this connection has not been shown directly.

APLYSIA. A neurotransmitter model for anxiety disorders is based on the study of *Aplysia californa,* by Nobel prize winner Eric Kandel, M.D. *Aplysia* is a sea snail that reacts to danger by moving away, withdrawing into its shell, and decreasing its feeding behavior. These behaviors can be classically conditioned, so that the snail responds to a neutral stimulus as if it were a dangerous stimulus. The snail can also be sensitized by random shocks, so that it exhibits a flight response in the absence of real danger. Parallels have previously been drawn between classical conditioning and human phobic anxiety. The classically conditioned *Aplysia* shows measurable changes in presynaptic facilitation, resulting in the release of increased amounts of neurotransmitter. Although the sea snail is a simple animal, this work shows an experimental approach to complex neurochemical processes potentially involved in anxiety disorders in humans.

Brain-Imaging Studies. A range of brain-imaging studies, almost always conducted with a specific anxiety disorder, has produced several possible leads in the understanding of anxiety disorders. Structural studies—for example, computed tomography (CT) and magnetic resonance imaging (MRI)—occasionally show some increase in the size of cerebral ventricles. In one study, the increase was correlated with the length of time patients had been taking benzodiazepines. In one MRI study, a specific defect in the right temporal lobe was noted in patients with panic disorder. Several other brain-imaging studies have reported abnormal findings in the right hemisphere but not the left hemisphere; this finding suggests that some types of cerebral asymmetries may be important in the development of anxiety disorder symptoms in specific patients. Functional brain-imaging studies—for example, positron emission tomography (PET), single photon emission computed tomography (SPECT), and electroencephalography (EEG)—of patients with anxiety disorder have variously reported abnormalities in the frontal cortex, the occipital and temporal areas, and, in a study of panic disorder, the parahippocampal gyrus. Several functional neuroimaging studies have implicated the caudate nucleus in the pathophysiology of obsessive-compulsive disorder. A conservative interpretation of these data is that some patients with anxiety disorders have a demonstrable functional cerebral pathological condition and that the condition may be causally relevant to their anxiety disorder symptoms.

Genetic Studies. Genetic studies have produced solid evidence that at least some genetic component contributes to the development of anxiety disorders. Almost half of all patients with panic disorder have at least one affected relative. The figures for other anxiety disorders, although not as high, also indicate a higher frequency of the illness in first-degree relatives of affected patients than in the relatives of nonaffected persons. Although adoption studies with anxiety disorders have not been reported, data from twin registers also support the hypothesis that anxiety disorders are at least partially genetically determined. Clearly, a linkage exists between genetics and anxiety disorders, but no anxiety disorder is likely to result from a simple Mendelian abnormality. A recent report has attributed about 4 percent of the intrinsic variability of anxiety within the general population to a polymorphic variant of the gene for the serotonin transporter, which is the site of action of many serotonergic drugs. Persons with the variant produce less transporter and have higher levels of anxiety.

Neuroanatomical Considerations. The locus ceruleus and the raphe nuclei project primarily to the limbic system and the cerebral cortex. In combination with the data from brain-imaging studies, these areas have become the focus of much hypothesis-building about the neuroanatomical substrates of anxiety disorders.

LIMBIC SYSTEM. In addition to receiving noradrenergic and serotonergic innervation, the limbic system also contains a high concentration of $GABA_A$ receptors. Ablation and stimulation studies in nonhuman primates have also implicated the limbic system in the generation of anxiety and fear responses. Two areas of the limbic system have received special attention in the literature: increased activity in the septohippocampal pathway, which may lead to anxiety, and the cingulate gyrus, which has been implicated particularly in the pathophysiology of obsessive-compulsive disorder.

CEREBRAL CORTEX. The frontal cerebral cortex is connected with the parahippocampal region, the cingulate gyrus, and the hypothalamus and thus may be involved in the production of anxiety disorders. The temporal cortex has also been implicated as a pathophysiological site in anxiety disorders. This association is based in part on the similarity in clinical presentation and electrophysiology between some patients with temporal lobe epilepsy and patients with obsessive-compulsive disorder.

DSM-IV-TR

DSM-IV-TR lists twelve anxiety disorders: (1) panic disorder with agoraphobia, (2) panic disorder without agoraphobia, (3) agoraphobia without history of panic disorder, (4) specific phobia, (5) social phobia, (6) obsessive-compulsive disorder, (7) posttraumatic stress disorder, (8) acute stress disorder, (9) generalized anxiety disorder, (10) anxiety disorder due to a general medical condition, (11) substance-induced anxiety disorder, and (12) anxiety disorder not otherwise specified. Each disorder is discussed in the sections that follow.

ICD-10

In the 10th revision of *International Statistical Classification of Diseases and Related Health Problems* (ICD-10), neurotic (anxiety) disorders are grouped with stress-related and somatoform disorders because of "their historical association with the concept of neurosis and the association of a substantial (though uncertain) proportion of these disorders with psychological causation." In ICD-10, mixtures of symp-

Table 16.1–2
ICD-10 Diagnostic Criteria for Phobic Anxiety Disorders

Agoraphobia

A. There is marked and consistently manifest fear in, or avoidance of, at least two of the following situations:
(1) crowds;
(2) public places;
(3) traveling alone;
(4) traveling away from home.

B. At least two symptoms of anxiety in the feared situation must have been present together, on at least one occasion since the onset of the disorder, and one of the symptoms must have been from items (1) to (4) listed below:

Autonomic arousal symptoms
(1) palpitations or pounding heart, or accelerated heart rate;
(2) sweating;
(3) trembling or shaking;
(4) dry mouth (not due to medication or dehydration);

Symptoms involving chest and abdomen
(5) difficulty in breathing;
(6) feeling of choking;
(7) chest pain or discomfort;
(8) nausea or abdominal distress (e.g., churning in stomach);

Symptoms involving mental state
(9) feeling dizzy, unsteady, faint, or light-headed;
(10) feelings that objects are unreal (derealization), or that the self is distant or "not really here" (depersonalization);
(11) fear of losing control, "going crazy," or passing out;
(12) fear of dying;

General symptoms
(13) hot flushes or cold chills;
(14) numbness or tingling sensations.

C. Significant emotional distress is caused by the avoidance or by the anxiety symptoms, and the individual recognizes that these are excessive or unreasonable.

D. Symptoms are restricted to, or predominate in, the feared situations or contemplation of the feared situations.

E. *Most commonly used exclusion clause.* Fear or avoidance of situations (Criterion A) is not the result of delusions, hallucinations, or other disorders such as organic mental disorders, schizophrenia and related disorders, mood [affective] disorders, or obsessive-compulsive disorder, and is not secondary to cultural beliefs.

The presence or absence of panic disorder in a majority of agoraphobic situations may be specified by using a fifth character:

Without panic disorder

With panic disorder

Options for rating severity

Severity in agoraphobia may be rated by indicating the degree of avoidance, taking into account the specific cultural setting. Severity in social phobias may be rated by counting the number of panic attacks.

Social phobias

A. Either of the following must be present:
(1) marked fear of being the focus of attention, or fear of behaving in a way that will be embarrassing or humiliating;
(2) marked avoidance of being the focus of attention, or of situations in which there is fear of behaving in an embarrassing or humiliating way.

These fears are manifested in social situations, such as eating or speaking in public, encountering known individuals in public, or entering or enduring small group situations (e.g., parties, meetings, classrooms).

B. At least two symptoms of anxiety in the feared situation as defined in agoraphobia, Criterion B, must have been manifest at some time since the onset of the disorder, together with at least one of the following symptoms:
(1) blushing or shaking;
(2) fear of vomiting;
(3) urgency or fear of micturition or defecation.

C. Significant emotional distress is caused by the symptoms or by the avoidance, and the individual recognizes that these are excessive or unreasonable.

D. Symptoms are restricted to, or predominate in, the feared situations or contemplation of the feared situations.

E. *Most commonly used exclusion clause.* The symptoms listed in Criteria A and B are not the result of delusions, hallucinations, or other disorders such as organic mental disorders, schizophrenia and related disorders, mood [affective] disorders, or obsessive-compulsive disorder, and are not secondary to cultural beliefs.

Specific (isolated) phobias

A. Either of the following must be present:
(1) marked fear of a specific object or situation not included in agoraphobia or social phobia;
(2) marked avoidance of a specific object or situation not included in agoraphobia or social phobia.

Among the most common objects and situations are animals, birds, insects, heights, thunder, flying, small enclosed spaces, the sight of blood or injury, injections, dentists, and hospitals.

B. Symptoms of anxiety in the feared situation as defined in agoraphobia, Criterion B, must have been manifest at some time since the onset of the disorder.

C. Significant emotional distress is caused by the symptoms or by the avoidance, and the individual recognizes that these are excessive or unreasonable.

D. Symptoms are restricted to the feared situation or contemplation of the feared situation.

If desired, the specific phobias may be subdivided as follows:
—animal type (e.g., insects, dogs)
—nature-forces type (e.g., storms, water)
—blood, injection, and injury type
—situational type (e.g., elevators, tunnels)
—other type

Other phobic anxiety disorders

Phobic anxiety disorder, unspecified

Reprinted with permission from World Health Organization. *The ICD-10 Classification of Mental and Behavioural Disorders: Diagnostic Criteria for Research.* Copyright, World Health Organization, Geneva, 1993.

toms are described as common, especially in less severe varieties of these disorders, and a category for cases that cannot be based on a single main syndrome is provided. Although the idea of neurosis is no longer the organizing principle, "care has been taken to allow the easy identification of disorders that some users still might wish to regard as neurotic in their own usage of the term."

Table 16.1–3
ICD-10 Diagnostic Criteria for Other Anxiety Disorders

Panic disorder [episodic paroxysmal anxiety]

A. The individual experiences recurrent panic attacks that are not consistently associated with a specific situation or object and that often occur spontaneously (i.e., the episodes are unpredictable). The panic attacks are not associated with marked exertion or with exposure to dangerous or life-threatening situations.

B. A panic attack is characterized by all of the following:

(1) it is a discrete episode of intense fear of discomfort;

(2) it starts abruptly;

(3) it reaches a maximum within a few minutes and lasts at least some minutes;

(4) at least four of the symptoms listed below must be present, one of which must be from items (a) to (d):

Autonomic arousal symptoms

(a) palpitations or pounding heart, or accelerated heart rate;

(b) sweating;

(c) trembling or shaking;

(d) dry mouth (not due to medication or dehydration);

Symptoms involving chest and abdomen

(e) difficulty in breathing;

(f) feeling of choking;

(g) chest pain or discomfort;

(h) nausea or abdominal distress (e.g., churning in stomach);

Symptoms involving mental state

(i) feeling dizzy, unsteady, faint, or light-headed;

(j) feelings that objects are unreal (derealization), or that the self is distant or "not really here" (depersonalization);

(k) fear of losing control, "going crazy," or passing out;

(l) fear of dying;

General symptoms

(m) hot flushes or cold chills;

(n) numbness or tingling sensations.

C. *Most commonly used exclusion clause.* Panic attacks are not due to a physical disorder, organic mental disorder, or other mental disorders, such as schizophrenia and related disorders, mood [affective] disorders, or somatoform disorders.

The range of individual variation in both content and severity is so great that two grades, moderate and severe, may be specified, if desired, with a fifth character.

Panic disorder, moderate

At least four panic attacks in a 4-week period.

Panic disorder, severe

At least four panic attacks per week over a 4-week period.

Generalized anxiety disorder

Note. In children and adolescents the range of complaints by which the general anxiety is manifest is often more limited than in adults, and the specific symptoms of autonomic arousal are often less prominent. For these individuals, an alternative set of criteria is provided for use (in generalized anxiety disorder of childhood) if preferred.

A. There must have been a period of at least 6 months with prominent tension, worry, and feelings of apprehension about everyday events and problems.

B. At least four of the symptoms listed below must be present, at least one of which must be from items (1) to (4):

Autonomic arousal symptoms

(1) palpitations or pounding heart, or accelerated heart rate;

(2) sweating;

(3) trembling or shaking;

(4) dry mouth (not due to medication or dehydration);

Symptoms involving chest and abdomen

(5) difficulty in breathing;

(6) feeling of choking;

(7) chest pain or discomfort;

(8) nausea or abdominal distress (e.g., churning in stomach);

Symptoms involving mental state

(9) feeling dizzy, unsteady, faint, or light-headed

(10) feelings that objects are unreal (derealization), or that the self is distant or "not really here" (depersonalization);

(11) fear of losing control, "going crazy," or passing out;

(12) fear of dying;

General symptoms

(13) hot flushes or cold chills;

(14) numbness or tingling sensations;

Symptoms of tension

(15) muscle tension or aches and pains;

(16) restlessness and inability to relax;

(17) feeling keyed up, on edge, or mentally tense;

(18) a sensation of a lump in the throat, or difficulty in swallowing;

Other nonspecific symptoms

(19) exaggerated response to minor surprise or being startled;

(20) difficulty in concentrating, or mind "going blank," because of worrying or anxiety;

(21) persistent irritability;

(22) difficulty in getting to sleep because of worrying.

C. The disorder does not meet the criteria for panic disorder, phobic anxiety disorders, obsessive-compulsive disorder, or hypochondriacal disorder.

D. *Most commonly used exclusion clause.* The anxiety disorder is not due to a physical disorder, such as hyperthyroidism, an organic mental disorder, or a psychoactive substance-related disorder, such as excess consumption of amphetaminelike substances or withdrawal from benzodiazepines.

Mixed anxiety and depressive disorder

There are so many possible combinations of comparatively mild symptoms for these disorders that specific criteria are not given, other than those already in *Clinical Descriptions and Diagnostic Guidelines.* It is suggested that researchers wishing to study patients with these disorders should arrive at their own criteria within the guidelines, depending upon the setting and purpose of their studies.

Other mixed anxiety disorders

Other specified anxiety disorders

Anxiety disorder, unspecified

The main ICD-10 categories for "neurotic" anxiety disorders are phobic anxiety disorders (agoraphobia, social phobias, and specific phobias); other anxiety disorders (panic disorder, generalized anxiety disorder, and mixed anxiety and depressive disorder); and obsessive-compulsive disorder (with predominantly obsessional thoughts, predominantly compulsive acts, or mixed obsessional thoughts and acts) (Tables 16.1–2 through 16.1–4).

Table 16.1–4
ICD-10 Diagnostic Criteria for Obsessive-Compulsive Disorder

A. Either obsessions or compulsions (or both) are present on most days for a period of at least 2 weeks.
B. Obsessions (thoughts, ideas, or images) and compulsions (acts) share the following features, all of which must be present:
   (1) They are acknowledged as originating in the mind of the patient and are not imposed by outside persons or influences.
   (2) They are repetitive and unpleasant, and at least one obsession or compulsion that is acknowledged as excessive or unreasonable must be present.
   (3) The patient tries to resist them (but resistance to very long-standing obsessions or compulsions may be minimal). At least one obsession or compulsion that is unsuccessfully resisted must be present.
   (4) Experiencing the obsessive thought or carrying out the compulsive act is not in itself pleasurable. (This should be distinguished from the temporary relief of tension or anxiety.)
C. The obsessions or compulsions cause distress or interfere with the patient's social or individual functioning, usually by wasting time.
D. *Most commonly used exclusion clause.* The obsessions or compulsions are not the result of other mental disorders, such as schizophrenia and related disorders or mood [affective] disorders.

The diagnosis may be further specified by the following four-character codes:

Predominantly obsessional thoughts and ruminations
Predominantly compulsive acts [obsessional rituals]
Mixed obsessional thoughts and acts
Other obsessive-compulsive disorders
Obsessive-compulsive disorder, unspecified

In ICD-10, reaction to severe stress and adjustment disorders are grouped into one category, which is classed together with neurotic and somatoform disorders. However, the stress-related category differs from the other two categories because it can be defined not only on the basis of symptoms but also on the basis of one of two causative influences: a stressful life event causing an acute stress reaction or a significant life change producing an adjustment disorder. Stress-related disorders in all age groups, including children, fall into this category.

In this group, ICD-10 classifies reactions to severe stress (acute stress reaction, posttraumatic distress disorder) and adjustment disorders (see Chapter 26). ICD-10 also includes the dissociative (conversion) disorders in the category of stress-related disorders. (For a discussion of dissociative disorders, see Chapter 20.) The criteria for reactions to severe stress are given in Table 16.1–5.

Table 16.1–5
ICD-10 Diagnostic Criteria for Reactions to Severe Stress

Acute stress reaction

A. The patient must have been exposed to an exceptional mental or physical stressor.
B. Exposure to the stressor is followed by an immediate onset of symptoms (within 1 hour).
C. Two groups of symptoms are given: the acute stress reaction is graded as:
   Mild
   Only Criterion (1) below is fulfilled.
   Moderate
   Criterion (1) is met, and there are any two symptoms from Criterion (2).
   Severe
   Either criterion (1) is met, and there are any four symptoms from criterion (2); *or* there is dissociative stupor.
   (1) Criteria B, C, and D for generalized anxiety disorder are met.
   (2) (a) Withdrawal from expected social interaction.
      (b) Narrowing of attention.
      (c) Apparent disorientation.
      (d) Anger or verbal aggression.
      (e) Despair or hopelessness.
      (f) Inappropriate or purposeless overactivity.
      (g) Uncontrollable and excessive grief (judged by local cultural standards).
D. If the stressor is transient or can be relieved, the symptoms must begin to diminish after not more than 8 hours. If exposure to the stressor continues, the symptoms must begin to diminish after not more than 48 hours.
E. *Most commonly used exclusion clause.* The reaction must occur in the absence of any other concurrent mental or behavioral disorder in ICD-10 (except generalized anxiety disorder and personality disorders) and not within 3 months of the end of an episode of any other mental or behavioral disorder.

Posttraumatic stress disorder

A. The patient must have been exposed to a stressful event or situation (either short- or long-lasting) of an exceptionally threatening or catastrophic nature, which would be likely to cause pervasive distress in almost anyone.
B. There must be persistent remembering or "reliving" of the stressor in intrusive "flashbacks," vivid memories, or recurring dreams or in experiencing distress when exposed to circumstances resembling or associated with the stressor.
C. The patient must exhibit an actual or preferred avoidance of circumstances resembling or associated with the stressor, which was not present before exposure to the stressor.
D. Either of the following must be present:
   (1) inability to recall, either partially or completely, some important aspects of the period of exposure to the stressor;
   (2) persistent symptoms of increased psychological sensitivity and arousal (not present before exposure to the stressor), shown by any two of the following:
      (a) difficulty in falling or staying asleep;
      (b) irritability or outbursts of anger;
      (c) difficulty in concentrating;
      (d) hypervigilance;
      (e) exaggerated startle response.
E. Criteria B, C, and D must all be met within 6 months of the stressful event or of the end of a period of stress. (For some purposes, onset delayed more than 6 months may be included, but this should be clearly specified.)

References

Cassem EH. Depression and anxiety secondary to medical illness. *Psychiatr Clin North Am.* 1990;13:597.

Charney DS, Nagy LM, Bremner JD, Goddard AW, Yehuda R, South SM. Neurobiologic mechanisms of human anxiety. In: Fogel BS, Schiffer RB, et al., eds. *Synopsis of Neuropsychiatry.* Philadelphia: Lippincott Williams & Wilkins; 2000:273.

Coryell W, Endicott J, Winokur G. Anxiety syndromes as epiphenomena of primary major depression: outcome and financial psychopathology. *Am J Psychiatry.* 1992;149:100.

Davis M. The role of the amygdala in fear-potentiated startle: implications for animal models of anxiety. *Trends Pharmacol Sci.* 1992;13:35.

Gabbard GO. *Psychodynamics Psychiatry in Clinical Practice: The DSM-IV Edition.* Washington, DC: American Psychiatric Press; 1994.

Gorman JM, section ed. Anxiety disorders. In: Sadock BJ, Sadock VA, eds. *Kaplan & Sadock's Comprehensive Textbook of Psychiatry.* 7th ed. Vol 1. Baltimore: Lippincott Williams & Wilkins; 2000:1441.

Gorman JM, Papp LA, eds. Anxiety disorders. In: Tasman A, Riba MB, eds. *American Psychiatric Press Review of Psychiatry.* Vol 11. Washington, DC: American Psychiatric Press; 1992:243.

Lucki I. Serotonin receptor specificity in anxiety disorders. *J Clin Psychiatry.* 1996;57(suppl 6):5.

Mennin DS, Heimberg RG, Holt CS. Panic, agoraphobia, phobias, and generalized anxiety disorder. In: Hersen M, Bellack AS, eds. *Psychopathology in Adulthood.* 2nd ed. Needham Heights, MA: Allyn & Bacon; 2000:169.

▲ 16.2 Panic Disorder and Agoraphobia

Panic disorder is characterized by the spontaneous, unexpected occurrence of panic attacks, that is, discrete periods of intense fear that can vary from several attacks during 1 day to only a few attacks during a year. Panic disorder is often accompanied by agoraphobia, the fear of being alone in public places (such as supermarkets), particularly places from which a rapid exit would be difficult in the course of a panic attack.

Agoraphobia can be the most disabling of the phobias, as it may significantly interfere with a person's ability to function in work and social situations outside the home. In the United States, most researchers of panic disorder believe that agoraphobia almost always develops as a complication in patients with panic disorder. That is, the fear of having a panic attack in a public place from which escape would be formidable is thought to cause the agoraphobia. Researchers in other countries as well as some U.S. researchers and clinicians disagree with this theory, but the text revision of the fourth edition of *Diagnostic and Statistical Manual of Mental Disorders* (DSM-IV-TR) establishes panic disorder as the predominant disorder in the dyad. DSM-IV-TR includes diagnoses for panic disorder with and without agoraphobia and also for agoraphobia without history of panic disorder. Panic attacks can also occur in many mental disorders (e.g., depressive disorders) and medical conditions (e.g., substance withdrawal or intoxication), and the presence of a panic attack does not in itself necessitate a diagnosis of panic disorder.

Because patients who have experienced panic attacks often go to medical clinics, the symptoms may be misdiagnosed as a serious medical condition (e.g., myocardial infarction) or as a so-called hysterical symptom. Nevertheless, since 1980, when the diagnosis was codified, clinicians have an increased ability to recognize the symptoms of panic disorder, and effective and specific treatments are available. Those who supply health care must be able to recognize the symptoms of panic disorder so that affected patients can receive appropriate therapy, including pharmacotherapeutic agents and psychotherapy.

HISTORY

The idea of panic disorder may have its roots in the concept of irritable heart syndrome, which the physician Jacob Mendes DaCosta (1833–1900) noted in soldiers in the American Civil War. DaCosta's syndrome included many psychological and somatic symptoms that have since been included among the diagnostic criteria for panic disorder. In 1895, Sigmund Freud introduced the concept of *anxiety neurosis*, consisting of acute and chronic psychological and somatic symptoms. Freud's acute anxiety neurosis was similar to panic disorder as defined in DSM-IV-TR, and Freud first noted the relation between panic attacks and agoraphobia. The term *agoraphobia* was coined in 1871 to describe the condition of patients who were afraid to venture alone into public places. The term is derived from the Greek words *agora* and *phobos,* meaning "fear of the marketplace."

EPIDEMIOLOGY

Epidemiological studies have reported lifetime prevalence rates of 1.5 to 5 percent for panic disorder and 3 to 5.6 percent for panic attacks. For example, one study of more than 1,600 randomly selected adults in Texas found a lifetime prevalence rate of 3.8 percent for panic disorder, 5.6 percent for panic attacks, and 2.2 percent for panic attacks with limited symptoms that did not meet the full diagnostic criteria.

Women are two to three times more likely to be affected than men, although underdiagnosis of panic disorder in men may contribute to the skewed distribution. The differences among Hispanics, whites, and blacks are small. The only social factor identified as contributing to the development of panic disorder is a recent history of divorce or separation. Panic disorder most commonly develops in young adulthood—the mean age of presentation is about 25 years—but both panic disorder and agoraphobia can develop at any age. Panic disorder has been reported in children and adolescents, and it is probably underdiagnosed in these age groups.

The lifetime prevalence of agoraphobia has been reported as ranging from as low as 0.6 percent to as high as 6 percent. The major factor leading to this wide range of estimates is the use of varying diagnostic criteria and assessment methods. Although studies of agoraphobia in psychiatric settings have reported that at least three fourths of the affected patients have panic disorder as well, studies of agoraphobia in community samples have found that as many as half the patients have agoraphobia without panic disorder. The reasons for these divergent findings are unknown but probably involve differences in ascertainment techniques. In many cases, the onset of agoraphobia follows a traumatic event.

COMORBIDITY

Ninety-one percent of patients with panic disorder and 84 percent of those with agoraphobia have at least one other psychiatric disorder. According to DSM-IV-TR, 10 to 15 percent of

persons with panic disorder have comorbid major depressive disorder. About one third of persons with both disorders have major depressive disorder before the onset of panic disorder; about two thirds first experience panic disorder during or after the onset of major depression.

Anxiety disorders also commonly occur in persons with panic disorder and agoraphobia. Fifteen to 30 percent of persons with panic disorder also have social phobia, 2 to 20 percent have specific phobia, 15 to 30 percent have generalized anxiety disorder, 2 to 10 percent have posttraumatic stress disorder, and up to 30 percent have obsessive-compulsive disorder. Other common comorbid conditions are hypochondriasis, personality disorders, and substance-related disorders.

ETIOLOGY

Biological Factors

Research on the biological basis of panic disorder has produced a range of findings; one interpretation is that the symptoms of panic disorder are related to a range of biological abnormalities in brain structure and function. Most work has used biological stimulants to induce panic attacks in patients with panic disorder. These and other studies have produced hypotheses implicating both peripheral and central nervous system dysregulation in the pathophysiology of panic disorder. The autonomic nervous systems of some patients with panic disorder have been reported to exhibit increased sympathetic tone, to adapt slowly to repeated stimuli, and to respond excessively to moderate stimuli. Studies of the neuroendocrine status of these patients have shown several abnormalities, although the studies have been inconsistent in their findings.

The major neurotransmitter systems that have been implicated are those for norepinephrine, serotonin, and γ-aminobutyric acid (GABA). Serotonergic dysfunction is quite evident in panic disorder and various studies with mixed serotonin agonist-antagonist drugs have demonstrated increased rates of anxiety. Such responses may be due to postsynaptic serotonin hypersensitivity in panic disorder. There is preclinical evidence that attenuation of local inhibitory GABAergic transmission in the basolateral amygdala, midbrain, and hypothalamus can elicit anxietylike physiological responses. The biological data has led to a focus on the brainstem (particularly the noradrenergic neurons of the locus ceruleus and the serotonergic neurons of the median raphe nucleus), the limbic system (possibly responsible for the generation of anticipatory anxiety), and the prefrontal cortex (possibly responsible for the generation of phobic avoidance). Among the various neurotransmitters involved, the noradrenergic system has also attracted much attention, with the presynaptic α_2-adrenergic receptors, particularly, playing a significant role. They have been identified by pharmacological challenges with the α_2-receptor agonist clonidine (Catapres) and the α_2-receptor antagonist yohimbine (Yocon), which stimulates firing of the locus ceruleus and elicits high rates of paniclike activity in panic disorder patients.

Panic-Inducing Substances. Panic-inducing substances (sometimes called panicogens) induce panic attacks in most patients with panic disorder and in a much smaller proportion of persons without panic disorder or a history of panic attacks. (The use of panic-inducing substances is strictly limited to research settings; there are no clinically indicated reasons to stimulate panic attacks in patients.) So-called respiratory panic-inducing substances cause respiratory stimulation and a shift in the acid–base balance. These substances include carbon dioxide (5 to 35 percent mixtures), sodium lactate, and bicarbonate. Neurochemical panic-inducing substances that act through specific neurotransmitter systems include yohimbine, an α_2-adrenergic receptor antagonist; *m*-chlorophenylpiperazine (mCPP), an agent with multiple serotonergic effects; μ-carboline drugs; $GABA_B$ receptor inverse agonists; flumazenil (Romazicon), a $GABA_B$ receptor antagonist; cholecystokinin; and caffeine. Isoproterenol (Isuprel) is also a panic-inducing substance, although its mechanism of action in inducing panic attacks is poorly understood. The respiratory panic-inducing substances may act initially at the peripheral cardiovascular baroreceptors and relay their signal by vagal afferents to the nucleus tractus solitarii and then on to the nucleus paragigantocellularis of the medulla. The hyperventilation in panic disorder patients may be due to a hypersensitive suffocation alarm system whereby increasing P_{CO_2} and brain lactate concentrations prematurely activate a physiological asphyxic monitor. The neurochemical panic-inducing substances are presumed to primarily affect the noradrenergic, serotonergic, and GABA receptors of the central nervous system directly.

Brain Imaging. Structural brain-imaging studies, for example, magnetic resonance imaging (MRI), in patients with panic disorder have implicated pathological involvement in the temporal lobes, particularly the hippocampus. One MRI study reported abnormalities, especially cortical atrophy, in the right temporal lobe of these patients. Functional brain-imaging studies, for example, positron emission tomography (PET), have implicated dysregulation of cerebral blood flow. Specifically, anxiety disorders and panic attacks are associated with cerebral vasoconstriction, which may result in central nervous system symptoms such as dizziness and in peripheral nervous system symptoms that may be induced by hyperventilation and hypocapnia. Most functional brain-imaging studies have used a specific panic-inducing substance (e.g., lactate, caffeine, or yohimbine) in combination with PET or single photon emission computed tomography to assess the effects of the panic-inducing substance and the induced panic attack on cerebral blood flow.

Mitral Valve Prolapse. Although great interest was formerly expressed in an association between mitral valve prolapse and panic disorder, research has almost completely erased any clinical significance or relevance to the association. Mitral valve prolapse is a heterogeneous syndrome consisting of the prolapse of one of the mitral valve leaflets, resulting in a midsystolic click on cardiac auscultation. Studies have found that the prevalence of panic disorder in patients with mitral valve prolapse is the same as the prevalence of panic disorder in patients without mitral valve prolapse.

Genetic Factors

Although the number of well-controlled studies of the genetic basis of panic disorder and agoraphobia is small, the data to date support the conclusion that the disorders have a distinct genetic component. In addition, some data indicate that panic

disorder with agoraphobia is a severe form of panic disorder and is thus more likely to be inherited. Various studies have found that the first-degree relatives of panic disorder patients have a fourfold to eightfold higher risk for panic disorder than first-degree relatives of other psychiatric patients. The twin studies conducted to date have generally reported that monozygotic twins are more likely to be concordant for panic disorder than are dizygotic twins. At this point, no data exist indicating association between a specific chromosomal location or mode of transmission and this disorder.

Psychosocial Factors

Both cognitive-behavioral and psychoanalytic theories have been developed to explain the pathogenesis of panic disorder and agoraphobia. The success of cognitive-behavioral approaches in the treatment of these disorders may add credence to the cognitive-behavioral theories.

Cognitive-Behavioral Theories. Behavioral theories posit that anxiety is a response learned either from parental behavior or through the process of classic conditioning. In a classic conditioning approach to panic disorder and agoraphobia, a noxious stimulus (e.g., a panic attack) that occurs with a neutral stimulus (e.g., a bus ride) can result in the avoidance of the neutral stimulus. Other behavioral theories posit a linkage between the sensation of minor somatic symptoms (e.g., palpitations) and generation of a panic attack. Although cognitive-behavioral theories can help explain the development of agoraphobia or an increase in the number or severity of panic attacks, they do not explain the occurrence of the first unprovoked and unexpected panic attack that an affected patient experiences.

Psychoanalytic Theories. Psychoanalytic theories conceptualize panic attacks as arising from an unsuccessful defense against anxiety-provoking impulses. What was previously a mild signal anxiety becomes an overwhelming feeling of apprehension, complete with somatic symptoms. To explain agoraphobia, psychoanalytic theories emphasize the loss of a parent in childhood and a history of separation anxiety. Being alone in public places revives the childhood anxiety about being abandoned. The defense mechanisms used include repression, displacement, avoidance, and symbolization. Traumatic separations during childhood may affect children's developing nervous systems in such a manner that they become susceptible to anxieties in adulthood. There may be a predisposing neurophysiological vulnerability that may interact with certain kinds of environmental stressors to produce the end result of a panic attack.

Many patients describe panic attacks as coming out of the blue, as though no psychological factors were involved, but psychodynamic exploration frequently reveals a clear psychological trigger for the panic attack. Although panic attacks are correlated neurophysiologically with the locus ceruleus, the onset of panic is generally related to environmental or psychological factors. Patients with panic disorder have a higher incidence of stressful life events (particularly loss) than control subjects in the months before the onset of panic disorder. Moreover, the patients typically experience greater distress about life events than control subjects do.

Table 16.2–1
Psychodynamic Themes in Panic Disorder

1. Difficulty tolerating anger
2. Physical or emotional separation from significant person both in childhood and in adult life
3. May be triggered by situations of increased work responsibilities
4. Perception of parents as controlling, frightening, critical, and demanding
5. Internal representations of relationships involving sexual or physical abuse
6. A chronic sense of feeling trapped
7. Vicious cycle of anger at parental rejecting behavior followed by anxiety that the fantasy will destroy the tie to parents
8. Failure of signal anxiety function in ego related to self fragmentation and self–other boundary confusion
9. Typical defense mechanisms: reaction formation, undoing, somatization, and externalization.

The hypothesis that stressful psychological events produce neurophysiological changes in panic disorder is supported by a study of female twins. The research findings revealed that panic disorder was strongly associated with both parental separation and parental death before children reached the age of 17. Separation from the mother early in life was clearly more likely to result in panic disorder than was paternal separation in the cohort of 1,018 pairs of female twins. Another etiological factor in adult female patients appears to be childhood physical and sexual abuse. Approximately 60 percent of women with panic disorder have a history of childhood sexual abuse, compared with 31 percent of women with other anxiety disorders. Further support for psychological mechanisms in panic disorder can be inferred from a study of panic disorder in which patients received successful treatment with cognitive therapy. Before the therapy, the patients responded to panic attack induction with lactate. After successful cognitive therapy, lactate infusion no longer produced a panic attack.

The research indicates that the cause of panic attacks is likely to involve the unconscious meaning of stressful events and that the pathogenesis of the panic attacks may be related to neurophysiological factors triggered by the psychological reactions. Psychodynamic clinicians should always do a thorough investigation of possible triggers whenever assessing a patient with panic disorder. The psychodynamics of panic disorder are summarized in Table 16.2–1.

DIAGNOSIS

Panic Attacks. In DSM-IV-TR, the criteria for a panic attack are listed as a separate set of criteria (Table 16.2–2). Panic attacks can occur in mental disorders other than panic disorder, particularly in specific phobia, social phobia, and posttraumatic stress disorder. Unexpected panic attacks occur at any time and are not associated with any identifiable situational stimulus, but panic attacks need not be unexpected. Attacks in patients with social and specific phobias are usually expected or cued to a recognized or specific stimulus. Some panic attacks do not fit easily into the distinction between unexpected and expected, and these attacks are referred to as situationally pre-

Table 16.2–2
DSM-IV-TR Criteria for Panic Attack

Note: A panic attack is not a codable disorder. Code the specific diagnosis in which the panic attack occurs (e.g., panic disorder with agoraphobia).

A discrete period of intense fear or discomfort, in which four (or more) of the following symptoms developed abruptly and reached a peak within 10 minutes:

(1) palpitations, pounding heart, or accelerated heart rate
(2) sweating
(3) trembling or shaking
(4) sensations of shortness of breath or smothering
(5) feeling of choking
(6) chest pain or discomfort
(7) nausea or abdominal distress
(8) feeling dizzy, unsteady, lightheaded, or faint
(9) derealization (feelings of unreality) or depersonalization (being detached from oneself)
(10) fear of losing control or going crazy
(11) fear of dying
(12) paresthesias (numbness or tingling sensations)
(13) chills or hot flushes

From American Psychiatric Association. *Diagnostic and Statistical Manual of Mental Disorders.* 4th ed. Text rev. Washington, DC: American Psychiatric Association; copyright 2000, with permission.

disposed panic attacks. They may or may not occur when a patient is exposed to a specific trigger, or they may occur either immediately after exposure or after a considerable delay.

Panic Disorder

DSM-IV-TR contains two diagnostic criteria for panic disorder, one without agoraphobia (Table 16.2–3) and the other with agoraphobia (Table 16.2–4), but both require the presence of panic attacks as described in Table 16.2–2. Some community surveys have indicated that panic attacks are common, and a major issue in developing diagnostic criteria for panic disorder was determining a threshold number or frequency of panic attacks required to meet the diagnosis. Setting the threshold too low results in the diagnosis of panic disorder in patients who do not have an impairment from an occasional panic attack; setting the threshold too high results in a situation in which patients who are impaired by their panic attacks do not meet the diagnostic criteria. The vagaries of setting a threshold are evidenced by the range of thresholds set in various diagnostic criteria. The Research Diagnostic Criteria require six panic attacks during a 6-week period. The 10th revision of the *International Statistical Classification of Diseases and Related Health Problems* (ICD-10) requires three attacks in 3 weeks (for moderate disease) or four attacks in 4 weeks (for severe disease). DSM-IV-TR does not specify a minimum number of panic attacks or a time frame but does require that at least one attack be followed by at least a month-long period of concern about having another panic attack or about the implications of the attack or a significant change in behavior. DSM-IV-TR also requires that the panic attacks generally be unexpected but allows for expected or situationally predisposed attacks.

Table 16.2–3
DSM-IV-TR Diagnostic Criteria for Panic Disorder without Agoraphobia

A. Both (1) and (2):
(1) recurrent unexpected panic attacks
(2) at least one of the attacks has been followed by 1 month (or more) of one (or more) of the following:
(a) persistent concern about having additional attacks
(b) worry about the implications of the attack or its consequences (e.g., losing control, having a heart attack, "going crazy")
(c) a significant change in behavior related to the attacks

B. Absence of agoraphobia

C. The panic attacks are not due to the direct physiological effects of a substance (e.g., a drug of abuse, a medication) or a general medical condition (e.g., hyperthyroidism).

D. The panic attacks are not better accounted for by another mental disorder, such as social phobia (e.g., occurring on exposure to feared social situations), specific phobia (e.g., on exposure to a specific phobic situation), obsessive-compulsive disorder (e.g., on exposure to dirt in someone with an obsession about contamination), posttraumatic stress disorder (e.g., in response to stimuli associated with a severe stressor), or separation anxiety disorder (e.g., in response to being away from home or close relatives).

From American Psychiatric Association. *Diagnostic and Statistical Manual of Mental Disorders.* 4th ed. Text rev. Washington, DC: American Psychiatric Association; copyright 2000, with permission.

Table 16.2–4
DSM-IV-TR Diagnostic Criteria for Panic Disorder with Agoraphobia

A. Both (1) and (2):
(1) recurrent unexpected panic attacks
(2) at least one of the attacks has been followed by 1 month (or more) of one (or more) of the following:
(a) persistent concern about having additional attacks
(b) worry about the implications of the attack or its consequences (e.g., losing control, having a heart attack, "going crazy")
(c) a significant change in behavior related to the attacks

B. The presence of agoraphobia

C. The panic attacks are not due to the direct physiological effects of a substance (e.g., a drug of abuse, a medication) or a general medical condition (e.g., hyperthyroidism).

D. The panic attacks are not better accounted for by another mental disorder, such as social phobia (e.g., occurring on exposure to feared social situations), specific phobia (e.g., on exposure to a specific phobic situation), obsessive-compulsive disorder (e.g., on exposure to dirt in someone with an obsession about contamination), posttraumatic stress disorder (e.g., in response to stimuli associated with a severe stressor), or separation anxiety disorder (e.g., in response to being away from home or close relatives).

From American Psychiatric Association. *Diagnostic and Statistical Manual of Mental Disorders.* 4th ed. Text rev. Washington, DC: American Psychiatric Association; copyright 2000, with permission.

Table 16.2–5
DSM-IV-TR Criteria for Agoraphobia

Note: Agoraphobia is not a codable disorder. Code the specific disorder in which the agoraphobia occurs (e.g., panic disorder with agoraphobia or agoraphobia without history of panic disorder.

A. Anxiety about being in places or situations from which escape might be difficult (or embarrassing) or in which help may not be available in the event of having an unexpected or situationally predisposed panic attack or paniclike symptoms. Agoraphobic fears typically involve characteristic clusters of situations that include being outside the home alone; being in a crowd or standing in a line; being on a bridge; and traveling in a bus, train, or automobile.

   Note: Consider the diagnosis of specific phobia if the avoidance is limited to one or only a few specific situations, or social phobia if the avoidance is limited to social situations.

B. The situations are avoided (e.g., travel is restricted) or else are endured with marked distress or with anxiety about having a panic attack or paniclike symptoms, or require the presence of a companion.

C. The anxiety or phobic avoidance is not better accounted for by another mental disorder, such as social phobia (e.g., avoidance limited to social situations because of fear of embarrassment), specific phobia (e.g., avoidance limited to a single situation like elevators), obsessive-compulsive disorder (e.g., avoidance of dirt in someone with an obsession about contamination), posttraumatic stress disorder (e.g., avoidance of stimuli associated with a severe stressor), or separation anxiety disorder (e.g., avoidance of leaving home or relatives).

From American Psychiatric Association. *Diagnostic and Statistical Manual of Mental Disorders.* 4th ed. Text rev. Washington, DC: American Psychiatric Association; copyright 2000, with permission.

Agoraphobia without History of Panic Disorder

Table 16.2–5 lists criteria for agoraphobia. The DSM-IV-TR diagnostic criteria for agoraphobia without history of panic disorder (Table 16.2–6) are based on the fear of a sudden incapacitating or embarrassing symptom. In contrast, the ICD-10 criteria require the presence of interrelated or overlapping phobias but do not require fear of incapacitating or embarrassing symptoms.

Table 16.2–6
DSM-IV-TR Diagnostic Criteria for Agoraphobia without History of Panic Disorder

A. The presence of agoraphobia related to fear of developing paniclike symptoms (e.g., dizziness or diarrhea).

B. Criteria have never been met for panic disorder.

C. The disturbance is not due to the direct physiological effects of a substance (e.g., a drug of abuse, a medication) or a general medical condition.

D. If an associated general medical condition is present, the fear described in Criterion A is clearly in excess of that usually associated with the condition.

From American Psychiatric Association. *Diagnostic and Statistical Manual of Mental Disorders.* 4th ed. Text rev. Washington, DC: American Psychiatric Association; copyright 2000, with permission.

The DSM-IV-TR criteria also address the avoidance of situations that are based on a concern related to a medical disorder (e.g., fear of a myocardial infarction in a patient with severe heart disease).

CLINICAL FEATURES

Panic Disorder

The first panic attack is often completely spontaneous, although panic attacks occasionally follow excitement, physical exertion, sexual activity, or moderate emotional trauma. DSM-IV-TR emphasizes that at least the first attacks must be unexpected (uncued) to meet the diagnostic criteria for panic disorder. Clinicians should attempt to ascertain any habit or situation that commonly precedes a patient's panic attacks. Such activities may include the use of caffeine, alcohol, nicotine, or other substances; unusual patterns of sleeping or eating; and specific environmental settings, such as harsh lighting at work.

The attack often begins with a 10-minute period of rapidly increasing symptoms. The major mental symptoms are extreme fear and a sense of impending death and doom. Patients usually cannot name the source of their fear; they may feel confused and have trouble concentrating. The physical signs often include tachycardia, palpitations, dyspnea, and sweating. Patients often try to leave whatever situation they are in to seek help. The attack generally lasts 20 to 30 minutes and rarely more than an hour. A formal mental status examination during a panic attack may reveal rumination, difficulty speaking (e.g., stammering), and impaired memory. Patients may experience depression or depersonalization during an attack. The symptoms may disappear quickly or gradually. Between attacks, patients may have anticipatory anxiety about having another attack. The differentiation between anticipatory anxiety and generalized anxiety disorder can be difficult, although pain disorder patients with anticipatory anxiety can name the focus of their anxiety.

Somatic concerns of death from a cardiac or respiratory problem may be the major focus of patients' attention during panic attacks. Patients may believe that the palpitations and chest pain indicate that they are about to die. As many as 20 percent of such patients actually have syncopal episodes during a panic attack. The patients may be seen in emergency rooms as young (20s), physically healthy persons who nevertheless insist that they are about to die from a heart attack. Rather than immediately diagnosing hypochondriasis, the emergency room physician should consider a diagnosis of panic disorder. Hyperventilation may produce respiratory alkalosis and other symptoms. The age-old treatment of breathing into a paper bag sometimes helps because it decreases alkalosis.

A 30-year-old college professor came to the clinic escorted by his wife. "I have to get my life back together. I have been out of work for nearly a month and, if it weren't for my wife accompanying me, I wouldn't be here now," he said.

About 4 months earlier, while attending a family picnic, he had suddenly become "nervous." His heart began to race "a mile a minute" and he began to perspire profusely, felt nau-

seated, experienced a tightness in his chest, and felt he was suffocating, "as if someone was smothering me with a pillow." The attack came on for no apparent reason and continued for about 15 minutes. It terrified him ("I thought that I was going to die"), so much so that he asked his wife to drive for fear that he might have another attack while driving. Later that day he experienced a second attack while sitting on the porch with a neighbor.

During the next 3 weeks he underwent numerous examinations by different specialists (cardiologists, endocrinologists, gastroenterologists, and so forth), but the results of all tests were negative.

The attacks continued at a rate of two or three a week. The patient noticed that the attacks were more likely to occur in trains, although they did not always occur in that situation. He had already stopped driving to work (for fear of having an attack) and needed the train to get to work. He began to take early trains (6:00 AM) to work and late trains (7:00 PM) from work to avoid crowds that might block his escape route. Also, he would limit himself to local trains (versus expresses) since they make more stops, and therefore the doors open more frequently." The anxiety experienced in anticipation of having an attack was almost as intense as the attacks themselves. Soon, he could no longer bear the extreme discomfort of riding in a train, and consequently took a leave of absence from work. In addition, his fear generalized to all crowded places (stores, banks, offices, streets) to the extent that he needed his wife to accompany him whenever he left the house.

When seen at the clinic, he was experiencing three or four attacks a week, was essentially housebound, and was in constant fear of having a fatal episode.

DISCUSSION

This case history exemplifies several of the features that are typically observed in the development of panic disorder with agoraphobia. Although the initial attacks were spontaneous, some of the later attacks were situationally predisposed. That is, the patient noticed that the likelihood of having an attack was increased when he was on a train, although the attacks did not occur invariably in that situation. Also, he altered his daily routine (taking early and late trains) to enable him to escape rapidly in the event of an attack. (Some individuals with panic disorder report sitting in an aisle seat that is close to an exit in a movie theater for the same reason.) In addition to avoidance of driving, trains, and crowds, the patient experienced extreme anticipatory anxiety (worry about what would happen if he had an attack driving or while on the train). His inability to leave home unaccompanied is observed in severe cases of the disorder. (Courtesy of Abby Fye, M.D., Salvatore Mannuzza, Ph.D., and Jeremy D. Coplan, M.D.)

Ms. B. is a 27-year-old businesswoman with a 3-year history of panic attacks. Her first panic attack occurred suddenly when Ms. B. was home watching television. This was about 3 months after her paternal grandfather died and 1 month after she announced her marriage plans. The attack began with the sensation of an electric shock going up her spine and a feeling of terror. Her heart raced, her hands tingled, and she could barely catch her breath. She felt hot, shaky, and disoriented and was convinced she was having a stroke and would soon die.

Although barely able to talk, Ms. B. placed an emergency call to her family physician. By the time the doctor returned her call 10 minutes later, the sensation of terror had passed and the other symptoms had abated but she still felt weak and fearful. A subsequent thorough medical workup indicated that she was a healthy young woman with low blood pressure (100/60) and normal resting heart rate (78 beats per minute). She had a soft heart murmur. An echocardiogram diagnosis of a slight mitral valve prolapse was made. Laboratory test results were normal, although they showed a mild reduction of plasma bicarbonate level.

During the next week the patient had five more panic episodes that occurred unexpectedly in different situations. The episodes were characterized by a rapid onset of electrical feelings in her spine, heart palpitations, dizziness, tingling in her fingers, fear of going crazy, and a sense of unreality.

Ms. B. accepted a prescription for a benzodiazepine, but she refused to see the psychiatrist recommended by her family doctor. She was convinced that psychiatrists had never helped her agoraphobic mother and could not help her and that seeing a psychiatrist would prove that she was losing control. Determined not to let her symptoms interfere with her life, she forced herself to continue working.

After a few weeks, the attacks began to diminish in frequency and intensity, but Ms. B. continued to experience intermittent episodes of panic several times a month for the next 2 years. These usually occurred when she was on a crowded subway or bus, was exercising on a stationary bike, was anticipating an interpersonal confrontation, or was relaxing in bed at night. On several occasions she awakened at night in the middle of a panic attack.

After a recent promotion at work, the frequency of Ms. B.'s panic attacks increased to several times a week. She began spending 14 hours a day at her job but felt that her anxiety was making her indecisive and reducing her efficiency. She worried constantly that her incompetence would be discovered and she would be fired. She also hated her boss and believed that he hated her, even though he had recommended her promotion. Although she is often uncomfortable in crowded, stores, movies, and restaurants, Ms. B. has forced herself to continue going to these places; however, she does avoid subways and driving by herself through a tunnel.

Ms. B. is a meticulous worker who takes her job very seriously. She is friendly but distant to coworkers and feels contempt for others who are less careful or waste their time gossiping or doing personal errands. Although she is engaged to be married and has several close women friends, she is generally isolated and tends to avoid people because she is afraid of being criticized, rejected, or burdened by other people's problems.

Ms. B. comes in for consultation because her symptoms have worsened and because her fiancé read that new treatment

methods were available for panic symptoms. Nevertheless, she appears to be an unwilling participant in the evaluation process. Guarded and mistrustful, she frequently replies to questions with "Why do you need to know that?" She seems sensitive to criticism and says she is fearful that discussing her problems with a therapist will only increase her anxiety.

DSM-IV DIAGNOSIS

Axis I:	Panic disorder without agoraphobia
Axis II:	Avoidant and compulsive personality traits
Axis III:	Possible mitral valve prolapse
Axis IV:	Job promotion, impending marriage
Axis V:	GAF = 60 (current); 85 (highest level in past year)

(From *DSM-IV Case Studies*.)

Agoraphobia

Patients with agoraphobia rigidly avoid situations in which it would be difficult to obtain help. They prefer to be accompanied by a friend or a family member in busy streets, crowded stores, closed-in spaces (e.g., tunnels, bridges, and elevators), and closed-in vehicles (e.g., subways, buses, and airplanes). Patients may insist that they be accompanied every time they leave the house. The behavior may result in marital discord, which may be misdiagnosed as the primary problem. Severely affected patients may simply refuse to leave the house. Particularly before a correct diagnosis is made, patients may be terrified that they are going crazy.

Associated Symptoms

Depressive symptoms are often present in panic disorder and agoraphobia, and in some patients, a depressive disorder coexists with the panic disorder. Some studies have found that the lifetime risk of suicide in persons with panic disorder is higher than it is in persons with no mental disorder. Clinicians should be alert to the risk of suicide. In addition to agoraphobia, other phobias and obsessive-compulsive disorder can coexist with panic disorder. The psychosocial consequences of panic disorder and agoraphobia, in addition to marital discord, can include time lost from work, financial difficulties related to the loss of work, and alcohol and other substance abuse.

DIFFERENTIAL DIAGNOSIS

Panic Disorder

The differential diagnosis for a patient with panic disorder includes a large number of medical disorders (Table 16.2–7), as well as many mental disorders.

Medical Disorders. Whenever a patient, regardless of age or risk factors, reports to an emergency room with symptoms of a potentially fatal condition (e.g., myocardial infarction), a complete medical history must be obtained, and a physical examination performed. Standard laboratory procedures include a complete blood count; studies of electrolytes, fasting glucose, calcium concentrations, liver function, urea, creatinine, and thyroid; a urinalysis; a drug screen; and an electrocardiogram (ECG). Once the presence of an immediately life-threatening condition is ruled out, the clinical suspicion is panic disorder. The possibility that additional medical diagnostic procedures will reveal a medical condition must be weighed against the potentially adverse effects of the procedure in helping the patient accept a diagnosis of panic disorder. Nevertheless, atypical symptoms (e.g., vertigo, loss of bladder control, and unconsciousness) or the late onset of the first panic attack (older than age 45 years) should cause clinicians to reconsider the presence of an underlying nonpsychiatric medical condition.

The standard workup helps clinicians evaluate patients for the presence of thyroid, parathyroid, adrenal, and substance-related causes of panic attacks. Symptoms of chest pain, especially in patients with cardiac risk factors (e.g., obesity and hypertension), may warrant further cardiac tests, including a 24-hour ECG, a stress test, a chest X-ray, and measurement of cardiac enzymes. Atypical neurological symptoms may warrant obtaining an electroencephalogram or an MRI to assess the possibility that the patient has temporal lobe epilepsy, multiple sclerosis, or a space-occupying brain lesion. The rare possibility that a patient has carcinoid syndrome or pheochromocytoma can best be checked by testing a 24-hour urine sample for serotonin metabolites or catecholamines.

Table 16.2–7
Organic Differential Diagnosis for Panic Disorder

Cardiovascular diseases	
Anemia	Hypertension
Angina	Mitral valve prolapse
Congestive heart failure	Myocardial infarction
Hyperactive β-adrenergic state	Paradoxical atrial tachycardia
Pulmonary diseases	
Asthma	Pulmonary embolus
Hyperventilation	
Neurological diseases	
Cerebrovascular disease	Migraine
Epilepsy	Multiple sclerosis
Huntington's disease	Transient ischemic attack
Infection	Tumor
Ménière's disease	Wilson's disease
Endocrine diseases	
Addison's disease	Hypoglycemia
Carcinoid syndrome	Hypoparathyroidism
Cushing's syndrome	Menopausal disorders
Diabetes	Pheochromocytoma
Hyperthyroidism	Premenstrual syndrome
Drug intoxications	
Amphetamine	Hallucinogens
Amyl nitrite	Marijuana
Anticholinergics	Nicotine
Cocaine	Theophylline
Drug withdrawal	
Alcohol	Opiates and opioids
Antihypertensives	Sedative-hypnotics
Other conditions	
Anaphylaxis	Systemic infections
B_{12} deficiency	Systemic lupus erythematosus
Electrolyte disturbances	Temporal arteritis
Heavy metal poisoning	Uremia

Mental Disorders. The psychiatric differential diagnosis for panic disorder includes malingering, factitious disorders, hypochondriasis, depersonalization disorder, social and specific phobias, posttraumatic stress disorder, depressive disorders, and schizophrenia. In the differential diagnosis, clinicians must determine whether a panic attack was unexpected, situationally bound, or situationally predisposed. Unexpected panic attacks are the hallmark of panic disorder; situationally bound panic attacks generally indicate a different condition, such as social phobia or specific phobia (when exposed to the phobic situation), obsessive-compulsive disorder (when trying to resist a compulsion), or a depressive disorder (when overwhelmed with anxiety). The focus of the anxiety or the fear is also important. Was there no focus (as in panic disorder), or was there a specific focus (e.g., a person with social phobia who fears becoming tongue-tied)? Somatoform disorders should also be considered in the differential diagnosis, although a patient may meet the criteria for both somatoform disorder and panic disorder.

SPECIFIC AND SOCIAL PHOBIAS. DSM-IV-TR addresses the sometimes difficult diagnostic task of distinguishing between panic disorder with agoraphobia, on the one hand, and specific and social phobias, on the other hand. Some patients who experience a single panic attack in a specific setting (e.g., an elevator) may go on to have long-lasting avoidance of the specific setting, regardless of whether they ever have another panic attack. These patients meet the diagnostic criteria for a specific phobia, and clinicians must use their judgment about what is the most appropriate diagnosis. In another example, a person who experiences one or more panic attacks may then fear speaking in public. Although the clinical picture is almost identical to the clinical picture in social phobia, a diagnosis of social phobia is excluded because the avoidance of the public situation is based on fear of having a panic attack, rather than on fear of the public speaking itself. Because empirical data on the distinctions are limited, DSM-IV-TR advises clinicians to use their clinical judgment to diagnose difficult cases.

Agoraphobia without History of Panic Disorder

The differential diagnosis for agoraphobia without a history of panic disorder includes all the medical disorders that may cause anxiety or depression. The psychiatric differential diagnosis includes major depressive disorder, schizophrenia, paranoid personality disorder, avoidance personality disorder, and dependent personality disorder.

COURSE AND PROGNOSIS

Panic Disorder

Panic disorder usually has its onset in late adolescence or early adulthood, although onset during childhood, early adolescence, and midlife does occur. Some data implicate increased psychosocial stressors with the onset of panic disorder, although no psychosocial stressor can be definitely identified in most cases.

Panic disorder, in general, is a chronic disorder, although its course is variable both among patients and within a single patient. The available long-term follow-up studies of panic disorder are difficult to interpret because they have not controlled for the effects of treatment. Nevertheless, about 30 to 40 percent of patients seem to be symptom free at long-term follow-up; about 50 percent have symptoms that are mild enough not to affect their lives significantly; and about 10 to 20 percent continue to have significant symptoms.

After the first one or two panic attacks, patients may be relatively unconcerned about their condition; with repeated attacks, however, the symptoms may become a major concern. Patients may attempt to keep the panic attacks secret and thereby cause their families and friends concern about unexplained changes in behavior. The frequency and severity of the attacks may fluctuate. Panic attacks may occur several times in a day or less than once a month. Excessive intake of caffeine or nicotine may exacerbate the symptoms.

Depression may complicate the symptom picture in anywhere from 40 to 80 percent of all patients, as estimated by various studies. Although the patients do not tend to talk about suicidal ideation, they are at increased risk for committing suicide. Alcohol and other substance dependence occurs in about 20 to 40 percent of all patients, and obsessive-compulsive disorder may also develop. Family interactions and performance in school and at work commonly suffer. Patients with good premorbid functioning and symptoms of brief duration tend to have good prognoses.

Agoraphobia

Most cases of agoraphobia are thought to be due to panic disorder. When the panic disorder is treated, the agoraphobia often improves with time. For rapid and complete reduction of agoraphobia, behavior therapy is sometimes indicated. Agoraphobia without a history of panic disorder is often incapacitating and chronic, and depressive disorders and alcohol dependence often complicate its course.

TREATMENT

With treatment, most patients exhibit dramatic improvement in the symptoms of panic disorder and agoraphobia. The two most effective treatments are pharmacotherapy and cognitive-behavioral therapy. Family and group therapy may help affected patients and their families adjust to the fact that the patients have the disorder and to the psychosocial difficulties that the disorder may have precipitated.

Pharmacotherapy

Overview. Alprazolam (Xanax) and paroxetine (Paxil) are the two drugs approved by the U.S. Food and Drug Administration (FDA) for the treatment of panic disorder. In general, experience is showing superiority of the selective serotonin reuptake inhibitors (SSRIs) and clomipramine (Anafranil) over the benzodiazepines, monoamine oxidase inhibitors (MAOIs), and tricyclic and tetracyclic drugs in terms of effectiveness and tolerance of adverse effects. A few reports have suggested a role for nefazodone (Serzone) and venlafaxine (Effexor), and buspirone (BuSpar) has been suggested as an additive medication in some cases. Venlafaxine is approved by the FDA for treatment of generalized anxiety disorder and it may be useful in panic disorder combined with depression. β-Adrenergic receptor antagonists have not been found to be particularly use-

Table 16.2–8
Recommended Dosages for Antipanic Drugs (Daily Unless Indicated Otherwise)

Drug	Starting (mg)	Maintenance (mg)
SSRIs		
Paroxetine	5–10	20–60
Fluoxetine	2–5	20–60
Sertraline	12.5–25	50–200
Fluvoxamine	12.5	100–150
Citalopram	10	20–40
Tricyclic antidepressants		
Clomipramine	5–12.5	50–125
Imipramine	10–25	150–500
Desipramine	10–25	150–200
Benzodiazepines		
Alprazolam	0.25–0.5 tid	0.5–2 tid
Clonazepam	0.25–0.5 bid	0.5–2 bid
Diazepam	2–5 bid	5–30 bid
Lorazepam	0.25–0.5 bid	0.5–2 bid
MAOIs		
Phenelzine	15 bid	15–45 bid
Tranylcypromine	10 bid	10–30 bid
RIMAs		
Moclobemide	50	300–600
Brofaromine	50	150–200
Atypical antidepressants		
Venlafaxine	6.25–25	50–150
Nefazodone	50 bid	100–300 bid
Other agents		
Valproic acid	125 bid	500–750 bid
Inositol	6,000 bid	6,000 bid

Courtesy of Laszlo Papp, M.D.

ful for panic disorder. A conservative approach is to begin treatment with paroxetine, sertraline (Zoloft), or fluvoxamine (Luvox) in isolated panic disorder. If rapid control of severe symptoms is desired, a brief course of alprazolam should be initiated concurrently with the SSRI, followed by slowly tapering use of the benzodiazepine. In long-term use, fluoxetine (Prozac) is an effective drug for panic with comorbid depression, although its initial activating properties may mimic panic symptoms for the first several weeks, and it may be poorly tolerated on this basis. Klonopin (Clonazepam) can be prescribed for patients who anticipate a situation in which panic may occur (0.5–1 mg prn) Common dosages for antipanic drugs are listed in Table 16.2–8.

Selective Serotonin Reuptake Inhibitors. All SSRIs are effective for panic disorder. Paroxetine has sedative effects and tends to calm patients immediately, which leads to greater compliance and less discontinuation. Fluvoxamine and sertraline are the next best tolerated. Anecdotal reports suggest that patients with panic disorder are particularly sensitive to the activating effects of SSRIs, particularly fluoxetine, so they should be given initially at small dosages and titrated up slowly. Once at therapeutic dosages—for example, 20 mg a day of paroxetine—some patients may experience increased sedation. One approach for patients with panic disorder is to give 5 or 10 mg a day of paroxetine for 1 to 2 weeks, then increase the dosage by 10 mg a day every 1 to 2 weeks to a maximum of 60 mg. If sedation becomes intolerable, then taper the paroxetine dosage down to 10 mg a day and switch to fluoxetine at 10 mg a day and titrate upward slowly. Other strategies can be used, based on the experience of the clinician.

Benzodiazepines. Benzodiazepines have the most rapid onset of action against panic, often within the first week, and they can be used for long periods without the development of tolerance to the antipanic effects. Alprazolam has been the most widely used benzodiazepine for panic disorder, but controlled studies have demonstrated equal efficacy for lorazepam (Ativan), and case reports have also indicated that clonazepam (Klonopin) may be effective. Some patients use benzodiazepines as needed when faced with a phobic stimulus. Benzodiazepines can reasonably be used as the first agent for treatment of panic disorder, while a serotonergic drug is being slowly titrated to a therapeutic dose. After 4 to 12 weeks, benzodiazepine use can be slowly tapered (over 4 to 10 weeks) while the serotonergic drug is continued. The major reservation among clinicians regarding the use of benzodiazepines for panic disorder is the potential for dependence, cognitive impairment, and abuse, especially after long-term use. Patients should be instructed not to drive or operate dangerous equipment while taking benzodiazepines. Benzodiazepines elicit a sense of well-being, whereas discontinuation of benzodiazepines produces a well-documented and unpleasant withdrawal syndrome. Anecdotal reports and small case series have indicated that addiction to alprazolam is one of the most difficult to overcome, and it may require a comprehensive program of detoxification. Benzodiazepine dosage should be tapered slowly, and all anticipated withdrawal effects should be thoroughly explained to the patient.

Tricyclic and Tetracyclic Drugs. The most robust data show that among tricyclic drugs, clomipramine and imipramine (Tofranil) are the most effective in the treatment of panic disorder. Clinical experience indicates that the dosages must be titrated slowly upward to avoid overstimulation and that the full clinical benefit requires full dosages and may not be achieved for 8 to 12 weeks. Some data support the efficacy of desipramine (Norpramin), and less evidence suggests a role for maprotiline (Ludiomil), trazodone (Desyrel), nortriptyline (Pamelor), amitriptyline (Elavil), and doxepin (Adapin). Tricyclic drugs are less widely used than SSRIs because the tricyclic drugs generally have more severe adverse effects at the higher dosages required for effective treatment of panic disorder.

Monoamine Oxidase Inhibitors. The most robust data support the effectiveness of phenelzine (Nardil), and some data also support the use of tranylcypromine (Parnate). MAOIs appear less likely to cause overstimulation than either SSRIs or tricyclic drugs, but they may require full dosages for at least 8 to 12 weeks to be effective. The need for dietary restrictions has limited the use of MAOIs, particularly since the appearance of the SSRIs.

Treatment Nonresponse. If patients fail to respond to one class of drugs, another should be tried. Recent data support

the effectiveness of nefazodone and venlafaxine. The combination of an SSRI or a tricyclic drug and a benzodiazepine or of an SSRI and lithium or a tricyclic drug can be tried. Case reports have suggested the effectiveness of carbamazepine (Tegretol), valproate (Depakene), and calcium channel inhibitors. Buspirone may have a role in the augmentation of other medications but has little effectiveness by itself. Clinicians should reassess the patient, particularly to establish the presence of comorbid conditions such as depression, alcohol use, or other substance use.

Duration of Pharmacotherapy. Once it becomes effective, pharmacological treatment should generally continue for 8 to 12 months. Data indicate that panic disorder is a chronic, perhaps lifelong condition that recurs when treatment is discontinued. Studies have reported that 30 to 90 percent of panic disorder patients who have received successful treatment have a relapse when their medication is discontinued. Patients may be likely to relapse if they have been given benzodiazepines and the benzodiazepine therapy is terminated in a way that causes withdrawal symptoms.

Cognitive and Behavior Therapies

Cognitive and behavior therapies are effective treatments for panic disorder. Various reports have concluded that cognitive and behavior therapies are superior to pharmacotherapy alone; other reports have concluded the opposite. Several studies and reports have found that the combination of cognitive or behavior therapy with pharmacotherapy is more effective than either approach alone. Several studies that included long-term follow-up of patients who received cognitive or behavior therapy showed that the therapies are effective in producing long-lasting remission of symptoms.

Cognitive Therapy. The two major foci of cognitive therapy for panic disorder are instruction about a patient's false beliefs and information about panic attacks. The instruction about false beliefs centers on the patient's tendency to misinterpret mild bodily sensations as indicating impending panic attacks, doom, or death. The information about panic attacks includes explanations that when panic attacks occur, they are time limited and not life threatening.

José was a 27-year-old laboratory technician who began having full-blown panic attacks 8 months prior to seeking help at our research clinic. While he was unable to identify specific situations that elicited attacks, he was particularly concerned about the possibility of their occurring while he was engaged in laboratory procedures with patients. His attacks typically involved a sudden explosion of autonomic arousal and included palpitations, sweating, dizziness, feelings of unreality, and tingling in his arms and legs. He dreaded the idea that the attacks might recur. In the beginning of his cognitive-behavioral program, he found an educational handout that described the myths of panic attacks (e.g., that they will lead to heart attacks, losing control, or going crazy) particularly reassuring. He began practicing diaphragmatic breathing each evening and, after several weeks, became effective in challenging his negative way of thinking about the consequences of panic attacks. In the latter few weeks of his 12-week program, he practiced exposing himself to physical sensations of panic by doing a variety of interoceptive exercises at home, including hyperventilating for 1 or 2 minutes at a time (designed to help José acclimate to the physical sensations associated with overbreathing), and spinning in a chair repeatedly (designed to help acclimate him to symptoms of dizziness and feelings of unreality). At the conclusion of the treatment program José's panic attacks had disappeared, and at 6-month follow-up he had maintained his treatment gains by attending "booster sessions" with his therapist once every 2 months.

Applied Relaxation. The goal of applied relaxation (e.g., Herbert Benson's relaxation training) is to instill in patients a sense of control over their levels of anxiety and relaxation. Through the use of standardized techniques for muscle relaxation and the imagining of relaxing situations, patients learn techniques that may help them through a panic attack.

Respiratory Training. Because the hyperventilation associated with panic attacks is probably related to some symptoms such as dizziness and faintness, one direct approach to control panic attacks is to train patients to control the urge to hyperventilate. After such training, patients can use the technique to help control hyperventilation during a panic attack.

In Vivo Exposure. In vivo exposure used to be the primary behavior treatment for panic disorder. The technique involves sequentially greater exposure of a patient to the feared stimulus; over time, the patient becomes desensitized to the experience. Previously, the focus was on external stimuli; recently, the technique has included exposure of the patient to internal feared sensations (e.g., tachypnea and fear of having a panic attack).

Other Psychosocial Therapies

Family Therapy. Families of patients with panic disorder and agoraphobia may also have been affected by the family member's disorder. Family therapy directed toward education and support is often beneficial.

Insight-Oriented Psychotherapy. Insight-oriented psychotherapy can be of benefit in the treatment of panic disorder and agoraphobia. Treatment focuses on helping patients understand the hypothesized unconscious meaning of the anxiety, the symbolism of the avoided situation, the need to repress impulses, and the secondary gains of the symptoms. A resolution of early infantile and oedipal conflicts is hypothesized to correlate with the resolution of current stresses.

Combined Psychotherapy and Pharmacotherapy

Even when pharmacotherapy is effective in eliminating the primary symptoms of panic disorder, psychotherapy may be needed to treat secondary symptoms. Glen O. Gabbard wrote:

Panic-disordered patients frequently require a combination of drug therapy and psychotherapy . . . Even when patients with panic attacks and agoraphobia have their symptoms pharmacologically controlled, they are often reluctant to venture out into the world again and may require psychotherapeutic interventions to help overcome this fear . . . Some patients will adamantly refuse any medication because they believe that it stigmatizes them as being mentally ill, so psychotherapeutic intervention is required to help them understand and eliminate their resistance to pharmacotherapy . . . For a comprehensive and effective treatment plan, these patients require psychotherapeutic approaches in addition to appropriate medications. In all patients with symptoms of panic disorder or agoraphobia, a careful psychodynamic evaluation will help weigh the contributions of biological and dynamic factors.

References

Charney DS, Woods SW, Krystal JH, Nagy LM, Heninger GR. Noradrenergic neuronal dysregulation in panic disorder: the effects of intravenous yohimbine and clonidine in panic disorder patients. *Acta Psychiatr Scand.* 1992;86:273.

Coplan JD, Gorman JM, Klein DF. Serotonin related functions in panic-anxiety: a critical overview. *Neuropsychopharmacology.* 1992;6:189.

Craske MG, Roy-Byrne P, Stein MB. Treating panic disorder in primary care: A collaborative care intervention. *Gen Hosp Psychiatry.* 2002;24:148.

Gabbard GO. *Psychodynamic Psychiatry in Clinical Practice: The DSM-IV Edition.* Washington, DC: American Psychiatric Press; 1994.

Gorman JM, section ed. Anxiety disorders. In: Sadock BJ, Sadock VA, eds. *Kaplan & Sadock's Comprehensive Textbook of Psychiatry.* 7th ed. Vol 1. Baltimore: Lippincott Williams & Wilkins; 2000;1441.

Hollifield M, Katon W, Skipper B, et al. Panic disorder and quality of life: variables predictive of functional impairment. *Am J Psychiatry.* 1997;154:766.

Jacob RG, Furman JM, Durrant JD, Turner SM. Panic, agoraphobia, and vestibular dysfunction. *Am J Psychiatry.* 1996;153:503.

Johnson MR, Lydiard RB, Ballenger JC. Panic disorder. Pathophysiology and drug treatment. *Drugs.* 1995;49:328.

Keller MB, Hanks DL. Course and outcome in panic disorder. *Prog Neuropsychopharmacol Biol Psychiatry.* 1993;17:551.

Klein DF. Panic disorder and agoraphobia: hypothesis hothouse. *J Clin Psychiatry.* 1996;57(suppl 6):21.

Levitt JT, Hoffman EC, Grisham JR, Barlow DH. Empirically supported treatments for panic disorder. *Psychiatr Ann.* 2001;31(8):478.

Lydiard RB, Lesser IM, Ballenger JC, Rubin RT, Laraia M, DuPont R. A fixed-dose study of alprazolam 2 mg, alprazolam 6 mg, and placebo in panic disorder. *J Clin Psychopharmacol.* 1992;12:96.

Maddock RJ. The lactic acid response to alkalosis in panic disorder: an integrative review. *J Neuropsychiatry Clin Neurosci.* 2001;13(1):22.

Mennin DS, Heimberg RG, Holt CS. Panic, agoraphobias, phobias, and generalized anxiety disorder. In: Hersen M, Bellack AS, eds. *Psychopathology in Adulthood.* 2nd ed. Needham Heights, MA: Allyn & Bacon; 2000:169.

Ost LG. Blood and injection phobia: background and cognitive, physiological, and behavioral variables. *J Abnorm Psychol.* 1992;101:68.

Persons JB. Understanding the exposure principle and using it to treat anxiety. *Psychiatr Ann.* 2001;31(8):472.

Pollard CA, Tait RC, Meldrum D, Dubinsky IH, Gall JS. Agoraphobia without panic: case illustrations of an overlooked syndrome. *J Nerv Ment Dis.* 1996;184:61.

Simon NM, Pollack MH. The current status of the treatment of panic disorder: pharmacotherapy and cognitive-behavioral therapy. *Psychiatr Ann.* 2000;30(11):689.

van den Heuvel OA, van de Wetering BJ, Veltman DJ, Pauls DL. Genetic studies of panic disorder: a review. *J Clin Psychiatry.* 2000;61(10):756.

▲ 16.3 Specific Phobia and Social Phobia

The term *phobia* refers to an excessive fear of a specific object, circumstance, or situation. A specific phobia is a strong, persisting fear of an object or situation, whereas a social phobia is a strong, persisting fear of situations in which embarrassment can occur. Persons with specific phobias may anticipate harm, such as being bitten by a dog, or may panic at the thought of losing control; for instance, if they fear being in an elevator, they may also worry about fainting after the door closes. Persons with social phobias (also called social anxiety disorder) have excessive fears of humiliation or embarrassment in various social settings, such as in speaking in public, urinating in a public rest room (also called shy bladder), and speaking to a date. A generalized social phobia, which is often a chronic and disabling condition characterized by a phobic avoidance of most social situations, can be difficult to distinguish from avoidant personality disorder.

A phobia is defined as an irrational fear that produces conscious avoidance of the feared subject, activity, or situation. Either the presence or the anticipation of the phobic entity elicits severe distress in an affected person, who usually recognizes that the reaction is excessive. These responses may take the form of a situationally bound or situationally predisposed panic attack. Phobic reactions usually disrupt a person's ability to function in life; however, some do not (e.g., fear of spiders).

EPIDEMIOLOGY

Recent epidemiological studies have shown that phobias are the single most common mental disorder in the United States, where approximately 5 to 10 percent of the population is estimated to be afflicted with these troubling and sometimes disabling disorders. Less-conservative estimates have ranged as high as 25 percent of the population. The distress associated with phobias, especially when they are not recognized or acknowledged as mental disorders, can lead to further psychiatric complications, including other anxiety disorders, major depressive disorder, and substance-related disorders, especially alcohol use disorders.

Although phobias are common mental disorders, a large percentage of persons with phobias either do not seek help to overcome their phobias or are misdiagnosed when they do seek psychiatric or medical attention. The lifetime prevalence of specific phobia is about 11 percent, and the lifetime prevalence of social phobia has been reported to be 3 to 13 percent.

Specific Phobia

Specific phobia is more common than social phobia. Specific phobia is the most common mental disorder among women and the second most common among men, second only to substance-related disorders. The 6-month prevalence of specific phobia is about 5 to 10 per 100 persons. The female-to-male ratio is about 2 to 1, although the ratio is closer to 1 to 1 for the fear of blood, injection, or injury type. (Types of phobias are discussed below in this section.) The peak age of onset for the natural environment type and the blood-injection-injury type is in the range of 5 to 9 years, although onset also occurs at older ages. In contrast, the peak age of onset for the situational type (except fear of heights) is higher, in the mid-20s, which is closer to the age of onset for agoraphobia. The feared objects and situations in specific phobias (listed in descending frequency of appearance) are animals, storms, heights, illness, injury, and death.

Table 16.3–1
Lifetime Prevalence Rates of Social Phobia per 100 Subjects

Site	Males	Females	Total
United States (ECA)	2.1	3.1	2.6
Edmonton, Canada	1.3	2.1	1.7
Puerto Rico	0.8	1.1	1.0
Korea	0.1	1.0	0.5
United States (NCS)	11.1	15.5	13.3

Adapted from Weissman MM, Bland RC, Canino GJ, et al. The cross-national epidemiology of social phobia: a preliminary report. *Int Clin Psychopharmacol.* 1996;11(suppl):9.

Social Phobia

Various studies have reported a lifetime prevalence ranging from 3 to 13 percent. The 6-month prevalence for social phobia is about 2 to 3 per 100 persons (Table 16.3–1). In epidemiological studies, females are affected more often than males, but in clinical samples, the reverse is often true. The reasons for these varying observations are unknown. The peak age of onset for social phobia is in the teens, although onset is common as young as 5 years of age and as old as 35.

COMORBIDITY

Persons with social phobia may have a history of other anxiety disorders, mood disorders, substance-related disorders, and bulimia nervosa. In addition, avoidant personality disorder frequently occurs in persons with generalized social phobia.

Reports of comorbidity in specific phobia range from 50 to 80 percent. Common comorbid disorders with specific phobia include anxiety, mood, and substance-related disorders.

ETIOLOGY

Both specific phobia and social phobia have types, and the precise causes of these types are likely to differ. Even within the types, as in all mental disorders, causative heterogeneity is found. The pathogenesis of the phobias, once it is understood, may prove to be a clear model for interactions between biological and genetic factors, on the one hand, and environmental events, on the other hand. In the blood-injection-injury type of specific phobia, affected persons may have inherited a particularly strong vasovagal reflex, which becomes associated with phobic emotions.

General Principles

Behavioral Factors. In 1920, John B. Watson wrote an article called "Conditioned Emotional Reactions," in which he recounted his experiences with Little Albert, an infant with a fear of rats and rabbits. Unlike Sigmund Freud's case of Little Hans, who had phobic symptoms (of horses) in the natural course of his maturation, Little Albert's difficulties were the direct result of the scientific experiments of two psychologists who used techniques that had successfully induced conditioned responses in laboratory animals.

Watson's hypothesis invoked the traditional pavlovian stimulus-response model of the conditioned reflex to account for the creation of the phobia: Anxiety is aroused by a naturally frightening stimulus that occurs in contiguity with a second inherently neutral stimulus. As a result of the contiguity, especially when the two stimuli are paired on several successive occasions, the originally neutral stimulus becomes capable of arousing anxiety by itself. The neutral stimulus, therefore, becomes a conditioned stimulus for anxiety production.

In the classic stimulus-response theory, the conditioned stimulus gradually loses its potency to arouse a response if it is not reinforced by periodic repetition of the unconditioned stimulus. In phobias, attenuation of the response to the stimulus does not occur; the symptom may last for years without any apparent external reinforcement. Operant conditioning theory provides a model to explain this phenomenon: Anxiety is a drive that motivates the organism to do whatever it can to obviate a painful affect. In the course of its random behavior, the organism learns that certain actions enable it to avoid the anxiety-provoking stimulus. These avoidance patterns remain stable for long periods as a result of the reinforcement they receive from their capacity to diminish anxiety. This model is readily applicable to phobias in that avoidance of the anxiety-provoking object or situation plays a central part. Such avoidance behavior becomes fixed as a stable symptom because of its effectiveness in protecting the person from the phobic anxiety.

Learning theory is particularly relevant to phobias and provides simple and intelligible explanations for many aspects of phobic symptoms. Critics contend, however, that learning theory deals mostly with surface mechanisms of symptom formation and is less useful than psychoanalytic theories in clarifying some of the complex underlying psychic processes involved.

Psychoanalytic Factors. Sigmund Freud's formulation of phobic neurosis is still the analytic explanation of specific phobia and social phobia. Freud hypothesized that the major function of anxiety is to signal the ego that a forbidden unconscious drive is pushing for conscious expression and to alert the ego to strengthen and marshall its defenses against the threatening instinctual force. Freud viewed the phobia—*anxiety hysteria,* as he continued to call it—as a result of conflicts centered on an unresolved childhood oedipal situation. Because sex drives continue to have a strong incestuous coloring in adults, sexual arousal can kindle an anxiety that is characteristically a fear of castration. When repression fails to be entirely successful, the ego must call on auxiliary defenses. In patients with phobias, the primary defense involved is displacement; that is, the sexual conflict is displaced from the person who evokes the conflict to a seemingly unimportant, irrelevant object or situation, which then has the power to arouse a constellation of affects, one of which is called signal anxiety. The phobic object or situation may have a direct associative connection with the primary source of the conflict and thus symbolizes it (the defense mechanism of symbolization).

Furthermore, the situation or the object is usually one that the person can avoid; with the additional defense mechanism of avoidance, the person can escape suffering serious anxiety. The end result is that the three combined defenses (repression, displacement, and symbolization) may eliminate the anxiety. However, the anxiety is controlled at the cost of creating a pho-

Table 16.3–2
Psychodynamic Themes in Phobias

- Principal defense mechanisms include: displacement, projection, and avoidance.
- Environmental stressors, including humiliation and criticism from an older sibling, parental fights, or loss and separation from parents, interact with a genetic-constitutional diathesis.
- A characteristic pattern of internal object relations is externalized in social situations in the case of social phobia.
- Anticipation of humiliation, criticism, and ridicule is projected onto individuals in the environment.
- Shame and embarrassment are the principal affect states.
- Family members may encourage phobic behavior and serve as obstacles to any treatment plan.
- Self-exposure to the feared situation is a basic principle of all treatment.

bic neurosis. Freud first discussed the theoretical formulation of phobia formation in his famous case history of Little Hans, a 5-year-old boy who feared horses.

Although psychiatrists followed Freud's thought that phobias resulted from castration anxiety, recent psychoanalytic theorists have suggested that other types of anxiety may be involved. In agoraphobia, for example, separation anxiety clearly plays a leading role, and in erythrophobia (a fear of red that can be manifested as a fear of blushing), the element of shame implies the involvement of superego anxiety. Clinical observations have led to the view that anxiety associated with phobias has a variety of sources and colorings.

Phobias illustrate the interaction between a genetic constitutional diathesis and environmental stressors. Longitudinal studies suggest that certain children are constitutionally predisposed to phobias because they are born with a specific temperament known as behavioral inhibition to the unfamiliar, but a chronic environmental stress must act on a child's temperamental disposition to create a full-blown phobia. Stressors such as the death of a parent, separation from a parent, criticism or humiliation by an older sibling, and violence in the household may activate the latent diathesis within the child, who then becomes symptomatic. An overview of psychodynamic aspects of phobias is summarized in Table 16.3–2.

COUNTERPHOBIC ATTITUDE. Otto Fenichel called attention to the fact that phobic anxiety can be hidden behind attitudes and behavior patterns that represent a denial, either that the dreaded object or situation is dangerous or that the person is afraid of it. Instead of being a passive victim of external circumstances, a person reverses the situation and actively attempts to confront and master whatever is feared. Persons with counterphobic attitudes seek out situations of danger and rush enthusiastically toward them. Devotees of potentially dangerous sports, such as parachute jumping and rock climbing, may be exhibiting counterphobic behavior. Such patterns may be secondary to phobic anxiety or may be normal means of dealing with a realistically dangerous situation. Children's play may exhibit counterphobic elements, as when children play doctor and give a doll the shot they received earlier that day in the pediatrician's office. This pattern of behavior may involve the related defense mechanism of identifying with the aggressor.

Specific Phobia

The development of specific phobia may result from the pairing of a specific object or situation with the emotions of fear and panic. Various mechanisms for the pairing have been postulated. In general, a nonspecific tendency to experience fear or anxiety forms the backdrop; when a specific event (e.g., driving) is paired with an emotional experience (e.g., an accident), the person is susceptible to a permanent emotional association between driving or cars and fear or anxiety. The emotional experience itself can be in response to an external incident, as a traffic accident, or to an internal incident, most commonly a panic attack. Although a person may never again experience a panic attack and may not meet the diagnostic criteria for panic disorder, he or she may have a generalized fear of driving, not an expressed fear of having a panic attack while driving. Other mechanisms of association between the phobic object and the phobic emotions include modeling, in which a person observes the reaction in another (e.g., a parent), and information transfer, in which a person is taught or warned about the dangers of specific objects (e.g., venomous snakes).

Genetic Factors. Specific phobia tends to run in families. The blood-injection-injury type has a particularly high familial tendency. Studies have reported that two thirds to three fourths of affected probands have at least one first-degree relative with specific phobia of the same type, but the necessary twin and adoption studies have not been conducted to rule out a significant contribution by nongenetic transmission of specific phobia.

Social Phobia

Several studies have reported that some children possibly have a trait characterized by a consistent pattern of behavioral inhibition. This trait may be particularly common in the children of parents who are affected with panic disorder, and it may develop into severe shyness as the children grow older. At least some persons with social phobia may have exhibited behavioral inhibition during childhood. Perhaps associated with this trait, which is thought to be biologically based, are the psychologically based data indicating that the parents of persons with social phobia were, as a group, less caring, more rejecting, and more overprotective of their children than were other parents. Some social phobia research has referred to the spectrum from dominance to submission observed in the animal kingdom. For example, dominant humans may tend to walk with their chins in the air and to make eye contact, whereas submissive humans may tend to walk with their chins down and to avoid eye contact.

Neurochemical Factors. The success of pharmacotherapies in treating social phobia has generated two specific neurochemical hypotheses about two types of social phobia. Specifically, the use of β-adrenergic receptor antagonists—for example, propranolol (Inderal)—for performance phobias (such as public speaking) has led to the development of an adrenergic theory for these phobias. Patients with performance phobias may release more norepinephrine or epinephrine, both centrally and peripherally, than do nonphobic persons, or such patients may be sensitive to a normal level of adrenergic stimulation. The observation that monoamine oxidase inhibitors

(MAOIs) may be more effective than tricyclic drugs in the treatment of generalized social phobia, in combination with preclinical data, has led some investigators to hypothesize that dopaminergic activity is related to the pathogenesis of the disorder. One study has shown significantly lower homovanillic acid concentrations. Another study using single photon emission computed tomography (SPECT) demonstrated decreased striatal dopamine reuptake site density. Thus, some evidence suggests dopaminergic dysfunction in social phobia.

Genetic Factors. First-degree relatives of persons with social phobia are about three times more likely to be affected with social phobia than are first-degree relatives of those without mental disorders. And some preliminary data indicate that monozygotic twins are more often concordant than are dizygotic twins, although in social phobia it is particularly important to study twins reared apart to help control for environmental factors.

DIAGNOSIS

Specific Phobia

The text revision of the fourth edition of the *Diagnostic and Statistical Manual of Mental Disorders* (DSM-IV-TR) uses the term *specific phobia* to match the nomenclature in the 10th revision of the *International Statistical Classification of Diseases and Related Health Problems* (ICD-10). Table 16.3–3 lists the diagnostic criteria. Criteria A (excessive fear) and B (stimulus exposure) have been carefully worded in DSM-IV-TR to allow for the possibility that exposure to a phobic stimulus may result in a panic attack. In contrast to panic disorder, however, in specific phobia, the panic attack is situationally bound to the specific phobic stimulus. Criterion G (the anxiety attack) in DSM-IV-TR includes the words "not better accounted for" to emphasize the need for clinicians' judgment about diagnosing the symptoms. The specific content of the phobia and the strength of the relation (e.g., cued or noncued) between the stimulus and a panic attack also need to be considered.

DSM-IV-TR includes distinctive types of specific phobia: animal type; natural environment type (e.g., storms); blood-injection-injury type; situational type (e.g., cars); and other type (for specific phobias that do not fit into the previous four types). Preliminary data indicate that the natural environment type is most common in children younger than 10 years old and the situational type most often occurs in persons in their early 20s. The blood-injection-injury type is differentiated from the others in that bradycardia and hypotension often follow the initial tachycardia that is common to all phobias. The blood-injection-injury type of specific phobia is particularly likely to affect many members and generations of a family. One type of recently reported specific phobia is space phobia, in which persons are afraid of falling when there is no nearby support like a wall or a chair. Some data indicate that affected persons may have abnormal right hemisphere function, possibly resulting in visual-spatial impairment. Balance disorders should also be ruled out in such patients.

FOCUS. Phobias have traditionally been classified according to the specific fear by means of Greek or Latin prefixes, as indicated by the following examples:

acrophobia	fear of heights
agoraphobia	fear of open places
ailurophobia	fear of cats
hydrophobia	fear of water
claustrophobia	fear of closed spaces
cynophobia	fear of dogs
mysophobia	fear of dirt and germs
pyrophobia	fear of fire
xenophobia	fear of strangers
zoophobia	fear of animals

Other phobias that are related to changes in the society are the fear of electromagnetic fields, of microwaves, and of society as a whole (amaxophobia).

Table 16.3–3
DSM-IV-TR Diagnostic Criteria for Specific Phobia

A. Marked and persistent fear that is excessive or unreasonable, cued by the presence or anticipation of a specific object or situation (e.g., flying, heights, animals, receiving an injection, seeing blood).

B. Exposure to the phobic stimulus almost invariably provokes an immediate anxiety response, which may take the form of a situationally bound or situationally predisposed panic attack. **Note:** In children, the anxiety may be expressed by crying, tantrums, freezing, or clinging.

C. The person recognizes that the fear is excessive or unreasonable. **Note:** In children, this feature may be absent.

D. The phobic situation(s) is avoided or else is endured with intense anxiety or distress.

E. The avoidance, anxious anticipation, or distress in the feared situation(s) interferes significantly with the person's normal routine, occupational (or academic) functioning, or social activities or relationships, or there is marked distress about having the phobia.

F. In individuals under age 18 years, the duration is at least 6 months.

G. The anxiety, panic attacks, or phobic avoidance associated with the specific object or situation are not better accounted for by another mental disorder, such as obsessive-compulsive disorder (e.g., fear of dirt in someone with an obsession about contamination), posttraumatic stress disorder (e.g., avoidance of stimuli associated with a severe stressor), separation anxiety disorder (e.g., avoidance of school), social phobia (e.g., avoidance of social situations because of fear of embarrassment), panic disorder with agoraphobia, or agoraphobia without history of panic disorder.

Specify type:

Animal type
Natural environment type (e.g., heights, storms, water)
Blood-injection-injury type
Situational type (e.g., airplanes, elevators, enclosed places)
Other type (e.g., fear of choking, vomiting, or contracting an illness; in children, fear of loud sounds or costumed characters)

From American Psychiatric Association. *Diagnostic and Statistical Manual of Mental Disorders.* 4th ed. Text rev. Washington, DC: American Psychiatric Association; copyright 2000, with permission.

Mr. M., a 28-year-old computer programmer, seeks treatment because of fears that prevent him from visiting his terminally ill father-in-law in the hospital. He explains that he is afraid of any situation even remotely associated with bodily injury or illness. For example, he cannot bear to have his blood drawn, or to see or even hear about sick people. These fears are the reason he avoids consulting a doctor even when he is sick and avoids visiting sick friends or family members and even listening to descriptions of medical procedures, physical trauma, or illness. He became a vegetarian 5 years ago to avoid thoughts of animals being killed.

The patient dates the onset of these fears to a particular incident when he was 9 and his Sunday school teacher gave a detailed account of a leg operation she had undergone. As he listened, he began to feel anxious and dizzy, he sweated profusely, and finally he fainted. He recalls great difficulty receiving immunizations and being subjected to other routine medical procedures through the rest of his school years, as well as numerous fainting and near-fainting episodes throughout his teenage and adult years whenever he witnessed the slightest physical trauma, heard of an injury or illness, or saw a sick or disfigured person. When he recently saw someone in a store in a wheelchair, he started wondering if the person was in pain and became so distressed that he fainted and fell to the floor. He was greatly embarrassed, when he regained consciousness, by the crowd of people surrounding him.

Mr. M. denies any other emotional problems. He enjoys his work, seems to get along well with his wife, and has many friends.

DISCUSSION

Mr. M. is afraid of thinking about or being near a situation involving bodily illness or injury. He recognizes that his fear is excessive and unreasonable, but nevertheless he avoids such situations. Although the fear and avoidance behavior apparently does not interfere with his normal routine or school activities, he is quite distressed about having the fear, which is the reason he now seeks treatment.

His fear is unrelated to obsessive-compulsive disorder (e.g., an obsession involving being infected with germs) and to any trauma that might precede posttraumatic stress disorder (e.g., having witnessed mutilation on the battlefield): therefore, neither of these diagnoses is made.

Mr. M. has a specific phobia called blood-injection-injury type. He feels faint in the presence of the phobic stimulus, as do many people with this type of phobia. Feeling faint is rarely seen in other specific phobias, such as fear of flying or of animals, or in social phobia or agoraphobia. (From *DSM-IV Casebook.*)

Social Phobia

The DSM-IV-TR diagnostic criteria for social phobia (Table 16.3–4) acknowledge that the disorder can be associated with panic attacks. DSM-IV-TR also includes a specifier for generalized type, which may be useful in predicting course, prognosis, and treatment response. DSM-IV-TR excludes a diagnosis of social phobia when the symptoms are a result of social avoidance stemming from embarrassment about another psychiatric or nonpsychiatric medical condition.

Table 16.3–4
DSM-IV-TR Diagnostic Criteria for Social Phobia

A. A marked and persistent fear of one or more social or performance situations in which the person is exposed to unfamiliar people or to possible scrutiny by others. The individual fears that he or she will act in a way (or show anxiety symptoms) that will be humiliating or embarrassing. **Note:** In children, there must be evidence of the capacity for age-appropriate social relationships with familiar people and the anxiety must occur in peer settings, not just in interactions with adults.

B. Exposure to the feared social situation almost invariably provokes anxiety, which may take the form of a situationally bound or situationally predisposed panic attack. **Note:** In children, the anxiety may be expressed by crying, tantrums, freezing, or shrinking from social situations with unfamiliar people.

C. The person recognizes that the fear is excessive or unreasonable. **Note:** In children, this feature may be absent.

D. The feared social or performance situations are avoided or else are endured with intense anxiety or distress.

E. The avoidance, anxious anticipation, or distress in the feared social or performance situation(s) interferes significantly with the person's normal routine, occupational (academic) functioning, or social activities or relationships, or there is marked distress about having the phobia.

F. In individuals under age 18 years, the duration is at least 6 months.

G. The fear or avoidance is not due to the direct physiological effects of a substance (e.g., a drug of abuse, a medication) or a general medical condition and is not better accounted for by another mental disorder (e.g., panic disorder with or without agoraphobia, separation anxiety disorder, body dysmorphic disorder, a pervasive developmental disorder, or schizoid personality disorder).

H. If a general medical condition or another mental disorder is present, the fear in Criterion A is unrelated to it, e.g., the fear is not of stuttering, trembling in Parkinson's disease, or exhibiting abnormal eating behavior in anorexia nervosa or bulimia nervosa.

Specify if:

Generalized: if the fears include most social situations (also consider the additional diagnosis of avoidant personality disorder)

From American Psychiatric Association. *Diagnostic and Statistical Manual of Mental Disorders.* 4th ed. Text rev. Washington, DC: American Psychiatric Association; copyright 2000, with permission.

Ms. M. was a successful secretary working in a law firm. While she reported a long history of feeling uncomfortable in social situations, Ms. M. came for treatment when she began to feel that her uneasiness was interfering with her social life and job performance. Ms. M. reported that she noticed herself feeling increasingly nervous whenever she met a new person. For example, upon meeting a new member of the law firm, she described feeling suddenly tense and sweaty, noticing that her heart was beating very fast. She had the sudden thought that she would say something foolish

in these situations or commit a terrible social gaffe that would make people laugh at her. At social gatherings she described similar feelings that led her to either leave the gathering early or decline invitations to attend. (Courtesy of Daniel S. Pine, M.D.)

CLINICAL FEATURES

Phobias are characterized by the arousal of severe anxiety when patients are exposed to specific situations or objects or when patients even anticipate exposure to the situations or objects. DSM-IV-TR emphasizes the possibility that panic attacks can and frequently do occur in patients with specific and social phobias, but the panic attacks, except perhaps for the first few, are expected. Exposure to the phobic stimulus or anticipation of it almost invariably results in a panic attack in a person who is susceptible to them.

Persons with phobias, by definition, try to avoid the phobic stimulus; some go to great trouble to avoid anxiety-provoking situations. For example, a phobic patient may take a bus across the United States, rather than fly, to avoid contact with the object of the patient's phobia, an airplane. Perhaps as another way to avoid the stress of the phobic stimulus, many phobic patients have substance-related disorders, particularly alcohol use disorders. Moreover, an estimated one third of patients with social phobia have major depressive disorder.

The major finding on the mental status examination is the presence of an irrational and ego-dystonic fear of a specific situation, activity, or object; patients are able to describe how they avoid contact with the phobia. Depression is commonly found on the mental status examination and may be present in as many as one third of all phobic patients.

DIFFERENTIAL DIAGNOSIS

Specific phobia and social phobia need to be differentiated from appropriate fear and normal shyness, respectively. DSM-IV-TR aids in the differentiation by requiring that the symptoms impair the patient's ability to function appropriately. Nonpsychiatric medical conditions that can result in the development of a phobia include the use of substances (particularly hallucinogens and sympathomimetics), central nervous system tumors, and cerebrovascular diseases. Phobic symptoms in these instances are unlikely in the absence of additional suggestive findings on physical, neurological, and mental status examinations. Schizophrenia is also in the differential diagnosis of both specific phobia and social phobia, since schizophrenic patients can have phobic symptoms as part of their psychoses. Unlike patients with schizophrenia, however, phobia patients have insight into the irrationality of their fears and lack the bizarre quality and other psychotic symptoms that accompany schizophrenia.

In the differential diagnosis of both specific phobia and social phobia, clinicians must consider panic disorder, agoraphobia, and avoidant personality disorder. Differentiation among panic disorder, agoraphobia, social phobia, and specific phobia can be difficult in individual cases. In general, however, patients with specific phobia or nongeneralized social phobia tend to experience anxiety immediately when presented with the phobic stimulus. Furthermore, the anxiety or panic is limited to the identified situation; patients are not abnormally anxious when they are neither confronted with the phobic stimulus nor caused to anticipate the stimulus.

A patient with agoraphobia is often comforted by the presence of another person in an anxiety-provoking situation, whereas a patient with social phobia is made more anxious than before by the presence of other persons. Whereas breathlessness, dizziness, a sense of suffocation, and a fear of dying are common in panic disorder and agoraphobia, the symptoms associated with social phobia usually involve blushing, muscle twitching, and anxiety about scrutiny. Differentiation between social phobia and avoidant personality disorder can be difficult and can require extensive interviews and psychiatric histories.

Specific Phobia

Other diagnoses to consider in the differential diagnosis of specific phobia are hypochondriasis, obsessive-compulsive disorder, and paranoid personality disorder. Hypochondriasis is the fear of having a disease, whereas specific phobia of the illness type is the fear of contracting the disease. Some patients with obsessive-compulsive disorder manifest behavior indistinguishable from that of a patient with specific phobia. For example, patients with obsessive-compulsive disorder may avoid knives because they have compulsive thoughts about killing their children, whereas patients with specific phobia about knives may avoid them for fear of cutting themselves. Patients with paranoid personality disorder have generalized fear that distinguishes them from those with specific phobia.

Social Phobia

Two additional differential diagnostic considerations for social phobia are major depressive disorder and schizoid personality disorder. The avoidance of social situations can often be a symptom in depression, but a psychiatric interview with the patient is likely to elicit a broad constellation of depressive symptoms. In patients with schizoid personality disorder, the lack of interest in socializing, not the fear of socializing, leads to the avoidant social behavior.

COURSE AND PROGNOSIS

Specific phobia exhibits a bimodal age of onset, with a childhood peak for animal phobia, natural environment phobia, and blood-injection-injury phobia and an early adulthood peak for other phobias, such as situational phobia. As with other anxiety disorders, limited prospective epidemiological data exist on the natural course of specific phobia. Because patients with isolated specific phobias rarely present for treatment, research on the course of the disorder in the clinic is limited. The available information suggests that most specific phobias that begin in childhood and persist into adulthood continue to persist for many years. The severity of the condition is thought to remain relatively constant, without the waxing and waning course seen with other anxiety disorders.

Mr. A. was a successful businessman who presented for treatment following a change in his business schedule. While he had formerly worked largely from an office near his home, a promotion led to a schedule of frequent out-of-town meetings, requiring weekly flights. Mr. A. reported being "deathly afraid" of flying. Even the thought of getting on an airplane led to thoughts of impending doom as he envisioned his airplane crashing to the ground. These thoughts were associated with intense fear, palpitations, sweating, clammy palms, and stomach upset. While the thought of flying was terrifying enough, Mr. A. became nearly incapacitated when he went to the airport. Immediately before boarding, Mr. A. often had to turn back from the plane and run to the bathroom to vomit. (Courtesy of Daniel S. Pine, M.D.)

Social phobia tends to have its onset in late childhood or early adolescence. Social phobia tends to be a chronic disorder, although as with the other anxiety disorders, prospective epidemiological data are limited. Both retrospective epidemiological studies and prospective clinical studies suggest that the disorder can profoundly disrupt the life of an individual over many years. This can include disruption in school or academic achievement and interference with job performance and social development.

TREATMENT

Behavior Therapy

The most studied and most effective treatment for phobias is probably behavior therapy. The key aspects of successful treatment are (1) the patient's commitment to treatment, (2) clearly identified problems and objectives, and (3) available alternative strategies for coping with the feelings. A variety of behavioral treatment techniques have been used, the most common being systematic desensitization, a method pioneered by Joseph Wolpe. In this method, the patient is exposed serially to a predetermined list of anxiety-provoking stimuli graded in a hierarchy from the least to the most frightening. Through the use of tranquilizing drugs, hypnosis, and instruction in muscle relaxation, patients are taught how to induce in themselves both mental and physical repose. Once they have mastered the techniques, patients are taught to use them to induce relaxation in the face of each anxiety-provoking stimulus. As they become desensitized to each stimulus in the scale, the patients move up to the next stimulus until, ultimately, what previously produced the most anxiety no longer elicits the painful affect.

Other behavioral techniques that have been used more recently involve intensive exposure to the phobic stimulus through either imagery or desensitization in vivo. In imaginal flooding, patients are exposed to the phobic stimulus for as long as they can tolerate the fear until they reach a point at which they can no longer feel it. Flooding (also known as implosion) in vivo requires patients to experience similar anxiety through exposure to the actual phobic stimulus.

Insight-Oriented Psychotherapy

Early in the development of psychoanalysis and the dynamically oriented psychotherapies, theorists believed that these methods were the treatments of choice for phobic neurosis, which was then thought to stem from oedipal-genital conflicts. Soon, however, therapists recognized that, despite progress in uncovering and analyzing unconscious conflicts, patients frequently failed to lose their phobic symptoms. Moreover, by continuing to avoid phobic situations, patients excluded a significant degree of anxiety and its related associations from the analytic process. Both Freud and his pupil Sandor Ferenczi recognized that if progress in analyzing these symptoms was to be made, therapists had to go beyond their analytic roles and actively urge phobic patients to seek the phobic situation and experience the anxiety and resultant insight. Since then, psychiatrists have generally agreed that a measure of activity on the therapist's part is often required to treat phobic anxiety successfully. The decision to apply the techniques of psychodynamic insight-oriented therapy should be based not on the presence of phobic symptoms alone but on positive indications from the patient's ego structure and life patterns for the use of this method of treatment. Insight-oriented therapy enables patients to understand the origin of the phobia, the phenomenon of secondary gain, and the role of resistance and enables them to seek healthy ways of dealing with anxiety-provoking stimuli.

Other Therapeutic Modalities

Hypnosis, supportive therapy, and family therapy may be useful in the treatment of phobic disorders. Hypnosis is used to enhance the therapist's suggestion that the phobic object is not dangerous, and self-hypnosis can be taught to the patient as a method of relaxation when confronted with the phobic object. Supportive psychotherapy and family therapy are often useful in helping the patient actively confront the phobic object during treatment. Not only can family therapy enlist the aid of the family in treating the patient, but also it may help the family understand the nature of the patient's problem.

Specific Phobia

The most commonly used treatment for specific phobia is exposure therapy. In this method therapists desensitize patients by using a series of gradual, self-paced exposures to the phobic stimuli, and they teach patients various techniques to deal with anxiety, including relaxation, breathing control, and cognitive approaches. The cognitive approaches include reinforcing the realization that the phobic situation is, in fact, safe. The key aspects of successful behavior therapy are the patient's commitment to treatment, clearly identified problems and objectives, and alternative strategies for coping with the patient's feelings. In the special situation of blood-injection-injury phobia, some therapists recommend that patients tense their bodies and remain seated during the exposure to help avoid the possibility of fainting from a vasovagal reaction to the phobic stimulation. β-Adrenergic receptor antagonists may be useful in the treatment of specific phobia, especially when the phobia is associated with panic attacks. Pharmacotherapy (e.g., benzodiazepines), psychotherapy, or combined therapy directed to the attacks may also be of benefit.

Social Phobia

Both psychotherapy and pharmacotherapy are useful in treating social phobias, and varying approaches are indicated for the generalized type and for performance situations. Some studies indicate that the use of both pharmacotherapy and psychotherapy produces better results than either therapy alone, although the finding may not be applicable to all situations and patients.

Effective drugs for the treatment of social phobia include (1) selective serotonin reuptake inhibitors (SSRIs), (2) the benzodiazepines, (3) venlafaxine (Effexor), and (4) buspirone (BuSpar). Most clinicians consider SSRIs the first-line treatment choice for patients with generalized social phobia. The benzodiazepines alprazolam (Xanax) and clonazepam (Klonopin) are also efficacious in both generalized and specific social phobia. Buspirone has shown additive effects when used to augment treatment with SSRIs.

In severe cases, successful treatment of social phobia with both irreversible MAOIs such as phenelzine (Nardil) and reversible inhibitors of monoamine oxidase such as moclobemide (Aurorix) and brofaromine (Consonar) (which are not available in the United States) has been reported. Therapeutic dosages of phenelzine range from 45 to 90 mg a day, with response rates ranging from 50 to 70 percent, and approximately 5 to 6 weeks are needed to assess the efficacy.

The treatment of social phobia associated with performance situations frequently involves the use of β-adrenergic receptor antagonists shortly before exposure to a phobic stimulus. The two compounds most widely used are atenolol (Tenormin), 50 to 100 mg every morning or 1 hour before the performance, and propranolol (20 to 40 mg). Cognitive, behavioral, and exposure techniques can also be useful in performance situations.

Psychotherapy for the generalized type of social phobia usually involves a combination of behavioral and cognitive methods, including cognitive retraining, desensitization, rehearsal during sessions, and a range of homework assignments.

References

Chapman TF, Fyer AJ, Mannuzza S, Klein DF. A comparison of treated and untreated simple phobia. *Am J Psychiatry.* 1993;150:816.

Coupland NJ. Social phobia: etiology, neurobiology, and treatment. *J Clin Psychiatry.* 2001;62(suppl 1):25.

Dilsaver SC, Qamar AB, Del Medico VJ. Secondary social phobia in patients with major depression. *Psychiatry Res.* 1992;44:33.

Francis G, Last CG, Strauss CC. Avoidant disorder and social phobia in children and adolescents. *J Am Acad Child Adolesc Psychiatry.* 1992;31:1086.

Fresco DM, Heimberg RG. Empirically supported psychological treatments for social phobia. *Psychiatr Ann.* 2001;31(8):489.

Gabbard GO. Psychodynamics of panic disorder and social phobia. *Bull Menninger Clin.* 1992;56(suppl 2):A3.

Gorman JM, section ed. Anxiety disorders. In: Sadock BJ, Sadock VA, eds. *Kaplan & Sadock's Comprehensive Textbook of Psychiatry.* 7th ed. Vol I. Baltimore: Lippincott Williams & Wilkins; 2000:1441.

Greist JH. The diagnosis of social phobia. *J Clin Psychiatry.* 1995;56:5.

Jefferson JW. Social phobia: everyone's disorder? *J Clin Psychiatry.* 1996; 57(suppl 6):28.

Magee WJ, Eaton WW, Wittchen HU, McGonagle KA, Kessler RC. Agoraphobia, simple phobia, and social phobia in the National Comorbidity Survey. *Arch Gen Psychiatry.* 1996;53:159.

Malis RW, Hartz AJ, Doebbling CC, Noyes RJR. Specific phobia of illness in the community. *Gen Hosp Psychiatry.* 2002;24:135.

Mennin DS, Heimberg RG, Craig S. Panic, agoraphobia, phobias, and generalized anxiety disorder. In: Hersen M, Bellack AS, eds. *Psychopathology in Adulthood.* 2nd ed. Needham Heights, MA: Allyn & Bacon; 2000:169.

Parker JDA, Taylor GJ, Bagby RM, Acklin MW. Alexithymia in panic disorder and simple phobia: a comparative study. *Am J Psychiatry.* 1993;150:1105.

Persons JB. Understanding the exposure principle and using it to treat anxiety. *Psychiatr Ann.* 2001;31(8):472.

Potts NLS, Davidson JRT. Social phobia: biological aspects and pharmacotherapy. *Prog Neuropsychopharmacol Biol Psychiatry.* 1992;16:635.

Schmidt NB, Koselka M, Woolaway-Bickel K. Combined treatments for phobic anxiety disorders. In: Sammons MT, Schmidt NB, eds. *Combined Treatment for Mental Disorders: A Guide to Psychological and Pharmacological Interventions.* Washington, DC: American Psychological Association; 2001:81.

Stein MB, Walker JR, Forde DR. Public-speaking fears in a community sample: prevalence, impact on functioning, and diagnostic classification. *Arch Gen Psychiatry.* 1995;53:169.

Tolin DF, Sawchuk CN, Thomas C. The role of disgust in blood-injection-injury phobia. *Behav Therap.* 1999;96:22.

Van Ameringen M, Mancini C, Streiner DL. Fluoxetine efficacy in social phobia. *J Clin Psychiatry.* 1993;54:27.

▲ 16.4 Obsessive-Compulsive Disorder

The essential feature of obsessive-compulsive disorder (OCD) is the symptom of recurrent obsessions or compulsions sufficiently severe to cause marked distress to the person. The obsessions or compulsions are time consuming and interfere significantly with the person's normal routine, occupational functioning, usual social activities, or relationships. A patient with OCD may have an obsession or a compulsion or both.

An *obsession* is a recurrent and intrusive thought, feeling, idea, or sensation. In contrast to an obsession, which is a mental event, a compulsion is a behavior. Specifically, a *compulsion* is a conscious, standardized, recurrent behavior, such as counting, checking, or avoiding. A patient with OCD realizes the irrationality of the obsession and experiences both the obsession and the compulsion as ego-dystonic (i.e., unwanted behavior).

Although the compulsive act may be carried out in an attempt to reduce the anxiety associated with the obsession, it does not always succeed in doing so. The completion of the compulsive act may not affect the anxiety, and it may even increase the anxiety. Anxiety is also increased when a person resists carrying out a compulsion.

EPIDEMIOLOGY

The lifetime prevalence of OCD in the general population is estimated at 2 to 3 percent. Some researchers have estimated that the disorder is found in as many as 10 percent of outpatients in psychiatric clinics. These figures make OCD the fourth most common psychiatric diagnosis after phobias, substance-related disorders, and major depressive disorder. Epidemiological studies in Europe, Asia, and Africa have confirmed these rates across cultural boundaries.

Among adults, men and women are equally likely to be affected, but among adolescents, boys are more commonly affected than girls. The mean age of onset is about 20 years, although men have a slightly earlier age of onset (mean about 19 years) than women (mean about 22 years). Overall, the symptoms of about two thirds of affected persons have an onset before age 25, and the symptoms of fewer than 15 percent have an onset after age 35. The onset of the disorder can occur in adolescence or childhood, in some cases as early as 2 years of age. Single persons are more frequently affected with OCD than are married persons, although this finding probably reflects the difficulty that persons with the disorder have maintaining a relationship. OCD occurs less often among blacks than among

whites, although access to health care rather than differences in prevalence may explain the variation.

COMORBIDITY

Persons with OCD are commonly affected by other mental disorders. The lifetime prevalence for major depressive disorder in persons with OCD is about 67 percent and for social phobia, about 25 percent. Other common comorbid psychiatric diagnoses in patients with OCD include alcohol use disorders, generalized anxiety disorder, specific phobia, panic disorder, eating disorders, and personality disorders. The incidence of Tourette's disorder in patients with OCD is 5 to 7 percent, and 20 to 30 percent of OCD patients have a history of tics.

ETIOLOGY

Biological Factors

Neurotransmitters. SEROTONERGIC SYSTEM. The many clinical drug trials that have been conducted support the hypothesis that dysregulation of serotonin is involved in the symptom formation of obsessions and compulsions in the disorder. Data show that serotonergic drugs are more effective than drugs that affect other neurotransmitter systems, but whether serotonin is involved in the cause of OCD is not clear. Clinical studies have assayed cerebrospinal fluid (CSF) concentrations of serotonin metabolites (e.g., 5-hydroxyindoleacetic acid [5-HIAA]) and affinities and numbers of platelet-binding sites of tritiated imipramine (Tofranil), which binds to serotonin reuptake sites, and have reported variable findings of these measures in patients with OCD. In one study, the CSF concentration of 5-HIAA decreased after treatment with clomipramine (Anafranil), focusing attention on the serotonergic system.

NORADRENERGIC SYSTEM. Currently, less evidence exists for dysfunction in the noradrenergic system in OCD. Anecdotal reports show some improvement in OCD symptoms with use of oral clonidine (Catapres), a drug that lowers the amount of norepinephrine released from the presynaptic nerve terminals.

NEUROIMMUNOLOGY. There has been some interest in a positive link between streptococcal infection and OCD. Group A β-hemolytic streptococcal infection can cause rheumatic fever, and approximately 10 to 30 percent of the patients develop Sydenham's chorea and show obsessive-compulsive symptoms.

Brain-Imaging Studies. Neuroimaging in OCD patients has produced converging data implicating altered function in the neurocircuitry between orbitofrontal cortex, caudate, and thalamus. Various functional brain-imaging studies—for example, positron emission tomography (PET)—have shown increased activity (e.g., metabolism and blood flow) in the frontal lobes, the basal ganglia (especially the caudate), and the cingulum of patients with OCD. The involvement of these areas in the pathology of OCD appears more associated with corticostriatal pathways than with the amygdala pathways that are the current focus of much anxiety disorder research. Pharmacological and behavioral treatments reportedly reverse these abnormalities (Fig. 16.4–1). Data from functional brain-imaging studies are consistent with data from structural brain-imaging studies. Both computed tomographic (CT) and magnetic resonance imaging (MRI) studies have found bilaterally smaller caudates in patients with OCD. Both functional and structural brain-imaging study results are also compatible with the observation that neurological procedures involving the cingulum are sometimes effective in the treatment of OCD patients. One recent MRI study reported increased T1 relaxation times in the frontal cortex, a finding consistent with the location of abnormalities discovered in PET studies.

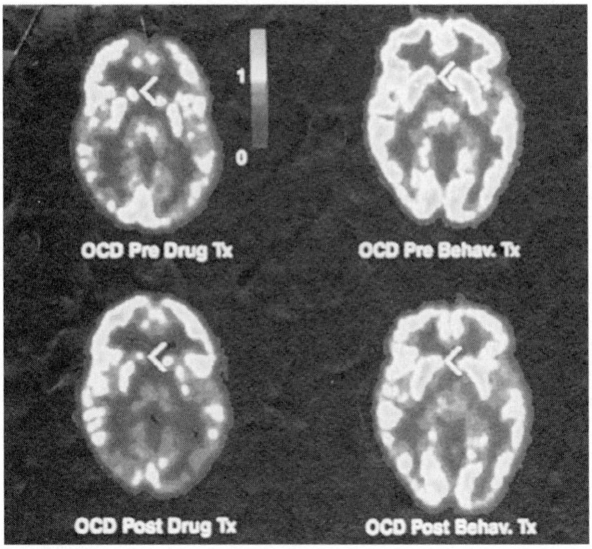

FIGURE 16.4–1

[^{18}F]Fluorodeoxyglucose positron emission tomographic scans of representative patients in a horizontal plane at a middle level of the head of the caudate nuclei before and after successful drug treatment (*Drug Tx*) or behavior therapy (*Behav. Tx*) for obsessive-compulsive disorder (*OCD*). Scans were processed to reflect the ratio of glucose metabolic rate registered by each pixel element, divided by that of the whole brain. *Arrowheads* indicate right head of caudate nucleus. (Display follows radiological and anatomical convention of displaying the right side on the viewer's left.) The examples were chosen for illustration because of exactness of scan repositioning and because they show various degrees of visible left-right asymmetry of caudate nucleus change from before to after treatment. (Reprinted with permission from Baxter LR Jr, Schwartz JM, Bergman KS, et al. Caudate glucose metabolic rate changes with both drug and behavior therapy for obsessive-compulsive disorder. *Arch Gen Psychiatry.* 1992;49:685.)

Genetics. Available genetic data on OCD support the hypothesis that the disorder has a significant genetic component. The data, however, do not yet distinguish the heritable factors from the influence of cultural and behavioral effects on the transmission of the disorder. Studies of concordance for the disorder in twins have consistently found a significantly higher concordance rate for monozygotic twins than for dizygotic twins. Family studies of these patients have shown that 35 percent of the first-degree relatives of OCD patients are also afflicted with the disorder.

Other Biological Data. Electrophysiological studies, sleep electroencephalogram (EEG) studies, and neuroendocrine studies have contributed data that indicate some commonalities between depressive disorders and OCD. A higher than usual incidence of nonspecific EEG abnormalities occurs in patients with OCD. Sleep EEG studies have found abnormalities similar

to those in depressive disorders, such as decreased rapid eye movement latency. Neuroendocrine studies have also produced some analogies to depressive disorders, such as nonsuppression on the dexamethasone-suppression test in about one third of patients and decreased growth hormone secretion with clonidine infusions.

As mentioned above, studies have suggested a possible link between a subset of OCD cases and certain types of motor tic syndromes (i.e., Tourette's disorder and chronic motor tics). There is a higher rate of OCD, Tourette's disorder, and chronic motor tics in relatives of Tourette's disorder patients than in relatives of controls, whether or not they had OCD. Most family studies of probands with OCD have found increased rates of Tourette's disorder and chronic motor tics only among the relatives of probands with OCD who also have some form of tic disorder. These data suggest a familial, and perhaps genetic, relationship between Tourette's disorder and chronic motor tics and some cases of OCD.

Behavioral Factors

According to learning theorists, obsessions are conditioned stimuli. A relatively neutral stimulus becomes associated with fear or anxiety through a process of respondent conditioning by being paired with events that are noxious or anxiety-producing. Thus, previously neutral objects and thoughts become conditioned stimuli capable of provoking anxiety or discomfort.

Compulsions are established in a different way. When a person discovers that a certain action reduces anxiety attached to an obsessional thought, he or she develops active avoidance strategies in the form of compulsions or ritualistic behaviors to control the anxiety. Gradually, because of their efficacy in reducing a painful secondary drive (anxiety), the avoidance strategies become fixed as learned patterns of compulsive behaviors. Learning theory provides useful concepts for explaining certain aspects of obsessive-compulsive phenomena—for example, the anxiety-provoking capacity of ideas not necessarily frightening in themselves and the establishment of compulsive patterns of behavior.

Psychosocial Factors

Personality Factors. OCD differs from obsessive-compulsive personality disorder. Most persons with OCD do not have premorbid compulsive symptoms, and such personality traits are neither necessary nor sufficient for the development of OCD. Only about 15 to 35 percent of OCD patients have had premorbid obsessional traits.

Psychodynamic Factors. Sigmund Freud originally conceptualized the condition we now call OCD as obsessional neurosis. He assumed there was a defensive retreat involved in the face of anxiety-provoking oedipal wishes. He postulated that the patient with an obsessive-compulsive neurosis regressed to the anal phase of psychosexual development. Freud's theories are discussed below.

Psychodynamic insight may be of great help in understanding problems with treatment compliance, interpersonal difficulties, and personality problems accompanying the Axis I disorder. Many patients with OCD may refuse to cooperate with effective treatments such as selective serotonin reuptake inhibitors (SSRIs) and behavior therapy. Even though the symptoms of OCD may be biologically driven, psychodynamic meanings may be attached to them. Patients may become invested in maintaining the symptomatology because of secondary gains. For example, a male patient, whose mother stays home to take care of him, may unconsciously wish to hang on to his OCD symptoms because they keep the attention of his mother.

Another contribution of psychodynamic understanding involves the interpersonal dimensions. Studies have shown that relatives will accommodate the patient through active participation in rituals or significant modifications of their daily routines. This form of family accommodation is correlated with stress in the family, rejecting attitudes toward the patient, and poor family functioning. Often the family members are involved in an effort to reduce the patient's anxiety or to control the patient's expressions of anger. This pattern of relatedness may become internalized and be recreated when the patient enters a treatment setting. By looking at recurring patterns of interpersonal relationships from a psychodynamic perspective, patients may learn how their illness affects others.

Finally, one other contribution of psychodynamic thinking is recognition of the precipitants that initiate or exacerbate symptoms. Often, interpersonal difficulties increase the patient's anxiety and thus increase the patient's symptomatology as well. Research suggests that OCD may be precipitated by a number of environmental stressors, especially those involving pregnancy, childbirth, or parental care of children. An understanding of the stressors may assist the clinician in an overall treatment plan that reduces the stressful events themselves or their meaning to the patient.

SIGMUND FREUD. In classic psychoanalytic theory, OCD was termed obsessive-compulsive neurosis and was considered a regression from the oedipal phase to the anal psychosexual phase of development. When patients with OCD feel threatened by anxiety about retaliation for unconscious impulses or by the loss of a significant object's love, they retreat from the oedipal position and regress to an intensely ambivalent emotional stage associated with the anal phase. The ambivalence is connected to the unraveling of the smooth fusion between sexual and aggressive drives characteristic of the oedipal phase. The coexistence of hatred and love toward the same person leaves patients paralyzed with doubt and indecision.

An example of how Freud viewed OCD symptoms is described by Otto Fenichel in the following case.

A patient, who was not analyzed, complained in the first interview that he suffered from the compulsion to look backward constantly, from fear that he might have overlooked something important behind him. These ideas were predominant; he might overlook a coin lying on the ground; he might have injured an insect by stepping on it; or an insect might have fallen on its back and need his help. The patient was also afraid of touching anything, and whenever he had touched an object he had to convince himself that he had not destroyed it. He had no vocation because the severe compulsions disturbed all his working activity; however, he had one passion: housecleaning. He liked to visit his neighbors

and clean their houses, just for fun. Another symptom was described by the patient as his "clothes consciousness"; he was constantly preoccupied with the question whether or not his suit fitted. He, too, stated that sexuality did not play an important part in his life. He had sexual intercourse two or three times a year only, and exclusively with girls in whom he had no personal interest. Later on, he mentioned another symptom. As a child, he had felt his mother to be disgusting and had been terribly afraid of touching her. There was no real reason whatsoever for such a disgust, for the mother had been a nice and popular person. (From Fenichel O. *The Psychoanalytic Theory of Neurosis*. New York: Norton; 1945:274, with permission.)

In this clinical picture, the need to be clean and not to touch is related to anal sexuality, and the disgust for the mother is a reaction against incestuous fears.

One of the striking features of patients with OCD is the degree to which they are preoccupied with aggression or cleanliness, either overtly in the content of their symptoms or in the associations that lie behind them. Therefore, the psychogenesis of OCD may lie in disturbances in normal growth and development related to the anal-sadistic phase of development.

Ambivalence. Ambivalence is the direct result of a change in the characteristics of the impulse life. It is an important feature of normal children during the anal-sadistic developmental phase; children feel both love and murderous hate toward the same object, sometimes simultaneously. Patients with OCD often consciously experience both love and hate toward an object. This conflict of opposing emotions is evident in a patient's doing and undoing patterns of behavior and in paralyzing doubt in the face of choices.

Magical Thinking. In magical thinking, regression uncovers early modes of thought rather than impulses; that is, ego functions, as well as id functions, are affected by regression. Inherent in magical thinking is omnipotence of thought. Persons believe that merely by thinking about an event in the external world they can cause the event to occur without intermediate physical actions. This feeling causes them to fear having an aggressive thought.

DIAGNOSIS

As part of the diagnostic criteria for OCD, the text revision of the fourth edition of *Diagnostic and Statistical Manual of Mental Disorders* (DSM-IV-TR) allows clinicians to specify that patients have the poor insight type of OCD if they generally do not recognize the excessiveness of their obsessions and compulsions (Table 16.4–1).

Table 16.4–1
DSM-IV-TR Diagnostic Criteria for Obsessive-Compulsive Disorder

A. Either obsessions or compulsions:

Obsessions as defined by (1), (2), (3), and (4):

(1) recurrent and persistent thoughts, impulses, or images that are experienced, at some time during the disturbance, as intrusive and inappropriate and that cause marked anxiety or distress

(2) the thoughts, impulses, or images are not simply excessive worries about real-life problems

(3) the person attempts to ignore or suppress such thoughts, impulses, or images, or to neutralize them with some other thought or action

(4) the person recognizes that the obsessional thoughts, impulses, or images are a product of his or her own mind (not imposed from without as in thought insertion)

Compulsions as defined by (1) and (2):

(1) repetitive behaviors (e.g., hand washing, ordering, checking) or mental acts (e.g., praying, counting, repeating words silently) that the person feels driven to perform in response to an obsession, or according to rules that must be applied rigidly

(2) the behaviors or mental acts are aimed at preventing or reducing distress or preventing some dreaded event or situation; however, these behaviors or mental acts either are not connected in a realistic way with what they are designed to neutralize or prevent or are clearly excessive

B. At some point during the course of the disorder, the person has recognized that the obsessions or compulsions are excessive or unreasonable. **Note:** This does not apply to children.

C. The obsessions or compulsions cause marked distress, are time consuming (take more than 1 hour a day), or significantly interfere with the person's normal routine, occupational (or academic) functioning, or usual social activities or relationships.

D. If another Axis I disorder is present, the content of the obsessions or compulsions is not restricted to it (e.g., preoccupation with food in the presence of an eating disorder; hair pulling in the presence of trichotillomania; concern with appearance in the presence of body dysmorphic disorder; preoccupation with drugs in the presence of a substance use disorder; preoccupation with having a serious illness in the presence of hypochondriasis; preoccupation with sexual urges or fantasies in the presence of a paraphilia; or guilty ruminations in the presence of major depressive disorder).

E. The disturbance is not due to the direct physiological effects of a substance (e.g., a drug of abuse, a medication) or a general medical condition.

Specify if:

With poor insight: if, for most of the time during the current episode, the person does not recognize that the obsessions and compulsions are excessive or unreasonable

From American Psychiatric Association. *Diagnostic and Statistical Manual of Mental Disorders.* 4th ed. Text rev. Washington, DC: American Psychiatric Association; copyright 2000, with permission.

CLINICAL FEATURES

Patients with OCD often take their complaints to physicians other than psychiatrists (Table 16.4–2). Most patients with OCD have both obsessions and compulsions—up to 75 percent in some surveys. Some researchers and clinicians believe that the number may be much closer to 100 percent if patients are carefully assessed for the presence of mental compulsions in addition to behavioral compulsions. For example, an obsession about hurting a child may be followed by a mental compulsion to repeat a specific prayer a specific number of times. Other researchers and clinicians, however, believe that some patients do have only obsessive thoughts without compulsions. Such patients are likely to have repetitious thoughts of a sexual or

Table 16.4–2
Nonpsychiatric Clinical Specialists Likely to See Obsessive-Compulsive Disorder Patients

Specialist	Presenting Problem
Dermatologist	Chapped hands, eczematoid appearance
Family practitioner	Family member washing excessively, may mention counting or checking compulsions
Oncologist, infectious disease internist	Insistent belief that person has acquired immune deficiency syndrome
Neurologist	Obsessive-compulsive disorder associated with Tourette's disorder, head injury, epilepsy, choreas, other basal ganglia lesions or disorders
Neurosurgeon	Severe, intractable obsessive-compulsive disorder
Obstetrician	Postpartum obsessive-compulsive disorder
Pediatrician	Parent's concern about child's behavior, usually excessive washing
Pediatric cardiologist	Obsessive-compulsive disorder secondary to Sydenham's chorea
Plastic surgeon	Repeated consultations for "abnormal" features
Dentist	Gum lesions from excessive teeth cleaning

Reprinted with permission from Rapoport JL. The neurobiology of obsessive-compulsive disorder. *JAMA.* 1988;260:2889.

Table 16.4–3
Obsessive-Compulsive Symptoms in Adults

Variable	%
Obsessions (*N* = 200)	
Contamination	45
Pathological doubt	42
Somatic	36
Need for symmetry	31
Aggressive	28
Sexual	26
Other	13
Multiple obsessions	60
Compulsions (*N* = 200)	
Checking	63
Washing	50
Counting	36
Need to ask or confess	31
Symmetry and precision	28
Hoarding	18
Multiple comparisons	48
Course of illness (*N* = 100)[a]	
Type	
Continuous	85
Deteriorative	10
Episodic	2
Not present	71
Present	29

[a]Age at onset: men, 17.5 ± 6.8 years; women, 20.8 ± 8.5 years.
Reprinted with permission from Rasmussen SA, Eiser JL. The epidemiology and differential diagnosis of obsessive compulsive disorder. *J Clin Psychiatry.* 1992;53(4 suppl):6.

aggressive act that is reprehensible to them. For clarity, it is best to conceptualize obsessions as thoughts and compulsions as behavior.

Obsessions and compulsions have certain features in common: An idea or an impulse intrudes itself insistently and persistently into a person's conscious awareness. A feeling of anxious dread accompanies the central manifestation and frequently leads the person to take countermeasures against the initial idea or impulse. The obsession or the compulsion is ego-alien; that is, it is experienced as foreign to the person's experience of himself or herself as a psychological being. No matter how vivid and compelling the obsession or compulsion, the person usually recognizes it as absurd and irrational. The person suffering from obsessions and compulsions usually feels a strong desire to resist them. Nevertheless, about half of all patients offer little resistance to compulsions, although about 80 percent of all patients believe that the compulsion is irrational. Sometimes patients overvalue obsessions and compulsions—for example, they may insist that compulsive cleanliness is morally correct, even though they have lost their jobs because of time spent cleaning.

Symptom Patterns

The presentation of obsessions and compulsions is heterogeneous in adults (Table 16.4–3) and in children and adolescents (Table 16.4–4). The symptoms of an individual patient may overlap and change with time, but OCD has four major symptom patterns.

Contamination. The most common pattern is an obsession of contamination, followed by washing or accompanied by compulsive avoidance of the presumably contaminated object. The feared object is often hard to avoid (e.g., feces, urine, dust, or germs). Patients may literally rub the skin off their hands by excessive hand washing or may be unable to leave their homes because of fear of germs. Although anxiety is the most common emotional response to the feared object, obsessive shame and disgust are also common. Patients with contamination obsessions usually believe that the contamination is spread from object to object or person to person by the slightest contact.

Pathological Doubt. The second most common pattern is an obsession of doubt, followed by a compulsion of checking. The obsession often implies some danger of violence (e.g., forgetting to turn off the stove or not locking a door). The checking may involve multiple trips back into the house to check the stove, for example. The patients have an obsessional self-doubt and always feel guilty about having forgotten or committed something.

Intrusive Thoughts. In the third most common pattern, there are intrusive obsessional thoughts without a compulsion. Such obsessions are usually repetitious thoughts of a sexual or aggressive act that is reprehensible to the patient. Patients obsessed with thoughts of aggressive or sexual acts may report themselves to police or confess to a priest.

Table 16.4–4
Reported Obsessions and Compulsions for 70 Consecutive Child and Adolescent Patients

Major Presenting Symptom	No. (%) Reporting Symptom at Initial Interview[a]
Obsession	
Concern or disgust with bodily wastes or secretions (urine, stool, saliva), dirt, germs, environmental toxins	30 (43)
Fear something terrible may happen (fire, death or illness of loved one, self, or others)	18 (24)
Concern or need for symmetry, order, or exactness	12 (17)
Scrupulosity (excessive praying or religious concerns out of keeping with patient's background)	9 (13)
Lucky and unlucky numbers	6 (8)
Forbidden or perverse sexual thoughts, images, or impulses	3 (4)
Intrusive nonsense sounds, words, or music	1 (1)
Compulsion	
Excessive or ritualized hand washing, showering, bathing, toothbrushing, or grooming	60 (85)
Repeating rituals (e.g., going in and out of door, up and down from chair)	36 (51)
Checking doors, locks, stove, appliances, car brakes	32 (46)
Cleaning and other rituals to remove contact with contaminants	16 (23)
Touching	14 (20)
Ordering and arranging	12 (17)
Measures to prevent harm to self or others (e.g., hanging clothes a certain way)	11 (16)
Counting	13 (18)
Hoarding and collecting	8 (11)
Miscellaneous rituals (e.g., licking, spitting, special dress pattern)	18 (26)

[a]Multiple symptoms recorded, so total exceeds 70.
Reprinted with permission from Rapoport JL. The neurobiology of obsessive-compulsive disorder. *JAMA.* 1988;260:2889.

Symmetry. The fourth most common pattern is the need for symmetry or precision, which can lead to a compulsion of slowness. Patients can literally take hours to eat a meal or shave their faces.

Other Symptom Patterns. Religious obsessions and compulsive hoarding are common in patients with OCD. Trichotillomania (compulsive hair pulling) and nail biting may be compulsions related to OCD.

Mental Status Examination

On mental status examinations, patients with OCD may show symptoms of depressive disorders. Such symptoms are present in about 50 percent of all patients. Some OCD patients have character traits suggesting obsessive-compulsive personality disorder (e.g., excessive need for preciseness and neatness), but most do not. Patients with OCD, especially men, have a higher than average celibacy rate. Married patients have a greater than usual amount of marital discord.

Ms. B. presented for psychiatric admission after being transferred from a medical floor where she had been treated for malnutrition. Ms. B. had been found unconscious in her apartment by a neighbor. When brought to the emergency room by ambulance, she was found to be hypotensive and hypokalemic. At psychiatric admission, Ms. B. described a long history of recurrent obsessions about cleanliness, particularly related to food items. She reported that it was difficult for her to eat any food unless she had washed it three to four times, since she often thought that a food item was dirty. She reported that washing her food decreased the anxiety she felt about the dirtiness of food. While Ms. B. reported that she occasionally tried to eat food that she did not wash (e.g., in a restaurant), she became so worried about contracting an illness from eating such food that she could no longer dine in restaurants. Ms. B. reported that her obsessions about the cleanliness of food had become so extreme over the past 3 months that she could eat very few foods, even if she washed them excessively. She recognized the irrational nature of these obsessive concerns but either could not bring herself to eat or became extremely nervous and nauseous after eating. (Courtesy of Daniel S. Pine, M.D.)

The DSM-IV-TR diagnostic requirement of personal distress and functional impairment differentiates OCD from ordinary or mildly excessive thoughts and habits.

DIFFERENTIAL DIAGNOSIS

Medical Conditions

The major neurological disorders to consider in the differential diagnosis are Tourette's disorder, other tic disorders, temporal lobe epilepsy, and, occasionally, trauma and postencephalitic complications.

Tourette's Disorder

The characteristic symptoms of Tourette's disorder are motor and vocal tics that occur frequently and virtually every day. Tourette's disorder and OCD have a similar age of onset and similar symptoms. About 90 percent of persons with Tourette's disorder have compulsive symptoms, and as many as two thirds meet the diagnostic criteria for OCD.

Other Psychiatric Conditions

The major psychiatric considerations in the differential diagnosis of OCD are schizophrenia, obsessive-compulsive personality disorder, phobias, and depressive disorders. OCD can usually be distinguished from schizophrenia by the absence of other schizophrenic symptoms, by the less bizarre nature of the symptoms, and by the patient's insight into the disorder. Obsessive-compulsive personality disorder does not have the degree of functional impairment associated with OCD. Phobias

are distinguished by the absence of a relation between obsessive thoughts and compulsions, usually a compulsion of avoidance. Major depressive disorder can sometimes be associated with obsessive ideas, but patients with only OCD fail to meet the diagnostic criteria for major depressive disorder.

Other psychiatric conditions that may be closely related to OCD are hypochondriasis, body dysmorphic disorder, and possibly other impulse-control disorders, such as kleptomania and pathological gambling. In all these disorders, patients have either a repetitious thought (e.g., concern about the body) or a repetitious behavior (e.g., stealing). Compulsive sexual behavior may bear a relation to OCD.

COURSE AND PROGNOSIS

More than half of patients with OCD have a sudden onset of symptoms. The onset of symptoms for about 50 to 70 percent of patients occurs after a stressful event, such as a pregnancy, a sexual problem, or the death of a relative. Because many persons manage to keep their symptoms secret, there is often a delay of 5 to 10 years before patients come to psychiatric attention, although the delay is probably shortening with increased awareness of the disorder. The course is usually long but variable; some patients experience a fluctuating course, and others experience a constant one.

About 20 to 30 percent of patients have significant improvement in their symptoms, and 40 to 50 percent have moderate improvement. The remaining 20 to 40 percent of patients either remain ill or their symptoms worsen.

About one third of patients with OCD have major depressive disorder, and suicide is a risk for all patients with OCD. A poor prognosis is indicated by yielding to (rather than resisting) compulsions, childhood onset, bizarre compulsions, the need for hospitalization, a coexisting major depressive disorder, delusional beliefs, the presence of overvalued ideas (i.e., some acceptance of obsessions and compulsions), and the presence of a personality disorder (especially schizotypal personality disorder). A good prognosis is indicated by good social and occupational adjustment, the presence of a precipitating event, and an episodic nature of the symptoms. The obsessional content does not seem to be related to the prognosis.

TREATMENT

With mounting evidence that OCD is largely determined by biological factors, classic psychoanalytic theory has fallen out of favor. Moreover, because OCD symptoms appear to be largely refractory to psychodynamic psychotherapy and psychoanalysis, pharmacological and behavioral treatments have become common. But psychodynamic factors may be of considerable benefit in understanding what precipitates exacerbations of the disorder and in treating various forms of resistance to treatment, such as noncompliance with medication.

Many patients with OCD tenaciously resist treatment efforts. They may refuse to take medication and may resist carrying out therapeutic homework assignments and other activities prescribed by behavior therapists. The obsessive-compulsive symptoms themselves, no matter how biologically based, may have important psychological meanings that make patients reluctant to give them up. Psychodynamic exploration of a patient's resistance to treatment may improve compliance.

Well-controlled studies have found that pharmacotherapy, behavior therapy, or a combination of both is effective in significantly reducing the symptoms of patients with OCD. The decision about which therapy to use is based on the clinician's judgment and experience and the patient's acceptance of the various modalities.

Pharmacotherapy

The efficacy of pharmacotherapy in OCD has been proved in many clinical trials and is enhanced by the observation that the studies find a placebo response rate of only about 5 percent.

The drugs, some of which are used to treat depressive disorders or other mental disorders, can be given in their usual dosage ranges. Initial effects are generally seen after 4 to 6 weeks of treatment, although 8 to 16 weeks are usually needed to obtain maximal therapeutic benefit. Treatment with antidepressant drugs is still controversial, and a significant proportion of patients with OCD who respond to treatment with antidepressant drugs seem to relapse if the drug therapy is discontinued.

The standard approach is to start treatment with an SSRI or clomipramine and then move to other pharmacological strategies if the serotonin-specific drugs are not effective. The serotonergic drugs have increased the percentage of patients with OCD who are likely to respond to treatment to the range of 50 to 70 percent.

Serotonin-Specific Reuptake Inhibitors. Each of the SSRIs available in the United States—fluoxetine (Prozac), fluvoxamine (Luvox), paroxetine (Paxil), sertraline (Zoloft)—has been approved by the Food and Drug Administration (FDA) for the treatment of OCD. Higher dosages have often been necessary for a beneficial effect, such as 80 mg a day of fluoxetine. Although the SSRIs may cause sleep disturbance, nausea and diarrhea, headache, anxiety, and restlessness, these adverse effects are often transient and are generally less troubling than the adverse effects associated with tricyclic drugs, such as clomipramine. The best clinical outcomes occur when SSRIs are used in combination with behavioral therapy.

Clomipramine. Of all the tricyclic and tetracyclic drugs, clomipramine is the most selective for serotonin reuptake versus norepinephrine reuptake and is exceeded in this respect only by the SSRIs. The potency of serotonin reuptake of clomipramine is exceeded only by sertraline and paroxetine. Clomipramine was the first drug to be FDA approved for the treatment of OCD. Its dosing must be titrated upward over 2 to 3 weeks to avoid gastrointestinal adverse effects and orthostatic hypotension, and like other tricyclic drugs, it causes significant sedation and anticholinergic effects, including dry mouth and constipation. As with SSRIs, the best outcomes result from a combination of drug and behavioral therapy.

Other Drugs. If treatment with clomipramine or an SSRI is unsuccessful, many therapists augment the first drug by the addition of valproate (Depakene), lithium (Eskalith), or carbamazepine (Tegretol). Other drugs that can be tried in the treatment of OCD are venlafaxine (Effexor), pindolol (Visken), and the monoamine oxidase inhibitors, especially phenelzine (Nardil). Other pharmacological agents for the treatment of

unresponsive patients include buspirone (BuSpar), 5-hydroxytryptamine (5-HT), L-tryptophan, and clonazepam (Klonopin).

Behavior Therapy

Although few head-to-head comparisons have been made, behavior therapy is as effective as pharmacotherapies in OCD, and some data indicate that the beneficial effects are longer lasting with behavior therapy. Therefore, many clinicians consider behavior therapy the treatment of choice for OCD. Behavior therapy can be conducted in both outpatient and inpatient settings. The principal behavioral approaches in OCD are exposure and response prevention. Desensitization, thought stopping, flooding, implosion therapy, and aversive conditioning have also been used in patients with OCD. In behavior therapy, patients must be truly committed to improvement.

Psychotherapy

In the absence of adequate studies of insight-oriented psychotherapy for OCD, any valid generalizations about its effectiveness are hard to make, although there are anecdotal reports of successes. Individual analysts have seen striking and lasting changes for the better in patients with obsessive-compulsive personality disorder, especially when they are able to come to terms with the aggressive impulses lying behind their character traits. Likewise, analysts and dynamically oriented psychiatrists have observed marked symptomatic improvement in patients with OCD in the course of analysis or prolonged insight psychotherapy.

Supportive psychotherapy undoubtedly has its place, especially for those OCD patients who, despite symptoms of varying degrees of severity, are able to work and make social adjustments. With continuous and regular contact with an interested, sympathetic, and encouraging professional person, patients may be able to function by virtue of this help, without which their symptoms would incapacitate them. Occasionally, when obsessional rituals and anxiety reach an intolerable intensity, it is necessary to hospitalize patients until the shelter of an institution and the removal from external environmental stresses diminish symptoms to a tolerable level.

A patient's family members are often driven to the verge of despair by the patient's behavior. Any psychotherapeutic endeavors must include attention to the family members through provision of emotional support, reassurance, explanation, and advice on how to manage and respond to the patient.

Other Therapies

Family therapy is often useful in supporting the family, helping reduce marital discord resulting from the disorder, and building a treatment alliance with the family members for the good of the patient. Group therapy is useful as a support system for some patients.

For extreme cases that are treatment resistant and chronically debilitating, electroconvulsive therapy (ECT) and psychosurgery may be considered. ECT is not as effective as psychosurgery, but it should be tried before surgery. The most common psychosurgical procedure for OCD is cingulotomy, which is successful in treating 25 to 30 percent of otherwise treatment-unresponsive patients. The most common complication of psychosurgery is the development of seizures, which are almost always controlled by treatment with phenytoin (Dilantin). Some patients who do not respond to psychosurgery alone and who did not respond to pharmacotherapy or behavior therapy before the operation do respond to pharmacotherapy or behavior therapy after psychosurgery.

References

Albert U, Maina G, Bogetto F. Obsessive-compulsive disorder (OCD) and triggering life events. *Eur J Psychiatry.* 2000;14(3):180.

Anthony MM, Swinson RP. Comparative and combined treatments for obsessive-compulsive disorder. In Sammons MT, Schmidt NB, eds. *Combined Treatment for Mental Disorders: A Guide to Psychological and Pharmacological Interventions.* Washington, DC: American Psychological Association; 2001:53.

Baxter LR, Schwartz JM, Bergman KS, et al. Caudate glucose metabolic rate changes with both drug and behavior therapy for obsessive-compulsive disorder. *Arch Gen Psychiatry.* 1992;49:681.

Black DW, Noyes R, Goldstein RB, Blum N. A family study of obsessive-compulsive disorder. *Arch Gen Psychiatry.* 1992;49:362.

Carter AS, Pollock RA. Obsessions and compulsions: the developmental and familial context. In: Sameroff AJ, Lewis M, et al., eds. *Handbook of Developmental Psychopathology.* 2nd ed. New York: Kluwer Academic/Plenum Publishers; 2000:549.

Fineberg NA, Bullock T, Montgomery DB, Montgomery SA. Serotonin reuptake inhibitors are the treatment of choice in obsessive compulsive disorder. *Int Clin Psychopharmacol.* 1992;7(suppl 1):43.

Franklin ME, Rynn M, March JS, Foa EB. Obsessive-compulsive disorder. In: Hersen M, ed. *Clinical Behavior Therapy: Adults and Children.* New York: John Wiley & Sons; 2002:276.

Gorman JM, section ed. Anxiety disorders. In: Sadock BJ, Sadock VA, eds. *Kaplan & Sadock's Comprehensive Textbook of Psychiatry.* 7th ed. Vol 1. Baltimore: Lippincott Williams & Wilkins; 2000:1441.

Greenberg BD, Murphy DL, Rasmussen SA. Neuroanatomically based approaches to obsessive-compulsive disorder: neurosurgery and transcranial magnetic stimulation. *Psychiatr Clin North Am.* 2000;23(3):671.

Hollander E, Kaplan A, Allen A, Cartwright C. Pharmacotherapy for obsessive-compulsive disorder. *Psychiatr Clin North Am.* 2000;23(3):643.

Insel TR. Toward a neuroanatomy of obsessive-compulsive disorder. *Arch Gen Psychiatry.* 1992;49:739.

Jenike MA, ed. Obsessional disorders. *Psychiatr Clin North Am.* 1992;15:743.

Matthew SJ, Simpson HB, Fallon BA. Treatment strategies for obsessive-compulsive disorder. *Psychiatr Ann.* 2000;30(11):699.

McDougle CJ, Gordman WK, Price LH. The pharmacotherapy of obsessive-compulsive disorder. *Pharmacopsychiatry.* 1993;26(suppl):24.

Micallef J, Blin O. Neurobiology and clinical pharmacology of obsessive-compulsive disorder. *Clin Neuropharmacol.* 2001;24(4):191.

Nelson E, Rice J. Stability of diagnosis of obsessive-compulsive disorder in the epidemiologic catchment area study. *Am J Psychiatry.* 1997;154:826.

Neziroglu F, Hsia C, Yaryura-Tobias JA. Behavioral, cognitive, and family therapy for obsessive-compulsive and related disorders. *Psychiatr Clin North Am.* 2000;23(3):657.

Pigott TA. OCD: where the serotonin selectivity story begins. *J Clin Psychiatry.* 1996;57(suppl 6):11.

Prather RC. Obsessive-compulsive disorder. In: Hersen M, Bellack AS, eds. *Psychopathology in Adulthood.* 2nd ed. Needham Heights, MA: Allyn & Bacon; 2000:232.

Saxena S, Bota RG, Brody AL. Brain-behavior relationships in obsessive-compulsive disorder. *Semin Clin Neuropsychiatry.* 2001;6(2):82. *Bull Menninger Clin* 2001;65(1):4.

Wolff M, Alsobrook JP II, Pauls DL. Genetic aspects of obsessive-compulsive disorder. *Psychiatr Clin North Am.* 2000;23(3):535.

▲ 16.5 Posttraumatic Stress Disorder and Acute Stress Disorder

Posttraumatic stress disorder (PTSD) is a syndrome that develops after a person sees, is involved in, or hears of an extreme traumatic stressor. The person reacts to this experience with fear and helplessness, persistently relives the event, and tries to avoid being reminded of it. To make the diagnosis, the symp-

toms must last for more than a month after the event and must significantly affect important areas of life such as family and work. The text revision of the fourth edition of *Diagnostic and Statistical Manual of Mental Disorders* (DSM-IV-TR) defines a disorder that is similar to PTSD called acute stress disorder, which occurs earlier than PTSD (within 4 weeks of the event) and remits within 2 days to 4 weeks. If symptoms persist after that time a diagnosis of PTSD is warranted.

The stressors causing both acute stress disorder and PTSD are overwhelming enough to affect almost anyone. They can arise from experiences in war, torture, natural catastrophes, assault, rape, and serious accidents, for example, in cars and in burning buildings. Persons reexperience the traumatic event in their dreams and their daily thoughts, they are determined to evade anything that would bring the event to mind, and they undergo a numbing of responsiveness along with a state of hyperarousal. Other symptoms are depression, anxiety, and cognitive difficulties such as poor concentration.

HISTORY

Because of the presence of autonomic cardiac symptoms, *soldier's heart* was the name given during the U.S. Civil War to a syndrome similar to PTSD. Jacob DaCosta's 1871 paper "On Irritable Heart," described soldiers with the syndrome. In the 1900s the influence of psychoanalysis was strong, particularly in the United States, and clinicians applied the diagnosis of traumatic neurosis to the condition. In World War I, the syndrome was called *shell shock* and was hypothesized to result from brain trauma caused by exploding shells. In 1941, the survivors of a fire in a crowded Boston nightclub, the Coconut Grove, showed increased nervousness, fatigue, and nightmares. World War II veterans, survivors of Nazi concentration camps, and survivors of the atomic bombings in Japan had similar symptoms, sometimes called *combat neurosis* or *operational fatigue.* The psychiatric morbidity associated with Vietnam War veterans finally brought the concept of *posttraumatic stress disorder,* as it is currently known, to fruition. In all these traumatic situations, the appearance of the disorder was roughly correlated with the severity of the stressor; the most severe stresses (e.g., incarceration in concentration camps) resulted in the occurrence of the syndrome in more than 75 percent of the victims.

EPIDEMIOLOGY

The lifetime prevalence of PTSD is estimated to be about 8 percent of the general population, although an additional 5 to 15 percent may experience subclinical forms of the disorder. Among high-risk groups whose members experienced traumatic events, the lifetime prevalence rates range from 5 to 75 percent. About 30 percent of Vietnam veterans experienced PTSD, and an additional 25 percent experienced subclinical forms of the disorder. The lifetime prevalence ranges from about 10 to 12 percent among women and 5 to 6 percent among men. Although PTSD can appear at any age, it is most prevalent in young adults, because they tend be more exposed to precipitating situations. Children can also have the disorder (discussed below). Men and women differ in the types of traumas to which they are exposed and their liability to develop PTSD. The lifetime prevalence is significantly higher in women, and a higher proportion of women go on to develop the disorder. Historically, men's trauma was usually combat experience, and women's trauma was most commonly assault or rape. The disorder is most likely to occur in those who are single, divorced, widowed, socially withdrawn, or of low socioeconomic level. The most important risk factors, however, for this disorder are the severity, duration, and proximity of a person's exposure to the actual trauma. There seems to be a familial pattern for this disorder, and first-degree biological relatives of persons with a history of depression have an increased risk for developing PTSD following a traumatic event.

COMORBIDITY

Comorbidity rates are high among patients with PTSD, with about two thirds having at least two other disorders. Common comorbid conditions include depressive disorders, substance-related disorders, other anxiety disorders, and bipolar disorders. Comorbid disorders make persons more vulnerable to developing PTSD.

ETIOLOGY

Stressor

By definition, the *stressor* is the prime causative factor in the development of PTSD. However, not everyone experiences the disorder after a traumatic event. The stressor alone does not suffice to cause the disorder. Clinicians must also consider individual preexisting biological and psychosocial factors and events that happened before and after the trauma. For example, a member of a group who lived through a disaster can sometimes deal with trauma because others shared the experience. The stressor's subjective meaning to a person is also important. For example, survivors of a catastrophe may experience guilt feelings (*survivor guilt*) that can predispose to, or exacerbate, PTSD.

Risk Factors

As mentioned above, even when faced with overwhelming trauma, most persons do not experience PTSD symptoms. The National Comorbidity Study found that 60 percent of males and 50 percent of females had experienced some significant trauma, while the reported lifetime prevalence of PTSD was only 6.7 percent. Similarly, events that may appear mundane or less than catastrophic to most persons may produce PTSD in some. Table 16.5–1 summarizes vulnerability factors that appear to play etiological roles in the disorder.

Table 16.5–1
Predisposing Vulnerability Factors in Posttraumatic Stress Disorder

Presence of childhood trauma
Borderline, paranoid, dependent, or antisocial personality disorder traits
Inadequate family or peer support system
Being female
Genetic vulnerability to psychiatric illness
Recent stressful life changes
Perception of an external locus of control (natural cause) rather than an internal one (human cause)
Recent excessive alcohol intake

Table 16.5–2
Psychodynamic Themes in Posttraumatic Stress Disorder

- The subjective meaning of a stressor may determine its traumatogenicity.
- Traumatic events may resonate with childhood traumas.
- Inability to regulate affect may result from trauma.
- Somatization and alexithymia may be among the aftereffects of trauma.
- Common defenses used include denial, minimization, splitting, projective disavowal, dissociation, and guilt (as a defense against underlying helplessness).
- Mode of object relatedness involves projection and introjection of the following roles: omnipotent rescuer, abuser, and victim.

Psychodynamic Factors

The psychoanalytic model of the disorder hypothesizes that the trauma has reactivated a previously quiescent, yet unresolved psychological conflict. The revival of the childhood trauma results in regression and the use of the defense mechanisms of repression, denial, reaction formation, and undoing. According to Freud, a splitting of consciousness occurs in patients who reported a history of childhood sexual trauma. A preexisting conflict might be symbolically reawakened by the new traumatic event. The ego relives and thereby tries to master and reduce the anxiety. Psychodynamic themes in PTSD are summarized in Table 16.5–2. Persons who suffer from alexithymia, the inability to identify or verbalize feeling states, are incapable of soothing themselves when under stress.

Cognitive-Behavioral Factors

The cognitive model of PTSD posits that affected persons cannot process or rationalize the trauma that precipitated the disorder. They continue to experience the stress and attempt to avoid experiencing it by avoidance techniques. Consistent with their partial ability to cope cognitively with the event, persons experience alternating periods of acknowledging and blocking the event. The attempt of the brain to process the massive amount of information provoked by the trauma is thought to produce these alternating periods. The behavioral model of PTSD emphasizes two phases in its development. First, the trauma (the unconditioned stimulus) that produces a fear response is paired, through classical conditioning, with a conditioned stimulus (physical or mental reminders of the trauma, such as sights, smells, or sounds). Second, through instrumental learning, the conditioned stimuli elicit the fear response independent of the original unconditioned stimulus, and persons develop a pattern of avoiding both the conditioned stimulus and the unconditioned stimulus. Some persons also receive secondary gains from the external world, commonly monetary compensation, increased attention or sympathy, and the satisfaction of dependency needs. These gains reinforce the disorder and its persistence.

Biological Factors

The biological theories of PTSD have developed from both preclinical studies of animal models of stress and from measures of biological variables in clinical populations with the disorder. Many neurotransmitter systems have been implicated by both sets of data. Preclinical models of learned helplessness, kindling, and sensitization in animals have led to theories about norepinephrine, dopamine, endogenous opioids, and benzodiazepine receptors and the hypothalamic-pituitary-adrenal (HPA) axis. In clinical populations, data have supported hypotheses that the noradrenergic and endogenous opiate systems, as well as the HPA axis, are hyperactive in at least some patients with PTSD. Other major biological findings are increased activity and responsiveness of the autonomic nervous system, as evidenced by elevated heart rates and blood pressure readings and by abnormal sleep architecture (e.g., sleep fragmentation and increased sleep latency). Some researchers have suggested a similarity between PTSD and two other psychiatric disorders, major depressive disorder and panic disorder.

NORADRENERGIC SYSTEM. Soldiers with PTSD-like symptoms exhibit nervousness, increased blood pressure and heart rate, palpitations, sweating, flushing, and tremors—symptoms associated with adrenergic drugs. Studies found increased 24-hour urine epinephrine concentrations in veterans with PTSD and increased urine catecholamine concentrations in sexually abused girls. Further, platelet α_2- and lymphocyte β-adrenergic receptors are downregulated in PTSD, possibly in response to chronically elevated catecholamine concentrations. About 30 to 40 percent of PTSD patients report flashbacks after yohimbine (Yocon) administration. Such findings are strong evidence for altered function in the noradrenergic system in PTSD.

OPIOID SYSTEM. Abnormality in the opioid system is suggested by low plasma beta-endorphin concentrations in PTSD. Combat veterans with PTSD demonstrate a naloxone (Narcan)-reversible analgesic response to combat-related stimuli, raising the possibility of opioid system hyperregulation similar to that in the HPA axis. One study showed that nalmefene (Revex), an opioid receptor antagonist, was of use in reducing symptoms of PTSD in combat veterans.

CORTICOTROPIN-RELEASING FACTOR (CRF) AND THE HPA AXIS. Several factors point to dysfunction of the HPA axis. Studies have demonstrated low plasma and urinary free cortisol concentrations in PTSD. There are more glucocorticoid receptors on lymphocytes, and challenge with exogenous CRF yields a blunted ACTH response. Further, suppression of cortisol by challenge with low-dose dexamethasone (Decadron) is enhanced in PTSD. This indicates hyperregulation of the HPA axis in PTSD. Also, some studies have revealed cortisol hypersuppression in trauma-exposed patients who develop PTSD, compared with patients exposed to trauma who do not develop PTSD, indicating that it might be specifically associated with PTSD and not just trauma. Overall, this hyperregulation of the HPA axis differs from the neuroendocrine activity usually seen during stress and in other disorders such as depression. Recently, the role of the hippocampus in PTSD has received increased attention, although the issue remains controversial. Animal studies have shown that stress is associated with structural changes in the hippocampus, and studies of combat veterans with PTSD have revealed lower average volume in the hippocampal region of the brain. Furthermore, researchers suggest that the hippocampus is not necessarily the only area of the

Table 16.5–3
DSM-IV-TR Diagnostic Criteria for Posttraumatic Stress Disorder

A. The person has been exposed to a traumatic event in which both of the following were present:
  (1) the person experienced, witnessed, or was confronted with an event or events that involved actual or threatened death or serious injury, or a threat to the physical integrity of self or others
  (2) the person's response involved intense fear, helplessness, or horror. **Note:** In children, this may be expressed instead by disorganized or agitated behavior

B. The traumatic event is persistently reexperienced in one (or more) of the following ways:
  (1) recurrent and intrusive distressing recollections of the event, including images, thoughts, or perceptions. **Note:** In young children, repetitive play may occur in which themes or aspects of the trauma are expressed.
  (2) recurrent distressing dreams of the event. **Note:** In children, there may be frightening dreams without recognizable content.
  (3) acting or feeling as if the traumatic event were recurring (includes a sense of reliving the experience, illusions, hallucinations, and dissociative flashback episodes, including those that occur on awakening or when intoxicated). **Note:** In young children, trauma-specific reenactment may occur.
  (4) intense psychological distress at exposure to internal or external cues that symbolize or resemble an aspect of the traumatic event
  (5) physiological reactivity on exposure to internal or external cues that symbolize or resemble an aspect of the traumatic event

C. Persistent avoidance of stimuli associated with the trauma and numbing of general responsiveness (not present before the trauma), as indicated by three (or more) of the following:
  (1) efforts to avoid thoughts, feelings, or conversations associated with the trauma
  (2) efforts to avoid activities, places, or people that arouse recollections of the trauma
  (3) inability to recall an important aspect of the trauma
  (4) markedly diminished interest or participation in significant activities
  (5) feeling of detachment or estrangement from others
  (6) restricted range of affect (e.g., unable to have loving feelings)
  (7) sense of a foreshortened future (e.g., does not expect to have a career, marriage, children, or a normal life span)

D. Persistent symptoms of increased arousal (not present before the trauma), as indicated by two (or more) of the following:
  (1) difficulty falling or staying asleep
  (2) irritability or outbursts of anger
  (3) difficulty concentrating
  (4) hypervigilance
  (5) exaggerated startle response

E. Duration of the disturbance (symptoms in Criteria B, C, and D) is more than 1 month.

F. The disturbance causes clinically significant distress or impairment in social, occupational, or other important areas of functioning.

Specify if:
  Acute: if duration of symptoms is less than 3 months
  Chronic: if duration of symptoms is 3 months or more

Specify if:
  With delayed onset: if onset of symptoms is at least 6 months after the stressor

From American Psychiatric Association. *Diagnostic and Statistical Manual of Mental Disorders.* 4th ed. Text rev. Washington, DC: American Psychiatric Association; copyright 2000, with permission.

brain to show structural changes in PTSD, since studies on depression have shown similar effects in the amygdala and prefrontal cortex.

DIAGNOSIS

The DSM-IV-TR diagnostic criteria for PTSD (Table 16.5–3) specify that the symptoms of experiencing, avoidance, and hyperarousal must have lasted more than 1 month. For patients whose symptoms have been present less than 1 month, the appropriate diagnosis may be acute stress disorder (Table 16.5–4). The

Table 16.5–4
DSM-IV-TR Diagnostic Criteria for Acute Stress Disorder

A. The person has been exposed to a traumatic event in which both of the following were present:
  (1) the person experienced, witnessed, or was confronted with an event or events that involved actual or threatened death or serious injury, or a threat to the physical integrity of self or others
  (2) the person's response involved intense fear, helplessness, or horror

B. Either while experiencing or after experiencing the distressing event, the individual has three (or more) of the following dissociative symptoms:
  (1) a subjective sense of numbing, detachment, or absence of emotional responsiveness
  (2) a reduction in awareness of his or her surroundings (e.g., "being in a daze")
  (3) derealization
  (4) depersonalization
  (5) dissociative amnesia (i.e., inability to recall an important aspect of the trauma)

C. The traumatic event is persistently reexperienced in at least one of the following ways: recurrent images, thoughts, dreams, illusions, flashback episodes, or a sense of reliving the experience; or distress on exposure to reminders of the traumatic event.

D. Marked avoidance of stimuli that arouse recollections of the trauma (e.g., thoughts, feelings, conversations, activities, places, people).

E. Marked symptoms of anxiety or increased arousal (e.g., difficulty sleeping, irritability, poor concentration, hypervigilance, exaggerated startle response, motor restlessness).

F. The disturbance causes clinically significant distress or impairment in social, occupational, or other important areas of functioning or impairs the individual's ability to pursue some necessary task, such as obtaining necessary assistance or mobilizing personal resources by telling family members about the traumatic experience.

G. The disturbance lasts for a minimum of 2 days and a maximum of 4 weeks and occurs within 4 weeks of the traumatic event.

H. The disturbance is not due to the direct physiological effects of a substance (e.g., a drug of abuse, a medication) or a general medical condition, is not better accounted for by brief psychotic disorder, and is not merely an exacerbation of a preexisting Axis I or Axis II disorder.

From American Psychiatric Association. *Diagnostic and Statistical Manual of Mental Disorders.* 4th ed. Text rev. Washington, DC: American Psychiatric Association; copyright 2000, with permission.

DSM-IV-TR diagnostic criteria for PTSD allow clinicians to specify whether the disorder is acute (if the symptoms have lasted less than 3 months) or chronic (if the symptoms have lasted 3 months or more). DSM-IV-TR also allows clinicians to specify that the disorder was with delayed onset if the onset of the symptoms was 6 months or more after the stressful event. An example of an acute stress disorder not progressing to PTSD as a result of timely therapy is given in the following vignette.

A 40-year-old man saw the September 11, 2001, terrorist attack on the World Trade Center (discussed below) on television. Immediately thereafter he developed feelings of panic associated with thoughts that he was going to die. The panic disappeared within a few hours; however, for the next few nights he had nightmares with obsessive thoughts about dying. He sought consultation and reported to the psychiatrist that his wife had been killed in a plane crash 10 years earlier. He described having adapted to the loss "normally" and was aware that his current symptoms were probably related to that traumatic event. On further exploration in brief psychotherapy, he realized that his reactions to his wife's death were muted and that his relationship with her was ambivalent. At the time of her death he was contemplating divorce and frequently had wished her dead. He had never fully worked through the mourning process for his wife, and his catastrophic reaction to the terrorist attack was, in part, related to those suppressed feelings. He was able to recognize his feelings of guilt related to his wife and his need for punishment manifested by thinking he was going to die.

CLINICAL FEATURES

The principal clinical features of PTSD are painful reexperiencing of the event, a pattern of avoidance and emotional numbing, and fairly constant hyperarousal. The disorder may not develop until months or even years after the event. The mental status examination often reveals feelings of guilt, rejection, and humiliation. Patients may also describe dissociative states and panic attacks, and illusions and hallucinations may be present. Associated symptoms can include aggression, violence, poor impulse control, depression, and substance-related disorders. Cognitive testing may reveal that patients have impaired memory and attention. Patients have elevated Sc, D, F, and Ps scores on the Minnesota Multiphasic Personality Inventory, and the Rorschach test findings often include aggressive and violent material.

Mr. F. sought treatment for symptoms that he developed in the wake of an automobile accident that had occurred about 6 weeks prior to his psychiatric evaluation. While driving to work on a mid-January morning, Mr. F. lost control of his car on an icy road. His car swerved out of control into oncoming traffic in another lane, collided with another car, and then hit a nearby pedestrian. Mr. F. was trapped in his car for 3 hours while rescue workers cut the door of his car. Upon referral, Mr. F. reported frequent intrusive thoughts about the accident, including nightmares of the event and recurrent intrusive visions of his car slamming into the pedestrian. He reported that he had altered his driving route to work to avoid the scene of the accident, and he found himself switching the television channel whenever a commercial for snow tires appeared. Mr. F. described frequent difficulty falling asleep, poor concentration, and an increased focus on his environment, particularly when he was driving.

Posttraumatic Stress Disorders in Children and Adolescents

PTSD occurs in children and adolescents but most studies of the disorder have focused on adults. DSM-IV-TR has little to say about PTSD as it effects young children except to describe symptoms such as repetitive dreams of the event, nightmares of monsters, and the development of physical symptoms such as stomachaches and headaches.

High rates of PTSD have been documented in children exposed to such life-threatening events as combat and other war-related trauma, kidnapping, severe illness or burns, bone marrow transplantation, and a number of natural and man-made disasters. Studies on young victims or witness to criminal assault, domestic violence, and community violence have revealed high psychiatric morbidity following exposure to violence. As might be expected, the prevalence of PTSD is higher in children than in adults exposed to the same stressor. In certain situations up to 90 percent of children will develop the disorder. In general PTSD has been underestimated in children and adolescents.

Child risk factors include demographic factors (e.g., age, sex, socioeconomic status), other life events (positive and negative), social and cultural cognitions, psychiatric comorbidity, and inherent coping strategies. Family factors (e.g., parental psychopathology and functioning, marital status, and education) play key roles in determining child symptoms. Parents' response to traumatic events particularly influence young children who may not completely understand the nature of the trauma or its inherent danger.

Stressor. Stressors in children may be sudden, single-incident trauma or ongoing or chronic trauma such as physical or sexual abuse. Children also suffer as the result of "indirect" exposure—that is, the unwitnessed death or injury of a loved one, as in situations of disaster, war, or community violence.

Reenactment and Reexperiencing. Children, like adults, reexperience the traumatic event in the form of distressing, intrusive thoughts or memories, flashbacks, and dreams. Children's nightmares may be linked specifically to a trauma theme or may generalize to other fears. Flashbacks occur in children as well as in their adolescent or adult victim counterparts. "Traumatic play," a specific form of reexperiencing seen in young children, consists of repetitive acting out of the trauma or trauma-related themes in play. Older children may incorporate aspects of the trauma into their lives in a process termed *reenactment.* Fantasized actions of intervention or revenge are common; adolescents should be considered at increased risk for

impulsive acting out secondary to anger and revenge fantasies. Related behaviors in child and adolescent victims of trauma include sexual acting out, substance use, and delinquency. Children often withdraw and show reduced interest in previously enjoyable activities. Regressive behaviors such as enuresis or fear of sleeping alone may also occur.

Gulf War Syndrome

In the Persian Gulf War against Iraq, which began in 1990 and ended in 1991, approximately 700,000 American soldiers served in the coalition forces. Although morbidity and mortality rates were minimal in comparison to previous wars, on their return, more than 100,000 U.S. veterans reported a vast array of health problems, including irritability, chronic fatigue, shortness of breath, muscle and joint pain, migraine headaches, digestive disturbances, rash, hair loss, forgetfulness, and difficulty concentrating. Collectively, these symptoms are called the Gulf War syndrome, but no government agency has identified the cause of these symptoms. Many veterans believe that their disorders were caused by exposure to biological and chemical agents such as fumes from burning oil wells and landfills or mustard and other nerve gases. The U.S. Department of Defense acknowledges that up to 20,000 troops serving in the combat area may have been exposed to chemical weapons but denies that those complaining of the syndrome are suffering from the effects of chemical exposure. The best evidence indicates that the condition is a disorder that in some cases may have been precipitated by exposure to an unidentified toxin (Table 16.5–5). One recent study of loss of memory found structural change in the right parietal lobe in 18 men with Gulf War syndrome with use of magnetic resonance spectroscopy. Such brain abnormalities have been found to correlate with specific clinical symptoms. New data show that damage to the basal ganglia and subsequent neurotransmitter dysfunction in veterans of the Gulf War may provide a neurological basis for this syndrome. A significant number of veterans have developed amyotrophic lateral sclerosis (ALS), thought to be the result of genetic mutations.

Several studies have found higher rates of physical complaints and psychological distress in veterans who were stationed in the Persian Gulf region than in those who were deployed to Germany or the United States during the war, even after controlling for the demographic effects. This, however, may also be due to toxins in the region and not simply the stress. PTSD (and its related symptoms) is a well-documented condition that occurs in wartime. It was first identified after the Civil War (Table 16.5–6) and has been noted in every war thereafter, although by different names. Yet many studies of Gulf War veterans have found lower rates of PTSD than were found among veterans of previous wars, which may lend some support to the notion of a separate syndrome. Likewise, however, some patients may in fact have treatable mood and anxiety disorders that are not diagnosed because their symptoms are primarily somatic.

Claims submitted by Gulf War veterans seeking disability payments from the U.S. Department of Veterans Affairs for this syndrome have been denied in over 90 percent of cases. Studies are ongoing to clarify the situation, but the morale of thousands of afflicted Gulf War veterans has seriously eroded, and confidence in the Department of Defense's concerns for illness among U.S. soldiers has been compromised among the public as a result. The Defense Department did agree to pay compensation to veterans who developed ALS.

In a 1997 editorial in the *Journal of the American Medical Association*, the relationship of the Persian Gulf War syndrome and stress was stated as follows:

> Physicians need to acknowledge that many Gulf War veterans are experiencing stress-related disorders and the physical consequences of

Table 16.5–5
Syndromes Associated with Toxic Exposure[a]

Syndrome	Characteristics	Possible Toxins
1	Impaired cognition	Insect repellant containing *N,N'*-diethyl-*m*-toluamide (DEET[b]) absorbed through skin
2	Confusion-ataxia	Exposure to chemical weapons, e.g., sarin
3	Arthromyoneuropathy	Insect repellant containing DEET[b] in combination with oral pyridostigmine[c]

[a]The three syndromes involve a relatively small group (*N* = 249) of veterans and are based on self-reported descriptions and selection. Data are from R. W. Haley and T. L. Kurt.
[b]DEET is a carbonate compound used as an insect repellant. Concentrations above 30 percent DEET are neurotoxic in children. The military repellant contained 75 percent. (DEET is available in 100 percent concentrations as an unregulated over-the-counter preparation usually sold in sports stores.)
[c]Most U.S. troops took low-dose pyridostigmine (Mestinon, 30 mg every 8 hours) for about 5 days in 1991 to protect against exposure to the nerve agent soman.

Table 16.5–6
Eponyms and Symptoms of Posttraumatic Stress Disorders in Various U.S. Wars

War	Disorder
Civil War	"Irritable heart": fatigue, shortness of breath, palpitations, headache, excessive sweating, dizziness, disturbed sleep, fainting
World War I	"Effort syndrome": fatigue, shortness of breath, palpitations, headache, excessive sweating, dizziness, disturbed sleep, fainting, difficulty concentrating
World War II	"Combat stress reaction": fatigue, shortness of breath, palpitations, headache, excessive sweating, dizziness, disturbed sleep, fainting, difficulty concentrating, forgetfulness
Vietnam War	"Posttraumatic stress disorder": fatigue, shortness of breath, palpitations, headache, muscle and joint pain, dizziness, disturbed sleep, difficulty concentrating, forgetfulness
Gulf War	"Gulf War syndrome": fatigue, shortness of breath, headache, muscle and joint pain, disturbed sleep, difficulty concentrating, forgetfulness

Adapted from Hymans KC, Wignall FS, Roswell P. War, syndromes and their evaluation: from the US Civil War to the Persian Gulf War. *Ann Intern Med.* 1996;125:398.

stress. These conditions should not be hidden or denied, but rather are well-recognized entities that have been studied extensively in survivors of past wars, most notably the Vietnam conflict. As physicians, we should not accept a diagnosis of stress-related disorder in veterans prior to excluding treatable physical factors, but at the same time, we need to recognize the pervasive presence of stress-related illness such as hypertension, fibromyalgia, and chronic fatigue among Persian Gulf War veterans and manage these illnesses appropriately. As a nation, we need to get beyond the fallacious idea that diseases of the mind either are not real or are shameful and to better recognize that the mind and the body are inextricably linked.

Torture

The intentional physical and psychological torture of one human by another can have emotionally damaging effects comparable to, and possibly worse than, those seen with combat and other types of trauma. As defined by the United Nations, torture is any deliberate infliction of severe mental pain or suffering, usually through cruel, inhuman, or degrading treatment or punishment. This broad definition includes various forms of interpersonal violence, from chronic domestic abuse to broad-scale genocide. According to Amnesty International, torture is common and widespread in most of the 150 countries worldwide where human rights violations have been documented. Recent figures estimate that between 5 and 35 percent of the world's 14 million refugees have had at least one torture experience, and these numbers do not even account for the consequences of the current political, regional, and religious disputes in Eastern Europe, the former Yugoslavia, and the Middle East.

Torture is distinct from most other types of trauma because it is human inflicted and intentional. One individual working for himself or for a higher authority may abuse another to punish, exact retribution, or obtain information from the victim. Methods can be physical (e.g., beatings, burning of the skin, electric shock, or asphyxiation) or psychological, through threats, humiliation, or being forced to watch others, often loved ones, being tortured. One distinct method of torture that may combine physical and psychological aspects is brainwashing (see section below). While many forms of torture can leave lasting physical scars, which themselves serve as constant reminders of the trauma, it seems that the true purpose is the psychological effect—the torturer invokes fear, helplessness, and, ultimately, physical and mental weakness in the victim. Reported prevalence rates of PTSD among survivors of torture are about 36 percent, much higher than the average lifetime prevalence, and researchers concur that the severity and duration of PTSD may be greater when the stressors are of human design. Studies have also revealed substantial comorbidity with depression and other anxiety disorders in victims of torture. Other common psychological complaints include somatization, obsessive-compulsive symptoms, anger-hostility, phobias, paranoid ideation, and psychotic episodes.

Treatment methods for survivors of torture are the same as those for other posttraumatic symptoms and disorders, but clinicians must be especially sensitive to the array of stressful life events that victims of torture have experienced. Many survivors who present for treatment are refugees who face new post-trauma stressors over and above the effects of torture, such as separation from family, difficulty finding work, difficulty obtaining health services, language barriers, loneliness, poverty, and racial discrimination. Religious faith, political education and commitment, strong social support, and mental preparedness for the possibility of torture seem to serve as protective factors against developing PTSD and other psychological consequences after torture. Moreover, cultural and religious factors that influence coping styles may also affect treatment response in survivors of torture.

Brainwashing

First practiced by the Chinese Communists on U.S. prisoners during the Korean War, brainwashing is the deliberate creation of cultural shock. A condition of isolation, alienation, and intimidation is developed for the express purpose of assaulting ego strengths and leaving the person to be brainwashed vulnerable to the imposition of alien ideas and behavior that would usually be rejected. Brainwashing relies on both mental and physical coercion. All persons are vulnerable to brainwashing if they are exposed to it long enough, if they are alone and without support, and if they are without hope of escape from the situation. Whether or not the psychological effects are permanent likely depends on the individual's strength of character and subsequent environment and support system. Help from the mental health care system, in the form of deprogramming, is usually necessary to help brainwashed persons readjust to their usual environments after the brainwashing experience. Supportive therapy is offered, with emphasis on reeducation, restitution of ego strengths that existed before the trauma, and alleviation of the guilt and depression that are remnants of the frightening experience and the lost confidence and confusion in identity that result from it.

DIFFERENTIAL DIAGNOSIS

A major consideration in the diagnosis of PTSD is the possibility that the patient also incurred a head injury during the trauma. Other organic considerations that can both cause and exacerbate the symptoms are epilepsy, alcohol use disorders, and other substance-related disorders. Acute intoxication or withdrawal from some substances may also present a clinical picture that is difficult to distinguish from the disorder until the effects of the substance have worn off.

PTSD is commonly misdiagnosed as another mental disorder and is then inappropriately treated. Clinicians must consider the diagnosis of PTSD in patients who have pain disorder, substance abuse, other anxiety disorders, and mood disorders. In general, PTSD can be distinguished from other mental disorders by interviewing a patient about previous traumatic experiences and by the nature of the current symptoms. Borderline personality disorder, dissociative disorders, factitious disorders, and malingering should also be considered. Borderline personality disorder can be difficult to distinguish from PTSD. The two disorders may coexist or even be causally related. Patients with dissociative disorders do not usually have the degree of avoidance behavior, the autonomic hyperarousal, or the history of trauma that patients with PTSD report. Partly because of the publicity that PTSD has received, clinicians should also consider the possibility of a factitious disorder and malingering.

COURSE AND PROGNOSIS

PTSD usually develops some time after the trauma. The delay can be as short as 1 week or as long as 30 years. Symptoms can fluctuate over time and may be most intense during periods of stress. Untreated, about 30 percent of patients recover completely, 40 percent continue to have mild symptoms, 20 percent continue to have moderate symptoms, and 10 percent remain unchanged or become worse. After 1 year, about 50 percent of patients will recover. A good prognosis is predicted by rapid onset of the symptoms, short duration of the symptoms (less than 6 months), good premorbid functioning, strong social supports, and the absence of other psychiatric, medical, or substance-related disorders or other risk factors.

In general, the very young and the very old have more difficulty with traumatic events than do those in midlife. For example, about 80 percent of young children who sustain a burn injury show symptoms of PTSD 1 or 2 years after the initial injury; only 30 percent of adults who suffer such an injury have a PTSD after 1 year. Presumably, young children do not yet have adequate coping mechanisms to deal with the physical and emotional insults of the trauma. Likewise, older persons are likely to have more rigid coping mechanisms than younger adults and to be less able to muster a flexible approach to dealing with the effects of trauma. Furthermore, the traumatic effects may be exacerbated by physical disabilities characteristic of late life, particularly disabilities of the nervous system and the cardiovascular system such as reduced cerebral blood flow, failing vision, palpitations, and arrhythmias. Preexisting psychiatric disability, whether a personality disorder or a more serious condition, also increases the effects of particular stressors. PTSD that is comorbid with other disorders is often more severe and perhaps more chronic and may be difficult to treat. The availability of social supports may also influence the development, severity, and duration of PTSD. In general, patients who have a good network of social support are less likely to have the disorder, are less likely to experience it in its severe forms, and are more likely to recover faster.

TREATMENT

When a clinician is faced with a patient who has experienced a significant trauma, the major approaches are support, encouragement to discuss the event, and education about a variety of coping mechanisms (e.g., relaxation). The use of sedatives and hypnotics can also be helpful. When a patient experienced a traumatic event in the past and now has PTSD, the emphasis should be on education about the disorder and its treatment, both pharmacological and psychotherapeutic. The clinician should also work to destigmatize the notion of mental illness and PTSD. Additional support for the patient and the family can be obtained through local and national support groups for patients with PTSD.

Pharmacotherapy

Selective serotonin reuptake inhibitors (SSRIs), such as sertraline (Zoloft) and paroxetine (Paxil), are considered first-line treatments for PTSD owing to their efficacy, tolerability, and safety ratings. SSRIs reduce symptoms from all PTSD symptom clusters and are effective in improving symptoms unique to PTSD, not just symptoms similar to those of depression or other anxiety disorders. Buspirone (BuSpar) is serotonergic and may also be of use.

The efficacy of imipramine (Tofranil) and amitriptyline (Elavil), two tricyclic drugs, in the treatment of PTSD is supported by a number of well-controlled clinical trials. Although some trials of the two drugs have had negative findings, most of these trials had serious design flaws, including too short a duration. Dosages of imipramine and amitriptyline should be the same as those used to treat depressive disorders, and an adequate trial should last at least 8 weeks. Patients who respond well should probably continue the pharmacotherapy for at least 1 year before an attempt is made to withdraw the drug. Some studies indicate that pharmacotherapy is more effective in treating the depression, anxiety, and hyperarousal than in treating the avoidance, denial, and emotional numbing.

Other drugs that may be useful in the treatment of PTSD include the monoamine oxidase inhibitors (e.g., phenelzine [Nardil]), trazodone (Desyrel), and the anticonvulsants (e.g., carbamazepine [Tegretol], valproate [Depakene]). Some studies have also revealed improvement in PTSD in patients treated with reversible monoamine oxidase inhibitors (RIMAs). Use of clonidine (Catapres) and propranolol (Inderal), which are antiadrenergic agents, is suggested by the theories about noradrenergic hyperactivity in the disorder. Almost no positive data concern the use of antipsychotic drugs in the disorder, so the use of drugs such as haloperidol (Haldol) should be reserved for the short-term control of severe aggression and agitation.

Psychotherapy

Psychodynamic psychotherapy may be useful in the treatment of many patients with PTSD. In some cases, reconstruction of the traumatic events with associated abreaction and catharsis may be therapeutic, but psychotherapy must be individualized because reexperiencing the trauma overwhelms some patients.

Psychotherapeutic interventions for PTSD include behavior therapy, cognitive therapy, and hypnosis. Many clinicians advocate time-limited psychotherapy for the victims of trauma. Such therapy usually takes a cognitive approach and also provides support and security. The short-term nature of the psychotherapy minimizes the risk of dependence and chronicity, but issues of suspicion, paranoia, and trust often adversely affect compliance. Therapists should overcome patients' denial of the traumatic event, encourage them to relax, and remove them from the source of the stress. Patients should be encouraged to sleep, using medication if necessary. Support from persons in their environment (such as friends and relatives) should be provided. Patients should be encouraged to review and abreact emotional feelings associated with the traumatic event and to plan for future recovery. Abreaction—experiencing the emotions associated with the event—may be helpful for some patients. The amobarbital (Amytal) interview has been used to facilitate this process.

Psychotherapy after a traumatic event should follow a model of crisis intervention with support, education, and the development of coping mechanisms and acceptance of the event. When PTSD has developed, two major psychotherapeutic approaches can be taken. The first is exposure therapy, in which the patient reexperiences the traumatic event through imaging techniques or in vivo exposure. The exposures can be intense, as in implosive therapy, or graded,

as in systematic desensitization. The second approach is to teach the patient methods of stress management, including relaxation techniques and cognitive approaches to coping with stress. Some preliminary data indicate that although stress management techniques are effective more rapidly than exposure techniques, the results of exposure techniques last longer.

Another psychotherapeutic technique that is relatively novel and somewhat controversial is eye movement desensitization and reprocessing (EMDR), in which the patient focuses on the lateral movement of the clinician's finger while maintaining a mental image of the trauma experience. The general belief is that symptoms can be relieved as patients work through the traumatic event while in a state of deep relaxation. Proponents of this treatment state it is as effective, and possibly more effective, than other treatments for PTSD and that it is preferred by both clinicians and patients who have tried it.

In addition to individual therapy techniques, group therapy and family therapy have been reported to be effective in cases of PTSD. The advantages of group therapy include sharing of traumatic experiences and support from other group members. Group therapy has been particularly successful with Vietnam veterans and survivors of catastrophic disasters such as earthquakes. Family therapy often helps sustain a marriage through periods of exacerbated symptoms. Hospitalization may be necessary when symptoms are particularly severe or when there is a risk of suicide or other violence.

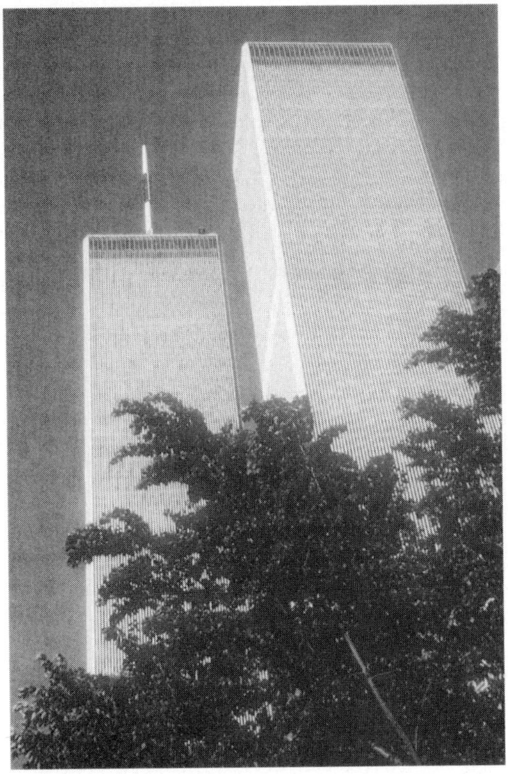

FIGURE 16.5–1
The World Trade Center, New York City, prior to 9/11/01. (Courtesy of Kimsamoon, Inc.)

Special Considerations

The terrorist activity of September 11, 2001, in which the World Trade Center (Fig. 16.5–1) in New York City and the Pentagon in Washington were destroyed and damaged, respectively, resulting in over 3,500 deaths and injuries, traumatized a nation, and many citizens required therapeutic intervention. A national survey of over 500 U.S. adults, taken less than one month after the event to assess their reactions and their children's reactions to the terrorist attacks, found evidence of psychologic sequelae.

Forty-five percent of adults reported one or more substantial symptoms of stress, such as distressing recollections of the event, insomnia, nightmares, fearfulness, and irritability, among others. Ninety percent of those interviewed reported minor degrees of symptoms. Susceptibility to symptoms was associated with being female, being nonwhite, having previous psychological illness, and being close to the disaster site. Most adults responded to the attack by talking to others about their feelings, attending religious services, and donating charitable gifts. Over 80 percent of parents reported that their children had one or more symptoms. Interestingly, the level of stress was associated with the extent of television viewing about the disaster.

In a later survey of Manhattan residents conducted 5 to 8 weeks after the World Trade Center collapse published in the *New England Journal of Medicine* in 2002, it was found that 9.8 percent or an estimated 90,000 people had PTSD or clinical depression. Another 3.7 percent—or an estimated 34,000 people—met the criteria for both diagnoses. Higher rates for both disorders were found among people who lived close to ground zero, who had suffered personal losses as a result of the attacks, who had endured other stressful events during the previous 12 months, or who had experienced extreme panic during or shortly after the attacks. The rates of both disorders were higher among Hispanic respondents than among whites, blacks or Asians, and higher among women than among men. Among people in upper income levels, the incidence was lower for both disorders.

Finally, in a study of over 8,000 children aged 10 through 13 who lived in New York at the time of the terrorist attacks it was found that 11 percent had symptoms compatible with a diagnosis of PTSD 9 months after the event. An additional 15 percent had signs of agoraphobia, e.g., fear of taking public transportation. Similar to the demographics in adults described above, Hispanic students and girls were disproportionally affected, as were those who were exposed to prior unrelated traumatic events.

Major public health efforts to provide psychological treatment for traumatized adults and children are under way. Longitudinal studies are needed to determine what, if any, long-term effects occur.

References

Axelrod BN, Milner IB. Gulf War illness research: separating the wheat from the chaff. *Clin Neuropsychol.* 2000;14:344.

Basoglu M, Jaranson JM, Mollica R, Kastrup M. Torture and mental health: a research overview. In: Gerrity E, Keane TM, Tuma F, eds. *The Mental Health Consequences of Torture.* Plenum Series on Stress and Coping. New York: Kluwer Academic/Plenum, 2001:35.

Bieliauskas LA, Turner RS. What Persian Gulf War syndrome? *Clin Neuropsychol.* 2000;14:341.

Bremme JD. Hypotheses and controversies related to effects of stress on the hippocampus: an argument for stress-induced damage to the hippocampus in patients with posttraumatic stress disorder. *Hippocampus.* 2001;11:75.

Chemtob, CM, Nakashima J, Carlson JG. Brief treatment for elementary school children with disaster-related posttraumatic stress disorder: A field study. *J Clin Psychol.* 2002;58:99.

Galea S, Ahern J, Resnick H, et al. Psychological sequelae of the September 11, 2001 terrorist attacks in New York City. *N Engl J Med.* 2002;346:982.

Gorman JM, section ed. Anxiety disorders. In: Sadock BJ, Sadock VA, eds. *Kaplan & Sadock's Comprehensive Textbook of Psychiatry.* 7th ed. Vol 1. Baltimore: Lippincott Williams & Wilkins; 2000:1441.
Harvey AG, Bryant RA. Memory for acute stress disorder symptoms: a two-year prospective study. *J Nerv Ment Dis.* 2000;188:602.
Harvey AG, Bryant RA. Two-year prospective evaluation of the relationship between acute stress disorder and posttraumatic stress disorder following mild traumatic brain injury. *Am J Psychiatry.* 2000;157:626.
Kaufman ML, Kimble MO, Kaloupek DG, et al. Peritraumatic dissociation and physiological response to trauma-relevant stimuli in Vietnam combat veterans with posttraumatic stress disorder. *J Nerv Ment Dis.* 2002;190:167.
McEwen BS. Commentary on PTSD discussion. *Hippocampus.* 2001;11:82.
McFarlane AC. Yehuda R. Clinical treatment of posttraumatic stress disorder: conceptual challenges raised by recent research. *Aust N Z J Psychiatry.* 2000;34:940.
Meltzer-Brody S, Connor KM, Churchill E, Davidson JRT. Symptom-specific effects of fluoxetine in post-traumatic stress disorder. *Int Clin Psychopharmacol.* 2000;15:227.
Meltzer-Brody S, Hidalgo R, Connor KM, Davidson JRT. Posttraumatic stress disorder: prevalence, health care use and costs, and pharmacologic considerations. *Psychiatr Ann.* 2000;30:722.
Perkonigg A, Kessler RC, Storz S, Wittchen H-U. Traumatic events and posttraumatic stress disorder in the community: prevalence, risk factors, and comorbidity. *Acta Psychiatr Scand.* 2000;101:46.
Pitman RK. Hippocampal diminution in PTSD: more (or less?) than meets the eye. *Hippocampus.* 2001;11:73.
Salmon K, Bryant RA. Posttraumatic stress disorder in children: the influence of developmental factors. *Clin Psychol Rev.* 2002;22:163.
Schuster MA, Stein BD, Jaycox LH, et al. A national survey of stress reactions after the September 11, 2001, terrorist attacks. *N Engl J Med.* 2001;345:1507.
Smyth NJ, Greenwald R, de Jongh A, Lee C. Letter to the editor: EMDR for treatment of PTSD. *J Clin Psychiatry.* 2000;61:784.
Wenzel T, Griengl H, Stompe T, Mirazaei S, Kieffer W. Psychological disorders in survivors of torture: exhaustion, impairment and depression. *Psychopathology.* 2000;33:292.

▲ 16.6 Generalized Anxiety Disorder

Persons who seem to be anxious about almost everything are likely to be classified as having generalized anxiety disorder. The text revision of the fourth edition of the *Diagnostic and Statistical Manual of Mental Disorders* (DSM-IV-TR) defines generalized anxiety disorder as excessive anxiety and worry about several events or activities for most days during at least a 6-month period. The worry is difficult to control and is associated with somatic symptoms such as muscle tension, irritability, difficulty sleeping, and restlessness. The anxiety is not focused on features of another Axis I disorder, is not caused by substance use or a general medical condition, and does not occur only during a mood or psychiatric disorder. The anxiety is difficult to control, is subjectively distressing, and produces impairment in important areas of a person's life.

EPIDEMIOLOGY

Generalized anxiety disorder is a common condition; reasonable estimates for its 1-year prevalence range from 3 to 8 percent. The ratio of women to men with the disorder is about 2 to 1, but the ratio of women to men who are receiving inpatient treatment for the disorder is about 1 to 1. There is a lifetime prevalence close to 5 percent. In anxiety disorder clinics about 25 percent of patients have generalized anxiety disorder.

COMORBIDITY

Generalized anxiety disorder is probably the disorder that most often coexists with another mental disorder, usually social phobia, specific phobia, panic disorder, or a depressive disorder. Perhaps 50 to 90 percent of patients with generalized anxiety disorder have another mental disorder. As many as 25 percent of patients eventually experience panic disorder. An additional high percentage of patients are likely to have major depressive disorder. Other common disorders associated with generalized anxiety disorder are dysthymic disorder and substance-related disorders.

ETIOLOGY

The cause of generalized anxiety disorder is not known. As currently defined, generalized anxiety disorder probably affects a heterogeneous group of persons. Perhaps because a certain degree of anxiety is normal and adaptive, differentiating normal anxiety from pathological anxiety and differentiating biological causative factors from psychosocial factors are difficult. Biological and psychological factors probably work together.

Biological Factors

The therapeutic efficacies of benzodiazepines and the azaspirones (e.g., buspirone [BuSpar]) have focused biological research efforts on the γ-aminobutyric acid and serotonin neurotransmitter systems. Benzodiazepines (which are benzodiazepine receptor agonists) are known to reduce anxiety, whereas flumazenil (Romazicon) (a benzodiazepine receptor antagonist) and the β-carbolines (benzodiazepine receptor reverse agonists) are known to induce anxiety. Although no convincing data indicate that the benzodiazepine receptors are abnormal in patients with generalized anxiety disorder, some researchers have focused on the occipital lobe, which has the highest concentrations of benzodiazepine receptors in the brain. Other brain areas that have been hypothesized to be involved in generalized anxiety disorder are the basal ganglia, the limbic system, and the frontal cortex. Because buspirone is an agonist at the serotonin 5-HT_{1A} receptor, there is the hypothesis that the regulation of the serotonergic system in generalized anxiety disorder is abnormal. Other neurotransmitter systems that have been the subject of research in generalized anxiety disorder include the norepinephrine, glutamate, and cholecystokinin systems. Some evidence indicates that patients with generalized anxiety disorder may have subsensitivity of their α_2-adrenergic receptors, as indicated by a blunted release of growth hormone after clonidine (Catapres) infusion.

Only a limited number of brain-imaging studies of patients with generalized anxiety disorder have been conducted. One positron emission tomography study reported a lower metabolic rate in basal ganglia and white matter in generalized anxiety disorder patients than in normal control subjects (Fig. 16.6–1). A few genetic studies have also been conducted in the field. One study found that a genetic relation might exist between generalized anxiety disorder and major depressive disorder in women. Another study showed a distinct, but difficult-to-quantitate, genetic component in generalized anxiety disorder. About 25 percent of first-degree relatives of patients with generalized anxiety disorder are also affected. Male relatives are likely to have an alcohol use disorder. Some twin studies report a concordance rate of 50 percent in monozygotic twins and 15 percent in dizygotic twins.

A variety of electroencephalogram (EEG) abnormalities have been noted in alpha rhythm and evoked potentials. Sleep

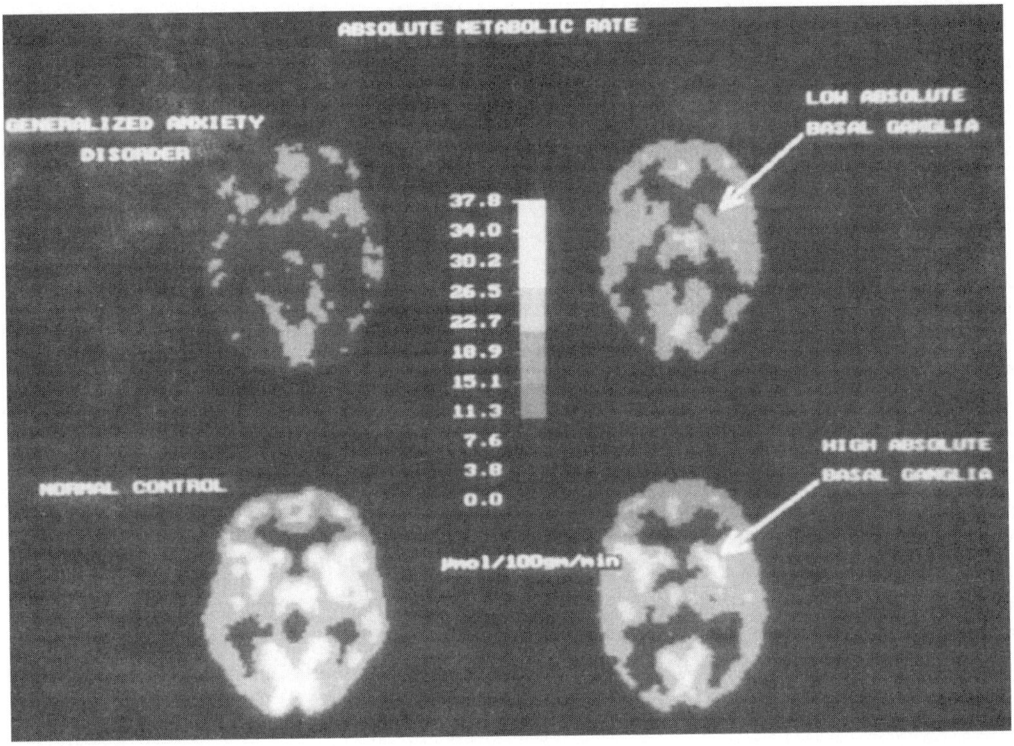

FIGURE 16.6–1
Basal ganglia metabolism. A common glucose scale shows the decrease in absolute glucose metabolic rate in the basal ganglia of two typical subjects with generalized anxiety disorder **(top row)** compared with two normal control subjects **(bottom row)**. (Reprinted with permission from Wu JC, Buchsbaum MS, Hershey TG, et al. PET in generalized anxiety disorder. *Biol Psychiatry.* 1991;29:1188.)

EEG studies have reported increased sleep discontinuity, decreased delta sleep, decreased stage 1 sleep, and reduced rapid eye movement sleep. These changes in sleep architecture differ from the changes seen in depressive disorders.

Psychosocial Factors

The two major schools of thought about psychosocial factors leading to the development of generalized anxiety disorder are the cognitive-behavioral school and the psychoanalytic school. According to the cognitive-behavioral school, patients with generalized anxiety disorder respond to incorrectly and inaccurately perceived dangers. The inaccuracy is generated by selective attention to negative details in the environment, by distortions in information processing, and by an overly negative view of the person's own ability to cope. The psychoanalytic school hypothesizes that anxiety is a symptom of unresolved unconscious conflicts. Sigmund Freud first presented this psychological theory in 1909 with his description of Little Hans; before then, Freud had conceptualized anxiety as having a physiological basis.

A hierarchy of anxieties is related to various developmental levels. At the most primitive level, anxiety may relate to the fear of annihilation or of fusion with another person. At a more mature level of development, anxiety is related to separation from a love object. At a still more mature level, anxiety is connected to the loss of love from an important object. Castration anxiety is related to the oedipal phase of development and is considered one of the highest levels of anxiety. Superego anxiety, a person's fear of disappointing his or her own ideals and values (derived from internalized parents), is the most mature form of anxiety.

DIAGNOSIS

The DSM-IV-TR diagnostic criteria (Table 16.6–1) include criteria to help clinicians differentiate among generalized anxiety disorder, normal anxiety, and other mental disorders. The distinction between generalized anxiety disorder and normal anxiety is emphasized by the use of the words "excessive" and "difficult to control" in the criteria and by the specification that the symptoms cause significant impairment or distress.

CLINICAL FEATURES

The primary symptoms of generalized anxiety disorder are anxiety, motor tension, autonomic hyperactivity, and cognitive vigilance. The anxiety is excessive and interferes with other aspects of a person's life. The motor tension is most commonly manifested as shakiness, restlessness, and headaches. The autonomic hyperactivity is commonly manifested by shortness of breath, excessive sweating, palpitations, and various gastrointestinal symptoms. The cognitive vigilance is evidenced by irritability and the ease with which patients are startled.

Patients with generalized anxiety disorder usually seek out a general practitioner or internist for help with a somatic symptom. Alternatively, the patients go to a specialist for a specific symptom (e.g., chronic diarrhea). A specific nonpsychiatric medical disorder is rarely found, and patients vary in their doctor-

Table 16.6–1
DSM-IV-TR Diagnostic Criteria for Generalized Anxiety Disorder

A. Excessive anxiety and worry (apprehensive expectation), occurring more days than not for at least 6 months, about a number of events or activities (such as work or school performance).
B. The person finds it difficult to control the worry.
C. The anxiety and worry are associated with three (or more) of the following six symptoms (with at least some symptoms present for more days than not for the past 6 months).
Note: Only one item is required in children.
(1) restlessness or feeling keyed up or on edge
(2) being easily fatigued
(3) difficulty concentrating or mind going blank
(4) irritability
(5) muscle tension
(6) sleep disturbance (difficulty falling or staying asleep, or restless unsatisfying sleep)
D. The focus of the anxiety and worry is not confined to features of an Axis I disorder, e.g., the anxiety or worry is not about having a panic attack (as in panic disorder), being embarrassed in public (as in social phobia), being contaminated (as in obsessive-compulsive disorder), being away from home or close relatives (as in separation anxiety disorder), gaining weight (as in anorexia nervosa), having multiple physical complaints (as in somatization disorder), or having a serious illness (as in hypochondriasis), and the anxiety and worry do not occur exclusively during posttraumatic stress disorder.
E. The anxiety, worry, or physical symptoms cause clinically significant distress or impairment in social, occupational, or other important areas of functioning.
F. The disturbance is not due to the direct physiological effects of a substance (e.g., a drug of abuse, a medication) or a general medical condition (e.g., hyperthyroidism) and does not occur exclusively during a mood disorder, a psychotic disorder, or a pervasive developmental disorder.

From American Psychiatric Association. *Diagnostic and Statistical Manual of Mental Disorders.* 4th ed. Text rev. Washington, DC: American Psychiatric Association; copyright 2000, with permission.

seeking behavior. Some patients accept a diagnosis of generalized anxiety disorder and the appropriate treatment; others seek additional medical consultations for their problems.

Ms. X. was a successful, married, 30-year-old attorney who presented for a psychiatric evaluation to treat growing symptoms of worry and anxiety. For the preceding 8 months, Ms. X. had noted increased worry about her job performance. For example, while she had always been a superb litigator, she increasingly found herself worrying about her ability to win each new case she was presented. Similarly, while she had always been in outstanding physical condition, she worried increasingly that her health had begun to deteriorate. Ms. X. noted frequent somatic symptoms that accompanied her worries. For example, she often felt restless while she worked and while she commuted to her office, thinking about the upcoming challenges of the day. She reported feeling increasingly fatigued, irritable, and tense. She noted that she had increasing difficulty falling asleep at night as she worried about her job performance and impending trials. (Courtesy of Daniel S. Pine, M.D.)

DIFFERENTIAL DIAGNOSIS

The differential diagnosis of generalized anxiety disorder includes all the medical disorders that may cause anxiety (see Table 16.1–2 in Section 16.1). The medical workup should include standard blood chemistry tests, an electrocardiogram, and thyroid function tests. Clinicians must rule out caffeine intoxication, stimulant abuse, alcohol withdrawal, and sedative, hypnotic, or anxiolytic withdrawal. The mental status examination and the history should explore the diagnostic possibilities of panic disorder, phobias, and obsessive-compulsive disorder. In general, patients with panic disorder seek treatment earlier, are more disabled by their disorder, had a sudden onset of symptoms, and are less troubled by their somatic symptoms than are patients with generalized anxiety disorder. Distinguishing generalized anxiety disorder from major depressive disorder and dysthymic disorder can be difficult; in fact, the disorders frequently coexist. Other diagnostic possibilities are adjustment disorder with anxiety, hypochondriasis, adult attention-deficit/hyperactivity disorder, somatization disorder, and personality disorders.

COURSE AND PROGNOSIS

The age of onset is difficult to specify; most patients with the disorder report that they have been anxious for as long as they can remember. Patients usually come to a clinician's attention in their 20s, although the first contact with a clinician can occur at virtually any age. Only one third of patients who have generalized anxiety disorder seek psychiatric treatment. Many go to general practitioners, internists, cardiologists, pulmonary specialists, or gastroenterologists, seeking treatment for the somatic component of the disorder. Because of the high incidence of comorbid mental disorders in patients with generalized anxiety disorder, the clinical course and prognosis of the disorder are difficult to predict. Nonetheless, some data indicate that life events are associated with the onset of generalized anxiety disorder: The occurrence of several negative life events greatly increases the likelihood that the disorder will develop. By definition, generalized anxiety disorder is a chronic condition that may well be lifelong.

TREATMENT

The most effective treatment of generalized anxiety disorder is probably one that combines psychotherapeutic, pharmacotherapeutic, and supportive approaches. The treatment may take a significant amount of time for the involved clinician, whether the clinician is a psychiatrist, a family practitioner, or another specialist.

Psychotherapy

The major psychotherapeutic approaches to generalized anxiety disorder are cognitive-behavioral, supportive, and insight oriented. Data are still limited on the relative merits of those approaches, although the most sophisticated studies have examined cognitive-behavioral techniques, which seem to have both short-term and long-term efficacy. Cognitive approaches address patients' hypothesized cognitive distortions directly,

and behavioral approaches address somatic symptoms directly. The major techniques used in behavioral approaches are relaxation and biofeedback. Some preliminary data indicate that the combination of cognitive and behavioral approaches is more effective than either technique used alone. Supportive therapy offers patients reassurance and comfort, although its long-term efficacy is doubtful. Insight-oriented psychotherapy focuses on uncovering unconscious conflicts and identifying ego strengths. The efficacy of insight-oriented psychotherapy for generalized anxiety disorder is reported in many anecdotal case reports, but large controlled studies are lacking.

Most patients experience a marked lessening of anxiety when given the opportunity to discuss their difficulties with a concerned and sympathetic physician. If clinicians discover external situations that are anxiety provoking, they may be able—alone or with the help of the patients or their families—to change the environment and thus reduce the stressful pressures. A reduction in symptoms often allows patients to function effectively in their daily work and relationships and thus gain new rewards and gratification that are themselves therapeutic.

In the psychoanalytic perspective, anxiety sometimes signals unconscious turmoil that deserves investigation. The anxiety can be normal, adaptive, maladaptive, too intense, or too mild, depending on the circumstances. Anxiety appears in numerous situations over the course of the life cycle; in many cases, symptom relief is not the most appropriate course of action.

For patients who are psychologically minded and motivated to understand the sources of their anxiety, psychotherapy may be the treatment of choice. Psychodynamic therapy proceeds with the assumption that anxiety may increase with effective treatment. The goal of the dynamic approach may be to increase the patient's anxiety tolerance (a capacity to experience anxiety without having to discharge it), rather than to eliminate anxiety. Empirical research indicates that many patients who have successful psychotherapeutic treatment may continue to experience anxiety after termination of the psychotherapy, but their increased ego mastery allows them to use the anxiety symptoms as a signal to reflect on internal struggles and to expand their insight and understanding. A psychodynamic approach to patients with generalized anxiety disorder involves a search for the patient's underlying fears.

Pharmacotherapy

The decision to prescribe an anxiolytic to patients with generalized anxiety disorder should rarely be made on the first visit. Because of the long-term nature of the disorder, a treatment plan must be carefully thought out. The three major drugs to be considered for the treatment of generalized anxiety disorder are buspirone, the benzodiazepines, and the serotonin-specific reuptake inhibitors (SSRIs). Other drugs that may be useful are the tricyclic drugs (e.g., imipramine [Tofranil]), antihistamines, and the β-adrenergic antagonists (e.g., propranolol [Inderal]).

Although drug treatment of generalized anxiety disorder is sometimes seen as a 6- to 12-month treatment, some evidence indicates that treatment should be long term, perhaps lifelong. About 25 percent of patients relapse in the first month after the discontinuation of therapy, and 60 to 80 percent relapse over the course of the next year. Although some patients become dependent on the benzodiazepines, tolerance rarely develops to the therapeutic effects of the benzodiazepines, buspirone, or the SSRIs.

Benzodiazepines. Benzodiazepines have been the drugs of choice for generalized anxiety disorder. They can be prescribed on an as-needed basis, so that patients take a rapidly acting benzodiazepine when they feel particularly anxious. The alternative approach is to prescribe benzodiazepines for a limited period, during which psychosocial therapeutic approaches are implemented.

Several problems are associated with the use of benzodiazepines in generalized anxiety disorder. About 25 to 30 percent of all patients fail to respond, and tolerance and dependence may occur. Some patients also experience impaired alertness while taking the drugs and are, therefore, at risk for accidents involving automobiles and machinery.

The clinical decision to initiate treatment with a benzodiazepine should be considered and specific. The patient's diagnosis, the specific target symptoms, and the duration of treatment should all be defined, and the information should be shared with patients. Treatment for most anxiety conditions lasts for 2 to 6 weeks, followed by 1 or 2 weeks of tapering drug use before it is discontinued. The most common clinical mistake with benzodiazepine treatment is to routinely continue treatment indefinitely.

For the treatment of anxiety, it is usual to begin giving a drug at the low end of its therapeutic range and to increase the dosage to achieve a therapeutic response. The use of a benzodiazepine with an intermediate half-life (8 to 15 hours) is likely to avoid some of the adverse effects associated with the use of benzodiazepines with long half-lives, and the use of divided doses prevents the development of adverse effects associated with high peak plasma levels. The improvement produced by benzodiazepines may go beyond a simple antianxiety effect. For example, the drugs may cause patients to regard various occurrences in a positive light. The drugs may also have a mild disinhibiting action, similar to that observed after ingesting modest amounts of alcohol.

Buspirone. Buspirone is a 5-HT_{1A} receptor partial agonist and is most likely effective in 60 to 80 percent of patients with generalized anxiety disorder. Data indicate that buspirone is more effective in reducing the cognitive symptoms of generalized anxiety disorder than in reducing the somatic symptoms. Evidence also indicates that patients who have previously undergone treatment with benzodiazepines are not likely to respond to treatment with buspirone. The lack of response may be due to the absence, with buspirone treatment, of some of the nonanxiolytic effects of benzodiazepines (such as muscle relaxation and the additional sense of well-being). The major disadvantage of buspirone is that its effects take 2 to 3 weeks to become evident, in contrast to the almost immediate anxiolytic effects of the benzodiazepines. One approach is to initiate benzodiazepine and buspirone use simultaneously, then taper off the benzodiazepine use after 2 to 3 weeks, at which point the buspirone should have reached its maximum effects. Some studies have also reported that long-term combined treatment with benzodiazepine and buspirone may be more effective than either drug alone. Buspirone is not an effective treatment for benzodiazepine withdrawal.

Venlafaxine. Venlafaxine is effective in treating the insomnia, poor concentration, restlessness, irritability, and excessive muscle tension associated with generalized anxiety disorder.

Selective Serotonin Reuptake Inhibitors. SSRIs may be effective, especially for patients with comorbid depression. The prominent disadvantage of SSRIs, especially fluoxetine (Prozac), is that they may transiently increase anxiety. For this reason, the SSRIs sertraline (Zoloft) or paroxetine (Paxil) are better choices. It is reasonable to begin treatment with sertraline or paroxetine plus a benzodiazepine, then to taper benzodiazepine use after 2 to 3 weeks. Further studies are needed to determine whether SSRIs are as effective for generalized anxiety disorder as they are for panic disorder and obsessive-compulsive disorder.

Other Drugs. If conventional pharmacological treatment (e.g., with buspirone or a benzodiazepine) is ineffective or not completely effective, then a clinical reassessment is indicated to rule out comorbid conditions, such as depression, or to better understand the patient's environmental stresses. Other drugs that have proven useful for generalized anxiety disorder include the tricyclic and tetracyclic drugs. The β-adrenergic receptor antagonists may reduce the somatic manifestations of anxiety but not the underlying condition, and their use is usually limited to situational anxieties, such as performance anxiety. Nefazodone (Serzone), also used in depression, has been shown to reduce anxiety and prevent panic disorder.

References

Astrom M. Generalized anxiety disorder in stroke patients. A 3-year longitudinal study. *Stroke.* 1996;27:270.

Borkovec TD, Roemer L. Perceived functions of worry among generalized anxiety disorder subjects: distraction from more emotionally distressing topics? *J Behav Ther Exp Psychiatry.* 1995;26:25.

Borkovec TD, Ruscio AM. Psychotherapy for generalized anxiety disorder. *J Clin Psychiatry.* 2001;62(suppl 11):37.

Butler G. Predicting outcome after treatment for generalized anxiety disorder. *Behav Res Ther.* 1993;31:211.

Butler G, Fennell M, Robson P, Gelder M. Comparison of behavior therapy and cognitive-behavior therapy in the treatment of generalized anxiety disorder. *J Consult Clin Psychol.* 1991;59:167.

Gabbard GO. Psychodynamic psychiatry in the "decade of the brain." *Am J Psychiatry.* 1992;149:991.

Gasperini M, Battaglia M, Diaferia G, Bellodi L. Personality features related to generalized anxiety disorder. *Compr Psychiatry.* 1990;31:363.

Gorman JM, section ed. Anxiety disorders. In: Sadock BJ, Sadock VA, eds. *Kaplan & Sadock's Comprehensive Textbook of Psychiatry.* 7th ed. Vol 1. Baltimore: Lippincott Williams & Wilkins; 2000:1441.

Kendler KS, Neale MC, Kessler RC, Health AC, Eaves LJ. Generalized anxiety disorder in women: a population-based twin study. *Arch Gen Psychiatry.* 1992;49:267.

Kollai M, Kollai B. Cardiac vagal tone in generalized anxiety disorder. *Br J Psychiatry.* 1992;161:831.

Massion AO, Warshaw MG, Keller MB. Quality of life and psychiatric morbidity in panic disorder and generalized anxiety disorder. *Am J Psychiatry.* 1993;150:600.

Mathews A, Mogg K, Kentish J, Eysenck M. Effect of psychological treatment on cognitive bias in generalized anxiety disorder. *Behav Res Ther.* 1995;33:293.

Mennin DS, Heimberg RG, Holt GS. Panic agoraphobia, phobias, and generalized anxiety disorder. In: Hersen M, Bellack AS, eds. *Psychopathology in Adulthood.* 2nd ed. Needham Heights, MA: Allyn & Bacon; 2000:169.

Noyes R Jr, Woodman C, Garvey MJ, et al. Generalized anxiety disorder vs panic disorder: distinguishing characteristics and patterns of comorbidity. *J Nerv Ment Dis.* 1992;180:369.

Rapee RM, Barlow DH. Generalized anxiety disorders, panic disorders, and phobias. In: Sutker PB, Adams HE, eds. *Comprehensive Handbook of Psychopathology.* 3rd ed. New York: Kluwer Academic/Plenum Publishers; 2001:131.

Rickels K, Schweizer E. The treatment of generalized anxiety disorder in patients with depression symptomatology. *J Clin Psychiatry.* 1993;54(suppl 1):20.

Thayer JF, Friedman BH, Borkovec TD. Autonomic characteristics of generalized anxiety disorder and worry. *Biol Psychiatry.* 1996;39:255.

▲ 16.7 Other Anxiety Disorders

ANXIETY DISORDER DUE TO A GENERAL MEDICAL CONDITION

Many medical disorders are associated with anxiety. Symptoms can include panic attacks, generalized anxiety, obsessions and compulsions, and other signs of distress. In all cases the signs and symptoms will be due to the direct physiological effects of the medical condition.

Epidemiology

The occurrence of anxiety symptoms related to general medical conditions is common, although the incidence of the disorder varies for each specific general medical condition.

Etiology

A wide range of medical conditions can cause symptoms similar to those of anxiety disorders (Table 16.7–1). Hyperthyroidism, hypothyroidism, hypoparathyroidism, and vitamin B_{12} deficiency are frequently associated with anxiety symptoms. A pheochromocytoma produces epinephrine, which can cause paroxysmal episodes of anxiety symptoms. Certain lesions of the brain and postencephalitic states reportedly produce symptoms identical to those seen in obsessive-compulsive disorder. Other medical conditions, such as cardiac arrhythmia, can produce physiological symptoms of panic disorder. Hypoglycemia can also mimic the symptoms of an anxiety disorder. The diverse medical conditions that can cause symptoms of anxiety disorder may do so through a common mechanism, the noradrenergic system, although the effects on the serotonergic system are also under study.

Diagnosis

The text revision of the fourth edition of *Diagnostic and Statistical Manual of Mental Disorders* (DSM-IV-TR) diagnosis of anxiety disorder due to a general medical condition (Table 16.7–2) requires the presence of symptoms of an anxiety disorder. DSM-IV-TR allows clinicians to specify whether the disorder is characterized by symptoms of generalized anxiety, panic attacks, or obsessive-compulsive symptoms.

Clinicians should have an increased level of suspicion for the diagnosis when chronic or paroxysmal anxiety is associated with a physical disease known to cause such symptoms in some patients. Paroxysmal bouts of hypertension in an anxious patient may indicate that a workup for a pheochromocytoma is appropriate. A general medical workup may reveal diabetes, an adrenal tumor, thyroid disease, or a neurological condition. For example, some patients with complex partial epilepsy have extreme episodes of anxiety or fear as their only manifestation of the epileptic activity.

Clinical Features

The symptoms of anxiety disorder due to a general medical condition can be identical to those of the primary anxiety disorders. A

Table 16.7–1
Disorders Associated with Anxiety

Neurological disorders	Miscellaneous conditions
Cerebral neoplasms	Hypoglycemia
Cerebral trauma and postconcussive syndromes	Carcinoid syndrome
Cerebrovascular disease	Systemic malignancies
Subarachnoid hemorrhage	Premenstrual syndrome
Migraine	Febrile illnesses and chronic infections
Encephalitis	Porphyria
Cerebral syphilis	Infectious mononucleosis
Multiple sclerosis	Posthepatitis syndrome
Wilson's disease	Uremia
Huntington's disease	Toxic conditions
Epilepsy	Alcohol and drug withdrawal
Systemic conditions	Amphetamines
Hypoxia	Sympathomimetic agents
Cardiovascular disease	Vasopressor agents
Cardiac arrhythmias	Caffeine and caffeine withdrawal
Pulmonary insufficiency	Penicillin
Anemia	Sulfonamides
Endocrine disturbances	Cannabis
Pituitary dysfunction	Mercury
Thyroid dysfunction	Arsenic
Parathyroid dysfunction	Phosphorus
Adrenal dysfunction	Organophosphates
Pheochromocytoma	Carbon disulfide
Virilization disorders of females	Benzene
Inflammatory disorders	Aspirin intolerance
Lupus erythematosus	Idiopathic psychiatric disorders
Rheumatoid arthritis	Depression
Polyarteritis nodosa	Mania
Temporal arteritis	Schizophrenia
Deficiency states	Anxiety disorders
Vitamin B_{12} deficiency	Generalized anxiety
Pellagra	Panic attacks
	Phobic disorders
	Posttraumatic stress disorder

Reprinted with permission from Cumming JL. *Clinical Neuropsychiatry.* Orlando, FL: Grune & Stratton; 1985:214.

Table 16.7–2
DSM-IV-TR Diagnostic Criteria for Anxiety Disorder Due to a General Medical Condition

A. Prominent anxiety, panic attacks, or obsessions or compulsions predominate in the clinical picture.

B. There is evidence from the history, physical examination, or laboratory findings that the disturbance is the direct physiological consequence of a general medical condition.

C. The disturbance is not better accounted for by another mental disorder (e.g., adjustment disorder with anxiety in which the stressor is a serious general medical condition).

D. The disturbance does not occur exclusively during the course of a delirium.

E. The disturbance causes clinically significant distress or impairment in social, occupational, or other important areas of functioning.

Specify if:

With generalized anxiety: if excessive anxiety or worry about a number of events or activities predominates in the clinical presentation

With panic attacks: if panic attacks predominate in the clinical presentation

With obsessive-compulsive symptoms: if obsessions or compulsions predominate in the clinical presentation

Coding note: Include the name of the general medical condition on Axis I, e.g., anxiety disorder due to pheochromocytoma, with generalized anxiety; also code the general medical condition on Axis III.

From American Psychiatric Association. *Diagnostic and Statistical Manual of Mental Disorders.* 4th ed. Text rev. Washington, DC: American Psychiatric Association; copyright 2000, with permission.

syndrome similar to panic disorder is the most common clinical picture, and a syndrome similar to a phobia is the least common.

Panic Attacks. Patients who have cardiomyopathy may have the highest incidence of panic disorder secondary to a general medical condition. One study reported that 83 percent of patients with cardiomyopathy awaiting cardiac transplantation had panic disorder symptoms. Increased noradrenergic tone in these patients may be the provoking stimulus for the panic attacks. In some studies, about 25 percent of patients with Parkinson's disease and chronic obstructive pulmonary disease have symptoms of panic disorder. Other medical disorders associated with panic disorder include chronic pain, primary biliary cirrhosis, and epilepsy, particularly when the focus is in the right parahippocampal gyrus.

Mr. A. was a 28-year-old electrician who developed panic attacks 6 months prior to evaluation. The first attack occurred shortly after he accidentally touched a live wire and received a moderately severe shock. It was thought initially that the panic attacks were causally related to that incident; however, as part of a medical workup he was found to have episodes of hypoglycemia (<50 mg/dL plasma glucose) that occurred 4 to 5 hours after eating, at which time he would become nervous and tremulous, feel faint, and have palpitations. A diagnosis of reactive hypoglycemia associated with early-onset type II diabetes mellitus was made.

Generalized Anxiety. A high prevalence of generalized anxiety disorder symptoms has been reported in patients with Sjögren's syndrome, and this rate may be related to the effects of Sjögren's syndrome on cortical and subcortical functions and thyroid function. The highest prevalence of generalized anxiety disorder symptoms in a medical disorder seems to be in Graves' disease (hyperthyroidism), in which as many as two thirds of all patients meet the criteria for generalized anxiety disorder.

Obsessive-Compulsive Symptoms. Reports have associated the development of obsessive-compulsive disorder symptoms with Sydenham's chorea and multiple sclerosis.

A 12-year-old girl had a sudden onset of high fever, lethargy, and sore throat with purulent tonsillar exudate. Streptococci were found in the infected site, and she was treated successfully with penicillin. Following recovery, mild athe-

toid movements of the upper torso and facial tics were noted and diagnosed as sequelae of the infection. She was kept on antibiotics (to prevent reinfection) until the neurological complication subsided spontaneously after 1 year.

Phobias. Symptoms of phobias appear to be uncommon, although one study reported a 17 percent prevalence of symptoms of social phobia in patients with Parkinson's disease.

Differential Diagnosis

Anxiety as a symptom can be associated with many psychiatric disorders in addition to the anxiety disorders themselves. A mental status examination is necessary to determine the presence of mood symptoms or psychotic symptoms that may suggest another psychiatric diagnosis. For a clinician to conclude that a patient has an anxiety disorder due to a general medical condition, the patient should clearly have anxiety as the predominant symptom and should have a specific causative nonpsychiatric medical disorder. To ascertain the degree to which a general medical condition is causative for the anxiety, the clinician should know whether the medical condition and the anxiety symptoms have been related closely in the literature, the age of onset (primary anxiety disorders usually have their onset before age 35), and the patient's family history of both anxiety disorders and relevant general medical conditions (e.g., hyperthyroidism). A diagnosis of adjustment disorder with anxiety must also be considered in the differential diagnosis.

Course and Prognosis

The unremitting experience of anxiety can be disabling and can interfere with every aspect of life, including social, occupational, and psychological functioning. A sudden increase in anxiety level may prompt an affected person to seek medical or psychiatric help more quickly than when the onset is insidious. The treatment or the removal of the primary medical cause of the anxiety usually initiates a clear course of improvement in the anxiety disorder symptoms. In some cases, however, the anxiety disorder symptoms continue even after the primary medical condition is treated (e.g., after an episode of encephalitis). Some symptoms, particularly obsessive-compulsive disorder symptoms, linger for a longer time than other anxiety disorder symptoms. When anxiety disorder symptoms are present for a significant period after the medical disorder has been treated, the remaining symptoms should probably be treated as if they were primary—that is, with psychotherapy or pharmacotherapy or both.

Treatment

The primary treatment for anxiety disorder due to a general medical condition is the treatment of the underlying medical condition. If a patient also has an alcohol or other substance use disorder, this disorder must also be addressed therapeutically to gain control of the anxiety disorder symptoms. If the removal of the primary medical condition does not reverse the anxiety disorder symptoms, treatment of these symptoms should follow the treatment guidelines for the specific mental disorder. In general, behavioral modification techniques, anxiolytic agents, and serotonergic antidepressants have been the most effective treatment modalities.

SUBSTANCE-INDUCED ANXIETY DISORDER

This disorder is the direct result of a toxic substance, including drugs of abuse, medication, poison, and alcohol, among others.

Epidemiology

Substance-induced anxiety disorder is common, both as the result of the ingestion of so-called recreational drugs and as the result of prescription drug use.

Etiology

A wide range of substances can cause symptoms of anxiety that may mimic any of the DSM-IV-TR anxiety disorders. Although sympathomimetics such as amphetamine, cocaine, and caffeine have been most associated with the production of anxiety disorder symptoms, many serotonergic drugs (e.g., lysergic acid diethylamide [LSD] and methylenedioxymethamphetamine [MDMA]) can also cause both acute and chronic anxiety syndromes in users. A wide range of prescription medications is also associated with the production of anxiety disorder symptoms in susceptible persons.

Diagnosis

The DSM-IV-TR diagnostic criteria for substance-induced anxiety disorder require the presence of prominent anxiety, panic attacks, obsessions, or compulsions (Table 16.7–3). The DSM-IV-TR guidelines state that the symptoms should have developed during the use of the substance or within a month of the cessation of substance use, but DSM-IV-TR encourages clinicians to use appropriate clinical judgment to assess the relation between substance exposure and anxiety symptoms. The structure of the diagnosis includes specification of the substance (e.g., cocaine), specification of the appropriate state during the onset (e.g., intoxication), and mention of the specific symptom pattern (e.g., panic attacks).

Clinical Features

The associated clinical features of substance-induced anxiety disorder vary with the particular substance involved. Even infrequent use of psychostimulants can result in anxiety disorder symptoms in some persons. Cognitive impairments in comprehension, calculation, and memory may be associated with anxiety disorder symptoms. These cognitive deficits are usually reversible when the substance use is stopped.

Virtually everyone who drinks alcohol has, on at least a few occasions, used it to reduce anxiety, most often social anxiety. In contrast, carefully controlled studies have found that the effects of alcohol on anxiety are variable and can be significantly affected by gender, the amount of alcohol ingested, and cultural attitudes. Nevertheless, alco-

Table 16.7–3
DSM-IV-TR Diagnostic Criteria for Substance-Induced Anxiety Disorder

A. Prominent anxiety, panic attacks, or obsessions or compulsions predominate in the clinical picture.
B. There is evidence from the history, physical examination, or laboratory findings of either (1) or (2):
   (1) the symptoms in Criterion A developed during, or within 1 month of, substance intoxication or withdrawal
   (2) medication use is etiologically related to the disturbance
C. The disturbance is not better accounted for by an anxiety disorder that is not substance induced. Evidence that the symptoms are better accounted for by an anxiety disorder that is not substance induced might include the following: the symptoms precede the onset of the substance use (or medication use); the symptoms persist for a substantial period of time (e.g., about a month) after the cessation of acute withdrawal or severe intoxication or are substantially in excess of what would be expected given the type or amount of the substance used or the duration of use; or there is other evidence suggesting the existence of an independent non-substance-induced anxiety disorder (e.g., a history of recurrent non-substance-related episodes).
D. The disturbance does not occur exclusively during the course of a delirium.
E. The disturbance causes clinically significant distress or impairment in social, occupational, or other important areas of functioning.

Note: This diagnosis should be made instead of a diagnosis of substance intoxication or substance withdrawal only when the anxiety symptoms are in excess of those usually associated with the intoxication or withdrawal syndrome and when the anxiety symptoms are sufficiently severe to warrant independent clinical attention.

Code [Specific substance]-induced anxiety disorder

Alcohol; amphetamine (or amphetaminelike substance); caffeine; cannabis; cocaine; hallucinogen; inhalant; phencyclidine (or phencyclidinelike substance); sedative, hypnotic, or anxiolytic; other [or unknown] substance

Specify if:

With generalized anxiety: if excessive anxiety or worry about a number of events or activities predominates in the clinical presentation

With panic attacks: if panic attacks predominate in the clinical presentation

With obsessive-compulsive symptoms: if obsessions or compulsions predominate in the clinical presentation

With phobic symptoms: if phobic symptoms predominate in the clinical presentation

Specify if:

With onset during intoxication: if the criteria are met for intoxication with the substance and the symptoms develop during the intoxication syndrome

With onset during withdrawal: if criteria are met for withdrawal from the substance and the symptoms develop during, or shortly after, a withdrawal syndrome

From American Psychiatric Association. *Diagnostic and Statistical Manual of Mental Disorders.* 4th ed. Text rev. Washington, DC: American Psychiatric Association; copyright 2000, with permission.

hol use disorders and other substance-related disorders are commonly associated with anxiety disorders. Alcohol use disorders are about 4 times more common among patients with panic disorder than among the general population, about 3.5 times more common among patients with obsessive-compulsive disorder, and about 2.5 times more common among patients with phobias. Several studies have reported data indicating that genetic diatheses for both anxiety disorders and alcohol use disorders may exist in some families.

Mr. B. was a 28-year-old single African American male graduate student who was in good health and had no history of previous psychiatric evaluation or treatment. He took no medications, did not smoke or consume alcohol, and had no current or past history of illicit drug use.

His chief complaint was that he had begun feeling mounting "anxiety" when working in the laboratory where he was pursuing his graduate studies. His work had been progressing well, he felt his relationship with his advisor was good and supportive, and he could not identify any problems with staff or peers that might explain his anxiety. He had been working long hours, but found the work interesting and had recently had his first paper accepted for publication.

Despite these successes, he reported feeling a "crescendoing anxiety" as his day progressed. He noted that by afternoon he would be experiencing palpitations, bursts of heart racing, tremors in his hands, and an overall feeling of "being on the edge." He also noted a nervous energy in the afternoons. These experiences were occurring daily and seemed confined to the laboratory (although he admitted he was in the laboratory every day of the week).

When reviewing Mr. B.'s caffeine intake, he was found to be consuming excessive amounts of coffee. Staff made a large urn of caffeinated coffee each morning, and Mr. B. routinely started with a large mug of coffee. Over the course of the morning he would consume three to four mugs of coffee (the equivalent of about six to eight 5-ounce cups of coffee), and he continued this level of use throughout the afternoon. He occasionally had a single can of caffeinated soda and used no other forms of caffeine on a regular basis. Mr. B. estimated he drank a total of six to eight or more mugs of coffee per day (which was estimated to be at least 1,200 mg of caffeine per day). Once it was pointed out to him, he realized that this level of caffeine consumption was considerably higher than at any other time in his life. He admitted he liked the taste of coffee and felt a burst of energy in the morning when he drank coffee, which helped him start his day.

Mr. B. and his physician developed a plan to decrease his caffeine use by tapering. Details of such a tapering schedule can be found in the section on treatment of caffeine dependence. Mr. B. successfully decreased his caffeine use, and he had good resolution of his anxiety symptoms once his daily caffeine use had been markedly decreased. (Courtesy of Eric C. Strain, M.D.)

Differential Diagnosis

The differential diagnosis for substance-induced anxiety disorder includes the primary anxiety disorders, anxiety disorder due to a general medical condition (for which the patient may be receiving an implicated drug), and mood disorders, which are frequently accompanied by symptoms of anxiety disor-

ders. Personality disorders and malingering must be considered in the differential diagnosis, particularly in some urban emergency rooms.

Course and Prognosis

The course and prognosis generally depend on removal of the causally involved substance and the long-term ability of the affected person to limit use of the substance. The anxiogenic effects of most drugs are reversible. When the anxiety does not reverse with cessation of the drug, clinicians should reconsider the diagnosis of substance-induced anxiety disorder or consider the possibility that the substance caused irreversible brain damage.

Treatment

The primary treatment for substance-induced anxiety disorder is the removal of the causally involved substance. Treatment then must focus on finding an alternative treatment if the substance was a medically indicated drug, on limiting the patient's exposure if the substance was introduced through environmental exposure, or on treating the underlying substance-related disorder. If anxiety disorder symptoms continue even though substance use has stopped, treatment of the anxiety disorder symptoms with appropriate psychotherapeutic or pharmacotherapeutic modalities may be appropriate.

Table 16.7–4
DSM-IV-TR Diagnostic Criteria for Anxiety Disorder Not Otherwise Specified

This category includes disorders with prominent anxiety or phobic avoidance that do not meet criteria for any specific anxiety disorder, adjustment disorder with anxiety, or adjustment disorder with mixed anxiety and depressed mood. Examples include

1. Mixed anxiety-depressive disorder: clinically significant symptoms of anxiety and depression, but the criteria are not met for either a specific mood disorder or a specific anxiety disorder
2. Clinically significant social phobic symptoms that are related to the social impact of having a general medical condition or mental disorder (e.g., Parkinson's disease, dermatological conditions, stuttering, anorexia nervosa, body dysmorphic disorder)
3. Situations in which the disturbance is severe enough to warrant a diagnosis of an anxiety disorder but the individual fails to report enough symptoms for the full criteria for any specific anxiety disorder to have been met; for example, an individual who reports all of the features of panic disorder without agoraphobia except that the panic attacks are all limited-symptom attacks
4. Situations in which the clinician has concluded that an anxiety disorder is present but is unable to determine whether it is primary, due to a general medical condition, or substance induced

From American Psychiatric Association. *Diagnostic and Statistical Manual of Mental Disorders.* 4th ed. Text rev. Washington, DC: American Psychiatric Association; copyright 2000, with permission.

ANXIETY DISORDER NOT OTHERWISE SPECIFIED

Some patients have symptoms of anxiety disorders that do not meet the criteria for any specific DSM-IV-TR anxiety disorder or adjustment disorder with anxiety or mixed anxiety and depressed mood. Such patients are most appropriately classified as having anxiety disorder not otherwise specified. DSM-IV-TR includes four examples of conditions that are appropriate for the diagnosis (Table 16.7–4). One of the examples is mixed anxiety-depressive disorder.

Mr. W. came into the emergency room of a New York hospital complaining of malaise, fever, and a cough. An upper respiratory infection was diagnosed. As the doctor was writing out a prescription. Mr. W. tearfully revealed that he had no home to go to, was depressed, and felt that life was not worth living. A psychiatric resident was called to see the patient and obtained the following additional information.

For the past month Mr. W. had been living in the basement of his apartment building, eating in restaurants, and using a health club for showers. He was eating and sleeping poorly. His own apartment was so full of newspapers, magazines, and books that he could no longer get in the door, but he could not bring himself to get rid of any of his "stuff."

When he was 12, Mr. W. began collecting baseball cards and then books and magazines. His parents were poor immigrants from Eastern Europe, and the idea of holding on to things that might someday be valuable was not strange to them. Eventually, however, the apartment became so cluttered that they threw out much of his collection. He retrieved it from the garbage, and from that point on his "collecting" became a focus of conflict with family and employers.

Mr. W. does not go out of his way to obtain things, but once he has a newspaper, book, or magazine, he cannot throw it away because "there might be something of value written in it." The thought of throwing things out makes him extremely anxious, and, in the end, he simply cannot do it.

For many years he worked as a doorman in elegant apartment buildings, but invariably was fired because he brought his "stuff" to store in his workplace, and sometimes got into fistfights with the building maintenance people who tried to throw it out. He was married for 10 years, and has a 25-year-old son. His wife finally left him, unable to tolerate his behavior. He rarely sees his son.

Mr. W. first entered treatment not because of his collecting, but because at age 20, "my mood took a turn for the worse. I had a breakdown." He stopped doing virtually everything—working, eating, sleeping. "It was an effort even to lift my leg." He began seeing a psychiatrist as an outpatient, and over the years has been in therapy much of the time, treated with a variety of antidepressants and anxiolytics.

After his divorce, 10 years ago, he moved some of his collection into his own apartment and rented storage space for the rest. Gradually his new apartment filled up with newspapers, magazines, and books, and it became a struggle

just to get in the front door and make his way to his bed. Finally, last month, he injured his shoulder trying to push things aside, and then abandoned the apartment for a cot in the basement of the building He understands that his inability to throw things out is irrational, but the thought of starting to do it makes him intolerably anxious.

DISCUSSION

Mr. W. presents with symptoms suggesting depression: depressed mood, difficulty eating and sleeping, and thoughts that life is not worth living. More information about the severity and persistence of these symptoms would rule out a diagnosis of major depressive disorder. However, what is most striking is that there is a long-standing problem with not being able to throw things out—hoarding—that has totally disrupted his life.

How to diagnose Mr. W.'s long-standing difficulty is not at all clear. Many people have trouble throwing things away that they think may be of potential value, but, if this trait does not cause significant distress or impairment, a diagnosis of a mental disorder is not appropriate. That is certainly not the case with Mr. W. One possibility is that the hoarding is part of a larger picture of obsessive-compulsive personality disorder, as hoarding behavior is actually one of the criteria for that disorder and is present in approximately half of the cases with the disorder. However, none of the other features of that disorder, such as perfectionism or excessive devotion to work, seems to be present.

Hoarding is sometimes seen as part of the disorganized or bizarre behavior of people with schizophrenia, but in this case none of the characteristic features of schizophrenia is present. Mr. W.'s anxiety, associated with the thought of throwing things away, suggests an obsession. However, in true obsessions such thoughts are ego-dystonic, whereas in Mr. W.'s case, they are not. Is the hoarding behavior a compulsion? Compulsions are repetitive behaviors or thoughts that the person engages in and that are done in a stereotyped manner or in response to an obsession. In contrast, Mr. W.'s hoarding is actually the failure to engage in an appropriate behavior (i.e., throwing out his junk). Furthermore, he does not follow any stereotyped rules in collecting his books and papers, and his hoarding is not in response to an obsession.

Experts in obsessive-compulsive disorder generally regard extreme hoarding as part of the spectrum of obsessive-compulsive disorder. They point out that many "hoarders" do in fact exhibit checking or other compulsive rituals that meet the criteria for compulsions even when the hoarding behavior is ego-syntonic. They also point to the extreme anxiety that these patients exhibit if the hoarding behavior is thwarted.

Because Mr. W. does not seem to have any strictly defined obsessions or compulsions, we would give the residual category of anxiety disorder not otherwise specified. An alternative way of viewing the hoarding is to consider it a maladaptive personality trait and make the diagnosis personality disorder not otherwise specified. (From *DSM-IV Casebook.*)

Mixed Anxiety-Depressive Disorder

This disorder describes patients with both anxiety and depressive symptoms who do not meet the diagnostic criteria for either an anxiety disorder or a mood disorder. The combination of depressive and anxiety symptoms results in significant functional impairment for the affected person. The condition may be particularly prevalent in primary care practices and outpatient mental health clinics. Opponents have argued that the availability of the diagnosis may discourage clinicians from taking the necessary time to obtain a complete psychiatric history to differentiate true depressive disorders from true anxiety disorders. In Europe and especially in China, many of these patients are given a diagnosis of neurasthenia (see Chapter 18).

Epidemiology. The coexistence of major depressive disorder and panic disorder is common. As many as two thirds of all patients with depressive symptoms have prominent anxiety symptoms, and one third may meet the diagnostic criteria for panic disorder. Researchers have reported that 20 to 90 percent of all patients with panic disorder have episodes of major depressive disorder. These data suggest that the coexistence of depressive and anxiety symptoms, neither of which meets the diagnostic criteria for other depressive or anxiety disorders, may be common. At this time, however, formal epidemiological data on mixed anxiety-depressive disorder are not available. Nevertheless, some clinicians and researchers have estimated that the prevalence of the disorder in the general population is as high as 10 percent and in primary care clinics, as high as 50 percent, although conservative estimates suggest a prevalence of about 1 percent in the general population.

Etiology. Four principal lines of evidence suggest that anxiety symptoms and depressive symptoms are causally linked in some affected patients. First, several investigators have reported similar neuroendocrine findings in depressive disorders and anxiety disorders, particularly panic disorder, including blunted cortisol response to adrenocorticotropic hormone, blunted growth hormone response to clonidine (Catapres), and blunted thyroid-stimulating hormone and prolactin responses to thyrotropin-releasing hormone. Second, several investigators have reported data indicating that hyperactivity of the noradrenergic system is causally relevant to some patients with depressive disorders and with panic disorder. Specifically, these studies have found elevated concentrations of the norepinephrine metabolite 3-methoxy-4-hydroxyphenyglycol (MHPG) in the urine, the plasma, or the cerebrospinal fluid (CSF) of depressed patients and panic disorder patients who were actively experiencing a panic attack. As with other anxiety and depressive disorders, serotonin and γ-aminobutyric acid (GABA) may also be causally involved in mixed anxiety-depressive disorder. Third, many studies have found that serotonergic drugs, such as fluoxetine (Prozac) and clomipramine (Anafranil), are useful in treating both depressive and anxiety disorders. Fourth, a number of family studies have reported data indicating that anxiety and depressive symptoms are genetically linked in at least some families.

Diagnosis. The DSM-IV-TR criteria (Table 16.7–5) require the presence of subsyndromal symptoms of both anxiety and

Table 16.7–5
DSM-IV-TR Research Criteria for Mixed Anxiety-Depressive Disorder

A. Persistent or recurrent dysphoric mood lasting at least 1 month.
B. The dysphoric mood is accompanied by at least 1 month of four (or more) of the following symptoms:
 (1) difficulty concentrating or mind going blank
 (2) sleep disturbance (difficulty falling or staying asleep, or restless, unsatisfying sleep)
 (3) fatigue or low energy
 (4) irritability
 (5) worry
 (6) being easily moved to tears
 (7) hypervigilance
 (8) anticipating the worst
 (9) hopelessness (pervasive pessimism about the future)
 (10) low self-esteem or feelings of worthlessness
C. The symptoms cause clinically significant distress or impairment in social, occupational, or other important areas of functioning.
D. The symptoms are not due to the direct physiological effects of a substance (e.g., a drug of abuse, a medication) or a general medical condition.
E. All of the following:
 (1) criteria have never been met for major depressive disorder, dysthymic disorder, panic disorder, or generalized anxiety disorder
 (2) criteria are not currently met for any other anxiety or mood disorder (including an anxiety or mood disorder, in partial remission)
 (3) the symptoms are not better accounted for by any other mental disorder

From American Psychiatric Association. *Diagnostic and Statistical Manual of Mental Disorders.* 4th ed. Text rev. Washington, DC: American Psychiatric Association; copyright 2000, with permission.

depression and the presence of some autonomic symptoms, such as tremor, palpitations, dry mouth, and the sensation of a churning stomach. Some preliminary studies have indicated that the sensitivity of general practitioners to a syndrome of mixed anxiety-depressive disorder is low, although this lack of recognition may reflect the lack of an appropriate diagnostic label for the patients.

Clinical Features. The clinical features of mixed anxiety-depressive disorder combine symptoms of anxiety disorders and some symptoms of depressive disorders. In addition, symptoms of autonomic nervous system hyperactivity, such as gastrointestinal complaints, are common and contribute to the high frequency with which the patients are seen in outpatient medical clinics.

Differential Diagnosis. The differential diagnosis includes other anxiety and depressive disorders and personality disorders. Among the anxiety disorders, generalized anxiety disorder is most likely to overlap with mixed anxiety-depressive disorder. Among the mood disorders, dysthymic disorder and minor depressive disorder are most likely to overlap with mixed anxiety-depressive disorder. Among the personality disorders, avoidant, dependent, and obsessive-compulsive personality disorders may have symptoms that resemble those of mixed anxiety-depressive disorder. A diagnosis of a somatoform disorder should also be considered. Only a psychiatric history, a mental status examination, and a working knowledge of the specific DSM-IV-TR criteria can help clinicians differentiate among these conditions.

Course and Prognosis. On the basis of clinical data to date, patients seem to be equally likely to have prominent anxiety symptoms, prominent depressive symptoms, or an equal mixture of the two symptoms at onset. During the course of the illness, anxiety or depressive symptoms may alternate in their predominance. The prognosis is not known.

Treatment. Because adequate studies comparing treatment modalities for mixed anxiety-depressive disorder are not available, clinicians are probably most likely to provide treatment based on the symptoms present, their severity, and the clinician's own level of experience with various treatment modalities. Psychotherapeutic approaches may involve time-limited approaches, such as cognitive therapy or behavior modification, although some clinicians use a less structured psychotherapeutic approach, such as insight-oriented psychotherapy. Pharmacotherapy for mixed anxiety-depressive disorder may include antianxiety drugs, antidepressant drugs, or both. Among the anxiolytic drugs, some data indicate that the use of triazolobenzodiazepines (e.g., alprazolam [Xanax]) may be indicated because of their effectiveness in treating depression associated with anxiety. A drug that affects the serotonin 5-HT_{1A} receptor, such as buspirone (BuSpar), may also be indicated. Among the antidepressants, despite the noradrenergic theories linking anxiety disorders and depressive disorders, the serotonergic antidepressants may be most effective in treating mixed anxiety-depressive disorder. Venlafaxine (Effexor) is an effective antidepressant that has been approved by the U.S. Food and Drug Administration (FDA) for the treatment of depression as well as generalized anxiety disorder and is a drug of choice in the combined disorder.

References

Cassem EH. Depression and anxiety secondary to medical illness. *Psychiatr Clin North Am.* 1990;13:597.

Coryell W, Endicott J, Winokur G. Anxiety syndromes as epiphenomena of primary major depression: outcome and financial psychopathology. *Am J Psychiatry.* 1992;149:100.

Davis M. The role of the amygdala in fear-potentiated startle: implications for animal models of anxiety. *Trends Pharmacol Sci.* 1992;13:35.

Gabbard GO. *Psychodynamics Psychiatry in Clinical Practice: The DSM-IV Edition.* Washington, DC: American Psychiatric Press; 1994.

Gorman JM, section ed. Anxiety disorders. In: Sadock BJ, Sadock VA, eds. *Kaplan & Sadock's Comprehensive Textbook of Psychiatry.* 7th ed. Vol 1. Baltimore: Lippincott Williams & Wilkins; 2000:1441.

Kara S, Yazici KM, Guelec C, Uensal I. Mixed anxiety-depressive disorder and major depressive disorder: comparison of the severity of illness and biological variables. *Psychiatry Res.* 2000;94(1):59.

Rouillon F. Anxiety with depression: a treatment need. *Eur Neuropsychopharmacol.* 1999;9(suppl 3):S87.

Wittchen H-U, Schuster P, Lieb R. Comorbidity and mixer anxiety-depressive disorder: clinical curiosity or pathophysiological need? *Hum Psychopharmacol.* 2001;16(suppl 1):S21.

17

Somatoform Disorders

The term *somatoform* derives from the Greek *soma* for body, and the somatoform disorders are a broad group of illnesses that have bodily signs and symptoms as a major component. These disorders encompass mind–body interactions in which the brain, in ways still not well understood, sends various signals that impinge on the patient's awareness, indicating a serious problem in the body. Additionally, minor or as yet undetectable changes in neurochemistry, neurophysiology, and neuroimmunology may result from unknown mental or brain mechanisms that cause illness.

From a nosological perspective somatoform disorders were grouped together for the first time in 1980 in the third edition of *Diagnostic and Statistical Manual of Mental Disorders* (DSM-III) as those disorders in which bodily sensations or functions, as the patient's predominant focus, are influenced by a disorder of the mind. This clustering was not based on theoretical construct or laboratory findings. In fact, physical and laboratory examinations persistently fail to show significant substantiating data about the patient's complaints, which are, nevertheless, vigorous and sincere. Patients with somatoform disorders are convinced that their suffering comes from some type of presumably undetected and untreated bodily derangement. As Charles Beard stated in 1881: "The complaints are not imaginary." The modern physician who dismisses his or her patient with the statement that the complaint is imaginary does a disservice to both the patient and the profession.

The text revision of the fourth edition of DSM (DSM-IV-TR) recognizes five specific somatoform disorders (Table 17–1): (1) somatization disorder, characterized by many physical complaints affecting many organ systems; (2) conversion disorder, characterized by one or two neurological complaints; (3) hypochondriasis, characterized less by a focus on symptoms than by patients' beliefs that they have a specific disease; (4) body dysmorphic disorder, characterized by a false belief or exaggerated perception that a body part is defective; and (5) pain disorder, characterized by symptoms of pain that are either solely related to, or significantly exacerbated by, psychological factors. DSM-IV-TR also has two residual diagnostic categories for somatoform disorders: (1) undifferentiated somatoform disorder, which includes somatoform disorders not otherwise described that have been present for 6 months or longer, and (2) somatoform disorder not otherwise specified, which is the category for somatoform symptoms that do not meet any of the somatoform disorder diagnoses mentioned above.

SOMATIZATION DISORDER

Somatization disorder is characterized by many somatic symptoms that cannot be explained adequately on the basis of physical and laboratory examinations. It usually begins before the age of 30, may continue for years, and is distinguished, according to DSM-IV-TR, by "a combination of pain, gastrointestinal, sexual, and pseudoneurological symptoms." Somatization disorder differs from other somatoform disorders because of the multiplicity of the complaints and the multiple organ systems (e.g., gastrointestinal and neurological) that are affected. The disorder is chronic and is associated with significant psychological distress, impaired social and occupational functioning, and excessive medical-help–seeking behavior.

Somatization disorder has been recognized since the time of ancient Egypt. An early name for somatization disorder was *hysteria,* a condition incorrectly thought to affect only women. (The word *hysteria* is derived from the Greek word for uterus, *hystera.*) In the 17th century, Thomas Sydenham recognized that psychological factors, which he called "antecedent sorrows," were involved in the pathogenesis of the symptoms. In 1859, Paul Briquet, a French physician, observed the multiplicity of symptoms and affected organ systems and commented on the usually chronic course of the disorder. Because of these astute clinical observations, the disorder was called Briquet's syndrome until the term *somatization disorder* became the standard in the United States.

Epidemiology

The lifetime prevalence of somatization disorder in the general population is estimated to be 0.2 percent to 2 percent in women and 0.2 percent in men. Women with somatization disorder outnumber men 5 to 20 times, but the highest estimates may be due to the early tendency not to diagnose somatization disorder in male patients. Nevertheless, it is not an uncommon disorder. With a 5-to-1 female-to-male ratio, the lifetime prevalence of somatization disorder among women in the general population may be 1 or 2 percent. Among patients in the offices of general practitioners and family practitioners, as many as 5 to 10 percent may meet the diagnostic criteria for somatization disorder. The disorder is inversely related to social position and occurs most often among patients who have little education and low incomes. Somatization disorder is defined as beginning before age 30; it usually begins during a person's teenage years.

Table 17–1
Clinical Features of Somatoform Disorders

Diagnosis	Clinical Presentation	Demographic and Epidemiological Features	Diagnostic Features	Management Strategy	Prognosis	Associated Disturbances	Primary Differential Presentation	Psychological Processes Contributing to Symptoms	Motivation for Symptom Production
Somatization disorder	Polysymptomatic Recurrent and chronic Sickly by history	Young age Female predominance 20 to 1 Familial pattern 5–10% incidence in primary care populations	Review of systems profusely positive Multiple clinical contacts Polysurgical	Therapeutic alliance Regular appointments Crisis intervention	Poor to fair	Histrionic personality disorder Antisocial personality disorder Alcohol and other substance abuse Many life problems Conversion disorder	Physical disease Depression	Unconscious Cultural and developmental	Unconscious psychological factors
Conversion disorder	Monosymptomatic Mostly acute Simulates disease	Highly prevalent Female predominance Young age Rural and low social class Little-educated and psychologically unsophisticated	Simulation incompatible with known physiological mechanisms or anatomy	Suggestion and persuasion Multiple techniques	Excellent except in chronic conversion disorder	Alcohol and other substance dependence Antisocial personality disorder Somatization disorder Histrionic personality disorder	Depression Schizophrenia Neurological disease	Unconscious Psychological stress or conflict may be present	Unconscious psychological factors
Hypochondriasis	Disease concern *or* preoccupation	Previous physical disease Middle or old age Male-female ratio equal	Disease conviction amplifies symptoms Obsessional	Document symptoms Psychosocial review Psychotherapeutic	Fair to good Waxes and wanes	Obsessive-compulsive personality disorder Depressive and anxiety disorders	Depression Physical disease Personality disorder Delusional disorder	Unconscious Stress—bereavement Developmental factors	Unconscious psychological factors
Body dysmorphic disorder	Subjective feelings of ugliness or concern with body defect	Adolescence or young adult ? Female predominance Largely unknown	Pervasive bodily concerns	Therapeutic alliance Stress management Psychotherapies Antidepressant medications	Unknown	Anorexia nervosa Psychosocial distress Avoidant or obsessive-compulsive personality disorder	Delusional disorder Depressive disorders Somatization disorder	Unconscious Self-esteem factors	Unconscious psychological factors
Pain disorder	Pain syndrome simulated	Female predominance 2 to 1 Older: 4th or 5th decade Familial pattern Up to 40% of pain populations	Simulation or intensity incompatible with known physiological mechanisms or anatomy	Therapeutic alliance Redefine goals of treatment Antidepressant medications	Guarded, variable	Depressive disorders Alcohol and other substance abuse Dependent or histrionic personality disorder	Depression Psychophysiological Physical disease Malingering and disability syndrome	Unconscious Acute stressor and developmental Physical trauma may predispose	Unconscious psychological factors

Adapted from Folks DG, Ford CV, Houck CA. Somatoform disorders, factitious disorders, and malingering. In: Stoudemire A, ed. *Clinical Psychiatry for Medical Students.* Philadelphia: JB Lippincott; 1990:233.

Several studies have noted that somatization disorder commonly coexists with other mental disorders. About two thirds of all patients with somatization disorder have identifiable psychiatric symptoms, and up to half have other mental disorders. Commonly associated personality traits or personality disorders are those characterized by avoidant, paranoid, self-defeating, and obsessive-compulsive features. Two disorders that are not seen more commonly in patients with somatization disorder than in the general population are bipolar I disorder and substance abuse.

Etiology

Psychosocial Factors. The cause of somatization disorder is unknown. Psychosocial formulations of the cause involve interpretations of the symptoms as social communication whose result is to avoid obligations (e.g., going to a job a person does not like), to express emotions (e.g., anger at a spouse), or to symbolize a feeling or a belief (e.g., a pain in the gut). Strict psychoanalytic interpretations of symptoms rest on the hypothesis that the symptoms substitute for repressed instinctual impulses.

A behavioral perspective on somatization disorder emphasizes that parental teaching, parental example, and ethnic mores may teach some children to somatize more than others. In addition, some patients with somatization disorder come from unstable homes and have been physically abused. Social, cultural, and ethnic factors may also be involved in the development of symptoms.

Biological Factors. Some studies point to a neuropsychological basis for somatization disorder. These studies propose that the patients have characteristic attention and cognitive impairments that result in the faulty perception and assessment of somatosensory inputs. The reported impairments include excessive distractibility, inability to habituate to repetitive stimuli, grouping of cognitive constructs on an impressionistic basis, partial and circumstantial associations, and lack of selectivity, as indicated in some studies of evoked potentials. A limited number of brain-imaging studies have reported decreased metabolism in the frontal lobes and the nondominant hemisphere.

Genetic data indicate that in at least some families, the transmission of somatization disorder has genetic components. Somatization disorder tends to run in families and occurs in 10 to 20 percent of the first-degree female relatives of probands of patients with somatization disorder. Within these families, first-degree male relatives are prone to substance abuse and antisocial personality disorder. One study also reported a concordance rate of 29 percent in monozygotic twins and 10 percent in dizygotic twins, an indication of a genetic effect.

Research into cytokines, a new area of basic neuroscience study, may be relevant to somatization disorder and other somatoform disorders. Cytokines are messenger molecules that the immune system uses to communicate within itself and with the nervous system, including the brain. Examples of cytokines are interleukins, tumor necrosis factor, and interferons. Some preliminary experiments indicate that cytokines may help cause some of the nonspecific symptoms of disease (especially infections), such as hypersomnia, anorexia, fatigue, and depression. Although no data yet support the hypothesis, abnormal regulation of the cytokine system may result in some of the symptoms seen in somatoform disorders.

Table 17–2
DSM-IV-TR Diagnostic Criteria for Somatization Disorder

A. A history of many physical complaints beginning before age 30 years that occur over a period of several years and result in treatment being sought or significant impairment in social, occupational, or other important areas of functioning.

B. Each of the following criteria must have been met, with individual symptoms occurring at any time during the course of the disturbance:

(1) *four pain symptoms:* a history of pain related to at least four different sites or functions (e.g., head, abdomen, back, joints, extremities, chest, rectum, during menstruation, during sexual intercourse, or during urination)

(2) *two gastrointestinal symptoms:* a history of at least two gastrointestinal symptoms other than pain (e.g., nausea, bloating, vomiting other than during pregnancy, diarrhea, or intolerance of several different foods)

(3) *one sexual symptom:* a history of at least one sexual or reproductive symptom other than pain (e.g., sexual indifference, erectile or ejaculatory dysfunction, irregular menses, excessive menstrual bleeding, vomiting throughout pregnancy)

(4) *one pseudoneurological symptom:* a history of at least one symptom or deficit suggesting a neurological condition not limited to pain (conversion symptoms such as impaired coordination or balance, paralysis or localized weakness, difficulty swallowing or lump in throat, aphonia, urinary retention, hallucinations, loss of touch or pain sensation, double vision, blindness, deafness, seizures; dissociative symptoms such as amnesia; or loss of consciousness other than fainting)

C. Either (1) or (2):

(1) after appropriate investigation, each of the symptoms in Criterion B cannot be fully explained by a known general medical condition or the direct effects of a substance (e.g., a drug of abuse, a medication)

(2) when there is a related general medical condition, the physical complaints or resulting social or occupational impairment are in excess of what would be expected from the history, physical examination, or laboratory findings

D. The symptoms are not intentionally produced or feigned (as in factitious disorder or malingering).

From American Psychiatric Association. *Diagnostic and Statistical Manual of Mental Disorders.* 4th ed. Text rev. Washington, DC: American Psychiatric Association; copyright 2000, with permission.

Diagnosis

For the diagnosis of somatization disorder, DSM-IV-TR requires onset of symptoms before age 30 (Table 17–2). During the course of the disorder, patients must have complained of at least four pain symptoms, two gastrointestinal symptoms, one sexual symptom, and one pseudoneurological symptom, none of which is completely explained by physical or laboratory examinations.

Clinical Features

Patients with somatization disorder have many somatic complaints and long, complicated medical histories. Nausea and

vomiting (other than during pregnancy), difficulty swallowing, pain in the arms and legs, shortness of breath unrelated to exertion, amnesia, and complications of pregnancy and menstruation are among the most common symptoms. Patients frequently believe that they have been sickly most of their lives. Pseudoneurological symptoms suggest, but are not pathognomonic of, a neurological disorder. According to DSM-IV-TR, they include impaired coordination or balance, paralysis or localized weakness, difficulty swallowing or lump in throat, aphonia, urinary retention, hallucinations, loss of touch or pain sensation, double vision, blindness, deafness, seizures, or loss of consciousness other than fainting.

Psychological distress and interpersonal problems are prominent; anxiety and depression are the most prevalent psychiatric conditions. Suicide threats are common, but actual suicide is rare. If suicide does occur, it is often associated with substance abuse. Patients' medical histories are often circumstantial, vague, imprecise, inconsistent, and disorganized. Patients classically (but not always) describe their complaints in a dramatic, emotional, and exaggerated fashion, with vivid and colorful language; they may confuse temporal sequences and cannot clearly distinguish current from past symptoms. Female patients with somatization disorder may dress in an exhibitionistic manner. Patients may be perceived as dependent, self-centered, hungry for admiration or praise, and manipulative.

Somatization disorder is commonly associated with other mental disorders, including major depressive disorder, personality disorders, substance-related disorders, generalized anxiety disorder, and phobias. The combination of these disorders and the chronic symptoms results in an increased incidence of marital, occupational, and social problems.

Ms. D. is a 52-year-old white woman who was referred to a general internist in the city for evaluation of persistent back pain and multiple other complaints. At hospitalization it was noted that the patient was disabled from her job as a machine operator at a shoe factory. Ms. D. gave a history of 10 operations: removal of a tumor from her right wrist, dilation and curettage, a hysterectomy, three abdominal gastric operations, three breast biopsies, and leg surgery. She had received care from five different hospitals and seven different physicians in the past 2 years.

On physical examination, Ms. D. was an obese, chronically ill-appearing woman who came to the hospital wearing her transcutaneous electrical nerve stimulation unit. She was cooperative and showed her various scars with a certain amount of enthusiasm. The remainder of her physical examination was within normal limits except for a decreased range of motion in the area of her lumbar spine and local muscle guarding, with some tenderness. Spinal radiographs revealed some degeneration of vertebral bodies L2 to L5. On mental status examination she was cooperative and pleasant, and her behavior was somewhat seductive. There was no pressure or eccentricities in her speech. She showed little hesitation in discussing intimate details of her life. Her mood was euthymic; her affect was appropriate to mood but possibly a little shallow. The remainder of her mental status examination was within normal limits.

Disallowing all back-related symptoms, Ms. D. was positive for eight pain symptoms: four gastrointestinal symptoms, two sexual symptoms, and two pseudoneurological symptoms with an age at onset of 26 years. During the previous 12 months, Ms. D. reported that she had been in bed 21 days, had made seven office visits to four physicians, and had been hospitalized for a total of 52 days.

Ms. D.'s case illustrates that the diagnosis of somatization disorder can and should be made in the presence of comorbid medical conditions. Patients with somatization disorder do become ill, and their problems need to be diagnosed and treated appropriately. However, the management of somatization disorder should continue unchanged. (Courtesy of Fredrick G. Guggenheim, M.D.)

Differential Diagnosis

Clinicians must always rule out nonpsychiatric medical conditions that may explain a patient's symptoms. Several medical disorders often show nonspecific, transient abnormalities in the same age group. These medical disorders include multiple sclerosis, myasthenia gravis, systemic lupus erythematosus, acquired immune deficiency syndrome (AIDS), acute intermittent porphyria, hyperparathyroidism, hyperthyroidism, and chronic systemic infections. The onset of multiple somatic symptoms in patients older than 40 should be presumed to be caused by a nonpsychiatric medical condition until an exhaustive medical workup has been completed.

Many mental disorders are considered in the differential diagnosis, which is complicated by the observation that at least 50 percent of patients with somatization disorder have a coexisting mental disorder. Patients with major depressive disorder, generalized anxiety disorder, and schizophrenia may all have an initial complaint that focuses on somatic symptoms. In all these disorders, however, the symptoms of depression, anxiety, or psychosis eventually predominate over the somatic complaints. Although patients with panic disorder may complain of many somatic symptoms related to their panic attacks, they are not bothered by somatic symptoms between panic attacks.

Among the other somatoform disorders, hypochondriasis, conversion disorder, and pain somatization disorder, patients with hypochondriasis falsely believe that they have a specific disease, whereas those with somatization disorder are concerned with many symptoms. The symptoms of conversion disorder are limited to one or two neurological symptoms rather than to the wide-ranging symptoms of somatization disorder. Pain disorder is limited to one or two complaints of pain symptoms.

Course and Prognosis

Somatization disorder is chronic and often debilitating. By definition, the symptoms should have begun before age 30 and have been present for several years. Episodes of increased symptom severity and the development of new symptoms are thought to last 6 to 9 months and may be separated by less symptomatic periods lasting 9 to 12 months. Rarely, however, does a patient with somatization disorder go for more than a year without seeking medical attention. Often, periods of increased stress are associated with the exacerbation of somatic symptoms.

Treatment

Somatization disorder is best treated when the patient has a single identified physician as primary caretaker. When more than one clinician is involved, patients have increased opportunities to express somatic complaints. Primary physicians should see patients during regularly scheduled visits, usually at monthly intervals. The visits should be relatively brief, although a partial physical examination should be conducted to respond to each new somatic complaint. Additional laboratory and diagnostic procedures should generally be avoided. Once somatization disorder has been diagnosed, the treating physician should listen to the somatic complaints as emotional expressions rather than as medical complaints. Nevertheless, patients with somatization disorder can also have bona fide physical illnesses; therefore, physicians must always use their judgment about what symptoms to work up and to what extent. A reasonable long-range strategy for a primary care physician who is treating a patient with somatization disorder is to increase the patient's awareness of the possibility that psychological factors are involved in the symptoms until the patient is willing to see a mental health clinician. In complex cases with many medical presentations, a psychiatrist is better able to judge whether or not to seek a medical or surgical consultation because of his or her medical training; however, a nonmedical mental health professional can explore the psychological antecedents of the disorder as well, especially if consulting closely with a physician.

Psychotherapy, both individual and group, decreases these patients' personal health care expenditures by 50 percent, largely by decreasing their rates of hospitalization. In psychotherapy settings, patients are helped to cope with their symptoms, to express underlying emotions, and to develop alternative strategies for expressing their feelings.

Giving psychotropic medications whenever somatization disorder coexists with a mood or anxiety disorder is always a risk, but psychopharmacological treatment, as well as psychotherapeutic treatment, of the coexisting disorder is indicated. Medication must be monitored, because patients with somatization disorder tend to use drugs erratically and unreliably. Few available data indicate that pharmacological treatment is effective in patients without coexisting mental disorders.

CONVERSION DISORDER

A conversion disorder is a disturbance of bodily functioning that does not conform to current concepts of the anatomy and physiology of the central or the peripheral nervous system. It typically occurs in a setting of stress and produces considerable dysfunction.

DSM-IV-TR defines conversion disorder as characterized by the presence of one or more neurological symptoms (e.g., paralysis, blindness, and paresthesias) that cannot be explained by a known neurological or medical disorder. In addition, the diagnosis requires association of psychological factors with the initiation or exacerbation of the symptoms (Table 17–3).

The syndrome currently known as conversion disorder was originally combined with the syndrome known as somatization disorder and was referred to as hysteria, conversion reaction, or dissociative reaction. Briquet and Jean-Martin Charcot contributed to the development of the concept of conversion disorder by noting the influence of heredity on the symptom and the common association with a traumatic event.

Table 17–3
Common Symptoms of Conversion Disorder

Motor symptoms	**Sensory deficits**
Involuntary movements	Anesthesia, especially of extremities
Tics	Midline anesthesia
Blepharospasm	Blindness
Torticollis	Tunnel vision
Opisthotonos	Deafness
Seizures	**Visceral symptoms**
Abnormal gait	Psychogenic vomiting
Falling	Pseudocyesis
Astasia-abasia	*Globus hystericus*
Paralysis	Swooning or syncope
Weakness	Urinary retention
Aphonia	Diarrhea

Courtesy of Frederick G. Guggenheim, M.D.

The term *conversion* was introduced by Sigmund Freud, who, based on his work with Anna O, hypothesized that the symptoms of conversion disorder reflect unconscious conflicts.

Epidemiology

Some symptoms of conversion disorder that are not severe enough to warrant the diagnosis may occur in up to one third of the general population sometime during their lives. One community reported an annual incidence of conversion disorder of 22 per 100,000. Among specific populations, the occurrence of conversion disorder may be even higher than that, perhaps making conversion disorder the most common somatoform disorder in some populations. Several studies have reported that 5 to 15 percent of psychiatric consultations in a general hospital and 25 to 30 percent of admissions to a Veterans Administration hospital involve patients with conversion disorder diagnoses. DSM-IV-TR gives a range from a low of 11 to a high of 500 cases per 100,000 population.

The ratio of women to men among adult patients is at least 2 to 1 and as much as 10 to 1; among children there is an even higher predominance in girls. Men with conversion disorder have often been involved in occupational or military accidents. Conversion disorder can have its onset at any time, from childhood to old age, but it is most common in adolescents and young adults. Data indicate that conversion disorder is most common among rural populations, persons with little education, those with low intelligence quotients, those in low socioeconomic groups, and military personnel who have been exposed to combat situations. Conversion disorder is commonly associated with comorbid diagnoses of major depressive disorder, anxiety disorders, and schizophrenia and shows an increased frequency in relatives of probands with conversion disorder.

Comorbidity

Medical and especially neurological disorders occur frequently among patients with conversion disorders. What is typically seen in these comorbid neurological or medical conditions is an elaboration of symptoms stemming from the original organic lesion.

group of college students found that more than 50 percent had at least some preoccupation with a particular aspect of their appearance, and in about 25 percent of the students, the concern had at least some significant effect on their feelings and functioning.

Available data indicate that the most common age of onset is between 15 and 30 years and that women are affected somewhat more often than men. Affected patients are also likely to be unmarried. Body dysmorphic disorder commonly coexists with other mental disorders. One study found that more than 90 percent of patients with body dysmorphic disorder had experienced a major depressive episode in their lifetimes; about 70 percent had experienced an anxiety disorder; and about 30 percent had experienced a psychotic disorder.

Etiology

The cause of body dysmorphic disorder is unknown. The high comorbidity with depressive disorders, a higher-than-expected family history of mood disorders and obsessive-compulsive disorder, and the reported responsiveness of the condition to serotonin-specific drugs indicate that in at least some patients, the pathophysiology of the disorder may involve serotonin and may be related to other mental disorders. Stereotyped concepts of beauty emphasized in certain families and within the culture at large may significantly affect patients with body dysmorphic disorder. In psychodynamic models, body dysmorphic disorder is seen as reflecting the displacement of a sexual or emotional conflict onto a nonrelated body part. Such an association occurs through the defense mechanisms of repression, dissociation, distortion, symbolization, and projection.

Diagnosis

The DSM-IV-TR diagnostic criteria for body dysmorphic disorder stipulate preoccupation with an imagined defect in appearance or overemphasis of a slight defect (Table 17–7). The preoccupation causes patients significant emotional distress or markedly impairs their ability to function in important areas.

Clinical Features

The most common concerns (Table 17–8) involve facial flaws, particularly those involving specific parts (e.g., the nose). Sometimes the concern is vague and difficult to understand, such as extreme concern over a "scrunchy" chin. One study found that, on average, patients had concerns about four body regions during the course of the disorder. Other body parts of concern are hair, breasts, and genitalia. A proposed variant of dysmorphic disorder among men is the desire to "bulk up" and develop large muscle mass, which can interfere with ordinary living, holding a job, or staying healthy. The specific body part may change during the time a patient is affected with the disorder. Common associated symptoms include ideas or frank delusions of reference (usually about persons' noticing the alleged body flaw), either excessive mirror checking or avoidance of reflective surfaces, and attempts to hide the presumed deformity (with makeup or clothing). The effects on a person's life can be significant; almost all affected patients avoid social and occupational exposure. As many as one third of the patients may be housebound because of worry about being ridiculed for the alleged deformities, and as many as one fifth attempt suicide. As discussed above, comorbid diagnoses of depressive disorders and anxiety disorders are common, and patients may also have traits of obsessive-compulsive, schizoid, and narcissistic personality disorders.

Table 17–7
DSM-IV-TR Diagnostic Criteria for Body Dysmorphic Disorder

A. Preoccupation with an imagined defect in appearance. If a slight physical anomaly is present, the person's concern is markedly excessive.
B. The preoccupation causes clinically significant distress or impairment in social, occupational, or other important areas of functioning.
C. The preoccupation is not better accounted for by another mental disorder (e.g., dissatisfaction with body shape and size in anorexia nervosa).

From American Psychiatric Association. *Diagnostic and Statistical Manual of Mental Disorders*. 4th ed. Text rev. Washington, DC: American Psychiatric Association; copyright 2000, with permission.

Table 17–8
Location of Imagined Defects in 30 Patients with Body Dysmorphic Disorder[a]

Location	*N*	%
Hair[b]	19	63
Nose	15	50
Skin[c]	15	50
Eyes	8	27
Head, face[d]	6	20
Overall body build, bone structure	6	20
Lips	5	17
Chin	5	17
Stomach, waist	5	17
Teeth	4	13
Legs, knees	4	13
Breasts, pectoral muscles	3	10
Ugly face (general)	3	10
Ears	2	7
Cheeks	2	7
Buttocks	2	7
Penis	2	7
Arms, wrists	2	7
Neck	1	3
Forehead	1	3
Facial muscles	1	3
Shoulders	1	3
Hips	1	3

[a]Total is greater than 100% because most patients had "defects" in more than one location.
[b]Involved head hair in 15 cases, beard growth in 2 cases, and other body hair in 3 cases.
[c]Involved acne in 7 cases, facial lines in 3 cases, and other skin concerns in 7 cases.
[d]Involved concerns with shape in 5 cases and size in 1 case.
Reprinted with permission from Phillips KA, McElroy SL, Keck PE Jr, Pope HG, Hudson JL. Body dysmorphic disorder: 30 cases of imagined ugliness. *Am J Psychiatry.* 1993;150:303.

Differential Diagnosis

Hypochondriasis must be differentiated from nonpsychiatric medical conditions, especially disorders that show symptoms that are not necessarily easily diagnosed. Such diseases include AIDS, endocrinopathies, myasthenia gravis, multiple sclerosis, degenerative diseases of the nervous system, systemic lupus erythematosus, and occult neoplastic disorders.

Hypochondriasis is differentiated from somatization disorder by the emphasis in hypochondriasis on fear of having a disease and emphasis in somatization disorder on concern about many symptoms. Patients with hypochondriasis usually complain about fewer symptoms than patients with somatization disorder. Somatization disorder usually has an onset before age 30, whereas hypochondriasis has a less specific age of onset. Patients with somatization disorder are more likely to be women; hypochondriasis is equally distributed among men and women.

Hypochondriasis must also be differentiated from the other somatoform disorders. Conversion disorder is acute and generally transient and usually involves a symptom rather than a particular disease. The presence or absence of *la belle indifférence* is an unreliable feature with which to differentiate the two conditions. Pain disorder is chronic, as is hypochondriasis, but the symptoms are limited to complaints of pain. Patients with body dysmorphic disorder wish to appear normal but believe that others notice that they are not, whereas those with hypochondriasis seek out attention for their presumed diseases.

Hypochondriacal symptoms can also occur in patients with depressive disorders and anxiety disorders. If a patient meets the full diagnostic criteria for both hypochondriasis and another major mental disorder, such as major depressive disorder or generalized anxiety disorder, the patient should receive both diagnoses, unless the hypochondriacal symptoms occur only during episodes of the other mental disorder. Patients with panic disorder may initially complain that they are affected by a disease (e.g., heart trouble), but careful questioning during the medical history usually uncovers the classic symptoms of a panic attack. Delusional hypochondriacal beliefs occur in schizophrenia and other psychotic disorders but can be differentiated from hypochondriasis by their delusional intensity and by the presence of other psychotic symptoms. In addition, schizophrenic patients' somatic delusions tend to be bizarre, idiosyncratic, and out of keeping with their cultural milieus.

Hypochondriasis is distinguished from factitious disorder with physical symptoms and from malingering in that patients with hypochondriasis actually experience and do not simulate the symptoms they report.

Course and Prognosis

The course of hypochondriasis is usually episodic; the episodes last from months to years and are separated by equally long quiescent periods. There may be an obvious association between exacerbations of hypochondriacal symptoms and psychosocial stressors. Although no well-conducted large outcome studies have been reported, an estimated one third to one half of all patients with hypochondriasis eventually improve significantly. A good prognosis is associated with high socioeconomic status, treatment-responsive anxiety or depression, sudden onset of symptoms, the absence of a personality disorder, and the absence of a related nonpsychiatric medical condition. Most children with hypochondriasis recover by late adolescence or early adulthood.

Treatment

Patients with hypochondriasis usually resist psychiatric treatment, although some accept this treatment if it takes place in a medical setting and focuses on stress reduction and education in coping with chronic illness. Group psychotherapy often benefits such patients, in part because it provides the social support and social interaction that seem to reduce their anxiety. Other forms of psychotherapy such as individual insight-oriented psychotherapy behavior therapy, cognitive therapy and hypnosis may be useful.

Frequent, regularly scheduled physical examinations help to reassure patients that their physicians are not abandoning them and that their complaints are being taken seriously. However, invasive diagnostic and therapeutic procedures should only be undertaken when objective evidence calls for them. When possible, the clinician should refrain from treating equivocal or incidental physical examination findings.

Pharmacotherapy alleviates hypochondriacal symptoms only when a patient has an underlying drug-responsive condition, such as an anxiety disorder or major depressive disorder. When hypochondriasis is secondary to another primary mental disorder, that disorder must be treated in its own right. When hypochondriasis is a transient situational reaction, clinicians must help patients cope with the stress without reinforcing their illness behavior and their use of the sick role as a solution to their problems.

BODY DYSMORPHIC DISORDER

Patients with body dysmorphic disorder have a pervasive subjective feeling of ugliness of some aspect of their appearance despite a normal or nearly normal appearance. The core of the disorder is the person's strong belief or fear that he or she is unattractive or even repulsive. This fear is rarely assuaged by reassurance or compliments, even though the typical patient with this disorder is quite normal in appearance.

The disorder was recognized and named dysmorphophobia more than 100 years ago by Emil Kraepelin, who considered it a compulsive neurosis; Pierre Janet called it *obsession de la honte du corps* (obsession with shame of the body). Freud wrote about the condition in his description of the Wolf-Man, who was excessively concerned about his nose. Although dysmorphophobia was widely recognized and studied in Europe, it was not until the publication of DSM-III in 1980 that dysmorphophobia, as an example of a typical somatoform disorder, was specifically mentioned in the U.S. diagnostic criteria. In DSM-IV-TR, the condition is known as body dysmorphic disorder, because the DSM editors believed that the term *dysmorphophobia* inaccurately implied the presence of a behavioral pattern of phobic avoidance.

Epidemiology

Body dysmorphic disorder is a poorly studied condition, partly because patients are more likely to go to dermatologists, internists, or plastic surgeons than to psychiatrists. One study of a

group of college students found that more than 50 percent had at least some preoccupation with a particular aspect of their appearance, and in about 25 percent of the students, the concern had at least some significant effect on their feelings and functioning.

Available data indicate that the most common age of onset is between 15 and 30 years and that women are affected somewhat more often than men. Affected patients are also likely to be unmarried. Body dysmorphic disorder commonly coexists with other mental disorders. One study found that more than 90 percent of patients with body dysmorphic disorder had experienced a major depressive episode in their lifetimes; about 70 percent had experienced an anxiety disorder; and about 30 percent had experienced a psychotic disorder.

Etiology

The cause of body dysmorphic disorder is unknown. The high comorbidity with depressive disorders, a higher-than-expected family history of mood disorders and obsessive-compulsive disorder, and the reported responsiveness of the condition to serotonin-specific drugs indicate that in at least some patients, the pathophysiology of the disorder may involve serotonin and may be related to other mental disorders. Stereotyped concepts of beauty emphasized in certain families and within the culture at large may significantly affect patients with body dysmorphic disorder. In psychodynamic models, body dysmorphic disorder is seen as reflecting the displacement of a sexual or emotional conflict onto a nonrelated body part. Such an association occurs through the defense mechanisms of repression, dissociation, distortion, symbolization, and projection.

Diagnosis

The DSM-IV-TR diagnostic criteria for body dysmorphic disorder stipulate preoccupation with an imagined defect in appearance or overemphasis of a slight defect (Table 17–7). The preoccupation causes patients significant emotional distress or markedly impairs their ability to function in important areas.

Clinical Features

The most common concerns (Table 17–8) involve facial flaws, particularly those involving specific parts (e.g., the nose). Sometimes the concern is vague and difficult to understand, such as extreme concern over a "scrunchy" chin. One study found that, on average, patients had concerns about four body regions during the course of the disorder. Other body parts of concern are hair, breasts, and genitalia. A proposed variant of dysmorphic disorder among men is the desire to "bulk up" and develop large muscle mass, which can interfere with ordinary living, holding a job, or staying healthy. The specific body part may change during the time a patient is affected with the disorder. Common associated symptoms include ideas or frank delusions of reference (usually about persons' noticing the alleged body flaw), either excessive mirror checking or avoidance of reflective surfaces, and attempts to hide the presumed deformity (with makeup or clothing). The effects on a person's life can be significant; almost all affected patients avoid social and occupational exposure. As many as one third of the patients may be housebound because of worry about being ridiculed for the alleged deformities, and as many as one fifth attempt suicide. As discussed above, comorbid diagnoses of depressive disorders and anxiety disorders are common, and patients may also have traits of obsessive-compulsive, schizoid, and narcissistic personality disorders.

Table 17–7
DSM-IV-TR Diagnostic Criteria for Body Dysmorphic Disorder

A. Preoccupation with an imagined defect in appearance. If a slight physical anomaly is present, the person's concern is markedly excessive.
B. The preoccupation causes clinically significant distress or impairment in social, occupational, or other important areas of functioning.
C. The preoccupation is not better accounted for by another mental disorder (e.g., dissatisfaction with body shape and size in anorexia nervosa).

From American Psychiatric Association. *Diagnostic and Statistical Manual of Mental Disorders.* 4th ed. Text rev. Washington, DC: American Psychiatric Association; copyright 2000, with permission.

Table 17–8
Location of Imagined Defects in 30 Patients with Body Dysmorphic Disorder[a]

Location	N	%
Hair[b]	19	63
Nose	15	50
Skin[c]	15	50
Eyes	8	27
Head, face[d]	6	20
Overall body build, bone structure	6	20
Lips	5	17
Chin	5	17
Stomach, waist	5	17
Teeth	4	13
Legs, knees	4	13
Breasts, pectoral muscles	3	10
Ugly face (general)	3	10
Ears	2	7
Cheeks	2	7
Buttocks	2	7
Penis	2	7
Arms, wrists	2	7
Neck	1	3
Forehead	1	3
Facial muscles	1	3
Shoulders	1	3
Hips	1	3

[a]Total is greater than 100% because most patients had "defects" in more than one location.
[b]Involved head hair in 15 cases, beard growth in 2 cases, and other body hair in 3 cases.
[c]Involved acne in 7 cases, facial lines in 3 cases, and other skin concerns in 7 cases.
[d]Involved concerns with shape in 5 cases and size in 1 case.
Reprinted with permission from Phillips KA, McElroy SL, Keck PE Jr, Pope HG, Hudson JL. Body dysmorphic disorder: 30 cases of imagined ugliness. *Am J Psychiatry.* 1993;150:303.

Clinical Features

Patients with hypochondriasis believe that they have a serious disease that has not yet been detected, and they cannot be persuaded to the contrary. They may maintain a belief that they have a particular disease, or as time progresses, they may transfer their belief to another disease. Their convictions persist despite negative laboratory results, the benign course of the alleged disease over time, and appropriate reassurances from physicians. Yet their beliefs are not fixed enough to be delusions. Hypochondriasis is often accompanied by symptoms of depression and anxiety and commonly coexists with a depressive or anxiety disorder.

Although DSM-IV-TR specifies that the symptoms must be present for at least 6 months, transient hypochondriacal states can occur after major stresses, most commonly the death or serious illness of someone important to the patient, or a serious (perhaps life-threatening) illness that has been resolved but that leaves the patient temporarily hypochondriacal in its wake. Such states that last fewer than 6 months should be diagnosed as somatoform disorder not otherwise specified. Transient hypochondriacal responses to external stress generally remit when the stress is resolved, but they can become chronic if reinforced by persons in the patient's social system or by health professionals.

A 38-year-old radiologist is evaluated after returning from a 10-day stay at a famous out-of-state diagnostic center to which he had been referred by a local gastroenterologist after "he reached the end of the line" with the radiologist. The patient reports that he underwent extensive physical and laboratory examinations, X-ray examinations of the entire gastrointestinal tract, esophagoscopy, gastroscopy, and colonoscopy at the center. Although he was told that the results of the examinations were negative for significant physical disease, he appears resentful and disappointed rather than relieved at the findings. He was seen briefly for a "routine" evaluation by a psychiatrist at the diagnostic center, but had difficulty relating to the psychiatrist on more than a superficial level.

On further inquiry concerning the patient's physical symptoms, he describes occasional twinges of mild abdominal pain, sensations of "fullness," "bowel rumblings," and a "firm abdominal mass" that he can sometimes feel in his left lower quadrant. Over the last few months he has gradually become more aware of these sensations and convinced that they may be the result of a carcinoma of the colon. He tests his stool for occult blood weekly and spends 15–20 minutes every 2 to 3 days carefully palpating his abdomen as he lies in bed at home. He has secretly performed several X-ray studies on himself in his own office after hours.

Although he is successful in his work, has an excellent attendance record, and is active in community life, the patient spends much of his leisure time at home alone in bed. His wife, an instructor at a local school of nursing, is angry and bitter about this behavior, which she describes as "robbing us of what we've worked so hard and postponed so much for." Although she and the patient share many values and genuinely love each other, his behavior causes a real strain on their marriage.

When the patient was 13, a heart murmur was detected on a school physical exam. Because a younger brother had died in early childhood of congenital heart disease, the patient was removed from gym class until the murmur could be evaluated. The evaluation proved the murmur to be benign, but the patient began to worry that the evaluation might have "missed something" and considered the occasional sensations of "skipping a beat" as evidence that this was so. He kept his fears to himself; they subsided over the next 2 years, but never entirely left him.

As a second-year medical student he was relieved to share some of his health concerns with his classmates, who also worried about having the diseases they were learning about in pathology. He realized, however, that he was much more preoccupied with and worried about his health than they were. Since graduating from medical school, he has repeatedly experienced a series of concerns, each following the same pattern: noticing a symptom, becoming increasingly preoccupied with what it might mean, and having a negative physical evaluation. At times he returns to an "old" concern, but is too embarrassed to pursue it with physicians he knows, as when he discovered a "suspicious" nevus only 1 week after he had persuaded a dermatologist to biopsy one that proved to be entirely benign.

The patient tells his story with a sincere, discouraged tone, brightened only by a note of genuine pleasure and enthusiasm as he provides a detailed account of the discovery of a genuine, but clinically insignificant, urethral anomaly as the result of an intravenous pyelogram he had ordered himself. Near the end of the interview, he explains that his coming in for evaluation now is largely at his own insistence, precipitated by an encounter with his 9-year-old son. The boy had accidentally walked in while he was palpating his own abdomen for "masses" and asked, "What do you think it is this time, Dad?" As he describes his shame and anger (mostly at himself) about this incident, his eyes fill with tears.

DISCUSSION

It is apparent that this doctor's symptoms are not caused by any general medical disorder. Preoccupation with physical symptoms can be seen in disorders such as schizophrenia, major depressive disorder, or anxiety disorders, but there is no evidence for any of these disorders in this case. This suggests, therefore, a somatoform disorder—mental disorder with physical symptoms suggesting a general medical disorder, but for which there is positive evidence, or a strong presumption, that the symptoms are linked to psychological factors.

A variety of physical symptoms not adequately explained by general medical conditions is seen in somatoform disorder. In this case the symptoms are few, whereas in somatoform disorder typically there are a large number of different symptoms that appear in many different organ systems. Furthermore, in somatoform disorder the preoccupation is generally with the symptoms themselves. In this case the disturbance is preoccupation with the fear of having a serious disease resulting from an unrealistic interpretation of physical signs or sensations. The persistence of this irrational fear for more than 6 months, despite medical reassurance, indicates hypochondriasis.

used to treat conversion disorder. The longer the duration of these patients' sick role and the more they have regressed, the more difficult the treatment.

HYPOCHONDRIASIS

Hypochondriasis is defined as a person's preoccupation with the fear of contracting, or the belief of having, a serious disease. This fear or belief arises when a person misinterprets bodily symptoms or functions. The term *hypochondriasis* is derived from the old medical term *hypochondrium,* ("below the ribs") and reflects the common abdominal complaints of many patients with the disorder. Hypochondriasis results from patients' unrealistic or inaccurate interpretations of physical symptoms or sensations, even though no known medical causes can be found. Patients' preoccupations result in significant distress to them and impair their ability to function in their personal, social, and occupational roles.

Epidemiology

One recent study reported a 6-month prevalence of hypochondriasis of 4 to 6 percent in a general medical clinic population, but it may be as high as 15 percent. Men and women are equally affected by hypochondriasis. Although the onset of symptoms can occur at any age, the disorder most commonly appears in persons 20 to 30 years of age. Some evidence indicates that the diagnosis is more common among blacks than among whites, but social position, education level, and marital status do not appear to affect the diagnosis. Hypochondriacal complaints reportedly occur in about 3 percent of medical students, usually in the first 2 years, but they are generally transient.

Etiology

In the diagnostic criteria for hypochondriasis, DSM-IV-TR indicates that the symptoms reflect a misinterpretation of bodily symptoms. A reasonable body of data indicates that persons with hypochondriasis augment and amplify their somatic sensations; they have low thresholds for, and low tolerance of, physical discomfort. For example, what persons normally perceive as abdominal pressure, persons with hypochondriasis experience as abdominal pain. They may focus on bodily sensations, misinterpret them, and become alarmed by them because of a faulty cognitive scheme.

A second theory is that hypochondriasis is understandable in terms of a social learning model. The symptoms of hypochondriasis are viewed as a request for admission to the sick role made by a person facing seemingly insurmountable and insolvable problems. The sick role offers an escape that allows a patient to avoid noxious obligations, to postpone unwelcome challenges, and to be excused from usual duties and obligations.

A third theory suggests that hypochondriasis is a variant form of other mental disorders, among which depressive disorders and anxiety disorders are most frequently included. An estimated 80 percent of patients with hypochondriasis may have coexisting depressive or anxiety disorders. Patients who meet the diagnostic criteria for hypochondriasis may be somatizing subtypes of these other disorders.

The psychodynamic school of thought has produced a fourth theory of hypochondriasis. According to this theory, aggressive and hostile wishes toward others are transferred (through repression and displacement) into physical complaints. The anger of patients with hypochondriasis originates in past disappointments, rejections, and losses, but the patients express their anger in the present by soliciting the help and concern of other persons and then rejecting them as ineffective. Hypochondriasis is also viewed as a defense against guilt, a sense of innate badness, an expression of low self-esteem, and a sign of excessive self-concern. Pain and somatic suffering thus become means of atonement and expiation (undoing) and can be experienced as deserved punishment for past wrongdoing (either real or imaginary) and for a person's sense of wickedness and sinfulness.

Diagnosis

The DSM-IV-TR diagnostic criteria for hypochondriasis require that patients be preoccupied with the false belief that they have a serious disease, based on their misinterpretation of physical signs or sensations (Table 17–6). The belief must last at least 6 months, despite the absence of pathological findings on medical and neurological examinations. The diagnostic criteria also stipulate that the belief cannot have the intensity of a delusion (more appropriately diagnosed as delusional disorder) and cannot be restricted to distress about appearance (more appropriately diagnosed as body dysmorphic disorder). The symptoms of hypochondriasis must be intense enough to cause emotional distress or impair the patient's ability to function in important areas of life. Clinicians may specify the presence of poor insight; patients do not consistently recognize that their concerns about disease are excessive.

Table 17–6
DSM-IV-TR Diagnostic Criteria for Hypochondriasis

A. Preoccupation with fears of having, or the idea that one has, a serious disease based on the person's misinterpretation of bodily symptoms.
B. The preoccupation persists despite appropriate medical evaluation and reassurance.
C. The belief in Criterion A is not of delusional intensity (as in delusional disorder, somatic type) and is not restricted to a circumscribed concern about appearance (as in body dysmorphic disorder).
D. The preoccupation causes clinically significant distress or impairment in social, occupational, or other important areas of functioning.
E. The duration of the disturbance is at least 6 months.
F. The preoccupation is not better accounted for by generalized anxiety disorder, obsessive-compulsive disorder, panic disorder, a major depressive episode, separation anxiety, or another somatoform disorder.

Specify if:

With poor insight: if, for most of the time during the current episode, the person does not recognize that the concern about having a serious illness is excessive or unreasonable

From American Psychiatric Association. *Diagnostic and Statistical Manual of Mental Disorders.* 4th ed. Text rev. Washington, DC: American Psychiatric Association; copyright 2000, with permission.

Table 17–5
Distinctive Physical Examination Findings in Conversion Disorder

Condition	Test	Conversion Findings
Anesthesia	Map dermatomes	Sensory loss does not conform to recognized pattern of distribution
Hemianesthesia	Check midline	Strict half-body split
Astasia-abasia	Walking, dancing	With suggestion, those who cannot walk may still be able to dance; alteration of sensory and motor findings with suggestion
Paralysis, paresis	Drop paralyzed hand onto face	Hand falls next to face, not on it
	Hoover test	Pressure noted in examiner's hand under paralyzed leg when attempting straight leg raising
	Check motor strength	Give-away weakness
Coma	Examiner attempts to open eyes	Resists opening; gaze preference is away from doctor
	Ocular cephalic maneuver	Eyes stare straight ahead, do not move from side to side
Aphonia	Request a cough	Essentially normal coughing sound indicates cords are closing
Intractable sneezing	Observe	Short nasal grunts with little or no sneezing on inspiratory phase; little or no aerosolization of secretions; minimal facial expression; eyes open; stops when asleep; abates when alone
Syncope	Head-up tilt test	Magnitude of changes in vital signs and venous pooling do not explain continuing symptoms
Tunnel vision	Visual fields	Changing pattern on multiple examinations
Profound monocular blindness	Swinging flashlight sign (Marcus Gunn)	Absence of relative afferent pupillary defect
	Binocular visual fields	Sufficient vision in "bad eye" precludes plotting normal physiological blind spot in good eye
Severe bilateral blindness	"Wiggle your fingers, I'm just testing coordination"	Patient may begin to mimic new movements before realizing the slip
	Sudden flash of bright light	Patient flinches
	"Look at your hand"	Patient does not look there
	"Touch your index fingers"	Even blind patients can do this by proprioception

Courtesy of Frederick G. Guggenheim, M.D.

symptoms occur in schizophrenia, depressive disorders, and anxiety disorders, but these other disorders are associated with their own distinct symptoms that eventually make differential diagnosis possible.

Sensorimotor symptoms also occur in somatization disorder. But somatization disorder is a chronic illness that begins early in life and includes symptoms in many other organ systems. In hypochondriasis, patients have no actual loss or distortion of function; the somatic complaints are chronic and are not limited to neurological symptoms, and the characteristic hypochondriacal attitudes and beliefs are present. If the patient's symptoms are limited to pain, pain disorder can be diagnosed. Patients whose complaints are limited to sexual function are classified as having a sexual dysfunction, rather than conversion disorder.

In both malingering and factitious disorder, the symptoms are under conscious, voluntary control. A malingerer's history is usually more inconsistent and contradictory than that of a patient with conversion disorder, and a malingerer's fraudulent behavior is clearly goal directed.

Table 17–5 lists examples of important tests that are relevant to conversion disorder symptoms.

Course and Prognosis

The initial symptoms of most patients with conversion disorder, perhaps 90 to 100 percent, resolve in a few days or less than a month. A reported 75 percent of patients may not experience another episode, but 25 percent have additional episodes during periods of stress. Associated with a good prognosis are a sudden onset, an easily identifiable stressor, good premorbid adjustment, no comorbid psychiatric or medical disorders, and no ongoing litigation. The longer the conversion disorder symptoms are present, the worse the prognosis. As discussed above, 25 to 50 percent of patients may later have neurological disorders or nonpsychiatric medical conditions affecting the nervous system; thus, patients with conversion disorder must have complete medical and neurological evaluations at the time of diagnosis.

Treatment

Resolution of the conversion disorder symptom is usually spontaneous, although probably facilitated by insight-oriented supportive or behavior therapy. The most important feature of the therapy is a relationship with a caring and confident therapist. With patients who are resistant to the idea of psychotherapy, physicians can suggest that the psychotherapy will focus on issues of stress and coping. Telling such patients that their symptoms are imaginary often makes them worse. Hypnosis, anxiolytics, and behavioral relaxation exercises are effective in some cases. Parenteral amobarbital or lorazepam may be helpful in obtaining additional historic information, especially when a patient has recently experienced a traumatic event. Psychodynamic approaches include psychoanalysis and insight-oriented psychotherapy, in which patients explore intrapsychic conflicts and the symbolism of the conversion disorder symptoms. Brief and direct forms of short-term psychotherapy have also been

Her demeanor had always been placid and unassuming. There was no family history of antisocial behavior or substance abuse.

On Thanksgiving Day, while taking her usual solitary afternoon walk along the creek behind the kitchen, she came upon the floating, lifeless bodies of two of her children. She shrieked, swooned, and fell to the ground. Relatives in the house rushed out to assist but could not revive the children. When she was helped up, she asked that her husband guide her back to her room. Later that afternoon she seemed calm, even detached, as others scurried about making arrangements. She admitted to a visitor that she seemed to have lost the gift of sight.

That evening the family physician was called to examine the newly sightless woman. He noted that her pupils were round, equal, and constricted briskly with a bright light; she could not touch the tips of her index fingers together in front of her; she failed to look at her own hands when instructed to do so; and she had no other neurological abnormalities, asymmetries, or complaints. The physician explained to the gathered family and patient that the woman was suffering from nervous shock, needed kind and quiet support, and should refrain from routine household chores for the moment. The physician also suggested that her eyesight would gradually return over the next week or so, perhaps following the funerals of her children. The patient's vision did slowly return over the next days, and she gradually resumed her usual level of care for the home, her surviving child, and other members of the family. (Courtesy of Frederick G. Guggenheim, M.D.)

Sensory Symptoms.

In conversion disorder, anesthesia and paresthesia are common, especially of the extremities. All sensory modalities can be involved, and the distribution of the disturbance is usually inconsistent with either central or peripheral neurological disease. Thus, clinicians may see the characteristic stocking-and-glove anesthesia of the hands or feet or the hemianesthesia of the body beginning precisely along the midline.

Conversion disorder symptoms may involve the organs of special sense and can produce deafness, blindness, and tunnel vision. These symptoms may be unilateral or bilateral, but neurological evaluation reveals intact sensory pathways. In conversion disorder blindness, for example, patients walk around without collisions or self-injury, their pupils react to light, and their cortical evoked potentials are normal.

Motor Symptoms.

The motor symptoms include abnormal movements, gait disturbance, weakness, and paralysis. Gross rhythmical tremors, choreiform movements, tics, and jerks may be present. The movements generally worsen when attention is called to them. One gait disturbance seen in conversion disorder is *astasia-abasia*, which is a wildly ataxic, staggering gait accompanied by gross, irregular, jerky truncal movements and thrashing and waving arm movements. Patients with the symptoms rarely fall; if they do, they are generally not injured.

Other common motor disturbances are paralysis and paresis involving one, two, or all four limbs, although the distribution of the involved muscles does not conform to the neural pathways. Reflexes remain normal; the patients have no fasciculations or muscle atrophy (except after long-standing conversion paralysis); electromyography findings are normal.

Seizure Symptoms.

Pseudoseizures are another symptom in conversion disorder. Clinicians may find it difficult to differentiate a pseudoseizure from an actual seizure by clinical observation alone. Moreover, about one third of the patient's pseudoseizures also have a coexisting epileptic disorder. Tongue biting, urinary incontinence, and injuries after falling can occur in pseudoseizures, although these symptoms are generally not present. Pupillary and gag reflexes are retained after pseudoseizure, and patients have no postseizure increase in prolactin concentrations.

Other Associated Features.

Several psychological symptoms have also been associated with conversion disorder.

PRIMARY GAIN. Patients achieve primary gain by keeping internal conflicts outside their awareness. Symptoms have symbolic value; they represent an unconscious psychological conflict.

SECONDARY GAIN. Patients accrue tangible advantages and benefits as a result of being sick, for example, being excused from obligations and difficult life situations, receiving support and assistance that might not otherwise be forthcoming, and controlling other persons' behavior.

LA BELLE INDIFFÉRENCE. La belle indifférence is a patient's inappropriately cavalier attitude toward serious symptoms; that is, the patient seems to be unconcerned about what appears to be a major impairment. That bland indifference may be lacking in some patients; it is also seen in some seriously ill medical patients who develop a stoic attitude. The presence or absence of la belle indifférence is an inaccurate measure of whether a patient has conversion disorder.

IDENTIFICATION. Patients with conversion disorder may unconsciously model their symptoms on those of someone important to them. For example, a parent or a person who has recently died may serve as a model for conversion disorder. During pathological grief reaction, bereaved persons commonly have symptoms of the deceased.

Differential Diagnosis

One of the major problems in diagnosing conversion disorder is the difficulty of definitively ruling out a medical disorder. Concomitant nonpsychiatric medical disorders are common in hospitalized patients with conversion disorder, and evidence of a current or previous neurological disorder or a systemic disease affecting the brain has been reported in 18 to 64 percent of such patients. An estimated 25 to 50 percent of patients classified as having conversion disorder eventually receive diagnoses of neurological or nonpsychiatric medical disorders that could have caused their earlier symptoms. Thus, a thorough medical and neurological workup is essential in all cases. If the symptoms can be resolved by suggestion, hypnosis, or parenteral amobarbital (Amytal) or lorazepam (Ativan), they are probably the result of conversion disorder.

Neurological disorders (such as dementia and other degenerative diseases), brain tumors, and basal ganglia disease must be considered in the differential diagnosis. For example, weakness may be confused with myasthenia gravis, polymyositis, acquired myopathies, or multiple sclerosis. Optic neuritis may be misdiagnosed as conversion disorder blindness. Other diseases that may cause confusing symptoms are Guillain-Barré syndrome, Creutzfeldt-Jakob disease, periodic paralysis, and early neurological manifestations of AIDS. Conversion disorder

Treatment

Somatization disorder is best treated when the patient has a single identified physician as primary caretaker. When more than one clinician is involved, patients have increased opportunities to express somatic complaints. Primary physicians should see patients during regularly scheduled visits, usually at monthly intervals. The visits should be relatively brief, although a partial physical examination should be conducted to respond to each new somatic complaint. Additional laboratory and diagnostic procedures should generally be avoided. Once somatization disorder has been diagnosed, the treating physician should listen to the somatic complaints as emotional expressions rather than as medical complaints. Nevertheless, patients with somatization disorder can also have bona fide physical illnesses; therefore, physicians must always use their judgment about what symptoms to work up and to what extent. A reasonable long-range strategy for a primary care physician who is treating a patient with somatization disorder is to increase the patient's awareness of the possibility that psychological factors are involved in the symptoms until the patient is willing to see a mental health clinician. In complex cases with many medical presentations, a psychiatrist is better able to judge whether or not to seek a medical or surgical consultation because of his or her medical training; however, a nonmedical mental health professional can explore the psychological antecedents of the disorder as well, especially if consulting closely with a physician.

Psychotherapy, both individual and group, decreases these patients' personal health care expenditures by 50 percent, largely by decreasing their rates of hospitalization. In psychotherapy settings, patients are helped to cope with their symptoms, to express underlying emotions, and to develop alternative strategies for expressing their feelings.

Giving psychotropic medications whenever somatization disorder coexists with a mood or anxiety disorder is always a risk, but psychopharmacological treatment, as well as psychotherapeutic treatment, of the coexisting disorder is indicated. Medication must be monitored, because patients with somatization disorder tend to use drugs erratically and unreliably. Few available data indicate that pharmacological treatment is effective in patients without coexisting mental disorders.

CONVERSION DISORDER

A conversion disorder is a disturbance of bodily functioning that does not conform to current concepts of the anatomy and physiology of the central or the peripheral nervous system. It typically occurs in a setting of stress and produces considerable dysfunction.

DSM-IV-TR defines conversion disorder as characterized by the presence of one or more neurological symptoms (e.g., paralysis, blindness, and paresthesias) that cannot be explained by a known neurological or medical disorder. In addition, the diagnosis requires association of psychological factors with the initiation or exacerbation of the symptoms (Table 17–3).

The syndrome currently known as conversion disorder was originally combined with the syndrome known as somatization disorder and was referred to as hysteria, conversion reaction, or dissociative reaction. Briquet and Jean-Martin Charcot contributed to the development of the concept of conversion disorder by noting the influence of heredity on the symptom and the common association with a traumatic event.

Table 17–3
Common Symptoms of Conversion Disorder

Motor symptoms	Sensory deficits
Involuntary movements	Anesthesia, especially of extremities
Tics	Midline anesthesia
Blepharospasm	Blindness
Torticollis	Tunnel vision
Opisthotonos	Deafness
Seizures	**Visceral symptoms**
Abnormal gait	Psychogenic vomiting
Falling	Pseudocyesis
Astasia-abasia	*Globus hystericus*
Paralysis	Swooning or syncope
Weakness	Urinary retention
Aphonia	Diarrhea

Courtesy of Frederick G. Guggenheim, M.D.

The term *conversion* was introduced by Sigmund Freud, who, based on his work with Anna O, hypothesized that the symptoms of conversion disorder reflect unconscious conflicts.

Epidemiology

Some symptoms of conversion disorder that are not severe enough to warrant the diagnosis may occur in up to one third of the general population sometime during their lives. One community reported an annual incidence of conversion disorder of 22 per 100,000. Among specific populations, the occurrence of conversion disorder may be even higher than that, perhaps making conversion disorder the most common somatoform disorder in some populations. Several studies have reported that 5 to 15 percent of psychiatric consultations in a general hospital and 25 to 30 percent of admissions to a Veterans Administration hospital involve patients with conversion disorder diagnoses. DSM-IV-TR gives a range from a low of 11 to a high of 500 cases per 100,000 population.

The ratio of women to men among adult patients is at least 2 to 1 and as much as 10 to 1; among children there is an even higher predominance in girls. Men with conversion disorder have often been involved in occupational or military accidents. Conversion disorder can have its onset at any time, from childhood to old age, but it is most common in adolescents and young adults. Data indicate that conversion disorder is most common among rural populations, persons with little education, those with low intelligence quotients, those in low socioeconomic groups, and military personnel who have been exposed to combat situations. Conversion disorder is commonly associated with comorbid diagnoses of major depressive disorder, anxiety disorders, and schizophrenia and shows an increased frequency in relatives of probands with conversion disorder.

Comorbidity

Medical and especially neurological disorders occur frequently among patients with conversion disorders. What is typically seen in these comorbid neurological or medical conditions is an elaboration of symptoms stemming from the original organic lesion.

Among the Axis I psychiatric conditions, depressive disorders, anxiety disorders, and somatization disorders are especially noted for their association with conversion disorder. Conversion in schizophrenia is reported but is very uncommon. Studies of patients admitted to a psychiatric hospital for conversion disorder reveal that on further study, one quarter to one half have a clinically significant mood disorder or schizophrenia.

Personality disorders also frequently accompany conversion disorder, especially the histrionic type (in 5 to 21 percent of cases) and the passive-dependent type (9 to 40 percent of cases). However, conversion disorders can occur in persons with no predisposing medical, neurological, or psychiatric disorder.

Table 17–4
DSM-IV-TR Diagnostic Criteria for Conversion Disorder

A. One or more symptoms or deficits affecting voluntary motor or sensory function that suggest a neurological or other general medical condition.
B. Psychological factors are judged to be associated with the symptom or deficit because the initiation or exacerbation of the symptom or deficit is preceded by conflicts or other stressors.
C. The symptom or deficit is not intentionally produced or feigned (as in factitious disorder or malingering).
D. The symptom or deficit cannot, after appropriate investigation, be fully explained by a general medical condition, or by the direct effects of a substance, or as a culturally sanctioned behavior or experience.
E. The symptom or deficit causes clinically significant distress or impairment in social, occupational, or other important areas of functioning or warrants medical evaluation.
F. The symptom or deficit is not limited to pain or sexual dysfunction, does not occur exclusively during the course of somatization disorder, and is not better accounted for by another mental disorder.

Specify type of symptom or deficit:
With motor symptom or deficit
With sensory symptom or deficit
With seizures or convulsions
With mixed presentation

From American Psychiatric Association. *Diagnostic and Statistical Manual of Mental Disorders.* 4th ed. Text rev. Washington, DC: American Psychiatric Association; copyright 2000, with permission.

Etiology

Psychoanalytic Factors. According to psychoanalytic theory, conversion disorder is caused by repression of unconscious intrapsychic conflict and conversion of anxiety into a physical symptom. The conflict is between an instinctual impulse (e.g., aggression or sexuality) and the prohibitions against its expression. The symptoms allow partial expression of the forbidden wish or urge but disguise it, so that patients can avoid consciously confronting their unacceptable impulses; that is, the conversion disorder symptom has a symbolic relation to the unconscious conflict—for example, vaginismus protects the patient from expressing unacceptable sexual wishes. Conversion disorder symptoms also let patients communicate that they need special consideration and special treatment. Such symptoms may function as a nonverbal means of controlling or manipulating others.

Learning Theory. In terms of conditioned learning theory, a conversion symptom can be seen as a piece of classically conditioned learned behavior; symptoms of illness, learned in childhood, are called forth as a means of coping with an otherwise impossible situation.

Biological Factors. Increasing data implicate biological and neuropsychological factors in the development of conversion disorder symptoms. Preliminary brain-imaging studies have found hypometabolism of the dominant hemisphere and hypermetabolism of the nondominant hemisphere and have implicated impaired hemispheric communication in the cause of conversion disorder. The symptoms may be caused by an excessive cortical arousal that sets off negative feedback loops between the cerebral cortex and the brainstem reticular formation. Elevated levels of corticofugal output, in turn, inhibit the patient's awareness of bodily sensation, which may explain the observed sensory deficits in some patients with conversion disorder. Neuropsychological tests sometimes reveal subtle cerebral impairments in verbal communication, memory, vigilance, affective incongruity, and attention in these patients.

Diagnosis

DSM-IV-TR limits the diagnosis of conversion disorder to those symptoms that affect a voluntary motor or sensory function, that is, neurological symptoms (Table 17–4). Physicians cannot explain the neurological symptoms solely on the basis of any known neurological condition.

The diagnosis of conversion disorder requires that clinicians find a necessary and critical association between the cause of the neurological symptoms and psychological factors, although the symptoms cannot result from malingering or factitious disorder. The diagnosis of conversion disorder also excludes symptoms of pain and sexual dysfunction and symptoms that occur only in somatization disorder. DSM-IV-TR allows specification of the type of symptom or deficit seen in conversion disorder (Table 17–4).

Clinical Features

Paralysis, blindness, and mutism are the most common conversion disorder symptoms. Conversion disorder may be most commonly associated with passive-aggressive, dependent, antisocial, and histrionic personality disorders. Depressive and anxiety disorder symptoms often accompany the symptoms of conversion disorder, and affected patients are at risk for suicide.

Mrs. A. was a 22-year-old right-handed fundamentalist farmer's wife, homemaker, and mother of three from a sparsely settled Western state. Her past medical history was benign except for a motor vehicle accident 2 years previously that produced a sharp blow to the right temporal area, resulting in several hours' loss of consciousness. She had an unremarkable behavioral history without substance abuse, prolonged depressions, or unexplained somatic symptoms.

Differential Diagnosis

Distortions of body image occur in anorexia nervosa, gender identity disorders, and some specific types of brain damage (e.g., neglect syndromes); body dysmorphic disorder should not be diagnosed in these situations. Body dysmorphic disorder must also be distinguished from a person's normal concern about appearance. In body dysmorphic disorder, however, a person experiences significant emotional distress and functional impairment because of the concern. Although distinguishing between a strongly held idea and a delusion is difficult, if a patient's preoccupation with the perceived body defect has delusional intensity, the appropriate diagnosis is delusional disorder, somatic type. Other diagnostic considerations are narcissistic personality disorder, depressive disorders, obsessive-compulsive disorder, and schizophrenia. In narcissistic personality disorder, concern about a body part is only a minor feature in the general constellation of personality traits. In depressive disorders, schizophrenia, and obsessive-compulsive disorder, the other symptoms of these disorders usually evidence themselves in short order, even when the initial symptom is excessive concern about a body part.

Course and Prognosis

The onset of body dysmorphic disorder is usually gradual. An affected person may become increasingly concerned about a particular body part until he or she notices that functioning is being affected. Then the person may seek medical or surgical help to address the presumed problem. The level of concern about the problem may wax and wane over time, although the disorder is usually chronic if left untreated.

Treatment

Treatment of patients with body dysmorphic disorder with surgical, dermatological, dental, and other medical procedures to address the alleged defects is almost invariably unsuccessful. Although tricyclic drugs, monoamine oxidase inhibitors, and pimozide (Orap) have reportedly been useful in individual cases, a larger body of data indicates that serotonin-specific drugs—for example, clomipramine (Anafranil) and fluoxetine (Prozac)—reduce symptoms in at least 50 percent of patients. In any patient with a coexisting mental disorder, such as a depressive disorder or an anxiety disorder, the coexisting disorder should be treated with the appropriate pharmacotherapy and psychotherapy. How long treatment should be continued after the symptoms of body dysmorphic disorder have remitted is unknown.

Relation to Plastic Surgery

Few data exist about the number of patients seeking plastic surgery who have body dysmorphic disorder. One study found that only 2 percent of the patients in a plastic surgery clinic had the diagnosis. The overall percentage may be much higher, however. Surgical requests are varied: removal of facial sags, jowls, wrinkles, or puffiness; rhinoplasty; breast reduction or enhancement; and penile enlargement, among others. Commonly associated with the belief about appearance is an unrealistic expectation of how much surgery will correct the defect. As reality sets in, the person realizes that life's problems are not solved by altering the perceived cosmetic defect. Ideally, such patients will seek out psychotherapy to understand the true nature of their neurotic feelings of inadequacy. Absent that, patients may take out their anger by suing their plastic surgeons—who have one of highest malpractice-suit rates of any specialty—or by developing a clinical depression.

PAIN DISORDER

DSM-IV-TR defines pain disorder as the presence of pain that is "the predominant focus of clinical attention." Psychological factors play an important role in the disorder. The primary symptom is pain in one or more sites that is not fully accounted for by a nonpsychiatric medical or neurological condition. The pain is associated with emotional distress and functional impairment. The disorder has been called *somatoform pain disorder, psychogenic pain disorder, idiopathic pain disorder,* and *atypical pain disorder.*

Epidemiology

Pain is perhaps the most frequent complaint in medical practice, and intractable pain syndromes are common. Low back pain has disabled an estimated 7 million persons in the United States and accounts for more than 8 million physician office visits annually. Pain disorder is diagnosed twice as frequently in women as in men. The peak ages of onset are in the fourth and fifth decades, perhaps because the tolerance for pain declines with age. Pain disorder is most common in persons with blue-collar occupations, perhaps because of increased likelihood of job-related injuries. First-degree relatives of patients with pain disorder have an increased likelihood of having the same disorder; thus genetic inheritance or behavioral mechanisms are possibly involved in its transmission. Depressive disorders, anxiety disorders, and substance abuse are also more common in the families of patients with pain disorder than in the general population.

Etiology

Psychodynamic Factors. Patients who experience bodily aches and pains without identifiable and adequate physical causes may be symbolically expressing an intrapsychic conflict through the body. Patients suffering from alexithymia, who are unable to articulate their internal feeling states in words, express their feelings with their bodies. Other patients may unconsciously regard emotional pain as weak and somehow lacking legitimacy. By displacing the problem to the body, they may feel that they have a legitimate claim to the fulfillment of their dependency needs. The symbolic meaning of body disturbances may also relate to atonement for perceived sin, to expiation of guilt, or to suppressed aggression. Many patients have intractable and unresponsive pain because they are convinced that they deserve to suffer.

Pain can function as a method of obtaining love, a punishment for wrongdoing, and a way of expiating guilt and atoning for an innate sense of badness. Among the defense mechanisms used by patients with pain disorder are displacement, substitution, and repression. Identification plays a part when a patient takes on the role of an ambivalent love object who also has pain, such as a parent.

Behavioral Factors. Pain behaviors are reinforced when rewarded and are inhibited when ignored or punished. For example, moderate pain symptoms may become intense when followed by the solicitous and attentive behavior of others, by monetary gain, or by the successful avoidance of distasteful activities.

Interpersonal Factors. Intractable pain has been conceptualized as a means for manipulation and gaining advantage in interpersonal relationships, for example, to ensure the devotion of a family member or to stabilize a fragile marriage. Such secondary gain is most important to patients with pain disorder.

Biological Factors. The cerebral cortex can inhibit the firing of afferent pain fibers. Serotonin is probably the main neurotransmitter in the descending inhibitory pathways, and endorphins also play a role in the central nervous system modulation of pain. Endorphin deficiency seems to correlate with augmentation of incoming sensory stimuli. Some patients may have pain disorder, rather than another mental disorder, because of sensory and limbic structural or chemical abnormalities that predispose them to experience pain.

Diagnosis

The DSM-IV-TR diagnostic criteria for pain disorder require the presence of clinically significant complaints of pain (Table 17–9). The complaints of pain must be judged to be significantly affected by psychological factors, and the symptoms must result in a patient's significant emotional distress or functional impairment (e.g., social or occupational). DSM-IV-TR requires that the pain disorder be associated primarily with psychological factors or with both psychological factors and a general medical condition. DSM-IV-TR further specifies that pain disorder associated solely with a general medical condition be diagnosed as an Axis III condition and also allows clinicians to specify whether the pain disorder is acute or chronic, depending on whether the duration of symptoms has been 6 months or more.

Clinical Features

Patients with pain disorder are not a uniform group but a heterogeneous collection of persons with low back pain, headache, atypical facial pain, chronic pelvic pain, and other kinds of pain. A patient's pain may be posttraumatic, neuropathic, neurological, iatrogenic, or musculoskeletal; to meet a diagnosis of pain disorder, however, the disorder must have a psychological factor judged to be significantly involved in the pain symptoms and their ramifications.

Patients with pain disorder often have long histories of medical and surgical care. They visit many physicians, request many medications, and may be especially insistent in their desire for surgery. Indeed, they can be completely preoccupied with their pain and cite it as the source of all their misery. Such patients often deny any other sources of emotional dysphoria and insist that their lives are blissful except for their pain. Their clinical picture can be complicated by substance-related disorders, because these patients attempt to reduce the pain through the use of alcohol and other substances.

Table 17–9
DSM-IV-TR Diagnostic Criteria for Pain Disorder

A. Pain in one or more anatomical sites is the predominant focus of the clinical presentation and is of sufficient severity to warrant clinical attention.

B. The pain causes clinically significant distress or impairment in social, occupational, or other important areas of functioning.

C. Psychological factors are judged to have an important role in the onset, severity, exacerbation, or maintenance of the pain.

D. The symptom or deficit is not intentionally produced or feigned (as in factitious disorder or malingering).

E. The pain is not better accounted for by a mood, anxiety, or psychotic disorder and does not meet criteria for dyspareunia.

Code as follows:

Pain disorder associated with psychological factors: psychological factors are judged to have the major role in the onset, severity, exacerbation, or maintenance of the pain. (If a general medical condition is present, it does not have a major role in the onset, severity, exacerbation, or maintenance of the pain.) This type of pain disorder is not diagnosed if criteria are also met for somatization disorder.

Specify if:

Acute: duration of less than 6 months

Chronic: duration of 6 months or longer

Pain disorder associated with both psychological factors and a general medical condition: both psychological factors and a general medical condition are judged to have important roles in the onset, severity, exacerbation, or maintenance of the pain. The associated general medical condition or anatomical site of the pain (see below) is coded on Axis III.

Specify if:

Acute: duration of less than 6 months

Chronic: duration of 6 months or longer

Note: The following is not considered to be a mental disorder and is included here to facilitate differential diagnosis.

Pain disorder associated with a general medical condition: a general medical condition has a major role in the onset, severity, exacerbation, or maintenance of the pain. (If psychological factors are present, they are not judged to have a major role in the onset, severity, exacerbation, or maintenance of the pain.) The diagnostic code for the pain is selected based on the associated general medical condition if one has been established or on the anatomical location of the pain if the underlying general medical condition is not yet clearly established—for example, low back, sciatic, pelvic, headache, facial, chest, joint, bone, abdominal, breast, renal, ear, eye, throat, tooth, and urinary.

From American Psychiatric Association. *Diagnostic and Statistical Manual of Mental Disorders.* 4th ed. Text rev. Washington, DC: American Psychiatric Association; copyright 2000, with permission.

At least one study has correlated the number of pain symptoms to the likelihood and severity of symptoms of somatization disorder, depressive disorders, and anxiety disorders. Major depressive disorder is present in about 25 to 50 percent of patients with pain disorder, and dysthymic disorder or depressive disorder symptoms are reported in 60 to 100 percent of the patients. Some investigators believe that chronic pain is almost always a variant of a depressive disorder, a masked or somatized form of depression. The most prominent depressive symptoms in patients with pain disorder are anergia, anhedonia, decreased libido, insomnia, and irritability; diurnal variation, weight loss, and psychomotor retardation appear to be less common.

Mr. L., a 72-year-old married, Ukrainian-born, pious, wealthy retailer and father of a large family from an east coast city was admitted to the orthopedic service of a general hospital for evaluation of unbearable pain in the arches of his feet. He had fled his native country following a pogrom when he was 9. During the year of flight he had endured enormous physical hardships, starvation, and beatings until the surviving family members finally were able to emigrate to the United States. With incessant hard work, he had prospered economically; married a patient, supportive wife; and witnessed his six children develop promising careers. He became the major contributor to his temple and gave unstintingly to local charities for the needy and unfortunate. He had little time for personal enjoyment. Over the years each time he and his wife had time alone together and she had been affectionate with him, he would develop some excruciating bodily pain shortly thereafter: blinding headache, severe back spasm, abdominal pain, facial pain, or pelvic pain. These pains usually receded several days after the weekend was over or the trip was completed. Some pains occurred more frequently than others. He sought medical attention rarely except for these pains, which occurred every few months. His mood varied from glum to gloomy, but he denied that he was depressed. He often claimed to have been blessed with good fortune. He led a temperate life, drank little, and had relatively good health between the episodes of pain.

Over the four decades that his physicians cared for him, they had become frustrated with this unassuming and humble man; his ardent complaints of pain were always so nonspecific and fluctuating that they could not devise any pathophysiological mechanisms to account for his pain. Their diagnostic tests were not revealing, and Mr. L. usually refused their offers of narcotic or other analgesic relief. Laboratory workup for pains in the arches was noncontributory, and he was discharged when his symptoms cleared in 3 days. Four months later he was readmitted to the surgical service of the general hospital with severe, unrelenting, left-side upper abdominal pain. This time Mr. L. described his new pain in meticulous detail. A brief workup revealed very advanced carcinoma of the tail of the pancreas. He took the news from his physician stoically and asked to be discharged home that day. (Courtesy of Frederick G. Guggenheim, M.D.)

Differential Diagnosis

Purely physical pain can be difficult to distinguish from purely psychogenic pain, especially because the two are not mutually exclusive. Physical pain fluctuates in intensity and is highly sensitive to emotional, cognitive, attentional, and situational influences. Pain that does not vary and is insensitive to any of these factors is likely to be psychogenic. When pain does not wax and wane and is not even temporarily relieved by distraction or analgesics, clinicians can suspect an important psychogenic component.

Pain disorder must be distinguished from other somatoform disorders, although some somatoform disorders can coexist. Patients with hypochondriacal preoccupations may complain of pain, and aspects of the clinical presentation of hypochondriasis, such as bodily preoccupation and disease conviction, can also be present in patients with pain disorder. Patients with hypochondriasis tend to have many more symptoms than patients with pain disorder, and their symptoms tend to fluctuate more than those of patients with pain disorder. Conversion disorder is generally short-lived, whereas pain disorder is chronic. In addition, pain is, by definition, not a symptom in conversion disorder. Malingering patients consciously provide false reports, and their complaints are usually connected to clearly recognizable goals.

The differential diagnosis can be difficult because patients with pain disorder often receive disability compensation or a litigation award. Muscle contraction (tension) headaches, for example, have a pathophysiological mechanism to account for the pain and so are not diagnosed as pain disorder. However, patients with pain disorder are not pretending to be in pain. As in all of the somatoform disorders, symptoms are not imaginary.

Course and Prognosis

The pain in pain disorder generally begins abruptly and increases in severity for a few weeks or months. The prognosis varies, although pain disorder can often be chronic, distressful, and completely disabling. When psychological factors predominate in pain disorder, the pain may subside with treatment or after the elimination of external reinforcement. The patients with the poorest prognoses, with or without treatment, have preexisting characterological problems, especially pronounced passivity; are involved in litigation or receive financial compensation; use addictive substances; and have long histories of pain.

Treatment

Because it may not be possible to reduce the pain, the treatment approach must address rehabilitation. Clinicians should discuss the issue of psychological factors early in treatment and should frankly tell patients that such factors are important in the cause and consequences of both physical and psychogenic pain. Therapists should also explain how various brain circuits that are involved with emotions (e.g., the limbic system) may influence the sensory pain pathways. For example, persons who hit their head while happy at a party can seem to experience less pain than when they hit their head while angry and at work. Nevertheless, therapists must fully understand that the patient's experiences of pain are real.

Pharmacotherapy. Analgesic medications do not generally benefit most patients with pain disorder. In addition, substance abuse and dependence are often major problems for patients who receive long-term analgesic treatment. Sedatives and antianxiety agents are not especially beneficial and are subject to abuse, misuse, and adverse effects.

Antidepressants, such as tricyclics and selective serotonin reuptake inhibitors (SSRIs), are the most effective pharmacological agents. Whether antidepressants reduce pain through their antidepressant action or exert an independent, direct analgesic effect (possibly by stimulating efferent inhibitory pain pathways) remains controversial. The success of SSRIs supports the hypothesis that serotonin is important in the pathophysiology of the disorder. Amphetamine, which has analgesic

effects, may benefit some patients, especially when used as an adjunct to SSRIs, but dosages must be monitored carefully.

Psychotherapy. Some outcome data indicate that psychodynamic psychotherapy benefits patients with pain disorder. The first step in psychotherapy is to develop a solid therapeutic alliance by empathizing with the patient's suffering. Clinicians should not confront somatizing patients with comments such as "This is all in your head." For the patient, the pain is real, and clinicians must acknowledge the reality of the pain, even as they understand that it is largely intrapsychic in origin. A useful entry point into the emotional aspects of the pain is to examine its interpersonal ramifications in the patient's life. In marital therapy, for example, the psychotherapist may soon get to the source of the patient's psychological pain and the function of the physical complaints in significant relationships. Cognitive therapy has been used to alter negative thoughts and to foster a positive attitude.

Other Therapies. Biofeedback can be helpful in the treatment of pain disorder, particularly with migraine pain, myofacial pain, and muscle tension states, such as tension headaches. Hypnosis, transcutaneous nerve stimulation, and dorsal column stimulation also have been used. Nerve blocks and surgical ablative procedures are effective for some patients with pain disorder; but these procedures must be repeated, since the pain returns after 6 to 18 months.

Pain Control Programs. It may sometimes be necessary to remove patients from their usual settings and place them in a comprehensive inpatient or outpatient pain control program or clinic. Multidisciplinary pain units use many modalities, such as cognitive, behavior, and group therapies. They provide extensive physical conditioning through physical therapy and exercise and offer vocational evaluation and rehabilitation. Concurrent mental disorders are diagnosed and treated, and patients who are dependent on analgesics and hypnotics are detoxified. Inpatient multimodal treatment programs generally report encouraging results.

UNDIFFERENTIATED SOMATOFORM DISORDER

According to DSM-IV-TR undifferentiated somatoform disorder is defined as unexplained physical effects that last for at least 6 months and are below the threshold for diagnosing somatization disorder. This diagnosis (Table 17–10) is appropriate for patients with one or more physical complaints that cannot be explained by a known medical condition or that grossly exceed the expected complaints in a medical condition but do not meet the diagnostic criteria for a specific somatoform disorder. The symptoms must cause patients significant emotional distress or impair their social or occupational functioning.

Two types of symptom patterns may be seen in patients with undifferentiated somatoform disorder: those involving the autonomic nervous system and those involving sensations of fatigue or weakness. In what is sometimes referred to as *autonomic arousal disorder,* some patients are affected with somatoform disorder symptoms that are limited to bodily functions innervated by the autonomic nervous system. Such patients have complaints involving the cardiovascular, respiratory, gastrointestinal, urogenital, and dermatological systems. Other patients complain of mental and physical fatigue, physical weakness and exhaustion, and inability to perform many everyday activities because of their symptoms. Some clinicians believe this syndrome is *neurasthenia,* a diagnosis used primarily in Europe and Asia. The syndrome may overlap chronic fatigue syndrome, which various research reports have hypoth-

Table 17–10
DSM-IV-TR Diagnostic Criteria for Undifferentiated Somatoform Disorder

A. One or more physical complaints (e.g., fatigue, loss of appetite, gastrointestinal or urinary complaints).
B. Either (1) or (2):
   (1) after appropriate investigation, the symptoms cannot be fully explained by a known general medical condition or the direct effects of a substance (e.g., a drug of abuse, a medication)
   (2) when there is a related general medical condition, the physical complaints or resulting social or occupational impairment is in excess of what would be expected from the history, physical examination, or laboratory findings
C. The symptoms cause clinically significant distress or impairment in social, occupational, or other important areas of functioning.
D. The duration of the disturbance is at least 6 months.
E. The disturbance is not better accounted for by another mental disorder (e.g., another somatoform disorder, sexual dysfunction, mood disorder, anxiety disorder, sleep disorder, or psychotic disorder).
F. The symptom is not intentionally produced or feigned (as in factitious disorder or malingering).

From American Psychiatric Association. *Diagnostic and Statistical Manual of Mental Disorders.* 4th ed. Text rev. Washington, DC: American Psychiatric Association; copyright 2000, with permission.

Table 17–11
DSM-IV-TR Diagnostic Criteria for Somatoform Disorder Not Otherwise Specified

This category includes disorders with somatoform symptoms that do not meet the criteria for any specific somatoform disorder. Examples include

1. Pseudocyesis: a false belief of being pregnant that is associated with objective signs of pregnancy, which may include abdominal enlargement (although the umbilicus does not become everted), reduced menstrual flow, amenorrhea, subjective sensation of fetal movement, nausea, breast engorgement and secretions, and labor pains at the expected date of delivery. Endocrine changes may be present, but the syndrome cannot be explained by a general medical condition that causes endocrine changes (e.g., a hormone-secreting tumor).
2. A disorder involving nonpsychotic hypochondriacal symptoms of less than 6 months' duration.
3. A disorder involving unexplained physical complaints (e.g., fatigue or body weakness) of less than 6 months' duration that are not due to another mental disorder.

From American Psychiatric Association. *Diagnostic and Statistical Manual of Mental Disorders.* 4th ed. Text rev. Washington, DC: American Psychiatric Association; copyright 2000, with permission.

esized to involve psychiatric, virological, and immunological factors. (The reader is referred to Chapter 18, which discusses chronic fatigue syndrome and neurasthenia in depth.)

SOMATOFORM DISORDER NOT OTHERWISE SPECIFIED

The DSM-IV-TR diagnostic category of somatoform disorder not otherwise specified (Table 17–11) is a residual category for patients who have symptoms suggesting a somatoform disorder but do not meet the specific diagnostic criteria for other somatoform disorders. Such patients may have a symptom not covered in the other somatoform disorders (e.g., pseudocyesis) or may not have met the 6-month criterion of the other somatoform disorders.

ICD-10

In the 10th revision of *International Statistical Classification of Diseases and Related Health Problems* (ICD-10), somatoform disorders are described as a "repeated presentation of physical symptoms, together with persistent requests for medical investigation," although patients have been reassured by their physicians that the symptoms have no physical basis. If physical disorders are present, they cannot account for patients' symptoms or for their distress.

The categories of somatoform disorders are similar in DSM-IV-TR and ICD-10, except that in ICD-10, body dysmorphic disorder is a subcategory (Table 17–12). ICD-10 also includes the diagnosis of neurasthenia, which has many signs and symptoms that overlap with the DSM-IV-TR categories of anxiety, depression, and somatization. (Neurasthenia is discussed in Chapter 18.)

Table 17–12
ICD-10 Diagnostic Criteria for Somatoform Disorders

Somatization disorder

A. There must be a history of at least 2 years' complaints of multiple and variable physical symptoms that cannot be explained by any detectable physical disorders. (Any physical disorders that are known to be present do not explain the severity, extent, variety, and persistence of the physical complaints, or the associated social disability.) If some symptoms clearly due to autonomic arousal are present, they are not a major feature of the disorder in that they are not particularly persistent or distressing.

B. Preoccupation with the symptoms causes persistent distress and leads the patient to seek repeated (three or more) consultations or sets of investigations with either primary care or specialist doctors. In the absence of medical services within either the financial or physical reach of the patient, there must be persistent self-medication or multiple consultations with local healers.

C. There is persistent refusal to accept medical reassurance that there is no adequate physical cause for the physical symptoms. (Short-term acceptance of such reassurance, i.e., for a few weeks during or immediately after investigations, does not exclude this diagnosis.)

D. There must be a total of six or more symptoms from the following list, with symptoms occurring in at least two separate groups:

Gastrointestinal symptoms

(1) abdominal pain;
(2) nausea;
(3) feeling bloated or full of gas;
(4) bad taste in mouth, or excessively coated tongue;
(5) complaints of vomiting or regurgitation of food;
(6) complaints of frequent and loose bowel motions or discharge of fluids from anus;

Cardiovascular symptoms

(7) breathlessness without exertion;
(8) chest pains;

Genitourinary symptoms

(9) dysuria or complaints of frequency of micturition;
(10) unpleasant sensations in or around the genitals;
(11) complaints of unusual or copious vaginal discharge;

Skin and pain symptoms

(12) blotchiness or discoloration of the skin;
(13) pain in the limbs, extremities, or joints;
(14) unpleasant numbness or tingling sensations.

E. *Most commonly used exclusion clause.* Symptoms do not occur only during any of the schizophrenic or related disorders, any of the mood [affective] disorders, or panic disorder.

Undifferentiated somatoform disorder

A. Criteria A, C, and E for somatization disorder are met, except that the duration of the disorder is at least 6 months.

B. One or both of Criteria B and D for somatization disorder are incompletely fulfilled.

Hypochondriacal disorder

A. Either of the following must be present:

(1) a persistent belief, of at least 5 months' duration, of the presence of a maximum of two serious physical diseases (of which at least one must be specifically named by the patient);
(2) a persistent preoccupation with a presumed deformity or disfigurement (body dysmorphic disorder).

B. Preoccupation with the belief and the symptoms causes persistent distress or interference with personal functioning in daily living and leads the patient to seek medical treatment or investigations (or equivalent help from local healers).

C. There is persistent refusal to accept medical reassurance that there is no physical cause for the symptoms or physical abnormality. (Short-term acceptance of such reassurance, i.e., for a few weeks during or immediately after investigations, does not exclude this diagnosis.)

D. *Most commonly used exclusion clause.* The symptoms do not occur only during any of the schizophrenic and related disorders or any of the mood [affective] disorders.

Somatoform autonomic dysfunction

A. There must be symptoms of autonomic arousal that are attributed by the patient to a physical disorder of one or more of the following systems or organs:

(1) heart and cardiovascular system;
(2) upper gastrointestinal tract (esophagus and stomach);
(3) lower gastrointestinal tract;

(*continued*)

Table 17–12 (*continued*)

(4) respiratory system;
(5) genitourinary system.

B. Two or more of the following autonomic symptoms must be present:
(1) palpitations;
(2) sweating (hot or cold);
(3) dry mouth;
(4) flushing or blushing;
(5) epigastric discomfort, "butterflies," or churning in the stomach.

C. One or more of the following symptoms must be present:
(1) chest pains or discomfort in and around the precordium;
(2) dyspnea or hyperventilation;
(3) excessive tiredness on mild exertion;
(4) aerophagy, hiccough, or burning sensations in chest or epigastrium;
(5) reported frequent bowel movements;
(6) increased frequency of micturition or dysuria;
(7) feeling of being bloated, distended, or heavy.

D. There is no evidence of a disturbance of structure or function in the organs or systems about which the patient is concerned.

E. *Most commonly used exclusion clause.* These symptoms do not occur only in the presence of phobic disorders or panic disorder.

A fifth character is to be used to classify the individual disorders in this group, indicating the organ or system regarded by the patient as the origin of the symptoms:

Heart and cardiovascular system

Includes: cardiac neurosis, neurocirculatory asthenia, da Costa's syndrome.

Upper gastrointestinal tract

Includes: psychogenic aerophagy, hiccough, gastric neurosis.

Lower gastrointestinal tract

Includes: psychogenic irritable bowel syndrome, psychogenic diarrhea, gas syndrome.

Respiratory system

Includes: hyperventilation.

Genitourinary system

Includes: psychogenic increase of frequency of micturition and dysuria.

Other organ or system

Persistent somatoform pain disorder

A. There is persistent severe and distressing pain (for at least 6 months, and continuously on most days), in any part of the body, which cannot be explained adequately by evidence of a physiological process or a physical disorder and which is consistently the main focus of the patient's attention.

B. *Most commonly used exclusion clause.* This disorder does not occur in the presence of schizophrenia or related disorders, or only during any of the mood [affective] disorders, somatization disorder, undifferentiated somatoform disorder, or hypochondriacal disorder.

Other somatoform disorders

In these disorders the presenting complaints are not mediated through the autonomic nervous system, and are limited to specific systems or parts of the body, such as the skin. This is in contrast to the multiple and often changing complaints of the origin of symptoms and distress found in somatization disorder and undifferentiated somatoform disorder. Tissue damage is not involved.

Any other disorder of sensation not due to physical disorder, which are closely associated in time with stressful events or problems, or which result in significantly increased attention for the patient, either personal or medical, should also be classified here.

Somatoform disorder, unspecified

References

Barsky AJ. Hypochondriasis: medical management and psychiatric treatment. *Psychosomatics.* 1996;37:48.

Barsky AJ, Cleary PD, Sarnie MK, Klerman GL. The course of transient hypochondriasis. *Psychiatry.* 1993;150:484.

Barsky AJ, Wyshak G, Klerman GL. Psychiatric comorbidity in DSM-III-R hypochondriasis. *Arch Gen Psychiatry.* 1992;49:101.

Carroll DH, Scahill L, Phillips KA. Current concepts in body dysmorphic disorder. *Arch Psychiatr Nurs.* 2002;16:72.

Guggenheim FG. Somatoform disorders. In: Sadock BJ, Sadock VA, eds. *Kaplan & Sadock's Comprehensive Textbook of Psychiatry.* 7th ed. Vol 1. Baltimore: Lippincott William & Wilkins; 2000:1504.

Hollander E, Neville D, Frenkel M, Josephson S, Liebowitz MR. Body dysmorphic disorder: diagnostic issues and related disorders. *Psychosomatics.* 1992;33:156.

Kirmayer LJ, Robbins JM, Dworkind M, Yaffe MJ. Somatization and the recognition of depression and anxiety in primary care. *Am J Psychiatry.* 1993;150:734.

Lesser RP. Psychogenic seizures. *Neurology.* 1996;46:1499.

Martin RL. Diagnostic issues for conversion disorder. *Hosp Community Psychiatry.* 1992;43:771.

Massive MJ, ed. Pain: what psychiatrists need to know. *Review of Psychiatry.* Vol. 19, no. 2. Washington, DC: American Psychiatric Press; 2000:89.

Phillip KA, ed. Somatoform and factitious disorders. *Review of Psychiatry.* Vol. 20, no. 3. Washington, DC: American Psychiatric Press; 2001:95.

Silver FW. Management of conversion disorder. *Am J Phys Med Rehabil.* 1996;75:134.

Simon GE. Management of somatoform and factitious disorders. In: Nathan PE, Gormon JM, eds. *A Guide to Treatments That Work.* 2nd ed. London: Oxford University Press; 2002:447.

Starcevic V, Lipsitt DR, eds. *Hypochondriasis: Modern Perspectives on an Ancient Malady.* New York: Oxford University Press; 2001:329.

18

Chronic Fatigue Syndrome and Neurasthenia

CHRONIC FATIGUE SYNDROME

Chronic fatigue syndrome (referred to as *myalgic encephalomyelitis* in the United Kingdom and Canada) is characterized by 6 months or more of severe, debilitating fatigue, often accompanied by myalgia, headaches, pharyngitis, low-grade fever, cognitive complaints, gastrointestinal symptoms, and tender lymph nodes. The search for an infectious cause of chronic fatigue syndrome has been active because of the high percentage of patients who report abrupt onset after a severe flulike illness.

In 1988, the U.S. Centers for Disease Control and Prevention (CDC) defined specific diagnostic criteria for chronic fatigue syndrome. Since then, the disorder has captured the attention of both the medical profession and the general public. The problems associated with studying chronic fatigue syndrome are of great interest in the United States today. The disorder is classified in the 10th revision of *International Statistical Classification of Diseases and Related Health Problems* (ICD-10) as an ill-defined condition of unknown etiology under the heading "Malaise and Fatigue" and is subdivided into asthenia and unspecified disability.

Epidemiology

The exact incidence and prevalence of chronic fatigue syndrome are unknown, but the incidence has been estimated at 1 per 1,000. The illness is observed primarily in young adults (ages 20 to 40). Women are at least twice as likely as men to be affected. In the United States, studies show that about 25 percent of the general adult population experiences fatigue lasting 2 weeks or longer. When the fatigue persists beyond 6 months, it is defined as chronic fatigue. Chronic fatigue syndrome reportedly has a prevalence of 0.52 percent in women and 0.29 percent in men. A study of patients in primary care clinics found that 24 percent had experienced fatigue lasting more than 1 year.

Etiology

The cause of the disorder is unknown. The diagnosis can be made only after all other medical and psychiatric causes of chronic fatiguing illness have been excluded. Scientific studies have validated no pathognomonic signs or diagnostic tests for this condition.

Investigators have tried to implicate the Epstein-Barr herpesvirus (EBV) as the etiological agent in chronic fatigue syndrome. EBV infection, however, is associated with specific antibodies and atypical lymphocytosis, which are absent in chronic fatigue syndrome. Results of tests for other viral agents, such as enteroviruses, herpesvirus, and retroviruses, have been negative. Some investigators have found nonspecific markers of immune abnormalities in patients with chronic fatigue syndrome, for example, reduced proliferation responses of peripheral blood lymphocytes, but these responses are similar to those detected in some patients with major depression.

Diagnosis and Clinical Features

Because chronic fatigue syndrome has no pathognomonic features, diagnosis is difficult. Physicians should attempt to delineate as many signs and symptoms as possible to facilitate the process. Even though chronic fatigue is the most common complaint, most patients have many other symptoms (Table 18–1). As a patient's history unfolds, clinicians are likely to think of a variety of disease states that fall within the range of neurological, metabolic, or psychiatric disorders to account for the patient's distress. In most cases, however, no picture of any disorder clearly emerges from history taking alone.

The physical examination is also an unreliable source of diagnostic certainty. In addition to chronic fatigue, for example, patients may complain of feeling warm or having chills with normal body temperature, and others may complain of lymph node tenderness in the absence of node enlargement. These and other equivocal findings neither confirm nor rule out the disorder.

The CDC diagnostic criteria for chronic fatigue syndrome are listed in Table 18–2 and include fatigue for at least 6 months, impaired memory or concentration, sore throat, tender or enlarged lymph nodes, muscle pain, arthralgias, headache, sleep disturbance, and postexertional malaise. Fatigue is the most obvious symptom and is characterized by severe mental and physical exhaustion, sufficient to cause a 50 percent reduction in patients' activities. The onset is usually gradual, but some patients have an acute onset that resembles a flulike illness.

Table 18–1
Signs and Symptoms Reported by Patients with Chronic Fatigue Syndrome

Fatigue or exhaustion	Double vision
Headache	Sensitivity to bright lights
Malaise	Numbness and/or tingling in extremities
Short-term memory loss	Fainting spells
Muscle pain	Light-headedness
Difficulty concentrating	Dizziness
Joint pain	Clumsiness
Depression	Insomnia
Abdominal pain	Fever or sensation of fever
Lymph node pain	Chills
Sore throat	Night sweats
Lack of restful sleep	Weight gain
Muscle weakness	Allergies
Bitter or metallic taste	Chemical sensitivities
Balance disturbance	Palpitations
Diarrhea	Shortness of breath
Constipation	Flushing rash of the face and cheeks
Bloating	Swelling of the extremities or eyelids
Panic attacks	Burning on urination
Eye pain	Sexual dysfunction
Scratchiness in eyes	Hair loss
Blurring of vision	

Adapted from Bell DS. *The Doctor's Guide to Chronic Fatigue Syndrome: Understanding, Treating, and Living with CFIDS.* Reading: Addison-Wesley; 1995:10.

The following case illustrates many of the uncertainties and difficulties involved in diagnosis and treatment.

Ms. J. was a 35-year-old single white librarian with a benign medical past and no psychiatric symptoms prior to developing a flulike illness. After 10 days the acute episode passed, but she continued to feel lethargic and fatigued readily. Two weeks after the onset of this illness, she returned to work but was unable to complete her usual 8-hour days because of increasing exhaustion and newly developed, gradually evolving, diffuse muscle and joint pain.

Her primary care physician suggested naproxen (Naprosyn) and encouraged her while counseling patience. The physician noted nothing unusual about her mood, and prescribed hypnotic agents to improve her sleep. There was no improvement, however, from 10 mg of zolpidem (Ambien). She then started having squeezing bitemporal headaches. After 3 months, she was referred to a rheumatologist who tried to give her amitriptyline (Elavil) 50 mg at night. She protested vehemently, saying that she was not depressed, just in pain.

Previously, she had been a conscientious employee and had rarely taken leave or missed work because of illness. After 3 months of this illness, however, she was forced to take a leave of absence, returning to live with her mother, since she no longer had any income. She continued to "hurt all over," was lethargic and irritable, and slept poorly because of pain. When she slept, she reported that she no longer awoke refreshed.

Table 18–2
CDC Criteria for Chronic Fatigue Syndrome

A. Severe unexplained fatigue for over 6 months that is:
  (1) of a new or definite onset
  (2) not due to continuing exertion
  (3) not resolved by rest
  (4) functionally impairing
B. The presence of four or more of the following new symptoms:
  (1) impaired memory or concentration
  (2) sore throat
  (3) tender lymph nodes
  (4) muscle pain
  (5) pain in several joints
  (6) new pattern of headaches
  (7) unrefreshing sleep
  (8) postexertional malaise lasting more than 24 hours

Six months after the onset of her original symptoms, she self-referred to an academic health center's rheumatology clinic, where she presented as an afebrile and otherwise healthy woman who was angry about her protracted illness and her living situation. She admitted to difficulty with concentration. Joint examination revealed full range of motion with no red, hot, or swollen joints; tender points were present at all 18 sites.

Her rheumatologist prescribed amitriptyline 25 mg at night for 4 days and then told her to increase the dose by one tablet until she achieved better sleep or reached a dosage of 150 mg. Still protesting that she was not depressed, she took the antidepressant medication because she was desperate for relief. A month later she returned to the rheumatology clinic, still hostile and impatient, with little change, and she was then prescribed 20 mg of fluoxetine (Prozac) in the morning in addition to the amitriptyline at night.

Within a month of this regimen, she was somewhat improved in her mood, sleep, and joint symptoms. However, she still continues to have episodes of fatigue, usually related to stressful life events. She had not yet returned to the work force. (Courtesy of Brian Anthony Fallan, M.D.)

Differential Diagnosis

Chronic fatigue must be differentiated from endocrine disorders (e.g., hypothyroidism), neurological disorders (e.g., multiple sclerosis), infectious disorders (e.g., acquired immune deficiency syndrome [AIDS], infectious mononucleosis), and psychiatric disorders (e.g., depressive disorders). The evaluation process is complex, and a diagnostic scheme is listed in Table 18–3.

Up to 80 percent of patients with chronic fatigue syndrome meet the diagnostic criteria for major depression. The correlation is so high that many psychiatrists believe that all cases of this syndrome are depressive disorders, yet patients with chronic fatigue syndrome rarely report feelings of guilt, suicidal ideation, or anhedonia and show little or no weight loss.

Table 18–3
Approach to the Assessment of Persistent Fatigue

History

- Record the medical and psychosocial circumstances at onset of symptoms.
- Assess previous physical and psychological health.
- Seek clues to an underlying medical disorder (e.g., fevers, weight loss, dyspnea).
- Assess the impact of the symptoms on the patient's lifestyle.

Characteristic symptoms of chronic fatigue syndrome (CFS) include fatigue, myalgia, arthralgia, impaired memory and concentration, and unrefreshing sleep.

↓ ↓

Physical examination

- Seek abnormalities to suggest an underlying medical disorder:
  —Hypothyroidism
  —Chronic hepatitis
  —Chronic anemia
  —Neuromuscular disease
  —Sleep apnea syndrome
  —Occult malignancy, etc.

The physical examination in patients with CFS characteristically shows no abnormalities.

Mental state examination

- Past or family history of psychiatric disorder, notably depression, anxiety
- Past history of frequent episodes of medically unexplained symptoms
- Past history of alcohol or substance abuse
- Current symptoms: depression, anxiety, self-destructive thoughts, and use of over-the-counter medications
- Current signs of psychomotor retardation
- Evaluate psychosocial support system

CFS patients have depressive symptoms, but not guilt, suicidal ideation, or observable psychomotor slowing.

↓ ↓

Laboratory investigation

- Screening tests:
  —Urinalysis
  —Blood count and differential
  —Erythrocyte sedimentation rate
  —Renal function tests
  —Liver function tests
  —Calcium, phosphate
  —Random blood glucose
  —Thyroid function tests (including thyroid stimulating hormone level)
- Additional investigations as clinically indicated (e.g., sleep study)

The diagnosis of CFS is primarily one of exclusion of alternative conditions.

↓

Chronic fatigue syndrome

- *Unexplained, persistent, or relapsing chronic fatigue lasting 6 or more consecutive months* that is of new or definite onset; is not the result of ongoing exertion; is not substantially relieved by rest; and results in substantial reduction in previous levels of occupational, educational, social, or personal activities; *and*
- *Four more of the following symptoms occurring concurrently:* (1) impairment of short-term memory or concentration; (2) sore throat; (3) tender cervical or axillary lymph nodes; (4) muscle pain, or multijoint pain; (5) headaches; (6) unrefreshing sleep; and (7) postexertional malaise.

Reprinted with permission from Hickie IB, Lloyd AR, Wakefield D. Chronic fatigue syndrome: current perspectives on evaluation and management. *Med J Aust.* 1995;163:315.

Also, there is usually no family history of depression or other genetic loading for psychiatric disorder and few if any stressful events in patients' lives that might precipitate or account for a depressive illness. In addition, although some patients respond to antidepressant medication, many eventually become refractory to all psychopharmacological agents. Regardless of diagnostic labeling, however, depressive comorbidity requires treatment with either antidepressants or cognitive-behavioral therapy or a combination of both.

Course and Prognosis

Spontaneous recovery is rare in patients with chronic fatigue syndrome, but improvement does occur. At present, most reports on course and prognosis are based on small samples. In one study, 63 percent of patients with the syndrome, followed for up to 4 years, reported improvement. Patients with the best prognosis have had no previous or concurrent psychiatric illness, are able to maintain social contacts, and continue to work, even at reduced levels.

Treatment

Treatment of chronic fatigue syndrome is mainly supportive. Physicians must first establish rapport and not dismiss patients' complaints as being without foundation. The complaints are not imaginary. A careful medical examination is necessary, and a psychiatric evaluation is indicated, both of which are geared to rule out other causes for the symptoms.

No effective medical treatment is known. Antiviral agents and corticosteroids are not useful, although a few patients have shown a lessening of fatigue with the antiviral drug amantadine (Symmetrel). Symptomatic treatment (e.g., analgesics for arthralgias and muscular pain) is the usual approach, but nonsteroidal antiinflammatory drugs (NSAIDs) are not effective. Patients must be encouraged to continue their daily activities and to resist their fatigue as much as possible. A reduced workload is far better than absence from work. Several studies have reported a positive effect from graded exercise therapy (GET).

Psychiatric treatment is desirable, especially when depression is present. In many cases, symptoms improve markedly

Table 18–4
Recommendations for a Logical Pharmacotherapy of Chronic Fatigue

- Establish a collaborative patient/physician treatment framework.
- Avoid premature diagnostic closure.
- Determine what self-administered, over-the-counter medications the patient is already taking and assess closely for interaction with the proposed medication.
- Discuss the role of medication and identify clear treatment goals:
  Psychiatric syndromes
  Domains of symptomatic distress (e.g., musculoskeletal pain, poor sleep quality, fatigue, subjective cognitive changes, and mood or anxiety symptoms)
- Choice of agent should be based on:
  The predicted side-effect profile
  The patient's preference
  Medical contraindications to the use of a particular medication
- Begin therapy at the lowest possible dose, and increase the dose gradually; observe and discuss side effects during treatment, clarifying issues of significant medical concern.
- Attempt thorough trial to known optimal target dose of drug or until maximum clinical effect is evident.
- Ongoing discussion of the patient's specific response pattern should occur, clarifying the patient's expectations about the treatment.
- Do not continue treatment indefinitely without evidence of clear clinical response; if necessary, discontinue treatment and reassess during medication-free state.
- Avoid polypharmacy; assess treatment response to one agent at a time.
- Frame pharmacotherapy with respect to other aspects of the treatment plan; use medication as setting a context for a multidimensional treatment framework.

Reprinted with permission from Demitrack MA. Psychopharmacological principles in the treatment of chronic fatigue syndrome. In: Demitrack MA, Abbey SE, eds. *Chronic Fatigue Syndrome.* New York: Guilford; 1996:281.

when patients are in supportive or insight-oriented psychotherapy. Cognitive-behavioral therapy is reportedly of use. Therapy is geared to helping patients overcome and correct mistaken beliefs, such as fear that any activity causing fatigue worsens the disorder. Pharmacological agents, especially antidepressants with nonsedating qualities, such as bupropion (Wellbutrin), may be helpful. Nefazodone (Serzone) was reported to decrease pain and improve sleep and memory in some patients. Analeptics (e.g., amphetamine or methylphenidate [Ritalin]) may help reduce fatigue. Table 18–4 contains recommendations for a general approach to pharmacotherapy.

Self-help groups have helped patients with chronic fatigue syndrome. They derive benefit from the group dynamic of instilling hope, offering identification, sharing experiences, and imparting information. The cohesion of members in such groups also raises self-esteem, which is usually impaired in these patients, who often feel that their physicians are not taking them seriously. For this reason, many persons with the syndrome rely on vitamins, minerals, and miscellaneous herbal products or treatment methods that fall under the rubric of alternative medicine. Neither these nor other unidentified general tonics have been peer reviewed in the medical literature, and they are of little or no benefit.

NEURASTHENIA

The term *neurasthenia* ("nervous exhaustion") was introduced in the 1860s by the American neuropsychiatrist George Miller Beard, who applied it to a condition characterized by chronic fatigue and disability (Fig. 18–1). This term is not used frequently now, but it does appear in the psychiatric literature, and it remains a diagnostic entity in ICD-10, where it is classified as one of the neurotic disorders. According to current nosology in the United States, the disorder is not considered a distinct diagnosis. The text revision of the fourth edition of *Diagnostic and Statistical Manual of Mental Disorders* (DSM-IV-TR) categorizes neurasthenia as undifferentiated somatoform disorder.

This disorder is a prime example of cultural differences influencing the classification and manifestations of diseases. Neurasthenia is an accepted condition in Europe and Asia, where it is characterized by fatigue, headache, insomnia, and other vague somatic complaints and is thought to result from chronic stress rather than from unconscious psychological conflicts. In many cultures (especially China), in which persons resist being categorized as having a mental disorder, neurasthenia is a preferred diagnosis. Thus, the disorder is most commonly diagnosed in eastern Asia.

Epidemiology

Difficulties investigating the epidemiology of neurasthenia stem from the fact that it occurs in connection with other conditions, such as anxiety, depression, and somatoform disorders, and it has not been studied sufficiently as an independent disorder. Beard considered neurasthenia one of the most frequently observed conditions in the 19th century United States, although no statistics were available to support his observation. A 1994

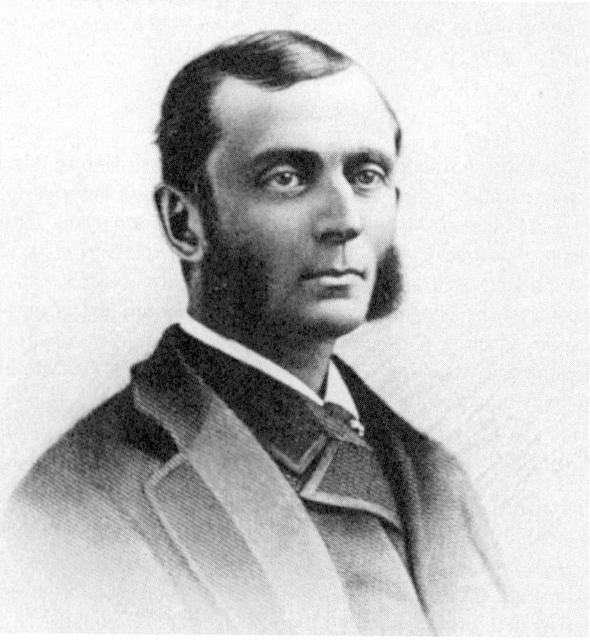

FIGURE 18–1
George Miller Beard. (Courtesy of New York Academy of Medicine, New York, NY.)

study in Switzerland (using ICD-10 criteria) found a prevalence rate of 12 percent.

Studies indicate that the major symptoms—fatigue and heightened concerns with bodily symptoms—are most commonly observed in persons who are socially and economically deprived, although the disorder is no more prevalent in this group than in others and may, in fact, occur more frequently in higher socioeconomic groups. Precursors of neurasthenia in the form of "growing pains," fatigue, and sleep disturbances appear in children. Beard believed childhood to be one of the peak periods for the onset of the disorder, the other being middle age (adults 40 to 65 years of age).

Etiology

According to Beard, the cause of neurasthenia was "nervous exhaustion," which referred to depletion of the "stored nutrient" in the nerve cell (neuron). This depletion resulted from stress, such as overwork. Beard considered the disorder to have a physiological cause in which (as described by Arthur Noyes) "the nervous system is drained of its energy in the manner of a partially discharged battery of low voltage." Beard postulated a "nervous diathesis" theory, in which a person has a specific vulnerability that, when acted on by a stressful environmental influence, allowed the symptoms of neurasthenia to develop. The environmental components could be either biological (infection) or psychological (death of a loved one).

Sigmund Freud was acquainted with the disorder. He agreed with Beard that stress was involved, but Freud thought that neurasthenia was produced by a disturbance in sexual functioning (one of the neuroses), specifically the inadequate discharge of sexual energy that occurred when masturbation replaced normal intercourse. Psychoanalysts after Freud considered neurasthenia a reaction to unconscious factors such as feelings of rejection, low self-esteem, a sense of worthlessness, and repressed anger.

Depletion Hypothesis. The present-day depletion hypothesis, which holds that prolonged stress lowers the levels of neurotransmitters in neurons, bears a striking resemblance to Beard's concept of nerve exhaustion. Depletion of brain amines causes symptoms of anxiety or depression. Low neuronal dopamine activity occurs in depression; the noradrenergic and adrenergic systems are affected in anxiety disorder and depression; and serotonin levels are low in depressive disorder.

A variety of neuroendocrine dysregulations have been reported in patients with mood and anxiety disorders, with the major ones affecting the adrenal, thyroid, and growth hormone axes. Other neuroendocrine abnormalities include decreased nocturnal secretion of melatonin, decreased basal levels of follicle-stimulating hormone (FSH) and luteinizing hormone (LH), and decreased testosterone levels. These hormones are also altered in prolonged stress states and, presumably, in neurasthenia as well.

Diagnosis and Clinical Features

According to ICD-10, neurasthenia is not used as a diagnostic category in all countries. In the United States, for example, many of the cases so diagnosed would meet the criteria for depressive disorder, somatoform disorder, or anxiety disorder. Some patients, however, have such varied symptoms that neurasthenia is the preferred diagnosis. These patients may be diagnosed using the ICD-10 diagnostic criteria (Table 18–5), or they may receive a diagnosis of undifferentiated somatoform disorder according to the DSM-IV-TR criteria (see Table 17–10).

Neurasthenia is characterized by a wide variety of signs and symptoms. The most common findings are chronic weakness and fatigue, aches and pains, and general anxiety or "nervousness." Beard, Freud, and others described a plethora of patients' complaints, which are listed in Table 18–6. These symptoms are real

Table 18–5
ICD-10 Diagnostic Criteria for Neurasthenia

A. Either of the following must be present:
  (1) persistent and distressing complaints of feelings of exhaustion after a minor mental effort (such as performing or attempting to perform everyday tasks that do not require unusual mental effort);
  (2) persistent and distressing complaints of feelings of fatigue and bodily weakness after minor physical effort;
  At least one of the following symptoms must be present:
  (1) feelings of muscular aches and pains;
  (2) dizziness;
  (3) tension headaches;
  (4) sleep disturbances;
  (5) inability to relax;
  (6) irritability;
The patient is unable to recover from the symptoms in Criterion A (1) or (2) by means of rest, relaxation, or entertainment.
The duration of the disorder is at least 3 months.
Most commonly used exclusion clause. The disorder does not occur in the presence of organic emotionally labile disorder, postencephalitic syndrome, postconcussional syndrome, mood disorders, panic disorder, or generalized anxiety disorder.

Table 18–6
Signs and Symptoms Reported by Patients with Neurasthenia

General fatigue	Sexual dysfunction, e.g., erectile disorder, anorgasmia
Exhaustion	Dysmenorrhea
General anxiety	Paresthesia
Difficulty concentrating	Insomnia
Physical aches and pains	Poor memory
Dizziness	Pessimism
Headache	Chronic worry
Intolerance of noise (hyperacusis) or bright lights	Fear of disease
Chills	Irritability
Indigestion	Feelings of hopelessness
Constipation or diarrhea	Dry mouth or hypersalivation
Flatulence	Arthralgias
Palpitations	Heat insensitivity
Extrasystole	Dysphagia
Tachycardia	Pruritus
Excess sweating	Tremors
Flushing of skin	Back pain

to patients. As Beard stated: "They are not imaginary. They have a real objective existence and cannot be willed away."

ICD-10 describes two types of the disorder, with substantial overlap between them. In one type, the main feature is increased fatigue after mental effort, often associated with some decrease in occupational performance or coping efficiency in daily tasks. The mental fatigability is typically described as an unpleasant intrusion of distracting association or recollections, difficulty concentrating, and generally inefficient thinking. The other type emphasizes feelings of bodily or physical weakness and exhaustion after only minimal effort, accompanied by muscular aches and pains and an inability to relax. In both types, other unpleasant physical feelings, such as dizziness, tension headaches, and a sense of general instability, are common. Worry about decreasing mental and physical well-being, irritability, anhedonia, and varying degrees of both depression and anxiety may be present. Sleep is frequently disturbed in its initial and middle phases, but hypersomnia may also be prominent.

If the DSM-IV-TR criteria are used, neurasthenia would be associated with one of the two forms of undifferentiated somatoform disorders, that is, with the group of physical complaints including chronic fatigue and loss of appetite.

Mr. W., a 36-year-old married technician, came to an outpatient psychiatric clinic in Hunan, People's Republic of China, complaining of easy fatigability. He also had insomnia, and his ability to work had decreased because of persistent weakness and tension headaches. These symptoms began about 12 years ago, without any evident cause. Mr. W. noticed that he began to tire easily and felt weak after exerting any mental or physical effort. He also had difficulty falling asleep and awakened many times during the night. He felt that his mental energy was insufficient during the day. He could not read or watch television for more than half an hour without feeling weary. Though he could perform his occupational tasks, he had difficulty concentrating and his memory was poor. In the past 12 years he has hardly ever been free of these symptoms, but they fluctuate in intensity over time. When his condition is really bad, he feels distressed, irritable, and nervous. It is not clear why he now comes for help. Mr. W. does not spontaneously complain about depression. How ever, when asked specifically about depressed mood, he says that sometimes he feels depressed and is unable to enjoy anything, which he attributes to his difficulty concentrating and his physical exhaustion. When he is feeling depressed, he experiences guilt, slowed thinking, appetite disturbance, and psychomotor retardation. The periods of depression never last more than 2 weeks and occur about five or six times a year.

Mr. W. has gone to the local hospital on many occasions, and has been treated with Chinese herbs and Western medicines. Once he went to see a psychiatrist, and an antidepressant was prescribed. All of these treatments were without effect.

Mr. W. describes himself as an "introverted person" since puberty, always preferring to stay home by himself. He obtained above-average grades in school. After graduating from college, he was hired as a technician in a factory. At the present time he is still working at his job.

In the interview, Mr. W. looks exhausted. There is no evidence of prominent anxiety or depression. Findings of a physical examination and laboratory tests are within normal limits.

DISCUSSION

Chinese-trained clinicians would have no difficulty in making a diagnosis of Mr. W.'s condition since he has the characteristic features of neurasthenia, one of the most commonly diagnosed disorders in the People's Republic of China. Mr. W. expresses almost all of his complaints in terms of somatic symptoms. For many years he has not had the energy and strength to function adequately. He also complains of difficulty sleeping and headaches. Although these symptoms, plus his poor concentration and memory, suggest a depressive syndrome, Mr. W. denies persistent depression or anhedonia. Therefore, the diagnosis of dysthymic disorder, which a Western-trained clinician might consider, cannot be made. The relative rarity of major depressive disorder and dysthymic disorder in China is probably due to the Chinese use of physical symptoms as a metaphor for expressing unpleasant mood states, whereas in this country it is more common for patients to report unpleasant mood states. There is also evidence, however, that when Chinese patients with neurasthenia are systematically interviewed about depressed mood their symptoms usually meet the criteria for major depressive disorder or dysthymic disorder.

Had a Western-trained clinician evaluated Mr. W., he or she might well have described him as appearing "depressed" rather than "exhausted," and would therefore have made a diagnosis of depressive disorder not otherwise specified since the recurrent short-lived periods of depression correspond neither to major depressive disorder nor to dysthymic disorder. However, if we accept the Chinese psychiatrist's description of Mr. W., then, according to DSM-IV-TR, his chronic physical complaints without any organic basis, and without a complaint of sustained depressed mood or anhedonia, indicate a diagnosis of undifferentiated somatoform disorder.

Differential Diagnosis

Neurasthenia must be distinguished from anxiety disorders, depressive disorder, and the somatoform disorders. Because so many signs and symptoms of neurasthenia overlap with, and appear in, each of these disorders, differential diagnosis may be exceedingly difficult. For example, patients with anxiety disorder do not uncommonly have depressive symptomatology; patients with hypochondriasis often complain of anxiety; and patients with body dysmorphic disorder can have somatic complaints.

Clinicians must rigorously apply the diagnostic criteria for anxiety, depressive, and somatoform disorders before making a diagnosis of neurasthenia. Hallmarks of neurasthenia are a patient's emphasis on fatigability and weakness and concern about lowered mental and physical efficiency (in contrast to the somatoform disorders, in which bodily complaints and preoccupation with physical disease dominate the picture). If the neurasthenic syndrome develops in the aftermath of a physical

illness (particularly influenza, viral hepatitis, or infectious mononucleosis), the diagnosis of the illness should also be recorded. Chronic fatigue syndrome must also be considered, and differentiating the two disorders is difficult.

Course and Prognosis

Neurasthenia most often occurs during adolescence or middle age. Untreated, the disorder is usually chronic, and patients may become incapacitated by one or more symptoms so that all areas of functioning become impaired. In childhood, difficulties in school functioning, including poor grades and truancy, are likely. In adulthood, work performance deteriorates, or patients may become so disabled that work is impossible. Similarly, social, marital, and interpersonal relationships suffer.

Beard believed that with treatment (such as it was in the 1860s) "the majority can be relieved or substantially cured." The range of therapeutic options now available is broad, and with treatment, the prognosis should be favorable; but the long-term prognosis is unknown. For patients first diagnosed in childhood, the prognosis without treatment is guarded, with chronic symptoms being the most likely outcome. Sometimes it is difficult to distinguish the prodromal signs of schizophrenia or bipolar disorder from neurasthenia.

Treatment

The key concept in the current treatment of neurasthenia is clinicians' understanding that a patient's symptoms are not imaginary. The symptoms are objective and are produced by emotions that influence the autonomic nervous system, which in turn affects bodily functions. Stress can cause structural change in an organ system, and the result can be life threatening. Therapy must therefore begin with a careful medical workup to determine whether the somatic symptoms are amenable to therapy, and if so, what treatment is likely to produce the best results. Patients should be reassured that the administration of medication (analgesics, laxatives, and so on) to relieve medical symptoms will be useful, but only when combined with concurrent psychotherapeutic intervention. Patients must be helped to recognize the stresses in their lives and the coping mechanisms they use to deal with these stresses, to gain insight into the interaction between mind and body. Without such insight-oriented psychotherapy, the neurasthenic condition is likely to continue unabated.

The availability of psychopharmacological agents has markedly improved therapeutic options. Serotonergic agents (e.g., fluoxetine), which have both antidepressant and antianxiety effects, are the most useful class of drugs. Other antidepressants, such as nefazodone and mirtazapine (Remeron), are also effective. Physicians should take care in prescribing drugs with abuse potential, such as benzodiazepines, because of these patients' predilection for self-medication and drug misuse. Such drugs may be useful, for brief periods and under careful supervision, to deal with overwhelming anxiety, phobias, or insomnia. Similarly, small doses of analeptics, such as amphetamine (Dexedrine) or methylphenidate, may help to treat chronic fatigue and anhedonia. In some cases, it may be necessary to prescribe these medications for long periods of time. In these situations, patients generally stabilize the dose of drugs taken (e.g., 15 mg of amphetamine per day in divided doses). Tolerance does not usually develop, and the clinician should rarely increase the dose lest drug dependence develop. Testosterone replacement can be tried in men with demonstrated low or borderline testosterone levels, but long-term treatment with testosterone may be associated with serious adverse effects, such as prostatic cancer.

References

Addington JW. Chronic fatigue syndrome: a dysfunction of the hypothalamus-pituitary-adrenal axis. *J Chronic Fatigue Syndrome*. 2000;7:63.

Ax S, Gregg VH, Jones D. Coping and illness cognitions: chronic fatigue syndrome. *Clin Psychol Rev*. 2001;21:161.

Bankier B, Aigner M, Bach M. Clinical validity of ICD-10 neurasthenia. *Psychopathology*. 2001;34:134.

Friedburg F, Jason LA. Chronic fatigue syndrome and fibromyalgia: clinical assessment and treatment. *J Clin Psychol*. 2001;57:433.

Jason LA, Taylor RR, Kennedy CL, et al. Subtypes of chronic fatigue syndrome: a review of findings. *J Chronic Fatigue Syndrome*. 2001;8:1.

Jason LA, Torres-Harding SR, Carrico AW, Taylor RR. Symptom occurrence in persons with chronic fatigue syndrome. *Biol Psychol*. 2002;59:15.

Jorge CM, Goodnick PJ. Chronic fatigue syndrome and depression: biological differentiation and treatment. *Psychiatr Ann*. 1997;17:365.

Lee S. The vicissitudes of neurasthenia in Chinese societies: where will it go from the ICD-10? *Transcult Psychiatr Res Rev*. 1994;31:153.

Lee S, Wong KC. Rethinking neurasthenia: the illness concepts of *shenjing shuairuo* among Chinese undergraduates in Hong Kong. *Cult Med Psychiatry*. 1995;19:91.

Merikangas K, Angst J. Neurasthenia in a longitudinal cohort study of young adults. *Psychol Med*. 1994;24:1013.

Price RK, North CS, Wessely S, Fraser VJ. Estimating the prevalence of chronic fatigue syndrome and associated symptoms in the community. *Public Health Rep*. 1992;107:514.

Richards J. Chronic fatigue syndrome in children and adolescents: a review article. *Clin Child Psychol Psychiatry*. 2000;5:31.

Schuepbach WMM, Adler RH, Sabbioni MEE. Accuracy of clinical diagnosis of "psychogenic disorders" in the presence of physical symptoms suggesting a general medical condition: a 5-year follow-up in 162 patients. *Psychother Psychosom*. 2002;71:11.

Taylor RR, Jason LA, Curie CJ. Prognosis of chronic fatigue in a community-based sample. *Psychosom Med*. 2002;64:319.

Vercouilen JH, Swanink CM, Fennis JF, Falama JM, van der Meer JW, Bleijenberg F. Dimensional assessment of chronic fatigue syndrome. *J Psychosom Res*. 1994;38:383.

Wessely A. Chronic fatigue syndrome—trials and tribulations. *JAMA*. 2001; 286:1378.

Wessely S. Neurasthenia and chronic fatigue: theory and practice in Britain and America. *Transcult Psychiatr Res Rev*. 1994;31:173.

Wessely S, Lutz T. Neurasthenia and fatigue syndromes. In: Berrios GE, Porter R, eds. *A History of Clinical Psychiatry: The Origin and History of Psychiatric Disorders*. New York: New York University Press; 1995:509.

19 Factitious Disorders

In factitious disorders, patients intentionally produce signs of medical or mental disorders and misrepresent their histories and symptoms. The only apparent objective of the behavior is to assume the role of a patient without an external incentive. For many persons, hospitalization itself is a primary objective and often a way of life. The disorders have a compulsive quality, but the behaviors are considered voluntary in that they are deliberate and purposeful, even if they cannot be controlled. Clinicians can assess whether a symptom is intentional both by direct evidence and by excluding other causes.

In a 1951 article in *Lancet*, Richard Asher coined the term "Munchausen syndrome" to refer to a syndrome in which patients embellish their personal history, chronically fabricate symptoms to gain hospital admission, and move from hospital to hospital. The syndrome was named after Baron Hieronymus Friedrich Freiherr von Munchausen (1720–1791), a German cavalry officer (Fig. 19–1).

EPIDEMIOLOGY

The prevalence of factitious disorders in the general population is unknown, although some clinicians believe that they are more common than acknowledged. They appear to occur more frequently in hospital and health care workers than the general population. The disorder occurs more frequently in females than in males, and the severe syndromes are more frequent in females. One study reported a 9 percent rate of factitious disorders among all patients admitted to a hospital; another study found factitious fever in 3 percent of all patients. According to the text revision of the fourth edition of *Diagnostic and Statistical Manual of Mental Disorders* (DSM-IV-TR), factitious disorder is diagnosed in about 1 percent of patients who are seen in psychiatric consultation in general hospitals. The prevalence appears to be greater in highly specialized treatment settings. Cases of feigned psychological signs and symptoms are reported much less commonly than those of physical signs and symptoms. A data bank of persons who feign illness has been established to alert hospitals about such patients, many of whom travel from place to place, seek admission under different names, or simulate different illnesses.

In the United States, factitious disorder by proxy (discussed separately below) accounts for fewer than 1,000 of the almost 3 million cases of child abuse reported annually.

COMORBIDITY

A large number of persons diagnosed with factitious disorder have comorbid psychiatric diagnoses (e.g., mood disorders, personality disorders, or substance-related disorders).

ETIOLOGY

Psychosocial Factors. The psychodynamic underpinnings of factitious disorders are poorly understood because the patients are difficult to engage in an exploratory psychotherapy process. They may insist that their symptoms are physical and that psychologically oriented treatment is therefore useless. Anecdotal case reports indicate that many of the patients suffered childhood abuse or deprivation, resulting in frequent hospitalizations during early development. In such circumstances, an inpatient stay may have been regarded as an escape from a traumatic home situation, and the patient may have found a series of caretakers (such as doctors, nurses, and hospital workers) to be loving and caring. In contrast, the patients' families of origin included a rejecting mother or an absent father. The usual history reveals that the patient perceives one or both parents as rejecting figures who are unable to form close relationships. The facsimile of genuine illness, therefore, is used to recreate the desired positive parent–child bond. The disorders are a form of repetition compulsion, repeating the basic conflict of needing and seeking acceptance and love while expecting that they will not be forthcoming. Hence, the patient transforms the physicians and staff members into rejecting parents.

Patients who seek out painful procedures, such as surgical operations and invasive diagnostic tests, may have a masochistic personality makeup in which pain serves as punishment for past sins, imagined or real. Some patients may attempt to master the past and the early trauma of serious medical illness or hospitalization by assuming the role of the patient and reliving the painful and frightening experience over and over again through multiple hospitalizations. Patients who feign psychiatric illness may have had a relative who was hospitalized with the illness they are simulating. Through identification, patients hope to reunite with the relative in a magical way.

Many patients have the poor identity formation and disturbed self-image that is characteristic of someone with borderline personality disorder. Some patients are as-if personalities who have assumed the identities of those around them. If these patients are health professionals, they are often unable to differ-

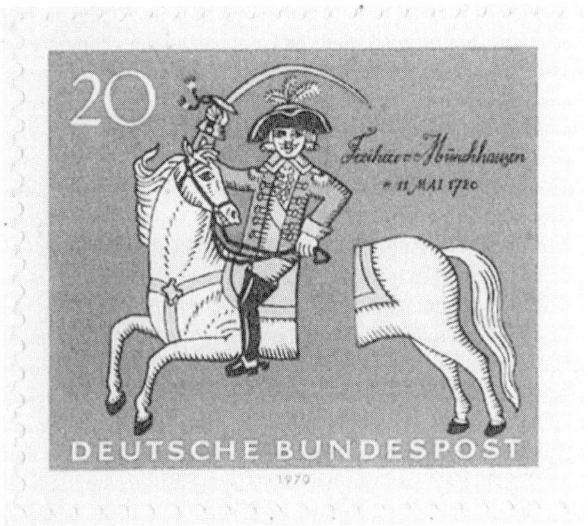

FIGURE 19–1
A commemorative stamp issued by Germany in 1970 to mark the two hundred fiftieth anniversary of Baron von Munchausen's birth. The Baron is depicted riding a severed horse into battle. (Courtesy of Marc D. Feldman and Charles V. Ford.)

Table 19–1
DSM-IV-TR Diagnostic Criteria for Factitious Disorder

A. Intentional production or feigning of physical or psychological signs or symptoms.
B. The motivation for the behavior is to assume the sick role.
C. External incentives for the behavior (such as economic gain, avoiding legal responsibility, or improving physical well-being, as in malingering) are absent.

Code based on type:

With predominantly psychological signs and symptoms: if psychological signs and symptoms predominate in the clinical presentation

With predominantly physical signs and symptoms: if physical signs and symptoms predominate in the clinical presentation

With combined psychological and physical signs and symptoms: if both psychological and physical signs and symptoms are present but neither predominates in the clinical presentation

From American Psychiatric Association. *Diagnostic and Statistical Manual of Mental Disorders.* 4th ed. Text rev. Washington, DC: American Psychiatric Association; copyright 2000, with permission.

entiate themselves from the patients with whom they come in contact. The cooperation or encouragement of other persons in simulating a factitious illness occurs in a rare variant of the disorder. Although most patients act alone, friends or relatives participate in fabricating the illness in some instances.

Significant defense mechanisms are repression, identification, identification with the aggressor, regression, and symbolization.

Biological Factors. Some researchers have proposed that brain dysfunction may be a factor in factitious disorders. It has been hypothesized that impaired information processing contributes to Munchausen patients' *pseudologia fantastica* and aberrant behavior; however, no genetic patterns have been established, and electroencephalographic (EEG) studies noted no specific abnormalities in patients with factitious disorders.

DIAGNOSIS AND CLINICAL FEATURES

The diagnostic criteria for factitious disorder in DSM-IV-TR are given in Table 19–1. The psychiatric examination should emphasize securing information from any available friends, relatives, or other informants, because interviews with reliable outside sources often reveal the false nature of the patient's illness. Although time consuming and tedious, verifying all the facts presented by the patient about previous hospitalizations and medical care is essential.

Psychiatric evaluation is requested on a consultation basis in about 50 percent of cases, usually after a simulated illness is suspected. The psychiatrist is often asked to confirm the diagnosis of factitious disorder. Under these circumstances, it is necessary to avoid pointed or accusatory questioning that may provoke truculence, evasion, or flight from the hospital. There may be a danger of provoking frank psychosis if vigorous confrontation is used; in some instances, the feigned illness serves an adaptive function and is a desperate attempt to ward off further disintegration.

Factitious Disorder with Predominantly Psychological Signs and Symptoms

Some patients show psychiatric symptoms judged to be feigned. This determination can be difficult and is often made only after a prolonged investigation (see Table 19–1). The feigned symptoms frequently include depression, hallucinations, dissociative and conversion symptoms, and bizarre behavior. Because the patient does not improve after routine therapeutic measures are administered, he or she may receive large doses of psychoactive drugs and may undergo electroconvulsive therapy.

Factitious psychological symptoms resemble the phenomenon of pseudomalingering, conceptualized as satisfying the need to maintain an intact self-image, which would be marred by admitting psychological problems that are beyond the person's capacity to master through conscious effort. In this case, deception is a transient ego-supporting device.

Recent findings indicate that factitious psychotic symptoms are more common than was previously suspected. The presence of simulated psychosis as a feature of other disorders, such as mood disorders, indicates a poor overall prognosis.

Psychotic inpatients found to have factitious disorder with predominantly psychological signs and symptoms—that is, exclusively simulated psychotic symptoms—generally have a concurrent diagnosis of borderline personality disorder. In these cases, the outcome appears to be worse than that of bipolar I disorder or schizoaffective disorder.

Patients may appear depressed and may explain their depression by offering a false history of the recent death of a significant friend or relative. Elements of the history that may suggest factitious bereavement include a violent or bloody

death, a death under dramatic circumstances, and the dead person's being a child or a young adult. Other patients may describe both recent and remote memory loss or both auditory and visual hallucinations. According to DSM-IV-TR:

> The individual may surreptitiously use psychoactive substances for the purpose of producing symptoms that suggest a mental disorder (e.g., stimulants to produce restlessness or insomnia, hallucinogens to induce altered perceptual states, analgesics to induce euphoria, and hypnotics to induce lethargy). Combinations of psychoactive substances can produce very unusual presentations.

Other symptoms, which also appear in the physical type of factitious disorder, include pseudologia fantastica and impostorship. In pseudologia fantastica, limited factual material is mixed with extensive and colorful fantasies. The listener's interest pleases the patient and thus reinforces the symptom. The history or the symptoms are not the only distortions of truth. Patients often give false and conflicting accounts about other areas of their lives (e.g., they may claim the death of a parent, to play on the sympathy of others). Imposture is commonly related to lying in these cases. Many patients assume the identity of a prestigious person. Men, for example, report being war heroes and attribute their surgical scars to wounds received during battle or in other dramatic and dangerous exploits. Similarly, they may say that they have ties to accomplished or renowned figures.

Table 19–2 lists various syndromes feigned by patients who want to be seen as having a mental illness.

Factitious Disorder with Predominantly Physical Signs and Symptoms

Factitious disorder with predominantly physical signs and symptoms is the best known type of Munchausen syndrome. The disorder has also been called hospital addiction, polysurgical addiction—producing the so-called washboard abdomen—and professional patient syndrome, among other names.

The essential feature of patients with the disorder is their ability to present physical symptoms so well that they can gain admission to, and stay in, a hospital (see Table 19–1). To support their history, these patients may feign symptoms suggesting a disorder involving any organ system. They are familiar with the diagnoses of most disorders that usually require hospital admission or medication and can give excellent histories capable of deceiving even experienced clinicians. Clinical presentations are myriad and include hematoma, hemoptysis, abdominal pain, fever, hypoglycemia, lupuslike syndromes, nausea, vomiting, dizziness, and seizures. Urine is contaminated with blood or feces, anticoagulants are taken to simulate bleeding disorders, insulin is used to produce hypoglycemia, and so on. Such patients often insist on surgery and claim adhesions from previous surgical procedures. They may acquire a "gridiron" or washboardlike abdomen from multiple procedures. Complaints of pain, especially that simulating renal colic, are common, with the patients wanting narcotics. In about half the reported cases, these patients demand treatment with specific medications, usually analgesics. Once in the hospital, they continue to be demanding and difficult. As each test is returned with a negative result, they may accuse doctors of incompetence, threaten litigation, and become generally abusive. Some may sign out abruptly shortly before they believe they are going to be confronted with their factitious behavior. They then go to another hospital in the same or another city and begin the cycle again. Specific predisposing factors are true physical disorders during childhood leading to extensive medical treatment, a grudge against the medical profession, employment as a medical paraprofessional, and an important relationship with a physician in the past.

Table 19–2
Presentations in Factitious Disorder with Predominantly Psychological Signs and Symptoms

Bereavement	Eating disorder
Depression	Amnesia
Posttraumatic stress disorder	Substance-related disorder
Pain disorder	Paraphilias
Psychosis	Hypersomnia
Bipolar I disorder	Transsexualism
Dissociative identity disorder	

Adapted with permission from Feldman MD, Eisendrath SJ. *The Spectrum of Factitious Disorders.* Washington, DC: American Psychiatric Press; 1996.

An orthopedic surgeon in Seattle requested a psychiatric consultation on Ms. S., a 28-year-old single graduate student who was recovering from a recent spinal fusion, because he thought she was not complying with physical therapy.

The psychiatrist noted that Ms. S. was an attractive young woman with a below-the-knee amputation of her left leg. She was oddly ingratiating and cheerful, and didn't seem to be appropriately troubled by her deteriorating medical condition. She reported that 5 years previously she had been thrown to the ground by a boyfriend, injuring her back. Over the next 2 years she had multiple surgical procedures on her back. Finally, a fusion left her pain free until 6 months ago, when she was diagnosed with spinal degenerative changes and was referred for physical therapy.

Amazed that she didn't volunteer any information about her amputation, the psychiatrist asked how it happened and learned that shortly after the original surgery to her back, she had been in a motorcycle accident, sustaining burns to her left ankle. This became a chronic injury and ultimately led to amputation of her leg, a year and a half ago. She reported this calmly and denied any distress over the disfigurement or disability. She also calmly reported that fluctuating swelling of her stump and recurrent ulcers had interfered with her being successfully fitted with a prosthesis. Thus, she had remained in a wheelchair. She had also been hospitalized several times many years earlier for colitis and kidney stones.

The psychiatrist called the surgeon who had performed her amputation. He reported that the original burn had quickly progressed to a chronic injury, with chronic pain and swelling of the left leg. When the leg proved unresponsive to medical management the patient received a series of

skin grafts, all of which failed because of infection and edema. She was instructed to keep her leg elevated, but did not comply, and her leg continued to deteriorate. She saw many doctors, and was followed in a pain clinic, but continued to experience pain, massive edema, and recurrent infections. Ms. S. repeatedly urged her surgeon to amputate her leg, claiming that it was painful and of no use to her. Ultimately he complied.

The surgeon who performed the amputation also reported that Ms. S. had recently had several admissions for left-sided weakness and numbness. Physical findings were inconsistent, the workup was negative and she was discharged with a diagnosis of "conversion disorder." It was shortly thereafter that her back pain recurred. The surgeon also commented that various physicians involved in the management of her leg injury had raised the possibility her symptoms might be self-induced.

Ms. S. is an only child, born to a middle-class family. By her own account after graduating from college, she moved from job to job for a number of years, generally leaving because of medical problems and repeated hospitalizations. At the time of admission, she was a part-time graduate student being supported by social security. No one had accompanied her to the hospital, and she had no visitors during her hospitalization. She asked that her doctors not contact her family.

Ms. S. was transferred to an inpatient rehabilitation unit, where she quickly developed a string of largely unexplained medical problems, including a urinary tract infection, gastroenteritis with diarrhea and fever, painful swelling of the right hand and wrist, a rash on her back and torso, and atypical mental status changes, including difficulty doing rudimentary calculations and inconsistent memory deficits. Meanwhile she repeatedly refused to comply with safety procedures on the unit, leaving her wheelchair unlocked and her bed rail down, despite constant reminders by the staff. Over time she generated a good deal of anger and frustration among most staff members, although a few found her a particularly sad and pathetic case.

After her previous surgeon had been contacted, the staff became suspicious about the role that she might be playing in the development of her symptoms. Ms. S.'s room was searched and furosemide (a diuretic), cathartics, and an exercise band that could serve as a tourniquet were found. These were believed possibly to explain many of her symptoms as well as the unexplained metabolic abnormalities that had been noted in her chart. Careful review of her chart revealed that her urinary tract infection had been diagnosed on the basis of positive cultures in the absence of cells in the urine, most consistent with a fecal contaminant. It remained unclear if or how she might have factitiously elevated her temperature, even while observed, or how she might have induced the bitelike lesions on her back and torso.

DISCUSSION

When a clinician attempts to obtain a history from a patient, there is a basic assumption that the patient is doing the best that he or she can do to provide accurate information. In this case, the referral was triggered by noncompliance with the surgeon's therapeutic recommendation. The first suggestion that things might not be as they appeared was the patient's striking nonchalance about her disability (the leg amputation)—referred to as *la belle indifférence.* Suspicions were further raised when additional history became available from her previous surgeon. Finally, compelling evidence was obtained that indicated that she had deliberately produced many of her puzzling physical symptoms and metabolic abnormalities, suggesting a diagnosis of either factitious disorder or malingering.

The distinction between these two conditions depends on the underlying motivation. In malingering, there are clear external incentives—for example, the man who, in order to avoid military service, puts sugar in his urine to simulate diabetes. In contrast, in factitious disorder the motivation is presumed to be a psychological need to assume the sick role. In this case there do not appear to be any clear external incentives, and one can only presume that, for unknown reasons, Ms. S. has a pathological need to perpetuate being a medical patient. Because her symptoms are primarily physical, the Axis I diagnosis would be factitious disorder with predominantly physical signs and symptoms, a disorder first called Munchausen syndrome, after an eighteenth-century baron who wrote fantastic tales.

We assume that people with factitious disorder also have severe personality disturbance. However, in the absence of any specific information about this patient's long-term personality functioning, we would note diagnosis deferred on Axis II. On Axis III we list the left leg amputation and her recent spinal fusion. Undoubtedly, Ms. S. has multiple psychosocial problems, but because of lack of any specific information, at this point we note deferred on Axis IV. Her Axis V GAF rating of 33 reflects her major impairment in thinking and judgment.

FOLLOW-UP

A team meeting was convened, and Ms. S. was told that it was suspected that she had factitious symptoms, implying that she was actively involved in inducing at least some of her symptoms. She was informed that this is a serious and potentially life-threatening mental illness, and that inpatient psychiatric hospitalization was recommended for further evaluation and management. She did not comment on the diagnosis, appeared unconcerned, and agreed to transfer to a psychiatric ward.

Ms. S. was in the acute psychiatric ward for 4 months. During that time, she developed no new medical problems and made no complaints of pain or physical discomfort. Instead she developed a series of psychiatric symptoms. She initially presented with rapid alternations of mood, appearing first hypomanic, racing around the unit in her wheelchair, and claiming to be up all night, then depressed, curling up on her bed with the lights out, refusing to eat or interact with others. Her presentation was thought by some staff members to result from factitious bipolar disorder, whereas others attributed her symptoms to genuine affective instability or true dissociative phenomena.

Ms. S.'s behavior on the unit was provocative and impulsive. She was liable and suspicious. She split staff, threw tantrums, said she was suicidal, and barricaded herself in her room. She improved on an anticonvulsive medication and an antipsychotic, but nevertheless spent the second half of her hospitalization refusing to participate in activities and with restricted privileges because of her threats of self-destructive behavior if she was allowed to leave the unit.

In psychotherapy, she gradually revealed a history of daily physical abuse at the hands of her parents throughout childhood and early adolescence. Her therapist believed that this history was genuine and diagnosed a dissociative disorder on the basis of the symptoms she described. Other staff members remained unconvinced of the veracity of her story of childhood abuse, but were impressed with the array of features characteristic of borderline personality disorder.

Ms. S. agreed to a voluntary transfer to long-term hospitalization. One day before the planned transfer, she changed her mind, saying she wanted to "get on with my life," and submitted a sign-out letter. She went to court, where she was granted discharge by the judge. She signed out against medical advice, and was lost to follow-up. (From *DSM-IV Casebook.*)

Baroreflex failure is characterized by episodes of severe hypertension and tachycardia, alternating with episodes of normal or even low blood pressure and bradycardia. It is often caused by interruption of the baroreflex arch as a result of bilateral damage to the glossopharyngeal and vagus nerves from trauma, radiation, or surgery. Less often, the lesion is in the brainstem, and in some cases, the primary cause is not found.

A 68-year-old woman was referred for evaluation of baroreflex failure because of a 4-year history of severe episodes of hypertension (systolic blood pressure >200 mm Hg for 2 to 4 days) alternating with periods of gradual onset hypotension (in which the systolic blood pressure dropped below 70 mm Hg over a period of hours), bradycardia (requiring a pacemaker), and extreme sleepiness.

Plasma norepinephrine levels were elevated (900 pg per milliliter) during the hypertensive episodes and inappropriately low (54 pg per milliliter) during the hypotensive episodes, changes consistent with the occurrence of baroreflex failure. However, there was no apparent cause, and baroreflex gain (the magnitude of proportional changes in heart rate per unit change in blood pressure) was only mildly reduced. A suppression test with 0.3 mg of clonidine reduced the blood pressure from 158/99 to 105/62 mm Hg, the heart rate from 93 to 66 beats per minute, and the plasma norepinephrine level from 961 to 93 pg per milliliter, reproducing the conditions recorded during spontaneous episodes.

The α_2-antagonist yohimbine, whose effects are the opposite of those of clonidine, reduced the severity and duration of the hypotensive episodes. Plasma samples obtained before and during a hypotensive episode revealed clonidine levels in the high therapeutic range, indicating that the cause of the episodes was Munchausen syndrome. The patient denied taking clonidine and refused psychiatric assistance, but the episodes did not recur during 9 months of follow-up with strict supervision of the patient by her family and the removal of all medications from the home. The severity of her disorder is underscored by her willingness to undergo invasive diagnostic procedures and treatments (arteriography, Swan-Ganz monitoring, placement of a pacemaker, and possible brainstem decompression surgery). The duration of her illness (4 years) emphasizes the difficulties in diagnosing this disease and its lack of recognition in the medical community. (From Tellioglue T, Oates JA, Biaggioni I. Munchausen's syndrome presenting as baroreflex failure [letter]. *N Engl J Med.* 2000;343:581.)

Factitious Disorder with Combined Psychological and Physical Signs and Symptoms

In combined forms of factitious disorder, both psychological and physical signs and symptoms are present. If neither type predominates in the clinical presentation, a diagnosis of factitious disorder with combined psychological and physical signs and symptoms should be made (see Table 19–1). In one representative report a patient alternated between feigned dementia, bereavement, rape, and seizures.

Factitious Disorder Not Otherwise Specified

Some patients with factitious signs and symptoms do not meet the DSM-IV-TR criteria for a specific factitious disorder and should be classified as having factitious disorder not otherwise specified (Table 19–3). The most notable example of the diagnosis is factitious disorder by proxy, which is also included in a DSM-IV-TR appendix (Table 19–4). In this diagnosis, a person intentionally produces physical signs or symptoms in another person who is under the first person's care. One apparent purpose of the behavior is for the caretaker to indirectly assume the sick role; another is to be relieved of the caretaking role by having the child hospitalized (Table 19–5). The most common case of factitious disorder by proxy involves a mother who deceives medical personnel into believing that her child is ill. The deception may involve a false medical history, contamination of labo-

Table 19–3
DSM-IV-TR Diagnostic Criteria for Factitious Disorder Not Otherwise Specified

This category includes disorders with factitious symptoms that do not meet the criteria for factitious disorder. An example is factitious disorder by proxy: the intentional production or feigning of physical or psychological signs or symptoms in another person who is under the individual's care for the purpose of indirectly assuming the sick role (see Table 19–4 for suggested research criteria).

From American Psychiatric Association. *Diagnostic and Statistical Manual of Mental Disorders.* 4th ed. Text rev. Washington, DC: American Psychiatric Association; copyright 2000, with permission.

Table 19–4
DSM-IV-TR Research Criteria for Factitious Disorder by Proxy

A. Intentional production or feigning of physical or psychological signs or symptoms in another person who is under the individual's care.
B. The motivation for the perpetrator's behavior is to assume the sick role by proxy.
C. External incentives for the behavior (such as economic gain) are absent.
D. The behavior is not better accounted for by another mental disorder.

ratory samples, alteration of records, or induction of injury and illness in the child.

ICD-10

The 10th revision of *International Statistical Classification of Diseases and Related Health Problems* (ICD-10) notes that "the condition is best interpreted as a disorder of illness behavior and the sick role. Individuals with this pattern of behavior usually show signs of . . . other marked abnormalities of personality and relationships." ICD-10 also includes a category called elaboration of physical symptoms for psychological reasons. The ICD-10 criteria for both conditions are presented in Table 19–6. In ICD-10 these conditions exclude factitious dermatitis, and "Munchausen by proxy" is classified under child abuse, not factitious disorders.

Table 19–5
Clinical Indicators That May Suggest Factitious Disorder by Proxy

The symptoms and pattern of illness are extremely unusual, or inexplicable physiologically.

Repeated hospitalizations and workups by numerous caregivers fail to reveal a conclusive diagnosis or cause.

Physiological parameters are consistent with induced illness; e.g., apnea monitor tracings disclose massive muscle artifact prior to respiratory arrest, suggesting that the child has been struggling against an obstruction to the airways.

The patient fails to respond to appropriate treatments.

The vitality of the patient is inconsistent with the laboratory findings.

The signs and symptoms abate when the mother has not had access to the child.

The mother is the only witness to the onset of signs and symptoms.

Unexplained illnesses have occurred in the mother or her other children.

The mother has had medical or nursing education, or exposure to models of the illnesses afflicting the child (e.g., a parent with sleep apnea).

The mother welcomes even invasive and painful tests.

The mother grows anxious if the child improves.

Maternal lying is proved.

Medical observations yield information that is inconsistent with parental reports.

Table 19–6
ICD-10 Diagnostic Criteria for Other Disorders of Adult Personality and Behavior

Elaboration of physical symptoms for psychological reasons

A. Physical symptoms originally due to a confirmed physical disorder, disease, or disability become exaggerated or prolonged in excess of what can be explained by the physical disorder itself.
B. There is evidence for a psychological causation for the excess symptoms (such as evident fear of disability or death, possible financial compensation, disappointment at the standard of care experienced).

Intentional production or feigning of symptoms or disabilities, either physical or psychological [factitious disorder]

A. The individual exhibits a persistent pattern of intentional production or feigning of symptoms and/or self-infliction of wounds in order to produce symptoms.
B. No evidence can be found for an external motivation such as financial compensation, escape from danger, or more medical care. (If such evidence can be found, the category, malingering, should be used.)
C. *Most commonly used exclusion clause.* There is no confirmed physical or mental disorder that could explain the symptoms.

Other specified disorders of adult personality and behavior

This category should be used for coding any specified disorder of adult personality and behavior that cannot be classified under any one of the preceding headings.

PATHOLOGY AND LABORATORY EXAMINATION

Psychological testing may reveal specific underlying pathology in individual patients. Features that are overrepresented in patients with factitious disorder include normal or above-average intelligence quotient (IQ); absence of a formal thought disorder; poor sense of identity, including confusion over sexual identity; poor sexual adjustment; poor frustration tolerance; strong dependence needs; and narcissism. An invalid test profile and elevations of all clinical scales on the Minnesota Multiphasic Personality Inventory-2 (MMPI-2) indicate an attempt to appear more disturbed than is the case ("fake bad").

There are no specific laboratory tests for factitious disorders. However, certain tests (e.g., drug screening) may help confirm or rule out specific mental or medical disorders.

DIFFERENTIAL DIAGNOSIS

Any disorder in which physical signs and symptoms are prominent should be considered in the differential diagnosis, and the possibility of authentic or concomitant physical illness must always be explored. Additionally, a history of many surgeries in factious disorder patients may predispose patients to complica-

tions or actual diseases, necessitating even further surgery. Factitious disorder is on a continuum between somatoform disorders and malingering, the goal being to assume the sick role. On one hand it is unconscious and nonvolitional (somatoform) and on the other hand it is conscious and willful (malingering).

Somatoform Disorders

A factitious disorder is differentiated from somatization disorder (Briquet's syndrome) by the voluntary production of factitious symptoms, the extreme course of multiple hospitalizations, and the seeming willingness of patients with a factitious disorder to undergo an extraordinary number of mutilating procedures. Patients with conversion disorder are not usually conversant with medical terminology and hospital routines, and their symptoms have a direct temporal relation or symbolic reference to specific emotional conflicts.

Hypochondriasis differs from factitious disorder in that the hypochondriacal patient does not voluntarily initiate the production of symptoms, and hypochondriasis typically has a later age of onset. As with somatization disorder, patients with hypochondriasis do not usually submit to potentially mutilating procedures. (Somatoform disorders are discussed in Chapter 17.)

Personality Disorders

Because of their pathological lying, lack of close relationships with others, hostile and manipulative manner, and associated substance abuse and criminal history, factitious disorder patients are often classified as having antisocial personality disorder. Antisocial persons, however, do not usually volunteer for invasive procedures or resort to a way of life marked by repeated or long-term hospitalization.

Because of attention seeking and an occasional flair for the dramatic, patients with factitious disorder may be classified as having histrionic personality disorder. But not all factitious disorder patients have a dramatic flair; many are withdrawn and bland.

Consideration of the patient's chaotic lifestyle, past history of disturbed interpersonal relationships, identity crisis, substance abuse, self-damaging acts, and manipulative tactics may lead to the diagnosis of borderline personality disorder. Persons with factitious disorder usually do not have the eccentricities of dress, thought, or communication that characterize schizotypal personality disorder patients. (Personality disorders are discussed in Chapter 27.)

Schizophrenia

The diagnosis of schizophrenia is often based on patients' admittedly bizarre lifestyles, but patients with factitious disorder do not usually meet the diagnostic criteria for schizophrenia unless they have the fixed delusion that they are actually ill and act on this belief by seeking hospitalization. Such a practice seems to be the exception; few patients with factitious disorder show evidence of a severe thought disorder or bizarre delusions.

Malingering

Factitious disorders must be distinguished from malingering. Malingerers have an obvious, recognizable environmental goal in producing signs and symptoms. They may seek hospitalization to secure financial compensation, evade the police, avoid work, or merely obtain free bed and board for the night, but they always have some apparent end for their behavior. Moreover, these patients can usually stop producing their signs and symptoms when they are no longer considered profitable or when the risk becomes too great. (Malingering is discussed in Chapter 32.)

Substance Abuse

Although patients with factitious disorders may have a complicating history of substance abuse, they should be considered not merely as substance abusers but as having coexisting diagnoses.

Ganser's Syndrome

Ganser's syndrome, a controversial condition most typically associated with prison inmates, is characterized by the use of approximate answers. Persons with the syndrome respond to simple questions with astonishingly incorrect answers. For example, when asked about the color of a blue car, the person answers "red" or answers "2 plus 2 equals 5." Ganser's syndrome may be a variant of malingering, in that the patients avoid punishment or responsibility for their actions. Ganser's syndrome is classified in DSM-IV-TR as a dissociative disorder not otherwise specified and in ICD-10 under other dissociative or conversion disorders. However, patients with factitious disorder with predominantly psychological signs and symptoms may intentionally give approximate answers. (See also page 689 for a further discussion.)

COURSE AND PROGNOSIS

Factitious disorders typically begin in early adulthood, although they may appear during childhood or adolescence. The onset of the disorder or of discrete episodes of seeking treatment may follow real illness, loss, rejection, or abandonment. Usually, the patient or a close relative had a hospitalization in childhood or early adolescence for a genuine physical illness. Thereafter, a long pattern of successive hospitalizations begins insidiously and evolves. As the disorder progresses, the patient becomes knowledgeable about medicine and hospitals. The onset of the disorder in patients who had early hospitalizations for actual illness is earlier than generally reported.

Factitious disorders are incapacitating to the patient and often produce severe trauma or untoward reactions related to treatment. A course of repeated or long-term hospitalization is obviously incompatible with meaningful vocational work and sustained interpersonal relationships. The prognosis in most cases is poor. A few patients occasionally spend time in jail, usually for minor crimes such as burglary, vagrancy, and disorderly conduct. Patients may also have a history of intermittent psychiatric hospitalization.

Although no adequate data are available about the ultimate outcome for the patients, a few of them probably die as a result of needless medication, instrumentation, or surgery. In view of the patients' often expert simulation and the risks that they take, some may die without the disorder being suspected. Possible features that indicate a favorable prognosis are (1) the presence of a

depressive-masochistic personality; (2) functioning at a borderline, not a continuously psychotic, level; and (3) the attributes of an antisocial personality disorder with minimal symptoms.

TREATMENT

No specific psychiatric therapy has been effective in treating factitious disorders. It is a clinical paradox that patients with the disorders simulate serious illness and seek and submit to unnecessary treatment while they deny to themselves and others their true illness and thus avoid possible treatment for it. Ultimately, the patients elude meaningful therapy by abruptly leaving the hospital or failing to keep follow-up appointments.

Treatment is thus best focused on management rather than on cure. Perhaps the single most important factor in successful management is a physician's early recognition of the disorder. In this way, physicians can forestall a multitude of painful and potentially dangerous diagnostic procedures for these patients. Good liaison between psychiatrists and the medical or surgical staff is strongly advised. Although a few cases of individual psychotherapy have been reported in the literature, there is no consensus about the best approach. In general, working in concert with the patient's primary care physician is more effective than working with the patient in isolation.

The personal reactions of physicians and staff members are of great significance in treating and establishing a working alliance with the patients, who invariably evoke feelings of futility, bewilderment, betrayal, hostility, and even contempt. In essence, staff members are forced to abandon a basic element of their relationship with patients—accepting the truthfulness of the patients' statements. One appropriate psychiatric intervention is to suggest to the staff ways of remaining aware that even though the patient's illness is factitious, the patient is ill.

Physicians should try not to feel resentment when patients humiliate their diagnostic prowess, and they should avoid any unmasking ceremony that sets up the patients as adversaries and precipitates their flight from the hospital. The staff should not perform unnecessary procedures or discharge patients abruptly, both of which are manifestations of anger.

Clinicians who find themselves involved with patients suffering from factitious disorders often become enraged at the patients for lying and deceiving them. Hence, therapists must be mindful of countertransference whenever they suspect factitious disorder. Often, the diagnosis is unclear because a definitive physical cause cannot be entirely ruled out. Although the use of confrontation is controversial, at some point in the treatment, patients must be made to face reality. Most patients simply leave treatment when their methods of gaining attention are identified and exposed. In some cases, clinicians should reframe the factitious disorder as a cry for help, so that patients do not view the clinicians' responses as punitive. A major role for psychiatrists working with factitious disorder patients is to help other staff members in the hospital deal with their own sense of outrage at having been duped. Education about the disorder and some attempt to understand the patient's motivations may help staff members maintain their professional conduct in the face of extreme frustration.

In cases of factitious disorder by proxy, legal intervention has been obtained in several instances, particularly with children. The senselessness of the disorder and the denial of false action by parents are obstacles to successful court action and often make conclusive proof unobtainable. In such cases, the child welfare services should be notified, and arrangements made for ongoing monitoring of the children's health.

Pharmacotherapy of factitious disorders is of limited use. Comorbid Axis I disorder (e.g., schizophrenia) will respond to antipsychotic medication, but in all cases medication should be administered carefully because of the potential for abuse. Selective serotonin reuptake inhibitors (SSRIs) may be useful in decreasing impulsive behavior when that is a major component in acting-out factitious behavior.

REFERENCES

Bauer M, Boegner F. Neurological syndromes in factitious disorder. *J Nerv Ment Dis*. 1996;184:28.

Feldman MD, Eisendrath SJ, eds. *The Spectrum of Factitious Disorders*. Washington, DC: American Psychiatric Press; 1996.

Feldman MD, Ford VF. Factitious disorders. In: Sadock BJ, Sadock VA, eds. *Kaplan & Sadock's Comprehensive Textbook of Psychiatry*. 7th ed. Vol 1. Baltimore: Lippincott Williams & Wilkins; 2000:1533.

Fliege H, Scholler G, Rose M, et al. Factitious disorders and pathological self-harm in a hospital population: an interdisciplinary challenge. *Gen Hosp Psychiatry*. 2002;24:164.

Folks DG. Munchausen's syndrome and other factitious disorders: malingering and conversion reactions. *Neurol Clin*. 1995;13(special issue):267.

French J. Pseudoseizures in the era of video-electroencephalogram monitoring. *Curr Opin Neurol*. 1995;8:117.

Hyler SE, Sussman N. Chronic factitious disorder with physical symptoms (the Munchausen syndrome). *Psychiatr Clin North Am*. 1981;4:365.

Iezzi T, Duckworth MP, Adams HE. Somatoform and factitious disorders. In: Stuker PB, Adams HE, eds. *Comprehensive Handbook of Psychopathology*. 3rd ed. New York: Kluwer Academic/Plenum Publishers; 2001:211.

Kinsella P. Factitious disorder: a cognitive behavioural perspective. *Behav Cogn Psychother*. 2001;29:195.

Ludviksson BR, Griffin J, Graziano FM. Münchausen's syndrome: the importance of a comprehensive medical history. *Wis Med J*. 1993;92:128.

Marmer S. Variations on a factitious theme. *J Psychiatry Law*. 1999;27:459.

Mountz JM, Parker PE, Liu HG, Bentley TW, Lill DW, Deutsch G. Tc-99m HMPAO brain SPECT scanning in Munchausen syndrome. *Psychiatry Neurosci*. 1996;21:49.

Phillips KA, ed. *Somatoform and Factitious Disorders. Review of Psychiatry*. Vol 20. No 3. Washington, DC: American Psychiatric Association; 2001.

Sanders MJ, Bursch B. Forensic assessment of illness falsification, Münchausen by proxy, and factitious disorder, NOS. *Child Maltreat*. 2002;7:112.

Siegel PT. Fischer H. Munchausen by proxy syndrome: barriers to detection, confirmation, and intervention. *Child Serv Soc Policy Res Pract*. 2001;41:31.

Songer DA. Factitious AIDS. A case reported and literature review. *Psychosomatics*. 1995;36:406.

20 Dissociative Disorders

Most persons see themselves as human beings with one basic personality; they experience a unitary sense of self. Persons with dissociative disorders, however, have lost the sense of having one consciousness. They feel as though they have no identity, they are confused about who they are, or they experience multiple identities. Everything that usually gives persons their unique personalities—their integrated thoughts, feelings, and actions—is abnormal in persons with dissociative disorders.

Dissociation arises as a self-defense against trauma. Dissociative defenses help persons remove themselves from trauma at the time that it occurs but also delay the working through needed to place the trauma in perspective within their lives. Unlike the phenomenon of repression, in which material is transferred to the dynamic unconscious, dissociation creates a situation in which mental contents coexist in parallel consciousness.

In most dissociative states, contradictory representations of the self, which conflict with each other, are kept in separate mental compartments. There are four types: (1) *dissociative amnesia* is characterized by an inability to remember information, usually related to a stressful or traumatic event, that cannot be explained by ordinary forgetfulness, the ingestion of substances, or a general medical condition; (2) *dissociative fugue* is characterized by sudden and unexpected travel away from home or work, associated with an inability to recall the past and with confusion about a person's personal identity or with adoption of a new identity; (3) *dissociative identity disorder* (also called *multiple personality disorder*), generally considered the most severe and chronic of the dissociative disorders, is characterized by the presence of two or more distinct personalities within a single person; and (4) *depersonalization disorder* is characterized by recurrent or persistent feelings of detachment from the body or mind. The text revision of the fourth edition of *Diagnostic and Statistical Manual of Mental Disorders* (DSM-IV-TR) includes the diagnostic category dissociative disorder not otherwise specified for dissociative disorders that do not meet the diagnostic criteria of the other dissociative disorders. DSM-IV-TR also includes in its appendix diagnostic guidelines for dissociative trance disorder, which is currently categorized as a dissociative disorder not otherwise specified. Mental contents coexist in parallel consciousness.

DISSOCIATIVE AMNESIA

The symptom amnesia is common to dissociative amnesia, dissociative fugue, and dissociative identity disorder. Dissociative amnesia is the appropriate diagnosis when the dissociative phenomena are limited to amnesia. Its key symptom is the inability to recall information, usually about stressful or traumatic events in persons' lives. This inability cannot be explained by ordinary forgetfulness, and there is no evidence of an underlying brain disorder. Persons retain the capacity to learn new information.

A common form of dissociative amnesia involves amnesia for personal identity but intact memory of general information. This clinical picture is exactly the reverse of the one seen in dementia, in which patients may remember their names but forget general information, such as what they had for lunch. Except for their amnesia, patients with dissociative amnesia seem completely intact and function coherently. By contrast, in most amnesias due to a general medical condition (such as postictal and toxic amnesias), patients may be confused and behave in a disorganized manner. Other types of amnesias (e.g., transient global amnesia and postconcussion amnesia) are associated with an ongoing anterograde amnesia, which does not occur in patients with dissociative amnesia.

Epidemiology

Amnesia is the most common dissociative symptom and occurs in almost all the dissociative disorders. Dissociative amnesia is thought to be the most common dissociative disorder, although epidemiological data for all the dissociative disorders are limited and uncertain. Dissociative amnesia is thought to occur more often in women than in men and more often in young adults than in older adults, but it can occur at any age. Since the disorder is usually associated with stressful and traumatic events, its incidence probably increases during times of war and natural disasters. Cases of dissociative amnesia related to domestic settings—for example, spousal abuse and child abuse—are probably constant in number. Most cases are seen in hospital emergency rooms, where amnesia patients are brought after being found on the street.

Etiology

The neuroanatomical, neurophysiological, and neurochemical processes of memory storage and retrieval are much better understood today than previously. The differentiation between short-term and long-term memory, the central role of the hippocampus, and the involvement of neurotransmitter systems have been clarified. The newly appreciated complexity of the formation and retrieval of memories may make dissociative amnesia intuitively understandable because of the many potential areas for dysfunction. Most patients with dissociative amnesia cannot retrieve painful memories of stressful and traumatic events, and thus the

emotional content of the memory is clearly related to the pathophysiology and the cause of the disorder.

One relevant observation about persons in general is that learning is often state dependent (i.e., dependent on the context in which it occurs). Information learned or experienced during a particular behavior (e.g., while driving a car), a pharmacological state (e.g., while drinking alcohol), a neurochemical state (e.g., associated with an emotion such as happiness), or in a particular physical setting (e.g., a garden) is often recalled only, or more easily, while reexperiencing the original state. Thus, persons can remember where a light switch is located in their car more easily while they are driving than when they are watching television. The theory of state-dependent learning applies to dissociative amnesia in that the memory of a traumatic event is laid down during the event, and the emotional state may be so extraordinary that it is hard for an affected person to remember information learned during that state.

In the psychoanalytic approach to dissociative amnesia, the disorder is considered primarily a defense mechanism whereby a person alters consciousness as a way of dealing with an emotional conflict or an external stressor. Secondary defenses involved in dissociative amnesia include repression (disturbing impulses are blocked from consciousness) and denial (an aspect of external reality is ignored by the conscious mind).

Table 20–1
DSM-IV-TR Diagnostic Criteria for Dissociative Amnesia

A. The predominant disturbance is one or more episodes of inability to recall important personal information, usually of a traumatic or stressful nature, that is too extensive to be explained by ordinary forgetfulness.

B. The disturbance does not occur exclusively during the course of dissociative identity disorder, dissociative fugue, posttraumatic stress disorder, acute stress disorder, or somatization disorder and is not due to the direct physiological effects of a substance (e.g., a drug of abuse, a medication) or a neurological or other general medical condition (e.g., amnestic disorder due to head trauma).

C. The symptoms cause clinically significant distress or impairment in social, occupational, or other important areas of functioning.

From American Psychiatric Association. *Diagnostic and Statistical Manual of Mental Disorders.* 4th ed. Text rev. Washington, DC: American Psychiatric Association; copyright 2000, with permission.

Diagnosis

The diagnostic criteria for dissociative amnesia in DSM-IV-TR (Table 20–1) emphasize that the forgotten information is usually of a traumatic or stressful nature. Dissociative amnesia can be diagnosed only when the symptoms are not limited to amnesia that occurs in the course of dissociative identity disorder and do not result from a general medical condition (e.g., head trauma) or ingestion of a substance.

Clinical Features

Although rare episodes of dissociative amnesia occur spontaneously, the history usually reveals a precipitating emotional trauma charged with painful emotions and psychological conflict—for example, a natural disaster in which persons witnessed severe injuries or feared for their lives. A fantasized or actual expression of an impulse (sexual or aggressive) with which a person cannot deal may also serve as a precipitant, and amnesia may follow behavior that a person later finds morally reprehensible, for example, violence or an extramarital affair.

Although not necessary for diagnosis, the onset of amnesia is often abrupt, and patients are usually aware that they have lost their memories. Some patients are upset by the memory loss, but others appear to be unconcerned or indifferent. When patients are not aware of their memory loss but a clinician suspects that they have dissociative amnesia, it is often useful to ask specific questions that may reveal the symptoms (Table 20–2). Amnestic patients are usually alert before and after the amnesia occurs. A few patients, however, report a slight clouding of consciousness during the period immediately surrounding the onset of amnesia. Depression and anxiety are common predisposing factors and frequently appear in a patient's mental status examination. Amnesia may provide a primary or a secondary gain. A woman who is amnestic about the birth of a dead infant achieves a primary gain by protecting herself from painful emotions. A soldier who has a sudden case of amnesia and is removed from combat as a result exemplifies a secondary gain.

Dissociative amnesia may take one of several forms: Localized amnesia, the most common type, is the loss of memory for the events of a short time (a few hours to a few days); generalized amnesia is the loss of memory for a whole lifetime of experience; selective (also known as systematized) amnesia is the failure to recall some but not all events that occurred during a short time.

Confabulation and Self-Monitoring. Because amnesia can have a disastrous effect on a patient's day-to-day life, many persons with chronic amnesia develop adaptive strategies. One such strategy is *confabulation,* the invention of false information to cover up a gap in memory. Other patients will resort to various forms of self-monitoring to protect themselves from memory loss, such as taking notes or ceasing regular activities.

Differential Diagnosis

The differential diagnosis of dissociative amnesia involves a consideration of both general medical conditions and other mental disorders (Table 20–3). Clinicians should conduct a medical history, a physical examination, a laboratory workup, a psychiatric history, and a mental status examination.

Amnesia associated with dementia and delirium is usually associated with many other easily recognized cognitive symptoms. When a patient has amnesia about personal information in these conditions, the dementia or delirium is usually advanced and easily differentiated from dissociative amnesia. Especially in a case of delirium, the patient may exhibit confabulation during the interview. In general a prompt return of memory usually indicates dissociative amnesia rather than amnestic disorder. Epilepsy can lead to sudden memory impairment associated with motor and electroencephalographic (EEG) abnormalities. Patients with epilepsy are prone to seizures during periods of stress, and some researchers have

Table 20–2
Questions to Reveal Dissociative Amnesia

If the answers to the mental status questions (below) are positive, the patient should be asked to describe in detail his or her experience of the symptom, including its relation to the use of psychoactive substances.

Blackouts or time loss
  Mental status questions: "Do you lose time?" "Do you have blackouts?"

Reports by others of disremembered behavior
  Mental status questions: "Are you told of things you say and do for which you have no memory? Out of character behavior? Childlike behavior?"

Appearance of unexplained possessions
  Mental status questions: "Do you find things in your possession that you cannot explain? For example, clothes, tools, weapons, artwork, writing, items in your shopping basket, receipts?"

Perplexing changes in relationships
  Mental status questions: "Do you find that your relationships with people seem influenced by factors that you cannot recall? For example, do you find that people are angry with you or act closer to you apparently based on events for which you have no memory?

Fuguelike episodes
  Mental status questions: "Do you find yourself in places with no idea how you got there? Do you set out to go somewhere but find yourself somewhere else without knowing how you got there? What is the longest period of time you have lost during such an experience?"

Evidence of unusual fluctuations in abilities, habits, tastes, knowledge
  Mental status questions: "Does your ability to do things—such as athletics, artistic endeavors, mechanical tasks, work tasks, and intellectual tasks—fluctuate markedly in ways you cannot explain? Are you told that you do things you didn't know you could do?"

Fragmentary recall of the life history
  Mental status questions: "Are you aware of gaps in your memory for your life? Are you missing memories for important events in your life, like a wedding or a graduation? For your childhood? For events in wartime? For other important aspects of your adult life?"

Chronic mistaken identity experiences
  Mental status questions: "Do you find that you are approached by people whom you don't know, who insist they know you? Who say they have met you before? Who say they have done things with you? Who even call you by another name?"

Brief (micro) amnesias during personal interactions
  Mental status questions: "Do you find that you do not remember all or part of your interactions or conversations with people? Like this interview? Do you or will you remember all or part of our conversation today?"

Reprinted with permission from Lowenstein RJ. Psychogenic amnesia and psychogenic fugue: a comprehensive review. In: Tasman A, Goldfinger SM, eds. *American Psychiatric Association Review of Psychiatry.* Vol 10. Washington, DC: American Psychiatric Press; 1991:189.

hypothesized that an epilepticlike cause may be involved in the dissociative disorders. A history of an aura, head trauma, or incontinence can help clinicians recognize amnesia related to epilepsy.

Transient Global Amnesia. Transient global amnesia is an acute and transient retrograde amnesia that affects recent, more than remote, memories. Although patients are usually aware of the amnesia, they may still perform highly complex mental and physical acts during the 6 to 24 hours that transient global amnesia episodes usually last. Recovery from the disorder is usually complete. Transient global amnesia is most often caused by transient ischemic attacks (TIAs) that affect limbic midline brain structures. It can also be associated with migraine headaches, seizures, and intoxication with sedative-hypnotic drugs.

Transient global amnesia can be differentiated from dissociative amnesia in several ways. Transient global amnesia is associated with anterograde amnesia during the episode; dissociative amnesia is not. Patients with transient global amnesia tend to be more upset and concerned about the symptoms than are patients with dissociative amnesia. The personal identity of a patient with dissociative amnesia is lost; that of a patient with transient global amnesia is retained. The memory loss of a patient with dissociative amnesia may be selective for certain areas and usually does not show a temporal gradient; the memory loss of a patient with transient global amnesia is generalized, and remote events are remembered better than recent events. Because of the association of transient global amnesia with vascular problems, the disorder is most common in patients in their 60s and 70s, whereas dissociative amnesia is most common in patients in their 20s to 40s, a period associated with the common psychological stressors seen in these patients. Other vasospastic events in the temporal lobe or thalamus have been reported in which transient amnestic attacks occur, even in young adults.

Table 20–3
Differential Diagnostic Considerations in Dissociative Amnesia

Dementia
Delirium
Anoxic amnesia
Cerebral infections (e.g., herpes simplex affecting temporal lobes)
Cerebral neoplasms (especially limbic and frontal)
Substance-induced (e.g., ethanol, sedative hypnotics, anticholinergics, steroids, lithium carbonate, β-adrenergic receptor antagonists, pentazocine, phencyclidine, hypoglycemic agents, marijuana, hallucinogens, methyldopa)
Electroconvulsive therapy (or other strong electric shock)
Epilepsy
Metabolic disorders (e.g., uremia, hypoglycemia, hypertensive encephalopathy, porphyria)
Postconcussion (posttraumatic) amnesia
Sleep-related amnesia (e.g., sleepwalking disorder)
Transient global amnesia
Wernicke-Korsakoff syndrome
Postoperative amnesia
Other dissociative disorders
Posttraumatic stress disorder
Acute stress disorder
Somatoform disorders (somatization disorder, conversion disorder)
Malingering (especially when associated with criminal activity)

Other Mental Disorders. Two other dissociative disorders, dissociative fugue and dissociative identity disorder, should be considered in the differential diagnosis. These disorders are distinguished on the basis of their additional symptoms.

In DSM-IV-TR, sleepwalking disorder is classified as a parasomnia, a type of sleep disorder. Patients suffering from sleepwalking disorder behave in a strange manner that resem-

bles the behavior of someone in a dissociative state. They exhibit an altered state of conscious awareness of their surroundings; they often have vivid hallucinatory recollections of an emotionally traumatic event in the past of which there is no memory during the usual waking state. Such patients are out of contact with the environment, appear preoccupied with a private world, and stare into space if their eyes are open. They may appear emotionally upset, speak excitedly in words and sentences that are frequently hard to understand, or engage in a pattern of seemingly meaningful activities repeated every time an episode occurs. The patient has amnesia for the sleepwalking episode once it has ended.

Although amnesia for a period of immediate past experience is found in patients with sleepwalking disorder and with localized and general amnesia, the state of consciousness during the period for which they are amnestic differs in character. Patients with sleepwalking disorder seem out of touch with the environment and appear to be dreaming. Patients with amnesia, by contrast, usually give no indication to observers that anything is amiss and seem entirely alert both before and after the amnesia occurs.

Posttraumatic stress disorder, acute stress disorder, and the somatoform disorders (especially somatization disorder and conversion disorder) should be considered in the differential diagnosis and may coexist with dissociative amnesia. The somatoform disorders may be associated with the same traumatic events that are usually seen in dissociative amnesia. Malingering, in this case a deliberate attempt to mimic amnesia, may be difficult to confirm. Any possible secondary gain, especially in regard to escaping punishment for criminal activity, should increase a clinician's suspicion, although such secondary gain does not rule out the diagnosis of dissociative amnesia.

Course and Prognosis

The symptoms of dissociative amnesia usually terminate abruptly, and recovery is generally complete, with few recurrences. In some patients, especially if there is secondary gain, the condition may last a long time. Clinicians should try to restore patients' lost memories to consciousness as soon as possible; otherwise, the repressed memory may form a nucleus in the unconscious mind around which future amnestic episodes may develop.

Treatment

Interviewing may give clinicians clues to the psychologically traumatic precipitant. Drug-assisted interviews with short-acting barbiturates, such as thiopental (Pentothal) and sodium amobarbital (Amytal), given intravenously and benzodiazepines may help patients recover their forgotten memories. Hypnosis can be used primarily as a means of relaxing patients enough for them to recall what has been forgotten. When a patient is placed in a somnolent state, mental inhibitions are diminished, and the amnestic material emerges into consciousness and is then recalled. Once the lost memories have been retrieved, psychotherapy is generally recommended to help patients incorporate the memories into their conscious states.

DISSOCIATIVE FUGUE

The behavior of patients with dissociative fugue is unusual and dramatic. The term *fugue* is used to reflect the fact that patients physically travel away from their customary homes or work situations and fail to remember important aspects of their previous identities (name, family, occupation). Such patients often, but not always, take on an entirely new identity and occupation, although the new identity is usually less complete than the alternate personalities in dissociative identity disorder, and the old and new identities do not alternate, as they do in dissociative identity disorder.

Epidemiology

Dissociative fugue is rare and, like dissociative amnesia, occurs most often during wartime, after natural disasters, and as a result of personal crises with intense internal conflicts. According to DSM-IV-TR there is a prevalence rate of 0.2 percent in the general population.

Etiology

Although heavy alcohol abuse may predispose persons to dissociative fugue, the cause of the disorder is thought to be basically psychological. The essential motivating factor seems to be a desire to withdraw from emotionally painful experiences. Patients with mood disorders and certain personality disorders (e.g., borderline, histrionic, and schizoid personality disorders) are predisposed to develop dissociative fugue.

A variety of stressors and personal factors predispose a person to the development of dissociative fugue. The psychosocial factors include marital, financial, occupational, and war-related stressors. Other associated predisposing features include depression, suicide attempts, organic disorders (especially epilepsy), and a history of substance abuse. A history of head trauma also predisposes a person to dissociative fugue.

Diagnosis and Clinical Features

DSM-IV-TR requires that a person either be confused about his or her identity or assume a new identity (Table 20–4).

Table 20–4
DSM-IV-TR Diagnostic Criteria for Dissociative Fugue

A. The predominant disturbance is sudden, unexpected travel away from home or one's customary place of work, with inability to recall one's past.
B. Confusion about personal identity or assumption of a new identity (partial or complete).
C. The disturbance does not occur exclusively during the course of dissociative identity disorder and is not due to the direct physiological effects of a substance (e.g., a drug of abuse, a medication) or a general medical condition (e.g., temporal lobe epilepsy).
D. The symptoms cause clinically significant distress or impairment in social, occupational, or other important areas of functioning.

From American Psychiatric Association. *Diagnostic and Statistical Manual of Mental Disorders.* 4th ed. Text rev. Washington, DC: American Psychiatric Association; copyright 2000, with permission.

Unlike dissociative amnesia, the diagnosis of dissociative fugue requires that the onset of the symptoms be sudden. The diagnosis is excluded if the symptoms occur only during the course of dissociative identity disorder or result from substance ingestion or a general medical condition (e.g., temporal lobe epilepsy).

Dissociative fugue has several typical features. Patients wander in a purposeful way, usually far from home and often for days at a time. During this period, they have complete amnesia for their past lives and associations, but unlike patients with dissociative amnesia, they are generally unaware that they have forgotten anything. Only when they suddenly return to their former selves do they recall the time antedating the onset of fugue, but then they remain amnestic for the period of the fugue itself. Patients with dissociative fugue do not seem to others to be behaving in extraordinary ways, nor do they give evidence of acting out any specific memory of a traumatic event. On the contrary, these patients lead quiet, prosaic, reclusive existences; work at simple occupations; live modestly; and, in general, do nothing to draw attention to themselves.

The patient was a 45-year-old man, an attorney, who was in the midst of bankruptcy proceedings and a deteriorating marriage. One day he suddenly disappeared from his office, much to the consternation of his law partners. Fearing foul play, his wife notified the police and an investigation was begun in an attempt to trace his whereabouts. A day later his car was found abandoned and out of gas at an interstate highway rest stop. Nothing was heard from the gentleman for almost a month, when he presented himself to a large inner city hospital emergency room several states away from his home. He remained amnesic for his identity and was admitted to the psychiatric unit. His picture and accompanying story were picked up by the wire services, and his wife recognized him on television. She was eventually summoned to the hospital where her husband was staying and in a collateral interview provided a full history of her husband to the attending psychiatrist. The patient was confronted with this information but remained amnesic until hypnosis was used to return him to his original personality state. Upon resuming this state, he was transported home and was hospitalized locally by his family physician. He continued to be amnesic for his fugue state. In consultation with a neurologist, a full physical and neurological examination was performed, which yielded normal results. An EEG and magnetic resonance imaging showed nothing abnormal. He was then referred to a psychologist who began psychodynamic psychotherapy. The precipitants, including the patient's failing marriage and poor financial status, were explored, and marital therapy was begun as an adjunct. Eventually his memory was restored. However, his financial problems remained unresolved, and he left on a shorter 5-day fugue but found his own way home. His treatment continued as the problems in his professional life, including gambling and misappropriation of funds from his legal clients, were explored. (Courtesy of Philip M. Coons, M.D.)

Differential Diagnosis

The differential diagnosis for dissociative fugue is similar to that for dissociative amnesia (Table 20–3). The wandering that is seen in dementia or delirium is usually distinguished from the traveling of a patient with dissociative fugue by the aimlessness of the former and the absence of complex and socially adaptive behaviors. Complex partial epilepsy may be associated with episodes of travel, but the patient does not usually assume a new identity, and the episodes are generally not precipitated by psychological stress. In dissociative amnesia, a loss of memory results from psychological stress, but without any episodes of purposeful travel or a new identity. Malingering may be difficult to distinguish from dissociative fugue; any evidence of a clear secondary gain should raise the clinician's suspicion.

Organic fugue states may be caused by a wide variety of medications including hallucinogenic drugs, steroids, barbiturates, phenothiazines, triazolam (Halcion), and L-asparaginase. An alcoholic blackout can be easily confused with dissociative fugue but can be easily differentiated through a good clinical history and alcohol concentrations in blood drawn during acute intoxication. The clinician should remember, however, that dissociative fugue and alcoholic blackouts can coexist in the same individual. There are reports of triazolam and alcohol together producing episodes of anterograde amnesia.

Course and Prognosis

The fugue is usually brief—hours to days. Less commonly, a fugue lasts many months and involves extensive travel covering thousands of miles. Generally, recovery is spontaneous and rapid. Recurrences are possible.

Treatment

Treatment of dissociative fugue is similar to that of dissociative amnesia. Psychiatric interviewing, drug-assisted interviewing, and hypnosis may help reveal to therapists and patients the psychological stressors that precipitated the fugue episode. Psychotherapy is indicated to help patients incorporate the precipitating stressors into their psyches in a healthy and integrated manner. The treatment of choice for dissociative fugue is expressive-supportive psychodynamic psychotherapy. The most widely accepted technique requires a mixture of abreaction of the past trauma and integration of the trauma into a cohesive self that no longer requires fragmentation to deal with the trauma.

DISSOCIATIVE IDENTITY DISORDER

Dissociative identity disorder is the name that DSM-IV-TR uses for what has been commonly known as multiple personality disorder. Dissociative identity disorder is a chronic dissociative disorder, and its cause typically involves a traumatic event, usually childhood physical or sexual abuse. The concept of personality conveys the sense of an integration of the way persons think, feel, and behave and the appreciation of themselves as a unitary being. Persons with dissociative identity disorder have two or more distinct personalities, each of which determines behavior and attitudes during any period in which it is dominant. Dissociative identity disorder is usually considered the

most serious of the dissociative disorders, although some clinicians who diagnose a variety of patients with the disorder have suggested that there may be a wider range of severity than was previously appreciated.

History

Until about 1800, patients with dissociative identity disorder were mainly considered to be suffering from various states of possession. In the early 1800s, Benjamin Rush, building on earlier clinical reports, provided a clinical description of the phenomenology of dissociative identity disorder. Subsequently, both Jean-Martin Charcot and Pierre Janet described the symptoms of the disorder and recognized the disease's dissociative nature. Both Sigmund Freud and Eugen Bleuler recognized the symptoms, although Freud attributed psychodynamic mechanisms to the symptoms and Bleuler thought that the symptoms reflected schizophrenia. Perhaps because of an increased appreciation of the problem of sexual and physical abuse of children and perhaps because of the cases described in the popular media (*The Three Faces of Eve, Sybil*), awareness of dissociative identity disorder increased. In 1980, with the inclusion of multiple personality disorder in the third edition of DSM (DSM-III), the stage was set for developing solid clinical research on the disorder.

Epidemiology

Anecdotal and research reports about dissociative identity disorder have varied in their estimates of the prevalence of the disorder. At one extreme, some investigators believe that dissociative identity disorder is extremely rare; at the other extreme, some believe that dissociative identity disorder is vastly underrecognized. Well-controlled studies have reported that 0.5 to 3 percent of general psychiatric hospital admissions meet the diagnostic criteria for dissociative identity disorder, as do perhaps as many as 5 percent of all psychiatric disorders. Patients who receive the diagnosis of dissociative identity disorder are overwhelmingly women—5:1 to 9:1 female-to-male ratios. Many clinicians and researchers, however, believe that men are underreported in clinical samples because, they believe, most men with the disorder enter the criminal justice system rather than the mental health system.

The disorder is most common in late adolescence and young adult life, with a mean age at diagnosis of 30 years, although patients have usually had symptoms for 5 to 10 years before the diagnosis. Several studies have found that the disorder is more common in first-degree biological relatives of persons with the disorder than in the general population.

Dissociative identity disorder frequently coexists with other mental disorders, including anxiety disorders, mood disorders, somatoform disorders, sexual dysfunctions, substance-related disorders, eating disorders, sleeping disorders, and posttraumatic stress disorder. The symptoms of dissociative identity disorder are similar to those seen in borderline personality disorder, and differentiating the two disorders can be difficult. Suicide attempts are common in patients with dissociative identity disorder; some studies have reported that as many as two thirds of all patients with dissociative identity disorder attempt suicide during the course of their illness.

Etiology

The cause of dissociative identity disorder is unknown, although the histories of the patients invariably (approaching 100 percent) involve a traumatic event, most often in childhood. In general, four types of causative factors have been identified: a traumatic life event, a vulnerability for the disorder to develop, environmental factors, and the absence of external support. The traumatic event is usually childhood physical or sexual abuse, commonly incestuous. Other traumatic events can include the death of a close relative or friend during childhood and witnessing a trauma or a death.

The tendency for the disorder to develop may be biologically or psychologically based. The variable ability of persons to be hypnotized may be one example of a risk factor for the development of dissociative identity disorder. Epilepsy has been hypothesized to be involved in the cause of dissociative identity disorder, and some studies of affected patients have reported a high percentage of abnormal EEG activity. One study of regional cerebral blood flow revealed temporal hyperperfusion in one of the subpersonalities but not in the main personality. Although several studies have found differences in pain sensitivity and other physiological measures among the personalities, the use of these data to prove the existence of dissociative identity disorder should be approached with great caution.

The environmental factors involved in the pathogenesis of dissociative identity disorder are nonspecific and are likely to include such factors as role models and the availability of other mechanisms for dealing with stress. In many cases, the development of dissociative identity seems to have involved the absence of support from significant others, such as parents, siblings, other relatives, and nonrelated persons, such as teachers.

Diagnosis and Clinical Features

In DSM-IV-TR, the name *dissociative identity disorder* replaces the earlier *multiple personality disorder*. As a diagnostic criterion (Table 20–5), DSM-IV-TR requires an amnestic component, which research has found to be essential to the complete clinical picture. The diagnosis also requires the presence of at least two distinct personality states. A diagnosis of dissociative personality disorder is excluded if the symptoms

Table 20–5
DSM-IV-TR Diagnostic Criteria for Dissociative Identity Disorder

A. The presence of two or more distinct identities or personality states (each with its own relatively enduring pattern of perceiving, relating to, and thinking about the environment and self).

B. At least two of these identities or personality states recurrently take control of the person's behavior.

C. Inability to recall important personal information that is too extensive to be explained by ordinary forgetfulness.

D. The disturbance is not due to the direct physiological effects of a substance (e.g., blackouts or chaotic behavior during alcohol intoxication) or a general medical condition (e.g., complex partial seizures). **Note:** In children, the symptoms are not attributable to imaginary playmates or other fantasy play.

From American Psychiatric Association. *Diagnostic and Statistical Manual of Mental Disorders*. 4th ed. Text rev. Washington, DC: American Psychiatric Association; copyright 2000, with permission.

Table 20–6
Signs of Multiplicity

1. Reports of time distortions, lapses, and discontinuities
2. Being told of behavioral episodes by others that are not remembered by the patient
3. Being recognized by others or called by another name by people whom the patient does not recognize
4. Notable changes in the patient's behavior reported by a reliable observer; the patient may call himself or herself by a different name or refer to himself or herself in the third person
5. Other personalities are elicited under hypnosis or during amobarbital interviews
6. Use of the word "we" in the course of an interview
7. Discovery of writings, drawings, or other productions or objects (identification cards, clothing, etc.) among the patient's personal belongings that are not recognized or cannot be accounted for
8. Headaches
9. Hearing voices originating from within and not identified as separate
10. History of severe emotional or physical trauma as a child (usually before the age of 5 years)

Reprinted with permission from Cummings JL. Dissociative states, depersonalization, multiple personality, episodic memory lapses. In: Cummings JL, ed. *Clinical Neuropsychiatry.* Orlando, FL: Grune & Stratton; 1985;122.

result from use of a substance (e.g., alcohol) or from a general medical condition (e.g., complex partial seizures).

Patients with dissociative identity disorder are often thought to have a personality disorder (commonly, borderline personality disorder), schizophrenia, or rapidly cycling bipolar disorder. Clinicians must be aware of the diagnostic category and must listen for specific suggestive features of dissociative identity disorder in the clinical interview (Table 20–6). The relative frequency of specific symptoms was reported in one study of 102 patients with dissociative identity disorder (Table 20–7). Despite stories in the popular press about patients with more than 20 personalities, the median number of personalities in dissociative identity disorder is in the range of 5 to 10. Often, only two or three of the personalities are evident at diagnosis; the others are recognized during the course of treatment. DSM-IV-TR reports an average of 8 identities for males and 15 for females, which may be somewhat high.

Table 20–7
Frequency of 16 Secondary Features of Dissociative Identity Disorder in 102 Patients

Item	Patients (*N*)
Another person existing inside	92
Voices talking	89
Voices coming from inside	84
Another person taking control	83
Amnesia for childhood	83
Referring to self as "we" or "us"	75
Person inside has a different name	72
Blank spells	69
Flashbacks	68
Being told by others of unremembered events	64
Feelings of unreality	58
Strangers know the patient	45
Noticing that objects are missing	43
Coming out of blank spell in a strange place	37
Objects are present that cannot be accounted for	32
Different handwriting styles	28

Reprinted with permission from Ross CA, Miller SD, Reagor P, Bjorns Fraser GA, Anderson G. Structured interview data from 102 cases of multiple personality disorder from four centers. *Am J Psychiatry.* 1990;14:596.

The transition from one personality to another is often sudden and dramatic. During each personality state, patients generally are amnestic about other states and the events that took place when another personality was dominant. Sometimes, however, one personality state is not bound by such amnesia and retains complete awareness of the existence, qualities, and activities of the other personalities. At other times, the personalities are aware of all or some of the others to varying degrees and may experience the others as friends, companions, or adversaries. In classic cases, each personality has a fully integrated, highly complex set of associated memories and characteristic attitudes, personal relationships, and behavior patterns. Most often, the personalities have proper names; occasionally, one or more is given the name of its function—for example, the protector. Although some clinicians have emphasized that one of the personalities tends to be dominant, this is not always the case. In fact, sometimes one personality masquerades as one of the others, but usually a host personality is the one who comes for treatment and carries the patient's legal name. This host personality is likely to be depressed or anxious, may have maso–chistic personality traits, and may seem overly moral.

The first appearance of the secondary personality or personalities may be spontaneous or may emerge in relation to what seems to be a precipitant (including hypnosis or a drug-assisted interview). The personalities may be of both sexes, of various races and ages, and from families different from the patient's family of origin. The most common subordinate personality is childlike. The personalities are often disparate and may even be opposites. In the same person, one of the personalities may be extroverted, even sexually promiscuous, and others may be introverted, withdrawn, and sexually inhibited.

On examination, patients frequently show nothing unusual in their mental status, other than a possible amnesia for periods of varying durations. Often, a clinician can detect the presence of multiple personalities only with prolonged interviews or many contacts with a patient with dissociative identity disorder. Sometimes, by having a patient keep a diary, the clinician finds the multiple personalities revealed in the diary entries. An estimated 60 percent of patients switch to alternate personalities only occasionally; another 20 percent of patients not only have rare episodes but also are adept at covering the switches.

Ms. A. is a 33-year-old married woman, employed as a librarian in a school for disturbed children. She presented to psychiatric attention after discovering her 5-year-old daughter "playing doctor" with several neighborhood children. Although this event was of little consequence, the patient

began to become fearful that her daughter would be molested. Ms. A. became panicked and increasingly obsessed with this idea, much to the bafflement of her husband. Ms. A. was seen by her internist and treated with antianxiety agents and antidepressants, but showed little improvement. She became increasingly anxious, phobic, depressed, and preoccupied. She sought psychiatric consultation from several clinicians, but repeated good trials of antidepressants, antianxiety agents, and supportive psychotherapy resulted in limited improvement. After the death of her father from complications of alcoholism, Ms. A. became more symptomatic. He had been estranged from the family since the patient was about 12 years old because of his drinking and associated antisocial behavior.

Ms. A. developed a variety of somatic complaints including headaches, abdominal pain, menstrual and gastrointestinal problems, back pain, and sleep difficulties. Repeated medical workup was unrevealing, leading to diagnoses such as fibromyalgia, irritable bowel syndrome, and premenstrual tension. Family and marital difficulties increased as the patient withdrew from her husband and was increasingly dysfunctional in taking care of her children; work function also deteriorated. Psychiatric hospitalization was precipitated by the patient's arrest for disorderly conduct in a nearby city. She was found in a hotel, dressed in revealing clothing, engaged in an altercation with a man. She denied knowledge of how she had come to this hotel, although the man insisted she had come there under a different name for a voluntary sexual encounter.

On psychiatric examination the patient described dense amnesia for the first 12 years of her life with the feeling that her "life started at 12 years old." She reported that for as long as she could remember she had had an imaginary companion, an elderly black woman, who advised her and kept her company. She reported hearing other voices in her head: several women and children, as well as her father's voice repeatedly speaking to her in a derogatory way. She reported that much of her life since age 12 was also punctuated by episodes of amnesia; for work, for her marriage, for the birth of her children, and for her sex life with her husband. She reported perplexing changes in skills; for example, she was often told she played the piano well, but had no conscious awareness that she could do so. Her husband reported that she had always been "forgetful" of conversations and family activities. He also noted that at times she would speak like a child, at times adopt a southern accent, and at other times be angry and provocative. She frequently had little recall of these episodes.

Questioned more closely about her early life, the patient appeared to enter a trance and stated: "I just don't want to be locked in the closet" in a childlike voice. Inquiry about this produced rapid shifts in state between alter identities who differed in manifest age, facial expression, voice tone, and knowledge of the patient's history. One identified itself by a diminutive of the patient's name and appeared childlike. Another spoke angrily, used expletives, and appeared irritable and preoccupied with sex. She discussed the episode with the man in the hotel and stated that it was she who had arranged it. A third alter personality identified itself as a protective entity, experiencing itself as an elderly African American woman who commented sadly and philosophically about "this whole situation." Gradually the alter identities described a history of family chaos, brutality, and neglect during the first 12 years of the patient's life, until her mother, also alcoholic, achieved sobriety and left her husband, taking her children with her. In the alter identities, the patient described episodes of physical abuse, sexual abuse, and emotional torment by her father, her siblings, and her mother.

Family sessions with the mother and siblings confirmed many of these reports, with the family recalling episodes of maltreatment that the patient did not recollect. The patient's mother had bid the family never to speak of the earlier difficulties, hoping that everyone would "just forget the whole thing." After additional assessment of family members, the patient's mother also met diagnostic criteria for dissociative identity disorder, as did her older sister, who also had been molested. A brother met diagnostic criteria for posttraumatic stress disorder, major depressive disorder, and alcohol dependence.

The patient improved significantly with psychotherapy directed at stabilization of her dissociative identity disorder and posttraumatic stress disorder. She responded well to clomipramine (Anafranil), with marked reduction in obsessive-compulsive and depressive symptoms. Family therapy was helpful in stabilizing the patient's marriage and helping her husband with the aftermath of the hospitalization and its precipitants. The husband also reported a family history of abuse, although primarily directed at his mother and siblings; he had always seen himself as the family protector. The patient's mother and siblings were already in treatment, but were helped by the opening up of the family history and clarification of their diagnoses. At 3-year follow-up the patient reported fusion of most alter identities and marked diminution of dissociative, somatoform, and posttraumatic stress disorder symptoms, but she still required clomipramine for stabilization of mood and for the symptoms of obsessive-compulsive disorder. (Courtesy of Frank W. Putnam, M.D., and Richard J. Loewenstein, M.D.)

Differential Diagnosis

The differential diagnosis includes two other dissociative disorders, dissociative amnesia and dissociative fugue. Both of those disorders, however, lack the shifts in identity and the awareness of the original identity that are seen in dissociative identity disorder. Psychotic disorders, notably schizophrenia, may be confused with dissociative identity disorder only because persons with schizophrenia may be delusional and believe that they have separate identities or report hearing other personalities' voices. In schizophrenia, a formal thought disorder, chronic social deterioration and other distinguishing signs are present. Recently, clinicians have increasingly appreciated rapidly cycling bipolar disorders, whose symptoms appear similar to those of dissociative identity disorder; interviewing, however, reveals the presence of *discrete* personalities in patients with dissociative identity disorder. Borderline personality disorder

may coexist with dissociative identity disorder, but the alteration of personalities in dissociative identity disorder may be mistakenly interpreted as nothing more than the irritability of mood and self-image problems characteristic of patients with borderline personality disorder. Malingering presents a difficult diagnostic problem. Clear secondary gain raises suspicion, and drug-assisted interviews may be helpful in making the diagnosis. Among the neurological disorders to consider, complex partial epilepsy is the most likely to imitate the symptoms of dissociative identity disorder (see Table 20–3).

Course and Prognosis

Dissociative identity disorder can develop in children as young as 3 years of age. In children, the symptoms may appear trancelike and may be accompanied by depressive disorder symptoms, amnestic periods, hallucinatory voices, disavowal of behaviors, changes in abilities, and suicidal or self-injurious behaviors. Although women are more likely to have the disorder than are men, affected children are more likely to be boys than girls; the female predominance develops only in adolescence. Two symptom patterns have been observed in affected female adolescents. One pattern is that of a chaotic life with promiscuity, drug use, somatic symptoms, and suicide attempts. Such patients may be misclassified as having an impulse control disorder, schizophrenia, rapidly cycling bipolar I disorder, or histrionic or borderline personality disorder. A second pattern is characterized by withdrawal and childlike behaviors. Sometimes, these patients are misclassified as having a mood disorder, a somatoform disorder, or generalized anxiety disorder. In male adolescents with dissociative identity disorder, the symptoms may cause them to have trouble with the law or school officials, and they may eventually end up in prison.

The earlier the onset of dissociative identity disorder, the worse the prognosis. One or more of the personalities may function relatively well while others function marginally. The level of impairment ranges from moderate to severe, the determining variables being the number, type, and chronicity of the various personalities. The disorder is considered the most severe and chronic of the dissociative disorders, and recovery is generally incomplete. In addition, individual personalities may have their own separate mental disorders; mood disorders, personality disorders, and other dissociative disorders are the most common.

Treatment

The most efficacious approaches to dissociative identity disorder involve insight-oriented psychotherapy, often in association with hypnotherapy or drug-assisted interviewing techniques. Hypnotherapy or drug-assisted interviewing can be useful in obtaining additional history, identifying previously unrecognized personalities, and fostering abreaction. A psychotherapeutic treatment plan should begin by confirming the diagnosis and by identifying and characterizing the various personalities. If any of the personalities is inclined toward self-destructive or otherwise violent behavior, the therapist should engage the patient and the appropriate personalities in treatment contracts about these dangerous behaviors. Hospitalization may be necessary in some cases.

Several clinicians and researchers have discussed psychotherapy with dissociative identity disorder patients. A summation of the basic principles (Table 20–8) and a description of the stages of therapy (Table 20–9) are useful guides in the difficult therapy for these patients. The initial therapy stage usually fosters communication between the personalities to begin reintegration and to help patients control their overall behavior. The

Table 20–8
Principles of Successful Therapy for Dissociative Identity Disorder

- Condition was created by broken boundaries. Therefore, a successful treatment has a secure treatment frame and firm, consistent boundaries.
- Condition is one of subjective dyscontrol and passively endured assaults and changes. Therefore, the focus must be on mastery and the patient's active participation in the treatment process.
- Condition is one of involuntariness. Its sufferers did not elect to be traumatized and find their symptoms are often beyond their control. Therefore, the therapy must be based on a strong therapeutic alliance, and efforts to establish that alliance must be undertaken throughout the process.
- Condition is one of buried traumata and sequestered affect. Therefore, what has been hidden away must be uncovered, and what feeling has been buried must be abreacted.
- Condition is one of perceived separateness and conflict among the alters. Therefore, the therapy must emphasize their collaboration, cooperation, empathy, and identification with one another so that their separateness becomes redundant and their conflicts are muted.
- Condition is one of hypnotic alternate realities. Therefore, the therapist's communication must be clear and straight. There is no room for confusing communication.
- Condition is related to the inconsistency of important others. Therefore, the therapist must be evenhanded with all the alters, avoiding playing favorites or dramatically altering his or her own behavior toward the various personalities. The therapist's consistency across all the alters is one of the most powerful assaults on the patient's dissociative defenses.
- Condition is one of shattered security, self-esteem, and future orientation. Therefore, the therapist must make efforts to restore morale and inculcate realistic hope.
- Condition stems from overwhelming experiences. Therefore, the pacing of the therapy is essential. Most treatment failures occur when the pace of the therapy outstrips the patient's capacity to tolerate the material under discussion. It is wise to adhere to the rule of thirds: if one cannot get into the difficult material one planned to address in the first third of the session, to work on it in the second, and process it and restabilize the patient in the third, not approaching the material, lest the patient leave the session in an overwhelmed state. Abreaction cannot be allowed to become retraumatization.
- Condition often results from the irresponsibility of others. Therefore, the therapist must be responsible and hold the patient to a high standard of responsibility once the therapist is confident that the patient, across alters, actually grasps what reasonable responsibility entails.
- Condition often results because people who could have protected a child did nothing. The therapist can anticipate that technical neutrality will be interpreted as uncaring and rejecting and is best served by taking a warm stance that allows for a latitude of affective expression.
- Patient has many cognitive errors. The therapy must address and correct them on an ongoing basis.

Adapted from Kluft RP. Multiple personality disorder. In: Tasman A, Goldfinger SM, eds. *American Psychiatric Association Review of Psychiatry.* Vol 10. Washington, DC: American Psychiatric Press; 1991:161.

Table 20–9
Stages of Therapy for Dissociative Identity Disorder

1. Establishing the psychotherapy involves the creation of an atmosphere of safety in which the diagnosis can be made, the security of the treatment frame can be assured, the patient begins to understand the concept of the treatment alliance in a preliminary way, the nature of the treatment is introduced to the patient, and sufficient hope and confidence are established so that the patient feels prepared to begin what may be a long and difficult process.
2. Preliminary interventions involve gaining access to the most readily reached personalities; establishing agreements or contracts with the alters against terminating treatment abruptly, self-harm, suicide, and as many other dysfunctional behaviors as the patient is able to agree to curtail; fostering communication and cooperation among the alters (a process that is the core of the treatment from here on); expanding the therapeutic alliance by gaining the patient's acceptance of the diagnosis across increasing numbers of the personalities (some deny it to the end); and offering what symptomatic relief is possible. Hypnosis may play a valuable role in facilitating those measures.
3. History gathering and mapping lead to learning more about the personalities, their origins, and their relationships with one another. The patient may be regarded as a system with its own rules of interaction. Here one learns the who, when, why, where, what, and how of the alters; their names (if any); age of onset and self-perceived age; the reasons for their creation and persistence; where they fit in the patient's overall history and in their relationships within the world of the personalities; and their particular problems, functions, and concerns. On that basis, one begins to work with their individual and interactional issues and presses for still more cooperation and collaboration.
4. Metabolism of the trauma refers to the often strenuous efforts needed to access and process the overwhelming events associated with the origins of the disorder. Such work should not be undertaken until one has some idea of the lay of the land in terms of the patient's system of personalities and at least some intellectual insight into what material is likely to be encountered. Negative therapeutic reactions are common. Precipitous or premature entry into this stage before stages 1 through 3 are achieved is a frequent cause of unnecessary crises and interruptions of therapy.
5. Moving toward integration-resolution involves the working through of recovered materials across the alters and facilitating still further cooperation, communication, and mutual awareness with enhanced mutual identification and empathy. Communication is increased, many internal conflicts become muted or resolved, and the alters begin to show some blurring of their once discrete characteristics. Some experience identity diffusion (e.g., "for a moment I wasn't sure who I was"; "I guess I am both Sally and Joanie").
6. Integration-resolution consists of the patient's coming to a new and more solid stance toward his or her self and the world. A smooth collaboration among the alters constitutes a resolution; their blending into a unity is an integration.
7. Learning new coping skills is important. The patient may have to face for the first time perspectives on his or her life that were not appreciable before and be helped to negotiate the circumstances that once were handled in a dissociative manner in constructive ways. Many important life decisions and relationships may require renegotiation.
8. Solidification of gains and working through may require as much therapy as reaching integration or resolution. The patient has to relearn how to live in the world. Often working through in the transference what has been learned about the past is valuable. Characterological issues that were inaccessible before or hidden behind a welter of symptoms must be addressed. Often extensive coaching on the management of relationships and intercurrent traumata is necessary.
9. Follow-up is advisable on several grounds. The stability of the outcome should be assessed, especially for those who opt for resolution rather than integration. Also, layers of personalities that had not entered the prior treatment may be encountered, and some apparent good results are flights into health.

Adapted from Kluft RP. Multiple personality disorder. In: Tasman A, Goldfinger SM, eds. *American Psychiatric Association Review of Psychiatry.* Vol 10. Washington, DC: American Psychiatric Press; 1991:161.

benefits of reintegration versus those of resolution continue to be disputed, and the relative benefits of each approach are unknown. Communication among the personalities also helps patients control their overall behavior. Clinicians must attempt to identify the personalities who remember the traumatic childhood events almost invariably associated with the disorder.

The use of antipsychotic medications is almost never indicated. Some data indicate that antidepressants and antianxiety medications may be useful as adjuvants to psychotherapy. A few uncontrolled studies report that anticonvulsant medications such as carbamazepine (Tegretol) help selected patients.

FORENSIC ISSUES

The intersection between the diagnosis dissociative identity disorder and the legal system has proved exceedingly controversial. The contentious dispute over its existence, the often-sensationalized media attention, and the need to rule out simulation or malingering have made the forensic evaluation of the disorder difficult to perform and to defend. Issues of competency to stand trial and degree of responsibility for the behavior of different alter personality states have received contradictory judicial opinions. The most common defenses are (1) dissociative defendants do not have control over, or are not conscious of, their alter personalities and therefore cannot be held responsible for their actions; (2) these defendants cannot recall the actions of their alter personalities and therefore cannot participate in their own defense; and (3) a diagnosis of dissociative identity disorder makes it impossible for a defendant to conform to the law or to know right from wrong. Evidentiary questions, such as the admissibility of hypnotic or amobarbital interviews and the independence of testimony by different alter personalities have proved problematic.

In general, most courts have not found dissociation sufficient grounds for a claim of legal incompetence. They have held the whole human being responsible for the behavior of any part.

DEPERSONALIZATION DISORDER

DSM-IV-TR characterizes depersonalization disorder as a persistent or recurrent alteration in the perception of the self to the extent that a person's sense of his or her own reality is temporarily lost. Patients with depersonalization disorder may feel that they are mechanical, in a dream, or detached from their bodies. The episodes are ego-dystonic, and the patients realize the unreality of the symptoms.

Some clinicians distinguish between depersonalization and derealization. *Depersonalization* is the feeling that the body or the personal self is strange and unreal; *derealization* is the per-

ception of objects in the external world as strange and unreal. The distinction provides a more accurate description of each phenomenon than is achieved by grouping them together under the rubric of depersonalization.

Epidemiology

As an occasional isolated experience in the lives of many persons, depersonalization is a common phenomenon and is not necessarily pathological. Studies indicate that transient depersonalization may occur in as many as 70 percent of a given population, with no significant difference between men and women. Children frequently experience depersonalization as they develop the capacity for self-awareness, and adults often undergo a temporary sense of unreality when they travel to new and strange places.

Information about the epidemiology of pathological depersonalization is scanty. In a few recent studies, depersonalization was found to occur in women at least twice as frequently as in men; it is rarely found in persons over 40 years of age. The mean age of onset is about 16 years.

Table 20–10
DSM-IV-TR Diagnostic Criteria for Depersonalization Disorder

A. Persistent or recurrent experiences of feeling detached from, and as if one is an outside observer of, one's mental processes or body (e.g., feeling like one is in a dream).
B. During the depersonalization experience, reality testing remains intact.
C. The depersonalization causes clinically significant distress or impairment in social, occupational, or other important areas of functioning.
D. The depersonalization experience does not occur exclusively during the course of another mental disorder, such as schizophrenia, panic disorder, acute stress disorder, or another dissociative disorder, and is not due to the direct physiological effects of a substance (e.g., a drug of abuse, a medication) or a general medical condition (e.g., temporal lobe epilepsy).

From American Psychiatric Association. *Diagnostic and Statistical Manual of Mental Disorders.* 4th ed. Text rev. Washington, DC: American Psychiatric Association; copyright 2000, with permission.

Etiology

Depersonalization may be caused by psychological, neurological, or systemic disease. Systemic causes include endocrine disorders of the thyroid and the pancreas. Experiences of depersonalization have been associated with epilepsy, brain tumors, sensory deprivation, and emotional trauma, and depersonalization phenomena have been caused by electrical stimulation of the cortex of the temporal lobes during neurosurgery. Depersonalization is associated with an array of substances, including alcohol, barbiturates, benzodiazepines, scopolamine, β-adrenergic receptor antagonists, marijuana, and virtually any phencyclidine (PCP)-like or hallucinogenic substance. Anxiety and depression are predisposing factors, as is severe stress experienced, for example, in combat or in an automobile accident. Depersonalization is a symptom frequently associated with anxiety disorders, depressive disorders, and schizophrenia.

Diagnosis and Clinical Features

The DSM-IV-TR diagnostic criteria for depersonalization disorder (Table 20–10) require persistent or recurrent episodes of depersonalization that result in significant distress to patients or in impairment of their ability to function in social, occupational, or interpersonal relationships. The disorder is largely differentiated from psychotic disorders by the diagnostic requirement that reality testing remain intact in depersonalization disorder. The disorder cannot be diagnosed if the symptoms are better accounted for by another mental disorder, substance ingestion, or a general medical condition.

The central characteristic of depersonalization is the quality of unreality and estrangement. Inner mental processes and external events seem to go on exactly as before, but they feel different and no longer seem to have any relation or significance to the person. Parts of the body or the entire physical being may seem foreign, as may mental operations and accustomed behavior. Particularly common is the sensation of a change in the patient's body; for instance, patients may feel that their extremities are bigger or smaller than usual. Hemidepersonalization, the patient's feeling that half of the body is unreal or does not exist, may be related to contralateral parietal lobe disease. Anxiety often accompanies the disorder, and many patients complain of distortion of their senses of time and space.

An occasional phenomenon is doubling; patients feel that the point of consciousness is outside their bodies, often a few feet overhead, and from there they observe themselves, as if they were totally separate persons. Sometimes, patients believe that they are in two places at the same time, a condition called *reduplicative paramnesia* or *double orientation.* Most patients are aware of their disturbed sense of reality; this awareness is considered one of the salient characteristics of the disorder.

Marlene Steinberg has reported the following examples from interviews with patients with this disorder.

FEELINGS OF UNREALITY

"It's really weird. It's sort of like I'm here, but I'm really not here and that I kind of stepped out of myself, like a ghost . . . I feel really light, you know. I feel kind of empty and light, like I'm going to float away . . . Sometimes I really look at myself that way . . . It's kind of a cold, eerie feeling. I'm just totally numbed by it."

BODILY PERCEPTIONS

"[I]t just doesn't seem real. Everything to me doesn't seem real, my body included . . . I was looking in the mirror and all of a sudden it just felt as if the image in the mirror was looking back out upon myself."

BEHAVIORAL PERCEPTIONS

"You just feel like you're never being yourself, uh, you're not thinking as you normally do. You just feel strange . . . I need to concentrate on things a lot more . . . I feel as if most

persons have their brain on automatic. I feel like I have to crank it, like I'm always working at it and always consciously trying to remember things, trying to concentrate . . . It's almost as if I can't visualize things in my mind the way you normally would, when you actually see things . . . I can't do that very well."

EXTERNAL PERCEPTIONS

"[Everything] just feels different, just like it's in a dream, in a daze, things are dulled . . . I remember when this first started and I was in college and I went home and the thing that kept going over in my mind was I want to go home, I want to go home and I was home, but that just kept coming into my mind . . . everything always seems unreal . . . other persons, myself, just everything."

Differential Diagnosis

Depersonalization may occur as a symptom in numerous other disorders (Table 20–11). The common occurrence of depersonalization in patients with depressive disorders and schizophrenia should alert clinicians to the possibility that a patient who initially complains of feelings of unreality and estrangement is suffering from one of these more common disorders. A history and the mental status examination usually should disclose the characteristic features of depressive disorders and schizophrenia. Because psychotomimetic drugs often induce long-lasting changes in the experience of the reality of the self and the environment, clinicians must inquire about the use of such substances. The presence of other clinical phenomena in patients complaining of a sense of unreality should usually take precedence in determining the diagnosis. In general, the diagnosis of depersonalization disorder is reserved for those conditions in which depersonalization constitutes the predominating symptom.

The fact that depersonalization phenomena may result from gross disturbances in brain function underlies the necessity for a neurological evaluation, especially when the depersonalization is not accompanied by common and obvious psychiatric symptoms. In particular, the possibility of a brain tumor or epilepsy should be considered. The experience of depersonalization may be the earliest presenting symptom of a neurological disorder.

Table 20–11
Causes of Depersonalization

- Neurological disorders
  - Epilepsy
  - Migraine
  - Brain tumors
  - Cerebrovascular disease
  - Cerebral trauma
  - Encephalitis
  - General paresis
  - Dementia of the Alzheimer's type
  - Huntington's disease
  - Spinocerebellar degeneration
- Toxic and metabolic disorders
  - Hypoglycemia
  - Hypoparathyroidism
  - Carbon monoxide poisoning
  - Mescaline intoxication
  - Botulism
  - Hyperventilation
  - Hypothyroidism
- Idiopathic mental disorders
  - Schizophrenia
  - Depressive disorders
  - Manic episodes
  - Conversion disorder
  - Anxiety disorders
  - Obsessive-compulsive disorder
  - Personality disorders
  - Phobic-anxiety depersonalization syndrome
- In normal persons
  - Exhaustion
  - Boredom; sensory deprivation
  - Emotional shock
- In hemidepersonalization
  - Lateralized (usually right parietal) focal brain lesion

Adapted from Cummings JL. Dissociative states, depersonalization, multiple personality, episodic memory lapses. In: Cummings JL, ed. *Clinical Neuropsychiatry.* Orlando, FL: Grune & Stratton; 1985:123.

Course and Prognosis

In most patients, the symptoms of depersonalization disorder first appear suddenly; only a few patients report a gradual onset. The disorder starts most often between the ages of 15 and 30 years, but it has been seen in patients as young as 10 years of age; it occurs less frequently after age 30 and almost never in the late decades of life. A few follow-up studies indicate that in more than 50 percent of cases, depersonalization tends to be a long-lasting condition. In many patients, the symptoms run a steady course without any significant fluctuation in intensity, or the symptoms may occur episodically, interspersed with symptom-free intervals. Little is known about precipitating factors, although the disorder has been observed to begin during a period of relaxation after a person has experienced fatiguing psychological stress. The disorder is sometimes ushered in by an attack of acute anxiety, frequently accompanied by hyperventilation.

Treatment

Little attention has been given to the treatment of patients with depersonalization disorder. At this time, too few data exist on which to base a specific pharmacological treatment, but the anxiety usually responds to antianxiety agents. An underlying disorder (e.g., schizophrenia) can also be treated pharmacologically. Psychotherapeutic approaches are equally untested. As with all patients with neurotic symptoms, the decision to use psychoanalysis or insight-oriented psychotherapy is determined not by the presence of the symptom itself but by a variety of positive indications derived from an assessment of the patient's personality, human relationships, and life situation.

DISSOCIATIVE DISORDER NOT OTHERWISE SPECIFIED

The diagnosis dissociative disorder not otherwise specified is applied to disorders with dissociative features that do not meet the diagnostic criteria for dissociative amnesia, dissociative fugue, dissociative identity disorder, or depersonalization disorder. The DSM-IV-TR examples of dissociative disorder not otherwise specified (Table 20–12) take into account changes in the diagnostic criteria for the other dissociative disorders. Specifically, example 1 describes patients who do not meet the diagnostic criteria for dissociative identity disorder because the second personality is not sufficiently distinct or because the patient has no amnestic period. According to DSM-IV-TR, derealization in the absence of depersonalization is an example of dissociative disorder not otherwise specified.

Table 20–12
DSM-IV-TR Diagnostic Criteria for Dissociative Disorder Not Otherwise Specified

This category is included for disorders in which the predominant feature is a dissociative symptom (i.e., a disruption in the usually integrated functions of consciousness, memory, identity, or perception of the environment) that does not meet the criteria for any specific dissociative disorder. Examples include

1. Clinical presentations similar to dissociative identity disorder that fail to meet full criteria for this disorder. Examples include presentations in which (a) there are not two or more distinct personality states, or (b) amnesia for important personal information does not occur.
2. Derealization unaccompanied by depersonalization in adults.
3. States of dissociation that occur in individuals who have been subjected to periods of prolonged and intense coercive persuasion (e.g., brainwashing, thought reform, or indoctrination while captive).
4. Dissociative trance disorder: single or episodic disturbances in the state of consciousness, identity, or memory that are indigenous to particular locations and cultures. Dissociative trance involves narrowing of awareness of immediate surroundings or stereotyped behaviors or movements that are experienced as being beyond one's control. Possession trance involves replacement of the customary sense of personal identity by a new identity, attributed to the influence of a spirit, power, deity, or other person, and associated with stereotyped "involuntary" movements or amnesia and is perhaps the most common dissociative disorder in Asia. Examples include *amok* (Indonesia), *bebainan* (Indonesia), *latah* (Malaysia), *pibloktoq* (Arctic), *ataque de nervios* (Latin America), and possession (India). The dissociative or trance disorder is not a normal part of a broadly accepted collective cultural or religious practice.
5. Loss of consciousness, stupor, or coma not attributable to a general medical condition.
6. Ganser syndrome: the giving of approximate answers to questions (e.g., "2 plus 2 equals 5") when not associated with dissociative amnesia or dissociative fugue.

From American Psychiatric Association. *Diagnostic and Statistical Manual of Mental Disorders.* 4th ed. Text rev. Washington, DC: American Psychiatric Association; copyright 2000, with permission.

Table 20–13
DSM-IV-TR Research Criteria for Dissociative Trance Disorder

A. Either (1) or (2):
   (1) trance, i.e., temporary marked alteration in the state of consciousness or loss of customary sense of personal identity without replacement by an alternate identity, associated with at least one of the following:
      (a) narrowing of awareness of immediate surroundings, or unusually narrow and selective focusing on environmental stimuli
      (b) stereotyped behaviors or movements that are experienced as being beyond one's control
   (2) possession trance, a single or episodic alteration in the state of consciousness characterized by the replacement of customary sense of personal identity by a new identity. This is attributed to the influence of a spirit, power, deity, or other person, as evidenced by one (or more) of the following:
      (a) stereotyped and culturally determined behaviors or movements that are experienced as being controlled by the possessing agent
      (b) full or partial amnesia for the event

B. The trance or possession trance state is not accepted as a normal part of a collective cultural or religious practice.

C. The trance or possession trance state causes clinically significant distress or impairment in social, occupational, or other important areas of functioning.

D. The trance or possession trance state does not occur exclusively during the course of a psychotic disorder (including mood disorder with psychotic features and brief psychotic disorder) or dissociative identity disorder and is not due to the direct physiological effects of a substance or a general medical condition.

From American Psychiatric Association. *Diagnostic and Statistical Manual of Mental Disorders.* 4th ed. Text rev. Washington, DC: American Psychiatric Association; copyright 2000, with permission.

Dissociative Trance Disorder

DSM-IV-TR adds, as an example of dissociative disorder not otherwise specified, patients with single or episodic alterations in consciousness that are limited to particular locations or cultures. The example states that the "dissociative or trance disorder is not a normal part of a broadly accepted collective cultural or religious practice." DSM-IV-TR includes in its appendixes a suggested set of diagnostic criteria for dissociative trance disorder (Table 20–13). The disorder is similar to the diagnosis of trance and possession disorder in the 10th revision of the *International Statistical Classification of Diseases and Related Health Problems* (ICD-10). The DSM-IV diagnostic criteria require that the symptoms cause a patient significant distress or an impairment in the ability to function.

Trance states are altered states of consciousness, and patients exhibit diminished responsivity to environmental stimuli. Children may have repeated amnestic periods or trancelike states after physical abuse or trauma. Possession and trance states are curious and imperfectly understood forms of dissociation. Apparently, trance states commonly appear in mediums who preside over seances. Mediums typically enter a dissociative state, during which a person from the so-called spirit world takes over much of the mediums' conscious awareness and influences their thoughts and speech.

Automatic writing and crystal gazing are less common manifestations of possession or trance states. In automatic writing, the dissociation affects only the arm and the hand that write the message, which often discloses mental contents of which the writer was unaware. Crystal gazing results in a trance state in which visual hallucinations are prominent.

Phenomena related to trance states include highway hypnosis and similar mental states experienced by airplane pilots. The monotony of moving at high speeds through environments that provide few distractions to the operator of the vehicle leads to a fixation on a single object, for example, a dial on the instrument panel or the never-ending horizon of a road running straight ahead for miles. When a trancelike state of consciousness results, visual hallucinations may occur, and the danger of a serious accident is always present. Possibly in the same category are the hallucinations and dissociated mental states of patients who have been confined to respirators for long periods without adequate environmental distractions.

The religions of many cultures recognize that the practice of concentration may lead to a variety of dissociative phenomena, such as hallucinations, paralyses, and other sensory disturbances.

Recovered Memory Syndrome

Under hypnosis or during psychotherapy, a patient may recover a memory of a painful experience or conflict—particularly of sexual or physical abuse—that is etiologically significant. When the repressed material is brought back to consciousness, the person not only may recall the experience but may relive it, accompanied by the appropriate affective response (a process called *abreaction*). If the event recalled never really happened but the person believes it to be true and reacts accordingly, it is known as *false memory syndrome*.

The recovered memory syndrome has been surrounded by controversy because victims of past abuse have sued perpetrators, many of whom have been convicted upon the recovered memory as the only evidence. Problems arise because memory is subject to distortion and retrospective falsification that may also be influenced by the therapist. In children, memories of abuse are often "recovered" by overzealous prosecuting attorneys or by so-called recovered memory experts, some of whom have no qualifications whatsoever. Such measures are often contaminated by the suggestibility of children and the prejudices of their adult interrogators.

Thomas E. Gutheil describes memory as a "slender reed—insufficiently strong to bear the weight of a court case." Even if the memory of abuse is real, the perpetrator is not the present person, but the person of the past. Gutheil does not believe that litigation usually serves the patient's psychological goals. Clinical attention should probably be directed toward helping patients cast aside the limiting restrictive role of victim and transcend their past traumas, work through them, and try to get on with their lives.

Ganser's Syndrome

Ganser's syndrome is the voluntary production of severe psychiatric symptoms, sometimes described as giving approximate answers or talking past the point (e.g., when asked to multiply 4 times 5, the patient answers 21). The syndrome may occur in persons with other mental disorders, such as schizophrenia, depressive disorders, toxic states, paresis, alcohol use disorders, and factitious disorder. The psychological symptoms generally represent the patient's sense of mental illness rather than any recognized diagnostic category. The syndrome is commonly associated with dissociative phenomena such as amnesia, fugue, perceptual disturbances, and conversion symptoms. Ganser's syndrome is apparently most common in men and in prisoners, although prevalence data and familial patterns are not established. A major predisposing factor is the existence of a severe personality disorder. The differential diagnosis may be extremely difficult. Unless a patient is able to admit the factitious nature of the presenting symptoms or unless conclusive evidence from objective psychological tests indicates that the symptoms are false, clinicians may be unable to determine whether the patient has a true disorder. The syndrome may be recognized by its pansymptomatic nature or by the fact that the symptoms are often worse when patients believe they are being watched. Recovery from the syndrome is sudden; patients claim amnesia for the events. Ganser's syndrome was previously classified as a factitious disorder.

BRAINWASHING

DSM-IV-TR describes this dissociative disorder not otherwise specified as "states of dissociation that occur in individuals who have been subjected to periods of prolonged and intense coercive persuasion (e.g., brainwashing, thought reform, or indoctrination while captive)." The term *brainwashing* was coined by an American journalist in the 1950s from Chinese ideographs that would more accurately have been translated as "thought reform." Indeed, the terms *brainwashing, thought reform, coercive persuasion,* and *mind control* are for all practical purposes used synonymously and interchangeably.

Brainwashing occurs largely in the setting of political reform, as has been described at length with the cultural revolution in communist China, war imprisonment, torture of political dissidents, terrorist hostages, and, more familiarly in Western culture: totalitarian cult indoctrination. It implies that under conditions of adequate stress and duress, individuals can be made to comply with the demands of those in power, thereby undergoing major changes in their personality, beliefs, and behaviors. Persons submitted to such conditions can undergo considerable harm, including loss of health and life, and they typically manifest a variety of posttraumatic and dissociative symptoms.

The first stage in coercive processes has been likened to the artificial creation of an identity crisis, with the emergence of a new pseudoidentity that manifests characteristics of a dissociative state. Under circumstances of extreme and malignant dependency, overwhelming vulnerability, and danger to one's existence, individuals develop a state characterized by extreme idealization of their captors, with ensuing identification with the aggressor and externalization of their superego, regressive adaptation known as traumatic infantilism, paralysis of will, and a state of frozen fright. The coercive techniques that are typically used to induce such a state in the victim have been amply described and include isolation of the subject, degradation, control over all communications and basic daily functions, induction of fear and confusion, peer pressure, assignment of repetitive and monotonous routines, unpredictability of environmental supplies, renunciation of past relationships and values, and various deprivations. Even though physical or sexual abuse, torture, and extreme sensory deprivation and physical neglect can be parts of this process, they are not required to define a coercive process. As a result, victims who have been studied extensively manifest extensive posttraumatic and dissociative symptomatology, including drastic alteration of their identity, values, and beliefs; reduction of cognitive flexibility with regression to simplistic perceptions of good–evil and dominance–submission; numbing of experience and blunting of affect; trancelike states and diminished environmental responsiveness; and in some cases more severe dissociative symptoms such as amnesia, depersonalization, and shifts in identity.

The treatment of the victims of coercion can vary considerably, depending on their particular background, the circumstances involved, and the setting in which help is sought. Although there are no systematic studies in this domain, basic principles involve validation of the traumatic experience and coercive techniques used, cognitive reframing of the events that transpired, exploration of preexisting psychopathology and vulnerabilities (when applicable), and general techniques used in treating posttraumatic and dissociative states. In addition, family interventions and therapy may be required, at least in cases of cult indoctrination, since significant family duress and disruption commonly occur.

ICD-10

ICD-10 organizes dissociative (conversion) disorders somewhat differently than does DSM-IV-TR. The dissociative disorders in ICD-10 include dissociative amnesia, dissociative fugue, dissociative stupor, trance and possession disorders, dissociative motor disorders, dissociative convulsions, dissociative anesthesia and sensory loss, mixed dissociative disorders, other dissociative disorders, and unspecified dissociative disorders (Table 20–14).

Table 20–14
ICD-10 Diagnostic Criteria for Dissociative [Conversion] Disorders

G1. There must be no evidence of a physical disorder that can explain the characteristic symptoms of this disorder (although physical disorders may be present that give rise to other symptoms).

G2. There are convincing associations in time between the onset of symptoms of the disorder and stressful events, problems, or needs.

Dissociative amnesia

A. The general criteria for dissociative disorder must be met.

B. There must be amnesia, either partial or complete, for recent events or problems that were or still are traumatic or stressful.

C. The amnesia is too extensive and persistent to be explained by ordinary forgetfulness (although its depth and extent may vary from one assessment to the next) or by intentional simulation.

Dissociative fugue

A. The general criteria for dissociative disorder must be met.

B. The individual undertakes an unexpected yet organized journey away from home or from the ordinary places of work and social activities, during which self-care is largely maintained.

C. There is amnesia, either partial or complete, for the journey, which also meets Criterion C for dissociative amnesia.

Dissociative stupor

A. The general criteria for dissociative disorder must be met.

B. There is profound diminution or absence of voluntary movements and speech and of normal responsiveness to light, noise, and touch.

C. Normal muscle tone, static posture, and breathing (and often limited coordinated eye movements) are maintained.

Trance and possession disorders

A. The general criteria for dissociative disorder must be met.

B. Either of the following must be present:

(1) *Trance.* There is temporary alteration of the state of consciousness, shown by any two of:

(a) loss of the usual sense of personal identity;

(b) narrowing of awareness of immediate surroundings, or unusually narrow and selective focusing on environmental stimuli;

(c) limitation of movements, postures, and speech to repetition of a small repertoire.

(2) *Possession disorder.* The individual is convinced that he or she has been taken over by a spirit, power, deity, or other person.

C. Both (1) and (2) of Criterion B must be unwanted and troublesome, occurring outside, or being a prolongation of, similar states in religious or other culturally accepted situations.

D. *Most commonly used exclusion clause.* The disorder does not occur at the same time as schizophrenia or related disorders, or mood [affective] disorders with hallucinations or delusions.

Dissociative motor disorders

A. The general criteria for dissociative disorder must be met.

B. Either of the following must be present:

(1) Complete or partial loss of the ability to perform movements that are normally under voluntary control (including speech);

(2) Various or variable degrees of incoordination or ataxia, or inability to stand unaided.

Dissociative convulsions

A. The general criteria for dissociative disorder must be met.

B. The individual exhibits sudden and unexpected spasmodic movements, closely resembling any of the varieties of epileptic seizure, but not followed by loss of consciousness.

C. The symptoms in Criterion B are not accompanied by tongue-biting, serious bruising or laceration due to falling, or urinary incontinence.

Dissociative anesthesia and sensory loss

A. The general criteria for dissociative disorder must be met.

B. Either of the following must be present:

(1) Partial or complete loss of any or all of the normal cutaneous sensations over part or all of the body (specify: touch, pinprick, vibration, heat, cold);

(2) Partial or complete loss of vision, hearing, or smell (specify).

Mixed dissociative [conversion] disorders

Other dissociative [conversion] disorders

This residual code may be used to indicate other dissociative and conversion states that meet Criteria G1 and G2 for dissociative [conversion] disorders but do not meet the criteria for the dissociative disorders listed above.

Ganser's syndrome (approximate answers)

Multiple personality disorder

A. Two or more distinct personalities exist within the individual, only one being evident at a time.

B. Each personality has its own memories, preferences, and behavior patterns, and at some time (and recurrently) takes full control of the individual's behavior.

C. There is inability to recall important personal information which is too extensive to be explained by ordinary forgetfulness.

D. The symptoms are not due to organic mental disorders (e.g., in epileptic disorders) or to psychoactive substance-related disorders (e.g., intoxication or withdrawal).

Transient dissociative [conversion] disorders occurring in childhood and adolescence

Other specified dissociative [conversion] disorders

Specific research criteria are not given for all disorders mentioned above, since these other dissociative states are rare and not well described. Research workers studying these conditions in detail should specify their own criteria according to the purpose of their studies.

Dissociative [conversion] disorder, unspecified

References

Boon S, Draijer N. Multiple personality disorder in The Netherlands: a clinical investigation of 71 patients. *Am J Psychiatry.* 1993;150:489.

Burton N, Lane RC. The relational treatment of dissociative identity disorder. *Clin Psychol Rev.* 2001;21:301.

Ellason JW, Ross CA. Two-year follow-up of inpatients with dissociative identity disorder. *Am J Psychiatry.* 1997;154:832.

Elzinga BM, Bermond B, van Dyck R. The relationship between dissociative proneness and alexithymia. *Psychother Psychosom.* 2002;71:104.

Fleisher WP, Anderson G. Dissociative disorders in adolescence. *Adolesc Psychiatry.* 1995;20:203.

Gabbard GO. *Psychodynamic Psychiatry in Clinical Practice: The DSM-IV Edition.* Washington, DC: American Psychiatric Press; 1994.

Hollander E, Liebowitz MR, DeCaria C, Fairbanks J, Fallon B, Klein DF. Treatment of depersonalization with serotonin reuptake blockers. *J Clin Psychopharmacol.* 1990;10:200.

Kapur N. Amnesia in relation to fugue states: distinguishing a neurological form from a psychogenic basis. *Br J Psychiatry.* 1991;159:872.

Loewenstein RJ. Multiple personality disorder. *Psychiatr Clin North Am.* 1991;14(3):489.

Merskey H. The manufacture of personalities: the production of multiple personality disorder. *Br J Psychiatry.* 1992;160:327.

Modestin J, Lotscher K, Erni T. Dissociative experiences and their correlates in young non-patients. *Psychol Psychother.* 2002;75:53.

Nijenhuis ERS. Somatoform dissociation. Major symptoms of dissociative disorders. *J Trauma Dissoc.* 2000;1:7.

Phillips ML, Sierra M, Hunter E, et al. Service innovations: a depersonalization research unit progress report. *Psychiatr Bull.* 2001;25:105.

Putnam FW, Loewenstein RJ. Treatment of multiple personality disorder: a survey of current practices. *Am J Psychiatry.* 1993;150:1048.

Ross CA, Anderson G, Fleischer WP, Norton GR. The frequency of multiple personality disorder among psychiatric inpatients. *Am J Psychiatry.* 1991;148:1717.

Ross CA, Miller SD, Reagor P, Bjornson L, Fraser GA, Anderson G. Structured interview data on 102 cases of multiple personality disorder from four centers. *Am J Psychiatry.* 1990;147:596.

Rossini ED, Schwartz DR, Braun BG. Intellectual functioning of inpatients with dissociative identity disorder and dissociative disorder not otherwise specified. *J Nerv Ment Dis.* 1996;184:289.

Rowan AJ, Soenbaum DH. Ictal amnesia and fugue states. *Adv Neurol.* 1991;55:357.

Sadock BJ, Sadock VA. Dissociative disorders. In: Sadock BJ, Sadock VA, eds. *Kaplan & Sadock's Comprehensive Textbook of Psychiatry.* 7th ed. Vol 1. Baltimore: Lippincott Williams & Wilkins; 2000:1544.

Sandberg DA, Lynn SJ. Dissociative experiences, psychopathology and adjustment, and child and adolescent maltreatment in female college students. *J Abnorm Psychol.* 1992;101:717.

Saxe GN, van der Kolk BA, Berkowitz R, et al. Dissociative disorders in psychiatric inpatients. *Am J Psychiatry.* 1993;150:1037.

Simeon D, Guralnik O, Knutelska M, Schmeidler J. Personality factors associated with dissociation: temperament, defenses, and cognitive schemata. *Am J Psychiatry.* 2002;159:489.

Simeon D, Hollander E. Depersonalization disorder. *Psychiatr Ann.* 1993; 23:382.

Spiegel D, ed. Dissociative disorders. In: Tasman A, Goldfinger SM, eds. *American Psychiatric Press Review of Psychiatry.* Vol 10. Washington, DC: American Psychiatric Press; 1991:141.

Steinberg M. *Handbook for the Assessment of Dissociation: A Clinical Guide.* Washington, DC: American Psychiatric Press; 1995.

Steinberg M, Rounsaville B, Cicchetti D. Detection of dissociative disorder in psychiatric patients by screening instrument and a structured diagnostic interview. *Am J Psychiatry.* 1991;48:1050.

Torch EM. The psychotherapeutic treatment of depersonalization disorder. *Hillside J Clin Psychiatry.* 1987;9:133.

21 Human Sexuality

▲ 21.1 Normal Sexuality

Sexuality is determined by anatomy, physiology, psychology, the culture in which one lives, one's relationship with others, and developmental experiences throughout the life cycle. It includes the perception of being male or female and all those thoughts, feelings, and behaviors connected with sexual gratification and reproduction, including the attraction of one person to another.

Normal sexuality involves feelings of desire, behavior that brings pleasure to oneself and one's partner, and stimulation of the primary sex organs including coitus; is devoid of inappropriate feelings of guilt or anxiety; and is not compulsive. In some contexts, sex outside a committed relationship, masturbation, and various forms of stimulation involving other than the primary sex organs constitute normal behavior.

PSYCHOSEXUALITY

Sexuality and total personality are so entwined that to speak of sexuality as a separate entity is virtually impossible. The term *psychosexual* is therefore used to describe personality development and functioning as these are affected by sexuality. The term *psychosexual* applies to more than sexual feelings and behavior, and it is not synonymous with *libido* in the broad freudian sense.

Sigmund Freud's generalization that all pleasurable impulses and activities are originally sexual has given laypersons a somewhat distorted view of sexual concepts and has presented psychiatrists a confused picture of motivation. For example, some oral activities are directed toward obtaining food, and others are directed toward achieving sexual gratification. Both activities are pleasure seeking and use the same organs, but they are not, as Freud contended, both necessarily sexual. Labeling all pleasure-seeking behaviors sexual makes it impossible to specify precise motivations. Persons may also use sexual activities for gratification of nonsexual needs, such as dependency, aggression, power, and status. Although sexual and nonsexual impulses may jointly motivate behavior, the analysis of behavior depends on understanding the underlying individual motivations and their interactions.

SEXUAL LEARNING IN CHILDHOOD

Before Freud described the effects of childhood experiences on adults' personalities, the universality of sexual activity and sexual learning in children was unrecognized. Most sexual learning experiences in childhood occur without the parents' knowledge, but awareness of a child's sex does influence parental behavior. Male infants, for instance, tend to be handled more vigorously and female infants tend to be cuddled more. Fathers spend more time with their infant sons than with their daughters, and they also tend to be more aware of their sons' adolescent concerns than of their daughters' anxieties. Boys are more likely than girls to be physically disciplined. A child's sex affects parental tolerance for aggression and reinforcement or extinction of activity and of intellectual, aesthetic, and athletic interests.

Observation of children reveals that genital play in infants is part of normal development. According to Harry Harlow, interaction with mothers and peers is necessary for the development of effective adult sexual behavior in monkeys, a finding that has relevance to the normal socialization of children. During a critical period in development, infants are especially susceptible to certain stimuli; later they may be immune to these stimuli. The detailed relation of critical periods to psychosexual development has yet to be established; Freud's stages of psychosexual development—oral, anal, phallic, latent, and genital—presumably provide a broad framework.

PSYCHOSEXUAL FACTORS

Sexuality depends on four interrelated psychosexual factors: sexual identity, gender identity, sexual orientation, and sexual behavior. These factors affect personality growth, development, and functioning. Sexuality is something more than physical sex, coital or noncoital, and something less than all behaviors directed toward attaining pleasure.

Sexual Identity and Gender Identity

Sexual identity is the pattern of a person's biological sexual characteristics: chromosomes, external genitalia, internal genitalia, hormonal composition, gonads, and secondary sex characteristics. In normal development, these characteristics form a cohesive pattern that leaves a person in no doubt about his or her sex. Gender identity is a person's sense of maleness or femaleness.

Sexual Identity. Modern embryological studies have shown that all mammalian embryos, whether genetically male (XY genotype) or genetically female (XX genotype) are anatomically female during the early stages of fetal life. Differentiation of the male from the female results from the action of fetal androgens; the action begins about the sixth week of embryonic life and is completed by the end of the third month

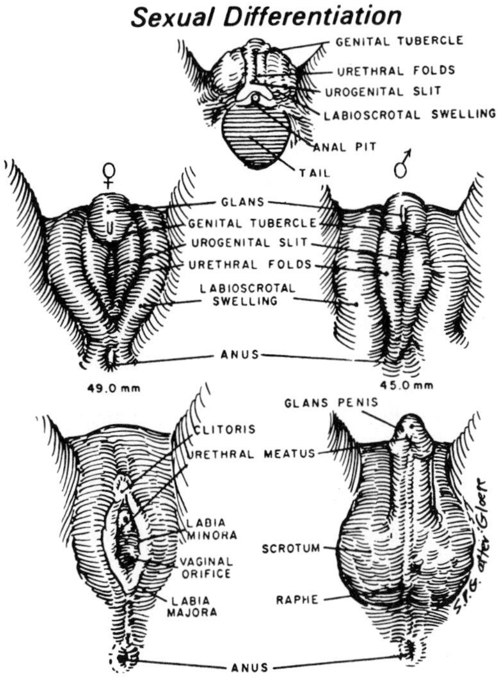

FIGURE 21.1–1
Differentiation of male and female external genitalia from indifferent primordia. Male differentiation occurs only in the presence of androgenic stimulation during the first 12 weeks of fetal life. (Redrawn from Van Wyk and Grumbach, 1968; reprinted with permission from Brobeck JR, ed. *Best & Taylor's Physiological Basis of Medical Practice*. 9th ed. Baltimore: Williams & Wilkins; 1973.)

(Fig. 21.1–1). Recent studies have explained the effects of fetal hormones on the masculinization or feminization of the brain. In animals, prenatal hormonal stimulation of the brain is necessary for male and female reproductive and copulatory behavior. The fetus is also vulnerable to exogenously administered androgens during that period. For instance, if a pregnant woman receives sufficient exogenous androgens, her female fetus possessing ovaries can develop external genitalia resembling those of a male (Table 21.1–1).

Gender Identity.

By the age of 2 to 3 years, almost everyone has a firm conviction that "I am male" or "I am female." Yet even if maleness and femaleness develop normally, persons must still develop a sense of masculinity or femininity.

Gender identity, according to Robert Stoller, "connotes psychological aspects of behavior related to masculinity and femininity." He considers gender social and sex biological: "Most often the two are relatively congruent, that is, males tend to be manly and females womanly." But sex and gender may develop in conflicting or even opposite ways. Gender identity results from an almost infinite series of cues derived from experiences with family members, teachers, friends, and coworkers and from cultural phenomena. Physical characteristics derived from a person's biological sex—such as physique, body shape, and physical dimensions—interrelate with an intricate system of stimuli, including rewards and punishment and parental gender labels, to establish gender identity.

Thus formation of gender identity arises from parental and cultural attitudes, the infant's external genitalia, and a genetic influence, which is physiologically active by the sixth week of fetal life. Even though family, cultural, and biological influences may complicate establishment of a sense of masculinity or femininity, persons usually develop a relatively secure sense of identification with their biological sex—a stable gender identity.

Table 21.1–1
Classification of Intersexual Disorders[a]

Syndrome	Description
Virilizing adrenal hyperplasia (adrenogenital syndrome)	Results from excess androgens in fetus with XX genotype; most common female intersex disorder; associated with enlarged clitoris, fused labia, hirsutism in adolescence
Turner's syndrome	Results from absence of second female sex chromosome (XO); associated with web neck, dwarfism, cubitus valgus; no sex hormones produced; infertile; usually assigned as females because of female-looking genitals
Klinefelter's syndrome	Genotype is XXY; male habitus present with small penis and rudimentary testes because of low androgen production; weak libido; usually assigned as male
Androgen insensitivity syndrome (testicular-feminizing syndrome)	Congenital X-linked recessive disorder that results in inability of tissues to respond to androgens; external genitals look female and cryptorchid testes present; assigned as females, even though they have XY genotype; in extreme form patient has breasts, normal external genitals, short blind vagina, and absence of pubic and axillary hair
Enzymatic defects in XY genotype (e.g., 5-α-reductase deficiency, 17-hydroxysteroid deficiency)	Congenital interruption in production of testosterone that produces ambiguous genitals and female habitus; usually assigned as female because of female-looking genitalia
Hermaphroditism	True hermaphrodite is rare and characterized by both testes and ovaries in same person (may be 46 XX or 46 XY)
Pseudohermaphroditism	Usually the result of endocrine or enzymatic defect (e.g., adrenal hyperplasia) in persons with normal chromosomes; female pseudohermaphrodites have masculine-looking genitals but are XX; male pseudohermaphrodites have rudimentary testes and external genitals and are XY; assigned as males or females, depending on morphology of genitals

[a]Intersexual disorders include a variety of syndromes that produce persons with gross anatomical or physiological aspects of the opposite sex.

GENDER ROLE. Related to, and in part derived from, gender identity is gender role behavior. John Money and Anke Ehrhardt described gender role behavior as all those things that a person says or does to disclose himself or herself as having the status of boy or man, girl or woman, respectively. A gender role is not established at birth but is built up cumulatively through experiences encountered and transacted through casual

and unplanned learning, through explicit instruction and inculcation, and through spontaneously putting two and two together to make sometimes four and sometimes five. The usual outcome is a congruence of gender identity and gender role. Although biological attributes are significant, the major factor in achieving the role appropriate to a person's sex is learning.

Research on sex differences in children's behavior reveals more psychological similarities than differences. However, girls are found to be less prone to tantrums after the age of 18 months than are boys, and boys generally are more physically and verbally aggressive than are girls from age 2 onward. Little girls and little boys are similarly active, but boys are more easily stimulated to sudden bursts of activity when they are in groups. Some researchers speculate that although aggression is a learned behavior, male hormones may have sensitized boys' neural organizations to absorb these lessons more easily than do girls.

Persons' gender roles can seem to be opposed to their gender identities. Persons may identify with their own sex and yet adopt the dress, hairstyle, or other characteristics of the opposite sex. Or they may identify with the opposite sex and yet for expediency adopt many behavioral characteristics of their own sex. A further discussion of gender issues appears in Chapter 22.

Sexual Orientation

Sexual orientation describes the object of a person's sexual impulses: heterosexual (opposite sex), homosexual (same sex), or bisexual (both sexes).

Sexual Behavior

Physiological Responses. Sexual response is a true psychophysiological experience. Arousal is triggered by both psychological and physical stimuli; levels of tension are experienced both physiologically and emotionally; and with orgasm, there is normally a subjective perception of a peak of physical reaction and release. Psychosexual development, psychological attitudes toward sexuality, and attitudes toward one's sexual partner are directly involved with, and affect, the physiology of human sexual response.

Table 21.1–2
Male Sexual Response Cycle[a]

Organ	Excitement Phase	Orgasmic Phase	Resolution Phase
	Lasts several minutes to several hours; heightened excitement before orgasm, 30 seconds to 3 minutes	3 to 15 seconds	10 to 15 minutes; if no orgasm, ½ to 1 day
Skin	Just before orgasm: sexual flush inconsistently appears; maculopapular rash originates on abdomen and spreads to anterior chest wall, face, and neck and can include shoulders and forearms	Well-developed flush	Flush disappears in reverse order of appearance; inconsistently appearing film of perspiration on soles of feet and palms of hands
Penis	Erection in 10 to 30 seconds caused by vasocongestion of erectile bodies of corpus cavernosa of shaft; loss of erection may occur with introduction of asexual stimulus, loud noise; with heightened excitement, size of glans and diameter of penile shaft increase further	Ejaculation; emission phase marked by three to four 0.8-second contractions of vas, seminal vesicles, prostate; ejaculation proper marked by 0.8-second contractions of urethra and ejaculatory spurt of 12 to 20 inches at age 18, decreasing with age to seepage at 70	Erection: partial involution in 5 to 10 seconds with variable refractory period; full detumescence in 5 to 30 minutes
Scrotum and testes	Tightening and lifting of scrotal sac and elevation of testes; with heightened excitement, 50% increase in size of testes over unstimulated state and flattening against perineum, signaling impending ejaculation	No change	Decrease to baseline size because of loss of vasocongestion; testicular and scrotal descent within 5 to 30 minutes after orgasm; involution may take several hours if no orgasmic release takes place
Cowper's glands	2 to 3 drops of mucoid fluid that contain viable sperm are secreted during heightened excitement	No change	No change
Other	Breasts: inconsistent nipple erection with heightened excitement before orgasm Myotonia: semispastic contractions of facial, abdominal, and intercostal muscles Tachycardia: up to 175 beats a minute Blood pressure: rise in systolic 20 to 80 mm; in diastolic 10 to 40 mm Respiration: increased	Loss of voluntary muscular control Rectum: rhythmical contractions of sphincter Heart rate: up to 180 beats a minute Blood pressure: up to 40 to 100 mm systolic; 20 to 50 mm diastolic Respiration: up to 40 respirations a minute	Return to baseline state in 5 to 10 minutes

[a]A desire phase consisting of sex fantasies and desire to have sex precedes excitement phase.
Table by Virginia Sadock, M.D.

Table 21.1–3
Female Sexual Response Cycle[a]

Organ	Excitement Phase	Orgasmic Phase	Resolution Phase
	Lasts several minutes to several hours; heightened excitement before orgasm, 30 seconds to 3 minutes	3 to 15 seconds	10 to 15 minutes; if no orgasm, ½ to 1 day
Skin	Just before orgasm: sexual flush inconsistently appears; maculopapular rash originates on abdomen and spreads to anterior chest wall, face, and neck; can include shoulders and forearms	Well-developed flush	Flush disappears in reverse order of appearance; inconsistently appearing film of perspiration on soles of feet and palms of hands
Breasts	Nipple erection in two thirds of women, venous congestion and areolar enlargement; size increases to one fourth over normal	Breasts may become tremulous	Return to normal in about ½ hour
Clitoris	Enlargement in diameter of glans and shaft; just before orgasm, shaft retracts into prepuce	No change	Shaft returns to normal position in 5 to 10 seconds; detumescence in 5 to 30 minutes; if no orgasm, detumescence takes several hours
Labia majora	Nullipara: elevate and flatten against perineum Multipara: congestion and edema	No change	Nullipara: increase to normal size in 1 to 2 minutes Multipara: decrease to normal size in 10 to 15 minutes
Labia minora	Size increased 2 to 3 times over normal; change to pink, red, deep red before orgasm	Contractions of proximal labia minora	Return to normal within 5 minutes
Vagina	Color change to dark purple; vaginal transudate appears 10 to 30 seconds after arousal; elongation and ballooning of vagina; lower third of vagina constricts before orgasm	3 to 15 contractions of lower third of vagina at intervals of 0.8 second	Ejaculate forms seminal pool in upper two thirds of vagina; congestion disappears in seconds or, if no orgasm, in 20 to 30 minutes
Uterus	Ascends into false pelvis; laborlike contractions begin in heightened excitement just before orgasm	Contractions throughout orgasm	Contractions cease, and uterus descends to normal position
Other	Myotonia A few drops of mucoid secretion from Bartholin's glands during heightened excitement Cervix swells slightly and is passively elevated with uterus	Loss of voluntary muscular control Rectum: rhythmical contractions of sphincter Hyperventilation and tachycardia	Return to baseline status in seconds to minutes Cervix color and size return to normal, and cervix descends into seminal pool

[a]A desire phase consisting of sex fantasies and desire to have sex precedes excitement phase.
Table by Virginia Sadock, M.D.

Normal men and women experience a sequence of physiological responses to sexual stimulation. In the first detailed description of these responses, William Masters and Virginia Johnson observed that the physiological process involves increasing levels of vasocongestion and myotonia (tumescence) and the subsequent release of the vascular activity and muscle tone as a result of orgasm (detumescence). Tables 21.1–2 and 21.1–3 describe the male and female sexual response cycles. The text revision of the fourth edition of *Diagnostic and Statistical Manual of Mental Disorders* (DSM-IV-TR) defines a four-phase response cycle: phase 1, desire; phase 2, excitement; phase 3, orgasm; phase 4, resolution.

PHASE 1: DESIRE. The classification of the desire (or appetitive) phase, which is distinct from any phase identified solely through physiology, reflects the psychiatric concern with motivations, drives, and personality. The phase is characterized by sexual fantasies and the desire to have sexual activity.

PHASE 2: EXCITEMENT. The excitement and arousal phase, brought on by psychological stimulation (fantasy or the presence of a love object) or physiological stimulation (stroking or kissing) or a combination of the two, consists of a subjective sense of pleasure. During this phase, penile tumescence leads to erection in men and vaginal lubrication occurs in women. The nipples of both sexes become erect, although nipple erection is more common in women than in men. A woman's clitoris becomes hard and turgid, and her labia minora become thicker as a result of venous engorgement. Initial excitement may last from several minutes to several hours. With continued stimulation, a man's testes increase 50 percent in size and elevate. A woman's vaginal barrel shows a characteristic constriction along the outer third, known as the orgasmic platform. The clitoris elevates and retracts behind the symphysis pubis, and as a result is not easily accessible. Stimulation of the area, however, causes traction on the labia minora and the prepuce and there is intrapreputial movement of the clitoral shaft. Women's breast size increases 25 percent. Continued engorgement of the penis and the vagina produces color changes, particularly in the labia minora, which become bright or deep red. Voluntary contractions of large muscle groups occur, heartbeat and respiration rates increase, and blood pressure rises. Heightened excitement lasts from 30 seconds to several minutes.

PHASE 3: ORGASM. The orgasm phase consists of a peaking of sexual pleasure, with the release of sexual tension and the rhythmic contraction of the perineal muscles and the pelvic reproductive organs. A subjective sense of ejaculatory inevitability triggers men's orgasms.

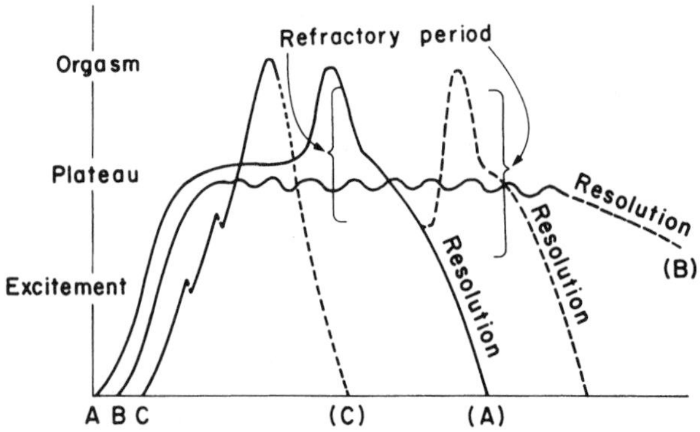

FIGURE 21.1–2
Male sexual response. An individual man may experience any of these three patterns (**A, B,** or **C**) during a particular sexual experience. (Reprinted with permission from Walker JI, ed. *Essentials of Clinical Psychiatry.* Philadelphia: JB Lippincott; 1985:276.)

The forceful emission of semen follows. The male orgasm is also associated with four to five rhythmic spasms of the prostate, seminal vesicles, vas, and urethra. In women, orgasm is characterized by 3 to 15 involuntary contractions of the lower third of the vagina and by strong sustained contractions of the uterus, flowing from the fundus downward to the cervix. Both men and women have involuntary contractions of the internal and external anal sphincters. These and the other contractions during orgasm occur at 0.8-second intervals. Other manifestations include voluntary and involuntary movements of the large muscle groups, including facial grimacing and carpopedal spasm. Blood pressure rises 20 to 40 mm (both systolic and diastolic), and the heart rate increases up to 160 beats a minute. Orgasm lasts from 3 to 25 seconds and is associated with a slight clouding of consciousness (Figs. 21.1–2 and 21.1–3).

PHASE 4: RESOLUTION. Resolution consists of the disgorgement of blood from the genitalia (detumescence), which brings the body back to its resting state. If orgasm occurs, resolution is rapid and is characterized by a subjective sense of well-being, general relaxation, and muscular relaxation. If orgasm does not occur, resolution may take from 2 to 6 hours and may be associated with irritability and discomfort. After orgasm, men have a refractory period that may last from several minutes to many hours; in that period they cannot be stimulated to further orgasm. Women do not have a refractory period and are capable of multiple and successive orgasms.

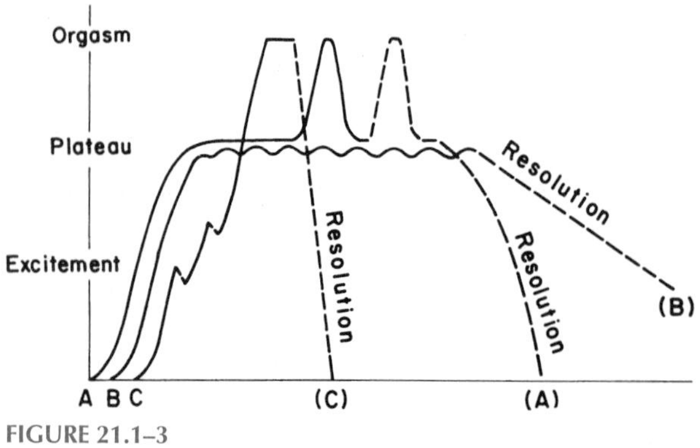

FIGURE 21.1–3
Female sexual response. An individual woman may experience any of these three patterns (**A, B,** or **C**) during a particular sexual experience. (Reprinted with permission from Walker JI, ed. *Essentials of Clinical Psychiatry.* Philadelphia: JB Lippincott; 1985:276.)

HORMONES AND NEUROHORMONES AND SEXUAL BEHAVIOR

In general, substances that increase dopamine levels in the brain increase desire, while substances that augment serotonin decrease desire. Testosterone increases libido in both men and women, although estrogen is a key factor in the lubrication involved in female arousal and may increase sensitivity in the woman to stimulation. Progesterone mildly depresses desire in men and women as do excessive prolactin and cortisol. Oxytocin is involved in pleasurable sensations during sex and is found in higher levels in men and women following orgasm.

Gender Differences in Desire and Erotic Stimuli

Sexual impulses and desire exist in men and women. However, if desire is measured by the frequency of spontaneous sexual thoughts, interest in participating in sexual activity, and alertness to sexual cues, males generally possess a higher baseline level of desire than women, which may be biologically determined.

Although explicit sexual fantasies are common to both sexes, the external stimuli for the fantasies frequently differ for men and women. Many men respond to visual stimuli of nude or barely dressed women, who are lust driven and interested only in physical satisfaction. Women report responding to romantic stories with a tender, demonstrative hero whose passion for the heroine impels him toward a lifetime commitment to her. A complicating factor is that a woman's subjective sense of arousal is not always congruent with her physiological state of arousal. Specifically, her sense of excitement may reflect a readiness to be aroused rather than physiological lubrication. Conversely she may experience the physical signs of arousal without being aware of them. This situation rarely occurs in men.

Masturbation

Masturbation is usually a normal precursor of object-related sexual behavior. No other form of sexual activity has been more frequently discussed, more roundly condemned, and more universally practiced than masturbation. Research by Alfred Kinsey into the prevalence of masturbation indicated that nearly all men and three fourths of all women masturbate sometime during their lives.

Longitudinal studies of development show that sexual self-stimulation is common in infancy and childhood. Just as infants learn to explore the functions of their fingers and mouths, they learn to do the same with their genitalia. At about 15 to 19 months of age, both sexes begin genital self-stimulation. Pleasurable sensations result from any gentle touch to the genital region. Those sensations, coupled with the ordinary desire for exploration of the body, produce a normal interest in masturbatory pleasure at that time. Children also develop an increased interest in the genitalia of others—parents, children, and even animals. As youngsters acquire playmates, the curiosity about their own and others' genitalia motivates episodes of exhibitionism or genital exploration. Such experiences, unless blocked by guilty fear, contribute to continued pleasure from sexual stimulation.

With the approach of puberty, the upsurge of sex hormones, and the development of secondary sex characteristics, sexual curiosity intensifies, and masturbation increases. Adolescents are physically capable of coitus and orgasm but are usually inhibited by social restraints. The dual and often conflicting pressures of establishing their sexual identities and controlling their sexual impulses produce a strong physiological sexual tension in teenagers that demands release, and masturbation is a normal way to reduce sexual tensions. In general, males learn to masturbate to orgasm earlier than females and masturbate more frequently. An important emotional difference between the adolescent and the youngster of earlier years is the presence of coital fantasies during masturbation in the adolescent. These fantasies are an important adjunct to the development of sexual identity; in the comparative safety of the imagination, the adolescent learns to perform the adult sex role. This autoerotic activity is usually maintained into the young adult years, when it is normally replaced by coitus.

Couples in a sexual relationship do not abandon masturbation entirely. When coitus is unsatisfactory or is unavailable because of illness or the absence of the partner, self-stimulation often serves an adaptive purpose, combining sensual pleasure and tension release. Kinsey reported that when women masturbate, most prefer clitoral stimulation. Masters and Johnson stated that women prefer the shaft of the clitoris to the glans because the glans is hypersensitive to intense stimulation. Most men masturbate by vigorously stroking the penile shaft and glans.

Moral taboos against masturbation have generated myths that masturbation causes mental illness or decreased sexual potency. No scientific evidence supports such claims. Masturbation is a psychopathological symptom only when it becomes a compulsion beyond a person's willful control. Then it is a symptom of emotional disturbance, not because it is sexual but because it is compulsive. Masturbation is probably a universal and inevitable aspect of psychosexual development, and in most cases it is adaptive.

HOMOSEXUALITY

In 1973 homosexuality was eliminated as a diagnostic category by the American Psychiatric Association, and in 1980, it was removed from DSM. The 10th revision of the *International Statistical Classification of Diseases and Related Health Problems* (ICD-10) states: "Sexual orientation alone is not to be regarded as a disorder." This change reflects a change in the understanding of homosexuality, which is now considered to occur with some regularity as a variant of human sexuality, not a pathological disorder. As David Hawkins wrote, "The presence of homosexuality does not appear to be a matter of choice; the expression of it is a matter of choice."

Definition

The term *homosexuality* often describes a person's overt behavior, sexual orientation, and sense of personal or social identity. Many persons prefer to identify sexual orientation by using terms like *lesbians* and *gay men,* rather than *homosexual,* which may imply pathology and etiology based on its origin as a medical term, and refer to sexual behavior with terms such as *same sex* and *male female*. Hawkins wrote that the terms *gay* and *lesbian* refer to a combination of self-perceived identity and social identity; they reflect a person's sense of belonging to a social group that is similarly labeled. *Homophobia* is a negative attitude toward or fear of homosexuality or homosexuals. *Heterosexism* is the belief that a heterosexual relationship is preferable to all others; it implies discrimination against those practicing other forms of sexuality.

Prevalence

When Kinsey conducted one of the first major studies of the incidence of homosexuality, in 1948, he reported that 10 percent of men and 5 percent of women were homosexual. Kinsey also found that 37 percent of all interviewees had had a homosexual experience at some time, including adolescent sexual activities.

Since 1948, these figures have been revised downward in many surveys. A 1994 survey by the U.S. Bureau of the Census concluded that the male prevalence rate for homosexuality is 2 to 3 percent. A 1989 University of Chicago study showed that less than 1 percent of both sexes are exclusively homosexual. The Alan Guttmacher Institute found in 1993 that 1 percent of men reported exclusively same-sex activity in the previous year and that 2 percent reported a lifetime history of homosexual experiences. Because sexual behavior surveys are unreliable, no accurate data are available, but government agencies such as the Centers for Disease Control and Prevention no longer use Kinsey's figures for national projections of homosexual behavior. Table 21.1–4 presents the worldwide estimates of homosexual behavior.

Some lesbians and gay men, particularly the latter, report being aware of same-sex romantic attractions before puberty. According to Kinsey's data, about half of all prepubertal boys have had some genital experience with a male partner. These experiences are often exploratory, particularly when shared with a peer, not an adult, and typically lack a strong affective component. Most gay men recall the onset of romantic and erotic attractions to same-sex partners during early adolescence. For women the onset of romantic feelings toward same-

Table 21.1–4
Estimates of Homosexual Behavior

Country	Sample	Findings
Canada	5,514 first-year college students under age 25	98% heterosexual 1% bisexual 1% homosexual
Norway	6,155 adults, ages 18–26	3.5% of males and 3% of females reported past homosexual experience
France	20,055 adults	Lifetime homosexual experience: 4.1% for men and 2.6% for women
Denmark	3,178 adults, ages 18–59	Less than 1% of men exclusively homosexual
Britain	18,876 adults, ages 16–59	6.1% of men reported past homosexual experience

Data reported by *The Wall Street Journal* (March 31, 1993) and *The New York Times* (April 15, 1993) from research studies on homosexual behavior.

sex partners may also be in preadolescence, but the clear recognition of a same-sex partner preference typically occurs in middle to late adolescence or in young adulthood. More lesbians than gay men appear to have engaged in heterosexual experiences. In one study, 56 percent of lesbians had experienced heterosexual intercourse before their first genital homosexual experience, compared with 19 percent of gay men who had sampled heterosexual intercourse first. Nearly 40 percent of the lesbians had had heterosexual intercourse during the year preceding the survey.

Theoretical Issues

Psychological Factors. The determinants of homosexual behavior are enigmatic. Freud viewed homosexuality as an arrest of psychosexual development and mentioned castration fears and fears of maternal engulfment in the preoedipal phase of psychosexual development. According to psychodynamic theory, early-life situations that can result in male homosexual behavior include a strong fixation on the mother; lack of effective fathering; inhibition of masculine development by the parents; fixation at, or regression to, the narcissistic stage of development; and losses when competing with brothers and sisters. Freud's views on the causes of female homosexuality included a lack of resolution of penis envy in association with unresolved oedipal conflicts.

Freud did not consider homosexuality a mental illness. In "Three Essays on the Theory of Sexuality," he wrote that homosexuality "is found in persons who exhibit no other serious deviations from normal whose efficiency is unimpaired and who are indeed distinguished by specially high intellectual development and ethical culture." In "Letter to an American Mother," Freud wrote, "Homosexuality is assuredly no advantage, but it is nothing to be ashamed of, no vice, no degradation, it cannot be classified as an illness; we consider it to be a variation of the sexual functions produced by a certain arrest of sexual development."

New Concepts of Psychoanalytic Factors. Some psychoanalysts have advanced new psychodynamic formulations that contrast with classic psychoanalytic theory. According to Richard Isay, gay men have described same-sex fantasies that occurred when they were 3 to 5 years old, at about the same age that heterosexuals have male–female fantasies.

Isay wrote that same-sex erotic fantasies in gay men center on the father or the father surrogate.

> The child's perception of and exposure to these erotic feelings may account for such "atypical" behavior as greater secretiveness than other boys, self-isolation, and excessive emotionality. Some "feminine" traits may also be caused by identification with the mother or a mother surrogate. Such characteristics usually develop as a way of attracting the father's love and attention in a manner similar to the way the heterosexual boy may pattern himself after his father to gain his mother's attention.
>
> The psychodynamics of homosexuality in women may be similar. The little girl does not give up her original fixation on the mother as a love object and continues to seek it in adulthood.

Biological Factors. Recent studies indicate that genetic and biological components may contribute to sexual orientation. Gay men reportedly exhibit lower levels of circulatory androgens than do heterosexual men. Prenatal hormones appear to play a role in the organization of the central nervous system: The effective presence of androgens in prenatal life is purported to contribute to a sexual orientation toward females, and a deficiency of prenatal androgens (or tissue insensitivity to them) may lead to a sexual orientation toward males. Preadolescent girls exposed to large amounts of androgens before birth are uncharacteristically aggressive, and boys exposed to excessive female hormones in utero are less athletic, less assertive, and less aggressive than other boys. Women with hyperadrenocorticalism are lesbian and bisexual in greater proportion than women in the general population.

Genetic studies have shown a higher incidence of homosexual concordance among monozygotic twins than among dizygotic twins; these results suggest a genetic predisposition, but chromosome studies have been unable to differentiate homosexuals from heterosexuals. Gay men show a familial distribution; they have more brothers who are gay than do heterosexual men. One study found that 33 of 40 pairs of gay brothers shared a genetic marker on the bottom half of the X chromosome. Another study found that a group of cells in the hypothalamus was smaller in women and in gay men than in heterosexual men. Neither of these studies has been replicated.

Sexual Behavior Patterns. The behavioral features of gay men and lesbian women are as varied as those of heterosexuals. Gay men and lesbians engage in the same sexual practices as heterosexuals, with the obvious differences imposed by anatomy.

Many ongoing relationship patterns occur among gay men and lesbians. Some same-sex pairs live in a common household in either a monogamous or a primary relationship for decades; other gay men and lesbians typically have only fleeting sexual contacts. Although many gay men form stable relationships, male–male relationships appear to be less stable and more fleeting than female–female relationships. Gay-male couples are subjected to civil and social discrimination and do not have the legal social support system of marriage or the biological capacity for childbearing that bonds some otherwise incompatible heterosexual couples. Lesbian couples appear to experience less social stigmatization and to have more-enduring monogamous or primary relationships.

Psychopathology. The range of psychopathology that may be found among distressed lesbians and gay men parallels that found among heterosexuals; some studies have reported a high suicide rate, however. Distress resulting only from conflict between gay men and lesbians and the societal value structure is not classifiable as a disorder. If the distress is severe enough to warrant a diagnosis, adjustment disorder or a depressive disorder should be considered. Some gay men and lesbians suffering from major depressive disorder may experience guilt and self-hatred that become directed toward their sexual orientation; then the desire for sexual reorientation is only a symptom of the depressive disorder. According to ICD-10 ego-dystonic sexual orientation occurs when

> The gender identity or sexual preference is not in doubt but the individual wishes it were different because of associated psychological and behavioural disorders and may seek treatment in order to change it.

Coming Out. According to Richelle Klinger and Robert Cabaj, coming out is a "process by which an individual acknowledges his or her sexual orientation in the face of societal stigma and with successful resolution accepts himself or herself." The authors wrote:

> Successful coming out involves the individual accepting his or her sexual orientation and integrating it into all spheres (e.g., social, vocational, and familial). Another milestone that individuals and couples must eventually confront is the degree of disclosure of sexual orientation to the external world. Some degree of disclosure is probably necessary for successful coming out.

Difficulty negotiating coming out and disclosure is a common cause of relationship difficulties. For each person, problems resolving the coming out process may contribute to poor self-esteem caused by internalized homophobia and lead to deleterious effects on the person's ability to function in the relationship. Conflict can also arise within a relationship when partners disagree on the degree of disclosure.

LOVE AND INTIMACY

Freud postulated that psychological health could be determined by a person's ability to function well in two spheres, work and love. A person able to give and receive love with a minimum of fear and conflict has the capacity to develop genuinely intimate relationships with others. A desire to maintain closeness to the love object typifies being in love. Mature love is marked by the intimacy that is a special attribute of the relationship between two persons. When involved in an intimate relationship, the person actively strives for the growth and happiness of the loved person. Sex frequently acts as a catalyst in forming and maintaining intimate relationships. The quality of intimacy in a mature sexual relationship is what Rollo May called "active receiving," in which a person, while loving, permits himself or herself to be loved. May describes the value of sexual love as an expansion of self-awareness, the experience of tenderness, an increase of self-affirmation and pride, and sometimes, at the moment of orgasm, loss of feeling of separateness. In that setting, sex and love are reciprocally enhancing and healthily fused.

Some persons suffer from conflicts that prevent them from fusing tender and passionate impulses. This can inhibit the expression of sexuality in a relationship, interfere with feelings of closeness to another person, and diminish a person's sense of adequacy and self-esteem. When these problems are severe they may prevent the formation of, or commitment to, an intimate relationship.

SEX AND THE LAW

Medicine and the law both assess the impact of sexuality on the individual and society and determine what is healthy or legal behavior. However, appropriateness or legality of sexual behavior is not always viewed the same way by both professions. The issues at the interface of sexual science and the law often are emotionally charged and reflect cultural divisions about acceptable sexual mores. They include abortion, pornography, prostitution, sex education, the treatment of sex offenders, and the right to sexual privacy, among other issues. Laws regarding these issues (e.g., criminalization of oral or anal sex by consenting adults, or the need for parental permission by minors requesting an abortion) vary from state to state.

TAKING A SEX HISTORY

A sex history provides important information about patients, regardless of the presence of a sexual disorder or whether that is the patient's chief complaint (Table 21.1–5). The information can be obtained gradually, through open-ended questions; however, the following outline provides a guide to the topics to be covered and a structure that can be used when time is limited.

Table 21.1–5
Taking a Sex History

I. Identifying data
  - A. Age
  - B. Sex
  - C. Occupation
  - D. Relationship status—single, married, number of times previously married, separated, divorced, cohabiting, serious involvement, casual dating (difficulty forming or keeping relationships should be assessed throughout the interview)
  - E. Sexual orientation—heterosexual, homosexual, or bisexual (this may also be ascertained later in the interview)

II. Current functioning
  - A. Unsatisfactory to highly satisfactory
  - B. If unsatisfactory, why?
  - C. Feeling about partner satisfaction
  - D. Dysfunctions?—e.g., lack of desire, erectile disorder, inhibited female arousal, anorgasmia, premature ejaculation, retarded ejaculation, pain associated with intercourse (dysfunction discussed below)
    1. Onset—lifelong or acquired
       - a. If acquired, when?
       - b. Did onset coincide with drug use (medications or illegal recreational drugs), life stresses (e.g., loss of job, birth of child), interpersonal difficulties
    2. Generalized—occurs in most situations or with most partners
    3. Situational
       - a. Only with current partner
       - b. In any committed relationship
       - c. Only with masturbation
       - d. In socially proscribed circumstance (e.g., affair)
       - e. In definable circumstance (e.g., very late at night, in parental home, when partner initiated sex play)
  - E. Frequency—partnered sex (coital and noncoital sex play)
  - F. Desire/libido—how often are sexual feelings, thoughts, fantasies, dreams, experienced? (per day, week, etc.)

(continued)

Table 21.1–5 (*continued*)

G. Description of typical sexual interaction
   1. Manner of initiation or invitation (e.g., verbal or physical? Does same person always initiate?)
   2. Presence, type, and extent of foreplay (e.g., kissing, caressing, manual or oral genital stimulation)
   3. Coitus? positions used?
   4. Verbalization during sex? if so, what kind?
   5. Afterplay? (whether sex act is completed or disrupted by dysfunction); typical activities (e.g., holding, talking, return to daily activities, sleeping)
   6. Feeling after sex: relaxed, tense, angry, loving

H. Sexual compulsivity?—intrusion of sexual thoughts or participation in sexual activities to a degree that interferes with relationships or work, requires deception and may endanger the patient

III. Past sexual history
 A. Childhood sexuality
   1. Parental attitudes about sex—degree of openness of reserve (assess unusual prudery or seductiveness)
   2. Parents' attitudes about nudity and modesty
   3. Learning about sex
      a. From parents? (initiated by child's questions or parent volunteering information? which parent? what was child's age?) subjects covered (e.g., pregnancy, birth, intercourse, menstruation, nocturnal emission, masturbation)
      b. From books, magazines, or friends at school or through religious group?
      c. Significant misinformation
      d. Feeling about information
   4. Viewing or hearing primal scene—reaction?
   5. Viewing sex play or intercourse of person other than parent
   6. Viewing sex between pets or other animals
 B. Childhood sex activities
   1. Genital self-stimulation before adolescence; age? reaction if apprehended?
   2. Awareness of self as boy or girl; bathroom sensual activities? (regarding urine, feces, odor, enemas)
   3. Sexual play or exploration with another child (playing doctor)—type of activity (e.g., looking, manual touching, genital touching); reactions or consequences if apprehended (by whom?)

IV. Adolescence
 A. Age of onset of puberty—development of secondary sex characteristics, age of menarche for girl, wet dreams or first ejaculation for boy (preparation for and reaction to)
 B. Sense of self as feminine or masculine—body image, acceptance by peers (opposite sex and same sex), sense of sexual desirability, onset of coital fantasies
 C. Sex activities
   1. Masturbation—age begun; ever punished or prohibited? method used, accompanying fantasies, frequency (questions about masturbation and fantasies are among the most sensitive for patients to answer)
   2. Homosexual activities—ongoing or rare and experimental episodes, approached by others? If homosexual, has there been any heterosexual experimentation?
   3. Dating—casual or steady, description of first crush, infatuation, or first love
   4. Experiences of kissing, necking, petting ("making out" or "fooling around"), age begun, frequency, number of partners, circumstances, type(s) of activity
   5. Orgasm—when first experienced? (may not be experienced during adolescence), with masturbation, during sleep, or with partner? with intercourse or other sex play? frequency?
   6. First coitus—age, circumstances, partner, reactions (may not be experienced during adolescence); contraception and/or safe sex precautions used

V. Adult sexual activities (may be experienced by some adolescents)
 A. Premarital sex
   1. Types of sex play experiences—frequency of sexual interactions, types and number of partners
   2. Contraception and/or safe sex precautions used
   3. First coitus (if not experienced in adolescence) age, circumstances, partner
   4. Cohabitation—age begun, duration, description of partner, sexual fidelity, types of sexual activity, frequency, satisfaction, number of cohabiting relationships, reasons for breakup(s)
   5. Engagement—age, activity during engagement period with fiancé(e), with others; length of engagement
 B. Marriage (if multiple marriages have occurred, explore sexual activity, reasons for marriage, and reasons for divorce in each marriage)
   1. Types and frequency of sexual interaction—describe typical sexual interaction (see above), satisfaction with sex life? view of partner's feeling
   2. First sexual experience with spouse—when? what were the circumstances? was it satisfying? disappointing?
   3. Honeymoon—setting, duration, pleasant or unpleasant, sexually active? frequency? problems? compatibility?
   4. Effect of pregnancies and children on marital sex
   5. Extramarital sex—number of incidents, partner; emotional attachment to extramarital partners? feelings about extramarital sex
   6. Postmarital masturbation—frequency? effect on marital sex?
   7. Extramarital sex by partner—effect on interviewee
   8. Ménage à trois or multiple sex (swinging)
   9. Areas of conflict in marriage (e.g., parenting, finances, division of responsibilities, priorities)

VI. Sex after widowhood, separation, divorce—celibacy, orgasms in sleep, masturbation, noncoital sex play, intercourse (number of and relationship to partners), other

VII. Special issues
 A. History of rape, incest, sexual or physical abuse
 B. Spousal abuse (current)
 C. Chronic illness (physical or psychiatric)
 D. History or presence of sexually transmitted diseases
 E. Fertility problems
 F. Abortions, miscarriages, or unwanted or illegitimate pregnancies
 G. Gender identity conflict—(e.g., transsexualism, wearing clothes of opposite sex)
 H. Paraphilias—(e.g., fetishes, voyeurism, sadomasochism)

References

Freud S. Letter to an American mother. *Am J Psychiatry.* 1951;102:786.

Freud S. Three essays on the theory of sexuality. In: *Standard Edition of the Complete Psychological Works of Sigmund Freud.* Vol 16. London: Hogarth Press; 1966:135.

Freud S. General theory of the neuroses. In: *Standard Edition of the Complete Psychological Works of Sigmund Freud.* Vol 16. London: Hogarth Press; 1966:241.

Harlow HF. The nature of love. *Am Psychol.* 1958;13:673.

Hawkins DM. Group psychotherapy with gay men and lesbians. In: Kaplan HI, Sadock BJ, editors. *Comprehensive Group Psychotherapy.* 3rd ed. Baltimore: Williams & Wilkins; 1993:506.

Hobbs K, Bramwell R, May K. Sexuality, sexual behaviour and pregnancy. *Sex Marital Ther.* 1999;14:371.

Kaplan MJ. Approaching sexual issues in primary care. *Prim Care.* 2002;29:113.

Kinsey AC, Pomeroy WB, Martin CE. *Sexual Behavior in the Human Male.* Philadelphia: WB Saunders; 1948.

Kinsey AC, Pomeroy WB, Martin CE, Gebbard PH. *Sexual Behavior in the Human Female.* Philadelphia: WB Saunders; 1953.

Masters WH, Johnson VE. *Human Sexual Response.* Boston: Little, Brown & Co; 1966.

Money J, Ehrhardt AA. *Man and Woman/Boy and Girl.* Baltimore: Johns Hopkins University Press; 1972.

Rowland DL. Issues in the laboratory study of human sexual response: a synthesis for the nontechnical sexologist. *J Sex Res.* 1999;36:3.

Sadock VA. Normal human sexuality and sexual dysfunctions. In: Sadock BJ, Sadock VA, eds. *Kaplan & Sadock's Comprehensive Textbook of Psychiatry.* 7th ed. Vol 1. Baltimore: Lippincott Williams & Wilkins; 2000;1577.

Sherfey MJ. *The Nature and Evolution of Female Sexuality.* New York: Random House; 1972.

Stein TS. Homosexuality and homosexual behavior. In: Sadock BJ, Sadock VA, eds. *Kaplan & Sadock's Comprehensive Textbook of Psychiatry.* 7th ed. Vol 1. Baltimore: Lippincott Williams & Wilkins; 2000;1608.

Stoller RJ. *Sex and Gender.* New York: Science House; 1968.

Wingood GM, DiClemente RJ, eds. *Handbook of Women's Sexual and Reproductive Health. Issues in Women's Health.* New York: Kluwer Academic/Plenum Publishers; 2002:303.

▲ 21.2 Abnormal Sexuality and Sexual Dysfunctions

In the text revision of the fourth edition of the *Diagnostic and Statistical Manual of Mental Disorders* (DSM-IV-TR), sexual dysfunctions are categorized as Axis I disorders. The syndromes listed are correlated with the sexual physiological response, which is divided into the four phases (Table 21.2–1). The essential feature of the sexual dysfunctions is inhibition in one or more of the phases, including disturbance in the subjective sense of pleasure or desire or in the objective performance. Either type of disturbance can occur alone or in combination. Sexual dysfunctions are diagnoses only when they are a major part of the clinical picture. They can be lifelong or acquired, generalized or situational, and due to psychological factors, physiological factors, or combined factors. If they are attributable entirely to a general medical condition, substance use, or adverse effects of medication, then sexual dysfunction due to a general medical condition or substance-induced sexual dysfunction is diagnosed. Sexual dysfunctions not associated with the sexual response cycle are listed in Table 21.2–2.

With the possible exception of premature ejaculation, sexual dysfunctions are rarely found separate from other psychiatric syndromes. Sexual disorders may lead to or result from relational problems, and patients invariably develop an increasing fear of failure and self-consciousness about their sexual performance. Sexual dysfunctions are frequently associated with other mental disorders, such as depressive disorders, anxiety disorders, personality disorders, and schizophrenia. In many instances, a sexual dysfunction may be diagnosed in conjunction with another psychiatric disorder; in other cases, however, it is only one of many signs or symptoms of the psychiatric disorder.

In DSM-IV-TR a *sexual dysfunction* is defined as a disturbance in the sexual response cycle or as pain with sexual intercourse. Seven major categories of sexual dysfunction are listed in DSM-IV-TR: sexual desire disorders, sexual arousal disorders, orgasm disorders, sexual pain disorders, sexual dysfunction caused by a general medical condition, substance-induced sexual dysfunction, and sexual dysfunction not otherwise specified.

Sexual dysfunctions can be symptomatic of biological (biogenic) problems or intrapsychic or interpersonal (psychogenic) conflicts or a combination of these factors. Sexual function can

Table 21.2–1
DSM-IV-TR Phases of the Sexual Response Cycle and Associated Sexual Dysfunctions[a]

Phases	Characteristics	Dysfunction
1. Desire	Distinct from any identified solely through physiology and reflects the patient's motivations, drives, and personality; characterized by sexual fantasies and the desire to have sex	Hypoactive sexual desire disorder; sexual aversion disorder; hypoactive sexual desire disorder due to a general medical condition (male or female); substance-induced sexual dysfunction with impaired desire
2. Excitement	Subjective sense of sexual pleasure and accompanying physiological changes; all physiological responses noted in Masters and Johnson's excitement and plateau phases are combined in this phase	Female sexual arousal disorder; male erectile disorder (may also occur in stages 3 and 4); male erectile disorder due to a general medical condition; dyspareunia due to a general medical condition (male or female); substance-induced sexual dysfunction with impaired arousal
3. Orgasm	Peaking of sexual pleasure, with release of sexual tension and rhythmic contraction of the perineal muscles and pelvic reproductive organs	Female orgasmic disorder; male orgasmic disorder; premature ejaculation; other sexual dysfunction due to a general medical condition (male or female); substance-induced sexual dysfunction with impaired orgasm
4. Resolution	A sense of general relaxation, well-being, and muscle relaxation; men are refractory to orgasm for a period of time that increases with age, whereas women can have multiple orgasms without a refractory period	Postcoital dysphoria; postcoital headache

[a]DSM-IV-TR consolidates the Masters and Johnson excitement and plateau phases into a single excitement phase, which is preceded by the desire (appetitive) phase. The orgasm and resolution phases remain the same as originally described by Masters and Johnson.

Table 21.2–2
Sexual Dysfunction Not Correlated with Phases of the Sexual Response Cycle

Category	Dysfunctions
Sexual pain disorders	Vaginismus (female) Dyspareunia (female and male)
Other	Sexual dysfunctions not otherwise specified Examples: 1. No erotic sensation despite normal physiological response to sexual stimulation (e.g., orgasmic anhedonia) 2. Female analogue of premature ejaculation 3. Genital pain occurring during masturbation

be adversely affected by stress of any kind, by emotional disorders, or by ignorance of sexual function and physiology. The dysfunction may be lifelong or acquired—that is, it can develop after a period of normal functioning. The dysfunction may be generalized or limited to a specific partner or a certain situation.

In considering each of the disorders, clinicians need to rule out an acquired medical condition and the use of a pharmacological substance that could account for, or contribute to, the dysfunction. If the disorder is biogenic, it is coded on Axis III unless there is substantial evidence of dysfunctional episodes apart from the onset of physiological or pharmacological influences. In some cases a patient suffers from more than one dysfunction—for example, premature ejaculation and male erectile disorder.

SEXUAL DESIRE DISORDERS

Sexual desire disorders are divided into two classes: hypoactive sexual desire disorder, characterized by a deficiency or absence of sexual fantasies and desire for sexual activity (Table 21.2–3); and sexual aversion disorder, characterized by an aversion to, and avoidance of, genital sexual contact with a sexual partner or by masturbation (Table 21.2–4). The former condition is more common than the latter and more common among women than among men. An estimated 20 percent of persons have hypoactive sexual desire disorder.

A variety of causative factors are associated with sexual desire disorders. Patients with desire problems often use inhibition of desire defensively, to protect against unconscious fears about sex. Sigmund Freud conceptualized low sexual desire as the result of inhibition during the phallic psychosexual phase of development and of unresolved oedipal conflicts. Some men, fixated at the phallic state of development, are fearful of the vagina and believe that they will be castrated if they approach it. Freud called this concept *vagina dentata;* because men unconsciously believe that the vagina has teeth, they avoid contact with the female genitalia. Equally, women may suffer from unresolved developmental conflicts that inhibit desire. Lack of desire can also result from chronic stress, anxiety, or depression.

Abstinence from sex for a prolonged period sometimes results in suppression of sexual impulses. Loss of desire may also be an expression of hostility to a partner or the sign of a deteriorating relationship. In one study of young married couples who ceased having sexual relations for 2 months, marital discord was the reason most frequently given for the cessation or inhibition of sexual activity.

The presence of desire depends on several factors: biological drive, adequate self-esteem, the ability to accept oneself as a sexual person, previous good experiences with sex, the avail-

Table 21.2–3
DSM-IV-TR Diagnostic Criteria for Hypoactive Sexual Desire Disorder

A. Persistently or recurrently deficient (or absent) sexual fantasies and desire for sexual activity. The judgment of deficiency or absence is made by the clinician, taking into account factors that affect sexual functioning, such as age and the context of the person's life.
B. The disturbance causes marked distress or interpersonal difficulty.
C. The sexual dysfunction is not better accounted for by another Axis I disorder (except another sexual dysfunction) and is not due exclusively to the direct physiological effects of a substance (e.g., a drug of abuse, a medication) or a general medical condition.

Specify type:
Lifelong type
Acquired type

Specify type:
Generalized type
Situational type

Specify:
Due to psychological factors
Due to combined factors

Table 21.2–4
DSM-IV-TR Diagnostic Criteria for Sexual Aversion Disorder

A. Persistent or recurrent extreme aversion to, and avoidance of, all (or almost all) genital sexual contact with a sexual partner.
B. The disturbance causes marked distress or interpersonal difficulty.
C. The sexual dysfunction is not better accounted for by another Axis I disorder (except another sexual dysfunction).

Specify type:
Lifelong type
Acquired type

Specify type:
Situational type
Generalized type

Specify:
Due to psychological factors
Due to combined factors

ability of an appropriate partner, and a good relationship in nonsexual areas with a partner. Damage to, or absence of, any of these factors may result in diminished desire.

In making the diagnosis, clinicians must evaluate a patient's age, general health, and life stresses and must attempt to establish a baseline of sexual interest before the disorder began. The need for sexual contact and satisfaction varies among persons and over time in any given person. In a group of 100 couples with stable marriages, 8 percent reported having intercourse less than once a month. In another group of couples, one third reported episodic lack of sexual relations for periods averaging 8 weeks. Married couples have coitus three times a month, on average. The diagnosis should not be made unless the lack of desire is a source of distress to a patient.

SEXUAL AROUSAL DISORDERS

The sexual arousal disorders are divided by DSM-IV-TR into female sexual arousal disorder, characterized by the persistent or recurrent partial or complete failure to attain or maintain the lubrication-swelling response of sexual excitement until the completion of the sexual act (Table 21.2–5), and male erectile disorder, characterized by the recurrent and persistent partial or complete failure to attain or maintain an erection to perform the sex act (Table 21.2–6). The diagnosis takes into account the focus, intensity, and duration of the sexual activity in which patients engage. If sexual stimulation is inadequate in focus, intensity, or duration, the diagnosis should not be made.

Female Sexual Arousal Disorder

The prevalence of female sexual arousal disorder is generally underestimated. Women who have excitement-phase dysfunction often have orgasm problems as well. In one study of relatively happily married couples, 33 percent of the women described difficulty maintaining sexual excitement. Many psychological factors (e.g., anxiety, guilt, and fear) are associated with female sexual arousal disorder. In many women, excitement-phase disorders are associated with dyspareunia and with lack of desire.

Table 21.2–5
DSM-IV-TR Diagnostic Criteria for Female Sexual Arousal Disorder

A. Persistent or recurrent inability to attain, or to maintain until completion of the sexual activity, an adequate lubrication-swelling response of sexual excitement.

B. The disturbance causes marked distress or interpersonal difficulty.

C. The sexual dysfunction is not better accounted for by another Axis I disorder (except another sexual dysfunction) and is not due exclusively to the direct physiological effects of a substance (e.g., a drug of abuse, a medication) or a general medical condition.

Specify type:
Lifelong type
Acquired type

Specify type:
Generalized type
Situational type

Specify:
Due to psychological factors
Due to combined factors

From American Psychiatric Association. *Diagnostic and Statistical Manual of Mental Disorders.* 4th ed. Text rev. Washington, DC: American Psychiatric Association; copyright 2000, with permission.

Table 21.2–6
DSM-IV-TR Diagnostic Criteria for Male Erectile Disorder

A. Persistent or recurrent inability to attain, or to maintain until completion of the sexual activity, an adequate erection.

B. The disturbance causes marked distress or interpersonal difficulty.

C. The erectile dysfunction is not better accounted for by another Axis I disorder (other than a sexual dysfunction) and is not due exclusively to the direct physiological effects of a substance (e.g., a drug of abuse, a medication) or a general medical condition.

Specify type:
Lifelong type
Acquired type

Specify type:
Generalized type
Situational type

Specify:
Due to psychological factors
Due to combined factors

From American Psychiatric Association. *Diagnostic and Statistical Manual of Mental Disorders.* 4th ed. Text rev. Washington, DC: American Psychiatric Association; copyright 2000, with permission.

Physiological studies of sexual dysfunctions indicate that a hormonal pattern may contribute to responsiveness in women who have excitement-phase dysfunction. William Masters and Virginia Johnson found women particularly desirous of sex before the onset of the menses. Other women report feeling the greatest sexual excitement immediately after the menses or at the time of ovulation. Alterations in testosterone, estrogen, prolactin, and thyroxin levels have been implicated in female sexual arousal disorder. Also, medications with antihistaminic or anticholinergic properties cause a decrease in vaginal lubrication. Some evidence indicates that women who are dysfunctional are less aware of the physiological arousal of their bodies and experience less warmth or less sensation in the genitalia.

Male Erectile Disorder

Male erectile disorder is also called erectile dysfunction and impotence. A man with lifelong male erectile disorder has never been able to obtain an erection sufficient for vaginal insertion. In acquired male erectile disorder a man has successfully achieved vaginal penetration at some time in his sexual life but is later unable to do so. In situational male erectile disorder a man is able to have coitus in certain circumstances but not in others; for example, he may function effectively with a prostitute but be impotent with his wife.

Acquired male erectile disorder has been reported in 10 to 20 percent of all men. Freud declared it common among his

patients. Impotence is the chief complaint of more than 50 percent of all men treated for sexual disorders. Lifelong male erectile disorder is rare; it occurs in about 1 percent of men under age 35, but the incidence increases with age. It has been reported in about 8 percent of the young adult population. Alfred Kinsey reported that 75 percent of all men were impotent at age 80. All men over 40, Masters and Johnson reported, have a fear of impotence, which the researchers believe reflects the masculine fear of loss of virility with advancing age. Male erectile disorder, however, is not universal in aging men; having an available sex partner is related to continuing potency, as is a history of consistent sexual activity and the absence of vascular disease.

The causes of male erectile disorder may be organic or psychological or a combination of both, but in young and middle-aged men the cause is usually psychological. A good history is of primary importance in determining the cause of the dysfunction. If a man reports having spontaneous erections at times when he does not plan to have intercourse, having morning erections, or having good erections with masturbation or with partners other than his usual one, the organic causes of his impotence can be considered negligible, and costly diagnostic procedures can be avoided. Male erectile disorder caused by a general medical condition or a pharmacological substance is discussed below in this section.

Freud ascribed one type of impotence to an inability to reconcile feelings of affection toward a woman with feelings of desire for her. Men with such conflicting feelings can function only with women whom they see as degraded (Madonna = Putana complex). Other factors that have been cited as contributing to impotence include a punitive superego, an inability to trust, and feelings of inadequacy or a sense of being undesirable as a partner. A man may be unable to express a sexual impulse because of fear, anxiety, anger, or moral prohibition. In an ongoing relationship, impotence may reflect difficulties between the partners, particularly when a man cannot communicate his needs or his anger in a direct and constructive way. In addition, episodes of impotence are reinforcing, with the man becoming increasingly anxious before each sexual encounter.

ORGASM DISORDERS

Female Orgasmic Disorder

Female orgasmic disorder, sometimes called inhibited female orgasm or anorgasmia, is defined as the recurrent or persistent inhibition of female orgasm, as manifested by the recurrent delay in, or absence of, orgasm after a normal sexual excitement phase that a clinician judges to be adequate in focus, intensity, and duration—in short, a woman's inability to achieve orgasm by masturbation or coitus (Table 21.2–7). Women who can achieve orgasm by one of these methods are not necessarily categorized as anorgasmic, although some sexual inhibition may be postulated.

Research on the physiology of the female sexual response has shown that orgasms caused by clitoral stimulation and those caused by vaginal stimulation are physiologically identical. Freud's theory that women must give up clitoral sensitivity for vaginal sensitivity to achieve sexual maturity is now considered misleading, but some women report that they gain a special sense of satisfaction from an orgasm precipitated by coitus.

Table 21.2–7
DSM-IV-TR Diagnostic Criteria for Female Orgasmic Disorder

A. Persistent or recurrent delay in, or absence of, orgasm following a normal sexual excitement phase. Women exhibit wide variability in the type or intensity of stimulation that triggers orgasm. The diagnosis of female orgasmic disorder should be based on the clinician's judgment that the woman's orgasmic capacity is less than would be reasonable for her age, sexual experience, and the adequacy of sexual stimulation she receives.

B. The disturbance causes marked distress or interpersonal difficulty.

C. The orgasmic dysfunction is not better accounted for by another Axis I disorder (except another sexual dysfunction) and is not due exclusively to the direct physiological effects of a substance (e.g., a drug of abuse, a medication) or a general medical condition.

Specify type:
Lifelong type
Acquired type

Specify type:
Generalized type
Situational type

Specify:
Due to psychological factors
Due to combined factors

From American Psychiatric Association. *Diagnostic and Statistical Manual of Mental Disorders.* 4th ed. Text rev. Washington, DC: American Psychiatric Association; copyright 2000, with permission.

Some researchers attribute this satisfaction to the psychological feeling of closeness engendered by the act of coitus, but others maintain that the coital orgasm is a physiologically different experience. Many women achieve orgasm during coitus by a combination of manual clitoral stimulation and penile vaginal stimulation.

A woman with lifelong female orgasmic disorder has never experienced orgasm by any kind of stimulation. A woman with acquired orgasmic disorder has previously experienced at least one orgasm, regardless of the circumstances or means of stimulation, whether by masturbation or while dreaming during sleep. Kinsey found that only 5 percent of married women over 35 years of age had never achieved orgasm by any means. The incidence of orgasm increases with age. According to Kinsey, the first orgasm occurs during adolescence in about 50 percent of women as a result of masturbation or genital caressing with a partner; the rest usually experience orgasm as they get older. Lifelong female orgasmic disorder is more common among unmarried women than married women. Increased orgasmic potential in women over 35 has been explained on the basis of less psychological inhibition, greater sexual experience, or both.

Acquired female orgasmic disorder is a common complaint in clinical populations. One clinical treatment facility reported having about four times as many nonorgasmic women in its practice as patients with all other sexual disorders. In another study, 46 percent of women complained of difficulty reaching orgasm. The true prevalence of problems maintaining excitement is not known, but inhibition of excitement and orgasmic problems often

occur together. The overall prevalence of female orgasmic disorder from all causes is estimated to be 30 percent.

Numerous psychological factors are associated with female orgasmic disorder. They include fears of impregnation, rejection by a sex partner, and damage to the vagina; hostility toward men; and feelings of guilt about sexual impulses. Some women equate orgasm with loss of control or with aggressive, destructive, or violent impulses; their fear of these impulses may be expressed through inhibition of excitement or orgasm. Cultural expectations and social restrictions on women are also relevant. Many women have grown up to believe that sexual pleasure is not a natural entitlement for so-called decent women. Nonorgasmic women may be otherwise symptom free or may experience frustration in a variety of ways; they may have such pelvic complaints as lower abdominal pain, itching, and vaginal discharge, as well as increased tension, irritability, and fatigue.

Male Orgasmic Disorder

In male orgasmic disorder, sometimes called inhibited orgasm or retarded ejaculation, a man achieves ejaculation during coitus with great difficulty, if at all (Table 21.2–8). A man with lifelong orgasmic disorder has never been able to ejaculate during coitus. The disorder is diagnosed as acquired if it develops after previously normal functioning. Some researchers think that orgasm and ejaculation should be differentiated, especially in the case of men who ejaculate but complain of a decreased or absent subjective sense of pleasure during the orgasmic experience (orgasmic anhedonia).

The incidence of male orgasmic disorder is much lower than the incidence of premature ejaculation or impotence. Masters and Johnson reported an incidence of male orgasmic disorder of only 3.8 percent in one group of 447 men with sexual dysfunctions. A general prevalence of 5 percent has been reported.

Lifelong male orgasmic disorder indicates severe psychopathology. A man may come from a rigid, puritanical background; he may perceive sex as sinful and the genitals as dirty; and he may have conscious or unconscious incest wishes and guilt. He usually has difficulty with closeness in areas beyond those of sexual relations. In a few cases the condition is aggravated by an attention-deficit disorder. A man's distractibility prevents sufficient arousal for climax to occur.

In an ongoing relationship, acquired male orgasmic disorder frequently reflects interpersonal difficulties. The disorder may be a man's way of coping with real or fantasized changes in the relationship, such as plans for pregnancy about which the man is ambivalent, the loss of sexual attraction to the partner, or demands by the partner for greater commitment as expressed by sexual performance. In some men the inability to ejaculate reflects unexpressed hostility toward a woman. The problem is more common among men with obsessive-compulsive disorder than among others.

Premature Ejaculation

In premature ejaculation men persistently or recurrently achieve orgasm and ejaculation before they wish to. There is no definite time frame within which to define the dysfunction; the diagnosis is made when a man regularly ejaculates before or immediately after entering the vagina. Clinicians need to consider factors that affect the duration of the excitement phase, such as age, the novelty of the sex partner, and the frequency and duration of coitus (Table 21.2–9). Masters and Johnson conceptualized the disorder

Table 21.2–8 DSM-IV-TR Diagnostic Criteria for Male Orgasmic Disorder

A. Persistent or recurrent delay in, or absence of, orgasm following a normal sexual excitement phase during sexual activity that the clinician, taking into account the person's age, judges to be adequate in focus, intensity, and duration.
B. The disturbance causes marked distress or interpersonal difficulty.
C. The orgasmic dysfunction is not better accounted for by another Axis I disorder (except another sexual dysfunction) and is not due exclusively to the direct physiological effects of a substance (e.g., a drug of abuse, a medication) or a general medical condition.

Specify type:
Lifelong type
Acquired type

Specify type:
Generalized type
Situational type

Specify:
Due to psychological factors
Due to combined factors

From American Psychiatric Association. *Diagnostic and Statistical Manual of Mental Disorders.* 4th ed. Text rev. Washington, DC: American Psychiatric Association; copyright 2000, with permission.

Table 21.2–9 DSM-IV-TR Diagnostic Criteria for Premature Ejaculation

A. Persistent or recurrent ejaculation with minimal sexual stimulation before, on, or shortly after penetration and before the person wishes it. The clinician must take into account factors that affect duration of the excitement phase, such as age, novelty of the sexual partner or situation, and recent frequency of sexual activity.
B. The disturbance causes marked distress or interpersonal difficulty.
C. The premature ejaculation is not due exclusively to the direct effects of a substance (e.g., withdrawal from opioids).

Specify type:
Lifelong type
Acquired type

Specify type:
Generalized type
Situational type

Specify:
Due to psychological factors
Due to combined factors

From American Psychiatric Association. *Diagnostic and Statistical Manual of Mental Disorders.* 4th ed. Text rev. Washington, DC: American Psychiatric Association; copyright 2000, with permission.

in terms of the couple and considered a man a premature ejaculator if he could not control ejaculation long enough during intravaginal containment to satisfy his partner in at least half their episodes of coitus. This definition assumes that the female partner is capable of an orgasmic response. Like the other dysfunctions, premature ejaculation is not diagnosed when it is caused exclusively by organic factors or when it is not symptomatic of any other clinical psychiatric syndrome.

Premature ejaculation is more commonly reported among college-educated men than among men with less education. The complaint is thought to be related to their concern for partner satisfaction, but the true cause of this increased frequency has not been determined. Premature ejaculation is the chief complaint of about 35 to 40 percent of men treated for sexual disorders. Some researchers divide men who experience premature ejaculation into two groups: those who are physiologically predisposed to climax quickly because of shorter nerve latency time and those with a psychogenic or behaviorally conditioned cause. Difficulty in ejaculatory control may be associated with anxiety regarding the sex act, with unconscious fears about the vagina, or with negative cultural conditioning. Men whose early sexual contacts occurred largely with prostitutes who demanded that the sex act proceed quickly or whose sexual contacts took place in situations in which discovery would be embarrassing (e.g., in the back seat of a car or in the parental home) might have been conditioned to achieve orgasm rapidly. With young, inexperienced men, who are more likely to have the problem, it may resolve in time. In ongoing relationships the partner has a great influence on a premature ejaculator, and a stressful marriage exacerbates the disorder. The developmental background and the psychodynamics found in premature ejaculation and in impotence are similar.

SEXUAL PAIN DISORDERS

Dyspareunia

Dyspareunia is recurrent or persistent genital pain occurring in either men or women before, during, or after intercourse. Much more common in women than in men, dyspareunia is related to, and often coincides with, vaginismus. Repeated episodes of vaginismus may lead to dyspareunia and vice versa; in either case, somatic causes must be ruled out. Dyspareunia should not be diagnosed when an organic basis for the pain is found or when, in a woman, it is caused exclusively by vaginismus or by a lack of lubrication (Table 21.2–10). The incidence of dyspareunia is unknown.

In most cases, dynamic factors are considered causative. Chronic pelvic pain is a common complaint in women with a history of rape or childhood sexual abuse. Painful coitus may result from tension and anxiety about the sex act that cause women to involuntarily contract their vaginal muscles. The pain is real and makes intercourse unpleasant or unbearable. Anticipation of further pain may cause women to avoid coitus altogether. If a partner proceeds with intercourse regardless of a woman's state of readiness, the condition is aggravated. Dyspareunia can also occur in men, but it is uncommon and is usually associated with an organic condition, such as herpes, prostatitis, or Peyronie's disease, which consists of sclerotic plaques on the penis that cause penile curvature.

Table 21.2–10
DSM-IV-TR Diagnostic Criteria for Dyspareunia

A. Recurrent or persistent genital pain associated with sexual intercourse in either a male or a female.
B. The disturbance causes marked distress or interpersonal difficulty.
C. The disturbance is not caused exclusively by vaginismus or lack of lubrication, is not better accounted for by another Axis I disorder (except another sexual dysfunction), and is not due exclusively to the direct physiological effects of a substance (e.g., a drug of abuse, a medication) or a general medical condition.

Specify type:
- **Lifelong type**
- **Acquired type**

Specify type:
- **Generalized type**
- **Situational type**

Specify:
- **Due to psychological factors**
- **Due to combined factors**

From American Psychiatric Association. *Diagnostic and Statistical Manual of Mental Disorders.* 4th ed. Text rev. Washington, DC: American Psychiatric Association; copyright 2000, with permission.

Vaginismus

Vaginismus is an involuntary muscle constriction of the outer third of the vagina that interferes with penile insertion and intercourse. This response may occur during a gynecological examination when involuntary vaginal constriction prevents the introduction of the speculum into the vagina. The diagnosis is not made when the dysfunction is caused exclusively by organic factors or when it is symptomatic of another Axis I mental disorder (Table 21.2–11).

Table 21.2–11
DSM-IV-TR Diagnostic Criteria for Vaginismus

A. Recurrent or persistent involuntary spasm of the musculature of the outer third of the vagina that interferes with sexual intercourse.
B. The disturbance causes marked distress or interpersonal difficulty.
C. The disturbance is not better accounted for by another Axis I disorder (e.g., somatization disorder) and is not due exclusively to the direct physiological effects of a general medical condition.

Specify type:
- **Lifelong type**
- **Acquired type**

Specify type:
- **Generalized type**
- **Situational type**

Specify:
- **Due to psychological factors**
- **Due to combined factors**

From American Psychiatric Association. *Diagnostic and Statistical Manual of Mental Disorders.* 4th ed. Text rev. Washington, DC: American Psychiatric Association; copyright 2000, with permission.

Vaginismus is less prevalent than female orgasmic disorder. It most often afflicts highly educated women and those in high socioeconomic groups. Women with vaginismus may consciously wish to have coitus but unconsciously wish to keep a penis from entering their bodies. A sexual trauma such as rape may cause vaginismus; women with psychosexual conflicts may perceive the penis as a weapon. In some cases, pain or the anticipation of pain at the first coital experience causes vaginismus. Clinicians have noted that a strict religious upbringing in which sex is associated with sin is frequent in these patients. Other women have problems in dyadic relationships; if women feel emotionally abused by their partners, they may protest in this nonverbal fashion.

SEXUAL DYSFUNCTION DUE TO A GENERAL MEDICAL CONDITION

The category sexual dysfunction due to a general medical condition covers sexual dysfunction that results in marked distress and interpersonal difficulty; the history, physical examination, or laboratory findings must provide evidence of a general medical condition judged to be causally related to the sexual dysfunction (Table 21.2–12).

Table 21.2–12
DSM-IV-TR Diagnostic Criteria for Sexual Dysfunction Due to a General Medical Condition

A. Clinically significant sexual dysfunction that results in marked distress or interpersonal difficulty predominates in the clinical picture.

B. There is evidence from the history, physical examination, or laboratory findings that the sexual dysfunction is fully explained by the direct physiological effects of a general medical condition.

C. The disturbance is not better accounted for by another mental disorder (e.g., major depressive disorder).

Select code and term based on the predominant sexual dysfunction:

Female hypoactive sexual desire disorder due to ... [indicate the general medical condition]: if deficient or absent sexual desire is the predominant feature

Male hypoactive sexual desire disorder due to ... [indicate the general medical condition]: if deficient or absent sexual desire is the predominant feature

Male erectile disorder due to ... [indicate the general medical condition]: if male erectile dysfunction is the predominant feature

Female dyspareunia due to ... [indicate the general medical condition]: if pain associated with intercourse is the predominant feature

Male dyspareunia due to ... [indicate the general medical condition]: if pain associated with intercourse is the predominant feature

Other female sexual dysfunction due to ... [indicate the general medical condition]: if some other feature is predominant (e.g., orgasmic disorder) or no feature predominates

Other male sexual dysfunction due to ... [indicate the general medical condition]: if some other feature is predominant (e.g., orgasmic disorder) or no feature predominates

Coding note: Include the name of the general medical condition on Axis I, e.g., male erectile disorder due to diabetes mellitus; also code the general medical condition on Axis III.

From American Psychiatric Association. *Diagnostic and Statistical Manual of Mental Disorders.* 4th ed. Text rev. Washington, DC: American Psychiatric Association; copyright 2000, with permission.

Male Erectile Disorder Due to a General Medical Condition

The incidence of psychological, as opposed to organic, male erectile disorder has been the focus of many studies. Statistics indicate that 20 to 50 percent of men with erectile disorder have an organic basis for the disorder. The organic causes of male erectile disorder are listed in Table 21.2–13. Side effects of medication may impair male sexual functioning in a variety of ways (Table 21.2–14). Castration (removal of the testes) does not always lead to sexual dysfunction, as erection may still occur. A reflex arc, fired when the inner thigh is stimulated, passes through the sacral cord erectile center to account for the phenomenon.

A number of procedures, benign and invasive, are used to help differentiate organically caused impotence from functional impotence. The procedures include monitoring nocturnal penile tumescence (erections that occur during sleep), normally associated with rapid eye movement; monitoring tumescence with a strain gauge; measuring blood pressure in the penis with a penile plethysmograph or an ultrasound (Doppler) flowmeter, both of which assess blood flow in the internal pudendal artery; and measuring pudendal nerve latency time. Other diagnostic tests that delineate organic bases for impotence include glucose tolerance tests, plasma hormone assays, liver and thyroid function tests, prolactin and follicle-stimulating hormone (FHS) determinations, and cystometric examinations. Invasive diagnostic studies include penile arteriography, infusion cavernosonography, and radioactive xenon penography. Invasive procedures require expert interpretation and are used only for patients who are candidates for vascular reconstructive procedures.

Dyspareunia Due to a General Medical Condition

An estimated 30 percent of all surgical procedures on the female genital area result in temporary dyspareunia. In addition, 30 to 40 percent of women with the complaint who are seen in sex therapy clinics have pelvic pathology. Organic abnormalities leading to dyspareunia and vaginismus include irritated or infected hymenal remnants, episiotomy scars, Bartholin's gland infection, various forms of vaginitis and cervicitis, and endometriosis. Postcoital pain has been reported by women with myomata and endometriosis and is attributed to the uterine contractions during orgasm. Postmenopausal women may have dyspareunia resulting from thinning of the vaginal mucosa and reduced lubrication.

Two conditions not readily apparent on physical examination that produce dyspareunia are vulvar vestibulitis and interstitial cystitis. The former may present with chronic vulvar pain and the latter produces pain most intensely following orgasm. Dyspareunia can also occur in men, but it is uncommon and is usually associated with an organic condition, such as Peyronie's disease, which consists of sclerotic plaques on the penis that cause penile curvature.

Table 21.2–13
Diseases and Other Medical Conditions Implicated in Male Erectile Disorder

Infectious and parasitic diseases
- Elephantiasis
- Mumps

Cardiovascular disease[a]
- Atherosclerotic disease
- Aortic aneurysm
- Leriche's syndrome
- Cardiac failure

Renal and urological disorders
- Peyronie's disease
- Chronic renal failure
- Hydrocele and varicocele

Hepatic disorders
- Cirrhosis (usually associated with alcohol dependence)

Pulmonary disorders
- Respiratory failure

Genetics
- Klinefelter's syndrome
- Congenital penile vascular and structural abnormalities

Nutritional disorders
- Malnutrition
- Vitamin deficiencies

Endocrine disorders[a]
- Diabetes mellitus
- Dysfunction of the pituitary-adrenal-testis axis
- Acromegaly
- Addison's disease
- Chromophobe adenoma
- Adrenal neoplasia
- Myxedema
- Hyperthyroidism

Neurological disorders
- Multiple sclerosis
- Transverse myelitis
- Parkinson's disease
- Temporal lobe epilepsy
- Traumatic and neoplastic spinal cord diseases[a]
- Central nervous system tumor
- Amyotrophic lateral sclerosis
- Peripheral neuropathy
- General paresis
- Tabes dorsalis

Pharmacological factors
- Alcohol and other dependence-inducing substances (heroin, methadone, morphine, cocaine, amphetamines, and barbiturates)
- Prescribed drugs (psychotropic drugs, antihypertensive drugs, estrogens, and antiandrogens)

Poisoning
- Lead (plumbism)
- Herbicides

Surgical procedures[a]
- Perineal prostatectomy
- Abdominal-perineal colon resection
- Sympathectomy (frequently interferes with ejaculation)
- Aortoiliac surgery
- Radical cystectomy
- Retroperitoneal lymphadenectomy

Miscellaneous
- Radiation therapy
- Pelvic fracture
- Any severe systemic disease or debilitating condition

[a]In the United States an estimated 2 million men are impotent because they suffer from diabetes mellitus; an additional 300,000 are impotent because of other endocrine diseases; 1.5 million are impotent as a result of vascular disease; 180,000 because of multiple sclerosis; 400,000 because of traumas and fractures leading to pelvic fractures or spinal cord injuries; and another 650,000 are impotent as a result of radical surgery, including prostatectomies, colostomies, and cystectomies.

Table 21.2–14
Some Pharmacological Agents Implicated in Male Sexual Dysfunctions

Drug	Impairs Erection	Impairs Ejaculation
Psychiatric drugs		
Cyclic drugs[a]		
Imipramine (Tofranil)	+	+
Protriptyline (Vivactil)	+	+
Desipramine (Pertofrane)	+	+
Clomipramine (Anafranil)	+	+
Amitriptyline (Elavil)	+	+
Trazodone (Desyrel)[b]	–	–
Monoamine oxidase inhibitors		
Tranylcypromine (Parnate)	+	
Phenelzine (Nardil)	+	+
Pargyline (Eutonyl)	–	+
Isocarboxazid (Marplan)	–	+
Other mood-active drugs		
Lithium (Eskalith)	+	
Amphetamines	+	+
Fluoxetine (Prozac)[e]	–	+
Antipsychotics[c]		
Fluphenazine (Prolixin)	+	
Thioridazine (Mellaril)	+	+
Chlorprothixene (Taractan)	–	+
Mesoridazine (Serentil)	–	+
Perphenazine (Trilafon)	–	+
Trifluoperazine (Stelazine)	–	+
Reserpine (Serpasil)	+	+
Haloperidol (Haldol)	–	+
Antianxiety agent[d]		
Chlordiazepoxide (Librium)	–	+
Antihypertensive drugs		
Clonidine (Catapres)	+	
Methyldopa (Aldomet)	+	+
Spironolactone (Aldactone)	+	–
Hydrochlorothiazide	+	–
Guanethidine (Ismelin)	+	+
Commonly abused substances		
Alcohol	+	+
Barbiturates	+	+
Cannabis	+	–
Cocaine	+	+
Heroin	+	+
Methadone	+	–
Morphine	+	+
Miscellaneous drugs		
Antiparkinsonian agents	+	+
Clofibrate (Atromid-S)	+	–
Digoxin (Lanoxin)	+	–
Glutethimide (Doriden)	+	+
Indomethacin (Indocin)	+	–
Phentolamine (Regitine)	–	+
Propranolol (Inderal)	+	–

[a]The incidence of male erectile disorder associated with the use of tricyclic drugs is low.
[b]Trazodone has been causative in some cases of priapism.
[c]Impairment of sexual function is not a common complication of the use of antipsychotics. Priapism has occasionally occurred in association with the use of antipsychotics.
[d]Benzodiazepines have been reported to decrease libido, but in some patients the diminution of anxiety caused by those drugs enhances sexual function.
[e]All selective serotonergic reuptake inhibitors can produce sexual dysfunction, more commonly, in men.

Table 21.2–15
Neurophysiology of Sexual Dysfunction

	DA	5-HT	NE	ACh	Clinical Correlation
Erection	↑	○	α, β ↓↑	M	Antipsychotics may lead to erectile dysfunction (DA block): DA agonists may lead to enhanced erection and libido; priapism with trazodone (α_1 block); β-blockers may lead to impotence
Ejaculation and orgasm	○	± ↓	α_1 ↑	M	α_1-Blockers (tricyclic drugs, MAOIs, thioridazine) may lead to impaired ejaculation; 5-HT agents may inhibit orgasm

↑, facilities; ↓, inhibits or decreases; ±, some; ACh, acetylcholine; DA, dopamine; 5-HT, serotonin; M, modulates; NE, norepinephrine; ○, minimal.
Reprinted with permission from Segraves R. *Psychiatric Times,* 1990.

Hypoactive Sexual Desire Disorder Due to a General Medical Condition

Desire commonly decreases after major illness or surgery, particularly when the body image is affected after such procedures as mastectomy, ileostomy, hysterectomy, and prostatectomy. Illnesses that deplete a person's energy, chronic conditions that require physical and psychological adaptation, and serious illnesses that may cause a person to become depressed can all markedly lessen sexual desire in both men and women.

In some cases, biochemical correlates are associated with hypoactive sexual desire disorder (Table 21.2–15). A recent study found markedly lower levels of serum testosterone in men complaining of low desire than in normal controls in a sleep-laboratory situation. Drugs that depress the central nervous system (CNS) or decrease testosterone production can decrease desire.

Other Male Sexual Dysfunction Due to a General Medical Condition

When another dysfunctional feature is predominant (e.g., orgasmic disorder) or when no feature predominates, the category other male sexual dysfunction due to a general medical condition is used.

Male orgasmic disorder may have physiological causes and can occur after surgery on the genitourinary tract, such as prostatectomy. It may also be associated with Parkinson's disease and other neurological disorders involving the lumbar or sacral sections of the spinal cord. The antihypertensive drug guanethidine monosulfate (Ismelin), methyldopa (Aldomet), the phenothiazines, the tricyclic drugs, and the selective serotonin reuptake inhibitors (SSRIs), among others, have been implicated in retarded ejaculation. Male orgasmic disorder must also be differentiated from retrograde ejaculation, in which ejaculation occurs but the seminal fluid passes backward into the bladder. Retrograde ejaculation always has an organic cause. It can develop after genitourinary surgery and is also associated with medications that have anticholinergic adverse effects, such as the phenothiazines, especially thioridazine (Mellaril).

Other Female Sexual Dysfunction Due to a General Medical Condition

Some medical conditions—specifically, endocrine diseases such as hypothyroidism, diabetes mellitus, and primary hyperprolactinemia—can affect a woman's ability to have orgasms. Several drugs also affect some women's capacity to have orgasms (Table 21.2–16). Antihypertensive medications, CNS stimulants, tricyclic drugs, SSRIs, and, frequently, monoamine oxidase inhibitors (MAOIs) have interfered with female orgasmic capacity. One study of women taking MAOIs, however, found that after 16 to 18 weeks of pharmacotherapy, the adverse effect of the medication disappeared and the women were able to reexperience orgasms, although they continued taking an undiminished dosage of the drug.

Table 21.2–16
Some Antipsychotic Drugs Implemented in Inhibited Female Orgasm[a]

Tricyclic antidepressants
Imipramine (Tofranil)
Clomipramine (Anafranil)
Nortriptyline (Aventyl)
Monoamine oxidase inhibitors
Tranylcypromine (Parnate)
Phenelzine (Nardil)
Isocarboxazid (Marplan)
Dopamine receptor antagonists
Thioridazine (Mellaril)
Trifluoperazine (Stelazine)
Selective serotonergic receptor inhibitors
Fluoxetine (Prozac)
Paroxetine (Paxil)
Sertraline (Zoloft)
Fluvoxamine (Luvox)
Citalopram (Celexa)

[a]The interrelation between female sexual dysfunction and pharmacological agents has been less extensively evaluated than male reactions. Oral contraceptives are reported to decrease libido in some women, and some drugs with anticholinergic side effects may impair arousal as well as orgasm. Benzodiazepines have been reported to decrease libido, but in some patients the diminution of anxiety caused by those drugs enhances sexual function. Both increase and decrease in libido have been reported with psychoactive agents. It is difficult to separate those effects from the underlying condition or from improvement of the condition. Sexual dysfunction associated with the use of a drug disappears when use of the drug is discontinued.

SUBSTANCE-INDUCED SEXUAL DYSFUNCTION

The diagnosis of substance-induced sexual dysfunction is used when evidence of substance intoxication or withdrawal is apparent from the history, physical examination, or laboratory findings. Distressing sexual dysfunction occurs within a month of significant substance intoxication or withdrawal (Table 21.2–17). Specified substances include alcohol; amphetamines or related substances; cocaine; opioids; sedatives, hypnotics, or anxiolytics; and other or unknown substances.

Abused recreational substances affect sexual function in various ways. In small doses, many substances enhance sexual performance by decreasing inhibition or anxiety or by causing a temporary elation of mood. With continued use, however, erectile engorgement, orgasmic, and ejaculatory capacities become impaired. The abuse of sedatives, anxiolytics, hypnotics, and particularly opiates and opioids nearly always depresses desire. Alcohol may foster the initiation of sexual activity by removing inhibition, but it also impairs performance. Cocaine and amphetamines produce similar effects. Although no direct evidence indicates that sexual drive is enhanced, users initially have feelings of increased energy and may become sexually active. Ultimately, dysfunction occurs. Men usually go through two stages: an experience of prolonged erection without ejaculation, then a gradual loss of erectile capability.

Patients recovering from substance dependency may need therapy to regain sexual function, partly because of psychological readjustment to a nondependent state. Many substance abusers have always had difficulty with intimate interactions. Others who spent their crucial developmental years under the influence of a substance have missed the experiences that would have enabled them to learn social and sexual skills.

Table 21.2–17
DSM-IV-TR Diagnostic Criteria for Substance-Induced Sexual Dysfunction

A. Clinically significant sexual dysfunction that results in marked distress or interpersonal difficulty predominates in the clinical picture.

B. There is evidence from the history, physical examination, or laboratory findings that the sexual dysfunction is fully explained by substance use as manifested by either (1) or (2):
 (1) the symptoms in Criterion A developed during, or within a month of, substance intoxication
 (2) medication use is etiologically related to the disturbance

C. The disturbance is not better accounted for by a sexual dysfunction that is not substance induced. Evidence that the symptoms are better accounted for by a sexual dysfunction that is not substance induced might include the following: the symptoms precede the onset of the substance use or dependence (or medication use); the symptoms persist for a substantial period of time (e.g., about a month) after the cessation of intoxication, or are substantially in excess of what would be expected given the type or amount of the substance used or the duration of use; or there is other evidence that suggests the existence of an independent non-substance-induced sexual dysfunction (e.g., a history of recurrent non-substance-related episodes).

Note: This diagnosis should be made instead of a diagnosis of substance intoxication only when the sexual dysfunction is in excess of that usually associated with the intoxication syndrome and when the dysfunction is sufficiently severe to warrant independent clinical attention.

Code [Specific substance]-induced sexual dysfunction:
 Alcohol; amphetamine [or amphetaminelike substance]; cocaine; opioid; sedative, hypnotic, or anxiolytic; other [or unknown] substance

Specify if:
 With impaired desire
 With impaired arousal
 With impaired orgasm
 With sexual pain

Specify if:
 With onset during intoxication: if the criteria are met for intoxication with the substance and the symptoms develop during the intoxication syndrome

From American Psychiatric Association. *Diagnostic and Statistical Manual of Mental Disorders.* 4th ed. Text rev. Washington, DC: American Psychiatric Association; copyright 2000, with permission.

PHARMACOLOGICAL AGENTS IMPLICATED IN SEX DYSFUNCTION

Almost every pharmacological agent, particularly those used in psychiatry, has been associated with an effect on sexuality. In men these effects include decreased sex drive, erectile failure (impotence), decreased volume of ejaculate, and delayed or retrograde ejaculation. In women decreased sex drive, decreased vaginal lubrication, inhibited or delayed orgasm, and decreased or absent vaginal contractions may occur. Drugs may also enhance the sexual responses and increase the sex drive, but this is less common than adverse effects (Table 21.2–18).

Table 21.2–18
Diagnostic Issues with Sex and Antipsychotic Drugs

Differential diagnosis of drug-induced sexual dysfunction	Problem after drug therapy started or drug overdose
	Problem not situation or partner specific
	Not a lifelong or recurrent problem
	No obvious nonpharmacological precipitant
	Dissipates with drug discontinuation
Antipsychotic drugs and ejaculatory problems	Perphenazine
	Chlorpromazine
	Trifluoperazine
	Haloperidol
	Mesoridazine
	Thioridazine
	Chlorprothixene
Antipsychotic drugs and priapism	Perphenazine
	Mesoridazine
	Chlorpromazine
	Thioridazine
	Fluphenazine
	Molindone
	Risperidone
	Clozapine

Table by R. T. Seagraves, M.D.

Psychoactive Drugs

Antipsychotic Drugs. Most antipsychotic drugs are dopamine receptor antagonists that also block adrenergic and cholinergic receptors, thus accounting for adverse sexual effects. Chlorpromazine (Thorazine), thioridazine, and trifluoperazine (Stelazine) are potent anticholinergics and impair erection and ejaculation, in which the seminal fluid backs up into the bladder rather than being propelled through the penile urethra. Patients still have a pleasurable sensation, but the orgasm is dry. When urinating after orgasm, the urine may be milky white because it contains the ejaculate. The condition is startling but harmless and may occur in up to 50 percent of patients taking the drug. Paradoxically, some rare cases of priapism have been reported with antipsychotics.

Antidepressant Drugs. The tricyclic and tetracyclic antidepressants have anticholinergic effects that interfere with erection and delay ejaculation. Since the anticholinergic effects vary among the cyclic antidepressants, those with the fewest effects (e.g., desipramine [Norpramin]) produce the fewest sexual adverse effects. The effects of the tricyclics and tetracyclics have not been documented sufficiently in women; however, few women seem to complain of any effects.

Some men report increased sensitivity of the glans that is pleasurable and that does not interfere with erection, although it delays ejaculation. In some cases, however, the tricyclic causes painful ejaculation, perhaps as the result of interference with seminal propulsion caused by interference with, in turn, urethral, prostatic, vas, and epididymal smooth muscle contractions. Clomipramine (Anafranil) has been reported to increase sex drive in some persons. Selegiline (Deprenyl), a selective MAO type B (MAO_B) inhibitor, and bupropion (Wellbutrin) have also been reported to increase sex drive, possibly by dopaminergic activity and increased production of norepinephrine.

Venlafaxine (Effexor) and the SSRIs most often have adverse effects because of the rise in serotonin levels. A lowering of the sex drive and difficulty reaching orgasm occur in both sexes. Reversal of those negative effects has been achieved with cyproheptadine (Periactin), an antihistamine with antiserotonergic effects, and with methylphenidate (Ritalin), which has adrenergic effects. Trazodone (Desyrel) is associated with the rare occurrence of priapism, the symptom of prolonged erection in the absence of sexual stimuli. That symptom appears to result from the α_2-adrenergic antagonism of trazodone.

The MAOIs affect biogenic amines broadly. Accordingly, they produce impaired erection, delayed or retrograde ejaculation, vaginal dryness, and inhibited orgasm. Tranylcypromine (Parnate) has a paradoxical sexually stimulating effect in some persons, possibly as a result of its amphetaminelike properties.

GENERAL EFFECTS. Since depression is associated with a decreased libido, varying levels of sexual dysfunction and anhedonia are part of the disease process. Some patients report improved sexual functioning as their depression improves as a result of antidepressant medication. The phenomenon makes the evaluation of sexual side effects difficult; also, the side effects may disappear with time, perhaps because a biogenic amine homeostatic mechanism comes into play.

Lithium. Lithium (Eskalith) regulates mood and in the manic state may reduce hypersexuality, possibly by a dopamine antagonist activity. In some patients, impaired erection has been reported.

Sympathomimetics. Psychostimulants are sometimes used in the treatment of depression and include amphetamines, methylphenidate, and pemoline (Cylert), which raise the plasma levels of norepinephrine and dopamine. Libido is increased; however, with prolonged use, men may experience a loss of desire and erections.

α-Adrenergic and β-Adrenergic Receptor Antagonists. α-Adrenergic and β-adrenergic receptor antagonists are used in the treatment of hypertension, angina, and certain cardiac arrhythmias. They diminish tonic sympathetic nerve outflow from vasomotor centers in the brain. As a result, they can cause impotence, decrease the volume of ejaculate, and produce retrograde ejaculation. Changes in libido have been reported in both sexes.

Suggestions have been made to use the side effects of drugs therapeutically. Thus a drug that delays or interferes with ejaculation (such as fluoxetine [Prozac]) might be used to treat premature ejaculation.

Anticholinergics. The anticholinergics block cholinergic receptors and include such drugs as amantadine (Symmetrel) and benztropine (Cogentin). They produce dryness of the mucous membranes (including those of the vagina) and impotence.

Antihistamines. Drugs such as diphenhydramine (Benadryl) have anticholinergic activity and are mildly hypnotic. They may inhibit sexual function as a result. Cyproheptadine, although an antihistamine, also has potent activity as a serotonin antagonist. It is used to block the serotonergic sexual adverse effects produced by SSRIs, such as delayed orgasm and impotence.

Antianxiety Agents. The major class of anxiolytics is the benzodiazepines (e.g., diazepam [Valium]). They act on the γ-aminobutyric acid (GABA) receptors, which are believed to be involved in cognition, memory, and motor control. Because they decrease plasma epinephrine concentrations, they diminish anxiety, and as a result they improve sexual function in persons inhibited by anxiety.

Alcohol. Alcohol suppresses CNS activity generally and can produce erectile disorders in men as a result. Alcohol has a direct gonadal effect that decreases testosterone levels in men; paradoxically, it can produce a slight rise in testosterone levels in women. The latter finding may account for women reporting increased libido after drinking small amounts of alcohol. The long-term use of alcohol reduces the ability of the liver to metabolize estrogenic compounds. In men that produces signs of feminization (such as gynecomastia as a result of testicular atrophy).

Opioids. Opioids, such as heroin, have adverse sexual effects, such as erectile failure and decreased libido. The alteration of consciousness may enhance the sexual experience in occasional users.

Hallucinogens. The hallucinogens include lysergic acid diethylamide (LSD), phencyclidine (PCP), psilocybin (from some mushrooms), and mescaline (from peyote cactus). In addition to inducing hallucinations, the drugs cause loss of contact with reality and an expanding and heightening of consciousness. Some users report that the sexual experience is similarly enhanced, but others experience anxiety, delirium, or psychosis, which clearly interferes with sexual function.

Cannabis. The altered state of consciousness produced by cannabis may enhance sexual pleasure for some persons. Its prolonged use depresses testosterone levels.

Barbiturates and Similarly Acting Drugs. Barbiturates and similarly acting sedative-hypnotic drugs may enhance sexual

responsiveness in persons who are sexually unresponsive as a result of anxiety. They have no direct effect on the sex organs; however, they do produce an alteration in consciousness that some persons find pleasurable. They are subject to abuse and may be fatal when combined with alcohol or other CNS depressants.

Methaqualone (Quaalude) acquired a reputation as a sexual enhancer, which had no biological basis in fact. It is no longer marketed in the United States.

SEXUAL DYSFUNCTION NOT OTHERWISE SPECIFIED

The category sexual dysfunction not otherwise specified covers sexual dysfunctions that cannot be classified under the categories described above (Table 21.2–19). Examples include persons who experience the physiological components of sexual excitement and orgasm but report no erotic sensation or even anesthesia (orgasmic anhedonia). Women with conditions analogous to premature ejaculation in men are classified here. Orgasmic women who desire, but have not experienced, multiple orgasms can be classified under this heading as well. Also, disorders of excessive, rather than inhibited, dysfunction, such as compulsive masturbation or coitus (sex addiction), or those with genital pain occurring during masturbation may be classified here. Other unspecified disorders are found in persons who have one or more sexual fantasies about which they feel guilty or otherwise dysphoric, but the range of common sexual fantasies is broad.

Female Premature Orgasm

Data on female premature orgasm are lacking; no separate category of premature orgasm for women is included in DSM-IV-TR. A case of multiple spontaneous orgasms without sexual stimulation was seen in a woman; the cause was an epileptogenic focus in the temporal lobe. Instances have been reported of women taking antidepressants (e.g., fluoxetine and clomipramine) who experience spontaneous orgasm associated with yawning.

Postcoital Headache

Postcoital headache, characterized by headache immediately after coitus, may last for several hours. It is usually described as throbbing and is localized in the occipital or frontal area. The cause is unknown. There may be vascular, muscle-contraction (tension), or psychogenic causes. Coitus may precipitate migraine or cluster headaches in predisposed persons.

Table 21.2–19
DSM-IV-TR Diagnostic Criteria for Sexual Dysfunction Not Otherwise Specified

This category includes sexual dysfunctions that do not meet criteria for any specific sexual dysfunction. Examples include

1. No (or substantially diminished) subjective erotic feelings despite otherwise normal arousal and orgasm
2. Situations in which the clinician has concluded that a sexual dysfunction is present but is unable to determine whether it is primary, due to a general medical condition, or substance induced

From American Psychiatric Association. *Diagnostic and Statistical Manual of Mental Disorders.* 4th ed. Text rev. Washington, DC: American Psychiatric Association; copyright 2000, with permission.

Orgasmic Anhedonia

Orgasmic anhedonia is a condition in which a person has no physical sensation of orgasm, even though the physiological component (e.g., ejaculation) remains intact. Organic causes, such as sacral and cephalic lesions that interfere with afferent pathways from the genitalia to the cortex, must be ruled out. Psychic causes usually relate to extreme guilt about experiencing sexual pleasure. These feelings produce a dissociative response that isolates the affective component of the orgasmic experience from consciousness.

Masturbatory Pain

Persons may experience pain during masturbation. Organic causes should always be ruled out; a small vaginal tear or early Peyronie's disease may produce a painful sensation. The condition should be differentiated from compulsive masturbation. Persons may masturbate to the extent that they do physical damage to their genitals and eventually experience pain during subsequent masturbatory acts. Such cases constitute a separate sexual disorder and should be so classified.

Certain masturbatory practices have resulted in what has been called autoerotic asphyxiation. The practices involve persons masturbating while hanging by the neck to heighten the erotic sensations and the orgasm's intensity through the mechanism of mild hypoxia. Although the persons intend to release themselves from the noose after orgasm, an estimated 500 to 1,000 persons a year accidentally kill themselves by hanging. Most who indulge in the practice are male; transvestism is often associated with the habit, and most deaths occur among adolescents. Such masochistic practices are usually associated with severe mental disorders, such as schizophrenia and major mood disorders.

TREATMENT

Before 1970 the most common treatment of sexual dysfunctions was individual psychotherapy. Classic psychodynamic theory holds that sexual inadequacy has its roots in early developmental conflicts, and the sexual disorder is treated as part of a pervasive emotional disturbance. Treatment focuses on the exploration of unconscious conflicts, motivation, fantasy, and various interpersonal difficulties. One of the assumptions of therapy is that removal of the conflicts allows the sexual impulse to become structurally acceptable to the ego, and thereby the patient finds appropriate means of satisfaction in the environment. Unfortunately, the symptoms of sexual dysfunctions frequently become secondarily autonomous and continue to persist, even when other problems evolving from the patients' pathology have been resolved. The addition of behavioral techniques is often necessary to cure the sexual problem.

Dual-Sex Therapy

The theoretical basis of dual-sex therapy is the concept of the marital unit or dyad as the object of therapy; the approach rep-

resents the major advance in the diagnosis and treatment of sexual disorders in this century. The methodology was originated and developed by Masters and Johnson. In dual-sex therapy, treatment is based on a concept that the couple must be treated when a dysfunctional person is in a relationship. Because both are involved in a sexually distressing situation, both must participate in the therapy program. The sexual problem often reflects other areas of disharmony or misunderstanding in the marriage so that the entire marital relationship is treated, with emphasis on sexual functioning as a part of the relationship. The keystone of the program is the roundtable session in which a male and female therapy team clarifies, discusses, and works through problems with the couple. The four-way sessions require active participation by the patients. Therapists and patients discuss the psychological and physiological aspects of sexual functioning, and therapists have an educative attitude. Therapists suggest specific sexual activities, which the couple follow in the privacy of their home. The aim of the therapy is to establish or reestablish communication within the marital unit. Sex is emphasized as a natural function that flourishes in the appropriate domestic climate, and improved communication is encouraged toward that end. In a variation of this therapy that has proved effective, one therapist may treat the couple. Treatment is short-term and behaviorally oriented. The therapists attempt to reflect the situation as they see it, rather than interpret underlying dynamics. An undistorted picture of the relationship presented by the therapists often corrects the myopic, narrow view held by each marriage partner. This new perspective can interrupt the couple's vicious circle of relating and can encourage improved, more effective communication. Specific exercises are prescribed for the couple to treat their particular problems. Sexual inadequacy often involves lack of information, misinformation, and performance fear. Therefore, the couple are specifically prohibited from any sexual play other than that prescribed by the therapists. Beginning exercises usually focus on heightening sensory awareness to touch, sight, sound, and smell. Initially, intercourse is interdicted, and the couple learn to give and receive bodily pleasure without the pressure of performance or penetration. At the same time, they learn how to communicate nonverbally in a mutually satisfactory way, and they learn that sexual foreplay is an enjoyable alternative to intercourse and orgasm.

During the sensate focus exercises, the couple receive much reinforcement to reduce their anxiety. They are urged to use fantasies to distract them from obsessive concerns about performance (spectatoring). The needs of both the dysfunctional partner and the nondysfunctional partner are considered. If either partner becomes sexually excited by the exercises, the other is encouraged to bring him or her to orgasm by manual or oral means. Open communication between the partners is urged, and the expression of mutual needs is encouraged. Resistances, such as claims of fatigue or not enough time to complete the exercises, are common and must be dealt with by the therapists. Genital stimulation is eventually added to general body stimulation. The couple are instructed sequentially to try various positions for intercourse, without necessarily completing the act, and to use varieties of stimulating techniques before they are instructed to proceed with intercourse.

Psychotherapy sessions follow each new exercise period, and problems and satisfactions, both sexual and in other areas of the couple's lives, are discussed. Specific instructions and the introduction of new exercises geared to the individual couple's progress are reviewed in each session. Gradually, the couple gain confidence and learn to communicate, verbally and sexually. Dual-sex therapy is most effective when the sexual dysfunction exists apart from other psychopathology.

Specific Techniques and Exercises

Various techniques are used to treat the various dysfunctions. In cases of vaginismus, a woman is advised to dilate her vaginal opening with her fingers or with graduated dilators.

In cases of premature ejaculation, an exercise known as the squeeze technique is used to raise the threshold of penile excitability. In this exercise the man or the woman stimulates the erect penis until the earliest sensations of impending ejaculation are felt. At this point, the woman forcefully squeezes the coronal ridge of the glans, the erection is diminished, and ejaculation is inhibited. The exercise program eventually raises the threshold of the sensation of ejaculatory inevitability and allows the man to become aware of his sexual sensations and confident about his sexual performance. A variant of the exercise is the stop–start technique developed by James H. Semans, in which the woman stops all stimulation of the penis when the man first senses an impending ejaculation. No squeeze is used. Research has shown that the presence or absence of circumcision has no bearing on a man's ejaculatory control; the glans is equally sensitive in the two states. Sex therapy has been most successful in the treatment of premature ejaculation.

A man with a sexual desire disorder or male erectile disorder is sometimes told to masturbate to prove that full erection and ejaculation are possible. Male orgasmic disorder is managed initially by extravaginal ejaculation and then by gradual vaginal entry after stimulation to a point near ejaculation.

In cases of lifelong female orgasmic disorder, the woman is directed to masturbate, sometimes using a vibrator. The shaft of the clitoris is the masturbatory site most preferred by women, and orgasm depends on adequate clitoral stimulation. An area on the anterior wall of the vagina has been identified in some women as a site of sexual excitation, known as the G-spot; but reports of an ejaculatory phenomenon at orgasm in women following the stimulation of the G-spot have not been satisfactorily verified.

Hypnotherapy

Hypnotherapists focus specifically on the anxiety-producing symptom—that is, the particular sexual dysfunction. The successful use of hypnosis enables patients to gain control over the symptom that has been lowering self-esteem and disrupting psychological homeostasis. The cooperation of the patient is first obtained and encouraged during a series of nonhypnotic sessions with the therapist. Those discussions permit the development of a secure doctor–patient relationship, a sense of physical and psychological comfort on the part of the patient, and the establishment of mutually desired treatment goals. During this time the therapist assesses the patient's capacity for the trance experience. The nonhypnotic sessions also permit the clinician to take a psychiatric history and perform a mental status examination before beginning hypnotherapy. The focus of

treatment is on symptom removal and attitude alteration. The patient is instructed in developing alternative means of dealing with the anxiety-provoking situation, the sexual encounter.

Patients are also taught relaxation techniques to use on themselves before sexual relations. With these methods to alleviate anxiety, the physiological responses to sexual stimulation can readily result in pleasurable excitation and discharge. Psychological impediments to vaginal lubrication, erection, and orgasms are removed, and normal sexual functioning ensues. Hypnosis may be added to a basic individual psychotherapy program to accelerate the effects of psychotherapeutic intervention.

Behavior Therapy

Behavioral approaches were initially designed for the treatment of phobias but are now used to treat other dysfunctions as well. Behavior therapists assume that sexual dysfunction is learned maladaptive behavior, which causes patients to be fearful of sexual interaction. Using traditional techniques, therapists set up a hierarchy of anxiety-provoking situations, ranging from least threatening (e.g., the thought of kissing) to most threatening (the thought of penile penetration). The behavior therapist enables the patient to master the anxiety through a standard program of systematic desensitization, which is designed to inhibit the learned anxious response by encouraging behaviors antithetical to anxiety. The patient first deals with the least anxiety-producing situation in fantasy and progresses by steps to the most anxiety-producing situation. Medication, hypnosis, and special training in deep muscle relaxation are sometimes used to help with the initial mastery of anxiety.

Assertiveness training is helpful in teaching patients to express sexual needs openly and without fear. Exercises in assertiveness are given in conjunction with sex therapy; patients are encouraged to make sexual requests and to refuse to comply with requests perceived as unreasonable. Sexual exercises may be prescribed for patients to perform at home, and a hierarchy may be established, starting with those activities that have proved most pleasurable and successful in the past.

One treatment variation involves the participation of the patient's sexual partner in the desensitization program. The partner, rather than the therapist, presents items of increasing stimulation value to the patient. In such situations, a cooperative partner is necessary to help the patient carry gains made during treatment sessions to sexual activity at home.

Group Therapy

Group therapy has been used to examine both intrapsychic and interpersonal problems in patients with sexual disorders. A therapy group provides a strong support system for a patient who feels ashamed, anxious, or guilty about a particular sexual problem. It is a useful forum in which to counteract sexual myths, correct misconceptions, and provide accurate information about sexual anatomy, physiology, and varieties of behavior.

Groups for the treatment of sexual disorders can be organized in several ways. Members may all share the same problem, such as premature ejaculation; members may all be of the same sex with different sexual problems; or groups may be composed of both men and women who are experiencing a variety of sexual problems. Group therapy may be an adjunct to other forms of therapy or the prime mode of treatment. Groups organized to treat a particular dysfunction are usually behavioral in approach.

Groups composed of married couples with sexual dysfunctions have also been effective. A group provides the opportunity to gather accurate information, offers consensual validation of individual preferences, and enhances self-esteem and self-acceptance. Techniques such as role playing and psychodrama may be used in treatment. Such groups are not indicated for couples when one partner is uncooperative, when a patient has a severe depressive disorder or psychosis, when a patient finds explicit sexual audiovisual material repugnant, or when a patient fears or dislikes groups.

Analytically Oriented Sex Therapy

One of the most effective treatment modalities is the use of sex therapy integrated with psychodynamic and psychoanalytically oriented psychotherapy. The sex therapy is conducted over a longer period than usual, which allows learning or relearning of sexual satisfaction under the realities of patients' day-to-day lives. The addition of psychodynamic conceptualizations to behavioral techniques used to treat sexual dysfunctions allows the treatment of patients with sexual disorders associated with other psychopathology.

The material and dynamics that emerge in patients in analytically oriented sex therapy are the same as those in psychoanalytic therapy, such as dreams, fear of punishment, aggressive feelings, difficulty trusting a partner, fear of intimacy, oedipal feelings, and fear of genital mutilation. The combined approach of analytically oriented sex therapy is used by the general psychiatrist who carefully judges the optimal timing of sex therapy and the ability of patients to tolerate the directive approach that focuses on their sexual difficulties.

Biological Treatments

Biological treatments, including pharmacotherapy, surgery, and mechanical devices, are used to treat specific cases of sexual disorder. Most of the recent advances involve male sexual dysfunction. Current studies are under way to test biological treatment of sexual dysfunction in women.

Pharmacotherapy. The major new medications to treatment of sexual dysfunction are sildenafil (Viagra) and its congeners; oral phentolamine (Vasomax); alprostadil (Caverject), an injectable prostaglandin; and a transurethral alprostadil (MUSE), all used to treat erectile disorder.

Sildenafil is a nitric oxide enhancer that facilitates the inflow of blood to the penis necessary for an erection. The drug takes effect about 1 hour after ingestion, and its effect can last up to 4 hours. Sildenafil is not effective in the absence of sexual stimulation. The most common adverse events associated with its use are headaches, flushing, and dyspepsia. The use of sildenafil is contraindicated for persons taking organic nitrates. The concomitant action of the two drugs can result in large, sudden, and sometimes fatal drops in systemic blood pressure. Sildenafil is not effective in all cases of erectile dysfunction. It fails to produce an erection rigid enough for penetration in about 50% of

men who have radical prostate surgery or in those with longstanding insulin-dependent diabetes. It is also ineffective in certain cases of nerve damage.

Sildenafil use in women results in vaginal lubrication, but not in increased desire. However, anecdotal reports describe individual women who have experienced intensified excitement with sildenafil.

Oral phentolamine and apomorphine are not FDA approved at present, but have proved effective as potency enhancers in men with minimal erectile dysfunction. Phentolamine reduces sympathetic tone and relaxes corporeal smooth muscle. Adverse events include hypotension, tachycardia, and dizziness. Apomorphine effects are mediated by the autonomic nervous system and result in vasodilatation that facilitates the inflow of blood to the penis. Adverse events include nausea and sweating.

In contrast to the oral medications, injectable and transurethral alprostadil act locally on the penis and can produce erections in the absence of sexual stimulation. Alprostadil contains a naturally occurring form of prostaglandin E, a vasodilating agent. Alprostadil may be administered by direct injection into the corpora cavernosa or by intraurethral insertion of a pellet through a canula. The firm erection produced within 2 to 3 minutes after administration of the drug may last as long as 1 hour. Infrequent and reversible adverse effects of injections include penile bruising and changes in liver function test results. However, possible hazardous sequelae exist, including priapism and sclerosis of the small veins of the penis. Users of transurethral alprostadil sometimes complain of burning sensations in the penis.

Two small trials found different topical agents effective in alleviating erectile dysfunction. One cream consists of three vasoactive substances known to be absorbed through the skin: aminophylline, isosorbide dinitrate, and co-dergocrine mesylate, which is a mixture of ergot alkaloids. The other is a gel containing alprostadil and an additional ingredient, which temporarily makes the outer layer of the skin more permeable.

A cream incorporating alprostadil also has been developed to treat female sexual arousal disorder. The initial results are promising. Also vaginally applied phentolamine mesylate, an α-receptor antagonist, significantly increased vasocongestion and a subjective sense of arousal in a trial of postmenopausal women with arousal problems who were already on hormonal therapy.

The pharmacological treatments described above are useful in the treatment of arousal dysfunction of various causes: neurogenic, arterial insufficiency, venous leakage, psychogenic, and mixed. When coupled with insight-oriented or behavioral sex therapy, the use of medications can reverse psychogenic arousal disorder resistant to psychotherapy alone, the ultimate goal being pharmacologically unassisted sexual functioning.

Other Pharmacological Agents

Numerous other pharmacological agents have been used to heal the various sexual disorders. Intravenous methohexital sodium (Brevital) has been used in desensitization therapy. Antianxiety agents may have some application in tense patients, although these drugs can also interfere with the sexual response. The side effects of antidepressants, in particular the SSRIs and tricyclic drugs, have been used to prolong the sexual response in patients with premature ejaculation. This approach is particularly useful in patients refractory to behavioral techniques who may fall into the category of physiologically determined premature ejaculation. The use of antidepressants has also been advocated in the treatment of patients who are phobic of sex and in those with a posttraumatic stress disorder following rape. Trazodone is an antidepressant that improves nocturnal erections. The risks of taking such medications must be carefully weighed against their possible benefits. Bromocriptine (Parlodel) is used in the treatment of hyperprolactinemia, which is frequently associated with hypogonadism. Such patients are first worked up to rule out pituitary tumors. Bromocriptine, a dopamine agonist, may improve sexual function impaired by hyperprolactinemia. Sometimes the problem requires androgen therapy.

A number of substances have popular standing as aphrodisiacs; for example, ginseng root and yohimbine (Yocon). However, studies have not confirmed any aphrodisiac properties. Yohimbine, an α-receptor antagonist, may cause dilation of the penile artery; however the American Urologic Association does not recommend its use to treat organic erectile dysfunction. Many recreational drugs, including cocaine, amphetamines, alcohol, and cannabis, are considered enhancers of sexual performance. Although they may provide the user with an initial benefit because of their tranquilizing, disinhibiting, or mood-elevating effects, consistent or prolonged use of any of these substances impairs sexual functioning.

Dopaminergic agents have been reported to increase libido and improve sex function. Those drugs include L-dopa, a dopamine precursor, and bromocriptine, a dopamine agonist. The antidepressant bupropion has dopaminergic effects and has increased sex drive in some patients. Selegiline, an MAOI, is selective for MAO_B and is dopaminergic. It improves sexual functioning in older persons.

Hormone Therapy. Androgens increase the sex drive in women and in men with low testosterone concentrations. Women may experience virilizing effects, some of which are irreversible (e.g., deepening of the voice). In men, prolonged use of androgens produces hypertension and prostatic enlargement. Testosterone is most effective when given parenterally; however, effective oral and transdermal preparations are available.

Women who use estrogens for replacement therapy or for contraception may report decreased libido; in such cases a combined preparation of estrogen and testosterone has been used effectively. Estrogen itself prevents thinning of the vaginal mucous membrane and facilitates lubrication. Two new forms of estrogen, vaginal rings and vaginal tablets, provide alternate administration routes to treat women with arousal problems or genital atrophy. Since tablets and rings do not increase circulating estrogen levels, these devices may be considered for breast cancer patients with arousal problems.

Antiandrogens and Antiestrogens. Estrogens and progesterone are antiandrogens that have been used to treat compulsive sexual behavior in men, usually in sex offenders. Clomiphene (Clomid) and tamoxifen (Nolvadex) are both antiestrogens, and both stimulate gonadotropin-releasing hormone (GnRH) secretion and increase testosterone concentrations,

thereby increasing libido. Women being treated for breast cancer with tamoxifen report an increased libido.

Mechanical Treatment Approaches

In male patients with arteriosclerosis (especially of the distal aorta, known as Leriche's syndrome), the erection may be lost during active pelvic thrusting. The need for increased blood in the gluteal muscles and others served by the ilial or hypogastric arteries takes blood away (steals) from the pudendal artery and thus interferes with penile blood flow. Relief may be obtained by decreasing pelvic thrusting, which is also aided by the woman's superior coital position.

Vacuum Pump. Vacuum pumps are mechanical devices that patients without vascular disease can use to obtain erections. The blood drawn into the penis following the creation of the vacuum is kept there by a ring placed around the base of the penis. This device has no adverse effects, but it is cumbersome, and partners must be willing to accept its use. Some women complain that the penis is redder and cooler than when erection is produced by natural circumstances, and they find the process and the result objectionable.

A similar device, called EROS, has been developed to create clitoral erections in women. EROS is a small suction cup that fits over the clitoral region and draws blood into the clitoris. There have been studies reporting its success in treating female sexual arousal disorder. Vibrators used to stimulate the clitoral area have been successful in treating anorgasmic women.

Surgical Treatment

Male Prostheses. Surgical treatment is infrequently advocated, but penile prosthetic devices are available for men with inadequate erectile responses who are resistant to other treatment methods or who have medically caused deficiencies. There are two main types of prostheses: a semirigid rod prosthesis that produces a permanent erection that can be positioned close to the body for concealment and an inflatable type that is implanted with its own reservoir and pump for inflation and deflation. The latter type is designed to mimic normal physiological functioning.

Outcome

The results of different treatment methods have varied considerably since Masters and Johnson first reported positive results for their treatment approach in 1970. Masters and Johnson studied the failure rates of their patients (defined as the failure to initiate reversal of the basic symptom of the presenting dysfunction). They compared initial failure rates with 5-year follow-up findings for the same couples. Although some have criticized their definition of the percentage of presumed successes, other studies have confirmed the effectiveness of their approach. Demonstrating the effectiveness of traditional outpatient psychotherapy is just as difficult when therapy is oriented to sexual problems as it is in general. The more severe the psychopathology associated with a problem of long duration, the more adverse the outcome is likely to be.

The more difficult treatment cases involve couples with severe marital discord. Desire disorders are particularly difficult to treat. They require longer, more intensive therapy than some other disorders, and their outcomes vary greatly.

When behavioral approaches are used, empirical criteria that predict outcome are more easily isolated. Using these criteria, for instance, couples who regularly practice assigned exercises appear to have a much greater likelihood of success than do more resistant couples or those whose interaction involves sadomasochistic or depressive features or mechanisms of blame and projection. Flexibility of attitude is also a positive prognostic factor. Overall, younger couples tend to complete sex therapy more often than older couples. Couples whose interactional difficulties center on their sex problems, such as inhibition, frustration, or fear of performance failure, are also likely to respond well to therapy.

In general, methods that have proved effective singly or in combination include training in behavioral sexual skills, systematic desensitization, directive marital counseling, traditional psychodynamic approaches, group therapy, and pharmacotherapy. Although most therapists prefer to treat a couple for sexual dysfunction, treatment of individual persons has also been successful.

ICD-10

According to the 10th revision of *International Statistical Classification of Diseases and Related Health Problems* (ICD-10), sexual dysfunction refers to a person's inability to "participate in a sexual relationship as he or she would wish." This dysfunction is expressed in various ways: a lack of desire or of pleasure or a physiological inability to begin, maintain, or complete sexual interaction. Because sexual response is psychosomatic, it may be difficult to determine "the relative importance of psychological and/or organic factors."

Sexual dysfunction such as lack of desire can occur in both men and women, but women complain more often of the "subjective quality" of the experience than of the "failure of a specific response." ICD-10 advises looking "beyond the presenting complaint to find the most appropriate diagnostic category." Table 21.2–20 presents the ICD-10 diagnostic criteria.

Table 21.2–20
ICD-10 Diagnostic Criteria for Sexual Dysfunction, Not Caused by Organic Disorder or Disease

G1. The subject is unable to participate in a sexual relationship as he or she would wish.

G2. The dysfunction occurs frequently, but may be absent on some occasions.

G3. The dysfunction has been present for at least 6 months.

G4. The dysfunction is not entirely attributable to any of the other mental and behavioral disorders in ICD-10, physical disorders (such as endocrine disorder), or drug treatment.

Comments

Measurement of each form of dysfunction can be based on rating scales that assess severity as well as frequency of the problem. More than one type of dysfunction can coexist.

Lack or loss of sexual desire

A. The general criteria for sexual dysfunction must be met.

B. There is a lack or loss of sexual desire, manifest by diminution of seeking out sexual cues, of thinking about sex with associated feelings of desire or appetite, or of sexual fantasies.

C. There is a lack of interest in initiating sexual activity either with a partner or as solitary masturbation, resulting in a frequency of activity clearly lower than expected, taking into account age and context, or in a frequency very clearly reduced from previous much higher levels.

Sexual aversion and lack of sexual enjoyment

Sexual aversion

A. The general criteria for sexual dysfunction must be met.

B. The prospect of sexual interaction with a partner produces sufficient aversion, fear, or anxiety that sexual activity is avoided, or, if it occurs, is associated with strong negative feelings and an inability to experience any pleasure.

C. The aversion is not the result of performance anxiety (reaction to previous failure of sexual response).

Lack of sexual enjoyment

A. The general criteria for sexual dysfunction must be met.

B. Genital response (orgasm and/or ejaculation) occurs during sexual stimulation, but is not accompanied by pleasurable sensations or feelings of pleasant excitement.

C. There is no manifest and persistent fear or anxiety during sexual activity (see sexual aversion).

Failure of genital response

A. The general criteria for sexual dysfunction must be met.

In addition, for men:

B. Erection sufficient for intercourse fails to occur when intercourse is attempted. The dysfunction takes one of the following forms:

(1) full erection occurs during the early stages of lovemaking but disappears or declines when intercourse is attempted (before ejaculation if it occurs);

(2) erection does occur, but only at times when intercourse is not being considered;

(3) partial erection, insufficient for intercourse, occurs, but not full erection;

(4) no penile tumescence occurs at all.

In addition, for women:

B. There is failure of genital response, experienced as failure of vaginal lubrication, together with inadequate tumescence of the labia. The dysfunction takes one of the following forms:

(1) general: lubrication fails in all relevant circumstances;

(2) lubrication may occur initially but fails to persist for long enough to allow comfortable penile entry;

(3) Situational: lubrication occurs only in some situations (e.g., with one partner but not another, or during masturbation, or when vaginal intercourse is not being contemplated).

Orgasmic dysfunction

A. The general criteria for sexual dysfunction must be met.

B. There is orgasmic dysfunction (either absence or marked delay of orgasm), which takes one of the following forms:

(1) orgasm has never been experienced in any situation;

(2) orgasmic dysfunction has developed after a period of relatively normal response:

(a) general: orgasmic dysfunction occurs in all situations and with any partner;

(b) situational:

For *women:* orgasm does occur in certain situations (e.g., when masturbating or with certain partners);

For *men,* one of the following can be applied:

i) orgasm occurs only during sleep, never during the waking state;

ii) orgasm never occurs in the presence of the partner;

iii) orgasm occurs in the presence of the partner but not during intercourse.

Premature ejaculation

A. The general criteria for sexual dysfunction must be met.

B. There is an inability to delay ejaculation sufficiently to enjoy lovemaking, manifest as either of the following:

(1) occurrence of ejaculation before or very soon after the beginning of intercourse (if a time limit is required: before or within 15 seconds of the beginning of intercourse);

(2) ejaculation occurs in the absence of sufficient erection to make intercourse possible.

C. The problem is not the result of prolonged abstinence from sexual activity.

Nonorganic vaginismus

A. The general criteria for sexual dysfunction must be met.

B. There is spasm of the perivaginal muscles, sufficient to prevent penile entry or make it uncomfortable. The dysfunction takes one of the following forms:

(1) normal response has never been experienced;

(2) vaginismus has developed after a period of relatively normal response;

(a) when vaginal entry is not attempted, a normal sexual response may occur;

(b) any attempt at sexual contact leads to generalized fear and efforts to avoid vaginal entry (e.g., spasm of the adductor muscles of the thighs).

Nonorganic dyspareunia

A. The general criteria for sexual dysfunction must be met.

In addition, for women:

B. Pain is experienced at the entry of the vagina, either throughout sexual intercourse or only when deep thrusting of the penis occurs.

C. The disorder is not attributable to vaginismus or failure of lubrication, dyspareunia of organic origin should be classified according to the underlying disorder.

(*continued*)

Table 21.2–20 (*continued*)

In addition, for men: B. Pain or discomfort is experienced during sexual response. (The timing of the pain and the exact localization should be carefully recorded.) C. The discomfort is not the result of local physical factors. If physical factors are found, the dysfunction should be classified elsewhere.	**Excessive sexual drive** No research criteria are attempted for this category. Researchers studying this category are recommended to design their own criteria. **Other sexual dysfunction, not caused by organic disorder or disease** **Unspecified sexual dysfunction, not caused by organic disorder or disease**

References

Bhugra D. Literature update: a critical review. *Sex Relat Ther.* 2001;16:407.
Everaerd W, Laan E. Drug treatments for women's sexual disorders. *J Sex Res.* 2000;37:195.
Fava M, Rankin M. Sexual functioning and SSRIs. *J Clin Psychiatry.* 2002;63(suppl 5):13.
Frank E. Frequency of sexual dysfunction in "normal" couples. *N Engl J Med.* 1978;299:111.
Freud S. Three essays on the theory of sexuality. In: *Standard Edition of the Complete Psychological Works of Sigmund Freud.* Vol 7. London: Hogarth Press; 1953:125.
Frohman EM. Sexual dysfunction in neurological disease. *Clin Neuropharmacol.* 2002;25:126.
Goldmeier D. "Responsive" sexual desire in women—managing the normal? *Sex Relat Ther.* 2001;16:381.
Graziottin A. Clinical approach to dyspareunia. *J Sex Marital Ther.* 2001;27:489.
Herman J, Lo Piccolo J. Clinical outcome of sex therapy. *Arch Gen Psychiatry.* 1983;40:443.
Linet OI, Ogrinc FG. Efficacy and safety of intracavernosal alprostadil in men with erectile dysfunction. The Alprostadil Study Group. *N Engl J Med.* 1996;334:873.
Masters WH, Johnson VE. *Human Sexual Inadequacy.* Boston: Little, Brown; 1970.
Rowland DL, Slob AK. Understanding and diagnosing sexual dysfunction: recent progress through psychophysiological and psychophysical methods. *Neurosci Biobehav Rev.* 1995;19:201.
Sadock BJ, Kaplan HI, Freedman AM, eds. *The Sexual Experience.* Baltimore: Williams & Wilkins; 1976.
Sadock VA. Normal human sexuality and sexual dysfunction. In: Sadock BJ, Sadock VA, eds. *Kaplan & Sadock's Comprehensive Textbook of Psychiatry.* 7th ed. Vol 1. Baltimore: Lippincott Williams & Wilkins; 2000:1577.
Schiavi RC, Karstaedt A, Schreiner-Engel P, Mandeli J. Psychometric characteristics of individuals with sexual dysfunction and their partners. *J Sex Marital Ther.* 1992;18:219.
Segraves RT. Effects of psychotropic drugs on human erections and ejaculation. *Arch Gen Psychiatry.* 1989;46:782.
Segraves RT. Historical and international context of nosology of female sexual disorders. *J Sex Marital Ther.* 2001;27:205.
Seidman SN. Exploring the relationship between depression and erectile dysfunction in aging men. *J Clin Psychiatry.* 2002;63(suppl 5):5.
Semans JH. Premature ejaculation: a new approach. *South Med J.* 1956;49:353.

▲ 21.3 Sexual Disorder Not Otherwise Specified and Paraphilias

PARAPHILIAS

Paraphilias are abnormal expressions of sexuality. They can range from nearly normal behavior to behavior that is destructive or hurtful only to a person's self or to a person's self and partner, and finally to behavior that is deemed destructive or threatening to the community at large. The text revision of the fourth edition of *Diagnostic and Statistical Manual of Mental Disorders* (DSM-IV-TR) addresses these differences by designating impulses toward pedophilia, frotteurism, voyeurism, exhibitionism, and sexual sadism clinically significant if the person has acted on these fantasies or if these fantasies cause marked distress or interpersonal difficulty. The remaining paraphilias, such as voyeurism, transvestic fetishism, sexual masochism, or those not otherwise specified such as zoophilia, meet the criteria for clinical significance only if they cause marked distress or impairment in social, occupational or other important areas of functioning, even if the urges have been expressed behaviorally. Paraphiliac urges may occur rarely, intermittently, or compulsively. They may be incidental or they may offer the only venue through which sexuality can be expressed.

A special fantasy with its unconscious and conscious components is the pathognomonic element of the paraphilia, with sexual arousal and orgasm being associated phenomena that *reinforce the fantasy or impulse.* The influence of these fantasies and their behavioral manifestations often extend beyond the sexual sphere to pervade people's lives.

The major functions of human sexual behavior are to assist in bonding, to create mutual pleasure in cooperation with a partner, to express and enhance love between two persons, and to procreate. Paraphilias are divergent behaviors in that those acts involve aggression, victimization, and extreme one-sidedness. The behaviors exclude or harm others and disrupt the potential for bonding between persons.

Epidemiology

Paraphilias are practiced by only a small percentage of the population, but the insistent, repetitive nature of the disorders results in a high frequency of such acts. Thus, a large proportion of the population has been victimized by persons with paraphilias. DSM-IV-TR suggests that the prevalence of paraphilias is significantly higher than the number of cases diagnosed in general clinical facilities, based on the large commercial market in paraphilic pornography and paraphernalia.

Among legally identified cases of paraphilias, pedophilia is most common. Ten to 20 percent of all children have been molested by age 18. Because a child is the object, the act is taken more seriously, and greater effort is spent tracking down

the culprit than in other paraphilias. Persons with exhibitionism who publicly display themselves to young children are also commonly apprehended. Those with voyeurism may be apprehended, but their risk is not great. Twenty percent of adult females have been the targets of persons with exhibitionism and voyeurism. Sexual masochism and sexual sadism are underrepresented in any prevalence estimates. Sexual sadism usually comes to attention only in sensational cases of rape, brutality, and lust murder. The excretory paraphilias are scarcely reported, as activity usually takes place between consenting adults or between prostitute and client. Persons with fetishism rarely become entangled in the legal system. Those with transvestic fetishism may be arrested occasionally for disturbing the peace or on other misdemeanor charges if they are obviously men dressed in women's clothes, but arrest is more common among those with gender identity disorders. Zoophilia as a true paraphilia is rare.

As usually defined, the paraphilias seem to be largely male conditions. Fetishism almost always occurs in men. More than 50 percent of all paraphilias have their onset before age 18. Patients with paraphilia frequently have three to five paraphilias, either concurrently or at different times in their lives. This pattern of occurrence is especially the case with exhibitionism, fetishism, sexual masochism, sexual sadism, transvestic fetishism, voyeurism, and zoophilia (Table 21.3–1). The occurrence of paraphiliac behavior peaks between ages 15 and 25 and gradually declines; in men of 50, criminal paraphiliac acts are rare. Those that occur are practiced in isolation or with a cooperative partner.

Etiology

Psychosocial Factors. In the classic psychoanalytic model, persons with a paraphilia have failed to complete the normal developmental process toward heterosexual adjustment, but the model has been modified by new psychoanalytic approaches. What distinguishes one paraphilia from another is the method chosen by a person (usually male) to cope with the anxiety caused by the threat of castration by the father and separation from the mother. However bizarre its manifestation, the resulting behavior provides an outlet for the sexual and aggressive drives that would otherwise have been channeled into proper sexual behavior.

Failure to resolve the oedipal crisis by identifying with the father-aggressor (for boys) or mother-aggressor (for girls) results either in improper identification with the opposite-sex parent or in an improper choice of object for libido cathexis. Classic psychoanalytic theory holds that transsexualism and transvestic fetishism are disorders because each involves identification with the opposite-sex parent instead of the same-sex parent; for instance, a man dressing in women's clothes is believed to identify with his mother. Exhibitionism and voyeurism may be attempts to calm anxiety about castration. Fetishism is an attempt to avoid anxiety by displacing libidinal impulses to inappropriate objects. A person with a shoe fetish unconsciously denies that women have lost their penises through castration by attaching libido to a phallic object, the shoe, which symbolizes the female penis. Persons with pedophilia and sexual sadism have a need to dominate and control their victims to compensate for their feelings of powerlessness during the oedipal crisis. Some theorists believe that choosing a child as a love object is a narcissistic act. Persons with sexual masochism overcome their fear of injury and their sense of powerlessness by showing that they are impervious to harm. Another theory proposes that the masochist directs the aggression inherent in all paraphilias toward herself or himself. Although recent developments in psychoanalysis place more emphasis on treating defense mechanisms than on oedipal traumas, psychoanalytic therapy for patients with a paraphilia remains consistent with Sigmund Freud's theory.

Other theories attribute the development of a paraphilia to early experiences that condition or socialize children into committing a paraphiliac act. The first shared sexual experience can be important in that regard. Molestation as a child can predispose a person to accept continued abuse as an adult or, conversely, to become an abuser of others. Also, early experiences of abuse that is not specifically sexual, such as spanking, enemas, or verbal humiliation, can be sexualized by a child and can form the basis for a paraphilia. Such experiences can result in the development of an *eroticized child.* The onset of paraphiliac acts can result from persons' modeling their behavior on the behavior of others who have carried out paraphiliac acts, mimicking sexual behavior depicted in the media, or recalling emotionally laden events from the past, such as their own molestation. Learning theory indicates that because the fantasizing of paraphiliac interests begins at an early age and because personal fantasies and thoughts are not shared with others (who could block or discourage them), the use and misuse of paraphiliac fantasies and urges continue uninhibited until late in life. Only then do persons begin to realize that such paraphiliac interests and urges are inconsistent with societal norms. Unfortunately, by that time the repetitive use of such fantasies has become ingrained, and the sexual thoughts and behaviors have become associated with, or conditioned to, paraphiliac fantasies.

Biological Factors. Several studies have identified abnormal organic findings in persons with paraphilias. None has used random samples of such persons; instead, they have extensively

Table 21.3–1
Frequency of Paraphiliac Acts Committed by Paraphilia Patients Seeking Outpatient Treatment

Diagnostic Category	Paraphilia Patients Seeking Outpatient Treatment (%)	Paraphiliac Acts per Paraphilia Patient[a]
Pedophilia	45	5
Exhibitionism	25	50
Voyeurism	12	17
Frotteurism	6	30
Sexual masochism	3	36
Transvestic fetishism	3	25
Sexual sadism	3	3
Fetishism	2	3
Zoophilia	1	2

[a]Median number.
Courtesy of Gene G. Abel, M.D.

investigated paraphilia patients who were referred to large medical centers. Among these patients, those with positive organic findings included 74 percent with abnormal hormone levels, 27 percent with hard or soft neurological signs, 24 percent with chromosomal abnormalities, 9 percent with seizures, 9 percent with dyslexia, 4 percent with abnormal electroencephalograms (EEGs), 4 percent with major mental disorders, and 4 percent with mental handicaps. The question is whether these abnormalities are causally related to paraphiliac interests or are incidental findings that bear no relevance to the development of paraphilia.

Psychophysiological tests have been developed to measure penile volumetric size in response to paraphiliac and nonparaphiliac stimuli. The procedures may be of use in diagnosis and treatment but are of questionable diagnostic validity because some men are able to suppress their erectile responses.

Table 21.3–3
DSM-IV-TR Diagnostic Criteria for Fetishism

A. Over a period of at least 6 months, recurrent, intense sexually arousing fantasies, sexual urges, or behaviors involving the use of nonliving objects (e.g., female undergarments).
B. The fantasies, sexual urges, or behaviors cause clinically significant distress or impairment in social, occupational, or other important areas of functioning.
C. The fetish objects are not limited to articles of female clothing used in cross-dressing (as in transvestic fetishism) or devices designed for the purpose of tactile genital stimulation (e.g., a vibrator).

From American Psychiatric Association. *Diagnostic and Statistical Manual of Mental Disorders.* 4th ed. Text rev. Washington, DC: American Psychiatric Association; copyright 2000, with permission.

Diagnosis and Clinical Features

In DSM-IV-TR the diagnostic criteria for paraphilias include the presence of a pathognomonic fantasy and an intense urge to act out the fantasy or its behavior elaboration. The fantasy, which may distress a patient, contains unusual sexual material that is relatively fixed and shows only minor variations. Arousal and orgasm depend on the mental elaboration or the behavioral playing out of the fantasy. Sexual activity is ritualized or stereotyped and makes use of degraded, reduced, or dehumanized objects.

Exhibitionism. Exhibitionism is the recurrent urge to expose the genitals to a stranger or to an unsuspecting person (Table 21.3–2). Sexual excitement occurs in anticipation of the exposure, and orgasm is brought about by masturbation during or after the event. In almost 100 percent of cases, those with exhibitionism are men exposing themselves to women. The dynamic of men with exhibitionism is to assert their masculinity by showing their penises and by watching the victims' reactions—fright, surprise, and disgust. In this situation, men unconsciously feel castrated and impotent. Wives of men with exhibitionism often substitute for the mothers to whom the men were excessively attached during childhood. In other related paraphilias the central themes involve derivatives of looking or showing.

Fetishism. In fetishism the sexual focus is on objects (e.g., shoes, gloves, pantyhose, and stockings) that are intimately associated with the human body (Table 21.3–3). The particular fetish is linked to someone closely involved with a patient during childhood and has a quality associated with this loved, needed, or even traumatizing person. Usually, the disorder begins by adolescence, although the fetish may have been established in childhood. Once established, the disorder tends to be chronic.

Sexual activity may be directed toward the fetish itself (e.g., masturbation with or into a shoe), or the fetish may be incorporated into sexual intercourse (e.g., the demand that high-heeled shoes be worn). The disorder is almost exclusively found in men. According to Freud, the fetish serves as a symbol of the phallus to persons with unconscious castration fears. Learning theorists believe that the object was associated with sexual stimulation at an early age.

Table 21.3–2
DSM-IV-TR Diagnostic Criteria for Exhibitionism

A. Over a period of at least 6 months, recurrent, intense sexually arousing fantasies, sexual urges, or behaviors involving the exposure of one's genitals to an unsuspecting stranger.
B. The person has acted on these sexual urges, or the sexual urges or fantasies cause marked distress or interpersonal difficulty.

From American Psychiatric Association. *Diagnostic and Statistical Manual of Mental Disorders.* 4th ed. Text rev. Washington, DC: American Psychiatric Association; copyright 2000, with permission.

A 53-year-old housebound man with agoraphobia who had been married four times sought help for a recent loss of control over his usual need for foot fetishism and fantasies of humiliation and domination. He claimed that his masochistic hunger dominated all his waking moments. He recalls being sexually aroused by women's feet since age 4. When his mother sat in a chair and placed her sole on his face, he developed an erection. He spent many of his childhood hours orchestrating games in which babysitters and neighbors placed their feet on his face. As an adult, he says he likes to be degraded and humiliated by a woman who leaves him with no decision-making capacities. He is excited by leather and the smell of a foot—particularly by being forced to endure disgusting odor from a foot. His new wife's insistence that he seek help came after he sought total domination from her and told her "I want to be broken, with no way out, then be used as a slave for sex and to cook and clean. I even want to watch you have sex with another man." She threatened to leave with their 4-year-old daughter and insisted that he seek professional help. When his first wife refused such behavior, he had an affair with a woman who whipped him. He and his second wife were "into bondage" until he became so obsessed that she became uncomfortable. His third marriage at age 50 was to a very aggressive thief who sexually dominated him but did not care about him outside their bedroom dramas. To conduct intercourse during the last decade, he has had to fantasize about being dominated. He has masturbated at least daily since age 17 and continues to attempt to regulate his frequent sexual tensions 3 to 4 times per day via masturbation or intercourse with his wife. (Courtesy of Stephen B. Levine, M.D.)

Table 21.3–4
DSM-IV-TR Diagnostic Criteria for Frotteurism

A. Over a period of at least 6 months, recurrent, intense sexually arousing fantasies, sexual urges, or behaviors involving touching and rubbing against a nonconsenting person.
B. The person has acted on these sexual urges, or the sexual urges or fantasies cause marked distress or interpersonal difficulty.

From American Psychiatric Association. *Diagnostic and Statistical Manual of Mental Disorders.* 4th ed. Text rev. Washington, DC: American Psychiatric Association; copyright 2000, with permission.

Frotteurism. Frotteurism is usually characterized by a man's rubbing his penis against the buttocks or other body parts of a fully clothed woman to achieve orgasm (Table 21.3–4). At other times, he may use his hands to rub an unsuspecting victim. The acts usually occur in crowded places, particularly in subways and buses. Those with frotteurism are extremely passive and isolated, and frottage is often their only source of sexual gratification. The expression of aggression in this paraphilia is readily apparent.

Pedophilia. Pedophilia involves recurrent intense sexual urges toward, or arousal by, children 13 years of age or younger, over a period of at least 6 months. Persons with pedophilia are at least 16 years of age and at least 5 years older than the victims. (Table 21.3–5). When a perpetrator is a late adolescent involved in an ongoing sexual relationship with a 12- or 13-year-old, the diagnosis is not warranted.

Most child molestations involve genital fondling or oral sex. Vaginal or anal penetration of children occurs infrequently except in cases of incest. Although most child victims coming to public attention are girls, this finding appears to be a product of the referral process. Offenders report that when they touch a child, most (60 percent) of the victims are boys. This figure is in sharp contrast to the figure for nontouching victimization of children, such as window peeping and exhibitionism; 99 percent of all such cases are perpetrated against girls. Of those with pedophilia, 95 percent are heterosexual, and 50 percent have consumed alcohol to excess at the time of the incident. In addition to their pedophilia, a significant number of the perpetrators are concomitantly or have previously been involved in exhibitionism, voyeurism, or rape.

Incest is related to pedophilia by the frequent selection of an immature child as a sex object, the subtle or overt element of coercion, and occasionally the preferential nature of the adult–child liaison.

Table 21.3–5
DSM-IV-TR Diagnostic Criteria for Pedophilia

A. Over a period of at least 6 months, recurrent, intense sexually arousing fantasies, sexual urges, or behaviors involving sexual activity with a prepubescent child or children (generally age 13 years or younger).
B. The person has acted on these sexual urges, or the sexual urges or fantasies cause marked distress or interpersonal difficulty.
C. The person is at least age 16 years and at least 5 years older than the child or children in Criterion A.

Note: Do not include an individual in late adolescence involved in an ongoing sexual relationship with a 12- or 13-year-old.

Specify if:
Sexually attracted to males
Sexually attracted to females
Sexually attracted to both

Specify if:
Limited to incest

Specify type:
Exclusive type (attracted only to children)
Nonexclusive type

From American Psychiatric Association. *Diagnostic and Statistical Manual of Mental Disorders.* 4th ed. Text rev. Washington, DC: American Psychiatric Association; copyright 2000, with permission.

A 67-year-old man with a doctorate degree whose aspiration for entrepreneurial success remained undaunted despite his lifetime of failures touched his 9-year-old granddaughter's genitals under the guise of teaching her what others should never do to her. The visibly disturbed child told her mother, who quickly called a family meeting to expose a previous secret she and her father had maintained: When she was between the ages of 13 and 16, her father had sexual intimacies with her and told her it would not be good for her depressed mother to know this. Her younger sister had also been approached when she was pubescent, but she had strongly rebuffed the father. The man said that he and his beloved granddaughter were having their usual warm affectionate time reading a story together when for "no good reason" he began educating her. He had not been erotically preoccupied with her; he was just in his ordinary state of sexual and financial frustration. Although potent, he had no interest in sex with his unemployable, dysthymic wife who could not stop complaining about her husband's vocational failures and their serious financial problems. (Courtesy of Stephen B. Levine, M.D.)

Sexual Masochism. Masochism takes its name from the activities of Leopold von Sacher-Masoch, a 19th century Austrian novelist whose characters derived sexual pleasure from being abused and dominated by women. According to DSM-IV-TR, persons with sexual masochism have a recurrent preoccupation with sexual urges and fantasies involving the act of being humiliated, beaten, bound, or otherwise made to suffer (Table 21.3–6). Sexual masochistic practices are more common among men that among women. Freud believed masochism resulted from destructive fantasies turned against the self. In some cases, persons can allow themselves to experience sexual feelings only when punishment for the feelings follows. Persons with sexual masochism may have had childhood experiences that convinced them that pain is a prerequisite for sexual pleasure. About 30 percent of those with sexual masochism also have sadistic fantasies. Moral masochism involves a need to suffer but is not accompanied by sexual fantasies.

Table 21.3–6
DSM-IV-TR Diagnostic Criteria for Sexual Masochism

A. Over a period of at least 6 months, recurrent, intense sexually arousing fantasies, sexual urges, or behaviors involving the act (real, not simulated) of being humiliated, beaten, bound, or otherwise made to suffer.

B. The fantasies, sexual urges, or behaviors cause clinically significant distress or impairment in social, occupational, or other important areas of functioning.

A 38-year-old thin, stylish mother of three, with lifelong inability to attain an orgasm with a partner, sought help for dysthymic disorder with recurrent suicidal ideation, sedative abuse, and aversion to sexual experience with her highly valued husband. She had masturbated almost every day of her life to orgasm to thoughts of being painfully penetrated with medical instruments, burned, or given painful enemas. The medical instrumentation fantasies began at age 19 when she worked in a urologist's office. She thought of her fantasies as "sick, uncontrollable, but necessary to relieve my tensions." A painfully shy child with school and social phobias until adult life, she was unable to recall any childhood medical procedure, burn experience, or physical or sexual abuse that might explain why her erotic life has been dominated by masochism. She was extremely close to her grossly obese mother, rarely saw her hard-working, idealized father, and was reluctant to discuss the possibility that she had experienced any pain and suffering in her home. (Courtesy of Stephen B. Levine, M.D.)

Sexual Sadism. The DSM-IV-TR diagnostic criteria for sexual sadism are presented in Table 21.3–7. The onset of the disorder is usually before the age of 18 years, and most persons with sexual sadism are male. According to psychoanalytic theory, sadism is a defense against fears of castration; persons with sexual sadism do to others what they fear will happen to them and derive pleasure from expressing their aggressive instincts. The disorder was named after the Marquis de Sade, an 18th century French author and military officer who was repeatedly imprisoned for his violent sexual acts against women. Sexual sadism is related to rape, although rape is more aptly considered an expression of power. Some sadistic rapists, however, kill their victims after having sex (so-called lust murders). In many cases, these persons have underlying schizophrenia. John Money believes that lust murderers have dissociative identity disorder and perhaps a history of head trauma. He lists five contributory causes of sexual sadism: hereditary predisposition, hormonal malfunctioning, pathological relationships, a history of sexual abuse, and the presence of other mental disorders.

Table 21.3–7
DSM-IV-TR Diagnostic Criteria for Sexual Sadism

A. Over a period of at least 6 months, recurrent, intense sexually arousing fantasies, sexual urges, or behaviors involving acts (real, not simulated) in which the psychological or physical suffering (including humiliation) of the victim is sexually exciting to the person.

B. The person has acted on these sexual urges with a nonconsenting person, or the sexual urges or fantasies cause marked distress or interpersonal difficulty.

A controlling, narcissistic physician, raised alone by his widowed mother since age 2, has been preoccupied with spanking's erotic charge for him since age 6. Socially awkward during adolescence and his 20s, he married the first woman he dated and gradually introduced her to his secret arousal pattern of imagining himself spanking women. Although horrified, she episodically agreed to indulge him on an infrequent schedule to supplement their frequent ordinary sexual behavior. He ejaculated only when imagining spanking. Following her sixth episode of anxious, sullen, depression in 20 years of marriage, her psychologist instructed her to tell him "No more." He fell into despair, was diagnosed with a major depressive disorder, and wrote a long letter to her about why he was entitled to spank her. He claimed to have had little idea that her participation in this humiliation was negatively affecting her mental health ("She even had orgasm sometimes after I spanked her!"). He became suicidal as a solution to the dilemma of choosing between his or her happiness and becoming conscious that what he was asking was abusive. He was shocked to discover that she had long considered suicide as a solution to her marital trap of loving an otherwise good husband and father who had an unexplained sick sexual need.

Voyeurism. Voyeurism, also known as scopophilia, is the recurrent preoccupation with fantasies and acts that involve observing persons who are naked or engaged in grooming or sexual activity (Table 21.3–8). Masturbation to orgasm usually accompanies or follows the event. The first voyeuristic act usually occurs during childhood and is most common in men. When persons with voyeurism are apprehended, the charge is usually loitering.

Transvestic Fetishism. Transvestic fetishism is described as fantasies and sexual urges to dress in opposite gender clothing as a means of arousal and as an adjunct to masturbation or coitus (Table 21.3–9). Transvestic fetishism typically begins in childhood or early adolescence. As years pass, some men with transvestic fetishism want to dress and live permanently as women. More rarely, women want to dress and live as men. These persons are classified in DSM-IV-TR as persons with transvestic fetishism and gender dysphoria. Usually a person

Table 21.3–8
DSM-IV-TR Diagnostic Criteria for Voyeurism

A. Over a period of at least 6 months, recurrent, intense sexually arousing fantasies, sexual urges, or behaviors involving the act of observing an unsuspecting person who is naked, in the process of disrobing, or engaging in sexual activity.

B. The person has acted on these sexual urges, or the sexual urges or fantasies cause marked distress or interpersonal difficulty.

From American Psychiatric Association. *Diagnostic and Statistical Manual of Mental Disorders.* 4th ed. Text rev. Washington, DC: American Psychiatric Association; copyright 2000, with permission.

Table 21.3–10
DSM-IV-TR Diagnostic Criteria for Paraphilia Not Otherwise Specified

This category is included for coding paraphilias that do not meet the criteria for any of the specific categories. Examples include, but are not limited to, telephone scatologia (obscene phone calls), necrophilia (corpses), partialism (exclusive focus on part of body), zoophilia (animals), coprophilia (feces), klismaphilia (enemas), and urophilia (urine).

From American Psychiatric Association. *Diagnostic and Statistical Manual of Mental Disorders.* 4th ed. Text rev. Washington, DC: American Psychiatric Association; copyright 2000, with permission.

wears more than one article of opposite sex clothing; frequently, an entire wardrobe is involved. When a man with transvestic fetishism is cross-dressed, the appearance of femininity may be striking, although not usually to the degree found in transsexualism. When not dressed in women's clothes, men with transvestic fetishism may be hypermasculine in appearance and occupation. Cross-dressing can be graded from solitary, depressed, guilt-ridden dressing to ego-syntonic, social membership in a transvestite subculture.

The overt clinical syndrome of transvestic fetishism may begin in latency but is more often seen around pubescence or in adolescence. Frank dressing in opposite sex clothing usually does not begin until mobility and relative independence from parents are well established.

A 15-year-old was brought for assessment to a residential setting by his third foster mother who could no longer tolerate his stealing of her underwear and his sexually provocative behavior with the two other foster children in the home. In the residential treatment center he constantly masturbated and repeatedly initiated sexual behaviors with staff and boy and girl residents. His developmental history was rife with early physical abuse, substance-abusing parents, paternal then maternal abandonment, and cross-dressing since age 6.

Table 21.3–9
DSM-IV-TR Diagnostic Criteria for Transvestic Fetishism

A. Over a period of at least 6 months, in a heterosexual male, recurrent, intense sexually arousing fantasies, sexual urges, or behaviors involving cross-dressing.

B. The fantasies, sexual urges, or behaviors cause clinically significant distress or impairment in social, occupational, or other important areas of functioning.

Specify if:

With gender dysphoria: if the person has persistent discomfort with gender role or identity

From American Psychiatric Association. *Diagnostic and Statistical Manual of Mental Disorders.* 4th ed. Text rev. Washington, DC: American Psychiatric Association; copyright 2000, with permission.

Paraphilia Not Otherwise Specified. The classification of paraphilia not otherwise specified includes varied paraphilias that do not meet the criteria for any of the aforementioned categories (Table 21.3–10).

TELEPHONE AND COMPUTER SCATOLOGIA. Telephone scatologia is characterized by obscene phone calling and involves an unsuspecting partner. Tension and arousal begin in anticipation of phoning; the recipient of the call listens while the telephoner (usually male) verbally exposes his preoccupations or induces her to talk about her sexual activity. The conversation is accompanied by masturbation, which is often completed after the contact is interrupted.

Persons also use interactive computer networks, sometimes compulsively, to send obscene messages by electronic mail and to transmit sexually explicit messages and video images. Because of the anonymity of the users in chat rooms who use aliases, on-line or computer sex (cybersex) allows some persons to play the role of the opposite sex ("genderbending"), which represents an alternative method of expressing transvestic or transsexual fantasies. A danger of on-line cybersex is that pedophiles often make contact with children or adolescents who are lured into meeting them and are then molested. Many on-line contacts develop into off-line liaisons. While some persons report that the off-line encounters develop into meaningful relationships, most such meetings are filled with disappointment and disillusionment, as the fantasized person fails to meet unconscious expectations of perfection. In other situations, when adults meet, rape or even homicide may occur.

NECROPHILIA. Necrophilia is an obsession with obtaining sexual gratification from cadavers. Most persons with this disorder find corpses in morgues, but some have been known to rob graves or even to murder to satisfy their sexual urges. In the few cases studied, those with necrophilia believed that they were inflicting the greatest conceivable humiliation on their lifeless victims. According to Richard von Krafft-Ebing, the diagnosis of psychosis is, under all circumstances, justified.

PARTIALISM. Persons with the disorder of partialism concentrate their sexual activity on one part of the body to the exclusion of all others. Mouth-genital contact—such as cunnilingus (oral contact with a woman's external genitals), fellatio (oral contact with the penis), and anilingus (oral contact with the anus)—is normally associated with foreplay; Freud recognized the mucosal surfaces of the body as erotogenic and capable of

producing pleasurable sensation. But when a person uses these activities as the sole source of sexual gratification and cannot have or refuses to have coitus, a paraphilia exists. It is also known as oralism.

ZOOPHILIA. In zoophilia, animals—which may be trained to participate—are preferentially incorporated into arousal fantasies or sexual activities, including intercourse, masturbation, and oral-genital contact. Zoophilia as an organized paraphilia is rare. For many persons, animals are the major source of relatedness, so it is not surprising that a broad variety of domestic animals are used sensually or sexually.

Sexual relations with animals may occasionally be an outgrowth of availability or convenience, especially in parts of the world where rigid convention precludes premarital sexuality and in situations of enforced isolation. Because masturbation is also available in such situations, however, a predilection for animal contact is probably present in opportunistic zoophilia.

COPROPHILIA AND KLISMAPHILIA. Coprophilia is sexual pleasure associated with the desire to defecate on a partner, to be defecated on, or to eat feces (coprophagia). A variant is the compulsive utterance of obscene words (coprolalia). These paraphilias are associated with fixation at the anal stage of psychosexual development. Similarly, klismaphilia, the use of enemas as part of sexual stimulation, is related to anal fixation.

UROPHILIA. Urophilia, a form of urethral eroticism, is interest in sexual pleasure associated with the desire to urinate on a partner or to be urinated on. In both men and women, the disorder may be associated with masturbatory techniques involving the insertion of foreign objects into the urethra for sexual stimulation.

MASTURBATION. Masturbation is a normal activity that is common in all stages of life from infancy to old age, but this viewpoint was not always accepted. Freud believed that neurasthenia was caused by excessive masturbation. In the early 1900s, masturbatory insanity was a common diagnosis in hospitals for the criminally insane in the United States. Masturbation can be defined as a person's achieving sexual pleasure—which usually results in orgasm—by himself or herself (autoeroticism). Alfred Kinsey found it to be more prevalent in males than in females, but this difference may no longer exist. The frequency of masturbation varies from three to four times a week in adolescence to one to two times a week in adulthood. It is common among married persons; Kinsey reported that it occurred on the average of once a month among married couples.

The techniques of masturbation vary in both sexes and among persons. The most common technique is direct stimulation of the clitoris or penis with the hand or the fingers. Indirect stimulation may also be used, such as rubbing against a pillow or squeezing the thighs. Kinsey found that 2 percent of women are capable of achieving orgasm through fantasy alone. Men and women have been known to insert objects in the urethra to achieve orgasm. The hand vibrator is now used as a masturbatory device by both sexes.

Masturbation is abnormal when it is the only type of sexual activity performed in adulthood, when its frequency indicates a compulsion or sexual dysfunction, or when it is consistently preferred to sex with a partner.

HYPOXYPHILIA. Hypoxyphilia is the desire to achieve an altered state of consciousness secondary to hypoxia while experiencing orgasm. Persons may use a drug (e.g., a volatile nitrite or nitrous oxide) to produce hypoxia. Autoerotic asphyxiation is also associated with hypoxic states, but it should be classified as a form of sexual masochism. (A discussion of autoerotic asphyxiation appears in Section 21.2 of this chapter.)

Differential Diagnosis

Clinicians must differentiate a paraphilia from an experimental act that is not recurrent or compulsive and that is done for its novelty. Paraphiliac activity is most likely to occur during adolescence. Some paraphilias (especially the bizarre types) are associated with other mental disorders, such as schizophrenia. Brain diseases may also release perverse impulses.

Course and Prognosis

A poor prognosis for paraphilias is associated with an early age of onset, a high frequency of acts, no guilt or shame about the act, and substance abuse. The course and the prognosis are good when patients have a history of coitus in addition to the paraphilia and when they are self-referred rather than referred by a legal agency.

Treatment

Five types of psychiatric interventions are used to treat persons with paraphilias: external control, reduction of sexual drives, treatment of comorbid conditions (e.g., depression or anxiety), cognitive-behavioral therapy, and dynamic psychotherapy.

Prison is an external control mechanism for sexual crimes that usually does not contain a treatment element. When victimization occurs in a family or work setting, the external control comes from letting supervisors, peers, or other adult family members know of the problem and advising them about eliminating opportunities for the perpetrator to act on his urges.

Drug therapy, including antipsychotic or antidepressant medication, is indicated for the treatment of schizophrenia or depressive disorders if the paraphilia is associated with these disorders. Antiandrogens, such as cyproterone acetate in Europe and medroxyprogesterone acetate (Depo-Provera) in the United States, may reduce the drive to behave sexually by decreasing serum testosterone levels to subnormal concentrations. Serotonergic agents such as fluoxetine (Prozac) have been used in some paraphilia patients with limited success.

Cognitive-behavioral therapy is used to disrupt learned paraphiliac patterns and modify behavior to make it socially acceptable. The interventions include social skills training, sex education, cognitive restructuring (confronting and destroying the rationalizations used to support victimization of others), and development of victim empathy. Imaginal desensitization, relaxation technique, and learning what triggers the paraphiliac impulse so that such stimuli can be avoided are also taught. In modified aversive behavior rehearsal the perpetrator is videotaped acting out his paraphilia with a mannequin. The paraphilia patient is then confronted by a therapist and a group of other offenders who ask questions about feelings, thoughts, motives associated with the act and repeatedly try to correct

cognitive distortions and point out lack of victim empathy to the patient.

Insight-oriented psychotherapy is a long-standing treatment approach. Patients have the opportunity to understand their dynamics and the events that caused the paraphilia to develop. In particular, they become aware of the daily events that cause them to act on their impulses (e.g., a real or fantasized rejection). Treatment helps them deal with life stresses better and enhances their capacity to relate to a life partner. Psychotherapy also allows patients to regain self-esteem, which in turn allows them to approach a partner in a more normal sexual manner. Sex therapy is an appropriate adjunct to the treatment of patients who suffer from specific sexual dysfunctions when they attempt nondeviant sexual activities.

Good prognostic indicators include the presence of only one paraphilia, normal intelligence, the absence of substance abuse, the absence of nonsexual antisocial personality traits, and the presence of a successful adult attachment. However, paraphilias remain significant treatment challenges even under these circumstances.

ICD-10

In the 10th revision of *International Statistical Classification of Diseases and Related Health Problems* (ICD-10), the paraphilias are classified as disorders of sexual preference. In ICD-10, six specific disorders—fetishism, fetishistic transvestism, exhibitionism, voyeurism, pedophilia, and sadomasochism—and three residual categories are listed (Table 21.3–11).

SEXUAL DISORDER NOT OTHERWISE SPECIFIED

Many sexual disorders are not classifiable as sexual dysfunctions or as paraphilias. These unclassified disorders are rare, poorly documented, not easily classified, or not specifically described in DSM-IV-TR (Table 21.3–12). ICD-10 has a similar residual category for problems related to sexual development or preference (Table 21.3–13).

Postcoital Dysphoria

Not listed in DSM-IV-TR, postcoital dysphoria occurs during the resolution phase of sexual activity, when persons normally experience a sense of general well-being and muscular and psychological relaxation. Some persons, however, undergo postcoital dysphoria at this time and, after an otherwise satisfactory sexual experience, become depressed, tense, anxious, and irritable and show psychomotor agitation. They often want to get away from their partners and may become verbally or even physically abusive. The incidence of the disorder is unknown, but it is more common in men than in women. The several causes relate to the person's attitude toward sex in general and toward the partner in particular. The disorder may occur in adulterous sex and in contacts with prostitutes. The fear of acquired immune deficiency syndrome (AIDS) causes some persons to experience postcoital dysphoria. Treatment requires insight-oriented psychotherapy to help patients understand the unconscious antecedents to their behavior and attitudes.

Couple Problems

At times, a complaint arises from the spousal unit or the couple, rather than from an individual dysfunction. For example, one partner may prefer morning sex, but the other functions more readily at night, or the partners have unequal frequencies of desire.

Unconsummated Marriage

A couple involved in an unconsummated marriage have never had coitus and are typically uninformed and inhibited about sexuality. Their feelings of guilt, shame, or inadequacy are increased by their problem, and they experience conflict between their need to seek help and their need to conceal their difficulty. Couples may seek help for the problem after having been married several months or several years. William Masters and Virginia Johnson reported one unconsummated marriage of 17 years' duration.

Frequently, the couple do not seek help directly; the woman may reveal the problem to her gynecologist on a visit ostensibly concerned with vague vaginal or other somatic complaints. On examining her, the gynecologist may find an intact hymen. In some cases, however, the wife may have undergone a hymenectomy to resolve the problem, but the surgery usually aggravates the situation without solving the basic problem. The surgical procedure is another stress and often increases the couple's feelings of inadequacy. The wife may feel put upon, abused, or mutilated, and the husband's concern about his manliness may increase. An inquiry by a physician who is comfortable dealing with sexual problems may be the first opening to a frank discussion of the couple's distress. Often, the pretext of the medical visit is a discussion of contraceptive methods or—even more ironically—a request for an infertility workup. Once presented, the complaint can often be treated successfully. The duration of the problem does not significantly affect the prognosis or the outcome of the case.

The causes of unconsummated marriage are varied: lack of sex education, sexual prohibitions overly stressed by parents or society, problems of an oedipal nature, immaturity in both partners, overdependence on primary families, and problems in sexual identification. Religious orthodoxy, with severe control of sexual and social development, and the equation of sexuality with sin or uncleanliness have also been cited as a dominant cause. Many women involved in an unconsummated marriage have distorted concepts about their vaginas. They may fear that it is too small or too soft, or they may confuse the vagina with the rectum and thus feel unclean. Men may share these distortions about the vagina and perceive it as dangerous to themselves. Similarly, both partners may have distortions about the man's penis and perceive it as a weapon, as too large, or as too small. Many patients can be helped by simple education about genital anatomy and physiology, by suggestions for self-exploration, and by correct information from a physician. The problem of unconsummated marriage is best treated by seeing both members of the couple. Dual-sex therapy involving a male-female cotherapist team has been markedly effective. Other forms of conjoint therapy, marital counseling, traditional psychotherapy on a one-to-one basis, and counseling from a sensitive family physician, gynecologist, or urologist are also helpful.

Table 21.3–11
ICD-10 Diagnostic Criteria for Disorders of Sexual Preference

G1. The individual experiences recurrent intense sexual urges and fantasies involving unusual objects or activities.
G2. The individual either acts on the urges or is markedly distressed by them.
G3. The preference has been present for at least 6 months.

Fetishism

A. The general criteria for disorders of sexual preference must be met.
B. The fetish (some nonliving object) is the most important source of sexual stimulation or is essential for satisfactory sexual response.

Fetishistic transvestism

A. The general criteria for disorders of sexual preference must be met.
B. The individual wears articles of clothing of the opposite sex in order to create the appearance and feeling of being a member of the opposite sex.
C. The cross-dressing is closely associated with sexual arousal. Once orgasm occurs and sexual arousal declines, there is a strong desire to remove the clothing.

Exhibitionism

A. The general criteria for disorders of sexual preference must be met.
B. There is either a recurrent or a persistent tendency to expose the genitalia to unsuspecting strangers (usually of the opposite sex), which is almost invariably associated with sexual arousal and masturbation.
C. There is no intention or invitation to have sexual intercourse with the "witness(es)."

Voyeurism

A. The general criteria for disorders of sexual preference must be met.
B. There is either a recurrent or a persistent tendency to look at people engaging in sexual or intimate behavior such as undressing, which is associated with sexual excitement and masturbation.
C. There is no intention to reveal one's presence.
D. There is no intention of sexual involvement with the person(s) observed.

Pedophilia

A. The general criteria for disorders of sexual preference must be met.
B. There is a persistent or predominant preference for sexual activity with a prepubescent child or children.
C. The individual is at least 16 years old and at least 5 years older than the child or children in Criterion B.

Sadomasochism

A. The general criteria for disorders of sexual preference must be met.
B. There is preference for sexual activity, as recipient (masochism) or provider (sadism), or both, which involves at least one of the following:
(1) pain;
(2) humiliation;
(3) bondage.
C. The sadomasochistic activity is the most important source of stimulation or is necessary for sexual gratification.

Multiple disorders of sexual preference

The likelihood of more than one abnormal sexual preference occurring in one individual is greater than would be expected by chance. For research purposes the different types of preference, and their relative importance to the individual, should be listed. The most common combination is fetishism, transvestism, and sadomasochism.

Other disorders of sexual preference

A variety of other patterns of sexual preference and activity may occur, each being relatively uncommon. These include such activities as making obscene telephone calls, rubbing up against people for sexual stimulation in crowded public places (frotteurism), sexual activity with animals, use of strangulation or anoxia for intensifying sexual excitement, and a preference for partners with some particular anatomical abnormality such as an amputated limb.

Erotic practices are too diverse and many too rare or idiosyncratic to justify a separate term for each. Swallowing urine, smearing feces, or piercing foreskin or nipples may be part of the behavioral repertoire in sadomasochism. Masturbatory rituals of various kinds are common, but the more extreme practices, such as the insertion of objects into the rectum or penile urethra, or partial self-strangulation, when they take the place of ordinary sexual contacts, amount to abnormalities. Necrophilia should also be coded here.

Disorder of sexual preference, unspecified

Body Image Problems

Some persons are ashamed of their bodies and experience feelings of inadequacy related to self-imposed standards of masculinity or femininity. They may insist on sex only during total darkness, not allow certain body parts to be seen or touched, or seek unnecessary operative procedures to deal with their imagined inadequacies. Body dysmorphic disorder should be ruled out.

Sex Addiction and Compulsivity

The concept of sex addiction developed over the past two decades to refer to persons who compulsively seek out sexual

Table 21.3–12
DSM-IV-TR Diagnostic Criteria for Sexual Disorder Not Otherwise Specified

This category is included for coding a sexual disturbance that does not meet the criteria for any specific sexual disorder and is neither a sexual dysfunction nor a paraphilia. Examples include

1. Marked feelings of inadequacy concerning sexual performance or other traits related to self-imposed standards of masculinity or femininity
2. Distress about a pattern of repeated sexual relationships involving a succession of lovers who are experienced by the individual only as things to be used
3. Persistent and marked distress about sexual orientation

From American Psychiatric Association. *Diagnostic and Statistical Manual of Mental Disorders.* 4th ed. Text rev. Washington, DC: American Psychiatric Association; copyright 2000, with permission.

experiences and whose behavior becomes impaired if they are unable to gratify their sexual impulses. The concept of sex addiction derived from the model of addiction to such drugs as heroin or addiction to behavioral patterns, such as gambling. Addiction implies psychological dependence, physical dependence, and the presence of a withdrawal syndrome if the substance (e.g., the drug) is unavailable or the behavior (e.g., gambling) is frustrated.

In DSM-IV-TR the term *sex addiction* is not used, nor is it a disorder that is universally recognized or accepted. Nevertheless, the phenomenon of a person whose entire life revolves around sex-seeking behavior and activities, who spends an excessive amount of time in such behavior, and who often tries to stop such behavior but is unable to do so is well known to clinicians. Such persons show repeated and increasingly frequent attempts to have a sexual experience, deprivation of which gives rise to symptoms of distress. Sex addiction is a useful concept heuristically, in that it can alert the clinician to seek an underlying cause for the manifest behavior. There is interest in making it a new official diagnostic category, which the authors support.

Table 21.3–13
ICD-10 Diagnostic Criteria for Psychological and Behavioral Disorders Associated with Sexual Development and Orientation

This section is intended to cover those types of problems that derive from variations of sexual development or orientation, when the sexual preference per se is not necessarily problematic or abnormal.

Sexual maturation disorder

The patient suffers from uncertainty about his or her gender identity or sexual orientation, which causes anxiety or depression.

Ego-dystonic sexual orientation

The gender identity or sexual preference is not in doubt, but the individual wishes it were different.

Sexual relationship disorder

The abnormality of gender identity or sexual preference is responsible for difficulties in forming or maintaining a relationship with a sexual partner.

Other psychosexual development disorders

Psychosexual development disorder, unspecified

Reprinted with permission from World Health Organization. *The ICD-10 Classification of Mental and Behavioural Disorders: Diagnostic Criteria for Research.* Copyright, World Health Organization, Geneva, 1993.

Diagnosis. Sex addicts are unable to control their sexual impulses, which can involve the entire spectrum of sexual fantasy or behavior. Eventually, the need for sexual activity increases, and the person's behavior is motivated solely by the persistent desire to experience the sex act. The history usually reveals a long-standing pattern of such behavior, which the person repeatedly has tried to stop, but without success. Although there may be feelings of guilt and remorse after the act, they do not suffice to prevent its recurrence. The patient may report that the need to act out is most severe during stressful periods or when angry, depressed, anxious, or otherwise dysphoric. Most acts culminate in a sexual orgasm. Eventually, the sexual activity interferes with the person's social, vocational, or marital life, which begins to deteriorate. The signs of sexual addictions are listed in Table 21.3–14.

Types of Behavioral Patterns. The paraphilias constitute the behavioral patterns most often found in the sex addict. As defined in DSM-IV-TR, the essential features of a paraphilia are recurrent intense sexual urges or behaviors, including exhibitionism, fetishism, frotteurism, sadomasochism, cross-dressing, voyeurism, and pedophilia. Paraphilias are associated with clinically significant distress and almost invariably interfere with interpersonal relationships, and they often lead to legal complications. In addition to the paraphilias, however, sex addiction can also include behavior that is considered normal, such as coitus and masturbation, except that it is promiscuous and uncontrolled.

In the 19th century, Krafft-Ebing reported on several cases of abnormally increased sexual desire. One involved a 36-year-old married teacher, the father of seven children, who masturbated repeatedly while sitting at his desk in front of his pupils, after which he was "penitent

Table 21.3–14
Signs of Sexual Addiction

1. Out-of-control behavior
2. Severe adverse consequences (medical, legal, interpersonal) due to sexual behavior
3. Persistent pursuit of self-destructive or high-risk sexual behavior
4. Repeated attempts to limit or stop sexual behavior
5. Sexual obsession and fantasy as a primary coping mechanism
6. The need for increasing amounts of sexual activity
7. Severe mood changes related to sexual activity (e.g., depression, euphoria)
8. Inordinate amount of time spent in obtaining sex, being sexual, or recovering from sexual experience
9. Interference of sexual behavior in social, occupational, or recreational activities

Data from Carnes P. *Don't Call It Love.* New York: Bantam Books; 1991.

and filled with shame." He indulged in coitus three or four times a day in addition to his repeated masturbatory act. In another case a young woman masturbated almost incessantly and was unable to control her impulses. She had frequent coitus with many men, but neither coitus nor masturbation sufficed, and she eventually was placed in an institution. Krafft-Ebing referred to the condition as "sexual hyperaesthesia," which he believed could occur in otherwise normal persons.

In many cases sex addiction is the final common pathway of a variety of other disorders. In addition to the paraphilias that are often present, there may be an associated major mental disorder or schizophrenia. Antisocial personality disorder and borderline personality disorder are common.

DON JUANISM. Some men who appear to be hypersexual, as manifested by their need to have many sexual encounters or conquests, use their sexual activities to mask deep feelings of inferiority. Some have unconscious homosexual impulses, which they deny by compulsive sexual contacts with women. After having sex, most Don Juans are no longer interested in the woman. The condition is sometimes referred to as satyriasis or sex addiction.

NYMPHOMANIA. Nymphomania signifies a woman's excessive or pathological desire for coitus. There have been few scientific studies of the condition, but those patients who have been studied usually have had one or more sexual disorders, often including female orgasmic disorder. The woman often has an intense fear of losing love and, through her actions, attempts to satisfy her dependence needs rather than gratify her sexual impulses. This disorder is a form of sex addiction.

Comorbidity. Comorbidity (dual diagnosis) refers to the presence of an addiction that coexists with another psychiatric disorder. For example, about 50 percent of patients with substance-use disorder also have an additional psychiatric disorder. Similarly, many sex addicts have an associated psychiatric disorder. Dual diagnosis implies that the psychiatric illness and the addiction are separate disorders; one does not cause the other. The diagnosis of comorbidity is often difficult to make because addictive behavior (of all types) can produce extreme anxiety and severe disturbances in mood and affect, especially while the addictive behavior is treated. If, after a period of abstinence, symptoms of a psychiatric disorder remain, the comorbid condition is more easily recognized and diagnosed than during the addictive period. Finally, there is a high correlation between sex addiction and substance-use disorders (up to 80 percent in some studies), which not only complicates the task of diagnosis, but also complicates treatment.

Treatment. Self-help groups based on the 12-step concept used in Alcoholics Anonymous (AA) have been used successfully with many sex addicts. They include such groups as Sexaholics Anonymous (SA), Sex and Love Addicts Anonymous (SLAA), and Sex Addicts Anonymous (SAA). The groups differ in that some are for men or women, or for married persons or couples. All advocate some abstinence from either the addictive behavior or sex in general. Should a substance-use disorder also be present, the patient often requires referral to AA or Narcotics Anonymous (NA) as well. Patients may enter an inpatient treatment unit when they lack sufficient motivation to control their behavior on an outpatient basis or may be a danger to themselves or others. Additionally, severe medical or psychiatric symptoms may require careful supervision and treatment best carried out in a hospital.

A 42-year-old married businessman with two children was considered a model of virtue in his community. He was active in his church and on the boards of several charitable organizations. He was living a secret life, however, and would lie to his wife, telling her that he was at a board meeting when he was actually visiting massage parlors for paid sex. He eventually was engaging in the behavior four to five times a day, and although he tried to quit many times, he was unable to do so. He knew that he was harming himself by putting his reputation and marriage at risk.

The patient presented himself to the psychiatric emergency room, stating that he would prefer to be dead rather than continue the behavior described. He was admitted with a diagnosis of major depressive disorder and started on a daily dose of 20 mg of fluoxetine. In addition, he received 100 mg of medroxyprogesterone intramuscularly once a day. His need to masturbate diminished markedly and ceased entirely on the third hospital day, as did his mental preoccupation with sex. The medroxyprogesterone was discontinued on the sixth day, when he was discharged. He continued to take fluoxetine, enrolled in a local SA group, and entered individual and couples psychotherapy. His addictive behavior eventually stopped, he was having satisfactory sexual relations with his wife, and he was no longer suicidal or depressed.

Psychotherapy. Insight-oriented psychotherapy may help patients understand the dynamics of their behavioral patterns. Supportive psychotherapy can help repair the interpersonal, social, or occupational damage that occurs. Cognitive behavioral therapy helps the patient recognize dysphoric states that precipitate sexual acting out. Marital therapy or couples therapy can help the patient regain self-esteem, which is severely impaired by the time a treatment program is begun. Finally, psychotherapy may be of help in the treatment of any associated psychiatric disorder.

Pharmacotherapy. Most specialists in general addiction avoid the use of psychotropic agents, especially in the early stages of treatment. Substance-dependent persons have a tendency to abuse those agents, especially agents with a high abuse potential, such as the benzodiazepines. Pharmacotherapy is of use in the treatment of associated psychiatric disorders, such as major depressive disorders and schizophrenia.

Certain medications may be of use to the sex addict, however, because of their specific effects on reducing the sex drive. Serotonin-specific reuptake inhibitors (SSRIs) reduce libido in some persons, a side effect that is used therapeutically. Compulsive masturbation is an example of a behavioral pattern that may benefit from such medication. Medroxyprogesterone acetate diminishes libido in men and thus makes it easier to control sexually addictive behavior.

The use of antiandrogens in women to control hypersexuality has not been tested sufficiently, but since androgenic compounds contribute to the sex drive in women, antiandrogens

could be of benefit. Antiandrogenic agents (cyproterone acetate) are not available in the United States but are used in Europe with varying success.

Persistent and Marked Distress about Sexual Orientation

Distress about sexual orientation is characterized by dissatisfaction with sexual arousal patterns and is usually applied to dissatisfaction with homosexual arousal patterns, a desire to increase heterosexual arousal, and strong negative feelings about being homosexual. Occasional statements to the effect that life would be easier if the speaker were not homosexual do not constitute persistent and marked distress about sexual orientation.

Treatment of sexual orientation distress is controversial. One study reported that with a minimum of 350 hours of psychoanalytic therapy, about a third of 100 bisexual and gay men achieved a heterosexual reorientation at a 5-year follow-up; but this study has been challenged. Behavior therapy and avoidance conditioning techniques have also been used, but these techniques may change behavior in the laboratory setting but not outside. Prognostic factors weighing in favor of heterosexual reorientation for men include being under 35 years of age, having some experience of heterosexual arousal, and feeling highly motivated to reorient.

Another and more prevalent style of intervention is directed at enabling persons with persistent and marked distress about sexual orientation to live comfortably with homosexuality without shame, guilt, anxiety, or depression. Gay counseling centers are engaged with patients in such treatment programs. At present, outcome studies of such centers have not been reported in detail.

Few data are available about the treatment of women with persistent and marked distress about sexual orientation, and these are primarily from single-case studies with variable outcomes. (Section 21.1 of this chapter presents a further discussion of sexual orientation, homosexuality, and coming out.)

References

Abel GG, Osborn C. The paraphilias: the extent and nature of sexually deviant and criminal behavior. *Psychiatr Clin North Am.* 1992;15:675.

Feierman JR, Feierman LA. Paraphilias. In: Szuchman LT, Muscarella F, eds. *Psychological Perspectives on Human Sexuality.* New York: John Wiley & Sons; 2000:480.

Freud S. Three essays on the theory of sexuality. In: *Standard Edition of the Complete Psychological Works of Sigmund Freud.* Vol 7. London: Hogarth Press; 1953:125.

Levine, SB. In: Sadock BJ, Sadock VA, eds. *Kaplan & Sadock's Comprehensive Textbook of Psychiatry.* 7th ed. Vol 1. Baltimore: Lippincott Williams & Wilkins; 2000:1631.

Meyer JK. Paraphilias. In: Kaplan HI, Sadock BJ, eds. *Comprehensive Textbook of Psychiatry.* 6th ed. Baltimore: Williams & Wilkins; 1995:1334.

Nurnberg HG, Hensley PL, Lauriello J. Sildenafil in the treatment of sexual dysfunction induced by selective serotonin reuptake inhibitors: an overview. *Cns Drugs.* 2000;13:321.

Santtila P, Sandnabba NK, Alison L, Nordling N. Investigating the underlying structure in sadomasochistically oriented behavior. *Arch Sex Behav.* 2002; 31:185.

Tierney DW, McCabe MP. The assessment of denial, cognitive distortions, and victim empathy among pedophilic sex offenders: an evaluation of the utility of self-report measures. *Trauma Violence Abuse.* 2001;2:259.

Travin S. Compulsive sexual behaviors. *Psychiatr Clin North Am.* 1995;18:155.

22

Gender Identity Disorders

Gender identity is a psychological state that reflects a person's sense of being male or female. It develops in most persons by the age of 2 or 3 years and usually corresponds to one's biological sex. Gender identity develops from an innumerable series of cues received from parents and the culture at large that are themselves reactions to the infant's genitalia. Gender role is the external behavioral pattern that reflects a person's inner sense of "I am male" or "I am female." While there is some flexibility regarding what behaviors are considered masculine or feminine, the culture expects men and women (or boys and girls) to have a sense of maleness or femaleness that reflects their anatomical sex. Gender identity disorders involve the persistent desire to be, or the insistence that one is, of the other sex and extreme discomfort with one's assigned sex and gender role.

The text revision of the fourth edition of *Diagnostic and Statistical Manual of Mental Disorders* (DSM-IV-TR) defines gender identity disorders as a heterogeneous group of disorders whose common feature is a strong and persistent preference for the status and role of the opposite sex. These disorders may be manifested verbally, in assertions that one properly belongs to the opposite sex, or nonverbally, in cross-sex behavior. The affective component of gender identity disorders is commonly referred to as *gender dysphoria,* which may be defined as discontent with one's biological sex, the desire to possess the body of the opposite sex, and the wish to be regarded as a member of the opposite sex. The extreme forms of gender identity disorders, collectively referred to as *transsexualism* in the third edition of DSM (DSM-III) and revised third edition (DSM-III-R), commonly involve attempts to pass as a member of the opposite sex in society and to obtain hormonal and surgical treatment to simulate the phenotype of the opposite biological sex. According to DSM-IV-TR, persons cannot be diagnosed with gender identity disorder when they have a concurrent physical intersex condition such as partial androgen insensitivity syndrome or congenital adrenal hyperplasia. DSM-IV-TR also requires specification of sexual orientation. A person with gender identity disorder may be attracted to persons of the opposite sex, of the same sex, or of both sexes or may not experience sexual attraction to others.

EPIDEMIOLOGY

Almost no information is available about the prevalence of gender identity disorders among children, teenagers, and adults. Most estimates of prevalence are based on the number of persons seeking sex-reassignment surgery, a number that indicates a male preponderance. The ratios of boys to girls reported in three child–gender-identity clinics were 30 to 1, 17 to 1, and 6 to 1; these clinics had little experience of girls. This disparity may indicate a greater male vulnerability to gender identity disorders or a greater sensitivity to, and worry about, cross-gender–identified boys than about cross-gender–identified girls in the United States. Studies of boys referred for outpatient psychiatric treatment revealed that up to about 50 percent had significant effeminate behavior. The boys were not referred primarily for problems with gender identity. How many met the criteria for gender identity disorders is unclear.

ETIOLOGY

Biological Factors

For mammals, the resting state of tissue is initially female; as the fetus develops, a male is produced only if androgen (set off by the Y chromosome, which is responsible for testicular development) is introduced. Without testes and androgen, female external genitalia develop. Thus, maleness and masculinity depend on fetal and perinatal androgens. Lower animals' sexual behavior is governed by sex steroids, but this effect diminishes as the evolutionary tree is scaled. Sex steroids influence the expression of sexual behavior in mature men or women; that is, testosterone can increase libido and aggressiveness in women, and estrogen can decrease libido and aggressiveness in men. But masculinity, femininity, and gender identity result more from postnatal life events than from prenatal hormonal organization.

The same principle of masculinization or feminization has been applied to the brain. Testosterone affects brain neurons that contribute to the masculinization of the brain in such areas as the hypothalamus. Whether testosterone contributes to so-called masculine or feminine behavioral patterns in gender identity disorders remains a controversial issue. Recent findings point to a difference in the brain of male-to-female transsexuals. In a postmortem sample of 6, the red nucleus corresponded in size to that of typical females rather than of typical males; independent of whether the male transsexual was heterosexual or homosexual.

Psychosocial Factors

Children develop a gender identity consonant with their sex of rearing (also known as assigned sex). The formation of gender identity is influenced by the interaction of children's temperament and parents' qualities and attitudes. There are culturally acceptable gender roles: Boys are not expected to be effeminate, and girls are not expected to be tomboys. There are boys'

games (e.g., cops and robbers) and girls' toys (e.g., dolls and dollhouses). These roles are learned, although some investigators believe that some boys are temperamentally delicate and sensitive and that some girls are aggressive and energized—traits that are stereotypically known in today's culture as feminine and masculine, respectively.

Sigmund Freud believed that gender identity problems resulted from conflicts experienced by children within the oedipal triangle. These conflicts are fueled by both real family events and children's fantasies. Whatever interferes with a child's loving the opposite-sex parent and identifying with the same-sex parent interferes with normal gender identity.

The quality of the mother–child relationship in the first years of life is paramount in establishing gender identity. During this period, mothers normally facilitate their children's awareness of, and pride in, their gender: Children are valued as little boys and girls, but devaluing, hostile mothering can result in gender problems. At the same time, the separation-individuation process is unfolding. When gender problems become associated with separation-individuation problems, the result can be the use of sexuality to remain in relationships characterized by shifts between a desperate infantile closeness and a hostile, devaluing distance.

Some children are given the message that they would be more valued if they adopted the gender identity of the opposite sex. Rejected or abused children may act on such a belief. Gender identity problems can also be triggered by a mother's death, extended absence, or depression, to which a young boy may react by totally identifying with her—that is, by becoming a mother to replace her.

The father's role is also important in the early years, and his presence normally helps the separation-individuation process. Without a father, mother and child may remain overly close. For a girl, the father is normally the prototype of future love objects; for a boy, the father is a model for male identification.

DIAGNOSIS

According to DSM-IV-TR, the essential feature of gender identity disorder is a person's persistent and intense distress about his or her assigned sex and a desire to be, or an insistence that he or she is, of the other sex. As children, both girls and boys show an aversion to normative, stereotypically feminine or masculine clothing and repudiate their respective anatomical characteristics. Table 22–1 lists the DSM-IV-TR criteria for the disorder.

Table 22–1
DSM-IV-TR Diagnostic Criteria for Gender Identity Disorder

A. A strong and persistent cross-gender identification (not merely a desire for any perceived cultural advantages of being the other sex).

In children, the disturbance is manifested by four (or more) of the following:

(1) repeatedly stated desire to be, or insistence that he or she is, the other sex

(2) in boys, preference for cross-dressing or simulating female attire; in girls, insistence on wearing only stereotypical masculine clothing

(3) strong and persistent preferences for cross-sex roles in make-believe play or persistent fantasies of being the other sex

(4) intense desire to participate in the stereotypical games and pastimes of the other sex

(5) strong preference for playmates of the other sex

In adolescents and adults, the disturbance is manifested by symptoms such as a stated desire to be the other sex, frequent passing as the other sex, desire to live or be treated as the other sex, or the conviction that he or she has the typical feelings and reactions of the other sex.

B. Persistent discomfort with his or her sex or sense of inappropriateness in the gender role of that sex.

In children, the disturbance is manifested by any of the following: in boys, assertion that his penis or testes are disgusting or will disappear or assertion that it would be better not to have a penis, or aversion toward rough-and-tumble play and rejection of male stereotypical toys, games, and activities; in girls, rejection of urinating in a sitting position, assertion that she has or will grow a penis, or assertion that she does not want to grow breasts or menstruate, or marked aversion toward normative feminine clothing.

In adolescents and adults, the disturbance is manifested by symptoms such as preoccupation with getting rid of primary and secondary sex characteristics (e.g., request for hormones, surgery, or other procedures to physically alter sexual characteristics to simulate the other sex) or belief that he or she was born the wrong sex.

C. The disturbance is not concurrent with a physical intersex condition.

D. The disturbance causes clinically significant distress or impairment in social, occupational, or other important areas of functioning.

Code based on current age:

Gender identity disorder in children

Gender identity disorder in adolescents or adults

Specify if (for sexually mature individuals):

Sexually attracted to males

Sexually attracted to females

Sexually attracted to both

Sexually attracted to neither

From American Psychiatric Association. *Diagnostic and Statistical Manual of Mental Disorders.* 4th ed. Text rev. Washington, DC: American Psychiatric Association; copyright 2000, with permission.

CLINICAL FEATURES

Children

At the extreme of gender identity disorder in children are boys who, by the standards of their cultures, are as feminine as the most feminine of girls and girls who are as masculine as the most masculine of boys. No sharp line can be drawn on the continuum of gender identity disorder between children who should receive a formal diagnosis and those who should not. Girls with the disorder regularly have male companions and an avid interest in sports and rough-and-tumble play; they show no interest in dolls or playing house (unless they play the father or another male role). They may refuse to urinate in a sitting position, claim that they have or will grow a penis, not want to grow breasts or to menstruate, and assert that they will grow up to become a man (not merely to play a man's role).

Boys with the disorder are usually preoccupied with stereotypically female activities. They may have a preference for dressing in girls' or women's clothes or may improvise such items from available material when the genuine articles are not available. (The cross-dressing typically does not cause sexual excitement, as in transvestic fetishism.) They often have a compelling desire to participate in the games and pastimes of girls. Female dolls are often their favorite toys, and girls are regularly their preferred playmates. When playing house, they take a girl's role. Their gestures and actions are often judged to be feminine, and they are usually subjected to male peer group teasing and rejection, a phenomenon that rarely occurs with boyish girls until adolescence. Boys with the disorder may assert that they will grow up to become a woman (not merely in role). They may claim that their penis or testes are disgusting or will disappear or that it would be better not to have a penis or testes. Some children refuse to attend school because of teasing or the pressure to dress in attire stereotypical of their assigned sex. Most children deny being disturbed by the disorder, except that it brings them into conflict with the expectations of their families or peers.

A 5-year-old boy, referred by his general practitioner, was brought for evaluation by both parents. He had been saying either he was a girl or had wanted to be one since age 3. His preferred clothing was that of his sister. He wanted to wear makeup and his mother's jewelry. His favorite toys were dress-up dolls, especially those with long hair. He refused to stand to urinate. In make-believe games he was usually the mommy or a female character. Most of his friends were girls. He showed no interest in sports. All the pictures he drew were of women. The cross-gender behavior was recalled by both parents since the boy was age 2. Neither attempted to interrupt it or redirect his interests until recently, and the boy met their efforts with resistance. They had been advised by a preschool teacher and a regular babysitter to ignore the behavior as it would go away. Neither parent expressed concern that their son would become homosexual, but they are concerned that he may be transsexual.

A 7-year-old girl, referred through her school, had been insisting to other children that she was a boy. Since the age of 2 years she has said that she was a boy and that she did not want to be a girl. Her clothing style preference is that of boys and attempts to make her wear a dress are met with refusal. She watches her father shave and ignores her mother applying makeup. Her friends are boys, and her favorite activity is sport. She has no interest in doll play but loves action and soldier toys and guns. She frequently attempts to urinate while standing.

Adolescents and Adults

There are similar signs and symptoms in adolescents and adults. Adolescents and adults with the disorder manifest a stated desire to be the other sex, they frequently try to pass as a member of the other sex, and they desire to live or to be treated as the other sex. In addition, they desire to acquire the sex characteristics of the opposite sex. They may believe that they were born the wrong sex and may make such characteristic statements as, "I feel that I'm a woman trapped in a male body" or vice versa.

Adolescents and adults frequently request medical or surgical procedures to alter their physical appearance. Although the term *transsexual* is not used in DSM-IV-TR, many clinicians find the term useful and will probably continue to use it. In addition, *transsexualism* appears in the 10th revision of *International Statistical Classification of Diseases and Related Health Problems* (ICD-10), and persons refer to themselves as transsexuals. Transsexual persons have a persistent preoccupation with getting rid of their primary and secondary sex characteristics and acquiring the sex characteristics of the other sex. The wish to dress and live as a member of the other sex is always present.

Most retrospective studies of transsexuals report gender identity problems during childhood, but prospective studies of children with gender identity disorders indicate that few become transsexuals and want to change their sex. The disorder is much more common in men (1 per 30,000) than in women (1 per 100,000). Adult transsexuals usually complain that they are uncomfortable wearing the clothes of their assigned sex; therefore, they dress the way the other sex dresses and engage in activities associated with the other sex. They find their genitals repugnant, a feeling that may lead to persistent requests for surgery. This desire may override all other wishes.

Men take estrogen to create breasts and other feminine contours, have electrolysis to remove their male hair, and have surgery to remove the testes and the penis and to create an artificial vagina. Women bind their breasts or have a double mastectomy, a hysterectomy, and an oophorectomy; take testosterone to build up muscle mass and deepen the voice; and have surgery in which an artificial phallus is created. These procedures may make a person indistinguishable from members of the other sex. Some investigators describe behavior in sex-reassigned persons as almost a caricature of the newly assumed male or female role.

A 37-year-old man presented with a request for sex reassignment surgery. He was dressed as a man, and he was masculine in his physical appearance and mannerisms. The patient had not been observably effeminate in boyhood. He had, however, been attracted to, and fascinated by, feminine activities from an early age. He particularly recalled having liked to watch women apply makeup. He began cross-dressing around puberty. During adolescence he sometimes stole women's underwear from clotheslines. At that stage he preferred women's clothes that had been worn because he felt that they were somehow infused with femininity. Cross-dressing was sexually arousing from puberty until his early 30s, when sexual excitement yielded to feelings of comfort and naturalness.

The patient married at 25. He initially hoped that marriage would cure his cross-dressing but that hope soon proved false. The couple's sex life was poor, and the marriage

dissolved after 8 years. He began another heterosexual relationship a few years after his divorce, but that relationship also failed in the face of his growing gender dysphoria.

Following clinical assessment, the patient began making systematic plans to move into the female role and began living and going to work as a woman full-time at 39. The attempt to live as a woman proved successful, and the patient underwent surgical sex reassignment at 41.

After moving into the female role, the patient went on a few dates with men but found that she could not really develop an interest in them. After surgery she began moving in lesbian social circles and having sexual relationships with women. She was content with her life in general and had no regrets about her decision to undergo sex reassignment.

Gender Identity Disorder Not Otherwise Specified

The diagnosis of gender identity disorder not otherwise specified is reserved for persons who cannot be classified as having a gender identity disorder with the characteristics described above (Table 22–2). Three examples are listed in DSM-IV-TR: persons with intersex conditions and gender dysphoria; adults with transient, stress-related cross-dressing behavior; and persons who have a persistent preoccupation with castration or penectomy without a desire to acquire the sex characteristics of the other sex.

Intersex Conditions. Intersex conditions include a variety of syndromes in which persons have gross anatomical or physiological aspects of the opposite sex.

TURNER'S SYNDROME. In Turner's syndrome (Fig. 22–1) one sex chromosome is missing (XO). The result is an absence (agenesis) or minimal development (dysgenesis) of the gonads; no significant sex hormones, male or female, are produced in fetal life or postnatally. The sexual tissues remain in a female resting state. Because the second X chromosome—which seems responsible for full femaleness—is missing, girls have incomplete sexual anatomy and, lacking adequate estrogens, develop no secondary sex characteristics without treatment. They often show other signs, such as webbed neck, low posterior hairline margin, short stature, and cubitus valgus. Infants are born with normal-appearing female external genitals and so are unequivocally assigned to the female sex and are reared as girls. All the children develop as unremarkably feminine, heterosexually oriented girls; but later medical management is necessary to assist them with their infertility and absence of secondary sex characteristics.

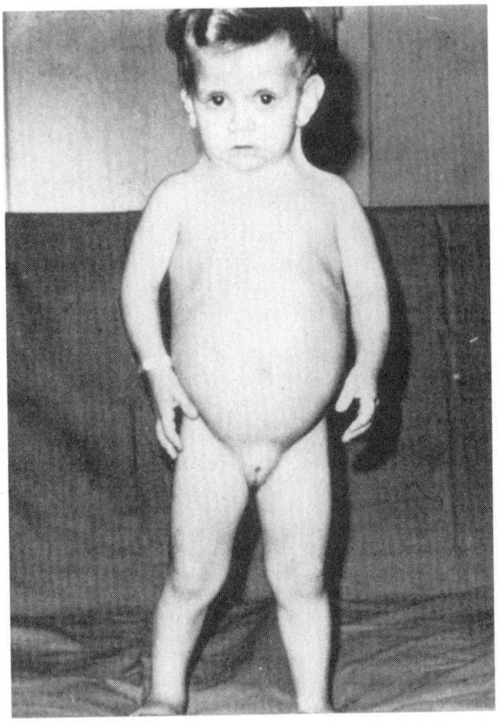

FIGURE 22–1

Photograph of patient with Turner's syndrome. The main characteristics are webbed neck, short stature, broad chest, and absence of sexual maturation. (Reprinted from Sadler T. *Langman's Medical Embryology.* 5th ed. Baltimore: Williams & Wilkins; 1985:121, with permission.)

Table 22–2
DSM-IV-TR Diagnostic Criteria for Gender Identity Disorder Not Otherwise Specified

This category is included for coding disorders in gender identity that are not classifiable as a specific gender identity disorder. Examples include

1. Intersex conditions (e.g., partial androgen insensitivity syndrome or congenital adrenal hyperplasia) and accompanying gender dysphoria
2. Transient, stress-related cross-dressing behavior
3. Persistent preoccupation with castration or penectomy without a desire to acquire the sex characteristics of the other sex

From American Psychiatric Association. *Diagnostic and Statistical Manual of Mental Disorders.* 4th ed. Text rev. Washington, DC: American Psychiatric Association; copyright 2000, with permission.

KLINEFELTER'S SYNDROME. Persons with Klinefelter's syndrome (usually XXY) have a male habitus under the influence of the Y chromosome, but the effect is weakened by the presence of the second X chromosome. Although patients are born with a penis and testes, the testes are small and infertile, and the penis may also be small. Beginning in adolescence, some patients develop gynecomastia and other feminine-appearing contours. Their sexual desire is usually weak. Sex assignment and rearing should lead to a clear sense of maleness, but the patients often have gender disturbances, ranging from a complete reversal, as in transsexualism, to an intermittent desire to put on women's clothes. As a result of lessened androgen production, the fetal hypogonadal condition in some patients seems to have interfered with the completion of the central nervous system organization that should underlie masculine behavior. In fact, many patients have a wide variability of psychopathology, ranging from emotional instability to mental retardation.

CONGENITAL VIRILIZING ADRENAL HYPERPLASIA (ADRENOGENITAL SYNDROME). Congenital virilizing adrenal hyperplasia results in an excess of androgen acting on the fetus. When the condition occurs in women, excessive fetal androgens from the adrenal gland have caused androgenization of the external genitals. The androgenization can range

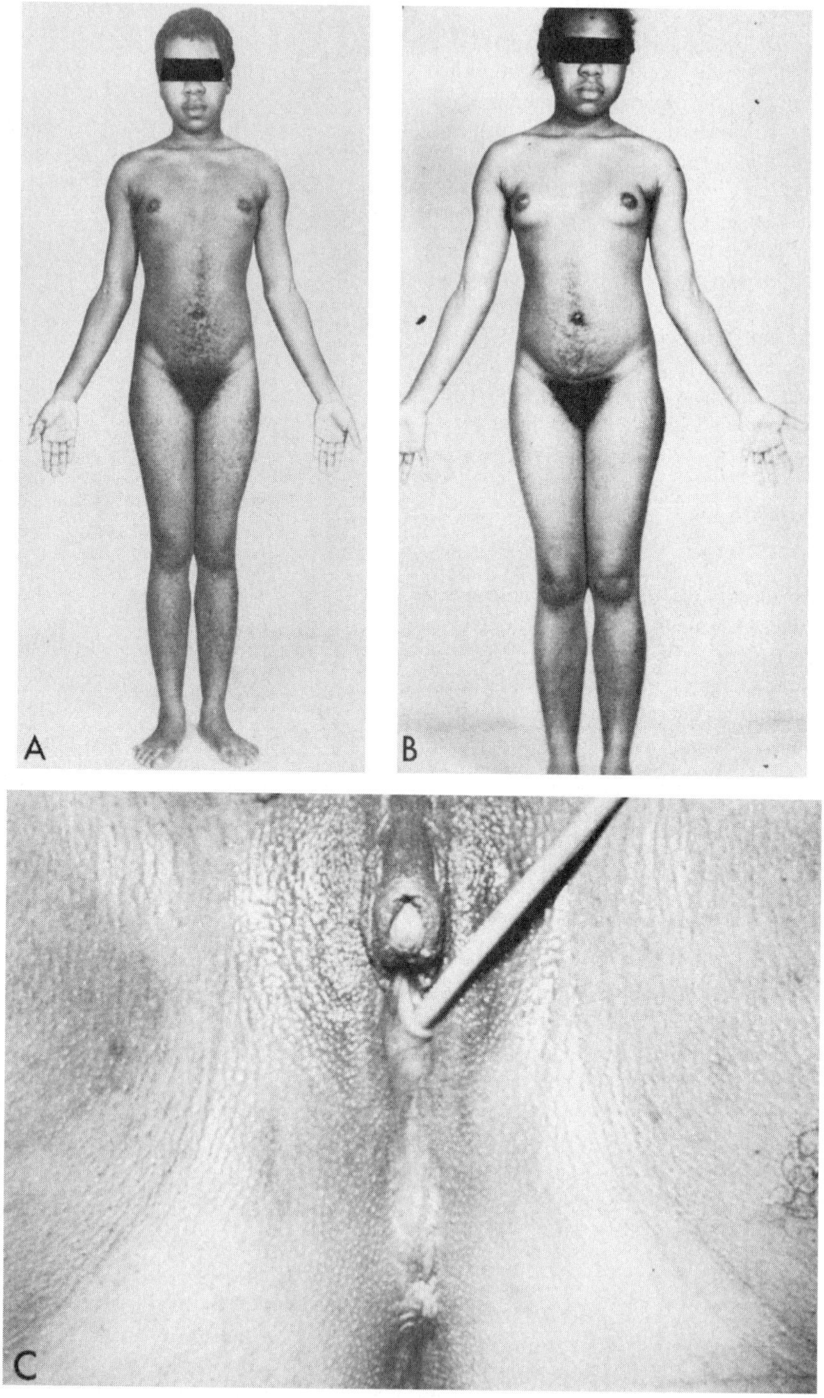

FIGURE 22–2

A. Female pseudohermaphroditism due to congenital adrenal hyperplasia. **B.** Note the breast development after 6 months of cortisone therapy; normal cyclic menses began within a few months. **C.** Note the enlarged clitoris and urogenital sinus. (Courtesy of Robert B. Greenblatt, M.D., and Virginia P. McNamara, M.D.)

from mild clitoral enlargement to external genitals that look like a normal scrotal sac, testes, and a penis, but hidden behind these external genitals are a vagina and a uterus (Fig. 22–2). The patients are otherwise normally female. At birth, if the genitals look male, children are assigned to the male sex and so reared; the result is usually a clear sense of maleness and unremarkable masculinity. If the children are assigned to the female sex and so reared, a sense of femaleness and femininity usually results. If the parents are uncertain about the sex of their child, a hermaphroditic identity results. The resultant gender identity usually reflects the rearing practices, but androgens may help determine behavior. Children raised unequivocally as girls have a more intense tomboy quality than that found in a control group. The girls

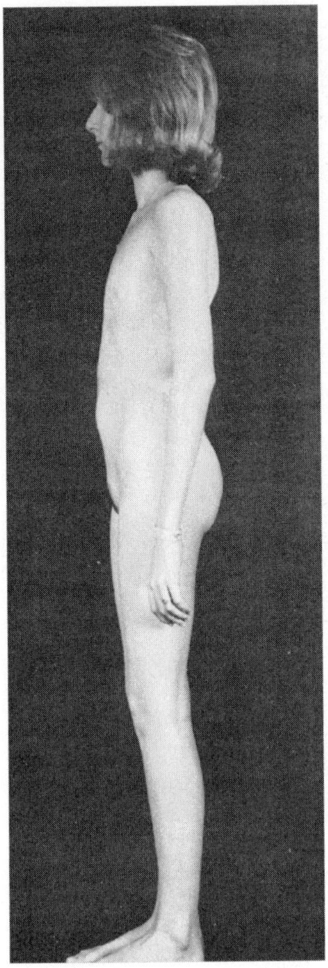

FIGURE 22–3
The vaginal canal was normal with clitoral enlargement. At laparotomy, dysgenetic gonads and a uterus with fallopian tubes were present. On cyclic estrogen-progestogen therapy, menses were induced at regular intervals, and good breast development resulted. (Courtesy of Robert B. Greenblatt, M.D., and Virginia P. McNamara, M.D.)

most often have a heterosexual orientation. Some of these children experience gender identity conflicts.

PSEUDOHERMAPHRODITISM. Infants born with ambiguous genitals are an obstetrical emergency. Sex assignment, based on the genitals' appearance at birth, determine gender identity, which is male, female, or hermaphroditic, depending on the family's conviction about the child's sex. Male pseudohermaphroditism is incomplete differentiation of the external genitalia even though a Y chromosome is present; testes are present but rudimentary. Female pseudohermaphroditism is the presence of virilized genitals in a person who is XX, the most common cause being the adrenogenital syndrome described above. Figure 22–3 illustrates a phenotypic female with an XY karyotype.

True hermaphroditism is characterized by the presence of both testes and ovaries in the same person. It is a rare condition (Fig. 22–4).

ANDROGEN INSENSITIVITY SYNDROME. Androgen insensitivity syndrome, a congenital X-linked recessive trait disorder (also known as testicular feminization syndrome), results from the inability of target tissues to respond to androgens. Unable to respond, the fetal tissues remain in their female resting state, and the central nervous system is not organized as masculine. At birth the infant appears unremarkably female, although she is later found to have cryptorchid testes, which produce the testosterone to which the tissues do not respond, and minimal or absent internal sexual organs. Secondary sex characteristics at puberty are female because of the small, but sufficient, amount of estrogens, which results from the conversion of testosterone into estradiol. The patients invariably sense themselves as females and are feminine.

Cross-Dressing. DSM-IV-TR lists cross-dressing—dressing in clothes of the opposite sex—as a gender identity disorder if it is transient and related to stress. If the disorder is not stress related, persons who cross-dress are classified as having transvestic fetishism, which is described as a paraphilia in DSM-IV-TR. An essential feature of transvestic fetishism is that it produces sexual excitement. Stress-related cross-dressing may sometimes produce sexual excitement, but it also reduces a patient's tension and anxiety. Patients may harbor fantasies of cross-dressing but act them out only under stress. Male adult cross-dressers may have the fantasy that they are female, in whole or in part.

Cross-dressing is commonly known as *transvestism,* and the cross-dresser as a *transvestite*. Although these terms are no longer used in DSM-IV-TR, they remain in common parlance. Cross-dressing phenomena range from the occasional solitary wearing of clothes of the other sex to extensive feminine identification in men and masculine identification in women, with involvement in a transvestic subculture. More than one article of clothing of the other sex is involved, and a person may dress entirely as a member of the opposite sex. The degree to which a cross-dressed person appears as a member of the other sex varies, depending on mannerisms, body habitus, and cross-dressing skill. When not cross-dressed, these persons usually appear as unremarkable members of their assigned sex. Cross-dressing may coexist with paraphilias, such as sexual sadism, sexual masochism, and pedophilia.

Cross-dressing differs from transsexualism in that the patients have no persistent preoccupation with getting rid of their primary and secondary sex characteristics and acquiring the sex characteristics of the other sex. Some persons with the disorder once had transvestic fetishism but no longer become sexually aroused by cross-dressing. Other persons with the disorder are homosexual men and women who cross-dress. The disorder is most common among female impersonators.

Preoccupation with Castration. The category of preoccupation with castration is reserved for men and women who have a persistent preoccupation with castration or penectomy without a desire to acquire the sex characteristics of the opposite sex. They are clearly uncomfortable with their assigned sex and live a life driven by the fantasy of what it would be like to be a different gender. They may be asexual and lack sexual interest in either men or women.

A 45-year-old married male was admitted to the hospital after amputating the glans of his penis with a carving knife. He claimed that he heard voices telling him to carry out the act. He had been diagnosed with schizophrenia at age 25 after an episode of paranoid ideation in which he felt that persons were going to harm him. Although married, he had

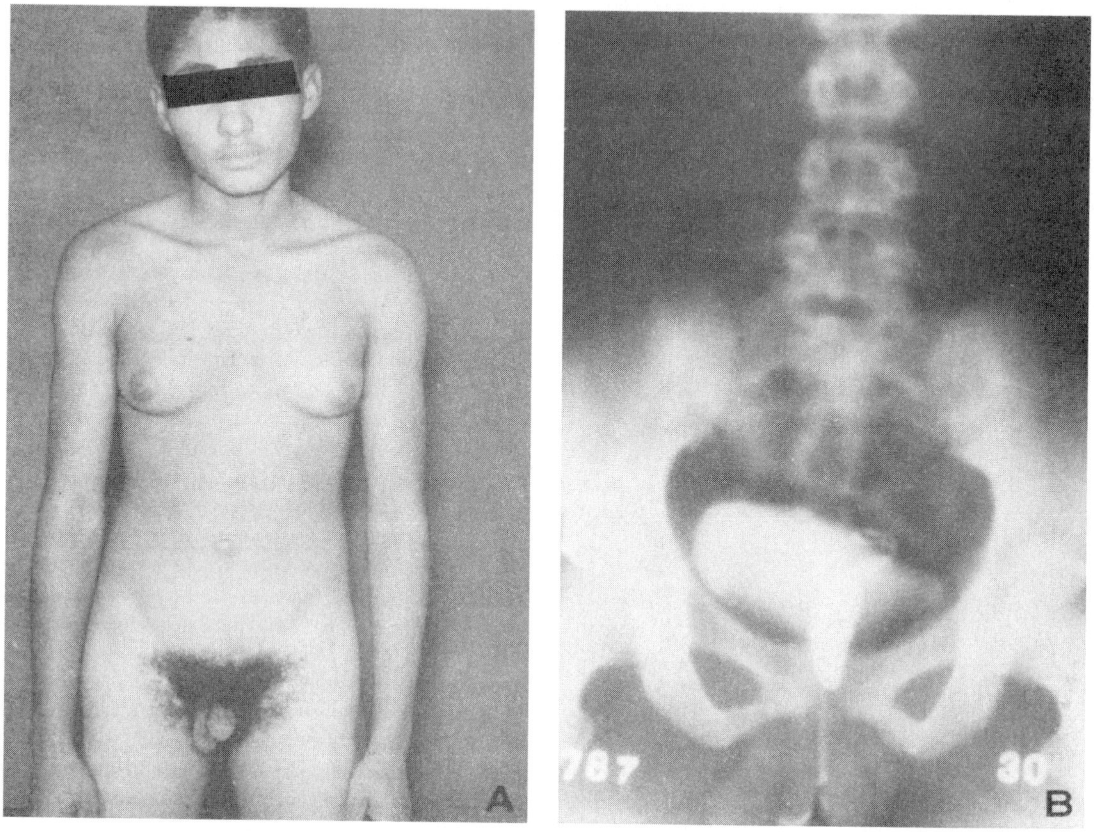

FIGURE 22–4
A true hermaphrodite. An abdominal ovary and a scrotal testis were found on biopsy of gonadal structures. Menses occurred each month from the urogenital sinus. **A.** Note gynecomastia. **B.** A cystogram and vaginal-uterosalpingogram revealed separate openings for the urethra and vaginal tract. The unicollis uterus and the fallopian tube are outlined. (Courtesy of Robert B. Greenblatt, M.D., and Virginia P. McNamara, M.D.)

had repeated homosexual encounters since adolescence. He was able to function in the community when taking antipsychotic medications, but at the time of the event, he had not taken medication for over 1 year.

COURSE AND PROGNOSIS

The prognosis for gender identity disorder depends on the age of onset and the intensity of the symptoms. Boys begin to have the disorder before the age of 4 years, and peer conflict develops during the early school years, at about the age of 7 or 8 years. Grossly feminine mannerisms may lessen as boys grow older, especially if attempts are made to discourage such behavior. Cross-dressing may be part of the disorder, and 75 percent of boys who cross-dress begin to do so before age 4. The age of onset is also early for girls, but most give up masculine behavior by adolescence.

In both sexes, homosexuality is likely to develop in one third to two thirds of all cases, although, for reasons that are unclear, fewer girls than boys have a homosexual orientation. Steven Levine reported that follow-up studies of gender-disturbed boys consistently indicated that homosexual orientation was the usual adolescent outcome. Transsexualism—that is, the desire for sex-reassignment surgery—occurs in less than 10 percent of cases. Retrospective data on homosexual men indicate a high frequency of cross-gender identifications and feminine gender role behavior during childhood.

Impaired social and occupational functioning as a result of a person's wanting to participate in the desired (and opposite) gender role is common. Depression is also a common problem, especially if a person feels hopeless about obtaining a sex change with surgery or hormones. Men have been known to castrate themselves, not as a suicide attempt but as a way of forcing a surgeon to deal with their problem.

TREATMENT

Treatment of gender identity disorders is complex and rarely successful when the goal is to reverse the disorder. Most persons with gender identity disorders have fixed ideas and values and are unwilling to change. If and when they enter psychotherapy, it is most often because of depression or anxiety that they attribute to their condition. Countertransference problems must be addressed assiduously by therapists, many of whom are uncomfortable with patients who have gender identity disorder.

Parents generally bring children with cross-gender behavior patterns to a psychiatrist. Richard Green developed a treatment program designed to inculcate culturally acceptable behavior patterns in boys. Green uses a one-to-one play relationship with

children in which adults or peers role-model masculine behavior. Parental counseling in conjunction with group meetings of parents and their children with gender identity disorder is also used. Parents' encouragement of children's atypical behavior (such as dressing a boy in girl's clothing or not cutting his hair) is examined when parents are unaware that they are fostering cross-gender behavior.

Adolescent patients are difficult to treat because of the coexistence of normal identity crises and gender identity confusion. Acting out is common, and adolescents rarely have a strong motivation to alter their cross-gender roles. Adult patients generally enter psychotherapy to learn how to deal with their disorder, not to alter it. Therapists usually set a goal of helping patients become comfortable with the gender identity they desire, not of creating a person with a conventional gender identity. Therapy also explores sex-reassignment surgery and the indications and contraindications for such procedures, which are often impulsively decided on by severely distressed and anxious patients.

Sex-Reassignment Surgery

Surgical treatment is definitive, and because there is no turning back, careful standards preceding the surgery have been developed. Among these standards are the following: Patients must go through a trial of cross-gender living for at least 3 months and sometimes up to 1 year. The real-life test may change the minds of some transsexuals, because they find it uncomfortable to relate to friends, workers, and lovers in this role. Patients must receive hormone treatments with estradiol and progesterone in male-to-female changes and testosterone in female-to-male changes. Many transsexuals like the changes that occur in their bodies as a result of this treatment and stop at this point. About 50 percent of transsexuals who meet these criteria go on to sex-reassignment surgery. Outcome studies are highly variable in terms of how success is defined and measured (e.g., successful intercourse and body image satisfaction).

About 70 percent of male-to-female and 80 percent of female-to-male sex reassignment surgery patients report satisfactory results. Unsatisfactory results correlate with a preexisting mental disorder. Suicide in postoperative sex-reassignment surgery patients has been reported in up to 2 percent of all cases. Sex-reassignment surgery is a highly controversial measure that is undergoing much scrutiny.

Hormonal Treatment

Both sexes may be treated with hormones in lieu of surgery. Those who are biologically male take estrogen, and those who are biologically female take testosterone. Patients who take estrogen usually report immediate psychological satisfaction, based on a sense of tranquility, less frequent erections, and fewer sexual drive manifestations than before the hormone treatment. Their new sterility is not of concern to them. After several months, bodily contours become rounded, a limited but pleasing breast enlargement develops, and testicular volume decreases. The quality of the voice does not change. Clinicians must monitor patients for hypertension, hyperglycemia, hepatic dysfunction, and thromboembolic phenomena.

Women who take androgens quickly notice an increased sexual drive, clitoral tingling and enlargement, and, after several months, amenorrhea and hoarseness. If patients undertake weight lifting, a pronounced increase in muscle mass may occur. Depending on the hair distribution already present, patients may have a moderate increase in the amount and coarseness of facial and body hair; some develop frontal balding. Thromboembolic phenomena, hepatic dysfunction, and elevations of cholesterol and triglyceride levels are possible.

Treatment of Intersex Conditions

Because intersex conditions are present at birth, treatment must be timely, and some physicians believe the conditions to be true medical emergencies. The appearance of the genitalia in diverse conditions is often ambiguous, and a decision must be made about the assigned sex (boy or girl) and how the child should be reared.

Problems should be addressed as early as possible, so that the entire family can regard the child in a consistent, relaxed manner. This is particularly important since intersex patients may have gender identity problems because of complicated biological influences and familial confusion about their actual sex. When intersex conditions are discovered, a panel of pediatric, urological, and psychiatric experts usually determines the sex of rearing on the basis of clinical examination, urological studies, buccal smears, chromosomal analyses, and assessment of the parental wishes.

Education of parents and presentation of the range of options open to them is essential, since parents respond to the infant's genitalia in ways that promote the formation of gender identity. One option is for parents to decide against immediate surgery for ambiguous genitalia, but assign the label of boy or girl to the infant on the basis of chromosomal and urological examination. They can then react to the child according to sex role assignment with leeway to adjust the sex assignment should the child act definitively as a member of the sex opposite to the one designated.

If the parents decide on surgery to normalize genital appearance, it is generally undertaken before the age of 3 years. It is easier to assign a child to be female than to assign one to be male, because male-to-female genital surgical procedures are far more advanced than female-to-male procedures. However, that is insufficient reason to assign a chromosomal male to be female.

Some believe that all surgery for intersex conditions is unethical because the infant cannot consent. About 2,000 babies in the United States each year have a surgical procedure performed for ambiguous genitalia. In many cases a markedly enlarged clitoris or an ambiguous penis may be plastically reshaped. Some groups (e.g., the Intersex Society of North America) oppose this practice on the grounds that it is only a cosmetic change that may interfere with later sexual functioning. In the view of most experts, however, such intervention contributes substantially to the well-being of both parents and child. To have genitals concordant with chromosomal, biological, physiological, and other genetic determinants allows the development of a person with a healthier gender identity than if the ambiguity is allowed to persist. Prohibiting doctors by law from performing such operations, as some congressional lobbying groups advocate, will do more harm than good. Cosmetic surgical techniques for ambiguous genitalia are sufficiently advanced that the risk of deformity or lack of future sexual response is practically nonexistent. The determination of whether or not to proceed with surgical intervention is ultimately the decision of the parents.

Table 22–3
ICD-10 Diagnostic Criteria for Gender Identity Disorders

Transsexualism

A. The individual desires to live and be accepted as a member of the opposite sex, usually accompanied by the wish to make his or her body as congruent as possible with the preferred sex through surgery and hormonal treatment.

B. The transsexual identity has been present persistently for at least 2 years.

C. The disorder is not a symptom of another mental disorder, such as schizophrenia, nor is it associated with chromosome abnormality.

Dual-role transvestism

A. The individual wears clothes of the opposite sex in order to experience temporarily membership of the opposite sex.

B. There is no sexual motivation for the cross-dressing.

C. The individual has no desire for a permanent change to the opposite sex.

Gender identity disorder of childhood

For girls:

A. The individual shows persistent and intense distress about being a girl, and has a stated desire to be a boy (not merely a desire for any perceived cultural advantages to being a boy), or insists that she is a boy.

B. Either of the following must be present:

(1) persistent marked aversion to normative feminine clothing and insistence on wearing stereotypical masculine clothing, e.g., boy's underwear and other accessories;

(2) persistent repudiation of female anatomical structures, as evidenced by at least one of the following:

(a) an assertion that she has, or will grow, a penis;

(b) rejection of urinating in a sitting position;

(c) assertion that she does not want to grow breasts or menstruate.

C. The girl has not yet reached puberty.

D. The disorder must have been present for at least 6 months.

For boys:

A. The individual shows persistent and intense distress about being a boy, and has an intense desire to be a girl or, more rarely, insists that he is a girl.

B. Either of the following must be present:

(1) preoccupation with stereotypical female activities, as shown by a preference for either cross-dressing or simulating female attire, or by an intense desire to participate in the games and pastimes of girls and rejection of stereotypical male toys, games, and activities;

(2) persistent repudiation of male anatomical structures, as indicated by at least one of the following repeated assertions:

(a) that he will grow up to become a woman (not merely in role);

(b) that his penis or testes are disgusting or will disappear;

(c) that it would be better not to have a penis or testes;

C. The boy has not yet reached puberty.

D. The disorder must have been present for at least 6 months.

Other gender identity disorders

Gender identity disorder, unspecified

Reprinted with permission from World Health Organization. *The ICD-10 Classification of Mental and Behavioural Disorders: Diagnostic Criteria for Research*. Copyright, World Health Organization, Geneva, 1993.

Treatment of Cross-Dressing

A combined approach, using psychotherapy and pharmacotherapy, is often useful in the treatment of cross-dressing. The stress factors that precipitate the behavior are identified in therapy. The goal is to help patients cope with the stressors appropriately and, if possible, eliminate them. Intrapsychic dynamics about attitudes toward men and women are examined, and unconscious conflicts are identified. Medication, such as antianxiety and antidepressant agents, is used to treat the symptoms. Because cross-dressing may occur impulsively, medications that reinforce impulse control may be helpful, such as fluoxetine (Prozac). Behavior therapy, aversive conditioning, and hypnosis are alternative methods that may be of use in selected patients.

ICD-10

ICD-10 lists five gender identity disorders: transsexualism, dual-role transvestism, gender identity disorder of childhood, other gender identity disorders, and gender identity disorders, unspecified (Table 22–3). Transsexualism, defined as a wish to be a member of the opposite sex, can be diagnosed when the transsexual identity has persisted for at least 2 years, is not a symptom of another mental disorder, and is not associated with intersex, genetic, or sex chromosome abnormality. In dual-role transvestism, a person wears opposite-sex clothing to temporarily change to the other sex but does not want a permanent change of sex and is not sexually excited by cross-dressing.

Childhood gender identity disorder, defined as a "persistent and intense distress about assigned sex . . . with a desire to be . . . of the other sex," must appear before puberty for a diagnosis to be made.

References

Bartlett NH, Vasey PL, Bukowski WM. Is gender identity disorder in children a mental disorder? *Sex Roles*. 2000;43:11.

Blanchard R, Steiner BW, eds. *Clinical Management of Gender Identity Disorders in Children and Adults*. Washington, DC: American Psychiatric Press; 1990.

Brown GR, Wise TN, Costa PT, et al. Personality characteristics and sexual functioning of 188 cross-dressing men. *J Nerv Ment Dis*. 1996;184:265.

Cohen-Kettenis PT, Gooren LJG. Transsexualism: a review of etiology, diagnosis, and treatment. *J Psychosom Res*. 1999;46:315.

Cole SS, Denny D, Eyler AE, Samons SL. Issues of transgender. In: Szuchman LT, Muscarella F, eds. *Psychological Perspectives on Human Sexuality*. New York: John Wiley & Sons; 2000:149.

Gonzalez T, Angel M. Transsexualism: some considerations on aggression, transference and countertransference. *Int Forum Psychoanal*. 1996;5:11.

Green R. Gender identity in childhood and later sexual orientation: followup of 78 males. *Am J Psychiatry*. 1985;142:399.

Green R, Blanchard R. Gender identity disorders. In: Sadock BJ, Sadock VA, eds. *Kaplan & Sadock's Comprehensive Textbook of Psychiatry*. 7th ed. Vol 1. Baltimore: Lippincott, Williams & Wilkins, 2000:1646.

Greenblatt RB, McNamara VP. Endocrinology of human sexuality. In: Sadock BJ, Kaplan HI, eds. *The Sexual Experience*. Baltimore: Williams & Wilkins; 1976:104.

Hirschfield M. *Transvestites: The Erotic Drive to Cross-Dress*. Buffalo, NY: Prometheus; 1991.

Jones BE, Hill MJ. Mental health issues in lesbian, gay, bisexual, and transgender communities. *Rev Psychiatry*. 2002;21:93.

Levine SB. Gender-disturbed males. *J Sex Marital Ther*. 1993;19:131.

Marantz S, Coates S. Mothers of boys with gender identity disorder: a comparison of matched controls. *J Am Acad Child Adolesc Psychiatry*. 1991;30:310.

Osbourne C, Wise TN. Split gender identity: problem or solution? Proposed parameters for addressing the gender dysphoric patient. *J Sex Marital Ther*. 2002;28:165.

Stoller RJ. *Presentations of Gender*. New Haven: Yale University Press; 1986.

Sugar M. A clinical approach to childhood gender identity disorder. *Am J Psychother*. 1995;49:260.

23 Eating Disorders

▲ 23.1 Anorexia Nervosa

Anorexia nervosa is characterized by willful and purposeful behavior directed toward losing weight, weight loss, preoccupation with body weight and food, peculiar patterns of handling food, intense fear of gaining weight, disturbance of body image, and amenorrhea. About half of these persons will lose weight by drastically reducing their total food intake, and some will also develop rigorous exercising programs. The other half of these patients will also rigorously diet but will lose control and regularly engage in binge eating followed by purging behaviors. Some patients routinely purge after eating small amounts of food. In the text revision of the fourth edition of *Diagnostic and Statistical Manual of Mental Disorders* (DSM-IV-TR), anorexia nervosa is characterized as a disorder in which persons refuse to maintain a minimally normal weight, intensely fear gaining weight, and significantly misinterpret their body and its shape. DSM-IV-TR also notes that the term *anorexia* ("lack of appetite") is misleading because loss of appetite rarely occurs in the early stage of the disorder. Anorexia nervosa is thus characterized by a profound disturbance of body image and the relentless pursuit of thinness, often to the point of starvation.

The disorder has been recognized for many decades and has been described in various persons with remarkable uniformity. Anorexia nervosa is much more prevalent in females than in males and usually has its onset in adolescence. Hypotheses of an underlying psychological disturbance in young women with the disorder include conflicts surrounding the transition from girlhood to womanhood. Psychological issues related to feelings of helplessness and difficulty establishing autonomy have also been suggested as contributing to the development of the disorder. Bulimic symptoms may occur as a separate disorder (bulimia nervosa, discussed in the next section) or as part of anorexia nervosa. Persons with either disorder are excessively preoccupied with weight, food, and body shape. The outcome of anorexia nervosa varies from spontaneous recovery to a waxing and waning course to death.

EPIDEMIOLOGY

Eating disorders of various kinds have been reported in up to 4 percent of adolescent and young adult students. Anorexia nervosa has been reported more frequently over the past several decades than in the past, with increasing reports of the disorder in prepubertal girls and in males. The most common ages of onset of anorexia nervosa are the midteens, but up to 5 percent of anorectic patients have the onset of the disorder in their early 20s. According to DSM-IV-TR the most common age is onset between 14 and 18 years. Anorexia nervosa is estimated to occur in about 0.5 to 1 percent of adolescent girls. It occurs 10 to 20 times more often in females than in males. The prevalence of young women with some symptoms of anorexia nervosa who do not meet the diagnostic criteria is estimated to be close to 5 percent. Although the disorder was initially reported most often among the upper classes, recent epidemiological surveys do not show that distribution. It seems to be most frequent in developed countries, and it may be seen with greatest frequency among young women in professions that require thinness, such as modeling and ballet.

COMORBIDITY

Anorexia nervosa is associated with depression in 65 percent of cases, social phobia in 34 percent of cases, and obsessive-compulsive disorder in 26 percent of cases.

ETIOLOGY

Biological, social, and psychological factors are implicated in the causes of anorexia nervosa. Some evidence points to higher concordance rates in monozygotic twins than in dizygotic twins. Sisters of patients with anorexia nervosa are likely to be afflicted, but this association may reflect social influences more than genetic factors. Major mood disorders are more common in family members than in the general population. Neurochemically, diminished norepinephrine turnover and activity are suggested by reduced 3-methoxy-4-hydroxyphenylglycol (MHPG) levels in the urine and the cerebrospinal fluid (CSF) of some patients with anorexia nervosa. An inverse relation is seen between MHPG and depression in these patients; an increase in MHPG is associated with a decrease in depression.

Biological Factors

Endogenous opioids may contribute to the denial of hunger in patients with anorexia nervosa. Preliminary studies show dramatic weight gains in some patients given opiate antagonists. Starvation results in many biochemical changes, some of which are also present in depression, such as hypercortisolemia and

Table 23.1–1
Neuroendocrine Changes in Anorexia Nervosa and Experimental Starvation

Hormone	Anorexia Nervosa	Weight Loss
Corticotropin-releasing hormone (CRH)	Increased	Increased
Plasma cortisol levels	Mildly increased	Mildly increased
Diurnal cortisol difference	Blunted	Blunted
Luteinizing hormone (LH)	Decreased, prepubertal pattern	Decreased
Follicle-stimulating hormone (FSH)	Decreased, prepubertal pattern	Decreased
Growth hormone (GH)	Impaired regulation	Same
	Increased basal levels and limited response to pharmacological probes	
Somatomedin C	Decreased	Decreased
Thyroxine (T_4)	Normal or slightly decreased	Normal or slightly decreased
Triiodothyronine (T_3)	Mildly decreased	Mildly decreased
Reverse T_3	Mildly increased	Mildly increased
Thyrotropin-stimulating hormone (TSH)	Normal	Normal
TSH response to thyrotropin-releasing hormone (TRH)	Delayed or blunted	Delayed or blunted
Insulin	Delayed release	—
C-peptide	Decreased	—
Vasopressin	Secretion uncoupled from osmotic challenge	—
Serotonin	Increased function with weight restoration	
Norepinephrine	Reduced turnover	Reduced turnover
Dopamine	Blunted response to pharmacological probes	—

nonsuppression by dexamethasone. Thyroid function is suppressed as well. These abnormalities are corrected by realimentation. Starvation produces amenorrhea, which reflects lowered hormonal levels (luteinizing, follicle-stimulating, and gonadotropin-releasing hormones). Some anorexia nervosa patients, however, become amenorrheic before significant weight loss. Several computed tomographic (CT) studies reveal enlarged CSF spaces (enlarged sulci and ventricles) in anorectic patients during starvation, a finding that is reversed by weight gain. In one positron emission tomographic (PET) scan study, caudate nucleus metabolism was higher in the anorectic state than after realimentation.

Some authors have proposed a hypothalamic-pituitary axis (neuroendocrine) dysfunction. Some studies have shown evidence for dysfunction in serotonin, dopamine, and norepinephrine, three neurotransmitters involved in regulating eating behavior in the paraventricular nucleus of the hypothalamus. Other humoral factors that may be involved include corticotropin-releasing factor (CRF), neuropeptide Y, gonadotropin-releasing hormone, and thyroid-stimulating hormone. Table 23.1–1 lists neuroendocrine changes associated with anorexia nervosa.

Social Factors

Patients with anorexia nervosa find support for their practices in society's emphasis on thinness and exercise. No family constellations are specific to anorexia nervosa, but some evidence indicates that these patients have close, but troubled, relationships with their parents. Families of children who present with eating disorders, especially binge eating or purging subtypes, may exhibit high levels of hostility, chaos, and isolation and low levels of nurturance and empathy. An adolescent with a severe eating disorder may tend to draw attention away from strained marital relationships.

Psychological and Psychodynamic Factors

Anorexia nervosa appears to be a reaction to the demand that adolescents behave more independently and increase their social and sexual functioning. Patients with the disorder substitute their preoccupations, which are similar to obsessions, with eating and weight gain for other, normal adolescent pursuits. These patients typically lack a sense of autonomy and selfhood. Many experience their bodies as somehow under the control of their parents, so that self-starvation may be an effort to gain validation as a unique and special person. Only through acts of extraordinary self-discipline can an anorectic patient develop a sense of autonomy and selfhood.

Psychoanalytic clinicians who treat patients with anorexia nervosa generally agree that these young patients have been unable to separate psychologically from their mothers. The body may be perceived as though it were inhabited by an introject of an intrusive and unempathic mother. Starvation may unconsciously mean arresting the growth of this intrusive internal object and thereby destroying it. Often, a projective identification process is involved in the interactions between the patient and the patient's family. Many anorectic patients feel that oral desires are greedy and unacceptable; therefore, these desires are projectively disavowed. Other theories have focused on fantasies of oral impregnation. Parents respond to the refusal to eat by becoming frantic about whether the patient is actually eating. The patient can then view the parents as the ones who have unacceptable desires and can projectively disavow them; that is, others may be voracious and ruled by desire but not the patient.

DIAGNOSIS AND CLINICAL FEATURES

The onset of anorexia nervosa usually occurs between the ages of 10 and 30 years. The DSM-IV-TR diagnostic criteria for anorexia nervosa are given in Table 23.1–2.

An intense fear of gaining weight and becoming obese is present in all patients with the disorder and undoubtedly contributes to their lack of interest in, and even resistance to, therapy. Most aberrant behavior directed toward losing weight occurs in secret. Patients with anorexia nervosa usually refuse to eat with their families or in public places. They lose weight by drastically reducing their total food intake, with a disproportionate decrease in high-carbohydrate and fatty foods.

As mentioned above, the term *anorexia* is a misnomer, because loss of appetite is usually rare until late in the disorder. Evidence that patients are constantly thinking about food is their passion for collecting recipes and for preparing elaborate meals for others. Some patients cannot continuously control their voluntary restriction of food intake and so have eating binges. These binges usually occur secretly and often at night and are frequently followed by self-induced vomiting. Patients abuse laxatives and even diuretics to lose weight, and ritualistic exercising, extensive cycling, walking, jogging, and running are common activities.

Patients with the disorder exhibit peculiar behavior about food. They hide food all over the house and frequently carry large quantities of candies in their pockets and purses. While eating meals, they try to dispose of food in their napkins or hide it in their pockets. They cut their meat into very small pieces and spend a great deal of time rearranging the pieces on their plates. If the patients are confronted with their peculiar behavior, they often deny that their behavior is unusual or flatly refuse to discuss it.

Obsessive-compulsive behavior, depression, and anxiety are other psychiatric symptoms of anorexia nervosa most frequently noted in the literature. Patients tend to be rigid and perfectionist, and somatic complaints, especially epigastric discomfort, are usual. Compulsive stealing, usually of candies and laxatives but occasionally of clothes and other items, is common.

Poor sexual adjustment is frequently described in patients with the disorder. Many adolescent patients with anorexia nervosa have delayed psychosocial sexual development; in adults, a markedly decreased interest in sex often accompanies onset of the disorder. An unusual minority of anorectic patients have a premorbid history of promiscuity, substance abuse, or both and during the disorder do not show a decreased interest in sex.

Patients usually come to medical attention when their weight loss becomes apparent. As the weight loss grows profound, physical signs such as hypothermia (as low as 35°C), dependent edema, bradycardia, hypotension, and lanugo (the appearance of neonatal-like hair) appear, and patients show a variety of metabolic changes (Fig. 23.1–1). Some female patients with anorexia nervosa come to medical attention because of amenorrhea, which often appears before their weight loss is noticeable. Some patients induce vomiting or abuse purgatives and diuretics; such behavior causes concern about hypokalemic alkalosis. Impaired water diuresis may be noted.

Electrocardiographic (ECG) changes, such as flattening or inversion of the T waves, ST segment depression, and lengthening of the QT interval, have been noted in the emaciated stage of anorexia nervosa. ECG changes may also result from potassium loss, which can lead to death. Gastric dilation is a rare complication of anorexia nervosa. In some patients, aortography has shown a superior mesenteric artery syndrome. Other medical complications of eating disorders are listed in Table 23.1–3.

Table 23.1–2
DSM-IV-TR Diagnostic Criteria for Anorexia Nervosa

A. Refusal to maintain body weight at or above a minimally normal weight for age and height (e.g., weight loss leading to maintenance of body weight less than 85% of that expected; or failure to make expected weight gain during period of growth, leading to body weight less than 85% of that expected).

B. Intense fear of gaining weight or becoming fat, even though underweight.

C. Disturbance in the way in which one's body weight or shape is experienced, undue influence of body weight or shape on self-evaluation, or denial of the seriousness of the current low body weight.

D. In postmenarcheal females, amenorrhea, i.e., the absence of at least three consecutive menstrual cycles. (A woman is considered to have amenorrhea if her periods occur only following hormone, e.g., estrogen, administration.)

Specify type:

Restricting type: during the current episode of anorexia nervosa, the person has not regularly engaged in binge-eating or purging behavior (i.e., self-induced vomiting or the misuse of laxatives, diuretics, or enemas)

Binge-eating/purging type: during the current episode of anorexia nervosa, the person has regularly engaged in binge-eating or purging behavior (i.e., self-induced vomiting or the misuse of laxatives, diuretics, or enemas)

From American Psychiatric Association. *Diagnostic and Statistical Manual of Mental Disorders.* 4th ed. Text rev. Washington, DC: American Psychiatric Association; copyright 2000, with permission.

Subtypes

DSM-IV-TR identifies two subtypes of anorexia nervosa—the restricting type and the binge eating–purging type. Binge eating–purging, common among anorectic patients, develops in up to 50 percent of them. Each type appears to have distinct historic and clinical features. Those who practice binge eating and purging share many features with persons who have bulimia nervosa without anorexia nervosa. Those who binge eat and purge tend to have families in which some members are obese, and they themselves have histories of heavier body weights before the disorder than do persons with the restricting type. Binge eating–purging persons are likely to be associated with substance abuse, impulse control disorders, and personality disorders. Persons with restricting anorexia nervosa limit their food selection, take in as few calories as possible, and often have obsessive-compulsive traits with respect to food and other matters. Both types of persons are preoccupied with weight and body image, and both may exercise for hours every day and exhibit bizarre eating behaviors. Both may be socially isolated and have depressive disorder symptoms and

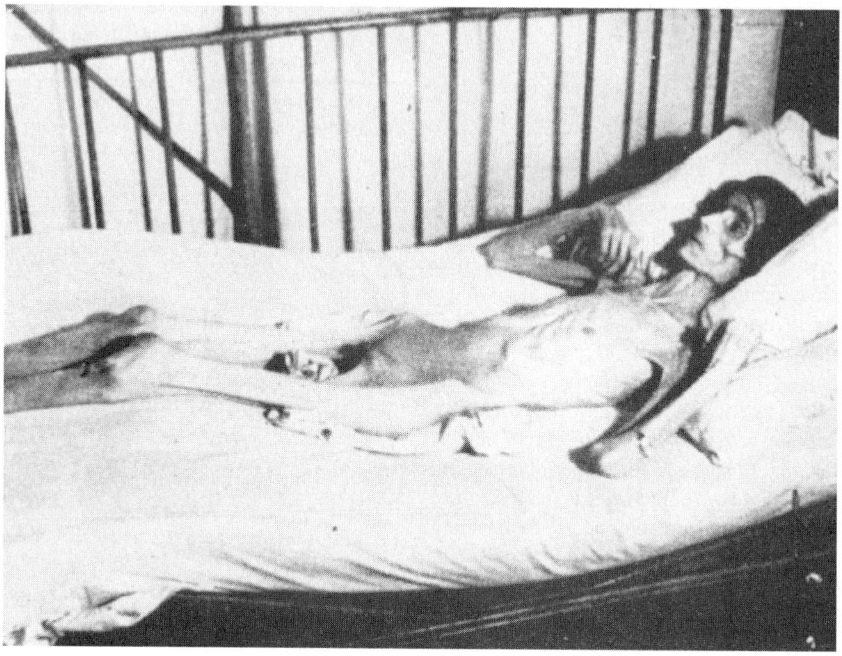

FIGURE 23.1–1
A patient with anorexia nervosa. (Courtesy of Katherine Halmi, M.D.)

Table 23.1–3
Medical Complications of Eating Disorders

Related to weight loss

Cachexia: Loss of fat, muscle mass, reduced thyroid metabolism (low T_3 syndrome), cold intolerance, and difficulty in maintaining core body temperature

Cardiac: Loss of cardiac muscle; small heart; cardiac arrhythmias, including atrial and ventricular premature contractions, prolonged His bundle transmission (prolonged QT interval), bradycardia, ventricular tachycardia; sudden death

Digestive-gastrointestinal: Delayed gastric emptying, bloating, constipation, abdominal pain

Reproductive: Amenorrhea, low levels of luteinizing hormone (LH) and follicle-stimulating hormone (FSH)

Dermatological: Lanugo (fine babylike hair over body), edema

Hematological: Leukopenia

Neuropsychiatric: Abnormal taste sensation (?zinc deficiency), apathetic depression, mild cognitive disorder

Skeletal: Osteoporosis

Related to purging (vomiting and laxative abuse)

Metabolic: Electrolyte abnormalities, particularly hypokalemic, hypochloremic alkalosis; hypomagnesemia

Digestive-gastrointestinal: Salivary gland and pancreatic inflammation and enlargement with increase in serum amylase, esophageal and gastric erosion, dysfunctional bowel with haustral dilation

Dental: Erosion of dental enamel, particularly of front teeth, with corresponding decay

Neuropsychiatric: Seizures (related to large fluid shifts and electrolyte disturbances), mild neuropathies, fatigue and weakness, mild cognitive disorder

Reprinted with permission from Yager I. Eating disorders. In: Stoudemire A, ed. *Clinical Psychiatry for Medical Students.* Philadelphia: JB Lippincott; 1990:324.

diminished sexual interest. Some persons with anorexia nervosa may purge but not binge.

Persons with anorexia nervosa have high rates of comorbid major depressive disorders; major depressive disorder or dysthymic disorder has been reported in up to 50 percent of anorexia nervosa patients. The suicide rate is higher in persons with the binge eating–purging type of anorexia nervosa than in those with the restricting type.

Patients with anorexia nervosa are often secretive, deny their symptoms, and resist treatment. In almost all cases, relatives or intimate acquaintances must confirm a patient's history. The mental status examination usually shows a patient who is alert and knowledgeable on the subject of nutrition and who is preoccupied with food and weight.

A patient must have a thorough general physical and neurological examination. If the patient is vomiting, a hypokalemic alkalosis may be present. Because most patients are dehydrated, serum electrolyte levels must be determined initially and periodically during hospitalization.

Sue, a 19-year-old single white female, has just completed 6 months in an eating disorder specialty unit for the treatment of anorexia nervosa and obsessive-compulsive disorder. She arrived weighing 30 kg (66 lb) and was 162 cm (5 ft 1 in.) tall.

Sue recalls that as early as age 4 she had to do everything "perfectly" and had rituals for putting things away and cleaning things thoroughly. These behaviors continued throughout grade school. In school she was extremely competitive and always got straight As. She began gymnastics when she was 8

years old and continued with this until the onset of her anorexia nervosa at age 12, when she began eating food slowly and gradually eating less food. She denies any reason for doing this or any stress at the time. The following summer she was hospitalized because of weight loss at a time when she should have been growing and gaining weight, and she was diagnosed as having anorexia nervosa. Her obsessions and compulsions became more severe as her anorexia worsened. She developed rituals around cleaning, straightening and arranging objects, counting, and exercising. She felt and continues to feel that she must be constantly industrious, moving and accomplishing things because she fears becoming "lazy." She often could not leave her home in the morning for hours because she had to touch objects and perform a number of rituals, which frequently made her late for school. The following year her weight dropped to 50 lb, and she was hospitalized again. This was the beginning of a series of repeated hospitalizations and weight losses up to the time she graduated from high school as valedictorian, despite her almost continual absence from school. After graduation she worked as a cashier in a grocery store for 1 year while living with her parents and was able to stay out of the hospital for 18 months. She then had a series of several hospitalizations and short-term jobs working as a copy center associate and as an aide in a nursing home.

Sue denies any binge eating, purging, illegal drug use, or use of alcohol, cigarettes, or caffeine. She only restricts her intake and vigorously exercises. She is distressed about her obsessions and compulsions but not about her eating behavior. She has never shown the signs and symptoms of depression. She has primary amenorrhea.

Sue stated she always had girlfriends throughout high school. She has never dated or had a boyfriend and has never been sexually active. She is extremely angry with her father and has an openly antagonistic relationship with him. She states that she has always wanted attention and approval from him but has never received it. She is the youngest of three children; her two older sisters have done well academically and professionally. She has a close, enmeshed relationship with her mother.

On admission to the specialized eating disorder program, Sue was placed on a liquid diet. She had enormous difficulty adhering to unit rules and procedures. She was perpetually in motion. She was upset and angry when confronted by staff and was extremely sensitive to criticism. She was exceedingly harsh, critical, and self-punishing. After 6 months of hospitalization, she was able to successfully maintain her weight within a normal range. Her confidence was greatly improved in her ability to eat three meals and maintain her weight. She stated that she actually enjoyed eating because she was allowed to be a vegetarian. She was much more sociable, interacting with peers and vocal in community meetings and groups. Her rituals had gradually decreased, and she was actually able to get through several days with no rituals. She found it more difficult to abstain from rituals in the evening, and she still felt very concerned about "being lazy." She was also more comfortable and open in talking with her father.

During her fifth month of hospitalization when she had reached her target weight, Sue was placed on 225 mg a day of clomipramine (Anafranil), which was helpful in reducing her obsessions and compulsions. Throughout her hospitalization Sue was treated with a cognitive-behavioral therapy program and family counseling. She was discharged to a specialized eating disorder outpatient program with cognitive psychotherapy, family counseling, and group therapy.

DISCUSSION

Sue had perfectionistic traits, a feature of obsessive-compulsive personality disorder, as a young child. There is growing evidence that this type of personality trait puts a young woman at risk for developing anorexia nervosa—restricting type, which is Sue's diagnosis. After several years, in addition to having an obsessive-compulsive personality disorder, Sue actually met diagnostic criteria for Axis I obsessive-compulsive disorder. These behaviors were not severe until she developed anorexia nervosa. Obsessions and compulsions such as counting and checking differ distinctly from eating disorder rituals and preoccupations. Sue was distressed by the former, which were ego-dystonic, but was not bothered by the eating disorder rituals, which were ego-syntonic. Because she failed to respond to fluoxetine (Prozac) in her previous hospitalizations she was placed on clomipramine and responded well to this drug, as evidenced by a decrease in obsessions and compulsions. (Courtesy of Katherine A. Halmi, M.D.)

PATHOLOGY AND LABORATORY EXAMINATION

A complete blood count often reveals leukopenia with a relative lymphocytosis in emaciated anorexia nervosa patients. If binge eating and purging are present, serum electrolyte determination reveals hypokalemic alkalosis. Fasting serum glucose concentrations are often low during the emaciated phase, and serum salivary amylase concentrations are often elevated if the patient is vomiting. The ECG may show S-T segment and T-wave changes, which are usually secondary to electrolyte disturbances; emaciated patients have hypotension and bradycardia. Young girls may have a high serum cholesterol level. All these values revert to normal with nutritional rehabilitation and cessation of purging behaviors. Endocrine changes that occur, such as amenorrhea, mild hypothyroidism, and hypersecretion of corticotrophin-releasing hormone are due to the underweight condition and revert to normal with weight gain.

DIFFERENTIAL DIAGNOSIS

The differential diagnosis of anorexia nervosa is complicated by patients' denial of the symptoms, the secrecy surrounding their bizarre eating rituals, and their resistance to seeking treatment. Thus, it may be difficult to identify the mechanism of

weight loss and the patient's associated ruminative thoughts about distortions of body image.

Clinicians must ascertain that a patient does not have a medical illness that can account for the weight loss (e.g., a brain tumor or cancer). Weight loss, peculiar eating behaviors, and vomiting can occur in several mental disorders. Depressive disorders and anorexia nervosa have several features in common, such as depressed feelings, crying spells, sleep disturbance, obsessive ruminations, and occasional suicidal thoughts. The two disorders, however, have several distinguishing features. Generally, a patient with a depressive disorder has decreased appetite, whereas a patient with anorexia nervosa claims to have normal appetite and to feel hungry; only in the severe stages of anorexia nervosa do patients actually have decreased appetite. In contrast to depressive agitation, the hyperactivity seen in anorexia nervosa is planned and ritualistic. The preoccupation with recipes, the caloric content of foods, and the preparation of gourmet feasts is typical of patients with anorexia nervosa but is absent in patients with a depressive disorder. In depressive disorders, patients have no intense fear of obesity or disturbance of body image.

Weight fluctuations, vomiting, and peculiar food handling may occur in somatization disorder. On rare occasions a patient fulfills the diagnostic criteria for both somatization disorder and anorexia nervosa; in such a case both diagnoses should be made. Generally, the weight loss in somatization disorder is not as severe as that in anorexia nervosa, nor does a patient with somatization disorder express a morbid fear of becoming overweight, as is common in the anorexia nervosa patient. Amenorrhea for 3 months or longer is unusual in somatization disorder.

In schizophrenia patients, delusions about food are seldom concerned with caloric content. More likely, they believe the food to be poisoned. Schizophrenia patients are rarely preoccupied with a fear of becoming obese and do not have the hyperactivity that is seen in patients with anorexia nervosa. Patients with schizophrenia have bizarre eating habits but not the entire syndrome of anorexia nervosa.

Anorexia nervosa must be differentiated from bulimia nervosa, a disorder in which episodic binge eating, followed by depressive moods, self-deprecating thoughts, and often self-induced vomiting, occurs while patients maintain their weight within a normal range. Patients with bulimia nervosa seldom lose 15 percent of their weight, but the two conditions frequently coexist.

COURSE AND PROGNOSIS

The course of anorexia nervosa varies greatly—spontaneous recovery without treatment, recovery after a variety of treatments, a fluctuating course of weight gains followed by relapses, a gradually deteriorating course resulting in death caused by complications of starvation. A recent study reviewing subtypes of anorectic patients found that restricting-type anorectic patients seemed less likely to recover than those of the binge eating–purging type. The short-term response of patients to almost all hospital treatment programs is good. Those who have regained sufficient weight, however, often continue their preoccupation with food and body weight, have poor social relationships, and exhibit depression. In general, the prognosis is not good. Studies have shown a range of mortality rates from 5 to 18 percent.

Indicators of a favorable outcome are admission of hunger, lessening of denial and immaturity, and improved self-esteem. Such factors as childhood neuroticism, parental conflict, bulimia nervosa, vomiting, laxative abuse, and various behavioral manifestations (e.g., obsessive-compulsive, hysterical, depressive, psychosomatic, neurotic, and denial symptoms) have been related to poor outcome in some studies but not in others.

Ten-year outcome studies in the United States have shown that about one fourth of patients recover completely and another one half are markedly improved and functioning fairly well. The other one fourth includes an overall 7 percent mortality rate and those who are functioning poorly with a chronic underweight condition. Swedish and English studies over a 20- and 30-year period show a mortality rate of 18 percent. About half of anorexia nervosa patients will eventually have the symptoms of bulimia, usually within the first year after the onset of anorexia nervosa.

TREATMENT

In view of the complicated psychological and medical implications of anorexia nervosa, a comprehensive treatment plan, including hospitalization when necessary and both individual and family therapy, is recommended. Behavioral, interpersonal, and cognitive approaches and, in some cases, medication should be considered.

Hospitalization

The first consideration in the treatment of anorexia nervosa is to restore patients' nutritional state; dehydration, starvation, and electrolyte imbalances can seriously compromise health and, in some cases, lead to death. The decision to hospitalize a patient is based on the patient's medical condition and the amount of structure needed to ensure patient cooperation. In general, anorexia nervosa patients who are 20 percent below the expected weight for their height are recommended for inpatient programs, and patients who are 30 percent below their expected weight require psychiatric hospitalization for 2 to 6 months.

Inpatient psychiatric programs for patients with anorexia nervosa generally use a combination of a behavioral management approach, individual psychotherapy, family education and therapy, and, in some cases, psychotropic medications. Successful treatment is promoted by the ability of staff members to maintain a firm yet supportive approach to patients, often through a combination of positive reinforcers (praise) and negative reinforcers (restriction of exercise and purging behavior). The program must have some flexibility for individualizing treatment to meet patients' needs and cognitive abilities. Patients must become willing participants for treatment to succeed in the long run.

Most patients are uninterested in psychiatric treatment and even resist it; they are brought to a doctor's office unwillingly by agonizing relatives or friends. The patients rarely accept the recommendation of hospitalization without arguing and criticizing the proposed program. Emphasizing the benefits, such as relief of insomnia and depressive signs and symptoms, may help persuade the patients to admit themselves willingly to the hospital. Relatives' support and confidence in the physicians

and treatment team are essential when firm recommendations must be carried out. Patients' families should be warned that the patients will resist admission and, for the several weeks of treatment, will make many dramatic pleas for the family's support to obtain release from the hospital program. Compulsory admission or commitment should be obtained only when the risk of death from the complications of malnutrition is likely. On rare occasions, patients prove that doctor's statements about the probable failure of outpatient treatment are wrong. Some patients may gain a specified amount of weight by the time of each outpatient visit, but such behavior is uncommon, and a period of inpatient care is usually necessary.

The following considerations apply to the general management of patients with anorexia nervosa during a hospitalized treatment program. Patients should be weighed daily, early in the morning after emptying the bladder. The daily fluid intake and urine output should be recorded. If vomiting is occurring, hospital staff members must monitor serum electrolyte levels regularly and watch for the development of hypokalemia. Because food is often regurgitated after meals, the staff may be able to control vomiting by making the bathroom inaccessible for at least 2 hours after meals or by having an attendant in the bathroom to prevent vomiting. Constipation in these patients is relieved when they begin to eat normally. Stool softeners may occasionally be given, but never laxatives. If diarrhea occurs, it usually means that patients are surreptitiously taking laxatives. Because of the rare complication of stomach dilation and the possibility of circulatory overload when patients immediately start eating an enormous number of calories, the hospital staff should give patients about 500 calories over the amount required to maintain their present weight (usually 1,500 to 2,000 calories a day). It is wise to give these calories in six equal feedings throughout the day, so that patients need not eat a large amount of food at one sitting. Giving patients a liquid food supplement such as Sustagen may be advisable, because they may be less apprehensive about gaining weight slowly with the formula than by eating food. After patients are discharged from the hospital, clinicians usually find it necessary to continue outpatient supervision of the problems identified in the patients and their families.

Psychotherapy

Cognitive-Behavioral Therapy. Cognitive and behavior therapy principles can be applied in both inpatient and outpatient settings. Behavior therapy has been found effective for inducing weight gain; no large-sample-size controlled studies of cognitive therapy with behavior therapy in anorexia nervosa patients have been reported. Monitoring is an essential component of cognitive-behavioral therapy. Patients are taught to monitor their food intake, their feelings and emotions, their bingeing and purging behaviors, and their problems in interpersonal relationships. Patients are taught cognitive restructuring to identify automatic thoughts and to challenge their core beliefs. Problem solving is a specific method whereby patients learn how to think through and devise strategies to cope with their food-related and interpersonal problems. Patients' vulnerability to rely on anorectic behavior as a means of coping can be addressed if they can learn to use these techniques effectively.

Dynamic Psychotherapy. Dynamic expressive-supportive psychotherapy is sometimes used in the treatment of patients with anorexia nervosa, but their resistance may make the process difficult and painstaking. Because patients view their symptoms as constituting the core of their specialness, therapists must avoid excessive investment in trying to change their eating behavior. The opening phase of the psychotherapy process must be geared to building a therapeutic alliance. Patients may experience early interpretations as though someone else were telling them what they really feel and thereby minimizing and invalidating their own experiences. Therapists who empathize with patients' points of view and take an active interest in what their patients think and feel, however, convey to patients that their autonomy is respected. Above all, psychotherapists must be flexible, persistent, and durable in the face of patients' tendencies to defeat any efforts to help them.

Family Therapy. A family analysis should be done on all anorexia nervosa patients who are living with their families, as a basis for a clinical judgment on what type of family therapy or counseling is advisable. In some cases family therapy is not possible; however, issues of family relationships can then be addressed in individual therapy. Sometimes, brief counseling sessions with immediate family members is the extent of family therapy required. In one controlled family therapy study in London, anorectic patients under the age of 18 benefited from family therapy, whereas patients over the age of 18 did worse in family therapy than with the control therapy. There are no controlled studies of the combination of individual and family therapy; however, in actual practice, most clinicians provide individual therapy and some form of family counseling in managing anorexia nervosa patients.

Pharmacotherapy

Pharmacological studies have not yet identified any medication that yields definitive improvement of the core symptoms of anorexia nervosa. Some reports support the use of cyproheptadine (Periactin), a drug with antihistaminic and antiserotonergic properties, for patients with the restricting type of anorexia nervosa. Amitriptyline (Elavil) has also been reported to have some benefit. Other medications that have been tried by patients with anorexia nervosa with variable results include clomipramine, pimozide (Orap), and chlorpromazine (Thorazine). Trials of fluoxetine have resulted in some reports of weight gain, and serotonergic agents may yield positive responses in the future. In anorexia nervosa patients with coexisting depressive disorders, the depressive condition should be treated. Concern exists about the use of tricyclic drugs in low-weight, depressed patients with anorexia nervosa, who may be vulnerable to hypotension, cardiac arrhythmia, and dehydration. Once an adequate nutritional status has been attained, the risk of serious adverse effects from the tricyclic drugs may decrease; in some patients the depression improves with weight gain and normalized nutritional status.

ICD-10

The 10th revision of the *International Statistical Classification of Diseases and Related Health Disorders* (ICD-10) describes anorexia ner-

Table 23.1–4
ICD-10 Diagnostic Criteria for Eating Disorders

Anorexia nervosa

A. There is weight loss or, in children, a lack of weight gain, leading to a body weight at least 15% below the normal or expected weight for age and height.

B. The weight loss is self-induced by avoidance of "fattening foods."

C. There is self-perception of being too fat, with an intrusive dread of fatness, which leads to a self-imposed low weight threshold.

D. A widespread endocrine disorder involving the hypothalamic-pituitary-gonadal axis is manifest in women as amenorrhea and in men as a loss of sexual interest and potency. (An apparent exception is the persistence of vaginal bleeding in anorexic women who are on replacement hormonal therapy, most commonly taken as a contraceptive pill.)

E. The disorder does not meet Criteria A and B for bulimia nervosa.

Comments

The following features support the diagnosis but are not essential elements: self-induced vomiting, self-induced purging, excessive exercise, and use of appetite suppressants and/or diuretics.

If onset is prepubertal, the sequence of pubertal events is delayed or even arrested (growth ceases; in girls the breasts do not develop, and there is a primary amenorrhea; in boys the genitals remain juvenile). With recovery, puberty is often completed normally, but the menarche is late.

Atypical anorexia nervosa

Researchers studying atypical forms of anorexia nervosa are recommended to make their own decisions about the number and type of criteria to be fulfilled.

Bulimia nervosa

A. There are recurrent episodes of overeating (at least twice a week over a period of 3 months) in which large amounts of food are consumed in short periods.

B. There is persistent preoccupation with eating and a strong desire or a sense of compulsion to eat (craving).

C. The patient attempts to counteract the "fattening" effects of food by one or more of the following:

(1) self-induced vomiting;

(2) self-induced purging;

(3) alternating periods of starvation;

(4) use of drugs such as appetite suppressants, thyroid preparations, or diuretics; when bulimia occurs in diabetic patients, they may choose to neglect their insulin treatment.

D. There is self-perception of being too fat, with an intrusive dread of fatness (usually leading to underweight).

Atypical bulimia nervosa

Researchers studying atypical forms of bulimia nervosa, such as those involving normal or excessive body weight, are recommended to make their own decisions about the number and type of criteria to be fulfilled.

Overeating associated with other psychological disturbances

Researchers wishing to use this category are recommended to design their own criteria.

Vomiting associated with other psychological disturbances

Researchers wishing to use this category are recommended to design their own criteria.

Other eating disorders

Eating disorder, unspecified

Adapted from World Health Organization. *The ICD-10 Classification of Mental and Behavioural Disorders: Diagnostic Criteria for Research.* Copyright, World Health Organization, Geneva, 1993.

vosa as a deliberate, severe weight loss caused by the patient. According to ICD-10, its causes remain unknown, but a combination of sociocultural and biological factors apparently contributes to the disorder, along with a vulnerable personality and other psychological processes. Undernutrition produces endocrine and metabolic changes and disturbs bodily functions. Whether the endocrine disorder is completely caused by the eating disorder or whether other factors are also at work is uncertain. The ICD-10 criteria for eating disorders are presented in Table 23.1–4.

References

American Psychiatric Association. Practice guidelines for eating disorders. *Am J Psychiatry.* 1993;150:212.

Bowers WA. Basic principles for applying cognitive-behavioral therapy to anorexia nervosa. *Psychiatr Clin North Am.* 2001;24:293.

Gabbard GO. *Psychodynamic Psychiatry in Clinical Practice: The DSM-IV Edition.* Washington, DC: American Psychiatric Press, 1994.

Garfinkel PE. Eating disorders. In: Kaplan HI, Sadock BJ, eds. *Comprehensive Textbook of Psychiatry.* 6th ed. Baltimore: Williams & Wilkins; 1995:1361.

Gillberg IC, Rastam M, Gillberg C. Anorexia nervosa outcomes: six-year controlled longitudinal study of 51 cases including a population cohort. *J Am Acad Child Adolesc Psychiatry.* 1994;33:729.

Harper-Giuffre H, MacKenzie KR, eds. *Group Psychotherapy for Eating Disorders.* Washington, DC: American Psychiatric Press; 1992.

Herzog DB, Field AE, Keller MB, et al. Subtyping eating disorders: is it justified? *J Am Acad Child Adolesc Psychiatry.* 1996;35:928.

Horesh N, Apter A, Ishai J, et al. Abnormal psychosocial situations and eating disorders in adolescence. *J Am Acad Child Adolesc Psychiatry.* 1996;35:921.

Jarry JL, Vaccarine FJ. Eating disorder and obsessive-compulsive disorder: neurochemical and phenomenological commonalities. *J Psychiatry Neurosci.* 1996;21:36.

Klump KL, Kaye WH, Strober M. The evolving genetic foundations of eating disorders. *Psychiatr Clin North Am.* 2001;24:215.

Kohn M, Golden NH. Eating disorders in children and adolescents: epidemiology, diagnosis and treatment. *Pediatr Drugs.* 2001;3:91.

Mitchell JE, Peterson CB, Myers T, Wonderlich S. Combining pharmacotherapy and psychotherapy in the treatment of patients with eating disorders. *Psychiatr Clin North Am.* 2001;24:315.

Polivy J, Herman CP. Causes of eating disorders [Review]. *Ann Rev Psychol.* 2002;53:187.

Romano SJ, Halmi KA. A placebo-controlled study of fluoxetine in continued treatment of bulimia nervosa after successful acute fluoxetine treatment. *Am J Psychiatry.* 2002;159:140.

Russell GF. Involuntary treatment in anorexia nervosa. *Psychiatr Clin North Am.* 2001;24:337.

Seidenfeld ME, Ricket VI. Impact of anorexia, bulimia and obesity on the gynecologic health of adolescents. *Am Fam Physician.* 2001;64:445.

Stoner SA, Fedoroff IC, Andersen AE, Rolls BJ. Food preferences and desire to eat in anorexia and bulimia nervosa. *Int J Eating Disord.* 1996;19:13.

Vanderlinden J, Vandereycken W, van Dyck R, Vertommen H. Dissociative experiences and trauma in eating disorders. *Int J Eating Disord.* 1993;13:195.

▲ 23.2 Bulimia Nervosa and Eating Disorder Not Otherwise Specified

BULIMIA NERVOSA

Bulimia is a term that means binge eating, which is defined as eating more food than most persons in similar circumstances and in a similar period of time, accompanied by a strong sense of losing control. When binge eating occurs in normal weight or overweight persons who are also excessively concerned with their body shape and weight and who regularly engage in behaviors to counteract the calorie gain in binges, the binge eating is in the context of the disorder known as *bulimia nervosa*.

In the text revision of the fourth edition of *Diagnostic and Statistical Manual of Mental Disorders* (DSM-IV-TR), bulimia

nervosa is defined as binge eating combined with inappropriate ways of stopping weight gain. The recurrent episodes of bulimia nervosa, which is more common than anorexia nervosa, are accompanied by feelings of being out of control. Social interruption or physical discomfort—that is, abdominal pain or nausea—terminates the binge eating, which is often followed by feelings of guilt, depression, or self-disgust. Persons with bulimia nervosa also show recurrent compensatory behaviors—such as purging (self-induced vomiting, repeated laxative or diuretic use), fasting, or excessive exercise—to prevent weight gain. Unlike patients with anorexia nervosa, those with bulimia nervosa may maintain a normal body weight.

Epidemiology

Bulimia nervosa is more prevalent than anorexia nervosa. Estimates of bulimia nervosa range from 1 to 3 percent of young women. Like anorexia nervosa, bulimia nervosa is significantly more common in women than in men, but its onset is often later in adolescence than that of anorexia nervosa. According to DSM-IV-TR, the rate of occurrence in males is one-tenth of that in females. The onset may even occur in early adulthood. Occasional symptoms of bulimia nervosa, such as isolated episodes of binge eating and purging, have been reported in up to 40 percent of college women. Although bulimia nervosa is often present in normal-weight young women, they sometimes have a history of obesity. In industrialized countries the prevalence is about 1 percent of the general population.

Etiology

Biological Factors. Some investigators have attempted to associate cycles of binging and purging with various neurotransmitters. Because antidepressants often benefit patients with bulimia nervosa and because serotonin has been linked to satiety, serotonin and norepinephrine have been implicated. Because plasma endorphin levels are raised in some bulimia nervosa patients who vomit, the feeling of well-being after vomiting that some of these patients experience may be mediated by raised endorphin levels. According to DSM-IV-TR, there is an increased frequency of bulimia nervosa in first-degree relatives of persons with the disorder.

Social Factors. Patients with bulimia nervosa, like those with anorexia nervosa, tend to be high achievers and to respond to societal pressures to be slender. As with anorexia nervosa patients, many patients with bulimia nervosa are depressed and have increased familial depression, but the families of patients with bulimia nervosa are generally less close and more conflictual than the families of anorexia nervosa patients. Patients with bulimia nervosa describe their parents as neglectful and rejecting.

Psychological Factors. Patients with bulimia nervosa, like those with anorexia nervosa, have difficulties with adolescent demands, but bulimia nervosa patients are more outgoing, angry, and impulsive than anorexia nervosa patients. Alcohol dependence, shoplifting, and emotional lability (including suicide attempts) are associated with bulimia nervosa. These patients generally experience their uncontrolled eating as more ego-dystonic than do anorexia nervosa patients and so seek help more readily.

Patients with bulimia nervosa lack superego control and the ego strength of their counterparts with anorexia nervosa. Their difficulties controlling their impulses are often manifested by substance dependence and self-destructive sexual relationships in addition to the binge eating and purging that characterize the disorder. Many bulimia nervosa patients have histories of difficulties separating from caretakers, as manifested by the absence of transitional objects during their early childhood years. Some clinicians have observed that patients with bulimia nervosa use their own bodies as transitional objects. The struggle for separation from a maternal figure is played out in the ambivalence toward food; eating may represent a wish to fuse with the caretaker, and regurgitating may unconsciously express a wish for separation.

Diagnosis and Clinical Features

According to DSM-IV-TR, the essential features of bulimia nervosa are recurrent episodes of binge eating; a sense of lack of control over eating during the eating binges; self-induced vomiting, the misuse of laxatives or diuretics, fasting, or excessive exercise to prevent weight gain; and persistent self-evaluation unduly influenced by body shape and weight (Table 23.2–1). Binging usually precedes vomiting by about 1 year.

Vomiting is common and is usually induced by sticking a finger down the throat, although some patients are able to vomit

Table 23.2–1
DSM-IV-TR Diagnostic Criteria for Bulimia Nervosa

A. Recurrent episodes of binge eating. An episode of binge eating is characterized by both of the following:
  (1) eating, in a discrete period of time (e.g., within any 2-hour period), an amount of food that is definitely larger than most people would eat during a similar period of time and under similar circumstances
  (2) a sense of lack of control over eating during the episode (e.g., a feeling that one cannot stop eating or control what or how much one is eating)

B. Recurrent inappropriate compensatory behavior in order to prevent weight gain, such as self-induced vomiting; misuse of laxatives, diuretics, enemas, or other medications; fasting; or excessive exercise.

C. The binge eating and inappropriate compensatory behaviors both occur, on average, at least twice a week for 3 months.

D. Self-evaluation is unduly influenced by body shape and weight.

E. The disturbance does not occur exclusively during episodes of anorexia nervosa.

Specify type:

Purging type: during the current episode of bulimia nervosa, the person has regularly engaged in self-induced vomiting or the misuse of laxatives, diuretics, or enemas

Nonpurging type: during the current episode of bulimia nervosa, the person has used other inappropriate compensatory behaviors, such as fasting or excessive exercise, but has not regularly engaged in self-induced vomiting or the misuse of laxatives, diuretics, or enemas

From American Psychiatric Association. *Diagnostic and Statistical Manual of Mental Disorders.* 4th ed. Text rev. Washington, DC: American Psychiatric Association; copyright 2000, with permission.

at will. Vomiting decreases the abdominal pain and the feeling of being bloated and allows patients to continue eating without fear of gaining weight. Depression, sometimes called *postbinge anguish,* often follows the episode. During binges, patients eat food that is sweet, high in calories, and generally soft or smooth textured, such as cakes and pastry. Some patients prefer bulky foods without regard to taste. The food is eaten secretly and rapidly and is sometimes not even chewed.

Most patients with bulimia nervosa are within their normal weight range, but some may be underweight or overweight. These patients are concerned about their body image and their appearance, worry about how others see them, and are concerned about their sexual attractiveness. Most are sexually active, compared with anorexia nervosa patients, who are not interested in sex. Pica and struggles during meals are sometimes revealed in the histories of patients with bulimia nervosa.

Bulimia nervosa occurs in persons with high rates of mood disorders and impulse control disorders. Bulimia nervosa is also reported to occur in those at risk for substance-related disorders and a variety of personality disorders. Patients with bulimia nervosa also have increased rates of anxiety disorders, bipolar I disorder, and dissociative disorders, and histories of sexual abuse.

Subtypes. Evidence indicates that bulimic persons who purge differ from binge eaters who do not purge in that the latter tend to have less body-image disturbance and less anxiety concerning eating. Bulimia nervosa patients who do not purge tend to be obese. Distinct physiological differences also exist between bulimia patients who purge and those who do not. Because of all these differences, the diagnosis of bulimia nervosa is subtyped into a purging type, for those who regularly engage in self-induced vomiting or the use of laxatives or diuretics, and a nonpurging type, for those who use strict dieting, fasting, or vigorous exercise but do not regularly engage in purging.

Patients with the purging type of bulimia nervosa may be at risk for certain medical complications, such as hypokalemia from vomiting or laxative abuse and hypochloremic alkalosis. Those who vomit repeatedly are at risk for gastric and esophageal tears, although these complications are rare. Patients who purge may have a different course from that of patients who binge and then diet or exercise.

Alice was 21 years old and had been binge eating and vomiting for 8 years before she was referred to an eating disorder treatment program. She had reached her greatest weight of 59 kg when she was a sophomore in high school and 15 years old. She had several stresses during that year—she did not make the cheerleading team; her grandfather, with whom she was very close, died; and some close friends moved away. She developed a general feeling of unhappiness, loneliness, and loss. Also that year, her parents had given away her pets because they were too much trouble. During this time Alice decided she wanted to lose weight and soon developed the habit of self-induced vomiting. She gradually increased the amount of vomiting until her senior year of high school, when she was vomiting four times a week. When Alice began to lose weight, she resorted to a series of fad diets. She refused to eat meals with her family and after about 6 months of dieting she began to get up at night for binge-eating episodes followed by self-induced vomiting, which she had perfected for the past several months.

After graduating from high school, Alice went to college for 1 year and majored in animal science. She did not like the curriculum and dropped out after a year. However, during that time her symptoms increased, and she actually wallpapered one of her walls with M&M wrappers. She then went back to live at home and had a series of jobs in food stores, such as a donut shop and a deli, as well as a clothing store. Finally, she was unable to hold a job for more than a few months because of her binge eating and vomiting. Her most stable relationship was with her boyfriend, with whom she was living a year before hospitalization.

During that time, at her boyfriend's insistence she saw a social worker weekly for several months but then stopped treatment abruptly. Her binge eating and vomiting got out of control, so her boyfriend took her to a local hospital. She was there for 3 months and then transferred directly to another program in a different hospital. During her initial hospitalization she was allowed to come and go as she pleased, and she continued her binge-eating and vomiting behavior. At the time of admission to the special eating disorder treatment program, Alice admitted to feeling depressed and having frequent crying spells. She also had difficulty falling asleep at night. She was totally preoccupied with thoughts of binge eating and of food. The significant findings on her physical examination were a slight scoliosis and marked deterioration of her teeth (Fig. 23.2–1).

Alice began her menses at age 14. At about the age of 16 she began to have irregular menses; however, she continued to menstruate. Her lowest weight was 50.9 kg, and that was just a few months before her admission to an eating disorder specialty unit. She was placed on a multifaceted treatment program with twice-weekly individual psychotherapy sessions, daily group therapies, and biweekly family sessions. Initially she expressed considerable denial and anger and was later able to describe feelings of emptiness, loneliness, and a sense of inadequacy. Response prevention techniques were used to stop the vomiting and binge-eating behavior, and she responded very well in a structured setting. She also received 60 mg of fluoxetine (Prozac) daily. Alice gradually gained control over the eating behavior and developed considerable insight into her problems and insecurities. During her 4 months in a special eating disorder treatment program, she responded well to the gradual introduction of responsibility for her eating behavior and other aspects of her life.

After discharge from the hospital, she continued her treatment in an outpatient setting and received individual and family therapy. She returned to live with her parents and brother, where she stayed for 6 months until she moved into a supportive apartment. Several months later she began attending a community college. Her binge eating and vomiting had stopped entirely, and she was eating normally and maintaining her weight within a normal range. Her prognosis, however, is guarded because of her long history of dysfunctional eating behavior.

DISCUSSION

Alice's dieting began when she had a series of stresses that challenged her feelings of competency and effectiveness. She was mildly overweight when she began dieting, which was not very effective until she started self-induced vomiting. Even with this behavior, as is typical in bulimia nervosa patients, she could not become emaciated. She was able to maintain a sexual relationship with her boyfriend, which contrasts with the more typical asexual nature of the anorexia nervosa patient. The rest of her life, however, was chaotic in that she could not keep a job for longer than a few months and was unable to have stable relationships with most persons. She suffered from depression, which responded to fluoxetine. Over the course of a year of cognitive psychotherapy, she ceased binging and vomiting. Although most bulimia nervosa patients have an immediate reduction in their binging and vomiting as a response to cognitive therapy, complete cessation of this behavior often occurs 1 or 2 years after the intensive therapy has occurred. (Courtesy of Katherine A. Halmi, M.D.)

Pathology and Laboratory Examinations

Bulimia nervosa can result in electrolyte abnormalities and various degrees of starvation, although it may not be as obvious as in low-weight patients with anorexia nervosa. Thus, even normal-weight patients with bulimia nervosa should have laboratory studies of electrolytes and metabolism. In general, thyroid function remains intact in bulimia nervosa, but patients may show nonsuppression on the dexamethasone-suppression test. Dehydration and electrolyte disturbances are likely to occur in bulimia nervosa patients who purge regularly. These patients commonly exhibit hypomagnesemia and hyperamylasemia. Although not a core diagnostic feature, many patients with bulimia nervosa have menstrual disturbances. Hypotension and bradycardia occur in some patients.

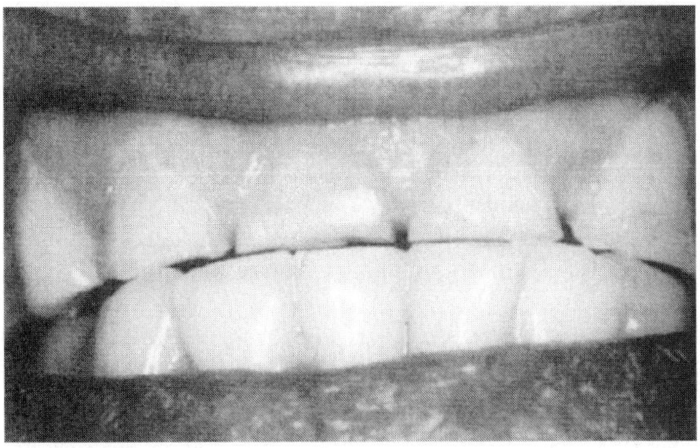

FIGURE 23.2–1

Dental erosion of upper front teeth of a patient with long-standing bulimia nervosa; binge eating/purging type. (Reprinted with permission from Walsh BT. Eating disorders. In: Tasman A, Kay J, Lieberman JA, eds. *Psychiatry.* Vol 2. Philadelphia: Saunders; 1997.)

Differential Diagnosis

The diagnosis of bulimia nervosa cannot be made if the binge-eating and purging behaviors occur exclusively during episodes of anorexia nervosa. In such cases the diagnosis is anorexia nervosa, binge eating–purging type.

Clinicians must ascertain that patients have no neurological disease, such as epileptic-equivalent seizures, central nervous system tumors, Klüver-Bucy syndrome, or Kleine-Levin syndrome. The pathological features manifested by Klüver-Bucy syndrome are visual agnosia, compulsive licking and biting, examination of objects by the mouth, inability to ignore any stimulus, placidity, altered sexual behavior (hypersexuality), and altered dietary habits, especially hyperphagia. The syndrome is exceedingly rare and is unlikely to cause a problem in differential diagnosis. Kleine-Levin syndrome consists of periodic hypersomnia lasting for 2 to 3 weeks and hyperphagia. As in bulimia nervosa, the onset is usually during adolescence, but the syndrome is more common in men than in women. Patients with borderline personality disorder sometimes binge eat, but the eating is associated with the other signs of the disorder.

Course and Prognosis

Little is known about the long-range course of bulimia nervosa, and the short-term outcome varies. Overall, bulimia nervosa seems to have a better prognosis than anorexia nervosa. In the short run, patients with bulimia nervosa who can engage in treatment have reported more than 50 percent improvement in binge eating and purging; among outpatients, improvement seems to last more than 5 years. The patients are not symptom free during periods of improvement, however; bulimia nervosa is a chronic disorder with a waxing and waning course. Some patients with mild courses have long-term remissions. Other patients are disabled by the disorder and have been hospitalized; less than one third of them are doing well at 3-year follow-up, more than one third have some improvement in their symptoms, and about one third have a poor outcome, with chronic symptoms. In a recent study, at 5 to 10 years, about half of patients recovered fully from the disorder, while 20 percent continued to meet full diagnostic criteria for bulimia nervosa. In some cases of untreated bulimia nervosa, spontaneous remission occurs in 1 to 2 years. The prognosis depends on the severity of the purging sequelae—that is, whether a patient has electrolyte imbalances and to what degree the frequent vomiting results in esophagitis, amylasemia, salivary gland enlargement, and dental caries.

Treatment

Most patients with uncomplicated bulimia nervosa do not require hospitalization. In general, patients with bulimia nervosa are not as secretive about their symptoms as patients with anorexia nervosa. Therefore, outpatient treatment is usually not difficult, but psychotherapy is frequently stormy and may be prolonged. Some obese patients with bulimia nervosa who have had prolonged psychotherapy do surprisingly well. In some cases—when eating binges are out of control, outpatient treatment does not work, or a patient exhibits such additional psychiatric symptoms as suicidality and substance abuse—hospitalization may become necessary. In addition, electrolyte and metabolic disturbances resulting from severe purging may necessitate hospitalization.

Psychotherapy. COGNITIVE-BEHAVIORAL THERAPY. Cognitive-behavioral therapy (CBT) should be considered the benchmark, first-line treatment for bulimia nervosa. The data supporting the efficacy of CBT are based upon strict adherence to rigorously implemented, highly detailed, manual-guided treatments that include about 18 to 20 sessions over 5 to 6 months. CBT implements a number of cognitive and behavioral procedures to (1) interrupt the self-maintaining behavioral cycle of bingeing and dieting and (2) alter the individual's dysfunctional cognitions; beliefs about food, weight, body image; and overall self-concept.

DYNAMIC PSYCHOTHERAPY. Psychodynamic treatment of patients with bulimia nervosa has revealed a tendency to concretize introjective and projective defense mechanisms. In a manner analogous to splitting, patients divide food into two categories: items that are nutritious and those that are unhealthy. Food that is designated nutritious may be ingested and retained because it unconsciously symbolizes good introjects. But junk food is unconsciously associated with bad introjects and is, therefore, expelled by vomiting, with the unconscious fantasy that all destructiveness, hate, and badness are being evacuated. Patients may temporarily feel good after vomiting because of the fantasized evacuation, but the associated feeling of "being all good" is short-lived because it is based on an unstable combination of splitting and projection.

Pharmacotherapy. Antidepressant medications have been shown to be helpful in bulimia. This includes the serotonin reuptake inhibitors such as fluoxetine. This may be based on elevating central 5-hydroxytryptamine levels. Antidepressant medications can reduce binge eating and purging independent of the presence of a mood disorder. Thus, antidepressants have been used successfully for particularly difficult binge–purge cycles that do not respond to psychotherapy alone. Imipramine (Tofranil), desipramine (Norpramin), trazodone (Desyrel), and monoamine oxidase inhibitors (MAOIs) have been helpful. In general, most of the antidepressants have been effective at dosages usually given in the treatment of depressive disorders. However, dosages of fluoxetine that are effective in decreasing binge eating may be higher (60 to 80 mg a day) than those used for depressive disorders. Medication is helpful in patients with comorbid depressive disorders and bulimia nervosa. Carbamazepine (Tegretol) and lithium (Eskalith) have not shown impressive results as treatments for binge eating, but they have been used in the treatment of bulimia nervosa patients with comorbid mood disorders, such as bipolar I disorder. Evidence indicates that the use of antidepressants alone results in a 22 percent rate of abstinence from bingeing and purging; other studies show that CBT and medications are the most effective combination.

Table 23.2–2
DSM-IV-TR Diagnostic Criteria for Eating Disorder Not Otherwise Specified

The eating disorder not otherwise specified category is for disorders of eating that do not meet the criteria for any specific eating disorder. Examples include

1. For females, all of the criteria for anorexia nervosa are met except that the individual has regular menses.
2. All of the criteria for anorexia nervosa are met except that, despite significant weight loss, the individual's current weight is in the normal range.
3. All of the criteria for bulimia nervosa are met except that the binge eating and inappropriate compensatory mechanisms occur at a frequency of less than twice a week or for a duration of less than 3 months.
4. The regular use of inappropriate compensatory behavior by an individual of normal body weight after eating small amounts of food (e.g., self-induced vomiting after the consumption of two cookies).
5. Repeatedly chewing and spitting out, but not swallowing, large amounts of food.
6. Binge-eating disorder: recurrent episodes of binge eating in the absence of the regular use of inappropriate compensatory behaviors characteristic of bulimia nervosa.

From American Psychiatric Association. *Diagnostic and Statistical Manual of Mental Disorders.* 4th ed. Text rev. Washington, DC: American Psychiatric Association; copyright 2000, with permission.

Table 23.2–3
DSM-IV-TR Research Criteria for Binge-Eating Disorder

A. Recurrent episodes of binge eating. An episode of binge eating is characterized by both of the following:
   (1) eating, in a discrete period of time (e.g., within any 2-hour period), an amount of food that is definitely larger than what most people would eat in a similar period of time under similar circumstances
   (2) a sense of lack of control over eating during the episode (e.g., a feeling that one cannot stop eating or control what or how much one is eating)
B. The binge-eating episodes are associated with three (or more) of the following:
   (1) eating much more rapidly than normal
   (2) eating until feeling uncomfortably full
   (3) eating large amounts of food when not feeling physically hungry
   (4) eating alone because of being embarrassed by how much one is eating
   (5) feeling disgusted with oneself, depressed, or very guilty after overeating
C. Marked distress regarding binge eating is present.
D. The binge eating occurs, on average, at least 2 days a week for 6 months.
   Note: The method of determining frequency differs from that used for bulimia nervosa; future research should address whether the preferred method of setting a frequency threshold is counting the number of days on which binges occur or counting the number of episodes of binge eating.
E. The binge eating is not associated with the regular use of inappropriate compensatory behaviors (e.g., purging, fasting, excessive exercise) and does not occur exclusively during the course of anorexia nervosa or bulimia nervosa.

From American Psychiatric Association. *Diagnostic and Statistical Manual of Mental Disorders.* 4th ed. Text rev. Washington, DC: American Psychiatric Association; copyright 2000, with permission.

EATING DISORDER NOT OTHERWISE SPECIFIED

The DSM-IV-TR diagnostic classification eating disorder not otherwise specified is a residual category used for eating disorders that do not meet the criteria for a specific eating disorder (Table 23.2–2). Binge-eating disorder—that is, recurrent episodes of binge eating in the absence of the inappropriate com-

pensatory behaviors characteristic of bulimia nervosa (Table 23.2–3)—falls into this category. Such patients are not fixated on body shape and weight.

ICD-10

The 10th revision of *International Statistical Classification of Diseases and Related Health Problems* (ICD-10) describes bulimia nervosa as repeated bouts of overeating and a preoccupation about controlling weight that lead to self-induced vomiting; in turn, vomiting produces physical complications, electrolyte disturbances, and severe weight loss (see Table 23.1–4 in Section 23.1).

In the category of eating disorders, ICD-10 also includes atypical anorexia, atypical bulimia nervosa, overeating associated with other psychological disturbances, vomiting associated with other psychological disturbances, other eating disorders, and eating disorders, unspecified (see Table 23.1–4).

References

Byrne S, McLean N. Eating disorders in athletes: a review of the literature. *J Sci Med Sport.* 2001;4:145.

Dalle Grave R, Ricca V, Todesco T. The stepped-care approach in anorexia nervosa and bulimia nervosa: progress and problems. *Eat Weight Disord.* 2001;6:81.

de Zwaan M. Binge eating disorder and obesity. *Int J Obes.* 2001;25(suppl 1):S51.

Devlin MJ. Binge-eating disorder and obesity. A combined treatment approach. *Psychiatr Clin North Am.* 2001;24:325.

Dingemans AE, Bruna MJ, van Furth EF. Binge eating disorder: a review. *Int J Obes Relat Metab Disord.* 2002;26:299.

Dorian BJ. An integration of feminist and self-psychological approaches to bulimia nervosa. *Eat Weight Disord.* 2001;6:107.

Garner DM, Rockert W, Davis R, Garner MV. Comparison of cognitive behavioral and supportive-expressive therapy for bulimia nervosa. *Am J Psychiatry.* 1993;150:37.

Keel PK, Dorer DJ, Eddy KT. Predictors of treatment utilization among women with anorexia and bulimia nervosa. *Am J Psychiatry.* 2002;159:96.

Keel PK, Mitchell JE. Outcome in bulimia nervosa. *Am J Psychiatry.* 1997;154:313.

Klump KL, Kaye WH, Strober M. The evolving genetic foundations of eating disorders. *Psychiatr Clin North Am.* 2001;24:215.

Mendell DA, Logermann JA. Bulimia and swallowing: cause for concern. *Int J Eat Disord.* 2001;30:252.

Mitchell JE, Peterson CB, Myers T, Wonderlich S. Combining pharmacotherapy and psychotherapy in the treatment of patients with eating disorders. *Psychiatr Clin North Am.* 2001;24:315.

Paul T, Schroeter K, Dahme B, Nutzinger DO. Self-injurious behavior in women with eating disorders. *Am J Psychiatry.* 2002;159:408.

Reas DL, Schoemaker C, Zipfel S, Williamson DA. Prognostic value of duration of illness and early intervention in bulimia nervosa: a systematic review of the outcome literature. *Int J Eat Disord.* 2001;30:1.

Seidenfeld M, Ricket VI. Impact of anorexia, bulimia and obesity on the gynecologic health of adolescents. *Am Fam Physician.* 2001;64:445.

Treasure J, Serpell L. Osteoporosis in young people. Research and treatment in eating disorders. *Psychiatr Clin North Am.* 2001;24:359.

▲ 23.3 Obesity

Obesity refers to an excess of body fat. In healthy individuals, body fat accounts for approximately 25 percent of body weight in women and 18 percent in men. *Overweight* refers to weight above some reference norm, typically standards derived from actuarial or epidemiological data. In most cases, increasing weight reflects increasing obesity, but not always. Muscular individuals might be overweight (weight might be high for height) but not be obese, and a person might have normal weight but have high body fat.

Indexes have been developed using height and weight to estimate level of obesity. The most common of these is the body mass index (BMI). BMI is calculated by dividing weight in kilograms by height in meters squared. Although there is debate about the ideal BMI, it is generally thought that a BMI of 20 to 25 kg/m^2 represents healthy weight, a BMI of 25 to 27 kg/m^2 is associated with somewhat elevated risk, a BMI above 27 kg/m^2 represents clearly increased risk, and a BMI above 30 kg/m^2 carries greatly increased risk.

In the United States approximately 35 percent of women and 31 percent of men are significantly overweight (BMI 27 or above, about 20 percent overweight). If one defines obesity as a BMI over 25, there are now more obese than nonobese Americans. Using a BMI over 31 (approximately 40 percent overweight), 11 percent of women and 8 percent of men are severely overweight. The prevalence of obesity in America has tripled since the early 1900s.

The prevalence of obesity is highest in minority populations, particularly among women. Fully 60 percent of African American women ages 45 years and older are overweight, as defined by a BMI of 27 or above. The high prevalence of obesity in minority populations appears to be attributable primarily to lower income and educational attainment rather than to race. Obesity is six times more prevalent in women of low socioeconomic status than in women of high socioeconomic status.

Weight gain is most pronounced in both sexes between the ages of 25 and 44. During this time, men gain an average of 4 kg, and women, 7 kg. Pregnancy probably contributes to the greater increase in women, who on average, begin each successive pregnancy approximately 2.5 kg heavier than at the last. After age 50, weights of men stabilize, and even decline slightly between ages 60 and 74. Women, in contrast, continue to increase in weight until age 60, at which time weight begins to decline.

ETIOLOGY

Persons accumulate fat by eating more calories than are expended as energy; thus intake of energy exceeds its dissipation. If fat is to be removed from the body, fewer calories must be put in or more calories must be taken out than are put in. An error of no more than 10 percent in either intake or output would lead to a 30-pound change in body weight in 1 year.

Satiety

Satiety is the feeling that results when hunger is satisfied. Persons stop eating at the end of a meal because they have replenished nutrients that had been depleted. Persons become hungry again when nutrients restored by earlier meals are once again depleted. It seems reasonable that a metabolic signal, derived from food that has been absorbed, is carried by the blood to the brain, where the signal activates receptor cells, probably in the hypothalamus, to produce satiety. Some studies have shown evidence for dysfunction in serotonin, dopamine, and norepinephrine involvement in regulating eating behavior through the hypothalamus. Other humoral factors that may be involved include corticotropin releasing factor (CRF), neuropeptide Y, gonadotropin-releasing hormone, and thyroid-stimulating hormone. Hunger results from a decrease in the strength of metabolic signals, secondary to the depletion of critical nutrients.

Satiety occurs soon after the beginning of a meal and before the total caloric content of the meal has been absorbed; therefore satiety is only one regulatory mechanism controlling food intake. Appetite, defined as the desire for food, is also involved. A hungry person may eat to full satisfaction when food is available, but appetite can also induce a person to overeat past the point of satiety. Appetite may be increased by psychological factors such as thoughts or feelings, and an abnormal appetite may result in an abnormal increase in food intake.

The olfactory system may play a role in satiety. Experiments have shown that strong stimulation of the olfactory bulbs in the nose with food odors by use of an inhaler saturated with a particular smell produces satiety for that food. This may have implications for therapy of obesity.

Genetic Factors

The existence of numerous forms of inherited obesity in animals and the ease with which adiposity can be produced by selective breeding make it clear that genetic factors can play a role in obesity. These factors must also be presumed to be important in human obesity.

About 80 percent of patients who are obese have a family history of obesity. This fact can be accounted for not only by genetic factors but also in part by identification with fat parents and by learned oral methods for coping with anxiety. Nonetheless, studies show that identical twins raised apart can both be obese, an observation that suggests a hereditary role. To date, no specific genetic marker of obesity has been found.

Developmental Factors

Early in life, adipose tissue grows by increases in both cell number and cell size. Once the number of adipocytes has been established, it does not seem to be susceptible to change. Obesity that begins early in life is characterized by adipose tissue with an increased number of adipocytes of increased size. Obesity that begins in adult life, on the other hand, results solely from an increase in the size of the adipocytes. In both instances, weight reduction produces a decrease in cell size. The greater number and size of adipocytes in patients with juvenile-onset diabetes may be a factor in their widely recognized difficulties with weight reduction and the persistence of their obesity.

The distribution and amount of fat vary in individuals, and fat in different body areas has different characteristics. Fat cells around the waist, flanks, and abdomen (the so-called potbelly) are more active metabolically than those in the thighs and buttocks. The former pattern is more common in men and has a higher correlation with cardiovascular disease than does the latter pattern. Women, whose fat distribution is in the thighs and buttocks, may become obsessed with nostrums that are advertised to reduce fat in these areas (so-called cellulite, which is not a medical term); but no externally applied preparation to reduce this fat pattern exists. Men with abdominal fat may attempt to reduce their girth with machines that exercise the abdominal muscles, but exercise has no effect on fat loss.

A hormone called *leptin*, made by fat cells, acts as a fat thermostat. When the blood level of leptin is low, more fat is consumed; when high, less fat is consumed. Further research is needed to determine whether this might lead to new ways of managing obesity.

Physical Activity Factors

The marked decrease in physical activity in affluent societies seems to be the major factor in the rise of obesity as a public health problem. Physical inactivity restricts energy expenditure and may contribute to increased food intake. Although food intake increases with increasing energy expenditure over a wide range of energy demands, intake does not decrease proportionately when physical activity falls below a certain minimum level.

Brain-Damage Factors

Destruction of the ventromedial hypothalamus can produce obesity in animals, but this is probably a very rare cause of obesity in humans. There is evidence that the central nervous system, particularly in the lateral and ventromedial hypothalamic areas, adjusts to food intake in response to changing energy requirements so as to maintain fat stores at a baseline determined by a specific set point. This set point varies from one person to another and depends on height and body build.

Other Clinical Factors

A variety of clinical disorders are associated with obesity. Cushing's disease is associated with a characteristic fat distribution (buffalo adiposity) (Fig. 23.3–1). Myxedema is associated with weight gain, although not invariably. Other neuroendocrine disorders include adiposogenital dystrophy (Fröhlich's syndrome), which is characterized by obesity and sexual and skeletal abnormalities.

Psychotropic Drugs

Among the atypical antipsychotics, olanzapine (Zyprexa), clozapine (Clozaril), and quetiapine (Seroquel) have weight gain as a known side effect; ziprasidone (Zeldox) shows promise of not interfering with weight. Among mood stabilizers, lithium (Eskalith), valproate (Depakene), and carbamazepine (Tegretol) are also associated with weight gain. Topiramate (Topamax), an anticonvulsant used for mood stabilization, tends not to increase weight and can act as an appetite suppressant in some patients. Selective serotonin reuptake inhibitors are also associated with weight gain with long-term use. Fluoxetine may cause an initial weight loss. Individual patients may respond idiosyncratically and should be individually monitored to determine if weight gain is an issue.

Psychological Factors

Although psychological factors are evidently crucial to the development of obesity, how such psychological factors result in obesity is not known. The food-regulating mechanism is susceptible to environmental influence, and cultural, family, and psychodynamic factors have all been shown to contribute to the development of obesity. Although many investigators have proposed that specific family histories, precipitating factors, per-

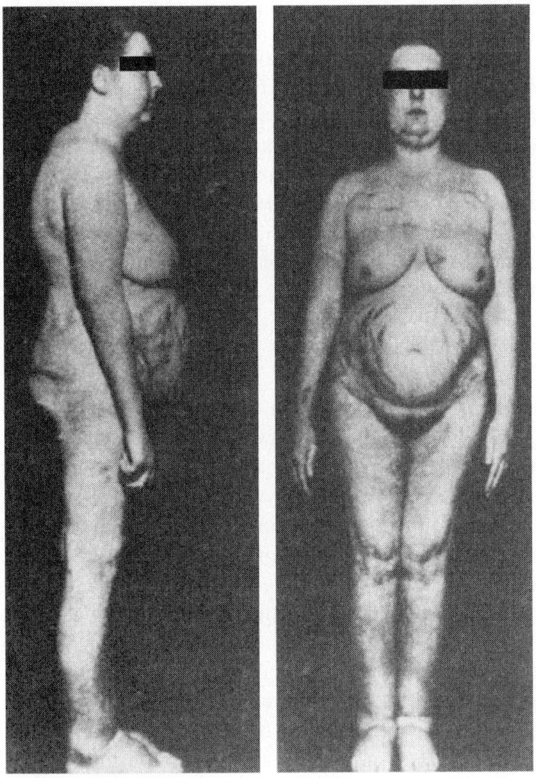

FIGURE 23.3–1
Cushing's syndrome. Obesity and round face are evident. Hirsutism and abdominal striae are noted. (Reprinted with permission from Spillane JD, Spillane JA. *An Atlas of Clinical Neurology,* 3rd ed. New York: Oxford University Press; 1982.)

sonality structures, or unconscious conflicts cause obesity, overweight persons may suffer from every conceivable psychiatric disorder and come from a variety of disturbed backgrounds. Many obese patients are emotionally disturbed persons who, because of the availability of the overeating mechanism in their environments, have learned to use hyperphagia as a means of coping with psychological problems. Some patients may show signs of serious mental disorder when they attain normal weight because they no longer have that coping mechanism.

CLINICAL FEATURES

Many obese persons report that they overeat when they are emotionally upset, often soon thereafter. But many nonobese persons report similar experiences, and it is difficult to ascertain the specificity for obesity of such short-term contingencies. Reports linking emotional factors and obesity over the long term seem more specific: Some obese persons lose large amounts of weight when they fall in love and gain weight when they lose a loved one.

The habitual eating patterns of many obese persons often seem similar to patterns found in experimental obesity. Impaired satiety is a particularly important problem. Obese persons seem inordinately susceptible to food cues in their environment, to the palatability of foods, and to the inability to stop eating if food is available. Obese persons are usually susceptible to all kinds of external stimuli to eating, but they remain relatively unresponsive to the usual internal signals of hunger. Some are unable to distinguish between hunger and other kinds of dysphoria.

DIFFERENTIAL DIAGNOSIS

Other Syndromes

The night-eating syndrome, in which persons eat excessively after they have had their evening meal, seems to be precipitated by stressful life circumstances and, once present, tends to recur daily until the stress is alleviated. The binge-eating syndrome (bulimia) is characterized by sudden, compulsive ingestion of very large amounts of food in a short time, usually with great subsequent agitation and self-condemnation. Binge eating also appears to represent a reaction to stress. In contrast to the night-eating syndrome, however, these bouts of overeating are not periodic, and they are far more often linked to specific precipitating circumstances. (See Chapter 23, Section 23.2, for a complete discussion of bulimia.) The *pickwickian syndrome* is said to exist when a person is 100 percent over desirable weight and has associated respiratory and cardiovascular pathology.

Body Dysmorphic Disorder (Dysmorphophobia)

Some obese persons feel that their bodies are grotesque and loathsome and that others view them with hostility and contempt. This feeling is closely associated with self-consciousness and impaired social functioning. Emotionally healthy obese persons have no body image disturbances, and only a minority of neurotic obese persons have such disturbances. The disorder is confined mainly to persons who have been obese since childhood; even among them, less than half suffer from it. (Body dysmorphic disorder is discussed further in Chapter 17 on somatoform disorders.)

COURSE AND PROGNOSIS

Effects on Health

Obesity has adverse effects on health and is associated with a broad range of illnesses (Table 23.3–1). There is a strong correlation between obesity and cardiovascular disorders. Hypertension (blood pressure higher than 160/95) is three times higher for persons who are overweight, and hypercholesterolemia (blood cholesterol over 250 mg/dL) is twice as common. Studies show that blood pressure and cholesterol levels can be reduced by weight reduction. Diabetes, which has clear genetic determinations, can often be reversed with weight reduction, especially type II diabetes (mature-onset or non–insulin-dependent diabetes mellitus).

According to National Institutes of Health data, obese men, regardless of smoking habits, have a higher mortality from colon, rectal, and prostate cancer than men of normal weight. Obese women have a higher mortality from cancer of the gallbladder, biliary passages, breast (postmenopause), uterus (including cervix and endometrium), and ovaries than women of normal weight.

Table 23.3–1
Health Disorders Thought to Be Caused or Exacerbated by Obesity

Heart
Premature coronary heart disease
Left ventricular hypertrophy
Angina pectoris
Sudden death (ventricular arrhythmia)
Congestive heart failure
Vascular system
Hypertension
Cerebrovascular disorder (cerebral infarction or hemorrhage)
Venous stasis (with lower-extremity edema, varicose veins)
Respiratory system
Obstructive sleep apnea
Pickwickian syndrome (alveolar hypoventilation)
Secondary polycythemia
Right ventricular hypertrophy (sometimes leading to failure)
Hepatobiliary system
Cholelithiasis and cholecystitis
Hepatic steatosis
Hormonal and metabolic functions
Diabetes mellitus (insulin independent)
Gout (hyperuricemia)
Hyperlipidemias (hypertriglyceridemia and hypercholesterolemia)
Kidney
Proteinuria and, in very severe obesity, nephrosis
Renal vein thrombosis
Joints, muscles, and connective tissue
Osteoarthritis of knees
Bone spurs of the heel
Osteoarthrosis of spine (in women)
Aggravation of preexisting postural faults
Neoplasia
In women: increased risk of cancer of endometrium, breast, cervix, ovary, gallbladder, and biliary passages
In men: increased risk of cancer of colon, rectum, and prostate

Reprinted with permission from Vanitallie TB. Obesity: adverse effects on health and longevity. *Am J Clin Nutr.* 1979;32:2723.

Longevity

Reliable studies indicate that the more overweight a person is, the higher is that person's risk for death. A person who reduces weight to acceptable levels has a mortality decline to normal rates. Weight reduction may be lifesaving for patients with extreme obesity, defined as weight that is twice the desirable weight. Such patients may have cardiorespiratory failure, especially when asleep (sleep apnea).

Prognosis

The prognosis for weight reduction is poor, and the course of obesity tends toward inexorable progression. Of patients who lose significant amounts of weight, 90 percent regain it eventually. The prognosis is particularly poor for those who become obese in childhood. Juvenile-onset obesity tends to be more severe, more resistant to treatment, and more likely to be associated with emotional disturbance than is adult obesity.

TREATMENT

As many as half of patients routinely treated for obesity by family physicians may develop mild anxiety and depression. In addition, a high incidence of emotional disturbances has been reported among obese persons undergoing long-term, in-hospital treatment by fasting or severe calorie restriction. Obese persons with extensive psychopathology, those with a history of emotional disturbance during dieting, and those in the midst of a life crisis should attempt weight reduction, if at all, cautiously and under careful supervision.

Diet

The basis of weight reduction is simple—establish a caloric deficit by bringing intake below output. The simplest way to reduce caloric intake is by means of a low-calorie diet. The best long-term effects are achieved with a balanced diet that contains readily available foods. For most persons, the most satisfactory reducing diet consists of their usual foods in amounts determined with the aid of tables of food values that are available in standard books on dieting. Such a diet gives the best chance of long-term maintenance of weight loss. Total unmodified fasts are used for short-term weight loss, but they have associated morbidity including orthostatic hypotension, sodium diuresis, and impaired nitrogen balance.

Ketogenic diets are high-protein, high-fat diets used to promote weight loss. They have a high cholesterol content and produce ketosis, which is associated with nausea, hypotension, and lethargy. Many obese persons find it tempting to use a novel or even bizarre diet. Whatever effectiveness these diets may have in large part results from their monotony. When a dieter stops the diet and returns to the usual fare, the incentives to overeat are multiplied.

In general, the best method of weight loss is a balanced diet of 1,100 to 1,200 calories. Such a diet can be followed for long periods but should be supplemented with vitamins, particularly iron, folic acid, zinc, and vitamin B_6.

Exercise

Increased physical activity is frequently recommended as part of a weight-reduction regimen. Because caloric expenditure in most forms of physical activity is directly proportional to body weight, obese persons expend more calories than persons of normal weight with the same amount of activity. Furthermore, increased physical activity may actually decrease food intake by formerly sedentary persons. This combination of increased caloric expenditure and decreased food intake makes an increase in physical activity a highly desirable feature of any weight-reduction program. Exercise also helps maintain weight loss.

Pharmacotherapy

Various drugs, some more effective than others, are used to treat obesity. Table 23.3–2 lists the drugs currently available. Drug treatment is effective because it suppresses appetite, but tolerance to this effect may develop after several weeks of use. An initial trial period of 4 weeks with a specific drug can be used; then, if the patient responds with weight loss, the drug

Table 23.3–2
Drugs for the Treatment of Obesity

Generic Name	Trade Name(s)	Usual Dosage Range (mg/day)
Amphetamine and dextroamphetamine	Biphetamine	12.5–20
Methamphetamine	Desoxyn	10–15
Benzphetamine	Didrex	75–150
Phendimetrazine	Bontril, Plegine, Prelu-2, X-Trozine	105
Phentermine		
Hydrochloride	Adipex-P, Fastin, Oby-trim	18.75–37.5
Resin	Ionamin	15–30
Diethylpropion hydrochloride	Tenuate	75
Mazindol	Sanorex, Mazanor	3–9
Sibutramine	Meridia	10–15
Orlistat	Xenical	360

can be continued to see whether tolerance develops. If a drug remains effective, it can be dispensed for a longer time until the desired weight is achieved.

The other weight-loss medication approved by the Food and Drug Administration (FDA) for long-term use (in 1999) is orlistat (Xenical), which is a selective gastric and pancreatic lipase inhibitor that reduces the absorption of dietary fat (which is then excreted in stool). In clinical trials orlistat (120 mg, three times a day), in combination with a low-calorie diet, induced losses of approximately 10 percent of initial weight in the first 6 months, which were generally well maintained for periods up to 24 months. Because of its peripheral mechanism of action, orlistat is generally free of the central nervous system effects (i.e., increased pulse, dry mouth, insomnia, etc.) that are associated with most weight-loss medications. The principal adverse effects of orlistat are gastrointestinal; patients must consume 30 percent or fewer calories from fat to prevent adverse events that include oily stool, flatulence with discharge, and fecal urgency.
Sibutramine (Meridia) is a β-phenylethylamine that inhibits the reuptake of serotonin and norepinephrine (and dopamine to a limited extent). It was approved by the FDA in 1997 for weight loss and the maintenance of weight loss (i.e., long-term use).

Surgery

Surgical methods that cause malabsorption of food or reduce gastric volume have been used in persons who are markedly obese. *Gastric bypass* is a procedure in which the stomach is made smaller by transecting or stapling one of the stomach curvatures. In *gastroplasty* the size of the stomach stoma is reduced so that the passage of food slows. Results are successful, although vomiting, electrolyte imbalance, and obstruction may occur. A syndrome called *dumping,* which consists of palpitations, weakness, and sweating may follow surgical procedures in some patients if they ingest large amounts of carbohydrates in a single meal. The surgical removal of fat (lipectomy) is used for cosmetic reasons and has no effect on weight loss in the long run.

Psychotherapy

The psychological problems of obese persons vary, and there is no particular personality type that is obese. Some patients may respond to insight-oriented psychodynamic therapy with weight loss, but this treatment has not had much success. No evidence indicates that uncovering the unconscious causes of overeating can alter the symptom choice of persons who overeat in response to stress. Years after successful psychotherapy and successful weight reduction, most persons who overeat under stress continue to do so. Furthermore, many obese persons seem particularly vulnerable to overdependency on a therapist and the inordinate regression that may occur during the uncovering psychotherapies.

Behavior modification has been the most successful of the psychotherapies and is considered the method of choice. Patients are taught to recognize external cues that are associated with eating and to keep diaries of foods consumed in particular circumstances, such as at the movies or while watching television, or during certain emotional states, such as anxiety or depression. Patients are also taught to develop new eating patterns, such as eating slowly, chewing food well, not reading while eating, and not eating between meals or when not seated. Operant conditioning therapies that use rewards such as praise or new clothes to reinforce weight loss have also been successful. Group therapy helps to maintain motivation, to promote identification among members who have lost weight, and to provide education about nutrition.

Comprehensive Approach

A truly comprehensive approach for managing obesity includes facilities (e.g., metabolic measurement rooms) and personnel (e.g., dietitians and exercise physiologists) at a single center; however, these are rarely available. High-quality programs can be devised with readily available resources (e.g., treatment manuals) and the judicious use of an integrated approach that combines exercise, psychotherapy, and pharmacotherapy. Deciding on the type of psychotherapy or weight management is an important task, as is deciding with the patient which combination of resources for weight control would be most suitable.

References

Crowley V, Vidal-Puig AJ. Mitochondrial uncoupling proteins (UCPs) and obesity. *Nutr Metab Cardiovasc Dis.* 2001;11:70.

Faggioni R, Feingold KR, Grunfeld C. Leptin regulation of the immune response and the immunodeficiency of malnutrition. *FASEB J.* 2001;15:2565.

Health Implication of Obesity. NIH Consensus Statement Online 1985, Feb 11–13 [cited 1997, Jan 7] 1997;5:1.

Jakicic JM, Clark K, Coleman E, et al. American College of Sports Medicine position stand. Appropriate intervention strategies for weight loss and prevention of weight regain for adults. *Med Sci Sports Exerc.* 2001;33:2145.

Malhotra S, McElroy SL. Medical management of obesity associated with mental disorders. *J Clin Psychiatry.* 2002;63(suppl 4):24.

Mayer J. *Overweight: Causes, Cost, and Control.* Englewood Cliffs, NJ: Prentice-Hall; 1968.

Shils ME, Olson JA, Shike M, eds. *Obesity in Modern Nutrition.* Malvern, PA: Lea & Febiger; 1994.

Shuldiner AR, Yang R, Gong DW. Resistin, obesity and insulin resistance—the emerging role of the adipocyte as an endocrine organ. *N Engl J Med.* 2001;345:1345.

Wieland HA, Hamilton BS. Weighing the options in the pharmacotherapy of obesity. *Int J Clin Pharmacol Ther.* 2001;39:406.

Yanovski SZ. Long-term pharmacotherapy in the management of obesity: National Task Force on Obesity. *JAMA.* 1996;276:1907.

24 Normal Sleep and Sleep Disorders

24.1 Normal Sleep

Sleep is a regular, recurrent, easily reversible state that is characterized by relative quiescence and a great increase in the threshold of response to external stimuli relative to the waking state. Close monitoring of sleep is an important part of clinical practice; sleep disturbance is often an early symptom of impending mental illness. Some mental disorders are associated with characteristic changes in sleep physiology.

The ancient Greeks ascribed the need for sleep to the god Hypnos (sleep) and his son Morpheus, also a creature of the night, who brought dreams in human forms (Fig. 24.1–1).

ELECTROPHYSIOLOGY OF SLEEP

Sleep is made up of two physiological states: non–rapid eye movement (NREM) sleep and rapid eye movement (REM) sleep. In NREM sleep, which is composed of stages 1 through 4, most physiological functions are markedly lower than in wakefulness. REM sleep is a qualitatively different kind of sleep, characterized by a high level of brain activity and physiological activity levels similar to those in wakefulness. About 90 minutes after sleep onset, NREM yields to the first REM episode of the night. This REM latency of 90 minutes is a consistent finding in normal adults; shortening of REM latency frequently occurs with such disorders as depressive disorders and narcolepsy. The electroencephalograph (EEG) records the rapid conjugate eye movements that are the identifying feature of the sleep state (there are no or few rapid eye movements in NREM sleep); the EEG pattern consists of low-voltage, random, fast activity with sawtooth waves; the electromyograph (EMG) shows a marked reduction in muscle tone (Fig. 24.1–2).

In normal persons, NREM sleep is a peaceful state relative to waking. The pulse rate is typically slowed 5 to 10 beats a minute below the level of restful waking and is very regular. Respiration is similarly affected, and blood pressure also tends to be low, with few minute-to-minute variations. The resting muscle potential of the body musculature is lower in REM sleep than in a waking state. Episodic, involuntary body movements are present in NREM sleep. There are few REMs, if any, and seldom any penile erections in men. Blood flow through most tissues, including cerebral blood flow, is slightly reduced.

The deepest portions of NREM sleep—stages 3 and 4—are sometimes associated with unusual arousal characteristics. When persons are aroused 1/2 to 1 hour after sleep onset—usually in slow-wave sleep—they are disoriented, and their thinking is disorganized. Brief arousals from slow-wave sleep are also associated with amnesia for events that occur during the arousal. The disorganization during arousal from stage 3 or stage 4 may result in specific problems, including enuresis, somnambulism, and stage 4 nightmares or night terrors.

Polygraphic measures during REM sleep show irregular patterns, sometimes close to aroused waking patterns. Otherwise, if researchers were unaware of the behavioral stage and happened to be recording a variety of physiological measures (aside from muscle tone) during REM periods, they would undoubtedly conclude that the person or animal they were studying was in an active waking state. Because of this observation, REM sleep has also been termed *paradoxical sleep*. Pulse, respiration, and blood pressure in humans are all high during REM sleep—much higher than during NREM sleep and often higher than during waking. Even more striking than the level or rate is the variability from minute to minute. Brain oxygen use increases during REM sleep. The ventilatory response to

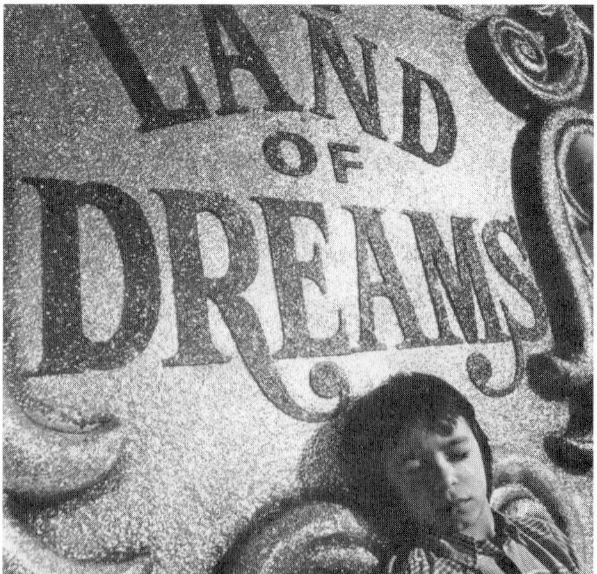

FIGURE 24.1–1
Dreams are the royal road to the unconscious, according to Sigmund Freud. They are also the guardians of sleep. (Courtesy of Arthur Tress for Magnum Photos, Inc.)

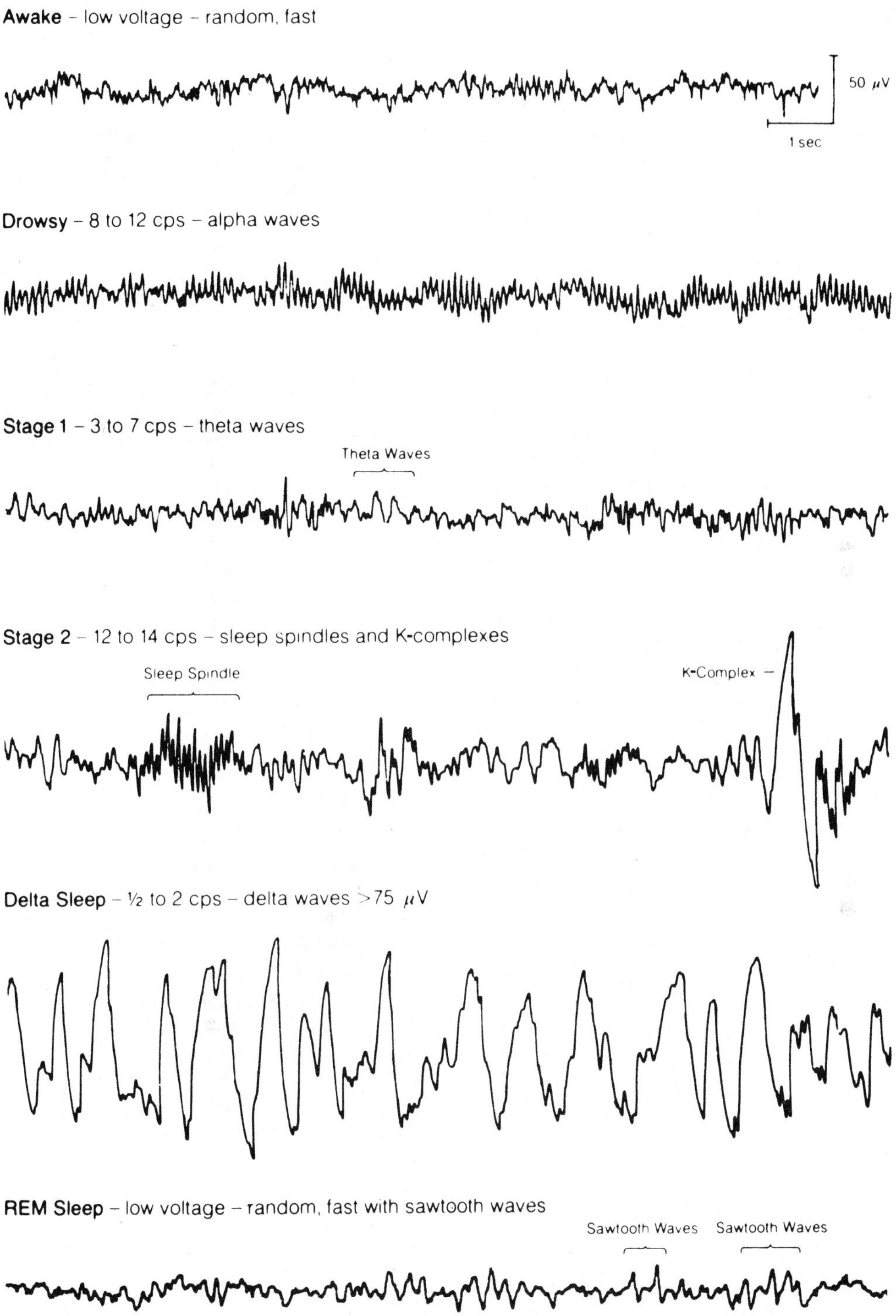

FIGURE 24.1–2
Human sleep stages. (Reproduced with permission from Hauri P. *The Sleep Disorders.* Current Concepts, Kalamazoo, MI: Upjohn; 1982:7.)

increased levels of carbon dioxide (CO_2) is depressed during REM sleep, so that there is no increase in tidal volume as the partial pressure of carbon dioxide (Pco_2) increases. Thermoregulation is altered during REM sleep. In contrast to the homeothermic condition of temperature regulation during wakefulness or NREM sleep, a poikilothermic condition (a state in which animal temperature varies with the changes in the temperature of the surrounding medium) prevails during REM sleep. Poikilothermia, which is characteristic of reptiles, results in a failure to respond to changes in ambient temperature with shivering or sweating, whichever is appropriate to maintaining body temperature. Almost every REM period in men is accompanied by a partial or full penile erection. This finding is clinically significant in evaluating the cause of impotence; the nocturnal penile

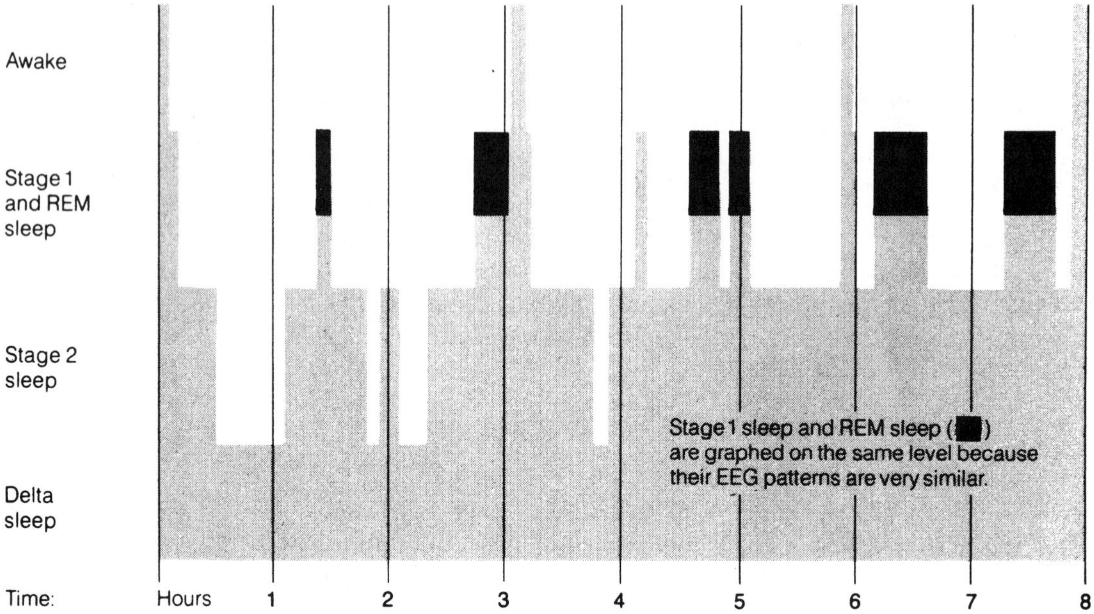

FIGURE 24.1–3

Typical sleep pattern of a young human adult. (Reproduced with permission from Hauri P. *The Sleep Disorders.* Current Concepts, Kalamazoo, MI: Upjohn; 1982:82.)

tumescence study is one of the most commonly requested sleep laboratory tests. Another physiological change that occurs during REM sleep is the near-total paralysis of the skeletal (postural) muscles. Because of this motor inhibition, body movement is absent during REM sleep. Probably the most distinctive feature of REM sleep is dreaming. Persons awakened during REM sleep frequently (60 to 90 percent of the time) report that they had been dreaming. Dreams during REM sleep are typically abstract and surreal. Dreaming does occur during NREM sleep, but it is typically lucid and purposeful.

The cyclical nature of sleep is regular and reliable; a REM period occurs about every 90 to 100 minutes during the night (Fig. 24.1–3). The first REM period tends to be the shortest, usually lasting less than 10 minutes; later REM periods may last 15 to 40 minutes each. Most REM periods occur in the last third of the night, whereas most stage 4 sleep occurs in the first third of the night.

These sleep patterns change over a person's life span. In the neonatal period, REM sleep represents more than 50 percent of total sleep time, and the EEG pattern moves from the alert state directly to the REM state without going through stages 1 through 4. Newborns sleep about 16 hours a day, with brief periods of wakefulness. By 4 months of age, the pattern shifts so that the total percentage of REM sleep drops to less than 40 percent, and entry into sleep occurs with an initial period of NREM sleep. By young adulthood, the distribution of sleep stages is as follows:

NREM (75 percent)
Stage 1: 5 percent
Stage 2: 45 percent
Stage 3: 12 percent
Stage 4: 13 percent
REM (25 percent)

This distribution remains relatively constant into old age, although a reduction occurs in both slow-wave sleep and REM sleep in older persons.

SLEEP REGULATION

Most researchers think that there is not one simple sleep control center but a small number of interconnecting systems or centers that are located chiefly in the brainstem and that mutually activate and inhibit one another. Many studies also support the role of serotonin in sleep regulation. Prevention of serotonin synthesis or destruction of the dorsal raphe nucleus of the brainstem, which contains nearly all the brain's serotonergic cell bodies, reduces sleep for a considerable time. Synthesis and release of serotonin by serotonergic neurons are influenced by the availability of amino acid precursors of this neurotransmitter, such as L-tryptophan. Ingestion of large amounts of L-tryptophan (1 to 15 g) reduces sleep latency and nocturnal awakenings. Conversely, L-tryptophan deficiency is associated with less time spent in REM sleep. Norepinephrine-containing neurons with cell bodies located in the locus ceruleus play an important role in controlling normal sleep patterns. Drugs and manipulations that increase the firing of these noradrenergic neurons markedly reduce REM sleep (REM-off neurons) and increase wakefulness. In humans with implanted electrodes (for the control of spasticity), electrical stimulation of the locus ceruleus profoundly disrupts all sleep parameters. Brain acetylcholine is also involved in sleep, particularly in the production of REM sleep. In animal studies, the injection of cholinergic-muscarinic agonists into pontine reticular formation neurons (REM-on neurons) results in a shift from wakefulness to REM sleep. Disturbances in central cholinergic activity are associated with the sleep changes observed in major depressive disorder. Compared with healthy persons and nondepressed psychiatric controls, patients who are depressed have

marked disruptions of REM sleep patterns. These disruptions include shortened REM latency (60 minutes or less), an increased percentage of REM sleep, and a shift in REM distribution from the last half to the first half of the night. Administration of a muscarinic agonist, such as arecoline, to depressed patients during the first or second NREM period results in a rapid onset of REM sleep. Depression may be associated with an underlying supersensitivity to acetylcholine. Drugs that reduce REM sleep, such as antidepressants, produce beneficial effects in depression. Indeed, about half the patients with major depressive disorder experience temporary improvement when they are deprived of sleep or when sleep is restricted. Conversely, reserpine (Serpasil), one of the few drugs that increase REM sleep, also produces depression. Patients with dementia of the Alzheimer's type have sleep disturbances characterized by reduced REM and slow-wave sleep. The loss of cholinergic neurons in the basal forebrain has been implicated as the cause of these changes. Melatonin secretion from the pineal gland is inhibited by bright light, so the lowest serum melatonin concentrations occur during the day. The suprachiasmatic nucleus of the hypothalamus may act as the anatomical site of a circadian pacemaker that regulates melatonin secretion and the entrainment of the brain to a 24-hour sleep–wake cycle. Evidence shows that dopamine has an alerting effect. Drugs that increase dopamine concentrations in the brain tend to produce arousal and wakefulness. In contrast, dopamine blockers, such as pimozide (Orap) and the phenothiazines, tend to increase sleep time. A hypothesized homeostatic drive to sleep, perhaps in the form of an endogenous substance—process S—may accumulate during wakefulness and act to induce sleep. Another compound—process C—may act as a regulator of body temperature and sleep duration.

FUNCTIONS OF SLEEP

The functions of sleep have been examined in a variety of ways. Most investigators conclude that sleep serves a restorative, homeostatic function and appears to be crucial for normal thermoregulation and energy conservation. As NREM sleep increases after exercise and starvation, this stage may be associated with satisfying metabolic needs.

Sleep Deprivation

Prolonged periods of sleep deprivation sometimes lead to ego disorganization, hallucinations, and delusions. Depriving persons of REM sleep by awakening them at the beginning of REM cycles increases the number of REM periods and the amount of REM sleep (rebound increase) when they are allowed to sleep without interruption. REM-deprived patients may exhibit irritability and lethargy. In studies with rats, sleep deprivation produces a syndrome that includes a debilitated appearance, skin lesions, increased food intake, weight loss, increased energy expenditure, decreased body temperature, and death. The neuroendocrine changes include increased plasma norepinephrine and decreased plasma thyroxine levels.

Sleep Requirements

Some persons are normally short sleepers who require fewer than 6 hours of sleep each night to function adequately. Long sleepers are those who sleep more than 9 hours each night to function adequately. Long sleepers have more REM periods and more rapid eye movements within each period (known as *REM density*) than short sleepers. These movements are sometimes considered a measure of the intensity of REM sleep and are related to the vividness of dreaming. Short sleepers are generally efficient, ambitious, socially adept, and content. Long sleepers tend to be mildly depressed, anxious, and socially withdrawn. Sleep needs increase with physical work, exercise, illness, pregnancy, general mental stress, and increased mental activity. REM periods increase after strong psychological stimuli, such as difficult learning situations and stress, and after the use of chemicals or drugs that decrease brain catecholamines.

SLEEP–WAKE RHYTHM

Without external clues, the natural body clock follows a 25-hour cycle. The influence of external factors—such as the light–dark cycle, daily routines, meal periods, and other external synchronizers—entrain persons to the 24-hour clock. Sleep is also influenced by biological rhythms. Within a 24-hour period, adults sleep once, sometimes twice. This rhythm is not present at birth but develops over the first 2 years of life. Some women exhibit sleep pattern changes during the phases of the menstrual cycle. Naps taken at different times of the day differ greatly in their proportions of REM and NREM sleep. In a normal nighttime sleeper, a nap taken in the morning or at noon includes a great deal of REM sleep, whereas a nap taken in the afternoon or the early evening has much less REM sleep. A circadian cycle apparently affects the tendency to have REM sleep. Sleep patterns are not physiologically the same when persons sleep in the daytime or during the time when they are accustomed to being awake; the psychological and behavioral effects of sleep differ as well. In a world of industry and communications that often functions 24 hours a day, these interactions are becoming increasingly significant. Even in persons who work at night, interference with the various rhythms can produce problems. The best-known example is jet lag, in which, after flying east to west, persons try to convince their bodies to go to sleep at a time that is out of phase with some body cycles. Most persons adapt within a few days, but some require more time. Conditions in these persons' bodies apparently involve long-term cycle disruption and interference.

REFERENCES

Cote KA, Etienne L, Campbell KB. Neurophysiological evidence for the detection of external stimuli during sleep. *Sleep.* 2001;24:791.

Dahl RE. The regulation of sleep and arousal: development and psychopathology. *Dev Psychopathol.* 1996;8:3.

Dement W, Kleitman N. Cyclic variations in EEG during sleep and their relation to eye movements, body motility, and dreaming. *Electroencephalogr Clin Neurophysiol.* 1975;9:673.

Douglas NJ. The sleep patient. *J Neurol Neurosurg Psychiatry.* 2001;71(suppl 1):13.

Edinger JD, Glenn DM, Bastian LA, et al. Sleep in the laboratory and sleep at home. II: Comparisons of middle-aged insomnia sufferers and normal sleepers. *Sleep.* 2001;24:761.

Gillin JC, Seifritz E, Zoltoski RK, Salin-Pascual R. Basic science of sleep. In: Sadock BJ, Sadock VA, eds. *Kaplan & Sadock's Comprehensive Textbook of Psychiatry.* 7th ed. Vol 1. Baltimore: Lippincott Williams & Wilkins; 2000:199.

Harrison Y, Bright V, Horne JA. Can normal subjects be motivated to fall asleep faster? *Physiol Behav.* 1996;60:681.

Johns MW. Sleep propensity varies with behaviour and the situation in which it is measured: the concept of somnificity. *J Sleep Research.* 2002;11:61.

Lamberg L. Medical news and perspectives. Dawn's early light to twilight's last gleaming. *JAMA*. 1998;280:1556.
Moore CA, Williams RL, Hirschkowitz M. Sleep disorders. In: Sadock BJ, Sadock VA, eds. *Kaplan & Sadock's Comprehensive Textbook of Psychiatry.* 7th ed. Vol 2. Baltimore: Lippincott Williams & Wilkins; 2000:1677.
O'Hara BF, Young KA, Watson FL, Heller HC, Kilduff T. Immediate early gene expression in brain during sleep deprivation. *Sleep*. 1993;16:1.
Santiage JR, Nolledo MS, Kinzler W, Santiago TV. Sleep and sleep disorders in pregnancy. *Ann Intern Med*. 2001;134:396.
Shapiro CM, Flanigan MJ. Function of sleep. *Br Med J*. 1993;306:383.
Smith A, Pollock J, Thomas M, et al. The relationship between subjective ratings of sleep and mental functioning in healthy subjects and patients with chronic fatigue syndrome. *Hum Psychopharmacol*. 1996;11:161.
Turek FW, Dugovic C, Zee PC. Current understanding of the circadian clock and the clinical implications for neurological disorders. *Arch Neurol*. 2001;58:1781.
Waterhouse J. Circadian rhythms. *Br Med J*. 1993;306:448.
Webb WB, ed. *Biological Rhythms, Sleep, and Performance.* New York: John Wiley & Sons; 1982.
Weinger MB, Ancoli-Israel S. Sleep deprivation and clinical performance. *JAMA*. 2002;287:955.

▲ 24.2 Sleep Disorders

MAJOR SYMPTOMS

Individual sleep requirements vary: Many persons are long sleepers and require 9 to 10 hours of sleep a night, and others are short sleepers, but length of sleep does not always correlate with a sleep disorder. However, a 2002 study of over 1 million men and women showed that persons who sleep more than 8.5 hours or less than 3.5 hours per night had a mortality risk 15 percent higher than those who slept an average of 7 hours per night. No reasons were given to explain this statistical finding. It was suggested that short sleepers may have comorbid conditions; but the explanation remains unknown. Four major symptoms characterize most sleep disorders: insomnia, hypersomnia, parasomnia, and sleep–wake schedule disturbance. The symptoms often overlap and are described below. Table 24.2–1 lists the terms used in this section to diagnose and describe sleep disorders.

Insomnia

Insomnia is difficulty initiating or maintaining sleep. It is the most common sleep complaint and may be transient or persistent. Population surveys show a 1-year prevalence rate of 30 to 45 percent in adults. Common causes of insomnia are given in Table 24.2–2.

A brief period of insomnia is most often associated with anxiety, either as a sequela to an anxious experience or in anticipation of an anxiety-provoking experience (e.g., an examination or an impending job interview). In some persons, transient insomnia of this kind may be related to grief, loss, or almost any life change or stress. The condition is not likely to be serious, although a psychotic episode or a severe depression sometimes begins with acute insomnia. Specific treatment for the condition is usually not required. When treatment with hypnotic medication is indicated, both the physician and the patient should be clear that the treatment is of short duration and that some symptoms, including a brief recurrence of the insomnia, may be expected when the medication is discontinued.

Persistent insomnia is a fairly common group of conditions in which the problem is most often difficulty falling asleep rather than remaining asleep. This insomnia involves two sometimes separable, but often intertwined, problems: somatized tension and anxiety, and a conditioned associative response. Patients often have no clear complaint other than insomnia. They may not experience anxiety per se but discharge the anxiety through physiological channels; they may complain chiefly of apprehensive feeling or ruminative thoughts that appear to keep them from falling asleep. Sometimes (but not always) a patient describes the condition's exacerbation at times of stress at work or at home and its remission during vacations.

Table 24.2–1
Common Polysomnographic Measures

Sleep latency: Period of time from turning out the lights until the appearance of stage 2 sleep
Early morning awakening: Time of being continuously awake from the last stage of the sleep until the end of the sleep record (usually at 7 AM)
Sleep efficiency: Total sleep time/total time of the sleep record × 100
Apnea index: Number of apneas longer than 10 seconds per hour of sleep
Nocturnal myoclonus index: Number of periodic leg movements per hour
REM latency: Period of time from the onset of sleep until the first REM period of the night
Sleep-onset REM period: REM sleep within the first 10 minutes of sleep.

Hypersomnia

Hypersomnia manifests as excessive amounts of sleep, excessive daytime sleepiness (somnolence), or sometimes both. The term *somnolence* should be reserved for patients who complain of sleepiness and have a clearly demonstrable tendency to fall asleep suddenly in the waking state, who have sleep attacks, and who cannot remain awake; it should not be used for persons who are simply physically tired or weary. The distinction, however, is not always clear. Complaints of hypersomnia are much less frequent (5 percent of adults) than complaints of insomnia, but they are by no means rare if clinicians are alert to them. More than 100,000 persons with narcolepsy are estimated to live in the United States, and narcolepsy is just one well-known condition that clearly produces hypersomnia. If substance-related conditions are included, hypersomnia is a common symptom.

Table 24.2–3 lists some common causes of hypersomnia. Like insomnia, hypersomnia is associated with conditions that are hard to classify and idiopathic cases. According to a recent survey, the most common conditions responsible for hypersomnia severe enough to be evaluated by all-night recordings at a sleep disorders center were sleep apnea and narcolepsy.

Transient and situational hypersomnia is a disruption of the normal sleep–wake pattern; it is marked by excessive difficulty in remaining awake and a tendency to remain in bed for unusually long periods or to return to bed to nap frequently during the day. The pattern is experienced suddenly in response to an identifiable recent life change, conflict, or loss and is much less common than insomnia. It is seldom marked by definite sleep attacks or unavoidable sleep but, rather, is characterized by

Table 24.2–2
Common Causes of Insomnia

Symptom	Insomnia Secondary to Medical Conditions	Insomnia Secondary to Psychiatric or Environmental Conditions
Difficulty falling asleep	Any painful or uncomfortable condition CNS lesions Conditions listed below, at times	Anxiety Tension anxiety, muscular Environmental changes Circadian rhythm sleep disorder
Difficulty remaining asleep	Sleep apnea syndromes Nocturnal myoclonus and restless legs syndrome Dietary factors (probably) Episodic events (parasomnias) Direct substance effects (including alcohol) Substance withdrawal effects (including alcohol) Substance interactions Endocrine or metabolic diseases Infectious, neoplastic, or other diseases Painful or uncomfortable conditions Brainstem or hypothalamic lesions or diseases Aging	Depression, especially primary depression Environmental changes Circadian rhythm sleep disorder Posttraumatic stress disorder Schizophrenia

Courtesy of Ernest L. Hartmann, M.D.

tiredness or by falling asleep sooner than usual and by difficulty arising in the morning.

Parasomnia

Parasomnia is an unusual or undesirable phenomenon that appears suddenly during sleep or that occurs at the threshold between waking and sleeping. Parasomnia usually occurs in stages 3 and 4 and is thus associated with poor recall of the disturbance.

SLEEP–WAKE SCHEDULE DISTURBANCE. Sleep–wake schedule disturbance involves the displacement of sleep from its desired circadian period. Patients commonly cannot sleep when they wish to sleep, although they are able to sleep at other times. Correspondingly, they cannot be fully awake when they want to be fully awake, but they are able to be awake at other times. The disturbance does not precisely produce insomnia or somnolence, although the initial complaint is often either insomnia or somnolence; the inabilities to sleep and be awake are elicited only on careful questioning. Sleep–wake schedule disturbance can be considered a misalignment between sleep and wake behaviors. A sleep history questionnaire is helpful in diagnosing a patient's sleep disorder (Table 24.2–4).

CLASSIFICATION

DSM-IV-TR

The text revision of the fourth edition of *Diagnostic and Statistical Manual of Mental Disorders* (DSM-IV-TR) classifies sleep disorders on the basis of clinical diagnostic criteria and presumed etiology. The three major categories of sleep disor-

Table 24.2–3
Common Causes of Hypersomnia

Symptom	Chiefly Medical	Chiefly Psychiatric or Environmental
Excessive sleep (hypersomnia)	Kleine-Levin syndrome Menstrual-associated somnolence Metabolic or toxic conditions Encephalitic conditions Alcohol and depressant medications Withdrawal from stimulants	Depression (some) Avoidance reactions
Excessive daytime sleepiness	Narcolepsy and narcolepsylike syndromes Sleep apneas Hypoventilation syndrome Hyperthyroidism and other metabolic and toxic conditions Alcohol and depressant medications Withdrawal from stimulants Sleep deprivation or insufficient sleep Any condition producing serious insomnia	Depression (some) Avoidance reactions Circadian rhythm sleep disorder

Courtesy of Ernest L. Hartmann, M.D.

Table 24.2–4
Sleep History Questionnaire

Patient name ______________________________

Date ______________________________

Please check the appropriate box or give short answers for the following:

	Yes	No
1. Do you feel sleepy or have sleep attacks during the day?	☐	☐
2. Do you nap during the day?	☐	☐
3. Do you have trouble concentrating during the day?	☐	☐
4. Do you have trouble falling asleep when you first go to bed?	☐	☐
5. Do you awaken during the night?	☐	☐
6. Do you awaken more than once?	☐	☐
7. Do you awaken too early in the morning?	☐	☐
8. How long have you had trouble sleeping? What do you think precipitated the problem? ______________________________		
9. How would you describe your usual night's sleep (hours of sleep, quality of sleep, etc.)? ______________________________		
10. Does your schedule for sleep and rising on the weekend differ from what it is during the week?	☐	☐
11. Do others live at home who interrupt your sleep?	☐	☐
12. Are you regularly awakened at night by pain or the need to use the bathroom?	☐	☐
13. Does your job require shift changes or travel?	☐	☐
14. Do you drink caffeinated beverages (coffee, tea, or soft drinks)?	☐	☐
15. Apart from difficulty in sleeping, what, if any, other medical problems do you have? ______________________________		
16. What sleep medications, prescription or nonprescription, do you take? (Please include the dosage, how often you take it, and for how many months or years you have taken it.) ______________________________		
17. What other prescription and over-the-counter medications do you regularly use? (Again, please include the dosage, the frequency, and the duration.) ______________________________		
18. Have you ever suffered from depression, anxiety, or similar problems?	☐	☐
19. Do you snore?	☐	☐
Questions for the sleep partner		
1. Does your sleep partner snore?	☐	☐
2. Does your sleep partner seem to stop breathing repeatedly during the night?	☐	☐
3. Does your sleep partner jerk his or her legs or kick you while he or she is sleeping?	☐	☐
4. Have you ever experienced trouble sleeping? Please explain. ______________________________	☐	☐

ders in DSM-IV-TR are primary sleep disorders, sleep disorders related to another mental disorder, and other sleep disorders (due to a general medical condition or substance induced). The disorders described in DSM-IV-TR are only a fraction of the known sleep disorders; they provide a framework for clinical assessment.

ICSD

The most detailed classification of sleep disorders appears in the American Sleep Disorders Association's *International Classification of Sleep Disorders: Diagnostic and Coding Manual* (ICSD). ICSD divides sleep disorders into four categories: dyssomnias, parasomnias, sleep disorders associated with medical-psychiatric disorders, and proposed sleep disorders. Table 24.2–5 presents an outline of ICSD.

ICD-10

In the 10th revision of *International Statistical Classification of Diseases and Related Health Problems* (ICD-10), the subject of sleep disorders covers only those of nonorganic type. These disorders are classified as *dyssomnias,* psychogenic conditions "in which the predominant disturbances . . . [are] in the amount, quality, or timing of sleep" because of emotional causes, and *parasomnias,* "abnormal episodic events occurring during sleep." The dyssomnias include insomnia, hypersomnia, and disorder of the sleep–wake schedule. The parasomnias in childhood are related to development; those in adulthood are psychogenic and include sleepwalking, sleep terrors, and nightmares. Sleep disorders of organic origin, nonpsychogenic disorders such as narcolepsy and cataplexy, and sleep apnea and episodic movement disorders are discussed under other categories.

ICD-10 notes that sleep disorders are often symptoms of other disorders, but even when they are not, the specific sleep disorder should be diagnosed along with as many other relevant diagnoses as necessary to describe the "psychopathology and/or pathophysiology involved in a given case." Table 24.2–6 presents the ICD-10 criteria for nonorganic sleep disorders.

PRIMARY SLEEP DISORDERS

DSM-IV-TR defines primary sleep disorders as those not caused by another mental disorder, a physical condition, or a substance but, rather, caused by an abnormal sleep–wake mechanism and often by conditioning. The two main primary sleep disorders are dyssomnias and parasomnias. Dyssomnias are a heterogeneous group of sleep disorders that includes primary insomnia, primary hypersomnia, narcolepsy, breathing-related sleep disorder, circadian rhythm sleep disorder (sleep–wake schedule disorder), and dyssomnia not otherwise specified. Parasomnias include nightmare disorder (dream anxiety disorder), sleep terror disorder, sleepwalking disorder, and parasomnia not otherwise specified.

Dyssomnias

Primary Insomnia. Primary insomnia is diagnosed when the chief complaint is nonrestorative sleep or difficulty in initiating or maintaining sleep, and the complaint continues for at least a month (Table 24.2–7). (According to ICD-10, the disturbance must occur at least 3 times a week for a month.) The term *primary* indicates that the insomnia is independent of any known physical or mental condition. Primary insomnia is often characterized by both difficulty falling asleep and by repeated awakening. Increased nighttime physiological or psychological arousal and negative conditioning for sleep are frequently evident. Patients with primary insomnia are generally preoccupied with getting enough sleep. The more they try to sleep, the greater the sense of frustration and distress and the more elusive sleep becomes.

Ms. W. was a 41-year-old, divorced, white female who presented with a 2½-year complaint of sleeplessness. She had some difficulty falling asleep (30- to 45-minute sleep-onset latency) and awakened every hour or two after sleep onset. These awakenings might last 15 minutes to several hours, and she estimated having approximately 4.5 hours of sleep on an average night. She rarely takes daytime naps, notwithstanding feeling tired and edgy. The patient described her sleep problem with the following words. "It seems like I never get into a deep sleep. I have never been a heavy sleeper, but now the slightest noise wakes me up. Sometimes I have a hard time getting my mind to shut down." She viewed the bedroom as an unpleasant place of sleeplessness and stated: "I tried staying at a friend's house where it is quiet, but then I couldn't sleep because of the silence. "

At times, Ms. W. was unsure whether she was asleep or awake. She had a history of clock watching (to time her wakefulness) but stopped doing this when she realized it was contributing to the problem. Reportedly, the insomnia is unrelated to seasonal changes, menstrual cycle, or time-zone translocation. Her basic sleep hygiene was good. Appetite and libido were unchanged. She denied mood disturbance, except for being quite frustrated and concerned about sleeplessness and its effect on her work. Her work involved sitting at a microscope for 6 hours of a 9-hour working day and meticulously documenting her findings. Her final output hadn't suffered, but she had to "double check" for accuracy.

She described herself as a worrier and a type A personality. She did not know how to relax. For example, on vacation she continually worried about things that could go wrong and would not even begin to unwind until she had arrived at the destination, checked in, and unpacked. Even then, she was unable to relax.

Medical history was unremarkable except for tonsillectomy (age 16 years), migraine headaches (current), and diet-controlled hypercholesterolemia. She took naproxen (Naprosyn) as needed for headache. She did not currently drink caffeinated beverages, smoke tobacco, or drink alcoholic beverages, and she did not use recreational drugs.

The problem with insomnia began after relocation to a new city and place of employment. She attributed her insomnia to the noisy neighborhood in which she lived. She first sought treatment 18 months earlier. Her family-practice physician diagnosed depression and fluoxetine (Prozac) therapy was started. This made her "climb the walls." Antihistamines were tried next with similar results. She was then switched to low-dose trazodone (Desyrel) (for sleep) and developed nausea. After these medical interventions, she sought medical care elsewhere. Zolpidem (Ambien), 5 mg, was prescribed, but it made her feel drugged, and upon discontinuation she had withdrawal effects. Another family-

Table 24.2–5
International Classification of Sleep Disorders (ICSD)

1. Dyssomnias
   A. Intrinsic sleep disorders
      1. Psychophysiological insomnia
      2. Sleep state misperception
      3. Idiopathic insomnia
      4. Narcolepsy
      5. Recurrent hypersomnia
      6. Idiopathic hypersomnia
      7. Posttraumatic hypersomnia
      8. Obstructive sleep apnea syndrome
      9. Central sleep apnea syndrome
      10. Central alveolar hypoventilation syndrome
      11. Periodic limb movement disorder
      12. Restless legs syndrome
      13. Intrinsic sleep disorder NOS
   B. Extrinsic sleep disorder
      1. Inadequate sleep hygiene
      2. Environmental sleep disorder
      3. Altitude insomnia
      4. Adjustment sleep disorder
      5. Insufficient sleep syndrome
      6. Limit-setting sleep disorder
      7. Sleep-onset association disorder
      8. Food allergy insomnia
      9. Nocturnal eating (drinking) syndrome
      10. Hypnotic-dependent sleep disorder
      11. Stimulant-dependent sleep disorder
      12. Alcohol-dependent sleep disorder
      13. Toxin-induced sleep disorder
      14. Extrinsic sleep disorder NOS
   C. Circadian rhythm sleep disorders
      1. Time zone change (jet lag) syndrome
      2. Shift work sleep disorder
      3. Irregular sleep–wake pattern
      4. Delayed sleep phase syndrome
      5. Advanced sleep phase syndrome
      6. Non-24-hour sleep–wake disorder
      7. Circadian rhythm sleep disorder NOS
2. Parasomnias
   A. Arousal disorders
      1. Confusional arousals
      2. Sleepwalking
      3. Sleep terrors
   B. Sleep–wake transition disorders
      1. Rhythmic movement disorder
      2. Sleep starts
      3. Sleep talking
      4. Nocturnal leg cramps
   C. Parasomnias usually associated with REM sleep
      1. Nightmares
      2. Sleep paralysis
      3. Impaired-sleep-related penile erections
      4. Sleep-related painful erections
      5. REM-sleep-related sinus arrest
      6. REM sleep behavior disorder
   D. Other parasomnias
      1. Sleep bruxism
      2. Sleep enuresis
      3. Sleep-related abnormal swallowing syndrome
      4. Nocturnal paroxysmal dystonia
      5. Sudden unexplained nocturnal death syndrome
      6. Primary snoring
      7. Infant sleep apnea
      8. Congenital central hypoventilation syndrome
      9. Sudden infant death syndrome
      10. Benign neonatal sleep myoclonus
      11. Other parasomnia NOS
3. Sleep disorders associated with medical-psychiatric disorders
   A. Associated with mental disorders
      1. Psychoses
      2. Mood disorders
      3. Anxiety disorders
      4. Panic disorders
      5. Alcoholism
   B. Associated with neurological disorders
      1. Cerebral degenerative disorders
      2. Dementia
      3. Parkinsonism
      4. Fatal familial insomnia
      5. Sleep-related epilepsy
      6. Electrical status epilepticus of sleep
      7. Sleep-related headaches
   C. Associated with other medical disorders
      1. Sleeping sickness
      2. Nocturnal cardiac ischemia
      3. Chronic obstructive pulmonary disease
      4. Sleep-related asthma
      5. Sleep-related gastroesophageal reflux
      6. Peptic ulcer disease
      7. Fibrositis syndrome
4. Proposed sleep disorders
      1. Short sleeper
      2. Long sleeper
      3. Subwakefulness syndrome
      4. Fragmentary myoclonus
      5. Sleep hyperhidrosis
      6. Menstrual-associated sleep disorder
      7. Pregnancy-associated sleep disorder
      8. Terrifying hypnagogic hallucinations
      9. Sleep-related neurogenic tachypnea
      10. Sleep-related laryngospasm
      11. Sleep choking syndrome

NOS, not otherwise specified.

practice physician diagnosed "nonspecific anxiety disorder" and began treating her with buspirone (BuSpar); an experience she described as "having an alien try to climb out of my skin." Buspirone treatment was discontinued. Paroxetine (Paxil) was tried for 8 weeks with no effect. Finally, a psychiatrist was consulted who diagnosed adult attention-deficit disorder (without hyperactivity) and suggested treatment with methylphenidate (Ritalin). At this point, the patient was convinced that a stimulant would not help her insomnia and demanded referral to a sleep disorders center.

DISCUSSION

Ms. W.'s symptoms fell into the broad category of insomnia, and the symptoms began after she moved from one city to another. Environmental sleep disorder (noise) and adjustment sleep disorder (new job, city, apartment) were likely initial diagnoses. However, a more-chronic, endogenous problem became operative. What was it? Ms. W. was a "worrier" and meticulous but did not meet diagnostic criteria for personality or anxiety disorders. Dyssomnia associated with mood disorder should be considered for any patient with sleep maintenance problems and early morning awakening insomnia. However, this patient did not have other significant signs of depression. Unfortunately, many patients are misdiagnosed with depression or "masked depression" on the sole basis of an insomnia complaint and are unsuccessfully treated with antidepressant medication. Ms. W.'s job demands long hours with focused concentration. Her job performance had been superior for many years, insomnia notwithstanding. Thus, a diagnosis of attention-deficit disorder is unlikely. Idiopathic insomnia implies a childhood complaint, which Ms. W. denied.

The likely working diagnosis was psychophysiological insomnia. She may have some sleep state misperception (sometimes unclear whether she was awake or asleep), but this cannot adequately account for the constellation of symptoms. An initial treatment plan should include further documentation of the sleep pattern with a sleep log. Behavioral treatments would likely benefit this patient. Medications with sedative effects are sometimes useful during initial treatment of psychophysiological insomnia. However, thus far in this patient they have done more harm than good. She is likely to be a challenging patient to treat. (Courtesy of Constance A. Moore, M.D., Robert L. Williams, M.D., and Max Hirshkowitz, Ph.D.)

TREATMENT. Treatment of primary insomnia is among the most difficult problems in sleep disorders. When the conditioned component is prominent, a deconditioning technique may be useful. Patients are asked to use their beds for sleeping and for nothing else; if they are not asleep after 5 minutes in bed, they are instructed to simply get up and do something else. Sometimes, changing to another bed or to another room is useful. When somatized tension or muscle tension is prominent, relaxation tapes, transcendental meditation, and practicing the relaxation response and biofeedback are occasionally helpful. Psychotherapy has not been very useful in the treatment of primary insomnia. Satisfying sexual experiences promote sleep, more so in men than in women.

THERAPY. Primary insomnia is commonly treated with benzodiazepines, zolpidem, zaleplon (Sonata), and other hypnotics. Hypnotic drugs should be used with care. Over-the-counter sleep aids have limited effectiveness. Long-acting sleep medications (e.g., flurazepam [Dalmane], quazepam [Doral]) are best for middle-of-the-night insomnia; short-acting drugs (e.g., zolpidem, triazolam [Halcion]) are useful for persons who have difficulty falling asleep. In general, sleep medications should not be prescribed for more than 2 weeks because tolerance and withdrawal may result.

Some dietary supplements used for insomnia include melatonin and L-tryptophan. Melatonin is an endogenous hormone produced by the pineal gland, which is linked to the regulation of sleep. Administration of exogenous melatonin has yielded mixed results, however, in clinical research. Melatonin's precursor L-tryptophan was used previously with the same rationale; however, in addition to having uncertain efficacy, it was found to be contaminated with a substance causing eosinophilic myalgia, a possibly deadly dyscrasia. However, these substances are available worldwide and may be obtained by patients in the United States. Other concerns with L-tryptophan include serotonin syndrome if used in conjunction with a selective serotonin reuptake inhibitor (SSRI). Dietary supplement use has increased during the past decade.

Various nonspecific measures—so-called sleep hygiene—can help improve sleep (Table 24.2–8). Physicians must reassure patients with insomnia that their health is not at risk if they do not get 6 to 8 hours of sleep. Light therapy is also used. In general, sleep medications should not be prescribed for more than 2 weeks because tolerance and withdrawal may result.

INADEQUATE SLEEP HYGIENE. DSM-IV-TR indicates that inadequate sleep hygiene sometimes falls within the primary insomnia classification, depending on the specific sleep hygiene factor involved. ICSD defines inadequate sleep hygiene as "a sleep disorder due to the performance of daily living activities that are inconsistent with the maintenance of good quality sleep and full daytime alertness." Many behaviors can interfere with sleep and may do so by increasing nervous system arousal near bedtime or by altering circadian rhythms. Treatment should focus on only two or three problem areas at a time. Overwhelming the patient with too many lifestyle changes or a complex regimen seldom succeeds. Some general "dos and don'ts" are instructive.

PSYCHOPHYSIOLOGICAL INSOMNIA. The patient with psychophysiological insomnia has developed a conditioned arousal associated with attempts to sleep. Objects associated with sleep (e.g., the bed, the bedroom) likewise become conditioned stimuli that evoke insomnia. Thus, psychophysiological insomnia is sometimes called *conditioned insomnia.* Psychophysiological insomnia often occurs in combination with other causes of insomnia, including episodes of stress and anxiety disorders, delayed sleep phase syndrome, and hypnotic drug use and withdrawal. In contrast to the insomnia in patients with psychiatric disorders, daytime adaptation is generally good. Work and rela-

Table 24.2–6
ICD-10 Diagnostic Criteria for Nonorganic Sleep Disorders

Note: A more comprehensive classification of sleep disorders is available (*International Classification of Sleep Disorders*[a]), but it should be noted that this is organized differently from ICD-10.

For some research purposes, where particularly homogeneous groups of sleep disorders are required, four or more events occurring within a 1-year period may be considered as a criterion for use of categories sleepwalking (somnambulism), sleep terrors (night terrors), and nightmares.

Nonorganic insomnia

A. The individual complains of difficulty falling asleep, difficulty maintaining sleep, or nonrefreshing sleep.
B. The sleep disturbance occurs at least 3 times a week for at least 1 month.
C. The sleep disturbance results in marked personal distress or interference with personal functioning in daily living.
D. There is no known causative organic factor, such as a neurological or other medical condition, psychoactive substance use disorder, or a medication.

Nonorganic hypersomnia

A. The individual complains of excessive daytime sleepiness or sleep attacks or of prolonged transition to the fully aroused state upon awakening (sleep drunkenness), which is not accounted for by an inadequate amount of sleep.
B. This sleep disturbance occurs nearly every day for at least 1 month or recurrently for shorter periods of time and causes either marked distress or interference with personal functioning in daily living.
C. There are no auxiliary symptoms of narcolepsy (cataplexy, sleep paralysis, hypnagogic hallucinations) and no clinical evidence for sleep apnea (nocturnal breath cessation, typical intermittent snorting sounds, etc.).
D. There is no known causative organic factor, such as a neurological or other medical condition, psychoactive substance use disorder, or a medication.

Nonorganic disorder of the sleep–wake schedule

A. The individual's sleep–wake pattern is out of synchrony with the desired sleep–wake schedule, as imposed by societal demands and shared by most people in the individual's environment.
B. As a result of disturbance of the sleep–wake schedule, the individual experiences insomnia during the major sleep period or hypersomnia during the waking period, nearly every day for at least 1 month or recurrently for shorter periods of time.
C. The unsatisfactory quantity, quality, and timing of sleep causes either marked personal distress or interference with personal functioning in daily living.
D. There is no known causative organic factor such as a neurological or other medical condition, psychoactive substance use disorder, or a medication.

Sleepwalking (somnambulism)

A. The predominant symptom is repeated (two or more) episodes of rising from bed, usually during the first third of nocturnal sleep, and walking about for between several minutes and half an hour.
B. During an episode, the individual has a blank, staring face, is relatively unresponsive to the efforts of others to influence the event or to communicate with him or her, and can be awakened only with considerable difficulty.
C. Upon awakening (either from an episode or the next morning), the individual has amnesia for the episode.
D. Within several minutes for awakening from the episode, there is no impairment of mental activity or behavior, although there may initially be a short period of some confusion and disorientation.
E. There is no evidence of an organic mental disorder, such as dementia, or a physical disorder, such as epilepsy.

Sleep terrors (night terrors)

A. Repeated (two or more) episodes in which the individual gets up from sleep with a panicky scream and intense anxiety, body motility, and autonomic hyperactivity (such as tachycardia, heart pounding, rapid breathing, and sweating).
B. The episodes occur mainly during the first third of sleep.
C. The duration of the episode is less than 10 minutes.
D. If others try to comfort the individual during the episode, there is a lack of response followed by disorientation and preservative movements.
E. The individual has limited recall of the event.
F. There is no known causative organic factor, such as neurological or other medical condition, psychoactive substance use disorder, or a medication.

Nightmares

A. The individual wakes from nocturnal sleep or naps with detailed and vivid recall or intensely frightening dreams, usually involving threats to survival, security, or self-esteem. The awakening may occur during any part of the sleep period, but typically during the second half.
B. Upon awakening from the frightening dreams, the individual rapidly becomes oriented and alert.
C. The dream experience itself and the disturbance of sleep resulting from the awakenings associated with the episodes cause marked distress to the individual.
D. There is no known causative organic factor, such as neurological or other medical condition, psychoactive substance use disorder, or a medication.

Other nonorganic sleep disorders

Nonorganic sleep disorder, unspecified

[a]Diagnostic Classification Steering Committee: *International Classification of Sleep Disorders: Diagnostic and Coding Manual.* Rochester, MN: American Sleep Disorders Association; 1990.

Reprinted with permission from World Health Organization. *The ICD-10 Classification of Mental and Behavioural Disorders: Diagnostic Criteria for Research.* Copyright, World Health Organization, Geneva, 1993.

tionships are satisfying; however, extreme tiredness can exist. Other features include (1) excessive worry about not being able to sleep; (2) trying too hard to sleep; (3) rumination, inability to clear one's mind while trying to sleep; (4) increased muscle tension when attempting to sleep; (5) other somatic manifestations of anxiety; (6) being able to sleep better away from one's own bedroom; and (7) being able to fall asleep when not trying (e.g., watching TV). The sleep complaint becomes fixed over time. Interestingly, many patients with psychophysiological insomnia sleep well in the laboratory.

Treatment can be difficult. Sleeping pills should be used sparingly and at the lowest effective dose. Sleeplessness during

Table 24.2–7
DSM-IV-TR Diagnostic Criteria for Primary Insomnia

A. The predominant complaint is difficulty initiating or maintaining sleep, or nonrestorative sleep, for at least 1 month.
B. The sleep disturbance (or associated daytime fatigue) causes clinically significant distress or impairment in social, occupational, or other important areas of functioning.
C. The sleep disturbance does not occur exclusively during the course of narcolepsy, breathing-related sleep disorder, circadian rhythm sleep disorder, or a parasomnia.
D. The disturbance does not exclusively occur during the course of another mental disorder (e.g., major depressive disorder, generalized anxiety disorder, a delirium).
E. The disturbance is not due to the direct physiological effects of a substance (e.g., a drug of abuse, a medication) or a general medical condition.

From American Psychiatric Association. *Diagnostic and Statistical Manual of Mental Disorders.* 4th ed. Text rev. Washington, DC: American Psychiatric Association; copyright 2000, with permission.

withdrawal from long-term sleeping pill use typically exacerbates the problem. Stimulus control therapy is recommended to break the conditioning and improve the association between going to bed and being able to fall asleep. Because many patients with psychophysiological insomnia have developed poor sleep habits, improving sleep hygiene is usually beneficial if muscle tension and rumination at bedtime are prominent features; relaxation therapy is a useful ancillary treatment.

SLEEP STATE MISPERCEPTION. For most persons, loss of awareness is a cognitive marker for sleep onset; however, under some circumstances, coordination between mental and biological processes is lost. Sleep state misperception is diagnosed when a patient complains of difficulty initiating or maintaining sleep and no objective evidence of sleep disruption is found. For example, a patient sleeping in the laboratory reports taking more than an hour to fall asleep, awakening more than 30 times, and sleeping less than 2 hours the entire night. By contrast, the polysomnogram shows sleep onset occurring within 15 minutes, few awakenings, a 90 percent sleep efficiency, and total sleep time exceeding 7 hours. Sleep state misperception can occur in individuals who are apparently free from psychopathology or can represent a somatic delusion or hypochondriasis. Some patients with sleep state misperception have obsessional features concerning somatic functions. Short-term sleep state misperception can occur during periods of stress, and some clinicians believe it can result from latent or ineffectively treated anxiety or depressive disorders. Cognitive relabeling, diffusing the worry about being unable to sleep, or both can help. Interestingly, anxiolytics can profoundly reduce the perception of sleeplessness without markedly changing sleep physiologically.

IDIOPATHIC INSOMNIA. Idiopathic insomnia typically starts early in life, sometimes at birth, and continues throughout life. As the name implies, its cause is unknown; suspected causes include neurochemical imbalance in brainstem reticular formation, impaired regulation of brainstem sleep generators (e.g., raphe nuclei, locus ceruleus), or basal forebrain dysfunction. Treatment is difficult, but improved sleep hygiene, relaxation therapy, and judicious use of hypnotic medicines are reportedly helpful.

Primary Hypersomnia.

Primary hypersomnia is diagnosed when no other cause for excessive somnolence occurring for at least 1 month can be found. Some persons are long sleepers who, like short sleepers, show a normal variation. Their sleep, although long, is normal in architecture and physiology. Sleep efficiency and the sleep–wake schedule are normal. This pattern

Table 24.2–8
Nonspecific Measures to Induce Sleep (Sleep Hygiene)

1. Arise at the same time daily.
2. Limit daily in-bed time to the usual amount present before the sleep disturbance.
3. Discontinue CNS-acting drugs (caffeine, nicotine, alcohol, stimulants).
4. Avoid daytime naps (except when sleep chart shows they induce better night sleep).
5. Establish physical fitness by means of a graded program of vigorous exercise early in the day.
6. Avoid evening stimulation; substitute radio or relaxed reading for television.
7. Try very hot, 20-minute, body-temperature-raising bath soaks near bedtime.
8. Eat at regular times daily; avoid large meals near bedtime.
9. Practice evening relaxation routines, such as progressive muscle relaxation or meditation.
10. Maintain comfortable sleeping conditions.

Table 24.2–9
DSM-IV-TR Diagnostic Criteria for Primary Hypersomnia

A. The predominant complaint is excessive sleepiness for at least 1 month (or less if recurrent) as evidenced by either prolonged sleep episodes or daytime sleep episodes that occur almost daily.
B. The excessive sleepiness causes clinically significant distress or impairment in social, occupational, or other important areas of functioning.
C. The excessive sleepiness is not better accounted for by insomnia and does not occur exclusively during the course of another sleep disorder (e.g., narcolepsy, breathing-related sleep disorder, circadian rhythm sleep disorder, or a parasomnia) and cannot be accounted for by an inadequate amount of sleep.
D. The disturbance does not occur exclusively during the course of another mental disorder.
E. The disturbance is not due to the direct physiological effects of a substance (e.g., a drug of abuse, a medication) or a general medical condition.

Specify if:

Recurrent: if there are periods of excessive sleepiness that last at least 3 days occurring several times a year for at least 2 years

From American Psychiatric Association. *Diagnostic and Statistical Manual of Mental Disorders.* 4th ed. Text rev. Washington, DC: American Psychiatric Association; copyright 2000, with permission.

is without complaints about the quality of sleep, daytime sleepiness, or difficulties with the awake mood, motivation, and performance. Long sleep may be a lifetime pattern, and it appears to have a familial incidence. Many persons are variable sleepers and may become long sleepers at certain times in their lives.

Some persons have subjective complaints of feeling sleepy without objective findings. They do not have a tendency to fall asleep more often than normal and do not have any objective signs. Clinicians should try to rule out clear-cut causes of excessive somnolence. According to DSM-IV-TR, the disorder should be coded as recurrent if patients have periods of excessive sleepiness lasting at least 3 days and occurring several times a year for at least 2 years (Table 24.2–9).

Mr. J. was a 28-year-old, single, African American male with an approximately 10-year history of fatigue and sleepiness in the daytime. He began to recognize the daytime sleepiness as a problem in his freshman year of college, when he would fall asleep in class or in the dormitory. He admitted that his sleep–wake schedule was disrupted during college because he took long naps and then had to stay up until 1:00 or 2:00 AM to complete his studies. His grades and social life suffered, and he described himself as depressed, isolated, and hopeless about his planned future as a certified public accountant (CPA).

Mr. J. said he slept "normally" as a child. In high school he felt best with 10 hours of sleep per night and was able to function well in the daytime. Mr. J. denied abuse of alcohol or drugs. He did not use tobacco and drank about 8 to 10 cups of coffee per day. Family history was negative for known sleep or psychiatric disorders. Physical examination findings were noncontributory except for a body mass index (BMI) of 0.29. Routine laboratory test results were normal, including thyroid-stimulating hormone (TSH).

Mr. J.'s excessive sleepiness continued, notwithstanding some improved sleep hygiene. Improvements included a more consistent bedtime, trying not to nap, and a torturous month-long trial without caffeine. He remained dysphoric and discouraged about his future, blaming his chronic sleepiness as the continuing impediment to his life plans. "I'm just tired of being tired," he said.

When last seen his bedtime was between 10:00 and 10:30 PM; his wake-up alarm was set for 6:30 AM. He oversleeps at least once a week on workdays and sleeps from 10:30 PM until 10:00 AM on weekends in an attempt to "catch up." He has difficulty awakening and feels unrefreshed or mildly refreshed. By drinking six to eight cups of coffee in the morning, he can usually avoid dozing during the morning. Luckily, he is an independent CPA and can schedule client appointments during this relatively alert time. After lunch, he routinely falls asleep at the computer while working. He sleeps for 20 to 60 minutes and is usually awakened by his secretary. He then drinks another two cups of coffee and continues with his work. Unexpected napping can also occur later in the afternoon or evening, and he has "nodded off" while driving. He sleeps alone; however, he has been told that he snores loudly. He does not awaken gasping or choking. He denied hypnagogic hallucinations and sleep paralysis but thought he might feel weak after the rare occasions when he participated in a heated argument.

DISCUSSION

Mr. J. had one of the hypersomnias. Most consistent with his history are obstructive sleep apnea syndrome, idiopathic hypersomnia, sleep deprivation in a long sleeper, dyssomnia associated with mood disorder, and narcolepsy. The ancillary symptoms of narcolepsy are absent, with the possible exception of cataplexy. When cataplexy occurs clearly, the diagnosis of narcolepsy is strongly indicated. However, Mr. J.'s possible infrequent weakness during heated arguments is equivocal for cataplexy. His persistent desire for a 10-hour sleep period would be unusual for a patient with narcolepsy.

A long sleeper (ICSD proposed sleep disorder) or an individual with idiopathic hypersomnia requires prolonged sleep periods and may awaken groggy as does Mr. J. The main differentiating feature is that whenever consistently given a chance to have a full nightly sleep period (usually 10 to 12 hours), the long sleeper does not experience excessive daytime sleepiness. Furthermore, patients with idiopathic hypersomnia may display associated autonomic nervous system dysfunction or polysomnographic evidence of elevated slow-wave sleep percentage.

Sleepiness associated with low-grade chronic depression may be difficult to differentiate from other causes of hypersomnia. Polysomnography, psychiatric interview, and psychometric testing can be helpful. Mr. J. related his dysphoria to sleepiness and not vice versa; nonetheless, dyssomnia associated with mood disorder should be considered.

Obstructive sleep apnea syndrome is a strong possibility. Mr. J. is overweight (BMI = 0.29) and snores loudly. Many patients are unaware of gasping or choking for breath. Often, family members witness cessation of breathing during sleep and urge patients to seek treatment. However, Mr. J. lives and sleeps alone.

Polysomnography is recommended for patients suspected of obstructive sleep apnea syndrome, narcolepsy, or idiopathic hypersomnia. These disorders usually require lifelong treatment and have significant morbidity and mortality if untreated. (Courtesy of Constance A. Moore, M.D., Robert L. Williams, M.D., and Max Hirshkowitz, Ph.D.)

TREATMENT. The treatment of primary hypersomnia consists mainly of stimulant drugs, such as amphetamines, given in the morning or evening. Nonsedating antidepressant drugs, such as SSRIs, may be of value in some patients.

Narcolepsy. Narcolepsy consists of excessive daytime sleepiness and abnormal manifestations of rapid eye movement (REM) sleep occurring daily for at least 3 months (Table 24.2–10). These sleep attacks typically occur two to six times a day and last 10 to 20 minutes. They may occur at inappropriate times (e.g., while eating, talking, or driving and during sex). The REM sleep includes hypnagogic and hypnopompic hallucinations, cataplexy, and sleep paralysis. The appearance of REM sleep within 10 minutes of sleep onset (sleep-onset REM periods) is also considered evidence of narcolepsy. The disorder can be dangerous because it can lead to automobile and industrial accidents.

Narcolepsy is not as rare as was once thought. It is estimated to occur in 0.02 to 0.16 percent of adults and shows some

Table 24.2–10
DSM-IV-TR Diagnostic Criteria for Narcolepsy

A. Irresistible attacks of refreshing sleep that occur daily over at least 3 months.
B. The presence of one or both of the following:
  (1) cataplexy (i.e., brief episodes of sudden bilateral loss of muscle tone, most often in association with intense emotion)
  (2) recurrent intrusions of elements of rapid eye movement (REM) sleep into the transition between sleep and wakefulness, as manifested by either hypnopompic or hypnagogic hallucinations or sleep paralysis at the beginning or end of sleep episodes
C. The disturbance is not due to the direct physiological effects of a substance (e.g., a drug of abuse, a medication) or another general medical condition.

From American Psychiatric Association. *Diagnostic and Statistical Manual of Mental Disorders.* 4th ed. Text rev. Washington, DC: American Psychiatric Association; copyright 2000, with permission.

familial incidence. Narcolepsy is neither a type of epilepsy nor a psychogenic disturbance. It is an abnormality of the sleep mechanisms—specifically, REM-inhibiting mechanisms—and it has been studied in dogs, sheep, and humans. Narcolepsy can occur at any age, but it most frequently begins in adolescence or young adulthood, generally before the age of 30. The disorder either progresses slowly or reaches a plateau that is maintained throughout life.

The most common symptom is sleep attacks: Patients cannot avoid falling asleep. Often associated with the problem (close to 50 percent of long-standing cases) is cataplexy, a sudden loss of muscle tone, such as jaw drop, head drop, weakness of the knees, or paralysis of all skeletal muscles with collapse. Patients often remain awake during brief cataplectic episodes; the long episodes usually merge with sleep and show the electroencephalographic (EEG) signs of REM sleep.

Other symptoms include hypnagogic or hypnopompic hallucinations: vivid perceptual experiences, either auditory or visual, occurring at sleep onset or on awakening. Patients are often momentarily frightened, but within a minute or two they return to an entirely normal frame of mind and are aware that nothing was actually there.

Another uncommon symptom is sleep paralysis, most often occurring on awakening in the morning; during the episode, patients are apparently awake and conscious but unable to move a muscle. If the symptom persists for more than a few seconds, as it often does in narcolepsy, it can become extremely uncomfortable. (Isolated brief episodes of sleep paralysis occur in many nonnarcoleptic persons.) Patients with narcolepsy report falling asleep quickly at night but often experience broken sleep.

When the diagnosis is not clinically clear, a nighttime polysomnographic recording reveals a characteristic sleep-onset REM period (Fig. 24.2–1). A test of daytime multiple sleep latency (several recorded naps at 2-hour intervals) shows rapid sleep onset and usually one or more sleep-onset REM periods. A type of human leukocyte antigen called HLA-DR2 is found in 90 to 100 percent of patients with narcolepsy and only 10 to 35 percent of unaffected persons. One recent study showed that narcolepsy patients are deficient in the neurotransmitter hypocretin, which stimulates appetite and alertness. Another study found that the number of hypocretin neurons (Hrct cells) in narcoleptics is 85 to 95 percent lower than in nonnarcoleptic brains.

TREATMENT. There is no cure for narcolepsy, but symptom management is possible. A regimen of forced naps at a regular time of day occasionally helps patients with narcolepsy, and in some cases, the regimen alone, without medication, can almost cure the patients. When medication is required, stimulants are most commonly used.

Modafinil (Provigil), an α_1-adrenergic receptor agonist, has been approved by the U.S. Food and Drug Administration (FDA) to reduce the number of sleep attacks and to improve psychomotor performance in narcolepsy. This observation suggests the involvement of noradrenergic mechanisms in the disorder. Modafinil lacks some of the adverse effects of traditional psychostimulants. Nonetheless, the clinician must monitor its use and be sensitive to developing tolerance.

Sleep specialists often prescribe tricyclic drugs or SSRIs to reduce cataplexy. This approach capitalizes on the REM sleep-suppressant properties of these drugs. Since cataplexy is presumably an intrusion of REM sleep phenomena into the awake state, the rationale is clear. Many reports indicate that imipramine (Tofranil), modafinil (Provigil), and fluoxetine are quite effective in reducing or eliminating cataplexy. Although drug therapy is the treatment of choice, the overall therapeutic approach should include scheduled naps, lifestyle adjustment, psychological counseling, drug holidays to reduce tolerance, and careful monitoring of drug refills, general health, and cardiac status.

Breathing-Related Sleep Disorder. Breathing-related sleep disorder is characterized by sleep disruption leading to

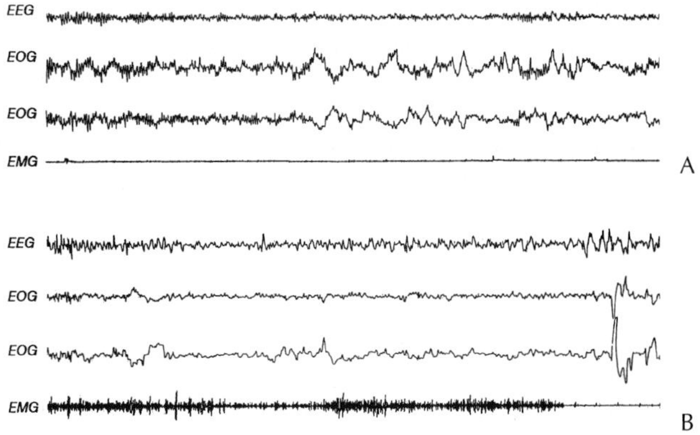

FIGURE 24.2–1

Polygraphic tracing comparing normal sleep onset with that of a patient with narcolepsy. Each panel illustrates approximately 30 seconds of polysomnographic recording beginning with relaxed wakefulness. **A** (normal sleep progression) shows reduced EEG alpha activity and development of slow rolling eye movements. **B** shows the normally expected abatement of EEG alpha activity associated with increased theta activity and the appearance of a few slow eye movements. However, within 25 seconds (*far right of figure*) a swift loss of muscle tone occurs accompanied by rapid eye movements. This appearance of sleep-onset REM sleep characterizes narcolepsy and is part of the diagnostic criteria. (Courtesy of Constance A. Moore, M.D., Robert W. Williams, M.D. and Max Hirschkowitz, Ph.D.)

Table 24.2–11
DSM-IV-TR Diagnostic Criteria for Breathing-Related Sleep Disorder

A. Sleep disruption, leading to excessive sleepiness or insomnia, that is judged to be due to a sleep-related breathing condition (e.g., obstructive or central sleep apnea syndrome or central alveolar hypoventilation syndrome).
B. The disturbance is not better accounted for by another mental disorder and is not due to the direct physiological effects of a substance (e.g., a drug of abuse, a medication) or another general medical condition (other than a breathing-related disorder).

Coding note: Also code sleep-related breathing disorder on Axis III.

From American Psychiatric Association. *Diagnostic and Statistical Manual of Mental Disorders.* 4th ed. Text rev. Washington, DC: American Psychiatric Association; copyright 2000, with permission.

excessive sleepiness or insomnia that is due to a sleep-related breathing disturbance (Table 24.2–11). Breathing disturbances that may occur during sleep include apneas, hypopneas, and oxygen desaturations. These disturbances invariably cause hypersomnia. Two disorders of the respiratory system that can produce hypersomnia are sleep apnea and central alveolar hypoventilation. Both disorders can also cause insomnia but more commonly produce hypersomnia.

Obstructive Sleep Apnea Syndrome. Many persons—older persons and obese persons, even those without clinical symptoms—are less likely to have apneic periods in sleep and, in general, more respiratory problems in sleep than when awake. Sleep apnea refers to the cessation of airflow at the nose or the mouth. By convention, an *apneic period* lasts 10 seconds or more. Sleep apnea can be of several distinct types. In pure central sleep apnea, both airflow and respiratory effort (abdomen and chest) cease during the apneic episodes and begin again during arousals. In pure obstructive sleep apnea, airflow ceases but respiratory effort increases during apneic periods; this pattern indicates an obstruction in the airway and increasing efforts by the abdominal and thoracic muscles to force air past the obstruction. Again, the episode ceases on arousal. The mixed types involve elements of both obstructive and central sleep apnea.

Sleep apnea usually is considered pathological if patients have at least five apneic episodes an hour or 30 apneic episodes during the night. In severe cases of obstructive sleep apnea, patients may have as many as 300 apneic episodes, each followed by an arousal. Thus almost no normal sleep occurs, even though patients have been in bed and often assume that they have been sleeping for the entire night.

Sleep apnea can be a dangerous condition. It is thought to account for a number of unexplained deaths and crib deaths of infants and children. It is probably also responsible for many pulmonary and cardiovascular deaths in adults and older persons. Episodes of sleep apnea can produce cardiovascular changes, including arrhythmias and transient alterations in blood pressure for each apneic episode. Long-standing sleep apnea is associated with increased pulmonary blood pressure and eventually increased systemic blood pressure as well. These cardiovascular changes in sleep apnea may account for a considerable number of cases in which the diagnosis is essential hypertension.

The prevalence of sleep apnea in the population has not been established, but an increasing number of cases are discovered as awareness of its existence grows. In a recent survey of patients with daytime sleepiness whose disorder was serious enough for them to be evaluated polygraphically at a sleep disorders center, 42 percent were found to be suffering from one of the variants of sleep apnea.

A tentative diagnosis of sleep apnea can be made even without polysomnographic recordings. The most characteristic picture is of middle-aged or older men who report tiredness and inability to stay awake in the daytime, sometimes associated with depression, mood changes, and daytime sleep attacks. They may or may not complain of anything unusual during sleep. When a history is obtained from a spouse or bed partner, it includes reports of loud, intermittent snoring, at times accompanied by gasping. Observers sometimes recall apneic periods when patients appeared to be trying to breathe but were unable to do so. Such patients almost certainly have obstructive sleep apnea. With central or mixed apnea, the complaints are of repeated awakenings during the night, associated with morning headaches and mood changes but with no difficulty of falling asleep. At onset, the patients may have no complaints at all, although bed partners or roommates report heavy snoring and restless sleep. Obese patients with the disorder are said to have *pickwickian syndrome*.

Patients suspected of having sleep apnea should undergo laboratory recordings. The usual all-night sleep recordings including EEG, electromyogram (EMG), electrocardiogram (ECG), and respiratory tracings of various kinds are useful (Fig. 24.2–2). Recording airflow and respiratory effort is usually necessary to make a diagnosis. The severity of apneic episodes is determined by using oximetry to measure oxygen saturation during the night. Twenty-four-hour ECG monitoring is sometimes useful to monitor cardiac changes.

Nasal continuous positive airway pressure (nCPAP) is the treatment of choice for obstructive sleep apnea (Fig. 24.2–3). Other procedures include weight loss, nasal surgery, tracheostomy, and uvulopalatoplasty. Some medications may normalize sleep in patients with apnea. SSRIs and heterocyclic antidepressant drugs sometimes help treat sleep apnea by decreasing the amount of time spent in REM sleep, the stage of sleep in which apneic episodes occur most often. In addition, theophylline has been shown to decrease the number of episodes of apnea; however, it may interfere with the overall quality of sleep, limiting its general utility. When sleep apnea is established or suspected, patients must avoid the use of sedative medication, including alcohol, because it can considerably exacerbate the condition, which may then become life threatening.

Central Alveolar Hypoventilation. Central alveolar hypoventilation refers to several conditions marked by impaired ventilation in which the respiratory abnormality appears or greatly worsens only during sleep and in which no significant apneic episodes are present. The ventilatory dysfunction is characterized by inadequate tidal volume or respiratory rate during sleep. Death may occur during sleep (Ondine's curse). Central alveolar hypoventilation is treated with some form of mechanical ventilation (e.g., nasal ventilation).

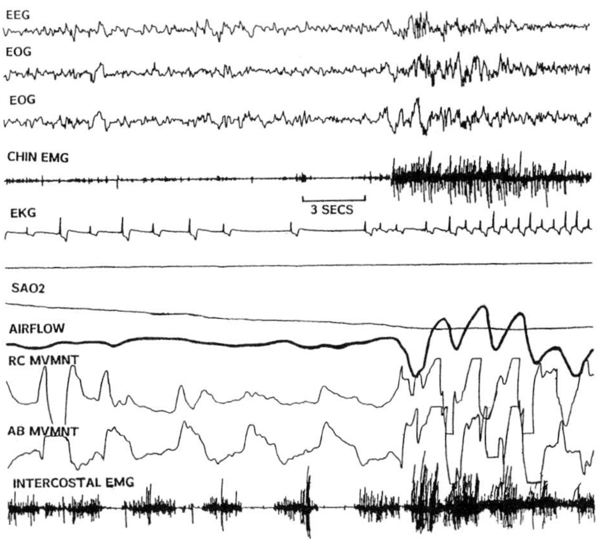

FIGURE 24.2–2

Obstructive sleep apnea. The airflow tracing shows cessation of breathing while the ribcage (*RC*) and abdominal (*AB*) movement (*MVMNT*) tracings clearly reveal respiratory effort. Intercostal EMG also confirms attempts to breathe. As blood oxygen saturation (*SAO2*) plummets, electrocardiographic abnormalities appear. Sinus pauses of more than 3 seconds' duration occurred. When the patient finally aroused (note *EEG-EOG-Chin EMG*), breathing resumed and was associated with a rebound tachycardia. The patient, whose chief complaint was excessive daytime sleepiness, had more than 200 similar events during a single night of sleep. (Courtesy of Constance A. Moore, M.D., Robert L. Williams, M.D., and Max Hirschkowitz, Ph.D.)

Circadian Rhythm Sleep Disorder. Circadian rhythm sleep disorder includes a wide range of conditions involving a misalignment between desired and actual sleep periods. DSM-IV-TR lists four types of circadian rhythm sleep disorders: delayed sleep phase type, jet lag type, shift work type, and unspecified (Table 24.2–12).

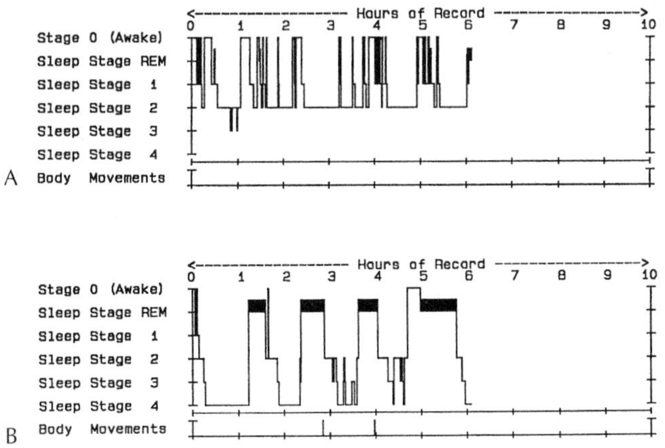

FIGURE 24.2–3

Sleep stage histogram illustrating the immediate, dramatic improvement in sleep architecture produced by treating obstructive sleep apnea with continuous positive airway pressure (CPAP) therapy. **A** illustrates the abnormal sleep pattern on a night when the patient had more than 200 episodes of obstructive sleep apnea. Sleep is disturbed by frequent awakenings while REM and slow-wave (stages 3 and 4) sleep are nearly absent. **B** shows data from the same patient being treated with CPAP on the next night. Normalization of sleep continuity with a massive rebound in REM and slow-wave sleep is evident. (Courtesy of Constance A. Moore, M.D., Robert L. Williams, M.D., and Max Hirschkowitz, Ph.D.)

Table 24.2–12
DSM-IV-TR Diagnostic Criteria for Circadian Rhythm Sleep Disorder

A. A persistent or recurrent pattern of sleep disruption leading to excessive sleepiness or insomnia that is due to a mismatch between the sleep–wake schedule required by a person's environment and his or her circadian sleep–wake pattern.
B. The sleep disturbance causes clinically significant distress or impairment in social, occupational, or other important areas of functioning.
C. The disturbance does not occur exclusively during the course of another sleep disorder or other mental disorder.
D. The disturbance is not due to the direct physiological effects of a substance (e.g., a drug of abuse, a medication) or a general medical condition.

Specify type:

Delayed sleep phase type: a persistent pattern of late sleep onset and late awakening times, with an inability to fall asleep and awaken at a desired earlier time

Jet lag type: sleepiness and alertness that occur at an inappropriate time of day relative to local time, occurring after repeated travel across more than one time zone

Shift work type: insomnia during the major sleep period or excessive sleepiness during the major awake period associated with night shift work or frequently changing shift work

Unspecified type

DELAYED SLEEP PHASE TYPE. The delayed sleep phase type of circadian rhythm sleep disorder is marked by sleep and wake times that are intractably later than desired, actual sleep times at virtually the same daily clock hour, no reported difficulty in maintaining sleep once begun, and an inability to advance the sleep phase by enforcing conventional sleep and wake times. The patients' major complaint is often the difficulty of falling asleep at a desired conventional time, and their disorder may appear to be similar to a sleep onset insomnia. Daytime sleepiness often occurs secondary to sleep loss.

Delayed sleep phase type can be treated by gradually delaying the hour of sleep over a period of several days until the desired sleep time is achieved. The strategy works when advancing the sleep time does not work. The process of sleep phase adjustment can be assisted by the brief use of short–half-life hypnotic agents, such as triazolam, to enforce sleep. Another approach to treating delayed sleep phase type is light therapy. Evening light therapy tends to delay sleep; regular morning light exposure tends to advance sleep.

JET LAG TYPE. Depending on the length of the east-to-west trip and individual sensitivity, jet lag type usually disappears spontaneously in 2 to 7 days; no specific treatment is required. Some persons find that they can prevent the symptoms by altering their mealtimes and sleep times in an appropriate direction before traveling. Others find that what appear to be symptoms of jet lag (fatigue and so on) are actually associated with sleep deprivation and that simply obtaining enough sleep helps. Melatonin taken orally at prescribed times is useful for some persons.

SHIFT WORK TYPE. The shift work type of circadian rhythm sleep disorder occurs in persons who change their work schedules repeatedly and rapidly and occasionally in persons with self-imposed chaotic sleep schedules. The most frequent symptom is a period of mixed insomnia and somnolence, but many other symptoms and somatic problems, including peptic ulcer, may be associated with the pattern after some time. Some adolescents and young adults appear to withstand such changes remarkably well and show few symptoms, but older persons and those with sensitivity to change are clearly affected.

The symptoms are generally worse the first few days after shifting to a new schedule, but in some persons the disrupted sleep–wake patterns persist for a long time. Enforcement of new sleep hours and light therapy may help workers adjust to their new schedules. Many persons never adapt completely to unusual shift schedules because they maintain the altered pattern only 5 days a week and return to the prevailing pattern of the rest of the population on days off and vacations.

Shift work schedules are an important area that has not received sufficient study, especially in view of the unusual shifts and changing shift schedules that a large proportion of the population now work. Persons' sensitivities to shifting schedules vary widely, but the bodies of a fair number of persons simply do not adapt to shift work; therefore, these persons should not be assigned to work in shifts. Temperamentally, some persons are "owls," who like to stay up at night and sleep during the day, and others are "larks," who rise early and retire early.

A particular problem occurs in the training of physicians, who are often required to work 36 to 48 hours without sleeping. This condition is dangerous to both doctors and their patients. It behooves medical educators to develop more shifts for doctors in training.

UNSPECIFIED. *Advanced Sleep Phase Syndrome.* The advanced sleep phase syndrome is characterized by sleep onsets and wake times that are intractably earlier than desired, actual sleep times at virtually the same daily clock hour, no reported difficulty in maintaining sleep once begun, and an inability to delay the sleep phase by enforcing conventional sleep and wake times. Unlike delayed sleep phase type, the condition does not interfere with the work or school day. The major presenting complaint is the inability to stay awake in the evening and to sleep in the morning until desired conventional times.

Disorganized Sleep–Wake Pattern. *Disorganized sleep–wake pattern* is defined as irregular, variable sleep and waking behavior that disrupts the regular sleep–wake pattern. The condition is associated with frequent daytime naps at irregular times and excessive bed rest. Sleep at night is not adequately long, and the

Table 24.2–13
DSM-IV-TR Diagnostic Criteria for Dyssomnia Not Otherwise Specified

The dyssomnia not otherwise specified category is for insomnias, hypersomnias, or circadian rhythm disturbances that do not meet criteria for any specific dyssomnia. Examples include

1. Complaints of clinically significant insomnia or hypersomnia that are attributable to environmental factors (e.g., noise, light, frequent interruptions).
2. Excessive sleepiness that is attributable to ongoing sleep deprivation.
3. "Restless legs syndrome": This syndrome is characterized by a desire to move the legs or arms, associated with uncomfortable sensations typically described as creeping, crawling, tingling, burning, or itching. Frequent movements of the limbs occur in an effort to relieve the uncomfortable sensations. Symptoms are worse when the individual is at rest and in the evening or night, and they are relieved temporarily by movement. The uncomfortable sensations and limb movements can delay sleep onset, awaken the individual from sleep, and lead to daytime sleepiness or fatigue. Sleep studies demonstrate involuntary periodic limb movements during sleep in a majority of individuals with restless legs syndrome. A minority of individuals have evidence of anemia or reduced serum iron stores. Peripheral nerve electrophysiological studies and gross brain morphology are usually normal. Restless legs syndrome can occur in an idiopathic form, or it can be associated with general medical or neurological conditions, including normal pregnancy, renal failure, rheumatoid arthritis, peripheral vascular disease, or peripheral nerve dysfunction. Phenomenologically, the two forms are indistinguishable. The onset of restless legs syndrome is typically in the second or third decade, although up to 20% of individuals with this syndrome may have symptoms before age 10. The prevalence of restless legs syndrome is between 2% and 10% in the general population and as high as 30% in general medical populations. Prevalence increases with age and is equal in males and females. Course is marked by stability or worsening of symptoms with age. There is a positive family history in 50–90% of individuals. The major differential diagnoses include medication-induced akathisia, peripheral neuropathy, and nocturnal leg cramps. Worsening at night and periodic limb movements are more common in restless legs syndrome than in medication-induced akathisia or peripheral neuropathy. Unlike restless legs syndrome, nocturnal leg cramps do not present with the desire to move the limbs nor are there frequent limb movements.
4. Periodic limb movements: Periodic limb movements are repeated low-amplitude brief limb jerks, particularly in the lower extremities. These movements begin near sleep onset and decrease during stage 3 or 4 non–rapid eye movement (NREM) and rapid eye movement (REM) sleep. Movements usually occur rhythmically every 20–60 seconds and are associated with repeated, brief arousals. Individuals are often unaware of the actual movements, but may complain of insomnia, frequent awakenings, or daytime sleepiness if the number of movements is very large. Individuals may have considerable variability in the number of periodic limb movements from night to night. Periodic limb movements occur in the majority of individuals with restless legs syndrome, but they may also occur without the other symptoms of restless legs syndrome. Individuals with normal pregnancy or with conditions such as renal failure, congestive heart failure, and posttraumatic stress disorder may also develop periodic limb movements. Although typical age at onset and prevalence in the general population are unknown, periodic limb movements increase with age and may occur in more than one-third of individuals over age 65. Men are more commonly affected than women.
5. Situations in which the clinician has concluded that a dyssomnia is present but is unable to determine whether it is primary, due to a general medical condition, or substance induced.

From American Psychiatric Association. *Diagnostic and Statistical Manual of Mental Disorders.* 4th ed. Text rev. Washington, DC: American Psychiatric Association; copyright 2000, with permission.

condition may seem to be insomnia, although the total amount of sleep in 24 hours is normal for the patient's age.

Dyssomnia Not Otherwise Specified. According to DSM-IV-TR, dyssomnia not otherwise specified includes insomnias, hypersomnias, and circadian rhythm disturbances that do not meet the criteria for any specific dyssomnia (Table 24.2–13).

NOCTURNAL MYOCLONUS. Nocturnal myoclonus consists of highly stereotyped abrupt contractions of certain leg muscles during sleep. Patients lack any subjective awareness of the leg jerks. The condition may be present in about 40 percent of persons over age 65.

The repetitive leg movements occur every 20 to 60 seconds, with extension of the large toe and flexion of the ankle, the knee, and the hips. Frequent awakenings, unrefreshing sleep, and daytime sleepiness are major symptoms. No treatment for nocturnal myoclonus is universally effective. Treatments that may be useful include benzodiazepines, levodopa (Larodopa), quinine, and, in rare cases, opioids.

RESTLESS LEGS SYNDROME. In restless legs syndrome, persons feel deep sensations of creeping inside the calves whenever sitting or lying down. The dysesthesias are rarely painful but are agonizingly relentless and cause an almost irresistible urge to move the legs; thus, this syndrome interferes with sleep and with falling asleep (Fig. 24.2–4). It peaks in middle age and occurs in 5 percent of the population.

The syndrome has no established treatment. Symptoms of restless legs syndrome are relieved by movement and by leg massage. When pharmacotherapy is required, the benzodiazepines, levodopa, quinine, opioids, propranolol (Inderal), valproate (Depakene), and carbamazepine (Tegretol) are of some benefit.

KLEINE-LEVIN SYNDROME. Kleine-Levin syndrome is a relatively rare condition consisting of recurrent periods of prolonged sleep (from which patients may be aroused) with intervening periods of normal sleep and alert waking. During the hypersomniac episodes, wakeful periods are usually marked by withdrawal from social contacts and return to bed at the first opportunity; patients may also display apathy, irritability, confusion, voracious eating, loss of sexual inhibitions, delusions, hallucinations, frank disorientation, memory impairment, incoherent speech, excitation or depression, and truculence. Unexplained fevers have occurred in a few patients.

Kleine-Levin syndrome is uncommon. About 100 cases with features suggesting the diagnosis have been reported. In most cases, several periods of hypersomnia, each lasting for one or several weeks, are experienced by patients over a year. With few exceptions the first attack occurs between the ages of 10 and 21 years. Rare instances of onset in the fourth and fifth decades of life have been reported. The syndrome appears to be almost invariably self-limited, and enduring remission occurs spontaneously before age 40 in early-onset cases.

MENSTRUAL-ASSOCIATED SYNDROME. Some women experience intermittent marked hypersomnia, altered behavioral patterns, and voracious eating at or shortly before the onset of their menses. Nonspecific EEG abnormalities similar to those associated with Kleine-Levin syndrome have been documented in several instances. Endocrine factors are probably involved, but no specific abnormalities in laboratory endocrine measures have been reported. Increased cerebrospinal fluid (CSF) serotonin levels were found in one patient.

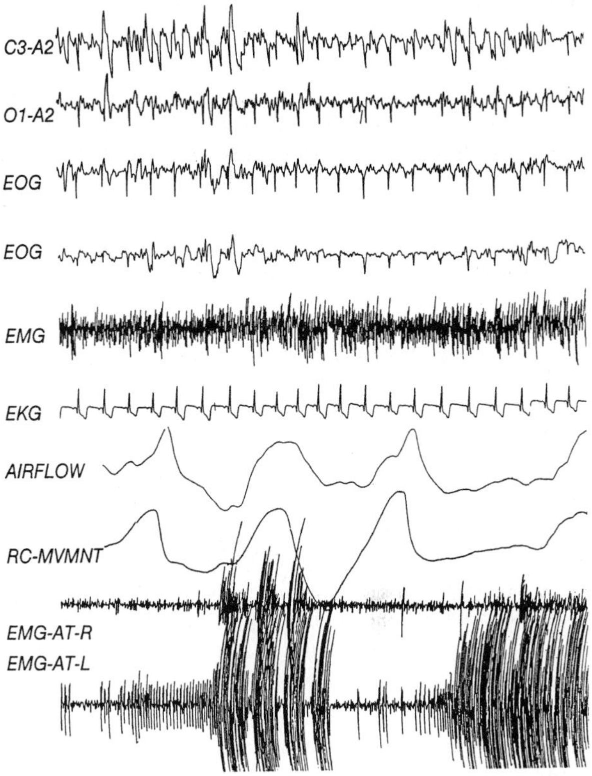

FIGURE 24.2–4

Restless legs syndrome. This patient presented with complaints of uncomfortable, crawling sensations in the legs when trying to fall asleep. Patients commonly report an urge to move the leg to dispel the sensation. This figure shows a bilateral pattern of leg EMG activity; however, the discharge is more pronounced in the left anterior tibialis (*EMG-AT-L*) than the right (*EMG-AT-R*). This pattern continued for more than an hour as the patient attempted to fall asleep; note that the sharp activity in central and occipital EEG (*C3-A2* and *O1-A2*, respectively) and EOG is an ECG artifact and not an EEG abnormality. (Courtesy of Constance A. Moore, M.D., Robert L. Williams, M.D., and Max Hirshkowitz, Ph.D.)

SLEEP DISTURBANCE IN PREGNANCY. Sleep disturbance is common in pregnant women. Several hormonal factors contribute to this disturbance, including changes in levels of estrogen, progesterone, cortisol, and melatonin from baseline. In addition, changes in maternal respiratory physiology, body habitus, and, in the third trimester, movements of the fetus can all act to diminish the quantity and quality of sleep.

INSUFFICIENT SLEEP. *Insufficient sleep* is defined as an earnest complaint of daytime sleepiness and associated waking symptoms by a person who persistently fails to obtain sufficient daily sleep to support alert wakefulness. The person is voluntarily, but often unwittingly, chronically sleep deprived. The diagnosis can usually be made on the basis of the history, including a sleep log. Some persons, especially students and shift workers, who want to maintain an active daytime life and perform their nighttime jobs, may seriously deprive themselves of sleep and thus produce somnolence during waking hours.

Table 24.2–14
DSM-IV-TR Diagnostic Criteria for Nightmare Disorder

A. Repeated awakenings from the major sleep period or naps with detailed recall of extended and extremely frightening dreams, usually involving threats to survival, security, or self-esteem. The awakenings generally occur during the second half of the sleep period.
B. On awakening from the frightening dreams, the person rapidly becomes oriented and alert (in contrast to the confusion and disorientation seen in sleep terror disorder and some forms of epilepsy).
C. The dream experience, or the sleep disturbance resulting from the awakening, causes clinically significant distress or impairment in social, occupational, or other important areas of functioning.
D. The nightmares do not occur exclusively during the course of another mental disorder (e.g., a delirium, posttraumatic stress disorder) and are not due to the direct physiological effects of a substance (e.g., a drug of abuse, a medication) or a general medical condition.

SLEEP DRUNKENNESS. Sleep drunkenness is an abnormal form of awakening in which the lack of a clear sensorium in the transition from sleep to full wakefulness is prolonged and exaggerated. A confusional state develops that often leads to individual or social inconvenience and sometimes to criminal acts. The diagnosis requires the absence of sleep deprivation. It is a rare condition, and there may be a familial tendency. Before making the diagnosis, clinicians should examine patients' sleep and rule out such conditions as apnea, nocturnal myoclonus, narcolepsy, and excessive use of alcohol and other substances.

Parasomnias

Nightmare Disorder. Nightmares are long, frightening dreams from which persons awaken scared (Table 24.2–14). Like other dreams, nightmares almost always occur during REM sleep and usually after a long REM period late in the night. Some persons have frequent nightmares as a lifelong condition; others experience them predominantly at times of stress and illness. About 50 percent of the adult population may report occasional nightmares. No specific treatment is usually required for nightmare disorder. Agents that suppress REM sleep, such as tricyclic drugs, may reduce the frequency of nightmares, and benzodiazepines have also been used. Contrary to popular belief, no harm results from awakening a person who is having a nightmare.

Ms. R. was a 20-year-old white woman who was referred with symptoms of talking, mumbling, and crying out during sleep. At least twice per week she screamed in her sleep. She was bothered by excessive sleepiness and falling asleep inappropriately (e.g., during a conversation). When inactive, she was tired and sleepy, even after a full 8-hour night of sleep. However, she had energy when motivated and led a vigorous life. Once, she awakened outside her apartment and her roommate had to let her back in because she had locked herself out. She did not recall the sleepwalking episode or other nocturnal wanderings but remembered yelling sometimes. From the history, crying seemed to occur in light sleep, but she rarely recalled any sleep-related thoughts or dreams. She had a history of occasional nightmares and bruxism. The patient used an oral appliance to protect her teeth. Leg kicking and mild snoring without gasping or choking were noted. The patient also complained of leg kicking during sleep. Her sleep–wake schedule was irregular, and she averaged between 5 and 7 hours of sleep per night. She occasionally awakened with a headache in the morning.

Previous health history included a hospitalization for febrile convulsions during infancy, ophthalmological surgery for strabismus during childhood, and tonsillectomy as a teenager. Health was otherwise excellent. The patient did not smoke tobacco or drink alcohol.

DISCUSSION

By history Ms. R. had one or more of the parasomnias. Sleep talking alone does not require a sleep study, but this patient had nocturnal wanderings. Polysomnography, with clinical EEG were indicated to rule out unrecognized nocturnal seizure disorder or other organic factors inducing sleepwalking. Sleepwalking is common and not necessarily considered abnormal in young children; however, it is rare in adults and merits careful evaluation. Ms. R.'s excessive daytime sleepiness was likely due to insufficient sleep (5 to 7 hours per night) and possibly parasomnia-related disruption. Interestingly, many parasomnias are exacerbated by sleep deprivation as is nocturnal seizure disorder.

Sleep studies were performed using comprehensive, attended, laboratory polysomnography. Prior to the overnight study, a clinical EEG was performed, which did not reveal any significant abnormal EEG activity during baseline, photic stimulation, or hyperventilation. An extended EEG montage was used during the sleep study. Overall sleep quality was within the normal range. Sleep efficiency was 96 percent, and latency to sleep was 1 minute. REM sleep percentage was high (31 percent), and latency to REM sleep was below normal (57 minutes). Slow-wave sleep was normal in percentage, but EEG delta activity was of very high amplitude. The overall macroarchitectural sleep pattern suggested rebound from sleep deprivation.

By contrast, sleep microarchitecture contained many abnormal features. We observed high-amplitude paroxysmal EEG bursts, excessively prolonged sleep spindles, and rhythmic K complexes. There was one arousal out of slow-wave sleep with rhythmic EEG discharges alternating with sharp waves. Sharps and spikes occurred several times; however, the focus was difficult to localize (possibly right temporal lobe). She exhibited frequent body movements and full body jerks, most of which occurred during NREM sleep. Episodes of moaning during slow-wave sleep and laughing

during stage 2 sleep were followed by high-amplitude theta bursts and REM sleep. Frequent movements and arousals from REM sleep were observed but no related spikes or sharp waves. Seizurelike EEG activity was noted during the night, predominantly during slow-wave sleep. However, the patient did not attempt to sleepwalk. Sharp wave and spike activity increased during the final 45 minutes of the sleep study.

The patient did not have any sleep-related breathing impairment and SaO_2 nadir was 90 percent. She had no periodic limb movements during sleep, and polygraphic features associated with restless legs syndrome were absent. (Courtesy of Constance A. Moore, M.D., Robert L. Williams, M.D., and Max Hirschkowitz, Ph.D.)

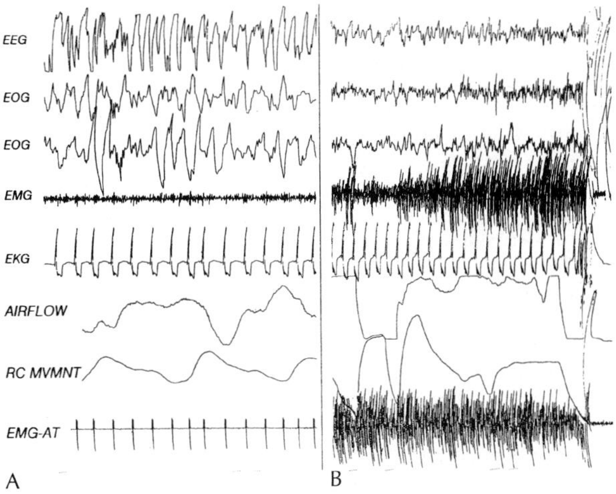

FIGURE 24.2–5

Polysomnogram of a sleep terror. **A** shows approximately 14 seconds of tracing occurring immediately before the sleep terror. Prominent EEG slow-wave activity and other characteristics of stage 4 sleep are seen. **B** shows the awakening, accompanied by tachycardia and movement. EEG activity is ambiguous, and the patient eventually disconnected his electrodes as he thrashed about in bed (visible at *far right of figure*). Although the patient was screaming and greatly agitated, no dreaming was reported. In the morning, he had little recollection of anything having occurred during the night. (Courtesy of Constance A. Moore, M.D., Robert L. Williams, M.D., and Max Hirschkowitz, Ph.D.)

Sleep Terror Disorder. Sleep terror disorder is an arousal in the first third of the night during deep NREM (stages 3 and 4) sleep. It is almost invariably inaugurated by a piercing scream or cry and accompanied by behavioral manifestations of intense anxiety bordering on panic (Table 24.2–15).

Typically, patients sit up in bed with a frightened expression, scream loudly, and sometimes awaken immediately with a sense of intense terror. Patients may remain awake in a disoriented state but more often fall asleep, and as with sleepwalking, they forget the episodes. A night terror episode after the original scream frequently develops into a sleepwalking episode. Polygraphic recordings of night terrors are somewhat like those of sleepwalking; in fact, the two conditions appear to be closely related. Night terrors, as isolated episodes, are especially frequent in children. About 1 to 6 percent of children have the disorder, which is more common in boys than in girls and which tends to run in families.

Night terrors may reflect a minor neurological abnormality, perhaps in the temporal lobe or underlying structures, because when night terrors begin in adolescence and young adulthood, they turn out to be the first symptom of temporal lobe epilepsy. In a typical case of night terrors, however, no signs of temporal lobe epilepsy or other seizure disorders are seen either clinically or on EEG recordings (Fig. 24.2–5).

Although night terrors are closely related to sleepwalking and are occasionally related to enuresis, they differ from nightmares. Night terrors are associated with simply awakening in terror. Patients generally have no dream recall but may occasionally recall a single frightening image.

Specific treatment for night terror disorder is seldom required. Investigation of stressful family situations may be important, and individual or family therapy is sometimes useful. In the rare cases when medication is required, diazepam (Valium) in small doses at bedtime improves the condition and sometimes completely eliminates the attacks.

Table 24.2–15
DSM-IV-TR Diagnostic Criteria for Sleep Terror Disorder

A. Recurrent episodes of abrupt awakening from sleep, usually occurring during the first third of the major sleep episode and beginning with a panicky scream.
B. Intense fear and signs of autonomic arousal, such as tachycardia, rapid breathing, and sweating, during each episode.
C. Relative unresponsiveness to efforts of others to comfort the person during the episode.
D. No detailed dream is recalled and there is amnesia for the episode.
E. The episodes cause clinically significant distress or impairment in social, occupational, or other important areas of functioning.
F. The disturbance is not due to the direct physiological effects of a substance (e.g., a drug of abuse, a medication) or a general medical condition.

From American Psychiatric Association. *Diagnostic and Statistical Manual of Mental Disorders.* 4th ed. Text rev. Washington, DC: American Psychiatric Association; copyright 2000, with permission.

Sleepwalking Disorder. Sleepwalking, also known as *somnambulism*, consists of a sequence of complex behaviors that are initiated in the first third of the night during deep NREM (stage 3 and 4) sleep and frequently, although not always, progress—without full consciousness or later memory of the episode—to leaving bed and walking about (Table 24.2–16).

Patients sit up and sometimes perform preservative motor acts, such as walking, dressing, going to the bathroom, talking, screaming, and even driving. The behavior occasionally terminates in awakening, with several minutes of confusion; more frequently, they return to sleep without any recollection of the sleepwalking event. An artificially induced arousal from stage 4 sleep can sometimes produce the condition. For instance, in children, especially those with a history of sleepwalking, an

Table 24.2–16
DSM-IV-TR Diagnostic Criteria for Sleepwalking Disorder

A. Repeated episodes of rising from bed during sleep and walking about, usually occurring during the first third of the major sleep episode.
B. While sleepwalking, the person has a blank, staring face, is relatively unresponsive to the efforts of others to communicate with him or her, and can be awakened only with great difficulty.
C. On awakening (either from the sleepwalking episode or the next morning), the person has amnesia for the episode.
D. Within several minutes after awakening from the sleepwalking episode, there is no impairment of mental activity or behavior (although there may initially be a short period of confusion or disorientation).
E. The sleepwalking causes clinically significant distress or impairment in social, occupational, or other important areas of functioning.
F. The disturbance is not due to the direct physiological effects of a substance (e.g., a drug of abuse, a medication) or a general medical condition.

From American Psychiatric Association. *Diagnostic and Statistical Manual of Mental Disorders.* 4th ed. Text rev. Washington, DC: American Psychiatric Association; copyright 2000, with permission.

attack can sometimes be provoked by standing them on their feet and thus producing a partial arousal during stage 4 sleep.

Sleepwalking usually begins between ages 4 and 8. Peak prevalence is at about 12 years of age. The disorder is more common in boys than in girls, and about 15 percent of children have an occasional episode. It tends to run in families. A minor neurological abnormality probably underlies the condition; the episodes should not be considered purely psychogenic, although stressful periods are associated with increased sleepwalking in affected persons. Extreme tiredness or previous sleep deprivation exacerbates attacks. The disorder is occasionally dangerous because of the possibility of accidental injury. Treatment consists of measures to prevent injury and drugs that suppress stages 3 and 4 sleep. The sleepwalker may be awakened during the episode without ill effects.

An 11-year-old girl asked her mother to take her to a psychiatrist because she feared she might be "going crazy." Several times during the last 2 months she had awakened confused about where she was until she realized she was on the living room couch or in her little sister's bed, even though she went to bed in her own room. When she recently woke up in her older brother's bedroom, she became very concerned and felt quite guilty about it. Her younger sister said that she had seen the patient walking during the night, looking like a "zombie," that she didn't answer when she called her, and that the patient had done that several times, but usually went back to her bed. The patient feared she might have "amnesia" because she had no memory of anything happening during the night.

There is no history of seizures or of similar episodes during the day. An EEG and physical examination proved normal. The patient's mental status was unremarkable except for some anxiety about her symptoms and the usual early adolescent concerns. School and family functioning were excellent.

DISCUSSION

This girl was not "going crazy" but, rather, was experiencing the characteristic features of sleepwalking disorder: episodes of arising from bed during sleep and walking about, appearing unresponsive during episodes, experiencing amnesia for the episode upon awakening, and exhibiting no evidence of impairment in consciousness several minutes after awakening. Psychomotor epileptic seizures were ruled out by the normal EEG and the absence of any seizurelike behavior during the waking state.

Although the process of dissociation is involved in sleepwalking disorder, because the disturbance begins during sleep, it was classified as a sleep disorder rather than as a dissociative disorder. (From *DSM-IV Casebook.*)

Parasomnia Not Otherwise Specified. The diagnostic criteria for parasomnia not otherwise specified are given in Table 24.2–17.

SLEEP-RELATED BRUXISM. Bruxism, tooth grinding, occurs throughout the night, most prominently in stage 2 sleep. According to dentists, 5 to 10 percent of the population suffer from bruxism severe enough to produce noticeable damage to teeth. The condition often goes unno-

Table 24.2–17
DSM-IV-TR Diagnostic Criteria for Parasomnia Not Otherwise Specified

The parasomnia not otherwise specified category is for disturbances that are characterized by abnormal behavioral or physiological events during sleep or sleep–wake transitions, but that do not meet criteria for a more specific parasomnia. Examples include

1. REM sleep behavior disorder: motor activity, often of a violent nature, that arises during rapid eye movement (REM) sleep. Unlike sleepwalking, these episodes tend to occur later in the night and are associated with vivid dream recall.
2. Sleep paralysis: an inability to perform voluntary movement during the transition between wakefulness and sleep. The episodes may occur at sleep onset (hypnagogic) or with awakening (hypnopompic). The episodes are usually associated with extreme anxiety and, in some cases, fear of impending death. Sleep paralysis occurs commonly as an ancillary symptom of narcolepsy and, in such cases, should not be coded separately.
3. Situations in which the clinician has concluded that a parasomnia is present but is unable to determine whether it is primary, due to a general medical condition, or substance induced.

From American Psychiatric Association. *Diagnostic and Statistical Manual of Mental Disorders.* 4th ed. Text rev. Washington, DC: American Psychiatric Association; copyright 2000, with permission.

ticed by the sleepers, except for an occasional jaw ache in the morning, but bed partners and roommates are consistently awakened by the sound. Treatment consists of a dental bite plate and corrective orthodontic procedures.

REM SLEEP BEHAVIOR DISORDER. REM sleep behavior disorder is a chronic, progressive condition found mainly in men. It is characterized by the loss of atonia during REM sleep and subsequent emergence of violent and complex behaviors. In essence, patients with the disorder are acting out their dreams. Serious injury to patients or their bed partners is a major risk. The development or aggravation of the disorder has been reported in patients with narcolepsy who have been treated with psychostimulants and tricyclic drugs and in patients with depression and obsessive-compulsive disorder who have been treated with fluoxetine. REM sleep behavior disorder is treated with clonazepam (Klonopin), 0.5 to 2.0 mg a day. Carbamazepine, 100 mg three times a day, is also effective in controlling the disorder.

SLEEPTALKING (SOMNILOQUY). Sleeptalking is common in children and adults. It has been studied extensively in the sleep laboratory and is found in all stages of sleep. The talking usually involves a few words that are difficult to distinguish. Long episodes of talking involve the sleeper's life and concerns, but sleeptalkers do not relate their dreams during sleep, nor do they often reveal deep secrets. Episodes of sleeptalking sometimes accompany night terrors and sleepwalking. Sleeptalking alone requires no treatment.

SLEEP-RELATED HEAD BANGING (JACTATIO CAPITIS NOCTURNA). *Sleep-related head banging* is the term for a sleep behavior consisting chiefly of rhythmic to-and-fro head rocking (less commonly, total body rocking) occurring just before or during sleep. Usually, it is observed in the immediate presleep period and is sustained into light sleep. It uncommonly persists into, or occurs in, deep NREM sleep. Treatment consists of measures to prevent injury.

SLEEP PARALYSIS. Familial sleep paralysis is characterized by a sudden inability to execute voluntary movements either just at the onset of sleep or on awakening during the night or in the morning.

SLEEP DISORDERS RELATED TO ANOTHER MENTAL DISORDER. DSM-IV-TR defines a sleep disorder related to another mental disorder as a complaint of sleep disturbance caused by a diagnosable mental disorder but severe enough to merit clinical attention on its own.

Insomnia Related to Axis I or Axis II Disorder

Insomnia that occurs for at least 1 month and is clearly related to the psychological and behavioral symptoms of the clinically well-known mental disorders is classified here (Table 24.2–18). The category consists of a heterogeneous group of conditions. The sleep problem is usually, but not always, difficulty falling asleep secondary to anxiety that is part of any of the various mental disorders listed. The insomnia is more common in women than in men. In clear-cut cases in which the anxiety has psychological roots, psychiatric treatment of the anxiety (e.g., individual psychotherapy, group psychotherapy, or family therapy) often relieves the insomnia.

The insomnia associated with major depressive disorder involves relatively normal sleep onset but repeated awakenings during the second half of the night and premature morning awakening (Fig. 24.2–6), usually with an uncomfortable mood in the morning. (Morning is the worst time of day for many patients with major depressive disorder.) Polysomnography shows reduced stage 3 and 4 sleep, often a short REM latency, and a long first REM period. The use of partial or total sleep deprivation can accelerate the response to antidepressant medication.

Table 24.2–18
DSM-IV-TR Diagnostic Criteria for Insomnia Related to Another Mental Disorder

A. The predominant complaint is difficulty initiating or maintaining sleep, or nonrestorative sleep, for at least 1 month that is associated with daytime fatigue or impaired daytime functioning.
B. The sleep disturbance (or daytime sequelae) causes clinically significant distress or impairment in social, occupational, or other important areas of functioning.
C. The insomnia is judged to be related to another Axis I or Axis II disorder (e.g., major depressive disorder, generalized anxiety disorder, adjustment disorder with anxiety) but is sufficiently severe to warrant independent clinical attention.
D. The disturbance is not better accounted for by another sleep disorder (e.g., narcolepsy, breathing-related sleep disorder, a parasomnia).
E. The disturbance is not due to the direct physiological effects of a substance (e.g., a drug of abuse, a medication) or a general medical condition.

From American Psychiatric Association. *Diagnostic and Statistical Manual of Mental Disorders.* 4th ed. Text rev. Washington, DC: American Psychiatric Association; copyright 2000, with permission.

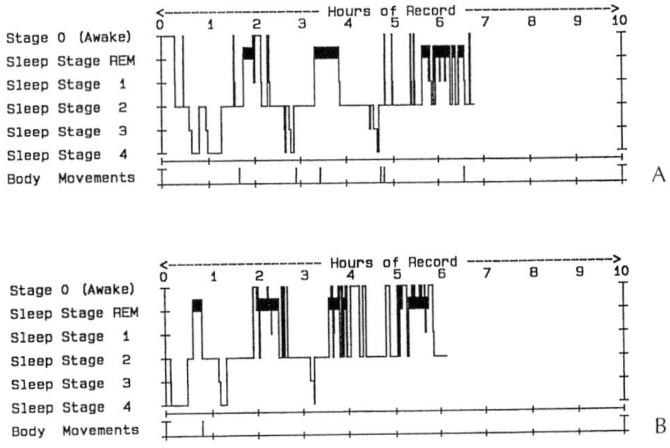

FIGURE 24.2–6

Sleep stage histograms comparing normal sleep **(A)** with that found in a patient with major depressive disorders **(B)**. Difficulty maintaining sleep and early morning awakenings are common complaints in patients with depression. **B** illustrates the electrophysiological correlates of these complaints beginning after approximately 2 hours of sleep. Sleep continuity becomes disrupted as morning approaches. Also present is a markedly reduced latency to REM sleep, a feature characteristic of this patient population and thought by some to reflect cholinergic-aminergic imbalance. (Courtesy of Constance A. Moore, M.D., Robert L. Williams, M.D., and Max Hirschkowitz, Ph.D.)

Ms. D. is a 36-year-old woman who complains of chronic insomnia. Although she has had sleep problems intermittently since her college years, she has developed more persistent problems over the past year and a half. This worsening coincided with several stresses, including a move to a new house, a change of jobs for her husband, her own decision to quit working, and her elderly and ill father's moving in with her family. She claims that she does not sleep at all some nights and is concerned that her sleeplessness will impair her ability to take care of her children and otherwise function during the day. She has been prescribed alprazolam and has used diphenhydramine and alcohol to help with her sleep problems, but the insomnia has always quickly returned upon discontinuation of each of these. In addition, she was treated by a psychologist with visualization and progressive relaxation techniques, but this resulted in only partial relief.

Ms. D. often falls asleep on the couch in the family room while watching television at night. She then wakes up, takes an alprazolam tablet, and goes back to bed at about 1:30 AM. She gets out of bed at approximately 8 AM. She acknowledges feeling physically and mentally tense about her sleep difficulty and notes that sometimes she clenches her jaw, grips her hands, or feels panicky at night. She also notes an increased heart rate and sweating on occasion at night but denies depersonalization or paresthesias. She denies other unusual behavior during sleep and daytime sleepiness, and she only rarely takes a daytime nap.

Upon further questioning, Ms. D. reveals that, although her sleep problem is the biggest difficulty she is having at the moment, it is only one of many symptoms that have been bothering her. She says that she can't stop herself from "worrying about everything": the health and safety of her family, their financial situation, the security of her husband's job, the possibility that their old oil furnace may explode, the state of the tires on the family car, the quality of her children's schools, filling out her tax forms, and so on. She constantly ruminates on these concerns and suffers from somatic tension manifested by tenseness in her neck, shoulder, and jaw muscles; digestive troubles; and general jumpiness. She denies abrupt episodes of panic but says that she does have intermittent episodes of severe anxiety that are characterized by palpitations, sweating, increased muscle tension, difficulty breathing, and a fear that she is losing her mind. She is meticulous about her work and appearance, but denies the presence of specific repeated intrusive thoughts or ritualistic behavior.

Ms. D. had one episode of major depressive disorder 8 years earlier that was characterized by low mood insomnia, decreased appetite and weight loss, poor concentration, and decreased enjoyment and interest, but no suicidal ideation. She saw a minister, and eventually these symptoms resolved. Ms. D. has a strong family history of insomnia, depression, and anxiety, and one of her sisters is currently being treated with an antidepressant medication. At the time of this evaluation, Ms. D. reports great interest and enthusiasm for her daily activities, although her energy is adversely affected by her sleep disturbance.

Ms. D. denies current alcohol or other substance abuse. She takes alprazolam 0.75 mg q.h.s. and drinks two cups of caffeinated coffee per day and approximately three alcoholic drinks per month. Her only current medical problem is endometriosis.

Ms. D. has been married for 10 years and has two children, ages 4 and 2. She worked as a dietitian but resigned after the birth of the second child to raise her family. She says that she has some marital stress because her husband works long hours and she communicates poorly with him.

On mental status examination, Ms. D. is awake, alert, and oriented and does not appear sleepy. She states that she feels anxious and nervous but denies depression. Her cognitive functions are well within normal limits. There is no evidence of psychotic symptoms or of clear-cut obsessions or compulsions. Her speech is normal in rate and rhythm but tends to include detailed answers to all questions.

DSM-IV Diagnosis

Axis I:	Insomnia related to generalized anxiety disorder
Axis II:	Generalized anxiety disorder, obsessive-compulsive personality traits
Axis III:	Endometriosis
Axis IV:	Marital stress, moving to a new house, father's illness
Axis V:	GAF = 65 (current); 75 (highest level in past year)

(From *DSM-IV Case Studies.*)

Panic disorder may be associated with paroxysmal awakenings or with entering stage 3 and 4 sleep. The emotional and cognitive symptoms of a panic attack are present, along with tachycardia and increased respiratory rate. Patients with manic episodes and bipolar II disorder appear to be extreme cases of short sleepers. They sometimes appear to have difficulty falling asleep but most often do not complain of sleep problems. They awaken refreshed after 2 to 4 hours of sleep and appear to have a true reduction in their need for sleep during the course of the manic or hypomanic episode. In schizophrenia, total sleep time and slow-wave sleep are reduced. REM sleep is often reduced early during an exacerbation. Other conditions associated with insomnia include posttraumatic stress disorder (nightmares), obsessive-compulsive disorder (rituals), and eating disorders. Attention-deficit/hyperactivity disorder (ADHD) has been linked to higher than normal rates of sleep disturbance (usually difficulty falling asleep). At times this can be exacerbated by the patient's schedule of stimulant administration; special care should be taken when designing a medication regimen.

Hypersomnia Related to Axis I or Axis II Disorder

Hypersomnia that occurs for at least 1 month and is associated with a mental disorder is found in a variety of conditions, including mood disorders. Excessive daytime sleepiness may be reported in the initial stages of many mild depressive disorders and characteristically in the depressed phase of bipolar I disorder. For a few weeks, hypersomnia may sometimes be

Table 24.2–19
DSM-IV-TR Diagnostic Criteria for Hypersomnia Related to Another Mental Disorder

A. The predominant complaint is excessive sleepiness for at least 1 month as evidenced by either prolonged sleep episodes or daytime sleep episodes that occur almost daily.
B. The excessive sleepiness causes clinically significant distress or impairment in social, occupational, or other important areas of functioning.
C. The hypersomnia is judged to be related to another Axis I or Axis II disorder (e.g., major depressive disorder, dysthymic disorder) but is sufficiently severe to warrant independent clinical attention.
D. The disturbance is not better accounted for by another sleep disorder (e.g., narcolepsy, breathing-related sleep disorder, a parasomnia) or by an inadequate amount of sleep.
E. The disturbance is not due to the direct physiological effects of a substance (e.g., a drug of abuse, a medication) or a general medical condition.

associated with uncomplicated grief. Other mental disorders—such as personality disorders, dissociative disorders, somatoform disorders, dissociative fugue, and amnestic disorders—can produce hypersomnia (Table 24.2–19). Treatment of the primary disorder should resolve the hypersomnia.

OTHER SLEEP DISORDERS

DSM-IV-TR defines a sleep disorder caused by a medical condition as a complaint of sleep disturbance produced by a physiological effect of the medical condition on the sleep–wake system. A substance-induced sleep disorder arises from the use, or the recently discontinued use, of a substance.

Sleep Disorder Due to a General Medical Condition

Any sleep disturbance (e.g., insomnia, hypersomnia, parasomnia, or a combination) can be caused by a general medical condition (Table 24.2–20). Almost any medical condition associated with pain and discomfort (e.g., arthritis or angina) can produce insomnia. Some conditions are associated with insomnia even when pain and discomfort are not specifically present. These conditions include neoplasms, vascular lesions, infections, and degenerative and traumatic conditions. Other conditions, especially endocrine and metabolic diseases, frequently involve some sleep disturbance.

Being aware of the possibility of such conditions and obtaining a good medical history usually lead to a correct diagnosis. The treatment, when possible, is treatment of the underlying medical condition.

Sleep-Related Epileptic Seizures. The relation of sleep and epilepsy is complex. Sleep disorders (sleep apnea in particular) can exacerbate seizures. Seizures, in turn, can disrupt sleep structure, particularly REM sleep. When seizures occur almost exclusively during sleep, the condition is called *sleep epilepsy.*

Table 24.2–20
DSM-IV-TR Diagnostic Criteria for Sleep Disorder Due to a General Medical Condition

A. A prominent disturbance in sleep that is sufficiently severe to warrant independent clinical attention.
B. There is evidence from the history, physical examination, or laboratory findings that the sleep disturbance is the direct physiological consequence of a general medical condition.
C. The disturbance is not better accounted for by another mental disorder (e.g., an adjustment disorder in which the stressor is a serious medical illness).
D. The disturbance does not occur exclusively during the course of a delirium.
E. The disturbance does not meet the criteria for breathing-related sleep disorder or narcolepsy.
F. The sleep disturbance causes clinically significant distress or impairment in social, occupational, or other important areas of functioning.

Specify type:

Insomnia type: if the predominant sleep disturbance is insomnia
Hypersomnia type: if the predominant sleep disturbance is hypersomnia
Parasomnia type: if the predominant sleep disturbance is a parasomnia
Mixed type: if more than one sleep disturbance is present and none predominates

Coding note: Include the name of the general medical condition on Axis I, e.g., sleep disorder due to chronic obstructive pulmonary disease, insomnia type; also code the general medical condition on Axis III.

Sleep-Related Cluster Headaches and Chronic Paroxysmal Hemicrania. Sleep-related cluster headaches are agonizingly severe unilateral headaches that often appear during sleep and are marked by an on–off pattern of attacks. Chronic paroxysmal hemicrania is a similar unilateral headache that occurs every day with more frequent, but short-lived onsets that are without a preponderant sleep distribution. Both types of vascular headaches are examples of sleep-exacerbated conditions and appear in association with REM sleep periods; paroxysmal hemicrania is virtually REM sleep locked.

Sleep-Related Abnormal Swallowing Syndrome. Abnormal swallowing syndrome is a condition during sleep in which inadequate swallowing results in aspiration of saliva, coughing, and choking. It is intermittently associated with brief arousals or awakenings.

Sleep-Related Asthma. Asthma that is exacerbated by sleep in some persons may result in significant sleep disturbances.

Sleep-Related Cardiovascular Symptoms. Sleep-related cardiovascular symptoms derive from disorders of cardiac rhythm, myocardial incompetence, coronary artery insufficiency, and blood pressure variability, which may be induced or exacerbated by sleep-altered or sleep-state–modified cardiovascular physiology.

Sleep-Related Gastroesophageal Reflux. Sleep-related gastroesophageal reflux is a disorder in which patients awaken from

sleep with burning, substernal pain or a feeling of general pain or tightness in the chest or a sour taste in the mouth. Coughing, choking, and vague respiratory discomfort may also occur repeatedly.

Sleep-Related Hemolysis (Paroxysmal Nocturnal Hemoglobinuria). Paroxysmal nocturnal hemoglobinuria is a rare, acquired, chronic hemolytic anemia in which intravascular hemolysis results in hemoglobinemia and hemoglobinuria. The hemolysis and consequent hemoglobinuria are accelerated during sleep, and the morning urine is brownish red. Hemolysis is linked to the sleep period, even when the period is shifted.

Substance-Induced Sleep Disorder

Any sleep disturbance (e.g., insomnia, hypersomnia, parasomnia, or a combination) can be caused by a substance (Table 24.2–21). According to DSM-IV-TR, clinicians should also specify whether the onset of the disorder occurred during intoxication or withdrawal.

Somnolence related to tolerance or withdrawal from a central nervous system (CNS) stimulant is common in persons withdrawing from amphetamines, cocaine, caffeine, and related substances. The somnolence may be associated with severe depression, which occasionally reaches suicidal proportions. Sustained use of a CNS depressant, such as alcohol, can cause somnolence. Heavy alcohol use in the evening produces sleepiness and difficulty arising the next day. This reaction may present a diagnostic problem when patients do not admit alcohol abuse.

Insomnia is associated with tolerance to, or withdrawal from, sedative-hypnotic drugs, such as benzodiazepines, barbiturates, and chloral hydrate. With the sustained use of such agents—usually undertaken to treat insomnia arising from a different source—tolerance increases, and the drugs lose their sleep-inducing effects; patients then often increase the dosage. On sudden discontinuation of the drug, severe sleeplessness supervenes, often accompanied by the general features of substance withdrawal. Typically, patients experience a temporary increase in the severity of the insomnia.

Long-term use (more than 30 days) of a hypnotic agent is well tolerated by some patients, but others begin to complain of sleep disturbance, most often multiple brief awakenings during the night. Recordings show a disruption of sleep architecture, reduced stage 3 and 4 sleep, increased stage 1 and 2 sleep, and fragmentation of sleep throughout the night.

Clinicians should be aware of CNS stimulants as a possible cause of insomnia and should remember that various medications for weight reduction, beverages containing caffeine, and, occasionally, adrenergic drugs taken by asthmatic patients may all produce this insomnia. Alcohol may help induce sleep but frequently results in nocturnal awakening. Alcohol use during the cocktail hour can produce difficulty falling asleep later in the evening.

For reasons that are not always clear, a wide variety of drugs occasionally produce sleep problems as a side effect. These drugs include antimetabolites and other cancer chemotherapeutic agents, thyroid preparations, anticonvulsant agents, antidepressant drugs, adrenocorticotropic hormone (ACTH)-like drugs, oral contraceptives, α-methyldopa, and β-adrenergic receptor antagonists.

Table 24.2–21
DSM-IV-TR Diagnostic Criteria for Substance-Induced Sleep Disorder

A. A prominent disturbance in sleep that is sufficiently severe to warrant independent clinical attention.

B. There is evidence from the history, physical examination, or laboratory findings of either (1) or (2):

(1) the symptoms in Criterion A developed during, or within a month of, substance intoxication or withdrawal

(2) medication use is etiologically related to the sleep disturbance

C. The disturbance is not better accounted for by a sleep disorder that is not substance induced. Evidence that the symptoms are better accounted for by a sleep disorder that is not substance induced might include the following: the symptoms precede the onset of the substance use (or medication use); the symptoms persist for a substantial period of time (e.g., about a month) after the cessation of acute withdrawal or severe intoxication or are substantially in excess of what would be expected given the type or amount of the substance used or the duration of use; or there is other evidence that suggests the existence of an independent non–substance-induced sleep disorder (e.g., a history of recurrent non–substance-related episodes).

D. The disturbance does not occur exclusively during the course of a delirium.

E. The sleep disturbance causes clinically significant distress or impairment in social, occupational, or other important areas of functioning.

Note: This diagnosis should be made instead of a diagnosis of substance intoxication or substance withdrawal only when the sleep symptoms are in excess of those usually associated with the intoxication or withdrawal syndrome and when the symptoms are sufficiently severe to warrant independent clinical attention.

Code [Specific substance]-induced sleep disorder:

Alcohol; amphetamine; caffeine; cocaine; opioid; sedative, hypnotic, or anxiolytic; other [or unknown] substance

Specify type:

Insomnia type: if the predominant sleep disturbance is insomnia

Hypersomnia type: if the predominant sleep disturbance is hypersomnia

Parasomnia type: if the predominant sleep disturbance is a parasomnia

Mixed type: if more than one sleep disturbance is present and none predominates

Specify if:

With onset during intoxication: if the criteria are met for intoxication with the substance and the symptoms develop during the intoxication syndrome

With onset during withdrawal: if criteria are met for withdrawal from the substance and the symptoms develop during, or shortly after, a withdrawal syndrome

From American Psychiatric Association. *Diagnostic and Statistical Manual of Mental Disorders.* 4th ed. Text rev. Washington, DC: American Psychiatric Association; copyright 2000, with permission.

Other agents do not produce sleep disturbance while being used but may have this effect after withdrawal. Almost any sedating or tranquilizing agents, including at times the benzodiazepines, the phenothiazines, the sedating tricyclic drugs, and various street drugs, including marijuana and opioids, can have this effect.

Alcohol is a CNS depressant and produces the serious problems of other CNS depressants, both during administration—perhaps related to the development of tolerance—and after withdrawal. The insomnia after long-term alcohol consumption is sometimes severe and lasts for weeks or longer. Clinicians should not give potentially addicting medications to patients who have just recovered from an addiction; if possible, sleeping medications should be avoided.

Among cigarette smokers, the combination of a relaxing ritual and the tendency of low doses of nicotine to cause sedation may actually help sleep, but high doses of nicotine can interfere with sleep, particularly sleep onset. Cigarette smokers typically sleep less than nonsmokers. Nicotine withdrawal may cause drowsiness or arousal.

References

Espie CA. Insomnia: conceptual issues in the development, persistence, and treatment of sleep disorder in adults. *Annu Rev Psychol.* 2002;53:215.

Farney RJ, Walker JM. Office management of common sleep–wake disorders. *Med Clin North Am.* 1995;79:391.

Greenhill LL, Pliszka S, Dulcan MK, et al. American Academy of Child and Adolescent Psychiatry practice parameter for the use of stimulant medications in the treatment of children, adolescents, and adults. *J Am Acad Child Adolesc Psychiatry.* 2002;41(2 suppl):26S.

Hartmann PM. Drug treatment of insomnia: indications and newer agents. *Am Fam Physician.* 1995;51:191.

Harvey AG. Identifying safety behaviors in insomnia. *J Nerv Ment Dis.* 2001;190:16.

Karacan I, ed. *Psychophysiological Aspects of Sleep.* Park Ridge, NJ: Noyes Medical; 1981.

Kripke DF, Garfinkel L, Wingard DL, Klauber MR, Marler MR. Mortality associated with sleep duration and insomnia. *Arch Gen Psychiatry.* 2002;59:131.

Kryger MH, Roth T, Dement WC, eds. *Principles and Practice of Sleep Medicine.* 2nd ed. Philadelphia: Saunders; 1993.

Mahowald MW. Diagnostic testing: sleep disorders. *Neurol Clin.* 1996;14:183.

Morin CM, Woote V. Psychological and pharmacological approaches to treating insomnia: critical issues in assessing their separate and combined effects. *Clin Psychol Rev.* 1996;16:521.

Silverberg DS, Iaina A, Oksenberg A. Treating obstructive sleep apnea improves essential hypertension and quality of life. *Am Fam Physician.* 2002;65:229.

Van Ommeren M, De Jong JTVM, Komproe I. Post-traumatic stress disorder and sleep. *N Engl J Med.* 2002;346:1334.

Weinger MB, Ancoli-Israel S. Sleep deprivation and clinical performance. *JAMA.* 2002;287:955.

Williams RL, Karacan I, Moore C, eds. *Sleep Disorders: Diagnosis and Treatment.* 2nd ed. New York: John Wiley & Sons; 1988.

Williams RL, Moore CA, Hirshkowitz M. Sleep disorders. In: Sadock BJ, Sadock VA, eds. *Kaplan & Sadock's Comprehensive Textbook of Psychiatry.* 7th ed. Vol 2. Baltimore: Lippincott Williams & Wilkins; 2000:1677.

25 Impulse-Control Disorders Not Elsewhere Classified

The text revision of the fourth edition of *Diagnostic and Statistical Manual of Mental Disorders* (DSM-IV-TR) lists six categories of impulse-control disorders not classified elsewhere: (1) intermittent explosive disorder, (2) kleptomania, (3) pyromania, (4) pathological gambling, (5) trichotillomania, and (6) impulse-control disorder not otherwise specified (NOS).

Disorders of impulse control have long been recognized. In 1838 Jean Etienne Esquirol proposed the term *monomanic instinctives* to describe behaviors characterized by irresistible urges without apparent motive. Patients with impulse-control disorders do not resist drives or enticements to do something harmful to themselves or to others. They are unable to resist impulses, although they may or may not consciously try to do so, and they may or may not plan their behaviors. Before they act there is a sense of increasing tension or arousal; afterward there is a sense of pleasure and satisfaction. On occasion, however, there may be feelings of remorse or guilt that disturb the sense of pleasure. Because their behaviors consciously coincide with their desires, their acts are considered ego-syntonic.

Etiology

Psychodynamic, psychosocial, and biological factors all play an important role in impulse-control disorders; however, the primary causal factor remains unknown. Some impulse-control disorders may have common underlying neurobiological mechanisms. Fatigue, incessant stimulation, and psychic trauma can lower a person's resistance to control impulses.

Psychodynamic Factors

An impulse is a disposition to act to decrease heightened tension caused by the buildup of instinctual drives or by diminished ego defenses against the drives. The impulse disorders have in common an attempt to bypass the experience of disabling symptoms or painful affects by acting on the environment. In his work with adolescents who were delinquent, August Aichhorn described impulsive behavior as related to a weak superego and weak ego structures associated with psychic trauma produced by childhood deprivation.

Otto Fenichel linked impulsive behavior to attempts to master anxiety, guilt, depression, and other painful affects by means of action. He thought that such actions defend against internal danger and that they produce a distorted aggressive or sexual gratification. To observers, impulsive behaviors may appear irrational and motivated by greed, but they may actually be endeavors to find relief from pain.

Heinz Kohut considered many forms of impulse-control problems, including gambling, kleptomania, and some paraphiliac behaviors, to be related to an incomplete sense of self. He observed that when patients do not receive the validating and affirming responses that they seek from persons in significant relationships with them, the self might fragment. As a way of dealing with this fragmentation and regaining a sense of wholeness or cohesion in the self, persons may engage in impulsive behaviors that to others appear self-destructive. Kohut's formulation has some similarities to Donald Winnicott's view that impulsive or deviant behavior in children is a way for them to try to recapture a primitive maternal relationship. Winnicott saw such behavior as hopeful in that the child searches for affirmation and love from the mother rather than abandoning any attempt to win her affection. Several therapists have stressed patients' fixation at the oral stage of development. Patients attempt to master anxiety, guilt, depression, and other painful affects by means of actions, but such actions aimed at obtaining relief seldom succeed even temporarily.

Psychosocial Factors

Psychosocial factors implicated causally in impulse-control disorders are related to early-life events. The growing child may have had improper models for identification, such as parents who had difficulty controlling impulses. Other psychosocial factors associated with the disorders include exposure to violence in the home, alcohol abuse, promiscuity, and antisocial behavior.

Biological Factors

Many investigators have focused on possible organic factors in the impulse-control disorders, especially for patients with overtly violent behavior. Experiments have shown that impulsive and violent activity is associated with specific brain regions such as the limbic system and that the inhibition of such behaviors is associated with other brain regions. A relation has been found between low cerebrospinal fluid (CSF) levels of 5-hydroxyindoleacetic acid (5-HIAA) and impulsive aggression. Certain hormones, especially testosterone, have also been associated with violent and aggressive behavior. Some reports have described a relation between temporal lobe epilepsy and certain

impulsive violent behaviors, as well as an association of aggressive behavior in patients who have histories of head trauma with increased numbers of emergency room visits and other potential organic antecedents. A high incidence of mixed cerebral dominance may be found in some violent populations.

Considerable evidence indicates that the serotonin neurotransmitter system mediates symptoms evident in impulse-control disorders. Brainstem and CSF levels of 5-HIAA are decreased, and serotonin-binding sites are increased in persons who have committed suicide. The dopaminergic and noradrenergic systems have also been implicated in impulsivity.

Impulse-control disorder symptoms may continue into adulthood in persons whose disorder has been diagnosed as childhood attention-deficit/hyperactivity disorder. Lifelong or acquired mental deficiency, epilepsy, and even reversible brain syndromes have long been implicated in lapses in impulse control.

INTERMITTENT EXPLOSIVE DISORDER

Intermittent explosive disorder manifests as discrete episodes of losing control of aggressive impulses; these episodes can result in serious assault or the destruction of property. The aggressiveness expressed is grossly out of proportion to any stressors that may have helped elicit the episodes. The symptoms, which patients may describe as spells or attacks, appear within minutes or hours and, regardless of duration, remit spontaneously and quickly. After each episode patients usually show genuine regret or self-reproach, and signs of generalized impulsivity or aggressiveness are absent between episodes. The diagnosis of intermittent explosive disorder should not be made if the loss of control can be accounted for by schizophrenia, antisocial or borderline personality disorder, attention-deficit/hyperactivity disorder, conduct disorder, or substance intoxication.

The term *epileptoid personality* has been used to convey the seizurelike quality of the characteristic outbursts, which are not typical of the patient's usual behavior, and to convey the suspicion of an organic disease process, for example, damage to the central nervous system. Several associated features suggest the possibility of an epileptoid state: the presence of auras; postictal-like changes in the sensorium, including partial or spotty amnesia; and hypersensitivity to photic, aural, or auditory stimuli.

Epidemiology

Intermittent explosive disorder is underreported. The disorder appears to be more common in men than in women. The men are likely to be found in correctional institutions and the women in psychiatric facilities. In one study, about 2 percent of all persons admitted to a university hospital psychiatric service had disorders that were diagnosed as intermittent explosive disorder; 80 percent were men.

Evidence indicates that intermittent explosive disorder is more common in first-degree biological relatives of persons with the disorder than in the general population. Many factors other than a simple genetic explanation may be responsible.

Comorbidity

High rates of fire setting in patients with intermittent explosive disorder have been reported. Other disorders of impulse control and substance use and mood, anxiety, and eating disorders have also been associated with intermittent explosive disorder.

Etiology

Psychodynamic Factors. Psychoanalysts have suggested that explosive outbursts occur as a defense against narcissistic injurious events. Rage outbursts serve as interpersonal distance and protect against any further narcissistic injury.

Psychosocial Factors. Typical patients have been described as physically large but dependent men whose sense of masculine identity is poor. A sense of being useless and impotent or of being unable to change the environment often precedes an episode of physical violence, and a high level of anxiety, guilt, and depression usually follows an episode.

An unfavorable childhood environment often filled with alcohol dependence, beatings, and threats to life is usual in these patients. Predisposing factors in infancy and childhood include perinatal trauma, infantile seizures, head trauma, encephalitis, minimal brain dysfunction, and hyperactivity. Workers who have concentrated on psychogenesis as causing episodic explosiveness have stressed identification with assaultive parental figures as symbols of the target for violence. Early frustration, oppression, and hostility have been noted as predisposing factors. Situations that are directly or symbolically reminiscent of early deprivations (e.g., persons who directly or indirectly evoke the image of the frustrating parent) become targets for destructive hostility.

Biological Factors. Some investigators suggest that disordered brain physiology, particularly in the limbic system, is involved in most cases of episodic violence. Compelling evidence indicates that serotonergic neurons mediate behavioral inhibition. Decreased serotonergic transmission, which can be induced by inhibiting serotonin synthesis or by antagonizing its effects, decreases the effect of punishment as a deterrent to behavior. The restoration of serotonin activity, by administering serotonin precursors such as L-tryptophan or drugs that increase synaptic serotonin levels, restores the behavioral effect of punishment. Restoring serotonergic activity by administration of L-tryptophan or drugs that increase synaptic serotonergic levels appears to restore control of episodic violent tendencies. Low levels of CSF 5-HIAA have been correlated with impulsive aggression. High CSF testosterone concentrations are correlated with aggressiveness and interpersonal violence in men. Antiandrogenic agents have been shown to decrease aggression.

Familial and Genetic Factors. First-degree relatives of intermittent explosive disorder patients have higher rates of impulse-control disorders, depressive disorders, and substance use disorders. Biological relatives of patients with the disorder were more likely to have histories of temper or explosive outbursts than the general population.

Diagnosis and Clinical Features

The diagnosis of intermittent explosive disorder should be the result of history-taking that reveals several episodes of loss of

control associated with aggressive outbursts (Table 25–1). One discrete episode does not justify the diagnosis. The histories typically describe a childhood in an atmosphere of alcohol dependence, violence, and emotional instability. Patients' work histories are poor; they report job losses, marital difficulties, and trouble with the law. Most patients have sought psychiatric help in the past but to no avail. Anxiety, guilt, and depression usually follow an outburst, but this is not a constant finding. Neurological examination sometimes reveals soft neurological signs such as left–right ambivalence and perceptual reversal. Electroencephalographic (EEG) findings are frequently normal or show nonspecific changes.

A 36-year-old real estate agent sought assistance for difficulty with his anger. He was quite competent at his job, though he frequently lost clients when he became enraged over their indecisiveness. On a number of occasions he became verbally abusive, leading clients to find ways out of escrow closings. The impulsive aggression also led to termination of multiple relationships because sudden angry outbursts contained demeaning accusations toward his girlfriends. This occurred frequently in the absence of any clear conflict. On multiple occasions, the patient became so uncontrollably enraged that he threw things across the room including books, his desk, and the contents of the refrigerator. Between episodes he was a kind and likable individual with many friends. He enjoyed drinking on the weekends and had a history of two arrests for driving while intoxicated. On one of these occasions he became involved in a verbal altercation with a police officer. He had a history of drug experimentation in college that included cocaine and marijuana.

Mental status examination revealed a generally cooperative patient. However, he became quite defensive when questioned about his anger and easily felt accused and blamed by the interviewer for his past behaviors. He had no significant medical history and no signs of neurological problems. He had never been in psychiatric treatment prior to this evaluation. He was on no medications. He denied any symptoms of a mood disorder or any other antisocial activity.

Treatment included the use of carbamazepine (Tegretol) and a combination of supportive and cognitive-behavioral psychotherapy. The patient's angry outbursts improved as he became aware of early signs that he was about to lose control. He learned techniques to avoid confrontation when he was faced with these warning signs. (Courtesy of Vivien K. Burt, M.D., Ph.D., and Jeffrey William Katzman, M.D.)

Physical Findings and Laboratory Examination

Persons with the disorder have a high incidence of soft neurological signs (e.g., reflex asymmetries), nonspecific EEG findings, abnormal neuropsychological testing results (e.g., letter reversal difficulties), and accident proneness. Blood chemistry (liver and thyroid function tests, fasting blood glucose, electrolytes), urinalysis (including drug toxicology), and syphilis serology may help rule out other causes of aggression. Magnetic resonance imagery (MRI) may reveal changes in the prefrontal cortex, which is associated with loss of impulse control.

Table 25–1
DSM-IV-TR Diagnostic Criteria for Intermittent Explosive Disorder

A. Several discrete episodes of failure to resist aggressive impulses that result in serious assaultive acts or destruction of property.

B. The degree of aggressiveness expressed during the episodes is grossly out of proportion to any precipitating psychosocial stressors.

C. The aggressive episodes are not better accounted for by another mental disorder (e.g., antisocial personality disorder, borderline personality disorder, a psychotic disorder, a manic episode, conduct disorder, or attention-deficit/hyperactivity disorder) and are not due to the direct physiological effects of a substance (e.g., a drug of abuse, a medication) or a general medical condition (e.g., head trauma, Alzheimer's disease).

From American Psychiatric Association. *Diagnostic and Statistical Manual of Mental Disorders.* 4th ed. Text rev. Washington, DC: American Psychiatric Association; copyright 2000, with permission.

Differential Diagnosis

The diagnosis of intermittent explosive disorder can be made only after disorders associated with the occasional loss of control of aggressive impulses have been ruled out as the primary cause. These other disorders include psychotic disorders, personality change due to a general medical condition, antisocial or borderline personality disorder, and substance intoxication (e.g., alcohol, barbiturates, hallucinogens, and amphetamines), epilepsy, brain tumors, degenerative diseases, and endocrine disorders.

Conduct disorder is distinguished from intermittent explosive disorder by its repetitive and resistant pattern of behavior, as opposed to an episodic pattern. Intermittent explosive disorder differs from the antisocial and borderline personality disorders because, in the personality disorders, aggressiveness and impulsivity are part of patients' characters and thus are present between outbursts. In paranoid and catatonic schizophrenia, patients may display violent behavior in response to delusions and hallucinations, and they show gross impairments in reality testing. Hostile patients with mania may be impulsively aggressive, but the underlying diagnosis is generally apparent from their mental status examinations and clinical presentations.

Amok is an episode of acute violent behavior for which the person claims amnesia. Amok is usually seen in southeastern Asia, but it has been reported in North America. Amok is distinguished from intermittent explosive disorder by a single episode and prominent dissociative features.

Course and Prognosis

Intermittent explosive disorder may begin at any stage of life but usually appears between late adolescence and early adulthood. The onset may be sudden or insidious, and the course may be episodic or chronic. In most cases the disorder decreases in severity with the onset of middle age, but heightened organic impairment can lead to frequent and severe episodes.

Treatment

A combined pharmacological and psychotherapeutic approach has the best chance of success. Psychotherapy with patients who have intermittent explosive disorder is difficult, however, because of their angry outbursts. Therapists may have problems with countertransference and limit setting. Group psychotherapy may be helpful, and family therapy is useful, particularly when the explosive patient is an adolescent or a young adult. A goal of therapy is to have the patient recognize and verbalize the thoughts or feelings that precede the explosive outbursts instead of acting them out.

Anticonvulsants have long been used, with mixed results, in treating explosive patients. Lithium (Eskalith) has been reported useful in generally lessening aggressive behavior, and carbamazepine, valproate (Depakene) or divalproex (Depakote), and phenytoin (Dilantin) have been reported helpful. Some clinicians have also used other anticonvulsants (e.g., gabapentin [Neurontin]). Benzodiazepines are sometimes used but have been reported to produce a paradoxical reaction of dyscontrol in some cases.

Antipsychotics (e.g., phenothiazines and serotonin-dopamine antagonists) and tricyclic drugs have been effective in some cases, but clinicians must then wonder whether schizophrenia or a mood disorder is the true diagnosis. When there is a likelihood of subcortical seizurelike activity, medications that lower the seizure threshold can aggravate the situation. Selective serotonin reuptake inhibitors (SSRIs), trazodone (Desyrel), and buspirone (BuSpar) are useful in reducing impulsivity and aggression.

Propranolol (Inderal) and other β-adrenergic receptor antagonists and calcium channel inhibitors have also been effective in some cases. Some neurosurgeons have performed operative treatments for intractable violence and aggression. No evidence indicates that such treatment is effective.

KLEPTOMANIA

The essential feature of kleptomania is a recurrent failure to resist impulses to steal objects not needed for personal use or for monetary value. The objects taken are often given away, returned surreptitiously, or kept and hidden. Persons with kleptomania usually have the money to pay for the objects they impulsively steal.

Like other impulse-control disorders, kleptomania is characterized by mounting tension before the act, followed by gratification and lessening of tension with or without guilt, remorse, or depression after the act. The stealing is not planned and does not involve others. Although the thefts do not occur when immediate arrest is probable, persons with kleptomania do not always consider their chances of being apprehended, even though repeated arrests lead to pain and humiliation. These persons may feel guilt and anxiety after the theft, but they do not feel anger or vengeance. Furthermore, when the object stolen is the goal, the diagnosis is not kleptomania; in kleptomania the act of stealing is itself the goal.

Epidemiology

The prevalence of kleptomania is not known but is estimated to be about 0.6 percent. The range varies from 3.8 to 24 percent of those arrested for shoplifting. DSM-IV-TR reports that it occurs in fewer than 5 percent of identified shoplifters. The male-to-female ratio is 1:3 in clinical samples.

Comorbidity

There is a high comorbidity with other disorders of impulse control, mood disorders, anxiety disorders, bulimia nervosa, and personality disorders. Many persons with kleptomania have obsessive-compulsive symptoms (e.g., cleaning, hand washing, collecting).

Etiology

Psychosocial Factors. The symptoms of kleptomania tend to appear in times of significant stress, for example, losses, separations, and endings of important relationships. Some psychoanalytic writers have stressed the expression of aggressive impulses in kleptomania; others have discerned a libidinal aspect. Those who focus on symbolism see meaning in the act itself, the object stolen, and the victim of the theft.

Analytic writers have focused on stealing by children and adolescents. Anna Freud pointed out that the first thefts from mother's purse indicate the degree to which all stealing is rooted in the oneness between mother and child. Karl Abraham wrote of the central feeling of being neglected, injured, or unwanted. One theoretician established seven categories of stealing in chronically acting-out children:

1. As a means of restoring the lost mother–child relationship
2. As an aggressive act
3. As a defense against fears of being damaged (perhaps a search by girls for a penis or a protection against castration anxiety in boys)
4. As a means of seeking punishment
5. As a means of restoring or adding to self-esteem
6. In connection with, and as a reaction to, a family secret
7. As excitement (lust angst) and a substitute for a sexual act

One or more of these categories can also apply to adult kleptomania.

Biological Factors. Brain diseases and mental retardation have been associated with kleptomania, as they have with other disorders of impulse control. Focal neurological signs, cortical atrophy, and enlarged lateral ventricles have been found in some patients. Disturbances in monoamine metabolism, particularly of serotonin, have been postulated.

Family and Genetic Factors. In one study, 7 percent of first-degree relatives had obsessive-compulsive disorder. In addition, a higher rate of mood disorders has been reported in family members.

Diagnosis and Clinical Features

The essential feature of kleptomania is recurrent, intrusive, and irresistible urges or impulses to steal unneeded objects (Table 25–2). Patients with kleptomania may also be distressed about the possibility or actuality of being apprehended and may manifest signs of depression and anxiety. Patients feel guilty, ashamed, and embarrassed about their behavior. They often

Table 25–2
DSM-IV-TR Diagnostic Criteria for Kleptomania

A. Recurrent failure to resist impulses to steal objects that are not needed for personal use or for their monetary value.
B. Increasing sense of tension immediately before committing the theft.
C. Pleasure, gratification, or relief at the time of committing the theft.
D. The stealing is not committed to express anger or vengeance and is not in response to a delusion or a hallucination.
E. The stealing is not better accounted for by conduct disorder, a manic episode, or antisocial personality disorder.

From American Psychiatric Association. *Diagnostic and Statistical Manual of Mental Disorders.* 4th ed. Text rev. Washington, DC: American Psychiatric Association; copyright 2000, with permission.

have serious problems with interpersonal relationships and often show signs of personality disturbance. In one study of patients with kleptomania, the frequency of stealing ranged from less than 1 to 120 episodes a month. Most kleptomaniac patients steal from retail stores, but they may also steal from family members in their own households.

Differential Diagnosis

Because most patients with kleptomania are referred for examination in connection with legal proceedings after apprehension, the clinical picture may be clouded by subsequent symptoms of depression and anxiety. Clinicians must differentiate between kleptomania and other forms of stealing. For a diagnosis of kleptomania, stealing must always follow a failure to resist the impulse and must be a solitary act, and the stolen articles must be without immediate usefulness or monetary gain. By contrast, ordinary stealing is usually planned, and the objects are stolen for their use or financial value. Malingerers may try to simulate kleptomania to avoid prosecution. Stealing that occurs in association with conduct disorder, antisocial personality disorder, or manic episodes is clearly related to the pervasive, underlying disorder. Persons with kleptomania do not typically display antisocial behavior other than stealing. Patients with schizophrenia may steal in response to hallucinations and delusions, and patients with cognitive disorders may be accused of stealing when they forget to pay for objects.

Course and Prognosis

Kleptomania may begin in childhood, although most children and adolescents who steal do not become kleptomaniac adults. The onset of the disorder generally is late adolescence. Women are more likely to present for psychiatric evaluation or treatment than are men. Men are more likely to be sent to prison. Men tend to present with the disorder at about 50 years of age and women, at about 35 years of age. In quiescent cases, new bouts of the disorder may be precipitated by loss or disappointment.

The course of the disorder waxes and wanes but tends to be chronic. Persons sometimes have bouts of being unable to resist the impulse to steal, followed by free periods that last for weeks or months. Its spontaneous recovery rate is unknown.

Serious impairment and complications are usually secondary to being caught, particularly to being arrested. Many persons seem never to have consciously considered the possibility of facing the consequences of their acts, a feature that agrees with some descriptions of patients with kleptomania (sometimes as persons who feel wronged and therefore entitled to steal). Often, the disorder in no way impairs a person's social or work functioning.

The prognosis with treatment can be good, but few patients come for help of their own accord.

Treatment

Because true kleptomania is rare, reports of treatment tend to be individual case descriptions or a short series of cases. Insight-oriented psychotherapy and psychoanalysis have been successful but depend on patients' motivations. Those who feel guilt and shame may be helped by insight-oriented psychotherapy because of their increased motivation to change their behavior.

Behavior therapy, including systematic desensitization, aversive conditioning, and a combination of aversive conditioning and altered social contingencies, has been reported successful, even when motivation was lacking. The reports cite follow-up studies of up to 2 years. SSRIs, such as fluoxetine (Prozac) and fluvoxamine (Luvox), appear to be effective in some patients with kleptomania. There have also been case reports of successful treatment with tricyclic drugs, trazodone, lithium, valproate, naltrexone (ReVia), and electroconvulsive therapy.

PYROMANIA

Pyromania is the recurrent, deliberate, and purposeful setting of fires. Associated features include tension or affective arousal before setting the fires; fascination with, interest in, curiosity about, or attraction to fire and the activities and equipment associated with fire fighting; and pleasure, gratification, or relief when setting fires or when witnessing or participating in their aftermath. Patients may make considerable advance preparations before starting a fire. Pyromania differs from arson in that the latter is done for financial gain, revenge, or other reasons and is planned beforehand.

Epidemiology

No information is available on the prevalence of pyromania, but only a small percentage of adults who set fires can be classified as having pyromania. The disorder is found far more often in men than in women. Among children who attend outpatient psychiatric clinics, about 20 percent have a history of occasional fire setting.

Comorbidity

Persons who set fires are more likely to be mildly retarded than are those in the general population. Some studies have noted an increased incidence of alcohol use disorders in persons who set fires. Fire setters also tend to have a history of antisocial traits, such as truancy, running away from home, and delinquency. Enuresis has been considered a common finding in the history of fire setters, although controlled studies have failed to confirm

this. Studies have, however, found an association between cruelty to animals and fire setting. Childhood and adolescent fire setting is often associated with attention-deficit/hyperactivity disorder or adjustment disorders.

Etiology

Psychosocial. Sigmund Freud saw fire as a symbol of sexuality. He believed the warmth radiated by fire evokes the same sensation that accompanies a state of sexual excitation, and a flame's shape and movements suggest a phallus in activity. Other psychoanalysts have associated pyromania with an abnormal craving for power and social prestige. Some patients with pyromania are volunteer firefighters who set fires to prove themselves brave, to force other firefighters into action, or to demonstrate their power to extinguish a blaze. The incendiary act is a way to vent accumulated rage over frustration caused by a sense of social, physical, or sexual inferiority. Several studies have noted that the fathers of patients with pyromania were absent from the home. Thus, one explanation of fire setting is that it represents a wish for the absent father to return home as a rescuer, to put out the fire, and to save the child from a difficult existence.

Female fire setters, in addition to being much fewer in number than male fire setters, do not start fires to put firefighters into action as men frequently do. Frequently noted delinquent trends in female fire setters include promiscuity without pleasure and petty stealing, often approaching kleptomania.

Biological Factors. Significantly low CSF levels of 5-HIAA and 3-methoxy-4-hydroxyphenylglycol (MHPG) have been found in fire setters, which suggests possible serotonergic or adrenergic involvement. The presence of reactive hypoglycemia, based on blood glucose concentrations on glucose tolerance tests, has been put forward as a cause of pyromania. Further studies are needed, however.

Diagnosis and Clinical Features

Persons with pyromania often regularly watch fires in their neighborhoods, frequently set off false alarms, and show interest in firefighting paraphernalia (Table 25–3). Their curiosity is evident, but they show no remorse and may be indifferent to the consequences for life or property. Fire setters may gain satisfaction from the resulting destruction; frequently, they leave obvious clues. Commonly associated features include alcohol intoxication, sexual dysfunctions, below-average intelligence quotient (IQ), chronic personal frustration, and resentment toward authority figures. Some fire setters become sexually aroused by the fire.

Table 25–3
DSM-IV-TR Diagnostic Criteria for Pyromania

A. Deliberate and purposeful fire setting on more than one occasion.
B. Tension or affective arousal before the act.
C. Fascination with, interest in, curiosity about, or attraction to fire and its situational contexts (e.g., paraphernalia, uses, consequences).
D. Pleasure, gratification, or relief when setting fires, or when witnessing or participating in their aftermath.
E. The fire setting is not done for monetary gain, as an expression of sociopolitical ideology, to conceal criminal activity, to express anger or vengeance, to improve one's living circumstances, in response to a delusion or hallucination, or as a result of impaired judgment (e.g., in dementia, mental retardation, substance intoxication).
F. The fire setting is not better accounted for by conduct disorder, a manic episode, or antisocial personality disorder.

From American Psychiatric Association. *Diagnostic and Statistical Manual of Mental Disorders.* 4th ed. Text rev. Washington, DC: American Psychiatric Association; copyright 2000, with permission.

Differential Diagnosis

Clinicians should have little trouble distinguishing between pyromania and the fascination of many young children with matches, lighters, and fire as part of the normal investigation of their environments. Pyromania must also be separated from incendiary acts of sabotage carried out by dissident political extremists or by paid torches, termed *arsonists* in the legal system.

When fire setting occurs in conduct disorder and antisocial personality disorder, it is a deliberate act, not a failure to resist an impulse. Fires may be set for profit, sabotage, or retaliation. Patients with schizophrenia or mania may set fires in response to delusions or hallucinations. Patients with brain dysfunction (e.g., dementia), mental retardation, or substance intoxication may set fires because of a failure to appreciate the consequences of the act.

Course and Prognosis

While fire setting often begins in childhood, the typical age of onset of pyromania is unknown. When the onset is in adolescence or adulthood, the fire setting tends to be deliberately destructive. Fire setting in pyromania is episodic and may wax and wane in frequency. The prognosis for treated children is good, and complete remission is a realistic goal. The prognosis for adults is guarded, because they frequently deny their actions, refuse to take responsibility, are dependent on alcohol, and lack insight.

Treatment

Little has been written about the treatment of pyromania, and treating fire setters has been difficult because of their lack of motivation. Until research reports the success of any single treatment, an appropriate approach is to use a number of modalities, including behavioral approaches. Because of the recurrent nature of pyromania, any treatment program should include supervision of patients to prevent a repeated episode of fire setting. Incarceration may be the only method of preventing a recurrence. Behavior therapy can then be administered in the institution.

Fire setting by children must be treated with the utmost seriousness. Intensive interventions should be undertaken when possible, but as therapeutic and preventive measures, not as punishment. In the case of children and adolescents, treatment of pyromania or fire setting should include family therapy.

PATHOLOGICAL GAMBLING

Pathological gambling is characterized by persistent and recurrent maladaptive gambling that causes economic problems and significant disturbances in personal, social, or occupational functioning. Aspects of the maladaptive behavior include (1) a preoccupation with gambling; (2) the need to gamble with increasing amounts of money to achieve the desired excitement; (3) repeated unsuccessful efforts to control, cut back, or stop gambling; (4) gambling as a way to escape from problems; (5) gambling to recoup losses; (6) lying to conceal the extent of the involvement with gambling; (7) the commission of illegal acts to finance gambling; (8) jeopardizing or losing personal and vocational relationships because of gambling; and (9) a reliance on others for money to pay off debts.

Epidemiology

Up to 3 percent of the general population may be classified as pathological gamblers. In addition, according to DSM-IV-TR, the prevalence of pathological gamblers has been reported to be from 2.8 to 8 percent in adolescents and college students. The disorder is more common in men than in women, and the rate is considerably higher in locations where gambling is legal. Approximately one fourth of pathological gamblers had a parent with a gambling problem; both the fathers of men and the mothers of women with the disorder are more likely to have the disorder than is the population at large. Alcohol dependence is also more common among the parents of pathological gamblers than in the overall population. Women with the disorder are more likely than those not so affected to be married to alcoholic men who are usually absent from the home.

Comorbidity

Rates of other impulse-control disorders, substance use disorders, mood disorders, attention-deficit/hyperactivity disorder, and antisocial, borderline, and narcissistic personality disorders are increased in persons with pathological gambling. Other associated disorders include panic disorder, agoraphobia, obsessive-compulsive disorder, and Tourette's disorder.

Etiology

Psychosocial Factors. Several factors may predispose persons to develop the disorder: loss of a parent by death, separation, divorce, or desertion before a child is 15 years of age; inappropriate parental discipline (absence, inconsistency, or harshness); exposure to, and availability of, gambling activities for adolescents; a family emphasis on material and financial symbols; and a lack of family emphasis on saving, planning, and budgeting.

Psychoanalytic theory has focused on a number of core character difficulties. Sigmund Freud suggested that compulsive gamblers have an unconscious desire to lose, and gamble to relieve unconscious feelings of guilt. Another suggestion is that the gamblers are narcissists whose grandiose and omnipotent fantasies lead them to believe they can control events and even predict their outcome. Learning theorists view uncontrolled gambling as resulting from erroneous perceptions regarding control of impulses.

Biological Factors. Several studies have suggested that gamblers' risk-taking behavior may have an underlying neurobiological cause. These theories have centered on both serotonergic and noradrenergic receptor systems. Male pathological gamblers may have subnormal MHPG concentrations in plasma, increased MHPG concentrations in the CSF, and increased urinary output of norepinephrine. Evidence also implicates serotonergic regulatory dysfunction in the pathological gambler. Chronic gamblers have low platelet monoamine oxidase (MAO) activity, a marker of serotonin activity, also linked to difficulties with inhibition. Further studies are needed to confirm these findings.

Diagnosis and Clinical Features

In addition to the features already described, pathological gamblers often appear overconfident, somewhat abrasive, energetic, and free spending. They often show obvious signs of personal stress, anxiety, and depression (Table 25–4). They commonly have the attitude that money is both the cause of, and the solution to, all their problems. As their gambling increases, they are usually forced to lie to obtain money and to continue gambling while hiding the extent of their gambling. They make no serious attempt to budget or save money. When their borrowing resources are strained, they are likely to engage in antisocial

Table 25–4
DSM-IV-TR Diagnostic Criteria for Pathological Gambling

A. Persistent and recurrent maladaptive gambling behavior as indicated by five (or more) of the following:
   (1) is preoccupied with gambling (e.g., preoccupied with reliving past gambling experiences, handicapping or planning the next venture, or thinking of ways to get money with which to gamble)
   (2) needs to gamble with increasing amounts of money in order to achieve the desired excitement
   (3) has repeated unsuccessful efforts to control, cut back, or stop gambling
   (4) is restless or irritable when attempting to cut down or stop gambling
   (5) gambles as a way of escaping from problems or of relieving a dysphoric mood (e.g., feelings of helplessness, guilt, anxiety, depression)
   (6) after losing money gambling, often returns another day to get even ("chasing" one's losses)
   (7) lies to family members, therapist, or others to conceal the extent of involvement with gambling
   (8) has committed illegal acts such as forgery, fraud, theft, or embezzlement to finance gambling
   (9) has jeopardized or lost a significant relationship, job, or educational or career opportunity because of gambling
   (10) relies on others to provide money to relieve a desperate financial situation caused by gambling

B. The gambling behavior is not better accounted for by a manic episode.

From American Psychiatric Association. *Diagnostic and Statistical Manual of Mental Disorders.* 4th ed. Text rev. Washington, DC: American Psychiatric Association; copyright 2000, with permission.

behavior to obtain money for gambling. Their criminal behavior is typically nonviolent, such as forgery, embezzlement, or fraud, and they consciously intend to return or repay the money. Complications include alienation from family members and acquaintances, the loss of life accomplishments, suicide attempts, and association with fringe and illegal groups. Arrest for nonviolent crimes may lead to imprisonment.

Mr. T. was a 47-year-old white male who presented to a community mental health center for evaluation of depression. In the course of the initial interview with the psychiatrist and social worker, he disclosed that he had previously been a quite successful manager of a restaurant in a Las Vegas hotel. He had been married, had two children, and supported a nice lifestyle. He became well known in several casinos and was given free nightly stays by a number of casinos. His gambling accelerated to the point at which he spent the entire family savings. He became unavailable at work because he spent his time around gambling activities. The business collapsed, and his wife later divorced him. He then moved to Los Angeles where he lived in an apartment while managing the other units in the building. He was responsible for collecting the rent from the tenants and turning it over to the building owner. However, on three occasions, he gambled a good portion of this money at the racetrack. The third episode involved a loss of $8,000. He was fired from this job and over the past year had been unable to find work because he had no references. Prior to his presentation to the mental health clinic, he was homeless for 6 months and was increasingly hopeless and suicidal.

An initial treatment plan involved mandatory daily attendance at Gamblers Anonymous and work with a sponsor in the 12-step model. He was started on a course of fluoxetine. He met weekly with his case manager in the clinic. His short-term goals involved acquiring housing and employment with continued abstinence from gambling. His long-term goals included reconnecting with his children whom he had not seen in many years. (Courtesy of Vivien K. Burt, M.D., and Jeffrey W. Katzman, M.D.)

Psychological Testing and Laboratory Examination

Males with the disorders have shown abnormalities in platelet MAO activity. Patients with pathological gambling often display high levels of impulsivity on neuropsychological tests. German studies have demonstrated increased cortisol levels in the saliva of gamblers while they gamble, which can account for the euphoria that occurs during the experience and its addictive potential.

Differential Diagnosis

Social gambling is distinguished from pathological gambling in that the former occurs with friends, on special occasions, and with predetermined acceptable and tolerable losses. Gambling that is symptomatic of a manic episode can usually be distinguished from pathological gambling by the history of a marked mood change and the loss of judgment preceding the gambling.

Maniclike mood changes are common in pathological gambling, but they always follow winning and are usually succeeded by depressive episodes because of subsequent losses. Persons with antisocial personality disorder may have problems with gambling. When both disorders are present, both should be diagnosed.

Course and Prognosis

Pathological gambling usually begins in adolescence for men and late in life for women. The disorder waxes and wanes and tends to be chronic. Four phases are seen in pathological gambling:

1. The winning phase, ending with a big win, equal to about a year's salary, which hooks patients. Women usually do not have a big win, but use gambling as an escape from problems.
2. The progressive-loss phase, in which patients structure their lives around gambling and then move from being excellent gamblers to being stupid ones who take considerable risks, cash in securities, borrow money, miss work, and lose jobs.
3. The desperate phase, with patients frenziedly gambling with large amounts of money, not paying debts, becoming involved with loan sharks, writing bad checks, and possibly embezzling.
4. The hopeless stage of accepting that losses can never be made up, but the gambling continues because of the associated arousal or excitement. The disorder may take up to 15 years to reach the last phase, but then, within a year or two, patients have deteriorated totally.

Treatment

Gamblers seldom come forward voluntarily to be treated. Legal difficulties, family pressures, or other psychiatric complaints bring gamblers to treatment. Gamblers Anonymous (GA) was founded in Los Angeles in 1957 and modeled on Alcoholics Anonymous (AA); it is accessible, at least in large cities, and is an effective treatment for gambling in some patients. GA is a method of inspirational group therapy that involves public confession, peer pressure, and the presence of reformed gamblers (like sponsors in AA) available to help members resist the impulse to gamble. However, the dropout rate from GA is high. In some cases, hospitalization may help by removing patients from their environments. Insight should not be sought until patients have been away from gambling for 3 months. At this point, patients who are pathological gamblers may become excellent candidates for insight-oriented psychotherapy. Family therapy is often valuable. Cognitive-behavioral therapy (e.g., relaxation techniques combined with visualization of gambling avoidance) have had some success.

Little is known about the efficacy of pharmacotherapy for treating patients with pathological gambling. One study reported that 7 of 10 patients remained completely abstinent over 8 weeks after taking fluvoxamine. There have also been case reports of successful treatment with lithium and clomipramine (Anafranil). If gambling is associated with depressive disorders, mania, anxiety, or other mental disorders, pharmacotherapy with antidepressants, lithium, or antianxiety agents is useful.

TRICHOTILLOMANIA

Trichotillomania was first described in 1889 by the French dermatologist François Hallopeau. According to DSM-IV-TR, the essential feature of trichotillomania is the recurrent pulling out of hair, which can result in noticeable hair loss. Other clinical symptoms include an increasing sense of tension before pulling the hair and a sense of pleasure, gratification, or relief when pulling out the hair. The diagnosis should not be made if hair pulling is the result of another mental disorder (e.g., disorders manifesting delusions or hallucinations) or a general medical disorder (e.g., a preexisting lesion of the skin).

Table 25–5
DSM-IV-TR Diagnostic Criteria for Trichotillomania

A. Recurrent pulling out of one's hair resulting in noticeable hair loss.
B. An increasing sense of tension immediately before pulling out the hair or when attempting to resist the behavior.
C. Pleasure, gratification, or relief when pulling out the hair.
D. The disturbance is not better accounted for by another mental disorder and is not due to a general medical condition (e.g., a dermatological condition).
E. The disturbance causes clinically significant distress or impairment in social, occupational, or other important areas of functioning.

From American Psychiatric Association. *Diagnostic and Statistical Manual of Mental Disorders.* 4th ed. Text rev. Washington, DC: American Psychiatric Association; copyright 2000, with permission.

Epidemiology

Trichotillomania is more common in women than in men but shows no sex difference in children. No information is available on familial patterns, but one study reported that 5 of 19 children had family histories of some form of alopecia. The lifetime prevalence according to DSM-IV-TR is below 1 percent, but this figure may be too low. Trichotillomania may be more common than is now believed, especially if hair pulling without the sense of tension before the pulling and without the sense of relief afterward is considered trichotillomania.

Comorbidity

Persons with trichotillomania have an increased prevalence of mood disorders (e.g., major depressive disorders), anxiety disorders (e.g., obsessive-compulsive disorders, generalized anxiety disorder, social phobia), substance use disorders, eating disorders, personality disorders (e.g., borderline and obsessive-compulsive), and mental retardation.

Etiology

Although trichotillomania is regarded as multidetermined, its onset has been linked to stressful situations in more than one fourth of all cases. Disturbances in mother–child relationships, fear of being left alone, and recent object loss are often cited as critical factors contributing to the condition. Substance abuse may encourage development of the disorder. Depressive dynamics are often cited as predisposing factors, but no particular personality trait or disorder characterizes patients. Some see self-stimulation as the primary goal of hair pulling.

Trichotillomania is increasingly being viewed as having a biologically determined substrate that may reflect inappropriately released motor activity or excessive grooming behaviors. Biological theories have also pointed to metabolic differences in the serotonin and opioid systems. Family members of trichotillomania patients often have a history of tics, impulse-control disorders, and obsessive-compulsive symptoms, further supporting a possible genetic predisposition.

Diagnosis and Clinical Features

Before engaging in the behavior, patients with trichotillomania experience an increasing sense of tension and achieve a sense of release or gratification from pulling out their hair (Table 25–5). All areas of the body may be affected, most commonly the scalp. Other areas involved are eyebrows, eyelashes, and beard; trunk, armpits, and pubic area are less commonly involved. Hair loss is often characterized by short, broken strands appearing together with long, normal hairs in the affected areas. No abnormalities of the skin or scalp are present. Hair pulling is not reported to be painful, although pruritus and tingling may occur in the involved area. Trichophagy, mouthing of the hair, may follow the hair plucking. Complications of trichophagy include trichobezoars, malnutrition, and intestinal obstruction. Patients usually deny the behavior and often try to hide the resultant alopecia. Head banging, nail biting, scratching, gnawing, excoriation, and other acts of self-mutilation may be present.

A 48-year-old woman presented to her internist for a routine physical examination. She became somewhat tearful during the interview, explaining that she was under tremendous pressure at home taking care of her three children and that she recently separated from her husband. During the physical examination, the patient pointed to her head saying that her hair had been falling out during this recent period of stress and that she was somewhat concerned about this. The physician noted that the patient had two distinct areas of hair thinning, one at the vertex of the scalp and one in the frontal region. He also noted that the eyebrow regions were covered with pencil. Otherwise results of the physical examination and routine blood work were normal. He suggested the possibility of a condition other than spontaneous stress-induced hair loss and referred her to a dermatologist. Quite reluctantly, she agreed to the referral.

The patient followed up with the dermatologist, who noted a mixture of long and short hairs in the thinning regions of the scalp. Specimens showed no pathology. When the dermatologist asked the woman whether she might be pulling out her hair, she hesitatingly disclosed that she was. Tearfully, she requested complete confidentiality and asked the physician if he had ever encountered this before. When he reassured her that he had numerous patients with her condition and that treatment was available, she was visibly relieved. (Courtesy of Vivien K. Burt, M.D., and Jeffrey W. Katzman, M.D.)

Pathology and Laboratory Examination

Characteristic histopathological changes in the hair follicle, known as trichomalacia, are demonstrated by biopsy and help distinguish trichotillomania from other causes of alopecia.

Differential Diagnosis

Hair pulling may be a wholly benign condition or it may occur in the context of several mental disorders. The phenomenology of trichotillomania and obsessive-compulsive disorder overlap. Like obsessive-compulsive disorder, trichotillomania is often chronic and recognized by patients as undesirable. Unlike those with obsessive-compulsive disorder, patients with trichotillomania do not experience obsessive thoughts, and the compulsive activity is limited to one act, hair pulling. Patients with factitious disorder with predominantly physical signs and symptoms actively seek medical attention and the patient role and deliberately simulate illness toward these ends. Patients who malinger or who have factitious disorder may mutilate themselves to get medical attention, but they do not acknowledge the self-inflicted nature of the lesions. Patients with stereotypic movement disorder have stereotypical and rhythmic movements, and they usually do not seem distressed by their behavior. A biopsy may be necessary to distinguish trichotillomania from alopecia areata and tinea capitis (Figs. 25–1 to 25–3).

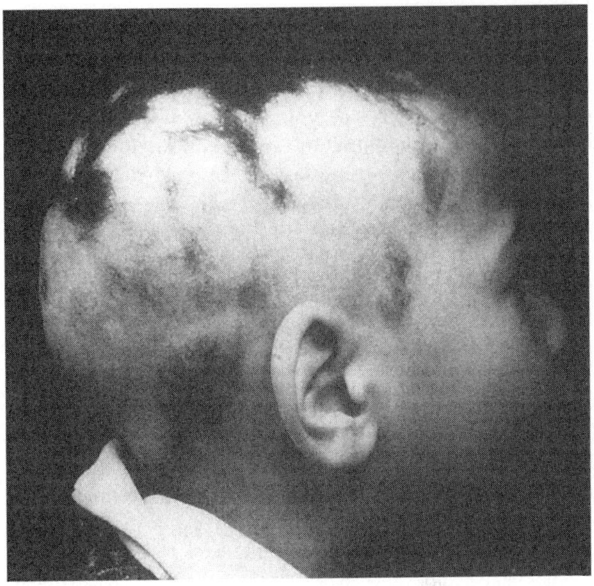

FIGURE 25–2
Alopecia areata. (Courtesy of Victor Newcomer, M.D.)

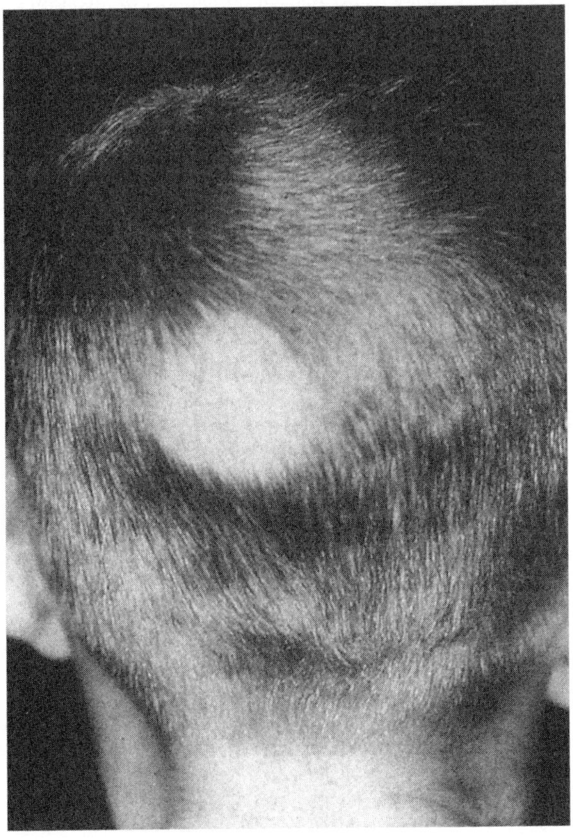

FIGURE 25–1
Tinea capitus in a young male due to *Microsporum audouinii*. (Courtesy of Victor Newcomer, M.D.)

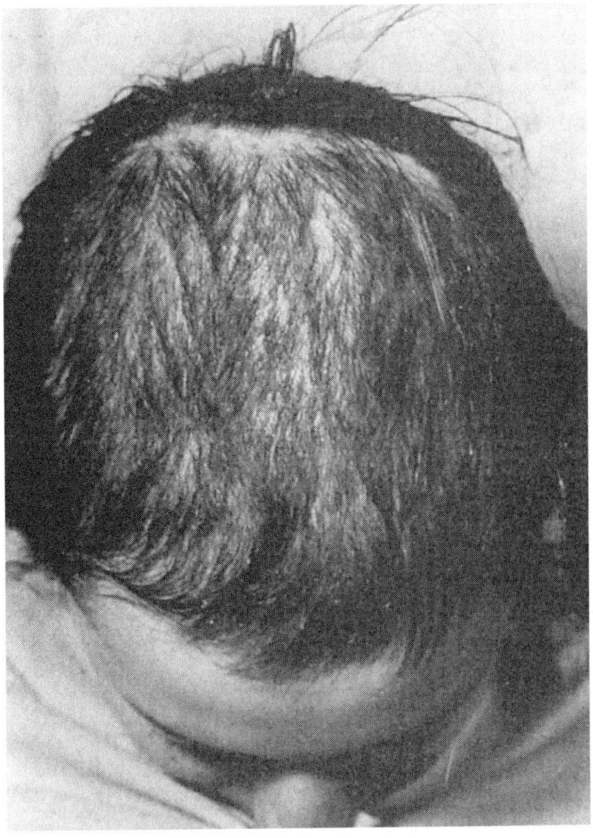

FIGURE 25–3
Trichotillomania with a mixture of short and long hairs with hair loss in a linear fashion. (Courtesy of Victor Newcomer, M.D.)

Course and Prognosis

The mean age at onset of trichotillomania is in the early teens, most frequently before age 17, but onsets have been reported much later in life. The course of the disorder is not well known; both chronic and remitting forms occur. An early onset (before age 6) tends to remit more readily and responds to suggestion, support, and behavioral strategies. Late onset (after age 13) is associated with an increased likelihood of chronicity and poorer prognosis than the early-onset form. About a third of persons presenting for treatment report a duration of 1 year or less, while in some cases the disorder has persisted for more than 2 decades.

Treatment

No consensus exists on the best treatment modality for trichotillomania. Treatment usually involves psychiatrists and dermatologists in a joint endeavor. Psychopharmacological methods that have been used to treat psychodermatological disorders include topical steroids and hydroxyzine hydrochloride (Vistaril), an anxiolytic with antihistamine properties; antidepressants; serotonergic agents; and antipsychotics. Whether depression is present or not, antidepressant agents may lead to dermatological improvement. Current evidence strongly points to the efficacy of drugs that alter central serotonin turnover. Patients who respond poorly to SSRIs may improve with augmentation with pimozide (Orap), a dopamine receptor antagonist. A report of successful lithium treatment for trichotillomania cited the possible effect of the drug on aggression, impulsivity, and mood instability as an explanation. Lithium also possesses serotonergic activity. There have been case reports of successful treatment with buspirone, clonazepam (Klonopin), and trazodone. In one placebo-controlled study, patients taking naltrexone had a reduction in symptom severity.

Successful behavioral treatments such as biofeedback, self-monitoring, covert desensitization, and habit reversal have been reported, but most studies have been based on individual cases or small series of cases with relatively short follow-up periods. Further controlled study of the treatments is warranted. Chronic trichotillomania has been treated successfully with insight-oriented psychotherapy. Hypnotherapy and behavior therapy have been mentioned as potentially effective in the treatment of dermatological disorders in which psychological factors may be involved; the skin has been shown to be susceptible to hypnotic suggestion. Most of the work has been research oriented, with little effect on clinical management.

IMPULSE-CONTROL DISORDER NOT OTHERWISE SPECIFIED

The DSM-IV-TR diagnostic category of impulse-control disorder not otherwise specified (Table 25–6) is a residual category for disorders of impulse control that do not meet the criteria for a specific impulse-control disorder. Some of the impulse disorders are listed below as compulsive disorders. There are important, although subtle, distinctions between the two terms. An *impulse* is a tension state that can exist without an action; a *compulsion* is a tension state that always has an action component. The disorders are classified here as compulsions because the patients feel "compelled" to act out their pathological behavior; they cannot resist the impulse to do so. Impulses are acted upon with the expectation of receiving pleasure; compulsions are usually ego-dystonic; for example, the patient does not like having to perform the act even though compelled to do so. An exception to the rule that impulses are associated with pleasure are those cases in which feelings of guilt follow the act and disturb the sense of pleasure. Similarly, not all compulsions are ego-dystonic; for example, certain compulsive video game playing may have a pleasurable component. Both impulsive and compulsive behaviors are characterized by their repetitive nature; however, the repeated acting out of impulses leads to psychosocial impairment, whereas compulsive behavior does not always carry that risk. Because of the repetitive and pleasurable nature of many of the behavioral patterns in this group of disorders they are often referred to as *addictions*.

Table 25–6
DSM-IV-TR Diagnostic Criteria for Impulse-Control Disorder Not Otherwise Specified

This category is for disorders of impulse control (e.g., skin picking) that do not meet the criteria for any specific impulse-control disorder or for another mental disorder having features involving impulse control described elsewhere in the manual (e.g., substance dependence, a paraphilia).

From American Psychiatric Association. *Diagnostic and Statistical Manual of Mental Disorders.* 4th ed. Text rev. Washington, DC: American Psychiatric Association; copyright 2000, with permission.

Compulsive Buying

Originally referred to as *oniomania* and recognized by Emil Kraeplin and Eugen Bleuler, compulsive buying is not listed as a separate diagnostic category in DSM-IV-TR and ICD-10. Proposed diagnostic criteria are listed in Table 25–7. Compulsive buying is estimated to affect 1.1 to 5.9 percent of the general population. It is more common in women than in men.

Table 25–7
Diagnostic Criteria for Compulsive Buying

A. Maladaptive preoccupation with buying or shopping, or maladaptive buying or shopping impulses or behavior, as indicated by at least one of the following:
   1. Frequent preoccupation with buying or impulses to buy that are experienced as irresistible, intrusive, and/or senseless.
   2. Frequent buying of more than can be afforded, frequent buying of items that are not needed, or shopping for longer periods of time than intended.

B. The buying preoccupations, impulses, or behaviors cause marked distress, are time consuming, significantly interfere with social or occupational functioning, or result in financial problems (e.g., indebtedness or bankruptcy).

C. The excessive buying or shopping behavior does not occur exclusively during periods of hypomania or mania.

Reprinted with permission from McElroy SL, Keck PE Jr, Pope HG Jr, Smith JM, Strakowski SM. Compulsive buying: a report of 20 cases. *J Clin Psychiatry.* 1994;55:242.

The cause of the disorder is unknown. Psychodynamic theories have implicated low self-esteem, anxiety, and the need to reduce stress. Comorbid conditions include other disorders of impulse control (e.g., kleptomania), mood disorders, and obsessive-compulsive disorders. A diagnosis of compulsive buying should not be made if the behavior occurs as part of a hypomanic or manic episode.

The onset of the disorder is usually about 18 years of age; however, patients do not seek treatment until their 20s or 30s, usually because they have developed serious financial problems. Compulsive buyers usually buy with credit and have many credit cards. Serious financial problems are usual, and some persons must declare bankruptcy. One study reported an average debt in compulsive shoppers of $23,000. The disorder may be chronic with urges to buy occurring hourly or as infrequently as once a month. Patients often try to limit their behavior but are unsuccessful.

Treatment of compulsive buying is difficult. Some patients are helped with supportive therapy, insight-oriented therapy, and self-help groups, such as Debtors Anonymous. Pharmacological therapies include antidepressants, antimanic drugs, anxiolytics, and antipsychotics to treat any comorbid conditions. The SSRIs have been used to limit compulsive behavior and may be of use in this condition, which has compulsive aspects.

Internet Compulsion

Also called *Internet addiction,* many persons spend almost all their waking hours at the computer terminal. Their patterns of use are repetitive and constant, and they are unable to resist strong urges to use the computer or to "surf the Web." Internet addicts may gravitate to certain sites that meet specific needs (e.g., shopping, sex, and interactive games, among others). Video game compulsive behavior is a variant behavioral pattern.

Cellular or Mobile Phone Compulsion

Some persons compulsively use mobile phones to call others—friends, acquaintances, or business associates. They justify their need to contact others by giving plausible reasons for calling; but there are underlying conflicts that may be expressed in the behavior, such as fear of being alone, the need to satisfy unconscious dependency needs, or undoing a hostile wish toward a loved one, among others.

Repetitive Self-Mutilation

Persons who repeatedly cut themselves or do damage to their bodies may do so in a compulsive manner. In all cases another disorder will be found. Parasuicidal behavior is common in borderline personality disorder. Compulsive body piercing or tattooing may be a symptom of a paraphilia or a depressive equivalent.

Compulsive Sexual Behavior

There are persons who repeatedly seek out sexual gratification, often in perverse ways (e.g., exhibitionism). They are unable to control their behavior and may not experience feelings of guilt after an episode of acting-out behavior. Sometimes called *sexual addiction,* this condition is discussed extensively in Chapter 21, "Human Sexuality."

Table 25–8
ICD-10 Diagnostic Criteria for Habit and Impulse Disorders

Pathological gambling

A. Two or more episodes of gambling occur over a period of at least 1 year.
B. These episodes do not have a profitable outcome for the individual but are continued despite personal distress and interference with personal functioning in daily living.
C. The individual describes an intense urge to gamble which is difficult to control and reports that he or she is unable to stop gambling by an effort of will.
D. The individual is preoccupied with thoughts or mental images of the act of gambling or the circumstances surrounding the act.

Pathological fire setting (pyromania)

A. There are two or more acts of fire setting without apparent motive.
B. The individual describes an intense urge to set fire to objects, with a feeling of tension before the act and relief afterward.
C. The individual is preoccupied with thoughts or mental images of fire setting or of the circumstances surrounding the act (e.g., abnormal interest in fire engines or in calling out the fire service).

Pathological stealing (kleptomania)

A. There are two or more thefts in which the individual steals without any apparent motive of personal gain or gain for another person.
B. The individual describes an intense urge to steal, with a feeling of tension before the act and relief afterward.

Trichotillomania

A. Noticeable hair loss is caused by the individual's persistent and recurrent failure to resist impulses to pull out hairs.
B. The individual describes an intense urge to pull out hairs, with mounting tension before the act and a sense of relief afterward.
C. There is no preexisting inflammation of the skin, and the hair pulling is not in response to a delusion or hallucination.

Other habit and impulse disorders

This category should be used for other kinds of persistently repeated maladaptive behaviors that are not secondary to a recognized psychiatric syndrome and in which it appears that there is repeated failure to resist impulses to carry out the behavior. There is a prodromal period of tension with a feeling of release at the time of the act.

Habit and impulse disorder, unspecified

Reprinted with permission from World Health Organization. *The ICD-10 Classification of Mental and Behavioural Disorders: Diagnostic Criteria for Research.* Copyright World Health Organization, Geneva, 1993.

ICD-10

In the 10th revision of the *International Statistical Classification of Diseases and Related Health Problems* (ICD-10), the categories listed in DSM-IV-TR under impulse control are discussed under habit and impulse disorders (Table 25–8). In this brief category, habit and impulse disorders are characterized by uncontrollable "repeated acts

that have no clear rational motivation and that generally harm the patient's own interests and those of other persons."

References

Aichhorn A. *Wayward Youth.* New York: Viking; 1935.

Allcock CC. Pathological gambling. *Aust N Z J Psychiatry.* 1986;20:259.

Benson AL, ed. *I Shop, Therefore I Am: Compulsive Buying and the Search for Self.* Northvale, NJ: Jason Aronson; 2000.

Black DW, Gabel J, Hansen J, Schlosser S. A double-blind comparison of fluvoxamine versus placebo in the treatment of compulsive buying disorder. *Ann Clin Psychiatry.* 2000;12:205.

Burt VK, Datzman JW. Impulse-control disorders not elsewhere classified. In: Sadock BJ, Sadock VA, eds. *Kaplan & Sadock's Comprehensive Textbook of Psychiatry.* 7th ed. Vol 1. Baltimore: Lippincott Williams & Wilkins; 2000:1701.

Campbell F, Lester D. The impact of gambling opportunities on compulsive gambling. *J Soc Psychol.* 1999;139:126.

Chong SA, Low BL. Treatment of kleptomania with fluvoxamine. *Acta Psychiatr Scand.* 1996;93:314.

Christenson GA, Crow SJ. The characterization and treatment of trichotillomania. *J Clin Psychiatry.* 1996;57(8 suppl):42.

DeCaria CM, Hollander E, Grossman R, Wong CM, Mosovich SA, Cherkasky S. Diagnosis, neurobiology, and treatment of pathological gambling. *J Clin Psychiatry.* 1996;57(8 suppl):80.

Greenberg HR, Sarner CA. Trichotillomania: symptom and syndrome. *Arch Gen Psychiatry.* 1965;12:482.

Hollander E, Rosen J. Impulsivity. *J Psychopharmacol.* 2000;14(2 suppl):S39.

Hollander E, Rosen J. Obsessive-compulsive spectrum disorders: a review. In: Maj M, Sartorius N, Okasha A, et al., eds. *Obsessive-Compulsive Disorder. WPA Series Evidence and Experience in Psychiatry.* Vol 4. New York: John Wiley & Sons; 2000:203.

Ibanez A, Blanco C, Saiz-Ruiz J. Neurobiology and genetics of pathological gambling. *Psychiatr Ann.* 2002;32:181.

Jaspers JPC. The diagnosis and psychopharmacological treatment of trichotillomania: a review. *Pharmacopsychiatry.* 1996;29:115.

Jenkins SC, Maruta T. Therapeutic use of propranolol for intermittent explosive disorder. *Mayo Clin Proc.* 1987;62:204.

Keuthen NJ, Savage CR, O'Sullivan RL, Brown H. Neuropsychological functioning in trichotillomania. *Biol Psychiatry.* 1996;39:747.

Lochner C, Simeon D, Niehaus DJ, Stein DJ. Trichotillomania and skin-picking: a phenomenological comparison. *Depress Anxiety.* 2002;15:83.

McElroy SL, Keck PE, Phillips KA. Kleptomania, compulsive buying, and binge eating disorder. *J Clin Psychiatry.* 1995;56(4 suppl):14.

McElroy SL, Pope HG, Hudson JI, Keck PE, White KL. Kleptomania: a report of 20 cases. *Am J Psychiatry.* 1991;148:652.

Milligan R-J, Waller G. Anger and impulsivity in non-clinical women. *Pers Individ Differ.* 2001;30:1073.

Rugle L, Melamed L. Neuropsychological assessment of attention problems in pathological gamblers. *J Nerv Ment Dis.* 1993;181:107.

Schultheiss OC, Rohde W. Implicit power motivation predicts men's testosterone changes and implicit learning in a contest situation. *Horm Behav.* 2002;41:195.

Vitulano LA, King RA, Scahill L, Cohen DS. Behavioral treatment of children and adolescents with trichotillomania. *J Am Acad Child Adolesc Psychiatry.* 1992;31:109.

26

Adjustment Disorders

Adjustment disorders are short-term maladaptive reactions to what a layperson would call a personal calamity but in psychiatric terms would be referred to as a *psychosocial stressor.* An adjustment disorder is expected to remit soon after the stressor ceases or, if it persists, a new level of adaptation is achieved.

According to the text revision of the fourth edition of *Diagnostic and Statistical Manual of Mental Disorders* (DSM-IV-TR), symptoms must appear within 3 months of a stressor's onset. The nature and severity of the stressors are not specified. However, the stressors are more often everyday events that are ubiquitous (e.g., loss of a loved one, change of employment or financial situation) rather than rare, catastrophic events (e.g., natural disasters, violent crimes). The disturbance must not fulfill the criteria for another major psychiatric disorder or bereavement (not considered a mental disorder, although it may be a focus of clinical attention). The symptoms of the disorder usually resolve within 6 months, although they may last longer if produced by a chronic stressor or one with long-lasting consequences.

EPIDEMIOLOGY

According to DSM-IV-TR, the prevalence of the disorder is estimated to be from 2 to 8 percent of the general population. Women are diagnosed twice as often as men, and single women are generally overly represented as most at risk. In children and adolescents, boys and girls are equally diagnosed with adjustment disorders. The disorders may occur at any age but are most frequently diagnosed in adolescents. Among adolescents of either sex, common precipitating stresses are school problems, parental rejection and divorce, and substance abuse. Among adults, common precipitating stresses are marital problems, divorce, moving to a new environment, and financial problems.

Adjustment disorders are one of the most common psychiatric diagnoses for disorders of patients hospitalized for medical and surgical problems. In one study, 5 percent of persons admitted to a hospital over a 3-year period were classified as having an adjustment disorder. Up to 50 percent of persons with specific medical problems or stressors have been diagnosed with adjustment disorders. Furthermore, 10 to 30 percent of mental health outpatients and up to 12 percent of general hospital inpatients referred for mental health consultations have been diagnosed with adjustment disorders.

ETIOLOGY

By definition, an adjustment disorder is precipitated by one or more stressors. The severity of the stressor or stressors does not always predict the severity of the disorder; the stressor severity is a complex function of degree, quantity, duration, reversibility, environment, and personal context. For example, the loss of a parent is different for a 10-year-old and a 40-year-old. Personality organization and cultural or group norms and values also contribute to the disproportionate responses to stressors.

Stressors may be single, such as a divorce or the loss of a job, or multiple, such as the death of a person important to a patient which coincides with the patient's own physical illness and loss of a job. Stressors may be recurrent, such as seasonal business difficulties, or continuous, such as chronic illness or poverty. A discordant intrafamilial relationship may produce an adjustment disorder that affects the entire family system, or the disorder may be limited to a patient who was perhaps the victim of a crime or who has a physical illness. Sometimes adjustment disorders occur in a group or community setting, and the stressors affect several persons, as in a natural disaster or in racial, social, or religious persecution. Specific developmental stages, such as beginning school, leaving home, getting married, becoming a parent, failing to achieve occupational goals, having the last child leave home, and retiring, are often associated with adjustment disorders.

Psychodynamic Factors

Pivotal to understanding adjustment disorders is an understanding of three factors: the nature of the stressor, the conscious and unconscious meanings of the stressor, and the patient's preexisting vulnerability. A concurrent personality disorder or organic impairment may make a person vulnerable to adjustment disorders. Vulnerability is also associated with the loss of a parent during infancy or being reared in a dysfunctional family. Actual or perceived support from key relationships may affect behavioral and emotional responses to stressors.

Several psychoanalytic researchers have pointed out that the same stress can produce a range of responses in various normal human beings. Throughout his life, Sigmund Freud remained interested in why the stresses of ordinary life produce illness in some and not in others, why an illness takes a particular form, and why some experiences and not others predispose a person to psychopathology. He gave considerable weight to constitutional factors and viewed them as interacting with a person's life experiences to produce fixation.

Psychoanalytic research has emphasized the role of the mother and the rearing environment in a person's later capacity to respond to stress. Particularly important was Donald Winni-

cott's concept of the *good-enough mother*, a person who adapts to the infant's needs and provides enough support to enable the growing child to tolerate the frustrations in life.

Clinicians must undertake a detailed exploration of a patient's experience of the stressor. Certain patients commonly place all the blame on a particular event when a less obvious event may have had more significant psychological meaning for the patient. Current events may reawaken past traumas or disappointments from childhood, so patients should be encouraged to think about how the current situation relates to similar past events.

Throughout early development, each child develops a unique set of defense mechanisms to deal with stressful events. Because of greater amounts of trauma or greater constitutional vulnerability, some children have less mature defensive constellations than other children. This disadvantage may cause them as adults to react with substantially impaired functioning when they are faced with a loss, a divorce, or a financial setback; those who have developed mature defense mechanisms are less vulnerable and bounce back more quickly from the stressor. Resilience is also crucially determined by the nature of children's early relationships with their parents. Studies of trauma repeatedly indicate that supportive, nurturant relationships prevent traumatic incidents from causing permanent psychological damage.

Psychodynamic clinicians must consider the relation between a stressor and the human developmental life cycle. When adolescents leave home for college, for example, they are at high developmental risk for reacting with a temporary symptomatic picture. Similarly, if the young person who leaves home is the last child in the family, the parents may be particularly vulnerable to a reaction of adjustment disorder. Moreover, middle-aged persons who are confronting their own mortality may be especially sensitive to the effects of loss or death.

Table 26–1
DSM-IV Diagnostic Criteria for Adjustment Disorders

A. The development of emotional or behavioral symptoms in response to an identifiable stressor(s) occurring within 3 months of the onset of the stressor(s).

B. These symptoms or behaviors are clinically significant as evidenced by either of the following:
  (1) marked distress that is in excess of what would be expected from exposure to the stressor
  (2) significant impairment in social or occupational (academic) functioning

C. The stress-related disturbance does not meet the criteria for another specific Axis I disorder and is not merely an exacerbation of a preexisting Axis I or Axis II disorder.

D. The symptoms do not represent bereavement.

E. Once the stressor (or its consequences) has terminated, the symptoms do not persist for more than an additional 6 months.

Specify if:

Acute: if the disturbance lasts less than 6 months

Chronic: if the disturbance lasts for 6 months or longer

Adjustment disorders are coded based on the subtype, which is selected according to the predominant symptoms. The specific stressor(s) can be specified on Axis IV.

With depressed mood
With anxiety
With mixed anxiety and depressed mood
With disturbance of conduct
With mixed disturbance of emotions and conduct
Unspecified

From American Psychiatric Association. *Diagnostic and Statistical Manual of Mental Disorders.* 4th ed. Text rev. Washington, DC: American Psychiatric Association; copyright 2000.

Family and Genetic Factors

Some studies suggest that certain persons appear to be at increased risk both for the occurrence of these adverse life events and for the development of pathology once they occur. Findings from a study of over 2,000 twin pairs indicate that life events and stressors are modestly correlated in twin pairs, with monozygotic twins showing greater concordance than dizygotic twins. Family-environmental and genetic factors each accounted for approximately 20 percent of the variance in that study. Another twin study, which examined genetic contributions to the development of posttraumatic stress disorder symptoms (not necessarily at the level of full disorder, and therefore relevant to adjustment disorders), also concluded that the likelihood of developing symptoms in response to traumatic life events is partially under genetic control.

DIAGNOSIS AND CLINICAL FEATURES

Although by definition adjustment disorders follow a stressor, the symptoms do not necessarily begin immediately. Up to 3 months may elapse between a stressor and the development of symptoms. Symptoms do not always subside as soon as the stressor ceases; if the stressor continues, the disorder may be chronic. The disorder may occur at any age, and its symptoms vary considerably, with depressive, anxious, and mixed features most common in adults. Physical symptoms are most common in children and the elderly but may occur in any age group. Manifestations may also include assaultive behavior and reckless driving, excessive drinking, defaulting on legal responsibilities, withdrawal, vegetative signs, insomnia, and suicidal behavior.

The clinical presentations of adjustment disorder can vary widely. DSM-IV-TR lists six adjustment disorders, including an unspecified category (Table 26–1).

Adjustment Disorder with Depressed Mood

In adjustment disorder with depressed mood, the predominant manifestations are depressed mood, tearfulness, and hopelessness. This type must be distinguished from major depressive disorder and uncomplicated bereavement. Adolescents with this type are at increased risk for major depressive disorder in young adulthood.

Adjustment Disorder with Anxiety

Symptoms of anxiety, such as palpitations, jitteriness, and agitation, are present in adjustment disorder with anxiety, which must be differentiated from anxiety disorders.

Adjustment Disorder with Mixed Anxiety and Depressed Mood

In adjustment disorder with mixed anxiety and depressed mood, patients exhibit features of both anxiety and depression that do not meet the criteria for an already established anxiety disorder or depressive disorder.

A 21-year-old college senior was in her usual state of health, vacationing with her aunt and uncle in Arizona during spring break. While she was away, a letter containing a copy of her full college transcript arrived at her parents' home. On reading the letter, her parents noticed that the grades on the transcript did not match those that they had previously seen at the end of each semester since freshman year. The mother called her daughter and confronted her with this information. During the conversation it became apparent that the daughter had been changing the grades on the transcripts that were sent home so that the grades her parents saw were better than was actually the case. An argument ensued and harsh words were exchanged. Following these events, the daughter became extremely upset and experienced feelings of anxiety and depressed mood. She felt ashamed about the situation and saw no way out. She spent most of the next 2 days in her room and did not participate in pleasurable activities; there were periods of crying as well as decreased eating and sleeping. Her aunt and uncle were only somewhat able to comfort her. Two days later, without warning, the patient ingested 10 tablets of an over-the-counter sleep preparation. Later that day, the aunt found the patient to be lethargic, and upon questioning, determined that she had made a suicide attempt. The patient was brought to a local emergency room, where she was admitted and retained in the psychiatric inpatient unit for several days. The patient's mother flew to Arizona to meet with her daughter and the hospital staff. Following crisis intervention, the patient was released with her mother to return home, where they consulted with another psychiatrist. By the time of this second evaluation, there were no longer signs of depressed or anxious mood, nor was there any suicidal ideation. The treatment plan consisted of crisis intervention, continued individual therapy for the patient on return to school, counseling for the parents, and conjoint family sessions to be held monthly during scheduled home visits. Despite continued individual and family upset over the precipitating event and the subsequent suicide attempt, the patient was able to return to school the following week to complete her spring semester. (Courtesy of Jeffrey H. Newcorn, M.D., James J. Strain, M.D., and Juan E. Mezzich, M.D., Ph.D.)

Adjustment Disorder with Disturbance of Conduct

In adjustment disorder with disturbance of conduct, the predominant manifestation involves conduct in which the rights of others are violated or age-appropriate societal norms and rules are disregarded. Examples of behavior in this category are truancy, vandalism, reckless driving, and fighting. The category must be differentiated from conduct disorder and antisocial personality disorder.

Adjustment Disorder with Mixed Disturbance of Emotions and Conduct

A combination of disturbances of emotions and of conduct sometimes occurs. Clinicians are encouraged to try to make one or the other diagnosis in the interest of clarity.

Adjustment Disorder Unspecified

Adjustment disorder unspecified is a residual category for atypical maladaptive reactions to stress. Examples include inappropriate responses to the diagnosis of physical illness, such as massive denial, severe noncompliance with treatment, and social withdrawal, without significant depressed or anxious mood.

ICD-10

The 10th revision of the *International Statistical Classification of Diseases and Related Health Problems* (ICD-10) places adjustment disorders in the same category as reactions to severe stress. ICD-10 also includes acute stress reaction and posttraumatic stress disorder in this category (see Table 16.1–11). ICD-10's time pattern for the disorders differs from that of DSM-IV, with an onset usually within a month of the stressful event or life change and a duration usually of no more than 6 months (Table 26–2). ICD also highlights particular features of maladjustment to stress in children, best exemplified by regressive behaviors such as bed-wetting, babyish speech, or thumb sucking. These behaviors are coded as adjustment disorders with predominant disturbance of other emotions.

DIFFERENTIAL DIAGNOSIS

Although uncomplicated bereavement can often produce temporarily impaired social and occupational functioning, the person's dysfunction remains within the expectable bounds of a reaction to the loss of a loved one and thus is not considered adjustment disorder. Other disorders from which adjustment disorder must be differentiated include major depressive disorder, brief psychotic disorder, generalized anxiety disorder, somatization disorder, substance-related disorder, conduct disorder, academic problem, occupational problem, identity problem, and posttraumatic stress disorder. These diagnoses should be given precedence in all cases that meet their criteria, even in the presence of a stressor or group of stressors that served as a precipitant. Patients with an adjustment disorder are impaired in social or occupational functioning and show symptoms beyond the normal and expectable reaction to the stressor. Because no absolute criteria help to distinguish an adjustment disorder from another condition, clinical judgment is necessary. Some patients may meet the criteria for both an adjustment disorder and a personality disorder. If the adjustment disorder follows a physical illness, the clinician must make sure that the symptoms are not a continuation or another manifestation of the illness or its treatment.

Acute and Posttraumatic Stress Disorders

In posttraumatic stress disorder or acute stress disorder, the symptoms develop after a traumatic event or events outside the

Table 26–2
ICD-10 Diagnostic Criteria for Adjustment Disorders

A. Onset of symptoms must occur within 1 month of exposure to an identifiable psychosocial stressor, not of an unusual or catastrophic type.

B. The individual manifests symptoms or behavior disturbance of the types found in any of the affective disorders (except for delusions and hallucinations), any disorder in neurotic, stress-related, and somatoform disorders, and conduct disorders, but the criteria for an individual disorder are not fulfilled. Symptoms may be variable in both form and severity.

The predominant feature of the symptoms may be further specified.

Brief depressive reaction

A transient mild depressive state of a duration not exceeding 1 month.

Prolonged depressive reaction

A mild depressive state occurring in response to a prolonged exposure to a stressful situation but of a duration not exceeding 2 years.

Mixed anxiety and depressive reaction

Both anxiety and depressive symptoms are prominent, but at levels no greater than those specified for mixed anxiety and depressive disorder or other mixed anxiety disorders.

With predominant disturbance of other emotions

The symptoms are usually of several types of emotions, such as anxiety, depression, worry, tensions, and anger. Symptoms of anxiety and depression may meet the criteria for mixed anxiety and depressive disorder or for other mixed anxiety disorders, but they are not so predominant that other more specific depressive or anxiety disorders can be diagnosed. This category should also be used for reactions in children in whom regressive behavior such as bed-wetting or thumb-sucking is also present.

With predominant disturbance of conduct

The main disturbance is one involving conduct, e.g., an adolescent grief reaction resulting in aggressive or dissocial behavior.

With mixed disturbance of emotions and conduct

Both emotional symptoms and disturbances of conduct are prominent features.

With other specified predominant symptoms

C. Except in prolonged depressive reaction, the symptoms do not persist for more than 6 months after the cessation of the stress or its consequences. However, this should not prevent a provisional diagnosis being made if this criterion is not yet fulfilled.

Reprinted with permission from World Health Organization. *The ICD-10 Classification of Mental and Behavioural Disorders: Diagnostic Criteria for Research.* Copyright, World Health Organization, Geneva, 1993.

range of normal human experience. The stressors producing this syndrome are expected to cause a psychological reaction in the average person. Persons may experience the stressor alone, as in rape or assault, or in groups, as in military combat or death camps. Mass catastrophes—such as hurricanes, floods, airplane crashes, and atomic bombings—are also identified as stressors. These stressors contain a psychological component and frequently a concomitant physical component that may directly damage persons' nervous systems. The disorder is more severe and longer lasting when the stressor is of human origin (e.g., rape) than when it is not (e.g., floods). In adjustment disorders, the precipitating stress need not be severe or unusual. Posttraumatic stress disorder is discussed fully in Chapter 16.5.

COURSE AND PROGNOSIS

With appropriate treatment, the overall prognosis of an adjustment disorder is generally favorable. Most patients return to their previous level of functioning within 3 months. Some persons (particularly adolescents) who receive a diagnosis of an adjustment disorder later have mood disorders or substance-related disorders. Adolescents usually require a longer time to recover than adults.

TREATMENT

Psychotherapy

Psychotherapy remains the treatment of choice for adjustment disorders. Group therapy can be particularly useful for patients who have undergone similar stresses—for example, a group of retired persons or patients undergoing renal dialysis. Individual psychotherapy offers the opportunity to explore the meaning of the stressor to the patient so that earlier traumas can be worked through. After successful therapy, patients sometimes emerge from an adjustment disorder stronger than in the premorbid period, although no pathology was evident during that period. Because a stressor can be clearly delineated in adjustment disorders, it is often believed that psychotherapy is not indicated and that the disorder will remit spontaneously. However, this viewpoint ignores the fact that many persons exposed to the same stressor experience different symptoms, and in adjustment disorders, the response is pathological. Psychotherapy can help persons adapt to stressors that are not reversible or time limited and can serve as a preventive intervention if the stressor does remit. Psychiatrists treating adjustment disorders must be particularly aware of problems of secondary gain. The illness role may be rewarding to some normal persons who have had little experience with illness's capacity to free them from responsibility. Thus, patients can find therapists' attention, empathy, and understanding, which are necessary for success, rewarding in their own right, and therapists may thereby reinforce patients' symptoms. Such considerations must be weighed before intensive psychotherapy is begun; when a secondary gain has already been established, therapy is difficult. Patients with an adjustment disorder that includes a conduct disturbance may have difficulties with the law, authorities, or school. Psychiatrists should not attempt to rescue such patients from the consequences of their actions. Too often, such kindness only reinforces socially unacceptable means of tension reduction and hinders the acquisition of insight and subsequent emotional growth. In these cases, family therapy can help.

Crisis Intervention. Crisis intervention and case management are short-term treatments aimed at helping persons with adjustment disorders resolve their situations quickly by supportive techniques, suggestion, reassurance, environmental modification, and even hospitalization, if necessary. The frequency and length of visits for crisis support vary according to

patients' needs; daily sessions may be necessary, sometimes 2 or 3 times each day. Flexibility is essential in this approach.

Pharmacotherapy

There are no studies assessing the efficacy of pharmacological interventions in individuals with adjustment disorder, but it may be reasonable to use medication to treat specific symptoms for a brief time. The judicious use of medications can help patients with adjustment disorders, but they should be prescribed for brief periods. Depending on the type of adjustment disorder, a patient may respond to an antianxiety agent or to an antidepressant. Patients with severe anxiety bordering on panic can benefit from anxiolytics such as diazepam (Valium), and those in withdrawn or inhibited states may be helped by a short course of psychostimulant medication. Antipsychotic drugs may be used if there are signs of decompensation or impending psychosis. Selective serotonin reuptake inhibitors have been found useful in treating symptoms of traumatic grief. Recently, there has been an increase in antidepressant use to augment psychotherapy in patients with adjustment disorders. However, pharmacological intervention in this population is most often used to augment psychosocial strategies rather than serving as the primary modality.

References

Bonelli RM, Bugram R. Additional A—Criterion for adjustment disorders? *Can J Psychiatry.* 2000;45:763.

Bronisch T. Adjustment reactions: a long-term prospective and retrospective follow-up of former patients in a crisis intervention ward. *Acta Psychiatr Scand.* 1991;84:86.

Giotakes O, Konstantakopoulos G. Parenting received in early childhood and early separation anxiety in male conscripts with adjustment disorder. *Mil Med.* 2002;167:28.

Holmes J, Raphe R. The social readjustment rating scale. *J Psychosom Res.* 1967;11:213.

Horowitz MJ. *Stress Response Syndromes.* New York: Aronson; 1976.

Newcorn JH, Strain JJ. Adjustment disorder in children and adolescents. *J Am Acad Child Adolesc Psychiatry.* 1991;31:318.

Newcorn JH, Strain JJ, Mezzich JE. Adjustment disorders. In: Sadock BJ, Sadock VA, eds. *Kaplan & Sadock's Comprehensive Textbook of Psychiatry.* 7th ed. Vol 2. Baltimore: Lippincott Williams & Wilkins; 2000:1714.

Pollock D. Structured ambiguity and the definition of psychiatric illness: adjustment among medical inpatients. *Soc Sci Med.* 1992;35:25.

Redd WH, DuHamel KN, Vickberg SMJ, et al. Long-term adjustment in cancer survivors: integration of classical-conditioning and cognitive-processing models. In: Baum A, Andersen BL, eds. *Psychosocial Interventions for Cancer.* Washington, DC: American Psychological Association; 2001:77.

Strain JW, Newcorn J, Wolf D, Fulop G, Davis W. Considering changes in adjustment disorder. *Hosp Community Psychiatry.* 1993;44:13.

27

Personality Disorders

Personality has generally been used as a global descriptive label for a person's observable behavior and his or her subjectively reportable inner experience. The wholeness of an individual described in this way represents both the public and the private aspects of his or her life. The word *personality* may have certain qualifying adjectives with psychiatric significance appended to it, such as *passive* or *aggressive*, or words without pathological overtones, such as *ambitious, religious,* or *friendly.* A coherent series of such qualifications making up a personality disorder diagnosis implies certain predictions about how a person will behave under given sets of circumstances. It also suggests the form that psychiatric illness may assume, should it develop. It offers the clinician clues about a person's disability and about how they may be approached for treatment purposes (i.e., if treatment should be conducted mainly through the use of drugs, surgery, or interviews). Whether used as a psychiatric diagnostic term or as a folk description, the personality label has value for the physician who must deal with the described individual.

Persons with personality disorders are far more likely to refuse psychiatric help and to deny their problems than persons with anxiety disorders, depressive disorders, or obsessive-compulsive disorder. Personality disorder symptoms are alloplastic (i.e., able to adapt to, and alter, the external environment) and ego-syntonic (i.e., acceptable to the ego). Persons with personality disorders do not feel anxiety about their maladaptive behavior. Because they do not routinely acknowledge pain from what others perceive as their symptoms, they often seem disinterested in treatment and impervious to recovery.

CLASSIFICATION

The text revision of the fourth edition of the *Diagnostic and Statistical Manual of Mental Disorders* (DSM-IV-TR) defines personality disorders as enduring subjective experiences and behavior that deviate from cultural standards, are rigidly pervasive, have an onset in adolescence or early adulthood, are stable through time, and lead to unhappiness and impairment. When personality traits are rigid and maladaptive and produce functional impairment or subjective distress, a personality disorder may be diagnosed (Table 27–1).

Personality disorders are grouped into three clusters in DSM-IV-TR. Cluster A covers the paranoid, schizoid, and schizotypal personality disorders; persons with these disorders are often perceived as odd and eccentric. Cluster B is made up of the antisocial, borderline, histrionic, and narcissistic personality disorders; persons with these disorders often seem dramatic, emotional, and erratic. Cluster C includes the avoidant, dependent, and obsessive-compulsive personality disorders and a category called personality disorder not otherwise specified (such as passive-aggressive personality disorder and depressive personality disorder); persons with those disorders often seem anxious or fearful. Many persons exhibit traits that are not limited to a single personality disorder. When a patient meets the criteria for more than one personality disorder, clinicians should diagnose each. Personality disorders are coded on Axis II of DSM-IV-TR.

ETIOLOGY

Genetic Factors

The best evidence that genetic factors contribute to personality disorders comes from investigations of 15,000 pairs of twins in the United States. Among monozygotic twins, the concordance for personality disorders was several times that among dizygotic twins. Moreover, according to one study, monozygotic twins reared apart are about as similar as monozygotic twins reared together. Similarities include multiple measures of personality and temperament, occupational and leisure-time interests, and social attitudes.

Cluster A personality disorders (paranoid, schizoid, and schizotypal) are more common in the biological relatives of patients with schizophrenia than in control groups. More relatives with schizotypal personality disorder occur in the family histories of persons with schizophrenia than in control groups. Less correlation exists between paranoid or schizoid personality disorder and schizophrenia.

Cluster B personality disorders (antisocial, borderline, histrionic, and narcissistic) apparently have a genetic base. Antisocial personality disorder is associated with alcohol use disorders. Depression is common in the family backgrounds of patients with borderline personality disorder. These patients have more relatives with mood disorders than do control groups, and persons with borderline personality disorder often have mood disorder as well. A strong association is found between histrionic personality disorder and somatization disorder (Briquet's syndrome); patients with each disorder show an overlap of symptoms.

Cluster C personality disorders (avoidant, dependent, obsessive-compulsive, and not otherwise specified) may also have a genetic base. Patients with avoidant personality disorder often

Table 27–1
DSM-IV-TR General Diagnostic Criteria for a Personality Disorder

A. An enduring pattern of inner experience and behavior that deviates markedly from the expectations of the individual's culture. This pattern is manifested in two (or more) of the following areas:
   (1) cognition (i.e., ways of perceiving and interpreting self, other people, and events)
   (2) affectivity (i.e., the range, intensity, lability, and appropriateness of emotional response)
   (3) interpersonal functioning
   (4) impulse control
B. The enduring pattern is inflexible and pervasive across a broad range of personal and social situations.
C. The enduring pattern leads to clinically significant distress or impairment in social, occupational, or other important areas of functioning.
D. The pattern is stable and of long duration, and its onset can be traced back at least to adolescence or early adulthood.
E. The enduring pattern is not better accounted for as a manifestation or consequence of another mental disorder.
F. The enduring pattern is not due to the direct physiological effects of a substance (e.g., a drug of abuse, a medication) or a general medical condition (e.g., head trauma).

From American Psychiatric Association. *Diagnostic and Statistical Manual of Mental Disorders.* 4th ed. Text rev. Washington, DC: American Psychiatric Association; copyright 2000, with permission.

have high anxiety levels. Obsessive-compulsive traits are more common in monozygotic twins than in dizygotic twins, and patients with obsessive-compulsive personality disorder show some signs associated with depression—for example, shortened rapid eye movement (REM) latency period and abnormal dexamethasone-suppression test (DST) results.

Biological Factors

Hormones. Persons who exhibit impulsive traits also often show high levels of testosterone, 17-estradiol, and estrone. In nonhuman primates, androgens increase the likelihood of aggression and sexual behavior, but the role of testosterone in human aggression is unclear. DST results are abnormal in some patients with borderline personality disorder who also have depressive symptoms.

Platelet Monoamine Oxidase. Low platelet monoamine oxidase (MAO) levels have been associated with activity and sociability in monkeys. College students with low platelet MAO levels report spending more time in social activities than students with high platelet MAO levels. Low platelet MAO levels have also been noted in some patients with schizotypal disorders.

Smooth Pursuit Eye Movements. Smooth pursuit eye movements are saccadic (i.e., jumpy) in persons who are introverted, who have low self-esteem and tend to withdraw, and who have schizotypal personality disorder. These findings have no clinical application, but they do indicate the role of inheritance.

Neurotransmitters. Endorphins have effects similar to those of exogenous morphine, such as analgesia and the suppression of arousal. High endogenous endorphin levels may be associated with persons who are phlegmatic. Studies of personality traits and the dopaminergic and serotonergic systems indicate an arousal-activating function for these neurotransmitters. Levels of 5-hydroxyindoleacetic acid (5-HIAA), a metabolite of serotonin, are low in persons who attempt suicide and in patients who are impulsive and aggressive.

Raising serotonin levels with serotonergic agents such as fluoxetine (Prozac) may produce dramatic changes in some character traits of personality. In many persons, serotonin reduces depression, impulsiveness, and rumination, and can produce a sense of general well-being. Increased dopamine concentrations in the central nervous system, produced by certain psychostimulants (e.g., amphetamines) can induce euphoria. The effects of neurotransmitters on personality traits have generated much interest and controversy about whether personality traits are inborn or acquired.

Electrophysiology. Changes in electrical conductance on the electroencephalogram (EEG) occur in some patients with personality disorders, most commonly antisocial and borderline types; these changes appear as slow-wave activity on EEGs.

Psychoanalytic Factors

Sigmund Freud suggested that personality traits are related to a fixation at one psychosexual stage of development. For example, those with an oral character are passive and dependent because they are fixated at the oral stage, when the dependence on others for food is prominent. Those with an anal character are stubborn, parsimonious, and highly conscientious because of struggles over toilet training during the anal period.

Wilhelm Reich subsequently coined the term *character armor* to describe persons' characteristic defensive styles for protecting themselves from internal impulses and from interpersonal anxiety in significant relationships. Reich's theory has had a broad influence on contemporary concepts of personality and personality disorders. For example, each human being's unique stamp of personality is considered largely determined by his or her characteristic defense mechanisms. Each personality disorder in Axis II has a cluster of defenses that help psychodynamic clinicians recognize the type of character pathology present. Persons with paranoid personality disorder, for instance, use projection, whereas schizoid personality disorder is associated with withdrawal.

When defenses work effectively, persons with personality disorders master feelings of anxiety, depression, anger, shame, guilt, and other affects. They often view their behavior as ego-syntonic; that is, it creates no distress for them, even though it may adversely affect others. They may also be reluctant to engage in a treatment process; because their defenses are important in controlling unpleasant affects, they are not interested in surrendering them.

In addition to characteristic defenses in personality disorders, another central feature is internal object relations. During development, particular patterns of self in relation to others are internalized. Through introjection, children internalize a parent or another significant person as an internal presence that contin-

ues to feel like an object rather than a self. Through identification, children internalize parents and others in such a way that the traits of the external object are incorporated into the self and the child "owns" the traits. These internal self-representations and object representations are crucial in developing the personality and, through externalization and projective identification, are played out in interpersonal scenarios in which others are coerced into playing a role in the person's internal life. Hence, persons with personality disorders are also identified by particular patterns of interpersonal relatedness that stem from these internal object relations patterns.

Defense Mechanisms. To help those with personality disorders, psychiatrists must appreciate patients' underlying defenses, the unconscious mental processes that the ego uses to resolve conflicts among the four lodestars of the inner life: instinct (wish or need), reality, important persons, and conscience. When defenses are most effective, especially in those with personality disorders, they can abolish anxiety and depression. Thus, abandoning a defense increases conscious anxiety and depression—a major reason that those with personality disorders are reluctant to alter their behavior.

Although patients with personality disorders may be characterized by their most dominant or rigid mechanism, each patient uses several defenses. Therefore, the management of defense mechanisms used by patients with personality disorders is discussed here as a general topic and not as an aspect of the specific disorders. Many formulations presented here in the language of psychoanalytic psychiatry can be translated into principles consistent with cognitive and behavioral approaches.

FANTASY. Many persons who are often labeled schizoid—those who are eccentric, lonely, or frightened—seek solace and satisfaction within themselves by creating imaginary lives, especially imaginary friends. In their extensive dependence on fantasy, these persons often seem to be strikingly aloof. Therapists must understand that the unsociableness of these patients rests on a fear of intimacy. Rather than criticizing them or feeling rebuffed by their rejection, therapists should maintain a quiet, reassuring, and considerate interest without insisting on reciprocal responses. Recognition of patients' fear of closeness and respect for their eccentric ways are both therapeutic and useful.

DISSOCIATION. Dissociation or denial is a Pollyanna-like replacement of unpleasant affects with pleasant ones. Persons who frequently dissociate are often seen as dramatizing and emotionally shallow; they may be labeled histrionic personalities. They behave like anxious adolescents who, to erase anxiety, carelessly expose themselves to exciting dangers. Accepting such patients as exuberant and seductive is to overlook their anxiety, but confronting them with their vulnerabilities and defects makes them still more defensive. Because they seek appreciation of their courage and attractiveness, therapists should not behave with inordinate reserve. While remaining calm and firm, clinicians should realize that these patients are often inadvertent liars, but they benefit from ventilating their own anxieties and may in the process "remember" what they "forgot." Often therapists deal best with dissociation and denial by using displacement. Thus, clinicians may talk with patients about an issue of denial in an unthreatening circumstance. Empathizing with the denied affect without directly confronting patients with the facts may allow them to raise the original topic themselves.

ISOLATION. Isolation is characteristic of the orderly, controlled persons who are often labeled obsessive-compulsive personalities. Unlike those with histrionic personality, persons with obsessive-compulsive personality remember the truth in fine detail but without affect. In a crisis patients may show intensified self-restraint, overly formal social behavior, and obstinacy. Patients' quests for control may annoy clinicians or make them anxious. Often, such patients respond well to precise, systematic, and rational explanations and value efficiency, cleanliness, and punctuality as much as they do clinicians' effective responsiveness. Whenever possible, therapists should allow such patients to control their own care and should not engage in a battle of wills.

PROJECTION. In projection, patients attribute their own unacknowledged feelings to others. Patients' excessive faultfinding and sensitivity to criticism may appear to therapists as prejudiced, hypervigilant injustice collecting, but should not be met by defensiveness and argument. Instead, clinicians should frankly acknowledge even minor mistakes on their part and should discuss the possibility of future difficulties. Strict honesty, concern for patients' rights, and maintaining the same formal, concerned distance as used with patients who use fantasy defenses are all helpful. Confrontation guarantees a lasting enemy and early termination of the interview. Therapists need not agree with patients' injustice collecting, but they should ask whether both can agree to disagree.

The technique of counterprojection is especially helpful. Clinicians acknowledge and give paranoid patients full credit for their feelings and perceptions; they neither dispute patients' complaints nor reinforce them but agree that the world described by patients is conceivable. Interviewers can then talk about real motives and feelings, misattributed to someone else, and begin to cement an alliance with patients.

SPLITTING. In splitting, persons toward whom patients' feelings are, or have been, ambivalent are divided into good and bad. For example, in an inpatient setting, a patient may idealize some staff members and uniformly disparage others. This defense behavior can be highly disruptive on a hospital ward and can ultimately provoke the staff to turn against the patient. When staff members anticipate the process, discuss it at staff meetings, and gently confront the patient with the fact that no one is all good or all bad, the phenomenon of splitting can be dealt with effectively.

PASSIVE AGGRESSION. Persons with passive-aggressive defense turn their anger against themselves. In psychoanalytic terms this phenomenon is called *masochism* and includes failure, procrastination, silly or provocative behavior, self-demeaning clowning, and frankly self-destructive acts. The hostility in such behavior is never entirely concealed. Indeed, in a mechanism such as wrist cutting, others feel as much anger as if they themselves had been assaulted and view the patient as a sadist, not a masochist. Therapists can best deal with passive aggression by helping patients to ventilate their anger.

ACTING OUT. In acting out, patients directly express unconscious wishes or conflicts through action to avoid being conscious of either the accompanying idea or the affect. Tantrums, apparently motiveless assaults, child abuse, and pleasureless promiscuity are common examples. Because the behavior occurs outside reflective awareness, acting out often appears to observers to be unaccompanied by guilt, but when acting out is impossible, the conflict behind the defense may be accessible. Faced with acting out, either aggressive or sexual, in an interview situation, a clinician must recognize that the patient has lost control, that anything the interviewer says will probably be misheard, and that getting the patient's attention is of paramount importance. Depending on the circumstances, a clinician's response may be, "How can I help you if you keep screaming?" or, if the patient's loss of control seems to be escalating, "If you continue screaming, I'll leave." An interviewer

who feels genuinely frightened of the patient can simply leave and, if necessary, ask for help from ward attendants or the police.

PROJECTIVE IDENTIFICATION. The defense mechanism of projective identification appears mainly in borderline personality disorder and consists of three steps. First, an aspect of the self is projected onto someone else. The projector then tries to coerce the other person into identifying with what has been projected. Finally, the recipient of the projection and the projector feel a sense of oneness or union.

PARANOID PERSONALITY DISORDER

Persons with paranoid personality disorder are characterized by long-standing suspiciousness and mistrust of persons in general. They refuse responsibility for their own feelings and assign responsibility to others. They are often hostile, irritable, and angry. Bigots, injustice collectors, pathologically jealous spouses, and litigious cranks often have paranoid personality disorder.

Epidemiology

The prevalence of paranoid personality disorder is 0.5 to 2.5 percent of the general population. Those with the disorder rarely seek treatment themselves; when referred to treatment by a spouse or an employer, they can often pull themselves together and appear undistressed. Relatives of patients with schizophrenia show a higher incidence of paranoid personality disorder than controls. The disorder is more common in men than in women and does not appear to have a familial pattern. The prevalence among persons who are homosexual is no higher than usual, as was once thought, but it is believed to be higher among minority groups, immigrants, and persons who are deaf than it is in the general population.

Diagnosis

On psychiatric examination, patients with paranoid personality disorder may be formal in manner and act baffled about having to seek psychiatric help. Muscular tension, an inability to relax, and a need to scan the environment for clues may be evident, and patients' manner is often humorless and serious. Although some premises of their arguments may be false, their speech is goal directed and logical. Their thought content shows evidence of projection, prejudice, and occasional ideas of reference. The DSM-IV-TR diagnostic criteria are listed in Table 27–2.

Table 27–2
DSM-IV-TR Diagnostic Criteria for Paranoid Personality Disorder

A. A pervasive distrust and suspiciousness of others such that their motives are interpreted as malevolent, beginning by early adulthood and present in a variety of contexts, as indicated by four (or more) of the following:
   (1) suspects, without sufficient basis, that others are exploiting, harming, or deceiving him or her
   (2) is preoccupied with unjustified doubts about the loyalty or trustworthiness of friends or associates
   (3) is reluctant to confide in others because of unwarranted fear that the information will be used maliciously against him or her
   (4) reads hidden demeaning or threatening meanings into benign remarks or events
   (5) persistently bears grudges, i.e., is unforgiving of insults, injuries, or slights
   (6) perceives attacks on his or her character or reputation that are not apparent to others and is quick to react angrily or to counterattack
   (7) has recurrent suspicions, without justification, regarding fidelity of spouse or sexual partner

B. Does not occur exclusively during the course of schizophrenia, a mood disorder with psychotic features, or another psychotic disorder and is not due to the direct physiological effects of a general medical condition.

Note: If criteria are met prior to the onset of schizophrenia, add "premorbid," e.g., "paranoid personality disorder (premorbid)."

From American Psychiatric Association. *Diagnostic and Statistical Manual of Mental Disorders.* 4th ed. Text rev. Washington, DC: American Psychiatric Association; copyright 2000, with permission.

Clinical Features

The essential feature of persons with paranoid personality disorder is a pervasive and unwarranted tendency to interpret other persons' actions as deliberately demeaning or threatening. This tendency begins by early adulthood and appears in a variety of contexts. Almost invariably, those with the disorder expect to be exploited or harmed by others in some way. They frequently dispute, without any justification, friends' or associates' loyalty or trustworthiness. Such persons are often pathologically jealous and for no reason question the fidelity of their spouses or sexual partners. Persons with this disorder externalize their own emotions and use the defense of projection; they attribute to others the impulses and thoughts that they cannot accept in themselves. Ideas of reference and logically defended illusions are common.

Persons with paranoid personality disorder are affectively restricted and appear to be unemotional. They pride themselves on being rational and objective, but such is not the case. They lack warmth and are impressed with, and pay close attention to, power and rank. They express disdain for those they see as weak, sickly, impaired, or in some way defective. In social situations, persons with paranoid personality disorder may appear businesslike and efficient, but they often generate fear or conflict in others.

Differential Diagnosis

Paranoid personality disorder can usually be differentiated from delusional disorder by the absence of fixed delusions. Unlike persons with paranoid schizophrenia, those with personality disorders have no hallucinations or formal thought disorder. Paranoid personality disorder can be distinguished from borderline personality disorder because paranoid patients are rarely capable of overly involved, tumultuous relationships with others. Paranoid patients lack the long history of antisocial behavior of persons with antisocial character. Persons with schizoid personality disorder are withdrawn and aloof and do not have paranoid ideation.

Course and Prognosis

No adequate, systematic long-term studies of paranoid personality disorder have been conducted. In some, paranoid personality disorder is lifelong; in others it is a harbinger of schizophrenia. In still others, paranoid traits give way to reaction formation, appropriate concern with morality, and altruistic concerns as they mature or as stress diminishes. In general, however, those with paranoid personality disorder have lifelong problems working and living with others. Occupational and marital problems are common.

Treatment

Psychotherapy. Psychotherapy is the treatment of choice. Therapists should be straightforward in all their dealings with these patients. If a therapist is accused of inconsistency or a fault, such as lateness for an appointment, honesty and an apology are preferable to a defensive explanation. Therapists must remember that trust and toleration of intimacy are troubled areas for patients with this disorder. Individual psychotherapy thus requires a professional and not overly warm style from therapists. Clinicians' overzealous use of interpretation—especially interpretation about deep feelings of dependence, sexual concerns, and wishes for intimacy—increase patients' mistrust significantly. Paranoid patients usually do not do well in group psychotherapy, although it can be useful for improving social skills and diminishing suspiciousness through role playing. Many cannot tolerate the intrusiveness of behavior therapy, also used for social skills training.

At times, patients with paranoid personality disorder behave so threateningly that therapists must control or set limits on their actions. Delusional accusations must be dealt with realistically but gently and without humiliating patients. Paranoid patients are profoundly frightened when they feel that those trying to help them are weak and helpless; therefore, therapists should never offer to take control unless they are willing and able to do so.

Pharmacotherapy. Pharmacotherapy is useful in dealing with agitation and anxiety. In most cases an antianxiety agent such as diazepam (Valium) suffices. But it may be necessary to use an antipsychotic such as haloperidol (Haldol) in small dosages and for brief periods to manage severe agitation or quasi-delusional thinking. The antipsychotic drug pimozide (Orap) has successfully reduced paranoid ideation in some patients.

SCHIZOID PERSONALITY DISORDER

Schizoid personality disorder is diagnosed in patients who display a lifelong pattern of social withdrawal. Their discomfort with human interaction, their introversion, and their bland, constricted affect are noteworthy. Persons with schizoid personality disorder are often seen by others as eccentric, isolated, or lonely.

Epidemiology

The prevalence of schizoid personality disorder is not clearly established, but the disorder may affect 7.5 percent of the general population. The sex ratio of the disorder is unknown; some studies report a 2-to-1 male-to-female ratio. Persons with the disorder tend to gravitate toward solitary jobs that involve little or no contact with others. Many prefer night work to day work, so that they need not deal with many persons.

Diagnosis

On an initial psychiatric examination, patients with schizoid personality disorder may appear ill at ease. They rarely tolerate eye contact, and interviewers may surmise that such patients are eager for the interview to end. Their affect may be constricted, aloof, or inappropriately serious, but underneath the aloofness, sensitive clinicians can recognize fear. These patients find it difficult to be lighthearted: Their efforts at humor may seem adolescent and off the mark. Their speech is goal-directed, but they are likely to give short answers to questions and to avoid spontaneous conversation. They may occasionally use unusual figures of speech, such as an odd metaphor, and may be fascinated with inanimate objects or metaphysical constructs. Their mental content may reveal an unwarranted sense of intimacy with persons they do not know well or whom they have not seen for a long time. Their sensorium is intact, their memory functions well, and their proverb interpretations are abstract. The DSM-IV-TR diagnostic criteria are listed in Table 27–3.

Clinical Features

Persons with schizoid personality disorder seem to be cold and aloof; they display a remote reserve and show no involve-

Table 27–3
DSM-IV-TR Diagnostic Criteria for Schizoid Personality Disorder

A. A pervasive pattern of detachment from social relationships and a restricted range of expression of emotions in interpersonal settings, beginning by early adulthood and present in a variety of contexts, as indicated by four (or more) of the following:
  (1) neither desires nor enjoys close relationships, including being part of a family
  (2) almost always chooses solitary activities
  (3) has little, if any, interest in having sexual experiences with another person
  (4) takes pleasure in few, if any, activities
  (5) lacks close friends or confidants other than first-degree relatives
  (6) appears indifferent to the praise or criticism of others
  (7) shows emotional coldness, detachment, or flattened affectivity

B. Does not occur exclusively during the course of schizophrenia, a mood disorder with psychotic features, another psychotic disorder, or a pervasive developmental disorder and is not due to the direct physiological effects of a general medical condition.

Note: If criteria are met prior to the onset of schizophrenia, add "premorbid," e.g., "schizoid personality disorder (premorbid)."

From American Psychiatric Association. *Diagnostic and Statistical Manual of Mental Disorders.* 4th ed. Text rev. Washington, DC: American Psychiatric Association; copyright 2000, with permission.

ment with everyday events and the concerns of others. They appear quiet, distant, seclusive, and unsociable. They may pursue their own lives with remarkably little need or longing for emotional ties, and they are the last to be aware of changes in popular fashion.

The life histories of such persons reflect solitary interests and success at noncompetitive, lonely jobs that others find difficult to tolerate. Their sexual lives may exist exclusively in fantasy, and they may postpone mature sexuality indefinitely. Men may not marry because they are unable to achieve intimacy; women may passively agree to marry an aggressive man who wants the marriage. Persons with schizoid personality disorder usually reveal a lifelong inability to express anger directly. They can invest enormous affective energy in nonhuman interests such as mathematics and astronomy, and they may be very attached to animals. Dietary and health fads, philosophical movements, and social improvement schemes, especially those that require no personal involvement, often engross them.

Although persons with schizoid personality disorder appear self-absorbed and lost in daydreams, they have a normal capacity to recognize reality. Because aggressive acts are rarely included in their repertoire of usual responses, most threats, real or imagined, are dealt with by fantasized omnipotence or resignation. They are often seen as aloof, yet such persons can sometimes conceive, develop, and give to the world genuinely original, creative ideas.

Mr. S. is a 38-year-old unmarried laboratory technician who is referred by his employer, a university scientist, because he is having difficulty being a team player on a project. For the past 5 years, Mr. S. has been employed in the laboratory working on a project more or less by himself and doing very well at it. The renewal grant that Mr. S.'s employer recently received, allowing for Mr. S.'s continued employment, involves a substantial expansion of the project. The scientist therefore hired a number of new employees to work in the lab, and he expected Mr. S. to train them. Several of the newly hired people quit within 3 weeks, saying that Mr. S. was impossible to learn from and to work with. They complained that he did not provide any guidance and that he was unfriendly and arrogant. When the scientist confronted Mr. S. with these charges after the third individual quit, Mr. S. was bland and surprised. He said that he was trying to do his best and that he could not understand the complaints. He did admit that he was somewhat annoyed at the change in his role and was not really clear about what was expected of him. His employer had previously been pleased with the thoroughness and accuracy of Mr. S.'s work and was reluctant to lose him, but he realized that the success of his expanded project was in jeopardy if Mr. S. was unable to learn to train and work with others. He therefore suggested to Mr. S. that he seek some professional help in dealing with his new duties and hence Mr. S. came in for evaluation.

During the initial interview, Mr. S. describes himself as a loner who has always felt awkward and unhappy when forced into relationships with others. He says that he has always been detached from the rest of his family. When asked to describe his life growing up, it becomes apparent that Mr. S. has never had a good friend, was never chosen to be on teams, and never participated in any school activities. Mr. S. describes these facts in a detached manner and does not appear at all distressed by them. He says that he has never dated or had any sexual experiences with others, nor does he express any desire to do so when asked. His interest in science began with a chemistry set he received for his 13th birthday, after which he spent long hours as a teenager conducting solitary experiments. When asked about how he spends his leisure time, he says that he mostly enjoys playing computer games. (From *DSM-IV-TR Case Studies.*)

Differential Diagnosis

In contrast to patients with schizophrenia and schizotypal personality disorder, patients with schizoid personality disorder do not have schizophrenic relatives, and they may have successful, if isolated, work histories. They also differ from patients with schizophrenia by exhibiting no thought disorder or delusional thinking. Although patients with paranoid personality disorder share many traits with those with schizoid personality disorder, the former exhibit more social engagement, a history of aggressive verbal behavior, and a greater tendency to project their feelings onto others. If just as emotionally constricted, patients with obsessive-compulsive and avoidant personality disorders experience loneliness as dysphoric, possess a richer history of past object relations, and do not engage as much in autistic reverie. Theoretically, the chief distinction between a patient with schizotypal personality disorder and one with schizoid personality disorder is that a schizotypal patient is more similar to a patient with schizophrenia in oddities of perception, thought, behavior, and communication. Patients with avoidant personality disorder are isolated but strongly wish to participate in activities, a characteristic absent in those with schizoid personality disorder.

Course and Prognosis

The onset of schizoid personality disorder usually occurs in early childhood. Like all personality disorders, schizoid personality disorder is long lasting, but not necessarily lifelong. The proportion of patients who incur schizophrenia is unknown.

Treatment

Psychotherapy. The treatment of patients with schizoid personality disorder is similar to that of those with paranoid personality disorder. Schizoid patients' tendencies toward introspection, however, are consistent with psychotherapists' expectations, and schizoid patients may become devoted, if distant, patients. As trust develops, schizoid patients may, with great trepidation, reveal a plethora of fantasies, imaginary friends, and fears of unbearable dependence—even of merging with the therapist.

In group therapy settings, patients with schizoid personality disorder may be silent for long periods; nonetheless, they do become involved. The patients should be protected against aggressive attack by group members for their proclivity to be

silent. With time the group members become important to schizoid patients and may provide the only social contact in their otherwise isolated existence.

Pharmacotherapy. Pharmacotherapy with small dosages of antipsychotics, antidepressants, and psychostimulants has benefitted some patients. Serotonergic agents may make patients less sensitive to rejection. Benzodiazepines may help diminish interpersonal anxiety.

SCHIZOTYPAL PERSONALITY DISORDER

Persons with schizotypal personality disorder are strikingly odd or strange, even to laypersons. Magical thinking, peculiar notions, ideas of reference, illusions, and derealization are part of a schizotypal person's everyday world.

Epidemiology

This disorder occurs in about 3 percent of the population. The sex ratio is unknown. There is a greater association of cases among the biological relatives of patients with schizophrenia than among controls, and a higher incidence among monozygotic twins than among dizygotic twins (33 percent versus 4 percent in one study).

Diagnosis

Schizotypal personality disorder is diagnosed on the basis of the patients' peculiarities of thinking, behavior, and appearance. Taking a history may be difficult because of the patients' unusual way of communicating. The DSM-IV-TR diagnostic criteria for schizotypal personality disorder are given in Table 27–4.

Table 27–4
DSM-IV-TR Diagnostic Criteria for Schizotypal Personality Disorder

A. A pervasive pattern of social and interpersonal deficits marked by acute discomfort with, and reduced capacity for, close relationships as well as by cognitive or perceptual distortions and eccentricities of behavior, beginning by early adulthood and present in a variety of contexts, as indicated by five (or more) of the following:
 (1) ideas of reference (excluding delusions of reference)
 (2) odd beliefs or magical thinking that influences behavior and is inconsistent with subcultural norms (e.g., superstitiousness, belief in clairvoyance, telepathy, or "sixth sense"; in children and adolescents, bizarre fantasies or preoccupations)
 (3) unusual perceptual experiences, including bodily illusions
 (4) odd thinking and speech (e.g., vague, circumstantial, metaphorical, overelaborate, or stereotyped)
 (5) suspiciousness or paranoid ideation
 (6) inappropriate or constricted affect
 (7) behavior or appearance that is odd, eccentric, or peculiar
 (8) lack of close friends or confidants other than first-degree relatives
 (9) excessive social anxiety that does not diminish with familiarity and tends to be associated with paranoid fears rather than negative judgments about self

B. Does not occur exclusively during the course of schizophrenia, a mood disorder with psychotic features, another psychotic disorder, or a pervasive developmental disorder.

Note: If criteria are met prior to the onset of schizophrenia, add "premorbid," e.g., "schizotypal personality disorder (premorbid)."

From American Psychiatric Association. *Diagnostic and Statistical Manual of Mental Disorders*. 4th ed. Text rev. Washington, DC: American Psychiatric Association; copyright 2000, with permission.

Clinical Features

Patients with schizotypal personality disorder exhibit disturbed thinking and communicating. Although frank thought disorder is absent, their speech may be distinctive or peculiar, may have meaning only to them, and may often need interpretation. Like patients with schizophrenia, those with schizotypal personality disorder may not know their own feelings and yet are exquisitely sensitive to, and aware of, the feelings of others, especially negative affects like anger. These patients may be superstitious or claim powers of clairvoyance and may believe that they have other special powers of thought and insight. Their inner world may be filled with vivid imaginary relationships and childlike fears and fantasies. They may admit to perceptual illusions or macropsia and confess that other persons seem wooden and all the same.

Because persons with schizotypal personality disorder have poor interpersonal relationships and may act inappropriately, they are isolated and have few, if any, friends. Patients may show features of borderline personality disorder, and indeed, both diagnoses can be made. Under stress, patients with schizotypal personality disorder may decompensate and have psychotic symptoms, but these are usually of brief duration. Patients with severe cases of the disorder may exhibit anhedonia and severe depression.

Differential Diagnosis

Theoretically, persons with schizotypal personality disorder can be distinguished from those with schizoid and avoidant personality disorders by the presence of oddities in their behavior, thinking, perception, and communication and perhaps by a clear family history of schizophrenia. Patients with schizotypal personality disorder can be distinguished from those with schizophrenia by their absence of psychosis. If psychotic symptoms do appear, they are brief and fragmentary. Some patients meet the criteria for both schizotypal personality disorder and borderline personality disorder. Patients with paranoid personality disorder are characterized by suspiciousness, but lack the odd behavior of patients with schizotypal personality disorder.

Course and Prognosis

A long-term study by Thomas McGlashan reported that 10 percent of those with schizotypal personality disorder eventually committed suicide. Retrospective studies have shown that many patients thought to have had schizophrenia actually had schizotypal personality disorder, and according to current clinical thinking, the schizotype is the premorbid personality of the patient with schizophrenia. Some, however, maintain a stable schizotypal personality throughout their lives and marry and work despite their oddities.

Treatment

Psychotherapy. The principles of treatment of schizotypal personality disorder do not differ from those of schizoid personality disorder, but clinicians must deal sensitively with the former. These patients have peculiar patterns of thinking, and some are involved in cults, strange religious practices, and the occult. Therapists must not ridicule such activities or be judgmental about these beliefs or activities.

Pharmacotherapy. Antipsychotic medication may be useful in dealing with ideas of reference, illusions, and other symptoms of the disorder and can be used in conjunction with psychotherapy. Antidepressants are useful when a depressive component of the personality is present.

ANTISOCIAL PERSONALITY DISORDER

Antisocial personality disorder is an inability to conform to the social norms that ordinarily govern many aspects of a person's adolescent and adult behavior. Although characterized by continual antisocial or criminal acts, the disorder is not synonymous with criminality (the 10th revision of *International Statistical Classification of Diseases and Related Health Problems* [ICD-10] uses the name *dissocial personality disorder*).

Table 27–5
DSM-IV-TR Diagnostic Criteria for Antisocial Personality Disorder

A. There is a pervasive pattern of disregard for and violation of the rights of others occurring since age 15 years, as indicated by three (or more) of the following:
   (1) failure to conform to social norms with respect to lawful behaviors as indicated by repeatedly performing acts that are grounds for arrest
   (2) deceitfulness, as indicated by repeated lying, use of aliases, or conning others for personal profit or pleasure
   (3) impulsivity or failure to plan ahead
   (4) irritability and aggressiveness, as indicated by repeated physical fights or assaults
   (5) reckless disregard for safety of self or others
   (6) consistent irresponsibility, as indicated by repeated failure to sustain consistent work behavior or honor financial obligations
   (7) lack of remorse, as indicated by being indifferent to or rationalizing having hurt, mistreated, or stolen from another

B. The individual is at least age 18 years.

C. There is evidence of conduct disorder with onset before age 15 years.

D. The occurrence of antisocial behavior is not exclusively during the course of schizophrenia or a manic episode.

From American Psychiatric Association. *Diagnostic and Statistical Manual of Mental Disorders.* 4th ed. Text rev. Washington, DC: American Psychiatric Association; copyright 2000, with permission.

Epidemiology

The prevalence of antisocial personality disorder is 3 percent in men and 1 percent in women. It is most common in poor urban areas and among mobile residents of these areas. Boys with the disorder come from larger families than girls with the disorder. The onset of the disorder is before the age of 15. Girls usually have symptoms before puberty, and boys even earlier. In prison populations the prevalence of antisocial personality disorder may be as high as 75 percent. A familial pattern is present; the disorder is 5 times more common among first-degree relatives of men with the disorder than among controls.

Diagnosis

Patients with antisocial personality disorder can fool even the most experienced clinicians. In an interview, patients can appear composed and credible, but beneath the veneer (or, to use Hervey Cleckley's term, *the mask of sanity*), there is tension, hostility, irritability, and rage. A stress interview, in which patients are vigorously confronted with inconsistencies in their histories, may be necessary to reveal the pathology.

A diagnostic workup should include a thorough neurological examination. Because patients often show abnormal EEG results and soft neurological signs suggesting minimal brain damage in childhood, these findings can be used to confirm the clinical impression. The DSM-IV-TR diagnostic criteria are listed in Table 27–5.

Clinical Features

Patients with antisocial personality disorder can often seem to be normal and even charming and ingratiating. Their histories, however, reveal many areas of disordered life functioning. Lying, truancy, running away from home, thefts, fights, substance abuse, and illegal activities are typical experiences that patients report as beginning in childhood. These patients often impress opposite-sex clinicians with the colorful, seductive aspects of their personalities, but same-sex clinicians may regard them as manipulative and demanding. Patients with antisocial personality disorder exhibit no anxiety or depression, a lack that may seem grossly incongruous with their situations, although suicide threats and somatic preoccupations may be common. Their own explanations of their antisocial behavior make it seem mindless, but their mental content reveals the complete absence of delusions and other signs of irrational thinking. In fact, they frequently have a heightened sense of reality testing and often impress observers as having good verbal intelligence.

Persons with antisocial personality disorder are highly represented by so-called con men. They are extremely manipulative and can frequently talk others into participating in schemes for easy ways to make money or to achieve fame or notoriety. These schemes may eventually lead the unwary to financial ruin or social embarrassment or both. Those with this disorder do not tell the truth and cannot be trusted to carry out any task or adhere to any conventional standard of morality. Promiscuity, spousal abuse, child abuse, and drunk driving are common events in their lives. A notable finding is a lack of remorse for these actions; that is, they appear to lack a conscience.

Mr. Y. is a 26-year-old man who is transferred from a prison to a psychiatric unit as a result of a suicide attempt. Mr. Y. has a history of three previous suicide attempts and multiple problems with the law. From information contained in the patient's social services, medical, and legal records, the clinician is able to piece together Mr. Y.'s history.

Mr. Y.'s mother was a prostitute and drug addict, and he never knew his father. He had a history of very serious conduct problems from a young age. He began getting into fights with other children almost from the day he began school and was caught torturing animals on a number of occasions when he was in elementary school. When he was 9 years old, Mr. Y. threw his baby brother out of the window of their first floor apartment, causing multiple fractures. During his childhood, Mr. Y. spent several years in a group home and stayed in many foster homes, but these placements were never successful. He would occasionally stay with his maternal grandmother, who was taking care of up to eight other grandchildren at the same time. Mr. Y. began using drugs at age 10.

In early adolescence, Mr. Y. joined a gang where he became involved in selling drugs and running numbers. He fathered his first child at the age of 13. Before he was 17, he was arrested on a variety of charges that included theft, possession of illegal drugs, and assault, but, because of his age, he received a series of suspended sentences. He was constantly truant from school and finally dropped out permanently at age 15. At that time, he began living on the street with other friends from his gang who were also engaged in using and selling drugs. At age 17, he was sentenced to 2 years in prison for stabbing someone in a fight in a bar. During this imprisonment, he attempted suicide by hanging himself with an article of clothing. As a result of this, he was transferred to the infirmary for several weeks and did not have to participate in his work detail.

By the time Mr. Y. was 23, he had fathered five children, none of whom he sees or supports. When he is not crossed, Mr. Y. is a manipulative person who can be charming, funny, and gregarious. When he is on drugs or when he does not get his way, however, he can become coldly furious and ruthlessly destructive.

Mr. Y. has been treated for a series of drug overdoses, several of which were intentional. He has been hospitalized in psychiatric facilities on three occasions because of depression and suicide attempts. This is the fourth such hospitalization. Mr. Y.'s behavior follows a characteristic pattern during these hospitalizations. Initially, he seems to blossom and get better right away and is helpful with staff and patients. Soon, however, Mr. Y. begins stirring up trouble on the ward and leading the other patients in revolt concerning smoking privileges, passes, and the need for medication. On one occasion during his most recent hospitalization, he was caught having intercourse with a 60-year-old female patient. (From *DSM-IV Case Studies.*)

Differential Diagnosis

Antisocial personality disorder can be distinguished from illegal behavior in that antisocial personality disorder involves many areas of a person's life. When antisocial behavior is the only manifestation, patients are classified in the DSM-IV-TR category of additional conditions that may be a focus of clinical attention—specifically, adult antisocial behavior. Dorothy Lewis found that many of these persons have a neurological or mental disorder that has been either overlooked or undiagnosed. More difficult is the differentiation of antisocial personality disorder from substance abuse. When both substance abuse and antisocial behavior begin in childhood and continue into adult life, both disorders should be diagnosed. When, however, the antisocial behavior is clearly secondary to premorbid alcohol abuse or other substance abuse, the diagnosis of antisocial personality disorder is not warranted.

In diagnosing antisocial personality disorder, clinicians must adjust for the distorting effects of socioeconomic status, cultural background, and sex. Furthermore, the diagnosis of antisocial personality disorder is not warranted when mental retardation, schizophrenia, or mania can explain the symptoms.

Course and Prognosis

Once an antisocial personality disorder develops, it runs an unremitting course, with the height of antisocial behavior usually occurring in late adolescence. The prognosis varies. Some reports indicate that symptoms decrease as persons grow older. Many patients have somatization disorder and multiple physical complaints. Depressive disorders, alcohol use disorders, and other substance abuse are common.

Treatment

Psychotherapy. If patients with antisocial personality disorder are immobilized (e.g., placed in hospitals), they often become amenable to psychotherapy. When patients feel that they are among peers, their lack of motivation for change disappears. Perhaps for this reason, self-help groups have been more useful than jails in alleviating the disorder.

Before treatment can begin, firm limits are essential. Therapists must find ways of dealing with patients' self-destructive behavior. And to overcome patients' fear of intimacy, therapists must frustrate patients' desire to run from honest human encounters. In doing so, a therapist faces the challenge of separating control from punishment and of separating help and confrontation from social isolation and retribution.

Pharmacotherapy. Pharmacotherapy is used to deal with incapacitating symptoms such as anxiety, rage, and depression, but because patients are often substance abusers, drugs must be used judiciously. If a patient shows evidence of attention-deficit/hyperactivity disorder, psychostimulants such as methylphenidate (Ritalin) may be useful. Attempts have been made to alter catecholamine metabolism with drugs and to control impulsive behavior with antiepileptic drugs, for example, carbamazepine (Tegretol) or valproate (Depakote), especially if abnormal waveforms are noted on an EEG. β-Adrenergic receptor antagonists have been used to reduce aggression.

BORDERLINE PERSONALITY DISORDER

Patients with borderline personality disorder stand on the border between neurosis and psychosis and are characterized by

extraordinarily unstable affect, mood, behavior, object relations, and self-image. The disorder has also been called *ambulatory schizophrenia, as-if personality* (a term coined by Helene Deutsch), *pseudoneurotic schizophrenia* (described by Paul Hoch and Phillip Politan), and *psychotic character disorder* (described by John Frosch). ICD-10 uses the name *emotionally unstable personality disorder.*

Epidemiology

No definitive prevalence studies are available, but borderline personality disorder is thought to be present in about 1 to 2 percent of the population and is twice as common in women as in men. An increased prevalence of major depressive disorder, alcohol use disorders, and substance abuse is found in first-degree relatives of persons with borderline personality disorder.

Diagnosis

According to DSM-IV-TR, the diagnosis of borderline personality disorder can made by early adulthood when patients show at least five of the criteria listed in Table 27–6. Biological studies may aid in the diagnosis; some patients with borderline personality disorder show shortened rapid eye movement (REM) latency and sleep continuity disturbances, abnormal DST results, and abnormal thyrotropin-releasing hormone test results. Those changes, however, are also seen in some patients with depressive disorders.

Table 27–6
DSM-IV-TR Diagnostic Criteria for Borderline Personality Disorder

A pervasive pattern of instability of interpersonal relationships, self-image, and affects, and marked impulsivity beginning by early adulthood and present in a variety of contexts, as indicated by five (or more) of the following:

(1) frantic efforts to avoid real or imagined abandonment. **Note:** Do not include suicidal or self-mutilating behavior covered in criterion 5.

(2) a pattern of unstable and intense interpersonal relationships characterized by alternating between extremes of idealization and devaluation

(3) identity disturbance: markedly and persistently unstable self-image or sense of self

(4) impulsivity in at least two areas that are potentially self-damaging (e.g., spending, sex, substance abuse, reckless driving, binge eating). **Note:** Do not include suicidal or self-mutilating behavior covered in criterion 5.

(5) recurrent suicidal behavior, gestures, or threats, or self-mutilating behavior

(6) affective instability due to a marked reactivity of mood (e.g., intense episodic dysphoria, irritability, or anxiety usually lasting a few hours and only hours and only rarely more than a few days)

(7) chronic feelings of emptiness

(8) inappropriate, intense anger or difficulty controlling anger (e.g., frequent displays of temper, constant anger, recurrent physical fights)

(9) transient, stress-related paranoid ideation or severe dissociative symptoms

From American Psychiatric Association. *Diagnostic and Statistical Manual of Mental Disorders.* 4th ed. Text rev. Washington, DC: American Psychiatric Association; copyright 2000, with permission.

Clinical Features

Persons with borderline personality disorder almost always appear to be in a state of crisis. Mood swings are common. Patients can be argumentative at one moment, depressed the next, and later complain of having no feelings. Patients may have short-lived psychotic episodes (so-called micropsychotic episodes) rather than full-blown psychotic breaks, and the psychotic symptoms of these patients are almost always circumscribed, fleeting, or doubtful. The behavior of patients with borderline personality disorder is highly unpredictable, and their achievements are rarely at the level of their abilities. The painful nature of their lives is reflected in repetitive self-destructive acts. Such patients may slash their wrists and perform other self-mutilations to elicit help from others, to express anger, or to numb themselves to overwhelming affect.

Because they feel both dependent and hostile, persons with this disorder have tumultuous interpersonal relationships. They can be dependent on those to whom they are close and when frustrated can express enormous anger toward their intimate friends. Patients with borderline personality disorder cannot tolerate being alone, and they prefer a frantic search for companionship, no matter how unsatisfactory, to their own company. To assuage loneliness, if only for brief periods, they accept a stranger as a friend or behave promiscuously. They often complain about chronic feelings of emptiness and boredom and the lack of a consistent sense of identity (identity diffusion); when pressed, they often complain about how depressed they usually feel despite the flurry of other affects.

Otto Kernberg described the defense mechanism of projective identification that occurs in patients with borderline personality disorder. In this primitive defense mechanism, intolerable aspects of the self are projected onto another; the other person is induced to play the projected role, and the two persons act in unison. Therapists must be aware of this process so that they can act neutrally toward such patients.

Most therapists agree that these patients show ordinary reasoning abilities on structured tests, such as the Wechsler adult intelligence scale, and show deviant processes only on unstructured projective tests, such as the Rorschach test.

Functionally, patients with borderline personality disorder distort their relationships by considering each person to be either all good or all bad. They see persons as either nurturing attachment figures or as hateful, sadistic figures who deprive them of security needs and threaten them with abandonment whenever they feel dependent. As a result of this splitting, the good person is idealized, and the bad person devalued. Shifts of allegiance from one person or group to another are frequent. Some clinicians use the concepts of panphobia, pananxiety, panambivalence, and chaotic sexuality to delineate these patients' characteristics.

Differential Diagnosis

The disorder is differentiated from schizophrenia on the basis of the borderline patient's lack of prolonged psychotic epi-

sodes, thought disorder, and other classic schizophrenic signs. Patients with schizotypal personality disorder show marked peculiarities of thinking, strange ideation, and recurrent ideas of reference. Those with paranoid personality disorder are marked by extreme suspiciousness. Patients with borderline personality disorder generally have chronic feelings of emptiness and short-lived psychotic episodes; they act impulsively and demand extraordinary relationships; they may mutilate themselves and make manipulative suicide attempts.

Course and Prognosis

This disorder is fairly stable; patients change little over time. Longitudinal studies show no progression toward schizophrenia, but patients have a high incidence of major depressive disorder episodes. The diagnosis is usually made before the age of 40, when patients are attempting to make occupational, marital, and other choices and are unable to deal with the normal stages of the life cycle.

Treatment

Table 27–7 summarizes the American Psychiatric Association guidelines for treating this disorder.

Psychotherapy. Psychotherapy for patients with borderline personality disorder is an area of intensive investigation and has been the treatment of choice. For best results, pharmacotherapy has been added to the treatment regimen.

Psychotherapy is difficult for patient and therapist alike. Patients regress easily, act out their impulses, and show labile or fixed negative or positive transferences, which are difficult to analyze. Projective identification may also cause countertransference problems when therapists are unaware that patients are unconsciously trying to coerce them to act out a particular behavior. The splitting defense mechanism causes patients to alternately love and hate therapists and others in the environment. A reality-oriented approach is more effective than in-depth interpretations of the unconscious.

Therapists have used behavior therapy to control patients' impulses and angry outbursts and to reduce their sensitivity to criticism and rejection. Social skills training, especially with videotape playback, helps enable patients see how their actions affect others and thereby improve their interpersonal behavior.

Patients with borderline personality disorder often do well in a hospital setting in which they receive intensive psychotherapy on both an individual basis and a group basis. In a hospital they can also interact with trained staff members from a variety of disciplines and can be provided with occupational, recreational, and vocational therapy. Such programs are especially helpful when the home environment is detrimental to a patient's rehabilitation because of intrafamilial conflicts or other stresses, such as parental abuse. Within the protected environment of the hospital, patients who are excessively impulsive, self-destructive, or self-mutilating can be given limits, and their actions can be observed. Under ideal circumstances, patients remain in the hospital until they show marked improvement, up to 1 year in some cases. Patients can then be discharged to special support systems such as day hospitals, night hospitals, and halfway houses.

A particular form of psychotherapy called *dialectical behavior therapy* (DBT) has been used for borderline patients, especially those with parasuicidal behavior such as frequent cutting. (For further discussion of DBT see Section 35.6 in Chapter 35.)

Pharmacotherapy. Pharmacotherapy is useful to deal with specific personality features that interfere with patients' overall functioning. Antipsychotics have been used to control anger, hostility, and brief psychotic episodes. Antidepressants improve the depressed mood common in patients with borderline personality disorder. The MAO inhibitors (MAOIs) have successfully modulated impulsive behavior in some patients. Benzodiazepines, particularly alprazolam (Xanax), help anxiety and depression, but some patients show a disinhibition with this class of drugs. Anticonvulsants such as carbamazepine may improve global functioning for some patients. Serotonergic agents such as selective serotonin reuptake inhibitors (SSRIs) have been helpful in some cases.

Table 27–7
Common Features of Recommended Psychotherapy for Borderline Personality Disorder

Therapy is not expected to be brief.
A strong helping relationship develops between patient and therapist.
Clear roles and responsibilities of patient and therapist are established.
Therapist is active and directive, not a passive listener.
Patient and therapist mutually develop a hierarchy of priorities.
Therapist conveys empathic validation plus the need for patient to control his/her behavior.
Flexibility is needed as new circumstances, including stresses, develop.
Limit setting, preferably mutually agreed upon, is used.
Concomitant individual and group approaches are used.

From Oldham JM. A 44-year-old woman with borderline personality disorder. *JAMA*. 2002;287:1034.

HISTRIONIC PERSONALITY DISORDER

Persons with histrionic personality disorder are excitable and emotional and behave in a colorful, dramatic, extroverted fashion. Accompanying their flamboyant aspects, however, is often an inability to maintain deep, long-lasting attachments.

Epidemiology

According to DSM-IV-TR, limited data from general population studies suggest a prevalence of histrionic personality disorder of about 2 to 3 percent. Rates of about 10 to 15 percent have been reported in inpatient and outpatient mental health settings when structured assessment is used. The disorder is diagnosed more frequently in women than in men. Some studies have found an association with somatization disorder and alcohol use disorders.

Diagnosis

In interviews, patients with histrionic personality disorder are generally cooperative and eager to give a detailed history. Ges-

Table 27–8
DSM-IV-TR Diagnostic Criteria for Histrionic Personality Disorder

A pervasive pattern of excessive emotionality and attention seeking, beginning by early adulthood and present in a variety of contexts, as indicated by five (or more) of the following:

(1) is uncomfortable in situations in which he or she is not the center of attention
(2) interaction with others is often characterized by inappropriate sexually seductive or provocative behavior
(3) displays rapidly shifting and shallow expression of emotions
(4) consistently uses physical appearance to draw attention to self
(5) has a style of speech that is excessively impressionistic and lacking in detail
(6) shows self-dramatization, theatricality, and exaggerated expression of emotion
(7) is suggestible, i.e., easily influenced by others or circumstances
(8) considers relationships to be more intimate than they actually are

From American Psychiatric Association. *Diagnostic and Statistical Manual of Mental Disorders.* 4th ed. Text rev. Washington, DC: American Psychiatric Association; copyright 2000, with permission.

tures and dramatic punctuation in their conversations are common; they may make frequent slips of the tongue, and their language is colorful. Affective display is common, but, when pressed to acknowledge certain feelings (e.g., anger, sadness, and sexual wishes), they may respond with surprise, indignation, or denial. The results of the cognitive examination are usually normal, although a lack of perseverance may be shown on arithmetic or concentration tasks, and the patients' forgetfulness of affect-laden material may be astonishing. The DSM-IV-TR diagnostic criteria are listed in Table 27–8.

Clinical Features

Persons with histrionic personality disorder show a high degree of attention-seeking behavior. They tend to exaggerate their thoughts and feelings and make everything sound more important than it really is. They display temper tantrums, tears, and accusations when they are not the center of attention or are not receiving praise or approval.

Seductive behavior is common in both sexes. Sexual fantasies about persons with whom patients are involved are common, but patients are inconsistent about verbalizing these fantasies and may be coy or flirtatious rather than sexually aggressive. In fact, histrionic patients may have a psychosexual dysfunction; women may be anorgasmic, and men may be impotent. Their need for reassurance is endless. They may act on their sexual impulses to reassure themselves that they are attractive to the other sex. Their relationships tend to be superficial, however, and they can be vain, self-absorbed, and fickle. Their strong dependence needs make them overly trusting and gullible.

The major defenses of patients with histrionic personality disorder are repression and dissociation. Accordingly, such patients are unaware of their true feelings and cannot explain their motivations. Under stress, reality testing easily becomes impaired.

Differential Diagnosis

Distinguishing between histrionic personality disorder and borderline personality disorder is difficult, but in borderline personality disorder, suicide attempts, identity diffusion, and brief psychotic episodes are more likely. Although both conditions may be diagnosed in the same patient, clinicians should separate the two. Somatization disorder (Briquet's syndrome) may occur in conjunction with histrionic personality disorder. Patients with brief psychotic disorder and dissociative disorders may warrant a coexisting diagnosis of histrionic personality disorder.

Course and Prognosis

With age, persons with histrionic personality disorder show fewer symptoms, but because they lack the energy of earlier years, the difference in number of symptoms may be more apparent than real. Persons with this disorder are sensation seekers, and they may get into trouble with the law, abuse substances, and act promiscuously.

Treatment

Psychotherapy. Patients with histrionic personality disorder are often unaware of their own real feelings; clarification of their inner feelings is an important therapeutic process. Psychoanalytically oriented psychotherapy, whether group or individual, is probably the treatment of choice for histrionic personality disorder.

Pharmacotherapy. Pharmacotherapy can be adjunctive when symptoms are targeted (e.g., the use of antidepressants for depression and somatic complaints, antianxiety agents for anxiety, and antipsychotics for derealization and illusions).

NARCISSISTIC PERSONALITY DISORDER

Persons with narcissistic personality disorder are characterized by a heightened sense of self-importance and grandiose feelings of uniqueness.

Epidemiology

According to DSM-IV-TR, estimates of the prevalence of narcissistic personality disorder range from 2 to 16 percent in the clinical population and less than 1 percent in the general population. Persons with the disorder may impart an unrealistic sense of omnipotence, grandiosity, beauty, and talent to their children; thus offspring of such parents may have a higher than usual risk for developing the disorder themselves. The number of cases of narcissistic personality disorder reported is increasing steadily.

Diagnosis

Table 27–9 gives the DSM-IV-TR diagnostic criteria for narcissistic personality disorder.

Clinical Features

Persons with narcissistic personality disorder have a grandiose sense of self-importance; they consider themselves special and

Table 27–9
DSM-IV-TR Diagnostic Criteria for Narcissistic Personality Disorder

A pervasive pattern of grandiosity (in fantasy or behavior), need for admiration, and lack of empathy, beginning by early adulthood and present in a variety of contexts, as indicated by five (or more) of the following:

(1) has a grandiose sense of self-importance (e.g., exaggerates achievements and talents, expects to be recognized as superior without commensurate achievements)
(2) is preoccupied with fantasies of unlimited success, power, brilliance, beauty, or ideal love
(3) believes that he or she is "special" and unique and can only be understood by, or should associate with, other special or high-status people (or institutions)
(4) requires excessive admiration
(5) has a sense of entitlement, i.e., unreasonable expectations of especially favorable treatment or automatic compliance with his or her expectations
(6) is interpersonally exploitative, i.e., takes advantage of others to achieve his or her own ends
(7) lacks empathy: is unwilling to recognize or identify with the feelings and needs of others
(8) is often envious of others or believes that others are envious of him or her
(9) shows arrogant, haughty behaviors or attitudes

From American Psychiatric Association. *Diagnostic and Statistical Manual of Mental Disorders.* 4th ed. Text rev. Washington, DC: American Psychiatric Association; copyright 2000, with permission.

expect special treatment. Their sense of entitlement is striking. They handle criticism poorly and may become enraged when someone dares to criticize them, or they may appear completely indifferent to criticism. Persons with this disorder want their own way and are frequently ambitious to achieve fame and fortune. Their relationships are fragile, and they can make others furious by their refusal to obey conventional rules of behavior. Interpersonal exploitiveness is commonplace. They cannot show empathy, and they feign sympathy only to achieve their selfish ends. Because of their fragile self-esteem, they are prone to depression. Interpersonal difficulties, occupational problems, rejection, and loss are among the stresses that narcissists commonly produce by their behavior—stresses they are least able to handle.

Differential Diagnosis

Borderline, histrionic, and antisocial personality disorders often accompany narcissistic personality disorder, so a differential diagnosis is difficult. Patients with narcissistic personality disorder have less anxiety than those with borderline personality disorder; their lives tend to be less chaotic, and they are less likely to attempt suicide. Patients with antisocial personality disorder have a history of impulsive behavior, often associated with alcohol or other substance abuse, which frequently gets them into trouble with the law. Patients with histrionic personality disorder show features of exhibitionism and interpersonal manipulativeness that resemble those of patients with narcissistic personality disorder.

Course and Prognosis

Narcissistic personality disorder is chronic and difficult to treat. Patients with the disorder must constantly deal with blows to their narcissism resulting from their own behavior or from life experience. Aging is handled poorly; patients value beauty, strength, and youthful attributes, to which they cling inappropriately. They may be more vulnerable, therefore, to midlife crises than are other groups.

Treatment

Psychotherapy. Because patients must renounce their narcissism to make progress, the treatment of narcissistic personality disorder is difficult. Psychiatrists such as Kernberg and Heinz Kohut have advocated using psychoanalytic approaches to effect change, but much research is required to validate the diagnosis and to determine the best treatment. Some clinicians advocate group therapy for their patients so they can learn how to share with others and, under ideal circumstances, can develop an empathic response to others.

Pharmacotherapy. Lithium (Eskalith) has been used with patients whose clinical picture includes mood swings. Because patients with narcissistic personality disorder tolerate rejection poorly and are prone to depression, antidepressants, especially serotonergic drugs, may also be of use.

AVOIDANT PERSONALITY DISORDER

Persons with avoidant personality disorder show extreme sensitivity to rejection and may lead a socially withdrawn life. Although shy, they are not asocial and show a great desire for companionship, but they need unusually strong guarantees of uncritical acceptance. Such persons are commonly described as having an inferiority complex. (ICD-10 uses the term *anxious personality disorder.*)

Epidemiology

Avoidant personality disorder is common: The prevalence of the disorder is 1 to 10 percent of the general population. No information is available on sex ratio or familial pattern. Infants classified as having a timid temperament may be more prone to the disorder than those who score high on activity–approach scales.

Diagnosis

In clinical interviews, patients' most striking aspect is anxiety about talking with an interviewer. Their nervous and tense manner appears to wax and wane with their perception of whether an interviewer likes them. They seem vulnerable to the interviewer's comments and suggestions and may regard a clarification or interpretation as criticism. The DSM-IV-TR diagnostic criteria for avoidant personality disorder are listed in Table 27–10.

Clinical Features

Hypersensitivity to rejection by others is the central clinical feature of avoidant personality disorder, and patients' main personal-

Table 27–10
DSM-IV-TR Diagnostic Criteria for Avoidant Personality Disorder

A pervasive pattern of social inhibition, feelings of inadequacy, and hypersensitivity to negative evaluation, beginning by early adulthood and present in a variety of contexts, as indicated by four (or more) of the following:

(1) avoids occupational activities that involve significant interpersonal contact, because of fears of criticism, disapproval, or rejection
(2) is unwilling to get involved with people unless certain of being liked
(3) shows restraint within intimate relationships because of the fear of being shamed or ridiculed
(4) is preoccupied with being criticized or rejected in social situations
(5) is inhibited in new interpersonal situations because of feelings of inadequacy
(6) views self as socially inept, personally unappealing, or inferior to others
(7) is unusually reluctant to take personal risks or to engage in any new activities because they may prove embarrassing

From American Psychiatric Association. *Diagnostic and Statistical Manual of Mental Disorders.* 4th ed. Text rev. Washington, DC: American Psychiatric Association; copyright 2000, with permission.

ity trait is timidity. These persons desire the warmth and security of human companionship but justify their avoidance of relationships by their alleged fear of rejection. When talking with someone, they express uncertainty, show a lack of self-confidence, and may speak in a self-effacing manner. Because they are hypervigilant about rejection, they are afraid to speak up in public or to make requests of others. They are apt to misinterpret other persons' comments as derogatory or ridiculing. The refusal of any request leads them to withdraw from others and to feel hurt.

In the vocational sphere, patients with avoidant personality disorder often take jobs on the sidelines. They rarely attain much personal advancement or exercise much authority but seem shy and eager to please. These persons are generally unwilling to enter relationships unless they are given an unusually strong guarantee of uncritical acceptance. Consequently, they often have no close friends or confidants.

Differential Diagnosis

Patients with avoidant personality disorder desire social interaction, unlike patients with schizoid personality disorder, who want to be alone. Patients with avoidant personality disorder are not as demanding, irritable, or unpredictable as those with borderline and histrionic personality disorders. Avoidant personality disorder and dependent personality disorder are similar. Patients with dependent personality disorder are presumed to have a greater fear of being abandoned or unloved than those with avoidant personality disorder, but the clinical picture may be indistinguishable.

Course and Prognosis

Many persons with avoidant personality disorder are able to function in a protected environment. Some marry, have children, and live their lives surrounded only by family members. Should their support system fail, however, they are subject to depression, anxiety, and anger. Phobic avoidance is common, and patients with the disorder may give histories of social phobia or incur social phobia in the course of their illness.

Treatment

Psychotherapy. Psychotherapeutic treatment depends on solidifying an alliance with patients. As trust develops, a therapist must convey an accepting attitude toward the patient's fears, especially the fear of rejection. The therapist eventually encourages a patient to move out into the world to take what are perceived as great risks of humiliation, rejection, and failure. But therapists should be cautious when giving assignments to exercise new social skills outside therapy; failure may reinforce a patient's already poor self-esteem. Group therapy may help patients understand how their sensitivity to rejection affects them and others. Assertiveness training is a form of behavior therapy that may teach patients to express their needs openly and to enlarge their self-esteem.

Pharmacotherapy. Pharmacotherapy has been used to manage anxiety and depression when they are associated with the disorder. Some patients are helped by β-adrenergic receptor antagonists, such as atenolol (Tenormin), to manage autonomic nervous system hyperactivity, which tends to be high in patients with avoidant personality disorder, especially when they approach feared situations. Serotonergic agents may help rejection sensitivity. Theoretically, dopaminergic drugs might engender novelty-seeking behavior in these patients; however, the patient must be psychologically prepared for any new experience that might result.

DEPENDENT PERSONALITY DISORDER

Persons with dependent personality disorder subordinate their own needs to those of others, get others to assume responsibility for major areas of their lives, lack self-confidence, and may experience intense discomfort when alone for more than a brief period. The disorder has been called *passive-dependent personality.* Freud described an oral-dependent personality dimension characterized by dependence, pessimism, fear of sexuality, self-doubt, passivity, suggestibility, and lack of perseverance; his description is similar to the DSM-IV-TR categorization of dependent personality disorder.

Epidemiology

Dependent personality disorder is more common in women than in men. One study diagnosed 2.5 percent of all personality disorders as falling into this category. It is more common in young children than in older ones. Persons with chronic physical illness in childhood may be most prone to the disorder.

Diagnosis

In interviews, patients appear compliant. They try to cooperate, welcome specific questions, and look for guidance. The DSM-IV-TR diagnostic criteria for dependent personality disorder are listed in Table 27–11.

Table 27–11
DSM-IV-TR Diagnostic Criteria for Dependent Personality Disorder

A pervasive and excessive need to be taken care of that leads to submissive and clinging behavior and fears of separation, beginning by early adulthood and present in a variety of contexts, as indicated by five (or more) of the following:

(1) has difficulty making everyday decisions without an excessive amount of advice and reassurance from others
(2) needs others to assume responsibility for most major areas of his or her life
(3) has difficulty expressing disagreement with others because of fear of loss of support or approval. **Note:** Do not include realistic fears of retribution
(4) has difficulty initiating projects or doing things on his or her own (because of a lack of self-confidence in judgment or abilities rather than a lack of motivation or energy)
(5) goes to excessive lengths to obtain nurturance and support from others, to the point of volunteering to do things that are unpleasant
(6) feels uncomfortable or helpless when alone because of exaggerated fears of being unable to care for himself or herself
(7) urgently seeks another relationship as a source of care and support when a close relationship ends
(8) is unrealistically preoccupied with fears of being left to take care of himself or herself

From American Psychiatric Association. *Diagnostic and Statistical Manual of Mental Disorders.* 4th ed. Text rev. Washington, DC: American Psychiatric Association; copyright 2000, with permission.

Clinical Features

Dependent personality disorder is characterized by a pervasive pattern of dependent and submissive behavior. Persons with the disorder cannot make decisions without an excessive amount of advice and reassurance from others. They avoid positions of responsibility and become anxious if asked to assume a leadership role. They prefer to be submissive. When on their own, they find it difficult to persevere at tasks but may find it easy to perform these tasks for someone else.

Because persons with the disorder do not like to be alone, they seek out others on whom they can depend; their relationships are thus distorted by their need to be attached to another person. In folie à deux (shared psychotic disorder), one member of the pair usually suffers from dependent personality disorder; the submissive partner takes on the delusional system of the more aggressive, assertive partner on whom he or she depends.

Pessimism, self-doubt, passivity, and fears of expressing sexual and aggressive feelings all typify the behavior of persons with dependent personality disorder. An abusive, unfaithful, or alcoholic spouse may be tolerated for long periods to avoid disturbing the sense of attachment.

Differential Diagnosis

The traits of dependence are found in many psychiatric disorders, so differential diagnosis is difficult. Dependence is a prominent factor in patients with histrionic and borderline personality disorders, but those with dependent personality disorder usually have a long-term relationship with one person, rather than a series of persons on whom they are dependent, and they do not tend to be overtly manipulative. Patients with schizoid and schizotypal personality disorders may be indistinguishable from those with avoidant personality disorder. Dependent behavior may occur in patients with agoraphobia, but these patients tend to have a high level of overt anxiety or even panic.

Course and Prognosis

Little is known about the course of dependent personality disorder. Occupational functioning tends to be impaired, as persons with the disorder cannot act independently and without close supervision. Social relationships are limited to those on whom they can depend, and many suffer physical or mental abuse because they cannot assert themselves. They risk major depressive disorder if they lose the person they depend on, but with treatment, the prognosis is favorable.

Treatment

Psychotherapy. The treatment of dependent personality disorder is often successful. Insight-oriented therapies enable patients to understand the antecedents of their behavior, and with the support of a therapist, patients can become more independent, assertive, and self-reliant. Behavioral therapy, assertiveness training, family therapy, and group therapy have all been used, with successful outcomes in many cases.

A pitfall may arise in treatment when a therapist encourages a patient to change the dynamics of a pathological relationship (e.g., supports a physically abused wife in seeking help from the police). At this point patients may become anxious and unable to cooperate in therapy; they may feel torn between complying with the therapist and losing a pathological external relationship. Therapists must show great respect for these patients' feelings of attachment, no matter how pathological these feelings may seem.

Pharmacotherapy. Pharmacotherapy has been used to deal with specific symptoms such as anxiety and depression, which are common associated features of dependent personality disorder. Patients who experience panic attacks or who have high levels of separation anxiety may be helped by imipramine (Tofranil). Benzodiazepines and serotonergic agents have also been useful. If a patient's depression or withdrawal symptoms respond to psychostimulants, they may be used.

OBSESSIVE-COMPULSIVE PERSONALITY DISORDER

Obsessive-compulsive personality disorder is characterized by emotional constriction, orderliness, perseverance, stubbornness, and indecisiveness. The essential feature of the disorder is a pervasive pattern of perfectionism and inflexibility. (ICD-10 uses the name *anancastic personality disorder.*)

Epidemiology

The prevalence of obsessive-compulsive personality disorder is unknown. It is more common in men than in women and is diagnosed most often in oldest children. The disorder also occurs more frequently in first-degree biological relatives of persons with the disorder than in the general population. Patients often

have backgrounds characterized by harsh discipline. Freud hypothesized that the disorder is associated with difficulties in the anal stage of psychosexual development, generally around the age of 2, but various studies have failed to validate this theory.

Diagnosis

In interviews, patients with obsessive-compulsive personality disorder may have a stiff, formal, and rigid demeanor. Their affect is not blunted or flat but can be described as constricted. They lack spontaneity, and their mood is usually serious. Such patients may be anxious about not being in control of the interview. Their answers to questions are unusually detailed. The defense mechanisms they use are rationalization, isolation, intellectualization, reaction formation, and undoing. The DSM-IV-TR diagnostic criteria for obsessive-compulsive personality disorder are listed in Table 27–12.

Clinical Features

Persons with obsessive-compulsive personality disorder are preoccupied with rules, regulations, orderliness, neatness, details, and the achievement of perfection. These traits account for the general constriction of the entire personality. They insist that rules be followed rigidly and cannot tolerate what they consider infractions. Accordingly, they lack flexibility and are intolerant. They are capable of prolonged work, provided it is routinized and does not require changes to which they cannot adapt.

Persons with obsessive-compulsive personality disorder have limited interpersonal skills. They are formal and serious and often lack a sense of humor. They alienate persons, are unable to compromise, and insist that others submit to their needs. They are, however, eager to please those whom they see as more powerful than they are, and they carry out these persons' wishes in an authoritarian manner. Because they fear making mistakes, they are indecisive and ruminate about making decisions. Although a stable marriage and occupational adequacy are common, persons with obsessive-compulsive personality disorder have few friends. Anything that threatens to upset their perceived stability or the routine of their lives can precipitate a great deal of anxiety otherwise bound up in the rituals that they impose on their lives and try to impose on others.

Table 27–12
DSM-IV-TR Diagnostic Criteria for Obsessive-Compulsive Personality Disorder

A pervasive pattern of preoccupation with orderliness, perfectionism, and mental and interpersonal control, at the expense of flexibility, openness, and efficiency, beginning by early adulthood and present in a variety of contexts, as indicated by four (or more) of the following:

(1) is preoccupied with details, rules, lists, order, organization, or schedules to the extent that the major point of the activity is lost
(2) shows perfectionism that interferes with task completion (e.g., is unable to complete a project because his or her own overly strict standards are not met)
(3) is excessively devoted to work and productivity to the exclusion of leisure activities and friendships (not accounted for by obvious economic necessity)
(4) is overconscientious, scrupulous, and inflexible about matters of morality, ethics, or values (not accounted for by cultural or religious identification)
(5) is unable to discard worn-out or worthless objects even when they have no sentimental value
(6) is reluctant to delegate tasks or to work with others unless they submit to exactly his or her way of doing things
(7) adopts a miserly spending style toward both self and others; money is viewed as something to be hoarded for future catastrophes
(8) shows rigidity and stubbornness

From American Psychiatric Association. *Diagnostic and Statistical Manual of Mental Disorders.* 4th ed. Text rev. Washington, DC: American Psychiatric Association; copyright 2000, with permission.

Ms. C., a 41-year-old grocery store manager, comes for an evaluation at the insistence of the regional manager of the chain for which she works. Ms. C. has failed to turn in the last four periodic reports on time, and her store has one of the lowest productivity ratings in the chain, even though she usually comes in earlier and stays later than any of the other managers and appears to be busy every minute of the day. Ms. C. has frequent battles with her employees and has the highest turnover rate of employees in the chain. When confronted with these problems, she insists that her store is being run "properly" and by the book—unlike the others in the chain, which are maintaining "shoddy" standards.

It is easy to identify the source of difficulty in the store. Ms. C. insists that her employees shelve and arrange goods in exquisitely straight lines. She checks, double-checks, triple-checks, and quadruple-checks all her figures, which is why her periodic reports never get in on time. She micromanages every aspect of the store's operation and, consequently, her meat produce managers are always transferring to other stores. Instead of appreciating Ms. C.'s constant supervision, her managers find it annoying and time consuming. She is constantly drawing up charts, tables, graphs, and employee directives. She spends much of her time each morning constructing an elaborate to-do list that she never finds time to complete.

Ms. C. has been married for 15 years and has two children in their early teens. Her husband is a postal worker. Mr. C. reported to the therapist that until Ms. C. began working at the store 6 years ago they had lots of marital struggles because of Ms. C.'s need to oversee and direct every aspect of his life. She had insisted on knowing where he was at every moment and had tried to plan all his leisure time activities. He said that it was a great relief to him when she began to work at the store and became too busy to pay so much attention to his life. Mr. C. says that he and the children have a hard time persuading his wife to take a vacation and that it generally does not turn out to be much fun when she does agree to go. Ms. C. plans their itinerary and activities minutely and insists that everyone must participate in what she has scheduled. Nothing is allowed to be spontaneous or unplanned, and everyone is expected to spend their time "productively," even when on vacation.

Ms. C. comes by her perfectionism honestly. Both her parents were austere, driven, and highly critical. No matter how hard she worked or what she achieved, it never seemed

like enough. She began being a maid in her own house at the age of 5 and began to do chores for others by the age of 9 so she could begin to save money ("a penny saved is a penny earned"). Nothing but As in school were acceptable to her parents. If she made a 95 on a test, her mother would ask her, "Where are the other 5 points?" Even though Ms. C. can admit that she often found her parents' attitude painful and frustrating, she finds herself reacting to her own children in much the same way. Although she tries to praise them for their accomplishments, she always finds herself demanding that they work harder and perform better, even when they have done very well. (From *DSM-IV Case Studies.*)

Differential Diagnosis

When recurrent obsessions or compulsions are present, obsessive-compulsive disorder should be noted on Axis I. Perhaps the most difficult distinction is between outpatients with some obsessive-compulsive traits and those with obsessive-compulsive personality disorder. The diagnosis of personality disorder is reserved for those with significant impairments in their occupational or social effectiveness. In some cases, delusional disorder coexists with personality disorders and should be noted.

Course and Prognosis

The course of obsessive-compulsive personality disorder is variable and unpredictable. From time to time, persons may develop obsessions or compulsions in the course of their disorder. Some adolescents with obsessive-compulsive personality disorder evolve into warm, open, and loving adults; in others, the disorder can be either the harbinger of schizophrenia or—decades later and exacerbated by the aging process—major depressive disorder.

Persons with obsessive-compulsive personality disorder may flourish in positions demanding methodical, deductive, or detailed work, but they are vulnerable to unexpected changes, and their personal lives may remain barren. Depressive disorders, especially those of late onset, are common.

Treatment

Psychotherapy. Unlike patients with the other personality disorders, those with obsessive-compulsive personality disorder are often aware of their suffering, and they seek treatment on their own. Overtrained and oversocialized, these patients value free association and no-directive therapy highly. Treatment, however, is often long and complex, and countertransference problems are common.

Group therapy and behavior therapy occasionally offer certain advantages. In both contexts it is easy to interrupt the patients in the midst of their maladaptive interactions or explanations. Preventing the completion of their habitual behavior raises patients' anxiety and leaves them susceptible to learning new coping strategies. Patients can also receive direct rewards for change in group therapy, something less often possible in individual psychotherapies.

Pharmacotherapy. Clonazepam (Klonopin), a benzodiazepine with anticonvulsant use, has reduced symptoms in patients with severe obsessive-compulsive disorder. Whether it is of use in the personality disorder is unknown. Clomipramine (Anafranil) and such serotonergic agents as fluoxetine, usually at dosages of 60 to 80 mg a day, may be useful if obsessive-compulsive signs and symptoms break through. Nefazodone (Serzone) may benefit some patients.

PERSONALITY DISORDER NOT OTHERWISE SPECIFIED

In DSM-IV-TR, the category personality disorder not otherwise specified is reserved for disorders that do not fit into any of the personality disorder categories described above. Passive-aggressive personality disorder and depressive personality disorder are now listed as examples of personality disorder not otherwise specified. A narrow spectrum of behavior or a particular trait—such as oppositionalism, sadism, or masochism—can also be classified in this category. A patient with features of more than one personality disorder but without the complete criteria of any one disorder can be assigned this classification. The DSM-IV-TR criteria for personality disorder not otherwise specified are presented in Table 27–13.

Passive-Aggressive Personality Disorder

Persons with passive-aggressive personality disorder are characterized by covert obstructionism, procrastination, stubbornness, and inefficiency. Such behavior is a manifestation of passively expressed underlying aggression. In DSM-IV-TR the disorder is also called *negativistic personality disorder.*

Epidemiology. No data are available about the epidemiology of the disorder. Sex ratio, familial patterns, and prevalence have not been adequately studied.

Diagnosis. The criteria for passive-aggressive personality disorder are presented in Table 27–14.

Clinical Features. Passive-aggressive personality disorder patients characteristically procrastinate, resist demands for adequate performance,

Table 27–13
DSM-IV-TR Diagnostic Criteria for Personality Disorder Not Otherwise Specified

This category is for disorders of personality functioning that do not meet criteria for any specific personality disorder. An example is the presence of features of more than one specific personality disorder that do not meet the full criteria for any one personality disorder ("mixed personality"), but that together cause clinically significant distress or impairment in one or more important areas of functioning (e.g., social or occupational). This category can also be used when the clinician judges that a specific personality disorder that is not included in the classification is appropriate. Examples include depressive personality disorder and passive-aggressive personality disorder.

From American Psychiatric Association. *Diagnostic and Statistical Manual of Mental Disorders.* 4th ed. Text rev. Washington, DC: American Psychiatric Association; copyright 2000, with permission.

Table 27–14
DSM-IV-TR Research Criteria for Passive-Aggressive Personality Disorder

A. A pervasive pattern of negativistic attitudes and passive resistance to demands for adequate performance, beginning by early adulthood and present in a variety of contexts, as indicated by four (or more) of the following:
   (1) passively resists fulfilling routine social and occupational tasks
   (2) complains of being misunderstood and unappreciated by others
   (3) is sullen and argumentative
   (4) unreasonably criticizes and scorns authority
   (5) expresses envy and resentment toward those apparently more fortunate
   (6) voices exaggerated and persistent complaints of personal misfortune
   (7) alternates between hostile defiance and contrition
B. Does not occur exclusively during major depressive episodes and is not better accounted for by dysthymic disorder.

find excuses for delays, and find fault with those on whom they depend; yet they refuse to extricate themselves from the dependent relationships. They usually lack assertiveness and are not direct about their own needs and wishes. They fail to ask needed questions about what is expected of them and may become anxious when forced to succeed or when their usual defense of turning anger against themselves is removed.

In interpersonal relationships, these persons attempt to manipulate themselves into a position of dependence, but others often experience this passive, self-detrimental behavior as punitive and manipulative. Persons with this disorder expect others to do their errands and to carry out their routine responsibilities. Friends and clinicians may become enmeshed in trying to assuage the patients' many claims of unjust treatment. The close relationships of persons with passive-aggressive personality disorder, however, are rarely tranquil or happy. Because they are bound to their resentment more closely than to their satisfaction, they may never even formulate goals for finding enjoyment in life. Persons with the disorder lack self-confidence and are typically pessimistic about the future.

Differential Diagnosis. Passive-aggressive personality disorders must be differentiated from histrionic and borderline personality disorders. Patients with passive-aggressive personality disorder, however, are less flamboyant, dramatic, affective, and openly aggressive than those with histrionic and borderline personality disorders.

Course and Prognosis. In a follow-up study averaging 11 years of 100 passive-aggressive inpatients, Ivor Small found that the primary diagnosis in 54 was passive-aggressive personality disorder; 18 were also alcohol abusers, and 30 could be clinically labeled as depressed. Of the 73 former patients located, 58 (79 percent) had persistent psychiatric difficulties, and 9 (12 percent) were considered symptom free. Most seemed irritable, anxious, and depressed; somatic complaints were numerous. Only 32 (44 percent) were employed full time as workers or homemakers. Although neglect of responsibility and suicide attempts were common, only one patient had committed suicide in the interim. Twenty-eight (38 percent) had been readmitted to a hospital, but only three had been diagnosed as having schizophrenia.

Treatment. Patients with passive-aggressive personality disorder who receive supportive psychotherapy have good outcomes, but psychotherapy for these patients has many pitfalls. Fulfilling their demands often supports their pathology, but refusing their demands rejects them. Therapy sessions can thus become a battleground on which a patient expresses feelings of resentment against a therapist on whom the patient wishes to become dependent. With these patients, clinicians must treat suicide gestures as any covert expression of anger, and not as object loss in major depressive disorder. Therapists must point out the probable consequences of passive-aggressive behaviors as they occur. Such confrontations may be more helpful than a correct interpretation in changing patients' behavior.

Antidepressants should be prescribed only when clinical indications of depression and the possibility of suicide exist. Depending on the clinical features, some patients have responded to benzodiazepines and psychostimulants.

Depressive Personality Disorder

Persons with depressive personality disorder are characterized by lifelong traits that fall along the depressive spectrum. They are pessimistic, anhedonic, duty bound, self-doubting, and chronically unhappy. The disorder is newly classified in DSM-IV-TR, but melancholic personality was described by early 20th century European psychiatrists such as Ernst Kretschmer.

Epidemiology. Because depressive personality disorder is a new category, no epidemiological data are available. On the basis of the prevalence of depressive disorders in the overall population, however, depressive personality disorder seems to be common, to occur equally in men and women, and to occur in families in which depressive disorders are found.

Etiology. The cause of depressive personality disorder is unknown, but the same factors involved in dysthymic disorder and major depressive disorder may be at work. Psychological theories involve early loss, poor parenting, punitive superegos, and extreme feelings of guilt. Biological theories involve the hypothalamic-pituitary-adrenal-thyroid axis, including the noradrenergic and serotonergic amine systems. Genetic predisposition, as indicated by Stella Chess's studies of temperament, may also play a role.

Diagnosis and Clinical Features. A classic description of depressive personality was provided in 1963 by Arthur Noyes and Laurence Kolb:

> They feel but little of the normal joy of living and are inclined to be lonely and solemn, to be gloomy, submissive, pessimistic, and self-deprecatory. They are prone to express regrets and feelings of inadequacy and hopelessness. They are often meticulous, perfectionistic, overconscientious, preoccupied with work, feel responsibility keenly, and are easily discouraged under new conditions. They are fearful of disapproval, tend to suffer in silence and perhaps to cry easily, although usually not in the presence of others. A tendency to hesitation, indecision, and caution betrays an inherent feeling of insecurity.

More recently, Hagop Akiskal described seven groups of depressive traits: quiet, introverted, passive, and nonassertive; gloomy, pessimistic, serious, and incapable of fun; self-critical, self-reproachful, and self-derogatory; skeptical, critical of others, and hard to please; conscientious, responsible, and self-disciplined; brooding and given to worry; and preoccupied with negative events, feelings of inadequacy, and personal shortcomings.

Table 27–15
DSM-IV-TR Research Criteria for Depressive Personality Disorder

A. A pervasive pattern of depressive cognitions and behaviors beginning by early adulthood and present in a variety of contexts, as indicated by five (or more) of the following:
   (1) usual mood is dominated by dejection, gloominess, cheerlessness, joylessness, unhappiness
   (2) self-concept centers around beliefs of inadequacy, worthlessness, and low self-esteem
   (3) is critical, blaming, and derogatory toward self
   (4) is brooding and given to worry
   (5) is negativistic, critical, and judgmental toward others
   (6) is pessimistic
   (7) is prone to feeling guilty or remorseful

B. Does not occur exclusively during major depressive episodes and is not better accounted for by dysthymic disorder.

Patients with depressive personality disorder complain of chronic feelings of unhappiness. They admit to low self-esteem and find it difficult to find anything in their lives about which they are joyful, hopeful, or optimistic. They are self-critical and derogatory and are likely to denigrate their work, themselves, and their relationships with others. Their physiognomy often reflects their mood—poor posture, depressed facies, hoarse voice, and psychomotor retardation. The DSM-IV-TR criteria are listed in Table 27–15.

Differential Diagnosis. Dysthymic disorder is a mood disorder characterized by greater fluctuation in mood than occurs in depressive personality disorder. The personality disorder is chronic and lifelong, whereas dysthymic disorder is episodic, can occur at any time, and usually has a precipitating stressor. The depressive personality can be conceptualized as part of a spectrum of affective conditions in which dysthymic disorder and major depressive disorder are more severe variants. Patients with avoidant personality disorder are introverted and dependent but tend to be more anxious than depressed, compared with persons with depressive personality disorder.

Course and Prognosis. Persons with depressive personality disorder may be at great risk for dysthymic disorder and major depressive disorder. In a recent study by Donald Klein and Gregory Mills, subjects with depressive personality exhibited significantly higher rates of current mood disorder, lifetime mood disorder, major depression, and dysthymia than subjects without depressive personality.

Treatment. Psychotherapy is the treatment of choice for depressive personality disorder. Patients respond to insight-oriented psychotherapy, and because their reality testing is good, they can gain insight into the psychodynamics of their illness and appreciate its effects on their interpersonal relationships. Treatment is likely to be long term. Cognitive therapy helps patients understand the cognitive manifestations of their low self-esteem and pessimism. Group psychotherapy and interpersonal therapy are also useful. Some persons respond to self-help measures.

Psychopharmacological approaches include the use of antidepressant medications, especially such serotonergic agents as sertraline (Zoloft), 50 mg a day. Some patients respond to small dosages of psychostimulants, such as amphetamine, 5 to 15 mg a day. In all cases, psychopharmacological agents should be combined with psychotherapy to achieve maximum effects.

Sadomasochistic Personality Disorder

Some personality types are characterized by elements of sadism or masochism or a combination of both. Sadomasochistic personality disorder is listed here because it is of major clinical and historical interest in psychiatry. It is not an official diagnostic category in DSM-IV-TR or its appendix, but it can be diagnosed as personality disorder not otherwise classified.

Sadism is the desire to cause others pain by being either sexually abusive or generally physically or psychologically abusive. It is named for the Marquis de Sade, a late 18th century writer of erotica describing persons who experienced sexual pleasure while inflicting pain on others. Freud believed that sadists ward off castration anxiety and are able to achieve sexual pleasure only when they can do to others what they fear will be done to them.

Masochism, named for Leopold von Sacher-Masoch, a 19th century German novelist, is the achievement of sexual gratification by inflicting pain on the self. So-called moral masochists generally seek humiliation and failure rather than physical pain. Freud believed that masochists' ability to achieve orgasm is disturbed by anxiety and guilt feelings about sex, which are alleviated by suffering and punishment.

Clinical observations indicate that elements of both sadistic and masochistic behavior are usually present in the same person. Treatment with insight-oriented psychotherapy, including psychoanalysis, has been effective in some cases. As a result of therapy, patients become aware of the need for self-punishment secondary to excessive unconscious guilt and also come to recognize their repressed aggressive impulses, which originate in early childhood.

Sadistic Personality Disorder

Sadistic personality disorder is not included in DSM-IV-TR, but it still appears in the literature and may be of descriptive use. Beginning in early adulthood, persons with sadistic personality disorder show a pervasive pattern of cruel, demeaning, and aggressive behavior that is directed toward others. Physical cruelty or violence is used to inflict pain on others, not to achieve another goal, such as mugging a person to steal. Persons with the disorder like to humiliate or demean persons in front of others and have usually treated or disciplined persons uncommonly harshly, especially children. In general, persons with sadistic personality disorder are fascinated by violence, weapons, injury, or torture. To be included in this category, such persons cannot be motivated solely by the desire to derive sexual arousal from their behavior; if they are so motivated, the paraphilia of sexual sadism should be diagnosed.

PERSONALITY CHANGE DUE TO A GENERAL MEDICAL CONDITION

Personality change due to a general medical condition (see Table 10.5–8 in Section 10.5) deserves some discussion here. ICD-10 includes the category personality and behavioral disorders due to brain disease, damage, and dysfunction, which includes organic personality disorder (see Table 10.5–13), postencephalitic syndrome, and postconcussional syndrome. Personality change due to a general medical condition is characterized by a marked change in personality style and traits from a previous level of functioning. Patients must show evidence of a causative organic factor antedating the onset of the personality change.

Table 27–16
Medical Conditions Associated with Personality Change

Head trauma
Cerebrovascular diseases
Cerebral tumors
Epilepsy (particularly complex partial epilepsy)
Huntington's disease
Multiple sclerosis
Endocrine disorders
Heavy metal poisoning (manganese, mercury)
Neurosyphilis
Acquired immune deficiency syndrome (AIDS)

Etiology

Structural damage to the brain is usually the cause of the personality change, and head trauma is probably the most common cause. Cerebral neoplasms and vascular accidents, particularly of the temporal and frontal lobes, are also common causes. The conditions most often associated with personality change are listed in Table 27–16.

Diagnosis and Clinical Features

A change in personality from previous patterns of behavior or an exacerbation of previous personality characteristics is notable. Impaired control of the expression of emotions and impulses is a cardinal feature. Emotions are characteristically labile and shallow, although euphoria or apathy may be prominent. The euphoria may mimic hypomania, but true elation is absent, and patients may admit to not really feeling happy. There is a hollow and silly ring to their excitement and facile jocularity, particularly when the frontal lobes are involved. Also associated with damage to the frontal lobes, the so-called frontal lobe syndrome, is prominent indifference and apathy, characterized by a lack of concern for events in the immediate environment. Temper outbursts may occur with little or no provocation, especially after alcohol ingestion, and may result in violent behavior. The expression of impulses may be manifested by inappropriate jokes, a coarse manner, improper sexual advances, and antisocial conduct resulting in conflicts with the law, such as assaults on others, sexual misdemeanors, and shoplifting. Foresight and the ability to anticipate the social or legal consequences of actions are typically diminished. Persons with temporal lobe epilepsy characteristically show humorlessness, hypergraphia, hyperreligiosity, and marked aggressiveness during seizures.

Persons with personality change due to a general medical condition have a clear sensorium. Mild disorders of cognitive function often coexist but do not amount to intellectual deterioration. Patients may be inattentive, which may account for disorders of recent memory. With some prodding, however, patients are likely to recall what they claim to have forgotten. The diagnosis should be suspected in patients who show marked changes in behavior or personality involving emotional lability and impaired impulse control, who have no history of mental disorder, and whose personality changes occur abruptly or over a relatively brief time. The DSM-IV-TR diagnostic criteria appear in Table 10.5–3.

Anabolic Steroids. An increasing number of high school and college athletes and bodybuilders are using anabolic steroids as a shortcut to maximize physical development. Anabolic steroids include oxymetholone (Anadrol), somatropin (Humatrope), stanozolol (Winstrol), and testosterone.

DSM-IV-TR does not include a diagnostic category for substance-induced personality disorder, so it is unclear whether a personality change caused by steroid abuse is better diagnosed as personality change due to a general medical condition or as one of the other (or unknown) substance use disorders. It is mentioned here because anabolic steroids can cause persistent alterations of personality and behavior. Anabolic steroid abuse is discussed in Section 12.13.

Differential Diagnosis

Dementia involves global deterioration in intellectual and behavioral capacities, of which personality change is just one category. A personality change may herald a cognitive disorder that will eventually evolve into dementia. In these cases, as deterioration begins to encompass significant memory and cognitive deficits, the diagnosis of the disorder changes from personality change caused by a general medical condition to dementia. In differentiating the specific syndrome from other disorders in which personality change may occur—such as schizophrenia, delusional disorder, mood disorders, and impulse control disorders—physicians must consider the most important factor, the presence in personality change disorder of a specific organic causative factor.

Course and Prognosis

Both the course and the prognosis of personality change due to a general medical condition depend on its cause. If the disorder results from structural damage to the brain, the disorder tends to persist. The disorder may follow a period of coma and delirium in cases of head trauma or vascular accident and may be permanent. The personality change may evolve into dementia in cases of brain tumor, multiple sclerosis, and Huntington's disease. Personality changes produced by chronic intoxication, medical illness, or drug therapy (such as levodopa [Larodopa] for parkinsonism) may be reversed if the underlying cause is treated. Some patients require custodial care or at least close supervision to meet their basic needs, avoid repeated conflicts with the law, and protect themselves and their families from the hostility of others and from destitution resulting from impulsive and ill-considered actions.

Treatment

Management of personality change disorder involves treatment of the underlying organic condition when possible. Psychopharmacological treatment of specific symptoms may be indicated in some cases, such as imipramine or fluoxetine for depression.

Patients with severe cognitive impairment or weakened behavioral controls may need counseling to help avoid difficulties at work or to prevent social embarrassment. As a rule, patients' families need emotional support and concrete advice on how to help minimize patients' undesirable conduct. Alcohol should be avoided, and social engagements should be curtailed when patients tend to act in a grossly offensive manner.

PSYCHOBIOLOGICAL MODEL OF TREATMENT

The psychobiological model of treatment combines psychotherapy and pharmacotherapy and is based on the established structural, clinical, and postulated neurochemical characteristics of temperament and character. Pharmacotherapy and

Table 27–17
Pharmacotherapy of Target Symptom Domains of Personality Disorders

Target Symptom	Drug of Choice	Contraindication[a]
I. Behavior dyscontrol		
Aggression/impulsivity		
Affective aggression (hot temper with normal EEG)	Lithium[a] Serotonergic drugs[a] Anticonvulsants[a] Low-dosage antipsychotics	? Benzodiazepines Stimulants
Predatory aggression (hostility/cruelty)	Antipsychotics[a] Lithium β-adrenergic receptor antagonists	Benzodiazepines Stimulants
Organiclike aggression	Imipramine[a] Cholinergic agonists (donepezil)	
Ictal aggression (abnormal EEG)	Carbamazepine[a] Diphenylhydantoin[a] Benzodiazepines	Antipsychotics Stimulants
II. Mood dysregulation		
Emotional lability	Lithium[a] Antipsychotics	? Tricyclic drugs
Depression		
Atypical depression, dysphoria	MAOIs[a] Serotonergic drugs[a] Antipsychotics	
Emotional detachment	Serotonin-dopamine antagonists[a] Atypical antipsychotics	? Tricyclic drugs
III. Anxiety		
Chronic cognitive	Serotonergic drugs[a] MAOIs[a] Benzodiazepines	Stimulants
Chronic somatic	MAOIs[a] β-adrenergic receptor antagonists	
Severe anxiety	Low-dose antipsychotics MAOIs	
IV. Psychotic symptoms		
Acute and psychosis	Antipsychotics[a]	Stimulants
Chronic and low-level psychoticlike symptoms	Low-dose antipsychotics[a]	

[a]Drug of choice or major contraindication.

psychotherapy can be systematically matched to the personality structure and stage of character development of each individual—clearly a unique advantage over other available approaches.

The newest development is treating personality disorders pharmacologically. Target symptoms are identified, and particular drugs with known effects on personality traits (e.g., harm avoidance) are used. Table 27–17 summarizes drug choices for various target symptoms of personality disorders.

In his book *Listening to Prozac*, Peter Kramer described dramatic personality changes when serotonin levels are raised by fluoxetine administration, such as decreased sensitivity to rejection, increased assertiveness, improved self-esteem, and the ability to tolerate stress. These changes in personality traits occur in patients with a wide range of psychiatric conditions as well as in persons without diagnosable mental disorders. Using medications to treat specific traits in a person who is otherwise normal (i.e., does not meet the criteria for a full-blown personality disorder) is controversial. It has been called "cosmetic psychopharmacology" by its critics.

Four character traits have been described (Table 27–18), each with certain neurochemical and neurophysiological substrates.

Harm Avoidance

Harm avoidance involves a heritable bias in the inhibition of behavior in response to signals of punishment and nonreward. High harm avoidance is observed as fear of uncertainty, social inhibition, shyness with strangers, rapid fatigability, and pessimistic worry in anticipation of problems, even in situations that do not worry other persons. Persons low in harm avoidance are carefree, courageous, energetic, outgoing, and optimistic, even in situations that worry most persons.

The psychobiology of harm avoidance is complex. Benzodiazepines disinhibit avoidance by γ-aminobutyric acid (GABA)-ergic inhibition of serotonergic neurons originating in the dorsal raphe nuclei.

Positron emission tomography (PET) at the National Institute of Mental Health (NIMH) with ^{18}F-deoxyglucose (FDG) in 31 healthy adult volunteers during a simple, continuous, perfor-

Table 27–18
Descriptors of Individuals Who Score High and Low on the Four Temperament Dimensions

Temperament Dimension	Descriptors of Extreme Variants: High	Low
Harm avoidance	Pessimistic Fearful Shy Fatigable	Optimistic Daring Outgoing Energetic
Novelty seeking	Exploratory Impulsive Extravagant Irritable	Reserved Deliberate Thrifty Stoical
Reward dependence	Sentimental Open Warm Affectionate	Detached Aloof Cold Independent
Persistence	Industrious Determined Enthusiastic Perfectionist	Lazy Spoiled Underachieving Pragmatic

mance task showed that harm avoidance was associated with increased activity in the anterior paralimbic circuit, specifically the right amygdala and insula, the right orbitofrontal cortex, and the left medial prefrontal cortex.

High GABA concentrations in plasma have also been correlated with low harm avoidance. Plasma GABA concentration has also been correlated with other measures of anxiety proneness, and it correlates highly with GABA concentration in the brain. Finally, a gene on chromosome 17q12 that regulates the expression of the serotonin transporter accounts for 4 to 9 percent of the total variance in harm avoidance. These findings support a role for both GABA and serotonergic projections from the dorsal raphe underlying individual differences in behavioral inhibition as measured by harm avoidance. Persons given serotonin drugs show decreased harm avoidance behavior.

Novelty Seeking

Novelty seeking reflects activation in response to novelty, approach to signals of reward, and active avoidance punishment. Individuals high in novelty seeking are quick-tempered, curious, easily bored, impulsive, extravagant, and disorderly. Persons low in novelty seeking are slow tempered, uninquiring, stoical, reflective, frugal, reserved, tolerant of monotony, and orderly.

Dopaminergic projections have a crucial role in novelty seeking. Novelty seeking involves increased reuptake of dopamine at presynaptic terminals, thereby requiring frequent stimulation to maintain optimal levels of postsynaptic dopaminergic stimulation. Novelty seeking leads to various pleasure-seeking behaviors, including cigarette smoking, which may explain the frequent observation of low platelet MAO type B (MAO_B) activity, because cigarette smoking inhibits MAO_B activity in platelets and brain.

Studies of genes involved in dopamine neurotransmission, such as the dopamine transporter gene (*DAT1*) and the type 4 dopamine receptor gene (*DRD4*) have provided evidence of association with novelty seeking.

Reward Dependence

Reward dependence reflects maintenance of behavior in response to cues of social reward. Individuals high in reward dependence are tender hearted, sensitive, socially dependent, and sociable. Individuals low in reward dependence are practical, tough minded, cold, socially insensitive, irresolute, and indifferent if alone.

Noradrenergic projections from the locus ceruleus and serotonergic projections from the median raphe are thought to influence such reward conditioning. High reward dependence is associated with increased activity in the thalamus. The 3-methoxy-4-hydroxyphenylglycol (MHPG) concentration is low in persons with high reward dependence.

Persistence

Persistence reflects maintenance of behavior despite frustration, fatigue, and intermittent reinforcement. Highly persistent persons are hard-working, perseverant, and ambitious overachievers who tend to intensify their effort in response to anticipated reward and view frustration and fatigue as a personal challenge. Individuals low in persistence are indolent, inactive, unstable, and erratic; they tend to give up easily when faced with frustration, rarely strive for higher accomplishments, and manifest little perseverance even in response to intermittent reward.

Recent work in rodents related the integrity of the partial reinforcement extinction effect to hippocampal connections and glutamate metabolism. Persistence may be enhanced by psychostimulants.

ICD-10

In ICD-10, personality disorders are described as severe disturbances of personality and behavior that are pronounced deviations from normal cultural patterns. ICD-10's diagnostic guidelines include disturbances of long-standing duration in several areas of functioning; pervasive and maladaptive behavior; onset in childhood or adolescence; continuation into adulthood; considerable personality distress (although sometimes apparent only late in the disorder's course); and usually, but not always, significant problems in work and in social behavior. ICD-10 also allows for the possibility of criteria developed to describe personality disorders in different cultures. The diagnostic criteria for specific personality disorders appear in Table 27–1.

References

Brown MZ, Comtois KA, Linehan MM. Reasons for suicide attempts and nonsuicidal self-injury in women with borderline personality disorder. *J Abnorm Psychol.* 2002;111:232.

Cloninger CR, Svrakic DM. Personality disorders. In: Sadock BJ, Sadock VA, eds. *Kaplan & Sadock's Comprehensive Textbook of Psychiatry.* 7th ed. Vol 2. Baltimore: Lippincott Williams & Wilkins; 2000:1723.

Dickey CC, McCarley RW, Shenton ME. The brain in schizotypal personality disorder: a review of structural MRI and CT findings. *Harv Rev Psychiatry.* 2002;10:1.

Mulder RT. Personality pathology and treatment outcome in major depression: a review. *Am J Psychiatry.* 2002;159:359.

Nickell AD, Waudby CJ, Trull TJ. Attachment, parental bonding and borderline personality disorder features in young adults. *J Personal Disord.* 2002;16:148.

Oldham JM. A 44-year-old woman with borderline personality disorder. *JAMA.* 2002;287:1029.

Rivas-Vazquez RA, Blais MA. Pharmacologic treatment of personality disorder. *Prof Psychol Res Pract.* 2002;33:104.

Sansone RA, Gaither GA, Songer DA. The relationships among childhood abuse, borderline personality and self-harm behavior in psychiatric inpatients. *Violence Vict.* 2002;17:49.

Teusch L, Boehme H, Finke J, Gastpar M. Effects of client-centered psychotherapy for personality disorder alone and in combination with psychopharmacological treatment. *Psychother Psychosom.* 2001;70:328.

28 Psychological Factors Affecting Medical Condition and Psychosomatic Medicine

▲ 28.1 Overview

Psychosomatic medicine emphasizes the unity of mind and body and the interaction between them (this is also the basis of complementary and alternative medicine). Overall, the conviction is that psychological factors are important in the development of all diseases. Whether that role is in the initiation, progression, aggravation, or exacerbation of a disease or in the predisposition or reaction to a disease is open to debate and varies from disorder to disorder. Psychosomatic medicine is now part of the larger field of behavioral medicine. In 1978 the National Academy of Sciences defined behavioral medicine as "the interdisciplinary field concerned with the development and integration of behavioral and biomedical science knowledge and techniques relevant to health and illness and the application of this knowledge and these techniques to prevention, diagnosis, and rehabilitation."

The revised fourth edition of *Diagnostic and Statistical Manual of Mental Disorders* (DSM-IV-TR) does not use the term *psychosomatic*. Instead it describes psychological factors affecting medical conditions as "one or more psychological or behavioral problems that adversely and significantly affect the course or outcome of a general medical condition, or that significantly increase a person's risk of an adverse outcome." Nevertheless, few would disagree that psychological or behavioral factors play a role in almost every medical condition.

CLASSIFICATION

The DSM-IV-TR diagnostic criteria for psychological factors affecting medical condition are presented in Table 28.1–1. Excluded are (1) classic mental disorders that have physical symptoms as part of the disorder (e.g., conversion disorder, in which a physical symptom is produced by psychological conflict); (2) somatization disorder, in which the physical symptoms are not based on organic pathology; (3) hypochondriasis, in which patients have an exaggerated concern with their health; (4) physical complaints that are frequently associated with mental disorders (e.g., dysthymic disorder, which usually has such somatic accompaniments as muscle weakness, asthenia, fatigue, and exhaustion); and (5) physical complaints associated with substance-related disorders (e.g., coughing associated with nicotine dependence). Criteria in the 10th revision of the *International Statistical Classification of Diseases and Related Health Problems* (ICD-10) are more general than the DSM-IV-TR criteria and are listed in Table 28.1–2.

HISTORY

The history of psychosomatic medicine dates to ancient beliefs that the body can be affected by external forces. Table 28.1–3 provides a survey of historical concepts of psychosomatic medicine. Over the years a great variety of conditions have been studied as having psychosomatic overtones (Table 28.1–4).

STRESS THEORY

In the 1920s, Walter Cannon (1875–1945) conducted the first systematic study of the relation of stress to disease. He demonstrated that stimulation of the autonomic nervous system, particularly the sympathetic system, readied the organism for the "fight or flight" response characterized by hypertension, tachycardia, and increased cardiac output. This was useful in the animal who could fight or flee; but in the person who could do neither by virtue of being civilized, the ensuing stress resulted in disease (e.g., produced a cardiovascular disorder).

In the 1950s, Harold Wolff (1898–1962) observed that the physiology of the gastrointestinal tract appeared to correlate with specific emotional states. Hyperfunction was associated with hostility, and hypofunction with sadness. Wolff regarded such reactions as nonspecific, believing that the patient's reaction is determined by the general life situation and perceptual appraisal of the stressful event. Earlier, William Beaumont (1785–1853), an American military surgeon, had a patient named Alexis St. Martin, who became famous because of a gunshot wound that resulted in a permanent gastric fistula. Beaumont noted that during highly charged emotional states the mucosa could become either hyperemic or blanch, indicating that blood flow to the stomach was influenced by emotions.

Hans Selye (1907–1982) developed a model of stress that he called the *general adaptation syndrome*. It consisted of three phases: (1) the alarm reaction; (2) the stage of resistance, in which adaptation is ideally achieved; and (3) the stage of exhaustion, in which acquired adaptation or resistance may be lost. He consid-

Table 28.1–1
DSM-IV-TR Diagnostic Criteria for Psychological Factors Affecting General Medical Condition

A. A general medical condition (coded on Axis III) is present.
B. Psychological factors adversely affect the general medical condition in one of the following ways:
  (1) the factors have influenced the course of the general medical condition as shown by a close temporal association between the psychological factors and the development or exacerbation of, or delayed recovery from, the general medical condition
  (2) the factors interfere with the treatment of the general medical condition
  (3) the factors constitute additional health risks for the individual
  (4) stress-related physiological responses precipitate or exacerbate symptoms of the general medical condition

Choose name based on the nature of the psychological factors (if more than one factor is present, indicate the most prominent):

Mental disorder affecting . . . [indicate the general medical condition] (e.g., an Axis I disorder such as major depressive disorder delaying recovery from a myocardial infarction)

Psychological symptoms affecting . . . [indicate the general medical condition] (e.g., depressive symptoms delaying recovery from surgery; anxiety exacerbating asthma)

Personality traits or coping style affecting . . . [indicate the general medical condition] (e.g., pathological denial of the need for surgery in a patient with cancer; hostile, pressured behavior contributing to cardiovascular disease)

Maladaptive health behaviors affecting . . . [indicate the general medical condition] (e.g., overeating; lack of exercise; unsafe sex)

Stress-related physiological response affecting . . . [indicate the general medical condition] (e.g., stress-related exacerbations of ulcer, hypertension, arrhythmia, or tension headache)

Other or unspecified psychological factors affecting . . . [indicate the general medical condition] (e.g., interpersonal, cultural, or religious factors)

Table 28.1–2
ICD-10 Diagnostic Criteria for Psychological and Behavioral Factors Associated with Disorders or Diseases Classified Elsewhere

This category should be used to record the presence of psychological or behavioral factors thought to have influenced the manifestation, or affected the course, of physical disorders that can be classified using other chapters of ICD-10. Any resulting mental disturbances are usually mild and often prolonged (such as worry, emotional conflict, apprehension) and do not of themselves justify the use of any of the categories described in the rest of this book. An additional code should be used to identify the physical disorder. (In the rare instances in which an overt psychiatric disorder is thought to have caused a physical disorder, a second additional code should be used to record the psychiatric disorder.)

ered stress a nonspecific bodily response to any demand caused by either pleasant or unpleasant conditions. Selye believed that stress, by definition, need not always be unpleasant. He called unpleasant stress *distress*. Accepting both types of stress requires adaptation.

The body reacts to stress—in this sense defined as anything (real, symbolic, or imagined) that threatens an individual's survival—by putting into motion a set of responses that seeks to diminish the impact of the stressor and restore homeostasis. Much is known about the physiological response to acute stress, but considerably less is known about the response to chronic stress. Many stressors occur over a prolonged period of time or have long-lasting repercussions. For example, the loss of a spouse may be followed by months or years of loneliness and a violent sexual assault may be followed by years of apprehension and worry. Neuroendocrine and immune responses to such events help explain why and how stress may have deleterious effects.

Neurotransmitter Responses to Stress. Stressors activate noradrenergic systems in the brain (most notably in the locus ceruleus) and cause release of catecholamines from the autonomic nervous system. Stressors also activate serotonergic systems in the brain, as evidenced by increased serotonin turnover. Recent evidence suggests that although glucocorticoids tend to enhance overall serotonin functioning, there may be differences in glucocorticoid regulation of serotonin-receptor subtypes, which may have implications for serotonergic functioning in depression and related illnesses. For example, glucocorticoids may increase serotonin 5-HT_2–mediated actions, thus contributing to the intensification of actions of these receptor types, which have been implicated in the pathophysiology of major depressive disorder. Stress also increases dopaminergic neurotransmission in mesoprefrontal pathways.

Clearly, amino acid and peptidergic neurotransmitters are also intricately involved in the stress response. Studies have shown that corticotropin-releasing factor (CRF) (as a neurotransmitter, not just as a hormonal regulator of hypothalamic-pituitary-adrenal axis functioning), glutamate (through *N*-methyl-D-aspartate [NMDA] receptors), and γ-aminobutyric acid (GABA) all play important roles in generating the stress response or in modulating other stress-responsive systems such as dopaminergic and noradrenergic brain circuitry.

Endocrine Responses to Stress. In response to stress, CRF is secreted from the hypothalamus into the hypophysial-pituitary-portal system. CRF acts at the anterior pituitary to trigger release of adrenocorticotropic hormone (ACTH). Once ACTH is released, it acts at the adrenal cortex to stimulate the synthesis and release of glucocorticoids. Glucocorticoids themselves have myriad effects within the body, but their actions can be summarized in the short term as promoting energy use, increasing cardiovascular activity (in the service of the "flight-or-fight" response), and inhibiting functions such as growth, reproduction, and immunity.

This hypothalamic-pituitary-adrenal axis is subject to tight negative feedback control by its own end products (i.e., ACTH and cortisol) at multiple levels, including the anterior pituitary, the hypothalamus, and such suprahypothalamic brain regions as the hippocampus. In addition to CRF, numerous secretagogues (i.e., substances that elicit ACTH release) exist that can bypass CRF release and act directly to initiate the glucocorticoid cascade. Examples of such secretagogues include catecholamines, vasopressin, and oxytocin. Interestingly, different stressors (e.g., cold stress versus hypotension) trigger different patterns of secretagogue release, again demonstrating that the notion of a uniform stress response to a generic stressor is an oversimplification.

Table 28.1–3
Major Conceptual Trends in Psychosomatic Medicine

I. Psychoanalytic

Sigmund Freud (1900) Somatic involvement occurs in conversion hysteria, which is psychogenic in origin—e.g., paralysis of an extremity. Conversion hysteria always has a primary psychic cause and meaning; i.e., it represents the symbolic substitutive expression of an unconscious conflict. It involves organs innervated only by the voluntary neuromuscular or the sensory-motor nervous system. Psychic energy that is dammed up is discharged through physiological outlets.

Sandor Ferenczi (1910) The concept of conversion hysteria is applied to organs innervated by the autonomic nervous system; e.g., the bleeding of ulcerative colitis may be described as representing a specific psychic fantasy. (Diseases, such as colitis, are known today as psychosomatic diseases that occur only in organs innervated by the autonomic nervous system.) Ferenczi's interpretation of psychosomatic symptoms as conversion reactions was the first application of the concept to diseases such as colitis.

Smith Ely Jelliffe, George Groddeck (1910) Clearly organic diseases, such as fever and hemorrhage, are held to have primary psychic meanings; i.e., they are interpreted as conversion symptoms that represent the expression of unconscious fantasies.

Franz Alexander (1934, 1968) Psychosomatic symptoms occur only in organs innervated by the autonomic nervous system and have no specific psychic meaning (as does conversion hysteria) but are end results of prolonged physiological states, which are the physiological accompaniments of certain specific unconscious repressed conflicts. In certain constitutional organic predisposing factors, in addition to the psychic factors involved, repressed psychic energy is discharged physiologically. Alexander's observations were supported by Herbert Weiner's 1957 study of pepsinogen hypersecretion. Presented first conceptualization of the biopsychosocial model.

Helen Flanders Dunbar (1936) Specific conscious personality pictures are associated with specific psychosomatic diseases, an idea similar to Meyer Friedman's 1959 theory of the type A coronary type.

Helen Deutsch (1939), Phyllis Greenacre (1949) Trauma during birth, infancy, and childhood predisposes to adult psychosomatic disease.

Angel Garma (1950) Peptic ulcer has a specific psychological meaning. Garma's idea is an extension of Sigmund Freud's conversion concept to an organ innervated by the autonomic nervous system. It is similar to Sandor Ferenczi's concept.

Jurgen Ruesch (1958) Importance of the interaction between persons—i.e., communication between the patient and the environment. A disturbance in communication results in psychosomatic illness, a regressive type of communication. Developed concept of "infantile personality" as vulnerable to psychosomatic illness.

Peter Sifneos, John C. Nemiah (1970) Elaborated the concept of alexithymia. Developmental arrests in the capacity and the ability to express conflict-related affect result in psychosomatic symptom formation. Concept of "alexithymia" modified later by Stoudemire, who advocated the term "somatothymia" emphasizing cultural influences on use of somatic language and somatic symptom to express affective distress.

II. Psychophysiological

Walter Cannon (1927) Demonstrated the physiological concomitants of some emotions and the important role of the autonomic nervous system in producing those reactions. The concept is based on pavlovian behavioral experimental designs.

Harold Wolff (1943) Attempted to correlate life stress (conscious) to physiological response, using objective laboratory tests. Physiological change, if prolonged, may lead to structural change. He established the basic research paradigm for the fields of psychoimmunology, psychocardiology, and psychoneuroendocrinology.

Hans Selye (1945) Under stress a general adaptation syndrome develops. Adrenal cortical hormones are responsible for the physiological reaction.

John Mason (1968) Individualized emotional responses are the dominant factor in determining the magnitude of stress-related physiological reactions and the role of intervening psychological variables or key factors in regulating reactions to stress. Mason's concepts presaged Richard Lazarus's 1984 emphasis on the person's cognitive appraisal of stressful stimuli as a critical factor determining stress reactions.

Meyer Friedman (1959) Theory of type A personality as a risk factor for cardiovascular disease. The concept has predominated much of psychosomatic research for the past 30 years. The basic concept was introduced by Helen Flanders Dunbar as early as 1936.

Robert Ader (1964) Established the basic concepts and the research methods for the field of psychoneuroimmunology.

III. Sociocultural

Karen Horney (1939), James Halliday (1948), Margaret Mead (1947) Emphasized the influence of the culture in the development of psychosomatic illness. They thought that culture influences the mother, who, in turn, affects the child in her relationship with the child—e.g., nursing, child rearing, anxiety transmission.

Thomas Holmes, Richard Rahe (1975) Correlated the severity and the number of recent stressful life events with the likelihood of disease.

John Cassel (1976) Psychosocial factors can serve as either stressors or buffers in determining vulnerability to disease.

IV. Systems theory

Adolph Meyer (1958) Formulated the psychobiological approach to patient assessment that emphasizes the integrated assessment of developmental, psychological, social, environmental, and biological aspects of the patient's condition. Basic concept of the biopsychosocial model implicit in his approach.

Zbigniew Lipowski (1970) A total approach to psychosomatic disease is necessary. External (ecological, infectious, cultural, environmental), internal (emotional), genetic, somatic, and constitutional factors as well as past and present history are important and should be studied by investigators working in the various fields in which they are trained.

George Engel (1977) Coined the term "biopsychosocial" derived from general systems theory and based on conceptual ideas introduced much earlier by Alexander and Meyer.

Herbert Weiner (1977) Integrative model of psychosomatic phenomena. He emphasized the need not only to integrate biological, social, and psychological factors contributing to disease vulnerability but also to understand such processes at the genetic, molecular, and neurophysiological levels.

Leon Eisenberg (1995) Contemporary psychiatric research demonstrates that the mind/brain responds to biological and social vectors while being jointly constructed of both. Major brain pathways are specified in the genome; detailed connections are fashioned by, and consequently reflect, socially mediated experience in the world.

Adapted from Harold I. Kaplan, M.D.

Table 28.1–4
Some Psychosomatic Disorders

Acne	Migraine
Allergic reactions	Mucous colitis
Angina pectoris	Nausea
Angioneurotic edema	Neurodermatitis
Arrhythmia	Obesity
Asthmatic wheezing	Painful menstruation
Bronchial asthma	Pruritus ani
Cardiospasm	Pylorospasm
Chronic pain syndromes	Regional enteritis
Coronary heart disease	Rheumatoid arthritis
Diabetes mellitus	Sacroiliac pain
Duodenal ulcer	Skin diseases, such as psoriasis
Essential hypertension	Spastic colitis
Gastric ulcer	Tachycardia
Headache	Tension headache
Herpes	Tuberculosis
Hyperinsulinism	Ulcerative colitis
Hyperthyroidism	Urticaria
Hypoglycemia	Vomiting
Immune diseases	Warts
Irritable colon	

Immune Response to Stress. Part of the stress response consists of the inhibition of immune functioning by glucocorticoids. This inhibition may reflect a compensatory action of the hypothalamic-pituitary-adrenal axis to mitigate other physiological effects of stress. Conversely, stress can also cause immune activation through a variety of pathways. CRF itself can stimulate norepinephrine release via CRF receptors located on the locus ceruleus, which activates the sympathetic nervous system, both centrally and peripherally, and increases epinephrine release from the adrenal medulla. In addition, there are direct links of norepinephrine neurons that synapse upon immune target cells. Thus, in the face of stressors there is also profound immune activation, including the release of humoral immune factors (cytokines) such as interleukin-1 (IL-1) and IL-6. These cytokines can themselves cause further release of CRF, which in theory serves to increase glucocorticoid effects and thereby self-limit the immune activation. An extensive discussion of the immune response can be found in Section 3.5.

Vicissitudes of Life

A life event or situation, favorable or unfavorable (Selye's distress), often occurring by chance, generates challenges to which the person must adequately respond. Thomas Holmes and Richard Rahe constructed a social readjustment rating scale after asking hundreds of persons from varying backgrounds to rank the relative degree of adjustment required by changing life events. Holmes and Rahe listed 43 life events associated with varying amounts of disruption and stress in average persons' lives: for example, the death of a spouse, 100 life-change units; divorce, 73 units; marital separations, 65 units; and the death of a close family member, 63 units (Table 28.1–5). Accumulation of 200 or more life-change units in a single year increases the risk of developing a psychosomatic disorder in that year. Of

Table 28.1–5
Social Readjustment Rating Scale

Life Event	Mean Value
1. Death of spouse	100
2. Divorce	73
3. Marital separation from mate	65
4. Detention in jail or other institution	63
5. Death of a close family member	63
6. Major personal injury or illness	53
7. Marriage	50
8. Being fired at work	47
9. Marital reconciliation with mate	45
10. Retirement from work	45
11. Major change in the health or behavior of a family member	44
12. Pregnancy	40
13. Sexual difficulties	39
14. Gaining a new family member (through birth, adoption, oldster moving in, etc.)	39
15. Major business readjustment (merger, reorganization, bankruptcy, etc.)	39
16. Major change in financial state (a lot worse off or a lot better off than usual)	38
17. Death of a close friend	37
18. Changing to a different line of work	36
19. Major change in the number of arguments with spouse (either a lot more or a lot less than usual regarding child rearing, personal habits, etc.)	35
20. Taking on a mortgage greater than $10,000 (purchasing a home, business, etc.)[a]	31
21. Foreclosure on a mortgage or loan	30
22. Major change in responsibilities at work (promotion, demotion, lateral transfer)	29
23. Son or daughter leaving home (marriage, attending college, etc.)	29
24. In-law troubles	29
25. Outstanding personal achievement	28
26. Wife beginning or ceasing work outside the home	26
27. Beginning or ceasing formal schooling	26
28. Major change in living conditions (building a new home, remodeling, deterioration of home or neighborhood)	25
29. Revision of personal habits (dress, manners, associations, etc.)	24
30. Troubles with the boss	23
31. Major change in working hours or conditions	20
32. Change in residence	20
33. Changing to a new school	20
34. Major change in usual type or amount of recreation	19
35. Major change in church activities (a lot more or a lot less than usual)	19
36. Major change in social activities (clubs, dancing, movies, visiting, etc.)	18
37. Taking on a mortgage or loan less than $10,000 (purchasing a car, TV, freezer, etc.)	17
38. Major change in sleeping habits (a lot more or a lot less sleep or change in part of day when asleep)	16
39. Major change in number of family get-togethers (a lot more or a lot less than usual)	15
40. Major change in eating habits (a lot more or a lot less food intake or very different meal hours or surroundings)	15
41. Vacation	15
42. Christmas	12
43. Minor violations of the law (traffic tickets, jaywalking, disturbing the peace, etc.)	11

[a]This figure no longer has any relevance in the light of inflation; what is significant is the total amount of debt from all sources.

Reprinted with permission from Holmes T. Life situations, emotions, and disease. *Psychosom Med.* 1978;9:747.

Table 28.1–6
Some Hypothesized Psychological Correlates of Psychophysiological Disorders

Disorder	Psychogenic Causes, Personality Characteristics, and Coping Aims
Peptic ulcer	Feels deprived of dependence needs; is resentful; represses anger; cannot vent hostility or actively seek dependence security; characterizes self-sufficient and responsible go-getter types who are compensating for dependence desires; has strong regressive wish to be nurtured and fed; revengeful feelings are repressed and kept unconscious
Colitis	Was intimidated in childhood into dependence and conformity; feels conflict over resentment and desire to please; anger restrained for fear of retaliation; is fretful, brooding, and depressive or passive; seeks to camouflage hostility by symbolic gesture of giving
Essential hypertension	Was forced in childhood to restrain resentments; inhibited rage; is threatened by and guilt-ridden over hostile impulses that may erupt; is a controlled, conforming, and "mature" personality; is hard-driving and conscientious; is guarded and tense; needs to control and direct anger into acceptable channels; wishes to gain approval from authority
Migraine	Is unable to fulfill excessive self-demands; feels intense resentment and envy toward intellectually or financially more successful competitors; has meticulous, scrupulous, perfectionistic, and ambitious personality; failure to attain perfectionist ambitions results in self-punishment
Bronchial asthma	Feels separation anxiety; was given inconsistent maternal affection; has fear and guilt that hostile impulses will be expressed toward loved persons; is clinging and dependent; symptom expresses suppressed cry for help and protection
Neurodermatitis	Has overprotective but ungiving parents; has craving for affection; has conflict regarding hostility and dependence; shows guilt and self-punishment for inadequacies; is a superficially friendly and oversensitive personality with depressive features and low self-image; symptoms are atonement for inadequacy and guilt by self-excoriation; displays oblique expression of hostility and exhibitionism in need for attention and soothing

Reprinted with permission from Millon T, Millon R. Psychophysiologic disorders. In: Millon T, ed. *Medical Behavioral Science.* Philadelphia: WB Saunders; 1975:211.

interest, persons who face general stresses optimistically, rather than pessimistically, are less apt to experience psychosomatic disorders; if they do, they are more apt to recover easily.

Specific versus Nonspecific Stress Factors

In addition to general stresses such as a divorce or the death of a spouse, some investigators have suggested that specific personalities and conflicts are associated with certain psychosomatic diseases. *Specific psychic stress* may be defined as a specific personality or a specific unconscious conflict that causes a homeostatic disequilibrium contributing to the development of a psychosomatic disorder. Researchers first identified specific personality types in connection with coronary disease. A coronary personality is a hard-driving, competitive, aggressive person who is predisposed to coronary disease. Meyer Friedman and Ray Rosenman first defined types A—similar to the coronary personality—and B personalities—calm, relaxed, and not prone to coronary disease. (Type A and type B personalities are discussed in Section 28.2.)

Franz Alexander hypothesized that specific unconscious conflicts are associated with specific psychosomatic disorders (e.g., unconscious dependence conflict may predispose persons to peptic ulcer). The specific psychic stress theory is no longer considered a reliable indicator of who will develop which disorder. Table 28.1–6 gives some psychological correlates of psychophysiological disorders.

The nonspecific stress theory is more acceptable to most workers in the field today than the specific stress theory. Chronic stress, usually with the intervening variable of anxiety, has physiological correlates that, combined with genetic organ vulnerability or debility, predispose certain persons to psychosomatic disorders. The vulnerable organ may be anywhere in the body. Some persons are "stomach reactors," others are "cardiovascular reactors," "skin reactors," and so on. The diathesis or susceptibility is probably of genetic origin; but it may also result from acquired vulnerability (e.g., lungs weakened by smoking). Another nonspecific factor is the concept of alexithymia, developed by Peter Sifneos and John Nemiah, in which persons cannot express feelings because they are unaware of their mood. Tension states leading to disease occur as a result.

References

Alexander F. *Psychosomatic Medicine.* New York: Norton; 1950.
Alexander F, French TM, Pollack GH. *Psychosomatic Specificity: Experimental Study and Results.* Chicago: University of Chicago Press; 1968.
Benson H. The relaxation response. In: Goleman D, Gurin J, eds. *Mind Body Medicine: How to Use Your Mind for Better Health.* Yonkers, NY: Consumer Reports; 1993:233.
Engel GH, Reichsman F, Siegel HL. A study of an infant with a gastric fistula. *Psychosom Med.* 1956;18:374.
Feifel H, Strack S, Nagy VT. Degree of life-threat and differential use of coping modes. *J Psychol Res.* 1987;31:91.
Frasure-Smith N, Lesperance F, Talajic M. Depression and 18-month prognosis after myocardial infarction. *Circulation* 1995;91:999.
Kiecolt-Glaser JK, Glaser R. Psychoneuroimmunology: can psychological interventions modulate immunity? *J Consult Clin Psychol.* 1992;60:569.
Nakano K. Application of self-control procedures to modifying type A behavior. *Psychol Rec.* 1996;46:595.
Larson MR, Ader R, Moynihan JA. Heart rate, neuroendocrine and immunological reactivity in response to an acute laboratory stressor. *Psychosom Med.* 2001;63:493.
Levenstein S, Ackerman S, Kiecolt-Glaser JK, Dubois A. Stress and peptic ulcer disease. *JAMA.* 1999;281:10.
Lipsitt DR. Consultation-liaison psychiatry and psychosomatic medicine. *Psychosom Med.* 2001;63:896.
Stoudemire A, McDaniel JS. History, classification, and current trends in psychosomatic medicine. In: Sadock BJ, Sadock VA, eds. *Kaplan & Sadock's Comprehensive Textbook of Psychiatry.* 7th ed. Vol 2. Baltimore: Lippincott Williams & Wilkins; 2000:1765.
Whitehead WE. Behavioral medicine approaches to gastrointestinal disorders. *J Consult Clin Psychol.* 1992;60:605.

▲ 28.2 Specific Disorders

GASTROINTESTINAL SYSTEM

There is a link between stress, anxiety, and physiological responsivity of the gastrointestinal system. Disturbances in gastrointestinal function occur through a central control mechanism or via

humoral effects such as the release of catecholamines. Sympathetic autonomic responses may be generated in the lateral hypothalamus, a region with neural interactions within the limbic forebrain. Parasympathetic autonomic responses also influence gastrointestinal function. Parasympathetic impulses originate in the periventricular and lateral hypothalamus and travel to the dorsal motor nucleus of the vagus, the main parasympathetic output pathway. The vagus is also modulated by the limbic brain, producing an emotional-gut pathway of response.

The enteric nervous system is exquisitely sensitive to emotional states. For example, in the esophagus, acute stress increases the resting tone of the upper esophageal sphincter and increases contraction amplitude in the distal esophagus. Such physiological responses may result in symptoms consistent with globus or esophageal spasm syndrome. In the stomach, acute stress decreases antral motor activity, potentially producing functional nausea and vomiting. Motor function is reduced in the small intestine and increased in the large intestine under acute stress, which may account for the bowel symptoms associated with irritable bowel syndrome.

Patients with contraction abnormalities and functional esophageal syndromes demonstrate high rates of psychiatric comorbidity. Anxiety disorders ranked high in a study of psychiatric comorbidity in functional esophageal spasm, being present in 67 percent of subjects referred to a gastrointestinal motility laboratory for testing. Many patients in this study had anxiety disorder symptoms prior to the onset of esophageal symptoms. This suggests that anxiety disorder may induce physiological changes in the esophagus that can produce functional esophageal symptoms.

Gastroesophageal Reflux Disease (GERD)

Gastrointestinal reflux disease (GERD) is the most common disorder of the esophagus and accounts for most over-the-counter antacid consumption. The predominant symptom is heartburn, which may be accompanied by regurgitation and pain. Multiple factors in addition to stress appear to be important in the generation of reflux: (1) presence of a hiatal hernia, (2) effectiveness of the lower esophageal sphincter in blocking the reflux of stomach acid, (3) effectiveness of the esophagus in clearing and neutralizing reflux, (4) ability of the esophagus to protect itself against acid and pepsin, and (5) delayed gastric emptying and acid hypersecretion. Up to 80 percent of patients with GERD have a hiatal hernia. However, 50 percent of patients with a hiatal hernia do not have GERD. Psychological distress increases symptom severity in patients prone to this disease. In a survey of GERD sufferers, excessive stress, too much excitement, family arguments, and temporary depression were felt to trigger symptoms.

Peptic Ulcer Disease

Peptic ulcer refers to mucosal ulceration involving the distal stomach or proximal duodenum. Symptoms of peptic ulcer disease include a gnawing or burning epigastric pain that occurs 1 to 3 hours after meals and is relieved by food or antacids. Accompanying symptoms can include nausea, vomiting, dyspepsia, or signs of gastrointestinal bleeding such as hematemesis or melena.

Early theories identified excess gastric acid secretion as the most important etiological factor, but the importance of infection with *Helicobacter pylori* is now acknowledged. *H. pylori* is associated with 95 to 99 percent of duodenal ulcers and 70 to 90 percent of gastric ulcers. Antibiotic therapy that targets *H. pylori* results in much higher healing and cure rates than antacid and histamine inhibitor therapy used alone.

Early studies of peptic ulcer disease suggested that psychological factors had a role in the production of ulcer vulnerability, mediated through the increased gastric acid excretion associated with psychological stress. Studies of prisoners of war during World War II documented rates of peptic ulcer formation twice as high as in controls. Psychosocial factors are involved in the clinical expression of symptoms, possibly by reducing immune responses, resulting in vulnerability to *H. pylori* infection.

Ulcerative Colitis

Ulcerative colitis is an inflammatory bowel disease of unknown cause affecting primarily the large intestine. The predominant symptom is bloody diarrhea. Extracolonic manifestations can include uveitis, iritis, skin diseases, and primary sclerosing cholangitis. Diagnosis is made mainly by colonoscopy or proctoscopy. Surgical resection of portions of the large bowel or entire bowel can result in cure for some patients. Studies of patients with ulcerative colitis have shown a predominance of obsessive-compulsive traits. They are neat, orderly, punctual, and have difficulty expressing anger. There is wide variation, however, in the psychiatric picture of patients with this disorder.

Crohn's Disease

Crohn's disease is an inflammatory bowel disease affecting primarily the small intestine and colon. Common symptoms include diarrhea, abdominal pain, and weight loss. It is less prevalent than ulcerative colitis. The course is chronic, often with periods of remission followed by periods of acute symptoms. Treatment consists of the use of antibiotic agents, immunosuppressive drugs, and corticosteroids. A study of psychiatric symptoms in Crohn's disease prior to the onset of physical symptoms found higher rates (23 percent) of preexisting panic disorder than in control subjects and subjects with ulcerative colitis.

A young woman from a small Midwestern town developed Crohn's disease while in high school. Her symptoms included intermittent abdominal pain and diarrhea. Prior to the onset of her inflammatory bowel disease, she had been obese, with a maximum weight of 225 pounds. She had no history of psychiatric illness prior to the development of Crohn's disease but had been a somewhat shy individual. Her family became quite distressed by the development of her medical illness. They developed a protective style of interacting with her, and she continued to live at home following completion of high school.

Her Crohn's disease became chronic, with intermittent periods of flare-up and remission. Over time her gastroenterologist noted that her complaints of abdominal pain did not

always correspond with periods of inflammatory disease activity. She developed a fear of eating and drinking and associated oral intake with abdominal pain. She became preoccupied with her weight and began vigorous dieting and restricting her oral fluid intake. By age 24 her weight began to drop, and over 6 months, she lost 100 pounds, down to a weight of 125. Her gastroenterologist suspected she might be developing an eating disorder, and she was referred for a psychiatric consultation.

The psychiatric consultant noted chronic low mood consistent with a diagnosis of dysthymia. She was preoccupied with concerns about her weight and had rigid rules about eating. Dieting complicated the medical management of her Crohn's disease. A diagnosis of eating disorder not otherwise specified along with dysthymic disorder was made, therapy with a selective serotonin reuptake inhibitor (SSRI) was started, and she was referred to an eating disorder partial hospitalization program. In the partial program her compliance was poor, and one day she collapsed in group therapy. Medical evaluation revealed orthostatic hypotension that resolved with hospitalization and intravenous fluid and electrolyte replacement. She was transferred to an inpatient eating disorder program; however, her family checked her out of the program against medical advice. The patient and family complained that a psychiatric disorder was not her problem and that the psychiatric treatment team did not understand her Crohn's disease and proper medical management.

DISCUSSION

This case illustrates the effect that chronic gastrointestinal disorders can have on individuals vulnerable to psychiatric illness. Chronic gastrointestinal illness can worsen abnormal family dynamics and stimulate development of psychiatric illnesses such as mood and eating disorders. When both a gastrointestinal illness and a psychiatric illness are present, the outcome and prognosis for each individual condition become complicated. Coordination of medical and psychiatric services is necessary to maximize the likelihood of a successful outcome. (Courtesy of William R. Yates, M.D.)

Table 28.2–1 lists other gastrointestinal disorders associated with high rates of psychiatric comorbidity. The term *functional* is sometimes applied to these disorders to indicate a change in function, which may or may not be associated with a change in structure.

Table 28.2–1
Gastrointestinal Disorders

Esophageal disorders	
Globus	Lump in throat, common transient response to emotional distress
Rumination	Repetitive regurgitation of gastric contents
Noncardiac chest pain	Anginalike chest pain thought to be esophageal in origin; motor abnormalities include nonspecific high-amplitude esophageal contractions, especially in the distal esophagus ("nutcracker esophagus") and diffuse esophageal motor spasms; symptoms particularly sensitive to emotional distress
Heartburn	Acid reflux without anatomical abnormality or esophagitis
Dysphagia	Difficulty swallowing solids or liquids in the absence of anatomical abnormality; intermittent esophageal motor disorder can be present
Gastroduodenal disorder	
Dyspepsia	Symptoms localized to epigastrium include pain, bloating, early satiety, nausea or vomiting, often associated with heartburn
Aerophagia	Repetitive air swallowing and belching
Bowel disorder	
Irritable-bowel syndrome	Abdominal pain, constipation, diarrhea, passage of bloody mucus
Burbulence	Bloating, fullness, borborygmi, and flatulence
Constipation	A wide range of patterns difficult to categorize; generally fewer than three bowel movements a week with hardened stools, causing discomfort in defecation; abdominal pain is variably present; diarrhea suggests diagnosis of irritable bowel syndrome
Diarrhea	Loose or watery stools more than 75% of time, often with urgency or incontinence; may or may not have pain, but lack other aspects of irritable bowel syndrome
Unspecified bowel disorder	Catchall category for symptoms not sufficient to allow clear diagnosis of another disorder; includes isolated symptomatic abdominal pain with or without change in stool habits, mucus, urgency, runny or loose stools, distention, heartburn, or borborygmi
Abdominal pain	
Abdominal pain	Diffuse abdominal pain without symptoms diagnostic of irritable bowel syndrome
Biliary pain	Right upper quadrant pain; sphincter of Oddi dyskinesia, fibrosis, or other anatomical abnormalities commonly identified
Anorectal disorder	
Incontinence	Commonly associated with fecal impaction; must differentiate from anatomical (scarring) or neurological disorders of rectum
Anorectal pain	Chronic severe persistent rectal pain (levator syndrome) or intermittent sharp pain lasting seconds to minutes and disappearing completely (proctalgia fugax)
Obstructed defecation	Due to spastic floor (pelvic floor dyssynergia; most common in young and middle-aged women)
Dyschezia	Difficulty with evacuation

Modified from Drossman DA, Thompson WG, Talley TJ, Funch-Jensen P, Janssens J, Whitehead WE. Identification of sub-groups of functional gastrointestinal disorders. *Gastroenterol Int.* 1990;3:159.

Psychiatric Adverse Effects Associated with Commonly Prescribed Drugs for Gastrointestinal Conditions

Gastrointestinal prescription drugs represent a significant percentage of all prescriptions. Several of these agents can produce psychiatric symptoms. Additionally, several gastrointestinal drugs can interact with common psychiatric prescription drugs (Table 28.2–2).

Table 28.2–2
Common Drugs Used for Gastrointestinal Disorders—Psychiatric Effects and Interactions with Psychiatric Drugs

Generic	Brand	Indications	Adverse Psychiatric Effects and Drug Interactions
Histamine receptor antagonists		Peptic ulcer disease	
Nizatidine	Axid		Cimetidine can cause delirium, especially in severely ill and hospitalized patients; cimetidine can increase blood levels of tricyclic drugs, carbamazepine, valproate, SSRI compounds; fewer CNS effects and metabolic disturbances are noted with other histamine receptor agonists
Famotidine	Pepcid		
Cimetidine	Tagamet		
Ranitidine	Zantac		
Proton pump inhibitor		Peptic ulcer disease	
Omeprazole	Prilosec		Can increase carbamazepine concentrations
Gastrointestinal stimulant		Gastroparesis	
Metoclopramide	Reglan		Can cause depression and less frequently dystonic reactions and parkinsonism
Antiemetics		Nausea	
Prochlorperazine	Compazine		Prochlorperazine is an phenothiazine and like others can increase tricyclic drug levels
Dronabinol	Marinol		A cannabinoid found in marijuana; can cause drowsiness, dizziness, euphoria
Ondansetron	Zofran		Interactions with SSRIs unclear
Antiinfective agents			
Interferon alpha	Intron A	Hepatitis C	Depression in up to 15%, also insomnia, anxiety, confusion
Metronidazole	Flagyl	Giardiasis, *Helicobacter*	Potential nephrotoxic effect when used with lithium; interacts with disulfiram

CARDIOVASCULAR SYSTEM

Coronary Heart Disease

Cardiovascular disease is the leading cause of death in the United States and most of the industrialized world. About one third of all adults over age 35 will ultimately die of cardiovascular disease. Behavioral risk factors such as smoking, overeating, physical inactivity, and poor compliance with management of diabetes, hypercholesterolemia, and hypertension are the main targets for primary preventive interventions, and achieving behavioral change with respect to these risk factors is a major challenge for medicine and psychiatry.

Psychiatric disorders frequently occur as complications or comorbid conditions in persons with cardiovascular disease. Depression, anxiety, delirium, and cognitive disorders are especially prevalent. Surveys of ambulatory cardiology patients with documented heart disease indicate that 5 to 10 percent have anxiety disorders (predominantly panic attacks and phobias) and 10 to 15 percent have mood disorders (predominantly depressive episodes, minor depression, or dysthymia). Major depressive disorder occurs in 15 to 20 percent of patients following myocardial infarction.

Because autonomic cardiac modulation is profoundly sensitive to acute emotional stress such as intense anger, fear, or sadness, it is not surprising that acute emotions, especially anxiety, affect the heart. Instances of sudden cardiac death related to sudden emotional distress have been noted throughout history in all cultures. High levels of anxiety symptoms are associated with a tripling of risk of sudden cardiac death and also raise the risk of future coronary events in patients with myocardial infarction by two to five times that for nonanxious patients who have had heart attacks. Risk is increased in both the immediate postinfarction period and over 18-month follow-up.

Hostility and Type A Behavior Pattern. The relation between a behavior pattern characterized by easily aroused anger, impatience, hostility, competitive striving, and time urgency (type A) and coronary heart disease dominated studies in psychosomatic cardiology in the 1970s and 1980s. Several large prospective epidemiological studies found the type A pattern to be associated with a nearly twofold increased risk of incident myocardial infarction and coronary disease–related mortality. Hostility as the core component of the type A concept has received considerable empirical support as the most important predictor of coronary heart disease; low hostility is associated with low coronary disease risk. Hostility is associated with increased levels of circulating catecholamines and increased lipid concentrations—risk factors for disease (Fig. 28.2–1). Adrenergic receptor function is down-regulated in hostile men, presumably an adaptive response to heightened sympathetic-adrenergic drive and chronic overproduction of catecholamines resulting from chronic and frequent anger. Conversely, submissiveness has been found to protect against coronary disease risk in women.

Acute Mental Stress. States of fear, excitement, and acute anger reduce blood flow through atherosclerotic coronary segments and provoke coronary spasm, thus causing abnormal left ventricular wall motion and electrocardiographic evidence of

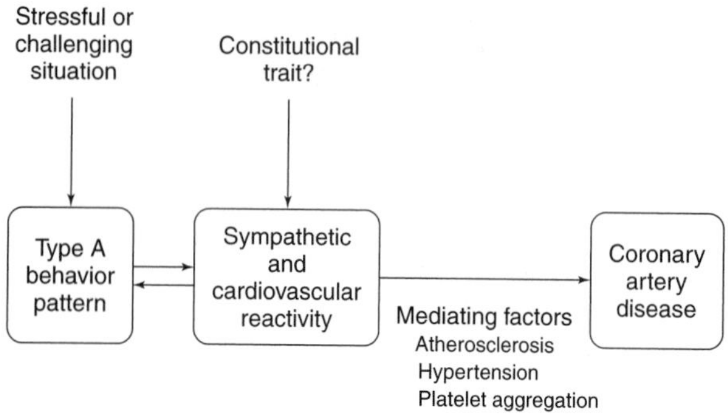

FIGURE 28.2–1

Conceptual model of type A behavior and the development of coronary artery disease. (Adapted from Goldstein MG, Niaura R. Cardiovascular disease, Part I: Coronary artery disease and sudden death. In *Psychological Factors Affecting Medical Conditions.* Stoudemire A, ed. Washington, DC: American Psychiatric Press; 1995:117.)

myocardial ischemia. Acute mental stress may cause angina in the presence of normal coronary arteries, as a result of coronary artery spasm. Studies indicate that relaxation training can alter autonomic activation during mental stress, implying a potential therapeutic role for such training in stress-induced ischemia.

Sudden cardiac death triggered by mental stress was demonstrated in a study of deaths in the aftermath of a major California earthquake. Following a surge of sudden deaths on the day of the earthquake, there was a several-day period of reduced incidence of sudden cardiac death, suggesting that only those predisposed to sudden cardiac death by underlying disease were affected by the monumental stressor. Deaths were primarily associated with emotional stress rather than physical exertion. Sudden death without antecedent angina, suggesting cardiac arrhythmia, as well as deaths preceded by chest pain, suggesting acute coronary occlusions, were observed. Other studies have led to estimates that between 20 and 40 percent of sudden cardiac deaths are precipitated by acute emotional stressors.

Valvular Heart Disease and Anxiety Disorders

The relation between valvular heart disease and psychiatric disorder has been of considerable interest over the past several decades. In panic disorder, mitral valve prolapse is detected in 10 to 25 percent of patients studied with echocardiography. However, prolapse also occurs in a substantial portion of the population without panic disorder, and the nature of the relation remains uncertain. The subjective experience of valve prolapse (palpitations, fluttering, and chest pressure) may trigger panic sensations; alternatively, the association may be purely coincidental.

Coronary Artery Bypass Graft Surgery

Coronary artery bypass graft surgery is one of the most frequently performed surgeries in the United States. Psychiatric complications after this surgery have been noted since its inception and persist despite improvements in cardiopulmonary bypass anesthetic and surgical technique. Persistent, subtle, memory and cognitive impairment may occur after this surgery. In a recent study of over 2,100 elective coronary artery bypass graft surgical patients at 24 centers, clinical observation yielded an adverse neurological event rate of 6.1 percent. Death, focal neurological impairment (stroke), or stupor occurred in 3.1 percent; these events were predicted by older age, proximal aortic atherosclerosis, and prior history of neurological disease. Nonspecific impairment in intellectual function occurred in 2.6 percent, and seizures in 0.4 percent. Risk factors for these events were older age, systolic hypertension at admission, pulmonary disease, and excessive alcohol use.

Mild to moderate depression occurs in approximately one third of patients after coronary bypass surgery but may remit within weeks to months. Depressive symptoms are present in almost 40 percent of coronary artery bypass graft patients 6 months after surgery. Patients who remain depressed exhibited increased mortality at 3-year follow-up.

Hypertension

Hypertension is a disease characterized by an elevated blood pressure of 160/95 mm Hg or above. It is primary (essential hypertension of unknown etiology) or secondary to a known medical illness. Some patients have labile blood pressure (e.g., "white coat" hypertension, in which elevations occur only in a physician's office and are related to anxiety). Personality profiles associated with essential hypertension include persons who have a general readiness to be aggressive which they try to control, albeit unsuccessfully. The psychoanalyst Otto Fenichel observed that the increase in essential hypertension is probably connected to the mental situation of persons who have learned that aggressiveness is bad and must live in a world in which an enormous amount of aggressiveness is called for.

Vasovagal Syncope

Vasovagal syncope is characterized by a sudden loss of consciousness (fainting) caused by a vasodepressor response decreasing cerebral perfusion. Sympathetic autonomic activity is inhibited, and parasympathetic vagal nerve activity is augmented; the result is decreased cardiac output, decreased vascular peripheral resistance, vasodilation, and bradycardia. This reaction decreases ventricular filling, lowers the blood supply to the brain, and leads to brain hypoxia and loss of consciousness. Because patients with vasomotor syncope normally put themselves, or fall into, a prone position, the decreased cardiac output is corrected. Raising the patient's legs also helps correct the physiological imbalance. When syncope is related to orthostatic hypotension, as an adverse effect of psychotropic medication, patients should be advised to shift slowly from a sitting to a standing position. The specific physiological triggers of vasovagal syncope have not been identified, but acutely stressful situations are known etiological factors.

Cardiovascular Presentations of Psychiatric Disorders

Somatization disorder, panic disorder, anxiety, and depression can all involve somatic complaints, and they represent a substantial issue in ambulatory and emergency cardiology practice. In studies, these diagnoses account for about 30 percent of patients presenting with the chief complaint of palpitations. In this population, psychiatric disorder is associated with more frequently

recurrent symptoms, emergency room visits, hypochondriacal concerns, and impairment in activities of daily living.

RESPIRATORY SYSTEM

Asthma

Asthma is a chronic, episodic illness characterized by extensive narrowing of the tracheobronchial tree. Symptoms include coughing, wheezing, chest tightness, and dyspnea. Nocturnal symptoms and exacerbations are common. Although patients with asthma are characterized as having excessive dependency needs, no specific personality type has been identified; however, up to 30 percent of persons with asthma meet the criteria for panic disorder or agoraphobia. The fear of dyspnea may directly trigger asthma attacks, and high levels of anxiety are associated with increased rates of hospitalization and asthma-associated mortality. Certain personality traits in asthma patients are associated with greater use of corticosteroids and bronchodilators and longer hospitalizations than would be predicted from pulmonary function alone. These traits include intense fear, emotional lability, sensitivity to rejection, and lack of persistence in difficult situations.

Family members of patients with severe asthma tend to have higher-than-predicted prevalence rates of mood disorders, posttraumatic stress disorder, substance use, and antisocial personality disorder. How these conditions contribute to the genesis or maintenance of asthma in an individual patient is unknown. The familial and current social environment may interact with a genetic predisposition for asthma to influence the timing and severity of the clinical picture. This interaction may be especially insidious in adolescents whose need for, and fear of, emotional separation from the family often become entangled in battles over medication adherence as well as other modes of diligent self-care.

Hyperventilation Syndrome

Patients with hyperventilation syndrome breathe rapidly and deeply for several minutes, often unaware that they are doing so. They soon complain of feelings of suffocation, anxiety, giddiness, and lightheadedness. Tetany, palpitations, chronic pain, and paresthesias about the mouth and in the fingers and toes are associated symptoms. Finally, syncope may occur. The symptoms are caused by an excessive loss of CO_2 resulting in respiratory alkalosis. Cerebral vasoconstriction results from low cerebral tissue P_{CO_2}.

The attack can be aborted by having patients breathe into a paper (not plastic) bag or hold their breath for as long as possible, which raises the plasma P_{CO_2}. Another useful treatment technique is to have patients deliberately hyperventilate for 1 or 2 minutes and then describe the syndrome to them. This can also be reassuring to patients who fear they have a progressive, if not fatal, disease.

ENDOCRINE SYSTEM

Hyperthyroidism

Hyperthyroidism, or thyrotoxicosis, results from overproduction of thyroid hormone by the thyroid gland. The most common cause is exophthalmic goiter, also called Graves' disease (Fig. 28.2–2). Toxic nodular goiter causes another 10 percent of cases among middle-aged and elderly patients. Physical signs of hyperthyroidism include increased pulse, arrhythmias, elevated blood pressure, fine tremor, heat intolerance, excessive sweating, weight loss, tachycardia, menstrual irregularities, muscle weakness, and exophthalmos. Psychiatric features include nervousness, fatigue, insomnia, mood lability, and dysphoria. Speech may be pressured, and patients may exhibit a heightened activity level. Cognitive symptoms include a short attention span, impaired recent memory, and an exaggerated startle response. Patients with severe cases may exhibit visual hallucinations, paranoid ideation, and delirium. While some symptoms of hyperthyroidism resemble those of a manic episode, an association between hyperthyroidism and mania has rarely been observed; however, both disorders may exist in the same patient.

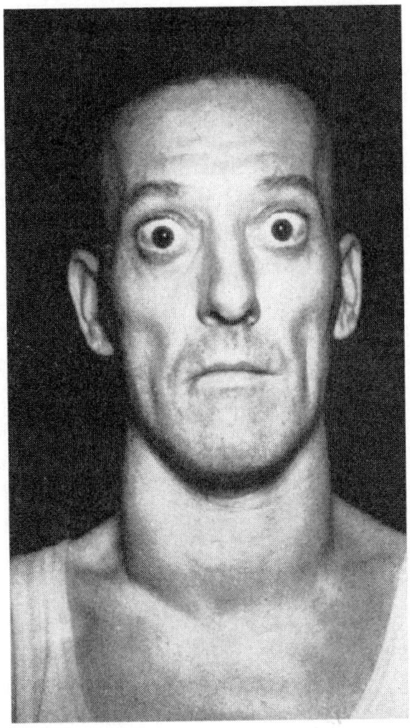

FIGURE 28.2–2
Exophthalmic goiter. Note lid retraction and enlarged thyroid. (Reprinted with permission from Douthwaite AH, ed. *French's Index of Differential Diagnosis.* 7th ed. Baltimore: Williams & Wilkins; 1954.)

Treatments for Graves' disease are (1) propylthiouracil (PTU) and antithyroid drugs, (2) radioactive iodine (RAI), and (3) surgical thyroidectomy. β-Adrenergic receptor antagonists (e.g., propranolol [Inderal]) can provide symptomatic relief.

Treatment of thyroid nodular goiter consists of β-adrenergic receptor antagonists and RAI. Treatment of thyroiditis consists of a brief course (a few weeks) of β-adrenergic receptor antagonists, as this condition is short-lived. For patients with psychotic symptoms, medium-potency antipsychotics are preferable to low-potency drugs, as the latter can worsen tachycardia. Tricyclic drugs should be used with caution, if at all, for the same reason. Depressed patients often respond to SSRIs. In general, the psychiatric symptoms resolve with successful treatment of the hyperthyroidism.

Hypothyroidism

Hypothyroidism results from inadequate synthesis of thyroid hormone and is categorized as either overt or subclinical. In overt hypothyroidism, thyroid hormone concentrations are abnormally low, thyroid-stimulating hormone (TSH) levels are elevated, and patients are symptomatic; in subclinical hypothyroidism, patients have normal thyroid hormone concentrations but elevated TSH levels.

Psychiatric symptoms of hypothyroidism include depressed mood, apathy, impaired memory and other cognitive defects. Also, hypothyroidism may contribute to treatment-refractory depression. A psychotic syndrome of auditory hallucinations and paranoia, named "myxedema madness," has been described in some patients. Urgent psychiatric treatment is necessary for patients presenting with severe psychiatric symptoms (e.g., psychosis or suicidal depression). Psychotropic agents should be given at low doses initially, as the reduced metabolic rate of hypothyroid patients may reduce breakdown and result in higher concentrations of medications in blood, as in the following case.

A 45-year-old male with bipolar I disorder had been well on lithium monotherapy for 5 years, but over the course of several months he became increasingly withdrawn and reported fatigue and poor concentration. The patient's family noted that he was forgetful and uncharacteristically listless and apathetic. No stressors were identified, and the patient's lithium concentration was therapeutic. His TSH concentration was elevated, at 14 mEq/L. The patient was treated with levothyroxine 0.05 mg and within 6 weeks experienced improved energy and a subjective return to baseline cognitive functioning. His TSH 8 weeks after initiation of thyroid replacement therapy was normal. (Courtesy of Victoria C. Hendrick, M.D., and Thomas R. Garrick, M.D.)

Subclinical Hypothyroidism. Subclinical hypothyroidism may produce depressive symptoms and cognitive deficits, although they are less severe than those produced by overt hypothyroidism. The lifetime prevalence of depression in patients with subclinical hypothyroidism is approximately double that in the general population. These patients display a lower response rate to antidepressants and a greater likelihood of responding to liothyronine (Cytomel) augmentation than euthyroid patients with depression.

Diabetes Mellitus

Diabetes mellitus is a disorder of metabolism and the vascular system, manifested by disturbances in the body's handling of glucose, lipid, and protein. It results from impaired insulin secretion or action. Heredity and family history are important in the onset of diabetes; however, sudden onset is often associated with emotional stress, which disturbs the homeostatic balance in persons who are predisposed to the disorder. Psychological factors that seem significant are those provoking feelings of frustration, loneliness, and dejection. Patients with diabetes must usually maintain some dietary control over their diabetes. When they are depressed and dejected, they often overeat or overdrink self-destructively and cause their diabetes to get out of control. This reaction is especially common in patients with juvenile, or type I, diabetes. Terms such as *oral, dependent, seeking maternal attention,* and *excessively passive* have been applied to persons with this condition.

Supportive psychotherapy helps achieve cooperation in the medical management of this complex disease. Therapists should encourage patients to lead as normal a life as possible, recognizing that they have a chronic but manageable disease. In known diabetes patients, ketoacidosis can produce some violence and confusion. More commonly, hypoglycemia (often occurring when a diabetic patient drinks alcohol) can produce severe anxiety states, confusion, and disturbed behavior. Inappropriate behavior due to hypoglycemia must be distinguished from that due to simple drunkenness.

ADRENAL DISORDERS

Hypercortisolism (Cushing's Syndrome)

Spontaneous Cushing's syndrome results from adrenocortical hyperfunction and can develop from either excessive secretion of ACTH (which stimulates the adrenal gland to produce cortisol) or from adrenal pathology (e.g., a cortisol-producing adrenal tumor). Cushing's disease, the most common form of spontaneous Cushing's syndrome, results from excessive pituitary secretion of ACTH, usually from a pituitary adenoma.

The clinical features of Cushing's disease include a characteristic "moon facies," or rounded face, from accumulation of adipose tissue around the zygomatic arch (Fig. 28.2–3). Truncal obesity, a "buffalo hump" appearance, results from cervicodorsal adipose tissue deposition. The catabolic effects of cortisol on protein produce muscle wasting, slow wound healing, easy bruising, and thinning of

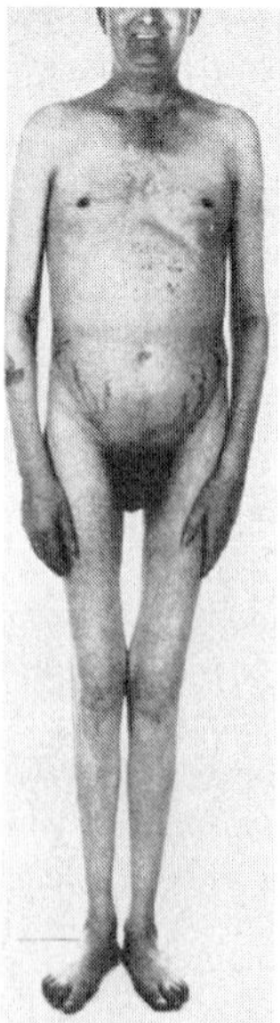

FIGURE 28.2–3

Cushing's syndrome. Legs thin owing to atrophy of thigh muscles. Some abdominal obesity with marked striae. (Reprinted with permission from Douthwaite AH, ed. *French's Index of Differential Diagnosis.* 7th ed. Baltimore: Williams & Wilkins; 1954.)

the skin leading to abdominal striae. Bones become osteoporotic, sometimes resulting in pathological fractures and loss of height. Psychiatric symptoms are common and vary from severe depression to elation with or without evidence of psychotic features.

The treatment of pituitary ACTH-producing tumors involves surgical resection or pituitary irradiation. Medications that antagonize cortisol production (e.g., metyrapone) or suppress ACTH (e.g., serotonin antagonists such as cyproheptadine [Periactin]) are sometimes used but have met with limited success.

Hyperprolactinemia

Prolactin, produced by the anterior pituitary, stimulates milk production from the breast and modulates maternal behavior. Its production is inhibited by dopamine (also known as prolactin-inhibiting factor) produced by the tuberoinfundibular neurons of the arcuate nucleus of the hypothalamus. Normal concentrations (5 to 25 ng/mL in women and 5 to 15 ng/mL in men) fluctuate during the day, peaking during sleep. Exercise and emotional stress can increase prolactin concentration. Medications that block dopamine action (e.g., antipsychotics) raise prolactin concentrations up to 20 times. All antipsychotics appear equally likely to raise prolactin concentrations, with the exception of clozapine (Clozaril) and olanzapine (Zyprexa). Other medications that may increase prolactin concentrations include oral contraceptives, estrogens, tricyclic drugs, serotonergic antidepressants, and propranolol. Hypothyroidism raises prolactin concentration because thyrotropin-releasing hormone (TRH) stimulates prolactin release. Physiological hyperprolactinemia occurs in pregnant and breast-feeding women; nipple stimulation also increases prolactin concentrations.

Traumatic childhood experiences such as separation from parents or living with an alcoholic father have been reported to predispose to hyperprolactinemia. Stressful life events are also associated with galactorrhea, even in the absence of increased prolactin concentrations. Low prolactin levels are associated with decreased libido.

SKIN DISORDERS

Atopic Dermatitis

Atopic dermatitis (also called *atopic eczema* or *neurodermatitis*) is a chronic skin disorder characterized by pruritus and inflammation (eczema), which often begins as an erythematous, pruritic, maculopapular eruption (Fig. 28.2–4). Atopic dermatitis patients tend to be more anxious and depressed than clinical and disease-free control groups. Anxiety or depression exacerbates atopic dermatitis by eliciting scratching behavior, and depressive symptoms appear to amplify the itch perception. Studies of children with atopic dermatitis found that those with behavior problems had more severe illness. In families that encouraged independence, children had less severe symptoms, whereas parental overprotectiveness reinforced scratching.

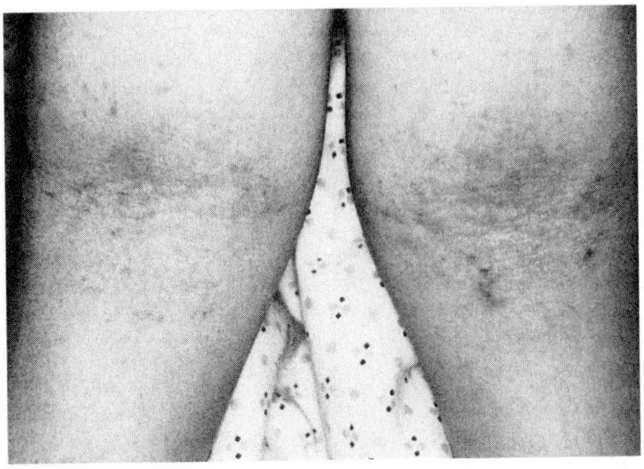

FIGURE 28.2–4
Atopic dermatitis. Note the maculopapular eruption behind the knees. (Courtesy of D. F. Mutasim.)

Psoriasis

Psoriasis is a chronic, relapsing disease of the skin, with lesions characterized by silvery scales with a glossy, homogeneous erythema under the scales. It is difficult to control the adverse effect of psoriasis on quality of life. It can lead to stress that can in turn trigger more psoriasis. Patients who report that stress triggered psoriasis often describe disease-related stress resulting from the cosmetic disfigurement and social stigma of psoriasis, rather than stressful major life events. Psoriasis-related stress may have more to do with psychosocial difficulties inherent in the interpersonal relationships of patients with psoriasis than with the severity or chronicity of psoriasis activity.

Controlled studies have found that psoriatic patients have high levels of anxiety and depression and significant comorbidity with a wide array of personality disorders including schizoid, avoidant, passive-aggressive, and obsessive-compulsive personality disorders. Patients' self-report of psoriasis severity correlated directly with depression and suicidal ideation, and comorbid depression reduced the threshold for pruritus in psoriasis patients. Heavy alcohol consumption (more than 80 grams of ethanol daily) by male psoriasis patients may predict a poor treatment outcome.

Psychogenic Excoriation

Psychogenic excoriations (also called *psychogenic pruritus*) are lesions caused by scratching or picking in response to an itch or other skin sensation or because of an urge to remove an irregularity on the skin from preexisting dermatoses such as acne. Lesions are typically found in areas that the patient can easily reach (e.g., the face, upper back, and the upper and lower extremities) and are a few millimeters in diameter and weeping, crusted, or scarred, with occasional postinflammatory hypopigmentation or hyperpigmentation (Fig. 28.2–5). The behavior in psychogenic excoriation sometimes resembles obsessive-compulsive disorder in that it is repetitive, ritualistic, and tension reducing, and patients attempt (often unsuccessfully) to resist excoriating. The skin is an important erogenous zone, and Freud believed it susceptible to unconscious sexual impulses.

Localized Pruritus

Pruritus Ani. The investigation of pruritus ani commonly yields a history of local irritation (e.g., threadworms, irritant dis-

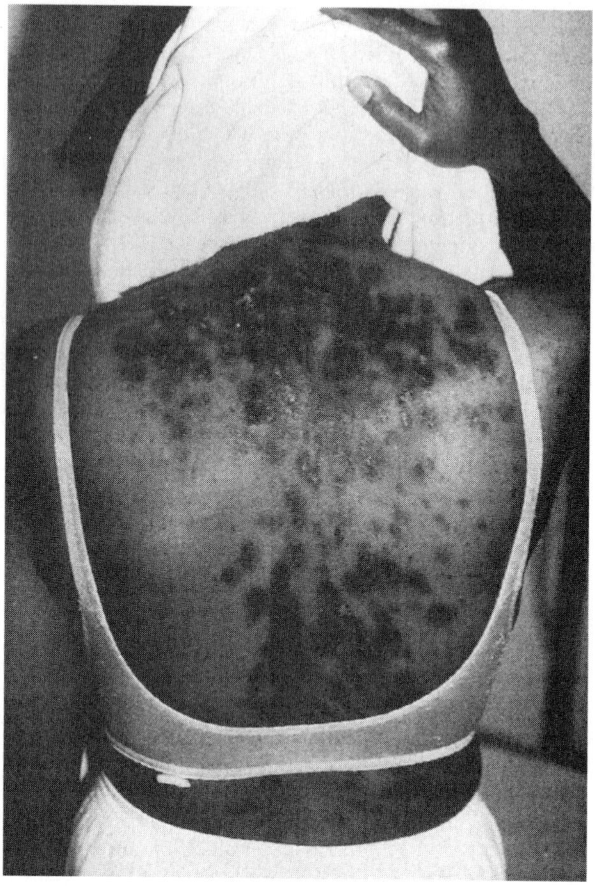

FIGURE 28.2–5
Psychogenic excoriation. The self-induced nature of the condition is suggested by the relative sparing of the lateral upper back, where the patient cannot easily reach.

charge, fungal infection) or general systemic factors (e.g., nutritional deficiencies, drug intoxication). After running a conventional course, however, pruritus ani often fails to respond to therapeutic measures and acquires a life of its own, apparently perpetuated by scratching and superimposed inflammation. It is a distressing complaint that often interferes with work and social activity. Investigation of large numbers of patients with the disorder has revealed that personality deviations often precede the condition and that emotional disturbances often precipitate and maintain it.

Pruritus Vulvae. As with pruritus ani, specific physical causes, either localized or generalized, may be demonstrable in pruritus vulvae, and the presence of glaring psychopathology in no way lessens the need for adequate medical investigation. In some patients, pleasure derived from rubbing and scratching is conscious—they realize it is a symbolic form of masturbation—but more often than not the pleasure element is repressed. Some patients may give a long history of sexual frustration, which was frequently intensified at the time of the onset of the pruritus.

Hyperhidrosis

States of fear, rage, and tension can induce increased sweat secretion that appears primarily on the palms, the soles, and the axillae. The sensitivity of sweating in response to emotion serves as the basis for measurement of sweat by the galvanic skin response (an important tool of psychosomatic research), biofeedback, and the polygraph (lie detector test). Under conditions of prolonged emotional stress, excessive sweating (hyperhidrosis) may lead to secondary skin changes, rashes, blisters, and infections; therefore, hyperhidrosis may underlie several other dermatological conditions that are not primarily related to emotions. Basically, hyperhidrosis may be viewed as an anxiety phenomenon mediated by the autonomic nervous system, and it must be differentiated from drug-induced states of hyperhidrosis.

MUSCULOSKELETAL SYSTEM

Rheumatoid Arthritis

Rheumatoid arthritis is a disease characterized by chronic musculoskeletal pain arising from inflammation of the joints. The disorder's significant causative factors are hereditary, allergic, immunological, and psychological.

Stress may predispose patients to rheumatoid arthritis and other autoimmune diseases by immune suppression. Depression is comorbid with rheumatoid arthritis in about 20 percent of individuals. Those who get depressed are more likely to be unmarried, have a longer duration of illness, and have a higher occurrence of medical comorbidities. Individuals with rheumatoid arthritis and depression commonly demonstrate poorer functional status, more reported painful joints, more pronounced experience of pain, more health care use, more bed days, and more inability to work than patients with similar objective measures of arthritic activity without depression.

Psychotropic agents may be of use in some patients. Sleep, which is often disrupted by pain, can be assisted by the combination of a nonsteroidal anti-inflammatory drug (NSAID) and trazodone (Desyrel) or mirtazapine (Remeron), with appropriate cautionary advice regarding orthostatic hypotension. Tricyclic drugs exert mild anti-inflammatory effects independent of their mood-altering benefit; however, anticholinergic effects (prominent among the tricyclic drugs and also present with some serotonergic agents) can aggravate dry oral and ocular membranes in some patients with the disorder.

Systemic Lupus Erythematosus

Systemic lupus erythematosus is a connective tissue disease of unclear etiology, characterized by recurrent episodes of destructive inflammation of several organs including the skin, joints, kidneys, blood vessels, and central nervous system (CNS) (see Color Plate 28.2–6 on page 835). This disorder is highly unpredictable, often incapacitating, and potentially disfiguring, and its treatment requires administration of potentially toxic drugs. The psychiatrist can assist in promoting positive interactions between patients and the program staff and ensuring a tolerant attitude on the part of these staff members. Supportive psychotherapy can help patients acquire the knowledge and maturity necessary to deal with the disorder as effectively as possible.

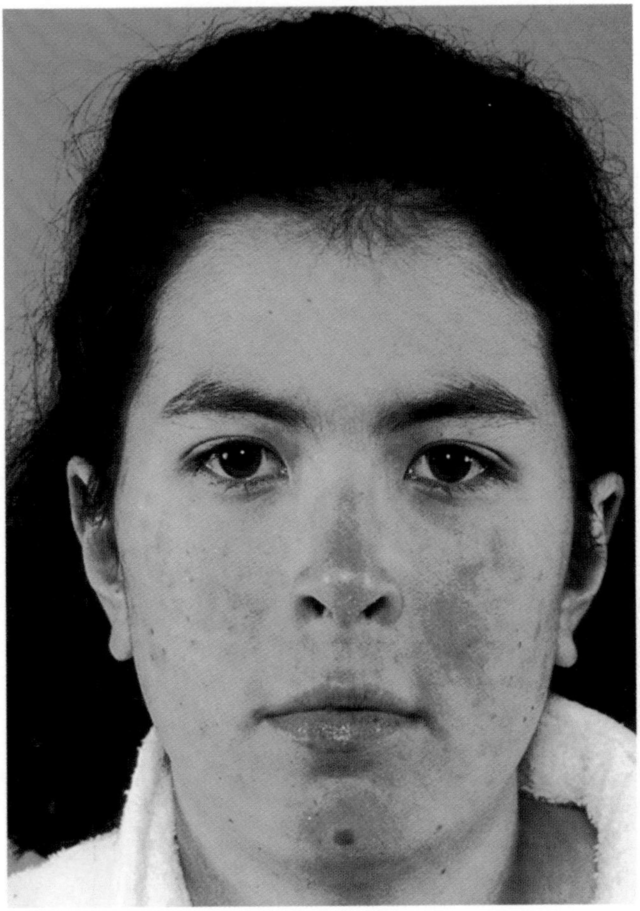

COLOR PLATE 28.2–6
Woman with lupus erythematosus malar rash. (Courtesy of M. Kevin O'Connor, M.D.)

Low Back Pain

Low back pain affects almost 15 million Americans and is one of the major reasons for days lost from work and for disability claims paid to workers by insurance companies. Signs and symptoms vary from patient to patient, most often consisting of excruciating pain, restricted movement, paresthesias, and weakness or numbness, all of which may be accompanied by anxiety, fear, or even panic. The areas most affected are the lower lumbar, lumbosacral, and sacroiliac regions. It is often accompanied by sciatica, with pain radiating down one or both buttocks or following the distribution of the sciatic nerve. Although low back pain may be caused by a ruptured intervertebral disk, a fracture of the back, congenital defects of the lower spine, or a ligamentous muscle strain, many instances are psychosomatic. Examining physicians should be particularly alert to patients who give a history of minor back trauma followed by severe disabling pain. Patients with low back pain often report that the pain began at a time of psychological trauma or stress, but others (perhaps 50 percent) develop pain gradually over a period of months. Patients' reaction to the pain is disproportionately emotional, with excessive anxiety and depression. Furthermore, the distribution of the pain rarely follows a normal neuroanatomical distribution and may vary in location and intensity.

There are two approaches to treatment. In the first or conventional method, treatment is symptomatic. Analgesics such as aspirin (up to 4 g a day) can be used for pain. Muscle relaxants such as diazepam (Valium; 2.5 to 5 mg every 4 to 6 hours for 2 or 3 days) are used to reduce muscle spasms and anxiety. Physical therapy is prescribed for the person in severe pain with restricted movement. Some patients respond to relaxation therapy and biofeedback. Many techniques have been proposed to treat low back pain, most of which are untested and unproved in overall effectiveness. These include various forms of massage, acupressure, acupuncture, injections of anesthetics or steroids, traction, bed rest, electrical stimulation, ultrasound, and hot packs and cold packs.

The second approach, developed by John Sarno, is psychoeducational. This treatment is based on the premise that the back is structurally sound without any abnormality to account for symptoms. To assure both patient and doctor, a careful physical examination is recommended, including a neurological examination and magnetic resonance imaging (MRI) if necessary. An MRI study that shows some abnormality does not automatically implicate it as the cause of the pain. To the contrary, normal changes in spinal morphology occur with age, and most such patients are asymptomatic. Additionally, many patients who have MRI studies show spinal abnormalities as an incidental finding and have never complained of back pain. These include bulging or herniated intravertebral disks, osteophytes, spinal stenosis, and other osteoarthritic changes, but they are not responsible for pain or any neurological symptom.

According to Sarno, the pathophysiology involved in TMS is vasospasm of blood vessels that supply the involved muscle, nerve, or tendon. Vasospasm is mediated by the autonomic nervous system, which is extraordinarily sensitive to changes in emotional tone, chronic emotional stress, and unconscious affects. The ischemia and oxygen deprivation cause pain in the areas involved. An analogy can be drawn to the vasospasm of coronary arteries that cause angina.

Table 28.2–3
The 1990 American College of Rheumatology Criteria for the Classification of Fibromyalgia

I. Widespread pain
   Pain must be present for 3 months, widespread and not localized to one area. Involvement includes left and right side of the body, above and below the waist, and axial-skeletal pain.

II. Presence of 11 of 18 tender-point sites
   Digital palpation must elicit pain in at least 11 of possible 18 tender-point sites. These bilateral sites include occiput, lower cervical, trapezius, supraspinatus, second rib, lateral epicondyle, gluteal, greater trochanter, and knees.

Treatment includes educating patients about the physiological component (vasospasm) and helping them understand the working of the unconscious mind and conflicts that arise from unconscious affects, especially that of rage. The patient understands that the mind is substituting physical pain for emotional pain so that the conscious mind does not have to deal with conflict. Physical activity should be resumed as quickly as possible, and treatments such as spinal manipulation and mandatory physical therapy sessions used minimally if it all.

Fibromyalgia

Fibromyalgia is characterized by pain and stiffness of the soft tissues, such as muscles, ligaments, and tendons. There are local areas of tenderness referred to as "trigger points." The cervical and thoracic areas are affected most often, but the pain may be located in the arms, shoulders, low back, or legs. It is more common in women than in men. The etiology is unknown; however, it is often precipitated by stress that causes localized arterial spasm that interferes with perfusion of oxygen in the affected areas. Pain results, with associated symptoms of anxiety, fatigue, and inability to sleep because of the pain. There are no pathognomonic laboratory findings. The diagnosis is made after excluding rheumatic disease or hypothyroidism (Table 28.2–3). Fibromyalgia is often present in chronic fatigue syndrome and depressive disorders.

Analgesics such as aspirin and acetaminophen are useful for pain. Narcotics should be avoided. Some patients may respond to NSAIDs. Patients with more severe cases may respond to injections of an anesthetic (e.g., procaine) into the affected area; steroid injections are usually unwarranted. The relation between stress, spasms, and pain should be explained. Relaxation exercises and massage of the trigger points may also be of use. Antidepressants, especially sertraline (Zoloft), have shown encouraging results. Psychotherapy may be warranted for patients who are able to gain insight into the nature of the disorder and also helps to identify and deal with psychosocial stressors.

HEADACHES

Headaches are the most common neurological symptom and one of the most common medical complaints. Every year

Table 28.2–4
Clinical Features of Episodic and Chronic Tension-Type Headache Compared with Migraine without Aura

Feature	Episodic Tension-Type Headache	Chronic Tension-Type Headache	Migraine/No Aura
Duration	30 min–7 days	>15 days/mo	4–72 h
Nausea/vomiting	Rare nausea	Occasional nausea	Nausea/vomiting
Pain	Bilateral/pressing, tightening/ mild to moderate	Bilateral/pressing, tightening/ moderate	Unilateral/pulsates/moderate to severe
Worse on activity	No	Occasionally	Yes
Age at onset	Usually over 18 years	Usually over 18 years	25% before 10 years
Onset on wakening	Uncommon	Common	Common
Medication overuse	No	Occasional opiate/barbiturate	No
Prevalence	Up to 80%	2–4%	11%

From Welch KM. A 47-year-old woman with tension-type headaches. *JAMA*. 2001;286:960.

about 80 percent of the population suffer from at least one headache, and 10 to 20 percent go to physicians with headache as their primary complaint. Headaches are also a major cause of absenteeism from work and avoidance of social and personal activities.

Most headaches are not associated with significant organic disease; many persons are susceptible to headaches at times of emotional stress. Moreover, in many psychiatric disorders, including anxiety and depressive disorders, headache is frequently a prominent symptom. Patients with headaches are often referred to psychiatrists by primary care physicians and neurologists after extensive biomedical workups, which often include MRI of the head. Most workups for common headache complaints have negative findings, and such results may be frustrating for both patient and physician. Physicians not well versed in psychological medicine may attempt to reassure such patients by telling them that there is no disease. But this reassurance may have the opposite effect—it may increase patients' anxiety and even escalate into a disagreement about whether the pain is real or imagined. Psychological stress usually exacerbates headaches, whether their primary underlying cause is physical or psychological.

Migraine (Vascular) and Cluster Headaches

Migraine (vascular) headache is a paroxysmal disorder characterized by recurrent unilateral headaches, with or without related visual and gastrointestinal disturbances (e.g., nausea, vomiting, and photophobia). They are probably caused by a functional disturbance in the cranial circulation. Migraines can be precipitated by cycling estrogen, which may account for their higher prevalence in women. Stress is also a precipitant, and many persons with migraine are overly controlled, perfectionists, and unable to suppress anger. Cluster headaches are related to migraines. They are unilateral, occur up to eight times a day, and are associated with miosis, ptosis, and diaphoresis.

Migraines and cluster headaches are best treated during the prodromal period with ergotamine tartrate (Cafergot) and analgesics. Prophylactic administration of propranolol or verapamil (Isoptin) is useful when the headaches are frequent. Sumatriptan (Imitrex) is indicated for the short-term treatment of migraine and can abort attacks. SSRIs are also useful for prophylaxis. Psychotherapy to diminish the effects of conflict and stress and certain behavioral techniques (e.g., biofeedback) have been reported to be useful.

Tension (Muscle Contraction) Headaches

Emotional stress is often associated with prolonged contraction of head and neck muscles, which over several hours may constrict the blood vessels and result in ischemia. A dull, aching pain, sometimes feeling like a tightening band, often begins suboccipitally and may spread over the head. The scalp may be tender to the touch, and in contrast to a migraine, the headache is usually bilateral and not associated with prodromata, nausea, or vomiting. Tension headaches may be episodic or chronic and need to be differentiated from migraine headaches, especially with and without aura (Table 28.2–4).

Tension headaches are frequently associated with anxiety and depression and occur to some degree in about 80 percent of persons during periods of emotional stress. Tense, high-strung, competitive personalities are especially prone to the disorder. In the initial stage persons may be treated with antianxiety agents, muscle relaxants, and massage or heat application to the head and the neck; antidepressants may be prescribed when an underlying depression is present. Psychotherapy is an effective treatment for persons chronically afflicted by tension headaches. Learning to avoid or cope better with tension is the most effective long-term management approach. Biofeedback using electromyogram (EMG) feedback from the frontal or temporal muscles may help some patients. Relaxation exercises and meditation also benefit some patients.

PSYCHO-ONCOLOGY

Psycho-oncology seeks to study both the impact of cancer on psychological functioning and the role that psychological and behavioral variables may play in cancer risk and survival. A hallmark of psycho-oncology research has been intervention studies that attempt to influence the course of illness in patients with cancer. A landmark study by David Spiegel found that women with metastatic breast cancer who received weekly group psychotherapy survived an average of 18 months longer than control patients randomly assigned to routine care. In another study, patients with malignant melanoma who received structured group intervention exhibited a statistically significant lower recurrence of cancer and a lower mortality rate than patients who did not receive such ther-

Table 28.2–5
Medical Conditions Associated with Delirium in Cancer Patients

Metabolic encephalopathy
Vital organ failure
Electrolyte imbalance (such as hypercalcemia in patients with bony metastases or those receiving tamoxifen, diethylstilbestrol, or chlorotrianisene)
Hypoxia, especially in patients with pulmonary involvement or severe anemia
Nutritional deficiencies, such as thiamine, folic acid, and B_{12}
Infections, especially in immunosuppressed hosts
Vascular disorders, especially in patients with coagulopathies
Endocrine and hormonal abnormalities

Courtesy of Marguerite S. Lederberg, M.D., and Jimmie C. Holland, M.D.

Table 28.2–7
Suicide Vulnerability Factors in Cancer Patients

Depression and hopelessness
Poorly controlled pain
Mild delirium (disinhibition)
Feeling of loss of control
Exhaustion
Anxiety
Preexisting psychopathology (substance abuse, character pathology, major psychiatric disorder)
Family problems
Threats and history of prior attempts of suicide
Positive family history of suicide
Other usually described risk factors in psychiatric patients

Adapted from Breitbart W. Suicide in cancer patients. *Oncology.* 1987;1:49.

apy. The malignant melanoma patients who received the group intervention also exhibited significantly more large granular lymphocytes and natural killer (NK) cells as well as indications of increased NK cell activity, suggesting an increased immune response. Another study used a group behavioral intervention (relaxation, guided imagery, and biofeedback training) for patients with breast cancer, who demonstrated higher NK cell activity and lymphocyte mitogen responses than the controls.

Because new treatment protocols have in many cases transformed cancer from an incurable to frequently chronic and often curable disease, the psychiatric aspects of cancer—the reactions to both the diagnosis and the treatment—are increasingly important. At least half of the 1 million persons who contracted cancer in the United States in 1987 were alive 5 years later. Currently, an estimated 3 million cancer survivors have no evidence of the disease.

About half of all cancer patients have mental disorders. The largest group are those with adjustment disorder (68 percent), and major depressive disorder (13 percent) and delirium (8 percent) are the next most common diagnoses. Most of these disorders are thought to be reactive to the knowledge of having cancer. Some of the most common causes of delirium are listed in Table 28.2–5, and some conditions associated with mood disorders in cancer patients are listed in Table 28.2–6.

Table 28.2–6
Causes of Mood Disorders Common in Cancer Patients

Drugs
Chemotherapeutic agents such as prednisone, dexamethasone, procarbazine, vincristine, vinblastine, L-asparaginase, tamoxifen, interferon
Additive effect of narcotics and many other drugs known to cause depression, such as antihypertensives, benzodiazepines, antiparkinson agents, and β-adrenergic receptor antagonists
Tumor effects
Hormone-secreting tumors
Central nervous system tumors
Associated medical conditions
Uremia
Viral encephalopathies
Electrolyte imbalances

Courtesy of Marguerite S. Lederberg, M.D., and Jimmie C. Holland, M.D.

When persons learn that they have cancer, their psychological reactions include fear of death, disfigurement, and disability; fear of abandonment and loss of independence; fear of disruption in relationships, role functioning, and financial standings; and denial, anxiety, anger, and guilt. Although suicidal thoughts and wishes are frequent in persons with cancer, the actual incidence of suicide is only slightly higher than that in the general population. Factors that signal vulnerability to suicide in persons with cancer are listed in Table 28.2–7.

Psychiatrists should make a careful assessment of psychiatric and medical issues in every patient. Special attention should be given to family factors, in particular, preexisting intrafamily conflicts, family abandonment, and family exhaustion.

References

Ader R, Cohen N. Behaviorally conditioned immunosuppression. *Psychosom Med.* 1995;37:333.

Ader R, Cohen N, Felten D. Brain, behavior, and immunity. *Brain Behav Immun.* 1987;1:1.

Berman WH, Berman ER, Heymsfield S, et al. The incidence and comorbidity of psychiatric disorders in obesity. *J Pers Disord.* 1992;6:168.

Blomhoff S, Spetalen S, Jacobsen MB, Malt UF. Phobic anxiety changes the function of brain-gut axis in irritable bowel syndrome. *Psychosom Med.* 2001;63:959.

Bovbjerg DH. Psychoneuroimmunology implications for oncology. *Cancer.* 1991;67:828.

Breitbart W. Psychiatric management of cancer pain. *Cancer.* 1989;63(suppl 11):2336.

Byrne DG. Personality, life events and cardiovascular disease. *J Psychosom Res.* 1987;31:661.

Case RB, Heller SS, Case NB. Type A behavior and survival after acute myocardial infarction. *N Engl J Med.* 1984;311:737.

Cassileth BR, Lusk EJ, Miller DS, Brown LL, Miller R. Psychosocial correlates of survival in advanced malignant disease. *N Engl J Med.* 1985;312:1551.

Dimsdale JE, Young D, Moore L, Strauss HW. Do plasma norepinephrine levels reflect behavioral stress? *Psychosom Med.* 1987;49:375.

Kubzansky LD, Sparrow D, Vokonas P, Kawachi I. Is the glass half empty or half full? A prospective study of optimism and coronary heart disease in the Normative Aging Study. *Psychosom Med.* 2001;63:910.

Starkman MN, Giordani B, Berent S, Schork MA, Schteingart DE. Elevated cortisol levels in Cushing's disease are associated with cognitive decrements. *Psychosom Med.* 2001;63:985.

Stoudemire A, section ed. Psychological factors affecting medical conditions. In: Sadock BJ, Sadock VA, eds. *Kaplan & Sadock's Comprehensive Textbook of Psychiatry.* Vol 2. Baltimore: Lippincott Williams & Wilkins; 2000:1765.

Stoudemire A, Fogel BS, Greenberg D, eds. *Psychiatric Care of the Medical Patient.* New York: Oxford University Press; 1999.

▲ 28.3 Treatment of Psychosomatic Disorders

From a multicausal point of view, all disease might be considered psychosomatic, because every disorder is affected by emotional factors. In varying ways, hostility, depression, and anxiety are to some degree at the root of most psychosomatic disorders. Psychosomatic medicine is concerned with those illnesses that present primarily somatic manifestations. The presenting complaint is usually physical; the patient rarely complains of anxiety, depression, or tension, but rather of vomiting, diarrhea, or anorexia. Such patients usually consult a primary care physician or internist before seeking psychiatric help. Surveys reveal that psychological disturbances accompany 50 percent of medical patients studied in medical and surgical outpatient departments.

COMBINED TREATMENT

The combined treatment approach, in which a psychiatrist handles the psychiatric aspects of the case and an internist or other specialist treats the somatic aspects, requires the closest collaboration between the two physicians. The purpose of the medical therapy is to build up the patient's physical state so that the patient can participate successfully in psychotherapy for a total cure.

Disorders such as bronchial asthma, in which psychosocial processes play a distinct role in the development and course, may respond well to the combined treatment approach. Although the asthmatic attacks themselves may be treated successfully by the internist, psychiatric treatment can be useful in the short run by helping to alleviate the anxiety associated with the attacks and in the long run by helping to uncover the stresses that may precipitate or be involved in the disorder.

In an acute somatic illness, such as an acute attack of ulcerative colitis, medical therapy is the primary form of treatment; at this stage, psychotherapy, with its long-range goals, consists of reassurance and support. As the pendulum of disease activity shifts and the illness becomes chronic, psychotherapy may assume the primary role, and medical therapy takes the less active position.

Sometimes, reassurance is all that is needed in the treatment of psychosomatic syndromes. Patients must participate in the process of improving their life situations. The symptoms themselves may be treated by the internist, if necessary. Usually, the psychiatrist can help patients focus on their feelings about the symptoms and gain understanding of the unconscious processes involved with symptom improvement. If patients are handled insensitively or if their illnesses are regarded unsympathetically, the results can be grave.

Indications for Combined Treatment

During an initial attack of a psychosomatic disorder, if patients respond to active medical therapy in association with the superficial support, ventilation, reassurance, and environmental manipulation provided by an internist, additional psychotherapy by a psychiatrist may not be required. Psychosomatic illness that is chronic or does not respond to medical treatment should receive psychosomatic evaluation by a psychiatrist, and combined therapy as indicated.

Goal of Treatment

It is useful to set up a tentative, flexible spectrum of therapeutic goals in the treatment of psychosomatic disorders. The desired end is a cure, which means resolution of any structural impairment and reorganization of the personality so that needs and tensions no longer produce pathophysiological results. Treatment should aim at a mature general life adjustment, increased capacity for physical and occupational activity, amelioration of the progression of the disease, reversal of the pathology, avoidance of complications of the basic disease process, decreased use of secondary gain associated with the illness, and increased capacity to adjust to the presence of the disease.

PSYCHIATRIC ASPECTS

Treatment of psychosomatic disorders from a psychiatric viewpoint is a difficult task. Psychiatrists must focus therapy on understanding the motivations and mechanisms of disturbed functioning and helping patients realize the nature of their illness and the implications of its costly adaptive patterns. These insights should produce changed and healthier patterns of behavior.

Patients with psychosomatic disorders are usually more reluctant to deal with their emotional problems than patients with other psychiatric problems. Psychosomatic patients try to avoid responsibility for their illness by isolating the diseased organ and presenting it to the doctor for diagnosis and cure. They may be satisfying an infantile need to be cared for passively, while denying that they are adults, with all the attendant stresses and conflicts.

DEVELOPMENT OF RELATIONSHIP AND TRANSFERENCE

Psychotherapy with psychosomatic patients must often proceed more slowly and cautiously than with other psychiatric patients. Positive transference should be developed gradually, and psychiatrists must be supportive and reassuring during the acute illness. As disorders become chronic, a psychiatrist may make exploratory interpretations, but a strong patient–physician relationship must precede any such exploration. Psychosomatic patients are dependent, and this characteristic can be used supportively and interpretatively at crucial periods in the treatment. Much hostility surfaces during therapy—first in the form of overt ventilation and then in the framework of the transference. Therapists must encourage free and appropriate expression of patients' hostility.

Interpretation

Therapists must pay particular attention to current problems in patients' immediate life situation and must deal with patients' reaction to the therapist and to treatment. Therapists should increasingly emphasize evaluation of patients' characterological difficulties and habitual reactions, particularly reactions to themselves (self-esteem, guilt) and reactions to their environment (dependence, submission, need for affection). Psychia-

trists should also analyze patients' anxieties and coping mechanisms for stress situations, such as requests for complete care, the need to always be right, lack of self-assertion, and suppression of all forbidden impulses.

Some psychoanalytic investigators have reported dramatic results when unconscious material was interpreted as a drastic measure during an acute illness. Although most freudian psychoanalysts seem to think that genetic material must eventually be interpreted for a complete cure, new approaches have shown that adequate results can be obtained when psychotherapy is limited to the analysis of characterological and ego defenses associated with disturbed interpersonal relationships.

Patients with psychosomatic disorders are often involved in a repetitious pattern of stress in their interpersonal relationships. Because such patients are usually unaware of the pattern, it is helpful to show them that it is not accidental but is determined by factors of which they are unaware. One must show patients how to change the disturbing pattern and act in a new and healthier manner.

Psychosomatic patients tend to drive toward psychologically regressed mental and physical behavior and usually regress to a traumatic or highly conflictual period. By reenacting certain specific attitudes of childhood or infancy, they are attempting to master the anxiety and illness first manifested during these earlier stages.

In the treatment of psychosomatic disorders, the key concept is flexibility in technique. Because of patients' lack of motivation and poor physical condition, it may be necessary to make frequent changes in the psychotherapeutic approach.

Resistance during Therapy

Because patients with psychosomatic disorders often strongly resist entering psychotherapy, resistance frequently continues unabated during therapy. Many patients have such poor motivation for entering treatment that frequently they drop out of therapy for minor reasons.

Interruption of Psychotherapy for a Medical Emergency

During a course of psychotherapy, a patient with a psychosomatic disorder may require medical or surgical treatment for the organic disorder. The psychiatrist should cooperate closely with the surgeon or medical personnel and should maintain contact with the patient—in person or by telephone—during the emergency. Such interest offers valuable emotional support in a time of crisis.

If a patient is hospitalized, the psychiatrist should help other hospital personnel recognize, and learn to tolerate, the frequently difficult and provocative behavior of some psychosomatic patients. The preparation can be of use to the patients as well; when they see their demands being met considerately, they may be less inclined to view their world as hostile and formidable.

Danger of Psychosis

There are no simple relations between psychosomatic disorders and psychoses. Some persons in whom physiological and psychological processes are poorly integrated manifest both psychosomatic disorders and psychoses. In other persons, the ego integration is such that stress produces a breakdown of bodily function rather than a psychotic maladjustment. Some nonpsychotic psychosomatic patients can become psychotic or exhibit psychotic symptoms if an interpretation is too active and defensive elements in the personality structure are removed.

MEDICAL ASPECTS

Internists' treatment of psychosomatic disorders should follow the established rules for medical management. Generally, internists should spend as much time as possible with a patient and listen sympathetically to the many complaints; they must be reassuring and supportive. Before performing a physically manipulative procedure—particularly if it is painful, such as a colonoscopy—the internist should explain to a patient just what to expect. The explanation allays the patient's anxiety, makes the patient more cooperative, and actually facilitates the examination.

Patients' attitudes toward taking drugs may also affect the outcome of the psychosomatic treatment. For example, patients with diabetes who do not accept their illness and who have self-destructive impulses of which they are unaware may purposely not control their diet and, as a result, end up in a hyperglycemic coma. Some cardiac patients refuse to curtail their physical activity after a myocardial infarction because of a reluctance to admit weakness or because of a fear that they will somehow be considered unsuccessful. Others use their illness as a welcome punishment for guilt or as a way to avoid responsibility. Therapy in such cases must strive to help patients minimize their fears and focus on self-care and reestablishment of a healthy body image.

BEHAVIORAL CHANGE

A major role of psychiatrists and other physicians working with psychosomatic patients is mobilizing the patient to change behavior in ways that optimize the process of healing. This may require a general change in lifestyle (e.g., taking vacations) or a more specific behavioral change (e.g., giving up smoking). Whether or not this occurs depends in large measure on the quality of the relationship between doctor and patient. Failure of the physician to establish good rapport accounts for much of the ineffectiveness in getting patients to change.

Rapport is the spontaneous, conscious feeling of harmonious responsiveness between patient and doctor. It implies understanding and trust between the two. With rapport, patients feel accepted, even though they may think their assets outnumber their liabilities. Frequently, the physician is the person to whom the patient can talk about things he or she cannot talk about with anyone else. Most patients feel that they can trust physicians, especially psychiatrists, to keep secrets. This confidence must not be betrayed. Feeling that someone knows, understands, and accepts them is a source of strength that may enable patients to embark on a healthy course of action such as enrolling in Alcoholics Anonymous (AA) or changing eating habits.

Ideally, both physician and patient collaborate and decide on a course of action. At times this may resemble a negotiation in which doctor and patient discuss various options and reach a compromise about an agreed-upon goal. Aaron Lazare described specific negotiating strategies to achieve behavioral changes:

1. Direct education. Explain the problem, goals, and methods to achieve goals. Education must be geared to the patient's socioeconomic level and cultural traditions. If the patient has questions, they should be answered frankly. Explanations in keeping with the patient's capacity to understand should be given. Such factors as intelligence, sophistication in regard to personality reactions, and degree and type of illness should influence the vocabulary and content of the physician's response. Every effort should be made to convey to belligerent patients both understanding and tolerance for their feelings.
2. Third-party intervention. Family members, friends, and other clinicians can provide support and encourage the patient to follow a course of action. This may occur in a group setting, which is especially effective in motivating patients who have substance abuse problems to obtain treatment (called an intervention).
3. Exploration of options. There may be alternative methods for achieving a desired goal. For example, quitting smoking can be done with support groups, nicotine patches or gum, psychotropic drugs, or "cold turkey," among others.
4. Provision of sample treatment. If a patient fears a particular course of action or considers change impossible, a treatment trial can be implemented. The patient always may opt out of the prescribed program.
5. Control sharing. Some patients resent any approach that appears to be authoritarian. They may wish to set the pace of a withdrawal program or titrate their medication depending on adverse effects.
6. Concession making. The clinician may grant the patient something that he or she wants (e.g., medication) as a bargaining chip to get the patient to comply with advice.
7. Empathic confrontation. Patients who resist change may do so because of fear or other uncomfortable emotions of which they are unaware. The doctor can try to "step into the patients' shoes" in an effort to raise their level of awareness. Doctors should be prepared to answer the patient's question: "What would you do if you were in my place?"
8. Standard setting. Guidelines or standards (sometimes called milestones) should be set to evaluate the progress of an agreed-upon program (e.g., the loss of 1 pound of weight every 2 weeks to achieve a weight loss of 10 pounds in 20 weeks.

In rare cases in which negotiations break down and an impasse is reached it may be necessary to threaten to terminate the relationship. As Lazare notes:

> This final stage may be unavoidable when a clinician believes that his or her professional standards are compromised or when the patient just cannot be satisfied regardless of the clinician's attempts.

Relapse

It is common for patients who embark upon a new or improved pattern of behavior to relapse. Physicians must not get angry with patients who have a recurrence of their previous maladaptive lifestyle. Relapse is sometimes a necessary part of the process of change, not a sign of failure. The doctor should explain that relapse may occur and support the patient in his or her effort to continue the program. Approaches to use in dealing with relapse behavior are outlined in Table 28.3–1.

Table 28.3–1
Approaches to Use with the Relapsing Patient

Approach	Comments
Cognitive	Provide information about high-risk situations (e.g., eating when anxious).
Attitudinal	Support motivation for change by emphasizing long-term benefits (e.g., lower risk of lung cancer with smoking cessation) and short-term benefits (e.g., decreased coughing).
Instrumental	Train and rehearse skills for coping with high-risk situations (e.g., chewing gum when anxious instead of eating); maintain a written log of when and where maladaptive behavior takes place; identify precipitating factors (e.g., anger).
Coping	Build strategies for minimizing or avoiding the occurrence of high-risk situations (e.g., have soft drinks instead of alcohol at parties); develop strategies for coping with relapse (e.g., do not shame patient, relapses are expected).
Social/environmental	Help patients find and build social support (e.g., AA, NA, OA).
Contact	Provide frequent follow-up visits to maintain doctor–patient relationship; use telephone, e-mail.

Modified after data from Grueninger UJ, Duffy FD, Goldstein MG. Patient education in the medical encounter: how to facilitate learning, behavior change and coping. In: Lipkin M, Putnam SM, Lazare A, eds. *The Medical Interview.* New York: Springer-Verlag; 1995.

OTHER TYPES OF THERAPY FOR PSYCHOSOMATIC DISORDERS

Group Psychotherapy and Family Therapy

The group approach offers interpersonal contact with others suffering from the same illness and provides support for patients who fear the threat of isolation and abandonment. Family therapy offers hope of a change in the relationship between family members who are often stressed and reactively hostile to the sick member.

Relaxation Techniques

Edmund Jacobson in 1938 developed a method called progressive muscle relaxation to teach relaxation without using instrumentation as is used in biofeedback. Patients were taught to relax muscle groups such as those involved in "tension headaches." When they encountered, and were aware of, situations that caused tension in their muscles, the patients were trained to relax. This method is a type of systematic desensitization—a type of behavior therapy.

Herbert Benson in 1975 used concepts developed from transcendental meditation in which a patient maintained a more passive attitude, allowing relaxation to occur on its own. Benson derived his techniques from various Eastern religions and practices, such as yoga. All of these techniques have in common a position of comfort, a peaceful environment, a passive approach, and a pleasant mental image on which one can concentrate.

Hypnosis

Hypnosis is effective in smoking cessation and dietary change augmentation. It is used in combination with aversive imagery (e.g., cigarettes taste obnoxious). Some patients exhibit a moderately high relapse rate and may require repeated programs of hypnotic therapy (usually three to four sessions).

Biofeedback

Neal Miller in 1969 published his pioneering paper "Learning of Visceral and Glandular Responses," in which he reported that in animals, various visceral responses regulated by the involuntary autonomic nervous system could be modified by learning accomplished through operant conditioning carried out in the laboratory. This led to humans being able to learn to control certain involuntary physiological responses (called *biofeedback*) such as blood vessel vasoconstriction, cardiac rhythm, and heart rate. These physiological changes seem to play a significant role in the development and treatment or cure of certain psychosomatic disorders. Such studies did, in fact, confirm that conscious learning could control heart rate and systolic pressure in humans.

Biofeedback and related techniques have been useful in tension headaches, migraine headaches, and Raynaud's disease. Although biofeedback techniques initially produced encouraging results in treating essential hypertension, relaxation therapy has produced more significant long-term effects than biofeedback.

References

Alexander F. *Psychosomatic Medicine*. New York: WW Norton; 1950.

Carney RM, Freedland KE, Stein PK, Skala JA, Hoffman P, Jaffe AS. Change in heart rate and heart rate variability during treatment for depression in patients with coronary heart disease. *Psychosom Med.* 2000;62:639.

Matheny KB, Brack GL, McCarthy CJ, Penick JM. The effectiveness of cognitively-based approaches in treating stress-related symptoms. *Psychotherapy.* 1996;33:305.

Sanders D. *Counselling for Psychosomatic Problems*. London: Sage Publications; 1996.

Speca M, Carlson LE, Goodey E, Angen M. A randomized, wait-list controlled clinical trial: the effect of a mindfulness meditation-based stress reduction program on mood and symptoms of stress in cancer outpatients. *Psychosom Med.* 2000;62:613.

Stoudemire A, section ed. Psychological factors affecting medical conditions. In: Sadock BJ, Sadock VA, eds. *Kaplan & Sadock's Comprehensive Textbook of Psychiatry.* 7th ed. Vol 2. Baltimore: Lippincott Williams & Wilkins; 2000:1765.

Stoudemire A, Fogel BS, Greenberg D, eds. *Psychiatric Care of the Medical Patient.* New York: Oxford University Press; 1999.

Temple N, Walker J, Evans M. Group psychotherapy with psychosomatic and somatizing patients in a general hospital. *Psychoanal Psychother.* 1996;10:251.

▲ 28.4 Consultation-Liaison Psychiatry

Consultation-liaison (C-L) psychiatry is the study, practice, and teaching of the relation between medical and psychiatric disorders. In C-L psychiatry, psychiatrists serve as consultants to medical colleagues (either another psychiatrist or, more commonly, a nonpsychiatric physician) or to other mental health professionals (psychologist, social worker, or psychiatric nurse). In addition, C-L psychiatrists consult regarding patients in medical or surgical settings and provide follow-up psychiatric treatment as needed. C-L psychiatry is associated with all the diagnostic, therapeutic, research, and teaching services that psychiatrists perform in the general hospital and serves as a bridge between psychiatry and other specialties.

In the medical wards of the hospital, C-L psychiatrists must play many roles: skillful and brief interviewer, good psychiatrist and psychotherapist, teacher, and knowledgeable physician who understands the medical aspects of the case. The C-L psychiatrist must be viewed as a part of the medical team, who makes a unique contribution to the patient's total medical treatment.

DIAGNOSIS

Knowledge of psychiatric diagnosis is essential to C-L psychiatrists. Both dementia and delirium frequently complicate medical illness, especially among hospital patients. Delirium occurs in 15 to 30 percent of hospitalized patients. Psychoses and other mental disorders often complicate the treatment of medical illness, and deviant illness behavior such as suicide is a common problem in patients who are organically ill. C-L psychiatrists must be aware of the many medical illnesses that can have psychiatric symptoms. Lifetime prevalence of mental illness in chronically physically ill patients is over 40 percent, particularly substance abuse and mood and anxiety disorders. (A list of such medical problems is presented in Table 28.4–1.) Interviews and serial clinical observations are the C-L psychiatrist's tools for diagnosis. The purposes of the diagnosis are to identify mental disorders and psychological responses to physical illness, identify patients' personality features, and identify patients' characteristic coping techniques to recommend the most appropriate therapeutic intervention for patients' needs.

TREATMENT

C-L psychiatrists' principal contribution to medical treatment is a comprehensive analysis of a patient's response to illness, psychological and social resources, coping style, and psychiatric illness, if any. This assessment is the basis of the patient treatment plan. In discussing the plan, C-L psychiatrists provide their patient assessment to nonpsychiatric health professionals. Psychiatrists' recommendations should be clear, concrete guidelines for action. A C-L psychiatrist may recommend a specific therapy, suggest areas for further medical inquiry, inform doctors and nurses of their roles in the patient's psychosocial care, recommend a transfer to a psychiatric facility for long-term psychiatric treatment, or suggest or undertake brief psychotherapy with the patient on the medical ward.

C-L psychiatrists must deal with a broad range of psychiatric disorders, the most common symptoms being anxiety, depression, and disorientation. Treatment problems account for 50 percent of the consultation requests made of psychiatrists. (Table 28.4–2 covers the most common C-L problems.)

One of the most critical areas for the C-L psychiatrist involves knowing the interaction of medical and psychiatric drugs. This includes knowledge about pharmacokinetics as it relates to end-organ dysfunction (kidney, liver, lung, heart) and the aging process. Drug–drug interactions are discussed in Section 36.1.

Table 28.4–1
Medical Conditions That Present with Psychiatric Symptoms

Disease	Common Medical Symptoms	Psychiatric Symptoms and Complaints	Impaired Performance and Behavior	Laboratory Tests and Findings	Diagnostic Problems
Hyperthyroidism (thyrotoxicosis)	Heat intolerance Excessive sweating Diarrhea Weight loss Tachycardia Palpitations Vomiting	Nervousness Excitability Irritability Pressured speech Insomnia May express fear of impending death Psychosis	Fine tremor Impaired cognition Decreased concentration Hyperactivity Intrusiveness	Free T_4 increased T_3 increased TSH decreased T_3 uptake decreased ECG: Tachycardia, atrial fibrillation, P and T wave changes	Full range of symptoms may not be present Hyperthyroidism and anxiety states may coexist Rule out occult malignancy, cardiovascular disease, amphetamine intoxication, cocaine intoxication, anxiety states, mania
Hypothyroidism (myxedema)	Cold intolerance Dry skin Constipation Weight gain Brittle hair Goiter	Lethargy Depressed affect Personality change Maniclike psychosis Paranoia Hallucinations	Muscle weakness Decreased concentration Psychomotor slowing Apathy Unusual sensitivity to barbiturates	TSH increased TSH low if pituitary disease Free T_4 decreased ECG: Bradycardia	More common in women Associated with lithium carbonate therapy Rule out pituitary disease, hypothalamic disease, major depressive disorder, bipolar I disorder
Hypoglycemia	Sweating Drowsiness Stupor Coma Tachycardia	Anxiety Confusion Agitation	Tremor Restlessness Seizures	Hypoglycemia Tachycardia	Excess insulin often complicated by exercise, alcohol, decreased food intake Rule out insulinoma, postictal states, agitated depression, paranoid psychosis
Hyperglycemia	Polyuria Anorexia Nausea Vomiting Dehydration Abdominal complaints	Anxiety Agitation Delirium	Acetone breath Seizures	Hyperglycemia Serum ketones Urine ketones Anion gap acidosis	Almost always associated with brittle diabetes in young juvenile diabetics and elderly non–insulin-dependent diabetics Rule out depressive disorders, anxiety disorders
Brain neoplasms	Headache Vomiting Papilledema Focal findings on neurology examination	Personality changes		Lumbar puncture: increased CSF pressure, skull X-ray, CT scan, EEG	40–50% gliomas most common in 40–50-year-olds Cerebellar tumors most common in children
Frontal lobe tumor		Mood changes Irritability Facetiousness Impaired judgment Impaired memory Delirium	Seizures Loss of speech Loss of smell	Angiogram: space-occupying lesion	Rule out intracranial abscess, aneurysm, subdural hematoma, seizure disorder, cerebrovascular disease, reactive depression, mania, schizophreniform disorder, dementia
Parietal lobe tumor	Hyperreflexia Babinski's sign Astereognosis		Sensory and motor abnormalities Contralateral hemiparesis Focal seizures		
Occipital lobe tumor	Headache Papilledema Homonymous hemianopsia	Aura Visual hallucinations	Visual problems Seizures		
Temporal lobe tumor	Contralateral homonymous field cut		Psychomotor seizures Aphasia		
Cerebellar tumor	Early evidence of increased intracranial pressure		Disturbed equilibrium Disturbed coordination		

(continued)

Table 28.4–1 (*continued*)

Disease	Common Medical Symptoms	Psychiatric Symptoms and Complaints	Impaired Performance and Behavior	Laboratory Tests and Findings	Diagnostic Problems
Head trauma	History or evidence of head trauma Headache Dizziness Bleeding from ear Altered level of consciousness Loss of consciousness Focal neurological findings	Confusion Personality changes Memory impairment	Seizures Paralysis	Lumbar puncture, skull X-rays, CT scan show evidence of bleeding or increased intracranial pressure Cerebral angiogram EEG	History of blow to head or bleeding confirms cause of ALS Rule out cerebrovascular disease, seizure disorder, alcohol dependence, diabetes mellitus, hepatic encephalopathy, depression, dementia
AIDS	Fever Weight loss Ataxia Incontinence Focal findings on neurological examination	Progressive dementia Personality changes Depression Loss of libido Psychosis Mutism	Impaired memory Decreased concentration Seizures	HIV testing CT, MRI, lumbar puncture, CSF, and blood cultures	>60% of patients have neuropsychiatric symptoms; always consider in high-risk populations and young patients with signs of dementia Rule out other infections, brain neoplasms, dementia, depression, schizophreniform disorder
Injuries requiring ambulatory surgical evaluation and treatment (for example, wrist slashing)	Alcohol abuse and other substance abuse Recent surgery Chronic pain Chronic illness Terminal illness	>90% have major psychiatric disease History of prior suicide attempts Depressed mood Postpartum psychosis in women	Frequent accidents Repeated emergency room visits Eager to leave emergency room before full evaluation		Suicidal behavior is a symptom of underlying psychiatric illness Knowledge of risk factors is helpful but not a substitute for good clinical judgment Prediction is best done through assessment of current risk projected into the immediate future
Hyponatremia	Excessive thirst Polydipsia Stupor Coma	Confusion Lethargy Personality changes	Seizures Speech abnormalities	Decreased serum Na^+ Serum Na^+ and osmolalities to document syndrome of inappropriate secretion of antidiuretic hormone (SIADH)	Caused by excessive free water for level of total body Na^+ Often abnormal SIADH May be psychogenic Rule out nephrotic syndrome, liver disease, congestive heart failure, schizophreniform disorder, schizotypal personality disorder
Pancreatic carcinoma	Weight loss Abdominal pain	Depression Lethargy Anhedonia	Apathy Decreased energy	Elevated amylase	Always consider in depressed middle-aged patients Rule out other GI illness, major depressive disorder
Cushing's syndrome	Central obesity Purple striae Easy bruising Osteoporosis Proximal muscle weakness Hirsutism	Depression Insomnia Emotional lability Suicidality Euphoria Mania Psychosis Delirium	Disturbed sleep Decreased energy Agitation Difficulty concentrating	Elevated blood pressure Poor glucose tolerance Dexamethasone-suppression test (may be falsely positive)	Must distinguish other causes—e.g., cancer from exogenous steroid excess Suicide rate in untreated cases is about 10% Rule out major depressive disorder, bipolar I disorder
Adrenocortical insufficiency (Addison's disease)	Nausea Vomiting Anorexia Stupor Coma Hyperpigmentation	Lethargy Depression Psychosis Delirium	Fatigue	Decreased blood pressure Decreased Na^+ Increased K^+ Eosinophilia	May be primary (Addison's disease) or secondary Rule out eating disorders, mood disorders

(*continued*)

Table 28.4–1 (*continued*)

Disease	Common Medical Symptoms	Psychiatric Symptoms and Complaints	Impaired Performance and Behavior	Laboratory Tests and Findings	Diagnostic Problems
Seizure disorder	Sensory distortions Aura	Confusion Psychosis Dissociative states Catatoniclike state	Violence Motor automatisms Belligerence Bizarre behavior	EEG, including NP leads	Consider complex partial seizures in all dissociative states Rule out postictal states, catatonic schizophrenia
Hyperparathyroidism	Constipation Polydipsia Nausea	Depression Paranoia Confusion		Increased Ca^{2-} PTH variable ECG: shortened QT interval	Causes hypercalcemia Rule out major depressive disorder, schizoaffective disorder
Hypoparathyroidism	Headache Paresthesias Tetany Carpopedal spasm Laryngeal spasm Abdominal pain	Anxiety Agitation Depression Confusion	Impaired memory	Low Ca^{2+}, normal albumin Low blood pressure ECG: QT prolongation, ventricular arrhythmias	Causes hypocalcemia Rule out anxiety disorders, mood disorders
Systemic lupus erythematosus	Fever Photosensitivity Butterfly rash Joint pains Headache	Depression Mood disturbances Psychosis Delusions Hallucinations	Fatigue	Positive ANA Positive lupus erythematosus test Anemia Thrombocytopenia Chest X-ray: pleural effusion, pericarditis	Multisystemic autoimmune disease most frequent in women Psychiatric symptoms are present in 50% of patients Steroid treatment can cause psychiatric symptoms Rule out depressive disorders, paranoid psychosis psychotic mood disorder
Multiple sclerosis	Sudden transient motor and sensory disturbances Impaired vision Diffuse neurological signs with remissions and exacerbations	Anxiety Euphoria Mania	Slurred speech Incontinence	CSF may show increased gamma globulin CT: degenerative patches in brain and spinal cord	Onset usually in young adults Rule out tertiary syphilis, other degenerative diseases, hysteria, mania (late)
Acute intermittent porphyria	Abdominal pain Fever Nausea Vomiting Constipation Peripheral neuropathy Paralysis	Acute depression Agitation Paranoia Visual hallucinations	Restlessness Diaphoresis Weakness	Leukocytosis Elevated δ-aminolevulinic acid Elevated porphobilinogen Tachycardia	Autosomal dominant More common in women ages 20–40 May be precipitated by a variety of drugs Rule out acute abdominal disease, acute psychiatric episode, schizophreniform disorder, major depressive disorder
Hepatic encephalopathy	Asterixis Hyperreflexia Spider angiomata Palmar erythema Ecchymoses Liver enlargement and atrophy	Euphoria Disinhibition Psychosis Depression	Restlessness Decreased activities of daily living (ADL) Impaired cognition Impaired concentration Ataxia Dysarthria	Abnormal liver function test results Abnormal albumin EEG: diffuse slowing	May be acute or chronic depending on cause Rule out substance intoxication, mania, depressive disorder, dementia
Injuries requiring inpatient surgical evaluation and treatment (e.g., suicide attempts, self-mutilation)	Alcohol abuse and other substance abuse Serious injury Major blood loss Damage to genitals, eyes, face, etc.	99% have severe psychiatric disease associated with psychosis, psychotic depression Impaired mental status secondary to substance intoxication Bizarre, inappropriate affect	Remain at great risk for suicide		Must assess and treat the underlying psychiatric condition on a priority basis Maintain a high index of suspicion for suicide risk

(*continued*)

Table 28.4–1 (*continued*)

Disease	Common Medical Symptoms	Psychiatric Symptoms and Complaints	Impaired Performance and Behavior	Laboratory Tests and Findings	Diagnostic Problems
Pheochromocytoma	Paroxysmal hypertension Headache	Anxiety Apprehension Feeling of impending doom	Panic Diaphoresis Tremor	Hypertension Elevated VMA in 24-h urine Tachycardia	Adrenal medulla secreting catecholamines Rule out anxiety disorders
Wilson's disease	Kayser-Fleischer corneal ring Hepatitislike picture	Mood disturbances Delusions Hallucinations	Choreoathetoid movements Gait disturbance Clumsiness Rigidity	Decreased serum ceruloplasmin Increased copper in urine	Hepatolenticular degeneration Autosomal recessive disorder of copper metabolism Often presents in adolescence, early adulthood Rule out extrapyramidal reactions, schizophreniform disorder, mood disorders
Huntington's disease	Family history	Depression Euphoria	Rigidity Choreoathetoid movements		Autosomal dominant Rule out mood disorders, mania, schizophrenia
Vitamin deficiencies					
Thiamine	Neuropathy Cardiomyopathy Wernicke-Korsakoff syndrome Nystagmus Headache Amnesia	Confusion Confabulation	General malaise Inability to sustain a conversation Poor concentration	Low thiamine level	Most common in alcoholic persons Rule out hypomania, depressive disorder, dementia
Nicotinamide	Diarrhea Stocking-glove dermatitis	Confusion Irritability Insomnia Depression Psychosis Dementia	Memory disturbances		Rule out mood disorders, mania, schizophreniform disorder, dementia
Pyridoxine		Apathy Irritability	Memory disturbance Muscle weakness Seizures		Often caused by medication: isoniazid Rule out mood disorders, dementia
Vitamin B_{12}	Pallor Dizziness Peripheral neuropathy Dorsal column signs	Irritability Inattentiveness Psychosis Dementia	Fatigue Ataxia	Low B_{12} level Schilling test Megaloblastic anemia	Often due to pernicious anemia Rule out dementia, mania, mood disorders
Tertiary syphilis	Skin lesions Leukoplakia Periostitis Arthritis Respiratory distress Progressive cardiovascular distress	Personality changes Irritability Confusion Psychosis	Irresponsible behavior Decreased attention to activities of daily living (ADLs)	VDRL, Treponema antibody test CSF abnormal	General paresis Rule out neoplasias, meningitis, dementia, psychotic mood disorder, schizophrenia

Permitting patients to make small choices restores some sense of control over the self and the future, gives them a symbolic sense of progress, and calms them far beyond the meaning of the specific choices. For example, allowing patients to control pain medications, the level of lighting, or the place where they sit reassures and relaxes them. Whether the disruptive behavior is hostility, dependence, or panic, allowing some behavior to be shown while setting limits on their extremes reassures patients. Thus, an independent patient can be allowed to move around but not too far; a dependent patient can make a limited number of interactions, such as using the call button; and a hostile patient can be permitted some disagreement and ventilation but be limited in disruptive acts.

All intensive care units (ICUs) deal mainly with anxiety, depression, and delirium. ICUs also impose extraordinarily high stress on staff and patients, related to the intensity of the problems. Patients and staff members alike frequently observe cardiac arrests, deaths, and medical disasters, which leave them all autonomically aroused and psychologically defensive. ICU nurses and their patients experience particularly high levels of anxiety and depression. As a result, nurse burnout and high turnover rates are common.

The problem of stress among ICU staff receives much attention, especially in the nursing literature. Much less attention is given to the house staff, especially those on the surgical services. All persons in ICUs must to be able to deal directly with their

Table 28.4–2
Common Consultation-Liaison Problems

Reason for Consultation	Comments
Suicide attempt or threat	High-risk factors: men over 45, no social support, alcohol dependence, previous attempt, incapacitating medical illness with pain, and suicidal ideation; if risk is present, transfer to psychiatric unit or start 24-h nursing care
Depression	Suicidal risks must be assessed in every depressed patient (see above); presence of cognitive defects in depression may cause diagnostic dilemma with dementia; check for history of substance abuse or depressant drugs (e.g., reserpine, propranolol); use antidepressants cautiously in cardiac patients because of conduction side effects, orthostatic hypotension
Agitation	Often related to cognitive disorder, withdrawal from drugs (e.g., opioids, alcohol, sedative-hypnotics); haloperidol most useful drug for excessive agitation; use physical restraints with great caution; examine for command hallucinations or paranoid ideation to which patient is responding in agitated manner; rule out toxic reaction to medication
Hallucinations	Most common cause in hospital is delirium tremens; onset 3 to 4 days after hospitalization; in intensive care units, check for sensory isolation; rule out brief psychotic disorder, schizophrenia, cognitive disorder; treat with antipsychotic medication
Sleep disorder	Common cause is pain; early morning awakening associated with depression; difficulty falling asleep associated with anxiety; use antianxiety or antidepressant agent, depending on cause (those drugs have no analgesic effect, so prescribe adequate painkillers); rule out early substance withdrawal
No organic basis for symptoms	Rule out conversion disorder, somatization disorder, factitious disorder, and malingering; glove and stocking anesthesia with autonomic nervous system symptoms seen in conversion disorder; multiple body complaints seen in somatization disorder; wish to be hospitalized seen in factitious disorder; obvious secondary gain in malingering (e.g., compensation case)
Disorientation	Delirium versus dementia; review metabolic status, neurological findings, substance history; prescribe small dose of antipsychotics for major agitation; benzodiazepines may worsen condition and cause sundowner syndrome (ataxia, confusion); modify environment so patient does not experience sensory deprivation
Noncompliance or refusal to consent to procedure	Explore relationship of patient and treating doctor; negative transference is most common cause of noncompliance; fears of medication or of procedure require education and reassurance; refusal to give consent is issue of judgment; if impaired, patient can be declared incompetent, but only by a judge; cognitive disorder is main cause of impaired judgment in hospitalized patients

feelings about their extraordinary experiences and difficult emotional and physical circumstances. Regular support groups in which persons can discuss their feelings are important to the ICU staff and the house staff. Such support groups protect staff members from the otherwise predictable psychiatric morbidity that some may experience and protect their patients from the loss of concentration, decreased energy, and psychomotor-retarded communications that some staff members otherwise exhibit.

Hemodialysis Units

Hemodialysis units present a paradigm of complex modern medical treatment settings. Patients are coping with lifelong, debilitating, and limiting disease; they are totally dependent on a multiplex group of caretakers for access to a machine controlling their well-being. Dialysis is scheduled three times a week and takes 4 to 6 hours; thus, it disrupts patients' previous living routines.

In this context, patients first and foremost fight the disease. Invariably, however, they also must come to terms with a level of dependence on others probably not experienced since childhood. Predictably, patients entering dialysis struggle for their independence; regress to childhood states; show denial by acting out against doctor's orders, by breaking their diet, or by missing sessions; show anger directed against staff members; bargain and plead or become infantilized and obsequious; but most often are accepting and courageous. The determinants of patients' responses to entering dialysis include personality styles and previous experiences with this or another chronic illness. Patients who have had time to react and adapt to their chronic renal failure face less new psychological work of adaptation than those with recent renal failure and machine dependence.

Although little has been written about social factors, the effect of cultural factors in reaction to dialysis and the management of the dialysis unit are known to be important. Units run with a firm hand, that are consistent in dealing with patients, have clear contingencies for behavioral failures, and have adequate psychological support for staff members tend to produce the best results.

Complications of dialysis treatment can include psychiatric problems such as depression, and suicide is not rare. Sexual problems can be neurogenic, psychogenic, or related to gonadal dysfunction and testicular atrophy. Dialysis dementia is a rare condition that evidences loss of memory, disorientation, dystonias, and seizures. The disorder occurs in patients who have been receiving dialysis treatment for many years. The cause is unknown.

The psychological treatment of dialysis patients falls into two areas. First, careful preparation before dialysis, including the work of adaptation to chronic illness, is important, especially in dealing with denial and unrealistic expectations. All predialysis patients should have a psychosocial evaluation. Second, once in a dialysis program, patients need periodic specific inquiries about adaptation that do not encourage dependence or the sick role. Staff members should be sensitive to the likelihood of depression and sexual problems. Group sessions function well for support, and patient self-help groups restore a useful social network, self-esteem, and self-mastery. When needed, tricyclic drugs or phenothiazines can be used for dialysis patients. Psychiatric care is most effective when brief and problem oriented.

The use of home dialysis units has improved treatment attitude. Home-treated patients can integrate the treatment into

Table 28.4–3
Transplantation and Surgical Problems

Organ	Biological Factors	Psychological Factors
Lung	One-year survival, 70%; risk of infectious pneumonitis high	Cadaveric lungs used; rejection is chronic; complex aftercare requires supportive psychotherapy
Kidney	70–90% success rate; may not be done if patient is over age 55; increasing use of cadaveric kidneys rather than those from living donors	Living donors must be emotionally stable; parents are best donors, siblings may be ambivalent; donors are subject to depression; patients who panic before surgery may have poor prognoses; altered body image with fear of organ rejection is common; group therapy for patients is helpful
Bone marrow	Used in aplastic anemias and immune system disease	Patients are usually ill and must deal with death and dying: compliance is important; commonly done in children who present problems of prolonged dependence; siblings are often donors and may be angry or ambivalent about procedure
Heart	End-stage coronary artery disease and cardiomyopathy	Donor is legally dead; relatives of the deceased may refuse permission or be ambivalent; no fall-back position is available if the organ is rejected; kidney rejection patient can go on hemodialysis; some patients seek transplantation hoping to die; postcardiotomy delirium occurs in 25% of patients
Breast	Radical mastectomy versus lumpectomy	Reconstruction of breast at time of surgery leads to postoperative adaptation; veteran patients are used to counsel new patients; lumpectomy patients are more open about surgery and sex than are mastectomy patients; group support is helpful
Uterus	Hysterectomy performed on 10% of women over 20	Fear of loss of sexual attractiveness with sexual dysfunction in a small percentage of women; loss of childbearing capacity is upsetting
Brain	Anatomical location of lesion determines behavioral change	Environmental dependence syndrome in frontal lobe tumors characterized by inability to show initiative; memory disturbances involved to periventricular surgery; hallucinations involved in parietooccipital area
Prostate	Cancer surgery has more negative psychobiological effects and is more technically difficult than surgery for benign hypertrophy	Sexual dysfunction is common except in transurethral prostatectomy; perineal prostatectomy produces absence of emission, ejaculation, and erection; penile implant may be of use; consider use of sildenafil (Viagra)
Colon and rectum	Colostomy and ostomy are common outcomes, especially for cancer	One third of patients with colostomies feel worse about themselves than before bowel surgery; shame and self-consciousness about the stoma can be alleviated by self-help groups that deal with those issues
Limbs	Amputation performed for massive injury, diabetes, or cancer	Phantom-limb phenomenon in 98% of cases; the experience may last for years; sometimes the sensation is painful, and neuroma at the stump should be ruled out; the condition has no known cause or treatment; it may stop spontaneously
Liver	One-year survival 25%; 5–15% receive second implant	Most common indication is hepatitis C; check history of alcohol abuse; complex postoperative course requires emotional support

their daily lives more easily, and they feel more autonomous and less dependent on others for their care than hospital-treated patients.

Surgical Units

Some surgeons believe that patients who expect to die during surgery will. This belief now seems less superstitious than it once did. Chase Patterson Kimball and others have studied the premorbid psychological adjustment of patients scheduled for surgery and have shown that those who show evident depression or anxiety and deny it have a higher risk for morbidity and mortality than those who, given similar depression or anxiety, can express it. Even better results occur in those with a positive attitude toward impending surgery. The factors that contribute to an improved outcome for surgery are informed consent and education so that patients know what they can expect to feel, where they will be (e.g., it is useful to show patients the recovery room), what loss of function to expect, what tubes and gadgets will be in place, and how to cope with the anticipated pain. If patients will not be able to talk or see after surgery, it is helpful to explain before surgery what they can do to compensate for these losses. If postoperative states such as confusion, delirium, and pain can be predicted, they should be discussed with patients in advance so they do not experience them as unwarranted or as signs of danger. Constructive family support members can help both before and after surgery.

Transplantation Issues

Transplantation programs have expanded over the past decade, and C-L psychiatrists play an important role in helping patients and their families deal with the many psychosocial issues involved: (1) which and when patients on a waiting list will receive organs, (2) anxiety about the procedure, (3) fear of death, (4) organ rejection, and (5) adaptation to life after successful transplantation. Posttransplant patients require complex aftercare, and achieving compliance with medication may be difficult without supportive psychotherapy. This is particularly relevant to patients who have received liver transplants as a result of hepatitis C brought on by promiscuous sexual behavior and to drug addicts who use contaminated needles.

Group therapy with patients who have had similar transplantation procedures benefits members who can support

one another and share information and feelings about particular stressors related to their disease. Groups may be conducted or supervised by the psychiatrist. Psychiatrists must be especially concerned about psychiatric complication. Within 1 year of transplant, almost 20 percent of patients experience a major depression or an adjustment disorder with depressed mood. In such cases evaluation for suicidal ideation and risk is important. In addition to depression, another 10 percent of patients experience signs of posttraumatic stress disorder, with nightmares and anxiety attacks related to the procedure. Other issues concern whether or not the transplanted organ came from a cadaver or from a living donor who may or may not be related to the patient. Pretransplant consulting sessions with potential organ donors helps to deal with fears about surgery and concerns about who will receive the donated organ. Sometimes the recipient may be counseled together with the donor, as in cases where one sibling is donating a kidney to another. Peer support groups with both donors and recipients have also been used to facilitate coping with transplantation issues. Table 28.4–3 lists various transplantation and surgical issues with which C-L psychiatrists must deal.

References

Cheng C. Seeking medical consultation: perceptual and behavioral characteristics distinguishing consulters and nonconsulters with functional dyspepsia. *Psychosom Med.* 2000;62:844.

Druss BG, Rohrbaugh RM, Rosenheck RA. Depressive symptoms and health costs in older medical patients. *Am J Psychiatry.* 1999;156:477.

Engle GL. The need for a new medical model: a challenge for biomedical science. *Science.* 1977;196:129.

Feifel H, Strack S, Nagy VT. Coping strategies and associated features of medically ill patients. *Psychosom Med.* 1987;49:545.

Field MJ, Lohr KN. *Guidelines for Clinical Practice: From Development to Use.* Washington, DC: National Academy Press; 1992.

Fink P, Ewald H, Jensen J, et al. Screening for somatization and hypochondriasis in primary care and neurological inpatients: a seven-item scale for hypochondriasis and somatization. *J Psychosom Res.* 1999;46:261.

Lipsitt DR. Consultation-liaison psychiatry and psychosomatic medicine: the company they keep. *Psychosom Med.* 2001;63:896.

Rundell JR, Wise MG, eds. *The American Psychiatric Press Textbook of Consultation-Liaison Psychiatry.* Washington, DC: American Psychiatric Press; 1996.

Strain JJ. Consultation-liaison psychiatry. In: Sadock BJ, Sadock VA, eds. *Kaplan & Sadock's Comprehensive Textbook of Psychiatry.* 7th ed. Vol 2. Baltimore: Lippincott Williams & Wilkins; 2000:1876.

29

Complementary and Alternative Medicine in Psychiatry

The term *complementary and alternative medicine* (CAM) refers to the various disease-treating or disease-preventing practices whose methods and efficacy differ from traditional or conventional biomedical treatment. Other terms used to describe these therapeutic approaches are *integrative medicine* and *holistic medicine*. In complementary medicine, some approaches can be used in conjunction with traditional therapeutic methods. In holistic medicine, a doctor treats the patient as a whole rather than focusing on a specific disease or disorder. This is not a new concept in psychiatry. The idea of emphasizing the whole patient and the need to evaluate psychosocial, environmental, and lifestyle factors in health and disease is subsumed under the heading of psychosomatic or mind–body medicine. The work of physician George Engel, who pioneered considering biological, psychological, and social factors in treating the patient, is entirely consistent with holistic medical approaches in which one treats the whole person and not simply the disease.

Traditional medicine, as practiced in the United States and elsewhere in the Western world, is based on the scientific method—the use of experiments to validate a hypothesis or determine the probability of a theory being correct. Traditional medicine presumes that the body is a biological and physiological system and that disorders have a cause that can be treated with medications, surgery, and complex technological methods to produce a cure. Traditional medicine is thus also referred to as *biomedicine* or *technomedicine*.

Traditional medicine is also known as allopathic medicine. The term *allopathy,* derived from the Greek word *allos* ("other"), refers to the use of outside agents or medications to counteract the signs and symptoms of disease. *Allopathy* is the type of medicine taught in U.S. medical schools. Samuel Hahnemann (1755–1843), a German physician, coined the term to distinguish this form of medicine from *homeopathy* (derived from the Greek word *homos* ["same"]), in which specially formulated medicinal remedies, different from allopathic medicine, are used. Allopathy is the most prevalent form of medicine practiced in the Western world. (Homeopathy is discussed more fully later in this chapter.)

Alternative medical therapy is increasingly popular. It is estimated that one person in three at some time uses these therapies for common ailments such as back problems, headaches, anxiety, and depression. These therapies are sought especially by persons with acquired immune deficiency syndrome (AIDS), cancer, and other life-threatening medical illnesses. More than $25 billion a year is spent on alternative medical therapies in the United States.

In 1991, the National Institutes of Health (NIH) established the Office of Alternative Medicine (OAM) now called the National Center for Complementary Medicine and Alternative Medicine (NCCAM or CAM) to evaluate the usefulness of a broad range of unrelated, nonorthodox therapeutic systems and provide scientific explanations for their possible effectiveness. CAM has compiled a classification of alternative medical practices (Table 29–1), designed to support research to investigate the effectiveness of these therapies. Including a treatment in the classification does not imply an endorsement of the method. Indeed, many complementary and alternative health practices are based on no known scientific principles and are considered quackery.

Some health maintenance organizations (HMOs) have approved alternative medical therapies for reimbursement. The HMOs claim to be responding to public pressure, but many health experts believe that these HMOs are motivated solely by financial consideration. Persons who visit alternative practitioners are reimbursed at lower rates than those who visit traditional practitioners. Some HMOs allow their members to self-refer to these practitioners. In contrast, referral to a traditional medical specialist may only be initiated by the patient's primary care physician. The practice of self-referral may endanger the health of the general public by encouraging persons to seek alternative treatment that may not help them.

Many systems of treatment discussed in this chapter are centuries old, and it would be presumptuous for traditional biomedical practitioners to dismiss them lightly as worthless. Nevertheless, without rigorous scientific evidence to the contrary, physicians must approach many of these treatments with skepticism. The influence of the mind on the body and the effect that psychological factors have in health and disease are well known to physicians, especially to psychiatrists. Suggestion is a potent remedy, and the well-established placebo effect, in which an inert substance is effective in curing a disorder, serves to confirm the importance of mind–body interaction in health and disease.

Currently, over half the medical schools in the United States offer courses in complementary and alternative medicine. Many have developed centers for alternative medicine research, with professors of mind–body or integrative medicine drawn largely

Table 29–1
Classification of Alternative and Complementary Medical Practices[a]

Diet, nutrition, lifestyle changes	
Changes in lifestyle	Gerson therapy
Diet	Macrobiotics
Nutritional supplements	Megavitamin
Mind/body control	
Art therapy, relaxation techniques	Guided imagery
	Humor therapy
Biofeedback	Psychotherapy
Counseling and prayer therapies	Sound, music therapy
	Support groups
Dance therapy	Yoga, meditation
Alternative systems of medical practice	
Acupuncture	Latin American rural practices
Anthroposophically extended medicine	Native American
	Natural products
Ayurveda	Naturopathic medicine
Community-based health care practices	Past life therapy
	Shamanism
Environmental medicine	Tibetan medicine
Homeopathic medicine	Traditional oriental medicine
Manual healing	
Acupressure	Osteopathy
Alexander technique	Reflexology
Aromatherapy	Rolfing
Biofield therapeutics	Therapeutic touch
Chiropractic medicine	Trager method
Feldenkrais method	Zone therapy
Massage therapy	
Pharmacological and biological treatments	
Antioxidizing agents	Metabolic therapy
Cell treatment	Oxidizing agents (ozone, hydrogen peroxide)
Chelation therapy	
Bioelectromagnetic applications	
Blue light treatment and artificial lighting	Electrostimulation and neuromagnetic stimulation devices
Electroacupuncture	Magnetoresonance spectroscopy
Electromagnetic fields	
Herbal medicine	
Echinacea (purple coneflower)	Ginseng root
	Wild chrysanthemum flower
Ginkgo biloba extract	Witch hazel
Ginger rhizome	Yellowdock

[a]This classification was developed by the ad hoc Advisory Panel to the Office of Alternative Medicine (OAM), National Institutes of Health (NIH), and further refined by the Workshop on Alternative Medicine as described in the report *Alternative Medicine: Expanding Medical Horizons.* This classification was designed to facilitate the grant review process and should not be considered definitive.

from the ranks of such traditional specialties as internal medicine and psychiatry. This trend is likely to continue, with the goal of determining which of the many existing alternative medical systems have scientific merit. Only when and if they can withstand rigorous clinical trials can certain of these techniques be integrated into traditional medicine. CAM is now funding studies on mind–body techniques and on each of the alternative systems discussed below (as well as many others not mentioned) to see if they withstand the rigors of controlled clinical trials, including precise outcome measures.

The following review lists some of the most visible complementary and alternative health practices that have been used in the treatment of (broadly defined) psychiatric conditions. They are listed in alphabetical order and described briefly. The discussion of therapies should not be considered definitive; new therapies continue to emerge. The number of alternative healing practices available in the United States is unknown and probably soars into the hundreds.

ACUPRESSURE AND ACUPUNCTURE

Acupressure and acupuncture are Chinese healing techniques that are mentioned in ancient medical texts dating back to 3000 BC. A basic tenet of Chinese medicine is the belief that vital energy (*qi* or *chi*) flows along specific pathways (meridians) that have about 350 points (acupoints) whose manipulation corrects imbalances by stimulating or removing blockages to energy flow. Another fundamental concept is the idea of two opposing energy fields (*yin* and *yang*) that must be in balance for health to be sustained. In acupressure, the acupoints are manipulated by the fingers; in acupuncture, sterilized silver or gold needles (some the diameter of a human hair) are inserted into the skin to varying depths (0.5 mm to 1.5 cm) and are rotated or left in place for varying periods to correct any imbalance of *qi*.

In the West, acupressure and acupuncture are explained on the basis of nerve stimulation that releases endogenous neurotransmitters and endorphins to help cure illness. Some of the conditions for which these techniques are applied are asthma, headaches, dysmenorrhea, cervical pain, insomnia, anxiety, depression, and substance abuse, including smoking cessation (see the description of moxibustion below). A variation of acupuncture uses mild electric current to augment therapeutic effects (electroacupuncture).

ALEXANDER TECHNIQUE

The Alexander technique was developed by F. M. Alexander (1869–1955), who was born in Tasmania and eventually became a well-known stage actor. After developing aphonia, he experimented on himself by changing his body posture and eventually regained his voice. Alexander developed a theory of the proper use of body musculature to help alleviate somatic and mental illness. Techniques involve corrective manipulation of the muscles involving the head and neck, torso, pelvis, and extremities to improve posture. Treatment improves cardiovascular, respiratory, and gastrointestinal functioning as well as mood. A small, devoted group of Alexander practitioners is found in the United States and throughout the world. The Alexander technique may deserve consideration, if for no other reason than that so many persons in the United States have poor posture (Fig. 29–1).

ANTHROPOSOPHICALLY EXTENDED MEDICINE

This form of healing was developed by the Austrian philosopher Rudolf Steiner (1861–1925). The healing process

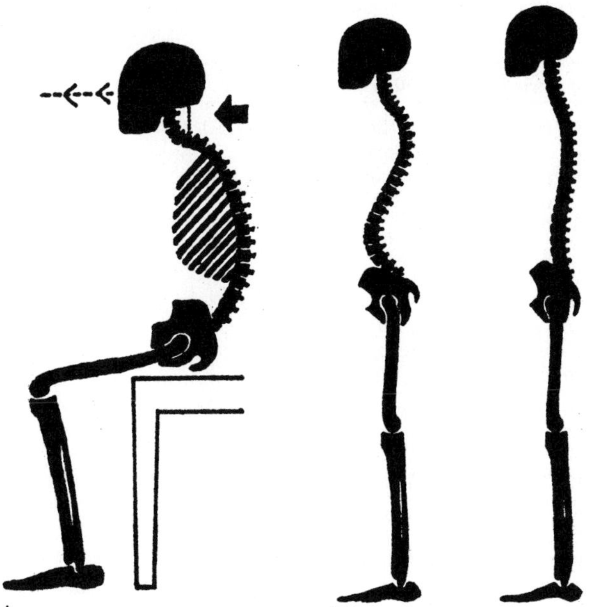

FIGURE 29–1
A. Position of pelvis, back, neck, and head in slumped position. **B**. Standing in hunched position (*left*) and well balanced (*right*). (Reprinted with permission from Barlow W. *The Alexander Principle*. London: Gollancz; 1973.)

involves the use of conscious understanding, which Steiner called *anthroposophy,* or the "wisdom of life." Anthroposophy focuses on mental exercises that enable persons to find a balance between mind and body to ensure health maintenance. Steiner founded a school of thought represented in this country by the Rudolf Steiner School, which teaches children these concepts as they apply to civilization, besides a standard educational curriculum.

AROMATHERAPY

Aromatherapy is the therapeutic use of plant oils. Named by the French chemist Maurice René-Maurice Gattefosse in 1928, aromatherapy is one of the fastest growing alternative therapies in the United States and Europe. The essential oils of plants are organic compounds that are benzene derivatives. Aromatic substances were used in ancient civilization as both medicines and perfumes. Today, plant oils are inhaled using atomizers or absorbed through the skin using massage (aromatherapy massage). Plant oils have many therapeutic effects—analgesic, psychological, antimicrobial—some of which have been demonstrated scientifically. Aromatherapy is used to reduce stress and anxiety and to alleviate gastrointestinal and musculoskeletal disorders. In psychiatry, olfactory stimulation has been used to elicit feeling tones, memories, and emotions during psychotherapy. Aromatherapy can cause skin irritation or allergic reactions in some people. Table 29–2 lists essential oils and their effects.

AYURVEDA

Ayurveda means "knowledge of life." The technique originated in India about 3000 BC and is believed to be one of the oldest and most comprehensive medical systems in the world. Ayurveda is similar to Chinese medicine in its beliefs about energy points on the body and a vital force (*prana*) that must be in balance to maintain health. Ayurveda practitioners diagnose illness by examining the pulse, the urine, and the heat or coldness of the body. Treatment relies on diet, medicines, purification, enemas, and bloodletting. (See also "Tibetan Medicine," on p. 866.)

BATES METHOD

The Bates method, designed to treat vision problems, was devised by William H. Bates. It is aimed at naturally strengthening the eye muscles and includes the following basic exercises: splashing closed eyes 20 times with warm water, then 20 times with cold water; alternately focusing on near and distant objects; focusing on an object while gently swaying the body; remembering objects in the mind's eye to facilitate the actual perception of these objects in reality; and closing the eyes, cupping them with the palms of both hands (without touching the eyes), and focusing on pleasant thoughts. Bates practitioners claim that persons who need glasses to correct refraction errors will not need them if these methods are followed rigorously.

BIOENERGETICS

Bioenergetics, based on the belief that dammed-up energy produces maladaptive behavioral patterns, evolved from the work of the Austrian psychoanalyst Wilhelm Reich (1897–1957), who studied with Sigmund Freud. Reich believed that energy fields were propelled by sexual impulses called *ergs* and that satisfactory orgasms indicated healthy bodily functioning. Modern-day practitioners look for areas of muscular tension in the body that are thought to be associated with repressed memories and emotions. Therapists try to bring these repressions to consciousness through a variety of relaxation techniques, including massage.

CHELATION

Chelation therapy is a traditional medical procedure used to treat accidental poisoning with heavy metals, such as lead, arsenic, and mercury. A chelating agent (ethylenediaminetetraacetic acid [EDTA]) is infused into the bloodstream and binds to the metal, which is then excreted from the body. As an alternative medical practice, chelation therapy is used as a form of preventive medicine to remove lead, cadmium, and aluminum from the body. These substances are presumed by some to be associated with premature aging, memory loss, and the symptoms of Alzheimer's disease. Chelation therapy has also been used to treat atherosclerosis and coronary artery disease.

CHIROPRACTIC

Chiropractic is concerned with the diagnosis and treatment of disorders of the musculoskeletal system, especially those of the spine. It was developed by a Canadian, Daniel David Palmer (1845–1913) (Fig. 29–2), who moved to the United States in 1895. Palmer believed that disease could be attributed to spinal misalignment leading to abnormal nerve transmission.

Table 29–2
Some Common Aromatherapies

Compound	Possible Properties	Purported Psychiatric Use	Other Purported Uses	Aroma
Angelica	Sedative, muscle relaxant, antibiotic, antifungal	Anorexia, anxiety, insomnia	GI spasm, ulcers, asthma, gout, bronchitis	Woody, pepper, sweet
Basil	Antispasmotic, active on sympathetic nervous system, narcotic, antiviral, insect repellant, aphrodisiac, antiinflammative, stimulant for the adrenal cortex, GI and urogenital tracts, cerebral/memory stimulator, hepatostimulative	Fatigue, memory problems, depression, anxiety, delirium, alcoholism	Prostatitis, hair loss, asthma, coronary spasm, epilepsy	Warm, spicy, sweet, woody
Bergamot	Antidepressant, sedative, antiseptic, antiinflammatory	Depression, hyperactivity, anxiety, insomnia	Acne, cold sores, eczema, psoriasis	Citrus, floral
Frankincense/ oil of olibanum	Antitumor, antidepressant, expectorant, immunostimulant, antiinflammatory	Depression	Asthma, bronchitis, pain relief	Woody, fruity
Geranium (*P.g* or *P.x a*) pelargonium	Pancreatic stimulant, antiinflammatory, antibiotic, relaxant, hemostatic	Anxiety, agitation, fatigue	PMS, menopause	Floral, dry
Jasmine	Antidepressant, stimulant, analgesic	Depression, stress, fatigue	Menstrual problems, headaches	Floral, musky
Lavender	Sedative, muscular relaxant, antiinflammatory	Depression, jet lag, insomnia, restlessness	Acne, burns, hiccups, ulcers	Powder, floral
Mandarin	Antispasmodic, sedative, hypnotic	Hyperactivity, anxiety, insomnia	Cardiovascular spasm, pain, dyspnea	Sweet, fruity
Marjoram	Diuretic, analgesic, spasmolytic, parasympathotonic	Anxiety, excessive sexual desire, psychosis, insomnia	Hyperthyroid, cardiovascular disease, vertigo, epilepsy	Nutty, woody, warm
Melissa	Sedative, antiinflammatory, antispasmodic	Anger, agitation, insomnia	Herpes, hypertension, asthma	Citrus, herb
Myrrh	Antiinflammatory, analgesic, antifungal	Sexual overexcitation	Dysentery, hemorrhoids	Fruity, clean
Neroli	Antidepressant, stimulant	Depression, fatigue, insomnia, anxiety, postpartum depression	Hemorrhoids, tuberculosis	Floral, powder, spicy
Spikenard	Sedative, antifungal, antiseptic, insect repellent	Insomnia, depression, anxiety	Psoriasis, epilepsy	Earthy, woody
Tuberose	Anxiety, sedative, analgesic	Agitation	Pain	Earthy, tropical

Table by Marissa Kaminsky.
References: Herbweb. *http://www.best.com/~timj/herbage/A337.htm*; Natural Resources Industries, Pure and Natural Essential Oils from Nepal. *http://www.msinp.com/herbs/index.html*; Ontario Ministry of Agriculture, Food and Rural Affairs. *http://gov.on.ca/OMAFRA/index.html*; Rose, Jeanne. *375 Essential Oils and Hydrosols.* Berkeley, CA: Frog, Ltd. North Atlantic Books, 1999; Schnaubelt, Kurt. *Medical Aromatherapy.* Berkeley, CA: Frog, Ltd. North Atlantic Books, 1999.

Chiropractors diagnose illness by clinical examination and X-ray. Treatment involves manual manipulation of bones, joints, and musculature to restore biomechanical function. Chiropractic is the largest independent alternative health profession in the Western world. There are over 50,000 chiropractors in the United States. They are recognized by government and insurance agencies and treat over 20 million persons in the United States annually.

COLOR THERAPY

In color therapy, different colors are thought to affect mood, and this has been used to address specific health problems. For example, blue is believed to be sedating, and red, excitatory. A Swiss psychologist, Max Lüscher, devised a color test in which a subject's mood at a particular time is determined by exposing the subject to various colors. Lüscher also experimented with the effect of color on the autonomic nervous system and found that pure red is sympathomimetic and can cause an increase in blood pressure, heart rate, and respiration. Blue is parasympathomimetic and produces opposite effects.

DANCE THERAPY

Dance therapy was formally recognized in 1942, with the hiring of pioneer dance therapist Marian Chace (1896–1990) at St. Elizabeth's Hospital in Washington, D.C. The terms *dance* and *movement* are used synonymously; however, each actually describes a point of view. *Movement* encompasses the world of physical motion, whereas *dance* is a specific creative act within that world. The American Dance Therapy Association defines *dance therapy* as "the psychotherapeutic use of movement which furthers the emotional and physical integration of the individual." Dance therapy sessions have four basic goals: the development of body awareness; the expression of feelings; the fostering of interaction and communication; and the integration

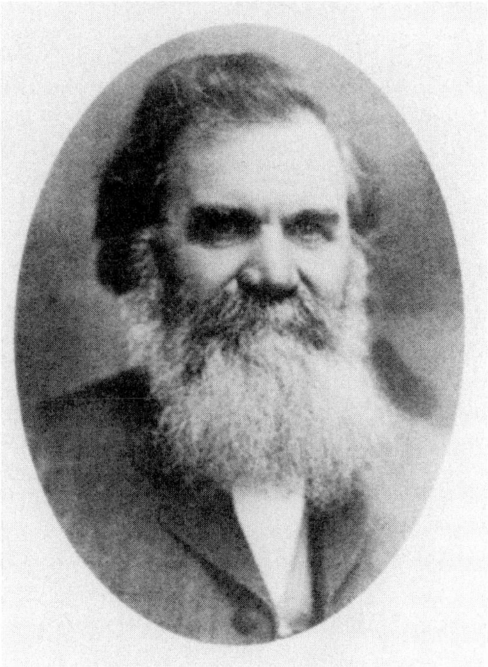

FIGURE 29–2
Daniel David Palmer (1845–1913), the founder of chiropractic. (Reprinted with permission from Shealy CN, ed. *The Complete Family Guide to Alternative Medicine: An Illustrated Encyclopedia of Natural Healing.* New York: Barnes & Noble Books; 1996:39.)

of the physical, emotional, and social experiences that result in a sense of increased self-confidence and contentment.

DIET AND NUTRITION

Nutritional methods to prevent or cure disease have an important place in modern medicine, and their efficacy has been proved by scientific evidence. The federal government has established recommended daily allowances (RDAs) to meet the nutritional needs of average persons in the United States, as illustrated in Figure 29–3, the food guide pyramid. There are many alternative diets, and specific vitamin and mineral supplementation programs have been developed to deal with specific diseases or bodily processes. Diets low in fat have been recommended for the treatment of cardiovascular disease and diabetes. The Pritikin diet developed by Nathan Pritikin is extremely low in fat (less than 10 percent of daily calories), high in complex carbohydrates, and high in fiber. The Ornish diet, developed by physician Dean Ornish, is vegetarian: No meat, poultry, or fish is allowed, and only 10 percent of calories are obtained from fat. Both diets include an exercise program. Studies have shown that these diets can reduce cholesterol, decrease blood pressure, and increase cardiac performance. They have also been effective in eliminating the need for drugs in newly diagnosed cases of adult-onset diabetes.

Diets from other cultures may have certain health benefits. In Asia, diets are low in fat, and there is a low incidence of cardiac disease; diets in Mediterranean countries are high in olive oil, garlic, and grains and are associated with a low incidence of colon cancer and cardiac disease. Food allergies have been implicated in many conditions: arthritis, asthma, hyperactivity, and ulcerative colitis, among others.

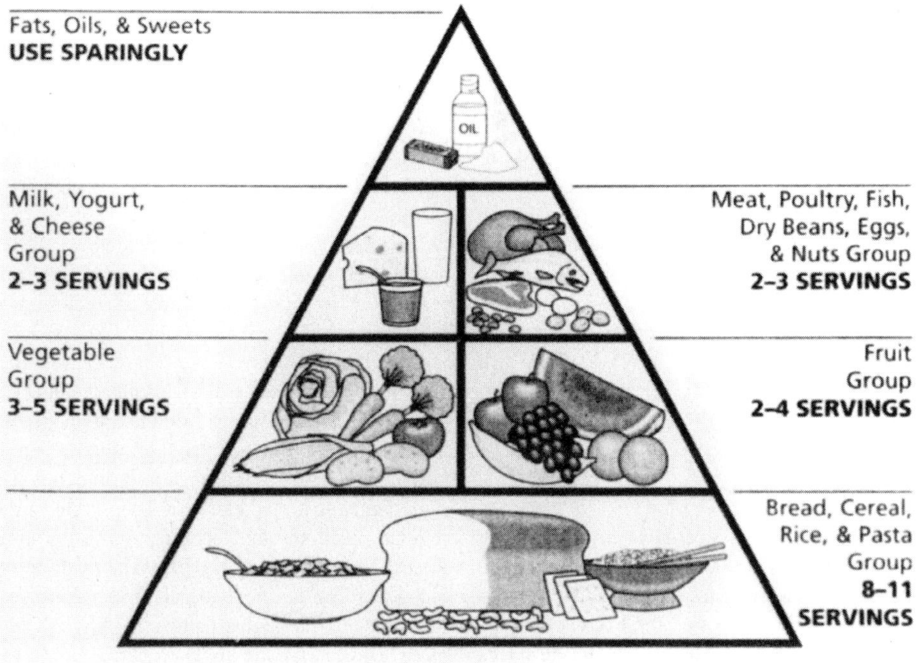

FIGURE 29–3
Food guide pyramid.

DIETARY SUPPLEMENTS

In addition to herbs (discussed below) a variety of dietary supplements are used to promote health. Dietary supplements are products that contain vitamins, minerals, or amino acids. In many cases, the supplement is actually an extract, metabolite, or combination of the above. They are intended to *supplement* a healthy diet; they do not comprise a diet or meal. Nutritional supplements have long been familiar to Americans in the form of multivitamins but are now available in a vast array of other compounds that can be purchased in grocery stores, pharmacies, health food stores, and over the Internet. In psychiatry, nutritional supplements are being used to treat a wide spectrum of illness including cognitive disorders, mood disorders, psychotic disorders, sleep disorders, and conduct disorders. Seventy-five percent of Americans currently use some form of nutritional supplement on a regular basis. While medicinal benefits are well documented in some supplements, especially vitamins, others vary greatly in safety and consistency. As a general rule, supplements should not be taken by pregnant or lactating women. Table 29–3 lists some of the more common supplements being used to treat psychiatric illness; however, there is little scientific evidence to support their efficacy. Table 29–4 lists available sources of Web-based data about dietary supplements.

ENVIRONMENTAL MEDICINE

The field of environmental medicine began to emerge in the 1950s when physicians such as Theron Randolf, professor of allergy and immunology at Northwestern University School of Medicine, began to examine some persons' allergic reactions to various foods. Other workers studied the effects on the body of pollutants in water and air, and eventually the field expanded to include the total environment in which humans exist. As a result, environmental medicine now concerns itself with issues such as food additives; electromagnetic fields from electric utility wires; fertilizers and hormones used in food production; microwaves from appliances such as microwave ovens, television sets, and cellular telephones; and nuclear radiation. Practitioners of environmental medicine believe that many persons are extraordinarily sensitive to environmental contaminants that can trigger a disease process. Some issues are highly controversial. For instance, in spite of claims to the contrary, studies fail to demonstrate a higher incidence of cancer in persons exposed to electromagnetic fields; however, a correlation exists between higher cancer rates and living near oil refineries and chemical plants. Environmental medicine is a form of preventative medicine that focuses on increased individual awareness of environmental hazards and the control or elimination of these hazards. (See also "Naturopathy," on p. 864.)

EXERCISE

A recent review of exercise as a treatment for depression included references to more than 1,000 trials and a meta-analysis of 80 studies. Generally, the evidence indicated that a statistically significant treatment effect favored the exercise groups over the comparison groups. This effect was found for all forms of regular exercise, was independent of age or sex, and increased with the duration of therapy. Exercise may increase serotonin levels in the brain.

FELDENKRAIS METHOD

The Feldenkrais method was developed by Moshe Feldenkrais (1904–1982), a Russian-born physicist who developed a theory evolved from Freud's work. Feldenkrais thought that the body should be emphasized as much as the mind and that proprioception (somatic sensations from muscles and other organs) can influence behavior. He believed that posture and the positions of the body reflected conflict; therefore, retraining the body was part of his treatment program (Fig. 29–4). Practitioners of the Feldenkrais method are active throughout the world. Those learning the Feldenkrais method are referred to as *students* rather than *patients,* to reinforce the view that the work is primarily an educational process. Lessons generally last from 30 to 60 minutes and consist of structured movement that involves thinking, sensing, moving, and imagining. The method has been used in central nervous system disorders such as multiple sclerosis, cerebral palsy, and stroke. Older persons who use the method claim that they retain or regain their ability to move without strain or discomfort.

HERBAL MEDICINE

Herbal medicine relies on plants to cure illnesses and to maintain health. It is probably the oldest known system of medicine and originated in China about 4000 BC. Ancient texts of Chinese medicine are still in use, and modern Chinese medicine relies on herbs in addition to other methods, such as acupuncture, massage, diet, and exercise, to correct imbalances in the body. A Greco-Roman medical text by Dioscorides, *De Materia Medica,* describes the use of over 500 plants and herbs to cure disease.

The decline of herbal medicine in the late 20th century was related to scientific and technological advances that led to the use of synthetic pharmaceuticals; nevertheless, according to some estimates, at least 25 percent of current medicines are derived from the active ingredients of plants. The examples are many: digitalis from foxglove; ephedrine from ephedra; morphine from the opium poppy; paclitaxel (Taxol) from the yew tree; and quinine from the bark of the cinchona tree.

Herbal medicine is becoming more and more popular. Western herbalists use plants to treat various disorders related to the respiratory, gastrointestinal, cardiovascular, and nervous systems; like most prescription medicines, these plants contain active compounds that produce physiological effects. As a result, they must be used in appropriate doses if toxic results are to be prevented.

About $1.5 billion a year is spent on herbal medicines, which are classified as dietary supplements. They are not subjected to Food and Drug Administration (FDA) approval, and there are no uniform standards for quality control or potency in herbal preparations. Indeed, some preparations have no active ingredients or are adulterated. The herbal industry attempts to regulate itself through organizations such as the Council for Responsible Nutrition and the American Herbal Association, but according to the Federal Trade Commission, fraudulent practices and false advertising still exist. There is now a *Physicians' Desk Reference* for both herbal products and nutritional supplements. NCAMM is conducting spectrographic and other analyses on herbal medicines to determine the active ingredients that may account for a particular herb's efficacy.

Table 29–3
Dietary Supplements

Name	Ingredients/What Is It?	Uses	Adverse Effects	Interactions	Dosage	Comments
Docosahexaenoic acid (DHA)	Omega-3 polyunsaturated fatty acid	ADD, dyslexia, cognitive impairment, dementia	Anticoagulant properties, mild GI distress	Warfarin	Varies with indication	Stop using prior to surgery
Choline	Choline	Fetal brain development, manic conditions, cognitive disorders, tardive dyskinesia, cancers	Restrict in patients with primary genetic trimethyluria, sweating, hypotension, depression	Methotrexate, works with B_6, B_{12}, and folic acid in metabolism of homocysteine	300–1,200 mg doses >3 g associated with fishy body odor	Needed for structure and function of all cells
L-α-Glyceryl-phosphorylcholine (α-GPC)	Derived from soy lecithin	To increase growth hormone secretion, cognitive disorders	None known	None known	500 mg–1 g daily	Remains poorly understood
Phosphatidylcholine	Phospholipid that is part of cell membranes	Manic conditions, Alzheimer's disease and cognitive disorders, tardive dyskinesia	Diarrhea, steatorrhea in those with malabsorption, avoid with antiphospholipid antibody syndrome	None known	3–9 g per day in divided doses	Soybeans, sunflower, rapeseed are major sources
Phosphatidylserine	Phospholipid isolated from soya and egg yolks	Cognitive impairment including Alzheimer's disease, may reverse memory problems	Avoid with antiphospholipid antibody syndrome, GI side effects	None known	For soya-derived variety, 100 mg tid	Type derived from bovine brain carries hypothetical risk of bovine spongiform encephalopathy
Zinc	Metallic element	Immune impairment, wound healing, cognitive disorders, prevention of neural tube defects	GI distress, high doses can cause copper deficiency, immunosuppression	Bisphosphonates, quinolones, tetracycline, penicillamine, copper, cysteine-containing foods, caffeine, iron	Typical dose 15 mg per day, adverse effects >30 mg	Claims that zinc can prevent and treat the common cold are supported in some studies but not in others; more research needed
Acetyl-L-carnitine	Acetyl ester of L-carnitine	Neuroprotection, Alzheimer's disease, Down's syndrome, strokes, antiaging, depression in geriatric patients	Mild GI distress, seizures, increased agitation in some with Alzheimer's disease	Nucleoside analogs, valproic acid and pivalic acid–containing antibiotics	500 mg–2 g daily in divided doses	Found in small amounts in milk and meat
Huperzine A	Plant alkaloid derived from Chinese club moss	Alzheimer's disease, age-related memory loss, inflammatory disorders	Seizures, arrhythmias, asthma, irritable bowel disease	Acetylcholinesterase inhibitors and cholinergic drugs	60 μg–200 μg per day	*Huperzia serrata* has been used in Chinese folk medicine for the treatment of fevers and inflammation
NADH (nicotinamide adenine dinucleotide)	Dinucleotide located in mitochondria and cytosol of cells	Parkinson's disease, Alzheimer's disease, chronic fatigue, CV disease	GI distress	None known	5 mg per day or 5 mg bid	Precursor of NADH is nicotinic acid
S-Adenosyl-L-methionine (SAMe)	Metabolite of essential amino acid L-methionine	Mood elevation, osteoarthritis	Hypomania, hyperactive muscle movement, caution in patients with cancer	None known	200–1,600 mg daily in divided doses	Several trials demonstrate some efficacy in the treatment of depression

(*continued*)

Table 29–3 (*continued*)

Name	Ingredients/What Is It?	Uses	Adverse Effects	Interactions	Dosage	Comments
5-Hydroxytryptophan (5-HTP)	Immediate precursor of serotonin	Depression, obesity, insomnia, fibromyalgia, headaches	Possible risk of serotonin syndrome in those with carcinoid tumors or taking MAOIs	SSRIs, MAOIs, methyldopa, St. John's wort, phenoxybenzamine, 5-HT antagonists, 5-HT receptor agonists	100 mg–2 g daily, safer with carbidopa	5-HTP along with carbidopa is used in Europe for the treatment of depression
Phenylalanine	Essential amino acid	Depression, analgesia, vitiligo	Contraindicated in patients with PKU, may exacerbate tardive dyskinesia or hypertension	MAOIs and neuroleptic drugs	Comes in 2 forms: 500 mg–1.5 g daily for L-phenylalanine, 375 mg–2.25 g for DL-phenylalanine	Found in vegetables, juices, yogurt, and miso
Myoinositol	Major nutritionally active form of inositol	Depression, panic attacks, OCD	Caution in patients with bipolar disorder, GI distress	Possible additive effects with SSRIs and 5-HT receptor agonists (sumatriptan)	12 g in divided doses for depression and panic attacks	Studies have *not* shown effectiveness in treating Alzheimer's disease, autism, or schizophrenia
Vinpocetine	Semisynthetic derivative of vincamine (plant derivative)	Cerebral ischemic stroke, dementias	GI distress, dizziness, insomnia, dry mouth, tachycardia, hypotension, flushing	Warfarin	5–10 mg daily with food, no more than 20 mg per day	Used in Europe, Mexico, and Japan as pharmaceutical agent for treatment of cerebrovascular and cognitive disorders
Vitamin E family	Essential fat-soluble vitamin, family made of tocopherols and tocotrienols	Immune-enhancing, antioxidant, some cancers, protection in CV disease, neurologic disorders, diabetes, premenstrual syndrome	May increase bleeding in those with propensity to bleed, possible increased risk of hemorrhagic stroke, thrombophlebitis	Warfarin, antiplatelet drugs, neomycin, may be additive with statins	Depends on form: tocotrienols, 200–300 mg daily with food; tocopherols, 200 mg per day	Stop members of vitamin E family 1 month prior to surgical procedures
Glycine	Amino acid	Schizophrenia, alleviating spasticity and seizures	Avoid in those who are anuric or have hepatic failure	Additive with antispasmodics	1 g per day in divided doses for supplement; 40–90 g per day for schizophrenia	
Melatonin	Hormone of pineal gland	Insomnia, sleep disturbances, jet lag, cancer	May inhibit ovulation in 1 g doses, seizures, grogginess, depression, headache, amnesia	Aspirin, NSAIDs, β-blockers, INH, sedating drugs, corticosteroids, valerian, kava kava, 5-HTP, alcohol	0.3–3 mg hs for short periods of time	Melatonin sets the timing of circadian rhythms and regulates seasonal responses
Fish oil	Lipids found in fish	Bipolar disorder, lowering triglycerides, hypertension, decrease blood clotting	Caution in hemophiliacs, mild GI upset, "fishy"-smelling excretions	Coumadin, aspirin, NSAIDs, garlic, ginkgo	Varies depending on form and indication—usually about 3–5 g daily	Stop prior to any surgical procedure

Table by Mercedes Blackstone, M.D.

Table 29–4
Herbal Medicine and Other Dietary Supplement–Related Sites on the World Wide Web

Organization	Web Address	Site Information
Center for Food Safety and Applied Nutrition, Food and Drug Administration	http://vm.cfsan.fda.gov/-dms/supplmnt.html	Clinicians should use this site to report adverse events associated with herbal medicines and other dietary supplements. Sections also contain safety, industry, and regulatory information.
National Center for Complementary and Alternative Medicine, National Institutes of Health	http://nccam.nlh.gov	This site contains fact sheets about alternative therapies, consensus reports, and databases.
Agricultural Research Service, United States Department of Agriculture	http://www.ars-grin.gov/duke	The site contains an extensive phytochemical database with search capabilities.
Quackwatch	http://www.quackwatch.com	Although this site addresses all aspects of health care, there is a considerable amount of information covering complementary and herbal therapies.
National Council Against Health Fraud	http://www.ncahf.org	This site focuses on health fraud with a position paper on over-the-counter herbal remedies.
HerbMed	http://www.herbmed.org	This site contains information on more than 120 herbal medications, with evidence for activity, warnings, preparations, mixtures, and mechanisms of action. There are short summaries of important research publications with MEDLINE links.
ConsumerLab	http://www.consumerlab.com	This site is maintained by a corporation that conducts independent laboratory investigations of dietary supplements and other health products.

From *JAMA*. 2001;286:213.

Psychoactive Herbs. Many phytomedicinals (from the Greek *phyto*, meaning "plant") have psychoactive properties that are used, or have been used, to treat a variety of psychiatric conditions. Adverse effects are possible, and toxic interactions with other drugs may occur with all phytomedicinals. Clinicians should always attempt to obtain a history of herbal use during the psychiatric evaluation. Adulteration is common, and there are no consistent standard preparations available for most herbs. Safety profiles and knowledge of adverse effects of most of these substances are lacking; many, if not all, of these herbs are secreted in breast milk and are contraindicated during lactation and should be avoided during pregnancy.

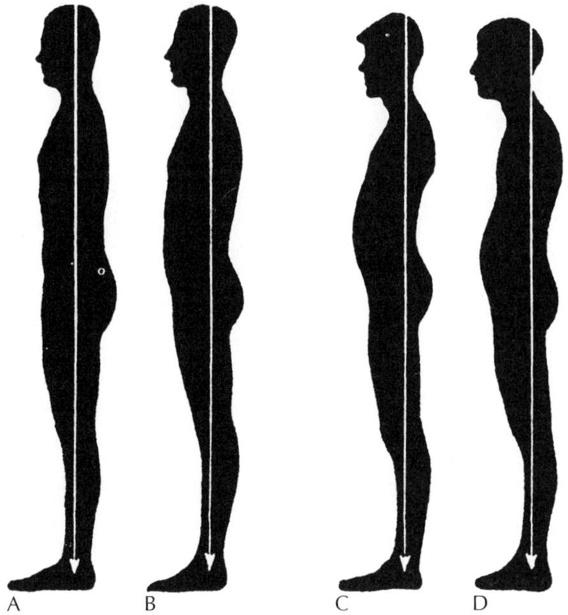

FIGURE 29–4
The Harvard University chart for grading body mechanics. The four figures represent (from left to right) excellent **(A)**, good **(B)**, poor **(C)**, and very poor **(D)** mechanical use of the body, determined by positions of head, chest, abdomen, and back. (Reprinted with permission from Feldenkrais M. *Body and Mature Behavior.* New York: International Universities Press; 1949:104.)

One must be nonjudgmental in dealing with patients who use phytomedicinals. Many do so, for various reasons: (1) as part of their cultural tradition, (2) because they mistrust physicians or are dissatisfied with conventional medicine, or (3) because they experience relief of symptoms. If psychotropic agents are prescribed, the clinician must be extraordinarily alert to the possibility of adverse effects as a result of drug–drug interactions, since many phytomedicinals have ingredients that produce physiological changes in the body. There are over 200 herbal drugs in use; only those with psychoactive properties are listed in Table 29–5.

HOMEOPATHY

Homeopathic healing was developed in the early 1800s by Samuel Hahnemann, a German physician (Fig. 29–5). It is based on the concept that self-healing is a basic characteristic of human life and that special medications can aid this inherent process. The homeopathic pharmacopoeia is unique in several ways. First, there are over 2,000 medications, including those from plants, such as aconite, ergot, and hellebore; minerals, such as silver, copper, gold, and iodine; and animals, such as snake and jellyfish venom and tissue extracts. Second, medica-

Table 29–5
Phytomedicinals with Psychoactive Effect

Name	Ingredients	Use	Adverse Effects[a]	Interactions	Dosage[a]	Comments
Areca, areca nut, betel nut, *L. Areca catechu*	Arecoline, guvacoline	For alteration of consciousness to reduce pain and elevate mood	Parasympathomimetic overload; increased salivation, tremors, bradycardia, spasms, gastrointestinal disturbances, ulcers of the mouth	Avoid with parasympathomimetic drugs; atropinelike compounds reduce effect	Undetermined; 8–10 g is toxic dose for humans	Used by chewing the nut; used in the past as a chewing balm for gum disease and as a vermifuge; long-term use may result in malignant tumors of the oral cavity
Belladonna, *L. Atropa belladonna,* deadly nightshade	Atropine, scopolamine, flavonoids[b]	Anxiolytic	Tachycardia, arrhythmias, xerostomia, mydriasis, difficulties with micturition and constipation	Synergistic with anticholinergic drugs; avoid with tricyclic antidepressants, amantadine, and quinidine	0.05–0.10 mg a day; maximum single dose is 0.20 mg	Has a strong smell, tastes sharp and bitter, and is poisonous
Bitter orange flower, *Citrus aurantium*	Flavonoids, limonene	Sedative, anxiolytic, hypnotic	Photosensitization	Undetermined	Tincture 2–3 g per day, drug 4–6 g per day, extract 1–2 g per day	Contradictory evidence; some refer to it as a gastric stimulant
Black cohosh, *L. Cimicifuga racemosa*	Triterpenes, isoferulic acid	For premenstrual syndrome, menopausal symptoms, dysmenorrhea	Weight gain, gastrointestinal disturbances	Possible adverse interaction with male or female hormones	1–2 g per day; over 5 g can cause vomiting, headache, dizziness, cardiovascular collapse	Estrogenlike effects questionable because root may act as estrogen-receptor blocker
Black haw, cramp bark, *L. Viburnum prunifolium*	Scopoletin, flavonoids, caffeic acids, triterpenes	Sedative, antispasmodic action on uterus; for dysmenorrhea	Undetermined	Anticoagulant-enhanced effects	1–3 g per day	
California poppy, *L. Eschscholtzia californica*	Isoquinoline alkaloids, cyanogenic glycosides	Sedative, hypnotic, anxiolytic; for depression	Lethargy	Combination of California poppy, valerian, St. John's wort, and passion flowers can result in agitation	2 g per day	Clinical or experimental documentation of effects is unavailable
Catnip, *L. Nepeta cataria*	Valeric acid	Sedative, antispasmodic; for migraine	Headache, malaise, nausea, hallucinogenic effects	Undetermined	Undetermined	Delirium produced in children
Chamomile, *L. Matricaria chamomilla*	Flavonoids	Sedative, anxiolytic	Allergic reaction	Undetermined	2–4 g per day	May be GABAergic
Corydalis, *L. Corydalis cava*	Isoquinoline alkaloids	Sedative, antidepressant; for mild depression	Hallucination, lethargy	Undetermined	Undetermined	Clonic spasms and muscular tremor with overdose
Cyclamen, *L. Cyclamen europaeum*	Triterpene	Anxiolytic; for menstrual complaints	Small doses (e.g., 300 mg) can lead to nausea, vomiting, and diarrhea	Undetermined	Undetermined	High doses can lead to respiratory collapse
Echinacea, *L. Echinacea purpurea*	Flavonoids, polysaccharides, caffeic acid derivatives, alkamides	Stimulates immune system; for lethargy, malaise, respiratory and lower urinary tract infections	Allergic reaction, fever, nausea, vomiting	Undetermined	1–3 g per day	Use in HIV and AIDS patients is controversial; potential for immunosuppression with long-term use

Ephedra, ma-huang *L. Ephedra sinica*	Ephedrine, pseudoephedrine	Stimulant; for lethargy, malaise, diseases of respiratory tract	Sympathomimetic overload; arrhythmias, increased blood pressure, headache, irritability, nausea, vomiting	Synergistic with sympathomimetics, serotonergic agents; avoid with MAOIs	1–2 g per day	Administer for short periods as tachyphylaxis and dependence can occur; risk of myocardial ischemia and stroke
Ginkgo, *L. Ginkgo biloba*	Flavonoids, ginkgolide A, B	Symptomatic relief of delirium, dementia; improves concentration and memory deficits; possible antidote to SSRI-induced sexual dysfunction	Allergic skin reactions, gastrointestinal upset, muscle spasms, headache	Anticoagulant: use with caution because of its inhibitory effect on platelet-activating factor (PAF); increased bleeding possible	120–240 mg per day	Studies indicate improved cognition in Alzheimer's patients after 4–5 weeks of use, possibly because of increased blood flow
Ginseng, *L. Panax ginseng*	Triterpenes, ginsenosides	Stimulant; for fatigue, elevation of mood, immune system	Insomnia, hypertonia, and edema (called ginseng abuse syndrome)	Not to be used with sedatives, hypnotic agents, MAOIs, antidiabetic agents, or steroids; has anticoagulant action (discontinue 7 days before surgery)	1–2 g per day	Several varieties exist: Korean (most highly valued), Chinese, Japanese, American (*Panax quinquefolius*)
Heather, *L. Calluna vulgaris*	Flavonoids, catechin, triterpenes, β-sitosterol	Anxiolytic, hypnotic	Undetermined	Undetermined	Undetermined	Efficacy for claimed uses is not documented
Hops, *L. Humulus lupulus*	Humulone, lupulone, flavonoids	Sedative, anxiolytic, hypnotic; for mood disturbances, restlessness	Contraindicated in patients with estrogen-dependent tumors (breast, uterine, cervical)	Hyperthermia effects with phenothiazine antipsychotics and with CNS depressants	0.5 g per day	May decrease plasma levels of drugs metabolized by CPY450 system
Horehound, *L. Ballota nigra*	Diterpenes, tannins	Sedative	Arrhythmias, diarrhea, hypoglycemia, possible spontaneous abortions	May enhance serotonergic drug effects, may augment hypoglycemic effects of drugs	1–4 g per day	May cause abortion
Jambolan, *L. Syzygium cumini*	Oleic acid, myristic acid, palmitic and linoleic acid, tannins	Anxiolytic, antidepressant	Undetermined	Undetermined	1–2 g per day	In folk medicine, a single dose is 30 seeds (1.9 g) of powder
Kava kava, *L. Piperis methysticum*	Kava lactones, kava pyrone	Sedative, hypnotic antispasmodic	Lethargy, impaired cognition, dermatitis with long-term unreported usage	Synergistic with anxiolytics, alcohol; avoid with levodopa and dopaminergic agents	600–800 mg per day	May be GABAergic; contraindicated in patients with endogenous depression; may increase the danger of suicide
Lavender, *L. Lavandula angustifolia*	Hydroxycoumarin, tannins, caffeic acid	Sedative, hypnotic	Headache, nausea, confusion	Synergistic with other sedatives	3–5 g per day	May cause death in overdose
Lemon balm, sweet Mary, *L. Melissa officinalis*	Flavonoids, caffeic acid, triterpenes	Hypnotic, anxiolytic, sedative	Undetermined	Potentiates CNS depressant; adverse reaction with thyroid hormone	8–10 g per day	
Mistletoe, *L. Viscum album*	Flavonoids, triterpenes, lectins, polypeptides	Anxiolytic; for mental and physical exhaustion	Berries said to have emetic and laxative effects	Contraindicated in patients with chronic infections, e.g., tuberculosis	10 per day	Berries have caused death in children

(*continued*)

Table 29–5 (*continued*)

Name	Ingredients	Use	Adverse Effects[a]	Interactions	Dosage[a]	Comments
Mugwort, *L. Artemisia vulgaris*	Sesquitemene lactones, flavonoids	Sedative, antidepressant, anxiolytic	Anaphylaxis, contact dermatitis	Potentiates anticoagulants	5–15 g per day	May stimulate uterine contractions
Nux vomica, *L. strychnos nux vomica,* poison nut	Indole alkaloids: strychnine and brucine, polysaccharides	Antidepressant; for migraine, menopausal symptoms	Convulsions, liver damage, death; severely toxic because of strychnine	Undetermined	0.02–0.05 g per day	Symptoms of poisoning can occur after ingestion of one bean; lethal dose is 1–2 g
Oats, *L. Avena sativa*	Flavonoids, oligo- and polysaccharides	Anxiolytic, hypnotic; for stress, insomnia, opium and tobacco withdrawal	Bowel obstruction or other bowel dysmotility syndromes, flatulence	Undetermined	3 g per day	Oats have sometimes been contaminated with aflatoxin, a fungal toxin linked with some cancers
Passion flower, *L. Passiflora incarnata*	Flavonoids, cyanogenic glycosides	Anxiolytic, sedative, hypnotic	Cognitive impairment	Undetermined	4–8 g per day	Overdose causes depression
St. John's wort, *L. Hypericum perforatum*	Hypericin, flavonoids, xanthones	Antidepressant, sedative, anxiolytic	Headaches, photosensitivity (may be severe), constipation	Report of manic reaction when used with sertraline (Zoloft); do not combine with SSRIs or MAOIs: possible serotonin syndrome; do not use with alcohol, opioids; discontinue 5 days before surgery	100–950 mg per day	Under investigation by the National Institutes of Health (NIH); may act as MAOI or SSRI; 4- to 6-week trial for mild depressive moods if no apparent improvement, another therapy should be tried
Scarlet pimpernel, *L. Anagallis arvensis*	Flavonoids, triterpenes, cucurbitacins, caffeic acids	Antidepressant	Overdose or long-term doses may lead to gastroenteritis and nephritis	Undetermined	1.8 g of powder 4 times a day	Flowers are poisonous
Skullcap, *L. Scutellaria lateriflora*	Flavonoid, monoterpenes	Anxiolytic, sedative, hypnotic	Cognitive impairment, hepatotoxicity	Disulfiramlike reaction may occur if used with alcohol	1–2 g per day	Little information exists to support the use of this herb in humans
Strawberry leaf, *L. Fragaria vesca*	Flavonoids, tannins	Anxiolytic	Contraindicated with strawberry allergy	Undetermined	1 g per day	Little information exists to support the use of this herb in humans
Tarragon, *L. Artemisia dracunculus*	Flavonoids, hydroxycoumarins	Hypnotic, appetite stimulant	Undetermined	Undetermined	Undetermined	Little information exists to support the use of this herb in humans
Valerian, *L. Valeriana officinalis*	Valepotriates, valerenic acid, caffeic acid	Sedative, muscle relaxant, hypnotic	Cognitive and motor impairment, gastrointestinal upset, hepatotoxicity; long-term use: contact allergy, headache, restlessness, insomnia, mydriasis, cardiac dysfunction	Avoid concomitant use with alcohol or CNS depressants	1–2 g per day	May be chemically unstable

[a]No reliable, consistent, or valid data exist on dosages or adverse affects of most phytomedicinals.
[b]Flavonoids are common to many herbs. They are plant by-products that act as antioxidants, i.e., agents that prevent the deterioration of material such as DNA via oxidation.

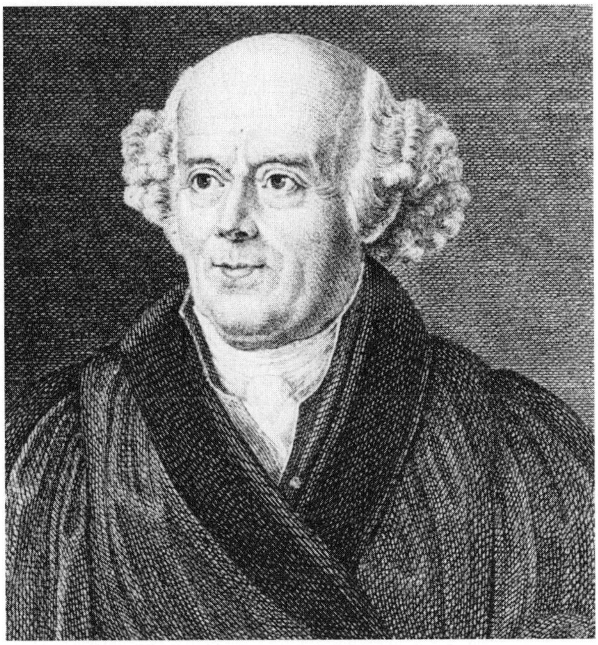

FIGURE 29–5
Samuel Hahnemann. (Reprinted with permission from the New York Academy of Medicine, New York, NY.)

tions are prepared as tinctures (i.e., mixed with 95 percent grain alcohol) or as pills with lactose fillers. Finally, medications are dispersed in infinitesimally dilute solutions, such as $1{:}10^{20,000}$, which prevents the medication from being detected by conventional chemical methods. Homeopaths claim that the therapeutic effect is based on "molecular medicine."

Hahnemann based his drug treatment on the following assumptions: medical substances elicit a standard array of signs and symptoms in healthy people and the medicine whose effect in normal persons most closely resembles the illness being treated is the one most likely to initiate a curative response. Thus, a medication that produces nausea would be used to treat nausea, except that it would be given in dilute amounts. This law of similars—*Similia similibus curantur* ("Let like be cured by like")—led to coining of the word *homeopathy* ("similar experiences"). In traditional medicine, such highly dilute substances are considered to have no effect, and no pharmacological research studies demonstrate otherwise.

There are no longer any homeopathic medical schools in the United States (the last one was Hahnemann University Medical School, which closed in 1994); nevertheless, the practice of homeopathy is increasing in this country and around the world. In Europe, homeopathy is extraordinarily popular. Homeopathic medicines are sold over the counter in the United States. Homeopathic remedies sold in the United States must meet the standards of monographs in the *Homeopathic Pharmacopoeia of the U.S.* (HPUS), which was recognized in the Food, Drug and Cosmetic Act with authority equivalent to that of the *United States Pharmacopeia* (USP).

LIGHT AND MELATONIN THERAPY

Light therapy is based on the concept that humans are subject to circadian rhythms (from the Latin words *circa* ["around"] and *dies* ["day"]) that affect physiological processes in predictable ways. There are 24-hour cycles of rest and activity that include changing levels of corticosteroids, electrolyte excretion, and physiological processes; for instance, blood pressure is higher during the day than at night. By varying light exposure, circadian rhythms can be altered. The concentration of the hormone melatonin, produced by the pineal gland, is highest in the bloodstream at night and is low or absent during the daylight. Melatonin is believed to regulate sleep, and exogenous melatonin (available over the counter) produces drowsiness in normal people. Artificial bright-light therapy (over 2,500 lux) is a proved method used to treat depressive disorder with seasonal pattern (see Section 15.2 in Chapter 15), which is seen during the winter months when daylight hours are reduced.

MACROBIOTICS

Macrobiotics (from the Greek words *makros* ["long"] and *bios* ["life"]) is a health practice that focuses on living in harmony with nature, using mainly a balanced diet. Macrobiotics became associated with the biblical patriarchs, the Chinese sages, and the Ethiopians of Africa, who were said to live 120 years or more. In 1797, a German physician and philosopher, Christoph W. Hufeland wrote an influential book on diet and health, *Macrobiotics or the Art of Prolonging Life.*

Macrobiotic foods are classified as *yin* (cold and wet) and *yang* (hot and dry); the goal is to keep *yin* and *yang* in balance. The diet consists of 50 percent grain products, 25 percent cooked or raw vegetables, 10 percent protein, 10 percent vegetable or fish soup, and 5 percent teas and fruits. Prolonged use of the diet may result in vitamin and mineral deficiencies.

MASSAGE

Massage is a treatment that involves manipulation of the soft tissues and the surfaces of the body. It was prescribed for the treatment of diseases over 5,000 years ago by Chinese physicians, and Hippocrates considered it to be a method of maintaining health.

Massage is believed to affect the body in several ways: it increases blood circulation, improves the flow of lymph through the lymphatic vessels, improves the tone of the musculoskeletal system, and has a tranquilizing effect on the mind. Massage techniques have been described in various ways: stroking, kneading, pinching, rubbing, knuckling, tapping, or applying friction. Massage is most often done with the hands and fingers, but vibrating machines and electrical stimulation are also used. The different types of massage therapies that have evolved over the years are more similar than different. These include Swedish, Oriental, Shiatsu, and Esalen massages. Most persons who experience massage find it physically and mentally restorative.

MEDITATION

Meditation is a technique that involves entering a trance state by focusing thought on a word or sound (a mantra), an object (e.g., a burning candle), or a movement (e.g., an oscillating disk). During the trance, the person experiences a state of calm. A meditative trance has physiological effects, all associated with decreased anxiety: heart and respiratory rates slow, blood pressure decreases, and alpha brain waves increase.

Transcendental meditation (TM), developed by the Indian mystic Maharishi Majesh Yogi, was introduced into the United States in the 1950s. TM uses mantras based on personal characteristics to induce a trance state. In the 1960s, a physician, Herbert Benson, developed the relaxation response, which used mantras and breath control as a treatment for stress and stress-related disorders.

MOXIBUSTION

Moxibustion is based on theories of Oriental medicine in which energy forces are balanced by applying heat to stimulate specific acupoints. The heat is generated by burning dry mugwort leaves (*Artemisia vulgaris*, known as moxa). Heat is applied either directly or indirectly. In the direct method, dried moxa is rolled into small cones and placed on the skin. The tops of the cones are lit, but they are extinguished as soon as heat is felt. In the indirect method, a burning cigarlike moxa is held near the skin at acupoints.

Moxibustion is used in musculoskeletal disorder, arthritis, asthma, and eczema. As with many other alternative therapies, however, no scientific clinical trials are available to show its effectiveness.

NATUROPATHY

Naturopathy is a health care system intended to ensure a healthy mind and body based on three principles: maintaining pollution-free air and water supplies; eating healthy foods; and exercising regularly. The treatment is based on the belief that the body has the power to heal itself; it requires the patient's active participation in the health maintenance program.

Naturopathy developed in Germany in the later 19th century under the guidance of Benedict Lusz, who prescribed hydrotherapy as a form of natural healing. Lusz came to the United States, became an osteopathic physician, and founded the American School of Naturopathy in 1902. Since then, naturopathic medicine has grown into a major form of health care, which uses an eclectic group of methods in addition to hydrotherapy. These methods include eating specialized diets, breathing ionized air, using fomentations (the application of hot and cold compresses), taking colonic irrigations and enemas, drinking pollution-free water, eating foods grown organically, and using massage therapy, herbs, and rest therapy. Naturopaths are licensed in several states (Alaska, Connecticut, New Hampshire, among others), but because there is no standard regulation of the field, persons with minimal or no educational background may call themselves naturopaths. This fact has contributed to the widespread belief that the field has many charlatans and quacks.

ORIENTAL MEDICINE

Oriental medicine is a broad term covering the traditional medicines of China, Korea, Japan, Vietnam, Tibet, and other Asian countries. In general, the techniques of Oriental medicine were first developed in China and include acupuncture, moxibustion, herbology, massage, cupping, *gwa sha,* breath work (*qi gong*), and exercise (*tai chi*). Chinese medicine is a coherent and independent system of thought and practice based on ancient texts. It is the result of a continuous process of critical thinking, extensive clinical observation, and testing and represents a thorough exposition of material by respected clinicians and theoreticians. It is rooted in philosophy, logic, sensibility, and habits of civilization foreign to Western civilization and is therefore difficult for Western physicians to understand. The basic theory is that there is a life force, called *chi* energy, and that this life force flows in us in a harmonious, balanced way. This harmony and balance signify health. When the life force does not flow properly, disharmony and imbalance, or illness, result.

OSTEOPATHIC MEDICINE

The scope of osteopathic medicine is similar to allopathic medicine and is best indicated by the fact that doctors of osteopathy (D.O.s) are licensed to practice in every state and are accepted into medical, surgical, and psychiatric residency programs and the military on the same basis as M.D.s; are qualified to practice in every branch of clinical medicine; and take the same licensure examinations as M.D.s. Their medical education is identical to that of medical doctors, except that they have additional training in disorders of the musculoskeletal system, in which D.O.s consider themselves more knowledgeable than M.D.s.

Nineteen osteopathic medical schools exist in the United States. Approximately 35,000 osteopaths treat about 20 million patients each year. Osteopathy was developed by Andrew Taylor Still, M.D. (1828–1917), who founded the American School of Osteopathy in Kirksville, Missouri (now Kirksville College of Osteopathic Medicine), in 1892. Disease is viewed in the same way as in allopathic medicine; however, special emphasis is placed on proper musculoskeletal alignment as a prerequisite for health maintenance. Osteopaths may rely on the manipulation of body parts, particularly the craniosacral spinal axis, as part of a treatment plan. Osteopathic manipulation therapy is perceived as an adjunct, not a substitute, to traditional medical, surgical, and pharmacological intervention.

OZONE THERAPY

Ozone acts as an antioxidant and disinfectant and is used conventionally for water purification, odor control, and air purification. Ozone therapy is based on the assumption that most illness is caused by viral and bacterial infection; ozone is used to treat medical conditions that range from influenza to cancer and AIDS. The first ozone generators were developed by Werner von Siemens in Germany in 1857, and ozone was used therapeutically to purify blood shortly thereafter in Germany and other European countries.

Ozone therapy introduces ozone into the body in various ways. These include drinking ozonated water; ozone limb bagging, in which ozone is pumped into an airtight bag that covers an arm or leg; breathing ozone bubbled through olive oil or topically applying ozonated olive oil; insufflations, in which a catheter is inserted into the rectum or vagina with ozone administered at a slow flow rate; and autohemotherapy, in which a person's own ozonized blood is reintroduced into the body.

PAST LIFE MEDICINE

In past life medicine, the healing process is aided by contact with spiritual beings who are believed to have the ability to

reverse illness and maintain health. The spirits are approached through the use of altered states of consciousness, so-called channeling, higher states of awareness, and transmissions from spiritually evolved beings. Past life regression using hypnosis allows a person to experience past life events (via imagery).

PRAYER

The pervasive interest in faith healing, the curative anecdotes of television evangelists, and the millions of hopeful individuals visiting religious shrines in search of relief give witness to the continuing interest in, and prevalence of, prayer and spirituality in the process of healing. Some religious groups specifically recommend against standard psychiatric therapies and offer their own approach as the only valid alternative for mental and spiritual health. Others view prayer as a form of distant healing defined by Elizabeth Targ as any purely mental effort undertaken by one person with the intention of improving the physical or emotional well-being of another (intercessory prayer). In a similar manner, the act of prayer can be self-administered and studied as part of the therapeutic process (personal or group prayer).

There are advocates for the use of shared prayer, silent prayer, and distant or "intercessory" prayer. One review concerning the use of prayer reported benefits experienced by patients dealing with terminal medical conditions.

Surveys indicate that 92 percent of a sample of inner city homeless women reported one or more spiritual or religious practices. Some 48 percent reported that prayer was significantly related to less use of alcohol or street drugs or both and fewer perceived worries and depression. Recent epidemiological research indicates that religious beliefs and practices are negatively correlated with substance abuse and positively correlated with health status. There is also a long history of 12-step programs successfully incorporating prayer and spirituality in the treatment of addictive behavior.

REFLEXOLOGY

Reflexology is the gentle massaging of the feet, hands, and ears to stimulate the body's natural healing power. It is used to alleviate tension by clearing crystalline deposits under the skin that may interfere with the natural flow of the body's energy. Reflexologists believe that all body parts can be mapped out on the soles or sides of the feet; for instance, the tip of the second toe represents the eye. Applying pressure to a particular area of the foot can relieve disorders related to the represented body parts.

REIKI

Reiki is a Japanese word with the general meaning of "healing." (*Rei* means "universal" or "spiritual," and *Ki* is "life force energy.") There are two degrees of Reiki healing. First-degree Reiki practitioners use light, nonmanipulative touch to precipitate a flow of healing energy, called *Reiki,* drawn through the practitioner and into the patient according to the recipient's needs. Second-degree healing enables practitioners to access this energy for distant healing when touch is impossible. Reiki treatment typically creates an almost immediate feeling of relaxation, which may reduce the biochemical effects of prolonged stress. First-degree Reiki is easily learned and is an effective method of self-healing patients can use to address anxiety, insomnia, and pain. Recipients may experience the energy as heat or cold, or as a sense of flow throughout the body, not limited to where the practitioner's hands are placed. Reiki is also used in hospices for pain management, to support a peaceful death, and to provide emotional support for family members.

ROLFING

Rolfing is a type of massage that was developed by an American biochemist, Ida Rolf (1896–1979), to relieve tension in muscle, connective tissue, and fascia, which she believed caused musculoskeletal diseases such as arthritis and fibromyalgia. Therapy consists of deep, sometimes painful, massage to produce flexible planes between muscle groups throughout the body. Rolf discovered that she could achieve remarkable changes in posture and structure by manipulating the body's myofascial system; as various parts of the body are massaged, past memories and emotional states are often released. In this sense rolfing is a psychophysiological experience.

SHAMANISM

A shaman is an individual who is believed to have the power to heal the sick and communicate with the spirit world. Individuals having this designation can be found in many parts of the world, including American aboriginal groups (Native Americans and Alaskan natives). Qualifications of a medicine man (or woman) are determined by a series of initiatory trials and teaching and "certification" by qualified, recognized elders. Shamanistic practices often include cleansing ceremonies such as fasting or sweating and so-called vision quests, which are accompanied by hallucinations. The ceremony is sometimes facilitated by rhythmic sounds, dancing, physical pain or privation, and the use of "spiritual herbs." Through this process the shaman escorts the soul of the dying to the afterlife. Shamanistic practices are also used to provide solutions to insolvable personal or social problems.

SOUND AND MUSIC THERAPY

Sound therapy is an ancient technique in which sounds (e.g., chants, bell rings, or drum beats) are used to create vibrations in the body and believed to have healing powers. Practitioners claim that a sense of relaxation can also be achieved. Sound therapy is used in Ayurveda to promote health, with claims of reducing tumor growth by using certain sounds known as Sama Veda.

Music therapy uses the sound of musical instruments, such as the flute, to achieve similar results. In the Bible, David attempted to treat King Saul's depression by playing the harp.

TAI CHI CHUAN

Tai chi chuan, or tai chi, is one of the most popular Asian movement arts used in the West. This ancient Chinese technique is designed to increase the life force in the body through a series of slow circular movements. It is a moving form of meditation and is based, like other Chinese methods, on the search for perfect balance between yin and yang energies.

The practitioner performs sequences of movements that last from 5 to 30 minutes. A session may last a couple of hours and is typically performed in early morning. The practitioner is expected to focus on breathing and its precise synchronization with the movements. Tai chi chuan is believed to help mainly stress-related problems and conditions and so is primarily used to treat anxiety, depression, muscular tension, high blood pressure, and other cardiovascular conditions.

THERAPEUTIC TOUCH

Therapeutic touch is the technique of healing with hands. It was developed by a nurse, Dolores Krieger, in the 1970s. Energy is believed to be transferred by laying the hands over specific parts of the body to aid in the process of healing. Therapeutic touch has gained popularity in the nursing profession as well as among some physicians.

TIBETAN MEDICINE

The Tibetan health system dates to about the 7th century AD. The Tibetan king Songsten Gampo is credited with its creation from the synthesis of various, more ancient sources. It has elements of Arabic, Indian, and Chinese health systems. In Tibet, its practice is closely related to religion and magic. Disease is believed to be the result of imbalance between the three components or humors of the living organism: wind (breathing and movement in general), bile (related to digestion and temperament), and phlegm (related to sleep, joint mobility, and skin elasticity). Imbalance can be caused by ignorance of health principles, environmental assaults, or improper diet. Treatment consists of restoring the balance between the different humors through the use of herbal medicine and accessory therapies, such as massage, moxibustion, acupuncture, appropriate diet, religious rituals, and purification techniques.

TRAGER METHOD

The Trager method, developed by Milton Trager, a Chicago physician, is a technique of movement reduction to aid individuals suffering from polio and other neuromuscular disorders. The client, typically in 60- to 90-minute sessions, is instructed to relax all conscious muscles and to allow the unconscious to choose natural, less restrictive body movements, as guided by the practitioner. This method is particularly suitable to individuals with back pain and severely restricted movement.

YOGA

Yoga ("yoking" or "union" in Sanskrit) is a comprehensive philosophical system with the goal of preparing an individual to unite with the supreme being. The technique of early Yoga seeks to bring into balance all the disparate aspects of body, mind, and personality. Early evidence of Yoga practice dates back to 5,000 years ago in India, and it has been practiced as a religion and health system ever since. Yoga is mainly known in the West for its physical component, the collection of postures known as Hatha Yoga; however, there are many forms that focus on meditation. Yoga is used to reduce stress and to treat anxiety, high blood pressure, and musculoskeletal conditions.

INTEGRATIVE PSYCHIATRY

A new type of psychiatry, called *integrative psychiatry,* selectively incorporates elements of complementary and alternative medicine into practice methods. It emphasizes treatment rather than diagnosis and views the patient holistically, taking into account not only mind–body issues and interactions but spiritual values as well. Integrative psychiatry also is concerned with prevention of illness, emphasized by having the patient pay attention to lifestyle factors such as diet and exercise. Stress reduction involves use of Yoga, meditation, or other relaxation exercises. Attention is paid to stress factors related to work and interpersonal relationships.

History

At one time, hypnosis and biofeedback were considered alternative therapies out of the mainstream of traditional psychiatric practice. These modalities are now incorporated into standard psychiatric practice. Hypnosis, for example, is used by psychiatrists for a variety of disorders, and dynamically oriented psychiatrists use hypnotherapy in their work to enable a patient to recover feelings and memories that are repressed and not otherwise available for analysis. In the middle of the 20th century, workers such as Paul Schilder, in his book *The Image and Appearance of the Human Body,* described how one's physiology and physiognomy could be influenced by psychological experiences during various developmental stages. More recently, mainstream psychiatrists such as Brian Weiss have described their use of past life regression as a therapeutic method and a means of accessing unconscious material.

Methods

Any of the complementary methods described in this section can be integrated into standard psychotherapeutic practice, although some lend themselves better than others. For example, during a Reiki treatment, a patient tends to be in a relaxed state and may have feeling tones, images, or thoughts that would not ordinarily be talked about. In an integrative therapy session, those mental and physical phenomena would be verbalized and subject to analysis and interpretation. Similarly, a patient undergoing past life regression may have an elaborate narrative about his or her past life that would be carefully examined by the integrative psychiatrist for its relevance to current life experiences. Most integrative psychiatrists view past-life narratives as dynamic representations of the patient's unconscious wishes and fears; some view them as representations of actual past lives lived. In either case, the material is used to help patients gain greater insight and understanding of themselves in their current life.

Complementary and alternative techniques that involve body manipulation (e.g., craniosacral manipulation, massage, or the Alexander technique) lend themselves to integrative psychiatric therapy. As mentioned above, the image persons have of their body and the way in which the body is held (e.g., stooped posture) are heavily influenced not only by genetics but also by life experiences. Depressive facies, Veraguth's folds, and other physiologic correlates of mood have long been recognized in the psychiatric literature. The integrative psychiatrist uses this and other bodily markers as a way to gain access to

previously unrecognized neurotic conflict. Patients with somatoform disorders such as dysmorphophobia are often helped by such approaches, as are patients with eating disorders who suffer from major body image distortions.

Any technique that involves manipulation of a body part can potentially elicit an image, thought, or feeling related to the experience. A patient experiencing a back rub may have myriad associations to the experience that are examined in the session. Some patients cannot tolerate being touched, a trait that is almost always related to some past traumatic experience. Body manipulation can be geared to correcting abnormalities. In the Alexander technique, careful attention is paid to posture and body alignment. As the corrective procedures unfold, patients may gain understanding and insight into what caused the defective or inefficient postural attitude in the first place.

Finally, spiritual beliefs derived from Judeo-Christian, Native American, and eastern religious thought can be integrated into traditional psychotherapy. Workers such as Alan Watts incorporated Zen Buddhism into Western psychotherapy more than 50 years ago. Psychiatrists are working with Native American healers to help patients diminish anxiety, especially regarding death and dying.

A 40-year-old man, in good health, with an obsessive fear of death was referred to an integrative psychiatrist to deal with his preoccupations about dying. The patient was placed in a trance state under hypnosis and asked to imagine and describe a past life. He described himself as an itinerant silk merchant living in 16th century France. He was married, had 8 children, and was content with his life. He was asked to describe his death and proceeded to do so. He was 90 years old when he died, surrounded by his family who were at his bedside. He knew he was dying and described the process as a "peaceful falling away." Following the session, his fears about dying diminished; when he became anxious about death he remembered the past life narrative and was able to relax.

Other Issues

Ideally, the psychiatrist practicing integrative therapy should be schooled in one or more of the complementary methods he or she plans to employ. In some cases, a complementary practitioner may work in conjunction with the psychiatrist, especially if the psychiatrist is not schooled in a particular method. At times, patients may be expert in a field (e.g., Yoga) and seek out the integrative psychiatrist to enlarge upon their experience. Integrative psychiatrists may use psychoactive herbs and homeopathic medicinals alone or in conjunction with traditional psychopharmacologic agents, mindful of the possibility of adverse drug–drug interactions.

Ethical Issues

The same standards that apply to traditional psychiatric practice and psychotherapy apply to this method. Because some of the techniques involve a laying on of hands or place the patient in a more dependent and vulnerable state than traditional psychotherapy techniques, so-called boundary issues must be carefully evaluated. Currently, there are no standards of practice for this method other than those to which physicians have always been held, including to do no harm. As in complementary and alternative medicine generally, careful outcome studies are needed if this new amalgam is to prove its worth.

References

Ai AL, Peterson C, Gillespie B, et al. Designing clinical trials on energy healing: ancient art meets medical science. *Alter Ther.* 2001;7:83.

Albert HC, Wong MD. Herbal remedies in psychiatric practice. *Arch Gen Psychiatry.* 1998;55:1033.

Anderson S, Lundeberg T. Acupuncture—from empiricism to science: functional background to acupuncture effects in pain and disease. *Med Hypotheses.* 1995;45:271.

Aular JJ. Alternative cancer treatments. *Sci Am.* 1996;275:162.

Beal MW, Nield-Anderson L. Acupuncture for symptom relief in HIV-positive adults: lessons learned from a pilot study. *Altern Ther Health Med.* 2000;6:33.

Beaubarn G, Grayu GE. A review of herbal medicine for psychiatric disorders. *Psychiatr Serv.* 2000;51:1130.

Engebretson J, Wind Wardell D. Experience of a Reiki session. *Alter Ther.* 2002;8:48.

Field T. Massage therapy for infants and children. *J Dev Behav Pediatr.* 1995;16:105.

Field T. Massage therapy. *Med Clin North Am.* 2002;86:163.

Gordon IS. The White House Commission and the future of healthcare. *Altern Ther Health Med* 2000;6:26.

Griffith JL, Griffith ME. *Encountering the Sacred in Psychotherapy: How to Talk with People about Their Spiritual Lives.* New York: The Guilford Press; 2002.

Kaptchuk TJ, Eisenberg DM. Varieties of healing: a taxonomy of unconventional healing practices. *Ann Intern Med.* 2001;135:189.

Kiresuk TJ, Trachtenberg A. Alternative and complimentary health practices. In: Sadock BJ, Sadock VA, eds. *Kaplan & Sadock's Comprehensive Textbook of Psychiatry.* 7th ed. Vol 2. Baltimore: Lippincott Williams & Wilkins; 2000.

Shannon S, ed. Handbook of Complementary and Alternative Therapies in Mental Health. San Diego: Academic Press; 2002.

Tyler VE. *Herbs of Choice: The Therapeutic Use of Phytomedicinals.* New York: Pharmaceutical Products Press; 1994.

Walsh R. Essential spirituality for healing professionals. *Alter Ther.* 2002;8:76.

Weiss B. *Many Lives, Many Masters.* New York: Guilford Press; 1988.

Woelk H. Comparison of St. John's wort and imipramine for treating depression: randomised controlled trial. *Br Med J.* 2000;321:536.

30 Psychiatry and Reproductive Medicine

Reproductive events and processes have profound psychological concomitants, some of which may progress to overt psychopathological states. This section addresses such events, including pregnancy, infertility, abortion, menopause, and sterilization, among others.

PREGNANCY

Biology of Pregnancy

The first presumptive sign of pregnancy is the absence of menses for 1 week. Other presumptive signs are breast engorgement and tenderness, changes in breast size and shape, nausea with or without vomiting (morning sickness), frequent urination, and fatigue. A diagnosis can be made 10 to 15 days after fertilization by testing for human chorionic gonadotropin (hCG), which is produced by the placenta. The definitive diagnosis requires a doubling of hCG levels and the presence of fetal heart sounds. Transvaginal ultrasound scanning can reveal a pregnant uterus as early as 4 weeks after fertilization, by visualization of a gestational sac.

Stages of Pregnancy

Pregnancy is commonly divided into three trimesters, starting from the first day of the last menstrual cycle and ending with the delivery of a baby. The estimated date of delivery (EDD) is calculated by subtracting 3 months from the first day of the last menses and adding 7 days and 1 year. Only about 10 percent of women are delivered on the EDD; the rest are delivered from 1 week early to 1 week late. A pregnant woman may experience considerable anxiety about various issues from one trimester to the next.

During the first trimester the woman must adapt to changes in her body. Many women experience profound fatigue. Increasing estrogen levels cause breast tenderness and mood lability. Constipation is caused by large amounts of progesterone, and nausea and vomiting occur in response to rising hCG levels. Early in pregnancy many women fear having a miscarriage and may choose not to tell family members and friends about being pregnant in case that occurs.

The second trimester is often the most rewarding for women. A return of energy and the end of nausea and vomiting allow women to feel better and experience the excitement of starting to look pregnant. Some, however, may consider their body unattractive at this time. A major event of the second trimester is quickening—the mother's perception of fetal movement that occurs between 16 and 20 weeks. Quickening reinforces the mother's mental picture of the child-to-be; many cultural beliefs relate the types of fetal movements to the sex of the baby and its personality. Such beliefs may create anxiety or depression in some women when those beliefs are at variance with their expectations. Most women, however, equate quickening with having a live fetus and find it an exhilarating experience that is commonly shared with their partner. If other children are in the household, allowing them to feel the fetal movements helps them prepare for the new sibling and work through issues of sibling rivalry.

The third trimester is associated with physical discomfort for many women. All systems—cardiovascular, renal, pulmonary, gastrointestinal, and endocrine—have undergone profound changes that may produce a heart murmur, weight gain, exertional dyspnea, and heartburn (pyrosis). Some women require reassurance that those changes are not evidence of disease and that they will return to normal shortly after delivery—generally in 4 to 6 weeks.

As delivery approaches, practical issues relate to the arrival of the baby (e.g., child care, baby clothes, and finances). In addition, preparations for the delivery and postnatal care are made (e.g., notifying the doctor, getting to the hospital, the use of an anesthetic, and breast versus bottle feeding). Parents often worry about specific health issues, such as whether the infant will be deformed, but in many cases the worries are not verbalized. If one or both partners show increasing anxiety as the EDD approaches, that and other issues may be provoking anxiety (e.g., vaginal delivery versus cesarean section) and should be discussed with the physician.

Psychology of Pregnancy

Pregnant women undergo marked psychological changes. Their attitudes toward pregnancy reflect deeply felt beliefs about all aspects of reproduction, including whether the pregnancy was planned and whether the baby is wanted. The relationship with the infant's father, the age of the mother, and her sense of identity also affect a woman's reaction to prospective motherhood. Prospective fathers also face psychological challenges.

Psychologically healthy women often find pregnancy a means of self-realization. Many women report that being pregnant is a creative act gratifying a fundamental need. Other women use pregnancy to diminish self-doubts about femininity or to reassure themselves that they can function as women in the most basic sense. Still others view pregnancy negatively; they may fear childbirth or feel inadequate about mothering.

During early stages of their own development, women must undergo the experience of separating from their mothers and of establishing an independent identity; this experience later affects their own success at mothering. If a woman's mother was a poor role model, a woman's sense of maternal competence may be impaired, and she may lack confidence before and after her baby's birth. Women's unconscious fears and fantasies during early pregnancy often center on the idea of fusion with their own mothers.

Psychological attachment to the fetus begins in utero, and by the beginning of the second trimester most women have a mental picture of the infant. Even before being born, the fetus is viewed as a separate being, endowed with a prenatal personality. Many mothers talk to their unborn children. Recent evidence suggests that emotional talk with the fetus is related not only to early mother–infant bonding but also to the mother's efforts to have a healthy pregnancy, for example, by giving up cigarettes and caffeine. According to psychoanalytic theorists, the child-to-be is a blank screen on which a mother projects her hopes and fears. In rare instances these projections account for postpartum pathological states, such as a mother's desire to harm her infant, whom she views as a hated part of herself. Normally, however, giving birth to a child fulfills a woman's need to create and nurture life.

Fathers are also profoundly affected by pregnancy. Impending parenthood demands a synthesis of such developmental issues as gender role and identity, separation-individuation from a man's own father, sexuality, and, as Erik Erikson proposed, generativity. Pregnancy fantasies in men and wishes to give birth in boys reflect early identification with their mothers as well as the wish to be as powerful and creative as they perceive mothers to be. For some men, getting a woman pregnant is proof of their potency, a dynamic that plays a large part in adolescent fatherhood.

Marriage and Pregnancy

The prospective mother-wife and father-husband must redefine their roles as a couple and as individuals. They face readjustments in their relationships with friends and relatives and must deal with new responsibilities as caretakers of the newborn and each other. Both parents may experience anxiety about their adequacy as parents; one or both partners may be consciously or unconsciously ambivalent about the addition of the child to the family and about the effects on the dyadic (two-person) relationship. A husband may feel guilty about his wife's discomfort during pregnancy and parturition, and some men experience jealousy or envy of the experience of pregnancy. Accustomed to gratifying each other's dependency needs, the couple must attend to the unremitting needs of a new infant and a developing child. Although most couples respond positively to these demands, some do not. Under ideal conditions the decision to become a parent and have a child should be agreed on by both partners, but sometimes parenthood is rationalized as a way to achieve intimacy in a conflicted marriage or to avoid having to deal with other life circumstance problems.

Attitudes toward the Pregnant Woman. In general, others' attitudes toward a pregnant woman reflect a variety of factors: intelligence, temperament, cultural practices, and myths of the society and the subculture into which the person was born. Married men's responses to pregnancy are generally positive. For some men, however, reactions vary from a misplaced sense of pride that they are able to impregnate the woman to fear of increased responsibility and subsequent termination of the relationship. The risk that a woman will be abused by her husband or boyfriend increases during pregnancy, particularly during the first trimester. One study found that 6 percent of pregnant women are abused. Domestic abuse adds significantly to the cost of health care during pregnancy, and abused women are more likely than nonabused controls to have histories of miscarriage, abortion, and neonatal death. The reasons for abuse vary. Some men fear being neglected and not having excessive dependency needs gratified; others may see the fetus as a rival. In most cases, however, one finds a history of abuse before the woman was pregnant.

Alternative Lifestyle Pregnancy

Some lesbian couples decide that one partner should become pregnant through artificial insemination. Societal attitudes may put stress on this arrangement, but if the two women have a secure relationship, they tend to bond strongly together as a family unit. Long-term follow-up studies have shown that children of lesbian mothers do not differ from children of heterosexual mothers in emotional health or interpersonal relationships, and the children are not more likely to be gay or lesbian themselves. Men in committed gay relationships are fathering children through artificial insemination with surrogate mothers. The long-term effects on children reared by gay men have not been determined; however, preliminary findings are similar to those with children who are raised in lesbian homes.

Some single, never-married women who do not wish to marry but do want to become pregnant may do so through artificial or natural insemination. Although few in number, such women constitute a group who believe that motherhood is the fulfillment of female identity, without which they view their lives to be incomplete and, in some cases, meaningless. Most of these women have considered the consequence of single parenthood and feel able to rise to the challenges.

Sexual Behavior

The effects of pregnancy on sexual behavior vary. Some women experience an increased sex drive as pelvic vasocongestion produces a more sexually responsive state. Others are more responsive than before the pregnancy because they no longer fear becoming pregnant. Some have diminished desire or lose interest in sexual activity altogether. A decrease in libido may be due to higher estrogen levels or feelings of unattractiveness. Avoidance of sex may also result from physical discomfort or an association of motherhood with asexuality. Men with a Madonna complex view pregnant women as sacred and not to be defiled by the sexual act. Either a man or a woman may erroneously consider intercourse potentially harmful to the developing fetus and thus something to be avoided. Men who have extramarital affairs during their wives' pregnancies usually do so during the last trimester.

Coitus. Most obstetricians place no prohibitions on coitus during pregnancy. Some suggest that sexual intercourse cease 4

to 5 weeks antepartum. If bleeding occurs early in pregnancy, an obstetrician may prohibit coitus temporarily as a therapeutic measure. Bleeding in the first 20 days of pregnancy occurs in 20 to 25 percent of women and approximately half experience spontaneous abortion. Maternal death resulting from forcibly blowing air into the vagina during cunnilingus has been reported; the deaths presumably result from air emboli in the placental–maternal circulation.

Parturition

Fears regarding pain and bodily harm during delivery are universal and to some extent, warranted. Preparation for childbirth affords a sense of familiarity and can ease anxieties, which facilitates delivery. Continuous emotional support during labor reduces the rate of cesarean section and forceps deliveries, the need for anesthesia, the use of oxytocin, and the duration of labor. A technically difficult or even painful delivery, however, does not appear to influence the decision to bear additional children.

Men's responses to pregnancy and labor have not been well studied, but the recent trend toward inclusion of fathers in the birth process eases their anxieties and elicits a fuller sense of participation. Fathers do not parent the same way as mothers, and new mothers often need to be encouraged to respect these differences and view them positively.

Lamaze Method. Also known as natural childbirth, the Lamaze method originated with the French obstetrician Fernand Lamaze. In this method, women are fully conscious during labor and delivery, and no analgesic or anesthetic is used. The expectant mother and father attend special classes, during which they are taught relaxation and breathing exercises designed to facilitate the birth process. Women who undergo such training often report minimal pain during labor and delivery. Participating in the birth process may help a fearful or ambivalent father bond to his newborn infant.

Depression and Psychosis in the Postpartum Period

About 20 to 40 percent of women report some emotional disturbance or cognitive dysfunction in the postpartum period. Many experience so-called baby blues, a normal state of sadness, dysphoria, frequent tearfulness, and clinging dependence. These feelings, which may last several days, have been ascribed to rapid changes in women's hormonal levels, the stress of childbirth, and the awareness of the increased responsibility that motherhood brings.

Postpartum depression is characterized by a depressed mood, excessive anxiety, and insomnia. The onset is within 3 to 6 months after delivery. Table 30–1 differentiates postpartum "baby blues" from postpartum depression.

In rare cases (1 to 2 in 1,000 deliveries), a woman's postpartum depression is characterized by depressed feelings and suicidal ideation. In severe cases the depression may reach psychotic proportions, with hallucinations, delusions, and thoughts of infanticide. Although previous psychiatric problems put women at risk for postpartum disturbances, some evidence suggests that postpartum mood disorder is a specific concept, distinct from other psychiatric diagnoses. Others argue that these mood disorders are not a distinct entity but part of a bipolar spectrum as reflected in the classification in the text revision of the fourth edition of *Diagnostic and Statistical Manual of Mental Disorders* (DSM-IV-TR). Women with severe postpartum depression are at high risk for future episodes, and failure to treat may contribute to long-term, treatment-refractory mood disorders.

A syndrome described in fathers is characterized by mood changes during their wives' pregnancies or after the babies are born. These fathers are affected by several factors: added responsibility, diminished sexual outlet, decreased attention from his wife, and the belief that the child is a binding force in an unsatisfactory marriage.

Table 30–1
Comparison of "Baby Blues" and Postpartum Depression

Characteristic	"Baby Blues"	Postpartum Depression
Incidence	50% of women who give birth	10% of women who give birth
Time of onset	3–5 days after delivery	Within 3–6 months after delivery
Duration	Days to weeks	Months to years, if untreated
Associated stressors	No	Yes, especially lack of support
Sociocultural influence	No; present in all cultures and socioeconomic classes	Strong association
History of mood disorder	No association	Strong association
Family history of mood disorder	No association	Some association
Tearfulness	Yes	Yes
Mood lability	Yes	Often present, but sometimes mood is uniformly depressed
Anhedonia	No	Often
Sleep disturbance	Sometimes	Nearly always
Suicidal thoughts	No	Sometimes
Thoughts of harming the baby	Rarely	Often
Feelings of guilt, inadequacy	Absent or mild	Often present and excessive

Reproduced with permission from Miller LJ. How "baby blues" and postpartum depression differ. *Women's Psychiatric Health.* 1995:13. © 1995, The KSF Group.

Prenatal Screening

Prenatal screening for potential or actual fetal malformation is conducted in most pregnant women. Sonograms are noninvasive and can detect structural fetal abnormalities Maternal α-fetoprotein (AFP) is measured between 15 and 20 weeks. An increase in concentration of this protein can indicate neural tube defects and a decrease may indicate Down syndrome. The sensitivity of Down syndrome testing is increased when a triple screen is done (AFP, hCG, and estriol). Amniocentesis is indicated for women over 35 years, those with a sibling or parent with a known chromosome anomaly, and those with abnormal AFP or any other risk for severe genetic disorder. Amniocentesis is usually done between 16 and 18 weeks and carries a risk that 1 in 300 women will miscarry after the procedure. In the first trimester chorionic villus sampling (CVS) can be done, which reveals the same information concerning chromosomal status, enzyme levels, and DNA patterns. There is a risk of 1 in 100 that a woman will have a spontaneous abortion after CVS. Screening in the first trimester allows women to choose early termination, which may be physically and emotionally easier on the woman. Profound ethical questions are involved in whether or not to abort a fetus with a known defect; some women choose not to terminate and report a strong loving bond that lasts throughout the life of the child, who usually predeceases the parent.

Lactation

Lactation occurs because of a complex psychoneuroendocrine cascade that is triggered by the abrupt decline in estrogen and progesterone concentrations at parturition. Lactation becomes established because of the neurological stimulation transmitted by suckling. The composition and amount of breast milk change as the infant grows. In general, babies should be fed as needed rather than by schedule. Currently more than 60 percent of babies are breast-fed; of this number about 25 percent are breast-fed for at least 6 months, and 15 percent for 5 years. In subsistence-level cultures in which children are allowed to nurse as long as they want (a practice supported by La Leche League, a breast-feeding advocacy group), most babies will wean themselves between 3 and 5 if not encouraged by the mother to do so earlier.

Breast-feeding has many benefits. The composition of breast milk supports timely neuronal development, confers passive immunity, and reduces food allergies in the child. Benefits for the mother are faster involution of the uterus and weight loss. Breast-feeding also promotes psychological attachment and facilitates positive self-esteem for the mother who views herself as a provider. Women who decide to breast-feed need good teaching and social support, which if lacking may lead to frustration and feelings of inadequacy. Women must not feel pressured or coerced into breast-feeding if they are opposed or ambivalent. In the long term, no discernible difference exists between bottle-fed and breast-fed children as adults.

An incidental finding about lactation is that some women experience sexual sensations during lactation, which in rare cases may lead to orgasm. In the early 1990s a woman who called a help line about such feelings was put in jail and had her infant taken from her on allegations of sexual abuse. Fortunately, common sense ultimately prevailed and they were reunited.

Teratogens

Teratogens are drugs or other agents that cause abnormal fetal development. Infections such as varicella, toxoplasmosis, and herpes simplex, among others, can interfere with normal development. Pregnant women who smoke are subject to premature births, and congenital defects are more common in smokers than in nonsmokers. Alcohol abuse is associated with fetal alcohol syndrome (see Section 12.2). Other drugs of abuse such as cocaine and heroin produce drug-dependent newborns. In general, pregnant women should not use prescription and over-the-counter drugs and phytomedicinals. Drugs given in the third trimester are rarely teratogenic. Retinoids (used to treat acne) taken early in pregnancy have been associated with fetal abnormalities. Anticonvulsants are especially teratogenic, as is lithium, which produces cardiovascular defects in almost 20 percent of fetuses.

Use of Psychotropic Medications. There are no definitive answers to the questions of which psychotropic medications are safest during pregnancy and lactation. In patients with worsening psychiatric illness during pregnancy, outpatient psychotherapy, hospitalization, and milieu therapy should be attempted before routine use of psychotropic medication. Before a planned pregnancy, withdrawal of psychotropic medications should be attempted under close supervision. The importance of close rapport between the treating physician and the pregnant or breastfeeding patient cannot be overstated and will obviate or decrease reliance on psychotropic medication in many cases. The U.S. Food and Drug Administration (FDA) rates drugs in five categories of safety for use in pregnancy (Table 30–2). In general, one wants to avoid all medications during pregnancy that are not absolutely essential.

Pseudocyesis

Pseudocyesis (false pregnancy) is the development of the classic symptoms of pregnancy—amenorrhea, nausea, breast enlargement and pigmentation, abdominal distention (Fig. 30–1), and labor pains—in a nonpregnant woman. Pseudocyesis demonstrates the ability of the psyche to dominate the soma, proba-

Table 30–2
FDA Rating of Drug Safety in Pregnancy

Category	Definition	Drug Examples
A	No fetal risks in controlled human studies	Iron
B	No fetal risk in animal studies but no controlled human studies or fetal risk in animals but no risk in well-controlled human studies	Acetaminophen
C	Adverse fetal effects in animals and no human data available	Aspirin, haloperidol, chlorpromazine
D	Human fetal risk seen (may be used in life-threatening situation)	Lithium, tetracycline, ethanol
X	Proved fetal risk in humans (no indication for use, even in life-threatening situations)	Valproic acid, thalidomide

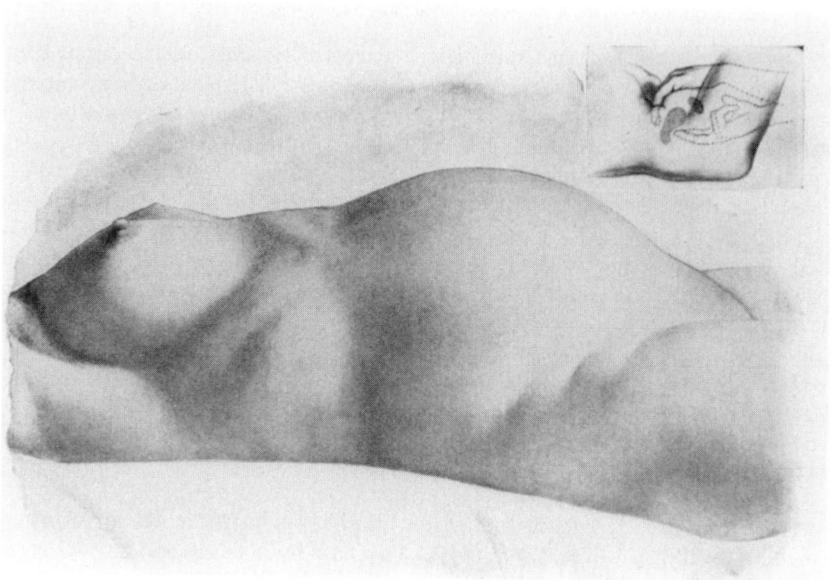

FIGURE 30–1
Patient at 36th (?) week. Bimanual examination revealed uterus normal in size and position.

bly via central input at the level of the hypothalamus. Predisposing psychological processes are thought to include a pathological wish for, and fear of, pregnancy; ambivalence or conflict regarding gender, sexuality, or childbearing; and a grief reaction to loss following a miscarriage, tubal ligation, or hysterectomy. The patient may have a true somatic delusion that is not subject to reality testing, but often a negative pregnancy test result or pelvic ultrasound scan leads to resolution. Psychotherapy is recommended during or after a presentation of pseudocyesis to evaluate and treat the underlying psychological dysfunction. A related event, *couvade,* occurs in some cultures in which the father of the child undergoes simulated labor, as though he were giving birth. In those societies *couvade* is a normal phenomenon.

Miss S., aged 16, thought she had become pregnant after her first coital experience, which occurred without contraception. Shortly after she read about the signs and symptoms of pregnancy, her menses stopped. She related that she felt tingling in her breasts, which she believed were enlarged. She also reported nausea and vomiting in the morning, which was observed by her mother. On examination, the uterus was enlarged, breasts were developed with dark areola and contained milk, and a pigmented line was observed from the umbilicus to the pubis. The abdomen was not enlarged, but she believed she felt fetal movement. A pregnancy test had negative results and the patient was so informed; however, she could not be dissuaded of her belief that she was pregnant. She entered psychotherapy, and within 2 months her menses returned and she accepted the fact that she was not pregnant.

Hyperemesis Gravidarum

Hyperemesis gravidarum is differentiated from morning sickness in that vomiting is chronic, persistent, and frequent, leading to ketosis, acidosis, weight loss, and dehydration. The prognosis is excellent for both mother and fetus with prompt treatment. Most women can be treated as outpatients, with changing to smaller meals, discontinuing iron supplements, and avoiding certain foods. In severe cases hospitalization may be necessary. Although the cause is unknown, there may be a psychological component. Women with histories of anorexia nervosa or bulimia nervosa may be at risk.

Pica

Pica is the repeated ingestion of nonnutritive substances such as dirt, clay, starch, sand, and feces. This eating disorder is most often seen in young children but is common in pregnant women in some subcultures, most notably among African American women in the rural South, who may eat clay or starch (e.g., Argo). The cause of pica is unknown.

Infertility

Infertility is the inability of a couple to conceive after 1 year of coitus without the use of a contraceptive. In the United States, about 15 percent of married couples are unable to have children. Until recently, women were blamed when couples did not have children, and feelings of guilt, depression, and inadequacy frequently accompanied the perception of being barren. Today, causes of infertility are attributed to disorders in women in 40 percent of cases, disorders in men in 40 percent, and disorders of both in 20 percent. Tests in an infertility workup usually reveal the specific cause; however, 10 to 20 percent of couples have no identifiable cause.

Common medical causes of infertility are irregular ovulation, endometriosis, impaired spermatogenesis, and damaged fallopian tubes. Current practice encourages a thorough sexual history of the couple, including frequency of coitus, erectile or ejaculatory dysfunction, and coital position. Frequently, conception is less likely simply because the woman rises to void, wash, or even douche immediately after coitus. Also, coitus with the woman in the superior position is not conducive to conception because less semen is retained. All of these factors must be considered.

The inability to have a child can produce severe psychological stress on one or both partners in a marriage. They may feel defective and undesirable, have low self-esteem, and become depressed. The couple must deal with a narcissistic blow to the sense of femininity or masculinity. Self-blame increases the likelihood of psychological problems. Women—but not men—are at increased risk for psychological distress if they are older and do not already have biological children. An infertile partner may fear abandonment or feel that the spouse resents remaining in the relationship. No statistics are available on infertility as a precipitating factor in divorce, but it does play a role. When one person in a couple (usually the woman) chooses adoption as an alternative but the other person (usually the man) is unwilling to do so, divorce may occur. Similarly, if one or both partners are unwilling to take advantage of assisted reproductive techniques, the marriage may falter.

A psychiatric evaluation of the couple may be advisable. Marital disharmony or emotional conflicts about intimacy, sexual relations, or parenting roles can directly affect endocrine function and such physiological processes as erection, ejaculation, and ovulation. There is no evidence, however, for any simple, causal relation between stress and infertility.

The stress of infertility itself in a couple who want children can lead to emotional disturbances. When preexisting conflict gives rise to problems of identity, self-esteem, and guilt, the disturbance may be severe and may manifest through regression; extreme dependence on a physician, mate, or parent; diffuse anger; impulsive behavior; or depression. The problem is further complicated when hormone therapy is used to treat the infertility, because the therapy may temporarily increase depression in some patients.

Mood and cognition may be altered by pharmacological agents used to treat disorders of ovulation or to hyperstimulate the ovaries. These agents include clomiphene citrate (Clomid) and other antiestrogens, gonadotropin-releasing hormone (GnRH) agonists, human chorionic gonadotropins (hCGs), progesterone, and bromocriptine (Parlodel). Danazol (Danocrine), a synthetic androgen, may be used to arrest the growth of endometriosis as a surgical or medical adjunct to later infertility therapy. Treatment of infertility itself provokes anxiety because of the uncertainty and sense of expectation. However, most of the agents also alter estradiol and progesterone levels, and the resultant hormonal fluctuations may trigger mood lability in sensitive individuals. Agents such as clomiphene, danazol, and bromocriptine may also have direct effects on the brain. If the use of these agents is indicated, psychological support should be offered in preference to anxiolytics and antidepressants.

Persons who have difficulty conceiving may experience shock, disbelief, and a general sense of helplessness, and they develop an understandable preoccupation with the problem. Involvement in the infertility workup and the development of expertise about infertility can be a constructive defense against feelings of inadequacy and the humiliating, sometimes painful aspects of the workup itself. Worries about attractiveness and sexual desirability are common. Partners may feel ugly or impotent, and episodes of sexual dysfunction and loss of desire are reported. These problems are aggravated when a couple is scheduling sexual relations according to temperature charts or ovulatory cycles.

Treatments for infertility (Table 30–3) are expensive and consume much time and energy. Both men and women can be overwhelmed by complexity, cost, invasiveness, and uncertainty associated with medical intervention. A loss of privacy and intimacy can threaten marital adjustment, especially if the partners react differently to challenges.

Table 30–3
Assisted Reproduction Techniques

Method	Comments
Ovulation induction or augmentation (multiple agents, particularly recombinant or highly purified gonadotropins)	Stimulates multifollicular development and ovulation; may produce multiple births; used in anovulation, luteal phase deficiency, unexplained infertility and assisted reproduction
Induction of spermatogenesis	Used in men with idiopathic hypothalamic hypogonadism of functional or organic nature
Artificial insemination	Donor sperm is injected into the uterine cavity or the fallopian tubes; the sperm of the husband may be used if healthy
Gamete intrafallopian transfer (GIFT)	Transfer of collected oocytes and sperm into the fallopian tubes; zygote may also be transferred (ZIFT); used for infertility from endometriosis and unexplained infertility
In vitro fertilization and embryo transfer (IVF-ET)	Transfer of developing embryos into the uterus after extracorporeal incubation of collected sperm with oocytes retrieved by laparoscopic surgery or by ultrasound-guided transvaginal aspiration; used with occlusion of the fallopian tubes or significant sperm dysfunction; permits preimplantation genetic diagnosis
Intracytoplasmic sperm injection (ICSI)	Injection in vitro of sperm head or sperm DNA to cause fertilization and production of embryos for transfer to receptive endometrium; may be used even if sperm are barely viable; genetic causes of male infertility may be transmitted to offspring
Gamete donors	Donation of sperm or oocytes to another couple. Donation can include oocytes only, oocyte cytoplasm only to restore reproductive competence to aged oocytes, donor sperm alone, or any combination
Surrogate mother	Surrogate mother receives donated embryo and carries the baby to term; a highly controversial technique with unclear legal ramifications

Data from Virginia Susman, M.D.

Single persons who are aware of their own infertility may shy away from relationships for fear of being rejected once their "defect" is known. Persons who are infertile may have particular difficulty in their adult relationships with their own parents. The identification and equality that come from sharing the experience of parenthood must be replaced by internal reserves and other generative aspects of their lives.

Professional intervention may be necessary to help infertile couples ventilate their feelings and go through the process of mourning for their lost biological functions and the children they cannot have. Couples who remain infertile must cope with an actual loss. Couples who decide not to pursue parenthood may develop a renewed sense of love, dedication, and identity as a pair. Others may need help in exploring the options of husband or donor insemination, laboratory implantation, and adoption.

Perinatal Death

Perinatal death is defined as death sometime between the 20th week of gestation and the first month of life and includes spontaneous abortion (miscarriage), fetal demise, stillbirth, and neonatal death. In previous years, the intense bond between the expectant or new parent and the fetus or neonate was underestimated, but perinatal loss is now recognized as a significant trauma for both parents. Parents who experience such a loss go through a period of mourning much like that experienced when any loved one is lost.

Intrauterine fetal death, which can occur at any time during the pregnancy, is an emotionally traumatic experience. In the early months of pregnancy, a woman is usually unaware of fetal death and learns of it only from her doctor. Later in pregnancy, after fetal movements and heart tones have been experienced, a woman may be able to detect fetal demise. When given the diagnosis of fetal death, most women want the dead fetus removed; depending on the trimester, labor may be induced, or the woman may have to wait for spontaneous expulsion of the uterine contents. Many couples consider sexual relations during the period of waiting not only undesirable but psychologically unacceptable as well.

A sense of loss also accompanies the birth of a stillborn child and induced abortion of an abnormal fetus detected by antenatal diagnosis. As mentioned above, attachment to an unborn child begins before birth, and grief and mourning occur after a loss at any time. The grief experienced after a third-trimester loss, however, is generally greater than that experienced after a first-trimester loss. Some parents do not wish to view a stillborn child, and their wishes should be respected. Others wish to hold the stillborn, and this act can assist the mourning process. A subsequent pregnancy may diminish overt feelings of grief, but it does not eliminate the need to mourn. So-called replacement children are at risk for overprotection and future emotional problems.

FAMILY PLANNING AND CONTRACEPTION

Family planning is the process of choosing when and if to bear children. One form of family planning is contraception, the prevention of fecundation, or fertilization of the ovum. The choice of a contraceptive method is a complex decision involving both women and their partners. Factors influencing the decision include a woman's age and medical condition, her access to medical care, the couple's religious beliefs, and the need for coital spontaneity. The woman and her partner can weigh the risks and benefits of the various forms of contraception and make their decision on the basis of their current lifestyle and other factors. The success of contraceptive technology has enabled career-minded couples to delay child-bearing into their 30s and 40s. Such a delay, however, may increase infertility problems. Consequently, many women with careers feel their biological clocks ticking and plan to have children while in their early 30s to avoid the risk of not being able to have them at all. Table 30–4 provides information on current methods of contraception, and Figure 30–2 shows some contraceptive modalities.

Induced Abortion

Induced abortion is the planned termination of a pregnancy. About 1.5 million abortions are performed in the United States each year—380 abortions for every 1,000 live births. Over the last decade the number of abortions has declined by about 5 percent. Family planning experts believe that more sex education and greater availability of contraceptive devices keep the number of abortions down. In Western countries, most women who obtain abortions are young, unmarried, and primiparous; in emerging countries, abortion is most common among married women with two or more children.

Fifty percent of abortions are performed before 8 weeks of gestation, 25 percent between 9 and 10 weeks, and 10 percent between 11 and 12 weeks. The remainder occur after 13 weeks, with 1 percent occurring after 21 weeks. Table 30–5 summarizes the most common abortion techniques.

Abortion has become a political and philosophical issue in the United States. The country is sharply divided between pro-choice (proabortion) and pro-life (antiabortion) factions. In recent years, antiabortion demonstrators have picketed abortion clinics and have provoked angry confrontations with patients. The atmosphere of moral condemnation and intimidation may make the decision to terminate a pregnancy difficult. Nonetheless, recent studies have shown that most women who undergo termination of pregnancy—particularly if they do so before the 12th week of gestation—do not suffer significant psychological sequelae. In fact, most women experience a sense of relief and have a less emotional reaction than those who maintain the pregnancy and give the baby up for adoption.

Second-trimester abortions are more psychologically traumatic than first-trimester abortions. The most common reason for late abortions is the discovery (via amniocentesis or ultrasound) of an abnormal karyotype or fetal anomaly. Thus, late abortions usually involve the loss of a wanted child with whom the mother has already formed a bond.

Before the legalization of abortion in the United States in 1973, many women sought illegal abortions, often performed by untrained practitioners under unsterile conditions. Considerable morbidity and mortality were associated with these abortions, and women who were denied abortion sometimes chose suicide over continuation of an unwanted pregnancy. When a woman is forced to carry a fetus to term, the risk of infanticide, abandonment, and neglect of the unwanted newborn increases.

Abortion can also be a significant experience for men. If a man has a close relationship with the woman, he may wish to

Table 30–4
Current Methods of Contraception

Type	Method of Action	Effectiveness	Advantages	Disadvantages	Potential Complications
Fertility awareness method (FAM); rhythm	Timed abstinence; couple abstains 7 days before and after ovulation	Low	No cost or health risks; always available; no professional help required	Imposed coital timing (lack of spontaneity); continuous recording of menstrual cycle necessary; must learn to take basal body temperature and check cervical mucus	Essentially none
Withdrawal; coitus interruptus	Prevention of insemination	Low (but theoretically high)	No cost; always available; no professional help required	Regular coital use required; requires considerable attention and control by man, which may interfere with pleasure for both partners	Essentially none
Diaphragm	Rubber dome inserted into vagina; works as sperm barrier; used with spermicidal jelly; must be left in place for 6 hours after coitus	Medium to high	Inexpensive	Regular coital use required; possible interference with enjoyment; requires professional fitting; not anatomically adaptable to everyone; repeated intercourse requires new application of spermicide	Essentially none, but diaphragm can dislodge during coitus; urinary tract infections; used by 3.4% of women
Cervical cap	Rubber cap covers only cervical os; works as sperm barrier; works best with spermicidal jelly	Medium to high	Inexpensive: does not cover anterior vaginal wall, so may be more pleasurable for both partners; allows repeated coitus without new application of spermicide	More difficult to fit and to insert than diaphragm; cannot be used if cervical lesions present	Essentially none, but may dislodge during coitus
Contraceptive sponge	Polyurethane sponge with spermicide inserted into vagina before intercourse; must be left in place for 6 hours after coitus	Medium	Easy to insert into vagina; vaginal walls not covered; must be left in place for 6 hours after intercourse; can be used for 24 hours with repeated coitus	Must be removed after 24 hours, or infection can develop	Chemical sensitivity to spermicide; sponge may break
Intravaginal foams, creams, jellies, and suppositories	Spermicidal	Low	Inexpensive; generally available; most effective when used with condom	Regular coital use required; possible messiness; possible interference with enjoyment	Essentially none; possible allergies
Condom	Sperm barrier (a female condom made of polyurethane is placed in the vaginal space before coitus and acts as a sperm barrier)	Medium	Inexpensive; latex condom protects against AIDS; generally available; no professional help required; decreased acquisition of coitally transmitted diseases	Regular coital use required; possible interference with enjoyment	Essentially none; may tear; 3 to 1,000 defective manufacture rate; allergy to latex is rare; used by 12.6% of couples
Intrauterine device (IUD)	Unknown (possibly prevents zygote implantation)	Medium	Inexpensive; only single decision required; not coitally connected; does not interfere with pleasure	Possible increase in bleeding and cramping; requires professional insertion; annual checkup required	Uterine perforation, pelvic infection, spontaneous expulsion; used by 10.2% of women
Oral (hormonal)	Prevention of ovulation (possible interference with sperm mobility); two types: (1) combined progesterone-estrogen, (2) progesterone only (minipill)	High (most commonly used method)	Inexpensive; potential absolute efficiency; not coitally connected	Possible side effects; daily ingestion; requires professional visit and prescription	Thromboembolism, hypertension, depression; used by 36.6% of women
Progestin implants (Norplant)	Suppresses ovulation; high change in cervical mucus	High	Effective for 5 years; no interference with spontaneity or pleasure	Requires minor surgery (local anesthesia) to implant and to remove	Menstrual irregularities, weight gain, headache
Male sterilization (vasectomy)	Surgical interruption of vas deferens so that sperm cannot travel from testes to penis	High	Failure very rare; 20-min office procedure	Morbidity in 1% to 2% of patients includes infections, clots	Can be reversed in only 80% of cases; rare neurotic impotence reaction; used by 10.4% of men
Female sterilization	Tubal ligation prevents transport of oocyte	High	Almost 100% protection; no impairment of sexual function or pleasure	More complex procedure than vasectomy; reversal is complicated and difficult	Surgical morbidity; used by 13.6% of women

Adapted and modified from data by Eugene C. Sandberg, M.D. Effectiveness is rated roughly as follows: low, more than 20 pregnancies for 100 women-years of use; medium, 1 to 20 pregnancies for 100 women-years of use; high, less than 1 pregnancy for 100 women-years of use.

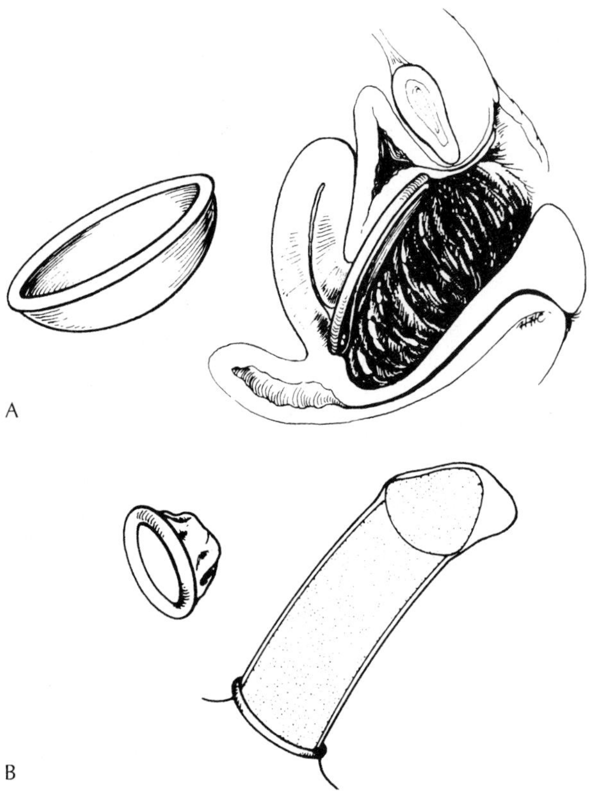

FIGURE 30–2

Pictorial representation of certain contraceptive modalities. **A**. Intravaginal diaphragm and its correct position as viewed during coition. **B**. Condom before and after being unrolled onto the erect penis.

play an active role in the abortion by accompanying her to the hospital or abortion clinic and providing emotional support. Fathers may experience considerable grief over the termination of a wanted pregnancy.

Sterilization

Sterilization is a procedure that prevents a man or a woman from producing offspring. In a woman the procedure is usually salpingectomy, ligation of the fallopian tubes, a procedure with low morbidity and low mortality. A man is usually sterilized by vasectomy, excision of part of the vas deferens. It is a simpler procedure than salpingectomy and may be performed in a physician's office. Voluntary sterilization, especially vasectomy, has become the most popular form of birth control in couples married for more than 10 years.

A small proportion of patients who elect sterilization may suffer a neurotic poststerilization syndrome, which may manifest through hypochondriasis, pain, loss of libido, sexual unresponsiveness, depression, and concerns about masculinity or femininity. One study of a group of women who regretted sterilization reported they had chosen the procedure while in poor relationships, frequently with abusing husbands. Regret is most prevalent when a woman forms a new relationship and wishes to have a child with a new partner. Psychiatric consultation may be necessary to separate persons seeking sterilization for irrational or psychotic reasons from those who have made the decision after some time and thought.

In the United States, involuntary sterilization procedures have been performed to prevent the reproduction of traits considered genetically undesirable, and various statutes allowed sterilization of hereditary criminals, sex offenders, syphilitic

Table 30–5
Abortion Techniques

Type	Benefits	Risks
Cervical dilation and evacuation of uterine contents by curettage or vacuum aspiration	Most commonly performed procedure for termination of pregnancy; can be done before 16 weeks' gestation	Uterine perforation Cervical incompetence Adhesions Hemorrhage Infection Incomplete removal of fetus and placenta
Menstrual aspiration (miniabortion)	Can be done within 1 to 3 weeks of missed period	Implanted zygote not removed Uterine perforation (rare) Failure to recognize ectopic pregnancy
Medical induction (cervical dilation with laminaria followed by high dose of IV oxytocin)	Can be used for second-trimester abortions	Water intoxication Rupture of uterus, cervix, or isthmus
Intraamniotic hyperosmotic solutions (salting out)	Can be used for second-trimester abortions	Hyperosmolar crisis Heart failure Peritonitis Hemorrhage Water intoxication Myometrial necrosis Accounts for only 2% of abortions
Prostaglandins (applied intravaginally, cervically, or intraamniotically)	Noninvasive procedure	Expulsion of live fetus
Mifepristone (Mifeprex), i.e., RU-486	Noninvasive procedure; can be used in pregnancies up to 49 days' duration	Excessive bleeding

patients, mentally retarded persons, and persons with epilepsy. Some of these statutes have been declared unconstitutional, and human rights and civil liberties groups have challenged the legality and ethical standing of such sterilization procedures with increasing vigor.

The operative procedures for sterilization have assumed less importance than in the past because of the advent of contraceptives and the relative ease of obtaining abortions. Nonetheless, sterilization procedures are still chosen by men and women who, for a variety of reasons, want to permanently end their ability to produce children.

Vasectomy. In a vasectomy a man's vas deferens is ligated bilaterally, and a segment is removed. The procedure is done under local anesthesia and takes about 20 minutes. The procedure can be reversed in 80 to 90 percent of cases. A few men experience a postvasectomy syndrome consisting of decreased libido, impotence, identity confusion, and signs of depression. Most of these men had been depressed prior to the vasectomy, however. No negative psychological sequelae are experienced in most cases of male sterilization.

Tubal Ligation. In tubal ligation the woman's fallopian tubes are cauterized by laparotomy. Reversal of the procedure is far less effective than reversal of vasectomy in men. A small proportion of women develop a poststerilization syndrome consisting of hypochondria, pain, loss of libido, and doubt about female identity; generally, this occurs in women with a preexisting psychopathological state. Psychiatric consultation before sterilization is useful for evaluating motivation for the procedure (e.g., coercion by a partner) and for ruling out preexisting psychopathology, such as depression, that may lead to poststerilization syndrome.

Reproductive Senescence

Both men and women age and experience an age-related decline in reproductive capacity, but only women experience complete gonadal cessation. Loss of reproductive capacity may present a psychological challenge to those who are not reconciled to the loss of fertility. However, even with gonadal failure, the availability of donor oocytes and sperm means that pregnancy can be initiated in a menopausal woman with an intact uterus who elects to pursue that option.

Menopause. Menopause, the cessation of ovulation, generally occurs between 47 and 53 years of age. The hypoestrogenism that follows can lead to hot flashes, sleep disturbances, vaginal atrophy and dryness, and cognitive and affective disturbances. Women are at increased risk for osteoporosis, dementia, and cardiovascular disease. Depression at menopause has been attributed to the empty nest syndrome. However, many women report an enhanced sense of well-being and enjoy opportunities to pursue goals postponed because of child rearing.

Hormone Replacement Therapy. The pros and cons of hormone replacement therapy have not been fully clarified; thus the question of whether to initiate or continue this therapy can pose a medical, financial, and philosophical challenge. There are studies that show estrogen use confers cardioprotection and neuroprotection, retards bone loss and urogenital atrophy, and stabilizes mood; however, other more recent studies have raised serious questions about some of these protective effects, especially on the cardiovascular system. Several studies have found that women who use hormone replacement therapy gain less weight, and the weight they do gain is deposited preferentially in a gynecoid (hips and thighs) rather than android (abdominal) pattern. Ongoing estrogen use may reduce the risk of Alzheimer's disease and other dementias. There is evidence of an association between estrogen use and breast cancer; therefore, hormone replacement therapy is problematic in women who have survived breast cancer. Hypoestrogenism can impair sexual enjoyment and libido and cause hot flashes, night sweats, and profound fatigue. These sequelae can generally be ameliorated or reversed with estrogen use.

Progestin use is generally recommended for women with a uterus to guard against development of endometrial hyperplasia and carcinoma; whether or to what degree progestin use compromises the beneficial effects of estrogen use needs clarification. The adverse effects that most limit progestin use are depression and bloating. Women who previously suffered from depression or premenstrual syndrome (PMS) are most prone to mood disturbances with progestin use.

In general, hormone replacement therapy enhances psychological functioning and promotes overall health. There are some data to support the notion that antidepressant and antidementia agents are more efficacious in women when they are taking hormone replacement therapy. Since hormone replacement may last well over 30 years, it is worth titrating and individualizing route, dosage, type, and regimen with the goal of maximizing benefit and minimizing adverse effects. The recent introduction of a wide range of estrogen and progestin products, including so-called designer estrogens or selective estrogen receptor modulators (SERMs), has expanded options; however, there is even less information about the long-term risks and benefits of partial estrogen agonists than about more conventional estrogen preparations.

Andropause, a term for the male climacteric, is caused by decreasing testosterone production. Inadequate testicular androgen production (hypogonadism) may be associated with loss of libido, fatigue, and depression, which can be reversed with testosterone therapy. Use of androgen replacement therapy in aging males is controversial because of cardiotoxicity and the risk of prostate cancer. Because of its catabolic effects growth hormone and growth hormone–releasing hormone (GHRH) have been used in aging males to increase muscle mass and general sense of well-being.

OTHER ISSUES

Sexually Transmitted Diseases

A sexually transmitted disease (STD) is a contagious disease acquired as a result of a physical sexual interaction. STDs always have been a reality, but from the 1950s through 1970s the infections were considered treatable and not life threatening. Acquired immune deficiency syndrome (AIDS), which is caused by infection with human immunodeficiency virus (HIV), is currently incurable, life threatening, and transmissible from mother to fetus. The specter of AIDS has captured the popular imagination.

Although it was initially found in male homosexuals and intravenous drug abusers, HIV knows no boundaries.

A sequela of STDs such as gonorrhea and chlamydia is pelvic inflammatory disease (PID). Untreated PID can develop into bilateral tuboovarian abscesses and necessitate hysterectomy and bilateral salpingo-oophorectomy. Early antibiotic treatment is advocated to prevent development of the abscesses and to reduce the likelihood of infertility, chronic pelvic pain, and ectopic pregnancy from tubal damage. These infections also can lead to obstruction of the vas deferens and chronic prostatitis and subsequent male infertility.

Another STD that can have serious consequences is venereal warts, or human papilloma virus (HPV). Genital infections with certain subtypes of HPV can lead to premalignant changes of the penis, vulva, vagina, and cervix and are thought to cause cervical cancer. Venereal warts can be removed chemically or surgically but are difficult to eradicate completely. Women who contract HPV are encouraged to have regular gynecological examinations and Papanicolaou smears to detect premalignant lesions.

Sexual monogamy and abstinence will prevent most STDs and are advocated as public health measures. However, libidinal impulses can be difficult to control and restrict. Therefore, measures such as condom use are strongly recommended as an alternative public health measure. Adolescents, in particular, need to know the potential consequences of sexual activity with regard to STDs and pregnancy. Admonishing teens to remain chaste is unlikely to be completely effective and may be counterproductive. The risks of sexual intercourse may be forgotten or seem minimal in comparison to the need for affection or escape. Persons with low self-esteem or under stress may view sex as a means of bolstering their self-image or escaping their stresses. The reinforcing properties of sex ensure that the problem of STDs will endure. Studies in Europe have shown that easy availability of condoms (such as in schools) reduces both STDs and unwanted pregnancies.

Pelvic Pain

Pelvic pain can have many causes, including endometriosis, pelvic adhesions, ovarian or adnexal masses, hernias, and bowel or rectal disease. Pelvic pain can also be secondary to psychogenic causes such as guilt, fertility, or infertility fears, and the emotional disturbances associated with ongoing or past incest or sexual abuse. Pelvic pain should not be attributed to psychogenic causes unless a thorough evaluation has excluded organic causes. In most instances, the evaluation should include a diagnostic laparoscopy. Likewise, dyspareunia or pain with intercourse should not be assumed to have a psychogenic origin unless all anatomical causes have been excluded.

Premenstrual Dysphoric Disorder

Premenstrual dysphoric disorder is a somatopsychic illness triggered by changing levels of sex steroids that accompany an ovulatory menstrual cycle (Fig. 30–3). It occurs about 1 week before the onset of menses and is characterized by irritability, emotional lability, headache, anxiety, and depression. Somatic symptoms include edema, weight gain, breast pain, syncope, and paresthesias. Approximately 5 percent of women have the disorder. Treatment is symptomatic and includes analgesics for pain and sedatives for anxiety and insomnia. Some patients respond to short courses of selective serotonin reuptake inhibitors (SSRIs). Fluid retention is relieved with diuretics. See Section 15.3 for a more complete discussion of this disorder.

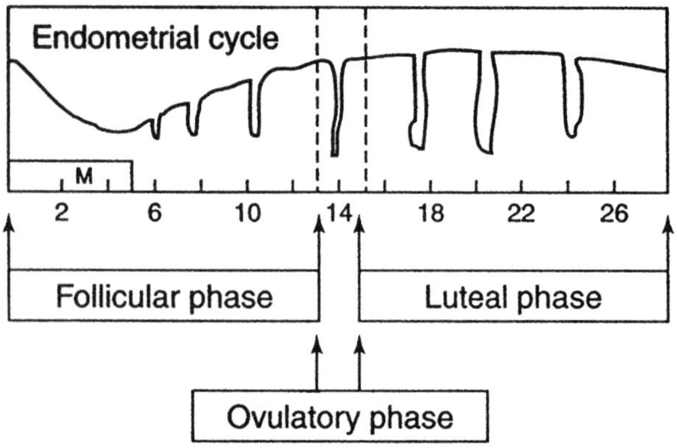

FIGURE 30–3
The idealized cyclic changes in uterine endometrium during the normal menstrual cycle. Days of menstrual bleeding are indicated by M. (From Beers MG, Berkow R, eds. *The Merck Manual of Diagnosis and Therapy.* 17th ed. Whitehouse Station, NJ: Merck Research Laboratories; 2000:1929, with permission.)

References

Adler B. Reproductive and obstetric issues. In: Johnston DW, Johnston M, eds. *Health Psychology.* Vol 8. *Comprehensive Clinical Psychology.* Amsterdam: Elsevier Science Publishers; 2001:383.

Annas GJ. Protecting the liberty of pregnant patients. *N Engl J Med.* 1987;316:1213.

Berga SL, Parry PL. Psychiatry and reproductive medicine. In: Sadock BJ, Sadock VA, eds. *Kaplan & Sadock's Comprehensive Textbook of Psychiatry.* 7th ed. Vol 1. Baltimore: Lippincott Williams & Wilkins; 2000:1935.

Freeman MP, Keck PE Jr, McElroy SL. Postpartum depression with bipolar disorder. *Am J Psychiatry.* 2001;158:652.

Hoffman NS. Stress factors related to antenatal testing during high-risk pregnancy. *J Perinatol.* 1990;10:195.

Hutchison KE, Stevens VM, Collins FL. Cigarette smoking and the intention to quit among pregnant smokers. *Behav Med.* 1996;19:307.

McDuffie RS Jr, Beck A, Bischoff K, Cross J, Orleans M. Effects of frequency of prenatal care visits on perinatal outcome among low-risk women: a randomized controlled trial. *JAMA.* 1996;275:847.

Nelson HD, Humphrey LL, Nygen P. Postmenopausal hormone replacement therapy: scientific review. *JAMA.* 2002;288:882.

Rofe Y, Blittner M, Lewin I. Emotional experiences during the three trimesters of pregnancy. *J Clin Psychol.* 1993;49:3.

Tasker F, Golumbok S. Adults raised as children in lesbian families. *Am J Orthopsychiatry.* 1995;65:203.

Victor SB, Fish MC. Lesbian mothers and the children: a review for school psychologists. *School Psychol Rev.* 1995;24:456.

Webster J, Chandler J, Battistutta D. Pregnancy outcomes and health care use: effects of abuse. *Am J Obstet Gynecol.* 1996;142:760.

Whiteford LM, Gonzoles L. Stigma: the hidden burden of infertility. *Soc Sci Med.* 1995;40:27.

31

Relational Problems

Most persons live in a matrix of relationships in which they find connection, comfort, intimacy, and happiness. However, they also experience obligation, responsibility, compromise, and friction. A person's psychological health and sense of well-being depends to a significant degree upon the qualities of one's relationships, that is, upon the patterns of interaction with one's partner and children, parents and siblings, friends and colleagues. The ability to function in a variety of relationships can be stressed by psychological problems as well as by external events such as illness, war, natural disaster, economic crisis, and social change. Persons can feel depressed or isolated at the loss or lack of relationships.

DEFINITION

According to the text revision of the fourth edition of *Diagnostic and Statistical Manual of Mental Disorders* (DSM-IV-TR), relational problems are patterns of interaction between members of a relational unit that are associated with symptoms or significantly impaired functioning in one or more individual members or with significantly impaired functioning of the relational unit itself. DSM-IV-TR distinguishes five categories of relational problems. The first category, relational problem related to a mental or general medical condition, deals with the association between relationships and health. The other categories focus on problems in specific relational units: parent–child relational problem, partner relational problem, sibling relational problem, and relational problem not otherwise specified.

EPIDEMIOLOGY

No reliable figures are available on the prevalence of relational problems. One can assume they are ubiquitous; however, most relational problems resolve without professional intervention. The nature, frequency, and effects of the problem on those involved are elements that must be considered before a diagnosis of relational problem is made. For example, divorce, which occurs in just under 50 percent of marriages, is a problem between partners that is resolved through the legal remedy of divorce and need not be diagnosed as a relational problem. However, if the persons cannot resolve the disputation between them and continue to live together in a sadomasochistic or pathologically depressed relationship with unhappiness and abuse, then they should be so labeled. Relationship problems that cannot be resolved by friends, family, or clergy of the persons involved will need professional intervention by psychiatrists, clinical psychologists, social workers, and other mental health professionals.

RELATIONAL PROBLEM RELATED TO A MENTAL DISORDER OR GENERAL MEDICAL CONDITION

According to DSM-IV-TR, clinicians should use the category relational problems related to a mental disorder or general medical condition when the focus of clinical attention is a pattern of impaired interaction associated with a mental disorder or a general medical condition in a family member.

Adults must often assume responsibility for caring for aging parents while they are still caring for their own children, and this dual obligation can create stress. When adults take care of their parents, both parties must adapt to a reversal of their former roles, and the caretakers not only face the potential loss of their parents, but also must cope with evidence of their own mortality.

Some caretakers abuse their aging parents—a problem that is now receiving attention. Abuse is most likely to occur when the caretaking offspring have substance abuse problems, are under economic stress, and have no relief from their caretaking duties, or when the parent is bedridden or has a chronic illness requiring constant nursing attention. More women are abused than men, and most abuse occurs in persons over age 75.

The development of a chronic illness in a family member stresses the family system and requires adaptation by both the sick person and the other family members. The person who has become sick must frequently face a loss of autonomy, an increased sense of vulnerability, and sometimes a taxing medical regimen. The other family members must experience the loss of the person as he or she was before the illness, and they usually have substantial caretaking responsibility—for example, in debilitating neurological diseases, including dementia of the Alzheimer's type, and in diseases such as acquired immune deficiency syndrome (AIDS) and cancer. In these cases, the whole family must deal with the stress of prospective death as well as the current illness. Some families use the anger engendered by such situations to create support organizations, increase public awareness of the disease, and rally around the sick member. But chronic illness frequently produces depression in family members and may cause them to withdraw from, or attack, one another. The burden of caring for ill family members falls disproportionately on the women in a family—mothers, daughters, and daughters-in-law.

Chronic emotional illness also requires major adaptations by families. For instance, family members may react with chaos or fear to the psychotic productions of a family member with

schizophrenia. The schizophrenic person's regression, exaggerated emotions, frequent hospitalizations, and economic and social dependence can stress the family system. Family members may react with hostile feelings (referred to as *expressed emotion*) that are associated with a poor prognosis for the person who is sick. Similarly, a family member with bipolar I disorder can disrupt a family, particularly during manic episodes.

Family devastation can occur when illness suddenly strikes a previously healthy person, when illness occurs earlier than expected in the life cycle (some impairment of physical capacities is expected in old age, although many older persons are healthy), when illness affects the economic stability of the family, and when little can be done to improve or ease the condition of the sick family member.

PARENT–CHILD RELATIONAL PROBLEM

Parents differ widely in sensing the needs of their infants. Some quickly note their child's moods and needs; others are slow to respond. Parental responsiveness interacts with the child's temperament to affect the quality of the attachment between child and parent.

According to DSM-IV-TR, this diagnosis applies when the focus of clinical attention is a pattern of interaction between parent and child that is associated with clinically significant impairment in individual or family functioning or with clinically significant symptoms. Examples include impaired communication, overprotection, and inadequate discipline.

Difficulties in many situations stress the usual parent–child interaction. In a family in which the parents are divorced, parent–child problems may arise in the relationship with either the custodial or the noncustodial parent. The remarriage of a divorced or widowed parent can also lead to a parent–child problem. The resentment of a stepparent by a stepchild and the favoring of a natural child are usual reactions in a new family's initial phases of adjustment. When a second child is born, both familial stress and happiness may result, although happiness is the dominant emotion in most families. The birth of a child can also be troublesome when parents had adopted a child in the belief that they were infertile.

Other situations that may produce a parent–child problem are the development of fatal, crippling, or chronic illness, such as leukemia, epilepsy, sickle-cell anemia, or spinal cord injury, in either parent or child. The birth of a child with congenital defects, such as cerebral palsy, blindness, and deafness, may also produce parent–child problems. These situations, which are not rare, challenge the emotional resources of those involved. Parents and child must face present and potential loss and must adjust their day-to-day lives physically, economically, and emotionally. These situations can strain the healthiest families and produce parent–child problems not only with the sick person but also with the unaffected family members. In a family with a severely sick child, parents may resent, prefer, or neglect the other children because the ill child requires so much time and attention.

Parents with children who have emotional disorders face particular problems, depending on the child's illness. In families with a child with schizophrenia, family treatment is beneficial and improves the social adjustment of the patient. Similarly, family therapy is useful if there is a child with mood disorder. In families with a substance-abusing child or adolescent, family involvement is crucial to help control the drug-seeking behavior and to allow family members to verbalize the feelings of frustration and anger that are invariably present.

Normal developmental crises can also be related to parent–child problems. For instance, adolescence is a time of frequent conflict, as the adolescent resists rules and demands increasing autonomy, while at the same time eliciting protective control by displaying immature and dangerous behavior.

The parents of sons aged 18, 15, and 11 years presented with distress about the behavior of their middle child. The family had been cohesive with satisfactory relationships among all members until 6 months prior to this consultation. At that time the 15-year-old began seeing a girl from a comparatively unsupervised household. Frequent arguments had developed between parents and son regarding going out on school nights, curfews, and neglect of schoolwork. The son's combativeness and lowered academic achievement upset his parents a great deal. They had not experienced similar conflicts with their oldest child. However, the adolescent maintained a good relationship with his siblings and friends, was not a behavior problem at school, continued to participate on the school basketball team, and was not a substance user.

Day Care Centers

Quality of care during the first 3 years of life is crucial to neuropsychological development. A 1997 study from the National Institute of Child Health and Human Development indicated that day care was not harmful to children, provided that the caregivers and day care teachers provided consistent, empathetic, nurturing care. Unfortunately, not all day care centers can meet that level of care, especially those located in poor urban areas. Children receiving less than optimal caring exhibit decreased intellectual and verbal skills that indicate delayed neurocognitive development. They may also become irritable, anxious, or depressed, which interferes with the parent–child bonding experience, and they are less assertive and less effectively toilet trained by the age of 5.

Currently, over 55 percent of women are in the work force, many of whom have no choice but to place their children in day care centers. Approximately 40 percent of entering medical students are women; unfortunately, few medical centers make adequate provisions for on-site day care centers for their students or staff. Similarly, corporations need to provide on-site, high-quality care for the children of their employees. Not only will that approach benefit the children, but also corporate economic benefits will accrue as a result of reduced absenteeism, increased productivity, and happier working mothers. Such programs have the added benefit of decreasing stresses on marriages.

PARTNER RELATIONAL PROBLEM

According to DSM-IV-TR, clinicians should use the category partner relational problem when the focus of clinical attention is a pattern of interaction between the spouses or partners.

These patterns are characterized by negative communication (e.g., criticisms), distorted communication (e.g., unrealistic expectations), or noncommunication (e.g., withdrawal), associated with clinically significant impairment in individual or family functioning or symptoms in one or both partners.

When persons have partner relational problems, psychiatrists must assess whether a patient's distress arises from the relationship or from a mental disorder. Mental disorders are more common in single persons—those who never married or who are widowed, separated, or divorced—than among married persons. Clinicians should evaluate developmental, sexual, and occupational and relationship histories, for purposes of diagnosis. (Divorce is discussed in Chapter 2, Section 2.4, and couples therapy is discussed in Chapter 35, Section 35.4.)

Marriage demands a sustained level of adaptation from both partners. In a troubled marriage, a therapist can encourage the partners to explore areas such as the extent of communication between the partners, their ways of solving disputes, their attitudes toward child-bearing and child rearing, their relationships with their in-laws, their attitudes toward social life, their handling of finances, and their sexual interaction. The birth of a child, an abortion or miscarriage, economic stresses, moves to new areas, episodes of illness, major career changes, and any situations that involve a significant change in marital roles can precipitate stressful periods in a relationship. Illness in a child exerts the greatest strain on a marriage, and marriages in which a child has died through illness or accident more often than not end in divorce. Complaints of lifelong anorgasmia or impotence by marital partners usually indicate intrapsychic problems, although sexual dissatisfaction is involved in many cases of marital maladjustment.

Adjustment to marital roles can be a problem when partners are from different backgrounds and have grown up with different value systems. For example, members of low socioeconomic status groups perceive a wife as making most of the decisions in the family, and they accept physical punishment as a way to discipline children. Middle-class persons perceive family decision-making processes as shared, with the husband often being the final arbiter, and they prefer to discipline children verbally. Problems involving conflicts in values, adjustment to new roles, and poor communication are handled most effectively when therapist and partners examine the couple's relationship, as in marital therapy.

Physician Marriages

Physicians have a higher risk of divorce than other occupational groups. A 1997 study reported in the *New England Journal of Medicine* found that the incidence of divorce among physicians was 29 percent. Specialty choice influenced divorce. The highest rate of divorce occurred in psychiatrists (50 percent), followed by surgeons (33 percent) and internists, pediatricians, and pathologists (31 percent). The average age at first marriage was 26 years among all groups.

It is not clear why physicians (including psychiatrists) are at high risk for divorce. Factors implicated include the stresses of dealing with dying patients, making life-and-death decisions, working long hours, and the constant risk of malpractice litigation. Such stressors may predispose physicians to a variety of emotional ills, with the most common being depression and substance abuse, including alcoholism. Such persons generally cannot deal with the complex interactions required to maintain successful long-term relationships of any kind, and marriage requires the most interpersonal skills of all.

SIBLING RELATIONAL PROBLEM

According to DSM-IV-TR, clinicians should use the category sibling relational problem when the focus of clinical attention is a pattern of sibling interaction associated with clinically significant impairment in individual or family functioning or symptoms in one or more siblings. Problems arising from sibling rivalry can occur with the birth of a child and can recur as children grow up. Competition among children for the attention, affection, and esteem of their parents is a fact of family life. This rivalry can extend to others who are not siblings and can remain a factor in normal and abnormal competitiveness throughout life. In some families, children receive labels early in life, such as "the good child" or "the black sheep," and they may turn these labels into self-fulfilling prophecies. In good sibling relationships, the pleasures of companionship and the bonds created by kinship and shared experiences outweigh feelings of rivalry.

RELATIONAL PROBLEM NOT OTHERWISE SPECIFIED

Racial and religious prejudices can cause problems in interpersonal relationships. Some social scientists believe that racism and religious bigotry have only a weak psychological base, and they emphasize social and class factors as causative. Other investigators view prejudice as a learned attitude and consider it a cultural variant. Several psychiatrists think that persons are motivated to change their prejudices only if they see them as part of a mental disorder. When prejudice is a maladaptive defense built to protect the prejudiced person from profound feelings of inadequacy, it involves the projection of unwanted and devalued attributes onto the blamed group.

In the workplace, sexual harassment is often a combination of inappropriate sexual interactions, displays of power and dominance, and expressions of negative gender stereotypes. Relational difficulties resulting from sexual harassment can be classified under this diagnosis.

References

Brody GH, Stoneman Z, Gauger K. Parent–child relationships, family problem-solving behavior, and sibling relationship quality: the moderating role of sibling temperaments. *Child Dev.* 1996;67:1289.

Cook WL. Interdependence and the interpersonal sense of control: an analysis of family relationships. *J Pers Soc Psychol.* 1993;64:587.

Cummings EM, Goeke-Morey MC, Graham MA. Interparental relations as a dimension of parenting. In: Borkowski JG, Ramey SL, eds. *Parenting and the Child's World: Influences on Academic, Intellectual, and Social-Emotional Development.* Monographs in parenting. Mahwah, NJ: Lawrence Erlbaum Associates; 2002:251.

Flanagan KM, Clements ML, Whitton SW, Portney MJ, Randall DW, Markman HJ. Retrospect and prospect in the psychological study of marital and couple relationships. In: McHale JP, Grolnick WS, eds. *Retrospect and Prospect in the Psychological Study of Families.* Mahwah, NJ: Lawrence Erlbaum Associates; 2002:99.

Galambos NL. Parent–adolescent relations. *Curr Direct Psychol Sci.* 1992;1:146.

Gonzales NA, Cauce AM, Friedman RJ, Mason CA. Family, peer, and neighborhood influences on academic achievement among African-American ado-

lescents: one-year prospective effects. *Am J Community Psychol.* 1996; 24:365.

Hibbs ED, Hamburger SD, Kruesi MJ, Lenane M. Factors affecting expressed emotion in parents of ill and normal children. *Am J Orthopsychiatry.* 1993;63:103.

Jouriles EN, Farris AM. Effects of marital conflict on subsequent parent–son interactions. *Behav Ther.* 1992;23:355.

Leach P, Eyer DE. Women's behavior: do mothers harm their children when they work outside the home? In: Walsh MR, ed. *Women, Men, & Gender: Ongoing Debates.* New Haven: Yale University Press; 1997:383.

Legazpi-Blair MC, Blair SL. Choice of child care and mother–child interaction: racial/ethnic distinctions in the maternal experience. In: Jacobson CK, ed. *American Families: Issues in Race and Ethnicity.* New York: Garland Publishing; 1995:261.

Newman J. The more the merrier? Effects of family size and sibling spacing on sibling relationships. *Child Care Health Dev.* 1996;22:285.

Robinson BE. Relationship between work addiction and family functioning: clinical implications for marriage and family therapists. *J Fam Psychother.* 1996;7:13.

Teti DM. Retrospect and prospect in the psychological study of sibling relationships. In: McHale JP, Grolnick WS, eds. *Retrospect and Prospect in the Psychological Study of Families.* Mahwah, NJ: Lawrence Erlbaum Associates; 2002:193.

Tuttle DH, Cornell DG. Maternal labeling of gifted children: effects on the sibling relationship. *Except Child.* 1993;59:402.

Van der Henst J-B, Sperber D, Politzer G. When is a conclusion worth deriving? A relevance-based analysis of indeterminate relational problems. *Thinking & Reasoning.* 2002;8:1.

Verhulst JMF. Relational problems. In: Sadock BJ, Sadock VA, eds. *Kaplan & Sadock's Comprehensive Textbook of Psychiatry.* 7th ed. Vol 2. Baltimore: Lippincott Williams & Wilkins; 2000:1888.

32 Problems Related to Abuse or Neglect

The text revision of the fourth edition of *Diagnostic and Statistical Manual of Mental Disorders* (DSM-IV-TR) specifies five problems related to abuse or neglect: (1) physical abuse of child, (2) sexual abuse of child, (3) neglect of child, and (4) physical abuse of adult, and (5) sexual abuse of adult (Table 32–1). Physical abuse of adult includes spouse or partner abuse and abuse of elderly persons. Sexual abuse of adult includes rape, sexual coercion, and sexual harassment.

CHILD ABUSE AND NEGLECT

Girls and boys of all ages, ethnic groups, and socioeconomic levels experience alarmingly high rates of child abuse and neglect, which are associated with a wide range of emotional problems and psychiatric symptoms. Children who are beaten or burned, repeatedly sexually assaulted, or deprived of food, clothing, and shelter may perish or may survive to struggle with the consequences. In most cases of persistent incest, sexually abused children are threatened with further abuse or abandonment if they disclose the family secrets; such treatment leaves them in the irreconcilable position of silently enduring continued abuse or risking the total loss of their families.

Children who have been physically or sexually abused exhibit many psychiatric disturbances, including anxiety, aggressive behavior, paranoid ideation, posttraumatic stress disorder, depressive disorders, and an increased risk of suicidal behavior. Abuse seems to increase the risk of psychiatric disturbances in already vulnerable children, and abused children of parents with psychopathology are more likely to experience a mental disorder than nonabused children of psychiatrically disturbed parents. Children who have been sexually abused reportedly have an increased frequency of poor self-esteem, depression, dissociative disorders, and substance abuse. Chronic maltreatment appears to promote aggressive and violent behavior in vulnerable children.

Epidemiology

According to the U.S. Department of Health and Human Services, about 2.9 million cases of possible child abuse and neglect were reported to public social service agencies in 1999, and about 826,000 of these cases were substantiated. In 1999, 58.4 percent of victims suffered neglect, 21.3 percent were physically abused, and 1.3 percent were sexually abused. In the United States, child abuse and neglect caused an estimated 1,100 deaths. An estimated one of every three to four girls and one of every seven to eight boys will be sexually assaulted by the age of 18 years. The actual occurrence rates are likely to be higher than these estimates, because many maltreated children go unrecognized, and many are reluctant to report the abuse. Of the children who are physically abused, 32 percent are less than 5 years of age; 27 percent are between 5 and 9 years; 27 percent are between 10 and 14 years; and 14 percent are between 15 and 18 years. More than 50 percent of all abused and neglected children were born prematurely or had low birth weights. Most child maltreatment is at the hands of parents (75 percent), other relatives (15 percent), or an unrelated caretaker (10 percent).

Sexual attacks on children by groups of other children have recently increased. Of 1,600 young offenders whose cases of sexual abuse of other children were analyzed by a university abuse-prevention center, more than 25 percent had started before the age of 12 years. Group leaders had often been abused themselves. However, followers seemed to succumb to peer pressure and to a society that glamorizes violence and links violence with sex.

Etiology

Many factors contribute to child abuse and neglect. Abusive parents have themselves often been victims of physical and sexual abuse and of long-term exposure to violent home lives of pain and physical torment, which are powerful promoters of aggression. Thus, parents brought up with harsh corporal punishment and cruel treatment by their own families may continue the abuse tradition with their children. In some cases, adults believe that their methods are acceptable ways of teaching discipline. In other cases, parents are ambivalent about their methods of abusive parenting but find themselves without coping mechanisms and so fall into behaviors similar to those of their own parents.

Stressful living conditions, such as overcrowding and poverty, can contribute to aggressive behavior and may contribute to physical abuse toward children. Social isolation, the lack of a support system, and parental substance abuse increase the potential for abusive and neglectful treatment of children. When such environmental crises as unemployment, housing problems, and financial need heighten stress levels in vulnera-

Table 32–1
DSM-IV-TR Problems Related to Abuse or Neglect

Physical abuse of child
This category should be used when the focus of clinical attention is physical abuse of a child.
Sexual abuse of child
This category should be used when the focus of clinical attention is sexual abuse of a child.
Neglect of child
This category should be used when the focus of clinical attention is child neglect.
Physical abuse of adult
This category should be used when the focus of clinical attention is physical abuse of an adult (e.g., spouse beating, abuse of elderly parent).
Sexual abuse of adult
This category should be used when the focus of clinical attention is sexual abuse of an adult (e.g., sexual coercion, rape).

ble families, neglect or abuse may ensue. Mental disorders can play a role in child abuse and neglect insofar as a parent's judgment and thought processes may be impaired. Parents who are depressed or psychotic or who have severe personality disorders may view their children as bad or as trying to drive them crazy.

Certain characteristics may increase a child's vulnerability to neglect and physical and sexual abuse. Children who are premature, mentally retarded, or physically disabled and those who cry excessively or are unusually demanding—the so-called difficult child—may be at high risk for abuse or neglect. Many abused children are perceived by their parents as different, slow in development, bad, selfish, or hard to discipline. Children who are hyperactive are particularly vulnerable to abuse, especially when they are born to parents with limited capacities for nurturant behavior. A child who is the object of physical abuse is also known as a *battered child.*

The perpetrator of physical abuse is more often the mother than the father. One parent is usually the active batterer, and the other passively accepts the battering. Of a group of perpetrators studied, 80 percent were regularly living in the homes of the children they abused. More than 80 percent of the children studied were living with married parents, and about 20 percent were living with a single parent. The average age of a mother who abuses her children is reportedly about 26 years; the father's average age is 30 years. Many abused children come from poor homes, and the families tend to be socially isolated.

Abusive parents have inappropriate expectations of their children, with a reversal of dependence needs. Parents treat an abused child as if the child were older than the parents. A parent often turns to the child for reassurance, nurturing, comfort, and protection and expects a loving response. Ninety percent of such parents were severely physically abused by their own mothers or fathers.

Men usually perpetrate sexual abuse, although women acting in concert with men or alone are also involved, especially in child pornography. Men are the perpetrators in about 95 percent of cases of sexual abuse of girls and about 80 percent of cases of sexual abuse of boys. Perpetrators of sexual abuse are usually known to the child and in many cases have been victims of physical or sexual abuse. In some circumstances, pedophilia is a factor; the adult perpetrator is more aroused by children than by adult partners. Many times, however, the perpetrator has no preference for child sexual partners. In some cases sexual abuse is mixed with physical abuse.

Diagnosis and Clinical Features

Physical Abuse of Child. Clinicians must always consider physical abuse when a child shows bruises or injuries that cannot be adequately explained or that are incompatible with the history that the parent gives. Suspicious physical indicators are bruises and marks that form symmetrical patterns, such as injuries to both sides of the face and regular patterns on the back, buttocks, and thighs; accidental injuries are unlikely to result in symmetrical patterns. Bruises may have the shape of the instrument used to make them, such as a belt buckle or a cord. Burns by cigarettes result in symmetrical, round scars, and immersions in boiling water produce burns that look like socks or gloves or that are doughnut-shaped. Physical aggression can cause multiple and spiral fractures, especially in a young baby; retinal hemorrhages in an infant may be due to shaking.

Children repeatedly brought to hospitals for treatment of peculiar or puzzling problems by overly cooperative parents may be victims of Munchausen syndrome by proxy, that is, factitious disorder. In this abuse scenario, a parent repeatedly inflicts illness on, or causes injury to, a child—by injecting toxins or by inducing the child to ingest drugs or toxins to cause diarrhea, dehydration, or other symptoms—and then eagerly seeks medical attention. Because the pathological parents are stealthy and superficially compliant, this diagnosis is difficult to make.

In hospital emergency rooms, severely abused children show external evidence of body trauma, bruises, abrasions, cuts, lacerations, burns, soft tissue swellings, and hematomas (Fig. 32–1). Hypernatremic dehydration, after periodic water deprivation of children by mothers who are usually psychotic, is another form of child abuse. Inability to move certain extremities because of dislocations and fractures associated with neurological signs of intracranial damage can also indicate inflicted trauma. Other clinical signs and symptoms attributed to inflicted abuse may include injury to the viscera. Abdominal trauma may result in unexplained ruptures of the stomach, the bowel, the liver, or the pancreas, with manifestations of an injured abdomen. Children with the most severe maltreatment injuries arrive at the hospital or physician's office in a coma or in convulsions; some arrive dead.

Behaviorally, abused children may appear withdrawn and frightened or may show aggressive behavior and labile mood. They often exhibit depression, poor self-esteem, and anxiety. They may try to physically cover up injuries and are usually reticent to disclose the abuse for fear of retaliation. Abused children often show some delay in developmental milestones, may

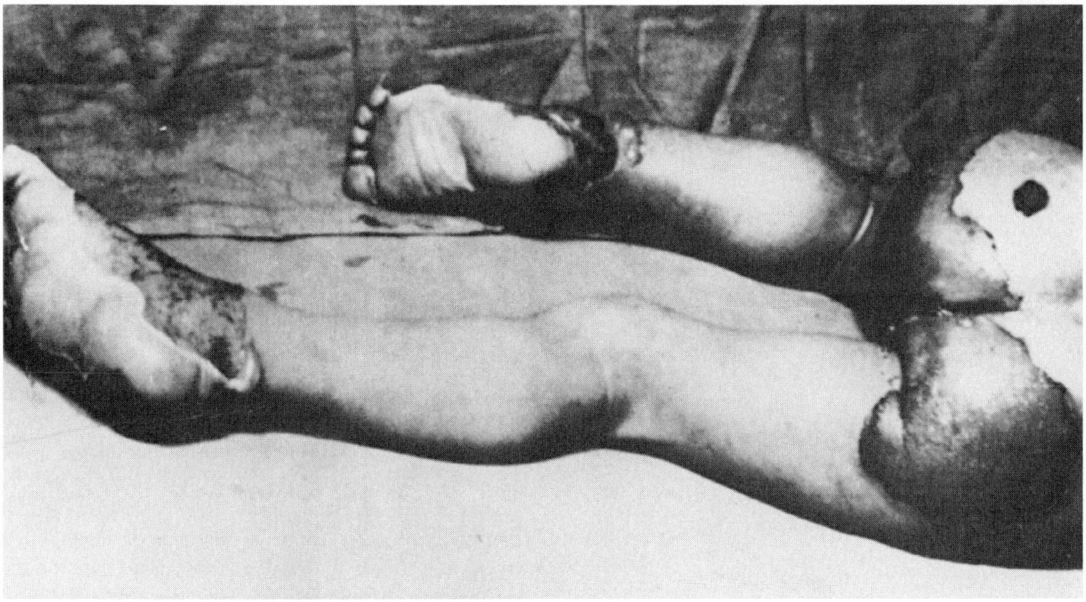

FIGURE 32–1
A $3\frac{1}{2}$-year-old boy, brought into an emergency room by his mother, had second-degree burns of his buttocks, perineum, hands, and feet. His mother related that the child accidentally fell into a tub of hot water while preparing to take a bath. Physical examination revealed no evidence of burns along the body area. The location of the burns led physicians to suspect that the child's buttocks were forced into boiling water, and, in an attempt to keep himself from being submerged, he extended his feet and hands into the water. Scalding injury to his feet, perineum, and buttocks caused burn areas corresponding to the child's posture on dunking. His mother later admitted that a boyfriend had placed the child into a tub of hot water while she was out shopping. (Courtesy of Vincent J. Fontana, M.D.)

have difficulties with peer relationships, and may engage in self-destructive or suicidal behaviors.

A 16-month-old boy was brought to the hospital emergency room because of burns from scalding water. The child had patches of erythema on his abdomen, down the sides of his legs, and on the medial aspect of his upper arms. The diapered area had been protected from the heat. While the emergency room staff proceeded with their assessment and treatment, the child abuse consultant interviewed the parents separately. The father reported that he had been trying to heat a baby bottle by placing it in the bathtub and running hot water on it. The father returned in a few minutes and found the toddler, who apparently had climbed into the tub, in about 2 inches of hot water. The mother confirmed that she had been busy and had asked the father to heat the bottle in the bathtub. The consultant thought that the pattern of the burns was consistent with the story; the pattern did not look like that seen in forcible submersion. Although the parents' accounts were unusual, they corroborated each other and were consistent with the injuries. The consultant concluded that this was not likely to be child abuse but might constitute negligence. The consultant notified child protective services. (Courtesy of Bessel A. van der Kolk, M.D.)

Sexual Abuse of Child. Adults within the immediate or extended family of a child perpetrate most child sexual abuse. Thus, children commonly know the sexual abuser, who is often a highly trusted family member with a position of authority and with wide access to the child (Table 32–2). Most cases of sexual abuse involving children are never revealed because of the victim's feelings of guilt, shame, ignorance, and tolerance, compounded by some physicians' reluctance to recognize and report sexual abuse, the court's insistence on strict rules of evidence, and families' fears of dissolution if the sexual abuse is discovered. Despite their familial roles, sexual abusers often threaten to hurt, kill, or abandon the children if the events are disclosed.

The incidence of sexual abuse and of child pornography, which is a form of sexual abuse, is much higher than was previously assumed. Children may be sexually abused as early as infancy and as late as adolescence. Sexual abuse has been reported in schools, day care centers, and group homes, where adult caretakers are the major offenders.

The overwhelming fear, shame, and guilt that contribute to a child's reticence to disclose sexual abuse also complicate identifying the abuse. Most often, no definitive physical evidence can prove the occurrence of sexual abuse. Physical indicators of sexual abuse include bruises, pain, and itching in the genital region. Genital or rectal bleeding may be a sign of sexual molestation. Recurrent urinary tract infections and vaginal discharges may be related to abuse. Sexually transmitted diseases and difficulty walking and sitting raise suspicions of sexual abuse.

No specific behavioral manifestations prove that sexual abuse has taken place, but children may exhibit many possible significant behaviors. Young children who have a detailed knowledge of sexual acts have usually witnessed or participated in sexual behavior. Young sexually abused children often exhibit their sexual knowledge through play and may initiate

Table 32–2
Sexual Abuse of Children

Reported cases in U.S., 1985[a]	123,000
Prevalence of male abuse	3–31%
Prevalence of female abuse	6–62%
Perpetrators	
Father or stepfather	7–8%
Uncles or older siblings	16–42%
Friends	32–60%
Strangers	1%
Sexual activity	
Coitus	16–29%
Oral sex and intercourse	3–11%
Touching genitals	13–33%
Age	Peak between ages 9 and 12 25% below age 8
High-risk factors	Child living in single-parent home Marital conflict History of physical abuse Increase in sexual abuse
Reported motivation of abuser	Pedophilic impulses No other sexual object Inability to delay gratification

[a]Current estimates are 150,000 to 200,000 new cases each year.
Data are from Finklehor D. The sexual abuse of children: current research reviewed. *Psychiatr Ann.* 1987;7:4. Percentages may total more than 100% because of overlapping studies.

sexual behaviors with their peers. Aggressive behavior is common among abused children. Children who are extremely fearful of adults, particularly men, may have been subjected to sexual abuse. Clinicians should listen carefully to children who report sexual assaults even when parts of their stories are not consistent. When a child begins to disclose information about sexual assaults, retractions and contradictions are typical, and anxiety may prevent full disclosure.

The diagnosis of sexual abuse in children is full of pitfalls. An estimated 2 to 8 percent of allegations of sexual abuse are false. A much higher percentage of reports cannot be substantiated. Many investigations are done hastily or are carried out by inexperienced evaluators. In custody cases, an allegation of sexual abuse can be a maneuver to limit a parent's visitation rights. Alleged sexual abuse of a preschool-age child is particularly difficult to evaluate because of the child's immature cognitive and language development. The use of anatomically correct dolls has grown in popularity but is controversial. Patient and careful evaluations by experienced, objective professionals are necessary, and leading questions must be avoided. Children under the age of 3 years are unlikely to produce a verbal memory of past trauma or abuses, but their experience may be reflected in play or fantasies. Some abused children meet the DSM-IV-TR diagnostic criteria for posttraumatic stress disorder.

No specific psychiatric symptom results universally from sexual abuse. Vulnerability to the sequelae of sexual abuse depends on the type of abuse, its chronicity, the age of the child, and the overall relationship of the victim and the abuser. The psychological and physical effects of sexual abuse can be devastating and long lasting. Children who are sexually stimulated by an adult feel anxiety and overexcitement, lose confidence in themselves, and become mistrustful of adults. Seduction, incest, and rape are important predisposing factors to later symptom formations such as phobias, anxiety, and depression. Abused children tend to be hyperalert to external aggression as shown by an inability to deal with their own aggressive impulses toward others or with others' hostility directed toward them.

Depressive feelings, usually combined with shame, guilt, and a sense of permanent damage, are commonly reported among children who have been sexually abused. Adolescents who have undergone sexual abuse are said to show high rates of poor impulse control and self-destructive and suicidal behaviors. Posttraumatic stress disorder and dissociative disorders are common in adults who have been sexually abused as children. Sexual abuse is a common preexisting factor in the development of dissociative identity disorder (also known as *multiple personality disorder*). Signs of dissociation include periods in which the children are amnestic, do not feel the pain, or feel that they are somewhere else. Borderline personality disorder has been reported in some patients with histories of sexual abuse. Substance abuse has also been reported with high frequency among adolescents and adults who were sexually abused as children.

INCEST. *Incest* is defined as the occurrence of sexual relations between close blood relatives. A broader definition describes incest as sexual intercourse between participants who are related to each other by a formal or informal kinship bond that is culturally regarded as a bar to sexual relations. For example, sexual relations between stepparents and stepchildren or among stepsiblings are usually considered incestuous, even though no blood relationships exist.

Sociologists have underlined the role of incest prohibitions as socialization factors, and biological factors also support the taboo. Inbreeding groups risk unmasking lethal or detrimental recessive genes and the progeny of inbred groups are generally less fit than less closely related offspring. Anthropologists have observed that different cultures have different types of incest taboos. In *Totem and Taboo*, Sigmund Freud developed the concept of the primal horde, in which young men collectively murdered the group's patriarch, who had kept all the women to himself. According to Freud, the incest taboo arose both from guilt about the murder and from a group's desire to prevent a repetition of the act, further rivalry after the murder, and subsequent disintegration of the horde.

Fathers, stepfathers, uncles, and older siblings most commonly abuse children. A passive, sick, absent, or somehow incapacitated mother, a daughter who takes on a maternal role in the family, a father who abuses alcohol, and overcrowding are features of father–daughter incest common in many homes. Mother–son incest is the strongest and most nearly universal taboo and is the rarest form of incest. Such behavior usually indicates more severe psychopathology in the participants than is the case in father–daughter and sibling incest.

Accurate figures on the incidence of incest are difficult to obtain because of families' shame and embarrassment. Girls are victims more often than are boys; in the United States, about 15 million women have been the objects of incestuous attention,

and one third of all sexually abused persons were molested before the age of 9.

Incestuous behavior is reported much more frequently among families of low socioeconomic status than among other families. This difference may be caused by greater contact with reporting officials such as welfare workers, public health personnel, and law enforcement agents and does not truly reflect a higher incidence in these families. Incest is more easily hidden by economically stable families than by those of low socioeconomic status.

Social, cultural, physiological, and psychological factors all contribute to the breakdown of the incest taboo. Incestuous behavior has been associated with alcohol abuse, overcrowding, increased physical proximity, and rural isolation that prevents adequate extrafamilial contacts. Some communities are more tolerant of incestuous behavior than the whole of society is. Major mental disorders and intellectual deficiencies can contribute to clinical incest. Some family therapists view incest as a defense designed to maintain a dysfunctional family unit. The older and stronger participant in incestuous behavior is usually male. Thus, incest may be viewed as a form of child abuse, a pedophilia, or a variant of rape.

About 75 percent of reported cases involve father–daughter incest, but parents often deny the occurrence of sibling incest. Other instances of sibling incest involve nearly normal interaction of prepubertal sexual play and exploration. In many cases of father–daughter incest, the daughter has had a close relationship with her father throughout her childhood and may appear to be pleased when he approaches her sexually. The incestuous behavior usually begins when the daughter is 10 years old. As the behavior continues, however, the abused daughter becomes bewildered, confused, and frightened, and when she nears adolescence, she undergoes physiological changes that add to her confusion. She never knows whether her father is a parent or sexual partner. Her mother may be alternately caring and competitive and may often refuse to believe her daughter's reports or to confront her husband with her suspicion. The daughter's relationships with her siblings are also affected; they sense her special position with her father and treat her as an outsider. The father, fearing that his daughter may expose their relationship and often jealously possessive of her, interferes with her development of normal peer relationships.

Physicians must be aware that intrafamilial sexual abuse can cause a wide variety of emotional and physical symptoms, including abdominal pain, genital irritations, separation anxiety disorder, phobias, nightmares, and school problems. When incest is suspected, clinicians must interview the child apart from the rest of the family.

Homosexual Incest. Father–son and mother–daughter incest are rarely reported, but a family in which same-sex incest occurs is usually highly disturbed, with a violent, alcohol-dependent, or antisocial father; a dependent or disabled mother who is unable to protect her children; and an absence of the usual family roles and individual identities. A son involved in father–son incest is frequently the eldest child, and, if there is a daughter, the father often sexually abuses her as well. Fathers in this situation do not necessarily have any other history of homosexual behavior. Sons may experience homicidal or suicidal ideation and may first consult or be sent to a psychiatrist because of self-destructive behavior.

STATUTORY RAPE. Intercourse is unlawful between a man over 16 years of age and a woman under the age of consent, which varies from 14 to 21 years, depending on the jurisdiction. Thus, a man of 18 and a girl of 15 may have consensual intercourse, yet the man may be held for statutory rape. Statutory rape may vary dramatically from other types of rape in being nonassaultive and nonviolent, and it is not a deviant act unless the age discrepancy is large enough for the man to be defined as a pedophile—that is, when the girl is less than 13 years old. Parents of a consenting girl, rather than the girl herself, usually press charges of statutory rape.

Neglect of Child.

A maltreated child often shows no obvious signs of being battered but has multiple minor physical evidences of emotional and, at times, nutritional deprivation, neglect, and abuse. A maltreated child, often brought to a hospital or to a private physician, has a history of failure to thrive, malnutrition, poor skin hygiene, irritability, withdrawal, and other signs of psychological and physical neglect.

Children who have been neglected may show overt failure to thrive at less than 1 year of age. Their physical and emotional development is drastically impaired; they may be physically small and unable to display appropriate social interaction. Hunger, chronic infections, poor hygiene, inappropriate dress, and eventual malnutrition may all be evident. Behaviorally, children who are chronically neglected can be indiscriminately affectionate, even with strangers, or socially unresponsive, even in familiar situations. Neglected children may be runaways or exhibit conduct disorder.

An extreme form of failure to thrive in children 5 years or older is psychosocial dwarfism, in which a chronically deprived child does not grow and develop, even when offered adequate amounts of food. Such children have normal proportions but are exceedingly small for their age. They often have reversible endocrinological changes resulting in decreased growth hormone, and they cease to grow for a time. Children with this disorder exhibit bizarre eating behaviors and disturbed social relationships. Binge eating, ingestion of garbage or inedible substances, drinking of toilet water, and induced vomiting have been reported.

Parents who neglect their children are often overwhelmed, depressed, isolated, and impoverished. Unemployment, the absence of a two-parent family, and substance abuse may exacerbate the situation. There are several possible prototypes of neglectful mothers. Some young, inexperienced, socially isolated, and ignorant mothers may temporarily be unable to care for their children. Other neglectful mothers are chronically passive and withdrawn women who may have been raised in chaotic, abusive, and neglectful homes. In these cases, once the situation comes to the attention of a child protective agency, the mother often accepts help. Mothers with major mental disorders who view their children as evil or as purposely driving them crazy are difficult to help.

Female Genital Mutilation.

Commonly called "female circumcision," female genital mutilation is performed on an estimated two million girls worldwide each year. It is practiced across diverse socioeconomic classes and different ethnic, cultural, and religious groups. Commonly, girls are circumcised between 4 and 10 years of age, but

vices to stressed families helps to prevent the problem in the first place.

PHYSICAL ABUSE OF ADULT

Spouse Abuse

Spouse abuse is estimated to occur in 2 to 12 million families in the United States. This aspect of domestic violence has been recognized as a severe problem, largely because of recent cultural emphasis on civil rights and the work of feminist groups, but the problem itself is long-standing.

The major problem in spouse abuse is wife abuse. One study estimated that there are 1.8 million battered wives in the United States, excluding divorced women and women battered on dates. Wife beating occurs in families of every racial and religious background and in all socioeconomic strata. It is most frequent in families with problems of substance abuse, particularly alcohol and crack abuse. Behavioral, cultural, intrapsychic, and interpersonal factors all contribute to the problem. Abusive men are likely to have come from violent homes where they witnessed wife beating or were abused themselves as children. The act itself is reinforcing; once a man has beaten his wife, he is likely to do so again. Abusive husbands tend to be immature, dependent, and nonassertive and to suffer from strong feelings of inadequacy.

The husbands' aggression is bullying behavior designed to humiliate their wives and to build up their own low self-esteem. Impatient, impulsive, abusive husbands physically displace aggression provoked by others onto their wives. The abuse is most likely to occur when a man feels threatened or frustrated at home, at work, or with his peers. The dynamics include identification with an aggressor (father, boss), testing behavior (Will she stay with me, no matter how I treat her?), distorted desires to express manhood, and dehumanization of women. As in rape, aggression is deemed permissible when a woman is perceived as property. About 50 percent of battered wives grew up in violent homes, and their most common trait is dependence.

The Surgeon General's Office has identified pregnancy as a high-risk period for battering; 15 to 25 percent of pregnant women are physically abused while pregnant, and the abuse often results in birth defects. Hot lines, emergency shelters for women, and other organizations (e.g., the National Coalition Against Domestic Violence) have been established to aid battered wives and to educate the public. One major problem of abused women is finding a place to go when they leave home, frequently in fear of their lives.

Battering is often severe, involving broken limbs, broken ribs, internal bleeding, and brain damage. When an abused wife tries to leave her husband, he often becomes doubly intimidating and threatens to "get" her. If the woman has small children to care for, her problem is compounded. The abusive husband wages a conscious campaign to isolate his wife and make her feel worthless. Women face risks when they leave an abusive husband; they have a 75 percent greater chance of being killed by their batterers than women who stay. New York State prepared a physician reference card to alert and guide doctors about domestic violence (Table 32–3).

Some men feel remorse and guilt after an episode of violent behavior and so become particularly loving. If this behavior gives the wife hope, she remains until the next, inevitable cycle of violence.

When a man is convinced that a woman will no longer tolerate the situation and when she begins to exert control over his behavior, change is initiated. By leaving for a prolonged period, if she is physically and economically able to do so, and by making therapy for the man a condition of return, a woman can begin a cycle of improvement. Family therapy is effective in treating the problem, usually in conjunction with social and legal agencies. With men who are relatively less impulsive, external controls, such as calling the neighbors or the police, may suffice to stop the behavior.

Some husband-beating wives have been also reported. Husbands complain of fear of ridicule if they expose the problem; they fear charges of counterassault and often feel unable to leave the situation because of financial difficulties. Husband abuse has also been reported when a frail, elderly man is married to a much younger woman.

Elder Abuse

Elder abuse is discussed in Chapter 54.

SEXUAL ABUSE OF ADULT

Rape

The conventional definition of *rape* is the perpetration of an act of sexual intercourse with a woman against her will and consent, whether her will is overcome by force or fear resulting from the threat of force or by drugs or intoxicants; or when, because of mental deficiency, she is incapable of exercising rational judgment, or when she is below an arbitrary age of consent. Rape, however, can occur between married partners and between persons of the same sex. The crime of rape requires only slight penile penetration of the victim's outer vulva; full erection and ejaculation are unnecessary for defining the crime. Forced acts of fellatio and anal penetration, although they frequently accompany rape, are legally considered sodomy.

The problem of rape is most appropriately discussed under the heading of aggression. Rape is an act of violence and humiliation that happens to be expressed through sexual means. Rape expresses power or anger; sex is rarely the dominant issue because sexuality is used in the service of nonsexual needs.

Rape of Women. Recent research categorizes male rapists in separate groups: sexual sadists, who are aroused by the pain of their victims; exploitive predators, who use their victims as objects for their gratification in an impulsive way; inadequate men, who believe that no woman would voluntarily sleep with them and who are obsessed with fantasies about sex; and men for whom rape is a displaced expression of anger and rage. Some believe that the anger was originally directed toward a wife or mother, but feminist theory proposes that a woman serves as an object for the displacement of aggression that a rapist cannot express directly toward other men. Women are considered men's property or vulnerable possessions, a rapist's instrument for revenge against other men.

Rape often accompanies another crime. Rapists always threaten their victims, with fists, a knife, or a gun, and fre-

children's veracity is being challenged. See Chapter 20 for a discussion of the recovered or false memory syndrome.

Course and Prognosis

The outcome of child physical and sexual abuse and neglect is multifactorial, depending on the severity, duration, and nature of the abuse, and on the child's vulnerabilities. Children who already suffer from mental retardation, pervasive developmental disorders, physical disabilities, disruptive behavior, and attention-deficit disorders are likely to have a poorer outcome than children who are unhampered by mental or physical disorders. Children who are abused for long periods, from the time they are babies or toddlers into adolescence, are likely to be more profoundly damaged than those who have experienced only brief episodes of abuse. The development of mental disorders—such as major depressive disorder, suicidal behavior, posttraumatic stress disorder, dissociative identity disorder, and substance abuse—further complicates the long-term prognosis, as does the nature of the relationship between victim and abuser and the adult support figures available to children after disclosure. The best outcomes occur when children are cognitively intact, the abuse is recognized and interrupted in an early phase, and the entire family is capable of participating in treatment.

Treatment

Child. The first part of treating child abuse and neglect is to ensure the child's safety and well-being. Children may need to be removed from abusive or neglectful families to ensure their protection; yet, on an emotional level, a child may feel additionally vulnerable in an unfamiliar setting. Because of the high risk for psychiatric symptoms in abused and neglected children, a comprehensive psychiatric evaluation is in order. Next, along with providing specific treatments for any mental disorders present, a therapist may have to deal with the immediate situation and the long-term implications of the abuse or neglect. Therapists must address several psychotherapeutic issues: dealing with the child's fears, anxieties, and self-esteem; building a trusting adult relationship in which the child is not exploited or betrayed; and ultimately gaining a helpful perspective of the factors contributing to the child's victimization at home.

Ideally, each abused and neglected child should receive an intervention plan based on the assessment of the factors responsible for the parental psychopathology. The plan should include an overall prognosis for parents' achieving adequate parenting skills; the time estimated to achieve meaningful change in their ability to parent; an estimate of whether the parental dysfunction is confined to this child or involves other children, whether the parents' overall malfunctioning, if that is the case, is short term or long term, and whether a mother's malfunctioning is confined to infants as opposed to older children (i.e., when the incidence of abuse is inversely related to a child's age); willingness of those involved to participate in the intervention plan; the availability of personnel and physical resources to implement the various intervention strategies; and the risk of the child sustaining additional physical or sexual abuse by remaining in the home.

Parents. On the basis of the information obtained, several options can be selected to improve parental functioning: eliminate or diminish the social or environmental stresses; lessen the adverse psychological effects of social factors on the parents; reduce the demands on the mother to a level within her capacity through day care placement of the child or provision of a housekeeper or baby-sitter; provide emotional support, encouragement, sympathy, stimulation, instruction in maternal care, and aid in learning to plan for, assess, and meet the needs of the infant (supportive casework); and resolve or diminish the parents' inner psychic conflicts (psychotherapy).

INCESTUOUS BEHAVIOR. The first step in the treatment of incestuous behavior is its disclosure. Once a breakthrough of family members' denial, collusion, and fear has been achieved, incest is unlikely to recur. When the participants suffer from severe psychopathology, treatment must be directed toward the underlying illness. Family therapy is useful to reestablish the group as a functioning unit and to develop healthier role definitions for each member. While the participants are learning to develop internal restraints and appropriate ways to gratify their needs, the external control provided by therapy helps prevent further incestuous behavior. At times, legal agencies must help enforce external controls.

Reporting. In cases of suspected child abuse and neglect, physicians should diagnose the suspected maltreatment; secure the child's safety by admitting the child to a hospital or arranging out-of-home placement; report the case to the appropriate social service department, child protection unit, or central registry; make an assessment with the help of a history, a physical examination, a skeletal survey, and photographs; request a social worker's report and appropriate surgical and medical consultations; confer with members of a child abuse committee within 72 hours; arrange a program of care for the child and the parents; and arrange for social service follow-up. Among those generally included as mandated child-abuse reporters are physicians, psychologists, school officials, police officers, hospital personnel engaged in the treatment of patients, district attorneys, and providers of child day care and foster care.

Prevention. To prevent child abuse and neglect, clinicians must identify those families at high risk and intervene before a child becomes a victim. Once high-risk families have been identified, a comprehensive program should include psychiatric monitoring of the families, including the identified high-risk child. Families can be educated to recognize when they are being neglectful or abusive, and alternative coping strategies can be suggested.

In general, child abuse and neglect prevention and treatment programs should try to prevent the separation of parents and children if possible, prevent the placement of children in institutions, encourage parental attainment of self-care status, and encourage the family's attainment of self-sufficiency. As a last resort and to prevent further abuse and neglect, children may have to be removed from families who are unwilling or unable to profit from the treatment program. In cases of sexual abuse, the licensing of day care centers and the psychological screening of persons who work in them should be mandatory to prevent further abuses. Education of the medical profession, members of allied health fields, and all who come in contact with children aid in early detection. And providing support ser-

vices to stressed families helps to prevent the problem in the first place.

PHYSICAL ABUSE OF ADULT

Spouse Abuse

Spouse abuse is estimated to occur in 2 to 12 million families in the United States. This aspect of domestic violence has been recognized as a severe problem, largely because of recent cultural emphasis on civil rights and the work of feminist groups, but the problem itself is long-standing.

The major problem in spouse abuse is wife abuse. One study estimated that there are 1.8 million battered wives in the United States, excluding divorced women and women battered on dates. Wife beating occurs in families of every racial and religious background and in all socioeconomic strata. It is most frequent in families with problems of substance abuse, particularly alcohol and crack abuse. Behavioral, cultural, intrapsychic, and interpersonal factors all contribute to the problem. Abusive men are likely to have come from violent homes where they witnessed wife beating or were abused themselves as children. The act itself is reinforcing; once a man has beaten his wife, he is likely to do so again. Abusive husbands tend to be immature, dependent, and nonassertive and to suffer from strong feelings of inadequacy.

The husbands' aggression is bullying behavior designed to humiliate their wives and to build up their own low self-esteem. Impatient, impulsive, abusive husbands physically displace aggression provoked by others onto their wives. The abuse is most likely to occur when a man feels threatened or frustrated at home, at work, or with his peers. The dynamics include identification with an aggressor (father, boss), testing behavior (Will she stay with me, no matter how I treat her?), distorted desires to express manhood, and dehumanization of women. As in rape, aggression is deemed permissible when a woman is perceived as property. About 50 percent of battered wives grew up in violent homes, and their most common trait is dependence.

The Surgeon General's Office has identified pregnancy as a high-risk period for battering; 15 to 25 percent of pregnant women are physically abused while pregnant, and the abuse often results in birth defects. Hot lines, emergency shelters for women, and other organizations (e.g., the National Coalition Against Domestic Violence) have been established to aid battered wives and to educate the public. One major problem of abused women is finding a place to go when they leave home, frequently in fear of their lives.

Battering is often severe, involving broken limbs, broken ribs, internal bleeding, and brain damage. When an abused wife tries to leave her husband, he often becomes doubly intimidating and threatens to "get" her. If the woman has small children to care for, her problem is compounded. The abusive husband wages a conscious campaign to isolate his wife and make her feel worthless. Women face risks when they leave an abusive husband; they have a 75 percent greater chance of being killed by their batterers than women who stay. New York State prepared a physician reference card to alert and guide doctors about domestic violence (Table 32–3).

Some men feel remorse and guilt after an episode of violent behavior and so become particularly loving. If this behavior gives the wife hope, she remains until the next, inevitable cycle of violence.

When a man is convinced that a woman will no longer tolerate the situation and when she begins to exert control over his behavior, change is initiated. By leaving for a prolonged period, if she is physically and economically able to do so, and by making therapy for the man a condition of return, a woman can begin a cycle of improvement. Family therapy is effective in treating the problem, usually in conjunction with social and legal agencies. With men who are relatively less impulsive, external controls, such as calling the neighbors or the police, may suffice to stop the behavior.

Some husband-beating wives have been also reported. Husbands complain of fear of ridicule if they expose the problem; they fear charges of counterassault and often feel unable to leave the situation because of financial difficulties. Husband abuse has also been reported when a frail, elderly man is married to a much younger woman.

Elder Abuse

Elder abuse is discussed in Chapter 54.

SEXUAL ABUSE OF ADULT

Rape

The conventional definition of *rape* is the perpetration of an act of sexual intercourse with a woman against her will and consent, whether her will is overcome by force or fear resulting from the threat of force or by drugs or intoxicants; or when, because of mental deficiency, she is incapable of exercising rational judgment, or when she is below an arbitrary age of consent. Rape, however, can occur between married partners and between persons of the same sex. The crime of rape requires only slight penile penetration of the victim's outer vulva; full erection and ejaculation are unnecessary for defining the crime. Forced acts of fellatio and anal penetration, although they frequently accompany rape, are legally considered sodomy.

The problem of rape is most appropriately discussed under the heading of aggression. Rape is an act of violence and humiliation that happens to be expressed through sexual means. Rape expresses power or anger; sex is rarely the dominant issue because sexuality is used in the service of nonsexual needs.

Rape of Women. Recent research categorizes male rapists in separate groups: sexual sadists, who are aroused by the pain of their victims; exploitive predators, who use their victims as objects for their gratification in an impulsive way; inadequate men, who believe that no woman would voluntarily sleep with them and who are obsessed with fantasies about sex; and men for whom rape is a displaced expression of anger and rage. Some believe that the anger was originally directed toward a wife or mother, but feminist theory proposes that a woman serves as an object for the displacement of aggression that a rapist cannot express directly toward other men. Women are considered men's property or vulnerable possessions, a rapist's instrument for revenge against other men.

Rape often accompanies another crime. Rapists always threaten their victims, with fists, a knife, or a gun, and fre-

and one third of all sexually abused persons were molested before the age of 9.

Incestuous behavior is reported much more frequently among families of low socioeconomic status than among other families. This difference may be caused by greater contact with reporting officials such as welfare workers, public health personnel, and law enforcement agents and does not truly reflect a higher incidence in these families. Incest is more easily hidden by economically stable families than by those of low socioeconomic status.

Social, cultural, physiological, and psychological factors all contribute to the breakdown of the incest taboo. Incestuous behavior has been associated with alcohol abuse, overcrowding, increased physical proximity, and rural isolation that prevents adequate extrafamilial contacts. Some communities are more tolerant of incestuous behavior than the whole of society is. Major mental disorders and intellectual deficiencies can contribute to clinical incest. Some family therapists view incest as a defense designed to maintain a dysfunctional family unit. The older and stronger participant in incestuous behavior is usually male. Thus, incest may be viewed as a form of child abuse, a pedophilia, or a variant of rape.

About 75 percent of reported cases involve father–daughter incest, but parents often deny the occurrence of sibling incest. Other instances of sibling incest involve nearly normal interaction of prepubertal sexual play and exploration. In many cases of father–daughter incest, the daughter has had a close relationship with her father throughout her childhood and may appear to be pleased when he approaches her sexually. The incestuous behavior usually begins when the daughter is 10 years old. As the behavior continues, however, the abused daughter becomes bewildered, confused, and frightened, and when she nears adolescence, she undergoes physiological changes that add to her confusion. She never knows whether her father is a parent or sexual partner. Her mother may be alternately caring and competitive and may often refuse to believe her daughter's reports or to confront her husband with her suspicion. The daughter's relationships with her siblings are also affected; they sense her special position with her father and treat her as an outsider. The father, fearing that his daughter may expose their relationship and often jealously possessive of her, interferes with her development of normal peer relationships.

Physicians must be aware that intrafamilial sexual abuse can cause a wide variety of emotional and physical symptoms, including abdominal pain, genital irritations, separation anxiety disorder, phobias, nightmares, and school problems. When incest is suspected, clinicians must interview the child apart from the rest of the family.

Homosexual Incest. Father–son and mother–daughter incest are rarely reported, but a family in which same-sex incest occurs is usually highly disturbed, with a violent, alcohol-dependent, or antisocial father; a dependent or disabled mother who is unable to protect her children; and an absence of the usual family roles and individual identities. A son involved in father–son incest is frequently the eldest child, and, if there is a daughter, the father often sexually abuses her as well. Fathers in this situation do not necessarily have any other history of homosexual behavior. Sons may experience homicidal or suicidal ideation and may first consult or be sent to a psychiatrist because of self-destructive behavior.

STATUTORY RAPE. Intercourse is unlawful between a man over 16 years of age and a woman under the age of consent, which varies from 14 to 21 years, depending on the jurisdiction. Thus, a man of 18 and a girl of 15 may have consensual intercourse, yet the man may be held for statutory rape. Statutory rape may vary dramatically from other types of rape in being nonassaultive and nonviolent, and it is not a deviant act unless the age discrepancy is large enough for the man to be defined as a pedophile—that is, when the girl is less than 13 years old. Parents of a consenting girl, rather than the girl herself, usually press charges of statutory rape.

Neglect of Child. A maltreated child often shows no obvious signs of being battered but has multiple minor physical evidences of emotional and, at times, nutritional deprivation, neglect, and abuse. A maltreated child, often brought to a hospital or to a private physician, has a history of failure to thrive, malnutrition, poor skin hygiene, irritability, withdrawal, and other signs of psychological and physical neglect.

Children who have been neglected may show overt failure to thrive at less than 1 year of age. Their physical and emotional development is drastically impaired; they may be physically small and unable to display appropriate social interaction. Hunger, chronic infections, poor hygiene, inappropriate dress, and eventual malnutrition may all be evident. Behaviorally, children who are chronically neglected can be indiscriminately affectionate, even with strangers, or socially unresponsive, even in familiar situations. Neglected children may be runaways or exhibit conduct disorder.

An extreme form of failure to thrive in children 5 years or older is psychosocial dwarfism, in which a chronically deprived child does not grow and develop, even when offered adequate amounts of food. Such children have normal proportions but are exceedingly small for their age. They often have reversible endocrinological changes resulting in decreased growth hormone, and they cease to grow for a time. Children with this disorder exhibit bizarre eating behaviors and disturbed social relationships. Binge eating, ingestion of garbage or inedible substances, drinking of toilet water, and induced vomiting have been reported.

Parents who neglect their children are often overwhelmed, depressed, isolated, and impoverished. Unemployment, the absence of a two-parent family, and substance abuse may exacerbate the situation. There are several possible prototypes of neglectful mothers. Some young, inexperienced, socially isolated, and ignorant mothers may temporarily be unable to care for their children. Other neglectful mothers are chronically passive and withdrawn women who may have been raised in chaotic, abusive, and neglectful homes. In these cases, once the situation comes to the attention of a child protective agency, the mother often accepts help. Mothers with major mental disorders who view their children as evil or as purposely driving them crazy are difficult to help.

Female Genital Mutilation. Commonly called "female circumcision," female genital mutilation is performed on an estimated two million girls worldwide each year. It is practiced across diverse socioeconomic classes and different ethnic, cultural, and religious groups. Commonly, girls are circumcised between 4 and 10 years of age, but

the procedure may be performed on infants, postponed until just before marriage, or done after the birth of the first child. Some cultures consider it part of a ceremonial induction into adult society. Female circumcision, in the mildest form, consists of clitoridectomy, the anatomical equivalent of penile amputation. In its most severe form, total infibulation involves removal of the clitoris and labia minora plus incision of the labia major to create raw surfaces that are then stitched together. This practice has been widely criticized, including opposition by the World Health Organization and other major health care groups. In the United States female circumcision is generally considered child abuse. Efforts have been made to educate immigrant communities about the health risks and legal liabilities of the practice. Compromise may be possible by finding a way to satisfy the cultural requirements without using mutilation such as adopting a nonmutilative ritual incision that results in only small scars on the labia.

Male genital mutilation (circumcision) is not usually considered child abuse, but it does have its critics. Although this simple procedure is one of the most common operations performed worldwide, serious complications may result. These complications include hemorrhage, infection, and penile amputation. In 1999, the American Academy of Pediatrics recommended it not be done as a routine procedure on newborns.

Pathology and Laboratory Examination. Although no definitive laboratory tests are available to help clinicians diagnose child physical or sexual abuse or neglect, a physical examination to detect physical stigmata is indicated when abuse is suspected. In cases of failure to thrive, endocrinological screening is indicated. An external genital examination is indicated in cases of suspected child sexual abuse to detect scars, tears, and genital infections. X-ray evidence of fractures may be present in various stages of reparative changes, but when no fractures or dislocations are apparent on examination, bone repair may become evident within weeks after the specific bone trauma.

Roentgenological examinations of unrecognized traumatic fractures reveal several unusual bone changes (Fig. 32–2). Metaphyseal fragmentation is caused by twisting or pulling of the afflicted extremity. There may be squaring of the long bones secondary to the new bone formation on the metaphyseal fragments. Periosteal hemorrhages are frequently noted because the periosteum of infants is not securely attached to the underlying bone. Periosteal calcification follows this hemorrhaging and begins to become apparent 5 to 7 days after the inflicted trauma. A layer of calcification around the shaft of the bone should cause suspicion of inflicted abuse. Epiphyseal separations and periosteal shearing usually result from traction and torsion of the affected extremity. X-ray findings of reparative changes involving excessive new bone formation or previously healed fractures with periosteal reactions may be diagnostic when correlated with other manifestations of child abuse.

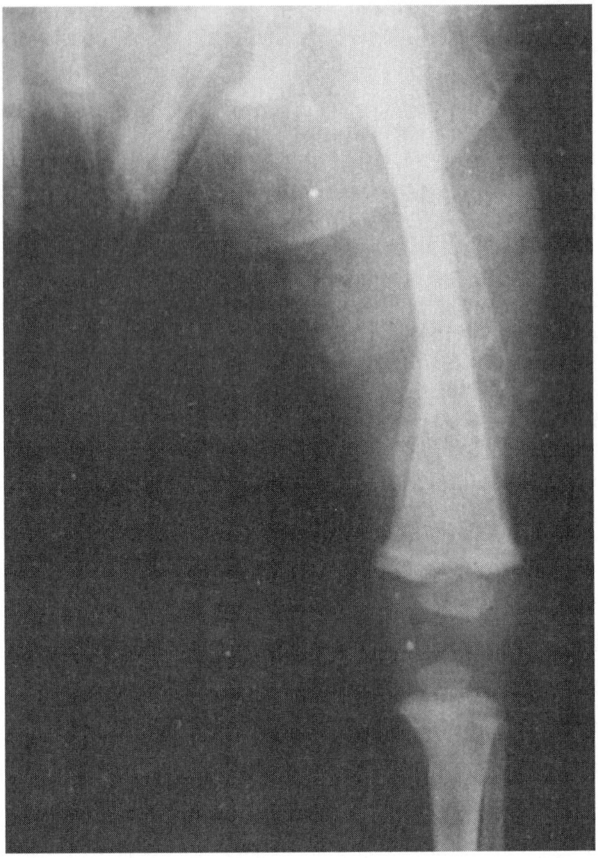

FIGURE 32–2

Follow-up X-ray of a maltreated 6-month-old infant taken 4 weeks after inflicted trauma to the upper thigh. Extensive reparative changes are noted in association with new bone formation, external cortical thickening, and squaring of the metaphysis—diagnostic evidence of bone changes after trauma. The layer of calcification around the shaft of the bone and the presence of bone fragments at the ends of the bone should be evidence for suspicion of inflicted trauma and should prompt further investigations into the causes of the X-ray findings. The X-ray changes may be diagnostic when correlated with other manifestations of physical abuse of child. (Courtesy of Vincent J. Fontana, M.D.)

Differential Diagnosis

Parental feuding and custody disputes are among the factors that complicate identifying and substantiating abuse and neglect situations. When marital discord is severe, children are often caught in the line of fire. A mother who is overwhelmingly hostile toward a separated father may be convinced and may convince a child that the father is abusive. In some cases, parents have gone so far as to fabricate entire abuse scenarios and coach children to repeat them. In other instances, parents may refuse to accept the possibility that a spouse or close relative is the perpetrator of abuse, may repeatedly insist that a child stop telling lies, and may coerce a child into retracting the disclosures. In either scenario, the child suffers profoundly, and the alleged abuse situation is never disentangled.

When a child speaks in a manner consistent with his or her language development stage, does not sound rehearsed, and does not use adultlike phrasing, the abuse allegations may be true. Distress, the display of precocious sexual behavior, and a knowledge of, or preoccupation with, sexual material also support the possibility of sexual abuse. A child who has not been abused but who is coached to report sexual or physical abuse is also placed under unbearable duress. Therefore, clinicians must recognize that severe chronic parental conflict in which a child is caught can be as destructive as physical and sexual abuse.

Controversies are now arising in the courts because children are accusing caretakers and teachers of sexual abuse, and the

Table 32–3
Physician Reference Card

PHYSICIAN REFERENCE CARD

RECOGNIZING AND TREATING VICTIMS OF DOMESTIC VIOLENCE BASED ON THE AMERICAN MEDICAL ASSOCIATION'S DIAGNOSTIC AND TREATMENT GUIDELINES ON DOMESTIC VIOLENCE

If you treat women, whether in private practice or a hospital setting, you are almost certainly treating some patients who are victims of domestic violence.

The following decision tree is designed to help you assess a patient's risk of domestic violence and offer appropriate help to those in need of it.

Identifying Victims of Domestic Violence

Although many women who are victims of abuse will not volunteer any information, they will discuss it if asked simple, direct questions in a nonjudgmental way and in a confidential setting. *The patient should be interviewed alone, without her partner present.*

You may want to offer a statement such as: "Because violence is so common in many women's lives, I've begun to ask about it routinely." Then you can ask a direct question, such as: "At any time, has your partner hit, kicked, or otherwise hurt or frightened you?"

IF PATIENT ANSWERS YES, THE FOLLOWING STEPS ARE SUGGESTED:

1. *Encourage her to talk about it:*
   "Would you like to talk about what has happened to you?"
   "How do you feel about it?"
   "What would you like to do about this?"
2. *Listen nonjudgmentally.*
   This serves both to begin the healing process for the woman and to give you an idea of what kind of referrals she needs.
3. *Validate:*
   Victims of domestic violence are frequently not believed, and the fear they report is minimized. The physician can express support through simple statements such as
   - You are not alone.
   - You don't deserve to be treated this way.
   - You are not to blame.
   - You are not crazy.
   - What happened to you is a crime.
   - Help is available for you.
4. *Document:*
   - The patient's complaints and symptoms as well as the results of the observation and assessment. (Complaints should be described in the patient's own words whenever possible.)
   - The patient's complete medical and trauma history and relevant social history.
   - A detailed description of the injuries, including type, number, size, location, resolution, possible causes, and explanations given.
   - An opinion on whether the injuries were inconsistent with the patient's explanation.
   - Results of all pertinent laboratory and other diagnostic procedures.
   - Color photographs and imaging studies, if applicable.
   - If the police are called, the name of the investigating officer and any action taken (the police should be called only if patient requests this or exhibits a reportable injury).
   - Child abuse and neglect is a reportable offense. If you suspect that children in the patient's home are also being abused, you are mandated to report the situation to the NYS Department of Social Services at 1-800-342-3720.
5. *Assess the danger to your patient:*
   Assess your patient's safety *before she leaves the medical setting.* The most important determinants of risk are the woman's level of fear and her appraisal of her immediate and future safety. Discussing the following indicators with the patient can help you determine if she is in escalating danger:
   - an increase in the frequency or severity of the assaults
   - increasing or new threats of homicide or suicide by the partner
   - threats to her children
   - the presence or availability of a firearm
6. *Provide appropriate treatment referral and support:*
   - Treat the patient's injuries as indicated. In prescribing medication, keep in mind that medications which hinder the patient's ability to protect herself or to flee from a violent partner may endanger her life.
   - If your patient is in imminent danger, determine if she has friends or family with whom she can stay. If this is not an option, ask if she wants immediate access to a shelter for battered women. If none is available, can she be admitted to the hospital?
   - If she doesn't need immediate access to a shelter, offer written information about shelters and other community resources. Remember that it may be dangerous for the woman to have these in her possession. Don't insist that she take them if she is reluctant to do so.

   Give your patient the telephone number of the local domestic violence hotline or the toll-free NYS Domestic Violence hotline (1-800-942-6906; 1-800-942-6908 for Spanish-speaking callers). It may be safest for your patient if you write the number on a prescription blank or an appointment card. You may wish to give her the opportunity to call from a private phone in your office.

IF THE PATIENT ANSWERS NO, OR WILL NOT DISCUSS THE TOPIC:

1. *Be aware of clinical findings that may indicate abuse:*
   - injury to the head, neck, torso, breasts, abdomen, or genitals
   - bilateral or multiple injuries
   - delay between onset of injury and seeking treatment
   - explanation by the patient which is inconsistent with the type of injury
   - any injury during pregnancy, especially to the abdomen or breasts
   - prior history of trauma
   - chronic pain symptoms for which no etiology is apparent
   - psychological distress, such as depression, suicidal ideation, anxiety, and/or sleep disorders
   - a partner who seems overly protective or who will not leave the woman's side
2. *If any of the above clinical signs is present, it is appropriate to ask more specific questions. Be sure that the patient's partner is not present.* Some examples of questions that may elicit more information about the patient's situation are:
   - It looks as though someone may have hurt you. Could you tell me how it happened?
   - Sometimes when people come for health care with physical symptoms like yours, we find that there may be trouble at home. We are concerned that someone is hurting or abusing you. Is this happening?
   - Sometimes when people feel the way you do, it's because they may have been hurt or abused at home. Is this happening to you?
3. *If patient answers YES:*
   See the suggestions for assessment and treatment that begin on the other side of this card.

   If patient answers NO:
   If the patient denies abuse, but you strongly suspect that it is taking place, you can let her know that your office can provide referrals to local programs, should she choose to pursue such options in the future.
   - You may want to write the Domestic Violence hotline number (1-800-942-6906 English; 1-800-942-6908 Spanish) on a prescription blank or on an appointment card.

   Don't judge the success of the intervention by the patient's action. A woman is most at risk of serious injury or even homicide when she attempts to leave an abusive partner, and it may take her a long time before she can finally do so. It is frustrating for the physician when a patient stays in an abusive situation. Be reassured that if you have acknowledged and validated her situation and offered appropriate referrals, you have done what you can to help her.

From Office for Prevention of Domestic Violence, Medical Society of the State of New York, New York State Department of Health.

quently harm them in nonsexual ways as well. Victims may be beaten, wounded, and killed.

Statistics show that most men who commit rapes are between 25 and 44 years of age; 51 percent are white and tend to rape white victims, 47 percent are black and tend to rape black victims, and the remaining 2 percent come from all other races. Alcohol is involved in 34 percent of all forcible rapes. A composite characterization of the archetypical rapist drawn from police statistics portrays a single 19-year-old man from a low socioeconomic group who has a police record of acquisitive offenses.

According to the Federal Bureau of Investigation (FBI), 97,464 forcible rapes were reported to law enforcement in the United States in 1995. Rape, however, is a highly underreported crime: An estimated 4 to 5 of 10 rapes is reported. The underreporting is attributed to victims' feelings of shame and to the belief that there is no recourse through the legal system. According to the FBI Uniform Crime Reporting program, in 1995, 72 of every 100,000 females in the United States were reported rape victims.

Persons who are raped can be of any age. Cases have been reported in which the victims were as young as 15 months and as old as 82 years, but women ages 16 to 24 are at highest risk. Rape most commonly occurs in a woman's own neighborhood, frequently inside or near her own home. Most rapes are premeditated; about half are committed by strangers and half by men known, to varying degrees, by the victims. Seven percent of all rapes are perpetrated by close relatives of the victim; 10 percent of rapes involve more than one attacker.

A woman being raped is frequently in a life-threatening situation. During the rape, she experiences shock and fright approaching panic; her prime motivation is to stay alive. In most cases, rapists choose victims slightly smaller than themselves. Rapists may urinate or defecate on their victims, ejaculate into their faces and hair, force anal intercourse, and insert foreign objects into their vaginas and rectums.

After a rape, a woman often experiences shame, humiliation, confusion, fear, and rage. The type and duration of the reaction vary, but women report that the effects last for a year or longer. Many women experience the symptoms of posttraumatic stress disorder. Some women, particularly those who have always felt sexually adequate, are able to resume sexual relations with men; but others become phobic about sexual interaction or exhibit such symptoms as vaginismus. Few women emerge from the assault completely unscathed. The manifestations and the degree of damage depend on the violence of the attack itself, the vulnerability of the woman, and the support system available to her immediately after the attack.

A rape victim fares best when she receives immediate support and can ventilate her fear and rage to loving family members, sympathetic physicians, and law enforcement officials. Knowing that she has socially acceptable means of recourse, such as the arrest and conviction of the rapist, can help a rape victim.

Unless a woman has a severe underlying disorder, therapy usually has a supportive approach and focuses on restoring a victim's sense of adequacy and control over her life; it also aims to relieve feelings of helplessness, dependence, and obsession with the assault, which frequently follow the rape. Group therapy with homogeneous groups of persons who have been raped is a particularly effective form of treatment.

In addition to the physical and psychological trauma experienced when they are assaulted, rape victims until recently also faced skepticism from those to whom they reported the crime (if they had sufficient strength to do so) or accusations of having provoked or desired the assault. In reality, the National Commission on the Causes and Prevention of Violence found discernible victim participation in rape in only 4.4 percent of all cases. This statistic is lower than that of any other crime of violence. Educating police officers and assigning policewomen to deal with rape victims have helped increase reporting of the crime. Rape crisis centers and telephone hot lines are available for immediate aid and information for victims. Volunteer groups work in emergency rooms in hospitals and with physician education programs to assist in the treatment of victims.

Legally, women no longer must prove in court that they actively struggled against a rapist, and testimony about a victim's previous sexual history has been declared inadmissible as evidence in several states. Because penalties for first-time rapists have been reduced, juries are likely to consider a conviction. In some states, wives can now prosecute husbands for rape.

DATE RAPE. *Date rape* and *acquaintance rape* are terms applied to rapes in which the rapist is known to the victim. The assault can occur on a first date or after the man and woman have known each other for many months. Considerable data on date rape have been gathered from college populations. In one study, 38 percent of male students said that they would commit rape if they thought they could get away with it, and 11 percent stated that they had committed rape; 16 percent of female students said that they had been raped by men they knew or were dating. In addition to suffering the symptoms of all rape survivors, victims of date rape berate themselves for exercising poor judgment in their choice of male friends and are more likely to blame themselves for provoking the rapist than are other victims. Many colleges and universities have set up programs for rape prevention and for counseling those who have been assaulted.

Rape of Men. In some states the definition of rape is being changed to substitute the word *person* for *female*. In most states, male rape is legally defined as sodomy. Homosexual rape is much more frequent among men than among women and occurs frequently in closed institutions such as prisons and maximum-security hospitals.

The dynamics are identical to those of heterosexual rape. The crime enables the rapist to discharge aggression and to aggrandize himself. The victim is usually smaller than the rapist, is always perceived as passive and unmanly (weaker), and is used as an object. A rapist selecting a male victim may be heterosexual, bisexual, or homosexual. The most common act is anal penetration of the victim; the second most common is fellatio.

Homosexual-rape victims often feel (as raped women do) that they have been ruined. Some also fear that they will become homosexual because of the attack.

Sexual Coercion

Sexual coercion is a term used in DSM-IV-TR for incidents in which one person dominates another by force or compels the other person to perform a sexual act.

Table 32–4
Educational Material to Reduce Sexual Harassment

WHAT YOU SHOULD KNOW ABOUT SEXUAL HARASSMENT
WHAT IS SEXUAL HARASSMENT?
WHAT IS PROHIBITED?

The 1980 Equal Opportunity Employment Commission Guidelines for Sexual Harassment encompass:

1. Unwelcomed sexual advances.
2. Requests for sexual favors.
3. Verbal conduct of a sexual nature.
4. Physical conduct of a sexual nature.

UNDER WHAT CONDITIONS?

When such conduct has the purpose or effect of:

1. Unreasonably interfering with an individual's work performance.
2. Creating an intimidating, hostile or offensive working environment. (This can be interpreted to include the "terms, conditions or privileges of unemployment" such as the psychological and emotional work environment and subjecting female employees to anxiety and debilitation.)
3. When submission to or rejection of the conduct is made either explicitly or implicitly a term or condition of an individual's employment or
4. Is the basis for employment decisions affecting the individual.

WHO IS RESPONSIBLE?

1. The employer who is committing the act.
2. The employer, even if its agents and supervisors committed the act regardless of whether the acts were authorized or even forbidden.
3. The employer for acts committed by an employee's co-worker.
4. The employer for conduct by a non-employee (such as a customer or supplier) if the employer "knows or should have known of the conduct and fails to take an immediate and appropriate action."
5. The employer, if timely corrective actions are not taken.

Reprinted with permission from Tulin DiversiTeam Associates, Philadelphia.

Stalking. *Stalking* is defined as a pattern of harassing or menacing behavior coupled with a threat to do harm. In 1990 California passed the first antistalking law, and most states now prohibit stalking, although some will not intervene unless an act of violence has occurred. In states with stalking laws the person can be arrested on the basis of a pattern of harassment and can be charged with either a misdemeanor or felony. Some stalkers continue the activity for years; others, for only a few months. The court may mandate that stalkers undergo counseling sessions. The best means of deterrent is to report all stalkers to law enforcement agencies. Most stalkers are men, but women who stalk are just as likely as men to attack their victims violently.

Sexual Harassment. *Sexual harassment* refers to sexual advances, requests for sexual favors, verbal or physical conduct of a sexual nature—all of which are unwelcomed by the victim. In over 95 percent of cases the perpetrator is a man and the victim, a woman. If a man is being harassed, it is almost always by another man. A woman sexually harassing a man is an extremely rare event. The victim of harassment reacts to the experience in various ways. Some blame themselves and become depressed; others become anxious or angry. In general, harassment most commonly occurs in the workplace, and many organizations have developed procedures to deal with the problem. All too often, however, the victim is unwilling to step forward and lodge a complaint because of fear of retribution, of being humiliated, of being accused of lying (which is exceedingly rare), or ultimately of being fired from the job.

The types of behaviors that make up sexual harassment are broad. They include abusive language, requests for sexual favors, sexual jokes, staring, ogling, and giving massages, among others.

To reduce harassment, organizations may distribute educational material (Table 32–4). Employers are obligated to investigate every complaint, which most often are addressed to the Equal Employment Opportunity Commission. Appropriate organizational responses range from a written reprimand to firing the offender.

REFERENCES

Acierno R, Gray M, Best C, et al. Rape and physical violence: comparison of assault characteristics in older and younger adults in the National Women's Study. *J Trauma Stress.* 2001;14:685.

Bernet W. Child maltreatment. In: Sadock BJ, Sadock VA, eds. *Kaplan & Sadock's Comprehensive Textbook of Psychiatry.* 7th ed. Vol 2. Baltimore: Lippincott Williams & Wilkins; 2000:2878.

Brownmiller S. *Against Our Will: Men, Women and Rape.* New York: Simon & Schuster; 1975.

Cash SJ. Risk assessment in child welfare: the art and science. *Child Youth Serv Rev.* 2001;23:811.

Cooke P, Standen PJ. Abuse and disabled children: hidden needs . . . ? *Child Abuse Rev.* 2002;11:1.

Donald T, Jureidini J. Munchausen syndrome by proxy. Child abuse in the medical system. *Arch Pediatr Adolesc Med.* 1996;150:753.

Dube SR, Anda RF, Felitti VJ, Edwards VJ, Williamson DF. Exposure to abuse, neglect and household dysfunction among adults who witnessed intimate partner violence as children: implications for health and social services. *Violence Vict.* 2002;17:3.

Follette VM, Polusny MA, Bechtle AE, Naugle AE. Cumulative trauma: the impact of child sexual abuse, adult sexual assault, and spouse abuse. *J Trauma Stress.* 1996;9:25.

Frazier PA. A comparative study of male and female rape victims seen at a hospital-based rape crisis program. *J Interpers Violence.* 1993;8:64.

Henderson DJ. Incest. In: Sadock BJ, Kaplan HI, Freedman AM, eds. *The Sexual Experience.* Baltimore: Williams & Wilkins; 1976:415.

Lewis DO. From abuse to violence: psychophysiological consequences of maltreatment. *J Am Acad Child Adolesc Psychiatry.* 1992;31:383.

McCoy M. Domestic violence: clues to victimization. *Ann Emerg Med.* 1996;27:764.

Reay AMC, Browne KD. The effectiveness of psychological interventions with individuals who physically abuse or neglect their elderly dependents. *J Interpers Violence.* 2002;17:416.

Resick PA. The psychological impact of rape. *J Interpers Violence.* 1993;8:223.

Salzinger S, Feldman RS, Hammer M, Rosario M. The effects of physical abuse on children's social relationships. *Child Dev.* 1993;64:169.

Schafran LH. Rape is a major public health issue. *Am J Public Health.* 1996;86:15.

Stermac L, Del Bove G, Addison M. Violence, injury, and presentation patterns in spousal sexual assaults. *Violence Women.* 2001;7:1218.

Ullman SE, Knight RA. The efficacy of women's resistance strategies in rape situations. *Psychol Women.* 1993;17:23.

Valle LA, Silovsky JF. Attributions and adjustment following child sexual and physical abuse. *Child Maltreat: J Am Prof Soc Abuse Child.* 2002;7:9.

van der Kolk BA. Physical and sexual abuse of adults. In: Sadock BJ, Sadock VA, eds. *Kaplan & Sadock's Comprehensive Textbook of Psychiatry.* 7th ed. Vol 2. Baltimore: Lippincott Williams & Wilkins; 2000:2002.

Vazquez CI. Spousal abuse and violence against women: the significance of understanding attachment. *Ann N Y Acad Sci.* 1996;789:119.

33

Additional Conditions That May Be a Focus of Clinical Attention

The conditions discussed in this section are not considered true mental disorders; they are problems that have brought persons into contact with the mental health care system. Once in the system, persons with a condition that may be a focus of clinical attention should have a thorough neuropsychiatric evaluation, which may or may not uncover a mental disorder. These categories are of clinical interest to psychiatrists because they may accompany mental illness or may be early harbingers of underlying mental disorders.

Thirteen conditions make up the diagnostic category of additional disorders that may be a focus of clinical attention. Nine of these conditions are discussed in this chapter: bereavement, occupational problems, adult antisocial behavior, malingering, phase of life problem, noncompliance with treatment for a mental disorder, religious or spiritual problem, acculturation problem, and age-associated memory decline. (Four other conditions included in the text revision of the fourth edition of *Diagnostic and Statistical Manual of Mental Disorders* [DSM-IV-TR] are discussed in Chapter 53: borderline intellectual functioning, academic problem, childhood or adolescent antisocial behavior, and identity problem.)

BEREAVEMENT

Normal bereavement begins immediately after, or within a few months of, the loss of a loved one. Typical signs and symptoms include feelings of sadness, preoccupation with thoughts about the deceased, tearfulness, irritability, insomnia, and difficulties concentrating and carrying out daily activities. On the basis of the cultural group, bereavement is limited to a varying time, usually 6 months, but it may be longer. Normal bereavement, however, can lead to a full depressive disorder that requires treatment.

DSM-IV-TR includes the following description of bereavement:

> This category can be used when the focus of clinical attention is a reaction to the death of a loved one. As part of their reaction to the loss, some grieving individuals present with symptoms characteristic of a Major Depressive Episode (e.g., feelings of sadness and associated symptoms such as insomnia, poor appetite, and weight loss). The bereaved individual typically regards the depressed mood as "normal," although the person may seek professional help for relief of associated symptoms such as insomnia or anorexia. The duration and expression of "normal" bereavement vary considerably among different cultural groups. The diagnosis of Major Depressive Disorder is generally not given unless the symptoms are still present 2 months after the loss. However, the presence of certain symptoms that are not characteristic of a "normal" grief reaction may be helpful in differentiating bereavement from a Major Depressive Episode. These include (1) guilt about things other than actions taken or not taken by the survivor at the time of the death; (2) thoughts of death other than the survivor feeling that he or she would be better off dead or should have died with the deceased person; (3) morbid preoccupation with worthlessness; (4) marked psychomotor retardation; (5) prolonged and marked functional impairment; and (6) hallucinatory experiences other than thinking that he or she hears the voice of, or transiently sees the image of, the deceased person. (Chapter 2, Section 2.6, presents a further discussion of bereavement.)

OCCUPATIONAL PROBLEM

Occupational or industrial psychiatry is that area of psychiatry specifically concerned with vocational maladjustment and the psychiatric aspects of problems at work. The practical symptoms of job dissatisfaction are mistakes at work, accident proneness, absenteeism, and sabotage. The psychiatric symptoms include insecurity, reduced self-esteem, anger, and resentment at having to work.

DSM-IV-TR includes the following statement about occupational problem:

> This category can be used when the focus of clinical attention is an occupational problem that is not due to a mental disorder or, if it is due to a mental disorder, is sufficiently severe to warrant independent clinical attention. Examples include job dissatisfaction and uncertainty about career choices.

Persons are particularly vulnerable to occupational problems at several points in their working lives—on entry into the working world, at times of promotion or transfer, during periods of unemployment, and at retirement. Specific situations—such as

having too much or too little to do, being subjected to conflicting demands, feeling distracted by family problems, having responsibility without authority, and working for demanding and unhelpful managers—also create occupational distress.

Career Choices and Changes

The choice of a career is a major life decision. A significant number of young persons follow in their parents' footsteps, but many others are unsure of what to do and try several jobs before settling on an occupation. Disadvantaged youngsters frequently have little choice about a career. When young adults have a poor education and lack training and skills, even overwhelming ambition rarely leads them out of poverty or into occupational satisfaction. When the disadvantaged are women or members of minority groups, they have even less chance of occupational success. In discussing career choices with a patient, a psychiatrist should explore special talents and interests, childhood goals, the patient's models, family influences, future expectations, work and academic histories, and motivation to work.

Distress about work is readily understood when an employee has been fired, demoted, or passed over for promotion. Minorities and those in low socioeconomic groups are particularly vulnerable to losing their jobs. Women are specifically at risk when they leave outside employment for homemaking, a transition that researchers have found to be extremely stressful. Some persons experience problems after they win professional advancement. Anxiety about assuming new responsibilities and the fact that persons may be promoted to jobs that are beyond their capacities are among the reasons for this reaction.

Adjusting to retirement is most difficult for those unprepared for it. Adverse reactions occur when a person is forced to retire prematurely or because of illness. Retirement is also a problem for persons whose identity is based primarily on occupational status and income. Women are reported to adjust faster to retirement than men. Some researchers, however, think that retirement poses a greater hardship for women than for men; women face a longer retirement period owing to their greater life expectancy, are more likely to be alone (widowed) during their retirement years, and are usually poorer and have lower retirement incomes than men.

Stress and the Workplace

Workplace distress is implicated in at least 15 percent of occupational disability claims. Expected distress follows recognized and uncontrollable work changes: downsizing, mergers and acquisitions, work overload, and chronic physical strains, including work noise, temperature, and injuries and strain due to computer work. According to one study the top ten most stressful jobs were (1) the U.S. president, (2) firefighter, (3) senior corporate executive, (4) race car driver, (5) taxi driver, (6) surgeon, (7) astronaut, (8) police officer, (9) football player, and (10) air traffic controller.

Work frustration can also arise from an individual worker's unrecognized (and therefore unresolved) psychodynamic issues, such as working appropriately with superiors and not relating to one's supervisor as a parent figure. Other developmental issues include unresolved problems with competition, assertiveness, envy, fear of success, and inability to communicate verbally in a constructive manner.

A 38-year-old white male has outbursts of anger when told to complete a day's tasks in a construction company. He complains to his union officer who, after investigating the worker's complaints, states that the work assignment is fair. The worker has never taken pride in completing assignments and has moved from company to company on average every 9 months since resigning from the military 6 years earlier because he tired of taking orders. (Courtesy of Leah J. Dickstein, M.D.)

Often work conflicts reflect similar conflicts in the worker's personal life, and referral for treatment is in order.

Career Problems of Women

During the past 25 years, the U.S. business world has undergone many changes. A significant number of women have entered the workforce; many corporations now employ a husband and a wife in the same organization; and teenagers have entered the labor force on a part-time basis on a large scale.

Ninety percent of all women today in the United States will have to work to support themselves and probably one or two others. Economic necessity now prompts homemakers to work, and rejection by employers on the basis of age, lack of recent experience, or insufficient training can cause dysphoria and depression. This is particularly true for recently divorced women in their 40s or 50s who have spent most of their adult lives as wives and mothers.

Young women have different stresses, primarily related to the conflicting demands of work and family responsibilities: More than 50 percent of all mothers in the workforce have children 1 year old or younger. But women's organizations and other critics charge that few corporations are removing barriers to women's advancement or are concerned about reducing the tension that arises when job and family demands conflict. Specific issues that need to be addressed are provisions for child care or for the care of elderly parents, the option of flexible work hours, and the availability and use of unpaid parental leaves. Studies reveal that when these leaves are made available to both parents, fathers rarely take them; that managers are more sensitive to crises in men's lives than to crises in the lives of female employees; and that managers respond to such major events as divorce and the death of a family member but ignore the stress placed on a worker by the illness of a child or a school closing because of a snow day. A few socially conscious corporations hold workshops to address the changes arising from the influx of women into the workforce and the issues of family responsibilities, sexual harassment in the workplace, personal safety during business travel, and rape prevention. Day-care facilities have been established on site in some organizations and have proved successful.

Dual-career families (in which both husband and wife have jobs) now constitute more than 50 percent of all families. Problems can arise when an employer wants one partner to make a geographical move to a new post. Even if the transfer is a promotion, the transfer can result in lower total income for the family because of the spouse's loss of job or career disruption. Some corporations offer new jobs to both spouses when one is asked to relocate, but such approaches are rare. A more

common advance is the acceptance of couples, married or unmarried, as employees of the same corporation. Couples employed by the same company seem to cause problems for themselves and others only when they compete with each other. The couples who fare best treat their spouses differently at the office than they do at home. Resentment from coworkers occurs when one spouse reports directly to the other; otherwise, no adverse responses from other employees have been noted.

Vocational Rehabilitation

Rehabilitation is often necessary for those traumatized by stresses in the workplace, those who had to take a leave of absence because of medical or psychiatric reasons, or those who have been fired. Individual or group counseling enables persons to improve personal relationships, raise self-esteem, or learn new work skills. Patients with schizophrenia may benefit from sheltered workshops in which they perform work that is geared to their level of function. Some patients with schizophrenia or autism do well in tasks that are repetitive or require obsessive concern with details.

ADULT ANTISOCIAL BEHAVIOR

Characterized by activities that are illegal, immoral, or both, antisocial behavior usually begins in childhood and often persists throughout life. DSM-IV-TR includes the following statements about adult antisocial behavior:

> This category can be used when the focus of clinical attention is adult antisocial behavior that is not due to a mental disorder (e.g., Conduct Disorder, Antisocial Personality Disorder, or an Impulse-Control Disorder). Examples include the behavior of some professional thieves, racketeers, or dealers in illegal substances.

The term *antisocial behavior* somewhat confusingly applies both to persons' actions that are not due to a mental disorder and to actions by those who never received a neuropsychiatric workup to determine the presence or absence of a mental disorder. As Dorothy Lewis noted, the term can apply to behavior by normal persons who "struggle to make a dishonest living."

Epidemiology

Depending on the criteria and the sampling, estimates of the prevalence of adult antisocial behavior range from 5 to 15 percent of the population. Within prison populations, investigators report prevalence figures between 20 and 80 percent. Men account for more adult antisocial behavior than women.

Etiology

Antisocial behaviors in adulthood are characteristic of a variety of persons, ranging from those with no demonstrable psychopathology to those who are severely impaired and suffer from psychotic disorders, cognitive disorders, and retardation, among other conditions. A comprehensive neuropsychiatric assessment of antisocial adults is indicated and may reveal potentially treatable psychiatric and neurological impairments that can easily be overlooked. Only in the absence of mental disorders can patients be categorized as displaying adult antisocial behavior. Adult antisocial behavior may be influenced by genetic and social factors.

Genetic Factors. Data supporting the genetic transmission of antisocial behavior are based on studies that find a 60 percent concordance rate in monozygotic twins and about a 30 percent concordance rate in dizygotic twins. Adoption studies show a high rate of antisocial behavior in the biological relatives of adoptees identified with antisocial behavior and a high incidence of antisocial behavior in the adopted-away offspring of those with antisocial behavior. The prenatal and perinatal periods of those who subsequently display antisocial behavior often are associated with low birth weight, mental retardation, and prenatal exposure to alcohol and other drugs of abuse.

Social Factors. Studies showed that in neighborhoods in which families with low socioeconomic status (SES) predominate, the sons of unskilled workers are more likely to commit more offenses and more serious criminal offenses than the sons of middle-class and skilled workers, at least during adolescence and early adulthood. These data are not as clear for women, but the findings are generally similar in studies from many countries. Areas of family training differ by SES group. Middle-SES parents use love-oriented techniques in discipline. They withdraw affection rather than impose physical punishment as in low-SES groups. Negative parental attitudes toward aggressive behavior, attempts to curb aggressive behavior, and the ability to communicate parental values are more characteristic of middle- and high-SES groups than of low ones. Adult antisocial behavior is associated with the use and abuse of alcohol and other substances and with the easy availability of handguns.

Diagnosis and Clinical Features

The diagnosis of adult antisocial behavior is one of exclusion. Substance dependence in such behavior often makes it difficult to separate the antisocial behavior related primarily to substance dependence from disordered behaviors that occurred either before substance use or during episodes unrelated to substance dependence.

During the manic phases of bipolar I disorder, certain aspects of behavior, such as wanderlust, sexual promiscuity, and financial difficulties, can be similar to adult antisocial behavior. Patients with schizophrenia may have episodes of adult antisocial behavior, but the symptom picture is usually clear, especially regarding thought disorder, delusions, and hallucinations on the mental status examination.

Neurological conditions may be associated with adult antisocial behavior, and electroencephalograms (EEGs), computed tomography (CT) scans, magnetic resonance imaging (MRI), and complete neurological examinations are indicated. Temporal lobe epilepsy should be considered in the differential diagnosis. When a clear-cut diagnosis of temporal lobe epilepsy or encephalitis can be made, the disorder may be considered to contribute to the adult antisocial behavior. Abnormal EEG findings are prevalent among violent offenders: An estimated 50 percent of aggressive criminals have abnormal EEG findings.

Persons with adult antisocial behavior have difficulties in work, marriage, and money matters and conflicts with various authorities. The symptoms of adult antisocial behavior are summarized in Table 33–1. (Antisocial personality disorder is discussed in Chapter 27.)

Table 33–1
Symptoms of Adult Antisocial Behavior

Life Area	Antisocial Patients with Significant Problems in Area (%)
Work problems	85
Marital problems	81
Financial dependence	79
Arrests	75
Alcohol abuse	72
School problems	71
Impulsiveness	67
Sexual behavior	64
Wild adolescence	62
Vagrancy	60
Belligerence	58
Social isolation	56
Military record (of those serving)	53
Lack of guilt	40
Somatic complaints	31
Use of aliases	29
Pathological lying	16
Drug abuse	15
Suicide attempts	11

Data are from Robins L. *Deviant Children Grown Up: A Sociological and Psychiatric Study of Sociopathic Personality.* Baltimore: Williams & Wilkins; 1966.

Treatment

In general, therapists are pessimistic about treating adult antisocial behavior. They have little hope of changing a pattern that has been present almost continuously throughout a person's life. Psychotherapy has not been effective, and no major breakthroughs with biological treatments, including medications, have occurred.

Therapists show more enthusiasm for the use of therapeutic communities and other forms of group treatment, even though the data provide little basis for optimism. Many adult criminals who are incarcerated in institutional settings have shown some response to group therapy approaches. The history of violence, criminality, and antisocial behavior has shown that such behaviors seem to decrease after age 40. Recidivism in criminals, which can reach 90 percent in some studies, also decreases in middle age.

Prevention. Because antisocial behavior often begins during childhood, the major focus must be on delinquency prevention. Any measures that improve the physical and mental health of socioeconomically disadvantaged children and their families are likely to reduce delinquency and violent crime. Often, recurrently violent persons have sustained many insults to the central nervous system (CNS), prenatally and throughout childhood and adolescence. Consequently, programs must be developed to educate parents about the dangers to their children of CNS injury from maltreatment, including the effects of psychoactive substances on the brain of the growing fetus. Public education about the releasing effect of alcohol on violent behaviors (not to mention its contribution to vehicular homicide) may also reduce crime.

In a *Surgeon General's Report on Violence and Public Health* issued over 15 years ago, the Committee on the Prevention of Assault and Homicide emphasized the importance of discouraging corporal punishment in the home, forbidding it in the schools, and even abolishing capital punishment by the state, saying that all are models and sanctions for violence. Since that time, capital punishment has been instituted in states that did not have it, such as New York. There is no evidence that capital punishment reduces crime in states that have it. Opponents of capital punishment see it as "vengeance," not punishment.

Although persons disagree about the contribution of violence in the media to violent crime, the propaganda potential of the media is universally recognized. The extent to which the media, such as television, can be used to transmit positive social values has not yet been realized. The guidelines issued by the television industry to indicate the amount of sex and violence in programs is an attempt to deal with the issue; however, program content that espouses traditional societal values would be beneficial.

The most successful preventive measures within the field of medicine have come from communitywide public health programs (e.g., campaigns against smoking) and from programs that detect individual vulnerabilities (e.g., individual monitoring of blood pressure). Studies of adult antisocial behavior reveal the contribution of broad cultural factors and constellations of individual biopsychosocial vulnerabilities. Prevention programs must recognize and address both kinds of factors.

MALINGERING

Malingering is characterized by the voluntary production and presentation of false or grossly exaggerated physical or psychological symptoms. Patients always have an external motivation that falls into one of three categories: to avoid difficult or dangerous situations, responsibilities, or punishment; to receive compensation, free hospital room and board, a source of drugs, or a haven from the police; and to retaliate when the patient feels guilt or suffers a financial loss, legal penalty, or job loss. The presence of a clearly definable goal is the main factor that differentiates malingering from factitious disorders.

Epidemiology

The incidence of malingering is unknown, but it is common and occurs most frequently in settings with a preponderance of men—the military, prisons, factories, and other industrial settings. The condition also occurs in women.

Diagnosis and Clinical Features

DSM-IV-TR includes the following remarks about malingering:

> The essential feature of malingering is the intentional production of false or grossly exaggerated physical or psychological symptoms, motivated by external incentives such as avoiding military duty, avoiding work, obtaining financial compensation, evading criminal prosecution, or obtaining drugs. Under some circumstances, malingering may represent adaptive behavior—for example, feigning illness while a captive of the enemy during wartime.

Malingering should be strongly suspected if any combination of the following is noted:

1. Medicolegal context of presentation (e.g., the person is referred by an attorney to the clinician for examination)
2. Marked discrepancy between the person's claimed stress or disability and the objective findings
3. Lack of cooperation during the diagnostic evaluation and in complying with the prescribed treatment regimen
4. Presence of antisocial personality disorder

Many malingerers express mostly subjective, vague, ill-defined symptoms—for example, headache; pains in the neck, lower back, chest, or abdomen; dizziness; vertigo; amnesia; anxiety; and depression—and the symptoms often have a family history, in all likelihood not medically caused but incredibly difficult to refute. Malingerers may complain bitterly and describe how much the symptoms impair their normal function and how much they dislike the symptoms. The patients may use the best doctors who are the most trusted (and perhaps most gullible) and promptly and willingly pay all their bills, even if excessive, to impress the doctors with their integrity. To seem credible, malingerers must report the symptoms but tell their physicians as little as possible. But often they complain of misery without objective signs or other symptoms congruent with recognized diseases and syndromes; if they do describe all the symptoms of a disease, the symptoms are said to "come and go." Malingerers are often preoccupied with compensation rather than cure and have a knowledge of the law and precedents relative to their claims. Objective tests—such as audiometry, brainstem audiometry, auditory and visually evoked potentials, galvanic skin response, electromyography, and nerve conduction studies—may be helpful in sorting out auditory, labyrinthine, ophthalmological, neurological, and other problems.

Differential Diagnosis

Malingering differs from factitious disorder in that the motivation for the symptom production in malingering is an external incentive (e.g., insurance payments); in factitious disorder external incentives are absent. Evidence of an intrapsychic need to maintain the sick role (e.g., to satisfy dependency needs) suggests factitious disorder. Malingering is differentiated from somatoform disorders by the intentional production of symptoms and by the obvious external incentives associated with it. In malingering, in contrast to some somatoform disorders such as conversion disorder, symptom relief is not often obtained by suggestion or hypnosis. Table 33–2 lists features that differentiate malingering from genuine illness.

Treatment

A patient suspected of malingering should be evaluated thoroughly and objectively, and the physician should refrain from showing any suspicion. If a clinician becomes angry (a common response to malingerers), a confrontation may occur, with two consequences: (1) the doctor–patient relationship is disrupted so that no further positive intervention is possible and (2) the patient becomes even more guarded, making proof of deception virtually impossible. If the patient is accepted and not discredited, subsequent patient hospital or outpatient observation may reveal the versatility of the symptoms, which are consistently present only when patients know that they are being observed. Preserving the doctor–patient relationship is often essential to diagnosis and long-term treatment. Careful evaluation usually reveals the relevant issue without the need for confrontation. It is usually best to use an intensive treatment approach as though the symptoms were real. The patient can then give up the symptoms in response to treatment without losing face.

Table 33–2
Malingering Features Usually Not Found in Genuine Illness

Symptoms are vague, ill-defined, overdramatized, and not in conformity with known clinical conditions.
The patient seeks addicting drugs, financial gain, the avoidance of onerous (e.g., jail) or other unwanted conditions.
History, examination, and evaluative data do not elucidate complaints.
The patient is uncooperative and refuses to accept a clean bill of health or an encouraging prognosis.
The findings appear compatible with self-inflicted injuries.
History or records reveal multiple past episodes of injury or undiagnosed illness.
Records or test data appear to have been tampered with (e.g., erasures, unprescribed substances in urine).

Courtesy of Arthur T. Meyerson, M.D.

PHASE OF LIFE PROBLEM

DSM-IV-TR includes the following description of phase of life problem:

> This category can be used when the focus of clinical attention is a problem associated with a particular developmental phase or some other life circumstance that is not due to a mental disorder or, if it is due to a mental disorder, is sufficiently severe to warrant independent clinical attention. Examples include problems associated with entering school, leaving parental control, starting a new career, and changes involved in marriage, divorce, and retirement.

External events are most likely to overwhelm a person's adaptive capacities when they are unexpected or numerous (i.e., a number of stresses occurring within a short time), when the strain is chronic and unremitting, or when one loss heralds a myriad of concomitant adjustments that strain the person's recuperative powers.

The strains most likely to produce anxiety and depression relate to major life-cycle changes: marriage, occupation, and parenthood. These events affect both men and women, but women, those in low socioeconomic groups, and minorities seem particularly vulnerable to adverse reactions. Again, the change creates significant strain when it is unexpected and when it involves not only adjustment to a loss (a spouse or a job) but also the need to adjust to a new status that entails further hardships and problems.

In general, persons are able to adjust to life changes if they have mature defense mechanisms such as altruism, humor, and capacity for sublimation. Flexibility, reliability, strong family ties, regular employment, adequate income, job satisfaction, a pattern of regular recreation and social participation, realistic

goals, and a history of adequate performance—in short, a full and satisfying life—create resilience to deal with life changes.

NONCOMPLIANCE WITH TREATMENT

DSM-IV-TR contains following statement:

> This category can be used when the focus of clinical attention is noncompliance with an important aspect of the treatment for a mental disorder or a general medical condition. The reasons for noncompliance may include discomfort resulting from treatment (e.g., medication side effects), expense of treatment, decisions based on personal value judgments, religious or cultural beliefs about the advantages and disadvantages of the proposed treatment, maladaptive personality traits or coping styles (e.g., denial of illness), or the presence of a mental disorder (e.g., Schizophrenia, Avoidant Personality Disorder). This category should be used only when the problem is sufficiently severe to warrant independent clinical attention.

Compliance is closely connected to the doctor–patient relationship, and a thorough discussion of noncompliance and compliance appears in Chapter 1.

RELIGIOUS AND SPIRITUAL PROBLEM

DSM-IV-TR contains the following statement:

> This category can be used when the focus of clinical attention is a religious or spiritual problem. Examples include distressing experiences that involve loss or questioning of faith, problems associated with conversion to a new faith, or questioning other spiritual values which may not necessarily be related to an organized church or religious institution.

From the psychological point of view, perhaps the most striking feature of religion is its universality. There are few societies in which religion plays no significant role, and there are relatively few persons who, at one time or another, have not experienced some religious stirring. From this universality one must infer that religion performs an adaptive function that is invoked to satisfy one or more universal human needs.

Pastoral Counseling

The pastoral function of the clergy in the United States extends to helping the individual members of the religious congregation deal with serious problems that they cannot resolve alone and that may cause anguish and damage. The pastoral function includes visiting the ill, comforting the mourner, encouraging the widow, and helping the orphan. The term *counseling* involves consultation for the purpose of helping the troubled person solve a specific presenting problem. It may be a marital problem, a parent–child problem, a problem of conflict among siblings, or a complaint of feeling guilt or anxiety.

Cults

Cults are charismatic groups that can affect participants in adverse ways, which may eventually bring them into contact with the mental health care system. Cults are characterized by an intensely held belief system and ideology imposed on members, by a high level of group cohesion serving to prevent members' freedom of choice to leave the group, and by a profound influence on the members' behavior, possibly inducing psychiatric symptoms and producing overt psychotic disorders.

Most potential cult members are in their adolescence or otherwise struggling to establish their own identities. They are drawn to a cult, which holds out the false promise of emotional well-being and purports to offer the sense of direction for which they are searching. Cult members are encouraged to proselytize and to draw new members into the group. They are often encouraged to break with family members and friends and to socialize only with other group members. Cults are invariably led by charismatic personalities, who are often ruthless in their quest for financial, sexual, and power gains. Cult leaders usually demand conformity to the cult's ideological belief system, which may have strong religious or quasi-religious overtones. Exit therapy has been developed to guide cult members out of the group when lingering emotional ties to persons outside the cult can be mobilized.

On March 28, 1997, the biggest group of suicides recorded in the United States was found in Rancho Santa Fe, California. Thirty-nine men and women who were members of a millennialist cult called Heaven's Gate killed themselves with lethal doses of phenobarbital combined with alcohol. Some suffocated themselves with plastic bags. Cult members believed that their human bodies were physical containers that had to be discarded so that their souls could be transported to a new level of being. Their souls were to rendezvous with an unidentified flying object that was trailing the Hale-Bopp comet passing Earth at that time and signaling for them to kill themselves. In their new plane of existence, they would inhabit new bodies and travel through different galaxies. The cult was made up primarily of young persons in their 20s who had left their parental homes for various reasons and who were seeking a sense of spiritual identity. The cult leader was an ex-minister who called himself "Bo" after Bo-Peep who shepherded sheep and, like most cult leaders, was charismatic and convincing to a group of psychologically vulnerable persons seeking an omnipotent godlike authority figure to diminish their sense of anxiety, depression, and alienation. The cult recruited its members through personal contacts and advertising on the Internet, where they had a site called Heaven's Gate.

ACCULTURATION PROBLEM

DSM-IV-TR contains the following statement about the acculturation problem:

> This category can be used when the focus of clinical attention is a problem involving adjustment to a different culture (e.g., following migration).

Periods of cultural transition, with changing mores and fluid role definition, may increase a person's vulnerability to life strain. Extreme cultural transition can create a condition of severe distress, also called *culture shock,* which occurs when a person is suddenly thrust into an alien culture or has divided loyalties to two different cultures. In a less extreme form, culture shock occurs when young men and women enter the army, when persons change jobs, when families move or undergo a significant change in income, when children first go to school, and when black inner-city children are bused to white middle-class schools. (Further discussion of culture change and culture shock appears in Chapter 4, Section 4.6.)

Brainwashing

First practiced by the Chinese Communists on U.S. prisoners during the Korean War, brainwashing is the deliberate creation of cultural shock. A condition of isolation, alienation, and intimidation is developed to assault ego strengths and leave the person to be brainwashed vulnerable to the imposition of alien ideas and behavior that he or she would usually reject. Brainwashing relies on both mental and physical coercion. All persons are vulnerable to brainwashing if they are exposed to it long enough, if they are alone and without support, and if they are without hope of escape from the situation. Help from the mental health care system, in the form of deprogramming, is usually necessary to help persons readjust to their usual environments after the brainwashing experience. Supportive therapy is offered, with emphasis on reeducation, restitution of ego strengths that existed before the trauma, and alleviation of the guilt and depression that are remnants of the frightening experience and the lost confidence and confusion in identity that resulted from it.

Prisoners of War and Torture Victims

Prisoners who survive war or torture experiences survive because of personal inner strengths developed in their earlier lives beginning within their emotionally strong and caring families; if from troubled families, they are at high risk for suicide. Prisoners must constantly cope with continued anxiety, fear, isolation from known lives, and complete loss of all control over their lives. Those who appear to cope best believe they must survive for a reason (e.g., to tell others what they experienced or to return to loved ones). Prisoners who cope best describe living simultaneously on two levels: coping in the here-and-now to survive the situation while maintaining constant mental connections to their past values and experiences and persons important to them.

Beyond the surviving prisoner's personal difficulties (including posttraumatic stress disorder), if and when their survival behavior continues, it can affect their consequent families, with inordinate fear of police and strangers, overprotection and overburdening of children to replace those lost, lack of sharing of the past, continued isolation from their current communities, or inappropriate expressed anger. Another generation can thus be affected in their personal development and psychological functioning and may require psychiatric evaluation and treatment.

A 72-year-old Jewish woman survivor of the Auschwitz Nazi concentration camp stated that as a 19-year-old married Hungarian who wanted to become a lawyer, she accepted the leadership of a women's barracks because she knew she could defend them as her father had helped the poor in their Hungarian city. She encouraged others to care for their bodies, share food and songs and stories at night, and maintain the hope they would survive to find some family and make a new life for themselves after the war. At liberation after the death march, she helped American soldiers translate, found her sister and husband, and built a new life, continuing her leadership in her new community at a hospital in Jerusalem.

AGE-RELATED COGNITIVE DECLINE

DSM-IV-TR includes the following comment:

> This category can be used when the focus of clinical attention is an objectively identified decline in cognitive functioning consequent to the aging process that is within normal limits given the person's age. Individuals with this condition may report problems remembering names or appointments or may experience difficulty in solving complex problems. This category should be considered only after it has been determined that the cognitive impairment is not attributable to a specific mental disorder or neurological condition.

Attempts to delay age-related cognitive decline are myriad. They include daily intake of vitamin E (200 to 600 mg), daily intake of nonsteroidal antiinflammatory drugs (NSAIDs), use of the herb ginkgo biloba, and use of male and female sex steroids. Cognitive decline is lower in persons who exercise, do not smoke, drink little or no alcohol, and who challenge their intellect at work or play (e.g., crossword puzzles). The ability to learn new material is maintained through old age; however, it takes longer and requires more practice than in young persons.

References

Bernard LC, Houston W, Natoli L. Malingering on neuropsychological memory tests: potential objective indicators. *J Clin Psychol.* 1993;49:45.

Blackwell B. Treatment compliance. In: Sadock BJ, Sadock VA, eds. *Kaplan & Sadock's Comprehensive Textbook of Psychiatry.* 7th ed. Vol 1. Baltimore: Lippincott Williams & Wilkins; 2000:1893.

Buckalew LW, Buckalew NM. Survey of the nature and prevalence of patients' noncompliance and implications for intervention. *Psychol Rep.* 1995;76:315.

Crittenden PM, Claussen AH, eds. *The Organization of Attachment Relationships: Maturation, Culture, and Context.* New York: Cambridge University Press; 2000.

Dickstein LJ. Other additional conditions that may be a focus of clinical attention. In: Sadock BJ, Sadock VA, eds. *Kaplan & Sadock's Comprehensive Textbook of Psychiatry.* 7th ed. Vol 1. Baltimore: Lippincott Williams & Wilkins; 2000:1918.

Everett B, Gallop R. *The Link Between Childhood Trauma and Mental Illness: Effective Interventions for Mental Health Professionals.* Thousand Oaks, CA: Sage Publications; 2001.

Holmes T. Life situations, emotions, and disease. *Psychosomatics.* 1978;19:747.

Hutri M. When careers reach a dead end: identification of occupational crisis states. *J Psychol.* 1996;130:383.

Kissane DW, Bloch S, Dowe DL, et al. The Melbourne Family Grief Study, I: perceptions of family functioning in bereavement. *Am J Psychiatry.* 1996;153:650.

Kissane DW, Bloch S, Onghena P, McKenzie DP, Snyder RD, Dowe DL. The Melbourne Family Grief Study, II: psychosocial morbidity and grief in bereaved families. *Am J Psychiatry.* 1996;153:659.

Lewis DO, Pincus JH, Feldman M, Jackson L, Bard B. Psychiatric, neurological, and psychoeducational characteristics of 15 death row inmates in the United States. *Am J Psychiatry.* 1986;143:7.

Lipian MS, Mills MJ. Malingering. In: Sadock BJ, Sadock VA, eds. *Kaplan & Sadock's Comprehensive Textbook of Psychiatry.* 7th ed. Vol 1. Baltimore: Lippincott Williams & Wilkins; 2000:1878.

Lukoff D, Lu FG, Turner R. Cultural considerations in the assessment and treatment of religious and spiritual problems. *Psychiatr Clin North Am.* 1995;18:467.

Pawliuk N, Grizenko N, Chan-Yip A, Gantous P, Mathew J, Nguyen D. Acculturation style and psychological functioning in children of immigrants. *Am J Orthopsychiatry.* 1996;66:111.

Repetti RL. Short-term effects of occupational stressors on daily mood and health complaints. *Health Psychol.* 1993;12:125.

Sadock VA. Other additional conditions that may be a focus of clinical attention. In: *Comprehensive Textbook of Psychiatry.* 6th ed. Kaplan HI, Sadock BJ, eds. Baltimore: Williams & Wilkins; 1995:1633.

Tardiff K. Adult antisocial behavior and criminality. In: Sadock BJ, Sadock VA, eds. *Kaplan & Sadock's Comprehensive Textbook of Psychiatry.* 7th ed. Vol 1. Baltimore: Lippincott Williams & Wilkins; 2000:1908.

34 Emergency Psychiatric Medicine

▲ 34.1 Psychiatric Emergencies

Emergency psychiatry has become a subspecialty of general psychiatry requiring specific skills to deal with situations for which immediate therapeutic intervention frequently is necessary. The widening scope of emergency psychiatry goes beyond general psychiatric practice to include such specialized problems as the abuse of substances, children, and spouses and the violence of suicide, homicide, and rape and such social issues as homelessness, aging, competence, and acquired immune deficiency syndrome (AIDS). Emergency psychiatrists must be up-to-date on medicolegal issues and managed care.

EPIDEMIOLOGY

Psychiatric emergency rooms are used equally by men and women and more by single than by married persons. About 20 percent of these patients are suicidal, and about 10 percent are violent. The most common diagnoses are mood disorders (including depressive disorders and manic episodes), schizophrenia, and alcohol dependence. About 40 percent of all patients seen in psychiatric emergency rooms require hospitalization. Most visits occur during the night hours, but there is no usage difference based on the day of the week or the month of the year. Contrary to popular belief, studies have not found that use of psychiatric emergency rooms increases during a full moon or the Christmas season.

EMERGENCY PSYCHIATRIC INTERVIEW

An emergency interview is similar to a standard psychiatric interview except for the time limitation imposed by other patients waiting to be seen and the potential sense of urgency in assessing the risk to the patient or others. Usually, a physician focuses on the presenting complaint and the reasons why the patient has come to the emergency room. The time constraint requires that a clinician structure the interview, particularly with patients who may respond with long, rambling accounts of their illnesses. If friends, relatives, or the police accompany the patient, a supplemental history should be obtained from them, especially if the patient is mute, negativistic, uncooperative, or otherwise unable to give a coherent history.

Patients may be highly motivated to reveal themselves to gain relief from suffering, but they may also be both consciously and unconsciously motivated to conceal innermost feelings that they perceive to be shameful or threatening. If a patient has been brought to the hospital involuntarily, willingness or ability to cooperate may be impaired. A psychiatrist's relationship with a patient strongly influences what the patient does and does not say, even within the context of a first interview in an emergency room; thus a large portion of the psychiatric emergency interview involves the specific and sophisticated techniques of listening, observation, and interpretation that provide the foundation of psychiatric training overall. A psychiatrist should be straightforward, honest, calm, and nonthreatening and convey to patients the idea that the clinician is in control and will act decisively to protect them from hurting themselves or others. Table 34.1–1 summarizes how to evaluate a psychiatric emergency.

Sometimes persons contact the emergency room by telephone. The psychiatrist should obtain the number from which the call is made and the exact address so that if the call is interrupted, the psychiatrist will be able to direct help to the patient. If the patient is alone and the psychiatrist ascertains that he or she is in danger, the police should be alerted. If possible, an assistant should call the police on another line while the psychiatrist keeps the patient engaged until help arrives. The patient should not be told to drive alone to the hospital; an emergency medical team or mobile crisis unit should be dispatched to bring the patient to the hospital.

The greatest potential error in emergency room psychiatry is overlooking a physical illness as the cause of an emotional illness. Head traumas, medical illnesses, substance abuse (including alcohol), cerebrovascular diseases, metabolic abnormalities, and medications may all cause abnormal behavior, and psychiatrists should take concise medical histories that concentrate on these areas.

Diagnosis

An emergency assessment is not expected to be complete, but it must address certain important questions. Toxicology screening, chest X-rays, an electrocardiogram (ECG), and other relevant laboratory tests (e.g., serum lithium [Eskalith] and phenytoin [Dilantin] levels) should be done as soon as possible for the most accurate information. Initial medical clearance and specialty consultations should be done in the emergency room whenever feasible. If available, old records should be reviewed,

Table 34.1–1
General Strategy in Evaluating Patients

I. Self-protection

A. Know as much as possible about the patients before meeting them.

B. Leave physical restraint procedures to those who are trained to handle them.

C. Be alert to risks for impending violence.

D. Attend to the safety of the physical surroundings (e.g., door access, room objects).

E. Have others present during the assessment if needed.

F. Have others in the vicinity.

G. Attend to developing an alliance with the patient (e.g., do not confront or threaten patients with paranoid psychoses).

II. Prevent harm

A. Prevent self-injury and suicide. Use whatever methods are necessary to prevent patients from hurting themselves during the evaluation.

B. Prevent violence toward others. During the evaluation, briefly assess the patient for the risk of violence. If the risk is deemed significant, consider the following options:

1. Inform the patient that violence is not acceptable.
2. Approach the patient in a nonthreatening manner.
3. Reassure and calm the patient or assist in reality testing.
4. Offer medication.
5. Inform the patient that restraint or seclusion will be used if necessary.
6. Have teams ready to restrain the patient.
7. When patients are restrained, always observe them closely, and frequently check their vital signs. Isolate restrained patients from agitating stimuli. Immediately plan a further approach—medication, reassurance, medical evaluation.

III. Rule out cognitive disorders caused by a general medical condition

IV. Rule out impending psychosis

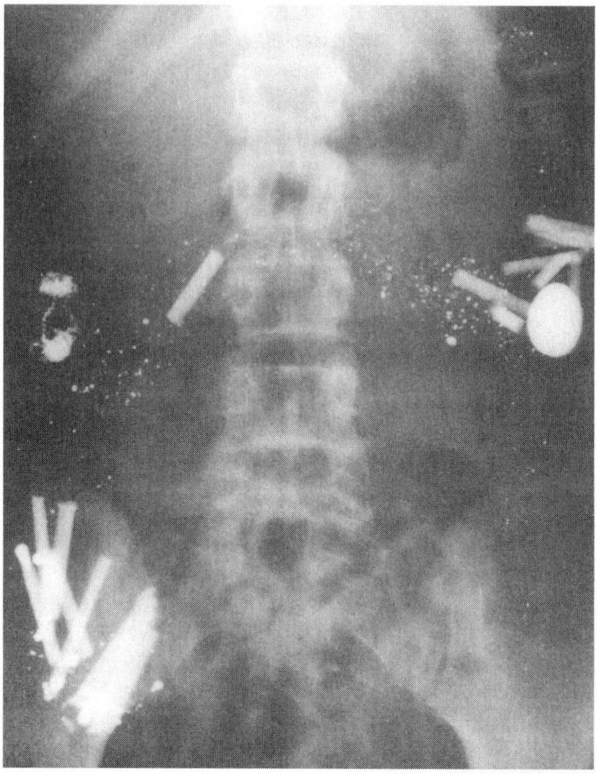

FIGURE 34.1–1
A mentally ill patient who is a habitual swallower of foreign objects. Included in his colonic lumen are 13 thermometers and 8 pennies. The dense, round, almost punctate densities are globules of liberated liquid mercury. (Courtesy of Stephen R. Baker, M.D., and Kyunghee C. Cho, M.D.)

and all information from outside sources, such as family members and the police, should be gathered before making a disposition. Although safety is always the highest priority, it should not unduly delay completion of the diagnostic evaluation. At times a medical emergency may be the direct result of severe mental illness. Patients may swallow foreign objects or deliberately cut or mutilate themselves among other dangerous practices (Figs. 34.1–1 and 34.1–2).

DIFFERENTIAL DIAGNOSIS

Emergency psychiatrists must consider a wide range of conditions that could account for the presenting signs and symptoms. The most common complaints fall within the categories of anxiety, depression, mania, and thought disorder. These conditions may overlap and have multiple causes.

The differential diagnoses of anxiety, depressive episodes, manic episodes, and thought disorders are listed in Tables 34.1–2 through 34.1–5. Anxiety differs from depression, mania, and thought disorder in that many illnesses that can cause anxiety are life threatening. Incipient myocardial infarctions, pulmonary emboli, cardiac arrhythmias, and internal hemorrhages can cause acute anxiety to the degree of panic. Untreated congestive heart failure secondary to a silent myocar-

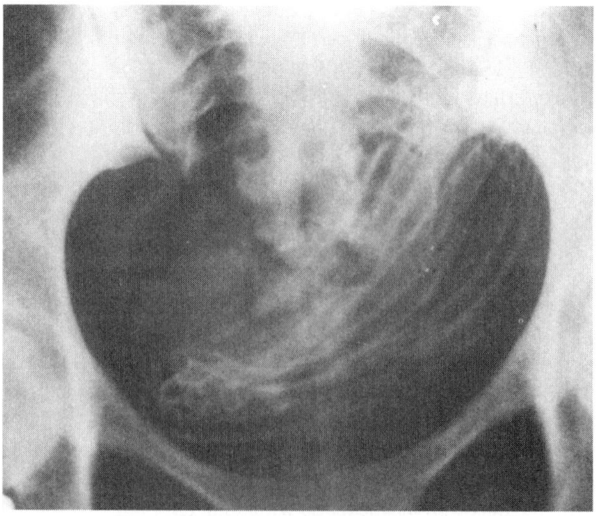

FIGURE 34.1–2
A patient brought to the emergency room with lower abdominal pain. X-ray shows a nasogastric tube folded into the bladder. The patient would insert the tube into his urethra as part of a masturbatory ritual (urethral eroticism). (Courtesy of Stephen R. Baker, M.D., and Kyunghee C. Cho, M.D.)

Table 34.1–2
Differential Diagnosis of Anxiety

Alcohol delirium and withdrawal
Amphetamine (or related substance) intoxication and withdrawal
Anxiety disorders
Bipolar I disorder
Borderline personality disorder
Caffeine intoxication
Cerebral arteriosclerosis
Cocaine intoxication
Encephalitis
Essential hypertension
Hyperthyroidism
Hyperventilation syndrome
Hypocalcemia
Hypoglycemia
Hypokalemia
Impending myocardial infarction
Internal hemorrhage
Major depressive disorder
Mitral valve prolapse
Normal anxiety
Other temporal lobe diseases
Panic disorder
Paroxysmal atrial tachycardia and other cardiac arrhythmias
Pheochromocytoma
Phobias
Postconcussion syndrome
Psychomotor epilepsy
Psychotic disorders
Pulmonary embolism
Schizophrenia
Sedative, hypnotic, or anxiolytic withdrawal and delirium
Sexual disorders
Subacute bacterial endocarditis

Adapted from Andrew Edmund Slaby, M.D., Ph.D.

Table 34.1–3
Differential Diagnosis of Depressive Episodes

Adjustment disorder with depressed mood
Dysthymic disorder
Schizoaffective disorder
Schizophrenia
Major depressive disorder
Bipolar I disorder
Borderline personality disorder
Hypokalemia
Brief psychotic disorder
Cyclothymic disorder
Antihypertensive toxicity
Steroid psychotic disorder
Hypothyroidism
Cerebral neoplasm
General paresis
Amphetamine use disorders
Cocaine use disorders
Carcinoma of pancreas
Hepatitis
Postviral infection syndrome
Dementia of the Alzheimer's type
Vascular dementia
Dementia of the Alzheimer's type with late onset
Dementia of the Alzheimer's type with early onset
Cirrhosis of the liver
Arteriosclerosis
Infectious mononucleosis
Hyperthyroidism
Occult malignancy
AIDS
Schizoid personality disorder
Schizotypal personality disorder

Adapted from Andrew Edmund Slaby, M.D., Ph.D.

dial infarction or malignant cardiac arrhythmia may be fatal. Older persons and those who have just suffered a loss may be perceived as having depressive or nihilistic ideation when, in fact, age or stress has propelled them into a life-threatening illness manifested by anxiety and a sense of impending doom. Persons who experience depression as an adverse effect of antihypertensive medications may perceive spouses, children, friends, or work in a negative light that changes with cessation of the medication.

Table 34.1–6 outlines features that should make emergency room clinicians consider an organic condition as the cause of the complaint. Table 34.1–7 lists the central nervous system (CNS) disorders that require immediate treatment. Table 34.1–8 lists the CNS disorders that present with behavioral features that require a careful neurological examination that may include neuroimaging.

The differential diagnosis of violent behavior includes substance-induced persisting dementia, antisocial personality disorder, catatonic schizophrenia, cerebral infection, cerebral neoplasm, obsessive-compulsive personality disorder, dissociative disorders, impulse-control disorders, sexual disorders, idiosyncratic alcohol intoxication, delusional disorder, paranoid personality disorder, schizophrenia, social maladjust-

Table 34.1–4
Differential Diagnosis of Manic Episodes

Bipolar I disorder
Schizoaffective disorder
Alcohol intoxication
Catatonic schizophrenia
Delirium
Hyperthyroidism
Postencephalitic syndrome
Steroid-induced mania
Antidepressant-induced mania
Decongestant-induced mania
Amphetamine-induced mania
Cocaine-induced mania
L-Dopa–induced mania
Bronchodilator-induced mania
Phencyclidine-induced mania
AIDS
Atypical psychosis

Courtesy of Andrew Edmund Slaby, M.D., Ph.D.

Table 34.1–5
Differential Diagnosis of Thought Disorders

Schizophrenia
Bipolar I disorder
Major depressive disorder
Alcohol psychotic disorder with hallucinations
Dementia of the Alzheimer's type with early onset
Frontal lobe neoplasm
Alcohol intoxication
Adjustment disorder
Dissociative disorders
Delusional disorder
Substance-induced (e.g., PCP, amphetamine) psychotic disorder
Steroid psychotic disorder
Syphilis
Endocrine diseases
Pernicious anemia
Temporal lobe epilepsy
Migraine equivalent
Cimetidine psychotic disorder
AIDS
Brief psychotic disorder
Schizophreniform disorder
Shared psychotic disorder
Atypical psychosis
Dementia of the Alzheimer's type
Vascular dementia
Dementia of the Alzheimer's type with late onset

Adapted from Andrew Edmund Slaby, M.D., Ph.D.

ment without mental disorder, temporal lobe epilepsy, bipolar I disorder, and uncontrollable violence secondary to interpersonal stress.

Violence and Assaultive Behavior

As mentioned above, the first task in evaluating violent behavior is to ascertain its cause. Cause directs treatment. Patients with thought disorders characterized by hallucinations commanding them to kill someone require psychiatric hospitalization and antipsychotic medication. If they are unwilling to accept treatment, certification is necessary to protect the intended victim and the patient. Those who take an extreme civil libertarian perspective fail to recognize that medical certification has evolved legally not only to protect society from violent patients, but also to protect patients from the consequences of their uncontrollable behavior. Psychotic patients who, while psychotic, destroy families' and friends' property or threaten to commit violent assaults destroy social supports that they need to help them function after the aberrant mood or delusional ideation is corrected.

Violence and assaultive behavior are difficult to predict (Table 34.1–9), but the fear with which some persons regard all psychiatric patients is completely out of proportion to the few who are an authentic danger to others. The best predictors of potential violent behavior are excessive alcohol intake, a history of violent acts with arrests or criminal activity, and a history of childhood abuse. Although violent patients can arouse a realistic fear in psychiatrists, they can also touch off irrational fears that impair clinical judgment and may lead to premature and excessive use of sedation or physical restraint. Violent patients are usually frightened by their own hostile impulses and desperately seek help to prevent loss of control. Nevertheless, restraints should be applied if there is a reasonable risk of violence.

Table 34.1–6
Features That Point to a Medical Cause of a Mental Disorder

Acute onset (within hours or minutes, with prevailing symptoms)
First episode
Geriatric age
Current medical illness or injury
Significant substance abuse
Nonauditory disturbances of perception
Neurological symptoms—loss of consciousness, seizures, head injury, change in headache pattern, change in vision
Classic mental status signs—diminished alertness, disorientation, memory impairment, impairment in concentration and attention, dyscalculia, concreteness
Other mental status signs—speech, movement, or gait disorders
Constructional apraxia—difficulties in drawing clock, cube, intersecting pentagons, Bender gestalt design

Table 34.1–7
Common Global Central Nervous System Disorders That Require Immediate Treatment

Hypoglycemia—dextrose 50% IV or juice orally, immediately; give to all diabetics
Wernicke's encephalopathy—thiamine, 100 mg IV, immediately
Opioid intoxication—naloxone (Narcan), 4 mg IV, immediately

Rape and Sexual Abuse

Rape is the forceful coercion of an unwilling victim to engage in a sexual act, usually sexual intercourse, although anal intercourse and fellatio can also be acts of rape. Like other acts of violence, rape is a psychiatric emergency that requires immediate, appropriate intervention. Rape victims may suffer sequelae that persist for a lifetime. Rape is a life-threatening experience

Table 34.1–8
Common Focal Central Nervous System Disorders with Behavioral Features

Aphasias—fluent or receptive aphasia results in patients' not understanding spoken word, although they have fluent but incoherent speech
Frontal lobe syndromes—changes in motor behavior, ability to concentrate, reasoning, thinking, social judgment, and impulse control
Temporal lobe syndromes—psychosis, seizure, personality and Klüver-Bucy features
Parietal lobe syndromes—right lesion with denial and hypomania
Occipital lobe syndromes—Anton's syndrome (cortical blindness with denial)

Table 34.1–9
Assessing and Predicting Violent Behavior

Signs of impending violence
- Recent acts of violence, including property violence
- Verbal or physical threats (menacing)
- Carrying weapons or other objects that may be used as weapons (e.g., forks, ashtrays)
- Progressive psychomotor agitation
- Alcohol or other substance intoxication
- Paranoid features in a psychotic patient
- Command violent auditory hallucinations—some but not all patients are at high risk
- Brain diseases, global or with frontal lobe findings; less commonly with temporal lobe findings (controversial)
- Catatonic excitement
- Certain manic episodes
- Certain agitated depressive episodes
- Personality disorders (rage, violence, or impulse dyscontrol)

Assess the risk for violence
- Consider violent ideation, wish, intention, plan, availability of means, implementation of plan, wish for help
- Consider demographics—sex (male), age (15–24), socioeconomic status (low), social supports (few)
- Consider the patient's history: violence, nonviolent antisocial acts, impulse dyscontrol (e.g., gambling, substance abuse, suicide or self-injury, psychosis)
- Consider overt stressors (e.g., marital conflict, real or symbolic loss)

in which the victim has almost always been threatened with physical harm, often with a weapon. In addition to rape, other forms of sexual abuse include genital manipulation with foreign objects, infliction of pain, and forced sexual activity.

The overwhelming majority of rapists are male, and most victims are female. However, male rape does occur, often in institutions where men are detained (e.g., prisons). Women between the ages of 16 and 24 years are in the highest risk category, but female victims as young as 15 months and as old as 82 years have been raped. More than a third of all rapes are committed by rapists known to the victim, 7 percent by close relatives. A fifth of all rapes involve more than one rapist (gang rape).

Typical reactions in both rape and sexual abuse victims include shame, humiliation, anxiety, confusion, and outrage. Many victims wonder whether they are partly responsible and somehow invited the assault. In fact, victim behavior is less important in precipitating a rape than it is in precipitating a homicide or a robbery. Rape and sexual abuse victims are often confused after the assault. Clinicians should be reassuring, supportive, and nonjudgmental. Inform the patient about the availability of medical and legal services and about rape crisis centers that provide multidisciplinary services.

If possible, a female clinician should evaluate the patient, since the victim may find it easier to talk with a woman than with a man. The evaluation should take place in private. When rape or sexual abuse has not been acknowledged openly, it is usually because many victims hesitate to discuss the assault and thus avoid the topic. If the patient appears to be anxious when questioned about sexual history and avoids the discussion, one must validate the patient's avoidance. Recognize that the rape victim has undergone an unanticipated, life-threatening stress. It is legally and therapeutically important to take a detailed and complete history of the attack.

With the patient's written consent, collect evidence such as semen and pubic hair that may be used to identify the rapist. Take photographs of the evidence if possible. The medical record may be used as evidence in criminal proceedings; therefore, meticulous objective documentation of all aspects of the evaluation is essential.

TREATMENT OF EMERGENCIES

Psychotherapy

In an emergency psychiatric intervention, all attempts are made to help patients' self-esteem. Empathy is critical to healing in a psychiatric emergency. The acquired knowledge of how biogenetic, situational, developmental, and existential forces converge at one point in history to create a psychiatric emergency is tantamount to the maturation of skill in emergency psychiatry. Adjustment disorder in all age groups may result in tantrumlike outbursts of rage. These outbursts are particularly common in marital quarrels, and police are often summoned by neighbors distressed by the sounds of a violent altercation. Such family quarrels should be approached with caution, because they may be complicated by alcohol use and the presence of dangerous weapons. The warring couple frequently turn their combined fury on an unwary outsider. Wounded self-esteem is a major issue, and clinicians must avoid patronizing or contemptuous attitudes and try to communicate an attitude of respect and an authentic peacemaking concern.

In family violence, psychiatrists should note the special vulnerability of selected close relatives. A wife or husband may have a curious masochistic attachment to the spouse and can provoke violence by taunting and otherwise undermining a partner's self-esteem. Such relationships often end in the murder of the provoking partner and sometimes in the suicide of the other partner—the dynamics behind most so-called suicide pacts. Like many suicidal patients, many violent patients require hospitalization and usually accept the offer of inpatient care with a sense of relief.

More than one psychotherapist or type of psychotherapy is frequently used in emergency therapy. For example, a 28-year-old man, depressed and suicidal after a colostomy for intractable colitis, whose wife was threatening to leave him because of his irritability and their constant altercations, may be referred to a psychiatrist for supportive psychotherapy and antidepressant medication, to a marital therapist with his wife to improve their marital functioning, and to a colostomy support group to learn ways of coping with a colostomy. Emergency psychiatric clinicians are pragmatic; they use every necessary mode of therapeutic intervention available to resolve the crisis and facilitate value exploration and growth, with less concern than usual about diluting a therapeutic relationship. Emergency therapy emphasizes how various psychiatric modalities act synergistically to enhance recovery.

No single approach is appropriate for all persons in similar situations. What does a doctor say to a patient and a family experiencing a psychiatric emergency such as a suicide attempt or a schizophrenic break? For some, a genetic rationale helps;

the information that an illness has a strong biological component relieves some persons. For others, however, this approach underlines a lack of control and increases depression and anxiety. All feel helpless because neither the family nor the patient can alter the behavior to minimize the likelihood of recurrence. Some persons may benefit from an explanation of family or individual dynamics. Others only want someone to listen to them; in time, they reach their own understanding.

In an emergency situation as in any other psychiatric situation, when a clinician does not know what to say, the best approach is to listen. Persons in crisis reveal how much they need support, denial, ventilation, and words to conceptualize the meaning of their crisis and to discover paths to resolution.

Pharmacotherapy

The major indications for the use of psychotropic medication in an emergency room include violent or assaultive behavior, massive anxiety or panic, and extrapyramidal reactions, such as dystonia and akathisia as adverse effects of psychiatric drugs. Laryngospasm is a rare form of dystonia, and psychiatrists should be prepared to maintain an open airway with intubation if necessary.

Persons who are paranoid or in a state of catatonic excitement require tranquilization. Episodic outbursts of violence respond to haloperidol (Haldol), β-adrenergic receptor antagonists (beta-blockers), carbamazepine (Tegretol), and lithium. If a history suggests a seizure disorder, use clinical studies to confirm the diagnosis and an evaluation to ascertain the cause. If the findings are positive, anticonvulsant therapy is initiated or appropriate surgery is provided (e.g., in the case of a cerebral mass). Conservative measures may suffice for intoxication from drugs of abuse. Sometimes, drugs such as haloperidol (5 to 10 mg every half-hour to an hour) are needed until a patient is stabilized. Benzodiazepines may be used instead of, or in addition to, antipsychotics (to reduce the antipsychotic dosage). When a recreational drug has strong anticholinergic properties, benzodiazepines are more appropriate than antipsychotics. Persons with allergic or aberrant responses to antipsychotics and benzodiazepines are treated with amobarbital (Amytal), 130 mg orally or intramuscularly (IM), paraldehyde, or diphenhydramine (Benadryl), 50 to 100 mg orally or IM.

Violent, struggling patients are subdued most effectively with an appropriate sedative or antipsychotic. Diazepam (Valium), 5 to 10 mg, or lorazepam (Ativan), 2 to 4 mg, may be given slowly intravenously (IV) over 2 minutes. Clinicians must give IV medication with great care to avoid respiratory arrest. Patients who require IM medication can be sedated with haloperidol, 5 to 10 mg IM, or with chlorpromazine (Thorazine), 25 mg IM. If the furor is due to alcohol or is part of a postseizure psychomotor disturbance, the sleep produced by a relatively small amount of an IV medication may go on for hours. On awakening, patients are often entirely alert and rational and typically have complete amnesia about the violent episode.

If the disturbance is part of an ongoing psychotic process, and returns as soon as the IV medication wears off, continuous medication may be given. It is sometimes better to use small IM or oral doses at half-hour to 1-hour intervals (e.g., haloperidol, 2 to 5 mg, or diazepam, 20 mg) until the patient is controlled than to use large dosages initially and end up with an overmedicated patient. As the disturbed behavior is brought under control, successively smaller and less frequent doses should be used. During the preliminary treatment, a patient's blood pressure and other vital signs should be monitored.

Rapid Tranquilization. Antipsychotic medication can be given rapidly at 30- to 60-minute intervals to achieve the quickest therapeutic result possible. The procedure is useful for agitated patients and those in excited states. The drugs of choice for rapid tranquilization are haloperidol and other high-potency antipsychotics. In adults, 5 to 10 mg of haloperidol can be given orally or IM and repeated in 20- to 30-minute intervals until a patient calms. Some patients may experience mild extrapyramidal symptoms within the first 24 hours after rapid tranquilization; although adverse effects are rare, psychiatrists should not overlook them. In general, most patients respond before a total dose of 50 mg is given. The goal is not to produce sedation or somnolence; a patient should be able to cooperate in the assessment process and, ideally, provide some explanation of the agitated behavior. Agitated or panic-stricken patients can be treated with small doses of lorazepam, 2 to 4 mg IV or IM, which can be repeated if necessary in 20 to 30 minutes until the patient quiets down. Extrapyramidal emergencies respond to benztropine (Cogentin), 2 mg orally or IM, or diphenhydramine, 50 mg IM or IV. Some patients respond to diazepam, 5 to 10 mg orally or IV.

Restraints

Restraints are used when patients are so dangerous to themselves or others that they pose a severe threat that cannot be controlled in any other way. Patients may be restrained temporarily to receive medication or for long periods if medication cannot be used. Usually, patients in restraints quiet down after a time. On a psychodynamic level, such patients may even welcome the control of their impulses provided by restraints. See Table 34.1–10 for a summary of the use of restraints.

Disposition

In some cases the usual option of admitting or discharging the patient is not considered optimal. Suspected toxic psychoses, brief decompensations in a patient with a personality disorder, and adjustment reactions to traumatic events, for example, may be best managed in an extended-observation setting. Allowing the patient additional time in a secure environment can result in sufficient improvement or clarification of the issues to make traditional inpatient treatment unnecessary. It can also spare the patient the trauma and stigma of a psychiatric admission and can free up bed space for needier patients. Crisis intervention for victims of rape and other traumas can also be done in an extended-observation setting.

When the decision is to admit the patient to the hospital, it is preferable to do so on a voluntary basis. Allowing patients that option gives them a sense of control over their lives and of participation in the treatment decisions. Patients who clearly meet involuntary admission criteria on the basis of dangerousness to themselves or to others cannot leave the hospital without further review and can always be converted to involuntary status if warranted.

Because the initial evaluation is often inconclusive, definitive treatment is best deferred until the patient can be further assessed

Table 34.1–10
Use of Restraints

Preferably five or a minimum of four persons should be used to restrain the patient. Leather restraints are the safest and surest type of restraint.

Explain to the patient why he or she is going into restraints.

A staff member should always be visible and reassuring the patient who is being restrained. Reassurance helps alleviate the patient's fear of helplessness, impotence, and loss of control.

Patients should be restrained with legs spread-eagled and one arm restrained to one side and the other arm restrained over the patient's head.

Restraints should be placed so that intravenous fluids can be given if necessary.

The patient's head is raised slightly to decrease the patient's feelings of vulnerability and to reduce the possibility of aspiration.

The restraints should be checked periodically for safety and comfort.

After the patient is in restraints, the clinician begins treatment, using verbal intervention.

Even in restraints, most patients still take antipsychotic medication in concentrated form.

After the patient is under control, one restraint at a time should be removed at 5-minute intervals until the patient has only two restraints on. Both of the remaining restraints should be removed at the same time, because it is inadvisable to keep a patient in only one restraint.

Always thoroughly document the reason for the restraints, the course of treatment, and the patient's response to treatment while in restraints.

Data from Dubin WR, Weiss KJ. Emergency psychiatry. In: Michaels R, Cooper A, Guze SB, et al., eds. *Psychiatry.* Vol 2. Philadelphia: JB Lippincott; 1991.

on the inpatient unit or in the outpatient department. However, when the diagnosis is clear and the patient's response to previous treatment is known, nothing is gained by delay. For example, a patient suffering from chronic schizophrenia who has decompensated after discontinuing the usual regimen of antipsychotic medication is best served by prompt resumption of treatment.

Even if patients feel comfortable coming to the emergency room in times of need, the emergency psychiatrist should always direct or redirect them to the most appropriate treatment setting. Patients in the psychopharmacology clinic who have missed their regular appointments should be given only enough medication to sustain them until they can be seen in the clinic. Feedback to others treating them should be a matter of course.

The emergency room is often the gateway to the department of psychiatry or the general hospital. First impressions carry a great deal of weight. The kind of attention and concern shown to patients on arrival in the emergency room strongly affects how they will respond to staff members and treatment recommendations and even their treatment compliance long after they have left the emergency room.

Documentation

In the interests of good care, respect for patients' rights, cost control, and medicolegal concerns, documentation has become a central focus for the emergency physician. The medical record should convey a concise picture of the patient, highlighting all pertinent positive and negative findings. Gaps in information and their reason should be mentioned. The names and the telephone numbers of interested parties should be noted. A provisional diagnosis or differential diagnosis must be made. An initial treatment plan or recommendations should clearly follow from the findings of the patient's history, mental status examination and other diagnostic tests, and the medical evaluation. The writing must be legible. The emergency physician has unusual latitude under the law to perform an adequate initial assessment; however, all interventions and decisions must be thought out, discussed, and documented in the patient's record.

Specific Psychiatric Emergencies

Table 34.1–11 outlines common psychiatric emergencies in alphabetical order. Readers are referred to the index and to specific chapters of this textbook for a thorough discussion of each disorder.

Table 34.1–11
Common Psychiatric Emergencies

Syndrome	Emergency Manifestations	Treatment Issues
Abuse of child or adult	Signs of physical trauma	Management of medical problems; psychiatric evaluation; report to authorities
Acquired immune deficiency syndrome (AIDS)	Changes in behavior secondary to organic causes; changes in behavior secondary to fear and anxiety; suicidal behavior	Management of neurological illness; management of psychological concomitants; reinforcement of social support
Adolescent crises	Suicidal attempts and ideation; substance abuse, truancy, trouble with law, pregnancy, running away; eating disorders; psychosis	Evaluation of suicidal potential, extent of substance abuse, family dynamics; crisis-oriented family and individual therapy; hospitalization if necessary; consultation with appropriate extrafamilial authorities
Agoraphobia	Panic; depression	Alprazolam (Xanax), 0.25 mg to 2 mg; propranolol (Inderal); antidepressant medication
Agranulocytosis (clozapine [Clozaril]-induced)	High fever, pharyngitis, oral and perianal ulcerations	Discontinue medication immediately; administer granulocyte colony-stimulating factor
Akathisia	Agitation, restlessness, muscle discomfort; dysphoria	Reduce antipsychotic dosage; propranolol (30 to 120 mg a day); benzodiazepines; diphenhydramine (Benadryl) orally or IV; benztropine (Cogentin) IM

(continued)

Table 34.1–11 (*continued*)

Syndrome	Emergency Manifestations	Treatment Issues
Alcohol-related emergencies		
Alcohol delirium	Confusion, disorientation, fluctuating consciousness and perception, autonomic hyperactivity; may be fatal	Chlordiazepoxide (Librium); haloperidol (Haldol) for psychotic symptoms may be added if necessary
Alcohol intoxication	Disinhibited behavior, sedation at high doses	With time and protective environment, symptoms abate
Alcohol persisting amnestic disorder	Confusion, loss of memory even for all personal identification data	Hospitalization; hypnosis; amobarbital (Amytal) interview; rule out organic cause
Alcohol persisting dementia	Confusion, agitation, impulsivity	Rule out other causes for dementia; no effective treatment; hospitalization if necessary
Alcohol psychotic disorder with hallucinations	Vivid auditory (at times visual) hallucinations with affect appropriate to content (often fearful); clear sensorium	Haloperidol for psychotic symptoms
Alcohol seizures	Grand mal seizures; rarely status epilepticus	Diazepam (Valium), phenytoin (Dilantin); prevent by using chlordiazepoxide (Librium) during detoxification
Alcohol withdrawal	Irritability, nausea, vomiting, insomnia, malaise, autonomic hyperactivity, shakiness	Fluid and electrolytes maintained; sedation with benzodiazepines; restraints; monitoring of vital signs; 100 mg thiamine IM
Idiosyncratic alcohol intoxication	Marked aggressive or assaultive behavior	Generally no treatment required other than protective environment
Korsakoff's syndrome	Alcohol stigmata, amnesia, confabulation	No effective treatment; institutionalization often needed
Wernicke's encephalopathy	Oculomotor disturbances, cerebellar ataxia; mental confusion	Thiamine, 100 mg IV or IM, with $MgSO_4$ given before glucose loading
Amphetamine (or related substance) intoxication	Delusions, paranoia; violence; depression (from withdrawal); anxiety, delirium	Antipsychotics; restraints; hospitalization if necessary; no need for gradual withdrawal; antidepressants may be necessary
Anorexia nervosa	Loss of 25% of body weight of the norm for age and sex	Hospitalization; electrocardiogram (ECG), fluid and electrolytes; neuroendocrine evaluation
Anticholinergic intoxication	Psychotic symptoms, dry skin and mouth, hyperpyrexia, mydriasis, tachycardia, restlessness, visual hallucinations	Discontinue drug, IV physostigmine (Antilirium), 0.5 to 2 mg, for severe agitation or fever, benzodiazepines; antipsychotics contraindicated
Anticonvulsant intoxication	Psychosis; delirium	Dosage of anticonvulsant is reduced
Benzodiazepine intoxication	Sedation, somnolence, and ataxia	Supportive measures; flumazenil (Romazicon), 7.5 to 45 mg a day, titrated as needed, should be used only by skilled personnel with resuscitative equipment available
Bereavement	Guilt feelings, irritability; insomnia; somatic complaints	Must be differentiated from major depressive disorder; antidepressants not indicated; benzodiazepines for sleep; encouragement of ventilation
Borderline personality disorder	Suicidal ideation and gestures; homicidal ideations and gestures; substance abuse; micropsychotic episodes; burns, cut marks on body	Suicidal and homicidal evaluation (if great, hospitalization); small dosages of antipsychotics; clear follow-up plan
Brief psychotic disorder	Emotional turmoil, extreme lability; acutely impaired reality testing after obvious psychosocial stress	Hospitalization often necessary; low dosage of antipsychotics may be necessary but often resolves spontaneously
Bromide intoxication	Delirium; mania; depression; psychosis	Serum levels obtained (>50 mg a day); bromide intake discontinued; large quantities of sodium chloride IV or orally; if agitation, paraldehyde or antipsychotic is used
Caffeine intoxication	Severe anxiety, resembling panic disorder; mania; delirium; agitated depression; sleep disturbance	Cessation of caffeine-containing substances; benzodiazepines
Cannabis intoxication	Delusions; panic; dysphoria; cognitive impairment	Benzodiazepines and antipsychotics as needed; evaluation of suicidal or homicidal risk; symptoms usually abate with time and reassurance
Catatonic schizophrenia	Marked psychomotor disturbance (either excitement or stupor); exhaustion; can be fatal	Rapid tranquilization with antipsychotics; monitor vital signs; amobarbital may release patient from catatonic mutism or stupor but can precipitate violent behavior
Cimetidine psychotic disorder	Delirium; delusions	Reduce dosage or discontinue drug

(*continued*)

Table 34.1–11 (*continued*)

Syndrome	Emergency Manifestations	Treatment Issues
Clonidine withdrawal	Irritability; psychosis; violence; seizures	Symptoms abate with time, but antipsychotics may be necessary; gradual lowering of dosage
Cocaine intoxication and withdrawal	Paranoia and violence; severe anxiety; manic state; delirium; schizophreniform psychosis; tachycardia, hypertension, myocardial infarction, cerebrovascular disease; depression and suicidal ideation	Antipsychotics and benzodiazepines; antidepressants or ECT for withdrawal depression if persistent; hospitalization
Delirium	Fluctuating sensorium; suicidal and homicidal risk; cognitive clouding; visual, tactile, and auditory hallucinations; paranoia	Evaluate all potential contributing factors and treat each accordingly; reassurance, structure, clues to orientation; benzodiazepines and low-dosage, high-potency antipsychotics must be used with extreme care because of their potential to act paradoxically and increase agitation
Delusional disorder	Most often brought in to emergency room involuntarily; threats directed toward others	Antipsychotics if patient will comply (IM if necessary); intensive family intervention; hospitalization if necessary
Dementia	Unable to care for self; violent outbursts; psychosis; depression and suicidal ideation; confusion	Small dosages of high-potency antipsychotics; clues to orientation; organic evaluation, including medication use; family intervention
Depressive disorders	Suicidal ideation and attempts; self-neglect; substance abuse	Assessment of danger to self; hospitalization if necessary; nonpsychiatric causes of depression must be evaluated
L-Dopa intoxication	Mania; depression; schizophreniform disorder; may induce rapid cycling in patients with bipolar I disorder	Lower dosage or discontinue drug
Dystonia, acute	Intense involuntary spasm of muscles of neck, tongue, face, jaw, eyes, or trunk	Decrease dosage of antipsychotic; benztropine or diphenhydramine IM
Group hysteria	Groups of people exhibit extremes of grief or other disruptive behavior	Group is dispersed with help of other health care workers; ventilation, crisis-oriented therapy; if necessary, small dosages of benzodiazepines
Hallucinogen-induced psychotic disorder with hallucinations	Symptom picture is result of interaction of type of substance, dose taken, duration of action, user's premorbid personality, setting; panic; agitation; atropine psychosis	Serum and urine screens; rule out underlying medical or mental disorder; benzodiazepines (2 to 20 mg) orally; reassurance and orientation; rapid tranquilization; often responds spontaneously
Homicidal and assaultive behavior	Marked agitation with verbal threats	Seclusion, restraints, medication
Homosexual panic	Not seen with men or women who are comfortable with their sexual orientation; occurs in those who adamantly deny having any homoerotic impulses; impulses are aroused by talk, a physical overture, or play among same-sex friends, such as wrestling, sleeping together, or touching each other in a shower or hot tub; panicked person sees others as sexually interested in him or her and defends against them	Ventilation, environmental structuring, and, in some instances, medication for acute panic (e.g., alprazolam, 0.25 to 2 mg) or antipsychotics may be required; opposite-sex clinician should evaluate the patient whenever possible, and the patient should not be touched save for the routine examination; patients have attacked physicians who were examining an abdomen or performing a rectal examination (e.g., on a man who harbors thinly veiled unintegrated homosexual impulses)
Hypertensive crisis	Life-threatening hypertensive reaction secondary to ingestion of tyramine-containing foods in combination with MAOIs; headache, stiff neck, sweating, nausea, vomiting	α-Adrenergic blockers (e.g., phentolamine [Regitine]); nifedipine (Procardia) 10 mg orally; chlorpromazine (Thorazine); make sure symptoms are not secondary to hypotension (side effect of monoamine oxidase inhibitors [MAOIs] alone)
Hyperthermia	Extreme excitement or catatonic stupor or both; extremely elevated temperature; violent hyperagitation	Hydrate and cool; may be drug reaction, so discontinue any drug; rule out infection
Hyperventilation	Anxiety, terror, clouded consciousness; giddiness, faintness; blurring vision	Shift alkalosis by having patient breathe into paper bag; patient education; antianxiety agents
Hypothermia	Confusion; lethargy; combativeness; low body temperature and shivering; paradoxical feeling of warmth	IV fluids and rewarming; cardiac status must be carefully monitored; avoidance of alcohol
Incest and sexual abuse of child	Suicidal behavior; adolescent crises; substance abuse	Corroboration of charge; protection of victim; contact social services; medical and psychiatric evaluation; crisis intervention

(*continued*)

Table 34.1–11 (*continued*)

Syndrome	Emergency Manifestations	Treatment Issues
Insomnia	Depression and irritability; early morning agitation; frightening dreams; fatigue	Hypnotics only in short term; e.g., triazolam (Halcion), 0.25 to 0.5 mg, at bedtime; treat any underlying mental disorder; rules of sleep hygiene
Intermittent explosive disorder	Brief outbursts of violence; periodic episodes of suicide attempts	Benzodiazepines or antipsychotics for short term; long-term evaluation with computed tomography (CT) scan, sleep-deprived electroencephalogram (EEG), glucose tolerance curve
Jaundice	Uncommon complication of low-potency phenothiazine use (e.g., chlorpromazine)	Change drug to low dosage of a low-potency agent in a different class
Leukopenia and agranulocytosis	Side effects within the first 2 months of treatment with antipsychotics	Patient should call immediately for sore throat, fever, etc., and obtain immediate blood count; discontinue drug; hospitalize if necessary
Lithium toxicity	Vomiting; abdominal pain; profuse diarrhea; severe tremor, ataxia; coma; seizures; confusion; dysarthria; focal neurological signs	Lavage with wide-bore tube; osmotic diuresis; medical consultation; may require ICU treatment
Major depressive episode with psychotic features	Major depressive episode symptoms with delusions; agitation, severe guilt; ideas of reference; suicide and homicide risk	Antipsychotics plus antidepressants; evaluation of suicide and homicide risk; hospitalization and ECT if necessary
Manic episode	Violent, impulsive behavior; indiscriminate sexual or spending behavior; psychosis; substance abuse	Hospitalization; restraints if necessary; rapid tranquilization with antipsychotics; restoration of lithium levels
Marital crises	Precipitant may be discovery of an extramarital affair, onset of serious illness, announcement of intent to divorce, or problems with children or work; one or both members of the couple may be in therapy or may be psychiatrically ill; one spouse may be seeking hospitalization for the other	Each should be questioned alone regarding extramarital affairs, consultations with lawyers regarding divorce, and willingness to work in crisis-oriented or long-term therapy to resolve the problem; sexual, financial, and psychiatric treatment histories from both, psychiatric evaluation at the time of presentation; may be precipitated by onset of untreated mood disorder or affective symptoms caused by medical illness or insidious-onset dementia; referral for management of the illness reduces immediate stress and enhances the healthier spouse's coping capacity; children may give insights available only to someone intimately involved in the social system
Migraine	Throbbing, unilateral headache	Sumatriptan (Imitrex) 6 mg IM
Mitral valve prolapse	Associated with panic disorder; dyspnea and palpitations; fear and anxiety	Echocardiogram; alprazolam or propranolol
Neuroleptic malignant syndrome	Hyperthermia; muscle rigidity; autonomic instability; parkinsonian symptoms; catatonic stupor; neurological signs; 10% to 30% fatality; elevated creatine phosphokinase	Discontinue antipsychotic; IV dantrolene (Dantrium); bromocriptine (Parlodel) orally; hydration and cooling; monitor CPK levels
Nitrous oxide toxicity	Euphoria and light-headedness	Symptoms abate without treatment within hours of use
Nutmeg intoxication	Agitation; hallucinations; severe headaches; numbness in extremities	Symptoms abate within hours of use without treatment
Opioid intoxication and withdrawal	Intoxication can lead to coma and death; withdrawal is not life-threatening	IV naloxone, narcotic antagonist; urine and serum screens; psychiatric and medical illnesses (e.g., AIDS) may complicate picture
Panic disorder	Panic, terror; acute onset	Must differentiate from other anxiety-producing disorders, both medical and psychiatric; ECG to rule out mitral valve prolapse; propranolol (10 to 30 mg); alprazolam (0.25 to 2.0 mg); long-term management may include an antidepressant
Paranoid schizophrenia	Command hallucinations; threat to others or themselves	Rapid tranquilization; hospitalization; long-acting depot medication; threatened persons must be notified and protected
Parkinsonism	Stiffness, tremor, bradykinesia, flattened affect, shuffling gait, salivation, secondary to antipsychotic medication	Oral antiparkinsonian drug for 4 weeks to 3 months; decrease dosage of the antipsychotic
Perioral (rabbit) tremor	Perioral tumor (rabbitlike facial grimacing) usually appearing after long-term therapy with antipsychotics	Decrease dosage or change to a medication in another class

(*continued*)

Table 34.1–11 (*continued*)

Syndrome	Emergency Manifestations	Treatment Issues
Phencyclidine (or phencyclidinelike intoxication)	Paranoid psychosis; can lead to death; acute danger to self and others	Serum and urine assay; benzodiazepines may interfere with excretion; antipsychotics may worsen symptoms because of anticholinergic side effects; medical monitoring and hospitalization for severe intoxication
Phenelzine-induced psychotic disorder	Psychosis and mania in predisposed people	Reduce dosage or discontinue drug
Phenylpropanolamine toxicity	Psychosis; paranoia; insomnia; restlessness; nervousness; headache	Symptoms abate with dosage reduction or discontinuation (found in over-the-counter diet aids and oral and nasal decongestants)
Phobias	Panic, anxiety; fear	Treatment same as for panic disorder
Photosensitivity	Easy sunburning secondary to use of antipsychotic medication	Patient should avoid strong sunlight and use high-level sunscreens
Pigmentary retinopathy	Reported with dosages of thioridazine (Mellaril) of 800 mg a day or above	Remain below 800 mg a day of thioridazine
Postpartum psychosis	Childbirth can precipitate schizophrenia, depression, reactive psychoses, mania, and depression; affective symptoms are most common; suicide risk is reduced during pregnancy but increased in the postpartum period	Danger to self and others (including infant) must be evaluated and proper precautions taken; medical illness presenting with behavioral aberrations is included in the differential diagnosis and must be sought and treated; care must be paid to the effects on father, infant, grandparents, and other children
Posttraumatic stress disorder	Panic, terror; suicidal ideation; flashbacks	Reassurance; encouragement of return to responsibilities; avoid hospitalization if possible to prevent chronic invalidism; monitor suicidal ideation
Priapism (trazodone [Desyrel]-induced)	Persistent penile erection accompanied by severe pain	Intracorporeal epinephrine; mechanical or surgical drainage
Propranolol toxicity	Profound depression; confusional states	Reduce dosage or discontinue drug; monitor suicidality
Rape	Not all sexual violations are reported; silent rape reaction is characterized by loss of appetite, sleep disturbance, anxiety, and, sometimes, agoraphobia; long periods of silence, mounting anxiety, stuttering, blocking, and physical symptoms during the interview when the sexual history is taken; fear of violence and death and of contracting a sexually transmitted disease or being pregnant	Rape is a major psychiatric emergency; victim may have enduring patterns of sexual dysfunction; crisis-oriented therapy, social support, ventilation, reinforcement of healthy traits, and encouragement to return to the previous level of functioning as rapidly as possible; legal counsel; thorough medical examination and tests to identify the assailant (e.g., obtaining samples of pubic hairs with a pubic hair comb, vaginal smear to identify blood antigens in semen); if a woman, methoxyprogesterone or diethylstilbestrol orally for 5 days to prevent pregnancy; if menstruation does not commence within one week of cessation of the estrogen, all alternatives to pregnancy, including abortion, should be offered; if the victim has contracted a venereal disease, appropriate antibiotics; witnessed written permission is required for the physician to examine, photograph, collect specimens, and release information to the authorities; obtain consent, record the history in the patient's own words, obtain required tests, record the results of the examination, save all clothing, defer diagnosis, and provide protection against disease, psychic trauma, and pregnancy; men's and women's responses to rape affectively are reported similarly, although men are more hesitant to talk about homosexual assault for fear they will be assumed to have consented
Reserpine intoxication	Major depressive episodes; suicidal ideation; nightmares	Evaluation of suicidal ideation; lower dosage or change drug; antidepressants or ECT may be indicated
Schizoaffective disorder	Severe depression; manic symptoms; paranoia	Evaluation of dangerousness to self or others; rapid tranquilization if necessary; treatment of depression (antidepressants alone can enhance schizophrenic symptoms); use of antimanic agents
Schizophrenia	Extreme self-neglect; severe paranoia; suicidal ideation or assaultiveness; extreme psychotic symptoms	Evaluation of suicidal and homicidal potential; identification of any illness other than schizophrenia; rapid tranquilization

(*continued*)

Table 34.1–11 (*continued*)

Syndrome	Emergency Manifestations	Treatment Issues
Schizophrenia in exacerbation	Withdrawn; agitation; suicidal and homicidal risk	Suicide and homicide evaluation; screen for medical illness; restraints and rapid tranquilization if necessary; hospitalization if necessary; reevaluation of medication regimen
Sedative, hypnotic, or anxiolytic intoxication and withdrawal	Alterations in mood, behavior, thought—delirium; derealization and depersonalization; untreated, can be fatal; seizures	Naloxone (Narcan) to differentiate from opioid intoxication; slow withdrawal with phenobarbital (Luminal) or sodium thiopental or benzodiazepine; hospitalization
Seizure disorder	Confusion; anxiety; derealization and depersonalization; feelings of impending doom; gustatory or olfactory hallucinations; fuguelike state	Immediate EEG; admission and sleep-deprived and 24-hour EEG; rule out pseudoseizures; anticonvulsants
Substance withdrawal	Abdominal pain; insomnia, drowsiness; delirium; seizures; symptoms of tardive dyskinesia may emerge; eruption of manic or schizophrenic symptoms	Symptoms of psychotropic drug withdrawal disappear with time or disappear with reinstitution of the substance; symptoms of antidepressant withdrawal can be successfully treated with anticholinergic agents, such as atropine; gradual withdrawal of psychotropic substances over two to four weeks generally obviates development of symptoms
Sudden death associated with antipsychotic medication	Seizures; asphyxiation; cardiovascular causes; postural hypotension; laryngeal-pharyngeal dystonia; suppression of gag reflex	Specific medical treatments
Sudden death of psychogenic origin	Myocardial infarction after sudden psychic stress; voodoo and hexes; hopelessness, especially associated with serious physical illness	Specific medical treatments; folk healers
Suicide	Suicidal ideation; hopelessness	Hospitalization, antidepressants
Sympathomimetic withdrawal	Paranoia; confusional states; depression	Most symptoms abate without treatment; antipsychotics; antidepressants if necessary
Tardive dyskinesia	Dyskinesia of mouth, tongue, face, neck, and trunk; choreoathetoid movements of extremities; usually but not always appearing after long-term treatment with antipsychotics, especially after a reduction in dosage; incidence highest in the elderly and brain-damaged; symptoms are intensified by antiparkinsonian drugs and masked but not cured by increased dosages of antipsychotic	No effective treatment reported; may be prevented by prescribing the least amount of drug possible for as little time as is clinically feasible and using drug-free holidays for patients who need to continue taking the drug; decrease or discontinue drug at first sign of dyskinetic movements
Thyrotoxicosis	Tachycardia; gastrointestinal dysfunction; hyperthermia; panic, anxiety, agitation; mania; dementia; psychosis	Thyroid function test (T_3, T_4, thyroid-stimulating hormone [TSH]); medical consultation
Toluene abuse	Anxiety; confusion; cognitive impairment	Neurological damage is nonprogressive and reversible if toluene use is discontinued early
Vitamin B_{12} deficiency	Confusion; mood and behavior changes; ataxia	Treatment with vitamin B_{12}
Volatile nitrates	Alternations of mood and behavior; light-headedness; pulsating headache	Symptoms abate with cessation of use

References

Breslow RE, Erickson BJ, Cavanaugh KC. The psychiatric emergency service: where we've been and where we're going. *Psychiatr Q.* 2000;71:101.

Fauman BJ. Other psychiatric emergencies. In: Sadock BJ, Sadock VA, eds. *Kaplan & Sadock's Comprehensive Textbook of Psychiatry.* 7th ed. Vol 2. Baltimore: Lippincott Williams & Wilkins; 2000:2040.

Kaplan HI, Sadock BJ. *Pocket Handbook of Emergency Psychiatric Medicine.* Baltimore: Williams & Wilkins; 1993.

Kleespies PM, Dettmer EL. An evidence-based approach to evaluating and managing suicidal emergencies. *J Clin Psychol.* 2000;56:1109.

Lejoyeux M, Boulenguiez S, Fichelle A, McLoughlin M, Claudon M, Ades J. Alcohol dependence among patients admitted to psychiatric emergency services. *Gen Hosp Psychiatry.* 2000;22:206.

Raphael B, Wilson JP, eds. *Psychological Debriefing: Theory, Practice and Evidence.* New York: Cambridge University Press; 2000.

Risser D, Hoenigschnabl S, Stichenwirth M, et al. Drug-related emergencies and drug-related deaths in Vienna, 1995–1997. *Drug Alcohol Depend.* 2001;61:307.

Roberts AR. *Crisis Intervention Handbook: Assessment, Treatment, and Research.* 2nd ed. New York: Oxford University Press; 2000.

Rosenberg RC, Kesselman M. The therapeutic alliance and the psychiatric emergency room. *Hosp Community Psychiatry.* 1993;44:78.

Schatzberg AF, Nemeroff CB, eds. *Essentials of Clinical Psychopharmacology.* Washington, DC: American Psychiatric Association; 2001.

Scott RL. Evaluation of a mobile crisis program: effectiveness, efficiency, and consumer satisfaction. *Psychiatr Serv.* 2000;51:1153.

Segal SP, Bola JR, Watson MA. Race, quality of care, and antipsychotic prescribing practices in psychiatric emergency services. *Psychiatr Serv.* 1996;47:282.

▲ 34.2 Suicide

Suicide has occurred since the beginning of recorded history, with attitudes toward it varying from condemnation to tolerance, depending on the time and the culture. The motives for suicide and its frequency have also varied. Today, in Western society, suicide is viewed as neither a random nor a pointless act. On the contrary, it is a way out of a problem or crisis that is invariably causing intense suffering. According to Edwin Shneidman suicide is associated with thwarted or unfulfilled needs, feelings of hopelessness and helplessness, ambivalent conflicts between survival and unbearable stress, a narrowing of perceived options, and a need for escape; the suicidal person sends out signals of distress. As Kay Redfield Jamison said:

> The suffering of the suicidal is private and inexpressible, leaving family members, friends, and colleagues to deal with an almost unfathomable kind of loss, as well as guilt. Suicide carries in its aftermath a level of confusion and devastation that is, for the most part, beyond description.

Suicide is derived from the Latin word for "self-murder." If successful, it is a fatal act that represents the person's wish to die. There is a range, however, between thinking about suicide and acting it out. Some persons have ideas of suicide that they will never act upon; some plan for days, weeks, or even years before acting; and others take their lives seemingly on impulse, without premeditation. Lost in the definition are intentional misclassifications of the cause of death, accidents of undetermined cause, and so-called chronic suicides—for example, death through alcohol and other substance abuse and consciously poor adherence to medical regimens for addiction, obesity, and hypertension.

EPIDEMIOLOGY

Each year more than 30,000 persons die by suicide in the United States. The number of attempted suicides is estimated to be 650,000. There are about 85 suicides a day in this country—about 1 every 20 minutes. The suicide rate in the United States has averaged 12.5 per 100,000 in the 20th century, with a high of 17.4 per 100,000 during the Great Depression of the 1930s. From 1983 to 1998, the overall suicide rate remained relatively stable, whereas the rate for 15- to 24-year-olds has increased two to threefold. Suicide is currently ranked the eighth overall cause of death in this country, after heart disease, cancer, cerebrovascular disease, chronic obstructive pulmonary disease, accidents, pneumonia and influenza, and diabetes mellitus.

U.S. suicide rates are at the midpoint of the rates for industrialized countries as reported to the United Nations. Internationally, suicide rates range from highs of more than 25 per 100,000 persons in Scandinavia, Switzerland, Germany, Austria, the Eastern European countries (the so-called suicide belt), and Japan, to fewer than 10 per 100,000 in Spain, Italy, Ireland, Egypt, and the Netherlands.

A state-by-state analysis of suicides in the last decade among persons between the ages of 15 and 44 revealed that New Jersey had the nation's lowest suicide rates for both sexes. Nevada and New Mexico had the highest rates for men, and Nevada and Wyoming had the highest rates for women. Women in Nevada killed themselves at a higher frequency than did men in New Jersey. The prime suicide site of the world is the Golden Gate Bridge in San Francisco, with more than 800 suicides since the bridge opened in 1937.

Table 34.2–1
Variables Enhancing Risk of Suicide among Vulnerable Groups

Adolescence and late life
Bisexual or homosexual gender identity
Criminal behavior
Cultural sanctions for suicide
Delusions
Disposition of personal property
Divorced, separated, or single marital status
Early loss or separation from parents
Family history of suicide
Hallucinations
Homicide
Hopelessness
Hypochondriasis
Impulsivity
Increasing agitation
Increasing stress
Insomnia
Lack of future plans
Lack of sleep
Lethality of previous attempt
Living alone
Low self-esteem
Male sex
Physical illness or impairment
Previous attempts that could have resulted in death
Protestant or nonreligious status
Recent childbirth
Recent loss
Repression as a defense
Secondary gain
Severe family pathology
Severe psychiatric illness
Sexual abuse
Signals of intent to die
Suicide epidemics
Unemployment
White race

From Slaby AE. Outpatient management of suicidal patients in the era of managed care. *Prim Psychiatry.* 1995;Apr:43, with permission.

Risk Factors

Table 34.2–1 lists variables that may increase the risk of suicide in vulnerable persons.

Sex. Men commit suicide more than four times as often as women, a rate that is stable over all ages. Women, however, are four times more likely to attempt suicide than men.

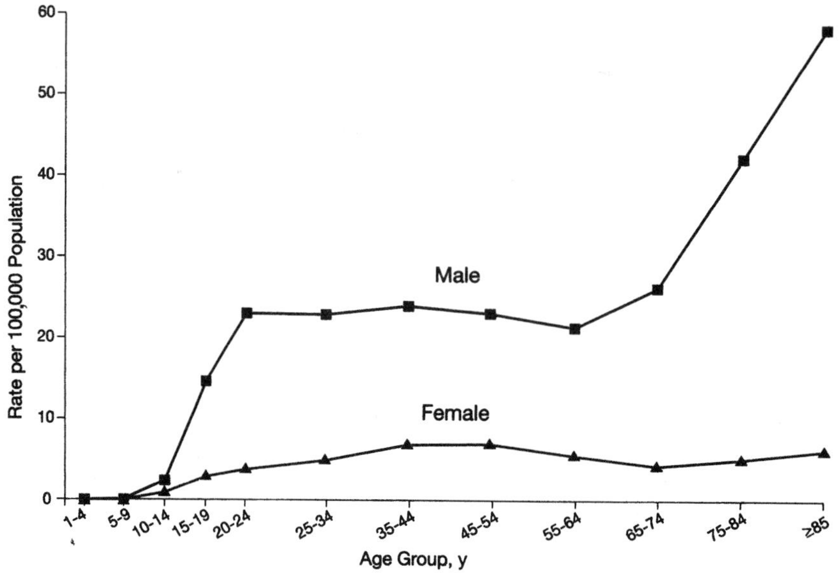

FIGURE 34.2–1
Suicide rates by age group and sex in the United States, 1998. (Reprinted with permission from *JAMA*. 2001;285:2701.)

Age. Suicide rates increase with age and underscore the significance of the midlife crisis. Among men, suicides peak after age 45; among women, the greatest number of completed suicides occurs after age 55. Rates of 40 per 100,000 population occur in men age 65 and older. Older persons attempt suicide less often than younger persons but are more often successful. Although they are only 10 percent of the total population, older persons account for 25 percent of suicides. The rate for those 75 or older is more than three times the rate among young persons.

The suicide rate, however, is rising most rapidly among young persons, particularly males 15 to 24 years old, and the rate is still rising. The suicide rate for females in the same age group is increasing more slowly than that for males. Among men 25 to 34 years old, the suicide rate increased almost 30 percent over the past decade. Suicide is the third leading cause of death in the 15- to 24-year-old age group, after accidents and homicides, and attempted suicides in this age group number between 1 million and 2 million annually. Most suicides now occur among those aged 15 to 44.

Suicide rates by age and sex in the United States are shown in Figure 34.2–1.

Race. Two of every three suicides are white males. The rate of suicide among whites has been nearly twice that among all other groups; these figures, however, are now questionable, as the suicide rate among blacks is rising. The suicide rate for white males (19.6 per 100,000 persons) is 1.6 times that for black males (12.5), 4 times that for white women (4.8), and 8.2 times that for black women (2.4). Among young persons who live in inner cities and certain Native American and Inuit groups, suicide rates have greatly exceeded the national rate. Suicide rates among immigrants are higher than those in the native-born population.

Religion. Historically, suicide rates among Roman Catholic populations have been lower than rates among Protestants and Jews. The degree of orthodoxy and integration may be a more accurate measure of risk in this category than simple institutional religious affiliation.

Marital Status. Marriage reinforced by children seems to lessen the risk of suicide significantly. The suicide rate is 11 per 100,000 for married persons; single, never-married persons register an overall rate nearly double that. Previously married persons, however, show sharply higher rates than those who never married: 24 per 100,000 among persons who are widowed, and 40 per 100,000 among those who are divorced, with divorced men registering 69 suicides per 100,000, compared with 18 per 100,000 for divorced women. Suicide occurs more frequently than usual in persons who are socially isolated and have a family history of suicide (attempted or real). Persons who commit so-called anniversary suicides take their lives on the day a member of their family did.

Occupation. The higher a person's social status, the greater the risk of suicide, but a fall in social status also increases the risk. Work, in general, protects against suicide. Among occupational rankings, professionals, particularly physicians, have traditionally been considered to be at the greatest risk of suicide, but the best recent studies have found no increased suicide risk for male physicians in the United States. Their annual suicide rate is about 36 per 100,000, which is the same as that for white men over 25 years of age. Recent U.K. and Scandinavian data, by contrast, show that the suicide rate for male physicians is two to three times that found in the general male population of the same age.

Studies agree that female physicians have a higher risk of suicide than other women. In the United States, the annual suicide rate for female physicians is about 41 per 100,000, compared with 12 per 100,000 among all white women over 25 years of age. Similarly, in England and Wales, the suicide rate for unmarried female physicians is 2.5 times that among unmarried women in the general population, although it is comparable to that of other groups of professional women.

Studies show that physicians who commit suicide have a mental disorder. The most common mental disorders among physicians and among physician suicide victims are depressive disorders and substance dependence. Often, a physician who commits suicide has experienced recent professional, personal, or family difficulties. Both male and female physicians commit suicide significantly more often by sub-

stance overdoses and less often by firearms than persons in the general population; drug availability and knowledge about toxicity are important factors in physician suicides. Some evidence indicates that female physicians have an unusually high lifetime risk for mood disorders, which may be the major determinant of the elevated suicide risk.

Among physicians, psychiatrists are considered to be at greatest risk, followed by ophthalmologists and anesthesiologists, but the trend is toward an equalization among all specialties. Special at-risk populations are musicians, dentists, law enforcement officers, lawyers, and insurance agents. Suicide is higher among the unemployed than among employed persons. The suicide rate increases during economic recessions and depressions and times of high unemployment and decreases during times of high employment and during wars.

Methods. Men's higher rate of successful suicide is related to the methods they use: firearms, hanging, or jumping from high places. Women more commonly take an overdose of psychoactive substances or a poison, but their use of firearms is increasing. In states with gun control laws, the use of firearms has decreased as a method of suicide. Globally, the most common method of suicide is hanging.

Climate. No significant seasonal correlation with suicide has been found. Suicides increase slightly in spring and fall but, contrary to popular belief, not during December and holiday periods.

Physical Health. The relation of physical health and illness to suicide is significant. Previous medical care appears to be a positively correlated risk indicator of suicide: 32 percent of all persons who commit suicide have had medical attention within 6 months of death. Postmortem studies show that a physical illness is present in some 25 to 75 percent of all suicide victims, and a physical illness is estimated to be an important contributing factor in 11 to 51 percent of suicides. In each instance, the percentage increases with age. For example, 50 percent of men with cancer who commit suicide do so within a year of receiving the diagnosis. Cancer of the breast or the genitals is found in 70 percent of all women with cancer who commit suicide. Seven diseases of the central nervous system (CNS) increase the risk of suicide: epilepsy, multiple sclerosis, head injury, cardiovascular disease, Huntington's disease, dementia, and acquired immune deficiency syndrome (AIDS). All these diseases are associated with mood disorders, and patients with epilepsy have available barbiturates and other medications with which to kill themselves.

Some endocrine conditions are associated with increased suicide risk: Cushing's disease, Klinefelter's syndrome, and porphyria. Mood disorders also attend these disorders. Two gastrointestinal disorders with an increased suicide risk are peptic ulcer and cirrhosis, both physical disorders found among persons who are alcohol dependent. Two urogenital problems that carry an increased suicide risk are prostatic hypertrophy treated with prostatectomy and renal disease treated with hemodialysis; mood changes may occur in both conditions.

Factors associated with illness and contributing to both suicides and suicide attempts are loss of mobility, especially when physical activity is important to occupation or recreation; disfigurement, particularly among women; and chronic, intractable pain. In addition to the direct effects of illness, the secondary effects—for example, disruption of relationships and loss of occupational status—are prognostic factors.

Certain drugs can produce depression, which may lead to suicide in some cases. Among these drugs are reserpine (Serpasil), corticosteroids, antihypertensives, and some anticancer agents.

Mental Health. Highly significant psychiatric factors in suicide include substance abuse, depressive disorders, schizophrenia, and other mental disorders. Almost 95 percent of all persons who commit or attempt suicide have a diagnosed mental disorder. Depressive disorders account for 80 percent of this figure, schizophrenia accounts for 10 percent, and dementia or delirium for 5 percent. Among all persons with mental disorders, 25 percent are also alcohol dependent and have dual diagnoses. Persons with delusional depression are at highest risk of suicide. The suicide risk in persons with depressive disorders is about 15 percent, and 25 percent of all those with a history of impulsive behavior or violent acts are also at high risk of suicide. Previous psychiatric hospitalization for any reason increases the risk of suicide.

Among adults who commit suicide, significant differences between young and old exist for both psychiatric diagnoses and antecedent stressors. A study in San Diego, California, showed that diagnoses of substance abuse and antisocial personality disorder occurred most often among suicides under 30 years of age, and diagnoses of mood disorders and cognitive disorders most often among suicides ages 30 and over. Stressors associated with suicide in those under 30 were separation, rejection, unemployment, and legal troubles; illness stressors most often occurred among suicide victims over 30.

Psychiatric Patients. Psychiatric patients' risk for suicide is 3 to 12 times that of nonpatients. The degree of risk varies, depending on age, sex, diagnosis, and inpatient or outpatient status. After adjustment for age, male and female psychiatric patients who have at some time been inpatients have 5 and 10 times higher suicide risks, respectively, than their counterparts in the general population. For male and female outpatients who have never been admitted to a hospital for psychiatric treatment, the suicide risks are 3 and 4 times greater, respectively, than those of their counterparts in the general population. The higher suicide risk for psychiatric patients who have been inpatients reflects the fact that patients with severe mental disorders tend to be hospitalized—for example, patients with depressive disorder who require electroconvulsive therapy (ECT). The psychiatric diagnosis with greatest risk of suicide in both sexes is a mood disorder.

Those in the general population who commit suicide tend to be middle aged or older, but studies increasingly report that psychiatric patients who commit suicide tend to be relatively young. In one study the mean age of male suicides was 29.5 years and that of women 38.4 years. The relative youthfulness of these suicide cases was due partly to the fact that two early-onset, chronic mental disorders—schizophrenia and recurrent major depressive disorder—accounted for just over half of these suicides and so reflected an age and diagnostic pattern found in most studies of psychiatric patient suicides.

A small, but significant, percentage of psychiatric patients who commit suicide do so while they are inpatients. Most of these do not kill themselves in the psychiatric ward itself but on the hospital grounds, while on a pass or weekend leave, or when absent without leave.

For both sexes, the suicide risk is highest in the first week of the psychiatric admission; after 3 to 5 weeks, inpatients have the same risk as the general population. The inpatient rates of suicide do not rise uniformly with age, as in the general population; in fact, the rates for female psychiatric patients fall with advancing age, mainly because older persons who are suicidal do not seek medical aid. Times of staff rotation, particularly of the psychiatric residents, are periods associated with inpatient suicides. Epidemics of inpatient suicides tend to be associated with periods of ideological change on the ward, staff disorganization, and staff demoralization.

Among psychiatric outpatients, the period after discharge is a time of increased suicide risk. A follow-up study of 5,000 patients discharged from an Iowa psychiatric hospital showed that in the first 3 months after discharge, the rate of suicide for female patients was 275 times that of all Iowa women; the rate of suicide for male patients was 70 times that of all Iowa men.

Patients, especially those with panic disorder, who frequent emergency services, also have an increased suicide risk. One study reported that such patients have a suicide rate more than 7 times the age-adjusted and sex-adjusted rate for the general population (but the rate is similar to that of other clinical psychiatric populations). The two main risk groups are patients with depressive disorders, schizophrenia, and substance abuse, and patients who make repeated visits to the emergency room. Thus, mental health professionals working in emergency services must be well trained in taking patients' psychiatric histories, examining their mental states, assessing suicidal risk, and making appropriate dispositions. They must also be aware of the need to contact patients at risk who fail to keep follow-up appointments.

DEPRESSIVE DISORDERS. Mood disorders are the diagnoses most commonly associated with suicide. As the suicide risk in depressive disorders rises mainly when patients are depressed, the psychopharmacological advances of the past 25 years may have reduced the suicide risk among patients with depressive disorder. Nevertheless, the age-adjusted suicide rates for patients with mood disorders have been estimated to be 400 per 100,000 for male patients and 180 per 100,000 for female patients.

More patients with depressive disorders commit suicide early in the illness than later; more men than women commit suicide; and the chance of depressed persons' killing themselves increases if they are single, separated, divorced, widowed, or recently bereaved. Depressive disorder patients in the community who commit suicide tend to be middle aged or older.

A few studies have investigated which patients with mood disorders have an increased suicide risk. These studies indicate that social isolation enhances suicidal tendencies among depressed patients. This finding is in accord with the data from epidemiological studies showing that persons who commit suicide may be poorly integrated into society. Suicide among depressed patients is likely at the onset or the end of a depressive episode. As with other psychiatric patients, the months after discharge from a hospital are a time of high risk. Studies show that one third or more of depressed patients who commit suicide do so within 6 months of leaving a hospital; presumably they have relapsed.

Regarding outpatient treatment, most depressed suicidal patients had a history of therapy; however, less than half were receiving psychiatric treatment at the time of suicide. Of those who were in treatment, studies have shown that it was less than adequate. For example, most patients who received antidepressants were prescribed subtherapeutic doses of the medication.

SCHIZOPHRENIA. The suicide risk is high among patients with schizophrenia: Up to 10 percent die by committing suicide. In the United States an estimated 4,000 schizophrenic patients commit suicide each year. The onset of schizophrenia is typically in adolescence or early adulthood, and most of these patients who commit suicide do so during the first few years of their illness; therefore, schizophrenic patients who commit suicide are young.

About 75 percent of all schizophrenic suicides are committed by unmarried men, and about 50 percent have made a previous suicide attempt. Depressive symptoms are closely associated with their suicides. Hospital-based studies have reported that depressive symptoms were present during the last period of contact in at least two thirds of patients with schizophrenia who committed suicide; only a small percentage committed suicide because of hallucinated instructions or a need to escape persecutory delusions. Up to 50 percent of suicides among patients with schizophrenia occur during the first few weeks and months after discharge from a hospital; only a minority commit suicide while inpatients.

Thus, the risk factors for suicide among patients with schizophrenia are young age, male gender, single marital status, a previous suicide attempt, a vulnerability to depressive symptoms, and a recent discharge from a hospital. Having three or four hospitalizations during their 20s probably undermines the social, occupational, and sexual adjustment of possibly suicidal schizophrenia patients. Consequently, potential suicide victims are likely to be male, unmarried, unemployed, socially isolated, and living alone—perhaps in a single room. After discharge from their last hospitalization, they may experience a new adversity or return to ongoing difficulties. As a result, they become dejected, experience feelings of helplessness and hopelessness, reach a depressed state, and have, and eventually act on, suicidal ideas.

ALCOHOL DEPENDENCE. Up to 15 percent of all alcohol-dependent persons commit suicide. The suicide rate for those who are alcoholic is estimated to be about 270 per 100,000 annually; in the United States, between 7,000 and 13,000 alcohol-dependent persons commit suicide each year.

About 80 percent of all alcohol-dependent suicide victims are male, a percentage that largely reflects the sex ratio for alcohol dependence. Alcohol-dependent suicide victims tend to be white, middle aged, unmarried, friendless, socially isolated, and currently drinking. Up to 40 percent have made a previous suicide attempt. Up to 40 percent of all suicides by persons who are alcohol dependent occur within a year of the patient's last hospitalization; older alcohol-dependent patients are at particular risk during the postdischarge period.

Studies show that many alcohol-dependent patients who eventually commit suicide are rated depressed during hospitalization and that up to two thirds are assessed as having mood disorder symptoms during the period in which they commit suicide. As many as 50 percent of all alcohol-dependent suicide victims have experienced the loss of a close, affectionate relationship during the previous year. Such interpersonal losses and other types of undesirable life events are probably brought about by the alcohol dependence and contribute to the development of the mood disorder symptoms, which are often present in the weeks and months before the suicide.

The largest group of male alcohol-dependent patients are those with an associated antisocial personality disorder. Studies show that such patients are particularly likely to attempt suicide; to abuse other substances; to exhibit impulsive, aggressive, and criminal behaviors; and to be found among alcohol-dependent suicide victims.

OTHER SUBSTANCE DEPENDENCE. Studies in various countries have found an increased suicide risk among those who abuse substances. The suicide rate for persons who are heroin dependent is about 20 times the rate for the general population. Adolescent girls who use intravenous substances also have a high suicide rate. The availability of a lethal amount of substances, intravenous use, associated antisocial personality disorder, a chaotic lifestyle, and impulsivity are some of the factors that predispose substance-dependent persons to suicidal behavior, particularly when they are dysphoric, depressed, or intoxicated.

PERSONALITY DISORDERS. A high proportion of those who commit suicide have various associated personality difficulties or disorders. Having a personality disorder may be a determinant of suicidal behavior in several ways: by predisposing to major mental disorders like depressive disorders or alcohol dependence; by leading to difficulties in relationships and social adjustment; by precipitating undesirable life events; by impairing the ability to cope with a mental or physical disorder; and by drawing persons into conflicts with those around them, including family members, physicians, and hospital staff members.

An estimated 5 percent of patients with antisocial personality disorder commit suicide. Suicide is 3 times more common among prisoners than among the general population. More than one third of prisoner suicides have had past psychiatric treatment, and half have made a previous suicide threat or attempt, often in the previous 6 months.

ANXIETY DISORDER. Unsuccessful suicide attempts are made by almost 20 percent of patients with a panic disorder and social phobia. If depression is an associated feature, however, the risk of success rises.

Previous Suicidal Behavior.

A past suicide attempt is perhaps the best indicator that a patient is at increased risk of suicide. Studies show that about 40 percent of depressed patients who commit suicide have made a previous attempt. The risk of a second suicide attempt is highest within 3 months of the first attempt. The relation between a mood disorder, completed suicide, and attempts at suicide is shown in Figure 34.2–2.

Depression is associated not only with completed suicide, but also with serious attempts at suicide. The clinical feature most often associated with the seriousness of the intent to die is a diagnosis of a depressive disorder. This is shown by studies that relate the clinical characteristics of suicidal patients with various measures of the medical seriousness of the attempt or of the intent to die. Also, intent-to-die scores correlate significantly with both suicide risk scores and the number and severity of depressive symptoms. The attempters rated as having high suicide intent are more often male, older, single or separated, and living alone than those with low intent. In other words, depressed patients who seriously attempt suicide more closely resemble suicide victims than they do suicide attempters.

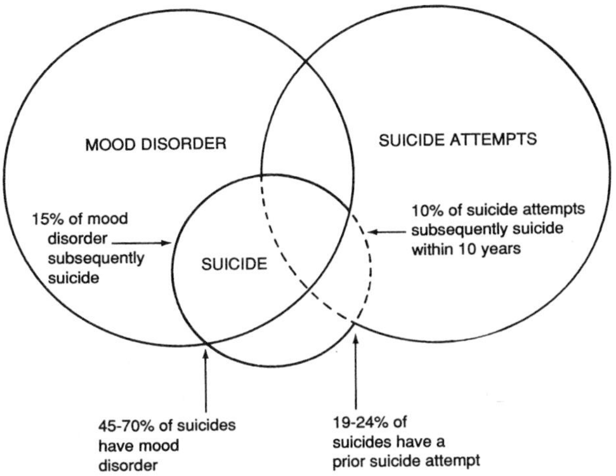

FIGURE 34.2–2
Venn diagram summarizing suicide data and its relation to mood disorder and suicide attempts. (Courtesy of Alec Roy, M.D.)

ETIOLOGY

Sociological Factors

Durkheim's Theory.

The first major contribution to the study of the social and cultural influences on suicide was made at the end of the 19th century by the French sociologist Émile Durkheim. In an attempt to explain statistical patterns, Durkheim divided suicides into three social categories: egoistic, altruistic, and anomic. Egoistic suicide applies to those who are not strongly integrated into any social group. The lack of family integration explains why unmarried persons are more vulnerable to suicide than married ones and why couples with children are the best protected group. Rural communities have more social integration than urban areas and thus less suicide. Protestantism is a less cohesive religion than Roman Catholicism, and so Protestants have a higher suicide rate than Catholics.

Altruistic suicide applies to those prone to suicide stemming from their excessive integration into a group, with suicide being the outgrowth of the integration—for example, a Japanese soldier who sacrifices his life in battle. Anomic suicide applies to persons whose integration into society is disturbed so that they cannot follow customary norms of behavior. Anomie explains why a drastic change in economic situation makes persons more vulnerable than they were before their change in fortune. In Durkheim's theory, anomie also refers to social instability, and a general breakdown of society's standards and values.

Psychological Factors

Freud's Theory.

Sigmund Freud offered the first important psychological insight into suicide. He described only one patient who made a suicide attempt, but he saw many depressed patients. In his paper "Mourning and Melancholia," Freud stated his belief that suicide represents aggression turned inward against an introjected, ambivalently cathected love object. Freud doubted that there would be a suicide without an earlier repressed desire to kill someone else.

Menninger's Theory.

Building on Freud's ideas, Karl Menninger, in *Man against Himself,* conceived of suicide as inverted homicide because of a patient's anger toward another person. This retroflexed murder is either turned inward or used as an excuse for punishment. He also described a self-directed death instinct (Freud's concept of Thanatos) plus three components of hostility in suicide: the wish to kill, the wish to be killed, and the wish to die.

Recent Theories.

Contemporary suicidologists are not persuaded that a specific psychodynamic or personality structure is

associated with suicide. They believe that much can be learned about the psychodynamics of suicidal patients from their fantasies about what would happen and what the consequences would be if they commit suicide. Such fantasies often include wishes for revenge, power, control, or punishment; atonement, sacrifice, or restitution; escape or sleep; rescue, rebirth, reunion with the dead; or a new life. The suicidal patients most likely to act out suicidal fantasies may have lost a love object or received a narcissistic injury, may experience overwhelming affects like rage and guilt, or may identify with a suicide victim. Group dynamics underlie mass suicides like those at Masada, at Jonestown, and by the Heaven's Gate cult.

Depressed persons may attempt suicide just as they appear to be recovering from their depression. A suicide attempt can cause a long-standing depression to disappear, especially if it fulfills a patient's need for punishment. Of equal relevance, many suicide patients use a preoccupation with suicide as a way of fighting off intolerable depression and a sense of hopelessness. In fact, a study by Aaron Beck showed that hopelessness was one of the most accurate indicators of long-term suicidal risk.

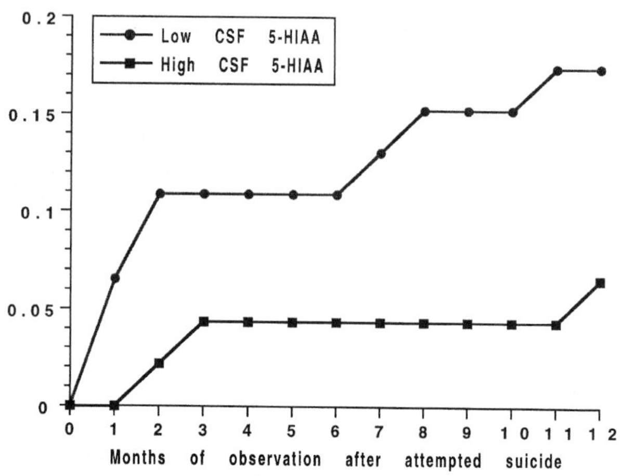

FIGURE 34.2–3

Cumulative suicide risk during first year after attempted suicide in patients with low versus high CSF concentrations of 5-HIAA. Filled circles indicate CSF 5-HIAA concentrations below the sample median and filled squares indicate concentrations above the sample median (87 nM). (Reprinted with permission from Nordstrom P, Samuelsson M, Asberg M, et al. CSF concentrations 5-HIAA predicts suicide risk after attempted suicide. *Suicide Life Threat Behav.* 1994;24:1.)

Biological Factors. Diminished central serotonin plays a role in suicidal behavior. A group at the Karolinska Institute in Sweden were the first to note that low concentrations of the serotonin metabolite 5-hydroxyindoleacetic acid (5-HIAA) in the lumbar cerebrospinal fluid (CSF) were associated with suicidal behavior. This finding has been replicated many times and in different diagnostic groups. Postmortem neurochemical studies have reported modest decreases in serotonin itself or 5-HIAA in either the brainstem or the frontal cortex of suicide victims. Postmortem receptor studies have reported significant changes in presynaptic and postsynaptic serotonin binding sites in suicide victims. Taken together, these CSF, neurochemical, and receptor studies support the hypothesis that reduced central serotonin is associated with suicide. Recent studies also report some changes in the noradrenergic system of suicide victims.

Low concentrations of 5-HIAA in CSF also predict future suicidal behavior. For example, the Karolinska group examined completed suicide in a sample of 92 depressed patients who had attempted suicide. They found that 8 of the 11 patients who committed suicide within 1 year belonged to the subgroup with below-median concentrations of 5-HIAA in CSF. The suicide risk in that subgroup was 17 percent, compared with 7 percent among those with above-median concentrations of 5-HIAA in CSF (Fig. 34.2–3). Also, the cumulative number of patient-months survived during the first year after attempted suicide was significantly lower in the subgroup with low 5-HIAA concentrations. The Karolinska group concluded that low 5-HIAA concentrations in CSF predict short-range suicide risk in the high-risk group of depressed patients who have attempted suicide. Low 5-HIAA concentrations in CSF have also been demonstrated in adolescents who kill themselves.

Genetic Factors. Suicidal behavior, like other psychiatric disorders, tends to run in families. For example, Margaux Hemingway's 1997 suicide was the fifth suicide among four generations of Ernest Hemingway's family. In psychiatric patients, a family history of suicide increases the risk of attempted suicide and that of completed suicide in most diagnostic groups. In medicine, the strongest evidence for involvement of genetic factors comes from twin and adoption studies and from molecular genetics. Such studies in suicide are reviewed below.

Twin Studies. A landmark study in 1991 investigated 176 twin pairs in which one twin had committed suicide. In nine of these twin pairs, both twins had committed suicide. Seven of these nine pairs concordant for suicide were found among the 62 monozygotic pairs, while two pairs concordant for suicide were found among the 114 dizygotic twin pairs. This twin group difference for concordance for suicide (11.3 versus 1.8 percent) is statistically significant ($P < .01$).

Another study collected a group of 35 twin pairs in which one twin had committed suicide, and the living co-twin was interviewed. Ten of the 26 living monozygotic co-twins had themselves attempted suicide, compared with 0 of the 9 living dizygotic co-twins ($P < .04$). Although monozygotic and dizygotic twins may have some differing developmental experiences, these results show that monozygotic twin pairs have significantly higher concordance for both suicide and attempted suicide, which suggests that genetic factors may play a role in suicidal behavior.

Danish-American Adoption Studies. The strongest evidence suggesting the presence of genetic factors in suicide comes from adoption studies carried out in Denmark. A screening of the registers of causes of death revealed that 57 of 5,483 adoptees in Copenhagen eventually committed suicide. They were matched with adopted controls. Searches of the causes of death revealed that 12 of the 269 biological relatives of these 57 adopted suicide victims had themselves committed suicide, compared with only 2 of the 269 biological relatives of the 57 adopted controls. This is a highly significant difference for suicide between the two groups of relatives. None of the adopting relatives of either the suicide or control group had committed suicide.

In a further study of 71 adoptees with mood disorder, adoptee suicide victims with a situational crisis or impulsive suicide

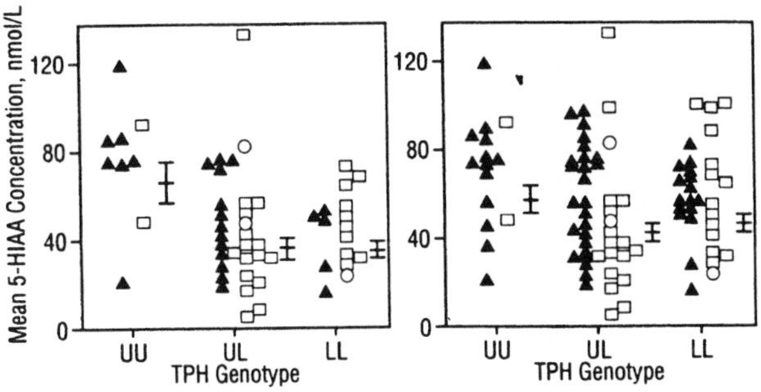

FIGURE 32.2–4

Relationship between tryptophan hydroxylase (TPH) genotype, mean (± SEM) 5-hydroxyindoleacetic acid (5-HIAA) concentration, and history of suicide attempts. The 5-HIAA concentrations of the subjects are plotted against their TPH geotypes for impulsive subjects (*left*) and all subjects (*right*). Triangles represent subjects who had never attempted suicide; squares, suicide attempters; and circles, those who had committed suicide. (Reprinted with permission from Nielsen D, Goldman D, Virkkunen M, et al. Suicidality and 5-hydroxyindoleacetic acid concentration associated with a tryptophan hydroxylase polymorphism. *Arch Gen Psychiatry.* 1994;51:34.)

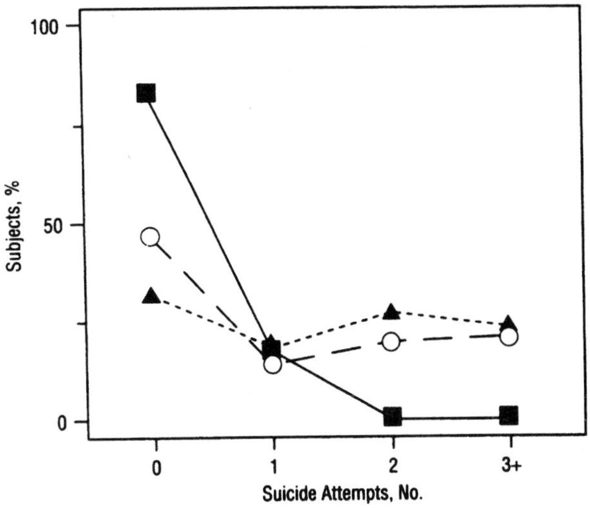

FIGURE 34.2–5

Relation between TPH genotype and lifetime history of multiple suicide attempts. For each genotype, the fraction of subjects having each genotype (UU, squares; UL, circles; LL, triangles) is plotted against the number of suicide attempts they have made in their lives. (Reprinted with permission from Nielsen D, Goldman D, Virkkunen M, et al. Suicidality and 5-hydroxyindoleacetic acid concentration associated with a tryptophan hydroxylase polymorphism. *Arch Gen Psychiatry.* 1994;51:34.)

attempt or both (particularly) had more biological relatives who had committed suicide than controls had. This led to the suggestion that a genetic factor lowering the threshold for suicidal behavior may lead to an inability to control impulsive behavior. Psychiatric disorder or environmental stress may serve "as potentiating mechanisms which foster or trigger the impulsive behavior, directing it toward a suicidal outcome."

Molecular Genetic Studies. Tryptophan hydroxylase (TPH) is an enzyme involved in the biosynthesis of serotonin. A polymorphism in the human *TPH* gene has been identified, with two alleles—*U* and *L*. Since low concentrations of 5-HIAA in CSF are associated with suicidal behavior, it was hypothesized that such individuals may have alterations in genes controlling serotonin synthesis and metabolism. It was found that impulsive alcoholics, who had low CSF 5-HIAA concentrations, had more *LL* and *UL* genotypes. Furthermore, a history of suicide attempts was significantly associated with *TPH* genotype in all the violent alcoholics (Fig. 34.2–4); 34 of the 36 violent subjects who attempted suicide had either the *UL* or *LL* genotype. Thus, it was concluded that the presence of the *L* allele was associated with an increased risk of suicide attempts.

Also, a history of multiple suicide attempts was found most often in subjects with the *LL* genotype and to a lesser extent among those with the *UL* genotype (Fig. 34.2–5). This led to the suggestion that the *L* allele was associated with repetitive suicidal behavior. The presence of one *TPH***L* allele may indicate a reduced capacity to hydroxylate tryptophan to 5-hydroxytryptophan in the synthesis of serotonin, producing low central serotonin turnover and thus a low concentration of 5-HIAA in CSF.

Parasuicidal Behavior. *Parasuicide* is a term introduced to describe patients who injure themselves by self-mutilation (e.g., cutting the skin) but who usually do not wish to die. Studies show that about 4 percent of all patients in psychiatric hospitals have cut themselves; the female-to-male ratio is almost 3 to 1. The incidence of self-injury in psychiatric patients is estimated to be more than 50 times that in the general population. Psychiatrists note that so-called cutters have cut themselves over several years. Self-injury is found in about 30 percent of all abusers of oral substances and 10 percent of all intravenous users admitted to substance-treatment units.

These patients are usually in their 20s and may be single or married. Most cut delicately, not coarsely, usually in private with a razor blade, knife, broken glass, or mirror. The wrists, arms, thighs, and legs are most commonly cut; the face, breasts, and abdomen are cut infrequently. Most persons who cut themselves claim to experience no pain and give reasons such as anger at themselves or others, relief of tension, and the wish to die. The great majority are classified as having personality disorders and are significantly more introverted, neurotic, and hostile than controls. Alcohol abuse and other substance abuse are common, and most cutters have attempted suicide. Self-mutilation has been viewed as localized self-destruction, with mishandling of aggressive impulses caused by a person's unconscious wish to punish himself or herself or an introjected object.

PREDICTION

Clinicians must assess an individual patient's risk for suicide on the basis of a clinical examination. The predictive items associated with suicide risk are listed in Table 34.2–1. Suicide is grouped into high-risk–related and low-risk–related factors (Table 34.2–2). High-risk characteristics include more than 45 years of age, male gender, alcohol dependence (the suicide rate is 50 times higher in alcohol-dependent persons than in those who are not alcohol dependent), violent behavior, previous suicidal behavior, and previous psychiatric hospitalization.

Table 34.2–2
Evaluation of Suicide Risk

Variable	High Risk	Low Risk
Demographic and social profile		
Age	Over 45 years	Below 45 years
Sex	Male	Female
Marital status	Divorced or widowed	Married
Employment	Unemployed	Employed
Interpersonal relationship	Conflictual	Stable
Family background	Chaotic or conflictual	Stable
Health		
Physical	Chronic illness	Good health
	Hypochondriac	Feels healthy
	Excessive substance intake	Low substance use
Mental	Severe depression	Mild depression
	Psychosis	Neurosis
	Severe personality disorder	Normal personality
	Substance abuse	Social drinker
	Hopelessness	Optimism
Suicidal activity		
Suicidal ideation	Frequent, intense, prolonged	Infrequent, low intensity, transient
Suicide attempt	Multiple attempts	First attempt
	Planned	Impulsive
	Rescue unlikely	Rescue inevitable
	Unambiguous wish to die	Primary wish for change
	Communication internalized (self-blame)	Communication externalized (anger)
	Method lethal and available	Method of low lethality or not readily available
Resources		
Personal	Poor achievement	Good achievement
	Poor insight	Insightful
	Affect unavailable or poorly controlled	Affect available and appropriately controlled
Social	Poor rapport	Good rapport
	Socially isolated	Socially integrated
	Unresponsive family	Concerned family

Reprinted with permission from Adam K. Attempted suicide. *Psychiatr Clin North Am.* 1985;8:183.

TREATMENT

Most suicides among psychiatric patients are preventable, as indicated by the evidence that inadequate assessment or treatment is often associated with suicide. Some patients experience suffering so great and intense, or so chronic and unresponsive to treatment, that their eventual suicides may be perceived as inevitable. Fortunately, such patients are relatively uncommon. Other patients have severe personality disorders, are highly impulsive, and commit suicide spontaneously, often when dysphoric or intoxicated or both.

The evaluation for suicide potential involves a complete psychiatric history; a thorough examination of the patient's mental state; and an inquiry about depressive symptoms, suicidal thoughts, intents, plans, and attempts. Taken together, a lack of future plans, giving away personal property, making a will, and having recently experienced a loss imply increased risk of suicide. The decision to hospitalize a patient depends on diagnosis, severity of the depression and suicidal ideation, the patient's and the family's coping abilities, the patient's living situation, availability of social support, and the absence or presence of risk factors for suicide.

Inpatient versus Outpatient Treatment

Whether to hospitalize patients with suicidal ideation is the most important clinical decision to be made. Not all such patients require hospitalization; some may be treated on an outpatient basis. But the absence of a strong social support system, a history of impulsive behavior, and a suicidal plan of action are indications for hospitalization. To decide whether outpatient treatment is feasible, clinicians should use a straightforward clinical approach: They should ask patients considered suicidal to agree to call when they become uncertain about their ability to control their suicidal impulses. Patients who can make such an agreement with a doctor with whom they have a relationship reaffirm the belief that they have sufficient strength to control such impulses and to seek help.

In return for a patient's commitment, clinicians should be available to the patient 24 hours a day. If a patient who is considered seriously suicidal cannot make the commitment, immediate emergency hospitalization is indicated; both the patient and the patient's family should be so advised. If, however, the patient is to be treated on an outpatient basis, the therapist

should note the patient's home and work telephone numbers for emergency reference; occasionally, a patient hangs up unexpectedly during a late night call or gives only a name to the answering service. If the patient refuses hospitalization, the family must take the responsibility to be with the patient 24 hours a day.

According to Shneidman, a clinician has several practical preventive measures for dealing with a suicidal person: reducing the psychological pain by modifying the patient's stressful environment, enlisting the aid of the spouse, the employer, or a friend; building realistic support by recognizing that the patient may have a legitimate complaint; and offering alternatives to suicide.

Many psychiatrists believe that any patient who has attempted suicide, despite its lethality, should be hospitalized. Although most of these patients voluntarily enter a hospital, the danger to self is one of the few clear-cut indications currently acceptable in all states for involuntary hospitalization. In a hospital, patients can receive antidepressant or antipsychotic medications as indicated; individual therapy, group therapy, and family therapy are available, and patients receive the hospital's social support and sense of security. Other therapeutic measures depend on patients' underlying diagnoses. For example, if alcohol dependence is an associated problem, treatment must be directed toward alleviating that condition.

Although patients classified as acutely suicidal may have favorable prognoses, chronically suicidal patients are difficult to treat, and they exhaust the caretakers. Constant observation by special nurses, seclusion, and restraints cannot prevent suicide when a patient is resolute. ECT may be necessary for some severely depressed patients, who may require several treatment courses.

Useful measures for the treatment of depressed suicidal inpatients include searching patients and their belongings on arrival in the ward for objects that may be used for suicide and repeating the search at times of exacerbation of the suicidal ideation. Ideally, suicidal depressed inpatients should be treated on a locked ward where the windows are shatterproof, and the patient's room should be located near the nursing station to maximize observation by the nursing staff. The treatment team must assess how much to restrict the patient and whether to make regular checks or use continuous direct observation.

Vigorous treatment with antidepressant or antipsychotic medication should be initiated, depending on the underlying disorder. Some medications (e.g., risperidone [Risperdal]) have both antipsychotic and antidepressant effects and are useful when the patient has signs and symptoms of both psychosis and depression.

Supportive psychotherapy by a psychiatrist shows concern and may alleviate some of a patient's intense suffering. Some patients may be able to accept the idea that they are suffering from a recognized illness and that they will probably make a complete recovery. Patients should be dissuaded from making major life decisions while they are suicidally depressed, because such decisions are often morbidly determined and may be irrevocable. The consequences of such bad decisions can cause further anguish and misery when the patient has recovered.

Patients recovering from a suicidal depression are at particular risk. As the depression lifts, patients become energized and are thus able to put their suicidal plans into action (paradoxical suicide). Sometimes, depressed patients, with or without treatment, suddenly appear to be at peace with themselves because they have reached a secret decision to commit suicide. Clinicians should be especially suspicious of such a dramatic clinical change, which may portend a suicide attempt. Although rare, some patients lie to the psychiatrist about their suicidal intent, thus subverting the most careful clinical assessment.

A patient may commit suicide even when in the hospital. According to one survey, about 1 percent of all suicides were committed by patients who were being treated in general medical-surgical or psychiatric hospitals, but the annual suicide rate in psychiatric hospitals is only 0.003 percent.

Legal and Ethical Factors. Liability issues stemming from suicides in psychiatric hospitals frequently involve questions about a patient's rate of deterioration, the presence during hospitalization of clinical signs indicating risk, and psychiatrists' and staff members' awareness of, and response to, these clinical signs.

In about half of cases in which suicides occur while patients are on a psychiatric unit, a lawsuit results. Courts do not require zero suicide rates, but do require periodic patient evaluation for suicidal risk, formulation of a treatment plan with a high level of security, and having staff members follow the treatment plan.

Currently, suicide and attempted suicide are variously viewed as a felony and a misdemeanor, respectively; in some states the acts are considered not crimes but unlawful under common law and statutes. Aiding and abetting a suicide adds another dimension to the legal morass; some court decisions have held that although neither suicide nor attempted suicide is punishable, anyone who assists in the act may be punished. (Doctor-assisted suicide is discussed in Chapter 2, Section 2.7.)

National Strategy for Suicide Prevention

In 2001, Surgeon General David Satcher organized the National Strategy for Suicide Prevention, under the auspices of the National Institutes of Health (NIH). The National Strategy of Suicide Prevention of NIH has set specific goals and objectives to reduce suicide. These include the following 11 goals:

1. Promote awareness that suicide is a public health problem that is preventable
2. Develop broad-based support for suicide prevention
3. Develop and implement strategies to reduce the stigma associated with being a consumer of mental health, substance abuse, and suicide prevention services
4. Develop and implement suicide prevention programs
5. Promote efforts to reduce access to lethal means and methods of self-harm
6. Implement training for recognition of at-risk behavior and delivery of effective treatment
7. Develop and promote effective clinical and professional practices
8. Improve access to, and community linkages with, mental health and substance abuse services
9. Improve reporting and portrayals of suicidal behavior, mental illness, and substance abuse in the entertainment and news media

10. Promote and support research on suicide and suicide prevention
11. Improve and expand surveillance systems

The *National Strategy for Suicide Prevention* creates a framework for suicide prevention for the nation. It is designed to encourage and empower groups and individuals to work together. The stronger and broader the support and collaboration on suicide prevention, the greater the chance of success for this public health initiative. Suicide and suicidal behaviors can be reduced as the general public gains more understanding about the extent to which suicide is a problem, about the ways in which it can be prevented, and about the roles individuals and groups can play in prevention efforts.

References

Allen M. *Emergency Psychiatry.* Washington, DC: American Psychiatric Publishing; 2002.

Barraclough B, Bunch J, Nelson B, Sainsbury P. A hundred cases of suicide. *Br J Psychiatry.* 1997;125:355.

de Wilde EJ, Kienhorst ICWM, Diekstra RFW, Goodyer IM, eds. *The Depressed Child and Adolescent.* 2nd ed. Cambridge child and adolescent psychiatry. New York: Cambridge University Press; 2001:267.

Duberstein PR, Conwell Y, Caine ED. Interpersonal stressors, substances abuse, and suicide. *J Nerv Ment Dis.* 1993;181:80.

Durkheim E. *Suicide.* Glencoe, IL: Free Press; 1951.

Hendin H, Mann JJ, eds. The clinical science of suicide prevention. *Ann N Y Acad Sci.* 2001;932:200.

Henry JA. Suicide risk and antidepressant treatment. *J Psychopharmacol.* 1996;10(suppl 1):39.

Kreitman N, ed. *Parasuicide.* New York: Wiley; 1977.

Mann JJ. A current perspective on suicide and attempted suicide. *Ann Intern Med.* 2002;136:302.

Meltzer HJ, Hendin H, eds. The clinical science of suicide prevention. *Ann N Y Acad Sci.* 2001;932:44.

Roy A. Suicide. In: Sadock BJ, Sadock VA, eds. *Kaplan & Sadock's Comprehensive Textbook of Psychiatry.* 7th ed. Vol 2. Baltimore: Lippincott Williams & Wilkins; 2001:2031.

Rud MDW, Canetto SS. *Review of Suicidology.* New York: Guilford Press; 2000:47.

Rudd MD, ed. *Suicide Science: Expanding the Boundaries.* Norwell, MA: Kluwer Academic Publishers; 2000:117.

Shneidman ES. *The Suicidal Mind.* New York: Oxford University Press; 1996.

35 Psychotherapies

▲ 35.1 Psychoanalysis and Psychoanalytic Psychotherapy

Sigmund Freud once noted that a treatment could be described as psychoanalytic if it involved the principles of transference and resistance. While those two principles (described below) remain of critical importance in psychoanalysis and psychoanalytic therapy, the distinguishing features of this approach are now much broader, as the field has moved more and more in the direction of acknowledging that the treatment involves a two-person field in which the analyst's or therapist's feelings must also be taken into account. Glen and Gabbard defines the essence of psychoanalysis and psychoanalytic therapy as "a therapy that involves careful attention to the therapist–patient interaction, with thoughtfully timed interpretation of transference and resistance embedded in a sophisticated appreciation of the therapist's contribution to the two-person field."

This definition subsumes both psychoanalysis and psychoanalytic psychotherapy because they are generally considered to reside on a continuum. Both derive from psychoanalytic theory (discussed in Chapter 6, Section 6.1), and both involve a focus on the patient's unconscious as it emerges in the treatment relationship with the clinician. Psychoanalytic psychotherapy is known by a number of different terms, including *insight-oriented psychotherapy, exploratory psychotherapy, expressive psychotherapy, psychodynamic psychotherapy,* and *uncovering psychotherapy.* Both psychoanalysis and psychoanalytic psychotherapy are generally considered extended, or long-term, treatments that go on for more than 6 months. However, some brief psychodynamic therapies that last for only a matter of weeks are based on psychoanalytic principles.

Psychoanalytic psychotherapy is often divided into expressive and supportive subtypes, with the recognition that most psychotherapies involve both expressive and supportive elements. The expressive interventions involve interpretation of unconscious conflict to produce insight in the patient. This form of intervention links it closely with psychoanalysis, which also emphasizes interpretation. Supportive psychotherapy focuses on strengthening the patients' defenses and helping them with problem solving and adaptation. In this regard, advice and praise may be given more frequently than in expressive therapy, and the therapist may focus more on practical coping skills to assist patients in daily living. Table 35.1–1 offers an outline of the distinguishing features of psychoanalysis, expressive psychoanalytic psychotherapy, and supportive psychoanalytic psychotherapy.

GOALS AND THERAPEUTIC ACTION

Any discussion of goals and therapeutic action must recognize that psychoanalysis and psychoanalytic psychotherapy are practiced today in an era of theoretical pluralism. When Freud first developed psychoanalysis at the end of the 19th century, he was primarily treating hysterical patients under the assumption that catharsis and abreaction connected with the lifting of repression of childhood memories would relieve symptoms. He ultimately found that this method was not as effective as he had hoped, so he developed the technique of *free association,* in which patients were instructed to say whatever came to mind without censoring. At this point, analysis began to shift from the excavation of deeply buried memories to an interpretation of the defenses and conflicts among ego, id, superego, and external reality.

Goals and therapeutic action also started to change according to new therapeutic models that emphasized analyzing the manifestations of a patient's internal object relations as they unfolded in the transference and countertransference of the analytic relationship. This approach, known as *object relations theory,* was influenced by Melanie Klein, D. W. Winnicott, Ronald Fairbairn, and others. In addition, Heinz Kohut's self psychology prompted more attention to another aspect of the patient's psychology—namely, the fragmentation of the self that occurs when the analyst fails to meet the patient's needs for mirroring, twinship, and idealization.

The therapeutic action itself varies in accord with specific goals. In other words, goals are to therapeutic action as the destination of a journey is to the vehicle designed to take one there. The analytic journey today has a multiplicity of destinations, and most analysts would agree that multiple modes of therapeutic action exist. The acquisition of understanding about oneself is a major goal of psychoanalysis and psychoanalytic psychotherapy, and interpretation of unconscious patterns that occur in the transference relationship with the analyst is one mode of therapeutic action. Through interpretation of the patient's transference, the superego is modified, the id is tamed, and the ego is expanded. Moreover, the patient begins to recognize that feelings arising in the present with the analyst stem from childhood experiences that have been internalized and that are repeated again and again in present-day relationships. Another major

Table 35.1–1
Scope of Psychoanalytic Practice: A Clinical Continuum[a]

Feature	Psychoanalysis	Psychoanalytic Psychotherapy: Expressive Mode	Psychoanalytic Psychotherapy: Supportive Mode
Frequency	Regular 4 to 5 times a week: 50-minute hour	Regular one to three times a week: half to full hour	Flexible once a week or less; or if needed, half to full hour
Duration	Long-term: usually 3 to 5+ years	Short-term or long-term: several sessions to months or years	Short-term or intermittent long-term; single session to lifetime
Setting	Patient primarily on couch with analyst out of view	Patient and therapist face to face; occasional use of couch	Patient and therapist face to face; couch contraindicated
Modus operandi	Systematic analysis of all (positive and negative) transference and resistance; primary focus on analyst and intrasession events; transference neurosis facilitated; regression encouraged	Partial analysis of dynamics and defenses; focus on current interpersonal events and transference to others outside sessions; analysis of negative transference; positive transference left unexplored unless it impedes progress; limited regression encouraged	Formation of therapeutic alliance and real object relationship; analysis of transference contraindicated with rare exceptions; focus on conscious external events; regression discouraged
Analyst-therapist role	Absolute neutrality; frustration of patient; reflector-mirror role	Modified neutrality; implicit gratification of patient and great activity	Neutrality suspended; limited explicit gratification, direction, and disclosure
Putative change agents	Insight predominates within relatively deprived environment	Insight within empathic environment; identification with benevolent object	Auxiliary or surrogate ego as temporary substitute; holding environment; insight to degree possible
Patient population	Neuroses; mild character psychopathology	Neuroses; mild to moderate character psychopathology, especially narcissistic and borderline personality disorders	Severe character disorders; latent or manifest psychoses; acute crises; physical illness
Patient requisites	High motivation; psychological-mindedness; good previous object relationships; ability to maintain transference neurosis; good frustration tolerance	High to moderate motivation and psychological-mindedness; ability to form therapeutic alliance; some frustration tolerance	Some motivation and ability to form therapeutic alliance
Basic goals	Structural reorganization of personality; resolution of unconscious conflicts; insight into intrapsychic events; symptom relief an indirect result	Partial reorganization of personality and defenses; resolution of preconscious and conscious derivatives of conflicts; insight into current interpersonal events; improved object relations; symptom relief a goal or prelude to further exploration	Reintegration of self and ability to cope; stabilization or restoration of preexisting equilibrium; strengthening of defenses; better adjustment or acceptance of pathology; symptom relief and environmental restructuring as primary goals
Major techniques	Free association method predominates; fully dynamic interpretation (including confrontation, clarification, and working through), with emphasis on genetic reconstruction	Limited free association; confrontation, clarification, and partial interpretation predominate, with emphasis on here-and-now interpretation and limited genetic interpretation	Free association method contraindicated; suggestion (advice) predominates; abreaction useful; confrontation, clarification, and interpretation in the here and now secondary; genetic interpretation contraindicated
Adjunct treatment	Primarily avoided; if applied, all negative and positive meanings and implications thoroughly analyzed	May be necessary (e.g., psychotropic drugs as temporary measure); if applied, negative implications explored and diffused	Often necessary (e.g., psychotropic drugs, family therapy, rehabilitative therapy, or hospitalization); if applied, positive implications are emphasized

[a]This division is not categorical; all practice resides on a clinical continuum.
Courtesy of Toksoz Byram Karasu, M.D.

mode of therapeutic action is the internalization of the new relationship with the analyst or therapist so that the patient begins to reflect and understand in the way the analyst does.

Object relations theorists stress the need for change in mental representation of self and object and in the affect linkage between these representations. They believed that such changes are brought about partly through interpretation but also through the analytic relationship, which provides a holding environment. They emphasized the process of containment in producing change. Through projective identification, the analyst becomes a container of patients' self-representations and object-representations, often in association with powerful affective states. Before these projected contents are returned to patients by the process of reintrojection, the analyst psychologically processes and thereby modifies patients' representations.

In self psychology, the goal of psychoanalytic treatment is to strengthen a weakened self so that it can move from dependence on archaic "selfobject" experiences to a position of greater self-cohesion that allows reliance on more mature selfobjects. Kohut asserted that the goal was accomplished by lay-

ing down psychic structure through optimal frustration and by transmuting internalizations. The essential curative aspect of the analytic process is the establishment of empathic attunement between the self and the selfobject on a mature level.

Analytic Setting

In the usual analytic setting, patients lie on a couch or sofa, and the analyst sits behind, partially or totally outside a patient's field of vision. The couch helps the analyst produce the controlled regression that favors the emergence of repressed material. The patient's reclining position in the presence of an attentive analyst almost recreates symbolically the early parent–child situation, which varies from patient to patient. The position also helps the patient focus on inner thoughts, feelings, and fantasies, which can then become the focus of free associations. Moreover, the use of the couch introduces an element of sensory deprivation; the patient's visual stimuli are limited, and the analyst's verbalizations are relatively few. This state promotes regression. There has been some disagreement, however, about the necessary use of the couch in psychoanalysis. Otto Fenichel stated that whether the patient lies down or sits and whether certain rituals of procedure are used do not matter. The best condition is the one most appropriate to the analytic task.

Duration of Treatment

The patient and the psychoanalyst must be prepared to persevere in the process indefinitely. Psychoanalysis takes time—between 3 and 6 years, sometimes even longer. Sessions are usually held 4 or more times a week for 45 to 50 minutes each.

Treatment Methods

Fundamental Rule of Psychoanalysis. According to the fundamental or basic rule, patients agree to be completely honest with their analysts and to tell everything without selection. Freud referred to the technique that allowed for such honesty as *free association*.

Free Association. In free association, patients attempt to comply with the fundamental rule by saying whatever comes to mind. Inevitably, they cannot accomplish this task because of embarrassment, concerns about what the analyst thinks, and their evaluations of whether an association is relevant. These resistances to the process of saying whatever comes to mind become a primary focus of analytic work. The analyst does not become more authoritarian in response to a patient's difficulties with free association but instead tries to understand the patient's obstacles in complying with the fundamental rule.

Free-Floating Attention. The analyst's counterpart to patients' free association is a particular way of listening, often referred to as free-floating or evenly suspended attention. An analyst avoids an intense focus on a patient's comments and instead allows the patient's associations to stimulate associations in the analyst. Similarly, analysts strive to attain a state of free-floating responsiveness, in which they allow themselves to be drawn into a patient's internal object world by identifying with the roles cast upon them by the patient's unconscious.

Analytic Process

Transference. *Transference* is a term that refers to the displacement of attitudes and feelings originally experienced in relationships with persons from the past onto the analyst. Modern analysts recognize that transference is also influenced by an analyst's *real* characteristics; thus transference is always to some extent an amalgam of old relationships and the new relationships with the analyst. Although Freud initially encouraged analysts to be opaque to their patients (the principle of anonymity), the contemporary view is that analysts' subjectivity is an ongoing influence to help shape the transference. Most analysts attempt to use restraint and avoid excessive self-disclosure, but they also recognize that the stereotype of the blank-screen analyst is no longer useful.

A major criterion by which psychoanalysis can, in principle, be differentiated from other forms of psychotherapy is its intensive focus on transference. To a considerable extent, psychoanalysis is defined by a much more systematic analysis of the transference than occurs in psychotherapy. In Freud's original formulation, a patient's infantile neurosis was revealed in the form of a transference neurosis to the analyst, in which a patient struggles to gratify unconscious infantile wishes through the analyst. The term *transference neurosis* has fallen out of favor as many analysts have become aware that speaking of multiple transferences is more accurate. Transference is the repetition of a patient's habitual modes of object relatedness in the analytic dyad. Because relationships are highly varied, transferences themselves are usually variable, though often they involve several core themes. For example, transferences may be idealizing, erotic, or hateful. However, labeling a transference as having one quality is perhaps oversimplified, because transferences are actually multilayered. An intensely loving transference may turn to hate if the analyst is perceived as unresponsive to the patient's love. With some narcissistic patients, there may appear to be an absence of any form of transference attachment. Freud believed that such patients could not be analyzed. Today analysts are more accustomed to narcissistic transferences and simply regard the apparent absence of transference as an example of how a narcissistic patient has brought a long-standing pattern of object relatedness into the analytic setting.

The analyst's role is to help a patient gain insight into the underlying wishes and conflicts inherent in transference and therefore make the unconscious conscious. By systematically understanding the nature of the relationship with the analyst, a patient also gains insight into characteristic patterns of relationships with others outside analysis.

Interpretation. In psychoanalysis, the analyst provides patients with interpretations about psychological events that were neither previously understood by, nor meaningful to, them. The transference constitutes a major frame of reference for interpretation. A complete psychoanalytic interpretation includes meaningful statements of current conflicts and the historical factors that influenced them. Such complete interpretations, however, constitute a relatively small part of analysis; most interpretations are limited in scope and deal with matters of immediate concern.

Interpretations must be well timed. An analyst may have a formulation in mind, but a patient may not be prepared to deal

with it directly because of factors such as anxiety level, negative transference, and external life stress. The analyst may decide to wait until the patient can fully understand the interpretation. The proper timing of interpretation requires great clinical skill.

DREAM INTERPRETATION. In his classic work *The Interpretation of Dreams,* Freud referred to the dream as the "royal road to the unconscious." The manifest content of a dream is what a dreamer reports. The latent content is a dream's unconscious meaning after the condensations, substitutions, and symbols are analyzed. Dreams arise from what Freud referred to as the day residue (the events of the preceding day, which stimulated the patient's unconscious mind). Dreaming may serve as a wish-fulfillment mechanism and a way of mastering anxiety about a life event.

Freud outlined several technical procedures to use in dream interpretation: Have a patient associate to elements of the dream in the order in which they occurred; have the patient associate to a particular dream element that the patient or the therapist chooses; disregard the content of the dream, and ask the patient what events of the previous day can be associated with the dream (the day residue); and avoid giving any instructions, and leave it to the dreamer to begin. Analysts use patients' associations to find a clue to the workings of the unconscious mind.

Countertransference. Freud originally understood countertransference as an analyst's transference to a patient. He viewed it as an obstacle, based on the analyst's own personal conflicts, that had to be removed so as not to interfere with the patient's analysis. This narrow or classical view has been superseded by the broad view of countertransference as an analyst's feelings that are thought to be related to what the patient is projecting onto the analyst. This formulation underscores the value of countertransference as a therapeutic tool; namely, it provides the analyst with clues about the nature of the patient's internal object world. The most widely held view of countertransference today is that it is a joint creation involving contributions from the analyst's past and the patient's internal world.

Therapeutic Alliance. In addition to transferential and countertransferential issues, the relationship between the analyst and the patient involves two adults entering into a joint venture, referred to as the therapeutic or working alliance. Both commit themselves to exploring the patient's problems, to establishing mutual trust, and to cooperating with each other to achieve a realistic goal of a cure or the amelioration of symptoms.

Resistance. Freud believed that unconscious ideas or impulses are repressed and prevented from reaching awareness because they are unacceptable to consciousness for some reason. He referred to this phenomenon as resistance, which must be overcome if the analysis is to proceed. Resistance may sometimes be a conscious process manifested by a patient's withholding relevant information. Other examples of patients' resistance are remaining silent for a long time, being late or missing appointments, and paying bills late or not at all. The signs of resistance are legion, and almost any feature of the analytic situation can be used in resistance. However, some psychoanalytic schools of thought view resistance quite differently. For example, self psychologists regard resistances as psychologically healthy activities that safeguard the self from narcissistic injury.

Indications for Psychoanalytic Treatment

The indications for psychoanalysis must consider generalized criteria for analyzability, which apply regardless of the diagnosis. There must be significant suffering so that patients are motivated to make the sacrifices of time and financial resources required for psychoanalysis. Patients who enter analysis must have a genuine wish to understand themselves, not a desperate hunger for symptomatic relief. They must be able to withstand frustration, anxiety, and other strong affects that emerge in analysis without fleeing or acting out their feelings in a self-destructive manner. They must also have a reasonable, mature superego that allows them to be honest with the analyst. Intelligence must be at least average, and above all, they must be psychologically minded in the sense that they can think abstractly and symbolically about the unconscious meanings of their behavior.

One survey of 580 analytic patients offers a basis for a general statement about indications for psychoanalysis. This survey found that 82 percent of patients currently in psychoanalysis had in the past undergone other forms of psychotherapy that had failed to address their problems. Hence, a common indication for psychoanalysis is failure of brief therapies or psychopharmacological interventions.

Contraindications for Treatment

Many contraindications for psychoanalysis are the flip side of the indications. The absence of suffering, poor impulse control, inability to tolerate frustration and anxiety, and low motivation to understand are all contraindications. The presence of extreme dishonesty or antisocial personality disorder contraindicates analytic treatment. Concrete thinking or the absence of psychological mindedness is another contraindication. Some patients who might ordinarily be psychologically minded are not suitable for analysis because they are in the midst of a major upheaval or life crisis, such as a job loss or a divorce. Serious physical illness may also interfere with a person's ability to invest in a long-term treatment process. Patients of low intelligence generally do not understand the procedure or cooperate in the process. An age older than 40 was once considered a contraindication, but today analysts recognize that patients are malleable and analyzable in their 60s or 70s. One final contraindication is a close relationship with the analyst. Analysts should avoid analyzing friends, relatives, or persons with whom they have other involvements.

PSYCHOANALYTIC PSYCHOTHERAPY

Psychoanalytic psychotherapy is based on psychoanalytic formulations that have been modified conceptually and technically. In highly expressive therapy, interpretation is still a commonly used intervention, but there is a less systematic analysis of the transference, there is only partial analysis of dynamics, and the couch is not generally used. More typically, patient and therapist sit opposite each other, a situation that can lend greater reality to the ther-

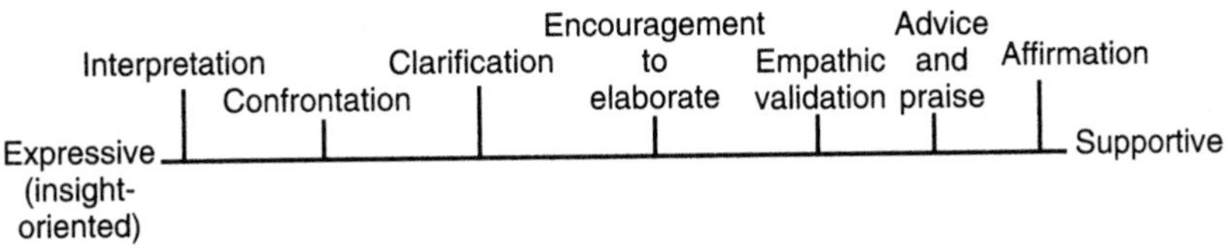

FIGURE 35.1–1
An expressive (insight-oriented)-supportive continuum of interventions. (Reproduced with permission from Gabbard GO. *Psychodynamic Psychiatry in Clinical Practice.* 3rd ed. Washington, DC: American Psychiatric Press; 2000:96.)

apist than a situation in which the therapist is out of view. Expressive psychotherapy is often conducted between 1 and 3 times a week for 45- or 50-minute sessions; sometimes 30-minute sessions are used as well. Supportive therapy is generally no more frequent than once a week and often even less frequent; sessions may last anywhere from 30 to 50 minutes.

Types

Many clinicians and researchers have conceptualized the types of psychotherapies as falling along a spectrum, with expressive (insight-oriented) therapies (e.g., psychoanalysis) and analytically oriented therapies at one end of the spectrum and supportive therapies at the other end. Most interventions of the therapist can be placed in seven categories along an expressive (or exploratory)-supportive continuum summarized in Figure 35.1–1. Table 35.1–2 summarizes the definitions of therapeutic interventions.

Expressive Psychotherapy. In expressive or insight-oriented therapy, therapists attempt to provide insight into the patients' unconscious processes. By systematically examining patterns of behavior, both in transference and in outside rela-

Table 35.1–2
Psychotherapeutic Interventions Defined

1. *Interpretation.* In the most expressive forms of treatment, interpretation is regarded as the therapist's ultimate decisive instrument. In its simplest form, interpretation involves making something conscious that was previously unconscious. An interpretation is an explanatory statement that links a feeling, thought, behavior, or symptom to its unconscious meaning or origin. For example, the therapist might say to a patient who is late, "Perhaps the reason you are late is that you were afraid I would react to the success you are now having the way your father reacted." Depending on the point in therapy and the patient's readiness to hear the interpretation, interpretations may focus on the transference (as in that example), extratransference issues, the patient's past or present situation, or the patient's resistances or fantasies. As a general rule, the therapist does not address unconscious content by interpretation until the material is almost conscious and, therefore, relatively accessible to the patient's awareness.
2. *Confrontation.* The next most expressive intervention is confrontation, which addresses something the patient does not want to accept or identifies the patient's avoidance or minimization. A confrontation may be geared to clarifying how the patient's behavior affects others or to reflecting back to the patient a denied or suppressed feeling. Confrontation, which is often gentle, carries the unfortunate connotation in common parlance of being aggressive or blunt. The following example illustrates that confrontation is not necessarily forceful or hostile. In the last session of a long-term therapy process, one patient talked at great length about car problems he encountered on the way to the session. The therapist commented, "I think you'd rather talk about your car than face the sadness you're feeling about our last session."
3. *Clarification.* Further along the continuum from expressive to supportive interventions, clarification involves a reformulation or pulling together of the patient's verbalizations to convey a coherent view of what is being communicated. Clarification differs from confrontation because it lacks the element of denial or minimization. A clarification is aimed at helping the patient articulate something that is difficult to put into words.
4. *Encouragement to elaborate.* Closer to the center of the continuum come interventions that are neither supportive nor expressive in and of themselves. Encouragement to elaborate may be broadly defined as a request for information about a topic brought up by the patient. It may be an open-ended question, such as, "What comes to mind about that?" or a more specific request, as in "Tell me more about your father." Such interventions are commonly used in both the most expressive and the most supportive treatments.
5. *Empathic validation.* This intervention is a demonstration of the therapist's empathic attunement with the patient's internal state. A typically validating comment is "I can understand why you feel depressed about that" or "It hurts when you're treated that way." In the view of the self psychologists, empathic immersion in the patient's internal experience is essential, regardless of the location of the therapy on the expressive-supportive continuum. When patients feel that the therapist understands their subjective experiences, they are likely to accept interpretations.
6. *Advice and praise.* This category really includes two interventions that are linked by the fact that they both prescribe and reinforce certain activities. Advice involves direct suggestions to the patient regarding how to behave; praise reinforces certain patient behaviors by expressing overt approval of them. An example of the former is, "I think you should stop going out with that man immediately." An example of the latter is, "I'm very pleased that you were able to tell him that you would not see him anymore." Those comments are on the opposite end of the continuum from traditional psychoanalytic interventions because they are departures from neutrality and to some extent compromise the patient's autonomy in making decisions.
7. *Affirmation.* This simple intervention involves succinct comments in support of the patient's comments or behaviors, such as "Uh-huh" and "Yes, I see what you mean."

Adapted from Gabbard GO. *Psychodynamic Psychiatry in Clinical Practice.* 3rd ed. Washington, DC: American Psychiatric Press; 2000:97.

tionships, patients become progressively aware of unconscious determinants of behavior.

Therapists rely on a range of interventions along the expressive-supportive continuum but emphasize interpretation, confrontation, and clarification much more than advice and praise. Interpretations often focus on linkages between relationships in childhood and the present. There is less emphasis on reconstructing childhood events in expressive psychotherapy than occurs in psychoanalysis and more focus on current functioning. Therapists create a nonjudgmental environment in which patients can talk about a wide range of issues. On the other hand, therapists might also set limits if self-destructive or aggressive behavior becomes a major issue.

Therapists also have the more limited goals of partially reorganizing patients' personality and defenses without completely resolving major conflicts. Object relations may improve, based partly on insight gained from interpretation and also on internalizing the therapeutic relationship. Much like psychoanalysts, expressive therapists point out how a patient's unconscious is observable through various behaviors and actions that go on outside the patient's awareness. The indications for expressive versus supportive emphasis in psychotherapy are outlined in Table 35.1–3.

Supportive Psychotherapy. Supportive psychotherapy offers patients the support of an authority figure during a period of illness, turmoil, or temporary decompensation. This treatment has the goal of restoring and strengthening patients' impaired defenses and integrating capacities. It provides a period of acceptance and dependence for a patient who needs help to deal with guilt, shame, and anxiety and to meet frustrations or external pressures that may be too great to handle.

Supportive therapy uses several methods, either singly or in combination, including warm, friendly, strong leadership; partial gratification of dependency needs; support in the ultimate development of legitimate independence; help in developing pleasurable activities (e.g., hobbies); adequate rest and diversion; removal of excessive strain when possible; hospitalization when indicated; medication to alleviate symptoms; and guidance and advice in dealing with current issues. This therapy uses techniques to help patients feel secure, accepted, protected, encouraged, safe, and not anxious.

One of the greatest dangers of supportive therapy is the possibility of an analyst fostering too great a regression and too strong a dependence. From the beginning, psychiatrists must plan to work persistently to enable patients to assume independence. Some patients, however, require supportive therapy indefinitely, often with the goal of maintaining a marginal adjustment that enables them to function in society.

The expression of emotion is an important part of supportive psychotherapy, and verbalizing unexpressed strong emotions may bring considerable relief. Talking things out is not primarily meant to gain insight into unconscious dynamic patterns that may be intensifying current responses. Rather, expressing emotion may reduce inner tension and anxiety, and subsequent discussion may lead to insight into a current problem and objectivity in evaluating it.

CORRECTIVE EMOTIONAL EXPERIENCE. The relationship between therapist and patient gives a therapist an opportunity to display behavior different from the destructive or unproductive behavior of a patient's parent. At times, such experiences seem to neutralize or reverse some effects of the parents' mistakes. If the patient had overly authoritarian parents, the therapist's friendly, flexible, nonjudgmental, nonauthoritarian—but at times firm and limit setting—attitude gives the patient an opportunity to adjust to, be led by, and identify with, a new parent figure. Franz Alexander described this process as a corrective emotional experience.

Table 35.1–3 summarizes indications for insight-oriented (expressive) therapy versus supportive therapy. Table 35.1–4 outlines supportive psychotherapy.

Table 35.1–3
Indications for Expressive or Supportive Emphasis in Psychotherapy

Insight-Oriented (Expressive)	Supportive
Strong motivation to understand	Significant ego defects of a long-term nature
Significant suffering	Severe life crisis
Ability to regress in the service of the ego	
Tolerance for frustration	Poor frustration tolerance
Capacity for insight (psychological-mindedness)	Lack of psychological-mindedness
Intact reality testing	Poor reality testing
Meaningful object relations	Severely impaired object relations
Good impulse control	Poor impulse control
Ability to sustain work	Low intelligence
Capacity to think in terms of analogy and metaphor	Little capacity for self-observation
Reflective responses to trial interpretations	Organically based cognitive dysfunction
	Tenuous ability to form a therapeutic alliance

Reprinted with permission from Gabbard GO. *Psychodynamic Psychotherapy in Clinical Practice.* 3rd ed. Washington, DC: American Psychiatric Press; 2000:108.

Table 35.1–4
Supportive Psychotherapy

Goal	Support reality testing
	Provide ego support
	Maintain or reestablish usual level of functioning
Selection criteria	Very healthy patient faced with overwhelming crises
	Patient with ego deficits
Duration	Days, months, or years—as needed
Technique	Therapist predictably available
	Interpretation used to strengthen defenses
	Therapist maintains working, reality-based relationship based on support, concern, and problem solving
	Suggestion, reinforcement, advice, reality testing, cognitive restructuring, and reassurance
	Psychodynamic life narrative
	Medication

Reprinted with permission from Ursano RJ, Silberman EK. Individual psychotherapies. In: Talbott JA, Hales RE, Yudofsky SC, eds. *The American Psychiatric Press Textbook of Psychiatry.* Washington, DC: American Psychiatric Press; 1988:878.

Table 35.1–5
Guidelines for Patient Referral

It is important to exhibit confidence and enthusiasm when making a referral for psychiatric evaluation or psychotherapy. Patients will detect ambivalence and skepticism on the physician's part about the need for such treatment. It is usually helpful to recommend a psychiatrist or other mental health professional who is known *personally* by the physician.

Always present the psychiatric referral as part of the patient's on-going medical care. Some patents view a psychiatric referral as a means to dump them onto another doctor or as a rejection. Patients should be reassured that any psychiatric treatment will be in parallel with their ongoing medical care.

Have the name and telephone number of your referral source readily available to give to the patient.

Call the psychiatrist to personally explain the reason and need for the referral and what role you would like to continue to play in the patient's care.

Make the appointment for the psychiatric evaluation while the patient is still in the office or clinic.

Be sure to schedule a follow-up appointment after the date of the psychiatric evaluation to check on the patient's reaction to the referral and his or her response to the initial treatment.

Reprinted with permission from Stoudemire A. *Clinical Psychiatry for Medical Students.* Philadelphia: JB Lippincott; 1990:457.

REFERRAL BY A NONPSYCHIATRIC PHYSICIAN

Nonpsychiatric physicians often treat psychiatric patients who may require referral to a psychiatrist for in-depth evaluation and treatment that cannot be provided in a nonpsychiatric setting. Sometimes a nonpsychiatric physician thinks that a patient would benefit from psychotherapy. Such a patient might or might not carry an Axis I or Axis II diagnosis. Table 35.1–5 summarizes a few key features involved in effectively referring a patient for psychotherapy.

CURRENT PROBLEMS

Managed care places increasing pressure on psychiatrists to provide psychotherapy that is short term and, theoretically, low cost. Short-term therapies—enthusiastically promoted by private insurance companies, health maintenance organizations, and several psychiatric residency programs—have explicitly delineated parameters about the number of sessions, concrete goals, and outcome evaluation criteria. These therapies are largely designed so that the techniques involved can be learned quickly and performed with the aid of instructional manuals by various practitioners other than psychiatrists.

The pressure to develop therapies that are less expensive, less training intensive, and less time consuming than psychoanalysis stems from some legitimate concerns about the accessibility of traditional insight-oriented approaches of psychoanalysis and analytically oriented psychotherapy. Nevertheless, the rush to relegate such treatments to the periphery seems shortsighted and ultimately impoverishes the field of psychiatry and those patients who respond only to extended treatment. The emphasis on empirically validated treatments has raised the clinical trial with randomized control design to the gold standard that determines whether or not a particular therapeutic modality is efficacious. Psychiatrists who ascribe to this view can now dismiss claims for therapeutic efficacy of psychoanalytic therapies in the absence of data that adhere to this standard.

The difficulty of conducting controlled clinical trials with psychoanalysis or long-term psychoanalytic therapy is obvious. Such a long-term study would be extraordinarily expensive. Uncontrolled variables such as life events, the emergence of Axis I disorders, medication changes, and illness would very likely influence the meaningfulness of the results. Randomization would interfere with self-selection of treatment, which is of critical importance in psychoanalytic treatments. Also, recruiting a suitably matched control group would be difficult.

Despite these difficulties, at least one randomized controlled trial of patients with borderline personality disorder treated with psychoanalytic psychotherapy in a partial hospital setting demonstrated impressive results. The patients who received the psychoanalytically oriented treatment showed significantly more improvements in depressive symptoms, social and interpersonal functioning, need for hospitalization, and suicidal and self-mutilating behavior than the control group who received no psychoanalytic psychotherapy.

Gender Issues in Psychotherapy

Few data are available about the influence of therapist gender on the therapeutic process. Most studies show a higher correlation between the therapist's experience and the outcome of psychotherapy or patient satisfaction with the therapist than between the patient's gender and the outcome. In general, patients of more experienced physicians fared better than those of less experienced clinicians, regardless of gender.

Nevertheless, the literature on gender issues in psychiatric treatment is growing. Carol Nadelson has pointed out that a patient's choosing to be treated by a woman may represent a search for the idealized mother, whether the patient is a man or a woman. Similarly, choosing a male therapist may represent a search for a father figure. A patient who has had traumatic experiences with persons of one gender may wish to avoid entering into a therapeutic relationship with someone who can evoke these experiences. It is not uncommon, for example, for women who have been sexually abused by men to request a female therapist. Women therapists are less likely to become sexually involved with their patients than are men, but such involvement does occur.

In a psychoanalytic situation, analysis of the transference is a basic issue. As the analytic process unfolds, patients can often perceive a psychotherapist as a member of the opposite sex: A woman may see a male therapist as a mother figure, and a man may perceive a female analyst as a father figure. These unconscious perceptions may shift as the analysis proceeds. These transference issues are analyzed in psychoanalysis. In supportive therapies, similar transference distortions may occur, but if they are discussed at all, they are not interpreted in the same way as in psychoanalysis. In any case, it is important to note that patients can view therapists as male or female regardless of the therapists' actual gender.

When patients identify with their therapists and rely on them as role models, as they often do, patients identify with therapists' value systems, not with their gender assignment. Under ideal circumstances, female therapists have worked through negative cul-

tural stereotypes of the female role and so can facilitate the same process in their female patients and can raise the consciousness of their male patients about prejudice toward females.

FUTURE DIRECTIONS

Psychoanalysis and psychoanalytic psychotherapy are facing a great challenge in this era of accountability. For them to gain credibility as treatments within psychiatry, more emphasis must be placed on systematic research. The distinguishing features of psychoanalytic treatments must be clearly defined. Indications and contraindications for psychoanalytic therapy require empirical underpinnings to validate them. Psychoanalysts and psychoanalytic therapists also must grow accustomed to defining treatment goals and measuring whether or not the treatment has attained those goals. Cost-benefit advantages must be factored in to determine in which cases the greater expense of intensive psychoanalytic therapy is warranted. Finally, as our understanding of neuroscience grows, imaging studies demonstrating the brain changes that accompany psychoanalytic treatments may also be useful in gaining credibility for these treatments.

References

Abend SM. Countertransference and psychoanalytic technique. *Psychoanal Q.* 1989;58:374.

Bateman A, Fonagy P. The effectiveness of partial hospitalization in the treatment of borderline personality disorder: a randomized controlled trial. *Am J Psychiatry.* 1999;156:1563.

Bateman A, Fonagy P. Treatment of borderline personality disorder with psychoanalytically oriented partial hospitalization: an 18-month follow-up. *Am J Psychiatry.* 2001;158:36.

Blechner J. Psychoanalysis and HIV disease. *Contemp Psychoanal.* 1993;29:61.

Bowden CL. Implications of psychopharmacological studies for the practice of psychoanalysis. *J Am Acad Psychoanal.* 1992;20:477.

Brenner C. *Psychoanalytic Technique and Psychic Conflict.* New York: International Universities Press; 1976.

Brown SD, Lent RW. *Handbook of Counseling Psychology.* 3rd ed. New York: John Wiley & Sons; 2000:711.

Crastnopol M. Convergence and divergence in the characters of analyst and patient: Fairbairn Guntrip. *Psychoanal Psychol.* 2001;18:120.

Etchegoyen A. Psychoanalysis of the child: psychic reality of the patient and the analyst. *Int J Psychoanal.* 1996;77:353.

Fenichel O. Problems of psychoanalytic technique. *Psychoanal Q.* 1941;10:84.

Fonagy P. The outcome of psychoanalysis: the hope of a future. *Psychologist.* 2000;13:620.

Freud A. *The Ego and Mechanisms of Defense.* New York: International Universities Press; 1966.

Gabbard GO. *Psychodynamic Psychiatry in Clinical Practice: The DSM-IV Edition.* Washington, DC: American Psychiatric Press; 1994.

Gabbard GO. Countertransference: the emerging common ground. *Int J Psychoanal.* 1995;76:475.

Gabbard GO. Psychoanalysis and psychoanalytic psychotherapy. In: Sadock BJ, Sadock VA, eds. *Kaplan & Sadock's Comprehensive Textbook of Psychiatry.* 7th ed. Vol 2. Baltimore: Lippincott Williams & Wilkins; 2000:2056.

Gabbard GO. Overview and commentary. *Psychoanal Q.* 2001;70:287.

Gill MM. *Psychoanalysis in Transition: A Personal View.* Hillsdale, NJ: Analytic Press; 1994.

Gunderson JG, Gabbard GO. Making the case for psychoanalytic therapies in the current psychiatric environment. *J Am Psychoanal Assoc.* 1999;47:679.

Hartmann H. *Ego Psychology and the Problem of Adaption.* New York: International Universities Press; 1959.

Hirsch I. An interpersonal perspective: the analyst's unwitting participation in the patient's change. *Psychoanal Psychol.* 1992;9:299.

Holinser PC. A developmental perspective on psychotherapy and psychoanalysis. *Am J Psychiatry.* 1989;146:1494.

Jones E. *The Life and Work of Sigmund Freud.* Vols 1–3. New York: Basic Books; 1953–1957.

Kay J, Gabbard GO, Greist J. Is psychoanalytic psychotherapy relevant to the treatment of OCD? *J Psychother Pract Res.* 1996;5:341.

Kernberg OF. *Object Relations Therapy and Clinical Psychoanalysis.* New York: Aronson; 1976.

Kernberg OF. The current status of psychoanalysis. *J Am Psychoanal Assoc.* 1993;41:45.

Klein M. *Contributions of Psychoanalysis.* London: Hogarth; 1948.

Kohut HH. *The Analysis of the Self.* New York: International Universities Press; 1984.

Lazar R. Psychotherapy and psychoanalysis: relations between the two modalities. *Contemp Psychoanal.* 1996;32:135.

Luborsky L. The meaning of empirically supported treatment research for psychoanalytic and other long-term therapies. *Psychoanal Dialog.* 2001;11:583.

Mahler M. *On Human Symbiosis and the Vicissitudes of Individuation.* New York: International Universities Press; 1968.

May R, Angel E, Ellenberger H. *Existence: A New Dimension in Psychiatry and Psychology.* New York: Basic Books; 1958.

Oremland JD. Interactive interventions in psychoanalytic psychotherapy and psychoanalysis: a critical review. *Psychoanal Inquiry.* 1996;16:67.

Reich W. *Character Analysis.* New York: Touchstone; 1974.

Sabo AN, Havens L, eds. *The Real World Guide to Psychotherapy Practice.* Cambridge, MA: Harvard University Press; 2000:163.

Schwaber EA. The conceptualization and communication of clinical facts in psychoanalysis: a discussion. *Int J Psychoanal.* 1996;77:235.

Shafer R. *A New Language for Psychoanalysis.* New Haven: Yale University Press; 1976.

Sullivan HS. *Interpersonal Theory of Psychiatry.* New York: WW Norton; 1953.

Wallerstein RS. Follow-up in psychoanalysis: what happens to treatment gains? *J Am Psychoanal Assoc.* 1992;40:665.

Yorke V. Boundaries, psychic structure, and time. *J Anal Psychol.* 1993;38:57.

▲ 35.2 Brief Psychotherapy

The brief psychotherapies are an important component of current methods to treat a variety of mental disorders. Short-term treatment methods (also called *time-limited psychotherapy*) not only help persons deal with current problems and crises but also are useful for major mental disorders such as depression, anxiety, and posttraumatic stress disorder, among others. Derived from psychoanalytic and learning theories, these therapies have their own treatment techniques and specific criteria for selecting patients. Short-term therapies have gained widespread popularity, partly because of the great pressure on health care professionals to contain treatment costs. It is also easier to evaluate treatment efficacy by comparing groups of persons who have undergone short-term therapy for mental illness with control groups than it is to measure the results of long-term psychotherapy. Thus short-term therapies have been the subject of much research, especially on outcome measures, which have found them to be effective.

BRIEF PSYCHOTHERAPY

History

In 1946, Franz Alexander and Thomas French identified most of the basic characteristics of brief psychotherapy. They described a therapeutic experience designed to put patients at ease, to manipulate the transference, and to use trial interpretations flexibly. Alexander and French emphasized developing a corrective emotional experience capable of repairing traumatic events of the past and convincing patients that new ways of thinking, feeling, and behaving are possible. At about the same time, Eric Lindemann established a consultation service at the Massachusetts General Hospital in Boston for persons experiencing a crisis. He developed new treatment methods to deal with these situations and eventually applied these techniques to persons who were not in crisis but who were experiencing various kinds of emotional distress. Since then the field has been influenced by many workers such as David Malan, Michael Balint in England, Peter Sifneos and Myrna Weissman in the

United States, and Habib Davanloo in Canada. Their work is discussed below.

Types

Brief Focal Psychotherapy (Tavistock–Malan).

Brief focal psychotherapy was originally developed in the 1950s by the Balint team at the Tavistock Clinic in London. Malan, a member of the team, reported the results of the therapy. Malan's selection criteria for treatment included eliminating absolute contraindications, rejecting patients for whom certain dangers seemed inevitable, clearly assessing patients' psychopathology, and determining patients' capacities to consider problems in emotional terms, face disturbing material, respond to interpretations, and endure the stress of the treatment. Malan found that high motivation invariably correlated with a successful outcome. Contraindications to treatment were serious suicide attempts, substance dependence, chronic alcohol abuse, incapacitating chronic obsessional symptoms, incapacitating chronic phobic symptoms, and gross destructive or self-destructive acting out.

REQUIREMENTS AND TECHNIQUES. In Malan's routine, therapists should identify the transference early and interpret it and the negative transference. They should then link the transferences to patients' relationships to their parents. Both patients and therapists should be willing to become deeply involved and to bear the ensuing tension. Therapists should formulate a circumscribed focus and set a termination date in advance, and patients should work through grief and anger about termination. An experienced therapist should allow about 20 sessions as an average length for the therapy; a trainee should allow about 30 sessions. Malan himself did not exceed 40 interviews with his patients. Tables 35.2–1 and 35.2–2 summarize Malan's techniques and exclusion criteria.

Table 35.2–1
Malan and the Tavistock Group: Brief Focal Psychotherapy

Goal	Clarify the nature of the defense, the anxiety, and the impulse
	Link the present, the past, and the transference
Selection criteria	Patient able to think in feeling terms
	High motivation
	Good response to trial interpretation
Duration	Up to one year
	Mean, 20 sessions
Focus	Internal conflict present since childhood
Termination	Set definite date at beginning of treatment

Reprinted with permission from Ursano RJ, Silberman EK. Individual psychotherapies. In: Talbott JA, Hales RE, Yudofsky SC, eds. *The American Psychiatric Press Textbook of Psychiatry.* Washington, DC: American Psychiatric Press; 1988:861.

Table 35.2–2
Malan and the Tavistock Group's Exclusion Criteria for Brief Focal Psychotherapy

1. Patient is unavailable to therapeutic contact.
2. Therapist anticipates that prolonged work will be needed to
   - generate motivation
   - penetrate rigid defenses
   - deal with complex or deep-seated issues
   - resolve unfavorable, intense transference, dependent or other, that may develop
3. Depressive or psychotic disturbance may intensify

Reprinted with permission from Ursano RJ, Silberman EK. Individual psychotherapies. In: Talbott JA, Hales RE, Yudofsky SC, eds. *The American Psychiatric Press Textbook of Psychiatry.* Washington, DC: American Psychiatric Press; 1988:861.

Time-Limited Psychotherapy (Boston University–Mann).

A psychotherapeutic model of exactly 12 interviews focusing on a specified central issue was developed at Boston University by James Mann and his colleagues in the early 1970s. In contrast with Malan's emphasis on clear-cut selection and rejection criteria, Mann has not been as explicit about the appropriate candidates for time-limited psychotherapy. Mann considered the major emphases of his theory to be determining a patient's central conflict reasonably correctly and exploring young persons' maturational crises with many psychological and somatic complaints. Mann's exceptions, similar to his rejection criteria, include persons with major depressive disorder that interferes with the treatment agreement, those with acute psychotic states, and desperate patients who need, but cannot tolerate, object relations.

REQUIREMENTS AND TECHNIQUES. Mann's technical requirements included strict limitation to 12 sessions, positive transference predominating early, specification and strict adherence to a central issue involving transference, positive identification, making separation a maturational event for patients, absolute prospect of termination to avoid development of dependence, clarification of present and past experiences and resistances, active therapists who support and encourage patients, and education of patients through direct information, reeducation, and manipulation. The conflicts likely to be encountered included independence versus dependence, activity versus passivity, unresolved or delayed grief, and adequate verses inadequate self-esteem. Table 35.2–3 summarizes the features of Mann's time-limited psychotherapy.

Short-Term Dynamic Psychotherapy (McGill University–Davanloo).

As conducted by Davanloo at McGill University, short-term dynamic psychotherapy encompasses nearly all varieties of brief psychotherapy and crisis intervention. Patients treated in Davanloo's series are classified as those whose psychological conflicts are predominantly oedipal, those whose conflicts are not oedipal, and those whose conflicts have more than one focus. Davanloo also devised a specific psychotherapeutic technique for patients with severe, long-standing neurotic problems, specifically those with incapacitating obsessive-compulsive disorders and phobias.

Davanloo's selection criteria emphasize evaluating those ego functions of primary importance to psychotherapeutic work: the establishment of a psychotherapeutic focus; the psychodynamic formulation of the patients' psychological problems; the ability

Table 35.2–3
Mann: Time-Limited Psychotherapy

Goal	Resolution of the present and chronically endured pain and the patient's negative self-image
Selection criteria	High ego strength
	Able to engage and disengage
	Therapist quickly able to identify a central issue
	Excludes major depressive disorder, acute psychosis, and borderline personality disorder
Duration	12 treatment hours
Focus	Present and chronically endured pain
	Particular image of the self
Termination	Specific last session set at beginning of treatment
	Termination a major focus of the therapy work

Reprinted with permission from Ursano RJ, Silberman EK. Individual psychotherapies. In: Talbott JA, Hales RE, Yudofsky SC, eds. *The American Psychiatric Press Textbook of Psychiatry.* Washington, DC: American Psychiatric Press; 1988:864.

to interact emotionally with evaluators; a history of give-and-take relationships with a significant person in patients' lives; patients' ability to experience and tolerate anxiety, guilt, and depression; their motivations for change; their psychological-mindedness; and their ability to respond to interpretation and to link evaluators with persons in the present and past. Both Malan and Davanloo emphasized patients' responses to interpretation as an important selection and prognostic criterion.

REQUIREMENTS AND TECHNIQUES. The highlights of Davanloo's psychotherapeutic approach are flexibility (therapists should adapt the technique to patients' needs), control of patients' regressive tendencies, active intervention to avoid having patients develop overdependence on a therapist, and patients' intellectual insight and emotional experiences in the transference. These emotional experiences become corrective as a result of the interpretation. Table 35.2–4 summarizes the features of Davanloo's short-term dynamic psychotherapy.

Table 35.2–4
Davanloo: Short-Term Dynamic Psychotherapy

Goal	Resolution of oedipal conflict, loss focus, or multiple foci
Selection criteria	Psychological-mindedness
	At least one past meaningful relationship
	Able to tolerate affect
	Good response to trial transference interpretation
	High motivation
	Flexible defenses
	Lack of projection, splitting, and denial
Duration	5–40 sessions, usually 5–25
	Longer durations for seriously ill
Termination	No specific termination date
	Patient is told that treatment will be short

Reprinted with permission from Ursano RJ, Silberman EK. Individual psychotherapies. In: Talbott JA, Hales RE, Yudofsky SC, eds. *The American Psychiatric Press Textbook of Psychiatry.* Washington, DC: American Psychiatric Press; 1988:865.

Short-Term Anxiety-Provoking Psychotherapy (Harvard University–Sifneos). Sifneos developed short-term anxiety-provoking psychotherapy at the Massachusetts General Hospital in Boston during the 1950s. He used the following criteria for selection: a circumscribed chief complaint (implying a patient's ability to select one of a variety of problems to be given top priority and the patient's desire to resolve the problem in treatment), one meaningful or give-and-take relationship during early childhood, the ability to interact flexibly with an evaluator and to express feelings appropriately, above-average psychological sophistication (implying not only above-average intelligence but also an ability to respond to interpretations), a specific psychodynamic formulation (usually a set of psychological conflicts underlying a patient's difficulties and centering on an oedipal focus), a contract between therapist and patient to work on the specified focus and the formulation of minimal expectations of outcome, and good to excellent motivation for change, not just for symptom relief.

REQUIREMENTS AND TECHNIQUES. Treatment can be divided into four major phases: patient–therapist encounter, early therapy, height of treatment, and evidence of change and termination. Therapists use the following techniques during the four phases.

Patient–Therapist Encounter. A therapist establishes a working alliance by using the patient's quick rapport with, and positive feelings for, the therapist that appear in this phase. Judicious use of open-ended and forced-choice questions enables the therapist to outline and concentrate on a therapeutic focus. The therapist specifies the minimum expectations of outcome to be achieved by the therapy.

Early Therapy. In transference, feelings for the therapist are clarified as soon as they appear, a technique that leads to the establishment of a true therapeutic alliance.

Height of the Treatment. This phase emphasizes active concentration on the oedipal conflicts that have been chosen as the therapeutic focus for the therapy; repeated use of anxiety-provoking questions and confrontations; avoidance of pregenital characterological issues, which the patient uses defensively to avoid dealing with the therapist's anxiety-provoking techniques; avoidance at all costs of a transference neurosis; repetitive demonstration of the patient's neurotic ways or maladaptive patterns of behavior; concentration on the anxiety-laden material, even before the defense mechanisms have been clarified; repeated demonstrations of parent-transference links by the use of properly timed interpretations based on material given by the patient; establishment of a corrective emotional experience; encouragement and support of the patient, who becomes anxious while struggling to understand the conflicts; new learning and problem-solving patterns; and repeated presentations and recapitulations of the patient's psychodynamics until the defense mechanisms used in dealing with oedipal conflicts are understood.

Evidence of Change and Termination of Psychotherapy. This phase emphasizes the tangible demonstration of change in the patient's behavior outside therapy, evidence that adaptive patterns of behavior are being used, and initiation of talk about terminating the treatment. Table 35.2–5 summarizes features of the Sifneos short-term anxiety-provoking psychotherapy.

Table 35.2–5
Short-Term Anxiety-Provoking Psychotherapy

Goal	Resolution of oedipal conflict
Selection criteria	Above-average intelligence
	At least one past meaningful relationship
	High motivation
	Specific chief complaint
	Able to interact with evaluator
	Able to express feelings
	Flexible
Duration	A few months
	Average 12–16 sessions
Focus	Oedipal (triangular) conflict
Termination	No specific date given

Reprinted with permission from Ursano RJ, Silberman EK. Individual psychotherapies. In: Talbott JA, Hales RE, Yudofsky SC, eds. *The American Psychiatric Press Textbook of Psychiatry.* Washington, DC: American Psychiatric Press; 1988:863.

Outcome

The shared techniques of all the brief psychotherapies described above outdistance their differences. They share the therapeutic alliance or dynamic interaction between therapist and patient, the use of transference, the active interpretation of a therapeutic focus or central issue, the repetitive links between parental and transference issues, and the early termination of therapy.

The outcomes of these brief treatments have been investigated more extensively than any other form of psychotherapy. Contrary to prevailing ideas that the therapeutic factors in psychotherapy are nonspecific, controlled studies and other assessment methods (e.g., interviews with unbiased evaluators, patients' self-evaluations) point to the importance of the specific techniques used. The capacity for genuine recovery in certain patients is far greater than was thought. A certain type of patient receiving brief psychotherapy can benefit greatly from a practical working through of his or her nuclear conflict in the transference. Such patients can be recognized in advance through a process of dynamic interaction, because they are responsive, motivated, and able to face disturbing feelings and because a circumscribed focus can be formulated for them. The more radical the technique in terms of transference, depth of interpretation, and the link to childhood, the more radical the therapeutic effects will be. For some disturbed patients, a carefully chosen partial focus can be therapeutically effective.

INTERPERSONAL PSYCHOTHERAPY

Interpersonal psychotherapy (ITP), a time-limited treatment for major depressive disorder, was developed in the 1970s, defined in a manual, and tested in randomized clinical trials by Gerald L. Klerman and Myrna Weissman. Based on the ideas of Harry Stack Sullivan and the interpersonal school, ITP generally deals with current, rather than past, interpersonal relationships, focusing on the patient's immediate social context. It attempts to intervene in symptom formation and social dysfunction associated with depression (Table 35.2–6). It assumes a connection between the onset of mood disorders (and perhaps other psychiatric disorders) and the interpersonal context in which they occur.

Table 35.2–6
Interpersonal Psychotherapy

Goal	Improvement in current interpersonal skills
Selection criteria	Outpatient, nonbipolar disorder, nonpsychotic depressive disorder
Duration	12–16 weeks, usually once-weekly meetings
Technique	Reassurance
	Clarification of feeling states
	Improvement of interpersonal communications
	Testing perceptions
	Development of interpersonal skills
	Medication

Reprinted with permission from Ursano RJ, Silberman EK. Individual psychotherapies. In: Talbott JA, Hales RE, Yudofsky SC, eds. *The American Psychiatric Press Textbook of Psychiatry.* Washington, DC: American Psychiatric Press; 1988:868.

Requirements and Techniques

As short-term treatment for depression, ITP consists of three phases. The first phase generally consists of the first one to three sessions. Its goals are to gather psychiatric history, establish a diagnosis, and introduce the framework for treatment. The psychiatric history explores current social functioning. Particular attention is paid to gathering extensive information about interpersonal events that may have precipitated the depressive episode. The patient's current and past significant interpersonal relationships, including the family of origin, friendships, and community relations, are also reviewed during this first phase. The data gleaned from this review are used to identify one of four problem areas that will guide the therapy: unresolved grief, social role disputes, social role transitions, and interpersonal deficits. Psychiatric diagnosis is informed by standard criteria. Decisions about the concomitant use of medication are based on the severity of the symptoms, past response to interventions, and patient preference. The patient is placed in the sick role; the therapist explicitly discusses the diagnosis of depression and its attendant symptoms and explains what the patient can expect from treatment. The depressive syndrome is then related to the patient's main interpersonal theme, which is related to the syndrome's onset.

The middle phase of treatment is directed toward resolving the problem area. Specific goals and strategies are used for each of the four areas. For a patient whose main problem area is unresolved grief, the goals of treatment are to facilitate the mourning process and assist the patient in finding new activities and relationships to offset the loss. In the treatment of interpersonal role disputes, the dispute is identified, a plan of action is chosen, and a satisfactory resolution is sought through modified expectations or improved communication. If resolution proves impossible, patients are encouraged to consider terminating that plan of action in favor of finding better ones. For depression associated with role transitions, the patient is helped to mourn and accept the loss of the old role.

Efforts are directed toward helping the patient regard the new role as more positive than the old one. Self-esteem is enhanced by focusing on the new skills that are mastered in learning the new role. Finally, when interpersonal deficits are the core theme, the therapist encourages the patient to establish relationships and diminish social isolation.

Each session begins with the question "How have things been since we last met?" to focus on current mood states and their association with recent interactions. The basic techniques for handling each problem area are clarifying positive and negative feeling states, identifying past models for relationships, and guiding and encouraging the patient in examining and choosing alternative courses of action.

ITP has been used across a variety of depressed populations: geriatric, adolescent, human immunodeficiency virus (HIV)–infected, dysthymic disorder, bipolar disorder, and depressed patients with marital problems. It has also been used for nonmood psychiatric conditions such as substance abuse and bulimia nervosa.

Ms. A., a 29-year-old never-married vice president in a successful business, presented with a 9-month history of depression complicated by panic attacks. She described her involvement in a relationship with her superior at work, which they both desired but which work policy forbade. Her symptoms emerged under the pressure she felt to resolve this situation, from which she saw no way out. Neither she nor her boyfriend, Bob, wanted to leave their jobs, and neither wanted to end the relationship. Yet exposure of their secret threatened both their jobs.

In this context Ms. A. developed the full spectrum of symptoms of major depressive disorder, with a Hamilton Rating Scale for Depression score of 28 on presentation, including intermittent panic attacks and suicidal ideation without attempts. Her work and mood suffered. She had a family history of depression and alcoholism but had no prior symptoms, and she did not drink. She had been in twice-weekly psychodynamic psychotherapy for 2 years, starting after the breakup of a previous relationship. She felt that this therapy had increased her self-understanding but had not helped her symptoms. She had considered but declined to take antidepressant medication, feeling it would not resolve her dilemma.

Although quite depressed, Ms. A. quickly agreed that she was in a depressive episode and was able to relate it to her interpersonal situation. This had some aspects of a role transition—a change in her personal and work roles—but was best characterized as a role dispute with Bob: What did she want to happen, and what options did she have to negotiate its happening? A 12-week time limit was set for treatment. Her interpersonal therapist focused on helping her explore various options. She developed a resume and went to a headhunter to seek new job possibilities, although she was ambivalent at leaving her hard-earned and promising post. Role-playing helped her discuss the situation and its possibilities with her lover. Subsequent encounters with Bob better defined the nature of their agreements and differences.

Simply defining the problem and mobilizing Ms. A. to constructive action improved her mood and yielded a greater sense of mastery of her situation. ITP also helped her develop interpersonal skills; although Ms. A. was appropriately assertive in her work role, she was far more pliant and submissive in her personal relationships, a problem that emerged in reviewing her interpersonal inventory of past romances. Depressive symptoms steadily subsided, but the turning point came in the sixth week of ITP when, after considerable exploration and role-playing in therapy, Ms. A. told her boyfriend that she had decided she could not give up her job; either they would have to end the relationship, or he would have to move. He initially said that his own job came first. But several days later he recanted, saying how much he loved her and that he would try to find a new job himself. Her symptoms resolved. Shortly thereafter, a wonderful prospect appeared for Ms. A., in effect giving her a promotion at a different, related company and allowing the relationship to continue overtly. She attributed her symptomatic improvement to her newly firm stand, not to the job change. On 6-month follow-up, she remained euthymic without panic attacks and felt she was holding her own in a relationship that was going more smoothly than previous relationships ever had. (Courtesy of Myrna M. Weissman, M.D., and John C. Markowitz, Ph.D.)

Results

The efficacy of ITP for the treatment of acute depression has been demonstrated in several randomized trials. In one study ITP was comparable to imipramine in depressed patients, and combined drug-ITP treatment was better than either alone. ITP also improves interpersonal relationships and social functioning, which are not addressed in psychopharmacological treatment. Trials are under way in other depressive disorders such as dysthymia, postpartum depression, eating disorders, and borderline personality disorders. ITP has not been efficacious compared with standard treatment for opioid- and cocaine-dependent patients. Monthly maintenance ITP has successfully prevented recurrences of depressive episodes in some patients.

References

Barber JP, Foltz C. Issues in research on short-term dynamic psychotherapy. *Clin Psychol Rev.* 1999;19:659.

Brom D, Kleber RJ, Defares PB. Brief psychotherapy for posttraumatic stress disorders. *J Consult Clin Psychol.* 1989;57:607.

Corcoran J, Roberts AR. Research on crisis intervention and recommendations for future research. In: Roberts AR, ed. *Crisis Intervention Handbook: Assessment, Treatment, and Research.* 2nd ed. New York: Oxford University Press; 2000:453.

Davanloo H. *Basic Principles and Technique of Short Term Dynamic Psychotherapy.* New York: Spectrum; 1978.

Everly GS Jr, Flannery RB Jr, Mitchell JT. Critical incident stress management (CISM): a review of the literature. *Aggress Violent Behav.* 2000;5:23.

France K. *Crisis Intervention: A Handbook of Immediate Person-to-Person Help.* 4th ed. Springfield, IL: Charles C Thomas; 2002.

Gingerich WJ, Eisengart S. *Fam Process.* 2000;39:477.

Gustafson JP. The field of brief psychotherapy. In: Sabo AN, Havens L, eds. *The Real World Guide to Psychotherapy Practice.* Cambridge, MA: Harvard University Press; 2000:214.

Hughes KH, Ashby C. Essential components of the short-term psychiatric unit. *Perspect Psychiatr Care.* 1996;32:20.

Mann J. *Time Limited Psychotherapy.* Cambridge, MA: Harvard University Press; 1973.

Sifneos PE. *Short-Term Dynamic Psychotherapy Evaluation and Technique.* 2nd ed. New York: Plenum; 1987.

Swenson CR, Torrey WC, Koerner K. Implementing dialectical behavior therapy. *Psychiatr Serv.* 2002;53:171.
Ursano RJ, Norwood AE. In: Sadock BJ, Sadock VA, eds. *Kaplan & Sadock's Comprehensive Textbook of Psychiatry.* 7th ed. Vol 2. Baltimore: Lippincott Williams & Wilkins; 2000:2187.
Wilborg IM, Dahl AA. Does brief dynamic psychotherapy reduce the relapse rate of panic disorder? *Arch Gen Psychiatry.* 1996;53:689.

▲ 35.3 Group Psychotherapy, Combined Individual and Group Psychotherapy, and Psychodrama

GROUP PSYCHOTHERAPY

Group psychotherapy is a treatment in which carefully selected persons who are emotionally ill meet in a group guided by a trained therapist and help one another effect personality change. By using a variety of technical maneuvers and theoretical constructs, the leader directs group members' interactions to bring about changes.

Group psychotherapy encompasses the theoretical spectrum of therapies in psychiatry: supportive, structured, limit setting (e.g., groups with chronically psychotic persons), cognitive-behavioral, interpersonal, family, and analytically oriented groups. Compared with individual therapies, two of the main strengths of group therapy are the opportunity for immediate feedback from a patient's peers and the chance for both patient and therapist to observe a patient's psychological, emotional, and behavioral responses to a variety of persons, who elicit a variety of transferences. Table 35.3–1 outlines some of the key features of group therapies.

Classification

Group therapy at present has many approaches. Some clinicians work within a psychoanalytic frame of reference. Others use therapy techniques such as transactional group therapy, which was devised by Eric Berne and emphasizes the here-and-now interactions among group members; behavioral group therapy, which relies on conditioning techniques based on learning theory; Gestalt group therapy, which was created from the theories of Frederick Perls and enables patients to abreact and express themselves fully; and client-centered group psychotherapy, which was developed by Carl Rogers and is based on the nonjudgmental expression of feelings among group members. Table 35.3–2 outlines the major group psychotherapy approaches.

Table 35.3–1
Group Therapies

Goal	Alleviation of symptoms
	Change interpersonal relations
	Alter specific family–couple dynamics
Selection	Varies greatly based on type of group
	Homogeneous groups target specific disorders
	Adolescents and patients with personality disorders may especially benefit
	Families and couples where the system needs change
	Contraindications: substantial suicide risk, sadomasochistic acting out in family or couple
Types	Directive-supportive group psychotherapy
	Psychodynamic-interpersonal group psychotherapy
	Psychoanalytic group psychotherapy
	Family therapy
	Couples therapy
Duration	Weeks to years; time limited and open-ended

Reprinted with permission from Stoudemire A. *Clinical Psychiatry for Medical Students.* Philadelphia: JB Lippincott; 1990:449.

Patient Selection

To determine a patient's suitability for group psychotherapy, a therapist needs a great deal of information, which is gathered in a screening interview. The psychiatrist should take a psychiatric history and perform a mental status examination to obtain certain dynamic, behavioral, and diagnostic information. Table 35.3–3 outlines the general criteria for the selection of patients for group therapy.

Authority Anxiety. Those patients whose primary problem is their relationship to authority and who are extremely anxious in the presence of authority figures may do well in group therapy because they are more comfortable in a group. But they are more likely to do better in a group than in a dyadic (one-to-one) setting. Patients with a great deal of authority anxiety may be blocked, anxious, resistant, and unwilling to verbalize thoughts and feelings in an individual setting, generally for fear of the therapist's censure or disapproval. Thus, they may welcome the suggestion of group psychotherapy to avoid the scrutiny of the dyadic situation. Conversely, if a patient reacts negatively to the suggestion of group psychotherapy or openly resists the idea, the therapist should consider the possibility that the patient has high peer anxiety.

Ms. B. was referred to group treatment after her fifth serious suicide attempt; each of which had occurred during the absence of her individual therapist. She came to the group most reluctantly, fearful that she was going to be dropped off in the group and abandoned. She viewed the group leader with much distrust but found three members of the group who could empathize with her plight and who had also suffered similar self-destructive incidents and could help her move away from taking action. Her presence in the group was stormy and embattled for years, but eventually she became a strong proponent of group treatment. Notably, she was never hospitalized after joining the group. Finally, she concluded her individual work and remained in the group with the full agreement of both therapists. (Courtesy of Anne Alonso, Ph.D.)

Peer Anxiety. Patients with conditions such as borderline and schizoid personality disorders who have destructive relationships with their peer groups or who have been extremely isolated from peer group contact generally react negatively or anxiously when placed in a group setting. When such patients

Table 35.3–2
Comparison of Types of Group Psychotherapy

Parameters	Supportive Group Therapy	Analytically Oriented Group Therapy	Psychoanalysis of Groups	Transactional Group Therapy	Behavioral Group Therapy
Frequency	Once a week	1–3 times a week	1–5 times a week	1–3 times a week	1–3 times a week
Duration	Up to 6 months	1–3+ years	1–3+ years	1–3 years	Up to 6 months
Primary indications	Psychotic and anxiety disorders	Anxiety disorders, borderline states, personality disorders	Anxiety disorders, personality disorders	Anxiety and psychotic disorders	Phobias, passivity, sexual problems
Individual screening interview	Usually	Always	Always	Usually	Usually
Communication content	Primarily environmental factors	Present and past life situations, intragroup and extragroup relationships	Primarily past life experiences, intragroup relationships	Primarily intragroup relationships; rarely, history; here and now stressed	Specific symptoms without focus on causality
Transference	Positive transference encouraged to promote improved functioning	Positive and negative transference evoked and analyzed	Transference neurosis evoked and analyzed	Positive relationships fostered, negative feelings analyzed	Positive relationships fostered, no examination of transference
Dreams	Not analyzed	Analyzed frequently	Always analyzed and encouraged	Analyzed rarely	Not used
Dependence	Intragroup dependence encouraged; members rely on leader to great extent	Intragroup dependence encouraged; dependence on leader variable	Intragroup dependence not encouraged; dependence on leader variable	Intragroup dependence encouraged; dependence on leader not encouraged	Intragroup dependence not encouraged; reliance on leader is high
Therapist activity	Strengthen existing defenses, active, give advice	Challenge defenses, active, give advice or personal response	Challenge defenses, passive, give no advice or personal response	Challenge defenses, active, give personal response, rather than advice	Create new defenses, active and directive
Interpretation	No interpretation of unconscious conflict	Interpretation of unconscious conflict	Interpretation of unconscious conflict extensive	Interpretation of current behavioral patterns in the here and now	Not used
Major group processes	Universalization, reality testing	Cohesion, transference, reality testing	Transference, ventilation, catharsis, reality testing	Abreaction, reality testing	Cohesion, reinforcement, conditioning
Socialization outside of group	Encouraged	Generally discouraged	Discouraged	Variable	Discouraged
Goals	Improved adaptation to environment	Moderate reconstruction of personality dynamics	Extensive reconstruction of personality dynamics	Alteration of behavior through mechanism of conscious control	Relief of specific psychiatric symptoms

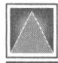

Table 35.3–3
General Membership Criteria for Group Therapy

Inclusion criteria
- Ability to perform the group task
- Problem areas compatible with goals of group
- Motivation to change

Exclusion criteria
- Marked incompatibility with group norms for acceptable behavior
- Inability to tolerate group setting
- Severe incompatibility with one or more of the other members
- Tendency to assume deviant role

Reprinted with permission from Vinogradov S, Yalom ID. Group therapy. In: Talbott JA, Hales RE, Yudofsky SC, eds. *The American Psychiatric Press Textbook of Psychiatry.* Washington, DC: American Psychiatric Press; 1988:956.

can work through their anxiety, however, group therapy can be beneficial.

Diagnosis. The diagnosis of patients' disorders is important in determining the best therapeutic approach and in evaluating patients' motivations for treatment, capacities for change, and personality structure strengths and weaknesses. There are few contraindications to group therapy. Antisocial patients generally do poorly in a heterogeneous group setting because they cannot adhere to group standards; but if the group is composed of other antisocial patients, they may respond better to peers than to perceived authority figures. Depressed patients profit from group therapy after they have established a trusting relationship with the therapist. Patients who are actively suicidal or severely depressed should not be treated solely in a group set-

Table 35.3–4
Therapist's Basic Tasks in Group Therapy

1. Decision to establish a therapy group:
   - Determine setting and size of the group
   - Choose frequency and length of group sessions
   - Decide on open versus closed group
   - Select a cotherapist for the group
   - Formulate policy on group therapy with other therapeutic modalities
2. Act of creating a therapy group:
   - Formulate appropriate goals
   - Select patients who can perform the group task
   - Prepare patients for group therapy
3. Construction and maintenance of a therapeutic environment:
   - Build the culture of the group explicitly and implicitly identify and resolve common problems (membership turnover, subgrouping, conflict)

Reprinted with permission from Vinogradov S, Yalom ID. Group therapy. In: Talbott JA, Hales RE, Yudofsky SC, eds. *The American Psychiatric Press Textbook of Psychiatry.* Washington, DC: American Psychiatric Press; 1988:964.

ting. Manic patients are disruptive but, once under pharmacological control, do well in the group setting. Patients who are delusional and who may incorporate the group into their delusional system should be excluded, as should patients who pose a physical threat to other members because of uncontrollable aggressive outbursts.

Preparation

Patients prepared by a therapist for a group experience tend to continue in treatment longer and report less initial anxiety than those who are not prepared. The preparation consists of having a therapist explain the procedure in as much detail as possible and answer the patient's questions before the first session.

Structural Organization

Table 35.3–4 summarizes some of the critical tasks that a group therapist must face when organizing a group.

Size. Group therapy has been successful with as few as 3 members and as many as 15, but most therapists consider 8 to 10 members the optimal size. There may be insufficient interaction with fewer members unless they are especially verbal, and with more than 10 members, the interaction may be too great for the members or the therapist to follow.

Frequency and Length of Sessions. Most group psychotherapists conduct group sessions once a week. Maintaining continuity in sessions is important. When there are alternate sessions, the group meets twice a week, once with and once without the therapist. Group sessions generally last anywhere from 1 to 2 hours, but the time limit should be constant.

Marathon groups were most popular in the 1970s but are much less common today. In time-extended therapy (marathon group therapy), the group meets continuously for 12 to 72 hours. Enforced interactional proximity and, during the longest time-extended sessions, sleep deprivation break down certain ego defenses, release affective processes, and theoretically promote open communication. Time-extended sessions, however, can be dangerous for patients with weak ego structures, such as persons with schizophrenia or borderline personality disorder.

Homogeneous versus Heterogeneous Groups. Most therapists believe that groups should be as heterogeneous as possible to ensure maximum interaction. Members with different diagnostic categories and varied behavioral patterns; from all races, social levels, and educational backgrounds; and of varying ages and both sexes should be brought together. Patients between ages 20 and 65 can be included effectively in the same group. Age differences help in developing parent–child and brother–sister models, and patients have the opportunity to relive and rectify interpersonal difficulties that may have appeared insurmountable.

Both children and adolescents are best treated in groups composed mostly of persons in their own age groups. Some adolescent patients are capable of assimilating the material of an adult group, regardless of content, but they should not be deprived of a constructive peer experience that they might otherwise not have.

Open versus Closed Groups. Closed groups have a set number and composition of patients. If members leave, no new members are accepted. In open groups membership is more fluid, and new members are taken on whenever old members leave.

Mechanisms

Group Formation. Each patient approaches group therapy differently, and in this sense groups are microcosms. Patients use typical adaptive abilities, defense mechanisms, and ways of relating, and when these tactics are ultimately reflected back to them by the group, they learn to be introspective about their personality functioning. A process inherent in group formation requires that patients suspend their previous ways of coping. In entering the group, they allow their executive ego functions—reality testing, adaptation to and mastery of the environment, and perception—to be assumed to some degree by the collective assessment provided by the total membership, including the leader.

Therapeutic Factors. Table 35.3–5 outlines 20 significant therapeutic factors that account for change in group psychotherapy. Table 35.3–6 summarizes the forces that shape learning and change secondary to the nature of the group as a social microcosm.

Role of the Therapist

Although opinions differ about how active or passive a group therapist should be, the consensus is that the therapist's role is primarily facilitative. Ideally, the group members themselves are the primary source of cure and change. The climate produced by the therapist's personality is a potent agent of change. The therapist is more than an expert applying techniques; he or

Table 35.3–5
Twenty Therapeutic Factors in Group Psychotherapy

Factor	Definition
Abreaction	A process by which repressed material, particularly a painful experience or conflict, is brought back to consciousness. In the process, the person not only recalls but relives the material, which is accompanied by the appropriate emotional response; insight usually results from the experience.
Acceptance	The feeling of being accepted by other members of the group; differences of opinion are tolerated, and there is an absence of censure.
Altruism	The act of one member helping another; putting another person's need before one's own and learning that there is value in giving to others. The term was originated by Auguste Comte (1798–1857), and Sigmund Freud believed it was a major factor in establishing group cohesion and community feeling.
Catharsis	The expression of ideas, thoughts, and suppressed material that is accompanied by an emotional response that produces a state of relief in the patient.
Cohesion	The sense that the group is working together toward a common goal; also referred to as a sense of "we-ness"; believed to be the most important factor related to positive therapeutic effects.
Consensual validation	Confirmation of reality by comparing one's own conceptualizations with those of other group members; interpersonal distortions are thereby corrected. The term was introduced by Harry Stack Sullivan; Trigant Burrow had used the phrase "consensual observation" to refer to the same phenomenon.
Contagion	The process in which the expression of emotion by one member stimulates the awareness of a similar emotion in another member.
Corrective familial experience	The group re-creates the family of origin for some members who can work through original conflicts psychologically through group interaction (e.g., sibling rivalry, anger toward parents).
Empathy	The capacity of a group member to put himself or herself into the psychological frame of reference of another group member and thereby understand his or her thinking, feeling, or behavior.
Identification	An unconscious defense mechanism in which the person incorporates the characteristics and the qualities of another person or object into his or her ego system.
Imitation	The conscious emulation or modeling of one's behavior after that of another (also called *role modeling*); also known as spectator therapy, as one patient learns from another.
Insight	Conscious awareness and understanding of one's own psychodynamics and symptoms of maladaptive behavior. Most therapists distinguish two types: (1) intellectual insight—knowledge and awareness without any changes in maladaptive behavior; (2) emotional insight—awareness and understanding leading to positive changes in personality and behavior.
Inspiration	The process of imparting a sense of optimism to group members; the ability to recognize that one has the capacity to overcome problems; also known as instillation of hope.
Interaction	The free and open exchange of ideas and feelings among group members; effective interaction is emotionally charged.
Interpretation	The process during which the group leader formulates the meaning or significance of a patient's resistance, defenses, and symbols; the result is that the patient has a cognitive framework within which to understand his or her behavior.
Learning	Patients acquire knowledge about new areas, such as social skills and sexual behavior; they receive advice, obtain guidance, and attempt to influence and are influenced by other group members.
Reality testing	Ability of the person to evaluate objectively the world outside the self; includes the capacity to perceive oneself and other group members accurately. *See also* Consensual validation.
Transference	Projection of feelings, thoughts, and wishes onto the therapist, who has come to represent an object from the patient's past. Such reactions, while perhaps appropriate for the condition prevailing in the patient's earlier life, are inappropriate and anachronistic when applied to the therapist in the present. Patients in the group may also direct such feelings toward one another, a process called *multiple transferences*.
Universalization	The awareness of the patient that he or she is not alone in having problems; others share similar complaints or difficulties in learning; the patient is not unique.
Ventilation	The expression of suppressed feelings, ideas, or events to other group members; the sharing of personal secrets that ameliorate a sense of sin or guilt (also referred to as *self-disclosure*).

she exerts a personal influence that taps such variables as empathy, warmth, and respect.

Inpatient Group Psychotherapy

Group therapy is an important part of hospitalized patients' therapeutic experiences. Groups may be organized in many ways on a ward. In a community meeting, an entire inpatient unit meets with all the staff members (e.g., psychiatrists, psychologists, and nurses). In team meetings, 15 to 20 patients and staff members meet; a regular or small group composed of 8 to 10 patients may meet with one or two therapists, as in traditional group therapy. Although the goals of each group vary, they all have common purposes: to increase patients' awareness of themselves through their interactions with the other group members, who provide feedback about their behavior; to provide patients with improved interpersonal and social skills; to help the members adapt to an inpatient setting; and to improve communication between patients and staff. In addition, one type of group meeting is attended only by inpatient hospital

Table 35.3–6
Learning from Behavioral Patterns in the Social Microcosm of the Therapy Group

Display of interpersonal pathology
↓
Feedback and self-observation
↓
Sharing reactions
↓
Examining the results of sharing reactions
↓
Understanding one's opinion of self
↓
Developing a sense of responsibility
↓
Realizing one's power to effect change
↓
High affect potentiates change

Reprinted with permission from Vinogradov S, Yalom ID. Group therapy. In: Talbott JA, Hales RE, Yudofsky SC, eds. *The American Psychiatric Press Textbook of Psychiatry.* Washington, DC: American Psychiatric Press; 1988:982.

staff and is meant to improve communication among the staff members and to provide mutual support and encouragement in their day-to-day work with patients. Community meetings and team meetings are more helpful for dealing with patient treatment problems than they are for providing insight-oriented therapy, which is the province of the small-group therapy meeting. Tables 35.3–7 and 35.3–8 summarize the goals and techniques for short-term inpatient therapy groups.

Group Composition. Two key factors of inpatient groups common to all short-term therapies are the heterogeneity of the members and the rapid turnover of patients. Outside the hospital, therapists have large caseloads from which to select patients for group therapy. On the ward, therapists have a limited number of patients to choose from and are further restricted to those patients who are both willing to participate and suitable for a small-group experience. In certain settings, group participation may be mandatory (e.g., in substance abuse and alcohol dependence units), but mandatory attendance does not usually apply in a general psychiatry unit. In fact, most group experiences are more productive when the patients themselves choose to enter them.

Table 35.3–7
Goals for Short-Term Inpatient Therapy Groups

Engaging patients in the therapeutic process
Teaching patients that talking helps
Problem spotting
Decreasing isolation
Allowing patients to be helpful
Alleviating hospital-related anxiety

Reprinted with permission from Vinogradov S, Yalom ID. Group therapy. In: Talbott JA, Hales RE, Yudofsky SC, eds. *The American Psychiatric Press Textbook of Psychiatry.* Washington, DC: American Psychiatric Press; 1988:980.

Table 35.3–8
Techniques for Short-Term Inpatient Therapy Groups

Use a shortened time frame.
Show direct support.
Emphasize the here and now.
Provide structure.

Reprinted with permission from Vinogradov S, Yalom ID. Group therapy. In: Talbott JA, Hales RE, Yudofsky SC, eds. *The American Psychiatric Press Textbook of Psychiatry.* Washington, DC: American Psychiatric Press; 1988:981.

More sessions are preferable to fewer. During patients' hospital stays, groups may meet daily to allow interactional continuity and the carryover of themes from one session to the next. A new member of a group can be brought up-to-date quickly, either by the therapist in an orientation meeting or by one of the members. A newly admitted patient has often learned many details about the small-group program from another patient before actually attending the first session. The less frequently the group sessions are held, the greater the need for a therapist to structure the group and be active in it.

Inpatient versus Outpatient Groups. Although the therapeutic factors that account for change in small inpatient groups are similar to those in the outpatient settings, there are qualitative differences. For example, the relatively high turnover of patients in inpatient groups complicates the process of cohesion. But the fact that all the group members are together in the hospital aids cohesion, as do the therapists' efforts to foster the process. Sharing of information, universalization, and catharsis are the main therapeutic factors at work in inpatient groups. Although insight is more likely to occur in outpatient groups because of their long-term nature, some patients can obtain a new understanding of their psychological makeup within the confines of a single group session. A unique quality of inpatient groups is the patients' extragroup contacts, which are extensive because they live together on the same ward. Verbalizing their thoughts and feelings about such contacts in the therapy sessions encourages interpersonal learning. In addition, conflicts between patients or between patients and staff members can be anticipated and resolved. Table 35.3–9 lists the differences between inpatient and outpatient groups.

Self-Help Groups

Self-help groups are composed of persons who are trying to cope with a specific problem or life crisis and are usually organized with a particular task in mind. Such groups do not attempt to explore individual psychodynamics in great depth or to change personality functioning significantly, but self-help groups have improved the emotional health and well-being of many persons.

A distinguishing characteristic of the self-help groups is their homogeneity. The members have the same disorders and share their experiences—good and bad, successful and unsuccessful—with one another. By so doing, they educate each other, provide mutual support, and alleviate the sense of alienation usually felt by persons drawn to this kind of group.

Self-help groups emphasize cohesion, which is exceptionally strong in these groups. Because the group members have

Table 35.4–2
Criteria for Treatment Termination

Treatment is completed:
- When family members can complete transactions, check, ask.
- When they can interpret hostility.
- When they can see how others see them.
- When they can see how they see themselves.
- When one member can tell others how they manifest themselves.
- When one member can tell others what is hoped, feared, and expected from them.
- When they can disagree.
- When they can make choices.
- When they can learn through practice.
- When they can free themselves from the harmful effects of past models.
- When they can give clear message—that is, be congruent in their behavior—with a minimum of difference between feelings and communication and with a minimum of hidden messages.

Adapted from Satir V. *Conjoint Family Therapy.* Palo Alto, CA: Science and Behavior; 1967:133.

member fills each role may change. Some families try to scapegoat one member by blaming him or her for the family's problems (the identified patient). If the identified patient improves, another family member may become the scapegoat. The family is defined as having external boundaries and internal rules. The general systems model overlaps with some of the other models presented, particularly the Bowen and structural models.

Modifications of Techniques

Family Group Therapy. Family group therapy combines several families into a single group. Families share mutual problems and compare their interactions with those of the other families in the group. Treatment of schizophrenia has been effective in multiple family groups. Parents of disturbed children may also meet together to share their situations.

Social Network Therapy. In social network therapy, the social community or network of a disturbed patient meets in group sessions with the patient. The network includes those

Table 35.4–3
Major Approaches to Family and Couple Therapy

Therapeutic Approach Examples	Core Concepts	Typical Goals	Common Strategies and Techniques	Comments
Behavioral/cognitive-behavioral (James Alexander, Neil Jacobson, Howard Markman, Gerald Patterson)	Functional analysis Social learning theory Communication and problem-solving Attributional style	Resolution of presenting problem Enhanced communication and problem-solving skills Balance between change and acceptance	Communication and problem-solving training Acceptance training/reattribution techniques Parent management, emphasis on behavior or consequences Therapist as educator	Functional analysis, not treatment techniques, is defining characteristic Arguably the most empirically supported of all family and couple methods
Bowen family systems (Murray Bowen, Edwin Friedman, Philip Guerin, Michael Kerr)	Differentiation of self Triangulation Emotional cutoffs Family emotional system Sibling position	Increased differentiation Detriangulation Cutoffs resolved Improved ability to manage anxiety	Use of genogram Therapist as coach Education about multigenerational family processes	Often conducted with only a single patient Influence continues but has waned since Bowen's death
Experimental-humanistic (Leslie Greenberg and Susan Johnson, Augustus Napier, Virginia Satir, Carl Whitaker)	Communication styles (e.g., placater-blamer) Psychotherapy of the absurd Attachment theory	Fostering creativity (comfort with "craziness") Increased family cohesion Personal growth, self-esteem Tolerance for conflict	Resolving the battle for structure and initiative Frequent use of cotherapists Family sculpture Use of self Family reconstruction	Since Whitaker's death, symbolic-experiential approach receding in visibility Greenberg and Johnson's emotionally focused therapy one of few nonbehavioral or psychodynamic couple methods increasing in influence
Integrative (Alan Gurman, William Pinsof)	Importance of and relationships among multiple levels of experience Theoretical and technical electicism	Improved communication and problem-solving Enhanced interactional insight Presenting problems	Combinations of cognitive-behavioral and psychodynamic methods, in general systems context	Along with behavioral and psychoeducational methods, the most sensitive to research findings Attempts to match interventions to problem and family
Mental Research Institute brief therapy (Don Jackson, John Weakland, Paul Watzlawick)	Distinction between "difficulties" and "problems" Communication processes Symptom as communication First- and second-order change	Resolution of presenting problem Second-order change	Reframing Therapist maneuverability	Historically overlaps strategic, but with important differences (e.g., "function" of symptoms)

(*continued*)

Table 35.4–1
Rationale for Family-Life Chronology

- The family therapist enters a session knowing little or nothing about the family.
  - The therapist may know who the identified patient is and what symptoms the patient manifests, but that is usually all. So the therapist must get clues about the meaning of the symptom.
  - The therapist may know that pain exists in the marital relationship but needs to get clues about how the pain shows itself.
  - The therapist needs to know how the mates have tried to cope with their problems.
  - The therapist may know that the mates both operate from models (from what they saw going on between their own parents) but needs to find out how those models have influenced each mate's expectations about how to be a mate and how to be a parent.
- The family therapist enters a session knowing that the family has, in fact, had a history, but that is usually all.
  - Every family, as a group, has gone through or jointly experienced many events. Certain events (such as deaths, childbirth, sickness, geographical moves, and job changes) occur in almost all families.
  - Certain events primarily affected the mates and only indirectly the children. (Maybe the children were not born yet or were too young to fully comprehend the nature of an event as it affected their parents. They may have only sensed periods of parental remoteness, distraction, anxiety, or annoyance.)
  - The therapist can profit from answers to just about every question asked.
- Family members enter therapy with a great deal of fear.
  - Therapist structuring helps decrease the threats. It says: "I am in charge of what will happen here. I will see to it that nothing catastrophic happens here."
  - All members are covertly feeling to blame for the fact that nothing seems to have turned out right (even though they may overtly blame the identified patient or the other mate).
  - Parents, especially, need to feel that they did the best they could as parents. They need to tell the therapist: "This is why I did what I did. This is what happened to me."
  - A family-life chronology that deals with such facts as names, dates, labeled relationships, and moves seems to appeal to the family. It asks questions that members can answer, questions that are relatively nonthreatening. It deals with life as the family understands it.
- Family members enter therapy with a great deal of despair.
  - Therapist structuring helps stimulate hope.
  - As far as family members are concerned, past events are part of them. They now can tell the therapist, "I existed." And they can also say: "I am not just a big blob of pathology. I succeeded in overcoming many handicaps."
  - If the family knew what questions needed asking, they would not need to be in therapy. So the therapist does not say, "Tell me what you want to tell me." Family members will simply tell the therapist what they have been telling themselves for years. The therapist's questions say: "I know what to ask. I take responsibility for understanding you. We are going to go somewhere."
- The family therapist also knows that, to some degree, the family has focused on the identified patient to relieve marital pain. The therapist also knows that, to some degree, the family will resist any effort to change that focus. A family-life chronology is an effective, nonthreatening way to change from an emphasis on the "sick" or "bad" family member to an emphasis on the marital relationship.
- The family-life chronology serves other useful therapy purposes, such as providing the framework within which a reeducation process can take place. The therapist serves as a model in checking out information or correcting communication techniques and placing questions and eliciting answers to begin the process. In addition, when taking the chronology, the therapist can introduce in a relatively nonfrightening way some of the crucial concepts to induce change.

Adapted from Satir V. *Conjoint Family Therapy.* Palo Alto, CA: Science and Behavior; 1967:57.

their enmeshment versus the degree of their ability to differentiate and the analysis of emotional triangles in the problem for which they seek help.

An emotional triangle is defined as a three-party system (and there can be many of these within a family) arranged so that the closeness of two members expressed as either love or repetitive conflict tends to exclude a third. When the excluded third person attempts to join with one of the other two or when one of the involved parties shifts in the direction of the excluded one, emotional cross-currents are activated. The therapist's role is, first, to stabilize or shift the "hot" triangle—the one producing the presenting symptoms—and, second, to work with the most psychologically available family members, individually if necessary, to achieve enough personal differentiation so that the hot triangle does not recur. To preserve his or her neutrality in the family's triangles, the therapist minimizes emotional contact with family members.

Bowen also originated the *genogram,* a theoretical tool that is a historical survey of the family, going back several generations.

Structural Model. In a structural model, families are viewed as single, interrelated systems assessed in terms of significant alliances and splits among family members, hierarchy of power (parents in charge of children), clarity and firmness of boundaries between the generations, and family tolerance for each other. The structural model uses concurrent individual and family therapy.

General Systems Model. Based on general systems theory, a general systems model holds that families are systems and that every action in a family produces a reaction in one or more of its members. Families have external boundaries and internal rules. Every member is presumed to play a role (e.g., spokesperson, persecutor, victim, rescuer, symptom bearer, nurturer), which is relatively stable, but which

Table 35.4–2
Criteria for Treatment Termination

Treatment is completed:
- When family members can complete transactions, check, ask.
- When they can interpret hostility.
- When they can see how others see them.
- When they can see how they see themselves.
- When one member can tell others how they manifest themselves.
- When one member can tell others what is hoped, feared, and expected from them.
- When they can disagree.
- When they can make choices.
- When they can learn through practice.
- When they can free themselves from the harmful effects of past models.
- When they can give clear message—that is, be congruent in their behavior—with a minimum of difference between feelings and communication and with a minimum of hidden messages.

Adapted from Satir V. *Conjoint Family Therapy.* Palo Alto, CA: Science and Behavior; 1967:133.

member fills each role may change. Some families try to scapegoat one member by blaming him or her for the family's problems (the identified patient). If the identified patient improves, another family member may become the scapegoat. The family is defined as having external boundaries and internal rules. The general systems model overlaps with some of the other models presented, particularly the Bowen and structural models.

Modifications of Techniques

Family Group Therapy. Family group therapy combines several families into a single group. Families share mutual problems and compare their interactions with those of the other families in the group. Treatment of schizophrenia has been effective in multiple family groups. Parents of disturbed children may also meet together to share their situations.

Social Network Therapy. In social network therapy, the social community or network of a disturbed patient meets in group sessions with the patient. The network includes those

Table 35.4–3
Major Approaches to Family and Couple Therapy

Therapeutic Approach Examples	Core Concepts	Typical Goals	Common Strategies and Techniques	Comments
Behavioral/cognitive-behavioral (James Alexander, Neil Jacobson, Howard Markman, Gerald Patterson)	Functional analysis Social learning theory Communication and problem-solving Attributional style	Resolution of presenting problem Enhanced communication and problem-solving skills Balance between change and acceptance	Communication and problem-solving training Acceptance training/reattribution techniques Parent management, emphasis on behavior or consequences Therapist as educator	Functional analysis, not treatment techniques, is defining characteristic Arguably the most empirically supported of all family and couple methods
Bowen family systems (Murray Bowen, Edwin Friedman, Philip Guerin, Michael Kerr)	Differentiation of self Triangulation Emotional cutoffs Family emotional system Sibling position	Increased differentiation Detriangulation Cutoffs resolved Improved ability to manage anxiety	Use of genogram Therapist as coach Education about multigenerational family processes	Often conducted with only a single patient Influence continues but has waned since Bowen's death
Experimental-humanistic (Leslie Greenberg and Susan Johnson, Augustus Napier, Virginia Satir, Carl Whitaker)	Communication styles (e.g., placater-blamer) Psychotherapy of the absurd Attachment theory	Fostering creativity (comfort with "craziness") Increased family cohesion Personal growth, self-esteem Tolerance for conflict	Resolving the battle for structure and initiative Frequent use of cotherapists Family sculpture Use of self Family reconstruction	Since Whitaker's death, symbolic-experiential approach receding in visibility Greenberg and Johnson's emotionally focused therapy one of few nonbehavioral or psychodynamic couple methods increasing in influence
Integrative (Alan Gurman, William Pinsof)	Importance of and relationships among multiple levels of experience Theoretical and technical electicism	Improved communication and problem-solving Enhanced interactional insight Presenting problems	Combinations of cognitive-behavioral and psychodynamic methods, in general systems context	Along with behavioral and psychoeducational methods, the most sensitive to research findings Attempts to match interventions to problem and family
Mental Research Institute brief therapy (Don Jackson, John Weakland, Paul Watzlawick)	Distinction between "difficulties" and "problems" Communication processes Symptom as communication First- and second-order change	Resolution of presenting problem Second-order change	Reframing Therapist maneuverability	Historically overlaps strategic, but with important differences (e.g., "function" of symptoms)

(*continued*)

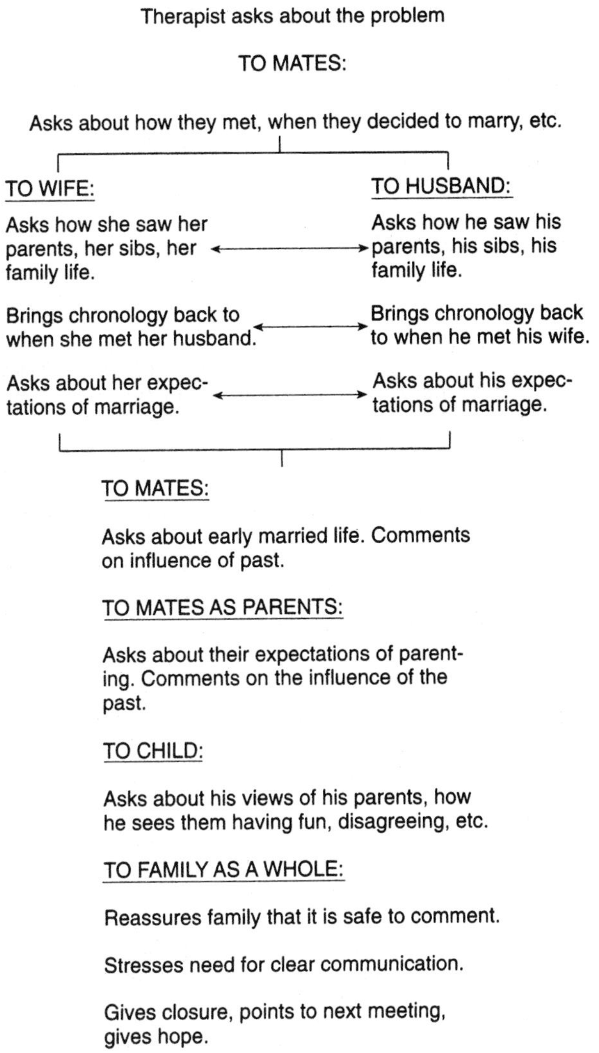
Therapist asks about the problem
TO MATES:
Asks about how they met, when they decided to marry, etc.
TO WIFE:
Asks how she saw her parents, her sibs, her family life.
TO HUSBAND:
Asks how he saw his parents, his sibs, his family life.
Brings chronology back to when she met her husband.
Brings chronology back to when he met his wife.
Asks about her expectations of marriage.
Asks about his expectations of marriage.
TO MATES:
Asks about early married life. Comments on influence of past.
TO MATES AS PARENTS:
Asks about their expectations of parenting. Comments on the influence of the past.
TO CHILD:
Asks about his views of his parents, how he sees them having fun, disagreeing, etc.
TO FAMILY AS A WHOLE:
Reassures family that it is safe to comment.
Stresses need for clear communication.
Gives closure, points to next meeting, gives hope.

FIGURE 35.4–1
Main flow of family-life chronology to family as a whole. (Reproduced with permission from Satir V. *Conjoint Family Therapy.* Palo Alto, CA: Science and Behavior; 1967:55.)

child's misbehavior will have a negative influence on siblings. Refusal by an adolescent or young adult patient to participate in family therapy is frequently a disguised collusion with the fears of one or both parents.

Interview Technique. The special quality of a family interview springs from two important facts. A family comes to treatment with its history and dynamics firmly in place. To a family therapist, the established nature of the group, more than the symptoms, constitutes the clinical problem. Family members usually live together and, at some level, depend on one another for their physical and emotional well-being. Whatever transpires in the therapy session is known to all. Central principles of technique also derive from these facts. For example, the therapist must carefully channel the catharsis of anger by one family member toward another. The person who is the object of the anger will react to the attack, and the anger may escalate into violence and fracture relationships, with one or more member withdrawing from therapy. For another example, free association is inappropriate in family therapy because it can encourage one person to dominate a session. Thus therapists must always control and direct the family interview.

Virginia Satir recommended initiating at least the first two sessions of family therapy with a family-life chronology. The technique reflects many family therapy paradigms. Figure 35.4–1 summarizes the key features of the family-life chronology, and Table 35.4–1 summarizes Satir's reasoning behind its use.

Frequency and Length of Treatment. Unless an emergency arises, sessions are usually held no more than once a week. Each session, however, may require as much as 2 hours. Long sessions can include an intermission to give the therapist time to organize the material and plan a response. A flexible schedule is necessary when geography or personal circumstances make it physically difficult for the family to get together. The length of treatment depends not only on the nature of the problem but also on the therapeutic model. Therapists who use problem-solving models exclusively may accomplish their goals in a few sessions, while therapists using growth-oriented models may work with a family for years and may schedule sessions at long intervals. Table 35.4–2 summarizes one model for treatment termination.

Models of Intervention

Many models of family therapy exist, none of which is superior to the others. An overview of family therapy models, techniques, and goals appears in Table 35.4–3. The particular model used depends on the training received, the context in which therapy occurs, and the personality of the therapist.

Psychodynamic-Experiential Models. Psychodynamic-experiential models emphasize individual maturation in the context of the family system and are free from unconscious patterns of anxiety and projection rooted in the past. Therapists seek to establish an intimate bond with each family member, and sessions alternate between the therapist's exchanges with the members and the members' exchanges with one another. Clarity of communication and honestly admitted feelings are given high priority. Toward this end, family members may be encouraged to change their seats, to touch each other, and to make direct eye contact. Their use of metaphor, body language, and parapraxes helps reveal the unconscious pattern of family relationships. The therapist may also use *family sculpting,* in which family members physically arrange one another in tableaus depicting their personal view of relationships, past or present. The therapist both interprets the living sculpture and modifies it in a way to suggest new relationships. In addition, the therapist's subjective responses to the family are given great importance. At appropriate moments, the therapist expresses these responses to the family to form yet another feedback loop of self-observation and change.

Bowen Model. Murray Bowen called his model family systems, but in the family therapy field it rightfully carries the name of its originator. The hallmark of the Bowen model is persons' differentiation from their family of origin, their ability to be their true selves in the face of familial or other pressures that threaten the loss of love or social position. Problem families are assessed on two levels: the degree of

members of the group to be spontaneous. The director must also be available to meet the group's needs without superimposing his or her values. Of all the group psychotherapies, psychodrama requires the most participation from the therapist and the greatest ability to lead.

Protagonist. The protagonist is the patient in conflict. The patient chooses the situation to portray in the dramatic scene, or the therapist chooses it if the patient so desires.

Auxiliary Ego. An auxiliary ego is another group member who represents something or someone in the protagonist's experience. The auxiliary egos help account for the great range of therapeutic effects available in psychodrama.

Group. The members of the psychodrama and the audience make up the group. Some are participants, and others are observers, but all benefit from the experience to the extent that they can identify with the ongoing events. The concept of spontaneity in psychodrama refers to the ability of each member of the group, especially the protagonist, to experience the thoughts and feelings of the moment and to communicate emotion as authentically as possible.

Techniques

The psychodrama may focus on any special area of functioning (a dream, a family, or a community situation), a symbolic role, an unconscious attitude, or an imagined future situation. Such symptoms as delusions and hallucinations can also be acted out in the group. Techniques to advance the therapeutic process and to increase productivity and creativity include the soliloquy (a recital of overt and hidden thoughts and feelings), role reversal (the exchange of the patient's role for the role of a significant person), the double (an auxiliary ego acting as the patient), the multiple double (several egos acting as the patient did on varying occasions), and the mirror technique (an ego imitating the patient and speaking for him or her). Other techniques include the use of hypnosis and psychoactive drugs to modify the acting behavior in various ways.

References

Alonso A. Group psychotherapy In: Sadock BJ, Sadock VA, eds. *Kaplan & Sadock's Comprehensive Textbook of Psychiatry.* 7th ed. Vol 2. Baltimore: Lippincott Williams & Wilkins; 2000:2146.

Cameron PM, Leszcz M, Bebchuk W, et al. The practice and roles of the psychotherapies: a discussion paper. *Can J Psychiatry.* 1999;44(suppl):18.

Carlin ME. Large group treatment of severely disturbed/conduct-disordered adolescents. *Int J Group Psychother.* 1996;46:379.

Cartwright D, Zander A, eds. *Group Dynamics and Research Theory.* New York: Harper & Row; 1960.

Erickson RC. *Inpatient Small Group Psychotherapy.* Springfield, IL: Charles C Thomas; 1984.

Frank JD. Some determinants, manifestations, and effects of cohesiveness in therapy groups. *J Psychother Pract Res.* 1997;6:59.

Freud S. Group psychology and analysis of the ego. In: *Standard Edition of the Complete Psychological Works of Sigmund Freud.* Vol 18. London: Hogarth Press; 1962:67.

Kaplan HI, Sadock BJ, eds. *Comprehensive Group Psychotherapy.* 3rd ed. Baltimore: Williams & Wilkins; 1993.

Kipper DA, Matsumoto M. From classical to eclectic psychodrama: conceptual similarities between psychodrama and interpersonal group treatments. *Int J Group Psychother.* 2002;52:111.

Lieberman MA, Yalom I. Brief group psychotherapy for the spousally bereaved: a controlled study. *Int J Group Psychother.* 1992;42:117.

Moreno JL. *Psychodrama.* Beacon, NY: Beacon Press; 1947.

Rosenthal L. Phenomena of resistance in modern group analysis. *Am J Psychother.* 1996;50:75.

Rothbaum BO, Astin MC. Integration of pharmacotherapy and psychotherapy for bipolar disorder. *J Clin Psychiatry.* 2000;6(suppl 9):68.

Rutan JS. Psychodynamic group psychotherapy. *Int J Group Psychother.* 1992;42:19.

Scheidlinger S. The concept of identification in group psychotherapy. *Am J Psychother.* 1996;50:529.

Steengarger BN, Budman SH. Group psychotherapy and managed behavioral health care: current trends and future challenges. *Int J Group Psychother.* 1996;46:297.

Weiner MF. Group therapy reduces medical and psychiatric hospitalization. *Int J Group Psychother.* 1992;42:267.

Wolf A, Schwartz M. *Psychoanalysis in Groups.* New York: Grune & Stratton; 1962.

Wolk DJ. The psychodramatic reenactment of a dream. *J Group Psychother Psychodrama Sociometry.* 1996;49:3.

Yalom ID. *The Theory and Practice of Group Psychotherapy.* 3rd ed. New York: Basic Books; 1985.

▲ 35.4 Family Therapy and Couples Therapy

FAMILY THERAPY

Family therapy is any intervention that focuses on altering the interactions among family members and attempts to improve the functioning of the family as a unit of individual members of the family. The clinician conducting family therapy attempts to interrupt rigid intergenerational patterns that cause distress within or between individuals. Family therapy can address the concerns of any family member, yet it is most likely to influence children, whose daily reality is directly affected by family context.

Theoretical Issues

According to family systems theory, family units act as though each has its own homeostasis of interacting that must be maintained at any cost. Family therapy aims to bring to light the often hidden patterns that maintain the group's balance and to help the group understand the purposes of the pattern. Family therapists generally think that one family member has been labeled the patient, whom the family identifies as "the one who is the problem, is to blame, and needs help." A family therapist's goal is to help a family understand that the identified patient's symptoms in fact serve the crucial function of maintaining the family's homeostasis. The process of family therapy helps reveal a family's repetitious and ultimately predictable communication patterns that sustain and reflect the identified patient's behavior.

Inherent in family systems theory is the belief, to one degree or another, that a marital relationship strongly influences the family's system of homeostasis. One influential family therapist has expressed this concept by describing the marital dyad as the "architects of the family."

Techniques

Initial Consultation. Family therapy is familiar enough to the general public for families with a high level of conflict to request it specifically. When the initial complaint is about an individual family member, however, pretreatment work may be needed. Underlying resistance to a family approach typically includes fears by parents that they will be blamed for their child's difficulties, that the entire family will be pronounced sick, that a spouse will object, and that open discussion of one

Table 35.3–6
Learning from Behavioral Patterns in the Social Microcosm of the Therapy Group

Display of interpersonal pathology
↓
Feedback and self-observation
↓
Sharing reactions
↓
Examining the results of sharing reactions
↓
Understanding one's opinion of self
↓
Developing a sense of responsibility
↓
Realizing one's power to effect change
↓
High affect potentiates change

Reprinted with permission from Vinogradov S, Yalom ID. Group therapy. In: Talbott JA, Hales RE, Yudofsky SC, eds. *The American Psychiatric Press Textbook of Psychiatry.* Washington, DC: American Psychiatric Press; 1988:982.

staff and is meant to improve communication among the staff members and to provide mutual support and encouragement in their day-to-day work with patients. Community meetings and team meetings are more helpful for dealing with patient treatment problems than they are for providing insight-oriented therapy, which is the province of the small-group therapy meeting. Tables 35.3–7 and 35.3–8 summarize the goals and techniques for short-term inpatient therapy groups.

Group Composition. Two key factors of inpatient groups common to all short-term therapies are the heterogeneity of the members and the rapid turnover of patients. Outside the hospital, therapists have large caseloads from which to select patients for group therapy. On the ward, therapists have a limited number of patients to choose from and are further restricted to those patients who are both willing to participate and suitable for a small-group experience. In certain settings, group participation may be mandatory (e.g., in substance abuse and alcohol dependence units), but mandatory attendance does not usually apply in a general psychiatry unit. In fact, most group experiences are more productive when the patients themselves choose to enter them.

Table 35.3–7
Goals for Short-Term Inpatient Therapy Groups

Engaging patients in the therapeutic process
Teaching patients that talking helps
Problem spotting
Decreasing isolation
Allowing patients to be helpful
Alleviating hospital-related anxiety

Reprinted with permission from Vinogradov S, Yalom ID. Group therapy. In: Talbott JA, Hales RE, Yudofsky SC, eds. *The American Psychiatric Press Textbook of Psychiatry.* Washington, DC: American Psychiatric Press; 1988:980.

Table 35.3–8
Techniques for Short-Term Inpatient Therapy Groups

Use a shortened time frame.
Show direct support.
Emphasize the here and now.
Provide structure.

Reprinted with permission from Vinogradov S, Yalom ID. Group therapy. In: Talbott JA, Hales RE, Yudofsky SC, eds. *The American Psychiatric Press Textbook of Psychiatry.* Washington, DC: American Psychiatric Press; 1988:981.

More sessions are preferable to fewer. During patients' hospital stays, groups may meet daily to allow interactional continuity and the carryover of themes from one session to the next. A new member of a group can be brought up-to-date quickly, either by the therapist in an orientation meeting or by one of the members. A newly admitted patient has often learned many details about the small-group program from another patient before actually attending the first session. The less frequently the group sessions are held, the greater the need for a therapist to structure the group and be active in it.

Inpatient versus Outpatient Groups. Although the therapeutic factors that account for change in small inpatient groups are similar to those in the outpatient settings, there are qualitative differences. For example, the relatively high turnover of patients in inpatient groups complicates the process of cohesion. But the fact that all the group members are together in the hospital aids cohesion, as do the therapists' efforts to foster the process. Sharing of information, universalization, and catharsis are the main therapeutic factors at work in inpatient groups. Although insight is more likely to occur in outpatient groups because of their long-term nature, some patients can obtain a new understanding of their psychological makeup within the confines of a single group session. A unique quality of inpatient groups is the patients' extragroup contacts, which are extensive because they live together on the same ward. Verbalizing their thoughts and feelings about such contacts in the therapy sessions encourages interpersonal learning. In addition, conflicts between patients or between patients and staff members can be anticipated and resolved. Table 35.3–9 lists the differences between inpatient and outpatient groups.

Self-Help Groups

Self-help groups are composed of persons who are trying to cope with a specific problem or life crisis and are usually organized with a particular task in mind. Such groups do not attempt to explore individual psychodynamics in great depth or to change personality functioning significantly, but self-help groups have improved the emotional health and well-being of many persons.

A distinguishing characteristic of the self-help groups is their homogeneity. The members have the same disorders and share their experiences—good and bad, successful and unsuccessful—with one another. By so doing, they educate each other, provide mutual support, and alleviate the sense of alienation usually felt by persons drawn to this kind of group.

Self-help groups emphasize cohesion, which is exceptionally strong in these groups. Because the group members have

Table 35.3–9
Differences between Outpatient Groups and Inpatient Groups

Outpatient Groups	Inpatient Groups
Stable composition	Rarely the same group for more than one or two meetings
Patients well selected and prepared	Patients admitted to the group with little prior selection or preparation
Group is homogeneous regarding ego function, although conflicts and issues differ	Heterogeneous level of ego functioning
Motivated, self-referred patients; growth-oriented	Ambivalent, often compulsory patients in crisis; relief-oriented
Treatment proceeds as long as required; 1 to 2 years; 50 to 100 meetings	Treatment limited to the hospitalization period; 1 to 3 weeks, with rapid patient turnover
Boundary of group well maintained with few external influences	Continuous boundary interface with the milieu
Group cohesion develops normally, given sufficient time in treatment	No time for cohesion to develop spontaneously; group development aborted in early phases
Therapy is private and unexposed	Exposed, open to observation and scrutiny by the milieu
Leader allows the process to unfold; there is ample time to set group norms	Group leader's structuring of the group is critical; passive analytic approaches lead to group disintegration
No extra group contact encouraged	Patients sleep, eat, and live together outside the group; extragroup contact endorsed

Reprinted with permission from Leszcz M. Inpatient groups. *Annu Rev Psychiatry.* 1986;5:729.

similar problems and symptoms, they develop a strong emotional bond. Each group may have its unique characteristics, to which the members can attribute magical qualities of healing. Examples of self-help groups are Alcoholics Anonymous (AA), Gamblers Anonymous (GA), and Overeaters Anonymous (OA).

The self-help group movement is presently in ascendancy. These groups meet their members' needs by providing acceptance, mutual support, and help in overcoming maladaptive patterns of behavior or states of feeling that traditional mental health and medical professionals have not generally dealt with successfully. Self-help groups and therapy groups have begun to converge. Self-help groups have enabled their members to give up patterns of unwanted behavior; therapy groups have helped their members understand why and how they got to be the way they were or are.

COMBINED INDIVIDUAL AND GROUP PSYCHOTHERAPY

In combined individual and group psychotherapy, patients see a therapist individually and also take part in group sessions. The therapist for the group and individual sessions is usually the same person. Groups can vary in size from 3 to 15 members, but the most helpful size is 8 to 10. Patients must attend all group sessions. Attendance at individual sessions is also important, and failure to attend either group or individual sessions should be examined as part of the therapeutic process.

Combined therapy is a particular treatment modality, not a system by which individual therapy is augmented by an occasional group session or a group therapy in which a participant meets alone with a therapist from time to time. Rather, it is an ongoing plan in which the group experience interacts meaningfully with the individual sessions and in which reciprocal feedback helps form an integrated therapeutic experience. Although the one-to-one doctor–patient relationship makes a deep examination of the transference reaction possible for some patients, it may not provide other patients with the corrective emotional experiences necessary for therapeutic change. The group gives patients a variety of persons with whom they can have transferential reactions. In the microcosm of the group, patients can relive and work through familial and other important influences.

Techniques

Differing techniques based on varying theoretical frameworks have been used in the combined therapy format. Some clinicians increase the frequency of individual sessions to encourage the emergence of the transference neurosis. In the behavioral model, individual sessions are scheduled regularly, but they tend to be less frequent than in other approaches. Whether patients use a couch or a chair during individual sessions depends on a therapist's orientation. Techniques such as alternate meetings or "aftersessions" without the therapist present may be used. A combined therapy approach called *structured interactional group psychotherapy* has a different group member as the focus of each weekly group session who is discussed in depth by the other members.

Results

Most workers in the field believe that combined therapy has the advantages of both dyadic and group settings, without sacrificing the qualities of either. Generally, the dropout rate in combined therapy is lower than that in group therapy alone. In many cases, combined therapy appears to bring problems to the surface and to resolve them more quickly than might be possible with either method alone.

PSYCHODRAMA

Psychodrama is a method of group psychotherapy originated by the Viennese-born psychiatrist Jacob Moreno in which personality makeup, interpersonal relationships, conflicts, and emotional problems are explored by means of special dramatic methods. Therapeutic dramatization of emotional problems includes the protagonist or patient, the person who acts out problems with the help of auxiliary egos, persons who enact varying aspects of the patient, and the director, psychodramatist, or therapist, the person who guides those in the drama toward the acquisition of insight.

Roles

Director. The director is the leader or therapist and so must be an active participant. He or she has a catalytic function by encouraging the

Table 35.4–3 (*continued*)

Therapeutic Approach Examples	Core Concepts	Typical Goals	Common Strategies and Techniques	Comments
Milan systemic (Luigi Boscolo, Gianfranco Cecchin, Mora Selvini-Palazzoli)	Therapeutic neutrality "Dirty games" Counterparadox "Long brief therapy"	Unmasking the family "game" Change symptom-bearer's self-sacrificing role	Therapeutic team (behind mirror) Circular questioning Hypothesizing Invariant prescriptions Counterparadoxical interventions Prescribed rituals	After flurry of worldwide interest for more than a decade, growth of approach has slowed of late
Narrative (David Epston, Michael White)	Constructivism Languaging Stories socially created Problem-saturated descriptions	Resolution of presenting problem Enhancing undiscovered parts of self	Externalization of problems Focusing on "unique outcomes" Creation of new meaning via "restorying" Therapeutic letters	Currently very popular, but rarely acknowledges overlaps with cognitive and behavioral theory
Psychodynamic-psychoanalytic (Nathan Ackerman)	Object relations Projective identification Splitting Scapegoating	Improved insight Genetic (historical) awareness Enhanced empathy Deemphasize presenting problem Disentangle interlocking pathologies	Transference, resistance, and countertransference analysis Creation of holding environment Interpretation Emphasis on therapeutic alliance	Probably influences family therapists' clinical work more than is usually acknowledged
Psychoeducational (Carol Anderson, Jan Falloon, Michael Goldstein, William McFarlane)	Biopsychosocial theory Stress-diathesis Expressed emotion	Enhanced family coping skills Improved communication and problem-solving skills Relapse prevention	Survival skills workshops Family management Family information and education Concurrent use of psychopharmacology	Without doubt, the most effective family-based approach for families with a member with major psychiatric disorder
Solution-focused (Steve de Shazar and Insoo Berg, William O'Hanlon, Michele Weiner-Davis)	Focus on solutions, not problems Unimportance of problem etiology Disbelief in resistance	Resolution of presenting problem Creation of solutions	Scaling questions Miracle questions Exception questions Client empowerment Coping questions Questions about presession change	Grows out of basic Mental Research Institute philosophy, emphasizing solutions more than problems Has made extraordinary claims of effectiveness
Strategic (Milton Erickson, Jay Haley, Cloe Madanes)	Power and control Family life cycle Symptom-maintaining sequences Function of problems	Resolve presenting problem Disruption of problem-maintaining sequences	Persuasion Paradoxical injections Insight downplayed Pretend and ordeal techniques	Unfortunate deemphasis on biology, psychiatric diagnosis, and personality theory
Structural (Henry Aponte, Salvador Minuchin, Braulios Montalvo)	Boundaries Hierarchies Coalitions and alliances Complementarity Engagement-enmeshment	Increased flexibility Adaptability to developmental change Balance between connectedness and differentiation Subsystem functioning	Multidirected Family of origin sessions Use of cotherapy	Arguably the most influential family therapy approach
Transgenerational (Iran Boszormenyi-Nagy, James Framo, Norman Paul, Donald Williamson)	Invisible loyalties Ledgers and debts Family mourning Personal authority	More universal than family-specific goals Increased trust Repair ruptured relationships	Multidirected partiality Family-of-origin sessions Use of cotherapy	Almost all multigenerational and transgenerational methods have significant psychodynamic underpinnings

Courtesy of Alan S. Gurman, Ph.D., and Jay L. Lebow, Ph.D.

with whom the patient comes into contact in daily life, not only the immediate family but also relatives, friends, tradespersons, teachers, and coworkers.

Paradoxical Therapy. In this approach, which evolved from the work of Gregory Bateson, a therapist suggests that the patient intentionally engage in the unwanted behavior (called the *paradoxical injunction*) and, for example, avoid a phobic object or perform a compulsive ritual. Although paradoxical therapy and the use of paradoxical injunctions are relatively new, the therapy can create new insights for some patients. It is used in individual therapy as well as in family therapy.

Reframing. Reframing, also known as *positive connotation,* is a relabeling of all negatively expressed feelings or behavior as positive. When the therapist attempts to get family members to view behavior from a new frame of reference, "This child is impossible" becomes "This child is desperately trying to distract and protect you from what he or she perceives as an unhappy marriage." Reframing is an important process that allows family members to view themselves in new ways that can produce change.

Goals

Family therapy has several goals: to resolve or reduce pathogenic conflict and anxiety within the matrix of interpersonal relationships; to enhance the perception and fulfillment by family members of one another's emotional needs; to promote appropriate role relationships between the sexes and generations; to strengthen the capacity of individual members and the family as a whole to cope with destructive forces inside and outside the surrounding environment; and to influence family identity and values so that members are oriented toward health and growth. The therapy ultimately aims to integrate families into the large systems of society, extended family, and community groups and social systems such as schools, medical facilities, and social, recreational, and welfare agencies.

COUPLES (MARITAL) THERAPY

Couples or marital therapy is a form of psychotherapy designed to psychologically modify the interaction of two persons who are in conflict with each other over one parameter or a variety of parameters—social, emotional, sexual, or economic. In couples therapy a trained person establishes a therapeutic contract with a patient-couple and, through definite types of communication, attempts to alleviate the disturbance, to reverse or change maladaptive patterns of behavior, and to encourage personality growth and development.

Marriage counseling may be considered more limited in scope than marriage therapy: Only a particular familial conflict is discussed, and the counseling is primarily task oriented, geared to solving a specific problem such as child rearing. Marriage therapy, by contrast, emphasizes restructuring a couple's interaction and sometimes explores the psychodynamics of each partner. Both therapy and counseling stress helping marital partners cope effectively with their problems. Most important is the definition of appropriate and realistic goals, which may involve extensive reconstruction of the union or problem-solving approaches or a combination of both.

Types of Therapies

Individual Therapy. In individual therapy, the partners may consult different therapists, who do not necessarily communicate with each other and indeed may not even know each other. The goal of treatment is to strengthen each partner's adaptive capacities. At times, only one of the partners is in treatment; and in such cases, it is often helpful for the person who is not in treatment to visit the therapist. The visiting partner may give the therapist data about the patient that may otherwise be overlooked, overt or covert anxiety in the visiting partner as a result of change in the patient can be identified and dealt with, irrational beliefs about treatment events can be corrected, and conscious or unconscious attempts by the partner to sabotage the patient's treatment can be examined.

Individual Couples Therapy. In individual couples therapy each partner is in therapy, which is either concurrent, with the same therapist, or collaborative, with each partner seeing a different therapist.

Conjoint Therapy. In conjoint therapy, the most common treatment method in couples therapy, either one or two therapists treat the partners in joint sessions. Cotherapy with therapists of both sexes prevents a particular patient from feeling ganged up on when confronted by two members of the opposite sex.

Four-Way Session. In a four-way session each partner is seen by a different therapist, with regular joint sessions in which all four persons participate. A variation of the four-way session is the roundtable interview, developed by William Masters and Virginia Johnson for the rapid treatment of sexually dysfunctional couples. Two patients and two opposite-sex therapists meet regularly.

Group Psychotherapy. Group therapy for couples allows a variety of group dynamics to affect the participants. Groups usually consist of three to four couples and one or two therapists. The couples identify with one another and recognize that others have similar problems, each gains support and empathy from fellow group members of the same or opposite sex, they explore sexual attitudes and have an opportunity to gain new information from their peer groups, and each receives specific feedback about his or her behavior, either negative or positive, which may have more meaning and be better assimilated coming from a neutral, nonspouse member, for example, than from the spouse or the therapist.

Combined Therapy. *Combined therapy* refers to all or any of the preceding techniques used concurrently or in combination. Thus, a particular patient-couple may begin treatment with one or both partners in individual psychotherapy, continue in conjoint therapy with the partner, and terminate therapy after a course of treatment in a married couples group. The rationale for combined therapy is that no single approach to marital problems has been shown to be superior to another. A familiarity with a variety of approaches thus allows therapists a flexibility that provides maximum benefit for couples in distress.

Indications

Whatever the specific therapeutic technique, initiation of couples therapy is indicated when individual therapy has failed to resolve the relationship difficulties, when the onset of distress in one or both partners is clearly a relational problem, and when couples therapy is requested by a couple in conflict. Problems in communication between partners are a prime indication for couples therapy. In such instances one spouse may be intimidated by the other, may become anxious when attempting to tell the other about thoughts or feelings, or may project unconscious expectations onto the other. The therapy is geared toward enabling each partner to see the other realistically.

Conflicts in one or several areas, such as the partners' sexual life, are also indications for treatment. Similarly, difficulty in establishing satisfactory social, economic, parental, or emotional roles implies that a couple needs help. Clinicians should evaluate all aspects of the marital relationship before attempting to treat only one problem, which could be a symptom of a pervasive marital disorder.

Contraindications

Contraindications for couples therapy include patients with severe forms of psychosis, particularly patients with paranoid elements and those in whom the marriage's homeostatic mechanism is a protection against psychosis, marriages in which one or both partners really want to divorce, and marriages in which one spouse refuses to participate because of anxiety or fear.

Goals

Nathan Ackerman defined the aims of couples therapy as follows: The goals of therapy for partner relational problems are to alleviate emotional distress and disability and to promote the levels of well-being of both partners together and of each as an individual. Ideally, therapists move toward these goals by strengthening the shared resources for problem solving, by encouraging the substitution of adequate controls and defenses for pathogenic ones, by enhancing both the immunity against the disintegrative effects of emotional upset and the complementarity of the relationship, and by promoting the growth of the relationship and of each partner.

Part of a therapist's task is to persuade each partner in the relationship to take responsibility in understanding the psychodynamic makeup of personality. Each person's accountability for the effects of behavior on his or her own life, the life of the partner, and the lives of others in the environment is emphasized, and the result is often a deep understanding of the problems that created the marital discord.

Couples therapy does not ensure the maintenance of any marriage or relationship. Indeed, in certain instances it may show the partners that they are in a nonviable union that should be dissolved. In these cases couples may continue to meet with therapists to work through the difficulties of separating and obtaining a divorce, a process that has been called *divorce therapy.*

Don and Kris, the 44-year-old parents of three children ages 19, 17, and 12, began contact with the therapist during Don's week-long hospitalization because of his intensifying depression and increased use of anxiolytics. Although he had had two brief psychiatric hospitalizations in his 20s and early 30s Don had generally functioned quite well for several years. But over the preceding several months, he had become easily fatigued, generally pessimistic, irritable, and "clingy."

These symptoms, among others, seemed to have arisen as Kris became increasingly less involved with Don's life. Kris, the eldest of three siblings, had a long history of self-sacrifice, originating in her family of origin, in which she was the "parentified child" of an alcoholic father and a passive, depression-prone mother. Although her father's alcohol problem had largely abated over the previous decade, the marriage between Kris's parents had never progressed much beyond becoming a "pseudo-civil, polite but distant" relationship. They had retired to the Sun Belt, hoping the change would allow them to "start over," but Kris's mother had become increasingly depressed of late as marital conflicts became more frequent.

Kris had recently become extremely involved in her parents' difficulties, especially as her mother's confidante, and less involved in her own family's life. In addition to this loss, Don, a generally avoidant man, felt more and more isolated from meaningful relationships, now that his 19-year-old son was away at college, and his 17-year-old son was "never around." Don was very dependent upon, and angry with, Kris, but he feared voicing his concerns about their disconnected lives. This dilemma was reminiscent of his relationship with his father, who had essentially abandoned the family when Don was 7 years old.

Over the next 5 months couples therapy addressed problematic patterns at several levels. Structural interventions included dislodging Kris from her therapist-like role with her parents, in part by helping her to help her parents identify a skilled couples therapist for them to see in their new location and by supporting her in setting and keeping appropriate boundaries in her conversations with her mother.

The sessions included cognitively oriented work on Kris's guilt about giving her own needs higher priority than connectedness to her husband and children, aided by bibliotherapy and other homework assignments. Don's normal adult attachment needs were validated, and he was also encouraged to explore new peer relationships in his community. Much therapy time was devoted to communication and problem-solving training. In this, Don had to address his anxiety about assertiveness and fear of conflict and abandonment, and Kris had to address her anxiety-guilt about "saying no" and expressing her own needs. (Courtesy of Alan S. Gurman, Ph.D., and Jay L. Lebow, Ph.D.)

References

Babcock JC, Waltz J, Jacobson NS, Gottman JM. Power and violence: the relation between communication patterns, power discrepancies, and domestic violence. *J Consult Clin Psychol.* 1993;61:40.

Bowen M. *Family Theory in Clinical Practice.* New York: Aronson; 1978.

Croake JW, Kelly FD. Structured group couples therapy with schizophrenic and bipolar patients and their wives. *J Individ Psychol.* 2002;58:76.

Diamond G, Liddle HA. Resolving a therapeutic impasse between parents and adolescents in multidimensional family therapy. *J Consult Clin Psychol.* 1996;64:481.

Diamond GS, Serrano AC, Dickey M, Sonis WA. Current status of family-based outcome and process research. *J Am Acad Child Adolesc Psychiatry.* 1996;35:6.

Glick ID. Family therapies: efficacy, indications, and treatment outcomes. In: Janowsky DS, ed. *Psychotherapy Indications and Outcomes.* Washington, DC: American Psychiatric Press; 1999:303.

Gurman AS, Lebow JL. Family therapy and couple therapy. In: Sadock BJ, Sadock VA, eds. *Kaplan & Sadock's Comprehensive Textbook of Psychiatry.* 7th ed. Vol 2. Baltimore: Lippincott Williams & Wilkins; 2000:2157.

Johnson S, Lebow J. The "coming of age" of couple therapy: a decade review. *J Marital Fam Ther.* 2000;26:23.

Kadis LB, McClendon RA. Couples and marital therapy. In: Kaplan HI, Sadock BJ, eds. *Comprehensive Textbook of Psychiatry.* 6th ed. Baltimore: Williams & Wilkins; 1995:1857.

Lidz T, Fleck S, Cornelison A. *Schizophrenia and the Family.* New York: International Universities Press; 1965.

Minuchin S. *Families and Family Therapy.* Cambridge, MA: Harvard University Press; 1974.
O'Leary KD, Beach SR. Marital therapy: a viable treatment for depression and marital discord. *Am J Psychiatry.* 1990;147:183.
Sadock V. Marital therapy. In: Kaplan HI, Sadock BJ, eds. *Comprehensive Textbook of Psychiatry.* 2nd ed. Baltimore: Williams & Wilkins; 1975:1886.
Satir V. *Conjoint Family Therapy.* Palo Alto, CA: Science & Behavior; 1967.
Scharff D, Scharff J. *Object Relations Family Therapy.* New York: Aronson; 1987.
Solomon P, Draine J, Mannion E, Meisel M. Impact of brief family psychoeducation on self-efficacy. *Schizophr Bull.* 1996;22:41.
Steinglass P. Family therapy. In: Kaplan HI, Sadock BJ, eds. *Comprehensive Textbook of Psychiatry.* 6th ed. Baltimore: Williams & Wilkins; 1995:1838.
Tatum DW, DelCampo RL. Selective mutism in children: a structural family therapy approach to treatment. *Contemp Fam Ther.* 1995;17:177.
Vansteenwegen A. Who benefits from couple therapy? A comparison of successful and failed couples. *J Sex Marital Ther.* 1996;22:63.

▲ 35.5 Biofeedback

Biofeedback relies on instrumentation to measure moment-to-moment feedback about physiological processes. It provides patients with information about their performance in various situations. Using this "feedback" it is possible to control physiological functions so as to change them. Biofeedback is based on the idea that the autonomic nervous system can come under voluntary control through operant conditioning. The benefits of biofeedback may be augmented by the relaxation that patients are trained to facilitate.

THEORY

Neal Miller demonstrated the medical potential of biofeedback by showing that the normally involuntary autonomic nervous system can be operantly conditioned by use of appropriate feedback. By means of instruments, patients acquire information about the status of involuntary biological functions, such as skin temperature and electrical conductivity, muscle tension, blood pressure, heart rate, and brain wave activity. Patients then learn to regulate one or more of these biological states that affect symptoms. For example, a person can learn to raise the temperature of his or her hands to reduce the frequency of migraines, palpitations, or angina pectoris. Presumably, patients lower the sympathetic activation and voluntarily self-regulate arterial smooth muscle vasoconstrictive tendencies.

METHODS

Instrumentation

The feedback instrument used depends on the patient and the specific problem. The most effective instruments are the electromyogram (EMG), which measures the electrical potentials of muscle fibers; the electroencephalogram (EEG), which measures alpha waves that occur in relaxed states; the galvanic skin response gauge (GSR), which shows decreased skin conductivity during a relaxed state; and the thermistor, which measures skin temperature (which drops during tension because of peripheral vasoconstriction). Patients are attached to one of the instruments that measures a physiological function and translates the measurement into an audible or visual signal that patients use to gauge their responses. For example, in the treatment of bruxism, an EMG is attached to the masseter muscle. The EMG emits a high tone when the muscle is contracted and a low tone when at rest. Patients can learn to alter the tone to indicate relaxation. Patients receive feedback about the masseter muscle, the tone reinforces the learning, and the condition ameliorates—all of these events interacting synergistically.

Many less specific clinical applications (e.g., treating insomnia, dysmenorrhea, and speech problems; improving athletic performance; treating volitional disorders; achieving altered states of consciousness; managing stress; and supplementing psychotherapy for anxiety associated with somatoform disorders) use a model in which frontalis muscle EMG biofeedback is combined with thermal biofeedback and verbal instructions in progressive relaxation. Table 35.5–1 outlines some important clinical applications of biofeedback and shows that a wide variety of biofeedback modalities have been used to treat numerous conditions.

Relaxation Therapy

Progressive relaxation was developed by Edmund Jacobson in 1929. Jacobson observed that

> When an individual lies "relaxed," in the ordinary sense, the following clinical signs reveal the presence of residual tension: respiration is slightly irregular in time or force; the pulse-rate, although often normal, is in some instances moderately increased as compared with later tests; voluntary or local reflex activities are revealed in such slight marks as wrinkling of the forehead, frowning, movements of the eye balls, frequent or rapid winking, restless shifting of the head, a limb or even a finger; finally, the mind continues to be active, and once started, worry or oppressive emotion will persist. It is amazing that a faint degree of tension can be responsible for all this.

Learning relaxation, therefore, involves cultivating a muscle sense. To develop the muscle sense further, patients are taught to isolate and contract specific muscles or muscle groups, one at a time. For example, patients flex the forearm while the therapist holds it back to observe tenseness in the biceps muscle. (Jacobson used the word "tenseness" rather than "tension" to emphasize the patient's role in tensing the muscles.) Once this sensation is reported, Jacobson would say, "This is your doing! What we wish is the reverse of this—simply not doing." Patients are repeatedly reminded that relaxation involves no effort. In fact "making an effort is being tense and therefore is not to relax." As the session progresses, patients are instructed to let go further and further, even past the point when the body part seemed perfectly relaxed.

Patients would work in this fashion with different muscle groups, often over more than 50 sessions. For example, an entire session might be devoted to relaxing the biceps muscle. Another feature of Jacobson's method was that instructions were given tersely so they would not interfere with the patients' focus on muscle sensations; suggestions commonly used today (e.g., "your arm is becoming limp") were avoided. Patients

Table 35.5–1
Biofeedback Applications

Condition	Effects
Asthma	Both frontal EMG and airway resistance biofeedback have been reported as producing relaxation from the panic associated with asthma, as well as improving air flow rate.
Cardiac arrhythmias	Specific biofeedback of the electrocardiogram has permitted patients to lower the frequency of premature ventricular contractions.
Fecal incontinence and enuresis	The timing sequence of internal and external anal sphincters has been measured, using triple lumen rectal catheters providing feedback to incontinent patients to allow them to reestablish normal bowel habits in a relatively small number of biofeedback sessions. An actual precursor of biofeedback dating to 1938 was a buzzer sounding for sleeping enuretic children at the first sign of moisture (the pad and bell).
Grand mal epilepsy	A number of EEG biofeedback procedures have been used experimentally to suppress seizure activity prophylactically in patients not responsive to anticonvulsant medication. The procedures permit patients to enhance the sensorimotor brain wave rhythm or to normalize brain activity as computed in real-time power spectrum displays.
Hyperactivity	EEG biofeedback procedures have been used on children with attention-deficit/hyperactivity disorder to train them to reduce their motor restlessness.
Idiopathic hypertension and orthostatic hypotension	A variety of specific (direct) and nonspecific biofeedback procedures—including blood pressure feedback, galvanic skin response, and foot-hand thermal feedback combined with relaxation procedures—have been used to teach patients to increase or decrease their blood pressure. Some follow-up data indicate that the changes may persist for years and often permit the reduction or elimination of antihypertensive medications.
Migraine	The most common biofeedback strategy with classic or common vascular headaches has been thermal biofeedback from a digit accompanied by autogenic self-suggestive phrases encouraging hand warming and head cooling. The mechanism is thought to help prevent excessive cerebral artery vasoconstriction, often accompanied by an ischemic prodromal symptom, such as scintillating scotomata, followed by rebound engorgement of arteries and stretching of vessel wall pain receptors.
Myofacial and temporomandibular joint (TMJ) pain	High levels of EMG activity over the powerful muscles associated with bilateral TMJs have been decreased, using biofeedback in patients who are jaw clenchers or have bruxism.
Neuromuscular rehabilitation	Mechanical devices or an EMG measurement of muscle activity displayed to a patient increases the effectiveness of traditional therapies, as documented by relatively long clinical histories in peripheral nerve-muscle damage, spasmodic torticollis, selected cases of tardive dyskinesia, cerebral palsy, and upper motor neuron hemiplegias.
Raynaud's syndrome	Cold hands and cold feet are frequent concomitants of anxiety and also occur in Raynaud's syndrome, caused by vasospasm of arterial smooth muscle. A number of studies report that thermal feedback from the hand, an inexpensive and benign procedure compared with surgical sympathectomy, is effective in about 70 percent of cases of Raynaud's syndrome.
Tension headaches	Muscle contraction headaches are most frequently treated with two large active electrodes spaced on the forehead to provide visual or auditory information about the levels of muscle tension. The frontal electrode placement is sensitive to EMG activity regarding the frontalis and occipital muscles, which the patient learns to relax.

were also frequently left alone, while the therapist attended to other patients.

Later Adaptation of Progressive Muscular Relaxation

Joseph Wolpe chose progressive relaxation as a response incompatible with anxiety when designing his systematic desensitization treatment (discussed below). For this purpose, Jacobson's original method was too lengthy to be practical. Wolpe abbreviated the program to 20 minutes during the first six sessions (devoting the remainder of these sessions to other things such as behavioral analysis). In a later modification of progressive relaxation, patients completed work with all the principal muscle groups in one session. The specific muscle groups and instructions for this type of progressive relaxation are listed in Table 35.5–2. Once the patients have mastered this procedure (typically after three sessions), these groups are combined into larger groups. Finally, patients practice relaxation by recall (i.e., without tensing the muscles).

Autogenic Training

Autogenic training is a method of self-suggestion that originated in Germany. It involves the patients directing their attention to specific bodily areas and hearing themselves think certain phrases reflecting a relaxed state. In the original German version patients progressed through six themes over many sessions. The six areas are listed in Table 35.5–3 along with representative autogenic phrases. Autogenic relaxation is an American modification of autogenic training, in which all six areas are covered in one session.

Applied Tension

Applied tension is a technique that is the opposite of relaxation; applied tension can be used to counteract the fainting response.

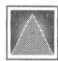

Table 35.5–2
Outline of Initial Progressive Relaxation Session, All Muscle Groups

Muscle Group	Instruction
Dominant hand and forearm	Make a tight fist, now
Dominant biceps, triceps	Make your upper arm tense by counterposing muscles
Nondominant arm, forearm	Make a tight fist, now
Nondominant biceps	Make your upper arm tense by counterposing muscles
Forehead	Lift eyebrows
Orbital and nose muscles	Squint and wrinkle your nose
Lower cheeks and jaws	Bite your teeth together and pull the corners of your mouth back
Neck and throat	Pull your chin toward your chest but prevent it from happening by counterposing muscles in front and back
Chest, shoulders, upper back	Take a deep breath, hold it, and pull the shoulder blades upward (if sitting) or backward (if supine)
Abdominal or stomach region	Make your stomach hard, as if you were going to hit yourself
Dominant thigh	Counterpose extensors and flexors
Dominant lower leg	Dorsiflex foot
Dominant foot	Curl toes upward (not down to avoid cramps)
Nondominant thigh	Counterpose extensors and flexors
Nondominant calf	Dorsiflex foot
Nondominant foot	Curl toes upward (not down, to avoid cramps)

Adapted from Bernstein DA, Borkovec TD. *Progressive Relaxation Training: A Manual for the Helping Professions.* Champaign, IL: Research Press; 1973.

The treatment extends over four sessions. In the first session patients learn to tense the muscles of the arms, legs, and torso for 10 to 15 seconds (as if they were bodybuilders). The tension is maintained long enough for a sensation of warmth to develop in the face. The patients then release the tension but do not progress to a state of relaxation. The maneuver is repeated five times at half-minute intervals. This method can be augmented with feedback of the patient's blood pressure during the muscle contraction; increased blood pressure suggests that appropriate muscle tension was achieved. The patients continue to practice the technique five times a day. An adverse effect of treatment that sometimes develops is headaches. In this case, the intensity of the muscle contraction and the frequency of treatment are reduced.

Table 35.5–3
Sample Autogenic Phrases

Theme	Examples of Self-Statements
Heaviness	"My left arm is heavy."
Warmth	"My left arm is warm."
Cardiac regulation	"My heartbeat is calm and regular."
Breathing adjustment	"It breathes me."
Solar plexus	"My solar plexus is warm."
Forehead	"My forehead is cool."

Patients with blood and injury phobia show a unique, biphasic response when exposed to a phobic stimulus. The first phase is associated with increased heart rate and blood pressure. In the second phase, however, blood pressure suddenly falls and the patient faints. To treat the problem, patients are shown a series of slides that are provocative (e.g., mutilated bodies). They are coached in identifying early warning signs of fainting, such as queasiness, cold sweats, or dizziness, and in applying the learned muscle tension response quickly, contingent on these warning signs. Patients can also perform applied tension while donating blood or watching a surgical operation. The technique of isometric tension raises blood pressure, which prevents fainting.

RESULTS

Biofeedback, progressive relaxation, and applied tension have been shown to be effective treatment methods for a broad range of disorders. They form one basis of behavioral medicine in which the patient changes (or learns how to change) behavior that contributes to illness. They form a basis upon which many complementary and alternative medical procedures are effective (e.g., yoga and Reiki) in which relaxation is an important component. Relaxation also informs more mainstream treatments such as hypnosis.

REFERENCES

Baddeley M. Brain wave states and hypnotherapy. *Aust J Clin Hynother Hypn.* 1999;20:108.

Berghmans LC, Frederiks CM, de Bie RA, et al. Efficacy of biofeedback, when included with pelvic floor muscle exercise treatment, for genuine stress incontinence. *Neurol Urodyn.* 1996;15:37.

Burish TG, Jenkins RA. Effectiveness of biofeedback and relaxation training in reducing the side effects of cancer chemotherapy. *Health Psychol.* 1992;11:17.

Linden M, Habib T, Radojevic V. A controlled study of the effects of EEG biofeedback on cognition and behavior of children with attention deficit disorder and learning disabilities. *Biofeedback Self Regul.* 1996;21:35.

McGrady A. A commentary of "Problems inherent in assessing biofeedback efficacy studies." *Appl Psychophysiol Biofeedback.* 2002;27:111.

McGrady A, Conran P, Dickey D, et al. The effects of biofeedback-assisted relaxation on cell-mediated immunity, cortisol, and white blood cell count in healthy and adult subjects. *J Behav Med.* 1992;15:343.

Plante TG. Could the perception of fitness account for many of the mental and physical health benefits of exercise? *Adv Mind Body Med.* 1999;15:291.

Sarafino EP, Goehring P. Age comparisons in acquiring biofeedback control and success in reducing headache pain. *Ann Behav Med.* 2000;22:10.

Wehck L, Leu PW, D'Amato RC. Evaluating the efficacy of a biofeedback intervention to reduce children's anxiety. *J Clin Psychol.* 1996;52:469.

Whitehead WE, Drossman DA. Biofeedback for disorders of elimination: fecal incontinence and pelvic floor dyssynergia. *Prof Psychol Res Pract.* 1996;27:234.

▲ 35.6 Behavior Therapy

Behavior therapy represents clinical applications of the principles developed in learning theory. Behavioral psychology, or behaviorism, arose in the early 20th century in reaction to the method of introspection that dominated psychology at the time. John B. Watson, the father of behaviorism, had initially studied animal psychology. This background made it a small conceptual leap to argue that psychology should concern itself only with publicly observable phenomena (i.e., overt behavior). According to behavioristic thinking, since mental content is not

publicly observable, it cannot be subjected to rigorous scientific inquiry. Consequently, behaviorists developed a focus on overt behaviors and their environmental influences.

Today different behavioral schools continue to share a focus on verifiable behavior. Behavioral views differ from cognitive views in holding that physical, rather than mental, events control behavior. According to behaviorism, mental phenomena or speculations about them are of little or no scientific interest.

HISTORY

As early as the 1920s, scattered reports about the application of learning principles to the treatment of behavioral disorders began to appear, but they had little effect on the mainstream of psychiatry and clinical psychology. Not until the 1960s did behavior therapy emerge as a systematic and comprehensive approach to psychiatric (behavioral) disorders, and at that time, it arose independently on three continents. Joseph Wolpe and his colleagues in Johannesburg, South Africa, used pavlovian techniques to produce and eliminate experimental neuroses in cats. From this research Wolpe developed systematic desensitization, the prototype of many current behavioral procedures for the treatment of maladaptive anxiety produced by identifiable stimuli in the environment. At about the same time a group at the Institute of Psychiatry of the University of London, particularly Hans Jurgen Eysenck and M. B. Shapiro, stressed the importance of an empirical, experimental approach to understanding and treating individual patients, using controlled, single-case experimental paradigms and modern learning theory. The third origin of behavior therapy was work inspired by the research of Harvard psychologist B. F. Skinner. Skinner's students began to apply his operant-conditioning technology developed in animal-conditioning laboratories to human beings in clinical settings.

SYSTEMATIC DESENSITIZATION

Developed by Wolpe, systematic desensitization is based on the behavioral principle of counterconditioning, whereby a person overcomes maladaptive anxiety elicited by a situation or an object by approaching the feared situation gradually, in a psychophysiological state that inhibits anxiety. In systematic desensitization, patients attain a state of complete relaxation and are then exposed to the stimulus that elicits the anxiety response. The negative reaction of anxiety is inhibited by the relaxed state, a process called *reciprocal inhibition.* Rather than use actual situations or objects that elicit fear, patients and therapists prepare a graded list or hierarchy of anxiety-provoking scenes associated with a patient's fears. The learned relaxation state and the anxiety-provoking scenes are systematically paired in treatment. Thus, systematic desensitization consists of three steps: relaxation training, hierarchy construction, and desensitization of the stimulus.

Relaxation Training

As described above (Section 35.5), relaxation produces physiological effects opposite to those of anxiety: slow heart rate, increased peripheral blood flow, and neuromuscular stability. A variety of relaxation methods have been developed. Some, such as yoga and Zen, have been known for centuries. Most methods use so-called progressive relaxation, developed by the psychiatrist Edmund Jacobson. Patients relax major muscle groups in a fixed order, beginning with the small muscle groups of the feet and working cephalad or vice versa. Some clinicians use hypnosis to facilitate relaxation or use tape-recorded exercise to allow patients to practice relaxation on their own. Mental imagery is a relaxation method in which patients are instructed to imagine themselves in a place associated with pleasant relaxed memories. Such images allow patients to enter a relaxed state or experience (as Herbert Benson termed it) the *relaxation response.*

The physiological changes that take place during relaxation are the opposite of those induced by the adrenergic stress responses that are part of many emotions. Muscle tension, respiration rate, heart rate, blood pressure, and skin conductance decrease. Finger temperature and blood flow to the finger usually increase. Relaxation increases respiratory heart rate variability, an index of parasympathetic tone.

Hierarchy Construction

When constructing a hierarchy, clinicians determine all the conditions that elicit anxiety, and then patients create a hierarchy list of 10 to 12 scenes in order of increasing anxiety. For example, an acrophobic hierarchy may begin with a patient's imagining standing near a window on the second floor and end with being on the roof of a 20-story building, leaning on a guard rail and looking straight down. Table 35.6–1 provides an example of a hierarchy construction for fear of water and heights.

Desensitization of the Stimulus

In the final step, called *desensitization,* patients proceed systematically through the list from the least, to the most, anxiety-provoking scene while in a deeply relaxed state. The rate at which patients progress through the list is determined by their responses to the stimuli. When patients can vividly imagine the most anxiety-provoking scene of the hierarchy with equanimity, they experience little anxiety in the corresponding real-life situation.

Adjunctive Use of Drugs

Clinicians have used various drugs to hasten relaxation, but drugs should be used cautiously and only by clinicians trained and experienced in potential adverse effects. Either the ultrarapidly acting barbiturate sodium methohexital (Brevital) or diazepam (Valium) is given intravenously in subanesthetic doses. If the procedural details are followed carefully, almost all patients find the procedure pleasant, with few unpleasant side effects. The advantages of pharmacological desensitization are that preliminary training in relaxation can be shortened, almost all patients can relax adequately, and the treatment itself seems to proceed more rapidly than without the drugs.

Indications

Systematic desensitization works best when there is a clearly identifiable anxiety-provoking stimulus. Phobias, obsessions, compulsions, and certain sexual disorders have been treated successfully with this technique.

Table 35.6–1
Hierarchy Construction (Least Anxious to Most Anxious): Fear of Water and Heights

1. Taking a bath at home.
2. Taking a shower at home.
3. Going into the shallow end of the swimming pool.
4. Starting to swim at the shallow end of the swimming pool, breaststroke only.
5. Swimming at the shallow end, doing the crawl.
6. Jumping into the swimming pool at the shallow end.
7. Jumping into the pool and then doing the crawl.
8. Swimming at the shallow end, first breaststroke, then the crawl.
9. Pushing away from the bars and causing a splash.
10. Swimming in the middle of the pool at a depth of 5 feet 3 inches.
11. Swimming at the shallow end and then at the deep end (10 feet 3 inches).
12. Going into the deep end of the swimming pool.
13. Watching people jump from the diving boards.
14. Standing on a step at the deep end of the pool and making a little jump into the water.
15. Backstroke at the shallow end of the pool.
16. Jumping into the water at the shallow end of the pool (belly-flop dive).
17. Belly-flop dive at the deep end of the pool.
18. Racing dive at the shallow end of the pool.
19. Racing dive at the deep end of the pool.
20. Swimming three times across the deep end of the pool without stopping:
    (a) breaststroke
    (b) crawl
    (c) backstroke
21. Jumping into the pool at a depth of:
    (a) 5 feet 3 inches
    (b) 6 feet
    (c) 7 feet
22. Several jumps at 6 feet and 7 feet, alternating them, and then remaining at the 7-foot depth.
23. Going onto the first diving board and jumping into the water.
24. Jumping off the first diving board, then diving from the first board.
25. Diving off the first board.
26. Jumping from the first diving board, jumping from the second diving board, then diving from the first diving board.
27. Jumping off the first, second, and third diving boards, then diving from the first diving board.
28. Jumping off the first, second, and third diving boards, then diving from the first and then the second diving board.
29. Jumping off the fourth diving board, then diving off the second diving board.
30. Jumping off the fifth diving board, then diving off the third diving board.
31. Jumping off the fifth diving board, then diving off the fourth diving board.
32. Jumping off the top board, then diving off the fourth diving board.
33. Jumping off the top board, then diving off the fifth diving board.
34. Diving off the top diving board.
35. Random stimuli.
36. Looking around before jumping off the third diving board.
37. Looking around before jumping off the fourth diving board.
38. Looking around before jumping off the fifth diving board.
39. Diving from the fifth diving board and looking around before diving.
40. Diving from the top board and looking around before diving.

Reprinted with permission from Kraft T. The use of behavior therapy in a psychotherapeutic context. In: Lazarus AA, ed. *Clinical Behavior Therapy.* New York: Brunner/Mazel; 1972:222.

THERAPEUTIC GRADED EXPOSURE

Therapeutic graded exposure is similar to systematic desensitization except that relaxation training is not involved and treatment is usually carried out in a real-life context. This means that the individual must be brought in contact with (i.e., be exposed to) the warning stimulus to learn firsthand that no dangerous consequences will ensue. Exposure is graded according to a hierarchy. Patients afraid of cats, for example, might progress from looking at a picture of a cat to holding one.

FLOODING

Flooding (sometimes called *implosion*) is similar to graded exposure in that it involves exposing the patient to the feared object in vivo; however, there is no hierarchy. Flooding is based on the premise that escaping from an anxiety-provoking experience reinforces the anxiety through conditioning. Thus, clinicians can extinguish the anxiety and prevent the conditioned avoidance behavior by not allowing patients to escape the situation. Clinicians encourage patients to confront feared situations directly, without a gradual buildup as in systematic desensitization or graded exposure. No relaxation exercises are used, as in systematic desensitization. Patients experience fear, which gradually subsides after a time. The success of the procedure depends on having patients remain in the fear-generating situation until they are calm and feel a sense of mastery. Prematurely withdrawing from the situation or prematurely terminating the fantasized scene is equivalent to an escape, which then reinforces both the conditioned anxiety and the avoidance behavior and produces the opposite of the desired effect. In a variant, called *imaginal flooding,* the feared object or situation is confronted only in the imagination, not in real life. Many patients refuse flooding because of the psychological discomfort involved. It is also contraindicated when intense anxiety would be hazardous to a patient (e.g., those with heart disease or fragile psychological adaptation). The technique works best with specific phobias. An example of in vivo flooding follows.

The patient was a 33-year-old female with social fears of eating in public. In particular, she was afraid of being observed by others when chewing and swallowing, particularly at dinner parties. A contrived situation was arranged in which the patient came to the session with a prepared meal and drink. She entered a conference room in which five persons in professional attire were already seated along a table. The patient was instructed to eat her meal in front of these individuals. Between bites, she was instructed to look at them often, and they had been instructed to avoid staring contests. She was not to distract herself from her anxiety symptoms. She was to eat her meal slowly, paying attention to the behavior of the observers and to her anxiety symptoms (e.g., dry mouth or difficulty swallowing). No conversation between the patient and observers was permitted. The observers would look at her and observe her chewing and swallowing behaviors, at times writing comments in a notebook. Occasionally observers would communicate by whispering to each other, exchanging written notes, or giving knowing glances and smiles.

The only other communication occurred between the patient and therapist, and this was limited to the patient providing her subjective units of distress rating. The session lasted 90 minutes. Note that this situation may seem quite traumatizing. However, because the exposure session is long and continues until ratings decline, the patient becomes desensitized. (Courtesy of Rolf G. Jacob, M.D., and William H. Pelham, M.D.)

PARTICIPANT MODELING

In participant modeling, patients learn a new behavior by imitation, primarily by observation, without having to perform the behavior until they feel ready. Just as irrational fears may be acquired by learning, they can be unlearned by observing a fearless model confront the feared object. The technique has been useful with phobic children who are placed with other children of their own age and sex who approach the feared object or situation. With adults, a therapist may describe the feared activity in a calm manner that a patient can identify. Or the therapist may act out the process of mastering the feared activity with a patient. Sometimes a hierarchy of activities is established, with the least anxiety-provoking activity being dealt with first. The participant-modeling technique has been used successfully with agoraphobia by having a therapist accompany a patient into the feared situation. In a variant of the procedure, called *behavior rehearsal,* real-life problems are acted out under a therapist's observation or direction.

The following is a self-report by a patient with a contamination phobia, who is afraid to touch objects for fear of being infected or contaminated. She describes her reactions.

> [The therapist] started touching everything very slowly. I was told to follow behind and touch everything she touched. It was like we were spreading the contamination. She touched doorknobs, light switches, walls, pictures, and woodwork. She opened drawers in each bedroom and touched the contents. She opened closets and touched clothes hanging on the rods. She touched the towels and sheets in the linen closet. She went through the children's rooms, touching dolls, stuffed animals, models, Star Wars figures, transformers, and books.
>
> [The therapist] kept talking to me quietly and calmly all the time we went along. I had been anxious when we started, but as we continued, my anxiety level decreased. At one point, when I had begun to think the worst was over, she pointed to the attic door and said we were going inside. I said, "No, that's where the mice were." She told me I didn't want to have a place in my home that was off limits. I agreed but became very anxious. It was very hard for me to go inside. I began touching the boxes too, but I was very upset. Then, she put her hands down on the floor and wanted me to do the same. I said, "I can't. I just can't." Julie said, "Yes you can."
>
> [The therapist] spent several hours with me that day. Before she left, she made a list of things for me to do by myself. Twice a day I was to go through the house touching everything the way she had done with me. I was to invite a friend of mine who had a pet to come and visit and also friends of my children who had pets. (Courtesy of Rolf G. Jacobs, M.D., and William H. Pelham, M.D.)

EXPOSURE TO STIMULI PRESENTED IN VIRTUAL REALITY

Advances in computer technology have made it possible to present environmental cues in virtual reality for exposure treatment. Beneficial effects have been reported with virtual reality exposure of patients with height phobia, fear of flying, spider phobia, and claustrophobia. A great deal of experimental work is being done in the field. One model uses an avatar of the patient walking through a crowded supermarket filled with other avatars (including one of the therapist) as a way of conquering agoraphobia.

ASSERTIVENESS TRAINING

To be assertive persons must have confidence in their judgment and sufficient self-esteem to express their opinions. Assertiveness and social skills training teach persons how to respond appropriately in social situations, to express their opinions in acceptable ways, and to achieve their goals. A variety of techniques including role modeling, desensitization, and positive reinforcement (reward of desired behavior) are used to increase assertiveness. Social skills training deals with assertiveness but also attends to a variety of real-life tasks, such as food shopping, looking for work, interacting with other persons, and overcoming shyness.

AVERSION THERAPY

When a noxious stimulus (punishment) is presented immediately after a specific behavioral response, theoretically the response is eventually inhibited and extinguished. Many types of noxious stimuli are used: electric shocks, substances that induce vomiting, corporal punishment, and social disapproval. The negative stimulus is paired with the behavior, which is thereby suppressed. The unwanted behavior may disappear after a series of such sequences. Aversion therapy has been used for alcohol abuse, paraphilias, and other behaviors with impulsive or compulsive qualities, but this therapy is controversial for many reasons. For example, punishment does not always lead to the expected decreased response and can sometimes be positively reinforcing. Aversion therapy has been used with good effect in some cultures in the treatment of opioid addicts (Fig. 35.6–1).

EYE MOVEMENT DESENSITIZATION AND REPROCESSING (EMDR)

Saccadic eye movements are rapid oscillations of the eyes that occur when a person tracks an object that is moved back and

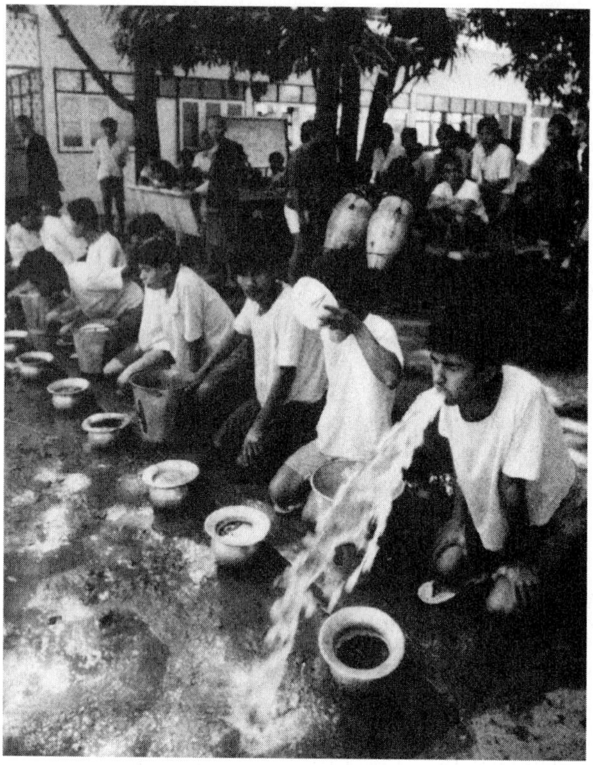

FIGURE 35.6–1
Treatment of addicts at Tham Krabok Monastery in Thailand results in a 70 percent success rate, according to its records. The 10-day free treatment begins with a vow to Buddha never to use narcotics again. Then patients are given an herbal medicine that makes them vomit immediately. (Reprinted with permission from White PT, Raymer S. The poppy—for good and evil. *Natl Geogr.* 1985;167:187.)

forth across the line of vision. A few studies have demonstrated that inducing saccades while a person is imagining or thinking about an anxiety-producing event can yield a positive thought or image that results in decreased anxiety. EMDR has been used in posttraumatic stress disorders and phobias.

POSITIVE REINFORCEMENT

When a behavioral response is followed by a generally rewarding event such as food, avoidance of pain, or praise, it tends to be strengthened and to occur more frequently than before the reward. This principle has been applied in a variety of situations. On inpatient hospital wards, patients with mental disorder receive a reward for performing a desired behavior, such as tokens that they may use to purchase luxury items or certain privileges. The process, known as *token economy,* has successfully altered behavior. Table 35.6–2 gives a summary of some clinical applications of behavior therapy.

Table 35.6–2
Some Common Clinical Applications of Behavior Therapy

Disorder	Comments
Agoraphobia	Graded exposure and flooding can reduce the fear of being in crowded places. About 60% of patients so treated improve. In some cases the spouse can serve as the model while accompanying the patient into the fear situation; however, the patient cannot get a secondary gain by keeping the spouse nearby and displaying symptoms.
Alcohol dependence	Aversion therapy in which the alcohol-dependent patient is made to vomit (by adding an emetic to the alcohol) every time a drink is ingested is effective in treating alcohol dependence. Disulfiram (Antabuse) can be given to alcohol-dependent patients when they are alcohol free. Such patients are warned of the severe physiological consequences of drinking (e.g., nausea, vomiting, hypotension, collapse) with disulfiram in the system.
Anorexia nervosa	Observe eating behavior; contingency management; record weight.
Bulimia nervosa	Record bulimic episodes; log moods.
Hyperventilation	Hyperventilation test; controlled breathing; direct observation.
Other phobias	Systematic desensitization has been effective in treating phobias, such as fears of heights, animals, and flying. Social skills training has also been used for shyness and fear of other people.
Paraphilias	Electric shocks or other noxious stimuli can be applied at the time of a paraphilic impulse, and eventually the impulse subsides. Shocks can be administered by either the therapist or the patient. The results are satisfactory but must be reinforced at regular intervals.
Schizophrenia	The token economy procedure, in which tokens are awarded for desirable behavior and can be used to buy ward privileges, has been useful in treating inpatient schizophrenia patients. Social skills training teaches schizophrenia patients how to interact with others in a socially acceptable way so that negative feedback is eliminated. In addition, the aggressive behavior of some schizophrenia patients can be diminished through those methods.
Sexual dysfunctions	Sex therapy, developed by William Masters and Virginia Johnson, is a behavior therapy technique used for various sexual dysfunctions, especially male erectile disorder, orgasm disorders, and premature ejaculation. It uses relaxation, desensitization, and graded exposure as the primary techniques.
Shy bladder	Inability to void in a public bathroom; relaxation exercises.
Type A behavior	Physiological assessment; muscle relaxation, biofeedback (on EMG)

DIALECTICAL BEHAVIOR THERAPY (DBT)

DBT has been used successfully in patients with borderline personality disorder and parasuicidal behavior. It is eclectic, drawing on methods from supportive, cognitive, and behavioral therapies. Some elements are derived from Franz Alexander's view of therapy as a corrective emotional experience, and some from certain Eastern philosophical schools (e.g., Zen). Patients are seen weekly, with the goal of improving interpersonal skills and decreasing self-destructive behavior by means of techniques involving advice, use of metaphor, storytelling, and con-

frontation, among others. Borderline patients especially are helped to deal with the ambivalent feelings that are characteristic of the disorder. Marsha Linehan, Ph.D., developed the treatment method, based on her theory that borderline patients cannot identify emotional experiences and cannot tolerate frustration or rejection. As with other behavioral approaches, DBT assumes all behavior (including thoughts and feelings) is learned and that borderline patients behave in ways that reinforce or even reward their behavior, regardless of how maladaptive it is.

Functions of DBT. As described by its originator there are five essential "functions" in treatment: (1) to enhance and expand the patient's repertoire of skillful behavioral patterns; (2) to improve patient motivation to change by reducing reinforcement of maladaptive behavior, including dysfunctional cognition and emotion; (3) to ensure that new behavioral patterns generalize from the therapeutic to the natural environment; (4) to structure the environment so that effective behaviors, rather than dysfunctional behaviors, are reinforced; and (5) to enhance the motivation and capabilities of the therapist so that effective treatment is rendered. Therapy is conducted in both individual or group behavioral skills training sessions. Homework assignments and coaching in person and by telephone are part of the treatment. Environmental structuring may occur by having family members come to treatment with the patient, by changing the environment to support and reinforce therapeutic improvements, or by training the patient how to intervene in his or her own environment. Finally, therapist capabilities and motivation are addressed through weekly team meetings aimed at improving their skills and motivation and reducing burnout.

In a study evaluating the effect of DBT for patients with borderline personality disorder there were positive findings. Patients had a low dropout rate from treatment; the incidence of parasuicidal behaviors declined; self-report of angry affect decreased; and social adjustment and work performance improved. The method is now being applied to other disorders including substance abuse, eating disorders, and posttraumatic stress disorder.

RESULTS

Behavior therapy has been successful in a variety of disorders (Table 35.6–2) and can be easily taught (Table 35.6–3). It requires less time than other therapies and is less expensive to administer. Although useful for circumscribed behavioral symptoms, the method cannot treat global areas of dysfunction (e.g., neurotic conflicts, personality disorders). There was and is controversy between behaviorists and psychoanalysts, which is epitomized by Eysenck's statement: "Learning theory regards neurotic symptoms as simply learned habits; there is no neurosis underlying the symptoms, but merely the symptom itself. Get rid of the symptom and you have eliminated the neurosis." Analytically oriented theorists have criticized behavior therapy by noting that simple symptom removal may lead to symptom substitution. In other words, when symptoms are not viewed as consequences of inner conflicts and the core cause of the symptoms is not addressed or altered, the result is the production of new symptoms. Whether or not this occurs remains open to question, however.

Table 35.6–3
Social Skills Competence Checklist of Therapist-Trainer Behaviors

1. Actively helps the patient set and elicit specific interpersonal goals.
2. Promotes favorable expectations, a therapeutic orientation, and motivation before role playing begins.
3. Assists the patient in building possible scenes in terms of "What emotion or communication?" "Who is the interpersonal target?" "Where and when?"
4. Structures the role playing by setting the scene and assigning roles to the patient and surrogates.
5. Engages the patient in behavioral rehearsal—getting the patient to role-play with others.
6. Uses self or other group members in modeling appropriate alternatives for the patient.
7. Prompts and cues the patient during the role playing.
8. Uses an active style of training through coaching, shadowing, being physically out of a seat, and closely monitoring and supporting the patient.
9. Gives the patient positive feedback for specific verbal and nonverbal behavioral skills.
10. Identifies the patient's specific verbal and nonverbal behavioral deficits or excesses and suggests constructive alternatives.
11. Ignores or suppresses inappropriate and interfering behavior.
12. Shapes behavioral improvements in small, attainable increments.
13. Solicits from the patient or suggests an alternative behavior for a problem situation that can be used and practiced during the behavioral rehearsal or role playing.
14. Evaluates deficits in social perception and problem solving and remedies them.
15. Gives specific attainable and functional homework assignments.

Courtesy of Robert Paul Liberman, M.D., and Jeffrey Bedell, Ph.D.

REFERENCES

Carr JE, Bailey JS. A brief behavior therapy protocol for Tourette syndrome. *J Behav Ther Exp Psychiatry.* 1996;27:33.

Cinciripini PM, Cinciripini LG, Wallfisch A, et al. Behavior therapy and the transdermal nicotine patch: effects on cessation outcome, affect, and coping. *J Consult Clin Psychol.* 1996;64:314.

Collins FL, Thompson JK. The integration of empirically derived personality assessment data into behavioral conceptualization and treatment plan: rationale, guidelines, and caveats. *Behav Modif.* 1993;17:58.

Frea WD, Vittimberga GL. Behavioral interventions for children with autism. In: Austin J, Carr JE, eds. *Handbook of Applied Behavior Analysis.* Reno, NV: Context Press; 2000:247.

Jacob RG, Pelham WH. Behavior therapy. In: Sadock BJ, Sadock VA, eds. *Kaplan & Sadock's Comprehensive Textbook of Psychiatry.* 7th ed. Vol 2. Baltimore: Lippincott Williams & Wilkins; 2000:2080.

Kellner R, Neidhardt J, Krakow B, Pathak D. Changes in chronic nightmares after one session of desensitization or rehearsal instructions. *Am J Psychiatry.* 1992;149:659.

Kohlenberg RJ, Tsai M, Kohlenberg BS. Functional analysis in behavior therapy. *Prog Behav Modif.* 1996;30:1.

Linehan MM. *Cognitive-Behavioral Treatment of Borderline Personality Disorder.* New York: Guilford Press; 1993.

Linehan MM. Behavioral treatments of suicidal behaviors: definitional obfuscation and treatment outcomes. In: Maris RW, Canetto SS, eds. *Review of Suicidology, 2000.* New York: Guilford Press; 2000:84.

McKee MG. Behavioral techniques in pain modification. *Cleve Clin J Med.* 1989;56:502.

Mohr B, Muller V, Mattes R, et al. Behavioral treatment of Parkinson's disease leads to improvement of motor skills and to tremor reduction. *Behav Ther.* 1996;27:235.

Muris P, Merckelbach H. Defense style and behavior therapy outcome in a specific phobia. *Psychol Med.* 1996;26:635.

Sayers JHR, Linehan MM. Treating borderline disorder: dialectical behavior therapy. *TEN.* 2001;3:57.

Stanley MA, Beck JG, Averill PM, Baldwin LE, Deagle EA III, Stadler JG. Patterns of change during cognitive behavioral treatment for panic disorder. *J Nerv Ment Dis.* 1996;184:567.

Waldron HB, Flicker SM. Alcohol and drug abuse. In: Hersen M, ed. *Clinical Behavior Therapy: Adults and Children*. New York: John Wiley & Sons; 2002:474.

▲ 35.7 Cognitive Therapy

Cognitive therapy—according to its originator, Aaron Beck—is "based on an underlying theoretical rationale that an individual's affect and behavior are largely determined by the way in which he structures the world." A person structures the world on the basis of cognitions (verbal or pictorial ideas available to consciousness) that are based on assumptions (schemas developed from previous experiences). According to Beck,

> If a person interprets all his experiences in terms of whether he is competent and adequate, his thinking may be dominated by the schema, "Unless I do everything perfectly, I'm a failure." Consequently, he reacts to situations in terms of adequacy even when they are unrelated to whether or not he is personally competent.

Table 35.7–1 summarizes the general assumptions underlying cognitive therapy.

GENERAL CONSIDERATIONS

Cognitive therapy is a short-term, structured therapy that uses active collaboration between patient and therapist to achieve its therapeutic goals, which are oriented toward current problems and their resolution. Therapy is usually conducted on an individual basis, although group methods are sometimes helpful. A therapist may also prescribe drugs in conjunction with therapy.

Depressive disorders (with or without suicidal ideation) have been the main focus of cognitive therapy; however, cognitive therapy is also used with other conditions, such as panic disorder, obsessive-compulsive disorder, paranoid personality disorder, and somatoform disorders. The treatment of depression can serve as a paradigm of the cognitive approach.

COGNITIVE THEORY OF DEPRESSION

According to the cognitive theory of depression, cognitive dysfunctions are the core of depression, and affective and physical changes and other associated features of depression are consequences of cognitive dysfunctions. For example, apathy and low energy result from a person's expectation of failure in all areas. Similarly, paralysis of will stems from a person's pessimism and feelings of hopelessness. The cognitive triad of depression is a negative self-perception whereby persons see themselves as defective, inadequate, deprived, worthless, and undesirable; they tend to experience the world as negative, demanding, and self-defeating and to expect failure and punishment; and they expect continued hardship, suffering, deprivation, and failure.

The goal of therapy is to alleviate depression and to prevent its recurrence by helping patients to identify and test negative cognitions, to develop alternative and more flexible schemas, and to rehearse both new cognitive and behavioral responses. Changing the way persons think can alleviate the depressive disorder. Table 35.7–2 contrasts examples of typical depressive thinking (termed *primitive thinking* by Beck) with the adaptive (mature) thinking that cognitive therapy attempts to foster.

STRATEGIES AND TECHNIQUES

Therapy is relatively short and lasts up to about 25 weeks. If a patient does not improve in this time, the diagnosis should be reevaluated. Maintenance therapy can be carried out over years. As with other psychotherapies, therapists' attributes are important to successful therapy. Therapists must exude warmth, understand the life experience of each patient, and be genuine and honest with themselves and with their patients. They must be

Table 35.7–1
General Assumptions of Cognitive Therapy

Perception and experiencing in general are active processes that involve both inspective and introspective data.
The patient's cognitions represent a synthesis of internal and external stimuli.
How persons appraise a situation is generally evident in their cognitions (thoughts and visual images).
Those cognitions constitute their stream of consciousness or phenomenal field, which reflects their configuration of themselves, their world, their past and future.
Alterations in the content of their underlying cognitive structures affect their affective state and behavioral pattern.
Through psychological therapy, patients can become aware of their cognitive distortions.
Correction of those faulty dysfunctional constructs can lead to clinical improvement.

Adapted from Beck AT, Rush AJ, Shaw BF, Emery G. *Cognitive Therapy of Depression*. New York: Guilford Press; 1979:47.

Table 35.7–2
Primitive versus Mature Thinking

Primitive Thinking	Mature Thinking
Nondimensional and global: I am fearful.	Multidimensional: I am moderately fearful, quite generous, and fairly intelligent.
Absolutistic and moralistic: I am a despicable coward.	Relativistic and nonjudgmental: I am more fearful than most people I know.
Invariant: I always have been and always will be a coward.	Variable: My fears vary from time to time and from situation to situation.
Character diagnosis: I have a defect in my character.	Behavioral diagnosis: I avoid situations too much, and I have many fears.
Irreversibility: Since I am basically weak, there's nothing that can be done about it.	Reversibility: I can learn ways of facing situations and fighting my fears.

Reprinted with permission from Beck AT, Rush AJ, Shaw BF, Emery G. *Cognitive Therapy of Depression*. New York: Guilford Press; 1979:31.

Table 35.7–3
Cognitive Psychotherapy

Goal	Identify and alter cognitive distortions that maintain symptoms
Selection criteria	Primarily used in dysthymic disorder Nonendogenous depressive disorders Symptoms not sustained by pathological family
Duration	Time-limited, usually 15–25 weeks, once-weekly meetings
Techniques	Collaborative empiricism Structured and directive Assigned readings Homework and behavioral techniques Identification of irrational beliefs and automatic thoughts Identification of attitudes and assumptions underlying negatively biased thoughts

Reprinted with permission from Ursano RJ, Silberman EK. Individual psychotherapies. In: Talbott JA, Hales RE, Yudofsky SC, eds. *The American Psychiatric Press Textbook of Psychiatry.* Washington, DC: American Psychiatric Press; 1988:872.

Table 35.7–4
Cognitive Profile of Psychiatric Disorders

Disorder	Specific Cognitive Content
Depressive disorder	Negative view of self, experience, and future
Hypomanic episode	Inflated view of self, experience, and future
Anxiety disorders	Fear of physical or psychological danger
Panic disorder	Catastrophic misinterpretation of bodily and mental experiences
Phobias	Danger in specific, avoidable situations
Paranoid personality disorder	Negative bias, interference, and so forth by others
Conversion disorder	Concept of motor or sensory abnormality
Obsessive-compulsive disorder	Repeated warning or doubting about safety and repetitive acts to ward off threat
Suicidal behavior	Hopelessness and deficit in problem solving
Anorexia nervosa	Fear of being fat or unshapely
Hypochondriasis	Attribution of serious medical disorder

Courtesy of Aaron Beck, M.D., and A. John Rush, M.D.

able to relate skillfully and interactively with their patients. Cognitive therapists set the agenda at the beginning of each session, assign homework to be performed between sessions, and teach new skills. Therapist and patient collaborate actively (Table 35.7–3). The three components of cognitive therapy are didactic aspects, cognitive techniques, and behavioral techniques.

Didactic Aspects

The therapy's didactic aspects include explaining to patients the cognitive triad, schemas, and faulty logic. Therapists must tell patients that they will formulate hypotheses together and test them over the course of the treatment. Cognitive therapy requires a full explanation of the relationship between depression and thinking, affect, and behavior, as well as the rationale for all aspects of treatment. This explanation contrasts with psychoanalytically oriented therapies, which require little explanation.

Cognitive Techniques

The therapy's cognitive approach includes four processes: eliciting automatic thoughts, testing automatic thoughts, identifying maladaptive underlying assumptions, and testing the validity of maladaptive assumptions.

Eliciting Automatic Thoughts. Automatic thoughts, also called *cognitive distortions,* are cognitions that intervene between external events and a person's emotional reaction to the event. For example, the belief that "people will laugh at me when they see how badly I bowl" is an automatic thought that occurs to someone who has been asked to go bowling and responds negatively. Another example is the thought "she doesn't like me" when someone passes in the hall without saying hello. Every psychopathological disorder has its own specific cognitive profile of distorted thought, which, if known, provides a framework for specific cognitive interventions (Table 35.7–4).

Testing Automatic Thoughts. Acting as a teacher, a therapist helps a patient test the validity of automatic thoughts. The goal is to encourage the patient to reject inaccurate or exaggerated automatic thoughts after careful examination. Patients often blame themselves when things that may well have been outside their control go awry. The therapist reviews the entire situation with the patient and helps reassign the blame or cause of the unpleasant events. Generating alternative explanations for events is another way of undermining inaccurate and distorted automatic thoughts.

Identifying Maladaptive Assumptions. As patient and therapist continue to identify automatic thoughts, patterns usually become apparent. The patterns represent rules or maladaptive general assumptions that guide a patient's life. Samples of such rules are "In order to be happy, I must be perfect" and "If anyone doesn't like me, I'm not lovable." Such rules inevitably lead to disappointments and failure and ultimately to depression (Fig. 35.7–1).

Testing the Validity of Maladaptive Assumptions. Testing the accuracy of maladaptive assumptions is similar to testing the validity of automatic thoughts. In a particularly effective test, therapists ask patients to defend the validity of their assumptions. For example, patients may state that they should always work up to their potential, and a therapist may ask, "Why is that so important to you?" Table 35.7–5 gives examples of some interventions designed to elicit, identify, test, and correct the cognitive distortions that lead to depressive and other painful affects.

Behavioral Techniques

Behavioral and cognitive techniques go hand in hand: Behavioral techniques test and change maladaptive and inaccurate cognitions. The overall purposes of such techniques are to help patients understand the inaccuracy of their cognitive assumptions and learn new strategies and ways of dealing with issues.

Among the behavioral techniques in cognitive therapy are scheduling activities, mastery and pleasure, graded task assign-

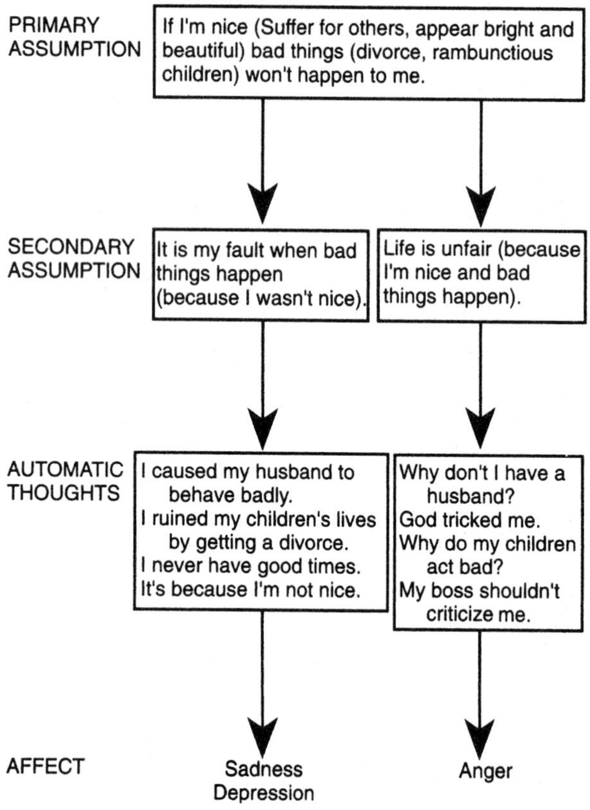

PRIMARY ASSUMPTION
If I'm nice (Suffer for others, appear bright and beautiful) bad things (divorce, rambunctious children) won't happen to me.
SECONDARY ASSUMPTION
It is my fault when bad things happen (because I wasn't nice).
Life is unfair (because I'm nice and bad things happen).
AUTOMATIC THOUGHTS
I caused my husband to behave badly.
I ruined my children's lives by getting a divorce.
I never have good times.
It's because I'm not nice.
Why don't I have a husband?
God tricked me.
Why do my children act bad?
My boss shouldn't criticize me.
AFFECT
Sadness
Depression
Anger

FIGURE 35.7–1

Cognition-affect flowchart. (Reproduced with permission from Beck AT, Rush AJ, Shaw BF, Emery C. *Cognitive Therapy of Depression.* New York: Guilford Press; 1979:33.)

ments, cognitive rehearsal, self-reliance training, role-playing, and diversion techniques. One of the first things done in therapy is scheduling activities on an hourly basis. Patients keep records of the activities and review them with the therapist. In addition to scheduling activities, patients are asked to rate the amount of mastery and pleasure their activities bring them. Patients are often surprised to learn that they have much more mastery of activities and enjoy them more than they had thought.

To simplify the situation and allow miniaccomplishments, therapists often break tasks into subtasks, as in graded task assignments, to show patients that they can succeed. Table 35.7–6 outlines the key features of a graded task assignment as described by Beck. In cognitive rehearsal, patients imagine and rehearse the various steps in meeting and mastering a challenge.

Patients (especially inpatients) are encouraged to become self-reliant by doing such simple things as making their own beds, doing their own shopping, and preparing their own meals. This process is called *self-reliance training.* Role-playing is a particularly powerful and useful technique to elicit automatic thoughts and to learn new behaviors. Diversion techniques are useful in helping patients get through difficult times and include physical activity, social contact, work, play, and visual imagery.

Imagery. The effect of imagery on behavior was first discussed by Paul Schilder in his book *The Image and Appearance of the Human Body.* Schilder described images as having physiological components. When persons visualize themselves running, they subliminally activate the same muscles used in running, which can be measured by electromyography. This phenomenon is used in sports training, in which athletes visualize every conceivable event in a performance and develop a muscle memory for each activity. A combination of behavioral and cognitive theories can help to master anxiety or to deal with feared situations.

Thought stoppage can treat impulsive or obsessive behavior For instance, patients imagine a stop sign with a police officer nearby or another image that evokes inhibition at the same time that they recognize an impulse or obsession that is alien to the ego. Similarly, obesity can be treated by having patients visualize themselves as thin, athletic, trim, and well muscled and then training them to evoke this image whenever they have an urge to eat. Hypnosis or autogenic training can enhance such imag-

Table 35.7–5
Cognitive Errors Derived from Assumptions

Cognitive Error	Assumption	Intervention
Overgeneralizing	If it's true in one case, it applies to any case that is even slightly similar.	Exposure of faulty logic. Establish criteria of which cases are similar to what degree.
Selective abstraction	The only events that matter are failures, deprivation, etc. Should measure self by errors, weaknesses, etc.	Use log to identify successes patient forgot.
Excessive responsibility (assuming personal causality)	I am responsible for all bad things, failures, etc.	Disattribution technique.
Assuming temporal causality (predicting without sufficient evidence)	If it has been true in the past, it's always going to be true.	Expose faulty logic. Specify factors that could influence outcome other than past events.
Self-references	I am the center of everyone's attention—especially my bad performances. I am the cause of misfortunes.	Establish criteria to determine when patient is the focus of attention and also the probable facts that cause bad experiences.
Catastrophizing	Always think of the worst. It's almost likely to happen to you.	Calculate real probabilities. Focus on evidence that the worst did not happen.
Dichotomous thinking	Everything is either one extreme or another (black or white, good or bad).	Demonstrate that events may be evaluated on a continuum.

Reprinted with permission from Beck AT, Rush AJ, Shaw BF, Emery G. *Cognitive Therapy of Depression.* New York: Guilford Press; 1979:48.

Table 35.7–6
Key Features of Graded Task Assignment

Problem definition—e.g., patients' beliefs that they are not capable of attaining goals that are important to them.
Formulation of a project. Stepwise assignment of tasks (or activities) from simple to complex.
Immediate and direct observation by patients that they are successful in reaching a specific objective (carrying out an assigned task). The continual concrete feedback provides patients with new corrective information regarding their functional capacity.
Ventilation of patients' doubts, cynical reactions, and belittling of their achievements.
Encouragement of realistic evaluation by patients of their actual performance.
Emphasis on the fact that patients reached goals as a result of their own efforts and skill.
Devising new, complex assignments in collaboration with the patients.

Adapted from Beck AT, Rush AJ, Shaw BF, Emery G. *Cognitive Therapy of Depression.* New York: Guilford Press; 1979:39.

ery. In a technique called *guided imagery,* therapists encourage patients to have fantasies that can be interpreted as wish fulfillments or attempts to master disturbing affects or impulses.

Table 35.7–7
Cognitions Contributing to Poor Adherence to Medication Prescription

Cognitions about the medication (before taking it):
- It's addicting.
- I am stronger if I don't need medicine.
- I am weak to need it (a crutch).
- It won't work for me.
- If I don't take medication, I'm not crazy.
- I can't stand side effects.
- I'll never get off medication once I start.
- There's nothing I need to do except take medicine.
- I only need to take medication on bad days.

Cognitions about medication (while taking it):
- Since I'm not perfectly well (any better) after days or weeks, the medicine isn't working.
- I should feel good right away.
- The medicine will solve all my problems.
- The medicine won't solve problems, so how can it help?
- I can't stand the dizziness (or fuzziness) or other side effects.
- It makes me into a zombie.

Cognitions about depression:
- I am not ill (I don't need help).
- Only weak people get depressed.
- I deserve to be depressed, since I am a burden to everybody.
- Isn't depression a normal reaction to the bad state of things?
- Depression is incurable.
- I am one of the small percentage who do not respond to any treatment.
- Life isn't worth living, so why should I try to get over my depression?

Reprinted with permission from Beck AT, Rush AJ, Shaw BF, Emery G. *Cognitive Therapy of Depression.* New York: Guilford Press; 1979:72.

Table 35.7–8
Indications for Cognitive Therapy

Criteria that justify the administration of cognitive therapy alone:
- Failure to respond to adequate trials of two antidepressants
- Partial response to adequate dosages of antidepressants
- Failure to respond or only a partial response to other psychotherapies
- Diagnosis of dysthymic disorder
- Variable mood reactive to environmental events
- Variable mood that correlates with negative cognitions
- Mild somatoform disorders (sleep, appetite, weight, libidinal)
- Adequate reality testing (i.e., no hallucinations or delusions), span of concentration, and memory function
- Inability to tolerate medication effects or evidence that excessive risk is associated with pharmacotherapy

Features that suggest cognitive therapy alone is not indicated:
- Evidence of coexisting schizophrenia, dementia, substance-related disorders, mental retardation
- Patient has medical illness or is taking medication that is likely to cause depression
- Obvious memory impairment or poor reality testing (hallucinations, delusions)
- History of manic episode (bipolar 1 disorder)
- History of family member who responded to antidepressant
- History of family member with bipolar 1 disorder
- Absence of precipitating or exacerbating environmental stresses
- Little evidence of cognitive distortions
- Presence of severe somatoform disorders (e.g., pain disorder)

Indications for combined therapies (medication plus cognitive therapy):
- Partial or no response to trial of cognitive therapy alone
- Partial but incomplete response to adequate pharmacotherapy alone
- Poor compliance with medication regimen
- Historical evidence of chronic maladaptive functioning with depressive syndrome on intermittent basis
- Presence of severe somatoform disorders and marked cognitive distortions (e.g., hopelessness)
- Impaired memory and concentration and marked psychomotor difficulty
- Major depressive disorder with suicidal danger
- History of first-degree relative who responded to antidepressants
- History of manic episode in relative or patient

Adapted from Beck AT, Rush AJ, Shaw BF, Emery G. *Cognitive Therapy of Depression.* New York: Guilford Press; 1979:42.

EFFICACY

Cognitive therapy can be used alone in the treatment of mild to moderate depressive disorders or in conjunction with antidepressant medication for major depressive disorder. Studies have clearly shown that cognitive therapy is effective and in some cases is superior or equal to medication alone. It is one of the most useful psychotherapeutic interventions currently available for depressive disorders, and it shows promise in the treatment of other disorders.

Cognitive therapy has also been studied as a way of increasing compliance with lithium (Eskalith) prescription by patients with bipolar I disorder and as an adjunct in treating withdrawal from heroin. Table 35.7–7 summarizes a number of negative cognitions that commonly produce noncompliance with medications. Table 35.7–8 outlines Beck's criteria for determining

Table 35.7–9
Major Features of Three Psychotherapeutic Approaches to Depression

Feature	Psychodynamic Approach	Cognitive Approach	Interpersonal Approach
Major theorists	Freud, Abraham, Jacobson, Kohut	Plato, Adler, Beck, Rush	Meyer, Sullivan, Klerman, Weissman
Concepts of pathology and causes	Ego regression: damaged self-esteem and unresolved conflict caused by childhood object loss and disappointment	Distorted thinking: dysphoria caused by learned negative views of self, others, and the world	Impaired interpersonal relationships: absent or unsatisfactory significant social bonds
Major goals and mechanisms of change	To promote personality change through understanding of past conflicts; to achieve insight into defenses, ego distortions, and superego defects; to provide a role model; to permit cathartic release of aggression	To provide symptomatic relief through alteration of target thoughts; to identify self-destructive cognitions; to modify specific erroneous assumptions; to promote self-control over thinking patterns	To provide symptomatic relief through solution of current interpersonal problems; to reduce stress involving family or work; to improve interpersonal communication skills
Primary techniques and practices	Expressive, empathic; fully or partially analyzing transference and resistance; confronting defenses; clarifying ego and superego distortions	Behavioral cognitive: recording and monitoring cognitions; correcting distorted themes with logic and experimental testing; providing alternative thought content; homework	Communicative, environmental: clarifying and managing maladaptive relationships and learning new ones through communication and social skills training; providing information on illness
Therapist role, therapeutic relationship	Interpreter, reflector: establishment and exploration of transference; therapeutic alliance for benign dependence and empathic understanding	Educator, shaper: positive relationship instead of transference; collaborative empiricism as basis for joint scientific (logical) task	Explorer, prescriber: positive relationship, transference without interpretation; active therapist role for influence and advocacy
Marital, family role	Full individual confidentiality; exclusion of significant others except in life-threatening situations	Use of spouse as objective reporter; couples therapy for disturbed cognitions sustained in marital relationship	Integral role of spouse in treatment: examination of spouse's role in patient's predisposition to depression and effect of illness on marriage

Reprinted with permission from Karasu TB. Psychotherapy for depression. *Am J Psychiatry.* 1990;147:141.

when cognitive therapy is and is not indicated. Table 35.7–9 summarizes and contrasts the major features of three of the most commonly used psychotherapeutic approaches to the treatment of depression, including the cognitive approach.

References

Arntz A, van den Hout M. Psychological treatments of panic disorder without agoraphobia: cognitive therapy versus applied relaxation. *Behav Res Ther.* 1996;34:113.

Asarnow JR, Scott CV, Mintz J. A combined cognitive-behavioral family education intervention for depression in children: a treatment development study. *Cognit Ther Res.* 2002;26:221.

Barlow DH. Cognitive-behavioral approaches to panic disorder and social phobia. *Bull Menninger Clin.* 1992;56(2 suppl A):14.

Beck AT. *Cognitive Therapy and the Emotional Disorders.* New York: International Universities Press; 1976.

Beck AT, Rush AJ, Shaw BF, Emery G. *Cognitive Therapy of Depression.* New York: Guilford Press; 1979.

Carroll KM. Behavioral and cognitive behavioral treatments. In: McCrady BS, Epstein EE, eds. *Addictions: A Comprehensive Guidebook.* New York: Oxford University Press; 1999:250.

Elliott CH, Adams RL, Hodge GK. Cognitive therapy: possible strategies for optimizing outcome. *Psychiatr Ann.* 1992;22:459.

Epstein N, Baucom DH, Rankin LA. Treatment of marital conflict: a cognitive-behavioral approach. *Clin Psychol Rev.* 1993;13:45.

Garner DM, Rockert W, Davis R, Garner MV, et al. Comparison of cognitive-behavioral and supportive-expressive therapy for bulimia nervosa. *Am J Psychiatry.* 1993;150:37.

Hoffart A. Cognitive treatments of agoraphobia: a critical evaluation of theoretical basis and outcome evidence. *J Anxiety Disord.* 1993;7:75.

Juster HR, Heimberg RG, Holt CS. Social phobia: diagnostic issues and review of cognitive behavioral treatment strategies. *Prog Behav Modif.* 1996;30:74.

Liberman RP, Green MF. Whither cognitive-behavioral therapy for schizophrenia? *Schizophr Bull.* 1992;18:27.

Pruitt D. Cognitive therapy: efficacy of current applications. *Psychiatr Ann.* 1992;22:474.

Rush AJ. Cognitive therapy in combination with antidepressant medication. In: Beitman BD, Klerman GL, eds. *Combining Psychotherapy and Drug Therapy in Clinical Practice.* New York: Spectrum; 1984:121.

Rush AJ, Beck AT. Cognitive therapy. In: Sadock BJ, Sadock VA, eds. *Kaplan & Sadock's Comprehensive Textbook of Psychiatry.* 7th ed. Vol 2. Baltimore: Lippincott Williams & Wilkins; 2000:2167.

Salkovskis PM, ed. *Frontiers of Cognitive Therapy.* New York: Guilford Press; 1996.

Scott J. Cognitive therapy of affective disorders: a review. *J Affect Disord.* 1996;37:1.

Thompson LW. Cognitive-behavioral therapy and treatment for late-life depression. *J Clin Psychiatry.* 1996;5:29.

Warwick HMC, Salkovskis PM. Cognitive-behavioral treatment of hypochondriasis. In: Starcevic V, Lipsitt DR, eds. *Hypochondriasis: Modern Perspectives on an Ancient Malady.* New York: Oxford University Press; 2001:314.

▲ 35.8 Hypnosis

Herbert Spiegel, who devised the eye-roll sign for hypnotizability (Fig. 35.8–1), defines *hypnosis* as a state of heightened focal concentration and receptivity. It is typified by a feeling of involuntariness; movements seem automatic, and suggested perceptions can alter or replace ordinary ones. *Hypnosis* has also been described as an altered state of consciousness, a dissociated state, and a state of regression.

Martin Orne defines *hypnosis* as a state or condition in which a person can respond to appropriate suggestions by experiencing altered perceptions, memory, or mood. The essential feature of hypnosis is the subjective experimental change. A pioneer in clinical hypnotic induction, Milton Erickson described the process of a clinical trance as "a free period in which individuality can flourish."

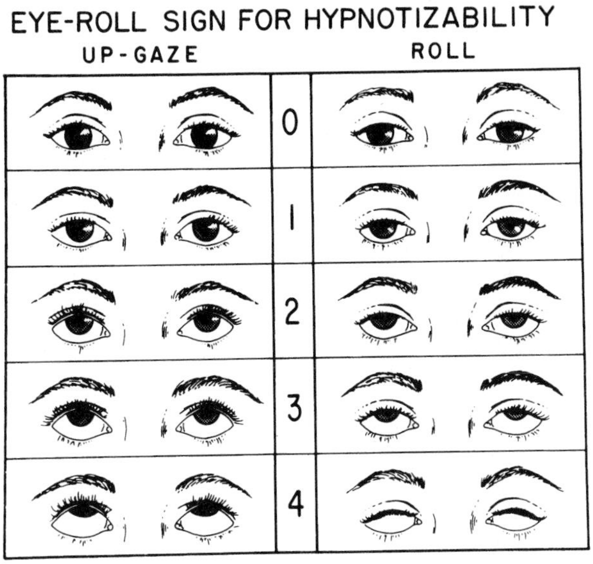

FIGURE 35.8–1

Administration of the Hypnotic Induction Profile can be a routine part of the initial visit and evaluation. The test begins with the eye-roll sign, a presumptive measure of biological ability to experience dissociation. In the test procedure for eye-roll sign measurement, the patient is told "Hold your head looking straight forward; while holding your head in that position, look upward, toward your eyebrows—now toward the top of your head [up-gaze]. While continuing to look upward, close your eyelids slowly [roll]."

The up-gaze and roll are scored on a 0 to 4 scale by observing the amount of sclera visible between the lower eyelid and the lower edge of the cornea. If an internal squint occurs, the degree is scored on a 1 to 3 scale. The squint score is added to the roll score. This procedure takes about 5 seconds. The eye-roll is a part of the hypnotic induction, which is also scored as an initial indicator of the potential for hypnotic experience. (Courtesy of Herbert Spiegel, M.D., Marcia Greenleaf, Ph.D., and David Spiegel, M.D.)

Hypnotherapists perceive clinical hypnosis and therapeutic trance as extensions of common processes in everyday life. Daydreaming and inner preoccupation, during which persons seem to go through the motions of a daily routine automatically, are typical examples. During such periods, persons spontaneously focus attention inward; just as in a trance state, a patient is induced to be receptive to inner experiences. The primary view shared by hypnotherapists and other psychotherapists is an appreciation and understanding of the dynamics of unconscious processes in behavior.

HISTORY

The Austrian physician Friedrich Anton Mesmer (1734–1815) originated the phenomenon of hypnosis, which he called *mesmerism* and believed to be the result of "animal magnetism" or an invisible fluid passing between subject and mesmerizer. A Scottish physician, James Braid (1795–1860), first used the term *hypnosis* (from *hypnos,* the Greek word for "sleep") in the 1840s, to refer to what he thought was a specific state of sleep. In the late 19th century the French neurologist Jean-Martin Charcot (1825–1893) considered hypnotism a special physiological state. His contemporary Hippolyte-Marie Bernheim (1840–1919) believed it to be a psychological state of heightened suggestibility.

Sigmund Freud, who had studied with Charcot, used hypnosis early in his career to help patients recover repressed memories. Freud noted that patients relived traumatic events while under hypnosis, a process known as *abreaction*. Freud later replaced hypnosis with the technique of free association.

Today, hypnosis is used as a form of therapy (hypnotherapy), a method of investigation to recover lost memories, and a research tool.

NEUROPHYSIOLOGICAL CORRELATES OF HYPNOSIS

There are no specific neurophysiological findings in a person who is in a hypnotized state. Unlike a sleeping person, who exhibits typical encephalographic (EEG) changes, a hypnotized person has an EEG that is more similar to that of a fully awake and attentive individual. Some researchers have found increased alpha activity, but this is not a consistent finding. Positron emission tomography (PET) studies have shown some poorly defined functional image changes in the frontal cortex of hypnotized subjects.

HYPNOTIC CAPACITY AND INDUCTION

Therapists can use several specific procedures to help patients be hypnotized and respond to suggestion. These procedures capitalize on naturally occurring hypnosislike phenomena that most persons have probably experienced. But because these experiences are rarely talked about, patients find them fascinating. For example, when discussing hypnosis with a patient, a therapist may ask: "Have you ever had the experience of driving home while thinking about an issue that preoccupies you and suddenly realize that, although you have arrived safe and sound, you can't recall having driven past familiar landmarks? It's as if you had been asleep, and yet you stopped at all the red lights, and you avoided collisions. You were somehow traveling on automatic pilot." Most persons resonate to this experience and are usually happy to describe similar personal experiences.

When patients realize that they have probably undergone hypnosislike episodes, they can understand that they have the capacity to use the hypnotic mode, which is merely an extension of such states. Although the episodes were not necessarily hypnotic states, the extent to which a person experiences them is correlated with hypnotizability. Table 35.8–1 lists a variety of naturally occurring trancelike experiences that can be discussed with patients and that point to the capacity to be hypnotized. Table 35.8–2 illustrates the indicators of trance induction, as set forth by Erickson.

The following is a typical induction protocol (courtesy of William Holt, M.D.) used to induce the trance state. There are many variations of the protocol, some less direct than this one. The one presented here is most likely to be effective in persons with a high hypnotizability potential.

> *Doctor:* Take a long, deep, breath—inhale and exhale; now close your eyes and relax. Pay particular attention to the muscles in and about your eyes—relax them to the point that they just won't work. Are you trying to do that? Good. If you really have them relaxed, right at this very moment, no matter how hard you try, they just won't open. Test them. The harder you try, the faster they stick together, just as if they were glued together. That's fine!

Table 35.8–1
Naturally Occurring Hypnoticlike Experiences and the Percentage of Persons Indicating That They Have Had Such Experiences

Have you ever been in a room full of people, ostensibly taking part in the group yet mentally being far away from it?	90%
Have you ever been unsure whether you did something or just thought about having to do it (e.g., not knowing whether you either mailed a certain letter or just thought about mailing it)?	87%
Have you ever been able to block out sounds from your mind so that they were no longer important to you? Or so that they seemed very far away? Or so that you no longer understood them? Or so that you did not hear them at all?	87%
Have you ever been so lost in thought that you did not understand what people said to you, even when they were talking directly to you and even when you nodded token agreement?	84%
Have you ever been staring off into space, actually thinking of nothing and hardly been aware of the passage of time?	81%
Have you ever had the experience of recollecting a past experience in your life with such clarity and vitality that it was almost like living it again? Or so that it actually seemed identical with living it again?	78%
Have you ever been able to shut out your surroundings from your mind by concentrating very hard on something else?	77%
Have you ever had the experience of reading a novel (or watching a play) and, while doing so, actually forgot yourself, your surroundings, and lived the story with such great reality and vividness that it became temporarily almost reality for you? Or actually seemed to become reality for you?	75%
Have you ever been lulled into a groggy state or put to sleep by a lecture or a concert, even though you were not otherwise fatigued or tired?	73%
Have you ever wandered off in your own thoughts while doing a routine task so that you actually forgot you were doing the task and then found, a few minutes later, that you had completed it without even being aware that you were doing it?	70%

Courtesy of Martin Orne, M.D., Ph.D., and David Dinges, Ph.D.

Now you can open your eyes; that's good. When I tell you to and not before, open and close your eyes once more, and, when you close them this time, you will be 10 times as relaxed as you are right now. Go ahead, open and close, and feel that surge of relaxation go through your whole body, from the top of your head to the tip of your toes. Very good!

Now once again, open and close your eyes, and this time, when you close them, you will double the relaxation that you now have. Fine.

If you have followed my suggestions, right at this very moment, when I lift your hand and let it drop into your lap, it will drop like a wet cloth, heavy and limp. That's very, very good.

You now have good physical relaxation, but medical relaxation consists of two phases: physical, which you now have, and mental, which I will now show you how to achieve.

When I ask you to and not before, I want you to start counting backward from 100. I know you can count; that is not what we're after. I just want you to relax mentally. As you say each number, pause momentarily until you feel a wave of relaxation cover your whole body, from the top of your head to the tip of your toes. When you feel this wave of relaxation, then say the next number, and each time you say a number, you will double the relaxation you had before you said the number. If you do this properly, an interesting thing will happen—as you say the numbers and relax, the succeeding numbers will start to disappear and vanish from your mind. Command your mind to dispel these numbers. Now, aloud and slowly, start counting backward from 100.

Patient: One hundred.

Doctor: Very good.

Patient: Ninety-nine.

Doctor: Make them start to disappear now.

Patient: Ninety-eight.

Doctor: Now they're fading away, and after the next number they'll all be gone. Make them disappear. Let the numbers go.

Patient: Ninety-seven.

Doctor: And now they're all gone. Are they gone? Fine. If there are any numbers still lurking in your mind, when I lift your hand and drop it, they will all disappear.

Table 35.8–2
Indicators of Trance Development

Autonomous ideation
Balanced tonicity (catalepsy)
Changed voice quality
Comfort, relaxation
Economy of movement
Eye changes and closure
Facial features ironed out
Feeling distant
Feeling good after trance
Lack of body movement
Lack of startle response
Literalism
Objective and impersonal ideation
Pupillary changes
Response attentiveness
Retardation of reflexes:
- Swallowing
- Blinking

Sensory, muscular, and body changes
Slowing and loss of blink reflex
Slowing pulse
Slowing respiration
Spontaneous hypnotic phenomena:
- Amnesia
- Anesthesia
- Catalepsy
- Regression

Time distortion
Time lag in motor and conceptual behavior

Reprinted with permission from Erickson M, Rossi EL, Rossi SI. *Hypnotic Realities: The Induction of Clinical Hypnosis and Forms of Indirect Suggestion.* New York: Irvington; 1976:98.

Table 35.8–3
Instructions for the Hypnotic Induction Profile

A. Up-gaze—Without moving your head, look toward me. As you hold your head in that position, look up toward your eyebrows—now, toward the top of your head.

B. Eye-roll—As you continue to look upward, close your eyelids slowly. That's right . . . close. Close, close, close.

C. Squint—(0-1-2-3-4)

D. Eye-roll sign (roll + squint) = (1-2-3-4)

E. Left arm levitation instruction—Take a deep breath, hold . . . Now, exhale, let your eyes relax while keeping the lids closed, and let your body float. Imagine yourself floating, floating right down through the chair . . . There will be something pleasant and welcome about this sensation of floating. As you concentrate on this imaginary floating, I am going to concentrate on your left arm and hand (*touch subject's arm and hand*).

In a while I am going to stroke the middle finger of your left hand. After I do, you will develop movement sensations in that finger, then these movements will spread, causing your left hand to feel light and buoyant, and you will let it float upward. Ready? (*Stroke finger and arm.*)

First one finger, then another. As these restless movements develop, your left hand will lift upward, your elbow bends, your forearm floats into an upright position—just like a balloon. (4) (3) (*You may need to gently encircle the subject's wrist for nonverbal encouragement for the forearm to lift.*) (2–3) Let your hand feel like a balloon. Just let it go. (2) You have the power to let it float upward. That's right. (1) Help it along. Just put it up there. (0) (0-1-2-3-4) × 1/2

Now I am going to position your arm in this manner, so . . . (*Arm is positioned with the elbow comfortably supported on the armrest of the chair and the forearm is in an upright position.*) It will remain in this position even after I give you the signal for your eyes to open. In fact, even after your eyes open, when I put your hand down, it will float right back up to where it is now. You'll find something amusing about this sensation. Later, when I touch your left elbow, your usual sensation and control will return.

In the future, each time you give yourself the signal for self-hypnosis, at the count of one your eyes will roll upward and by three your eyelids will close and you'll be in a relaxed trance state. Each time you'll find the experience easier and easier.

Now, I am going to count backward. At two, again your eyes will roll upward with your eyelids closed. At one let them open very slowly. Ready . . . three . . . two, with your eyelids closed, roll up your eyes and one, let them open slowly. All right, stay in this position and describe what physical sensations you're aware of now in your left hand and arm.

F. Is it comfortable? Are you aware of any tingling sensations?

G. Dissociation—Does your left hand feel *as if* it is not as much a part of your body as your right hand? (Yes = 2) *If patient says "no" ask:* Does your left hand feel as connected to the wrist as your right hand feels connected to the wrist? Is there a difference? (Yes = 1, No = 0)

H. Levitation—postinduction—Now note this—(*gently pull hand down*). (If hand levitates right away = 4) *Continue with reinforcements as needed in 3-second intervals* (*First reinforcement*) Turn your head, look at your left hand, and watch what is going to happen. (3) (*Second reinforcement*) While concentrating on your left hand, imagine it to be a huge buoyant balloon. (2) (*Third reinforcement*) Now, while imagining it to be a balloon, permit it to act out if it were a balloon. That's right, be "big" about it. (1) (*Fourth reinforcement*) This is your chance to be a method actor or dancer. Pretend it's a balloon. If necessary, fake it. That's right, just put it up there. (0)

I. Control differential—While it remains in an upright position, by way of comparison, raise your right hand. Now put your right arm down. Are you aware of a difference in sensation in your right arm going up, compared to your left? For example, does one arm feel lighter or heavier than the other? Are you aware of a relative difference in your sense of control in one arm compared to the other as it goes up? In which arm did you feel more control? *Optional:* On a more or less basis, do you feel a difference in control? (Yes = 2) *If uncertain, ask:* Is it exactly the same, or is there a difference? (Yes = 1) (*If no or still uncertain, re-test.*) (Yes = 1) (No = 0)

J. Cut-off—Now, note this (*touch elbow and lower arm, then tap back of hand while giving instruction*): Make a tight fist, real tight, and now open your fist. Are you aware (*touch elbow second time and stroke arm*) of any change in sensation *now* (*firm pressure on hand*) in your left hand and arm? Lift them both up together and put them both down. Before there was a difference in control. Is that difference still there or is the control becoming equal? (Yes = 2) (*In the event that the cut-off is not complete, continue.*) Make a fist a few times. That's right. Open your fist and now put your hand down. Now, make fists with both hands at the same time. Lift your forearms up a few times and tell me when you feel that your control is equal. (Yes = 1) (*If still No, repeat a few times, score 0.*)

K. Amnesia to cut-off—You see that the relative difference in control that was in your arms is gone. Do you have any idea why? Is there anything I said or did that might account for it? *No or Yes with wrong answer = 2. If patient mentions "elbow," ask:* What about it? *If patient doesn't remember being touched, score 1. If patient specifies "elbow touch" and being touched, ask:* Are you inferring that I touched your elbow or do you remember whether or not I did? *If "infers," score 1. If remembers, ask:* How many times? *If remembers one elbow touch, score 1. If remembers two elbow touches, score 0.*

L. Floating sensation—When your left arm went up before, did you feel a physical sensation that you can describe as a lightness, floating or "buoyancy" in your left arm or hand? Were you aware of similar sensations in any other part of your body—such as your head, neck, chest, abdomen, thighs, legs, or all over—or just in your left hand or arm? *If floating in other parts of body in addition to left hand and arm, score 2. If floating in left hand and/or arm only, score 1. If no floating, score 0.*

Score_____

Profile Grade Score (Eye-Roll Sign Score)_____

_____Intact: ER = 1–4, Lev & CD 1 or more

_____Incremental Intact: Lev 2 pts higher than ER

_____Soft: ER greater than 0, Lev 0, CD 1 or 2

_____Decrement: ER greater than 0, CD = 0

_____Zero: ER = 0, Lev = 0, CD = 0

_____Special Zero: ER = 0, Lev and or CD 1 or more

Courtesy of Herbert Spiegel, M.D., Marcia Greenleaf, Ph.D., and David Spiegel, M.D.

Another technique, used by Herbert Spiegel, is given in Table 35.8–3.

TRANCE STATE

Persons under hypnosis are said to be in a trance state, which may be light, medium, or heavy (deep). In a light trance there are changes in motor activity—persons' muscles can feel relaxed, the hands can levitate, and paresthesia can be induced. A medium trance is characterized by diminished pain sensation and partial or complete amnesia. A deep trance is associated with induced visual or auditory experiences and deep anesthesia. Time distortion occurs at all trance levels but is most profound in the deep trance. Table 35.8–3 summarizes a number of the indicators of a developing and deepening trance state. Patients manifest the indications to differing degrees and in differing combinations.

In posthypnotic suggestion a person is instructed to perform a simple act or experience a particular sensation after awakening from the trance state. The suggestion may cause a person to perceive a bad taste to cigarettes or a particular food and thus can aid in treating nicotine dependence or obesity. Posthypnotic suggestions are associated with deep trance states.

HYPNOTHERAPY

Patients in hypnotic trances can recall memories that are unavailable to consciousness in the nonhypnotic state. In therapy such memories can corroborate psychoanalytic hypotheses about a patient's dynamics or can enable a patient to use such memories as a catalyst for new associations. Some patients can induce age regression, during which they reexperience events that occurred earlier in life. Whether the patient experiences the events as they actually occurred is controversial, but the material elicited can be used to further the therapy. Patients in a trance state may describe an event with an intensity similar to its original occurrence (abreaction) and can feel a sense of relief as a result. Trance states play a role in treating amnestic disorders and dissociative fugue, although clinicians should be aware that bringing repressed memory into consciousness quickly may be hazardous and may overwhelm the patient with anxiety.

Indications and Uses

Hypnosis has been used, with varying degrees of success, to control obesity and substance-related disorders such as alcohol abuse and nicotine dependence. Major surgery has been performed with no anesthetic except hypnosis. Hypnosis has also been applied to managing chronic pain disorder, asthma, warts, pruritus, aphonia, and conversion disorder. Patients can easily achieve relaxation with hypnosis, so they can deal with phobias by controlling their anxiety. Hypnosis can also induce relaxation in systematic desensitization.

Contraindications

Hypnotized patients are in a state of atypical dependence on a therapist; they may develop a strong transference, characterized by a positive attachment that must be respected and interpreted. In other instances a negative transference may erupt in patients who are fragile or who have difficulty testing reality. Patients who have problems about basic trust, such as those with paranoia or patients who dislike giving up control, such as those who are obsessive-compulsive, are not good candidates for hypnosis. A secure ethical value system is important to all therapy, particularly to hypnotherapy, in which patients (especially those in a deep trance) are extremely suggestible and malleable. There is controversy about whether patients can perform acts during a trance state that they otherwise find repugnant or that run contrary to their moral code. Fears about hypnosis still exist, generally due to misinformation.

References

Allison DB, Faith MS. Hypnosis as an adjunct to cognitive-behavioral psychotherapy for obesity: a meta-analytic reappraisal. *J Consult Clin Psychol.* 1996;64:513.

Benson H. Hypnosis and the relaxation response. *Gastroenterology.* 1989;96:1609.

Chaves JF. Hypnosis in the management of anxiety associated with medical conditions and their treatment. In: Mostofsky DI, Barlow DH, eds. *The Management of Stress and Anxiety in Medical Disorders.* Needham Heights, MA: Allyn & Bacon; 2000:119.

Council JR. Hypnosis and response expectancies. In: Kirsch I, ed. *How Expectancies Shape Experience.* Washington, DC: American Psychological Association; 1999:383.

Eisen ML, Quas JA, eds. *Memory and Suggestibility in the Forensic Interview.* Personality and Clinical Psychology Series. Mahwah, NJ: Lawrence Erlbaum Associates; 2002:287.

Erickson M, Rossi EL, Rossi SI. *Hypnotic Realities: The Induction of Clinical Hypnosis and Forms of Indirect Suggestion.* New York: Irvington; 1976.

Gruzelier J. The state of hypnosis: evidence and applications. *Q J Med.* 1996;89:313.

Hilgard E, Hilgard J. *Hypnosis in the Relief of Pain.* Los Altos, CA: Kaufmann; 1983.

Lynn SJ, Vanderhoff H, Shindler K, Stafford J. Defining hypnosis as a trance vs. cooperation: hypnotic inductions, suggestibility, and performance standards. *Am J Clin Hypn.* 2002;44:231.

MacHovec F. Hypnosis complications, risk factors, and prevention. *Am J Clin Hypn.* 1988;31:40.

Orne MT, Dinges DF. Hypnosis. In: Kaplan HI, Sadock BJ, eds. *Comprehensive Textbook of Psychiatry.* 6th ed. Baltimore: Williams & Wilkins, 1996:1807.

Patterson DR, Everett JJ, Burns GL, Marvin JA. Hypnosis for the treatment of burn pain. *J Consult Clin Psychol.* 1992;60:713.

Roelofs K, Hoogduin KA, Keijsers GP, et al. Hypnotic susceptibility in patients with conversion disorder. *J Abnorm Psychol.* 2002;111:390.

Spiegel H, Greenleaf M, Spiegel D. Hypnosis. In: Sadock BJ, Sadock VA, eds. *Kaplan & Sadock's Comprehensive Textbook of Psychiatry.* 7th ed. Vol 2. Baltimore: Lippincott Williams & Wilkins; 2000:2128.

Valbo A, Eide T. Smoking cessation in pregnancy: the effect of hypnosis in a randomized study. *Addict Behav.* 1996;21:29.

▲ 35.9 Psychosocial Treatment and Rehabilitation

Psychosocial treatment and rehabilitation refer to the use of various methods to enable persons who are severely mentally ill to develop social and vocational skills for independent living. Such treatment is carried out at many sites: hospitals, outpatient clinics, mental health centers, day hospitals, and home or social clubs.

SOCIAL SKILLS TRAINING

Social skills are interpersonal behaviors required for community survival, for independence, and for establishing, maintaining, and deepening supportive, socially rewarding relationships. Severe mental disorders such as schizophrenia disrupt one or more affective, cognitive, verbal, and behavioral domains of functioning and impair a person's potential for enjoying and sustaining interpersonal relationships, which are the essence of social life. Clinicians have developed treatment packages

termed *social skills training,* which have proved effective for patients with schizophrenia to remediate deficits in social behaviors.

Methods

Role-playing is the vehicle used to assess a patient's pretreatment social competence and to train targeted behavioral excesses or deficits during treatment. Training scenes are selected on the basis of either an individual's past difficulties or problems that apply to most of the psychiatric population to which the patient belongs. Training sessions vary in length from 45 to 90 minutes, depending on the number of patients participating and their levels of functioning. Although the group format provides both vicarious learning opportunities through observation of other patients' behavior and reinforcement by peers, the group experience is sometimes supplemented by individual training, which allows more intensive focus on a single patient's behavior and an opportunity for more practice in sessions.

Social skills training programs for schizophrenia patients cover skills needed for conversation, conflict management, assertiveness, community living, friendship and dating, work and vocations, and medication management. Each of these skills has several components. For example, assertiveness skills include making requests, refusing requests, making complaints, responding to complaints, expressing unpleasant feelings, asking for information, making apologies, letting someone know you are afraid, and refusing alcohol and street drugs. Each component involves specific steps. Conflict management includes skills in negotiating, compromising, tactful disagreeing, responding to untrue accusations, and leaving overly stressful situations. Table 35.9–1 outlines social skills training for schizophrenia patients.

Table 35.9–1
Social Skills Training in Schizophrenia Patients

Skills	Component Behaviors
Initiating positive comments	
Listening empathically	
Making positive requests for action	
Expressing negative feelings directly	
Coping with unexpected hostility and withdrawal	
Acknowledging pleasing events	Look at the other person
	Pleasant facial expression
	Warm tone of voice
	Say what the other person did or said and how that pleased you
Problem solving	Pinpoint the problem
	Share ownership of the problem
	Generate alternatives
	Weigh pros and cons of each alternative
	Choose a reasonable alternative
	Plan how to implement
	Review and reward progress and efforts

Courtesy of Robert Paul Liberman, M.D.

Goals

In a treatment setting, there are four major goals of social skills training: (1) improved social skills in specific situations, (2) moderate generalization of acquired skills to similar situations, (3) acquisition or relearning of social and conversational skills, and (4) decreased social anxiety. Learning, however, is tedious or almost nonexistent when patients are floridly ill with positive symptoms and high levels of distractibility.

Some findings limit the applicability of social skills training. It is more difficult to teach complex conversational skills than to teach briefer, more discrete verbal and nonverbal responses in social situations. Because complex behaviors are more critical for generating social support in the community, methods have been developed to improve the learning and durability of conversational skills. These training methods, focusing on training in social skills and information-processing skills, are discussed below.

Training in Social Perception Skills. Recently efforts have been made to develop strategies for training patients in affect and social cue recognition. Patients with chronic psychotic disorders such as schizophrenia often have difficulty perceiving and interpreting the subtle affective and cognitive cues that are critical elements of communication. Social perception abilities are considered the first step in effective interpersonal problem solving; difficulties in this area are likely to lead to a cascade of deficits in social behavior. Training skills in social perception address these deficits and help provide a foundation for developing more specific social and coping skills.

Despite attending several social gatherings, Matt felt apart from the rest of the group. He reported that these events seemed like "a jumble of sights and sounds." His therapist, recognizing Matt's difficulty with social perception, gave him a series of questions designed to help him organize and give meaning to the social stimuli he encountered. For example, when Matt was confused about a conversation someone was having with him, he would ask himself, "What is this person's short-term goal? At what level of disclosure should I be? Should I be talking now or listening?" Identifying the rules and goals of a particular social interaction provided a template for Matt to recognize and react to a greater variety of social cues, thus enhancing his behavioral repertoire. (Courtesy of Robert Paul Liberman, M.D., Alex Kopelowicz, M.D., and Thomas E. Smith, M.D.)

Information-Processing Model of Training. Methods of training that follow a cognitive perspective teach patients to use a set of generative rules that can be adapted for use in various situations. For example, a six-step problem-solving strategy has developed as an outline for helping patients overcome interpersonal dilemmas: (1) adopt a problem-solving attitude, (2) identify the problem, (3) brainstorm alternative solutions, (4) evaluate

solutions and pick one to implement, (5) plan the implementation and carry it out, and (6) evaluate the efficacy of the effort and, if ineffective, choose another alternative. While the stepwise, structured, linear process of problem solving occurs intuitively, without conscious awareness in normal persons, it can be a useful interpersonal crutch to help cognitively impaired mental patients cope with the information needed to fill their social and personal needs.

MILIEU THERAPY

The locus of milieu is a living, learning, or working environment. The defining characteristics of treatment are the use of a team to provide treatment and the time the patient spends in the environment. Recent adaptations of milieu therapy include 24-hour-a-day programs situated in community locales frequented by patients, which provide in vivo support, case management, and training in living skills.

Table 35.9–2
Contingencies of Reinforcement in the Token Economy Used at the Camarillo-UCLA Clinical Research Unit[a]

Token earnings	
Morning rising from bed and getting dressed on time	3
Satisfactory completion of morning activities of daily living	3
Satisfactory participation in a social skills training group or recreational therapy activity	10
Satisfactory participation in individual behavioral therapy session	10
Satisfactory participation in leisure time activities (per activity)	5
Meets criteria for dress and grooming checks during day (per check)	3
Showers satisfactorily	3
Completes assigned jobs or tasks on unit (per job or task)	4
Participates in off-unit vocational rehabilitation or adult education activity (per half-day)	10
Token fines	
Smoking rule violation	5
Lying on floor	5
Stealing	10
Forgery of token credit card	10
Assault or property destruction	20
Late return from grounds privileges	20
Reinforcers available for tokens	
Cigarettes	4
Drinks (coffee, tea, sodas, hot chocolate)	10
Snacks (potato chips, pretzels, ice cream, candy)	10
Grounds privileges (per half-hour)	4
Music time (per half-hour)	4
Private room time (per half-hour)	4
Nintendo, Walkman stereo, private TV (per half-hour)	4

[a]This token economy uses a card that can be punched with holes to document token earnings and purchases. The token economy has three levels, which differ in the immediacy and type of reinforcement and privileges. At the highest level of performance, the patient carries a "credit card" and has full access to all unit privileges and rewards without having to pay with tokens.
Courtesy of Robert Paul Liberman, M.D.

Most milieu therapy programs emphasize group and social interaction; rules and expectations are mediated by peer pressure for normalization of adaptation. When patients are viewed as responsible human beings, the patient role becomes blurred. Milieu therapy stresses a patient's rights to goals and to have freedom of movement and informal relationship with staff; it also emphasizes interdisciplinary participation and goal-oriented, clear communication.

Token Economy. The use of tokens, points, or credits as secondary or generalized reinforcers can be seen as normalizing a mental hospital or day hospital environment with a program mimicking society's use of money to meet instrumental needs. Token economies establish the rules and culture of a hospital inpatient unit or partial hospitalization program, offering coherence and consistency to the interdisciplinary team as it struggles to promote therapeutic progress in difficult patients. These programs are challenging to establish, however, and their widespread dissemination has suffered because of the organizational prerequisites and the additional resources and rewards needed to create a truly positively reinforcing environment. Table 35.9–2 lists behaviors that are reinforced by tokens.

PSYCHOSOCIAL CLUBHOUSES AND SELF-HELP PROGRAMS

Psychosocial self-help programs emerged during the late 1940s when expatients began to meet together in so-called social clubs to satisfy their needs for acceptance and emotional support. Emphasizing self-help, mutual interdependence, and reliance on assets, the movement led to the establishment of Fountain House and hundreds of similar programs throughout the United States. Instead of thinking of themselves as patients, these expatients became members and formed groups and teams to accomplish tasks, plan activities, and solve problems, and in so doing, they improved the quality of their lives. Creating their own social support network, members of psychosocial clubs design activities that build experiences of mutual ownership and needs. Staff members, primarily nonprofessionals or those trained in vocational rehabilitation, provide positive, accepting reactions and require members to obtain psychiatric treatment, such as medication, elsewhere. Thus, the club has rehabilitation goals, not clinical goals. During the day, members of the club spend time engaging in activities such as chores, operating a snack bar, assisting each other in banking and budgeting, visiting friends who are hospitalized, printing a newspaper, helping each other with entitlements from social agencies, manning a thrift shop, working the switchboard, or refurbishing cooperative apartments.

VOCATIONAL TRAINING

An important part of psychosocial rehabilitation is enabling persons to work. Job placements are located in normal places of business, from large corporations to small businesses; they are at the entry level and require minimal training or skills. These jobs are opportunities to work temporarily en route to full-time employment elsewhere or longer-term employment in the entry-level position. The number of transitional employment programs for mentally ill persons in the United States has grown, with over 500 employers involved in providing wages in excess of $4 mil-

lion. An 18-month follow-up evaluation of persons working in transitional jobs revealed that 16 percent were employed independently on a full-time basis, and an additional 45 percent continued part-time work in the transitional program or were attending school or other training programs. Only 2 percent were in psychiatric hospitals at the 18-month follow-up.

COMBINING PSYCHOSOCIAL AND DRUG THERAPIES

In a disorder such as schizophrenia, where the biological diathesis runs deep, most patients need combined drug and psychosocial treatments. Evidence from many studies supports the conclusion that when combined with antipsychotic drugs, psychosocial treatments offer greater protection against relapse and better social adjustment than either drugs or psychosocial treatment alone. The consensus of these studies is that drugs have a primary effect on cognitive disorganization and positive symptoms of schizophrenia and less impact on psychosocial functioning. The opposite seems to be the case with social and psychosocial therapies. In combination, their beneficial impact on the comprehensive needs of patients with schizophrenia is additive. A therapist, therefore, must be able to provide both biological and psychosocial care to respond professionally to the needs of schizophrenic patients. If a therapist is not a psychiatrist, close collaboration with a psychiatrist is necessary so that medication may be managed appropriately.

Bill was a 23-year-old man with a 5-year history of schizophrenia. He had been resistant to taking medication due to the adverse effects he had experienced, including severe akathisia, tremors, and muscle stiffness. He acknowledged that these medications had diminished his psychotic symptoms and improved his attention and concentration but resisted efforts to become more compliant with prescribed regimens. He also related that some of his psychotic symptoms, particularly auditory hallucinations, persisted at a low level despite altered dosages and types of medications. Bill had been hospitalized an average of three times a year for psychotic exacerbations since the onset of his illness. He said that all efforts to treat him "missed the boat" and that staff had not attended to his own goals and ambitions.

At this point, staff engaged Bill in a goal-setting process, in which he identified targets of living independently without being hospitalized, taking little or no medication, and eventually getting a job. His psychiatrist and social worker accepted these goals as laudable and set out to establish clear and measurable landmarks to gauge his success in pursuing these aims. They then worked with Bill to identify his personal resources and the obstacles he faced in attaining his goals. Bill said that the most frustrating problem was his lack of understanding about his illness and its treatment, because this led to frequent relapses and concomitant life disruption.

Bill's psychiatrist and social worker next enrolled him in a class designed to increase his understanding of his illness and the medications used to treat it. He gained a good working knowledge of how these medications caused the adverse effects he found so intolerable, and he learned communication skills that would help him effectively negotiate the type and dosage of his medication. Following this, he worked with his psychiatrist and agreed to a trial of an atypical antipsychotic. He noticed that the new medication resulted in much less discomfort from extrapyramidal adverse effects. Finally, he was taught coping methods—such as humming and reducing social stimulation—to manage the persisting auditory hallucinations he experienced. This gave Bill a sense of mastery over his illness, and he adhered to his medication regimen. During the next year, he experienced two minor relapses but sought help from treatment personnel early in the prodromes of these relapses and did not require rehospitalization. (Courtesy of Robert Paul Liberman, M.D., Alex Kopelowicz, M.D., and Thomas E. Smith, M.D.)

REFERENCES

Beitchman PD. Psychosocial rehabilitation in residential programs for adults. *Int J Ment Health.* 1996;24:52.

Chwalisz K, Vaux A. Social support and adjustment to disability. In: Frank RG, Elliott TR, eds. *Handbook of Rehabilitation Psychology.* Washington, DC: American Psychological Association; 2000:537.

DeLeon G, Melnick G, Tims FM. The role of motivation and readiness in treatment and recovery. In: Tims FM, Leukefeld CG, eds. *Relapse and Recovery in Addictions.* New Haven: Yale University Press; 2001:143.

Dobson DJ, McDougall G, Busheikin J, Aldous J. Effects of social skills training and social milieu treatment on symptoms of schizophrenia. *Psychiatr Serv.* 1995;46:376.

Dowdy A. Vocational rehabilitation and special education: partners in transition for individuals with learning disabilities. *J Learn Disabil.* 1996;29:137.

Fisher DB. Health care reform based on an empowerment model of recovery of people with psychiatric disabilities. *Hosp Community Psychiatry.* 1994;45:913.

Glueckauf RL, Liss HJ, McQuillen DE, et al. Therapeutic alliance in family therapy for adolescents with epilepsy: an exploratory study. *Am J Fam Ther.* 2002;30:125.

Green MF. Cognitive remediation in schizophrenia: is it time yet? *Am J Psychiatry.* 1993;150:178.

Liberman RP, Kopelowicz A, Smith TE. In: Sadock BJ, Sadock VA, eds. *Kaplan & Sadock's Comprehensive Textbook of Psychiatry.* 7th ed. Vol 2. Baltimore: Lippincott Williams & Wilkins; 2000:3218.

Littrell KH. Psychopharmacology and social reintegration. In: Breier A, Tran PV, eds. *Current Issues in the Psychopharmacology of Schizophrenia.* Philadelphia: Lippincott Williams & Wilkins; 2001:556.

Lynch TR, Morse JQ, Vitt CM. Dialectical behavior therapy for depressed older adults. *Behav Ther.* 2002;25:7.

Penk W, Flannery RB Jr. Psychosocial rehabilitation. In: Foa EB, Keane TM, eds. *Effective Treatments for PTSD: Practice Guidelines from the International Society for Traumatic Stress Studies.* New York: Guilford Press; 2000:224.

Piper WE, Joyce AS. Psychosocial treatment outcome. In: Livesey WJ, ed. *Handbook of Personality Disorders: Theory, Research, and Treatment.* New York: Guilford Press; 2001:323.

Reddon JR, Pope GA, Dorias S, Pullan MD. Improvement in psychosocial adjustment for psychiatric patients after a 16-week life skills education program. *J Clin Psychol.* 1996;52:169.

Sinha R, Schottenfeld R. The role of comorbidity in relapse and recovery. In: Tims FM, Leukefeld CG, eds. *Relapse and Recovery in Addictions.* New Haven: Yale University Press; 2001:172.

Weiden P, Havens L. Psychotherapeutic management techniques in the treatment of outpatients with schizophrenia. *Hosp Community Psychiatry.* 1994;45:549.

▲ 35.10 Combined Psychotherapy and Pharmacotherapy

Surveys of psychiatrists in clinical practice suggest that most psychiatric patients receive both medication and psychotherapy. These two modalities are often administered by two separate clinicians because of managed care arrangements that tend to reim-

burse a psychiatrist for medication management and a nonpsychiatrist mental health professional for psychotherapy. In other cases a psychiatrist may provide both psychotherapy and pharmacotherapy. Few residency training programs teach integrated treatment in a systematic way, however, so often the psychiatrist who combines the treatments in a one-person model may have little instruction about the optimal approach to integration.

Psychiatry is the ultimate biopsychosocial specialty, and regardless of whether psychiatrists are involved in one-person or two-person models of treatment, they should have an overarching view of the patient that takes into account biology, psychology, and sociocultural aspects of both diagnosis and treatment. In practice, the biological and the psychosocial often intersect in the thoughtful combination of psychotherapeutic and pharmacotherapeutic approaches. Psychotherapeutic interventions and medication often interact in highly complex ways. In the ensuing discussion, these interactions are explored, and the practical clinical implications are outlined. In addition, the literature on combined treatment for a variety of disorders is reviewed, and the economics of divided versus integrated treatment is considered.

PSYCHOTHERAPEUTIC MANAGEMENT

In conceptualizing how psychotherapeutic intervention and medication work together, two general strategies can be delineated. One is the psychotherapeutic management inherent in skilled pharmacotherapy practice. The other is the combination of formal psychotherapy and the prescription of medication.

In considering the former, a good starting point is the *American Psychiatric Association Practice Guidelines on Depression,* which points out that "psychotherapeutic management" is an essential component of every medication-based treatment plan. In fact, one indication that good clinical management has psychotherapeutic effects is the recurrent finding that a placebo condition in a controlled trial is often an effective treatment for a significant number of patients. Simply by asking about symptoms and taking a history, clinicians often help patients become aware of connections among external events, the meaning of these events, and symptoms, which lead them to insight about their illness. In addition, having a caring physician listen and provide help may be a powerful corrective emotional experience for some patients. Another mechanism of action may involve the so-called transference cure, in which a patient gets better to please the physician.

Many psychodynamic principles derived from psychotherapy apply equally to pharmacotherapy practice. A pharmacotherapeutic alliance is essential to ensure that a patient understands the reason for medication and complies with the treatment plan, just as a psychotherapeutic alliance is essential to enlist a patient as a collaborator in psychotherapy. Other dynamic principles, such as transference, resistance, and countertransference, are also integral parts of the pharmacotherapy practice. Many problems with noncompliance can be traced to these principles. The application of psychodynamic constructs to compliance problems in pharmacotherapy is often referred to as *dynamic pharmacotherapy.*

The phenomenon of transference is not limited to psychotherapy. In clinical practice, patients routinely attribute qualities that stem from figures in their past to the prescribing physician. Patients may perceive a psychiatrist as authoritarian and refuse to cooperate with the prescribed treatment plan because he or she reminds them of a parent barking orders and trying to control them. If the psychiatrist feels irritated with patients for not cooperating and becomes more insistent, the problem may worsen because the clinician is behaving in the authoritarian manner the patient fears. In this case, the psychiatrist's countertransference has entered into the equation and has affected the patient's capacity to collaborate in a good alliance.

Resistance to taking medication can often relate to issues of transference and countertransference or to a fundamental ambivalence about getting better. In particular, some patients with depression may feel that they have committed such sinful and evil acts that they deserve to be punished by remaining depressed. For them, an antidepressant medication may have a specific meaning, such as the potential to relieve suffering, and they may not fill their prescription or take the tablets as prescribed.

Medication may be imbued with a myriad of other meanings. Many patients think of medication as a crutch. They may make no distinction between being addicted to a narcotic and taking a maintenance dose of antidepressant medication. Some patients interpret needing the medication as a sign of weakness and will discontinue taking it on their own as soon as their symptoms start to lift. For still other patients, the medication has meaning connected with a family member.

Optimal psychotherapeutic management of a pharmacotherapy patient involves attention to these psychological dimensions of the relationship and to the medication itself. In addition, clinicians must empathize with patients' perceptions of medication and try to appreciate its meaning for each patient. Good listening skills, attention to rapport, and a systematic effort to establish a good alliance based on careful explanations are all integral parts of this approach to pharmacotherapy.

MEDICATION IN COMBINATION WITH FORMAL PSYCHOTHERAPY

In clinical practice today, the combined use of medication and psychotherapy is widely accepted. Even among psychoanalysts, who were once the most vocal critics of combined treatment, prescribing is commonplace. In a survey of members of the American Academy of Psychoanalysts, 90 percent of respondents said they were prescribing medications. In a study of psychoanalytic candidate training cases at the Columbia University Center for Psychoanalytic Training and Research, medication was combined with psychoanalysis in 29 percent of cases. This fact indicates that medication is no longer seen as a contaminant that interferes with certification or graduation.

Many analysts and other therapists have noted that medication and psychotherapy work synergistically to improve outcomes in a wide variety of illnesses. Investigations of outcome geared to specific disorders generally demonstrate advantages to combined approaches.

Specific Diagnostic Categories

Schizophrenia. An extensive series of studies has examined the rate of relapse when a specific form of psychoeducational family therapy is combined with antipsychotic

medication. This intervention is based on the observation that high levels of expressed emotion (EE) in the families of patients with schizophrenia predicted a relapse following hospital discharge. High EE families have been characterized as excessively intrusive, critical, and overinvolved with the patient who suffers from schizophrenia. Psychoeducational family therapy is aimed at helping the family reduce the factors that constitute EE and educating the family about the disease of schizophrenia and the need to continue antipsychotic medication indefinitely.

In a follow-up study by a team of investigators led by Gerald Hogarty, the impact of family therapy on relapse prevention was just as significant as the impact of antipsychotic medication. In other words, the relapse rate was cut in half by the addition of antipsychotic drugs and was reduced by half again when family psychoeducational therapy was combined with drugs. The relapse rate was even further reduced at 1-year follow-up when social skills training was added to family therapy and medication. Recent research has suggested that group treatment involving families is also successful in reducing relapse rates and is even more cost-effective than single-family therapy.

Major Depressive Disorder. Combined psychotherapy and medication has been most extensively studied in persons suffering from major depression. A study of 107 elderly patients who were randomly assigned to either nortriptyline (Aventyl), placebo, monthly maintenance interpersonal therapy with placebo, or monthly maintenance interpersonal therapy and nortriptyline, found a clear advantage for combined treatment. Recurrence rates over the 3-year period of the study were only 20 percent when interpersonal therapy and nortriptyline were combined, compared with 64 percent in the group that received interpersonal therapy and placebo, and 43 percent in the group that received medication alone.

In a large study of persons with chronic nonpsychotic major depression, 519 subjects were randomly assigned to either nefazodone (Serzone), the cognitive-behavioral analysis system of psychotherapy, or the combination of the two. Eighty-five percent in the combined treatment group had positive responses, compared with only 52 percent in the group who received psychotherapy alone and 55 percent in the group who received nefazodone alone.

Some data suggest that medication and psychotherapy may work on different target symptoms and at different rates. Patients in both interpersonal therapy and cognitive-behavior therapy report significantly greater capacity to establish and maintain interpersonal relationships and to recognize and understand sources of their depression than patients on antidepressant medication or placebo alone. Hence, use of both modalities may increase the breadth of the response. The combination appears to be particularly effective in more severely distressed patients; it is more difficult to demonstrate a clear advantage of combined treatment over either modality alone in patients with mild to moderate depression.

Bipolar I Disorder. Much less controlled research has been conducted on combined treatments of bipolar I disorder, although there is a growing consensus that psychosocial interventions are essential in treating most patients. A German study looked at the relapse rates in 20 patients with bipolar disorder and in 10 patients with schizoaffective disorder before and after treatment with systemic family therapy in conjunction with medication. The average duration of treatment was 14.7 months, with a range of 0 to 35 months, and the average number of sessions was 6.60, with a range of 1 to 19. The relapse rate was measured by the number of hospitalizations during the observation period. Following family therapy, there was a 77.6 percent reduction of relapse in the total sample (67.8 percent for patients with bipolar disorder and 89.8 percent for patients with schizoaffective disorder).

This statistically significant reduction in relapse rate was accompanied by a low rate of hospitalization. Before family therapy, only 1 of 30 patients required no hospitalization whatsoever. After family therapy, 14 of 30 patients required no hospitalization. Because only an average 6.6 sessions of family therapy were required, this intervention was also highly effective in reducing hospital costs.

Several characteristics were noted in the families with improved relapse rates. Most significantly, no longer did either the patients or their family members view the patients as victims of an illness beyond their control. Both family members and patients felt empowered and had gained a sense of mastery over the illness.

With the increasing awareness that lithium (Eskalith) alone is not effective prophylaxis for many patients with bipolar disorders, individual psychotherapy has been added to increase occupational and social functioning, encourage compliance with lithium or other mood stabilizers, and cut through the denial that is so common in bipolar patients. Many patients deny that their mania or hypomania is part of their illness and insist that it is simply part of who they are. Others manifest a form of psychic discontinuity in which the manic "self" is split from the euthymic "self," as though the two are in no way connected. Some clinicians use video- or audiotapes of patients during a manic episode to help them integrate this aspect of themselves as part of the illness and overcome their denial. Bipolar disorder patients may also need assistance in mourning losses they have incurred through their erratic behavior during manic episodes.

Two studies have demonstrated that addition of a psychotherapeutic intervention improves compliance with medication. Many patients have acknowledged that psychotherapy has been an important adjunct in their overall treatment.

Panic Disorder. An elegantly conducted randomized controlled trial demonstrated that combining cognitive-behavioral therapy and imipramine (Tofranil) for the treatment of panic disorder provides clear advantage at long-term follow-up, compared with either treatment alone. No advantage of combining treatments is demonstrable when a combination of behavior therapy and benzodiazepines is compared with either modality alone.

A Scandinavian study compared clomipramine (Anafranil) alone for patients with panic disorder with clomipramine and 15 weekly sessions of dynamic psychotherapy. All patients in both treatment groups were panic free within 26 weeks. On termination of clomipramine after 9 months, the relapse rate was significantly lower in the clomipramine-psychotherapy group. The investigators concluded that dynamic therapy reduces psychosocial vulnerability associated with panic disorder.

Selected patients may require couples or family therapy in combination with medication, behavior therapy, or both.

A middle-aged woman was virtually housebound because of her anxiety about having a panic attack in the shopping mall. Her husband had adapted to her disorder to a large extent, and he frequently performed routine tasks such as grocery shopping for her. When she was successfully treated with exposure plus imipramine, she described deterioration in her marital relationship. The treating psychiatrist asked her to bring her husband with her to the sessions. It soon became apparent that her husband was highly ambivalent about her improvement because he was convinced that she would be attracted to another man when she went out shopping and would have an extramarital affair. His jealous rage had led him to become extremely controlling of his wife at home, and she was wondering whether it would be better if she just returned to being housebound again.

This case vignette reflects how a couple can reach an equilibrium around an illness. Without attention to the marital issues that support and maintain a disorder, there is little likelihood that improvement will be lasting.

Obsessive-Compulsive Disorder. Treatment of obsessive-compulsive disorder usually takes one of two directions. Selective serotonin reuptake inhibitors (SSRIs) often make significant symptomatic improvements in patients. Clomipramine is also useful, but troublesome adverse effects make SSRIs the preferred agents. About three quarters of patients who comply with behavior therapy and consciously apply the techniques show sustained improvement in symptoms.

Because the improvements effected by SSRIs are limited in terms of overall symptom reduction in patients who relapse rapidly when the agents are discontinued, a strong case can be made for combining behavior therapy and SSRIs. Some studies suggest both short-term and long-term improvements as well as more rapid response when both treatments are used. Behavior therapy, of course, also holds out the possibility of stopping the medication without relapsing.

Despite some suggestive data, however, the reports published so far are not entirely convincing about the advantages of combined medication and behavior therapy. Overall, combining treatments appears to yield a better outcome than medication alone but not necessarily than behavior therapy alone. Nevertheless, behavior therapy to maintain robust results costs the patient time, energy, and money. Daily therapy sessions are usually conducted for several weeks. When the sessions are over, patients are expected to devote a good deal of their day to exposure work. Hence, it may not always be practical to provide behavior therapy at this intensity, and many patients may benefit with less intense exposure accompanied by the use of SSRIs.

Substance Dependence. Both psychotherapy and methadone (Dolophine) have shown encouraging success with opioid-dependent patients. Data are also accumulating that indicate even better outcomes with the combination of the two approaches. In a randomized, controlled trial comparing treatments, opioid-dependent patients were assigned to one of three groups. One group had only methadone and virtually no psychotherapy. The second group had methadone along with meetings with a counselor, which were oriented toward behavioral interventions. The third group had enhanced services involving the same dose of methadone and the same form of counseling, but patients also received additional resources, including a half-time employment counselor, a full-time psychiatrist, and a half-time family therapist.

Analysis of the results of this trial showed that the groups receiving psychotherapy had greater earning power, less welfare income, and strikingly lower hospital rates than the group that did not receive psychotherapy. In addition, a beneficial impact on costs could be inferred because of the reduced rate of hospitalization when psychotherapy was added. The investigators also noted that the incremental value of enhanced services over simple counseling in the second group indicated that family therapy, the presence of a psychiatrist, and employment counseling were highly useful interventions.

Attention-Deficit/Hyperactivity Disorder (ADHD). The combination of methylphenidate (Ritalin) and intensive behavioral treatment was recently tested in a randomized controlled trial, which used methylphenidate alone as the control treatment. While the combination did not necessarily display significantly greater benefits than methylphenidate alone for the core symptoms of ADHD, it provided modest advantages for positive functioning outcomes and for non-ADHD symptoms.

Eating Disorders. Both medication and psychotherapy are commonly used in the treatment of patients with eating disorders. A study comparing cognitive-behavioral therapy plus an antidepressant with each treatment alone found that the combined treatment resulted in greater improvement in binge eating and depression than a placebo and psychological treatment or an antidepressant alone.

Borderline Personality Disorder. Although both psychotherapy and pharmacotherapy have been shown to be effective in the treatment of symptoms associated with borderline personality disorder, the combination of the two approaches has not been systematically investigated. Nevertheless, an evolving clinical literature suggests that the optimal strategy with such patients is to combine psychotherapy and medication.

Psychopharmacological intervention with borderline personality disorder is a new field of study, and some preliminary data indicate that certain medications may serve as valuable adjuncts to psychotherapy. Because the symptoms of the disorder vary, a target-symptom approach is generally recommended. Problems of cognitive dyscontrol, such as brief paranoid states, often respond well to low-dose neuroleptics. Problems related to impulsivity and behavioral dyscontrol may respond well to carbamazepine (Tegretol) or perhaps lithium carbonate.

Many patients with borderline personality disorder are comorbid for major depressive disorder on Axis I. Tricyclic drugs have not been shown to be effective with these patients, but monoamine oxidase inhibitors have shown some promise, particularly for patients with atypical depression involving so-called paradoxical symptoms, such as hyperphagia and hypersomnia. In addition, recent double-blind controlled studies are highly encouraging about the use of SSRIs. In one study,

patients receiving fluoxetine (Prozac) showed improvement in a wide range of areas, including depression, anxiety, paranoia, psychoticism, interpersonal sensitivity, obsessionality, hostility, and global functioning, compared with the placebo group.

A second study using fluoxetine indicated that the intense anger of patients with borderline personality disorder appears to be positively affected by the medication. Hence, when SSRIs are used in conjunction with psychotherapy, patients may be able to reflect and think more clearly because the anger and other intense affects are toned down by the medication. This improvement in affective regulation may allow patients to collaborate with therapists more effectively.

One of the central features of borderline psychopathology is difficulty tolerating aloneness. During a therapist's vacations, some borderline patients begin to deteriorate: Because of a lack of object constancy, they develop anxieties that their therapist has disappeared and will never come back. Pills prescribed by the psychotherapist may serve as a transitional object that represents the therapist during his or her absence. Some patients will look at the pill or the name of the therapist on the label and experience a soothing effect.

Finally, the literature suggests that at least half of borderline patients misuse prescription drugs. Psychotherapy in combination with medication may be effective in uncovering the meanings of the medication misuse and in exploring the transference manifestations of these forms of acting-out behavior. Because suicidality is a frequent problem with these patients, a therapist's psychotherapeutic understanding may also help prevent overdoses with prescribed medication.

CLINICAL CONSIDERATIONS

In considering various combinations of pharmacotherapy and psychotherapy, two models are commonly used in clinical practice today. The one-person model involves a psychiatrist conducting the psychotherapy and prescribing medication for the same patient at the same time. The two-person model divides the functions so that the clinician conducting psychotherapy and the physician prescribing medication are separate individuals. There are, of course, practical considerations in deciding which model to use. If a psychotherapist does not feel competent to prescribe certain medications, a psychopharmacology consultant must be involved. Conversely, if a psychopharmacologist does not feel sufficiently skilled to provide the psychotherapy, the patient must be referred to a separate psychotherapist. A managed care company may stipulate for economic reasons that a psychotherapist can see the patient for only 15 minutes to prescribe while psychotherapy is carried out with a less expensive nonmedical therapist. In another common situation, psychotherapy begins with a nonmedical therapist, the patient becomes depressed, and a consultation by a psychopharmacologist is then requested. Assuming, however, for purposes of discussion, that a psychiatrist is the primary treater and is competent at both treatment modalities, several factors must be taken into account in deciding which approach to recommend.

One-Person Model

Just like a physicist who simultaneously thinks in terms of particles and waves, a psychiatrist must think about a dysfunctional brain and a distressed mind as part of a unified whole. In practice, this may require flexible shifting back and forth between an empathic, introspective, subjective approach on the one hand and an objective, descriptive approach on the other. Although psychotherapy often encourages verbalization as opposed to action, prescription of medication requires clear action on the part of the clinician (and the patient). Moreover, direct questions must be asked to elicit information about symptoms and adverse effects in contrast to a more open-ended approach of allowing the patient to set the agenda in a dynamic therapy process.

In addition, whereas a dynamic therapist may eschew an authoritarian posture vis-à-vis a patient, this position may shift when discussing medication and citing the literature on such things as maintenance doses and prevention of relapse. Both patient and clinician may need to shift mental sets in the course of a session.

One strategy for managing these difficulties is to set aside a few minutes at the beginning or end of each session to review how the medication is affecting the symptoms and to write a prescription, if necessary. During the remainder of the session, the medication may be discussed from the standpoint of its meaning to the patient. Indeed, one of the advantages in this arrangement is that the prescribing and the psychotherapy do not get split from one another in a way that fragments treatment. All transferences and resistances are dealt with by one clinician. Compliance problems may be readily linked to specific transference paradigms because of the clinician's intimate knowledge of the patient's internal object relations.

Two-Person Model

Surveys have shown that approximately 65 percent of psychiatrists have provided medication for patients who are in psychotherapy with other clinicians. In some cases, of course, two clinicians must be involved because one is a nonmedical therapist. In other cases, however, psychiatrists who are conducting psychotherapy do not feel comfortable with the kind of bimodal thinking necessary to prescribe medication as well. They may prefer to keep the transference uncontaminated by feelings about the medication, and they may also not feel qualified to prescribe because they have not kept up with psychopharmacology data.

The two-person model may be effective for some patients, but it also runs the risk of serving as a nidus for splitting, particularly, although not exclusively, with borderline patients.

A 27-year-old woman with a diagnosis of borderline personality disorder had been seeing a psychotherapist once weekly for 1 year. She and her therapist had felt that they were at an impasse, and the therapist suggested that she might seek consultation with a local psychopharmacologist. She saw the psychopharmacologist for 30 minutes, and he diagnosed her disorder as major depression. He explained the illness to her and prescribed fluoxetine.

The patient felt an almost immediate positive response to the medication, and at her next psychotherapy appointment, she blasted her psychotherapist with a long tirade about her

inadequacies: "You sit there for 1 year, just listening and trying to understand me. All this time I had a depression that needed drug treatment. Dr. A. (her psychopharmacologist) was so helpful. He took my complaints seriously, and for God's sake, he took some action! All you do is talk, talk, talk. Why didn't it occur to you sooner that something needed to be done?"

In this brief vignette, the psychopharmacologist becomes the idealized object who was responsive to the patient's needs, in contrast to the psychotherapist, who is seen as the bad object, almost sadistic in her perceived refusal to "do something." The individual prescribing the medication may contribute to the split by implying either directly or indirectly that the psychotherapist was derelict in her duty by not sending the patient for medication sooner.

The cleavage may occur along opposite lines as well. Some borderline patients feel that the prescribing psychiatrist is eager to get rid of them because the appointment is scheduled for only 15 minutes. They may object to being "thrown out" of the doctor's office without the opportunity to talk more about what they are experiencing. In this case, the prescriber becomes the bad object, while the therapist is idealized because he or she takes the time to listen and to express great concern about the patient's internal experiences.

Splitting of this nature cannot be entirely prevented, but steps can be taken to minimize the potential destructiveness of such behavior. From the beginning, a patient should understand that the psychotherapist and the prescribing psychiatrist must be given permission to communicate about diagnosis and treatment. They should consider themselves part of a treatment team rather than isolated individuals. Often, discussing the patient's perceptions about the other clinician openly and honestly reduces a great deal of the tension created by such splits. In addition, the two clinicians should have an agreement about which one has responsibility for making decisions about hospitalization, vacation coverage, changes in medication, and the investigation of any potential medical problems.

Although the frequency and duration of communication between clinicians cannot be arbitrarily established, it must take place often enough so each has a clear understanding of the other's treatment approach. Often a critical factor in the evolution of splitting is that the patient distorts to one clinician what the other is saying or doing. If the clinician hearing this report simply takes it at face value without calling and checking the veracity of the account with the other clinician, the situation may rapidly deteriorate. The clinician hearing the report may subsequently collude with the patient's feeling of being victimized by the other clinician. When communication finally occurs, the colluding clinician may confront the colleague in an accusatory tone that creates greater defensiveness. A tactful inquiry about whether the patient's account is accurate is generally much more productive.

COST-EFFECTIVENESS

Many managed care companies insist that psychiatrists do not need to conduct psychotherapy because nonmedical therapists can do just as well at a cheaper price. Hence, they allow a psychiatrist to see a patient for a 15-minute medication check while referring the psychotherapy to someone whose time is much less expensive, often a counselor with a bachelor's degree, who is not well trained in psychotherapy. Although this approach seems to be cost-effective, the treatment may become so fragmented that the patient's condition deteriorates and hospitalization is necessary. In this event, the hospital costs far outweigh the added expense of one clinician who serves both functions. Moreover, the division of labor between two clinicians requires extremely close collaboration. The time spent in communication between the two is often a hidden cost, not generally reimbursed, which must ultimately be factored into a comprehensive consideration of cost-effectiveness. Meanwhile, data are needed on the two alternative arrangements for systematic study of whether one is ultimately more cost-effective than the other.

In the absence of definitive data, clinical experiences suggest that in many situations there are advantages to having a psychiatrist perform both roles. Patients with severe psychotic disorders who are not compliant with prescribed medication, patients with bipolar affective disorder who deny illness, those with schizoaffective disorder, and patients with schizophrenia all may require one central clinician who works with them around the issue of medication as well as psychological and family issues to ensure adherence to the treatment plan. Patients with severe or unstable medical conditions may also require a combined approach in which a psychiatrist's medical knowledge is important in the overall management. Because of the potential for splitting, many patients with borderline personality disorder will also do better with one central clinician performing both roles. Finally, patients who are likely to require hospitalization because of severe suicidality and impulse control problems may be treated most beneficially by a psychiatrist attentive to both psychotherapeutic and pharmacotherapeutic issues.

In many discussions of the value of combined psychotherapy and pharmacotherapy, dissenters argue that the combination of the two treatments may be unduly expensive and that the benefits are not commensurate with the additional cost. This perspective has left some to suggest innovative means of gaining benefit from both modalities. For example, for patients with agoraphobia, some have suggested that prescription of imipramine with instructions for systematic self-directed exposure may be a cost-efficient way to derive benefits from both treatments. Similar efforts have been made to assist patients with obsessive-compulsive disorder with self-administered exposure in vivo practice.

The assumption that dividing treatment between a psychiatrist and a nonpsychiatrist psychotherapist is more cost-effective may not be warranted. Few data are available to test this assumption. In one quasi-experimental retrospective design that compared claims data from a national managed mental health care organization, integrated treatment by one psychiatrist was compared with split treatment administered by two professionals for depressed patients. Over an 18-month period, the patients who received integrated treatment had significantly lower treatment costs because fewer outpatient sessions were necessary. Another study examined fee schedules of seven large managed care organizations from 1998 and compared psychotherapy alone, medication alone, and combined treatment pro-

vided by a psychiatrist working with a social worker or psychologist. When treatment required both modalities, combined treatment by a psychiatrist cost roughly the same or less than divided treatment with a social worker psychotherapist. Combined treatment was generally *less* expensive than divided treatment when a psychologist was doing the therapy. Both these studies are modest and far from definitive, but they suggest that more empirical data are needed to guide practitioners in identifying patients who may actually do better with integrated treatment conducted by one psychiatrist and to decide whether divided or integrated treatment is more cost-effective.

References

Barlow DH, Gorman JM, Shear MK, Woods SW. Cognitive-behavioral therapy, imipramine, or their combination for panic disorder: a randomized controlled trial. *JAMA.* 2000;283:2529.

Blatt SJ, Zuroff DC, Bondi CM, Sanislow CA. Short- and long-term effects of medication and psychotherapy in the brief treatment of depression: further analyses of data from the NIMH TDCRP. *Psychother Res.* 2000;10:215.

Clarkin JF, Carpenter D, Hull J, Wilner P, Glick I. Effects of psychoeducational intervention for married patients with bipolar disorder and their spouses. *Psychiatr Serv.* 1998;49:531.

Dewan M. Are psychiatrists cost-effective: an analysis of integrated versus split treatment. *Am J Psychiatry.* 1999;156:324.

Faloon IR, Boyd JL, McGill CW, et al. Family management in the prevention of morbidity of schizophrenia: clinical outcome of a two-year longitudinal study. *Arch Gen Psychiatry.* 1985;42:887.

Gabbard GO. Combining medication with psychotherapy in the treatment of personality disorders. In: Gunderson JG , Gabbard GO, eds. *Psychotherapy for Personality Disorders.* Washington, DC: American Psychiatric Press; 2000:65.

Gabbard GO. Combined psychotherapy and psychopharmacology. In: Sadock BJ, Sadock VA, eds. *Kaplan & Sadock's Comprehensive Textbook of Psychiatry.* 7th ed. Vol 2. Baltimore: Lippincott Williams & Wilkins; 2000:2225.

Gabbard GO, Kay J. The fate of integrated treatment: whatever happened to the biopsychosocial psychiatrists? *Am J Psychiatry.* 2001;158:12.

Goldman W, McCulloch J, Cuffel B, Zarin DA, Suarez A, Burns BJ. Outpatient utilization patterns of integrated and split psychotherapy and pharmacotherapy for depression. *Psychiatr Serv.* 1998;49:477.

Greist JH, Jefferson JW. Obsessive-compulsive disorder. In: Gabbard GO, ed. *Treatment of Psychiatric Disorders: The Second Edition.* Vol 2. Washington, DC: American Psychiatric Press; 2001:1515.

Hollon SD, Fawcett J. Combined medication and psychotherapy. In: Gabbard GO, ed. *Treatment of Psychiatric Disorders: The Second Edition.* Vol 2. Washington, DC: American Psychiatric Press; 1995:1221.

Keller MB, McCullough JP, Klein DN, et al. A comparison of nefazodone, the cognitive behavioral-analysis system of psychotherapy, and their combination for the treatment of chronic depression. *N Engl J Med.* 2000;342:1462.

Linehan MM, Armstrong HE, Suarez A, Allmon D, Heard HL. Cognitive-behavioral treatment of chronically parasuicidal borderline patients. *Arch Gen Psychiatry.* 1991;48:1060.

Mavissakalian MR. Combined behavioral and pharmacological treatment of anxiety disorders. In: Oldham JM, Riba MB, Tasman A, eds. *American Psychiatric Press Review of Psychiatry.* Vol 12. Washington, DC: American Psychiatric Press; 1993:565.

MTA Cooperative Group. A 14-month randomized clinical trial of treatment strategies for attention-deficit/hyperactivity disorder. *Arch Gen Psychiatry.* 1999;56:1073.

Reynolds CF 3rd, Frank E, Perel JM, et al. Nortriptyline and interpersonal psychotherapy as maintenance therapies for recurrent major depression: a randomized controlled trial in patients older than 59 years. *JAMA.* 1999;281:39.

Roose SP. Psychodynamic therapy and medication: can treatments in conflict be integrated? In: Kay J, ed. *Integrated Treatment of Psychiatric Disorders. Rev Psychiatry.* 2001;20:31.

Sammons MT, Schmidt NB, eds. *Combined Treatment for Mental Disorders: A Guide to Psychological and Pharmacological Interventions.* Washington, DC: American Psychological Association; 2001:111.

Woodward B, Duckworth KS, Gutheil TG. The pharmacotherapist–psychotherapist collaboration. In: Oldham JM, Riba MB, Tasman A, eds. *American Psychiatric Press Review of Psychiatry.* Vol 12. Washington, DC: American Psychiatric Press; 1993:631.

36 Biological Therapies

▲ 36.1 GENERAL PRINCIPLES OF PSYCHOPHARMACOLOGY

The use of drugs to treat psychiatric disorders is often the foundation for a successful treatment approach that can also include other types of interventions such as psychotherapy or behavioral therapies. As knowledge about the biology of normal and abnormal brain function continues to grow, the practice of clinical psychopharmacology continues to evolve in scope and effectiveness. Those involved in the prescribing and clinical follow-up of psychiatric drug treatments must remain current with the research literature, including the emergence of new agents, the demonstration of new indications for existing agents, and the identification and treatment of drug-related adverse effects. The emergence of new drugs and new indications is one of the most exciting areas of psychiatry.

The practice of pharmacotherapy in psychiatry should not be oversimplified—for example, it should not be reduced to a one-diagnosis–one-drug approach. Many variables affect the practice of psychopharmacology, including drug selection and administration; the psychodynamic meaning to the patient; and family and environmental influences. Some patients may view drug treatment as a panacea; others may view it as an assault. The patient, the patient's relatives, and the nursing staff must be instructed on the reasons for the drug treatment as well as the expected benefits and potential risks. In addition, the clinician may find it useful to explain the theoretical basis for pharmacotherapy to the patient and other involved parties.

Drugs must be used in effective dosages for sufficient periods, as determined by previous clinical investigations and clinical experience. Subtherapeutic doses and incomplete therapeutic trials should not be used simply because the psychiatrist is excessively concerned that the patient will develop adverse effects. The use of dosages that are too low or durations that are too short merely exposes patients to some risk, without providing them the maximum chance of therapeutic benefit. Treatment response and the emergence of adverse effects must be monitored closely; drug dosage should be adjusted accordingly, and appropriate treatments for emergent adverse effects must be instituted as quickly as possible.

CLASSIFICATION OF DRUGS

The numerous pharmacological agents used to treat psychiatric disorders are referred to by three general terms that are used interchangeably: *psychotropic drugs, psychoactive drugs,* and *psychotherapeutic drugs.* Traditionally, those agents were divided into four categories: (1) antipsychotic drugs or neuroleptics, used to treat psychosis; (2) antidepressant drugs, used to treat depression; (3) antimanic drugs, or mood stabilizers, used to treat bipolar disorder; and (4) antianxiety drugs, or anxiolytics, used to treat anxious states (which were also effective as hypnotics in high dosages). That division, however, is less valid now than it was in the past for the following reasons:

1. Many drugs of one class are used to treat disorders previously assigned to another class. For example, many antidepressant drugs are used to treat anxiety disorders, and some antianxiety drugs are used to treat psychoses, depressive disorders, and bipolar disorders.
2. Drugs from all four categories are used to treat disorders not previously treatable by drugs—for example, eating disorders, panic disorder, and impulse-control disorders.
3. Drugs such as clonidine (Catapres), propranolol (Inderal), verapamil (Isoptin, Calan), and gabapentin (Neurontin) can treat a variety of psychiatric disorders effectively and do not fit easily into the traditional classification of drugs.
4. Some descriptive psychopharmacological terms overlap in meaning. For example, anxiolytics decrease anxiety, sedatives produce a calming or relaxing effect, and hypnotics produce sleep. However, most anxiolytics function as sedatives and at high doses can be used as hypnotics, and all hypnotics can be used for daytime sedation at low doses.

For these reasons, in the sections that follow, each drug is discussed according to its pharmacological category. Each drug is described in terms of its pharmacological actions, including pharmacodynamics and pharmacokinetics. Indications, contraindications, drug–drug interactions, and adverse effects are also discussed.

PHARMACOLOGICAL ACTIONS

Pharmacokinetic interactions concern how the body handles a drug. Pharmacodynamic interactions concern the effects of drugs on the biological activities of the body.

Pharmacodynamics

The major pharmacodynamic considerations include receptor mechanisms, the dose-response curve, the therapeutic index, and the development of tolerance, dependence, and withdrawal phenomena. The *receptor* for a drug can be defined generally as the

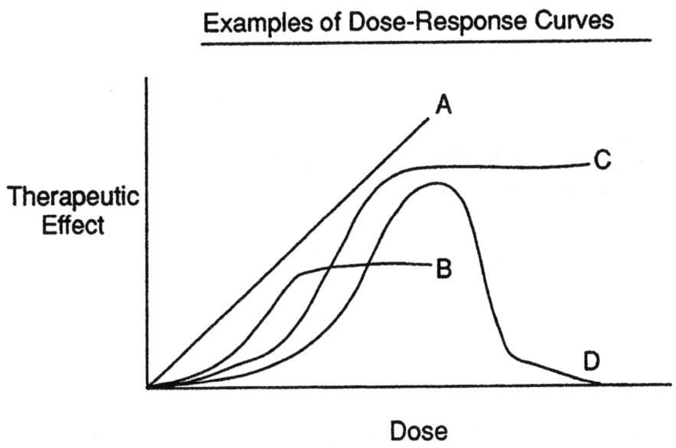

FIGURE 36.1–1

These dose-response curves plot the therapeutic effect as a function of increasing the dose, often calculated as the log on the dose. Drug *A* has a linear dose response; drugs *B* and *C* have sigmoidal curves; and drug *D* has a curvilinear dose-response curve. Although doses of drug *B* are more potent than equal doses of drug *C*, drug *C* has a higher maximum efficacy than drug *B*. Drug *D* has a therapeutic window such that both low and high doses are less effective than midrange doses.

cellular component to which the drug binds and through which the drug initiates its pharmacodynamic effects on the body. A drug can be an agonist for a receptor and stimulate the specific biological activity of the receptor or an antagonist that inhibits the biological activity. Some drugs are classified as partial agonists because they cannot fully activate a specific receptor. The receptor site for a psychopharmacological drug is often the receptor for an endogenous neurotransmitter. For example, most antipsychotic medications are receptor antagonists at the dopamine type 2 (D_2) receptor. However, this may not be true for other psychotherapeutic drugs (e.g., lithium [Eskalith], which may act by inhibiting the enzyme inositol 1-phosphatase).

The dose-response curve plots the drug concentration against the effects of the drug (Fig. 36.1–1). The *potency* of a drug refers to the relative dose required to achieve certain effects. Haloperidol (Haldol), for example, is more potent than chlorpromazine (Thorazine) because approximately 5 mg of haloperidol is required to achieve the same therapeutic effect as 100 mg of chlorpromazine. However, both these drugs are equal in their *clinical efficacy*—that is, the maximum clinical response achievable by administration of a drug.

The adverse effects of most drugs are often a direct result of their primary pharmacodynamic effects. *Therapeutic index* is a relative measure of the toxicity or safety of a drug and is defined as the ratio of the median toxic dose to the median effective dose. The *median toxic dose* is the dose at which 50 percent of patients experience a specific toxic effect, and the *median effective dose* is the dose at which 50 percent of patients have a specified therapeutic effect. The therapeutic index for haloperidol and cardiovascular effects is quite high, as evidenced by the wide range of dosages in which haloperidol is prescribed. Conversely, the therapeutic index for lithium is quite low, thus requiring careful monitoring of serum lithium levels in patients given the drug. Both interindividual and intraindividual variations can affect the response to a specific drug. An individual patient may be hyporeactive, normally reactive, or hyperreactive to a drug. For example, some patients require 150 mg a day of imipramine (Tofranil) whereas others may require 300 mg a day. Idiosyncratic drug responses occur when a patient experiences a particularly unusual or rare effect from a drug. For example, some patients become quite agitated when given a benzodiazepine, such as diazepam (Valium).

A person may become less responsive to a particular drug as it is administered over time, a process that is referred to as the development of *tolerance*. The development of tolerance may sometimes be associated with the appearance of physical dependence on the drug. In a parallel fashion, pharmacokinetic drug interactions concern the effects of drugs on the plasma concentrations of one other, and pharmacodynamic drug interactions concern the effects of drugs on the receptor activities of one other.

Pharmacokinetics

Absorption. Psychotherapeutic drugs reach the brain through the bloodstream. Orally administered drugs dissolve in the fluid of the gastrointestinal (GI) tract, depending on their lipid solubility and the GI tract's local pH, motility, and surface area, and are then absorbed into the blood.

Stomach acidity may be reduced by gastric ion pump inhibitors, such as omeprazole (Prilosec) and lansoprazole (Prevacid); by histamine H_2 receptor blockers, such as cimetidine (Tagamet), famotidine (Pepcid), nizatidine (Axid), and ranitidine (Zantac); or by antacids. Gastric and intestinal motility may be slowed by anticholinergic drugs or increased by dopamine receptor antagonists, such as metoclopramide (Reglan).

Under favorable conditions, parenteral administration can achieve therapeutic plasma concentrations more rapidly than oral administration. However, if a drug is emulsified in an insoluble carrier matrix, intramuscular administration can sustain the drug's gradual release for several weeks. Such formulations are called *depot* preparations. Intravenous administration is the quickest route for achieving therapeutic blood concentrations, but it also carries the highest risk of sudden and life-threatening adverse effects.

Distribution and Bioavailability. Drugs that circulate bound to plasma proteins are called *protein bound*, and those that circulate unbound are called *free*. Only the free fraction can pass through the blood–brain barrier. The *distribution* of a drug to the brain is governed by the brain's regional blood flow, the blood–brain barrier, and the drug's affinity for its receptors in the brain. High cerebral blood flow, high lipid solubility, and high receptor affinity promote the therapeutic actions of the drug. A drug's *volume of distribution* is a measure of the apparent space in the body available to contain the drug, which can vary with age, sex, adipose tissue content, and disease state.

Bioavailability refers to the fraction of the total amount of administered drug that can subsequently be recovered from the bloodstream. Bioavailability is an important variable, because Food and Drug Administration (FDA) regulations specify that the bioavailability of a generic formulation can differ from that of the brand-name formulation by no more than a specific amount.

Metabolism and Excretion

Metabolic Routes. The four major metabolic routes for drugs are *oxidation, reduction, hydrolysis,* and *conjugation.* Metabolism usually yields inactive metabolites that are more

polar and therefore more readily excreted. However, metabolism also transforms many inactive prodrugs into therapeutically active metabolites. The liver is the principal site of *metabolism,* and bile, feces, and urine are the major routes of *excretion.* Psychotherapeutic drugs are also excreted in sweat, saliva, tears, and breast milk.

Quantitation of Metabolism and Excretion. Four important quantities regarding metabolism and excretion are time of peak plasma concentration, half-life, first-pass effect, and clearance. The time between the administration of a drug and the appearance of *peak plasma concentrations* varies depending on the route of administration and rate of absorption. A drug's *half-life* is the amount of time it takes for metabolism and excretion to reduce a particular plasma concentration by half. A drug administered steadily at time intervals shorter than its half-life will reach 97 percent of its steady-state plasma concentration after five half-lives. The *first-pass effect* refers to the initial metabolism of orally administered drugs within the portal circulation of the liver and is quantitated as the fraction of absorbed drug reaching the systemic circulation unmetabolized. *Clearance* is a measure of the amount of the drug excreted from the body in a specific period of time.

Cytochrome P450 Enzymes. Most psychotherapeutic drugs are oxidized by the hepatic cytochrome P450 (CYP) enzyme system, which is so named because it absorbs light strongly at a wavelength of 450 nm. The human CYP enzymes comprise several distinct families and subfamilies. In the CYP nomenclature, the family is denoted by a numeral, the subfamily by a capital letter, and the individual member of the subfamily by a second numeral (e.g., 2D6). Persons with genetic polymorphisms in the CYP genes that encode inefficient versions of CYP enzymes are considered "poor metabolizers" (Table 36.1–1).

The CYP enzymes are responsible for the inactivation of most psychotherapeutic drugs. These enzymes act primarily in the endoplasmic reticulum of the hepatocytes and the cells of the intestine. Thus, cellular pathophysiology, such as that caused by viral hepatitis or cirrhosis, may affect the efficiency of drug metabolism by the CYP enzymes.

There are three ways in which drug interactions influence the CYP system:

1. Induction. Expression of the CYP genes may be induced by alcohol, by certain drugs (barbiturates, anticonvulsants), or by smoking. For example, an inducer of CYP 3A4, such as cimetidine, may increase the metabolism and decrease the plasma concentrations of a substrate of 3A4, such as alprazolam (Xanax).
2. Noncompetitive inhibition. Certain drugs that are not substrates for a particular enzyme may nonetheless indirectly inhibit the enzyme and slow its metabolism of other drug substrates. For example, concurrent administration of a CYP 2D6 inhibitor, such as fluoxetine (Prozac), may inhibit the metabolism and thus raise the plasma concentrations of CYP 2D6 substrates, including amitriptyline (Elavil). If one CYP enzyme is inhibited, then its substrate accumulates until it is metabolized by an alternate CYP enzyme.
3. Competitive inhibition. Concurrent administration of two or more substrates for a particular enzyme may produce competitive inhibition of the enzyme, but such interactions are not usually clinically relevant. For example, clomipramine (Anafranil) and theophylline (Theo-Dur, Slo-bid) are both substrates of CYP 1A2, but their concurrent administration has little effect on their respective plasma concentrations.

Table 36.1–1
Genetic Polymorphisms

P450 Isoenzymes	Percentage of Poor Metabolizers
2C19	3–5% of whites, 15–20% of Asians
2C9	1–3% of whites
2D6	5–10% of whites

Clinically Relevant CYP-Induced Drug Interactions. With respect to CYP 2D6, tricyclic and tetracyclic drugs, dopamine receptor antagonists, and type 1C antiarrhythmic drugs should be used cautiously or avoided with certain selective serotonin reuptake inhibitors (SSRIs).

Because of inhibition of CYP 3A4, fluvoxamine (Luvox), nefazodone (Serzone), and fluoxetine should not be used together with alprazolam, triazolam (Halcion), or carbamazepine (Tegretol).

Due to interactions with CYP 1A2, fluvoxamine should not be used with theophylline or clozapine (Clozaril).

Also, the long half-lives of certain psychotherapeutic drugs, especially fluoxetine, may prolong their inhibition of the CYP enzymes. Table 36.1–2 lists some psychotropics with CYP drug interactions.

CLINICAL GUIDELINES

Physicians who practice clinical psychopharmacology require skill as both diagnosticians and psychotherapists, knowledge of the available drugs, and the ability to plan a pharmacotherapeutic regimen. The selection and initiation of drug treatment should be based on patients' history, current clinical state, and the treatment plan. Psychiatrists should know the purpose or goal of a drug trial, the length of time that the drug must be administered to assess its efficacy, the approach to be taken to reduce any adverse effects that may occur, alternative drug strategies should the current one fail, and indications for long-term maintenance of the patient on the drug. In almost all cases, psychiatrists should explain the treatment plan to patients and often to families and other caretakers. A patient's reaction to and ideas about a proposed drug trial should be considered, but if a psychiatrist thinks that accommodating the patient's wishes would hinder treatment, this fact should be explained to the patient.

Choice of Drug

The first two steps in selecting drug treatment, diagnosis and identification of the target symptoms, should ideally be carried out when the patient has been in a drug-free state for 1 to 2 weeks. The drug-free state should include the absence of medications for sleep (e.g., hypnotics), because the quality of sleep can be both an important diagnostic guide and a target symptom. If a patient is hospitalized, however, insurance guidelines may make a drug-free period difficult or even impossible to obtain. Psychiatrists often evaluate symptomatic patients who are already receiving one or more psychoactive medications and must usually wean patients from the current medication and then make the assessment. One must note not only the drugs currently taken but also those recently discontinued, which could be producing

Table 36.1–2
Cytochrome P450 Drug Interactions

Substrates	Fluoxetine	**Inhibitors**
1A2	Fluvoxamine	**1A2**
Amitriptyline	Methoxyamphetamine	Fluvoxamine
Clomipramine	Nortriptyline	**2C19**
Clozapine	Paroxetine	Fluoxetine
Fluvoxamine	Propranolol	Fluvoxamine
Haloperidol	Venlafaxine	Paroxetine
Imipramine	**3A3,4,5,7**	Topiramate
Propranolol	Alprazolam	**2C9**
Tacrine	Amitriptyline	Fluvoxamine
Verapamil	Carbamazepine	Paroxetine
2C19	Clomipramine	**2D6**
Amitriptyline	Clonazepam	Chlorpheniramine
Citalopram	Clozapine	Cimetidine
Clomipramine	Diazepam	Clomipramine
Diazepam	Imipramine	Fluoxetine
Hexobarbital	Midazolam	Haloperidol
Imipramine	Triazolam	Methadone
Mephobarbital	Astemizole	Moclobemide
Moclobemide	Chlorpheniramine	Paroxetine
Propranolol	Diltiazem	**2E1**
2C9	Loratadine	Disulfiram
Amitriptyline	Nefazodone	**3A3,4,5,7**
Fluoxetine	Nifedipine	Fluvoxamine
2D6	Nisoldipine	Grapefruit juice
Metoprolol	Nitrendipine	Nefazodone
Timolol	Verapamil	Norfluoxetine
Amitriptyline	Haloperidol	**Inducers**
Clomipramine	Methadone	**2C19**
Desipramine	Sertraline	Carbamazepine
Imipramine	Sildenafil	**2C9**
Haloperidol	Terfenadine	Secobarbital
Perphenazine	Trazodone	**3A3,4,5,7**
Risperidone	Verapamil	Barbiturates
Thioridazine	Zaleplon	Carbamazepine
Amphetamine	Zolpidem	Phenobarbital

symptoms of withdrawal. An exception to this practice occurs when a patient is taking a suboptimal dosage of an otherwise appropriate drug. In such cases a psychiatrist may decide to continue giving the drug at a higher dosage to complete a full therapeutic trial. The importance of an accurate and complete diagnostic evaluation cannot be overstated. It is no longer reasonable to try all available agents. Rather, the choice of drug and nondrug interventions should be based on careful and thorough review of all the patient's problems and resources. Failure to diagnose a treatable condition accurately is a common reason for unsatisfactory clinical outcomes.

From among the drugs appropriate to a particular diagnosis, a specific drug should be selected on the basis of a patient's history of drug response (compliance, therapeutic response, and adverse effects), the patient's family history of drug response, the profile of adverse effects for the drug with regard to the particular patient, and the psychiatrist's usual practice. If a drug has previously been effective in treating a patient or a family member, the same drug should be used again unless there is a specific reason not to use it. A history of severe adverse effects from a specific drug is a strong indicator that the patient would not be compliant with this drug regimen. Patients and their families are often ignorant about what drugs have been used before, in what dosages, and for how long. This ignorance may reflect the tendency of psychiatrists not to explain drug trials to their patients. Psychiatrists should consider giving their patients written records of drug trials for their personal medical records. A caveat in obtaining a history of drug response from patients is that, because of their mental disorders, they may report the effects of a previous drug trial inaccurately. If possible, therefore, the patients' medical records should be obtained to confirm their reports. Most psychotherapeutic drugs of a single class are equally efficacious; but drugs do differ in their adverse effects on individual patients. A selected drug should exacerbate any preexisting medical problems of the patient only minimally.

Off-Label Use and Nonapproved Dosages. The federal Food, Drug, and Cosmetic (FDC) Act authorizes the FDA to control the initial availability of a drug by approving only those new drugs that demonstrate both safety and effectiveness and then to ensure that the drug's proposed labeling is truthful and contains all pertinent information for the safe and effective use of the drug. An additional level of government regulation is directed by the Drug Enforcement Agency, which has classified drugs according to their abuse potential (Table 36.1–3). Clinicians are advised to exercise extra caution when prescribing controlled substances.

According to the Medical Liability Mutual Insurance Company, a malpractice insurance company in New York State, once a drug is approved for commercial use, physicians may, as part of the practice of medicine, lawfully prescribe a different dosage for a patient or otherwise vary the conditions of use from those approved in the package labeling without notifying the FDA or obtaining its approval. Specifically, the FDC Act does not limit the manner in which physicians may use an approved drug. Although physicians may treat patients with an approved drug for unapproved purposes—that is, indications not included on the drug's official labeling—without violating the FDC Act, patients may have a right to redress for possible medical malpractice. Patients' rights are a significant concern, because failure to follow the FDA-approved label may allow an inference that a physician was departing from the prevailing standard of care. Although failure to follow the contents of the drug label does not impose liability per se and should not preclude physicians from using good clinical judgment in patients' interest, physicians should be aware that the drug label presents important information about the safe and effective use of the drug.

Psychiatrists may prescribe medication for any reason that they believe is medically indicated for patients' welfare. This clarification is important in view of the increasing regulation of physicians by federal, state, and local government agencies and the intimidation experienced by many physicians in exercising their best medical judgment. When using a drug for an unapproved indication or in a dosage outside the usual range, physicians should document the reasons for their treatment decisions in patients' charts. If clinicians are in doubt about a treatment plan, they should consult a colleague or suggest that the patient obtain a second opinion.

Therapeutic Trials. A drug's therapeutic trial with a particular patient should last for a previously determined time. Because behavioral symptoms are more difficult to assess than physiolog-

Table 36.1–3
Characteristics of Drugs at Each DEA Level

Schedule (Control Level)	Characteristics of Drug at Each Schedule	Examples of Drugs at Each Schedule
I	High abuse potential No accepted use in medical treatment in the United States at the present time and, therefore, not for prescription use Can be used for research	Lysergic acid diethylamide (LSD), heroin, marijuana, peyote, phencyclidine (PCP), mescaline, psilocybin, nicocodeine, nicomorphine
II	High abuse potential Severe physical dependence liability Severe psychological dependence liability No refills; no telephone prescriptions	Amphetamine, opium, morphine, codeine, hydromorphine, phenmetrazine, amobarbital, secobarbital, pentobarbital, glutethimide, methylphenidate
III	Abuse potential lower than levels I and II Moderate or low physical dependence liability High psychological liability Prescriptions must be rewritten after 6 months or five refills	Ketamine, methyprylon; nalorphine; sulfonmethane; benzphetamine; phendimetrazine; chlorphentermine; compounds containing codeine, morphine, opium, hydrocodone, dihydrocodeine; diethylpropion; dronabinol
IV	Low abuse potential Limited physical dependence liability Limited psychological dependence liability Prescriptions must be rewritten after 6 months or five refills	Phenobarbital, benzodiazepines,[a] chloral hydrate, ethchlorvynol, ethinamate, meprobamate, paraldehyde, sibutramine
V	Lowest abuse potential of all controlled substances	Narcotic preparations containing limited amounts of nonnarcotic active medicinal ingredients

[a]In New York State benzodiazepines are treated as schedule II substances, which require an official state government prescription for a maximum of 3 months' supply.

ical symptoms such as hypertension, it is particularly important to identify specific target symptoms at the initiation of a drug trial. The psychiatrist and the patient can then assess the target symptom over the course of the drug trial to help determine whether the drug has been effective. Several objective rating scales, such as the Brief Psychiatric Rating Scale and the Hamilton Rating Scale for Depression, are available to help assess a patient's progress over the course of a drug trial. If a drug has not been effective in reducing target symptoms in the specified time and if other reasons for the lack of response can be eliminated, use of the drug should be tapered and stopped. The brain is not a group of on-off neurochemical switches; rather, it is an interactive network of neurons in complex homeostasis. Thus, the abrupt discontinuation of virtually any psychoactive drug is likely to disrupt the brain's functioning. For example, lithium discontinuation may lead to rebound mania; dopamine receptor antagonist discontinuation may lead to tardive dyskinesias; serotonergic drug discontinuation may lead to agitation, nausea, dysequilibrium, and dysphoria; and benzodiazepine discontinuation may lead to anxiety and insomnia. Another common clinical mistake is routinely adding medications without discontinuing a previously prescribed drug. Although this practice is indicated in specific circumstances, such as lithium potentiation of an unsuccessful trial of antidepressants, it often results in increased noncompliance and adverse effects. A clinician may also not know whether the second drug alone or the combination of drugs resulted in a therapeutic success or adverse effect.

Therapeutic Failures. The failure of a specific drug trial should prompt clinicians to reconsider several possibilities. First, was the original diagnosis correct? This reconsideration should include the possibility of an undiagnosed cognitive disorder, including illicit drug abuse. Second, are the observed remaining symptoms the drug's adverse effects and not related to the original disease? Antipsychotic drugs, for example, can produce akinesia, which resembles psychotic withdrawal; akathisia and neuroleptic malignant syndrome resemble increased psychotic agitation. Third, was the drug administered in sufficient dosage for an appropriate time? Patients can have varying drug absorption and metabolic rates for the same drug, and plasma drug concentrations should be determined to assess this variable. Fourth, did a pharmacokinetic or pharmacodynamic interaction with another drug the patient was taking reduce the efficacy of the psychotherapeutic drug? Fifth, did the patient take the drug as directed? Drug noncompliance is a common clinical problem. The reasons for drug noncompliance include complicated drug regimens (more than one drug in more than one daily dose), adverse effects (especially if unnoticed by a clinician), and poor patient education about the drug treatment plan (Table 36.1–4). Drug compliance improves if the clinician explains the use of the drug and the expected responses fully, if

Table 36.1–4
Conditions That May Reduce Adherence to Recommended Treatment

Excessively complex regimen (multiple agents, multiple small doses)
Early onset and persistence of side effects
Slow onset of beneficial effects
Low apparent relapse risk experienced if treatment is interrupted
Psychosis, confusion, dementia, pseudodementia, low intelligence, impaired hearing or vision, illiteracy
Simple lack of information, need for patient education
Financial hardship, conflicting obligations of time or money
Resentment, lack of confidence or trust
Specific psychopathology: paranoid delusions, hopelessness, masochism, anxiety and fear, ambivalence, control, splitting, passive aggression, passive dependence, denial, sociopathy, substance abuse
Involvement of multiple clinicians
Poor clinician–patient relationship
Inevitable human error

Adapted from Baldessarini RJ, Cole JO. Chemotherapy. In: Nicholi AM, ed. *The New Harvard Guide to Psychiatry.* Cambridge, MA: Belknap; 1988:530.

the patient has a positive transference toward the clinician, and if the patient does not have to wait in the waiting room to see the clinician. Patients should be warned in particular about the potential adverse consequences of missing even one dose of medication.

SPECIAL TREATMENT CONSIDERATIONS

Children

Special care must be taken when administering psychotherapeutic drugs to children. Although the small volume of distribution suggests the use of lower dosages than in adults, children's higher rate of metabolism indicates that the ratio of milligrams of drug to kilograms of body weight should be higher. In practice, it is best to begin with a small dose and increase the dosage until clinical effects are observed. Clinicians should not hesitate to use adult dosages in children if the dosages are effective and the adverse effects are acceptable.

Geriatric Patients

The two major concerns when treating geriatric patients with psychotherapeutic drugs are that older persons may be especially susceptible to adverse effects (particularly cardiac effects) and may metabolize drugs slowly (Table 36.1–5). Thus, geriatric patients may require low dosages of medication. Further, geriatric patients are often taking other medications, and psychiatrists must consider possible drug interactions.

Table 36.1–5
Pharmacokinetics and Aging

Phase	Change	Effect
Absorption	Gastric pH increases Decreased surface villi Decreased gastric motility and delayed gastric emptying Intestinal perfusion decreases	Little overall change Absorption is slowed but just as complete
Distribution	Total body water and lean body mass decrease Increased total body fat, more marked in women than in men Albumin decreases, gamma globulin increases, alpha globulin, acid glycoprotein unchanged	V_d increases for lipid-soluble drugs, decreases for water-soluble drugs The free or unbound percentage of albumin-bound drugs increases
Metabolism	Renal: renal blood flow and glomerular filtration rates decrease Hepatic: decreased enzyme activity and perfusion	Decreased metabolism leads to prolonged half-lives, if V_d remains the same
Total body weight	Decreases	Think on a mg/kg basis
Receptor sensitivity	May increase	Increased effect

V_d, volume of distribution.
Reprinted with permission from Guttmacher LB. *Concise Guide to Somatic Therapies in Psychiatry.* Washington, DC: American Psychiatric Press; 1988:126.

In practice, psychiatrists should begin treating geriatric patients with a small dose, usually approximately one half the usual dose. The dosage should be raised in small amounts more slowly than in younger adults until either a clinical benefit is achieved or unacceptable adverse effects appear. Although many geriatric patients require a small dosage of medication, others require the usual adult dosage.

Pregnant and Nursing Women

The basic rule is to avoid administering any drug to a woman who is pregnant (particularly during the first trimester) or breast-feeding a child. This rule, however, is broken occasionally when a women's mental disorder is severe. If psychotherapeutic medications must be administered during a pregnancy, the possibility of therapeutic abortion should be discussed. The two most teratogenic drugs in the psychopharmacopoeia are lithium and the anticonvulsants. Lithium administration during pregnancy is associated with a high incidence of birth abnormalities, including Ebstein's anomaly, a serious abnormality in cardiac development. Anticonvulsants used during pregnancy are associated with fetal craniofacial and neural tube abnormalities in less than 10 percent of infants. The risk of teratogenicity can be reduced by the administration of folic acid. Other psychoactive drugs (antidepressants, antipsychotics, and anxiolytics), although less clearly associated with birth defects, should also be avoided during pregnancy if at all possible. The most common clinical situation is a pregnant woman's becoming psychotic. If a decision is made not to terminate the pregnancy, electroconvulsive therapy (ECT) or antipsychotics are preferable to lithium.

The administration of psychotherapeutic drugs at or near delivery may cause a baby to be overly sedated at delivery, to need a respirator, or to be physically dependent on the drug and require detoxification and treatment of a withdrawal syndrome. Virtually all psychotropic drugs are secreted in the milk of a nursing women; therefore, mothers taking these agents should not breast-feed their infants.

Persons with Hepatic or Renal Insufficiency

Drugs that are metabolized in the liver may accumulate to toxic concentrations in persons with hepatocellular insufficiency of any cause, including cirrhosis, hepatitis, metabolic disorders, and bile duct obstruction. Drugs that are excreted by the kidneys may accumulate to toxic concentrations in persons with renal insufficiency of any cause, including atherosclerosis, nephrosis, nephritis, infiltrative disorders, and outflow obstruction. Hepatocellular or renal insufficiency requires administration of a reduced dosage, usually half of the recommended dosage for healthy persons. Clinicians should be particularly alert to signs and symptoms of adverse drug effects in persons with hepatic or renal disorders. Monitoring plasma drug concentrations may help guide dosage adjustments.

Persons with Other Medical Illnesses

Considerations in administering psychotherapeutic drugs to medically ill persons include a potentially increased sensitivity to the drug's adverse effects, either increased or decreased metabolism and excretion of the drug, and interactions with other medications. As with children and geriatric persons, the most reasonable clinical practice is to begin with a low dosage, increase it slowly, and watch for both clinical and adverse effects.

ADVERSE EFFECTS

Most psychotherapeutic drugs do not affect a single neurotransmitter system, and their effects are not localized to the brain.

verify that patients are taking the medication and not hoarding the pills for a later overdose attempt. Patients may attempt suicide just as they appear to be getting better. Clinicians, therefore, should continue to be careful about prescribing large quantities of medication until the patient has almost completely recovered.

Another consideration is the possibility of an accidental overdose, particularly by children in the household. Patients should be advised to keep psychotherapeutic medications clearly labeled and in a safe place. A guide to the signs and symptoms and the treatment of overdose with psychotherapeutic drugs is contained in Table 36.1–9.

Table 36.1–9
Intoxication and Overdose with Psychotherapeutic Drugs[a]

Drug	Toxic/Lethal Dose	Signs and Symptoms	Treatment
β-Adrenergic receptor antagonists	Toxic effects with 0.8–6 g of propranolol	Hypotension, bradycardia, cardiac failure, bronchospasm, loss of consciousness, seizures	Emesis or gastric lavage; supportive care; norepinephrine or dopamine for severe hypotension; glucagon for hypotension and myocardial depression; IV atropine for symptomatic bradycardia, IV isoproterenol for persistent cases, pacemaker if refractory; diuretic or cardiac glycoside for heart failure; theophylline or β_2 agonist for bronchospasm; IV diazepam for seizures
Amantadine	Lethal dose of 2 g reported	Arrhythmia, tachycardia, hypertension, disorientation, lethargy, confusion, visual hallucinations, aggressive behavior, anxiety, minimally reactive and dilated pupils, ataxia, tremor, hypertonia, seizure exacerbation, coma, edema and respiratory distress, renal insufficiency, urinary retention, acid–base disturbances	Emesis or gastric lavage; supportive measures including cardiovascular monitoring, airway maintenance, and control of respiration and oxygen administration; avoid adrenergic agents as they may predispose to ventricular arrhythmias; IV physostigmine to treat CNS toxicity, chlorpromazine for toxic psychosis, sedation and anticonvulsants as needed; monitor urine pH, urinary output, serum electrolytes, urine acidifying agents increase rate of excretion, IV fluids, catheter for urinary retention
Amphetamines	Toxic effects at 30 mg, idiosyncratic toxicity as low as 2 mg, survival reported after 500 mg	Elation, irritability, hyperactivity, psychotic symptoms, depression, panic, rapid speech, confusion, anorexia, insomnia, hyperreflexia, tremor, dry mouth, hyperpyrexia, convulsions, coma, chest pain, arrhythmia, heart block, hyper/hypotension, shock, nausea, vomiting, diarrhea, abdominal cramps, tachypnea, rhabdomyolysis	Emesis or lavage, activated charcoal, cathartic (can be effective long after ingestion because of recycling through gastric mucosa); supportive care; reduce external stimuli, sedate with chlorpromazine; IV phentolamine for severe HTN; acidification of urine
Anticholinergics	700 mg to 7 g (doses vary depending on agent involved)	Hot, dry, flushed skin; dry mucous membranes, hyperthermia, rash, shock, tachycardia, unreactive dilated pupils, blurred vision; delirium, delusions, ataxia, hallucinations, convulsions, coma, dysphagia, nausea, vomiting, hypoactive bowel sounds, respiratory arrest, urinary retention	Emesis or lavage, activated charcoal, saline cathartics; supportive and symptomatic therapy; 1–2 mg physostigmine can reverse anticholinergic effects; cold packs, mechanical cooling devices, or sponging with tepid water for hyperthermia; continuous ECG monitoring; vasopressors and fluid therapy for shock, IV propranolol for supraventricular tachyarrhythmias, avoid dopamine receptor antagonists; local miotics for mydriasis; diazepam for agitation
Antihistamines	2.8 g diphenhydramine, 1.75–17.5 g hydroxyzine	Disorientation, drowsiness, excitation, depression, hallucinations, anxiety, delirium, hyperthermia, tachycardia, hypotension, arrhythmias, seizures	Emesis or lavage; support cardiorespiratory function; IV fluids and vasopressors for hypotension; caffeine and sodium benzoate to counteract CNS depressant effects, physostigmine for anticholinergic effects; diazepam for seizures; sponge baths with tepid water (not alcohol) or cold packs for hyperthermia
Barbiturates	10 times the daily dose or 1 g of most barbiturates causes severe toxicity, 2–10 g fatal	Delirium, confusion, excitement, headache, CNS and respiratory depression (somnolence to coma), Cheyne-Stokes respiration, areflexia, shock, miosis, oliguria, tachycardia, hypotension, hypothermia	Emesis or lavage, activated charcoal, saline cathartics; supportive treatment, including maintaining airway and respiration and treating shock as needed; maintain vital signs and fluid balance; alkalinizing the urine increases excretion; forced diuresis if renal function is normal; hemodialysis in severe cases

(continued)

syndrome. It consists of agitation, nausea, dysequilibrium, and dysphoria. The syndrome is more likely to occur if the plasma half-life of the agent is brief, if the drug is taken for at least 2 months, or if higher dosages are used. The symptoms are time limited and can be minimized by gradually reducing the dosage.

DRUG INTERACTIONS

In addition to the CYP-induced drug interactions mentioned above, drug interactions with other causes may increase or decrease the activity of both the psychiatric drug and any other medications the patient is taking. In some cases, this may increase the risk of adverse reactions, and clinicians should be fully aware of all of the possible interactions before exposing patients to more than one drug at a time. Drug interactions are frequently used to augment the desired therapeutic benefit by influencing distinct pharmacodynamic sites of action. For example, in the treatment of depression, SSRIs, which raise synaptic serotonin levels, may be mixed with bupropion, which has little serotonergic activity but is highly active on the norepinephrine and dopamine systems. The resulting mixture of activities may be more powerfully antidepressant than either drug alone. Augmentation strategies should avoid duplication of pharmacodynamic activity, should not pair an agonist with an antagonist of the same receptor, and should be approached with caution to avoid potentially dangerous adverse effects. For example, mixing a tricyclic drug and an MAOI is reasonable, since each drug affects distinct cellular sites, but it is also perilous because it may cause a hypertensive crisis. In general, drugs with few adverse effects make the best candidates for augmentation strategies.

Drug interactions may be either pharmacokinetic or pharmacodynamic, and they vary greatly in their potential to cause serious problems. An additional consideration is phantom drug interactions. A patient who was taking only drug A may later receive both drug A and drug B. The clinician may notice some effect and attribute it to the induction of metabolism. What may have happened is that the patient was more compliant at one point in the observation period than in another, or there may have been some other effect of which the clinician was unaware. The clinical literature can contain reports of phantom drug interactions that are rare or nonexistent.

Other interactions are true but unproved, although reasonably plausible. Still other interactions have some modest effects and are well documented, and some clinically important drug interactions are well studied and well proved. But clinicians must remember that animal pharmacokinetic data cannot always be generalized readily to humans; in vitro data do not necessarily replicate the results obtained under in vivo conditions; single-case reports can contain misleading information; and studies of acute conditions should not be regarded uncritically as relevant to chronic, steady-state conditions.

Informed clinicians need to keep these considerations in mind and focus on clinically important interactions, not on those that may be mild, unproved, or entirely phantom. At the same time, clinicians should maintain an open and receptive attitude toward the possibility of pharmacokinetic and pharmacodynamic drug interactions.

DEVELOPMENT OF NEW DRUGS

The first stage in the development of a new drug involves identifying a compound that for theoretical reasons may be effective in treating a disorder. Techniques under development, called *combinatorial chemistry*, promise to generate several times the existing number of drugs for testing in the near future. The compound is then studied in a wide variety of in vitro and in vivo tests that may predict the clinical drug effects. Compounds found to be of potential importance in these tests then undergo studies of their toxicity and pharmacokinetics in animals. If these preliminary preclinical tests are thought to merit the costs of further drug development, a pharmaceutical company in the United States can file an Investigational New Drug Application with the FDA. If the application is granted, the compound can then be used in humans for research purposes. Only 1 in 1,000 compounds examined in preclinical testing proceeds to human testing.

The first such experiments are called phase I experiments, in which the drug is administered to about 100 normal persons to assess its pharmacokinetic effects and its potential for adverse effects. Phase I studies are conducted primarily to determine the safety and tolerability of a new compound. The information from the phase I trials is then used to help decide on a dosage of the new drug in phase II trials, which involve using the new compound in a patient population of 100 to 300 volunteers. The primary purpose of phase II trials is to assess the efficacy of the new drug in the treatment of specific disorders. If the phase II trials indicate that a drug is efficacious, safe, and well tolerated, much larger phase III trials are conducted on 1,000 to 3,000 patients to validate the findings of the phase II studies. Phase III studies also require gathering detailed information about optimum dosage schedules and the use of the drug in elderly and young populations and in persons with impaired hepatic or renal function. After completion of the phase III trials, the pharmaceutical company can apply to the FDA to market the drug commercially. The total elapsed time from initial identification of a drug to FDA approval is usually 15 years, and the cost averages $500 million per approved drug. In 1997, the FDA proposed a New Use Initiative, which will permit approval of new drugs or new indications for existing drugs based on fewer trials or on existing data that were collected for other reasons. Once marketed, a drug enters phase IV, in which postmarketing experience on a far larger patient population is monitored for the emergence of adverse effects. On occasion, the FDA has withdrawn approval of a drug for a certain indication because of severe toxicity.

INTOXICATION AND OVERDOSE

Adverse effects may occur with any drug. Although most are mild and transitory, some are severe and lethal. The prescribing psychiatrist or physician must be vigilant in determining the emergence of toxicity or signs of overdose. The toxic dose for one person may be lethal in another person, depending on such factors as route of administration, rate of absorption, interaction with other drugs, and age and general health of the patient. One must also remember that a patient may have ingested more than one substance, so the clinical picture may represent polysubstance abuse. Treatment must be adjusted accordingly, and a history (from other persons) should be obtained and all drugs should be inspected. The beginning of this book contains illustrations of the various drugs used in psychiatry, which can be useful.

An attempt by a patient to commit suicide by taking an overdose of a prescribed medication is an extreme event. Some are more lethal than others in overdose. Barbiturates, for example, have a higher potential for lethality than SSRIs, and the doctor must be aware of which drugs are more potentially lethal. It is good clinical practice to write nonrefillable prescriptions for small quantities of drugs when suicide is a consideration. In extreme cases the doctor should

verify that patients are taking the medication and not hoarding the pills for a later overdose attempt. Patients may attempt suicide just as they appear to be getting better. Clinicians, therefore, should continue to be careful about prescribing large quantities of medication until the patient has almost completely recovered.

Another consideration is the possibility of an accidental overdose, particularly by children in the household. Patients should be advised to keep psychotherapeutic medications clearly labeled and in a safe place. A guide to the signs and symptoms and the treatment of overdose with psychotherapeutic drugs is contained in Table 36.1–9.

Table 36.1–9
Intoxication and Overdose with Psychotherapeutic Drugs[a]

Drug	Toxic/Lethal Dose	Signs and Symptoms	Treatment
β-Adrenergic receptor antagonists	Toxic effects with 0.8–6 g of propranolol	Hypotension, bradycardia, cardiac failure, bronchospasm, loss of consciousness, seizures	Emesis or gastric lavage; supportive care; norepinephrine or dopamine for severe hypotension; glucagon for hypotension and myocardial depression; IV atropine for symptomatic bradycardia, IV isoproterenol for persistent cases, pacemaker if refractory; diuretic or cardiac glycoside for heart failure; theophylline or β_2 agonist for bronchospasm; IV diazepam for seizures
Amantadine	Lethal dose of 2 g reported	Arrhythmia, tachycardia, hypertension, disorientation, lethargy, confusion, visual hallucinations, aggressive behavior, anxiety, minimally reactive and dilated pupils, ataxia, tremor, hypertonia, seizure exacerbation, coma, edema and respiratory distress, renal insufficiency, urinary retention, acid–base disturbances	Emesis or gastric lavage; supportive measures including cardiovascular monitoring, airway maintenance, and control of respiration and oxygen administration; avoid adrenergic agents as they may predispose to ventricular arrhythmias; IV physostigmine to treat CNS toxicity, chlorpromazine for toxic psychosis, sedation and anticonvulsants as needed; monitor urine pH, urinary output, serum electrolytes, urine acidifying agents increase rate of excretion, IV fluids, catheter for urinary retention
Amphetamines	Toxic effects at 30 mg, idiosyncratic toxicity as low as 2 mg, survival reported after 500 mg	Elation, irritability, hyperactivity, psychotic symptoms, depression, panic, rapid speech, confusion, anorexia, insomnia, hyperreflexia, tremor, dry mouth, hyperpyrexia, convulsions, coma, chest pain, arrhythmia, heart block, hyper/hypotension, shock, nausea, vomiting, diarrhea, abdominal cramps, tachypnea, rhabdomyolysis	Emesis or lavage, activated charcoal, cathartic (can be effective long after ingestion because of recycling through gastric mucosa); supportive care; reduce external stimuli, sedate with chlorpromazine; IV phentolamine for severe HTN; acidification of urine
Anticholinergics	700 mg to 7 g (doses vary depending on agent involved)	Hot, dry, flushed skin; dry mucous membranes, hyperthermia, rash, shock, tachycardia, unreactive dilated pupils, blurred vision; delirium, delusions, ataxia, hallucinations, convulsions, coma, dysphagia, nausea, vomiting, hypoactive bowel sounds, respiratory arrest, urinary retention	Emesis or lavage, activated charcoal, saline cathartics; supportive and symptomatic therapy; 1–2 mg physostigmine can reverse anticholinergic effects; cold packs, mechanical cooling devices, or sponging with tepid water for hyperthermia; continuous ECG monitoring; vasopressors and fluid therapy for shock, IV propranolol for supraventricular tachyarrhythmias, avoid dopamine receptor antagonists; local miotics for mydriasis; diazepam for agitation
Antihistamines	2.8 g diphenhydramine, 1.75–17.5 g hydroxyzine	Disorientation, drowsiness, excitation, depression, hallucinations, anxiety, delirium, hyperthermia, tachycardia, hypotension, arrhythmias, seizures	Emesis or lavage; support cardiorespiratory function; IV fluids and vasopressors for hypotension; caffeine and sodium benzoate to counteract CNS depressant effects, physostigmine for anticholinergic effects; diazepam for seizures; sponge baths with tepid water (not alcohol) or cold packs for hyperthermia
Barbiturates	10 times the daily dose or 1 g of most barbiturates causes severe toxicity, 2–10 g fatal	Delirium, confusion, excitement, headache, CNS and respiratory depression (somnolence to coma), Cheyne-Stokes respiration, areflexia, shock, miosis, oliguria, tachycardia, hypotension, hypothermia	Emesis or lavage, activated charcoal, saline cathartics; supportive treatment, including maintaining airway and respiration and treating shock as needed; maintain vital signs and fluid balance; alkalinizing the urine increases excretion; forced diuresis if renal function is normal; hemodialysis in severe cases

(*continued*)

analgesics, but some persons may have to switch to another antidepressant. Although SSRIs may cause headache, they much more commonly provide relief from headache. SSRIs are an effective treatment for chronic tension-type headache and for migraine headache.

Anorexia. SSRI-associated appetite suppression is more pronounced in obese persons and persons with carbohydrate craving and may therefore be desirable. However, other persons may gain weight while taking SSRIs. Clinicians can reassure persons who experience SSRI-associated weight changes that most persons return to their pretreatment weight by the end of the first year.

Fluoxetine (60 mg per day) in the context of a comprehensive program of behavioral management is an approved treatment for bulimia and is also useful for treatment of anorexia nervosa. However, persons with eating disorders may abuse fluoxetine if use is not monitored. Unless a comprehensive therapeutic program is available, SSRIs should be used cautiously by persons with eating disorders.

Weight Gain. Many psychotherapeutic drugs cause weight gain as a result of either fluid retention or increased caloric intake. The atypical antipsychotics have been shown to cause weight gain possibly because of a disturbance in glucose or insulin metabolism. Edema can be treated by elevating the affected body parts or by administering a diuretic. If a diuretic is added to a regimen of lithium or cardiac medications, the clinician must monitor blood concentrations, blood chemistries, and vital signs. Increased caloric intake is safely managed only through dietary regulation. No drug has yet been shown to suppress the appetite safely in all persons. The most effective appetite suppressants, the amphetamines, are not used generally because of concerns about abuse.

Sibutramine (Meridia) causes modest weight loss in some persons through inhibition of reuptake of serotonin and norepinephrine. Thus, it should not be used by persons taking any type of antidepressant drug, including SSRIs, bupropion, venlafaxine (Effexor), nefazodone, trazodone, mirtazapine (Remeron), reboxetine (Vestra), tricyclic and tetracyclic drugs, and monoamine oxidase inhibitors (MAOIs).

Orlistat (Xenical) does not suppress the appetite; instead it blocks absorption of fat from the intestine. Thus, it reduces caloric intake from fatty foods but not from carbohydrates or proteins. Because orlistat causes retention of dietary fats in the intestines, it frequently causes excessive flatulence. Most overweight persons misperceive their daily caloric intake as considerably lower than it actually is. Persons wishing to lose weight must adhere strictly to a reduced-calorie diet and must assiduously document every calorie of food they consume.

Somnolence. Many psychotropic drugs cause sedation. Some persons may self-medicate this adverse effect with caffeine, but this practice may worsen orthostatic hypotension. The clinician must alert the person to the possibility of sedation and must document advising the person not to drive or operate dangerous equipment if sedated by medications. Fortunately, newer generations of antidepressant and antipsychotic drugs are much less likely to cause sedation than their predecessors, and the newer drugs should be substituted for the sedating medications when possible.

Dry Mouth. Dry mouth is caused by the blockade of muscarinic acetylcholine receptors. When persons attempt to relieve the dry mouth by constantly sucking on sugar-containing hard candies, they increase their risk for dental caries. They can avoid the problem by chewing sugarless gum or sucking on sugarless hard candies. Some clinicians recommend the use of a 1 percent solution of pilocarpine (Salagen), a cholinergic agonist, as a mouthwash three times daily. Other clinicians suggest bethanechol tablets, another cholinergic agonist, 10 to 30 mg, once or twice daily. It is best to start with 10 mg once a day and to increase the dosage slowly. Adverse effects of cholinomimetic drugs, such as bethanechol, include tremor, diarrhea, abdominal cramps, and excessive eye watering.

Blurred Vision. The blockage of muscarinic acetylcholine receptors causes mydriasis (pupillary dilation) and cycloplegia (ciliary muscle paresis), resulting in blurred vision. The symptom can be relieved by cholinomimetic eyedrops. A 1 percent solution of pilocarpine can be prescribed as one drop four times daily. Alternatively, bethanecol can be used as it is used for dry mouth.

Urinary Retention. The anticholinergic activity of many psychotherapeutic drugs can lead to urinary hesitation, dribbling, urinary retention, and increased urinary tract infections. Elderly men with prostatic enlargement are at increased risk for these adverse effects. Ten to 30 mg of bethanechol three to four times daily is usually effective in the treatment of the urological adverse effects.

Constipation. The anticholinergic activity of psychotherapeutic drugs can cause constipation. The first line of treatment involves the prescribing of bulk laxatives, such as Citrucel, Fiber-Con, Konsyl, Metamucil, Perdiem, and Unifiber. If this treatment fails, cathartic laxatives, such as milk of magnesia, or other laxative preparations can be tried. Prolonged use of cathartic laxatives can result in a loss of their effectiveness. Bethanechol, 10 to 30 mg three to four times daily, can also be used.

Orthostatic Hypotension. Orthostatic hypotension is caused by the blockade of α_1-adrenergic receptors. The elderly are at particular risk for development of orthostatic hypotension. The risk of hip fractures from falls is significantly increased in persons taking psychotherapeutic drugs. Most simply, the person can be instructed to get up slowly and to sit down immediately if dizziness is experienced. Treatments for orthostatic hypotension include avoiding caffeine, drinking at least 2 L of fluid per day, adding salt to food (unless prescribed by a physician), reassessing the dosages of any antihypertensive medications, and wearing support hose. Fludrocortisone (Florinef) is rarely needed.

DISCONTINUATION (WITHDRAWAL) SYNDROMES

The transient emergence of mild symptoms upon discontinuation or reduction of dosage is associated with a number of drugs, including paroxetine (Paxil), venlafaxine, sertraline, fluvoxamine, and the tricyclic and tetracyclic drugs. More severe discontinuation symptoms are associated with lithium (rebound mania), dopamine-receptor antagonists (tardive dyskinesias), and benzodiazepines (anxiety and insomnia). One such syndrome occurs with the withdrawal of SSRIs—the serotonin discontinuation

Table 36.1–8
Adverse Effects of Antidepressants

Drugs	Sedation	Anticholinergic	Orthostatic Hypotension	Cardiac Conduction Effects
Heterocyclics				
Amitriptyline	High	High	Moderate	High
Imipramine	Moderate	Moderate	High	High
Doxepin	High	Moderate	Moderate	Moderate
Desipramine	Low	Low	Low	Moderate
Nortriptyline	Moderate	Moderate	Low	Moderate
Trimipramine	High	High	Moderate	High
Protriptyline	Low	Moderate	Low	Moderate
Clomipramine	High	High	Low	Moderate
Maprotiline	Moderate	Moderate	Low	Moderate
Serotonin reuptake inhibitors				
Fluoxetine	Very low	None	Very low	Very low
Sertraline	Low	None	None	Very low
Paroxetine	Low	Low	None	Very low
Fluvoxamine	Low	None	None	Very low
Citalopram	Low	None	None	Very low
Escitalopram	Low	None	None	Very low
Phenylethylamine				
Venlafaxine	Low	None	Very low	Very low
Dibenzoxazepines				
Amoxapine	Low	Low	Low	Low
Triazolopyridines				
Trazodone	High	Very low	Moderate	Low
Phenylpiperazines				
Nefazodone	Moderate	None	Low	Low
Piperazinoazepines				
Mirtazapine	High	Moderate	Low	Low
Aminoketones				
Bupropion	Low	Very low	Very low	0
Triazolobenzodiazepines				
Alprazolam	High	Very low	Very low	0
Monoamine oxidase inhibitors				
Phenelzine Tranylcypromine Isocarboxazid	As a class, orthostatic hypotension, dizziness, headache, drowsiness, overstimulation (hypomania, insomnia, anxiety), constipation, nausea, diarrhea, abdominal pain			

Adapted from Janicak PG, Davis JM, Preskorn SH, Ayd FJ. *Principles and Practice of Psychopharmacology.* Baltimore: Williams & Wilkins; 1993:272.

(Yocon). Cyproheptadine (Periactin) can be used for inhibited female orgasm, 4 mg every morning, and for inhibited male orgasm secondary to serotonergic agents, 4 to 8 mg orally taken 1 to 2 hours before anticipated sexual activity.

Anxiety, Akathisia, Agitation, and Insomnia. As many as one quarter of persons initiating treatment with serotonergic antidepressants, especially fluoxetine, experience a transient increase in psychomotor activation in the first 2 to 3 weeks of use. Antipsychotic medication can produce movement-related disorders that are discussed extensively in Section 36.3.

The agitating effects of SSRIs modestly increase the risk of persons at risk for suicide acting out their suicidal impulses. During the initial period of SSRI treatment, persons at risk for self-injury should maintain close contact with the clinician or should be hospitalized, depending on the clinician's assessment of the risk for suicide.

Insomnia and anxiety associated with use of serotonergic drugs may be counteracted by administration of a benzodiazepine or trazodone (Desyrel) for the first several weeks. A small number of persons experience increased anxiety beyond the initial 3-week period; these persons may require a nonserotonergic antidepressant drug.

GI Upset and Diarrhea. Most of the body's serotonin is in the GI tract, and serotonergic drugs, particularly sertraline (Zoloft) and fluvoxamine, may therefore produce mildly to moderately severe stomach pain, nausea, and diarrhea, usually only for the first few weeks of therapy. Sertraline is most likely to cause loose stools, and fluvoxamine is most likely to cause nausea. These symptoms may be minimized by initiating treatment with a very small dosage and administering the drug after eating. Dietary alteration, such as the BRAT diet (*b*ananas, *r*ice, *a*pples, and *t*oast), may reduce loose stools. These symptoms usually abate over time, but some persons never accommodate and must switch to another drug.

Headache. A small fraction of persons initiating therapy with an SSRI experience mildly to moderately severe headache. SSRI-associated headaches often respond to over-the-counter

the patient has a positive transference toward the clinician, and if the patient does not have to wait in the waiting room to see the clinician. Patients should be warned in particular about the potential adverse consequences of missing even one dose of medication.

SPECIAL TREATMENT CONSIDERATIONS

Children

Special care must be taken when administering psychotherapeutic drugs to children. Although the small volume of distribution suggests the use of lower dosages than in adults, children's higher rate of metabolism indicates that the ratio of milligrams of drug to kilograms of body weight should be higher. In practice, it is best to begin with a small dose and increase the dosage until clinical effects are observed. Clinicians should not hesitate to use adult dosages in children if the dosages are effective and the adverse effects are acceptable.

Geriatric Patients

The two major concerns when treating geriatric patients with psychotherapeutic drugs are that older persons may be especially susceptible to adverse effects (particularly cardiac effects) and may metabolize drugs slowly (Table 36.1–5). Thus, geriatric patients may require low dosages of medication. Further, geriatric patients are often taking other medications, and psychiatrists must consider possible drug interactions.

Table 36.1–5
Pharmacokinetics and Aging

Phase	Change	Effect
Absorption	Gastric pH increases Decreased surface villi Decreased gastric motility and delayed gastric emptying Intestinal perfusion decreases	Little overall change Absorption is slowed but just as complete
Distribution	Total body water and lean body mass decrease Increased total body fat, more marked in women than in men Albumin decreases, gamma globulin increases, alpha globulin, acid glycoprotein unchanged	V_d increases for lipid-soluble drugs, decreases for water-soluble drugs The free or unbound percentage of albumin-bound drugs increases
Metabolism	Renal: renal blood flow and glomerular filtration rates decrease Hepatic: decreased enzyme activity and perfusion	Decreased metabolism leads to prolonged half-lives, if V_d remains the same
Total body weight	Decreases	Think on a mg/kg basis
Receptor sensitivity	May increase	Increased effect

V_d, volume of distribution.
Reprinted with permission from Guttmacher LB. *Concise Guide to Somatic Therapies in Psychiatry.* Washington, DC: American Psychiatric Press; 1988:126.

In practice, psychiatrists should begin treating geriatric patients with a small dose, usually approximately one half the usual dose. The dosage should be raised in small amounts more slowly than in younger adults until either a clinical benefit is achieved or unacceptable adverse effects appear. Although many geriatric patients require a small dosage of medication, others require the usual adult dosage.

Pregnant and Nursing Women

The basic rule is to avoid administering any drug to a woman who is pregnant (particularly during the first trimester) or breast-feeding a child. This rule, however, is broken occasionally when a women's mental disorder is severe. If psychotherapeutic medications must be administered during a pregnancy, the possibility of therapeutic abortion should be discussed. The two most teratogenic drugs in the psychopharmacopoeia are lithium and the anticonvulsants. Lithium administration during pregnancy is associated with a high incidence of birth abnormalities, including Ebstein's anomaly, a serious abnormality in cardiac development. Anticonvulsants used during pregnancy are associated with fetal craniofacial and neural tube abnormalities in less than 10 percent of infants. The risk of teratogenicity can be reduced by the administration of folic acid. Other psychoactive drugs (antidepressants, antipsychotics, and anxiolytics), although less clearly associated with birth defects, should also be avoided during pregnancy if at all possible. The most common clinical situation is a pregnant woman's becoming psychotic. If a decision is made not to terminate the pregnancy, electroconvulsive therapy (ECT) or antipsychotics are preferable to lithium.

The administration of psychotherapeutic drugs at or near delivery may cause a baby to be overly sedated at delivery, to need a respirator, or to be physically dependent on the drug and require detoxification and treatment of a withdrawal syndrome. Virtually all psychotropic drugs are secreted in the milk of a nursing women; therefore, mothers taking these agents should not breast-feed their infants.

Persons with Hepatic or Renal Insufficiency

Drugs that are metabolized in the liver may accumulate to toxic concentrations in persons with hepatocellular insufficiency of any cause, including cirrhosis, hepatitis, metabolic disorders, and bile duct obstruction. Drugs that are excreted by the kidneys may accumulate to toxic concentrations in persons with renal insufficiency of any cause, including atherosclerosis, nephrosis, nephritis, infiltrative disorders, and outflow obstruction. Hepatocellular or renal insufficiency requires administration of a reduced dosage, usually half of the recommended dosage for healthy persons. Clinicians should be particularly alert to signs and symptoms of adverse drug effects in persons with hepatic or renal disorders. Monitoring plasma drug concentrations may help guide dosage adjustments.

Persons with Other Medical Illnesses

Considerations in administering psychotherapeutic drugs to medically ill persons include a potentially increased sensitivity to the drug's adverse effects, either increased or decreased metabolism and excretion of the drug, and interactions with other medications. As with children and geriatric persons, the most reasonable clinical practice is to begin with a low dosage, increase it slowly, and watch for both clinical and adverse effects.

ADVERSE EFFECTS

Most psychotherapeutic drugs do not affect a single neurotransmitter system, and their effects are not localized to the brain.

Table 36.1–6
Potential Adverse Effects Caused by Blockade of Muscarinic Acetylcholine Receptors

Blurred vision
Constipation
Decreased salivation
Decreased sweating
Delayed or retrograde ejaculation
Delirium
Exacerbation of asthma (through decreased bronchial secretions)
Hyperthermia (through decreased sweating)
Memory problems
Narrow-angle glaucoma
Photophobia
Sinus tachycardia
Urinary retention

Psychotherapeutic drugs produce a wide range of adverse effects on neurotransmitter systems. For example, some of the most common adverse effects of psychotherapeutic drugs are caused by the blockade of muscarinic acetylcholine receptors (Table 36.1–6). Many psychotherapeutic drugs antagonize dopaminergic, histaminergic, and adrenergic neurons or excessively activate serotonergic neurons, resulting in the adverse effects listed in Table 36.1–7. There are also several commonly observed adverse effects for which the neurotransmitters involved have not been specifically identified.

Patients generally have less trouble with adverse effects if they have been told to expect them. Psychiatrists can explain the appearance of adverse effects as evidence that the drug is working. But clinicians should distinguish between probable or expected adverse effects and rare or unexpected ones.

Table 36.1–7
Potential Adverse Effects of Psychotherapeutic Drugs and Associated Neurotransmitter Systems

Antidopaminergic
Endocrine dysfunction
Hyperprolactinemia
Menstrual dysfunction
Sexual dysfunction
Movement disorders
Akathisia
Dystonia
Parkinsonism
Tardive dyskinesia
Antiadrenergic (primarily α_1)
Dizziness
Postural hypotension
Reflex tachycardia
Antihistaminergic
Hypotension
Sedation
Weight gain
Excessive serotonergic
Akathisia and agitation
Anxiety
GI upset and diarrhea
Headache
Insomnia or somnolence
Nausea and vomiting
Sexual dysfunction
Multiple neurotransmitter systems
Agranulocytosis (and other blood dyscrasias)
Allergic reactions
Anorexia
Cardiac conduction abnormalities
Nausea and vomiting
Seizures

Treatment of Common Adverse Effects

Many adverse effects occur with psychotherapeutic drugs. The management of the adverse effects is similar, regardless of which psychotherapeutic drug a patient is taking. If possible, another drug with similar benefits but fewer or less undesirable adverse effects should be substituted. For example, common adverse effects of antidepressant drugs are listed in Table 36.1–8. In addition to those listed here, common antidopaminergic effects are discussed in Section 36.3 on medication-induced movement disorders.

Sexual Dysfunction. Psychotherapeutic drug use can be associated with sexual dysfunction—specifically, decreased libido, impaired ejaculation and erection, and inhibition of female orgasm. This is by far the most common adverse effect associated with use of SSRIs. Fifty to 80 percent of persons taking an SSRI experience some sexual dysfunction, although few complain of severe dysfunction.

The pharmacological management of sexual dysfunction involves either switching from the SSRI to nefazodone or bupropion (Wellbutrin), which are much less likely to cause sexual dysfunction, or adding a prosexual agent. Merely administering bupropion concurrently may be enough to reverse the sexual inhibition caused by SSRIs.

Specific pharmacological strategies are available for treating dysfunctions of each stage of the sexual response cycle, but improvement of any stage of sexual function can be reassuring and may stimulate full endogenous sexual functioning. The best tolerated and most potent prosexual drug currently available is sildenafil (Viagra). Taken 1 hour before intercourse, it increases blood flow to the genital erectile tissues in both men and women. In men, it improves erectile function, and in women, it may promote engorgement of the clitoris and labia minora. Sildenafil not only improves the arousal phase of the sexual response cycle, but it may also stimulate the desire and orgasm phases in both men and women.

Alprostadil (Muse, Caverject) is an alternative treatment for male erectile dysfunction. Alprostadil improves the arousal phase of the sexual response cycle and may also stimulate the desire and orgasm phases in men. Other, less effective prosexual agents include neostigmine (Prostigmin) for impaired ejaculation, 7.5 to 15 mg taken orally 30 minutes before sexual intercourse. Erectile function may be improved with bethanechol (Urecholine), dopamine receptor agonists, amantadine (Symmetrel), or yohimbine

Table 36.1–9 (*continued*)

Drug	Toxic/Lethal Dose	Signs and Symptoms	Treatment
Benzodiazepines	Toxic dose; diazepam 2 g, chlordiazepoxide 6 g	CNS depression ranging from drowsiness to coma, slurred speech, ataxia, confusion, hyporeflexia, hypotension, hypotonia	Emesis or lavage, saline cathartic and activated charcoal; supportive care, monitor vital signs, maintain airway; IV fluids and norepinephrine for hypotension; the benzodiazepine antagonist flumazenil can be used with caution and only in hospitalized patients
Bromocriptine	Survival after 225 mg; 1 death of unknown dosage	Severe hypotension, nausea, vomiting, psychosis	Lavage and aspiration; IV fluids for hypotension
Bupropion	Survival after 0.85–4.2 g; deaths reported in massive overdoses	Seizures, loss of consciousness, hallucinations, tachycardia	Lavage and activated charcoal, emesis not recommended; supportive care, maintain airway and respiration, EEG, ECG, and vital signs monitoring for 48 hours, provide fluids; IV benzodiazepines for seizures
Buspirone	Toxicity at 375 mg; fatal dose unknown	Dizziness, drowsiness, nausea, vomiting, miosis, gastric distress	Emesis or lavage; symptomatic and supportive care, monitor vital signs
Calcium channel inhibitors	10.8 g diltiazem and 9 g of nifedipine has been survived; 9.6 g verapamil—fatal	Confusion, headache, nausea, vomiting, seizures, flushing, constipation, hyperglycemia, metabolic acidosis, hypotension, bradycardia, AV block, cardiac failure, arrhythmias, noncardiogenic pulmonary edema with verapamil	Emesis or lavage, activated charcoal; supportive care, monitor cardiovascular and respiratory function, observation for at least 48 hours; IV calcium chloride 10–20 mg/kg in 10% solution with normal saline over 30 min and repeated as needed; atropine or isoproterenol for bradycardia or AV block, a pacemaker may be needed; inotropes and diuretics for cardiac failure, CPR for asystole; fluid and vasopressors for hypotension
Carbamazepine	30 g in adults and 10 g in children have been survived; lethal doses of 3.2 g in adults and 1.6 g in children reported	Drowsiness, coma, seizures, dizziness, ataxia, agitation, tremor, athetoid movements, opisthotonos, ballism, abnormal reflexes, adiadochokinesis, nystagmus, mydriasis, nausea, vomiting, flushing, cyanosis, urinary retention, hypo/hypertension, arrhythmias, tachycardia, shock, respiratory depression	Emesis or lavage, activated charcoal and laxatives; supportive care, respiratory support; monitor vital signs, ECG, kidney function, and pupillary reflexes; forced diuresis, dialysis in severe poisoning with renal failure; IV fluids and vasopressors for hypotension; diazepam for seizures
Chloral hydrate	30 g has been survived; lethal dose of 10 g reported	Coma, confusion, drowsiness, miosis, respiratory depression, hypotension, hypothermia, vomiting, gastric necrosis and perforation, esophageal stricture, hepatic and renal injury	Lavage: supportive care, maintain airway, cardiorespiratory function, and body temperature; hemodialysis or peritoneal dialysis may be of use; saline enema if drug was administered rectally
Clonidine	100 mg has been survived, 0.1 mg toxic in children; no deaths with clonidine alone, 2 deaths from mixed overdoses	Hypertension (followed by hypotension), bradycardia, arrhythmia, cardiac conduction defects, respiratory depression, apnea, hyporeflexia or areflexia, seizures, miosis, weakness, irritability, sedation, coma, hypothermia	Lavage, activated charcoal, and a saline cathartic, emesis not recommended; supportive treatment, maintain airway and respiration; IV furosemide, β-adrenergic receptor antagonists, or diazoxide for hypertension; IV fluids, vasopressors, and Trendelenburg's position for hypotension; IV atropine for symptomatic bradycardia; naloxone for respiratory depression, hypotension, and coma; IV benzodiazepines for seizures
Clozapine	>4 g has been survived; lethal dose >2.5 g	Delirium, drowsiness, coma, respiratory depression, tachycardia, arrhythmias, hypotension, hypersalivation, seizures	Activated charcoal with sorbitol (may be as or more effective than lavage or emesis); supportive and symptomatic treatment, maintain airway and respiration; cardiac and vital signs monitoring; epinephrine, quinidine, and procainamide are to be avoided; patient should be observed for several days for delayed effects
Dantrolene	No overdose data available	Muscular weakness, lethargy, coma, crystalluria, diarrhea	Lavage; supportive care, maintain airway and respiration, careful observation of patient; ECG monitoring; large quantities of IV fluids to avert crystalluria

(*continued*)

Table 36.1–9 (*continued*)

Drug	Toxic/Lethal Dose	Signs and Symptoms	Treatment
Disulfiram	≥6 deaths with 0.5–1 g disulfiram with BAL of 1 mg/mL; 30 g ingestion produces serious toxicity	Headache, peripheral or optic neuropathy, psychotic behavior, mucous membrane injury, rash, respiratory depression, cardiovascular collapse, arrhythmias, myocardial infarction, acute CHF, unconsciousness, convulsions, death	Lavage; supportive care; restore blood pressure and treat shock; monitor potassium levels; maintain airway and respiration; IV antihistamines, vitamin C, and ephedrine sulfate may be of benefit
Dopamine receptor antagonists	Chlorpromazine: 26 g adult fatality, 0.35 g child fatality; thiothixene: 2.5–4 g fatal; phenothiazines: 1.05–10.5 g fatal	CNS depression from somnolence to coma, extrapyramidal symptoms, agitation, restlessness, convulsions, fever, dry mouth, ileus, hypotension, tachycardia, arrhythmias, ECG changes (prolonged QT interval and wide QRS complexes with Risperdal)	Lavage, saline cathartic, activated charcoal; emesis is not recommended; symptomatic and supportive care, monitor vital signs and ECG; maintain airway and respiration; IV fluids and norepinephrine or phenylephrine for hypotension, avoid dopamine and epinephrine; antiparkinsonism drugs, anticholinergics, and diphenhydramine (Benadryl) may be useful for extrapyramidal symptoms; stimulants such as amphetamines or caffeine with sodium benzoate if desired, avoid picrotoxin and pentylenetetrazol; antiarrhythmics such as neostigmine, pyridostigmine, propranolol, disopyramide, procainamide, and quinidine should be avoided; diazepam for convulsions
Ethchlorvynol	50–100 g has been survived; 6 g lethal	Hypotension, hypothermia, severe respiratory depression, apnea, prolonged coma (can last days to weeks), areflexia, mydriasis, bradycardia, nystagmus, pancytopenia	Lavage; supportive treatment; maintain airway and respiration, maintain cardiorespiratory function and body temperature; monitor blood gases and vital signs; hemoperfusion using Amberlite column technique hastens drug elimination; hemodialysis, peritoneal dialysis, or forced diuresis may be useful in increasing urinary output
Fluoxetine	3 g has been survived; lethal dose unknown, 2 deaths in combination with other drugs	Nausea, vomiting, CNS excitation, restlessness, agitation, hypomania, tachycardia, hypertension, seizures	Lavage and activated charcoal, emesis not recommended; supportive and symptomatic care; maintain airway and respiration; monitor ECG and vital signs; IV diazepam for ongoing seizures
Fluvoxamine	10 g has been survived; 2 deaths of unknown dosages solely due to fluvoxamine	Drowsiness, vomiting, diarrhea, dizziness, coma, tachycardia, bradycardia, hypotension, ECG abnormalities, liver function abnormalities, convulsions	Lavage and activated charcoal; supportive care; maintain airway and respiration; monitor ECG and vital signs
Glutethimide	5 g severe intoxication, but survived; 10–20 g fatal	Hypotension, prolonged coma, shock, respiratory depression, hypothermia, fever, inadequate ventilation, apnea, cyanosis, fixed and dilated pupils, ileus, bladder atony, dry mouth, hyporeflexia, areflexia, intermittent spasticity or flaccidity	Lavage using 1:1 mixture of castor oil and water may be more effective than aqueous lavage, leave 50 mL castor oil in stomach as a cathartic, activated charcoal; maintain airway and cardiorespiratory function; hemodialysis with activated charcoal or soybean dialysate; hemoperfusion with Amberlite XAD-2 resin; charcoal hemoperfusion; continue drug removal for at least 2 hours after the patient regains consciousness; maintain urinary output but avoid overhydration
Levodopa	≥8 a day causes toxicity	Palpitations, arrhythmias, spasm or closing of eyes, psychosis	Lavage; supportive and symptomatic treatment; maintain airway; ECG monitoring; IV fluids; treat arrhythmias as necessary
Lithium	Lethal dose produces serum levels >3.5 mEq/L 12 hours after ingestion	Diarrhea, nausea, vomiting, drowsiness, tremor, muscle weakness, giddiness, ataxia, vertical nystagmus, tinnitus, diabetes insipidus, multiorgan toxicity	Emesis or lavage; infuse 0.9% sodium chloride IV if toxicity is due to sodium depletion; hemodialysis for 8–12 hours if fluid and electrolyte imbalance does not respond to supportive measures; repeated courses of dialysis are needed if level >3 mEq/L or if level is 2–3 mEq/L and patient is deteriorating, or if level has not decreased 20% in 6 hours; goal is level <1 mEq/L 8 hours after dialysis is completed; urea, mannitol, and aminophylline increase lithium excretion

(*continued*)

Table 36.1–9 (*continued*)

Drug	Toxic/Lethal Dose	Signs and Symptoms	Treatment
Meprobamate	40 g has been survived; 12 g lethal	Stupor, drowsiness, lethargy, ataxia, coma, respiratory depression, hypotension, shock	Emesis or lavage and activated charcoal; supportive care; maintain airway, respiration, and blood pressure; pressor agents if necessary; CNS stimulants; elimination may be enhanced by forced diuresis, hemodialysis, peritoneal dialysis, or osmotic diuresis; monitor urine output
Methadone	40–60 mg lethal in nontolerant persons	CNS depression (stupor to coma), pinpoint pupils, cold and clammy skin, bradycardia, hypotension, cardiac arrest, shock, respiratory depression, Cheyne-Stokes respiration, cyanosis, apnea, skeletal muscle flaccidity	Lavage; supportive care; IV fluids and vasopressors; maintain airway and respiration; IV naloxone to treat clinically significant respiratory or cardiovascular depression, monitor continuously for recurrence of respiratory depression, treat repeatedly with naloxone until patient's status is stable (initial adult dose of naloxone is 0.4–2 mg IV every 2–3 minutes)
Methylphenidate	2 g	Delirium, confusion, agitation, hallucinations, hyperpyrexia, mydriasis, tremors, muscle twitching, seizures, coma, hyperreflexia, euphoria, headache, palpitations, tachycardia, arrhythmias, hypertension, vomiting, sweating, flushing, dry mucous membranes	Lavage, activated charcoal, and cathartics; in severe toxicity use a carefully titrated dose of short-acting barbiturate before lavage; supportive care; maintain respiratory and circulatory function; isolation to reduce external stimuli; protection against self-harm; external cooling procedures for hyperpyrexia
Mirtazapine	No deaths reported solely due to mirtazapine	Disorientation, drowsiness, impaired memory, tachycardia	Emesis or lavage and activated charcoal; supportive care; monitor cardiac and vital signs, maintain airway and respiration
Monoamine oxidase inhibitors (MAOIs)	600 mg severe toxicity; single doses of 1.75–7 g fatal	Dizziness, drowsiness, irritability, insomnia, headache, confusion, hyperactivity, agitation, anxiety, hallucinations, trismus, opisthotonus, rigidity, convulsions, coma, hypertensive crisis (mainly seen in conjunction with tyramine), tachycardia, hypotension, arrhythmia, diaphoresis, chest pain, shock, hypertension, respiratory depression, faintness, hyperpyrexia	Emesis or lavage and activated charcoal; symptomatic and supportive care; maintain airway and respiration; monitor vital signs; maintain fluid and electrolyte balance; treat hypotension and shock with IV fluids and vasopressors (adrenergics may produce a markedly increased pressor response, therefore administer carefully); IV diazepam for convulsions; phenothiazine derivatives and CNS stimulants should be avoided; manage hyperpyrexia intensively with external cooling; hypertensive crisis; discontinue MAOIs and treat with 5 mg IV phentolamine by slow injection; toxic effects may be delayed—therefore, observe patient for at least 1 week; never use meperidine (Demerol)
Naltrexone	≥1,000 mg/kg toxic	Salivation, depression, convulsions, tremors, reduced activity	Supportive care and symptomatic treatment
Nefazodone	1–11.2 g toxicity; death reported in combination with alcohol	Nausea, vomiting, somnolence	Lavage (emesis not recommended); supportive care; maintain airway and respiration; monitor ECG and vital signs
Olanzapine	300 mg has been survived	Drowsiness, slurred speech, shock	Lavage, activated charcoal, and laxatives (emesis not recommended); maintain airway and respiration; continuous cardiovascular and ECG monitoring; IV fluids and vasopressors for hypotension and shock, avoid beta agonists; avoid epinephrine and dopamine in the presence of α-adrenergic blockade
Paroxetine	2 g has been survived	Nausea, vomiting, sedation, dizziness, sweating, facial flush	Lavage and activated charcoal (emesis not recommended); maintain airway and respiration; monitor ECG and vital signs
Pemoline	2 g	Agitation, euphoria, delirium, hallucinations, tremors, hyperreflexia, convulsions, coma, headache, mydriasis, flushing, hyperpyrexia, vomiting, hypertension, tachycardia; hepatic effects not due to overdose	Lavage, activated charcoal, and cathartic; symptomatic treatment; chlorpromazine to decrease CNS stimulation and sympathomimetic effects; protect against self-injury and external stimuli that would aggravate overstimulation

(*continued*)

Table 36.1–9 (*continued*)

Drug	Toxic/Lethal Dose	Signs and Symptoms	Treatment
Risperidone	20–300 mg has been survived	Drowsiness, sedation, tachycardia, hypotension, extrapyramidal symptoms, hyponatremia, hypokalemia, prolonged QT interval, widened QRS complex conversions	Establish and maintain airway; gastric lavage; activated charcoal; continuous cardiovascular monitoring; disopyramide, procainamide, and quinidine should be avoided in the presence of arrhythmias; fluid management of hypotension; avoid epinephrine and dopamine in the presence of α-adrenergic receptor blockade; anticholinergics for extrapyramidal symptoms
Sertraline	0.5–6 g toxicity; no deaths with sertraline alone, 4 deaths in combination with other drugs and alcohol	Somnolence, nausea, vomiting, tachycardia, ECG changes, anxiety, mydriasis	Lavage, charcoal, and cathartics; supportive care; maintain airway and respiration; monitor vital signs and cardiac function; hydration
Tacrine	2 g toxic	Cholinergic crisis: nausea, vomiting, salivation, perspiration, bradycardia, hypotension, collapse, convulsions, increasing muscle weakness (death if respiratory muscles involved)	Supportive care; tertiary anticholinergics such as IV atropine titrated to effect, initial dose 1–2 mg in adults, 0.05 mg/kg in children, subsequent dosing every 10–30 minutes
Thyroid hormones	0.3 g/kg desiccated thyroid—severe toxicity	Thyrotoxicosis: nervousness, sweating, palpitations, abdominal cramps, diarrhea, tachycardia, hypertension, headache, arrhythmias, tremors, cardiac failure, angina, insomnia, increased appetite, weight loss, heat intolerance, fever, menstrual irregularities	Emesis or lavage, charcoal and cholestyramine to interfere with thyroxine absorption; supportive care; control fluid loss, fever, hypoglycemia; maintain airway and respiration; β-adrenergic receptor antagonists such as propranolol (1–3 mg IV over 10 minutes) can be used to counteract increased sympathetic activity
Trazodone	7.5–9.2 g has been survived	Lethargy, vomiting, drowsiness, headache, orthostasis, dizziness, dyspnea, tinnitus, myalgias, tachycardia, incontinence, shivering, coma	Emesis or lavage; supportive care; forced diuresis may enhance elimination; treat hypotension and sedation as appropriate; acute liver failure reported
Tricyclics and tetracyclics	0.7–1.4 g: toxicity; 2.1–2.8 g: fatal; amitriptyline: 10 g has been survived, 0.5 g lowest known fatality; imipramine: 0.5 g fatal (30 mg/kg average lethal dose)	Initial CNS stimulation, confusion, agitation, hallucinations, hyperpyrexia, nystagmus, hyperreflexia, parkinsonian symptoms, mydriasis, seizures, CNS stimulation followed by depression, hypothermia, respiratory depression, hypotension, coma, arrhythmias, QRS prolongation (degree indicates severity of the overdose), impaired cardiac contractility, vomiting, polyradiculoneuropathy, stupor, drowsiness	Lavage and activated charcoal, emesis is not recommended; symptomatic and supportive care; monitor ECG and vital signs; maintain airway and respiration; minimum of 6 hours' observation with cardiac monitoring; IV diazepam for seizures; IV sodium bicarbonate to maintain pH of 7.45–7.55 to help treat arrhythmias, hyperventilation and/or antiarrhythmics such as lidocaine may be needed, type 1A and 1C antiarrhythmics contraindicated; physostigmine not recommended except for life-threatening treatment-refractory anticholinergic toxicity and then only in consultation with poison control center
Valproic acid	36 g has been survived, patients with blood levels of 2,120 μg/mL have survived; fatalities of unknown dose reported	Somnolence, coma, heart block	Value of emesis or lavage varies with time since the drug has rapid absorption; supportive measures; maintain adequate urinary output; naloxone may reverse CNS depressant effects of overdose but may also reverse anticonvulsant effects and should be used with caution
Venlafaxine	6.75 g has been survived; fatalities reported in combination with other drugs and alcohol	Somnolence, convulsions, prolonged QT interval, mild sinus tachycardia	Lavage and activated charcoal, emesis not recommended; supportive and symptomatic care; maintain airway and respiration; monitor vital signs and cardiac rhythm

[a]The clinician should always consult *Physicians' Desk Reference* (PDR) or contact the manufacturer of the drug for the latest information on toxicity and lethality.

REFERENCES

Armstrong SC, Cozza KL, Oesterheld JR. Med-psych drug-drug interactions update. *Psychosomatics*. 2002;43:77.

Baker CB, Coutts RT, Greenshaw AJ. Neurochemical and metabolic aspects of antidepressants: an overview. *J Psychiatry Neurosci*. 2000;25:481.

Breier A, Tran PV, eds. *Current Issues in the Psychopharmacology of Schizophrenia*. Philadelphia: Lippincott Williams & Wilkins; 2001:556.

Dahl ML, Bertilsson L. Genetically variable metabolism of antidepressants and neuroleptic drugs in man. *Pharmacogenetics*. 1993;3:61.

Delva NH, Chang A, Hawken ER, et al. Effects of clonidine in schizophrenic patients with primary polydipsia: three single case studies. *Prog Neuropsychopharmacol Biol Psychiatry*. 2002;26:387.

Gabbard G, Kay J. The fate of integrated treatment: whatever happened to the biopsychosocial psychiatrist? *Am J Psychiatry*. 2001;158:12.

Grebb JA. General principles of psychopharmacology. In: Sadock BJ, Sadock VA,

eds. *Kaplan & Sadock's Comprehensive Textbook of Psychiatry.* 7th ed. Vol 2. Baltimore: Lippincott Williams & Wilkins; 2000:2235.
Hardman, JG, Limbird LE, Goodman Gilman A, eds. *Goodman & Gilman's The Pharmacological Basis of Therapeutics.* 10th ed. New York: McGraw-Hill; 2001.
Hirschfeld RMA. Clinical importance of long-term antidepressant treatment. *Br J Psychiatry.* 2001;179(suppl 42):S4.
Hyman SE, Arana GW, Rosenbaum JF. *Handbook of Psychiatry Drug Therapy.* 3rd ed. Boston: Little, Brown; 1996.
Janicak PG, Davis JM. Pharmacokinetics and drug interactions. In: Sadock BJ, Sadock VA, eds. *Kaplan & Sadock's Comprehensive Textbook of Psychiatry.* 7th ed. Vol 2. Baltimore: Lippincott Williams & Wilkins; 2000:2250.
Leber P. Drug development and approval process in the United States. In: Sadock BJ, Sadock VA, eds. *Kaplan & Sadock's Comprehensive Textbook of Psychiatry.* 7th ed. Vol 2. Baltimore: Lippincott Williams & Wilkins; 2000:2259.
Sadock BJ, Sadock VA. *Pocket Handbook of Psychiatry Drug Treatment.* Philadelphia: Lippincott Williams & Wilkins; 2001.
Stable SM. *Essential Psychopharmacology.* Cambridge: Cambridge University Press; 2001.

▲ 36.2 DRUG AUGMENTATION THERAPY

Combination drug therapy is often used to achieve optimal response in the treatment of mental disorders. Reasons for use of combination therapy include nonresponse, partial response, delay in onset of response, intolerance of adverse effects, and the presence of comorbid disorders. Drug combination strategies may involve the combination of two or more agents with the same therapeutic indication. For example, there may be simultaneous use of two different classes of antidepressants (e.g., a selective serotonin reuptake inhibitor [SSRI] and bupropion [Wellbutrin]). Other strategies consist of the addition of a second agent with an unrelated indication. One such combination is the addition of thyroid hormone to an antidepressant.

Some drugs are extensively, and almost exclusively, used in an adjunct role. Antiparkinsonian drugs, for example, are routinely prescribed by psychiatrists to treat extrapyramidal adverse effects of dopamine receptor agonists. Coadministration of benzodiazepine agonists may improve treatment outcome by enhancing the effects of the primary medication or may help manage particular symptoms, such as anxiety and insomnia, which accompany most psychiatric disorders.

While complex combination therapy is common, it has not been studied systematically. Often-used strategies are either discovered by accident or are based on the application of theoretical neurochemical synergies. Augmentation should be considered only when conventional treatment has failed and in the context of clinical circumstances. Each additional agent increases the possibility of an adverse interaction. It also gives a message that the person being treated may interpret—often correctly—as desperation. In terms of compliance, the more medications that are used, the more reluctant a patient may be to continue treatment.

Primary considerations when using drug augmentation include the potential for enhanced response and possible risks. It is wise to inform patients of the risks and benefits involved with drug combinations (Table 36.2–1) and to document clearly the rationale for using a combination strategy. Selected combination strategies used in the treatment of common mental disorders are described below.

Table 36.2–1
Advantages and Disadvantages of Drug Augmentation or Combination

Advantages
Novel mechanisms
Treatment of residual symptoms
Continuity of treatment
Reduced adverse effects
Treatment of comorbid disorders
Disadvantages
Off-label use
Lack of extensive database
Medicolegal concerns
Drug interactions
Possible increase in severity or frequency of side effects
Reduced compliance because of complexity, apprehension
Cost

DEPRESSION

Most antidepressants have been described as part of a successful combination strategy (Table 36.2–2). No antidepressant augmentation strategy has been proved more effective than another. In the absence of standard algorithms for choice of augmentation agent, one must consider such factors as the level of supporting evidence, safety, tolerability, or concerns about special cautions or clinical monitoring (Table 36.2–3).

Antidepressant Supplementation

A standard warning states that other antidepressants should not be used in combination with a monoamine oxidase inhibitor (MAOI) or within 2 to 4 weeks of discontinuing MAOI use. However, it has been the practice, in extremely refractory cases of depression, to combine an MAOI with a tricyclic antidepressant (TCA). MAOI-TCA combinations are used with greater comfort in the United Kingdom than in the United States. If this strategy is selected, use of both drugs is started concurrently or TCA use is started before that of the MAOI. MAOIs should not be added to ongoing therapy with another class of antidepressant. Given the risks involved and the lack of data showing this combination to be more effective than other approaches, the reluctance

Table 36.2–2
Antidepressant Combinations

MAOI + TCA
TCA + SSRI
SSRI + bupropion
SSRI + venlafaxine
Venlafaxine + bupropion
Nefazodone + bupropion
Nefazodone + SSRI
Mirtazapine + bupropion
Mirtazapine + SSRI

Table 36.2–3
Clinical Considerations for Selecting Antidepressant Augmentation Strategies

Treatment	Level of Supporting Evidence	Safety	Tolerability	Cautions or Special Monitoring
Lithium	+++	++	++	Lithium levels, thyroid function, and renal function monitoring
Thyroid	+++	++	++	Thyroid function monitoring
Buspirone	++	+++	+++	No specific safety concerns or need for special laboratory monitoring
Pindolol	++	+	++	Blood pressure and heart rate monitoring; caution in patients with asthma, severe allergies, and cardiac conduction problems
Dopamine agonists and stimulants	+	+	+	Abuse, regulatory concerns; activation, nausea, blood pressure changes
Anticonvulsants	+	+	++	Pharmacokinetic interactions
Antidepressant combinations	+	+	+	Safety varies according to combination; risk of drug interactions requires plasma monitoring

+++, very positive; ++, positive; +, problematic.

of American clinicians to use MAOI-TCA combinations is understandable. MAOIs and SSRIs should not be combined because of the risks of hypertension and serotonin syndrome.

Clinical studies show an enhanced response rate when noradrenergic TCAs, such as desipramine (Norpramin, Pertofrane) and nortriptyline (Aventyl, Pamelor), are used with an SSRI. The risks of this approach include potentially dangerous increases in TCA plasma concentrations, caused by inhibition of hepatic metabolism, and an overall increase in adverse effects. Among the SSRIs, sertraline (Zoloft) and citalopram (Celexa) are least likely to increase TCA plasma concentrations. It is advisable to monitor TCA plasma concentrations whenever SSRI-TCA combinations are used. Venlafaxine (Effexor) may be used instead of a TCA because of its lack of TCA-like cardiovascular effects and its favorable cytochrome P450 profile.

SSRIs may also be combined with bupropion, which has no independent effects on serotonergic neurotransmission. This combination exemplifies the broad-spectrum approach to antidepressant drug combinations, since this mixture contains agents that are selective for different neurotransmitters. There is a strong theoretical argument for this strategy, mainly that there is targeting of all the monoamine systems that have been implicated in the pathophysiology of depression. A few case series have reported improved rates of response with addition of bupropion to ongoing treatment with fluoxetine (Prozac), sertraline, and paroxetine (Paxil).

Another reason to combine antidepressant drugs is the mitigation of adverse effects. Mirtazapine (Remeron) is especially well suited for blocking some common SSRI adverse effects. Its serotonin 5-HT_3 antagonist properties reduce nausea and diarrhea, while its histamine H_1 antagonist properties help normalize sleep. Bupropion may be useful to counteract sedation caused by other drugs.

Lithium

Controlled trials support the clinical experience that lithium (Eskalith) augmentation of a variety of antidepressants converts 30 to 65 percent of nonresponders into responders. Dosages of 600 to 1,200 mg a day (or blood levels of 0.4 to 0.8 mmol) have been used to augment antidepressant response. Serum lithium levels do not appear to be tightly correlated with responsiveness of depressive symptoms to lithium augmentation. Patients with first-degree relatives with bipolar disorders should be considered candidates for lithium augmentation.

Thyroid Hormones

The addition of small doses (25 to 50 μg) of the thyroid hormone liothyronine (Cytomel) has been used to augment response to TCAs and MAOIs. Fewer controlled studies have been conducted than with lithium. Liothyronine augmentation of TCAs was shown to be effective in approximately 50 to 60 percent of patients. The efficacy of liothyronine augmentation of MAOIs and the SSRI fluoxetine has been limited to evaluation of case reports, but preliminary evidence suggests that liothyronine may be effective with a wide range of antidepressants. Although levothyroxine (Levoxyl, Levothroid, Synthroid) is a precursor of liothyronine, levothyroxine appears to be less effective as an augmenting agent. Doses of 25 to 50 μg have been used to augment antidepressant response.

Sympathomimetics

Sympathomimetics, such as dextroamphetamine (Dexedrine), modafinil (Provigil), and methylphenidate (Ritalin), have been used in patients with depression. Persons who do not respond to SSRIs, TCAs, and even MAOIs may be treated successfully with the addition of a stimulant drug. Persons who exhibit sluggishness, apathy, and fatigue despite otherwise good antidepressant response, or perhaps because of their primary antidepressant, may benefit from the addition of a sympathomimetic. However, there are no controlled studies of sympathomimetic augmentation therapy, and abuse potential makes use of sympathomimetics a less desirable strategy than other options.

Pindolol

Pindolol (Visken) is an antagonist of β-adrenergic receptors and 5-HT_{1A} serotonin receptors. Pindolol reportedly reduces the latency period of antidepressant response in persons with

depression and in those who are resistant to treatment with SSRIs. In controlled studies, however, pindolol has been no more effective than placebo.

Benzodiazepines

Augmentation with a benzodiazepine during the first weeks of antidepressant treatment may provide a more rapid anxiolytic response. Drawbacks include sedation, psychomotor impairment, small risk of withdrawal phenomena, and long-term dependence if the benzodiazepine, especially alprazolam (Xanax), is used for more than 2 months. Benzodiazepines have been used to augment antipsychotic effects of neuroleptics in schizophrenia patients.

Buspirone

Case reports and open-label clinical trials have noted positive responses to buspirone (BuSpar) augmentation at dosages between 20 and 50 mg a day. The addition of buspirone to nefazodone (Serzone) or fluvoxamine (Luvox) may result in higher than expected plasma levels of buspirone. It is thus best to lower the initial dosage of buspirone (e.g., to 2.5 mg twice daily) when it is used in combination with nefazodone or fluvoxamine. Buspirone has been reported to reverse SSRI-induced bruxism and sexual dysfunction.

Dopamine Receptor Antagonists and Other Antipsychotic Agents

Persons with depression who exhibit psychotic symptoms may benefit from the addition of drugs that are used primarily to treat schizophrenia. These include dopamine receptor antagonists and the serotonin-dopamine antagonists (SDAs), such as risperidone (Risperdal), olanzapine (Zyprexa), and quetiapine (Seroquel). There have also been reports of nonpsychotic depressed patients, unresponsive to conventional treatment, who benefited from this strategy.

BIPOLAR DISORDER

Many patients with bipolar disorder cannot be stabilized with a single mood stabilizer. Combination therapy is thus common in the management of bipolar disorders. Typically, patients take a primary mood stabilizer, such as lithium, carbamazepine (Tegretol), or divalproex (Depakote), or a combination of these drugs (Table 36.2–4). In addition, a dopamine receptor agonist, an SDA, or clonazepam (Klonopin) may be used simultaneously, particularly during the treatment of acute mania. Patients with depressed-phase bipolar disorder may also be treated with an antidepressant.

Lamotrigine (Lamictal) is an anticonvulsant that is increasingly being used alone and as an adjunct in the treatment of bipolar disorders and resistant unipolar depression. Case reports and clinical trials suggest that it has both mood-stabilizing and antidepressant activity. Potentially life-threatening rashes are associated with use of the drug. The risk of rash is concentration dependent, especially early in treatment, and occurs more often when lamotrigine is administered along with valproic acid (Depakene). Coadministration of lamotrigine and valproic acid increases lamotrigine concentrations, necessitating a reduction in lamotrigine dosage.

Table 36.2–4
Mood Stabilizer Combinations in Refractory Bipolar Disorder

Lithium + divalproex
Lithium + gabapentin
Lithium + tiagabine
Divalproex + carbamazepine
Divalproex + gabapentin
Divalproex + topiramate
Carbamazepine + gabapentin

Other anticonvulsant drugs, such as gabapentin (Neurontin), topiramate (Topamax), and tiagabine (Gabitril), are also being used as adjuncts in the treatment of bipolar disorders. However, in contrast to lamotrigine, currently no significant drug interaction concerns have been noted with these drugs. Topiramate may offer a particular advantage when combined with other mood stabilizers in that it may both enhance efficacy and also counteract drug-induced weight gain, although it may also impair cognition.

OBSESSIVE-COMPULSIVE DISORDER (OCD)

SSRIs and clomipramine (Anafranil) are the only proved treatments for OCD, but only 40 percent of patients respond to these agents. Few patients demonstrate complete remission with monotherapy while using these drugs. Commonly used add-on agents include valproate, gabapentin, and clonazepam. SDAs such as risperidone have recently been reported to be effective. Comorbid tics may require the coadministration of an SDA, pimozide (Orap), or haloperidol (Haldol). Buspirone may be useful in some patients. Patients with body dysmorphic disorder, which has been broadly conceptualized as a form of OCD and which responds to treatment with SSRIs, may also respond to buspirone augmentation. Patients who have a partial response to the antidepressant before augmentation exhibit the best response following the addition of buspirone.

SCHIZOPHRENIA

Two different antipsychotic drugs may be combined for the purpose of enhancing efficacy. Usually these combinations result from attempts to make a transition from one agent to another, in which the patient shows improvement in the midst of the conversion. Some clinicians choose to leave well enough alone and maintain the patient on the combination. The most common combination involving a dopamine receptor antagonist is the addition of an antiparkinsonian agent. The use of these drugs to treat movement disorders caused by antipsychotics is discussed in other sections of this book.

SSRIs are used to treat secondary depression in schizophrenia patients already stabilized on a neuroleptic and to treat residual negative symptoms, with some patients exhibiting improvement, including reduction in positive and negative

symptoms and decreased frequency of aggressive incidents. Reported adverse effects of SSRI–dopamine receptor antagonist treatment include worsening of psychosis and aggressiveness and worsening of extrapyramidal symptoms. The effects of combining an SSRI with a dopamine receptor antagonist may result from pharmacokinetic interactions. For example, fluoxetine may produce a 65 percent elevation in fluphenazine (Prolixin) concentrations and a 20 percent increase in haloperidol concentrations.

Patients may experience either improvement or worsening of psychosis when clozapine (Clozaril) and SSRIs are combined. Special caution is needed when combining some SSRIs with clozapine. Seizure is a serious, concentration-dependent adverse effect of clozapine, and SSRIs can significantly elevate concentrations of clozapine and its primary metabolite. Fluvoxamine may be more likely than other SSRIs to produce marked increases in these plasma concentrations.

ATTENTION-DEFICIT/HYPERACTIVITY DISORDER (ADHD)

The combination of clonidine (Catapres) with sympathomimetics is sometimes helpful in treating children with ADHD who are unresponsive to other interventions. A potential benefit of combining clonidine with sympathomimetics is improvement of sleep difficulties. For this purpose, daily dosages range from 0.05 to 0.8 mg of clonidine.

Sudden deaths have been reported in children taking the clonidine-methylphenidate combination. The mechanism causing these deaths is unknown, and evidence that these deaths were related to this combination of drugs is still viewed as tenuous. Electrocardiograms (ECGs) should be obtained, whether clonidine is used alone or in combination with other drugs, if abnormalities are found during the physical examination or if there is evidence or a history of preexisting heart disease. It is advisable to monitor vital signs whenever clonidine is used because of its hypotensive effects. Alternatives to the clonidine-methylphenidate combination may also be considered. Dextroamphetamine can be substituted for methylphenidate, and guanfacine (Tenex) for clonidine.

REFERENCES

Gabbay V, O'Dowd MA, Asnis GM. Combined antidepressant treatment: a risk factor for switching in bipolar patients. *J Clin Psychiatry.* 2002;63:367.

Grebb JA. General principles of psychopharmacology. In: Sadock BJ, Sadock VA, eds. *Kaplan & Sadock's Comprehensive Textbook of Psychiatry.* 7th ed. Vol 1. Baltimore: Lippincott Williams & Wilkins; 2000:2235.

Papp LA. Anxiety disorders: somatic treatment. In: Sadock BJ, Sadock VA, eds. *Kaplan & Sadock's Comprehensive Textbook of Psychiatry.* 7th ed. Vol 1. Baltimore: Lippincott Williams & Wilkins; 2000:1490.

Post RM. Mood disorders: treatment of bipolar disorders. In: Sadock BJ, Sadock VA, eds. *Kaplan & Sadock's Comprehensive Textbook of Psychiatry.* 7th ed. Vol 1. Baltimore: Lippincott Williams & Wilkins; 2000:1385.

Post RM, Keck P Jr, Rush AJ. New design for studies of the prophylaxis of bipolar disorder. *J Clin Psychopharmacol.* 2002;22:1.

Rush AJ. Mood disorders: treatment of depression. In: Sadock BJ, Sadock VA, eds. *Kaplan & Sadock's Comprehensive Textbook of Psychiatry.* 7th ed. Vol 1. Baltimore: Lippincott Williams & Wilkins; 2000:1377.

Spina E, Perucca E. Clinical pharmacokinetic interactions between antiepileptic and psychotropic drugs. *Epilepsia.* 2002;43(suppl 2):37.

Weiss E, Hummer M, Koller D, Ulmer H, Fleischhacker WW. Off-label use of antipsychotic drugs. *J Clin Psychopharmacol.* 2001;21:695.

Wheeler Vega JA, Mortimer AM, Tyson PJ. Somatic treatment of psychotic depression: review and recommendations for practice. *J Clin Psychopharmacol.* 2000;20:504.

▲ 36.3 MEDICATION-INDUCED MOVEMENT DISORDERS

Clinicians who alter brain chemistry with drugs in an effort to treat mental illness are aware of the possible unintended consequences of the pharmacological approach. Adverse drug effects must be distinguished from features of the underlying disease, and effects ascribed to the drugs must be skillfully managed by changing dosing, adding adjunct medications, or substituting other agents. Clinicians should use the lowest effective dosage of any psychotropic medication, to reduce the risk of adverse effects, but this desire should be tempered by the need to prevent relapse of illness.

The most common medication-induced movement disorders in psychiatry are those attributed to the dopamine receptor antagonist antipsychotic drugs. These drugs act by blocking the binding of dopamine to the dopamine D_2 receptors, some of which are located in the caudate nucleus and other nuclei in the basal ganglia that belong to the extrapyramidal motor system. It is thought that D_2 receptor blockade disables crucial neural pathways in the basal ganglia that are involved in the control of movements, both voluntary and involuntary; it also disinhibits primitive circuits that coarsely determine "extrapyramidal" abnormalities of muscle tone and movement. The clinical expression of the disarrayed loops of feedback and feed-forward regulation in the basal ganglia may include dystonic posturing, features of parkinsonism (tremor, rigidity, and bradykinesia), akathisia (restlessness), and choreiform ("dancing") or athetoid (writhing) movements. The association between D_2 blockade and the extrapyramidal system is not straightforward: There is no immediate and direct temporal association between the administration of the drugs and the appearance of the various symptom patterns, which occur at different times after the administration of dopamine receptor antagonists.

The newer antipsychotics, the serotonin-dopamine antagonists (SDAs) are much less likely to produce movement disorders. Nonetheless, there have been a few case reports of more severe movement disorders even in patients on these newer agents. Because the natural history of psychotic disorders may include features of parkinsonism, dystonia, akathisia, and tardive dyskinesia, the contribution of specified drugs to movement disorders must be carefully assessed by withdrawing and rechallenging with the agent presumed responsible. Other psychotherapeutic agents, including antidepressants and antianxiety agents, have been occasionally reported to be associated with movement disorders. For example, selective serotonin reuptake inhibitors (SSRIs) may cause akathisia and in rare cases, tardive dyskinesia mainly of the oral–buccal type.

The text revision of the fourth edition of *Diagnostic and Statistical Manual of Mental Disorders* (DSM-IV-TR) includes in the category of "medication-induced movement disorders" not only such disorders but also any medication-induced adverse effect that becomes a focus of clinical attention. When one of these diagnoses is made and included as a focus of treatment, the movement disorder or adverse effect diagnosis should be listed on Axis I of the DSM-IV-TR multiaxial diagnostic formulation.

When faced with a patient on medication who develops a movement disorder, clinicians should consider the differential diagnosis for these symptoms. For example, anxiety needs to be distinguished from akathisia, catatonia from neuroleptic malignant syndrome, parkinsonism from depression, and tardive dyskinesia from other basal ganglia–related movement disorders.

NEUROLEPTIC-INDUCED MOVEMENT DISORDERS

The most common neuroleptic-related movement disorders are parkinsonism, acute dystonia, and acute akathisia. Neuroleptic malignant syndrome is a life-threatening and often misdiagnosed condition. Neuroleptic-induced tardive dyskinesia is a late-appearing adverse effect of neuroleptic drugs and can be irreversible; but recent data indicate that the syndrome, although still serious and potentially disabling, is less pernicious than was previously thought in patients taking dopamine receptor antagonists and occurs only rarely in patients taking SDAs.

Neuroleptic-Induced Parkinsonism

Neuroleptic-induced parkinsonism is characterized principally by the triad of resting tremor, rigidity, and bradykinesia (referred to in DSM-IV-TR as *akinesia*) (Table 36.3–1). The typical parkinsonian tremor oscillates at a steady rate of 3 to 6 cycles per second, and it may be suppressed by intended movement. Rigidity is a disorder of muscle tone—that is, the underlying tension involuntarily present in the muscles. Disorders of tone can result in either hypertonia (rigidity) or hypotonia. The hypertonia associated with neuroleptic-induced parkinsonism is of either the lead-pipe type, in which tone is continuously elevated, or the cogwheel type, in which a tremor is superimposed on rigidity. Cogwheel rigidity is revealed when an examiner rotates the hand around the axis of the wrist and encounters a regular rhythmical, ratchetlike resistance. The syndrome of bradykinesia can include a patient's masklike facial appearance, decreased accessory arm movements when the patient walks, and a characteristic difficulty in initiating movement. The so-called rabbit syndrome is a tremor affecting the lips and perioral muscles; it is most commonly considered part of the syndrome of neuroleptic-induced parkinsonism, although it often appears later in treatment than other symptoms. Other parkinsonian features include slowed thinking, worsening of negative symptoms, excessive salivation, drooling, shuffling gait, micrographia, seborrhea, and dysphoria.

The pathophysiology of neuroleptic-induced parkinsonism involves the blockade of D_2 receptors in the caudate at the termination of the nigrostriatal dopamine neurons, the same neurons that degenerate in idiopathic Parkinson's disease. Patients who are elderly and female are at the highest risk for neuroleptic-induced parkinsonism. More than 50 percent of patients treated with long-term, high-potency dopamine receptor antagonists may develop neuroleptic-induced parkinsonism at some point in their course of medication. Functional neuroimaging studies have shown that parkinsonism is seen with 80 percent or higher occupancy of D_2 receptors in the caudate. By the same method, antipsychotic efficacy was seen with only 50 to 75 percent D_2 receptor occupancy.

Treatment. The benefits and risks of prophylactic treatment with antiextrapyramidal system medications—for example, anticholinergics and amantadine (Symmetrel) or antihistamines—continue to be debated. Once parkinsonian symptoms appear, the three steps in treatment are reducing the dosage of the neuroleptic, instituting antiextrapyramidal system medications, and (possibly) changing the neuroleptic. The SDAs are a recommended alternative to the dopamine receptor antagonists for patients with neuroleptic-induced movement disorders. Studies show that the incidence of drug-induced parkinsonism is low for the SDAs and for low-potency dopamine receptor antagonists, such as thioridazine (Mellaril). Extrapyramidal symptoms are associated with dosages of risperidone (Risperdal) in excess of the recommended maximum dose of 4 to 6 mg a day. The common development of tolerance to the parkinsonian adverse effects of these drugs is poorly understood. Once treatment is initiated, therefore, clinicians should attempt to reduce or stop the antiextrapyramidal system medications after 14 to 21 days of treatment to assess whether the medications are still necessary.

Table 36.3–1
DSM-IV-TR Research Criteria for Neuroleptic-Induced Parkinsonism

A. One (or more) of the following signs or symptoms has developed in association with the use of neuroleptic medication:
  (1) parkinsonian tremor (i.e., a coarse, rhythmic, resting tremor with a frequency between 3 and 6 cycles per second, affecting the limbs, head, mouth, or tongue)
  (2) parkinsonian muscular rigidity (i.e., cogwheel rigidity or continuous "lead-pipe" rigidity)
  (3) akinesia (i.e., a decrease in spontaneous facial expressions, gestures, speech, or body movements)

B. The symptoms in Criterion A developed within a few weeks of starting or raising the dose of a neuroleptic medication, or of reducing a medication used to treat (or prevent) acute extrapyramidal symptoms (e.g., anticholinergic agents).

C. The symptoms in Criterion A are not better accounted for by a mental disorder (e.g., catatonic or negative symptoms in schizophrenia, psychomotor retardation in a major depressive episode). Evidence that the symptoms are better accounted for by a mental disorder might include the following: the symptoms precede the exposure to neuroleptic medication or are not compatible with the pattern of pharmacological intervention (e.g., no improvement after lowering the neuroleptic dose or administering anticholinergic medication).

D. The symptoms in Criterion A are not due to a nonneuroleptic substance or to a neurological or other general medical condition (e.g., Parkinson's disease, Wilson's disease). Evidence that the symptoms are due to a general medical condition might include the following: the symptoms precede exposure to neuroleptic medication, unexplained focal neurological signs are present, or the symptoms progress despite a stable medication regimen.

From American Psychiatric Association. *Diagnostic and Statistical Manual of Mental Disorders.* 4th ed. Text rev. Washington, DC: American Psychiatric Association; copyright 2000, with permission.

Neuroleptic Malignant Syndrome

Neuroleptic malignant syndrome is a life-threatening complication of antipsychotic treatment and can occur anytime during

Table 36.3–2
DSM-IV-TR Research Criteria for Neuroleptic Malignant Syndrome

A. The development of severe muscle rigidity and elevated temperature associated with the use of neuroleptic medication.
B. Two (or more) of the following:
 (1) diaphoresis
 (2) dysphagia
 (3) tremor
 (4) incontinence
 (5) changes in level of consciousness ranging from confusion to coma
 (6) mutism
 (7) tachycardia
 (8) elevated or labile blood pressure
 (9) leukocytosis
 (10) laboratory evidence of muscle injury (e.g., elevated CPK)
C. The symptoms in Criteria A and B are not due to another substance (e.g., phencyclidine) or a neurological or other general medical condition (e.g., viral encephalitis).
D. The symptoms in Criteria A and B are not better accounted for by a mental disorder (e.g., mood disorder with catatonic features).

From American Psychiatric Association. *Diagnostic and Statistical Manual of Mental Disorders.* 4th ed. Text rev. Washington, DC: American Psychiatric Association; copyright 2000, with permission.

Table 36.3–3
DSM-IV-TR Research Criteria for Neuroleptic-Induced Acute Dystonia

A. One (or more) of the following signs or symptoms has developed in association with the use of neuroleptic medication:
 (1) abnormal positioning of the head and neck in relation to the body (e.g., retrocollis, torticollis)
 (2) spasms of the jaw muscles (trismus, gaping, grimacing)
 (3) impaired swallowing (dysphagia), speaking, or breathing (laryngeal-pharyngeal spasm, dysphonia)
 (4) thickened or slurred speech due to hypertonic or enlarged tongue (dysarthria, macroglossia)
 (5) tongue protrusion or tongue dysfunction
 (6) eyes deviated up, down, or sideward (oculogyric crisis)
 (7) abnormal positioning of the distal limbs or trunk
B. The signs or symptoms in Criterion A developed within 7 days of starting or rapidly raising the dose of neuroleptic medication, or of reducing a medication used to treat (or prevent) acute extrapyramidal symptoms (e.g., anticholinergic agents).
C. The symptoms in Criterion A are not better accounted for by a mental disorder (e.g., catatonic symptoms in schizophrenia). Evidence that the symptoms are better accounted for by a mental disorder might include the following: the symptoms precede the exposure to neuroleptic medication or are not compatible with the pattern of pharmacological intervention (e.g., no improvement after neuroleptic lowering or anticholinergic administration).
D. The symptoms in Criterion A are not due to a nonneuroleptic substance or to a neurological or other general medical condition. Evidence that the symptoms are due to a general medical condition might include the following: the symptoms precede the exposure to the neuroleptic medication, unexplained focal neurological signs are present, or the symptoms progress in the absence of change in medication.

From American Psychiatric Association. *Diagnostic and Statistical Manual of Mental Disorders.* 4th ed. Text rev. Washington, DC: American Psychiatric Association; copyright 2000, with permission.

the course of treatment (Table 36.3–2). The symptoms include muscular rigidity and dystonia (hence the classification of the disorder as a movement disorder), akinesia, mutism, obtundation, and agitation. The autonomic symptoms include high fever, sweating, and increased blood pressure and heart rate. The neuroleptic malignant syndrome may also be precipitated in patients with Parkinson's disease by abrupt withdrawal of the dopamine precursor levodopa, which suggests that the syndrome may be one possible result of a precipitous reduction in dopamine receptor activation. The prevalence of neuroleptic malignant syndrome is estimated to be 0.02 to 2.4 percent of patients exposed to dopamine receptor antagonists. In addition to supportive medical treatment, the most commonly used medications for the condition are dantrolene (Dantrium) and bromocriptine (Parlodel), although amantadine is sometimes used. Bromocriptine and amantadine possess direct dopamine receptor agonist effects and may serve to overcome the antipsychotic-induced dopamine receptor blockade. Mortality rates are reported to be 10 to 20 percent. The lowest effective dosage of antipsychotic drug should be used to reduce the chance of neuroleptic malignant syndrome. Antipsychotic drugs with anticholinergic effects seem less likely to cause neuroleptic malignant syndrome.

Neuroleptic-Induced Acute Dystonia

Dystonias are brief or prolonged contractions of muscles that result in obviously abnormal movements or postures, including oculogyric crises, tongue protrusion, trismus, torticollis, laryngeal-pharyngeal dystonias, and dystonic postures of the limbs and trunk (Table 36.3–3). The development of dystonic symptoms is characterized by their early onset during the course of treatment with neuroleptics and their high incidence in men, in patients under age 30, and in patients given high dosages of high-potency medications. The pathophysiological mechanism for dystonias is not clearly understood, although changes in neuroleptic concentrations and the resulting changes in homeostatic mechanisms within the basal ganglia may be the major causes of dystonias.

Treatment. Treatment of dystonias should be immediate; the most common agents are anticholinergic or antihistaminergic drugs. If a patient fails to respond to three doses of these drugs within 2 hours, the clinician should consider other causes for the dystonic movements. After resolution of the acute episode, oral anticholinergic agents should be given, and their effects reassessed every 2 weeks.

Neuroleptic-Induced Acute Akathisia

Akathisia is characterized by subjective feelings of restlessness, objective signs of restlessness, or both. Examples include a sense of anxiety, inability to relax, jitteriness, pacing, rocking motions while sitting, and rapid alternation of sitting and standing (Table 36.3–4). Akathisia can often be misdiagnosed as anxiety or as increased psychotic agitation, and it may result in an increase in

Table 36.3–4
DSM-IV-TR Research Criteria for Neuroleptic-Induced Acute Akathisia

A. The development of subjective complaints of restlessness after exposure to a neuroleptic medication.
B. At least one of the following is observed:
 (1) fidgety movements or swinging of the legs
 (2) rocking from foot to foot while standing
 (3) pacing to relieve restlessness
 (4) inability to sit or stand still for at least several minutes
C. The onset of the symptoms in Criteria A and B occurs within 4 weeks of initiating or increasing the dose of the neuroleptic, or of reducing medication used to treat (or prevent) acute extrapyramidal symptoms (e.g., anticholinergic agents).
D. The symptoms in Criterion A are not better accounted for by a mental disorder (e.g., schizophrenia, substance withdrawal, agitation from a major depressive or manic episode, hyperactivity in attention-deficit/hyperactivity disorder). Evidence that symptoms may be better accounted for by a mental disorder might include the following: the onset of symptoms preceding the exposure to the neuroleptics, the absence of increasing restlessness with increasing neuroleptic doses, and the absence of relief with pharmacological interventions (e.g., no improvement after decreasing the neuroleptic dose or treatment with medication intended to treat the akathisia).
E. The symptoms in Criterion A are not due to a nonneuroleptic substance or to a neurological or other general medical condition. Evidence that symptoms are due to a general medical condition might include the onset of the symptoms preceding the exposure to neuroleptics or the progression of symptoms in the absence of a change in medication.

Table 36.3–5
DSM-IV-TR Research Criteria for Neuroleptic-Induced Tardive Dyskinesia

A. Involuntary movements of the tongue, jaw, trunk, or extremities have developed in association with the use of neuroleptic medication.
B. The involuntary movements are present over a period of at least 4 weeks and occur in any of the following patterns:
 (1) choreiform movements (i.e., rapid, jerky, nonrepetitive)
 (2) athetoid movements (i.e., slow, sinuous, continual)
 (3) rhythmic movements (i.e., stereotypies)
C. The signs or symptoms in Criteria A and B develop during exposure to a neuroleptic medication or within 4 weeks of withdrawal from an oral (or within 8 weeks of withdrawal from a depot) neuroleptic medication.
D. There has been exposure to neuroleptic medication for at least 3 months (1 month if age 60 years or older).
E. The symptoms are not due to a neurological or general medical condition (e.g., Huntington's disease, Sydenham's chorea, spontaneous dyskinesia, hyperthyroidism, Wilson's disease), ill-fitting dentures, or exposure to other medications that cause acute reversible dyskinesia (e.g., L-dopa, bromocriptine). Evidence that the symptoms are due to one of these etiologies might include the following: the symptoms precede the exposure to the neuroleptic medication or unexplained focal neurological signs are present.
F. The symptoms are not better accounted for by a neuroleptic-induced acute movement disorder (e.g., neuroleptic-induced acute dystonia, neuroleptic-induced acute akathisia).

the dosage of antipsychotic medication, which actually exacerbates the condition. Middle-aged women are at increased risk of akathisia, and the time course is similar to that for neuroleptic-induced parkinsonism. Akathisia has been associated with the use of a wide range of psychiatric drugs, including antipsychotics, antidepressants, and sympathomimetics. A recent report associates akathisia with a poor treatment outcome.

Treatment. The three basic steps in the treatment of akathisia are reducing neuroleptic medication dosage, attempting treatment with appropriate drugs, and considering changing the neuroleptic. The most efficacious drugs in the treatment of akathisia are the β-adrenergic receptor antagonists, although anticholinergic drugs, benzodiazepines, and cyproheptadine (Periactin) may benefit some patients. Patients may be less likely to experience akathisia while receiving low-potency neuroleptics—for example, thioridazine—than while receiving high-potency neuroleptics—for example, haloperidol (Haldol); the SDAs are associated with a low incidence of akathisia.

Neuroleptic-Induced Tardive Dyskinesia

Neuroleptic-induced tardive dyskinesia is a late-appearing disorder of involuntary, choreoathetoid movements (Table 36.3–5). The most common movements involve the orofacial region along with choreoathetoid movements of the fingers and toes. Athetoid movements of the head, neck, and hips also occur in seriously affected patients. In the most serious cases, patients may have breathing and swallowing irregularities that result in aerophagia, belching, and grunting. The Abnormal Involuntary Movement Scale (AIMS), administered every 3 to 6 months to patients who are taking antipsychotic drugs, is an effective diagnostic tool for tardive dyskinesia (Table 36.3–6).

The risk factors for tardive dyskinesia, which occurs in up to 25 percent of patients treated with dopamine receptor antagonists for over 4 years, include long-term treatment with neuroleptics, increasing age, female sex, the presence of a mood disorder, and the presence of a cognitive disorder. Tardive dystonia may appear after several years of exposure to neuroleptics, is more common in younger patients, and may coexist with tardive dyskinesia. It is characterized by sustained or slow involuntary movements of the neck, trunk, face, or limbs.

Although various treatments for tardive dyskinesia have been unsuccessful, the course of tardive dyskinesia is considered less relentless than was previously thought. The SDAs are associated with an extremely low risk of developing tardive dyskinesia and therefore present an effective treatment approach. Patients with tardive dyskinesia frequently experience an exacerbation of their symptoms when the dopamine receptor antagonist is withheld, whereas substitution of an SDA may limit the abnormal movements without worsening the progression of the dyskinesia. Before the appearance of the antipsychotics in the 1950s, clini-

Table 36.3–6
Abnormal Involuntary Movement Scale (AIMS) Examination Procedure

Patient identification:__________________________ Date_____

Rated by:

Either before or after completing the examination procedure, observe the patient unobtrusively at rest (e.g., in waiting room).

The chair to be used in this examination should be a hard, firm one without arms.

After observing the patient, he or she may be rated on a scale of 0 (none), 1 (minimal), 2 (mild), 3 (moderate), and 4 (severe) according to the severity of symptoms.

Ask the patient whether there is anything in his/her mouth (i.e., gum, candy, etc.) and if there is to remove it.

Ask patient about the current condition of his/her teeth. Ask patient if he/she wears dentures. Do teeth or dentures bother patient now?

Ask patient whether he/she notices any movement in mouth, face, hands, or feet. If yes, ask to describe and to what extent they currently bother patient or interfere with his/her activities.

0 1 2 3 4	Have patient sit in chair with hands on knees, legs slightly apart, and feet flat on floor. (Look at entire body for movements while in this position.)
0 1 2 3 4	Ask patient to sit with hands hanging unsupported. If male, between legs; if female and wearing a dress, hanging over knees. (Observe hands and other body areas.)
0 1 2 3 4	Ask patient to open mouth. (Observe tongue at rest within mouth.) Do this twice.
0 1 2 3 4	Ask patient to protrude tongue. (Observe abnormalities of tongue movement.) Do this twice.
0 1 2 3 4	Ask the patient to tap thumb, with each finger, as rapidly as possible for 10–15 seconds; separately with right hand, then with left hand. (Observe facial and leg movements.)
0 1 2 3 4	Flex and extend patient's left and right arms. (One at a time.)
0 1 2 3 4	Ask patient to stand up. (Observe in profile. Observe all body areas again, hips included.)
0 1 2 3 4	Ask patient to extend both arms outstretched in front with palms down. (Observe trunk, legs, and mouth.)[a]
0 1 2 3 4	Have patient walk a few paces, turn and walk back to chair. (Observe hands and gait.) Do this twice.[a]

[a]Activated movements.

Table 36.3–7
Research Criteria for Medication-Induced Postural Tremor

A. A fine postural tremor that has developed in association with the use of a medication (e.g., lithium, antidepressant medication, valproic acid).

B. The tremor (i.e., a regular, rhythmic oscillation of the limbs, head, mouth, or tongue) has a frequency between 8 and 12 cycles per second.

C. The symptoms are not due to a preexisting nonpharmacologically induced tremor. Evidence that the symptoms are due to a preexisting tremor might include the following: the tremor was present prior to the introduction of the medication, the tremor does not correlate with serum levels of the medication, and the tremor persists after discontinuation of the medication.

D. The symptoms are not better accounted for by neuroleptic-induced parkinsonism.

From American Psychiatric Association. *Diagnostic and Statistical Manual of Mental Disorders.* 4th ed. Text rev. Washington, DC: American Psychiatric Association; copyright 2000, with permission.

cians noted that 1 to 5 percent of psychiatric inpatients with schizophrenia developed movements resembling tardive dyskinesia. This observation suggests that not all cases of tardive dyskinesia should necessarily be attributed to antipsychotics. Nevertheless, the treatment is the same whatever the cause.

MEDICATION-INDUCED POSTURAL TREMOR

Tremor is defined as a rhythmical alteration in movement that usually exceeds 1 beat per second (Table 36.3–7). Typically, tremors decrease during periods of relaxation and sleep and increase during periods of anger and increased tension. These characteristics sometimes mistakenly lead inexperienced clinicians to assume that a patient is faking the tremor. Whereas all the DSM-IV-TR diagnoses previously discussed specifically include an association with neuroleptics, DSM-IV-TR acknowledges that a range of psychiatric medications can produce tremor—most notably lithium (Eskalith), antidepressants, and valproate (Depakene)—and still other psychiatric medications are associated with the induction of tremor.

The treatment of tremor involves four general steps. First, the lowest possible dosage of the psychiatric drug should be used. Second, patients should minimize their caffeine and alcohol consumption. Third, the psychiatric drug should be taken at bedtime to minimize the amount of daytime tremor. Fourth, β-adrenergic receptor antagonists can be given to treat drug-induced tremors.

MEDICATION-INDUCED MOVEMENT DISORDER NOT OTHERWISE SPECIFIED

Although neuroleptics are the psychiatric drugs most commonly associated with movement disorders, almost all the most commonly used psychiatric drugs can produce movement disorders in some patients (Table 36.3–8). Furthermore, many nonpsychiatric drugs can produce movement disorders, and patients who are treated with both psychiatric and nonpsychiatric drugs may experience additive effects of these medications

Table 36.3–8
DSM-IV-TR Research Criteria for Medication-Induced Movement Disorder Not Otherwise Specified

This category is for medication-induced movement disorders that do not meet criteria for any of the specific disorders listed above. Examples include (1) parkinsonism, acute akathisia, acute dystonia, or dyskinetic movement that is associated with a medication other than a neuroleptic; (2) a presentation that resembles neuroleptic malignant syndrome that is associated with a medication other than a neuroleptic; or (3) tardive dystonia.

From American Psychiatric Association. *Diagnostic and Statistical Manual of Mental Disorders.* 4th ed. Text rev. Washington, DC: American Psychiatric Association; copyright 2000, with permission.

on their movement disorders. DSM-IV-TR also defines the diagnostic category as including movement disorders other than those already specified. Such movement disorders include tardive dystonia, tardive Tourette's syndrome, tardive myoclonus, tardive akathisia, and tardive parkinsonism. Table 36.3–9 lists several movement disorders and the drugs that induce them.

Table 36.3–9
Drug-Induced Movement Disorders

Syndrome	Drugs Responsible	Degree
Postural tremor	Sympathomimetics	++
	Levodopa	++
	Amphetamines	++
	Bronchodilators	++
	Tricyclic drugs	++
	Lithium carbonate	++
	Caffeine	++
	Thyroid hormone	++
	Sodium valproate	++
	APDs	++
	Hypoglycemic agents	++
	Adrenocorticosteroids	++
	Alcohol withdrawal	++
	Amiodarone	+
	Cyclosporine	+
	MAOIs	++
Acute dystonic reactions	APDs	++
	Metoclopramide	++
	Antimalarial agents	+
	Tetrabenazine	+/–
	Diphenhydramine	+/–
	Mefenamic acid	+/–
	Oxatomide	+/–
	Tricyclic drugs	+/–
	Flunarizine and cinnarizine	+/–
Akathisia	APDs	++
	Metoclopramide	++
	Reserpine	++
	Tetrabenazine	++
	Levodopa and dopamine agonists[a,b]	+
	Flunarizine and cinnarizine	+/–
	Ethosuximide	+/–
	Methysergide	+/–
	Amoxapine	+/–
Parkinsonism, including perioral tremor	APDs	++
	Metoclopramide	++
	Reserpine	++
	Tetrabenazine	++
	Methyldopa	+
	Flunarizine and cinnarizine	+/–
	Fluoxetine	+/–
	Lithium	+/–
	Phenelzine	+/–
	Phenytoin	+/–
	Captopril	+/–
	Alcohol withdrawal	+
	MPTP	+
	Other toxins (manganese, carbon disulfide, cyanide)	+
	Cytosine arabinoside	+/–
Chorea, including tardive dyskinesia and orofacial dyskinesia	APDs	++
	Metoclopramide	++
	Levodopa	++
	Direct dopamine agonists	++
	Indirect dopamine agonists and other catecholaminergic drugs[a]	++
	Anticholinergics	+
	Antihistaminics	+
	Oral contraceptives	+
	Phenytoin (T)	+
	Carbamazepine (T)	+/–
	Ethosuximide	+/–
	Phenobarbital (T)	+/–
	Lithium carbonate (T)	+/–
	Benzodiazepines	+/–
	MAOIs	+/–
	Tricyclic drugs	+/–
	Methyldopa	+/–
	Methadone	+/–
	Digoxin	+/–
	Alcohol withdrawal	+/–
	Toluene (glue-sniffing)	+/–
	Flunarizine and cinnarizine	+/–
Dystonia, including tardive dystonia (excluding acute dystonic reactions)	APDs	++
	Metoclopramide	++
	Levodopa	++
	Direct dopamine agonists[a]	+
	Phenytoin (T)	+
	Carbamazepine (T)	+/–
	Flunarizine and cinnarizine	+/–
	Trazodone	+/–
	Lithium	+/–
Neuroleptic malignant syndrome	APDs	+
	Tetrabenazine with AMPT	+/–
Tics (simple and complex), including aggravation of preexisting tic disorders	Withdrawal of antiparkinsonian drugs in Parkinson's disease	+/–
	Levodopa	+
	Direct dopamine agonists	+
	Indirect dopamine agonists	++
	APDs	+
	Carbamazepine	+/–
Myoclonus	Levodopa	++
	Anticonvulsants[c] (T)	++
	MAOIs	++
	Lithium	++
	Tricyclic drugs	++
	APDs	+/–
Asterixis	Anticonvulsants[c] (T)	++
	Levodopa	+/–
	Hepatotoxins (T)	++
	Respiratory depressants (T)	++

++, well documented, common or not infrequent; +, relatively well documented, uncommon; +/–, not well documented or only small number of cases in literature; AMPT, α-methyl-paratyrosine; APD, antipsychotic drug; MAOI, monoamine oxidase inhibitor; MPTP, 1-methyl-4-phenyl-1,2,3,6-tetrahydropyridine; T, usually evidence of drug toxicity present (including serum drug levels).

[a]Includes apomorphine, bromocriptine, lisuride, pergolide.

[b]Includes amphetamines, methylphenidate, amantadine, pemoline, fenfluramine.

[c]Includes most categories of anticonvulsant drugs.

Adapted from Gershanil OS. Drug-induced movement disorders. *Curr Opin Neurol Neurosurg.* 1993;6:369.

Table 36.3–10
DSM-IV-TR Diagnostic Criteria for Adverse Effects of Medication Not Otherwise Specified

This category is available for optional use by clinicians to code side effects of medication (other than movement symptoms) when these adverse effects become a main focus of clinical attention. Examples include severe hypotension, cardiac arrhythmias, and priapism.

From American Psychiatric Association. *Diagnostic and Statistical Manual of Mental Disorders.* 4th ed. Text rev. Washington, DC: American Psychiatric Association; copyright 2000, with permission.

ADVERSE EFFECTS OF MEDICATION NOT OTHERWISE SPECIFIED

This category allows clinicians to record the adverse effects of medications, other than movement symptoms, which become a focus of treatment (Table 36.3–10). Examples of such adverse effects include priapism, severe hypotension, and cardiac abnormalities.

HYPERTHERMIC SYNDROMES

Many drugs used in psychiatry and all of the medication-induced movement disorders may be associated with hyperthermia. Table 36.3–11 summarizes various conditions and agents associated with hyperthermia.

References

Arya DK. Extrapyramidal symptoms with selective serotonin reuptake inhibitors. *Br J Psychiatry.* 1994;165:728.

Ballesteros J, González-Pinto A, Bulbena A. Tardive dyskinesia associated with higher mortality in psychiatric patients: result of a meta-analysis of seven independent studies. *J Clin Psychopharmacol.* 2000;20:188.

Casey DE. Neuroleptic drug-induced extrapyramidal syndromes and tardive dyskinesia. *Schizophr Res.* 1991;4:109.

Dursun SM, Burke JG, Reveley MA. Toxic serotonin syndrome or extrapyramidal side-effects? *Br J Psychiatry.* 1995;166:401.

Gershanik OS. Drug-induced movement disorders. *Curr Opin Neurol Neurosurg.* 1993;6:369.

Glazer WM, Morgenstern H, Doucette JT. Predicting long-term risk of tardive dyskinesia in outpatients maintained on neuroleptic medications. *J Clin Psychiatry.* 1993;54:133.

Hsin-Tung P, Simpson GM. Medication-induced movement disorders. In: Sadock BJ, Sadock VA, eds. *Kaplan & Sadock's Comprehensive Textbook of Psychiatry.* 7th ed. Vol 2. Baltimore: Lippincott Williams & Wilkins; 2000:2265.

Table 36.3–11
Drug-Induced Central Hyperthermic Syndromes[a]

Condition (and Mechanism)	Common Drug Causes	Frequent Symptoms	Possible Treatment[b]	Clinical Course
Hyperthermia (↓ heat dissipation) (↑ heat production)	Atropine, lidocaine, meperidine NSAID toxicity, pheochromocytoma, thyrotoxicosis	Hyperthermia, diaphoresis, malaise	Acetaminophen per rectum (325 mg every 4 h), diazepam oral or per rectum (5 mg every 8 h) for febrile seizures	Benign, febrile seizures in children
Malignant hyperthermia (↑ heat production)	NMJ blockers (succinylcholine), halothane (1:50,000)	Hyperthermia, **muscle rigidity, arrhythmias,** ischemia,[c] hypotension, **rhabdomyolysis;** disseminated intravascular coagulation	Dantrolene sodium (1–2 mg/kg/min IV infusion)[d]	Familial, 10% mortality if untreated
Tricyclic overdose (↑ heat production)	Tricyclic antidepressants, cocaine	Hyperthermia, confusion, visual hallucinations, agitation, **hyperreflexia, muscle relaxation, anticholinergic effects** (dry skin, pupil dilation), arrhythmias	**Sodium bicarbonate** (1 mEq/kg IV bolus) if arrhythmias are present, physostigmine (1–3 mg IV) with cardiac monitoring	Fatalities have occurred if untreated
Autonomic hyperreflexia (↑ heat production)	CNS stimulants (amphetamines)	Hyperthermia excitement, **hyperreflexia**	Trimethaphan (0.3–7 mg/min IV infusion)	Reversible
Lethal catatonia (↓ heat dissipation)	Lead poisoning	Hyperthermia, intense anxiety, **destructive behavior, psychosis**	Lorazepam (1–2 mg IV every 4 h), antipsychotics may be contraindicated	High mortality if untreated
Neuroleptic malignant syndrome (mixed: hypothalamic, ↓ heat dissipation, ↑ heat production)	Antipsychotics (neuroleptics), methyldopa, reserpine	Hyperthermia, **muscle rigidity, diaphoresis (60%), leukocytosis, delirium, rhabdomyolysis, elevated CPK,** autonomic deregulation, **extrapyramidal symptoms**	**Bromocriptine (2–10 mg every 8 h po or NG tube),** lisuride (0.02–0.1 mg/h IV infusion). Sinemet (carbidopa: levodopa 25/100 po every 8 h), dantrolene sodium (0.3–1 mg/kg IV every 6 h)	Rapid onset, 20% mortality if untreated

[a]Boldface indicates features that may be used to distinguish one syndrome from another. NSAID, nonsteroidal antiinflammatory drugs; MAOI, monoamine oxidase inhibitors; NMJ, neuromuscular junction; CNS, central nervous system; DO, dopamine; CPK, creatine phosphokinase; IV, intravenously; po, orally; NG, nasogastric.
[b]Gastric lavage and supportive measures, including cooling, are required in most cases.
[c]Oxygen consumption increases by 7% for every 1°F up in body temperature.
[d]Has been associated with idiosyncratic hepatocellular injury, as well as severe hypotension in one case.
From Theocharides TC, Harris RS, Weckstein D. Neuroleptic malignant-like syndrome due to cyclobenzapine? (letter). *J Clin Psychopharmacol.* 1995;15:80, with permission.

Lang AE, Weiner WJ. *Drug-Induced Movement Disorders*. Mount Kisco, NY: Futura; 1992.
Meltzer HY. Pre-clinical pharmacology of atypical antipsychotic drugs: a selective review. *Br J Psychiatry*. 1996;168(29 suppl):23.
McGreadie RG, Thara R. Abnormal movements in never-medicated Indian patients with schizophrenia. *Br J Psychiatry*. 1996;168:221.
van Harten PN, Kamphuis DJ, Matroos GE. Use of clozapine in tardive dystonia. *Prog Neuropsychopharmacol Biol Psychiatry*. 1996;20:263.
van Harten PN, Matroos GE, Kahn RS. The prevalence of tardive dystonia, tardive dyskinesia, parkinsonism and akathisia. The Curacao extrapyramidal syndromes study: I. *Schizophr Res*. 1996;19:195.

▲ 36.4 PSYCHOTHERAPEUTIC DRUGS

The use of pharmacological agents or psychotherapeutic drugs can be defined as an attempt to modify or correct pathological behavior by chemical means. The relation between the physical state of the brain and behavior is highly complex and imperfectly understood. Clearly, however, the various parameters of both normal and deviant behavior, such as perception, consciousness, affect, and the cognitive functions, may be profoundly affected by certain physiological changes in the central nervous system. Pharmacological treatment of psychiatric disorders is largely empirical. The underlying mechanisms by which a chemical or physical change in the brain changes abnormal behavior has not been completely delineated. Nevertheless, many drugs have proved highly effective and may constitute the treatment of choice for certain psychopathological conditions. As such, they form an important part of the treatment armamentarium of the psychiatrist and of practitioners in other medical specialties as well.

As knowledge about the brain has increased, investigators have developed novel chemical compounds to influence one or more of the receptor systems that have thus far been identified, e.g., dopamine, serotonin, γ-aminobutyric acid (GABA), among others. This approach, called *rational drug design,* has yielded agents that are highly specific for the desired neurotransmitter systems yet lack interactions with other receptors that are normally associated with adverse effects. Such rational drug design is likely to yield many interesting and safe new agents in the coming years. The field of psychopharmacology is expanding rapidly and will probably be ever more widely practiced by nonpsychiatric physicians, who will require expert advice and continuing education about adverse effects and drug–drug interactions.

A trend in psychopharmacological practice is the use of a particular class of medications in a wide variety of clinical conditions, thus expanding the array of useful indications for a specific drug. It is no longer practical to discuss psychopharmacological drugs only according to their therapeutic indication. In this book each drug is discussed on the basis of its pharmacological category, as is done in textbooks of general pharmacology. Moreover, this organization anticipates the development of newer agents through rational drug design, which is grounded in established and emerging insights into the neurobiological basis of mental illness.

GUIDE TO USE

The table of contents for this chapter lists the 36 groups into which drugs used in psychiatry have been divided for discussion in this textbook. An alphabetical list of generic names of drugs discussed in this book is presented in Table 36.4–1, with cross-references to the subsections in which they are discussed. In addition, a list of therapeutic indications and the drugs commonly used for these indications is presented in Table 36.4–2, with cross-references to the appropriate subsections.

Table 36.4–1
Index to Section by Generic Name of Drug

Generic Name	Brand Name	Subsection Title	Subsection Number
Acebutolol	Sectral	β-Adrenergic Receptor Antagonists	36.4.2
Acetophenazine	Tindal	Dopamine Receptor Antagonists	36.4.17
Alprazolam	Xanax	Benzodiazepines	36.4.7
Amantadine	Symmetrel	Amantadine	36.4.3
Amitriptyline	Elavil, Endep	Tricyclics and Tetracyclics	36.4.33
Amlodipine	Lotrel, Norvasc	Calcium Channel Inhibitors	36.4.10
Amobarbital	Amytal	Barbiturates and Similarly Acting Substances	36.4.6
Amoxapine	Asendin	Tricyclics and Tetracyclics	36.4.33
Amphetamine	—	Sympathomimetics and Related Drugs	36.4.30
Apomorphine	Uprima	Dopamine Receptor Agonists and Precursors	36.4.16
Aprobarbital	Alurate	Barbiturates and Similarly Acting Substances	36.4.6
Aripiprazole	Abilify	Serotonin-Dopamine antagonists	36.4.27
Atenolol	Tenormin	β-Adrenergic Receptor Antagonists	36.4.2
Befloxatone	—	Monoamine Oxidase Inhibitors	36.4.20
Benzphetamine	Didrex	Sympathomimetics and Related Drugs	36.4.30
Benztropine	Cogentin	Anticholinergics	36.4.4
Biperiden	Akineton	Anticholinergics	36.4.4
Bromocriptine	Parlodel	Dopamine Receptor Agonists and Precursors	36.4.16
Buprenorphine	Buprenex	Opioid Receptor Agonists	36.4.22

(continued)

Table 36.4–1 (*continued*)

Generic Name	Brand Name	Subsection Title	Subsection Number
Bupropion	Wellbutrin, Zyban	Bupropion	36.4.8
Buspirone	BuSpar	Buspirone	36.4.9
Butabarbital	Butisol	Barbiturates and Similarly Acting Substances	36.4.6
Butaperazine[b]	Repoise	Dopamine Receptor Antagonists	36.4.17
Carbamazepine	Tegretol	Carbamazepine	36.4.11
Carbidopa	Lodosyn	Dopamine Receptor Agonists and Precursors	36.4.16
Carphenazine	Proketazine	Dopamine Receptor Antagonists	36.4.17
Chloral hydrate	Somnote	Chloral Hydrate	36.4.12
Chlorpromazine	Thorazine	Dopamine Receptor Antagonists	36.4.17
Chlorprothixene	Taractan	Dopamine Receptor Antagonists	36.4.17
Citalopram	Celexa	Selective Serotonin Reuptake Inhibitors	36.4.26
Clomipramine	Anafranil	Tricyclics and Tetracyclics	36.4.33
Clonazepam	Klonopin	Benzodiazepines	36.4.7
Clonidine	Catapres	α_2-Adrenergic Receptor Agonists	36.4.1
Clozapine	Clozaril	Serotonin-Dopamine Antagonists	36.4.27
Cyproheptadine	Periactin	Antihistamines	36.4.5
Dantrolene	Dantrium	Dantrolene	36.4.14
Desipramine	Norpramin, Pertofrane	Tricyclics and Tetracyclics	36.4.33
Dextroamphetamine	Dexedrine	Sympathomimetics and Related Drugs	36.4.30
Diazepam	Valium	Benzodiazepines	36.4.7
Dexmethylphenidate	Focalin	Sympathomimetics and Related Drugs	36.4.30
Diethylpropion	Tenuate	Sympathomimetics and Related Drugs	36.4.30
Disulfiram	Antabuse	Disulfiram	36.4.15
Diphenhydramine	Benadryl	Antihistamines	36.4.5
Divalproex	Depakote	Valproate	36.4.34
Donepezil	Aricept	Cholinesterase Inhibitors	36.4.13
Doxepin	Adapin, Sinequan	Tricyclics and Tetracyclics	36.4.33
Droperidol	Inapsine	Dopamine Receptor Antagonists	36.4.17
Duloxetine	Cymbalta	Venlafaxine	36.4.35
Escitalopram	Lexapro	Selective Serotonin Reuptake Inhibitors	36.4.26
Estazolam	ProSom	Benzodiazepines	36.4.7
Ethopropazine	Parsidol	Anticholinergics	36.4.4
Ethchlorvynol	Placidyl	Barbiturates and Similarly Acting Substances	36.4.6
Flumazenil	Romazicon	Benzodiazepines	36.4.7
Fluoxetine	Prozac, Sarafem	Selective Serotonin Reuptake Inhibitors	36.4.26
Fluphenazine	Prolixin, Permitil	Dopamine Receptor Antagonists	36.4.17
Flurazepam	Dalmane	Benzodiazepines	36.4.7
Fluvoxamine	Luvox	Selective Serotonin Reuptake Inhibitors	36.4.26
Gabapentin	Neurontin	Other Anticonvulsants	36.4.24
Galantamine	Reminyl	Cholinesterase Inhibitors	36.4.13
Gepirone	Ariza	Buspirone	36.4.9
Glutethimide	Doriden	Barbiturates and Similarly Acting Substances	36.4.6
Guanfacine	Tenex	α_2-Adrenergic Receptor Agonists	36.4.1
Halazepam	Paxipam	Benzodiazepines	36.4.7
Haloperidol	Haldol	Dopamine Receptor Antagonists	36.4.17
Hydroxyzine	Atarax, Vistaril	Antihistamines	36.4.5
Imipramine	Tofranil	Tricyclics and Tetracyclics	36.4.33
Iproniazid	Marsilid	Monoamine Oxidase Inhibitors	36.4.20
Isocarboxazid	Marplan	Monoamine Oxidase Inhibitors	36.4.20
Isradipine	DynaCirc	Calcium Channel Inhibitors	36.4.10
Labetalol	Normodyne, Trandate	β-Adrenergic Receptor Antagonists	36.4.2
Lamotrigine	Lamictal	Other Anticonvulsants	36.4.24
Levodopa	Larodopa	Dopamine Receptor Agonists and Precursors	36.4.16
Levomethadyl	ORLAAM	Opioid Receptor Agonists	36.4.22

(*continued*)

Table 36.4–1 (*continued*)

Generic Name	Brand Name	Subsection Title	Subsection Number
Levothyroxine	Levoxine, Levothroid, Synthroid	Thyroid Hormones	36.4.31
Liothyronine	Cytomel	Thyroid Hormones	36.4.31
Lithium	Eskalith, Lithobid, Lithonate	Lithium	36.4.18
Lorazepam	Ativan	Benzodiazepines	36.4.7
Loxapine	Loxitane	Dopamine Receptor Antagonists	36.4.17
Mazindol	Mazanor, Sanorex	Sympathomimetics and Related Drugs	36.4.30
Memantine	—	Cholinesterase Inhibitors	36.4.13
Mephobarbital	Mebaral	Barbiturates and Similarly Acting Substances	36.4.6
Meprobamate	Miltown	Barbiturates and Similarly Acting Substances	36.4.6
Mesoridazine	Serentil	Dopamine Receptor Antagonists	36.4.17
Methadone	Dolophine, Methadose	Opioid Receptor Agonists	36.4.22
Methamphetamine	Desoxyn	Sympathomimetics and Related Drugs	36.4.30
Methohexital	Brevital	Barbiturates and Similarly Acting Substances	36.4.6
Methylphenidate	Ritalin	Sympathomimetics and Related Drugs	36.4.30
Metoprolol	Lopressor, Toprol	β-Adrenergic Receptor Antagonists	36.4.2
Midazolam	Versed	Benzodiazepine Receptor Agonists	36.4.7
Mirtazapine	Remeron	Mirtazapine	36.4.19
Moclobemide	Manerix	Monoamine Oxidase Inhibitors	36.4.20
Modafinil	Provigil	Sympathomimetics and Related Drugs	36.4.30
Molindone	Moban	Dopamine Receptor Antagonists	36.4.17
Nadolol	Corgard	β-Adrenergic Receptor Antagonists	36.4.2
Nalmefene	Revex	Opioid Receptor Antagonists	36.4.23
Naltrexone	ReVia	Opioid Receptor Antagonists	36.4.23
Nefazodone	Serzone	Nefazodone	36.4.21
Nicardipine	Cardene	Calcium Channel Inhibitors	36.4.10
Nifedipine	Adalat, Procardia	Calcium Channel Inhibitors	36.4.10
Nimodipine	Nimotop	Calcium Channel Inhibitors	36.4.10
Nisoldipine	Sular	Calcium Channel Inhibitors	36.4.10
Nitrendipine	—	Calcium Channel Inhibitors	36.4.10
Nortriptyline	Pamelor, Aventyl	Tricyclics and Tetracyclics	36.4.33
Olanzapine	Zyprexa	Serotonin Dopamine Antagonists	36.4.27
Orphenadrine	Norflex, Dispal	Anticholinergics	36.4.4
Oxazepam	Serax	Benzodiazepine Receptor Agonists	36.4.7
Oxcarbazepine	Trileptal	Carbamazepine	36.4.11
Paraldehyde	—	Barbiturates and Similarly Acting Substances	36.4.6
Paroxetine	Paxil	Selective Serotonin Reuptake Inhibitors	36.4.2
Pemoline	Cylert	Sympathomimetics and Related Drugs	36.4.30
Pentobarbital	Nembutal	Barbiturates and Similarly Acting Substances	36.4.6
Pergolide	Permax	Dopamine Receptor Agonists and Precursors	36.4.16
Perphenazine	Trilafon	Dopamine Receptor Antagonists	36.4.17
Phendimetrazine	Adipost, Bontril	Sympathomimetics and Related Drugs	36.4.30
Phenelzine	Nardil	Monoamine Oxidase Inhibitors	36.4.20
Phenmetrazine	Prelude	Sympathomimetics and Related Drugs	36.4.30
Phenobarbital	Solfoton, Luminal	Barbiturates and Similarly Acting Substances	36.4.6
Phentermine	Adipex-P, Fastin, Ionamin	Sympathomimetics and Related Drugs	36.4.30
Pimozide	Orap	Dopamine Receptor Antagonists	36.4.17
Pindolol	Visken	β-Adrenergic Receptor Antagonists	36.4.2
Piperacetazine	Quide	Dopamine Receptor Antagonists	36.4.17
Pramipexole	Mirapex	Dopamine Receptor Agonists and Precursors	36.4.16
Prazepam	Centrax	Benzodiazepines	36.4.7
Prochlorperazine	Compazine	Dopamine Receptor Antagonists	36.4.17
Procyclidine	Kemadrin	Anticholinergics	36.4.4
Promazine	Sparine	Dopamine Receptor Antagonists	36.4.17
Promethazine	Phenergan	Antihistamines	36.4.5

(*continued*)

Table 36.4–1 (*continued*)

Generic Name	Brand Name	Subsection Title	Subsection Number
Propranolol	Inderal	β-Adrenergic Receptor Antagonists	36.4.2
Protriptyline	Vivactil	Tricyclics and Tetracyclics	36.4.33
Quazepam	Doral	Benzodiazepines	36.4.7
Quetiapine	Seroquel	Serotonin-Dopamine Antagonists	36.4.27
Reboxetine	Vestra	Reboxetine	36.4.25
Reserpine	Diupres	Dopamine Receptor Antagonists	36.4.17
Risperidone	Risperdal	Serotonin-Dopamine Antagonists	36.4.27
Rivastigmine	Exelon	Cholinesterase Inhibitors	36.4.13
Ropinirole	Requip	Dopamine Receptor Agonists and Precursors	36.4.16
Secobarbital	Seconal	Barbiturates and Similarly Acting Substances	36.4.6
Selegiline	Eldepryl	Monoamine Oxidase Inhibitors	36.4.20
Sertraline	Zoloft	Selective Serotonin Reuptake Inhibitors	36.4.26
Sibutramine	Meridia	Sibutramine	36.4.28
Sildenafil	Viagra	Sildenafil	36.4.29
Tacrine	Cognex	Cholinesterase Inhibitors	36.4.13
Temazepam	Restoril	Benzodiazepines	36.4.7
Thiopental	Pentothal	Barbiturates and Similarly Acting Substances	36.4.6
Thioridazine	Mellaril	Dopamine Receptor Antagonists	36.4.17
Thiothixene	Navane	Dopamine Receptor Antagonists	36.4.17
Topiramate	Topamax	Other Anticonvulsants	36.4.24
Tranylcypromine	Parnate	Monoamine Oxidase Inhibitors	36.4.20
Trazodone	Desyrel	Trazodone	36.4.32
Triazolam	Halcion	Benzodiazepines	36.4.7
Trihexyphenidyl	Artane	Anticholinergics	36.4.4
Trifluoperazine	Stelazine	Dopamine Receptor Antagonists	36.4.17
Triflupromazine	Vesprin	Dopamine Receptor Antagonists	36.4.17
Trimipramine	Surmontil	Tricyclics and Tetracyclics	36.4.33
Valproate	Depakene	Valproate	36.4.34
Valproic Acid	Depakene	Valproate	36.4.34
Venlafaxine	Effexor	Venlafaxine	36.3.35
Verapamil	Calan, Isoptin	Calcium Channel Inhibitors	36.4.10
Yohimbine	Yocon	Yohimbine	36.4.36
Ziprasidone	Geodon	Serotonin-Dopamine Antagonists	36.4.27
Zaleplon	Sonata	Benzodiazepines	36.4.7
Zolpidem	Ambien	Benzodiazepines	36.4.7

COMBINATION DRUGS

In addition to the drugs that contain a single active component, a few combination drugs are available in the United States. The use of such drugs may increase patient compliance by simplifying the drug regimen. A problem with combination drugs, however, is that clinicians have little flexibility in adjusting the dosage of one of the components; that is, the use of combination drugs may cause two drugs to be administered when only one drug continues to be necessary for therapeutic efficacy. For that reason combination drugs are not recommended as a first-line approach to management.

Table 36.4–2
Major Mental Disorders and Common Drugs and Classes of Drugs Used in Their Treatment

Disorder	Subsection Number	Disorder	Subsection Number
Aggression and agitation (see Intermittent explosive disorder)		Alcohol dependence and withdrawal	
Akathisia (see Medication-induced movement disorders)		α_2-Adrenergic receptor agonists	36.4.1
		β-Adrenergic receptor antagonists	36.4.2
		Benzodiazepines	36.4.7

(*continued*)

Table 36.4–2 (*continued*)

Disorder	Subsection Number
Carbamazepine	36.4.11
Disulfiram	36.4.15
Opioid receptor antagonists	36.4.23
Other anticonvulsants (gabapentin)	36.4.24
Valproate	36.4.34
Anorexia nervosa (see Eating disorders)	
Anxiety (see also specific anxiety disorders)	
Antihistamines	36.4.5
Benzodiazepines	36.4.7
Buspirone	36.4.9
Selective serotonin reuptake inhibitors	36.4.26
Tricyclics and tetracyclics	36.4.33
Venlafaxine	36.4.35
Attention-deficit disorders	
α_2-Adrenergic receptor agonists	36.4.1
Bupropion	36.4.8
Buspirone	36.4.9
Selective serotonin reuptake inhibitors	36.4.26
Sympathomimetics and related drugs	36.4.30
Tricyclics and tetracyclics	36.4.33
Benzodiazepine dependence and withdrawal (see Sedative, hypnotic, and anxiolytic dependence and withdrawal)	
Bipolar disorders	
Benzodiazepines (especially clonazepam, lorazepam, and alprazolam)	36.4.7
Calcium channel inhibitors	36.4.10
Dopamine receptor antagonists	36.4.17
Other anticonvulsants	36.4.24
Lithium	36.4.18
Serotonin-dopamine antagonists	36.4.27
Valproate	36.4.34
Bulimia nervosa (see Eating disorders)	
Cocaine dependence and withdrawal	
Bupropion	36.4.8
Other anticonvulsants (gabapentin)	36.4.24
Valproate	36.4.34
Cyclothymic disorder (see Bipolar disorders)	
Delusional disorder (see Schizophrenia)	
Dementia	
Cholinesterase inhibitors	36.4.13
Dopamine receptor antagonists	36.4.17
Serotonin-dopamine antagonists	36.4.27
Depression	
Benzodiazepines (especially alprazolam)	36.4.7
Bupropion	36.4.8
Calcium channel inhibitors	36.4.10
Carbamazepine	36.4.11
Dopamine receptor agonists and precursors (bromocriptine)	36.4.16
Lithium	36.4.18
Mirtazapine	36.4.19
Monoamine oxidase inhibitors	36.4.20
Nefazodone	36.4.21
Reboxetine	36.4.25
Selective serotonin reuptake inhibitors	36.4.26
Sympathomimetics and related drugs	36.4.30
Thyroid hormones	36.4.31
Trazodone	36.4.32
Tricyclics and tetracyclics	36.4.33
Valproate	36.4.34
Venlafaxine	36.4.35
Dysthymic disorder (see Depression)	
Dystonia (see Medication-induced movement disorders)	
Eating disorders and obesity	
Antihistamines (cyproheptadine)	36.4.5
Lithium	36.4.18
Monoamine oxidase inhibitors	36.4.20
Other anticonvulsants (topiramate)	36.4.24
Selective serotonin reuptake inhibitors	36.4.26
Sibutramine	36.4.28
Sympathomimetics and Related Drugs	36.4.30
Trazodone	36.4.32
Tricyclics and tetracyclics	36.4.33
Valproate	36.4.34
Generalized anxiety disorder	
α_2-Adrenergic receptor antagonists	36.4.1
Barbiturates and similarly acting drugs	36.4.6
Benzodiazepines	36.4.7
Buspirone	36.4.9
Nefazodone	36.4.21
Selective serotonin reuptake inhibitors	36.4.26
Trazodone	36.4.32
Tricyclics and tetracyclics	36.4.33
Venlafaxine	36.4.34
Intermittent explosive disorder	
β-Adrenergic receptor antagonists	36.4.2
Carbamazepine	36.4.11
Buspirone	36.4.9
Calcium channel inhibitors	36.4.10
Dopamine receptor antagonists	36.4.17
Lithium	36.4.18
Other anticonvulsants	36.4.24
Serotonin-dopamine antagonists	36.4.27
Valproate	36.4.34
Medication-induced movement disorders (see Neuroleptic malignant syndrome)	
β-Adrenergic receptor antagonists	36.4.2
Amantadine	36.4.3
Anticholinergics	36.4.4
Antihistamines	36.4.5
Benzodiazepines	36.4.7
Dopamine receptor antagonists	36.4.16
Other anticonvulsants (gabapentin)	36.4.24
Serotonin-dopamine antagonists	36.4.27

(*continued*)

Table 36.4–2 (*continued*)

Disorder	Subsection Number
Neuroleptic malignant syndrome	
Dopamine receptor agonists and precursors (bromocriptine)	36.4.16
Dantrolene	36.4.14
Nicotine dependence and withdrawal	
α_2-Adrenergic receptor antagonists	36.4.1
Bupropion	36.4.8
Obsessive-compulsive disorder	
α_2-Adrenergic receptor agonists	36.4.1
Selective serotonin reuptake inhibitors	36.4.26
Trazodone	36.4.32
Tricyclics and tetracyclics	36.4.33
Valproate	36.4.34
Opioid dependence and withdrawal	
α_2-Adrenergic receptor agonists	36.4.1
Opioid receptor antagonists	36.4.23
Opioid receptor agonists	36.4.22
Other anticonvulsants (gabapentin)	36.4.24
Panic disorder (with or without agoraphobia)	
α_2-Adrenergic receptor agonists	36.4.1
β-Adrenergic receptor antagonists	36.4.2
Benzodiazepines (especially alprazolam and clonazepam)	36.4.7
Monoamine oxidase inhibitors	36.4.20
Nefazodone	36.4.21
Other anticonvulsants (gabapentin)	36.4.24
Selective serotonin reuptake inhibitors	36.4.26
Trazodone	36.4.32
Tricyclics and tetracyclics	36.4.33
Valproate	36.4.34
Parkinsonism (see Medication-induced movement disorders)	
Phobias (see Panic disorder)	
α_2-Adrenergic receptor agonists	36.4.1
β-Adrenergic receptor antagonists	36.4.2
Benzodiazepines	36.4.7
Monoamine oxidase inhibitors	36.4.20
Other anticonvulsants (gabapentin)	36.4.24
Reboxetine	36.4.25
Selective serotonin reuptake inhibitors	36.4.26
Posttraumatic stress disorder	
α_2-Adrenergic receptor agonists	36.4.1
β-Adrenergic receptor antagonists	36.4.2
Antihistamines (cyproheptadine)	36.4.5
Benzodiazepines	36.4.7
Carbamazepine	36.4.11
Monoamine oxidase inhibitors	36.4.20
Nefazodone	36.4.21
Other anticonvulsants (lamotrigine)	36.4.24
Selective serotonin reuptake inhibitors	36.4.26
Tricyclics and tetracyclics	36.4.33
Valproate	36.4.34
Premenstrual dysphoric disorder and premenstrual syndrome	
Buspirone	36.4.9
Nefazodone	36.4.21
Selective serotonin reuptake inhibitors	36.4.26
Psychosis (see Schizophrenia)	
Rabbit syndrome (see Medication-induced movement disorders)	
Schizoaffective disorder (see Depression, Bipolar I disorder, and Schizophrenia)	
Schizophrenia	
Benzodiazepines	36.4.7
Carbamazepine	36.4.11
Dopamine receptor antagonists	36.4.17
Lithium	36.4.18
Other anticonvulsants (lamotrigine)	36.4.24
Serotonin-dopamine antagonists	36.4.27
Sedative, hypnotic, and anxiolytic dependence and withdrawal	
α_2-Adrenergic receptor agonists	36.4.1
Barbiturates and similarly acting drugs	36.4.6
Carbamazepine	36.4.11
Other anticonvulsants (gabapentin)	36.4.24
Valproate	36.4.34
Sexual dysfunctions	
Amantadine	36.4.3
Antihistamines (cyproheptadine)	36.4.5
Bupropion	36.4.8
Buspirone	36.4.9
Dopamine receptor agonists and precursors	36.4.16
Selective serotonin reuptake inhibitors	36.4.26
Sildenafil	36.4.29
Sympathomimetics and related drugs	36.4.30
Trazodone	36.4.32
Tricyclics and tetracyclics (clomipramine)	36.4.33
Yohimbine	36.4.36
Sleep disorders	
Antihistamines	36.4.5
Barbiturates and similarly acting drugs	36.4.6
Benzodiazepines	36.4.7
Chloral hydrate	36.4.12
Sympathomimetics and related drugs	36.4.30
Trazodone	36.4.32
Tricyclics and tetracyclics	36.4.33
Tourette's and other tic disorders	
α_2-Adrenergic receptor agonists	36.4.1
Calcium channel inhibitors	36.4.10
Dopamine receptor agonists	36.4.17
Violence (see Intermittent explosive disorder)	

▲ 36.4.1 α_2-Adrenergic Receptor Agonists: Clonidine and Guanfacine

Clonidine (Catapres) and guanfacine (Tenex) are presynaptic α_2-adrenergic receptor agonists approved for use as antihypertensive agents. Stimulation of α_2-adrenergic receptors reduces the firing rate of noradrenergic neurons and reduces plasma concentrations of norepinephrine. Because of the widespread actions of the noradrenergic system, clonidine has also been adopted for use as a psychopharmacological agent. The most important clinical applications in psychiatry are as therapy for attention-deficit/hyperactivity disorder, opioid withdrawal, Tourette's disorder, and suppression of agitation in posttraumatic stress disorder.

Their role as a treatment for selected mental disorders is generally limited to instances in which other interventions have failed to ameliorate symptoms adequately. The frequent development of tolerance tends to limit their long-term effectiveness, making them more useful in short-term therapy. There is also uncertainty about cardiovascular risks with their use in children. Guanfacine appears to offer some advantages over clonidine. It is less sedating than clonidine and has a longer half-life. There is, however, less clinical experience with guanfacine, and fewer controlled studies involve its use in psychiatric disorders than use of clonidine.

CHEMISTRY

The molecular structures of clonidine and guanfacine are shown in Figure 36.4.1–1.

PHARMACOLOGICAL ACTIONS

Clonidine and guanfacine are well absorbed from the gastrointestinal (GI) tract and reach peak plasma levels 1 to 3 hours after oral administration. The half-life of clonidine is 6 to 20 hours and that of guanfacine is 10 to 30 hours.

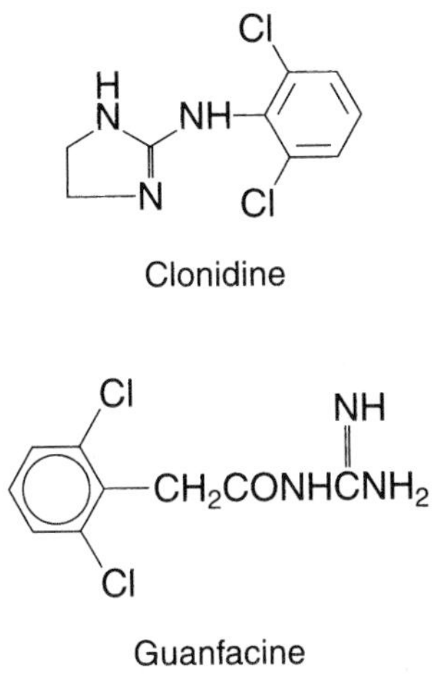

FIGURE 36.4.1–1
Molecular structures of clonidine and guanfacine.

The agonist effects of clonidine and guanfacine on presynaptic α_2-adrenergic receptors in the sympathetic nuclei of the brain result in a decrease in the amount of norepinephrine released from the presynaptic nerve terminals. This generally resets the body's sympathetic tone to a lower level and decreases arousal.

EFFECTS ON SPECIFIC ORGANS AND SYSTEMS

Both clonidine and guanfacine reduce peripheral sympathetic tone, lower diastolic and systolic blood pressure, and cause bradycardia. Activation of central α_2-receptors results in a sleeplike state in animal studies. Both cause sedation and sleep in humans. Both increase slow-wave sleep, reduce rapid eye movement (REM) sleep time and percentage, and increase REM latency. The effects on the GI tract are minimal, with some reduction in basal gastric acid secretion. There is little effect on renal function.

THERAPEUTIC INDICATIONS

Withdrawal from Opioids, Alcohol, Benzodiazepines, or Nicotine

Clonidine and guanfacine are effective in reducing the autonomic symptoms of rapid opioid withdrawal (e.g., hypertension, tachycardia, dilated pupils, sweating, lacrimation, and rhinorrhea) but not the associated subjective sensations. Clonidine administration (0.1 to 0.2 mg two to four times a day) is initiated prior to detoxification and is then tapered off over 1 to 2 weeks (Table 36.4.1–1).

Clonidine and guanfacine can reduce symptoms of alcohol and benzodiazepine withdrawal, including anxiety, diarrhea, and tachycardia. Clonidine and guanfacine can reduce craving, anxiety, and irritability symptoms of nicotine withdrawal. The transdermal patch formulation of clonidine is associated with better long-term compliance for purposes of detoxification than the tablet formulation is.

Tourette's Disorder

Clonidine and guanfacine are effective drugs for the treatment of Tourette's disorder. Most clinicians begin treatment for Tourette's disorder with the standard dopamine receptor antagonists, haloperidol (Haldol) and pimozide (Orap), and the serotonin-dopamine antagonists, risperidone (Risperdal) and olanzapine (Zyprexa). However, if concerned about the adverse effects of these drugs, the clinician may begin treatment with clonidine or guanfacine. The starting dosage of clonidine for a child is 0.05 mg a day; it can be raised to 0.3 mg a day in divided doses. Three months are needed before the beneficial effects of clonidine can be seen in Tourette's disorder. Response rates of 0 to 70 percent have been reported.

Other Tic Disorders

Clonidine and guanfacine reduce the frequency and severity of tics in persons with tic disorder, with or without comorbid attention-deficit/hyperactivity symptoms.

Table 36.4.1–1
Oral Clonidine Protocols for Opioid Detoxification

Clonidine 0.1–0.2 mg po 4 times a day; hold for systolic blood pressure <90 mm Hg or bradycardia; stabilize for 2–3 days, then taper over 5–10 days

OR

Clonidine 0.1–0.2 mg po q4–6h as needed for withdrawal signs or symptoms; stabilize for 2–3 days, then taper over 5–10 days

OR

Test dose with clonidine 0.1–0.2 mg po or sublingually (for patients weighing over 200 lb) check blood pressure after 1 h if diastolic BP >70 mm Hg and no symptoms of hypotension, begin treatment as follows

Weight (lb)	Number of clonidine patches
<110	2–3 TTS-1 patches
110–160	1 TTS-2 and 2 TTS-1 patches
160–200	2 TTS-2 patches
>200	2–3 TTS-2 patches

OR

Test dose of oral clonidine 0.1 mg; check BP after 1 h (if systolic blood pressure <90, do not give patch)

Place 2 TTS-2 clonidine patches (or 3 patches if patient weighs >150 lb) on hairless area of upper body; then

For first 23 h after patch application, give oral clonidine 0.2 mg q6h; then

For next 24 h, give oral clonidine 0.1 mg q6h

Change patches weekly

After 2 weeks of 2 patches, switch to 1 TTS-2 patch (or 2 TTS-2 patches if patient weighs >150 lb)

After 1 week of 1 patch, discontinue patches

From American Society of Addiction Medicine. Detoxification: principles and protocols. In: *The Principles Update Series: Topics in Addiction Medicine*, section 11. American Society of Addiction; 1997, with permission.

Hyperactivity and Aggression in Children

Clonidine and guanfacine can be useful alternatives for the treatment of attention-deficit/hyperactivity disorder. They are used in place of sympathomimetics and antidepressants, which may produce paradoxical worsening of hyperactivity in some children with mental retardation, aggression, or features on the spectrum of autism. Clonidine and guanfacine can improve mood, reduce activity level, and improve social adaptation. Some multiply impaired children may respond favorably to clonidine, while others may simply become sedated. The starting dosage is 0.05 mg a day; it can be raised to 0.3 mg a day in divided doses. The efficacy of clonidine and guanfacine for control of hyperactivity and aggression often diminishes over several months of use.

Clonidine or guanfacine can be combined with methylphenidate (Ritalin) or dextroamphetamine (Dexedrine, Dextrostat) to treat hyperactivity and inattentiveness, respectively. A small number of cases have been reported of sudden death of children taking clonidine together with methylphenidate; however, it has not been conclusively demonstrated that these medications contributed to those deaths. Clinicians should explain to the family that the efficacy and safety of this combination have not been investigated in controlled trials. Periodic cardiovascular assessments, including vital signs and electrocardiograms, are warranted if this combination is used.

Posttraumatic Stress Disorder

Acute exacerbations of posttraumatic stress disorder may be associated with hyperadrenergic symptoms, such as hyperarousal, exaggerated startle response, insomnia, vivid nightmares, tachycardia, agitation, hypertension, and perspiration. These symptoms may respond to the use of clonidine or (especially for overnight benefit) guanfacine.

Other Disorders

Other potential indications for clonidine include other anxiety disorders (panic disorder, phobias, obsessive-compulsive disorder, and generalized anxiety disorder) and mania, in which it may be synergistic with lithium (Eskalith) or carbamazepine (Tegretol). Anecdotal reports have noted the efficacy of clonidine in schizophrenia and tardive dyskinesia. A clonidine patch can reduce the hypersalivation and dysphagia caused by clozapine (Clozaril). Isolated reports describe successful use of clonidine in premenstrual syndrome and restless legs syndrome.

PRECAUTIONS AND ADVERSE REACTIONS

The most common adverse effects associated with clonidine are dry mouth and eyes, fatigue, sedation, dizziness, nausea, hypotension, and constipation, which result in discontinuation of therapy by about 10 percent of all persons taking the drug. Some persons also experience sexual dysfunction. Tolerance may develop to these adverse effects. A similar but milder adverse effect profile is seen with guanfacine, especially at doses of 3 mg or more per day. Clonidine and guanfacine should not be taken by adults with a blood pressure below 90/60 or with cardiac arrhythmias, especially bradycardia. Development of bradycardia warrants gradual, tapered discontinuation of the drug. Clonidine in particular is associated with sedation, and tolerance does not usually develop to this adverse effect. Uncommon central nervous system (CNS) adverse effects of clonidine include insomnia, anxiety, and depression; rare CNS adverse effects include vivid dreams, nightmares, and hallucinations. Fluid retention associated with clonidine treatment can be treated with diuretics. The transdermal patch formulation of clonidine can cause local skin irritation, which can be minimized by rotating the sites of application.

Overdose

Persons who take an overdose of clonidine can present with coma and constricted pupils, symptoms similar to those of an opioid overdose. Other symptoms of overdose are decreased blood pressure, pulse, and respiratory rates. Guanfacine overdose produces a milder version of these symptoms. Clonidine and guanfacine should be used with caution in persons with heart disease, any type of vascular disease, renal disease, Raynaud's syndrome, or a history of depression. Clonidine and guanfacine should be avoided during pregnancy and by nursing mothers. Elderly persons are more sensitive to the drug than younger adults. Children are susceptible to the same adverse effects as adults.

Table 36.4.1–2
α_2-Adrenergic Receptor Agonists Used in Psychiatry[a]

Drug	Preparations	Usual Child Starting Dosage	Usual Child Dosage Range	Usual Starting Adult Dosage	Usual Adult Dosage
Clonidine tablets (Catapres)	0.1, 0.2, 0.3 mg	0.05 mg a day	Up to 0.3 mg a day tablets in divided doses	0.1–0.2 mg 2–4 times a day (0.2–0.8 mg a day)	0.3–1.2 mg a day, 2–3 times a day (1.2 mg a day maximal dosage)
Clonidine transdermal system (Catapres-TTS)	0.1, 0.2, 0.3 mg a day	0.05 mg a day	Up to 0.3 mg a day patch every 5 days (0.5 mg a day every 5 days maximal dosage)	0.1 mg a day every 7 days	0.1 mg a day patch per week (0.6 mg a day every 7 days)
Guanfacine (Tenex)	1-, 2-mg tablets	1 mg a day at bedtime	1–2 mg a day at bedtime (3 mg a day maximal dosage)	1 mg a day at bedtime	1–2 mg at bedtime (3 mg a day maximal dosage)

[a]Dosages for medical indications, such as hypertension, vary.

Withdrawal

Abrupt discontinuation of clonidine use can cause anxiety, restlessness, perspiration, tremor, abdominal pain, palpitations, headache, and a dramatic rise in blood pressure. These symptoms may appear about 20 hours after the last dose of clonidine and thus may be seen if one or two doses are skipped. A similar set of symptoms occasionally occurs 2 to 4 days after discontinuation of guanfacine, but the usual course is a gradual return to baseline blood pressure over 2 to 4 days. Because of the possibility of discontinuation symptoms, dosages of clonidine and guanfacine should be tapered down slowly.

DRUG–DRUG INTERACTIONS

Coadministration of clonidine or guanfacine and tricyclic drugs can inhibit the hypotensive effects of both. Trazodone (Desyrel) can potentially produce hypotension and sedation when combined with clonidine. Any antihypertensive agent or drug that causes hypotension as a side effect may amplify blood pressure drops if coadministered with these drugs. They may also enhance the CNS depressive effects of barbiturates, alcohol, and other sedative-hypnotic agents. Concomitant use of β-adrenergic receptor antagonists can increase the severity of rebound phenomena, including hypertension, when clonidine use is discontinued. Yohimbine, an α_2-adrenergic receptor antagonist, blocks the pharmacological effects of clonidine. The reported sudden deaths of children taking concurrent methylphenidate and clonidine remains unexplained. They may represent isolated instances of children with preexisting cardiovascular abnormalities who either experienced adverse events unrelated to medication or had reactions to the clonidine alone.

LABORATORY INTERFERENCES

No known laboratory interferences are associated with the use of clonidine or guanfacine.

Dosage and Clinical Guidelines

Clonidine is available in 0.1-, 0.2-, and 0.3-mg tablets. The usual starting dosage is 0.1 mg orally twice a day; the dosage can be raised by 0.1 mg a day to an appropriate level (up to 1.2 mg per day). Clonidine must be always be tapered when it is discontinued, to avoid rebound hypertension, which may occur about 20 hours after the last clonidine dose. A weekly transdermal formulation of clonidine is available at doses of 0.1, 0.2, and 0.3 mg per day. The usual starting dosage is a 0.1-mg-per-day patch, which is changed each week for adults and every 5 days for children; the dosage can be increased every 1 to 2 weeks. Transition from the oral to the transdermal formulations should be accomplished gradually, by overlapping them for 3 to 4 days.

Guanfacine is available in 1- and 2-mg tablets. The usual starting dose is 1 mg before sleep, and this may be increased to 2 mg before sleep after 3 to 4 weeks, if necessary. Regardless of the indication for which clonidine or guanfacine is being used, the drug should be withheld if a person becomes hypotensive (blood pressure below 90/60).

Table 36.4.1–2 provides a summary of the α_2-adrenergic receptor agonists used in psychiatry.

REFERENCES

Ahmed I, Takeshita J. Clonidine: a critical review of its role in the treatment of psychiatric disorders. *CNS Drugs*. 1996;6:53.

Bremner JD, Krystal JH, Southwick SM, Charney DS. Noradrenergic mechanisms in stress and anxiety, II. Clinical studies. *Synapse*. 1996;23:39.

Connor DF, Barkley RA, Davis HT. A pilot study of methylphenidate, clonidine, or the combination in ADHD comorbid with aggressive oppositional defiant or conduct disorder. *Clin Pediatr*. 2000;39:15.

Fahlke C, Berggren U, Balldin J. Cardiovascular responses to clonidine in alcohol withdrawal: are they related to psychopathology and mental well-being? *Alcohol*. 2000;21:231.

Harmon RJ, Riggs PD. Clonidine for posttraumatic stress disorder in preschool children. *J Am Acad Child Adolesc Psychiatry*. 1996;35:1247.

Hoffman BB. Catecholamines, sympathomimetic drugs, and adrenergic receptor antagonists. In: Hardman JG, Limbird LE, Goodman Gilman A, eds. *Goodman & Gilman's the Pharmacological Basis of Therapeutics*. 10th ed. New York: McGraw-Hill; 2001:215.

Mokrani M-C, Duval F, Diep TS, Bailey PE, Macher JP. Multihormonal response to clonidine in patients with affective and psychotic symptoms. *Psychoneuroendocrinology*. 2000;25:741.

Oesterheld J, Tervo R. Clonidine: a practical guide for usage in children. *SD J Med*. 1996;49:234.

Sallee FR, Richman H, Sethuraman G, Dougherty D, Sine L, Altman-Hamamdzic S. Clonidine challenge in childhood anxiety disorder. *J Am Acad Child Adolesc Psychiatry*. 1998;37:655.

Schmidt ME, Matochik JA, Goldstein DS, Schouten JL, Zametkin AJ, Potteer WZ. Gender differences in brain metabolic and plasma catecholamine responses to alpha2-adrenoreceptor blockade. *Neuropsychopharmacology*. 1997;16:298.

Sussman N. Clonidine. In: Sadock BJ, Sadock VA, eds. *Kaplan & Sadock's Comprehensive Textbook of Psychiatry.* 7th ed. Vol 2. Baltimore: Lippincott Williams & Wilkins; 2000:2352.

Tallarida RJ, Stone DJ Jr, McCary JD, Raffa RB. Response surface analysis of synergism between morphine and clonidine. *J Pharmacol Exp Ther.* 1999;289:8.

▲ 36.4.2 β-Adrenergic Receptor Antagonists

The β-adrenergic receptor antagonists, which are variously referred to as beta-blockers and β-antagonists, represent an important psychopharmacological intervention—the reduction of adrenergic receptor activation. β-Adrenergic receptor antagonists are commonly used in medical practice for their peripheral effects in the treatment of hypertension, angina, certain cardiac arrhythmias, and the symptoms of hyperthyroidism, but the drugs are also used for their central actions in the treatment of migraine. Their effectiveness as peripherally and centrally acting agents has been well demonstrated for social phobia (e.g., performance anxiety), lithium-induced postural tremor, control of aggressive behavior, and neuroleptic-induced acute akathisia (Table 36.4.2–1).

Table 36.4.2–1
Psychiatric Uses for β-Adrenergic Receptor Antagonists

Definitely effective
Performance anxiety
Lithium-induced tremor
Neuroleptic-induced akathisia
Probably effective
Adjunctive therapy for alcohol withdrawal and other substance-related disorders
Adjunctive therapy for aggressive or violent behavior
Possibly effective
Antipsychotic augmentation
Antidepressant augmentation

CHEMISTRY

The seven β-adrenergic receptor antagonists most commonly studied for psychiatric indications in the United States are atenolol (Tenormin), metoprolol (Lopressor), labetalol (Normodyne, Trandate), acebutolol (Sectral), nadolol (Corgard), propranolol (Inderal) and pindolol (Visken). The molecular structures of these drugs are shown in Figure 36.4.2–1.

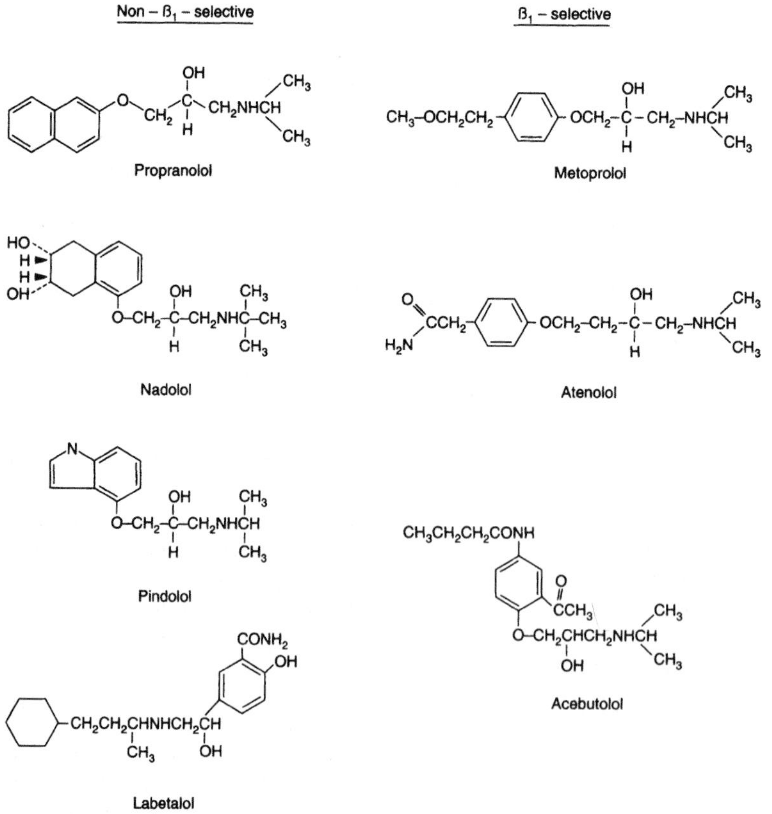

FIGURE 36.4.2–1

Molecular structures of β-adrenergic receptor antagonists.

Table 36.4.2–2
β-Adrenergic Drugs Used in Psychiatry

Generic Name	Trade Name	Lipophilic	Metabolism	Receptor Selectivity	Half-Life (h)	Usual Starting Dosage (mg)	Usual Maximum Dosage (mg)
Propranolol	Inderal	Yes	Hepatic	$\beta_1 = \beta_2$	3–6	10–20 bid or tid	30–140 bid
Nadolol	Corgard	No	Renal	$\beta_1 = \beta_2$	14–24	40 od	30–240 od
Pindolol	Visken	Intermediate	Hepatic	$\beta_1 = \beta_2$	3–4	5 bid	30 bid
Labetalol	Normodyne, Trandate	Intermediate	Hepatic	$\beta_1 = \beta_2$	4–6	100 bid	400–800 tid
Metoprolol	Lopressor	Yes	Hepatic	$\beta_1 > \beta_2$	3–4	50 bid	75–150 bid
Atenolol	Tenormin	No	Renal	$\beta_1 > \beta_2$	5–8	50 od	50–100 od
Acebutolol	Sectral	No	Hepatic	$\beta_1 > \beta_2$	3–4	400 od	600 bid

PHARMACOLOGICAL ACTIONS

The β-adrenergic receptor antagonists differ with regard to lipophilicities, metabolic routes, β-receptor selectivity, and half-lives (Table 36.4.2–2). The absorption of β-receptor antagonists from the gastrointestinal tract is variable. The agents that are most soluble in lipids (i.e., are lipophilic) are likely to cross the blood–brain barrier and enter the brain; agents that are least lipophilic are less likely to enter the brain. When central nervous system (CNS) effects are desired, a lipophilic drug may be preferred; when only peripheral effects are desired, a less lipophilic drug may be indicated.

Propranolol, nadolol, pindolol, and labetalol have essentially equal potency at both the β_1- and β_2-receptors, whereas metoprolol, atenolol, and acebutolol have greater affinity for the β_1-receptor than for the β_2-receptor. Relative β_1 selectivity confers few pulmonary and vascular effects on these drugs, although they must be used with caution in asthmatic persons, because the drugs retain some activity at the β_2-receptors.

Pindolol has sympathomimetic effects in addition to its β-adrenergic receptor antagonist effects, which permits its use to augment antidepressant drugs. Pindolol, propranolol, and nadolol possess some antagonist activity at the serotonin 5-HT_{1A} receptors.

EFFECTS ON SPECIFIC ORGANS AND SYSTEMS

β_1-Receptors modulate chronotropic and inotropic cardiac functions. They have a marked blood-pressure-lowering effect in patients with hypertension and produce bradycardia. β_2-Receptors modulate bronchodilatation and vasodilation. For this reason, β_1-selective drugs are preferable in the treatment of patients with asthma and other obstructive pulmonary diseases; the blockade of the pulmonary β_2-receptors blocks the bronchodilating effects of epinephrine. Some experts, however, would never use β-adrenergic receptor antagonists in patients with asthma but might substitute a benzodiazepine for the same indication.

THERAPEUTIC INDICATIONS

Anxiety Disorders

Propranolol is useful for the treatment of social phobia, primarily of the performance type (e.g., disabling anxiety before a musical performance). Data are also available for its use in treatment of panic disorder, posttraumatic stress disorder, and generalized anxiety disorder. In social phobia, the common treatment approach is to take 10 to 40 mg of propranolol 20 to 30 minutes before the anxiety-provoking situation. Persons may try a test run of one of the β-adrenergic receptor antagonists before using it to prepare for an anxiety-provoking situation to ensure that they do not experience any adverse effects from the drug or the dose. β-Adrenergic receptor antagonists may blunt cognition in some persons. They are less effective for the treatment of panic disorder than benzodiazepines or selective serotonin reuptake inhibitors (SSRIs).

Lithium-Induced Postural Tremor

β-Adrenergic receptor antagonists are beneficial for lithium-induced postural tremor and other medication-induced postural tremors—for example, those induced by the tricyclic drugs and valproate (Depakene). The initial approach to this movement disorder includes lowering the dose of lithium, eliminating aggravating factors such as caffeine, and administering lithium at bedtime. However, if these interventions are inadequate, propranolol in the range of 20 to 160 mg a day, given two or three times daily, is generally effective for the treatment of lithium-induced postural tremor.

Neuroleptic-Induced Acute Akathisia

Many studies have shown that β-adrenergic receptor antagonists can be effective in the treatment of neuroleptic-induced acute akathisia. Most clinicians believe that β-adrenergic receptor antagonists are more effective for this indication than anticholinergics and benzodiazepines. β-Adrenergic receptor antagonists are not effective in the treatment of such neuroleptic-induced movement disorders as acute dystonia and parkinsonism.

Aggression and Violent Behavior

β-Adrenergic receptor antagonists may be effective in reducing the number of aggressive and violent outbursts in persons with impulse disorders, schizophrenia, and aggression associated with brain injuries such as trauma, tumors, anoxic injury, encephalitis, alcohol dependence, and degenerative disorders (e.g., Huntington's disease). Many studies have added a β-

adrenergic receptor antagonist to the ongoing therapy (e.g., antipsychotics, anticonvulsants, lithium), making it difficult to distinguish additive effects from independent effects. Propranolol dosages for this indication range from 50 to 800 mg a day.

Alcohol Withdrawal

Propranolol has been reported to be useful as an adjuvant to benzodiazepines but not as a sole agent in the treatment of alcohol withdrawal. The following dose schedule is suggested: no propranolol for a pulse rate below 50; 50 mg of propranolol for a pulse rate between 50 and 80; and 100 mg of propranolol for a pulse rate of 80 or above.

Antidepressant Augmentation

Pindolol has been used to augment and hasten the antidepressant effects of SSRIs, tricyclic drugs, and electroconvulsive therapy. Small studies have shown that pindolol administered at the onset of antidepressant therapy may shorten the usual 2- to 4-week latency of antidepressant response by several days. Because the β-adrenergic receptor antagonists may induce depression in some persons, augmentation strategies with these drugs must be further clarified in controlled trials.

Other Disorders

A number of case reports and controlled studies have reported data indicating that β-adrenergic receptor antagonists may be of modest benefit to persons with schizophrenia and with manic symptoms. It has also been used in some patients with stuttering.

PRECAUTIONS AND ADVERSE REACTIONS

The β-adrenergic receptor antagonists are contraindicated for use in persons with asthma, insulin-dependent diabetes, congestive heart failure, significant vascular disease, persistent angina, and hyperthyroidism. They are contraindicated in diabetic persons because the drugs antagonize the normal physiological response to hypoglycemia. The β-adrenergic receptor antagonists can worsen atrioventricular (A-V) conduction defects and lead to complete A-V heart block and death. If the clinician decides that the risk-benefit ratio warrants a trial of a β-adrenergic receptor antagonist in a person with one of these coexisting medical conditions, a β_1-selective agent should be the first choice. All currently available β-adrenergic receptor antagonists are excreted in breast milk and should be administered with caution to nursing women.

The most common adverse effects of β-adrenergic receptor antagonists are hypotension and bradycardia. In persons at risk for these adverse effects, a test dosage of 20 mg a day of propranolol can be given to assess their reaction to the drug. Depression has been associated with lipophilic β-receptor antagonists such as propranolol, but it is probably rare. Nausea, vomiting, diarrhea, and constipation may also be caused by treatment with these agents. Serious CNS adverse effects (e.g., agitation, confusion, and hallucinations) are rare. Table 36.4.2–3 lists the possible adverse affects of β-adrenergic receptor antagonists.

Table 36.4.2–3
Adverse Effects and Toxicity of β-Adrenergic Receptor Antagonists

Cardiovascular
Hypotension
Bradycardia
Dizziness
Congestive failure (in patients with compromised myocardial function)
Respiratory
Asthma (less risk with β_1-selective drugs)
Metabolic
Worsened hypoglycemia in diabetic patients on insulin or oral agents
Gastrointestinal
Nausea
Diarrhea
Abdominal pain
Sexual function
Impotence
Neuropsychiatric
Lassitude
Fatigue
Dysphoria
Insomnia
Vivid nightmares
Depression (rare)
Psychosis (rare)
Other (rare)
Raynaud's phenomenon
Peyronie's disease
Withdrawal syndrome
Rebound worsening of preexisting angina pectoris when β-adrenergic receptor antagonists are discontinued

DRUG–DRUG INTERACTIONS

Concomitant administration of propranolol results in increased plasma concentrations of antipsychotics, anticonvulsants, theophylline (Theo-Dur, Slo-Bid), and levothyroxine (Synthroid). Other β-adrenergic receptor antagonists possibly have similar effects. The β-adrenergic receptor antagonists that are eliminated by the kidneys may have similar effects on drugs that are also eliminated by the renal route. Barbiturates, phenytoin (Dilantin), and cigarette smoking increase the elimination of β-adrenergic receptor antagonists that are metabolized by the liver. Several reports have associated hypertensive crises and bradycardia with the coadministration of β-adrenergic receptor antagonists and monoamine oxidase inhibitors. Depressed myocardial contractility and A-V nodal conduction may occur from concomitant administration of a β-adrenergic receptor antagonist and calcium channel inhibitors.

LABORATORY INTERFERENCES

The β-adrenergic receptor antagonists do not interfere with standard laboratory tests.

Dosage and Clinical Guidelines

Propranolol is available in 10-, 20-, 40-, 60-, 80-, and 90-mg tablets; 4-, 8-, and 80-mg/mL solutions; and 60-, 80-, 120-, and 160-mg sustained-release capsules. Nadolol is available in 20-, 40-, 80-, 120-, and 160-mg tablets. Pindolol is available in 5- and 10-mg tablets. Labetalol is available in 100-, 200-, and 300-mg tablets. Metoprolol is available in 50- and 100-mg tablets; and in 50-, 100-, and 200-mg sustained-release tablets. Atenolol is available in 25-, 50-, and 100-mg tablets. Acebutolol is available in 200- and 400-mg capsules.

For the treatment of chronic disorders, propranolol administration is usually initiated at 10 mg by mouth three times a day or 20 mg by mouth twice daily. The dosage can be raised by 20 to 30 mg a day until a therapeutic effect begins to emerge. The dosage should be leveled off at the appropriate range for the disorder under treatment. The treatment of aggressive behavior sometimes requires dosages up to 800 mg a day, and therapeutic effects may not be seen until the person has been receiving the maximal dosage for 4 to 8 weeks. As mentioned, for treatment of social phobia, primarily the performance type, the patient should take 10 to 40 mg of propranolol 20 to 30 minutes before the performance.

Pulse and blood pressure should be taken regularly, and the drug should be withheld if the pulse rate is below 50 or the systolic blood pressure is below 90. Drug use should be temporarily discontinued if it produces severe dizziness, ataxia, or wheezing. Treatment with β-adrenergic receptor antagonists should never be discontinued abruptly. Propranolol use should be tapered by 60 mg a day until a dosage of 60 mg a day is reached, after which the dosage should be tapered by 10 to 20 mg a day every 3 or 4 days.

References

Bright RA, Everitt DE. β-Blockers and depression. *JAMA*. 1992;267:1783.

Concores JA, Dackis CA, Davies RK, Gold MS. Propranolol and stuttering. *Am J Psychiatry*. 1986;143:1071.

Granville-Grossman KL. Propranolol, anxiety, and the central nervous system. *Br J Clin Pharmacol*. 1974;1:361.

Hoffman BB. Catecholamines, sympathomimetic drugs, and adrenergic receptor antagonists. In: Hardman JG, Limbird LE, Goodman Gilman A, eds. *Goodman & Gilman's the Pharmacological Basis of Therapeutics*. 10th ed. New York: McGraw-Hill; 2001:215.

Jonas DL, Blumenthal JA, Madden DJ, Serra M. Cognitive consequences of antihypertensive medications. In: Waldstein SR, Elias MF, eds. *Neuropsychology of Cardiovascular Disease*. Mahwah, NJ: Lawrence Erlbaum Associates; 2001:167.

Kraus ML, Gottlieb LD, Horwitz RI, Anscher M. Randomized clinical trial of atenolol in patients with alcohol withdrawal. *N Engl J Med*. 1985;313:905.

Lader M. β-Adrenoceptor antagonists in neuropsychiatry: an update. *J Clin Psychiatry*. 1988;49:213.

Ma YC. Huang XY. Novel signaling pathway through the beta-adrenergic receptor. *Trends Cardiovasc Med*. 2002;12:46.

Mattes JA. Metoprolol for intermittent explosive disorder. *Am J Psychiatry*. 1985;142:1108.

McAllister-Williams RH, Young AH. Pindolol augmentation of antidepressant therapy. *Br J Psychiatry*. 1999;173:536.

Ratey JJ, Prough EE. The current status of β-blockers in psychiatric practice. *Dir Psychiatry*. 1996;16:16.

Ratey JJ, Sorgi P, O'Driscoll GA, et al. Nadolol to treat aggression and psychiatric symptomatology in chronic psychiatric inpatients: a double-blind, placebo-controlled study. *J Clin Psychiatry*. 1992;53:41.

Reist C, Duffy JG, Fujimoto K, Cahill L. β-Adrenergic blockade and emotional memory in PTSD. *Int J Neuropsychopharmacol*. 2001;4:377.

Ruedrich S, Erhardt L. Beta-adrenergic blockers in mental retardation and developmental disabilities. *Ment Retard Dev Disabil Res Rev*. 1999;5:290.

Simpson GM, Flowers CJ. β-Adrenergic receptor antagonists. In: Sadock BJ, Sadock VA, eds. *Kaplan & Sadock's Comprehensive Textbook of Psychiatry*. 7th ed. Vol 2. Baltimore: Lippincott Williams & Wilkins; 2000:2271.

Yudofsky SC, Silver JM, Hales RE. Pharmacologic management of aggression in the elderly. *J Clin Psychiatry*. 1990;51(suppl):22.

▲ 36.4.3 Amantadine

Amantadine (Symmetrel) is used primarily for the treatment of medication-induced movement disorders, such as neuroleptic-induced parkinsonism. It is also used as an antiviral agent for the prophylaxis and treatment of influenza A infection.

CHEMISTRY

Amantadine's molecular structure is given in Figure 36.4.3–1.

PHARMACOLOGICAL ACTIONS

Amantadine is well absorbed from the gastrointestinal (GI) tract after oral administration, reaches peak plasma concentrations in approximately 2 to 3 hours, has a half-life of about 12 to 18 hours, and attains steady-state concentrations after approximately 4 to 5 days of therapy. Amantadine is excreted unmetabolized in the urine. Plasma concentrations of amantadine can be as much as twice as high in elderly persons as in younger adults. Patients with renal failure accumulate amantadine in their bodies.

Amantadine augments dopaminergic neurotransmission in the central nervous system (CNS). The precise mechanism for this effect is unknown, but it may involve dopamine release from presynaptic vesicles, blocking reuptake of dopamine into presynaptic nerve terminals, or an agonist effect on postsynaptic dopamine receptors.

EFFECTS ON SPECIFIC ORGANS AND SYSTEMS

Amantadine is associated with CNS and GI adverse effects at high doses.

THERAPEUTIC INDICATIONS

The primary indication for amantadine in psychiatry is for the treatment of extrapyramidal signs and symptoms, such as parkinsonism, akinesia, and so-called rabbit syndrome (focal perioral tremor of the choreoathetoid type) caused by the administration of dopamine receptor antagonist drugs (e.g., haloperidol [Haldol]). Amantadine is as effective as the anticholinergics (e.g., benztropine [Cogentin]) for these indications and results in improvement in approximately one half of all persons who take it. However, amantadine is not generally considered as effective as the anticholinergics for the treatment of acute dystonic reactions and is not effective in treating tardive dyskinesia and akathisia.

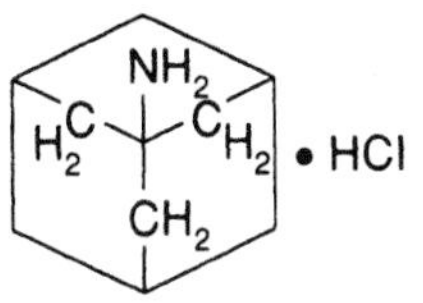

FIGURE 36.4.3–1
Molecular structure of amantadine.

Amantadine is a reasonable compromise for persons with extrapyramidal symptoms who would be sensitive to additional anticholinergic effects, particularly those taking a low-potency dopamine receptor antagonist or the elderly. Elderly persons are prone to anticholinergic adverse effects in both the CNS, such as anticholinergic delirium, and in the peripheral nervous system, such as urinary retention. Amantadine is associated with less memory impairment than the anticholinergics are. Amantadine is reportedly of benefit in treating some selective serotonin reuptake inhibitor–associated side effects, such as lethargy, fatigue, anorgasmia, and ejaculatory inhibition. It is used in general medical practice for the treatment of parkinsonism of all causes, including idiopathic parkinsonism.

PRECAUTIONS AND ADVERSE EFFECTS

The most common CNS effects are mild dizziness, insomnia, and impaired concentration (dosage related), which occur in 5 to 10 percent of persons. Irritability, depression, anxiety, dysarthria, and ataxia occur in 1 to 5 percent of persons. More severe CNS adverse effects, including seizures and psychotic symptoms, have been reported. Nausea is the most common peripheral adverse effect of amantadine. Headache, loss of appetite, and blotchy spots on the skin have also been reported.

Livedo reticularis of the legs (a purple discoloration of the skin, caused by dilation of blood vessels) has been reported in up to 5 percent of persons who take the drug for over a month. It usually diminishes with elevation of the legs and resolves in almost all cases when drug use is terminated.

Amantadine is relatively contraindicated in persons with renal disease or a seizure disorder. It should be used with caution in persons with edema or cardiovascular disease. Some evidence indicates that amantadine is teratogenic, and thus it should not be taken by pregnant women. Because amantadine is excreted in milk, women who are breast-feeding should not take the drug.

Suicide attempts with amantadine overdosages are life threatening. Symptoms can include toxic psychoses (confusion, hallucinations, aggressiveness) and cardiopulmonary arrest. Emergency treatment beginning with gastric lavage is indicated.

DRUG INTERACTIONS

Coadministration of amantadine with phenelzine (Nardil) or other monoamine oxidase inhibitors (MAOIs) may significantly increase resting blood pressure. The coadministration of amantadine with CNS stimulants can result in insomnia, irritability, nervousness, and possibly seizures or irregular heartbeat. Amantadine should not be coadministered with anticholinergics because adverse effects such as confusion, hallucinations, nightmares, dryness of mouth, and blurred vision may be exacerbated.

DOSAGE AND CLINICAL GUIDELINES

Amantadine is available in 100-mg capsules and as a 50 mg/5 mL syrup. The usual starting dosage of amantadine is 100 mg given orally twice a day, although the dosage can be cautiously increased up to 200 mg given orally twice a day if indicated. Amantadine should be used in persons with renal impairment only in consultation with the physician treating the renal condition. If amantadine is successful in the treatment of the drug-induced extrapyramidal symptoms, it should be continued for 4 to 6 weeks and then discontinued to see whether the person has become tolerant to the neurological adverse effects of the antipsychotic medication. Amantadine use should be tapered over 1 to 2 weeks once a decision has been made to discontinue use of the drug. Persons taking amantadine should not drink alcoholic beverages.

REFERENCES

Bennett VL, Juorio AV, Li XM. Possible new mechanism for the antiparkinsonian effect of amantadine. *J Psychiatry Neurosci.* 1999;24:52.

DiMascio A, Diosdado BL, Greenblatt DJ, Marder JE. A controlled trial of amantadine in drug-induced extrapyramidal disorders. *Arch Gen Psychiatry.* 1976;33:599.

Meyer JM, Simpson GM. Anticholinergics and amantadine. In: Sadock BJ, Sadock VA, eds. *Kaplan & Sadock's Comprehensive Textbook of Psychiatry.* 7th ed. Vol 2. Baltimore: Lippincott Williams & Wilkins; 2000:2276.

Miyasaki JM, Grimes D, Lang AE. Acute delirium after withdrawal of amantadine in Parkinson's disease. *Neurology.* 1999;52:1720.

Paci C, Thomas A, Onofrj M. Amantadine for dyskinesia in patients affected by severe Parkinson's disease. *Neurol Sci.* 2001;22:75.

Silver H, Geraisy N. Effects of biperiden and amantadine on memory in medicated chronic schizophrenic patients. A double-blind cross-over study. *Br J Psychiatry.* 1995;166:241.

Standaert DG, Young AB. Treatment of central nervous system degenerative disorders. In: Hardman JG, Limbird LE, Goodman Gilman A, eds. *Goodman & Gilman's the Pharmacological Basis of Therapeutics.* 10th ed. New York: McGraw-Hill; 2001:549.

Terao T. Female sexual dysfunction and antidepressant use. *Am J Psychiatry.* 2001;158:326.

Wilcox JA, Tsuang J. Psychological effects of amantadine on psychotic subjects. *Neuropsychobiology.* 1990;23:144.

Yang CC, Deng JF. Anticholinergic syndrome with severe rhabdomyolysis—an unusual feature of amantadine toxicity [letter]. *Intensive Care Med.* 1997;23:355.

▲ 36.4.4 Anticholinergics

In the clinical practice of psychiatry, the anticholinergic drugs have their primary use as treatments for medication-induced movement disorders, particularly neuroleptic-induced parkinsonism, neuroleptic-induced acute dystonia, and medication-induced postural tremor. The anticholinergic drugs may also be of limited use in the treatment of neuroleptic-induced acute akathisia. Before the introduction of levodopa (Larodopa), the anticholinergic drugs were commonly used in the treatment of idiopathic Parkinson's disease.

The common use of the term *anticholinergic drugs* is misleading. There are two general types of acetylcholine receptors: the muscarinic receptors and the nicotinic receptors. The muscarinic receptors are G protein–linked receptors, and the nicotinic receptors are ligand-gated ion channels. The anticholinergic drugs discussed in this section are specific for the muscarinic receptors and thus are also referred to as *antimuscarinic drugs*.

CHEMISTRY

The molecular structures of representative anticholinergic drugs are shown in Figure 36.4.4–1.

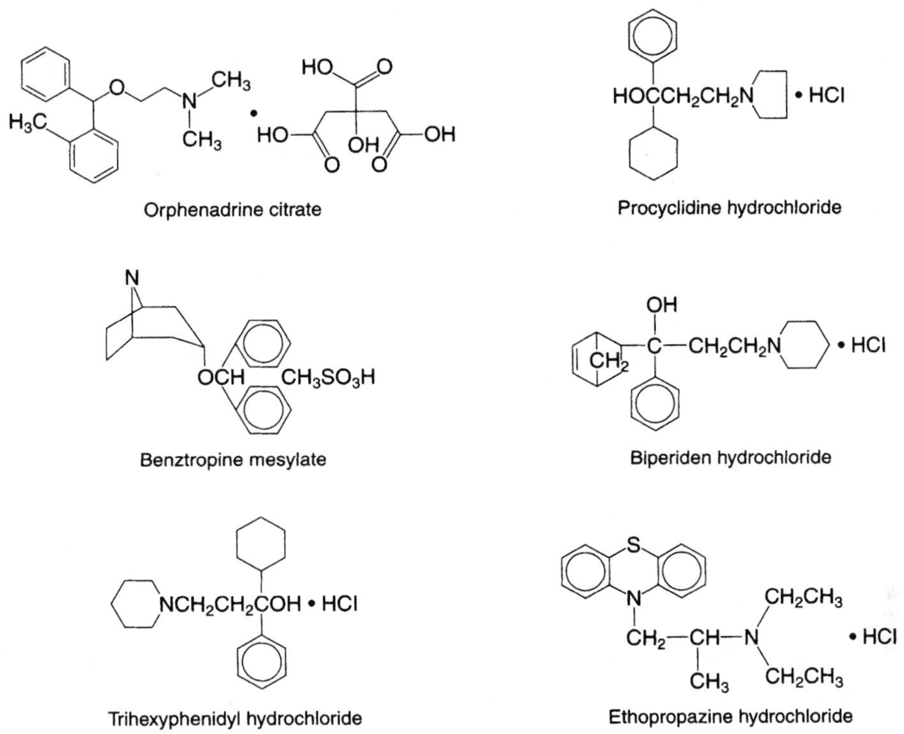

FIGURE 36.4.4–1
Molecular structures of selected anticholinergic drugs.

PHARMACOLOGICAL ACTIONS

All anticholinergic drugs are well absorbed from the gastrointestinal tract after oral administration, and all are lipophilic enough to enter the central nervous system (CNS). Trihexyphenidyl (Artane) and benztropine (Cogentin) reach peak plasma concentrations in 2 to 3 hours after oral administration and have a duration of action of 1 to 12 hours. Benztropine is absorbed equally rapidly by intramuscular (IM) and intravenous (IV) administration; intramuscular administration is preferred because of its low risk for adverse effects.

All six anticholinergic drugs listed in this chapter block muscarinic acetylcholine receptors, and benztropine and ethopropazine (Parsidol) also have some antihistaminergic effects. None of the available anticholinergic drugs has any effects on the nicotinic acetylcholine receptors. Of the six drugs, trihexyphenidyl is the most stimulating, perhaps acting through dopaminergic neurons, and benztropine is the least stimulating and thus carries the least abuse potential.

EFFECTS ON SPECIFIC ORGANS AND SYSTEMS

The antimuscarinic activity of the anticholinergic drugs discussed here affects the functioning of the autonomic ganglia and most commonly affects the gastrointestinal tract, the heart, the bladder, and other parasympathetic functions.

THERAPEUTIC INDICATIONS

The primary indication for the use of anticholinergics in psychiatric practice is for the treatment of *neuroleptic-induced parkinsonism,* characterized by tremor, rigidity, cogwheeling, bradykinesia, sialorrhea, stooped posture, and festination. All the available anticholinergics are equally effective in the treatment of parkinsonian symptoms. Neuroleptic-induced parkinsonism is most common in the elderly and is most frequently seen with high-potency dopamine receptor antagonists, for example, haloperidol (Haldol). The onset of symptoms usually occurs after 2 or 3 weeks of treatment. The incidence of neuroleptic-induced parkinsonism is significantly lower with the newer antipsychotic drugs of the serotonin-dopamine antagonist (SDA) class.

Another indication is for the treatment of *neuroleptic-induced acute dystonia,* which is most common in young men. The syndrome often occurs early in the course of treatment, is commonly associated with high-potency dopamine receptor antagonists (e.g., haloperidol), and most commonly affects the muscles of the neck, tongue, face, and back. Anticholinergic drugs are effective in both short-term treatment of dystonias and prophylaxis against neuroleptic-induced acute dystonias.

Akathisia is characterized by a subjective and objective sense of restlessness, anxiety, and agitation. Although a trial of anticholinergics for the treatment of neuroleptic-induced acute akathisia is reasonable, these drugs are not generally considered as effective as the β-adrenergic receptor antagonists, the benzodiazepines, and clonidine (Catapres).

Table 36.4.4–1
Anticholinergic Drugs

Generic Name	Brand Name	Tablet Size	Injectable	Usual Daily Oral Dose	Short-Term IM or IV Dose
Benztropine	Cogentin	0.5, 1, 2 mg	1 mg/mL	1–4 mg one to three times	1–2 mg
Biperiden	Akineton	2 mg	5 mg/mL	2 mg one to three times	2 mg
Ethopropazine	Parsidol	10, 50 mg	—	50–100 mg one to three times	—
Orphenadrine	Norflex, Dispal	100 mg	30 mg/mL	50–100 mg three times	60 mg IV given over 5 min
Procyclidine	Kemadrin	5 mg	—	2.5–5 mg three times	—
Trihexyphenidyl	Artane, Trihexane, Trihexy-5	2.5 mg elixir 2 mg per 5 mL	—	2–5 mg two to four times	—

PRECAUTIONS AND ADVERSE REACTIONS

The adverse effects of the anticholinergic drugs result from blockade of muscarinic acetylcholine receptors. Anticholinergic drugs should be used cautiously, if at all, by persons with prostatic hypertrophy, urinary retention, and narrow-angle glaucoma. The anticholinergics are occasionally used as drugs of abuse because of their mild mood-elevating properties.

The most serious adverse effect associated with anticholinergic toxicity is anticholinergic intoxication, which can be characterized by delirium, coma, seizures, agitation, hallucinations, severe hypotension, supraventricular tachycardia, and peripheral manifestations—flushing, mydriasis, dry skin, hyperthermia, and decreased bowel sounds. Treatment should begin by immediate discontinuation of all anticholinergic drugs. The syndrome of anticholinergic intoxication can be diagnosed and treated with physostigmine (Antilirium, Eserine), an inhibitor of anticholinesterase, 1 to 2 mg IV (1 mg every 2 minutes) or IM every 30 or 60 minutes. Treatment with physostigmine should be used only in severe cases and only when emergency cardiac monitoring and life-support services are available, because physostigmine can lead to severe hypotension and bronchial constriction.

DRUG–DRUG INTERACTIONS

The most common drug–drug interactions with the anticholinergics occur when they are coadministered with psychotropics that also have high anticholinergic activity, such as dopamine receptor antagonists, tricyclic and tetracyclic drugs, and monoamine oxidase inhibitors (MAOIs). Many other prescription drugs and over-the-counter cold preparations also induce significant anticholinergic activity. The coadministration of those drugs can result in a life-threatening anticholinergic intoxication syndrome. Anticholinergic drugs can also delay gastric emptying, thereby decreasing the absorption of drugs that are broken down in the stomach and usually absorbed in the duodenum (e.g., levodopa and dopamine receptor antagonists).

LABORATORY INTERFERENCES

No laboratory interferences have been associated with anticholinergics.

DOSAGE AND CLINICAL GUIDELINES

The six anticholinergic drugs discussed in this chapter are available in a range of preparations (Table 36.4.4–1).

Neuroleptic-Induced Parkinsonism

For the treatment of neuroleptic-induced parkinsonism, the equivalent of 1 to 4 mg of benztropine should be given one to four times daily. The anticholinergic drug should be administered for 4 to 8 weeks, then it should be discontinued to assess whether it is still required. Anticholinergic drug use should be tapered over 1 to 2 weeks.

Treatment with anticholinergics as prophylaxis against the development of neuroleptic-induced parkinsonism is usually not indicated, since the symptoms of neuroleptic-induced parkinsonism are usually mild enough and gradual enough in onset to allow the clinician to initiate treatment only after it is clearly indicated. However, in young men, prophylaxis may be indicated, especially if a high-potency dopamine receptor antagonist is being used. The clinician should attempt to discontinue the antiparkinsonian agent in 4 to 6 weeks to assess whether its continued use is necessary.

Neuroleptic-Induced Acute Dystonia

For the short-term treatment and prophylaxis of neuroleptic-induced acute dystonia, 1 to 2 mg of benztropine or its equivalent in another drug should be given IM. The dose can be repeated in 20 to 30 minutes as needed. If the person still does not improve in another 20 to 30 minutes, a benzodiazepine (e.g., 1 mg of lorazepam [Ativan]) should be given IM or IV. Laryngeal dystonia is a medical emergency and should be treated with benztropine, up to 4 mg in a 10-minute period, followed by 1 to 2 mg of lorazepam, administered slowly by the IV route.

Prophylaxis against dystonias is indicated in persons who have had one episode or in persons at high risk (young men taking high-potency dopamine receptor antagonists). Prophylactic treatment is given for 4 to 8 weeks and then gradually tapered over 1 to 2 weeks to allow assessment of its continued need. The prophylactic use of anticholinergics in persons requiring antipsychotic drugs has largely become a moot issue because of the availability of SDAs, which are relatively free of parkinsonian effects.

Akathisia

As mentioned above, anticholinergics are not the drugs of choice for this syndrome. The β-adrenergic receptor antagonists (Section 36.4.2) and perhaps the benzodiazepines (Section 36.4.7) and clonidine (Section 36.4.1) are preferable and should be tried first.

References

Baker LA, Cheng LY, Amara IB. The withdrawal of benztropine mesylate in chronic schizophrenic patients. *Br J Psychiatry.* 1983;143:584.

Bergen J, Kitchin R, Berry G. Predictors of the course of tardive dyskinesia in patients receiving neuroleptics. *Biol Psychiatry.* 1992;32:580.

Blaisdell GD. Akathisia: a comprehensive review and treatment summary. *Pharmacopsychiatry.* 1994;27:139.

de Leon J, Canuso C, White AO, Simpson GM. A pilot effort to determine benztropine equivalents of anticholinergic medications. *Hosp Community Psychiatry.* 1994;45:606.

Elliott KJ, Lewis S, el Mallakh RS, Looney SW, Caudill R, Bacani Oropilla T. The role of parkinsonism and antiparkinsonian therapy in the subsequent development of tardive dyskinesia. *Ann Clin Psychiatry.* 1994;6:197.

Goff DC, Amico E, Dreyfuss D, Ciraulo D. A placebo-controlled trial of trihexyphenidyl in unmedicated patients with schizophrenia. *Am J Psychiatry.* 1994;151:429.

Katz IR, Sands LP, Bilker W, DiFilippo S, Boyce A, D'Angelo K. Identification of medications that cause cognitive impairment in older people: the case of oxybutynin chloride. *J Am Geriatr Soc.* 1998;46:8.

Manos N, Gkiouzepas J, Logothetis J. The need for continuous use of antiparkinsonian medication with chronic schizophrenic patients receiving long-term neuroleptic therapy. *Am J Psychiatry.* 1981;138:184.

Meyer JM, Simpson GM. Anticholinergics and amantadine. In: Sadock BJ, Sadock VA, eds. *Kaplan & Sadock's Comprehensive Textbook of Psychiatry.* 7th ed. Vol 2. Baltimore: Lippincott Williams & Wilkins; 2000:2276.

Mori K, Yamashita H, Nagao M, Horiguchi J, Yamawaki S. Effects of anticholinergic drug withdrawal on memory, regional cerebral blood flow and extrapyramidal side effects in schizophrenic patients. *Pharmacopsychiatry.* 2002;35:6.

Roe CM, Anderson MJ, Spivack B. Use of anticholinergic medications by older adults with dementia. *J Am Geriatr Soc.* 2002;50:836.

Standaert DG, Young AB. Treatment of central nervous system degenerative disorders. In: Hardman JG, Limbird LE, Goodman Gilman A, eds. *Goodman & Gilman's the Pharmacological Basis of Therapeutics.* 10th ed. New York: McGraw-Hill; 2001:549.

Tandon R, DeQuardo JR, Goodson J, Mann NA, Greden JF. Effect of anticholinergics on positive and negative symptoms in schizophrenia. *Psychopharmacol Bull.* 1992;28:297.

Tune LE. Anticholinergic effects of medication in elderly patients. *J Clin Psychiatry.* 2001;62:11.

Tune LE, Strauss ME, Lew MF, Breitlinger E, Coyle JT. Serum levels of anticholinergic drugs and impaired recent memory in chronic schizophrenic patients. *Am J Psychiatry.* 1982;139:1460.

Vitiello B, Martin A, Hill J, et al. Cognitive and behavioral effects of cholinergic, dopaminergic, and serotonergic blockade in humans. *Neuropsychopharmacology.* 1997;16:15.

World Health Organization. Prophylactic use of anticholinergics in patients on long-term neuroleptic treatment. *Br J Psychiatry.* 1990;156:412.

▲ 36.4.5 Antihistamines

Certain antihistamines (antagonists of histamine H_1 receptors) are used in clinical psychiatry to treat neuroleptic-induced parkinsonism and neuroleptic-induced acute dystonia and also as hypnotics and anxiolytics. Diphenhydramine (Benadryl) is used to treat neuroleptic-induced parkinsonism and neuroleptic-induced acute dystonia and sometimes as a hypnotic. Hydroxyzine hydrochloride (Atarax) and hydroxyzine pamoate (Vistaril) are used as anxiolytics. Promethazine (Phenergan) is used for its sedative and anxiolytic effects. Cyproheptadine (Periactin) has been used for the treatment of anorexia nervosa and inhibited male and female orgasm caused by serotonergic agents.

Table 36.4.5–1
Other Antihistamines with Relevance to Psychiatry

Class	Generic Name	Brand Name	Comments
H_2 receptor antagonist	Cimetidine Ranitidine Famotidine Nizatidine	Tagamet Zantac Pepcid Axid	Widely prescribed for treatment of ulcers and gastroesophageal reflux. All have the potential for CNS toxicities, including psychosis and delirium
Second-generation (nonsedating) H_1 receptor antagonists	Loratadine Cetirizine Fexofenadine	Claritin Zyrtec Allegra	No apparent cardiotoxicity, but increased levels can occur when administered with CYP 3A4 inhibitors

So-called second-generation H_1 receptor antagonists fexofenadine (Allegra), loratadine (Claritin), and cetirizine (Zyrtec) are not used in psychiatry. Terfenadine (Seldane) and astemizole (Hismanal) were available in the 1990s but were withdrawn from commercial availability because they were associated with serious cardiac arrhythmias when coadministered with some drugs (e.g., nefazodone [Serzone], selective serotonin reuptake inhibitors [SSRIs]); these drugs can cause serious and life-threatening cardiac toxicity.

Table 36.4.5–1 lists antihistaminic drugs used for nonpsychiatric disorders (e.g., gastric reflux), which may have psychiatric adverse effects or drug–drug interactions.

CHEMISTRY

The molecular structures of representative first-generation antihistamines used in psychiatry are shown in Figure 36.4.5–1.

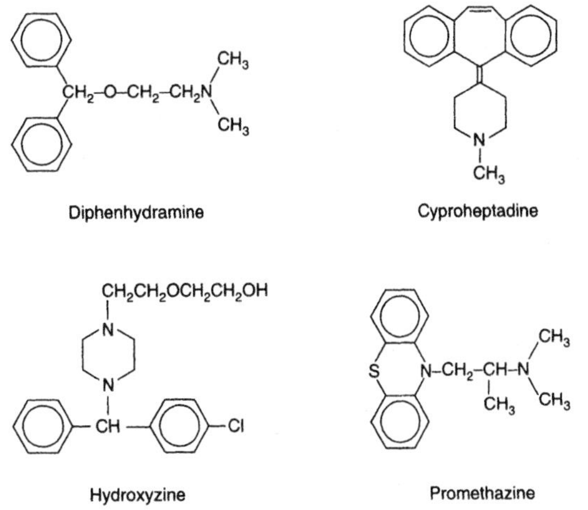

FIGURE 36.4.5–1
Molecular structures of antihistamines used in psychiatry.

PHARMACOLOGICAL ACTIONS

The H_1 antagonists used in psychiatry are well absorbed from the gastrointestinal (GI) tract. The antiparkinsonian effects of intramuscular (IM) diphenhydramine have their onset in 15 to 30 minutes, and the sedative effects of diphenhydramine peak in 1 to 3 hours. The sedative effects of hydroxyzine and promethazine begin after 20 to 60 minutes and last for 4 to 6 hours. Because all three drugs are metabolized in the liver, persons with hepatic disease, such as cirrhosis, may attain high plasma concentrations with long-term administration. Cyproheptadine is well absorbed after oral administration, and its metabolites are excreted in the urine.

Activation of H_1 receptors stimulates wakefulness; therefore, receptor antagonism causes sedation. All four agents also possess some antimuscarinic cholinergic activity. Cyproheptadine is unique among the drugs, since it has both potent antihistamine and serotonin 5-HT_2 receptor antagonist properties.

EFFECTS ON SPECIFIC ORGANS AND SYSTEMS

The effects of the antihistamines on the central nervous system (CNS) include sedation and antagonism of dopamine D_2 receptor blockade–induced movement disorders. The antihistamines may also reduce the symptoms of motion sickness in some patients. Peripherally, histamine triggers capillary permeability and stimulates the release of mediators of inflammation.

THERAPEUTIC INDICATIONS

Antihistamines are useful as a treatment for neuroleptic-induced parkinsonism, neuroleptic-induced acute dystonia, and neuroleptic-induced akathisia. They are an alternative to anticholinergics and amantadine for these purposes. The antihistamines are relatively safe hypnotics, but they are not superior to the benzodiazepines, which have been much better studied in terms of efficacy and safety. The antihistamines have not been proved effective for long-term anxiolytic therapy; therefore, either the benzodiazepines, buspirone (BuSpar), or SSRIs are preferable for such treatment. Cyproheptadine is sometimes used to treat impaired orgasms, especially delayed orgasm resulting from treatment with serotonergic drugs.

Because it promotes weight gain, cyproheptadine may be of some use in the treatment of eating disorders, such as anorexia nervosa. Cyproheptadine can reduce recurrent nightmares with posttraumatic themes. The antiserotonergic activity of cyproheptadine may counteract the serotonin syndrome caused by concomitant use of multiple serotonin-activating drugs, such as SSRIs and monoamine oxidase inhibitors.

PRECAUTIONS AND ADVERSE REACTIONS

Antihistamines are commonly associated with sedation, dizziness, and hypotension, all of which can be severe in elderly persons, who are also likely to suffer from the anticholinergic effects of those drugs. Paradoxical excitement and agitation are adverse effects seen in a small number of persons. Poor motor coordination can result in accidents; therefore, persons should be warned about driving and operating machinery. Other common adverse effects include epigastric distress, nausea, vomiting, diarrhea, and constipation. Because of mild anticholinergic activity, some persons experience dry mouth, urinary retention, blurred vision, and constipation. For this reason also, antihistamines should be used only at very low doses, if at all, by persons with narrow-angle glaucoma or obstructive GI, prostate, or bladder conditions. A central anticholinergic syndrome with psychosis may be induced by either cyproheptadine or diphenhydramine. The use of cyproheptadine in some persons has been associated with weight gain, which may contribute to its reported efficacy in some persons with anorexia nervosa.

In addition to the above adverse effects, antihistamines have some potential for abuse. The coadministration of antihistamines and opioids can increase the euphoria experienced by persons with substance dependence. Overdoses of antihistamines can be fatal. Antihistamines are excreted in breast milk, so their use should be avoided by nursing mothers. Because of some potential for teratogenicity, pregnant women should also avoid use of antihistamines.

DRUG–DRUG INTERACTIONS

The sedative property of antihistamines can be additive with that of other CNS depressants, such as alcohol, other sedative-hypnotic drugs, and many psychotropic drugs, including tricyclic drugs and dopamine receptor antagonists. The anticholinergic activity can also be additive with that of other anticholinergic drugs and can sometimes result in severe anticholinergic symptoms or intoxication. The beneficial effects of SSRIs can be antagonized by cyproheptadine.

LABORATORY INTERFERENCES

H_1 antagonists may eliminate the wheal and induration that form the basis of allergy skin tests. Promethazine may interfere with pregnancy tests and may increase blood glucose concentrations. Diphenhydramine may yield a false-positive urine test result for phencyclidine (PCP). Hydroxyzine use can falsely elevate the results of certain tests for urinary 17-hydroxycorticosteroids.

DOSAGE AND CLINICAL GUIDELINES

The antihistamines are available in a variety of preparations (Table 36.4.5–2). IM injections should be deep, since superficial administration can cause local irritation.

Intravenous (IV) administration of 25 to 50 mg of diphenhydramine is an effective treatment for neuroleptic-induced acute dystonia, which may immediately disappear. Treatment with 25 mg three times a day—up to 50 mg four times a day if necessary—can be used for neuroleptic-induced parkinsonism, akinesia, and buccal movements. Diphenhydramine can be used as a hypnotic at a 50-mg dose for mild transient insomnia. Doses of 100 mg have not been shown to be superior to doses of 50 mg, but they produce more anticholinergic effects than doses of 50 mg.

Hydroxyzine is most commonly used as a short-term anxiolytic. Hydroxyzine should not be given IV, since it is irritating to the blood vessels. Dosages of 50 to 100 mg given orally four

Table 36.4.5–2
Dosage and Administration of Traditional Antihistamines Used in Psychiatry

Drugs	Route	Preparation	Dosage
Diphenhydramine (Benadryl)	po	Capsules and tablets: 25 mg, 50 mg elixir and syrup: 12.5 mg/5 mL	Adults: 25–50 mg 3–4 times daily Usual sleep-aid dose: 50 mg hs Children: 5 mg/kg/24 h in 4 divided doses, not to exceed 300 mg/day
	IM (deep)	Solution: 10 mg/mL, 50 mg/mL	Adults: 10–50 mg IV or deep IM may use 100 mg if required, maximum daily dose 400 mg: for dystonic reactions, 50 mg IV over 2–3 min Children: 5 mg/kg/24 h (maximum 300 mg/day)
Hydroxyzine (Atarax, Vistaril)	po	Hydrochloride syrup: 10 mg/5 mL Tablets: 10 mg, 25 mg, 50 mg, 100 mg Pamoate suspension: 25 mg/5 mL Capsules: 25 mg, 50 mg, 100 mg	Adults: 25–100 mg qid Children: under 6: 50 mg/24 h in 3–4 divided doses over 6: 50–100 mg/day in 3–4 divided doses
	IM	Hydrochloride solution: 25 mg/mL, 50 mg/mL	Adults: 50–100 mg q4–6h prn for sedation Children: 0.5 mg/lb of body weight
Promethazine (Phenergan)	po	Syrup: 6.25 mg/5 mL, 25 mg/5 mL Tablets: 12.5 mg, 25 mg, 50 mg	Adults: 25–50 mg for sedation Children: 12.5–25 mg hs for nighttime and preoperative sedation
	pr	Suppositories: 50 mg, 25 mg, 12.5 mg	
	IM	Solution: 25 mg/mL and 50 mg/mL	
Cyproheptadine (Periactin)	po	Tablets: 4 mg Syrup: 2 mg/5 mL	Adult: usually 4–20 mg/day (may require up to 32 mg/day) for allergies, not to exceed 0.5 mg/kg/day: for antidepressant-induced anorgasmia: 4–16 mg, either in divided daily doses or approximately 1–2 h prior to coitus Children: for allergies, approximately 0.25 mg/kg/day 2–6 yr old: 2 mg po 2–3 times daily; maximum 12 mg/day 7–14 yr old: 4 mg po 2–3 times daily; maximum 16 mg/day

times a day for long-term treatment or 50 to 100 mg IM every 4 to 6 hours for short-term treatment are usually effective.

SSRI-induced anorgasmia may sometimes be reversed with 4 to 16 mg a day of cyproheptadine taken by mouth 1 or 2 hours before anticipated sexual activity. A number of case reports have reported that cyproheptadine may be of some use in the treatment of eating disorders, such as anorexia nervosa. Cyproheptadine is available in 4-mg tablets and a 2 mg/5 mL solution. Children and elderly patients are more sensitive to the effects of antihistamines than are young adults.

References

Aizenberg D, Zemishlany Z, Weizman A. Cyproheptadine treatment of sexual dysfunction induced by serotonin reuptake inhibitors. *Clin Neuropharmacol.* 1995;18:320.

Ashton AK, Weinstein WL. Cyproheptadine for drug-induced sweating. *Am J Psychiatry.* 2002;159:874.

De Nesnera AP. Diphenhydramine dependence: a need for awareness [letter]. *J Clin Psychiatry.* 1996;57:136.

Halpert AG, Olmstead MC, Beninger RJ. Mechanisms and abuse liability of the anti-histamine dimenhydrinate. *Neurosci Biobehav Rev.* 2002;26:61.

Hardman JG, Limbird LE, Goodman Gilman A, eds. *Goodman & Gilman's the Pharmacological Basis of Therapeutics.* 10th ed. New York: McGraw-Hill; 2001.

Labbate LA, Arana GW, Ballenger JC. Antihistamines. In: Sadock BJ, Sadock VA, eds. *Kaplan & Sadock's Comprehensive Textbook of Psychiatry.* 7th ed. Vol 2. Baltimore: Lippincott Williams & Wilkins; 2000:2304.

Nemeroff CB, DeVane CL, Pollock BG. Newer antidepressants and the cytochrome P450 system. *Am J Psychiatry.* 1996;153:311.

Ninn PT, Cole JO, Yonkers KA. Nonbenzodiazepine anxiolytics. In: Schatzberg AF, Nemeroff CB, eds. *Essentials of Clinical Psychopharmacology.* Washington, DC: American Psychiatric Association; 2001:93.

Qidwai JC, Watson GS, Weiler JM. Sedation, cognition, and antihistamines. *Curr Allergy Asthma Rep.* 2002;2:216.

Shamsi Z, Hindmarch I. Sedation and antihistamines: a review of inter-drug differences using proportional impairment ratios. *Hum Psychopharmacol Clin Exp.* 2000;15(suppl 1):S3.

Weiss D, Aizenberg D, Hermesh H, et al. Cyproheptadine treatment in neuroleptic-induced akathisia. *Br J Psychiatry.* 1995;167:483.

Yap YG, Camm AJ. The current cardiac safety situation with antihistamines. *Clin Exp Allergy.* 1999;29:15.

▲ 36.4.6 Barbiturates and Similarly Acting Drugs

The use of barbiturates and similar compounds such as meprobamate (Miltown) has been practically eliminated by the benzodiazepines, other anxiolytics such as buspirone (BuSpar), and the hypnotics zolpidem (Ambien) and zaleplon (Sonata). The newer agents have a lower abuse potential and a higher therapeutic index than the barbiturates; nevertheless, the barbiturates and similarly acting drugs still have a role in the treatment of certain mental disorders.

BARBITURATES

Chemistry

The various clinically available barbiturates are derived from the same barbituric acid substrate and differ primarily in their substitutions at the C5 position of the parent molecule (Fig. 36.4.6–1). These C5 molecular substitutions are the primary basis for the differing lipid solubilities and half-lives of the various resulting molecules.

General Formula:

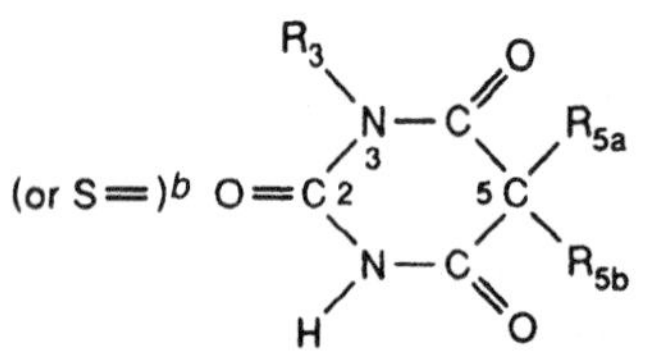

Barbiturate	R_{5a}	R_{5b}
Amobarbital	Ethyl	Isopentyl
Aprobarbital	Allyl	Isopropyl
Butabarbital	Ethyl	*Sec*-Butyl
Butalbital	Allyl	Isobutyl
Mephobarbital[a]	Ethyl	Phenyl
Methohexital[a]	Allyl	1-Methyl-2-Pentynyl
Pentobarbital	Ethyl	1-Methylbutyl
Phenobarbital	Ethyl	Phenyl
Secobarbital	Allyl	1-Methylbutyl
Thiamylal[b]	Allyl	1-Methylbutyl
Thiopental[b]	Ethyl	1-Methylbutyl

[a] R_3 = H_1 except in mephobarbital and methohexital, where it is replaced by CH_3.
[b] O, except in thiamylal and thiopental, where it is replaced by S.

FIGURE 36.4.6–1

Molecular structures and names of barbiturates available in the United States. (From Rall TW. Hypnotics and sedatives: ethanol. In: Goodman A, Gilman AG, Rall TW, et al., eds. *Goodman and Gilman's The Pharmacological Basis of Therapeutics.* 8th ed. New York: McGraw-Hill; 1990:752, with permission.)

PHARMACOLOGICAL ACTIONS

The barbiturates are well absorbed after oral administration. The binding of barbiturates to plasma proteins is high, but lipid solubility varies. The individual barbiturates are metabolized by the liver and excreted by the kidneys. The half-lives of specific barbiturates range from 1 to 120 hours. The mechanism of action of barbiturates involves the γ-aminobutyric acid (GABA) receptor–benzodiazepine receptor–chloride ion channel complex.

Effects on Specific Organs and Systems

The barbiturates have their major effects on the central nervous system (CNS), although significant effects also occur in the liver and can occur in the cardiovascular system. In the CNS, barbiturates are associated with the inhibition of the reticular activating system. Respiratory depression can arise, which can be additive to that of other respiratory depressants (e.g., alcohol). In the liver, barbiturate use can double the induction of metabolic liver enzymes and thus lower the plasma levels of both the barbiturates and other drugs metabolized in the liver. Although at low dosages barbiturates have a relatively safe cardiovascular profile, at high dosages they may impair cardiac contractility or evoke cardiac arrhythmias. Barbiturate administration rarely causes potentially fatal laryngospasm, a potential adverse event that may guide clinicians to use benzodiazepines, rather than barbiturates, in most situations (e.g., drug-assisted interviewing).

THERAPEUTIC INDICATIONS

Electroconvulsive Therapy

Methohexital (Brevital) is commonly used as an anesthetic agent for electroconvulsive therapy (ECT). It carries lower cardiac risks than other barbiturate anesthetics. Used intravenously, methohexital produces rapid unconsciousness and because of rapid redistribution has a brief duration of action (5 to 7 minutes). Typical dosing for ECT is 0.7 to 1.2 mg/kg. Methohexital may also be used to abort prolonged seizures in ECT or to limit postictal agitation.

Seizures

Phenobarbital (Solfoton, Luminal), the most commonly used barbiturate for treatment of seizures, has indications for the treatment of generalized tonic-clonic and simple partial seizures. Parenteral barbiturates are used in the emergency management of seizures independent of cause. Intravenous phenobarbital should be administered slowly, 10 to 20 mg/kg, for status epilepticus.

Narcoanalysis

Amobarbital (Amytal) has been used historically as a diagnostic aid in a number of clinical conditions, including conversion reactions, catatonia, hysterical stupor, and unexplained muteness, and to differentiate stupor of depression, schizophrenia, and structural brain lesions.

The "Amytal interview" is performed by placing the patient in a reclining position and administering amobarbital intravenously, 50 mg a minute. Infusion is continued until lateral nystagmus is sustained or drowsiness is noted, usually at 75 to 150 mg. Following this, 25 to 50 mg may be administered every 5 minutes to maintain narcosis. The patient should rest for 15 to 30 minutes after the interview before attempting to walk.

Sleep

The barbiturates reduce sleep latency and the number of awakenings during sleep, though tolerance to these effects generally develops within 2 weeks. Discontinuation of barbiturates often leads to rebound increases on electroencephalogram (EEG) measures of sleep and worsening of the insomnia.

Withdrawal from Sedative Hypnotics

Barbiturates are sometimes used to determine the extent of tolerance to barbiturates or other hypnotics to guide detoxification. Once intoxication has resolved, a test dose of pentobarbital (200 mg) is given orally. An hour later the patient is examined. Tolerance and dose requirements are determined by the extent to which the patient is affected. If the patient is not sedated, another 100 mg of pentobarbital may be administered every 2 hours, up to three times (maximum, 500 mg over 6 hours). The amount needed for mild intoxication corresponds to the approximate daily dose of barbiturate used. Phenobarbital (30 mg) may then be substituted for each 100 mg of pentobarbital. This daily dose requirement may be administered in divided doses and gradually tapered by 10 percent a day, with adjustments made according to withdrawal signs (Table 36.4.6–1).

Table 36.4.6–1
Pentobarbital Challenge Test

1. Give pentobarbital 200 mg orally.
2. Observe for intoxication after 1 h (e.g., sleepiness, slurred speech, or nystagmus).
3. If patient is not intoxicated, give another 100 mg of pentobarbital every 2 h (maximum 500 mg over 6 h).
4. Total dose given to produce mild intoxication is equivalent to daily abuse level of barbiturates.
5. Substitute phenobarbital 30 mg (longer half-life) for each 100 mg of pentobarbital.
6. Reduce dosage by about 10 percent a day.
7. Adjust rate if signs of intoxication or withdrawal are present.

PRECAUTIONS AND ADVERSE REACTIONS

Some adverse effects of barbiturates are similar to those of benzodiazepines, including paradoxical dysphoria, hyperactivity, and cognitive disorganization. Rare adverse effects associated with barbiturate use include the development of Stevens-Johnson syndrome, megaloblastic anemia, and neutropenia.

A major difference between the barbiturates and the benzodiazepines is the low therapeutic index of the barbiturates. An overdose of barbiturates can easily prove fatal. In addition to narrow therapeutic indexes, the barbiturates are associated with a significant risk of abuse potential and the development of tolerance and dependence. Barbiturate intoxication is manifested by confusion, drowsiness, irritability, hyporeflexia or areflexia, ataxia, and nystagmus. The symptoms of barbiturate withdrawal are similar to, but more marked than, those of benzodiazepine withdrawal.

Because of some evidence of teratogenicity, barbiturates should not be used by pregnant women or women who are breast-feeding. Barbiturates should be used with caution by patients with a history of substance abuse, depression, diabetes, hepatic impairment, renal disease, severe anemia, pain, hyperthyroidism, or hypoadrenalism. Barbiturates are also contraindicated in patients with acute intermittent porphyria, impaired respiratory drive, or limited respiratory reserve.

DRUG–DRUG INTERACTIONS

The primary area for concern about drug interactions is the potentially additive effects of respiratory depression. Barbiturates should be used with great caution with other prescribed CNS drugs (including antipsychotic and antidepressant drugs) and nonprescribed CNS agents (e.g., alcohol). Caution must also be exercised when prescribing barbiturates to patients who are taking other drugs that are metabolized in the liver, especially cardiac drugs and anticonvulsants. Because individual patients have a wide range of sensitivities to barbiturate-induced enzyme induction, one cannot predict how much the metabolism of concurrently administered medications will be affected. Drugs that may have their metabolism enhanced by barbiturate administration include opioids, antiarrhythmic agents, antibiotics, anticoagulants, anticonvulsants, antidepressants, β-adrenergic receptor antagonists, dopamine receptor antagonists, contraceptives, and immunosuppressants (Table 36.4.6–2).

Table 36.4.6–2
Drug Interactions

The metabolism of the following drugs is reportedly increased with long-term use of barbiturates. Others unlisted may also be affected.

Analgesics—acetaminophen, fenoprofen
Antiarrhythmics—digitalis, lidocaine, mexiletine
Antibiotics—chloramphenicol, metronidazole, rifampin, tetracycline, griseofulvin
Anticoagulants—warfarin
Anticonvulsants—carbamazepine, phenytoin
Antidepressants—amitriptyline, desipramine, paroxetine, protriptyline
Antihypertensives—methyldopa
Antipsychotics—haloperidol, thioridazine, loxapine
β-Adrenergic receptor antagonists—labetalol, propranolol, metoprolol
Benzodiazepines—clonazepam, diazepam
Contraceptives—all containing estrogens
Immunosuppressants—corticosteroids, cyclophosphamide, cyclosporine, dacarbazine
Xanthines—aminophylline, caffeine, theophylline

LABORATORY INTERFERENCES

No known laboratory interferences are associated with the administration of barbiturates.

DOSAGE AND CLINICAL GUIDELINES

Barbiturates and other drugs described below begin to act within 1 to 2 hours of administration. The dosages of barbiturates vary (Table 36.4.6–3), and treatment should begin with low dosages that are increased to achieve a clinical effect. Children and older persons are more sensitive to the effects of barbiturates than young adults. The most commonly used barbiturates are available in a variety of dose forms. Barbiturates with half-lives in the 15- to 40-hour range are preferable, because long-acting drugs tend to accumulate in the body. Clinicians should instruct patients clearly about the adverse effects and the potential for dependence associated with barbiturates.

Although determining plasma concentrations of barbiturates is rarely necessary in psychiatry, monitoring phenobarbital concentrations is standard practice when the drug is used as an anticonvulsant. The therapeutic blood concentrations for phenobarbital in this indication range from 15 to 40 mg/L, although some patients may experience significant adverse effects in that range.

Barbiturates are contained in combination products with which the clinician should be familiar (Table 36.4.6–4).

OTHER SIMILARLY ACTING DRUGS

A number of agents that act similarly to the barbiturates are used in the treatment of anxiety and insomnia. Four such available drugs are paraldehyde (Paral), ethchlorvynol (Placidyl), meprobamate, and glutethimide (Doriden). These drugs are

Table 36.4.6–3
Barbiturate Dosages

Drug	Selected Preparations[a]	Daily Dosage Range[b] (Sedative[c]/Hypnotic)	Anticonvulsant	Pediatric
Amobarbital	30, 200 mg	100–200 mg[c]/50–300 mg	65–500 mg (IV)	2–6 mg/kg up to 100 mg
Aprobarbital	40 mg/5 mL (e)	40–160 mg[c]/40–120 mg	Not established	Not established
Butabarbital	30 mg/5 mL (e) 15, 30, 50, 100 mg	45–120 mg[c]/50–100 mg	Not established	2–6 mg/kg (max 100 mg)
Mephobarbital	32, 50, 100 mg	66–300 mg[c]/100 mg	200–600 mg	16–32 mg three to four times daily (≤ age 5) 32–64 mg three to four times daily (> age 5)
Methohexital	500 mg/50 mL (I)	0.7–1.2 mg/kg for ECT	Not established	Not established
Pentobarbital	50, 100 mg 50 mg/mL (I) 20 mg/mL (e) 30, 60, 120, 200 mg (r)	60–100 mg[c]/100–150 mg	100 mg IV at 1-min intervals up to 500 mg	2–6 mg/kg up to 100 mg
Phenobarbital	8, 15, 30, 60, 100 mg 30, 60, 65, 130 mg/mL (I) 20 mg/5 mL (e)	30–120 mg[c]/100–300 mg	100–300 mg IV up to 600 mg/day 60–250 mg/day oral	1–3 mg/kg
Secobarbital	100 mg 50 mg/mL (I)	100–300 mg[c]/100 mg	5.5 mg/kg intravenous, may repeat every 3–4 hours	3–5 mg/kg

[a]Other preparations are available.
[b]Dosages are oral form (tablets or capsules) unless specified: I, injection; r, rectal suppository.
[c]Sedative dosage is equal to the hypnotic dosage, but should be split 3 to 4 times daily.

rarely used because of their abuse potential and potentially toxic effects.

Paraldehyde

Paraldehyde is a cyclic ether, first used in 1882 as a hypnotic. It has also been used to treat epilepsy, alcohol withdrawal symptoms, and delirium tremens. Because of its low therapeutic index it has been supplanted by the benzodiazepines and other anticonvulsants.

Chemistry. The molecular structure of paraldehyde is shown in Figure 36.4.6–2.

Pharmacological Actions. Paraldehyde is rapidly absorbed from the gastrointestinal (GI) tract and from intramuscular injections. It is primarily metabolized to acetaldehyde by the liver, and unmetabolized drug is expired by the lungs. Reported half-lives range from 3.4 to 9.8 hours. Onset of action is 15 to 30 minutes.

Therapeutic Indications. Paraldehyde is not indicated as an anxiolytic or hypnotic and has little place in current psychopharmacology.

Precautions and Adverse Reactions. Paraldehyde frequently causes foul breath because of expired unmetabolized drug. It may inflame pulmonary capillaries and cause coughing. It may also cause local thrombophlebitis with intravenous use. Patients may experience nausea and vomiting with oral use. Overdose leads to metabolic acidosis and decreased renal output. There is risk of abuse among drug addicts.

Drug Interactions. Disulfiram (Antabuse) inhibits acetaldehyde dehydrogenase and reduces metabolism of paraldehyde, leading to a possibly toxic concentration of paraldehyde. Paral-

Table 36.4.6–4
Barbiturates Contained in Combination Products

Product Name	Barbiturate	Other Content
Floricet with Codeine	Butalbital, 50 mg	Caffeine, 40 mg; codeine, 30 mg; acetaminophen, 325 mg
Florinal with Codeine	Butalbital, 50 mg	Caffeine, 40 mg; codeine, 30 mg; aspirin, 325 mg
Cafatine-PB	Phenobarbital, 30 mg	Caffeine, 100 mg; ergotamine tartrate, 1 mg; alkaloid of belladonna, 0.125 mg
Barbidonna	Phenobarbital, 32 mg	Atropine sulfate, 0.025 mg; scopolamine, 0.0074 mg; hyoscyamine, 0.1286 mg
Butibel	Butabarbital, 15 mg	Belladonna extract, 15 mg
Donnatal Extentabs	Phenobarbital, 48.6 mg	Atropine sulfate, 0.0582 mg; scopolamine, 0.0195 mg; hyoscyamine, 0.311 mg
Phenerbel-S	Phenobarbital, 40 mg	Alkaloid of belladonna, 0.2 mg; ergotamine tartrate, 0.6 mg

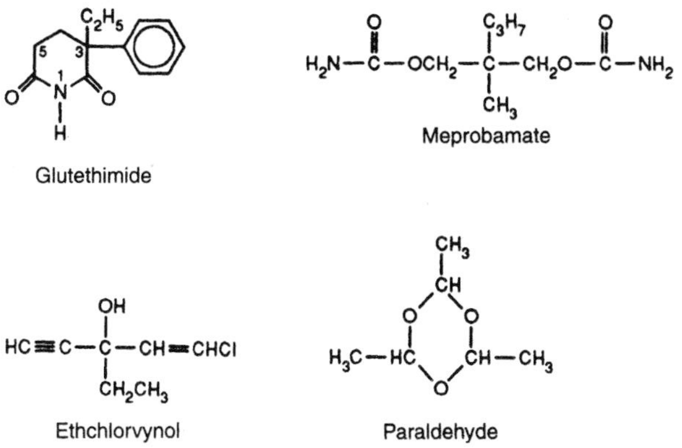

FIGURE 36.4.6–2
Molecular structures of similarly acting drugs.

dehyde has addictive sedating effects in combination with other CNS depressants such as alcohol or benzodiazepines.

Laboratory Interferences. Paraldehyde may interfere with phentolamine or urinary 17-hydroxycorticosteroid tests.

Dosage and Clinical Guidelines. Paraldehyde is available in 30-mL vials for oral, intravenous, or rectal use. For seizures in adults, up to 12 mL (diluted to a 10 percent solution) may be administered by gastric tube every 4 hours. For children the oral dose is 0.3 mg/kg.

Meprobamate

Meprobamate, a carbamate, was introduced shortly before the benzodiazepines, specifically to treat anxiety. It is also used for muscle relaxant effects.

Chemistry. The molecular structure of meprobamate is shown in Figure 36.4.6–2.

Pharmacological Actions. Meprobamate is rapidly absorbed from the GI tract and from intramuscular injections. It is primarily metabolized by the liver, and a small portion is excreted unchanged in urine. The plasma half-life is approximately 10 hours.

Therapeutic Indications. Meprobamate is indicated for short-term treatment of anxiety disorders. It has also been used as a hypnotic and is prescribed as a muscle relaxant.

Precautions and Adverse Reactions. Meprobamate may cause CNS depression and death in overdose and carries the risk of abuse by patients with drug or alcohol dependence. Abrupt cessation following long-term use may lead to a withdrawal syndrome including seizures and hallucinations. Meprobamate may exacerbate acute intermittent porphyria. Other rare side effects include hypersensitivity reactions, wheezing, hives, paradoxical excitement, and leukopenia. It should not be given to patients with hepatic damage.

Drug Interactions. Meprobamate has additive sedating effects in combination with other CNS depressants such as alcohol, barbiturates, or benzodiazepines.

Laboratory Interferences. Meprobamate may interfere with phentolamine or urinary 17-hydroxycorticosteroid tests.

Dosage and Clinical Guidelines. Meprobamate is available in 200-, 400-, and 600-mg tablets, 200- and 400-mg extended-release capsules, and various combinations (e.g., aspirin, 325 mg, and 200 mg of meprobamate [Equagesic] for oral use). For adults, the usual dosage is 400 to 800 mg twice daily. Elderly patients and children age 6 to 12 require half the adult dose.

Ethchlorvynol

Ethchlorvynol, a tertiary carbinol, was marketed to treat insomnia and anxiety. It has been replaced by the benzodiazepines and other safer agents in the treatment of anxiety and sleep disturbance. It has a low therapeutic index.

Chemistry. The molecular structure of ethchlorvynol is shown in Figure 36.4.6–2.

Pharmacological Action. Ethchlorvynol is rapidly absorbed from the GI tract. It is primarily metabolized by the liver, and a small portion is metabolized by the kidney. Metabolites are excreted in the urine. Elimination half-life is approximately 10 to 20 hours.

Therapeutic Indications. Ethchlorvynol is indicated for up to 1-week treatment of insomnia.

Precautions and Adverse Reactions. Ethchlorvynol may cause CNS depression, slurred speech, double vision, confusion, and death in overdose. There is risk of abuse by patients with drug or alcohol dependence. Abrupt cessation following long-term use may lead to a withdrawal syndrome including seizures and hallucinations. Ethchlorvynol may exacerbate acute intermittent porphyria or cause cholestatic jaundice. Hypersensitivity reactions are uncommon. Paradoxical excitement is rare. It should not be given to patients with hepatic compromise.

Drug Interactions. In combination with other CNS drugs including tricyclic drugs, alcohol, barbiturates or benzodiazepines, ethchlorvynol has additive sedating effects. Ethchlorvynol stimulates hepatic microenzymes and may increase metabolism of many drugs, most notably warfarin (Coumadin).

Laboratory Interferences. Ethchlorvynol may cause a false-positive phentolamine test result.

Dosage and Clinical Guidelines. Ethchlorvynol is available in 200-, 500-, and 750-mg capsules. For adults, the usual dose is 500 to 750 mg at bedtime. It is best taken with food to limit rate of onset for patients in whom ataxia is of concern. Patients requiring withdrawal should be switched to a barbi-

turate such as phenobarbital and gradually tapered. Safety and efficacy in children or elderly patients have not been established.

Glutethimide

Chemistry. The molecular structure of glutethimide is shown in Figure 36.4.6–2.

Pharmacological Action. Glutethimide is absorbed erratically from the GI tract, is metabolized by the liver, and has an onset of action of 30 minutes. Its elimination half-life is 10 to 12 hours, and it is known to induce hepatic microsomal enzymes. It has potent anticholinergic activity.

Therapeutic Indications. Glutethimide has been used to treat insomnia.

Precautions and Adverse Reactions. Glutethimide may cause CNS depression, slurred speech, double vision, confusion, and death in overdose. There is a risk of abuse by patients with drug or alcohol dependence. Abrupt cessation following long-term use may lead to a withdrawal syndrome including seizures and hallucinations. Glutethimide may exacerbate acute intermittent porphyria. Because of its potent anticholinergic effects it should be used cautiously in patients with prostatic hypertrophy or narrow-angle glaucoma. Hypersensitivity reactions are uncommon. Paradoxical excitement is rare. It should not be given to patients with hepatic damage.

Drug Interactions. Glutethimide has additive sedating effects in combination with other CNS drugs including alcohol, barbiturates, and benzodiazepines. Glutethimide induces hepatic microenzymes and may increase metabolism of many drugs, most notably warfarin.

Laboratory Interferences. Glutethimide may cause a false-positive phentolamine test result or interfere with urine assays for 17-ketosteroids.

Dosage and Clinical Guidelines. Glutethimide is available in 500-mg tablets. For adults, the usual dose for insomnia is 250 to 500 mg at bedtime. For elderly patients the recommended dose is 250 mg. Safety and efficacy in children have not been established. Patients requiring withdrawal should be switched to a barbiturate such as phenobarbital and gradually tapered.

References

Hardman JG, Limbird LE, Goodman Gilman A, eds. *Goodman & Gilman's the Pharmacological Basis of Therapeutics.* 10th ed. New York: McGraw-Hill; 2001.

Kavirajan H. The amobarbital interview revisited: a review of the literature since 1966. *Harvard Rev Psychiatry.* 1999;7:153.

Labbate LA, Arana GW, Ballenger JC. Barbiturates and similarly acting substances. In: Sadock BJ, Sadock VA, eds. *Kaplan & Sadock's Comprehensive Textbook of Psychiatry.* 7th ed. Vol 2. Baltimore: Lippincott Williams & Wilkins; 2000:2309.

Macdonald RL, Kelly KM. Antiepileptic drug mechanisms of action. *Epilepsia.* 1995;36(suppl):S2.

Matthew H. Barbiturates. *Clin Toxicol.* 1975;8:495.

McNutt LA, Coles FB, McAuliffe T, et al. Impact of regulation on benzodiazepine prescribing to a low income elderly population, New York State. *J Clin Epidemiol.* 1994;47:613.

Miller LG. Herbal medicinals: selected clinical considerations focusing on known or potential drug-herb interactions. *Arch Intern Med.* 1998;158:2200.

Reinisch JM, Sanders SA, Mortensen EL, Rubin DB. In utero exposure to phenobarbital and intelligence deficits in adult men. *JAMA.* 1995;274:1518.

Roberts I, Schierhout G, Alderson P. Absence of evidence for the effectiveness of five interventions routinely used in the intensive care management of severe head injury: a systematic review. *J Neurol Neurosurg Psychiatry.* 1998;65:729.

Swanson RA, Seid LL. Barbiturates impair astrocyte glutamate uptake. *Glia.* 1998;24:365.

Tietjen CS, Hurn PD, Ulatowski JA, Kirsch JR. Treatment modalities for hypertensive patients with intracranial pathology: options and risks. *Crit Care Med.* 1996;24:311.

United States Pharmacopeial Convention. Barbiturates. In: *United States Pharmacopeial Dispensing Information—Drug Information for the Health Care Professional.* 19th ed. Rockville, MD: United States Pharmacopeial Convention; 1999.

▲ 36.4.7 Benzodiazepines

This section covers three areas: (1) the benzodiazepines, a group of compounds that enhance the activity of the $GABA_A$ receptor by binding to the benzodiazepine receptor site; (2) zolpidem (Ambien) and zaleplon (Sonata), benzodiazepine agonists at the type 2 benzodiazepine receptor (BZ_2) site; and (3) flumazenil (Romazicon), a benzodiazepine receptor antagonist. The benzodiazepine receptor agonists are primarily indicated for treating anxiety and insomnia; flumazenil is primarily indicated for treating benzodiazepine overdose.

Benzodiazepines are sometimes classified as sedative-hypnotics, although other drugs can also be classified in this group (e.g., barbiturates). A sedative drug reduces daytime anxiety, tempers excessive excitement, and generally quiets or calms persons. One distinction sometimes drawn between sedatives and anxiolytics is that sedatives treat less pathological conditions than anxiolytics, but this poorly defined distinction should be avoided. A hypnotic drug produces drowsiness and facilitates the onset and maintenance of sleep. In general, benzodiazepines act as hypnotics in high doses and as anxiolytics or sedatives in low doses.

Benzodiazepines are the drugs of choice for management of acute anxiety and agitation. Because of the risk of psychological dependence, long-term use of benzodiazepines should be carefully monitored.

CHEMISTRY

The structural formulas of the benzodiazepines are shown in Figure 36.4.7–1. The formulas for zolpidem and zaleplon are shown in Figure 36.4.7–2, and the formula for flumazenil, in Figure 36.4.7–3.

PHARMACOLOGICAL ACTIONS

With the exception of clorazepate (Tranxene), all the benzodiazepines are completely absorbed unchanged from the gastrointestinal (GI) tract. The absorption, the attainment of peak concentrations, and the onset of action are quickest for diazepam (Valium), lorazepam (Ativan), alprazolam (Xanax), triazolam (Halcion), and estazolam (ProSom). The rapid onset of effects is important to persons who take a single dose of a benzodiazepine to calm an episodic burst of anxiety or to fall asleep rapidly. Several benzodiazepines are effective following

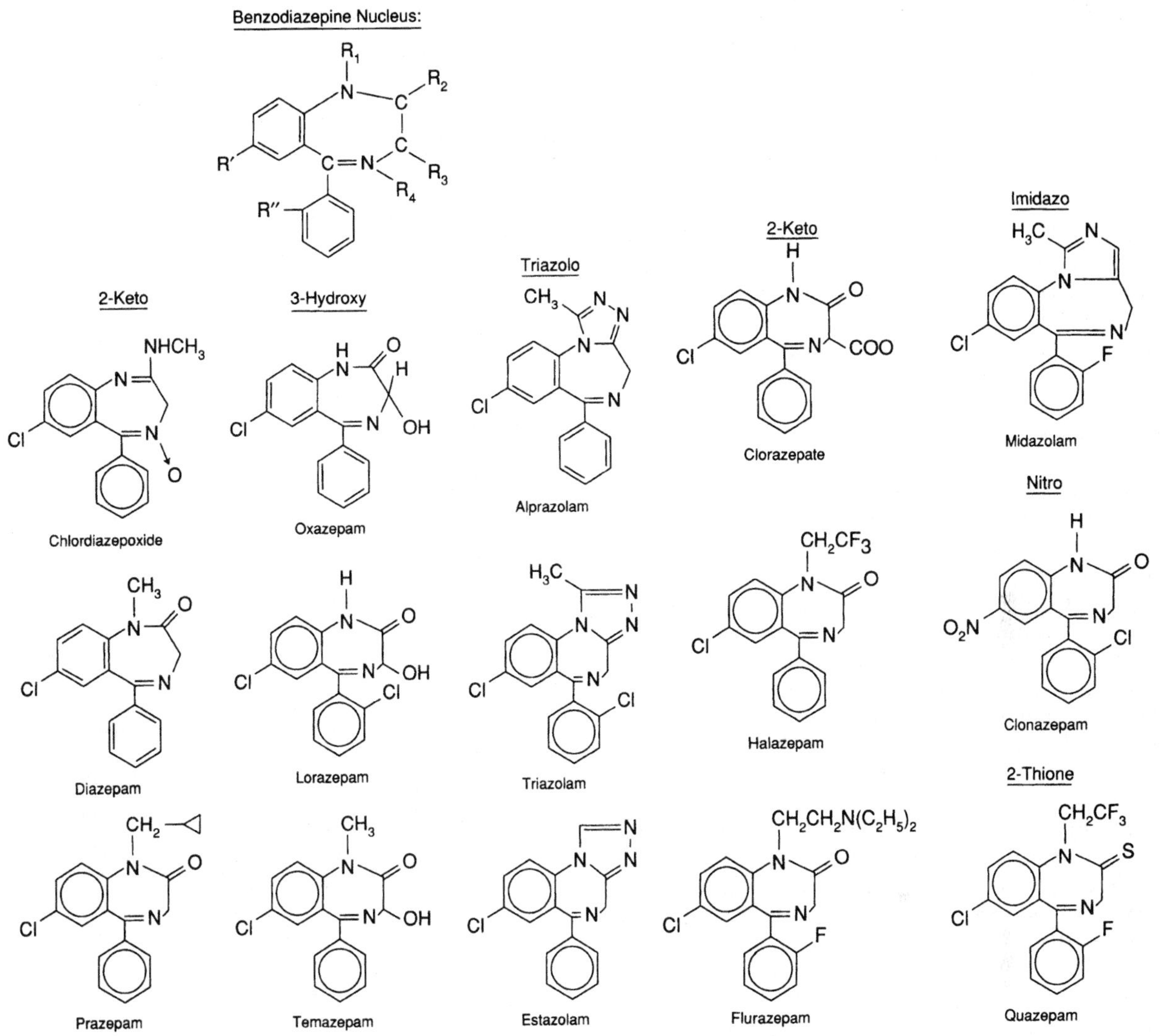

FIGURE 36.4.7–1
Molecular structures of benzodiazepines.

intravenous (IV) injection, whereas only lorazepam and midazolam (Versed) have rapid and reliable absorption following intramuscular (IM) administration.

Diazepam, chlordiazepoxide (Librium), clonazepam (Klonopin), clorazepate, flurazepam (Dalmane), prazepam (Centrax), quazepam (Doral), and halazepam (Paxipam) have plasma half-lives of 30 to more than 100 hours and are, therefore, the longest-acting benzodiazepines. The plasma half-life of these compounds can be as high as 200 hours in persons whose metabolism is genetically slow. Because attainment of steady-state plasma concentrations of the drugs can take up to 2 weeks, persons may experience symptoms and signs of toxicity after only 7 to 10 days of treatment with a dosage that seemed initially to be in the therapeutic range.

The half-lives of lorazepam, oxazepam (Serax), temazepam (Restoril), and estazolam are between 8 and 30 hours. Alprazolam has a half-life of 10 to 15 hours, and triazolam has the shortest half-life (2 to 3 hours) of all the orally administered benzodiazepines.

The advantages of long–half-life drugs over short–half-life drugs include less frequent dosing, less variation in plasma concentration, and less severe withdrawal phenomena. The disadvantages include drug accumulation, increased risk of daytime psychomotor impairment, and increased daytime sedation. The advantages of the short–half-life drugs over the long–half-life drugs include no drug accumulation and less daytime sedation. The disadvantages include more frequent dosing and earlier and more severe withdrawal syndromes. Rebound insomnia and anterograde amnesia are considered more of a problem with the short–half-life drugs than with the long–half-life drugs. (Table 36.4.7–1 lists the half-lives of the drugs.)

Zolpidem and zaleplon are rapidly and well absorbed after oral administration, though absorption can be delayed by as much as 1 hour if they are taken with food. Zolpidem reaches peak plasma concentrations in 1.6 hours and has a half-life of 2.6 hours. Zaleplon reaches peak plasma concentrations in 1 hour and has a half-life of 1 hour. The rapid metabolism and lack of active metabolites of zolpidem and zaleplon avoid the

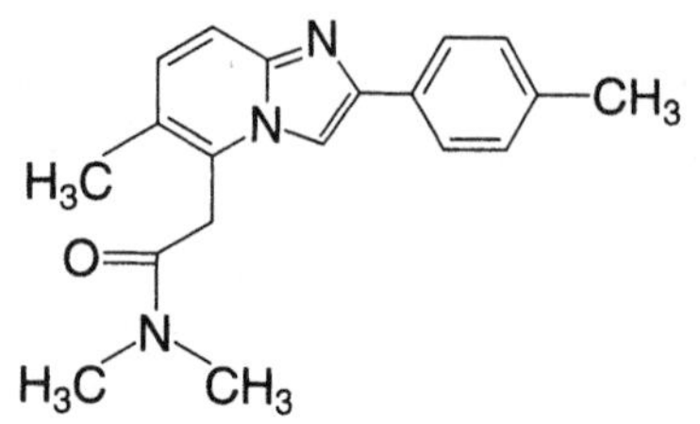

Zolpidem

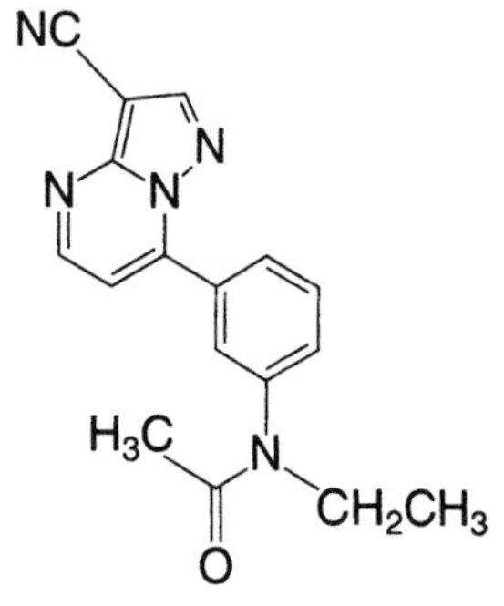

Zaleplon

FIGURE 36.4.7–2
Molecular structures of zolpidem and zaleplon.

accumulation of potentially toxic compounds often seen with long-term use of benzodiazepines.

Benzodiazepines activate all three specific γ-aminobutyric acid–benzodiazepine (GABA-BZ) binding sites of the $GABA_A$ receptor, which opens chloride channels and reduces the rate of neuronal and muscle firing. Because of the wide tissue distribution of $GABA_A$ receptors, benzodiazepines have sedative, muscle relaxant, and anticonvulsant effects. Zolpidem and zaleplon selectively activate only one of the benzodiazepine binding sites, which may account for their selective sedative effects and relative lack of muscle relaxant and anticonvulsant effects.

EFFECTS ON SPECIFIC ORGANS AND SYSTEMS

In addition to the central nervous system (CNS) effects on anxiety and sleep, benzodiazepines are effective anticonvulsants. They are also effective skeletal muscle relaxants, primarily through their ability to inhibit spinal polysynaptic afferent pathways, although monosynaptic afferent pathways may also be affected.

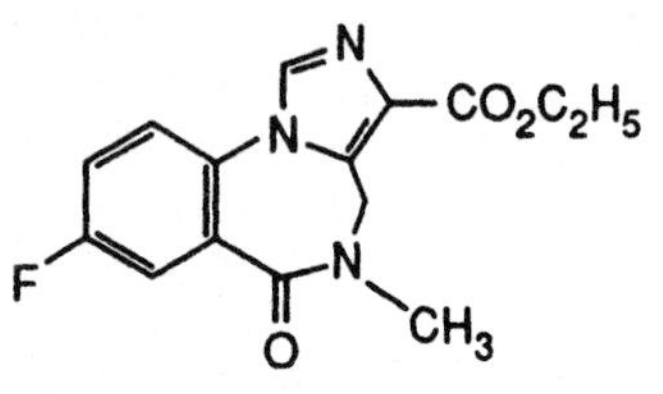

FIGURE 36.4.7–3
Molecular structure of flumazenil.

THERAPEUTIC INDICATIONS

Anxiety

Generalized anxiety disorder, adjustment disorder with anxiety, and other anxiety states are the major clinical applications for benzodiazepines in psychiatry and general medical practice. Most patients should be treated for a predetermined, specific, and relatively brief period. Some patients with generalized anxiety disorder may warrant maintenance treatment with benzodiazepines. The serotonin-specific reuptake inhibitors (SSRIs) are effective antianxiety agents that lack abuse potential, although their antianxiety effects require 2 to 4 weeks to develop.

Mixed Anxiety-Depressive Disorder

Alprazolam is indicated for the treatment of anxiety associated with depression. The availability of several antidepressant drugs with more favorable safety profiles makes alprazolam a second-line drug for this indication; however, some patients respond to this medication when other drugs have had minimal effects.

Panic Disorder and Social Phobia

The two high-potency benzodiazepines, alprazolam and clonazepam, are effective for two anxiety disorders, panic disorder with or without agoraphobia and social phobia. The Food and Drug Administration (FDA) has approved the use of alprazolam for the treatment of panic disorder. The dosage guidelines for the use of alprazolam in panic disorder are similar to those for depression, discussed below. Paroxetine (Paxil) and sertraline (Zoloft) have also been approved by the FDA for treatment of panic disorder. Because SSRIs may not be fully effective for 2 to 4 weeks after initiation of treatment, coadministration of a high-potency benzodiazepine for the first 2 to 4 weeks of use of the SSRI can provide rapid control of anxiety.

Obsessive-Compulsive Disorder and Posttraumatic Stress Disorder

Benzodiazepines, especially clonazepam, which has serotonergic properties, may treat the anxiety component of obsessive-compulsive disorder. Clonazepam may be effective for certain patients who do not respond to clomipramine (Anafranil). Benzodiazepines may also be used to augment clomipramine or the SSRIs, and they may help reduce hyperarousal in posttraumatic stress disorder.

Insomnia. Flurazepam, temazepam, quazepam, estazolam, and triazolam are the benzodiazepines approved for use as hypnotics. The benzodiazepine hypnotics differ principally in their half-lives; flurazepam has the longest half-life, and triazolam has the shortest. Flurazepam may be associated with minor cognitive impairment on the day after its administration, and triazolam may be associated with mild rebound anxiety. Temazepam or estazolam may be a reasonable compromise for the average adult patient. Because of its high specificity for the BZ_1 receptor, quazepam may be associated with few adverse cognitive effects, but quazepam shares the final metabolite with flurazepam—desalkylflurazepam (half-life of about 100

Table 36.4.7–1
Half-Lives, Doses, and Preparations of Benzodiazepine Receptor Agonists and Antagonists

Drug	Dose Equivalents	Half-Life (h)	Rate of Absorption	Usual Adult Dosage	Dose Preparations
Agonists					
Clonazepam	0.5	Long (metabolite, >20)	Rapid	1–6 mg/d bid	0.5-, 1.0-, and 2.0-mg tablets
Diazepam	5	Long (>20) (Nordazepam—long, >20)	Rapid	4–40 mg/d bid to qid	2-, 5-, and 10-mg tablets (slow-release 15-mg capsules)
Alprazolam	0.25	Intermediate (6–20)	Medium	0.5–10 mg/d bid to qid	0.25-, 0.5-, 1.0-, and 2.0-mg tablets
Lorazepam	1	Intermediate (6–20)	Medium	1–6 mg/d tid	0.5-, 1.0-, and 2.0-mg tablets; 2, 4 mg/mL parenteral
Oxazepam	15	Intermediate (6–20)	Slow	30–120 mg/d tid or qid	10-, 15-, and 30-mg capsules (15-mg tablets)
Temazepam	5	Intermediate (6–20)	Medium	7.5–30 mg/d hs	7.5-, 15-, and 30-mg capsules
Chlordiazepoxide	10	Intermediate (6–20) (Demethylchlordiazepoxide—intermediate, 6–20) (Demoxepam—long, >20) (Nordazepam—long, >20)	Medium	10–150 mg tid or qid	5-, 10-, and 25-mg tablets or capsules
Flurazepam	5	Short (<6) (*N*-hydroxyethylflurazepam—short, <6) (*N*-desalkylflurazepam—long, >20)	Rapid	15–30 mg hs	15- and 30-mg capsules
Triazolam	0.1–0.03	Short (<6)	Rapid	0.125 mg or 0.250 mg hs	0.125- or 0.250-mg tablets
Clorazepate	7.5	Short (<6) Nordazepam—long, >20)	Rapid	15–60 mg bid or qid	3.75-, 7.5-, and 15-mg tablets (slow-release 11.25- and 22.5-mg tablets)
Halazepam	20	Short (<6) (Nordazepam—long, >20)	Medium	60–160 mg/d tid or qid	20- and 40-mg tablets
Prazepam	10	Short (<6) (Nordazepam—long, >20)	Slow	30 mg/d (20–60 mg/d) qid or tid	5-, 10-, or 20-mg capsules
Estazolam	0.33	Intermediate (6–20) (4-hydroxyestazolam—intermediate 6–20)	Rapid	1.0 or 2.0 hs	1- and 2-mg tablets
Quazepam	5	Long (>20) (2-oxoquazepam-*N*-desalkylflurazepam—long, >20)	Rapid	7.5 or 15 mg hs	7.5- and 15-mg tablets
Midazolam	1.25–1.7	Short (<6)	Rapid	5 to 50 mg parenteral	5 mg/mL parenteral, 1-, 2-, 5-, and 10-mL vials
Zolpidem	2.5	Short (<6)	Rapid	5 mg or 10 mg hs	5- and 10-mg tablets
Zaleplon	2.5	Short (1)	Rapid	10 mg hs	5- and 10-mg capsules
Antagonist					
Flumazenil	0.05	Short (<6)	Rapid	0.2 to 0.5 mg/min injection over 3–10 min (total, 1–5 mg)	0.1 mg/mL (5- and 10-mL vials)

hours)—and, therefore, may be associated with daytime impairment when used for a long time. Estazolam produces rapid onset of sleep and a hypnotic effect for 6 to 8 hours. All the benzodiazepines produce a moderate decrease in rapid eye movement (REM) sleep, although their use is not associated with REM rebound. Generally, the benzodiazepines are associated with a decrease in stage 3 and stage 4 sleep, although the significance of this is not known. Benzodiazepines alone generally should not be taken for long periods of time, to limit the risk of development of dependence. Longer-term treatment of insomnia should include behavioral modification, relaxation techniques, and exploration of the underlying causes of insomnia, such as anxiety or depression.

The sole indication for zolpidem and zaleplon is insomnia, but the spectrum of their psychological effects closely resembles that of benzodiazepines. Zolpidem and particularly zaleplon are usually not associated with rebound insomnia after the discontinuation of their use for short periods. Use of zolpidem

and zaleplon for periods longer than 1 month is not associated with delayed emergence of adverse effects.

Depression

Unique among the benzodiazepines, alprazolam has antidepressant effects equal to those of the tricyclic drugs, but alprazolam is not effective with seriously depressed inpatients. The efficacy of alprazolam in depressive disorders may reflect its potency; the antidepressant effects of other benzodiazepines may be evident only at doses that also induce sedation or sleep. The starting dosage of alprazolam for the treatment of depression should be 1 to 1.5 mg a day and should be raised by 0.5 mg a day every 3 or 4 days. The maximal dosage is usually 4 mg a day, although some investigators and clinicians have used dosages as high as 10 mg a day. The use of high dosages is controversial because of the possibility of withdrawal symptoms. Clinicians must taper, rather than abruptly stop, alprazolam use, usually at the rate of 0.5 mg a day every 3 to 4 days.

Bipolar I Disorder

Clonazepam is effective in the management of manic episodes and as an adjuvant to lithium (Eskalith) therapy in lieu of antipsychotics. As an adjuvant to lithium, clonazepam may result in increased time between cycles and fewer-than-usual depressive episodes. The other high-potency benzodiazepine, alprazolam, may be as effective as clonazepam for this indication, which is not recognized by the FDA, and alprazolam should be considered a second-line treatment.

Akathisia

Standard anticholinergic drugs—for example, benztropine (Cogentin)—are often ineffective in treating neuroleptic-induced acute akathisia. The first-line drug for akathisia is most commonly a β-adrenergic receptor antagonist—for example, propranolol (Inderal). Several studies have found, however, that benzodiazepines are also effective in treating some patients with akathisia.

Parkinson's Disease

A small number of persons with idiopathic Parkinson's disease will respond to long-term use of zolpidem with reduced bradykinesia and rigidity. Zolpidem dosages of 10 mg four times daily may be tolerated without sedation for several years.

Other Psychiatric Indications

Clonazepam augmentation may accelerate, but not potentiate, the antidepressant effects of fluoxetine (Prozac). Chlordiazepoxide is used to manage the symptoms of alcohol withdrawal. The benzodiazepines (especially IM lorazepam) are used to manage both substance-induced (except amphetamine) and psychotic agitation in the emergency room. A few studies report the use of high dosages of benzodiazepines in schizophrenia patients who had not responded to antipsychotics or who were unable to take the traditional drugs because of adverse effects. The successful use of IM lorazepam for the treatment of catatonia has been reported. Benzodiazepines have also been used instead of amobarbital (Amytal) for drug-assisted interviewing.

Flumazenil for Benzodiazepine Overdose

Flumazenil is used to reverse the adverse psychomotor, amnestic, and sedative effects of benzodiazepine receptor agonists, including benzodiazepines, zolpidem, and zaleplon. Flumazenil is administered IV and has a half-life of 7 to 15 minutes. The most common adverse effects of flumazenil are nausea, vomiting, dizziness, agitation, emotional lability, cutaneous vasodilation, injection-site pain, fatigue, impaired vision, and headache. The most common serious adverse effect associated with use of flumazenil is the precipitation of seizures, which is especially likely to occur in persons with seizure disorders, those who are physically dependent on benzodiazepines, or those who have ingested large quantities of benzodiazepines. Flumazenil alone may impair memory retrieval.

In mixed-drug overdosage the toxic effects (e.g., seizures and cardiac arrhythmias) of other drugs (e.g., tricyclic drugs) may emerge with the reversal of the benzodiazepine effects of flumazenil. For example, seizures caused by an overdosage of tricyclic drugs may have been partially treated in a person who had also taken an overdosage of benzodiazepines. With flumazenil treatment, the tricyclic-induced seizures or cardiac arrhythmias may appear and result in a fatal outcome. Flumazenil does not reverse the effects of ethanol, barbiturates, or opioids.

For initial management of a known or suspected benzodiazepine overdosage, the recommended initial dosage of flumazenil is 0.2 mg (2 mL) administered IV over 30 seconds. If the desired consciousness is not obtained after 30 seconds, a further dose of 0.3 mg (3 mL) can be administered over 30 seconds. Further doses of 0.5 mg (5 mL) can be administered over 30 seconds at 1-minute intervals up to a cumulative dose of 3.0 mg. The clinician should not rush the administration of flumazenil. A secure airway and intravenous access should be established before administration of the drug. Persons should be awakened gradually.

Most persons with a benzodiazepine overdosage respond to a cumulative dose of 1 to 3 mg of flumazenil; doses above 3 mg of flumazenil do not reliably produce additional effects. If a person has not responded 5 minutes after receiving a cumulative dose of 5 mg of flumazenil, the major cause of sedation is probably not benzodiazepine-receptor agonists, and additional flumazenil is unlikely to have an effect.

Sedation can return in 1 to 3 percent of persons treated with flumazenil. It can be prevented or treated by giving repeated doses of flumazenil at 20-minute intervals. For repeat treatment, no more than 1 mg (given as 0.5 mg a minute) should be given at any one time, and no more than 3 mg should be given in any 1 hour.

PRECAUTIONS AND ADVERSE REACTIONS

The most common adverse effect of benzodiazepines is drowsiness, which occurs in about 10 percent of all patients. Because of this adverse effect, patients should be advised to be careful while driving or using machinery when taking the drugs. Drowsiness can occur the day after the use of a benzo-

diazepine for insomnia the previous night, so-called residual daytime sedation. Some patients also experience dizziness (less than 1 percent) and ataxia (less than 2 percent). These symptoms can result in falls and hip fractures, especially in elderly patients. The most serious adverse effects of benzodiazepines occur when other sedative substances, such as alcohol, are taken concurrently. The combinations can result in marked drowsiness, disinhibition, or even respiratory depression. Other relatively rare adverse effects have been mild cognitive deficits that may impair job performance in patients who are taking benzodiazepines. Anterograde amnesia has also been associated with benzodiazepines, particularly high-potency benzodiazepines. A rare, paradoxical increase in aggression has been reported in patients given benzodiazepines, although this effect may be most common in patients with brain damage. Allergic reactions to the drugs are also rare, but a few studies report maculopapular rashes and generalized itching. The symptoms of benzodiazepine intoxication include confusion, slurred speech, ataxia, drowsiness, dyspnea, and hyporeflexia.

Triazolam has received significant attention in the media because of an alleged association with serious aggressive behavioral manifestations, which were associated with doses greater than 1 mg, which is twice the recommended maximum dose. Although little evidence supports the association, the Upjohn Company, which manufactures triazolam, has issued a statement emphasizing that the drug is best used as a short-term (fewer than 10 days) treatment of insomnia, that physicians should carefully evaluate the emergence of any abnormal thinking or behavioral changes in patients treated with triazolam, and that they should consider all appropriate potential causes.

Patients with hepatic disease and elderly patients are particularly likely to have adverse effects and toxicity from the benzodiazepines, especially when the drugs are administered in repeated or high doses, because of these patients' impaired metabolism of the compounds. Benzodiazepines can significantly impair respiration in patients with chronic obstructive pulmonary disease and sleep apnea. Benzodiazepines should be used with caution in patients with a history of substance abuse, cognitive disorders, renal disease, hepatic disease, porphyria, CNS depression, and myasthenia gravis.

Some data indicate that benzodiazepines are teratogenic; therefore, their use during pregnancy is not advised. Moreover, the use of benzodiazepines in the third trimester can precipitate a withdrawal syndrome in newborns. The drugs are secreted in the breast milk in sufficient concentrations to affect neonates. Benzodiazepines may cause dyspnea, bradycardia, and drowsiness in nursing babies.

Zolpidem and zaleplon are generally well tolerated. At zolpidem dosages of 10 mg per day and zaleplon dosages above 10 mg per day, a small number of persons experience dizziness, drowsiness, dyspepsia, or diarrhea. Zolpidem and zaleplon are secreted in breast milk and are, therefore, contraindicated for use by nursing mothers. The dosage of zolpidem and zaleplon should be reduced in the elderly and in persons with hepatic impairment. In rare cases, zolpidem may cause hallucinations, which can last up to 1 hour in some persons. Coadministration of zolpidem and SSRIs may extend the duration of hallucinations in susceptible patients to 1 to 7 hours.

Table 36.4.7–2
Commonly Observed Withdrawal Symptoms (Benzodiazepine Withdrawal Syndrome)

Anxiety
Irritability
Insomnia
Fatigue
Headache
Muscle twitching or aching
Tremor, shakiness
Sweating
Dizziness
Concentration difficulties
Nausea, loss of appetite[a]
Observable depression[a]
Depersonalization, derealization[a]
Increased sensory perception (smell, sight, taste, touch)[a]
Abnormal perception or sensation of movement[a]

[a]Symptoms likely to represent true withdrawal, rather than an exacerbation or return of original anxiety.
Reprinted with permission from Roy-Byrne PP, Hommer D. Benzodiazepine withdrawal: overview and implications for the treatment of anxiety. *Am J Med.* 1988;84:1041.

Tolerance, Dependence, and Withdrawal

When benzodiazepines are used for short periods (1 to 2 weeks) in moderate dosages, they usually cause no significant tolerance, dependence, or withdrawal effects. The short-acting benzodiazepines (e.g., triazolam) may be an exception, as some patients have reported increased anxiety the day after taking a single dose of the drug. Some patients also report a tolerance for the anxiolytic effects of benzodiazepines and require increased dosages to maintain the clinical remission of symptoms. There is also a cross-tolerance among most of the classes of antianxiety drugs, with the notable exception of buspirone (BuSpar) and the SSRIs.

The appearance of a withdrawal syndrome, also called a *discontinuation syndrome* (Table 36.4.7–2), depends on the length of time a patient has taken a benzodiazepine, the dosage the patient has been taking, the rate at which drug use is tapered, and the half-life of the compound. Abrupt discontinuation of benzodiazepine use, particularly those with short half-lives, is associated with severe withdrawal symptoms. Serious symptoms may include depression, paranoia, delirium, and seizures. The incidence of the syndrome is controversial, but some features of the syndrome may occur in as many as 50 percent of patients treated with the drugs. A severe withdrawal syndrome develops only in patients who have taken high dosages for long periods. The appearance of the syndrome may be delayed for 1 or 2 weeks in patients who had been taking 2-keto benzodiazepines with long half-lives.

Alprazolam use seems to be particularly associated with an immediate, severe withdrawal syndrome, and it should be tapered gradually. A recent study comparing simple tapering of alprazolam use with tapering plus cognitive, anticipatory guidance regarding the alprazolam discontinuation effects found that patients were much more likely to remain off alprazolam indefinitely if they have been fully warned to expect the signs

and symptoms of discontinuation. This is important because a significant percentage of patients who use alprazolam for long periods cannot successfully discontinue taking it.

Zolpidem and zaleplon can produce a mild withdrawal syndrome lasting 1 day after prolonged use at higher therapeutic dosages. Rarely, a person taking zolpidem has self-titrated the daily dosage up to 300 to 400 mg a day. Abrupt discontinuation of such a high dosage of zolpidem may cause withdrawal symptoms for 4 or more days. Tolerance does not develop to the sedative effects of zolpidem and zaleplon.

DRUG–DRUG INTERACTIONS

The most common and potentially serious benzodiazepine receptor agonist interaction is excessive sedation and respiratory depression occurring when benzodiazepines, zolpidem, or zaleplon are administered concomitantly with other CNS depressants, such as alcohol, barbiturates, tricyclic and tetracyclic drugs, dopamine receptor antagonists, opioids, and antihistamines. Ataxia and dysarthria may be likely to occur when lithium, antipsychotics, and clonazepam are combined. The combination of benzodiazepines and clozapine (Clozaril) has been reported to cause delirium and should be avoided. Cimetidine (Tagamet), disulfiram (Antabuse), isoniazid (Nydrazid), estrogen, and oral contraceptives increase the plasma concentrations of diazepam, chlordiazepoxide, clorazepate, flurazepam, prazepam, and halazepam. Cimetidine increases the plasma concentrations of zaleplon. The plasma concentrations of triazolam and alprazolam are increased to potentially toxic concentrations by nefazodone (Serzone) and fluvoxamine (Luvox). The manufacturer of nefazodone recommends that the dosage of triazolam be lowered by 75 percent and the dosage of alprazolam lowered by 50 percent, when given concomitantly with nefazodone. Over-the-counter preparations of kava plant, advertised as a "natural tranquilizer," can potentiate the action of benzodiazepine receptor agonists through synergistic overactivation of GABA receptors. Carbamazepine (Tegretol) can lower the plasma concentration of alprazolam. Antacids and food may decrease the plasma concentrations of benzodiazepines, and smoking may increase the metabolism of benzodiazepines. Rifampin (Rifadin), phenytoin (Dilantin), carbamazepine, and phenobarbital (Solfoton, Luminal) significantly increase the metabolism of zaleplon. The benzodiazepines may increase the plasma concentrations of phenytoin and digoxin (Lanoxin). SSRIs may prolong and exacerbate the severity of zolpidem-induced hallucinations.

Laboratory Interferences

No known laboratory interferences are associated with the use of benzodiazepine receptor agonists or antagonists.

DOSAGE AND ADMINISTRATION

Benzodiazepines

Benzodiazepines are categorized as short-, intermediate-, or long-acting drugs. Their sedative and anxiolytic effects appear within 30 to 60 minutes of administration and terminate as soon as the drugs are excreted. This is in contrast to the antianxiety effects of the serotonergic drugs, which may take 2 to 4 weeks to develop.

The clinical decision to treat an anxious patient with a benzodiazepine should be carefully considered. Medical causes of anxiety (e.g., thyroid dysfunction, caffeinism, and medications) should be ruled out. Benzodiazepine use should be started at a low dosage, and the patient should be instructed about the drug's sedative properties and abuse potential. An estimated length of therapy should be decided at the beginning of therapy, and the need for continued therapy should be reevaluated at least monthly because of the problems associated with long-term use.

Duration of Treatment. Benzodiazepines can be used to treat illnesses other than anxiety disorders. In such cases the duration of treatment should generally be similar to that for the standard drugs used to treat these disorders. The use of benzodiazepines over a long period for chronically anxious patients is often valuable, although controversial. In his 1980 textbook on drug treatment in psychiatry, Donald Klein stated, "There are many reports of patients maintained on benzodiazepines for years with apparent benefit and without the development of tolerance. Nonetheless, it is dubious practice to prescribe such medications indefinitely without accompanying psychotherapy."

Discontinuation of Therapy. Benzodiazepine withdrawal syndrome occurs when patients discontinue benzodiazepines abruptly; 90 percent of patients after long-term use experience some symptoms of withdrawal on discontinuation if the drug is tapered slowly. Benzodiazepine withdrawal syndrome consists of anxiety, nervousness, diaphoresis, restlessness, irritability, fatigue, light-headedness, tremor, insomnia, and weakness. The higher the dose and the shorter the half-life, the more severe the withdrawal symptoms can be.

When the medication is to be discontinued, drug use must be tapered slowly (25 percent a week); otherwise, symptoms are likely to recur or rebound. Monitoring of any withdrawal symptoms (possibly with a standardized rating scale) and psychological support for the patient aid successful discontinuation of benzodiazepine use. Concurrent use of carbamazepine during discontinuation of benzodiazepine use reportedly permits more rapid and better tolerated withdrawal than a gradual taper alone. The dosage range of carbamazepine used to facilitate withdrawal is 400 to 500 mg a day. Some clinicians report particular difficulty in tapering and discontinuing alprazolam use, particularly with patients who have been receiving high dosages for long periods. There have been reports of successful discontinuation of alprazolam use by switching to clonazepam, which is then gradually withdrawn.

Choice of Drug and Potency. The wide range of benzodiazepines is available in an equally wide range of formulations (Table 36.4.7–1). The drugs differ primarily in their half-lives. Another difference is in the rate of onset of their potency and anxiolytic effects. *Potency* is a general term used to express the pharmacological activity of a drug. Some benzodiazepines are more potent than others, in that a relatively smaller dose of one compound will achieve the same effect as a larger dose of another. For example, 0.25 mg of clonazepam achieves the same effect as 5 mg of diazepam; thus, clonazepam is consid-

ered a high-potency benzodiazepine. Conversely, oxazepam has an approximate dose equivalence of 15 mg and is a low-potency drug. The four high-potency benzodiazepines—alprazolam, triazolam, estazolam, and clonazepam—are the drugs most likely to be effective for new applications such as depression, bipolar I disorder, panic disorder, and the phobias.

Drug Combinations. The most common drug combinations with benzodiazepines involve antipsychotics and antidepressants, in addition to the benzodiazepines' obvious use as adjuvant hypnotics. The combination of a benzodiazepine and an antidepressant may be indicated in the treatment of markedly anxious depressed patients and patients with panic disorder. Several reports indicate that the combined use of alprazolam and an antipsychotic may further reduce psychotic symptoms in patients who did not respond adequately to the antipsychotic alone. The combined use of benzodiazepines and tricyclic drugs may improve compliance by reducing the subjective side effects and immediately reducing anxiety and insomnia. The combination, however, may also cause excessive sedation and cognitive impairment and may even exacerbate the depression, and it adds significantly to the lethality of an overdose.

Zolpidem and Zaleplon

Zolpidem is available in 5- and 10-mg tablets. A single 10-mg dose is the usual dose for the treatment of insomnia and is also the maximum daily dose. A single dose of zolpidem can be expected to provide 5 hours of sleep with minimal residual impairment. For persons over age 65 or persons with hepatic impairment, an initial dose of 5 mg is advised.

Zaleplon is available in 5- and 10-mg capsules. A single 10-mg dose is the usual adult dose. The dose can be increased to a maximum of 20 mg as tolerated. A single dose of zaleplon can be expected to provide 4 hours of sleep with minimal residual impairment. For persons over age 65 or persons with or hepatic impairment, an initial dose of 5 mg is advised.

References

Balkin TJ, O'Donnell VM, Wesenten N, McCann U, Belenky G. Comparison of the daytime sleep and performance effects of zolpidem versus triazolam. *Psychopharmacology.* 1992;107:83.

Ballenger JC. Benzodiazepine receptor agonists and antagonists. In: Sadock BJ, Sadock VA, eds. *Kaplan & Sadock's Comprehensive Textbook of Psychiatry.* 7th ed. Vol 2. Baltimore: Lippincott Williams & Wilkins; 2000:2317.

Begg A, Drummond G, Tiplady B. Effects of temazepam on memory and psychomotor performance: a dose-response study. *Hum Psychopharmacol.* 2001;166:6.

Bishop KI, Curran HV. Psychopharmacological analysis of implicit and explicit memory: a study with lorazepam and the benzodiazepine antagonist flumazenil. *Psychopharmacology.* 1995;121:267.

Duka T, Krause W, Dorow R, Rohloff A, Ott H, Voet B. Abecarnil: a new beta-carboline anxiolytic preliminary clinical pharmacology. *Psychopharmacol Ser.* 1993;11:132.

Endeshaw Y. The role of benzodiazepines in the treatment of insomnia: meta-analysis of benzodiazepines in the treatment of insomnia. *J Am Geriatr Soc.* 2001;49:824.

Hardman JG, Limbird LE, Goodman Gilman A, eds. *Goodman & Gilman's the Pharmacological Basis of Therapeutics.* 10th ed. New York: McGraw-Hill; 2001.

Kapczinski F, Sherman D, Williams R, Lader M. Differential effects of flumazenil in alcoholic and nonalcoholic cirrhotic patients. *Psychopharmacology (Berl).* 1995;120:220.

Kasper S, Resinger E. Panic disorder: the place of benzodiazepines and selective serotonin reuptake inhibitors. *Eur Neuropsychopharmacol.* 2001;11:307.

Laurijssens BE, Greenblatt DJ. Pharmacokinetic-pharmacodynamic relationships for benzodiazepines. *Clin Pharmacokinet.* 1996;30:52.

Mumford GK, Rush CR, Griffiths RR. Abecarnil and alprazolam in humans: behavioral, subjective and reinforcing effects. *J Pharmacol Exp Ther.* 1995;272:570.

Noyes R Jr, Burrows GD, Reich JH, et al. Diazepam versus alprazolam for the treatment of panic disorder. *J Clin Psychiatry.* 1996;57:349.

Roth T, Roehrs TA. The use of benzodiazepine hypnotics: a scientific examination of a clinical controversy. *J Clin Psychiatry.* 1992;53(suppl 12):2.

Roy-Byrne P, Fleishaker J, Arnett C, et al. Effects of acute and chronic alprazolam treatment on cerebral blood flow, memory, sedation, and plasma catecholamines. *Neuropsychopharmacology.* 1993;8:161.

Roy-Byrne P, Wingerson DK, Radant A, Greenblatt DJ, Cowley DS. Reduced benzodiazepine sensitivity in patients with panic disorder: comparison with patients with obsessive-compulsive disorder and normal subjects. *Am J Psychiatry.* 1006;153:1444.

Simpson CA, Rush CR. Acute performance-impairing and subject-rated effects of triazolam and temazepam, alone and in combination with ethanol, in humans. *J Psychopharmacol.* 2002;16:23.

Song C. Anxiety and the immune system: the modulation of benzodiazepines. *Stress Health.* 2001;17:129.

Zandstra SM, Furer JW, van de Lisdonk EH, et al. Different study criteria affect the prevalence of benzodiazepine use. *Soc Psychiatry Psychiatr Epidemiol.* 2002;37:139.

▲ 36.4.8 Bupropion

Bupropion (Wellbutrin, Zyban) is a first-line agent for treatment of depression and smoking cessation. It generally is more effective against symptoms of depression than those of anxiety, and it is quite effective in combination with selective serotonin reuptake inhibitors (SSRIs). Despite early warnings that it could cause seizures, clinical experience shows that when used at recommended doses, bupropion is no more likely to cause seizures than any other antidepressant drug. Smoking cessation is most successful when bupropion (called Zyban for this indication) is used in combination with behavioral modification techniques.

Bupropion is a unique antidepressant in the available armamentarium of drugs, with a highly favorable profile of adverse effects. Of particular note among antidepressants, it is associated with little inhibition of sexual function. It also carries a higher likelihood of weight loss than weight gain. It possesses some dopaminergic effects and may serve as a mild psychostimulant as well as an antidepressant.

CHEMISTRY

Bupropion is a unicyclic aminoketone that resembles amphetamine and the anorectic diethylpropion (Tenuate) in its molecular structure (Fig. 36.4.8–1). It is structurally unrelated to any other antidepressant available in the United States.

PHARMACOLOGICAL ACTIONS

Bupropion is well absorbed from the gastrointestinal (GI) tract. Peak plasma concentrations of bupropion are usually reached

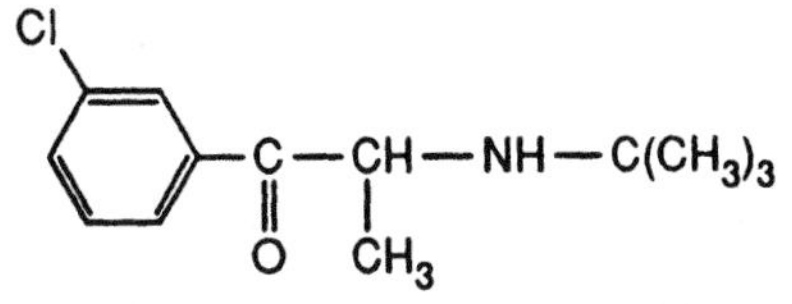

FIGURE 36.4.8–1
Molecular structure of bupropion.

within 2 hours of oral administration, and peak levels of the sustained-release version are seen after 3 hours. The mean half-life of the compound is 12 hours, ranging from 8 to 40 hours.

The mechanism of action for the antidepressant effects of bupropion is poorly understood. It was initially thought that bupropion acts through the blockade of dopamine reuptake. However, central nervous system (CNS) concentrations of bupropion are probably not sufficient to result in significant dopamine reuptake inhibition. Nonetheless, some data indicate that bupropion exerts its antidepressant effects by increasing the functional efficiency of noradrenergic systems. Regarding the effects of bupropion on smoking cessation, it is a noncompetitive inhibitor of nicotinic acetylcholine receptors and thus may interfere with the addictive actions of nicotine.

EFFECTS ON SPECIFIC ORGANS AND SYSTEMS

Except for its CNS effects, bupropion is nearly devoid of activity in human organs. No evidence has been found for significant effects of bupropion on liver, cardiac, or renal function, although the dosage of bupropion should be adjusted downward in patients with liver and renal impairment. It may increase blood pressure in previously hypertensive patients. Rare cases of lymphadenopathy, anemia, and pancytopenia have been reported, although their association with bupropion use is uncertain and routine monitoring of blood is not indicated. Bupropion does not affect sexual functioning. It has been associated with weight changes, more often with weight loss than with weight gain. There have been reports of rashes and pruritus in a few patients

THERAPEUTIC INDICATIONS

Depression

The therapeutic efficacy of bupropion in depression is well established in both outpatient and inpatient settings. Improved sleep early in the course of treatment is seen less often with bupropion than with some other antidepressants, because of its lack of sedation; however, it does not disrupt sleep architecture as much as the SSRIs. It is also of use in hypoactive sexual desire that may accompany depression.

Bupropion in combination with lithium (Eskalith) is effective and well tolerated in some persons with refractory depression, but this combination may rarely cause CNS toxicity, including seizures.

Bipolar Disorders

Bupropion may be less likely than tricyclics to precipitate mania in persons with bipolar I disorder, although it is not free of this risk. It may be less likely than other antidepressants to exacerbate or induce rapid-cycling bipolar II disorder.

Attention-Deficit/Hyperactivity Disorder

Bupropion is a major second-line agent, after the sympathomimetics, for treatment of attention-deficit/hyperactivity disorder (ADHD). It can be nearly as efficacious as methylphenidate (Ritalin) for childhood and adult ADHD. Bupropion is an appropriate choice for persons with comorbid ADHD and depression or persons with comorbid ADHD, conduct disorder, or substance abuse.

Cocaine Detoxification

Some clinicians have reported that bupropion can be used to reduce the cravings for cocaine in persons who have withdrawn from the substance.

Smoking Cessation

Bupropion is indicated for use in combination with behavioral modification programs for smoking cessation. Success of smoking cessation efforts is best associated with a high degree of motivation and structured behavioral support. Bupropion and nicotine substitutes (Nicoderm, Nicotrol) individually increase the success rate, and they act synergistically in combination.

PRECAUTIONS AND ADVERSE REACTIONS

The most common adverse effects associated with use of bupropion are headache, insomnia, upper respiratory complaints, and nausea. Restlessness, agitation, and irritability may also occur. Most likely because of its potentiating effects on dopaminergic neurotransmission, bupropion has rarely been associated with psychotic symptoms, including hallucinations, delusions, and catatonia, as well as delirium. Most notable about bupropion is the absence of significant drug-induced orthostatic hypotension, weight gain, daytime drowsiness, and anticholinergic effects. Some persons, however, may experience dry mouth or constipation, and weight loss may occur in about 25 percent of persons. Bupropion causes no significant cardiovascular or clinical laboratory changes.

A major advantage of bupropion over SSRIs is that bupropion is virtually devoid of any adverse effects on sexual functioning, whereas the SSRIs are associated with such effects in up to 80 percent of persons. Some persons taking bupropion experience increased sexual responsiveness and even spontaneous orgasm.

At dosages of 300 mg a day or less of the sustained-release preparation, the incidence of seizures is 0.05 percent, which is no worse than the incidence of seizures with other antidepressants. The risk of seizures increases to about 0.1 percent with doses above 400 mg a day. Risk factors for seizures, such as past history of seizures, use of alcohol, recent benzodiazepine withdrawal, organic brain disease, head trauma, or epileptiform discharges on electroencephalography (EEG), warrant critical examination of the decision to use bupropion.

Because high dosages (more than 400 mg a day) of bupropion may be associated with a euphoric feeling, bupropion may be relatively contraindicated in persons with histories of substance abuse. The use of bupropion by pregnant women has not been studied and is not recommended. Because bupropion is secreted in breast milk, the use of bupropion by nursing women is not recommended.

Overdoses with bupropion are associated with a generally favorable outcome, except in the cases of huge doses and mixed-drug overdoses. Seizures occur in about a third of all

overdoses, and fatalities can involve uncontrollable seizures, bradycardia, and cardiac arrest. In general, however, bupropion is safer in overdose cases than other antidepressants are, with the possible exception of the SSRIs.

DRUG–DRUG INTERACTIONS

Bupropion should not be used concurrently with monoamine oxidase inhibitors (MAOIs) because of the possibility of inducing a hypertensive crisis, and at least 14 days should pass after discontinuation of MAOI use before treatment with bupropion is initiated. Addition of bupropion may permit persons taking antiparkinsonian medications to lower the doses of their dopaminergic drugs. However, delirium, psychotic symptoms, and dyskinetic movements may be associated with coadministration of bupropion and dopaminergic agents such as levodopa (Larodopa), pergolide (Permax), ropinirole (Requip), pramipexole (Mirapex), amantadine (Symmetrel), and bromocriptine (Parlodel).

The combination of bupropion and fluoxetine (Prozac) is one of the most effective and well-tolerated treatments for all types of depression, but a few case reports indicate that panic, delirium, or seizures may be associated with this combination. Patients with panic disorder are sensitive to the activating effects of bupropion and may have their anxiety exacerbated.

Carbamazepine (Tegretol) may decrease plasma concentrations of bupropion, and bupropion may increase plasma concentrations of valproic acid (Depakene).

LABORATORY INTERFERENCES

Bupropion may give a false-positive result on urinary amphetamine screens. No other reports have appeared of laboratory interferences clearly associated with bupropion treatment. Clinically nonsignificant changes in the electrocardiogram (ECG) (premature beats and nonspecific ST-T changes) and decreases in the white blood cell count (by about 10 percent) have been reported in a small number of persons.

DOSAGE AND CLINICAL GUIDELINES

Bupropion is available in 75- and 100-mg tablets, and sustained-release bupropion is available in 100-, 150-, and 200-mg tablets. Treatment should be initiated in the average adult with 100 mg orally twice a day or 150 mg of the sustained-release version once a day. On the fourth day of treatment, the dosage can be raised to 100 mg three times a day or 300 mg a day of the sustained-release formulation taken in the morning or in two divided doses. Since 300 mg is the recommended dosage, the person should be maintained on this dosage for several weeks before increasing the dosage further. Because of the risk of seizures, dosage increases should never exceed 100 mg in a 3-day period; a single dose of bupropion should never exceed 150 mg, and a single dose of sustained-release bupropion should never exceed 300 mg. The total daily dosage should not exceed 450 mg of the immediate-release formulation or 400 mg of the sustained-release version.

For smoking cessation, the patient should start taking 150 mg a day of sustained-release bupropion 10 to 14 days before quitting smoking. On the fourth day, the dosage should be increased to 150 mg twice daily. Treatment generally lasts 7 to 12 weeks.

REFERENCES

Ansari A. The efficacy of newer antidepressants in the treatment of chronic pain: a review of current literature. *Harvard Rev Psychiatry.* 2000;7:257.

Ascher J, Cole JO, Colin J, et al. Bupropion: a review of its mechanism of antidepressant activity. *J Clin Psychiatry.* 1995;56:395.

Ashton AK, Rosen RC. Bupropion as an antidote for serotonin reuptake inhibitor-induced sexual dysfunction. *J Clin Psychiatry.* 1998;59:112.

Baldessarini RJ. Drugs and the treatment of psychiatric disorders: depression and anxiety disorders. In: Hardman JG, Limbird LE, Goodman Gilman A, eds. *Goodman & Gilman's the Pharmacological Basis of Therapeutics.* 10th ed. New York: McGraw-Hill; 2001:447.

Berigan TR, Deagle EA III. Treatment of smokeless tobacco addiction with bupropion and behavior modification [letter]. *JAMA.* 1999;281:233.

Conners CK, Casat CD, Gualtieri CT, et al. Bupropion hydrochloride in attention deficit disorder with hyperactivity. *J Am Acad Child Adolesc Psychiatry.* 1996;34:1314.

Golden RN, Nicholas LM. Bupropion. In: Sadock BJ, Sadock VA, eds. *Kaplan & Sadock's Comprehensive Textbook of Psychiatry.* 7th ed. Vol 2. Baltimore: Lippincott Williams & Wilkins; 2000:2324.

Goodnick PJ, Dominguez RA, De Vane CL, Bowden CL. Bupropion slow-release response in depression: diagnosis and biochemistry. *Biol Psychiatry.* 1998;44:629.

Hebert S. Bupropion (Zyban, sustained-release tablets): reported adverse reactions. *Can Med Assoc J.* 1999;160:1050.

Montoya ID, Preston KL, Rothman R, Gorelick DA. Open-label pilot study of bupropion plus bromocriptine for treatment of cocaine dependence. *Am J Drug Alcohol Abuse.* 2002;28:189.

Namerow LB. Seizure associated with bupropion and guanfacine. *J Am Acad Child Adolesc Psychiatry.* 1999;38:2.

Neumann JK, Peeples B, East J, Ellis AR. Nicotine reduction: effectiveness of bupropion. *Br J Psychiatry.* 2000;177:87.

Raymond E, Bahdai Z, Waters H, et al. What's new in smoking cessation: Zyban. *Can Fam Physician.* 1999;45:633.

Riggs PD, Leon SL, Mikulich SK, Pottle LC. An open trial of bupropion for ADHD in adolescents with substance use disorders and conduct disorder. *J Am Acad Child Adolesc Psychiatry.* 1998;37:1271.

Shiffman S, Johnston J, Andrew K, et al. The effect of bupropion on nicotine craving and withdrawal. *Psychopharmacology.* 2000;148:33.

Trappler B, Miyashiro AM. Bupropion-amantadine-associated neurotoxicity. *J Clin Psychiatry.* 2000;61:61.

▲ 36.4.9 Buspirone

Buspirone (BuSpar) is indicated for the treatment of anxiety disorders. Unlike the benzodiazepines and the barbiturates, buspirone does not have sedative, hypnotic, muscle-relaxant, or anticonvulsant effects; carries a low potential for abuse; and is not associated with withdrawal phenomena or cognitive impairment.

CHEMISTRY

The molecular structure of buspirone is chemically distinct from currently available benzodiazepines, barbiturates, and antidepressants (Fig. 36.4.9–1). It is an azaspirone-class drug.

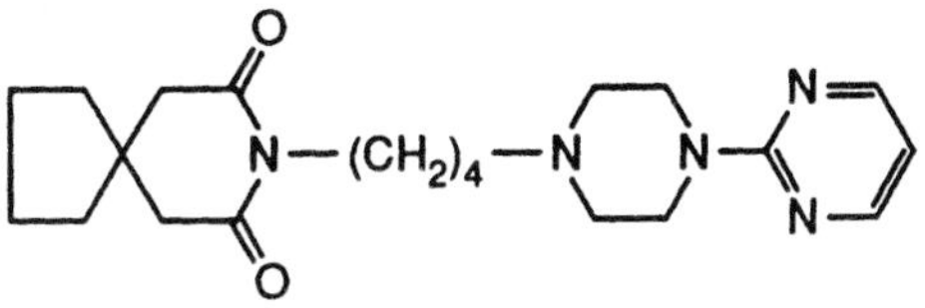

FIGURE 36.4.9–1
Molecular structure of buspirone.

PHARMACOLOGICAL ACTIONS

Buspirone is well absorbed from the gastrointestinal (GI) tract and is unaffected by food intake. The drug reaches peak plasma levels in 60 to 90 minutes after oral administration. The short half-life (2 to 11 hours) necessitates dosing three times daily.

In contrast to benzodiazepines and barbiturates, which act on the γ-aminobutyric acid (GABA)-associated chloride ion channel, buspirone has no effect on that receptor mechanism. Rather, buspirone acts as an agonist or partial agonist on serotonin 5-HT_{1A}-receptors. Buspirone also has activity at 5-HT_2 and dopamine D_2 receptors, although the significance of the effects at these receptors is unknown. At D_2 receptors, it has properties of both an agonist and an antagonist. The fact that buspirone takes 2 to 3 weeks to exert its therapeutic effects implies that whatever its initial effects, the therapeutic effects may involve the modulation of several neurotransmitters and intraneuronal mechanisms.

Table 36.4.9–1
Comparison of Benzodiazepines and Buspirone

	Benzodiazepine	Buspirone
Effect of single dose	Yes	No
Full therapeutic action	Days	Weeks
Sedating	Yes	No
Dependence liability	Yes	No
Impair performance	Yes	No
Suppress sedative withdrawal symptoms	Yes	No
History of previous benzodiazepine response	Good response	Poor response
Side effects	Sedation, memory impairment	Restlessness, nervousness

From Silver JM, Yudofsky SC, Hurowitz G. Psychopharmacology and electroconvulsive therapy. In: *The American Psychiatric Press Textbook of Psychiatry.* 2nd ed. Washington, DC: American Psychiatric Press; 1994, with permission.

EFFECTS ON SPECIFIC ORGANS AND SYSTEMS

The effects of buspirone on organs other than the brain are minimal. The drug has no significant effects on the respiratory system, heart, vascular system, blood, smooth muscles, or autonomic nervous system.

THERAPEUTIC INDICATIONS

Generalized Anxiety Disorder

Buspirone is safe and effective for treatment of generalized anxiety disorder. Compared with benzodiazepines, buspirone is generally more effective for symptoms of anger and hostility, equally effective for psychic symptoms of anxiety, and less effective for somatic symptoms of anxiety. The full benefit of buspirone is evident only at dosages above 30 mg a day. Buspirone offers several advantages over the benzodiazepines in long-term use, including lack of development of withdrawal symptoms upon discontinuation and less need to return to benzodiazepines once the initial course of drug treatment is terminated (Table 36.4.9–1). Buspirone is not associated with any abuse potential, even in groups at high risk for addictive behavior.

Compared with the benzodiazepines, buspirone has a delayed onset of action and lacks any euphoric effect. Unlike benzodiazepines, buspirone has no immediate effects, and the patient should be told that a full clinical response may take 2 to 4 weeks. If an immediate response is needed, the patient can start treatment with a benzodiazepine and then be withdrawn from the drug after buspirone's effects begin. Sometimes the sedative effects of benzodiazepines, which are not found with buspirone, are desirable; however, these sedative effects may impair motor performance and cause cognitive deficits.

Other Disorders

Buspirone is not effective in the treatment of panic disorder or social phobia; however, it may reduce the increased arousal and flashbacks associated with posttraumatic stress disorder. Evidence of the efficacy of high-dosage buspirone (30 to 90 mg a day) for depressive disorders is mixed. Buspirone is sometimes used to augment serotonergic antidepressant drugs for major depressive and obsessive-compulsive disorders.

Because buspirone does not act on the GABA-chloride ion channel complex, the drug is not recommended for the treatment of withdrawal from benzodiazepines, alcohol, or sedative-hypnotic drugs, except as treatment of comorbid anxiety symptoms.

Buspirone can effectively reduce aggression and anxiety in persons with organic brain disease or traumatic brain injury. It may also reduce comorbid oppositional-defiant symptoms, aggressive behavior, hyperactivity, impulsivity, inattention, and mood in children with attention-deficit/hyperactivity disorder (ADHD). Buspirone may also reduce hyperactivity associated with autistic spectrum disorders.

Buspirone may be beneficial for treatment of the physical and psychic symptoms of premenstrual dysphoric disorder. At higher dosages, buspirone may ameliorate the sexual inhibition of the selective serotonin reuptake inhibitors (SSRIs). It is also used to treat SSRI-induced bruxism.

PRECAUTIONS AND ADVERSE REACTIONS

The most common adverse effects of buspirone are headache, nausea, dizziness, and (rarely) insomnia. No sedation is associated with buspirone. Some persons may report a minor feeling of restlessness, although that symptom may reflect an incompletely treated anxiety disorder. No deaths have been reported from overdoses of buspirone, and the median lethal dose (LD_{50}) is estimated to be 160 to 550 times the recommended daily dose. Buspirone should be used with caution by persons with hepatic and renal impairment, pregnant women, and nursing mothers. It can be used safely by the elderly.

DRUG–DRUG INTERACTIONS

Coadministration of buspirone and haloperidol (Haldol) results in increased blood concentrations of haloperidol. Buspirone should not be used with monoamine oxidase inhibitors (MAOIs) to avoid hypertensive episodes, and a 2-week washout period should pass between the discontinuation of MAOI use

and the initiation of treatment with buspirone. Erythromycin (E-mycin), itraconazole (Sporanox), nefazodone (Serzone), and grapefruit juice may raise plasma concentrations of buspirone.

LABORATORY INTERFERENCES

Single doses of buspirone can cause transient elevations in growth hormone, prolactin, and cortisol concentrations, although the effects are not clinically significant.

DOSAGE AND CLINICAL GUIDELINES

Buspirone is available in single-scored 5- and 10-mg tablets and triple-scored 15- and 30-mg tablets; treatment is usually initiated with either 5 mg orally three times daily or 7.5 mg orally twice daily. The dosage can be raised 5 mg every 2 to 4 days to the usual dosage range of 15 to 60 mg a day.

Switching from a Benzodiazepine to Buspirone

Buspirone is as effective as the benzodiazepines in the treatment of anxiety in persons who have never received benzodiazepines; however, buspirone does not achieve the same response in patients who have received benzodiazepines in the past. This is probably due to the absence of the immediate mildly euphoric and sedative effects of the benzodiazepines. The most common clinical problem, therefore, is how to initiate buspirone therapy in a person who is currently taking benzodiazepines. There are two alternatives. First, the clinician can start buspirone treatment gradually while the benzodiazepine is being withdrawn. Second, the clinician can start buspirone treatment and bring the person up to a therapeutic dosage for 2 to 3 weeks while that person is still receiving the regular dosage of the benzodiazepine, and then slowly taper the benzodiazepine dosage. Coadministration of buspirone and benzodiazepines may be effective in the treatment of anxiety disorders that have not responded to treatment with either drug alone.

GEPIRONE

Gepirone (Ariza) is a pyridinyl piperazine partial 5-HT_{1A} receptor agonist related to buspirone that is awaiting approval as an antidepressant. Studies of gepirone in generalized anxiety disorder patients showed a delayed anxiolytic response similar to that seen with buspirone. Mechanism-of-action studies have demonstrated that gepirone, compared to buspirone, possesses a much greater selectivity for 5-HT_{1A} receptors over D_2 receptors. Long-term studies have shown that gepirone has a differential action at presynaptic (agonist) and postsynaptic (partial agonist) 5-HT_{1A} receptors. It has minimal receptor affinity for histamine and other receptor types.

Common adverse events include dizziness, paresthesias, palpitations, headache, nausea, nervousness, and insomnia. There are no clinically relevant changes in blood pressure, heart rate, cardiac conduction, or laboratory parameters. Gepirone has no detectable inhibition of CYP 450 enzymes.

Gepirone is used once daily in the form of extended-release tablets. Dose titration is necessary, with a starting dosage of 20 mg a day, increased over several weeks up to 80 mg a day if necessary.

References

Algeri S, De Luigi A, De Simoni MG, et al. Multiple and complex effects of buspirone on central dopaminergic system. *Pharmacol Biochem Behav.* 1988;29:823.

Apter JT, Allen LA. Buspirone: future directions. *J Clin Psychopharmacol.* 1999;19:86.

Baldessarini RJ, Tarazi RI. Drugs and the treatment of psychiatric disorders: psychosis and mania. In: Hardman JG, Limbird LE, Goodman Gilman A, eds. *Goodman & Gilman's the Pharmacological Basis of Therapeutics.* 10th ed. New York: McGraw-Hill; 2001:485.

Brawman-Mintzer O, Lydiard RB, Ballenger JC. Buspirone. In: Sadock BJ, Sadock VA, eds. *Kaplan & Sadock's Comprehensive Textbook of Psychiatry.* 7th ed. Vol 2. Baltimore: Lippincott Williams & Wilkins; 2000:2329.

Buitelaar JK, van der Gaag RJ, van der Hoeven J. Buspirone in the management of anxiety and irritability in children with pervasive developmental disorders: results of an open-label study. *J Clin Psychiatry.* 1998;59:56.

Dimitriou EC, Dimitriou CE. Buspirone augmentation of antidepressant therapy. *J Clin Psychopharmacol.* 1998;18:465.

McEvoy GK, ed. *AHFS Drug Information.* Bethesda, MD: American Society of Hospital Pharmacists; 2002.

Montoya ID, Preston KL, Rothman R, Gorelick DA. Open-label pilot study of bupropion plus bromocriptine for treatment of cocaine dependence. *Am J Drug Alcohol Abuse.* 2002;28:189.

Rickels K, DeMartinis N, Garcia-Espana F, Greenblatt DJ, Mandos LA, Rynn M. Imipramine and buspirone in treatment of patients with generalized anxiety disorder who are discontinuing long-term benzodiazepine therapy. *Am J Psychiatry.* 2000;157:1973.

Trappler B, Miyashiro AM. Bupropion-amantadine-associated neurotoxicity. *J Clin Psychiatry.* 2000;61:61.

Van Vliet IM, den Boer JA, Westenberg HG, Pian KL. Clinical effects of buspirone in social phobia: a double-blind placebo-controlled study. *J Clin Psychiatry.* 1997;58:164.

▲ 36.4.10 Calcium Channel Inhibitors

The calcium channel inhibitors are variously referred to as *calcium channel antagonists, calcium channel blockers,* and *organic calcium channel inhibitors.* The calcium channel inhibitors were first developed as cardiac drugs to treat hypertension, angina, and specific types of cardiac arrhythmias.

Calcium channel inhibitors are used in psychiatry as antimanic agents for persons who do not respond well to first-line agents such as lithium (Eskalith), valproic acid (Depakene), carbamazepine (Tegretol), or other anticonvulsants. Calcium channel inhibitors include nifedipine (Procardia, Adalat), nimodipine (Nimotop), isradipine (DynaCirc), amlodipine (Norvasc, Lotrel), nicardipine (Cardene), nisoldipine (Sular), nitrendipine, and verapamil (Calan). They are used for control of mania and ultradian bipolar disorder (mood cycling in less than 24 hours).

CHEMISTRY

The molecular structures of the calcium channel inhibitors that are most relevant to psychiatry are shown in Figure 36.4.10–1.

PHARMACOLOGICAL ACTIONS

The calcium channel inhibitors are well absorbed from the gastrointestinal (GI) tract, with significant first-pass hepatic metabolism. Considerable intraindividual and interindividual variations are seen in the plasma concentrations of the drugs after a single dose. The half-life of verapamil after the first dose is 2 to 8 hours; the half-life increases to 5 to 12 hours after the first few days of therapy. The half-lives of the other calcium channel blockers range from 1 to 2 hours for nimo-

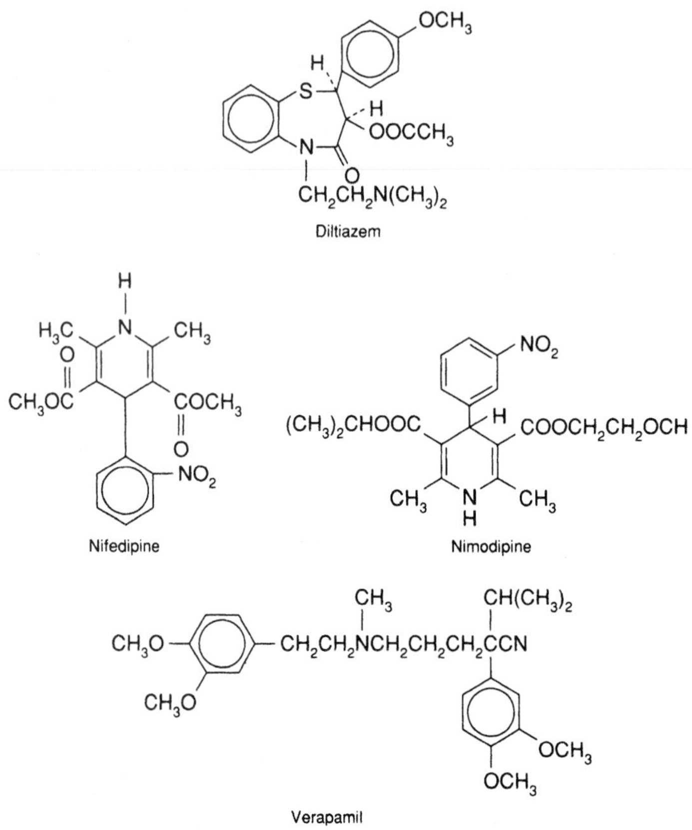

FIGURE 36.4.10–1
Molecular structures of calcium channel inhibitors.

dipine and isradipine, to 30 to 50 hours for amlodipine (Table 36.4.10–1).

The calcium channel inhibitors discussed in this section inhibit the influx of calcium into neurons through L-type (long-acting) voltage-dependent calcium channels. The calcium ion is a major intracellular second messenger. Intraneuronal calcium has many functions, including the activation of calcium-dependent protein kinases. Calcium influx may be one step in the cascade of molecular events that trigger excitotoxic cellular damage of the type postulated to lead to neuronal death, for example, in Alzheimer's disease.

EFFECTS OF SPECIFIC ORGANS AND SYSTEMS

The major effects of calcium channel inhibitors are on the vasculature, which responds with vasodilation to the calcium channel inhibitors. Diuresis has also been associated with the use of calcium channel inhibitors. The calcium channel inhibitors interfere with atrioventricular (AV) conduction and can lead to AV heart block, especially in elderly patients. Calcium channel blockers may also regulate ion flux directly in neurons.

Table 36.4.10–1
Half-Lives, Dosages, and Effectiveness of Selected Calcium Channel Inhibitors in Psychiatric Disorders

	Verapamil (Calan, Isoptin)	Nimodipine (Nimotop)	Isradipine (DynaCirc)	Amlodipine (Norvasc)
Half-life	Short (5–12 h)	Short (1–2 h)	Short (1½–2 h)	Long (30–50 h)
Starting dosage	30 mg tid	30 mg tid	2.5 mg bid	5 mg hs
Peak daily dosage	480 mg	240–450 mg	15 mg	10–15 mg
Antimanic	++	++	(++)	[a]
Antidepressant	±	+	(+)	[a]
Antiultradian[b]	±	++	(++)	[a]

[a]No systematic studies, only case reports.
[b]Rapid-cycling bipolar disorder.
Table adapted from Robert M. Post, M.D.

THERAPEUTIC INDICATIONS

Bipolar Disorder

There are mixed reports about the efficacy of verapamil for both short-term and maintenance treatment of bipolar disorders, to be used following trials of lithium, carbamazepine, and valproate. The other drugs, such as nimodipine, isradipine, and amlodipine, may be particularly effective in the treatment of manic episodes and of rapid-cycling or ultrarapid-cycling bipolar disorders. The clinician should begin treatment with a short-acting drug such as nimodipine or isradipine, beginning with a low dosage and increasing the dosage every 4 to 5 days until a clinical response is seen or adverse effects appear. Once symptoms are controlled, a longer-acting drug, such as amlodipine, can be substituted as maintenance therapy. Failure to respond to verapamil does not exclude a favorable response to one of the other drugs.

Recurrent Brief Depressive Disorder

This disorder, characterized by brief (1 to 3 days), but possibly severe, depressive episodes, may not be affected by standard antidepressants or lithium. Early experience shows that the calcium channel inhibitors may be effective for persons with recurrent brief depressive disorder; however, more trials are needed.

Other Psychiatric Indications

Calcium channel inhibitors may be beneficial in Tourette's disorder, Huntington's disease, Alzheimer's disease, panic disorder, premenstrual dysphoric disorder, and intermittent explosive disorder. Well-controlled studies have found a lack of efficacy for calcium channel inhibitors in schizophrenia, tardive dyskinesia, and major depression.

PRECAUTIONS AND ADVERSE REACTIONS

The most common adverse effects associated with calcium channel inhibitors are those due to vasodilation: dizziness, headache, tachycardia, nausea, dysesthesias, and peripheral edema. Verapamil and diltiazem (Cardizem) in particular can cause hypotension, bradycardia, and AV heart block, which necessitates close monitoring and sometimes discontinuation of the drugs. In all patients with cardiovascular disease, the drugs should be used with caution. Other common adverse effects include constipation, fatigue, rash, coughing, and wheezing. Adverse effects noted with diltiazem include hyperactivity, akathisia, and parkinsonism; with verapamil, delirium, hyperprolactinemia, and galactorrhea; with nimodipine, a subjective sense of chest tightness and skin flushing; and with nifedipine, depression. The drugs have not been evaluated for safety in pregnant women and are best avoided. Because the drugs are secreted in breast milk, nursing mothers should also avoid the drugs.

DRUG–DRUG INTERACTIONS

Calcium channel inhibitors should not be used by persons taking β-adrenergic receptor antagonists, hypotensives (e.g., diuretics, vasodilators, and angiotensin-converting enzyme inhibitors), or antiarrhythmic drugs (e.g., quinidine [Cardioquin] and digoxin [Lanoxin]) without consultation with an internist or cardiologist. Verapamil and diltiazem but not nifedipine have been reported to precipitate carbamazepine-induced neurotoxicity. Cimetidine (Tagamet) has been reported to increase plasma concentrations of nifedipine and diltiazem. Some patients who are treated with lithium and calcium channel inhibitors concurrently may be at increased risk for the signs and symptoms of neurotoxicity, and deaths have occurred.

LABORATORY INTERFERENCES

No known laboratory interferences are associated with the use of calcium channel inhibitors.

DOSAGE AND CLINICAL GUIDELINES

Verapamil is available in 40-, 80-, and 120-mg tablets; 120-, 180-, and 240-mg sustained-release tablets; and 100-, 120-, 180-, 200-, 240-, 300-, and 360-mg sustained-release capsules. The starting dosage is 40 mg orally three times a day and can be raised in increments every 4 to 5 days up to 80 to 120 mg three times a day. The patient's blood pressure, pulse, and electrocardiogram (ECG) (in patients more than 40 years old or with a history of cardiac illness) should be routinely monitored.

Nifedipine is available in 10- and 20-mg capsules and 30-, 60-, and 90-mg extended-release tablets. Administration should be started at 10 mg orally three or four times a day and can be increased up to a maximum dosage of 120 mg a day.

Nimodipine is available in 30-mg capsules. It has been used at 60 mg every 4 hours for ultrarapid-cycling bipolar disorder, and sometimes briefly at up to 630 mg per day.

Isradipine is available in 2.5- and 5-mg capsules and 5- or 10-mg controlled-release tablets. Administration should be started at 2.5 mg a day and can be increased up to a maximum of 15 mg a day in divided doses.

Amlodipine is available in 2.5-, 5-, and 10-mg tablets. Administration should start at 5 mg once at night and can be increased to a maximum dosage of 10 to 15 mg a day.

Diltiazem is available in 30-, 60-, 90-, and 120-mg tablets; 60-, 90-, 120-, 180-, 240-, 300-, and 360-mg extended-release capsules; and 60-, 90-, 120-, 180-, 240-, 300-, and 360-mg extended-release tablets. Administration should start with 30 mg orally four times a day and can be increased up to a maximum of 360 mg a day.

Elderly persons are more sensitive to the calcium channel inhibitors than younger adults. No specific information is available regarding the use of the agents for children.

References

Baldessarini RJ, Tarazi RI. Drugs and the treatment of psychiatric disorders: psychosis and mania. In: Hardman JG, Limbird LE, Goodman Gilman A, eds. *Goodman & Gilman's the Pharmacological Basis of Therapeutics.* 10th ed. New York: McGraw-Hill; 2001:485.

Delisi SM, Konopka LM, O'Connor FL, Crayton JW. Platelet cytosolic calcium responses to serotonin in depressed patients and controls: relationship to symptomatology and medication. *Biol Psychiatry.* 1998;43:327.

de Vry J, Fritze J, Post RM. The management of coexisting depression in patients with dementia: potential of calcium channel antagonists. *Clin Neuropharmacol.* 1977;20:22.

Dubovsky SL, Buzan RD. Novel alternatives and supplements to lithium and anticonvulsants for bipolar affective disorder. *J Clin Psychiatry.* 1997;58:224.

Dunn RT, Frye MS, Kimbrell TA, Denicoff KD, Leverich GS, Post RM. The efficacy and use of anticonvulsants in mood disorders. *Clin Neuropharmacol.* 1998;21:215.

Emamghoreishi M, Schlichter L, Li PP, et al. High intracellular calcium concentrations in transformed lymphoblasts from subjects with bipolar I disorder. *Am J Psychiatry.* 1997;154:976.

Janicak PG, Sharma RP, Pandey G, Davis JM. Verapamil for the treatment of acute mania: a double-blind, placebo-controlled trial. *Am J Psychiatry.* 1998;155:972.

Nonaka S, Hough CJ, Chuang DM. Chronic lithium treatment robustly protects neurons in the central nervous system against excitotoxicity by inhibiting *N*-methyl-D-aspartate receptor-mediated calcium influx. *Proc Natl Acad Sci U S A.* 1998;95:2642.

Pazzaglia PJ, Post RM, Ketter T, et al. Nimodipine monotherapy and carbamazepine augmentation in patients with refractory recurrent affective illness. *J Clin Psychopharmacol.* 1998;18:404.

Post RM. Calcium channel inhibitors. In: Sadock BJ, Sadock VA, eds. *Kaplan & Sadock's Comprehensive Textbook of Psychiatry.* 7th ed. Vol 2. Baltimore: Lippincott Williams & Wilkins; 2000:2334.

Post RM, Pazzaglia PJ, Ketter TA, et al. Carbamazepine and nimodipine in affective illness: efficacy, mechanisms of action, and interactions. In: Montgomery S, Halbreich U, eds. *Pharmacotherapy of Mood and Cognition.* Vol 4. Washington, DC: American Psychiatric Press; 1999:432.

Post RM, Weiss SRB, Clark M, Chuang DM, Hough C, Li H. Lithium, carbamazepine, and valproate in affective illness: biochemical and neurobiological mechanisms. In: Manji H, ed. *Mechanisms of Action of the Mood Stabilizers Lithium, Carbamazepine, and Valproate in Affective Illness.* Washington, DC: American Psychiatric Press; 1999:278.

Schumacher TB, Beck H, Steinhauser C, Schramm J, Elger CE. Effects of phenytoin, carbamazepine, and gabapentin on calcium channels in hippocampal granule cells from patients with temporal lobe epilepsy. *Epilepsia.* 1998;39:355.

Sze KH, Sim TC, Wong E, Cheng S, Woo J. Effect of nimodipine on memory after cerebral infarction. *Acta Neurol Scand.* 1998;97:386.

Taragano FE, Allegri R, Vicario A, Bagnatti P, Lyketsos CG. A double blind, randomized clinical trial assessing the efficacy and safety of augmenting standard antidepressant therapy with nimodipine in the treatment of "vascular depression." *Int J Geriatr Psychiatry.* 2001;16:254.

▲ 36.4.11 Carbamazepine

Carbamazepine (Tegretol) is effective for the treatment of acute mania and for the prophylactic treatment of bipolar I disorder. It is a first-line agent for these disorders along with lithium (Eskalith) and valproic acid (Depakene). Carbamazepine is also used to treat partial and generalized-onset epilepsy and trigeminal neuralgia. A congener, oxcarbazepine (Trileptal), is also available for use in bipolar disorder.

CHEMISTRY

The molecular structure of carbamazepine (Fig. 36.4.11–1) is similar to the tricyclic structure of imipramine (Tofranil).

PHARMACOLOGICAL ACTIONS

Carbamazepine is absorbed slowly and erratically from the gastrointestinal (GI) tract, and absorption is enhanced when the drug is taken with meals. Peak plasma concentrations are reached 2 to 8 hours after a single dose, and steady-state levels are reached after 2 to 4 days on a steady dosage. The suspension formulation is absorbed somewhat faster, and the extended-release formulation somewhat slower, than the standard formulation. The half-life of carbamazepine at the initiation of treatment has a wide range; after 1 month of administration the half-life decreases to a range of 12 to 17 hours because of the induction of hepatic enzymes, which reach their maximum level after about 1 month of therapy. The extended-release formulation permits achievement of smooth steady-state concentrations with twice-daily dosing. Carbamazepine is metabolized in the liver, and the 10,11-epoxide metabolite is active as an anticonvulsant; its activity in the treatment of bipolar disorders is unknown.

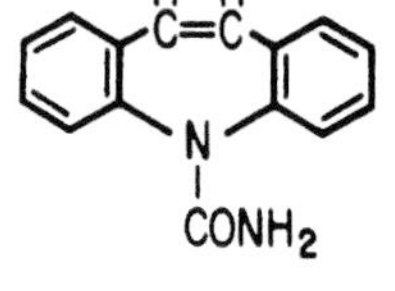

FIGURE 36.4.11–1
Molecular structure of carbamazepine.

The anticonvulsant effects of carbamazepine are attributed mainly to binding to voltage-dependent sodium channels in the inactive state and prolonging their inactivation. This secondarily reduces voltage-dependent calcium channel activation and, therefore, synaptic transmission. Additional effects include reduction of currents through *N*-methyl-D-aspartate (NMDA) glutamate-receptor channels, competitive antagonism of adenosine A_1 receptors, and potentiation of central nervous system (CNS) catecholamine neurotransmission. Whether any or all of these mechanisms also result in mood stabilization is not known.

EFFECTS ON SPECIFIC ORGANS AND SYSTEMS

Besides the effects on the CNS, carbamazepine has its most significant effects on the hematopoietic system. Carbamazepine is associated with a benign and often transient decrease in the white blood cell count, with values usually remaining above 3,000. The decrease is thought to be due to the inhibition of colony-stimulating factor in bone marrow, an effect that can be reversed by the coadministration of lithium, which stimulates the colony-stimulating factor. The benign suppression of white blood cell production must be differentiated from the potentially fatal adverse effects of agranulocytosis, pancytopenia, and aplastic anemia.

As reflected by its use in treating diabetes insipidus, carbamazepine apparently has a vasopressinlike effect on the vasopressin receptor and sometimes causes the development of water intoxication or hyponatremia, particularly in elderly patients. This adverse effect can be treated with demeclocycline (Declomycin) or lithium. Another endocrine effect associated with carbamazepine is an increase in urinary free cortisol.

Carbamazepine induces several hepatic enzymes and may thus interfere with the metabolism of various other drugs. The effects of carbamazepine on the cardiovascular system are minimal. It does decrease atrioventricular (A-V) conduction, and thus the use of carbamazepine is contraindicated in patients with A-V heart blocks.

Carbamazepine may cause a rash, which may be transient even if the drug is continued, but may lead to serious and potentially life-threatening dermatological conditions on rare occasions. Other system-specific allergic reactions have been reported, and rarely, a lupuslike disorder has been associated with use of carbamazepine.

THERAPEUTIC INDICATIONS

Bipolar Disorder

Manic Episodes. Carbamazepine is effective in the treatment of acute mania, with efficacy comparable to that of lithium and antipsychotics. Carbamazepine is also effective as a second-line agent in the prophylaxis of both manic and depressive episodes in bipolar disorders, after lithium and valproic acid. Carbamazepine is an effective antimanic agent in 50 to 70 percent of persons within 2 to 3 weeks of initiation, and it may be effective in some persons who are not responsive to lithium, such as those with dysphoric mania, rapid cycling, or a negative family history of mood disorders. The antimanic effects of carbamazepine can be augmented by concomitant administration of lithium, valproic acid, thyroid hormones, dopamine receptor antagonists, or serotonin-dopamine antagonists. Some persons may respond to carbamazepine but not lithium or valproic acid, and vice versa. Tolerance for the antimanic effects of carbamazepine can develop in some persons.

Depressive Episodes. The available data indicate that carbamazepine is an effective treatment for depression in some persons. About 25 to 33 percent of depressed persons respond to carbamazepine. That percentage is significantly smaller than the 60 to 70 percent response rate for standard antidepressants. Nevertheless, carbamazepine is an alternative drug for depressed persons who have not responded to conventional treatments, including electroconvulsive therapy (ECT) or who have marked or rapid periodicity in their depressive episodes.

Schizophrenia and Schizoaffective Disorder

Carbamazepine is effective in the treatment of schizophrenia and schizoaffective disorder. Persons with prominent positive symptoms (e.g., hallucinations) may be likely to respond, as are persons who display impulsive aggressive outbursts.

Impulse-Control Disorders

Several studies have reported that carbamazepine is effective in controlling impulsive, aggressive behavior in nonpsychotic persons of all ages, including children and the elderly. Other drugs for impulse-control disorders, particularly intermittent explosive disorder, include lithium, propranolol (Inderal), and antipsychotics. Because of the risk of serious adverse effects with carbamazepine, treatment with other agents is warranted before initiating a trial with carbamazepine.

Carbamazepine is also effective in controlling nonacute agitation and aggressive behavior in schizophrenic persons. Diagnoses to be ruled out before initiating treatment with carbamazepine include akathisia and neuroleptic malignant syndrome. Lorazepam (Ativan) is more effective than carbamazepine for the control of acute agitation.

Posttraumatic Stress Disorder

Carbamazepine has been suggested, along with antidepressants, benzodiazepines, lithium, β-adrenergic receptor antagonists, and α_2-adrenergic receptor agonists, as a treatment for posttraumatic stress disorder (PTSD). Carbamazepine is particularly useful for management of agitation and aggression in PTSD.

Table 36.4.11–1
Adverse Events Associated with Carbamazepine

Dosage-Related Adverse Effects	Idiosyncratic Adverse Effects
Double or blurred vision	Agranulocytosis
Vertigo	Stevens-Johnson syndrome
Gastrointestinal disturbances	Aplastic anemia
Task performance impairment	Hepatic failure
Hematological effects	Rash
	Pancreatitis

Alcohol and Benzodiazepine Withdrawal

According to several studies, carbamazepine is as effective as the benzodiazepines in the control of symptoms associated with alcohol withdrawal. It may also assist in withdrawal from chronic alcohol or benzodiazepine use, especially in seizure-prone persons. However, the lack of any advantage of carbamazepine over the benzodiazepines for alcohol withdrawal and the potential risk of adverse effects with carbamazepine limit the clinical usefulness of this application.

PRECAUTIONS AND ADVERSE REACTIONS

Although the drug's hematological effects are not dose related, most of the adverse effects of carbamazepine are correlated with plasma concentrations above 9 μg/mL. The rarest but most serious adverse effects of carbamazepine are blood dyscrasias, hepatitis, and exfoliative dermatitis (Table 36.4.11–1). Otherwise, carbamazepine is relatively well tolerated by persons except for mild GI and CNS effects that can be significantly reduced if the dosage is increased slowly and minimal effective plasma concentrations are maintained.

Blood Dyscrasias

Severe blood dyscrasias (aplastic anemia, agranulocytosis) occur in about 1 in 125,000 persons treated with carbamazepine. There does not appear to be a correlation between the degree of benign white blood cell suppression (leukopenia), which is seen in 1 to 2 percent of persons, and the emergence of life-threatening blood dyscrasias. Persons should be warned that the emergence of such symptoms as fever, sore throat, rash, petechiae, bruising, and easy bleeding can potentially herald a serious dyscrasia and should cause them to seek medical evaluation immediately. Routine hematological monitoring in carbamazepine-treated persons is recommended at 3, 6, 9, and 12 months. If there is no significant evidence of bone marrow suppression by that time, many experts would reduce the monitoring interval. However, even assiduous monitoring may fail to detect severe blood dyscrasias before they cause symptoms.

Hepatitis

Within the first few weeks of therapy, carbamazepine can cause both a hepatitis associated with increases in liver enzymes, particularly transaminases, and a cholestasis associated with elevated bilirubin and alkaline phosphatase. Mild transaminase elevations warrant observation only, but persistent elevations that exceed three times the upper limit of normal indicate discontinuation of carbamazepine. Hepatitis can recur if the drug is reintroduced to the person and can result in death.

Exfoliative Dermatitis

A benign pruritic rash occurs in 10 to 15 percent of persons treated with carbamazepine, usually within the first few weeks of treatment. Approximately three persons per million per week may experience life-threatening dermatological syndromes, including exfoliative dermatitis, erythema multiforme, Stevens-Johnson syndrome, and toxic epidermal necrolysis. The possible emergence of these serious dermatological problems causes most clinicians to discontinue carbamazepine use in a person who develops any type of rash. If carbamazepine seems to be the only effective drug for a person who has a benign rash with carbamazepine treatment, a retrial of the drug can be undertaken with pretreatment of the person with prednisone (40 mg a day) in an attempt to treat the rash, although other symptoms of an allergic reaction (e.g., fever and pneumonitis) may develop, even with steroid pretreatment. The risk of drug rash is about equal between valproic acid and carbamazepine in the first 2 months of use but is subsequently much higher for carbamazepine.

Gastrointestinal Effects

The most common adverse effects of carbamazepine are nausea, vomiting, gastric distress, constipation, diarrhea, and anorexia. The severity of the adverse effects is reduced if the dosage of carbamazepine is increased slowly and kept at the minimal effective plasma concentration. Unlike lithium and valproate, carbamazepine does not appear to cause weight gain.

Central Nervous System Effects

Acute confusional states can occur with carbamazepine alone but occur most often in combination with lithium or antipsychotic drugs. Elderly persons and persons with cognitive disorders are at increased risk for CNS toxicity from carbamazepine. The symptoms of CNS toxicity include dizziness, ataxia, clumsiness, sedation, diplopia, hyperreflexia, clonus, and tremor. These symptoms can be reduced by slow upward titration of the dosage. The incidence of cognitive disturbances about equals that with carbamazepine, lithium, and valproic acid.

Other Adverse Effects

Carbamazepine decreases cardiac conduction (although less than the tricyclic drugs do) and thus can exacerbate preexisting cardiac disease. Carbamazepine should be used with caution in persons with glaucoma, prostatic hypertrophy, diabetes, or a history of alcohol abuse. Carbamazepine occasionally activates vasopressin-receptor function, which results in a condition resembling the syndrome of secretion of inappropriate antidiuretic hormone (SIADH), characterized by hyponatremia and (rarely) water intoxication. This is the opposite of the renal effects of lithium (i.e., nephrogenic diabetes insipidus). Augmentation of lithium with carbamazepine does not reverse the lithium effect, however. Emergence of confusion, severe weakness, or headache in a person taking carbamazepine should prompt measurement of serum electrolytes. Carbamazepine use (rarely) elicits an immune hypersensitivity response consisting of fever, rash, eosinophilia, and possibly fatal myocarditis.

Some evidence indicates that minor cranial facial abnormalities, fingernail hypoplasia, and spina bifida in infants may be associated with maternal use of carbamazepine during pregnancy. Therefore, pregnant women should not use carbamazepine unless absolutely necessary. The risk of neural tube defects can be reduced by maternal intake of folic acid 1 to 4 mg daily for at least 3 months prior to conception. Carbamazepine is secreted in breast milk, but its use during breast-feeding is considered safe by the American Academy of Pediatrics.

DRUG–DRUG INTERACTIONS

Principally because it induces several hepatic enzymes, carbamazepine may interact with many drugs (Table 36.4.11–2). For the most part, addition of carbamazepine lowers the plasma concentrations of affected drugs, and monitoring for decreased clinical effects is frequently indicated. Coadministration with lithium, antipsychotic drugs, verapamil (Calan), or nifedipine (Procardia) can precipitate carbamazepine-induced CNS adverse effects. Carbamazepine can decrease the concentrations of oral contraceptives in blood, resulting in breakthrough bleeding and uncertain prophylaxis against pregnancy. Carbamazepine should not be administered with monoamine oxidase inhibitors (MAOIs), which should be discontinued at least 2 weeks before initiating treatment with carbamazepine. Carbamazepine may significantly induce the metabolism of bupropion (Wellbutrin).

LABORATORY INTERFERENCES

Carbamazepine treatment is associated with a transient decrease in thyroid hormones (thyroxine [T_4] and triiodothyronine [T_3]) without an associated increase in thyroid-stimulating hormone (TSH). Carbamazepine is also associated with an increase in total serum cholesterol, primarily by increasing high-density lipoproteins. The thyroid and cholesterol effects are not clinically significant. Carbamazepine may interfere with the dexamethasone suppression test and may also cause false-positive pregnancy test results.

DOSAGE AND CLINICAL GUIDELINES

Carbamazepine can be used alone or with an antipsychotic drug for the treatment of manic episodes, although carbamazepine-induced CNS adverse effects (drowsiness, dizziness, ataxia) are likely to occur with this combination of drugs. Persons who do not respond to lithium alone may respond when carbamazepine is added to the lithium treatment. If a person then responds, an attempt should be made to withdraw the lithium to assess

Table 36.4.11–2
Carbamazepine–Drug Interactions

Effect of Carbamazepine on Plasma Concentrations of Concomitant Agents		Agents That May Affect Carbamazepine Plasma Concentrations	
Carbamazepine may decrease drug plasma concentration of		*Agents that may increase carbamazepine plasma concentration*	
Acetaminophen	Haloperidol	Allopurinol	Itraconazole
Alprazolam	Hormonal contraceptives	Cimetidine	Lamotrigine
Amitriptyline	Imipramine	Clarithromycin	Loratadine
Bupropion	Lamotrigine	Danazol	Macrolides
Clomipramine	Methadone	Diltiazem	Nefazodone
Clonazepam	Methsuximide	Erythromycin	Nicotinamide
Clozapine	Methylprednisolone	Fluoxetine	Propoxyphene
Cyclosporine	Nimodipine	Fluvoxamine	Terfenadine
Desipramine	Pancuronium	Gemfibrozil	Troleandomycin
Dicumarol	Phensuximide	Itraconazole	Valproate[a]
Doxepin	Phenytoin	Ketoconazole	Verapamil
Doxycycline	Primidone	Isoniazid[a]	Viloxazine
Ethosuximide	Theophylline	*Drugs that may decrease carbamazepine plasma concentrations*	
Felbamate	Valproate	Carbamazepine (autoinduction)	Phenytoin
Fentanyl	Warfarin	Cisplatin	Primidone
Fluphenazine		Doxorubicin HCl	Rifampin[b]
Carbamazepine may increase drug plasma concentrations of		Felbamate	Theophylline
Clomipramine	Primidone	Phenobarbital	Valproate
Phenytoin			

[a]Increased concentrations of the active 10, 11-epoxide.
[b]Decreased concentrations of carbamazepine and increased concentrations of the 10, 11-epoxide.
Table by Carlos A. Zarate, Jr., M.D., and Mauricio Tohen, M.D.

whether the person can be treated successfully with carbamazepine alone. When lithium and carbamazepine are used together, the clinician should minimize or discontinue any antipsychotics, sedatives, or anticholinergic drugs the person may be taking, to reduce the risks for adverse effects associated with taking multiple drugs. The combination of lithium and carbamazepine must be monitored closely for CNS toxicity, which may be fatal if not properly treated. Lithium and the carbamazepine should both be used at standard therapeutic plasma concentrations before a trial of combined therapy is considered to have been a therapeutic failure. A 3-week trial of carbamazepine at therapeutic plasma concentrations usually suffices to determine whether the drug will be effective in the treatment of acute mania; a longer trial is necessary to assess efficacy in the treatment of depression. Carbamazepine is also used in combination with valproic acid, another anticonvulsant that is effective in bipolar disorders. When carbamazepine and valproate are used in combination, the dosage of carbamazepine should be decreased, because valproate displaces carbamazepine binding on proteins, and the dosage of valproate may need to be increased.

Pretreatment Medical Evaluation

The person's medical history should include information about preexisting hematological, hepatic, and cardiac diseases, because all three can be relative contraindications for carbamazepine treatment. Persons with hepatic disease require only one third to one half the usual dosage; the clinician should be cautious about raising the dosage in such persons and should do so only slowly and gradually. The laboratory examination should include a complete blood count with platelet count, liver function tests, serum electrolytes, and an electrocardiogram in persons more than 40 years of age or with a preexisting cardiac disease. An electroencephalogram (EEG) is not necessary before the initiation of treatment, but it may be helpful in some cases for the documentation of objective changes correlated with clinical improvement.

Initiation of Treatment

Carbamazepine is available in 100- and 200-mg tablets and as a 100 mg/5 mL suspension. The usual starting dosage is 200 mg orally two times a day; however, with titration, three-times-a-day dosing is optimal. An extended-release version suitable for twice-a-day maintenance dosing is available in 100-, 200-, and 400-mg tablets. Carbamazepine should be taken with meals, and the drug should be stored in a cool, dry place. Carbamazepine can lose one third of its potency when stored in a humid environment, such as a bathroom. In a hospital setting with seriously ill persons, the dosage can be raised by not more than 200 mg a day until a dosage of 600 to 1,200 mg a day is reached. This relatively rapid titration, however, is often associated with adverse effects and may adversely affect compliance with the drug. In less ill persons and in outpatients, the dosage should be raised no more quickly than 200 mg every 2 to 7 days to minimize the occurrence of minor adverse effects such as nausea, vomiting, drowsiness, and dizziness. When discontinuing treatment with carbamazepine, the clinician generally

Table 36.4.11–3
Laboratory Monitoring of Carbamazepine for Adult Psychiatric Disorders

	Baseline	Weekly to Stability	Monthly for 6 Mo	6–12 Mo
CBC[a]	+	+	+	+
Bilirubin	+		+	+
Alanine aminotransferase	+		+	+
Aspartate aminotransferase	+		+	+
Alkaline phosphatase	+		+	+
Carbamazepine level		+		+

[a]Complete blood count.

should taper the dosage, although the drug can safely be stopped abruptly in most persons.

Blood Concentrations

The anticonvulsant blood concentration range for carbamazepine is 4 to 12 μg/mL, and this range should be reached before determining that carbamazepine is not effective in the treatment of a mood disorder. It is clinically prudent to come up to that range gradually, since the person is likely to tolerate a gradual increase of carbamazepine better than a rapid increase. The clinician should titrate carbamazepine up to the highest well-tolerated dosage before deciding that the drug is ineffective. Plasma concentrations should be determined when a person has been receiving a steady dosage for at least 5 days. Blood for the determination of plasma levels is drawn in the morning, before the first daily dose of carbamazepine is taken. The total daily dosage necessary to achieve plasma concentrations in the usual therapeutic range varies from 400 to 1,600 mg a day, with a mean around 1,000 mg a day.

Routine Laboratory Monitoring

The most serious potential effects of carbamazepine are agranulocytosis and aplastic anemia. Although it has been suggested that complete laboratory blood assessments be performed every 2 weeks for the first 2 months of treatment and quarterly thereafter, this conservative approach may not be justified by a cost-benefit analysis and may not detect a serious blood dyscrasia before it occurs. The Food and Drug Administration (FDA) has revised the package insert for carbamazepine to suggest that blood monitoring be performed at the discretion of the physician. Education about the signs and the symptoms of a developing hematological problem is probably more effective than frequent blood monitoring in protecting against blood dyscrasias. It has also been suggested that liver and renal function tests be conducted quarterly, although the benefit of conducting tests this frequently has been questioned. It seems reasonable, however, to assess hematological status, along with liver and renal functions, whenever a routine examination of the person is being conducted. A monitoring protocol is listed in Table 36.4.11–3.

The following laboratory values should prompt the physician to discontinue carbamazepine treatment and to consult a hematologist: total white blood cell count below 3,000/mm^3, erythrocyte count below 4.0×10^6 per mm^3, neutrophil count below 1,500/mm^3, hematocrit less than 32 percent, hemoglobin less than 11 g per 100 mL, platelet count below 100,000/mm^3, reticulocyte count below 0.3 percent, and a serum iron concentration below 150 mg per 100 mL.

References

Bernus I, Dickinson RG, Hooper WD, Eadie MJ. The mechanism of the carbamazepine-valproate interaction in humans. *Br J Clin Pharmacol.* 1997;44:21.

Denicoff KD, Smith-Jackson EE, Disney ER, Ali SO, Leverich GS, Post RM. Comparative prophylactic efficacy of lithium, carbamazepine, and the combination in bipolar disorder. *J Clin Psychiatry.* 1997;58:470.

Greil W, Ludwig-Mayerhofer W, Erazo N, et al. Lithium versus carbamazepine in the maintenance treatment of bipolar disorders—a randomized study. *J Affect Disord.* 1997;43:151.

Hardman JG, Limbird LE, Goodman Gilman A, eds. *Goodman & Gilman's the Pharmacological Basis of Therapeutics.* 10th ed. New York: McGraw-Hill; 2001.

Keck PE Jr, Mendlwicz J, Calabrese JR, et al. A review of randomized controlled clinical trials in acute mania. *J Affect Disord.* 2000;59:S31.

Leucht S, McGrath J, White P, Kissling W. Carbamazepine augmentation for schizophrenia: how good is the evidence? *J Clin Psychiatry.* 2002;63:218.

Tariot PN, Porteinsson AP. Anticonvulsants to treat agitation in dementia. *Int Psychogeriatr.* 2000;12:237.

Woolston JL. Case-study: carbamazepine treatment of juvenile-onset bipolar disorder. *J Am Acad Child Adolesc Psychiatry.* 1999;38:335.

Yukawa E, Honda T, Ohdo S, Higuchi S, Aoyama T. Detection of carbamazepine-induced changes in valproic acid relative clearance in man by simple pharmacokinetic screening. *J Pharm Pharmacol.* 1997;49:751.

Zarate CA, Tohen M. Carbamazepine. In: Sadock BJ, Sadock VA, eds. *Kaplan & Sadock's Comprehensive Textbook of Psychiatry.* 7th ed. Vol 2. Baltimore: Lippincott Williams & Wilkins; 2000:2329.

▲ 36.4.12 Chloral Hydrate

Chloral hydrate, in use since 1869, is one of the oldest sedative-hypnotic drugs. Because many compounds were later introduced, chloral hydrate is now prescribed only as a short-term (2- or 3-day) hypnotic. It is rarely used because there are safer options, such as the benzodiazepines.

CHEMISTRY

Chloral hydrate's molecular structure is shown in Figure 36.4.12–1.

PHARMACOLOGICAL ACTIONS

Chloral hydrate is well absorbed from the gastrointestinal (GI) tract. The parent compound is metabolized within minutes by

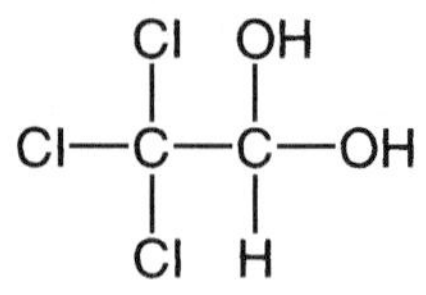

FIGURE 36.4.12–1
Molecular structure of chloral hydrate.

the liver to the active metabolite trichloroethanol, which has a half-life of 8 to 11 hours. A dose of chloral hydrate induces sleep in about 30 to 60 minutes and maintains sleep for 4 to 8 hours. It probably potentiates γ-aminobutyric (GABAergic) neurotransmission, which suppresses neuronal excitability.

EFFECTS ON SPECIFIC ORGANS AND SYSTEMS

In addition to its central nervous system (CNS) effects, chloral hydrate has effects on the GI system and the skin. The GI effects include nonspecific irritation, nausea, vomiting, flatulence, and an unpleasant taste. The dermatological effects, although uncommon, include rashes, urticaria, purpura, eczema, and erythema multiforme. The dermatological lesions are sometimes accompanied by fever.

THERAPEUTIC INDICATIONS

The major indication for chloral hydrate is insomnia. Whether chloral hydrate affects rapid eye movement (REM) sleep is controversial, but patients experience no REM rebound after discontinuation of chloral hydrate therapy. Long-term treatment with chloral hydrate is associated with an increased incidence and severity of adverse effects. Tolerance develops to the hypnotic effects of chloral hydrate after 2 weeks of treatment.

PRECAUTIONS AND ADVERSE REACTIONS

The most common GI adverse effects are nausea, vomiting, and diarrhea. Patients should be warned that they may experience residual daytime sedation and impaired motor coordination. Chloral hydrate should be avoided in patients with severe renal, cardiac, or hepatic disease or with porphyria. The drug may aggravate GI inflammatory conditions. Chloral hydrate should not be used during pregnancy or by nursing women. It is not expected to cause particular difficulties in children or older adults. It may be used as a sedative for diagnostic procedures in children weighing up to 25 kg.

In addition to the development of tolerance, chloral hydrate dependence can occur, with symptoms similar to those of alcohol dependence. The symptoms of intoxication include confusion, ataxia, dysarthria, bradycardia, arrhythmia, and severe drowsiness. The lethal adult dose of chloral hydrate has ranged between 5 and 40 g; thus the drug is a particularly poor choice for potentially suicidal patients. The lethality of the drug is potentiated by other CNS depressants, including alcohol. With long-term use and overdose, gastritis and gastric ulceration can develop. Hepatic and renal damage can follow overdose attempts, which may result in jaundice and albuminuria.

DRUG–DRUG INTERACTIONS

Chloral hydrate sedation occurs in addition to sedation due to other centrally acting agents. Because of metabolic interference, chloral hydrate should be strictly avoided with alcohol, a notorious concoction known as a "Mickey Finn." Use of chloral hydrate less than 24 hours before receiving intravenous furosemide (Lasix) can cause diaphoresis, flushes, and unsteady blood pressure. Chloral hydrate may displace warfarin (Coumadin) from plasma proteins and enhance anticoagulant activity; this combination should be avoided.

LABORATORY INTERFERENCES

Chloral hydrate administration can lead to false-positive results for urine glucose determinations that use cupric sulfate (e.g., Clinitest) but not in tests that use glucose oxidase (e.g., Clinistix and Tes-Tape). Chloral hydrate may also interfere with the determination of urinary catecholamines and 17-hydroxycorticosteroids.

DOSAGE AND CLINICAL GUIDELINES

Chloral hydrate is available in 500-mg capsules, 500 mg/5 mL solution, and 324-, 500-, and 648-mg rectal suppositories. The standard dose of chloral hydrate is 500 to 2,000 mg at bedtime. Because the drug is a GI irritant, it should be administered with excess water, milk, other liquids, or antacids to decrease gastric irritation.

References

Charney DS, Mihic SJ, Harris RA. In: Hardman JG, Limbird LE, Goodman Gilman A, eds. *Goodman & Gilman's the Pharmacological Basis of Therapeutics.* 10th ed. New York: McGraw-Hill; 2001:399.

Labbate LA, Arana GW, Ballenger JC. Chloral hydrate. In: Sadock BJ, Sadock VA, eds. *Kaplan & Sadock's Comprehensive Textbook of Psychiatry.* 7th ed. Vol 2. Baltimore: Lippincott Williams & Wilkins; 2000:2343.

Lovinger DM, Zimmerman SA, Levitan M, Harrison NL. Trichloroethanol potentiates synaptic transmission mediated by gamma-aminobutyric acid A receptors in hippocampal neurons. *J Pharmacol Exp Ther.* 1993;264:1097.

McEvoy GK, ed. *AHFS 2002 Drug Information.* Bethesda, MD: American Society of Health-System Pharmacists; 2002.

Solt K, Johansson JS. Binding of the active metabolite of chloral hydrate, 2,2,2-trichloroethanol, to serum albumin demonstrated using tryptophan fluorescence quenching. *Pharmacology.* 2002;64:152.

Vade A, Sukhani R, Dolenga M, Habisohn-Schuck C. Chloral hydrate sedation of children undergoing CT and MR imaging: safety as judged by American Academy of Pediatrics guidelines. *Am Roentgenol.* 1995;165:905.

Yamada A, Ohshima Y, Tsukahara H, et al. Two cases of anaphylactic reaction to gelatin induced by a chloral hydrate suppository. *Pediatr Int.* 2002;44:87.

▲ 36.4.13 Cholinesterase Inhibitors

Four drugs have been approved by the Federal Drug Administration (FDA) for treatment of Alzheimer's disease and similar disorders with cognitive deficits; tacrine (Cognex), rivastigmine (Exelon), galantamine (Reminyl), and donepezil (Aricept). These drugs are cholinesterase inhibitors, which reduce intrasynaptic cleavage and inactivation of acetylcholine and thus potentiate cholinergic neurotransmission (Fig. 36.4.13–1), which in turn tends to produce modest improvement in memory and goal-directed thought.

At one time tacrine was the only drug available, but several untoward effects, especially hepatic toxicity that required weekly blood tests, rendered it useful to only a minority of patients with Alzheimer's disease. Later, donepezil, was approved, which has a simpler dosage regimen, has fewer adverse effects, and does not require weekly blood tests. Rivastigmine and galantamine followed, also with a safer profile. Other similar agents are in the investigational stages of development but are not yet available for use in the United States, including sustained-release physostigmine salicylate

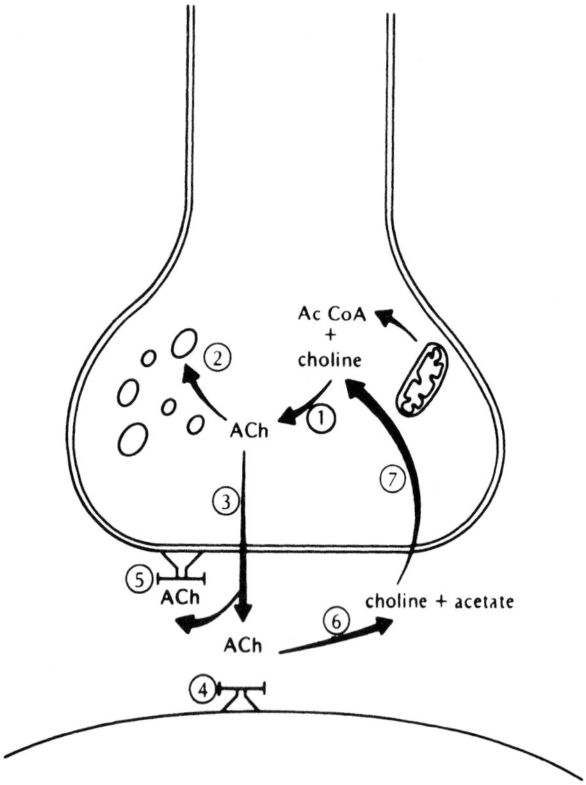

FIGURE 36.4.13–1
Potential sites of drug action at cholinergic synapses. Acetylcholinesterase inhibitors, such as donepezil and tacrine, block the hydrolysis of acetylcholine (*Ach*) in the synaptic cleft (*6*) and therefore prolong the action of secreted Ach. Anticholinergic drugs, such as benztropine and trihexyphenidyl, block presynaptic (*5*) and postsynaptic (*4*) muscarinic receptors and therefore reduce the action of intrasynaptic ACh. Other sites of potential drug action for which no clinical agents are yet available include synthesis of ACh (*1*), transport of ACh into vesicles (*2*), secretion of ACh into the synaptic cleft (*3*), and reuptake of choline (*7*). (Reprinted with permission from Cooper JR, Bloom FE, Roth RH. *The Biochemical Basis of Neuropharmacology.* 7th ed. New York: Oxford University Press; 1996:221.)

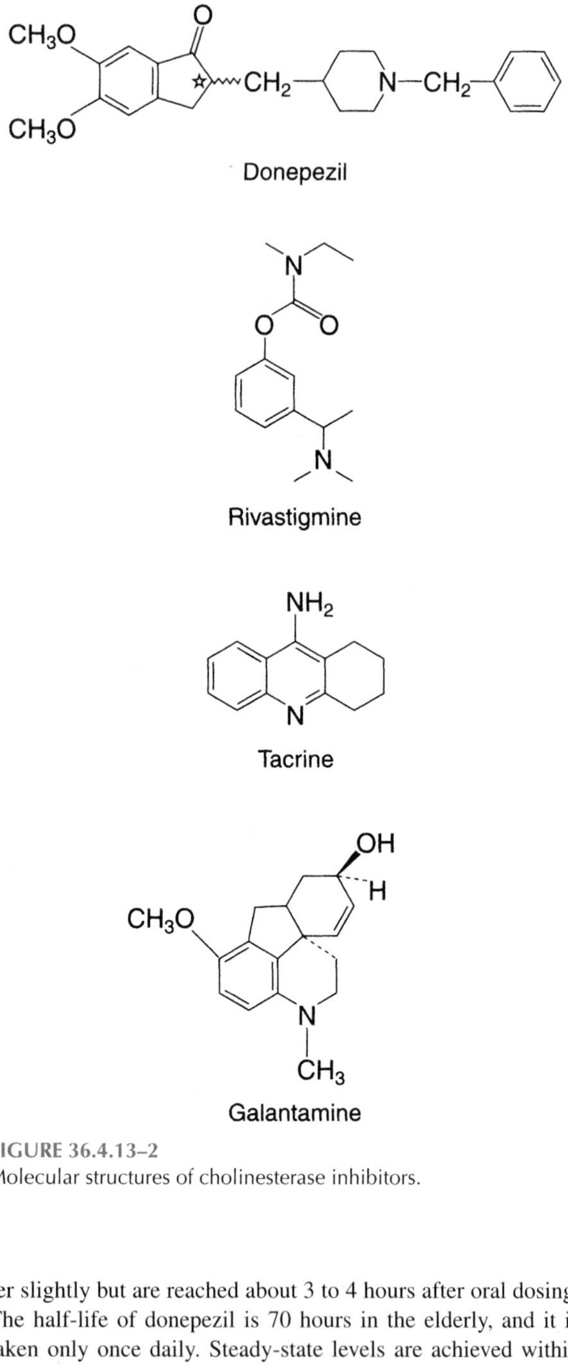

FIGURE 36.4.13–2
Molecular structures of cholinesterase inhibitors.

(Synapton), suronacrine, eptastigmine, and metrifonate. These drugs are considered most useful for patients who have mild to moderate memory loss but nevertheless have enough of their basal forebrain cholinergic neurons to benefit from augmentation of cholinergic neurotransmission.

Memantine, an *N*-methyl-D-aspartate (NMDA) receptor antagonist is under investigation. It is not a cholinesterase inhibitor and works by protecting neurons from excessive stimulation by glutamate, a possible factor in the cause of Alzheimer's disease.

Memantine is discussed separately below.

CHEMISTRY

The molecular structures of donepezil, rivastigmine, tacrine, and galantamine are shown in Figure 36.4.13–2.

PHARMACOLOGICAL ACTIONS

All of the cholinesterase inhibiters are readily absorbed from the gastrointestinal (GI) tract. Peak plasma concentrations differ slightly but are reached about 3 to 4 hours after oral dosing. The half-life of donepezil is 70 hours in the elderly, and it is taken only once daily. Steady-state levels are achieved within about 2 weeks. Presence of stable alcoholic cirrhosis reduces clearance of donepezil by 20 percent. Rivastigmine and galantamine reach peak plasma concentrations in 1 hour. The actions of both drugs may be delayed by up to 90 minutes if taken with food. The half-life of rivastigmine is 1 hour, but because it remains bound to cholinesterases, a single dose is therapeutically active for 10 hours, and it is taken twice daily.

Peak plasma concentrations of tacrine are reached about 90 minutes after oral dosing. The half-life of tacrine is about 2 to 4 hours, thereby necessitating four-times-daily dosing; galantamine has a half-life of about 7 hours and is given twice daily.

Galantamine is an agonist at nicotinic sites without producing desensitization, as well as a cholinesterase inhibitor. This

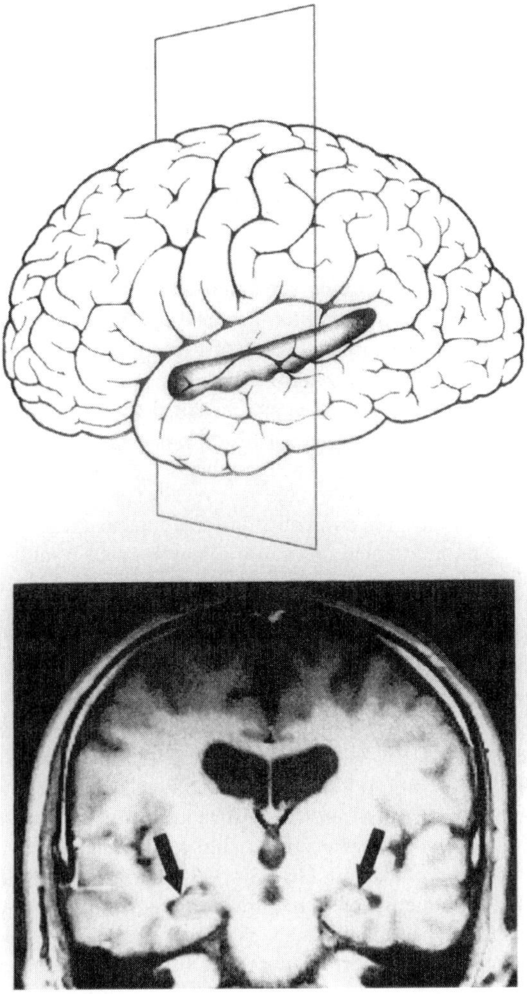

FIGURE 36.4.13–3

The hippocampus is a major site of action of memory-enhancing acetylcholinesterase inhibitors. **Upper:** Schematic depiction of the hippocampus in the temporal lobe. **Lower:** Magnetic resonance image in the coronal plane at the level indicated in the upper drawing. *Arrows* denote the hippocampi at the inner border of the temporal lobes. (Reprinted with permission from Spitzer M. *Geist im Netz.* Heidelberg: Spektrum Akdademischer Verlag; 1996:215.)

ability to enhance the sensitivity of the acetylcholine receptor is possessed only by galantamine and physostigmine. The mechanism of action is analogous to that of benzodiazepines at the γ-aminobutyric acid (GABA) A site. Consequently, the drug has an in vivo cholinomimetic activity that is even stronger than its acetylcholinesterase inhibitory properties alone would predict.

The primary mechanism of action of cholinesterase inhibitors is reversible, nonacylating inhibition of acetylcholinesterase and butyrylcholinesterase, the enzymes that catabolize acetylcholine in the central nervous system (CNS). The enzyme inhibition increases synaptic concentrations of acetylcholine, especially in hippocampus and cerebral cortex (Fig. 36.4.13–3). Unlike tacrine, which is nonselective for all forms of acetylcholinesterase, donepezil appears to be selectively active within the CNS and to have little activity in the periphery. Donepezil's favorable adverse effect profile appears to correlate with its lack of inhibition of cholinesterases in the GI tract. Rivastigmine and galantamine appear to have somewhat more peripheral activity than donepezil and are thus more likely to cause GI adverse effects than donepezil is.

Effects on Specific Organs and Systems

In addition to its effects on cognitive performance, tacrine affects the liver and the parasympathetic nervous system. Tacrine is associated with an increase in hepatic enzymes—serum glutamic-oxaloacetic transaminase (SGOT) and serum glutamic-pyruvic transaminase (SGPT)—in 25 to 30 percent of patients. Because of its cholinomimetic properties, tacrine causes activation of the parasympathetic nervous system, which results in all the usual signs and symptoms of muscarinic activity: nausea, vomiting, diarrhea, and other autonomic symptoms. The other drugs in this class have little or no hepatotoxic effect, although they may produce GI activation with nausea, vomiting, and anorexia.

THERAPEUTIC INDICATIONS

Donepezil, rivastigmine, galantamine, and tacrine are effective for the treatment of cognitive impairment in dementia of the Alzheimer's type. Based on numerous well-controlled studies, the cholinesterase inhibitors in long-term use slow the progression of memory loss and diminish apathy, depression, hallucinations, anxiety, euphoria, and purposeless motor behaviors. Functional autonomy (i.e., the ability to carry out the activities of daily living) is less well preserved. Some persons note immediate improvement in memory, mood, psychotic symptoms, and interpersonal skills. Others note little initial benefit but are able to retain their cognitive and adaptive faculties at a relatively stable level for many months. Use of cholinesterase inhibitors may delay or reduce the need for nursing home placement.

Donepezil may be beneficial for the treatment of dementia due to diffuse Lewy body disease and for treatment of cognitive deficits due to traumatic brain injury. Donepezil is under study for treatment of cognitive impairment less severe than that due to Alzheimer's disease. People with multiinfarction and other types of dementia may not respond to acetylcholinesterase inhibitors. Occasionally, cholinesterase inhibitors elicit an idiosyncratic catastrophic reaction, with signs of grief and agitation, which is self-limited once the drug is discontinued. Use of cholinesterase inhibitors to improve cognition by nondemented individuals should be discouraged.

PRECAUTIONS AND ADVERSE REACTIONS

Donepezil

Donepezil is generally well tolerated at recommended dosages. Less than 3 percent of persons taking donepezil experience nausea, diarrhea, and vomiting. These mild symptoms are more common with a 10-mg dose than with a 5-mg dose, and they tend to resolve after 3 weeks of continued use. Donepezil may cause weight loss. Donepezil treatment has been infrequently associated with bradyarrhythmias, especially in persons with underlying cardiac disease. A small number of persons experience syncope.

Rivastigmine

Rivastigmine is generally well tolerated, but recommended dosages may need to be scaled back in the initial period of treatment to limit GI and CNS adverse effects. These mild symptoms are more common at dosages above 6 mg a day, and they tend to resolve once the dosage is lowered. The most common adverse effects associated with rivastigmine are nausea, vomiting, dizziness, headache, diarrhea, abdominal pain, anorexia, fatigue, and somnolence. Rivastigmine may cause weight loss, but it does not appear to cause hepatic, renal, hematological, or electrolyte abnormalities.

Galantamine

Galantamine is well tolerated and at 8 mg a day produced improved cognition in patients with mild or moderate impairment. With higher doses (24 mg a day) the risk of adverse effects, including syncope, increases. Adverse effects are primarily GI, are dose related, and in about 5 percent of patients lead to discontinuation of use of the drug.

Tacrine

Tacrine is cumbersome to titrate and use, and it poses the risk of potentially significant elevations in hepatic transaminase levels in 25 to 30 percent of persons, nausea and vomiting in about 20 percent of persons, and diarrhea and other cholinergic symptoms in about 11 percent of persons. Aside from elevated transaminase levels, the most common specific adverse effects associated with tacrine treatment are nausea, vomiting, myalgia, anorexia, and rash, but only nausea, vomiting, and anorexia are clearly related to the dosage. Transaminase elevations characteristically develop during the first 6 to 12 weeks of treatment, and cholinergically mediated events are dosage related. Because of the high risk of hepatotoxicity and the availability of newer and safer drugs in this class, tacrine is rarely, if ever, used.

DRUG–DRUG INTERACTIONS

The metabolism of donepezil may be increased by phenytoin (Dilantin), carbamazepine (Tegretol), dexamethasone (Decadron), rifampin (Rifadin), or phenobarbital (Solfoton). All cholinesterase inhibitors should be used cautiously with drugs that also possess cholinomimetic activity, such as succinylcholine (Anectine) or bethanechol (Urecholine). Coadministration of cholinesterase inhibitors and drugs that have cholinergic antagonist activity (e.g., tricyclic drugs) is probably counterproductive. Donepezil is highly protein bound, but it does not displace other protein-bound drugs, such as furosemide (Lasix), digoxin (Lanoxin), or warfarin (Coumadin). Rivastigmine circulates mostly unbound to serum proteins and has no significant known drug interactions. Coadministration of paroxetine (Paxil) and erythromycin increases the blood level of galantamine. Except for tacrine, some of these drugs inhibit the metabolic pathways of the cytochrome P450 isoenzymes, but this has no clinical significance.

LABORATORY INTERFERENCES

No laboratory interferences have been associated with any of the cholinesterase inhibitors.

DOSAGE AND CLINICAL GUIDELINES

Before the initiation of treatment with cholinesterase inhibitors, potentially treatable causes of dementia should be ruled out and the diagnosis of dementia of the Alzheimer's type should be established with a thorough neurological evaluation. Detailed neuropsychological testing can detect early signs of Alzheimer's disease. Psychiatric evaluation also should focus on depression, anxiety, and psychosis.

Donepezil is available in 5- and 10-mg tablets. Treatment should be initiated at 5-mg each night. If well tolerated and of some discernible benefit after 4 weeks, the dosage should be increased to a maintenance dosage of 10 mg each night. Donepezil absorption is unaffected by meals.

Rivastigmine is available in 1.5-, 3-, 4.5-, and 6-mg capsules. The recommended initial dosage is 1.5 mg twice daily for a minimum of 2 weeks, after which increases of 1.5 mg a day can be made at intervals of at least 2 weeks to a target dosage of 6 mg a day, taken in two equal doses. If tolerated, the dosage may be further titrated upward to a maximum of 6 mg twice daily. The risk of adverse GI events can be reduced by administration of rivastigmine with food.

Galantamine is available in 4-, 8-, and 12-mg tablets and a 4-mg/mL oral solution. The recommended starting dose is 4 mg twice a day. After 4 weeks the dose should be increased to 8 mg twice a day (16 mg per day). If tolerated, a further increase to 12 mg twice a day may be attempted after a minimum of 4 weeks of the previous dose. Administration with meals may limit adverse GI complaints. For patients with renal impairment a dose greater than 16 mg a day should be avoided.

Tacrine is available in 10-, 20-, 30-, and 40-mg capsules. Before the initiation of tacrine treatment, a complete physical and laboratory examination should be conducted, with special attention to liver function tests and baseline hematological indexes. Treatment should be initiated at 10 mg four times a day and then raised by increments of 10 mg a dose every 6 weeks up to 160 mg a day; the person's tolerance of each dosage is indicated by the absence of unacceptable adverse effects and lack of elevation of alanine aminotransferase (ALT) activity. Tacrine should be given four times daily—ideally 1 hour before meals, since the absorption of tacrine is reduced by about 25 percent when it is taken during the first 2 hours after meals. As mentioned above, because of the high risk of hepatotoxicity, tacrine is no longer recommended, especially since the newer compounds are equally effective and without risk.

MEMANTINE

Memantine is an NMDA receptor antagonist. The mechanism of action by which memantine is thought to produce clinical effects is distinctly different from the agents currently available to treat Alzheimer's disease, all of which modulate concentrations of the neurotransmitter acetylcholine.

By blocking the *N*-methyl-D-aspartate (NMDA) receptor, the investigational agent memantine is able to protect neurons from excessive stimulation by the excitatory neurotransmitter glutamate, without interfering with the role of glutamate in normal neuronal functioning—unlike certain other investigational NMDA antagonists. Glutamate plays an integral role in neural pathways associated with learning and memory, perhaps affecting

the movement of electrical signals across nearly 70 percent of the central nervous system's excitatory synapses. Excessive amounts of glutamate can, however, damage cells by causing too much excitation. The excitotoxicity produced by glutamate is hypothesized to be responsible for the neuronal cell death observed in Alzheimer's as well as other neurodegenerative disorders. Memantine, known as Akatinol, is currently used in Europe.

References

Corey-Bloom J, Anand R, Veach J. A randomized trial evaluating the efficacy and safety of ENA-713 (rivastigmine tartrate), a new acetylcholinesterase inhibitor, in patients with mild to moderately severe Alzheimer's disease. *Int J Geriatr Psychopharmacol.* 1998;1:55.

Cummings JL, Askin-Edgar S. Evidence for psychotropic effects of acetylcholinesterase inhibitors. *CNS Drugs.* 2000;13:385.

Cummings JL, Cyrus PA, Bieber F, Mas J, Orazem J, Gulanski B. Metrifonate treatment of the cognitive deficits of Alzheimer's disease. Metrifonate Study Group. *Neurology.* 1998;50:1214.

Dunn NR, Pearce GL, Shakir SAW. Adverse effects associated with the use of donepezil in general practice in England. *J Psychopharmacol.* 2000;14:406.

Hardman JG, Limbird LE, Goodman Gilman A, eds. *Goodman & Gilman's the Pharmacological Basis of Therapeutics.* 10th ed. New York: McGraw-Hill; 2001.

Knapp MJ, Knopman DS, Solomon PR, Pendlebury WW, Davis CS, Gracon SI. A 30-week randomized controlled trial of high-dose tacrine in patients with Alzheimer's disease. The Tacrine Study Group. *JAMA.* 1994;271:985.

Knopman D, Schneider L, Davis K, et al. Long-term tacrine (Cognex) treatment: effects on nursing home placement and mortality. Tacrine Study Group. *Neurology.* 1996;47:166.

Morris JC, Cyrus PA, Orazem J, et al. Metrifonate benefits cognitive, behavioral, and global function in patients with Alzheimer's disease. *Neurology.* 1998;50:1222.

Rocca P, Cocuzza E, Marchiaro L, Bogetto F. Donepezil in the treatment of Alzheimer's disease: long-term efficacy and safety. *Prog Neuropsychopharmacol Biol Psychiatry.* 2002;26:369.

Rogers SL, Doody RS, Mohs RC, Friedhoff LT. Donepezil improves cognitive and global function in Alzheimer disease: a 15-week, double-blind, placebo-controlled study. Donepezil Study Group. *Arch Intern Med.* 1998;158:1021.

Rogers SL, Farlow MR, Doody RS, Mohs R, Friedhoff LT. A 24-week, double-blind, placebo-controlled trial of donepezil in patients with Alzheimer's disease. Donepezil Study Group. *Neurology.* 1998;50:136.

Samuels SC, Davis KL. Cholinesterase inhibitors. In: Sadock BJ, Sadock VA, eds. *Kaplan & Sadock's Comprehensive Textbook of Psychiatry.* 7th ed. Vol 2. Baltimore: Lippincott Williams & Wilkins; 2000:2346.

Taylor P. Anticholinesterase agents. In: Hardman JG, Limbird LE, Goodman Gilman A, eds. *Goodman & Gilman's the Pharmacological Basis of Therapeutics.* 10th ed. New York: McGraw-Hill; 2001:175.

van Gool WA. Efficacy of donepezil in Alzheimer's disease: fact or artifact? *Neurology.* 1999;52:218.

Watkins PB, Zimmerman HJ, Knapp MJ, Gracon SI, Lewis KW. Hepatotoxic effects of tacrine administration in patients with Alzheimer's disease. *JAMA.* 1994;271:992.

▲ 34.4.14 Dantrolene

Dantrolene (Dantrium) is a direct-acting skeletal muscle relaxant. In contemporary clinical psychiatry, dantrolene is one of the potentially effective treatments for neuroleptic malignant syndrome, catatonia, and serotonin syndrome.

CHEMISTRY

Dantrolene is derived from hydantoin, as indicated in its molecular structure (Fig. 36.4.14–1). Dantrolene is structurally and pharmacologically unrelated to other skeletal muscle relaxants.

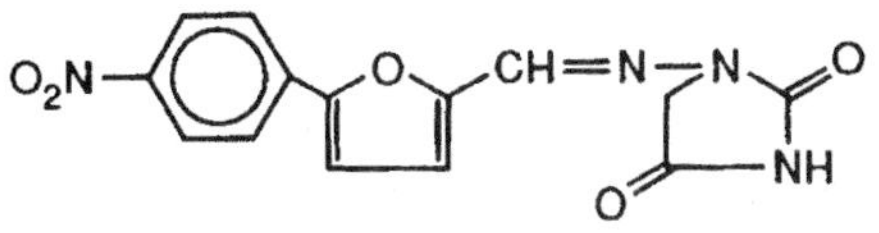

FIGURE 36.4.14–1
Molecular structure of dantrolene.

PHARMACOLOGICAL ACTIONS

About one third of orally administered dantrolene is slowly absorbed from the gastrointestinal (GI) tract. At sufficient dosages, consistent plasma concentrations can be maintained. Peak blood concentrations are seen about 5 hours after oral administration. The elimination half-life of dantrolene is about 9 hours. Dantrolene is largely protein bound, metabolized by the liver, and excreted in the urine. Dantrolene produces skeletal muscle relaxation by directly affecting the contractile response of the muscles at the site beyond the myoneural junction. The skeletal muscle relaxant effect is the basis of its efficacy in reducing the muscle destruction and hyperthermia associated with neuroleptic malignant syndrome.

EFFECTS ON SPECIFIC ORGANS AND SYSTEMS

The skeletal muscle relaxant effect of dantrolene can cause muscle weakness and such symptoms as slurring of speech and drooling. Dantrolene also has effects on the GI system (e.g., diarrhea) and the nervous system (e.g., headache and depression) and possibly toxic effects on hepatocytes, as indicated by an association with elevated liver function test results.

THERAPEUTIC INDICATIONS

The primary psychiatric indication for intravenous (IV) dantrolene is muscle rigidity in neuroleptic malignant syndrome. Dantrolene is almost always used in conjunction with appropriate supportive measures and a dopamine receptor agonist—for example, bromocriptine (Parlodel). If all available case reports and studies are summarized, about 80 percent of all patients with neuroleptic malignant syndrome who received dantrolene apparently benefited clinically from the drug. Muscle relaxation and general and dramatic improvement in symptoms can appear within minutes of IV administration, although in most cases the beneficial effects can take several hours to appear. Some evidence indicates that dantrolene treatment must be continued for some time, perhaps days to a week or more, to minimize the risk of symptoms recurring, although the data for this clinical opinion are limited. Dantrolene has been used in efforts to treat other psychiatric conditions characterized by life-threatening muscle rigidity, such as catatonia and serotonin syndrome.

PRECAUTIONS AND ADVERSE REACTIONS

Muscle weakness, drowsiness, dizziness, light-headedness, nausea, diarrhea, malaise, and fatigue are the most common adverse effects of dantrolene. These effects are generally transient. The central nervous system (CNS) effects of dantrolene can include speech disturbances (which may also reflect its effects on the muscles of speech), headaches, visual disturbances, altered taste, depression, confusion, hallucinations, nervousness, and insomnia. Many serious adverse effects of

dantrolene are associated with long-term treatment, rather than with its short-term use in treating neuroleptic malignant syndrome. They include hepatitis, seizures, and pleural effusion with pericarditis. Because of its potential for severe adverse effects, dantrolene should not be used by psychiatric patients for any long-term treatment. Dantrolene should be used with caution by patients with hepatic, renal, and chronic lung diseases. Dantrolene can cross the placenta and is thus contraindicated for pregnant women and should not be used by nursing mothers except in emergency situations, such as neuroleptic malignant syndrome. Data are not available about the use of dantrolene by older patients, and no unique problems have been associated with its use by children.

DRUG–DRUG INTERACTIONS

The risk of liver toxicity may be increased for patients also taking estrogens. Dantrolene should be used with caution by patients who are using other drugs that produce drowsiness, most notably the benzodiazepines. In the case of neuroleptic malignant syndrome, however, the general guidelines for dantrolene must be weighed against the severity of the syndrome. Dantrolene should not be given intravenously in combination with calcium channel inhibitors. Concomitant administration of dantrolene and theophylline in animals has caused seizures and death.

LABORATORY INTERFERENCES

No known laboratory interferences are associated with dantrolene, although experience with its use in patients with neuroleptic malignant syndrome is still limited.

DOSAGE AND ADMINISTRATION

In addition to the immediate discontinuation of antipsychotic drugs, medical support to cool the patient, and monitoring of vital signs and renal output, dantrolene can be given in dosages of 1 mg/kg orally 4 times daily or 1 to 5 mg/kg IV to reduce muscle spasms in patients with neuroleptic malignant syndrome. Although some clinicians have recommended low dosages because of the adverse effects, other clinicians indicate that dosages of 10 mg/kg a day are most likely to be effective. Intravenous administration of dantrolene relaxes muscle tension within several minutes. Dantrolene is supplied as 25-, 50-, and 100-mg capsules and in a 20-mg parenteral preparation for reconstitution with 60 mL of sterile water.

REFERENCES

DeBattista C, Shatzberg AF. Other pharmacological and biological therapies. In: Sadock BJ, Sadock VA, eds. *Kaplan & Sadock's Comprehensive Textbook of Psychiatry.* 7th ed. Vol 2. Baltimore: Lippincott Williams & Wilkins; 2000:2521.

Hardman JG, Limbird LE, Goodman Gilman A, eds. *Goodman & Gilman's the Pharmacological Basis of Therapeutics.* 10th ed. New York: McGraw-Hill; 2001.

Mercadante S. Dantrolene treatment of opioid-induced myoclonus. *Anesth Analg.* 1995;18:1307.

Nisijima K, Ishigura T. Does dantrolene influence central dopamine and serotonin metabolism in the neuroleptic malignant syndrome? A retrospective study. *Biol Psychiatry.* 1993;33:45.

Otani K, Mihara K, Kondo T, et al. Treatment of neuroleptic malignant syndrome with levodopa. *Hum Psychopharmacol.* 1992;7:217.

Rice J, Lebowitz PW, Bailine SH, Mowerman A. Malignant hyperthermia and electroconvulsive therapy. *Convuls Ther.* 1993;9:45.

Scheftner WA, Shulman RB. Treatment choice in neuroleptic malignant syndrome. *Convuls Ther.* 1992;8:267.

Susman VL. Clinical management of neuroleptic malignant syndrome. *Psychiatr Q.* 2000;72:325.

Tsai G, Crisostomo G, Rosenblatt ML, Stern TA. Neuroleptic malignant syndrome associated with clozapine treatment. *Ann Clin Psychiatry.* 1995;7:91.

Waldman HJ. Centrally acting skeletal muscle relaxants and associated drugs. *J Pain Symptom Manage.* 1994;9:434.

▲ 36.4.15 Disulfiram

Disulfiram (Antabuse) is used to ensure abstinence in the treatment of alcohol dependence. Its main effect is to produce a rapid and violently unpleasant reaction in a person who ingests even a small amount of alcohol while taking disulfiram. Because of the risk of severe and even fatal disulfiram–alcohol reactions, disulfiram therapy is used less often today than previously.

CHEMISTRY

The molecular structure of disulfiram is presented in Figure 36.4.15–1.

PHARMACOLOGICAL ACTIONS

Disulfiram is almost completely absorbed from the gastrointestinal tract after oral administration. It is metabolized in the liver and excreted in the urine. It is lipid soluble and has an estimated half-life of 60 to 120 hours. One or 2 weeks may be needed before disulfiram is totally eliminated from the body after the last dose has been taken.

The metabolism of ethanol proceeds through oxidation via alcohol dehydrogenase to the formation of acetaldehyde, which is further metabolized to acetylcoenzyme A (acetyl-CoA) by aldehyde dehydrogenase. Acetyl-CoA proceeds down the citric acid cycle and other metabolic pathways. Disulfiram is an aldehyde dehydrogenase inhibitor that interferes with the metabolism of alcohol and produces a marked increase in blood acetaldehyde levels. The accumulation of acetaldehyde (to a level up to 10 times higher than occurs in the normal metabolism of alcohol) produces a wide array of unpleasant reactions called the *disulfiram–alcohol reaction,* characterized by nausea, throbbing headache, vomiting, hypotension, flushing, sweating, thirst, dyspnea, tachycardia, chest pain, vertigo, and blurred vision. The reaction occurs almost immediately after the ingestion of one alcoholic drink and may last up to 30 minutes.

THERAPEUTIC INDICATIONS

The primary indication for disulfiram use is as an aversive conditioning treatment for alcohol dependence. Either the fear of having a disulfiram–alcohol reaction or the memory of having

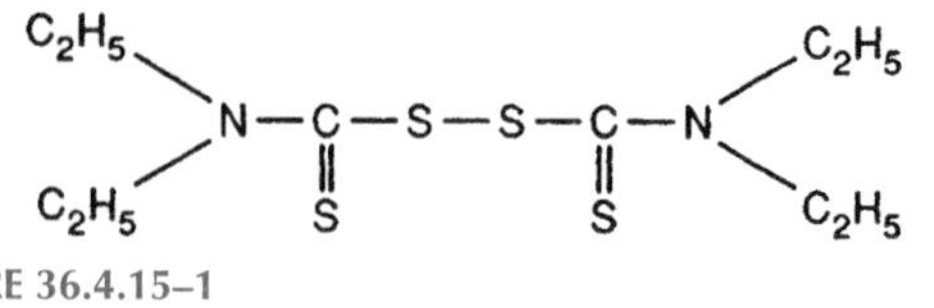

FIGURE 36.4.15–1
Molecular formula of disulfiram.

had one is meant to condition the patient not to use alcohol. Some clinicians induce a disulfiram–alcohol reaction in patients at the beginning of therapy to convince the patients of the severe unpleasantness of the symptoms. This practice is not recommended, however, as a disulfiram–alcohol reaction can lead to cardiovascular collapse. A graphic description of the severity and unpleasantness of the disulfiram–alcohol reaction usually suffices to discourage patients from imbibing alcohol. Disulfiram treatment should be combined with such treatments as psychotherapy, group therapy, and support groups like Alcoholics Anonymous. The treatment of alcohol dependence requires careful monitoring, since a patient can simply decide not to take the disulfiram; compliance with the medication should be checked if possible.

PRECAUTIONS AND ADVERSE REACTIONS

With Alcohol Consumption

The intensity of the disulfiram–alcohol reaction varies with each patient. In extreme cases it is marked by respiratory depression, cardiovascular collapse, myocardial infarction, convulsions, and death. Therefore, disulfiram is contraindicated for patients with a significant pulmonary or cardiovascular disease. In addition, disulfiram should be used with caution, if at all, by patients with nephritis, brain damage, hypothyroidism, diabetes, hepatic disease, seizures, polydrug dependence, or an abnormal electroencephalogram. Most fatal reactions occur in patients who are taking more than 500 mg a day of disulfiram and who consume more than 3 ounces of alcohol. The treatment of a severe disulfiram–alcohol reaction is primarily supportive to prevent shock.

Without Alcohol Consumption

The adverse effects of disulfiram in the absence of alcohol consumption include fatigue, dermatitis, impotence, optic neuritis, a variety of mental changes, acute polyneuropathy, and hepatic damage. A metabolite of disulfiram inhibits dopamine hydroxylase and thus potentially exacerbates psychosis in patients with psychotic disorders.

DRUG–DRUG INTERACTIONS

Disulfiram increases the blood concentration of diazepam (Valium), chlordiazepoxide (Librium), paraldehyde (Paral), phenytoin (Dilantin), caffeine, theophylline (Theo-Dur, Slo-Bid), tetrahydrocannabinol (the active ingredient in marijuana), barbiturates, anticoagulants, isoniazid (Nydrazid, Rifamate), and tricyclic drugs. Concomitant administration of disulfiram and tranylcypromine (Parnate) causes seizures and death in animals.

LABORATORY INTERFERENCES

In rare instances, disulfiram has been reported to decrease the uptake of iodine-131 (^{131}I) and protein-bound iodine test results. In research settings, disulfiram may reduce urinary concentrations of homovanillic acid, the major metabolite of dopamine, because of its inhibition of dopamine hydroxylase.

DOSAGE AND ADMINISTRATION

Disulfiram is supplied in tablets of 250 and 500 mg. The usual initial dosage is 500 mg a day taken by mouth for the first 1 or 2 weeks, followed by a maintenance dosage of 250 mg a day. The dosage should not exceed 500 mg a day. The maintenance dosage range is 125 to 500 mg a day.

Patients must be instructed that the ingestion of even the smallest amount of alcohol brings on a disulfiram–alcohol reaction, with all its unpleasant effects. Patients should also be warned against ingesting any alcohol-containing preparations, such as cough drops, tonics of any kind, and alcohol-containing foods and sauces. Some reactions have occurred in men who used alcohol-based aftershave lotions and inhaled the fumes; therefore, precautions must be explicit and should include any topically applied preparations containing alcohol, such as perfume.

Disulfiram should not be administered until patients have abstained from alcohol for at least 12 hours. Disulfiram can cause an unpleasant reaction within 15 minutes after the first dose in a person who has even tiny serum concentrations of unmetabolized alcohol. Patients should be warned that the disulfiram–alcohol reaction may occur as long as 1 or 2 weeks after the last dose of disulfiram. Patients should carry identification cards describing the disulfiram–alcohol reaction and listing the name and the telephone number of the physician to be called.

References

Anton RF. Pharmacologic approaches to the management of alcoholism. *J Clin Psychiatry.* 2001;62:11.

DeBattista C, Shatzberg AF. Other pharmacological and biological therapies. In: Sadock BJ, Sadock VA, eds. *Kaplan & Sadock's Comprehensive Textbook of Psychiatry.* 7th ed. Vol 2. Baltimore: Lippincott Williams & Wilkins; 2000:2521.

Hameedi FA, Rosen MI, McCance-Katz EF, et al. Behavioral, physiological, and pharmacological interaction of cocaine and disulfiram in humans. *Biol Psychiatry.* 1995;37:560.

Hardman JG, Limbird LE, Goodman Gilman A, eds. *Goodman & Gilman's the Pharmacological Basis of Therapeutics.* 10th ed. New York: McGraw-Hill; 2001.

Kaminer Y. Disulfiram in adolescents? *J Am Acad Child Adolesc Psychiatry.* 1995;34:2.

Masia M, Gutierrez F, Jimeno A, et al. Fulminant hepatitis and fatal toxic epidermal necrolysis (Lyell disease) coincident with clarithromycin administration in an alcholic patient receiving disulfiram therapy. *Arch Intern Med.* 2002;162:474.

Miller NS. Pharmacotherapy in alcoholism. *Alcohol Treat Q.* 1995;12:129.

Miller NS. Pharmacotherapy in alcoholism. *J Addict Dis.* 1995;14:23.

Schuckit MA. Recent developments in the pharmacotherapy of alcohol dependence. *J Consult Clin Psychol.* 1996;64:669.

Smith JE, Meyers RJ. The community reinforcement approach. In: Hester RK, Miller WR, eds. *Handbook of Alcoholism Treatment Approaches: Effective Alternatives.* 2nd ed. Boston: Allyn & Bacon; 1995:251.

Thas ME, Salloum IM, Cornelius JD. Comorbid alcoholism and depression: treatment issues. *J Clin Psychiatry.* 2001;62:32.

▲ 36.4.16 Dopamine Receptor Agonists and Precursors: Bromocriptine, Levodopa, Pergolide, Pramipexole, and Ropinirole

Dopamine receptor agonists and precursors increase the amount of dopamine in the brain. They are used by psychiatrists to treat various adverse effects of antipsychotic drugs, including (1) par-

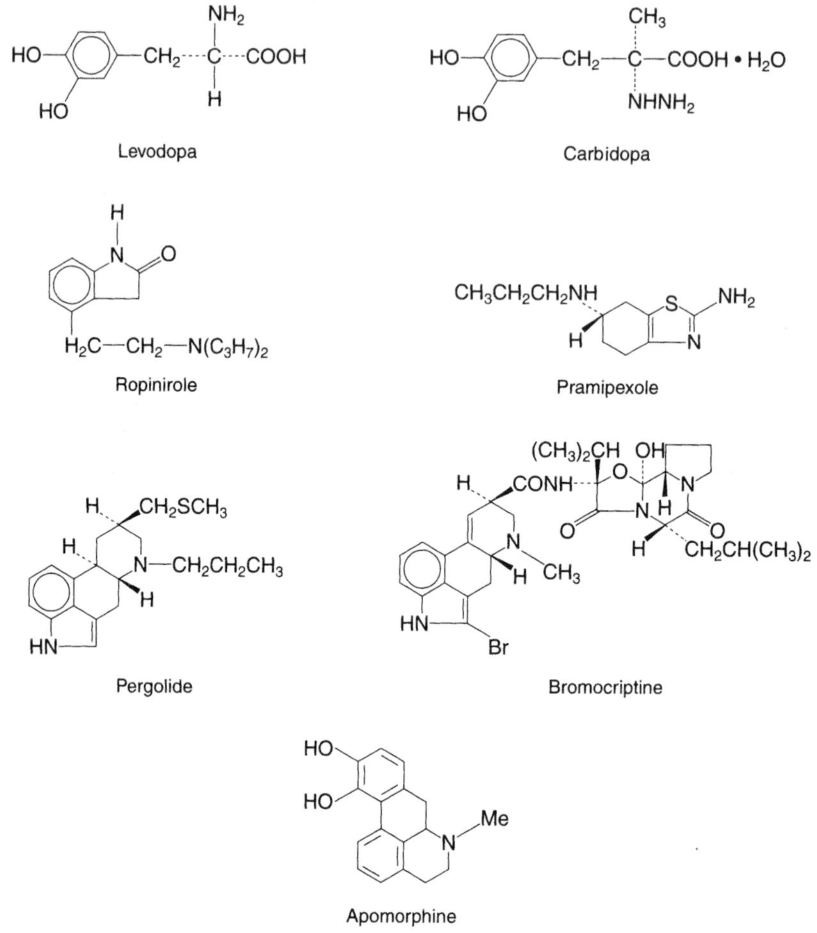

FIGURE 36.4.16–1
Molecular structures of dopamine receptor agonists and carbidopa.

kinsonism, (2) extrapyramidal symptoms, (3) akinesia, (4) focal perioral tremors, (5) hyperprolactinemia, (6) galactorrhea, (7) and neuroleptic malignant syndrome. The drugs in this class most commonly prescribed are bromocriptine (Parlodel), levodopa (Larodopa), and carbidopa-levodopa (Sinemet). New dopamine receptor agonists include ropinirole (Requip), pramipexole (Mirapex), and pergolide (Permax), which are better tolerated than bromocriptine.

CHEMISTRY

Levodopa is the natural precursor of dopamine. The formulation of levodopa combined with carbidopa reduces the incidence of non–central nervous system (CNS) adverse effects experienced with use of levodopa alone. Bromocriptine and pergolide are ergotamine derivatives. The molecular structures of dopamine receptor agonists and carbidopa (Lodosyn) are shown in Figure 36.4.16–1.

PHARMACOLOGICAL ACTIONS

Levodopa, or L-dopa, is rapidly absorbed after oral administration, and peak plasma levels are reached after 30 to 120 minutes. The half-life of levodopa is 90 minutes. Absorption of levodopa can be significantly reduced by changes in gastric pH and by ingestion with meals. Bromocriptine, pergolide, and ropinirole are rapidly absorbed but undergo first-pass metabolism such that only about 30 to 55 percent of the dosage is bioavailable. Peak concentrations are achieved $1\frac{1}{2}$ to 3 hours after oral administration. Pergolide has a half-life of about 27 hours, and a single dose has 5 to 6 hours of clinical activity. The half-life of ropinirole is 6 hours. Pramipexole is rapidly absorbed with little first-pass metabolism and reaches peak concentrations in 2 hours. Its half-life is 8 hours.

Once levodopa enters the dopaminergic neurons of the CNS, it is converted by dopa decarboxylase into the neurotransmitter dopamine. Bromocriptine, pergolide, ropinirole, and pramipexole act directly on dopamine receptors. Dopamine, pramipexole, and ropinirole bind about 20 times more selectively to dopamine D_3 than D_2 receptors; the corresponding ratio for pergolide is 5, and for bromocriptine is less than 2. Levodopa, pramipexole, and ropinirole have no significant activity at nondopaminergic receptors, but pergolide and bromocriptine bind to serotonin 5-HT_1 and 5-HT_2, and α_1-, α_2-, and β-adrenergic receptors.

EFFECTS ON SPECIFIC ORGANS AND SYSTEMS

Dopamine activity affects many organ systems in addition to the CNS. Because of the role of dopamine in the maintenance of blood pressure, these drugs are commonly associated with hypertension, although hypotension has been reported in some patients. Dopaminergic activity can also affect heart rate and rhythm. The gastrointestinal (GI) system is also sensitive to dopaminergic drugs and frequently causes symptoms of GI distress, especially nausea.

THERAPEUTIC INDICATIONS

Medication-Induced Movement Disorders

In present day clinical psychiatry, dopamine receptor agonists are used for the treatment of medication-induced parkinsonism, extrapyramidal symptoms, akinesia, and focal perioral tremors. Their use has diminished sharply, however, because the incidence of medication-induced movement disorders is much lower with the use of the newer, atypical antipsychotics (serotonin-dopamine antagonists [SDAs]).

For the treatment of medication-induced movement disorders, most clinicians rely on anticholinergics, amantadine (Symmetrel), and antihistamines because they are equally effective and have few adverse effects. Bromocriptine remains in use in the treatment of neuroleptic malignant syndrome; however, the incidence of this disorder is diminishing with the decreasing use of dopamine receptor antagonists.

Dopamine receptor agonists are also used to counteract the hyperprolactinemic effects of dopamine receptor antagonists, which result in the side effects of amenorrhea and galactorrhea. Dopamine receptor agonists may reduce the pharmacological effects of cocaine but are not effective in reducing the craving for cocaine associated with withdrawal.

Sexual Dysfunction

All dopamine receptor agonists can improve erectile dysfunction. However, they are rarely used because therapeutic dosages frequently cause intolerable adverse effects and sildenafil (Viagra) is better tolerated and more effective. Sublingual apomorphine may find a therapeutic niche in treatment of erectile dysfunction in men in whom sildenafil is contraindicated due to use of nitrate-containing medications. However, the safety of coadministration of apomorphine and nitrates has not yet been determined.

PRECAUTIONS AND ADVERSE REACTIONS

Adverse effects are common with dopamine receptor agonists, thus limiting the usefulness of these drugs. Adverse effects are dosage dependent and include nausea, vomiting, orthostatic hypotension, headache, dizziness, and cardiac arrhythmias. To reduce the risk of orthostatic hypotension, the initial dosage of all dopamine receptor agonists should be quite low, with incremental increases in dosage at intervals of at least 1 week. These drugs should be used with caution in persons with hypertension, cardiovascular disease, and hepatic disease. After long-term use, persons and particularly elderly persons may experience choreiform and dystonic movements and psychiatric disturbances, including hallucinations, delusions, confusion, depression, and mania and other behavioral changes.

Long-term use of bromocriptine and pergolide can produce retroperitoneal and pulmonary fibrosis, pleural effusions, and pleural thickening. In general, ropinirole and pramipexole have a similar but much milder adverse effect profile than levodopa, bromocriptine, and pergolide. Pramipexole and ropinirole may cause irresistible sleep attacks that occur suddenly, without warning and have caused motor vehicle accidents. The most common adverse effects of apomorphine are nausea, orthostatic hypotension, sedation, bradycardia, syncope, perspiration, and vomiting. Apomorphine's sedative effects are exacerbated by concurrent use of alcohol or other CNS depressants. Dopamine receptor agonists are contraindicated during pregnancy and for nursing mothers especially, because they inhibit lactation.

DRUG–DRUG INTERACTIONS

Dopamine receptor antagonists are capable of reversing the effects of dopamine receptor agonists, but this is not usually clinically significant. The concurrent use of tricyclic drugs and dopamine receptor agonists has been reported to cause symptoms of neurotoxicity, such as rigidity, agitation, and tremor. They may also potentiate the hypotensive effects of diuretics and other antihypertensive medications. Dopamine receptor agonists should not be used in conjunction with monoamine oxidase inhibitors (MAOIs), including selegiline (Eldepryl), and MAOI use should be discontinued at least 2 weeks before the initiation of dopamine receptor agonist therapy.

Benzodiazepines, phenytoin (Dilantin), and pyridoxine may interfere with the therapeutic effects of dopamine receptor agonists. Ergot alkaloids and bromocriptine should not be used concurrently, as they may cause hypertension and myocardial infarction. Progestins, estrogens, and oral contraceptives may interfere with the effects of bromocriptine and may raise plasma concentrations of ropinirole. Ciprofloxacin (Cipro) can raise plasma concentrations of ropinirole, and cimetidine (Tagamet) can raise plasma concentrations of pramipexole.

LABORATORY INTERFERENCES

Levodopa administration has been associated with false reports of elevated serum and urinary uric acid concentrations, urinary glucose test results, urinary ketone test results, and urinary catecholamine concentrations. No laboratory interferences have been associated with the administration of the other dopamine receptor agonists.

DOSAGE AND CLINICAL GUIDELINES

Table 36.4.16–1 lists the various dopamine receptor agonists and their formulations. For the treatment of antipsychotic-induced parkinsonism the clinician should start with a 100-mg dose of levodopa three times a day, which may be increased until the person has functionally improved. The maximum dosage of levodopa is 2,000 mg a day, but most persons respond to dosages below 1,000 mg per day. The dosage of the carbidopa component of the levodopa-carbidopa formulation should total at least 75 mg a day.

Table 36.4.16–1
Available Preparations of Dopamine Receptor Agonists and Carbidopa

Generic Name	Trade Name	Preparations
Bromocriptine	Parlodel	2.5-, 5-mg tablets
Carbidopa	Lodosyn	25 mg[a]
Levodopa	Larodopa	100-, 250-, 500-mg tablets
Levodopa-carbidopa (cocareldopa)	Sinemet, Atamet	100/10-, 100/25-, 250/25-mg tablets, 100/25-, 200/50-mg extended-release tablets
Pergolide	Permax	0.05-, 0.25-, and 1-mg tablets
Pramipexole	Mirapex	0.125-, 0.25-, 0.5-, 1-, 1.5-mg tablets
Ropinirole	Requip	0.25-, 0.5-, 1-, 2-, 5-mg tablets

[a]Drug only available directly through the manufacturer.

The dosage of bromocriptine for mental disorders is uncertain, although it seems prudent to begin with low dosages (1.25 mg twice daily) and to increase the dosage gradually. Bromocriptine is usually taken with meals to help reduce the likelihood of nausea.

The starting dosage of pergolide is 0.05 mg daily, which can be increased by 0.1 to 0.15 mg a day every 3 days for four increments, then by 0.25 mg per day every 3 days divided into three equal daily dosages, until therapeutic benefit or adverse effects emerge. The average dosage for treatment of idiopathic Parkinson's disease is 3 mg per day, and the maximum dosage is 5 mg per day.

The starting dosage of pramipexole is 0.125 mg three times daily, which is increased to 0.25 mg three times daily in the second week and is increased by 0.25 mg per dose each week until therapeutic benefit or adverse effects emerge. Persons with idiopathic Parkinson's disease usually experience benefit at a total daily dose of 1.5 mg, and the maximum daily dose is 4.5 mg.

For ropinirole, the starting dosage is 0.25 mg three times daily and is increased by 0.25 mg per dose each week to a total daily dose of 3 mg, then by 0.5 mg per dosage each week to a total daily dose of 9 mg, then by 1 mg per dose each week to a maximum dosage of 24 mg a day, until therapeutic benefit or adverse effects emerge. The average daily dose for persons with idiopathic Parkinson's disease is about 16 mg.

Sublingual apomorphine for treatment of erectile dysfunction has been tested in 2- and 4-mg formulations. It is taken at least 15 minutes before initiation of sexual intercourse. Clinical guidelines regarding the minimum time interval between doses are not yet available.

References

DeBattista C, Schatzberg AF. Other pharmacological and biological therapies. In: Sadock BJ, Sadock VA, eds. *Kaplan & Sadock's Comprehensive Textbook of Psychiatry.* 7th ed. Vol 2. Baltimore: Lippincott Williams & Wilkins; 2000:2521.

Dooneief G, Mirabello E. An estimate of the incidence of depression in idiopathic Parkinson's disease. *Arch Neurol* 1992;49:305.

Doraiswamy M, Martin W, Metz A. Psychosis of Parkinson's disease: diagnosis and treatment. *Prog Neuropsychopharmacol Biol Psychiatry.* 1995;19:835.

Hubble JP. Long-term studies of dopamine agonists. *Neurology.* 2002;58(suppl 1):S42.

Jankovic J. Parkinson's disease therapy: tailoring choices for early and late disease, young and old patients. *Clin Neuropharmacol.* 2000;23:252.

Kaplan B, Mason NA. Levodopa in restless legs syndrome. *Ann Pharmacother.* 1992;26:214.

Kaplan HI, Sadock BJ. Other pharmacological therapies. In: Kaplan HI, Sadock BJ, eds. *Comprehensive Textbook of Psychiatry.* 6th ed. Baltimore: Williams & Wilkins; 1995.

Pahwa R, Koller WC. Treatment of Parkinson's disease with controlled-release carbidopa/L-DOPA. *Adv Neurol.* 1996;69:487.

Standaert DG, Young AB. Treatment of central nervous system degenerative disorders. In: Hardman JG, Limbird LE, Goodman Gilman A, eds. *Goodman & Gilman's the Pharmacological Basis of Therapeutics.* 10th ed. New York: McGraw-Hill; 2001:5498.

Swerdlow NR, Eastvold A, Karban B, et al. Dopamine agonist effects on startle and sensorimotor gating in normal male subjects: time course studies. *Psychopharmacology.* 2002;161:189.

Wada T, Kanno M, Aoshima T, Otani K. Dose-dependent augmentation effect of bromocriptine in a case with refractory depression. *Prog Neuropsychopharmacol Biol Psychiatry.* 2001;25:457.

Wagner ML, Defilippi JL, Menzo MA, Sage JI. Clozapine for the treatment of psychosis in Parkinson's disease: chart review of 49 patients. *J Neuropsychiatry Clin Neurosci.* 1996;8:276.

▲ 36.4.17 Dopamine Receptor Antagonists: Typical Antipsychotics

The dopamine receptor antagonists discussed in this section are so named because they are high-affinity antagonists of dopamine receptors. Other terms used to refer to these drugs are *typical, traditional,* or *conventional antipsychotics.* They are used in the treatment of schizophrenia and other psychotic disorders. The dopamine receptor antagonists include chlorpromazine (Thorazine), thioridazine (Mellaril), fluphenazine (Prolixin), and haloperidol (Haldol) among many others (Table 36.4.17–1).

A new class of antipsychotic agents, the serotonin-dopamine antagonists (SDAs), also called *newer, novel,* or *atypical antipsychotics,* has appeared, which has fewer neurological adverse effects than the dopamine receptor antagonists and is effective against a broader range of psychotic symptoms. Differentiating the two classes of antipsychotics—dopamine receptor antagonists and SDAs—is increasingly important, since they have different mechanisms of action and different clinical effects. The SDAs are covered in Section 36.4.27.

HISTORY

The first antipsychotic drugs were the phenothiazines. Drugs from this class were originally used as antihelmintics in veterinary medicine and as urinary antiseptics in humans. In 1950, Paul Charpentier at the Rhone-Poulenc Laboratories in Paris synthesized chlorpromazine, a mild antihistaminic that appeared notable as a sedating agent. Henri Laborit, a surgeon interested in drugs that would decrease preoperative anxiety and prevent postsurgical shock, convinced the Rhone-Poulenc Laboratories of the importance of identifying compounds that would relax patients and make surgical shock less likely. Chlorpromazine appeared to fulfill these criteria, and also appeared qualitatively different from other sedating drugs. Patients appeared indifferent toward the environment and more tranquil. These properties led Laborit to attempt to convince psychiatrists, including Jean Delay and Pierre Deniker, to administer chlorpromazine to patients with mania. In 1952, they reported that chlorpromazine was effective in treating mania and schizophrenia. Within a year, the atmosphere in Paris psychiatric hospitals had improved substantially. The discovery of chlorpromazine's

Table 36.4.17–1
Dopamine Receptor Antagonist Drugs, Trade Names, Potencies, and Dosages

Generic Name	Trade Name	Potency[a] (mg of drug equivalent to 100 mg chlorpromazine)	Usual Adult Dosage Range (mg/day)	Usual Single IM Dosage (mg)
Phenothiazines				
Aliphatic				
Chlorpromazine	Thorazine	100—low	300–800	25–50
Triflupromazine	Vesprin	25–50—low	100–150	20–60
Promazine	Sparine	40—low	40–800	50–150
Piperazine				
Prochlorperazine	Compazine	15—medium	40–150	10–20
Perphenazine	Trilafon	10—medium	8–40	5–10
Trifluoperazine	Stelazine	3–5—high	6–20	1–2
Fluphenazine	Prolixin, Permitil	1.5–3—high	1–20	2–5
Acetophenazine	Tindal (no longer manufactured)	25—medium	60–120	—
Butaperazine	Repoise (not sold in U.S.)	10—medium	—	—
Carphenazine	Proketazine (not sold in U.S.)	25—medium	—	—
Piperidine				
Thioridazine[c]	Mellaril	100—low	200–700[b]	—
Mesoridazine	Serentil	50—low	75–300	25
Piperacetazine	Quide (not sold in U.S.)	10—medium	—	—
Thioxanthenes				
Chlorprothixene	Taractan (no longer manufactured)	50—low	50–400	25–50
Thiothixene	Navane	2–5—high	6–30	2–4
Dibenzoxazepine				
Loxapine	Loxitane	10–15—medium	60–100	12.5–50
Dihydroindole				
Molindone	Moban	6–10—medium	50–100	—
Butyrophenones				
Haloperidol	Haldol	2–5—high	6–20	2–6
Droperidol	Inapsine	10—medium	—	—
Diphenylbutylpiperidine				
Pimozide[c]	Orap	1—high	1–10	—

[a]Recommended adult dosages are 200 to 400 mg per day of chlorpromazine or an equivalent amount of another drug.
[b]Maximum 800 mg.
[c]Second-line drug because of cardiotoxicity.

effectiveness for psychosis marked the beginning of modern psychopharmacology by showing that drugs could have specific effects on the symptoms of mental disorders that went beyond sedation. Moreover, the availability of drugs with direct effects on mental disorders became a powerful tool for laboratory studies with animals; that is, understanding how drugs affect the brain could provide information on the illnesses that were affected.

The use of chlorpromazine was reported by Heinz Lehman from Montreal in 1954, and it rapidly captured the interest of U.S. psychiatrists. In 1955, Henry Brill, the assistant state mental health commissioner in New York, initiated the general use of chlorpromazine and reserpine (Serpasil) in state hospitals in that state. Although reserpine was also an effective antipsychotic, its adverse effects led clinicians to prefer chlorpromazine. Reserpine is rarely used for treating psychosis.

In 1953, reports surfaced indicating that chlorpromazine caused parkinsonian symptoms. Although some individuals warned that these symptoms evidenced neural toxicity, others suggested that the dosage should be increased until patients experienced a mild form of parkinsonism. Later that year, clinicians noted that chlorpromazine could also elicit forms of persistent dyskinesia, a syndrome later called *tardive dyskinesia.*

The introduction of chlorpromazine was followed by the introduction of other phenothiazines including perphenazine (Trilafon) and fluphenazine (Prolixin). In 1958, the first effective butyrophenone, haloperidol (Haldol), was introduced by Paul Janssen from Belgium. The first thioxanthene antipsychotics were introduced the same year by P. V. Peterson and his coworkers.

Although many other dopamine receptor antagonists were introduced in subsequent years, they were all similar in effectiveness and differed only in their adverse-effect profiles. The first long-acting antipsychotic, fluphenazine enanthate, was introduced in the early 1960s. Although this and subsequent long-acting agents were similar to other antipsychotics in effectiveness and adverse effects, they provided a way to administer an antipsychotic without requiring patients to take daily oral medication.

CLASSIFICATION AND CHEMISTRY

The dopamine receptor antagonists have been referred to by a number of names including *neuroleptics, antipsychotics,* and *major tranquilizers.* The designation *neuroleptic* was suggested

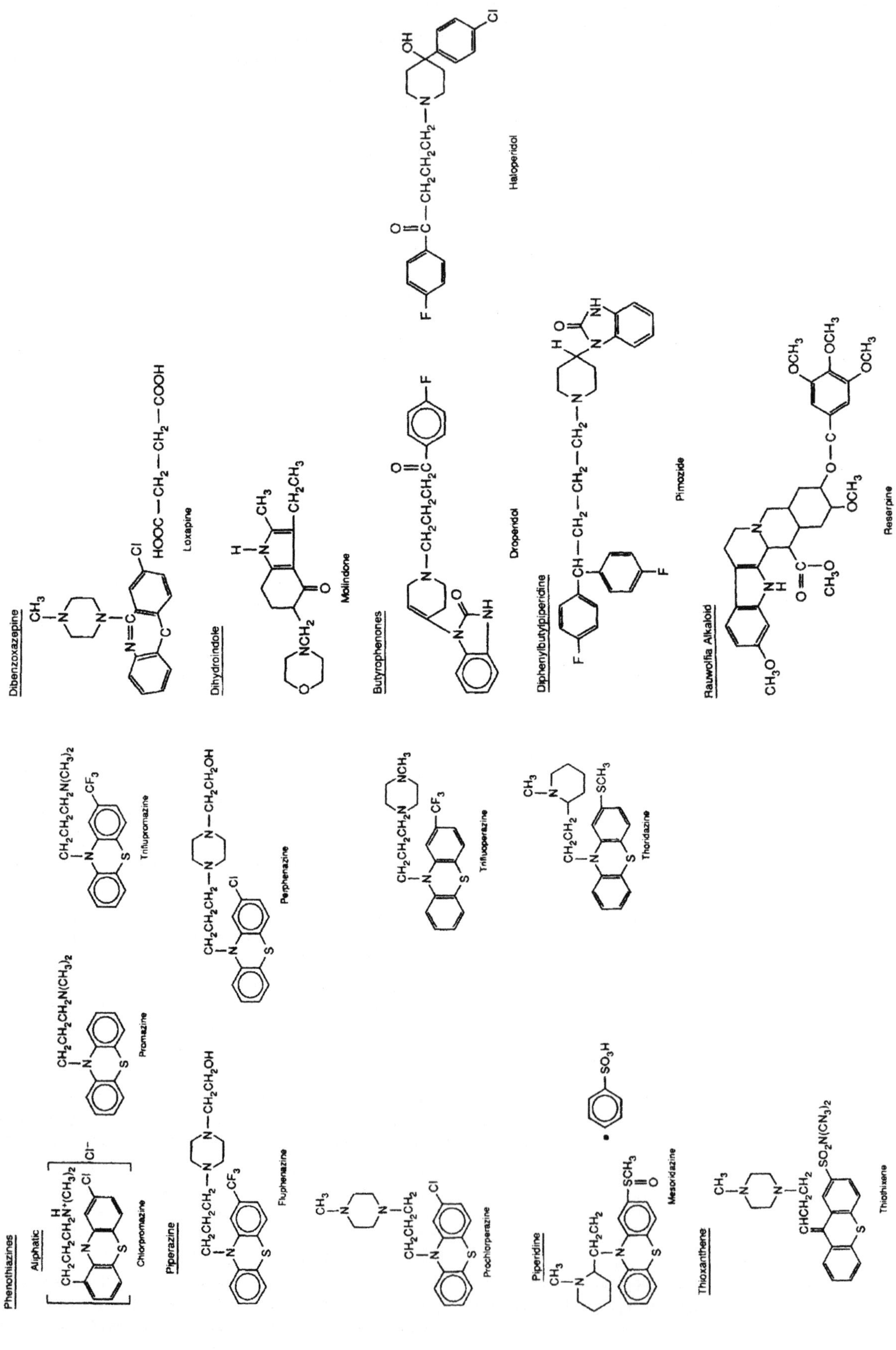

FIGURE 36.4.17–1
Molecular structures of dopamine receptor antagonists and reserpine.

because of the tendency of these agents to have neurological adverse effects and thus to appear to "seize the neuron." This term is based on the observation that neurological adverse effects are inevitably associated with the antipsychotic activity of these agents. However, the effectiveness of drugs such as clozapine (Clozaril) suggests that neurological adverse effects are not necessary to treat psychosis; thus, referring to an adverse effect of these agents rather than the primary clinical effect may be misleading. The term *major tranquilizer* referred to the strange quietness or blandness (or ataraxia) that had been associated with these agents. However, the suggestion that these agents function by their tranquilizing effects is also misleading. These agents, as a group, can be most economically called *antipsychotic drugs*, thus referring to their target symptoms. Differentiating two classes of antipsychotics, the dopamine receptor antagonists and the SDAs, appears to be meaningful, since it suggests a mechanism that underlines important clinical differences between these two groups of agents.

The dopamine receptor antagonists may be subclassified according to either their chemical structure (Fig. 36.4.17–1) or their clinical effects. In the section that follows, these agents are classified according to their chemical structure. Another system for subclassifying this group uses the antipsychotic potency of these agents. According to this system, agents are classified as low-, mild-, or high-potency agents. This method is probably more useful to clinicians because it provides information about the amount of drug required for a clinical effect and the likelihood of important adverse effects.

Phenothiazines

All the phenothiazines have the same three-ring phenothiazine nucleus but differ in the side chains joined to the nitrogen atom of the middle ring. The phenothiazines are typed according to the nature of their side chain: aliphatic (e.g., chlorpromazine), piperazine (e.g., fluphenazine), or piperidine (e.g., thioridazine).

Thioxanthenes

The thioxanthene three-ring nucleus differs from the phenothiazine nucleus by the substitution of a carbon atom for the nitrogen atom in the middle ring. The available thioxanthene has a piperazine (thiothixene [Navane]) side chain.

Dibenzoxazepines

The dibenzoxazepines are based on another modification of the three-ring phenothiazine nucleus. The only dibenzoxazepine available in the United States is loxapine (Loxitane), which has a piperazine side chain. Although loxapine is similar in structure to clozapine, the two compounds have dramatically different pharmacodynamic properties, and loxapine is clearly classifiable with the dopamine receptor antagonists, whereas clozapine is not.

Dihydroindoles

The only dihydroindole available in the United States, molindone (Moban, Lidone), has unusual clinical properties, such as not inducing weight gain and perhaps being less epileptogenic than the other dopamine receptor antagonist antipsychotics.

Butyrophenones

The two butyrophenones available in the United States are haloperidol and droperidol (Inapsine). Haloperidol is one of the most widely used antipsychotics. Although droperidol is approved only for use as an adjuvant to anesthetics, some researchers and clinicians have used droperidol as an intravenous (IV) antipsychotic drug in emergency settings. Spiroperidol, also called *spiperone,* is a butyrophenone compound that can be labeled with a radioactive atom and used in basic and clinical research studies (e.g., positron emission tomography [PET]) to mark dopamine receptors.

Diphenylbutylpiperidines

Diphenylbutylpiperidines are structurally similar to the butyrophenones. Only one diphenylbutylpiperidine, pimozide (Orap), is available in the United States; it is approved for the treatment of Tourette's disorder, although haloperidol is also widely used for this indication, and the other agents are probably equally effective. In Europe, however, pimozide has been shown to be an effective antipsychotic agent. A controversial clinical and research observation about pimozide indicates that it may be more effective than the other antipsychotics in reducing the deficit or negative symptoms of schizophrenia; strongly supportive data for this impression are lacking.

Benzamides

Sulpiride (Dogmatil) and raclopride are available in some countries outside the United States and have been found to be effective antipsychotic drugs. Like spiperone, raclopride has been used as a radiolabeled ligand in research studies, particularly in PET studies of schizophrenic patients, because of its specificity for D_2 receptors.

PHARMACOLOGICAL ACTIONS

Most dopamine receptor antagonists are incompletely absorbed after oral administration, although liquid preparations are absorbed more efficiently than other formulations. The half-lives of the these drugs range from 10 to 20 hours, and all can be given in one daily oral dose once the person is in a stable condition and has adjusted to any adverse effects. Many drugs are also available in parenteral forms that can be given intramuscularly in emergency situations, resulting in more rapid and more reliable attainment of therapeutic plasma concentrations than is possible with oral administration. Peak plasma concentrations are usually reached 1 to 4 hours after oral administration and 30 to 60 minutes after parenteral administration.

In the United States, two antipsychotics, haloperidol and fluphenazine, are available in long-acting depot parenteral formulations for administration once every 1 to 4 weeks, depending on the dose and the person. It can take up to 6 months of treatment with depot formulations to reach steady-state plasma levels, indicating that oral therapy should perhaps be continued during the first month or so of depot antipsychotic treatment. The long half-life of the depot formulation also means that detectable concentrations of the antipsychotic are present long after the last administration of the drug.

The typical antipsychotic drugs appear to reduce psychotic symptoms by inhibiting dopamine binding to dopamine D_2 receptors. The antipsychotic effects appear to derive from inhi-

bition of dopaminergic neurotransmission in the mesocortical dopamine projection, while the parkinsonian adverse effects result from blockade of the nigrostriatal pathway. Inhibition of the tuberoinfundibular tract is responsible for the endocrine effects of the drugs. The drugs reduce psychotic symptoms due to either a primary psychiatric disorder, such as schizophrenia, or another medical condition.

Most of the neurological and endocrinological adverse effects can be explained by their blockade of dopamine receptors. In addition, various antipsychotics also block noradrenergic, cholinergic, and histaminergic receptors, thus accounting for the variation in adverse-effect profiles seen among these drugs. The drugs fall on a spectrum of potency, which ranges from high-potency drugs, which are more likely to cause parkinsonian adverse effects, to low-potency drugs, which are more likely to interact with nondopaminergic receptors and thus have cardiotoxic, epileptogenic, and anticholinergic adverse effects.

EFFECTS ON SPECIFIC ORGANS AND SYSTEMS

Most dopamine receptor antagonists have significant effects on other receptors, including adrenergic, cholinergic, and histaminergic receptors. The other receptor effects affect organs and systems in various ways in addition to the brain. Perhaps the most significant effects involve the heart and the vascular system. Many dopamine receptor antagonist drugs, particularly the low-potency drugs, decrease cardiac contractility, increase atrial and ventricular conduction times, and increase the length of refractory periods. The α_1-adrenergic antagonist activity can result in vasodilation and orthostatic (postural) hypotension. The major effect on the gastrointestinal system is mediated by the drugs' blockade of muscarinic cholinergic receptors, which results in dry mouth and constipation, especially with clozapine and the low-potency drugs. The dopamine receptor antagonist drugs as a class can have various effects on the skin (e.g., rashes, photosensitivities, and discoloring), although these effects are uncommon. A transient decrease in leukopoiesis commonly results from dopamine receptor antagonist treatment. Chlorpromazine has weak diuretic effects, but the predominant genitourinary effects are those affecting sexual function. The effects on sexual function are mediated primarily through the resulting imbalances in adrenergic and cholinergic activities, decreases in catecholamine activity, and endocrine effects of the dopamine receptor antagonists (e.g., increased prolactin).

THERAPEUTIC INDICATIONS

Primary Psychotic Disorders

Dopamine receptor antagonists are effective in both short-term and long-term management of schizophrenia, schizophreniform disorder, schizoaffective disorder, delusional disorder, brief psychotic disorder, manic episodes, and major depressive disorder with psychotic features. They both reduce acute symptoms and prevent future exacerbations.

Schizophrenia. About 75 percent of all persons with schizophrenia relapse over the course of 1 year if treated with a placebo; by comparison, only 15 to 25 percent relapse after taking dopamine receptor antagonists. Furthermore, the symptoms during the relapses are less severe in persons receiving maintenance treatment than in those not receiving antipsychotic treatment.

In general, the dopamine receptor antagonists are thought to be more effective in the treatment of the positive symptoms of schizophrenia (e.g., hallucinations, delusions, and agitation) than in the treatment of the negative symptoms (e.g., emotional withdrawal and ambivalence) or the cognitive dissociations. The dopamine receptor antagonists themselves may also contribute to the negative symptoms. It is also generally believed that paranoid symptoms are treated more effectively than nonparanoid symptoms and that women are more responsive than men. Some persons do not respond to any of the dopamine receptor antagonists but may show improvement with the SDAs, which also have been demonstrated to improve negative and cognitive as well as positive symptoms.

Bipolar Disorders. Antipsychotics are often used in combination with antimanic drugs to treat psychosis or manic excitement in bipolar I disorder. The standard drugs for treatment of bipolar disorder, lithium (Eskalith), carbamazepine (Tegretol), and valproate (Depakene), generally have a slower onset of action than do antipsychotics in the treatment of the acute symptoms. The general practice is to use combination therapy at the initiation of treatment and then gradually withdraw the antipsychotics.

Combination treatment with an antipsychotic and an antidepressant is one of the treatments of choice for major depressive disorder with psychotic features; the other is electroconvulsive therapy (ECT). These patients tend to exhibit faster improvement when an antipsychotic is added to an antidepressant agent. No evidence suggests that any dopamine receptor antagonist is more effective than any other for this indication. The added benefits of dopamine receptor antagonists are most apparent for patients tormented by severe delusions. When the psychotic symptoms have remitted, antipsychotic use should be discontinued.

Persons with schizoaffective disorder and delusional disorder often respond favorably to treatment with dopamine receptor antagonists. Some persons with borderline personality disorder who have marked psychotic symptoms as part of their disorder respond at least partially to antipsychotic drugs, although these persons in particular also require psychotherapeutic treatment.

Secondary Psychoses

Secondary psychoses are psychotic syndromes that are associated with an identified organic cause, such as a brain tumor, a dementing disorder (e.g., dementia of the Alzheimer's type), or substance abuse. The dopamine receptor antagonists are generally effective in the treatment of psychotic symptoms associated with these syndromes. The high-potency dopamine receptor antagonists are usually safer than the low-potency dopamine receptor antagonists in such persons because the high-potency drugs have lower cardiotoxic, epileptogenic, and anticholinergic activities. Dopamine receptor antagonists should not be used to treat withdrawal symptoms associated with ethanol or barbiturate intoxication because of the risk that

such treatment will cause withdrawal seizures. The drug of choice in such patients is usually a benzodiazepine. Agitation and psychosis associated with such neurological conditions as dementia of the Alzheimer's type also respond to antipsychotic treatment. High-potency drugs and low dosages are generally preferable; however, even with high-potency drugs, as many as 25 percent of elderly persons may experience episodes of hypotension. Low dosages of high-potency drugs, such as 0.5 to 5 mg a day of haloperidol, usually suffice for the treatment of these persons.

Severe Agitation and Violent Behavior

Dopamine receptor antagonists are used to treat persons who are severely agitated and violent, although other drugs such as benzodiazepines are also effective for the immediate control of such behavior. Symptoms such as extreme irritability, lack of impulse control, severe hostility, gross hyperactivity, and agitation respond to short-term treatment with dopamine receptor antagonists. Mentally handicapped children, especially those with profound mental retardation and autistic disorder, often have associated episodes of violence, aggression, and agitation that respond to treatment with antipsychotic drugs; however, the repeated administration of antipsychotics to control disruptive behavior in children is controversial. If dopamine receptor antagonists are used, the high-potency drugs, which cause little sedation (e.g., 0.5 to 1 mg a day of haloperidol), are preferred to the more sedating low-potency drugs.

Tourette's Disorder

Dopamine receptor antagonists are used to treat Tourette's disorder. Haloperidol and pimozide are the most frequently used drugs in this class. Many clinicians prefer to use clonidine (Catapres) for this indication because of the lower risk of neurological adverse effects.

Other Psychiatric and Nonpsychiatric Indications

Some clinicians use low dosages of typical antipsychotic drugs (0.5 mg of haloperidol daily) to treat severe anxiety. The risk of inducing neurological adverse effects must be carefully weighed against the potential therapeutic benefits in such cases. Other miscellaneous indications for the use of dopamine receptor antagonists include the treatment of nausea, emesis, intractable hiccups, and pruritus. The rare neurological disorders ballismus and hemiballismus (which affects only one side of the body), characterized by propulsive movements of the limbs away from the body, also respond to treatment with antipsychotic agents.

PRECAUTIONS AND ADVERSE REACTIONS

One generalization about the adverse effects of dopamine receptor antagonists is that low-potency drugs cause most nonneurological adverse effects and high-potency drugs cause most neurological extrapyramidal adverse events (Table 36.4.17–2).

Table 36.4.17–2
Potencies and Adverse Effect Profiles of Dopamine Receptor Antagonists

Drug	Potency	Sedative Effect	Hypotensive Effect	Anticholinergic Effect	Extrapyramidal Effect
Phenothiazines					
Aliphatic					
Chlorpromazine (Thorazine)	Low	High	High	Medium	Low
Piperidines					
Mesoridazine (Serentil)	Low	Medium	Medium	Medium	Medium
Thioridazine (Mellaril)	Low	High	High	High	Low
Piperazines					
Fluphenazine (Prolixin, Permitil)	High	Medium	Low	Low	High
Perphenazine (Trilafon)	Medium	Low	Low	Low	High
Trifluoperazine (Stelazine)	High	Medium	Low	Low	High
Thioxanthene					
Thiothixene (Navane)	High	Low	Low	Low	High
Dibenzodiazepines					
Loxapine (Loxitane)	Medium	Medium	Medium	Medium	High
Butyrophenones					
Droperidol (Inapsine—Injection only)	Medium	Low	Low	Low	High
Haloperidol (Haldol)	High	Low	Low	Low	High
Indolone					
Molindone (Moban)	Medium	Medium	Low	Medium	High
Diphenylbutylpiperidine					
Pimozide (Orap)	High	Low	Low	Low	High

From Hyman SE, Arana GW, Rosenbaum JF. *Handbook of Psychiatric Drug Therapy.* 3rd ed. Boston: Little, Brown; 1996, with permission.

Nonneurological Adverse Effects

Cardiac Effects. Low-potency dopamine receptor antagonists are more cardiotoxic than high-potency dopamine receptor antagonists are. Chlorpromazine use prolongs the QT and PR intervals, blunts the T waves, and depresses the ST segment. Thioridazine use, in particular, markedly affects the T wave and is associated with malignant arrhythmias, such as torsade de pointes, perhaps explaining why overdoses of piperidine phenothiazines may be the most lethal of this group of drugs. When QT intervals exceed 0.44 ms, there is some correlation with an increased risk for sudden death, possibly secondary to ventricular tachycardia or ventricular fibrillation.

Sudden Death. The cardiac effects of dopamine receptor antagonists have been hypothesized to be related to sudden death in patients treated with the drugs. But careful evaluation of the literature indicates that it is premature to attribute the sudden deaths to dopamine receptor antagonist drugs used alone. Supporting this view is the observation that the introduction of dopamine receptor antagonists had no effect on the incidence of sudden death in patients with schizophrenia. In addition, both low-potency and high-potency drugs were involved in the reported cases. Furthermore, many reports concerned patients with other medical problems who were also treated with several other drugs. Pimozide use prolongs the QT interval, an effect that is potentiated during concomitant administration of macrolide antibiotics, which inhibit the metabolism of pimozide by the hepatic enzyme cytochrome P450 isoenzyme 3A3/4 (CYP 3A3/4). At least 2 deaths have been attributed to cardiotoxicity as a result of simultaneous administration of pimozide and clarithromycin (Biaxin). The Food and Drug Administration (FDA) has therefore recently contraindicated the use of pimozide with clarithromycin (Biaxin), erythromycin, azithromycin (Zithromax), and dirithromycin (Dynabac).

Orthostatic (Postural) Hypotension. Orthostatic (postural) hypotension is mediated by adrenergic blockade and is most common with low-potency dopamine receptor antagonists, particularly chlorpromazine, thioridazine, chlorprothixene (Taractan), and clozapine. It occurs most frequently during the first few days of treatment, and tolerance is rapidly developed for the adverse effects. The chief dangers of orthostatic hypotension are that the patients may faint, fall, and injure themselves, although such occurrences are uncommon.

When using intramuscular (IM) low-potency dopamine receptor antagonists, clinicians should measure patients' blood pressure (lying and standing) before and after the first dose and during the first few days of treatment. When appropriate, patients should be warned of the possibility of fainting and should be given the usual instructions to rise from bed gradually, sit at first with their legs dangling, wait for a minute, and sit or lie down if they feel faint. Support hose may help some patients. Patients with orthostatic hypotension should avoid caffeine, drink at least 2 liters of fluid per day, and add salt to food, if they are not already hypertensive.

If hypotension does occur in patients receiving the medications, the symptoms can usually be managed by having the patients lie down with the feet higher than the head. On rare occasions, volume expansion or vasopressor agents, such as norepinephrine (Levophed), may be indicated. Because hypotension is produced by α-adrenergic blockade, the drugs also block the α-adrenergic stimulating properties of epinephrine and leave the β-adrenergic stimulating effects untouched. Therefore, administration of epinephrine results in a paradoxical worsening of hypotension and is contraindicated in cases of dopamine receptor antagonist–induced hypotension. Pure α-adrenergic pressor agents, such as metaraminol (Aramine) and norepinephrine, are the drugs of choice in the treatment of the disorder.

Hematological Effects. An often transient leukopenia with a white blood cell (WBC) count of about 3,500 is a common but not serious problem. Agranulocytosis is a life-threatening hematological problem that occurs most often with chlorpromazine use but is seen with almost all dopamine receptor antagonists. Agranulocytosis occurs most frequently during the first 3 months of treatment and with an incidence of about 1 in 10,000 patients treated with dopamine receptor antagonists. Routine complete blood counts (CBCs) are not indicated, but if a patient reports a sore throat and fever, a CBC should be done immediately to check for the possibility. If the blood indexes are low, use of the dopamine receptor antagonist should be stopped, and the patient should be transferred to a medical facility. The mortality rate for the complication may be as high as 30 percent. Thrombocytopenic or nonthrombocytopenic purpura, hemolytic anemias, and pancytopenia may occur rarely in patients treated with dopamine receptor antagonists.

Peripheral Anticholinergic Effects. Peripheral anticholinergic effects are common and consist of dry mouth and nose, blurred vision, constipation, urinary retention, and mydriasis. Some patients also have nausea and vomiting. Chlorpromazine, mesoridazine (Serentil), and loxapine are potent anticholinergics (Table 36.4.17–2). Anticholinergic effects can be particularly severe if a low-potency dopamine receptor antagonist is used with a tricyclic drug and an anticholinergic drug; this practice is seldom warranted.

Dry mouth can be a troubling symptom for some patients and can endanger continued compliance. Patients can be advised to rinse out their mouths frequently with water and not to chew gum or candy containing sugar, which can result in fungal infections of the mouth or an increased incidence of dental caries. Constipation should be treated with the usual laxative preparations, but the condition can still progress to paralytic ileus in some patients. A decrease in the dopamine receptor antagonist dosage or a change to another less anticholinergic drug is warranted in such a case. Pilocarpine (Salagen) may be used to treat paralytic ileus, although the relief is only transitory. Bethanechol (Urecholine) (20 to 40 mg a day) may be useful in some patients with urinary retention.

Endocrine Effects. Blockade of the dopamine receptors in the tuberoinfundibular tract results in the increased secretion of prolactin, which can result in breast enlargement, galactorrhea, and impotence in men and amenorrhea and inhibited orgasm in women. The SDAs, in contrast, are not particularly associated with increased prolactin levels and may be the drug of choice for patients in whom increased prolactin release results in disturbing effects.

Sexual Adverse Effects. Psychiatrists may not find out about the disturbing sexual effects of a dopamine receptor antagonist if they do not specifically ask about the effects. The incidence of these effects is believed to be significantly underestimated. Up to 50 percent of men taking dopamine receptor antagonists may experience ejaculatory and erectile dysfunction. Several reports have stated that treatment of the condition with sildenafil (Viagra) has been successful. Bromocriptine (Parlodel) or yohimbine (Yocon) may also work in some patients, although the risk of exacerbating the underlying psychosis must be considered with both drugs. Both men and women taking dopamine receptor antagonists can experience anorgasmia and decreased libido. Thioridazine is particularly associated with decreased libido and retrograde ejaculation in men. The latter is harmless, but patients should be advised that voiding after orgasm may be characterized by milky white urine. Other dopamine receptor antagonists have been associated with both delayed and retrograde ejaculation, although some therapeutic success has been reported after treatment with brompheniramine (Dimetane), ephedrine, phenylpropanolamine, and imipramine (Tofranil) for the condition. Priapism and painful orgasms have also been described, both of which possibly result from α_1-adrenergic antagonist activity.

Weight Gain. A common adverse effect of treatment with dopamine receptor antagonists is weight gain, which can be significant in some cases. Molindone and, perhaps, loxapine are not associated with the symptom and may be indicated when weight gain is a serious health hazard or a reason for noncompliance.

Dermatological Effects. Allergic dermatitis and photosensitivity occur in a small percentage of patients, most commonly in those taking low-potency drugs, particularly chlorpromazine. A variety of skin eruptions—urticarial, maculopapular, petechial, and edematous—have been reported. The eruptions occur early in treatment, generally in the first few weeks, and remit spontaneously. A photosensitivity reaction that resembles severe sunburn also occurs in some patients taking chlorpromazine. Patients should be warned of this adverse effect, should spend no more than 30 to 60 minutes in the sun, and should use sunscreens. Chlorpromazine is also associated with some cases of a blue-gray discoloration of the skin over areas exposed to sunlight. The skin changes often begin with a tan or golden brown color and progress to such colors as slate gray, metallic blue, and purple.

Ophthalmological Effects. Thioridazine is associated with irreversible pigmentation of the retina when given in dosages of more than 800 mg a day. An early symptom of this effect can sometimes be nocturnal confusion related to difficulty with night vision. The pigmentation is similar to that seen in retinitis pigmentosa; it can progress even after the thioridazine is stopped and can finally result in blindness. The pigmentation is not reversible.

In contrast, chlorpromazine is associated with a relatively benign pigmentation of the eyes, characterized by whitish brown granular deposits concentrated in the anterior lens and posterior cornea and visible only by slit-lens examination. The deposits can progress to opaque white and yellow-brown granules, often stellate. Occasionally, the conjunctiva is discolored by a brown pigment. Retinal damage does not occur in the patients, and their vision is almost never impaired. Most patients who show the deposits have ingested 1 to 3 kg of chlorpromazine throughout their lives.

Jaundice. Obstructive or cholestatic jaundice is a rare adverse effect of dopamine receptor antagonist treatment. The adverse effect usually occurs in the first month of treatment and is heralded by symptoms of upper abdominal pain, nausea and vomiting, a flulike syndrome, fever, rash, eosinophilia, bilirubin in the urine, and increased serum bilirubin, alkaline phosphatase, and hepatic transaminases. In the early days of chlorpromazine treatment, jaundice was not unusual; it occurred in about 1 of every 100 patients treated. Currently, the incidence is about 1 in 1,000. The drop in the incidence is perhaps caused by a reduction in impurities in the manufacturing of the compound, although the definitive reason for the drop in incidence is unknown.

If jaundice occurs, clinicians generally discontinue the medication, although the value of this practice is unproved. Indeed, patients have continued to receive chlorpromazine throughout the illness without adverse effects, although this approach seems unwarranted in view of the wide range of alternative treatments available. Jaundice has also been reported with use of promazine, thioridazine, and prochlorperazine (Compazine) and very rarely with fluphenazine and trifluoperazine (Stelazine). No convincing evidence indicates that haloperidol or many of the other nonphenothiazine dopamine receptor antagonists can produce jaundice.

Overdoses of Antipsychotics. The symptoms of dopamine receptor antagonist overdose include extrapyramidal symptoms (discussed below), mydriasis, decreased deep tendon reflexes, tachycardia, and hypotension. With the exception of overdoses of thioridazine and mesoridazine, the outcome of dopamine receptor antagonist overdose is generally favorable unless a patient has also ingested other central nervous system (CNS) depressants, such as alcohol or benzodiazepines. The severe symptoms of overdose include delirium, coma, respiratory depression, and seizures. Haloperidol may be among the safest dopamine receptor antagonists in overdose. After an overdose, the electroencephalogram (EEG) shows diffuse slowing and low voltage. Overdose of the piperazine phenothiazines (e.g., thioridazine) can lead to heart block, ventricular fibrillation, and death.

The treatment of dopamine receptor antagonist overdose should include the use of activated charcoal, if possible, and gastric lavage. The use of emetics is not indicated, as the antiemetic actions of the dopamine receptor antagonists inhibit their efficacy. Seizures can be treated with IV diazepam (Valium) or phenytoin (Dilantin). Hypotension can be treated with either norepinephrine or dopamine (Dopastat) but not epinephrine.

Neurological Adverse Effects

The dopamine receptor antagonist drugs, especially the typical or old ones, are associated with a number of uncomfortable extrapyramidal neurological adverse effects and several potentially serious ones. Many of the neurological adverse effects are severe enough to warrant attention as separate problems that

require their own treatment plans. The recognition that the treatment-emergent adverse effects are of significant clinical importance is reflected in the text revision of the fourth edition of *Diagnostic and Statistical Manual of Mental Disorders* (DSM-IV-TR) by the inclusion of a separate group of medication-induced movement disorders (see Section 36.3). The common occurrence of uncomfortable neurological adverse effects—particularly parkinsonism, tremor, akathisia, and dystonia—prompted the search for new antipsychotic drugs that are not likely to cause medication-induced movement disorders. The SDAs are less likely than the dopamine receptor antagonists drugs to cause these movement disorders. Of the adverse effects next described, for example, only akathisia is significantly more common in patients treated with SDAs than in patients treated with placebo.

Neuroleptic-Induced Parkinsonism. Parkinsonian adverse effects occur in about 15 percent of patients treated with dopamine receptor antagonists, usually within 5 to 90 days of the initiation of treatment. Symptoms include muscle stiffness (lead-pipe rigidity), cogwheel rigidity, shuffling gait, stooped posture, and drooling. The pill-rolling tremor of idiopathic parkinsonism is rare, but a regular, coarse tremor similar to essential tremor may be present and is referred to as *medication-induced postural tremor* in DSM-IV-TR. A focal, perioral tremor, sometimes referred to as *rabbit syndrome* (a term that is best avoided because of its insensitive comparison between the movement disorder and the masticatory movements of a rabbit), is another parkinsonian effect of dopamine receptor antagonists, although perioral tremor is more likely than other tremors to occur late in the course of treatment. A physical sign of parkinsonism is a positive glabella tap reflex, elicited by tapping the forehead between the eyebrows. Normal subjects habituate to the tap to the extent that they no longer blink after a couple of taps. A positive glabellar sign consists of continuous blinking in response to repeated taps. The masklike facies, bradykinesia, akinesia (lack of initiative), and ataraxia (indifference toward the environment) that are also symptoms of the parkinsonian syndrome are often misdiagnosed as part of the negative or deficit symptom picture of schizophrenia. This misdiagnosis results in the incorrect clinical decision not to attempt to treat the symptoms with anticholinergic drugs or similarly effective drugs for the treatment of neuroleptic-induced movement disorders.

Women are affected by neuroleptic-induced parkinsonism about twice as often as men; the disorder can occur at all ages, although it is most common after age 40. All dopamine receptor antagonists can cause the symptoms, especially the high-potency drugs with low anticholinergic activity. Chlorpromazine and thioridazine are not likely to be involved. The blockade of dopaminergic transmission in the nigrostriatal tract is the cause of neuroleptic-induced parkinsonism. The differential diagnosis of the parkinsonian symptoms should include idiopathic parkinsonism, other organic causes of parkinsonism, and depression, which can also be associated with parkinsonian symptoms.

The disorder can be treated with anticholinergic agents such as benztropine (Cogentin), amantadine (Symadine, Symmetrel), or diphenhydramine (Benadryl). Although amantadine may have fewer adverse effects than anticholinergics do, it may be less effective in reducing muscular rigidity. Anticholinergics should be withdrawn after 4 to 6 weeks to assess whether a patient has developed a tolerance for the parkinsonian effects; about 50 percent of patients with neuroleptic-induced parkinsonism need continued treatment. Even after the dopamine receptor antagonists are withdrawn, parkinsonian symptoms may last up to 2 weeks and even up to 3 months in elderly patients. With such patients, clinicians may continue the anticholinergic drug after stopping the dopamine receptor antagonist until the parkinsonian symptoms have completely resolved.

Neuroleptic-Induced Acute Dystonia. About 10 percent of all patients experience dystonia as an adverse effect of dopamine receptor antagonists, usually in the first few hours or days of treatment. Dystonic movements result from a slow, sustained muscular contraction or spasm that can result in an involuntary movement. Dystonia can involve the neck (spasmodic torticollis or retrocollis), the jaw (forced opening resulting in a dislocation of the jaw or trismus), the tongue (protrusions, twisting), and the entire body (opisthotonos). Involvement of the eyes can result in an oculogyric crisis, characterized by the eyes' upward lateral movement. Unlike other types of dystonia, an oculogyric crisis may also occur late in treatment. Other dystonias include blepharospasm and glossopharyngeal dystonia, which can result in dysarthria, dysphagia, and even trouble breathing, which can cause cyanosis. Children are particularly likely to exhibit opisthotonos, scoliosis, lordosis, and writhing movements. Dystonia can be painful and frightening and often results in noncompliance with the drug treatment regimen.

Dystonia is most common in young men (less than 40 years old) but can occur at any age in either sex. Although it is most common with IM dosages of high-potency dopamine receptor antagonists, dystonia can occur with any dopamine receptor antagonist. The mechanism of action is thought to be the dopaminergic hyperactivity in the basal ganglia that occurs when the CNS levels of the dopamine receptor antagonist drug begin to fall between doses. Dystonia can fluctuate spontaneously, can respond to reassurance, and can result in a clinician's false impression that the movement is hysterical or completely under conscious control. The differential diagnosis of a dystonic movement should include seizures and tardive dyskinesia.

Prophylaxis with anticholinergics or related drugs (Table 36.4.17–3) usually prevents the development of dystonia, although the risks of prophylactic treatment weigh against this benefit. Treatment with IM anticholinergics or IV or IM diphenhydramine (50 mg) almost always relieves the symptoms. Diazepam (10 mg IV), amobarbital (Amytal), caffeine sodium benzoate, and hypnosis are also reportedly effective. Although tolerance for the adverse effect usually develops, it is sometimes prudent to change the dopamine receptor antagonist if a patient is particularly concerned that the reaction may recur.

Neuroleptic-Induced Acute Akathisia. Akathisia is a subjective feeling of muscular discomfort that can cause patients to be agitated, pace relentlessly, alternately sit and stand in rapid succession, and feel generally dysphoric. The symptoms are primarily motor and cannot be controlled by a patient's will. Akathisia can appear at any time during treatment. The disorder is probably underdiagnosed because the symptoms are mistakenly attributed to psychosis, agitation, or lack of cooperation. The mechanism underlying akathisia is poorly understood, although the disorder may represent an

Table 36.4.17–3
Drug Treatment of Extrapyramidal Disorders

Generic Name	Trade Name	Usual Daily Dosage	Indications
Anticholinergic			
Benztropine	Cogentin	PO 1–4 mg bid; IM or IV 1–2 mg	Acute dystonic reaction, parkinsonism, akinesia, akathisia
Biperiden	Akineton	PO 2–6 mg tid; IM or IV 2 mg	
Procyclidine	Kemadrin	PO 2.5–5 mg bid-qid	
Trihexyphenidyl	Artane, Tremin, Pipanol	PO 2–5 mg tid	
Orphenadrine	Norflex	PO 50–100 mg bid; IV 60 mg	
Antihistaminergic			
Diphenhydramine	Benadryl	PO 25 mg qid; IM or IV 25 mg	Acute dystonic reaction, parkinsonism, akinesia, rabbit syndrome
Dopamine agonists			
Amantadine	Symmetrel	PO 100–200 mg bid (max 300 mg)	Parkinsonism, akinesia, rabbit syndrome
β-Adrenergic antagonists			
Propranolol	Inderal	PO 20–40 mg tid	Akathisia, tremor
α-Adrenergic antagonists			
Clonidine	Catapres	PO 0.1 mg tid	Akathisia
Benzodiazepines			
Clonazepam	Klonopin	PO 1 mg bid	Akathisia, acute dystonic reactions
Lorazepam	Ativan	PO 1 mg tid	

imbalance between the noradrenergic and dopaminergic systems caused by the dopamine receptor antagonists.

Once akathisia is recognized and diagnosed, the dopamine receptor antagonist dosage should be reduced to the minimal effective level. Treatment can be attempted with anticholinergics or amantadine, although these drugs are not particularly effective for akathisia. Drugs that may be more effective include propranolol (Inderal, 30 to 120 mg a day), benzodiazepines, and clonidine. In some cases of akathisia, no treatment seems to be effective.

Neuroleptic-Induced Tardive Dyskinesia. The word *tardive,* like *tardy,* implies *late*. Tardive dyskinesia is a delayed effect of antipsychotics; it rarely occurs until after 6 months of treatment. The disorder consists of abnormal, involuntary, irregular choreoathetoid movements of the muscles of the head, limbs, and trunk. The severity of the movements ranges from minimal—often missed by patients and their families—to grossly incapacitating. Perioral movements are the most common and include darting, twisting, and protruding movements of the tongue; chewing and lateral jaw movements; lip puckering; and facial grimacing. Finger movements and hand clenching are also common. Torticollis, retrocollis, trunk twisting, and pelvic thrusting occur in severe cases. Respiratory dyskinesia has also been reported. Dyskinesia is exacerbated by stress and disappears during sleep. Other late-appearing movement disorders have been noted and have been referred to, depending on the symptoms, as *tardive dystonia, tardive parkinsonism,* and *tardive Tourette's disorder.*

All of the dopamine receptor antagonists have been associated with tardive dyskinesia. The longer patients take dopamine receptor antagonists, the more likely they are to experience tardive dyskinesia. About 10 to 20 percent of patients who are treated for more than 1 year have tardive dyskinesia. About 15 to 20 percent of long-term hospital patients have tardive dyskinesia. Women are more likely to be affected than men, and patients over 50 years of age, patients with brain damage, children, and patients with mood disorders are also at high risk. Before the introduction of antipsychotics in the early 1950s, 1 to 5 percent of patients with schizophrenia had similar abnormal movements. Thus the pattern of movement disorders can be related to the underlying pathophysiology of schizophrenia itself. Tardive dyskinesia may be caused by dopaminergic receptor supersensitivity in the basal ganglia resulting from chronic blockade of dopamine receptors by dopamine receptor antagonists.

The three basic approaches to tardive dyskinesia are prevention, diagnosis, and management. Prevention is best achieved by using dopamine receptor antagonist medications only when clearly indicated and in the lowest effective dosages. Early experience suggests that the SDAs carry a lower risk for development of tardive dyskinesias than the dopamine receptor antagonists. Patients who are receiving dopamine receptor antagonists should be examined regularly for the appearance of abnormal movements, preferably by using a standardized rating scale (see Table 36.3–9 in Section 36). When abnormal movements are detected, a differential diagnosis should be considered (Table 36.4.17–4).

Once a diagnosis of tardive dyskinesia is made, clinicians must regularly conduct objective ratings of the movement disorder. Although tardive dyskinesia often emerges while patients are taking a steady dosage of medication, it is even more likely to emerge when the dosage is reduced. Some investigators have referred to this effect as *withdrawal dyskinesia,* although differentiating withdrawal dyskinesia from tardive dyskinesia is impossible. Once tardive dyskinesia is recognized, clinicians should consider reducing the dosage of the dopamine receptor antagonist or even stopping use of the medication altogether. The SDAs may be used in patients with tardive dyskinesias, since they reduce the movements and have the lowest risk of exacerbating the condition.

Table 36.4.17–4
Differential Diagnosis for Tardive Dyskinesia–Like Movements

Common: schizophrenic mannerisms and stereotypies
Dental problems (e.g., ill-fitting dentures)
Meige's syndrome and other senile dyskinesias
Drug-induced: antidepressants
Antihistamines
Antimalarials
Antipsychotics
Diphenylhydantoin
Heavy metals
Levodopa
Sympathomimetics
CNS: anoxia induced
Hepatic failure
Huntington's disease
Parathyroid hypoactivity
Postencephalitic
Pregnancy (chorea gravidarum)
Renal failure
Sydenham's chorea
Systemic lupus erythematosus
Thyroid hyperactivity
Torsion dystonia
Tumors
Wilson's disease

When tardive dyskinesia was first recognized and until recently, the movement disorder was believed to be chronic and progressive. Recent surveys conclude that tardive dyskinesia develops rapidly, stabilizes, and then often remits, sometimes even while the patient continues the same drug treatment. Nonetheless, continuing to use the same drug does not seem necessary when potentially better drugs are available. Between 5 and 40 percent of all cases of tardive dyskinesia eventually remit, and between 50 and 90 percent of all mild cases remit; but tardive dyskinesia is less likely to remit in elderly patients than in young ones.

Tardive dyskinesia has no single effective treatment. Lowering the dosage of the dopamine receptor antagonist and switching to an SDA are the primary treatment strategies. In patients who cannot continue taking any dopamine receptor antagonist medication, lithium, carbamazepine, or benzodiazepines may be effective in reducing both the movement disorder symptoms and the psychotic symptoms, although these drugs are less effective than the dopamine receptor antagonists in treating the psychiatric symptoms. Various small studies have reported that cholinergic agonists and antagonists, dopaminergic agonists, and γ-aminobutyric acid (GABA)-ergic drugs—for example, valproic acid (Depakene)—may be helpful, although the use of these drugs should be considered experimental and should be started only after a review of the most recent literature.

Neuroleptic Malignant Syndrome. Neuroleptic malignant syndrome is a life-threatening complication that can occur any time during the course of dopamine receptor antagonist treatment. The motor and behavioral symptoms include muscular rigidity and dystonia, akinesia, mutism, obtundation, and agitation. The autonomic symptoms include hyperpyrexia (up to 107°F), sweating, and increased pulse and blood pressure. Laboratory findings include increased WBC count, creatinine phosphokinase, liver enzymes, plasma myoglobin, and myoglobinuria, occasionally associated with renal failure. The symptoms usually evolve over 24 to 72 hours, and the untreated syndrome lasts 10 to 14 days. The diagnosis is often missed in the early stages, and the withdrawal or agitation may mistakenly be considered to reflect increased psychosis. Men are affected more frequently than women, and young patients are affected more commonly than elderly patients. The mortality rate can reach 20 to 30 percent or even higher when depot dopamine receptor antagonist medications are involved. The pathophysiology is unknown.

The first steps in treatment are immediate discontinuation of dopamine receptor antagonist drug use; medical support to cool the patient; monitoring of vital signs, electrolytes, fluid balance, and renal output; and symptomatic treatment of fevers. Antiparkinsonian medications may reduce some of the muscle rigidity. Intravenous dantrolene (Dantrium), a skeletal muscle relaxant (0.8 to 2.5 mg/kg every 6 hours, up to a total dosage of 10 mg a day), may be useful in the treatment of the disorder. Once the patient can take oral medications, the dantrolene can be given in doses of 100 to 200 mg a day. Bromocriptine (20 to 30 mg a day in four divided doses) or perhaps amantadine can be added to the regimen. Treatment should usually be continued for 5 to 10 days. When dopamine receptor antagonist treatment is restarted, clinicians should consider switching to a low-potency drug or to an SDA, although neuroleptic malignant syndrome has also been reported to be associated with both clozapine and risperidone (Risperdal).

Epileptogenic Effects. Dopamine receptor antagonist administration is associated with slowing and increased synchronization of the EEG. This effect may be the mechanism by which some dopamine receptor antagonists decrease the seizure threshold. Chlorpromazine, loxapine, and other low-potency dopamine receptor antagonists are thought to be more epileptogenic than high-potency drugs. Animal data and in vitro experimental data indicate that molindone may be the least epileptogenic of the dopamine receptor antagonist drugs. The risk of inducing a seizure by drug administration warrants consideration when a patient already has a seizure disorder or an organic brain lesion.

Sedation. Sedation is primarily a result of the blockade of histamine type 1 receptors. Chlorpromazine is the most sedating dopamine receptor antagonist; thioridazine, chlorprothixene, and loxapine are also sedating; the high-potency dopamine receptor antagonists are much less sedating than are these drugs (Table 36.4.17–2). When first treated with dopamine receptor antagonists, patients should be warned about driving and operating machinery. Giving the entire daily dopamine receptor antagonist dose at bedtime usually eliminates any problems with sedation, and tolerance for this adverse effect often develops.

Central Anticholinergic Effects. The symptoms of central anticholinergic activity include severe agitation; disorientation to time, person, and place; hallucinations; seizures; high

fever; and dilated pupils. Stupor and coma may ensue. The treatment of anticholinergic toxicity consists of discontinuing the causal agent or agents, close medical supervision, and physostigmine (Antilirium, Eserine), 2 mg by slow IV infusion, repeated within 1 hour as necessary. Too much physostigmine is dangerous, and symptoms of physostigmine toxicity include hypersalivation and sweating. Atropine sulfate (0.5 mg) can reverse the effects of physostigmine toxicity.

Prevention and Treatment of Some Neuroleptic-Induced Movement Disorders. A variety of drugs (Table 36.4.17–3) may be used to prevent and treat medication-induced movement disorders, particularly neuroleptic-induced parkinsonism and neuroleptic-induced acute dystonia. The drugs include anticholinergics, amantadine, antihistamines, benzodiazepines, β-adrenergic receptor antagonists, and clonidine. Most acute dystonia and parkinsonism symptoms are treated effectively by these drugs, and acute akathisia may also respond in some cases.

It remains controversial whether prophylactic treatment with these drugs is warranted when starting a patient on dopamine receptor antagonist use. The proponents of prophylactic treatment argue that the increased likelihood of avoiding adverse neurological effects is humane to the patient and increases the possibility of future compliance. The opponents of the practice argue that a large proportion (30 to 50 percent) of patients do not need antiparkinsonian drugs, that their use may increase the likelihood of tardive dyskinesia, autonomic adverse effects, cognitive impairment, hyperthermia, and anticholinergic toxicity. Many drugs used to treat parkinsonian symptoms also have some abuse liability and may be associated with changes in the plasma concentrations of the dopamine receptor antagonists. A reasonable compromise is to use the drugs prophylactically in patients under the age of 45 who are at risk for adverse effects, particularly dystonia, and not to use the drugs prophylactically in patients over 45 who are at increased risk for anticholinergic toxicity.

Once patients start taking drugs to treat a movement disorder, they should be treated for 4 to 6 weeks. Then clinicians should attempt to taper and stop use of the medication over a 1-month period. Many patients become tolerant for the neurological adverse effects and no longer require treatment for the neuroleptic-induced movement disorder. Some patients experience the return of neurological symptoms and should be restarted on use of the appropriate drugs.

Most clinicians use one of the anticholinergic drugs (e.g., benztropine) or diphenhydramine to provide prophylaxis for, or treatment of, neurological adverse effects. Of these drugs, diphenhydramine is the most sedating; biperiden (Akineton) is neither sedating nor stimulating; and trihexyphenidyl (Artane) may be slightly stimulating. Amantadine is most often used when one of the anticholinergic drugs is ineffective. Although amantadine does not typically exacerbate the psychosis of schizophrenia, some patients become tolerant of its antiparkinsonian effects. Amantadine is also a sedating drug for some patients.

Pregnancy and Lactation

If possible, dopamine receptor antagonists should be avoided during pregnancy, particularly in the first trimester, unless the benefit outweighs the risk. In fact, however, very few data indicate a correlation between the presence of congenital malformations in infants and the use of dopamine receptor antagonists during pregnancy, except perhaps for chlorpromazine. Some data do indicate that the use of dopamine receptor antagonists during pregnancy may result in decreased dopamine receptors in the neonate, increased cholesterol, and perhaps behavioral disturbances. Nevertheless, dopamine receptor antagonist use in the second and third trimesters is probably relatively safe. High-potency dopamine receptor antagonists are preferable to low-potency drugs, as the low-potency drugs are associated with hypotension.

Haloperidol and phenothiazines pass into breast milk. Whether loxapine, molindone, and pimozide pass into breast milk is not known, although they probably do. Women who are taking dopamine receptor antagonists should not breastfeed their infants, as the available data do not prove the practice safe.

DRUG INTERACTIONS

Because of their many receptor effects and because the metabolism of most dopamine receptor antagonists is in the liver, many pharmacokinetic and pharmacodynamic drug interactions are associated with these drugs (Table 36.4.17–5).

Antacids

Antacids, cimetidine (Tagamet), ranitidine (Zantac), famotidine (Pepcid), and nizatidine (Axid), administered within 2 hours of dopamine receptor antagonist administration, can reduce the absorption of dopamine receptor antagonist drugs.

Anticholinergics

Anticholinergics may decrease the absorption of dopamine receptor antagonists. The additive anticholinergic activity of dopamine receptor antagonists, anticholinergics, and tricyclic drugs may result in anticholinergic toxicity.

Anticonvulsants

Phenothiazines, especially thioridazine, may decrease the metabolism of diphenylhydantoin and can result in toxic levels of diphenylhydantoin. Barbiturates may increase the metabolism of dopamine receptor antagonists, and the dopamine receptor antagonists may lower a patient's seizure threshold.

Antidepressants

Tricyclic drugs and dopamine receptor antagonists may decrease each other's metabolism, resulting in increased plasma concentrations of both drugs. The anticholinergic, sedative, and hypotensive effects of the drugs may also be additive.

Haloperidol, perphenazine, thioridazine, and other dopamine receptor antagonists are metabolized by the hepatic enzyme CYP 2D6. Drugs that inhibit CYP 2D6, such as fluoxetine (Prozac) and paroxetine (Paxil), may increase antipsychotic levels when administered concomitantly.

Table 36.4.17–5
Antipsychotic Drug Interactions

Interacting Medication	Mechanism	Clinical Effect
Drug interactions assessed to have major severity		
β-Adrenergic receptor antagonists	Synergistic pharmacologic effect; antipsychotic inhibits metabolism of propranolol; antipsychotic increases plasma concentrations	Severe hypotension
Anticholinergics	Pharmacodynamic effects	Decreased antipsychotic effect
	Additive anticholinergic effect	Anticholinergic toxicity
Barbiturates	Phenobarbital induces antipsychotic metabolism	Decreased antipsychotic concentrations
Carbamazepine	Induces antipsychotic metabolism	Up to 50% reduction in antipsychotic concentrations
Charcoal	Reduces GI absorption of antipsychotic and adsorbs drug during enterohepatic circulation	May reduce antipsychotic effect or cause toxicity during overdose or for GI disturbances
Cigarette smoking	Induction of microsomal enzymes	Reduced plasma concentrations of antipsychotic agents
Epinephrine, norepinephrine	Antipsychotic antagonizes pressor effect	Hypotension
Ethanol	Additive CNS depression	Impaired psychomotor skills
Fluvoxamine	Fluvoxamine inhibits metabolism of haloperidol and clozapine	Increased concentrations of haloperidol and clozapine
Guanethidine	Antipsychotic antagonizes guanethidine reuptake	Impaired antihypertensive effect
Lithium	Unknown	Rare reports of neurotoxicity
Meperidine	Additive CNS depression	Hypotension and sedation
Drug interactions assessed to have minor or moderate severity		
Amphetamines, anorexiants	Decreased pharmacological effect of amphetamine; drug-disease state interaction	Diminished weight loss effect; amphetamines may exacerbate psychosis; treatment-refractory schizophrenics may improve
Angiotensin-converting enzyme inhibitors	Additive hypotensive crisis	Hypotension, postural intolerance
Antacids containing aluminum	Insoluble complex formed in GI tract	Possible reduced antipsychotic effect
Antidepressants (AD) nonspecific	Decreased metabolism of AD through competitive inhibition	Increased AD concentration
Benzodiazepines	Increased pharmacological effect of the benzodiazepine	Respiratory depression, stupor, hypotension
Bromocriptine	Antipsychotic antagonizes dopamine receptor stimulation	Increased prolactin
Caffeinated beverages	Form precipitate with antipsychotic solutions	Possible diminished antipsychotic effect
Cimetidine	Reduced antipsychotic absorption and clearance	Decreased antipsychotic effect
Clonidine	Antipsychotic potentiates α-adrenergic hypotensive effect	Hypotension or hypertension
Disulfiram	Impairs antipsychotic metabolism	Increased antipsychotic concentrations
Methyldopa	Unknown	Blood pressure elevations
Phenytoin	Induction of antipsychotic metabolism; decreased phenytoin metabolism	Decreased antipsychotic concentrations; increased phenytoin levels
Serotonin-specific reuptake inhibitors	Impair antipsychotic metabolism; pharmacodynamic interaction	Sudden onset of extrapyramidal symptoms
Valproic acid	Antipsychotic inhibits valproic acid metabolism	Increased valproic acid half-life and levels

From Ereshosky L, Overman GP, Karp JK. Current psychotropic dosing and monitoring guidelines. *Prim Psychiatry.* 1996;3:21, with permission.

Antihypertensives

Dopamine receptor antagonists may inhibit the uptake of guanethidine (Esimil, Ismelin) in the synapse and may also inhibit the hypotensive effects of clonidine and methyldopa (Aldomet). Conversely, dopamine receptor antagonists may have an additive effect on some hypotensive drugs. Dopamine receptor antagonist drugs have a variable effect on the hypotensive effects of clonidine. Propranolol coadministration with dopamine receptor antagonists increases the blood concentrations of both drugs. Coadministration of captopril (Capoten), hydralazine (Apresoline), minoxidil (Loniten, Rogaine) opioids, trazodone (Desyrel), and tricyclics can worsen hypotension.

Central Nervous System Depressants

Dopamine receptor antagonists potentiate the CNS depressant effects of sedatives, antihistamines, opiates, opioids, and alcohol, particularly in patients with impaired respiratory status. When these agents are taken with alcohol, the risk for heat stroke may be increased.

Other Substances

Cigarette smoking may decrease the plasma levels of dopamine receptor antagonist drugs. Epinephrine has a paradoxical hypotensive effect in patients taking dopamine receptor antagonists. Dopamine

receptor antagonist drugs may decrease the blood concentration of warfarin (Coumadin) and result in decreased bleeding time. Phenothiazines and pimozide should not be coadministered with other agents that prolong the QT interval, particularly macrolide antibiotics (e.g., erythromycin, clarithromycin, azithromycin, and dirithromycin). Hydroxyzine (Atarax, Vistaril) may potentiate mesoridazine and thioridazine toxicity.

LABORATORY INTERFERENCES

Dopamine receptor antagonists may have a calming and sedating effect within 1 hour of administration, but improvement in the full range of positive psychotic symptoms usually appears within 1 to 2 weeks of onset of treatment, and a therapeutic trial in severely or chronically ill patients requires 6 weeks. Continuing improvement in symptoms is seen over the first 3 to 12 months of use. Dopamine receptor antagonist drugs have been reported to interfere with some laboratory tests. Chlorpromazine and perphenazine have been reported to cause both false-positive and false-negative results in immunological pregnancy tests and falsely elevated bilirubin (with reagent test strips) and urobilinogen (with Ehrlich's reagent test) values. Dopamine receptor antagonist drugs have also been associated with an abnormal shift in results of the glucose tolerance test, although this shift may reflect the effects of the drugs on the glucose-regulating system.

Phenothiazines have been reported to interfere with the measurement of 17-ketosteroids (with the Haltorff-Koch modification of the Zimmerman reaction) and 17-hydroxycorticosteroids (with the modified Glenn-Nelson reaction).

DOSAGE AND ADMINISTRATION

Dopamine receptor antagonists may have a calming and sedating effect within 1 hour of administration, but improvement in the full range of positive psychotic symptoms usually appears within 1 to 2 weeks of onset of treatment, and a therapeutic trial in severely or chronically ill patients requires 6 weeks. Continuing improvement in symptoms is seen over the first 3 to 12 months of use. These drugs are remarkably safe in short-term use, and, if necessary, clinicians can administer the drugs without conducting a physical or laboratory examination of the patient. The major contraindications for dopamine receptor antagonists are a history of a serious allergic response, the possibility that the patient has ingested a substance that will interact with the antipsychotic to induce CNS depression (e.g., alcohol, opiates, opioids, barbiturates, and benzodiazepines) or anticholinergic delirium (e.g., scopolamine [Donnagel] and possibly phencyclidine [PCP]), the presence of a severe cardiac abnormality, a high risk for seizures from organic and idiopathic causes, the presence of narrow-angle glaucoma or prostatic hypertrophy if a dopamine receptor antagonist with high anticholinergic activity is to be used, and the presence, or a history, of tardive dyskinesia. Dopamine receptor antagonists should be administered with caution in patients with hepatic disease, as impaired hepatic metabolism may result in high plasma concentrations of the dopamine receptor antagonists. In the usual assessment, clinicians should obtain a CBC with white blood cell indexes, liver function tests, and an electrocardiogram (ECG), especially in women over 40 and men over 30. Older adults and children are more sensitive to adverse effects than young adults are, and the dosage of the drug should be adjusted accordingly.

Choice of Drug

Although the potencies of the dopamine receptor antagonists vary widely, all available typical dopamine receptor antagonists are equally efficacious in the treatment of schizophrenia. The dopamine receptor antagonists are available in a wide range of formulations and dose sizes (Table 36.4.17–6). Data support the conclusion that SDAs may be more effective than other antipsychotic drugs for the treatment of the negative symptoms of schizophrenia. With the dopamine receptor antagonist drugs, no type of schizophrenia and no particular symptoms are most effectively treated by any single class of dopamine receptor antagonists. The SDAs may become the drugs of first choice in the treatment of schizophrenia if their possibly superior efficacies with negative symptoms and their superior safety profiles are confirmed in wide clinical testing.

The general guidelines for choosing a particular psychotherapeutic drug should be followed when choosing a dopamine receptor antagonist drug (see Section 36.1). If no other rationale prevails, the choice should be based on adverse-effect profiles and the clinician's preference. Although high-potency dopamine receptor antagonists are associated with increased neurological adverse effects, current clinical practice favors using them because of the high incidence of other adverse effects (e.g., cardiac, hypotensive, epileptogenic, sexual, and allergic) with the low-potency drugs. A myth in psychiatry is that hyperexcitable patients respond best to chlorpromazine because it is highly sedating, whereas withdrawn patients respond best to high-potency dopamine receptor antagonists, such as fluphenazine. This has never been proved; if sedation is a desired goal, either the dopamine receptor antagonist can be given in divided doses or a sedative drug, such as a benzodiazepine, can also be administered.

The SDAs offer many advantages over the dopamine receptor antagonists and have been increasingly chosen as first-line agents. The most prominent advantages of the SDAs are their low risk of extrapyramidal symptoms and the therapeutic benefit for both positive and negative symptoms. Clozapine, olanzapine (Zyprexa), sertindole (Serlect), and others are less likely to raise prolactin levels than are dopamine receptor antagonists. Clozapine and olanzapine have significant anticholinergic effects, however, and may cause sedation. In the future, the dopamine receptor antagonists may be reserved for those patients who tolerate them with minimal adverse effects, for economic reasons, or for the fact that they are available in depot forms.

A clinical observation supported by some research is that a patient's unpleasant reaction to the first dose of a dopamine receptor antagonist drug correlates highly with future poor response and noncompliance. Such experiences include a subjective negative feeling, oversedation, and acute dystonia. If a patient reports such a reaction, the clinician may be well advised to switch the patient to a different antipsychotic. Similarly, if patients have reported that they did not feel well while taking a particular drug in the past, clinicians are well advised not to initiate treatment with this drug again.

Table 36.4.17–6
Dopamine Receptor Antagonist Preparations

	Tablets	Capsules	Solution	Parenteral	Rectal Suppositories
Acetophenazine	20 mg	—	—	—	—
Chlorpromazine	10, 25, 50, 100, 200 mg	30, 75, 150, 200, 300 mg	10 mg/5 mL, 30 mg/mL, 100 mg/mL	25 mg/mL	25, 100 mg
Droperidol	—	—	—	2.5 mg/mL	—
Fluphenazine	1, 2.5, 5, 10 mg	—	2.5 mg/5 mL, 5 mg/mL	2.5 mg/mL (IM only)	—
Fluphenazine decanoate	—	—	—	25 mg/mL	—
Fluphenazine enanthate	—	—	—	25 mg/mL	—
Haloperidol	0.5, 1, 2, 10, 20 mg	—	2 mg/mL	5 mg/mL (IM only)	—
Haloperidol decanoate	—	—	—	50 mg/mL, 100 mg/mL (IM only)	—
Loxapine	—	5, 10, 25, 50 mg	25 mg/mL	50 mg/mL	—
Mesoridazine	10, 25, 50, 100 mg	—	25 mg/mL	25 mg/mL	—
Molindone	5, 10, 25, 50, 100 mg	—	20 mg/mL	—	—
Perphenazine	2, 4, 8, 16 mg	—	16 mg/5 mL	5 mg/mL	—
Pimozide	2 mg	—	—	—	—
Prochlorperazine	5, 10, 25 mg	10, 15, 30 mg (SR)	5 mg/5 mL	5 mg/mL	2.5, 5, 25 mg
Promazine	25, 50, 100 mg	—	—	25 mg/mL, 50 mg/mL	—
Thioridazine	10, 15, 25, 50, 100, 150, 200 mg	—	25 mg/5 mL, 100 mg/5 mL, 30 mg/mL, 100 mg/mL	—	—
Thiothixene	—	1, 2, 5, 10, 20 mg	5 mg/mL	10 mg (IM only), 2 mg/mL (IM only)	—
Trifluoperazine	1, 2, 5, 10 mg	—	10 mg/mL	2 mg/mL	—
Triflupromazine	—	—	—	10 mg/mL, 20 mg/mL	—

Dosage and Schedule

The therapeutic index for dopamine receptor antagonists is favorable and has contributed to the unfortunate practice of routinely using high dosages of the drugs. Because of this common practice, physicians may be pressured by staff members to use very high dosages. Recent investigations of the dose-response curve for dopamine receptor antagonists indicate that the equivalent of 10 to 20 mg of haloperidol is usually efficacious for either short-term or long-term treatment of schizophrenia. Some clinicians and researchers recommend that dosages equivalent to 5 to 10 mg of haloperidol be used before going to higher dosages. Dopamine receptor antagonist drugs may have a bell-shaped dose-response curve. In general, the dosage of a dopamine receptor antagonist drug should be evaluated over a 6-week period before increasing it or switching to another antipsychotic drug. Overly high dosages of dopamine receptor antagonists may lead to adverse neurological effects, such as akinesia and akathisia, which are difficult to distinguish from exacerbations of psychosis.

Although patients can build up a tolerance for most adverse effects caused by dopamine receptor antagonists, they do not build up a tolerance for the antipsychotic effect. Nevertheless, clinicians should taper the dosage when a drug is being discontinued, as patients may experience rebound effects from the other neurotransmitter systems that the drug may have blocked. Cholinergic rebound, for example, can produce a flulike syndrome in patients.

Short-Term Treatment. The equivalent of 5 to 10 mg of haloperidol is a reasonable dose for an adult patient in an acute state. A geriatric patient may benefit from as little as 1 mg of haloperidol. The administration of more than 50 mg of chlorpromazine in one injection may result in serious hypotension. IM administration of the dopamine receptor antagonists results in peak plasma levels in about 30 minutes, versus 90 minutes by the oral route. Doses of dopamine receptor antagonists for IM administration are about half the doses given by the oral route. In a short-term treatment setting, patients should be observed for 1 hour after the first dose of dopamine receptor antagonist medication. After that time, most clinicians administer a second dose of a dopamine receptor antagonist or a sedative agent (e.g., a benzodiazepine) to achieve effective behavioral control. Possible sedatives include lorazepam (Ativan, 2 mg IM) and amobarbital (50 to 250 mg IM).

RAPID NEUROLEPTIZATION. Rapid neuroleptization (also called *psychotolysis*) is the practice of administering hourly IM doses of dopamine receptor antagonist medications until marked sedation of a patient is achieved. Several research studies have shown, however, that merely waiting several more hours after one dose of a dopamine receptor antagonist results in the same clinical improvement as occurs with repeated doses of dopamine receptor antagonists. Nevertheless, clinicians must be careful to keep patients from becoming violent while they are psychotic. Clinicians can help prevent violent episodes by using adjuvant sedatives or by temporarily using physical restraints until patients can control their behavior.

Early Treatment. Agitation and excitement are usually the first symptoms to improve with dopamine receptor antagonist treatment. About 75 percent of patients with a short history of illness have significant improvement in their psychosis. Patients with a long history of illness may need a full 6 weeks of treatment to evaluate the extent of the improvement in psychotic symptoms. Data indicate that psychotic symptoms, both positive and negative, continue to improve 3 to 12 months after the initiation of treatment.

The equivalent of 10 to 20 mg of haloperidol or 400 mg of chlorpromazine a day is adequate treatment for most patients with schizophrenia. Some research studies indicate that in a significant proportion of patients, 5 mg of haloperidol or 200 mg of chlorpromazine may, in fact, be just as effective as higher doses. It is reasonable to give dopamine receptor antagonist drugs in divided doses when initiating treatment, to minimize the peak plasma levels and to reduce the incidence of adverse effects. The total daily dose can subsequently be consolidated into a single daily dose after the first or second week of treatment. The single daily dose is usually given at bedtime to help induce sleep and to reduce the incidence of adverse effects. This practice may increase the risk of elderly patients falling if they get out of bed during the night. The sedative effects of dopamine receptor antagonists last only a few hours, in contrast to the antipsychotic effects, which last for 1 to 3 days.

"AS-NEEDED" MEDICATIONS. It is common clinical practice to order medications to be given as needed (prn). Although this practice may be reasonable during the first few days that a patient is hospitalized, the length of time the patient takes antipsychotic drugs, not an increase in dosage, is what produces therapeutic improvement. Clinicians may feel pressured by their staff members to write prn antipsychotic orders. Orders for prn medications should include specific symptoms, how often the drugs should be given, and how many doses can be given each day. Clinicians may choose to use small doses for the prn doses (e.g., 2 mg of haloperidol) or to use a benzodiazepine instead (e.g., 2 mg of lorazepam IM). If prn doses of a dopamine receptor antagonist are necessary after the first week of treatment, the clinician may want to consider increasing the standing daily dosage of the drug.

Maintenance Treatment. The first 3 to 6 months after a psychotic episode are usually considered a period of stabilization for the patient. After that time, the dosage of the dopamine receptor antagonist can be decreased about 20 percent every 6 months until the minimum effective dosage is found. A patient is usually maintained on antipsychotic medications for 1 to 2 years after the first psychotic episode. Antipsychotic treatment is often continued for 5 years after a second psychotic episode, and lifetime maintenance is considered after the third psychotic episode, although attempts to reduce the daily dosage can be made every 6 to 12 months.

Dopamine receptor antagonist drugs are effective in controlling psychotic symptoms, but patients may report that they prefer being off the drugs, because they feel better without them. This problem may be less common with the new antipsychotic drugs, such as clozapine, risperidone, and olanzapine. Normal persons who have taken dopamine receptor antagonist drugs report a sense of dysphoria. Clinicians must discuss maintenance medication with patients and take into account the patients' wishes, the severity of their illnesses, and the quality of their support systems.

Alternative Maintenance Regimens. Alternative maintenance regimens have been designed to reduce both the risk of long-term adverse effects and any unpleasantness associated with taking dopamine receptor antagonist medications. Intermittent medication is the use of antipsychotics only when patients require them. This arrangement requires that patients or their caretakers be both willing and able to watch carefully for early signs of clinical exacerbations. At the earliest signs of such problems, use of antipsychotic medications should be reinstituted for a reasonable period, usually 1 to 3 months. Although this treatment approach is not indicated for most patients, it is a safe and effective treatment approach for some.

Drug holidays are regular 2- to 7-day periods during which a patient is not given antipsychotic medications. Currently, no evidence indicates that drug holidays reduce the risk of long-term adverse effects from antipsychotics, and drug holidays may increase the incidence of noncompliance.

Long-Acting Depot Medications. Because some patients with schizophrenia do not comply with oral dopamine receptor antagonist regimens, long-acting depot preparations may be needed (Table 36.4.17–7). A clinician usually administers the IM

Table 36.4.17–7
Use of Long-Acting Dopamine Receptor Antagonists

Dosage
- a. Stabilize patient on lowest effective dose of oral preparation.
- b. Usual dosage conversion:
  - 10 mg/day oral fluphenazine = 12.5–25 mg/2 weeks fluphenazine decanoate
  - 10 mg/day oral haloperidol = 100–200 mg/4 weeks haloperidol decanoate
- c. As with all other antipsychotic medications, the lowest effective dose should be used. Note that patients with chronic schizophrenia have been adequately maintained on doses of fluphenazine decanoate as low as 5 mg/2 weeks.
- d. Supplementation with oral medication may be necessary for the first several months until the optimum dosage regimen has been determined.

Techniques of injection
- a. Using a 2-inch needle, inject no more than 3 mL of medication per injection into upper quadrant of buttock (to inject more than 3 mL, use alternate buttocks and vary injection sites).
- b. After drawing up medication, draw a small air bubble of 0.1 mL into syringe and change needle for injection.
- c. Wipe injection site with alcohol swab and allow to dry before giving injection; otherwise alcohol may infiltrate subcutaneous tissue and cause local irritation.
- d. Stretch the skin over the injection site to one side and hold firmly.
- e. Inject medication slowly, including air bubble, which forces last drop from needle into the muscle and prevents any medication from being deposited in subcutaneous tissue as needle is withdrawn.
- f. Wait about 10 seconds before withdrawing needle, then do so quickly and release skin.
- g. Do not massage injection site, as this may force medication to ooze from muscle and infiltrate subcutaneous tissue.
- h. Precautions should also be taken with glass ampules to avoid injection of glass particles.

Technique for injecting long-acting neuroleptics. *Br J Psychiatry.* 1982;144:316, with permission.

preparations once every 1 to 4 weeks, and thus knows immediately when a patient has missed a dose of medication. Depot dopamine receptor antagonist may be associated with increased adverse effects, including tardive dyskinesia, although the data for this increased association are controversial. Some researchers and clinicians limit their use of depot dopamine receptor antagonists to patients who are not compliant with oral medications; other researchers and clinicians, particularly in Europe, consider depot dopamine receptor antagonists the formulation of choice for the treatment of schizophrenia.

Two depot preparations (a decanoate and an enanthate) of fluphenazine and a decanoate preparation of haloperidol are available in the United States. The preparations are injected IM into an area of large muscle tissue, from which they are absorbed slowly into the blood. Decanoate preparations can be given less frequently than enanthate preparations because they are absorbed more slowly. Although stabilizing a patient on the oral preparation of the specific drugs is not necessary before initiating the depot form, it is good practice to give at least one oral dose of the drug to assess the possibility of an adverse effect, such as severe extrapyramidal symptoms or an allergic reaction.

The correct dosage and time interval for depot preparations are difficult to predict. It is reasonable to begin with 12.5 mg (0.5 mL) of fluphenazine preparation or 25 mg (0.5 mL) of haloperidol decanoate. If symptoms emerge in the next 2 to 4 weeks, a patient can be treated temporarily with additional oral medications or with additional small depot injections. After 3 to 4 weeks the depot injection can be increased to include the supplemental doses given during the initial period.

A good reason to initiate depot treatment with low doses is that absorption of the preparations may be faster than usual at the onset of treatment, which can result in frightening episodes of dystonia that eventually discourage compliance with the medication. Some clinicians keep patients drug free for 3 to 7 days before initiating depot treatment and then give very small doses of the depot preparations (3.125 mg of fluphenazine or 6.25 mg of haloperidol) every few days to avoid these initial problems. Because the major indication for depot medication is poor compliance with oral forms, clinicians should go slowly with what is practically the last method of achieving compliance.

Plasma Concentrations. Interindividual variation in the metabolism of the antipsychotics is significant and arises in part from genetic differences among patients and from pharmacokinetic interactions with other drugs. In patients who have not improved after 4 to 6 weeks of dopamine receptor antagonist treatment, the plasma concentration of the drug should be determined if such a test is available. Other possible indications for obtaining a plasma concentration are questions regarding compliance, concern about pharmacokinetic interactions, and the development of significant akathisia or akinesia.

The blood sample must be obtained after a patient has been taking a particular dosage for at least 5 times the half-life of the drug, so as to approach steady-state concentrations. It is also standard practice to obtain plasma samples at trough levels—that is, just before the daily dose is given, usually at least 12 hours after the previous dose and most commonly 20 to 24 hours after the previous dose. Unfortunately, the quality of the laboratories that perform the analyses varies significantly; thus clinicians must obtain the normal ranges for a particular laboratory and must test the laboratory with multiple plasma samples from well-controlled patients. Having taken all these precautions, clinicians are still left with the reality that most dopamine receptor antagonists have no well-defined dose-response curve. The best studied drug is haloperidol, which may have a therapeutic window ranging from 2 to 15 ng/mL. Other therapeutic ranges that have been reasonably well documented are 30 to 100 ng/mL for chlorpromazine and 0.8 to 2.4 ng/mL for perphenazine.

Treatment-Resistant Persons. Various studies indicate that 10 to 35 percent of persons with schizophrenia fail to obtain significant benefit from the antipsychotic drugs. Persons are often defined as treatment-resistant if they have failed at least two adequate trials of antipsychotics from two pharmacological classes. Adequate trials are usually defined as at least 6 weeks of daily doses equivalent to 20 mg of haloperidol or 1000 mg of chlorpromazine. It is useful to determine plasma concentrations for such persons, since one possibility is that they are slow metabolizers who are grossly overmedicated with a particular drug. More likely, however, they simply do not respond to the typical antipsychotic drugs. Studies have shown that up to two thirds of nonresponders to typical antipsychotic drugs may respond to SDAs.

Adjuvant Treatments. Medications that have been reported to be useful adjuvants to antipsychotics include lithium, carbamazepine, β-adrenergic receptor antagonists, antidepressants, and benzodiazepines. Of these medications, the most robust data support the use of lithium as an adjuvant medication. When using the combination of lithium and antipsychotics, the clinician should use slightly lower dosages of each initially to avoid the development of delirium or neurotoxicity. Carbamazepine has also been reported to be an effective addition to antipsychotic drug treatment, although the coadministration of carbamazepine can lower the plasma concentrations of the antipsychotic as much as 50 percent because of the induction of hepatic enzymes. Benzodiazepines have been reported to be effective as an adjuvant treatment; however, their withdrawal must be monitored carefully to avoid significant worsening of symptoms. An increasing body of data supports the use of antidepressants in schizophrenic persons who have significant depressive symptoms.

References

Baldessarini RJ, Tarazi A. Drugs and the treatment of psychiatric disorders: psychosis and mania. In: Hardman JG, Limbird LE, Goodman Gilman A, eds. *Goodman & Gilman's the Pharmacological Basis of Therapeutics.* 10th ed. New York: McGraw-Hill; 2001:485.

Blin O, Azorin JM, Bouhours P. Antipsychotic and anxiolytic properties of risperidone, haloperidol and methotrimeprazine in schizophrenic patients. *J Clin Psychopharmacol.* 1996;16:38.

Brauer LH, de Wit H. Subjective responses to D-amphetamine alone and after pimozide pretreatment in normal, healthy volunteers. *Biol Psychiatry.* 1996;39:26.

Breier A, Tram PV, eds. *Current Issues in the Psychopharmacology of Schizophrenia.* Philadelphia: Lippincott Williams & Wilkins; 2001:534.

Crescimanno G, Mannino M, Casarrubea M, Amato G. Effects of sulpiride on the orienting movement evoked by acoustic stimulation in the rat. *Pharmacol Biochem Behav.* 2000;66:747.

Czobor P, Volavka J. Dimensions of the Brief Psychiatric Rating Scale: an examination of stability during haloperidol treatment. *Comp Psychiatry.* 1996;37:205.

de la Fuente FR. Drug-induced motor complications in dopa-responsive dystonia: implications for the pathogenesis of dyskinesias and motor fluctuations. *Clin Neuropharmacol.* 1999;22:216.

Deleu D, Hanssens Y. Aging and neuroleptic-induced acute dystonia. *Am J Psychiatry.* 1996;153:447.

Finlay WML, Bernal SJ. Tourette's syndrome and challenging behaviour: a case study. *Ment Handicap.* 1996;24:80.
Huang HF, Jann MW, Tseng Y-T, et al. Ketone reductase activity and reduced haloperidol ratios in haloperidol-treated schizophrenic patients. *Psychiatry Res.* 1995;57:101.
Huttunen MO, Tuhkanen H, Haavisto E, et al. Low- and standard-dose depot haloperidol combined with targeted oral neuroleptics. *Psychiatr Serv.* 1996;47:83.
Keshavan MS, Aguilar EJ. Aging and neuroleptic-induced acute dystonia: reply. *Am J Psychiatry.* 1996;153:448.
Marder SR, van Kammen DP. Dopamine receptor antagonists (typical antipsychotics). In: Sadock BJ, Sadock VA, eds. *Kaplan & Sadock's Comprehensive Textbook of Psychiatry.* 7th ed. Vol 2. Baltimore: Lippincott Williams & Wilkins; 2000:2356.
Markianos M, Hatzimanolos J, Lykouras L. Neuroendocrine responsivities of the pituitary dopamine system in male schizophrenia during treatment with clozapine, olanzapine, risperidone, sulpiride, or haloperidol. *Eur Arch Psychiatry Clin Neurosci.* 2001;251:141.
Oosthuizen P, Emsley RA, Turner J, Keyter N. Determining the optimal dose of haloperidol in first-episode psychosis. *J Psychopharmacol.* 2001;15:251.
Volavka J, Czobor P, Sheitman B, et al. Clozapine, olanzapine, risperidone, and haloperidol in the treatment of patients with chronic schizophrenia and schizoaffective disorder. *Am J Psychiatry.* 2002;159:255.
Xiberas X, Martinot JL, Mallet L, et al. Extrastriatal and striatal D_2 dopamine receptor blockade with haloperidol or new antipsychotic drugs in patients with schizophrenia. *Br J Psychiatry.* 2001;179:503.

▲ 36.4.18 Lithium

Lithium (Eskalith, Lithobid, Lithonate) is the most commonly used short-term, long-term, and prophylactic treatment for bipolar I disorder. It is also used as an adjunctive medication in the treatment of major depressive disorder, schizoaffective disorder, therapy-resistant schizophrenia, anorexia nervosa, and bulimia nervosa and for control of chronic aggression in both children and adults.

HISTORY

Building on the discoveries of others, Humphry Davy isolated metallic lithium in 1818. Lithium was introduced into medicine in the 1840s by Alexander Ure for the treatment of bladder stones and by Alfred Garrod for the treatment of gout. In 1873, in the United States, William Hammond described the use of lithium bromide to treat manic episodes, although bromide was considered the active ingredient. In 1886 in Denmark, Carl Lange and Fritz Lange described the prophylactic and short-term effects of lithium for depression. In the late 1880s and early 1900s, the general public in the United States was enthusiastically endorsing "taking the waters," the use of mineral spring waters that supposedly contained lithium (Fig. 36.4.18–1). The waters, in which only vanishingly small concentrations of lithium were dissolved, were misleadingly advertised as being beneficial for a wide variety of aches, pains, and ills. In the United States in the 1940s, lithium chloride was used as a replacement for sodium chloride in hypertensive patients with low-salt diets; this practice resulted in lithium toxicity and death for some patients, and lithium-related products were withdrawn from the marketplace. In 1949, an Australian, John F. J. Cade, noticed that lithium urate caused lethargy when injected into animals. He later reported the successful therapeutic effects of lithium in a patient with manic episodes. In the 1950s and the 1960s, Mogens Schou conducted the critical experiments demonstrating short-term prophylactic efficacy of lithium for bipolar I disorder. Eventually, the U.S. Food and Drug Administration (FDA) approved lithium for the treatment of bipolar I disorder.

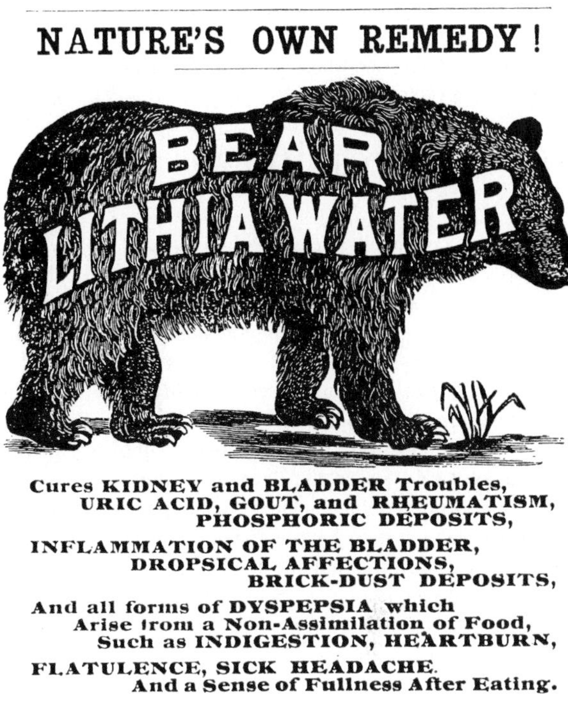

FIGURE 36.4.18–1
Advertisement for Bear Lithia Water.

CHEMISTRY

Lithium (Li), a monovalent ion, is an element and the lightest of the alkali metals (group IA of the periodic table), and is similar to sodium, potassium, and rubidium. Lithium exists as both ^{6}Li and ^{7}Li. The latter isotope allows the imaging of lithium by magnetic resonance spectroscopy.

PHARMACOLOGICAL ACTIONS

After ingestion, lithium is completely absorbed by the gastrointestinal (GI) tract. Serum levels peak in 1 to 1½ hours for standard preparations and in 4 to 4½ hours for controlled-release preparations. Lithium does not bind to plasma proteins, is not metabolized, and is distributed nonuniformly throughout body water. Lithium does not cross the blood–brain barrier rapidly, a fact that perhaps explains why an overdose is not usually a problem and why long-term lithium intoxication takes time to resolve completely. The half-life of lithium is about 20 hours, and equilibrium is reached after 5 to 7 hours of regular intake. Lithium is almost entirely eliminated by the kidneys. Because lithium is absorbed by the proximal tubules, lithium clearance is about one fifth of creatinine clearance. Renal clearance of lithium decreases with renal insufficiency (common in older persons) and in the puerperium and increases during pregnancy. Lithium is excreted in breast milk and in insignificant amounts in the feces and perspiration.

The therapeutic mechanism of action for lithium remains uncertain. The similarity of the lithium ion to the sodium, potassium, calcium, and magnesium ions may be related to its therapeutic effects.

EFFECTS ON SPECIFIC ORGANS AND SYSTEMS

Lithium most commonly affects the thyroid, heart, kidneys, and hematopoietic system. Lithium impedes the release of thyroid hormones from the thyroid and can result in hypothyroidism or goiter; the disorder affects women more than men. Lithium also impairs sinus node function, which can result in heart block in susceptible persons. Lithium reduces the ability of the kidneys to concentrate urine. Although this effect is usually not clinically significant, it is not always reversible after discontinuing lithium use. Pathological nonspecific interstitial fibrosis has been reported as a postmortem finding in some persons who were treated with lithium for a long time, but this is an unusual outcome. The major effect of lithium on the hematopoietic system is a clinically nonsignificant increase in leukocyte production.

THERAPEUTIC INDICATIONS

Bipolar I Disorder

Lithium has proved effective in both the short-term treatment and the prophylaxis of bipolar I disorder in about 70 to 80 percent of patients. Both manic and depressive episodes respond to lithium treatment alone. Lithium should also be considered as a potential treatment for patients with severe cyclothymic disorder.

Manic Episodes. About 80 percent of manic patients respond to lithium treatment, although the response to lithium alone can take 1 to 3 weeks of treatment at therapeutic concentrations. Because of the delay in response to lithium alone, benzodiazepines—for example, clonazepam (Klonopin) and lorazepam (Ativan)—or antipsychotics are used for the first 1 to 3 weeks to obtain immediate relief from the mania. Predictors of a poor response to lithium in the treatment of manic episodes include mixed and dysphoric manic episodes (which may occur in up to 40 percent of patients), rapid cycling, and coexisting substance-related disorders (Table 36.4.18–1). Lithium is effective as long-term prophylaxis of both manic and depressive episodes in about 70 to 80 percent of persons with bipolar I disorder.

Depressive Episodes. Lithium is effective in the treatment of major depressive disorder and depression associated with bipolar I disorder. Because antidepressants can trigger mania in persons with bipolar disorders, lithium monotherapy is an ideal treatment for both mania and depression in persons with bipolar disorder. Lithium may also be prescribed with an antidepressant for long-term maintenance of persons with bipolar disorder. Tricyclic and tetracyclic drugs are considered more likely to trigger severe mania than are bupropion (Wellbutrin) or selective serotonin reuptake inhibitors (SSRIs). Augmentation of lithium therapy with valproate (Depakene) or carbamazepine (Tegretol) is usually well tolerated, with little risk of precipitation of mania.

Table 36.4.18–1
Factors Hypothesized to Predict Response to Lithium

Negative or Unfavorable Response	Positive or Favorable Response
Borderline features	Prior long-term response to lithium
Neuroticism	Classic euphoric or pure mania
Rapid cycling	Family history of bipolar disorder
Mixed manic/depressive symptoms	Secondary mania
Substance abuse	Family history of response to lithium
Psychosis	Obsessional features
Depression is followed by mania	Mania is followed by depression

Reprinted with permission from Krishnan KRR, Davidson JRT, Doraiswamy PM. Pharmacotherapy of depression in bipolar disorder. *Prim Psychiatry.* 1996;3:45.

Schizophrenia. The symptoms of one fifth to one half of all patients with schizophrenia are further reduced when lithium is coadministered with their antipsychotic drug. The therapeutic benefit of lithium does not seem to be correlated with the absence or presence of affective symptoms in these patients. Some schizophrenia patients who cannot take antipsychotic drugs may benefit from lithium treatment alone. The intermittent aggressive outbursts of some patients with schizophrenia may also be reduced by lithium treatment.

Schizoaffective Disorder and Schizophrenia

Among persons with schizoaffective disorder, those with predominant mood symptoms—either bipolar type or depressive type—are more likely to respond to lithium than those with predominant psychotic symptoms. Serotonin-dopamine antagonists (SDAs) and dopamine receptor antagonists are the treatments of choice for persons with schizoaffective disorder, whereas lithium is a useful augmentation agent, particularly for persons whose symptoms are resistant to treatment with SDAs and dopamine receptor antagonists. Lithium augmentation of SDA or dopamine receptor antagonist treatment, however, may be effective for persons with schizoaffective disorder, even in the absence of a prominent mood disorder component.

Aggression

Lithium has been used to treat aggressive outbursts in patients with schizophrenia, prison inmates, children with conduct disorder, and mentally retarded patients. Less success has been reported in the treatment of aggressiveness associated with head trauma and epilepsy. Other drugs for the treatment of aggression include anticonvulsants, β-adrenergic receptor antagonists, and antipsychotics. The treatment of aggressive patients requires a flexible approach in the use of these drugs along with psychosocial and behavioral treatment strategies.

Other Disorders

A few studies have reported that the episodic disorder characterizing premenstrual dysphoric disorder, the intermittent

behaviors of borderline personality disorder, bulimia nervosa, and episodes of binge drinking respond to lithium treatment. Animal models of alcohol dependence have shown that lithium intake can reduce the intake of alcohol. In spite of these basic data, at least one large study has shown no benefit of lithium treatment in alcohol dependence, although anecdotal case reports and small studies in the literature are hopeful. Alcohol use disorder partly caused by an underlying bipolar disorder, for example, may be particularly amenable to lithium treatment. The same treatment may be appropriate for a patient with bipolar disorder who abuses cocaine.

Lithium has been used for treatment-refractory obsessive-compulsive disorder, trichotillomania, and posttraumatic stress disorder. Each of these indications, however, remains to be tested in a placebo-controlled trial. Lithium is particularly effective for the short-term treatment of cluster headaches in some patients.

Maintenance. Maintenance treatment with lithium markedly decreases the frequency, the severity, and the duration of manic and depressive episodes in persons with bipolar I disorder. Lithium provides relatively more effective prophylaxis for mania than for depression, and supplemental antidepressant strategies may be necessary either intermittently or continuously. Lithium maintenance is almost always indicated after the second episode of bipolar I disorder depression or mania and should be considered after the first episode for adolescents or for persons who have a family history of bipolar I disorder. Others who benefit from lithium maintenance are those who have poor support systems, had no precipitating factors for the first episode, have a high suicide risk, had a sudden onset of the first episode, or had a first episode of mania. Clinical studies have shown that lithium reduces the incidence of suicide in bipolar I disorder patients sixfold or sevenfold. Lithium is also effective treatment for persons with severe cyclothymic disorder.

Initiating maintenance therapy after the first manic episode is considered wise on the basis of several observations. First, each episode of mania increases the risk of subsequent episodes. Second, among persons responsive to lithium, relapses are 30 times more likely after lithium use is discontinued. Third, case reports describe persons who initially responded to lithium, discontinued taking it, and then had a relapse but no longer responded to lithium in subsequent episodes. Continued maintenance treatment with lithium is often associated with increasing efficacy and reduced mortality. Therefore, an episode of depression or mania that occurs after a relatively short time of lithium maintenance does not necessarily represent treatment failure. However, lithium treatment alone may begin to lose its effectiveness after several years of successful use. If this occurs, then supplemental treatment with an anticonvulsant may be useful.

Maintenance lithium dosages often can be adjusted to achieve a plasma concentration somewhat lower than that needed for treatment of acute mania. If lithium use is to be discontinued, then the dosage should be slowly tapered. Abrupt discontinuation of lithium therapy is associated with increased risk of recurrence of manic and depressive episodes.

Table 36.4.18–2
Adverse Effects of Lithium

Neurological
Benign, nontoxic: dysphoria, lack of spontaneity, slowed reaction time, memory difficulties
Tremor: postural, occasional extrapyramidal
Toxic: coarse tremor, dysarthria, ataxia, neuromuscular irritability, seizures, coma, death
Miscellaneous: peripheral neuropathy, benign intracranial hypertension, myasthenia gravis–like syndrome, altered creativity, lowered seizure threshold
Endocrine
Thyroid: goiter, hypothyroidism, exophthalmos, hyperthyroidism (rare)
Parathyroid: hyperparathyroidism, adenoma
Cardiovascular
Benign T-wave changes, sinus node dysfunction
Renal
Concentrating defect, morphological changes, polyuria (nephrogenic diabetes insipidus), reduced GFR, nephrotic syndrome, renal tubular acidosis
Dermatological
Acne, hair loss, psoriasis, rash
Gastrointestinal
Appetite loss, nausea, vomiting, diarrhea
Miscellaneous
Altered carbohydrate metabolism, weight gain, fluid retention

PRECAUTIONS AND ADVERSE EFFECTS

The most common adverse effects from lithium treatment are increased thirst, polyuria, gastric distress, weight gain, tremor, fatigue, and mild cognitive impairment (Table 36.4.18–2). Gastric distress may include nausea, vomiting, and diarrhea and can often be reduced by further dividing the dosage, administering the lithium with food, or switching among the various lithium preparations. Weight gain and edema can be impossible to treat except by encouraging the patient to eat less and to exercise moderately. The tremor affects mostly the fingers and sometimes can be worse at peak levels of the drug. It can be reduced by further dividing the dosage. Propranolol (Inderal) (30 to 160 mg a day in divided doses) reduces the tremor significantly in most patients. The fatigue and mild cognitive impairment may decrease with time. Rare neurological adverse effects include symptoms of mild parkinsonism, ataxia, and dysarthria. Patients with brain impairment are at risk of neurotoxicity. Lithium may exacerbate Parkinson's disease. Lithium should be used with caution in diabetic patients, as it may induce seizures or exacerbate a seizure disorder. Dehydrated, debilitated, and medically ill patients are susceptible to adverse effects and toxicity. Leukocytosis is a common benign effect of lithium treatment.

Gastrointestinal Effects

GI symptoms can include nausea, decreased appetite, vomiting, and diarrhea and can be diminished by dividing the dosage, administering the lithium with food, or switching to another

lithium preparation. The lithium preparation least likely to cause diarrhea is lithium citrate. Some lithium preparations contain lactose, which can cause diarrhea in lactose-intolerant persons. Persons taking slow-release formulations of lithium who experience diarrhea due to unabsorbed medication in the lower part of the GI tract may experience less diarrhea with standard-release preparations. Diarrhea may also respond to antidiarrheal preparations such as loperamide (Imodium, Kaopectate), bismuth subsalicylate (Pepto-Bismol), or diphenoxylate with atropine (Lomotil). Weight gain results from a poorly understood effect of lithium on carbohydrate metabolism and can also result from lithium-induced edema.

Neurological Effects

Tremor. A lithium-induced postural tremor may occur that is usually 8 to 12 Hz and is most notable in outstretched hands, especially in the fingers, and during tasks involving fine manipulations. The tremor can be reduced by dividing the daily dosage, using a sustained-release formulation, reducing caffeine intake, reassessing the concomitant use of other medicines, and treating comorbid anxiety. β-Adrenergic receptor antagonists, such as propranolol, 30 to 120 mg a day in divided doses, and primidone (Mysoline), 50 to 250 mg a day, are usually effective in reducing the tremor. In persons with hypokalemia, potassium supplementation may improve the tremor. When a person taking lithium has a severe tremor, the possibility of lithium toxicity should be suspected and evaluated.

After 19 years of successful lithium maintenance, a 37-year-old woman was switched to carbamazepine because of polyuria and proteinuria. Only in retrospect did she and her physicians become aware of the cognitive dulling and impaired concentration that had been present during her many years of lithium use.

Cognitive Effects. Lithium use has been associated with dysphoria, lack of spontaneity, slowed reaction times, and impaired memory. The presence of these symptoms should be noted carefully, because they are a frequent cause of noncompliance. The differential diagnosis for such symptoms should include depressive disorders, hypothyroidism, hypercalcemia, other illnesses, and other drugs. Some, but not all, persons have reported that fatigue and mild cognitive impairment decrease with time.

Other Neurological Effects. Uncommon neurological adverse effects include symptoms of mild parkinsonism, ataxia, and dysarthria, although the last two symptoms may also be due to lithium intoxication. Lithium is (rarely) associated with development of peripheral neuropathy, benign intracranial hypertension (pseudotumor cerebri), findings resembling myasthenia gravis, and increased risk of seizures.

Renal Effects

The most common adverse renal effect of lithium is polyuria with secondary polydipsia. The symptom is a particular problem in 25 to 35 percent of persons taking lithium, who may have a urine output of more than 3 L a day (normal, 1 to 2 L a day). The polyuria primarily results from lithium antagonism to the effects of antidiuretic hormone, which thus causes diuresis. When polyuria is a significant problem, the person's renal function should be evaluated and followed up with 24-hour urine collections for creatinine clearance determinations. Treatment consists of fluid replacement, the use of the lowest effective dosage of lithium, and single daily dosing of lithium.

The most serious renal adverse effects, which are rare and associated with continuous lithium administration for 10 years or more, involve appearance of nonspecific interstitial fibrosis, associated with a gradual decrease in glomerular filtration rate, increased serum creatinine concentrations, and (rarely) renal failure. Lithium occasionally is associated with nephrotic syndrome and features of distal renal tubular acidosis. It is prudent to check the serum creatinine concentration, urine chemistries, and 24-hour urine volume of persons taking lithium, annually.

A 55-year-old man, successfully stabilized on lithium for 22 years, experienced a gradual increase in serum creatinine to 2.4 mg/dL (normal range, 0.6 to 1.3 mg/dL). A thorough evaluation by a nephrologist produced no another explanation, and lithium was felt to be the most likely cause.

Thyroid Effects

Lithium affects thyroid function, causing a generally benign and often transient diminution in the concentrations of circulating thyroid hormones. Reports have attributed goiter (5 percent of persons), benign reversible exophthalmos, hyperthyroidism, and hypothyroidism (7 to 10 percent of persons) to lithium treatment. Lithium-induced hypothyroidism is more common in women (14 percent) than in men (4.5 percent). Women are at highest risk during the first 2 years of treatment. Persons taking lithium to treat bipolar disorder are twice as likely to develop hypothyroidism if they develop rapid cycling. About 50 percent of persons receiving long-term lithium treatment have laboratory abnormalities, such as an abnormal thyrotropin-releasing hormone (TRH) response, and about 30 percent have elevated concentrations of thyroid-stimulating hormone (TSH). If symptoms of hypothyroidism are present, replacement with levothyroxine (Synthroid) is indicated. Even in the absence of hypothyroid symptoms, some clinicians treat persons with significantly elevated TSH concentrations with levothyroxine. In lithium-treated persons, TSH concentrations should be measured every 6 to 12 months. Lithium-induced hypothyroidism should be considered when evaluating depressive episodes that emerge during lithium therapy.

Cardiac Effects

The cardiac effects of lithium, which resemble those of hypokalemia on the electrocardiogram (ECG), are caused by the displacement of intracellular potassium by the lithium ion. The most common changes on the ECG are T wave flattening or inversion. The changes are benign and disappear after the lithium is excreted from the body. Nevertheless, baseline ECGs are essential and should be repeated annually.

Because lithium also depresses the pacemaking activity of the sinus node, lithium treatment can result in sinus dysrhythmias, heart block, and episodes of syncope. Lithium treatment, therefore, is contraindicated in persons with sick sinus syndrome. In rare cases, ventricular arrhythmias and congestive heart failure have been associated with lithium therapy. Lithium cardiotoxicity is more prevalent in persons on a low-salt diet, those taking certain diuretics or angiotensin-converting enzyme inhibitors, and those with fluid-electrolyte imbalances or any renal insufficiency.

Dermatological Effects

Several cutaneous adverse effects, which may be dose dependent, have been associated with lithium treatment. The most prevalent effects include acneiform, follicular, and maculopapular eruptions; pretibial ulcerations; and worsening of psoriasis. Alopecia has also been reported. Many of those conditions respond favorably to changing to another lithium preparation and taking the usual dermatological measures. Lithium concentrations should be monitored if tetracycline is used for the treatment of acne, because it can increase the retention of lithium. Occasionally, aggravated psoriasis or acneiform eruptions may force the discontinuation of lithium treatment.

Lithium Toxicity and Overdoses

The early signs and symptoms of lithium toxicity include neurological symptoms, such as coarse tremor, dysarthria, and ataxia; GI symptoms; cardiovascular changes; and renal dysfunction. The later signs and symptoms include impaired consciousness, muscular fasciculations, myoclonus, seizures, and coma (Table 36.4.18–3). Risk factors include exceeding the recommended dosage; reduced excretion due to renal impairment, a low-sodium diet, or drug interaction; and dehydration. Elderly persons are more vulnerable to the effects of increased serum lithium concentrations. The higher the lithium concentration and the longer the lithium concentration has been high, the worse are the symptoms of lithium toxicity. Lithium toxicity is a medical emergency, since it can result in permanent neuronal damage and death.

The treatment of lithium toxicity (Table 36.4.18–4) involves discontinuing the lithium and treating the dehydration. Unabsorbed lithium can be removed from the GI tract by ingestion of polystyrene sulfonate (Kayexalate) or polyethylene glycol solution (GoLYTELY) but not activated charcoal. Ingestion of a single large dose may create clumps of medication in the stomach, which can be removed by gastric lavage with a wide-bore tube. The value of forced diuresis is still debated. In the most serious cases, hemodialysis is the most effective means of rapid removal of excessive amounts of serum lithium. Postdialysis serum lithium concentrations may rise as lithium is redistributed from tissues to blood, and repeat dialysis may be needed. Neurological improvement may lag behind clearance of serum lithium by several days, because lithium crosses the blood–brain barrier slowly.

Adolescents

The serum lithium concentration for adolescents is similar to that for adults. Although the adverse-effect profile is similar in adolescents and adults, weight gain and acne associated with lithium use can be particularly troublesome to an adolescent.

Table 36.4.18–3
Signs and Symptoms of Lithium Toxicity

Mild to moderate intoxication (lithium level = 1.5–2.0 mEq/L)		
	Gastrointestinal	Vomiting
		Abdominal pain
		Dryness of mouth
	Neurological	Ataxia
		Dizziness
		Slurred speech
		Nystagmus
		Lethargy or excitement
		Muscle weakness
Moderate to severe intoxication (lithium level = 2.0–2.5 mEq/L)		
	Gastrointestinal	Anorexia
		Persistent nausea and vomiting
	Neurological	Blurred vision
		Muscle fasciculations
		Clonic limb movements
		Hyperactive deep tendon reflexes
		Choreoathetoid movements
		Convulsions
		Delirium
		Syncope
		Electroencephalographic changes
		Stupor
		Coma
		Circulatory failure (lowered blood pressure, cardiac arrhythmias, and conduction abnormalities)
Severe lithium intoxication (lithium level >2.5 mEq/L)		
	Generalized convulsions	
	Oliguria and renal failure	
	Death	

From Marangeli LB, Silver JM, Yudofsky SC. Psychopharmacology and electroconvulsive therapy. In: *The American Psychiatric Press Textbook of Psychiatry.* 3rd ed. Washington, DC: American Psychiatric Press; 1999, with permission.

Elderly Persons

Lithium is a safe and effective drug for the elderly. However, the treatment of elderly persons taking lithium may be complicated by the presence of other medical illnesses, decreased renal function, special diets that affect lithium clearance, and generally increased sensitivity to lithium. Elderly persons should initially be given low dosages, their dosages should be switched less frequently than those of younger persons, and a longer time must be allowed for renal excretion to equilibrate with absorption before lithium can be assumed to have reached its steady-state concentrations.

In general, the elderly should be started on lower-than-usual dosages, with dosage changes occurring less frequently than in younger patients. The elimination half-life of lithium increases with age, and the time required to reach steady state is much longer in the elderly. If lithium use is stopped, levels fall more slowly and the resolution of adverse effects and toxicity may be prolonged.

Table 36.4.18–4
Drug Interactions with Lithium

Drug Class	Reaction
Antipsychotics	Case reports of encephalopathy, worsening of extrapyramidal adverse effects, and neuroleptic malignant syndrome; inconsistent reports of altered red blood cell and plasma concentrations of lithium, antipsychotic drug, or both
Antidepressants	Occasional reports of a serotoninlike syndrome with potent serotonin reuptake inhibitors
Anticonvulsants	No significant pharmacokinetic interactions with carbamazepine or valproate; reports of neurotoxicity with carbamazepine; combinations helpful for treatment resistance
Nonsteroidal anti-inflammatory drugs	May reduce renal lithium clearance and increase serum concentration; toxicity reported (exception is aspirin)
Diuretics	
Thiazides	Well-documented reduced renal lithium clearance and increased serum concentration; toxicity reported
Potassium sparing	Limited data, may increase lithium concentration
Loop	Lithium clearance unchanged (some case reports of increased lithium concentration)
Osmotic (mannitol, urea)	Increase renal lithium clearance and decrease lithium concentration
Xanthine (aminophylline, caffeine, theophylline)	Increase renal lithium clearance and decrease lithium concentration
Carbonic anhydrase inhibitors (acetazolamide)	Increase renal lithium clearance
Angiotensin-converting enzyme (ACE) inhibitors	Reports of reduced lithium clearance, increased concentrations, and toxicity
Calcium channel inhibitors	Case reports of neurotoxicity; no consistent pharmacokinetic interactions
Miscellaneous	
Succinylcholine, pancuronium	Reports of prolonged neuromuscular blockade
Metronidazole	Increased lithium concentration
Methyldopa	Few reports of neurotoxicity
Sodium bicarbonate	Increased renal lithium clearance
Iodides	Additive antithyroid effects
Propranolol	Used for lithium tremor. Possible slight increase in lithium concentration

A 60-year-old man was treated with 900 mg a day of lithium carbonate. The dosage was continued unchanged for 10 years, despite laboratory evidence of gradually increasing serum lithium and creatinine concentrations. Even as the clinical symptoms of toxicity were being reported, a thiazide diuretic was added to treat hypertension. Three weeks later, the patient was hospitalized with a serum lithium concentration of 4.2 mEq/L and marked neurological impairment that never fully resolved.

Pregnant Women

Lithium should not be administered to pregnant women in the first trimester because of the risk of birth defects. The most common malformations involve the cardiovascular system, most commonly Ebstein's anomaly of the tricuspid valves. The risk of Ebstein's malformation in lithium-exposed fetuses is 1 in 1,000, which is 20 times the risk in the general population. The possibility of fetal cardiac anomalies can be evaluated with fetal echocardiography. The teratogenic risk of lithium (4 to 12 percent) is higher than that for the general population (2 to 3 percent) but appears to be lower than that associated with use of valproate or carbamazepine. A woman who continues to take lithium during pregnancy should use the lowest effective dosage. The maternal lithium concentration must be monitored closely during pregnancy and especially after pregnancy, because of the significant decrease in renal lithium excretion in the first few days after delivery. Adequate hydration can reduce the risk of lithium toxicity during labor. Lithium prophylaxis is recommended for all women with bipolar disorder as they enter the postpartum period. Lithium is excreted into breast milk and should be taken by a nursing mother only after careful evaluation of potential risks and benefits. Signs of lithium toxicity in infants include lethargy, cyanosis, abnormal reflexes, and sometimes hepatomegaly.

Miscellaneous Effects

Lithium should be used with caution in diabetic persons, who should monitor their blood glucose concentrations carefully to avoid diabetic ketoacidosis. Benign, reversible leukocytosis is commonly associated with lithium treatment. Dehydrated, debilitated, and medically ill persons are most susceptible to adverse effects and toxicity.

DRUG INTERACTIONS

Lithium drug interactions are summarized in Table 36.4.18–4. Lithium has been used successfully with dopamine receptor antagonists for many years. However, coadministration of higher dosages of dopamine receptor antagonists and lithium may result in a synergistic increase in the symptoms of lithium-induced neurological adverse effects. This interaction may occur with use of any dopamine receptor antagonist.

Coadministration of lithium and anticonvulsants—including carbamazepine, valproate, and clonazepam—may increase lithium concentrations and aggravate lithium-induced neurological adverse effects. Used wisely, however, the coadministration of lithium and anticonvulsants can benefit some persons therapeutically. Treatment with the combination should be initiated at slightly lower dosages than usual, and dosages should be increased gradually. Changes from one treatment for mania to another should be made carefully, with as little temporal overlap between the drugs as possible.

Most diuretics (e.g., thiazide and potassium sparing) can increase lithium concentrations; when treatment with such a diuretic is stopped, the clinician may need to increase the person's daily lithium dose. Osmotic and loop diuretics, carbonic anhydrase inhibitors, and xanthines (including caffeine) may reduce lithium concentrations below therapeutic concentra-

Table 36.4.18–5
Possible Effects of Lithium on Laboratory Values

Laboratory Value	Possible Effect
White blood cells (WBCs)	Increased count
Serum glucose	Increased level
Serum magnesium	Increased level
Serum potassium	Decreased level
Serum uric acid	Decreased level
Serum thyroxine	Decreased level
Serum cortisol	Decreased AM levels
Serum parathyroid hormone	Increased level due to adenoma
Serum calcium	Increased level due to increased parathyroid hormone level
Serum phosphorus	Decreased level due to increased parathyroid hormone level

Reprinted with permission from Doupe A, Szuba M. Lithium and other antimanic agents. In: *The Handbook of Psychiatry,* Residents of the UCLA Department of Psychiatry. Chicago: Year Book Medical; 1990:366.

tions. Angiotensin-converting enzyme inhibitors may cause an increase in lithium concentrations, whereas the AT_1 angiotensin II receptor inhibitors losartan (Cozaar) and irbesartan (Avapro) do not alter lithium concentrations. A wide range of nonsteroidal antiinflammatory drugs can decrease lithium clearance, thereby increasing lithium concentrations. These drugs include indomethacin (Indocin), phenylbutazone (Azolid), diclofenac (Voltaren), ketoprofen (Orudis), oxyphenbutazone (Oxalid), ibuprofen (Motrin, Advil, Nuprin), piroxicam (Feldene), and naproxen (Naprosyn). Aspirin and sulindac (Clinoril) do not affect lithium concentrations.

Coadministration of lithium and quetiapine (Seroquel) may cause somnolence but is otherwise well tolerated. Coadministration of lithium and ziprasidone may modestly increase the incidence of tremor. Coadministration of lithium and calcium channel inhibitors should be avoided because of potentially fatal neurotoxicity.

A person taking lithium who is about to undergo ECT should discontinue taking lithium 2 days before beginning ECT, to reduce the risk of delirium resulting from the coadministration of these two treatments.

LABORATORY INTERFERENCES

Lithium is not known to interfere with any laboratory tests. However, lithium treatment does affect a number of commonly obtained laboratory values (Table 36.4.18–5).

DOSAGE AND CLINICAL GUIDELINES

Initial Medical Workup

Before a clinician administers lithium, the patient should have a routine laboratory workup and physical examination. The laboratory tests should include serum creatinine concentration (or a 24-hour urine creatinine if the clinician has any reason to be concerned about renal function), electrolytes, thyroid function (TSH, T_3, and T_4), a complete blood count (CBC), ECG, and a pregnancy test in women of child-bearing age.

Dosage Recommendations

Lithium formulations include 150-, 300-, and 600-mg lithium carbonate capsules (Eskalith, Lithonate, and generic), 300-mg lithium carbonate tablets (Lithotabs), 450-mg controlled-release lithium carbonate capsules (Eskalith CR), and 8-mEq/mL lithium citrate syrup.

If a person has previously been treated with lithium and the previous dosage is known, then the same dosage should be used for the current episode unless changes in the person's pharmacokinetic parameters have affected lithium clearance. The starting dosage for most adults is 300 mg of the regular-release formulation three times daily. The starting dosage for elderly persons or persons with renal impairment should be 300 mg once or twice daily. An eventual dosage between 900 and 1,200 mg a day usually produces a therapeutic plasma concentration of 0.6 to 1 mEq/L, and a daily dose of 1,200 to 1,800 mg usually produces a therapeutic concentration of 0.8 to 1.2 mEq/L. Maintenance dosing can be given either in two or three divided doses of the regular-release formulation or in a single dose of the sustained-release formulation equivalent to the combined daily dose of the regular-release formulation. The use of divided doses reduces gastric upset and avoids single high-peak lithium concentrations. No data show a difference in clinical efficacy between the regular- and sustained-release formulations.

Serum and Plasma Concentrations

Serum and plasma concentrations of lithium are the standard methods of assessing lithium concentrations, and they serve as the basis for titrating the dosages. Lithium concentrations should be determined routinely every 2 to 6 months and promptly in persons suspected to be noncompliant with the prescribed dosages, in persons who exhibit signs of toxicity, and during dosage adjustments. Although reports have noted the measurement of lithium concentrations in saliva, tears, and red blood cells, these methods have no clinical superiority to analysis of serum or plasma.

A consensus method for sample collection specifies that the person must be at steady-state lithium dosing (usually after 5 days of constant dosing), preferably using a twice- or thrice-daily dosing regimen, and that the blood sample must be drawn 12 hours (plus or minus 30 minutes) after a given dose. Lithium concentrations 12 hours postdose in persons treated with sustained-release preparations are generally about 30 percent higher than the corresponding concentrations obtained from those taking the regular-release preparations. Because available data are based on a sample population following a multiple-dosage regimen, regular-release formulations given at least twice daily should be used for initial determination of the appropriate dosages.

Two technical considerations should be considered if laboratory values do not seem to correspond to clinical status. First, collection of blood in a tube with a lithium-heparin anticoagulant can give results falsely elevated by as much as 1 mEq/L. Second, aging of the lithium ion-selective electrode can cause inaccuracies of up to 0.5 mEq/L. Once the daily dose has been set, it is reasonable to change to the sustained-release formulation given once daily.

The most common guidelines are 1.0 to 1.5 mEq/L for the treatment of acute mania and 0.4 to 0.8 mEq/L for maintenance treatment. Biological variations in regulation of mood and in lithium metabolism bolster the universal maxim "treat the patient, not the laboratory results." A small number of persons will not achieve therapeutic benefit with a lithium concentration of 1.5 mEq/L yet will have no signs of toxicity. For such persons, titration of the lithium dosage to achieve a concentration above 1.5 mEq/L may be warranted. If there is no response after 2 weeks at a concentration that is beginning to cause adverse effects, then the person should taper off lithium use over 1 to 2 weeks and should try other mood-stabilizing drugs. Other therapeutic options include carbamazepine, valproate, other anticonvulsants, thyroid hormones, ECT, calcium channel inhibitors, monoamine oxidase inhibitors, dopamine receptor antagonists, and SDAs.

Discontinuation

Lithium use is discontinued if it is ineffective or tolerated. Patients may stop the drug for other reasons, such as a perceived or real loss in creativity, feeling cured, or a dislike for feeling controlled by a medicine. After a period of stability with maintenance therapy, a trial off lithium may be considered, although the risk of recurrence is considerable (especially if there have been several prior episodes), and there have been reports of failure to respond to lithium when treatment is reinstituted. Discontinuation should be gradual over many weeks, because more abrupt discontinuation appears to be associated with a higher likelihood of early recurrence of mania or depression. Teaching patients and significant others to recognize early signs of recurrence is an important part of the discontinuation process.

Patient Education

Persons taking lithium should be advised that changes in the body's water and salt content can affect the amount of lithium excreted, resulting in either increased or decreased lithium concentrations. Excessive sodium intake (e.g., a dramatic dietary change) lowers lithium concentrations. Conversely, too little sodium (e.g., fad diets) can lead to potentially toxic concentrations of lithium. Decreases in body fluid (e.g., excessive perspiration) can lead to dehydration and lithium intoxication.

References

Baldessarini RJ, Tarazi RI. Drugs and the treatment of psychiatric disorders: psychosis and mania. In: Hardman JG, Limbird LE, Goodman Gilman A, eds. *Goodman & Gilman's the Pharmacological Basis of Therapeutics.* 10th ed. New York: McGraw-Hill; 2001:485.

Baldessarini RJ, Tondo L. Does lithium treatment still work? Evidence of stable responses over three decades. *Arch Gen Psychiatry.* 2000;57:187.

Bouman TK, de Vries J, Koopmans IH. Lithium prophylaxis and inter-episode mood: a prospective longitudinal comparison of euthymic bipolars and non-patient controls. *J Affect Disord.* 1002;24:199.

Bowden CL. Efficacy of lithium in mania and maintenance therapy of bipolar disorder. *J Clin Psychiatry.* 2000;61(suppl 9):35.

Campbell M, Katantaris V, Cueva JE. An update on the use of lithium carbonate in aggressive children and adolescents with conduct disorder. *Psychopharmacol Bull.* 1995;31:93.

Carpenter LL, Yasmin S, Price LH. A double-blind, placebo-controlled study of antidepressant augmentation with mirtazapine. *Biol Psychiatry.* 2002; 51:183.

Coppen A. Lithium in unipolar depression and the prevention of suicide. *J Clin Psychiatry.* 2000;61(suppl 9):52.

Dinan TG. Lithium in bipolar mood disorder. *BMJ.* 2002;324:989.

Granneman GR, Schneck DW, Cavanaugh JH, Witt GF. Pharmacokinetic interactions and side effects resulting from concomitant administration of lithium and divalproex sodium. *J Clin Psychiatry.* 1996;57:204.

Grounds D. Connection between lithium and muscular incoordination. *Aust N Z J Psychiatry.* 2002;36:142.

Hoffman L, Halmi KA. Psychopharmacology in the treatment of anorexia nervosa and bulimia nervosa. *Psychiatr Clin North Am.* 1993;16:767.

Jefferson JW, Greist JH. Lithium. In: Sadock BJ, Sadock VA, eds. *Kaplan & Sadock's Comprehensive Textbook of Psychiatry.* 7th ed. Vol 2. Baltimore: Lippincott Williams & Wilkins; 2000:2377.

Kane JM. Drug therapy: schizophrenia. *N Engl J Med.* 1996;334:34.

Katona CLE. Refractory depression: a review with particular reference to the use of lithium augmentation. *Eur Neuropsychopharmacol.* 1995;5(suppl):109.

Keck PE, McElroy SL. Outcome in the pharmacologic treatment of bipolar disorder. *J Clin Psychopharmacol.* 1996;16(suppl 1):15S.

Lenox RH, Hahn C-G. Overview of the mechanism of action of lithium in the brain: fifty-year update. *J Clin Psychiatry.* 2000;61(suppl 9):5.

Markoff RA, King M Jr. Does lithium dose prediction improve treatment efficiency? Prospective evaluation of a mathematical method. *J Clin Psychopharmacol.* 1992;12:305.

O'Brien G. Treatment of patients with learning disabilities and schizoaffective illness. *Hum Psychopharmacol.* 1995;10:491.

Pantelis C, Barnes TRE. Drug strategies and treatment-resistant schizophrenia. *Aust N Z J Psychiatry.* 1996;30:20.

Pert M, Pratt JP. Lithium: current status in psychiatric disorders. *Drugs.* 1993;46:7.

Reischer H, Pfeffer CR. Lithium pharmacokinetics. *Am Acad Child Adolesc Psychiatry.* 1996;35:130.

Schou M. Forty years of lithium treatment. *Arch Gen Psychiatry.* 1997;54:9.

Sharpley AL, Walsh AES, Cowen PJ. Effect of nefazodone and lithium on sleep architecture in healthy men. *J Psychopharmacol.* 1996;10(suppl 1):26.

Solomon DA, Ristow WR, Keller JM, Goldberg AJ, Rosenbaum JF, Warshaw MG. Serum lithium levels and psychosocial function in patients with bipolar I disorder. *Am J Psychiatry.* 1996;153:1301.

Stein G, Bernadt M. Lithium augmentation therapy in tricyclic-resistant depression: a controlled trial using lithium in low and normal doses. *Br J Psychiatry.* 1993;162:634.

Stoll AL, Locke CA, Vuckovic A, Mayer PV. Lithium-associated cognitive and functional deficits reduced by a switch to divalproex sodium: a case series. *J Clin Psychiatry.* 1996;57:356.

Swanson CL, Price WA, McEvoy JP. Effects of concomitant risperidone and lithium treatment. *Am J Psychiatry.* 1995;152:1096.

Tariot PN, Schneider LS. Anticonvulsant and other non-neuroleptic treatment of agitation in dementia. *J Geriatr Psychiatry Neurol.* 1995;8(suppl 1):S28.

▲ 36.4.19 Mirtazapine

Mirtazapine (Remeron) is an effective medication used to treat depression. It lacks the annoying anticholinergic effects of the tricyclic antidepressants.

CHEMISTRY

The molecular structure of mirtazapine is shown in Figure 36.4.19–1.

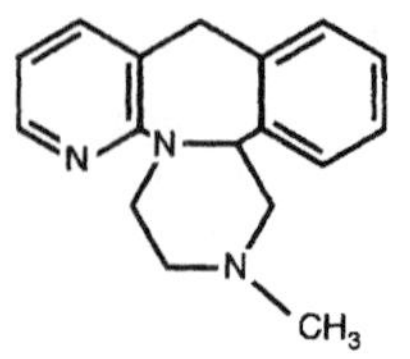

FIGURE 36.4.19–1
The molecular structure of mirtazapine.

PHARMACOLOGICAL ACTIONS

Mirtazapine is rapidly and completely absorbed from the gastrointestinal (GI) tract. Peak concentration is achieved within 2 hours of ingestion. Plasma clearance may be slowed up to 30 percent in persons with impaired hepatic function and up to 50 percent in those with impaired renal function. Clearance may be up to 40 percent slower in elderly males and up to 10 percent slower in elderly females. The mean elimination half-life is 20 to 40 hours, and steady-state levels are achieved within about 5 days. A clinical response may require 2 to 4 weeks.

Mirtazapine acts as an antagonist of central presynaptic α_2-adrenergic receptors within the central nervous system (CNS), where it has a net effect of increasing synaptic levels of noradrenaline and serotonin. It is a potent antagonist of serotonin 5-HT_2 and 5-HT_3 receptors but has little effect on 5-HT_1 receptors. This appears to bias the activation of serotonin receptors in favor of the 5-HT_1 family, whose activation is thought to reduce anxiety and depression. Mirtazapine is a potent antagonist of histamine H_1 receptors and is a moderately potent antagonist at α_1-adrenergic and muscarinic-cholinergic receptors.

EFFECTS ON SPECIFIC ORGANS AND SYSTEMS

Mirtazapine exerts most of its effects in the CNS, and the principal non-CNS effects are in the GI system (e.g., weight gain, increased appetite).

THERAPEUTIC INDICATIONS

Mirtazapine is effective for the treatment of depression. It is highly sedating, in the same range as amitriptyline (Elavil, Endep), clomipramine (Anafranil), and trazodone (Desyrel), and is thus useful for treatment of sleep disturbances. However, some of the sedating effects generally lessen within the first week of treatment. In direct comparison, it causes somewhat less somnolence, weight gain, and constipation than amitriptyline and less headache and nausea than fluoxetine (Prozac). It also appears to reduce somatic and psychological symptoms of anxiety and agitation.

PRECAUTIONS AND ADVERSE REACTIONS

The most common adverse effect of mirtazapine is somnolence, which may occur in over 50 percent of persons (Table 36.4.19–1). Therefore, when persons start to take mirtazapine, they should exercise caution when driving or operating dangerous machinery. This adverse effect may be minimized by giving the dose before sleep. Mirtazapine also causes dizziness in 7 percent of persons. It does not appear to increase the risk for seizures. Mania or hypomania occurred in 0.2 percent of persons in clinical trials, a rate similar to that of other antidepressant drugs. Mirtazapine potentiates the sedative effects of alcohol.

Mirtazapine increases appetite in about 15 percent of patients. Mirtazapine may also increase serum cholesterol concentration to 20 percent or more above the upper limit of normal in 15 percent of persons and increase triglycerides to 500 mg/dL or more in 6 percent of persons. Elevations of alanine transaminase (ALT) levels to more than three times the upper limit of normal were seen in 2 percent of mirtazapine-treated persons, as opposed to 0.3 percent of placebo controls.

Table 36.4.19–1
Adverse Reactions Reported with Mirtazapine

Event	Percentage (%)
Somnolence	54
Dry mouth	25
Increased appetite	17
Constipation	13
Weight gain	12
Dizziness	7
Myalgias	5
Disturbing dreams	4

In limited premarketing experience, the absolute neutrophil count dropped to 500/mm^3 or less within 2 months of onset of use in 0.3 percent of persons, some of whom developed symptomatic infections. This hematological condition was reversible in all cases and was more likely to occur when other risk factors for neutropenia were present. In postmarketing experience, no increases in the frequency of neutropenia have been reported. The manufacturer recommends instructing all persons to seek medical attention if they develop fever, chills, sore throat, mucous membrane ulceration, or other signs of infection. If a low white blood cell count is found, mirtazapine should be discontinued immediately, and the infectious disease status should be followed closely.

A small number of persons experience orthostatic hypotension while taking mirtazapine. Although no human data exist regarding effects on fetal development, mirtazapine should be used with caution during pregnancy. Because the drug may be excreted in breast milk, it should not be taken by nursing mothers. Because of the risk of agranulocytosis associated with mirtazapine use, persons should be attuned to signs of infection (see above). Because of the sedating effects of mirtazapine, persons should determine the degree to which they are affected prior to driving or engaging in other potentially dangerous activities. Other potentially sedating prescription or over-the-counter drugs and alcohol should be avoided during use of mirtazapine.

DRUG INTERACTIONS

Mirtazapine can potentiate the sedation of alcohol and benzodiazepines. Mirtazapine should not be used within 14 days of a monoamine oxidase inhibitor.

LABORATORY INTERFERENCES

No laboratory interferences have been described for mirtazapine.

DOSAGE AND ADMINISTRATION

Mirtazapine is available in 15-, 30- and 45-mg scored tablets. If persons fail to respond to an initial dose of mirtazapine of 15 mg before sleep, the dose may be increased in 15-mg increments every 5 days to a maximum of 45 mg before sleep. Lower dosages may be necessary in elderly persons or those with renal or hepatic insufficiency.

References

Baldessarini RJ. Drug and the treatment of psychiatric disorders: depression and anxiety disorders. In: Hardman JG, Limbird LE, Goodman Gilman A, eds. *Goodman & Gilman's the Pharmacological Basis of Therapeutics*. 10th ed. New York: McGraw-Hill; 2001:447.

Claghorn JL. Mirtazapine. In: Sadock BJ, Sadock VA, eds. *Kaplan & Sadock's Comprehensive Textbook of Psychiatry*. 7th ed. Vol 2. Baltimore: Lippincott Williams & Wilkins; 2000:2390.

Claghorn JL, Lesem MD. A double-blind placebo-controlled study of Org 3770 in depressed outpatients. *J Affect Disord*. 1995;34:165.

Davis R, Wilde MI. Mirtazapine: a review of its pharmacology and therapeutic potential in the management of major depression. *CNS Drugs*. 1996;5:389.

de Boer T. The effects of mirtazapine on central noradrenergic and serotonergic neurotransmission. *Int Clin Psychopharmacol*. 1995;10(suppl 4):19.

Kasper S. Clinical efficacy of mirtazapine: a review of meta-analyses of pooled data. *Int Clin Psychopharmacol*. 1995;10(suppl 4):25.

Kehoe WA, Schorr RB. Focus on mirtazapine: a new antidepressant with noradrenergic and specific serotonergic activity. *Formulary*. 1996;31:455.

Montgomery SA. Safety of mirtazapine: a review. *Int Clin Psychopharmacol*. 1995;10(suppl 4):37.

Nierenberg AA. Do some antidepressants work faster than others? *J Clin Psychiatry*. 2001;62(suppl 15):22.

Schittecatte M, Dumont F, Machowski R. Mirtazapine, but not fluvoxamine, normalizes the blunted REM sleep response to clonidine in depressed patients: implications for subsensitivity of alpha(2)-adrenergic receptors in depression. *Psychiatry Res*. 2002;109:1.

van Moffaert M, Dierick M. Noradrenaline (norepinephrine) and depression: role in aetiology and therapeutic implications. *CNS Drugs*. 1999;12:293.

▲ 36.4.20 Monoamine Oxidase Inhibitors

The monoamine oxidase (MAO) inhibitors (MAOIs) are highly effective antidepressants and anxiolytics, but they are used less frequently than other antidepressants because of the dietary precautions that must be followed to avoid tyramine-induced hypertensive crises. MAOIs increase biogenic amine neurotransmitter levels by inhibiting their degradation. The degradation of the biogenic amines, serotonin, norepinephrine, and dopamine, occurs by only two mechanisms. The more important pathway involves the presynaptic reuptake of these neurotransmitters through specific transporter molecules, followed by deamination in mitochondria by the enzyme MAO. MAOIs, however, are generally considered equal in efficacy to other antidepressant drugs. The transporters may be inhibited, for example, by the tricyclic antidepressants and the serotonin-specific reuptake inhibitors (SSRIs), which form the mainstay of current antidepressant drugs.

The currently available MAOIs include phenelzine (Nardil), isocarboxazid (Marplan), tranylcypromine (Parnate), and selegiline (Eldepryl). Selegiline is a selective inhibitor of type B MAO (MAO_B) used for the treatment of parkinsonism. A newer class of reversible inhibitors of MAO_A (RIMAs), not available in the United States (e.g., moclobemide [Aurorix, Manerix] and befloxatone), require few dietary restrictions. Some clinicians believe that MAOIs are underused as effective antidepressant treatment.

HISTORY

Iproniazid (Marsilid), a derivative of the antituberculosis drug isoniazid (Nydrazid, Rifamate), was abandoned as a potential treatment for tuberculosis and introduced as a treatment for depression in 1952, when its stimulatory effects in tubercular patients were noted. This discovery led to the development of several MAOIs that were effective in treating depression. In 1962, however, a case report described a patient's death from a hypertensive crisis. The patient, who was being treated with an MAOI, had ingested a tyramine-rich cheese. This report led to the brief withdrawal in the United States of the MAOIs. After the drugs were reintroduced, they had a negative image and were used minimally for a long time. The disuse of MAOIs was further driven by the introduction of the tricyclic drugs, which were judged to have a more favorable adverse-effect profile, a judgment that many clinicians and researchers consider not entirely accurate. The use of MAOIs has decreased in the past decade because of the appearance of several safer alternatives. Several research groups observed that MAOIs may have superior efficacy in the treatment of specific groups of patients—for example, depressed patients with marked anxiety or phobic symptoms. In addition, clinicians now realize that the dietary restrictions that must be followed by patients taking MAOIs are not as difficult or as extensive as was previously thought and that large amounts of tyramine-containing foods must generally be consumed to induce a serious hypertensive crisis. The use of classic MAOIs and tricyclic drugs has declined, as they have been replaced by the SSRIs and other, new antidepressants, which have significantly more favorable adverse-effect profiles. As mentioned above, RIMAs are used in Europe and may become available in the United States. This class of drugs includes moclobemide, befloxatone, brofaromine (Consonar), tetrindole, pyrasidol, and E2011.

CHEMISTRY

Isocarboxazid and phenelzine are derivatives of hydrazine, and tranylcypromine is a derivative of amphetamine. The molecular structures of phenelzine, isocarboxazid, tranylcypromine, and moclobemide are shown in Figure 36.4.20–1.

PHARMACOLOGICAL ACTIONS

Phenelzine, tranylcypromine, and isocarboxazid are readily absorbed through the gastrointestinal (GI) tract and reach peak plasma concentrations within 2 hours. Their plasma half-lives are in the range of 2 to 3 hours; their tissue half-lives are consider-

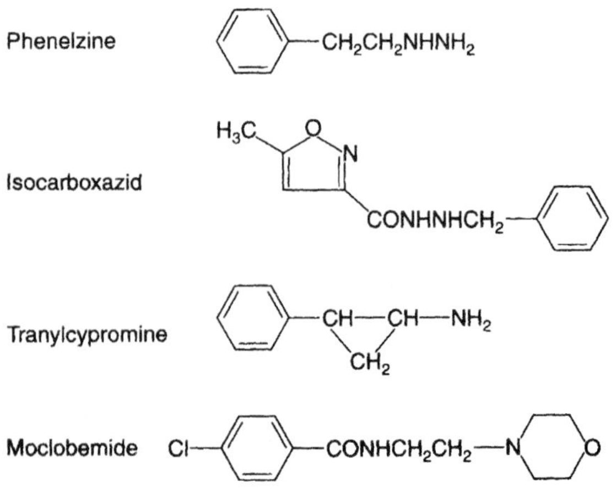

FIGURE 36.4.20–1
Molecular structures of MAOIs used in psychiatry.

Table 36.4.20–1
Comparison of Monoamine Oxidase A and B

Type	Location	Preferred Substrates	Selective Inhibitors
A	Central nervous system, sympathetic terminals, liver, gut, skin	Norepinephrine, serotonin, dopamine, tyramine, octopamine, tryptamine	Clorgyline
B	Central nervous system, liver, platelets	Dopamine, tyramine, tryptamine, phenylethylamine, benzylamine, *N*-methylhistamine	Selegiline[a] (Eldepryl)

[a]Selectivity lost at higher doses (≥10 mg/day).
From Arano GW, Hymar SE. *Handbook of Psychiatric Drug Therapy.* 3rd ed. Boston: Little, Brown; 1995, with permission.

ably longer. Because they irreversibly inactivate MAOs, the therapeutic effect of a single dose of irreversible MAOIs may persist for as long as 2 weeks. The RIMA moclobemide is rapidly absorbed and has a half-life of 0.5 to 3.5 hours. Because it is a reversible inhibitor, moclobemide has a much briefer clinical effect following a single dose than irreversible MAOIs have.

MAO is an enzyme found intracellularly on the outer mitochondrial membrane, which degrades cytoplasmic monoamines, including norepinephrine, serotonin, dopamine, epinephrine, and tyramine. There are two types of MAOs: MAO_A and MAO_B. MAO_A primarily metabolizes norepinephrine, serotonin, and epinephrine; dopamine and tyramine are metabolized by both MAO_A and MAO_B. MAOIs act in the central nervous system (CNS), the sympathetic nervous system, the liver, and the GI tract (Table 36.4.20–1). At dosages above 60 mg per day, tranylcypromine may inhibit the reuptake or increase the release of dopamine and norepinephrine and, to a lesser extent, serotonin.

When GI metabolism of dietary tyramine by MAOs is inactivated by an irreversible MAOI, intact tyramine can enter the circulation and exert a potent pressor effect, resulting in a hypertensive crisis. Tyramine-containing foods must therefore be avoided for 2 weeks after the last dose of an irreversible MAOI to permit resynthesis of adequate concentrations of MAOs. In contrast, RIMAs have relatively little inhibitory activity for MAO_B, and because they are reversible, normal activity of existing MAO_A returns within 16 to 48 hours of the last dose of a RIMA. Therefore, the dietary restrictions are less stringent for RIMAs, applying only to foods containing high concentrations of tyramine, which need be avoided for only 3 days after the last dose of a RIMA.

EFFECTS ON SPECIFIC ORGANS AND SYSTEMS

The primary effects of the MAOIs in psychiatry are on the CNS. In addition to their effects on depressed mood, the MAOIs are associated with potentially clinically significant disturbances in sleep and sleep architecture. MAOI use is frequently associated with decreased sleep and insomnia and sometimes results in daytime drowsiness. Furthermore, the sleep of MAOI-treated patients is characterized by significantly less rapid eye movement (REM) sleep. RIMAs lack an effect on, or may improve, sleep.

The other principal concerns when treating patients with MAOIs are the cardiovascular system and the liver. MAOIs are commonly associated with hypotension because of their effects on vascular tone, which may be mediated both centrally and peripherally. In rare cases, MAOI use alone (without tyramine) is associated with episodes of acute hypertension. With regard to the liver, phenelzine and isocarboxazid are associated with a significant liability for hepatotoxicity.

THERAPEUTIC INDICATIONS

The indications for MAOIs are similar to those for tricyclic and tetracyclic drugs. MAOIs may be particularly effective in panic disorder with agoraphobia, posttraumatic stress disorder, eating disorders, social phobia, and pain disorder. Some investigators have reported that MAOIs may be preferable to tricyclic drugs in the treatment of atypical depression characterized by hypersomnia, hyperphagia, anxiety, and the absence of vegetative symptoms. Patients with this symptom pattern are often less severely depressed than patients with classic symptoms of depression, which is often evidenced by less functional impairment. The failure of a patient to improve after treatment with an SSRI and a tricyclic or tetracyclic drug may be the most common reason that a patient is given a therapeutic trial of an MAOI.

Although depression is not an approved indication for selegiline, some positive results have been reported. A possible advantage of selegiline is that its primary effect in low dosages is on MAO_B; thus the risk of an MAO_A-associated, tyramine-induced hypertensive crisis is lessened. Unfortunately, many of the positive results with selegiline for depression have been at higher dosages (20 to 60 mg a day) than the dosages used to treat Parkinson's disease (10 mg a day). At these higher dosages, selegiline loses a significant amount of its specificity for MAO_B and requires that patients follow the guidelines for a restricted tyramine diet.

PRECAUTIONS AND ADVERSE REACTIONS

The most frequent adverse effects of MAOIs are orthostatic hypotension, insomnia, weight gain, edema, and sexual dysfunction. The initial appearance of signs of orthostatic hypotension in the course of a cautious upward tapering of the dosage determines the maximum tolerable dosage. Treatment for orthostatic hypotension includes avoidance of caffeine, intake of 2 L of fluid per day, addition of dietary salt or adjustment of antihypertensive drugs (if applicable), support stockings, and in severe cases, treatment with fludrocortisone (Florinef), a mineralocorticoid, 0.1 to 0.2 mg a day. Orthostatic hypotension asso-

ciated with tranylcypromine use can usually be relieved by dividing the daily dose.

A rare adverse effect of MAOIs, most commonly of tranylcypromine, is a spontaneous, non-tyramine-induced hypertensive crisis occurring shortly after the first exposure to the drug. Persons experiencing such a crisis should avoid MAOIs altogether. Insomnia and behavioral activation can be treated by dividing the dose, not giving the medication after dinner, and using trazodone (Desyrel) or a benzodiazepine hypnotic if necessary. Weight gain, edema, and sexual dysfunction often do not respond to any treatment and may warrant switching to another agent. When switching from one MAOI to another, the clinician should taper and stop use of the first drug for 10 to 14 days before beginning use of the second drug.

Paresthesias, myoclonus, and muscle pains are occasionally seen in persons treated with MAOIs. Paresthesias may be secondary to MAOI-induced pyridoxine deficiency, which may respond to supplementation with pyridoxine, 50 to 150 mg orally each day. Occasionally, persons complain of feeling drunk or confused, perhaps indicating that the dosage should be reduced and then increased gradually. Reports that the hydrazine MAOIs are associated with hepatotoxic effects are relatively uncommon. MAOIs are less cardiotoxic and less epileptogenic than the tricyclic and tetracyclic drugs.

The most common adverse effects of the RIMA moclobemide are dizziness, nausea, and insomnia or sleep disturbance. RIMAs cause fewer GI adverse effects than SSRIs. Moclobemide does not have adverse anticholinergic or cardiovascular effects, and it has not been reported to interfere with sexual function.

MAOIs should be used with caution by persons with renal disease, cardiovascular disease, or hyperthyroidism. MAOIs may alter the dosage of a hypoglycemic agent required by diabetic persons. MAOIs have been particularly associated with inducing mania in persons in the depressed phase of bipolar I disorder and triggering psychotic decompensation in persons with schizophrenia. MAOIs are contraindicated during pregnancy, although data on their teratogenic risk are minimal. MAOIs should not be taken by nursing women because the drugs can pass into the breast milk.

Table 36.4.20–2
Tyramine-Rich Foods to Be Avoided in Planning MAOI Diets

High tyramine content[a] ($\geq$2 mg of tyramine a serving)
Cheese: English Stilton; blue cheese; white (3 years old); extra old; old cheddar; Danish blue; mozzarella; cheese snack spreads
Fish, cured meats, sausage; pates and organs; salami; mortadella; air-dried sausage
Alcoholic beverages[b]: Liqueurs and concentrated after-dinner drinks
Marmite (concentrated yeast extract)
Sauerkraut (Krakus)
Moderate tyramine content[a] (0.5–1.99 mg of tyramine a serving)
Cheese: Swiss Gruyere; Muenster; feta; parmesan; gorgonzola; blue cheese dressing; Black Diamond
Fish, cured meats, sausage, pates, and organs: Chicken liver (5 days old); bologna; aged sausage; smoked meat; salmon mousse
Alcoholic beverages: Beer and ale (12 oz per bottle)—Amstel, Export Draft, Blue Light, Guinness Extra Stout, Old Vienna, Canadian, Miller Light, Export, Heineken, Blue Wines (per 4 oz glass)—Rioja (red wine)
Low tyramine content[b] (0.01 ta >0.49 mg of tyramine a serving)
Cheese: Brie, Camembert, Cambozola with or without rind
Fish, cured meat, sausage, organs, and pates: Pickled herring; smoked fish; kielbasa sausage; chicken livers, liverwurst (<2 days old)
Alcoholic beverages: red wines; sherry; scotch[c]
Others: Banana or avocado (ripe or not); banana peel

[a]Any food left out to age or spoil can spontaneously develop tyramine through fermentation.
[b]Alcohol can produce profound orthostasis interacting with MAOIs, but cannot produce direct hypertensive reactions.
[c]White wines, gin, and vodka have no tyramine content.
Table by Jonathan M. Himmelhoch, M.D.

Tyramine-Induced Hypertensive Crisis

Foods rich in tyramine (Table 36.4.20–2) or other sympathomimetic amines should be avoided by persons who are taking irreversible MAOIs to avoid significant risk of potentially life-threatening hypertension. Persons should be warned about the dangers of ingesting tyramine-rich foods while taking MAOIs, and they should be advised to continue the dietary restrictions for 2 weeks after they stop MAOI treatment, to allow the body to resynthesize the enzyme. Patients should also be warned that bee stings may cause a hypertensive crisis. The prodromal signs and symptoms of a hypertensive crisis may include headache, stiff neck, sweating, nausea, and vomiting. If these signs and symptoms occur, the patient should seek immediate medical treatment. An MAOI-induced hypertensive crisis should be treated with α-adrenergic antagonists—for example, phentolamine (Regitine) or chlorpromazine (Thorazine)—which lower blood pressure within 5 minutes. A diuretic to reduce fluid load and a β-adrenergic receptor antagonist to control tachycardia may also be necessary. Acute lowering of blood pressure with use of nifedipine (Procardia) is not recommended, because a person who mistakes a headache resulting from the rebound of MAOI-induced orthostatic hypotension for a hypertensive crisis–related headache and therefore takes nifedipine runs a high risk of causing signs and symptoms of hypotensive shock. MAOIs should not be used by persons with thyrotoxicosis or pheochromocytoma. The risk of tyramine-induced hypertensive crises is relatively low for persons who are taking RIMAs, such as moclobemide and befloxatone. A reasonable dietary recommendation for persons taking RIMAs is not to eat tyramine-containing foods for a period from 1 hour before to 2 hours after taking a RIMA.

Withdrawal

Persons taking regular doses of MAOIs who cease administration abruptly may experience a self-limited discontinuation syndrome consisting of arousal, mood disturbances, and somatic symptoms. To avoid these symptoms when discontinuing use of an MAOI, dosages should be gradually tapered over several weeks.

Overdose

In general, intoxication caused by MAOIs is characterized by agitation that progresses to coma with hyperthermia, hyper-

Table 36.4.20–3
Drugs to Be Avoided during MAOI Treatment (Partial Listing)

Never use	
	Antiasthmatics
	Antihypertensives (methyldopa, guanethidine, reserpine)
	Buspirone
	Levodopa
	Opioids (especially meperidine, dextromethorphan, propoxyphene, tramadol; morphine or codeine may be less dangerous)
	Cold, allergy, or sinus medications containing dextromethorphan or sympathomimetics
	SSRIs, clomipramine, venlafaxine, sibutramine
	Sympathomimetics (amphetamines, cocaine, methylphenidate, dopamine, metaraminol, epinephrine, norepinephrine, isoproterenol, ephedrine, pseudoephedrine, phenylpropanolamine)
	L-Tryptophan
Use carefully	
	Anticholinergics (propanolol)
	Antihistamines
	Disulfiram
	Bromocriptine
	Hydralazine
	Sedative-hypnotics
	Terpin hydrate with codeine
	Tricyclics and tetracyclics (avoid clomipramine)

tension, tachypnea, tachycardia, dilated pupils, and hyperactive deep tendon reflexes. Involuntary movements may be present, particularly in the face and the jaw. There is often an asymptomatic period of 1 to 6 hours after the ingestion of the drugs before the symptoms of toxicity occur. Acidification of the urine markedly hastens the excretion of MAOIs, and dialysis can be of some use. Phentolamine or chlorpromazine may be useful if hypertension is a problem. Moclobemide alone in overdosage causes relatively mild and reversible symptoms. The toxicity of all MAOIs is potentially increased in multidrug overdosages, especially if the overdosage includes serotonergic agents.

DRUG INTERACTIONS

The inhibition of MAO can cause severe and even fatal interactions with various other drugs (Table 36.4.20–3). In particular, because MAOIs serve to increase intrasynaptic concentrations of biogenic amine neurotransmitters, they should never be administered simultaneously with drugs with a similar effect on these neurotransmitters. This includes most antidepressants as well as precursor agents. Persons should be instructed to tell any other physicians or dentists who are treating them that they are taking an MAOI. MAOIs may potentiate the action of CNS depressants, including alcohol and barbiturates. MAOIs should not be coadministered with serotonergic drugs such as SSRIs and clomipramine (Anafranil) because this combination can trigger a serotonin syndrome. The initial symptoms of a serotonin syndrome can include tremor, hypertonicity, myoclonus, and autonomic signs, which can then progress to hallucinosis, hyperthermia, and even death. Fatal reactions have occurred when MAOIs were combined with meperidine (Demerol) or fentanyl (Sublimaze).

As mentioned, when switching from an irreversible MAOI to any other type of antidepressant drug, persons should wait at least 14 days after the last dose of the MAOI before beginning use of the next drug, to allow replenishment of the body's MAOs. When switching from an antidepressant to an irreversible MAOI, persons should wait 10 to 14 days (or 5 weeks for fluoxetine [Prozac]) before starting use of the MAOI, to avoid drug–drug interactions. In contrast, MAO activity recovers completely 24 to 48 hours after the last dose of a RIMA.

Cimetidine (Tagamet) and fluoxetine significantly reduce the elimination of moclobemide. Modest doses of fluoxetine and moclobemide administered concurrently may be well tolerated, with no significant pharmacodynamic or pharmacokinetic interactions.

LABORATORY INTERFERENCES

The MAOIs are associated with lowering blood glucose concentrations, which are accurately reflected by laboratory analysis. MAOIs artificially raise urinary metanephrine concentrations and may cause a false-positive test result for pheochromocytoma or neuroblastoma. MAOIs have been reported to be associated with a minimal false elevation in thyroid function test results.

DOSAGE AND CLINICAL GUIDELINES

Table 36.4.20–4 lists MAOI preparations and typical dosages. There is no definitive rationale for choosing one of the currently available irreversible MAOIs over another, although some clinicians recommend tranylcypromine because of its activating qualities, possibly associated with a fast onset of action, and its low hepatotoxic potential. Phenelzine use should begin with a test dose of 15 mg on the first day. The dosage can be increased to 15 mg three times daily during the first week and increased by 15 mg a day each week thereafter until the dosage of 90 mg a day, in divided doses, is reached by the end of the fourth week. Tranylcypromine and isocarboxazid use should begin with a test dosage of 10 mg and may be increased to 10 mg three times daily by the end of the first week. Many clinicians and researchers have recommended upper limits of 50 mg a day for isocarboxazid and 40 mg a day for tranylcypromine. Administration of tranylcypromine in multiple small daily doses may reduce its hypotensive effects. If an MAOI trial is not successful after 6 weeks, lithium (Eskalith) or liothyronine (Cytomel) augmentation is warranted.

Hepatic transaminase serum concentrations should be monitored periodically because of the potential for hepatotoxicity, especially with phenelzine and isocarboxazid. Elderly persons may be more sensitive to MAOI adverse effects than younger adults. MAO activity increases with age, so MAOI dosages for elderly persons are the same as those required for younger adults. The use of MAOIs in children has had minimal study.

Moclobemide use is initiated at 300 to 450 mg a day, divided three times per day, and it may be increased to a maximum of 600 mg a day after several weeks. Dietary restrictions consist of avoidance of only large quantities of tyramine-containing foods, and the administration of moclobemide after, rather than before, tyramine-containing meals. RIMAs may be

Table 36.4.20–4
Available Preparations and Typical Dosages of MAOIs

Generic Name	Trade Name	Preparations	Usual Daily Dose (mg)	Usual Maximum Daily Dose (mg)
Isocarboxazid[a]	Marplan	10-mg tablets	20–40	60
Moclobemide[b]	Manerix	100-, 150-mg tablets	300–600	600
Phenelzine	Nardil	15-mg tablets	30–60	90
Selegiline	Eldepryl, Atapryl	5-mg capsules, 5-mg tablets	10	30
Tranylcypromine	Parnate	10-mg tablets	20–60	60

[a]Available directly from the manufacturer.
[b]Not available in the United States.

used in combination with other antidepressants with somewhat less concern for hypertensive crises, but still with caution.

References

Amsterdam JD, Chopra M. Monoamine oxidase inhibitors revisited. *Psychiatr Ann.* 2001;31:361.

Baldessarini RJ. Drugs and the treatment of psychiatric disorders: depression and anxiety disorders. In: Hardman JG, Limbird LE, Goodman Gilman A, eds. *Goodman & Gilman's the Pharmacological Basis of Therapeutics.* 10th ed. New York: McGraw-Hill; 2001:447.

Coupland NJ, Wilson SJ, Potokar JP, et al. A comparison of the effects of phenelzine treatment with moclobemide treatment on cardiovascular reflexes. *Int Clin Psychopharmacol.* 1995;10:229.

Fischer P. Serotonin syndrome in the elderly after antidepressive monotherapy. *J Clin Psychopharmacol.* 1995;15:440.

Fitton A, Faulds D, Goa KL. Moclobemide: a review of its pharmacological properties and therapeutic use in depressive illness. *Drugs.* 1992;43:561.

Flint AJ, Rifat SL. The effect of sequential antidepressant treatment on geriatric depression. *J Affect Disord.* 1996;36:95.

Hammerness P, Parada H, Abrams A. Linezolid: MAOI activity and potential drug interactions. *Psychosomatics.* 2002;43:248.

Hawley CJ, Ratnam S, Pattinson HA, et al. Safety and tolerability of combined treatment with moclobemide and SSRIs: a preliminary study of 19 patients. *J Psychopharmacol.* 1996;10:241.

Kennedy SH, McKenna KF, Baker GB. Monoamine oxidase inhibitors. In: Sadock BJ, Sadock VA, eds. *Kaplan & Sadock's Comprehensive Textbook of Psychiatry.* 7th ed. Vol 2. Baltimore: Lippincott Williams & Wilkins; 2000:2397.

Merikangas KR, Merikangas JR. Combination monoamine oxidase inhibitor and β-blocker treatment of migraine, with anxiety and depression. *Biol Psychiatry.* 1995;38:603.

Reynaert C, Parent M, Mirel J, et al. Moclobemide versus fluoxetine for a major depressive episode. *Psychopharmacology.* 1995;118:183.

Thase ME, Mallinger AG, McKnight D, Himmelhoch JM. Treatment of imipramine-resistant recurrent depression: IV. A double-blind cross-over study of tranylcypromine for anergic bipolar depression. *Am J Psychiatry.* 1992; 149:195.

Thase ME, Trivedi MH, Rush AJ. MAOIs in the contemporary treatment of depression. *Neuropsychopharmacology.* 1995;12:185.

Thomas T. Monoamine oxidase-B inhibitors in the treatment of Alzheimer's disease. *Neurobiol Aging.* 2000;21:343.

▲ 36.4.21 Nefazodone

Nefazodone (Serzone) has antidepressant and antianxiety effects. It is structurally related to trazodone (Desyrel) and unrelated to the classical tricyclic and tetracyclic drugs, the monoamine oxidase inhibitors (MAOIs), serotonin-specific reuptake inhibitors (SSRIs), and other available antidepressant drugs. Although trazodone is distinctive in having more marked sedative effects than most other antidepressants, nefazodone is relatively free of this adverse effect and generally well tolerated. Nefazodone is less likely than the SSRIs to adversely affect sexual functioning.

CHEMISTRY

Nefazodone is a phenylpiperazine analogue of trazodone. Its molecular structure is shown in Figure 36.4.21–1.

PHARMACOLOGICAL ACTIONS

Nefazodone is rapidly and completely absorbed but is then extensively metabolized, so the bioavailability of active compounds is about 20 percent of the oral dose. Its half-life is 2 to 4 hours. Steady-state concentrations of nefazodone and its principal active metabolite, hydroxynefazodone, are achieved within 4 to 5 days. Metabolism of nefazodone in the elderly, especially women, is about half that seen in younger persons, so that lowered doses are recommended for elderly persons. An important metabolite of nefazodone is methchlorophenylpiperazine (mCPP), which has some serotonergic effects and may cause migraine, anxiety, and weight loss.

Nefazodone is an inhibitor of serotonin uptake and, more weakly, of norepinephrine reuptake. Its antagonism of type 2A serotonin 5-HT_{2A} receptors is thought to lessen anxiety and depression. By both inhibiting serotonin reuptake, which raises synaptic serotonin concentrations, and blocking 5-HT_{2A} receptors, nefazodone may selectively activate 5-HT_{1A} receptors, which gives additional antidepressant and anxiolytic effects. Nefazodone is a mild antagonist of the α_1-adrenergic receptors, which predisposes some persons to orthostatic hypotension but is not sufficiently potent to produce priapism. There is no significant direct activity at α_2- and β-adrenergic, 5-HT_{1A}, cholinergic, opioid, dopaminergic, or benzodiazepine receptors.

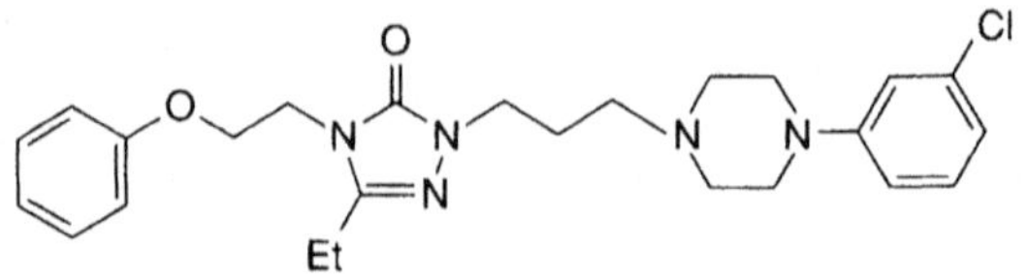

FIGURE 36.4.21–1
Molecular structure of nefazodone.

EFFECTS ON SPECIFIC ORGANS AND SYSTEMS

The main effects of nefazodone are on the central nervous system (CNS). The main extra-CNS effects are related to α_1-adrenergic antagonism, which may cause orthostatic hypotension. Unlike its structural relative trazodone, nefazodone has not been reported to cause priapism. There have been reports of liver failure in some patients taking nefazodone, prompting warnings about this risk factor.

Cardiovascular Effects

In premarketing trials, 5.1 percent of patients taking nefazodone experienced a significant drop in blood pressure, compared with 2.5 percent of patients receiving placebo. Although there was no increase in true syncopal events, symptoms of postural hypotension were experienced by 2.8 percent of patients treated with nefazodone. This rate compares with postural hypotension in 0.8 percent of placebo-treated, 1.1 percent of SSRI-treated, and 10.8 percent of tricyclic antidepressant-treated patients. Sinus bradycardia was seen in 1.5 percent of nefazodone-treated patients and 0.4 percent of placebo-treated patients. Nefazodone should thus be used with caution in patients with underlying cardiac conditions, history of stroke or heart attack, dehydration, and hypovolemia and in patients under treatment with antihypertensive medications.

Activation of Mania

In patients with known bipolar illness, 1.6 percent of those treated with nefazodone experienced mania, compared with 5.1 percent of tricyclic-treated patients and 0 percent of placebo-treated patients. The activation of mania in unipolar illness patients was no higher with nefazodone than with placebo. Therefore, nefazodone may be a drug to try earlier in the treatment of patients with a history of manic episodes. Electroconvulsive therapy and the antidepressant lithium (Eskalith) are least likely to activate mania.

THERAPEUTIC INDICATIONS

Nefazodone has been approved for the treatment of depression on the basis of data from several large clinical trials. Nefazodone has been shown to be as efficacious as imipramine (Tofranil), fluoxetine (Prozac), and paroxetine (Paxil) for treatment of moderate, severe, melancholic, nonmelancholic, chronic, and recurrent depression. Clinical reports indicate that nefazodone is also an effective treatment for depression accompanied by anxiety, such as panic disorder and panic with comorbid depression or depressive symptoms, for obsessive-compulsive disorder, for premenstrual dysphoric disorder, and for the management of chronic pain of neuropathic or non-neuropathic origin. Nefazodone also may help reduce obsessive thoughts in obsessive-compulsive disorders; however, one case report documents the initial appearance of obsessive thoughts during nefazodone treatment, which ceased when the drug was discontinued. More data are needed to establish whether nefazodone is as effective for obsessive-compulsive disorder as the SSRIs and clomipramine.

PRECAUTIONS AND ADVERSE REACTIONS

The most common adverse reactions to nefazodone use are nausea, dizziness, insomnia, weakness, and agitation. Patients with any degree of liver function impairment should not take nefazodone.

Cardiovascular Effects

Some patients taking nefazodone may experience a drop in blood pressure that can cause episodes of postural hypotension. Nefazodone should therefore be used with caution by persons with underlying cardiac conditions, history of stroke or heart attack, dehydration, or hypovolemia or by persons being treated with antihypertensive medications.

Activation of Mania

Some 1.6 percent of persons with known bipolar disorder treated with nefazodone experienced mania, compared with 5.1 percent of tricyclic-treated persons. The activation of mania in persons with unipolar depression was no higher with nefazodone than with placebo. Nonetheless, nefazodone, like other antidepressant medications, should be used with caution in persons with a history of manic episodes.

Other Precautions

The effects of nefazodone in human mothers are not yet as well understood as those of the SSRIs. Nefazodone should thus be used during pregnancy only if the potential benefit to the mother outweighs the potential risks to the fetus. It is not known whether nefazodone is excreted in human breast milk. Therefore, it should be used with caution by lactating mothers. As mentioned above, because of the risk of liver failure, nefazodone should not be used in persons with hepatic disease, but no adjustment is necessary for persons with renal disease.

DRUG INTERACTIONS

Nefazodone should not be given concomitantly with MAOIs. In addition, nefazodone has particular drug–drug interactions with the triazolobenzodiazepines triazolam (Halcion) and alprazolam (Xanax) because of the inhibition of cytochrome P450 isoenzyme 3A4 (CYP 3A4) by nefazodone. Potentially elevated levels of each of these drugs can develop after administration of nefazodone, whereas the levels of nefazodone are generally not affected. The manufacturer recommends lowering the dose of triazolam by 75 percent and the dose of alprazolam by 50 percent when given concomitantly with nefazodone.

Nefazodone may slow the metabolism of digoxin (Lanoxin); therefore, digoxin levels should be monitored carefully in persons taking both medications. Nefazodone also slows the metabolism of haloperidol (Haldol), so that the dosage of haloperidol should be reduced in persons taking both medications. Addition of nefazodone may also exacerbate the adverse effects of lithium.

LABORATORY INTERFERENCES

There are no known laboratory interferences associated with nefazodone.

DOSAGE AND CLINICAL GUIDELINES

Nefazodone is available in 50-, 200-, and 250-mg unscored tablets and 100- and 150-mg scored tablets. The recommended starting dosage of nefazodone is 100 mg twice a day, but 50 mg twice a day may be better tolerated, especially by elderly persons. To limit the development of adverse effects, the dosage should be slowly tapered up in increments of 100 to 200 mg a day at intervals of no less than 1 week per increase. The optimal dosage is 300 to 600 mg daily in two divided doses. However, some studies report that nefazodone is effective when taken once a day, especially at bedtime. Geriatric persons should receive dosages about two thirds of the usual nongeriatric dosages, with a maximum of 400 mg a day. In common with other antidepressants, clinical benefit of nefazodone usually appears after 2 to 4 weeks of treatment. Patients with premenstrual syndrome are treated with a flexible dosage that averages about 250 mg a day.

References

Ansari A. The efficacy of newer antidepressants in the treatment of chronic pain: a review of current literature. *Harvard Rev Psychiatry.* 2000;7:257.

Baldessarini RJ. Drugs and the treatment of psychiatric disorders: depression and anxiety disorders. In: Hardman JG, Limbird LE, Goodman Gilman A, eds. *Goodman & Gilman's the Pharmacological Basis of Therapeutics.* 10th ed. New York: McGraw-Hill; 2001: 447.

Baldwin DS, Hawley CJ, Abed RT, et al. A multicenter double-blind comparison of nefazodone and paroxetine in the treatment of outpatients with moderate-to-severe depression. *J Clin Psychiatry.* 1996;57(suppl 2):46.

DeMartinis NA, Schweizer E, Rickels K. An open-label trial of nefazodone in high comorbidity panic disorder. *J Clin Psychiatry.* 1996;57:245.

Dunner DL, Laird LK, Zajecka J, et al. Six-year perspectives on the safety and tolerability of nefazodone. *J Clin Psychiatry.* 2002;63:32.

Ellingrod VL, Perry PJ. Nefazodone: a new antidepressant. *Am J Health System Pharm.* 1995;52:2799.

Feiger A, Kiev A, Shrivastava RK, Wisselink PG, Wilcox CS. Nefazodone versus sertraline in outpatients with major depression: focus on efficacy, tolerability, and effects on sexual function and satisfaction. *J Clin Psychiatry.* 1996;57(suppl 2):53.

Garlow SJ, Owens MJ, Nemeroff CB. Nefazodone. In: Sadock BJ, Sadock VA, eds. *Kaplan & Sadock's Comprehensive Textbook of Psychiatry.* 7th ed. Vol 2. Baltimore: Lippincott Williams & Wilkins; 2000:2412.

Lader MH. Tolerability and safety: essentials in antidepressant pharmacotherapy. *J Clin Psychiatry.* 1996;57(suppl 2):39.

Marcus RN, Mendels J. Nefazodone in the treatment of severe, melancholic, and recurrent depression. *J Clin Psychiatry.* 1996;57(suppl 2):19.

Nemeroff CB, DeVane CL, Pollock BG. Newer antidepressants and the cytochrome P450 system. *Am J Psychiatry.* 1996;153:311.

Robinson DS, Marcus RN, Archibald DG, Hardy SA. Therapeutic dose range of nefazodone in the treatment of major depression. *J Clin Psychiatry.* 1996;57(suppl 2):6.

▲ 36.4.22 Opioid Receptor Agonists: Methadone, Levomethadyl, and Buprenorphine

Opioid receptor agonists are used in psychiatry for detoxification from heroin and other opioids and in maintenance opioid detoxification programs. Maintenance therapy is used in addicted patients who are unable to remain abstinent from opioids. Persons who switch from use of heroin to one of these drugs continue to satisfy their acute physical craving for opioids but are gradually weaned from their crippling psychological dependence on heroin. The drugs in this class include methadone (Dolophine), buprenorphine (Buprenex), and levomethadyl acetate (ORLAAM), also called L-α-acetylmethadol or LAAM. The most clinical experience is available for methadone; levomethadyl and buprenorphine are relatively new and are still being evaluated in various clinical and research settings.

CHEMISTRY

The structural formulas of the synthetic opioid receptor agonists methadone, levomethadyl, and buprenorphine are shown in Figure 36.4.22–1.

PHARMACOLOGICAL ACTIONS

Methadone, levomethadyl, and buprenorphine are absorbed rapidly from the gastrointestinal (GI) tract. Hepatic first-pass metabolism significantly affects the bioavailability of each of the drugs but in markedly different ways. For methadone, hepatic enzymes reduce the bioavailability of an oral dosage by about half, an effect that is easily managed with dosage adjustments. For levomethadyl, hepatic enzymes metabolize an oral dosage into normethyl-LAAM and dinormethyl-LAAM, which are actually several times more potent μ-opioid receptor agonists than levomethadyl itself. For buprenorphine, in contrast, first-pass intestinal and hepatic metabolism eliminates oral bioavailability almost completely; thus for use in opioid detoxification buprenorphine is given sublingually, in either a liquid or a tablet formulation.

The peak plasma concentrations of oral methadone are reached within 2 to 6 hours, and the plasma half-life initially is 4 to 6 hours in opioid-naive persons and 24 to 36 hours after steady dosing of any type of opioid. Methadone is highly protein bound and equilibrates widely throughout the body, which ensures little postdosage variation in steady-state plasma concentrations. The peak plasma concentrations of oral levomethadyl are reached within 1.5 to 2 hours, and the plasma half-lives of levomethadyl and its active metabolites range from 2 to 4 days. Elimination of a sublingual dosage of buprenorphine occurs in two phases, an initial phase with a half-life of 3 to 5 hours and a terminal phase with a half-life of more than 24 hours. Buprenorphine dissociates from its receptor binding site slowly, which permits an every-other-day dosing schedule.

EFFECTS ON ORGANS AND SYSTEMS

The relative safety of long-term methadone maintenance has been established through prospective and retrospective studies. No evidence of methadone toxicity for organ systems has been found during three decades of widespread clinical use. Less information is available regarding the long-term safety of levomethadyl acetate or buprenorphine. Levomethadyl acetate prolongs the QT interval in some patients, so patients entering methadone maintenance programs need careful monitoring, since many suffer from a number of chronic diseases, including (most commonly) human immunodeficiency virus (HIV) infection, hepatitis, tuberculosis, other infectious diseases, and cardiac or renal disorders. Methadone maintenance is associated with improved health and decreased risk of HIV transmission, largely as a result of reducing drug use and facilitating appropriate use of medical services.

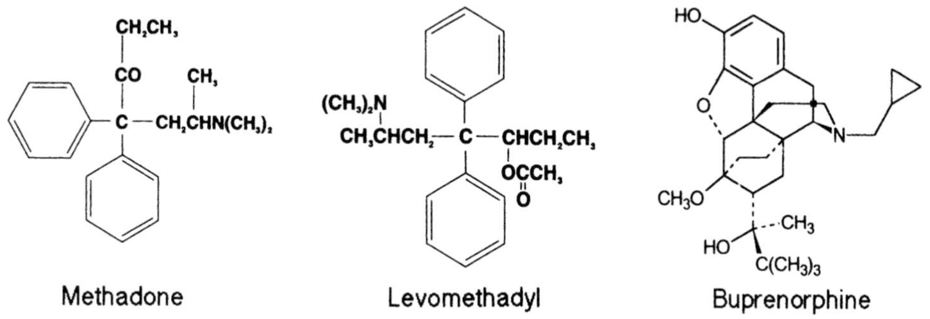

FIGURE 36.4.22–1
Molecular structures of opioid agonists.

THERAPEUTIC INDICATIONS

Methadone

Methadone is used for short-term detoxification (7 to 30 days), long-term detoxification (up to 180 days), and maintenance (treatment beyond 180 days), of opioid-dependent individuals. For these purposes, it is only available through designated clinics called *methadone maintenance treatment programs* (MMTPs) and in hospitals and prisons. Methadone is a Schedule II drug, which means that its administration is tightly governed by specific federal laws and regulations.

Enrollment in a methadone program reduces the risk of death by 70 percent; reduces illicit use of opioids and other substances of abuse; reduces criminal activity; reduces the risk of infectious diseases of all types, most importantly HIV and hepatitis B and C infection; and, in pregnant women, reduces the risk of fetal and neonatal morbidity and mortality. The use of methadone maintenance frequently requires lifelong treatment.

Some opioid-dependence treatment programs use a stepwise detoxification protocol in which a person addicted to heroin switches first to the strong agonist methadone, then to the weaker agonist buprenorphine, and finally to maintenance on an opioid receptor antagonist, such as naltrexone (ReVia). This approach minimizes the appearance of opioid withdrawal effects, which, if they occur, are mitigated with clonidine (Catapres). However, compliance with opioid receptor antagonist treatment is poor outside settings using intensive cognitive-behavioral techniques. In contrast, noncompliance with methadone maintenance precipitates opioid withdrawal symptoms, which serve to reinforce use of methadone and make cognitive-behavioral therapy less than essential. Thus, some well-motivated, socially integrated former heroin addicts are able to use methadone for years without participation in a psychosocial support program.

Data pooled from many reports indicate that methadone is more effective when taken at dosages in excess of 60 mg a day. The analgesic effects of methadone are sometimes used in the management of chronic pain when less addictive agents are ineffective.

Pregnancy. Methadone maintenance, combined with effective psychosocial services and regular obstetrical monitoring, significantly improves obstetrical and neonatal outcomes for women addicted to heroin. Enrollment of a heroin-addicted pregnant woman in such a maintenance program reduces the risk of malnutrition, infection, preterm labor, spontaneous abortion, preeclampsia, eclampsia, abruptio placenta, and septic thrombophlebitis.

The dosage of methadone during pregnancy should be the lowest effective dosage, and no withdrawal to abstinence should be attempted during pregnancy. Methadone is metabolized more rapidly in the third trimester, which may necessitate higher dosages. To avoid potentially sedating postdose peak plasma concentrations, the daily dose can be administered in two divided doses during the third trimester. Methadone treatment has no known teratogenic effects.

Neonatal Methadone Withdrawal Symptoms. Withdrawal symptoms in newborns frequently include tremor, high-pitched cry, increased muscle tone and activity, poor sleep and eating, mottling, yawning, perspiration, and skin excoriation. Convulsions that require aggressive anticonvulsant therapy may also occur. Withdrawal symptoms may be delayed in onset and prolonged in neonates because of their immature hepatic metabolism. Women taking methadone are sometimes counseled to initiate breast-feeding as a means of gently weaning their infants from methadone dependence, but they should not breast-feed their babies while still taking methadone.

Levomethadyl

Levomethadyl is used only for maintenance treatment of opioid-dependent patients. It is not used for detoxification treatment or for analgesia. Thrice-weekly levomethadyl dosing, consisting of 100 mg on Monday, 100 mg on Wednesday, and 140 mg on Friday, is more effective for opioid maintenance than smaller doses. Daily dosing of levomethadyl may cause overdosage.

Buprenorphine

Buprenorphine is an analgesic approved only for treatment of moderate to severe pain. Buprenorphine at a dosage of 8 to 16 mg a day appears to reduce heroin use. Buprenorphine also is effective in thrice-weekly dosing because of its slow dissociation from opioid receptors. The analgesic effects of buprenorphine are sometimes used in the management of chronic pain when less addictive agents are ineffective. There are some

reports of depressed patients responding to buprenorphine when other agents have failed.

PRECAUTIONS AND ADVERSE REACTIONS

The most common adverse effects of opioid receptor agonists are lightheadedness, dizziness, sedation, nausea, constipation, vomiting, perspiration, weight gain, decreased libido, inhibition of orgasm, and insomnia or sleep irregularities. Opioid receptor agonists can induce tolerance and can produce physiological and psychological dependence. Other central nervous system (CNS) adverse effects include dizziness, depression, sedation, euphoria, dysphoria, agitation, and seizures. Delirium and insomnia have also been reported in rare cases. Occasional non-CNS adverse effects include peripheral edema, urinary retention, rash, arthralgia, dry mouth, anorexia, biliary tract spasm, bradycardia, hypotension, hypoventilation, syncope, antidiuretic hormone–like activity, pruritus, urticaria, and visual disturbances. Menstrual irregularities are common in women, especially in the first 6 months of use. Various abnormal endocrine laboratory indexes of little clinical significance may also be seen. Most persons develop tolerance to the pharmacological adverse effects of opioid agonists during long-term maintenance, and relatively few adverse effects are experienced after the induction period.

Overdosage

The acute effects of opioid receptor agonist overdosage include sedation, hypotension, bradycardia, hypothermia, respiratory suppression, miosis, and decreased GI motility. Severe effects include coma, cardiac arrest, shock, and death. The risk of overdosage is greatest in the induction stage of treatment and in persons with slow drug metabolism due to preexisting hepatic insufficiency. Deaths have been caused during the first week of induction by methadone dosages of only 50 to 60 mg a day.

Because the therapeutic effects of levomethadyl may not appear in the first few days of treatment, addicted persons sometimes continue to administer doses of illicit opioids during this time and may experience symptoms of overdosage. Also, because of the long half-lives of levomethadyl and its active metabolites, daily dosing of levomethadyl causes excessive drug accumulation and is to be avoided in favor of thrice-weekly dosing.

The risk of overdosage with buprenorphine appears to be lower than that with methadone or levomethadyl. However, deaths have been caused by use of buprenorphine in combination with benzodiazepines.

Withdrawal Symptoms

Abrupt cessation of methadone use triggers withdrawal symptoms within 3 to 4 days, which usually reach peak intensity on the sixth day. Withdrawal symptoms include weakness, anxiety, anorexia, insomnia, gastric distress, headache, sweating, and hot and cold flashes. The withdrawal symptoms usually resolve after 2 weeks. However, a protracted methadone abstinence syndrome is possible that may include restlessness and insomnia.

The withdrawal symptoms associated with levomethadyl and buprenorphine are similar to, but less marked than, those due to methadone. In particular, buprenorphine is sometimes used to ease the transition from methadone to opioid receptor antagonists or abstinence, because of the relatively mild withdrawal reaction associated with discontinuation of buprenorphine.

DRUG–DRUG INTERACTIONS

Opioid receptor agonists can potentiate the CNS-depressant effects of alcohol, barbiturates, benzodiazepines, other opioids, low-potency dopamine receptor antagonists, tricyclic and tetracyclic drugs, and monoamine oxidase inhibitors (MAOIs). Carbamazepine (Tegretol), phenytoin (Dilantin), barbiturates, rifampin (Rimactane, Rifadin), and heavy long-term consumption of alcohol may induce hepatic enzymes, which may lower the plasma concentration of methadone or buprenorphine and thus precipitate withdrawal symptoms. In contrast, however, hepatic enzyme induction may raise the plasma concentration of active levomethadyl metabolites and cause toxicity.

Acute opioid withdrawal symptoms may be precipitated in persons on methadone maintenance therapy who take pure opioid receptor antagonists such as naltrexone, nalmefene (Revex), and naloxone (Narcan); partial agonists such as buprenorphine; or mixed agonist-antagonists such as pentazocine (Talwin). These symptoms may be mitigated by use of clonidine, a benzodiazepine, or both.

Competitive inhibition of methadone or buprenorphine metabolism following short-term use of alcohol or administration of cimetidine (Tagamet), erythromycin, ketoconazole (Nizoral), fluoxetine (Prozac), fluvoxamine (Luvox) loratadine (Claritin), quinidine (Quinidex), and alprazolam (Xanax) may increase plasma concentrations or prolong the duration of action of methadone or buprenorphine. Inhibition of levomethadyl metabolism by the same agents, however, may lower plasma concentrations, delay the onset of action, or prolong the duration of action. Medications that alkalinize the urine may reduce methadone excretion.

Methadone maintenance may also increase plasma concentrations of desipramine (Norpramin, Pertofrane) and fluvoxamine. Use of methadone may increase zidovudine (Retrovir) concentrations, which increases the possibility of zidovudine toxicity at otherwise standard dosages. In vitro human liver microsome studies, moreover ,demonstrate competitive inhibition of methadone demethylation by several protease inhibitors including ritonavir (Norvir), indinavir (Crixivan), and saquinavir (Invirase). The clinical relevance of this finding is unknown.

Fatal drug–drug interactions with the MAOIs are associated with use of the opioids fentanyl (Sublimaze) and meperidine (Demerol) but not with use of methadone, levomethadyl, or buprenorphine.

LABORATORY INTERFERENCES

Methadone, levomethadyl, and buprenorphine can be tested for separately in urine toxicology to distinguish them from other opioids. No known laboratory interferences are associated with use of methadone, levomethadyl, or buprenorphine.

DOSAGE AND CLINICAL GUIDELINES

Methadone

Methadone is supplied in 5-, 10-, and 40-mg dispersible scored tablets; 40-mg scored wafers; 5 mg/5 mL, 10 mg/5 mL, and 10 mg/mL solutions; and a 10-mg/mL parenteral form. In maintenance programs, methadone is usually dissolved in water or juice, and dose administration is observed directly to ensure compliance. For induction of opioid detoxification, an initial methadone dose of 15 to 20 mg will usually suppress craving and withdrawal symptoms. However, some individuals may require up to 40 mg a day in single or divided doses. Higher dosages should be avoided during induction of treatment to reduce the risk of acute overdosage.

Over several weeks, the dosage should be raised to at least 70 mg a day. The maximum dosage is usually 120 mg a day, and higher dosages require prior approval from regulatory agencies. Dosages above 60 mg a day are associated with much more complete abstinence from use of illicit opioids than are dosages below 60 mg a day.

The duration of treatment should not be predetermined but should be based on response to treatment and assessment of psychosocial factors. All studies of methadone maintenance programs endorse long-term treatment (i.e., several years) as more effective than short-term programs (i.e., less than 1 year) for prevention of relapse into opioid abuse. In actual practice, however, a minority of programs are permitted by policy or approved by insurers to provide even 6 months of continuous maintenance treatment. Moreover, some programs actually encourage withdrawal from methadone in less than 6 months after induction. This is quite ill conceived, because over 80 percent of persons who terminate methadone maintenance treatment eventually return to illicit drug use within 2 years. In programs that offer both maintenance and withdrawal treatments, the overwhelming majority of participants enroll in the maintenance treatment. These programs should be encouraged and expanded.

Levomethadyl

Levomethadyl is supplied as a 10-mg/mL oral solution and is usually administered thrice weekly. Because of the tendency of levomethadyl to accumulate to toxic concentrations if taken daily, it should not be taken more frequently than every other day. The initial dose in persons not known to have tolerance to opioids is 20 or 40 mg. Each subsequent dose may be increased by 5 or 10 mg, and steady state for a given dosage is achieved in no less than 2 weeks. Persons already dependent on methadone should receive a starting dosage of levomethadyl acetate that is 1.2 to 1.3 times the dosage of methadone being replaced but not more than 120 mg. It is unnecessary to taper or overlap dosages during the crossover from methadone to levomethadyl, which can be accomplished over 2 consecutive days. Subsequent dosages of levomethadyl should be adjusted according to clinical response.

Most persons require levomethadyl doses of 60 to 90 mg, thrice weekly. The clinical dose range is 10 to 140 mg thrice weekly. The maximum recommended weekly dose is 440 mg.

Buprenorphine

Buprenorphine is supplied as a 0.3-mg/mL solution in 1-mL ampules for use as an analgesic. Sublingual preparations of buprenorphine appropriate for use in opioid maintenance programs are not currently available in the United States. Sublingual tablet formulations of buprenorphine containing buprenorphine only or buprenorphine combined with naloxone in a 4:1 ratio are used outside the United States for opioid maintenance treatment. Buprenorphine is not used for short-term opioid detoxification. Maintenance dosages of 8 to 16 mg thrice weekly have effectively reduced heroin use in clinical trials.

References

Comer SD, Collins ED, Fischman MW. Intravenous buprenorphine self-administration by detoxified heroin abusers. *J Pharmacol Exp Ther.* 2002;301:266.

Cone EJ, Preston KL. Toxicologic aspects of heroin substitution treatment. *Ther Drug Monit.* 2002;24:193.

Farrell M, Strang J. Compressed opiate withdrawal syndrome and naltrexone. *J Psychopharmacol.* 1995;9:383.

Greif GL, Drechsler M. Common issues for parents in a methadone maintenance group. *J Subst Abuse Treat.* 1993;10:339.

Hardman JG, Limbird LE, Goodman Gilman A, eds. *Goodman & Gilman's the Pharmacological Basis of Therapeutics.* 10th ed. New York: McGraw-Hill; 2001.

Keller MB. Efficacy of nefazodone in chronic depression. *J Clin Psychiatry.* 2002;63:24.

Ling W, Wesson DR. A controlled trial comparing buprenorphine and methadone maintenance in opioid dependence. *Arch Gen Psychiatry.* 1996;53:401.

Milby JB, Sims MK, Khuder S, et al. Psychiatric comorbidity: prevalence in methadone maintenance treatment. *Am J Drug Alcohol Abuse.* 1996;22:95.

Nanovskaya T, Deshmukh S, Brooks M, Ahmed MS. Transplacental transfer and metabolism of buprenorphine. *J Pharmacol Exp Ther.* 2002;300:26.

Prendergast ML, Grella C, Perry SM, Anglin MD. Levo-alpha-acetylmethadol (LAAM): clinical, research, and policy issues of a new pharmacotherapy for opioid addiction. *J Psychoactive Drugs.* 1995;27:239.

Schottenfeld RS, Kleber HD. Methadone. In: Kaplan HI, Sadock BJ, eds. *Comprehensive Textbook of Psychiatry.* 6th ed. Baltimore: Williams & Wilkins; 1995:2031.

Schottenfeld RS, Kleber HD. Opioid agonists. In: Sadock BJ, Sadock VA, eds. *Kaplan & Sadock's Comprehensive Textbook of Psychiatry.* 7th ed. Vol 2. Baltimore: Lippincott Williams & Wilkins; 2000:2419.

Strain EC, Stitzer ML, Liebson IA, Bigelow GE. Buprenorphine versus methadone in the treatment of opioid dependence: self-reports, urinalysis and addiction severity index. *J Clin Psychopharmacol.* 1996;16:58.

Weinrich M, Stuart M. Provision of methadone treatment in primary care medical practices: review of the Scottish experience and implications for US policy. *JAMA.* 2000;283:1343.

▲ 36.4.23 Opioid Receptor Antagonists: Naltrexone and Nalmefene

The oral opioid receptor antagonists naltrexone (ReVia) and nalmefene (Revex) are effective treatments for opioid dependence when used in combination with structured cognitive-behavioral therapy. They may also be of use in alcohol dependence. Opioid receptor antagonists appear to reduce or eliminate the subjective "high" associated with consumption of opioids, thus interrupting their reinforcing effects. Opioid receptor antagonists also reduce or eliminate the craving associated with withdrawal from chronic opioid abuse.

Of these two opioid receptor antagonists, at present only oral naltrexone is Food and Drug Administration (FDA)-approved for treatment of opioid dependence or for blockade of

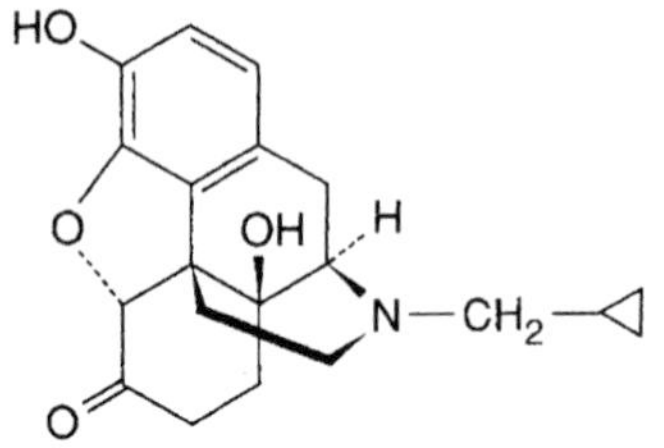

FIGURE 36.4.23–1
Molecular structure of naltrexone.

the effects of exogenously administered opioids. Currently, the only commercially available formulation of nalmefene is for intravenous administration, but at least one manufacturer has an oral formulation of nalmefene in clinical trials. Naloxone (Narcan), another opioid receptor antagonist, is not discussed in detail because it is available only for intravenous use. Its use is covered under treatment for opioid overdose in Section 12.10 of Chapter 12.

CHEMISTRY

The molecular structure of naltrexone is shown in Figure 36.4.23–1. The molecular structure of nalmefene in shown in Figure 30.4.23–2.

PHARMACOLOGICAL ACTIONS

Oral opioid receptor antagonists are rapidly absorbed from the gastrointestinal (GI) tract, but because of first-pass hepatic metabolism, only 60 percent of a dose of naltrexone and 40 to 50 percent of a dose of nalmefene reach the systemic circulation unchanged. Peak concentrations of naltrexone and its active metabolite, 6-β-naltrexol, are achieved within 1 hour of ingestion. The half-life of naltrexone is 1 to 3 hours, and the half-life of 6-β-naltrexol is 13 hours. Peak concentrations of nalmefene are achieved in about 1 to 2 hours, and the half-life is 8 to 10 hours. Clinically, a single dose of naltrexone effectively blocks the rewarding effects of opioids for 72 hours. Traces of 6-β-naltrexol may linger for up to 125 hours after a single dose.

Naltrexone and nalmefene are competitive antagonists of opioid receptors. Understanding the pharmacology of opioid receptors can explain the difference in adverse effects caused by naltrexone and nalmefene. Opioid receptors in the body are typed pharmacologically as either μ, κ, or δ. Activation of the κ- and δ-receptors is thought to reinforce opioid and alcohol consumption centrally, whereas activation of μ-receptors is more closely associated with central and peripheral antiemetic effects. Because naltrexone is a relatively weak antagonist of κ- and δ-receptors and a potent μ-receptor antagonist, dosages of naltrexone that effectively reduce opioid and alcohol consumption also strongly block μ-receptors and therefore may cause nausea. Nalmefene, in contrast, is an equally potent antagonist of all three opioid receptor types, and dosages of nalmefene that effectively reduce opioid and alcohol consumption have no particularly increased effect on μ-receptors. Thus, nalmefene is associated clinically with few GI adverse effects.

Whereas the effects of opioid receptor antagonists on opioid use are easily understood in terms of competitive inhibition of opioid receptors, the effects of opioid receptor antagonists on alcohol dependence are less straightforward and probably relate to the fact that the desire for, and effects of, alcohol consumption appear to be regulated by several neurotransmitter systems, both opioid and nonopioid.

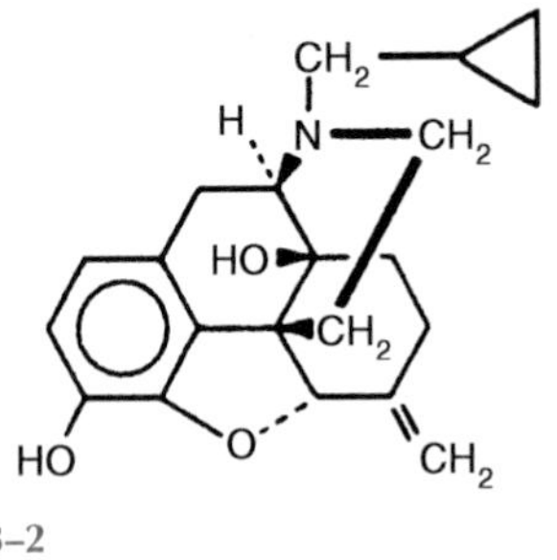

FIGURE 36.4.23–2
Molecular structure of nalmefene.

THERAPEUTIC INDICATIONS

Opioid receptor antagonists are most effective when combined with cognitive-behavioral therapy. This combination is more successful than either a cognitive-behavioral program or use of opioid receptor antagonists alone.

Opioid Dependence

Patients in detoxification programs are usually weaned from potent opioid agonists such as heroin over a period of days to weeks, during which emergent adrenergic withdrawal effects are treated as needed with clonidine (Catapres). A serial protocol is sometimes used in which potent agonists are gradually replaced by weaker agonists, followed by mixed agonist-antagonists, and finally by pure antagonists. For example, an abuser of the potent agonist heroin would switch first to the weaker agonist methadone (Dolophine), then to the partial agonist buprenorphine (Buprenex) or levomethadyl acetate (ORLAAM)—commonly called *LAAM*—and finally, following a 7- to 10-day washout period, to a pure antagonist, such as naltrexone or nalmefene. However, even with gradual detoxification, some persons continue to experience mild adverse effects or opioid withdrawal symptoms for the first several weeks of treatment with naltrexone.

As the opioid receptor agonist potency diminishes, so do the adverse consequences of discontinuing the drug. Thus, because there are no pharmacological barriers to discontinuation of pure opioid receptor antagonists, the social environment and frequent cognitive-behavioral intervention become extremely important factors supporting continued opioid abstinence. Because of poorly tolerated adverse symptoms, most persons not simultaneously enrolled in a cognitive-behavioral program stop taking opioid receptor antagonists within 3 months. Compliance with administration of an opioid receptor antagonist regimen can also be increased with participation in a well-conceived voucher program in which the patient is rewarded for taking the drug.

Issues of medication compliance should be a central focus of treatment. If a person with a history of opioid addiction stops taking a pure opioid receptor antagonist, the person's risk of

relapse into opioid abuse is exceedingly high, because reintroduction of a potent opioid agonist would yield a very rewarding subjective "high." In contrast, compliant persons do not develop tolerance to the therapeutic benefits of naltrexone, even if it is administered continuously for 1 year or longer. Individuals may undergo several relapses and remissions before achieving long-term abstinence.

Persons taking opioid receptor antagonists should also be warned that sufficiently high dosages of opioid agonists can overcome the receptor antagonism of naltrexone or nalmefene, which may lead to hazardous and unpredictable levels of receptor activation.

Rapid Detoxification. To avoid the 7- to 10-day period of opioid abstinence generally recommended prior to use of opioid receptor antagonists, rapid detoxification protocols have been developed. Continuous administration of adjunct clonidine—to reduce the adrenergic withdrawal symptoms—and adjunct benzodiazepines, such as oxazepam (Serax)—to reduce muscle spasms and insomnia—can permit use of oral opioid receptor antagonists on the first day of opioid cessation. Detoxification can thus be completed within 48 to 72 hours, at which point opioid receptor antagonist maintenance is initiated. Moderately severe withdrawal symptoms may be experienced on the first day, but they tail off rapidly thereafter.

Because of the potential hypotensive effects of clonidine, the blood pressure of persons undergoing rapid detoxification must be closely monitored for the first 8 hours. Outpatient rapid detoxification settings must thus be adequately prepared to administer emergency care.

The main advantage of rapid detoxification is that the transition from opioid abuse to maintenance treatment occurs over just 2 or 3 days. Completion of detoxification in as little time as possible minimizes the risk that a person will relapse into opioid abuse during the detoxification protocol.

Ultrarapid Detoxification. In a variant technique called ultrarapid opioid detoxification, the body is cleared of opioid agonist activity over a period of only a few hours by infusion of naloxone. In this controversial approach, the severe withdrawal symptoms that are triggered by the sudden naloxone-mediated reversal of opioid agonist activity are mitigated with clonidine and benzodiazepines, while the person is partially or fully anesthetized. Naltrexone or nalmefene maintenance is then initiated before the anesthesia is reversed.

Aside from the potential for morbidity and mortality associated with administration of general anesthesia, the main pitfall of ultrarapid detoxification is its high rate of relapse, most likely because naloxone-mediated opioid withdrawal does nothing to eliminate the disabling psychological need for opioids, and psychosocial support is not necessarily an integral part of the technique. Extreme caution is further warranted because the dosages of the required combination of drugs frequently affect the cardiovascular and respiratory systems adversely.

An estimated 10,000 persons worldwide have undergone anesthetized ultrarapid opioid detoxification since its introduction in the 1980s. Practitioners have been disappointed by the very high rate of relapse into opioid abuse soon after the technique is completed. Moreover, at least 10 deaths have been associated with administration of this technique. Because the known risks of the technique appear to outweigh the potential benefits, ultrarapid detoxification cannot be recommended at present.

Alcohol Dependence

Opioid receptor antagonists are also used as adjuncts to cognitive-behavioral programs for treatment of alcohol dependence. Opioid receptor antagonists reduce alcohol craving and alcohol consumption, and they ameliorate the severity of relapses. The risk of relapse into heavy consumption of alcohol attributable to an effective cognitive-behavioral program alone may be halved with concomitant use of opioid receptor antagonists.

The newer agent nalmefene has a number of potential pharmacological and clinical advantages over its predecessor naltrexone for treatment of alcohol dependence. Whereas naltrexone may cause reversible transaminase elevations in persons who take dosages of 300 mg a day (which is 6 times the recommended dosage for treatment of alcohol and opioid dependence [50 mg a day]), nalmefene has not been associated with any hepatotoxicity. Clinically effective dosages of naltrexone are discontinued by 10 to 15 percent of persons because of adverse effects, most commonly nausea. In contrast, discontinuation of nalmefene because of an adverse event is rare at the clinically effective dosage of 20 mg a day and in the range of 10 percent at excessive dosages (i.e., 80 mg a day). Because of its pharmacokinetic profile, a given dosage of nalmefene may also produce a more sustained opioid antagonist effect than naltrexone. The efficacy of opioid receptor antagonists in reducing alcohol craving may be augmented with a selective serotonin reuptake inhibitor, although data from large trials are needed to assess this potential synergistic effect more fully.

PRECAUTIONS AND ADVERSE REACTIONS

Because opioid receptor antagonists are used to maintain a drug-free state after opioid detoxification, great care must be taken to ensure that an adequate washout period elapses after the last dose of opioids before the first dose of an opioid receptor antagonist is taken: at least 5 days for a short-acting opioid such as heroin, and at least 10 days for longer-acting opioids such as methadone. The opioid-free state should be determined by self-report and urine toxicology screens. If any question persists of whether opioids are in the body despite a negative urine screen result, then a naloxone challenge test should be performed. Naloxone challenge is used because its opioid antagonism lasts less than 1 hour, whereas those of naltrexone and nalmefene may persist for more than 24 hours. Thus any withdrawal effects elicited by naloxone will be relatively short-lived. Symptoms of acute opioid withdrawal include drug craving, feeling of temperature change, musculoskeletal pain, and GI distress. Signs of opioid withdrawal include confusion, drowsiness, vomiting, and diarrhea. Naltrexone and nalmefene should not taken be if naloxone infusion causes any signs of opioid withdrawal, except as part of a supervised rapid detoxification protocol.

A set of adverse effects, resembling a vestigial withdrawal syndrome, tends to affect up to 10 percent of persons who take opioid receptor antagonists. Up to 15 percent of persons taking naltrexone may experience abdominal pain, cramps, nausea, and vomiting, which may be limited by transiently halving the dosage or altering the time of administration. Adverse central nervous system effects of naltrexone, experienced by up to 10

percent of persons, include headache, low energy, insomnia, anxiety, and nervousness. Joint and muscle pains may occur in up to 10 percent of persons taking naltrexone, as may rash.

Naltrexone may cause dosage-related hepatic toxicity at dosages well in excess of 50 mg a day: 20 percent of persons taking 300 mg a day of naltrexone may experience serum aminotransferase concentrations 3 to 19 times the upper limit of normal. The hepatocellular injury of naltrexone appears to be a dose-related toxic effect rather than an idiosyncratic reaction. At the lowest dosages of naltrexone required for effective opioid antagonism, hepatocellular injury is not typically observed. However, naltrexone dosages as low as 50 mg a day may be hepatotoxic in persons with underlying liver disease, such as cirrhosis of the liver due to chronic alcohol abuse. Serum aminotransferase concentrations should be monitored monthly for the first 6 months of naltrexone therapy and thereafter on the basis of clinical suspicion. Hepatic enzyme concentrations usually return to normal after discontinuation of naltrexone therapy.

If analgesia is required while a dose of an opioid receptor antagonist is pharmacologically active, opioid agonists should be avoided in favor of benzodiazepines or other nonopioid analgesics. Persons taking opioid receptor antagonists should be instructed that low dosages of opioids will have no effect, but larger dosages could overcome the receptor blockade and suddenly produce symptoms of profound opioid overdosage, with sedation possibly progressing to coma or death. Use of opioid receptor antagonists is contraindicated in persons who are taking opioid agonists (small amounts of which may be present in over-the-counter antiemetic and antitussive preparations), persons with acute hepatitis or hepatic failure, and those who are hypersensitive to the drugs.

Because naltrexone is transported across the placenta, opioid receptor antagonists should only be taken by pregnant women if a compelling need outweighs the potential risks to the fetus. It is not known whether opioid receptor antagonists are distributed into maternal milk.

Opioid receptor antagonists are relatively safe drugs, and ingestion of high doses of them should be treated with supportive measures combined with efforts to decrease GI absorption.

DRUG–DRUG INTERACTIONS

Many drug interactions involving opioid receptor antagonists are discussed above, including those with opioid agonists associated with drug abuse as well as those involving antiemetics and antitussives. Because of its extensive hepatic metabolism, naltrexone may affect or be affected by other drugs that influence hepatic enzyme levels. However, the clinical importance of these potential interactions is not known.

One potentially hepatotoxic drug that has been used in some cases with opioid receptor antagonists is disulfiram (Antabuse). Although no adverse effects were observed, frequent laboratory monitoring is indicated when such combination therapy is contemplated. Opioid receptor antagonists have been reported to potentiate the sedation associated with use of thioridazine (Mellaril), an interaction that probably applies equally to all low-potency dopamine receptor antagonists.

LABORATORY INTERFERENCES

No laboratory interferences have been described for opioid receptor antagonists, although relatively nonspecific immune-based toxicology screens for opioids could potentially yield positive results in persons taking only opioid receptor antagonists, because of their structural similarities to other opioids.

DOSAGE AND CLINICAL GUIDELINES

To avoid the possibility of precipitating an acute opioid withdrawal syndrome, several steps should be taken to ensure that the person is opioid free. Within a supervised detoxification setting, at least 5 days should elapse following the last dose of short-acting opioids such as heroin, hydromorphone (Dilaudid), meperidine (Demerol), or morphine, and at least 10 days should elapse after the last dose of longer-acting opioids, such as methadone, before opioid antagonist use is initiated. Briefer periods off opioid use have been used in rapid detoxification protocols. To confirm that opioid detoxification is complete, urine toxicological screens should demonstrate no opioid metabolites. However, an individual may have a negative urine opioid screen result yet still be physically dependent on opioids and thus susceptible to antagonist-induced withdrawal effects. Thus once the urine screen result is negative, a naloxone challenge test is recommended, unless reliable observers can confirm an adequate period of opioid abstinence (Table 36.4.23–1).

Table 36.4.23–1
Naloxone (Narcan) Challenge Test

The naloxone challenge test should not be performed in a patient showing clinical signs or symptoms of opioid withdrawal or in one whose urine contains opioids. The naloxone challenge test may be administered by either the intravenous or subcutaneous route.

Intravenous challenge: Following appropriate screening of the patient, 0.8 mg of naloxone should be drawn into a sterile syringe. If the intravenous route of administration is selected, 0.2 mg of naloxone should be injected, and while the needle is still in the patient's vein, the patient should be observed for 30 seconds for evidence of withdrawal signs or symptoms. If there is no evidence of withdrawal, the remaining 0.6 mg of naloxone should be injected, and the patient observed for an additional 20 minutes for signs and symptoms of withdrawal.

Subcutaneous challenge: If the subcutaneous route is selected, 0.8 mg should be administered subcutaneously, and the patient observed for signs and symptoms of withdrawal for 20 minutes.

Conditions and technique for observation of patient: During the appropriate period of observation, the patient's vital signs should be monitored, and the patient should be monitored for signs of withdrawal. It is also important to question the patient carefully. The signs and symptoms of opioid withdrawal include, but are not limited to, the following:

- **Withdrawal signs:** stuffiness or running nose, tearing, yawning, sweating, tremor, vomiting, or piloerection
- **Withdrawal symptoms:** feeling of temperature change, joint or bone and muscle pain, abdominal cramps, and formication (feeling of bugs crawling under skin)

Interpretation of the challenge: Warning—elicitation of the enumerated signs or symptoms indicates a potential risk for the subject, and naltrexone should not be administered. If no signs or symptoms of withdrawal are observed, elicited, or reported, naltrexone may be administered. If there is any doubt in the observer's mind that the patient is not in an opioid-free state or is in continuing withdrawal, naltrexone should be withheld for 24 hours and the challenge repeated.

The initial dosage of naltrexone for treatment of opioid or alcohol dependence is 50 mg a day, which should be achieved through gradual introduction, even when the naloxone challenge test result is negative. Various authorities begin with 5, 10, 12.5, or 25 mg and titrate up to the 50-mg dosage over a period ranging from 1 hour to 2 weeks, while constantly monitoring for evidence of opioid withdrawal. Once a daily dose of 50 mg is well tolerated, it may be averaged over a week by giving 100 mg on alternate days or 150 mg every third day. Such schedules may increase compliance. The corresponding therapeutic dosage of nalmefene is 20 mg a day, divided into two equal doses. Gradual titration of nalmefene to this daily dose is probably a wise strategy, although clinical data on dosage strategies for nalmefene are not yet available.

To maximize compliance, it is recommended that ingestion of each dose be directly observed either in a facility or by family members, and that random urine tests for opioid receptor antagonists and their metabolites as well as for ethanol or opioid metabolites be taken. Opioid receptor antagonist use should be continued until the person is no longer considered psychologically at risk for relapse into opioid or alcohol abuse. This generally requires at least 6 months but may take longer, particularly if there are external stresses.

Rapid Detoxification

Rapid detoxification has been standardized using naltrexone, although nalmefene would be expected to be equally effective with fewer adverse effects. In rapid detoxification protocols, the addicted person stops opioid use abruptly and begins the first opioid-free day by taking clonidine 0.2 mg orally every 2 hours for nine doses, to a maximum dose of 1.8 mg, during which time blood pressure is monitored every 30 to 60 minutes for the first 8 hours. Naltrexone 12.5 mg is administered 1 to 3 hours after the first dose of clonidine. To reduce muscle cramps and later insomnia, a short-acting benzodiazepine, such as oxazepam 30 to 60 mg, is administered simultaneously with the first dose of clonidine, and half of the initial dose is readministered every 4 to 6 hours as needed. The maximum daily dosage of oxazepam should not exceed 180 mg. The person undergoing rapid detoxification should be accompanied home by a reliable escort. On the second day, similar doses of clonidine and the benzodiazepine are administered, but with a single 25-mg dose of naltrexone taken in the morning. Relatively asymptomatic persons may return home after 3 to 4 hours. Administration of the daily maintenance dose of 50 mg of naltrexone is begun on the third day, and the dosages of clonidine and the benzodiazepine are gradually tapered off over 5 to 10 days.

References

Comer SD, Collins ED, Kleber HD, et al. Depot naltrexone: long-lasting antagonism of the effects of heroin in humans. *Psychopharmacology.* 2002;159:351.

Hardman JG, Limbird LE, Goodman Gilman A, eds. *Goodman & Gilman's the Pharmacological Basis of Therapeutics.* 10th ed. New York: McGraw-Hill; 2001.

Johnson BA, Alit-Daoud N. Medication to treat alcoholism. *Alcohol Res Health.* 1999;23:99.

Johnson BA, Alit-Daoud N. Neuropharmacological treatment for alcoholism: scientific basis and clinical findings. *Psychopharmacology.* 2000;149:327.

Jones HE, Johnson RE, Fudala PJ, Henningfield JE, Heishman SJ. Nalmefene: blockade of intravenous morphine challenge effects in opioid abusing humans. *Drug Alcohol Depend.* 2000;60:29.

O'Malley SS, Krishnan-Sarin S, Rounsavile BJ. Naltrexone. In: Sadock BJ, Sadock VA, eds. *Kaplan & Sadock's Comprehensive Textbook of Psychiatry.* 7th ed. Vol 2. Baltimore: Lippincott Williams & Wilkins; 2000:2407.

O'Mara NB, Wesley LC. Naltrexone in the treatment of alcohol dependence. *Ann Pharmacother.* 1994;28:210.

Rabinowitz J, Cohen H, Atias S. Outcomes of naltrexone maintenance following ultra rapid opiate detoxification versus intensive inpaient detoxification. *Am J Addict.* 2002;11:52.

Sax DS, Kornetsky C, Kim A. Lack of hepatotoxicity with naltrexone treatment. *J Clin Pharmacol.* 1994;34:898.

Shufman EN, Porat S, Witztum E, Gandaeu D, Bar-Hamburger R, Ginath Y. The efficacy of naltrexone in preventing reabuse of heroin after detoxification. *Biol Psychiatry.* 1994;35:935.

Sinclair JD. Evidence about the use of naltrexone and for different ways of using it in the treatment of alcoholism. *Alcohol Alcohol.* 2001;36:362.

▲ 36.4.24 Other Anticonvulsants: Gabapentin, Lamotrigine, and Topiramate

Initially developed as anticonvulsant drugs, gabapentin (Neurontin), lamotrigine (Lamictal), and topiramate (Topamax) appear to have therapeutic spectra that extend to other conditions seen in psychiatric practice. Like valproate (Depakene) and carbamazepine (Tegretol), they represent possible alternatives or adjuncts for the treatment of bipolar disorders, anxiety disorders, agitation, pain, and substance abuse.

The newer antiepileptic agents are structurally diverse and have multiple central nervous system effects. They differ in metabolism, drug interactions, and adverse effects. The clinical significance of the neurochemical mechanisms associated with these drugs is not fully understood. None of them has an identical combination of neurochemical actions.

Another approved anticonvulsant, tiagabine (Gabitril), has been studied in psychiatric disorders but to a much smaller extent than gabapentin, lamotrigine, and topiramate. A new anticonvulsant pregabalin, which is related to gabapentin, is in phase III clinical development. Research reports of pregabalin in generalized anxiety disorder have found it to be as effective as some benzodiazepines and antidepressants.

CHEMISTRY

Gabapentin is chemically related to γ-aminobutyric acid (GABA) and is structurally similar to L-leucine. Lamotrigine and topiramate are each novel three-ringed compounds. Their molecular structures are shown in Figure 36.4.24–1.

PHARMACOLOGICAL ACTIONS

Gabapentin

Gabapentin is absorbed by the neutral amino acid membrane transporter system in the gut, and it crosses the blood–brain barrier. Bioavailability of 300- or 600-mg doses is 60 percent, whereas bioavailability of a 1,600-mg dose is 35 percent. Because higher amounts are not absorbed, doses should not exceed 1,800 mg per single dose or 5,400 mg a day. Food has no effect on gabapentin absorption, and it does not bind to plasma proteins. The steady-state half-life of 5 to 9 hours is reached in 2 days if thrice-daily dosing is used. Gabapentin is not metabolized and is excreted unchanged in the urine.

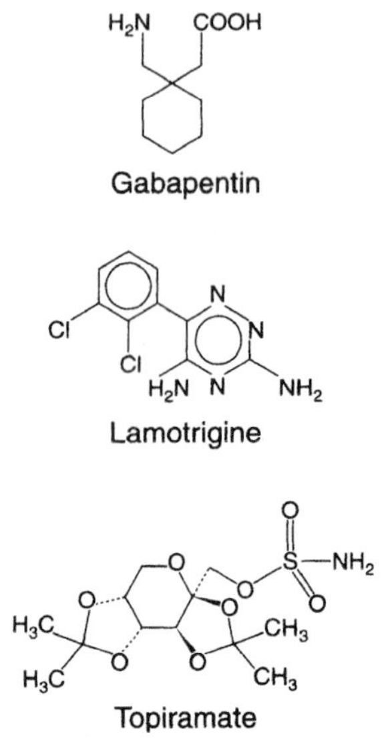

FIGURE 36.3.24–1
Molecular structure of other anticonvulsants used in psychiatry.

Lamotrigine

Lamotrigine is completely absorbed, and its steady-state plasma half-life is 25 hours. However, the rate of lamotrigine's metabolism varies over a sixfold range, depending on which other drugs are administered concomitantly. Dosing is escalated slowly to twice-a-day maintenance dosing. Food does not affect its absorption, and it is 55 percent protein bound in the plasma; 94 percent of lamotrigine and its inactive metabolites is excreted in the urine. Lamotrigine has an anticonvulsant profile similar to that of carbamazepine and phenytoin (Dilantin). Lamotrigine inhibits dihydrofolate reductase, the enzyme responsible for generation of folic acid, which is necessary for proper fetal development. Lamotrigine increases plasma serotonin concentrations modestly and is a weak inhibitor of serotonin 5-HT_3 receptors.

Topiramate

Topiramate is rapidly and completely absorbed, and its steady-state half-life is 21 hours. Food does not affect its absorption. It is 15 percent protein bound in the plasma, and 70 percent of an oral dose of topiramate is excreted unchanged in the urine, together with small amounts of several inactive metabolites. Topiramate is an inhibitor of state-dependent sodium channels. It potentiates the action of GABA at a non-benzodiazepine-, non-barbiturate-sensitive $GABA_A$ receptor.

THERAPEUTIC INDICATIONS

Gabapentin, lamotrigine, and topiramate are indicated by the Food and Drug Administration (FDA) in the treatment of seizure disorders. Gabapentin is also widely used to treat chronic pain, particularly that of polyneuropathy. Many prescriptions for these drugs are written for the nonepileptic indications listed below.

Bipolar Disorder

Each of these drugs has been used as monotherapy and adjunctive medication for treatment-refractory persons with bipolar disorders, including bipolar I, bipolar II, cyclothymic disorder, and bipolar disorder not otherwise specified. These drugs appear to have both mood-stabilizing and antidepressant effects. Generally, they have been added when persons have not responded satisfactorily to first-line agents such as lithium (Eskalith), valproic acid, or carbamazepine. Some clinicians have used these drugs successfully as monotherapy. There are many positive clinical trials of lamotrigine use for acute and prophylactic treatment in patients with depressive episodes of bipolar I disorder and in those with rapid cycling variants.

Chronic Pain

Gabapentin is effective for treatment of postherpetic neuralgia and painful diabetic neuropathy, and lamotrigine has been shown to be effective for treatment of human immunodeficiency virus (HIV)–associated peripheral neuropathy and reduction of postoperative analgesic use. Other conditions responsive to gabapentin and lamotrigine include trigeminal neuralgia; central pain syndromes; compression neuropathies, such as carpal tunnel syndrome, radiculopathies, and meralgia paresthetica; and painful neuropathies due to other causes. The pain-reduction response for these conditions is similar to that with selective serotonin reuptake inhibitors and tricyclic antidepressants and superior to that with intravenous and topical lidocaine (Xylocaine), carbamazepine, topical aspirin, mexiletine (Mexitil), phenytoin, topical capsaicin (Double Cap Cream), oral nonsteroidal antiinflammatory drugs (NSAIDs), opioids, propranolol (Inderal), lorazepam (Ativan), and phentolamine (Regitine). Because of their distinct mechanisms of action and absence of interactions, gabapentin and antidepressants are often used in combination for treatment of neuropathic pain.

Other Indications

Gabapentin appears to reduce the frequency and intensity of explosive outbursts in persons with dyscontrol disorders, including children, persons with dementia, and persons with traumatic brain injury. It is also an effective treatment for social phobia and panic disorder in some persons. Because of its mildly sedating properties, gabapentin can treat insomnia and agitation due to withdrawal from benzodiazepines, alcohol, and cocaine. Gabapentin is also an effective treatment for tremor and parkinsonism.

Lamotrigine has antipsychotic effects in persons with epilepsy. This is important for those comorbid for epilepsy and psychosis, because many antipsychotic medications lower the seizure threshold. Lamotrigine may reduce intrusive and avoidance or numbing symptoms of posttraumatic stress disorder.

Topiramate can markedly reduce appetite and may have other metabolic properties. It is being used as a treatment for obesity, binge eating, and migraine prophylaxis.

PRECAUTIONS AND ADVERSE REACTIONS

Gabapentin

Gabapentin is well tolerated, and the dosage can be escalated to the maintenance range within 2 to 3 days. There are almost no

dose-related adverse effects, even at doses of 5 g per day, which far exceeds the absorptive capacity of the intestines. The most frequent adverse effects of gabapentin, like other antiepileptic drugs, are somnolence, dizziness, ataxia, fatigue, and nystagmus, which are usually transient.

Lamotrigine

The most common adverse effects associated with use of lamotrigine, especially when used in combination with other antiepileptic drugs for the treatment of epilepsy, are dizziness, ataxia, somnolence, headache, diplopia, blurred vision, nausea, vomiting, and rash. Lamotrigine accumulates in melanin-rich tissues including the pigmented retina. The long-term effect on vision is unknown.

Skin Conditions. Lamotrigine is significantly associated with development of potentially life-threatening skin conditions, such as toxic epidermal necrolysis and Stevens-Johnson syndrome, in 0.1 percent of adults and 1 to 2 percent of children. These are more likely to appear if the starting dosage is too high, if the dosage is escalated too rapidly, or during concomitant administration of valproic acid. Most cases appear after 2 to 8 weeks of therapy, but cases have been reported in the absence of any of the above risk factors. The character of the rash is not a clue to the severity of the condition. Thus, lamotrigine use should be discontinued immediately upon development of any rash or other sign of hypersensitivity reaction. This may not prevent subsequent development of life-threatening rash or permanent disfiguration.

Topiramate

The most common non-dose-related adverse effects of topiramate used in combination with other antiepileptic drugs include psychomotor slowing, speech and language problems (especially word-finding difficulties), somnolence, dizziness, ataxia, nystagmus, and paresthesias. The most common dose-related adverse effects are fatigue, nervousness, poor concentration, confusion, depression, anorexia, visual problems, mood problems, weight loss, and tremor. Some 1.5 percent of persons taking topiramate develop renal calculi, a rate ten times that associated with placebo. Patients at risk for calculi should be encouraged to drink plenty of fluids.

DRUG–DRUG INTERACTIONS

Gabapentin

Gabapentin has no significant hepatic cytochrome P450 or pharmacodynamic interactions. Antacids containing aluminum hydroxide and magnesium hydroxide (Maalox) decrease gabapentin absorption by 20 percent if administered concurrently but negligibly if administered 2 hours prior to the dose of gabapentin.

Lamotrigine

Lamotrigine has significant, well-characterized drug interactions involving other anticonvulsants. Lamotrigine decreases the plasma concentration of valproic acid by 25 percent; may increase the concentration of the epoxide metabolite of carbamazepine; and may increase the incidence of carbamazepine-induced dizziness, diplopia, ataxia, and blurred vision. It has no effect on phenytoin concentrations. Lamotrigine concentrations are decreased 40 to 50 percent with concomitant administration of carbamazepine, phenytoin, or phenobarbital, whereas lamotrigine concentration is at least doubled with concurrent administration of valproic acid. Sertraline (Zoloft) also increases plasma lamotrigine concentrations, but to a lesser extent than valproic acid does. Combinations of lamotrigine and other anticonvulsants have complex effects on the time of peak plasma concentration and the plasma half-life of lamotrigine.

Topiramate

Topiramate has a few well-characterized drug interactions with other anticonvulsant drugs. Topiramate may increase phenytoin concentrations up to 25 percent and valproic acid concentrations, 11 percent; it does not affect the concentrations of carbamazepine or its epoxide, phenobarbital (Luminal), or primidone (Mysoline). Topiramate concentrations are decreased by 40 to 48 percent with concomitant administration of carbamazepine or phenytoin and by 14 percent with concurrent administration of valproic acid. Topiramate also slightly decreases digoxin (Lanoxin) bioavailability and the efficacy of estrogenic oral contraceptives. Addition of topiramate, a weak inhibitor of carbonic anhydrase, to other inhibitors of carbonic anhydrase, such as acetazolamide (Diamox) or dichlorphenamide (Daranide), may promote development of renal calculi and should be avoided.

LABORATORY INTERFERENCES

Gabapentin can cause false-positive readings with the Ames N-Multistix SG dipstick test for urinary protein. Lamotrigine and topiramate do not interfere with any laboratory tests.

DOSAGE AND CLINICAL GUIDELINES

Gabapentin

Gabapentin is available as 100-, 300-, and 400-mg capsules and as 600- and 800-mg tablets. The starting dose of gabapentin is 300 mg three times a day, and the dose can be rapidly titrated to a maximum of 1,800 mg three times a day over a period of a few days. Efficacy is broadly dose dependent, and most persons achieve satisfactory benefit within the range of 600 to 900 mg three times a day. Rapid advancement of the dosage and high doses are limited by sedation, which is usually mild. Although abrupt discontinuation of gabapentin does not cause withdrawal effects, use of all anticonvulsant drugs should be gradually tapered.

Lamotrigine

Lamotrigine is available as unscored 25-, 100-, 150-, and 200-mg tablets. The major determinant of lamotrigine dosing is minimization of the risk of rash. Lamotrigine should not be taken by anyone under the age of 16 years. Because valproic acid markedly slows the elimination of lamotrigine, concomitant administration of these two drugs necessitates a much slower titration (Table 36.4.24–1). Persons with renal insufficiency should aim for a lower maintenance dosage. Appearance

Table 36.4.24–1
Lamotrigine Dosing (mg/day)

Treatment	Weeks 1–2	Weeks 3–4	Weeks 4–5
Lamotrigine monotherapy	25	50	100–200 (500 maximum)
Lamotrigine plus carbamazepine	50	100	200–500 (700 maximum)
Lamotrigine plus valproate	25 every other day	25	50–200 (200 maximum)

of any type of rash necessitates immediate discontinuation of lamotrigine use. Lamotrigine should usually be discontinued gradually, over 2 weeks, unless a rash emerges, in which case it should be discontinued over 1 to 2 days.

Topiramate

Topiramate is available as unscored 25-, 100-, and 200-mg tablets. To reduce the risk of adverse cognitive and sedating effects, topiramate dosage is titrated gradually over 8 weeks to a maximum of 200 mg twice a day. Higher doses are not associated with increased efficacy. Persons with renal insufficiency should reduce doses by half.

References

Boyd RA, Turck D, Abel RB, Sedman AJ, Bockbrader HN. Effects of age and gender on single-dose pharmacokinetics of gabapentin. *Epilepsia*. 1999;40:474.

Burgess LH. Gabapentin: an alternative mood stabilizer for patients with developmental disabilities? *Mental Health Aspects of Developmental Disabilities*. 2002;5:22.

Ghaemi SN, Goodwin FK. Gabapentin treatment of the non-refractory bipolar spectrum: an open case series. *J Affect Disord*. 2001;65:167.

Hardman JG, Limbird LE, Goodman Gilman A, eds. *Goodman & Gilman's the Pharmacological Basis of Therapeutics*. 10th ed. New York: McGraw-Hill; 2001.

Jensen TS. Anticonvulsants in neuropathic pain: rationale and clinical evidence. *Eur J Pain*. 2002;6(suppl A):61.

Keck PE Jr, Mendlwicz J, Calabrese JR, et al. A review of randomized, controlled clinical trials in acute mania. *J Affect Disord*. 2000;59(suppl 1):S31.

Ketter TA, Malow BA, Flamini RKD, White SR, Post RM, Theodore WH. Felbamate monotherapy has stimulant-like effects in patients with epilepsy. *Epilepsy Res*. 1996;23:129.

Knoll J, Stegman K, Suppes T. Clinical experience using gabapentin adjunctively in patients with a history of mania or hypomania. *J Affect Disord*. 1998;49:229.

Kotler M, Matar M. Lamotrigine in the treatment of resistant bipolar disorder. *Clin Neuropharmacol*. 1998;21:65.

Kushnir MM, Crossett J, Brown PI, Urry FM. Analysis of gabapentin in serum and plasma by solid-phase extraction and gas chromatography-mass spectrometry for therapeutic drug monitoring. *J Anal Toxicol*. 1999;23:6.

Martin R, Kuzniecky R, Ho S, et al. Cognitive effects of topiramate, gabapentin, and lamotrigine in healthy young adults. *Neurology*. 1999;52:321.

Petroff OA, Hyder F, Mattson RH, Rothman DL. Topiramate increases brain GABA, homocarnosine, and pyrrolidinone in patients with epilepsy. *Neurology*. 1999;52:473.

Pollack MH, Matthews J, Scott EL. Gabapentin as a potential treatment for anxiety disorders. *Am J Psychiatry*. 1998;155:992.

Stephen LJ, Maxwell JE, Brodie MJ. Transient hemiparesis with topiramate. *Br Med J*. 1999;318:845.

Sussman N. Other anticonvulsants. In: Sadock BJ, Sadock VA, eds. *Kaplan & Sadock's Comprehensive Textbook of Psychiatry*. 7th ed. Vol 2. Baltimore: Lippincott Williams & Wilkins; 2000:2299.

▲ 36.4.25 Reboxetine

Reboxetine (Vestra) is an effective antidepressant of a novel pharmacological class that selectively inhibits norepinephrine reuptake but has little effect on serotonin reuptake. It is thus the pharmacodynamic mirror image of the selective serotonin reuptake inhibitors (SSRIs), which inhibit the reuptake of serotonin but not of norepinephrine. Reboxetine is used in Europe but is not marketed in the United States.

CHEMISTRY

Reboxetine is structurally related to fluoxetine (Prozac). The structural formula of reboxetine is shown in Figure 36.4.25–1.

Pharmacological Actions

Reboxetine is rapidly absorbed and reaches peak plasma concentrations in 2 hours. Food does not affect the rate of absorption. The half-life is 13 hours, which permits twice-daily dosing. Steady-state concentrations are achieved in 5 days. Reboxetine is extensively metabolized in the liver (primarily via the cytochrome P450 3A4 isoenzyme [CYP 3A4]) and mostly excreted in the urine.

Reboxetine selectively inhibits norepinephrine reuptake, with little inhibition of serotonin or dopamine reuptake. It is highly selective for norepinephrine and lacks direct effects on serotonin metabolism. Reboxetine has a low affinity for muscarinic or cholinergic receptors and does not interact with α_1-, α_2-, or β-adrenergic; serotonergic; dopaminergic; or histaminic receptors.

THERAPEUTIC INDICATIONS

Reboxetine is effective for treatment of acute and chronic depressive disorders, such as major depression and dysthymia. Reboxetine is as effective as imipramine (Tofranil) and may be more effective than fluoxetine for treatment of persons with severe (melancholic) depression. Reboxetine promotes sleep but is not associated with daytime somnolence. Patients show improved energy, interest, and concentration and decreased anxiety. Reboxetine can also produce relatively rapid improvement in symptoms of social phobia. Social impairments, particularly those revolving around negative self-perception and a low level of social activity, appear to respond positively to reboxetine.

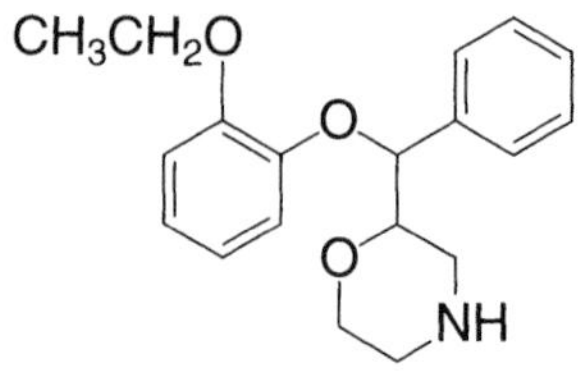

FIGURE 36.4.25–1
Molecular structure of reboxetine.

PRECAUTIONS AND ADVERSE REACTIONS

Reboxetine is overall as well tolerated as SSRIs. The most common adverse effects are urinary hesitancy, headache, constipation, nasal congestion, perspiration, dizziness, dry mouth, decreased libido, and insomnia. Urinary hesitancy may respond to augmentation with doxazosin (Cardura). Hypertension and tachycardia may be of clinical relevance, especially at higher doses. Reboxetine is less likely than SSRIs to cause anxiety or nausea or to inhibit sexual functioning. Limited data suggest that reboxetine, like fluoxetine, may rarely cause the syndrome of inappropriate secretion of antidiuretic hormone (SIADH). In long-term use, persons taking reboxetine experience no more adverse effects than those taking a placebo. Reboxetine at 4 mg twice a day does not produce psychomotor slowing and does not act synergistically with alcohol. Reboxetine is not cardiotoxic and does not increase the risk of seizures.

No data exist on the effects of reboxetine on embryonic and fetal development, and it is not known whether reboxetine is secreted into breast milk. Currently, women who are pregnant or breast-feeding should not take reboxetine.

DRUG–DRUG INTERACTIONS

Reboxetine has few significant drug interactions and does not inhibit hepatic metabolic enzymes. Until further data are available, reboxetine should not be taken concurrently with monoamine oxidase inhibitors (MAOIs).

LABORATORY INTERFERENCE

Reboxetine is not known to interfere with any clinical laboratory tests.

DOSAGE AND CLINICAL GUIDELINES

Reboxetine is available in 4-mg scored tablets. The usual starting dosage is 4 mg twice a day. Most patients do not require an increase in dosage; however, if needed, the dosage may be increased to a total of 10 mg a day in two divided doses after 3 weeks. In elderly persons and persons with severe renal impairment, therapy may be initiated at 2 mg twice a day and increased to a maximum of 6 mg a day in two divided doses after 3 weeks.

Because reboxetine and SSRIs act on nonoverlapping neurotransmitter systems, some clinicians combine them to treat persons whose depression does not respond to either agent alone.

REFERENCES

Baldessarini RJ. Drugs and the treatment of psychiatric disorders: depression and anxiety disorders. In: Hardman JG, Limbird LE, Goodman Gilman A, eds. *Goodman & Gilman's the Pharmacological Basis of Therapeutics*. 10th ed. New York: McGraw-Hill; 2001:447.

De Battista C, Schatzberg AF. Other pharmacological and biological therapies. In: Sadock BJ, Sadock VA, editors. *Kaplan & Sadock's Comprehensive Textbook of Psychiatry*. 7th ed. Vol 2. Baltimore: Lippincott Williams & Wilkins; 2000: 2521.

Kasper S. Managing reboxetine-associated urinary hesitancy in a patient with major depressive disorder: a case study. *Psychopharmacology*. 2002;159:445.

Schueler P, Seibel K, Chevts V, Schaffler K. Analgesic effect of the selective noradrenaline reuptake inhibitor, reboxetine: objective and subjective appraisal. *Nervenarzt*. 2002;73:149.

Versiani M, Cassano G, Perugi G, et al. Reboxetine, a selective norepinephrine reuptake inhibitor, is an effective and well-tolerated treatment for panic disorder. *J Clin Psychiatry*. 2002;63:31.

▲ 36.4.26 Selective Serotonin Reuptake Inhibitors

Selective serotonin reuptake inhibitors (SSRIs) are first-line agents for treatment of depression, obsessive-compulsive disorder (OCD), and panic disorder, as well as many other disorders. Currently, five SSRIs are available. Fluoxetine (Prozac) was introduced in 1988, and it has since become the single most widely prescribed antidepressant in the world. In the subsequent years, sertraline (Zoloft) and paroxetine (Paxil) have become nearly as widely prescribed as fluoxetine. Fluvoxamine (Luvox) has gained its own smaller niche, particularly for treating OCD. Citalopram (Celexa) has been used in Europe since 1989 and was introduced into the United States in 1998, where it has already gained acceptance. Escitalopram, (Lexapro) the *S*(+) enantiomer of citalopram, is being studied in clinical trials.

Although depressive disorders were the initial indications for these drugs, they are effective in a wide range of disorders, including eating disorders, panic disorder, OCD, and borderline personality disorder. These drugs are called SSRIs because they share the pharmacodynamic property of specifically inhibiting serotonin reuptake by presynaptic neurons, with relatively little effect on the reuptake of norepinephrine and almost no effect on the reuptake of dopamine.

Clomipramine (Anafranil) is another serotonin-specific drug sometimes considered in the same category as SSRIs. However, because its structure and adverse effect profile are more similar to those of the tricyclic antidepressant drugs, it is discussed with the tricyclic and tetracyclic drugs (see Section 36.4.33).

CHEMISTRY

The SSRIs share almost no molecular features, which explains why certain individuals may respond to one SSRI but not to another. The structural formulas of citalopram, fluoxetine, fluvoxamine, paroxetine, and sertraline are shown in Figure 36.4.26–1.

PHARMACOLOGICAL ACTIONS

Pharmacokinetics

The major differences among the available SSRIs lie primarily in their pharmacokinetic profiles (Table 36.4.26–1), specifically their half-lives. Fluoxetine has the longest half-life, 2 to 3 days; its active metabolite has a half-life of 7 to 9 days. The half-lives of the other SSRIs are much shorter, about 20 hours, and these SSRIs have no major active metabolites. All SSRIs are well absorbed after oral administration and reach their peak concentrations in 4 to 8 hours. All SSRIs are metabolized in the liver. Paroxetine and fluoxetine are metabolized in the liver by cytochrome P450 (CYP) isoenzyme CYP 2D6, a

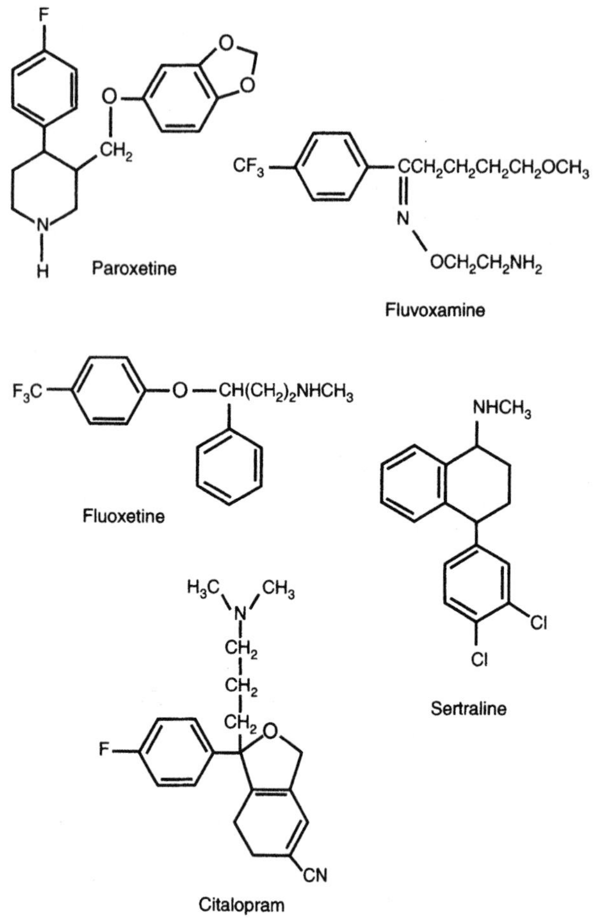

FIGURE 36.4.26–1
Molecular structures of SSRIs.

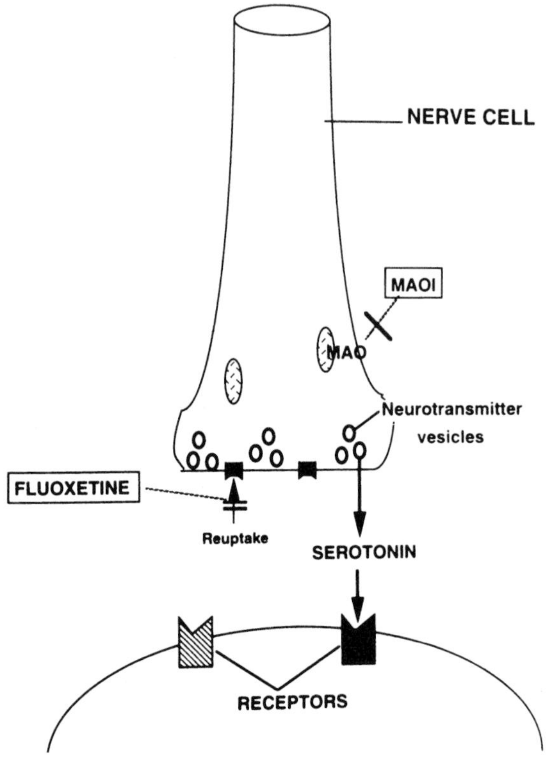

FIGURE 36.4.26–2
SSRIs, such as fluoxetine, block the reuptake of serotonin into the presynaptic nerve terminal. This increases the synaptic concentrations of serotonin, which permits increased activation of receptors, and it also prevents serotonin from being metabolized by MAO. MAOIs also prevent the degradation of serotonin. When MAOIs are used in conjunction with SSRIs, the massive excess of synaptic serotonin may produce a toxic serotonin syndrome. (Reprinted with permission from Hyman SE, Arana GW, Rosenbaum JF. *Handbook of Psychiatric Drug Therapy.* 3rd ed. Boston: Little, Brown; 1996:45.)

specific subtype of the enzyme, which may indicate that clinicians should be careful in the coadministration of other drugs that are also metabolized by CYP 2D6. Fluvoxamine inhibits the CYP 3A4 enzyme, which also metabolizes terfenadine (Seldane) and astemizole (Hismanal) and has led the FDA to recommend that fluvoxamine not be given with these agents. In general, food does not have a large effect on the absorption of SSRIs; in fact, administration of SSRIs with food often reduces the incidence of the nausea and diarrhea commonly associated with SSRI use.

Pharmacodynamics

SSRIs share two common features. First, they have specific activity in the inhibition of serotonin reuptake without effects on norepinephrine and dopamine reuptake (Fig. 36.4.26–2). Clinical efficacy is associated with 70 to 80 percent occupancy of the serotonin transporters. Inhibition of reuptake raises synaptic concentrations of serotonin, which binds to and activates at least 14 distinct receptors (Fig. 36.4.26–3). It is tempting to assume that like the tricyclic antidepressants, the SSRIs have a

Table 36.4.26–1
Pharmacokinetic Profiles of the SSRIs

Drug	Time to Peak Plasma Concentration (h)	Half-Life	Half-Life Metabolite	Time to Steady State (d)	Plasma Protein Binding (%)
Fluoxetine	6–8	4–6 days	4–16 days	28–35	95
Fluvoxamine	3–8	15 h	—	5–7	80
Paroxetine	5–6	21 h	—	5–10	95
Sertraline	4.5–8.5	26 h	62–104 h	5–7	95
Citalopram	4	35 h	3 h	7	80
Escitalopram	4	30 h	—	10	55

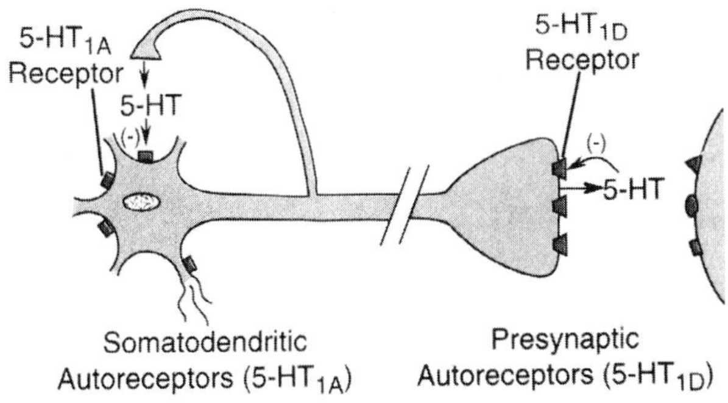

FIGURE 36.4.26–3

Two classes of 5-hydroxytryptamine (5-HT) autoreceptors with differential localizations. Somatodendritic 5-HT_{1A} autoreceptors decrease raphe cell firing when activated by 5-HT released from axon collaterals of the same or adjacent neurons. The receptor subtype of the presynaptic autoreceptor on axon terminals in the forebrain has different pharmacological properties and has been classified as 5-HT_{1D} (in human beings) or 5-HT_{1B} (in rodents). This receptor modulates the release of 5-HT. Postsynaptic 5-HT_1 receptors are also indicated. (Reprinted with permission from Sanders Bush E, Mayer SE. 5-Hydroxytryptamine [serotonin] receptor agonists and antagonists. In: Hardman JG, Limbird LE, Mollinoff PB, Ruddon RW, eds. *Goodman & Gilman's The Pharmacological Basis of Therapeutics*. 9th ed. New York: McGraw-Hill; 1996:253.)

linear dose-response curve and thus higher dosages will yield increased clinical effectiveness. In fact, however, at least 90 percent of clinical response to the SSRIs occurs at the starting doses, and higher doses tend mainly to increase adverse effects, without much additional clinical benefit. In clinical use, sertraline is most commonly raised above its usual starting dosage (50 mg a day, raised to 150 to 200 mg a day), followed by fluoxetine (starting dosage 20 mg a day, raised to 40 to 80 mg a day). Paroxetine is the most likely to be continued at its starting dosage (20 mg a day), and although it may be raised to 30 to 60 mg a day, anticholinergic effects may predominate at higher dosages. Although the available compounds differ in their specific potencies (Table 36.4.26–2), the differences do not result in any meaningful clinical differences.

Second, SSRIs are essentially devoid of agonist and antagonist activities on any neurotransmitter receptor. The lack of antihistaminergic and anti-α_1-adrenergic receptor activities is the pharmacodynamic basis for the low incidence of adverse

Table 36.4.26–2
Approximate Potency of Inhibition of ^{3}H Biogenic Amine Uptake[a]

Compound	Serotonin	K_i (nM) Norepinephrine	Dopamine
Citalopram	4	6,000	>20,000
Fluoxetine	6	1,000	>10,000
Fluvoxamine	25	500	4,200
Paroxetine	1	350	2,000
Sertraline	7	1,400	230

[a]In vitro rat brain tissue preparation. Lower K_i values indicate higher potency. All five compounds are potent inhibitors of serotonin reuptake.

effects with SSRI administration. SSRIs have very mild anticholinergic effects in some patients, usually minimal and far less than the tricyclic and tetracyclic drugs.

THERAPEUTIC INDICATIONS

Depression

Fluoxetine, sertraline, paroxetine, and citalopram are indicated for treatment of depression. SSRIs are first-line agents for depression in the general population, the elderly, the medically ill, and those who are pregnant. SSRIs are as effective as any other class of antidepressants for mild and moderate depression. For severe depression and melancholia, several studies have found that the efficacy of serotonin-norepinephrine reuptake inhibitors, such as venlafaxine (Effexor), mirtazapine (Remeron), or tricyclic drugs, often exceeds that of SSRIs. However, sertraline may be more effective than the other SSRIs for treatment of severe depression with melancholia. It is appropriate to initiate antidepressant therapy with SSRIs for all degrees of depression.

Direct comparison of the benefits of specific SSRIs has not shown any one to be generally superior to the others. However, a given individual can exhibit considerable diversity in response to the various SSRIs. Over 50 percent of persons who respond poorly to one SSRI will respond favorably to another. Thus before shifting to non-SSRI antidepressants, one should try other agents in the SSRI class for persons who did not respond to the first SSRI.

Studies have shown that SSRIs have a similar efficacy but markedly more favorable adverse effect profile than the tricyclic antidepressants. These studies have also shown that some nervousness or agitation, sleep disturbances, gastrointestinal (GI) symptoms, and sexual adverse effects are more common in SSRI-treated patients than in tricyclic-treated patients.

Some clinicians have attempted to select a particular SSRI for a specific person on the basis of the drug's unique adverse-effect profile. For example, since fluoxetine is a more activating and stimulating SSRI, they may consider it a better choice for an abulic person than paroxetine, which is presumed to be a sedating SSRI. These differences, however, usually vary from person to person.

Augmentation Strategies. In depressed persons with a partial response to an SSRI, augmentation strategies have generally not proved superior to simply increasing the SSRI dosage. However, one such drug combination, an SSRI plus bupropion (Wellbutrin), has marked added benefits. The noradrenergic and dopaminergic actions of bupropion dovetail nicely with the serotonergic actions of the SSRIs and pose a low risk of pharmacodynamic interactions. The addition of bupropion can elicit an antidepressant response in up to 70 percent of SSRI nonresponders. Bupropion has the additional advantage of tending to counteract the antiorgasmic adverse effects of SSRIs. Some evidence indicates that lithium (Eskalith), levothyroxine (Synthroid), sympathomimetics, pindolol (Visken), or clonazepam (Klonopin) can also augment the antidepressant effects of SSRIs.

Suicide. SSRIs markedly reduce the risk of suicide. When first introduced, a widely publicized report suggested an association between fluoxetine use and violent acts, including suicide,

but many subsequent reviews have clearly refuted this association. A few patients, however, become especially anxious and agitated when given fluoxetine. The appearance of these symptoms in suicidal persons could conceivably aggravate the seriousness of the suicidal ideation. In addition, suicidal persons may attempt to act out their suicidal thoughts more effectively as they rise out of their depression. Thus, potentially suicidal persons should be closely monitored during the first few weeks they are taking SSRIs.

Antidepressant drugs are an essential component of the current treatment of suicidally depressed persons. A recent assessment of the use of drugs for treatment of persons with a history of prior suicide attempts concluded that a large majority received inadequate dosages of antidepressants.

Depression during Pregnancy and Postpartum. Many studies, including one that followed children into their early school years, have failed to find any perinatal complications, congenital fetal anomalies, decreases in global intelligence quotient (IQ), language delays, or specific behavioral problems attributable to the use of fluoxetine during pregnancy. Emerging data for sertraline, paroxetine, and fluvoxamine suggest that taking these agents during pregnancy also does not increase the risk of major congenital malformations.

Prospective studies have found that the risk of relapse into depression when a newly pregnant mother is taken off SSRI use is severalfold higher than the risk to the fetus of exposure to SSRIs. Since maternal depression is an independent risk factor for fetal morbidity, the clinician may want to continue the SSRI without interruption during pregnancy. SSRIs may produce a self-limited neonatal withdrawal syndrome that consists of jitteriness and mild tachypnea; it begins several hours after birth and may persist for days to a few weeks. The syndrome is rare and does not interfere with feeding.

Postpartum depression (with or without psychotic features) affects a small percentage of mothers. Some clinicians start administering SSRIs if the postpartum blues extend beyond a few weeks or if a woman becomes depressed during pregnancy. The head start afforded by starting SSRI administration during pregnancy if a woman is at risk for postpartum depression also protects the newborn, toward whom the woman may have harmful thoughts after parturition.

Whether or not SSRIs appear in the plasma of babies breastfeeding from mothers who are taking them is controversial. In one study, however, a breast-fed infant was reported to have a plasma concentration of sertraline equal to one half of the maternal concentration; however, this infant showed no abnormal behavior. Citalopram is also excreted in breast milk. Further studies are needed and physicians should be alert to potential problems whenever prescribing drugs to nursing women.

Depression in the Elderly and Medically Ill. Behavioral disturbances in the elderly, particularly those with medical illnesses, require a thorough diagnostic evaluation to rule out delirium or dementia. Diagnosis and treatment of depression significantly reduce the risk of excessive physical morbidity, myocardial infarction, prolonged hospitalization, and death. The ideal antidepressant in this population would have no cognitive, cardiotoxic, anticholinergic, antihistaminergic, or α-adrenergic adverse effects. Of the SSRIs, only paroxetine has some anticholinergic activity, though this is clinically relevant only at higher doses. All SSRIs are useful for elderly, medically frail persons. They are less well tolerated by persons with preexisting GI symptoms.

Chronic Depression. Several studies have shown that nortriptyline (Aventyl, Pamelor) and monthly interpersonal psychotherapy markedly reduced the rate of relapse of depression over a 3-year period. Similar results have been reported with sertraline and would be expected with other SSRIs. The natural history of major depression consists of waxing and waning of symptoms over periods lasting several months. Many studies indicate that discontinuation of SSRI use only 6 months after a depressive episode is associated with a high rate of relapse. It is therefore prudent for a person with chronic depression to continue taking SSRIs for at least 1 year and preferably longer. SSRIs are well tolerated in long-term use.

Depression in Children. Children of depressed adults are at increased risk of depression. Case reports and small series have reported that SSRIs reduce childhood depressive symptoms and may prevent efforts by children and adolescents to self-medicate their sadness with alcohol or illicit drugs. The adverse effect profile of SSRIs in children includes GI symptoms, insomnia, motor restlessness, social disinhibition, and hypomania or mania. It is therefore critical to determine that the child is truly depressed and to initiate SSRI use with small doses. There are anecdotal reports of successful treatment of children with depression together with another disorder (e.g., attention-deficit/hyperactivity disorder [ADHD]) when SSRIs are combined with other psychotropic drugs.

Anxiety Disorders

Obsessive-Compulsive Disorder. Fluvoxamine, paroxetine, sertraline, and fluoxetine are indicated for treatment of OCD in persons over the age of 18. Fluvoxamine and sertraline have also been approved for treatment of pediatric OCD (ages 6 to 17). About 50 percent of persons with OCD begin to show symptoms in childhood or adolescence, and over half of these respond favorably to medication. Beneficial responses can be dramatic. Long-term data support the model of OCD as a genetically determined, lifelong condition that is best treated continuously with drugs and cognitive-behavioral therapy from the onset of symptoms in childhood throughout the life span.

In general, effective SSRI dosages for OCD are higher than those required to treat depression. Fluoxetine is effective for OCD at 20, 40, and 60 mg a day, with a dose-dependent gradation of response. The 60-mg dose is significantly more effective than the 20-mg dose. Response of OCD to sertraline is less clearly dose dependent, with efficacy demonstrated at dosages from 50 to 200 mg a day. Paroxetine is effective at 40 and 60 mg; 20 mg is not better than placebo. Response can be seen in the first few weeks of treatment, but 15 to 20 percent of persons respond only after prolonged treatment.

Comorbid depressive symptoms respond significantly better to SSRIs than to clomipramine, nortriptyline, or amitriptyline (Elavil, Endep). Comorbid tics, as in tic disorders and Tourette's syndrome, respond to the addition of dopamine receptor antagonists or serotonin-dopamine receptor antagonists such as risperidone (Risperdal). In contrast, clozapine

(Clozaril) and buspirone (BuSpar) can worsen tics. There appears to be no role for lithium augmentation for OCD treatment. The combination of SSRIs and clomipramine is potentially hazardous because of the potential for cardiotoxicity.

Panic Disorder. The SSRIs are effective for treatment of panic disorder, with or without agoraphobia. These agents work less rapidly than the benzodiazepines alprazolam (Xanax) or clonazepam, but they are better tolerated in long-term use and do not cause dependence. Citalopram, fluvoxamine, and fluoxetine also may reduce spontaneous or induced panic attacks. Because fluoxetine can initially heighten anxiety symptoms, persons with panic disorder must begin taking small dosages (5 mg a day) and raise the dosage slowly. SSRIs are far superior to benzodiazepines for treatment of panic disorder with comorbid depression.

SSRIs are effective for childhood panic symptoms. If it is well tolerated, SSRI treatment of childhood panic disorder should be continued at least for 1 year. Additional benefit and maintenance of remission would be expected well into adulthood following treatment with medication for at least 1 year.

Social Phobia. Paroxetine is an effective agent in the treatment of social phobia. Paroxetine reduces both symptoms and disability. This response rate was comparable to that seen with the monoamine oxidase inhibitor (MAOI) phenelzine (Nardil), the previous standard treatment. SSRIs are safer to use than MAOIs or benzodiazepines. All SSRIs are probably effective for social phobia.

Posttraumatic Stress Disorder. Pharmacotherapy for posttraumatic stress disorder (PTSD) must target specific symptoms in three clusters: reexperiencing, avoidance, and hyperarousal. For long-term treatment, SSRIs appear to have a broader spectrum of therapeutic effects on specific PTSD symptom clusters than tricyclic antidepressants and MAOIs do. Benzodiazepine augmentation is useful in the acute symptomatic state. SSRIs are associated with marked improvement of both intrusive and avoidant symptoms.

Other Anxiety Disorders. SSRIs may be useful for the treatment of specific phobias, generalized anxiety disorder, and separation anxiety disorder. A thorough, individualized evaluation is the first approach, with particular attention to identifying conditions amenable to drug therapy. Cognitive-behavioral or other psychotherapies can be added for greater efficacy.

Bulimia Nervosa and Other Eating Disorders

Fluoxetine is indicated for treatment of bulimia, which is best done in the context of psychotherapy. Doses of 60 mg a day are significantly more effective than 20 mg a day. In several well-controlled studies, fluoxetine 60 mg a day was superior to placebo in reducing binge eating and induced vomiting. Some experts recommend an initial course of cognitive-behavioral therapy alone. If there is no response in 3 to 6 weeks, then fluoxetine administration is added. The appropriate duration of treatment with fluoxetine and psychotherapy has not been determined.

Fluvoxamine was not effective at a statistically significant level in one double-blind, placebo-controlled trial for inpatients with bulimia.

Anorexia Nervosa. Fluoxetine has been used in inpatient treatment of anorexia nervosa to attempt to control comorbid mood disturbances and obsessive-compulsive symptoms. However, at least two careful studies, one of 7 months and one of 24 months, failed to find that fluoxetine affected the overall outcome and the maintenance of weight. Effective treatments for anorexia include cognitive-behavioral, interpersonal, psychodynamic, and family therapies in addition to a trial with SSRIs.

Obesity. Fluoxetine, in combination with a behavioral program, has only a modest benefit for weight loss. A significant percentage of all persons who take SSRIs, including fluoxetine, lose weight initially, but later they may gain weight. However, all SSRIs may cause initial weight gain.

DEXFENFLURAMINE. In 1997 the serotonin-releasing agent dexfenfluramine (Redux) was withdrawn from the market because it produced heart valve defects. This raised concern about the long-term consequences of SSRI use. Specifically, since both dexfenfluramine and SSRIs increase serotonin activity in some way, would SSRIs cause the same heart-valve defects, primary pulmonary hypertension, and loss of serotonergic fibers caused by dexfenfluramine?

All available evidence indicates that SSRIs *do not* cause the same adverse consequences caused by dexfenfluramine. Dexfenfluramine causes a massive release of serotonin throughout the body, particularly from nerve terminals, far in excess of that required for neurotransmission. The resulting elevated plasma serotonin concentration is thought to contribute to the cardiac and pulmonary damage. In contrast, SSRIs prolong the activity of serotonin released into the synaptic cleft in the course of normal neurotransmission. SSRIs do not damage serotonergic fibers or raise plasma serotonin concentrations.

Clinically, SSRIs have been taken by tens of millions of persons worldwide and have been subjected to intense scrutiny. They have not been associated with an increased risk of heart valve damage or pulmonary hypertension.

Premenstrual Dysphoric Disorder

Premenstrual dysphoric disorder is characterized by debilitating mood and behavioral changes in the week preceding menstruation that interfere with normal functioning. Sertraline, paroxetine, fluoxetine, and fluvoxamine have been reported to reduce the symptoms of premenstrual dysphoric disorder. Controlled trials of fluoxetine and sertraline administered either throughout the cycle or only during the luteal phase (the 2-week period between ovulation and menstruation) showed both schedules to be equally effective.

An additional observation of unclear significance was that fluoxetine was associated with changing the duration of the menstrual period by more than 4 days, either lengthening or shortening. The effects of SSRIs on menstrual cycle length are mostly unknown and may warrant careful monitoring in women of reproductive age.

Premature Ejaculation

The antiorgasmic effects of SSRIs make them useful as a treatment for men with premature ejaculation. SSRIs permit intercourse for a significantly longer period and are reported to improve sexual satisfaction in couples in which the man has

premature ejaculation. Fluoxetine and sertraline have been shown to be effective for this purpose.

Paraphilias

SSRIs reduce obsessive-compulsive behavior in persons with paraphilias. SSRIs diminish unconventional total sexual activity and average time per day spent in unconventional sexual fantasies, urges, and activities. Evidence suggests a greater response for sexual obsessions than for paraphilias. The data support the hypothesis that paraphilias and related disorders are on the impulsive rather than the compulsive end of the obsessive-compulsive spectrum.

Attention-Deficit/Hyperactivity Disorder

Sympathomimetic drugs are the first-line agents for ADHD in children, followed by bupropion, then SSRIs. In adults, sympathomimetics and antidepressants are reported to be equally effective.

Autistic Disorder

Obsessive-compulsive behavior, poor social relatedness, and aggression are prominent autistic features that respond to serotonergic agents such as SSRIs and clomipramine. Sertraline and fluvoxamine have been shown in controlled and open-label trials to mitigate aggressiveness, self-injurious behavior, repetitive behaviors, some degree of language delay, and (rarely) lack of social relatedness in adults with autistic spectrum disorders. These agents were generally well tolerated. In contrast, a controlled trial of fluvoxamine in autistic children found it to be less well tolerated in this group. Fluoxetine has been reported to be effective for features of autism in children, adolescents, and adults.

Chronic Pain Syndromes

Neuropathic Pain. Pain due to nerve damage, typically described as tingling, numb, or burning pain, often responds to SSRIs and other antidepressants. In contrast, nonsteroidal anti-inflammatory agents and opioids have little effect on neuropathic pain. The most common causes of neuropathic pain are diabetes, trauma, herpes zoster, and chronic nerve compression.

Fibromyalgia. Pain syndromes in which the complaints of pain and distress appear excessive for the amount of demonstrable tissue injury are highly associated with comorbid affective disorders. SSRIs and older antidepressants have been reported to reduce subjective complaints of chronic pain.

Headache. Tricyclic drugs have long been used to reduce the frequency and intensity of both migrainous and nonmigrainous headaches. More recently, studies have shown that SSRIs are equally efficacious, with a more favorable adverse effect profile. In addition, persons with chronic or recurrent headaches have a high incidence of comorbid depression and may require antidepressant drug therapy specifically to treat depression.

Concomitant use of SSRIs and drugs in the triptan class (sumatriptan [Imitrex], naratriptan [Amerge], rizatriptan [Maxalt], and zolmitriptan [Zomig]) may (rarely) result in development of a reversible serotonin syndrome (see "Precautions and Adverse Reactions"). However, many persons use triptans while taking a low dose of an SSRI for headache prophylaxis without adverse reaction.

Psychosomatic Conditions

Mood and the propensity for panic regulate the autonomic nervous system and may trigger paroxysmal somatic events. SSRIs modulate the incidence of psychogenic symptoms. Some patients with chronic fatigue syndrome have benefited from long-term use of SSRIs, particularly fluoxetine.

Syncope. Excessive vagal tone may cause bradycardia, hypotension, and syncope. This sequence is called *neurocardiogenic syncope*. Medical causes of syncope to be ruled out include acute dehydration, excessive caffeine intake, overly aggressive treatment of hypertension, parkinsonism and related neurodegenerative disorders, and inadequate fluid and salt intake. Sertraline has been reported to reduce the risk of idiopathic and neurocardiogenic syncope in some persons. Other SSRIs are also effective for neurocardiogenic symptoms such as dizziness.

Respiratory Conditions. The use of psychotropic medications for pulmonary disorders in persons without psychiatric illness has received little attention. Airway reactivity is closely modulated by fear and panic in individuals with asthma or chronic obstructive airway disease (COPD). As many as one fourth of persons with COPD also meet criteria for panic disorder. Increased carbon dioxide (CO_2) sensitivity and dyspnea are cardinal features of both panic attacks and COPD. Persons with COPD often must use daily steroids and bronchodilators, which can have serious adverse effects.

In a small case series of persons with COPD, sertraline use was reported to significantly decrease subjective breathlessness after 3 to 4 weeks of treatment, even in persons who did not meet criteria for diagnosable psychiatric illness. SSRIs are much better tolerated than steroids and bronchodilators. In contrast to the results with SSRIs, results have been mixed or contradictory with buspirone and tricyclic drugs in persons with obstructive airway disease.

PRECAUTIONS AND ADVERSE REACTIONS

Three fourths of persons experience no side effects at low starting dosages of SSRIs, and dosages may be increased relatively rapidly (i.e., on the order of an increase every 1 to 2 weeks) in this group. In the remaining one fourth of patients, most of the adverse effects of the SSRIs appear within the first 1 to 2 weeks, and they generally subside or resolve spontaneously if the drugs are continued at the same dosage. However, 10 to 15 percent of persons will not be able to tolerate even a low dosage of a particular SSRI and may discontinue taking the drug after only a few doses. One approach for such individuals is to fractionate the dosage over a week, with one dose every 2, 3, or 4 days. Some persons may tolerate a different SSRI or another class of antidepressant, such as a tricyclic drug or one of the other newer agents. Some persons appear unable to tolerate even tiny doses of any antidepressant drug.

Because of the unfortunate possibility that adverse effects may reduce compliance, some clinicians administer a low dos-

age for the first 3 to 6 weeks of therapy and then increase it gradually once a therapeutic benefit is seen. Because of the long half-life of the SSRIs, especially fluoxetine, and the even longer time it may take for the full benefit of a particular dose to be appreciated, steep increases in dose are to be avoided. For example, the lowest dosage may provide over 90 percent of the benefit of the highest dosage, if enough time is allowed. On the other hand, adverse effects are much more predictably dose dependent, and increasing the dosage too rapidly may provoke an aversive response in a sensitive person.

Sexual Dysfunction

Sexual inhibition is the most common adverse effect of SSRIs, with an incidence between 50 and 80 percent. All SSRIs appear to be equally likely to cause sexual dysfunction. The most common complaints are inhibited orgasm and decreased libido, which are dose dependent. Unlike most of the other adverse effects of SSRIs, sexual inhibition does not resolve in the first few weeks of use but usually continues as long as the drug is taken.

Treatment for SSRI-induced sexual dysfunction includes decreasing the dosage; switching to bupropion or nefazodone (Serzone), which cause much less sexual dysfunction; addition of bupropion; and addition of yohimbine (Yocon), cyproheptadine (Periactin), or dopamine receptor agonists. The combination of an SSRI with bupropion is particularly effective for both the antidepressant effect and the reduced sexual inhibition.

Recent reports have described successful treatment of SSRI-induced sexual dysfunction with sildenafil (Viagra). It is not immediately obvious why sildenafil, which works in the excitement phase of the sexual cycle, would counteract the orgasm-phase inhibition of SSRIs. Possibly, the positive reinforcement of robust sexual excitement due to sildenafil permits a mental state more conducive to orgasm. Amphetamine (5 mg) has also been reported to reverse anorgasmia.

Gastrointestinal Adverse Effects

Sertraline, fluvoxamine, and citalopram have the highest rates of GI adverse effects, but they are also caused by fluoxetine and paroxetine. The most common GI complaints are nausea, diarrhea, anorexia, vomiting, and dyspepsia. Data indicate that the nausea and loose stools are dose related and transient, resolving usually within a few weeks. Anorexia is most common with fluoxetine, but some persons gain weight while taking fluoxetine. Fluoxetine-induced appetite loss and weight loss begin as soon as the drug is taken and peak at 20 weeks, after which weight often returns to baseline.

Weight Gain. Although most patients initially lose weight, up to one third of persons taking SSRIs will gain weight, sometimes more than 20 pounds. Paroxetine has anticholinergic activity and is the SSRI most often associated with weight gain. In some cases, weight gain results from the drug use itself or the increased appetite associated with better mood.

Headaches

The incidence of headache in SSRI trials was 18 to 20 percent, only 1 percentage point higher than the placebo rate. Fluoxetine is the most likely to cause headache. On the other hand, all SSRIs are effective prophylaxis against both migraine and tension-type headaches in many persons.

Central Nervous System Adverse Effects

Anxiety. Fluoxetine is the SSRI most likely to cause anxiety, particularly in the first few weeks; however, these initial effects usually give way to an overall reduction in anxiety after a few weeks. Increased anxiety is caused considerably less frequently by the other SSRIs, which may be a better choice if sedation is desired, as in mixed anxiety and depressive disorders.

Insomnia and Sedation. The major effect SSRIs exert in the area of insomnia and sedation is improved sleep resulting from treatment of depression and anxiety. However, as many as one fourth of persons taking SSRIs note either trouble sleeping or excessive somnolence. Fluoxetine is the most likely to cause insomnia, for which reason it is often taken in the morning. Sertraline and fluvoxamine are about equally likely to cause insomnia as to cause somnolence, and citalopram and especially paroxetine are more likely to cause somnolence than insomnia. With the latter agents, persons usually report that taking the dose before retiring to bed helps them sleep better, without residual daytime somnolence.

SSRI-induced insomnia can be treated with benzodiazepines, trazodone (Desyrel) (clinicians must explain the risk of priapism), or other sedating medicines. Significant SSRI-induced somnolence often requires switching to use of another SSRI or bupropion.

Vivid Dreams and Nightmares. A minority of persons taking SSRIs report recalling extremely vivid dreams or nightmares. An individual experiencing such dreams with one SSRI may get the same therapeutic benefit without the disturbing dream images by switching to use of another SSRI. This adverse effect often resolves spontaneously over several weeks.

Seizures. Seizures have been reported in 0.1 to 0.2 percent of patients treated with SSRIs, an incidence comparable to that reported with other antidepressants and not significantly different from that with placebo. Seizures are more frequent at the highest doses of SSRIs (e.g., fluoxetine 100 mg a day or higher).

Extrapyramidal Symptoms. Tremor is seen in 5 to 10 percent of persons taking SSRIs, a frequency 2 to 4 times that seen with placebo. SSRIs may rarely cause akathisia, dystonia, tremor, cogwheel rigidity, torticollis, opisthotonos, gait disorders, and bradykinesia. Rare cases of tardive dyskinesia have been reported. Persons with well-controlled Parkinson's disease may experience acute worsening of their motor symptoms when they take SSRIs. Extrapyramidal adverse effects are most closely associated with use of fluoxetine, particularly at dosages in excess of 40 mg per day, but may occur at any time during the course of therapy. Bruxism has also been reported, which responds to small doses of buspirone.

Anticholinergic Effects

Paroxetine has mild anticholinergic activity that causes dry mouth, constipation, and sedation in a dose-dependent fashion. However, the anticholinergic activity of paroxetine is perhaps

only one fifth that of nortriptyline, and most persons taking paroxetine do not experience cholinergic adverse effects. Although not considered to have anticholinergic activity, the other SSRIs are associated with dry mouth in 15 to 20 percent of patients.

Hematological Adverse Effects

SSRIs affect platelet function and may increase bruisability. Paroxetine and fluoxetine are (rarely) associated with development of reversible neutropenia, particularly if administered concurrently with clozapine.

Electrolyte and Glucose Disturbances

SSRIs are (rarely) associated with a decrease in glucose concentrations; therefore, diabetic patients should be carefully monitored. Rare cases of SSRI-associated hyponatremia and the secretion of inappropriate antidiuretic hormone (SIADH) have been seen in patients treated with diuretics who are also water deprived.

Endocrine and Allergic Reactions

SSRIs can increase prolactin levels and cause mammoplasia and galactorrhea in both men and women. Breast changes are reversible upon discontinuation of the drug, but this may take several months to occur.

Various types of rashes appear in about 4 percent of all patients; in a small subset of these patients, the allergic reaction may generalize and involve the pulmonary system, resulting rarely in fibrotic damage and dyspnea. SSRI treatment may have to be discontinued in patients with drug-related rashes.

Galactorrhea

SSRIs may cause reversible galactorrhea, presumably because of interference with regulation of prolactin secretion.

Serotonin Syndrome

Concurrent administration of an SSRI with an MAOI, L-tryptophan, or lithium can raise plasma serotonin concentrations to toxic levels, producing a constellation of symptoms called the *serotonin syndrome* (Table 36.4.26–3). This serious and possibly fatal syndrome of serotonin overstimulation comprises, in order of appearance as the condition worsens, (1) diarrhea; (2) restlessness; (3) extreme agitation, hyperreflexia, and autonomic instability with possible rapid fluctuations in vital signs; (4) myoclonus, seizures, hyperthermia, uncontrollable shivering, and rigidity; and (5) delirium, coma, status epilepticus, cardiovascular collapse, and death.

Treatment of the serotonin syndrome consists of removing the offending agents and promptly instituting comprehensive supportive care with nitroglycerine, cyproheptadine, methysergide (Sansert), cooling blankets, chlorpromazine (Thorazine), dantrolene (Dantrium), benzodiazepines, anticonvulsants, mechanical ventilation, and paralyzing agents.

Table 36.4.26–3
Serotonin Syndrome

Diarrhea
Diaphoresis
Tremor
Ataxia
Myoclonus
Hyperactive reflexes
Disorientation
Uncontrollable shivering
Rigidity
Hyperthermia
Delirium
Coma
Status epilepticus
Cardiovascular collapse
Death

SSRI Withdrawal

The abrupt discontinuation of SSRI use, especially one with a shorter half-life, such as paroxetine or fluvoxamine, has been associated with a withdrawal syndrome that may include dizziness, weakness, nausea, headache, rebound depression, anxiety, insomnia, poor concentration, upper respiratory symptoms, paresthesias, and migrainelike symptoms. It usually does not appear until after at least 6 weeks of treatment and usually resolves spontaneously in 3 weeks. Persons who experienced transient adverse effects in the first weeks of taking an SSRI are more likely to experience discontinuation symptoms.

Fluoxetine is the SSRI least likely to be associated with this syndrome, because the half-life of its metabolite is more than 1 week and it effectively tapers itself. Fluoxetine has therefore been used in some cases to treat the discontinuation syndrome caused by termination of other SSRIs.

DRUG–DRUG INTERACTIONS

SSRIs do not interfere with most other drugs. A serotonin syndrome (Table 36.4.26–3) can develop with concurrent administration of MAOIs, tryptophan, lithium, or other antidepressants that inhibit reuptake of serotonin. Fluoxetine, sertraline, and paroxetine can raise plasma concentrations of tricyclic antidepressants, which can cause clinical toxicity. A number of potential pharmacokinetic interactions have been described on the basis of in vitro analyses of the CYP enzymes (see Table 36.1–2 in Section 36.1), but clinically relevant interactions are rare (Table 36.4.26–4).

The combination of lithium and any serotonergic drug should be used with caution, because of the possibility of precipitating seizures. SSRIs, particularly fluvoxamine, should not be used with clozapine because it raises clozapine concentrations and seizures may result. SSRIs may increase the duration and severity of zolpidem (Ambien)-induced hallucinations.

Fluoxetine

Fluoxetine can be administered with tricyclic drugs, but the clinician should use low dosages of the tricyclic drug. Because it is metabolized by the hepatic CYP 2D6, fluoxetine may interfere with the metabolism of other drugs in the 7 percent of the

Table 36.4.26–4
Interactions of Drugs with the SSRIs Fluoxetine, Fluvoxamine, Paroxetine, and Sertraline

SSRI	Other Drugs	Effect	Clinical Importance
Fluoxetine	Desipramine	Inhibits metabolism	Possible
	Carbamazepine	Inhibits metabolism	Possible
	Diazepam	Inhibits metabolism	Not important
	Haloperidol	Inhibits metabolism	Possible
	Warfarin	No interaction	—
	Tolbutamide	No interaction	—
Fluvoxamine	Antipyrine	Inhibits metabolism	Not important
	Propranolol	Inhibits metabolism	Unlikely
	Tricyclics	Inhibits metabolism	Unlikely
	Warfarin	Inhibits metabolism	Possible
	Atenolol	No interaction	—
	Digoxin	No interaction	—
Paroxetine	Phenytoin	AUC increases by 12%	Possible
	Procyclidine	AUC increases by 39%	Possible
	Cimetidine	Paroxetine AUC increases by 50%	Possible
	Antipyrine	No interaction	—
	Digoxin	No interaction	—
	Propranolol	No interaction	—
	Tranylcypromine	No interaction	Caution with combined treatment
	Warfarin	No interaction	
Sertraline	Antipyrine	Increased clearance	Not important
	Diazepam	13% decreased clearance	Not important
	Tolbutamide	16% decreased clearance	Not important
	Digoxin	No interaction	—
	Lithium	No pharmacokinetic interaction	Caution with combined treatment
	Desipramine	No interaction	—
	Atenolol	No pharmacodynamic interaction	—
Citalopram	Cimetidine	Increased clearance	—
	Digoxin	No interaction	—
	Lithium	No interaction	—

From Warrington SJ. Clinical implications of the pharmacology of serotonin reuptake inhibitors. *Int J Clin Psychopharmacol.* 1962;7(suppl 2):13, with permission.

population that has an inefficient isoform of this enzyme, the so-called poor metabolizers. Fluoxetine may slow the metabolism of carbamazepine (Tegretol), antineoplastic agents, diazepam (Valium), and phenytoin (Dilantin). Possibly significant drug interactions have been described for fluoxetine with benzodiazepines, antipsychotics, and lithium. Fluoxetine has no interactions with warfarin (Coumadin), tolbutamide (Orinase), or chlorothiazide (Diuril).

Sertraline

Sertraline may displace warfarin from plasma proteins and may increase the prothrombin time. The drug interaction data on sertraline support a generally similar profile to that of fluoxetine, although sertraline does not interact as strongly with the CYP 2D6 enzyme.

Paroxetine

Paroxetine carries a higher risk for drug interactions than either fluoxetine or sertraline because it is a more potent inhibitor of the CYP 2D6 enzyme. Cimetidine (Tagamet) can increase the concentration of sertraline and paroxetine, and phenobarbital (Luminal) and phenytoin can decrease the concentration of paroxetine. Because of the potential for interference with the CYP 2D6 enzyme, coadministration of paroxetine with other antidepressants, phenothiazines, and antiarrhythmic drugs should be undertaken with caution. Paroxetine may increase the anticoagulant effect of warfarin. Coadministration of paroxetine and tramadol (Ultram) may precipitate a serotonin syndrome in elderly persons.

Fluvoxamine

Among the SSRIs, fluvoxamine appears to present the most risk for drug–drug interactions. Fluvoxamine is metabolized by the enzyme CYP 3A4, which may be inhibited by ketoconazole (Nizoral). Administration of terfenadine (no longer manufactured) to patients in whom the CYP 3A4 enzyme is inhibited may produce cardiotoxicity, which has been fatal in several cases. Fluvoxamine may increase the half-life of alprazolam, triazolam (Halcion), and diazepam, and it should

not be coadministered with these agents. Fluvoxamine may increase theophylline (Slo-Bid, Theo-Dur) levels threefold and warfarin levels twofold, with important clinical consequences; thus the serum levels of the latter drugs should be closely monitored, and the doses adjusted accordingly. Fluvoxamine raises concentrations and may increase the activity of clozapine, carbamazepine, methadone (Dolophine, Methadose), propranolol (Inderal), and diltiazem (Cardizem). Fluvoxamine has no significant interactions with lorazepam (Ativan) or digoxin (Lanoxin).

Citalopram

Citalopram is not a potent inhibitor of any CYP enzymes. Concurrent administration of cimetidine increases concentrations of citalopram about 40 percent. Citalopram does not significantly affect the metabolism of, nor is its metabolism significantly affected by, digoxin, lithium, warfarin, carbamazepine, or imipramine (Tofranil). Citalopram increases the plasma concentrations of metoprolol (Lopressor) twofold, but this usually has no effect on blood pressure or heart rate. Data on coadministration of citalopram and potent inhibitors of CYP 3A4 or CYP 2D6 are not available.

LABORATORY INTERFERENCES

SSRIs do not interfere with any laboratory tests.

DOSAGE AND CLINICAL GUIDELINES

Fluoxetine

Fluoxetine is available in 10- and 20-mg capsules, in a scored 10-mg tablet, and as a liquid (20 mg/5 mL). There is also a 90-mg long-acting tablet used for once-a-week dosing that delivers the equivalent of once-daily dosing with 20 mg. For depression, the initial dosage is usually 10 or 20 mg orally each day, usually given in the morning, because insomnia is a potential adverse effect of the drug. Fluoxetine should be taken with food to minimize the possible nausea. The long half-lives of the drug and its metabolite contribute to a 4-week period to reach steady-state concentrations. As with all available antidepressants, the antidepressant effects of fluoxetine may be seen in the first weeks, but the clinician should wait until the patient has been taking the drug for 4 to 6 weeks before definitively evaluating its antidepressant activity. Several studies indicate that 20 mg is often as effective as higher doses for treating depression. The maximum dosage recommended by the manufacturer is 80 mg a day, and higher dosages may cause seizures. A reasonable strategy is to maintain a patient with 20 mg a day for 3 weeks. If the patient shows no signs of clinical improvement at that time, an increase to 40 mg may be warranted, although at least one study has found that continuing use of 20 mg a day is as effective as increasing the dosage.

To minimize the early side effects of anxiety and restlessness, some clinicians initiate fluoxetine use at 5 to 10 mg a day, either with the scored 10-mg tablet or by using the liquid preparation. Alternatively, because of the long half-life of fluoxetine, its use can be initiated with an every-other-day administration schedule.

At least 2 weeks should elapse between the discontinuation of MAOI use and the administration of fluoxetine. Fluoxetine use must be discontinued at least 5 weeks before the initiation of MAOI treatment.

The dosage of fluoxetine that is effective in other indications may differ from the 20 mg a day that is generally used for depression. A dosage of 60 mg a day has been reported to be the most effective for the treatment of obsessive-compulsive disorder, obesity, and bulimia nervosa. Fluoxetine is also marketed as Sarafem for premenstrual dysphoric disorder.

Sertraline

Sertraline is available in scored 25-, 50-, and 100-mg tablets. For the initial treatment of depression, sertraline use should be initiated with a dose of 50 mg once daily. To limit the GI effects, some clinicians begin treatment using 25 mg a day, and increase to 50 mg a day after 3 weeks. Patients who do not respond after 1 to 3 weeks may benefit from dosage increases of 50 mg every week up to a maximum of 200 mg, given once daily. Sertraline generally is given in the evening, because it is slightly more likely to cause sedation than insomnia. However, it can be administered in the morning or the evening. Administration after eating may reduce the GI adverse effects. Sertraline concentrate is now available (1 mL = 20 mg).

Guidelines regarding the logic of dosage increases for sertraline are similar to those for fluoxetine. Several studies suggest that maintaining the dosage at 50 mg a day for many weeks may be as beneficial as rapidly increasing the dosage. Nevertheless, many clinicians maintain their patients on doses of 100 to 200 mg a day.

Paroxetine

Paroxetine is available in scored 20-mg tablets, in unscored 10-, 30-, and 40-mg tablets, and as an orange-flavored 10 mg/5 mL oral suspension. It is also available in a controlled-release preparation (CR) in doses of 12.5 and 25 mg. Paroxetine use for the treatment of depression is usually initiated at a dosage of 10 or 20 mg a day. An increase in the dosage should be considered when an adequate response is not seen in 1 to 3 weeks. The CR preparation is also taken once daily. At that point, the clinician can initiate upward dose titration in 10-mg increments at weekly intervals to a maximum of 50 mg a day. Dosages of 60, 70, and 80 mg a day have been tolerated by certain individuals but have not been studied in controlled trials. Persons who experience GI upset may benefit from taking the drug with food. Paroxetine should be taken initially as a single daily dose in the evening; higher dosages may be divided into two doses per day. Patients with melancholic features may require dosages exceeding 20 mg a day. The suggested therapeutic dosage range for elderly patients is 10 to 20 mg a day, as the elderly have been found to have higher mean plasma concentrations than younger adults.

Paroxetine is the SSRI most likely to produce a discontinuation syndrome, because plasma concentrations drop rapidly in the absence of continuous dosing. To limit the development of symptoms of abrupt discontinuation, paroxetine use should be tapered gradually in increments of 10 mg a day each week until the daily dose is 10 mg, at which point its use may be stopped either directly or after an additional increment of 5 mg a day.

Fluvoxamine

Fluvoxamine is available in unscored 25-mg tablets and scored 50- and 100-mg tablets. The effective daily dosage range is 50 to 300 mg a day. A usual starting dosage is 50 mg once a day at bedtime for the first week, after which the dosage can be adjusted according to the adverse effects and clinical response. Dosages above 100 mg a day may be divided into twice-daily dosing. A temporary dosage reduction or slower upward titration may be necessary if nausea develops over the first 2 weeks of therapy. Fluvoxamine can also be administered as a single evening dose to minimize its adverse effects. Tablets should be swallowed with food, without chewing the tablet.

Fluvoxamine is relatively likely to cause a discontinuation syndrome.

Citalopram

Citalopram is available in 20- and 40-mg tablets and as a liquid (10 mg/5 mL). The usual starting dosage is 20 mg a day for the first week, after which it usually is increased to 40 mg a day. Some persons may require 60 mg a day, but there are no controlled trials supporting this dose. For elderly persons or persons with hepatic impairment, 20 mg a day is recommended, with an increase to 40 mg a day only if there is no response to 20 mg a day. Tablets should be taken once daily, in either the morning or the evening, with or without food.

Loss of Efficacy

Some patients report a lessened response to SSRIs with recurrence of depressive symptoms after a period of time (e.g., 4 to 6 months). The exact mechanism is unknown; however, data from an open-label trial suggest that persons with moderate to severe depression who respond rapidly to fluoxetine use are unlikely to experience recurrence of depression while taking fluoxetine, whereas one third of those with milder depression whose initial response to fluoxetine was slower and less robust experienced recurrence of depression within 3 months.

Potential responses to the attenuation of response to SSRIs include increasing or decreasing the dosage; tapering drug use, then rechallenging with the same medication; switching to another SSRI or non-SSRI antidepressant; and augmenting with bupropion, sympathomimetics, buspirone, lithium, anticonvulsants, naltrexone (ReVia), or another non-SSRI antidepressant. A change in response to an SSRI should be explored in psychotherapy, which may reveal the underlying conflicts causing an increase in depressive symptoms.

Escitalopram

Escitalopram (Lexapro) is a new SSRI antidepressant approved by the FDA for the treatment of major depressive disorder. Escitalopram has a broad spectrum of anxiolytic effects as well, as indicated by its efficacy in clinical trials of panic disorder, generalized anxiety disorder, social anxiety disorder, and in relieving the anxiety symptoms associated with depression.

Chemistry. Escitalopram's molecular structure is given in the following figure:

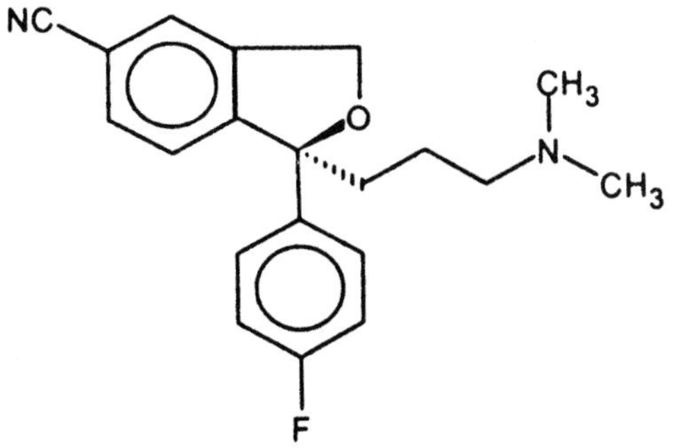

Pharmacological Actions. The kinetics of escitalopram in humans are characterized by rapid absorption with an average time to peak plasma or serum concentrations (T_{max}) of 4 hours, following single or multiple dose administration. Steady-state levels of escitalopram are achieved within 10 days of dosing. In humans, unchanged escitalopram is the predominant compound in plasma. *S*-demethylcitalopram (*S*-DCT) is the principal metabolite. In vitro studies have shown that *S*-DCT is a weak inhibitor of serotonin reuptake and thus does not contribute to clinical efficacy. The pharmacokinetics of escitalopram and *S*-DCT are linear and dose proportional over the therapeutic dosing range. The percentage of escitalopram bound to plasma proteins is in the range of 50 to 59 percent. The terminal half-life of escitalopram is about 27 to 32 hours, consistent with once-daily dosing.

The mechanism of antidepressant action of escitalopram, the *S*(+) enantiomer of racemic citalopram, is presumed to be linked to potentiation of serotonergic activity in the central nervous system resulting from its inhibition of central nervous system neuronal uptake of serotonin (5-HT). Escitalopram is the most selective SSRI with minimal effects on norepinephrine and dopamine neuronal uptake. Escitalopram is at least 100-fold more potent than the *R*-enantiomer with respect to inhibition of 5-HT reuptake and inhibition of 5-HT neuronal firing rate. Escitalopram has no or very low affinity for serotonergic (5-HT_{1-7}) or other receptors including α- and β-adrenergic, dopamine (D_{1-5}), histamine (H_{1-3}), muscarinic (M_{1-5}), and benzodiazepine receptors. Antagonism of muscarinic, histaminergic, and adrenergic receptors has been hypothesized to be associated with various anticholinergic, sedative, and cardiovascular side effects of other psychotropic drugs.

Therapeutic Indications. Escitalopram is expected to be indicated initially for the treatment of major depressive disorder. However, other uses in psychiatry may be expected. Clinical trial results have already demonstrated that escitalopram has a broad spectrum of anxiolytic activity. Several investigators have reported that escitalopram effectively relieves anxiety symptoms associated with major depression.

Precautions and Adverse Events. The most common adverse events are nausea, insomnia, ejaculation disorder, diarrhea, and dry mouth. These events are typical of SSRI treatment; however, the incidence of the individual events compares favorably to the rest of the class in general; of the most common adverse events, only nausea occurs in more than 10 percent of patients.

The 10-mg-a-day dose is particularly well tolerated. Overall, the incidence of adverse events reported by patients treated with 10 mg a day was not statistically different from those treated with placebo. Furthermore, in fixed-dose trials of 8-week duration, the incidence of discontinuation because of adverse events was not different for escitalopram 10 mg a day and placebo.

Drug Interactions. Studies in human liver microsomes have shown that escitalopram is a weak to negligible inhibitor of CYP enzymes, indicating that at therapeutic doses, escitalopram and its metabolites are not very likely to cause clinically significant drug–drug interactions. Furthermore, escitalopram is not highly protein bound.

As with all SSRIs, concomitant use in patients taking monoamine oxidase inhibitors (MAOIs) is contraindicated.

Dosage and Clinical Guidelines. The recommended dose of escitalopram is 10 mg once daily for all patients. Patients not responding to a 10-mg dose may benefit from a dose increase to 20 mg. In a fixed-dose trial, there was a trend toward greater improvement in patients with severe major depressive disorder receiving 20-mg-a-day escitalopram as compared to 10-mg-a-day escitalopram; in this trial, no differences were found in the improvement seen in the 10 mg a day escitalopram group compared to the 40-mg-a-day citalopram group. A minimum of 1 week of treatment at a dose of 10 mg a day is recommended before upward titration to 20 mg a day. Escitalopram should be administered once daily, in the morning or evening, with or without food. Ten mg a day is the recommended dose for most elderly patients and patients with hepatic impairment, with titration to 20 mg a day only for nonresponding patients. No dosage adjustment is necessary for patients with mild or moderate renal impairment. It is generally agreed that acute episodes of depression require several months or longer of sustained pharmacological therapy beyond response to the acute episode. Such long-term, or continuation, treatment with escitalopram has been shown to effectively prevent relapse of depressive episodes. Patients should be periodically reassessed to determine the need for maintenance treatment and the appropriate dose for such treatment.

References

American College of Neuropsychopharmacology Council. Suicidal behavior and psychotropic medication. *Neuropsychopharmacology.* 1993;8:177.

Baldessarini RJ. Drugs and the treatment of psychiatric disorders: depression and anxiety disorders. In: Hardman JG, Limbird LE, Goodman Gilman A, eds. *Goodman & Gilman's the Pharmacological Basis of Therapeutics.* 10th ed. New York: McGraw-Hill; 2001:447.

Black DW, Monahan P, Wesner R. The effect of fluvoxamine, cognitive therapy, and placebo on abnormal personality traits in 44 patients with panic disorder. *J Pers Disord.* 1996;10:185.

Bodkin JA, Lasser RA, Wines JD, Gardner DM, Baldessarini RJ. Combining serotonin reuptake inhibitors and bupropion in partial responders to antidepressant monotherapy. *J Clin Psychiatry.* 1997;58:137.

Bogenschutz MP, Nurnberg HG. Effects of sertraline in the treatment of alcoholism. *Am J Addict.* 1996;5:91.

Burke D, Fanker S. Fluoxetine and the syndrome of inappropriate secretion of antidiuretic hormone (SIADH). *Aust N Z J Psychiatry.* 1996;30:295.

De Wilde J, Spieres R, Mertens C, Bartholome BF, Schotte G, Leyman S. A double-blind, comparative, multicentre study comparing paroxetine with fluoxetine in depressed patients. *Acta Psychiatr Scand.* 1993;87:141.

Den Boer JA, Westenberg HGM. Serotonergic compounds in panic disorder, obsessive-compulsive disorder and anxious depression: a concise review. *Hum Psychopharmacol.* 1995;10(suppl 3):S173.

Golden RN, Nicholas LM. Bupropion. In: Sadock BJ, Sadock VA, eds. *Kaplan & Sadock's Comprehensive Textbook of Psychiatry.* 7th ed. Vol 2. Baltimore: Lippincott Williams & Wilkins; 2000:2324.

Golding M, Kotlyar M, Garbutt JC, et al. Paroxetine modulates psychological and sympathetic responses during public speaking. *J Clin Psychopharmacol.* 2002;22:98.

Hellings JA, Kelley LA, Gabrielli WF, et al. Sertraline response in adults with mental retardation and autistic disorder. *J Clin Psychiatry.* 1996;57:333.

Judd FK, Mijch AM, Cockram A. Fluoxetine treatment of depressed patients with HIV infection. *Aust N Z J Psychiatry.* 1995;29:433.

Kelsey JE, Nemeroff CB. Citalopram. In: Sadock BJ, Sadock VA, eds. *Kaplan & Sadock's Comprehensive Textbook of Psychiatry.* 7th ed. Vol 2. Baltimore: Lippincott Williams & Wilkins; 2000:2435.

Kelsey JE, Nemeroff CB. Fluoxetine. In: Sadock BJ, Sadock VA, eds. *Kaplan & Sadock's Comprehensive Textbook of Psychiatry.* 7th ed. Vol 2. Baltimore: Lippincott Williams & Wilkins; 2000:2438.

Kelsey JE, Nemeroff CB. Fluvoxamine. In: Sadock BJ, Sadock VA, eds. *Kaplan & Sadock's Comprehensive Textbook of Psychiatry.* 7th ed. Vol 2. Baltimore: Lippincott Williams & Wilkins; 2000:2444.

Kelsey JE, Nemeroff CB. Paroxetine. In: Sadock BJ, Sadock VA, eds. *Kaplan & Sadock's Comprehensive Textbook of Psychiatry.* 7th ed. Vol 2. Baltimore: Lippincott Williams & Wilkins; 2000:2447.

Kelsey JE, Nemeroff CB. Sertraline. In: Sadock BJ, Sadock VA, eds. *Kaplan & Sadock's Comprehensive Textbook of Psychiatry.* 7th ed. Vol 2. Baltimore: Lippincott Williams & Wilkins; 2000:2451.

Kosten TR, McCance E. A review of pharmacotherapies for substance abuse. *Am J Addict.* 1996;5:58.

Kroenke K, West SL, Gilsenan A, et al. Similar effectiveness of paroxetine, fluoxetine, and sertraline in primary care: a randomized trial. *JAMA.* 2001;286:2947.

Laird LK, Lydiard RB, Morton WA, et al. Cardiovascular effects of imipramine, fluvoxamine, and placebo in depressed outpatients. *J Clin Psychiatry.* 1993;54:224.

Lejoyeux M. Use of serotonin (5-hydroxytryptamine) reuptake inhibitors in the treatment of alcoholism. *Alcohol Alcohol.* 1996;31(suppl 1):69.

Liebowitz MR, Stein MB, Tancer M, Carpenter D, Oakes R, Pitts CD. A randomized, double-blind, fixed-dose comparison of paroxetine and placebo in treatment of generalized social anxiety disorder. *J Clin Psychiatry.* 2002;63:66.

Meijer WEE, Heerdink ER, Egberts ACG, Leufkens HGM, Waldinger MD. Is sexual dysfunctioning a reason for discontinuation in users of selective serotonin reuptake inhibitors? *J Clin Psychopharmacol.* 2002;22:96.

Patel RM, Grossberg GT. The use of selective serotonin reuptake inhibitors in geriatric depression: a review of the literature. *Rev Clin Gerontol.* 1995;5:442.

Perlis RH, Fava M, Nierenberg AA, et al. Strategies for treatment of SSRI-associated sexual dysfunction: a survey of an academic psychopharmacology practice. *Harv Rev Psychiatry.* 2002;10:109.

Rapaport MH, Endicott J, Clary CM. Posttraumatic stress disorder and quality of life: results across 64 weeks of sertraline treatment. *J Clin Psychiatry.* 2002;63:59.

Reist C, Helmeste D, Albers L, et al. Serotonin indices and impulsivity in normal volunteers. *Psychiatry Res.* 1996;60:177.

Sandor P. Clinical management of Tourette's syndrome and associated disorders. *Can J Psychiatry.* 1995;40:577.

Schatzberg AF. Fluoxetine in the treatment of comorbid anxiety and depression. *J Clin Psychiatry.* 1995;13:2.

Sonawalla SB. Citalopram in the maintenance treatment of major depressive disorder. *J Clin Psychiatry.* 2001;62:993.

Song F, Freemantle N, Sheldon TA, et al. Selective serotonin reuptake inhibitors: meta-analysis of efficacy and acceptability. *BMJ.* 1993;306:683.

Tam EM, Lam RW, Levitt AJ. Treatment of seasonal affective disorder: a review. *Can J Psychiatry.* 1995;40:457.

Varia IM, Cloutier CA, Doraiswamy PM. Treatment of anxiety disorder with citalopram. *Prog Neuropsychopharmacol Biol Psychiatry.* 2002;26:205.

▲ 36.4.27 Serotonin-Dopamine Antagonists: Atypical Antipsychotics

The serotonin-dopamine antagonists (SDAs) are also referred to as *novel* or *atypical antipsychotic drugs* and include risperidone (Risperdal), olanzapine (Zyprexa), quetiapine (Seroquel), clozapine (Clozaril), and ziprasidone (Geodon). These drugs improve two classes of disabilities typical of schizophrenia: (1) positive symptoms such as hallucinations, delusions, disordered thoughts, and agitation and (2) negative symptoms such as withdrawal, flat affect, anhedonia, poverty of speech, catatonia, and cognitive impairment. SDAs carry a smaller risk of extrapyramidal symptoms than the

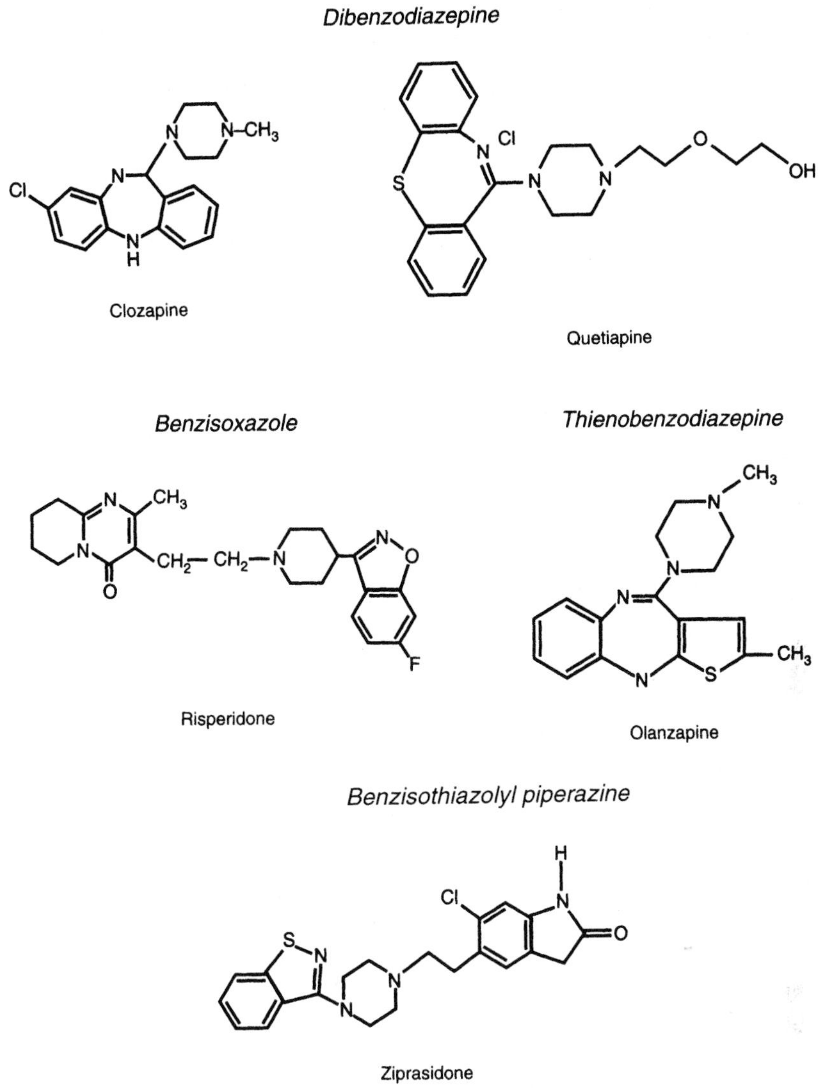

FIGURE 36.4.27–1
Molecular structures of serotonin-dopamine antagonists.

dopamine receptor antagonists, which eliminates the need for concurrent anticholinergic drug use with their annoying adverse effects.

SDAs are also effective for the treatment of mood disorders with psychotic or manic features and for behavioral disturbances associated with dementia. Olanzapine is indicated for short-term treatment of acute manic episodes associated with bipolar I disorders. All these agents are considered first-line drugs except clozapine, which causes adverse hematological effects that require weekly blood sampling.

A new atypical antipsychotic, aripiprazole, with a different mechanism of action, partial dopamine agonism, has an efficacy and safety profile very similar to the SDA's.

CHEMISTRY

Clozapine is a dibenzodiazepine. Risperidone is a benzisoxazole. Olanzapine is a thienobenzodiazepine derivative of clozapine. Quetiapine is a dibenzothiazepine structurally related to clozapine. Ziprasidone is a benzisothiazolyl piperazine. The molecular structures of these compounds are shown in Figure 36.4.27–1.

PHARMACOLOGICAL ACTIONS

These drugs are called *serotonin-dopamine antagonists,* because they block not only dopamine receptors, as do the typical antipsychotic drugs (dopamine receptor antagonists), but also serotonin receptors. These drugs possess a diverse combination of receptor affinities, and the relative contribution of each receptor interaction to the clinical effects is unknown. Dosage changes for special populations are shown in Table 36.4.27–1.

Risperidone

Between 70 and 85 percent of risperidone is absorbed from the gastrointestinal (GI) tract, and it undergoes extensive first-pass

Table 36.4.27–1
Changes in Pharmacokinetics: Special Populations

Drug	Elderly	Renal Impairment	Hepatic Impairment	Ethnic
Clozapine	↓↓ dosage	No Δ dosage	↓ dosage	↓ dosage women
Risperidone	↓↓ dosage	↓ dosage	↓ dosage	↓ dosage Asians?
Olanzapine	↓ dosage (35%)	No Δ dosage	No Δ dosage (preliminary)	↓ dosage women ↓ dosage Asians?
Sertindole	No Δ dosage PD concerns	No Δ dosage	↓ dosage (1/2)	↓ dosage women
Quetiapine	No PK Δ[a] ↓ dosage secondary PD	No Δ dosage	Slight ↓ dosage	No Δ dosage
Ziprasidone	No Δ dosage	No Δ dosage	No Δ dosage	?

Abbreviations: PD, pharmacodynamic; PK, pharmacokinetic; Δ, change in.
[a]Increased adverse reactions (α_1-blockade).
From Ereshásky L. Pharmacokinetics and drug interactions: update for new antipsychotics. *J Clin Psychiatry.* 1996;7(suppl):12, with permission.

hepatic metabolism to 9-hydroxyrisperidone, a metabolite with comparable biological activity. The combined half-life of risperidone and 9-hydroxyrisperidone averages 20 hours, so that it is effective in once-daily dosing. Risperidone is an antagonist of the serotonin 5-HT_{2A}, dopamine D_2, α_1- and α_2-adrenergic, and histamine H_1 receptors. It has a low affinity for β-adrenergic and muscarinic cholinergic receptors. Although it is as potent an antagonist of D_2 receptors as haloperidol (Haldol) is, risperidone is much less likely than haloperidol to cause extrapyramidal symptoms in humans.

Olanzapine

Approximately 85 percent of olanzapine is absorbed from the GI tract, and about 40 percent of the dosage is inactivated by first-pass hepatic metabolism. Peak concentrations are achieved within 6 hours, and the half-life averages 30 hours. Therefore, it is effective in once-daily dosing. Olanzapine is an effective antagonist of the 5-HT_{2A}; D_1, D_2, and D_4; α_1; muscarinic M_1 through M_5; and H_1 receptors.

Quetiapine

Quetiapine is rapidly absorbed from the GI tract. Peak plasma concentrations are reached in 1 to 2 hours. Steady-state half-life is about 6 hours, and optimal dosing is two or three times per day. Quetiapine is an antagonist of 5-HT_2 and 5-HT_6, D_1 and D_2, H_1, and α_1 and α_2 receptors. It does not block muscarinic or benzodiazepine receptors. The receptor antagonism for quetiapine is generally lower than that for other antipsychotic drugs, and it is not associated with extrapyramidal symptoms.

Clozapine

Clozapine is rapidly absorbed from the GI tract, and peak plasma levels are reached in 1 to 4 hours. The steady-state half-life of 10 to 16 hours is usually reached in 3 to 4 days if twice-daily dosing is used. The two major metabolites have minimal pharmacological activity. Clozapine is an antagonist of 5-HT_{2A}; D_1, D_3, and D_4; and α (especially α_1) receptors. It has relatively low potency as a D_2-receptor antagonist. Data from positron emission tomography (PET) scanning show that 10 mg of haloperidol produces 80 percent occupancy of striatal D_2 receptors, whereas clinically effective dosages of clozapine occupy only 40 to 50 percent of striatal D_2 receptors. This difference in D_2 receptor occupancy is probably why clozapine does not cause extrapyramidal adverse effects.

Ziprasidone

Peak plasma concentrations of ziprasidone are reached in 2 to 6 hours. The steady-state half-life of 5 to 10 hours is reached by the third day, and twice-daily dosing is necessary. Ziprasidone is an antagonist of 5-HT_{1D}, 5-HT_{2A}, and 5-HT_{2C}; D_2, D_3, and D_4; α_1; and H_1 receptors. It has very low affinity for D_1, M_1, and α_2-receptors. Ziprasidone also has agonist activity at the serotonin 5-HT_{1A} receptors and is a serotonin reuptake inhibitor and a norepinephrine reuptake inhibitor. This suggests that it could possess antidepressant effects.

Aripiprazole

Aripiprazole is not a serotonin-dopamine antagonist; rather, it is a partial agonist at the dopamine D_2 receptor.

THERAPEUTIC INDICATIONS

Psychotic Disorders

SDAs are effective for treating acute and chronic psychoses such as schizophrenia and schizoaffective disorders, in both adults and adolescents. They are also effective for treating psychotic depression and for psychosis secondary to head trauma, dementia, or treatment drugs. SDAs are as good as, or better than, typical antipsychotics (dopamine receptor antagonists) for the treatment of positive symptoms in schizophrenia and clearly superior to dopamine receptor antagonists for the treatment of negative symptoms. Compared with persons treated with dopamine receptor antagonists, those treated with SDAs have fewer relapses and require less frequent hospitalization, fewer emergency room visits, less phone contact with mental health professionals, and less treatment in day programs.

Because clozapine has potentially life-threatening adverse effects, it is now appropriate only for patients with schizophrenia resistant to all other antipsychotics, and it retains a therapeutic niche for patients who are treatment resistant. Other indications for clozapine include treatment of persons with severe tardive dyskinesia and those with a low threshold for extrapyramidal symptoms. Persons who tolerate clozapine have done well on long-term therapy. The effectiveness of clozapine may be increased by augmentation with risperidone, which raises clozapine concentrations and sometimes results in dramatic clinical improvement.

The studies done for the regulatory approval of aripiprazole were done with patients with schizophrenia and schizoaffective disorder. Studies using aripiprazole in other disorders are under way.

Mood Disorders

SDAs are useful for the initial control of agitation during a manic episode, but they are less effective for long-term control of bipolar disorders than lithium (Eskalith), valproate (Depakene), and carbamazepine (Tegretol). Olanzapine is Food and Drug Administration (FDA)–approved for treatment of acute mania at dosages of 10 or 15 mg a day. In preclinical trials, olanzapine was an effective treatment for manic persons with or without psychotic features. Olanzapine and risperidone can be used to augment antidepressants in the short-term management of major depression with psychotic features. SDAs are effective in the treatment of schizoaffective disorder, although risperidone has been reported to precipitate mania in persons with schizoaffective disorder. Olanzapine and clozapine augmentation can improve up to two thirds of persons with refractory bipolar disorder, and risperidone has been used to reduce mood swings in persons with rapid-cycling bipolar disorder. Olanzapine, but not clozapine, is effective for treatment of depressive symptoms in persons with bipolar disorders.

Other Indications

SDAs are effective for treatment of acquired immune deficiency syndrome (AIDS) dementia, autistic spectrum disorders, dementia-related psychosis, Tourette's disorder, Huntington's disease, and Lesch-Nyhan syndrome. Risperidone and olanzapine have been used to control aggression and self-injury in children. These drugs have also been coadministered with sympathomimetics, such as methylphenidate (Ritalin) or dextroamphetamine (Dexedrine, Dextrostat), to children with attention-deficit/hyperactivity disorder who are comorbid for either opposition-defiant disorder or conduct disorder. SDAs, especially olanzapine, quetiapine, and clozapine, are useful in persons who have severe tardive dyskinesia. SDA treatment suppresses the abnormal movements of tardive dyskinesia but does not appear to worsen the movement disorder.

Treatment with olanzapine and ziprasidone decreases depressive symptoms in persons with schizophrenia to a greater extent than haloperidol does. In depressed persons without psychotic features who respond only partially to antidepressants, augmentation with olanzapine can improve treatment efficacy.

Treatment with SDAs decreases the risk of suicide and water intoxication in patients with schizophrenia. Patients with treatment-resistant obsessive-compulsive disorder have responded to SDAs; however, a few persons treated with SDAs have noted treatment-emergent symptoms of obsessive-compulsive disorder. Some patients with borderline personality disorder may improve with SDAs.

ADVERSE EFFECTS

The adverse reactions reported with SDAs are listed in Table 36.4.27–2.

Risperidone

There is evidence that risperidone-induced extrapyramidal effects may be dosage dependent. Weight gain, anxiety, nausea and vomiting, rhinitis, erectile dysfunction, orgasmic dysfunction, and increased pigmentation are associated with risperidone use. The most common drug-related reasons for discontinuation of risperidone use are extrapyramidal symptoms, dizziness, hyperkinesia, somnolence, and nausea.

Olanzapine

Somnolence, dry mouth, dizziness, constipation, dyspepsia, increased appetite, and tremor are associated with olanzapine use. Olanzapine is somewhat more likely than risperidone to cause weight gain. A small number of patients (2 percent) may need to discontinue use of the drug because of transaminase elevation.

Quetiapine

The most common adverse effects of quetiapine are somnolence, postural hypotension, and dizziness, which are usually transient and are best managed with initial gradual upward titration of the dosage. Quetiapine appears not to cause extrapyramidal symptoms. Quetiapine is associated with modest transient weight gain in 23 percent of persons, small increases in heart rate, constipation, and a transient rise in liver transaminases.

Clozapine

The most common drug-related adverse effects are sedation, dizziness, syncope, tachycardia, hypotension, electrocardiogram (ECG) changes, nausea, and vomiting. Leukopenia, granulocytopenia, agranulocytosis, and fever occur in about 1 percent of patients. Other common adverse effects include fatigue, sialorrhea, weight gain, various GI symptoms (most commonly, constipation), anticholinergic effects, and subjective muscle weakness. Changes in insulin metabolism have been reported. The risk of seizures is about 4 percent in patients taking dosages above 600 mg a day. Myocarditis and cardiomyopathy are also adverse events reported.

Ziprasidone

In early clinical trials involving persons with schizophrenia or schizoaffective disorder, no adverse effects were reported more frequently by persons taking ziprasidone than by those taking

Table 36.4.27–2
Adverse Effects of SDAs

Item	Conventional Antipsychotics[a]	Clozapine	Risperidone	Olanzapine	Quetiapine	Ziprasidone
Central nervous system						
Extrapyramidal symptoms (EPS)	0 to ++	0	0[b,c]	0[b] to +[c]	0[b]	0[b]
Tardive dyskinesia	+++	0	(+)	+	?	?
Seizures	0 to +	+++	0	+	0	0
Sedation, somnolence	+ to +++	+++	+[d]	+	+[d]	+[d]
Other						
Neuroleptic malignant syndrome	+	+	+	+	?	?
Orthostatic hypotension	+ to +++	0 to +++	+	+[d]	0	0
QT_c	0 to ++	0	0 to +	0	0 to +	+
Liver transaminase increase	0 to ++	0 to +	0 to +	0 to +	0 to +	0 to +
Anticholinergic adverse effects	0 to +++	+++	0	+	0	0
Agranulocytosis	0	+++	0	0	0	0
Prolactin increase	++ to +++	0	+ to ++	0	0[d]	0[e]
Decreased ejaculatory volume	0 to +	0	0	0	0	0
Weight gain	0 to ++	+++	+	++	+	0
Nasal congestion	0 to +	0 to +	0 to +	0 to +	0 to +	0

[a]0, None or not significantly different from placebo; +, mild; ++, moderate; +++, marked; ?, insufficient data.
[b]Not significantly different from placebo-treated group, which may have received conventional antipsychotic before entering the study and could have EPS carried forward into the initial weeks of the investigation.
[c]Dosage-related EPS above 6 mg/day.
[d]Transient.
[e]Dosage-related increases within the normal range.
Modified from Casey DE. Side effect profiles of new antipsychotic agents. *J Clin Psychiatry.* 1996;57(suppl):40, with permission.

placebo. The most common adverse effects in patients taking ziprasidone were somnolence, headache, dizziness, nausea, and lightheadedness. Ziprasidone has almost no significant effects outside the central nervous system (CNS) and is associated with almost no weight gain; however, QT prolongation is potentially fatal in patients with a history of cardiac arrhythmia.

Aripiprazole

Because aripiprazole is a new typical antipsychotic, its adverse effect profile is not well known. Based on limited data, aripiprazole appears to be associated with low risk of extrapyramidal symptoms, low sedation, minimal weight gain, no QT prolongation, and no prolactin elevation. Additional information about adverse effects is needed.

Neuroleptic Malignant Syndrome

Although rare with use of SDAs, all antipsychotic drugs may cause neuroleptic malignant syndrome. This syndrome consists of muscular rigidity, fever, dystonia, akinesia, mutism, shifting between obtundation and agitation, diaphoresis, dysphagia, tremor, incontinence, labile blood pressure, leukocytosis, and elevated creatine phosphokinase (CPK). Neuroleptic malignant syndrome has been reported with clozapine, risperidone, and olanzapine and must be considered in the differential diagnosis of fever in a clozapine-treated person. Clozapine may be associated with reversible elevations of serum CPK concentrations that do not involve rhabdomyolysis and do not lead to neuroleptic malignant syndrome. Neuroleptic malignant syndrome is more likely to occur if clozapine is given together with lithium.

Tardive Dyskinesia

SDAs are much less likely than dopamine receptor antagonists to be associated with treatment-emergent tardive dyskinesias. Moreover, SDAs ameliorate the symptoms of tardive dyskinesias and are especially indicated for psychotic persons with preexisting tardive dyskinesias. Tardive dyskinesias can occur in persons treated with dopamine receptor antagonists for as little as 1 month. Therefore, use of dopamine receptor antagonists for long-term maintenance of patients with psychosis has become a questionable practice. SDAs should replace dopamine receptor antagonists for long-term treatment.

Although rare, treatment-emergent cases of tardive dyskinesia have been associated with risperidone, to a lesser degree with olanzapine, and very rarely with clozapine and quetiapine. Many of these persons were previously exposed to dopamine receptor antagonists, though some only briefly. Clozapine is the drug of choice for persons with severe tardive dyskinesia. A reduction in symptoms is usually seen in 1 to 4 weeks.

Orthostatic Hypotension, Syncope, and Tachycardia

All SDAs, but most frequently quetiapine, are associated with orthostatic hypotension, particularly if dosages are escalated rapidly. SDAs should be used with caution in persons with hypotension, diabetes mellitus, or myocardial infarction and those who are taking antihypertensive medications. The risk of hypotension and syncope can be minimized with gradual upward titration of dosages. To determine whether the dosage can be increased, a comparison should be made between blood

pressure supine and standing after 10 deep knee bends. Evidence of orthostatic hypotension includes a mean arterial pressure drop of 20 mm Hg or more, a pulse rate increase of 20 beats per minute or more, and/or subjective dizziness. Dosage escalation should be delayed until any signs of orthostatic hypotension resolve. The tachycardia, which is due to vagal inhibition, can be treated with peripherally acting β-adrenergic antagonists, such as atenolol (Tenormin), although this treatment may aggravate the hypotensive effects of SDAs. Additional treatment measures for hypotension include avoidance of caffeine and alcohol, increased sodium intake, adequate fluid intake, support stockings, and (rarely) fludrocortisone (Florinef) treatment. SDAs should not be used with other drugs that may cause orthostatic hypotension, such as benzodiazepines or antihypertensives. Clozapine is associated with paradoxical hypertension in 4 percent of persons.

Cardiac Changes

Potential ECG changes include nonspecific ST-T wave changes, T wave flattening, or T wave inversions, although these changes are usually not clinically significant. Olanzapine, quetiapine, ziprasidone, and clozapine are not associated with significant changes in QT or PR intervals; however, ziprasidone may have clinically significant QT prolongation in susceptible patients. Because of the variety of cardiac changes associated with SDA use, the drugs should be used with caution by persons with preexisting cardiac disease or in combination with drugs that prolong the QT interval significantly, such as quinidine (Cardioquin).

Agranulocytosis

Agranulocytosis is a potentially fatal condition defined as a decrease in the absolute neutrophil count (ANC) to less than 500/mm^3 in association with infectious disease. With recommended laboratory monitoring, it occurs in 0.38 percent of all persons treated with clozapine, compared with an incidence of 0.04 to 0.05 percent in persons treated with standard antipsychotics. Careful clinical monitoring of the hematological status of clozapine-treated persons can prevent fatalities by early recognition of hematological problems and subsequent cessation of clozapine use. Agranulocytosis can appear precipitously or gradually and most often develops in the first 6 months of treatment. Increased age and female sex are additional risk factors. Clozapine is also associated with the development of benign cases of leukocytosis (0.6 percent of persons), leukopenia (3 percent), eosinophilia (1 percent), and elevated erythrocyte sedimentation rates. Clozapine should not be used by persons with white blood cell (WBC) counts below 3,500, a history of a bone marrow disorder, or a history of clozapine-induced agranulocytosis. A case report describes successful treatment of clozapine-induced neutropenia with granulocyte colony-stimulating factor (G-CSF) without discontinuation of clozapine, which was the only antipsychotic drug to which the person responded. This technique requires further study before it can be recommended.

Seizures

The risk of seizures is less than 1 percent with risperidone, olanzapine, quetiapine, and ziprasidone. About 5 percent of persons taking more than 600 mg a day of clozapine, 3 to 4 percent of persons taking 300 to 600 mg a day, and 1 to 2 percent of persons taking less than 300 mg a day have clozapine-associated seizures. If seizures develop, clozapine use should be temporarily stopped. Anticonvulsant treatment can be initiated, and clozapine use can be resumed at about 50 percent of the previous dosage, then gradually raised again. Carbamazepine and phenytoin (Dilantin) should not be used in combination with clozapine because of their association with agranulocytosis. The plasma concentrations of other anticonvulsants must be monitored carefully because of the possibility of pharmacokinetic interactions with clozapine. Persons with preexisting seizure disorders or histories of significant head trauma are at greater risk for seizures while taking clozapine.

Hyperprolactinemia

The D_2 receptor antagonist activity of antipsychotic drugs causes a rise in prolactin levels for the duration of the therapy. Of the SDAs, risperidone is most strongly associated with hyperprolactinemia, followed by olanzapine and ziprasidone. Clozapine and quetiapine do not increase prolactin secretion. Hyperprolactinemia can cause galactorrhea, amenorrhea, gynecomastia, and impotence. Aripiprazole does not increase prolactin release.

Cognitive and Motor Impairment

All currently available SDAs cause sedation. Therefore, persons who take SDAs should exercise caution when driving or operating dangerous machinery. This adverse effect may be minimized by giving most of the dosage before sleep. Somnolence can occur in 30 percent of persons on the usual maintenance dosage of olanzapine (10 mg a day); dizziness and akathisia have also been reported in persons taking olanzapine. Somnolence due to quetiapine occurs in 18 percent of patients. Somnolence due to risperidone is dosage dependent; it is relatively infrequent at dosages below 6 mg a day, but it may occur in over 40 percent of persons taking 16 mg a day. Clozapine is associated with sedation in 40 percent of persons taking therapeutic dosages.

Body Temperature Regulation

Because SDAs alter the ability of the body to regulate temperature, persons taking them should avoid strenuous exercise, exposure to extreme heat, concomitant administration of anticholinergic drugs, and dehydration. With clozapine, fevers 1 to 2°F above normal may develop, usually during the first month of treatment, often causing concern about the development of an infection because of agranulocytosis. Clozapine should be withheld in these cases; if the WBC count is normal, clozapine use can be reinstituted slowly at a low dosage.

Extrapyramidal Symptoms

All SDAs are much less likely than dopamine receptor antagonists to produce extrapyramidal symptoms, such as acute dystonia, parkinsonism, rabbit syndrome, and akinesia. Risperidone induces extrapyramidal symptoms in a dose-dependent manner

at dosages above 6 mg a day. Olanzapine is occasionally associated with extrapyramidal symptoms at dosages above 15 mg a day. The ziprasidone-aripiprazole–associated risk of extrapyramidal symptoms is low. Quetiapine and clozapine do not increase the risk of extrapyramidal symptoms. There are reports that risperidone, olanzapine, quetiapine, ziprasidone, aripiprazole, and clozapine may be associated with akathisia.

Weight Gain

Risperidone, olanzapine, quetiapine, and clozapine are associated with weight gain, which can be controlled with strict adherence to a planned diet. Clozapine and olanzapine in particular may be associated with a gain of as much as 30 to 50 pounds with short-term use. Significant weight gain may induce or exacerbate diabetes mellitus, and olanzapine and clozapine should therefore be used with caution by persons who have, or are at risk for, diabetes. Ziprasidone and quetiapine appear not to cause significant weight gain. One approach to management of weight gain associated with use of clozapine or olanzapine is to switch over gradually to ziprasidone, quetiapine, or risperidone.

Anticholinergic Symptoms

Clozapine and, to a lesser extent, olanzapine, are associated with anticholinergic symptoms, such as dry mouth, blurred vision, constipation, and urinary retention. This may necessitate transient addition of an anticholinergic agent when switching from clozapine or olanzapine to a less anticholinergic antipsychotic drug.

Sialorrhea

Clozapine can cause sialorrhea, which may place the patient at risk for aspiration of saliva and gagging, particularly during sleep. Clozapine is thought to produce sialorrhea by inhibiting swallowing rather than by increasing salivation. Treatment options include the clonidine patch, 0.1 or 0.2 mg each week, or amitriptyline (Elavil, Endep) or clomipramine (Anafranil), 75 to 100 mg, before sleep. Anticholinergic drugs, such as atropine, should not be used because they can exacerbate the anticholinergic activity of clozapine. Clozapine-induced sialorrhea may resolve spontaneously in a small number of patients after several months.

Obsessive-Compulsive Symptoms

Treatment-emergent obsessive-compulsive symptoms have been reported in patients with a favorable antipsychotic response to clozapine, risperidone, and olanzapine. Controlled trials have not established a clear causal relationship. When used by persons with a prior diagnosis of obsessive-compulsive disorder, on the other hand, SDAs have been successful in augmenting the anti-obsessional effects of serotonin reuptake inhibitors.

Priapism

The α-receptor antagonism of SDAs can induce priapism. There are a few isolated case reports of priapism during treatment with risperidone, olanzapine, quetiapine, and clozapine.

Genitourinary Symptoms

Enuresis, urinary frequency or urgency, and urinary hesitancy or retention have been seen with use of clozapine. These problems may respond to desmopressin (DDAVP), oxybutynin (Ditropan), or timed interruption of sleep.

Dysphagia

Antipsychotic drug use is infrequently associated with esophageal dysmotility and aspiration, which can cause aspiration pneumonia.

Transaminase Elevations and Hepatic Dysfunction

About 6 percent of persons who take quetiapine and 2 percent of those who take olanzapine have serum transaminase concentrations more than three times the upper limit of normal in the first 3 weeks of treatment. This has no clinical significance and is transient; however, quetiapine and olanzapine should be used with caution by persons with underlying liver disease.

Risperidone use is (rarely) associated with reversible hepatotoxicity in adults and children. Obesity is a risk factor for risperidone-induced hepatotoxicity. Clozapine use is frequently associated with elevated transaminase concentrations that usually resolve within 3 months and is rarely associated with serious, possibly fatal hepatotoxicity.

Cholesterol and Triglyceride Elevations

Quetiapine and olanzapine use may increase serum cholesterol and triglyceride concentrations by 11 to 17 percent.

Hypothyroidism

A small number of persons taking higher dosages of quetiapine have decreased serum concentrations of total and free thyroxine. This usually has no clinical significance.

Use in Pregnancy and Lactation

SDA use by pregnant women has not been studied, but consideration should be given to the potential of risperidone to raise prolactin concentrations, sometimes to three to four times the upper limit of the normal range. Because the drugs can be excreted in breast milk, they should not be taken by nursing mothers.

DRUG–DRUG INTERACTIONS

CNS depressants, alcohol, or tricyclic drugs coadministered with SDAs may increase the risk for seizures, sedation, and cardiac effects. Antihypertensive medications may potentiate the orthostatic hypotension caused by SDAs. Coadministration of benzodiazepines and SDAs may be associated with an increased incidence of orthostasis, syncope, and respiratory depression. Risperidone, olanzapine, quetiapine, and ziprasidone can antagonize the effects of levodopa (Larodopa) and dopamine agonists. Long-term use of SDAs with drugs that induce cytochrome P450 isoenzymes, such as carbamazepine,

barbiturates, omeprazole (Prilosec), rifampin (Rifadin, Rifamate), or glucocorticoids, may increase the clearance of the SDAs by 50 percent or more.

Risperidone

Concurrent use of risperidone and phenytoin or serotonin reuptake inhibitors may produce extrapyramidal symptoms. Use of risperidone by persons with opioid dependence may precipitate opioid withdrawal symptoms. Addition of risperidone to the regimen of a person taking clozapine can raise clozapine plasma concentrations by 75 percent. Otherwise, risperidone use has little effect on other drugs.

Olanzapine

Cimetidine (Tagamet) and warfarin (Coumadin) do not influence olanzapine metabolism. Olanzapine use does not affect the metabolism of imipramine (Tofranil), desipramine (Norpramin), warfarin, diazepam (Valium), lithium, or biperiden (Akineton). Fluvoxamine (Luvox) use increases serum concentrations of olanzapine.

Quetiapine

Phenytoin use increases quetiapine clearance fivefold, and thioridazine (Mellaril) use increases quetiapine clearance by 65 percent. Cimetidine use reduces quetiapine clearance by 20 percent. Fluoxetine, imipramine, haloperidol, or risperidone use does not influence quetiapine metabolism. Quetiapine use reduces lorazepam (Ativan) clearance by 20 percent and does not affect lithium clearance.

Clozapine

Clozapine should not be used with any other drug that is associated with the development of agranulocytosis or bone marrow suppression. Such drugs include carbamazepine, phenytoin, propylthiouracil, sulfonamides, and captopril (Capoten). Addition of paroxetine (Paxil) may precipitate clozapine-associated neutropenia. Lithium combined with clozapine may increase the risk of seizures, confusion, and movement disorders. Lithium should not be used in combination with clozapine by persons who have experienced an episode of neuroleptic malignant syndrome. Use of risperidone, fluoxetine, paroxetine, or fluvoxamine increases serum concentrations of clozapine.

Ziprasidone

Ziprasidone appears to have low potential for clinically significant drug interactions. It should be avoided in combination with drugs that prolong the QT interval, however.

DOSAGE AND CLINICAL GUIDELINES

Risperidone, olanzapine, quetiapine, and ziprasidone are appropriate for the management of an initial psychotic episode, whereas clozapine is reserved for persons refractory to all other antipsychotic drugs. If a person does not respond to the first SDA, other SDAs or aripiprazole should be tried. Olanzapine and clozapine have some initial calming effects due to their anticholinergic activity. The SDAs are less effective sedatives for treatment of acute psychosis than dopamine receptor antagonists or benzodiazepines. It is thus sometimes necessary to augment an SDA with a high-potency dopamine receptor antagonist or benzodiazepine in the first few weeks of use. Lorazepam 1 to 2 mg orally or intramuscularly (IM) can be used as needed for acute agitation. SDAs usually require 4 to 6 weeks to reach full effectiveness. Once effective, dosages can be lowered as tolerated. Clinical improvement may take 6 months of treatment with SDAs in some particularly treatment-refractory persons.

Use of all SDAs must be initiated at low dosages and gradually tapered upward to therapeutic dosages. The gradual increase in dosage is necessitated by the potential development of hypotension, syncope, and sedation; patients can usually develop tolerance to these adverse effects if the dosage titration is gradual enough. If a person stops taking an SDA for more than 36 hours, drug use should be resumed at the initial titration schedule. After a decision to terminate olanzapine or clozapine use, dosages should be tapered whenever possible, to avoid cholinergic rebound symptoms such as diaphoresis, flushing, diarrhea, and hyperactivity.

Once a clinician has determined that a trial of an SDA is warranted for a particular person, the risks and the benefits of SDA treatment must be explained to the person and the family. In the case of clozapine, an informed consent procedure should be documented in the person's chart. The patient's history should include information about blood disorders, epilepsy, cardiovascular disease, hepatic and renal diseases, and drug abuse. The presence of a hepatic or renal disease necessitates using low starting dosages. Physical examination should include supine and standing blood pressure measurements to screen for orthostatic hypotension. The laboratory examination should include an ECG; several complete blood counts (CBCs) with WBC counts, which can then be averaged; and liver and renal function tests (Table 36.4.27–3).

Risperidone

Risperidone is available in 1-, 2-, 3-, and 4-mg tablets, and a 1-mg/mL oral solution. The initial dosage is usually 1 to 2 mg at night. The dosage can then be raised gradually (1 mg per dose every 2 or 3 days) to 4 to 6 mg at night. Risperidone was initially given twice a day, but several studies have shown equal efficacy with once-a-day dosing. Dosages above 6 mg a day are associated with a higher incidence of adverse effects. Dosages below 6 mg a day have generally not been associated with extrapyramidal symptoms, but dystonic reactions have been seen at dosages from 4 to 16 mg a day.

Olanzapine

Olanzapine is available in 2.5-, 5-, 7.5-, 10-, and 15-mg tablets. The initial dosage for treatment of psychosis is usually 5 or 10 mg and for treatment of acute mania is usually 10 or 15 mg, given once daily. A starting daily dose of 5 mg is recommended for elderly and medically ill persons and those with hepatic impairment or hypotension; after 1 week the dosage can be raised to 10 mg a day. Given the long half-life, 1 week must be allowed to achieve each new steady-state blood level. Dosages in clinical use range from 5 to 20 mg a day, but a beneficial response usually occurs at dosages of 10 mg a day. The higher

Table 36.4.27–3
Guidelines for the Management of Patients on Clozapine[a]

1. Patients should have a thorough medical history and physical examination prior to initiation of treatment.
2. Testing for tuberculosis should be performed and testing for HIV offered to any patient with risks for either disease. Risk factors include prolonged residence in an institutional facility, group home, shelter, etc. Treatment with clozapine may begin before test results are available if the patient lacks physical signs or symptoms of illness. If either condition is diagnosed, appropriate consultation should be obtained regarding the risks and benefits of continuing clozapine.
3. It is advisable to begin clozapine therapy with a small dose (e.g., 25 mg) and build up gradually, over a 30-day period, to a therapeutic level of 500 mg or more per day.
4. The physician must complete a three-part National Registry WBC Reporting Form (provided by Sandoz). The physician keeps one copy and forwards the remaining two copies to the patient's pharmacist.
5. The pharmacist may dispense a maximum of 7 days' supply of medication, provided three criteria are met:
   a. The patient's current WBC is recorded.
   b. The initial WBC is at least 3,500 per mm^3.
   c. Subsequent WBCs, obtained weekly, are at least 3,000 per mm^3.
6. Benign neutropenia is not typical with clozapine. The following thresholds must be observed in monitoring WBC levels:
   a. Treatment should not be initiated if the WBC is less than 3,500 per mm^3.
   b. If subsequent WBCs are between 3,000 and 3,500 per mm^3, twice-weekly WBCs with differentials should be obtained.
   c. If the total WBC falls below 3,000 per mm^3, therapy should be interrupted and the patient closely monitored.
   d. If the total WBC falls below 2,000 per mm^3, therapy should be discontinued, and the patient should never be rechallenged with clozapine.
   e. If a weekly WBC falls 30% from the previous level, the WBC should be repeated. If the repeat level shows the WBC continuing to fall significantly, appropriate consultation from Sandoz and/or another expert (i.e., psychiatrist, hematologist, or infectious disease specialist) should be obtained.
   f. A gradual progressive decrease in the WBC from the time of initiation of therapy with clozapine should be monitored closely, and consideration should be given to obtaining consultation as above.

[a]These guidelines are based on the requirements set forth by Sandoz (through items 6a, b, and c) and the procedures of the Psychiatry Department of Columbia-Presbyterian Medical Center (items 6d and e).
Reprinted with permission from Silver JM, Yudofsky SC, Hurowitz GI. Psychopharmacology and electroconvulsive therapy. In: Hales RE, Yudofsky SC, Talbott JA, eds. *The American Psychiatric Press Textbook of Psychiatry.* 2nd ed. Washington, DC: American Psychiatric Press; 1994:920.

dosages are associated with increased extrapyramidal and other adverse effects. The manufacturer recommends "periodic" assessment of transaminases during treatment with olanzapine.

Olanzapine will shortly be available in the United States as an IM formulation for administration in acute care situations.

Quetiapine

Quetiapine is available in 25-, 100-, and 200-mg tablets. Dosing should begin at 25 mg twice daily, and dosages can be raised by 25 to 50 mg per dose every 2 to 3 days up to a target of 300 to 400 mg a day, divided into two or three daily doses. Studies have shown efficacy in the range of 300 to 800 mg a day, with most persons receiving maximum benefit at 300 to 500 mg a day.

Clozapine

Clozapine is available in 25- and 100-mg tablets. The initial dosage is usually 25 mg one or two times daily, although a conservative initial dosage is 12.5 mg twice daily. The dosage can then be raised gradually (25 mg a day every 2 or 3 days) to 300 mg a day in divided dosages, usually two or three times daily. Dosages up to 900 mg a day can be used.

Weekly WBC counts are indicated to monitor the patient for the development of agranulocytosis. Although monitoring is expensive, early indication of agranulocytosis can prevent a fatal outcome. If the WBC count is below 2,000 cells per mm^3 or the granulocyte count is below 1,000 per mm^3, clozapine use should be discontinued, a hematological consultation should be obtained, and obtaining a bone marrow sample should be considered. Persons with agranulocytosis should not be reexposed to the drug. Persons can obtain the WBC count through any laboratory. Proof of monitoring must be presented to the pharmacist to obtain the medication.

Ziprasidone

Ziprasidone dosing should be initiated at 40 mg a day, divided into two daily doses. Studies have shown efficacy in the range of 80 to 160 mg a day, divided twice daily. Ziprasidone is expected to be the first SDA to be available in both oral and long-acting (depot) injectable formulations.

Aripiprazole

The dose of aripiprazole is estimated to be between 15 and 30 mg given once daily; however, physicians should follow the drug labeling for this new drug for initial guidance.

Switching from Typical to Atypical Antipsychotic Drugs

Although the transition from a dopamine receptor antagonist to an SDA may be made abruptly, it is probably wiser to taper off use of the dopamine receptor antagonist slowly while titrating up the SDA. Clozapine and olanzapine both have anticholinergic effects, and the transition from one to the other can usually be accomplished with little risk of cholinergic rebound. The transition from risperidone to olanzapine is best accomplished by tapering off risperidone use over 3 weeks while simultaneously beginning olanzapine use directly at 10 mg a day. Risperidone, quetiapine, and ziprasidone lack anticholinergic effects, and the abrupt transition from a dopamine receptor antagonist, olanzapine, or clozapine to one of these agents may cause cholinergic rebound, which consists of excessive salivation, nausea, vomiting, and diarrhea. The risk of cholinergic rebound can be mitigated by initially augmenting risperidone, quetiapine, or ziprasidone with an anticholinergic drug, which is then tapered off slowly. Any initiation and termination of SDA use should be accomplished gradually.

It is wise to overlap administration of the new drug with the old drug. Of interest, some persons have a more robust clinical response while taking the two agents during the transition, then regress on monotherapy with the newer drug. Little is known about the effectiveness and safety of a strategy of combining use of one SDA with another SDA or with a dopamine receptor antagonist.

Persons receiving regular injections of depot formulations of a dopamine receptor antagonist who are to switch to SDA use are given the first dose of the SDA on the day the next injection is due. At present, SDAs are only available in oral formulations.

Persons who developed agranulocytosis while taking clozapine can safely switch to olanzapine use, although initiation of olanzapine use in the midst of clozapine-induced agranulocytosis can prolong the time of recovery from the usual 3 to 4 days up to 11 to 12 days. It is prudent to wait for resolution of agranulocytosis before initiating olanzapine use. Emergence or recurrence of agranulocytosis has not been reported with olanzapine, even in persons who developed it while taking clozapine.

References

Baldessarini RJ, Tarazi RI. Drugs and the treatment of psychiatric disorders: psychosis and mania. In: Hardman JG, Limbird LE, Goodman Gilman A, eds. *Goodman & Gilman's the Pharmacological Basis of Therapeutics.* 10th ed. New York: McGraw-Hill; 2001:485.

Meltzer HY. Serotonin as a target for antipsychotic drug action. In: Breier A, Tran PV, eds. *Current Issues in the Psychopharmacology of Schizophrenia.* Philadelphia: Lippincott Williams & Wilkins; 2001:289.

Millan MJ. Improving the treatment of schizophrenia: focus on serotonin (5-HT_{1A}) receptors. *J Pharmacol Exp Ther.* 2000;295:853.

Parker G, Malhi G. Are the atypical antipsychotic drugs antidepressants? *J Clin Psychopharmacol.* 2002;22:94.

Sartorius A, Hewer W, Zink M, Henn FA. High-dose clozapine intoxication. *J Clin Psychopharmacol.* 2002;22:91.

Thase ME. What role do atypical antipsychotic drugs have in treatment-resistant depression? *J Clin Psychiatry.* 2002;63:95.

Van Kammen DP, Marder SR. Serotonin-dopamine antagonists. In: Sadock BJ, Sadock VA, eds. *Kaplan & Sadock's Comprehensive Textbook of Psychiatry.* 7th ed. Vol 2. Baltimore: Lippincott Williams & Wilkins; 2000:2455.

Vieta E, Goikolea JM, Corbella B, et al. Correction: risperidone safety and efficacy in the treatment of bipolar and schizoaffective disorders: results from a 6-month, multicenter, open study. *J Clin Psychiatry.* 2002;63:79.

▲ 36.4.28 Sibutramine

Sibutramine (Meridia) is a novel appetite suppressant used to treat obesity and is pharmacologically similar to several antidepressant drugs, especially venlafaxine (Effexor). Sibutramine is a reuptake inhibitor of serotonin, norepinephrine, and, to a lesser extent, dopamine, but it lacks any clinical antidepressant effect.

CHEMISTRY

The structural formula of sibutramine is shown in Figure 36.4.28–1.

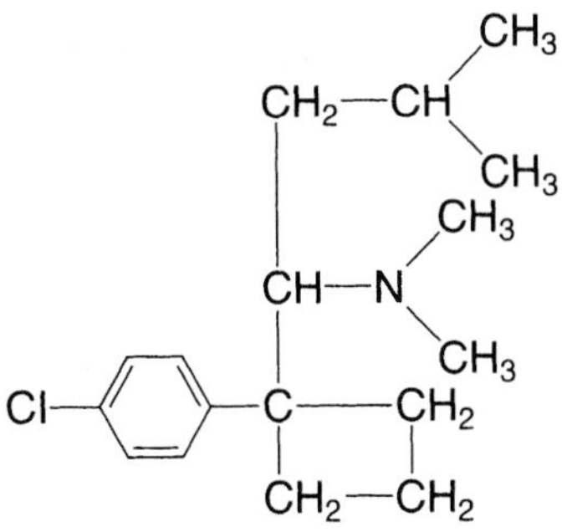

FIGURE 36.4.28–1
Molecular structure of sibutramine.

PHARMACOLOGICAL ACTIONS

Sibutramine is rapidly absorbed after oral administration and promptly metabolized to its active metabolites, called M_1 and M_2, which reach their peak plasma concentrations in 3 to 4 hours. The half-lives of M_1 and M_2 are 14 to 16 hours, which permits once-daily dosing.

Sibutramine's active metabolites are inhibitors of reuptake of serotonin, norepinephrine, and, to a lesser degree, dopamine. Sibutramine prolongs the action of monoamines released normally into the synaptic cleft in the process of neurotransmission.

THERAPEUTIC INDICATIONS

Sibutramine is indicated for use as part of a supervised weight loss and maintenance program that includes dietary restrictions. Sibutramine is indicated for use by persons with a body-mass index (BMI) of 30 or above or a BMI of 27 or above in the presence of atherosclerosis risk factors such as hypertension, diabetes mellitus, or hypercholesterolemia. Sibutramine is effective only while it is being taken, provided that dietary guidelines are strictly followed.

Sibutramine responsiveness is defined as loss of 4 or more pounds in the first 4 weeks of use. Some 60 percent of sibutramine responders who continue to take the drug for at least 6 months will lose at least 5 percent of their initial body weight. The weight loss can be maintained for at least 12 months with continuous use of the drug. Sibutramine may also improve glucose tolerance in persons with non–insulin-dependent diabetes mellitus.

Some clinicians promote the combined use of sibutramine and phentermine (Ionamin, Adipex-P) or the use of sibutramine together with orlistat (Xenical). However, no controlled trials support these combinations.

PRECAUTIONS AND ADVERSE EFFECTS

The most common adverse effects associated with use of sibutramine are headache, dry mouth, anorexia, insomnia, and constipation. The most serious effects associated with its use are elevations of blood pressure and pulse rate. On average, persons who take 5 to 20 mg a day of sibutramine experience a rise in mean systolic and diastolic blood pressure of 1 to 3 mm Hg and a rise in pulse rate of 4 to 5 beats per minute. The elevations in blood pressure and pulse are dose dependent and may reach clinically significant levels (15 mm Hg systolic and 10 mm Hg diastolic) at dosages exceeding 10 mg a day. Because of these cardiovascular effects, sibutramine should be used cautiously by persons with a history of hypertension, atherosclerotic heart disease, myocardial infarction, congestive heart failure, arrhythmias, or stroke. Because of the reported elevations in blood pressure and the risk of cerebrovascular accidents, sibutramine

use is being carefully monitored by the Food and Drug Administration (FDA). Sibutramine may also cause mydriasis, which could exacerbate narrow-angle glaucoma.

DRUG–DRUG INTERACTIONS

Sibutramine should not be taken within 14 days of use of a monoamine oxidase inhibitor. Sibutramine could potentially precipitate a serotonin syndrome if used concurrently with serotonin-specific reuptake inhibitors, tricyclic antidepressants, triptan antimigraine drugs, dihydroergotamine (D.H.T. 45), dextromethorphan, meperidine (Demerol), pentazocine (Talwin, Talacen), fentanyl (Duragesic), lithium (Eskalith), or tryptophan, but no reports of sibutramine-associated serotonin syndrome exist at this time. Sibutramine could raise blood pressure if used together with prescription or nonprescription preparations containing phenylpropanolamine (Entex, others), ephedrine (Rynatuss, others), or pseudoephedrine (numerous combination products). Ketoconazole (Nizoral), erythromycin (several), and cimetidine (Tagamet) may raise plasma concentrations of sibutramine modestly.

LABORATORY INTERFERENCES

Sibutramine has not been reported to interfere with any laboratory tests. However, some patients may exhibit a transient elevation of hepatic transaminase concentration.

DOSAGE AND CLINICAL GUIDELINES

Pretreatment evaluation for use of sibutramine should include a review of the cardiovascular system and identification of risk factors for atherosclerosis as well as a complete drug history. Physical examination should include a series of at least three separate determinations of blood pressure and pulse and should focus on signs of atherosclerosis. Laboratory examination should focus on evidence for diabetes mellitus. Documentation should include evidence that the pretreatment weight falls into the category defined in the product literature as obese. (A full discussion on obesity appears in Section 23.3.)

Sibutramine is available in 5-, 10-, and 15-mg capsules. The starting dosage of sibutramine is 10 mg once a day. If no weight loss occurs after 4 weeks, then sibutramine probably will not be effective. If weight loss is less than 4 pounds in the first 4 weeks, then the dosage may be increased to 15 to 20 mg a day. If the 10-mg daily dose is not tolerated, then the dosage should be lowered to 5 mg a day.

REFERENCES

Brownell KD, Wadden TA. Obesity. In: Sadock BJ, Sadock VA, eds. *Kaplan & Sadock's Comprehensive Textbook of Psychiatry.* 7th ed. Vol 2. Baltimore: Lippincott Williams & Wilkins; 2000:1787.

Chapelot D, Marmonier C, Thomas F, Hanotin C. Modalities of the food intake-reducing effect of sibutramine in humans. *Physiol Behav.* 2000;68:299.

Cole JO, Levin A, Beake B, Kaiser PE, Scheinbaum ML. Sibutramine: a new weight loss agent without evidence of the abuse potential associated with amphetamines. *J Clin Psychopharmacol.* 1998;18:231.

Hardman, JG, Limbird LE, Goodman Gilman A, eds. *Goodman & Gilman's the Pharmacological Basis of Therapeutics.* 10th ed. New York: McGraw-Hill; 2001.

Wirth A, Krause J. Long-term weight loss with sibutramine: a randomized controlled trial. *JAMA.* 2001;286:1331.

▲ 36.4.29 Sildenafil

Sildenafil (Viagra) has revolutionized the treatment of erectile disorder (impotence) and has rapidly created its own therapeutic niche. Although indicated only for treatment of male erectile dysfunction, sildenafil has been used to improve the sexual functioning of both men and women. It is effective whether or not erectile disorder is caused by medical, surgical, or psychological factors.

CHEMISTRY

Sildenafil is a heterocyclic piperazine derivative of zaprinast, a weak and nonselective phosphodiesterase (PDE) inhibitor. Pure sildenafil is poorly soluble in water. Its structural formula is shown in Figure 36.4.29–1.

PHARMACOLOGICAL ACTIONS

Sildenafil is fairly rapidly absorbed from the gastrointestinal (GI) tract, and its bioavailability is 40 percent. Maximum plasma concentrations of oral sildenafil are reached in 30 to 120 minutes (median, 60 minutes) in the fasting state. Because of its lipophilicity, concomitant ingestion with a high-fat meal delays the rate of absorption by up to 60 minutes and reduces the peak concentration by one quarter. Sildenafil is principally metabolized by the cytochrome P450 (CYP) 3A4 system, which may lead to clinically significant drug–drug interactions, not all of which have been documented. Excretion of 80 percent of the dose is via feces, and another 13 percent is eliminated in the urine. Elimination is reduced in persons over age 65, which results in plasma concentrations 40 percent higher than in persons aged 18 to 45. Elimination is also reduced in the presence of severe renal or hepatic insufficiency.

The principal cellular site of action of sildenafil is the enzyme PDE5, which acts on arteriolar smooth muscle cells of the corpus cavernosum of the penis. PDE5 is efficiently and selectively inhibited by sildenafil, which allows blood to fill the corpus cavernosum and cause an erection.

The clinician needs to be aware of the important clinical observation that sildenafil does not by itself create an erection. Rather, the mental state of sexual arousal brought on by erotic

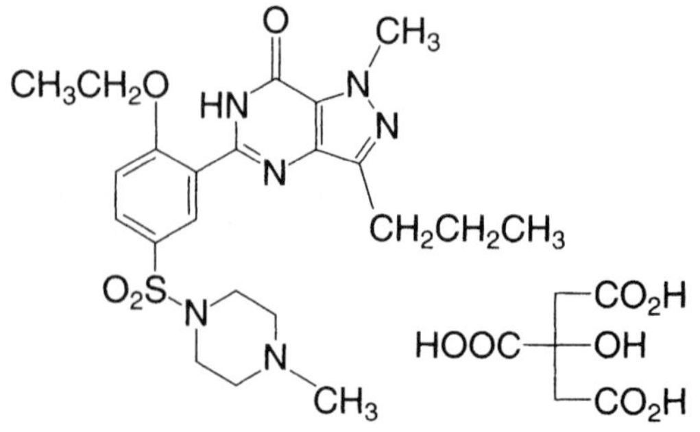

FIGURE 36.4.29–1
Molecular structure of sildenafil.

stimulation of any kind—tactile, visual, auditory, olfactory, or fantasy—must first lead to activity in the penile nerves. Excited nerve endings then release nitric oxide into the cavernosum, triggering the erectile cascade. Sildenafil maintains the resulting erection by its enzymatic action. Thus, sildenafil permits full advantage to be taken of a sexually exciting stimulus, but it is not a substitute for foreplay and emotional arousal.

THERAPEUTIC INDICATIONS

Erectile dysfunctions have traditionally been classified as organic, psychogenic, or mixed. Over the last 20 years, the prevailing view of the cause of erectile dysfunction has shifted away from the psychological cause toward the organic. Organic causes include diabetes mellitus, hypertension, hypercholesterolemia, cigarette smoking, peripheral vascular disease, pelvic or spinal cord injury, pelvic or abdominal surgery (especially prostate surgery), multiple sclerosis, peripheral neuropathy, and Parkinson's disease. Erectile dysfunction is often induced by alcohol, other substances of abuse, and prescription drugs.

Sildenafil is effective regardless of the baseline severity of erectile dysfunction, cause of erectile dysfunction, race, or age. Among those responding to sildenafil are men with coronary artery disease, hypertension, other cardiac disease, peripheral vascular disease, diabetes mellitus, depression, coronary artery bypass graft (CABG), radical prostatectomy, transurethral resection of the prostate, spina bifida, and spinal cord injury, as well as persons taking antidepressants, antipsychotics, antihypertensives, and diuretics.

Sildenafil has been reported to reverse selective serotonin reuptake inhibitor (SSRI)–induced anorgasmia in both men and women. There are reports of a therapeutic effect on sexual inhibition in women as well.

Table 36.4.29–1
Generic and Trade Names of Some Commonly Used Organic Nitrates

Nitroglycerin
Deponit (transdermal)
Minitran
Nitrek
Nitro-Bid
Nitrodisc
Nitro-Dur
Nitrogard
Nitroglyn
Nitrolingual Spray
Nitrol Ointment (Appli-Kit)
Nitrong
Nitro-Par
Nitrostat
Nitro-Time
Transderm-Nitro
Isosorbide mononitrate
Imdur
Ismo
Monoket Tablets
Isosorbide dinitrate
Dilatrate-SR
Isordil
Sorbitrate
Erythatyl tetranitrate
Pentaerythritol tetranitrate
Sodium nitroprusside

PRECAUTIONS AND ADVERSE REACTIONS

The most important potential adverse effect associated with use of sildenafil is myocardial infarction (MI). The manufacturer and the U.S. Food and Drug Administration (FDA) distinguished the risk of MI due directly to sildenafil from that due to underlying conditions such as hypertension, atherosclerotic heart disease, diabetes mellitus, and other atherogenic conditions. The FDA concluded that when used according to the approved labeling, sildenafil does not by itself confer an increased risk of death. In addition to the increased oxygen demand and the stress placed on the cardiac muscle by sexual intercourse, which is facilitated by sildenafil, coronary perfusion may be severely compromised by the combined actions of sildenafil and nitrates, but not by sildenafil used alone. Any person with a history of MI, stroke, renal failure, hypertension, or diabetes mellitus and any person over the age of 70 should discuss plans to use sildenafil with an internist or a cardiologist. The cardiac evaluation should specifically address exercise tolerance and the use of nitrates. Most deaths associated with the use of sildenafil have occurred during or after sexual intercourse and are related to the amount of exertion used in the act of coitus in a person with preexisting cardiovascular disease.

Use of sildenafil is contraindicated in persons who are taking organic nitrates in any form. These medications include nitroglycerin, isosorbide mononitrate (Imdur, ISMO, Monoket), isosorbide dinitrate (Isordil, Sorbitrate), erythatyl tetranitrate, pentaerythritol tetranitrate, and sodium nitroprusside (Nipride). These agents are listed in Table 36.4.29–1. Amyl nitrate ("poppers"), a popular substance of abuse used by gay men and other persons to enhance the intensity of orgasm, should not be used with sildenafil. This combination has caused several deaths. Organic nitrates raise circulating nitric oxide concentrations and potentiate the nitric oxide signaling pathway that causes vasodilation. Use of 100 mg of sildenafil caused an average drop in blood pressure of 10 mm Hg in normal volunteers; more significant drops in blood pressure occur in patients concurrently taking organic nitrates. Precipitous lowering of blood pressure can reduce coronary perfusion to the point of causing MI.

Adverse effects are dose dependent, occurring at a higher rate with a dose of 100 mg than with 25 or 50 mg. The most common adverse effects are headache, flushing, and stomach pain. Other less common adverse effects include nasal congestion, urinary tract infection, abnormal vision (colored tinge [usually blue], increased sensitivity to light, or blurred vision), diarrhea, dizziness, and rash. No cases of priapism were reported in premarketing trials. Supportive management is indicated in cases of overdosage.

Even though no data are available on the effects of sildenafil on human fetal growth and development, it should not be used during pregnancy.

DRUG–DRUG INTERACTIONS

The major route of sildenafil metabolism is through CYP 3A4; the minor route is through CYP 2C9. Inducers or inhibitors of these enzymes will therefore affect the plasma concentration and half-life of sildenafil. For example, 800 mg of cimetidine (Tagamet), a nonspecific CYP inhibitor, increases plasma sildenafil concentrations by 56 percent, and erythromycin (E-mycin) increases plasma sildenafil concentrations by 182 percent. Other stronger inhibitors of CYP 3A4 include ketoconazole (Nizoral), itraconazole (Sporanox), and mibefradil (Posicor). In contrast, rifampicin, a CYP 3A4 inducer, decreases plasma concentrations of sildenafil.

LABORATORY INTERFERENCES

No laboratory interferences have been described for sildenafil.

DOSAGE AND CLINICAL GUIDELINES

Sildenafil is available in 25-, 50-, and 100-mg tablets. The recommended dose of sildenafil is 50 mg taken by mouth 1 hour prior to intercourse. However, sildenafil may take effect within 30 minutes. The duration of the effect is usually 4 hours, but in healthy young men, the effect may persist for 8 to 12 hours. Based on effectiveness and adverse effects, the dose should be titrated between 25 and 100 mg. Sildenafil is recommended for use no more than once a day, although in the earliest clinical trials for treatment of angina, doses up to 50 mg every 8 hours for 10 consecutive days were generally well tolerated. The dosing guidelines for use by women, an off-label use, are the same as those for men.

Increased plasma concentrations of sildenafil may occur in persons over 65 years of age and those with cirrhosis or severe renal impairment or using CYP 3A4 inhibitors. A starting dose of 25 mg should be used in these circumstances.

An investigational nasal spray formulation of sildenafil has been developed that acts within 5 to 15 minutes of administration. This formulation is highly water soluble, and it is rapidly absorbed directly into the bloodstream. Such a formulation would permit more ease of use. Congeners of sildenafil are being developed at a rapid rate.

REFERENCES

Andersson KE, Hedlund P. New directions for erectile dysfunction therapies. *Int J Impot Res.* 2002;14(suppl 1):S82.

Berman JR, Berman LA, Lin H, et al. Effect of sildenafil on subjective and physiologic parameters of the female sexual response in women with sexual arousal disorder. *J Sex Marital Ther.* 2001;27:411.

Hardman JG, Limbird LE, Goodman Gilman A, eds. *Goodman & Gilman's the Pharmacological Basis of Therapeutics.* 10th ed. New York: McGraw-Hill; 2001.

Nurnberg HG, Gelenberg A, Hargreave TB, Harrison WM, Siegel RL, Smith MD. Efficacy of sildenafil citrate for the treatment of erectile dysfunction in men taking serotonin reuptake inhibitors. *Am J Psychiatry.* 2001;158:1926.

Rosenberg KP. Sildenafil. *J Sex Marital Ther.* 1999;25:271.

Sadock VA. Normal human sexuality and sexual dysfunctions. In: Sadock BJ, Sadock VA, eds. *Kaplan & Sadock's Comprehensive Textbook of Psychiatry.* 7th ed. Vol 1. Baltimore: Lippincott Williams & Wilkins; 2000:1577.

Seidman SN, Roose SP, Menza MA, Shabsigh R, Rosen RC. Treatment of erectile dysfunction in men with depressive symptoms: results of a placebo-controlled trial with sildenafil citrate. *Am J Psychiatry.* 2001;158:1623.

▲ 36.4.30 Sympathomimetics and Related Drugs

Sympathomimetic drugs cause the stimulation of α- and β-adrenergic receptors directly as agonists and, indirectly, cause the release of dopamine and norepinephrine from presynaptic terminals. They are variously referred to as *stimulants, psychostimulants,* or *analeptics.* While these drugs act specifically on symptoms of poor concentration and hyperactivity in children and adults, as well as increasing alertness in narcolepsy, they are also used to maintain wakefulness, alertness, and energy. Because of their rapid onset, immediate behavioral effects and the propensity to develop tolerance, which leads to the risk of abuse and dependence in vulnerable individuals, they have been classified as controlled drugs, and their manufacture, distribution, and use are regulated by state and federal agencies.

Despite these caveats, they are valuable agents and their use persists and may be increasing in medicine and psychiatry in specific clinical situations. Stimulants can be of great help, if appropriately prescribed and monitored, because of their effectiveness in disorders in which no other drug has been helpful. Sympathomimetics have been widely used in attention-deficit/hyperactivity disorder (ADHD) and narcolepsy because no other equally effective agent exists. They are effective in medical or surgical disorders that result in secondary depression or profound apathy (e.g., acquired immune deficiency syndrome [AIDS] and also are used to augment antidepressant medications in treatment-refractory depressions).

The sympathomimetics used in psychiatry include methylphenidate (Ritalin, Concerta), dexmethylphenidate (Focalin), dextroamphetamine (Dexedrine), a combination of amphetamine and dextroamphetamine (Adderall), methamphetamine (Desoxyn), and pemoline (Cylert), the last now considered a second-line agent, because of rare but potentially fatal hepatic toxicity. The drugs are indicated for the treatment of ADHD and narcolepsy and are also effective in the treatment of depressive disorders in special populations (e.g., the medically ill).

Both amphetamine and nonamphetamine sympathomimetics have been used as appetite suppressants. Other sympathomimetics used for appetite suppression include methamphetamine (Desoxyn), benzphetamine (Didrex), phentermine (Adipex-P, Fastin, Ionamin), diethylpropion (Tenuate), phenmetrazine (Preludin), phendimetrazine (Bontril, Adipost), and mazindol (Sanorex, Mazanor). A novel stimulant approved for treatment of narcolepsy in the United States, modafinil (Provigil), is discussed at the end of this section.

CHEMISTRY

The molecular structures of dextroamphetamine, methylphenidate, pemoline, methamphetamine, phentermine, and modafinil are shown in Figure 36.4.30–1. Amphetamine is similar in structure to methylphenidate.

PHARMACOLOGICAL ACTIONS

All of these drugs are well absorbed from the gastrointestinal tract. Dextroamphetamine reaches peak plasma concentrations

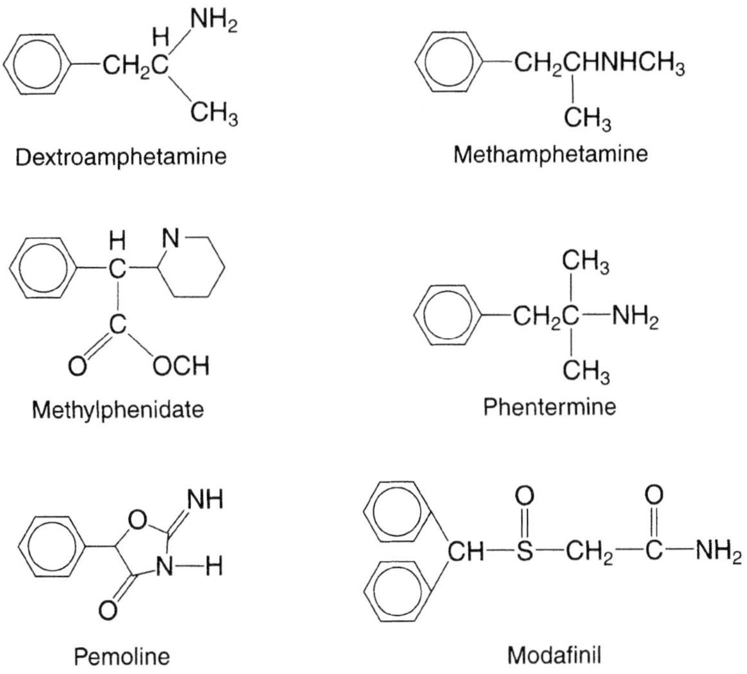

FIGURE 36.4.30–1
Molecular structures of selected sympathomimetics. Dexmethylphenidate is the D-threo-enantiomer of methylphenidate.

in 2 to 3 hours and has a half-life of about 6 hours, thereby necessitating twice- or thrice-daily dosing.

Methylphenidate is available in immediate-release (Ritalin), sustained-release (Ritalin SR), and extended-release (Concerta) formulations. Immediate-release methylphenidate reaches peak plasma concentrations in 1 to 2 hours and has a short half-life of 2 to 3 hours, thereby necessitating multiple-daily dosing. The sustained-release formulation reaches peak plasma concentrations in 4 to 5 hours and doubles the effective half-life of methylphenidate. The extended-release formulation reaches peak plasma concentrations in 6 to 8 hours and is designed to be effective for 12 hours in once-daily dosing. Dexmethylphenidate reaches peak plasma level in about 7 hours and is given twice daily.

Pemoline reaches peak plasma concentrations in 2 to 4 hours and has a half-life of about 12 hours, and modafinil reaches peak plasma concentrations in 2 to 4 hours and has a half-life of 15 hours, thereby allowing once-daily dosing of these two agents.

Adderall is available in immediate-release and sustained-release (Adderall XR) formulations. The immediate-release drug reaches peak plasma concentrations in about 3 hours. The time to peak concentration for the extended-release drug is about 7 hours and provides effective full-day symptom control in a single morning dose; the immediate-release preparation requires multiple dosing.

Methylphenidate, dexmethylphenidate, dextroamphetamine, and amphetamine are indirectly acting sympathomimetics, with the primary effect of causing the release of catecholamines from presynaptic neurons. Clinical effectiveness is associated with increased release of both dopamine and norepinephrine. Dextroamphetamine and methylphenidate are also weak inhibitors of catecholamine reuptake and inhibitors of monoamine oxidase. Pemoline may indirectly stimulate dopaminergic activity by a poorly understood mechanism, but it has little actual sympathomimetic activity.

EFFECTS ON SPECIFIC ORGANS AND SYSTEMS

Central Nervous System. Amphetamine stimulates the medullary respiratory center and has excitatory effects on cortical function. Depending on personality and contextual factors, amphetamine in adults can increase wakefulness, energy, alertness, initiative, self-confidence, and physical and mental performance, lessen fatigue, and produce euphoria. These effects occur shortly after dosing.

Cardiovascular System. Amphetamines can raise blood pressure (particularly in patients with hypertension), and high doses can lead to cardiac arrhythmias (especially in patients with cardiovascular disease). Such effects are not likely at usual clinical doses in a patient without cardiovascular disease or hypertension. Amphetamine is more potent in producing cardiovascular effects than dextroamphetamine because of stronger effects on norepinephrine.

Endocrine Effects. Early reports suggested that both dextroamphetamine and methylphenidate might suppress growth in children. A recent controlled study of children and young adolescents found small but significant height differences evident in early (but not late) adolescent children with ADHD, unrelated to the use of psychotropic medications. This study concluded that the effects on growth seemed to be related to the disorder, not its treatment.

THERAPEUTIC INDICATIONS

Attention-Deficit/Hyperactivity Disorder

Sympathomimetics are the first-line drugs for treatment of ADHD in children and are effective about 75 percent of the time. Methylphenidate and dextroamphetamine are equally effective and work within 15 to 30 minutes. Pemoline requires 3 to 4 weeks to reach its full efficacy, which nevertheless may be less than that of methylphenidate and dextroamphetamine. The drugs decrease hyperactivity, increase attentiveness, and reduce impulsivity. They may also reduce comorbid oppositional behaviors associated with ADHD. Many persons take these drugs throughout their schooling and beyond. In responsive persons, use of a sympathomimetic may be a critical determinant of scholastic success.

Sympathomimetics improve the core ADHD symptoms of hyperactivity, impulsivity, and inattentiveness and permit improved social interactions with teachers, family, other adults, and peers. The success of long-term treatment of ADHD with sympathomimetics, which are efficacious for most of the various constellations of ADHD symptoms present from childhood to adulthood, supports a model in which ADHD results from a genetically determined neurochemical imbalance that requires lifelong pharmacological management.

Methylphenidate is the most commonly used initial agent, at a dosage of 5 to 10 mg every 3 to 4 hours. Dosages may be increased to a maximum of 20 mg four times daily or 1 mg/kg a day. Use of the 20-mg sustained-release formulation to achieve 6 hours of benefit and eliminate the need for dosing at school is supported by many experts, although other authorities feel it is less effective than the immediate-release formulation. Dexmethylphenidate is prescribed at an initial dose of 2.5 mg and increased in 2.5- to 5-mg increments to a maximum of 10 mg twice a day.

Dextroamphetamine is about twice as potent as methylphenidate on a per-milligram basis and provides 6 to 8 hours of benefit. Some 70 percent of nonresponders to one sympathomimetic may benefit from another. All the sympathomimetic drugs should be tried before switching to drugs of a different class. The previous dictum that sympathomimetics worsen tics and therefore should be avoided by persons with comorbid ADHD and tic disorders has been questioned more recently because of reports that small to moderate dosages of sympathomimetics may be well tolerated without causing an increase in the frequency and severity of the tics. Alternatives to sympathomimetics for ADHD include bupropion (Wellbutrin), venlafaxine (Effexor), guanfacine (Tenex), clonidine (Catapres), and tricyclic drugs.

Short-term use of the sympathomimetics induces a euphoric feeling; however, tolerance can develop for both the euphoric feeling and the sympathomimetic activity. Tolerance does not develop for the therapeutic effects in ADHD.

Narcolepsy

Narcolepsy consists of sudden sleep attacks, sudden loss of postural tone (cataplexy), loss of voluntary motor control going into (hypnagogic) or coming out of (hypnopompic) sleep (sleep paralysis), and hypnagogic or hypnopompic hallucinations. Sympathomimetics reduce narcoleptic sleep attacks and also improve wakefulness in other types of hypersomnolent states. Sympathomimetics are used to maintain wakefulness and accuracy of motor performance in persons subject to sleep deprivation, such as pilots and military personnel. Persons with narcolepsy, unlike persons with ADHD, may develop tolerance for the therapeutic effects of the sympathomimetics.

Depressive Disorders

Sympathomimetics may be used for treatment-resistant depressive disorders, usually to augment standard antidepressant drug therapy. Possible indications for use of sympathomimetics as monotherapy include depression in the elderly, who are at increased risk for adverse effects from standard antidepressant drugs; depression in medically ill persons, especially persons with AIDS; obtundation due to chronic use of opioids; and clinical situations in which a rapid response is important but electroconvulsive therapy (ECT) is contraindicated. Depressed patients with abulia and anergia may also benefit.

Dextroamphetamine may be useful in differentiating pseudodementia of depression from dementia. A depressed person generally responds to a 5-mg dose with increased alertness and improved cognition. Sympathomimetics are thought to provide only short-term benefit (2 to 4 weeks) for depression, because most persons rapidly develop tolerance for the antidepressant effects of the drugs. However, some clinicians report that long-term treatment with sympathomimetics can benefit some persons.

Encephalopathy Due to Brain Injury

Sympathomimetics increase alertness, cognition, motivation, and motor performance in persons with neurological deficits caused by strokes, trauma, tumors, or chronic infections. Treatment with sympathomimetics may permit earlier and more robust participation in rehabilitative programs. Poststroke lethargy and apathy may respond to long-term use of sympathomimetics.

Obesity

Sympathomimetics are used in the treatment of obesity because of their anorexia-inducing effects. Because tolerance develops for the anorectic effects and because of the drugs' high abuse potential, their use for this indication is limited. Of the sympathomimetic drugs, phentermine is the most widely used for appetite suppression. Phentermine was the second half of "fen-phen," an off-label combination of fenfluramine and phentermine, widely used to promote weight loss until fenfluramine and dexfenfluramine were withdrawn from commercial availability because of an association with cardiac valvular insufficiency, primary pulmonary hypertension, and irreversible loss of cerebral serotoninergic nerve fibers. The toxicity of fenfluramine is attributed to the fact that it stimulates release of massive amounts of serotonin from nerve endings, a mechanism of action not shared by phentermine. Use of phentermine alone has not been reported to cause the same adverse effects as fenfluramine or dexfenfluramine.

Careful limitation of caloric intake and judicious exercise are at the core of any successful weight loss program. Sympathomimetic drugs facilitate loss of, at most, an additional fraction of a pound per week. Sympathomimetic drugs are effective appetite suppressants only for the first few weeks of use; then the anorexigenic effects tend to decrease.

Other Disorders

As mentioned above, patients suffering from abulia or anergia as part of a depressive syndrome may benefit from sympathomimetics. These symptoms are also found in other conditions such as chronic fatigue syndrome, neurasthenia, fibromyalgia, dysthymia and depressive personality disorder. In each of these conditions, psychostimulants have benefited individual patients. A daily dose of dextroamphetamine (5 to 15 mg) may enable patients to overcome their lethargy and engage in constructive activity. When using these medications, the potential development of tolerance and dependence must be considered and discussed with the patient, and drug use must be closely monitored. When prescribed appropriately, many patients are able to maintain the use of amphetamine at a daily stable dosage level for long periods.

PRECAUTIONS AND ADVERSE REACTIONS

The most common adverse effects associated with amphetamine-like drugs are stomach pain, anxiety, irritability, insomnia, tachycardia, cardiac arrhythmias, and dysphoria. Sympathomimetics decrease appetite, although tolerance usually develops for this effect. The treatment of common adverse effects in children with ADHD is usually straightforward (Table 36.4.30–1). Use of these drugs can also increase the heart rate and the blood pressure and may cause palpitations. Less common adverse effects include the induction of movement disorders, such as tics, Tourette's disorder–like symptoms, and dyskinesias, which are often self-limited over 7 to 10 days. If a person taking a sympathomimetic develops one of these movement disorders, a correlation between the dose of the medication and the severity of the disorder must be firmly established prior to adjustments in the medication dosage. In severe cases, augmentation with risperidone (Risperdal), clonidine, or guanfacine is necessary. Methylphenidate may worsen tics in one third of persons; these persons fall into two groups: those whose methylphenidate-induced tics resolve immediately upon metabolism of the dosage and a smaller group in whom methylphenidate appears to trigger tics that persist for several months but eventually resolve spontaneously.

Longitudinal studies do not indicate that sympathomimetics cause growth suppression. Sympathomimetics may exacerbate glaucoma, hypertension, cardiovascular disorders, hyperthyroidism, anxiety disorders, psychotic disorders, and seizure disorders.

High dosages of sympathomimetics can cause dry mouth, pupillary dilation, bruxism, formication, excessive ebullience, restlessness, and emotional lability. Long-term use of high dosages can cause a delusional disorder that resembles paranoid schizophrenia. Overdoses of sympathomimetics result in hypertension, tachycardia, hyperthermia, toxic psychosis, delirium, and occasionally seizures. Overdoses of sympathomimetics can also result in death, often due to cardiac arrhythmias. Seizures can be treated with benzodiazepines, cardiac effects with β-adrenergic receptor antagonists, fever with cooling blankets, and delirium with dopamine receptor antagonists.

The most limiting adverse effect of sympathomimetics is their association with psychological and physical dependence. At the doses used for treatment of ADHD, psychological dependence virtually never develops. A larger concern is the presence of adolescent or adult cohabitants who might confiscate the supply of sympathomimetics for abuse or sale.

Table 36.4.30–1
Management of Common Stimulant-Induced Adverse Effects in Attention-Deficit/Hyperactivity Disorder

Adverse Effect	Management
Anorexia, nausea, weight loss	• Administer stimulant with meals. • Use caloric-enhanced supplements. Discourage forcing meals. • If using pemoline, check liver function tests.
Insomnia, nightmares	• Administer stimulants earlier in day. • Change to short-acting preparations. • Discontinue afternoon or evening dosing. • Consider adjunctive treatment (e.g., antihistamines, clonidine, antidepressants).
Dizziness	• Monitor blood pressure. • Encourage fluid intake. • Change to long-acting form.
Rebound phenomena	• Overlap stimulant dosing. • Change to long-acting preparation or combine long- and short-acting preparations. • Consider adjunctive or alternative treatment (e.g., clonidine, antidepressants).
Irritability	• Assess timing of phenomena (during peak or withdrawal phase). • Evaluate comorbid symptoms. • Reduce dose. • Consider adjunctive or alternative treatment (e.g., lithium, antidepressants, anticonvulsants).
Dysphoria, moodiness, agitation	• Consider comorbid diagnosis (e.g., mood disorder). • Reduce dose or change to long-acting preparation. • Consider adjunctive or alternative treatment (e.g., lithium, anticonvulsants, antidepressants).

From Wilens TE, Biederman J. The stimulants. In: Shatter D, ed. *The Psychiatric Clinics of North America: Pediatric Psychopharmacology.* Philadelphia: WB Saunders; 1992, with permission.

The use of sympathomimetics should be avoided during pregnancy, especially during the first trimester. Dextroamphetamine and methylphenidate pass into the breast milk, and it is not known whether pemoline and modafinil do.

A review of postmarketing experience with pemoline from 1975 to 1996 found 13 cases of acute hepatic failure, 10 of which were in children. This prompted the Food and Drug Administration (FDA) to change the package insert to recommend that pemoline no longer be considered first-line therapy for ADHD.

DRUG–DRUG INTERACTIONS

Coadministration of sympathomimetics and tricyclic or tetracyclic antidepressants, warfarin (Coumadin), primidone (Mysoline), phenobarbital (Luminal), phenytoin (Dilantin), or phenylbutazone (Butazolidin) decreases the metabolism of these compounds, resulting in increased plasma levels. Sympathomimetics decrease the therapeutic efficacy of many antihypertensive drugs, especially

Table 36.4.30–2
Sympathomimetics Commonly Used in Psychiatry

Generic Name	Trade Name	Preparations	Initial Daily Dose	Usual Daily Dose for ADHD[a]	Usual Daily Dose for Narcolepsy	Maximum Daily Dose
Amphetamine-dextro-amphetamine	Adderall	5-, 10-, 20-, 30-mg tablets; 10-, 20-, 30-mg extended-release (ER) tablets	5–10 mg	20–30 mg	5–60 mg	Children: 40 mg Adults: 60 mg
Dextroamphetamine	Dexedrine, DextroStat	5-, 10-, 15-mg ER capsules; 5-, 10-mg tablets	5–10 mg	20–30 mg	5–60 mg	Children: 40 mg Adults: 60 mg
Modafinil	Provigil	100-, 200-mg tablets	100 mg	Not used	400 mg	400 mg
Methamphetamine	Desoxyn	5-mg tablets; 5-, 10-, 15-mg ER tablets	5–10 mg	20–25 mg	Not generally used	45 mg
Methylphenidate	Ritalin, Methidate, Methylin, Attenade	5-, 10-, 15-, 20-mg tablets; 10-, 20-mg SR tablets	5–10 mg	5–60 mg	20–30 mg	Children: 80 mg Adults: 90 mg
	Concerta	18-, 36-, 54-mg ER tablets	18 mg	18–54 mg	Not yet established	54 mg
Dexmethylphenidate	Focalin	2.5-, 5-, 10-mg tablets	2.5 mg	5–20 mg	Not yet established	60 mg
Pemoline	Cylert	18.75-, 37.5-, 75-mg tablets; 37.5 chewable tablets	37.5 mg	56.25–75 mg	Not used	112.5 mg

[a]For children 6 years of age or older.

guanethidine (Esimil, Ismelin). The sympathomimetics should be used with extreme caution with monoamine oxidase inhibitors.

LABORATORY INTERFERENCES

Dextroamphetamine may elevate plasma corticosteroid levels and interfere falsely with some assay methods for urinary corticosteroids.

DOSAGE AND ADMINISTRATION

The dosage ranges and the available preparations for sympathomimetics are presented in Table 36.4.30–2. Dextroamphetamine, dexmethylphenidate, methylphenidate, amphetamine, benzphetamine, and methamphetamine are Schedule II drugs and in some states require official government-regulated prescriptions. Phendimetrazine and phenmetrazine are Schedule III drugs, and modafinil, phentermine, diethylpropion, and mazindol are Schedule IV drugs.

Pretreatment evaluation should include an evaluation of the person's cardiac function, with particular attention to the presence of hypertension or tachyarrhythmias. The clinician should also examine the person for the presence of movement disorders, such as tics and dyskinesia, because these conditions can be exacerbated by the use of sympathomimetics. If tics are present, many experts will not use sympathomimetics, but will instead choose clonidine or an antidepressant. However, recent data indicate that sympathomimetics may cause only a mild increase in motor tics and may actually suppress vocal tics. Liver function and renal function should be assessed, and dosages of sympathomimetics should be reduced for persons with impaired metabolism. In the case of pemoline, any elevation of liver enzymes is a compelling reason to discontinue use of the medication.

Persons with ADHD can take immediate-release methylphenidate at 8 AM, 12 noon, and 4 PM. Sustained-released amphetamine, sustained-release methylphenidate, or extended-release methylphenidate may be taken once at 8 AM. The starting dosage of methylphenidate ranges from 2.5 to 20 mg daily. If this is inadequate, the dosage may be increased to a maximum of 80 mg. Dexmethylphenidate is given twice daily, starting at 5 mg per day and increasing to 20 mg per day. The dosage of dextroamphetamine is 2.5 to 40 mg a day. Pemoline is given in dosages of 18.75 to 112.5 mg a day. Liver function tests should be monitored when using pemoline. Although it is not clear that routine liver screening can predict acute liver failure due to pemoline, it is certainly necessary to stop pemoline use if screening tests give any hint of hepatic dysfunction. Children are generally more sensitive to adverse effects than adults are. Dosing for treatment of narcolepsy and depression is comparable to that for treatment of ADHD.

Many psychiatrists believe that amphetamine use has been overly regulated by governmental authorities. Amphetamines are listed as Schedule II drugs by the U.S. Drug Enforcement Agency (DEA). In some states physicians must use official prescriptions for such drugs, with a copy filed with a state government agency. Such mandates worry both patients and physicians about breaches in confidentiality, and physicians are concerned that their prescribing practices may be misinterpreted by official agencies. Consequently, some physicians may withhold prescriptions of sympathomimetics, even from persons who may benefit from the medications.

MODAFINIL

Modafinil (Provigil) is a unique compound among the currently approved psychostimulant drugs. Modafinil is approved for use

in improving wakefulness in patients with excessive daytime sleepiness associated with narcolepsy. The mechanism of action is unknown, but the novel effects of modafinil are prompting clinicians to use the drug to treat daytime sleepiness in other neurologic and psychiatric conditions.

Chemistry

The molecular structure of modafinil is shown in Fig. 36.4.30–1.

Pharmacological Actions

Modafinil is rapidly absorbed from the gastrointestinal tract and reaches peak plasma concentrations in 2 to 4 hours, has a half-life of about 15 hours, and reaches steady state after 2 to 4 days of daily dosing. Food does not affect the bioavailability of modafinil, but may delay its rate of absorption, which could be clinically meaningful if the patient is in need of therapeutic effects early in the morning. Modafinil is metabolized in the liver and the metabolites are secreted primarily through the kidney.

The mechanism of action for the wakefulness-inducing properties of modafinil is not known. One possibility is that modafinil acts as a weak inhibitor of dopamine reuptake. This is supported in in vitro models by the observation of an increase in extracellular dopamine levels without an increase in dopamine release.

Therapeutic Indications

The only approved indication for modafinil is to reduce the daytime sleepiness in patients with narcolepsy. It is important to note that modafinil does not treat the underlying narcolepsy itself. The studies done for approval of modafinil were 9 weeks in duration, but patients were also continued in open-label studies, which demonstrated continued benefit of the drug in studies up to four years long.

Since the launch of modafinil, clinicians have used modafinil to treat daytime sedation in other neurological and psychiatric disorders. The neurological disorders that have been studied include Parkinson's disease and multiple sclerosis, both of which are associated with daytime sedation in many patients. The fatigue associated with depression has also been reported to be improved with the use of modafinil. The use of modafinil in these indications is currently under investigation in larger, well-controlled studies. Because of the effect on alertness, modafinil has also been studied in children with ADHD, and some of the preliminary studies in this disorder have been positive.

Effects on Specific Organs and Systems

Central Nervous System. In in vitro studies modafinil shows some characteristics of sympathomimetic drugs, including self-administration of modafinil by a monkey previously trained to self-administer cocaine, and also some evidence that it was partially discriminated by animals as stimulantlike. In humans, modafinil has been reported to be associated with euphoric effects, alterations in mood, perception, and thinking.

Cardiovascular System. There were a small number of cardiovascular-related adverse effects in the narcolepsy clinical studies; therefore, it is currently not recommended that modafinil be used in combination with sympathomimetic drugs in patients who are at increased risk of cardiovascular disorders (e.g., history of left ventricular hypertrophy, ischemic ECG changes, recent history of myocardial infarction).

Precautions and Adverse Effects

The most common adverse effects associated with modafinil use are headache and nausea. Modafinil is not associated with changes in vital signs, ECG measurements, or weight. In general, modafinil is a well-tolerated drug.

Abuse Potential. Because modafinil has some properties somewhat similar to the sympathomimetic drugs, use of modafinil in patients with a history of stimulant abuse should be avoided or carefully monitored if prescribed. In clinical studies, no withdrawal symptoms were seen related to the discontinuation of modafinil use.

Pregnancy. As with most other psychoactive drugs, modafinil should not be used in women who are pregnant. It is not known whether or not modafinil is excreted in human milk; therefore, nursing mothers should not be prescribed modafinil at this time.

Drug–Drug Interactions

Modafinil is metabolized by cytochrome P450 (CYP) isoenzyme 2C9 and also causes a modest induction of CYP 3A4 with chronic administration. An important result of the CYP 3A4 induction is that plasma concentrations of low-dose steroidal contraceptives may be reduced to levels below therapeutic effectiveness. Upward adjustment of the dose of low-dose steroidal contraceptives and some other drugs metabolized by CYP 3A4 (e.g., cyclosporine, theophylline) might be warranted. The competitive effects of modafinil on the enzyme CYP 2C9 could result in increased plasma concentrations of other CYP 2C9 substrates such as diazepam, phenytoin, and propranolol.

Laboratory Interferences

There have been no laboratory interferences reported for modafinil.

Dosage and Administration

Modafinil is supplied as 100- and 200-mg tablets. The starting dosage is 200 mg a day given once in the morning. Some patients may require 300 to 400 mg a day, also given once in the morning. These doses are for the approved indication in narcolepsy, but these are also the range of doses that have been used by clinicians in other indications as well.

References

Fawcett J. Sympathomimetics. In: Sadock BJ, Sadock VA, eds. *Kaplan & Sadock's Comprehensive Textbook of Psychiatry.* 7th ed. Vol 2. Baltimore: Lippincott Williams & Wilkins; 2000:2474.

Fawcett J, Busch KA. Stimulants in psychiatry. In: Schatzberg AF, Nemeroff CB, eds. *Essentials of Clinical Psychopharmacology.* Washington, DC: American Psychiatric Association; 2001:303.

Greenhill LL, Ford RE. Childhood attention-deficit hyperactivity disorder: pharmacological treatments. In: Nathan PE, Gorman JM, eds. *A Guide to Treatments That Work.* 2nd ed. London: Oxford University Press; 2002:25.

Hoffman BB. Catecholamines, sympathomimetic drugs, and adrenergic receptor antagonists. In: Hardman JG, Limbird LE, Goodman Gilman A, eds. *Goodman & Gilman's the Pharmacological Basis of Therapeutics.* 10th ed. New York: McGraw-Hill; 2001:215.
Levy F, Hobbes G. Does haloperidol block methylphenidate? *Psychopharmacology.* 1996;126:70.
Littner M, Johnson SF, McCall V, et al. Practice parameters for the treatment of narcolepsy: an update for 2000. *Sleep.* 2001;24:451.
Mattay VS, Berman KF, Ostrem JL, et al. Dextroamphetamine enhances "neural network-specific" physiological signals: a positron-emission tomography rCBF study. *J Neurosci.* 1996;16:4816.
Nieves AV, Lang AE. Treatment of excessive daytime sleepiness in patients with Parkinson's disease with modafinil. *Clin Neuropharmacol.* 2002;25:111.
Olin J, Masand P. Psychostimulants for depression in hospitalized cancer patients. *Psychosomatics.* 1996;37:57.
Ross DC, Fischhoff J, Davenport B. Treatment of ADHD when tolerance to methylphenidate develops. *Psychiatr Serv.* 2002;53:102.
Scammel TE, Estabrooke IV, McCarthy MT, et al. Hypothalamic arousal regions are activated during modafinil-induced wakefulness. *J Neurosci.* 2000;10:8620.
Spiga R, Pearson DA, Broitman M, Santos CW. Effects of methylphenidate on cooperative responding in children with attention-deficit hyperactivity disorder. *Exp Clin Psychopharmacol.* 1996;4:451.
Stoll AL, Pillay SS, Diamond L, Workum A. Methylphenidate augmentation of serotonin selective reuptake inhibitors: a case series. *J Clin Psychiatry.* 1996;57:72.
Taylor FB, Russo J. Efficacy of modafinil compared to dextroamphetamine for the treatment of attention deficit hyperactivity disorder in adults. *J Child Adolesc Psychopharmacol.* 2000;10:311.
Teitelman E. Modafinil for narcolepsy. *Am J Psychiatry.* 2001;158:970.
US Modafinil in Narcolepsy Multicenter Study Group: Randomized trial of modafinil for the treatment of pathological somnolence in narcolepsy. *Ann Neurol.* 1997;43:88.
Wagner GJ, Rabkin R. Effects of dextroamphetamine on depression and fatigue in men with HIV: a double-blind, placebo-controlled trial. *J Clin Psychiatry.* 2000;61:436.
Wensten NJ, Belenky G, Kautz MA, Thorne DR, Reichardt RM, Balkin TJ. Maintaining alertness and performance during sleep deprivation: modafinil versus caffeine. *Psychopharmacology.* 2002;159:238.

▲ 36.4.31 Thyroid Hormones

Thyroid hormones—levothyroxine (Synthroid, Levothroid, Levoxine) and liothyronine (Cytomel)—are used in psychiatry either alone or as augmentation to treat persons with depression or rapid-cycling bipolar I disorder. They can convert an antidepressant-nonresponsive person into an antidepressant-responsive person. Thyroid hormones are also used as replacement therapy for persons who have developed a hypothyroid state due to lithium (Eskalith) treatment.

CHEMISTRY

The molecular structures of levothyroxine and liothyronine are shown in Figure 36.4.31–1. Both endogenous levothyroxine and exogenous liothyronine are converted into triiodothyronine in the body.

PHARMACOLOGICAL ACTIONS

Thyroid hormones are administered orally, and their absorption from the gastrointestinal tract is variable. Absorption is increased if the drug is administered while the patient's stomach is empty. The half-life of levothyroxine is 6 to 7 days, and the half-life of liothyronine is 1 to 2 days.

The mechanism of action for thyroid hormone effects on antidepressant efficacy is unknown, but interactions with the β-adrenergic receptors may be involved. Thyroid hormone is essential to the proper functioning of all neurons. It binds to intracellular

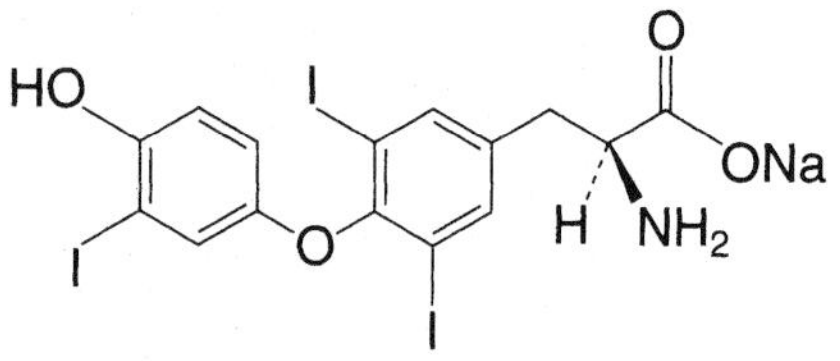

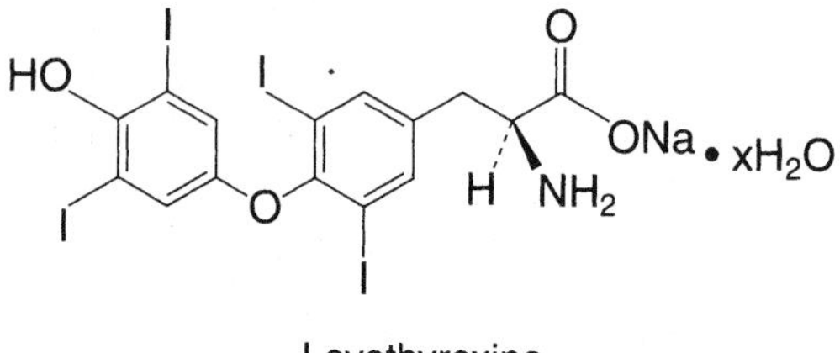

FIGURE 36.4.31–1
Molecular structures of liothyronine and levothyroxine.

receptors that regulate the transcription of a wide range of genes, including several receptors for neurotransmitters.

EFFECTS ON SPECIFIC ORGANS AND SYSTEMS

The effects of the drugs levothyroxine and liothyronine on specific organs and systems are the same as the effects of endogenous thyroid hormones, and the symptoms of toxicity and overdose are the symptoms of hyperthyroidism. Thyroid hormones affect most of the body's organs and systems, especially the cardiovascular system.

THERAPEUTIC INDICATIONS

The major indication for thyroid hormones in psychiatry is as an adjuvant to antidepressants. There is no clear correlation between the laboratory measures of thyroid function and the response to thyroid hormone supplementation of antidepressants. If a patient has not responded to a 6-week course of antidepressants at appropriate dosages, adjuvant therapy with either lithium or a thyroid hormone is an alternative. Most clinicians use adjuvant lithium before trying a thyroid hormone. Several controlled trials have indicated that liothyronine use converts about 50 percent of antidepressant nonresponders to responders.

Thyroid hormones have not been shown to cause particular problems in pediatric or geriatric patients; however, the hormones should be used with caution in the elderly, who may have occult heart disease.

PRECAUTIONS AND ADVERSE REACTIONS

The most common adverse effects associated with thyroid hormones are weight loss, palpitations, nervousness, diarrhea, abdominal cramps, sweating, tachycardia, increased blood pressure, tremors, headache, and insomnia. Osteoporosis may also occur with long-term treatment. Overdoses of thyroid hormones can lead to cardiac failure and death.

Thyroid hormones should not be administered to patients with cardiac disease, angina, or hypertension. The hormones are contraindicated in thyrotoxicosis and uncorrected adrenal insufficiency and in patients with acute myocardial infarctions. Because thyroid hormones do not cross the placenta, they can be administered safely to pregnant women. Thyroid hormones are minimally excreted in the breast milk and have not been shown to cause problems to women who are nursing infants.

DRUG–DRUG INTERACTIONS

Thyroid hormones can potentiate the effects of warfarin (Coumadin) and other anticoagulants by increasing the catabolism of clotting factors. Thyroid hormones may increase the insulin requirement for patients with diabetes. Sympathomimetics and thyroid hormones should not be coadministered because of the risk of cardiac decompensation.

LABORATORY INTERFERENCES

Levothyroxine has not been reported to interfere with any laboratory test. Liothyronine use, however, suppresses the release of endogenous T_4, thus lowering the value of any thyroid function test that depends on measuring T_4. The value for TSH is not affected by either levothyroxine or liothyronine administration.

DOSAGE AND ADMINISTRATION

Liothyronine is available in 5-, 25-, and 50-μg tablets. Levothyroxine is available in 12.5-, 25-, 50-, 75-, 88-, 100-, 112-, 125-, 137-, 150-, 175-, 200-, and 300-μg tablets; it is also available in a 200- and 500-μg parenteral form. The dosage of liothyronine is 25 or 50 μg a day added to the patient's antidepressant regimen. Liothyronine has been used as an adjuvant for all the available antidepressant drugs. An adequate trial of liothyronine supplementation should last 7 to 14 days. If liothyronine supplementation is successful, it should be continued for 2 months and then tapered at the rate of 12.5 μg a day every 3 to 7 days.

REFERENCES

Aronson R, Offman HJ, Joffe RT, Naylor CD. Triiodothyronine augmentation in the treatment of refractory depression: a meta-analysis. *Arch Gen Psychiatry.* 1996;53:842.

Baumgartner A, Bauer M, Hellweg R. Treatment of intractable non–rapid cycling bipolar affective disorder with high-dose thyroxine: an open clinical trial. *Neuropsychopharmacology.* 1994;10:183.

Gitlin MJ. Treatment-resistant bipolar disorder. *Bull Menninger Clin.* 2000;65:26.

Harris B. Hormonal aspects of postnatal depression. *Int Rev Psychiatry.* 1996;8:27.

Hopkins HS, Gelenberg AJ. Treatment of bipolar disorder: how far have we gone? *Psychopharmacol Bull.* 1994;30:27.

Joffe RT. Thyroid hormones. In: Sadock BJ, Sadock VA, eds. *Kaplan & Sadock's Comprehensive Textbook of Psychiatry.* 7th ed. Vol 2. Baltimore: Lippincott Williams & Wilkins; 2000:2478.

Joffe RT, Sokolov STH. Thyroid hormone treatment of primary unipolar depression: a review. *Int J Neuropsychopharmacol.* 2000;3:143.

Prohaska ML. Thyroid, lithium, and cognition: the use of thyroid hormone augmentation in the reduction of cognitive side effects associated with lithium maintenance. *Diss Abstr Int B Sci Eng.* 1994;55:603.

Prohaska ML, Stern RA, Nevels CT, et al. The relationship between thyroid status and neuropsychological performance in psychiatric outpatients maintained on lithium. *Neuropsychiatry Neuropsychol Behav Neurol.* 1996;9:30.

Suzuki K, Kusumi I, Inoue T, et al. Effect of thyroxine for treatment-resistant affective disorder [Japanese]. *Seishin Igaku (Clin Psychiatry).* 1995;37:477.

Terao T, Oga T, Nozaki S, et al. Possible inhibitory effect of lithium on peripheral conversion of thyroxine to triiodothyronine: a prospective study. *Int Clin Psychopharmacol.* 1995;10:103.

Verdoux H, Mury M, Bourgeois M. Comorbidity of bipolar disorder and bulimia nervosa. *Eur Psychiatry.* 1994;9:315.

▲ 36.4.32 Trazodone

Trazodone (Desyrel) is effective in the treatment of depressive disorders. It is structurally unrelated to the tricyclic and tetracyclic drugs used to treat depressive disorders, the monoamine oxidase inhibitors (MAOIs), selective serotonin reuptake inhibitors (SSRIs), and other currently available antidepressant drugs. Trazodone may have benefit in anxiety disorders such as panic disorder and obsessive-compulsive disorder. It is chemically related to nefazodone (Serzone), which is discussed in Section 36.4.21.

Trazodone differs from tricyclic and tetracyclic drugs and from MAOIs in having almost no anticholinergic adverse effects. It is also distinctive in having more marked sedative effects than are found with other antidepressants. For this reason it is used to treat insomnia.

CHEMISTRY

Trazodone is a triazolopyridine derivative that shares the triazolo ring structure with alprazolam (Xanax), a benzodiazepine with possible antidepressant effects (Fig. 36.4.32–1).

Trazodone is readily absorbed from the gastrointestinal tract, reaches peak plasma levels in 1 to 2 hours, and has a half-life of 6 to 11 hours. It is metabolized in the liver, and 75 percent of its metabolites are excreted in the urine. The active metabolite of trazodone is *m*-chlorophenylpiperazine (mCPP).

Trazodone has its therapeutic effects as a relatively specific inhibitor of serotonin reuptake; mCPP also possesses some postsynaptic serotonin activity. The adverse effects of trazodone are partially mediated by α_1-adrenergic antagonism and antihistaminergic activity. Long-term administration of trazodone appears to decrease the number of postsynaptic serotonin type 2A ($5\text{-}HT_{2A}$) and β-adrenergic receptors.

EFFECTS ON SPECIFIC ORGANS AND SYSTEMS

Aside from its effects on the central nervous system (CNS), trazodone has relatively few effects on organs and systems. The effects it does have are primarily the result of its α_1-adrenergic antagonism, which can affect vascular tone and result in ortho-

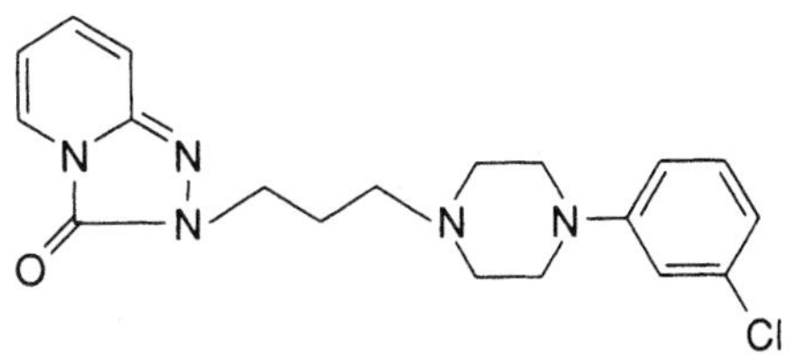

FIGURE 36.4.32–1
Molecular structure of trazodone.

static hypotension. The drug is also associated with gastric irritation. Relatively rare among the antidepressants is trazodone's association with priapism, which is also probably a result of its α_1-adrenergic antagonist activity. Trazodone has weak activity as a relaxer of skeletal muscles.

THERAPEUTIC INDICATIONS

Depressive Disorders

The primary indication for the use of trazodone is major depressive disorder. Trazodone is as effective as the standard antidepressants in short-term and long-term treatment of major depressive disorder. The drug is particularly effective at improving sleep quality—increasing total sleep time, decreasing the number and duration of nighttime awakenings, and decreasing the amount of rapid eye movement (REM) sleep. Unlike tricyclic drugs, trazodone does not decrease stage 4 sleep. Trazodone may be less likely than tricyclic drugs to precipitate mania.

Insomnia

The marked sedative qualities of trazodone and its favorable effects on sleep architecture have suggested to many clinicians that it would be effective as a hypnotic, and a number of clinicians have used trazodone effectively for this purpose. A recent controlled study confirmed that trazodone is superior to placebo for treatment of insomnia. It has also been used effectively as a hypnotic in combination with less sedating psychotropic drugs. Trazodone has been reported to be useful in treating fluoxetine (Prozac)-induced insomnia. The usual dosage is 50 to 100 mg at bedtime.

Other Indications

Some data indicate that trazodone may be useful in low dosages (50 mg a day) for controlling severe agitation in elderly patients, particularly those with personality change due to a general medical condition. A few case reports and uncontrolled trials of trazodone have indicated its usefulness in the treatment of depression with marked anxiety symptoms, of posttraumatic stress disorder, and of panic disorder with agoraphobia. Because it does not worsen psychotic symptoms, trazodone is preferable to tricyclic drugs as adjunctive treatment for schizophrenia. Limited data support an adjunctive role for trazodone in treatment of alcohol-induced tremor, alcohol-induced depressive disorder, and alcohol-induced anxiety disorder; anxiety; obsessive-compulsive disorder; eating disorders; chronic pain; autistic disorder; male erectile disorder; and paraphilias. The final evaluation of the use of trazodone in the treatment of these disorders requires further research.

PRECAUTIONS AND ADVERSE REACTIONS

The most common adverse effects associated with trazodone are sedation, orthostatic hypotension, dizziness, headache, and nausea. As a result of α_1-adrenergic blockade, dry mouth is present in some patients. Trazodone may also cause gastric irritation. The drug is not associated with the usual anticholinergic adverse effects, such as urinary retention and constipation. A few case reports have noted an association between trazodone and arrhythmias in patients with preexisting premature ventricular contractions or mitral valve prolapse. Neutropenia, usually not clinically significant, may develop and should be considered if patients have fever or sore throat.

Trazodone is relatively safe in overdose attempts. No fatalities from trazodone overdoses have been reported when the drug was taken alone, but there have been fatalities when trazodone was taken with other drugs. The symptoms of overdose include priapism, loss of muscle coordination, nausea and vomiting, and drowsiness. Trazodone does not have the quinidine-like antiarrhythmic effects of imipramine (Tofranil).

As mentioned above, trazodone is associated with the rare occurrence of priapism, prolonged erection in the absence of sexual stimuli. Patients should be advised to tell their clinicians if erections are gradually becoming frequent or prolonged. Physicians should strongly consider switching these patients to another antidepressant medication. Other forms of sexual dysfunction may also occur with trazodone treatment. The use of trazodone is contraindicated in pregnant and nursing women, and it should be used with caution in patients with hepatic and renal diseases.

DRUG–DRUG INTERACTIONS

Trazodone potentiates the CNS depressant effects of other centrally acting drugs and alcohol. The combination of MAOIs and trazodone should be avoided. Trazodone concentrations are increased by fluoxetine, and trazodone increases concentrations of digoxin (Lanoxin) and phenytoin (Dilantin). Concurrent use of trazodone and antihypertensives may cause hypotension. Electroconvulsive therapy concurrent with trazodone administration should also be avoided.

LABORATORY INTERFERENCES

No known laboratory interferences are associated with the use of trazodone.

DOSAGE AND ADMINISTRATION

The sedative effects of trazodone appear within 1 hour of administration, whereas the antidepressant effects usually appear after 2 to 4 weeks of treatment. Trazodone is available in tablets that can be divided into 50-, 100-, 150-, and 300-mg amounts. The usual starting dose is 50 mg orally the first day. The dosage can be increased to 50 mg orally twice daily on the second day and possibly 50 mg orally 3 times daily on the third and fourth days if sedation or orthostatic hypotension does not become a problem. The therapeutic range for trazodone is 200 to 600 mg a day in divided doses. Some reports indicate that dosages of 400 to 600 mg a day are required for maximal therapeutic effects; other reports indicate that 300 to 400 mg a day is sufficient. The dosage may be titrated up to 300 mg a day; then the patient can be evaluated for the need for further dosage increases on the basis of the presence or the absence of signs of clinical improvement.

References

Baldessarini RJ. Drugs and the treatment of psychiatric disorders: depression and anxiety disorders. In: Hardman JG, Limbird LE, Goodman Gilman A, eds. *Goodman & Gilman's the Pharmacological Basis of Therapeutics.* 10th ed. New York: McGraw-Hill; 2001:447.

Balon R. Sleep terror disorder and insomnia treated with trazodone: a case report. *Ann Clin Psychiatry.* 1994;6:161.
Cunningham LA, Borison RL, Carman JS, et al. A comparison of venlafaxine, trazodone, and placebo in major depression. *J Clin Psychopharmacol.* 1994;14:99.
Garlow SJ, Nemeroff GB. Trazodone. In: Sadock BJ, Sadock VA, eds. *Kaplan & Sadock's Comprehensive Textbook of Psychiatry.* 7th ed. Vol 2. Baltimore: Lippincott Williams & Wilkins; 2000:2482.
Khouzam HR, Mayo-Smith MF, Bernard DR, et al. Treatment of crack-cocaine-induced compulsive behavior with trazodone. *J Subst Abuse Treat.* 1995;12:85.
Otani K, Yasui N, Kaneko S, et al. Trazodone treatment increases plasma prolactin concentrations in depressed patients. *Int Clin Psychopharmacol.* 1995;10:115.
Reeves RR, Bullen JA. Serotonin syndrome produced by paroxetine and low-dose trazodone. *Psychosomatics.* 1995;36:159.
Staner L, Luthringer R, Macher JP. Effects of antidepressant drugs on sleep EEG inpatients with major depression: mechanisms and therapeutic implications. *CNS Drugs.* 1999;11:49.
Sultzer DL. Selective serotonin reuptake inhibitors and trazodone for treatment of depression, psychosis and behavioral symptoms in patients with dementia. *Int Psychogeriatr.* 2000;12(suppl 1):245.
Ware JC, Rose FV, McBrayer RH. The acute effects of nefazodone, trazodone and buspirone on sleep and sleep-related penile tumescence in normal subjects. *Sleep.* 1994;17:544.
Zarate CA, Tohen M, Baraibar G. Prescribing trends of antidepressants in bipolar depression. *J Clin Psychiatry.* 1995;56:260.

▲ 36.4.33 Tricyclics and Tetracyclics

The tricyclic antidepressants and the tetracyclic antidepressants (commonly abbreviated *TCAs*) are effective treatments for persons with a wide range of disorders, including depression, panic disorder, generalized anxiety disorder, posttraumatic stress disorder, obsessive-compulsive disorder, eating disorders, and pain syndromes. With the current availability of several less toxic alternatives, including the selective serotonin reuptake inhibitors (SSRIs), bupropion (Wellbutrin), nefazodone (Serzone), venlafaxine (Effexor), trazodone (Desyrel), and mirtazapine (Remeron), the TCAs are no longer widely used for these indications.

CHEMISTRY

All tricyclics have a three-ring nucleus in their molecular structures (Fig. 36.4.33–1). Imipramine (Tofranil), amitriptyline (Elavil), clomipramine (Anafranil), trimipramine (Surmontil), and doxepin (Adapin, Sinequan) are called *tertiary amines* because two methyl groups are on the nitrogen atom of the side chain. Desipramine (Norpramin), nortriptyline (Pamelor, Aventyl), and protriptyline (Vivactil) are called *secondary amines* because only one methyl group is in the position. The tertiary amines are metabolized into their corresponding secondary amines in the body.

The arbitrary classification of tetracyclic drugs is based on a gross count of the number of rings in their molecular structures. Amoxapine (Asendin), a dibenzoxazepine, is a derivative of the antipsychotic drug loxapine (Loxitane) and has a cyclic side chain off the three-ring nucleus, for a total of four rings. Maprotiline (Ludiomil) is a tetracyclic with the same side chain as desipramine; its fourth ring bridges the center of the standard tricyclic nucleus. Mianserin is a tetracyclic drug whose side chain has been cyclized to form a fourth ring; mianserin is not currently available for clinical use in the United States.

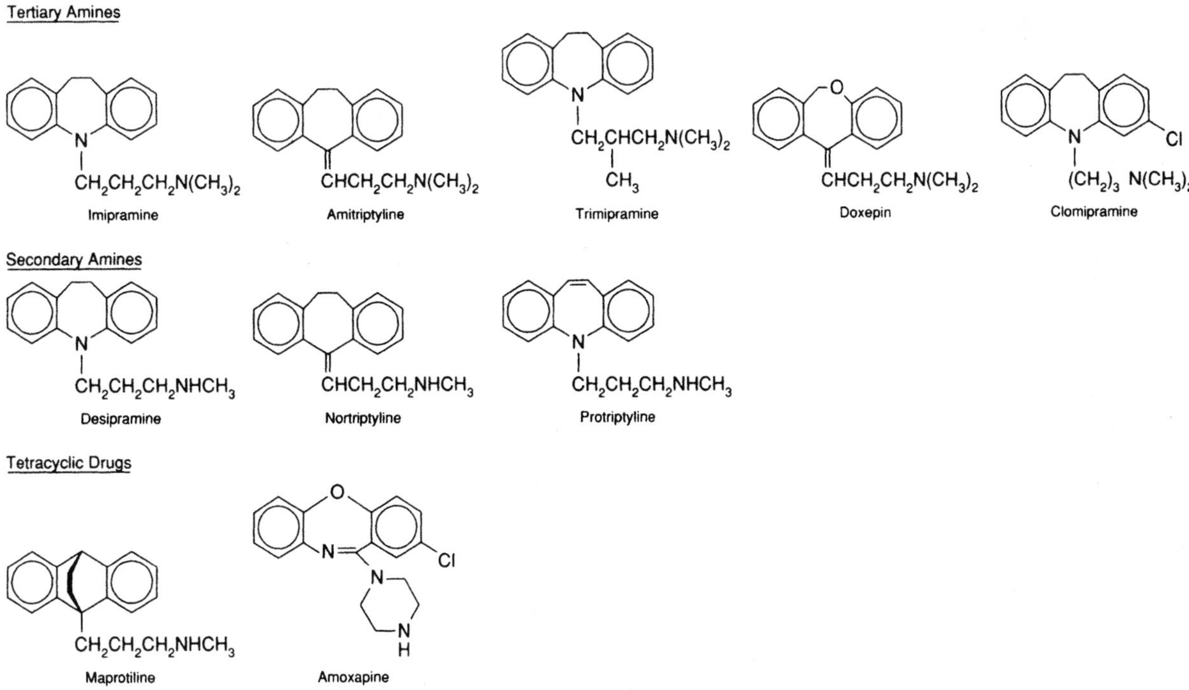

FIGURE 36.4.33–1
Molecular structures of tricyclic and tetracyclic drugs.

PHARMACOLOGICAL ACTIONS

Most TCAs are completely absorbed from oral administration, and there is significant metabolism from the first-pass effect. Peak plasma concentrations occur within 2 to 8 hours, and the half-lives of the TCAs vary from 10 to 70 hours; nortriptyline, maprotiline, and particularly protriptyline can have longer half-lives. The long half-lives allow all these compounds to be given once daily; 5 to 7 days are needed to reach steady-state plasma concentrations. Imipramine pamoate is a depot form of the drug for intramuscular (IM) administration; indications for the use of this preparation are limited.

TCAs undergo hepatic metabolism by the cytochrome P450 enzyme system. Clinically relevant drug interactions may result from competition for enzyme P450 (CYP) 2D6 between TCAs and quinidine (Cardioquin), cimetidine (Tagamet), fluoxetine (Prozac), sertraline (Zoloft), paroxetine (Paxil), phenothiazines, carbamazepine (Tegretol), and the type IC antiarrhythmics propafenone (Rythmol) and flecainide (Tambocor). Concomitant administration of TCAs and these inhibitors may slow the metabolism and raise the plasma concentrations of TCAs. Additionally, genetic variations in the activity of CYP 2D6 may account for up to a 40-fold difference in plasma TCA concentrations in different persons. The dosage of the TCA may need to be adjusted to correct changes in the rate of hepatic TCA metabolism.

TCAs block the reuptake of norepinephrine and serotonin and are competitive antagonists at the muscarinic acetylcholine, histamine H_1, and α_1- and α_2-adrenergic receptors (Table 36.4.33–1). Amoxapine, nortriptyline, desipramine, and maprotiline have the least anticholinergic activity; doxepin has the most antihistaminergic activity; clomipramine is the most serotonin-selective of the TCAs. A metabolite of amoxapine has potent dopamine-blocking activity, thus causing antipsychotic-like neurological and endocrinological adverse effects.

EFFECTS ON SPECIFIC ORGANS AND SYSTEMS

The major effects of the TCAs are on the central nervous system (CNS), although the anticholinergic effects of these drugs produce a diverse range of adverse effects mediated by the autonomic nervous system (Table 36.4.33–2). In addition to these effects, the TCAs have significant effects on the cardiovascular system. In therapeutic dosages, the drugs are classified as type 1A antiarrhythmic drugs, as they terminate ventricular fibrillation and can increase the collateral blood supply to an ischemic heart. In overdoses, however, the drugs are highly cardiotoxic and cause decreased contractility, increased myocardial irritability, hypotension, and tachycardia.

THERAPEUTIC INDICATIONS

Major Depressive Disorder

The treatment of a major depressive episode and the prophylactic treatment of major depressive disorder are the principal indications for using TCAs. The drugs are also effective in treating depression in patients with bipolar I disorder. Melancholic features, previous major depressive episodes, and a family history of depressive disorders increase the likelihood of a therapeutic response. The treatment of a major depressive episode with psychotic features almost always requires coadministration of an antipsychotic drug and an antidepressant.

Mood Disorder Due to a General Medical Condition with Depressive Features

Depression associated with a general medical condition (secondary depression) may respond to TCA treatment. Depression is associated with dementias and with movement disorders such as Parkinson's disease. Depression associated with acquired immune deficiency syndrome (AIDS) may respond to the drugs.

Panic Disorder with Agoraphobia

Imipramine is the tricyclic most studied for panic disorder with agoraphobia, but other TCAs are also effective. Early reports indicated that small dosages of imipramine (50 mg a day) were often effective; recent studies, however, indicate that the usual

Table 36.4.33–1
Neurotransmitter Effects of Tricyclic and Tetracyclic Drugs

	Reuptake Blockade		Receptor Blockade		
Drug	NE	5-HT	Muscarinic Ach	H_1	H_2
Imipramine	+	+	++	±	±
Desipramine	+++	±	±	–	–
Trimipramine	±	±	++	++	?
Amitriptyline	±	++	+++	++	++
Nortriptyline	++	±	+	±	±
Protriptyline	+++	±	+	+++	–
Amoxapine	++	±	+	±	?
Doxepin	+	±	++	+++	+
Maprotiline	+++	–	+	±	?
Clomipramine	±	++	+	?	?

NE, norepinephrine; 5-HT, serotonin; ACh, acetylcholine; H_1, histamine type 1; H_2, histamine type 2.

Table 36.4.33–2
Side-Effect Profile of Tricyclic and Tetracyclic Antidepressants

Drug	Anticholinergic Effects	Sedation	Orthostatic Hypotension	Seizures	Conduction Abnormalities
Tertiary amines					
Amitriptyline	++++	++++	+++	+++	++++
Clomipramine	++++	++++	+++	+++	++++
Doxepin	+++	++++	++	+++	++
Imipramine	+++	+++	++++	+++	++++
Trimipramine	++++	++++	+++	+++	+++++
Secondary amines					
Desipramine	++	++	+++	++	+++
Nortriptyline	+++	+++	+	++	+++
Protriptyline	+++	+	++	++	++++
Tetracyclics					
Amoxapine	+++	++	+	+++	++
Maprotiline	++	+++	++	++++	+++

++++, high; +++, moderate; ++, low; +, very low.

antidepressant dosages are usually required. In the past few years, SSRIs, especially paroxetine, have become additional agents for treatment of panic disorder.

Generalized Anxiety Disorder

The use of doxepin to treat anxiety disorders is approved by the U.S. Food and Drug Administration (FDA). Some research data show that imipramine may also be useful, and some clinicians use a drug containing a combination of chlordiazepoxide and amitriptyline (Limbitrol) for mixed anxiety and depressive disorders.

Obsessive-Compulsive Disorder

Obsessive-compulsive disorder is classified as an anxiety disorder. The disorder appears to respond specifically to clomipramine and SSRIs. None of the other TCAs appears to be nearly as effective as clomipramine for the disorder. Multicenter, placebo-controlled trials found clomipramine to be superior to SSRIs, and another controlled trial found paroxetine to be equal in efficacy to clomipramine for treatment of obsessive-compulsive disorder.

Eating Disorders

Both anorexia nervosa and bulimia nervosa have been treated successfully with imipramine and desipramine, although other TCAs may also be effective.

Pain Disorder

Chronic pain disorder, including headache (such as migraine), is often treated with TCAs.

Other Disorders

Childhood enuresis is often treated with imipramine. Peptic ulcer disease can be treated with doxepin, which has marked antihistaminergic effects. Other indications for tricyclics and tetracyclics are narcolepsy, nightmare disorder, and posttraumatic stress disorder. The drugs are sometimes used for children and adolescents with attention-deficit/hyperactivity disorder, sleepwalking disorder, separation anxiety disorder, and sleep terror disorder. Clomipramine has been used to treat premature ejaculation, movement disorders, and compulsive behavior in children with autistic disorder.

PRECAUTIONS AND ADVERSE REACTIONS

The relative concentrations at which therapeutic and adverse effects appear for TCAs are presented in Figure 36.4.33–2.

Psychiatric Effects

A major adverse effect of all TCAs and other antidepressants is the possibility of inducing a manic episode in patients with and without a history of bipolar I disorder. Clinicians should watch for this effect in patients with bipolar I disorder, especially if substance-induced mania has been a problem in the past. It is prudent to use low dosages of TCAs in such patients or to use an agent such as fluoxetine or bupropion, which may be less likely to induce a manic episode. TCAs have also been reported to exacerbate psychotic disorders in susceptible patients.

Anticholinergic Effects

Clinicians should warn patients that anticholinergic effects are common but that patients may develop a tolerance for these effects with continued treatment. Amitriptyline, imipramine, trimipramine, and doxepin are the most anticholinergic drugs; amoxapine, nortriptyline, and maprotiline are less anticholinergic; and desipramine may be the least anticholinergic. Anticholinergic effects include dry mouth, constipation, blurred vision, and urinary retention. Sugarless gum, candy, or fluoride lozenges can alleviate the dry mouth. Bethanechol (Urecholine), 25 to 50 mg three or four times a day, may reduce urinary hesi-

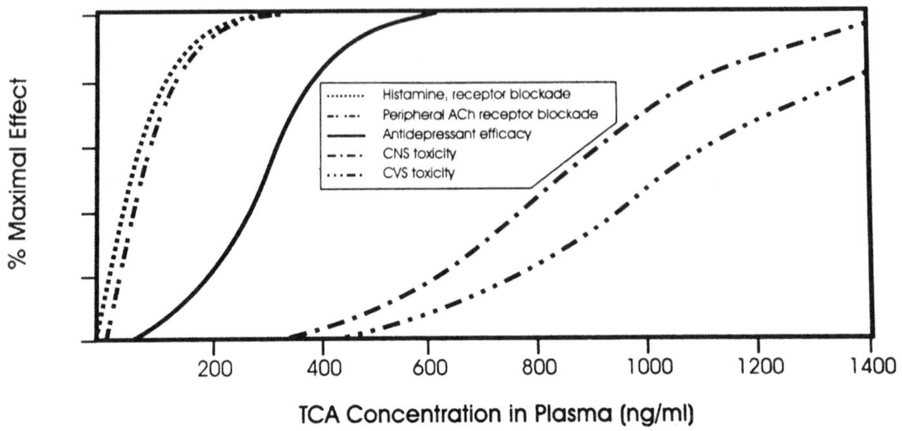

FIGURE 36.4.33–2
Multiple concentration:response curves of tertiary amine tricyclic drugs. ACh, acetylcholine; CNS, central nervous system; CVS, cardiovascular system. (Reprinted with permission from Preskorn SH. *Clinical Pharmacology of Selective Serotonin Reuptake Inhibitors*. Caddo, OK: Professional Communications; 1996:54.)

tancy and may help patients with impotence if the drug is taken 30 minutes before sexual intercourse. Narrow-angle glaucoma can also be aggravated by anticholinergic drugs, and precipitation of glaucoma requires emergency treatment with a miotic agent. TCAs can be used in patients with narrow-angle glaucoma, provided pilocarpine eyedrops are administered concurrently. Severe anticholinergic effects can lead to a CNS anticholinergic syndrome with confusion and delirium, especially if TCAs are administered with antipsychotics or anticholinergic drugs. Some clinicians have used intramuscular or intravenous physostigmine (Antilirium) as a diagnostic tool to confirm the presence of anticholinergic delirium.

Sedation

Sedation is a common effect of TCAs and may be welcomed if sleeplessness has been a problem. The sedative effect of TCAs results from serotonergic, cholinergic, and histaminergic (H_1) activities. Amitriptyline, trimipramine, and doxepin are the most sedating agents; imipramine, amoxapine, nortriptyline, and maprotiline have some sedating effects; and desipramine and protriptyline are the least sedating agents.

Autonomic Effects

The most common autonomic effect, partly because of α_1-adrenergic blockade, is orthostatic hypotension, which can result in falls and injuries in affected patients. Nortriptyline may be the drug least likely to cause the problem, and some patients respond to fludrocortisone (Florinef), 0.05 mg twice a day. Other possible autonomic effects are profuse sweating, palpitations, and increased blood pressure.

Cardiac Effects

When administered in their usual therapeutic dosages, the TCAs may cause tachycardia, flattened T waves, prolonged QT intervals, and depressed ST segments on electrocardiograms (ECGs). Imipramine has a quinidinelike effect at therapeutic plasma concentrations and may reduce the number of premature ventricular contractions. Because the drugs prolong conduction time, their use in patients with preexisting conduction defects is contraindicated. In patients with cardiac histories, TCAs should be initiated at low dosages, with gradual increases in dosage and monitoring of cardiac functions. At high plasma concentrations, as occur in overdoses, the drugs become arrhythmogenic. The agents should be discontinued several days before elective surgery because of the occurrence of hypertensive episodes during surgery in patients receiving TCAs.

Neurological Effects

In addition to the sedation induced by TCAs and the possibility of anticholinergic-induced delirium, two tricyclics—desipramine and protriptyline—are associated with psychomotor stimulation. Myoclonic twitches and tremors of the tongue and the upper extremities are common. Rare effects include speech blockage, paresthesia, peroneal palsies, and ataxia.

Amoxapine is unique in causing parkinsonian symptoms, akathisia, and even dyskinesia because of the dopaminergic blocking activity of one of its metabolites. Amoxapine may also cause neuroleptic malignant syndrome in rare cases. Maprotiline may cause seizures when the dosage is increased too quickly or is kept at high levels for too long. Clomipramine and amoxapine may lower the seizure threshold more than other drugs in the class. As a class, however, the TCAs have a relatively low risk for inducing seizures, except in patients who are at risk for seizures (e.g., patients with epilepsy or brain lesions). Although TCAs can still be used in such patients, the initial dosages should be lower than usual, and subsequent dosage increases should be gradual.

Allergic and Hematological Effects

Exanthematous rashes are seen in 4 to 5 percent of all patients treated with maprotiline. Jaundice is rare. Agranulocytosis, leukocytosis, leukopenia, and eosinophilia are rare complications of tetracyclic drug treatment. A patient who has a sore throat or a fever during the first few months of TCA treatment, however, should have a complete blood count (CBC) done immediately.

Other Adverse Effects

Weight gain, primarily an effect of the blockade of histamine type 2 (H_2) receptors, is common. If weight gain is a major problem, changing to a different class of antidepressants may help. Impotence, an occasional problem, is perhaps most often associated with amoxapine because of the drug's blockade of dopamine receptors in the tuberoinfundibular tract. Amoxapine can also cause hyperprolactinemia, galactorrhea, anorgasmia, and ejaculatory disturbances. Other TCAs have also been associated with gynecomastia and amenorrhea. Inappropriate secretion of antidiuretic hormone has also been reported with TCAs. Other effects include nausea, vomiting, and hepatitis.

Precautions

The TCAs should be avoided during pregnancy. The drugs pass into breast milk and can potentially cause serious adverse reactions in nursing infants. A case series suggested, however, that clomipramine at therapeutic concentrations in women who are breast-feeding does not produce detectable concentrations in the infant. The drugs should be used with caution in patients with hepatic and renal diseases. TCAs should not be administered during a course of electroconvulsive therapy, primarily because of the risk of serious adverse cardiac effects.

DRUG–DRUG INTERACTIONS

Antihypertensives

TCAs block the neuronal reuptake of guanethidine (Ismelin), which is required for antihypertensive activity. The antihypertensive effects of β-adrenergic receptor antagonists (e.g., propranolol [Inderal]) and clonidine (Catapres) may also be blocked by TCAs. Coadministration of a TCA and methyldopa (Aldomet) may cause behavioral agitation.

Antipsychotics

The plasma concentrations of TCAs and antipsychotics are increased by their coadministration. Antipsychotics also add to the anticholinergic and sedative effects of the TCAs.

Central Nervous System Depressants

Opioids, alcohol, anxiolytics, hypnotics, and over-the-counter cold medications have additive effects by causing CNS depression when coadministered with TCAs.

Sympathomimetics

Tricyclic drug use with sympathomimetic drugs may cause serious cardiovascular effects.

Oral Contraceptives

Birth control pills may decrease TCA plasma concentrations via the induction of hepatic enzymes.

Other Interactions

TCA plasma concentrations may also be increased by acetazolamide (Diamox), aspirin, cimetidine, thiazide diuretics, fluoxetine, and sodium bicarbonate. Decreased plasma concentrations may be caused by ascorbic acid, ammonium chloride, barbiturates, cigarette smoking, chloral hydrate, lithium (Eskalith), and primidone (Mysoline). Tricyclic drugs that are metabolized by CYP 2D6 may interfere with the metabolism of other drugs metabolized by the hepatic enzyme.

LABORATORY INTERFERENCES

Laboratory interferences with the TCAs have not been reported.

DOSAGE AND CLINICAL GUIDELINES

Persons who intend to take TCAs should undergo routine physical and laboratory examination, including a complete blood count, a white blood cell (WBC) count with differential, and serum electrolytes with liver function tests. An ECG should be obtained for all persons, especially women over 40 and men over 30. TCAs are contraindicated in persons with a QTc above 450 milliseconds. The initial dose should be small and should be raised gradually. Because of the availability of highly effective alternatives to TCAs, a newer agent should be used if there is any medical condition that may interact adversely with the TCAs. Elderly persons and children are more sensitive to TCA adverse effects than are young adults. In children, the ECG should be monitored regularly during use of a TCA.

The available preparations of TCAs are presented in Table 36.4.33–3. The dosages for the TCAs vary among the drugs (Table 36.4.33–4). Imipramine, amitriptyline, doxepin, desipramine, clomipramine, and trimipramine use can be started at 75 mg a day. Divided doses at first reduce the severity of the adverse effects, although most of the dosage should be given at night to help induce sleep if a sedating drug such as amitriptyline is used. Eventually, the entire daily dose can be given at bedtime. Protriptyline and less sedating drugs should be given at least 2 to 3 hours before a person goes to sleep. The dosage can be raised to 150 mg a day the second week, 225 mg a day the third week, and 300 mg a day the fourth week. A common clinical mistake is to stop increasing the dosage when the person is taking less than 250 mg a day and does not show clinical improvement. Doing so can result in further delay in obtaining a therapeutic response, disenchantment with the treatment, and premature discontinuation of drug use. The clinician should routinely assess the person's pulse and orthostatic changes in blood pressure while the dosage is being increased.

Nortriptyline use should be started at 50 mg a day and raised to 150 mg a day over 3 or 4 weeks unless a response occurs at a lower dosage, such as 100 mg a day. Amoxapine use should be started at 150 mg a day and raised to 400 mg a day. Protriptyline use should be started at 15 mg a day and raised to 60 mg a day. Maprotiline has been associated with an increased incidence of seizures if the dosage is raised too quickly or is maintained at too high a level. Maprotiline use should be started at 75 mg a day and maintained at that level for 2 weeks. The dosage can be increased over 4 weeks to 225 mg a day but should be kept at that level for only 6 weeks and then be reduced to 175 to 200 mg a day.

Table 36.4.33–3
Tricyclic and Tetracyclic Antidepressant Preparations

Drug	Tablets	Capsules	Parenteral	Solution
Imipramine	10, 25, 50 mg	75, 100, 125, 150 mg	12.5 mg/mL	—
Desipramine	10, 25, 50, 75, 100, 150 mg	25, 50 mg	—	—
Trimipramine	—	25, 50, 100 mg	—	—
Amitriptyline	10, 25, 50, 75, 100, 150 mg	—	10 mg/mL	—
Nortriptyline	—	10, 25, 50, 75 mg	—	10 mg/5 mL
Protriptyline	5, 10 mg	—	—	—
Amoxapine	25, 50, 100, 150 mg	—	—	—
Doxepin	—	10, 25, 50, 75, 100, 150 mg	—	10 mg/mL
Maprotiline	25, 50, 75 mg	—	—	—
Clomipramine	—	25, 50, 75 mg	—	—

Persons with chronic pain may be particularly sensitive to adverse effects when TCA use is started. Therefore, treatment should begin with low dosages that are raised in small increments. However, persons with chronic pain may experience relief on long-term low-dosage therapy, such as amitriptyline or nortriptyline at 10 to 75 mg a day.

TCAs should be avoided in children, except as a last resort. Dosing guidelines in children for imipramine include initiation at 1.5 mg/kg a day. The dosage can be titrated to no more than 5 mg/kg a day. In enuresis the dosage is usually 50 to 100 mg a day taken at bedtime. Clomipramine use can be initiated at 50 mg a day and increased to no more than 3 mg/kg a day or 200 mg a day.

Plasma Concentrations and Therapeutic Drug Monitoring

Research has defined the dose-response curves for a number of the TCAs when given to treat depressive disorders. Clinical determinations of plasma concentrations should be conducted after 5 to 7 days on the same dosage of medication and 8 to 12 hours after the last dose. Because of variations in absorption and metabolism, there may be a 30- to 50-fold difference in the plasma concentrations in persons given the same dosage of a TCA. The therapeutic ranges for plasma concentrations have been determined (Table 36.4.33–4). Nortriptyline is unique in its association with a therapeutic window; that is, plasma concentrations below 50 ng/mL or above 150 ng/mL may reduce its efficacy. Clinicians must follow the directions for collection from the testing laboratory and have confidence in the assay procedure used at a particular laboratory.

The use of plasma concentrations in clinical practice is still an evolving skill. Plasma concentrations may be useful in confirming compliance, assessing reasons for drug failures, and documenting effective plasma concentrations for future treatment. Clinicians should always treat the person and not the plasma concentration. Some persons have adequate clinical responses with seemingly subtherapeutic plasma concentrations, and other persons only respond at supratherapeutic plasma concentrations, without experiencing adverse effects. The latter situation, however, should alert the clinician to monitor the person's condition with, for example, serial ECG recordings.

Table 36.4.33–4
General Information for the Tricyclic and Tetracyclic Antidepressants

Generic Name	Trade Name	Usual Adult Dosage Range (mg a day)	Therapeutic Plasma Concentrations (μg per mL)
Imipramine	Tofranil	150–300	150–300[a]
Desipramine	Norpramin, Pertofrane	150–300	150–300[a]
Trimipramine	Surmontil	150–300	?
Amitriptyline	Elavil, Endep	150–300	100–250[b]
Nortriptyline	Pamelor, Aventyl	50–150	50–150[a] (maximum)
Protriptyline	Vivactil	15–60	75–250
Amoxapine	Asendin	150–400	?
Doxepin	Adapin, Sinequan	150–300	100–250[a]
Maprotiline	Ludiomil	150–230	150–300[a]
Clomipramine	Anafranil	130–250	?

[a]Exact range may vary among laboratories.
[b]Includes parent compound and desmethyl metabolite.

Overdose Attempts

Overdose attempts with TCAs are serious and can often be fatal. Prescriptions for these drugs should be nonrefillable and for no longer than a week at a time for patients at risk for suicide. Amoxapine may be more likely than the other TCAs to result in death when taken in overdose. The newer antidepressants are safer in overdose.

Symptoms of overdose include agitation, delirium, convulsions, hyperactive deep tendon reflexes, bowel and bladder paralysis, dysregulation of blood pressure and temperature, and mydriasis. The patient then progresses to coma and perhaps respiratory depression. Cardiac arrhythmias may not respond to treatment. Because of the long half-lives of TCAs, the patients are at risk of cardiac arrhythmias for 3 to 4 days after the overdose, so they should be monitored in an intensive care medical setting.

Failure of Drug Trial and Treatment-Resistant Depression

If a TCA has been used for 4 weeks at maximal dosages without a therapeutic effect, the clinician should obtain a plasma concentration and adjust the dosage accordingly. If plasma concentrations are adequate, supplementation with lithium or liothyronine (T_3) (Cytomel) should be considered. Alternatively, an SSRI or other antidepressant can be substituted.

Lithium. Lithium (900 to 1,200 mg a day, serum concentration between 0.6 and 0.8 mEq/L) can be added to the TCA dosage for 7 to 14 days. This approach converts a significant number of nonresponders into responders. The mechanism of action is unknown, but the lithium may potentiate the serotonergic neuronal system.

Liothyronine. The addition of 25 to 50 μg a day of liothyronine, the levorotatory isomer of triiodothyronine (T_3), to the regimen for 7 to 14 days may convert a tricyclic or tetracyclic nonresponder into a responder. The mechanism of action for liothyronine augmentation is unknown. Empirical data indicate that liothyronine is more effective than levothyroxine, the levorotatory isomer of thyroxine (T_4), as an adjunct to TCAs. If liothyronine augmentation is successful, the liothyronine should be continued for 2 months and then tapered at the rate of 12.5 μg a day every 3 to 7 days.

Monoamine Oxidase Inhibitors (MAOIs). MAOIs should be discontinued for 2 weeks before initiating treatment with a TCA. A minimum of a 1-week washout is needed when switching from a TCA tetracyclic to an MAOI.

Termination of Short-Term Treatment

TCAs effectively resolve the acute symptoms of depression. If treatment is stopped prematurely, symptoms are likely to reemerge. To minimize the risk for recurrence or relapse, clinicians should continue the TCA at the same treatment dosage throughout the course of treatment. When treatment is discontinued, clinicians may reasonably reduce the dosage to three fourths of the maximal dosage for another month. At this time, if no symptoms are present, the drug can be tapered by 25 mg (5 mg for protriptyline) every 2 to 3 days. The slow tapering process is indicated for most psychotherapeutic drugs; in the case of most TCAs, slow tapering avoids a cholinergic rebound syndrome, consisting of nausea, upset stomach, sweating, headache, neck pain, and vomiting. This syndrome can be treated by reinstituting a small dosage of the drug and tapering use more slowly than before. Several case reports note the appearance of rebound mania or hypomania after abrupt discontinuation of TCAs. If a patient has been treated with lithium augmentation, the clinician should probably taper and stop use of the lithium first and then the tricyclic or tetracyclic drug. But clinical studies supporting this approach are lacking, and the guidelines may change as more physicians report their experience with this drug combination.

References

Baldessarini RJ. Drugs and the treatment of psychiatric disorders: depression and anxiety disorders. In: Hardman JG, Limbird LE, Goodman Gilman A, eds. *Goodman & Gilman's the Pharmacological Basis of Therapeutics.* 10th ed. New York: McGraw-Hill; 2001:447.

Boyce P, Judd F. The place for tricyclic antidepressants in the treatment of depression. *Aust N Z J Psychiatry.* 1999;33:323.

Bruijn JA, Moleman P, Mulder PGH, van den Broek WW. Treatment of mood-congruent psychotic depression with imipramine. *J Affect Disord.* 2001;66:165.

Buysee DJ, Reynolds CF III, Hoch CG, et al. Longitudinal effects of nortriptyline on EEG sleep and the likelihood of recurrence in elderly depressed patients. *Neuropsychopharmacology.* 1996;14:243.

Dahl M-L, Bertilsson L, Nordin C. Steady-state plasma levels of nortriptyline and its 10-hydroxy metabolite: relationship to the CYP2D6 genotype. *Psychopharmacology.* 1996;123:315.

Greil W, Ludwig-Mayerhofer W, Erazo N, et al. Comparative efficacy of lithium and amitriptyline in the maintenance treatment of recurrent unipolar depression: a randomized study. *J Affect Disord.* 1996;40:179.

Kocsis JH, Friedman RA, Markowitz JC, et al. Maintenance therapy for chronic depression: a controlled clinical trial of desipramine. *Arch Gen Psychiatry.* 1996;53:769.

Koran LM, Gelenberg AJ, Kornstein SG, et al. Sertraline versus imipramine to prevent relapse in chronic depression. *J Affect Disord.* 2001;65:27.

Kuhs H, Farber D, Borgstadt S, et al. Amitriptyline in combination with repeated late sleep deprivation versus amitriptyline alone in major depression. A randomized study. *J Affect Disord.* 1996;37:31.

Kye CH, Waterman GS, Ryan ND, et al. A randomized, controlled trial of amitriptyline in the acute treatment of adolescent major depression. *J Am Acad Child Adolesc Psychiatry.* 1996;35:1139.

Leonard BE. Tricyclic antidepressants: effective, cheap but are they safe? *J Psychopharmacol.* 1996;10(suppl 1):35.

Lotufo-Neto F, Bernik M, Ramos RT, et al. A dose-finding and discontinuation study of clomipramine in panic disorder. *J Psychopharmacol.* 2001;15:13.

Nelson JC. Tricyclics and tetracyclics. In: Sadock BJ, Sadock VA, eds. *Kaplan & Sadock's Comprehensive Textbook of Psychiatry.* 7th ed. Vol 2. Baltimore: Lippincott Williams & Wilkins; 2000:2491.

Oesterheld J. TCA cardiotoxicity: the latest. *J Am Acad Child Adolesc Psychiatry.* 1996;35:701.

Sanchez LE, Campbell M, Small AM, et al. A pilot study of clomipramine in young autistic children. *J Am Acad Child Adolesc Psychiatry.* 1996;35:537.

Schindler KM, Pato MT. Clomipramine. In: Pato MT, Zohar J, eds. *Current Treatments of Obsessive-Compulsive Disorder.* 2nd ed. Clinical practice; no. 51. Washington, DC: American Psychiatric Association; 2001:19.

▲ 36.4.34 Valproate

Valproate (Depakene), also called valproic acid (because it is rapidly converted to the acid form in the stomach) and divalproex (Depakote), has been shown to be effective for absence seizures, generalized epilepsy, and partial epilepsy with or without secondary generalization and for prophylaxis against migraine headaches. In addition, valproate and two other anticonvulsant drugs, carbamazepine (Tegretol) and clonazepam (Klonopin), have been shown to be effective in treating bipolar I disorder. Commercially available antiepileptic drugs that are being studied for treatment of rapid-cycling bipolar disorder include gabapentin (Neurontin), lamotrigine (Lamictal), vigabatrin (Sabril), tiagabine (Gabitril), and topiramate (Topamax). Although lithium (Eskalith) is still the most widely used drug in the treatment of bipolar I disorder, valproate is considered equal in efficacy and safety.

CHEMISTRY

The molecular structures of valproate and valproic acid are shown in Figure 36.4.34–1. Valproic acid is a simple, branched-chain, carboxylic *n*-dipropylacetic acid.

PHARMACOLOGICAL ACTIONS

All valproate formulations are rapidly and completely absorbed after oral administration. The steady-state half-life of valproate

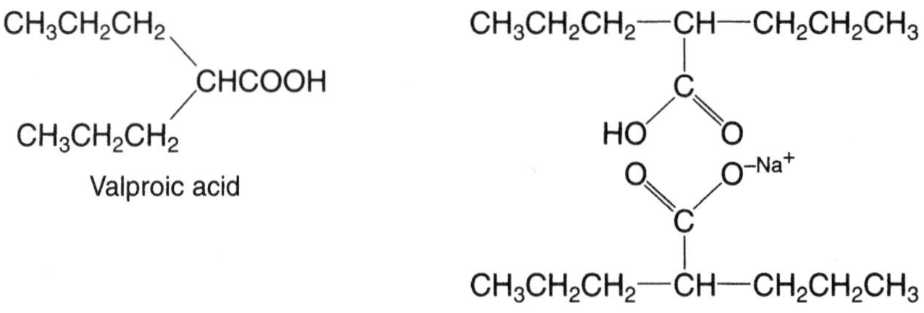

Valproic acid

Valproate

FIGURE 36.4.34–1
Molecular structure of valproic acid and valproate.

is about 8 to 17 hours, and clinically effective plasma concentrations can usually be maintained with dosing one to four times a day. Protein binding becomes saturated and concentrations of therapeutically effective free valproate increase at serum concentrations above 50 to 100 μg/mL.

The therapeutic effects of valproate in bipolar I disorder may be mediated by as yet undefined effects of the drug on the γ-aminobutyric acid (GABA) neurotransmitter system.

THERAPEUTIC INDICATIONS

Bipolar I Disorder

Acute Episodes. Valproate controls manic symptoms in about two thirds of persons with acute mania. Valproate also reduces overall psychiatric symptoms and the need for supplemental doses of benzodiazepines or dopamine receptor antagonists. Persons with mania usually respond 1 to 4 days after valproate serum concentrations rise above 50 μg/mL. Using gradual dosing strategies, this serum concentration may be achieved within 1 week of initiation of dosing, but newer, rapid oral-loading strategies achieve therapeutic serum concentrations in 1 day and can control manic symptoms within 5 days. The short-term antimanic effects of valproate can be augmented with addition of lithium, carbamazepine, or dopamine receptor antagonists. Serotonin-dopamine antagonists and gabapentin may also potentiate the effects of valproate, albeit less rapidly. Because of its more favorable profile of cognitive, dermatological, thyroid, and renal adverse effects, valproate is preferred to lithium for treatment of acute mania in children and elderly persons.

Valproate alone is less effective for the short-term treatment of depressive episodes in bipolar I disorder than for treatment of manic episodes. Among depressive symptoms, valproate is more effective for treatment of agitation than dysphoria.

Prophylaxis. Valproate is effective in the prophylactic treatment of bipolar I disorder, resulting in fewer, less severe, and shorter manic episodes. In direct comparison, valproate is at least as effective as lithium and is better tolerated than lithium. Compared with lithium, valproate may be particularly effective in persons with rapid-cycling and ultrarapid-cycling bipolar disorders, dysphoric or mixed mania, and mania due to a general medical condition and in persons who have comorbid substance abuse or panic attacks or who have not had completely favorable responses to lithium treatment. Addition of valproate to lithium may be more effective than use of lithium alone.

In persons with bipolar I disorder, maintenance valproate treatment markedly reduces the frequency and severity of manic episodes but is only mildly to moderately effective in the prophylactic treatment of depressive episodes. The prophylactic effectiveness of valproate can be augmented by addition of lithium, carbamazepine, dopamine receptor antagonists, serotonin-dopamine antagonists, antidepressant drugs, gabapentin, or lamotrigine.

Schizoaffective Disorder

Valproate is effective in treating the short-term phase of the bipolar type of schizoaffective disorder, but valproate alone is generally less effective in schizoaffective disorder than in bipolar I disorder. Valproate may be an effective adjunct agent for use with lithium, carbamazepine, or a serotonin-dopamine antagonist by persons with schizoaffective disorder. Valproate alone is ineffective for treatment of psychotic symptoms.

Other Mental Disorders

Valproate can be effective for treatment of intermittent explosive disorder, kleptomania, and other behavioral dyscontrol syndromes, particularly if these disorders are comorbid with bipolar symptoms. Valproate can control physical aggression, restlessness, agitation, and (to a lesser degree) verbal aggression associated with dementia, organic brain diseases, or traumatic brain injury, although it should be considered for use only after therapeutic trials of benzodiazepines and serotonin-dopamine antagonists have failed. Valproate may be effective alone or in combination with other psychotropic drugs in treatment of other mental disorders, including major depressive disorder; panic disorder; posttraumatic stress disorder; obsessive-compulsive disorder; bulimia nervosa; alcohol and sedative, hypnotic, or anxiolytic (particularly benzodiazepine) withdrawal; symptoms of borderline personality disorder; and cocaine detoxification.

PRECAUTIONS AND ADVERSE REACTIONS

Valproate treatment is generally well tolerated and safe and is less likely than lithium to trigger medication discontinuation because of adverse effects. The common adverse effects associated with valproate (Table 36.4.34–1) are those affecting the

Table 36.4.34–1
Adverse Effects of Valproate

- Common
  - Gastrointestinal irritation
  - Nausea
  - Sedation
  - Tremor
  - Weight gain
  - Hair loss
- Uncommon
  - Vomiting
  - Diarrhea
  - Ataxia
  - Dysarthria
  - Persistent elevation of hepatic transaminases
- Rare
  - Fatal hepatotoxicity (primarily in pediatric patients)
  - Reversible thrombocytopenia
  - Platelet dysfunction
  - Coagulation disturbances
  - Edema
  - Hemorrhagic pancreatitis
  - Agranulocytosis
  - Encephalopathy and coma
  - Respiratory muscle weakness and respiratory failure

gastrointestinal (GI) system, such as nausea, vomiting, dyspepsia, and diarrhea. The GI effects are generally most common in the first month of treatment, particularly if the dosage is increased rapidly. Unbuffered valproic acid is more likely to cause GI symptoms than the enteric-coated "sprinkle" or the delayed-release divalproex sodium formulations. GI symptoms may respond to histamine H_2 receptor antagonists. Other common adverse effects involve the nervous system, such as sedation, ataxia, dysarthria, and tremor. Valproate-induced tremor may respond well to treatment with β-adrenergic receptor antagonists or gabapentin. Treatment of the other neurological adverse effects usually requires lowering the valproate dosage.

Weight gain is a common adverse effect, especially in long-term treatment, and can best be treated by strict limitation of caloric intake. Hair loss may occur in 5 to 10 percent of all persons treated, and rare cases of complete loss of body hair have been reported. Some clinicians have recommended treatment of valproate-associated hair loss with vitamin supplements that contain zinc and selenium. Five to 40 percent of persons experience a persistent but clinically insignificant elevation in liver transaminases to three times the upper limit of normal, which is usually asymptomatic and resolves after discontinuation of the drug. Other rare adverse events include effects on the hematopoietic system, including thrombocytopenia and platelet dysfunction, occurring most commonly at high dosages and resulting in prolonged bleeding times. High dosages of valproate (above 1,000 mg a day) may rarely produce mild to moderate hyponatremia, most likely because of some degree of the syndrome of secretion of inappropriate antidiuretic hormone (SIADH), which is reversible upon lowering of the dosage. Overdoses of valproate can lead to coma and death. There are reports that valproate-induced coma can be successfully treated with naloxone (Narcan) and that hemodialysis and hemoperfusion can be useful in the treatment of valproate overdoses.

The two most serious adverse effects of valproate treatment affect the pancreas and the liver. Risk factors for potentially fatal hepatotoxicity include young age (less than 3 years), concurrent use of phenobarbital (Luminal, Solfoton), and the presence of neurological disorders, especially inborn errors of metabolism. The rate of fatal hepatotoxicity in persons who have been treated with only valproate is 0.85 per 100,000 persons; no persons over the age of 10 years are reported to have died from fatal hepatotoxicity. Therefore, the risk of this adverse reaction in adult psychiatric persons seems low. Nevertheless, if symptoms of lethargy, malaise, anorexia, nausea and vomiting, edema, and abdominal pain occur in a person treated with valproate, the clinician must consider the possibility of severe hepatotoxicity. A modest increase in liver function test results does not correlate with the development of serious hepatotoxicity. Rare cases of pancreatitis have been reported; they occur most often in the first 6 months of treatment, and the condition occasionally results in death. Pancreatic function can be assessed and followed with serum amylase determinations.

Valproate should not be used by pregnant or nursing women. The drug is associated with neural tube defects (e.g., spina bifida) in about 1 to 2 percent of all women who take valproate during the first trimester of the pregnancy. The risk of valproate-induced neural tube defects can be reduced with daily folic acid supplements (1 to 4 mg a day) taken continuously for at least 3 months prior to conception and throughout pregnancy. Women who require valproate therapy should therefore inform their physicians if they intend to become pregnant. Infants breast-fed by mothers taking valproate develop serum valproate concentrations 1 to 10 percent of maternal serum concentrations, and no data suggest that this poses a risk to the infant. Thus, valproate is relatively contraindicated in nursing mothers. Clinicians should not administer the drug to persons with hepatic diseases. Rare cases of polycystic ovary disease have been reported in woman using valproate.

EFFECTS ON SPECIFIC ORGANS AND SYSTEMS

Although the principal effects of valproate are on the central nervous system (CNS), the drug also affects the GI and hematopoietic systems. The effects on the GI system lead both to common adverse effects (e.g., nausea) and to serious but rare effects (e.g., fatal hepatotoxicity). A comparison of the use of lithium, valproate, and carbamazepine in bipolar disorder is presented in Table 36.4.34–2.

DRUG–DRUG INTERACTIONS

Valproate is commonly coadministered with lithium, carbamazepine, and dopamine receptor antagonists. The only consistent drug interaction with lithium, if both drugs are maintained in their respective therapeutic ranges, is the exacerbation of drug-induced tremors, which can usually be treated with β-receptor antagonists. The combination of valproate and dopa-

Table 36.4.34–2
Comparison of Lithium, Valproic Acid, and Carbamazepine for Bipolar I Disorder

	Lithium (Cibalith-S, Eskalith, Lithane, Lithobid, Lithonate, Lithotabs)	Valproic Acid (Depakene, Depakote)	Carbamazepine (Epitol, Tegretol)
Serum plasma levels	0.6–1.2 mEq/L (acute)	50–100 μg/mL	4–12 μg/mL
Usual adult daily dose	600–1,800 mg	750–4,200 mg	400–1,600 mg
Onset of action	5–14 days	5–15 days	3–15 days
Protein binding	Not bound to plasma proteins	90% concentration dependent ↓ with high concentration (variable due to saturation)	76%
$t_{1/2}$	24 h (average) Increases with age and/or with decreased renal function	6–16 hours (average) Increases with age and/or decreased hepatic function	Initial range 25–65 hours; with repeated dosing, 12–17 hours; 10,11-epoxide (active), approximately 5–8 hours
Metabolic pathway(s)	Not metabolized, primarily excreted unchanged in urine	Hepatic (glucuronidation, mitochondrial B oxidation, microsomal oxidation)	Hepatic: CYP 3A, possibly 2D6
Route(s) of elimination	Renal	Renal, glucuronidation	Renal (72%), fecal (28%)
Common drug interactions	↑ Lithium serum concentrations (fluoxetine, ACE inhibitors, diuretics, NSAIDs) ↓ Lithium serum concentrations (acetazolamide, osmotic diuretics, theophylline, urinary alkalinizers) Antipsychotics may increase lithium neurotoxicity	Interacts with many drugs that are hepatically metabolized; enzyme inducers can decrease concentrations of valproic acid; valproic acid can increase phenobarbital by impairment of nonrenal clearance (severe CNS depression)	Interacts with drugs that are hepatically metabolized; shortens the half-life of certain drugs that are hepatically metabolized (e.g., phenytoin, warfarin, doxycycline, theophylline); carbamazepine levels can be markedly decreased by phenobarbital, phenytoin, or primidone; valproic acid can cause an increase in 10,11-epoxide: parent drug ratio; carbamazepine reduces plasma levels of haloperidol and valproic acid
Common adverse effects	Nausea, vomiting, diarrhea, polyuria, polydipsia, tremor, hypothyroidism	GI distress, diplopia, sedation, tremor, edema, weight gain, alopecia, and thrombocytopenia	Dizziness, drowsiness, unsteadiness
Indication(s)	Manic episodes of bipolar disorder Bipolar disorder maintenance	Bipolar disorder, acute mania (and seizure disorders)	Bipolar disorder (and seizure disorders)

ACE, angiotensin-converting enzyme; NSAIDs, nonsteroidal antiinflammatory drugs.
Reprinted with permission from Ereshefsky L, Overman GP, Karp JK. Current psychotropic dosing and monitoring guidelines. *Prim Psychiatry.* 1996;3:21.

mine receptor antagonists may result in increased sedation, as can be seen when valproate is added to any CNS depressant (e.g., alcohol), and increased severity of extrapyramidal symptoms, which generally respond to treatment with the usual antiparkinsonian drugs. Valproate can usually be safely combined with carbamazepine or serotonin-dopamine antagonists. The plasma concentrations of carbamazepine, lamotrigine, diazepam (Valium), amitriptyline (Elavil), nortriptyline (Pamelor), and phenobarbital may be increased when these drugs are coadministered with valproate, and the plasma concentrations of phenytoin (Dilantin) and desipramine (Norpramin) may be decreased when they are combined with valproate. Plasma concentrations of valproate may be decreased when the drug is coadministered with carbamazepine and may be increased when coadministered with guanfacine (Tenex), amitriptyline, or fluoxetine (Prozac). Valproate can be displaced from plasma proteins by carbamazepine, diazepam, and aspirin. Persons who are treated with anticoagulants (e.g., aspirin and warfarin [Coumadin]) should also be monitored when valproate use is initiated, to detect the development of any undesired augmentation of the anticoagulation effects. Interactions of valproate with other drugs are listed in Table 36.4.34–3.

Table 36.4.34–3
Interactions of Valproate with Other Drugs

Drug	Interactions Reported with Valproate
Lithium	Increased tremor
Antipsychotics	Increased sedation; increased extrapyramidal effects; delirium and stupor (single report)
Clozapine	Increased sedation; confusional syndrome (single report)
Carbamazepine	Acute psychosis (single report); ataxia, nausea, lethargy (single report); may decrease valproate serum concentrations
Antidepressants	Amitriptyline and fluoxetine may increase valproate serum concentrations
Diazepam	Serum concentration increased by valproate
Clonazepam	Absence status (rare; reported only in patients with preexisting epilepsy)
Phenytoin	Serum concentration decreased by valproate
Phenobarbital	Serum, concentration increased by valproate; increased sedation
Other CNS depressants	Increased sedation
Anticoagulants	Possible potentiation of effect

Table 36.4.34–4
Valproate Preparations Available in the United States

Generic Name	Trade Name, Form (doses)	Time to Peak
Valproate sodium injection	Depacon injection (100 mg valproic acid/mL)	1 h
Valproic acid	Depakene, syrup (250 mg/5 mL)	1–2 h
	Depakene, capsules (250 mg)	1–2 h
Divalproex sodium	Depakote, delayed-released tablets (125, 250, 500 mg)	3–8 h
Divalproex sodium-coated particles in capsules	Depakote, sprinkle capsules (125 mg)	Compared with divalproex tablets, divalproex sprinkle has earlier onset and slower absorption, with slightly lower peak plasma concentration

LABORATORY INTERFERENCES

Valproate use has been reported to cause an overestimation of serum free fatty acids in almost half of the patients tested. Valproate use has also been reported to elevate urinary ketone estimations falsely and to result in falsely abnormal thyroid function test results.

DOSAGE AND ADMINISTRATION

Prior to administration of valproate, hepatic and pancreatic disease should be ruled out by a combination of clinical and laboratory evaluations. Valproate is available in a number of formulations and dosages (Table 36.4.36–4). It is best to initiate drug treatment gradually to minimize the common adverse effects of nausea, vomiting, and sedation. The dose on the first day should be 250 mg administered with a meal. The dosage can be raised to 250 mg orally 3 times daily over the course of 3 to 6 days. Plasma concentrations can be assessed in the morning before the first daily dose of the drug is administered. Therapeutic plasma concentrations for the control of seizures range between 50 and 100 mg/mL, although some physicians use 125 or even 150 mg/mL if the drug is well tolerated. It is reasonable to use the same range for the treatment of mental disorders; most of the controlled studies have used 50 to 100 mg/mL. Most patients attain therapeutic plasma concentrations on a daily dose between 1,200 and 1,500 mg in divided doses. The mood-stabilizing effects of valproate appear between 5 and 15 days after initiation of treatment.

REFERENCES

Baldessarini RJ, Tarazi RI. Drugs and the treatment of psychiatric disorders: psychosis and mania. In: Hardman JG, Limbird LE, Goodman Gilman A, eds. *Goodman & Gilman's the Pharmacological Basis of Therapeutics*. 10th ed. New York: McGraw-Hill; 2001:485.

Bowden CL, Janicak PG, Orsulak P, et al. Relation of serum valproate concentration to response in mania. *Am J Psychiatry*. 1996;153:765.

Kando JC, Tohen M, Castillo J, Zarate CA Jr. The use of valproate in an elderly population with affective symptoms. *J Clin Psychiatry*. 1996;57:238.

Keck PE, McElroy SL, Tugrul KC, Bennett JA. Valproate oral loading in the treatment of acute mania. *J Clin Psychiatry*. 1993;54:305.

Lennkh C, Simhandl C. Current aspects of valproate in bipolar disorders. *Int Clin Psychopharmacol*. 2000;15:1.

Lindenmayer JP, Kotsaftis A. Use of sodium valproate in violent and aggressive behaviors: a critical review. *J Clin Psychiatry*. 2000;61:123.

Lott AD, McElroy SL, Keys MA. Valproate in the treatment of behavioral agitation in elderly patients with dementia. *J Neuropsychiatry Clin Neurosci*. 1995;7:314.

McElroy SL, Pope HG Jr, Keck PE. Valproate. In: Sadock BJ, Sadock VA, eds. *Kaplan & Sadock's Comprehensive Textbook of Psychiatry*. 7th ed. Vol 2. Baltimore: Lippincott Williams & Wilkins; 2000:2289.

Minuk GY, Rockman GE, German GB, et al. The use of sodium valproate in the treatment of alcoholism. *J Addict Dis*. 1995;14:67.

Stoll AL, Locke CA, Vuckovic A, Mayer PV. Lithium-associated cognitive and functional deficits reduced by a switch to divalproex sodium: a case series. *J Clin Psychiatry*. 1996;57:356.

West SA, Keck PE, McElroy SL, et al. Open trial of valproate in the treatment of adolescent mania. *J Child Adolesc Psychopharmacol*. 1994;4:263.

Vasudev K, Das S, Goswami U, Tayal G. Pharmacokinetics of valproic acid in patients with bipolar disorder. *J Psychopharmacol*. 2001;5:87.

▲ 36.4.35 Venlafaxine

Venlafaxine (Effexor) is an effective antidepressant drug that may have a faster onset of action than other antidepressant drugs when the dosage is increased rapidly. Venlafaxine is among the most efficacious drugs for treatment of severe depression with melancholic features. Venlafaxine has also been approved by the Food and Drug Administration (FDA) for treatment of generalized anxiety disorder. A related drug, duloxetine, is discussed at the end of this section.

CHEMISTRY

Venlafaxine is structurally distinct from other antidepressant drugs. Its structural formula is shown in Figure 36.4.35–1.

PHARMACOLOGICAL ACTIONS

Venlafaxine is well absorbed from the gastrointestinal tract. The immediate-release formulation of venlafaxine and the sustained-release formulation reach peak plasma concentrations in 5.5 hours and 9 hours, respectively. Venlafaxine has a half-life of about 3.5 hours, and the sustained-release form has a half-life of 9 hours.

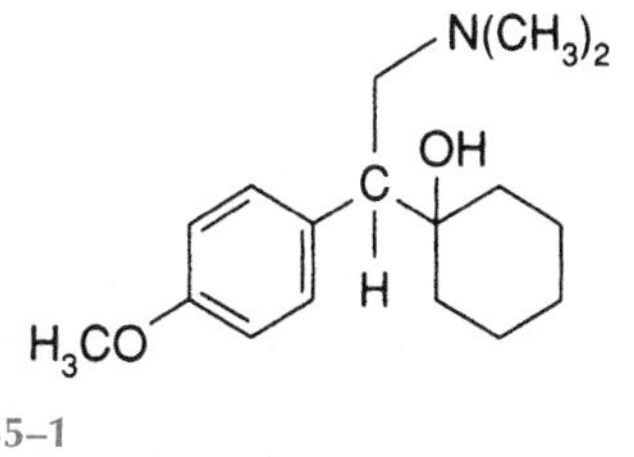

FIGURE 36.4.35–1
Molecular structure of venlafaxine.

Venlafaxine is a potent inhibitor of serotonin and norepinephrine reuptake and a weak inhibitor of dopamine reuptake. Venlafaxine does not have activity at muscarinic, nicotinic, histaminergic, opioid, or adrenergic receptors, and it is not active as a monoamine oxidase inhibitor. It is metabolized in the liver by cytochrome P450 isoenzyme 2D6 (CYP 2D6).

THERAPEUTIC INDICATIONS

Depression

Venlafaxine is used for the treatment of major depressive disorder. Severely depressed persons may respond within 2 weeks to 200 mg a day of venlafaxine, which is somewhat faster than the 2 to 4 weeks usually required for the serotonin-specific reuptake inhibitors (SSRIs). Therefore, high-dosage venlafaxine may become a preferred drug to use for seriously ill persons when a rapid response is desired. In studies directly comparing fluoxetine (Prozac) with venlafaxine for the treatment of seriously depressed persons with melancholic features, venlafaxine has consistently been superior in terms of rate of response, percentage response, and completeness of response. No direct comparisons of venlafaxine and sertraline (Zoloft), the most effective SSRI for treatment of seriously depressed persons with melancholic features, have been described.

Generalized Anxiety Disorder

The extended-release formulation of venlafaxine is approved for treatment of generalized anxiety disorder. In clinical trials, dosages of 75 to 225 mg a day were effective against insomnia, poor concentration, restlessness, irritability, and excessive muscle tension related to generalized anxiety disorder.

Other Indications

Case reports and uncontrolled studies have indicated that venlafaxine may be beneficial in the treatment of obsessive-compulsive disorder, panic disorder, agoraphobia, social phobia, and attention-deficit/hyperactivity disorder. It has also been used in chronic pain syndromes with good effect.

PRECAUTIONS AND ADVERSE REACTIONS

Venlafaxine has generally been reported to be well tolerated. The most common adverse reactions are nausea, somnolence, dry mouth, dizziness, nervousness, constipation, asthenia, anxiety, anorexia, blurred vision, abnormal ejaculation or orgasm, erectile disturbances, and impotence. The incidence of nausea is reduced considerably with use of the extended-release capsules. Abrupt discontinuation of venlafaxine use may produce a discontinuation syndrome consisting of nausea, somnolence, and insomnia. Therefore, venlafaxine use should be tapered gradually over 2 to 4 weeks.

The most potentially worrisome adverse effect associated with venlafaxine is an increase in blood pressure in some persons, particularly those who are treated with more than 300 mg a day. In clinical trials a mean increase of 7.2 mm Hg in diastolic blood pressure was observed in persons who were receiving 375 mg a day of venlafaxine, in contrast to no significant change in persons receiving 75 or 225 mg a day. Thus, the drug should be used cautiously by persons with preexisting hypertension and then only at lower dosages.

No information concerning use of venlafaxine by pregnant and nursing women is available at this time. Clinicians should avoid the use of venlafaxine by pregnant and nursing women until more clinical experience has been gained.

DRUG–DRUG INTERACTIONS

Cimetidine (Tagamet) appears to inhibit the first-pass hepatic metabolism of venlafaxine and to raise the levels of the unmetabolized drug. However, since the metabolite is mainly responsible for the therapeutic effect, this interaction is of concern only in persons with preexisting hypertension or hepatic disease, in whom this combination should be avoided. Venlafaxine may raise plasma concentrations of concurrently administered haloperidol (Haldol). Like all antidepressant medications, venlafaxine should not be used within 14 days of use of monoamine oxidase inhibitors, and it may potentiate the sedative effects of other drugs that act on the central nervous system.

LABORATORY INTERFERENCES

Data are not currently available on laboratory interferences with venlafaxine.

DOSAGE AND ADMINISTRATION

Venlafaxine is available in 25-, 37.5-, 50-, 75-, and 100-mg tablets and 37.5-, 75-, and 150-mg extended-release capsules. The tablets should be given in two or three daily doses, and the extended-release capsules are to be taken in a single dose before sleep, up to a maximum of 225 mg a day. The tablets and the extended-release capsules are equally potent, and persons stabilized with one can switch to an equivalent dosage of the other. The usual starting dosage in depressed persons is 75 mg a day, given as tablets in two to three divided doses or as extended-release capsules in a single dose before sleep. Some persons require a starting dosage of 37.5 mg for 4 to 7 days to minimize adverse effects, particularly nausea, prior to titration up to 75 mg a day. In persons with depression, the dosage can be raised to 150 mg a day, given as tablets in two or three divided doses or as extended-release capsules once at night, after an appropriate period of clinical assessment at the lower dosage (usually 2 to 3 weeks). The dosage can be raised in increments of 75 mg a day every 4 or more days. Moderately depressed persons probably do not need dosages above 225 mg a day, whereas severely depressed persons may require 300 to 375 mg a day for a satisfactory response. Rapid antidepressant response—within 1 to 2 weeks—may result from administration of dosages of 200 mg per day from the beginning. The maximum dosage of venlafaxine is 375 mg a day. The dosage of venlafaxine should be halved in persons with significantly diminished hepatic or renal function. If discontinued, venlafaxine use should be gradually tapered over 2 to 4 weeks.

DULOXETINE

Duloxetine hydrochloride (Cymbalta) is a dual reuptake inhibitor of serotonin and norepinephrine that acts as an anti-

depressant. It is chemically unrelated to venlafaxine. Duloxetine has minimal receptor affinity for dopamine, histamine or other receptor types. Limited information is available about its clinical profile. Doses used in clinical trials ranged from 60 mg once a day to 60 mg twice a day. At lower doses, duloxetine is used once a day, but at higher doses it is used twice a day. In clinical trials, duloxetine demonstrates a similar side effect profile to SSRIs. Discontinuation due to adverse events was similar to SSRIs (15 percent for fluoxetine versus 5 percent for placebo). The most common side effects are nausea, dry mouth, fatigue, dizziness, constipation, somnolence and sweating. Duloxetine is a moderate inhibitor of CYP450 2D6 enzyme.

References

Baldessarini RJ. Drugs and the treatment of psychiatric disorders: depression and anxiety disorders. In: Hardman JG, Limbird LE, Goodman Gilman A, eds. *Goodman & Gilman's the Pharmacological Basis of Therapeutics.* 10th ed. New York: McGraw-Hill; 2001:447.

Beauclair L, Radoi-Andraous D, Chouinard G. Selective serotonin-noradrenaline reuptake inhibitors. In: Sadock BJ, Sadock VA, eds. *Kaplan & Sadock's Comprehensive Textbook of Psychiatry.* 7th ed. Vol 2. Baltimore: Lippincott Williams & Wilkins; 2000:1132.

Bray GA, Ryan DH, Gordon D, Heidingsfelder S, Cerise F, Wilson K. A double-blind randomized placebo-controlled trial of sibutramine. *Obes Res.* 1996;4:263.

Findling RL, Schwartz MA, Flannery DJ, Manos MJ. Venlafaxine in adults with attention-deficit/hyperactivity disorder: an open clinical trial. *J Clin Psychiatry.* 1996;57:184.

Katz IR, Reynolds CF III, Alexopoulos GS, Hackett D. Venlafaxine ER as a treatment for generalized anxiety disorder in older adults: pooled analysis of five randomized placebo-controlled trials. *J Am Geriatr Soc.* 2002;50:18.

Meoni P, Salinas E, Brault Y, Hackett D. Pattern of symptom improvement following treatment with venlafaxine XR in patients with generalized anxiety disorder. *J Clin Psychiatry.* 2001;62:888.

Russell JL. Relatively low doses of cisapride in the treatment of nausea in patients with venlafaxine for treatment-refractory depression. *J Clin Psychopharmacol.* 1996;16:35.

Saletu B, Grunberger J, Anderer P, Linzmayer L, Semlitsch HV, Magni G. Pharmacodynamics of venlafaxine evaluated by EEG brain mapping, psychometry, and psychophysiology. *Br J Clin Pharmacol.* 1992;33:589.

Scott MA, Shelton PS, Gattis W. Therapeutic options for treating major depression, and the role of venlafaxine. *Pharmacotherapy.* 1996;16:352.

Sheehan DV. Attaining remission in generalized anxiety disorder: venlafaxine extended release comparative data. *J Clin Psychiatry.* 2001;62(suppl 19):26.

Silverstone PH, Salinas E. Efficacy of venlafaxine extended release in patients with major depressive disorder and comorbid generalized anxiety disorder. *J Clin Psychiatry.* 2001;62:523.

▲ 36.4.36 Yohimbine

Yohimbine (Yocon, Aphrodyne) is an α_2-adrenergic receptor antagonist that is used to treat both idiopathic and medication-induced male sexual dysfunction. Currently, sildenafil (Viagra) and alprostadil (Muse, Caverject) are generally considered more efficacious for this indication than yohimbine.

CHEMISTRY

Yohimbine hydrochloride is derived from an alkaloid found in *Rubaceae* and related trees and in the *Rauwolfia serpentina* plant. Its molecular structure is shown in Figure 36.4.36–1.

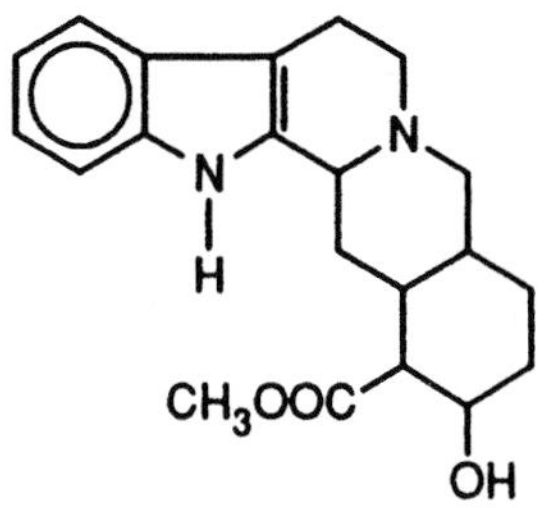

FIGURE 36.4.36–1
Molecular structure of yohimbine.

PHARMACOLOGICAL ACTIONS

Yohimbine is absorbed erratically following oral administration, with bioavailablity ranging from 7 to 87 percent. There is extensive hepatic first-pass metabolism. Yohimbine affects the sympathomimetic autonomic nervous system by increasing plasma concentrations of norepinephrine. The half-life of yohimbine is 0.5 to 2 hours.

Yohimbine is an antagonist of α_2-receptors located both presynaptically and postsynaptically on noradrenergic neurons. α_2-Receptors are also located on synaptic terminals of some serotonergic neurons. Stimulation of presynaptic α_2-receptors decreases the release of neurotransmitters from the neuron; therefore, blockade of the receptors increases the release of neurotransmitters. Both norepinephrine and serotonin are involved in the physiology of the male sexual response. Clinically, yohimbine produces increased parasympathetic (cholinergic) tone.

THERAPEUTIC INDICATIONS

In psychiatry, yohimbine has been used to treat medical, psychogenic, and substance-induced erectile dysfunction. Penile erection has been linked to cholinergic activity and to α_2-adrenergic blockade, which theoretically increases penile inflow of blood or decreases penile outflow of blood or both. Urologists have used yohimbine for diagnostic classification of certain types of male impotence.

Yohimbine is reported to help counteract the loss of sexual desire and the orgasmic inhibition caused by some serotonergic antidepressants (e.g., selective serotonin reuptake inhibitors). It has not been found useful in women for these indications.

EFFECTS ON SPECIFIC ORGANS AND SYSTEMS

Yohimbine primarily affects the peripheral nervous system through its effects on adrenergic neurotransmission. The peripheral nervous system effects influence vascular, cardiac, and gastrointestinal functions.

PRECAUTIONS AND ADVERSE EFFECTS

The adverse effects of yohimbine include anxiety, elevated blood pressure and heart rate, increased psychomotor activity, irritability, tremor, headache, flushing, dizziness, urinary frequency, nausea, vomiting, and sweating. Patients with panic disorder show heightened sensitivity to yohimbine and experience increased anxiety, increased blood pressure, and increased plasma 3-methoxy-4-hydroxyphenylglycol (MHPG).

Yohimbine should be used with caution in female patients and should not be used in patients with renal disease, cardiac disease, glaucoma, or a history of gastric or duodenal ulcer.

DRUG INTERACTIONS

Yohimbine blocks the effect of clonidine (Catapres), guanfacine (Tenex), and other α_2-receptor agonists.

LABORATORY INTERFERENCES

No known laboratory interferences are associated with yohimbine use.

DOSAGE AND CLINICAL GUIDELINES

Yohimbine is available in 5.4-mg tablets. The dosage of yohimbine in the treatment of impotence is approximately 18 mg a day given in doses that range from 2.7 to 5.4 mg three times a day. In the event of significant adverse effects, dosage should first be reduced then gradually increased again. Yohimbine should be used judiciously in psychiatric patients because it may have an adverse effect on their mental status. Because yohimbine has no consistent effects on erectile dysfunction and more effective drugs now exist, its use has diminished considerably.

References

Ashton AK. Yohimbine in the treatment of male erectile dysfunction. *Am J Psychiatry.* 1994;151:1397.

Cameron OG, Zubiete JK, Grunhaus L, Minoshima S. Effects of yohimbine on cerebral blood flow, symptoms, and physiological functions in humans. *Psychosom Med.* 2000;62:549.

Cappiello A, McDougle CJ, Malison RT, et al. Yohimbine augmentation of fluvoxamine in refractory depression: a single-blind study. *Biol Psychiatry.* 1995;38:765.

DeBattista C, Shatzberg AF. Other pharmacological and biological therapies. In: Sadock BJ, Sadock VA, eds. *Kaplan & Sadock's Comprehensive Textbook of Psychiatry.* 7th ed. Vol 2. Baltimore: Lippincott Williams & Wilkins; 2000:2521.

Hoffman BB. Catecholamines, sympathomimetic drugs, and adrenergic receptor antagonists. In: Hardman JG, Limbird LE, Goodman Gilman A, eds. *Goodman & Gilman's the Pharmacological Basis of Therapeutics.* 10th ed. New York: McGraw-Hill; 2001:215.

Gitlin MJ. Psychotropic medications and their effects on sexual function: diagnosis, biology, and treatment approaches. *J Clin Psychiatry.* 1994;55:406.

Goddard AW, Charney DS, Germine M, et al. Effects of tryptophan depletion on responses to yohimbine in healthy human subjects. *Biol Psychiatry.* 1995;38:74.

Knoll LD, Benson RC Jr, Bilhartz DL, Minich PJ, Furlow WL. A randomized crossover study using yohimbine and isoxsuprine versus pentoxifylline in the management of vasculogenic impotence. *J Urol.* 1996;155:144.

Mann K, Klingler T, Noe S, et al. Effects of yohimbine on sexual experiences and nocturnal penile tumescence and rigidity in erectile dysfunction. *Arch Sex Behav.* 1996;25:1.

McDougle CJ, Krystal JH, Price LH, et al. Noradrenergic response to acute ethanol administration in healthy subjects: comparison with intravenous yohimbine. *Psychopharmacology.* 1995;118:127.

Morgan CA, Grillon C, Southwick SM, et al. Yohimbine facilitated acoustic startle in combat veterans with post-traumatic stress disorder. *Psychopharmacology.* 1995;117:466.

Morgan CA, Southwick SM, Grillon C, et al. Yohimbine—facilitated acoustic startle reflex in humans. *Psychopharmacology.* 1993;110:342.

Peskind ER, Wingerson D, Murray S, et al. Effects of Alzheimer's disease and normal aging on cerebrospinal fluid norepinephrine response to yohimbine and clonidine. *Arch Gen Psychiatry.* 1995;52:774.

▲ 36.5 ELECTROCONVULSIVE THERAPY

More than 50 years after it was developed, electroconvulsive therapy (ECT) remains an important, effective, and safe treatment for a variety of neuropsychiatric disorders. Major depression, especially in the elderly, is presently the most common indication for the treatment; however, it is used in other serious mental disorders such as schizophrenia and bipolar I illness. The invasiveness of the procedure and the major adverse effects of memory loss and confusion are limiting variables in the use of ECT. However, cognitive adverse effects of ECT clearly have nothing to do with therapeutic benefits. Most major innovations in ECT technique over the past 20 years have sought to diminish cognitive effects while maintaining benefits. New developments in ECT technique offer the hope that this form of treatment will find better acceptance among psychiatrists and patients.

HISTORY

Although camphor-induced seizures were used as early as the 16th century to treat psychosis, most histories of ECT start in 1934, when Ladislas J. von Meduna reported the successful treatment of catatonia and other schizophrenic symptoms with pharmacologically induced seizures. Von Meduna began by using intramuscular injections of camphor suspended in oil but quickly switched to intravenously administered pentylenetetrazol. Von Meduna attempted the treatment method on the basis of two observations. First, schizophrenic symptoms often decrease after a seizure; seizures were often accidentally or iatrogenically induced in psychiatric patients secondary to withdrawal from medications (e.g., barbiturates). Second, schizophrenia and epilepsy, it was incorrectly believed, cannot coexist in the same patient; therefore, the induction of seizures might rid patients of schizophrenia. Pentylenetetrazol-induced seizures were used as an effective treatment for 4 years before the introduction of electrically induced seizures. Primarily on the basis of the work of von Meduna, Ugo Cerletti and Lucio Bini administered the first electroconvulsive treatment in Rome in April 1938. Initially, the treatment was referred to as *electroshock therapy* (EST), but it later became known as *electroconvulsive therapy.*

The major problems associated with ECT were patients' discomfort caused by the procedure and the bone fractures resulting from the motor activity of the seizure. These problems were eventually eliminated by the use of general anesthetics and pharmacological muscle relaxation during treatment. An American psychiatrist, Abram E. Bennett, helped develop the method for extracting pure curare from plant material. Bennett suggested the use of spinal anesthetics and the use of curare (to paralyze the muscles to prevent fractures) during ECT. In 1951, succinylcholine (Anectine) was introduced and became the most widely used muscle relaxant for ECT. Currently, about 100,000 patients annually receive ECT in the United States.

ELECTROPHYSIOLOGY IN ECT

Neurons maintain a resting potential across the plasma membrane and may propagate an action potential, which is a transient reversal of the membrane potential. Normal brain activity is desynchronized; that is, neurons fire action potentials asynchronously. A convulsion, or seizure, occurs when a large percentage of neurons fire in unison. Such rhythmical changes in the extracellular potential entrain neighboring neurons, propagate the seizure activity across the cortex and into deeper structures, and eventually engulf the entire brain in high-voltage synchronous neuronal firing. Cellular mechanisms work to contain the seizure activity and to maintain cellular homeostasis, and the seizure eventually ends. In epilepsy, any of possibly several hundred genetic defects can alter the balance in favor of

unrestrained activity. In ECT, seizures are triggered in normal neurons by application through the scalp of pulses of current, under conditions that are carefully controlled to create a seizure of a particular duration over the entire brain.

The qualities of the electricity used in ECT can be described by Ohm's law, $E = IR$, or $I = E/R$, in which E is voltage, I is current, and R is resistance. The intensity or dose of electricity in ECT is measured in terms of charge (milliampere-seconds or millicoulombs) or energy (watt-seconds or joules). Resistance is synonymous with impedance, and in the case of ECT, the electrode's contact with the body and the nature of the bodily tissues are the major determinants of resistance. The skull has a high impedance; the brain has a low impedance. Because scalp tissues are much better conductors of electricity than bone, only about 20 percent of the applied charge actually enters the skull to excite neurons. The ECT machines that are now widely used can be adjusted to administer the electricity under conditions of constant current, voltage, or energy.

MECHANISM OF ACTION

The induction of a bilateral generalized seizure is necessary for both the beneficial and the adverse effects of ECT. Although a seizure superficially seems like an all-or-none event, some data indicate that not all generalized seizures involve all the neurons in deep brain structures (e.g., the basal ganglia and the thalamus); recruitment of these deep neurons may be necessary for full therapeutic benefit. After the generalized seizure, the electroencephalogram (EEG) shows about 60 to 90 seconds of postictal suppression. This period is followed by the appearance of high-voltage delta and theta waves and a return of the EEG to preseizure appearance in about 30 minutes. During the course of a series of ECT treatments, the interictal EEG is generally slower and of greater amplitude than usual, but the EEG returns to pretreatment appearance 1 month to 1 year after the end of the course of treatment.

One research approach to the mechanism of action for ECT has been to study the neurophysiological effects of treatment. Positron emission tomography (PET) studies of both cerebral blood flow and glucose use have shown that during seizures, cerebral blood flow, use of glucose and oxygen, and permeability of the blood–brain barrier increase. After the seizure, blood flow and glucose metabolism are decreased, perhaps most markedly in the frontal lobes. Some research indicates that the degree of decrease in cerebral metabolism is correlated with therapeutic response.

Seizure foci in idiopathic epilepsy are hypometabolic during interictal periods; ECT itself acts as an anticonvulsant because its administration is associated with an increase in the seizure threshold as treatment progresses. Recent data suggest that for 1 to 2 months following a session of ECT, EEGs record a large increase in slow-wave activity located over the prefrontal cortex in patients who responded well to the ECT. High-intensity bilateral stimulation produced the best response; low-intensity unilateral stimulation, the weakest. These data are of unclear significance, however, as the specific EEG correlate disappeared 2 months after ECT, whereas the clinical benefit persisted.

ECT affects the cellular mechanisms of memory and mood regulation and raises the seizure threshold. The latter effect may be blocked by the opiate antagonist naloxone (Narcan).

Neurochemical research into the mechanisms of action of ECT has focused on changes in neurotransmitter receptors and, recently, changes in second-messenger systems. Virtually every neurotransmitter system is affected by ECT, but a series of ECT sessions results in downregulation of postsynaptic β-adrenergic receptors, the same receptor change observed with virtually all antidepressant treatments. The effects of ECT on serotonergic neurons remain controversial. Various research studies have reported an increase in postsynaptic serotonin receptors, no change in serotonin receptors, and a change in the presynaptic regulation of serotonin release. ECT has also been reported to effect changes in the muscarinic, cholinergic, and dopaminergic neuronal systems. In second-messenger systems, ECT has been reported to affect the coupling of G proteins to receptors, the activity of adenylyl cyclase and phospholipase C, and the regulation of calcium entry into neurons.

INDICATIONS

Major Depressive Disorder

The most common indication for ECT is major depressive disorder, for which ECT is the fastest and most effective available therapy. ECT should be considered for use in patients who have failed medication trials, have not tolerated medications, have severe or psychotic symptoms, are acutely suicidal or homicidal, or have marked symptoms of agitation or stupor. Controlled studies have shown that up to 70 percent of patients who fail to respond to antidepressant medications may respond positively to ECT.

ECT is effective for depression in both major depressive disorder and bipolar I disorder. Delusional or psychotic depression has long been considered particularly responsive to ECT; but recent studies have indicated that major depressive episodes with psychotic features are no more responsive to ECT than nonpsychotic depressive disorders. Nevertheless, because major depressive episodes with psychotic features respond poorly to antidepressant pharmacotherapy alone, ECT should be considered much more often as the first-line treatment for patients with the disorder. Major depressive disorder with melancholic features (such as markedly severe symptoms, psychomotor retardation, early morning awakening, diurnal variation, decreased appetite and weight, and agitation) is considered likely to respond to ECT. ECT is particularly indicated for persons who are severely depressed, who have psychotic symptoms, who show suicidal intent, or who refuse to eat. Depressed patients less likely to respond to ECT include those with somatization disorder. Elderly patients tend to respond to ECT more slowly than young patients. ECT is a treatment for major depressive episode and does not provide prophylaxis unless it is administered on a long-term maintenance basis.

Manic Episodes

ECT is at least equal to lithium (Eskalith) in the treatment of acute manic episodes. The pharmacological treatment of manic episodes, however, is so effective in the short term and for prophylaxis that the use of ECT to treat manic episodes is generally limited to situations with specific contraindications to all available pharmacological approaches. The relative rapidity of

the ECT response indicates its usefulness for patients whose manic behavior has produced dangerous levels of exhaustion. ECT should not be used for a patient who is receiving lithium, because lithium may lower the seizure threshold and cause a prolonged seizure.

Schizophrenia

ECT is an effective treatment for the symptoms of acute schizophrenia but not for those of chronic schizophrenia. Patients with schizophrenia who have marked positive symptoms, catatonia, or affective symptoms are considered most likely to respond to ECT. In such patients, the efficacy of ECT is about equal to that of antipsychotics but improvement may occur faster.

Other Indications

Small studies have found ECT effective in the treatment of catatonia, a symptom associated with mood disorders, schizophrenia, and medical and neurological disorders. ECT is also reportedly useful to treat episodic psychoses, atypical psychoses, obsessive-compulsive disorder, and delirium and such medical conditions as neuroleptic malignant syndrome, hypopituitarism, intractable seizure disorders, and the on-off phenomenon of Parkinson's disease. ECT may also be the treatment of choice for depressed suicidal pregnant women who require treatment and cannot take medication, for geriatric and medically ill patients who cannot take antidepressant drugs safely, and perhaps even for severely depressed and suicidal children and adolescents who may be less likely to respond to antidepressant drugs than are adults. ECT is not effective in somatization disorder (unless accompanied by depression), personality disorders, and anxiety disorders.

CLINICAL GUIDELINES

Patients and their families are often apprehensive about ECT; therefore, clinicians must explain both beneficial and adverse effects and alternative treatment approaches. The informed-consent process should be documented in the patients' medical records and should include a discussion of the disorder, its natural course, and the option of receiving no treatment. Printed literature and videotapes about ECT may be useful in attempting to obtain a truly informed consent. The use of involuntary ECT is rare today and should be reserved for patients who urgently need treatment and who have a legally appointed guardian who has agreed to its use. Clinicians must know local, state, and federal laws about the use of ECT.

Pretreatment Evaluation

Pretreatment evaluation should include standard physical, neurological, and preanesthesia examinations and a complete medical history. Laboratory evaluations should include blood and urine chemistries, a chest X-ray, and an electrocardiogram (ECG). A dental examination to assess the state of patients' dentition is advisable for elderly patients and patients who have had inadequate dental care. An X-ray of the spine is needed if there is other evidence of a spinal disorder. Computed tomography (CT) or magnetic resonance imaging (MRI) should be performed if a clinician suspects the presence of a seizure disorder or a space-occupying lesion. Practitioners of ECT no longer consider even a space-occupying lesion to be an absolute contraindication to ECT, but with such patients the procedure should be performed only by experts.

Concomitant Medications. Patients' ongoing medications should be assessed for possible interactions with the induction of a seizure, for effects (both positive and negative) on the seizure threshold, and for drug interactions with the medications used during ECT. The use of tricyclic and tetracyclic drugs, monoamine oxidase inhibitors, and antipsychotics is generally considered acceptable. Benzodiazepines used for anxiety should be withdrawn because of their anticonvulsant activity; lithium should be withdrawn because it can result in increased postictal delirium and can prolong seizure activity; clozapine (Clozaril) and bupropion (Wellbutrin) should be withdrawn because they are associated with the development of late-appearing seizures. Lidocaine (Xylocaine) should not be administered during ECT because it markedly increases the seizure threshold; theophylline (Theo-Dur) is contraindicated because it increases the duration of seizures. Reserpine (Serpasil) is also contraindicated because it is associated with further compromise of the respiratory and cardiovascular systems during ECT.

Premedications, Anesthetics, and Muscle Relaxants

Patients should not be given anything orally for 6 hours before treatment. Just before the procedure, the patient's mouth should be checked for dentures and other foreign objects, and an intravenous (IV) line should be established. A bite block is inserted in the mouth just before the treatment is administered to protect the patient's teeth and tongue during the seizure. Except for the brief interval of electrical stimulation, 100 percent oxygen is administered at a rate of 5 L a minute during the procedure until spontaneous respiration returns. Emergency equipment for establishing an airway should be immediately available in case it is needed.

Muscarinic Anticholinergic Drugs. Muscarinic anticholinergic drugs are administered before ECT to minimize oral and respiratory secretions and to block bradycardias and asystoles, unless the resting heart rate is above 90 beats a minute. Some ECT centers have stopped the routine use of anticholinergics as premedications, although their use is still indicated for patients taking β-adrenergic receptor antagonists and those with ventricular ectopic beats. The most commonly used drug is atropine, which can be administered 0.3 to 0.6 mg intramuscularly (IM) or subcutaneously (SC) 30 to 60 minutes before the anesthetic or 0.4 to 1.0 mg IV 2 or 3 minutes before the anesthetic. An option is to use glycopyrrolate (Robinul) (0.2 to 0.4 mg IM, IV, or SC), which is less likely to cross the blood–brain barrier and less likely to cause cognitive dysfunction and nausea, although it is thought to have less cardiovascular protective activity than does atropine.

ECT Anesthesia. Administration of ECT requires general anesthesia and oxygenation. The depth of anesthesia should be as light as possible, not only to minimize adverse effects but also to avoid elevating the seizure threshold associated with

many anesthetics. Methohexital (Brevital) (0.75 to 1.0 mg/kg IV bolus) is the most commonly used anesthetic because of its shorter duration of action and lower association with postictal arrhythmias than thiopental (Pentothal) (usual dose 2 to 3 mg/kg IV), although this difference in cardiac effects is not universally accepted. Four other anesthetic alternatives are etomidate (Amidate), ketamine (Ketalar), alfentanil (Alfenta), and propofol (Diprivan). Etomidate (0.15 to 0.3 mg/kg IV) is sometimes used because it does not increase the seizure threshold; this effect is particularly useful for elderly patients because the seizure threshold increases with age. Ketamine (6 to 10 mg/kg IM) is sometimes used because it does not increase the seizure threshold, although its use is limited by the frequent association of psychotic symptoms with emergence from anesthesia with this drug. Alfentanil (2 to 9 mg/kg IV) is sometimes coadministered with barbiturates to allow the use of low doses of the barbiturate anesthetics and thus reduce the seizure threshold less than usual, although its use may be associated with an increased incidence of nausea. Propofol (0.5 to 3.5 mg/kg IV) is less useful because of its strong anticonvulsant properties.

Muscle Relaxants. After the onset of the anesthetic effect, usually within a minute, a muscle relaxant is administered to minimize the risk of bone fractures and other injuries resulting from motor activity during the seizure. The goal is to produce profound relaxation of the muscles, not necessarily to paralyze them, unless the patient has a history of osteoporosis or spinal injury or has a pacemaker and is, therefore, at risk for injury related to motor activity during the seizure. Succinylcholine, an ultrafast-acting depolarizing blocking agent, has gained virtually universal acceptance for the purpose. Succinylcholine is usually administered in a dose of 0.5 to 1 mg/kg as an IV bolus or drip. Because succinylcholine is a depolarizing agent, its action is marked by the presence of muscle fasciculations, which move in a rostrocaudal progression. The disappearance of these movements in the feet or the absence of muscle contractions after peripheral nerve stimulation indicates maximal muscle relaxation. In some patients, tubocurarine (3 mg IV) is administered to prevent myoclonus and increases in potassium and muscle enzymes; these reactions may be a problem in patients with musculoskeletal or cardiac disease. To monitor the duration of the convulsion, a blood pressure cuff may be inflated at the ankle to a pressure in excess of the systolic pressure before infusion of the muscle relaxant, to allow observation of relatively innocuous seizure activity in the foot muscles.

If a patient has a known history of pseudocholinesterase deficiency, atracurium (Tracrium) (0.5 to 1 mg/kg IV) or curare can be used instead of succinylcholine. In such a patient, the metabolism of succinylcholine is disrupted, and prolonged apnea may necessitate emergency airway management. In general, however, because of the short half-life of succinylcholine, the duration of apnea after its administration is generally shorter than the delay in regaining consciousness caused by the anesthetic and the postictal state. Table 36.5–1 summarizes medications used in ECT.

Table 36.5–1
Medications Used in the Administration of ECT

Drug	Dose
Anticholinergics	
Atropine	0.4–1.0 mg IV or IM
Glycopyrrolate	0.2–0.4 mg IV or IM
Anesthetics	
Methohexital	0.5–1.0 mg/kg IV
Thiopental	1.5–2.5 mg/kg IV
Etomidate	0.1–0.3 mg/kg IV
Alfentanil	0.2–0.3 μg/kg IV
Ketamine	0.5–1.0 mg/kg IV
Propofol	0.75–1.5 mg/kg IV
Midazolam	0.15–0.3 mg/kg IV
Muscle relaxants	
Depolarizing	
Succinylcholine	0.75–1.5 mg/kg IV
Nondepolarizing	
Mivacurium	0.1–0.2 mg/kg IV
Atracurium	0.3–0.4 mg/kg IV
Antihypertensives	
Esmolol	0.05–0.1 mg/kg IV
Labetalol	0.04–0.2 mg/kg IV
Nifedipine	10–30 mg PO

Table by K. E. Isenberg, M.D., and C. F. Zorumski, M.D.

Electrode Placement

ECT can be conducted with either bilaterally or unilaterally placed electrodes. Bilateral placement usually yields a more rapid therapeutic response, and unilateral placement results in less marked cognitive adverse effects in the first week or weeks after treatment, although this difference between placements is absent 2 months after treatment. In bilateral placement, which was introduced first, one stimulating electrode is placed several centimeters apart over each hemisphere of the brain. In unilateral ECT, both electrodes are placed several centimeters apart over the nondominant hemisphere, almost always the right hemisphere. Some attempts have been made to vary the location of the electrodes in unilateral ECT, but these attempts have not obtained the rapidity of response seen with bilateral ECT or further reduced the cognitive adverse effects. The most common approach is to initiate treatment with unilateral ECT because of its more favorable adverse effect profile. If a patient does not improve after four to six unilateral treatments, bilateral placement is used. Initial bilateral placement of the electrodes may be indicated in the following situations: severe depressive symptoms, marked agitation, immediate suicide risk, manic symptoms, catatonic stupor, and treatment-resistant schizophrenia. Some patients are particularly at risk for anesthetic-related adverse effects, and these patients may also be treated with bilateral placement from the beginning to minimize the number of treatments and exposure to anesthetics.

In traditional bilateral ECT, the electrodes are placed bifrontotemporally with the center of each electrode about 1 inch above the midpoint of an imaginary line drawn from the tragus to the external canthus. With unilateral ECT, one stimulus electrode is typically placed over the nondominant frontotemporal area. Although several locations for the second stimulus electrode have been proposed, placement on the nondominant cen-

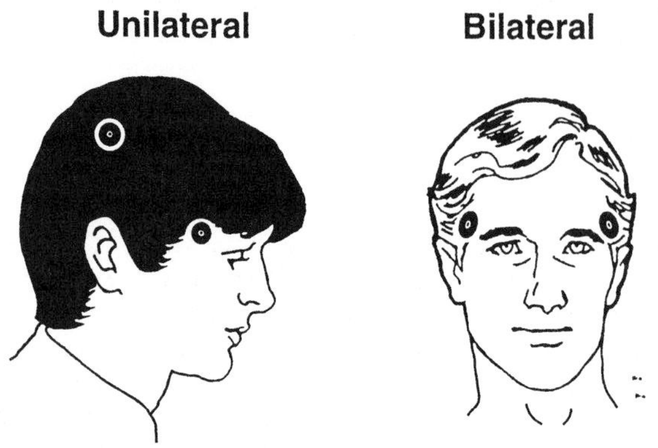

FIGURE 36.5–1

Types of electrode placements used with ECT—bilateral (*right*) and right unilateral nondominant (*left*). In the latter case, a wide centroparietal-frontotemporal placement is depicted. (Courtesy of K. E. Isenberg, M.D., and C. F. Zuronski, M.D.)

troparietal scalp, just lateral to the midline vertex, appears to provide the most effective configuration (Fig. 36.5–1).

Which cerebral hemisphere is dominant can generally be determined by a simple series of performance tasks (e.g., for handedness and footedness) and stated preference. Right body responses correlate highly with left brain dominance. If the responses are mixed or if they clearly indicate left body dominance, clinicians should alternate the polarity of unilateral stimulation during successive treatments. Clinicians should also monitor the time that it takes for patients to recover consciousness and to answer simple orientation and naming questions. The side of stimulation associated with less rapid recovery and return of function is considered dominant. The left hemisphere is dominant in most persons; therefore, unilateral electrode placement is almost always over the right hemisphere.

Electrical Stimulus

The electrical stimulus must be strong enough to reach the seizure threshold (the level of intensity needed to produce a seizure). The electrical stimulus is given in cycles, and each cycle contains a positive and a negative wave. Old machines use a sine wave; however, this type of machine is now considered obsolete because of the inefficiency of that wave shape. When a sine wave is delivered, the electrical stimulus in the sine wave before the seizure threshold is reached and after the seizure is activated is unnecessary and excessive. Modern ECT machines use a brief pulse waveform that administers the electrical stimulus usually in 1 to 2 ms at a rate of 30 to 100 pulses a second. Machines that use an ultrabrief pulse (0.5 ms) are not as effective as brief pulse machines.

Establishing a patient's seizure threshold is not straightforward. A 40-fold variability in seizure thresholds occurs among patients. In addition, during the course of ECT treatment, a patient's seizure threshold may increase 25 to 200 percent. The seizure threshold is also higher in men than in women and higher in older than in younger adults. A common technique is to initiate treatment at an electrical stimulus that is thought to be below the seizure threshold for a particular patient and then to increase this intensity by 100 percent for unilateral placement and by 50 percent for bilateral placement until the seizure threshold is reached. A debate in the literature concerns whether a minimally suprathreshold dose, a moderately suprathreshold dose (1 1/2 times the threshold), or a high suprathreshold dose (3 times the threshold) is preferable. The debate about stimulus intensity resembles the debate about electrode placement. Essentially, the data support the conclusion that doses of 3 times the threshold are the most rapidly effective and that minimal suprathreshold doses are associated with the fewest and least severe cognitive adverse effects.

Induced Seizures

A brief muscular contraction, usually strongest in a patient's jaw and facial muscles, is seen concurrently with the flow of stimulus current, regardless of whether a seizure occurs. The first behavioral sign of the seizure is often a plantar extension, which lasts 10 to 20 seconds and marks the tonic phase. This phase is followed by rhythmic (i.e., clonic) contractions that decrease in frequency and finally disappear. The tonic phase is marked by high-frequency, sharp EEG activity on which a higher-frequency muscle artifact may be superimposed. During the clonic phase, bursts of polyspike activity occur simultaneously with the muscular contractions but usually persist for at least a few seconds after the clonic movements stop.

Monitoring Seizures. A physician must have an objective measure that a bilateral generalized seizure has occurred after the stimulation. The physician should be able to observe either some evidence of tonic-clonic movements or electrophysiological evidence of seizure activity from the EEG or electromyogram (EMG). Seizures with unilateral ECT are asymmetrical, with higher ictal EEG amplitudes over the stimulated hemisphere than over the nonstimulated hemisphere. Occasionally, unilateral seizures are induced; for this reason, at least a single pair of EEG electrodes should be placed over the contralateral hemisphere when using unilateral ECT. For a seizure to be effective in the course of ECT, it should last at least 25 seconds.

Failure to Induce Seizures. If a particular stimulus fails to cause a seizure of sufficient duration, up to four attempts at seizure induction can be tried during a course of treatment. The onset of seizure activity is sometimes delayed as long as 20 to 40 seconds after the stimulus administration. If a stimulus fails to result in a seizure, the contact between the electrodes and the skin should be checked, and the intensity of the stimulus should be increased by 25 to 100 percent. The clinician can also change the anesthetic agent to minimize increases in the seizure threshold caused by the anesthetic. Additional procedures to lower the seizure threshold include hyperventilation and administration of 500 to 2,000 mg IV of caffeine sodium benzoate 5 to 10 minutes before the stimulus.

Prolonged and Tardive Seizures. Prolonged seizures (seizures lasting more than 180 seconds) and status epilepticus can be terminated either with additional doses of the barbiturate anesthetic agent or with intravenous diazepam (Valium) (5 to 10 mg). Management of such complications should be accompanied by intubation, because the oral airway is insufficient to maintain adequate ventilation over an extended apneic period.

Tardive seizures—that is, additional seizures appearing some time after the ECT treatment—may develop in patients with preexisting seizure disorders. In rare patients, ECT precipitates the development of an epileptic disorder. Such situations should be managed clinically as if they were pure epileptic disorders.

Number and Spacing of ECT Treatments

ECT treatments are usually administered two to three times a week; twice-weekly treatments are associated with less memory impairment than thrice-weekly treatments. In general, the course of treatment of major depressive disorder can take 6 to 12 treatments (although up to 20 sessions are possible); the treatment of manic episodes can take 8 to 20 treatments; the treatment of schizophrenia can take more than 15 treatments; and the treatment of catatonia and delirium can take as few as 1 to 4 treatments. Treatment should continue until the patient achieves what is considered the maximum therapeutic response. Further treatment does not yield any therapeutic benefit but increases the severity and duration of the adverse effects. The point of maximal improvement is usually thought to occur when a patient fails to continue to improve after two consecutive treatments. If a patient is not improving after 6 to 10 sessions, bilateral placement and high-density treatment (three times the seizure threshold) should be attempted before ECT is abandoned.

Multiple Monitored ECT. Multiple monitored ECT (MMECT) involves giving multiple ECT stimuli during a single session, most commonly two bilateral stimuli within 2 minutes. This approach may be warranted in severely ill patients and in those at especially high risk from the anesthetic procedures. MMECT is associated with the most frequent occurrences of serious cognitive adverse effects.

Maintenance Treatment

A short-term course of ECT induces a remission in symptoms but does not, of itself, prevent a relapse. Post-ECT maintenance treatment should always be considered. Maintenance therapy is generally pharmacological, but maintenance ECT treatments (weekly, biweekly, or monthly) have been reported to be effective relapse prevention treatments, although data from large studies are lacking. Indications for maintenance ECT treatments may include rapid relapse after initial ECT, severe symptoms, psychotic symptoms, and the inability to tolerate medications. If ECT was used because a patient was unresponsive to a specific medication, then, following ECT, the patient should be given a trial of a different medication.

Failure of ECT Trial

Patients who fail to improve after a trial of ECT should again be treated with the pharmacological agents that failed in the past. Although the data are primarily anecdotal, many reports indicate that patients who had previously failed to improve while taking an antidepressant drug do improve while taking the same drug after receiving a course of ECT treatments, even if the ECT seemed to be a therapeutic failure. Nonetheless, with the increased availability of drugs that act at diverse receptor sites, it is less often necessary to return to a drug that has failed than it was formerly.

ADVERSE EFFECTS

Contraindications

ECT has no absolute contraindications, only situations in which a patient is at increased risk and has an increased need for close monitoring. Pregnancy is not a contraindication for ECT, and fetal monitoring is generally considered unnecessary unless the pregnancy is high risk or complicated. Patients with space-occupying central nervous system lesions are at increased risk for edema and brain herniation after ECT. But if the lesion is small, pretreatment with dexamethasone (Decadron) is given, and hypertension is controlled during the seizure, the risk of serious complications can be minimized for these patients. Patients who have increased intracerebral pressure or are at risk for cerebral bleeding (e.g., those with cerebrovascular diseases and aneurysms) are at risk during ECT because of the increased cerebral blood flow during the seizure. This risk can be lessened, although not eliminated, by control of the patient's blood pressure during the treatment. Patients with recent myocardial infarctions are another high-risk group, although the risk is greatly diminished 2 weeks after the myocardial infarction and is even further reduced 3 months after the infarction. Patients with hypertension should be stabilized on their antihypertensive medications before ECT is administered. Propranolol (Inderal) and sublingual nitroglycerin can also be used to protect such patients during treatment.

Mortality

The mortality rate with ECT is about 0.002 percent per treatment and 0.01 percent for each patient. These numbers compare favorably with the risks associated with general anesthesia and childbirth. ECT death is usually from cardiovascular complications and is most likely to occur in patients whose cardiac status is already compromised.

Central Nervous System Effects

Common adverse effects associated with ECT are headache, confusion, and delirium shortly after the seizure while the patient is coming out of anesthesia. Marked confusion may occur in up to 10 percent of patients within 30 minutes of the seizure and can be treated with barbiturates and benzodiazepines. Delirium is usually most pronounced after the first few treatments and in patients who receive bilateral ECT or who have coexisting neurological disorders. The delirium characteristically clears within days or a few weeks at the longest.

Memory. The greatest concern about ECT is the association between ECT and memory loss. About 75 percent of all patients given ECT say that the memory impairment is the worst adverse effect. Although memory impairment during a course of treatment is almost the rule, follow-up data indicate that almost all patients are back to their cognitive baselines after 6 months. Some patients, however, complain of persistent memory difficulties. For example, a patient may not remember

the events leading up to the hospitalization and ECT, and such autobiographical memories may never be recalled. The degree of cognitive impairment during treatment and the time it takes to return to baseline are related in part to the amount of electrical stimulation used during treatment. Memory impairment is most often reported by patients who have experienced little improvement with ECT. In spite of the memory impairment, which usually resolves, there is no evidence of brain damage caused by ECT. This subject has been the focus of several brain-imaging studies, using a variety of modalities; virtually all concluded that permanent brain damage is not an adverse effect of ECT. Neurologists and epileptologists generally agree that seizures that last less than 30 minutes do not cause permanent neuronal damage.

Other Adverse Effects of ECT

Fractures often accompanied treatments in the early days of ECT. With routine use of muscle relaxants, fractures of long bones or vertebrae should not occur. However, some patients may break teeth or experience back pain because of contractions during the procedure. Muscle soreness may occur in some individuals but often results from the effects of muscle depolarization by succinylcholine and is most likely to be particularly troublesome after the first session in a series. This soreness can be treated with mild analgesics, including nonsteroidal anti-inflammatory drugs (NSAIDs). A significant minority of patients experience nausea, vomiting, and headaches following an ECT treatment. Nausea and vomiting can be prevented by treatment with antiemetics at the time of ECT (e.g., metoclopramide [Reglan], 10 mg IV, or prochlorperazine [Compazine], 10 mg IV; ondansetron [Zofran] is an acceptable alternative if adverse effects preclude use of dopamine receptor antagonists).

ECT can be associated with headaches, although this effect is usually readily manageable. Headaches often respond to NSAIDs given in the ECT recovery period. In patients with severe headaches, pretreatment with ketorolac (Toradol) (30 to 60 mg IV), an NSAID approved for brief parenteral use, can be helpful. Acetaminophen (Tylenol), tramadol (Ultram), propoxyphene (Darvon), and more potent analgesia provided by opioids can be used individually or in various combinations (e.g., pretreatment with ketorolac and postseizure management with acetaminophen-propoxyphene) to manage more intractable headache. ECT can induce migrainous headache and related symptoms; sumatriptan (Imitrex) (6 mg subcutaneously or 25 mg orally) may be a useful addition to the agents described above. Ergot compounds can exacerbate cardiovascular changes observed during ECT and probably should not be a component of ECT pretreatment.

References

Abrams R. *Electroconvulsive Therapy.* 2nd ed. Oxford: Oxford University Press; 1992.

Beale MD, Bernstein HJ, Kellner CH. Maintenance electroconvulsive therapy for geriatric depression: a one-year follow-up. *Clin Gerontol.* 1996;16:86.

Colenda CC, McCall WV. A statistical model predicting the seizure threshold for right unilateral ECT in 106 patients. *Convuls Ther.* 1996;12:3.

Ding Z, White PF. Anesthesia for electroconvulsive therapy. *Anesth Analg.* 2002;94:1351.

George MS, Lisanby SH, Sackeim HA. Transcranial magnetic stimulation. *Arch Gen Psychiatry.* 1999;56:300.

Hamner M, Huber M. Discontinuation of antidepressant medications before ECT. *Convuls Ther.* 1996;12:125.

Helsley S, Sheikh T, Kim KY, Park SK. ECT therapy in PTSD. *Am J Psychiatry.* 1999;156:94.

Jha AK, Stein GS, Fenwick P. Negative interaction between lithium and electroconvulsive therapy: a case-control study. *Br J Psychiatry.* 1996;168:241.

Kellner CH, Pritchett JT, Beale MD, Coffey CE. *Handbook of ECT.* Washington, DC: American Psychiatric Press; 1997.

Klein E, Kreinin I, Chistyakov A, et al. Therapeutic efficacy of right prefrontal slow repetitive transcranial magnetic stimulation in major depression: a double-blind controlled study. *Arch Gen Psychiatry.* 1999;56:315.

Prudic J, Sackeim HA. Electroconvulsive therapy and suicide risk. *J Clin Psychiatry.* 1999;60:104.

▲ 36.6 OTHER BIOLOGICAL AND PHARMACOLOGICAL THERAPIES

TRANSCRANIAL MAGNETIC STIMULATION

Transcranial magnetic stimulation (TMS) is a noninvasive technique for stimulating cells of the cerebral cortex. It does not cause generalized seizures as in electroconvulsive therapy (ECT). TMS uses a magnet to allow focused electrical stimulation across the scalp and cranium without the pain associated with percutaneous electrical stimulation. TMS was originally used to map cortical motor control and hemisphere dominance. Stimulating the motor cortex with TMS results in a contralateral motor response. Likewise, stimulating Broca's area with TMS has resulted in speech blockage. Currently, the potential use of TMS for the treatment of neurological and psychiatric disorders is being explored actively.

In TMS a powerful electrical current is passed through a small coil applied to the scalp. This current generates a focused magnetic field of 1.5 to 2 teslas that passes through the scalp and is largely unimpeded by bone or tissue. The magnetic field in turn depolarizes brain cells to a depth of 2 cm from the coil. Cortical interneurons are more likely to be stimulated than cortical output cells are because the interneurons tend to lie parallel to the brain surface. TMS uses magnetic stimulators with multiple capacitors capable of generating very rapid pulses up to 60 Hz. Low-frequency pulses in the range of 1 Hz may have an inhibitory effect on cortical cells, while higher frequencies have an excitatory effect.

A number of small, open-labeled studies have suggested that TMS may be effective in some patients with treatment-resistant major depressive disorder as well as in those with milder major depressive disorder. Recent functional imaging studies have suggested that the baseline hypofrontality associated with major depressive disorder can be reversed. In addition to major depressive disorder, TMS has shown some preliminary efficacy in obsessive-compulsive disorder and in posttraumatic stress disorder.

TMS has been used to map the motor cortex, help determine hemispheric dominance, and probe short-term memory. In some symptoms of Parkinson's disease, including bradykinesia, diminished reaction time has improved transiently with TMS. Finally, TMS has been used to help elucidate the pathophysiology of migraine headache, and some patients have had temporary symptomatic relief with TMS. The application of TMS to psychiatric conditions has lagged behind its neurological appli-

cations. It is used primarily as a research tool, but its clinical use is increasing steadily.

PHOTOTHERAPY

Phototherapy (light therapy) was introduced in 1984 as a treatment for seasonal affective disorder (mood disorder with seasonal pattern). In this disorder, patients typically experience depression as the photoperiod of the day decreases with advancing winter. Women represent at least 75 percent of all patients with seasonal depression, and the mean age of presentation is 40. Patients rarely present over the age of 55 with seasonal affective disorder.

Phototherapy typically involves exposing the afflicted patient to bright light in the range of 1,500 to 10,000 lux or more, typically with a light box that sits on a table or desk. Patients sit in front of the box for approximately 1 to 2 hours before dawn each day, although some patients may also benefit from exposure after dusk. Alternatively, some manufacturers have developed light visors, with a light source built into the brim of the hat. These light visors allow mobility, but recent controlled studies have questioned the use of this type of light exposure. Trials have typically lasted 1 week, but longer treatment durations may be associated with greater response.

Phototherapy tends to be well tolerated. Newer light sources tend to use lower light intensities and come equipped with filters; patients are instructed not to look directly at the light source. As with any effective antidepressant, phototherapy has on rare occasions been implicated in switching some depressed patients into mania or hypomania.

In addition to seasonal depression, the other major indication for phototherapy may be in sleep disorders. Phototherapy has been used to decrease the irritability and diminished functioning associated with shift work. Sleep disorders in geriatric patients have reportedly improved with exposure to bright light during the day. Likewise, some evidence suggests that jet lag might respond to light therapy. Preliminary data indicate that phototherapy may benefit some patients with obsessive-compulsive disorder that has a seasonal variation.

VAGAL NERVE STIMULATION (VNS)

Experimental stimulation of the vagus nerve in several studies designed for the treatment of epilepsy found that patients showed improved mood. This observation led to the use of left vagal nerve stimulation using an electronic device implanted in the skin, similar to a cardiac pacemaker. Preliminary studies have shown that a significant number of patients with chronic, recurrent major depressive disorder went into remission when treated with VNS. The mechanism of action of VNS to account for improvement is unknown. The vagus nerve connects to the enteric nervous system and when stimulated may cause release of peptides that act as neurotransmitters. Extensive clinical trials are being conducted to determine the efficacy of VNS.

ACUPUNCTURE

Acupuncture originated in China about 5,000 years ago and continues to be an important medical intervention in the East. America was first exposed to acupuncture by Chinese immigrants in the 1800s. The practice involves inserting fine needles at specific points in the body to relieve pain and other ailments. In the East, acupuncture is used to treat mental disturbances, including agitation, depression, insomnia, and anxiety states. Unfortunately, these indications have not been fully investigated in the West. The two indications for acupuncture that have been best studied in the West are pain management and the treatment of substance abuse.

Abundant data from both animal and human studies suggest that acupuncture can modulate pain responses. Clinically, acupuncture has been used to treat a variety of pain conditions including trigeminal neuralgia, neuropathies, chronic back pain, and headache. The analgesic effects of acupuncture appear to be at least partly mediated by endorphins and enkephalins. Multiple studies have reported that naloxone (Narcan) appears to block the analgesic effects of acupuncture.

A number of studies in the past 25 years suggest that acupuncture may be beneficial in the treatment of alcohol, cocaine, and opioid dependence. Studies in rats and humans suggest that acupuncture may limit narcotic withdrawal symptoms. Among alcoholic patients, acupuncture appears to improve the rate at which they complete detoxification programs and may reduce the frequency of alcohol cravings when used as a maintenance treatment. The reader is referred to Chapter 29, Complementary and Alternative Medicine in Psychiatry, for further information on this subject.

SLEEP DEPRIVATION

Mood disorders are characterized by sleep disturbance. Mania tends to be characterized by a decreased need for sleep, while depression may be associated with either hypersomnia or insomnia. Sleep deprivation may precipitate mania in bipolar I patients and temporarily relieve depression in unipolar patients. Approximately 60 percent of depressive disorder patients exhibit significant but transient benefit from total sleep deprivation. The positive results are typically reversed by the next night of sleep. Several strategies have been used in an attempt to achieve a more sustained response to sleep deprivation. One method used serial total sleep deprivation with a day or two of normal sleep in between. This method does not achieve a sustained antidepressant response since the depression tends to return with normal sleep cycles. Another approach used phase delay in the time patients go to sleep each night, or partial sleep deprivation. In this method, patients may stay awake from 2 AM to 10 PM daily. Up to 50 percent of patients get same-day antidepressant effects from partial sleep deprivation, but this benefit also tends to wear off in time. However, in some reports serial partial sleep deprivation has successfully treated insomnia associated with depression. The third, and probably most effective, strategy combines sleep deprivation with pharmacological treatment of depression. A number of studies have suggested that total and partial sleep deprivation followed by immediate treatment with an antidepressant or lithium (Eskalith) sustains the antidepressant effects of sleep deprivation. Likewise, several recent reports have suggested that sleep deprivation accelerates the response to antidepressants including fluoxetine (Prozac) and nortriptyline (Aventyl, Pamelor). Sleep deprivation has also been noted to improve premenstrual dysphoria.

HERBS, VITAMINS, AND AMINO ACIDS

Nutritional status has long been deemed important in mental health, and certain, now rare, vitamin deficiencies can produce

psychiatric symptoms. For example, severe niacin deficiency results in pellagra with its characteristic triad of skin lesions, gastrointestinal disorder, and psychiatric symptoms. The psychiatric symptoms include irritability and emotional instability progressing to severe depression and then to disorientation, memory impairment, hallucinations, and paranoia. Folic acid deficiency is associated with depression and dementia, while B_{12} deficiency is associated with cognitive impairment, depression, and other affective symptoms. Severe malnutrition can result in apathy and emotional instability.

In 1968 the eminent chemist Linus Pauling coined the term *orthomolecular* to refer to the connection between the mind and nutrition. In his book *Orthomolecular Psychiatry,* research articles were compiled supporting the notion that taking many times the recommended minimum daily dose of vitamins is useful in the treatment of schizophrenia and other psychiatric disorders. While some severe vitamin deficiencies may result in syndromes with a psychiatric component (i.e., niacin deficiency resulting in pellagra), empirical data and an American Psychiatric Association (APA) task force have failed to find evidence supporting the notion that schizophrenia and other disorders respond to vitamin therapies. However, that is not to say that vitamins and amino acids are of no importance in preserving mental health. Evidence indicates that severe vitamin deficiencies can result in psychiatric symptoms and that amino acid supplements may be pharmacologically useful in the treatment of some disorders. These are briefly reviewed below.

Thiamine, Vitamin B_{12}, and Folate

In industrialized societies, severe vitamin deficiencies are rarely encountered except in certain populations. Those who are elderly, alcohol dependent, or chronically ill or who have certain types of gastrointestinal surgeries are at greatest risk. Among the forms of vitamin deficiency most commonly encountered in the emergency room is acute thiamine depletion from alcohol dependence. While the chronic forms of thiamine deficiency that lead to beriberi are rarely seen in the Western world, the fulminant depletion of already low stores of thiamine result in Wernicke's encephalopathy and Korsakoff's syndrome.

Wernicke's encephalopathy classically presents with the triad of ataxia, ophthalmoplegia, and mental confusion, but confusion and a staggering gait are perhaps most common. While Wernicke's encephalopathy is an acute process, Korsakoff's syndrome may be the permanent residue of this encephalopathy. Patients with Korsakoff's syndrome exhibit a well-circumscribed retrograde and anterograde amnesia that results from destruction of the mamillary bodies, and psychotic symptoms are also reported. Wernicke's encephalopathy is a medical emergency that responds to short-term treatment with 50 mg of thiamine intravenously followed by 250-mg intramuscular injections daily until a normal diet is attained. The treatment of uncomplicated acute thiamine deficiencies usually involves 100 mg given orally one to three times a day.

Vitamin B_{12} deficiency or pernicious anemia is often seen in elderly adults, patients with gastric surgery, and malnourished depressed patients. The most typical psychiatric presentations include apathy, malaise, depressed mood, confusion, and memory deficits. B_{12} concentrations of 150 mg/mL of serum are sometimes associated with these symptoms. B_{12} deficiency is a more common cause of reversible dementia and is typically assessed in dementia evaluations. The treatment of pernicious anemia usually involves daily intramuscular injections of 1,000 mg of B_{12} for approximately 1 week, followed by maintenance doses of 1,000 mg every 1 to 2 months.

Folate deficiency has been associated with depression and dementia. Other psychiatric symptoms occasionally associated with depression include paranoia, psychosis, agitation, and confusion. The relation of folate to depression has been debated over the years. Folate deficiency may result from anorexia in depressed patients and may also contribute to depression by interfering with the synthesis of norepinephrine and serotonin. Folate deficiency has been associated with anticonvulsant use, particularly phenytoin (Dilantin), primidone (Mysoline), and phenobarbital (Solfoton), and the sex steroids, including oral contraceptives and estrogen replacement. Perhaps the most common cause of folate deficiency is the malnourishment associated with alcoholism. Many folate deficiencies respond to 1 mg of folate orally per day; however, some more severe forms may require dosages of 5 mg up to three times a day.

Amino Acids

Amino acids provide the substrate for neurotransmitters and have been used as adjunctive agents in the treatment of depression and sleep. L-Tryptophan was used for many years in this country and elsewhere to treat insomnia and augment standard antidepressants. L-Tryptophan, the precursor to serotonin, must be obtained from the diet. Patients who respond to serotonergic antidepressants may relapse rapidly into depression on a diet that is deficient in L-tryptophan. Interestingly, patients who respond to more noradrenergic antidepressants appear less vulnerable to relapse with an L-tryptophan–free diet. In the 1970s and 1980s, L-tryptophan was used to augment standard antidepressants. It was part of the Newcastle cocktail for refractory depression, which included clomipramine (Anafranil) or phenelzine (Nardil), lithium, and L-tryptophan. A number of small studies have suggested that it did have some effect on augmenting antidepressants; however, it has little antidepressant effect of its own.

L-Tryptophan was also used as an over-the-counter treatment of insomnia in the United States. A number of studies suggested that L-tryptophan in doses of 1 to 4 g before bedtime decreased sleep latency. L-Tryptophan has been unavailable in the United States since 1989, because of its association with the eosinophilia-myalgia syndrome, which may have been secondary to an impurity resulting from the processing of the compound.

Another amino acid that has been examined as an augmentor of antidepressants is phenylalanine. Phenylalanine is converted to tyrosine as a catecholamine precursor. Phenylalanine has been used with selegiline (Eldepryl) successfully in the treatment of some patients with refractory major depression. Tyrosine has been investigated as an augmentor of tricyclic drugs and may also have some mild antidepressant activity itself.

Herbs

Over the years many herbs have been purported to affect mood and mental health. Homeopathic practitioners in many parts of the world, particularly Europe, use plant derivatives such as belladonna to treat a variety of emotional maladies. Herbalists recommend *Valeriana officinalis* (valerian) for insomnia, *Passiflora incarnata* (passion flower) for nervous unrest, and *Ginkgo biloba* (ginkgo) for memory problems and anxiety. Ginkgo is currently being investigated in the treatment of selective serotonin reuptake inhibitor (SSRI)-induced sexual dysfunction.

However, few herbs have been subjected to any systematic investigation. One herb that has caught the attention of Western psychiatry recently is *Hypericum perforatum* (St. John's wort) for the treatment of major depressive disorders. St. John's wort has been used in folk medicine for hundreds of years and is still commonly used in Europe. In Germany, it is estimated that several million prescriptions for hypericum are obtained annually for the treatment of depression, anxiety, and sleep problems. Many studies have compared hypericum extracts with placebo and tricyclic drugs. Metaanalyses of these studies found that hypericum extracts were more effective than placebo in the treatment of mild to moderate depression. The major problem with these studies has been the lack of rigor in the diagnosis of depression and the assessment of efficacy. (See Chapter 29, Alternative Medicine and Psychiatry, for further information).

ENDOCRINE THERAPIES

Hormones may act directly as neurotransmitters and also indirectly influence the activity of some neurotransmitters. For example, T_3 has numerous cortical receptors, and this thyroid hormone may also modulate central and peripheral noradrenergic activity. These actions may be the basis for liothyronine's (Cytomel) use to augment antidepressants. In addition to thyroid hormone, the psychotropic effects of a number of other hormones remain under investigation.

Estrogen

Estrogen has been used for many years to relieve menopausal symptoms and as hormone replacement therapy after menopause. Some evidence suggests that estrogens may have some antidepressant effects in postmenopausal women and that progesterone may be depressogenic. Estrogens appear to lower monoamine oxidase (MAO) concentrations and increase synaptic availability of monoamines. In addition, estrogen displaces tryptophan from its albumin binding site and enhances the availability of this precursor to serotonin synthesis. Attempts to augment tricyclic drugs with estrogen have been mixed. Some studies have indicated that estradiol in dosages of 15 to 25 mg a day does augment tricyclic drug response in some women; other studies have failed to find any benefit. Other data suggest that estrogens modulate the effect of serotonin agonists. For example, estrogen appears to enhance the hormonal response of the serotonin agonist methylchlorophenyl piperazine (mCPP). Recent reports of increased risk of breast cancer and cardiovascular disease in women receiving estrogen replacement therapy have limited its use.

Dehydroepiandrosterone

Dehydroepiandrosterone (DHEA), a precursor hormone for both estrogens and androgens, is available over the counter. Recent years have seen an interest in DHEA for improving cognition, depression, sex drive, and general well-being in elderly adults. Some reports suggest that DHEA in dosages of 50 to 100 mg per day increases the sense of physical and social well-being in women aged 40 to 70 years. Reports also exist of androgenic effects, including irreversible hirsutism, hair loss, voice deepening, and other undesirable sequelae. In addition, DHEA has at least a theoretical potential of enhancing tumor growth in persons with latent, hormone-sensitive malignancies such as prostate, cervical, and breast cancer. Despite its significant popularity, few controlled data exist on the safety or efficacy of DHEA.

Melatonin

Melatonin is another popular over-the-counter hormone used by many Americans on a regular basis for insomnia and jet lag. Melatonin is produced by the pineal gland, and commercially available supplies are derived synthetically or from hog pineal glands. The hormone is released naturally by the pineal gland early in the sleep cycle and appears to contribute to natural sleep cycles. A number of small, brief studies have suggested that melatonin can act as a hypnotic in doses of 0.2 and 5 mg at night. Mostly anecdotal reports suggest that melatonin can also reduce the insomnia associated with jet lag. Some uncontrolled reports suggest that melatonin has mild antidepressant effects. However, because of its reciprocal relationship to β-adrenergic receptor activity, it may worsen depression in some patients. The long-term effects of melatonin use are unknown, and the efficacy of melatonin has been poorly studied at this time, given the widespread use of the drug.

Testosterone

Testosterone derivatives are anabolic-androgenic steroids that appear to have psychotropic effects in both men and women. Testosterone is sometimes given to postmenopausal women to enhance libido, since this hormone appears to have significant effects on libido in both men and women. In hypogonadal men, testosterone may improve sexual dysfunction, mood, energy, muscle-to-fat ratio, and sex drive. High doses of testosterone derivatives are sometimes abused by bodybuilders, football players, and even teenagers trying to increase muscle bulk. Anabolic steroids have sometimes been associated with rage attacks, aggressive behavior, and untoward physical effects including accelerated atherosclerosis, testicular atrophy, alopecia, and enhanced tumor growth. Women who use testosterone at high doses also may experience irreversible virilization. Testosterone is now available in a transdermal patch and has been marketed fairly aggressively, resulting in a recent increase in prescriptions for both men and women.

PSYCHOSURGERY

Psychosurgery involves surgical modification of the brain with the goal of reducing the symptoms of the most severely ill psychiatric patients who have not responded adequately to less radical treatments. Psychosurgical procedures focus on lesion-specific brain regions (e.g., lobotomies and cingulotomies) or their connecting tracts (e.g., tractotomies and leukotomies). Psychosurgical techniques are also used in the treatment of neurological disorders such as epilepsy and chronic pain disorder.

The interest in psychosurgical approaches to mental disorders has only recently been rekindled. The renewed interest is based on several factors, including much-improved techniques that allow neurosurgeons to make exact stereotactically placed lesions, improved preoperative diagnoses, and comprehensive preoperative and postoperative psychological assessments. New techniques also facilitate gathering complete follow-up data and enable a growing understanding of the neuroanatomical basis of some mental disorders.

In 1935, after C. F. Jacobsen and John F. Fulton at Yale University in New Haven, Connecticut, demonstrated that frontal lobe ablation in

a monkey had a calming effect, Antonio Egas Moniz, working in Portugal, severed frontal lobe white matter in 20 psychotic patients and reported a decrease in their tension and psychotic symptoms. In 1936, Walter Freeman and James Watts at George Washington University in Washington, DC, introduced the psychosurgical technique of prefrontal lobotomy to the United States. Although early procedures required burr holes or other exposure of the brain, Freeman eventually developed the technique of transorbital leukotomy, which involved the introduction and lateral movement of a sharp instrument (actually an ice pick) through the eye socket as a method of sectioning the white matter of the frontal lobes. By the late 1940s, psychosurgery was being performed worldwide, and an estimated 5,000 patients were being operated on each year. In 1949, Egas Moniz won the Nobel prize for his work in developing psychosurgical techniques. Shortly thereafter, the introduction of antipsychotic drugs and the increasing public concern about the ethics of psychosurgery led to a near abandonment of these techniques for the treatment of psychiatric patients, although psychosurgical procedures for pain control and epilepsy continued to be used.

Stereotactic neurosurgical equipment now allows neurosurgeons to place discrete lesions in the brain. Radioactive implants, cryoprobes, electrical coagulation, proton beams, and ultrasonic waves are used to make the actual lesions.

The major indication for psychosurgery is the presence of a debilitating, chronic mental disorder that has not responded to any other treatment. A reasonable guideline is that the disorder should have been present for 5 years, during which a wide variety of alternative treatment approaches was attempted. Chronic intractable major depressive disorder and obsessive-compulsive disorder are the two disorders reportedly most responsive to psychosurgery. These two disorders have been influenced by TMS of the prefrontal cortex. The presence of vegetative symptoms and marked anxiety further increases the likelihood of a successful therapeutic outcome. Whether psychosurgery is a reasonable treatment for intractable and extreme aggression is still controversial. Psychosurgery is not indicated for the treatment of schizophrenia, and data about manic episodes are controversial.

When patients are carefully selected, between 50 and 70 percent have significant therapeutic improvement with psychosurgery. Fewer than 3 percent become worse. Continued improvement is often noted from 1 to 2 years after surgery, and patients often respond better to traditional pharmacological and behavioral treatment approaches than they did before psychosurgery. Postoperative seizures are present in fewer than 1 percent of patients, and these seizures are usually controlled with phenytoin. As measured by intelligence quotient (IQ) scores, cognitive abilities improve after surgery, probably because of patients' increased ability to attend to cognitive tasks. No undesired changes in personality have been noted with modern limited procedures.

DRUG-ASSISTED INTERVIEWING

The use of amobarbital (Amytal) and other sedative-hypnotic agents to facilitate interviewing in some patients has become uncommon but is still used in some settings. The primary indication for drug-assisted interviewing is ostensibly to recover repressed material in amnesiac patients and as a diagnostic probe in assessing conversion disorder, catatonia, confusion, and mutism. For example, if a patient is mute because of severe anxiety, use of a sedative-hypnotic agent may facilitate gaining access to traumatic material. Catatonic patients anecdotally may become more activated when a hypnotic agent is administered. Confusion due to functional causes such as schizophrenia may improve with drug-assisted interviewing, while confusion due to organic causes may worsen. Despite the use of drug-assisted interviewing for over 60 years, there is very little evidence that interviewing with a sedative-hypnotic agent is any better than skillful interviewing without drugs. In some instances, memories are inhibited by the concurrent use of a sedative-hypnotic agent.

The amobarbital interview involves administering a 10 percent solution of sodium amobarbital at 0.5 to 1.0 mL per minute until mild sedation is achieved. Alternatively, intravenous diazepam (Valium) or lorazepam (Ativan) have been used as safer alternatives to barbiturates. Respiratory suppression is the most serious complication of drug-assisted interviewing, and the clinician must be prepared to take emergency measures as needed.

Given the risks of Amytal interviews, drug-assisted interviewing using safer agents, such as benzodiazepines, has emerged as an alternative. Diazepam, lorazepam, and other benzodiazepines have been used for this purpose. One of the most recent studies on drug-assisted interviewing used the very short-acting benzodiazepine midazolam (Versed) and a pulse oximeter to decrease the risk of respiratory suppression. Patients are treated with midazolam, 1 mg/mL given up to every minute depending on the levels of sedation observed and oxygen saturation. In addition to having a wider therapeutic index than barbiturates, benzodiazepines have the added advantage of having an effective antagonist available, flumazenil (Romazicon), which can quickly reverse the effects if necessary.

PLACEBOS

Pharmacologically inactive substances have long been known to sometimes produce significant clinical benefits. A patient who believes that a compound is helpful may often derive considerable benefit from taking that substance, whether it is known to be pharmacologically active or not. For many psychiatric disorders, including mild to moderate depression and some anxiety disorders, well over 30 percent of patients can exhibit significant improvement or remission of symptoms on a placebo. For other conditions, such as schizophrenia, manic episodes, and psychotic depression, the placebo response rate is very low. While suggestion is undoubtedly important in the efficacy of placebos (and active drugs), placebos may produce biological effects. For example, placebo-induced analgesia may sometimes be blocked by naloxone, which suggests that endorphins may mediate the analgesia derived from taking a placebo. It is conceivable that placebos may also stimulate endogenous anxiolytic and antidepressant factors, resulting in clinical improvement in patients with depression and anxiety disorders.

Just as placebos may produce benefit, they may also have adverse effects. In many studies, some adverse effects are likely to be more common with placebos than with the active drug. Some patients will not tolerate placebos despite the fact that they are supposedly inert, and they exhibit adverse effects (called the *nocebo phenomenon*). It is easy to discount such patients as overly suggestible; however, if beneficial endogenous factors can be stimulated by placebos, perhaps toxic endogenous factors may also be produced.

Prudence is needed in contemplating the use of a placebo in clinical practice. Treating a patient with a placebo without consent can seriously undermine a patient's confidence in the physician if, and when, it is discovered.

TREATMENTS OF HISTORICAL OR OTHER INTEREST

Chemical Convulsive Therapies

Convulsive therapies for the treatment of serious psychiatric disorders date back hundreds of years, with the Swiss physician Paracelsus reportedly giving camphor by mouth to induce seizures and treat lunacy in the 16th century. Several European manuscripts from the 1700s describe the benefits of camphor-induced seizures for the treatment of mania and other forms of insanity. These manuscripts were largely forgotten until the work of Ladislas von Meduna in the 1930s. Von Meduna had experimented with intramuscular camphor monobromide, caffeine, strychnine, brucine, and other compounds before settling on pentylenetetrazol as a more reliable convulsant for the treatment of dementia precox. Pentylenetetrazol was more soluble than many other compounds and also had a quicker onset of action. Meduna typically used an initial dose of 5 mL of a 10 percent solution of pentylenetetrazol, followed by additional doses every minute if convulsions were not achieved. The major drawbacks of these chemical convulsions are that seizures sometimes did not occur and that patients would experience significant preictal discomfort including nausea and anxiety and, thus, tend to decline further treatment. In the late 1930s and early 1940s, chemical convulsive therapy was replaced by the considerably more reliable electroconvulsive therapy (ECT).

Coma-Inducing Therapies

Insulin coma therapy emerged approximately the same time in the 1930s as ECT. As von Meduna observed that epilepsy and dementia praecox were incompatible, Manfred Sakel observed that dementia praecox patients who went into a coma tended to come out less symptomatic. The treatment involved using incrementally higher doses of intramuscular insulin until the patient became comatose. Comas were initially terminated with glucagon after approximately 15 minutes, but an attempt was made to increase subsequent comas to a maximum of 60 minutes. Patients often required 60 or more treatments before results were seen. Complications including arrhythmias and laryngeal spasms were not uncommon, and insulin coma therapy had a fatality rate of at least 1 percent and in some samples considerably higher. The danger of the procedure and a controlled study in 1962 that suggested that it was no more effective than a similar period of unconsciousness induced by barbiturates hastened the demise of the procedure. However, some patients who did not respond to other available treatments clearly appeared to respond to insulin coma therapy.

Variations of insulin coma therapy included atropine coma therapy used briefly in the 1950s. Atropine in dosages up to 200 mg a day was given to induce comas lasting 6 to 8 hours. If the patient did not wake up spontaneously, the coma was aborted by intramuscular physostigmine (Antilirium). Like insulin coma therapy, atropine coma therapy was said to be effective for the treatment of schizophrenia and mania. The most serious complications were hyperthermia and rhabdomyolysis. By the late 1950s, coma therapies had been all but abandoned for safer treatments, including ECT and effective antipsychotic drugs.

Continuous Sleep Therapy

In the 1930s, therapies that altered consciousness for extended periods by seizure or coma were thought to be effective in the treatment of psychosis. Even earlier, psychosis was treated by inducing a state of continuous sleep for 10 days or more. Continuous sleep therapy was introduced for the treatment of psychosis in the early 1920s. This intervention originally involved the use of barbiturates to keep patients asleep 20 hours or more a day with brief interruptions for the patient to eat and use the bathroom. Complications of barbiturate-induced continuous sleep included allergic reactions, seizures on withdrawal, and respiratory depression ending in death. Later the combination of chlorpromazine (Thorazine) with benzodiazepines and other hypnotics was used to keep patients asleep for therapeutic purposes. Although there are some reports of improvement in anxiety states, obsessive-compulsive disorder, and schizophrenia, no controlled data are available to support these claims. Given the significant morbidity and clear lack of efficacy of this method, it was largely abandoned in the United States by the 1960s.

Hallucinogen Therapy

Many cultures have used hallucinogens, including mescaline, psilocybin, and ergots, for thousands of years to gain spiritual and personal insight. Lysergic acid diethylamide (LSD) was synthesized in the 1930s and was marketed to psychiatrists and other practitioners in the late 1940s under the trade name Delysid as a tool for understanding psychosis and for facilitating psychotherapy. Using LSD reportedly helped patients capture repressed memories and deal with anxiety, and it allowed patients to gain insight through an analysis of the primary process induced by the hallucinogen. Oral doses of 150 to 250 mg were administered occasionally by psychiatrists throughout the 1950s and early 1960s to facilitate psychotherapy with some patients. In the 1960s Timothy Leary advocated the widespread use of hallucinogens, but the drugs were outlawed as class I controlled substances in 1965.

While no longer used for therapeutic purposes in this country, LSD has fulfilled part of its early promise as a probe for psychosis. More recent understanding of the pharmacology of LSD and its affinity to serotonin (5-HT) type 2 (5-HT_2) receptors has supported the interest in developing serotonin-dopamine antagonists (atypical antipsychotics) with the 5-HT_2–receptor blocking properties. Recently, studies using methylenedioxymethamphetamine (MDMA, "ecstasy") have been approved by the National Institutes of Health (NIH) to determine whether psychotherapy is facilitated when the patient is under the influence of the drug, which can affect interpersonal relationships positively by promoting feeling of empathy.

References

Barbini B, Bertelli S, Colombo C, Smeraldi E. Sleep loss, a possible factor in augmenting manic episode. *Psychiatry Res*. 1996;65:121.

Benedetti F, Barbini B, Lucca A, Campori E, Colombo C, Smeraldi E. Sleep deprivation hastens the antidepressant action of fluoxetine. *Eur Arch Psychiatry Clin Neurosci*. 1997;247:100.

Ernst E. Acupuncture/acupressure for weight reduction? A systematic review. *Wien Klin Wochenschr*. 1997;109:60.

Feinsod M, Kreinin B, Chistyakov A, Klein E. Preliminary evidence for a beneficial effect of low-frequency, repetitive transcranial magnetic stimulation in patients with major depression and schizophrenia. *Depress Anxiety*. 1998;7:65.

Gross F, Gysin F. Phototherapy in psychiatry: clinical update and review of indications. *Encephale*. 1996;22:143.

Harvey AG. Sleep hygiene and sleep onset insomnia. *J Nerv Mental Disease*. 2000;1:53.

Klein E, Kreinin I, Chistyakov A. Therapeutic efficacy of right prefrontal slow

repetitive transcranial magnetic stimulation in major depression: a double-blind controlled study. *Arch Gen Psychiatry.* 1999;56:315.

Linde K, Ramirez G, Mulraw CD, Pauls A, Weidenhammer W, Melchart D. St. John's wort for depression—an overview and meta-analysis of randomized clinical trials [see comments]. *Br Med J.* 1996;313:253.

Nahas Z, Bohning DE, Molloy MA, Ovotz JA, Risch SC, George MS. Safety and feasibility of repetitive transcranial magnetic stimulation in the treatment of anxious depression in pregnancy: a case report. *J Clin Psychiatry.* 1999;60:50.

Neary JT, Bu Y. Hypericum LI 160 inhibits uptake of serotonin and norepinephrine in astrocytes. *Brain Res.* 1999;816:358.

Palmer ME, Rao RB. Problems evaluating contamination of dietary supplements. *N Engl J Med.* 1999;340:568.

Pascual-Leone A, Rubio B, Pallardo F, Catala MD. Rapid-rate transcranial magnetic stimulation of left dorsolateral prefrontal cortex in drug-resistant depression. *Lancet.* 1996;348:233.

Rush AJ, George MS, Sackeim HA. Vagus nerve stimulation (VNS) for treatment-resistant depressions: a multicenter study. *Biol Psychiatry.* 2000; 47:276.

Sartori S, Poirrier R. Seasonal affective syndrome and phototherapy: theoretical concepts and clinical applications. *Encephale.* 1996;22:7.

37

Child Psychiatry: Assessment, Examination, and Psychological Testing

Psychiatric evaluation of a child is initiated to develop a formulation of the child's overall functioning including long-standing and current behavioral and emotional difficulties. It is essential to assess the developmental patterns of a child during an evaluation, since psychiatric disorders in this age group often emerge as a failure to achieve developmental milestones. Developmental considerations include expected skills in social, motor, language, and intellectual domains. During the evaluation, the clinician must integrate the contributions of many different factors that have affected the child, including biological growth and health, mood and behavioral symptoms, and family, school and environmental factors. At the end of the evaluation, the extent to which the child's development has not met expectations for his or her chronological age is determined, and the degree of impairment due to behavioral and emotional factors is established. In addition, an assessment of environmental factors that may either exacerbate or improve the child's overall functioning is considered.

A comprehensive evaluation of a child includes interviews with the parents, the child, and other family members; gathering information regarding the child's current school functioning; and often, a standardized assessment of the child's intellectual level and academic achievement. In some cases, standardized measures of developmental level and neuropsychological assessments are useful. Psychiatric evaluations of children are rarely initiated by the child, so clinicians must obtain information from the family and the school to understand the reasons for the evaluation. In some cases, the court, or a child protective service agency may initiate a psychiatric evaluation. Children can be excellent informants about symptoms related to mood and inner experiences such as psychotic phenomena, sadness, fears, and anxiety, but they often have difficulty with the chronology of symptoms and are sometimes reticent about reporting behaviors that have gotten them into trouble. Very young children often cannot articulate their experiences verbally and do better showing their feelings and preoccupations in a play situation.

The first step in the comprehensive evaluation of a child or adolescent is to obtain a full description of the current concerns and a history of the child's past psychiatric and medical problems. This is often done with the parents for school-aged children, while adolescents may be seen alone first, to get their perception of the situation. Direct interview and observation of the child is usually next, followed by psychological testing, when indicated.

Clinical interviews offer the most flexibility in understanding the evolution of problems and in establishing the role of environmental factors and life events, but they may not systematically cover all psychiatric diagnostic categories. To increase the breath of information generated, the clinician may use semistructured interviews such as the Kiddie Schedule for Affective Disorders and Schizophrenia for School-Age Children (K-SADS), structured interviews such as the National Institute for Mental Health Diagnostic Interview Schedule for Children Version IV (NIMH DISC-IV), and rating scales, such as the Child Behavior Checklist and Connors Parent or Teacher Rating Scale for ADHD.

It is not uncommon for interviews from different sources, such as parents, teachers, and school counselors, to reflect different or even contradictory information about a given child. When faced with conflictual ınformation, the clinician must determine whether apparent contradictions actually reflect an accurate picture of the child in different settings. Once a complete history is obtained from the parents, the child is examined, the child's current functioning at home and at school is assessed, and psychological testing is completed, the clinician can use all the available information to make a best-estimate diagnosis and can then make recommendations.

CLINICAL INTERVIEWS

To conduct a useful interview with a child of any age, clinicians must be familiar with normal development to place the child's responses in the proper perspective. For example, a young child's discomfort on separation from a parent and a school-age child's lack of clarity about the purpose of the interview are both perfectly normal and should not be misconstrued as psychiatric symptoms. Furthermore, behavior that is normal in a child at one age, such as temper tantrums in a 2-year-old, takes on a different meaning, for example, in a 17-year-old.

The interviewer's first task is to engage the child and develop a rapport so that the child is comfortable. The interviewer should inquire about the child's concept of the purpose of the interview and should ask what the parents have told the child. If the child appears to be confused about the reason for

trained "laypersons." It is available in parallel child and parent forms. The parent form can be used for children from 6 to 17 years of age, and the direct child form of the instrument was designed for children from 9 to 17 years of age. It is applicable for a multitude of diagnoses keyed to DSM-IV-TR. A computer scoring algorithm is available. This instrument assesses the presence of diagnoses that have been present within the last 4 weeks, and also within the last year. Because it is a fully structured interview, the instructions serve as a complete guide for the questions, and the examiner need not have any knowledge of child psychiatry to administer the interview correctly.

Children's Interview for Psychiatric Syndromes (ChIPS). The ChIPS is a highly structured interview designed for use by trained interviewers with children from 6 to 18 years of age. It is composed of 15 sections, and it elicits information on psychiatric symptoms as well as psychosocial stressors targeting 20 psychiatric disorders, according to DSM-IV criteria. There are parent and child forms. It takes approximately 40 minutes to administer the ChIPS. Diagnoses covered include depression, mania, attention-deficit/hyperactivity disorder, separation disorder, obsessive-compulsive disorder, conduct disorder, substance use disorder, anorexia, and bulimia. The ChIPS was designed for use as a screening instrument for clinicians and a diagnostic instrument for clinical and epidemiological research.

Diagnostic Interview for Children and Adolescents (DICA). The current version of the DICA was developed in 1997 to assess information resulting in diagnoses according to either DSM-IV or DSM-III-R. Although it was originally designed to be a highly structured interview, it can now be used in a semistructured format. This means that although interviewers are allowed to use additional questions and probes to clarify elicited information, the method of probing is standardized so that all interviewers will follow a specific pattern. When using the interview with younger children, more flexibility is built in, allowing interviewers to deviate from written questions to ensure that the child understands the question. Parent and child interviews are expected to be used. It covers children 6 to 17 years of age and generally takes 1 to 2 hours to administer. It covers externalizing behavior disorders, anxiety disorders, depressive disorders, and substance abuse disorders, among others.

Pictorial Diagnostic Instruments

Dominic-R. The Dominic-R is a pictorial fully structured interview designed to elicit psychiatric symptoms from children from 6 to 11 years of age. The pictures illustrate abstract emotional and behavioral content of diagnostic entities according to DSM-III-R. The instrument uses a picture of a child called "Dominic" who is experiencing the symptom in question. Some symptoms have more than one picture, with a brief story that is read to the child. Along with each picture is a sentence asking about the situation being shown and asking the child if he or she has experiences similar to the one that Dominic is having. Diagnostic entities covered by the Dominic-R include separation anxiety, generalized anxiety, depression and dysthymia, attention-deficit/hyperactivity disorder, oppositional defiant disorder, conduct disorder, and specific phobia. Although symptoms of the above diagnoses can be fully elicited from the Dominic-R, there is no specific provision within the instrument to inquire about frequency of the symptom, duration, or age of onset. The paper version of this interview takes about 20 minutes, and the computerized version of this instrument takes about 15 minutes. Trained lay-interviewers administer this interview. Computerized versions of this interview are available with pictures of a child who is white, black, Latino, or Asian.

Pictorial Instrument for Children and Adolescents (PICA-III-R). PICA-III-R comprises 137 pictures organized in modules and designed to cover five diagnostic categories including disorders of anxiety, mood, psychosis, disruptive disorders, and substance use disorder. It is designed to be administered by clinicians and can be used for children and adolescents ranging from 6 to 16 years of age. It provides a categorical (diagnosis present or absent) and a dimensional (range of severity) assessment. This instrument presents pictures of a child experiencing emotional, behavioral, and cognitive symptoms. The child is asked "How much are you like him/her?" and a 5-point rating scale with pictures of a person with open arms in increasing degrees is shown to the child to help him or her identify the severity of the symptoms. It takes about 40 minutes to 1 hour to administer the interview. This instrument is currently keyed to DSM-III-R. It can be used to aid in clinical interviews and in research diagnostic protocols.

QUESTIONNAIRES AND RATING SCALES

Child Behavior Checklist

The parent and teacher versions of the Child Behavior Checklist were developed to cover a broad range of symptoms and several positive attributes related to academic and social competence. The checklist presents items related to mood, frustration tolerance, hyperactivity, oppositional behavior, anxiety, and various other behaviors. The parent version consists of 118 items to be rated 0 (not true), 1 (sometimes true), or 2 (very true). The teacher version is similar but without the items that apply only to home life. Profiles were developed based on normal children of three different age groups (4 to 5, 6 to 11, and 12 to 16).

Such a checklist identifies specific problem areas that might otherwise be overlooked, and it may point out areas in which the child's behavior deviates from that of normal children of the same age group. The checklist is not used specifically to make diagnoses.

Revised Behavior Problem Checklist

Consisting of 150 items that cover a variety of childhood behavioral and emotional symptoms, the Revised Behavior Problem Checklist discriminates between clinic-referred and nonreferred children. Separate subscales have been found to correlate in the appropriate direction with other measures of intelligence, academic achievement, clinical observations, and peer popularity. Like the other broad rating scales, this instrument can help one gain a comprehensive view of a multitude of behavioral areas, but it is not designed to make psychiatric diagnoses.

Connors Abbreviated Parent-Teacher Rating Scale for ADHD

In its original form, the Connors Abbreviated Parent-Teacher Rating Scale for ADHD consisted of 93 items rated on a 0 to 3 scale and was subgrouped into 25 clusters including problems with restlessness, temper, school, stealing, eating, and sleeping. Over the years, multiple versions of this scale were developed and used to aid in systematic identification of children with attention-deficit/hyperactivity disorder. A highly abbreviated form of this rating scale, the Connors Abbreviated Parent-Teacher Questionnaire, was developed for use with both parents

tinue an interview if they feel threatened or if patients become destructive to property or engage in self-injurious behavior. Every interview should include an exploration of suicidal thoughts, assaultive behavior, psychotic symptoms, substance use, and knowledge of safe sexual practices along with a sexual history. Once rapport has been established, many adolescents appreciate the opportunity to tell their side of the story and may reveal things that they have not disclosed to anyone else.

Family Interview

An interview with parents and the patient may take place first or may occur later in the evaluation. Sometimes an interview with the entire family, including siblings, can be enlightening. The purpose is to observe the attitudes and behavior of the parents toward the patient and the responses of the children to their parents. The clinician's job is to maintain a nonthreatening atmosphere in which each member of the family can speak freely without feeling that the clinician is taking sides with any particular member. Although child psychiatrists generally function as advocates for the child, the clinician must validate each family member's feelings in this setting, because lack of communication often contributes to the patient's problems.

Parents

The interview with the patient's parents or caretakers is necessary to get a chronological picture of the child's growth and development. A thorough developmental history and details of any stressors or important events that have influenced the child's development must be elicited. The parents' view of the family dynamics, their marital history, and their own emotional adjustment are also elicited. The family's psychiatric history and the upbringing of the parents are pertinent. Parents are usually the best informants about the child's early development and previous psychiatric and medical illnesses. They may be better able to provide an accurate chronology of past evaluations and treatment. In some cases, especially with older children and adolescents, the parents may be unaware of significant current symptoms or social difficulties of the child. Clinicians elicit the parents' formulation of the causes and nature of their child's problems and ask about expectations about the current assessment.

DIAGNOSTIC INSTRUMENTS

The two main types of diagnostic instruments used by clinicians and researchers are diagnostic interviews and questionnaires. Diagnostic interviews are administered to either children or their parents and are often designed to elicit enough information on numerous aspects of functioning to determine whether criteria are met from the text revision of the fourth edition of the *Diagnostic and Statistical Manual of Mental Disorders* (DSM-IV-TR).

Semistructured interviews, or "interviewer-based" interviews, such as K-SADS and the Child and Adolescent Psychiatric Assessment (CAPA) serve as guides for the clinician. They help the clinician clarify answers to questions about symptoms. Structured interviews, or "respondent-based" interviews, such as NIMH DISC-IV, the Children's Interview for Psychiatric Syndromes (ChIPS), and the Diagnostic Interview for Children and Adolescents (DICA), basically provide a script for the interviewer without interpretation of the subject's responses. There are also two diagnostic instruments that use pictures, the Dominic-R and the Pictorial Instrument for Children and Adolescents (PICA-III-R). These instruments use pictures as cues along with an accompanying question to elicit information about symptoms, especially for young children as well as for adolescents.

Diagnostic instruments aid the collection of information in a systematic way. Diagnostic instruments, even the most comprehensive, however, cannot replace clinical interviews, because clinical interviews are superior in understanding the chronology of symptoms, the interplay between environmental stressors and emotional responses, and developmental issues. Clinicians often find it helpful to combine the data from diagnostic instruments with clinical material gathered in a comprehensive evaluation.

Questionnaires can cover a broad range of symptom areas, such as the Child Behavior Checklist, or they can be focused on a particular type of symptomatology and are often called rating scales, such as the Connors Parent Rating Scale for ADHD.

Semi-Structured "Interviewer-Based" Interviews

Kiddie Schedule for Affective Disorders and Schizophrenia for School-Age Children (K-SADS). K-SADS can be used for children from 6 years to 18 years of age. It presents multiple items with some space for further clarification of symptoms. It elicits information on current diagnosis and on symptoms present in the previous year. There is also a version that can ascertain lifetime diagnoses. It assesses diagnoses according to both DSM-IV and DSM-III-R. This instrument has been used extensively, especially in evaluation of mood disorders, and includes measures of impairment due to symptoms. The schedule comes in a form for parents to give information about their child and in a version for use directly with the child. The schedule takes about 1 to 1½ hours to administer. The interviewer should have some training in the field of child psychiatry, but need not be a psychiatrist.

Child and Adolescent Psychiatric Assessment (CAPA). The CAPA is an "interviewer-based" interview that can be used for children from 9 to 17 years of age. It comes in modular form so that certain diagnostic entities can be administered without having to give the entire interview. It covers disruptive behavior disorders, mood disorders, anxiety disorders, eating disorders, sleep disorders, elimination disorders, substance use disorders, tic disorders, schizophrenia, posttraumatic stress disorder, and somatization symptoms. It focuses on the 3 months prior to the interview, called the "primary period." In general, it takes about 1 hour to administer. It has a glossary to aid in decision making regarding symptoms and provides separate ratings of presence of symptoms and severity of symptoms. It can be used to determine diagnoses according to the fourth edition of DSM (DSM-IV), the revised third edition of DSM (DSM-III-R), or the 10th revision of *International Statistical Classification of Diseases and Related Health Problems* (ICD-10). Training is necessary to administer this interview, and the interviewer must be prepared to use some clinical judgment in interpreting elicited symptoms.

Structured "Respondent-Based" Interviews

National Institute of Mental Health Interview Schedule for Children Version IV (NIMH DISC-IV). The NIMH DISC-IV is a highly structured interview designed to assess more than 30 DSM-IV diagnostic entities administered by

trained "laypersons." It is available in parallel child and parent forms. The parent form can be used for children from 6 to 17 years of age, and the direct child form of the instrument was designed for children from 9 to 17 years of age. It is applicable for a multitude of diagnoses keyed to DSM-IV-TR. A computer scoring algorithm is available. This instrument assesses the presence of diagnoses that have been present within the last 4 weeks, and also within the last year. Because it is a fully structured interview, the instructions serve as a complete guide for the questions, and the examiner need not have any knowledge of child psychiatry to administer the interview correctly.

Children's Interview for Psychiatric Syndromes (ChIPS). The ChIPS is a highly structured interview designed for use by trained interviewers with children from 6 to 18 years of age. It is composed of 15 sections, and it elicits information on psychiatric symptoms as well as psychosocial stressors targeting 20 psychiatric disorders, according to DSM-IV criteria. There are parent and child forms. It takes approximately 40 minutes to administer the ChIPS. Diagnoses covered include depression, mania, attention-deficit/hyperactivity disorder, separation disorder, obsessive-compulsive disorder, conduct disorder, substance use disorder, anorexia, and bulimia. The ChIPS was designed for use as a screening instrument for clinicians and a diagnostic instrument for clinical and epidemiological research.

Diagnostic Interview for Children and Adolescents (DICA). The current version of the DICA was developed in 1997 to assess information resulting in diagnoses according to either DSM-IV or DSM-III-R. Although it was originally designed to be a highly structured interview, it can now be used in a semistructured format. This means that although interviewers are allowed to use additional questions and probes to clarify elicited information, the method of probing is standardized so that all interviewers will follow a specific pattern. When using the interview with younger children, more flexibility is built in, allowing interviewers to deviate from written questions to ensure that the child understands the question. Parent and child interviews are expected to be used. It covers children 6 to 17 years of age and generally takes 1 to 2 hours to administer. It covers externalizing behavior disorders, anxiety disorders, depressive disorders, and substance abuse disorders, among others.

Pictorial Diagnostic Instruments

Dominic-R. The Dominic-R is a pictorial fully structured interview designed to elicit psychiatric symptoms from children from 6 to 11 years of age. The pictures illustrate abstract emotional and behavioral content of diagnostic entities according to DSM-III-R. The instrument uses a picture of a child called "Dominic" who is experiencing the symptom in question. Some symptoms have more than one picture, with a brief story that is read to the child. Along with each picture is a sentence asking about the situation being shown and asking the child if he or she has experiences similar to the one that Dominic is having. Diagnostic entities covered by the Dominic-R include separation anxiety, generalized anxiety, depression and dysthymia, attention-deficit/hyperactivity disorder, oppositional defiant disorder, conduct disorder, and specific phobia. Although symptoms of the above diagnoses can be fully elicited from the Dominic-R, there is no specific provision within the instrument to inquire about frequency of the symptom, duration, or age of onset. The paper version of this interview takes about 20 minutes, and the computerized version of this instrument takes about 15 minutes. Trained lay-interviewers administer this interview. Computerized versions of this interview are available with pictures of a child who is white, black, Latino, or Asian.

Pictorial Instrument for Children and Adolescents (PICA-III-R). PICA-III-R comprises 137 pictures organized in modules and designed to cover five diagnostic categories including disorders of anxiety, mood, psychosis, disruptive disorders, and substance use disorder. It is designed to be administered by clinicians and can be used for children and adolescents ranging from 6 to 16 years of age. It provides a categorical (diagnosis present or absent) and a dimensional (range of severity) assessment. This instrument presents pictures of a child experiencing emotional, behavioral, and cognitive symptoms. The child is asked "How much are you like him/her?" and a 5-point rating scale with pictures of a person with open arms in increasing degrees is shown to the child to help him or her identify the severity of the symptoms. It takes about 40 minutes to 1 hour to administer the interview. This instrument is currently keyed to DSM-III-R. It can be used to aid in clinical interviews and in research diagnostic protocols.

QUESTIONNAIRES AND RATING SCALES

Child Behavior Checklist

The parent and teacher versions of the Child Behavior Checklist were developed to cover a broad range of symptoms and several positive attributes related to academic and social competence. The checklist presents items related to mood, frustration tolerance, hyperactivity, oppositional behavior, anxiety, and various other behaviors. The parent version consists of 118 items to be rated 0 (not true), 1 (sometimes true), or 2 (very true). The teacher version is similar but without the items that apply only to home life. Profiles were developed based on normal children of three different age groups (4 to 5, 6 to 11, and 12 to 16).

Such a checklist identifies specific problem areas that might otherwise be overlooked, and it may point out areas in which the child's behavior deviates from that of normal children of the same age group. The checklist is not used specifically to make diagnoses.

Revised Behavior Problem Checklist

Consisting of 150 items that cover a variety of childhood behavioral and emotional symptoms, the Revised Behavior Problem Checklist discriminates between clinic-referred and nonreferred children. Separate subscales have been found to correlate in the appropriate direction with other measures of intelligence, academic achievement, clinical observations, and peer popularity. Like the other broad rating scales, this instrument can help one gain a comprehensive view of a multitude of behavioral areas, but it is not designed to make psychiatric diagnoses.

Connors Abbreviated Parent-Teacher Rating Scale for ADHD

In its original form, the Connors Abbreviated Parent-Teacher Rating Scale for ADHD consisted of 93 items rated on a 0 to 3 scale and was subgrouped into 25 clusters including problems with restlessness, temper, school, stealing, eating, and sleeping. Over the years, multiple versions of this scale were developed and used to aid in systematic identification of children with attention-deficit/hyperactivity disorder. A highly abbreviated form of this rating scale, the Connors Abbreviated Parent-Teacher Questionnaire, was developed for use with both parents

37

Child Psychiatry: Assessment, Examination, and Psychological Testing

Psychiatric evaluation of a child is initiated to develop a formulation of the child's overall functioning including long-standing and current behavioral and emotional difficulties. It is essential to assess the developmental patterns of a child during an evaluation, since psychiatric disorders in this age group often emerge as a failure to achieve developmental milestones. Developmental considerations include expected skills in social, motor, language, and intellectual domains. During the evaluation, the clinician must integrate the contributions of many different factors that have affected the child, including biological growth and health, mood and behavioral symptoms, and family, school and environmental factors. At the end of the evaluation, the extent to which the child's development has not met expectations for his or her chronological age is determined, and the degree of impairment due to behavioral and emotional factors is established. In addition, an assessment of environmental factors that may either exacerbate or improve the child's overall functioning is considered.

A comprehensive evaluation of a child includes interviews with the parents, the child, and other family members; gathering information regarding the child's current school functioning; and often, a standardized assessment of the child's intellectual level and academic achievement. In some cases, standardized measures of developmental level and neuropsychological assessments are useful. Psychiatric evaluations of children are rarely initiated by the child, so clinicians must obtain information from the family and the school to understand the reasons for the evaluation. In some cases, the court, or a child protective service agency may initiate a psychiatric evaluation. Children can be excellent informants about symptoms related to mood and inner experiences such as psychotic phenomena, sadness, fears, and anxiety, but they often have difficulty with the chronology of symptoms and are sometimes reticent about reporting behaviors that have gotten them into trouble. Very young children often cannot articulate their experiences verbally and do better showing their feelings and preoccupations in a play situation.

The first step in the comprehensive evaluation of a child or adolescent is to obtain a full description of the current concerns and a history of the child's past psychiatric and medical problems. This is often done with the parents for school-aged children, while adolescents may be seen alone first, to get their perception of the situation. Direct interview and observation of the child is usually next, followed by psychological testing, when indicated.

Clinical interviews offer the most flexibility in understanding the evolution of problems and in establishing the role of environmental factors and life events, but they may not systematically cover all psychiatric diagnostic categories. To increase the breath of information generated, the clinician may use semistructured interviews such as the Kiddie Schedule for Affective Disorders and Schizophrenia for School-Age Children (K-SADS), structured interviews such as the National Institute for Mental Health Diagnostic Interview Schedule for Children Version IV (NIMH DISC-IV), and rating scales, such as the Child Behavior Checklist and Connors Parent or Teacher Rating Scale for ADHD.

It is not uncommon for interviews from different sources, such as parents, teachers, and school counselors, to reflect different or even contradictory information about a given child. When faced with conflictual information, the clinician must determine whether apparent contradictions actually reflect an accurate picture of the child in different settings. Once a complete history is obtained from the parents, the child is examined, the child's current functioning at home and at school is assessed, and psychological testing is completed, the clinician can use all the available information to make a best-estimate diagnosis and can then make recommendations.

CLINICAL INTERVIEWS

To conduct a useful interview with a child of any age, clinicians must be familiar with normal development to place the child's responses in the proper perspective. For example, a young child's discomfort on separation from a parent and a school-age child's lack of clarity about the purpose of the interview are both perfectly normal and should not be misconstrued as psychiatric symptoms. Furthermore, behavior that is normal in a child at one age, such as temper tantrums in a 2-year-old, takes on a different meaning, for example, in a 17-year-old.

The interviewer's first task is to engage the child and develop a rapport so that the child is comfortable. The interviewer should inquire about the child's concept of the purpose of the interview and should ask what the parents have told the child. If the child appears to be confused about the reason for

the interview, the examiner may opt to summarize the parents' concerns in a developmentally appropriate and supportive manner. During the interview with the child, the clinician seeks to learn about the child's relationships with family members and peers, academic achievement and peer relationships in school, and the child's pleasurable activities. An estimate of the child's cognitive functioning is a part of the mental status examination.

The extent of confidentiality in child assessment is correlated with the age of the child. In most cases, almost all specific information can appropriately be shared with the parents of a very young child, whereas privacy and permission of an older child or adolescent are mandated before sharing information with parents. School-age and older children are informed that if the clinician becomes concerned that any child is dangerous to himself or herself or to others, this information must be shared with parents and at times additional adults. As part of a psychiatric assessment of a child of any age, the clinician must determine whether that child is safe in his or her environment and must develop an index of suspicion about whether the child is a victim of abuse or neglect. Whenever there is a suspicion of child maltreatment, the local child protective service agency must be notified.

Toward the end of the interview, the child may be asked in an open-ended manner whether he or she would like to bring up anything else. Each child should be complimented for his or her cooperation and thanked for participating in the interview, and the interview should end on a positive note.

Infants and Young Children

Assessments of infants usually begin with the parents present, as very young children may be frightened by the interview situation; the interview with the parents present also allows the clinician to assess the parent–infant interaction. Infants may be referred for a variety of reasons, including high levels of irritability, difficulty being consoled, eating disturbances, poor weight gain, sleep disturbances, withdrawn behavior, lack of engagement in play, and developmental delay. The clinician assesses areas of functioning that include motor development, activity level, verbal communication, ability to engage in play, problem-solving skills, adaptation to daily routines, relationships, and social responsiveness.

The child's developmental level of functioning is determined by combining observations made during the interview with standardized developmental measures. Observations of play reveal a child's developmental level and reflect the child's emotional state and preoccupations. The examiner can interact with an infant age 18 months or younger in a playful manner by using such games as peekaboo. Children between the ages of 18 months and 3 years can be observed in a playroom. Children ages 2 years or older may exhibit symbolic play with toys, revealing more in this mode than through conversation. The use of puppets and dolls with children under 6 years of age is often an effective way to elicit information, especially if questions are directed to the dolls, rather than to the child.

School-Age Children

Some school-age children are at ease when conversing with an adult; others are hampered by fear, anxiety, poor verbal skills, or oppositional behavior. School-age children can usually tolerate a 45-minute session. The room should be spacious enough for the child to move around, but not large enough to reduce intimate contact between the examiner and the child. Part of the interview can be reserved for unstructured play, and various toys can be made available to capture the child's interest and to elicit themes and feelings. Children in lower grades may be more interested in the toys in the room, whereas by the sixth grade, children may be more comfortable with the interview process and less likely to show spontaneous play.

The initial part of the interview explores the child's understanding of the reasons for the meeting. The clinician should confirm the fact that the interview was not set up because the child is "in trouble" or as a punishment for "bad" behavior. Techniques that can facilitate disclosure of feelings include asking the child to draw peers, family members, a house, or anything else that comes to mind. The child can then be questioned about the drawings. Children may be asked to reveal three wishes, to describe the best and worst events of their lives, and to name a favorite person to be stranded with on a desert island. Games such as Donald W. Winnicott's "squiggle," in which the examiner draws a curved line and then the child and the examiner take turns continuing the drawing, may facilitate conversation.

Questions that are partially open-ended with some multiple choices may elicit the most complete answers from school-age children. Simple, closed (yes/no) questions may not elicit enough information, and completely open-ended questions can overwhelm a school-age child who cannot construct a chronological narrative. These techniques often result in a shoulder shrug from the child. The use of indirect commentary—such as, "I once knew a child who felt very sad when he moved away from all his friends"—is helpful, although the clinician must be careful not to lead the child into confirming what the child thinks the clinician wants to hear. School-age children respond well to clinicians who help them compare moods or feelings by asking them to rate feelings on a scale of 1 to 10.

Adolescents

Adolescents usually have distinct ideas about why the evaluation was initiated, and can usually give a chronological account of the recent events leading to the evaluation, although some may disagree with the need for the evaluation. The clinician should clearly communicate the value of hearing the story from an adolescent's point of view and must be careful to reserve judgment and not assign blame. Adolescents may be concerned about confidentiality, and clinicians can assure them that permission will be requested from them before any specific information is shared with parents, except situations involving danger to the adolescent or others, in which case confidentiality must be sacrificed. Adolescents can be approached in an open-ended manner; however, when silences occur during the interview, the clinician should attempt to reengage the patient. Clinicians can explore what the adolescent believes the outcome of the evaluation will be (change of school, hospitalization, removal from home, removal of privileges).

Some adolescents approach the interview with apprehension or hostility, but open up when it becomes evident that the clinician is neither punitive nor judgmental. Clinicians must be aware of their own responses to adolescents' behavior (countertransference) and stay focused on the therapeutic process even in the face of defiant, angry, or difficult teenagers. Clinicians should set appropriate limits and should postpone or discon-

and teachers by Keith Connors in 1973. It consists of 10 items that assess both hyperactivity and inattention.

COMPONENTS OF THE CHILD PSYCHIATRIC EVALUATION

Psychiatric evaluation of a child includes a description of the reason for the referral, the child's past and present functioning, and any test results. An outline of the evaluation is given in Table 37–1.

Identifying Data

To understand the clinical problems to be evaluated, the clinician must first identify the patient and keep in mind the family constellation surrounding the child. The clinician must also pay attention to the source of the referral—that is, whether it is the child's family, school, or another agency—as this influences the family's attitude toward the evaluation. Finally, many informants contribute to the child's evaluation, and each must be identified to gain insight into the child's functioning in different settings.

History

A comprehensive history contains information about the child's current and past functioning, from the child's report, from clinical and structured interviews with the parents, and from information from teachers and previous treating clinicians. The chief complaint and the history of the present illness are generally obtained from both the child and the parents. Naturally, the child will articulate the situation according to his or her developmental level. The developmental history is more accurately obtained from the parents. Psychiatric and medical histories, current physical examination findings, and immunization histories can be augmented with reports from psychiatrists and pediatricians who have treated the child in the past. The child's report is critical in understanding the current situation regarding peer relationships and adjustment to school. Adolescents are the best informants regarding knowledge of safe sexual practices, drug or alcohol use, and suicidal ideation. The family's psychiatric and social histories, and family function are best obtained from the parents.

Table 37–1
Child Psychiatric Evaluation

Identifying data
- Identified patient and family members
- Source of referral
- Informants

History
- Chief complaint
- History of present illness
- Developmental history and milestones
- Psychiatric history
- Medical history, including immunizations
- Family social history and parents' marital status
- Educational history and current school functioning
- Peer relationship history
- Current family functioning
- Family psychiatric and medical histories
- Current physical examination

Mental status examination
Neuropsychiatric examination (when applicable)
Developmental, psychological, and educational testing
Formulation and summary
DSM-IV-TR diagnosis
Recommendations and treatment plan

Table 37-2
Mental Status Examination for Children

1. Physical appearance
2. Parent–child interaction
3. Separation and reunion
4. Orientation to time, place, and person
5. Speech and language
6. Mood
7. Affect
8. Thought process and content
9. Social relatedness
10. Motor behavior
11. Cognition
12. Memory
13. Judgment and insight

Mental Status Examination

A detailed description of the child's current mental functioning can be obtained through observation and specific questioning. An outline of the mental status examination is presented in Table 37–2.

Physical Appearances. The examiner should document the child's size, grooming, nutritional state, bruising, head circumference, physical signs of anxiety, facial expressions, and mannerisms.

Parent-Child Interaction. The examiner can observe the interactions between parents and child in the waiting area before the interview and in the family session. The manner in which parents and child converse and the emotional overtones are pertinent.

Separation and Reunion. The examiner should note both the manner in which the child responds to the separation from a parent for an individual interview and the reunion behavior. Either lack of affect at separation and reunion or severe distress on separation or reunion can indicate problems in the parent–child relationship or other psychiatric disturbances.

Orientation to Time, Place, and Persons. Impairments in orientation can reflect organic damage, low intelligence, or a thought disorder. The age of the child must be kept in mind, however, because very young children are not expected to know the date, other chronological information, or the name of the interview site.

Speech and Language. The examiner should evaluate the child's speech and language acquisition. Is it appropriate for the child's age? A disparity between expressive language usage and receptive language is notable. The examiner should also note the child's rate of speech, rhythm, latency to answer, spontaneity of speech, intonation, articulation of words, and prosody. Echolalia, repetitive stereotypical phrases, and unusual syntax are important psychiatric findings. Children who do not use words by age 18 months or who do not use phrases by age 2½ to 3 years, but who have a history of normal babbling and responding appropriately to nonverbal cues are probably developing normally. The examiner should consider the possibility that a hearing loss is contributing to a speech and language deficit.

Mood. A child's sad expression, lack of appropriate smiling, tearfulness, anxiety, euphoria, and anger are valid indicators of mood, as are verbal admissions of feelings. Persistent themes in play and fantasy also reflect the child's mood.

Affect. The examiner should note the child's range of emotional expressivity, appropriateness of affect to thought content, ability to move smoothly from one affect to another, and sudden labile emotional shifts.

Thought Process and Content. In evaluating a thought disorder in a child, the clinician must always consider what is developmentally expected for the child's age and what is deviant for any age group. The evaluation of the form of thought considers loosening of associations, excessive magical thinking, perseveration, echolalia, the ability to distinguish fantasy from reality, sentence coherence, and the ability to reason logically. The evaluation of thought content considers delusions, obsessions, themes, fears, wishes, preoccupations, and interests.

Suicidal ideation is always a part of the mental status examination for children who are verbal enough to understand the questions and old enough to understand the concept. Children of average intelligence more than 4 years of age usually have some understanding of what is real and what is make-believe and may be asked about suicidal ideation, although a firm concept of the permanence of death may not be present until several years later.

Aggressive thoughts and homicidal ideation are assessed here. Perceptual disturbances, such as hallucinations, are also assessed. Very young children are expected to have short attention spans and may change the topic and conversation abruptly without exhibiting a symptomatic flight of ideas. Transient visual and auditory hallucinations in very young children do not necessarily represent major psychotic illnesses, but they do deserve further investigation.

Social Relatedness. The examiner assesses the appropriateness of the child's response to the interviewer, general level of social skills, eye contact, and degree of familiarity or withdrawal in the interview process. Overly friendly or familiar behavior may be as troublesome as extremely retiring and withdrawn responses. The examiner assesses the child's self-esteem, general and specific areas of confidence, and success with family and peer relationships.

Motor Behavior. The motor behavior part of the mental status examination includes observations of the child's coordination and activity level and ability to pay attention and carry out developmentally appropriate tasks. It also involves involuntary movements, tremors, motor hyperactivity, and any unusual focal asymmetries of muscle movement.

Cognition. The examiner assesses the child's intellectual functioning and problem-solving abilities. An approximate level of intelligence can be estimated by the child's general information, vocabulary, and comprehension. For a specific assessment of the child's cognitive abilities, the examiner can use a standardized test.

Memory. School-age children should be able to remember three objects after 5 minutes and to repeat five digits forward and three digits backward. Anxiety may interfere with the child's performance, but an obvious inability to repeat digits or to add simple numbers may reflect brain damage, mental retardation, or learning disabilities.

Judgment and Insight. The child's view of the problems, reactions to them, and suggested solutions may give the clinician a good idea of the child's judgment and insight. In addition, the child's understanding of what he or she can realistically do to help and what the clinician can do adds to the assessment of the child's judgment.

Neuropsychiatric Assessment

A neuropsychiatric assessment is appropriate for children who are suspected of having a neurological disorder, a psychiatric impairment that coexists with neurological signs, or psychiatric symptoms that may be due to neuropathology. The neuropsychiatric evaluation combines information from neurological, physical, and mental status examinations. The neurological examination can identify asymmetrical abnormal signs (hard signs) that may indicate lesions in the brain. A physical examination can evaluate the presence of physical stigmata of particular syndromes in which neuropsychiatric symptoms or developmental aberrations play a role (e.g., fetal alcohol syndrome, Down syndrome).

An important part of the neuropsychiatric examination is the assessment of neurological soft signs and minor physical anomalies. The term *neurological soft signs* was first noted by Loretta Bender in the 1940s in reference to nondiagnostic abnormalities in the neurological examinations of children with schizophrenia. Soft signs do not indicate focal neurological disorders, but they are associated with a wide variety of developmental disabilities and occur frequently in children with low intelligence, learning disabilities, and behavioral disturbances. Soft signs may refer to both behavioral symptoms (which are sometimes associated with brain damage, such as severe impulsivity and hyperactivity), physical findings (including contralateral overflow movements), and a variety of nonfocal signs (such as mild choreiform movements, poor balance, mild incoordination, asymmetry of gait, nystagmus, and the persistence of infantile reflexes). Soft signs can be divided into those that are normal in a young child but become abnormal when they persist in an older child and those that are abnormal at any age. The Physical and Neurological Examination for Soft Signs (PANESS) is an instrument used with children up to the age of 15 years. It consists of 15 questions about general physical status and medical history and 43 physical tasks (e.g., touch your finger to your nose, hop on one foot to the end of the line, tap quickly with

your finger). Neurological soft signs are important to note, but they are not useful in making a specific psychiatric diagnosis.

Minor physical anomalies or dysmorphic features occur with a higher than usual frequency in children with developmental disabilities, learning disabilities, speech and language disorders, and hyperactivity. As with soft signs, the documentation of minor physical anomalies is part of the neuropsychiatric assessment, but it is rarely helpful in the diagnostic process and does not imply a good or bad prognosis. Minor physical anomalies include a high-arched palate, epicanthal folds, hypertelorism, low-set ears, transverse palmar creases, multiple hair whorls, a large head, a furrowed tongue, and partial syndactyly of several toes.

When a seizure disorder is being considered in the differential diagnosis or a structural abnormality in the brain is suspected, an electroencephalogram (EEG), computed tomography (CT), or magnetic resonance imaging (MRI) may be indicated.

Developmental, Psychological, and Educational Testing

Psychological tests are not always required to assess psychiatric symptoms, but they are valuable in determining a child's developmental level, intellectual functioning, and academic difficulties. A measure of adaptive functioning (including the child's competence in communication, daily living skills, socialization, and motor skills) is a prerequisite when a diagnosis of mental retardation is being considered. Table 37–3 outlines the general categories of psychological tests.

Table 37–3
Commonly Used Child and Adolescent Psychological Assessment Instruments

Test	Age/Grades	Data Generated and Comments
Intellectual ability		
Wechsler Intelligence Scale for Children—Third Edition (WISC-III-R)	6–16	Standard scores: verbal, performance and full-scale IQ: scaled subtest scores permitting specific skill assessment.
Wechsler Adult Intelligence Scale—(WAIS-III)	16–adult	Same as WISC-III-R.
Wechsler Preschool and Primary Scale of Intelligence—Revised (WPPSI-R)	3–7	Same as WISC-III-R.
Kaufman Assessment Battery for Children (K-ABC)	2.6–12.6	Well grounded in theories of cognitive psychology and neuropsychology. Allows immediate comparison of intellectual capacity with acquired knowledge. Scores: Mental Processing Composite (IQ equivalent); sequential and simultaneous processing and achievement standard scores; scaled mental processing and achievement subtest scores; age equivalents; percentiles.
Kaufman Adolescent and Adult Intelligence Test (KAIT)	11–85+	Composed of separate Crystallized and Fluid scales. Scores: Composite Intelligence Scale; Crystallized and Fluid IQ; scaled subtest scores; percentiles.
Stanford-Binet, 4th Edition (SB:FE)	2–23	Scores: IQ; verbal, abstract/visual, and quantitative reasoning; short-term memory; standard age.
Peabody Picture Vocabulary Test—III (PPVT-III)	4–adult	Measures receptive vocabulary acquisition; standard scores, percentiles, age equivalents.
Achievement		
Woodcock-Johnson Psycho-Educational Battery—Revised (W-J)	K–12	Scores: reading and mathematics (mechanics and comprehension), written language, other academic achievement; grade and age scores, standard scores, percentiles.
Wide Range Achievement Test—3, Levels 1 and 2 (WRAT-3)	Level 1: 1–5 Level 2: 12–75	Permits screening for deficits in reading, spelling, and arithmetic; grade levels, percentiles, stanines, standard scores.
Kaufman Test of Educational Achievement, Brief and Comprehensive Forms (K-TEA)	1–12	Standard scores: reading, mathematics, and spelling; grade and age equivalents, percentiles, stanines. Brief Form is sufficient for most clinical applications; Comprehensive Form allows error analysis and more detailed curriculum planning.
Wechsler Individual Achievement Test (WIAT)	K–12	Standard scores: basic reading, mathematics reasoning, spelling (constituting Screener); reading comprehension, numerical operations, listening comprehension, oral expression, written expression. Conormal with WISC-III-R.
Adaptive behavior		
Vineland Adaptive Behavior Scales	Normal: 0–19 Retarded: All ages	Standard scores: adaptive behavior composite and communication, daily living skills, socialization and motor domains; percentiles, age equivalents, developmental age scores. Separate standardization groups for normal, visually handicapped, hearing impaired, emotionally disturbed, and retarded.
Scales of Independent Behavior—Revised	Newborn–adult	Standard scores: four adaptive (motor, social interaction, communication, personal living, community living) and three maladaptive (internalized, asocial, and externalized) areas; General Maladaptive Index and Broad Independence cluster.

(continued)

Table 37–3 (*continued*)

Test	Age/Grades	Data Generated and Comments
Attentional capacity		
Trail Making Test	8–adult	Standard scores, standard deviations, ranges; corrections for age and education.
Wisconsin Card Sorting Test	6.6–adult	Standard scores, standard deviations, T-scores, percentiles, developmental norms for number of categories achieved, perseverative errors, and failures to maintain set; computer measures.
Behavior Assessment System for Children (BASC)	4–18	Teacher and parent rating scales and child self-report of personality permitting multireporter assessment across a variety of domains in home, school, and community. Provides validity, clinical, and adaptive scales. ADHD component avails.
Home Situations Questionnaire—Revised (HSQ-R)	6–12	Permits parents to rate child's specific problems with attention or concentration. Scores for number of problem settings, mean severity, and factor scores for compliance and leisure situations.
ADHD Rating Scale	6–12	Score for number of symptoms keyed to DSM cutoff for diagnosis of ADHD; standard scores permit derivation of clinical significance for total score and two factors (Inattentive-Hyperactive and Impulsive-Hyperactive).
School Situations Questionnaire (SSQ-R)	6–12	Permits teachers to rate a child's specific problems with attention or concentration. Scores for number of problem settings and mean severity.
Child Attention Profile (CAP)	6–12	Brief measure allowing teachers' weekly ratings of presence and degree of child's inattention and overactivity. Normative scores for inattention, overactivity, and total score.
Projective tests		
Rorschach Inkblots	3–adult	Special scoring systems. Most recently developed and increasingly universally accepted is John Exner's Comprehensive System (1974). Assesses perceptual accuracy, integration of affective and intellectual functioning, reality testing, and other psychological processes.
Thematic Apperception Test (TAT)	6–adult	Generates stories which are analyzed qualitatively. Assumed to provide especially rich data regarding interpersonal functioning.
Machover Draw-A-Person Test (DAP)	3–adult	Qualitative analysis and hypothesis generation, especially regarding subject's feelings about self and significant others.
Kinetic Family Drawing (KFD)	3–adult	Qualitative analysis and hypothesis generation regarding an individual's perception of family structure and sentient environment. Some objective scoring systems in existence.
Rotter Incomplete Sentences Blank	Child, adolescent, and adult forms	Primarily qualitative analysis, although some objective scoring systems have been developed.
Personality tests		
Minnesota Multiphasic Personality Inventory-Adolescent (MMPI-A)	14–18	1992 version of widely used personality measure, developed specifically for use with adolescents. Standard scores: 3 validity scales, 14 clinical scales, additional content and supplementary scales.
Million Adolescent Personality Inventory (MAPI)	13–18	Standard scores for 20 scales grouped into three categories: Personality styles; expressed concerns; behavioral correlates. Normed on adolescent population. Focuses on broad functional spectrum, not just problem areas. Measures 14 primary personality traits, including emotional stability, self-concept level, excitability, and self-assurance.
Children's Personality Questionnaire	8–12	Generates combined broad trait patterns including extraversion and anxiety.
Neuropsychological screening tests and test batteries		
Developmental Test of Visual-Motor Integration (VMI)	2–16	Screening instrument for visual motor deficits. Standard scores, age equivalents, percentiles.
Benton Visual Retention Test	6–adult	Assesses presence of deficits in visual-figure memory. Mean scores by age.
Benton Visual Motor Gestalt Test	5–adult	Assesses visual-motor deficits and visual-figural retention. Age equivalents.
Reitan-Indiana Neuropsychological Test Battery for Children	5–8	Cognitive and perceptual-motor tests for children with suspected brain damage.
Halstead-Reitan Neuropsychological Test Battery for Older Children	9–14	Same as Reitan-Indiana.
Luria-Nebraska Neuropsychological Battery: Children's Revision LNNB:C	8–12	Sensory-motor, perceptual, cognitive tests measuring 11 clinical and 2 additional domains of neuropsychological functioning. Provides standard scores.
Developmental status		
Bayley Scales of Infant Development-Second Edition	16 days–42 months	Mental, motor, and behavior scales measuring infant, development. Provides standard scores.
Mullen Scales of Early Learning	Newborn–5 years	Language and visual scales for receptive and expressive ability. Yields age scores and T scores.

Adapted from Racusin G, Moss N. Psychological assessment of children and adolescents. In: Lewis M, ed. *Child and Adolescent Psychiatry: A Comprehensive Textbook.* Baltimore: Williams & Wilkins; 1991.

Development Tests for Infants and Preschoolers. The Gesell Infant Scale, the Cattell Infant Intelligence Scale, Bayley Scales of Infant Development, and the Denver Developmental Screening Test include developmental assessments of infants as young as 2 months of age. When used with very young infants, the tests focus on sensorimotor and social responses to a variety of objects and interactions. When these instruments are used with older infants and preschoolers, emphasis is placed on language acquisition. The Gesell Infant Scale measures development in four areas: motor, adaptive functioning, language, and social.

An infant's score on one of these developmental assessments is not a reliable way to predict a child's future intelligence quotient (IQ) in most cases. Infant assessments are valuable, however, in detecting developmental deviation and mental retardation and in raising suspicions of a developmental disorder. Whereas infant assessments rely heavily on sensorimotor functions, intelligence testing in older children and adolescents includes later-developing functions, including verbal, social, and abstract cognitive abilities.

Intelligence Tests for School-Age Children and Adolescents. The most widely used test of intelligence for school-age children and adolescents is the third edition of the Wechsler Intelligence Scale for Children (WISC-III-R). It can be given to children from 6 to 17 years old and yields a verbal IQ, a performance IQ, and a combined full-scale IQ. The verbal subtests consist of vocabulary, information, arithmetic, similarities, comprehension, and digit span (supplemental) categories. The performance subtests include block design, picture completion, picture arrangement, object assembly, coding, mazes (supplemental), and symbol search (supplemental). The scores of the supplemental subtests are not included in the computation of IQ.

Each subcategory is scored from 1 to 19, with 10 being the average score. An average full-scale IQ is 100; 70 to 80 represents borderline intellectual function; 80 to 90 is in the low average range; 90 to 109 is average; 110 to 119 is high average; and above 120 is in the superior or very superior range. The multiple breakdowns of the performance and verbal subscales allow great flexibility in identifying specific areas of deficit and scatter in intellectual abilities. Because a large part of intelligence testing measures abilities used in academic settings, the breakdown of the WISC-III-R can also be helpful in pointing out skills in which a child is weak and may benefit from remedial education.

The Stanford-Binet Intelligence Scale covers an age range from 2 to 24 years. It relies on pictures, drawings, and objects for very young children and on verbal performance for older children and adolescents. This intelligence scale, the earliest version of an intelligence test of its kind, leads to a mental age score as well as an intelligence quotient.

The McCarthy Scales of Children's Abilities and the Kaufman Assessment Battery for Children are two other intelligence tests that are available for preschool and school-age children. They do not cover the adolescent age group.

LONG-TERM STABILITY OF INTELLIGENCE. Although a child's intelligence is relatively stable throughout the school-age years and adolescence, some factors can influence intelligence and a child's score on an intelligence test. The intellectual functions of children with severe mental illnesses and of those from low socioeconomic levels may decrease over time, whereas the IQs of children whose environments have been enriched may increase over time. Factors that influence a child's score on a given test of intellectual functioning and thus affect the accuracy of the test are motivation, emotional state, anxiety, and cultural milieu.

Perceptual and Perceptual Motor Tests. The Bender Visual Motor Gestalt test can be given to children between the ages of 4 and 12 years. The test consists of a set of spatially related figures that the child is asked to copy. The scores are based on the number of errors. Although not a diagnostic test, it is useful in identifying developmentally age-inappropriate perceptual performances.

Personality Tests. Personality tests are not of much use in making diagnoses, and they are less satisfactory than intelligence tests in regard to norms, reliability, and validity, but they can be helpful in eliciting themes and fantasies.

The Rorschach test is a projective technique in which ambiguous stimuli—a set of bilaterally symmetrical inkblots—are shown to a child, who is then asked to describe what he or she sees in each. The hypothesis is that the child's interpretation of the vague stimuli reflects basic characteristics of personality. The examiner notes the themes and patterns. Two sets of norms have been established for the Rorschach test, one for children between 2 and 10 years and one for adolescents between 10 and 17 years.

A more structured projective test is the Children's Apperception Test (CAT), which is an adaptation of the Thematic Apperception Test (TAT). The CAT consists of cards with pictures of animals in scenes that are somewhat ambiguous but are related to parent–child and sibling issues, caretaking, and other relationships. The child is asked to describe what is happening and to tell a story about the scene. Animals are used because it was hypothesized that children might respond more readily to animal images than to human figures.

Drawings, toys, and play are also applications of projective techniques that can be used during the evaluation of children. Dollhouses, dolls, and puppets have been especially helpful in allowing a child a nonconversational mode in which to express a variety of attitudes and feelings. Play materials that reflect household situations are likely to elicit a child's fears, hopes, and conflicts about the family.

Projective techniques have not fared well as standardized instruments. Rather than being considered tests, projective techniques are best considered as additional clinical modalities.

Educational Tests. Achievement tests measure the attainment of knowledge and skills in a particular academic curriculum. The Wide-Range Achievement Test–Revised (WRAT-R) consists of tests of knowledge and skills and timed performances of reading, spelling, and mathematics. It is used with children from 5 years of age to adulthood. The test yields a score that is compared with the average expected score for the child's chronological age and grade level.

The Peabody Individual Achievement Test (PIAT) includes word identification, spelling, mathematics, and reading comprehension.

The Kaufman Test of Educational Achievement, the Gray Oral Reading Test–Revised (GORT-R), and the Sequential Tests of Educational Progress (STEP) are achievement tests that determine whether a child has achieved the educational level expected for his or her grade level. Children with an average IQ, whose achievement is significantly lower than expected for their grade level in one or more subjects, are considered to be learning disabled. Thus, achievement testing, combined with a measure of intellectual function, can identify specific learning disabilities for which remediation is recommended. Children who do not reach their grade level according to their chronological age, but who function intellectually in the borderline range or lower, are not necessarily learning disabled unless a disparity exists between their IQs and their levels of achievement.

Biopsychosocial Formulation. The clinician's task is to integrate all of the information obtained into a formulation that takes into account the biological predisposition, psychodynamic factors, environmental stressors, and life events that have led to the child's current level of functioning. Psychiatric disorders and any specific physical, neuromotor, or developmental abnormalities must be considered in the formulation of etiologic factors for current impairment. The clinician's conclusions are an integration of clinical information along with data from standardized psychological and developmental assessments. The psychiatric formulation includes an assessment of family function as well as the appropriateness of the child's educational setting. A determination of the child's overall safety in his or her current situation is made. Any suspected maltreatment must be reported to the local child protective service agency. The child's overall well-being regarding growth, development, and academic and play activities is considered.

Diagnosis

The clinician's task includes making all appropriate diagnoses according to DSM-IV-TR. Some clinical situations do not fulfill criteria for DSM-IV-TR diagnoses but cause impairment and require psychiatric attention and intervention. Clinicians who evaluate children are frequently in the position of determining the impact of behavior of family members on the child's well-being. In many cases, a child's level of impairment is related to factors extending beyond a psychiatric diagnosis, such as the child's adjustment to his or her family life, peer relationships, and educational placement.

RECOMMENDATIONS AND TREATMENT PLAN

Recommendations and a treatment plan following an evaluation of a child most often include the cooperation of family members. The treatment of a given psychiatric disorder in a child often includes direct family and environmental interventions. The clinician's recommendations may include, for example, family psychotherapy, a change in the child's school setting, or (in rare cases) having the child live outside the family setting for some period. The safety of the child is always a consideration when devising a set of recommendations. The clinician must communicate the recommendations and proposed treatment plan to both the parents and the child, since without parental cooperation, treatment may be compromised or not obtained.

A clinician seeks to give feedback to whomever has referred the child for the evaluation, with appropriate permission. Thus, when a child is referred for evaluation by an outside agency, such as a school, therapist, or protective service agency, permission is generally obtained to provide information to those who made the referral.

References

Adams RL, Culbertson JL. Neuropsychological and intellectual assessment of children. In: Sadock BJ, Sadock VA, eds. *Kaplan & Sadock's Comprehensive Textbook of Psychiatry.* 7th ed. Vol 1. Baltimore: Lippincott Williams & Wilkins; 2000:722.

Ambrosini PJ. Historical development and present status of the Schedule for Affective Disorders and Schizophrenia for School-Age Children (K-SADS). *J Am Acad Child Adolesc Psychiatry.* 2000;39:49.

Angold A, Costello EJ. The Child and Adolescent Psychiatric Assessment (CAPA). *J Am Acad Child Adolesc Psychiatry.* 2000;39:39.

Barber CC, Neese DT, Coyne L, et al. The Target Symptom Rating: a brief clinical measure of acute psychiatric symptoms in children and adolescents. *J Clin Child Adolesc Psychol.* 2002;31:181.

Bender L. Childhood schizophrenia: clinical study of 100 schizophrenic children. *Am J Orthopsychiatry.* 1947;17:40.

Chandler MC, Gualtieri CT, Barnhill LJ. The neuropsychiatric examination of the child. In: Tonge BJ, Burrows GD, Werry JC, eds. *Handbook of Studies on Child Psychiatry.* Amsterdam: Elsevier; 1990:91.

Ernst M, Cookus BA, Moravec BC. Pictorial Instrument for Children and Adolescents (PICA-III-R). *J Am Acad Child Adolesc Psychiatry.* 2000;39:94.

Jensen PS, Watanabe H. Sherlock Holmes and child psychopathology assessment approaches: the case of the false-positive. *J Am Acad Child Adolesc Psychiatry.* 1999;38:138.

King RA, Hodapp RM, Schwab-Stone ME, Peterson BS, Thies AP. Psychiatric examination of the infant, child, and adolescent. In: Sadock BJ, Sadock VA, eds. *Kaplan & Sadock's Comprehensive Textbook of Psychiatry.* 7th ed. Vol 2. Baltimore: Lippincott Williams & Wilkins; 2000:2558.

Ollendick TH, Hersen M, eds. *Handbook of Child and Adolescent Assessment.* Boston: Allyn & Bacon; 1993.

Pataki CS. Child psychiatry: introduction and overview. In: Sadock BJ, Sadock VA, eds. *Kaplan & Sadock's Comprehensive Textbook of Psychiatry.* 7th ed. Vol 2. Baltimore: Lippincott Williams & Wilkins; 2000:2532.

Practice parameters for the psychiatric assessment of children and adolescents. *J Am Acad Child Adolesc Psychiatry.* 1997;36:4S.

Reich W. Diagnostic Interview for Children and Adolescents (DICA). *J Am Acad Child Adolesc Psychiatry.* 2000;39:59.

Schetky DH, Benedek EP, eds. *Principles and Practice of Child and Adolescent Forensic Psychiatry.* Washington, DC: American Psychiatric Publishing; 2002.

Shaffer D, Fisher P, Lucas CP, Dulcan MK, Schwab-Stone ME. NIMH Diagnostic Interview Schedule for Children (Version IV): description, differences from previous versions, and reliability of some common diagnoses. *J Am Acad Child Adolesc Psychiatry.* 2000;39:28.

Storch EA. Prescriptions of medications to youths. *Psychiatr Serv.* 2002;53:214.

Valla JP, Bergeron L, Smolla N. The Dominic-R: a pictorial interview for 6- to 11-year-old children. *J Am Acad Child Adolesc Psychiatry.* 2000;39:85.

Weller EB, Weller, RA, Fristad MA, Rooney MT, Schecter J. Children's Interview for Psychiatric Syndromes (ChIPS). *J Am Acad Child Adolesc Psychiatry.* 2000;39:76.

38

Mental Retardation

Mental retardation is not a disease; rather it is the result of a pathological process in the brain characterized by limitations in intellectual and adaptive function. The cause of mental retardation is often unidentified, and the consequences become evident by a person's difficulty with intellectual functioning and living skills.

In the mid-1800s many children with mental retardation were placed in residential educational facilities with the belief that if these children received enough intensive training, they would be able to return to their families and function in society at a higher level. The original plan of educating the children so they could overcome their disabilities was not realized. Gradually, these residential programs became larger, and eventually the focus began to shift from intensive education to custodial care. These residential institutional settings for children with mental retardation received their maximum use in the mid-1900s, until public awareness of the crowded, unsanitary, and in some cases abusive conditions sparked the movement toward "deinstitutionalization." Since the late 1960s, few children with mental retardation have been placed in institutional settings, and the concept of "inclusion" in school settings, and "normalization" in living situations became prominent among advocacy groups and most citizens. Since the passage of Public Law 94-142 (the Education for all Handicapped Children Act) in 1975, the public school system has been mandated to provide appropriate educational service to all children with disabilities. The Individuals with Disabilities Act in 1990 extended and modified the above legislation. Currently, provision of public education for all children, including those with disabilities, is mandated by law and is to be provided "within the least restrictive environment."

In addition to the educational system, many organizations have developed to advocate for persons with mental retardation. Among them, the Council for Exceptional Children (CEC) and the National Association for Retarded Citizens (NARC) are well known. The NARC functions as the main parental lobbying organization for children with mental retardation and was instrumental in advocating for Public Law 94-142. The most prominent advocacy organization in this field is the American Association on Mental Retardation (AAMR), which has been most influential in educating the public about mental retardation as well as in its support of research and legislation relating to mental retardation.

The AAMR, currently promotes a view of mental retardation as a functional interaction between an individual and the environment instead of a static description of a person's limitations. Within this conceptual framework, a person is designated as needing intermittent, limited, extensive, or pervasive "environmental support" with respect to a specific set of adaptive function domains. These areas of function are communication, self-care, home living, social/interpersonal skills, use of community resources, self-direction, functional academic skills, work, leisure, health, and safety.

The AAMR criteria also promote allowing an IQ of 75, rather than 70, to be considered in the mild mental retardation range, thereby enabling many more persons to receive services as mentally retarded. The advantage of the AAMR view is that instead of defining a person's degree of mental retardation by the level of cognitive and adaptive impairment, the degree of "support" necessary for functioning becomes the defining feature. The disadvantage of this nomenclature is that it is difficult to quantify the "supports" and it would be problematic to match new research with the existing body of research using an IQ cutoff of 70. The decision of the work group of the fourth edition of *Diagnostic and Statistical Manual of Mental Disorders* (DSM-IV) and its text revision (DSM-IV-TR) was that an IQ cutoff of 70 would be retained, and the adaptive function domains recommended by the AAMR would be included in the diagnostic criteria for mental retardation.

NOMENCLATURE

Accurately defining *mental retardation* has challenged clinicians over the centuries. In the 1800s the notion that mental retardation was based primarily on a deficit in social or moral reasoning was promoted. Since then, the addition of intellectual deficit was added to the concept of inadequate social function. All current classification systems retain the understanding that mental retardation is based on more than intellectual deficits, that is, it also depends upon a lower than expected level of adaptive function. According to DSM-IV-TR, a diagnosis of mental retardation can be made only when both the IQ, as measured by a standardized test, is subaverage and a measure of adaptive function reveals deficits in at least two of the areas of adaptive function. Mental retardation diagnoses are coded on Axis II in the DSM-IV-TR.

CLASSIFICATION

According to the DSM-IV-TR, mental retardation is defined as significantly subaverage general intellectual functioning resulting in, or associated with, concurrent impairment in adaptive behavior and manifested during the developmental period, before the age of 18. The diagnosis is made regardless of

Table 38–1
Developmental Characteristics of Mentally Retarded Persons

Degree of Mental Retardation	Preschool Age (0–5) Maturation and Development	School Age (6–20) Training and Education	Adult (21 and Over) Social and Vocational Adequacy
Profound	Gross retardation; minimal capacity for functioning in sensorimotor areas; needs nursing care; constant aid and supervision required	Some motor development present; may respond to minimal or limited training in self-help	Some motor and speech development; may achieve very limited self-care; needs nursing care
Severe	Poor motor development; speech minimal; generally unable to profit from training in self-help; little or no communication skills	Can talk or learn to communicate; can be trained in elemental health habits; profits from systematic habit training; unable to profit from vocational training	May contribute partially to self-maintenance under complete supervision; can develop self-protection skills to a minimal useful level in controlled environment
Moderate	Can talk or learn to communicate; poor social awareness; fair motor development; profits from training in self-help; can be managed with moderate supervision	Can profit from training in social and occupational skills; unlikely to progress beyond second-grade level in academic subjects; may learn to travel alone in familiar places	May achieve self-maintenance in unskilled or semiskilled work under sheltered conditions; needs supervision and guidance when under mild social or economic stress
Mild	Can develop social and communication skills; minimal retardation in sensorimotor areas; often not distinguished from normal until later age	Can learn academic skills up to approximately sixth-grade level by late teens; can be guided toward social conformity	Can usually achieve social and vocational skills adequate to minimum self-support but may need guidance and assistance when under unusual social or economic stress

Adapted from *Mental Retarded Activities of the U.S. Department of Health, Education and Welfare.* Washington, DC: US Government Printing Office; 1989:2. Used with permission. DSM-IV criteria are adapted essentially from this chart.

whether the person has a coexisting physical disorder or other mental disorder. Table 38–1 presents an overview of developmental levels in communication, academic functioning, and vocational skills expected of persons with various degrees of mental retardation.

General intellectual functioning is determined by the use of standardized tests of intelligence, and the term *significantly subaverage* is defined as an IQ of approximately 70 or below or two standard deviations below the mean for the particular test. Adaptive functioning can be measured by using a standardized scale, such as the Vineland Adaptive Behavior Scale. This scale scores communications, daily living skills, socialization, and motor skills (up to 4 years, 11 months) and generates an adaptive behavior composite that is correlated with the expected skills at a given age.

Approximately 85 percent of persons who are mentally retarded fall within the mild mental retardation category (IQ between 50 and 70). The adaptive functions of mildly retarded persons are effective in several areas, such as communications, self-care, social skills, work, leisure, and safety. Mental retardation is influenced by genetic, environmental, and psychosocial factors, and in past years, the development of mild retardation was often attributed to severe psychosocial deprivation. More recently, however, researchers have increasingly recognized the likely contribution of a host of subtle biological factors including chromosomal abnormalities, subclinical lead intoxication, and prenatal exposure to drugs, alcohol, and other toxins. Furthermore, evidence is increasing that subgroups of persons who are mentally retarded, such as those with fragile X syndrome, Down syndrome, and Prader-Willi syndrome, have characteristic patterns of social, linguistic, and cognitive development and typical behavioral manifestations.

The DSM-IV-TR has included in its text on mental retardation additional information regarding etiological factors and their association with mental retardation syndromes (e.g., fragile X syndrome).

DEGREES OF SEVERITY OF MENTAL RETARDATION

The degrees, or levels, of mental retardation are expressed in various terms. DSM-IV-TR presents four levels of mental retardation: mild, moderate, severe, and profound. The category borderline mental retardation (between one and two standard deviations below the test mean) was eliminated in 1973. Borderline intellectual functioning, according to DSM-IV-TR, is not within the diagnostic boundary of mental retardation and refers to a full-scale IQ in the 71 to 84 range that is a focus of psychiatric attention.

Mild mental retardation (IQ range, 50–55 to 70) represents approximately 85 percent of persons with mental retardation. In general, children with mild mental retardation are not identified until after first or second grade, when academic demands increase. By late adolescence they often acquire academic skills at approximately a sixth grade level. Specific causes for the mental retardation are often unidentified in this group. Many adults with mild mental retardation can live independently with appropriate support and raise their own families.

Moderate mental retardation (IQ range, 35–40 to 50–55) represents about 10 percent of persons with mental retardation. Most children with moderate mental retardation acquire language and can communicate adequately during early childhood. They are challenged academically and often are not able to achieve academically above a second to third grade level. During adoles-

cence, socialization difficulties often set these persons apart, and a great deal of social and vocational support is beneficial. As adults, persons with moderate mental retardation may be able to perform semiskilled work under appropriate supervision.

Severe mental retardation (IQ range, 20–25 to 35–40) comprises about 4 percent of individuals with mental retardation. They may be able to develop communication skills in childhood and often can learn to count as well as recognize words that are critical to functioning. In this group, the cause for the mental retardation is more likely to be identified than it is in milder forms of mental retardation. In adulthood, persons with severe mental retardation may adapt well to supervised living situations such as group homes and may be able to perform work-related tasks under supervision.

Profound mental retardation (IQ range below 20 or 25) constitutes approximately 1 to 2 percent of persons with mental retardation. Most individuals with profound mental retardation have identifiable causes for their condition. Children with profound mental retardation may be taught some self-care skills and learn to communicate their needs given the appropriate training.

DSM-IV-TR lists mental retardation, severity unspecified, as a type reserved for persons who are strongly suspected of having mental retardation but who cannot be tested by standard intelligence tests or are too impaired or uncooperative to be tested. This type may be applicable to infants whose significantly subaverage intellectual functioning is clinically judged but for whom the available tests (e.g., Bayley Scales of Infant Development and Cattell Infant Scale) do not yield numerical IQ values. This type should not be used when the intellectual level is presumed to be above 70.

EPIDEMIOLOGY

The prevalence of mental retardation at any one time is estimated to be about 1 percent of the population. The incidence of mental retardation is difficult to calculate because mental retardation sometimes goes unrecognized until middle childhood, when it is mild. In some cases, even when intellectual function is limited, good adaptive skills are not challenged until late childhood or early adolescence, and the diagnosis is not made until that time. The highest incidence is in school-age children, with the peak at ages 10 to 14. Mental retardation is about 1.5 times more common among men than among women. In older persons, prevalence is lower; those with severe or profound mental retardation have high mortality rates due to the complications of associated physical disorders.

COMORBIDITY

Prevalence

Epidemiological surveys indicate that up to two thirds of children and adults with mental retardation have comorbid mental disorders; this rate is several times higher than that in non–mentally retarded community samples. The prevalence of psychopathology seems to be correlated with the severity of mental retardation; the more severe the mental retardation, the higher the risk for other mental disorders. A recent epidemiological study found that 40.7 percent of intellectually disabled children between 4 and 18 years of age met criteria for at least one psychiatric disorder. The severity of retardation affected the type of psychiatric disorder. Disruptive and conduct-disorder behaviors occurred more commonly in the mildly retarded group; the more severely retarded group exhibited psychiatric problems more often associated with autistic disorder such as self-stimulation and self-mutilation. In contrast to the epidemiology of psychopathology in children in general, age and sex did not affect the prevalence of psychiatric disorders in this study. Those with profound mental retardation were less likely to exhibit psychiatric symptoms.

The mental disorders that occur among persons who are mentally retarded appear to run the gamut of those seen in non–mentally retarded persons, including mood disorders, schizophrenia, attention-deficit/hyperactivity disorder, and conduct disorder. Those with severe mental retardation have a particularly high rate of autistic disorder and pervasive developmental disorders. About 2 to 3 percent of mentally retarded persons meet the criteria for schizophrenia; this percentage is several times higher than the rate for the general population. Up to 50 percent of mentally retarded children and adults had a mood disorder when such instruments as the Kiddie Schedule for Affective Disorders and Schizophrenia, the Beck Depression Inventory, and the Children's Depression Inventory were used in pilot studies, but since these instruments have not been standardized within the mentally retarded population, these findings must be considered preliminary.

Highly prevalent psychiatric symptoms that can occur in mentally retarded persons outside the context of a mental disorder include hyperactivity and short attention span, self-injurious behaviors (e.g., head banging and self-biting), and repetitive stereotypical behaviors (hand flapping and toe walking). Personality styles and traits in mentally retarded persons are not unique to them, but negative self-image, low self-esteem, poor frustration tolerance, interpersonal dependence, and a rigid problem-solving style are overrepresented. Specific causal syndromes seen in mental retardation may also predispose affected persons to various types of psychopathologies.

Neurological Disorders

Comorbid psychiatric disorders are increased in individuals with mental retardation who also have known neurological conditions, such as seizure disorders. Rates of psychopathology increase with the severity of mental retardation; thus neurological impairment increases as intellectual impairment increases. In a recent review of psychiatric disorders in children and adolescents with mental retardation and epilepsy, approximately one third also had autistic disorder or an autisticlike condition. The combination of mental retardation, active epilepsy, and autism or an autisticlike condition occurs at a rate of 0.07 percent in the general population.

Genetic Syndromes

Some evidence indicates that genetically based syndromes such as fragile X syndrome, Prader-Willi syndrome, and Down syndrome are associated with comorbid specific behavioral manifestations (Fig. 38–1). Persons with fragile X syndrome have extremely high rates (up to three fourths of those studied) of attention-deficit/hyperactivity disorders. High

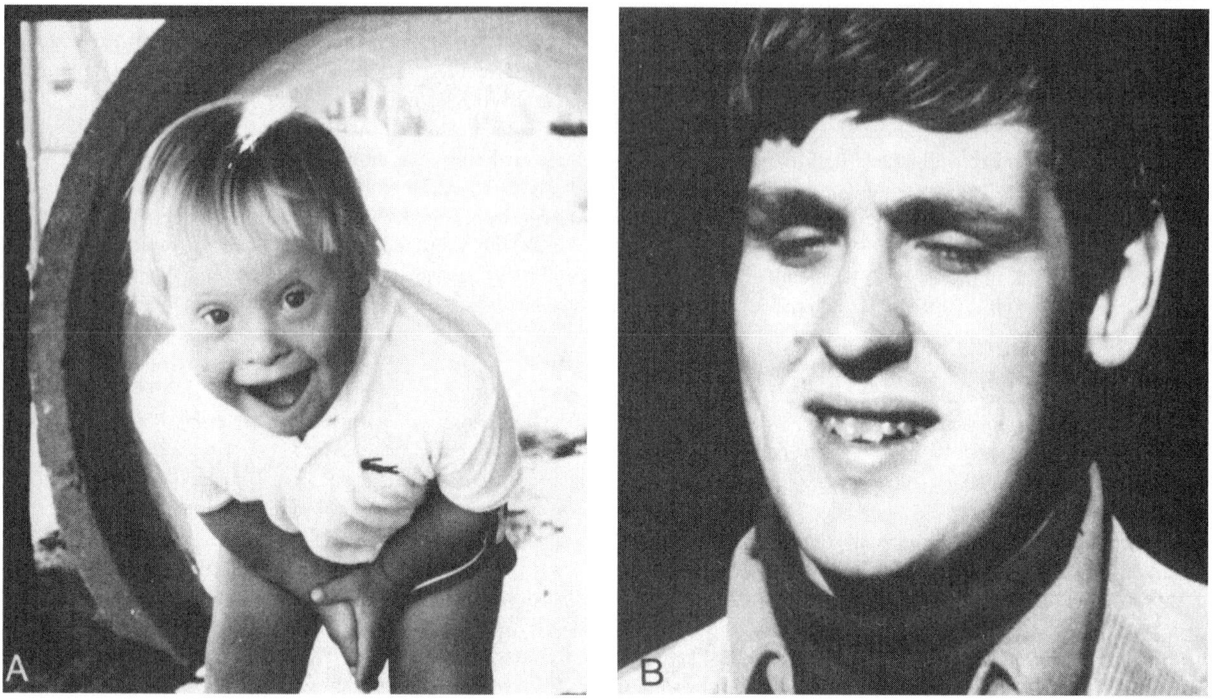

FIGURE 38–1
A. A young child with Down syndrome. **B**. A young adult with fragile X syndrome. (Courtesy of L. S. Syzmanski, M.D., and A. C. Crocker, M.D.)

rates of aberrant interpersonal behavior and language function often meet the criteria for autistic disorder and avoidant personality disorder. Prader-Willi syndrome is almost always associated with compulsive eating disturbances, hyperphagia, and obesity. Children with the syndrome have been described as oppositional and defiant. Socialization is an area of weakness, especially in coping skills. Externalizing behavior problems—such as temper tantrums, irritability, and arguing—seem to be heightened in adolescence.

In Down syndrome, language function is a relative weakness, whereas sociability and social skills, such as interpersonal cooperation and conformity with social conventions, are relative strengths. Most studies have noted muted affect in children with Down syndrome relative to nonretarded children of the same mental age. Those with Down syndrome also manifest deficiencies in scanning the environment; they are likely to focus on a single stimulus and have difficulty noticing environmental changes. A variety of mental disorders occur in persons with Down syndrome, but the rates appear to be lower than those of other mental retardation syndromes, especially autistic disorder.

Psychosocial Syndromes

A negative self-image and poor self-esteem are common features of mildly and moderately mentally retarded persons, who are well aware of being different from others. They experience repeated failure and disappointment in not meeting their parents' and society's expectations and in falling progressively behind their peers and even their younger siblings. Communication difficulties further increase their vulnerability to feelings of ineptness and frustration. Inappropriate behaviors, such as withdrawal, are common. The perpetual sense of isolation and inadequacy has been linked to feelings of anxiety, anger, dysphoria, and depression.

ETIOLOGY

Etiological factors in mental retardation may be primarily genetic, developmental, acquired, or a combination. Genetic causes include chromosomal and inherited conditions, developmental factors include prenatal exposure to infections and toxins, and acquired syndromes include perinatal trauma (such as prematurity) and sociocultural factors. The severity of the resulting mental retardation is related to the timing and duration of the trauma as well as the degree of exposure to the central nervous system. The more severe the mental retardation, the more likely it is that the cause is evident. In about three fourths of persons with severe mental retardation, the cause is known, whereas the cause is apparent in only half of those with mild mental retardation. No cause is known for three fourths of persons with borderline intellectual functioning. Overall, in up to two thirds of all mentally retarded persons, the probable cause can be identified. Among chromosomal and metabolic disorders, Down syndrome, fragile X syndrome, and phenylketonuria (PKU) are the most common disorders that usually produce at least moderate mental retardation. Those with mild mental retardation sometimes have a familial pattern apparent in parents and siblings. Deprivation of nutrition, nurturance, and social stimulation may contribute to the development of mental retardation. Current knowledge suggests that genetic, envi-

ronmental, biological, and psychosocial factors work additively in mental retardation.

Genetic Factors

Abnormalities in autosomal chromosomes are associated with mental retardation, although aberrations in sex chromosomes are not always associated with mental retardation (such as Turner's syndrome with XO and Klinefelter's syndrome with XXY, XXXY, and XXYY variations). Some children with Turner's syndrome have normal to superior intelligence. There is agreement on a few predisposing factors for chromosomal disorders—among them, advanced maternal age, increased age of the father, and X-ray radiation.

Down Syndrome. The description of Down syndrome, first made by the English physician Langdon Down in 1866, was based on the physical characteristics associated with subnormal mental functioning. Since then, Down syndrome has been the most investigated, and most discussed, syndrome in mental retardation. Children with this syndrome were originally called *mongoloid* because of their physical characteristics of slanted eyes, epicanthal folds, and flat nose. Despite a plethora of theories and hypotheses advanced in the past 100 years, the cause of Down syndrome is still unknown.

The problem of cause is complicated even further by the recent recognition of three types of chromosomal aberrations in Down syndrome:

1. Patients with trisomy 21 (three chromosome 21s, instead of the usual two) represent the overwhelming majority; they have 47 chromosomes, with an extra chromosome 21. The mothers' karyotypes are normal. A nondisjunction during meiosis, occurring for unknown reasons, is held responsible for the disorder.
2. Nondisjunction occurring after fertilization in any cell division results in mosaicism, a condition in which both normal and trisomic cells are found in various tissues.
3. In translocation there is a fusion of two chromosomes, usually 21 and 15, resulting in a total of 46 chromosomes, despite the presence of an extra chromosome 21. The disorder, unlike trisomy 21, is usually inherited, and the translocated chromosome may be found in unaffected parents and siblings. The asymptomatic carriers have only 45 chromosomes.

The incidence of Down syndrome in the United States is about 1 in every 700 births. In his original description, Down mentioned the frequency of 10 percent among all mentally retarded patients. For a middle-aged mother (more than 32 years old), the risk of having a child with Down syndrome with trisomy 21 is about 1 in 100 births, but when translocation is present, the risk is about 1 in 3. These facts assume special importance in genetic counseling.

Mental retardation is the overriding feature of Down syndrome. Most persons with the syndrome are moderately or severely retarded, with only a minority having an IQ above 50. Mental development seems to progress normally from birth to 6 months of age; IQ scores gradually decrease from near normal at 1 year of age to about 30 at older ages. The decline in intelligence may not be readily apparent. Infantile tests may not reveal the full extent of the defect, which may become manifest when sophisticated tests are used in early childhood. According to many sources, children with Down syndrome are placid, cheerful, and cooperative and adapt easily at home. With adolescence, the picture changes: Youngsters may experience various emotional difficulties, behavior disorders, and (rarely) psychotic disorders.

The diagnosis of Down syndrome is made with relative ease in an older child but is often difficult in newborn infants. The most important signs in a newborn include general hypotonia, oblique palpebral fissures, abundant neck skin, a small, flattened skull, high cheekbones, and a protruding tongue. The hands are broad and thick, with a single palmar transversal crease, and the little fingers are short and curved inward. Moro reflex is weak or absent. More than 100 signs or stigmata are described in Down syndrome, but rarely are all found in one person. Life expectancy was once about 12 years; with the advent of antibiotics, few young patients succumb to infections, but many do not live beyond the age of 40. Life expectancy is increasing, however.

Persons with Down syndrome tend to exhibit marked deterioration in language, memory, self-care skills, and problem solving in their 30s. Postmortem studies of those with Down syndrome over the age of 40 have shown a high incidence of senile plaques and neurofibrillary tangles, as seen in Alzheimer's disease. Neurofibrillary tangles are known to occur in a variety of degenerative diseases, whereas senile plaques seem to be found most often in Alzheimer's disease and in Down syndrome. Thus the two disorders may share some pathophysiology.

Fragile X Syndrome. Fragile X syndrome is the second most common single cause of mental retardation. The syndrome results from a mutation on the X chromosome at what is known as the fragile site (Xq27.3). The fragile site is expressed in only some cells, and it may be absent in asymptomatic males and female carriers. Much variability is present in both genetic and phenotypic expression. Fragile X syndrome is believed to occur in about 1 in every 1,000 males and 1 in every 2,000 females. The typical phenotype includes a large, long head and ears, short stature, hyperextensible joints, and postpubertal macroorchidism. The mental retardation ranges from mild to severe. The behavioral profile of persons with the syndrome includes a high rate of attention-deficit/hyperactivity disorder, learning disorders, and pervasive developmental disorders, such as autism. Deficits in language function include rapid perseverative speech with abnormalities in combining words into phrases and sentences. Persons with fragile X syndrome seem to have relatively strong skills in communication and socialization; their intellectual functions seem to decline in the pubertal period. Female carriers are often less impaired than males with fragile X syndrome, but females can also manifest the typical physical characteristics and can be mildly retarded.

Prader-Willi Syndrome. Prader-Willi syndrome is postulated to result from a small deletion involving chromosome 15, usually occurring sporadically. Its prevalence is less than 1 in 10,000. Persons with the syndrome exhibit compulsive eating behavior and often obesity, mental retardation, hypogonadism, small stature, hypotonia, and small hands and feet. Children with the syndrome often have oppositional and defiant behavior.

Cat's Cry (Cri-du-Chat) Syndrome. Children with cat's cry syndrome lack part of chromosome 5. They are severely retarded and show many signs often associated with chromosomal aberrations, such as microcephaly, low-set ears, oblique palpebral fissures, hypertelorism, and micrognathia. The characteristic catlike cry caused by laryngeal abnormalities that gave the syndrome its name gradually changes and disappears with increasing age.

Other Chromosomal Abnormalities. Other syndromes of autosomal aberrations associated with mental retardation are much less prevalent than Down syndrome.

Phenylketonuria. PKU was first described by Ivar Asbjörn Fölling in 1934 as the paradigmatic inborn error of metabolism. PKU is transmitted as a simple recessive autosomal mendelian trait and occurs in about 1 in every 10,000 to 15,000 live births. For parents who have already had a child with PKU, the chance of having another child with PKU is 1 in every 4 to 5 successive pregnancies. Although the disease is reported predominantly in persons of North European origin, a few cases have been described in blacks, Yemenite Jews, and Asians. The frequency among institutionalized retarded patients is about 1 percent. The basic metabolic defect in PKU is an inability to convert phenylalanine, an essential amino acid, to paratyrosine because of the absence or inactivity of the liver enzyme phenylalanine hydroxylase, which catalyzes the conversion. Two other types of hyperphenylalaninemia have recently been described. One is due to a deficiency of the enzyme dihydropteridine reductase, and the other to a deficiency of a cofactor, biopterin. The first defect can be detected in fibroblasts, and biopterin can be measured in body fluids. Both these rare disorders carry a high risk of fatality.

Most patients with PKU are severely retarded, but some are reported to have borderline or normal intelligence. Eczema, vomiting, and convulsions occur in about a third of all patients. Although the clinical picture varies, typical children with PKU are hyperactive; they exhibit erratic, unpredictable behavior, and are difficult to manage. They frequently have temper tantrums and often display bizarre movements of their bodies and upper extremities, including twisting hand mannerisms; their behavior sometimes resembles that of children with autism or schizophrenia. Verbal and nonverbal communication is usually severely impaired or nonexistent. The children's coordination is poor, and they have many perceptual difficulties.

The disease was previously diagnosed on the basis of a urine test: Phenylpyruvic acid in the urine reacts with ferric chloride solution to yield a vivid green color. The test, however, has its limitations; it may not detect the presence of phenylpyruvic acid in urine before a baby is 5 or 6 weeks old, and it may give positive responses with other aminoacidurias. Currently, a more reliable screening test, the Guthrie inhibition assay, is more widely used, which uses a bacteriological procedure to detect phenylalanine in the blood.

In the United States, newborn infants are now routinely screened for PKU. Early diagnosis is important, because a low-phenylalanine diet, in use since 1955, significantly improves both behavior and developmental progress. The best results seem to be obtained with early diagnosis and the start of dietary treatment before the child is 6 months of age. Dietary treatment, however, is not without risk. Phenylalanine is an essential amino acid, and its omission from the diet may lead to such severe complications as anemia, hypoglycemia, edema, and even death. Dietary treatment of PKU should be continued indefinitely. Children who receive a diagnosis before the age of 3 months and are placed on an optimal dietary regimen may have normal intelligence. A low-phenylalanine diet does not influence the level of mental retardation in untreated older children and adolescents with PKU, but the diet does decrease irritability and abnormal electroencephalogram (EEG) changes and does increase social responsiveness and attention span. The parents of children with PKU and some of the children's normal siblings are heterozygous carriers. The disease can be detected by a phenylalanine tolerance test, which may be important in genetic counseling of the family members.

Rett's Disorder. Rett's disorder is hypothesized to be an X-linked dominant mental retardation syndrome that is degenerative and affects only females. In 1966, Andreas Rett reported on 22 girls with a serious progressive neurological disability. Deterioration in communications skills, motor behavior, and social functioning starts at about 1 year of age. Autisticlike symptoms are common, as are ataxia, facial grimacing, teeth grinding, and loss of speech. Intermittent hyperventilation and a disorganized breathing pattern are characteristic while the child is awake. Stereotypical hand movements, including hand wringing, are typical. Progressive gait disturbance, scoliosis, and seizures occur. Severe spasticity is usually present by middle childhood. Cerebral atrophy occurs with decreased pigmentation of the substantia nigra, which suggests abnormalities of the dopaminergic nigrostriatal system. (The disorder is discussed further in Chapter 41.)

Neurofibromatosis. Also called *von Recklinghausen's disease,* neurofibromatosis is the most common of the neurocutaneous syndromes caused by a single dominant gene, which may be inherited or may be a new mutation. The disorder occurs in about 1 in 5,000 births and is characterized by café au lait spots on the skin and by neurofibromas, including optic gliomas and acoustic neuromas, caused by abnormal cell migration. Mild mental retardation occurs in up to one third of those with the disease.

Tuberous Sclerosis. Tuberous sclerosis is the second most common of the neurocutaneous syndromes; a progressive mental retardation occurs in up to two thirds of all affected persons. It occurs in about 1 in 15,000 persons and is inherited by autosomal dominant transmission. Seizures are present in all those who are mentally retarded and in two thirds of those who are not. Infantile spasms may occur as early as 6 months of age. The phenotypic presentation includes adenoma sebaceum and ash-leaf spots that can be identified with a slit lamp.

Lesch-Nyhan Syndrome. Lesch-Nyhan syndrome is a rare disorder caused by a deficiency of an enzyme involved in purine metabolism. The disorder is X-linked; patients have mental retardation, microcephaly, seizures, choreoathetosis, and spasticity. The syndrome is also associated with severe compulsive self-mutilation by biting the mouth and fingers. Lesch-Nyhan syndrome is another example of a genetically determined syndrome with a specific, predictable behavioral pattern.

Adrenoleukodystrophy. The most common of several disorders of sudanophilic cerebral sclerosis, adrenoleukodystrophy is characterized by diffuse demyelination of the cerebral white matter resulting in visual and intellectual impairment, seizures, spasticity, and progression to death. The cerebral degeneration in adrenoleukodystrophy is accompanied by adrenocortical insufficiency. The disorder is transmitted by a sex-linked gene located on the distal end of the long arm of the X chromosome. The clinical onset is generally between 5 and 8 years of age, with early seizures, disturbances in gait, and mild intellectual impairment. Abnormal pigmentation reflecting adrenal insufficiency sometimes precedes the neurological symptoms, and attacks of crying are common. Spastic contractures, ataxia, and swallowing disturbances are also frequent. Although the course is often rapidly progressive, some patients may have a relapsing and remitting course. The story of a child with the disorder was presented in the 1992 film *Lorenzo's Oil.*

Maple Syrup Urine Disease. The clinical symptoms of maple syrup urine disease appear during the first week of life. The

infant deteriorates rapidly and has decerebrate rigidity, seizures, respiratory irregularity, and hypoglycemia. If untreated, most patients die in the first months of life, and the survivors are severely retarded. Some variants have been reported with transient ataxia and only mild retardation. Treatment follows the general principles established for PKU and consists of a diet very low in the three involved amino acids—leucine, isoleucine, and valine.

Other Enzyme Deficiency Disorders. Several enzyme deficiency disorders associated with mental retardation have been identified, and still more diseases are being added as new discoveries are made, including Hartnup disease, galactosemia, and glycogen-storage disease. Thirty important disorders with inborn errors of metabolism, hereditary transmission patterns, defective enzymes, clinical signs, and relation to mental retardation are listed in Table 38–2.

Table 38–2
Thirty Impairment Disorders with Inborn Errors of Metabolism

Disorder	Hereditary Transmission[a]	Enzyme Defect	Prenatal Diagnosis	Mental Retardation	Clinical Signs
I. LIPID METABOLISM					
Niemann-Pick disease					
Group A, infantile		Unknown			Hepatomegaly
Group B, adult	A.R.	Sphingomyelinase	+	±	Hepatosplenomegaly
Groups C and D, intermediate		Unknown	–	+	Pulmonary infiltration
Infantile Gaucher's disease	A.R.	β-Glucosidase	+	±	Hepatosplenomegaly, pseudobulbar palsy
Tay-Sachs disease	A.R.	Hexosaminidase A	+	+	Macular changes, seizures, spasticity
Generalized gangliosidosis	A.R.	β-Galactosidase	+	+	Hepatosplenomegaly, bone changes
Krabbe's disease	A.R.	Galactocerebroside β-Galactosidase	+	+	Stiffness, seizures
Metachromatic leukodystrophy	A.R.	Cerebroside sulfatase	+	+	Stiffness, developmental failure
Wolman's disease	A.R.	Acid lipase	+	–	Hepatosplenomegaly, adrenal calcification, vomiting, diarrhea
Farber's lipogranulomatosis	A.R.	Acid ceramidase	+	+	Hoarseness, arthropathy, subcutaneous nodules
Fabry's disease	X.R.	α-Galactosidase	+	–	Angiokeratomas, renal failure
II. MUCOPOLYSACCHARIDE METABOLISM					
Hurler's syndrome MPS I	A.R.	Iduronidase	+	+	?
Hurler's disease II	X.R.	Iduronate sulfatase	+	+	?
Sanfilippo's syndrome III	A.R.	Various sulfatases (types A–D)	+	+	Varying degrees of bone changes, hepatosplenomegaly, joint restriction, etc.
Morquio's disease IV	A.R.	*N*-Acetylgalactosamine-6-sulfate sulfatase	+	–	?
Maroteaux-Lamy syndrome VI	A.R.	Arylsulfatase B	+	±	?
III. OLIGOSACCHARIDE AND GLYCOPROTEIN METABOLISM					
I-cell disease	A.R.	Glycoprotein *N*-acetylglucosaminyl-phosphotransferase	+	+	Hepatomegaly, bone changes, swollen gingivae
Mannosidosis	A.R.	Mannosidase	+	+	Hepatomegaly, bone changes, facial coarsening
Fucosidosis	A.R.	Fucosidase	+	+	Same as above
IV. AMINO ACID METABOLISM					
Phenylketonuria	A.R.	Phenylalanine hydroxylase	–	+	Eczema, blonde hair, musty odor
Hemocystinuria	A.R.	Cystathionine β-synthetase	+	+	Ectopia lentis, Marfanlike phenotype, cardiovascular anomalies
Tyrosinosis	A.R.	Tyrosine amine transaminase	–	+	Hyperkeratotic skin lesions, conjunctivitis
Maple syrup urine disease	A.R.	Branched-chain ketoacid decarboxylase	+	+	Recurrent ketoacidosis

(*continued*)

Table 38–2 (*continued*)

Disorder	Hereditary Transmission[a]	Enzyme Defect	Prenatal Diagnosis	Mental Retardation	Clinical Signs
Methylmalonic acidemia	A.R.	Methylmalonyl-CoA mutase	+	+	Recurrent ketoacidosis, hepatomegaly, growth retardation
Propionic acidemia	A.R.	Propionyl-CoA carboxylase	+	+	Same as above
Nonketotic hyperglycinemia	A.R.	Glycine cleavage enzyme	+	+	Seizures
Urea cycle disorders	Mostly A.R.	Urea cycle enzymes	+	+	Recurrent acute encephalopathy, vomiting
Hartnup disease	A.R.	Renal transport disorder	–	–	None consistent
V. OTHERS					
Galactosemia	A.R.	Galactose-1-phosphate uridyltransferase	+	+	Hepatomegaly, cataracts, ovarian failure
Wilson's hepatolenticular degeneration	A.R.	Unknown factor in copper metabolism	–	±	Liver disease, Kayser-Fleischer ring, neurological problems
Menkes' kinky-hair disease	X.R.	Same as above	+	–	Abnormal hair, cerebral degeneration
Lesch-Nyhan syndrome	X.R.	Hypoxanthine guanine phosphoribosyltransferase	+	+	Behavioral abnormalities

[a]A.R., autosomal recessive transmission; X.R., X-linked recessive transmission.
Adapted from Leroy JC. Hereditary, development, and behavior. In: Levine MD, Carey WB, Crocker AC, eds. *Developmental-Behavioral Pediatrics*. Philadelphia: WB Saunders; 1983:315.

Acquired and Developmental Factors

Prenatal Period. Important prerequisites for the overall development of the fetus include the mother's physical, psychological, and nutritional health during pregnancy. Maternal chronic illnesses and conditions affecting the normal development of the fetus's central nervous system include uncontrolled diabetes, anemia, emphysema, hypertension, and long-term use of alcohol and narcotic substances. Maternal infections during pregnancy, especially viral infections, have been known to cause fetal damage and mental retardation. The extent of fetal damage depends on such variables as the type of viral infection, the gestational age of the fetus, and the severity of the illness. Although numerous infectious diseases have been reported to affect the fetus's central nervous system, the following medical disorders have been definitely identified as high-risk conditions for mental retardation.

Rubella (German Measles). Rubella has replaced syphilis as the major cause of congenital malformations and mental retardation caused by maternal infection. The children of affected mothers may show several abnormalities, including congenital heart disease, mental retardation, cataracts, deafness, microcephaly, and microphthalmia. Timing is crucial, as the extent and frequency of the complications are inversely related to the duration of the pregnancy at the time of maternal infection. When mothers are infected in the first trimester of pregnancy, 10 to 15 percent of the children are affected, but the incidence rises to almost 50 percent when the infection occurs in the first month of pregnancy. The situation is often complicated by subclinical forms of maternal infection that often go undetected. Maternal rubella can be prevented by immunization.

Cytomegalic Inclusion Disease. In many cases, cytomegalic inclusion disease remains dormant in the mother. Some children are stillborn, and others have jaundice, microcephaly, hepatosplenomegaly, and radiographic findings of intracerebral calcification. Children with mental retardation from the disease frequently have cerebral calcification, microcephaly, or hydrocephalus. The diagnosis is confirmed by positive findings of the virus in throat and urine cultures and the recovery of inclusion-bearing cells in the urine.

Syphilis. Syphilis in pregnant women was once the main cause of various neuropathological changes in their offspring, including mental retardation. Today, the incidence of syphilitic complications of pregnancy fluctuates with the incidence of syphilis in the general population. Some recent alarming statistics from several major cities in the United States indicate that there is still no room for complacency.

Toxoplasmosis. Toxoplasmosis can be transmitted by the mother to the fetus. It causes mild or severe mental retardation and, in severe cases, hydrocephalus, seizures, microcephaly, and chorioretinitis.

Herpes Simplex. The herpes simplex virus can be transmitted transplacentally, although the most common mode of infection is during birth. Microcephaly, mental retardation, intracranial calcification, and ocular abnormalities may result.

Acquired Immune Deficiency Syndrome (AIDS). Many fetuses of mothers with AIDS never come to term because of stillbirth or spontaneous abortion. Of those who are born infected with the human immunodeficiency virus (HIV), up to half have progressive encephalopathy, mental retardation, and seizures within the first year of life. Children born with HIV infection often live only a few years; however, most babies born to HIV-infected mothers are not infected with the virus.

Fetal Alcohol Syndrome. Fetal alcohol syndrome results in mental retardation and a typical phenotypic picture of facial dysmor-

phism that includes hypertelorism, microcephaly, short palpebral fissures, inner epicanthal folds, and a short, turned-up nose. Often, the affected children have learning disorders and attention-deficit/hyperactivity disorder. Cardiac defects are also frequent. The entire syndrome occurs in up to 15 percent of babies born to women who regularly ingest large amounts of alcohol. Babies born to women who consume alcohol regularly during pregnancy have a high incidence of attention-deficit/hyperactivity disorder, learning disorders, and mental retardation without the facial dysmorphism.

Prenatal Drug Exposure. Prenatal exposure to opioids, such as heroin, often results in infants who are small for their gestational age, with a head circumference below the 10th percentile and withdrawal symptoms that appear within the first two days of life. The withdrawal symptoms of infants include irritability, hypertonia, tremor, vomiting, a high-pitched cry, and an abnormal sleep pattern. Seizures are unusual, but the withdrawal syndrome can be life threatening to infants if it is untreated. Diazepam (Valium), phenobarbital (Luminal), chlorpromazine (Thorazine), and paregoric have been used to treat neonatal opioid withdrawal. The long-term sequelae of prenatal opioid exposure are not fully known; the children's developmental milestones and intellectual functions may be within the normal range, but they have an increased risk for impulsivity and behavioral problems. Infants prenatally exposed to cocaine are at high risk for low birth weight and premature delivery. In the early neonatal period, they may have transient neurological and behavioral abnormalities, including abnormal results on EEGs, tachycardia, poor feeding patterns, irritability, and excessive drowsiness. Rather than a withdrawal reaction, the physiological and behavioral abnormalities are a response to the cocaine, which may be excreted for up to a week postnatally.

Complications of Pregnancy. Toxemia of pregnancy and uncontrolled maternal diabetes present hazards to the fetus and sometimes result in mental retardation. Maternal malnutrition during pregnancy often results in prematurity and other obstetrical complications. Vaginal hemorrhage, placenta previa, premature separation of the placenta, and prolapse of the cord may damage the fetal brain by causing anoxia. The potential teratogenic effect of pharmacological agents administered during pregnancy was widely publicized after the thalidomide tragedy (the drug produced a high percentage of deformed babies when given to pregnant women). So far, with the exception of metabolites used in cancer chemotherapy, no usual dosages of medications are known to damage the fetus's central nervous system, but caution and restraint in prescribing drugs to pregnant women are certainly indicated. The use of lithium during pregnancy was recently implicated in some congenital malformations, especially of the cardiovascular system (e.g., Ebstein's anomaly).

Perinatal Period. Some evidence indicates that premature infants and infants with low birth weight are at high risk for neurological and intellectual impairments that appear during their school years. Infants who sustain intracranial hemorrhages or show evidence of cerebral ischemia are especially vulnerable to cognitive abnormalities. The degree of neurodevelopmental impairment generally correlates with the severity of the intracranial hemorrhage. Recent studies have documented that among children with very low birth weight (less than 1,000 g), 20 percent had significant disabilities including cerebral palsy, mental retardation, autism, and low intelligence with severe learning problems. Very premature children and those who suffered intrauterine growth retardation were found to be at high risk for developing both social problems and academic difficulties. Socioeconomic deprivation can also affect the adaptive function of these vulnerable infants. Early intervention may improve their cognitive, language, and perceptual abilities.

Acquired Childhood Disorders. Occasionally, a child's developmental status changes dramatically as a result of a specific disease or physical trauma. In retrospect, it is sometimes difficult to ascertain the full picture of the child's developmental progress before the insult, but the adverse effects on the child's development or skills are apparent afterward.

Infection. The most serious infections affecting cerebral integrity are encephalitis and meningitis. Measles encephalitis has been virtually eliminated by the universal use of measles vaccine, and the incidence of other bacterial infections of the central nervous system has been markedly reduced with antibacterial agents. Most episodes of encephalitis are caused by viruses. Sometimes a clinician must retrospectively consider a probable encephalitic component in a past obscure illness with high fever. Meningitis that was diagnosed late, even when followed by antibiotic treatment, can seriously affect a child's cognitive development. Thrombotic and purulent intracranial phenomena secondary to septicemia are rarely seen today except in small infants.

Head Trauma. The best-known causes of head injury in children that produces developmental handicaps, including seizures, are motor vehicle accidents, but more head injuries are caused by household accidents, such as falls from tables, from open windows, and on stairways. Child abuse is also a cause of head injury.

Other Issues. Brain damage from cardiac arrest during anesthesia is rare. One cause of complete or partial brain damage is asphyxia associated with near drowning. Long-term exposure to lead is a well-established cause of compromised intelligence and learning skills. Intracranial tumors of various types and origins, surgery, and chemotherapy can also adversely affect brain function.

Environmental and Sociocultural Factors

Mild retardation may result from significant deprivation of nutrition and nurturance. Children who have endured these conditions are subject to long-lasting damage to their physical and emotional development. Prenatal environment compromised by poor medical care and poor maternal nutrition can be contributing factors in the development of mild mental retardation. Teenage pregnancies are risk factors and are associated with obstetrical complications, prematurity, and low birth weight. Poor postnatal medical care, malnutrition, exposure to such toxic substances as lead, and physical trauma are risk factors for mild mental retardation. Family instability, frequent moves, and multiple but inadequate caretakers may deprive an infant of necessary emotional relationships, leading to failure to thrive and potential risk to the developing brain.

An incapacitating mental disorder in a parent may interfere with appropriate child care and stimulation and cause develop-

Table 38–3
DSM-IV-TR Diagnostic Criteria for Mental Retardation

A. Significantly subaverage intellectual functioning: an IQ of approximately 70 or below on an individually administered IQ test (for infants, a clinical judgment of significantly subaverage intellectual functioning).

B. Concurrent deficits or impairments in present adaptive functioning (i.e., the person's effectiveness in meeting the standards expected for his or her age by his or her cultural group) in at least two of the following areas: communication, self-care, home living, social/interpersonal skills, use of community resources, self-direction, functional academic skills, work, leisure, health, and safety.

C. The onset is before age 18 years.

Code based on degree of severity reflecting level of intellectual impairment:

Mild mental retardation:	IQ level 50–55 to approximately 70
Moderate mental retardation:	IQ level 35–40 to 50–55
Severe mental retardation:	IQ level 20–25 to 35–40
Profound mental retardation:	IQ level below 20 or 25
Mental retardation, severity unspecified:	When there is strong presumption of mental retardation but the person's intelligence is untestable by standard tests

From American Psychiatric Association. *Diagnostic and Statistical Manual of Mental Disorders.* 4th ed. Text rev. Washington, DC: American Psychiatric Association; copyright 2000, with permission.

mental risk. Children of parents with mood disorders and schizophrenia are known to be at risk for these and related disorders. Some studies indicate a higher than expected prevalence of motor skills disorder and developmental disorders, but not necessarily mental retardation, among the children of parents with chronic mental disorders.

DIAGNOSIS

The diagnosis of mental retardation can be made after the history, a standardized intellectual assessment, and a measure of adaptive function indicate that a child's current behavior is significantly below the expected level (Table 38–3). The diagnosis itself does not specify either the cause or the prognosis. A history and psychiatric interview are useful in obtaining a longitudinal picture of the child's development and functioning, and examination of physical signs, neurological abnormalities, and laboratory tests can be used to ascertain the cause and prognosis.

History

The history is most often obtained from the parents or the caretaker, with particular attention to the mother's pregnancy, labor, and delivery; the presence of a family history of mental retardation; consanguinity of the parents; and hereditary disorders. As part of the history, the clinician assesses the overall level of functioning and intellectual capacity of the parents and the emotional climate of the home.

Psychiatric Interview

Two factors are of paramount importance when interviewing the patient: the interviewer's attitude and manner of communicating. The interviewer should not be guided by the patient's mental age, which cannot fully characterize the person. A mildly retarded adult with a mental age of 10 is not a 10-year-old child. When addressed as if they were children, some retarded persons become justifiably insulted, angry, and uncooperative. Passive and dependent persons, alternatively, may assume the child's role that they think is expected of them. In neither case can valid diagnostic data be obtained.

The patient's verbal abilities, including receptive and expressive language, should be assessed as soon as possible by observing the communication between the caretakers and the patient and by taking the history. The clinician often finds it helpful to see the patient and the caretakers together. If the patient uses sign language, the caretaker may have to stay during the interview as an interpreter. Retarded persons often have the lifelong experience of failing in many areas, and they may be anxious about seeing an interviewer. The interviewer and the caretaker should attempt to give such patients a clear, supportive, concrete explanation of the diagnostic process, particularly patients with sufficiently receptive language. Giving patients the impression that their bad behavior is the cause of the referral should be avoided. Support and praise should be offered in language appropriate to the patient's age and understanding. Leading questions should be avoided, as retarded persons may be suggestible and wish to please others. Subtle direction, structure, and reinforcement may be necessary to keep them focused on the task or topic.

The patient's control over motility patterns should be ascertained, and clinical evidence of distractibility and distortions in perception and memory may be evaluated. The use of speech, reality testing, and the ability to generalize from experiences should be noted. The nature and maturity of the patient's defenses—particularly exaggerated or self-defeating uses of avoidance, repression, denial, introjection, and isolation—should be observed. Frustration tolerance, and impulse control—especially over motor, aggressive, and sexual drives—should be assessed. Also important are self-image and its role in the development of self-confidence, as well as an assessment of tenacity, persistence, curiosity, and willingness to explore the unknown. In general, the psychiatric examination of a retarded person should reveal how the patient has coped with the stages of development.

Physical Examination

Various parts of the body may have certain characteristics that have prenatal causes and are commonly found in persons who are mentally retarded. For example, the configuration and the size of the head offer clues to a variety of conditions, such as microcephaly, hydrocephalus, and Down syndrome. The patient's face may have some signs of mental retardation that greatly facilitate the diagnosis, such as hypertelorism, a flat nasal bridge, prominent eyebrows, epicanthal folds, corneal opacities, retinal changes, low-set and small or misshapen ears, a protruding tongue, and a disturbance in dentition. Facial expression, such as a dull appearance, may be misleading and should not be relied on without other supporting evidence. The color and texture of the skin and hair, a high-arched

palate, the size of the thyroid gland, and the size of the child and his or her trunk and extremities should also be explored. The circumference of the head should be measured as part of the clinical investigation. Dermatoglyphics may offer another diagnostic tool, as uncommon ridge patterns and flexion creases on the hand are often found in persons who are retarded. Abnormal dermatoglyphics occur in chromosomal disorders and in persons who were prenatally infected with rubella. Table 38–4 lists the multiple

Table 38–4
Representative Sample of Mental Retardation Syndromes and Behavioral Phenotypes

Disorder	Pathophysiology	Clinical Features and Behavioral Phenotype
Down syndrome	Trisomy 21, 95% nondisjunction, approx. 4% translocation; 1/1,000 live births: 1:2,500 in women less than 30 years old, 1:80 over 40 years old, 1:32 at 45 years old; possible overproduction of β-amyloid due to defect at 21q 21.1	Hypotonia, upward-slanted palpebral fissures, midface depression, flat wide nasal bridge, simian crease, short stature, increased incidence of thyroid abnormalities and congenital heart disease Passive, affable, hyperactivity in childhood, stubborn; verbal > auditory processing, increased risk of depression, and dementia of the Alzheimer type in adulthood
Fragile X syndrome	Inactivation of *FMR-1* gene at X q27.3 due to CGG base repeats, methylation; recessive; 1:1,000 male births, 1:3,000 female; accounts for 10–12% of mental retardation in males	Long face, large ears, midface hypoplasia, high arched palate, short stature, macroorchidism, mitral valve prolapse, joint laxity, strabismus Hyperactivity, inattention, anxiety, stereotypies, speech and language delays, IQ decline, gaze aversion, social avoidance, shyness, irritability, learning disorder in some females; mild mental retardation in affected females, moderate to severe in males; verbal IQ > performance IQ
Prader-Willi syndrome	Deletion in 15q12 (15q11–15q13) of paternal origin; some cases of maternal uniparental disomy; dominant 1/10,000 live births; 90% sporadic; candidate gene: small nuclear ribonucleoprotein polypeptide (SNRPN)	Hypotonia, failure to thrive in infancy, obesity, small hands and feet, microorchidism, cryptorchidism, short stature, almond-shaped eyes, fair hair and light skin, flat face, scoliosis, orthopedic problems, prominent forehead and bitemporal narrowing Compulsive behavior, hyperphagia, hoarding, impulsivity, borderline to moderate mental retardation, emotional lability, tantrums, excess daytime sleepiness, skin picking, anxiety, aggression
Angelman syndrome	Deletion in 15q12 (15q11–15q13) of maternal origin; dominant; frequent deletion of GABA B-3 receptor subunit, prevalence unknown but rare, estimated 1/20,000–1/30,000	Fair hair and blue eyes (66%); dysmorphic faces including wide smiling mouth, thin upper lip, and pointed chin; epilepsy (90%) with characteristic EEG; ataxia; small head circumference, 25% microcephalic Happy disposition, paroxysmal laughter, hand flapping, clapping; profound mental retardation; sleep disturbance with nighttime waking; possible increased incidence of autistic features; anecdotal love of water and music
Cornelia de Lange syndrome	Lack of pregnancy associated plasma protein A (PAPPA) linked to chromosome 9q33; similar phenotype associated with trisomy 5p, ring chromosome 3; rare (1/40,000–1/100,000 live births); possible association with 3q26.3	Continuous eyebrows, thin downturning upper lip, microcephaly, short stature, small hands and feet, small upturned nose, anteverted nostrils, malformed upper limbs, failure to thrive Self-injury, limited speech in severe cases, language delays, avoidance of being held, stereotypic movements, twirling, severe to profound mental retardation
Williams syndrome	1/20,000 births; hemizygous deletion that includes elastin locus chromosome 7q11–23; autosomal dominant	Short stature, unusual facial features including broad forehead, depressed nasal bridge, stellate pattern of the iris, widely spaced teeth, and full lips; elfinlike facies; renal and cardiovascular abnormalities; thyroid abnormalities; hypercalcemia Anxiety, hyperactivity, fears, outgoing, sociable, verbal skills > visual spatial skills
Cri-du-chat syndrome	Partial deletion 5p; 1/50,000; region may be 5p15.2	Round face with hypertelorism, epicanthal folds, slanting palpebral fissures, broad flat nose, low-set ears, micrognathia; prenatal growth retardation; respiratory and ear infections; congenital heart disease; gastrointestinal abnormalities Severe mental retardation, infantile catlike cry, hyperactivity, stereotypies, self-injury
Smith-Magenis syndrome	Incidence unknown, estimated 1/25,000 live births; complete or partial deletion of 17p11.2	Broad face; flat midface; short, broad hands; small toes; hoarse, deep voice. Severe mental retardation; hyperactivity; severe self-injury including hand biting, head banging, and pulling out finger- and toenails; stereotyped self-hugging; attention seeking; aggression; sleep disturbance (decreased REM)

(*continued*)

Table 38–4 (*continued*)

Disorder	Pathophysiology	Clinical Features and Behavioral Phenotype
Rubinstein-Taybi syndrome	1/250,000, approx. male = female; sporadic; likely autosomal dominant; documented microdeletions in some cases at 16p13.3	Short stature and microcephaly, broad thumb and big toes, prominent nose, broad nasal bridge, hypertelorism, ptosis, frequent fractures, feeding difficulties in infancy, congenital heart disease, EEG abnormalities, seizures Poor concentration, distractible, expressive language difficulties, performance IQ > verbal IQ; anecdotally happy, loving, sociable, responsive to music, self-stimulating behavior; older patients have mood lability and temper tantrums
Tuberous sclerosis complex 1 and 2	Benign tumors (hamartomas) and malformations (hamartias) of CNS, skin, kidney, heart; dominant; 1/10,000 births; 50% TSC 1, 9q34; 50% TSC 2, 16p13	Epilepsy, autism, hyperactivity, impulsivity, aggression; spectrum of mental retardation from none (30%) to profound; self-injurious behaviors, sleep disturbances
Neurofibromatosis type 1 (NF1)	1/2,500–1/4,000; male = female; autosomal dominant; 50% new mutations; more than 90% paternal NF1 allele mutated; *NFI* gene 17q11.2; gene product is neurofibromin thought to be tumor suppressor gene	Variable manifestations; café au lait spots, cutaneous neurofibromas, Lisch nodules; short stature and macrocephaly in 30–45% Half with speech and language difficulties; 10% with moderate to profound mental retardation; verbal IQ > performance IQ; distractible, impulsive, hyperactive, anxious; possibly associated with increased incidence of mood and anxiety disorders
Lesch-Nyhan syndrome	Defect in hypoxanthine guanine phosphoribosyltransferase with accumulation of uric acid; Xq26–27; recessive; rare (1/10,000–1/38,000)	Ataxia, chorea, kidney failure, gout Often severe self-biting behavior; aggression; anxiety; mild to moderate mental retardation
Galactosemia	Defect in galactose-1-phosphate uridyltransferase or galactokinase or empiramase; autosomal recessive; 1/62,000 births in the U.S.	Vomiting in early infancy, jaundice, hepatosplenomegaly; later cataracts, weight loss, food refusal, increased intracranial pressure and increased risk for sepsis, ovarian failure, failure to thrive, renal tubular damage Possible mental retardation even with treatment, visuospatial deficits, language disorders, reports of increased behavioral problems, anxiety, social withdrawal, and shyness
Phenylketonuria	Defect in phenylalanine hydroxylase (PAH) or cofactor (biopterin) with accumulation of phenylalanine; approximately 1/11,500 births; varies with geographical location; gene for PAH, 12q22–24.1; autosomal recessive	Symptoms absent neonatally, later development of seizures (25% generalized), fair skin, blue eyes, blond hair, rash Untreated: mild to profound mental retardation, language delay, destructiveness, self-injury, hyperactivity
Hurler's syndrome	1/100,000; deficiency in α-L-iduronidase activity; autosomal recessive	Early onset; short stature, hepatosplenomegaly; hirsutism, corneal clouding, death before age 10 years, dwarfism, coarse facial features, recurrent respiratory infections Moderate-to-severe mental retardation, anxious, fearful, rarely aggressive
Hunter's syndrome	1/100,000, X-linked recessive; iduronate sulfatase deficiency; X q28	Normal infancy; symptom onset at age 2–4 years; typical coarse faces with flat nasal bridge, flaring nostrils; hearing loss, ataxia, hernia common; enlarged liver and spleen, joint stiffness, recurrent infections, growth retardation, cardiovascular abnormality Hyperactivity, mental retardation by 2 years; speech delay; loss of speech at 8–10 years; restless, aggressive, inattentive, sleep abnormalities; apathetic, sedentary with disease progression
Fetal alcohol syndrome	Maternal alcohol consumption (trimester III>II>I); 1/3,000 live births in Western countries; 1/300 with fetal alcohol effects	Microcephaly, short stature, midface hypoplasia, short palpebral fissure, thin upper lip, retrognathia in infancy, micrognathia in adolescence, hypoplastic long or smooth philtrum Mild to moderate mental retardation, irritability, inattention, memory impairment

Table by B. H. King, M.D., R. M. Hodapp, Ph.D., and E. M. Dykens, Ph.D.

handicaps associated with various mental retardation syndromes. The clinician should bear in mind during the examination that mentally retarded children, particularly those with associated behavioral problems, are at increased risk for child abuse.

Neurological Examination

Sensory impairments occur frequently among persons who are mentally retarded; for example, up to 10 percent are hearing impaired, a rate that is four times that of the general population. Sensory disturbances may include hearing difficulties, ranging from cortical deafness to mild hearing deficits. Visual disturbances may range from blindness to disturbances of spatial concepts, design recognition, and concepts of body image. Various other neurological impairments also occur frequently in mentally retarded persons; seizure disorders occur in about 10 percent of all mentally retarded persons and in one third of those with severe retardation. When neurological abnormalities

are present, their incidence and severity generally rise in direct proportion to the degree of retardation. Many severely retarded children, however, have no neurological abnormalities; conversely, about 25 percent of all children with cerebral palsy have normal intelligence. Disturbances in motor areas are manifested in abnormalities of muscle tone (spasticity or hypotonia), reflexes (hyperreflexia), and involuntary movements (choreoathetosis). Less disability is revealed in clumsiness and poor coordination.

The infants with the poorest prognoses are those who manifest a combination of inactivity, general hypotonia, and exaggerated response to stimuli. In older children, hyperactivity, short attention span, distractibility, and a low frustration tolerance are often signs of brain damage. In general, the younger the child at the time of investigation, the more caution is indicated in predicting future ability, as the recovery potential of the infantile brain is very good. Observing the child's development at regular intervals is probably the most reliable approach.

Skull X-rays are usually taken routinely but are illuminating in only a relatively few conditions, such as craniosynostosis, hydrocephalus, and other disorders that result in intracranial calcifications (e.g., toxoplasmosis, tuberous sclerosis, cerebral angiomatosis, and hypoparathyroidism). Computed tomography (CT) scans and magnetic resonance imaging (MRI) have become important tools for uncovering central nervous system pathology associated with mental retardation. There are occasional findings of internal hydrocephalus, cortical atrophy, or porencephaly in severely retarded, brain-damaged children. An EEG is best interpreted with caution in cases of mental retardation. The exceptions are patients with hypsarhythmia and grand mal seizures, in whom the EEG may help establish the diagnosis and suggest treatment. In most other conditions, a diffuse cerebral disorder produces nonspecific EEG changes, characterized by slow frequencies with bursts of spikes and sharp or blunt wave complexes. The confusion over the significance of the EEG in the diagnosis of mental retardation is best illustrated by the reports of frequent EEG abnormalities in Down syndrome, which range from 25 percent to most patients examined.

CLINICAL FEATURES

Mild mental retardation may not be diagnosed until the affected children enter school; their social skills and communication may be adequate in the preschool years. As they get older, however, such cognitive deficits as poor ability to abstract and egocentric thinking may distinguish them from others of their age. Although mildly retarded persons can function academically at the high elementary level and their vocational skills suffice to support themselves in some cases, social assimilation may be difficult. Communication deficits, poor self-esteem, and dependence may contribute to their relative lack of social spontaneity. Some persons who are mildly retarded may fall into relationships with peers who exploit their shortcomings. In most cases, persons with mild mental retardation can achieve some social and vocational success in a supportive environment.

Moderate mental retardation is likely to be diagnosed at a younger age than mild mental retardation; communication skills develop more slowly in persons who are moderately retarded, and their social isolation may begin in the elementary school years. Although academic achievement is usually limited to the middle-elementary level, moderately retarded children benefit from individual attention focused on the development of self-help skills. Children with moderate mental retardation are aware of their deficits and often feel alienated from their peers and frustrated by their limitations. They continue to require a relatively high level of supervision but can become competent at occupational tasks in supportive settings.

Severe mental retardation is generally obvious in the preschool years; affected children's speech is minimal, and their motor development is poor. Some language development may occur in the school-age years. By adolescence, if language is poor, nonverbal forms of communication may have evolved; the inability to articulate needs fully may reinforce the physical means of communicating. Behavioral approaches can help promote some self-care, although those with severe mental retardation generally need extensive supervision.

Children with profound mental retardation require constant supervision and are severely limited in communication and motor skills. By adulthood, some speech development may be present, and simple self-help skills may be acquired. Even in adulthood, nursing care is needed.

Surveys have identified several clinical features that occur with greater frequency in persons who are mentally retarded than in the general population. These features, which may occur in isolation or as part of a mental disorder, include hyperactivity, low frustration tolerance, aggression, affective instability, repetitive and stereotypic motor behaviors, and various self-injurious behaviors. Self-injurious behaviors seem to be more frequent and more intense with increasingly severe mental retardation. It is often difficult to decide whether these clinical features are comorbid mental disorders or direct sequelae of the developmental limitations imposed by mental retardation.

Joseph is an 8-year-old boy who was brought for psychiatric evaluation because of increasing problems in school and at home with temper tantrums, oppositional behavior, and aggression. Joseph is in a self-contained special education class and is considered a third grader, although he is functioning at a first-grade level academically.

Joseph, according to his mother, has had problems since the day she took him home from the hospital. Although there were no complications during the pregnancy, Joseph was felt to be hypotonic at birth and did not gain appropriate weight in the first 6 months of his life because of his poor suck reflex, in spite of his mother's efforts to feed him constantly. Otherwise, he appeared healthy; he did not get sick often and was up-to-date on his immunizations. When he reached preschool age, Joseph began to "make up" for his poor eating early in life and began to "eat everything in sight." He became very strong-willed and oppositional with frequent temper outbursts. Joseph's mother felt that he was just making up for lost time, since he seemed to be sleepy and weak as an infant and young toddler.

As he got older, Joseph began to gain weight and was currently obese for his age. Joseph's mother is now wondering if there is something wrong with his eating habits, since Joseph seems to be obsessed with food. She has even found him eating out of the garbage can at times. He also takes food

from the dinner table and hides it in his room. Other than hoarding food, Joseph seems to like order, and he keeps his things neatly lined up. Lately, since he has been getting into trouble in school, Joseph has started picking on his skin and has many scabs on his arms. Joseph is currently an obese boy with light blond hair and fair skin who appears to have small hands and feet for his size. In an interview, Joseph reports that he only gets into trouble in school and at home because his teacher and his mother try to stop him from eating so much. He says that whenever he is prevented from finding additional food because he is still hungry, he gets very angry, cannot control himself, and will hit his mother and his teacher. Joseph's mother and his teacher feel that he should be able to find alternatives to his aggression. Joseph's mother believes that Joseph is a little slow in school but not mentally retarded. When asked about his social skills, Joseph's teacher reports that Joseph seems to be moody with his peers and does not really have any friends in class. Joseph's mother concurs that Joseph has seemed more moody and socially withdrawn since school began this year. Joseph was referred for psychological testing, particularly for intellectual function.

Joseph's WISC-III reveals a full-scale IQ of 68 with a verbal IQ of 62 and a performance IQ of 69. A Vineland Test of Adaptive Function shows adaptive weaknesses, resulting in function that would be expected of a 6-year-old boy. Joseph's mother and school are given the information that his IQ and adaptive function scores place Joseph in the mild mental retardation range and that he may require a more structured and supportive school environment. Given the combination of Joseph's early history of hypotonia, current obesity in conjunction with small hands and feet, compulsive eating behavior, and skin picking, chromosome analysis was recommended. Joseph's chromosome analysis revealed that he had a deletion on the long arm of chromosome 15. A diagnosis of Prader-Willi syndrome was made.

Joseph was given paroxetine (Paxil) 10 mg. Since he tolerated the medication well, the dose was increased to 20 mg. Joseph was also referred for cognitive behavioral therapy through which a simple behavioral program was instituted to reinforce behavior showing cooperation with redirection from his mother and his teacher to do another activity when it was not time to eat. He also could earn a reward for inhibiting aggressive behavior when angry. Over the next 2 months Joseph's skin picking behaviors diminished considerably, and his mood was more stable and improved. He had improvement in his food seeking, he was engaged in the treatment, and the reward system had resulted in a decrease in the frequency and intensity of his temper tantrums. Joseph's mother requested a meeting of the Individualized Educational Plan (IEP) committee, through his public school, and it was decided that he required a more structured school placement in which he could receive more individualized education.

LABORATORY EXAMINATION

Laboratory tests used to elucidate the causes of mental retardation include chromosomal analysis, urine and blood testing for metabolic disorders, and neuroimaging. Chromosomal abnormalities are the single most common cause of mental retardation found in individuals for whom a cause can be identified.

Chromosome Studies

The determination of the karyotype in a genetic laboratory is considered whenever a chromosomal disorder is suspected or when the cause of the mental retardation is unknown. Amniocentesis, in which a small amount of amniotic fluid is removed from the amniotic cavity transabdominally at about the 15th week of gestation has been useful in diagnosing prenatal chromosomal abnormalities. It is often considered when there is increased fetal risk, such as with increased maternal age, of Down syndrome. Amniotic fluid cells, mostly fetal in origin, are cultured for cytogenetic and biochemical studies. Many serious hereditary disorders can be predicted with amniocentesis, and it should be considered by pregnant women over the age of 35.

Chronic villi sampling (CVS) is a screening technique to determine fetal chromosomal abnormalities. It is done at 8 to 10 weeks of gestation, 6 weeks earlier than amniocentesis is done. The results are available in a short time (hours or days), and if the result is abnormal, the decision to terminate the pregnancy can be made within the first trimester. The procedure has a miscarriage risk between 2 and 5 percent; the risk in amniocentesis is lower (1 in 200).

Urine and Blood Analysis

Lesch-Nyhan syndrome, galactosemia, PKU, Hurler's syndrome, and Hunter's syndrome (Figs. 38–2 and 38–3) are examples of disorders that include mental retardation and can be identified through assays of the appropriate enzyme or organic or amino acids. Enzymatic abnormalities in chromosomal disorders, particularly Down syndrome, promise to become useful diagnostic tools. Unexplained growth abnormality, seizure disorder, poor muscle tone, ataxia, bone or skin abnormalities, and eye abnormalities are some indications for testing metabolic function.

Electroencephalography (EEG)

EEG is indicated whenever there is a consideration of a seizure disorder.

Neuroimaging

Neuroimaging studies may in some cases render etiologic information in some individuals with mental retardation. MRI is generally superior to CT, since MRI provides finer resolution and can identify subtler abnormalities in the brain such as myelination patterns. MRI studies can provide a baseline for comparison of a later, potentially degenerative process in the brain.

Hearing and Speech Evaluations

Hearing and speech should be evaluated routinely. Speech development may be the most reliable criterion in investigating mental retardation. Various hearing impairments often occur in

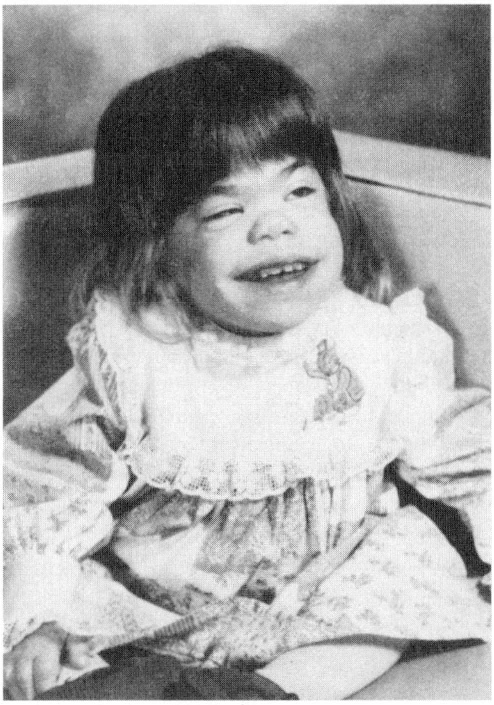

FIGURE 38–2

A 6-year-old girl with Hurler's syndrome. Her care has involved a class for seriously multihandicapped children, attention to cardiac problems, and special counseling for the parents. (Courtesy of L. S. Syzmanski, M.D., and A. C. Croker, M.D.)

persons who are mentally retarded, but in some instances impairments can simulate mental retardation. Unfortunately, the commonly used methods of hearing and speech evaluation require the patient's cooperation and, thus, are often unreliable in severely retarded persons.

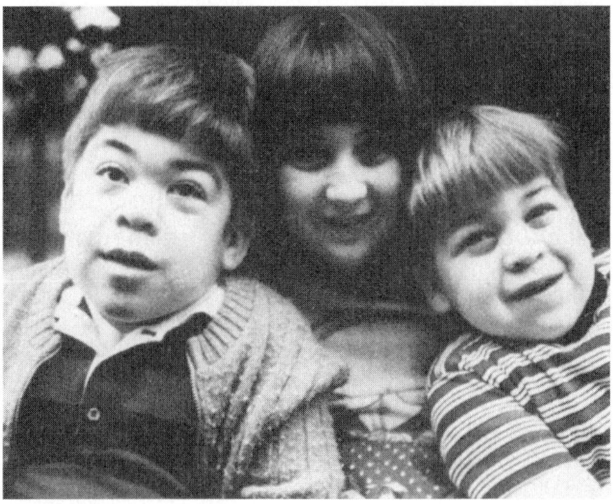

FIGURE 38–3

Two brothers, age 6 and 8 years, with Hunter's syndrome, shown with their normal older sister. They have had significant developmental delay, trouble with recurrent respiratory infection, and behavioral abnormalities. (Courtesy of L. S. Syzmanski, M.D., and A. C. Crocker, M.D.)

Psychological Assessment

Examining clinicians may use several screening instruments for infants and toddlers. As in many areas of mental retardation, the controversy over the predictive value of infant psychological tests is heated. Some report the correlation of abnormalities during infancy with later abnormal functioning as very low, and others report it to be very high. The correlation rises in direct proportion to the age of the child at the time of the developmental examination; however, copying geometric figures, the Goodenough Draw-a-Person test, the Kohs Block Test, and geometric puzzles all may be used as quick screening tests of visual-motor coordination. Psychological testing, performed by an experienced psychologist, is a standard part of an evaluation for mental retardation. The Gesell and Bayley scales and the Cattell Infant Intelligence Scale are most commonly used with infants. For children, the Stanford-Binet Intelligence Scale and the third edition of the Wechsler Intelligence Scale for Children (WISC-III) are the most widely used in the United States. Both tests have been criticized for penalizing culturally deprived children, for being culturally biased, for testing mainly the potential for academic achievement and not for adequate social functioning, and for their unreliability in children with IQs below 50. Some persons have tried to overcome the language barrier of persons who are mentally retarded by devising picture vocabulary tests, of which the Peabody Vocabulary Test is the most widely used. The tests often found useful in detecting brain damage are the Bender gestalt test and the Benton Visual Retention Test (see Figs. 5.2–1 and 5.2–3 in Section 5.2 of Chapter 5). These tests are also useful for mildly retarded children. In addition, a psychological evaluation should assess perceptual, motor, linguistic, and cognitive abilities. Information about motivational, emotional, and interpersonal factors is also important.

COURSE AND PROGNOSIS

In most cases of mental retardation, the underlying intellectual impairment does not improve, yet the affected person's level of adaptation can be influenced positively by an enriched and supportive environment. In general, persons with mild and moderate mental retardation have the most flexibility in adapting to various environmental conditions. As in those who are not mentally retarded, the more comorbid mental disorders there are, the more guarded is the overall prognosis. When clear-cut mental disorders are superimposed on mental retardation, standard treatments for the comorbid mental disorders are often beneficial. Yet there is still a lack of clarity about the classification of such aberrant behaviors as hyperactivity, emotional lability, and social dysfunction.

DIFFERENTIAL DIAGNOSIS

By definition, mental retardation must begin before the age of 18. A mentally retarded child has to cope with so many difficult social and academic situations that maladaptive patterns often complicate the diagnostic process. Children whose family life provides inadequate stimulation may manifest motor and mental retardation that can be reversed if an enriched, stimulating environment is provided in early childhood. Several sensory

disabilities, especially deafness and blindness, may be mistaken for mental retardation if no compensation is allowed during testing. Speech deficits and cerebral palsy often make a child seem retarded, even in the presence of borderline or normal intelligence. Chronic, debilitating diseases of any kind may depress a child's functioning in all areas. Convulsive disorders may give an impression of mental retardation, especially in the presence of uncontrolled seizures. Chronic brain syndromes may result in isolated handicaps—failure to read (alexia), failure to write (agraphia), failure to communicate (aphasia), and several others—that may exist in a person of normal and even superior intelligence. Children with learning disorders (which can coexist with mental retardation) experience a delay or failure of development in a specific area, such as reading or mathematics, but they develop normally in other areas. In contrast, children with mental retardation show general delays in most areas of development.

Mental retardation and pervasive developmental disorders often coexist; 70 to 75 percent of those with pervasive developmental disorders have an IQ below 70. A pervasive developmental disorder results in distortion of the timing, rate, and sequence of many basic psychological functions necessary for social development. Because of their general level of functioning, children with pervasive developmental disorders have more problems with social relatedness and more deviant language than those with mental retardation. In mental retardation, generalized delays in development are present, and mentally retarded children behave in some ways as though they were passing through an earlier normal developmental stage, rather than one with completely aberrant behavior.

A most difficult differential diagnostic problem concerns children with severe mental retardation, brain damage, autistic disorder, schizophrenia with childhood onset, or, according to some, Heller's disease. The confusion stems from the fact that details of the child's early history are often unavailable or unreliable. In addition, when the children are evaluated, many with these conditions display similar bizarre and stereotyped behavior—mutism, echolalia, or functioning on a retarded level. By the time the children are usually seen, it does not matter from a practical point of view whether their retardation is secondary to a primary early infantile autistic disorder or schizophrenia or whether the personality and behavioral distortions are secondary to brain damage or mental retardation. In a recent epidemiological study, pervasive developmental disorders (such as autistic disorder) were found in 19.8 percent of children with mental retardation.

Children under the age of 18 years who meet the diagnostic criteria for dementia and who have an IQ below 70 are given the diagnoses of dementia and mental retardation. Those whose IQs drop below 70 after the age of 18 years and who have new onsets of cognitive disorders are not given the diagnosis of mental retardation but only the diagnosis of dementia.

TREATMENT

Mental retardation is associated with a variety of comorbid psychiatric disorders and usually requires many psychosocial supports. The treatment of individuals with mental retardation is based on an assessment of social and environmental needs as well as attention to comorbid conditions. The optimal treatment of conditions that could lead to mental retardation is primary, secondary, and tertiary prevention.

Primary Prevention

Primary prevention concerns actions taken to eliminate or reduce the conditions that lead to development of the disorders associated with mental retardation. Such measures include education to increase the general public's knowledge and awareness of mental retardation; continuing efforts of health professionals to ensure and upgrade public health policies; legislation to provide optimal maternal and child health care; and eradication of the known disorders associated with central nervous system damage. Family and genetic counseling helps reduce the incidence of mental retardation in a family with a history of a genetic disorder associated with mental retardation. For the children and the mothers of low socioeconomic status, proper prenatal and postnatal medical care and various supplementary enrichment programs and social service assistance may help minimize medical and psychosocial complications.

Secondary and Tertiary Prevention

Once a disorder associated with mental retardation has been identified, the disorder should be treated to shorten the course of the illness (secondary prevention) and to minimize the sequelae or consequent disabilities (tertiary prevention). Hereditary metabolic and endocrine disorders, such as PKU and hypothyroidism, can be treated effectively in an early stage by dietary control or hormone replacement therapy. Mentally retarded children frequently have emotional and behavioral difficulties requiring psychiatric treatment. Their limited cognitive and social capabilities require modified psychiatric treatment modalities based on their level of intelligence.

Education for the Child. Educational settings for children who are mentally retarded should include a comprehensive program that addresses adaptive skills training, social skills training, and vocational training. Particular attention should be focused on communication and efforts to improve the quality of life. Group therapy has often been a successful format in which mentally retarded children can learn and practice hypothetical real-life situations and receive supportive feedback.

Behavioral, Cognitive, and Psychodynamic Therapies. The difficulties in adaptation among mentally retarded persons are widespread and so varied that several interventions alone or in combination may be beneficial. Behavior therapy has been used for many years to shape and enhance social behaviors and to control and minimize aggressive and destructive behaviors. Positive reinforcement for desired behaviors and benign punishment (such as loss of privileges) for objectionable behaviors have been helpful. Cognitive therapy, such as dispelling false beliefs and relaxation exercises with self-instruction, has also been recommended for mentally retarded persons who can follow the instructions. Psychodynamic therapy has been used with patients and their families to decrease conflicts about expectations that result in persistent anxiety, rage, and depression.

Table 38–5
Service Needs and Resources for Families of Disabled Children at Different Ages

	Needs	Resources
Age 0–3 years		
Child	Evaluation: physical, motor, cognitive, linguistic, social-emotional; early intervention services	Multidisciplinary evaluation, which results in an Individualized Family Service Plan (IFSP), with child and family receiving either center- or home-based early intervention services for set number of hours per week
Mother	Emotional support; caregiving behaviors	Support groups by disability, region, and etiology; part of early intervention evaluation, intervention, and IFSP
Family	Support; financial assistance; information	Support groups; depending on problem, state developmental disabilities or insurance payment for some services; hospitals, agencies, groups
Age 3–21 years		
Child	Evaluation, referral, and Individualized Educational Program (IEP)	School system: involves legal process of evaluation and placement (notification, hearings, appeals if necessary); information on transition to adult services as child nears age 21 (and school services end)
Family	Information; financial assistance; support	Local and national groups; state departments in some states; includes respite care, camps, art (Very Special Arts) or athletic activities (Special Olympics), scholarships for adolescents with some disabilities (deafness, blindness)
Above 21 years		
Offspring	Residential services; work	Both run by state developmental disability departments (parents and offspring have major say concerning whether residential or work placements are appropriate)
Family	Support; information; guardianship issues	Continuation of many of the services provided during the school years; particularly for individuals with severe disabilities, provisions for residential and work status after parents can no longer serve as legal guardians

Adapted from Hodapp RD. *Development and Disabilities.* New York: Cambridge University Press; 1998.

Family Education. One of the most important areas that a clinician can address is educating the family of a mentally retarded patient about ways to enhance competence and self-esteem while maintaining realistic expectations for the patient. The family often finds it difficult to balance the fostering of independence and the providing of a nurturing and supportive environment for a mentally retarded child, who is likely to experience some rejection and failure outside the family context. The parents may benefit from continuous counseling or family therapy and should be allowed opportunities to express their feelings of guilt, despair, anguish, recurring denial, and anger about their child's disorder and future. The psychiatrist should be prepared to give the parents all the basic and current medical information regarding causes, treatment, and other pertinent areas (such as special training and the correction of sensory defects). Table 38–5 lists some important needs of families of children with mental retardation and resources for them.

Social Intervention. One of the most prevalent problems among persons who are mentally retarded is a sense of social isolation and social skills deficits. Thus, improving the quantity and quality of social competence is a critical part of their care. Special Olympics International is the largest recreational sports program geared for this population. In addition to providing a forum to develop physical fitness, Special Olympics also enhances social interactions, friendships, and (it is hoped) general self-esteem. A recent study confirmed positive effects of the Special Olympics on the social competence of the mentally retarded adults who participated.

Pharmacology. Pharmacological approaches to the treatment of comorbid mental disorders in mentally retarded patients is much the same as it is for patients who are not mentally retarded. Increasing data support the use of a variety of medications for patients with mental disorders who are not mentally retarded, and some studies have focused on the use of medications for the following behavioral syndromes that are frequent among persons who are mentally retarded.

ATTENTION-DEFICIT/HYPERACTIVITY DISORDER. Studies of methylphenidate (Ritalin) treatment in mildly retarded patients with attention-deficit/ hyperactivity disorder have shown significant improvement in the ability to maintain attention and to stay focused on tasks. Methylphenidate treatment studies have not shown evidence of long-term improvement in social skills or learning.

AGGRESSION AND SELF-INJURIOUS BEHAVIOR. There are few well-controlled clinical trials to guide optimal treatment of aggression and self-injurious behavior. Some evidence from controlled and uncontrolled studies indicates that lithium (Eskalith) has been useful in decreasing aggression and self-injurious behavior. Narcotic antagonists such as naltrexone (ReVia, Trexan) have not been systematically shown to diminish aggression or self-injurious behaviors. Anticonvulsants including carbamazepine (Tegretol) and valproic acid (Depakene) are currently under investigation as medications for these behaviors in children and adolescents, whether they are mentally retarded or not. Double-blind placebo-controlled studies in mentally retarded adults and open clinical trials in mentally retarded children and adolescents have indicated that risperidone (Risperdal), an antipsychotic with potent dopamine D_2 and serotonin 5-HT_2, is efficacious in decreasing aggression and self-injurious behavior. Persons with mental retardation appear to be at higher risk for the development of tardive dyski-

Table 38–6
ICD-10 Diagnostic Criteria for Mental Retardation

Detailed clinical diagnostic criteria that can be used internationally for research cannot be specified for mental retardation in the same way as they can for most of the other disorders in Chapter V(F) of ICD-10. This is because manifestations of the two main components of mental retardation, namely low cognitive ability and diminished social competence, are profoundly affected by social and cultural influences. Only general guidance can be given here about the most appropriate methods of assessment to use.

Level of cognitive abilities

Depending upon the cultural norms and expectations of the individuals being studied, research workers must make their own judgments as to how best to estimate the intelligence quotient (IQ) or mental age according to the bands given below:

Category	Mental retardation	IQ range	Mental age (years)
F70	Mild	50–69	9 to under 12
F71	Moderate	35–49	6 to under 9
F72	Severe	20–34	3 to under 6
F73	Profound	Below 20	Less than 3

Level of social competence

Within most European and North American cultures, the Vineland Social Maturity Scale[a] is recommended for use, if it is judged to be appropriate. Modified versions or equivalent scales should be developed for use in other cultures.

A fourth character may be used to specify the extent of associated impairment of behaviour:

No, or minimal, impairment of behaviour

Significant impairment of behaviour requiring attention or treatment

Other impairments of behaviour

Without mention of impairment of behaviour

Comments

A specially designed multi-axial system is required to do justice to the variety of personal, clinical, and social statements needed for the comprehensive assessment of the causes and consequences of mental retardation. One such system is now in preparation for this section of Chapter V(F) of ICD-10.

[a]Doll EA. *Vineland Social Maturity Scale, Condensed Manual of Directions.* Circle Pines, MN: American Guidance Service; 1965.

nesia after use of a variety of antipsychotic medications. The atypical antipsychotics, including risperidone (Risperdal) and clozapine (Clozaril), may provide some relief with a decreased risk of tardive dyskinesia.

DEPRESSIVE DISORDERS. The diagnosis of depressive disorders among individuals with mental retardation may be overlooked when behavioral problems are prominent, and the need for antidepressant treatment for individuals with mental retardation may be underestimated. There have been some reports of disinhibition in response to serotonin reuptake inhibitors (such as fluoxetine [Prozac], paroxetine, sertraline [Zoloft]) in mentally retarded individuals who also have a diagnosis of pervasive developmental disorder. In general, given the relative safety of these medications, their use is indicated when a depressive disorder is diagnosed.

STEREOTYPICAL MOTOR MOVEMENTS. Antipsychotic medications, such as haloperidol (Haldol) and chlorpromazine, decrease repetitive self-stimulatory behaviors in mentally retarded patients, but these medications have not increased adaptive behavior. Some mentally retarded children and adults (up to one third) face a high risk for tardive dyskinesia with the continued use of antipsychotic medications. Obsessive-compulsive symptoms often overlap with the repetitive stereotypical behaviors seen in mentally retarded children and adolescents and in those with mental retardation and a pervasive developmental disorder. Serotonin reuptake inhibitors, such as fluoxetine, fluvoxamine (Luvox), paroxetine, and sertraline, have been shown to have efficacy in treating obsessive-compulsive symptoms in children and adolescents and thus may have some efficacy for stereotyped motor movements.

EXPLOSIVE RAGE BEHAVIOR. β-Adrenergic receptor antagonists (beta-blockers) such as propranolol (Inderal) reportedly result in fewer explosive rages in patients with mental retardation and autistic disorder. Antipsychotic medications have also been used in the treatment of explosive rage. Systematic controlled studies are indicated to confirm the efficacy of these drugs in the treatment of rage outbursts.

ICD-10

The 10th revision of *International Statistical Classification of Diseases and Related Health Problems* (ICD-10) approaches the diagnosis of mental retardation from a somewhat different viewpoint than DSM-IV-TR. According to ICD-10, mental retardation is a condition of "arrested or incomplete development of the mind" characterized by impaired developmental skills that "contribute to the overall level of intelligence." ICD-10 offers categories for specifying the extent of behavior impairment: none or minimal; significant, requiring treatment or attention; other impairments; no mention of impairments (Table 38–6).

References

Copeland SR, Hughes C. Effects of goal setting on task performance of persons with mental retardation. *Educ Train Ment Retard.* 2002;37:40.

Dykens EM, Cohen DJ. Effects of Special Olympics International on social competence in persons of mental retardation. *J Am Acad Child Adolesc Psychiatry.* 1996;35:223.

Einfeld SL, Tonge BJ. Population prevalence of psychopathology in children and

adolescents with intellectual disability: II. epidemiological findings. *J Intellect Disabil Res*. 1996;40:99.

Hagerman RJ. Biomedical advances in developmental psychology: the case of fragile X syndrome. *Dev Psychol*. 1996;32:416.

Halsey CL, Collins ME, Anderson CL. Extremely low-birth-weight children and their peers: a comparison of school-age outcomes. *Arch Pediatr Adolesc Med*. 1996;150:790.

Handen BL, Breaux AM, Janosky J, McAuliffe S, Feldman H, Gosling A. Effects and noneffects of methylphenidate in children with mental retardation and ADHD. *J Am Acad Child Adolesc Psychiatry*. 1992;31:455.

Healy DL, Saunders K. Follow-up of children born after in-vitro fertilisation. *Lancet*. 2002;359:459.

Hendren RL, De Backer I, Pandina GJ. Review of neuroimaging studies of child and adolescent psychiatric disorders from the past 10 years. *J Am Acad Child Adolesc Psychiatry*. 2000;39:815.

King BH, Hodapp RM, Dykens EM. Mental retardation. In: Sadock BJ, Sadock VA, eds. *Kaplan & Sadock's Comprehensive Textbook of Psychiatry*. 7th ed. Vol 2. Baltimore: Lippincott Williams & Wilkins; 2000:2587.

King BH, State MW, Shah B, Davanzo P, Dykens E. Mental retardation: a review of the past 10 years. Part I. *J Am Acad Child Adolesc Psychiatry*. 1997;36:1656.

Nordin V, Gillberg C. Autism spectrum disorders in children with physical or mental disability or both. I. Clinical and epidemiological aspects. *Dev Med Child Neurol*. 1996;38:297.

Perry R, Pataki C, Munoz-Silva DM, Armenteros J, Silva R. Pilot trial of risperidone in pervasive developmental disorders. In: Scientific proceedings of the 149th American Psychiatric Association meeting, 1996.

Pulsifer MB. The neuropsychology of mental retardation. *J Int Neuropsychol Soc*. 1996;2:159.

Ross E, Oliver C. The relationship between levels of mood, interest and pleasure and "challenging behaviour" in adults with severe and profound intellectual disability. *J Intellect Disabil Res*. 2002;46:191.

State MW, King BH, Dykens E. Mental retardation: a review of the past 10 years. Part II. *J Am Acad Child Adolesc Psychiatry*. 1997;36:1664.

State MW, Lombroso PJ, Pauls DL, Leckman JF. The genetics of childhood psychiatric disorders: a decade of progress. *J Am Acad Child Adolesc Psychiatry*. 2000;39:946.

Szymanski L, King BH. Practice parameters for the assessment and treatment of children, adolescents, and adults with mental retardation and comorbid mental disorders. *J Am Acad Child Adolesc Psychiatry*. 1999;38(suppl 12):5S.

39 Learning Disorders

Learning disorders refer to a child's or adolescent's deficits in acquiring expected skills in reading, writing, speaking, use of listening, reasoning, or mathematics, compared with other children of the same age and intellectual capacity. Learning disorders are not uncommon; they affect at least 5 percent of school-age children. This represents approximately half of all public school children who receive special education services in the United States. In 1975, Public Law 94-142, the "Education for All Handicapped Children Act," mandated all states to provide free and appropriate educational services to all children. Since that time, the number of children identified with learning disorders has increased, and a variety of definitions of learning disabilities has arisen. The fourth edition of *Diagnostic and Statistical Manual of Mental Disorders* (DSM-IV) introduced the term *learning disorders,* formerly called *academic skills disorders.* All of the current learning disorder diagnoses require that the child's achievement in that particular learning disorder is significantly lower than expected and that the learning problems interfere with academic achievement or activities of daily living.

The text revision of DSM-IV (DSM-IV-TR) includes four diagnostic categories in the chapter on learning disorders: reading disorder, mathematics disorder, disorder of written expression, and learning disorder not otherwise specified. Children with a learning disorder, such as reading disorder, for example, can be identified in two different ways: children who read poorly compared with most other children of the same age and children whose achievement in reading is significantly lower than their overall IQ would predict. DSM-IV-TR criteria for learning disorders require a substantial IQ-achievement discrepancy and significantly poor achievement in reading compared with that of most children of the same age. Research studies have led to questions regarding inclusion of an IQ-achievement discrepancy component in the definition of a learning disorder, since current data suggest that most children with reading disorders, for example, have similar deficits in phonological processing skills, regardless of their IQ. That is, most children with reading disorders have trouble with word recognition and "sounding out" words because they cannot understand and use phonemes, the smaller bits of words that are associated with particular sounds.

Learning disorders often make it agonizing for a child to succeed in school and, in some cases, lead to eventual demoralization, low self-esteem, chronic frustration, and poor peer relationships. Learning disorders are associated with higher than average risk of a variety of comorbid disorders including attention-deficit/hyperactivity disorder (ADHD), communication disorders, conduct disorders, and depressive disorders. Adolescents with learning disorders are about 1 1/2 times more likely to drop out of school, approximating rates of 40 percent. Adults with learning disorders are at increased risk for difficulties in employment and social adjustment. Learning disorders can be associated with other developmental disorders, major depressive disorder, and dysthymic disorder.

Genetic predisposition, perinatal injury, and neurological and other medical conditions may contribute to the development of learning disorders, but many children and adolescents with learning disorders have no specific risk factors. Learning disorders are, nevertheless, frequently found in association with conditions such as lead poisoning, fetal alcohol syndrome, and in utero drug exposure.

READING DISORDER

In DSM-IV-TR, reading disorder is defined as reading achievement below the expected level for a child's age, education, and intelligence, with the impairment interfering significantly with academic success or the daily activities that involve reading. According to DSM-IV-TR, if a neurological condition or sensory disturbance is present, the reading disability exhibited exceeds that usually associated with the other condition.

Reading disorder is associated with reading achievement below the expected level for a child's age, intelligence, and education. It is characterized by an impaired ability to recognize words, slow and inaccurate reading, and poor comprehension. In addition, children with ADHD are at high risk for reading disorder. Historically, many different labels have been used to describe reading disabilities including *word blindness, reading backward, learning disability, alexia,* and *developmental word blindness.* The term *developmental alexia* was accepted and defined as a developmental deficit in the recognition of printed symbols. This term was simplified by adopting the term *dyslexia* in the 1960s. *Dyslexia* was used extensively for many years to describe a reading disability syndrome that often included speech and language deficits and right–left confusion. Reading disorder is frequently accompanied by disabilities in other academic skills, and the term *dyslexia* has been replaced by broader terms, such as *learning disorder.*

Epidemiology

An estimated 4 percent of school-age children in the United States have reading disorder; prevalence studies find rates ranging between 2 and 8 percent. Three to four times as many boys

as girls are reported to have reading disability in clinically referred samples. Careful epidemiological studies have found closer to equal rates of reading disorder among boys and girls. Boys with reading disorder may be referred for evaluation more often than girls because of frequently associated behavior problems. There is no clear gender differential among adults who report reading difficulties.

Comorbidity

Children with reading disorder are at higher than average risk for attentional problems, disruptive behavior disorders (e.g., conduct disorder) and depressive disorders, particularly older children and adolescents. Data suggest that up to 25 percent of children with reading disorder also have ADHD. Family studies indicate that there may be some common genetic factors producing both reading disorder and attentional syndromes. Some evidence shows a higher than random incidence of aggression in young children with reading disorders and a higher than average rate of conduct disorders among adolescents with reading disorders. The increased risk may be attributed to comorbid ADHD as well as to independent factors that make adolescents with reading disorders more susceptible to engaging in antisocial behaviors. Children with reading disorders have higher than average rates of depression on self-report measures and experience higher levels of anxiety symptoms than children without learning disorders. Furthermore, children with reading disorders tend to have difficulties with peer relationships and less skill in responding sensitively in ambiguous social situations.

Etiology

There is no single identified cause of reading disorder; factors including genetic, developmental, and environmental attributes may contribute to the core deficits in reading disorders. Current research on reading disorders indicates that in most cases, children who struggle with reading have a deficit in phonological processing skills. These children cannot identify effectively the parts of words that denote specific sounds, which leads to grave difficulty in recognizing and sounding out words. Children with reading disorders are slower than average in naming letters and numbers, even when controlling for IQ. Thus, the core deficit for children with reading disorders lies within the domain of language use.

Given that reading disorder is essentially a language deficit, the left brain has been hypothesized to be the anatomical site of the dysfunction. Several research studies using magnetic resonance imaging studies have suggested that the planum temporale in the left brain shows less asymmetry than the same site in the right brain in children with both language and learning disorders. Positron emission tomographic (PET) studies have led some researchers to conclude that left temporal blood flow patterns during language tasks differ between children with and without learning disorders. Also, some cell analysis studies suggest that in reading-disordered persons, the visual magnocellular system (which normally contains large cells) contains more disorganized and smaller cell bodies than expected. None of the above studies provides conclusive evidence regarding brain differences between reading-disordered and normal individuals.

Many studies support the hypothesis that genetic factors play a major role in the presence of reading disorders. Studies indicate that 35 to 40 percent of first-degree relatives of children with reading disorder also have some reading disability. Several recent studies have suggested that phonological awareness (i.e., the ability to decode sounds and sound out words) is linked to chromosome 6. Furthermore, the ability to identify single words has been linked to chromosome 15.

Several historical hypotheses about the origin of reading disorders are now known to be untrue. The first myth is that reading disorders are primarily due to visual-motor problems, or what has been termed *scotopic sensitivity syndrome*. There is no evidence that children with reading disorders have visual problems or difficulties with their visual-motor system. The second theory with no supporting evidence is that allergies can cause, or contribute to, reading disabilities. Finally, unsubstantiated theories have implicated the cerebellar-vestibular system as the source of reading disorder.

Research in the fields of cognitive neuroscience and neuropsychology supports the hypothesis that encoding processes and working memory, rather than attention or long-term memory, are areas of weakness for children with reading disorder. Developmental factors have been hypothesized to play a role in reading disorders. One recent study found an association between dyslexia and birth in the months of May, June, and July, which suggests that prenatal exposure to a maternal infectious illness, such as influenza, in the winter months may contribute to reading disorder.

Studies in the 1930s attempted to explain reading disorder according to the cerebral hemispheric function model, which suggested positive correlations of reading disorder with left-handedness, left-eyedness, or mixed laterality. Subsequent epidemiological studies did not find any consistent association between reading disorder and laterality of handedness or eyedness, but right–left confusion has been shown to be associated with reading difficulties.

Complications during pregnancy and prenatal and perinatal difficulties are common in the histories of children with reading disorder. Extremely low birth weight and severely premature children are at higher risk for reading disorder and other learning disorders than children who are born full term and have normal birth weight. A higher than average incidence of reading disorder occurs among children of normal intelligence who have cerebral palsy, and epileptic children exhibit a slightly increased incidence of reading disorder. Children with postnatal brain lesions in the left occipital lobe, which results in right visual-field blindness, may have secondary reading disorder, as may children with lesions in the splenium of the corpus callosum that blocks transmission of visual information from the intact right hemisphere to the language areas of the left hemisphere.

Some studies suggest an association between malnutrition and subsequent reading disorder. Children who were malnourished for long periods during early childhood are at increased risk of subaverage performance in many cognitive areas, including reading. Their cognitive performances appear to be lower than those of siblings who were not subjected to the same degree of malnutrition.

Diagnosis

Reading disorder is diagnosed when a child's reading achievement is significantly below that expected of a child of the same age and intellectual capacity (Table 39–1). Characteristic diag-

Table 39–1
DSM-IV-TR Diagnostic Criteria for Reading Disorder

A. Reading achievement, as measured by individually administered standardized tests of reading accuracy or comprehension, is substantially below that expected given the person's chronological age, measured intelligence, and age-appropriate education.
B. The disturbance in Criterion A significantly interferes with academic achievement or activities of daily living that require reading skills.
C. If a sensory deficit is present, the reading difficulties are in excess of those usually associated with it.

Coding note: If a general medical (e.g., neurological) condition or sensory deficit is present, code the condition on Axis III.

From American Psychiatric Association. *Diagnostic and Statistical Manual of Mental Disorders.* 4th ed. Text rev. Washington, DC: American Psychiatric Association; copyright 2000, with permission.

nostic features include difficulty recalling, evoking, and sequencing printed letters and words; processing sophisticated grammatical constructions; and making inferences. Clinically, a child may be first identified with a reading disorder after becoming demoralized or exhibiting symptoms of depression related to being unable to succeed in school. School failure and ensuing poor self-esteem may exacerbate the problems as the child becomes more consumed with a sense of failure and spends less time focusing on academic work. Students suspected of having reading disorders are entitled to an educational evaluation through the school district to determine eligibility for special education services. Special education classification, however, is not uniform across states or regions, and students with identical reading difficulties may be eligible for services in one region but ineligible in another. In some cases, an evaluation is requested on the basis of disruptive behavioral problems that occur in conjunction with the reading disorder.

Clinical Features

Children who have reading disorder can usually be identified by the age of 7 years (second grade). Reading difficulty may be apparent among students in classrooms where reading skills are expected as early as the first grade. Children can sometimes compensate for reading disorder in the early elementary grades by the use of memory and inference, particularly when the disorder is associated with high intelligence. In such instances, the disorder may not be apparent until age 9 (fourth grade) or later. Children with reading disorder make many errors in their oral reading. The errors are characterized by omissions, additions, and distortions of words. Such children have difficulty in distinguishing between printed letter characters and sizes, especially those that differ only in spatial orientation and length of line. The problems in managing printed or written language may pertain to individual letters, sentences, and even a page. The child's reading speed is slow, often with minimal comprehension. Most children with reading disorder have an age-appropriate ability to copy from a written or printed text, but nearly all spell poorly.

Associated problems include language difficulties, exhibited often as impaired sound discrimination and difficulty in sequencing words properly. A child with disorders may start a word either in the middle or at the end of a printed or written sentence. At times, because of a poorly established left–right tracking sequence, such children transpose letters to be read. Failures in both memory recall and sustained elicitation result in poor recall of letter names and sounds.

Most children with reading disorder dislike and avoid reading and writing. Their anxiety is heightened when they are confronted with demands that involve printed language. Many children with the disorder who do not receive remedial education have a sense of shame and humiliation because of their continuing failure and subsequent frustration. These feelings grow more intense with time. Older children tend to be angry and depressed and exhibit poor self-esteem.

B.C. was a 12-year-old male student who presented for evaluation of problems in school. He attended an academic preschool and was presently enrolled in a regular sixth-grade class at a public school.

Current evaluation revealed no history of neurological, visual, or hearing problems that could explain B.C.'s school difficulties. Intelligence testing revealed high-average scores in both the verbal and performance subtests of the Wechsler Intelligence Scale for Children-III (WISC-III). Reading and mathematical scores on standardized tests of academic performance were consistent with his intelligence and chronological age; however, spelling scores were significantly below the predicted level of performance. Multiple misspellings occurred. Although the examiner noted adequate handwriting, B.C. appeared unable to express thoughts in complete sentences. His sentences were short and failed to state intended points clearly. Careful study of B.C.'s written paragraphs revealed numerous grammatical and syntactic errors as well as errors in punctuation and capitalization.

The clinical picture of an inability to compose, poor spelling, and grammatical errors in the absence of low intelligence, problems with reading or mathematics, or pervasive attentional problems led to a diagnosis of disorder of written expression. (Courtesy of Michael E. Spagna, Ph.D., Dennis P. Cantwell, M.D., and Lorian Baker, Ph.D.)

Pathology and Laboratory Examination

No specific physical signs or laboratory measures are helpful in the diagnosis of reading disorder. Psychoeducational testing, however, is critical in determining this diagnosis. The diagnosis of reading disorder is made after collecting data from a standardized intelligence test and an educational assessment of achievement. The diagnostic battery generally includes a standardized spelling test, written composition, processing and using oral language, design copying, and judgment of the adequacy of pencil use. The reading subtests of the Woodcock-Johnson Psycho-Educational Battery–Revised, and the Peabody Individual Achievement Test–Revised are useful in identifying reading disability. A screening projective battery may include

human-figure drawings, picture-story tests, and sentence completion. The evaluation should also include systematic observation of behavioral variables.

Course and Prognosis

Many children with reading disorder gain some knowledge of printed language during their first 2 years in grade school, even without any remedial assistance. By the end of the first grade, many children with reading disorder have, in fact, learned how to read a few words; however, by the time a child with a reading disorder reaches the third grade, keeping up with classmates is exceedingly difficult without remedial educational intervention. In the best circumstances, a child is recognized as being at risk for a reading disorder during the kindergarten year or early in the first grade. When remediation is instituted early, in milder cases, it is no longer necessary by the end of the first or second grade. In severe cases and depending on the pattern of deficits and strengths, remediation may be continued into the middle and high school years.

Differential Diagnosis

Reading disorder is often accompanied by comorbid disorders, such as expressive language disorder, disorder of written expression, and ADHD. A recent study indicates that children with reading disorder consistently present difficulties with linguistic abilities, while children with ADHD do not. Children with reading disorder who do not qualify for a diagnosis of ADHD, however, were shown to have some overlapping deficits in the area of cognitive inhibition such that they perform impulsively on continuous performance tasks. Deficits in expressive language and speech discrimination in reading disorder may be severe enough to warrant the additional diagnosis of expressive language disorder or mixed receptive-expressive language disorder. Some children exhibit a discrepancy between scores on verbal and performance intelligence. Visual perceptual deficits occur in only about 10 percent of cases. Reading disorder must be differentiated from mental retardation syndromes in which reading, along with other skills, is below the achievement expected for a child's chronological age. Intellectual testing helps to differentiate global deficits from more specific reading difficulties.

Poor reading skills resulting from inadequate schooling can be detected by finding out whether other children in the same school have similarly poor reading performances on standardized reading tests. Hearing and visual impairments should be ruled out with screening tests.

Treatment

Most current remediation strategies for children with reading disorder focus on direct instruction of the various components of reading. Many effective remediation programs begin by teaching the child to make accurate associations between letters and sounds. This approach is based on the current consensus that in most cases, the core deficits in reading disorders are related to difficulty recognizing and remembering the associations between letters and sounds. After individual letter-sound associations have been mastered, remediation can target larger components of reading such as syllables and words. The exact focus of any reading program can only be determined after accurate assessment of a child's specific deficits and weaknesses. Positive coping strategies include small, structured reading groups that offer individual attention and make it easier for a child to ask for help.

Reading instruction programs such as the Orton Gillingham and DISTAR approaches begin by concentrating on individual letters and sounds, advance to the mastery of simple phonetic units, and then blend these units into words and sentences. Thus, if children are taught to cope with graphemes, they will learn to read. Other reading remediation programs, such as the Merill program, and the SRA Basic Reading Program, begin by introducing whole words first and then teach children how to break them down and recognize the sounds of the syllables and the individual letters in the word. Another approach teaches children with reading disorders to recognize whole words through the use of visual aids and bypasses the sounding-out process. One such program is called the Bridge Reading Program. The Fernald Method uses a multisensory approach that combines teaching whole words with a tracing technique so that the child has kinesthetic stimulation while learning to read the words.

As in psychotherapy, the therapist–patient relationship is important to a successful treatment outcome in remedial educational therapy. Children should be placed in a grade as close as possible to their social functional level and given special remedial work in reading. Coexisting emotional and behavioral problems should be treated by appropriate psychotherapeutic means. Parental counseling may also be helpful. Approximately 75 percent of children with learning disorders can be differentiated from comparison samples by lower measures of social competence. Therefore, it is important to include social skills improvement as a therapeutic component of a treatment program for children with reading disorders.

MATHEMATICS DISORDER

Children with mathematics disorder have difficulty learning and remembering numerals, cannot remember basic facts about numbers, and are slow and inaccurate in computation. Poor achievement in four groups of skills have been identified in mathematics disorder: linguistic skills (those related to understanding mathematical terms and converting written problems into mathematical symbols), perceptual skills (the ability to recognize and understand symbols and order clusters of numbers), mathematical skills (basic addition, subtraction, multiplication, division, and following sequencing of basic operations), and attentional skills (copying figures correctly and observing operational symbols correctly). A variety of terms over the years, including *dyscalculia, congenital arithmetic disorder, acalculia, Gerstmann syndrome*, and *developmental arithmetic disorder* have been used to denote the difficulties present in mathematics disorder.

Mathematics disorder can occur in isolation or in conjunction with language and reading disorders. The diagnosis of mathematics disorder consists of deficits in arithmetic skills expected for a child's intellectual capacity and educational level, as measured by standardized, individually administered tests. This lack of expected mathematics ability must interfere

with school performance or daily life activities, and the difficulties must exceed impairment associated with any existing neurological or sensory deficits.

Epidemiology

Mathematics disorder alone is estimated to occur in about 1 percent of school-age children, that is, approximately one of every five children with learning disorder. Epidemiological studies have indicated that up to 6 percent of school-age children have some difficulty with mathematics. Mathematics disorder may occur with greater frequency in girls. Many studies of learning disorders in children have lumped several disorders together rather than separating them into individual disorders, which makes it more difficult to ascertain the precise prevalence of mathematics disorder.

Table 39–2
DSM-IV-TR Diagnostic Criteria for Mathematics Disorder

A. Mathematical ability, as measured by individually administered standardized tests, is substantially below that expected given the person's chronological age, measured intelligence, and age-appropriate education.
B. The disturbance in Criterion A significantly interferes with academic achievement or activities of daily living that require mathematical ability.
C. If a sensory deficit is present, the difficulties in mathematical ability are in excess of those usually associated with it.

Coding note: If a general medical (e.g., neurological) condition or sensory deficit is present, code the condition on Axis III.

From American Psychiatric Association. *Diagnostic and Statistical Manual of Mental Disorders*. 4th ed. Text rev. Washington, DC: American Psychiatric Association; copyright 2000, with permission.

Comorbidity

Mathematics disorder is commonly found comorbid with reading disorder and disorder of written expression. Children with mathematics disorder may also be at higher risk for expressive language disorder, mixed receptive-expressive language disorder, and developmental coordination disorder.

Etiology

Mathematics disorder, like other learning disorders, is probably due at least in part to genetic factors. An early theory proposed a neurological deficit in the right cerebral hemisphere, particularly in the occipital lobe areas. These regions are responsible for processing visual-spatial stimuli that, in turn, are responsible for mathematical skills. This theory, however, has received little support in subsequent neuropsychiatric studies.

Currently the cause is thought to be multifactorial, so that maturational, cognitive, emotional, educational, and socioeconomic factors account in varying degrees and combinations for mathematics disorder. Compared with reading, arithmetic abilities seem to depend more on the amount and quality of instruction.

Diagnosis

The diagnosis of mathematics disorder is made when a child's skills in mathematics fall significantly below what is expected for that child's age, intellectual ability, and education. Many different skills are needed for mathematics proficiency. These include linguistic skills, conceptual skills, and computational skills. Linguistic skills are being able to understand mathematical terms, understand word problems, and translate them into the proper mathematical process. Conceptual skills involve recognition of mathematical symbols and being able to use mathematical signs correctly. Computational skills include the ability to line up numbers correctly and to follow the "rules" of the mathematical operation. A definitive diagnosis can be made only after a child takes an individually administered standardized arithmetic test and scores markedly below the level expected in view of the child's schooling and intellectual capacity as measured by a standardized intelligence test. A pervasive developmental disorder and mental retardation should also be ruled out before confirming the diagnosis of mathematics disorder. The DSM-IV-TR diagnostic criteria for mathematics disorder are given in Table 39–2.

Clinical Features

Common features of mathematics disorder include difficulty with various components of mathematics, such as learning number names, remembering the signs for addition and subtraction, learning multiplication tables, translating word problems into computations, and doing calculations at the expected pace. Most children with mathematics disorder can be detected during the second and third grades in elementary school. A child with mathematics disorder generally has significant problems with concepts such as counting and adding even one-digit numbers, compared with classmates of the same age. During the first 2 or 3 years of elementary school, a child with mathematics disorder may scrape by in mathematics by relying on rote memory. But soon, as math problems require discrimination and manipulation of spatial and numerical relations, a child with mathematics disorder is overwhelmed.

Some investigators have classified mathematics disorder into the following categories: difficulty learning to count meaningfully; difficulty mastering cardinal and ordinal systems; difficulty performing arithmetic operations; and difficulty envisioning clusters of objects as groups. Children with the disorder may have trouble associating auditory and visual symbols, understanding the conservation of quantity, remembering sequences of arithmetic steps, and choosing principles for problem-solving activities. Children with these problems are presumed to have good auditory and verbal abilities.

Mathematics disorder often coexists with other disorders affecting reading, expressive writing, coordination, and expressive and receptive language. Spelling problems, deficits in memory or attention, and emotional or behavioral problems may be present. Young grade-school children often first show other learning disorders and should be checked for mathematics disorder. Children with cerebral palsy may have mathematics disorder with normal overall intelligence.

The relation between mathematics disorder and other communication and learning disorders is not clear. Although children with mixed receptive-expressive language disorder and

expressive language disorder are not necessarily affected by mathematics disorder, the conditions often coexist, as they are associated with impairments in both decoding and encoding processes.

Janet, age 13, has a long history of school problems. She failed first grade, supposedly because her teacher was "mean," and was removed from a special classroom after she kept getting into fights with the other children. Currently in a normal sixth-grade classroom, she is failing reading, barely passing English, arithmetic, and spelling, but doing satisfactory work in art and sports. Her teacher describes Janet as a "slow learner with a poor memory" and states that she doesn't learn in a group setting and requires a great deal of individual attention.

Janet's medical history is unremarkable except for a tonsillectomy at age 5 and an early history of chronic otitis. She sat up at 6 months, walked at 12 months, and began talking at 18 months. Examination revealed an open and friendly girl who was very touchy about her academic problems. She stated that she was "bossed around" at school, but had good friends in the neighborhood. Intelligence testing produced grade-level scores of 4.8 for reading, 5.3 for spelling, and 6.3 for arithmetic.

DISCUSSION

The differential diagnosis of academic problems includes consideration of poor schooling, mental retardation, ADHD, oppositional defiant disorder, conduct disorder, and learning disorders. In this case, because other children in her class are apparently passing when she is not, it is reasonable to rule out inadequate schooling as an explanation for Janet's academic difficulties. Her average intelligence rules out a diagnosis of mental retardation. Although there is a mention of "fights with other children" and inability to "learn in a group setting," there is certainly no description of other behaviors that would justify a diagnosis of either ADHD, oppositional defiant disorder, or conduct disorder.

There is positive evidence suggesting a learning disorder: She not only seems to have particular difficulty with reading in school but also performs significantly below her expected level on a reading achievement test. Her reading score of 4.8 is more than 1 year below her expected reading level. We thus gave Janet the diagnosis of reading disorder. Given this diagnosis, it is reasonable to regard the fighting and difficulty learning in a group as associated features of the learning disorder.

There is now considerable research evidence suggesting that early, chronic otitis may be associated with later learning or language difficulties. (From *DSM-IV Casebook.*)

Pathology and Laboratory Examination

No physical signs or symptoms indicate mathematics disorder, but educational testing and standardized measurement of intellectual function are necessary to make this diagnosis. The Keymath Diagnostic Arithmetic Test measures several areas of mathematics including knowledge of mathematical content, function, and computation. It is used to assess ability in mathematics of children in grades 1 to 6.

Course and Prognosis

A child with a mathematics disorder can usually be identified by the age of 8 years (third grade). In some children the disorder is apparent as early as 6 years (first grade); in others it may not occur until age 10 (fifth grade) or later. Too few data are currently available from longitudinal studies to predict clear patterns of developmental and academic progress of children classified as having mathematics disorder in early school grades. On the other hand, children with a moderate mathematics disorder who do not receive intervention may have complications, including continuing academic difficulties, shame, poor self-concept, frustration, and depression. These complications may lead to reluctance to attend school, truancy, and eventual hopelessness about academic success.

Differential Diagnosis

Mathematics disorder must be differentiated from global causes of impaired functioning such as mental retardation syndromes. Arithmetic difficulties in mental retardation are accompanied by generalized impairment in overall intellectual functioning. In unusual cases of mild mental retardation, arithmetic skills may be significantly below the level expected on the basis of a person's schooling and level of mental retardation. In such cases, an additional diagnosis of mathematics disorder should be made. Treatment of the arithmetic difficulties can particularly help a child's chances for employment in adulthood. Inadequate schooling can often affect a child's poor arithmetic performance on a standardized arithmetic test. Conduct disorder or ADHD may occur with mathematics disorder, and in these cases, both diagnoses should be made.

Treatment

Currently, the most effective treatments for mathematics disorder combine teaching mathematics concepts with continuous practice in solving math problems. Flash cards, wordbooks, and computer games can be a viable part of this treatment. A recent report indicates that math instruction is most helpful when the focus is on problem-solving activities, including word problems, rather than only computation. Project MATH, a multimedia self-instructional or group-instructional in-service training program, has been successful for some children with mathematics disorder. Computer programs can be helpful and can increase compliance with remediation efforts.

Social skills deficits may contribute to a child's hesitation in asking for help, so a child identified with a mathematics disorder may benefit from gaining positive problem-solving skills in a social arena as well as in mathematics.

DISORDER OF WRITTEN EXPRESSION

Disorder of written expression is characterized by writing skills that are significantly below the expected level for a child's age

and intellectual capacity. These difficulties impair the child's academic performance and writing in everyday life. The many components of writing disorder include poor spelling, errors in grammar and punctuation, and poor handwriting. Spelling errors are among the most common difficulties for a child with a writing disorder. Spelling mistakes are most often phonetic errors, that is, an erroneous spelling that sounds like the correct spelling. Examples of common types of spelling errors are *fone* for *phone,* or *beleeve* for *believe.*

In the past, it was believed that dysgraphia (i.e., poor writing skills) did not occur in the absence of a reading disorder; however, evidence indicates that disorder of written expression can occur on its own. Terms once used to describe writing disability include *spelling disorder* and *spelling dyslexia.* Writing disabilities are often associated with other learning disorders, but they may be diagnosed later because expressive writing is acquired later than language and reading.

In addition to a disorder similar to DSM-IV-TR's disorder of written expression, the 10th revision of *International Statistical Classification of Diseases and Related Health Problems* (ICD-10) includes a separate specific spelling disorder.

Epidemiology

The prevalence of disorder of written expression alone has not been studied, but like reading disorder, it is estimated to occur in approximately 4 percent of school-age children. The gender ratio in writing disorder is believed to be like that of reading disorder, occurring in about three times as many boys. Disorder of written expression often occurs along with reading disorder, but not always.

Comorbidity

Children with writing disorder are at higher risk for a variety of other learning and language disorders including reading disorder, mathematics disorder, and expressive and receptive language disorders. ADHD occurs with greater frequency in children with writing disorders than in the general population. Finally, children with writing disorders are believed to be at higher risk for social skills difficulties, and some go on to develop poor self-esteem and depressive symptoms.

Etiology

Causes of writing disorders are believed to be similar to those of reading disorder, that is, a deficit in the use of the components of language related to letter sounds. It is likely that genetic factors play a role in the development of writing disorder. Writing difficulties often accompany language disorders in which a given child may have trouble understanding grammatical rules, finding words, and expressing ideas clearly. According to one hypothesis, a disorder of written expression may result from the combined effects of one or more of the following: expressive language disorder, mixed receptive-expressive language disorder, and reading disorder. Hereditary predisposition to the disorder is supported by findings that most children with disorder of written expression have first-degree relatives with the disorder. Children with limited attention spans and high levels of distractibility may find writing an arduous task.

Diagnosis

A diagnosis of disorder of written expression is based on a child's poor performance on composing written text, including handwriting and impaired ability to spell and to place words sequentially in coherent sentences, compared with most other children of the same age and intellectual ability. In addition to spelling mistakes, a child with writing disorder may have serious grammatical mistakes, such as using incorrect tenses, forgetting words in sentences, and placing words in the wrong order. Punctuation may be incorrect, and the child may have poor ability to remember which words begin with capital letters. Poor handwriting may also contribute to writing disorder, including letters that are not legible, inverted letters, and mixtures of capital and lowercase letters in a given word. Other features of writing disorders include poor organization of written stories, which lack critical elements such as "where," "when," and "who" or clear expression of the plot.

Clinical Features

Children with disorder of written expression have difficulties early in grade school in spelling words and expressing their thoughts according to age-appropriate grammatical norms. Their spoken and written sentences contain an unusually large number of grammatical errors and poor paragraph organization. During and after the second grade, these children commonly make simple grammatical errors in writing a short sentence. For example, despite constant reminders, they frequently fail to capitalize the first letter of the first word in a sentence and to end the sentence with a period. Common features of the disorder of written expression are spelling errors, grammatical errors, punctuation errors, poor paragraph organization, and poor handwriting.

As they grow older and progress into higher grades in school, such children's spoken and written sentences become more conspicuously primitive, odd, and inferior to what is expected of students at their grade level. Their word choices are erroneous and inappropriate; their paragraphs are disorganized and not in proper sequence; and spelling correctly becomes increasingly difficult as their vocabulary becomes larger and more abstract. Associated features of disorder of written expression include refusal or reluctance to go to school and to do assigned written homework, poor academic performance in other areas (e.g., mathematics), general avoidance of school work, truancy, attention deficit, and conduct disturbance.

Many children with disorder of written expression become frustrated and angry because of feelings of inadequacy and failure in their academic performance. In severe cases, depressive disorders may result from a growing sense of isolation, estrangement, and despair. Young adults with disorder of written expression who do not receive remedial intervention continue to have difficulties in social adaptation involving writing skills and a continuing sense of incompetence, inferiority, isolation, and estrangement. Some even try to avoid writing a

response letter or a simple greeting card for fear of exposing their writing incompetence.

Ryan was a 9-year-old boy who was referred by his teacher for evaluation of his poor classwork production. The teacher reported to Ryan's parents that he was not disruptive in class, but never seemed to know exactly what was going on. He often seemed to be preoccupied or daydreaming. He had good ideas when he spoke up in class but did not volunteer to answer questions verbally most of the time. When he was given written assignments in class, he rushed through them and could not remember how to spell even simple words correctly. His stories often did not make sense, since he often left out important verbs, the names of the main subjects, or critical parts of the plot. Ryan's teacher reported that she used to get frustrated with Ryan because she felt that he wasn't paying attention because he just didn't care, but even after she moved his seat to the front of the room, his work did not improve. Ryan always did well on assignments that involved drawing, which he did quickly and effortlessly.

Ryan was given a standardized test of intelligence (WISC-III), the Test of Written Language (TOWL), and the Diagnostic Evaluation of Writing Skills (DEWS) and had a clinical psychiatric interview with a child and adolescent psychiatrist. Ryan's full-scale intellectual quotient was in the superior range, 122, with a verbal scale of 112, and a performance scale of 128. His tests of written language revealed that he had significant deficits in spelling, use of punctuation, and applying grammatical rules. A diagnosis of disorder of written expression was made. Ryan's psychiatric interview revealed that he also met criteria for ADHD, inattentive type.

Ryan was referred for resource room remediation in writing for one period each day in school and was given a trial of stimulant medication. Ryan's attention improved modestly in the classroom, and he began to demonstrate more motivation to write carefully, especially while he was with his resource room teacher. His self-esteem improved as his problems were being addressed.

Pathology and Laboratory Examination

While no physical stigmata of a writing disorder exist, educational testing is used in making a diagnosis of writing disorder. Diagnosis is based on a child's writing performance being markedly below his or her intellectual capacity, as confirmed by an individually administered standardized expressive writing test (Table 39–3). Currently available tests of written language include the TOWL, the DEWS, and the Test of Early Written Language (TEWL). The presence of a major disorder such as a pervasive developmental disorder or mental retardation may obviate the diagnosis of disorder of written expression. Other disorders to be differentiated from disorder of written expression are communication disorders, reading disorder, and impaired vision and hearing.

A child suspected of having disorder of written expression should first be given a standardized intelligence test, such as WISC-III or the revised Wechsler Adult Intelligence Scale (WAIS-R) to determine the child's overall intellectual capacity.

Table 39–3
DSM-IV-TR Diagnostic Criteria for Disorder of Written Expression

A. Writing skills, as measured by individually administered standardized tests (or functional assessments of writing skills), are substantially below those expected given the person's chronological age, measured intelligence, and age-appropriate education.
B. The disturbance in Criterion A significantly interferes with academic achievement or activities of daily living that require the composition of written texts (e.g., writing grammatically correct sentences and organized paragraphs).
C. If a sensory deficit is present, the difficulties in writing skills are in excess of those usually associated with it.

Coding note: If a general medical (e.g., neurological) condition or sensory deficit is present, code the condition on Axis III.

From American Psychiatric Association. *Diagnostic and Statistical Manual of Mental Disorders.* 4th ed. Text rev. Washington, DC: American Psychiatric Association; copyright 2000, with permission.

Course and Prognosis

Because writing, language, and reading disorders often coexist and because a child normally speaks well before learning to read and learns to read well before writing well, a child with all these disorders has expressive language disorder diagnosed first and disorder of written expression diagnosed last. In severe cases, a disorder of written expression is apparent by age 7 (second grade); in less severe cases, the disorder may not be apparent until age 10 (fifth grade) or later. Most persons with mild and moderate disorder of written expression fare well if they receive timely remedial education early in grade school. Severe disorder of written expression requires continual, extensive remedial treatment through the late part of high school and even into college.

The prognosis depends on the severity of the disorder, the age or grade when the remedial intervention is started, the length and continuity of treatment, and presence or absence of associated or secondary emotional or behavioral problems. Those who later become well compensated or who recover from disorder of written expression are often from families with high socioeconomic backgrounds.

Differential Diagnosis

One must determine whether another disorder such as ADHD or a depressive disorder is preventing a child from being able to concentrate on writing tasks in the absence of writing disorder itself. If this is the case, treatment for the above disorder should improve a child's writing performance. Disorder of written expression may also occur with a variety of other language and learning disorders. Common associated disorders are reading disorder, mixed receptive-expressive language disorder, expressive language disorder, mathematics disorder, developmental coordination disorder, and disruptive behavior and attention-deficit disorders.

Treatment

Remedial treatment for writing disorder includes direct practice in spelling and sentence writing as well as a review of grammatical rules. Intensive and continuous administration of individually tailored, one-on-one expressive and creative writing therapy appears to effect favorable outcome. Teachers in some special schools devote as much as 2 hours a day to such writing instruction. The effectiveness of a writing intervention largely depends on an optimal relationship between the child and the writing specialist. Success or failure in sustaining the patient's motivation greatly affects the treatment's long-term efficacy. Associated secondary emotional and behavioral problems should be given prompt attention, with appropriate psychiatric treatment and parental counseling.

Table 39–4
DSM-IV-TR Diagnostic Criteria for Learning Disorder Not Otherwise Specified

This category is for disorders in learning that do not meet criteria for any specific learning disorder. This category might include problems in all three areas (reading, mathematics, written expression) that together significantly interfere with academic achievement even though performance on tests measuring each individual skill is not substantially below that expected given the person's chronological age, measured intelligence, and age-appropriate education.

From American Psychiatric Association. *Diagnostic and Statistical Manual of Mental Disorders.* 4th ed. Text rev. Washington, DC: American Psychiatric Association; copyright 2000, with permission.

LEARNING DISORDER NOT OTHERWISE SPECIFIED

Learning disorder not otherwise specified is a new category in DSM-IV-TR for disorders that do not meet the criteria for any specific learning disorder but cause impairment and reflect learning abilities below those expected for a person's intelligence, education, and age (Table 39–4). An example of a disability that could be placed in this category is a spelling skills deficit.

ICD-10

ICD-10 classifies specific developmental disorders of scholastic skills learning disorders under the category disorders of psychological development, which must have an onset during infancy or childhood, must show a delay or impairment in developing functions strongly related to the biological maturation of the central nervous system, and must undergo a steady course without remissions and relapses typical of many mental disorders. Scholastic skills learning disorders are usually of unknown cause but often have a family history of similar or related disorders, lending support to the probability of genetic influences. Environmental factors may play a part but are often not identified as major factors.

Specific developmental disorders of scholastic skills include specific reading disorder; specific spelling disorder; specific disorder of arithmetic skills; mixed disorder of scholastic skills; other developmental disorders of scholastic skills; and developmental disorder of scholastic skills, unspecified (Table 39–5). Normal patterns of skill acquisition are disturbed because of abnormalities in cognitive processing that derive largely from biological dysfunction. Diagnostic difficulties can arise from the need to differentiate the disorders from normal variations, the need to consider developmental course, the fact that these skills must be taught and learned and are not simply a function of biological maturation, and the difficulty in distinguishing between cognitive abnormalities that cause reading problems and those that arise from reading problems.

Table 39–5
ICD-10 Diagnostic Criteria for Specific Developmental Disorders of Scholastic Skills

Specific reading disorder

A. Either of the following must be present:
   (1) A score on reading accuracy and/or comprehension that is at least 2 standard errors of prediction below the level expected on the basis of the child's chronological age and general intelligence, with both reading skills and IQ assessed on an individually administered test standardized for the child's culture and educational system.
   (2) A history of serious reading difficulties, or test scores that met Criterion A(1) at an earlier age, plus a score on a spelling test that is at least 2 standard errors of prediction below the level expected on the basis of the child's chronological age and IQ.

B. The disturbance described in Criterion A significantly interferes with academic achievement or with activities of daily living that require reading skills.

C. The disorder is not the direct result of a defect in visual or hearing acuity, or of a neurological disorder.

D. School experiences are within the average expectable range (i.e., there have been no extreme inadequacies in educational experiences).

E. *Most commonly used exclusion clause.* IQ is below 70 on an individually administered standardized test.

Possible additional inclusion criterion

For some research purposes, investigators may wish to specify a history of some level of impairment during the preschool years in speech, language, sound categorization, motor coordination, visual processing, attention, or control or modulation of activity.

Comments

The above criteria would not include general reading backwardness of a type that would fall within the clinical guidelines. The research diagnostic criteria for general reading backwardness would be the same as for specific reading disorder except that Criterion A(1) would specify reading skills 2 standard errors of prediction below the level expected on the basis of chronological age (i.e., not taking IQ into account), and Criterion A(2) would follow the same principle for spelling. The validity of the differentiation between these two varieties of reading problem is not unequivocally established, but it seems that the specific type has a more specific association with language retardation (whereas general reading backwardness is associated with a wider range of developmental disabilities), and is more prevalent in boys than in girls.

(*continued*)

Table 39–5 (*continued*)

There are further research differentiations that are based on analyses of the types of spelling error.

Specific spelling disorder

A. The score on a standardized spelling test is at least 2 standard errors of prediction below the level expected on the basis of the child's chronological age and general intelligence.

B. Scores on reading accuracy and comprehension and on arithmetic are within the normal range (±2 standard deviations from the mean).

C. There is no history of significant reading difficulties.

D. School experience is within the average expectable range (i.e., there have been no extreme inadequacies in educational experiences).

E. Spelling difficulties have been present from the early stages of learning to spell.

F. The disturbance described in Criterion A significantly interferes with academic achievement or with activities of daily living that require spelling skills.

G. *Most commonly used exclusion clause.* IQ is below 70 on an individually administered standardized test.

Specific disorder of arithmetical skills

A. The score on a standardized arithmetic test is at least 2 standard errors of prediction below the level expected on the basis of the child's chronological age and general intelligence.

B. Scores on reading accuracy and comprehension and on spelling are within the normal range (±2 standard deviations from the mean).

C. There is no history of significant reading or spelling difficulties.

D. School experience is within the average expectable range (i.e., there have been no extreme inadequacies in educational experiences).

E. Arithmetical difficulties have been present from the early stages of learning arithmetic.

F. The disturbance described in Criterion A significantly interferes with academic achievement or with activities of daily living that require arithmetical skills.

G. *Most commonly used exclusion clause.* IQ is below 70 on an individually administered standardized test.

Mixed disorder of scholastic skills

This is an ill-defined, inadequately conceptualized (but necessary) residual category of disorders in which both arithmetical and reading or spelling skills are significantly impaired, but in which the disorder is not solely explicable in terms of general mental retardation or inadequate schooling. It should be used for disorders meeting the criteria for specific disorder of arithmetical skills and either specific reading disorder or specific spelling disorder.

Other developmental disorders of scholastic skills

Developmental disorder of scholastic skills, unspecified

This category should be avoided as far as possible and should be used only for unspecified disorders in which there is a significant disability of learning that cannot be solely accounted for by mental retardation, visual acuity problems, or inadequate schooling.

Reprinted with permission from World Health Organization. *The ICD-10 Classification of Mental and Behavioural Disorders: Diagnostic Criteria for Research.* Copyright, World Health Organization, Geneva, 1993.

References

Beitchman J, Cantwell DP, Forness SR, Kavale K, Kaufman JM. Practice parameters for the assessment and treatment of children and adolescents with language and learning disorders. *J Am Acad Child Adolesc Psychiatry.* 1998;37:46S.

Beitchman J, Young AR. Learning disorders with a special emphasis on reading disorders: a review of the past 10 years. *J Am Acad Child Adolesc Psychiatry.* 1997;36:1020.

Bussing R, Zima BT, Perwien AR. Self-esteem in special education children with ADHD: relationship to disorder characteristics and medication use. *J Am Acad Child Adolesc Psychiatry.* 2000;39:1260.

Glisky EL, Glisky ML. Learning and memory impairments. In: Eslinger RJ, ed. *Neuropsychological Interventions: Clinical Research and Practice.* New York: Guilford Press; 2002:137.

Goldstein S. *Managing Attention and Learning Disorders in Late Adolescence and Adulthood: A Guide for Practitioners.* New York: John Wiley & Sons; 1997.

Grant ML, Ilai D, Nussbaum NL, Bigler ED. The relationship between continuous performance tasks and neuropsychological tests in children with attention-deficit/hyperactivity disorder. *Percept Mot Skills.* 1990;70:435.

Livingston R, Adam BS, Bracha HS. Season of birth and neurodevelopmental disorder: summer birth is associated with dyslexia. *J Am Acad Child Adolesc Psychiatry.* 1993;32:612.

Mayer R. Understanding individual differences in mathematical problem solving. *Learn Disabil Q.* 1993;16:2.

Nussbaum NL, Grant ML, Roman MJ, Poole JH, Bigler ED. Attention-deficit disorder and the mediating effect of age on academic and behavioral variables. *J Dev Behav Pediatr.* 1990;11:22.

Orton S. *Reading, Writing, and Speech Problems in Children.* New York: WW Norton; 1937.

Poduska JM. Parents' perceptions of their first graders' need for mental health and educational services. *J Am Acad Child Adolesc Psychiatry.* 2000; 39:584.

Purvis KL, Tannock R. Phonological processing, not inhibitory control, differentiates ADHD and reading disability. *J Am Acad Child Adolesc Psychiatry.* 2000;39:485.

Rourke BP, Ahmad SA, Collins DW, et al. Child clinical/pediatric neuropsychology: some recent advances. *Annu Rev Psychol.* 2002;53:309.

Semrod-Clikeman E, Biederman J, Sprich-Buckminster S, Lehman BK, Faraone SV, Norman D. Comorbidity between ADDH and learning disability: a review and report in a clinically referred sample. *J Am Acad Child Adolesc Psychiatry.* 1992;31:439.

Smith SD, Pennington BF, Kimberling WJ, Ing PS. Familial dyslexia: use of genetic linkage data to define subtypes. *J Am Acad Child Adolesc Psychiatry.* 1990;29:204.

Spagna ME, Cantwell DP, Baker L. Reading disorder. In: Sadock BJ, Sadock VA, eds. *Kaplan & Sadock's Comprehensive Textbook of Psychiatry.* 7th ed. Vol 2. Baltimore: Lippincott Williams & Wilkins; 2000:2614.

Spagna ME, Cantwell DP, Baker L. Mathematics disorder. In: Sadock BJ, Sadock VA, eds. *Kaplan & Sadock's Comprehensive Textbook of Psychiatry.* 7th ed. Vol 2. Baltimore: Lippincott Williams & Wilkins; 2000:2620.

Spagna ME, Cantwell DP, Baker L. Disorder of written expression and learning disorder not otherwise specified. In: Sadock BJ, Sadock VA, eds. *Kaplan & Sadock's Comprehensive Textbook of Psychiatry.* 7th ed. Vol 2. Baltimore: Lippincott Williams & Wilkins; 2000:2625.

Vaughn S, Elbaum BE, Schumm JS. The effects of inclusion on the social functioning of students with learning disabilities. *J Learn Disabil.* 1996;29:598.

40 Motor Skills Disorder: Developmental Coordination Disorder

Developmental coordination disorder is a condition characterized by low performance in daily activities that require coordination below what is expected for age and intellectual level. According to the text revision of the fourth edition of *Diagnostic and Statistical Manual of Mental Disorders* (DSM-IV-TR), the disorder may present with delays in achieving motor milestones such as sitting, crawling, and walking.

Developmental coordination disorder may also be manifested by clumsy gross and fine motor skills, resulting in poor performance in sports and even poor handwriting. A child with developmental coordination disorder may bump into things more often than siblings or drop things. In the 1930s, the term *clumsy child syndrome* began to be used in the literature to denote a condition of awkward motor behaviors that could not be correlated with any specific neurological disorder or damage. This term continues to be used to identify imprecise or delayed gross and fine motor behavior in children, resulting in subtle motor inabilities, but often significant social rejection. Currently, there are indications that perinatal problems such as prematurity, low birth weight, and hypoxia may contribute to the emergence of developmental coordination disorders. Children with developmental coordination disorder are at higher risk for language and learning disorders. There is a strong association between speech and language problems and coordination problems, as well as an association of coordination difficulties with hyperactivity, impulsivity, and poor attention span.

Children with developmental coordination disorder may resemble younger children because of their inability to master motor activities typical for their age group. For example, children with developmental coordination disorder in elementary school may not be adept at bicycle riding, skateboarding, running, skipping, or hopping. In the middle school years, children with this disorder may have trouble in team sports such as soccer, baseball, or basketball. Fine motor skill manifestations of developmental coordination disorder typically include clumsiness using utensils and difficulty with buttons and zippers in the preschool age group. In older children, using scissors and more complex grooming skills such as styling hair and putting on makeup is difficult. Children with developmental coordination disorder are often ostracized by peers because of their poor skills in many sports, and they often have long-standing difficulties with peer relationships. Developmental coordination disorder is the sole disorder in the DSM-IV-TR category motor skills disorder. Gross and fine motor impairment in this disorder cannot be explained on the basis of a medical condition, such as cerebral palsy, muscular dystrophy, or any other neuromuscular disorder.

Epidemiology

The prevalence of developmental coordination disorder has been estimated at about 5 percent of school-age children. The male-to-female ratio in referred populations tends to show increased rates of the disorder in males, but schools refer boys more often for testing and special education evaluations. Reports in the literature of the male-to-female ratio have ranged from 2 to 1 to as much as 4 to 1. These rates may also be inflated because motor behaviors in male children are scrutinized more closely than those in female children.

Comorbidity

Developmental coordination disorder is strongly associated with speech and language disorders. Children with coordination difficulties have higher than expected rates of speech and language disorders, and studies of children with speech disorders report very high rates of "clumsiness." Some studies have found associations between fine motor skills in the upper arms and expressive and receptive language disorders, whereas gross motor problems and visual motor coordination problems were not associated with language disturbance. Developmental coordination disorder is also associated with reading disorders, mathematics disorder, and disorder of written expression. Higher than expected rates of attention-deficit/hyperactivity disorders are also associated with developmental coordination disorder.

Secondary peer relationship problems are common among children with developmental coordination disorders, because of the rejection that occurs along with their poor performance in sports and games that require good motor skill. Adolescents with coordination problems often exhibit poor self-esteem and academic difficulties.

Etiology

The causes of developmental coordination disorder are unknown, and are believed to include both "organic" and "developmental" factors. Risk factors postulated to contribute to this disorder include prematurity, hypoxia, perinatal malnutrition, and low birth weight. Prenatal exposure to alcohol, cocaine, and nicotine have also been hypothesized to contribute to both low birth weight and cognitive and behavioral abnormalities. Neurochemical abnormalities and parietal lobe lesions have also been suggested to contribute to coordination deficits. Developmental coordination disorder and communication disorders have strong associations, although the specific causative agents are unknown for both. Coordination problems are also more frequently found in children with hyperactivity syndromes and learning disorders. Developmental coordination disorder probably has a multifactorial cause.

Diagnosis

The diagnosis of developmental coordination disorder depends on poor performance, for a child's age and intellectual level, in activities requiring coordination. Diagnosis is based on a history of the child's delay in achieving early motor milestones as well as direct observation of current deficits in coordination. An informal screen for developmental coordination disorder involves asking the child to perform tasks involving gross motor coordination (e.g., hopping, jumping, and standing on one foot); fine motor coordination (e.g., finger tapping and shoelace tying); and hand–eye coordination (e.g., catching a ball and copying letters). Judgments regarding poor performance must be based on what is expected for a child's age. A child who is mildly clumsy but whose functioning is not impaired does not qualify for a diagnosis of developmental coordination disorder.

The diagnosis may be associated with below-normal scores on performance subtests of standardized intelligence tests and by normal or above-normal scores on verbal subtests. Specialized tests of motor coordination can be useful, such as the Bender Visual Motor Gestalt test, the Frostig Movement Skills Test Battery, and the Bruininks-Oseretsky Test of Motor Development. The child's chronological age and intellectual capacity must be taken into account, and the disorder cannot be caused by a neurological or neuromuscular condition. Examination, however, may occasionally reveal slight reflex abnormalities and other soft neurological signs. The DSM-IV-TR diagnostic criteria are given in Table 40–1.

Table 40–1
DSM-IV-TR Diagnostic Criteria for Developmental Coordination Disorder

A. Performance in daily activities that require motor coordination is substantially below that expected given the person's chronological age and measured intelligence. This may be manifested by marked delays in achieving motor milestones (e.g., walking, crawling, sitting), dropping things, "clumsiness," poor performance in sports, or poor handwriting.

B. The disturbance in Criterion A significantly interferes with academic achievement or activities of daily living.

C. The disturbance is not due to a general medical condition (e.g., cerebral palsy, hemiplegia, or muscular dystrophy) and does not meet criteria for a pervasive developmental disorder.

D. If mental retardation is present, the motor difficulties are in excess of those usually associated with it.

Coding note: If a general medical (e.g., neurological) condition or sensory deficit is present, code the condition on Axis III.

From American Psychiatric Association. *Diagnostic and Statistical Manual of Mental Disorders.* 4th ed. Text rev. Washington, DC: American Psychiatric Association; copyright 2000, with permission.

Clinical Features

The clinical signs suggesting the existence of developmental coordination disorder are evident as early as infancy in some cases, when a child begins to attempt tasks requiring motor coordination. The essential clinical feature is significantly impaired performance in motor coordination. The difficulties in motor coordination may vary with a child's age and developmental stage.

In infancy and early childhood the disorder may be manifested by delays in developmental motor milestones, such as turning over, crawling, sitting, standing, walking, buttoning shirts, and zipping up pants. Between the ages of 2 and 4 years, clumsiness appears in almost all activities requiring motor coordination. Affected children cannot hold objects and drop them easily, their gait may be unsteady, they often trip over their own feet, and they may bump into other children while attempting to go around them. Older children may display impaired motor coordination in table games, such as putting together puzzles or building blocks, and in any type of ball game. Although no specific features are pathognomonic of developmental coordination disorder, developmental milestones are frequently delayed. Many children with the disorder also have speech and language difficulties. Older children may have secondary problems including academic difficulties, as well as poor peer relationships based on social rejection.

Johnny, age 8, was brought to a clinic for evaluation by his mother, who said, "There is something wrong with his brain." When asked to be more specific, she replied with a vague litany of complaints that were frequently self-contradictory.

> He was always slow to learn things, slower than any of my other children. But I know he's really very smart. Sometimes he just amazes me with what he remembers or can figure out. He doesn't do much, for example, at school or with activities outside school. Sometimes I think it's because he's lazy, and other times I think he's depressed, and other times I think maybe it's because he is sick a lot. He gets a lot of stomachaches. He's really such a sweet boy. I mean he's so nice with his four sisters and our pets. But sometimes he's so nasty I get afraid. For example, he gets frustrated with some of his toys, and then he gets destructive. He's broken more toys than all of my other three children put together. He seems to like people, but he only has one friend at school. He refuses to try out for soccer or anything like that where he could play with the other boys. Sometimes I think

he just doesn't care about anything. He's always dropping dishes and things around the house.

A more detailed history revealed that the pregnancy, birth, and early medical history had been unremarkable, but minor problems had appeared in his first year of life. These included being slow to sit up, crawl, and walk. Because Johnny was the fourth child in the family, the mother had not "had time" to record the actual ages when these milestones were reached. She could only pinpoint that "he was much older than any of the other children when he did finally manage to do those things," adding that the pediatrician had nonetheless assured her that Johnny was not retarded. "A good thing he did," she laughed, "because later when Johnny had so much trouble learning to use the knife and fork, and to tie his shoelaces, and to button his shirts, I did worry about that."

Asked if there were any remaining concerns along these lines, the mother replied "none at all." Apparently, Johnny excelled in reading and did well in all his school subjects except handwriting and physical education.

His medical history was also unremarkable. During the preschool years there had been only "the normal childhood illnesses" (chicken pox, earaches, and flu) and "an awful lot of bruises and scraped knees." The stomachaches had started "some time around age 7," but again, the pediatrician had assured the mother that they were not cause for concern.

Examination revealed a pleasant but rather quiet boy with appropriate affect, good concentration, and apparently normal cognitive skills. Although quiet and reserved, Johnny did not appear apathetic; indeed, he became quite enthusiastic when describing a book he had just read. During the interview, Johnny denied any problems in school or with peers. When specifically asked, he did admit to occasional stomachaches and to nonparticipation in group activities, which he attributed to simply "not liking that stuff."

Psychological testing performed in the school setting revealed above-average intelligence and academic performance. However, Johnny scored well below the norm on a test of motor development requiring tasks involving running, balancing, coordination, and motor speed. The psychologist noted that he showed good concentration and attention during the testing.

DISCUSSION

Many features of this case are typical of developmental coordination disorder. These include late gross motor milestones (standing, sitting, walking), early history of bruises (from bumping into things) and falls, reported "destructiveness" (dropping things or breaking toys when trying to manipulate them), difficulty with tasks requiring fine motor coordination (buttoning clothes, tying shoelaces, and handwriting) and with sports, such as ball games.

The stomachaches, "laziness," "depression," and "apathy" probably represent Johnny's efforts to avoid physical education class, tests in which handwriting is necessary, and the embarrassment of repeated failures in team sports situations. Similarly, Johnny's "bad temper" and "frustration" are probably not evidence of disturbed attention or conduct, but rather a manifestation of his motor difficulties. As often happens, it is these secondary problems that have brought him to professional attention.

One may wonder why a disorder of physical coordination appears in a classification of mental disorders. It is true that the defining features of the disorder are more physical than behavioral or psychological, and therefore one could argue that the disorder is more properly a physical, not a mental, disorder. However, it seems reasonable to classify it with the other developmental disorders of childhood because of the absence of a specific known cause and because the behavioral consequences of the disorder (e.g., irritability and avoidance behavior) are treated by mental health professionals. (From *DSM-IV Casebook.*)

Differential Diagnosis

The differential diagnosis includes medical conditions that produce coordination difficulties (such as cerebral palsy and muscular dystrophy), pervasive developmental disorders, and mental retardation. In mental retardation and in the pervasive developmental disorders, coordination usually does not stand out as a significant deficit compared with other skills. Children with neuromuscular disorders may exhibit more global muscle impairment rather than clumsiness and delayed motor milestones. Neurological examination and workups usually reveal more extensive deficits in neurological conditions than in developmental coordination disorder. Extremely hyperactive and impulsive children may be physically careless because of their high levels of motor activity. Clumsy gross and fine motor behavior and attention-deficit/hyperactivity disorder seem to be associated.

Course and Prognosis

Few data are available on the prospective longitudinal outcomes of both treated and untreated children with developmental coordination disorder. For the most part, while clumsiness may continue, some children can compensate by developing interests in other skills. Some studies suggest a favorable outcome for children who have an average or above-average intellectual capacity, in that they come up with strategies to develop friendships that do not depend upon physical activities. Clumsiness generally persists into adolescence and adult life. One study following a group of children with developmental coordination problems over a decade found that the clumsy children remained less dexterous, showed poor balance, and continued to be physically awkward. The affected children were also more likely to have both academic problems and poor self-esteem. Commonly associated features include delays in nonmotor milestones, expressive language disorder, and mixed receptive-expressive language disorder.

Treatment

The treatment of developmental coordination disorder generally includes versions of sensory-integration programs and

modified physical education. Sensory integration programs are usually administered by occupational therapists and consist of physical activities that increase awareness of motor and sensory function. For example, a child who bumps into objects often might be given the task of trying to balance on a scooter, under supervision, to improve balance and body awareness. Children who have difficulty writing letters are often given tasks to increase awareness of hand movements. Currently, many schools encourage children with coordination difficulties that affect writing to use computers to aid in writing reports and long papers.

Adaptive physical education programs are designed to help children enjoy exercise and physical activities without the pressures of team sports. These programs generally incorporate certain sports actions such as kicking a soccer ball or throwing a basketball. Children with coordination disorder may also benefit from social skills groups and other prosocial interventions. The Montessori technique (developed by Maria Montessori) may be useful with preschool children since this educational program emphasizes the development of motor skills. Secondary academic problems, emotional problems, and coexisting communication disorders should be considered in children with coordination problems as these associated problems often warrant individual treatments.

No large-scale controlled studies have reported on the effects of treatment, although small studies have suggested that exercise in rhythmic coordination, practicing motor movements, and learning to use word processing keyboards may be beneficial. Parental counseling may help reduce parents' anxiety and guilt about their child's impairment, increase their awareness, and facilitate their confidence to cope with the child.

Table 40–2
ICD-10 Diagnostic Criteria for Specific Developmental Disorder of Motor Function

A. The score on a standardized test of fine or gross motor coordination is at least 2 standard deviations below the level expected for the child's chronological age.

B. The disturbance described in Criterion A significantly interferes with academic achievement or with activities of daily living.

C. There is no diagnosable neurological disorder.

D. *Most commonly used exclusion clause.* IQ is below 70 on an individually administered standardized test.

ICD-10

According to the 10th revision of *International Statistical Classification of Diseases and Related Health Problems* (ICD-10), the main feature of specific developmental disorder of motor function (sometimes called *clumsy child syndrome*) is a "serious impairment in the development of motor coordination that is not solely explicable in terms of general intellectual retardation or of any specific congenital or acquired neurological disorder (other than the one that may be implicit in the coordination abnormality)." The motor clumsiness is usually associated with "impaired performance on visuo-spatial cognitive tasks." The ICD-10 diagnostic criteria are presented in Table 40–2.

References

Ernst M, Moolchan ET, Robinson ML. Behavioral and neural consequences of prenatal exposure to nicotine. *Am J Child Adolesc Psychiatry.* 2001;40:630.

Estil B, Whiting A. The validity of the inter- and/or intrahemispheric deficit hypothesis as an explanation of the co-occurrence of motor and language impairments. *Exp Brain Res.* 2002;143:126.

Henderson L, Rose P, Henderson S. Reaction time and movement time in children with a developmental coordination disorder. *J Child Psychol Psychiatry.* 1992;33:895.

Holsti L, Grunau RV, Whitfield MF. Developmental coordination disorder in extremely low birth weight children at nine years. *J Dev Behav Pediatr.* 2002;23:9.

Hutton JL, Pharoah PO. Effects of cognitive, motor, and sensory disabilities on survival in cerebral palsy. *Arch Dis Child.* 2002;86:84.

Kadesjo B, Gillberg C. Attention deficits and clumsiness in Swedish 7-year-old children. *Dev Med Child Neurol.* 1998;40:796.

Little RE, Northstone K, Golding J, ALSPAC Study Team. Alcohol, breastfeeding, and development at 18 months. *Pediatrics.* 2002;109:72.

Losse A, Henderson SE, Elliman D, Hall D, Knight E, Jongmans M. Clumsiness in children: do they grow out of it? A ten-year follow-up study. *Dev Med Child Neurol.* 1991;33:55.

Pine DS, Scott MR, Busner C, et al. Psychometrics of neurological soft signs. *J Am Acad Child Adolesc Psychiatry.* 1996;35:509.

Prechtl HF, Stemmer CJ. The choreiform syndrome in children. *Dev Med Child Neurol.* 1962;4:119.

Robinson RJ. Causes and associations of severe and persistent specific speech and language disorders in children. *Dev Med Child Neurol.* 1991;33:943.

Roussonis SH, Gaussen TH, Stratton R. A 2-year follow-up study of children with motor coordination problems identified at school entry age. *Child Care Health Dev.* 1987;13:377.

Smyth MM, Mason UC. Use of proprioception in normal and clumsy children. *Dev Med Child Neurol.* 1998;40:672.

Smyth TR. Abnormal clumsiness in children: a defect of motor programming? *Child Care Health Dev.* 1991;17:283.

Spagna ME, Cantwell DP, Baker L. Motor skills disorder: developmental coordination disorder. In: Sadock BJ, Sadock VA, eds. *Kaplan & Sadock's Comprehensive Textbook of Psychiatry.* 7th ed. Vol 2. Baltimore: Lippincott Williams & Wilkins; 2000:2629.

Willoughby C, Polatajko HJ. Motor problems in children with developmental coordination disorder: review of the literature. *Am J Occup Ther.* 1995;49:787.

Wilson BN, Kaplan BJ, Crawford SG, Campbell A, Dewey D. Reliability and validity of a parent questionnaire on childhood motor skills. *Am J Occup Ther.* 2000;54:484.

Wilson PH, McKenzie BE. Information processing deficits associated with developmental coordination disorder: a meta-analysis of research findings. *J Child Psychol Psychiatry.* 1998;39:829.

Wright HC, Sugden DA. The nature of developmental coordination disorder: inter- and intragroup differences. *Adapt Phys Activ Q.* 1996;13:357.

41 Communication Disorders

Spoken language is an essential part of communicating ideas, social interactions, and academic understanding. Effective communication for a child or adolescent includes proficiency in both language and speech skills. The text revision of the fourth edition of *Diagnostic and Statistical Manual of Mental Disorders* (DSM-IV-TR) includes four specific communication disorders and one residual category. Two of the communication disorders (expressive and mixed receptive-expressive communication disorder) are language disorders; the other two (phonological disorder and stuttering) are speech disorders. A child with a language disorder may have a limited vocabulary, speak in short simple sentences, and tell stories in a disorganized and incomplete manner. A child with a speech disorder may attempt to use appropriate descriptive words but has difficulty pronouncing the speech sounds correctly and may either omit sounds or pronounce sounds in an unusual way. A child with stuttering generally has acquired a normal vocabulary but speech fluency is disrupted by pauses, sound repetitions, or sound prolongations.

Language usage includes four components: phonology, grammar, semantics, and pragmatics. *Phonology* refers to the ability to produce sounds that constitute words in a given language and the skills to discriminate the various phonemes (sounds that are made by a letter or group of letters in a language). To imitate words, a child must be able to produce the sounds of a word. *Grammar* designates the organization of words and the rules for placing words in an order that makes sense in that language. *Semantics* refers to the organization of concepts and the acquisition of words themselves. A child draws from a mental list of words to produce sentences. *Pragmatics* has to do with skill in the actual use of language and the "rules" of conversation, including pausing so that a listener can answer a question and knowing when to change the topic when there is a break in a conversation. By age 2 years, toddlers may know up to 200 words, and by age 3 years, most children understand the basic rules of language and can converse effectively. Table 41–1 provides an overview of typical milestones in language and nonverbal development.

EXPRESSIVE LANGUAGE DISORDER

Expressive language disorder is present when a child's skills are below the expected levels of vocabulary, use of correct tenses, production of complex sentences, and recall of words. Language disability can be acquired at any time during childhood (e.g., secondary to a trauma or a neurological disorder) or it can be developmental; it is usually congenital, without an obvious cause. Most childhood language disorders fall in the developmental category. In either case, deficits in receptive skills (language comprehension) or expressive skills (ability to use language) can occur. Expressive language disturbance often appears in the absence of comprehension difficulties, whereas receptive dysfunction generally diminishes proficiency in the expression of language. Children with expressive language disorder alone have courses and prognoses that differ from children with mixed receptive-expressive language disorder.

In DSM-IV-TR, the diagnosis of expressive language disorder can be made in the absence of receptive language disorder. Mixed receptive-expressive language disorder is diagnosed according to DSM-IV-TR when both receptive and expressive language syndromes are present, and mixed receptive-expressive language disorder is an exclusionary criterion for expressive language disorder. In general, whenever receptive skills are impaired enough to warrant a diagnosis, expressive skills are also impaired. In DSM-IV-TR, expressive language disorder and mixed receptive-expressive language disorder are not limited to developmental language disabilities; acquired forms of language disturbances are included. To meet the criteria for expressive language disorder, patients must have scores on standardized measures of expressive language markedly below those of standardized nonverbal intelligence quotient (IQ) subtests and standardized tests of receptive language.

Epidemiology

The prevalence of expressive language disorder is estimated to be between 3 and 5 percent of all school-age children. Some have estimated the prevalence of combined language disorders to be up to 10 percent. According to DSM-IV-TR it can be as high as 15 percent in children under age 3. The disorder is two to three times more common in boys than in girls and is most prevalent among children whose relatives have a family history of phonological disorder or other communication disorders.

Comorbidity

Children with developmental language disorders such as expressive language disorder have above-average rates of comorbid psychiatric disorders. In one large study of children with speech and language disorders by Cantwell and Baker, the

Table 41–1
Normal Development of Speech, Language, and Nonverbal Skills in Children

Speech and Language Development	Nonverbal Development
1 year	
Recognizes own name	Stands alone
Follows simple directions accompanied by gestures (e.g., bye-bye)	Takes first steps with support
Speaks 1 or 2 words	Uses common objects (e.g., spoon, cup)
Mixes words and jargon sounds	Releases objects willfully
Uses communicative gestures (e.g., showing, pointing)	Searches for object in location where last seen
2 years	
Uses 200–300 words	Walks up and down stairs alone but without alternating feet
Names most common objects	Runs rhythmically but is unable to stop or start smoothly
Uses 2-word or longer phrases	Eats with a fork
Uses a few prepositions (e.g., in, on), pronouns (e.g., you, me), verb endings (e.g., -ing, -s, -ed) and plurals (-s), but not always correctly	Cooperates with adult in simple household tasks
Follows simple commands not accompanied by gestures	Enjoys play with action toys
3 years	
Uses 900–1,000 words	Rides tricycle
Creates 3- to 4-word sentences, usually with subject and verb but simple structure	Enjoys simple "make-believe" play
Follows 2-step commands	Matches primary colors
Repeats 5- to 7-syllable sentences	Balances momentarily on one foot
Speech is usually understood by family members	Shares toys with others for short periods
4 years	
Uses 1,500–1,600 words	Walks up and down stairs with alternating feet
Recounts stories and events from recent past	Hops on one foot
Understands most questions about immediate environment	Copies block letters
Uses conjunctions (e.g., if, but, because)	Role-plays with others
Speech is usually understood by strangers	Categorizes familiar objects
5 years	
Uses 2,100–2,300 words	Dresses self without assistance
Discusses feelings	Cuts own meat with knife
Understands most prepositions referring to space (e.g., above, beside, toward) and time (e.g., before, after, until)	Draws a recognizable person
Follows 3-step commands	Plays purposefully and constructively
Prints own name	Recognizes part-whole relationships
6 years	
Defines words by function and attributes	Rides a bicycle
Uses a variety of well-formed complex sentences	Throws a ball well
Uses all parts of speech (e.g., verbs, nouns, adverbs, adjectives, conjunctions, prepositions)	Sustains attention to motivating tasks
Understands letter-sound associations in reading	Enjoys competitive games
8 years	
Reads simple books for pleasure	Understands conservation of liquid, number, length, etc.
Enjoys riddles and jokes	Knows left and right of others
Verbalizes ideas and problems readily	Knows differences and similarities
Understands indirect requests (e.g., "It's hot in here" understood as request to open window)	Appreciates that others have different perspectives
Produces all speech sounds in an adultlike manner	Categorizes same object into multiple categories

Adapted from Owens RE. *Language Development: An Introduction.* 4th ed. Needham Heights, MA: Allyn & Bacon; 1996.

most common comorbid disorders were attention-deficit/hyperactivity disorder (19 percent), anxiety disorders (10 percent), and oppositional defiant disorder and conduct disorder (7 percent). Children with expressive language disorder are also at higher risk for a speech disorder, receptive difficulties, and other learning disorders. Many disorders—such as reading disorder, developmental coordination disorder, and other communication disorders—are associated with expressive language disorder. Children with expressive language disorder often have some receptive impairment, although not always significant enough for the diagnosis of mixed receptive-expressive language disorder. Delayed motor milestones and a history of

enuresis are common in children with expressive language disorder. Phonological disorder is commonly found in young children with the disorder, and neurological abnormalities have been reported in a number of children, including soft neurological signs, depressed vestibular responses, and electroencephalogram (EEG) abnormalities.

Etiology

The specific cause of developmental expressive language disorder is unknown. Subtle cerebral damage and maturational lags in cerebral development have been postulated as underlying causes. Some children with language disorders have difficulty processing information in a time-limited manner. Scant data are available on the specific brain structure of children with language disorder, but limited magnetic resonance imaging (MRI) studies suggest that language disorders are associated with a loss of the normal left–right brain asymmetry in the perisylvian and planum temporale regions. Results of one small MRI study suggested possible inversion of brain asymmetry (right>left). Left-handedness or ambilaterality appears to be associated with expressive language problems. There is good evidence showing that language disorders occur with higher frequency in certain families. Genetic factors have been suspected to play a role, and several studies of twins show significant concordance for monozygotic twins for developmental language disorders. Environmental and educational factors are also postulated to contribute to developmental language disorders.

Table 41–2
DSM-IV-TR Diagnostic Criteria for Expressive Language Disorder

A. The scores obtained from standardized individually administered measures of expressive language development are substantially below those obtained from standardized measures of both nonverbal intellectual capacity and receptive language development. The disturbance may be manifest clinically by symptoms that include having a markedly limited vocabulary, making errors in tense, or having difficulty recalling words or producing sentences with developmentally appropriate length or complexity.
B. The difficulties with expressive language interfere with academic or occupational achievement or with social communication.
C. Criteria are not met for mixed receptive-expressive language disorder or a pervasive developmental disorder.
D. If mental retardation, a speech-motor or sensory deficit, or environmental deprivation is present, the language difficulties are in excess of those usually associated with these problems.

Coding note: If a speech-motor or sensory deficit or a neurological condition is present, code the condition on Axis III.

From American Psychiatric Association. *Diagnostic and Statistical Manual of Mental Disorders.* 4th ed. Text rev. Washington, DC: American Psychiatric Association; copyright 2000, with permission.

Diagnosis

Expressive language disorder is present when a child has a selective deficit in language skills and is functioning well in nonverbal areas and in receptive skills. Markedly below-age-level verbal or sign language, accompanied by a low score on standardized expressive verbal tests, is diagnostic of expressive language disorder (Table 41–2). The disorder is not caused by a pervasive developmental disorder, and a child with an expressive language disorder usually develops some nonverbal strategies to aid in socialization. A child with an expressive language disorder exhibits the following features: limited vocabulary, simple grammar, and variable articulation. "Inner language" or the appropriate use of toys and household objects is present.

To confirm the diagnosis, a child is given standardized expressive language and nonverbal intelligence tests. Observations of children's verbal and sign language patterns in various settings (e.g., school yard, classroom, home, and playroom) and during interactions with other children help ascertain the severity and specific areas of a child's impairment and aid in early detection of behavioral and emotional complications. Family history should include the presence or absence of expressive language disorder among relatives.

Clinical Features

Children with expressive language disorders may be ostracized by peers because of their poor ability to explain what they are talking about. They may appear vague when telling a story and use many filler words such as *stuff* and *things* instead of naming specific objects.

The essential feature of expressive language disorder is marked impairment in the development of age-appropriate expressive language, which results in the use of verbal or sign language markedly below the expected level in view of a child's nonverbal intellectual capacity. Language understanding (decoding) skills remain relatively intact. When severe, the disorder becomes recognizable by about the age of 18 months, when a child fails to utter spontaneously or even echo single words or sounds. Even simple words, such as *Mama* and *Dada*, are absent from the child's active vocabulary, and the child points or uses gestures to indicate desires. The child seems to want to communicate, maintains eye contact, relates well to the mother, and enjoys games such as pat-a-cake and peekaboo. The child's vocabulary is severely limited. At 18 months the child may be limited to pointing to common objects when they are named.

When a child with expressive language disorder begins to speak, the language impairment gradually becomes apparent. Articulation is often immature; numerous articulation errors occur but are inconsistent, particularly with such sounds as *th, r, s, z, y,* and *l,* which are either omitted or are substituted for other sounds.

By the age of 4 years, most children with expressive language disorder can speak in short phrases but may have difficulty retaining new words. After beginning to speak, they acquire language more slowly than normal children. Their use of various grammatical structures is also markedly below the age-expected level, and their developmental milestones may be slightly delayed.

Emotional problems involving poor self-image, frustration, and depression may develop in school-age children.

Jennifer was a sociable, active 5-year-old who was diagnosed with expressive language disorder. She often played with her best friend, Sarah. One day, in the course of pretend play, each girl told the story of Little Red Riding Hood to her doll. Sarah's story began: "Little Red Riding Hood was taking a basket of food to her grandmother who was sick. A bad wolf stopped Riding Hood in the forest. He tried to get the basket away from her but she wouldn't give it to him." By contrast, Jennifer's story illustrated her marked difficulties in verbal expression: "Riding Hood going to grandma house. Her taking food. Bad wolf in a bed. Riding Hood say, what big ears, grandma? Hear you, dear. What big eyes, grandma? See you, dear. What big mouth, grandma? Eat you all up!"

Many features of Jennifer's story were characteristic of children with expressive language disorder, including the short, incomplete sentences; simple sentence structure; omission of grammatical function words (e.g., *is, the*) and endings (e.g., possessive *–'s*, present tense verb *–s*); problems in question formation; and incorrect use of pronouns (e.g., *her* for *she*). Nonetheless, testing by methods that did not require verbal responding showed clearly that Jennifer understood the details and plot of the Riding Hood tale as well as Sarah did. Jennifer also demonstrated adequate comprehensive skills in her kindergarten classroom, where she readily followed the teacher's complex, multistep verbal instructions (e.g., "Before you get ready for recess, make sure that you draw a green circle around all the animals, put your library books under your chair, and line up at the back of the room). (Courtesy of Carla J. Johnson, Ph.D., and Joseph H. Beitchman, M.D.)

Differential Diagnosis

Language disorders are associated with many other psychiatric disorders, and thus the language disorder itself may be difficult to separate from other difficulties. In mental retardation, patients have an overall impairment in intellectual functioning, as shown by below-normal intelligence test scores in all areas, but the nonverbal intellectual capacity and functioning of children with expressive language disorder are within normal limits. In mixed receptive-expressive language disorder, language comprehension (decoding) is markedly below the expected age-appropriate level, whereas in expressive language disorder, language comprehension remains within normal limits.

In pervasive developmental disorders, in addition to the cardinal cognitive characteristics, affected children have no inner language, symbolic or imagery play, appropriate use of gesture, or capacity to form warm and meaningful social relationships. Moreover, children show little or no frustration with the inability to communicate verbally. In contrast, all these characteristics are present in children with expressive language disorder.

Children with acquired aphasia or dysphasia have a history of early normal language development; the disordered language had its onset after a head trauma or other neurological disorder (e.g., a seizure disorder). Children with selective mutism have a history of normal language development. Often these children will speak only in front of family members (e.g., mother, father, and siblings). Children affected by selective mutism are socially anxious and withdrawn outside the family.

Pathology and Laboratory Examination

Children with speech and language disorders should have an audiogram to rule out hearing loss.

Course and Prognosis

The prognosis for expressive language disorder is related to the severity of the disorder. Studies of "late talkers" concur that 50 to 80 percent of these children master language skills that are within the expected level during the preschool years. Most children who begin to talk later than average but catch up during preschool years are not at high risk to develop further language or learning disorders. Outcome of expressive language disorder is influenced by other comorbid disorders. If children do not develop mood disorders or disruptive behavior problems, the prognosis is better. The rapidity and extent of recovery depend on the severity of the disorder, the child's motivation to participate in therapy, and the timely institution of speech and other therapeutic interventions. The presence or absence of other factors—such as moderate to severe hearing loss, mild mental retardation, and severe emotional problems—also affects the prognosis for recovery. As many as 50 percent of children with mild expressive language disorder recover spontaneously without any sign of language impairment, but children with severe expressive language disorder may later display features of mild to moderate language impairment.

Recent literature has shown that children who demonstrate poor comprehension, poor articulation, or poor academic performance tend to continue to have problems in these areas at follow-up 7 years later. There is also an association between particular language impairment profiles and persistent mood and behavior problems. Children who have poor comprehension associated with expressive difficulties seem to be the most socially isolated and impaired with respect to peer relationships.

Expressive language level and many nonverbal and communication skills are strongly related in children with language impairment. Expressive language may be seen as an index of general development or as a marker of social and other communication skills. Especially in preschool age groups, expressive language appears to be related to social and nonverbal communication skills as much as it is simply a measure of knowledge of words.

Treatment

Treatment for expressive language disorder is generally initiated when it persists after the preschool years. Various techniques have been used to help a child improve use of such parts of speech as pronouns, correct tenses, and question forms. Direct interventions use a speech and language pathologist who works directly with the child. Mediated interventions, in which a speech and language professional teaches a child's teacher or parent to promote therapeutic language techniques have also been efficacious. Language therapy is often aimed at using words to improve communication strategies and social interactions as well. Such therapy consists of behaviorally reinforced

exercises and practice with phonemes (sound units), vocabulary, and sentence construction. The goal is to increase the number of phrases by using block-building methods and conventional speech therapies.

Psychotherapy may be useful for children whose language impairment has affected their self-esteem, insofar as it can be used as a positive model for more effective communication and broadening social skills. Supportive parental counseling may be indicated in some cases. Parents may need help to reduce intrafamilial tensions arising from difficulties in rearing language-disordered children and to increase their awareness and understanding of the disorder.

MIXED RECEPTIVE-EXPRESSIVE LANGUAGE DISORDER

In mixed receptive-expressive language disorder, children are impaired in both understanding and expressing language. DSM-IV-TR combines receptive and expressive language disorders. The implication is that clinically significant receptive language impairment is believed to be accompanied by expressive language dysfunction. According to DSM-IV-TR, it is advised not to diagnose receptive language disorder in the absence of expressive language disorder.

The essential features of mixed receptive-expressive language disorder are shown by scores on standardized tests; both receptive (comprehension) and expressive language development scores fall substantially below those obtained from standardized measures of nonverbal intellectual capacity. Language difficulties must be severe enough to impair academic achievement or daily social communication. A patient with this disorder must not meet the criteria for a pervasive developmental disorder, and the language dysfunctions must exceed those usually associated with mental retardation and other neurological and sensory-deficit syndromes.

Epidemiology

Mixed receptive-expressive language disorder is believed to occur in about 3 percent of school-age children, and the combination is less common than expressive language disorder alone. Mixed receptive-expressive language disorder is believed to be at least twice as prevalent in boys as in girls.

Comorbidity

Children with mixed receptive-expressive disorder are at high risk for additional speech and language disorders, learning disorders, and additional psychiatric disorders. About half of children with this disorder also have pronunciation difficulties leading to phonological disorder, and about half also have reading disorder. The above rates are significantly higher than the comorbidity found in children with expressive language disorder alone. Attention-deficit/hyperactivity disorder is present in at least one third of children with mixed receptive-expressive language disorder.

Etiology

The cause of mixed receptive-expressive language disorder is unknown. As with expressive language disorder alone, there is evidence of familial aggregation of mixed receptive-expressive language disorder. Genetic contribution to this disorder is implicated by twin studies, but no mode of genetic transmission has been proved. Some studies of children with various speech and language disorders have also shown cognitive deficits, particularly slower processing of tasks involving naming objects, as well as fine motor tasks. Slower myelinization of neural pathways has been hypothesized to account for the slow processing found in children with developmental language disorders. Several studies suggest an underlying impairment of auditory discrimination, as most children with the disorder are more responsive to environmental sounds than to speech sounds.

Diagnosis

Children with mixed receptive-expressive language disorder develop language more slowly than their peers and have trouble understanding conversations that peers can follow. In mixed receptive-expressive language disorder, receptive dysfunction coexists with expressive dysfunction. Therefore, standardized tests for both receptive and expressive language abilities must be given to anyone suspected of having mixed receptive-expressive language disorder.

A markedly below-expected level of comprehension of verbal or sign language with intact age-appropriate nonverbal intellectual capacity, confirmation of language difficulties by standardized receptive language tests, and the absence of pervasive developmental disorders confirm the diagnosis of mixed receptive-expressive language disorder (Table 41–3).

Clinical Features

The essential clinical feature of the disorder is significant impairment in both language comprehension and language expression. In the mixed disorder, the expressive impairments are similar to those of expressive language disorder but can be

Table 41–3
DSM-IV-TR Diagnostic Criteria for Mixed Receptive-Expressive Language Disorder

A. The scores obtained from a battery of standardized individually administered measures of both receptive and expressive language development are substantially below those obtained from standardized measures of nonverbal intellectual capacity. Symptoms include those for expressive language disorder as well as difficulty understanding words, sentences, or specific types of words, such as spatial terms.

B. The difficulties with receptive and expressive language significantly interfere with academic or occupational achievement or with social communication.

C. Criteria are not met for a pervasive developmental disorder.

D. If mental retardation, a speech-motor or sensory deficit, or environmental deprivation is present, the language difficulties are in excess of those usually associated with these problems.

Coding note: If a speech-motor or sensory deficit or a neurological condition is present, code the condition on Axis III.

From American Psychiatric Association. *Diagnostic and Statistical Manual of Mental Disorders.* 4th ed. Text rev. Washington, DC: American Psychiatric Association; copyright 2000, with permission.

more severe. The clinical features of the receptive component of the disorder typically appear before the age of 4 years. Severe forms are apparent by the age of 2 years; mild forms may not become evident until age 7 (second grade) or older, when language becomes complex. Children with mixed receptive-expressive language disorder show markedly delayed and below-normal ability to comprehend (decode) verbal or sign language, although they have age-appropriate nonverbal intellectual capacity. In most cases of receptive dysfunction, verbal or sign expression (encoding) of language is also impaired. The clinical features of mixed receptive-expressive language disorder in children between the ages of 18 and 24 months result from a child's failure to utter a single phoneme spontaneously or to mimic another person's words.

Many children with mixed receptive-expressive language disorder have auditory sensory difficulties or cannot process visual symbols, such as explaining the meaning of a picture. They have deficits in integrating both auditory and visual symbols—for example, recognizing the basic common attributes of a toy truck and a toy passenger car. Whereas at 18 months, a child with expressive language disorder only can comprehend simple commands and can point to familiar household objects when told to do so, a child of the same age with mixed receptive-expressive language disorder cannot either point to common objects or obey simple commands. A child with mixed receptive-expressive language disorder usually appears to be deaf, but the child can hear. He or she responds normally to nonlanguage sounds from the environment but not to spoken language. If the child later starts to speak, the speech contains numerous articulation errors, such as omissions, distortions, and substitutions of phonemes. Language acquisition is much slower for children with mixed receptive-expressive language disorder than for normal children.

Children with mixed receptive-expressive language disorder have difficulty recalling early visual and auditory memories and recognizing and reproducing symbols in proper sequence. In some cases bilateral EEG abnormalities are seen. Some children with mixed receptive-expressive language disorder have a partial hearing defect for true tones, an increased threshold of auditory arousal, and an inability to localize sound sources. Seizure disorders and reading disorder are more common among the relatives of children with mixed receptive-expressive language disorder than they are in the general population.

Most children with mixed receptive-expressive language disorder are impaired socially and in terms of nonverbal communication. This impairment causes a variety of additional difficulties and often results in poor self-esteem and feelings of inferiority that in turn can further prevent the child from succeeding in the usual developmental tasks.

Pathology and Laboratory Examination

An audiogram is indicated for all children thought to have mixed receptive-expressive language disorder, to rule out or confirm the presence of deafness and to determine the types of auditory deficits. A history of the child and family and observation of the child in various settings help to clarify the diagnosis.

Differential Diagnosis

Children with significant mixed receptive-expressive language disorder have a deficit in language comprehension. This deficit may at first be overlooked, since the expressive language deficit may be more obvious. In expressive language disorder alone, comprehension of spoken language (decoding) remains within age norms. Children with phonological disorder or stuttering have normal expressive and receptive language competence, despite the speech impairments. Hearing impairment should be ruled out.

Most children with mixed receptive-expressive language disorder have a history of variable and inconsistent responses to sounds; they respond more often to environmental sounds than to speech sounds (Table 41–4). Mental retardation, selective mutism, acquired aphasia, and pervasive developmental disorders should also be ruled out. Hearing impairment, pervasive developmental disorders, and severe environmental deprivation may contribute significantly to language impairment.

Course and Prognosis

The overall prognosis for mixed receptive-expressive language disorder is less favorable than that for expressive language disorder alone. When the mixed disorder is identified in a young child, it is usually severe, and the short-term prognosis is poor. Language develops at a rapid rate in early childhood, and young children with the disorder may appear to be falling behind. In view of the likelihood of comorbid learning disorders and other mental disorders, the prognosis is guarded. Young children with severe mixed receptive-expressive language disorder are likely to have learning disorders in the future. In children with mild versions, mixed disorder may not be identified for several years, and the disruption in everyday life may be less overwhelming than that in severe forms of the disorder. Over the long run, some children with mixed receptive-expressive language disorder achieve close to normal language functions. The prognosis for children who acquire mixed receptive-expressive language disorder varies widely and depends on the nature and severity of the damage.

Treatment

A comprehensive speech and language evaluation is recommended for children with mixed receptive-expressive language disorder, before embarking on a speech and language remediation program. Some language therapists favor a low-stimuli setting, in which children are given individual linguistic instruction. Others recommend that speech and language instruction be integrated into a varied setting with several children who are taught several language structures simultaneously. Often, a child with mixed receptive-expressive language disorder will benefit from a small, special-educational setting that allows more individualized learning.

Psychotherapy may be helpful for children with mixed receptive-expressive language disorder who have associated emotional and behavioral problems. Particular attention should be paid to evaluating the child's self-image and social skills. Family counseling in which parents and children can develop more effective, less frustrating means of communicating may be beneficial.

PHONOLOGICAL DISORDER

Children with a phonological disorder may be mistaken for younger children because of their difficulties in producing speech sounds correctly. Phonological disorder includes poor sound pro-

Table 41–4
Differential Diagnosis of Language Disorders

	Hearing Impairment	Mental Retardation	Infantile Autism	Expressive Language Disorder	Mixed Receptive-Expressive Language Disorder	Selective Mutism	Phonological Disorder
Language comprehension	–	–	–	+	–	+	+
Expressive language	–	–	–	–	–	Variable	+
Audiogram	–	+	+	+	Variable	+	+
Articulation	–	–	– (Variable)	– (Variable)	– (Variable)	+	–
Inner language	+	+ (Limited)	–	+	+ (Slightly limited)	+	+
Uses gestures	+	+ (Limited)	–	+	+	+ (Variable)	+
Echoes	–	+	+ (Inappropriate)	+	+	+	+
Attends to sounds	Loud or low frequency only	+	–	+	Variable	+	+
Watches faces	+	+	–	+	+	+	+
Performance	+	–	+	+	+	+	+

+, normal; –, abnormal.
Courtesy of Lorian Baker, Ph.D., and Dennis Cantwell, M.D.

duction, substitutions of one sound for another, and omissions of sounds that are part of words. The diagnosis of a phonological disorder is made by comparing the skills of a given child with the expected skill level of others of the same age. The disorder results in errors in whole words due to incorrect pronunciation of consonants, substitution of one sound for another, omission of entire phonemes, and in some cases dysarthria (slurred speech due to incoordination of speech muscles) or dyspraxia (difficulty planning and executing speech). Speech sound development is believed to be based on both linguistic and motor development that must be integrated to produce sounds. According to DSM-IV-TR, if mental retardation, a speech-motor or sensory deficit, or environmental deprivation is present, the language dysfunction must exceed that associated with those problems.

Components of phonological disorder such as dysarthria and dyspraxia, are more likely to have a neurological basis. Developmental articulation disorder, however, is the most common phonological disorder in children. Developmental phonological disorder, characterized by frequent misarticulation, sound substitution, and speech sound omission, gives the impression of "baby talk." The developmental form of this disorder is not caused by anatomical, structural, physiological, auditory, or neurological abnormalities. It varies from mild to severe and results in speech that ranges from completely intelligible to unintelligible.

Epidemiology

The reported prevalence rates of phonological disorders in children have varied because of the age of the children surveyed and the methods used to identify the disorder. Several studies have found the prevalence rates of developmental phonological disorder to be 7 to 8 percent in children under 12 years. The studies further indicate that about 5 percent of children over the age of 8 years persist with distortions of certain speech sounds. The disorder is 2 to 3 times more common in boys than in girls. It is also more common among first-degree relatives of patients with the disorder than in the general population. According to DSM-IV-TR the prevalence falls to 0.5 percent by mid- to late adolescence.

Comorbidity

More than half of children with developmental phonological disorder have some difficulty with expressive language. Disorders commonly present with phonological disorder are expressive language disorder, mixed receptive-expressive language disorder, reading disorder, and developmental coordination disorder. Enuresis may also accompany the disorder. A delay in reaching speech milestones (such as first word and first sentence) has been reported in some children with phonological disorder, but most children with the disorder begin speaking at the appropriate age. Children with phonological disorder who also have language disorders are at greatest risk for attentional problems and learning disorders. Children with phonological disorder who do not have language dysfunction have lower risk of comorbid psychiatric or behavioral problems.

Etiology

The causes of phonological disturbance are likely to include multiple variables including perinatal problems, genetic factors,

auditory processing problems, hearing impairment, and structural abnormalities related to speech. A developmental lag or maturational delay in the neurological process underlying speech has been postulated in some cases. The likelihood of a subtle brain abnormality is supported by the observation that children with phonological disorder are also more likely to manifest "soft neurological signs" as well as additional disorders, including receptive and expressive language difficulties and a higher-than-expected rate of reading disorder. Genetic factors are implicated by data from twin studies that show concordance rates for monozygotic twins that are higher than chance.

Articulation disorders caused by structural or mechanical problems are quite rare. Phonological disorders caused by neurological impairment can be divided into dysarthria and apraxia or dyspraxia. Dysarthria results from an impairment in the neural mechanisms regulating the muscular control of speech. This may occur in congenital conditions such as cerebral palsy, muscular dystrophy, or head injury or infectious processes. Apraxia or dyspraxia is characterized by difficulty in the execution of speech even when there is no obvious paralysis or weakness of the muscles used in speech.

Environmental factors may play a role in developmental phonological disorder, but constitutional factors seem to make the most significant contribution. The high proportion of phonological disorder in certain families implies a genetic component in the development of this disorder. Poor motor coordination, laterality, and handedness are not associated with phonological disorder.

Diagnosis

The essential feature of phonological disorder is a child's delay or failure to produce developmentally expected speech sounds, especially consonants, resulting in sound omissions, substitutions, and distortions of phonemes. A rough guideline for clinical assessment of children's articulation is that normal 3-year-olds correctly articulate *m, n, ng, b, p, h, t, k, q,* and *d;* normal 4-year-olds correctly articulate *f, y, ch, sh,* and *z;* and normal 5-years-olds correctly articulate *th, s,* and *r.*

Phonological disorder cannot be attributed to structural or neurological abnormalities, and it is accompanied by normal language development. The DSM-IV-TR diagnostic criteria for phonological disorder are given in Table 41–5.

Table 41–5
DSM-IV-TR Diagnostic Criteria for Phonological Disorder

A. Failure to use developmentally expected speech sounds that are appropriate for age and dialect (e.g., errors in sound production, use, representation, or organization such as, but not limited to, substitutions of one sound for another [use of /t/ for target /k/ sound] or omissions of sounds such as final consonants).

B. The difficulties in speech sound production interfere with academic or occupational achievement or with social communication.

C. If mental retardation, a speech-motor or sensory deficit, or environmental deprivation is present, the speech difficulties are in excess of those usually associated with these problems.

Coding note: If a speech-motor or sensory deficit or a neurological condition is present, code the condition on Axis III.

From American Psychiatric Association. *Diagnostic and Statistical Manual of Mental Disorders.* 4th ed. Text rev. Washington, DC: American Psychiatric Association; copyright 2000, with permission.

Clinical Features

Children with phonological disorder are delayed in, or incapable of, producing speech sounds that are expected for their age, intelligence, and dialect. The sounds are often substitutions—for example, the use of *t* instead of *k*—and omissions, such as leaving off the final consonants of words. Phonological disorder can be recognized in early childhood. In severe cases the disorder is first recognized at about 3 years of age. In less severe cases the disorder may not be apparent until the age of 6 years. A child's articulation is judged disordered when it is significantly behind that of most children at the same age level, intellectual level, and educational level.

In very mild cases, a single speech sound (i.e., phoneme) may be affected. When a single phoneme is affected, it is usually one that is acquired late in normal language acquisition. The speech sounds most frequently misarticulated are also those acquired late in the developmental sequence, including *r, sh, th, f, z, l,* and *ch.* In severe cases and in young children, sounds such as *b, m, t, d, n,* and *h* may be mispronounced. One or many speech sounds may be affected, but vowel sounds are not among them.

Children with phonological disorder cannot articulate certain phonemes correctly and may distort, substitute, or even omit the affected phonemes. With omissions, the phonemes are absent entirely—for example, *bu* for *blue, ca* for *car,* or *whaa*? for *what's that*? With substitutions, difficult phonemes are replaced with incorrect ones—for example, *wabbit* for *rabbit, fum* for *thumb,* or *whath dat*? for *what's that*? With distortions, the correct phoneme is approximated but is articulated incorrectly. Rarely, additions (usually of the vowel *uh*) occur—for example, *puhretty* for *pretty, what's uh that uh*? for *what's that*?

Omissions are thought to be the most serious type of misarticulation, with substitutions the next most serious, and distortions the least serious type. Omissions are most frequent in the speech of young children and usually occur at the ends of words or in clusters of consonants (*ka* for *car, scisso* for *scissors*). Distortions, which are found mainly in the speech of older children, result in a sound that is not part of the speaker's dialect. Distortions may be the last type of misarticulation remaining in the speech of children whose articulation problems have mostly remitted. The most common types of distortions are the *lateral slip*—in which a child pronounces *s* sounds with the airstream going across the tongue, producing a whistling effect—and the palatal\lisp—in which the *s* sound, formed with the tongue too close to the palate, produces a *ssh* sound effect.

The misarticulations of children with phonological disorder are often inconsistent and random. A phoneme may be pronounced correctly one time and incorrectly another time. Misarticulations are most common at the ends of words, in long and syntactically complex sentences, and during rapid speech.

Omissions, distortions, and substitutions also occur normally in the speech of young children learning to talk. But, whereas young, normally speaking children soon replace these misarticulations, children with phonological disorder do not. Even as children with phonological disorder grow and finally acquire the correct phoneme, they may use it

only in newly acquired words and may not correct the words learned earlier that they have been mispronouncing for some time.

Most children eventually outgrow phonological disorder, usually by the third grade. After the fourth grade, however, spontaneous recovery is unlikely, and so it is important to try to remediate the disorder before the development of complications. Often, beginning kindergarten or school precipitates the improvement when recovery from phonological disorder is spontaneous. Speech therapy is clearly indicated for children who have not shown spontaneous improvement by the third or fourth grade. Speech therapy should be initiated at an early age for children whose articulation is significantly unintelligible and who are clearly troubled by their inability to speak clearly.

Children with phonological disorder may have various concomitant social, emotional, and behavioral problems, particularly when there are comorbid expressive language problems. Children with expressive language disorder and severe articulation impairment and those whose disorder is chronic and nonremitting are the ones most likely to suffer from psychiatric problems.

Sasha was a talkative, likable 3-year-old whose speech was virtually unintelligible. He had normal hearing and language comprehension skills. No firm conclusion about his level of expressive language development could be made because he was so difficult to understand. He did, however, seem to be producing multiword utterances. Sasha produced only a small number of early-developing consonants (*lml, lnl, ldl, ltl, lbl, lhl, lwl*), vowels (*leel, lahlm, lool*), and syllable shapes (V, CV, CVCV). As a result, many of his spoken words were indistinguishable from each other (e.g., he said "bahbah" for *baby bottle* and *bubble*; he used "nee" for *knee, need*, and *Anita* [his sister]). Moreover, he never produced consonant sounds at the end of words or used consonant cluster sequences (e.g., *ltr-l, lst-l, l-ntl, l-mpl*). On occasion, Sasha reacted with frustration and tantrums to his difficulties making himself understood. (Courtesy of Carla J. Johnson, Ph.D., and Joseph H. Beitchman, M.D.)

Differential Diagnosis

The differential diagnosis of phonological disorder includes a careful determination of the severity of the symptoms and possible medical conditions that might be producing the symptoms. First, the clinician must determine that the misarticulations are severe enough to be considered impairing, rather than a normative developmental process of learning to speak. Second, the clinician must determine that no physical abnormalities account for the articulation errors and must rule out neurological disorders that may cause dysarthria, hearing impairment, mental retardation, and pervasive developmental disorders. Third, the clinician must obtain an evaluation of receptive and expressive language to determine that the speech difficulty is not solely attributable to the above disorders.

Neurological, oral structural, and audiometric examinations may be necessary to rule out physical factors that cause certain types of articulation abnormalities. Children with dysarthria, a disorder caused by structural or neurological abnormalities, differ from children with developmental phonological disorder in that dysarthria is less likely to remit spontaneously and may be more difficult to remediate. Drooling, slow, or uncoordinated motor behavior, abnormal chewing or swallowing, and awkward or slow protrusion and retraction of the tongue indicate dysarthria. A slow rate of speech also indicates dysarthria (Table 41–6).

Course and Prognosis

Spontaneous remission of symptoms is common in children whose misarticulations involve only a few phonemes. Children who persist in exhibiting articulation problems after the age of 5 years may be experiencing a myriad of other speech and language impairments, so that a comprehensive evaluation may be indicated at this time. Children over the age of 5 with articulation problems are at higher risk for auditory perceptual problems. Spontaneous recovery is rare after the age of 8 years.

Treatment

Speech therapy, provided by a speech and language therapist is considered the most successful treatment for most phonological errors. Speech therapy is indicated when a child's articulation intelligibility is poor; when an affected child is over 8 years of age; when a speech problem apparently causes problems with peers, learning, and self-image; when the disorder is so severe that many consonants are misarticulated; and when errors involve omissions and substitutions of phonemes, rather than distortions.

Children with persistent articulation problems are likely to be teased or ostracized by peers and may become isolated and demoralized. Therefore, it is important to give support to children with phonological disorders and whenever possible to support prosocial activities and social interactions with peers. Parental counseling and monitoring of child-peer relationships and school behavior can help minimize the social impairment with speech and language disorder.

STUTTERING

Stuttering is a condition characterized by involuntary disruptions in the flow of speech. Various speech motor events may occur that result in dysfluency in speaking. Stuttering may consist of one or more of the following phenomena: sound repetitions, prolongations, interjections, pauses within words, observable word substitutions to avoid blocking, and audible or silent blocking. Severe stuttering typically contains secondary features that may include disordered breathing, lip pursing, and tongue clicking. Additional behaviors such as facial grimacing, head jerks, or abnormal body movements are not uncommon during the disrupted speech. The disorder usually originates in childhood.

There has been controversy among speech and language experts as to whether stuttering should be considered an independent entity or part of a broader speech and language disorder. Some question whether stuttering should be considered a psychiatric condition at all. Many children who stutter do endure significant psychological distress, and stuttering does cause impairment in everyday life for many children with this condition.

Table 41–6
Differential Diagnosis of Phonological Dysfunctions

Criteria	Phonological Dysfunction Due to Structural or Neurological Abnormalities (Dysarthria)	Phonological Dysfunction Due to Hearing Impairment	Phonological Disorder	Phonological Dysfunction Associated with Mental Retardation, Infantile Autism, Developmental Dysphasia, Acquired Aphasia, or Deafness
Language development	Within normal limits	Within normal limits unless hearing impairment is serious	Within normal limits	Not within normal limits
Examination	Possible abnormalities of lips, tongue, or palate; muscular weakness, incoordination, or disturbance of vegetative functions, such as sucking or chewing	Hearing impairment shown on audiometric testing	Normal	
Rate of speech	Slow; marked deterioration of articulation with increased rate	Normal	Normal; possible deterioration of articulation with increased rate	
Phonemes affected	Any phonemes, even vowels	*F, th, sh,* and *s*	*R, sh, th, ch, dg, j, f, v, s,* and *z* are most commonly affected	

Courtesy of Lorian Baker, Ph.D., and Dennis Cantwell, M.D.

Epidemiology

In the general population the prevalence of stuttering is about 1 percent. Stuttering tends to be most common in young children and has often resolved spontaneously in older children. The typical age of onset is 2 to 7 years old with a peak at age 5. It has been estimated that up to 3 to 4 percent of individuals may have stuttered at some time in their lives. Approximately 80 percent of young children who stutter are likely to have a spontaneous remission over time. According to DSM-IV-TR, it dips to 0.8 percent by adolescence. Stuttering affects about three to four males for every female. The disorder is significantly more common among family members of affected children than in the general population. According to DSM-IV-TR, for male persons who stutter, 20 percent of their male children and 10 percent of their female children will also stutter.

Comorbidity

Very young children who stutter typically show some delay in the development of language and articulation without additional disorders of speech and language. Preschoolers and school-age children who stutter exhibit an increased incidence of social anxiety, school refusal, and other anxiety symptoms. Older children who stutter also do not necessarily have comorbid speech and language disorders, but often manifest anxiety symptoms and disorders. When stuttering persists into adolescence, social isolation occurs at higher rates than in the general adolescent population. Stuttering is also associated with a variety of abnormal motor movements, upper body tics, and facial grimaces. Other disorders that coexist with stuttering include phonological disorder, expressive language disorder, mixed receptive-expressive language disorder, and attention-deficit/hyperactivity disorder.

Etiology

The precise cause of stuttering is unknown, and various theories have been proposed. In the past, psychoanalytic theory suggested that stuttering occurs as a response to conflicts, fears, or neurosis. No evidence indicates that anxiety or conflicts cause stuttering or that persons who stutter have more psychiatric disturbances than those with other forms of speech and language disorders. Stuttering, however, may be exacerbated by certain stressful situations.

Other theories about the cause of stuttering include organic models and learning models. Organic models include those that focus on incomplete lateralization or abnormal cerebral dominance. Several studies using electroencephalography found that stuttering males had right-hemispheric alpha suppression across stimulus words and tasks; nonstutterers had left-hemispheric suppression. Some studies of stutterers have noted an overrepresentation of left-handedness and ambidexterity. Twin studies and striking gender differences in stuttering indicate that stuttering has some genetic basis.

Learning theories about the cause of stuttering include the semantogenic theory, in which stuttering is basically a learned response to normative early childhood dysfluencies. Another learning model focuses on classical conditioning, in which the stuttering becomes conditioned to environmental factors. In the cybernetic model, speech is viewed as a process that depends on appropriate feedback for regulation; stuttering is hypothesized to occur because of a breakdown in the feedback loop. The observations that stuttering is reduced by white noise and that delayed auditory feedback produces stuttering in normal speakers lend support to the feedback theory.

The motor functioning of some children who stutter appears to be delayed or slightly abnormal. The observation of difficulties in speech planning exhibited by some children who stutter suggests that higher-level cognitive dysfunction may contribute

to stuttering. Although children who stutter do not routinely exhibit other speech and language disorders, family members of these children often exhibit an increased incidence of a variety of speech and language disorders. Stuttering is most likely to be caused by a set of interacting variables that include both genetic and environmental factors.

Diagnosis

The diagnosis of stuttering is not difficult when the clinical features are apparent and well developed and each of the four phases (described in the next section) can be readily recognized. Diagnostic difficulties may arise when one is trying to determine the existence of stuttering in young children, as some preschool children experience transient dysfluency. It may not be clear whether the nonfluent pattern is part of normal speech and language development or whether it represents the initial stage in the development of stuttering. If incipient stuttering is suspected, referral to a speech pathologist is indicated. Table 41–7 presents the DSM-IV-TR diagnostic criteria for stuttering.

Clinical Features

Stuttering usually appears between the ages of 18 months and 9 years, with two sharp peaks of onset between the ages of 2 to 3 1/2 years and 5 to 7 years. Some, but not all, stutterers have other speech and language problems, such as phonological disorder and expressive language disorder. Stuttering does not begin suddenly; it typically develops over weeks or months with a repetition of initial consonants, whole words that are usually the first words of a phrase, or long words. As the disorder progresses, the repetitions become more frequent, with consistent stuttering on the most important words or phrases. Even after it develops, stuttering may be absent during oral readings, singing, and talking to pets or inanimate objects.

Four gradually evolving phases in the development of stuttering have been identified:

- Phase 1 occurs during the preschool period. Initially, the difficulty tends to be episodic and appears for weeks or months between long interludes of normal speech. A high percentage of recovery from these periods of stuttering occurs. During this phase, children stutter most often when excited or upset, when they seem to have a great deal to say, and under other conditions of communicative pressure.
- Phase 2 usually occurs in the elementary school years. The disorder is chronic, with few if any intervals of normal speech. Affected children become aware of their speech difficulties and regard themselves as stutterers. In phase 2, the stuttering occurs mainly with the major parts of speech—nouns, verbs, adjectives, and adverbs.
- Phase 3 usually appears after the age of 8 and up to adulthood, most often in late childhood and early adolescence. During phase 3, stuttering comes and goes largely in response to specific situations, such as reciting in class, speaking to strangers, making purchases in stores, and using the telephone. Some words and sounds are regarded as more difficult than others.
- Phase 4 typically appears in late adolescence and adulthood.

Stutterers show a vivid, fearful anticipation of stuttering. They fear words, sounds, and situations. Word substitutions and circumlocutions are common. Stutterers avoid situations requiring speech and show other evidence of fear and embarrassment.

Stutterers may have associated clinical features: vivid, fearful anticipation of stuttering, with avoidance of particular words, sounds, or situations in which stuttering is anticipated; eye blinks; tics; and tremors of the lips or jaw. Frustration, anxiety, and depression are common among those with chronic stuttering.

Table 41–7
DSM-IV-TR Diagnostic Criteria for Stuttering

A. Disturbance in the normal fluency and time patterning of speech (inappropriate for the individual's age), characterized by frequent occurrences of one or more of the following:
   (1) sound and syllable repetitions
   (2) sound prolongations
   (3) interjections
   (4) broken words (e.g., pauses within a word)
   (5) audible or silent blocking (filled or unfilled pauses in speech)
   (6) circumlocutions (word substitutions to avoid problematic words)
   (7) words produced with an excess of physical tension
   (8) monosyllabic whole-word repetitions (e.g., "I-I-I-I see him")

B. The disturbance in fluency interferes with academic or occupational achievement or with social communication.

C. If a speech-motor or sensory deficit is present, the speech difficulties are in excess of those usually associated with these problems.

Coding note: If a speech-motor or sensory deficit or a neurological condition is present, code the condition on Axis III.

From American Psychiatric Association. *Diagnostic and Statistical Manual of Mental Disorders.* 4th ed. Text rev. Washington, DC: American Psychiatric Association; copyright 2000, with permission.

Differential Diagnosis

Normal speech dysfluency in preschool years is difficult to differentiate from incipient stuttering. In stuttering there are more nonfluencies, part-word repetitions, sound prolongations, and disruptions in voice airflow through the vocal track. Children who stutter appear to be tense and uncomfortable with their speech pattern, in contrast to young children who are nonfluent in their speech but seem to be at ease. Spastic dysphonia is a stuttering-like speech disorder distinguished from stuttering by the presence of an abnormal breathing pattern.

Cluttering is a speech disorder characterized by erratic and dysrhythmic speech patterns of rapid and jerky spurts of words and phrases. In cluttering, those affected are usually unaware of the disturbance, whereas, after the initial phase of the disorder, stutterers are aware of their speech difficulties. Cluttering is often an associated feature of expressive language disorder.

Course and Prognosis

The course of stuttering is usually long term, with some periods of partial remission lasting for weeks or months and exacerbations occurring most frequently when a stutterer is under pres-

sure to communicate. Fifty to 80 percent of all children who stutter, mostly those with mild cases, recover spontaneously. School-age children who stutter chronically may have impaired peer relationships as a result of testing and social ostracism. The children may face academic difficulties if they avoid speaking in class. Later major complications include an affected person's limitations in occupational choice and advancement.

Treatment

Treatment entails breathing exercises, relaxation techniques, and speech therapy to help children slow the rate of speaking and modulate speech volume. Until the end of the 19th century, the most common treatments for stuttering were distraction, suggestion, and relaxation. Recent approaches using distraction include teaching stutterers to talk in time to rhythmic movements of the arm, hand, or fingers. Stutterers are also advised to speak slowly in a sing-song or monotone manner. However, these approaches remove stuttering only temporarily. Suggestion techniques, such as hypnosis, also stop stuttering but, again, only temporarily. Relaxation techniques are based on the premise that it is almost impossible to be relaxed and stutter in the usual manner at the same time. Because of their lack of long-term benefits, distraction, suggestion, and relaxation approaches as such are not currently used.

Classic psychoanalysis, insight-oriented psychotherapy, group therapy, and other psychotherapeutic modalities have not been successful in treating stuttering. But if stutterers have a poor self-image, are anxious or depressed, or show evidence of an established emotional disorder, individual psychotherapy is indicated and effective for the associated condition. One study found that nonstuttering listeners reacted more positively to stutterers who acknowledged their stuttering than to stutterers who did not. Family therapy should also be considered if there is evidence of family dysfunction, a family contribution to a stutterer's symptoms, or family stress caused by trying to cope with, or help, the stutterer.

Most modern treatments of stuttering are based on the view that stuttering is essentially a learned form of behavior not necessarily associated with a basic mental disorder or neurological abnormality. The approaches work directly with the speech difficulty to minimize the issues that maintain and strengthen stuttering, to modify or decrease the severity of stuttering by eliminating the secondary symptoms, and to encourage stutterers to speak, even when stuttering, in a relatively easy and effortless fashion that thereby avoids fears and blocks.

One example of this approach is the self-therapy proposed by the Speech Foundation of America. Self-therapy is based on the premise that stuttering is not a symptom but a behavior that can be modified. Stutterers are told that they can learn to control their difficulty partly by modifying their feelings about stuttering and attitudes toward it and partly by modifying the deviant behaviors associated with their stuttering blocks. The approach includes desensitizing; reducing the emotional reaction to, and fears of, stuttering; and substituting positive action to control the moment of stuttering.

Recently developed therapies focus on restructuring fluency. The entire speech production pattern is reshaped, with emphasis on a variety of target behaviors, including rate reduction, easy or gentle onset of voicing, and smooth transitions between sounds, syllables, and words. The approaches have met with substantial success in establishing perceptually fluent speech in adults, but fluency maintenance over long periods and relapses remain problems for all involved in adult-stuttering treatment.

Psychopharmacological intervention such as treatment with haloperidol (Haldol) has been used in an attempt increase relaxation; there are no data to assess the efficacy of this approach. Whichever therapeutic approach is used, individual and family assessments and supportive interventions may be helpful. A team assessment of a child or adolescent and his or her family should be made before any approaches to treatment are begun.

Table 41–8
DSM-IV-TR Diagnostic Criteria for Communication Disorder Not Otherwise Specified

This category is for disorders in communication that do not meet criteria for any specific communication disorder; for example, a voice disorder (i.e., an abnormality of vocal pitch, loudness, quality, tone, or resonance).

From American Psychiatric Association. *Diagnostic and Statistical Manual of Mental Disorders.* 4th ed. Text rev. Washington, DC: American Psychiatric Association; copyright 2000, with permission.

COMMUNICATION DISORDER NOT OTHERWISE SPECIFIED

Disorders that do not meet the diagnostic criteria for any specific communication disorder fall into the category of communication disorder not otherwise specified. An example is voice disorder, in which the patient has an abnormality in pitch, loudness, quality, tone, or resonance. To be coded as a disorder, the voice abnormality must be severe enough to impair academic achievement or social communication (Table 41–8).

Cluttering is not listed as a disorder in DSM-IV-TR, but it is an associated speech abnormality in which the disturbed rate and rhythm of speech impair intelligibility. Speech is erratic and dysrhythmic and consists of rapid, jerky spurts that are inconsistent with normal phrasing patterns. The disorder usually occurs in children between 2 and 8 years of age; in two thirds of cases, the patient recovers spontaneously by early adolescence. Cluttering is associated with learning disorders and other communication disorders.

ICD-10

The 10th revision of *International Statistical Classification of Diseases and Related Health Problems* (ICD-10) includes four disorders of speech and language as well as two residual categories (Table 41–9). ICD-10 defines *cluttering* as a "rapid rate of speech with breakdown in fluency, but no repetitions or hesitations, of a severity to give rise to reduced speech intelligibility. Speech is erratic and dysrhythmic, with rapid, jerky spurts that usually involve faulty phrasing patterns." The faulty speech patterns may include using groups of words unrelated to the sentence's grammar. According to ICD-10, cluttering must be distinguished from stuttering. ICD-10 defines *stuttering* as speech "characterized by frequent repetition or prolongation of sounds or syllables or words, or by frequent hesitations or pauses that disrupt the rhythmic flow of speech." Minor stuttering is common throughout life, but persistent, severe stuttering that destroys the fluency of speech must be

Table 41–9
ICD-10 Diagnostic Criteria for Specific Developmental Disorders of Speech and Language

Specific speech articulation disorder

Note. This disorder is also referred to as specific speech phonological disorder.

A. Articulation (phonological) skills, as assessed on standardized tests, are below the 2 standard deviations limit for the child's age.
B. Articulation (phonological) skills are at least 1 standard deviation below nonverbal IQ as assessed on standardized tests.
C. Language expression and comprehension, as assessed on standardized tests, are within the 2 standard deviations limit for the child's age.
D. There are no neurological, sensory, or physical impairments that directly affect speech sound production, nor is there a pervasive developmental disorder.
E. *Most commonly used exclusion clause.* Nonverbal IQ is below 70 on a standardized test.

Expressive language disorder

A. Expressive language skills, as assessed on standardized tests, are below the 2 standard deviations limit for the child's age.
B. Expressive language skills are at least 1 standard deviation below nonverbal IQ as assessed on standardized tests.
C. Receptive language skills, as assessed on standardized tests, are within the 2 standard deviations limit for the child's age.
D. Use and understanding of nonverbal communication and imaginative language functions are within the normal range.
E. There are no neurological, sensory, or physical impairments that directly affect use of spoken language, nor is there a pervasive developmental disorder.
F. *Most commonly used exclusion clause.* Nonverbal IQ is below 70 on a standardized test.

Receptive language disorder

Note. This disorder is also referred to as mixed receptive/expressive disorder.

A. Language comprehension, as assessed on standardized tests, is below the 2 standard deviations limit for the child's age.
B. Receptive language skills are at least 1 standard deviation below nonverbal IQ as assessed on standardized tests.
C. There are no neurological, sensory, or physical impairments that directly affect receptive language, nor is there a pervasive developmental disorder.
D. *Most commonly used exclusion clause.* Nonverbal IQ is below 70 on a standardized test.

Acquired aphasia with epilepsy [Landau-Kleffner syndrome]

A. Severe loss of expressive and receptive language skills occurs over a period of time not exceeding 6 months.
B. Language development was normal before the loss.
C. Paroxysmal EEG abnormalities affecting one or both temporal lobes become apparent within a time span extending from 2 years before to 2 years after the initial loss of language.
D. Hearing is within the normal range.
E. A level of nonverbal intelligence within the normal range is retained.
F. There is no diagnosable neurological condition other than that implicit in the abnormal EEG and presence of epileptic seizures (when they occur).
G. The disorder does not meet the criteria for a pervasive developmental disorder.

Other developmental disorders of speech and language

Developmental disorder of speech and language, unspecified

This category should be avoided as far as possible and should be used only for unspecified disorders in which there is significant impairment in the development of speech or language that cannot be accounted for by mental retardation, or by neurological, sensory, or physical impairments that directly affect speech or language.

Reprinted with permission from World Health Organization. *The ICD-10 Classification of Mental and Behavioural Disorders: Diagnostic Criteria for Research.* Copyright, World Health Organization, Geneva, 1993.

present for stuttering to be diagnosed. The disorder may be accompanied by movements of the face or body that coincide with speech.

References

Beitchman JH, Cohen NJ, Konstantareas MM, Tannock R, eds. *Language, Learning, and Behavior Disorders: Developmental, Biological, and Clinical Perspectives.* New York: Cambridge University Press; 1996.

Beitchman JH, Wilson B, Brownlie EB, Walters H, Inglis A, Lancee W. Long-term consistency in speech/language profiles. II. Behavioral, emotional, and social outcomes. *J Am Acad Child Adolesc Psychiatry.* 1996;35:815.

Beitchman JH, Wilson B, Brownlie EB, Walters H, Lancee W. Long-term consistency in speech/language profiles: developmental and academic outcomes. *J Am Acad Child Adolesc Psychiatry.* 1996;35:804.

Beitchman JH, Wilson B, Johnson CJ, et al. Fourteen-year follow-up of speech/language-impaired and control children: psychiatric outcome. *J Am Acad Child Adolesc Psychiatry.* 2001;40:75.

Cleary P, McFadden S. Helping children with communication deficits in the classroom. *Int J Lang Commun Disord.* 2001;36(suppl):31.

Cohen NJ, Davine M, Horodezky N, Lipsett L, Isaacson L. Unsuspected language impairment in psychiatrically disturbed children: prevalence and language and behavioral characteristics. *J Am Acad Child Adolesc Psychiatry.* 1993;32:595.

Cordes AK, Ingham RJ. The reliability of observational data. II. Issues in the identification and measurement of stuttering events. *J Speech Hear Res.* 1994;37:2.

Detweiler RF, Beitchman JH. Communication disorder not otherwise specified. In: Sadock BJ, Sadock VA, eds. *Kaplan & Sadock's Comprehensive Textbook of Psychiatry.* 7th ed. Vol 2. Baltimore: Lippincott Williams & Wilkins; 2000:2655.

Duchan JF. A situated pragmatics approach for supporting children with severe communication disorders. *Top Lang Disord.* 1997;17:1.

Gow ML, Ingham RJ. Stuttering modification and changes in phonation: observations of findings from recent reports. *J Speech Hear Res.* 1994;37:2.

Guralnick MJ, Connor RT, Neville B, Hammond MA. Mothers' perspectives of the peer-related social development of young children with developmental delays and communication disorders. *Early Educ Dev.* 2002;13:59.

Hoit J, Watson P, Hixon K, McMahon P, Johnson C. Age and velopharyngeal function during speech production. *J Speech Hear Res*. 1994;37:295.
Johnson CJ, Beitchman JH. Expressive language disorder. In: Sadock BJ, Sadock VA, eds. *Kaplan & Sadock's Comprehensive Textbook of Psychiatry*. 7th ed. Vol 2. Baltimore: Lippincott Williams & Wilkins; 2000:2634.
Johnson CJ, Beitchman JH. Mixed receptive-expressive language disorder. In: Sadock BJ, Sadock VA, eds. *Kaplan & Sadock's Comprehensive Textbook of Psychiatry*. 7th ed. Vol 2. Baltimore: Lippincott Williams & Wilkins; 2000:2639.
Johnson CJ, Beitchman JH. Phonological disorder. In: Sadock BJ, Sadock VA, eds. *Kaplan & Sadock's Comprehensive Textbook of Psychiatry*. 7th ed. Vol 2. Baltimore: Lippincott Williams & Wilkins; 2000:2645.
Kroll R, Beitchman JH. Stuttering. In: Sadock BJ, Sadock VA, eds. *Kaplan & Sadock's Comprehensive Textbook of Psychiatry*. 7th ed. Vol 2. Baltimore: Lippincott Williams & Wilkins; 2000:2651.
Nash P, Stengelhofen J, Toombs L, Brown J, Kellow B. An alternative management of older children with persisting communication problems. *Int J Lang Commun Dis*. 2001;36(suppl):179.
Rvachew S. Speech perception training can facilitate sound production learning. *J Speech Hear Res*. 1994;37:347.
Snowling MJ. From language to reading and dyslexia. *Dyslexia*. 2001;7:37.
Stallard P, Williams L, Velleman R, Lenton S, McGrath PJ. Intervening factors in caregivers' assessments of pain in non-communicating children. *Dev Med Child Neurol*. 2002;44:213.
Stallard P, Williams L, Velleman R, Lenton S, McGrath PJ. Brief report: behaviors identified by caregivers to detect pain in noncommunicating children. *J Pediatr Psychol*. 2002;27:209.
Throneburg RN, Yairi E, Paden E. Relation between phonological difficulty and the occurrence of dysfluencies in the early stage of stuttering. *J Speech Hear Res*. 1994;37:504.
Toppelberg CO, Shapiro T. Language disorders: a 10-year research update review. *J Am Acad Child Adolesc Psychiatry*. 2000;39:143.

42 Pervasive Developmental Disorders

The pervasive developmental disorders include a group of conditions in which there are delay and deviance in the development of social skills, language and communication, and behavioral repertoire. Children with pervasive developmental disorders often exhibit idiosyncratic intense interest in a narrow range of activities, resist change, and are not appropriately responsive to the social environment. These disorders affect multiple areas of development, are manifested early in life, and cause persistent dysfunction. Autistic disorder, the best known of these disorders, is characterized by sustained impairment in comprehending and responding to social cues, aberrant language development and usage, and restricted, stereotypical behavioral patterns. According to the text revision of the fourth edition of *Diagnostic and Statistical Manual of Mental Disorders* (DSM-IV-TR), to meet criteria for autistic behavior, abnormal functioning in at least one of the above areas must be present by age 3. More than two thirds of children with autistic disorder have mental retardation, although it is not required for the diagnosis.

DSM-IV-TR includes five pervasive developmental disorders: autistic disorder, Rett's disorder, childhood disintegrative disorder, Asperger's disorder, and pervasive developmental disorder not otherwise specified. Rett's disorder appears to occur exclusively in girls; it is characterized by normal development for at least 6 months, stereotyped hand movements, a loss of purposeful motions, diminishing social engagement, poor coordination, and decreasing language use. In childhood disintegrative disorder, development progresses normally for the first 2 years, after which the child shows a loss of previously acquired skills in two or more of the following areas: language use, social responsiveness, play, motor skills, and bladder or bowel control. Asperger's disorder is a condition in which the child is markedly impaired in social relatedness and shows repetitive and stereotyped patterns of behavior without a delay in language development. In Asperger's disorder, a child's cognitive abilities and adaptive skills are normal.

AUTISTIC DISORDER

Autistic disorder (historically called *early infantile autism, childhood autism,* or *Kanner's autism*) is characterized by deviant reciprocal social interaction, delayed and aberrant communication skills, and a restricted repertoire of activities and interests.

History

As early as 1867, Henry Maudsley, a psychiatrist, noted a group of very young children with severe mental disorders who had marked deviation, delay, and distortion in development. In that era, most serious disturbance in young children was believed to fall within the category of psychoses. In 1943 Leo Kanner, in his classic paper "Autistic Disturbances of Affective Contact," coined the term *infantile autism* and provided a clear, comprehensive account of the early childhood syndrome. He described children who exhibited extreme autistic aloneness; failure to assume an anticipatory posture; delayed or deviant language development with echolalia and pronominal reversal (using *you* for *I*); monotonous repetitions of noises or verbal utterances; excellent rote memory; limited range of spontaneous activities, stereotypies, and mannerisms; anxiously obsessive desire for the maintenance of sameness and dread of change; poor eye contact; abnormal relationships with persons; and a preference for pictures and inanimate objects. Kanner suspected that the syndrome was more frequent than it seemed and suggested that some children had been misclassified as mentally retarded or schizophrenic. Before 1980, children with pervasive developmental disorders were generally diagnosed with childhood schizophrenia. Over time, it became evident that autistic disorder and schizophrenia were two distinct psychiatric entities. In some cases, however, a child with autistic disorder may develop a comorbid schizophrenic disorder later in childhood.

Epidemiology

Prevalence. Autistic disorder is believed to occur at a rate of about 5 cases per 10,000 children (0.05 percent). Reports of the rate of autistic disorder have ranged from 2 to 20 cases per 10,000. By definition, the onset of autistic disorder is before the age of 3 years, although in some cases, it is not recognized until a child is much older.

Sex Distribution. Autistic disorder is four to five times more frequent in boys than in girls. Girls with autistic disorder are more likely to have more severe mental retardation.

Socioeconomic Status. Early studies suggested that a high socioeconomic status was more common in families with autistic children; however, these findings were probably based on referral bias. Over the past 25 years, no epidemiological studies have demonstrated an association between autistic disorder and any socioeconomic status.

Etiology and Pathogenesis

Autistic disorder is a developmental behavioral disorder. Although Kanner initially hypothesized that autism disorder

was due to emotionally unresponsive "refrigerator" mothers, there is no validity to this hypothesis. On the other hand, much evidence supports a biological substrate for this disorder.

Psychosocial and Family Factors. In his initial report, Kanner indicated that few parents of autistic children were warmhearted and that, for the most part, parents were preoccupied with intellectual abstractions, and mothers' lack of emotional responsivity was held accountable for the autism. No evidence has been found to support this theory. Other theories, such as parental rage and rejection and parental reinforcement of autistic symptoms are also unsubstantiated. More recent studies comparing parents of autistic children with parents of normal children have shown no significant differences in child-rearing skills.

Children with autistic disorder, like children with other disorders, can respond with exacerbated symptoms to psychosocial stressors including family discord, the birth of a new sibling, or a family move. Some children with autistic disorder may be excruciatingly sensitive to even small changes in their families and immediate environment.

Biological Factors. The high rate of mental retardation among children with autistic disorder and the higher-than-expected rates of seizure disorders suggest a biological basis for autistic disorder. Approximately 75 percent of children with autistic disorder have mental retardation. About one third of these children have mild to moderate mental retardation, and close to half of these children are severely or profoundly mentally retarded. Children with autistic disorder and mental retardation typically show more marked deficits in abstract reasoning, social understanding, and verbal tasks than in performance tasks such as block design and digit recall, in which details can be remembered without reference to the "gestalt" meaning.

Four to 32 percent of persons with autism have grand mal seizures at some time, and about 20 to 25 percent show ventricular enlargement on computed tomography (CT) scans. Various electroencephalogram (EEG) abnormalities are found in 10 to 83 percent of autistic children, and although no EEG finding is specific to autistic disorder, there is some indication of failed cerebral lateralization. Recently, one magnetic resonance imaging (MRI) study revealed hypoplasia of cerebellar vermal lobules VI and VII, and another MRI study revealed cortical abnormalities, particularly polymicrogyria, in some autistic patients. Those abnormalities may reflect abnormal cell migrations in the first 6 months of gestation. An autopsy study revealed fewer Purkinje's cells, and another study found increased diffuse cortical metabolism during positron emission tomography (PET) scanning.

Autistic disorder is also associated with neurological conditions, notably congenital rubella, phenylketonuria (PKU), tuberous sclerosis, and Rett's disorder. Autistic children show more evidence of perinatal complications than comparison groups of normal children and those with other disorders. The finding that autistic children have significantly more minor congenital physical anomalies than expected suggests abnormal development within the first trimester of pregnancy.

Genetic Factors. In several surveys, between 2 and 4 percent of siblings of autistic children also had autistic disorder, a rate 50 times that in the general population. The concordance rate of autistic disorder in the two largest twin studies was 36 percent in monozygotic pairs versus 0 percent in dizygotic pairs in one study and about 96 percent in monozygotic pairs versus about 27 percent in dizygotic pairs in the second study. High rates of cognitive difficulties, even in the nonautistic twin in monozygotic twins with perinatal complications, suggest that contributions of perinatal insult along with genetic vulnerability may lead to autistic disorder.

Clinical reports suggest that the nonautistic members of families with autistic members have higher rates of less pronounced language or other cognitive problems. Fragile X syndrome, a genetic disorder in which a portion of the X chromosome fractures, appears to be associated with autistic disorder. Approximately 1 percent of children with autistic disorder also have fragile X syndrome. Tuberous sclerosis, a genetic disorder characterized by multiple benign tumors, with autosomal dominant transmission is found with greater frequency among children with autistic disorder. Up to 2 percent of children with autistic disorder may also have tuberous sclerosis.

Recently, researchers screened the DNA of more than 150 pairs of siblings with autism. They found extremely strong evidence that two regions on chromosomes 2 and 7 contain genes involved with autism. Likely locations for autism-related genes were also found on chromosomes 16 and 17, although the strength of the correlation was somewhat weaker.

Immunological Factors. Several reports have suggested that immunological incompatibility (i.e., maternal antibodies directed at the fetus) may contribute to autistic disorder. The lymphocytes of some autistic children react with maternal antibodies, which raises the possibility that embryonic neural, or extraembryonic, tissues may be damaged during gestation.

Perinatal Factors. A higher-than-expected incidence of perinatal complications seems to occur in infants who are later diagnosed with autistic disorder. Maternal bleeding after the first trimester and meconium in the amniotic fluid have been reported in the histories of autistic children more often than in the general population. In the neonatal period, autistic children have a high incidence of respiratory distress syndrome and neonatal anemia.

Neuroanatomical Factors. MRI studies comparing autistic subjects and normal controls have shown that the total brain volume was larger in those with autism, although autistic children with severe mental retardation generally have smaller heads. The greatest average percentage increase in size occurred in the occipital lobe, parietal lobe, and temporal lobe. No differences were found in the frontal lobes. Specific origins of this enlargement are unknown. The increased volume can arise from three different possible mechanisms: increased neurogenesis, decreased neuronal death, and increased production of nonneuronal brain tissue such as glial cells or blood vessels. Brain enlargement has been suggested as a possible biological marker for autistic disorder.

The temporal lobe is believed to be a critical area of brain abnormality in autistic disorder. This suggestion is based on reports of autistic-like syndromes in some persons with temporal lobe damage. When the temporal region of animals is damaged, normal social behavior is lost, and restlessness, repetitive motor behavior, and a limited behavioral repertoire are seen.

References

Dawson G, Munson J, Estes A, et al. Neurocognitive function and joint attention ability in young children with autism spectrum disorder versus developmental delay. *Child Dev.* 2002;73:345.

Frazier JA, Doyle R, Chiu S, Coyle JT. Treating a child with Asperger's disorder and comorbid bipolar disorder. *Am J Psychiatry.* 2002;159:13.

Hardan A, Johnson K, Johnson C, Hrecznyi B. Case study: risperidone treatment of children and adolescents with developmental disorders. *J Am Acad Child Adolesc Psychiatry.* 1996;35:1551.

Hendren RL, De Backer I, Pandina GJ. Review of neuroimaging studies of child and adolescent psychiatric disorders from the past 10 years. *J Am Acad Child Adolesc Psychiatry.* 2000;39:815.

King BH, Wright DM, Handen BL, et al. Double-blind, placebo-controlled study of amantadine hydrochloride in the treatment of children with autistic disorder. *J Am Acad Child Adolesc Psychiatry.* 2001;40:658.

Kristensen H. Selective mutism and comorbidity with developmental disorder/delay, anxiety disorder and elimination disorder. *J Am Acad Child Adolesc Psychiatry.* 2000;39:249.

Lord C, Pickles A. Language level and nonverbal social-communicative behaviors in autistic and language delayed children. *J Am Acad Child Adolesc Psychiatry.* 1996;35:1542.

Lord C, Risi S, Labrecht L, et al. The ADOS-G (Autistic Diagnostic Observation Schedule-Generic): a standard measure of social and communication deficits associated with autism spectrum disorder. *J Autism Dev Disord.* 2000;30:205.

Ozonoff S, Strayer DL. Inhibitory function in nonretarded children with autism. *J Autism Dev Disord.* 1997;27:59.

Perry A. Rett's syndrome: a comprehensive review of the literature. *Am J Ment Retard.* 1991;96:275.

Perry RI, Pataki CS, Munoz DM, Armenteros JL, Silva RR. Pilot trial of risperidone in children with pervasive developmental disorder. Abstract, Proceedings of the American Psychiatric Association annual meeting, 1996.

Pisen J, Berthier ML, Sharkstein SE, Nehme E, Pearlson G, Folstein S. Magnetic resonance imaging: evidence for a defect of cerebral cortical development in autism. *Am J Psychiatry.* 1990;147:734.

Rogers SJ, Di Lalla DL. Age of symptom onset in young children with pervasive developmental disorders. *J Am Acad Child Adolesc Psychiatry.* 1990;29:863.

Sanchez LE, Campbell M, Small AM, Cueva JE, Armenteros JL, Adams PB. A pilot study of clomipramine in young autistic children. *J Am Acad Child Adolesc Psychiatry.* 1996;35:537.

Schuntermann P. Pervasive developmental disorder and parental adaptation: previewing and reviewing atypical development with parents in child psychiatric consultation. *Harv Rev Psychiatry.* 2002;10:16.

Sponheim E. Changing criteria of autistic disorders: a comparison of the ICD-10 research criteria and DSM-IV with DSM-IIIBR, CARS, and ABC. *J Autism Dev Disord.* 1996;26:513.

Tanguay PE. Pervasive developmental disorders: a 10-year review. *J Am Acad Child Adolesc Psychiatry.* 2000;39:1079.

Volkmar F, Cook DH, Pomeroy J, Realmuto Tanguay P. Practice parameters for the assessment of and treatment of children, adolescents and adults with autism and other pervasive developmental disorders. *J Am Acad Child Adolesc Psychiatry.* 1999;38(suppl 12):32S.

Waterhouse L, Morris R, Allen D, et al. Diagnosis and classification in autism. *J Autism Dev Disord.* 1996;26:59.

Table 42–9 (*continued*)

C. There is severe impairment of expressive and receptive language, together with severe psychomotor retardation.

D. There are stereotyped midline hand movements (such as hand-wringing or "hand-washing") with an onset at or after the time when purposeful hand movements are lost.

Other childhood disintegrative disorder

A. Development is apparently normal up to the age of at least 2 years. The presence of normal age-appropriate skills in communication, social relationships, play, and adaptive behavior at age 2 years or later is required for diagnosis.

B. There is a definite loss of previously acquired skills at about the time of onset of the disorder. The diagnosis requires a clinically significant loss of skills (not just a failure to use them in certain situations) in at least two of the following areas:

(1) expressive or receptive language;

(2) play;

(3) social skills or adaptive behavior;

(4) bowel or bladder control;

(5) motor skills.

C. Qualitatively abnormal social functioning is manifest in at least two of the following areas:

(1) qualitative abnormalities in reciprocal social interaction (of the type defined for autism);

(2) qualitative abnormalities in communication (of the type defined for autism);

(3) restricted, repetitive, and stereotyped patterns of behavior, interests, and activities, including motor stereotypies and mannerisms;

(4) a general loss of interest in objects and in the environment.

D. The disorder is not attributable to the other varieties of pervasive developmental disorder; acquired aphasia with epilepsy; elective mutism; Rett's syndrome; or schizophrenia.

Overactive disorder associated with mental retardation and stereotyped movements

A. Severe motor hyperactivity is manifest by at least two of the following problems in activity and attention:

(1) continuous motor restlessness, manifest in running, jumping, and other movements of the whole body;

(2) marked difficulty in remaining seated: the child will ordinarily remain seated for a few seconds at most except when engaged in a stereotypic activity (see Criterion B);

(3) grossly excessive activity in situations where relative stillness is expected;

(4) very rapid changes of activity, so that activities generally last for less than a minute (occasional longer periods spent in highly favored activities do not exclude this, and very long periods spent in stereotypic activities can also be compatible with the presence of this problem at other times).

B. Repetitive and stereotyped patterns of behavior and activity are manifest by at least one of the following:

(1) fixed and frequently repeated motor mannerisms: these may involve either complex movements of the whole body or partial movements such as hand-flapping;

(2) excessive and nonfunctional repetition of activities that are constant in form: this may be play with a single object (e.g., running water) or a ritual of activities (either alone or involving other people);

(3) repetitive self-injury.

C. IQ is less than 50.

D. There is no social impairment of the autistic type, i.e., the child must show at least three of the following:

(1) developmentally appropriate use of eye gaze, expression, and posture to regulate social interaction;

(2) developmentally appropriate peer relationships that include sharing of interests, activities, etc.;

(3) approaches to other people, at least sometimes, for comfort and affection;

(4) ability to share other people's enjoyment at times; other forms of social impairment, e.g., a disinhibited approach to strangers, are compatible with the diagnosis.

E. The disorder does not meet diagnostic criteria for autism, childhood disintegrative disorder, or hyperkinetic disorders.

Asperger's syndrome

A. There is no clinically significant general delay in spoken or receptive language or cognitive development. Diagnosis requires that single words should have developed by 2 years of age or earlier and that communicative phrases be used by 3 years of age or earlier. Self-help skills, adaptive behavior, and curiosity about the environment during the first 3 years should be at a level consistent with normal intellectual development. However, motor milestones may be somewhat delayed and motor clumsiness is usual (although not a necessary diagnostic feature). Isolated special skills, often related to abnormal preoccupations, are common, but are not required for diagnosis.

B. There are qualitative abnormalities in reciprocal social interaction (criteria as for autism).

C. The individual exhibits an unusually intense, circumscribed interest or restricted, repetitive, and stereotyped patterns of behavior, interests, and activities (criteria as for autism; however, it would be less usual for these to include either motor mannerisms or preoccupations with part-objects or nonfunctional elements of play materials).

D. The disorder is not attributable to the other varieties of pervasive developmental disorder: simple schizophrenia; schizotypal disorder; obsessive-compulsive disorder; anankastic personality disorder; reactive and disinhibited attachment disorders of childhood.

Other pervasive developmental disorders

Pervasive developmental disorder, unspecified

This is a residual diagnostic category that should be used for disorders which fit the general description for pervasive developmental disorders but in which contradictory findings or a lack of adequate information mean that the criteria for any of the other pervasive developmental disorders codes cannot be met.

References

Dawson G, Munson J, Estes A, et al. Neurocognitive function and joint attention ability in young children with autism spectrum disorder versus developmental delay. *Child Dev.* 2002;73:345.

Frazier JA, Doyle R, Chiu S, Coyle JT. Treating a child with Asperger's disorder and comorbid bipolar disorder. *Am J Psychiatry.* 2002;159:13.

Hardan A, Johnson K, Johnson C, Hrecznyi B. Case study: risperidone treatment of children and adolescents with developmental disorders. *J Am Acad Child Adolesc Psychiatry.* 1996;35:1551.

Hendren RL, De Backer I, Pandina GJ. Review of neuroimaging studies of child and adolescent psychiatric disorders from the past 10 years. *J Am Acad Child Adolesc Psychiatry.* 2000;39:815.

King BH, Wright DM, Handen BL, et al. Double-blind, placebo-controlled study of amantadine hydrochloride in the treatment of children with autistic disorder. *J Am Acad Child Adolesc Psychiatry.* 2001;40:658.

Kristensen H. Selective mutism and comorbidity with developmental disorder/delay, anxiety disorder and elimination disorder. *J Am Acad Child Adolesc Psychiatry.* 2000;39:249.

Lord C, Pickles A. Language level and nonverbal social-communicative behaviors in autistic and language delayed children. *J Am Acad Child Adolesc Psychiatry.* 1996;35:1542.

Lord C, Risi S, Labrecht L, et al. The ADOS-G (Autistic Diagnostic Observation Schedule-Generic): a standard measure of social and communication deficits associated with autism spectrum disorder. *J Autism Dev Disord.* 2000;30:205.

Ozonoff S, Strayer DL. Inhibitory function in nonretarded children with autism. *J Autism Dev Disord.* 1997;27:59.

Perry A. Rett's syndrome: a comprehensive review of the literature. *Am J Ment Retard.* 1991;96:275.

Perry RI, Pataki CS, Munoz DM, Armenteros JL, Silva RR. Pilot trial of risperidone in children with pervasive developmental disorder. Abstract, Proceedings of the American Psychiatric Association annual meeting, 1996.

Pisen J, Berthier ML, Sharkstein SE, Nehme E, Pearlson G, Folstein S. Magnetic resonance imaging: evidence for a defect of cerebral cortical development in autism. *Am J Psychiatry.* 1990;147:734.

Rogers SJ, Di Lalla DL. Age of symptom onset in young children with pervasive developmental disorders. *J Am Acad Child Adolesc Psychiatry.* 1990; 29:863.

Sanchez LE, Campbell M, Small AM, Cueva JE, Armenteros JL, Adams PB. A pilot study of clomipramine in young autistic children. *J Am Acad Child Adolesc Psychiatry.* 1996;35:537.

Schuntermann P. Pervasive developmental disorder and parental adaptation: previewing and reviewing atypical development with parents in child psychiatric consultation. *Harv Rev Psychiatry.* 2002;10:16.

Sponheim E. Changing criteria of autistic disorders: a comparison of the ICD-10 research criteria and DSM-IV with DSM-IIIBR, CARS, and ABC. *J Autism Dev Disord.* 1996;26:513.

Tanguay PE. Pervasive developmental disorders: a 10-year review. *J Am Acad Child Adolesc Psychiatry.* 2000;39:1079.

Volkmar F, Cook DH, Pomeroy J, Realmuto Tanguay P. Practice parameters for the assessment of and treatment of children, adolescents and adults with autism and other pervasive developmental disorders. *J Am Acad Child Adolesc Psychiatry.* 1999;38(suppl 12):32S.

Waterhouse L, Morris R, Allen D, et al. Diagnosis and classification in autism. *J Autism Dev Disord.* 1996;26:59.

Table 42–9
ICD-10 Diagnostic Criteria for Pervasive Developmental Disorders

Childhood autism

A. Abnormal or impaired development is evident before the age of 3 years in at least one of the following areas:
  (1) receptive or expressive language as used in social communication;
  (2) the development of selective social attachments or of reciprocal social interaction;
  (3) functional or symbolic play.

B. A total of at least six symptoms from (1), (2), and (3) must be present, with at least two from (1) and at least one from each of (2) and (3):
  (1) Qualitative abnormalities in reciprocal social interaction are manifest in at least two of the following areas:
    (a) failure adequately to use eye-to-eye gaze, facial expression, body posture, and gesture to regulate social interaction;
    (b) failure to develop (in a manner appropriate to mental age, and despite ample opportunities) peer relationships that involve a mutual sharing of interests, activities, and emotions;
    (c) lack of socioemotional reciprocity as shown by an impaired or deviant response to other people's emotions; or lack of modulation of behavior according to social context; or a weak integration of social, emotional, and communicative behaviors;
    (d) lack of spontaneous seeking to share enjoyment, interests, or achievements with other people (e.g., a lack of showing, bringing, or pointing out to other people objects of interest to the individual).
  (2) Qualitative abnormalities in communication are manifest in at least one of the following areas:
    (a) a delay in, or total lack of, development of spoken language that is *not* accompanied by an attempt to compensate through the use of gesture or mime as an alternative mode of communication (often preceded by a lack of communicative babbling);
    (b) relative failure to initiate or sustain conversational interchange (at whatever level of language skills is present), in which there is reciprocal responsiveness to the communications of the other person;
    (c) stereotyped and repetitive use of language or idiosyncratic use of words or phrases;
    (d) lack of varied spontaneous make-believe or (when young) social imitative play.
  (3) Restricted, repetitive, and stereotyped patterns of behavior, interests, and activities are manifest in at least one of the following areas:
    (a) an encompassing preoccupation with one or more stereotyped and restricted patterns of interest that are abnormal in content or focus; or one or more interests that are abnormal in their intensity and circumscribed nature though not in their content or focus;
    (b) apparently compulsive adherence to specific, nonfunctional routines or rituals;
    (c) stereotyped and repetitive motor mannerisms that involve either hand or finger flapping or twisting, or complex whole body movements;
    (d) preoccupations with part-objects or nonfunctional elements of play materials (such as their odor, the feel of their surface, or the noise or vibration that they generate).

C. The clinical picture is not attributable to the other varieties of pervasive developmental disorder: specific developmental disorder of receptive language with secondary socioemotional problems; reactive attachment disorder or disinhibited attachment disorder, mental retardation with some associated emotional or behavioral disorder; schizophrenia of unusually early onset; and Rett's syndrome.

Atypical autism

A. Abnormal or impaired development is evident at or after the age of 3 years (criteria as for autism except for age of manifestation).

B. There are qualitative abnormalities in reciprocal social interaction or in communication, or restricted, repetitive, and stereotyped patterns of behavior, interests, and activities. (Criteria as for autism except that it is unnecessary to meet the criteria for number of areas of abnormality.)

C. The disorder does not meet the diagnostic criteria for autism. Autism may be atypical in either age of onset or symptomatology; the two types are differentiated with a fifth character for research purposes. Syndromes that are atypical in both respects should be coded. Atypicality in both ages of onset and symptomatology.

Atypicality in age of onset

A. The disorder does not meet Criterion A for autism; that is, abnormal or impaired development is evident only at or after the age of 3 years.

B. The disorder meets Criteria B and C for autism.

Atypicality in symptomatology

A. The disorder meets Criterion A for autism; that is, abnormal or impaired development is evident before the age of 3 years.

B. There are qualitative abnormalities in reciprocal social interactions or in communication, or restricted, repetitive, and stereotyped patterns of behavior, interests, and activities. (Criteria as for autism except that it is unnecessary to meet the criteria for number of areas of abnormality.)

C. The disorder meets Criterion C for autism.

D. The disorder does not fully meet Criterion B for autism.

Atypicality in both age of onset and symptomatology

A. The disorder does not meet Criterion A for autism; that is, abnormal or impaired development is evident only at or after the age of 3 years.

B. There are qualitative abnormalities in reciprocal social interactions or in communication, or restricted, repetitive, and stereotyped patterns of behavior, interests, and activities. (Criteria as for autism except that it is unnecessary to meet the criteria for number of areas of abnormality.)

C. The disorder meets Criterion C for autism.

D. The disorder does not fully meet Criterion B for autism.

Rett's syndrome

A. There is an apparently normal prenatal and perinatal period *and* apparently normal psychomotor development through the first 5 months *and* normal head circumference at birth.

B. There is deceleration of head growth between 5 months and 4 years *and* loss of acquired purposeful hand skills between 5 and 30 months of age that is associated with concurrent communication dysfunction and impaired social interactions *and* the appearance of poorly coordinated/unstable gait and/or trunk movements.

(*continued*)

Table 42–8
DSM-IV-TR Diagnostic Criteria for Pervasive Developmental Disorder Not Otherwise Specified (Including Atypical Autism)

This category should be used when there is a severe and pervasive impairment in the development of reciprocal social interaction associated with impairment in either verbal or nonverbal communication skills or with the presence of stereotyped behavior, interests, and activities, but the criteria are not met for a specific pervasive developmental disorder, schizophrenia, schizotypal personality disorder, or avoidant personality disorder. For example, this category includes "atypical autism"—presentations that do not meet the criteria for autistic disorder because of late age at onset, atypical symptomatology, or subthreshold symptomatology, or all of these.

From American Psychiatric Association. *Diagnostic and Statistical Manual of Mental Disorders.* 4th ed. Text rev. Washington, DC: American Psychiatric Association; copyright 2000, with permission.

appear socially uncomfortable and shy, and often exhibit illogical thinking.

Treatment

Treatment depends on the patient's level of adaptive functioning. Some of the same techniques used for autistic disorder are likely to benefit Asperger's disorder patients with severe social impairment.

PERVASIVE DEVELOPMENTAL DISORDER NOT OTHERWISE SPECIFIED

DSM-IV-TR defines pervasive disorder not otherwise specified as severe, pervasive impairment in communication skills or the presence of stereotyped behavior, interests, and activities with associated impairment in social interactions. However, the criteria for a specific pervasive developmental disorder, schizophrenia, and schizotypal and avoidant personality disorders are not met (Table 42–8). Some children who receive the diagnosis exhibit a markedly restricted repertoire of activities and interest. The condition usually shows a better outcome than autistic disorder.

Leslie was the oldest of two children. She had been a difficult baby who was not easy to console but whose motor and communicative development seemed appropriate. She was socially related and sometimes enjoyed interaction, but was easily overstimulated. She exhibited some hand flapping. Her parents sought evaluation when she was 4 years of age because of difficulties in nursery school. Leslie had problems with peer interaction. She was often preoccupied with possible adverse events. At evaluation she displayed both communicative and cognitive functions within the normal range. Although differential social relatedness was present, Leslie had difficulty using her parents as sources of support and comfort. She displayed behavioral rigidity and a tendency to impose routines on social skills. Subsequently, she was placed in a transitional kindergarten and did well academically although problems in peer interactions and unusual affective responses persisted. As an adolescent, she describes herself as a "loner" who has difficulties with social interaction and tends to enjoy solitary activities. (Reprinted with permission from Volkmar F. Autism and the pervasive developmental disorders. In: Lewis M, ed. *Child and Adolescent Psychiatry: A Comprehensive Approach.* 2nd ed. Baltimore: Williams & Wilkins; 1996.)

Treatment

The treatment approach is basically the same as in autistic disorder. Mainstreaming in school may be possible. Compared with autistic children, those with pervasive developmental disorder not otherwise specified generally have better language skills and more self-awareness, so they are better candidates for psychotherapy.

ICD-10

Like the description of pervasive developmental disorders in DSM-IV-TR, in the 10th revision of *International Statistical Classification of Diseases and Related Health Problems* (ICD-10), these disorders are described as characterized by "qualitative abnormalities in reciprocal social interactions and in patterns of communications, and by a restricted, stereotyped, repetitive repertoire of interests and activities." Although cognitive impairment is frequently present, the disorders are defined in terms of behavior "that is deviant in relation to mental age (whether the individual is retarded or not)."

Among these disorders, ICD-10 includes childhood autism, atypical autism, Rett's syndrome, other childhood disintegrative disorder, overactive disorder associated with mental retardation and stereotyped movements, Asperger's syndrome, other pervasive developmental disorders, and pervasive developmental disorder, unspecified. The ICD-10 childhood autism category corresponds to autistic disorder in DSM-IV-TR. According to ICD-10, however, atypical autism differs from childhood autism in age or onset or in failure to fulfill all three sets of diagnostic criteria. It first becomes apparent only after the age of 3 years, shows fewer abnormalities in the areas required for diagnosing autism, and generally occurs in children who are profoundly retarded or who have a severe "specific developmental disorder of receptive language."

According to ICD-10, overactive disorder associated with mental retardation and stereotyped movements is "an ill-defined disorder of uncertain nosological validity." ICD-10 includes this diagnosis because children with severe mental retardation who have hyperactivity and inattention problems also frequently show stereotyped behaviors. Their overactivity tends not to benefit from stimulant drugs as does that of children with a normal IQ; in adolescents, these children tend toward underactivity. They may also display developmental delays. (In ICD-10, cases of mild retardation with hyperkinetic syndrome are classified in the category of hyperkinetic disorders.) The ICD-10 criteria are presented in Table 42–9.

course in rare cases, and some improvement in occasional cases to the point of regaining the ability to speak in sentences. Most patients are left with at least moderate mental retardation.

Treatment

Because of the clinical similarity to autistic disorder, the treatment of childhood disintegrative disorder includes the same components available in the treatment of autistic disorder.

ASPERGER'S DISORDER

According to DSM-IV-TR, those with Asperger's disorder show severe, sustained impairment in social interaction and restricted, repetitive patterns of behavior, interests, and activities. Unlike autistic disorder, in Asperger's disorder there are no significant delays in language, cognitive development, or age-appropriate self-help skills. In 1944, Hans Asperger, an Austrian physician, described a syndrome that he named *autistic psychopathy.* His original description of the syndrome applied to persons with normal intelligence who exhibit a qualitative impairment in reciprocal social interaction and behavioral oddities without delays in language development. Since that time, a person with mental retardation but without language delay has received a diagnosis of Asperger's disorder, and a person with language delay but without mental retardation has also been given that diagnosis.

Etiology

The cause of Asperger's disorder is unknown, but family studies suggest a possible relationship to autistic disorder. The similarity of Asperger's disorder to autistic disorder supports the presence of genetic, metabolic, infectious, and perinatal contributing factors.

Diagnosis and Clinical Features

The clinical features include at least two of the following indications of qualitative social impairment: markedly abnormal nonverbal communicative gestures, the failure to develop peer relationships, the lack of social or emotional reciprocity, and an impaired ability to express pleasure in other persons' happiness. Restricted interests and patterns of behavior are always present. According to DSM-IV-TR, the patient shows no language delay, clinically significant cognitive delay, or adaptive impairment (Table 42–7).

Table 42–7
DSM-IV-TR Diagnostic Criteria for Asperger's Disorder

A. Qualitative impairment in social interaction, as manifested by at least two of the following:
   (1) marked impairment in the use of multiple nonverbal behaviors such as eye-to-eye gaze, facial expression, body postures, and gestures to regulate social interaction
   (2) failure to develop peer relationships appropriate to developmental level
   (3) a lack of spontaneous seeking to share enjoyment, interests, or achievements with other people (e.g., by a lack of showing, bringing, or pointing out objects of interest to other people)
   (4) lack of social or emotional reciprocity

B. Restricted repetitive and stereotyped patterns of behavior, interests, and activities, as manifested by at least one of the following:
   (1) encompassing preoccupation with one or more stereotyped and restricted patterns of interest that is abnormal either in intensity or focus
   (2) apparently inflexible adherence to specific, nonfunctional routines or rituals
   (3) stereotyped and repetitive motor mannerisms (e.g., hand or finger flapping or twisting, or complex whole-body movements)
   (4) persistent preoccupation with parts of objects

C. The disturbance causes clinically significant impairment in social, occupational, or other important areas of functioning.

D. There is no clinically significant general delay in language (e.g., single words used by age 2 years, communicative phrases used by age 3 years).

E. There is no clinically significant delay in cognitive development or in the development of age-appropriate self-help skills, adaptive behavior (other than in social interaction), and curiosity about the environment in childhood.

F. Criteria are not met for another specific pervasive developmental disorder or schizophrenia.

From American Psychiatric Association. *Diagnostic and Statistical Manual of Mental Disorders.* 4th ed. Text rev. Washington, DC: American Psychiatric Association; copyright 2000, with permission.

Differential Diagnosis

The differential diagnosis includes autistic disorder, pervasive development disorder not otherwise specified, and, in patients approaching adulthood, schizoid personality disorder. According to DSM-IV-TR, the most obvious distinctions between Asperger's disorder and autistic disorder are the criteria about language delay and dysfunction. The lack of language delay is a requirement for Asperger's disorder, while language impairment is a core feature in autistic disorder. Recent studies comparing children with Asperger's disorder and autistic disorder find that children with Asperger's disorder were more likely to look for social interaction and sought more vigorously to make friends. More efforts seem to be made on the part of those with Asperger's disorder to engage in an activity with another child. Although significant general delay in language is an exclusionary criterion in the diagnosis of Asperger's disorder, some delay in the acquisition of language has been seen in over one third of clinical samples.

Course and Prognosis

Although little is known about the cohort described by the DSM-IV-TR diagnostic criteria, past case reports have shown variable courses and prognoses for patients who have received diagnoses of Asperger's disorder. The factors associated with a good prognosis are a normal IQ and high-level social skills. Anecdotal reports of some adults diagnosed with Asperger's disorder as children show them to be verbal and intelligent; however, they relate in an awkward way to other adults,

language function occurring in 3- and 4-year-olds with previously normal functions. After the deterioration, the children closely resembled children with autistic disorder.

Epidemiology

Epidemiological data have been complicated by the variable diagnostic criteria used, but childhood disintegrative disorder is estimated to be at least one tenth as common as autistic disorder, and the prevalence has been estimated to be about one case in 100,000 boys. The ratio of boys to girls is estimated to be between 4 and 8 boys to 1 girl.

Etiology

The cause of childhood disintegrative disorder is unknown, but it has been associated with other neurological conditions, including seizure disorders, tuberous sclerosis, and various metabolic disorders.

Diagnosis and Clinical Features

The diagnosis is made on the basis of features that fit a characteristic age of onset, clinical picture, and course. Cases reported have ranged in onset from ages 1 to 9 years, but in the vast majority, the onset is between 3 and 4 years; according to DSM-IV-TR, the minimum age of onset is 2 years (Table 42–6). The onset may be insidious over several months or relatively abrupt, with abilities diminishing in days or weeks. In some cases, a child displays restlessness, increased activity level, and anxiety before the loss of function. The core features of the disorder include loss of communication skills, marked regression of reciprocal interactions, and the onset of stereotyped movements and compulsive behavior. Affective symptoms are common, particularly anxiety, as is the regression of self-help skills, such as bowel and bladder control.

To receive the diagnosis, a child must exhibit loss of skills in two of the following areas: language, social or adaptive behavior, bowel or bladder control, play, and motor skills. Abnormalities must be present in at least two of the following categories: reciprocal social interaction, communication skills, and stereotyped or restricted behavior. The main neurological associated feature is seizure disorder.

Table 42–6
DSM-IV-TR Diagnostic Criteria for Childhood Disintegrative Disorder

A. Apparently normal development for at least the first 2 years after birth as manifested by the presence of age-appropriate verbal and nonverbal communication, social relationships, play, and adaptive behavior.

B. Clinically significant loss of previously acquired skills (before age 10 years) in at least two of the following areas:
   (1) expressive or receptive language
   (2) social skills or adaptive behavior
   (3) bowel or bladder control
   (4) play
   (5) motor skills

C. Abnormalities of functioning in at least two of the following areas:
   (1) qualitative impairment in social interaction (e.g., impairment in nonverbal behaviors, failure to develop peer relationships, lack of social or emotional reciprocity)
   (2) qualitative impairments in communication (e.g., delay or lack of spoken language, inability to initiate or sustain a conversation, stereotyped and repetitive use of language, lack of varied make-believe play)
   (3) restricted, repetitive, and stereotyped patterns of behavior, interests, and activities, including motor stereotypies and mannerisms

D. The disturbance is not better accounted for by another specific pervasive developmental disorder or by schizophrenia.

From American Psychiatric Association. *Diagnostic and Statistical Manual of Mental Disorders.* 4th ed. Text rev. Washington, DC: American Psychiatric Association; copyright 2000, with permission.

Bob's early history was within normal limits. By age 2, he was speaking in sentences, and his development appeared to be proceeding appropriately. At age 40 months he abruptly exhibited a period of marked behavioral regression shortly after the birth of a sibling. He lost previously acquired skills in communication and was no longer toilet trained. He became uninterested in social interaction, and various unusual self-stimulatory behaviors became evident. Comprehensive medical examination failed to reveal any conditions that might account for this developmental regression. Behaviorally, he exhibited features of autistic disorder. At follow-up at age 12 he spoke only an occasional single word and was severely retarded. (Reprinted with permission from Volkmar F. Autism and the pervasive developmental disorders. In: Lewis M, ed. *Child and Adolescent Psychiatry: A Comprehensive Approach.* 2nd ed. Baltimore: Williams & Wilkins; 1996.)

Differential Diagnosis

The differential diagnosis of childhood disintegrative disorder includes autistic disorder and Rett's disorder. In many cases the clinical features overlap with autistic disorder, but childhood disintegrative disorder is distinguished from autistic disorder by the loss of previously acquired development. Before the onset of childhood disintegrative disorder (occurring at 2 years or older), language has usually progressed to sentence formation. This skill is strikingly different from the premorbid history of even high-functioning autistic disorder patients, in whom language generally does not exceed single words or phrases before diagnosis of the disorder. Once the disorder occurs, however, those with childhood disintegrative disorder are more likely to have no language abilities than are high-functioning autistic disorder patients. In Rett's disorder, the deterioration occurs much earlier than in childhood disintegrative disorder, and the characteristic hand stereotypies of Rett's disorder do not occur in childhood disintegrative disorder.

Course and Prognosis

The course of childhood disintegrative disorder is variable, with a plateau reached in most cases, a progressive deteriorating

been done, available data indicate a prevalence of 6 to 7 cases of Rett's disorder per 100,000 girls.

Etiology

The cause of Rett's disorder is unknown, although the progressive deteriorating course after an initial normal period is compatible with a metabolic disorder. In some patients with Rett's disorder, the presence of hyperammonemia has led to postulation that an enzyme metabolizing ammonia is deficient, but hyperammonemia has not been found in most patients with Rett's disorder. It is likely that Rett's disorder has a genetic basis. It has been seen only in girls, and case reports so far indicate complete concordance in monozygotic twins.

Diagnosis and Clinical Features

During the first 5 months after birth, infants have age-appropriate motor skills, normal head circumference, and normal growth. Social interactions show the expected reciprocal quality. At 6 months to 2 years of age, however, these children develop progressive encephalopathy with a number of characteristic features. The signs often include the loss of purposeful hand movements, which are replaced by stereotypic motions such as hand-wringing, the loss of previously acquired speech, psychomotor retardation, and ataxia. Other stereotypical hand movements may occur, such as licking or biting the fingers and tapping or slapping. The head-circumference growth decelerates and produces microcephaly. All language skills are lost, and both receptive and expressive communicative and social skills seem to plateau at developmental levels between 6 months and 1 year. Poor muscle coordination and an apraxic gait with an unsteady and stiff quality develop. All of these clinical features are diagnostic criteria for the disorder (Table 42–5).

Associated features include seizures in up to 75 percent of affected children and disorganized EEGs with some epileptiform discharges in almost all young children with Rett's disorder, even in the absence of clinical seizures. An additional associated feature is irregular respiration, with episodes of hyperventilation, apnea, and breath holding. The disorganized breathing occurs in most patients while they are awake; during sleep the breathing usually normalizes. Many patients with Rett's disorder also have scoliosis. As the disorder progresses, muscle tone seems to increase from an initial hypotonic condition to spasticity to rigidity.

Although children with Rett's disorder may live for well over a decade after the onset of the disorder, after 10 years, many patients are wheelchair-bound, with muscle wasting, rigidity, and virtually no language ability. Long-term receptive and expressive communication and socialization abilities remain at a developmental level of less than 1 year.

Table 42–5
DSM-IV-TR Diagnostic Criteria for Rett's Disorder

A. All of the following:
  (1) apparently normal prenatal and perinatal development
  (2) apparently normal psychomotor development through the first 5 months after birth
  (3) normal head circumference at birth
B. Onset of all of the following after the period of normal development:
  (1) deceleration of head growth between ages 5 and 48 months
  (2) loss of previously acquired purposeful hand skills between ages 5 and 30 months with the subsequent development of stereotyped hand movements (e.g., hand wringing or hand washing)
  (3) loss of social engagement early in the course (although often social interaction develops later)
  (4) appearance of poorly coordinated gait or trunk movements
  (5) severely impaired expressive and receptive language development with severe psychomotor retardation

From American Psychiatric Association. *Diagnostic and Statistical Manual of Mental Disorders.* 4th ed. Text rev. Washington, DC: American Psychiatric Association; copyright 2000, with permission.

Differential Diagnosis

Some children with Rett's disorder receive initial diagnoses of autistic disorder because of the marked disability in social interactions in both disorders, but the two disorders have some predictable differences. In Rett's disorder, a child shows deterioration of developmental milestones, head circumference, and overall growth; in autistic disorder, aberrant development is usually present from early on. In Rett's disorder, specific and characteristic hand motions are always present; in autistic disorder, hand mannerisms may or may not appear. Poor coordination, ataxia, and apraxia are predictably part of Rett's disorder; many persons with autistic disorder have unremarkable gross motor function. In Rett's disorder, verbal abilities are usually lost completely; in autistic disorder, patients use characteristically aberrant language. Respiratory irregularity is characteristic of Rett's disorder, and seizures often appear early; in autistic disorder, no respiratory disorganization is seen, and seizures do not develop in most patients; when seizures do develop, they are more likely in adolescence than in childhood.

Course and Prognosis

Rett's disorder is progressive. The prognosis is not fully known, but patients who live into adulthood remain at a cognitive and social level equivalent to that in the first year of life.

Treatment

Treatment is symptomatic. Physiotherapy has been beneficial for the muscular dysfunction, and anticonvulsant treatment is usually necessary to control the seizures. Behavior therapy, along with medication, may help control self-injurious behaviors, as it does in the treatment of autistic disorder, and it may help regulate the breathing disorganization.

CHILDHOOD DISINTEGRATIVE DISORDER

According to DSM-IV-TR, childhood disintegrative disorder is characterized by marked regression in several areas of functioning after at least 2 years of apparently normal development. Childhood disintegrative disorder, also called *Heller's syndrome* and *disintegrative psychosis,* was described in 1908 as a deterioration over several months of intellectual, social, and

in eliciting language to produce messages demonstrating a child's ability to read and write, to do mathematics, to express feelings, and even to write poetry. Although these techniques are risky because the facilitator may need to inject much interpretation to produce typical communication, some families of autistic children support this technique and continue to use it.

There are no specific medications to treat the core symptoms of autistic disorder; however, psychopharmacotherapy is a valuable adjunctive treatment to ameliorate associated behavioral symptoms. Medication has been reported to improve associated symptoms including aggression, severe temper tantrums, self-injurious behaviors, hyperactivity, and obsessive-compulsive behaviors and stereotypies. The administration of antipsychotic medication may reduce aggressive or self-injurious behavior. One early study indicated that haloperidol (Haldol) reduced behavioral symptoms such as hyperactivity, stereotypies, withdrawal, fidgetiness, irritability, and labile affect and accelerated learning. There have been no additional studies replicating these findings, and because of its potentially serious adverse effects, haloperidol is no longer the drug of choice in the treatment of self-injurious behaviors in children with autistic disorder. Although the serious adverse effects of antipsychotic medications, such as tardive and withdrawal dyskinesias and neuroleptic malignant syndrome, can occur with use of any antipsychotic medication, the newer, safer atypical antipsychotics (i.e., the serotonin-dopamine antagonists [SDAs]) have generally replaced the older typical antipsychotic agents (i.e., the dopamine receptor antagonists).

SDAs carry a lower risk of causing extrapyramidal adverse effects, although some sensitive individuals cannot tolerate the extrapyramidal or anticholinergic adverse effects of the atypical antipsychotic agents. The SDAs include risperidone (Risperdal), olanzapine (Zyprexa), quetiapine (Seroquel), clozapine (Clozaril), and ziprasidone (Geodon).

Risperidone, a high-potency antipsychotic with combined dopamine D_2 and serotonin 5-HT_2 receptor antagonist properties, has been used to subdue aggressive or self-injurious behaviors. Several reports have suggested that risperidone is effective in diminishing aggressiveness, hyperactivity, and self-injurious behavior in children with autistic disorder. In some cases it reportedly encouraged socially acceptable behaviors. Studies of risperidone use in the treatment of adult psychosis indicate that a dosage up to 6 mg per day is generally effective. For children with autism, lower dosages ranging from 0.5 to 4 mg per day are generally used. Extrapyramidal effects and akathisia are not uncommon adverse effects, as well as sedation, dizziness, or weight gain.

Olanzapine specifically blocks 5-HT_{2A} and D_2 receptors and also blocks muscarinic receptors. No studies provide specific guidelines regarding the use of olanzapine in children with autism. Dosages that have been used clinically to target aggression and self-injurious behaviors range from 2.5 to about 10 mg per day. Among olanzapine's most common adverse effects are sedation, orthostatic hypotension, and (over time) weight gain.

Quetiapine is an antipsychotic with more potent 5-H_2 than D_2 receptor blocking properties. Although there are no data on its effectiveness on aggression in children with autism, it is sometimes tried when risperidone and olanzapine are not efficacious or well tolerated. There are no guidelines about best dosage; it has been used in clinical practice at dosages ranging from 50 to 200 mg per day. Adverse effects include drowsiness, tachycardia, agitation, and weight gain.

Clozapine has a heterocyclic chemical structure that is related to certain conventional antipsychotics such as loxapine (Loxitane), though clozapine carries a lower risk of extrapyramidal symptoms. It is not generally used in the treatment of aggression and self-injurious behavior unless those behaviors coexist with psychotic symptoms. Its most serious adverse effect is agranulocytosis, which necessitates monitoring white blood cell count weekly during clozapine's use. Its use is generally limited to treatment-resistant psychotic patients.

Ziprasidone has receptor-blocking properties at the 5-HT_{2A} and D_2 receptor sites and carries little risk of extrapyramidal and antihistaminic effects. There are no guidelines for its use in autistic children with aggressive and self-injurious behaviors, but it has been used clinically to treat the latter behaviors in children who are treatment resistant. In studies of its use in adults with schizophrenia, dosage ranges of 40 to 160 mg were found to be effective. Adverse effects include sedation, dizziness, and lightheadedness. An electrocardiogram (ECG) is generally obtained prior to use of this medication.

The selective serotonin reuptake inhibitors (SSRIs) have been used as adjunctive treatments to diminish and modify obsessive-compulsive and stereotypical behaviors. The amount of improvement attained with use of these medications for autistic children with the above behaviors is still not clear.

A recent double-blind study investigated the efficacy of amantadine (Symmetrel), which blocks *N*-methyl-D-aspartate (NMDA) receptors, in the treatment of behavioral disturbance such as irritability, aggression, and hyperactivity in children with autism. Some have suggested that abnormalities of the glutamatergic system may contribute to the emergence of pervasive developmental disorders. High glutamate levels have been found in children with Rett's syndrome. In the above study, 47 percent of children on amantadine were rated "improved" by their parents, and 37 percent of children on placebo were rated "improved" by parents in irritability and hyperactivity, although this difference was not statistically significant. Investigators rated the children on amantadine "significantly improved" with respect to hyperactivity. A double-blind, placebo-controlled study of the efficacy of the anticonvulsant lamotrigine (Lamictal) on hyperactivity in children with autism showed high rates of placebo improvement in ratings of hyperactivity.

Clomipramine (Anafranil) has been used in autistic disorders but without positive results. Fenfluramine (Pondimin), which reduces blood serotonin levels, was reported anecdotally to be effective in a few autistic children. Improvement does not seem to be associated with a reduction in blood serotonin level. Naltrexone (ReVia), an opioid receptor antagonist, has been investigated without much success, based on the notion that blocking endogenous opioids would reduce autistic symptoms. Lithium (Eskalith) use can be tried for aggressive or self-injurious behaviors when other medications fail.

RETT'S DISORDER

Rett's disorder is described by DSM-IV-TR as a development of several specific deficits following a period of normal functioning after birth. In 1965, Andreas Rett, an Australian physician, identified a syndrome in 22 girls who appeared to have developed normally for at least 6 months, followed by devastating developmental deterioration. Although few surveys have

Table 42–4
Autistic Disorder versus Mixed Receptive-Expressive Language Disorder

Criteria	Autistic Disorder	Mixed Receptive-Expressive Language Disorder
Incidence	2–5 in 10,000	5 in 10,000
Sex ratio (M:F)	3–4:1	Equal or almost equal sex ratio
Family history of speech delay or language problems	Present in about 25 percent of cases	Present in about 25 percent of cases
Associated deafness	Very infrequent	Not infrequent
Nonverbal communication (gestures, etc.)	Absent or rudimentary	Present
Language abnormalities (e.g., echolalia, stereotyped phrases out of context)	More common	Less common
Articulatory problems	Less frequent	More frequent
Level of intelligence	Often severely impaired	Though may be impaired, less frequently severe
Patterns of IQ tests	Uneven, lower on verbal scores than dysphasic patients, lower on comprehension subtest than dysphasic patients	More even, though verbal IQ lower than performance IQ
Autistic behaviors, impaired social life, stereotypies, and ritualistic activities	More common and more severe	Absent or, if present, less severe
Imaginative play	Absent or rudimentary	Usually present

Adapted from Magda Campbell, M.D., and Wayne Green, M.D.

only infrequently, whereas deaf infants have a history of relatively normal babbling that then gradually tapers off and may stop at 6 months to 1 year of age. Deaf children respond only to loud sounds, whereas autistic children may ignore loud or normal sounds and respond to soft or low sounds. Most importantly, audiogram or auditory-evoked potentials indicate significant hearing loss in deaf children. Unlike autistic children, deaf children usually relate to their parents, seek their affection, and enjoy being held as infants.

Psychosocial Deprivation. Severe disturbances in the physical and emotional environment (e.g., maternal deprivation, psychosocial dwarfism, hospitalism, and failure to thrive) can cause children to appear apathetic, withdrawn, and alienated. Language and motor skills can be delayed. Children with these signs almost always improve rapidly when placed in a favorable and enriched psychosocial environment, but such improvement is not the case with autistic children.

Course and Prognosis

Autistic disorder is generally a lifelong disorder with a guarded prognosis. Autistic children with IQs above 70 and those who use communicative language by ages 5 to 7 tend to have the best prognoses. Recent follow-up data comparing high-IQ autistic children at the age of 5 years with their current symptomatology at ages 13 through young adulthood found that a small proportion no longer met criteria for autism, although they still exhibited some features of the disorder. Most demonstrated positive changes in communication and social domains over time.

The symptom areas that did not seem to improve over time were those related to ritualistic and repetitive behaviors. In general, adult-outcome studies indicate that about two thirds of autistic adults remain severely handicapped and live in complete dependence or semidependence, either with their relatives or in long-term institutions. Only 1 to 2 percent acquire a normal, independent status with gainful employment, and 5 to 20 percent achieve a borderline normal status. The prognosis is improved if the environment or home is supportive and capable of meeting the extensive needs of such a child. Although symptoms decrease in many cases, severe self-mutilation or aggressiveness and regression may develop in others. About 4 to 32 percent have grand mal seizures in late childhood or adolescence, and the seizures adversely affect the prognosis.

Treatment

The goals of treatment for children with autistic disorder are to increase socially acceptable and prosocial behavior, to decrease odd behavioral symptoms, and to improve verbal and nonverbal communication. Both language remediation and academic remediation are often required. Children with mental retardation need intellectually appropriate behavioral interventions to reinforce socially acceptable behaviors and encourage self-care skills. In addition, parents, often distraught, need support and counseling. Insight-oriented individual psychotherapy has proved ineffective. Educational and behavioral interventions are currently considered the treatments of choice. Structured classroom training in combination with behavioral methods is the most effective treatment for many autistic children.

Well-controlled studies indicate that gains in the areas of language and cognition and decreases in maladaptive behaviors are achieved by consistent behavioral programs. Careful training of parents in the concepts and skills of behavior modification and resolution of the parents' concerns may yield considerable gains in children's language, cognitive, and social areas of behavior. These training programs, however, are rigorous and require much parental time. An autistic child requires as much structure as possible, and a daily program for as many hours as feasible is desirable.

Facilitated communication is a technique by which an autistic or a mentally retarded child with some language is aided in communication by a teacher who helps the child pick out letters on a computer or letter board. Some facilitators have reported success

Table 42–2
Procedure for Differential Diagnosis on a Multiaxial System

1. Determine intellectual level
2. Determine level of language development
3. Consider whether child's behavior is appropriate for
   (i) chronological age
   (ii) mental age
   (iii) language age
4. If not appropriate, consider differential diagnosis of psychiatric disorder according to
   (i) pattern of social interaction
   (ii) pattern of language
   (iii) pattern of play
   (iv) other behaviors
5. Identify any relevant medical conditions
6. Consider whether there are any relevant psychosocial factors

Reprinted with permission from Rutter M, Hersov I. *Child and Adolescent Psychiatry: Modern Approaches.* 2nd ed. Oxford: Blackwell; 1985:73.

mixed receptive-expressive language disorder, congenital deafness or severe hearing disorder, psychosocial deprivation, and disintegrative (regressive) psychoses. Because children with a pervasive developmental disorder usually have many concurrent problems, Michael Rutter and Lionel Hersov suggested a stepwise approach to the differential diagnosis (Table 42–2).

Schizophrenia with Childhood Onset. Although a wealth of literature on autistic disorder is available, few data exist on children under age 12 who meet the diagnostic criteria for schizophrenia. Schizophrenia is rare in children under the age of 5. It is accompanied by hallucinations or delusions, with a lower incidence of seizures and mental retardation and a more even IQ than autistic children exhibit. Table 42–3 compares autistic disorder and schizophrenia with childhood onset.

Mental Retardation with Behavioral Symptoms. About 40 percent of autistic children are moderately, severely, or profoundly retarded, and retarded children may have behavioral symptoms that include autistic features. When both disorders are present, both should be diagnosed. The main differentiating features between autistic disorder and mental retardation are that mentally retarded children usually relate to adults and other children in accordance with their mental age, use the language they do have to communicate with others, and exhibit a relatively even profile of impairments without splinter functions.

Mixed Receptive-Expressive Language Disorder. Some children with mixed receptive-expressive language disorder have mild autistic-like features and may present a diagnostic problem. Table 42–4 summarizes the major differences between autistic disorder and mixed receptive-expressive language disorder.

Acquired Aphasia with Convulsion. Acquired aphasia with convulsion is a rare condition that is sometimes difficult to differentiate from autistic disorder and childhood disintegrative disorder. Children with the condition are normal for several years before losing both their receptive and their expressive language over a period of weeks or months. Most have a few seizures and generalized EEG abnormalities at the onset, but these signs usually do not persist. A profound language comprehension disorder then follows, characterized by a deviant speech pattern and speech impairment. Some children recover but with considerable residual language impairment.

Congenital Deafness or Severe Hearing Impairment. Because autistic children are often mute or show a selective disinterest in spoken language, they are often thought to be deaf. Differentiating factors include the following. Autistic infants may babble

Table 42–3
Autistic Disorder versus Schizophrenia with Childhood Onset

Criteria	Autistic Disorder	Schizophrenia (with Onset before Puberty)
Age of onset	Before 38 months	Not under 5 years of age
Incidence	2–5 in 10,000	Unknown, possibly same or even rarer
Sex ratio (M:F)	3–4:1	1.67:1 (nearly equal, or slight preponderance of males)
Family history of schizophrenia	Not raised or probably not raised	Raised
Socioeconomic status (SES)	Overrepresentation of upper SES groups (artifact)	More common in lower SES groups
Prenatal and perinatal complications and cerebral dysfunction	More common in autistic disorder	Less common in schizophrenia
Behavioral characteristics	Failure to develop relatedness; absence of speech or echolalia; stereotyped phrases; language comprehension absent or poor; insistence on sameness and stereotypies	Hallucinations and delusions; thought disorder
Adaptive functioning	Usually always impaired	Deterioration in functioning
Level of intelligence	In majority of cases subnormal, frequently severely impaired (70% ≤ 70)	Usually within normal range, mostly dull normal (15% ≤ 70)
Pattern of IQ	Marked unevenness	More even
Grand mal seizures	4–32%	Absent or lower incidence

Courtesy of Magda Campbell, M.D., and Wayne Green, M.D.

has had trouble following directions since he started preschool at age 3 years, but he had never been described as aggressive until this year. According to his teacher, Roy is picked on often by his classmates, who think he is "weird."

Roy was the product of a normal pregnancy but was treated for 10 days with antibiotics in the neonatal intensive care unit after birth because he developed bacterial meningitis after delivery. Fortunately, it was caught early, and the doctors had assured his mother that there was no permanent damage. He was healthy after being discharged from the hospital.

Roy's parents began to get concerned about his language development because he could only say "dada" at 18 months. The pediatrician was very reassuring, stating that some children develop language later than others and that there were no signs of any neurological disease. Roy's mother had his hearing tested, since she had read that babies who were treated with antibiotics as newborns might develop hearing loss. Roy's hearing was normal, but his mother continued to notice that he did not usually turn his head toward her when she spoke to him. Roy's mother assumed that he had a poor attention span, like his older brother, and was not too worried about his lack of attention to adults. She continued to be concerned that his language was not developing appropriately.

When Roy started preschool, it became clear that he did not play with toys the same way as the other children. He did not seem to understand how to use the toys and would use a truck, for example, to bang on the floor. He had acquired more words by now, but his sentences were often incomprehensible. He often said "You" when he meant "I" and repeated verbatim phrases that he had heard earlier in the day. He was unable to share toys and never joined in group activities that required the class to sit in a circle. Instead, he stayed in the corner of the room playing by himself. He would not let the teacher know when he was thirsty or had to go to the bathroom. He would not answer questions; sometimes he became overly excited and hyperactive and ran around the room with no apparent goal. Most of the time he did not make eye contact and was isolated from others. Roy usually did not do much with the other children, so the teacher only had difficulty managing him when he became hyperactive and resisted sitting down. The teacher did mention that Roy was a creature of habit, he played with the same toy every single day, and he would get extremely upset if any other child tried to touch his favorite toy.

By the time Roy reached first grade, it was clear that he was not socializing with any of his classmates, and his language was still poor. He also did not seem to understand what was expected of him in class, and he often appeared distracted and distant.

An evaluation was initiated with psychological testing. On intellectual testing, Roy's full-scale intelligence quotient (IQ) was 68, with a verbal IQ of 61 and a performance IQ of 75, placing him in the range of probable mild mental retardation. Roy's language skills were an area of major weakness. Although Roy had now learned many words, he exhibited great difficulty making himself understood and responding to his peers. Roy's language problems included pronoun reversals, echolalia, and unusual syntax. Roy's social problems were as much a problem as his language. He had few interests and was rejected by his peers. He seemed fixated on running water and would spend up to an hour, if allowed, watching water run out of the faucet. Roy did not understand his schoolwork and continued to have periods of overactivity in which he would run around the classroom aimlessly.

DISCUSSION

Given the combination of aberrant language development, significant inability to relate to peers or adults, and a very restricted range of interests, a diagnosis of autistic disorder was made. In addition, after evaluating his "living skills," such as dressing himself and communicating with others, along with his intellectual testing, it was determined that Roy also had mild mental retardation. Furthermore, he also had frequent periods of hyperactivity, poor attention, and distractibility in school and at home, causing significant problems for him, which led to a diagnosis of attention-deficit/hyperactivity disorder. It was recommended that Roy's family request initiation of an Individualized Educational Plan by his school so that he could be placed in a smaller, more structured special education classroom. A referral was made for a behavioral program to reinforce both appropriate social and task-oriented behaviors. A trial of methylphenidate (Ritalin) was recommended to target Roy's hyperactivity and poor attention.

Intellectual Functioning. About 75 percent of children with autistic disorder function in the mentally retarded range of intellectual function. About 30 percent of children function in the mild to moderate range, and about 45 to 50 percent are severely to profoundly mentally retarded. Epidemiological and clinical studies show that the risk for autistic disorder increases as the IQ decreases. About one fifth of all autistic children have a normal nonverbal intelligence. The IQ scores of autistic children tend to reflect most severe problems with verbal sequencing and abstraction skills, with relative strengths in visuospatial or rote memory skills. This finding suggests the importance of defects in language-related functions.

Unusual or precocious cognitive or visuomotor abilities occur in some autistic children. The abilities, which may exist even in the overall retarded functioning, are referred to as *splinter functions* or *islets of precocity.* Perhaps the most striking examples are idiot or autistic savants, who have prodigious rote memories or calculating abilities, usually beyond the capabilities of their normal peers. Other precocious abilities in young autistic children include hyperlexia, an early ability to read well (although they cannot understand what they read), memorizing and reciting, and musical abilities (singing or playing tunes or recognizing musical pieces).

Differential Diagnosis

The major differential diagnoses are schizophrenia with childhood onset, mental retardation with behavioral symptoms,

responding to another's interests, emotions, and feelings are major obstacles in developing them. Autistic adolescents and adults experience sexual feelings, but their lack of social competence and skills prevents many of them from developing sexual relationships.

DISTURBANCES OF COMMUNICATION AND LANGUAGE. Deficits in language development and difficulty using language to communicate ideas are among the principal criteria for diagnosing autistic disorder. Autistic children are not simply reluctant to speak, and their speech abnormalities are not due to lack of motivation. Language deviance, as much as language delay, is characteristic of autistic disorder. In contrast to normal and mentally retarded children, autistic children have significant difficulty putting meaningful sentences together even when they have large vocabularies. When children with autistic disorder do learn to converse fluently, their conversations may impart information without providing a sense of acknowledging how the other person is responding. In children with autism and nonautistic children with language disorders, nonverbal communication skills may also be impaired when there is significant difficulty with expressive language.

In the first year of life, an autistic child's pattern of babbling may be minimal or abnormal. Some children emit noises—clicks, sounds, screeches, and nonsense syllables—in a stereotyped fashion, without a seeming intent of communication. Unlike normal young children, who generally have better receptive language skills than expressive ones, verbal autistic children may say more than they understand. Words and even entire sentences may drop in and out of a child's vocabulary. It is not atypical for a child with autistic disorder to use a word once and then not use it again for a week, a month, or years. Children with autistic disorder typically exhibit speech that contains echolalia, both immediate and delayed, or stereotyped phrases that seem out of context. These language patterns are frequently associated with pronoun reversals. A child with autistic disorder might say, "You want the toy" when she means that she wants it. Difficulties in articulation are also common. Many children with autistic disorder use peculiar voice quality and rhythm. About 50 percent of autistic children never develop useful speech. Some of the brightest children show a particular fascination with letters and numbers. Children with autistic disorder sometimes excel in certain tasks or have special abilities; for example, a child may learn to read fluently at preschool age (hyperlexia), often astonishingly well. Very young autistic children who can read many words, however, have little comprehension of the words read.

STEREOTYPED BEHAVIOR. In the first years of an autistic child's life, much of the expected spontaneous exploratory play is absent. Toys and objects are often manipulated in a ritualistic manner, with few symbolic features. Autistic children generally do not show imitative play or use abstract pantomime. The activities and play of these children are often rigid, repetitive, and monotonous. Ritualistic and compulsive phenomena are common in early and middle childhood. Children often spin, bang, and line up objects and may exhibit an attachment to a particular inanimate object. Many autistic children, especially those who are severely mentally retarded, exhibit movement abnormalities. Stereotypies, mannerisms, and grimacing are most frequent when a child is left alone and may decrease in a structured situation. Autistic children are generally resistant to transition and change. Moving to a new house, moving furniture in a room, or a change such as having breakfast before a bath when the reverse was the routine may evoke panic, fear, or temper tantrums.

INSTABILITY OF MOOD AND AFFECT. Some children with autistic disorder exhibit sudden mood changes, with bursts of laughing or crying without an obvious reason. It is difficult to learn more about these episodes if the child cannot express the thoughts related to the affect.

RESPONSE TO SENSORY STIMULI. Autistic children have been observed to overrespond to some stimuli and underrespond to other sensory stimuli (e.g., to sound and pain). It is not uncommon for a child with autistic disorder to appear deaf, at times showing little response to a normal speaking voice; on the other hand, the same child may show intent interest in the sound of a wristwatch. Some children with autistic disorder have a heightened pain threshold or an altered response to pain. Indeed, some autistic children do not respond to an injury by crying or seeking comfort. Many autistic children reportedly enjoy music. They frequently hum a tune or sing a song or commercial jingle before saying words or using speech. Some particularly enjoy vestibular stimulation—spinning, swinging, and up-and-down movements.

ASSOCIATED BEHAVIORAL SYMPTOMS. Hyperkinesis is a common behavior problem in young autistic children. Hypokinesis is less frequent; when present, it often alternates with hyperactivity. Aggression and temper tantrums are observed, often prompted by change or demands. Self-injurious behavior includes head banging, biting, scratching, and hair pulling. Short attention span, poor ability to focus on a task, insomnia, feeding and eating problems, and enuresis are also common among children with autism.

ASSOCIATED PHYSICAL ILLNESS. Young children with autistic disorder have a higher-than-expected incidence of upper respiratory infections and other minor infections. Gastrointestinal symptoms commonly found among children with autistic disorder include excessive burping, constipation, and loose bowel movements. There is also an increased incidence of febrile seizures in children with autistic disorder. Some autistic children do not show temperature elevations with minor infectious illnesses and may not show the typical malaise of ill children. In some children, behavior problems and relatedness seem to improve noticeably during a minor illness, and in some, such changes are a clue to physical illness.

A standardized instrument that can be very helpful in eliciting comprehensive information regarding developmental disorders is the Autism Diagnostic Observation Schedule-Generic (ADOS-G).

Roy, a 6-year-old boy, was referred for a psychiatric evaluation by his first-grade teacher, who reported that Roy was disruptive in class, was unable to follow directions, had not really made any friends, and, at unpredictable times, was hyperactive and aggressive. Roy had never had a psychiatric evaluation, but his mother suspects that, like his older brother, he probably has attention-deficit/hyperactivity disorder. Roy

was due to emotionally unresponsive "refrigerator" mothers, there is no validity to this hypothesis. On the other hand, much evidence supports a biological substrate for this disorder.

Psychosocial and Family Factors. In his initial report, Kanner indicated that few parents of autistic children were warmhearted and that, for the most part, parents were preoccupied with intellectual abstractions, and mothers' lack of emotional responsivity was held accountable for the autism. No evidence has been found to support this theory. Other theories, such as parental rage and rejection and parental reinforcement of autistic symptoms are also unsubstantiated. More recent studies comparing parents of autistic children with parents of normal children have shown no significant differences in child-rearing skills.

Children with autistic disorder, like children with other disorders, can respond with exacerbated symptoms to psychosocial stressors including family discord, the birth of a new sibling, or a family move. Some children with autistic disorder may be excruciatingly sensitive to even small changes in their families and immediate environment.

Biological Factors. The high rate of mental retardation among children with autistic disorder and the higher-than-expected rates of seizure disorders suggest a biological basis for autistic disorder. Approximately 75 percent of children with autistic disorder have mental retardation. About one third of these children have mild to moderate mental retardation, and close to half of these children are severely or profoundly mentally retarded. Children with autistic disorder and mental retardation typically show more marked deficits in abstract reasoning, social understanding, and verbal tasks than in performance tasks such as block design and digit recall, in which details can be remembered without reference to the "gestalt" meaning.

Four to 32 percent of persons with autism have grand mal seizures at some time, and about 20 to 25 percent show ventricular enlargement on computed tomography (CT) scans. Various electroencephalogram (EEG) abnormalities are found in 10 to 83 percent of autistic children, and although no EEG finding is specific to autistic disorder, there is some indication of failed cerebral lateralization. Recently, one magnetic resonance imaging (MRI) study revealed hypoplasia of cerebellar vermal lobules VI and VII, and another MRI study revealed cortical abnormalities, particularly polymicrogyria, in some autistic patients. Those abnormalities may reflect abnormal cell migrations in the first 6 months of gestation. An autopsy study revealed fewer Purkinje's cells, and another study found increased diffuse cortical metabolism during positron emission tomography (PET) scanning.

Autistic disorder is also associated with neurological conditions, notably congenital rubella, phenylketonuria (PKU), tuberous sclerosis, and Rett's disorder. Autistic children show more evidence of perinatal complications than comparison groups of normal children and those with other disorders. The finding that autistic children have significantly more minor congenital physical anomalies than expected suggests abnormal development within the first trimester of pregnancy.

Genetic Factors. In several surveys, between 2 and 4 percent of siblings of autistic children also had autistic disorder, a rate 50 times that in the general population. The concordance rate of autistic disorder in the two largest twin studies was 36 percent in monozygotic pairs versus 0 percent in dizygotic pairs in one study and about 96 percent in monozygotic pairs versus about 27 percent in dizygotic pairs in the second study. High rates of cognitive difficulties, even in the nonautistic twin in monozygotic twins with perinatal complications, suggest that contributions of perinatal insult along with genetic vulnerability may lead to autistic disorder.

Clinical reports suggest that the nonautistic members of families with autistic members have higher rates of less pronounced language or other cognitive problems. Fragile X syndrome, a genetic disorder in which a portion of the X chromosome fractures, appears to be associated with autistic disorder. Approximately 1 percent of children with autistic disorder also have fragile X syndrome. Tuberous sclerosis, a genetic disorder characterized by multiple benign tumors, with autosomal dominant transmission is found with greater frequency among children with autistic disorder. Up to 2 percent of children with autistic disorder may also have tuberous sclerosis.

Recently, researchers screened the DNA of more than 150 pairs of siblings with autism. They found extremely strong evidence that two regions on chromosomes 2 and 7 contain genes involved with autism. Likely locations for autism-related genes were also found on chromosomes 16 and 17, although the strength of the correlation was somewhat weaker.

Immunological Factors. Several reports have suggested that immunological incompatibility (i.e., maternal antibodies directed at the fetus) may contribute to autistic disorder. The lymphocytes of some autistic children react with maternal antibodies, which raises the possibility that embryonic neural, or extraembryonic, tissues may be damaged during gestation.

Perinatal Factors. A higher-than-expected incidence of perinatal complications seems to occur in infants who are later diagnosed with autistic disorder. Maternal bleeding after the first trimester and meconium in the amniotic fluid have been reported in the histories of autistic children more often than in the general population. In the neonatal period, autistic children have a high incidence of respiratory distress syndrome and neonatal anemia.

Neuroanatomical Factors. MRI studies comparing autistic subjects and normal controls have shown that the total brain volume was larger in those with autism, although autistic children with severe mental retardation generally have smaller heads. The greatest average percentage increase in size occurred in the occipital lobe, parietal lobe, and temporal lobe. No differences were found in the frontal lobes. Specific origins of this enlargement are unknown. The increased volume can arise from three different possible mechanisms: increased neurogenesis, decreased neuronal death, and increased production of nonneuronal brain tissue such as glial cells or blood vessels. Brain enlargement has been suggested as a possible biological marker for autistic disorder.

The temporal lobe is believed to be a critical area of brain abnormality in autistic disorder. This suggestion is based on reports of autistic-like syndromes in some persons with temporal lobe damage. When the temporal region of animals is damaged, normal social behavior is lost, and restlessness, repetitive motor behavior, and a limited behavioral repertoire are seen.

Some brains of autistic individuals exhibit a decrease in cerebellar Purkinje's cells, which is believed to potentially account for abnormalities of attention, arousal, and sensory processes.

Biochemical Factors. A number of studies in the last few decades have demonstrated that about one third of patients with autistic disorder have high plasma serotonin concentrations. This finding, however, is not specific to autistic disorder, and persons with mental retardation without autistic disorder also display this trait. Several studies have reported that autistic individuals without mental retardation have a high incidence of hyperserotonemia. In some autistic children, high concentrations of homovanillic acid (the major dopamine metabolite) in cerebrospinal fluid (CSF) is associated with increased withdrawal and stereotypes. Some evidence indicates that symptom severity decreases as the ratio of 5-hydroxyindoleacetic acid (5-HIAA, metabolite of serotonin) to homovanillic acid in CSF increases. The 5-HIAA concentration in CSF may be inversely proportional to blood serotonin concentrations, which are increased in one third of autistic disorder patients, a nonspecific finding that also occurs in mentally retarded persons.

Diagnosis and Clinical Features

The DSM-IV-TR diagnostic criteria for autistic disorder are given in Table 42–1.

Table 42–1
DSM-IV-TR Diagnostic Criteria for Autistic Disorder

A. A total of six (or more) items from (1), (2), and (3), with at least two from (1), and one each from (2) and (3):
   (1) qualitative impairment in social interaction, as manifested by at least two of the following:
      (a) marked impairment in the use of multiple nonverbal behaviors such as eye-to-eye gaze, facial expression, body postures, and gestures to regulate social interaction
      (b) failure to develop peer relationships appropriate to developmental level
      (c) a lack of spontaneous seeking to share enjoyment, interests, or achievements with other people (e.g., by a lack of showing, bringing, or pointing out objects of interest)
      (d) lack of social or emotional reciprocity
   (2) qualitative impairments in communication as manifested by at least one of the following:
      (a) delay in, or total lack of, the development of spoken language (not accompanied by an attempt to compensate through alternative modes of communication such as gesture or mime)
      (b) in individuals with adequate speech, marked impairment in the ability to initiate or sustain a conversation with others
      (c) stereotyped and repetitive use of language or idiosyncratic language
      (d) lack of varied, spontaneous make-believe play or social imitative play appropriate to developmental level
   (3) restricted repetitive and stereotyped patterns of behavior, interests, and activities, as manifested by at least one of the following:
      (a) encompassing preoccupation with one or more stereotyped and restricted patterns of interest that is abnormal either in intensity or focus
      (b) apparently inflexible adherence to specific, nonfunctional routines or rituals
      (c) stereotyped and repetitive motor mannerisms (e.g., hand or finger flapping or twisting, or complex whole-body movements)
      (d) persistent preoccupation with parts of objects

B. Delays or abnormal functioning in at least one of the following areas, with onset prior to age 3 years: (1) social interaction, (2) language as used in social communication, or (3) symbolic or imaginative play.

C. The disturbance is not better accounted for by Rett's disorder or childhood disintegrative disorder.

From American Psychiatric Association. *Diagnostic and Statistical Manual of Mental Disorders.* 4th ed. Text rev. Washington, DC: American Psychiatric Association; copyright 2000, with permission.

Physical Characteristics. Children with autistic disorder are often described as attractive and, on first glance, do not show any physical signs indicating autistic disorder. These children do have high rates of minor physical anomalies, such as ear malformations. The minor physical anomalies may reflect the particular fetal developmental period in which the abnormalities arose, since ear formation occurs at approximately the same time as portions of the brain.

Many autistic children do not show lateralization and remain ambidextrous at an age when cerebral dominance is established in normal children. Autistic children also have a higher incidence of abnormal dermatoglyphics (e.g., fingerprints) than those in the general population. This finding may suggest a disturbance in neuroectodermal development.

Behavioral Characteristics. QUALITATIVE IMPAIRMENTS IN SOCIAL INTERACTION. Autistic children fail to show the subtle signs of social relatedness to their parents and other persons. As infants, many lack a social smile and anticipatory posture for being picked up as an adult approaches. Less frequent or poor eye contact is common. The social development of autistic children is characterized by impaired, but not usually totally absent, attachment behavior. Autistic children often do not acknowledge or differentiate the most important persons in their lives—parents, siblings, and teachers—and may show extreme anxiety when their usual routine is disrupted, but they may not react overtly to being left with a stranger. When autistic children have reached school age, their withdrawal may have diminished and be less obvious, particularly in higher-functioning children. There is a notable deficit in ability to play with peers and to make friends; their social behavior is awkward and may be inappropriate. Cognitively, children with autistic disorder are more skilled in visual-spatial tasks than in tasks requiring skill in verbal reasoning.

One description of the cognitive style of children with autism is that they cannot infer the feelings or mental state of others around them. That is, they cannot make attributions about the motivation or intentions of others and thus cannot develop empathy. This lack of a "theory of mind" leaves them unable to interpret the social behavior of others and leads to a lack of social reciprocation.

In late adolescence, autistic persons who make the most progress often desire friendships, but their difficulties in

43

Attention-Deficit Disorders

ATTENTION-DEFICIT/HYPERACTIVITY DISORDER

Attention-deficit/hyperactivity disorder (ADHD) consists of a persistent pattern of inattention and/or hyperactive and impulsive behavior that is more severe than expected in children of that age and level of development. To meet the criteria for the diagnosis of ADHD, some symptoms must be present before the age of 7 years, although many children are not diagnosed until they are older than 7 years when their behaviors cause problems in school and other places. To meet diagnostic criteria for ADHD, impairment from inattention and/or hyperactivity-impulsivity must be present in at least two settings and interfere with developmentally appropriate functioning socially, academically, and in extracurricular activities. The disorder must not take place in the course of a pervasive developmental disorder, schizophrenia, or other psychotic disorder and must not be better accounted for by another mental disorder.

The disorder has been identified in the literature for many years under a variety of terms. In the early 1900s, impulsive, disinhibited, and hyperactive children—many of whom had neurological damage caused by encephalitis—were grouped under the label *hyperactive syndrome*. In the 1960s, a heterogeneous group of children with poor coordination, learning disabilities, and emotional lability but without specific neurological damage were described as having minimal brain damage. Since then, other hypotheses have been put forth to explain the origin of the disorder, such as genetically based condition involving abnormal arousal and poor ability to modulate emotions. This theory was initially supported by the observation that stimulant medications help produce sustained attention and improve these children's ability to focus on a given task. Currently, no single factor is believed to cause the disorder, although many environmental variables may contribute to it and many predictable clinical features are associated with it.

Epidemiology

Reports on the incidence of ADHD in the United States have varied from 2 to 20 percent of grade-school children. A conservative figure is about 3 to 7 percent of prepubertal elementary school children. In Great Britain a lower incidence is reported than in the United States, less than 1 percent. ADHD is more prevalent in boys than in girls, with the ratio ranging from 2 to 1 to as much as 9 to 1. First-degree biological relatives, e.g., siblings of probands with ADHD are at high risk to develop it as well as to develop other disorders, including disruptive behavior disorders, anxiety disorders, and depressive disorders. Siblings of children with ADHD are also at higher risk than the general population to have learning disorders and academic difficulties. The parents of children with ADHD show an increased incidence of hyperkinesis, sociopathy, alcohol use disorders, and conversion disorder. Symptoms of ADHD are often present by age 3 years, but the diagnosis is generally not made until the child is in a structured school setting, such as preschool or kindergarten, when teacher information is available comparing the attention and impulsivity of the child in question with peers of the same age.

Etiology

The causes of ADHD are unknown. Most children with ADHD have no evidence of gross structural damage in the central nervous system (CNS). Conversely, most children with known neurological disorders caused by brain injuries do not display attention deficits and hyperactivity. Despite the lack of a specific neurophysiological or neurochemical basis for the disorder, it is predictably associated with a variety of other disorders that affect brain function, such as learning disorders. The suggested contributory factors for ADHD include prenatal toxic exposures, prematurity, and prenatal mechanical insult to the fetal nervous system. Food additives, colorings, preservatives, and sugar have also been proposed as possible causes of hyperactive behavior. No scientific evidence indicates that these factors cause ADHD.

Genetic Factors. Evidence for a genetic basis for ADHD includes greater concordance in monozygotic than in dizygotic twins. Also, siblings of hyperactive children have about twice the risk of having the disorder as those in the general population. One sibling may have predominantly hyperactivity symptoms, and others may have predominantly inattention symptoms. Biological parents of children with the disorder have a higher risk for ADHD than adoptive parents. Children with ADHD are at higher risk of developing conduct disorders, and alcohol use disorders and antisocial personality disorder are more common in their parents than in those in the general population.

Developmental Factors. Reports in the literature state that September is the peak month for births of ADHD children with and without comorbid learning disorders. The implication is that prenatal exposure to winter infections during the first tri-

mester may contribute to the emergence of ADHD symptoms in some susceptible children.

BRAIN DAMAGE. It has been speculated that some children affected by ADHD suffered subtle damage to the CNS and brain development during their fetal and perinatal periods. The hypothesized brain damage may potentially be associated with circulatory, toxic, metabolic, mechanical, or physical insult to the brain during early infancy caused by infection, inflammation, and trauma. Children with ADHD exhibit nonfocal (soft) neurological signs at higher rates than those in the general population.

Neurochemical Factors. Many neurotransmitters have been associated with ADHD symptoms. Animal studies have shown that the locus ceruleus, consisting of mainly noradrenergic neurons, plays a major role in attention. The noradrenergic system consists of the central system (originating in the locus ceruleus) and the peripheral sympathetic system. The peripheral noradrenergic system may be of more importance in ADHD. Thus, a dysfunction in peripheral epinephrine, which causes the hormone to accumulate peripherally, could potentially feed back to the central system and "reset" the locus ceruleus to a lower level. In part, hypotheses about the neurochemistry of the disorder have arisen from the impact of many medications that exert a positive effect on it. The most widely studied drugs in the treatment of ADHD, the stimulants, affect both dopamine and norepinephrine, leading to neurotransmitter hypotheses that include possible dysfunction in both the adrenergic and the dopaminergic systems. Stimulants increase catecholamine concentrations by promoting their release and blocking their uptake. Stimulants and some tricyclic drugs—for example, desipramine (Norpramin)—reduce levels of urinary 3-methoxy-4-hydroxyphenylglycol (MHPG), a metabolite of norepinephrine. Clonidine (Catapres), a norepinephrine agonist, has been helpful in treating hyperactivity. Other drugs that have reduced hyperactivity include tricyclic drugs and monoamine oxidase inhibitors (MAOIs). Overall, no clear-cut evidence implicates a single neurotransmitter in the development of ADHD, but many neurotransmitters may be involved in the process.

Neurophysiological Factors. The human brain normally undergoes major growth spurts at several ages: 3 to 10 months, 2 to 4 years, 6 to 8 years, 10 to 12 years, and 14 to 16 years. Some children have a maturational delay in the sequence and manifest symptoms of ADHD that appear to normalize by about age 5. A physiological correlate is the presence of a variety of nonspecific abnormal electroencephalogram (EEG) patterns that are disorganized and characteristic of young children. In some cases the EEG findings normalize over time. A recent study of quantitative EEGs in children with ADHD, in children with undifferentiated attentional problems, and in normal controls indicates that both groups with attentional problems evince increased beta band relative percentages and decreased rare tone P3000 amplitudes. Increased beta band percentage or decreased delta band percentage is associated with increased arousal.

Computed tomographic (CT) head scans of children with ADHD show no consistent findings. Studies using positron emission tomography (PET) have found lower cerebral blood flow and metabolic rates in the frontal lobe areas of children with ADHD than in controls. PET scans have also shown that adolescent females with the disorder have globally lower glucose metabolism than both normal control females and males and males with the disorder. One theory explains these findings by supposing that the frontal lobes in children with ADHD are not adequately performing their inhibitory mechanism on lower structures, an effect leading to disinhibition.

Psychosocial Factors. Children in institutions are frequently overactive and have poor attention spans. These signs result from prolonged emotional deprivation, and they disappear when deprivational factors are removed, such as through adoption or placement in a foster home. Stressful psychic events, disruption of family equilibrium, and other anxiety-inducing factors contribute to the initiation or perpetuation of ADHD. Predisposing factors may include the child's temperament, genetic-familial factors, and the demands of society to adhere to a routinized way of behaving and performing. Socioeconomic status does not seem to be a predisposing factor.

Diagnosis

The principal signs of hyperactivity and impulsivity are based on detailed prenatal history of a child's early developmental patterns along with direct observation of the child, especially in situations that require attention. Hyperactivity may be more severe in some situations (e.g., school) and less marked in others (e.g., one-on-one interviews), and it may be less obvious in pleasant structured activities (sports). The diagnosis of ADHD requires persistent, impairing symptoms of either hyperactivity/impulsivity or inattention that cause impairment in at least two different settings. For example, many children with ADHD have difficulties in school and at home. The diagnostic criteria for ADHD are outlined in Table 43–1.

Other distinguishing features of ADHD are short attention span and easy distractibility. In school, children with ADHD cannot follow instructions and often demand extra attention from their teachers. At home, they often do not comply with their parents' requests. They act impulsively, show emotional lability, and are explosive and irritable.

Children who have hyperactivity as a predominant feature are more likely to be referred for treatment than are children with primarily symptoms of attention deficit. Children with the predominantly hyperactive-impulsive type are more likely to have a stable diagnosis over time and to have concurrent conduct disorder than are children with the predominantly inattentive type without hyperactivity. Disorders involving reading, arithmetic, language, and coordination may occur in association with ADHD. A child's history may give clues to prenatal (including genetic), natal, and postnatal factors that may have affected the CNS structure or function. Rates of development, deviations in development, and parental reactions to significant or stressful behavioral transitions should be ascertained, as they may help clinicians determine the degree to which parents have contributed or reacted to a child's inefficiencies and dysfunctions.

School history and teachers' reports are important in evaluating whether a child's difficulties in learning and school behavior are primarily due to the child's attitudinal or maturational problems or to poor self-image because of felt inadequacies. These reports may also reveal how the child has handled

Table 43–1
DSM-IV-TR Diagnostic Criteria for Attention-Deficit/Hyperactivity Disorder

A. Either (1) or (2):
(1) six (or more) of the following symptoms of **inattention** have persisted for at least 6 months to a degree that is maladaptive and inconsistent with developmental level:
Inattention
(a) often fails to give close attention to details or makes careless mistakes in schoolwork, work, or other activities
(b) often has difficulty sustaining attention in tasks or play activities
(c) often does not seem to listen when spoken to directly
(d) often does not follow through on instructions and fails to finish schoolwork, chores, or duties in the workplace (not due to oppositional behavior or failure to understand instructions)
(e) often has difficulty organizing tasks and activities
(f) often avoids, dislikes, or is reluctant to engage in tasks that require sustained mental effort (such as schoolwork or homework)
(g) often loses things necessary for tasks or activities (e.g., toys, school assignments, pencils, books, or tools)
(h) is often easily distracted by extraneous stimuli
(i) is often forgetful in daily activities
(2) six (or more) of the following symptoms of **hyperactivity-impulsivity** have persisted for at least 6 months to a degree that is maladaptive and inconsistent with developmental level:
Hyperactivity
(a) often fidgets with hands or feet or squirms in seat
(b) often leaves seat in classroom or in other situations in which remaining seated is expected
(c) often runs about or climbs excessively in situations in which it is inappropriate (in adolescents or adults, may be limited to subjective feelings of restlessness)
(d) often has difficulty playing or engaging in leisure activities quietly
(e) is often "on the go" or often acts as if "driven by a motor"
(f) often talks excessively
Impulsivity
(g) often blurts out answers before questions have been completed
(h) often has difficulty awaiting turn
(i) often interrupts or intrudes on others (e.g., butts into conversations or games)

B. Some hyperactive-impulsive or inattentive symptoms that caused impairment were present before age 7 years.
C. Some impairment from the symptoms is present in two or more settings (e.g., at school [or work] and at home).
D. There must be clear evidence of clinically significant impairment in social, academic, or occupational functioning.
E. The symptoms do not occur exclusively during the course of a pervasive developmental disorder, schizophrenia, or other psychotic disorder and are not better accounted for by another mental disorder (e.g., mood disorder, anxiety disorder, dissociative disorder, or a personality disorder).

Code based on type:
Attention-deficit/hyperactivity disorder, combined type: if both Criteria A1 and A2 are met for the past 6 months
Attention-deficit/hyperactivity disorder, predominantly inattentive type: if Criterion A1 is met but Criterion A2 is not met for the past 6 months
Attention-deficit/hyperactivity disorder, predominantly hyperactive-impulsive type: if Criterion A2 is met but Criterion A1 is not met for the past 6 months
Coding note: For individuals (especially adolescents and adults) who currently have symptoms that no longer meet full criteria, "in partial remission" should be specified.

From American Psychiatric Association. *Diagnostic and Statistical Manual of Mental Disorders.* 4th ed. Text rev. Washington, DC: American Psychiatric Association; copyright 2000, with permission.

these problems. How the child has related to siblings, to peers, to adults, and to free and structured activities gives valuable diagnostic clues to the presence of ADHD and helps identify the complications of the disorder.

The mental status examination may show a secondarily depressed mood but no thought disturbance, impaired reality testing, or inappropriate affect. A child may show great distractibility, perseveration, and a concrete and literal mode of thinking. Indications of visual-perceptual, auditory-perceptual, language, or cognition problems may be present. Occasionally, evidence appears of a basic, pervasive, organically based anxiety, often referred to as *body anxiety.* A neurological examination may reveal visual, motor, perceptual, or auditory discriminatory immaturity or impairments without overt signs of visual or auditory acuity disorders. Children may have problems with motor coordination and difficulty copying age-appropriate figures, rapid alternating movements, right–left discrimination, ambidexterity, reflex asymmetries, and a variety of subtle nonfocal neurological signs (soft signs).

Clinicians should obtain an EEG to recognize the child with frequent bilaterally synchronous discharges resulting in short absence spells. Such a child may react in school with hyperactivity out of sheer frustration. The child with an unrecognized temporal lobe seizure focus can have a secondary behavior disorder. In these instances, several features of ADHD are often present. Identification of the focus requires an EEG obtained during drowsiness and during sleep.

Clinical Features

ADHD may have its onset in infancy, although it is rarely recognized until a child is at least toddler age. Infants with the disorder are unduly sensitive to stimuli and are easily upset by noise, light, temperature, and other environmental changes. At times, the reverse occurs, and the children are placid and limp, sleep much of the time, and appear to develop slowly in the first months of life. More commonly, however, infants with ADHD are active in the crib, sleep little, and cry a great deal. They are far less likely than normal children to reduce their locomotor activity when their environment is structured by social limits.

In school, ADHD children may attack a test rapidly but answer only the first two questions. They may be unable to wait to be called on in school and may respond before everyone else. At home, they cannot be put off for even a minute. Children with ADHD are often explosive or irritable. The irritability may be set off by relatively minor stimuli, which may puzzle and dismay the children. They are frequently emotionally labile and easily set off to laughter or to tears; their mood and performance are apt to be variable and unpredictable. Impulsiveness and an inability to delay gratification are characteristic. Children are often accident-prone.

Concomitant emotional difficulties are frequent. The fact that other children grow out of this behavior but children with ADHD do not grow out of it at the same time and rate may engender adults' dissatisfaction and pressure. The resulting negative self-concept and reactive hostility are worsened by the children's recognition that they have problems.

The most cited characteristics of children with ADHD are, in order of frequency, hyperactivity, perceptual motor impairment, emotional lability, general coordination deficit, attention deficit (short attention span, distractibility, perseveration, failure to fin-

ish tasks, inattention, poor concentration), impulsivity (action before thought, abrupt shifts in activity, lack of organization, jumping up in class), memory and thinking deficits, specific learning disabilities, speech and hearing deficits, and equivocal neurological signs and EEG irregularities. About 75 percent of children with ADHD show behavioral symptoms of aggression and defiance fairly consistently. But, whereas defiance and aggression are generally associated with adverse intrafamily relationships, hyperactivity is more closely related to impaired performance on cognitive tests requiring concentration.

School difficulties, both learning and behavioral, commonly coexist with ADHD. They sometimes come from concomitant communication disorders or learning disorders or from the child's distractibility and fluctuating attention, which hampers the acquisition, retention, and display of knowledge. These difficulties are noted especially on group tests. The adverse reactions of school personnel to the behavior characteristics of ADHD and the lowering of self-regard because of felt inadequacies may combine with the adverse comments of peers to make school a place of unhappy defeat. This situation may lead to acting-out antisocial behavior and self-defeating, self-punitive behaviors.

Sean was a 5-year-old boy who was referred for evaluation when his kindergarten teacher found that he was unable to stay on any tasks, and he would run around the room disrupting the other children. Sean was also oppositional with the teacher and unable to sit in his seat, although he was good-natured and rarely had a physical altercation with a peer. Sean was an athletic and active child who appeared to be below most of his classmates in his ability to recognize letters, numbers, and shapes. Although his teacher felt that Sean was rejected by his peers occasionally because of his impulsive nature, Sean felt that nobody liked him. At home, Sean was much more active than his two sisters, and his siblings often gave in to him, to be left alone. He was the middle child, with one sister 2 years older and the other sister 1 year younger.

Sean's mother reported that in the third month of her pregnancy with Sean, she had had some bleeding, but otherwise there were no complications. Sean was a full-term baby, who seemed robust and went home from the hospital without problems. He was healthy throughout the neonatal period but had been a poor sleeper, never sleeping more than 4 hours without waking. He was usually awake between 5 and 6 in the morning, and he was just not tired. In preschool, Sean was reported to be one of the most active and impulsive children, but his teacher had taken a liking to him, and she gave him a lot of one-on-one attention to keep him under control. In spite of the extra attention, Sean seemed to be a little slower than his classmates in learning new words and overall use of language. On intellectual testing, Sean had a full-scale intelligence quotient (IQ) of 105, with slightly higher performance than verbal score. Sean was referred for a psychiatric evaluation with a child psychiatrist, who diagnosed ADHD, combined type; oppositional-defiant disorder; and reading disorder according to the text revision of the fourth edition of *Diagnostic and Statistical Manual of Mental Disorders* (DSM-IV-TR). It was also noted that Sean seemed to be "down-on-himself" and felt socially rejected. The initial treatment plan for Sean included a trial of methylphenidate (Concerta), 18 mg per day, and a therapeutic social skills group, along with a parent-training component for his parents. On medication, Sean's teacher reported significant improvement in remaining on-task and a diminished activity level.

Over time, Sean sustained his good response to the methylphenidate, with minimal adverse effects that included decreased appetite at lunchtime but increased hunger in the evening. He was able to benefit from the practice that he had during his social skills group, and within 2 months, he made a friend from school who came to his house to play. Finally, Sean's family gained competence in managing his oppositional behaviors and impulsivity by instituting a reward system for listening to them. Sean was able to follow his teacher's instructions, mastered the expected kindergarten curriculum, and was recommended for a regular education class for the first grade.

Pathology and Laboratory Examination

No specific laboratory measures are pathognomonic of ADHD. Several laboratory measures often yield nonspecific abnormal results in hyperactive children, such as a disorganized, immature result on an EEG, and PET may show decreased cerebral blood flow in the frontal regions. Cognitive testing that helps to confirm a child's inattention and impulsivity includes the continuous performance task, in which a child is asked to press a button each time a particular sequence of letters or numbers is flashed on a screen. Children with poor attention make errors of omission—that is, they fail to press the button, even when the sequence has flashed. Impulsivity is manifested by errors of commission, in which children cannot resist pushing the button, even though the desired sequence has not yet appeared on the screen.

Differential Diagnosis

A temperamental constellation consisting of high activity level and short attention span but in the normal range of expectation for a child's age should be considered first. Differentiating these temperamental characteristics from the cardinal symptoms of ADHD before the age of 3 is difficult, mainly because of the overlapping features of a normally immature nervous system and the emerging signs of visual-motor-perceptual impairments frequently seen in ADHD. Anxiety in a child needs to be evaluated. Anxiety may accompany ADHD as a secondary feature, and anxiety alone may be manifested by overactivity and easy distractibility.

Many children with ADHD have secondary depression in reaction to their continuing frustration over their failure to learn and their consequent low self-esteem. This condition must be distinguished from a primary depressive disorder, which is likely to be characterized by hypoactivity and withdrawal. Mania and ADHD share many core features such as excessive verbalization, motoric hyperactivity, and high levels of distractibility. Additionally, in children with mania, irritability seems to be more common than euphoria. Although mania and ADHD can coexist,

children with bipolar I disorder exhibit more waxing and waning of symptoms than those with ADHD. Recent follow-up data for children who met the criteria for ADHD and subsequently developed bipolar disorder suggest that certain clinical features occurring during the course of ADHD predict future mania. Children with ADHD who had developed bipolar I disorder at 4-year follow-up had a greater co-occurrence of additional disorders and a greater family history of bipolar disorders and other mood disorders than children without bipolar disorder.

Frequently, conduct disorder and ADHD coexist, and both must be diagnosed. Learning disorders of various kinds must also be distinguished from ADHD; a child may be unable to read or do mathematics because of a learning disorder, rather than because of inattention. ADHD often coexists with one or more learning disorders, including reading disorder, mathematics disorder, and disorder of written expression.

Course and Prognosis

The course of ADHD is variable. Symptoms may persist into adolescence or adult life, they may remit at puberty, or the hyperactivity may disappear, but the decreased attention span and impulse-control problems persist. Overactivity is usually the first symptom to remit, and distractibility is the last. In a recent 4-year follow-up study, ADHD was generally persistent. Persistence was predicted by a family history of the disorder, negative life events, and comorbidity with conduct symptoms, depression, and anxiety disorders. Remission is unlikely before the age of 12. When remission does occur, it is usually between the ages of 12 and 20. Remission may be accompanied by a productive adolescence and adult life, satisfying interpersonal relationships, and few significant sequelae. Most patients with the disorder, however, undergo partial remission and are vulnerable to antisocial behavior, substance use disorders, and mood disorders. Learning problems often continue throughout life.

In about 15 to 20 percent of cases, symptoms persist into adulthood. Those with the disorder may show diminished hyperactivity but remain impulsive and accident-prone. Although their educational attainments are lower than those of people without ADHD, their early employment histories do not differ from those of people with similar educations.

Children with the disorder whose symptoms persist into adolescence are at risk for developing conduct disorder. Children with both ADHD and conduct disorder are also at risk for developing a substance-related disorder. The development of substance abuse disorders during adolescence appears to be related to the presence of conduct disorder rather than to ADHD alone.

Most children with ADHD have some social difficulties. Socially dysfunctional children with ADHD have significantly higher rates of comorbid psychiatric disorders and experience more problems with behavior in school as well as with peers and family members. Overall, the outcome of ADHD in childhood seems to be related to the amount of persistent comorbid psychopathology, especially conduct disorder, social disability, and chaotic family factors. Optimal outcomes may be promoted by ameliorating children's social functioning, diminishing aggression, and improving family situations as early as possible.

Treatment

Pharmacotherapy. Pharmacological agents shown to have significant efficacy, and excellent safety records in the treatment of ADHD are the CNS stimulants, including short- and sustained-release preparations of methylphenidate (Ritalin, Ritalin-SR, Concerta, Metadate CD, Metadate ER), dextroamphetamine (Dexedrine, Dexedrine spansules), and dextroamphetamine and amphetamine salt combinations (Adderall, Adderall XR). One additional form of methylphenidate, containing only the *d*-enantiomer, dexmethylphenidate (Focalin), was recently placed on the market, aimed at maximizing the target effects and minimizing the adverse effects in individuals with ADHD who obtain partial response from methylphenidate. One of the advantages of the sustained-release preparations for many children is that one dose in the morning will sustain the effects all day, and the child is no longer required to interrupt his or her school day to take a second or third dose. Another advantage of the sustained-release preparations of the above stimulants for some children is that the medication is sustained at an approximately even level in the body throughout the day so that periods of rebound and irritability are avoided. Table 43–2 contains comparative information on the

Table 43–2
Stimulant Medications in the Treatment of ADHD

Medication	Preparation (mg)	Approx. Duration (h)	Recommended Dose
Methylphenidate preparations			
Ritalin	5, 10, 15, 20	3–4	0.3–1 mg/kg tid; up to 60 mg/d
Ritalin-SR	20	8	Up to 60 mg/d
Concerta	18, 36, 54	12	Up to 54 mg/q AM
Metadate ER	10, 20	8	Up to 60 mg/d
Metadate CD	20	12	Up to 60 mg/q AM
Dexmethylphenidate preparation			
Focalin	2.5, 5, 10	3–4	Up to 10 mg
Dextroamphetamine preparations			
Dexedrine	5, 10	3–4	0.15–0.5 mg/kg bid; up to 40 mg/d
Dexedrine Spansule	5, 10, 15	8	Up to 40 mg/d
Dextroamphetamine and amphetamine salt preparations			
Adderall	5, 10, 20, 30	4–6	0.15–0.5 mg/kg bid; up to 40 mg/d
Adderall XR	10, 20, 30	12	Up to 40 mg q AM

Table 43–3
Nonstimulant Medications for ADHD

Medication	Preparation (mg)	Recommended Dose
Bupropion preparations		
Wellbutrin	75, 100	(3–6 mg/kg) 150–300 mg/d; up to 150 mg/dose bid
Wellbutrin SR	100, 150	(3–6 mg/kg) 150–300 mg/d; up to 150 mg q AM; >150 mg/d, use bid dosing
Venlafaxine		
Effexor	25, 37.5, 50, 75, 100	25–150 mg/d; use bid dosing
Effexor XR	37.5, 75, 150	37.5–150 mg q AM
α-Adrenergic agonists		
Clonidine (Catapres)	0.1, 0.2, 0.3	3–10 μg/kg/d divided tid; up to 0.1 mg tid
Guanfacine (Tenex)	1, 2	0.5–1.5 mg/d

above medications. Second-line agents with evidence of efficacy for some children and adolescents with ADHD include antidepressants such as bupropion (Wellbutrin, Wellbutrin SR), venlafaxine (Effexor, Effexor XR), and the α-adrenergic receptor agonists clonidine (Catapres), and guanfacine (Tenex). (Table 43–3 contains comparative information on the nonstimulant medications.) The Food and Drug Administration (FDA) approves the use of dextroamphetamine in children 3 years old and older and methylphenidate in children 6 years old and older. These are the two most commonly used treatments for children.

The precise mechanism of the stimulant's central action remains unknown. The idea of paradoxical response by hyperactive children is no longer accepted. Methylphenidate has been shown to be highly effective in up to three quarters of all children with ADHD with relatively few adverse effects. Methylphenidate is a short-acting medication that is generally used to be effective during school hours, so that children with the disorder can attend to tasks and remain in the classroom. The drug's most common adverse effects include headaches, stomachaches, nausea, and insomnia. Some children experience a rebound effect, in which they become mildly irritable and appear to be slightly hyperactive for a brief period when the medication wears off. In children with a history of motor tics, some caution must be used; in some cases, methylphenidate may exacerbate the tic disorder. Another common concern about methylphenidate is whether it causes some growth suppression. During periods of use, methylphenidate is associated with growth suppression, but children tend to make up the growth when they are given drug holidays in the summer or on weekends. An important question about using methylphenidate is how much it normalizes school performance. A recent study found that about 75 percent of a group of hyperactive children exhibited significant improvement in their ability to pay attention in class and on measures of academic efficiency when treated with methylphenidate. The drug has been shown to improve hyperactive children's scores on tasks of vigilance, such as the continuous performance task and paired associations. Dextroamphetamine and dextroamphetamine/amphetamine salt combinations are usually the second drugs of choice when methylphenidate is not effective.

Bupropion has been used as both an antidepressant and in the treatment of the disorder. A recent multisite, double-blind, placebo-controlled study confirmed the efficacy of bupropion. No further studies have compared bupropion with other stimulants. Although there was initial concern about the risk for seizures, these risks do not differ significantly from those of other antidepressants when the drug is used in dosages of less than 450 mg per day. Venlafaxine has been used in clinical practice, especially for children and adolescents with combinations of ADHD and depression or anxiety features. There is no clear empirical evidence to support the use of venlafaxine in the treatment of ADHD. Clonidine has also been used in the treatment of ADHD with some success, according to case reports. It may be helpful when patients also have tic disorders. There are few data to confirm the efficacy of selective serotonin reuptake inhibitors (SSRIs) in the treatment of ADHD, but because of the comorbidity of depression and anxiety with the disorder, these drugs are sometimes considered.

Other classes of medications, tricyclic drugs and pemoline (Cylert), previously used to treat ADHD are no longer recommended because of potential adverse effects on liver function (pemoline) and potential cardiac arrhythmia effects (tricyclic drugs). The report of sudden death in at least four children with ADHD who were being treated with desipramine (Norpramin, Pertofrane) has made the tricyclic antidepressants a less likely choice. Why the deaths occurred is unclear, but they reinforce the need for close follow-up of any child receiving a tricyclic drug. Antipsychotics are occasionally used to treat refractory hyperactivity in children and adolescents who are severely impaired and do not respond to other treatments. Antipsychotics may be efficacious for some children with the disorder, but with the alternative medications available and the risk for tardive dyskinesia, withdrawal dyskinesia, and neuroleptic malignant syndrome, antipsychotics are less desirable.

Modafinil (Provigil), another type of CNS stimulant, originally developed to reduce daytime sleepiness in patients with narcolepsy, has been tried clinically in the treatment of adults with ADHD, but controlled trials are needed to document its efficacy. Overall, stimulants remain the drugs of choice in the pharmacological treatment of ADHD.

Monitoring Stimulant Treatment

At baseline, the most recent American Academy of Child and Adolescent Psychiatry (AACAP) practice parameters recom-

mend the following workup prior to starting use of stimulant medications:

- Physical examination
- Blood pressure
- Pulse
- Weight
- Height

It is recommended that children and adolescents being treated with stimulants have their height, weight, blood pressure, and pulse checked on a quarterly basis and have a physical examination annually.

EVALUATION OF THERAPEUTIC PROGRESS. Monitoring starts with the initiation of medication. Because school performance is most markedly affected, special attention and effort should be given to establishing and maintaining a close collaborative working relation with a child's school. In most patients, stimulants reduce overactivity, distractibility, impulsiveness, explosiveness, and irritability. No evidence indicates that medications directly improve any existing impairments in learning, although, when the attention deficits diminish, children can learn more effectively than in the past. In addition, medication can improve self-esteem when children are no longer constantly reprimanded for their behavior.

Psychosocial Interventions. Medication alone is often not enough to satisfy the comprehensive therapeutic needs of children with the disorder and is usually but one facet of a multimodality regimen. Social skills groups, training for parents of children with ADHD, and behavioral interventions at school and at home are often efficacious in the overall management of children with ADHD. Evaluation and treatment of coexisting learning disorders or additional psychiatric disorders is important.

Children who are prescribed medications should be taught the purpose of the medication and given the opportunity to reveal their feelings about it. Doing so helps dispel misconceptions about medication use (such as "I'm crazy") and makes it clear that the medication helps the child handle situations better than before. When children are helped to structure their environment, their anxiety diminishes. It is often beneficial for parents and teachers to work together to develop a concrete set of expectations for the child and a system of rewards for the child when the expectations are met.

A common goal of therapy is to help parents of children with ADHD recognize and promote the notion that while the child may not "voluntarily" exhibit symptoms of ADHD, he or she is still capable of being responsible for meeting reasonable expectations. Parents should also be helped to recognize that in spite of their child's difficulties, all children face the normal tasks of maturation, including significant building of self-esteem when he or she develops a sense of mastery. Therefore, children with ADHD do not benefit from being exempted from the requirements, expectations, and planning applicable to other children. Parental training is an integral part of the psychotherapeutic interventions for ADHD. Most parental training is based on helping parents develop usable behavioral interventions with positive reinforcement that targets both social and academic behaviors.

Group therapy aimed at both refining social skills and increasing self-esteem and a sense of success may be very useful for children with ADHD who have great difficulty functioning in group settings, especially in school. A recent year-long group therapy intervention in a clinical setting for boys with the disorder described the goals as helping the boys improve skills in game playing and feeling a sense of mastery with peers. The boys were first asked to do a task that was fun, in pairs, and then were gradually asked to do projects in a group. They were directed in following instructions, waiting, and paying attention and were praised for successful cooperation. This level of highly structured group therapeutic "play" is developmentally appropriate for these children, who benefit from an increased ability to participate in any group activities.

ATTENTION-DEFICIT/HYPERACTIVITY DISORDER NOT OTHERWISE SPECIFIED

DSM-IV includes attention-deficit/hyperactivity disorder not otherwise specified as a residual category for disturbances with prominent symptoms of inattention or hyperactivity that do not meet the criteria for ADHD (Table 43–4).

The incidence of adult manifestations of ADHD is unknown, but there are many more cases than were previously thought or diagnosed. This illness is being more frequently diagnosed and requires much greater attention and study. In adults, residual signs of the disorder include impulsivity and attention deficit (e.g., difficulty in organizing and completing work, inability to concentrate, increased distractibility, and sudden decision making without thought of the consequences). Many people with the disorder suffer from a secondary depressive disorder associated with low self-esteem related to their impaired performance and that affects both occupational and social functioning. Treatment of the disorder involves the use of amphetamines (5 to 60 mg a day) or methylphenidate (5 to 60 mg a day). Signs of a positive response are an increased attention span, decreased impulsiveness, and improved mood. Psychopharmacological therapy may be needed indefinitely. Because of the abuse potential of the drugs, clinicians should monitor drug response and patient compliance.

ICD-10

In the 10th revision of *International Statistical Classification of Diseases and Related Health Problems* (ICD-10), the category hyperkinetic disor-

Table 43–4
DSM-IV-TR Diagnostic Criteria for Attention-Deficit/Hyperactivity Disorder Not Otherwise Specified

This category is for disorders with prominent symptoms of inattention or hyperactivity-impulsivity that do not meet criteria for attention-deficit/hyperactivity disorder. Examples include

1. Individuals whose symptoms and impairment meet the criteria for attention-deficit/hyperactivity disorder, predominantly inattentive type but whose age at onset is 7 years or after
2. Individuals with clinically significant impairment who present with inattention and whose symptom pattern does not meet the full criteria for the disorder but have a behavioral pattern marked by sluggishness, daydreaming, and hypoactivity

From American Psychiatric Association. *Diagnostic and Statistical Manual of Mental Disorders.* 4th ed. Text rev. Washington, DC: American Psychiatric Association; copyright 2000, with permission.

Table 43–5
ICD-10 Diagnostic Criteria for Hyperkinetic Disorders

Note: The research diagnosis of hyperkinetic disorder requires the definite presence of abnormal levels of inattention, hyperactivity, and restlessness that are pervasive across situations and persistent over time and that are not caused by other disorders such as autism or affective disorders.

G1. *Inattention.* At least six of the following symptoms of inattention have persisted for at least 6 months, to a degree that is maladaptive and inconsistent with the developmental level of the child:
- (1) often fails to give close attention to details, or makes careless errors in schoolwork, work, or other activities;
- (2) often fails to sustain attention in tasks or play activities;
- (3) often appears not to listen to what is being said to him or her;
- (4) often fails to follow through on instructions or to finish schoolwork, chores, or duties in the workplace (not because of oppositional behavior or failure to understand instructions);
- (5) is often impaired in organizing tasks and activities;
- (6) often avoids or strongly dislikes tasks, such as homework, that require sustained mental effort;
- (7) often loses things necessary for certain tasks or activities, such as school assignments, pencils, books, toys, or tools;
- (8) is often easily distracted by external stimuli;
- (9) is often forgetful in the course of daily activities.

G2. *Hyperactivity.* At least three of the following symptoms of hyperactivity have persisted for at least 6 months, to a degree that is maladaptive and inconsistent with the developmental level of the child:
- (1) often fidgets with hands or feet or squirms on seat;
- (2) leaves seat in classroom or in other situations in which remaining seated is expected;
- (3) often runs about or climbs excessively in situations in which it is inappropriate (in adolescents or adults, only feelings of restlessness may be present);
- (4) is often unduly noisy in playing or has difficulty in engaging quietly in leisure activities;
- (5) exhibits a persistent pattern of excessive motor activity that is not substantially modified by social context or demands.

G3. *Impulsivity.* At least one of the following symptoms of impulsivity has persisted for at least 6 months, to a degree that is maladaptive and inconsistent with the developmental level of the child:
- (1) often blurts out answers before questions have been completed;
- (2) often fails to wait in lines or await turns in games or group situations;
- (3) often interrupts or intrudes on others (e.g., butts into others' conversations or games);
- (4) often talks excessively without appropriate response to social constraints.

G4. Onset of the disorder is no later than the age of 7 years.

G5. *Pervasiveness.* The criteria should be met for more than a single situation, e.g., the combination of inattention and hyperactivity should be present both at home and at school, or at both school and another setting where children are observed, such as a clinic. (Evidence for cross-situationality will ordinarily require information from more than one source; parental reports about classroom behavior, for instance, are unlikely to be sufficient.)

G6. The symptoms in G1–G3 cause clinically significant distress or impairment in social, academic, or occupational functioning.

G7. The disorder does not meet the criteria for pervasive developmental disorders, manic episode, depressive episode, or anxiety disorders.

Comments

Many authorities also recognize conditions that are subthreshold for hyperkinetic disorder. Children who meet criteria in other ways but do not show abnormalities of hyperactivity-impulsiveness may be recognized as showing *attention deficit*; conversely, children who fall short of criteria for attention problems but meet criteria in other respects may be recognized as showing *activity disorder.* In the same way, children who meet criteria for only one situation (e.g., only the home or only the classroom) may be regarded as showing a *home-specific* or *classroom-specific disorder.* These conditions are not yet included in the main classification because of insufficient empirical predictive validation, and because many children with subthreshold disorders show other syndromes (such as oppositional defiant disorder) and should be classified in the appropriate category.

Disturbance of activity and attention

The general criteria for hyperkinetic disorder must be met, but not those for conduct disorders.

Hyperkinetic conduct disorder

The general criteria for both hyperkinetic disorder and conduct disorders must be met.

Other hyperkinetic disorders

Hyperkinetic disorder, unspecified

This residual category is not recommended and should be used only when there is a lack of differentiation between disturbance of activity and attention and hyperkinetic conduct disorder but the overall criteria for hyperkinetic disorders are fulfilled.

ders includes disturbance of activity and attention (which in turn encompasses attention-deficit disorder or syndrome with hyperactivity, ADHD), hyperkinetic conduct disorder, other hyperkinetic disorders, and hyperkinetic disorder, unspecified. According to ICD-10, hyperkinetic disorders are characterized by "early onset; a combination of overactive, poorly modulated behavior with marked inattention and lack of persistent task involvement; and pervasiveness over situations and persistence over time." The ICD-10 criteria for hyperkinetic disorders are given in Table 43–5.

References

Arnold LE, Jensen PS. Attention-deficit hyperactivity disorders: adult manifestations. In: Kaplan HI, Sadock BJ, eds. *Comprehensive Textbook of Psychiatry.* 6th ed. Baltimore: Williams & Wilkins; 1995:2295.

Bagwell CL, Molina BSG, Pelham WE, Hoza B. Attention-deficit hyperactivity and problems in peer relations: predictors from childhood to adolescence. *J Am Acad Child Adolesc Psychiatry.* 2001;40:1285.

Biederman J, Faraone S, Mick E, et al. Attention-deficit hyperactivity disorder and juvenile mania: an overlooked comorbidity? *J Am Acad Child Adolesc Psychiatry.* 1996;35:997.

Biederman J, Wilens T, Mick E, et al. Is ADHD a risk factor for psychoactive substance use disorders? Findings from a four-year prospective follow-up study. *J Am Acad Child Adolesc Psychiatry.* 1997;36:21.

DuPaul GJ, McGuey KE, Eckert TL, VanBrackle J. Preschool children with attention-deficit/hyperactivity disorder: impairments in behavioral, social and school functioning. *J Am Acad Child Adolesc Psychiatry.* 2001;40:508.

DuPaul GJ, Rapport MD. Does methylphenidate normalize the classroom performance of children with attention deficit disorders? *J Am Acad Child Adolesc Psychiatry.* 1993;32:190.

Fischer M, Barkley RA, Fletcher KE, Smallish L. The adolescent outcome of hyperactive children: predictors of psychiatric, academic, social and emotional adjustment. *J Am Acad Child Adolesc Psychiatry.* 1993;32:324.

Garfinkel BD, Wender PH. Attention-deficit hyperactivity disorder. In: Kaplan HI, Sadock BJ, eds. *Comprehensive Textbook of Psychiatry.* 6th ed. Baltimore: Williams & Wilkins; 1995:1828.

Greenhill LL, Pliszka S, Dulcan M. Practice parameters for the use of stimulant medications in the treatment of children, adolescents and adults. *J Am Acad Child Adolesc Psychiatry.* 2002;41(suppl):26.

Horner BR, Scheibe K. Prevalence and implications of attention-deficit hyperactivity disorder among adolescents in treatment for substance abuse. *J Am Acad Child Adolesc Psychiatry.* 1997;36:30.

James RS, Sharp WS, Bastain TM, et al. Double-blind-controlled study of single-dose amphetamine formulations in ADHD. *J Am Acad Child Adolesc Psychiatry.* 2001;40:1268.

Kuperman S, Johnson B, Arndt A, Lindgren A, Wolraich M. Quantitative EEG differences in a nonclinical sample of children with ADHD and undifferentiated ADD. *J Am Acad Child Adolesc Psychiatry.* 1996;35:1009.

Nigg JT, Blaskey LG, Huang-Pollock CL, Rappley MD. Neuropsychological executive functions and DSM-IV ADHD subtypes. *J Am Acad Child Adolesc Psychiatry.* 2002;41:59.

Rapport MD, Carlson GA, Kelly KL, Pataki C. Methylphenidate and desipramine in hospitalized children. I. Separate and combined effects on cognitive function. *J Am Acad Child Adolesc Psychiatry.* 1993;32:333.

Sonuga-Barke EJS, Daley D, Thompson M, Lauer-Bradbury C, Weeks A. Parent-based therapies for pre-school attention-deficit/hyperactivity disorder: a randomized, controlled trial with a community sample. *J Am Acad Child Adolesc Psychiatry.* 2001;40:402.

Spencer T, Biederman J, Wilens T, Harding M, O'Donnell D, Griffin S. Pharmacotherapy of attention-deficit hyperactivity disorder across the life cycle. *J Am Acad Child Adolesc Psychiatry.* 1996;35:409.

Steingard R, Biederman J, Spender T, Wilens T, Gonzales A. Comparison of clonidine response in the treatment of attention-deficit hyperactivity disorder with and without comorbid tic disorders. *J Am Acad Child Adolesc Psychiatry.* 1993;32:350.

Strayhorn JM. Self-control: theory and research. *J Am Acad Child Adolesc Psychiatry.* 2002;41:7.

Wilens TE, Biederman J, Geist DE, Steingard R, Spencer T. Nortriptyline in the treatment of ADHD: a chart review of 58 cases. *J Am Acad Child Adolesc Psychiatry.* 1993;32:343.

44

Disruptive Behavior Disorders

Disruptive behavior disorders include two persistent constellations of disruptive symptoms categorized as oppositional defiant disorder and conduct disorder, which result in impaired social or academic function in a child. Some defiance and refusal to comply with adult requests is developmentally appropriate and marks growth in all children, yet children with the following disorders are themselves impaired by the frequency and severity of their disruptive behaviors.

Oppositional defiant disorder is characterized by enduring patterns of negativistic, disobedient, and hostile behavior toward authority figures as well as an inability to take responsibility for mistakes, leading to placing blame on others. Children with oppositional defiant disorder frequently argue with adults and become easily annoyed by others, leading to a state of anger and resentment. Children with oppositional defiant disorder may have difficulty in the classroom and with peer relationships but generally do not resort to physical aggression or significantly destructive behavior.

In contrast, children with conduct disorder engage in severe repeated acts of aggression that may cause physical harm to themselves and others and frequently violate the rights of others. Children with conduct disorder usually have behaviors characterized by aggression to persons or animals, destruction of property, deceitfulness or theft, and multiple violations of rules such as truancy from school. These behavior patterns cause distinct difficulties in school life as well as in peer relationships. Conduct disorder has been divided into a childhood-onset subtype, in which at least one symptom has emerged repeatedly before age 10 years, and adolescent-onset type, in which there were no characteristic persistent symptoms until after age 10 years. While some young children show persistent patterns of behavior consistent with violating the rights of others or destroying property, the diagnosis of conduct disorder in children appears to increase with age.

OPPOSITIONAL DEFIANT DISORDER

In oppositional defiant disorder, a child's temper outbursts, active refusal to comply with rules, and annoying behaviors exceed expectations for these behaviors for children of that age. The disorder is an enduring pattern of negativistic, hostile, and defiant behaviors in the absence of serious violations of social norms or of the rights of others.

Epidemiology

Oppositional, negativistic behavior, in moderation, is developmentally normal in early childhood and adolescence. Epidemiological studies of negativistic traits in nonclinical populations found such behavior in 16 to 22 percent of school-age children. According to DSM-IV-TR, prevalence rates for this disorder range from 2 to 16 percent. Although oppositional defiant disorder can begin as early as 3 years of age, it typically is noted by 8 years of age and usually not later than adolescence. Oppositional defiant disorder has been reported to occur at rates ranging from 2 to 16 percent. The disorder seems more prevalent in boys than in girls before puberty, and the sex ratio appears to be equal after puberty. One authority suggests that girls are classified as having oppositional disorder more frequently than boys, since boys more often receive the diagnosis of conduct disorder. There are no distinct family patterns, but many parents of children with the disorder are themselves overly concerned with issues of power, control, and autonomy.

Etiology

The ability of a child to communicate his or her own will and opposing others' will is crucial to normal development as a route toward establishing autonomy, forming an identity, and setting inner standards and controls. The most dramatic example of normal oppositional behavior peaks between 18 and 24 months, the "terrible twos," when toddlers behave negativistically as an expression of growing autonomy. Pathology begins when this developmental phase persists abnormally, authority figures overreact, or oppositional behavior recurs considerably more frequently than in most children of the same mental age.

Children exhibit a range of temperamental predispositions to strong will, strong preferences, or great assertiveness. Parents who model more extreme ways of expressing and enforcing their own will may contribute to the development of chronic struggles with their children that are then reenacted with other authority figures. What begins for an infant as an effort to establish self-determination may end up transformed into an exaggerated behavioral pattern. In late childhood, environmental trauma, illness, or chronic incapacity, such as mental retardation, may trigger oppositionalism as a defense against helplessness, anxiety, and loss of self-esteem. Another normative oppositional stage occurs in adolescence as an expression of the need to separate from the parents and establish an autonomous identity.

Classical psychoanalytic theory implicates unresolved conflicts that are being expressed with all authority figures. Behaviorists have suggested that oppositionalism is a reinforced, learned behavior through which a child exerts control over authority figures; for example, by having a temper tantrum when an undesired act is requested, a child coerces the parents to withdraw their request. In addition, increased parental attention—for example, long discussions about the behavior—may reinforce the behavior.

Diagnosis and Clinical Features

Children with oppositional defiant disorder often argue with adults, lose their temper, and are angry, resentful, and easily annoyed by others. Frequently they actively defy adults' requests or rules and deliberately annoy other persons. They tend to blame others for their own mistakes and misbehavior. Manifestations of the disorder are almost invariably present in the home, but they may not be present at school or with other adults or peers. In some cases, features of the disorder from the beginning of the disturbance are displayed outside the home; in other cases, the behavior starts in the home but is later displayed outside. Typically, symptoms of the disorder are most evident in interactions with adults or peers whom the child knows well. Thus, a child with the disorder is likely to show little or no sign of the disorder when examined clinically. Usually, these children do not regard themselves as oppositional or defiant but justify their behavior as a response to unreasonable circumstances. The disorder appears to cause more distress to those around the child than to the child. Diagnostic criteria for oppositional defiant disorder from the text revision of the fourth edition of *Diagnostic and Statistical Manual of Mental Disorders* (DSM-IV-TR) are given in Table 44–1.

Chronic oppositional defiant disorder almost always interferes with interpersonal relationships and school performance. These children are often friendless and perceive human relationships as unsatisfactory. Despite adequate intelligence, they do poorly or fail in school, as they withhold participation, resist external demands, and insist on solving problems without others' help. Secondary to these difficulties are low self-esteem, poor frustration tolerance, depressed mood, and temper outbursts. Adolescents may abuse alcohol and illegal substances. Often, the disturbance evolves into a conduct disorder or a mood disorder.

Table 44–1
DSM-IV-TR Diagnostic Criteria for Oppositional Defiant Disorder

A. A pattern of negativistic, hostile, and defiant behavior lasting at least 6 months, during which four (or more) of the following are present:
(1) often loses temper
(2) often argues with adults
(3) often actively defies or refuses to comply with adults' requests or rules
(4) often deliberately annoys people
(5) often blames others for his or her mistakes or misbehavior
(6) is often touchy or easily annoyed by others
(7) is often angry and resentful
(8) is often spiteful or vindictive
Note: Consider a criterion met only if the behavior occurs more frequently than is typically observed in individuals of comparable age and developmental level.

B. The disturbance in behavior causes clinically significant impairment in social, academic, or occupational functioning.

C. The behaviors do not occur exclusively during the course of a psychotic or mood disorder.

D. Criteria are not met for conduct disorder, and, if the individual is age 18 years or older, criteria are not met for antisocial personality disorder.

From American Psychiatric Association. *Diagnostic and Statistical Manual of Mental Disorders.* 4th ed. Text rev. Washington, DC: American Psychiatric Association; copyright 2000, with permission.

Pathology and Laboratory Examination. No specific laboratory tests or pathological findings help diagnose oppositional defiant disorder. Because some children with the disorder become physically aggressive and violate the rights of others as they get older, they may share some of the same characteristics under investigation in violent people, such as low serotonin levels in the central nervous system (CNS).

Differential Diagnosis

Because oppositional behavior is both normal and adaptive at specific developmental stages, these periods of negativism must be distinguished from oppositional defiant disorder. Developmental-stage oppositional behavior, which is of shorter duration than oppositional defiant disorder, is neither considerably more frequent nor more intense than that seen in other children of the same mental age.

Oppositional defiant behavior occurring temporarily in reaction to a stress should be diagnosed as an adjustment disorder. When features of oppositional defiant disorder appear during the course of conduct disorder, schizophrenia, or a mood disorder, the diagnosis of oppositional defiant disorder should not be made. Oppositional and negativistic behaviors may also be present in attention-deficit/hyperactivity disorder, cognitive disorders, and mental retardation. Whether a concomitant diagnosis of oppositional defiant disorder should be made depends on the severity, pervasiveness, and duration of such behavior. Some young children who receive a diagnosis of oppositional defiant disorder go on in several years to meet the criteria for conduct disorder. Some investigators believe that the two disorders may be developmental variants of each other, with conduct disorder being the natural progression of oppositional defiant behavior when a child matures. Most children with oppositional defiant disorder, however, do not later meet the criteria for conduct disorder, and up to one quarter of children with oppositional defiant disorder may not meet the diagnosis several years later.

The subtype of oppositional defiant disorder that tends to progress to conduct disorder is one in which aggression is prominent. Most children who have attention-deficit/hyperactivity disorder and conduct disorder develop conduct disorder before the age of 12. Most children who develop conduct disorder have a previous history of oppositional defiant disorder. Overall, the current consensus is that two subtypes of oppositional defiant disorder may exist. One type is likely to progress to conduct disorder and includes certain symptoms of conduct disorder (e.g., fighting, bullying). The other type is characterized by less aggression and fewer antisocial traits and does not progress to conduct disorder.

Robert, age 7, presented to the consultation-liaison team. He suffered from leukemia and was extremely difficult to manage. He would refuse all necessary blood work and repeatedly ran away from the clinic when asked to cooperate

with requests for X-rays, blood tests, etc. He was sullen, argumentative, and irritable. The behavior was unchanged when his mother was used as a "filter" for the demands. He was a chronically cranky child, although his illness was in remission and he was mostly medication free at the time of consultation. His care was severely compromised. At home his behavior was very similar and had been so for several months. He argued continuously with his single mother about any kind of request, such as cleaning up his room. Prior to his difficulties at the hospital, he began to exhibit similar problems at school. He was suspended for 1 week for being verbally abusive and out of control with his teacher. His mother had been diagnosed with acquired immune deficiency syndrome (AIDS) 2 years ago, having become infected by her drug-abusing husband who had died about 3 years ago from the effects of AIDS. She seemed dysphoric, passive, and extremely permissive with the child. She had no additional help because her own mother was also gravely ill, and she had no current social support network. Robert would often scream at his mother at the top of his voice without her evincing any reaction or making any attempt to contain him. Testing showed him to have normal intelligence, without symptoms of attention-deficit/hyperactivity disorder or learning disabilities. He knew of his father's death and his mother's illness. His mood remained dysphoric for many weeks when discussing this. He had never exhibited other reactions to being told about the illnesses of his parents. His mother described his early development as unremarkable except for his tendencies to have irregular sleep and eating patterns and his propensity to be cranky. His mother had intermittently taken drugs while pregnant with him, her only child. (Courtesy of Hans Steiner, M.D.)

Course and Prognosis

The course of oppositional defiant disorder depends largely on the severity of the symptoms and the ability of the child to develop more adaptive responses to authority. The stability of oppositional defiant disorder over time varies. Persistence of oppositional defiant symptoms poses an increased risk of additional disorders such as conduct disorder and substance use disorders. Positive outcomes are more likely for intact families who can modify their own expression of demands and give less attention to the child's argumentative behaviors.

About one quarter of all children who receive the diagnosis of oppositional defiant disorder do not continue to meet diagnostic criteria over the next several years. It is not clear in these cases whether the criteria captured children whose behavior was not developmentally abnormal or whether the disorder spontaneously remitted. Patients in whom the diagnosis persists may remain stable or go on to violate the rights of others and thus develop conduct disorder. Such patients should receive guarded prognoses.

There is an association between conduct disorder and later substance use disorders, as well as elevated rates of mood disorders, in children with oppositional defiant disorder, conduct disorder, and attention-deficit/hyperactivity disorder. Parental psychopathology, such as antisocial personality disorder and substance abuse, appears to be more common in families with children who have oppositional defiant disorder than in the general population, which creates additional risks for chaotic and troubled home environments. The prognosis for oppositional defiant disorder in a child depends somewhat on family functioning and the development of comorbid psychopathology.

Treatment

The primary treatment of oppositional defiant disorder is family intervention using both direct training of the parents in child management skills and careful assessment of family interactions. Behavior therapists emphasize teaching parents how to alter their behavior to discourage the child's oppositional behavior and encourage appropriate behavior. Behavior therapy focuses on selectively reinforcing and praising appropriate behavior and ignoring or not reinforcing undesired behavior.

Children with oppositional defiant behavior may also benefit from individual psychotherapy insofar as the child is exposed to a situation with an adult in which to "practice" more adaptive responses. In the therapeutic relationship, the child can learn new strategies to develop a sense of mastery and success in social situations with peers and families. In the safety of a more "neutral" relationship, children may discover that they are capable of less provocative behavior. Often, self-esteem must be restored before a child with oppositional defiant disorder can make more positive responses to external control. Parent–child conflict strongly predicts conduct problems; patterns of harsh physical and verbal punishment particularly evoke the emergence of aggression and deviance in children. Thus, it is likely that eliminating harsh, punitive parenting and increasing positive parent–child interactions may positively influence the course of oppositional and defiant behaviors.

CONDUCT DISORDER

Conduct disorder is an enduring set of behaviors that evolves over time, usually characterized by aggression and violation of the rights of others. Conduct disorder is associated with many other psychiatric disorders including attention-deficit/hyperactivity disorder, depression, and learning disorders, and it is also associated with several psychosocial factors such as low socioeconomic level; harsh, punitive parenting; family discord; lack of appropriate parental supervision; and lack of social competence. The DSM-IV-TR criteria require three specific behaviors of the 15 listed, which include bullying, threatening, or intimidating others and staying out at night despite parental prohibitions, beginning before 13 years of age. DSM-IV-TR also specifies that truancy from school must begin before 13 years of age to be considered a symptom of conduct disorder. The disorder can be diagnosed in a person older than 18 years only if the criteria for antisocial personality disorder are not met. DSM-IV-TR describes a mild level of the disorder as showing few if any conduct problems in excess of those needed to make the diagnosis and conduct problems that cause only minor harm to others. According to DSM-IV-TR, the severe level shows many conduct problems in excess of the minimal diagnostic criteria or conduct problems that cause considerable harm to others.

Epidemiology

Conduct disturbance is common during childhood and adolescence. Estimated rates of conduct disorder among the general population range from 1 to 10 percent. The disorder is more common among boys than girls, and the ratio ranges from 4 to 1 to as much as 12 to 1. Conduct disorder is more common in the children of parents with antisocial personality disorder and alcohol dependence than it is in the general population. The prevalence of conduct disorder and antisocial behavior is significantly related to socioeconomic factors.

Etiology

No single factor can account for a child's antisocial behavior and conduct disorder. Rather, many biopsychosocial factors contribute to development of the disorder.

Parental Factors. Harsh, punitive parenting characterized by severe physical and verbal aggression is associated with the development of children's maladaptive aggressive behaviors. Chaotic home conditions are associated with conduct disorder and delinquency. Divorce itself is considered a risk factor, but the persistence of hostility, resentment, and bitterness between divorced parents may be the more important contributor to maladaptive behavior. Parental psychopathology, child abuse, and negligence often contribute to conduct disorder. Sociopathy, alcohol dependence, and substance abuse in the parents are associated with conduct disorder in their children. Parents may be so negligent that a child's care is shared by relatives or assumed by foster parents. Many such parents were scarred by their own upbringing and tend to be abusive, negligent, or engrossed in getting their own personal needs met.

In the 1980s, particularly in urban areas, cocaine abuse and AIDS increased family dysfunction. Recent studies suggest that many parents of children with conduct disorder have serious psychopathology, including psychotic disorders. Psychodynamic hypotheses suggest that children with conduct disorder unconsciously act out their parents' antisocial wishes.

Sociocultural Factors. Socioeconomically deprived children are at higher risk for the development of conduct disorder, as are children and adolescents who grow up in urban environments. Unemployed parents, lack of a supportive social network, and lack of positive participation in community activities seem to predict conduct disorder. Associated findings that may influence the development of conduct disorder in urban areas are increased rates and prevalence of substance use. Although drug and alcohol use does not contribute to the onset of conduct disorder, it possibly makes it more difficult to remit from it. Drug use may also aggravate the symptoms. Thus, factors that increase the likelihood of regular substance use may in fact prolong the disorder.

Psychological Factors. Children brought up in chaotic, negligent conditions often express poor emotional modulation of emotions including anger, frustration, and sadness. Poor modeling of impulse control and the chronic lack of having their own needs met leads to a less well developed sense of empathy.

Neurobiological Factors. Neurobiological factors in conduct disorder have been little studied, but research in attention-deficit/hyperactivity disorder yields some important findings, and this disorder often coexists with conduct disorder. In some children with conduct disorder, a low level of plasma dopamine β-hydroxylase, an enzyme that converts dopamine to norepinephrine, has been found. This finding supports a theory of decreased noradrenergic functioning in conduct disorder. Some conduct-disordered juvenile offenders have high serotonin levels in blood. Evidence indicates that blood serotonin levels correlate inversely with levels of the serotonin metabolite 5-hydroxyindoleacetic acid (5-HIAA) in the cerebrospinal fluid (CSF) and that low 5-HIAA levels in CSF correlates with aggression and violence.

Child Abuse and Maltreatment. Children chronically exposed to violence, especially those who endure physically abusive treatment, often behave aggressively. Such children may have difficulty verbalizing their feelings, and this difficulty increases their tendency to express themselves physically. In addition, severely abused children and adolescents tend to be hypervigilant; in some cases they misperceive benign situations and respond with violence. Not all physical behavior is synonymous with conduct disorder, but children with a pattern of hypervigilance and violent responses are likely to violate the rights of others.

Other Factors. Attention-deficit/hyperactivity disorder, CNS dysfunction or damage, and early extremes of temperament can predispose a child to conduct disorder. Propensity to violence correlates with CNS dysfunction and signs of severe psychopathology, such as delusional tendencies. Longitudinal temperament studies suggest that many behavioral deviations are initially a straightforward response to a poor fit between a child's temperament and emotional needs, on one hand, and parental attitudes and child-rearing practices, on the other.

Diagnosis and Clinical Features

Conduct disorder does not develop overnight; instead, many symptoms evolve over time until a consistent pattern develops that involves violating the rights of others. Very young children are unlikely to meet the criteria for the disorder, as they are not developmentally able to exhibit the symptoms typical of older children with conduct disorder. A 3-year-old does not break into someone's home, steal with confrontation, force someone into sexual activity, or deliberately use a weapon that can cause serious harm. School-age children, however, may become bullies, initiate physical fights, destroy property, or set fires. The DSM-IV-TR diagnostic criteria for conduct disorder are given in Table 44–2.

The average age of onset of conduct disorder is younger in boys than in girls. Boys most commonly meet the diagnostic criteria by 10 to 12 years of age, whereas girls often reach 14 to 16 years of age before the criteria are met.

Children who meet the criteria for conduct disorder express their overt aggressive behavior in various forms. Aggressive antisocial behavior may take the form of bullying, physical aggression, and cruel behavior toward peers. Children may be hostile, verbally abusive, impudent, defiant, and negativistic toward adults. Persistent lying, frequent truancy, and vandalism are common. In severe cases, destructiveness, stealing, and physical violence often occur. Children usually make little attempt to conceal their antisocial behavior. Sexual behavior and regular use of tobacco, liquor, or nonprescribed psychoactive substances begin unusually early for such children and adolescents. Suicidal thoughts, gestures, and acts are frequent.

Table 44–2
DSM-IV-TR Diagnostic Criteria for Conduct Disorder

A. A repetitive and persistent pattern of behavior in which the basic rights of others or major age-appropriate societal norms or rules are violated, as manifested by the presence of three (or more) of the following criteria in the past 12 months, with at least one criterion present in the past 6 months:

Aggression to people and animals

(1) often bullies, threatens, or intimidates others
(2) often initiates physical fights
(3) has used a weapon that can cause serious physical harm to others (e.g., a bat, brick, broken bottle, knife, gun)
(4) has been physically cruel to people
(5) has been physically cruel to animals
(6) has stolen while confronting a victim (e.g., mugging, purse snatching, extortion, armed robbery)
(7) has forced someone into sexual activity

Destruction of property

(8) has deliberately engaged in fire setting with the intention of causing serious damage
(9) has deliberately destroyed others' property (other than by fire setting)

Deceitfulness or theft

(10) has broken into someone else's house, building, or car
(11) often lies to obtain goods or favors or to avoid obligations (i.e., "cons" others)
(12) has stolen items of nontrivial value without confronting a victim (e.g., shoplifting, but without breaking and entering; forgery)

Serious violations of rules

(13) often stays out at night despite parental prohibitions, beginning before age 13 years
(14) has run away from home overnight at least twice while living in parental or parental surrogate home (or once without returning for a lengthy period)
(15) is often truant from school, beginning before age 13 years

B. The disturbance in behavior causes clinically significant impairment in social, academic, or occupational functioning.

C. If the individual is age 18 years or older, criteria are not met for antisocial personality disorder.

Code based on age at onset:

Conduct disorder, childhood-onset type: onset of at least one criterion characteristic of conduct disorder prior to age 10 years

Conduct disorder, adolescent-onset type: absence of any criteria characteristic of conduct disorder prior to age 10 years

Conduct disorder, unspecified onset: age at onset is not known

Specify severity:

Mild: few if any conduct problems in excess of those required to make the diagnosis **and** conduct problems cause only minor harm to others

Moderate: number of conduct problems and effect on others intermediate between "mild" and "severe"

Severe: many conduct problems in excess of those required to make the diagnosis **or** conduct problems cause considerable harm to others

From American Psychiatric Association. *Diagnostic and Statistical Manual of Mental Disorders.* 4th ed. Text rev. Washington, DC: American Psychiatric Association; copyright 2000, with permission.

Some children with aggressive behavioral patterns have impaired social attachments, as evinced by their difficulties with peer relationships. Some may befriend a much older or younger person or have superficial relationships with other antisocial youngsters. Many children with conduct problems have poor self-esteem, although they may project an image of toughness. They may lack the skills to communicate in socially acceptable ways and appear to have little regard for the feelings, wishes, and welfare of others. Children and adolescents with conduct disorders often feel guilt or remorse for some of their behaviors but try to blame others to stay out of trouble.

Many children and adolescents with conduct disorder suffer from the deprivation of having few of their dependency needs met and may have had either overly harsh parenting or a lack of appropriate supervision. The deficient socialization of many children and adolescents with conduct disorder may be expressed in physical violation of others and, for some, in sexual violation of others. Severe punishments for behavior in children with conduct disorder almost invariably increases their maladaptive expression of rage and frustration rather than ameliorating the problem.

In evaluation interviews, children with aggressive conduct disorders are typically uncooperative, hostile, and provocative. Some have a superficial charm and compliance until they are urged to talk about their problem behaviors. Then they often deny any problems. If the interviewer persists, the child may attempt to justify misbehavior or become suspicious and angry about the source of the examiner's information and perhaps bolt from the room. Most often, the child becomes angry with the examiner and expresses resentment of the examination with open belligerence or sullen withdrawal. Their hostility is not limited to adult authority figures but is expressed with equal venom toward their age-mates and younger children. In fact, they often bully those who are smaller and weaker than they. By boasting, lying, and expressing little interest in a listener's responses, such children reveal their lack of trust in adults to understand their position.

Evaluation of the family situation often reveals severe marital disharmony, which initially may center on disagreements about management of the child. Because of a tendency toward family instability, parent surrogates are often in the picture. Children with conduct disorder are more likely to be unplanned or unwanted babies. The parents of children with conduct disorder, especially the father, have higher rates of antisocial personality disorder or alcohol dependence. Aggressive children and their family show a stereotyped pattern of impulsive and unpredictable verbal and physical hostility. A child's aggressive behavior rarely seems directed toward any definable goal and offers little pleasure, success, or even sustained advantages with peers or authority figures.

In other cases, conduct disorder includes repeated truancy, vandalism, and serious physical aggression or assault against others by a gang, such as mugging, gang fighting, and beating. Children who become part of a gang usually have the skills for age-appropriate friendships. They are likely to show concern for the welfare of their friends or their own gang members and are unlikely to blame them or inform on them. In most cases, gang members have a history of adequate or even excessive conformity during early childhood that ended when the youngster became a member of the delinquent peer group, usually in pread-

olescence or during adolescence. Also present in the history is some evidence of early problems, such as marginal or poor school performance, mild behavior problems, anxiety, and depressive symptoms. Some family social or psychological pathology is usually evident. Patterns of paternal discipline are rarely ideal and may vary from harshness and excessive strictness to inconsistency or relative absence of supervision and control. The mother has often protected the child from the consequences of early mild misbehavior but does not seem to encourage delinquency actively. Delinquency, also called *juvenile delinquency,* is most often associated with conduct disorder but may also result from other psychological or neurological disorders.

Pathology and Laboratory Examination

No specific laboratory test or neurological pathology helps make the diagnosis of conduct disorder. Some evidence indicates that amounts of certain neurotransmitters, such as serotonin in the CNS, are low in some persons with a history of violent or aggressive behavior toward others or themselves. Whether this association is related to the cause, or is the effect, of violence or is unrelated to the violence is not clear.

Differential Diagnosis

Disturbances of conduct may be part of many childhood psychiatric conditions, ranging from mood disorders to psychotic disorders to learning disorders. Therefore, clinicians must obtain a history of the chronology of the symptoms to determine whether the conduct disturbance is a transient or reactive phenomenon or an enduring pattern. Isolated acts of antisocial behavior do not justify a diagnosis of conduct disorder; an enduring pattern must be present. The relation of conduct disorder to oppositional defiant disorder is still under debate. Historically, oppositional defiant disorder has been conceptualized as a mild precursor of conduct disorder, which is likely to be diagnosed in young children at risk for conduct disorder. Children who progress from oppositional defiant disorder to conduct disorder do maintain their oppositional characteristics, but some evidence indicates that the two disorders are independent. Many children with oppositional defiant disorder never go on to have conduct disorder, and when conduct disorder first appears in adolescence, it may be unrelated to oppositional defiant disorder. The main distinguishing clinical feature of the two disorders is that in conduct disorder, the basic rights of others are violated, whereas in oppositional defiant disorder, hostility and negativism fall short of seriously violating the rights of others.

Mood disorders are often present in children who exhibit irritability and aggressive behavior. Both major depressive disorder and bipolar disorders must be ruled out, but the full syndrome of conduct disorder may occur and be diagnosed during the onset of a mood disorder. There is a substantial comorbidity of conduct disorder and depressive disorders. A recent report concludes that the high correlation between the two disorders arises from shared risk factors for both disorders rather than a causal relation. Thus, a series of factors including family conflict, negative life events, early history of conduct disturbance, level of parental involvement, and affiliation with delinquent peers contribute to the development of affective disorders and conduct disorder. This is not the case with oppositional defiant disorder, which cannot be diagnosed if it occurs exclusively during a mood disorder.

Attention-deficit/hyperactivity disorder and learning disorders are commonly associated with conduct disorder. Usually, the symptoms of these disorders predate the diagnosis of conduct disorder. Substance abuse disorders are also more common in adolescents with conduct disorder than in the general population. There is evidence of an association between fighting behaviors as a child and substance use as an adolescent. Once a pattern of drug use is formed, this pattern may interfere with the development of positive mediators, such as social skills and problem solving, which could enhance remission of the conduct disorder. Thus, once substance abuse develops, it may promote continuation of the conduct disorder. Obsessive-compulsive disorder also frequently seems to coexist with disruptive behavior disorders. All the disorders described here should be noted when they co-occur. Children with attention-deficit/hyperactivity disorder often exhibit impulsive and aggressive behaviors that may not meet the full criteria for conduct disorder.

Course and Prognosis

In general, the prognosis for children with conduct disorder is most guarded in those who have symptoms at a young age, exhibit the greatest number of symptoms, and express them most frequently. This finding is true partly because those with severe conduct disorder seem to be most vulnerable to comorbid disorders later in life, such as mood disorders and substance use disorders. It stands to reason that the more concurrent mental disorders a person has, the more troublesome life will be. A recent report found that although assaultive behavior in childhood and parental criminality predict a high risk for incarceration later in life, the diagnosis of conduct disorder per se was not correlated with imprisonment. A good prognosis is predicted for mild conduct disorder in the absence of coexisting psychopathology and the presence of normal intellectual functioning.

Treatment

Treatment programs have been more successful in decreasing overt symptoms of conduct disorder than the covert symptoms. Multimodality treatment programs that use all the available family and community resources are likely to bring about the best results in efforts to control conduct-disordered behavior. No treatment is considered curative for the entire spectrum of behaviors that contribute to conduct disorder, but a variety of treatments may be helpful in containing symptoms and promoting prosocial behavior.

An environmental structure that provides support, along with consistent rules and expected consequences, can help control a variety of problem behaviors. The structure can be applied to family life in some cases, so that parents become aware of behavioral techniques and grow proficient at using them to foster appropriate behaviors. Families in which psychopathology or environmental stressors prevent parental understanding of the techniques may require parental psychiatric evaluation and treatment before making such an endeavor. When a family is abusive or chaotic, the child may have to be removed from the home to benefit from a consistent and structured environment. School settings can also use behavioral

techniques to promote socially acceptable behavior toward peers and to discourage covert antisocial incidents.

Individual psychotherapy oriented toward improving problem-solving skills can be useful, as children with conduct disorder may have a long-standing pattern of maladaptive responses to daily situations. The age at which treatment begins is important, because the longer the maladaptive behaviors continue, the more entrenched they become.

Medication can be a useful adjunctive treatment for symptoms that often contribute to conduct disorder. Overt explosive aggression responds to several medications. Antipsychotics, most notably haloperidol (Haldol), have reportedly helped children control aggressive and assaultive behaviors that may be present in various disorders. Currently, the newer antipsychotics such as risperidone (Risperdal), and olanzapine (Zyprexa) have replaced haloperidol because they carry a lower risk of extrapyramidal symptoms. Lithium (Eskalith) has been reported to have efficacy for some aggressive children with or without comorbid bipolar disorders. Some trials suggest that carbamazepine (Tegretol) may help control aggression, but a double-blind, placebo-controlled study did not show superiority of carbamazepine over placebo in decreasing aggression. A recent pilot study found that clonidine (Catapres) may decrease aggression. The selective serotonin reuptake inhibitors (SSRIs), such as fluoxetine (Prozac), sertraline (Zoloft), paroxetine (Paxil), and citalopram (Celexa) have been used in an attempt to diminish impulsivity, irritability, and lability of mood, which often occur with conduct disorder. Conduct disorder frequently coexists with attention-deficit/hyperactivity disorder, learning disorders, and, over time, mood disorders and substance-related disorders; thus, the treatment of any concurrent disorders must also be addressed.

DISRUPTIVE BEHAVIOR DISORDER NOT OTHERWISE SPECIFIED

According to DSM-IV-TR, the category of disruptive behavior disorder not otherwise specified can be used for disorders of conduct or oppositional-defiant behaviors that do not meet the diagnostic criteria for either conduct disorder or oppositional defiant disorder but in which there is notable impairment (Table 44–3).

Table 44–3
DSM-IV-TR Diagnostic Criteria for Disruptive Behavior Disorder Not Otherwise Specified

This category is for disorders characterized by conduct or oppositional defiant behaviors that do not meet the criteria for conduct disorder or oppositional defiant disorder. For example, include clinical presentations that do not meet full criteria either for oppositional defiant disorder or conduct disorder, but in which there is clinically significant impairment.

From American Psychiatric Association. *Diagnostic and Statistical Manual of Mental Disorders.* 4th ed. Text rev. Washington, DC: American Psychiatric Association; copyright 2000, with permission.

ICD-10

In the 10th revision of *International Statistical Classification of Diseases and Related Health Problems* (ICD-10), conduct disorders include disorder confined to the family context, unsocialized conduct disorder, socialized conduct disorder, oppositional defiant behavior, other conduct disorders, and conduct disorder, unspecified. ICD-10 characterizes conduct disorders as repetitive and persistent patterns of "dissocial, aggressive, or defiant conduct."

In ICD-10, oppositional defiant disorder is sometimes considered a less severe variant of conduct disorder rather than a distinct type. Although, according to ICD-10, it is uncertain whether the distinction is qualitative or quantitative, findings suggest that it is distinctive "mainly or only in younger children." In older children, conduct disorders generally include behavior that is aggressive or dissocial beyond defiance, even when it was preceded by oppositional defiant behaviors. Thus, this disorder accommodates "common diagnostic practice" and facilitates "the classification of disorders occurring in younger children."

The ICD-10 criteria for conduct disorders are listed in Table 44–4. The criteria for mixed disorders of conduct and emotions are listed in Table 44–5.

Table 44–4
ICD-10 Diagnostic Criteria for Conduct Disorders

G1. There is a repetitive and persistent pattern of behavior, in which either the basic rights of others or major age-appropriate societal norms or rules are violated, lasting at least 6 months, during which some of the following symptoms are present (see individual subcategories for rules or numbers of symptoms).

Note: The symptoms in 11, 13, 15, 16, 20, 21, and 23 need only have occurred once for the criterion to be fulfilled.

The individual:

(1) has unusually frequent or severe temper tantrums for his or her developmental level;
(2) often argues with adults;
(3) often actively refuses adults' requests or defies rules;
(4) often, apparently deliberately, does things that annoy other people;
(5) often blames others for his or her own mistakes or misbehavior;
(6) is often "touchy" or easily annoyed by others;
(7) is often angry or resentful;
(8) is often spiteful or vindictive;
(9) often lies or breaks promises to obtain goods or favors or to avoid obligations;
(10) frequently initiates physical fights (this does not include fights with siblings);
(11) has used a weapon that can cause serious physical harm to others (e.g., bat, brick, broken bottle, knife, gun);
(12) often stays out after dark despite parental prohibition (beginning before 13 years of age);
(13) exhibits physical cruelty to other people (e.g., ties up, cuts, or burns a victim);

(*continued*)

Table 44–4 (*continued*)

(14) exhibits physical cruelty to animals;
(15) deliberately destroys the property of others (other than by fire-setting);
(16) deliberately sets fires with a risk or intention of causing serious damage;
(17) steals objects of nontrivial value without confronting the victim, either within the home or outside (e.g., shoplifting, burglary, forgery);
(18) is frequently truant from school, beginning before 13 years of age;
(19) has run away from parental or parental surrogate home at least twice or has run away once for more than a single night (this does not include leaving to avoid physical or sexual abuse);
(20) commits a crime involving confrontation with the victim (including purse-snatching, extortion, mugging);
(21) forces another person into sexual activity;
(22) frequently bullies others (e.g., deliberate infliction of pain or hurt, including persistent intimidation, tormenting, or molestation);
(23) breaks into someone else's house, building, or car.

G2. The disorder does not meet the criteria for dissocial personality disorder, schizophrenia, manic episode, depressive episode, pervasive developmental disorders, or hyperkinetic disorder. (If criteria for emotional disorder are met, the diagnosis should be mixed disorder of conduct and emotions.)

It is recommended that the age of onset be specified:

— *childhood-onset type:* onset of at least one conduct problem before the age of 10 years;

— *adolescent-onset type:* no conduct problems before the age of 10 years.

Specification for possible subdivisions

Authorities differ on the best way of subdividing the conduct disorders, although most agree that the disorders are heterogeneous. For determining prognosis, the severity (indexed by number of symptoms) is a better guide than the precise type of symptomatology. The best-validated distinction is that between *socialized* and *unsocialized* disorders, defined by the presence or absence of lasting peer friendships. However, it seems that disorders confined to the family context may also constitute an important variety, and a category is provided for this purpose. It is clear that further research is needed to test the validity of all proposed subdivisions of conduct disorder.

In addition to these categorizations, it is recommended that cases be described in terms of their scores on three dimensions of disturbance:

(1) hyperactivity (inattentive, restless behavior);
(2) emotional disturbance (anxiety, depression, obsessionality, hypochondriasis); and
(3) severity of conduct disorder:
 (a) *mild:* few if any conduct problems are in excess of those required to make the diagnosis, *and* conduct problems cause only minor harm to others;
 (b) *moderate:* the number of conduct problems and the effects on others are intermediate between "mild" and "severe";
 (c) *severe:* there are many conduct problems in excess of those required to make the diagnosis, *or* the conduct problems cause considerable harm to others, e.g., severe physical injury, vandalism, or theft.

Conduct disorder confined to the family context

A. The general criteria for conduct disorder must be met.
B. Three or more of the symptoms listed for criterion G1 must be present, with at least three from items (9)–(23).
C. At least one of the symptoms from items (9)–(23) must have been present for at least 6 months.
D. Conduct disturbance must be limited to the family context.

Unsocialized conduct disorder

A. The general criteria for conduct disorder must be met.
B. Three or more of the symptoms listed for conduct disorder criterion G1 must be present, with at least three from items (9)–(23).
C. At least one of the symptoms from items (9)–(23) must have been present for at least 6 months.
D. There must be definitely poor relationships with the individual's peer group, as shown by isolation, rejection, or unpopularity, and by a lack of lasting close reciprocal friendships.

Socialized conduct disorder

A. The general criteria for conduct disorder must be met.
B. Three or more of the symptoms listed for criterion G1 must be present, with at least three from items (9)–(23).
C. At least one of the symptoms from items (9)–(23) must have been present for at least 6 months.
D. Conduct disturbance must include settings outside the home or family context.
E. Peer relationships are within normal limits.

Oppositional defiant disorder

A. The general criteria for conduct disorder must be met.
B. Four or more of the symptoms listed for criterion G1 must be present, but with no more than two symptoms from items (9)–(23).
C. The symptoms in criterion B must be maladaptive and inconsistent with the developmental level.
D. At least four of the symptoms must have been present for at least 6 months.

Other conduct disorders

Conduct disorder, unspecified

This residual category is not recommended and should be used only for disorders that meet the general criteria for conduct disorder but that have not been specified as to subtype or that do not fulfill the criteria for any of the specified subtypes.

Table 44–5
ICD-10 Diagnostic Criteria for Mixed Disorders of Conduct and Emotions

Depressive conduct disorder

A. The general criteria for conduct disorders must be met.

B. Criteria for one of the mood (affective) disorders must be met.

Other mixed disorders of conduct and emotions

A. The general criteria for conduct disorders must be met.

B. Criteria for one of the neurotic, stress-related, and somatoform disorders or childhood emotional disorders must be met.

Mixed disorder of conduct and emotions, unspecified

Reprinted with permission from World Health Organization. *The ICD-10 Classification of Mental and Behavioural Disorders: Diagnostic Criteria for Research.* Copyright, World Health Organization, Geneva, 1993.

References

Butler SM, Seto MC. Distinguishing two types of adolescent sex offenders. *J Am Acad Child Adolesc Psychiatry.* 2002;41:83.

Cueva JE, Overall JE, Small AM, Armenteros JL, Perry R, Campbell M. Carbamazepine in aggressive children with conduct disorder: a double-blind and placebo-controlled study. *J Am Acad Child Adolesc Psychiatry.* 1996;35:480.

Geller DA, Biederman J, Griffin S, Jones J, Lefkowitz TR. Co-morbidity of juvenile obsessive-compulsive disorder with disruptive behavior disorders. *J Am Acad Child Adolesc Psychiatry.* 1996;35:1637.

Kemph JP, DeVane CL, Levin GM, Jarecke R, Miller RL. Treatment of aggressive children with clonidine: results of an open pilot study. *J Am Acad Child Adolesc Psychiatry.* 1993;32:577.

Lahey BB, Applegate B, Barkley RA, et al. DSM-IV field trials for oppositional defiant disorder and conduct disorder in children and adolescents. *Am J Psychiatry.* 1994;151:1163.

Lahey BB, Loeber R, Quay HC, Frick PJ, Grimm J. Oppositional defiant disorder and conduct disorders: issues to be resolved for DSM-IV. *J Am Acad Child Adolesc Psychiatry.* 1992;31:539.

Lewis DO. From abuse to violence: psychophysiological consequences of maltreatment. *J Am Acad Child Adolesc Psychiatry.* 1992;31:383.

Lewis DO, Lovely R, Yeager C, et al. Intrinsic and environmental characteristics of juvenile murderers. *J Am Acad Child Adolesc Psychiatry.* 1988; 27:582.

Lipman EL, Boyle MH, Dooley MD, Offord DR. Child well-being in single-mother families. *J Am Acad Child Adolesc Psychiatry.* 2002;41:75.

Masters KJ, Bellonci C. Practice parameters for the prevention and management of aggressive behavior in child and adolescent psychiatric institutions, with special reference to seclusion and restraint. *J Am Acad Child Adolesc Psychiatry.* 2002;41(suppl):4.

Robins L. *Deviant Children Grown Up.* Baltimore: Williams & Wilkins; 1966.

Steiner H. Disruptive behavior disorders. In: Sadock BJ, Sadock VA, eds. *Kaplan and Sadock's Comprehensive Textbook of Psychiatry.* 7th ed. Vol 2. Baltimore: Lippincott Williams & Wilkins; 2000:2693.

Vance JE, Bowen NK, Fernandez G, Thompson S. Risk and protective factors as predictors of outcome in adolescents with psychiatric disorder and aggression. *J Am Acad Child Adolesc Psychiatry.* 2002;41:36.

Wasserman GA, Miller LS, Pinner E, Jaramillo B. Parenting predictors of early conduct problems in urban, high-risk boys. *J Am Acad Child Adolesc Psychiatry.* 1996;35:1227.

Wichtrom L, Skogen K, Oia T. Increased rate of conduct problems in urban areas: what is the mechanism? *J Am Acad Child Adolesc Psychiatry.* 1996; 35:471.

45

Feeding and Eating Disorders of Infancy or Early Childhood

Feeding and eating disorders of infancy or early childhood include persistent symptoms of inadequate food intake, recurrent regurgitation and rechewing of food, or repeated ingestion of nonnutritive substances. Since very young children depend upon parents or caregivers to feed them and provide meals, these disorders are often conceptualized as reflecting, in part, an interaction between the child and parent. The text revision of the fourth edition of *Diagnostic and Statistical Manual of Mental Disorders* (DSM-IV-TR) includes three distinct disorders of feeding and eating in this age group: pica, rumination disorder, and feeding disorder of infancy or early childhood. There is a high rate of spontaneous recovery from all of these feeding disorders, although a subset of infants refuses to eat and has persistent eating problems throughout childhood.

PICA

In DSM-IV-TR, pica is described as persistent eating of nonnutritive substances for at least 1 month. The behavior must be developmentally inappropriate, not culturally sanctioned, and sufficiently severe to merit clinical attention. Pica is diagnosed even when these symptoms occur in the context of another disorder such as autistic disorder, schizophrenia, or Kleine-Levin syndrome. Pica appears much more frequently in young children than in adults; it also occurs in persons who are mentally retarded. Among adults, certain forms of pica, including geophagia (clay eating) and amylophagia (starch eating), have been reported in pregnant women.

Epidemiology

Few data confirm the prevalence of pica among children, and it is rare among older children and adolescents. Pica is more common among children and adolescents with mental retardation. It has been reported in up to 15 percent of persons with severe mental retardation. Pica appears to affect both sexes equally.

Etiology

Several theories have been proposed to explain the phenomenon of pica, but none has been universally accepted. A higher than expected incidence of pica seems to occur in the relatives of persons with the symptoms. Nutritional deficiencies have been postulated as causes of pica; in particular circumstances, cravings for nonedible substances have been produced by dietary insufficiencies. For example, cravings for dirt and ice are sometimes associated with iron and zinc deficiencies, which are corrected by their administration. A high incidence of parental neglect and deprivation has been associated with cases of pica. Theories relating children's psychological deprivation and subsequent ingestion of inedible substances have suggested that pica is a compensatory mechanism to satisfy oral needs.

Diagnosis and Clinical Features

Eating nonedible substances repeatedly after 18 months of age is usually considered abnormal. The onset of pica is usually between ages 12 and 24 months, and the incidence declines with age. The specific substances ingested vary with their accessibility, and they increase with a child's mastery of locomotion and the resultant increased independence and decreased parental supervision. Typically, young children ingest paint, plaster, string, hair, and cloth; older children have access to dirt, animal feces, stones, and paper. The clinical implications can be benign or life-threatening, depending on the objects ingested. Among the most serious complications are lead poisoning (usually from lead-based paint), intestinal parasites after ingestion of soil or feces, anemia and zinc deficiency after ingestion of clay, severe iron deficiency after ingestion of large quantities of starch, and intestinal obstruction from the ingestion of hair balls, stones, or gravel. Except in persons who are mentally retarded, pica usually remits by adolescence. Pica associated with pregnancy is usually limited to the pregnancy itself. The DSM-IV-TR diagnostic criteria for pica are given in Table 45–1.

George, a thin, pale, 5-year-old boy, was admitted to the hospital for a nutritional anemia that seemed to result from his ingestion of paint, plaster, dirt, wood, and paste. He had had numerous hospitalizations under similar circumstances, beginning at age 19 months, when he had ingested lighter fluid.

George's parents subsisted on welfare, and were described as immature. He was the product of an unplanned but normal pregnancy. His mother began eating dirt when she was pregnant, at age 16. His father periodically abused drugs and alcohol.

DISCUSSION

Eating of nonnutritive substances may be developmentally appropriate for an infant, but its persistence up to age 5

warrants a diagnosis of pica. As in this case, it is commonly associated with a similar history in the mother and low socioeconomic status.

In some cultural settings, the eating of nonnutritive substances, such as clay, may be a sanctioned practice, in which case the diagnosis would not apply but that certainly is not the case here. In other cases the disturbance may be associated with other disorders, such as autistic disorder, schizophrenia, or the neurological disorder Kleine-Levin syndrome. (From *DSM-IV Casebook.*)

Pathology and Laboratory Examination

No single laboratory test confirms or rules out a diagnosis of pica, but several laboratory tests are useful because pica has frequently been associated with abnormal indexes. Levels of iron and zinc in serum should always be determined; in many cases of pica, these levels are low and may contribute to the development of pica. Pica may disappear when oral iron and zinc are administered. A patient's hemoglobin level should be determined; if the level is low, anemia can result. In children with pica, the lead level in serum should be determined; lead poisoning can result from ingesting lead. When a child's lead level is high, this condition must be treated.

Differential Diagnosis

The differential diagnosis of pica includes iron and zinc deficiencies. Pica also may occur in conjunction with failure to thrive and several other mental and medical disorders, including schizophrenia, autistic disorder, anorexia nervosa, and Kleine-Levin syndrome. In psychosocial dwarfism, a dramatic but reversible endocrinological and behavioral form of failure to thrive, children often show bizarre behaviors, including ingesting toilet water, garbage, and other nonnutritive substances. A recent case report presented an association of pica with hypersomnolence, lead intoxication, and precocious puberty. Precocious puberty implicates the hypothalamus as a site for at least part of the dysfunction. Lead intoxication is known to be associated with pica as well as several other neuropsychiatric abnormalities in memory and cognitive performance. A small minority of children with autistic disorder and schizophrenia may have pica. For children who exhibit pica along with another medical disorder, both disorders should be coded according to DSM-IV-TR.

In certain regions of the world and among certain cultures, such as the Australian aborigines, rates of pica in pregnant women are reportedly high. According to DSM-IV-TR, however, if such practices are culturally accepted, the diagnostic criteria for pica are not met.

Table 45–1
DSM-IV-TR Diagnostic Criteria for Pica

A. Persistent eating of nonnutritive substances for a period of at least 1 month.
B. The eating of nonnutritive substances is inappropriate to the developmental level.
C. The eating behavior is not part of a culturally sanctioned practice.
D. If the eating behavior occurs exclusively during the course of another mental disorder (e.g., mental retardation, pervasive developmental disorder, schizophrenia), it is sufficiently severe to warrant independent clinical attention.

From American Psychiatric Association. *Diagnostic and Statistical Manual of Mental Disorders.* 4th ed. Text rev. Washington, DC: American Psychiatric Association; copyright 2000, with permission.

Course and Prognosis

The prognosis for pica varies, though in children of normal intelligence it usually remits spontaneously. In children, pica usually resolves with increasing age; in pregnant women, pica is usually limited to the term of the pregnancy. In some adults, however, especially those who are mentally retarded, pica may continue for years. Follow-up data on these populations are too limited to permit conclusions.

Treatment

The first step in the treatment of pica is determining the cause whenever possible. When pica is associated with situations of neglect or maltreatment, these circumstances naturally need to be altered. Exposure to toxic substances, such as lead, must also be eliminated. No definitive treatment exists for pica; most treatment is aimed at education and behavior modification. Treatments emphasize psychosocial, environmental, behavioral, and family guidance approaches. An effort should be made to ameliorate any significant psychosocial stressors. When lead is present in the surroundings, it must be eliminated or rendered inaccessible or the child must be moved to new surroundings.

Several behavioral techniques have been used with some effect. The most rapidly successful technique seems to be mild aversion therapy or negative reinforcement (e.g., a mild electric shock, an unpleasant noise, or an emetic drug). Positive reinforcement, modeling, behavioral shaping, and overcorrection treatment have also been used. Increasing parental attention, stimulation, and emotional nurturance may yield positive results. One study found that pica was negatively correlated with involvement with play materials and occurred most frequently in impoverished environments. In some patients, correcting an iron or zinc deficiency has eliminated pica. Medical complications (e.g., lead poisoning) that develop secondarily to the pica must also be treated.

RUMINATION DISORDER

In DSM-IV-TR rumination disorder is described as an infant's or child's repeated regurgitation and rechewing of food, after a period of normal functioning. The symptoms last for at least 1 month, are not caused by a medical condition, and are severe enough to merit clinical attention. The onset of the disorder generally occurs after 3 months of age; once the regurgitation occurs, the food may be swallowed or spit out. Infants who ruminate are observed to strain to bring the food back into their mouths and appear to find the experience pleasurable. The infants are often brought for evaluation because of failure to

thrive. The disorder is rare in older children, adolescents, and adults. It varies in severity and is sometimes associated with medical conditions, such as hiatal hernia, that result in esophageal reflux. In its most severe form, the disorder can be fatal.

The diagnosis of rumination disorder can be made whether or not an infant has attained a normal weight for his or her age. Failure to thrive, therefore, is not a necessary criterion of this disorder, but it is sometimes a sequela. According to DSM-IV-TR, the disorder must be present for at least 1 month after a period of normal functioning, and it is not associated with gastrointestinal illness or other general medical conditions.

Rumination has been recognized for hundreds of years. An awareness of the disorder is important, so that it is correctly diagnosed and so that unnecessary surgical procedures and inappropriate treatment are avoided. *Rumination* is derived from the Latin word *ruminare,* meaning "to chew the cud." The Greek equivalent is *merycism,* the act of regurgitating food from the stomach into the mouth, rechewing the food, and reswallowing it.

Epidemiology

Rumination is a rare disorder. It seems to be more common among infants between 3 months and 1 year of age and among children and adults who are mentally retarded. Adults with rumination usually maintain a normal weight. The disorder may be more common in males. No reliable figures on predisposing factors or familial patterns are available.

Etiology

Several causes of rumination have been proposed. In those who are mentally retarded, the disorder may simply be self-stimulatory behavior. In those who are nonretarded, psychodynamic theories hypothesize various disturbances in the mother–child relationship. The mothers of infants with the disorder are usually immature, involved in a marital conflict, and unable to give much attention to the baby. These factors result in insufficient emotional gratification and stimulation for the infant, who seeks gratification from within. The rumination is interpreted as the infant's attempt to recreate the feeding process and to provide gratification that the mother does not provide.

Overstimulation and tension have also been suggested as causes of rumination. A dysfunctional autonomic nervous system may be implicated. As sophisticated and accurate investigative techniques are refined, a substantial number of children classified as ruminators are shown to have gastroesophageal reflux or hiatal hernia.

Behaviorists attribute rumination to the positive reinforcement of pleasurable self-stimulation and to the attention the baby receives from others as a consequence of the disorder.

Diagnosis and Clinical Features

The DSM-IV-TR diagnostic criteria for rumination disorder are given in Table 45–2. DSM-IV-TR notes that the essential feature of the disorder is repeated regurgitation and rechewing of food for a period of at least 1 month after a period of normal functioning. Partially digested food is brought up into the mouth without nausea, retching, disgust, or associated gastrointestinal disorder. This activity can be distinguished from vomiting by the clear, purposeful movements the infant makes to induce it. The food is then ejected from the mouth or reswallowed. A characteristic position of straining and arching of the back, with the head held back, is observed. The infant makes sucking movements with the tongue and gives the impression of gaining considerable satisfaction from the activity. Usually, the infant is irritable and hungry between episodes of rumination.

Table 45–2
DSM-IV-TR Diagnostic Criteria for Rumination Disorder

A. Repeated regurgitation and rechewing of food for a period of at least 1 month following a period of normal functioning.
B. The behavior is not due to an associated gastrointestinal or other general medical condition (e.g., esophageal reflux).
C. The behavior does not occur exclusively during the course of anorexia nervosa or bulimia nervosa. If the symptoms occur exclusively during the course of mental retardation or a pervasive developmental disorder, they are sufficiently severe to warrant independent clinical attention.

From American Psychiatric Association. *Diagnostic and Statistical Manual of Mental Disorders.* 4th ed. Text rev. Washington, DC: American Psychiatric Association; copyright 2000, with permission.

Initially, rumination may be difficult to distinguish from the regurgitation that frequently occurs in normal infants. In fully developed cases, however, the diagnosis is obvious. Food or milk is regurgitated without nausea, retching, or disgust and is subjected to what appears to be innumerable pleasurable sucking and chewing movements. The food is then reswallowed or ejected from the mouth.

Although spontaneous remissions are common, severe secondary complications may develop, such as progressive malnutrition, dehydration, and lowered resistance to disease. Failure to thrive, with absence of growth and developmental delays in all areas, may occur. Mortality as high as 25 percent has been reported in severe cases. An additional complication is that the mother or caretaker is often discouraged by failure to feed the infant successfully and may become alienated, if she is not already so. Further alienation often occurs as the noxious odor of the regurgitated material leads to avoidance of the infant.

Pathology and Laboratory Examination

No specific laboratory examination is pathognomonic of rumination disorder. Clinicians must rule out physical causes of vomiting, such as pyloric stenosis and hiatal hernia, before making the diagnosis of rumination disorder. Rumination disorder can be associated with failure to thrive and varying degrees of starvation. Thus, laboratory measures of endocrinological function (thyroid function tests, dexamethasone-suppression test), serum electrolytes, and a hematological workup help determine the severity of the effects of rumination disorder.

Differential Diagnosis

To make the diagnosis of rumination disorder, clinicians must rule out gastrointestinal congenital anomalies, infections, and other medical illnesses. Pyloric stenosis is usually associated with projectile vomiting and is generally evident before 3 months of age, when rumination has its onset. Rumination has

been associated with various mental retardation syndromes in which other stereotypic behaviors and eating disturbances, such as pica, are present. Rumination disorder may occur in patients with other eating disorders, such as bulimia nervosa.

Course and Prognosis

Rumination disorder is believed to have a high rate of spontaneous remission. Indeed, many cases of rumination disorder may develop and remit without ever being diagnosed. Only limited data are available about the prognosis of rumination disorder in adults.

Treatment

The treatment of rumination disorder is often a combination of education and behavioral techniques. Sometimes an evaluation of the mother–child relationship reveals deficits that can be influenced by offering guidance to the mother. Behavioral interventions, such as squirting lemon juice into the infant's mouth whenever rumination occurs, can be effective in diminishing the behavior. This practice appears to be the most rapidly effective treatment; rumination is eliminated in 3 to 5 days. In the aversive-conditioning reports on rumination disorder, infants were doing well at 9- or 12-month follow-up, with no recurrence of the rumination and with weight gains, increased activity levels, and increased responsiveness to persons. Rumination may be decreased by the technique of withdrawing attention from the child whenever this behavior occurs. The effectiveness of treatments is difficult to evaluate. Most reported are single-case studies; patients are not randomly assigned to controlled studies.

Any concomitant medical complications must also be treated. Treatments include improvement of the child's psychosocial environment, increased tender loving care from the mother or caretakers, and psychotherapy for the mother or both parents. When anatomical abnormalities such as hiatal hernia are present, surgical repair may be necessary. Medications including metoclopramide (Reglan), cimetidine (Tagamet), and antipsychotics such as haloperidol (Haldol) and thioridazine (Mellaril) have been successful according to anecdotal reports. One study showed that when infants were allowed to eat as much as they wanted, the rate of rumination decreased.

FEEDING DISORDER OF INFANCY OR EARLY CHILDHOOD

According to DSM-IV-TR, feeding disorder of infancy or early childhood is a persistent failure to eat adequately, reflected in significant failure to gain weight or in significant weight loss over 1 month. The symptoms are not better accounted for by a medical condition or by another mental disorder and are not caused by lack of food (Table 45–3). The disorder has its onset before the age of 6 years.

Epidemiology

It is estimated that between 15 and 35 percent of infants and young children have some feeding difficulties. Data from community samples estimate a prevalence of the disorder, however, in about 3 percent of infants with failure to thrive syndromes, with approximately half of those infants exhibiting feeding disorders.

Table 45–3
DSM-IV-TR Diagnostic Criteria for Feeding Disorder of Infancy or Early Childhood

A. Feeding disturbance as manifested by persistent failure to eat adequately with significant failure to gain weight or significant loss of weight over at least 1 month.
B. The disturbance is not due to an associated gastrointestinal or other general medical condition (e.g., esophageal reflux).
C. The disturbance is not better accounted for by another mental disorder (e.g., rumination disorder) or by lack of available food.
D. The onset is before age 6 years.

From American Psychiatric Association. *Diagnostic and Statistical Manual of Mental Disorders.* 4th ed. Text rev. Washington, DC: American Psychiatric Association; copyright 2000, with permission.

Differential Diagnosis

Feeding disorder of infancy must be differentiated from structural problems with the infants' gastrointestinal tract that may be contributing to discomfort during the feeding process.

Course and Prognosis

Most infants exhibit feeding disorders within the first year of life and, with appropriate recognition and intervention, do not go on to develop failure to thrive. When feeding disorders have their onset later, in children 2 to 3 years of age, growth and development may be affected when the disorder lasts for several months. It is estimated that about 70 percent of infants who persistently refuse food in the first year of life continue to have some feeding problems during childhood.

Table 45–4
ICD-10 Diagnostic Criteria for Feeding Disorder of Infancy and Childhood

A. There is persistent failure to eat adequately, or persistent rumination or regurgitation of food.
B. The child fails to gain weight, loses weight, or exhibits some other significant health problem over a period of at least 1 month. (In view of the frequency of transient eating difficulties, researchers may prefer a minimum duration of 3 months for some purposes.)
C. Onset of the disorder is before the age of 6 years.
D. The child exhibits no other mental or behavioral disorder in the ICD-10 classification (other than mental retardation).
E. There is no evidence of organic disease sufficient to account for the failure to eat.

Reprinted with permission from World Health Organization. *The ICD-10 Classification of Mental and Behavioural Disorders: Diagnostic Criteria for Research.* Copyright, World Health Organization, Geneva, 1993.

Table 45–5
ICD-10 Diagnostic Criteria for Pica of Infancy and Childhood

A. There is persistent or recurrent eating of nonnutritive substances, at least twice a week.
B. Duration of the disorder is at least 1 month. (For some purposes, researchers may prefer a minimum period of 3 months.)
C. The child exhibits no other mental or behavioral disorder in the ICD-10 classification (other than mental retardation).
D. The child's chronological and mental age is at least 2 years.
E. The eating behavior is not part of a culturally sanctioned practice.

Reprinted with permission from World Health Organization. *The ICD-10 Classification of Mental and Behavioural Disorders: Diagnostic Criteria for Research.* Copyright, World Health Organization, Geneva, 1993.

Treatment

Interventions for feeding disorders are aimed at evaluating the interaction between the mother and infant during feedings, and identifying any factors that can be changed to promote greater ingestion. The mother is helped to become more aware of the infant's stamina for length of individual feedings, the infant's biological regulation patterns, and when the infant is fatigued, with a goal of increasing the level of engagement between mother and infant during feeding.

ICD-10

In the 10th revision of *International Statistical Classification of Diseases and Related Health Problems* (ICD-10), feeding disorder of infancy and childhood, which also includes rumination disorder (Table 45–4), and pica of infancy and childhood (Table 45–5) are included in the category other emotional and behavioral disorders with onset usually occurring in childhood and adolescence.

References

Benoit D. Phenomenology and treatment of failure to thrive. *Child Adolesc Psychiatry Clin North Am.* 1993;2:61.

Boris NW, Hagino OR, Steiner GP. Case study: hypersomnolence and precocious puberty in a child with pica and chronic lead intoxication. *J Am Acad Adolesc Psychiatry.* 1996;35:1050.

Carter AS, Garrity-Rokous FE, Chazan-Cohen R, Little C, Briggs-Gowan MJ. Maternal depression and comorbidity: predicting early parenting, attachment security, and toddler social-emotional problems and competencies. *J Am Acad Child Adolesc Psychiatry.* 2001;40:18.

Chatoor I. Feeding and eating disorders of infancy or early childhood. In: Sadock BJ, Sadock VA, eds. *Comprehensive Textbook of Psychiatry.* Vol 2. Baltimore: Lippincott Williams & Wilkins; 2000:2704.

Connors ME, Morse W. Sexual abuse and eating disorders: a review. *Int J Eat Disord.* 1993;13:1.

Davis PK, Cuvo AJ. Chronic vomiting and rumination in intellectually normal and retarded individuals: review and evaluation of behavioral research. *Behav Res Severe Dev Disabil.* 1980;1:31.

DelCarmen-Wiggins R, Carter AS. Assessment of infant and toddler mental health: advances and challenges. *Am J Child Adolesc Psychiatry.* 2001;40:8.

Franco K, Campbell N, Tamburrino M, Evans C. Rumination: the eating disorder of infancy. *Child Psychiatry Hum Dev.* 1993;24:91.

Hodes M, Le Grange D. Expressed emotion in the investigation of eating disorders: a review. *Int J Eat Disord.* 1993;13:279.

Keren M, Feldman R, Tyano S. Diagnoses and interactive patterns of infants referred to a community-based infant mental health clinic. *J Am Acad Child Adolesc Psychiatry.* 2001;40:27.

Kramer SS, Eicher PM. The evaluation of pediatric feeding abnormalities. *Dysphagia.* 1993;8:215.

Mayes SD, Humphrey FJ, Handford HA, Mitchell JF. Rumination disorder: differential diagnosis. *J Am Acad Child Adolesc Psychiatry.* 1988;27:300.

Millican FK, Lourie RS, Laymen EM. Emotional factors in the etiology and treatment of lead poisoning. *Am J Dis Child.* 1956;91:144.

Nasser M. A prescription of vomiting: historical footnotes. *Int J Eat Disord.* 1993;13:129.

Provence S, Lipton RC. *Infants and Institutions.* New York: International Universities Press; 1962.

Rast J, Johnston JM, Drum C, Conrin J. The relation of food quantity to rumination behavior. *J Appl Behav Anal.* 1981;14:221.

Steiner H, Lock J. Anorexia nervosa and bulimia nervosa in children and adolescents: a review of the past 10 years. *J Am Acad Child Adolesc Psychiatry.* 1998;37:352.

Stunkard AJ, Stellar E, eds. *Eating and Its Disorders.* New York: Raven Press; 1984.

Vanderlinden J, Vanderecycken W, van Dyck R, Vertommen H. Dissociative experience and trauma in eating disorders. *Int J Eat Disord.* 1993;13:187.

Zeanah CH, Larrieu JA, Heller SS, et al. Evaluation of a preventive intervention for maltreated infants and toddlers in foster care. *J Am Acad Child Adolesc Psychiatry.* 2001;40:214.

46 Tic Disorders

Tics are defined as rapid and repetitive muscle contractions resulting in movements or vocalizations that are experienced as involuntary. Children and adolescents may exhibit tic behaviors that occur after a stimulus or in response to an internal urge. Tic disorders are a group of neuropsychiatric disorders that generally begin in childhood or adolescence and may be constant or wax and wane over time. Although tics are not volitional, in some individuals they may be suppressed for periods. The most widely known and most severe tic disorder is Gilles de la Tourette syndrome, also known as Tourette's disorder. The text revision of the fourth edition of the *Diagnostic and Statistical Manual of Mental Disorders* (DSM-IV-TR) includes several other tic disorders such as chronic motor or vocal tic disorder, transient tic disorder, and tic disorder not otherwise specified. While tics have no particular purpose, they often consist of motions that are used in volitional movements.

Motor and vocal tics are divided into simple and complex types. *Simple motor tics* are those composed of repetitive, rapid contractions of functionally similar muscle groups—for example, eye blinking, neck jerking, shoulder shrugging, and facial grimacing. Common *simple vocal tics* include coughing, throat clearing, grunting, sniffing, snorting, and barking. *Complex motor tics* appear to be more purposeful and ritualistic than simple tics. Common *complex motor tics* include grooming behaviors, the smelling of objects, jumping, touching behaviors, echopraxia (imitation of observed behavior), and copropraxia (display of obscene gestures). *Complex vocal tics* include repeating words or phrases out of context, coprolalia (use of obscene words or phrases), palilalia (a person's repeating his or her words), and echolalia (repetition of the last-heard words of others).

Some persons with tic disorders can suppress the tics for minutes or hours, but others, especially young children, either are not cognizant of their tics or experience their tics as irresistible. Tics may be attenuated by sleep, relaxation, or absorption in an activity. Tics often, but not always, disappear during sleep.

TOURETTE'S DISORDER

According to DSM-IV-TR, tics in Tourette's disorder are multiple motor tics and one or more vocal tics. The tics occur many times a day for more than 1 year. Tourette's disorder causes distress or significant impairment in important areas of functioning. The disorder has an onset before the age of 18 years, and it is not caused by a substance or by a general medical condition.

Georges Gilles de la Tourette first described a patient with what was later known as Tourette's disorder in 1885, while he was studying with Jean-Martin Charcot in France. De la Tourette noted a syndrome in several patients that included multiple motor tics, coprolalia, and echolalia.

Epidemiology

The lifetime prevalence of Tourette's disorder is estimated to be 4 to 5 per 10,000. More children exhibit this disorder than adults, such that 5 to 30 of 10,000 children are affected, but by adulthood, only 1 to 2 of 10,000 meet diagnostic criteria. The onset of the motor component of the disorder generally occurs by the age of 7 years; vocal tics emerge on average by the age of 11 years. Tourette's disorder occurs about 3 times more often in boys than in girls.

Etiology

Genetic Factors. Twin studies, adoption studies, and segregation analysis studies all support a genetic cause for Tourette's disorder. Twin studies indicate that concordance for the disorder in monozygotic twins is significantly greater than that in dizygotic twins. The fact that Tourette's disorder and chronic motor or vocal tic disorder are likely to occur in the same families lends support to the view that the disorders are part of a genetically determined spectrum. The sons of mothers with Tourette's disorder seem to be at the highest risk for the disorder. Evidence in some families indicates that Tourette's disorder is transmitted in an autosomal dominant fashion. Recent studies of a long family pedigree suggest that Tourette's disorder may be transmitted in a bilinear mode; that is, Tourette's disorder appears to be inherited through an autosomal pattern intermediate between dominant and recessive.

A relation is found between Tourette's disorder and attention-deficit/hyperactivity disorder; up to half of all Tourette's disorder patients also have attention-deficit/hyperactivity disorder. A relation also appears between Tourette's disorder and obsessive-compulsive disorder; up to 40 percent of all those with Tourette's disorder also have obsessive-compulsive disorder. In addition, first-degree relatives of persons with Tourette's disorder are at high risk for the development of the disorder, of chronic motor or vocal tic disorder, and of obsessive-compulsive disorder. The presence of symptoms of attention-deficit/hyperactivity disorder in more than half of persons with Tourette's disorder raises questions about a genetic relation between these two disorders.

Neurochemical and Neuroanatomical Factors. Compelling evidence of dopamine system involvement in tic disorders includes the observations that pharmacological agents that antagonize

dopamine (haloperidol [Haldol], pimozide [Orap], and fluphenazine [Prolixin]) suppress tics and that agents that increase central dopaminergic activity (methylphenidate [Ritalin], amphetamines, pemoline [Cylert], and cocaine) tend to exacerbate tics. The relation of tics to the dopamine system is not simple, because in some cases antipsychotic medications, such as haloperidol, are not effective in reducing tics and the effect of stimulants on tic disorders reportedly varies. In some cases, Tourette's disorder has emerged during treatment with antipsychotic medications. Thus, the term *tardive Tourette's disorder* refers to the disorder's similarity to tardive dyskinesia.

Endogenous opioids may be involved in tic disorders and obsessive-compulsive disorder. Some evidence indicates that pharmacological agents that antagonize endogenous opiates—for example, naltrexone (ReVia)—reduce tics and attention deficits in Tourette's disorder patients. Abnormalities in the noradrenergic system have been implicated in some cases by the reduction of tics with clonidine (Catapres). This adrenergic agonist reduces the release of norepinephrine in the central nervous system and thus may reduce activity in the dopaminergic system. Abnormalities in the basal ganglia result in various movement disorders, such as Huntington's disease, and are implicated as possible sites of disturbance in Tourette's disorder, obsessive-compulsive disorder, and attention-deficit/hyperactivity disorder.

Immunological Factors and Postinfection. An autoimmune process that is secondary to streptococcal infections is a potential mechanism for Tourette's disorder. Such a process could act synergistically with a genetic vulnerability for this disorder. Poststreptococcal syndromes have also been associated with one potential causative factor in the development of obsessive-compulsive disorder in children.

Diagnosis and Clinical Features

To make a diagnosis of Tourette's disorder, clinicians must obtain a history of multiple motor tics and the emergence of at least one vocal tic at some point in the disorder. According to DSM-IV-TR, the tics must occur many times a day nearly every day or intermittently for more than 1 year. The average age of onset of tics is 7 years, but tics may occur as early as age 2 years. The onset must occur before the age of 18 years (Table 46–1).

In Tourette's disorder, the initial tics are in the face and neck. Over time, the tics tend to occur in a downward progression. The most commonly described tics are those affecting the face and head, the arms and hands, the body and lower extremities, and the respiratory and alimentary systems. In these areas, the tics take the form of grimacing; forehead puckering; eyebrow raising; eyelid blinking; winking; nose wrinkling; nostril trembling; mouth twitching; displaying the teeth; biting the lips and other parts; tongue extruding; protracting the lower jaw; nodding, jerking, or shaking the head; twisting the neck; looking sideways; head rolling; hand jerking; arm jerking; plucking fingers; writhing fingers; fist clenching; shoulder shrugging; foot, knee, or toe shaking; walking peculiarly; body writhing; jumping; hiccuping; sighing; yawning; snuffing; blowing through the nostrils; whistling inspiration; exaggerated; belching; sucking or smacking sounds; and clearing the throat.

Typically, prodromal behavioral symptoms (e.g., irritability, attention difficulties, and poor frustration tolerance) are evident before, or coincide with the onset of, tics. More than 25 percent of persons in some studies received stimulants for a diagnosis of attention-deficit/hyperactivity disorder before receiving a diagnosis of Tourette's disorder. The most frequent initial symptom is an eye-blink tic, followed by a head tic or a facial grimace. Most complex motor and vocal symptoms emerge several years after the initial symptoms. Coprolalia usually begins in early adolescence and occurs in about one third of all patients. Mental coprolalia—in which a patient thinks a sudden, intrusive, socially unacceptable thought or obscene word—may also occur. In some severe cases, physical injuries, including retinal detachment and orthopedic problems, have resulted from severe tics.

Obsessions, compulsions, attention difficulties, impulsivity, and personality problems have been associated with Tourette's disorder. Attention difficulties often precede the onset of tics, whereas obsessive-compulsive symptoms often occur after their onset. Whether these problems usually develop secondarily to a patient's tics or are caused primarily by the same underlying pathological condition is still being debated. Many tics have an aggressive or sexual component that may result in serious social consequences for the patient. Phenomenologically, tics resemble a failure of censorship, both conscious and unconscious, with increased impulsivity and inability to inhibit a thought from being put into action.

Table 46–1
DSM-IV-TR Diagnostic Criteria for Tourette's Disorder

A. Both multiple motor and one or more vocal tics have been present at some time during the illness, although not necessarily concurrently. (A *tic* is a sudden, rapid, recurrent, nonrhythmic, stereotyped motor movement or vocalization.)

B. The tics occur many times a day (usually in bouts) nearly every day or intermittently throughout a period of more than 1 year, and during this period there was never a tic-free period of more than 3 consecutive months.

C. The onset is before age 18 years.

D. The disturbance is not due to the direct physiological effects of a substance (e.g., stimulants) or a general medical condition (e.g., Huntington's disease or postviral encephalitis).

From American Psychiatric Association. *Diagnostic and Statistical Manual of Mental Disorders.* 4th ed. Text rev. Washington, DC: American Psychiatric Association; copyright 2000, with permission.

Sam is a 10-year-old boy who was referred for a psychiatric inpatient admission because of persistent refusal to attend school. Sam has a past history of attention-deficit/hyperactivity disorder, diagnosed at age 7 years and has responded well to methylphenidate, most recently Concerta, 36 mg each morning. He is in a regular class in the fifth grade, and his parents report that since age 6 years, he has had numerous motor and vocal tics, but that they have not interfered with his social life or academic achievement until the present time. Sam first began to have repetitive eye blinking during the first grade, but he did not seem to be aware of it, and these tics did not interfere with his friendships, sports, or social life. After several months, he experienced some jerking movements of his head and shoulder, though he no longer had the eye-blinking tic. Again, Sam did not seem to be bothered by these, and none of his friends noticed either. Sam was being treated with methylphenidate

at this time, because he has always had a short attention span and would find it impossible to remain in his seat or raise his hand in class. The methylphenidate has controlled his symptoms of hyperactivity and inattention.

Sam began to refuse to attend school after he developed a repetitive complex motor tic that involved walking forward, then retracing his steps and twirling around in a circle. He did this at least once every hour, and some of his peers began to tease him. Sam reported that he "couldn't help it" and felt that he had to do this. Sam became extremely upset and decided that he would no longer attend school, since everybody was making fun of him. Examination revealed that Sam did exhibit a complex tic as he described as well as repeated soft grunting that occurred several times per minute. Sam's tics were causing him to be self-conscious and preventing him from being able to socialize with peers. A diagnosis of Tourette's disorder was made.

Sam was admitted to the children's psychiatric inpatient unit and a trial of risperidone was started with 0.5 mg orally daily. This was increased to 0.5 mg orally twice a day, and titrated upward in accordance with his ability to tolerate the medication. Initially, Sam felt sleepy during the day, but after a few days, he had adjusted to the medication and could tolerate this dose well. His risperidone dose was increased every 3 days by 0.5 mg, until he reached a dosage of 1 mg orally each morning and 2 mg orally at bedtime. Sam tolerated this dosage and did not experience any extrapyramidal symptoms. After a week at the highest dose, Sam began to feel less compelled to retrace his steps and twirl, and he started to have sessions with a behavioral psychologist who helped him become more aware of his urges to twirl around in a circle. He practiced turning that "motion" into a useful movement, so that others would be less likely to notice it. Sam continued taking Concerta, 36 mg, because he reported that without it, he was unable to focus on any school work. After leaving the hospital, Sam returned to school and continued his medication and sessions with the psychologist. Although he still retraced his steps and twirled occasionally, the frequency of this complex behavior had diminished, and he was usually able to transform the behavior into a movement that appeared to be purposeful and useful.

Pathology and Laboratory Examination

No specific laboratory diagnostic test exists for Tourette's disorder, but many patients with Tourette's disorder have nonspecific abnormal electroencephalographic findings. Computed tomography (CT) and magnetic resonance imaging (MRI) scans have revealed no specific structural lesions, although about 10 percent of all patients with Tourette's disorder show some nonspecific abnormality on CT scans.

Differential Diagnosis

Tics must be differentiated from other disordered movements (e.g., dystonic, choreiform, athetoid, myoclonic, and hemiballismic movements) and the neurological diseases which they characterize (e.g., Huntington's disease, parkinsonism, Sydenham's chorea, and Wilson's disease), as listed in Table 46–2. Tremors, mannerisms, and stereotypic movement disorder (e.g., head banging or body rocking) must also be distinguished from tic disorders. Stereotypic movement disorders, including movements such as rocking, hand gazing, and other self-stimulatory behaviors, seem to be voluntary and often produce a sense of comfort, in contrast to tic disorders. Although tics in children and adolescents may or may not feel controllable, they rarely produce a sense of well-being. Compulsions are sometimes difficult to distinguish from complex tics and may be on the same continuum biologically. Tic disorders also occur comorbidly with multiple behavioral and mood disturbances. In a recent survey, the greater the severity of tics, the higher the probability of both aggressive and depressive symptoms in children. Even in a given child with Tourette's disorder, it has been reported that when there is exacerbation of tic symptoms, behavior and mood also seem to deteriorate. This phenomenon occurs with children who have Tourette's disorder and attention-deficit/hyperactivity disorder and also those who have depression or oppositional-defiant disorders. In children with Tourette's disorder and attention-deficit/hyperactivity disorder, even when the tic disorder had always been mild, a high frequency of disruptive behavior problems and mood disorder still exists. Both autistic and mentally retarded children may exhibit symptoms similar to those seen in tic disorders, including Tourette's disorder. A greater than expected occurrence of Tourette's disorder, autistic disorder, and bipolar disorder also is present.

Before instituting treatment with an antipsychotic medication, clinicians must make a baseline evaluation of preexisting abnormal movements; such medication can mask abnormal movements, and if the movements occur later, they can be mistaken for tardive dyskinesia. Stimulant medications (e.g., methylphenidate, amphetamines, and pemoline) have reportedly exacerbated preexisting tics in some cases. These effects have been reported primarily in some children and adolescents being treated for attention-deficit/hyperactivity disorder. In most but not all cases, after the drug was discontinued, the tics remitted or returned to premedication levels. Most experts suggest that children and adolescents who experience tics while receiving stimulants are probably genetically predisposed and would have experienced tics regardless of their treatment with stimulants. Until the situation is clarified, clinicians should use great caution and should frequently monitor children at risk for tics who are given stimulants.

Course and Prognosis

Untreated, Tourette's disorder is usually a chronic, lifelong disease with relative remissions and exacerbations. Initial symptoms may decrease, persist, or increase, and old symptoms may be replaced by new ones. Severely afflicted persons may have serious emotional problems, including major depressive disorder. Some of these difficulties appear to be associated with Tourette's disorder, whereas others result from severe social, academic, and vocational consequences, which are frequent sequelae of the disorder. In some cases, despair over the disruption of social and occupational functioning is so severe that persons contemplate and attempt suicide. But, some children with Tourette's disorder have satisfactory peer relationships, function well in school, and have adequate self-esteem; they may need no treatment and can be monitored by their pediatricians.

Table 46–2
Differential Diagnosis of Tic Disorders

Disease or Syndrome	Age at Onset	Associated Features	Course	Predominant Type of Movement
Hallervorden-Spatz	Childhood-adolescence	May be associated with optic atrophy, club feet, retinitis pigmentosa, dysarthria, dementia, ataxia, emotional lability, spasticity, autosomal recessive inheritance	Progressive to death in 5 to 20 years	Choreic, athetoid, myoclonic
Dystonia musculorum deformans	Childhood-adolescence	Autosomal recessive inheritance commonly, primarily among Ashkenazi Jews; a more benign autosomal dominant form also occurs	Variable course, often progressive but with rare remissions	Dystonia
Sydenham's chorea	Childhood, usually 5–15 years	More common in females, usually associated with rheumatic fever (carditis elevated ASLO titers)	Usually self-limited	Choreiform
Huntington's disease	Usually 30–50 years, but childhood forms are known	Autosomal dominant inheritance, dementia, caudate atrophy on CT scan	Progressive to death in 10 to 15 years after onset	Choreiform
Wilson's disease (hepatolenticular degeneration)	Usually 10–25 years	Kayser-Fleischer rings, liver dysfunction, inborn error of copper metabolism; autosomal recessive inheritance	Progressive to death without chelating therapy	Wing-beating tremor, dystonia
Hyperreflexias (including latah, myriachit, jumper disease of Maine)	Generally in childhood (dominant inheritance)	Familial; may have generalized rigidity and autosomal inheritance	Nonprogressive	Excessive startle response; may have echolalia, coprolalia, and forced obedience
Myoclonic disorders	Any age	Numerous causes, some familial, usually no vocalizations	Variable, depending on cause	Myoclonus
Myoclonic dystonia	5–47 years	Nonfamilial, no vocalizations	Nonprogressive	Torsion dystonia with myoclonic jerks
Paroxysmal myoclonic dystonia with vocalization	Childhood	Attention, hyperactive, and learning disorders; movements interfere with ongoing activity	Nonprogressive	Bursts of regular, repetitive clonic (less tonic) movements and vocalizations
Tardive Tourette's disorder syndromes	Variable (after antipsychotic medication use)	Reported to be precipitated by discontinuation or reduction of medication	May terminate after increase or decrease of dosage	Orofacial dyskinesias, choreoathetosis, tics, vocalization
Neuroacanthocytosis	Third or fourth decade	Acanthocytosis, muscle wasting, parkinsonism, autosomal recessive inheritance	Variable	Orofacial dyskinesia and limb chorea, tics, vocalization
Encephalitis lethargica	Variable	Shouting fits, bizarre behavior, psychosis, Parkinson's disease	Variable	Simple and complex motor and vocal tics, coprolalia, echolalia, echopraxia, palilalia
Gasoline inhalation	Variable	Abnormal EEG; symmetrical theta and theta bursts frontocentrally	Variable	Simple motor and vocal tics
Postangiographic complications	Variable	Emotional lability, amnestic syndrome	Variable	Simple motor and complex vocal tics, palilalia
Postinfectious	Variable	EEG: occasional asymmetrical theta bursts before movements, elevated ASLO titers	Variable	Simple motor and vocal tics, echopraxia
Posttraumatic	Variable	Asymmetrical tic distribution	Variable	Complex motor tics
Carbon monoxide poisoning	Variable	Inappropriate sexual behavior	Variable	Simple and complex motor and vocal tics, coprolalia, echolalia, palilalia
XYY genetic disorder	Infancy	Aggressive behavior	Static	Simple motor and vocal tics
XXY and 9_p mosaicism	Infancy	Multiple physical anomalies, mental retardation	Static	Simple motor and vocal tics
Duchenne's muscular dystrophy (X-linked recessive)	Childhood	Mild mental retardation	Progressive	Motor and vocal tics
Fragile X syndrome	Childhood	Mental retardation, facial dysmorphism, seizures, autistic features	Static	Simple motor and vocal tics, coprolalia
Developmental and perinatal disorders	Infancy, childhood	Seizures, EEG and CT abnormalities, psychosis, aggressivity, hyperactivity, Ganser's syndrome, compulsivity, torticollis	Variable	Motor and vocal tics, echolalia

Treatment

Consideration of a child or adolescent's overall functioning is the first step in determining the most appropriate treatments for tic disorders. Families, teachers, and peers sometimes misinterpret tics as purposeful behaviors, and a child may be treated as if he or she has a "behavior" problem when the tics are actually experienced as involuntary. Treatment should begin with comprehensive education for families so that children are not unwittingly punished for their tic behaviors. Families must also understand the waxing and waning nature of many tic disorders. In mild cases, children with tic disorders who are functioning well socially and academically may not require treatment. In more severe cases, children with tic disorders may be ostracized by peers and have academic work compromised by the disruptive nature of tics, and a variety of treatments must be considered.

Pharmacological interventions have some efficacy in tic suppression, and behavioral interventions such as "habit reversal" techniques are being used to help children and adolescents become more aware of their tics and initiate voluntary movements that can "counter" tics. Other behavioral techniques—including massed (negative) practice, self-monitoring, incompatible response training, presentation and removal of positive reinforcement, as well as habit reversal treatment—were reviewed by Stanley A. Hobbs. He reported that tic frequency was reduced in many cases, particularly with habit reversal treatment; currently, additional studies are under way to replicate the efficacy of these techniques. Behavioral techniques, including relaxation, may reduce stress that often exacerbates Tourette's disorder. It is hypothesized that behavioral techniques and pharmacotherapy together have a synergistic effect.

Pharmacotherapy. Historically, high-potency dopamine receptor antagonists (typical antipsychotics), such as haloperidol, trifluoperazine (Stelazine), and pimozide, have been shown to reduce tics significantly. Up to 80 percent of patients have some favorable response; their symptoms decrease by as much as 70 to 90 percent of baseline frequency. Follow-up studies, however, indicate that only 20 to 30 percent of these patients continue to take long-term maintenance therapy. Discontinuation is often based on the drug's adverse effects, including extrapyramidal effects and dysphoria. The initial daily haloperidol dose for adolescents and adults is usually between 0.25 and 0.5 mg. Haloperidol is not approved for use in children less than 3 years of age. For children between 3 and 12 years of age, the recommended total daily dose is between 0.05 and 0.075 mg/kg, administered in divided doses either two or three times a day. This dosage imposes a daily limit of 3 mg of haloperidol for a 40-kg child.

The initial dosage of pimozide is usually 1 to 2 mg daily in divided doses; the dosage may be increased every other day. Most patients are maintained on less than 0.2 mg/kg a day or 10 mg a day, whichever is less. A dosage of 0.3 mg/kg a day or 20 mg a day should never be exceeded because of cardiotoxic adverse effects. Pimozide appears to be relatively safe at recommended dosages, with cardiotoxicity limited to prolonged QT wave intervals. Electrocardiography is needed at baseline and periodically during treatment. There is little experience in administering pimozide to children less than 12 years of age

Clinicians must forewarn patients and families of the possibility of acute dystonic reactions and parkinsonian symptoms when use of a conventional or atypical antipsychotic medication is to be initiated. The more recently marketed "atypical" antipsychotics (serotonin-dopamine antagonists), including risperidone and olanzapine (Zyprexa), are often chosen as a treatment option instead of the conventional antipsychotics in the hope that adverse effects will be less pervasive. Risperidone has been used in the treatment of Tourette's disorder in doses ranging from 1 to 6 mg per day with some success. Adverse effects include weight gain, sedation, and extrapyramidal adverse effects. Olanzapine is generally well tolerated, although weight gain and reports of cognitive dulling have limited its use. Even with the serotonin-dopamine antagonists, diphenhydramine (Benadryl) or benztropine (Cogentin) are not infrequently required to control extrapyramidal adverse effects.

Although not presently approved by the Food and Drug Administration (FDA) for use in Tourette's disorder, several studies reported that clonidine, an α_2-adrenergic agonist, was efficacious; 40 to 70 percent of patients benefited from the medication. In addition to the improvement in tic symptoms, patients may experience less tension and improved attention span. Another α_2-adrenergic agonist, guanfacine (Tenex), has also been used in the treatment of tic disorders. Clonidine has generally been used in dosages ranging from 0.05 mg orally thrice daily to 0.1 mg four times daily; and guanfacine is usually used in dosages ranging from 1 to 4 mg per day. When used in these dosage ranges, adverse effects of the α-adrenergic agents include drowsiness, headache, irritability, and occasional hypotension.

In view of the frequent comorbidity of tic behaviors and obsessive-compulsive symptoms or disorders, the selective reuptake inhibitors (SSRIs) have been used alone or in combination with antipsychotics in the treatment of Tourette's disorder. Some data suggest that SSRIs, such as fluoxetine (Prozac), may be helpful.

Although clinicians must weigh the risks and benefits of using stimulants in cases of severe hyperactivity and comorbid tics, a recent study reports that methylphenidate does not increase the rate or intensity of motor or vocal tics in most children with hyperactivity and tic disorders. There was one case report that use of bupropion (Wellbutrin), an antidepressant of the aminoketone class, increased tic behavior in several children being treated for Tourette's disorder and attention-deficit/hyperactivity disorder. Other antidepressants, such as imipramine (Tofranil) and desipramine (Norpramin, Pertofrane), may decrease disruptive behavior in children with Tourette's disorder but are no longer widely used because of their potentially serious cardiac adverse effects.

CHRONIC MOTOR OR VOCAL TIC DISORDER

In DSM-IV-TR, chronic motor or vocal tic disorder is defined as the presence of either motor tics or vocal tics but not both. The other features are the same as those of Tourette's disorder, but chronic motor or vocal tic disorder cannot be diagnosed if the criteria for Tourette's disorder have ever been met. According to DSM-IV-TR criteria, the disorder must have its onset before the age of 18 years.

Epidemiology

The rate of chronic motor or vocal tic disorder has been estimated to be from 100 to 1,000 times greater than that of Tourette's disorder. School-age boys are at highest risk, but the incidence is unknown. Although the disorder was once believed to be rare, current estimates of the prevalence of chronic motor or vocal tic disorder range from 1 to 2 percent.

Etiology

Tourette's disorder and chronic motor or vocal tic disorder aggregate in the same families. Twin studies have found a high concordance for either Tourette's disorder or chronic motor tics in monozygotic twins. This finding supports the importance of hereditary factors in the transmission of at least some tic disorders.

Diagnosis and Clinical Features

The onset of chronic motor or vocal tic disorder appears to be in early childhood. The types of tics and their locations are similar to those in transient tic disorder. Chronic vocal tics are considerably rarer than chronic motor tics. The chronic vocal tics are usually much less conspicuous than those in Tourette's disorder. The vocal tics are usually not loud or intense and are not primarily produced by the vocal cords; they consist of grunts or other noises caused by thoracic, abdominal, or diaphragmatic contractions. The DSM-IV-TR diagnostic criteria are given in Table 46–3.

Differential Diagnosis

Chronic motor tics must be differentiated from a variety of other motor movements, including choreiform movements, myoclonus, restless legs syndrome, akathisia, and dystonias. Involuntary vocal utterances can occur in certain neurological disorders, such as Huntington's disease and Parkinson's disease.

Course and Prognosis

Children whose tics start between the ages of 6 and 8 years seem to have the best outcomes. Symptoms usually last for 4 to 6 years and stop in early adolescence. Children whose tics involve the limbs or trunk tend to do less well than those with only facial tics.

Table 46–3
DSM-IV-TR Diagnostic Criteria for Chronic Motor or Vocal Tic Disorder

A. Single or multiple motor or vocal tics (i.e., sudden, rapid, recurrent, nonrhythmic, stereotyped motor movements or vocalizations), but not both, have been present at some time during the illness.
B. The tics occur many times a day nearly every day or intermittently throughout a period of more than 1 year, and during this period there was never a tic-free period of more than 3 consecutive months.
C. The onset is before age 18 years.
D. The disturbance is not due to the direct physiological effects of a substance (e.g., stimulants) or a general medical condition (e.g., Huntington's disease or postviral encephalitis).
E. Criteria have never been met for Tourette's disorder.

From American Psychiatric Association. *Diagnostic and Statistical Manual of Mental Disorders.* 4th ed. Text rev. Washington, DC: American Psychiatric Association; copyright 2000, with permission.

Treatment

The treatment of chronic motor or vocal tic disorder depends on the severity and frequency of the tics; the patient's subjective distress; the effects of the tics on school or work, job performance, and socialization; and the presence of any other concomitant mental disorder. Psychotherapy may be indicated to minimize the secondary emotional problems caused by the tics. Several studies found that behavioral techniques, particularly habit reversal treatments, were effective in treating chronic motor or vocal tic disorder. Antianxiety agents have been unsuccessful. Haloperidol has been helpful in some cases, but the risks must be weighed against the possible clinical benefits because of the drug's adverse effects, including the development of tardive dyskinesia.

TRANSIENT TIC DISORDER

DSM-IV-TR defines transient tic disorder as the presence of a single tic or multiple motor or vocal tics or both. The tics occur many times a day for at least 4 weeks but no longer than 12 months. The other features are the same as those for Tourette's disorder, but transient tic disorder cannot be diagnosed if the criteria for Tourette's disorder or chronic motor or vocal tic disorder have ever been met. According to DSM-IV-TR, the disorder must have its onset before the age of 18 years.

Epidemiology

Transient ticlike movements and nervous muscular twitches are common in children. From 5 to 24 percent of all school-age children have a history of tics. The prevalence of tics as defined here is unknown.

Etiology

Transient tic disorder probably has either organic or psychogenic origins, with some tics combining elements of both. Organic tics, which are probably most likely to progress to Tourette's disorder, have an increased family history of tics, whereas psychogenic tics are most likely to remit spontaneously. Tics that progress to chronic motor or vocal tic disorder are most likely to have components of both organic and psychogenic origin. Tics of all sorts are exacerbated by stress and anxiety, but no evidence indicates that tics are caused by stress or anxiety.

Diagnosis and Clinical Features

The DSM-IV-TR criteria for establishing the diagnosis of transient tic disorder are as follows. The tics are single or multiple, motor or vocal. They occur many times a day nearly every day for at least 4 weeks but no longer than 12 consecutive months. The patient has no history of Tourette's disorder or chronic motor or vocal tic disorder. The onset is before age 18. The tics do not occur exclusively during substance intoxication, and they are not caused by a general medical condition. The diagnosis should specify whether a single episode or recurrent episodes are present (Table 46–4). Transient tic disorder can be

Table 46–4
DSM-IV-TR Diagnostic Criteria for Transient Tic Disorder

A. Single or multiple motor and/or vocal tics (i.e., sudden, rapid, recurrent, nonrhythmic, stereotyped motor movements or vocalizations)
B. The tics occur many times a day, nearly every day for at least 4 weeks, but for no longer than 12 consecutive months.
C. The onset is before age 18 years.
D. The disturbance is not due to the direct physiological effects of a substance (e.g., stimulants) or a general medical condition (e.g., Huntington's disease or postviral encephalitis).
E. Criteria have never been met for Tourette's Disorder or Chronic Motor or Vocal Tic Disorder.

Specify if:
Single episode or **Recurrent**

From American Psychiatric Association. *Diagnostic and Statistical Manual of Mental Disorders.* 4th ed. Text rev. Washington, DC: American Psychiatric Association; copyright 2000, with permission.

distinguished from chronic motor or vocal tic disorder and Tourette's disorder only by observing the symptoms' progression over time.

Course and Prognosis

Most persons with transient tic disorder do not progress to a more serious tic disorder. Their tics either disappear permanently or recur during periods of special stress. Only a small percentage develop chronic motor or vocal tic disorder or Tourette's disorder.

Treatment

Whether the tics will disappear spontaneously, progress, or become chronic is unclear at the beginning of treatment. Focusing attention on tics may exacerbate them; thus, clinicians often recommend that, at first, the family disregard the tics as much as possible. But if the tics are so severe that they impair the patient or if they are accompanied by significant emotional disturbance, complete psychiatric and pediatric neurological examinations are recommended. Treatment depends on the results of the evaluations. Psychopharmacology is not recommended unless the symptoms are unusually severe and disabling. Several studies have found that behavioral techniques, particularly habit reversal treatment, are effective in treating transient tics.

Table 46–5
DSM-IV-TR Diagnostic Criteria for Tic Disorder Not Otherwise Specified

This category is for disorders characterized by tics that do not meet criteria for a specific tic disorder. Examples include tics lasting less than 4 weeks or tics with an onset after age 18 years.

From American Psychiatric Association. *Diagnostic and Statistical Manual of Mental Disorders.* 4th ed. Text rev. Washington, DC: American Psychiatric Association; copyright 2000, with permission.

Table 46–6
ICD-10 Diagnostic Criteria for Tic Disorders

Note: A tic is an involuntary, sudden, rapid, recurrent, nonrhythmic, stereotyped motor movement or vocalization.

Transient tic disorder

A. Single or multiple motor or vocal tic(s) or both occur many times a day, on most days, over a period of at least 4 weeks.
B. Duration of the disorder is 12 months or less.
C. There is no history of Tourette's syndrome, and the disorder is not the result of physical conditions or side effects of medication.
D. Onset is before the age of 18 years.

Chronic motor or vocal tic disorder

A. Motor or vocal tics, but not both, occur many times per day, on most days, over a period of at least 12 months.
B. No period of remission during that year lasts longer than 2 months.
C. There is no history of Tourette's syndrome, and the disorder is not the result of physical conditions or side effects of medication.
D. Onset is before the age of 18 years.

Combined vocal and multiple motor tic disorder (de la Tourette's syndrome)

A. Multiple motor tics and one or more vocal tics have been present at some time during the disorder, but not necessarily concurrently.
B. The frequency of tics must be many times a day, nearly every day, for more than 1 year, with no period of remission during that year lasting longer than 2 months.
C. Onset is before the age of 18 years.

Other tic disorders

Tic disorder, unspecified

A nonrecommended residual category for a disorder that fulfills the general criteria for a tic disorder but in which the specific subcategory is not specified or in which the features do not fulfill the criteria for transient tic disorders, chronic motor or vocal tic disorder, combined vocal and multiple motor tic disorder (de la Tourette's syndrome).

Reprinted with permission from World Health Organization. *The ICD-10 Classification of Mental and Behavioural Disorders: Diagnostic Criteria for Research.* Copyright, World Health Organization, Geneva, 1993.

TIC DISORDER NOT OTHERWISE SPECIFIED

According to DSM-IV-TR, tic disorder not otherwise specified refers to disorders characterized by tics but not otherwise meeting the criteria for a specific tic disorder (Table 46–5).

ICD-10

In the 10th revision of *International Statistical Classification of Diseases and Related Health Problems* (ICD-10), tic disorders form a category under disorders of childhood and adolescence. ICD-10 includes the same tic disorders as DSM-IV-TR and adds another, other tic disorders. Tics—motor movements or vocal productions that serve no apparent purpose and are of sudden onset—are described as the predominant manifestation in these syndromes. The severity of tics varies greatly, from near normal, with 1 in 5 or 1 in 10 children occasionally manifesting tics, to Tourette's syndrome, which is rare, severe, and incapacitating. Tic disorders are more common in boys than in girls, and a family history of tics is frequent (Table 46–6).

References

Hawkridge S, Stein DJ, Bouwer C. Combined pharmacotherapy for TS and OCD. *J Am Acad Child Adolesc Psychiatry.* 1996;35:703.

Kerbeshian J, Burd L. Case study: comorbidity among Tourette's syndrome, autistic disorder, and bipolar disorder. *J Am Acad Child Adolesc Psychiatry.* 1996;35:681.

Law SF, Schachar RJ. Do typical clinical doses of methylphenidate cause tics in children treated for attention-deficit hyperactivity disorder? *J Am Acad Child Adolesc Psychiatry.* 1999;38:944.

McCracken JT. Tic disorders. In: Sadock BJ, Sadock VA, editors. *Kaplan & Sadock's Comprehensive Textbook of Psychiatry.* 7th ed. Vol 2. Baltimore: Lippincott Williams & Wilkins; 2000:2711.

McMahon WM, van de Weterin BJM, Filloux F, Betit K, Coon H, Leppert M. Bilineal transmission and phenotypic variation of Tourette's disorder in a large pedigree. *J Am Acad Child Adolesc Psychiatry.* 1996;35:672.

Nolan EE, Sverd J, Gadow KD, Sprafkin J, Ezor SN. Associated psychopathology in children with both ADHD and chronic tic disorder. *J Am Acad Child Adolesc Psychiatry.* 1996;35:1622.

Peterson BS, Pine DS, Cohen P, Brook J. Prospective, longitudinal study of tic, obsessive-compulsive, and attention-deficit/hyperactivity disorders in an epidemiological sample. *J Am Acad Child Adolesc Psychiatry.* 2001;40:685.

Piacentini J, Chang S. Behavior therapy: state of the art. In: Cohen D, Jankovic H, Goetz C, eds. *Advances in Neurology.* Vol 85. Philadelphia: Lippincott Williams & Wilkins; 2001:319.

Segal NL, Dysken MW, Bouchard TJ, Petersen NL, Eckert ED, Heston LL. Tourette's disorder in a set of reared-apart triplets: genetic and environmental influences. *Am J Psychiatry.* 1990;147:196.

Spencer T, Biederman J, Steingard R, Wilens T. Bupropion exacerbates tics in children with attention-deficit hyperactivity disorder and Tourette's syndrome. *J Am Acad Child Adolesc Psychiatry.* 1993;32:211.

Spencer T, Biederman J, Wilens T, Steingard R, Geist D. Nortriptyline treatment of children with attention-deficit hyperactivity disorder and tic disorder or Tourette's syndrome. *J Am Acad Child Adolesc Psychiatry.* 1993;32:205.

Steingard R, Biederman J, Spencer T, Wilens T, Gonzalez A. Comparison of clonidine response in the treatment of attention-deficit hyperactivity disorder with and without comorbid tic disorders. *J Am Acad Child Adolesc Psychiatry.* 1993;32:350.

Tucker DM, Leckman JF, Scahill L, et al. A putative poststreptococcal case of OCD with chronic tic disorder, not otherwise specified. *J Am Acad Child Adolesc Psychiatry.* 1996;35:1684.

47

Elimination Disorders

Enuresis and encopresis are the two elimination disorders described in the text revision of the fourth edition of *Diagnostic and Statistical Manual of Mental Disorders* (DSM-IV-TR). These disorders are considered only when a child is chronologically and developmentally beyond the point at which it is expected that these functions can be mastered. Normal development encompasses a range of time in which a given child is able to devote the attention, motivation, and physiological skills to exhibit competency in elimination processes. *Encopresis* is defined as a pattern of passing feces into inappropriate places, whether the passage is involuntary or intentional. The pattern must be present for at least 3 months; the child's chronological age must be at least 4 years. *Enuresis* is the repeated voiding of urine into clothes or bed, whether the voiding is involuntary or intentional. The behavior must occur twice weekly for at least 3 months or must cause clinically significant distress or impairment socially or academically. The child's chronological or developmental age must be at least 5 years.

Bowel and bladder control develops gradually over time. Toilet training is affected by many factors, such as a child's intellectual capacity and social maturity, cultural determinants, and the psychological interactions between child and parents. The normal sequence of developing control over bowel and bladder functions is the development of nocturnal fecal continence, diurnal fecal continence, diurnal bladder control, and nocturnal bladder control.

ENCOPRESIS

Epidemiology

In Western cultures, bowel control is established in more than 95 percent of children by the fourth birthday and in 99 percent by the fifth birthday. Thereafter, frequency decreases to virtual absence by the age of 16. After the age of 4, encopresis at all ages is three to four times as common in boys as in girls. At the ages of 7 to 8, frequency is about 1.5 percent in boys and about 0.5 percent in girls. By the ages of 10 to 12, once-a-month soiling occurs in 1.3 percent of boys and in 0.3 percent of girls. A significant relation exists between encopresis and enuresis.

Etiology

Encopresis involves an often complicated interplay between physiological and psychological factors. Inadequate training or the lack of appropriate toilet training may delay a child's attainment of continence. Evidence indicates that some encopretic children suffer from lifelong inefficient and ineffective sphincter control. Thus, encopresis may occur in children with adequate bowel control who, for a variety of emotional reasons, including anger, anxiety, fear, or some combination of these, do not deposit the feces appropriately. Other children may soil involuntarily, either because of an inability to control the sphincter adequately or because of excessive fluid caused by a retentive overflow. Up to 75 percent of children with encopresis are constipated and have excessive fluid overflow.

Any combination of these factors may promote a power struggle between child and parent over issues of autonomy and control. Perpetual battles often aggravate the disorder and frequently cause secondary behavioral difficulties. Many encopretic children, however, do not have behavioral problems. When behavioral problems do occur, they are the social consequences of soiling. Encopretic children who clearly can control their bowel function adequately and who deposit feces of relatively normal consistency in abnormal places usually have a psychiatric difficulty. Encopresis may be associated with other neurodevelopmental problems, including easy distractibility, short attention span, low frustration tolerance, hyperactivity, and poor coordination. Occasionally, the child has a special fear of using the toilet. Encopresis may also be precipitated by life events, such as the birth of a sibling or a move to a new home. Encopresis after a long period of fecal continence sometimes appears to be a regression after such stresses as a parental separation, a change in domicile, or the start of school.

Psychogenic Megacolon. Many encopretic children also retain feces and become constipated, either voluntarily or secondarily to painful defecation. In these cases, no clear evidence indicates that preexisting anorectal dysfunction contributes to the constipation. The resulting chronic rectal distention from large, hard fecal masses may cause loss of tone in the rectal wall and desensitization to pressure. Thus, many children become unaware of the need to defecate, and overflow encopresis occurs, usually with relatively small amounts of liquid or soft stool leaking out.

Olfactory accommodation may diminish or eliminate sensory cues. Children whose parenting has been harsh and punitive and who have been severely punished for "accidents" during toilet training may also develop encopresis.

Diagnosis and Clinical Features

According to DSM-IV-TR, encopresis is diagnosed when feces are passed into inappropriate places on a regular basis

Table 47–1
DSM-IV-TR Diagnostic Criteria for Encopresis

A. Repeated passage of feces into inappropriate places (e.g., clothing or floor) whether involuntary or intentional.
B. At least one such event a month for at least 3 months.
C. Chronological age is at least 4 years (or equivalent developmental level).
D. The behavior is not due exclusively to the direct physiological effects of a substance (e.g., laxatives) or a general medical condition except through a mechanism involving constipation.

Code as follows:

With constipation and overflow incontinence
Without constipation and overflow incontinence

From American Psychiatric Association. *Diagnostic and Statistical Manual of Mental Disorders.* 4th ed. Text rev. Washington, DC: American Psychiatric Association; copyright 2000, with permission.

(at least once a month) for 3 months (Table 47–1). Encopresis may be present in children who have bowel control and intentionally deposit feces in their clothes or other places for a variety of emotional reasons. Some children engage in the inappropriate behavior when angry at parental figures or as part of a pattern of oppositional defiant disorder. The children often develop repetitive behaviors that seem to seek negative attention. In other children, sporadic episodes of encopresis may occur during times of stress—for example, proximal to the birth of a new sibling—but in such cases, the behavior is usually transient and does not fulfill the diagnostic criteria for the disorder.

Encopresis may also be present on an involuntary basis in the absence of physiological abnormalities. In these cases, a child may not exhibit adequate control over the sphincter muscles, either because the child is absorbed in another activity or because he or she is unaware of the process. The feces may be of normal, near-normal, or liquid consistency. Some involuntary soiling is due to chronic retaining of stool, which results in liquid overflow. In rare cases, the involuntary overflow of stool results from psychological causes of diarrhea or anxiety disorder symptoms.

DSM-IV-TR breaks down the types of encopresis into with constipation and overflow incontinence and without constipation and overflow incontinence. To receive a diagnosis of encopresis, a child must have a developmental or chronological level of at least 4 years. If the fecal incontinence is directly related to a medical condition, encopresis is not diagnosed.

Studies have indicated that children with encopresis who do not have gastrointestinal illnesses have high rates of abnormal anal sphincter contractions. This finding is particularly prevalent among children with encopresis with constipation and overflow incontinence who have difficulty relaxing their anal sphincter muscles when trying to defecate. Children with constipation who have difficulties with sphincter relaxation are not likely to respond well to laxatives in the treatment of their encopresis. Encopretic children without abnormal sphincter tone are likely to improve over a short period.

Henry was an 11-year-old male with almost-daily encopresis and a number of associated behaviors including hiding the feces around the house. He resided in a specialized foster care setting, having been removed from his biological parents at age 7 because of physical and sexual abuse. Both parents were involved with substance abuse, and his early history is not well documented. However, a parent did indicate that he had not exhibited sustained bowel continence for several months. Henry had also been enuretic until age 6, but this had resolved to an occasional nocturnal episode every 4 to 6 months. Henry also qualified for a diagnosis of oppositional-defiant disorder. Although he had experienced physical and sexual abuse, he did not have flashbacks or other symptoms that would meet the criteria for posttraumatic stress disorder. Henry also had an attention-deficit/hyperactivity disorder and was being treated effectively with 10 mg of methylphenidate (Ritalin) twice a day.

The foster family resided in an urban area that had access to a nationally recognized children's hospital. The Ambulatory Care Department had a specialized behavioral encopresis program that coupled the bowel training method with a psychoeducational component and psychotherapy. The psychiatric consultant to the specialized foster care program doubted that this program would be successful for Henry since he had so much associated psychopathology and the feces were often deposited around the house in a symbolic manner. Also, the encopresis was not of the retentive-overflow type, and the feces were always well formed. However, since no apparent harm could come from the referral, the consulting child psychiatrist agreed it. Much to the surprise of the consultant, the several-week outpatient bowel training course coupled with the psychoeducational component and psychotherapy resulted in complete cessation of the encopresis. On one of her visits to the home, Henry proudly showed his case manger a diagram of the functioning of the digestive system that was part of the psychoeducational program. In retrospect, it appeared that although there were symbolic aspects to Henry's encopretic behavior, the soiling was ego-dystonic, and he was motivated to change the behavior, although this motivation could not be prospectively detected by the treatment team because of his oppositional-defiant manner of responding to adults. (Courtesy of Edwin J. Mikkelsen, M.D.)

Pathology and Laboratory Examination

Although no specific test indicates a diagnosis of encopresis, clinicians must rule out medical illnesses, such as Hirschsprung's disease, before making a diagnosis. If it is unclear whether fecal retention is responsible for encopresis with constipation and overflow incontinence, a physical examination of the abdomen is indicated, and an abdominal X-ray can help determine the degree of constipation present. Sophisticated tests to determine whether sphincter tone is abnormal are generally not conducted in simple cases of encopresis.

Differential Diagnosis

In encopresis with constipation and overflow incontinence, constipation can begin as early as the child's first year and can peak between the second and fourth years. Soiling usually begins at age 4. Frequent liquid stools and hard fecal masses are found in the colon and the rectum on abdominal palpation and rectal examination. Complications include impaction, megacolon, and anal fissures.

Encopresis with constipation and overflow incontinence can be caused by faulty nutrition; structural disease of the anus, rectum, and colon; medicinal adverse effects; or nongastrointestinal medical (endocrine or neurological) disorders. The chief differential problem is aganglionic megacolon or Hirschsprung's disease, in which a patient may have an empty rectum and no desire to defecate but may still have an overflow of feces. The disorder occurs in 1 in 5,000 children; signs appear shortly after birth.

Course and Prognosis

The outcome of encopresis depends on the cause, the chronicity of the symptoms, and coexisting behavioral problems. In many cases, encopresis is self-limiting, and it rarely continues beyond middle adolescence. Children who have contributing physiological factors, such as poor gastric motility and an inability to relax the anal sphincter muscles, are more difficult to treat than those with constipation but normal sphincter tone.

Encopresis is a particularly repugnant disorder to most persons, including family members; thus, family tension is often high. The child's peers are also sensitive to the developmentally inappropriate behavior and often ostracize the child. An encopretic child is often scapegoated by peers and shunned by adults. Many encopretic children have abysmally low self-esteem and are aware of their constant rejection. Psychologically, the child may appear blunted toward the symptoms or may be entrenched in a pattern of encopresis as a mode of expressing anger. The outcome of cases of encopresis is affected by the family's willingness and ability to participate in treatment without being overly punitive and by the child's awareness of when the passage of feces is about to occur.

Treatment

By the time a child is brought for treatment, considerable family discord and distress are common. Family tensions about the symptom must be reduced, and a nonpunitive atmosphere established. Similar efforts should be made to reduce the child's embarrassment at school. Many changes of underwear with a minimum of fuss should be arranged. Education of the family and correction of misperceptions that a family may have about soiling must occur before treatment. A useful physiological approach involves a combination of daily laxatives or mineral oil along with a behavioral intervention in which the child sits on the toilet for timed intervals daily and is rewarded for successful defecation. Laxatives are not necessary for children who are not constipated and do have good bowel control, but regular, timed intervals on the toilet may be useful with these children as well.

Supportive psychotherapy and relaxation techniques may be useful in treating encopretic children's anxieties and other sequelae, such as low self-esteem and social isolation. Family interventions can be helpful for children who have bowel control but continue to deposit their feces in inappropriate locations. A good outcome occurs when a child feels in control of life events. Coexisting behavior problems predict a poorer outcome. In all cases, proper bowel habits may need to be taught. In some cases biofeedback techniques have been of benefit.

ENURESIS

Epidemiology

The prevalence of enuresis decreases with increasing age. Thus, 82 percent of 2-year-olds, 49 percent of 3-year-olds, 26 percent of 4-year-olds, and 7 percent of 5-year-olds are reportedly enuretic on a regular basis. Prevalence rates vary, however, on the basis of the population studied and the tolerance for the symptoms in various cultures and socioeconomic groups.

The Isle of Wight study reported that 15.2 percent of 7-year-old boys were enuretic occasionally and that 6.7 percent of them were enuretic at least once a week. The study reported that 3.3 percent of girls at the age of 7 years were enuretic at least once a week. By age 10, the overall prevalence of enuresis was reported to be 3 percent. The rate drops drastically for teenagers; a prevalence of 1.5 percent has been reported for 14-year-olds. Enuresis affects about 1 percent of adults.

Mental disorders are present in only about 20 percent of enuretic children; they are most common in enuretic girls, in children with symptoms during the day and night, and in children who maintain the symptoms into older childhood.

Etiology

Most children are not enuretic by intention or even with awareness until after they are wet. Physiological factors are likely to play a major role in most cases of enuresis. Normal bladder control, which is acquired gradually, is influenced by neuromuscular and cognitive development, socioemotional factors, toilet training, and possible genetic factors. Difficulties in one or more of these areas may delay urinary continence.

Although a specific organic cause precludes a diagnosis of enuresis, correcting an anatomical defect or curing an infection does not always cure the enuresis. In a longitudinal study of child development, enuretic children were about twice as likely to have concomitant developmental delays as nonenuretic children. About 75 percent of enuretic children have a first-degree relative who is or was enuretic. A child's risk for enuresis has been found to be more than 7 times greater if the father was enuretic. The concordance rate is higher in monozygotic twins than in dizygotic twins. There is a strong suggestion of a genetic component, and much can be accounted for by tolerance for enuresis in some families and by other psychosocial factors.

Some studies report that enuretic children have a bladder with a normal anatomic capacity when anesthetized but a functionally small bladder, so that the child feels an urge to void with little urine in the bladder. Other studies report that bedwetting occurs because the bladder is full and there is a lack of high levels of nighttime antidiuretic hormone. These factors

allow a higher-than-usual urine output. Enuresis does not appear to be related to a specific stage of sleep or time of night; rather, bed-wetting appears randomly. In most cases, the quality of sleep is normal. Little evidence indicates that enuretic children sleep more soundly than other children.

Psychosocial stressors appear to precipitate some cases of enuresis. In young children, the disorder has been particularly associated with the birth of a sibling, hospitalization between the ages of 2 and 4, the start of school, the breakup of a family because of divorce or death, and a move to a new domicile.

Diagnosis and Clinical Features

Enuresis is the repeated voiding of urine into a child's clothes or bed; the voiding may be involuntary or intentional. For the diagnosis to be made, a child must exhibit a developmental or chronological age of at least 5 years. According to DSM-IV-TR, the behavior must occur twice weekly for a period of at least 3 months or must cause distress and impairment in functioning to meet the diagnostic criteria. Enuresis is diagnosed only if the behavior is not due to a medical condition. DSM-IV-TR and the 10th revision of *International Statistical Classification of Diseases and Related Health Problems* (ICD-10) break down the disorder into three types: nocturnal only, diurnal only, and nocturnal and diurnal (Table 47–2).

Pathology and Laboratory Examination

No single laboratory finding is pathognomonic of enuresis; but clinicians must rule out organic factors, such as the presence of urinary tract infections, that may predispose a child to enuresis. Structural obstructive abnormalities may be present in up to 3 percent of children with apparent enuresis. Sophisticated radiographic studies are usually deferred in simple cases of enuresis with no signs of repeated infections or other medical problems.

Table 47–2
DSM-IV-TR Diagnostic Criteria for Enuresis

A. Repeated voiding of urine into bed or clothes (whether involuntary or intentional).

B. The behavior is clinically significant as manifested by either a frequency of twice a week for at least 3 consecutive months or the presence of clinically significant distress or impairment in social, academic (occupational), or other important areas of functioning.

C. Chronological age is at least 5 years (or equivalent developmental level).

D. The behavior is not due exclusively to the direct physiological effect of a substance (e.g., a diuretic) or a general medical condition (e.g., diabetes, spina bifida, a seizure disorder).

Specify type:

Nocturnal only
Diurnal only
Nocturnal and diurnal

From American Psychiatric Association. *Diagnostic and Statistical Manual of Mental Disorders*. 4th ed. Text rev. Washington, DC: American Psychiatric Association; copyright 2002, with permission.

Differential Diagnosis

Possible organic causes of bed-wetting must be ruled out. Organic features occur most often in children with both nocturnal and diurnal enuresis combined with urinary frequency and urgency. The organic features include genitourinary pathology—structural, neurological, and infectious—such as obstructive uropathy, spina bifida occulta, and cystitis; other organic disorders that may cause polyuria and enuresis, such as diabetes mellitus and diabetes insipidus; disturbances of consciousness and sleep, such as seizures, intoxication, and sleepwalking disorder, during which a child urinates; and adverse effects from treatment with antipsychotics (e.g., thioridazine [Mellaril]).

Course and Prognosis

Enuresis is usually self-limited, and a child can eventually remain dry without psychiatric sequelae. Most enuretic children find their symptoms ego-dystonic and enjoy enhanced self-esteem and improved social confidence when they become continent. About 80 percent of affected children have never achieved a year-long period of dryness. Enuresis after at least 1 dry year usually begins between the ages of 5 and 8 years; if it occurs much later, especially during adulthood, organic causes must be investigated. Some evidence indicates that late onset of enuresis in children is more frequently associated with a concomitant psychiatric difficulty than is enuresis without at least 1 dry year. Relapses occur in enuretic children who are becoming dry spontaneously and in those who are being treated. The significant emotional and social difficulties of enuretic children usually include poor self-image, decreased self-esteem, social embarrassment and restriction, and intrafamilial conflict.

Treatment

Treatment modalities that have been used successfully for enuresis include behavioral and pharmacological interventions. A relatively high rate of spontaneous remission over long periods also occurs. The first step in any treatment plan is to review appropriate toilet training. If toilet training was not attempted, the parents and the patient should be guided in this undertaking. Record keeping is helpful in determining a baseline and following the child's progress and may itself be a reinforcer. A star chart may be particularly helpful. Other useful techniques include restricting fluids before bed and night lifting to toilet train the child.

Behavioral Therapy. Classic conditioning with the bell (or buzzer) and pad apparatus is generally the most effective treatment for enuresis, with dryness resulting in more than 50 percent of cases. The treatment is equally effective in children with and without concomitant mental disorders, and there is no evidence of symptom substitution. Difficulties may include child and family noncompliance, improper use of the apparatus, and relapse. Bladder training—encouragement or reward for delaying micturition for increasing times during waking hours—has also been used. Although sometimes effective, this method is decidedly inferior to the bell and pad.

Table 47–3
ICD-10 Diagnostic Criteria for Nonorganic Encopresis

A. The child repeatedly passes feces in places that are inappropriate for the purpose (e.g., clothing, floor), either involuntarily or intentionally. (The disorder may involve overflow incontinence secondary to functional fecal retention.)
B. The child's chronological and mental age is at least 4 years.
C. There is at least one encopretic event per month.
D. Duration of the disorder is at least 6 months.
E. There is no organic condition that constitutes a sufficient cause for the encopretic events.

Table 47–4
ICD-10 Diagnostic Criteria for Nonorganic Enuresis

A. The child's chronological and mental age is at least 5 years.
B. Involuntary or intentional voiding of urine into bed or clothes occurs at least twice a month in children aged under 7 years, and at least once a month in children aged 7 years or more.
C. The enuresis is not a consequence of epileptic attacks or of neurological incontinence, and not a direct consequence of structural abnormalities of the urinary tract or any other nonpsychiatric medical condition.
D. There is no evidence of any other psychiatric disorder that meets the criteria for other ICD-10 categories.
E. Duration of the disorder is at least 3 months.

Pharmacotherapy. Medication is not the first line of treatment for enuresis and is often not warranted at all. When the problem interferes significantly with a child's functioning, several medications can be considered, although the problem often recurs as soon as medications are withdrawn. Imipramine (Tofranil) is efficacious and has been approved for use in treating childhood enuresis, primarily on a short-term basis. Initially, up to 30 percent of enuretic patients stay dry, and up to 85 percent wet less frequently than before treatment. The success often does not last, however, and tolerance can develop after 6 weeks of therapy. Once the drug is discontinued, relapse and enuresis at former frequencies usually occur within a few months. The drug's adverse effects, which include cardiotoxicity, are also a serious problem.

The tricyclic drugs are not currently used frequently for enuresis because of their risks and reports of sudden death in several children with attention-deficit/hyperactivity disorder who were taking desipramine (Norpramin, Pertofrane). Desmopressin (DDAVP), an antidiuretic compound that is available as an intranasal spray, has shown some initial success in reducing enuresis. Reduction of enuresis has varied from 10 to 90 percent with the use of desmopressin. In most studies, enuresis recurred shortly after discontinuation of this medication. Adverse effects that can occur with desmopressin include headache, nasal congestion, epistaxis, and stomachache. The most serious adverse effect reported with the use of desmopressin to treat enuresis was a hyponatremic seizure experienced by a child.

Psychotherapy. Although many psychological and psychoanalytic theories regarding enuresis have been advanced, controlled studies have found that psychotherapy alone is not an effective treatment of enuresis. Psychotherapy, however, may be useful in dealing with the coexisting psychiatric problems and the emotional and family difficulties that arise secondary to the disorder.

ICD-10

In ICD-10, nonorganic encopresis (Table 47–3) and nonorganic enuresis (Table 47–4) are classified as other behavioral and emotional disorders with onset usually occurring in childhood or adolescence.

References

Beach PS, Beach RE, Smith LR. Hyponatremic seizures in a child treated with desmopressin to control enuresis: a rational approach to fluid intake. *Clin Pediatr.* 1992;31:566.
Cossio SE. Enuresis. *South Med J.* 2002;95:183.
Eggert P. What's new in enuresis? *Acta Paediatr Taiwan.* 2002;43:6.
Loening-Baucke V. Modulation of abnormal defecation dynamics by biofeedback treatment in chronically constipated children with encopresis. *J Pediatr.* 1990;116:214.
Mikkelsen EJ. Elimination disorders. In: Sadock BJ, Sadock VA, eds. *Kaplan & Sadock's Comprehensive Textbook of Psychiatry.* 7th ed. Vol 2. Baltimore: Lippincott Williams & Wilkins; 2000:2720.
Mikkelsen EJ. Enuresis and encopresis: ten years of progress. *J Am Acad Child Adolesc Psychiatry.* 2001;40:1456.
Rolands D, Stathopulu E. Social deprivation affects outcome of nocturnal enuresis. *Br Med J.* 2002;324:677A.
Thompson S, Rey JM. Functional enuresis: is desmopressin the answer? *J Am Acad Child Adolesc Psychiatry.* 1995;34:266.
Van Kerrebropeck PE. Experience with the long-term use of desmopressin for nocturnal enuresis in children and adolescents. *BJU Int.* 2002;89:420.
Von Gontard A, Lehmkuh A. Desmopressin side effects. *J Am Acad Child Adolesc Psychiatry.* 1996;35:129.

48

Other Disorders of Infancy, Childhood, and Adolescence

▲ 48.1 Separation Anxiety Disorder

Separation anxiety is a universal human developmental phenomenon emerging in infants less than 1 year of age and marking the child's awareness of a separation from his or her mother or primary caregiver. Separation anxiety, or *stranger anxiety* as it has been termed during infancy, is an expected part of normal development and most likely evolved as a human response that has survival value. The expression of some separation anxiety is also normal in young children entering school for the first time. Separation anxiety disorder, however, is diagnosed when developmentally inappropriate and excessive anxiety emerges related to separation from the major attachment figure. According to the text revision of the fourth edition of *Diagnostic and Statistical Manual of Mental Disorders* (DSM-IV-TR), separation anxiety disorder requires the presence of at least three symptoms related to excessive worry about separation from the major attachment figures. The worries may take the form of refusal to go to school, fears and distress upon separation, repeated complaints of such physical symptoms as headaches and stomachaches when separation is anticipated and nightmares related to separation issues.

Separation anxiety disorder is the only anxiety disorder currently found in the child and adolescent section of DSM-IV-TR. Children who are persistently more anxious in multiple settings than other children of the same age usually meet the DSM-IV-TR criteria for generalized anxiety disorder. Children who experience significant anxiety and avoidance of social situations in which they fear scrutiny, generally meet the DSM-IV-TR diagnostic criteria for social phobia, which is also used for adults. Children and adolescents may also have other anxiety disorders described among the adult disorders of DSM-IV-TR, including specific phobia, panic disorder, obsessive-compulsive disorder, and posttraumatic stress disorder.

EPIDEMIOLOGY

The prevalence of separation anxiety disorder is estimated to be about 4 percent in children and young adolescents. Separation anxiety disorder is more common in young children than in adolescents and has been reported to occur equally in boys and girls. The onset may occur during preschool years but is most common in 7- to 8-year-olds The rate of generalized anxiety disorder in school-age children is estimated to be approximately 3 percent, the rate of social phobia is 1 percent, and the rate of simple phobias is 2.4 percent. In adolescents, a lifetime prevalence for panic disorder was found to be 0.6 percent; the prevalence for generalized anxiety disorder was 3.7 percent.

ETIOLOGY

Biopsychosocial Factors

Young children, immature and dependent on a mothering figure, are particularly prone to excessive anxiety related to separation. The relation between temperamental traits and the predisposition to develop anxiety symptoms has been investigated. The temperamental tendency to be unusually shy or to withdraw in unfamiliar situations seems to be an enduring response pattern, and young children with this propensity are at higher risk of developing anxiety disorders during their next few years of life.

There is neurophysiological correlation of *behavioral inhibition* (extreme shyness); children with this constellation are shown to have a higher resting heart rate and an acceleration of heart rate with tasks requiring cognitive concentration. Additional physiological correlates of behavioral inhibition include elevated salivary cortisol levels, elevated urinary catecholamine levels, and greater papillary dilation during cognitive tasks. The quality of maternal attachment also appears to play a role in the development of anxiety disorder in children. Mothers with anxiety disorders who are observed to show insecure attachment to their children tend to have children with higher rates of anxiety disorders. It is difficult to separate the contribution of the relationship between mother and child from the mother's potential genetic contribution to anxiety. Families in which a child manifests separation anxiety disorder may be close-knit and caring, and the children often seem to be the objects of parental overconcern. External life stresses often coincide with development of the disorder. The death of a relative, a child's illness, a change in a child's environment, or a move to a new neighborhood or school is frequently noted in the histories of children with separation anxiety disorder. In a vulnerable child, these changes probably intensify anxiety.

Learning Factors

Phobic anxiety may be communicated from parents to children by direct modeling. If a parent is fearful, the child will probably have a phobic adaptation to new situations, especially to a school environment. Some parents appear to teach their children to be anxious by overprotecting them from expected dangers or by exaggerating the dangers. For example, a parent who cringes in a room during a lightning storm teaches a child to do the same. A parent who is afraid of mice or insects conveys the affect of fright to a child. Conversely, a parent who becomes angry with a child during an incipient phobic concern about animals may inculcate a phobic concern in the child by the very intensity of the anger expressed.

Genetic Factors

The temperamental constellation of behavioral inhibition, excessive shyness, the tendency to withdraw from unfamiliar situations, and separation anxiety are all likely to have a genetic contribution. Family studies have shown that the biological offspring of adults with anxiety disorders are prone to suffer from separation anxiety disorder in childhood. Parents who have panic disorder with agoraphobia appear to have an increased risk of having a child with separation anxiety disorder. Separation anxiety disorder and depression in children overlap, and some clinicians view separation anxiety disorder as a feature of a depressive disorder.

DIAGNOSIS AND CLINICAL FEATURES

Separation anxiety disorder is the most common anxiety disorder in childhood. To meet the diagnostic criteria, according to DSM-IV-TR, the disorder must be characterized by three of the following symptoms for at least 4 weeks: persistent and excessive worry about losing, or possible harm befalling, major attachment figures; persistent and excessive worry that an untoward event can lead to separation from a major attachment figure; persistent reluctance or refusal to go to school or elsewhere because of fear of separation; persistent and excessive fear or reluctance to be alone or without major attachment figures at home or without significant adults in other settings; persistent reluctance or refusal to go to sleep without being near a major attachment figure or to sleep away from home; repeated nightmares involving the theme of separation; repeated complaints of physical symptoms, including headaches and stomachaches, when separation from major attachment figures is anticipated; and recurrent excessive distress when separation from home or major attachment figures is anticipated or involved. According to DSM-IV-TR, the disturbance must also cause significant distress or impairment in functioning (Table 48.1–1).

Table 48.1–1
DSM-IV-TR Diagnostic Criteria for Separation Anxiety Disorder

A. Developmentally inappropriate and excessive anxiety concerning separation from home or from those to whom the individual is attached, as evidenced by three (or more) of the following:
   (1) recurrent excessive distress when separation from home or major attachment figures occurs or is anticipated
   (2) persistent and excessive worry about losing, or about possible harm befalling, major attachment figures
   (3) persistent and excessive worry that an untoward event will lead to separation from a major attachment figure (e.g., getting lost or being kidnapped)
   (4) persistent reluctance or refusal to go to school or elsewhere because of fear of separation
   (5) persistently and excessively fearful or reluctant to be alone or without major attachment figures at home or without significant adults in other settings
   (6) persistent reluctance or refusal to go to sleep without being near a major attachment figure or to sleep away from home
   (7) repeated nightmares involving the theme of separation
   (8) repeated complaints of physical symptoms (such as headaches, stomachaches, nausea, or vomiting) when separation from major attachment figures occurs or is anticipated

B. The duration of the disturbance is at least 4 weeks.

C. The onset is before age 18 years.

D. The disturbance causes clinically significant distress or impairment in social, academic (occupational), or other important areas of functioning.

E. The disturbance does not occur exclusively during the course of a pervasive developmental disorder, schizophrenia, or other psychotic disorder and, in adolescents and adults, is not better accounted for by panic disorder with agoraphobia.

Specify if:
Early onset: if onset occurs before age 6 years

From American Psychiatric Association. *Diagnostic and Statistical Manual of Mental Disorders.* 4th ed. Text rev. Washington, DC: American Psychiatric Association; copyright 2000, with permission.

A patient's history may reveal important episodes of separation in the child's life, particularly because of illness and hospitalization, illness or loss of a parent, or geographical relocation. Clinicians should scrutinize the period of infancy for evidence of separation-individuation disorders or lack of an adequate mothering figure. Using fantasies, dreams, and play materials and observing the child help greatly in making the diagnosis. Clinicians should examine not only thought content but also the way in which thoughts are expressed. For example, children may express fears that their parents will die, even when their behavior does not show evidence of anxiety. Similarly, a child's difficulty in describing events or bland denial of obviously anxiety-provoking events may indicate a separation anxiety disorder. Difficulty with memory in expressing separation themes and patent distortions in the recital of such themes may give clues to the disorder's presence.

The essential feature of separation anxiety disorder is extreme anxiety precipitated by separation from parents, home, or other familiar surroundings. A child's anxiety may approach terror or panic. The distress is greater than that normally expected for the child's developmental level and cannot be explained by any other disorder. Morbid fears, preoccupations, and ruminations characterize separation anxiety disorder. Children with the disorder become fearful that someone close to them will be hurt or that something terrible will happen to them when they are away from important caring figures. Many children worry that they or their parents will have an accident or become ill. Fears about getting lost and about being kidnapped and never again finding their parents are common.

Adolescents may not directly express any anxious concern about separation from mothering figures. However, their behavior patterns often reflect a separation anxiety in that they express discomfort about leaving home, engage in solitary activities, and continue to use mothering figures as helpers in buying clothes and entering social and recreational activities. Separation anxiety disorder in children is often manifested at the thought of travel or in the course of travel away from home. Children may refuse to go to camp, a new school, or even a friend's house. Frequently, a continuum exists between mild anticipatory anxiety before separation from an important figure and pervasive anxiety after the separation has occurred. Premonitory signs include irritability, difficulty eating, whining, staying in a room alone, clinging to parents, and following a parent everywhere. Often, when a family moves, a child displays separation anxiety by intense clinging to the mother figure. Sometimes, geographical relocation anxiety is expressed in feelings of acute homesickness or psychophysiological symptoms that break out when the child is away from home or is going to a new country. The child yearns to return home and becomes preoccupied with fantasies of how much better the old home was. Integration into the new life situation may become extremely difficult.

Sleep difficulties are frequent and may require having someone remain with a child until he or she falls asleep. A child often goes to the parent's bed or even sleeps at the parents' door when the bedroom is barred to him or her. Nightmares and morbid fears are other expressions of anxiety.

Associated features include fear of the dark and imaginary, bizarre worries. Children may see eyes staring at them and become preoccupied with mythical figures or monsters reaching out for them in their bedrooms. Many children are demanding, intrude in adult affairs, and require constant attention to allay their anxieties. Symptoms emerge when separation from an important parent figure becomes necessary. If separation is threatened, many children with the disorder do not experience interpersonal difficulties. They may, however, look sad and may cry easily. They sometimes complain that they are not loved, express a wish to die, or complain that siblings are favored over them. They frequently experience gastrointestinal symptoms, nausea, vomiting, and stomachaches, and have pains in various parts of the body, sore throats, and flulike symptoms. In older children, typical cardiovascular and respiratory symptoms—palpitations, dizziness, faintness, and strangulation—are reported. The most common anxiety disorder that coexists with separation anxiety disorder is specific phobia, which occurs in about one third of referred cases of separation anxiety disorder.

Tony was a 6-year-old boy referred by his school because of persistent refusal to attend school. He had always been a somewhat "clingy" child, but his difficulties had intensified in the past 4 months. He would follow his parents around the house and refuse to leave their sides in playgrounds or other situations where separating would be age appropriate. That behavior was worse if he could not keep them in clear sight. He said that he might be kidnapped or lost if he ever got out of their sight. He would tantrum whenever they would try to go out for the evening, saying that they were not coming back. When forced to engage in any of the distressing activities, he would complain of various somatic symptoms until one of his parents remained.

He was the product of a pregnancy marred by caesarean section for premature rupture of membranes at 34 weeks' gestation. The perinatal course was complicated by moderate respiratory distress necessitating hospitalization for more than 3 weeks. Evaluation of the recent somatic symptoms revealed a child who was normal except for the psychiatric complaints.

His early development had been normal. He attempted preschool, but his mother had removed him because he cried at the beginning of each day, followed by aggression toward smaller peers. She participated as a parent aide in his kindergarten classroom, stating that she was trying to help him adjust to school. He was in grade school with peers who were after-school playmates in his home but would only go to their homes with a parent.

Family history was positive for maternal recurrent major depressive disorder, in remission, and a history of panic disorder in Tony's maternal grandmother. His maternal grandfather and a paternal uncle had alcoholism. Tony's parents were both in their early 30s, with some college education. His father worked as an assistant manager in a small service firm; his mother had worked as a bookkeeper until Tony was born. They said that his mother would have returned to work if he had liked preschool. His difficulties were straining their marriage, as he frequently insisted on sleeping in their bed. His mother insisted that she wanted to return to the workforce and that Tony's separation anxiety prevented it. There was no suggestion of domestic violence.

Mental status examination revealed a thin, nicely attired boy who had great difficulty allowing his mother to go beyond a chair outside the office door. He insisted on checking twice to see if she was there. He was fidgety and admitted feeling very worried about his mother leaving. He said that kind of worry was bad enough that he has trouble thinking. He denied depressed mood or symptoms including irritability. He denied hallucinations and did not voice any delusional ideas. He said that he enjoyed his friends and that his teacher was "nice" but that he worried about his mother when he was away from her.

Further exploration of the family situation revealed that his maternal grandfather had died 2 years earlier. His grandmother, who lived nearby, had been very agoraphobic until recently and had depended on the patient's mother, which had caused significant marital friction. Tony's father had hoped that the mother would return to work so that he could complete college and leave a job he hated. When she tried to force Tony to go to school, grandmother would come to the home to help and would then encourage mother to "go easy on the child." Mother would become angry, relent, and feel guilty about her interactions with her mother and her child. Grandmother further lectured mother that she needed to stay at home to care for her needy and delicate child because he had been premature.

Treatment focused on bringing the adults together to develop a supportive program for the child and to enlist grandmother in an appropriate role helping her daughter and son-in-law move forward with their lives. Grandmother supported Tony's return to the classroom once she understood the issues and approach. That was accomplished without directly addressing or interpreting her significant identification

with her separation-anxious grandchild. Mother returned to work, with grandmother providing after-school care. Tony also responded well to a simple reward program for sleeping in his own room. Unfortunately, he presented again 7 years later as a popular, very good student and athlete who developed major depressive disorder. He responded well to fluoxetine (Prozac) and cognitive therapy. (Courtesy of Carrie Sylvester, M.D.)

Pathology and Laboratory Examination

No specific laboratory measures help in the diagnosis of separation anxiety disorder.

DIFFERENTIAL DIAGNOSIS

Some separation anxiety is a normal phenomenon, and clinical judgment must be used in distinguishing that normal anxiety from separation anxiety disorder. In generalized anxiety disorder, anxiety is not focused on separation. In pervasive developmental disorders and schizophrenia, anxiety about separation may occur but is viewed as caused by these conditions rather than being a separate disorder. In depressive disorders occurring in children, the diagnosis of separation anxiety disorder should also be made when the criteria for both disorders are met; the two diagnoses often coexist. Panic disorder with agoraphobia is uncommon before 18 years of age; the fear is of being incapacitated by a panic attack rather than of separation from parental figures. In some adult cases, however, many symptoms of separation anxiety disorder may be present. In conduct disorder, truancy is common, but children stay away from home and do not have anxiety about separation. School refusal is a frequent symptom in separation anxiety disorder but is not pathognomonic of it. Children with other diagnoses, such as phobias, also evince school refusal; in these disorders, the age of onset may be later and the school refusal may be more severe than in separation anxiety disorder. Common characteristics of selected anxiety disorders that occur in children are presented in Table 48.1–2.

COURSE AND PROGNOSIS

The course and the prognosis of separation anxiety disorder are varied and are related to the age of onset, the duration of the symptoms, and the development of comorbid anxiety and depressive disorders. Young children who experience the disorder but can maintain attendance in school generally have a better prognosis than adolescents with the disorder who refuse to attend school for long periods. A follow-up study of children and adolescents with anxiety disorders over a 3-year period reported that up to 82 percent no longer met criteria for the anxiety disorder at follow-up. Of the group followed, 96 percent of those with separation anxiety disorder had a remission at follow-up. Most children who recovered did so within the first year. Early age of onset and later age at diagnosis were factors that predicted slower recovery. Close to one third of the group studied, however, had developed another psychiatric disorder within the follow-up period, and 50 percent of these children developed another anxiety disorder. Reports have indicated a significant overlap of separation anxiety disorder and depressive disorders. In these complicated cases, the prognosis is guarded. Most follow-up studies have methodological problems and are limited to hospitalized, school-phobic children, not children with separation anxiety disorder per se. Little is reported about the outcome

Table 48.1–2
Common Characteristics of Selected Anxiety Disorders That Occur in Children

Criteria	Separation Anxiety Disorder	Social Phobia	Generalized Anxiety Disorder
Minimum duration to establish diagnosis	At least 4 weeks	No minimum	At least 6 months
Age of onset	Preschool to 18 years	Not specified	Not specified
Precipitating stresses	Separation from significant parental figures, other losses, travel	Pressure for social participation with peers	Unusual pressure for performance, damage to self-esteem, feelings of lack of competence
Peer relationships	Good when no separation is involved	Tentative, overly inhibited	Overly eager to please, peers sought out and dependent relationships established
Sleep	Reluctance or refusal to go to sleep, fear of dark, nightmares	Difficulty in falling asleep at times	Difficulty in falling asleep
Psychophysiological symptoms	Complaints of stomachaches, nausea, vomiting, flulike symptoms, headaches, palpitations, dizziness, faintness	Blushing, body tension	Stomachaches, nausea, vomiting, lump in the throat, shortness of breath, dizziness, palpitations
Differential diagnosis	Generalized anxiety disorder, schizophrenia, depressive disorders, conduct disorder, pervasive developmental disorders, major depressive disorder, panic disorder with agoraphobia	Adjustment disorder with depressed mood, generalized anxiety disorder, separation anxiety disorder, major depressive disorder, dysthymic disorder, avoidant personality disorder, borderline personality disorder	Separation anxiety disorder, attention-deficit/hyperactivity disorder, social phobia, adjustment disorder with anxiety, obsessive-compulsive disorder, psychotic disorders, mood disorders

Adapted from Sidney Werkman, M.D.

of mild cases, whether children are seen in outpatient treatment or receive no treatment. Notwithstanding the limitations of the studies, reports indicate that some children with severe school phobia continue to resist attending school for many years.

During the 1970s, it was reported that many adult women with agoraphobia had suffered from separation anxiety disorder in childhood. Although research indicates that many children with an anxiety disorder are at increased risk for an adult anxiety disorder, the specific link between separation anxiety disorder in childhood and agoraphobia in adulthood has not been established clearly. Studies do indicate that anxious parents are at increased risk of having children with anxiety disorders. In addition, in recent years, some cases of children with both panic disorder and separation anxiety disorder have been reported.

TREATMENT

A multimodal treatment plan including cognitive-behavioral therapy, family education, and family psychosocial intervention is recommended in the initial management of separation anxiety disorder. Pharmacological interventions are recommended when additional strategies are needed to control the symptoms. Cognitive-behavioral therapy is currently widely recommended as a first-line treatment for a variety of anxiety disorders for children, including separation anxiety disorder. Specific cognitive strategies and relaxation exercises are also components of treatment for some children to provide them with mechanisms that they can incorporate to control their anxiety. Family interventions can be critical in the management of separation anxiety disorder, especially in children who refuse to attend school, so that firm encouragement of school attendance is maintained while appropriate support is also provided.

A recent placebo-controlled study found pharmacotherapy with selective serotonin reuptake inhibitors (SSRIs) efficacious in the treatment of anxiety disorders in children. First-line pharmacological agents currently widely recommended are the SSRIs including fluoxetine, fluvoxamine (Luvox), sertraline (Zoloft), paroxetine (Paxil), and citalopram (Celexa). Tricyclic drugs are not currently recommended as first-line treatments for disorders because of their potentially serious cardiac adverse effects. β-Adrenergic receptor antagonists, such as propranolol (Inderal), and buspirone (BuSpar) have been used clinically in children with anxiety disorders, but currently no data support their efficacy. Diphenhydramine (Benadryl) may be used in the short term to control sleep disturbances in children with anxiety disorders. Open trials and one double-blind, placebo-controlled study suggested that alprazolam (Xanax), a benzodiazepine, may help to control anxiety symptoms in separation anxiety disorder. Clonazepam (Klonopin) has been studied in open trials and may be useful in controlling symptoms of panic and other anxiety symptoms.

School refusal associated with separation anxiety disorder may be viewed as a psychiatric emergency. A comprehensive treatment plan involves the child, the parents, and the child's peers and school. The child should be encouraged to attend school, but when a return to a full school day is overwhelming, a program should be arranged so the child can progressively increase the time spent at school. Graded contact with an object of anxiety is a form of behavior modification that can be applied to any type of separation anxiety. Some severe cases of school refusal require hospitalization. Cognitive-behavioral modalities can be used in psychotherapy, including exposure to feared separations and cognitive strategies such as coping self-statements aimed at increasing a sense of autonomy and mastery.

ICD-10

The 10th revision of *International Statistical Classification of Diseases and Related Health Problems* (ICD-10) includes a category for emotional disorders with onset specific to childhood. This category contains five specific childhood-onset anxiety disorders and one residual diagnosis (Table 48.1–3). According to ICD-10, several reasons exist for tradi-

Table 48.1–3
ICD-10 Diagnostic Criteria for Emotional Disorders with Onset Specific to Childhood

Note. Phobic anxiety disorder of childhood, social anxiety disorder of childhood, and general anxiety disorder of childhood have obvious similarities to some of the disorders in neurotic, stress-related and somatoform disorders, but current evidence and opinion suggest that there are sufficient differences in the ways that anxiety disorders present in children for additional categories to be provided. Further studies should show whether descriptions and definitions can be developed that can be used satisfactorily for both adults and children, or whether the present distinction should be preserved.

Separation anxiety disorder of childhood

A. At least three of the following must be present:
- (1) unrealistic and persistent worry about possible harm befalling major attachment figures or about the loss of such figures (e.g., fear that they will leave and not return or that the child will not see them again), or persistent concerns about the death of attachment figures;
- (2) unrealistic and persistent worry that some untoward event will separate the child from a major attachment figure (e.g., the child getting lost, being kidnapped, admitted to hospital, or killed);
- (3) persistent reluctance or refusal to go to school because of fear over separation from a major attachment figure or in order to stay at home (rather than for other reasons such as fear over events at school);
- (4) difficulty in separating at night, as manifested by any of the following:
  - (a) persistent reluctance or refusal to go to sleep without being near an attachment figure;
  - (b) getting up frequently during the night to check on, or to sleep near, an attachment figure;
  - (c) persistent reluctance or refusal to sleep away from home
- (5) persistent inappropriate fear of being alone, or otherwise without the major attachment figure, at home during the day;
- (6) repeated nightmares involving themes of separation;
- (7) repeated occurrence of physical symptoms (such as nausea, stomachache, headache, or vomiting) on occasions that involve separation from a major attachment figure, such as leaving home to go to school or on other occasions involving separation (holidays, camps, etc.).

(*continued*)

Table 48.1–3 (*continued*)

(8) excessive, recurrent distress in anticipation of, during, or immediately after separation from a major attachment figure (as shown by: anxiety, crying, tantrums; persistent reluctance to go away from home; excessive need to talk with parents or desire to return home; misery, apathy, or social withdrawal).

B. The criteria for generalized anxiety disorder of childhood are not met.

C. Onset is before the age of 6 years.

D. The disorder does not occur as part of a broader disturbance of emotions, conduct, or personality or of a pervasive developmental disorder, psychotic disorder, or psychoactive substance use disorder.

E. Duration of the disorder is at least 4 weeks.

Phobic anxiety disorder of childhood

A. The individual manifests a persistent or recurrent fear (phobia) that is developmentally phase-appropriate (or was so at the time of onset) but that is abnormal in degree and is associated with significant social impairment.

B. The criteria for generalized anxiety disorder of childhood are not met.

C. The disorder does not occur as part of a broader disturbance of emotions, conduct, or personality or of a pervasive developmental disorder, psychotic disorder, or psychoactive substance use disorder.

D. Duration of the disorder is at least 4 weeks.

Social anxiety disorder of childhood

A. Persistent anxiety in social situations in which the child is exposed to unfamiliar people, including peers, is manifested by socially avoidant behavior.

B. The child exhibits self-consciousness, embarrassment, or overconcern about the appropriateness of his or her behavior when interacting with unfamiliar figures.

C. There is significant interference with social (including peer) relationships, which are consequently restricted; when new or forced social situations are experienced, they cause marked distress and discomfort as manifested by crying, lack of spontaneous speech, or withdrawal from the social situation.

D. The child has satisfying social relationships with familiar figures (family members or peers that he or she knows well).

E. Onset of the disorder generally coincides with a developmental phase in which these anxiety reactions are considered appropriate. The abnormal degree, persistence over time, and associated impairment must be manifest before the age of 6 years.

F. The criteria for generalized anxiety disorder of childhood are not met.

G. The disorder does not occur as part of broader disturbances of emotions, conduct, or personality or of a pervasive developmental disorder, psychotic disorder, or psychoactive substance use disorder.

H. Duration of the disorder is at least 4 weeks.

Sibling rivalry disorder

A. The child has abnormally intense negative feelings toward an immediately younger sibling.

B. Emotional disturbance is shown by regression, tantrums, dysphoria, sleep difficulties, oppositional behavior, or attention-seeking behavior with one or both parents (two or more of these must be present).

C. Onset is within 6 months of the birth of an immediately younger sibling.

D. Duration of the disorder is at least 4 weeks.

Other childhood emotional disorders

Generalized anxiety disorder of childhood

Note: In children and adolescents, the range of complaints by which the general anxiety is manifest is often more limited than in adults (see Generalized anxiety disorder), and the specific symptoms of autonomic arousal are often less prominent. For these individuals, the following alternative set of criteria can be used if preferred:

A. Extensive anxiety and worry (apprehensive expectation) occur on at least half of the total number of days over a period of at least 6 months, the anxiety and worry referring to at least several events or activities (such as work or school performance).

B. The individual finds it difficult to control the worry.

C. The anxiety and worry are associated with at least three of the following symptoms (with at least two symptoms present on at least half of the total number of days):

(1) restlessness, feeling "keyed up" or "on edge" (as shown, for example, by feelings of mental tension combined with an inability to relax);

(2) feeling tired, "worn out," or easily fatigued because of worry or anxiety;

(3) difficulty in concentrating, or mind "going blank";

(4) irritability;

(5) muscle tension;

(6) sleep disturbance (difficulty in falling or staying asleep, or restless, unsatisfying sleep) because of worry or anxiety.

D. The multiple anxieties and worries occur across at least two situations, activities, contexts, or circumstances. Generalized anxiety does not present as discrete paroxysmal episodes (as in panic disorder), nor are the main worries confined to a single, major theme (as in separation anxiety disorder or phobic disorder of childhood). (When more focused anxiety is identified in the broader context of a generalized anxiety, generalized anxiety disorder takes precedence over other anxiety disorders.)

E. Onset occurs in childhood or adolescence (before the age of 18 years).

F. The anxiety, worry, or physical symptoms cause clinically significant distress or impairment in social, occupational, or other important areas of functioning.

G. The disorder is not due to the direct effects of a substance (e.g., psychoactive substances, medication) or a general medical condition (e.g., hyperthyroidism) and does not occur exclusively during a mood disorder, psychotic disorder, or pervasive developmental disorder.

Childhood emotional disorder, unspecified

Reprinted with permission from World Health Organization. *The ICD-10 Classification of Mental and Behavioural Disorders: Diagnostic Criteria for Research.* Copyright, World Health Organization, Geneva, 1993.

tionally differentiating emotional disorders specific to childhood and adolescence from those of adulthood. First, research has consistently shown that most children with emotional disorders become normal adults and that many adult emotional disorders have an onset in adult life and lack precursors in childhood. Second, many emotional disorders of childhood appear to be exaggerations of normal developmental trends rather than abnormalities. Third, the mental mechanisms of childhood emotional disorders are believed to often differ from those of adult disorders; this point, however, has not been verified empirically. Finally, childhood emotional disorders are less clearly separated into specific categories

such as phobic or obsessional disorders, but epidemiological data suggest that this distinction is only relative because it is often difficult to differentiate adult disorders as well. Thus, the second feature, developmental appropriateness, is the key factor in diagnosing differences between disorders with specific childhood onset and the neurotic disorders in general; some empirical evidence supports this hypothesis.

References

Allen AJ, Leonard H, Swedo SE. Current knowledge of medications for the treatment of childhood anxiety disorders. *J Am Acad Child Adolesc Psychiatry.* 1995;34:976.

Barrett PM, Duffy Al, Dadds MR, Rapee RM. Cognitive-behavioral treatment of anxiety disorders in children: long-term (6 year) follow-up. *J Consult Clin Psychol.* 2001;69:135.

Bernstein GA, Borchardt CM, Perwien AR. Anxiety disorders in children and adolescents: a review of the past 10 years. *J Am Acad Child Adolesc Psychiatry.* 1996;35:1110.

Birmaher B, Waterman GS, Ryan N. Fluoxetine for childhood anxiety disorders. *J Am Acad Child Adolesc Psychiatry.* 1994;33:993.

Bradley SJ, Hood L. Psychiatrically referred adolescents with panic attacks: presenting symptoms, stressors, and comorbidity. *J Am Acad Child Adolesc Psychiatry.* 1993;32:826.

Cheer SM, Figgitt DP. Spotlight on fluvoxamine in anxiety disorders in children and adolescents. *CNS Drugs.* 2002;16:139.

Coyle JT. Drug treatment of anxiety disorders in children. *N Engl J Med.* 2001;344:1326.

Gittelman R, ed. *Anxiety Disorders of Children.* New York: Guilford Press; 1986.

Kashani JH, Orveschel H. A community study of anxiety in children and adolescents. *Am J Psychiatry.* 1990;147:313.

Kranzler HR. Use of buspirone in an adolescent with overanxious disorder. *J Am Acad Child Adolesc Psychiatry.* 1988;27:789.

Last CG, Perrin S, Hersen M, Krazdin AE. DSM-III-R anxiety disorders in children: sociodemographic and clinical characteristics. *J Am Acad Child Adolesc Psychiatry.* 1992;31:1070.

Last CG, Strauss CC. School refusal in anxiety-disordered children and adolescents. *J Am Acad Child Adolesc Psychiatry.* 1990;29:31.

Liebowitz MR, Stein MG, Tancer M, Carpenter D, Oakes R, Pitts CD. A randomized, double-blind, fixed dose comparison of paroxetine and placebo in the treatment of generalized social anxiety disorder. *J Clin Psychiatry.* 2002;63:66.

Manassis K, Bradley S, Goldberg S, Hood J, Swinson RP. Behavioral inhibition, attachment and anxiety in children of mothers with anxiety disorders. *Can J Psychiatry.* 1995;40:87.

The Research Unit on Pediatric Psychopharmacology Anxiety Study Group. Fluvoxamine for the treatment of anxiety disorders in children. *N Engl J Med.* 2001;344:1279.

Sylvester C. Separation anxiety disorder and other anxiety disorders. In: Sadock BJ, Sadock VA, eds. *Kaplan & Sadock's Comprehensive Textbook of Psychiatry.* 7th ed. Vol 2. Baltimore: Lippincott Williams & Wilkins; 2000:2770.

▲ 48.2 Selective Mutism

Selective mutism is a childhood condition in which a child remains completely silent or near silent in social situations, most typically in school. Most children with the disorder are completely silent during the stressful situations, while others whisper or use single-syllable words. Children with selective mutism can speak competently when not in a socially stressful situation. Some children with the disorder communicate with eye contact or nonverbal gestures. These children speak fluently in other situations, such as at home and in certain familiar settings. Selective mutism is believed to be a form of social phobia because of its expression in selective social situations.

EPIDEMIOLOGY

The prevalence of selective mutism has been estimated to range between 3 and 8 per 10,000 children. More recent surveys indicate that it may be more common, emerging in more than 0.5 percent of schoolchildren in the community. Young children are more vulnerable to the disorder than older ones. Selective mutism appears to be more common in girls than in boys.

Etiology

Although selective mutism is a psychologically determined inhibition or refusal to speak, many children with the disorder have histories of delayed onset of speech or speech abnormalities that may be contributory. In a recent survey, 90 percent of children with selective mutism met diagnostic criteria for social phobia. These children showed high levels of social anxiety without notable psychopathology in other areas, according to parent and teacher ratings. Thus, selective mutism may not represent a distinct disorder but may be better conceptualized as a subtype of social phobia. Similar to families with children who exhibit other anxiety disorders, maternal anxiety, depression, and heightened dependence needs are often noted in families of children with selective mutism. These factors may result in maternal overprotection and an overly close, but ambivalent, relationship between a mother and her selectively mute child. Children with selective mutism usually speak freely at home; they have no significant biological disability. Some children seem predisposed to selective mutism after early emotional or physical trauma; thus, some clinicians refer to the phenomenon as traumatic mutism rather than selective mutism.

DIAGNOSIS AND CLINICAL FEATURES

The diagnostic criteria from the text revision of the fourth edition of *Diagnosis and Statistical Manual of Mental Disorders* (DSM-IV-TR) appear in Table 48.2–1. The diagnosis of selective mutism is not difficult to make after it is clear that a child has adequate language skills in some environments but not in others. The mutism may have developed gradually or suddenly after a disturbing experience. The age of onset can range from 4 to 8 years. Mute periods are most commonly manifested in school or outside the home; in rare cases, a child is mute at home but not in school. Children who exhibit selective mutism

Table 48.2–1
DSM-IV-TR Diagnostic Criteria for Selective Mutism

A. Consistent failure to speak in specific social situations (in which there is an expectation for speaking, e.g., at school) despite speaking in other situations.

B. The disturbance interferes with educational or occupational achievement or with social communication.

C. The duration of the disturbance is at least 1 month (not limited to the first month of school).

D. The failure to speak is not due to a lack of knowledge of, or comfort with, the spoken language required in the social situation.

E. The disturbance is not better accounted for by a communication disorder (e.g., stuttering) and does not occur exclusively during the course of a pervasive developmental disorder, schizophrenia, or other psychotic disorder.

From American Psychiatric Association. *Diagnostic and Statistical Manual of Mental Disorders.* 4th ed. Text rev. Washington, DC: American Psychiatric Association; copyright 2000, with permission.

may also have symptoms of separation anxiety disorder, school refusal, and delayed language acquisition. Because social anxiety is almost always present in children with selective mutism, behavioral disturbances, such as temper tantrums and oppositional behaviors, may also occur in the home.

Pathology and Laboratory Examination

No specific laboratory measures are useful in the diagnosis or treatment of selective mutism.

DIFFERENTIAL DIAGNOSIS

Shy children may exhibit a transient muteness in new, anxiety-provoking situations. These children often have histories of not speaking in the presence of strangers and of clinging to their mothers. Most children who are mute upon entering school improve spontaneously and may be described as having transient adaptational shyness. Selective mutism must also be distinguished from mental retardation, pervasive developmental disorders, and expressive language disorder. In these disorders, the symptoms are widespread, and there is not one situation in which the child communicates normally; the child may have an inability, rather than a refusal, to speak. In mutism secondary to conversion disorder, the mutism is pervasive. Children introduced into an environment in which a different language is spoken may be reticent to begin using the new language. Selective mutism should be diagnosed only when children also refuse to converse in their native language and when they have gained communicative competence in the new language but refuse to speak it.

COURSE AND PROGNOSIS

Although children with selective mutism are often abnormally shy during preschool years, the onset of the disorder is usually at age 5 or 6. The most common pattern is that children speak almost exclusively at home with the nuclear family but not elsewhere, especially not at school. Consequently, they may have academic difficulties and even failure. Children with selective mutism are generally shy, anxious, and vulnerable to the development of depression. Most children with mild forms of anxiety disorder, including selective mutism, remit with or without treatment. With recent data suggesting that fluoxetine (Prozac) may influence the course of selective mutism, recovery may be enhanced. Children in whom the disorder persists often have difficulty forming social relationships. Teasing and scapegoating by peers may induce them to refuse to go to school. Some children with this severe social phobia are characterized by rigidity, compulsive traits, negativism, temper tantrums, and oppositional and aggressive behavior at home. Other children with the disorder tolerate the feared situation better by communicating with gestures, such as nodding, shaking the head, and saying "Um-hum" or "No." Most cases last for only a few weeks or months, but some cases persist for years. In one follow-up study, about one half of the children improved within 5 to 10 years. Children who do not improve by age 10 appear to have a long-term course and a worse prognosis than those who do improve by age 10. As many as one third of children with selective mutism, with or without treatment, may develop other psychiatric disorders, particularly other anxiety disorders and depression.

TREATMENT

A multimodal approach using individual, cognitive-behavioral, behavioral, and family interventions is recommended. Preschool children may also benefit from a therapeutic nursery. For school-age children, individual cognitive-behavioral therapy is recommended as a first-line treatment. Family education and cooperation are beneficial. Selective serotonin reuptake inhibitor (SSRI) medication is now an accepted component of treatment when psychosocial interventions do not suffice to manage symptoms.

A recent report of 21 children with selective mutism treated in an open trial with fluoxetine suggested that this medication may be effective for childhood selective mutism. Reports have confirmed the efficacy of fluoxetine in the treatment of adult social phobia and in at least one double-blind, placebo-controlled study using fluoxetine with children with mutism. Other medications such as phenelzine (Nardil) also reportedly improve symptoms of social phobia adults but are rarely recommended for mutism in school-age children.

ICD-10

The 10th revision of *International Statistical Classification of Diseases and Related Health Problems* (ICD-10) contains the diagnosis *elective mutism* for children who fail to speak in specific situations. In ICD-10, elective mutism is classified with the attachment disorders (see Table 48.3–2 in Section 48.3 of this chapter).

References

Black B, Uhde TW. Treatment of elective mutism with fluoxetine: a double-blind placebo controlled study. *J Am Acad Adolesc Psychiatry.* 1994;33:1000.
Black B, Uhde TW. Psychiatric characteristics of children with selective mutism: a pilot study. *J Am Acad Adolesc Psychiatry.* 1995;34:847.
Cheer SM, Figgitt DP. Fluvoxamine: a review of its therapeutic potential in the management of anxiety disorders in children and adolescents. *Paediatr Drugs.* 2001;3:763.
Coupland NJ. Social phobia: etiology, neurobiology, and treatment. *J Clin Psychiatry.* 2001;62(suppl):25.
Dummit ES III, Klein RG, Tancer NK, Asche B, Martin J. Fluoxetine treatment of children with selective mutism: an open trial. *J Am Acad Adolesc Psychiatry.* 1996;35:615.
Isaacs E. Fluvoxamine for the treatment of anxiety disorders in children and adolescents. *N Engl J Med.* 2001;345:466.
Last CG, Perrin S, Hersen M, Kazdin A. A prospective study of childhood anxiety disorders. *J Am Acad Adolesc Psychiatry.* 1996;35:1502.
Leonard HL. Selective mutism. In: Sadock BJ, Sadock VA, eds. *Kaplan & Sadock's Comprehensive Textbook of Psychiatry.* 7th ed. Vol 2. Baltimore: Lippincott Williams & Wilkins; 2000:2777.
Mancini C, Van Amerigen M, Szatmari P, Fugere C, Boyle M. A high-risk pilot study of the children of adults with social phobia. *J Am Acad Adolesc Psychiatry.* 1996;35:11.
Schill MT, Kratochwill TR, Gardner WI. An assessment protocol for selective mutism: analogue assessment using parents as facilitators. *J School Psychol.* 1996;34:1.
Shortt AL, Barrett PM, Fox TL. Evaluating the FRIENDS program: a cognitive-behavioral group treatment for anxious children and their parents. *J Clin Child Psychol.* 2001;30:525.

▲ 48.3 Reactive Attachment Disorder of Infancy or Early Childhood

According to the text revision of the fourth edition of *Diagnostic and Statistical Manual of Mental Disorders* (DSM-IV-TR), reactive attachment disorder of infancy or early childhood is marked by an inappropriate social relatedness that occurs in

most contexts. The disorder appears before the age of 5 and is associated with "grossly pathological care." It is not accounted for solely by a developmental delay and does not meet the criteria for pervasive developmental disorder. The pattern of care may exhibit lasting disregard for a child's emotional or physical needs or repeated changes of caregivers as when a child is frequently relocated during foster care. The pathological care pattern is believed to cause the disturbance in social relatedness.

The disorder has two subtypes: the inhibited type, in which the disturbance takes the form of constantly failing to initiate and respond to most social interactions in a developmentally normal way; and the disinhibited type, in which the disturbance takes the form of undifferentiated, unselective social relatedness. These developmentally inappropriate behaviors are presumed to be due to a large degree to pathogenic caregiving, but less severe disturbances in parenting may also be associated with infants who exhibit the disorder.

The disorder may result in a picture of failure to thrive, in which an infant shows physical signs of malnourishment and does not exhibit the expected developmental motor and verbal milestones. When this is the case, the failure to thrive is coded on Axis III.

EPIDEMIOLOGY

No specific data on the prevalence, sex ratio, or familial pattern are currently available. Although patients with reactive attachment disorder of infancy or early childhood come from all socioeconomic groups, studies of some patients (e.g., infants with failure to thrive) indicate increased vulnerability among those from low socioeconomic levels. This finding is congruent with the likelihood of psychosocial deprivation, single-parent households, family disorganization, and economic difficulties. A caregiver may be fully satisfactory for one child, while another child under the same care has a reactive attachment disorder of infancy or early childhood.

ETIOLOGY

The cause of reactive attachment disorder of infancy or early childhood is included in the disorder's definition. Reactive attachment disorder is linked to maltreatment, including neglect and possible physical abuse as well. Grossly pathogenic care of an infant or young child by the caregiver presumably causes the markedly disturbed social relatedness that is usually evident. The emphasis is on the unidirectional cause; that is, the caregiver does something inimical or neglects to do something essential for the infant or child. In evaluating a patient for whom such a diagnosis is appropriate, however, clinicians should consider the contributions of each member of the caregiver-dyad and their interactions. Clinicians should weigh such things as infant or child temperament, deficient or defective bonding, a developmentally disabled or sensorially impaired child, and a particular caregiver-child mismatch. The likelihood of neglect increases with parental mental retardation; lack of parenting skills because of personal upbringing, social isolation, or deprivation and lack of opportunities to learn about caregiving behavior; and premature parenthood (during early and middle adolescence), in which parents are unable to respond to, and care for, an infant's needs and in which the parents' own needs take precedence over their infant's or child's needs. Frequent changes of the primary caregiver—as may occur in institutionalization, repeated lengthy hospitalizations, and multiple foster care placements—may also cause a reactive attachment disorder of infancy or early childhood.

DIAGNOSIS AND CLINICAL FEATURES

Children with reactive attachment disorder of infancy or early childhood often first come to the attention of a pediatrician. The clinical picture varies greatly depending on a child's chronological and mental ages, but expected social interaction and liveliness are not present. Often, the child is developmentally not progressing or is frankly malnourished. Perhaps the most typical clinical picture of an infant with the disorder is the nonorganic failure to thrive. Such infants usually exhibit hypokinesis, dullness, listlessness, and apathy with a poverty of spontaneous activity. Infants look sad, joyless, and miserable. Some infants also appear frightened and watchful, with a radarlike gaze. Nevertheless, they may exhibit delayed responsiveness to a stimulus that would elicit fright or withdrawal from a normal infant (Table 48.3–1). Most infants appear significantly malnourished, and many have

Table 48.3–1
DSM-IV-TR Diagnostic Criteria for Reactive Attachment Disorder of Infancy or Early Childhood

A. Markedly disturbed and developmentally inappropriate social relatedness in most contexts, beginning before age 5 years, as evidenced by either (1) or (2):
   (1) persistent failure to initiate or respond in a developmentally appropriate fashion to most social interactions, as manifest by excessively inhibited, hypervigilant, or highly ambivalent and contradictory responses (e.g., the child may respond to caregivers with a mixture of approach, avoidance, and resistance to comforting, or may exhibit frozen watchfulness)
   (2) diffuse attachments as manifest by indiscriminate sociability with marked inability to exhibit appropriate selective attachments (e.g., excessive familiarity with relative strangers or lack of selectivity in choice of attachment figures)
B. The disturbance in Criterion A is not accounted for solely by developmental delay (as in mental retardation) and does not meet criteria for a pervasive developmental disorder.
C. Pathogenic care as evidenced by at least one of the following:
   (1) persistent disregard of the child's basic emotional needs for comfort, stimulation, and affection
   (2) persistent disregard of the child's basic physical needs
   (3) repeated changes of primary caregiver that prevent formation of stable attachments (e.g., frequent changes in foster care)
D. There is a presumption that the care in Criterion C is responsible for the disturbed behavior in Criterion A (e.g., the disturbances in Criterion A began following the pathogenic care in Criterion C).

Specify type:

Inhibited type: if Criterion A1 predominates in the clinical presentation

Disinhibited type: if Criterion A2 predominates in the clinical presentation

From American Psychiatric Association. *Diagnostic and Statistical Manual of Mental Disorders.* 4th ed. Text rev. Washington, DC: American Psychiatric Association; copyright 2000, with permission.

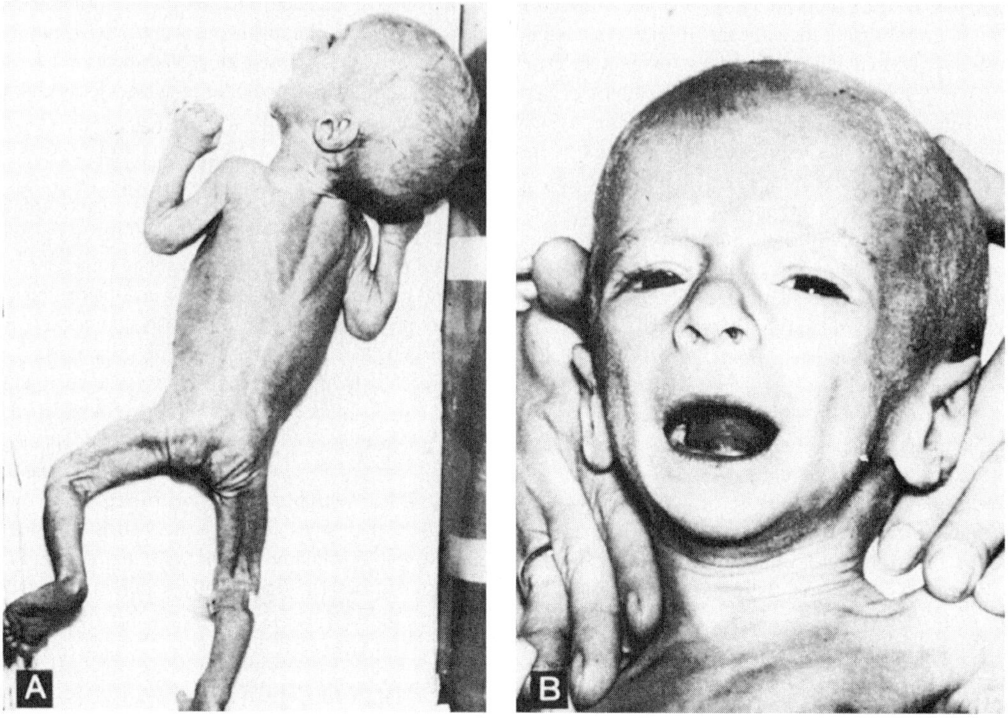

FIGURE 48.3–1
Three-month-old baby boy suffering from failure to thrive secondary to caloric deprivation. Weight is only 1 ounce over birth weight. (Courtesy of Barton Schmitt, M.D., Children's Hospital, Denver, CO.)

protruding abdomens (Figs. 48.3–1 and 48.3–2). Occasionally, foul-smelling, celiaclike stools are reported. In unusually severe cases, a clinical picture of marasmus appears.

The infant's weight is often below the third percentile and markedly below the appropriate weight for his or her height. If serial weights are available, the weight percentiles may have

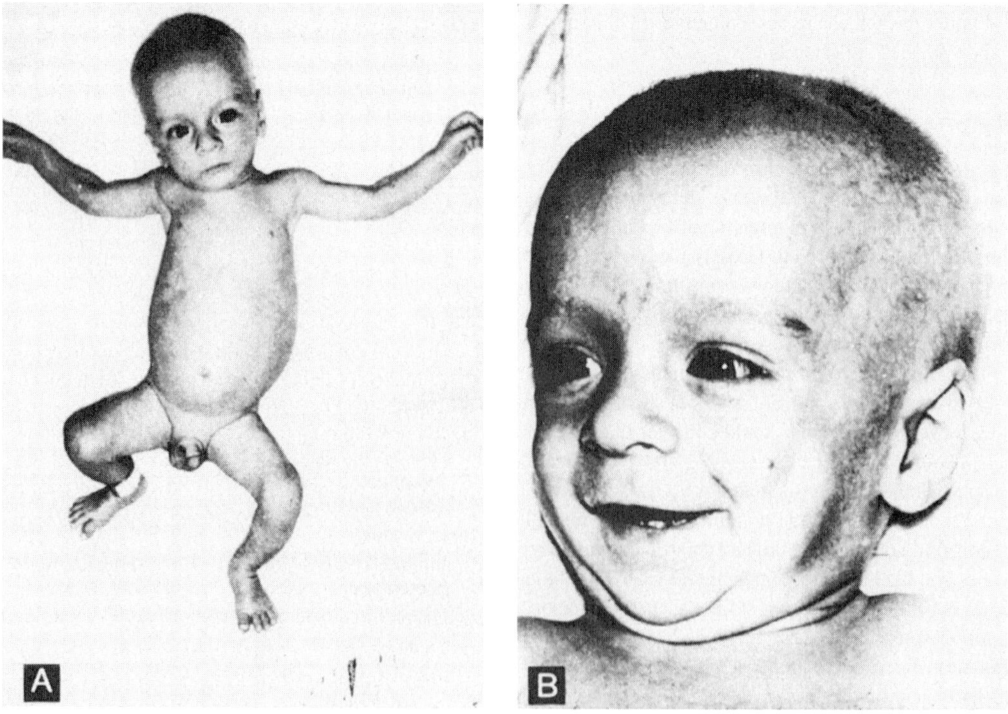

FIGURE 48.3–2
The same infant as in Figure 48.3–1, 3 weeks later, after hospitalization. (Courtesy of Barton Schmitt, M.D., Children's Hospital, Denver, CO.)

decreased progressively because of an actual weight loss or a failure to gain weight as height increases. Head circumference is usually normal for the infant's age. Muscle tone may be poor. The skin may be colder and paler or more mottled than skin of a normal child. Laboratory findings are usually within normal limits, except for abnormal findings coincident with any malnutrition, dehydration, or concurrent illness. Bone age is usually retarded. Growth hormone levels are usually normal or elevated, a finding suggesting that growth failure in these children is secondary to caloric deprivation and malnutrition. The children improve physically and gain weight rapidly after they are hospitalized.

Socially, the infants usually show little spontaneous activity and a marked diminution of both initiative toward others and reciprocity in response to the caregiving adult or examiner. Both mother and infant may be indifferent to separation on hospitalization or to termination of subsequent hospital visits. The infants frequently show none of the normal upset, fretting, or protest about hospitalization. Older infants usually show little interest in their environment. They may not play with toys, even if encouraged; however, they rapidly or gradually take an interest in, and relate to, their caregivers in the hospital.

Classic psychosocial dwarfism or psychosocially determined short stature is a syndrome that usually is first manifest in children 2 to 3 years of age. The children are typically unusually short and have frequent growth hormone abnormalities and severe behavioral disturbances. All of these symptoms result from an inimical caregiver–child relationship. The affectionless character may appear when there is a failure, or lack of opportunity, to form attachments before the age of 2 to 3 years. Children cannot form lasting relationships, and their inability is sometimes accompanied by a lack of guilt, an inability to obey rules, and a need for attention and affection. Some children are indiscriminately friendly.

A 26-month-old girl, recently placed in foster care, was referred by state child protective services with her biological and foster families to assist with long-term case management. Her history included two admissions for failure to thrive in the first year of life and a third admission at 13 months that revealed retinal hemorrhage and a subdural hematoma from suspected shaken baby syndrome. No perpetrator was conclusively identified. When seen with her biological mother in a comfortable, toy-filled room, she stood completely still and maintained little facial expression. She complied completely and in rote fashion with her mother's often-angry instructions, maintaining no sustained eye contact with either her mother or the examiner. When briefly separated from her mother, she showed little reaction, looking up briefly with an odd grimace when her mother returned to the room. Her mother confirmed that her behavior had been similar when she had lived in her home; the child spoke infrequently and rarely sought comfort when distressed. When seen with her foster mother of 3 months, she was markedly more animated, though frequently irritable. She engaged in play freely and referenced both her foster mother and the examiner during play. She stopped playing and stared blankly when separated from her foster mother, though she actively reengaged her foster mother upon her return. The biological mother's parental rights were eventually terminated and though the child was placed in two more homes, she showed the capacity to engage with her new caregivers each time. The girl was diagnosed with reactive attachment disorder, inhibited type. (Courtesy of Neil W. Boris, M.D., and Charles H. Zeanah, M.D.)

Pathology and Laboratory Examination

Although no single specific laboratory test is used to make a diagnosis, many children with the disorder have disturbances of growth and development. Thus, establishing a growth curve and examining the progression of developmental milestones may be helpful in determining whether associated phenomena, such as failure to thrive, are present.

DIFFERENTIAL DIAGNOSIS

Metabolic disorders, pervasive developmental disorders, mental retardation, various severe neurological abnormalities, and psychosocial dwarfism are the primary considerations in the differential diagnosis. Children with autistic disorder are typically well nourished and of age-appropriate size and weight; they are generally alert and active, despite their impairments in reciprocal social interactions. Moderate, severe, or profound mental retardation is present in about 50 percent of children with autistic disorder, whereas most children with reactive attachment disorder of infancy or early childhood are only mildly retarded or have normal intelligence. No evidence indicates that autistic disorder is caused by parental pathology, and most parents of autistic children do not differ significantly from the parents of normal children. Unlike most children with reactive attachment disorder, children with autistic disorder do not improve rapidly if they are removed from their homes and placed in a hospital or other favorable environment. Mentally retarded children may show delays in all social skills. Such children, unlike children with reactive attachment disorder, are usually adequately nourished, their social relatedness is appropriate to their mental age, and they show a sequence of development similar to that seen in normal children.

COURSE AND PROGNOSIS

The course and prognosis of reactive attachment disorder depend on the duration and severity of the neglectful and pathogenic parenting and on associated complications such as failure to thrive. Constitutional and nutritional factors interact in children, who may either respond resiliently to treatment or continue to fail to thrive. Outcomes range from the extremes of death to the developmentally healthy child. In general, the longer a child remains in the adverse environment without adequate intervention, the more the physical and emotional damage and the worse the prognosis. After the pathological environmental situation has been recognized, the amount of treatment and rehabilitation that the family receives affects the child who returns to this family. Children who have multiple problems stemming from pathogenic caregiving may recover physically faster and more completely than they do emotionally.

Table 48.3–2
ICD-10 Diagnostic Criteria for Disorders of Social Functioning with Onset Specific to Childhood or Adolescence

Elective mutism

Note. This disorder is also referred to as selective mutism.

A. Language expression and comprehension, as assessed on individually administered standardized tests, is within the 2 standard deviations limit for the child's age.

B. There is demonstrable evidence of a consistent failure to speak in specific social situations in which the child would be expected to speak (e.g., in school), despite speaking in other situations.

C. Duration of the elective mutism exceeds 4 weeks.

D. There is no pervasive developmental disorder.

E. The disorder is not accounted for by a lack of knowledge of the spoken language required in the social situation in which there is a failure to speak.

Reactive attachment disorder of childhood

A. Onset is before the age of 5 years.

B. The child exhibits strongly contradictory or ambivalent social responses that extend across social situations (but that may show variability from relationship to relationship).

C. Emotional disturbance is shown by lack of emotional responsiveness, withdrawal reactions, aggressive responses to the child's own or other's distress, and/or fearful hypervigilance.

D. Some capacity for social reciprocity and responsiveness is evident in interactions with normal adults.

E. The criteria for pervasive developmental disorders are not met.

Disinhibited attachment disorder of childhood

A. Diffuse attachments are a persistent feature during the first 5 years of life (but do not necessarily persist into middle childhood). Diagnosis requires a relative failure to show selective social attachments manifest by:

(1) a normal tendency to seek comfort from others when distressed and

(2) an abnormal (relative) lack of selectivity in the people from whom comfort is sought

B. Social interactions with unfamiliar people are poorly modulated.

C. At least one of the following must be present:

(1) generally clinging behavior in infancy

(2) attention-seeking and indiscriminately friendly behavior in early or middle childhood

D. The general lack of situation-specificity in the above features must be clear. Diagnosis requires that the symptoms in Criteria A and B above are manifest across the range of social contacts experienced by the child.

Other childhood disorders of social functioning

Childhood disorder of social functioning, unspecified

Reprinted with permission from World Health Organization. *The ICD-10 Classification of Mental and Behavioural Disorders: Diagnostic Criteria for Research.* Copyright, World Health Organization, Geneva, 1993.

TREATMENT

The first consideration in treating reactive attachment disorder is a child's safety. The first decision is often whether to hospitalize the child or to attempt treatment while the child remains in the home. Usually, the severity of the child's physical and emotional state or the severity of the pathological caregiving determines the strategy. A determination must be made regarding the nutritional status of the child and the presence of ongoing physical abuse or threat. Hospitalization is necessary for children with malnourishment. Along with an assessment of the child's physical well-being, an evaluation of the child's emotional condition is important. Immediate intervention must address the parents' awareness and capacity to participate in altering the injurious patterns that have ensued. The treatment team must begin to alter the unsatisfactory relationship between the caregiver and child, which usually requires extensive and intensive intervention and education with the mother or with both parents when possible.

Possible interventions include, but are not limited to, the following: (1) psychosocial support services, including hiring a homemaker, improving the physical condition of the apartment, or obtaining more adequate housing; improving the family's financial status; and decreasing the family's isolation; (2) psychotherapeutic interventions, including individual psychotherapy, psychotropic medications, and family or marital therapy; (3) educational counseling services, including mother–infant or mother–toddler groups, and counseling to increase awareness and understanding of the child's needs and to increase parenting skills; and (4) provisions for close monitoring of the progression of the patient's emotional and physical well-being. Sometimes, separating a child from the stressful home environment temporarily, as in hospitalization, allows the child to break out of the accustomed pattern. A neutral setting such as the hospital is the best place to start with families who are genuinely available emotionally and physically for intervention. If interventions are unfeasible or inadequate or if they fail, placement with relatives or in foster care, adoption, or a group home or residential treatment facility must be considered.

ICD-10

The 10th revision of *International Statistical Classification of Diseases and Related Health Problems* (ICD-10) includes a category for disorders of social functioning. This category includes reactive attachment disorders of childhood, disinhibited attachment disorder of childhood, elective mutism, and two residual categories (Table 48.3–2).

ICD-10 describes the disorders of social functioning with onset specific to childhood and adolescence as a rather heterogeneous group that shares common abnormalities in social functioning arising during the developmental period but that is not mainly characterized by social incapacity or deficit impairing all areas of functioning. Severe environmental "distortions or privations are commonly associated and are thought to play a crucial etiological role in many instances." Although the disorders are well known, they are not clearly defined diagnostically, and workers disagree about the appropriate classifications.

References

Ainsworth MDS. The development of infant–mother attachment. In: Caldwen BM, Ricciuhi HN, eds. *Review of Child Development Research.* Vol 3. Chicago: University of Chicago Press; 1973:1.

Benedersky M, Lewis M. Environmental risks, biological risks, and developmental outcome. *Dev Psychol.* 1994;30:484.

Boris NW, Zeanah CH. Reactive attachment disorder of infancy and early childhood. In: Sadock BJ, Sadock VA, eds. *Kaplan & Sadock's Comprehensive Textbook of Psychiatry.* 7th ed. Vol 2. Baltimore: Lippincott Williams & Wilkins; 2000:2729.

Campbell M, Green WH, Caplon R, David R. Psychiatry and endocrinology in children: early infantile autism and psychosocial dwarfism. In: Beumont PJV,

Burrows GD, eds. *Handbook of Psychiatry and Endocrinology.* Amsterdam: Elsevier; 1982:15.
Cicetti D, Toth S. A developmental psychology perspective on child abuse and neglect. *J Am Acad Child Adolesc Psychiatry.* 1995;34:541.
Ferholt JB. A psychodynamic study of psychosomatic dwarfism. *J Am Acad Child Adolesc Psychiatry.* 1985;14:49.
Klaus MH, Kennell JM. *Parent–Infant Bonding.* 2nd ed. St. Louis: Mosby; 1982.
Lamb ME. Social development. *Pediatr Ann.* 1989;18:292.
Nachmias M, Gunnar MR, Mangelsdorf S, Paritz RH, Buss K. Behavioral inhibition and stress reactivity: moderating role of attachment security. *Child Dev.* 1996;67:508.
Rutter M. *Maternal Deprivation Reassessed.* 2nd ed. Middlesex, England: Penguin, 1981.
Shaw DS, Vondra JI. Infant attachment security and maternal predictors of early behavior problems: a longitudinal study of low income families. *J Child Psychol Psychiatry.* 1995;23:355.
Terwogt MM, Schene J, Koops W. Concepts of motion in institutionalized children. *J Child Psychol Psychiatry.* 1990;31:1131.
Zeanah CH, Larrieu JA. Infant development and developmental risk: a review of the past 10 years. *J Am Acad Child Adolesc Psychiatry.* 1997;36:165.

▲ 48.4 Stereotypic Movement Disorder and Disorder of Infancy, Childhood, or Adolescence Not Otherwise Specified

STEREOTYPIC MOVEMENT DISORDER

According to the text revision of the fourth edition of *Diagnostic and Statistical Manual of Mental Disorders* (DSM-IV-TR), stereotypic movement disorder is repetitive, nonfunctional motor behavior that seems to be compulsive. The behavior significantly interferes with normal activities or produces self-inflicted bodily injuries severe enough to need medical care unless the child is protected. For children with mental retardation, the injurious behavior is dangerous enough to become the focus of treatment.

Epidemiology

The prevalence of stereotypic movement disorder is unknown, but according to DSM-IV-TR, the prevalence of self-injurious behavior is about 2 to 3 percent of children and adolescents. Behaviors such as nail biting are common and affect as many as one half of all school-age children; behaviors such as thumb sucking and rocking are normal in young children but are often maladaptive in older children and adolescents. These behaviors usually do not constitute a stereotypic movement disorder; most children who bite their nails function in daily activities without impairment or self-injury. In one pediatric clinic, as many as 20 percent of children had a history of rocking, head banging, or swaying in one form or another.

Deciding which cases are severe enough to confirm a diagnosis of stereotypic movement disorder may be difficult. The diagnosis is a compilation of many symptoms, and various behaviors must be studied separately to obtain data about prevalence, sex ratio, and familial patterns. It is clear, however, that stereotypic movement disorder is more prevalent in boys than in girls. Stereotypic behaviors are common among children who are mentally retarded; 10 to 20 percent are affected. Self-injurious behaviors occur in some genetic syndromes, such as Lesch-Nyhan syndrome, and also occur in some patients with Tourette's disorder. Self-injurious stereotypic behaviors are increasingly common in persons with severe mental retardation. Stereotypic behaviors are also common in children with sensory impairments such as blindness and deafness.

Etiology

The cause of stereotypic movements is unknown; it is likely to have multiple determinants because of the wide range of behaviors that fall into this category. Many stereotypic behaviors may be associated with normal development. For example, as many as 80 percent of all normal children show rhythmic activities that phase out by 4 years of age. These rhythmic patterns seem to be purposeful, to provide sensorimotor stimulation and tension release, and to be satisfying and pleasurable to the children. The movements may increase at times of frustration, boredom, and tension.

The progression from what are perhaps vicissitudes of normal development to stereotypic movement disorder is believed to reflect disordered development, as in mental retardation or a pervasive developmental disorder. Genetic factors are likely to play a role in some stereotypic movements such as the X-linked recessive deficiency of enzymes leading to Lesch-Nyhan syndrome, which has predictable features including mental retardation, hyperuricemia, spasticity, and self-injurious behaviors. Other stereotypic movements (such as nail biting), although often causing minimal or no impairment, seem to run in families. Some stereotypic behaviors seem to emerge or become exaggerated in situations of neglect or deprivation; such behaviors as head banging have been associated with psychosocial deprivation.

Stereotypic movements seem to be associated with dopamine activity. Neurobiological factors may contribute to the development of stereotypic movement disorders. Dopamine agonists induce or increase stereotypic behaviors, whereas dopamine antagonists decrease them. In one report, four children with attention-deficit/hyperactivity disorder who were treated with a stimulant medication began to bite their nails and fingertips. The nail biting ceased when the medication was eliminated. Endogenous opioids also have been implicated in producing self-injurious behaviors.

Diagnosis and Clinical Features

Affected persons may suffer from one or more symptoms of stereotypic movement disorder; thus, the clinical picture varies considerably. Most commonly, one symptom predominates. The presence of several severe symptoms tends to occur among those most severely afflicted with mental retardation or a pervasive development disorder. Patients frequently have other significant mental disorders, especially disruptive behavior disorders. In extreme cases, severe mutilation and life-threatening injuries may result, and secondary infection and septicemia may follow self-inflicted trauma. The DSM-IV-TR diagnostic criteria for stereotypic movement disorder are listed in Table 48.4–1.

Head Banging. Head banging exemplifies a stereotypic movement disorder that can result in functional impairment. According to the DSM-IV-TR, the male-to-female ratio is 3 to

Table 48.4–1
DSM-IV-TR Diagnostic Criteria for Stereotypic Movement Disorder

A. Repetitive, seemingly driven, and nonfunctional motor behavior (e.g., hand shaking or waving, body rocking, head banging, mouthing of objects, self-biting, picking at skin or bodily orifices, hitting own body).
B. The behavior markedly interferes with normal activities or results in self-inflicted bodily injury that requires medical treatment (or would result in an injury if preventive measures were not used).
C. If mental retardation is present, the stereotypic or self-injurious behavior is of sufficient severity to become a focus of treatment.
D. The behavior is not better accounted for by a compulsion (as in obsessive-compulsive disorder), a tic (as in tic disorder), a stereotypy that is part of a pervasive developmental disorder, or hair pulling (as in trichotillomania).
E. The behavior is not due to the direct physiological effects of a substance or a general medical condition.
F. The behavior persists for 4 weeks or longer.

Specify if:

With self-injurious behavior: if the behavior results in bodily damage that requires specific treatment (or that would result in bodily damage if protective measures were not used)

1. Typically, head banging begins during infancy, between 6 and 12 months of age. Infants strike their heads with a definite rhythmic and monotonous continuity against the crib or another hard surface. They seem to be absorbed in the activity, which may persist until they become exhausted and fall asleep. The head banging is often transitory but sometimes persists into middle childhood. Head banging that is a component of temper tantrums differs from stereotypic head banging and ceases after the tantrums and their secondary gains have been controlled.

Nail Biting. Nail biting begins as early as 1 year of age and increases in incidence until age 12. All nails are usually bitten. Most cases are not severe enough to meet the DSM-IV-TR diagnostic criteria. In other cases, children cause physical damage to the fingers themselves, usually by associated biting of the cuticles, which leads to secondary infections of the fingers and nail beds. Nail biting seems to occur or increase in intensity when a person is either anxious or bored. Some of the most severe nail biting occurs in those who are severely and profoundly mentally retarded and some patients with paranoid schizophrenia; however, some nail biters have no obvious emotional disturbance.

Pathology and Laboratory Examination

No specific laboratory measures are helpful in the diagnosis of stereotypic movement disorder.

Differential Diagnosis

The differential diagnosis of stereotypic movement disorder includes obsessive-compulsive disorder and tic disorders, both of which are exclusionary criteria in DSM-IV-TR. Although stereotypic movements are voluntary and not spasmodic, it is difficult to differentiate these features from tics in all cases. Stereotypic movements are likely to be comforting, whereas tics are often associated with distress. In obsessive-compulsive disorder, the compulsions must be ego-dystonic, although this, too, is difficult to discern in young children.

Differentiating dyskinetic movements from stereotypic movements can be difficult. Because antipsychotic medications can suppress stereotypic movements, clinicians must note any stereotypic movements before initiating treatment with an antipsychotic agent. Stereotypic movement disorder may be diagnosed concurrently with substance-related disorders (e.g., amphetamine use disorders), severe sensory impairments, central nervous system and degenerative disorders (e.g., Lesch-Nyhan syndrome), and severe schizophrenia.

Course and Prognosis

The duration and course of stereotypic movement disorder vary, and the symptoms may wax and wane. As many as 80 percent of normal children show rhythmic activities that seem purposeful and comforting and tend to disappear by 4 years of age. When stereotypic movements are present or emerge more severely later in childhood or in a noncomforting manner, they range from brief episodes occurring under stress to an ongoing pattern in the context of a chronic condition such as mental retardation or a pervasive developmental disorder. Even in chronic conditions, stereotypic behaviors may come and go. In some cases, stereotypic movements are prominent in early childhood and diminish as a child gets older.

The severity of the dysfunction caused by stereotypic movements also varies with the associated frequency, amount, and degree of self-injury. Children who exhibit frequent, severe, self-injurious stereotypic behaviors have the poorest prognosis. Repetitive episodes of head banging, self-biting, and eye poking may be difficult to control without physical restraints. Most nail biting is benign and often does not meet the diagnostic criteria for stereotypic movement disorder. In severe cases in which the nail beds are repetitively damaged, bacterial and fungal infections can occur. Although chronic stereotypic movement disorders can severely impair daily functioning, several treatments help control the symptoms.

Treatment

Treatment should be related to the specific symptom or symptoms being treated, their causes, and the patient's mental age. Treatment modalities yielding the most promising effects have been behavioral and pharmacological, sometimes in combination. In extreme situations in which environmental deprivation is deemed a factor, the psychosocial environment must be adjusted. Behavioral techniques, including reinforcement and behavioral shaping, are successful in some cases. For instances in which severe physical damage occurs, especially in persons who are severely retarded, psychopharmacology must be considered.

The dopamine antagonists are the most commonly used medications for treating stereotypic movements and self-injurious behavior. Phenothiazines have been the most frequently used drugs. Opiate antagonists have reduced self-injurious behav-

Table 48.4–2
DSM-IV-TR Diagnostic Criteria for Disorder of Infancy, Childhood, or Adolescence Not Otherwise Specified

This category is a residual category for disorders with onset in infancy, childhood, or adolescence that do not meet criteria for any specific disorder in the classification.

From American Psychiatric Association. *Diagnostic and Statistical Manual of Mental Disorders.* 4th ed. Text rev. Washington, DC: American Psychiatric Association; copyright 2000, with permission.

Table 48.4–3
ICD-10 Diagnostic Criteria for Stereotyped Movement Disorders

A. The child exhibits stereotyped movements to an extent that either causes physical injury or markedly interferes with normal activities.
B. Duration of the disorder is at least 1 month.
C. The child exhibits no other mental or behavioral disorder in the ICD-10 classification (other than mental retardation).

Reprinted with permission from World Health Organization. *The ICD-10 Classification of Mental and Behavioural Disorders: Diagnostic Criteria for Research,* Copyright, World Health Organization, Geneva, 1993.

iors in some patients without exposing them to tardive dyskinesia or impaired cognition. Additional pharmacological agents that have been tried in the treatment of stereotypic movement disorder include fenfluramine (Pondimin), clomipramine (Anafranil), and fluoxetine (Prozac). In some reports, fenfluramine diminished stereotypic behaviors in children with autistic disorder; in other studies, the results were less encouraging. Open trials indicate that both clomipramine and fluoxetine may decrease self-injurious behaviors and other stereotypic movements in some patients. Trazodone (Desyrel) and buspirone (BuSpar) have also been tried, with unclear results.

DISORDER OF INFANCY, CHILDHOOD, OR ADOLESCENCE NOT OTHERWISE SPECIFIED

DSM-IV-TR describes disorder of infancy, childhood, or adolescence not otherwise specified as a category including disorders with onset in infancy, childhood, or adolescence that do not meet the criteria for any specific disorder. The DSM-IV-TR diagnostic criteria are shown in Table 48.4–2.

ICD-10

The criteria for stereotyped movement disorders from the 10th revision of *International Statistical Classification of Diseases and Related Health Problems* (ICD-10) are listed in Table 48.4–3. ICD-10 also includes two residual categories for childhood mental disorders: (1) other specified behavioral and emotional disorders with onset usually occurring in childhood and adolescence and (2) unspecified behavioral and emotional disorders with onset usually occurring in childhood and adolescence.

REFERENCES

Buitelaar K. Self-injurious behavior in retarded children: clinical phenomena and biological mechanisms. *Acta Paedopsychiatr.* 1993;56:105.

Hanna GL. Stereotypic movement disorder of infancy, childhood, or adolescence NOS. In: Kaplan HI, Sadock BJ, eds. *Comprehensive Textbook of Psychiatry.* 6th ed. Baltimore: Williams & Wilkins; 1995:2359.

King BH. Self-injury by people with mental retardation: a compulsive behavior hypothesis. *Am J Ment Retard.* 1993;98:93.

Leonard HL, Lenane MC, Swedo SE, Rettew DC, Rapoport JL. A double-blind comparison of clomipramine and desipramine treatment of severe onychophagia (nail biting). *Arch Gen Psychiatry.* 1992;48:821.

Linsceid TR, Pejeau C, Cohen S, Footo-Lenz M. Positive side effects in the treatment of SIB using the Self-Injurious Behavior Inhibiting System (SIBIS): implications for operant and biochemical explanations of SIB. *Res Dev Disabil.* 1994;15:81.

Luby JL. Stereotypic movement disorder of infancy and early childhood and disorders of infancy and early childhood not otherwise specified. In: Sadock BJ, Sadock VA, eds. *Kaplan & Sadock's Comprehensive Textbook of Psychiatry.* 7th ed. Vol 2. Baltimore: Lippincott Williams & Wilkins; 2000:2735.

Meiselas KD, Spencer EK, Oberfield R, Peselow ED, Angrist B, Campbell M. Differentiation of stereotypies from neuroleptic-related dyskinesias in autistic children. *J Clin Psychopharmacol.* 1989;9:207.

Ratey JJ. *Mental Retardation: Developing Pharmacotherapies.* Washington, DC: American Psychiatric Press; 1991.

Ricketts RW, Goza AB, Ellis CR, Singh YN, Singh NN, Cooke JC III. Fluoxetine treatment of severe self-injury in young adults with mental retardation. *J Am Acad Child Adolesc Psychiatry.* 1993;32:865.

Silberstein RM, Blackman S, Mandell W. Autoerotic head banging: a reflection of the opportunism of infants. *J Am Acad Child Adolesc Psychiatry.* 1966;5:235.

Sokol MS, Campbell M, Goldstein M, Kriechman AM. Attention deficit disorder with hyperactivity and the dopamine hypothesis: case presentations with theoretical background. *J Am Acad Child Adolesc Psychiatry.* 1987;26:428.

Troster H. Prevalence and functions of stereotyped behaviors in nonhandicapped children in residential care. *J Abnorm Child Psychol.* 1994;22:79.

49

Mood Disorders and Suicide in Children and Adolescents

MOOD DISORDERS

Mood disorders appear in children of all ages, consisting of enduring patterns of disturbed mood; diminished enthusiasm in play activities, sports, friendships, or school; and a general feeling of worthlessness. The core features of major depression are similar in children, adolescents, and adults, with the expression of these features modified to match the age and maturity of the individual.

Mood disorders among children and adolescents have been increasingly diagnosed and treated with a variety of modalities. Although clinicians and parents have always recognized that children and adolescents may experience transient sadness and despair, it has become clear that persistent disorders of mood occur in children of all ages and under many different circumstances. Two criteria for mood disorders in childhood and adolescence are a disturbance of mood, such as depression or elation, and irritability. (Mood disorders in adults are reviewed in detail in Chapter 15. Only those issues that pertain specifically to children and adolescents are discussed here.)

Although diagnostic criteria for mood disorders in the text revision of the fourth edition of *Diagnostic and Statistical Manual of Mental Disorders* (DSM-IV-TR) are almost identical across all age groups, the expression of disturbed mood varies in children according to their age. Young, depressed children commonly show symptoms that appear less often as they grow older, including mood-congruent auditory hallucinations, somatic complaints, withdrawn and sad appearance, and poor self-esteem. Symptoms that are more common among depressed youngsters in late adolescence than in young childhood are pervasive anhedonia, severe psychomotor retardation, delusions, and a sense of hopelessness. Symptoms that appear with the same frequency regardless of age and developmental status include suicidal ideation, depressed or irritable mood, insomnia, and diminished ability to concentrate.

Developmental issues, however, influence the expression of all symptoms. For example, unhappy young children who exhibit recurrent suicidal ideation are generally unable to think of a realistic suicide plan or to put their ideas into action. Children's moods are especially vulnerable to the influences of severe social stressors, such as chronic family discord, abuse and neglect, and academic failure. Most young children with major depressive disorder have histories of abuse or neglect. Children with depressive disorders in the midst of toxic environments may have remission of some or many depressive symptoms when the stressors diminish or when the children are removed from the stressful environment. Bereavement often becomes a focus of psychiatric treatment when children have lost a loved one, even when a depressive disorder is not present.

Depressive disorders and bipolar I disorder are generally episodic, although their onset may be insidious. Manic episodes are rare in prepubertal children but fairly common in adolescents. Attention-deficit/hyperactivity disorder (ADHD), oppositional defiant disorder, and conduct disorder may occur among children who later experience depression. In some cases, conduct disturbances or disorders may occur in the context of a major depressive episode and resolve with the resolution of the depressive episode. Clinicians must clarify the chronology of the symptoms to determine whether a given behavior (such as poor concentration, defiance, or temper tantrums) was present before the depressive episode and is unrelated to it or whether the behavior is occurring for the first time and is related to the depressive episode.

Epidemiology

Mood disorders increase with increasing age, and prevalence in any age group is drastically higher in psychiatrically referred groups than in the general population. Mood disorders in preschool-age children are extremely rare; the rate of major depressive disorder in preschoolers has been estimated to be about 0.3 percent in the community and 0.9 percent in a clinic setting. Among school-age children in the community, about 2 percent have major depressive disorder. Depression is more common in boys than in girls among school-age children, but some bias may be present in the clinic reports, as boys outnumber girls in psychiatric clinics. Among adolescents, about 5 percent in the community have major depressive disorder. Among hospitalized children and adolescents, the rates of major depressive disorder are much higher than in the general community; as many as 20 percent of children and 40 percent of adolescents are depressed. Dysthymic disorder is estimated to be more common than major depressive disorder among school-age children, with rates up to 2.5 percent, compared with 2 percent for major depressive disorder. School-age children with dysthymic disorder have a high likelihood of developing major depressive disorder at some point after 1 year of the dysthymic disorder. In adolescents, as in adults, dysthymic

disorder is less common than major depressive disorder; the prevalence rate for dysthymic disorder is about 3.3 percent, compared with about 5 percent for major depressive disorder.

The rate of bipolar I disorder is exceedingly low in prepubertal children and may take years to be diagnosed, because mania typically appears for the first time in adolescence. The lifetime rate of bipolar I disorder has been estimated to be 0.6 percent in a community study of adolescents. Adolescents with clinical variants of mania (some manic symptoms but without the full diagnostic criteria [bipolar II disorder]) have rates up to about 10 percent, according to some studies.

Etiology

Considerable evidence indicates that the mood disorders in childhood are the same fundamental diseases experienced by adults.

Genetic Factors. Mood disorders in children, adolescents, and adult patients tend to cluster in the same families. An increased incidence of mood disorders is generally found among children of parents with mood disorders and relatives of children with mood disorders, and having one depressed parent probably doubles the risk for offspring. Having two depressed parents probably quadruples the risk of a child having a mood disorder before age 18 compared with the risk for children with two unaffected parents. Some evidence indicates that the number of recurrences of parental depression increases the likelihood that the children will be affected, but this increase may be at least partly related to the affective loading of the parent's own family tree. Similarly, children with the largest number of severe episodes have shown much evidence of dense and deep familial aggregation for major depressive disorder.

Other Biological Factors. Studies of prepubertal major depressive disorder and adolescent mood disorder have revealed biological abnormalities. Prepubertal children in an episode of depressive disorder secrete significantly more growth hormone during sleep than normal children and those with nondepressed mental disorders. These children also secrete significantly less growth hormone in response to insulin-induced hypoglycemia than nondepressed patients. Both abnormalities persist for at least 4 months of full, sustained clinical response, with the last month in a drug-free state. In contrast, the data conflict regarding cortisol hypersecretion during major depressive disorder; some workers report hypersecretion, and others report normal secretion.

The dexamethasone-suppression test is used in children and adolescents but not as frequently or as reliably as in adults. Sleep studies are inconclusive in depressed children and adolescents. Polysomnography shows either no change or changes characteristic of adults with major depressive disorder: reduced rapid eye movement (REM) latency and an increased number of REM periods. A recent study evaluating magnetic resonance imaging (MRI) scans in more than 100 psychiatrically hospitalized children with mood disturbances showed a low frontal lobe volume and a high ventricular volume. These results are consistent with MRI findings in adults with major depression insofar as postmortem studies of depressed adults have demonstrated selective loss of frontal lobe cells and frontal lobe serotonin. Damage to the frontal lobes has also been associated with depressive symptoms in poststroke patients. The frontal lobes seem to have multiple connections with the basal ganglia and the limbic system and are also believed to be involved in the neuropathology of depressive symptomatology.

Thyroid hormone studies have found lower free total thyroxine (FT_4) levels in depressed adolescents than in a matched control group. These values were associated with normal thyroid-stimulating hormone (TSH). This finding suggests that although values of thyroid function remain in the normative range, FT_4 levels have been shifted downward. These downward shifts in thyroid hormone possibly contribute to the clinical manifestations of depression. Some data suggest that the addition of exogenous thyroid hormone can potentiate the effects of antidepressant medication in adults with depression. It has also been shown that mood and cognitive function can be impaired in adults with subclinical hypothyroidism and that the impairment can be corrected with exogenous thyroid hormone. The evidence for adolescents is still only speculative, but dysfunction of the hypothalamic pituitary axis may also contribute to the development and maintenance of depression in certain teenagers.

Social Factors. The finding that identical twins do not have 100 percent concordance suggests a role for nongenetic factors. So far, little evidence indicates that parental marital status, number of siblings, family's socioeconomic status, parental separation, divorce, marital functioning, or familial constellation or structure plays much of a role in causing depressive disorders in children. However, some evidence indicates that boys whose fathers died before they were 13 years of age are more likely than controls to have depression.

The psychosocial deficits in depressed children improve after sustained recovery from the depression. These deficits seem to be secondary to the depression itself and may be compounded by the long duration of most dysthymic or depressive episodes, during which poorly accomplished or unaccomplished developmental tasks accumulate. Among preschoolers with described depressive clinical presentations, the role of environmental influences will probably receive experimental support in the future.

Diagnosis and Clinical Features

Major Depressive Disorder. Major depressive disorder in children is diagnosed most easily when it is acute and occurs in a child without previous psychiatric symptoms. Often, however, the onset is insidious, and the disorder occurs in a child who has had several years of difficulties with hyperactivity, separation anxiety disorder, or intermittent depressive symptoms.

According to the DSM-IV-TR diagnostic criteria for major depressive episode, at least five symptoms must be present for a period of 2 weeks, and there must be a change from previous functioning (see Table 15.2–3 in Chapter 15). Among the necessary symptoms is either a depressed or irritable mood or a loss of interest or pleasure. Other symptoms from which the other four diagnostic criteria are drawn include a child's failure to make expected weight gains, daily insomnia or hypersomnia, psychomotor agitation or retardation, daily fatigue or loss of energy, feelings of worthlessness or inappropriate guilt, diminished ability to think or concentrate, and recurrent thoughts of death. These symptoms must produce social or academic impairment. To meet

the diagnostic criteria for major depressive disorder, the symptoms cannot be the direct effects of a substance (e.g., alcohol) or a general medical condition. A diagnosis of major depressive disorder is not made within 2 months of the loss of a loved one, except when marked functional impairment, morbid preoccupation with worthlessness, suicidal ideation, psychotic symptoms, or psychomotor retardation is present.

A major depressive episode in a prepubertal child is likely to be manifest by somatic complaints, psychomotor agitation, and mood-congruent hallucinations. Anhedonia is also frequent, but anhedonia, as well as hopelessness, psychomotor retardation, and delusions, is more common in adolescent and adult major depressive episodes than in those of young children. Adults have more problems with sleep and appetite than depressed children and adolescents. In adolescence, negativistic or frankly antisocial behavior and the use of alcohol or illicit substances may occur and may justify the additional diagnoses of oppositional defiant disorder, conduct disorder, and substance abuse or dependence. Feelings of restlessness, grouchiness, aggression, sulkiness, reluctance to cooperate in family ventures, withdrawal from social activities, and a desire to leave home are all common in adolescent depression. School difficulties are likely. Adolescents may be inattentive to personal appearance and show increased emotionality, with particular sensitivity to rejection in love relationships.

Children can be reliable reporters about their own behavior, emotions, relationships, and difficulties in psychosocial functions. They may, however, refer to their feelings by many names. Therefore, clinicians must ask children about feeling sad, empty, low, down, blue, or very unhappy, about feeling like crying, or about having a bad feeling that is present most of the time. Depressed children usually identify one or more of these terms as their persistent feeling. Clinicians should assess the duration and periodicity of the depressive mood to differentiate relatively universal, short-lived, and sometimes frequent periods of sadness, usually after a frustrating event, from a true, persistent depressive mood. The younger the child, the more imprecise his or her time estimates are likely to be.

Mood disorders tend to be chronic if they begin early. Childhood onset may be the most severe form of mood disorder and tends to appear in families with a high incidence of mood disorders and alcohol abuse. The children are likely to have such secondary complications as conduct disorder, alcohol and other substance abuse, and antisocial behavior. Functional impairment associated with a depressive disorder in childhood extends to practically all areas of a child's psychosocial world; school performance and behavior, peer relationships, and family relationships all suffer. Only highly intelligent and academically oriented children with no more than a moderate depression can compensate for their difficulties in learning by substantially increasing their time and effort. Otherwise, school performance is invariably affected by a combination of difficulty concentrating, slowed thinking, lack of interest and motivation, fatigue, sleepiness, depressive ruminations, and preoccupations. Depression in a child may be misdiagnosed as a learning disorder. Learning problems secondary to depression, even when long-standing, are corrected rapidly after a child's recovery from the depressive episode.

Children and adolescents with major depressive disorder may have hallucinations and delusions. Usually, these psychotic symptoms are thematically consistent with the depressed mood, occur with the depressive episode (usually at its worst), and do not include certain types of hallucinations (such as conversing voices and a commenting voice, which are specific to schizophrenia). Depressive hallucinations usually consist of a single voice speaking to the person from outside his or her head, with derogatory or suicidal content. Depressive delusions center on themes of guilt, physical disease, death, nihilism, deserved punishment, personal inadequacy, and (sometimes) persecution. These delusions are rare in prepuberty, probably because of cognitive immaturity, but are present in about one half of psychotically depressed adolescents.

Adolescent onset of a mood disorder may be difficult to diagnose when first seen if the adolescent has attempted self-medication with alcohol or other illicit substances. In a recent study, 17 percent of young persons with a mood disorder first received medical attention because of substance abuse. Only after detoxification could the psychiatric symptoms be assessed properly and the mood disorder be diagnosed correctly.

Dysthymic Disorder. Dysthymic disorder in children and adolescents consists of a depressed or irritable mood for most of the day, for more days than not, over a period of at least 1 year. DSM-IV-TR notes that in children and adolescents, irritable mood can replace the depressed mood criterion for adults and that the duration criterion is not 2 years but 1 year for children and adolescents. According to the DSM-IV-TR diagnostic criteria, at least three of the following symptoms must accompany the depressed or irritable mood: poor self-esteem, pessimism or hopelessness, loss of interest, social withdrawal, chronic fatigue, feelings of guilt or brooding about the past, irritability or excessive anger, decreased activity or productivity, and poor concentration or memory. During the year of the disturbance, these symptoms do not resolve for more than 2 months at a time. In addition, no major depressive episode is present during the first year of the disturbance. To meet the DSM-IV-TR diagnostic criteria for dysthymic disorder, a child must not have a history of a manic or hypomanic episode. Dysthymic disorder is also not diagnosed if the symptoms occur exclusively during a chronic psychotic disorder or if they are the direct effects of a substance or a general medical condition. DSM-IV-TR provides for specification of early onset (before 21 years of age) or late onset (after 21 years of age) (see Table 15.2–1).

A child or adolescent with dysthymic disorder may have had a major depressive episode before the onset of dysthymic disorder, but it is much more common for a child with dysthymic disorder for more than 1 year to have major depressive disorder. In this case, both depressive diagnoses are given (*double depression*). Dysthymic disorder in children is known to have an average age of onset that is several years earlier than the age of onset of major depressive disorder. Clinicians disagree about whether dysthymic disorder is a chronic, insidious version of major depressive disorder or a separate disorder. Occasionally, young persons fulfill the criteria for dysthymic disorder, except that their episodes last only 2 weeks to several months, with symptom-free intervals lasting for 2 to 3 months. These minor mood presentations in children are likely to indicate severe mood disorder episodes in the future. Current knowledge suggests that the longer, the more recurrent, the more frequent, and perhaps the less related to social stress these episodes are, the greater the like-

lihood of a severe mood disorder in the future. When minor depressive episodes follow a significant stressful life event by less than 3 months, however, they do not indicate future mood disorder episodes and therefore should be diagnosed as adjustment disorder with depressed mood or bereavement.

Bipolar I Disorder. Bipolar I disorder is being diagnosed with increasing frequency in prepubertal children, with the caveat that "classic" manic episodes are uncommon in this age group, even when depressive symptoms have already appeared. Since prepubertal children with features of depression and mania or hypomania do not usually exhibit discrete mood "cycles," whether these children actually meet diagnostic criteria for bipolar disorder remains controversial. These "atypical" manic episodes among prepubertal children are sometimes associated with family histories of classic bipolar I disorder. Features of the mood and behavior disturbances among prepubertal children who are currently diagnosed with bipolar disorder by some clinicians include extreme mood variability, intermittent aggressive behavior, high levels of distractibility, and poor attention span. These episodes are not likely to be clearly episodic, but show fluctuations, and they seem less responsive to mood-stabilizing agents. Children with atypical hypomanic episodes often have past histories of severe ADHD, making the diagnosis of bipolar disorder even more complicated. In general, families with many relatives with ADHD do not have family histories with an increased rate of bipolar I disorder. The group of children who are currently diagnosed by some clinicians with bipolar disorder function poorly, often require hospitalization, exhibit symptoms of depression, and often have a history of attention-deficit/hyperactivity disorder. Whether these children will develop more discrete mood cycling as they mature or whether their clinical pictures will remain the same over time remains under investigation.

Usually, a major depressive episode precedes a manic episode in an adolescent who develops bipolar I disorder. But when a classic manic episode occurs in an adolescent, it emerges as a definitive change from a preexisting state and often appears with grandiose and paranoid delusions and hallucinatory phenomena. According to DSM-IV-TR, the diagnostic criteria for a manic episode are the same for children and adolescents as for adults (see Table 15.1–6). The diagnostic criteria for a manic episode include a distinct period of an abnormally elevated, expansive, or irritable mood that lasts at least 1 week or for any duration if hospitalization is necessary. In addition, during periods of mood disturbance, at least three of the following significant and persistent symptoms must be present: inflated self-esteem or grandiosity, decreased need for sleep, pressure to talk, flight of ideas or racing thoughts, distractibility, an increase in goal-directed activity, and excessive involvement in pleasurable activities that may result in painful consequences. The mood disturbance suffices to cause marked impairment, and it is not due to the direct effect of a substance or a general medical condition. Thus, manic states precipitated by somatic medications (e.g., antidepressants) cannot be interpreted as indicating a diagnosis of bipolar I disorder.

When mania appears in an adolescent, there is a higher incidence than in adults of psychotic features, and hospitalization is often necessary. Delusions and hallucinations of adolescents may involve grandiose notions about their power, worth, knowledge, family, or relationships. Persecutory delusions and flight of ideas are common. Overall, gross impairment of reality testing is common in adolescent manic episodes. In adolescents with major depressive disorder destined for bipolar I disorder, those at highest risk have family histories of bipolar I disorder and exhibit acute severe depressive episodes with psychosis, hypersomnia, and psychomotor retardation.

Cyclothymic Disorder. The only difference in the DSM-IV-TR diagnostic criteria for child or adolescent cyclothymic disorder is that a period of 1 year of numerous mood swings is necessary instead of the adult criterion of 2 years. Some adolescents with cyclothymic disorder probably experience bipolar I disorder.

Schizoaffective Disorder. The criteria for schizoaffective disorder in children and adolescents are identical to those in adults. Although some adolescents and probably some children do fit the criteria for schizoaffective disorder, little is known about the natural course of their illness, family history, psychobiology, and treatment. In DSM-IV-TR, schizoaffective disorder in children is classified as a psychotic disorder.

Bereavement. Bereavement is a state of grief related to the death of a loved one, which may occur with symptoms characteristic of a major depressive episode. Typical depressive symptoms associated with bereavement include feelings of sadness, insomnia, diminished appetite, and, in some cases, weight loss. Grieving children may become withdrawn and appear sad, and they are not easily drawn into even favorite activities.

In DSM-IV-TR, bereavement is not a mental disorder but is in the category of additional conditions that may be a focus of clinical attention. Children in the midst of a typical bereavement period may also meet the criteria for major depressive disorder when the symptoms persist longer than 2 months after the loss. In some instances, severe depressive symptoms within 2 months of the loss are considered to be beyond the scope of normal grieving, and a diagnosis of major depressive disorder is warranted. Symptoms indicating major depressive disorder exceeding usual bereavement include guilt related to issues beyond those surrounding the death of the loved one, preoccupation with death other than thoughts about being dead to be with the deceased person, morbid preoccupation with worthlessness, marked psychomotor retardation, prolonged serious functional impairment, and hallucinations other than transient perceptions of the voice of the deceased person.

The duration of a normal period of bereavement varies; in children, the duration may depend partly on the support system in place. For example, a child who must be removed from home because of the death of the only parent in the home may feel devastated and abandoned for a long time. Children who lose loved ones may feel that the death occurred because they were bad or did not perform as expected. The reaction to the loss of a loved one may be influenced partly by the child's being prepared for the death because of chronic illness. (Bereavement is also discussed in Chapter 33 and Chapter 2, Section 2.6.)

Pathology and Laboratory Examination. No single laboratory test is useful in making a diagnosis of a mood disorder. A screening test for thyroid function can rule out the possibility of an endocrinological contribution to a mood disorder.

Dexamethasone-suppression tests may be performed serially in cases of major depressive disorder to document whether an initial nonsuppressor becomes a suppressor with treatment or with resolution of the symptoms.

Differential Diagnosis

Psychotic forms of depressive and manic episodes must be differentiated from schizophrenia. Substance-induced mood disorder can sometimes be differentiated from other mood disorders only after detoxification. Anxiety symptoms and conduct-disordered behavior can coexist with depressive disorders and frequently can pose problems in differentiating those disorders from nondepressed emotional and conduct disorders.

Of particular importance is the distinction between agitated depressive or manic episodes and ADHD, in which the persistent excessive activity and restlessness can cause confusion. Prepubertal children do not show classic forms of agitated depression, such as hand wringing and pacing. Instead, an inability to sit still and frequent temper tantrums are the most common symptoms. Sometimes, the correct diagnosis becomes evident only after remission of the depressive episode. If a child has no difficulty concentrating, is not hyperactive when recovered from a depressive episode, and is in a drug-free state, ADHD probably is not present.

Course and Prognosis

The course and prognosis of mood disorders in children and adolescents depend on the age of onset, the severity of the episode, and the presence of comorbid disorders; a young age of onset and multiple disorders predict a poorer prognosis. The mean length of an episode of major depression in children and adolescents is about 9 months; the cumulative probability of recurrence is 40 percent by 2 years and 70 percent by 5 years. Reportedly, depressed children who live in families with high levels of chronic conflict are more likely to have relapses. Follow-up studies have found that in 20 to 40 percent of adolescents who have a major depression, bipolar I disorder will develop in a period of 5 years after the index depression. Clinical characteristics of the depressive episode that suggest the highest risk of developing bipolar I disorder include delusionality and psychomotor retardation in addition to a family history of bipolar illness. Depressive disorders are associated with short-term and long-term peer relationship difficulties and complications, poor academic achievement, and persistently poor self-esteem. Dysthymic disorder has an even more protracted recovery than major depression; the mean episode length is about 4 years. Early-onset dysthymic disorder is associated with significant risks of comorbidity with major depression (70 percent), bipolar disorder (13 percent), and eventual substance abuse (15 percent). The risk of suicide, which represents 12 percent of mortalities in the adolescent age range, is significant among adolescents with depressive disorders.

Treatment

Hospitalization. The important immediate consideration is often whether hospitalization is indicated to keep the child or adolescent safe or whether it is the only setting in which it is possible to initiate treatment. When a patient is suicidal, hospitalization is indicated to provide maximum protection against the patient's own self-destructive impulses and behavior. Hospitalization also may be needed when a child or adolescent has coexisting substance abuse or dependence.

Psychotherapy. Cognitive-behavioral therapy is now widely recognized as an efficacious intervention for the treatment of moderately severe depression in children and adolescents. Cognitive-behavioral therapy aims to challenge maladaptive beliefs and enhance problem-solving abilities and social competence. A recent review of controlled cognitive-behavioral studies in children and adolescents revealed that like adults, both children and adolescents showed consistent improvement with these methods. Other "active" treatments, including relaxation techniques, were also shown to be helpful as adjunctive treatment for mild to moderate depression. Findings from one large controlled study comparing cognitive-behavioral interventions with nondirective supportive psychotherapy and systemic behavioral family therapy showed that 70 percent of adolescents had some improvement with each of the interventions; cognitive-behavioral intervention had the most rapid effect. Another controlled study comparing a brief course of cognitive-behavioral therapy with relaxation therapy favored the cognitive-behavioral intervention. At a 3- to 6-month follow-up, however, no significant differences existed between the two treatment groups. This effect was due to relapse in the cognitive-behavioral group, along with continued recovery in some patients in the relaxation group. Factors that seem to interfere with treatment responsiveness include the presence of comorbid anxiety disorder that probably was present before the depressive episode.

Family education and participation are necessary components of treatment for children with depression, especially to promote more effective conflict resolution. As depressed children's psychosocial function may remain impaired for long periods, even after the depressive episode has remitted, long-term social support from families and (in some cases) social skills interventions are helpful. Modeling and role-playing techniques can be useful in fostering good problem-solving skills.

Pharmacotherapy. The selective serotonin reuptake inhibitors (SSRIs) are widely accepted as a first-line pharmacological intervention for moderate to severe depressive disorders in children and adolescents. Controlled double-blind studies found SSRIs to have efficacy in children and adolescents with depression, and they have a benign adverse effect profile with relatively low lethality potential in overdose. Currently, two double-blind, placebo-controlled studies of an adolescent sample show statistically significant improvement with fluoxetine compared to paroxetine. There were no differences between males and females. All of the available SSRI medications, including fluoxetine (Prozac), sertraline (Zoloft), paroxetine (Paxil), fluvoxamine (Luvox), and citalopram (Celexa) are favorable choices in the treatment of depression for children and adolescents. Starting doses for prepubertal children are lower than doses recommended for adults, and adolescents are generally treated at the same dosages recommended for adults.

Bupropion (Wellbutrin) has stimulant properties as well as antidepressant efficacy and has been used for youth with both

ADHD and depression. It is a useful antidepressant with few anticholinergic properties or other adverse effects such as sedation. Venlafaxine (Effexor), which blocks both serotonin and norepinephrine uptake is also used clinically in the treatment of depression in adolescents. Adverse effects are usually mild, and include agitation, nervousness, and nausea. Mirtazapine (Remeron) is a also a serotonin and norepinephrine uptake inhibitor with a relatively safe adverse-effect profile, but it has not been used as frequently because of its adverse effect of sedation.

No other controlled studies show the efficacy of other antidepressants for depressive disorders in children and adolescents. Tricyclic drugs have not been generally recommended as a treatment for depression in children and adolescents since the SSRIs came on the market. The use of tricyclic antidepressants requires baseline studies, gradual titration of the drug, and monitoring of electrocardiogram (ECG) changes, blood pressure, adverse effects, and, whenever possible, serum levels. Because toxicity produces serious cardiac arrhythmias, seizures, coma, and death, monitoring is essential. The clinical response may be correlated with plasma level. One uncontrolled study using imipramine (Tofranil) to treat prepubertal major depressive disorder obtained good responses when blood levels were 140 to 150 ng/mL. Because some children and adolescents who have depressive episodes eventually experience bipolar II disorder, clinicians must note hypomanic symptoms that may occur during the use of fluoxetine and other antidepressants. In these cases, the medication should be discontinued to determine whether the hypomanic episode then resolves. Hypomanic responses to antidepressants, however, do not necessarily predict that bipolar disorder has emerged.

Bipolar I disorder and bipolar II disorder in childhood and adolescence are treated with lithium (Eskalith) with good results. Children with early-onset bipolar disorder and preexisting disruptive behavior disorders (e.g., conduct disorder and ADHD) who experience bipolar disorders early in adolescence are less likely to respond well to lithium than those without the behavior disorders.

Electroconvulsive Therapy. Electroconvulsive therapy (ECT) has been used for a variety of psychiatric illnesses in adults, primarily severe depressive and manic mood disorders and catatonia. ECT rarely is used for adolescents, although there have been published case reports of its efficacy in adolescents with depression and mania. Currently, case reports suggest that ECT may be a relatively safe and useful treatment for adolescents with severe treatment-resistant affective disorders with psychosis, catatonic symptoms, and persistent suicidality.

SUICIDE

The suicide rate among adolescents has quadrupled since 1950, from 2.5 to 11.2 per 100,000 adolescents. Suicide currently accounts for 12 percent of deaths in the adolescent age group. Adolescent suicide attempts have also increased in recent years; 1-year prevalence rates range from 1.7 to 5.9 percent, and lifetime prevalence rates range from 3.0 to 7.1 percent. Suicidal ideation, gestures, and attempts frequently are associated with depressive disorders, and these suicidal phenomena, particularly in adolescents, are a growing public mental health problem.

Suicidal ideation occurs in all age groups and with greatest frequency when the depressive disorder is severe. More than 12,000 children and adolescents are hospitalized in the United States each year because of suicidal threats or behavior, but completed suicide is rare in children younger than 12 years of age. A young child is hardly capable of designing and carrying out a realistic suicide plan. Cognitive immaturity seems to play a protective role in preventing even children who wish they were dead from committing suicide. Completed suicide occurs about 5 times more often in adolescent boys than in girls, although the rate of suicide attempts is at least 3 times higher among adolescent girls than among boys. Suicidal ideation is not a static phenomenon; it may wax and wane with time. The decision to engage in suicidal behavior may be made impulsively without much forethought or the decision may be the culmination of prolonged rumination.

The method of the suicide attempt influences the morbidity and completion rates independent of the severity of the intent to die at the time of the suicidal behavior. The most common method of completed suicide in children and adolescents is the use of firearms, which accounts for about two thirds of all suicides in boys and almost one half of suicides in girls. The second most common method of suicide in boys, occurring in about one fourth of all cases, is hanging; in girls, about one fourth commit suicide through ingestion of toxic substances. Carbon monoxide poisoning is the next most common method of suicide in boys, but it occurs in less than 10 percent; suicide by hanging and carbon monoxide poisoning are equally frequent among girls and account for about 10 percent each. Additional risk factors in suicide include a family history of suicidal behavior, exposure to family violence, impulsivity, substance abuse, and availability of lethal methods.

Epidemiology

Recently, the suicide rate among adolescents in the United States has risen dramatically, although this is not the case in some other countries. There has been a steady increase in the suicide rate for persons 15 to 19 years of age in the United States. The rate is currently 13.6 per 100,000 for boys and 3.6 per 100,000 for girls. More than 5,000 adolescents commit suicide each year in the United States—1 every 90 minutes. These increased suicide rates are believed to reflect changes in the social environment, changing attitudes toward suicide, and the increasing availability of the means to commit suicide; for example, in the United States, 66 percent of adolescent suicides by boys are committed with firearms, compared with 6 percent in the United Kingdom. Suicide is the third leading cause of death in the United States for persons 15 to 24 years of age and is second among white males in this age group. The rates for suicide depend on age, and they increase significantly after puberty. Whereas fewer than 1 completed suicide per 100,000 occurs in persons younger than 14 years of age, about 10 per 100,000 completed suicides occur in adolescents between 15 and 19 years of age. In adolescents younger than 14 years of age, suicide attempts are at least 50 times more common than suicide completions. Between 15 and 19 years of age, however, the rate of suicide attempts is about 15 times greater than the rate of suicide completions. The number of adolescent suicides over the past several decades has tripled or quadrupled.

Etiology

Universal features in suicidal adolescents are the inability to synthesize solutions to problems and the lack of coping strategies to deal with immediate stressors. Therefore, a narrow view of the options available to deal with recurrent family discord, rejection, or failure contributes to a decision to commit suicide.

Genetic Factors. Evidence of a genetic contribution to suicidal behavior is based on family suicide risk studies and the higher concordance for suicide among monozygotic twins than dizygotic twins. Although the risk for suicide is high in persons with mental disorders—including schizophrenia, major depressive disorder, and bipolar I disorder—the risk for suicide is much higher in relatives of those with mood disorders than in relatives of persons with schizophrenia.

Other Biological Factors. Neurochemical findings show some overlap between persons with aggressive, impulsive behaviors and those who complete suicide. Low levels of serotonin and its major metabolite, 5-hydroxyindoleacetic acid (5-HIAA), have been found postmortem in the brains of persons who completed suicide. Low levels of 5-HIAA have been found in the cerebrospinal fluid of depressed persons who attempted suicide by violent methods. Alcohol and other psychoactive substances may lower 5-HIAA levels, perhaps by increasing the vulnerability for suicidal behavior in an already predisposed person. The mechanism linking low serotonergic function and aggressive or suicidal behavior is unknown, and low serotonin may turn out to be a marker, rather than a cause, of aggression and suicidal propensity. The dexamethasone-suppression test has produced less reliable findings in depressed children and adolescents than in adults, but some studies of children and adolescents indicate an association of nonsuppression on the dexamethasone-suppression test and potentially lethal suicide attempts. In children and adolescents, the association between suicidality and nonsuppression is not necessarily in the context of a major mood disorder.

Social Factors. Children and adolescents are vulnerable to overwhelmingly chaotic, abusive, and neglectful environments. A wide range of psychopathological symptoms may result from exposure to violent and abusive homes. Aggressive, self-destructive, and suicidal behaviors seem to occur with greatest frequency in those who have endured chronically stressful family lives.

Diagnosis and Clinical Features

Direct questioning of children and adolescents about suicidal thoughts is necessary, because studies have consistently shown that parents are frequently unaware of such ideas in their children. Suicidal thoughts (i.e., children talking about wanting to harm themselves) and suicidal threats (e.g., children stating that they want to jump in front of a car) are more common than suicide completion.

The characteristics of adolescents who attempt suicide and those who complete suicide are similar, and about one third of those who complete suicide had made previous attempts. Mental disorders in some persons who attempt or complete suicide include major depressive disorder, manic episodes, and psychotic disorders. Those with mood disorders in combination with substance abuse and a history of aggressive behavior are particularly high-risk adolescents. Those without mood disorders who are violent, aggressive, and impulsive may be prone to suicide during family or peer conflicts. High levels of hopelessness, poor problem-solving skills, and a history of aggressive behavior are risk factors for suicide. Depression alone is a more serious risk factor for suicide in girls than in boys, but boys often have more severe psychopathology than girls who commit suicide. The profile of an adolescent who commits suicide is occasionally one of high achievement and perfectionistic character traits; such an adolescent may have been humiliated recently by a perceived failure, such as diminished academic performance.

In psychiatrically disturbed and vulnerable adolescents, suicide attempts are often related to recent stressors. The precipitants of suicidal behavior include conflicts and arguments with family members and boyfriends or girlfriends. Alcohol and other substance use may further predispose an already vulnerable adolescent to suicidal behavior. In other cases, an adolescent attempts suicide in anticipation of punishment after being caught by the police or other authority figures for a forbidden behavior.

About 40 percent of youthful persons who complete suicide had previous psychiatric treatment, and about 40 percent had made a previous suicide attempt. A child who has lost a parent by any means before age 13 is at high risk for mood disorders and suicide. The precipitating factors include loss of face with peers, a broken romance, school difficulties, unemployment, bereavement, separation, and rejection. Clusters of suicides among adolescents who know one another and go to the same school have been reported. Suicidal behavior may precipitate other such attempts within a peer group through identification—so-called copycat suicides. Some studies have found an increase in adolescent suicide after television programs in which the main theme was the suicide of a teenager. In general, however, many other factors are involved, including a necessary substrate of psychopathology.

One recent study investigated two clusters of teenage suicide in Texas. The researchers found that indirect exposure to suicide through the media was not significantly associated with suicide. Factors that were associated included previous suicidal threats or attempts, self-injury, exposure to someone who had died violently, recent romantic breakups, and a high frequency of moves and changes in schools attended and parental figures lived with.

The tendency of disturbed young persons to imitate highly publicized suicides has been called the *Werther syndrome,* after the protagonist in Johann Wolfgang von Goethe's novel, *The Sorrows of Young Werther.* The novel, in which the hero kills himself, was banned in some European countries after its publication more than 200 years ago because of a rash of suicides by young men who read it; some dressed like Werther before killing themselves or left the book open at the passage describing his death. In general, although imitation may play a role in the timing of suicide attempts by vulnerable adolescents, the overall suicide rate does not seem to increase when media exposure increases.

Treatment

Adolescents who attempt suicide must be evaluated before the decision is made regarding hospitalization or return home. Those who fall into high-risk groups should be hospitalized until the sui-

cidality is no longer present. High-risk persons include those who have made previous suicide attempts; boys older than 12 years of age with histories of aggressive behavior or substance abuse; those who have made an attempt with a lethal method, such as a gun or a toxic ingested substance; those with major depressive disorder characterized by social withdrawal, hopelessness, and a lack of energy; girls who have run away from home, are pregnant, or have made an attempt with a method other than ingesting a toxic substance; and any person who exhibits persistent suicidal ideation. A child or an adolescent with suicidal ideation must be hospitalized if a clinician has any doubt about the family's ability to supervise the child or to cooperate with treatment in an outpatient setting. In such a situation, child protective services must be involved before the child can be discharged. When adolescents with suicidal ideation report that they are no longer suicidal, discharge can be considered only after a complete discharge plan is in place. The plan must include psychotherapy, pharmacotherapy, and family therapy as indicated. A written contract with the adolescent, outlining the adolescent's agreement not to engage in suicidal behavior and providing an alternative if suicidal ideation reoccurs, should be in place. In addition, a follow-up outpatient appointment should be made before the discharge, and a telephone hot-line number should be provided to the adolescent and the family in case suicidal ideation reappears before treatment begins.

References

Dorn LD, Burgess ES, Dichek HL, Putnam FW, Chrousos GP, Gold PW. Thyroid hormone concentrations in depressed and nondepressed adolescents: group differences and behavioral relations. *J Am Acad Child Adolesc Psychiatry.* 1996;35:299.

Esposito CL, Clum GA. Psychiatric symptoms and their relationship to suicidal ideation in a high-risk adolescent community sample. *J Am Acad Child Adolesc Psychiatry.* 2002;41:44.

Kovacs M, Goldston D, Gatsonis C. Suicidal behaviors and childhood-onset depressive disorders: a longitudinal investigation. *J Am Acad Child Adolesc Psychiatry.* 1993;32:8.

Lewinsohn PM, Rohde P, Seeley JR. Psychosocial characteristics of adolescents with a history of suicide attempt. *J Am Acad Child Adolesc Psychiatry.* 1993;32:60.

McLennan JD, Offord DR. Should postpartum depression be targeted to improve child mental health? *J Am Acad Child Adolesc Psychiatry.* 2002;41:28.

Moise FN, Petrides G. Case study: electroconvulsive therapy in adolescents. *J Am Acad Child Adolesc Psychiatry.* 1996;35:312.

Pataki CS. Mood disorders and suicide in children and adolescents. In: Sadock BJ, Sadock VA, eds. *Kaplan & Sadock's Comprehensive Textbook of Psychiatry.* 7th ed. Vol 2. Baltimore: Lippincott Williams & Wilkins; 2000:2740.

Pataki CS, Carlson GA. Bipolar disorder in children and adolescents. In: Shafii M, Shafii S, eds. *Clinical Guide to Depression in Children and Adolescents.* Washington, DC: American Psychiatric Press; 1992:269.

Pfeffer CR, Klerman GL, Hurt SW, et al. Suicidal children grow up: rates and psychosocial risk factors for suicide attempts during follow-up. *J Am Acad Child Adolesc Psychiatry.* 1993;32:106.

Rushton JL, Forcier M, Schectman RM. Epidemiology of depressive symptoms in the National Longitudinal Study of Adolescent Health. *J Am Acad Child Adolesc Psychiatry.* 2002;41:199.

Shaffer D, Garland A, Gould M, Fisher P, Trautman P. Preventing teenage suicide: a critical review. *J Am Acad Child Adolesc Psychiatry.* 1988;27:675.

Steingard RJ, Renshaw PF, Yurgelun-Todd D, et al. Structural abnormalities in brain magnetic resonance images in depressed children. *J Am Acad Child Adolesc Psychiatry.* 1996;35:307.

Vance JE, Bowen NK, Fernandez G, Thompson S. Risk and protective factors as predictors of outcome in adolescents with psychiatric disorder and aggression. *J Am Acad Child Adolesc Psychiatry.* 2002;41:36.

Varanka TM, Weller RA, Weller EB, Fristad MA. Lithium treatment of manic episodes with psychotic features in prepubertal children. *Am J Psychiatry.* 1988;145:1557.

Wade TJ, Cairney J, Pevalin DJ. Emergence of gender differences in depression during adolescence: national panel results from three countries. *J Am Acad Child Adolesc Psychiatry.* 2002;41:190.

50

Early-Onset Schizophrenia

Schizophrenia usually has its onset in late adolescence or early adulthood, but it does (rarely) present in children 10 years of age or younger. Schizophrenia with childhood onset is conceptually the same as schizophrenia in adolescence and adulthood. When schizophrenia occurs in prepubertal children, it more commonly occurs in males. Psychosocial stressors are known to influence the course of schizophrenia, and the same stressors may possibly interact with biological risk factors in the emergence of the disorder. Schizophrenia in prepubertal children includes the presence of at least two of the following: hallucinations, delusions, grossly disorganized speech or behavior, and severe withdrawal for at least 1 month. Social or academic dysfunction must be present, and continuous signs of the disturbance must persist for at least 6 months. The diagnostic criteria for schizophrenia in children are identical to the criteria for the adult form, except that instead of showing deteriorating functioning, children may fail to achieve their expected levels of social and academic functioning.

Before the 1960s, the term *childhood psychosis* was applied to a heterogeneous group of pervasive developmental disorders without hallucinations and delusions. In the 1960s and 1970s, children with evidence of a profound psychotic disturbance early in life often were observed to be mentally retarded, socially dysfunctional with severe communication and language impairments, and without a family history of schizophrenia. In children with psychoses that emerged after the age of 5, however, auditory hallucinations, delusions, inappropriate affects, thought disorder, and normal intelligence were manifest, and these children often had a family history of schizophrenia; they were viewed as exhibiting schizophrenia, whereas the younger children were identified as having an entirely different disorder, either autistic disorder or a pervasive developmental disorder.

In the 1980s, schizophrenia with childhood onset was formally separated from autistic disorder. This change reflected evidence accrued during the 1960s and 1970s that the clinical picture, family history, age of onset, and course of the two disorders differed. After the separation of the disorders, two controversies ensued. First, a minority of researchers remained of the opinion that a subgroup of autistic children will eventually have schizophrenia, as evidence shows for a small group. In general, schizophrenia is easily differentiated from autistic disorder (Table 42–1 in Chapter 42). Most children with autistic disorder are impaired in all areas of adaptive functioning from early life onward. The onset is almost always before 3 years of age, whereas the onset of schizophrenia usually is in adolescence or young adulthood. Schizophrenia in prepubertal children is much rarer than in adolescence and young adulthood, and there are practically no reports of an onset of schizophrenia before 5 years of age. According to the text revision of the fourth edition of *Diagnostic and Statistical Manual of Mental Disorders* (DSM-IV-TR), schizophrenia can be diagnosed in the presence of autistic disorder.

The second controversy concerned applying adult diagnostic criteria for schizophrenia to children. Several reports indicate that some children do have hallucinations, delusions, and thought disorders typical of schizophrenia, but normal developmental immaturities in language development and in separating reality from fantasy sometimes make it difficult to diagnose schizophrenia in children ages 5 to 7 years.

EPIDEMIOLOGY

Schizophrenia in prepubertal children is exceedingly rare; it is estimated to occur less frequently than autistic disorder. In adolescents, the prevalence of schizophrenia is estimated to be 50 times that in younger children, with probable rates of 1 to 2 per 1,000. Boys seem to have a slight preponderance among children with schizophrenia, with an estimated ratio of about 1.67 boys to 1 girl. Boys often become symptomatic at a younger age than girls. It has been estimated that 0.1 to 1 percent present before age 10 years with 4 percent before 15 years of age. The rate of onset increases sharply during adolescence. Schizophrenia rarely is diagnosed in children younger than 5 years of age. The symptoms usually emerge insidiously, and the diagnostic criteria are met gradually over time. Occasionally, the onset of schizophrenia is sudden and occurs in a previously well-functioning child. Schizophrenia also may be diagnosed in a child who has had chronic difficulties and then experiences a significant exacerbation. The prevalence of schizophrenia among the parents of children with schizophrenia is about 8 percent, which is close to twice the prevalence in the parents of patients with adult-onset schizophrenia.

Schizotypal personality disorder is similar to schizophrenia in its inappropriate affects, excessive magical thinking, odd beliefs, social isolation, ideas of reference, and unusual perceptual experiences, such as illusions. Schizotypal personality disorder, however, does not have psychotic features; still, the disorder seems to aggregate in families with adult-onset schizophrenia. Therefore, there is an unclear relation between the two disorders.

ETIOLOGY

Although family and genetic studies provide substantial evidence for a biological contribution to the development of

schizophrenia, no specific biological markers have been identified, and the precise mechanisms of transmission of schizophrenia are not understood. Schizophrenia is significantly more prevalent among first-degree relatives of those with schizophrenia than in the general population. Adoption studies of patients with adult-onset schizophrenia have shown that schizophrenia occurs in the biological relatives, not the adoptive relatives. Additional genetic evidence is supported by higher concordance rates for schizophrenia in monozygotic twins than in dizygotic twins. The genetic transmission pattern of schizophrenia remains unknown, but more genetic loading is seen in the relatives of those with childhood-onset schizophrenia than in the relatives of those with adult-onset schizophrenia.

Currently, no reliable method can identify persons at the highest risk for schizophrenia in a given family. Nevertheless, higher-than-expected rates of neurological soft signs and impairments in sustaining attention and in strategies for information processing appear among high-risk groups of children. Increased rates of disturbed communication styles are found in families with a member with schizophrenia. High expressed emotion, characterized by overly critical responses in families, negatively affects the prognosis of patients with schizophrenia.

Various abnormal, nonspecific results on computed tomography (CT) scans and electroencephalograms (EEGs) have been noted in patients with schizophrenia. Children and adolescents with schizophrenia are more apt to have a premorbid history of social rejection, poor peer relationships, clingy withdrawn behavior, and academic trouble than those with adult-onset schizophrenia. Some children with schizophrenia first seen in middle childhood have early histories of motor milestones and delayed language acquisition that are similar to some symptoms of autistic disorder. The mechanisms of biological vulnerability and environmental influences producing manifestations of schizophrenia remain under investigation.

DIAGNOSIS AND CLINICAL FEATURES

All of the symptoms included in adult-onset schizophrenia may be manifest in children with the disorder. The onset is frequently insidious; after first exhibiting inappropriate affects of unusual behavior, a child may take months or years to meet all of the diagnostic criteria for schizophrenia. Children who eventually meet the criteria often are socially rejected and clingy and have limited social skills. They may have histories of delayed motor and verbal milestones and do poorly in school despite normal intelligence. Although children with schizophrenia and autistic disorder may be similar in their early histories, children with schizophrenia have normal intelligence and do not meet the criteria for a pervasive developmental disorder.

According to DSM-IV-TR, a child with schizophrenia may experience deterioration of function, along with the emergence of psychotic symptoms, or the child may never achieve the expected level of functioning (see Table 13–3 in Chapter 13). Auditory hallucinations commonly occur in children with schizophrenia. They may hear several voices making an ongoing critical commentary, or command hallucinations may tell children to kill themselves or others. The voices may be bizarre, identified as "a computer in my head," Martians, or the voice of someone familiar, such as a relative. Visual hallucinations are experienced by a significant number of children with schizophrenia and often are frightening; the children may see the devil, skeletons, scary faces, or space creatures. Transient phobic visual hallucinations also occur in traumatized children who do not eventually have a major psychotic disorder.

Delusions are present in more than one half of children with schizophrenia; the delusions take various forms, including persecutory, grandiose, and religious. Delusions increase in frequency with increased age. Blunted or inappropriate affects appear almost universally in children with schizophrenia. Children with schizophrenia may giggle inappropriately or cry without being able to explain why. Formal thought disorders, including loosening of associations and thought blocking, are common features among children with schizophrenia. Illogical thinking and poverty of thought are also often present. Unlike adults with schizophrenia, children with schizophrenia do not have poverty of content of speech, but they speak less than other children of the same intelligence and are ambiguous in the way they refer to persons, objects, and events. The communication deficits observable in children with schizophrenia include unpredictably changing the topic of conversation without introducing the new topic to the listener (loose associations). Children with schizophrenia also exhibit illogical thinking and speaking and tend to underuse self-initiated repair strategies to aid in their communication. When an utterance is unclear or vague, normal children attempt to clarify their communication with repetitions, revision, and more detail. Children with schizophrenia, on the other hand, fail to aid communication with revision, fillers, or starting over. These deficits may be conceptualized as negative symptoms in childhood schizophrenia.

The core phenomena for schizophrenia seem to be the same among various age groups, but a child's developmental level influences the presentation of the symptoms. Therefore, delusions of young children are less complex than those of older children. Age-appropriate content, such as animal imagery and monsters, is likely to be a source of delusional fear in children. Other features that seem to occur frequently in children with schizophrenia are poor motor functioning, visuospatial impairments, and attention deficits.

DSM-IV-TR delineates five types of schizophrenia: paranoid, disorganized, catatonic, undifferentiated, and residual.

Tom was a 10-year-old boy who was referred for evaluation after he was found repeatedly dressing in his mother's clothing and demanding that he be taken to nightclubs that he believed wanted him to perform. Tom had always been a talkative child with few friends his own age, but his parents believed he was highly intelligent. As a young child, he had been socially rejected by peers but was able to relate to his teachers and other adults. When he entered the fourth grade, he began to be actively teased by his classmates, who considered him strange. Tom could still attend school, but his grades started to deteriorate because he was not as attentive as he used to be. At home, he became more and more obsessed with being a nightclub performer and seemed to be deep in thought most of the time.

Tom began to warn his mother not to go outside and believed that he and his mother were being followed. He increasingly resisted leaving his mother and began to refuse

to go to school. He explained that he had been communicating with God and that he was here for a larger purpose. He admitted to hearing several voices that would argue and warn him when there was danger. He began to mistrust everyone, including his mother, but at the same time, he would not "allow" her to go to work. Tom was admitted to the children's psychiatric inpatient unit because of his inability to be separated from his mother and his persistent school refusal.

He was started on a trial of risperidone (Risperdal), 0.5 mg twice daily, which was increased to 1 mg twice daily. Tom seemed to be responding over a period of 10 days, the voices were less predominant, and he seemed to be less paranoid. He still seemed to be responding to internal stimuli and held on to the belief that he was a nightclub performer. He had developed troubling akathisia and required benztropine (Cogentin), 0.5 mg twice daily, in addition to the risperidone. After continuing his titration of risperidone and benztropine for approximately 2 weeks, Tom developed a severe dystonic reaction. After the dystonic reaction, Tom's mother refused to allow him to receive risperidone again and requested that another medication be tried. The treatment team agreed that Tom was unable to tolerate a therapeutic dose of risperidone, and use of olanzapine (Zyprexa) was started at 2.5 mg per day. Tom did well on olanzapine, which was increased over time to 7.5 mg per day with good response and virtually no adverse effects aside from mild sedation. Given Tom's deterioration in function over the last year, persistence of auditory hallucinations, and the delusion that he was a performer for more than a 6-month period, a diagnosis of schizophrenia was made. Tom was referred to attend a small, structured, therapeutic day-treatment school program in which he received more individualized educational programming and social skills interventions. Tom was able to attend this school, since he liked the staff, and over time, he improved his social skills with his classmates.

PATHOLOGY AND LABORATORY EXAMINATIONS

No specific laboratory tests are helpful in the diagnosis of schizophrenia with childhood onset. High incidences of pregnancy and birth complications have been reported in the histories of children with schizophrenia, but presently, no specificity has been found in these risks for childhood schizophrenia. EEG studies have not been helpful in distinguishing children with schizophrenia from other children. A recent report of endocrine and neuroimaging tests in adolescents with first-time psychosis did not reveal any specific use of these tests either in making a diagnosis of schizophrenia or in detecting occult medical causes for the psychosis.

DIFFERENTIAL DIAGNOSIS

Children with schizotypal personality disorder have some traits in common with children who meet diagnostic criteria for schizophrenia. Blunted affect, social isolation, eccentric thoughts, ideas of reference, and bizarre behavior may be seen in both disorders; however, in schizophrenia, overt psychotic symptoms such as hallucinations, delusions, and incoherence must be present at some point. When they are present, they exclude a diagnosis of schizotypal personality disorder. Hallucinations alone, however, are not evidence of schizophrenia; patients must show either a deterioration of function or an inability to meet an expected developmental level to warrant the diagnosis of schizophrenia. Auditory and visual hallucinations can appear as self-limited events in nonpsychotic young children who are faced with extreme psychosocial stressors, such as the breakup of their parents, and in children experiencing a major loss or significant change in lifestyle.

Psychotic phenomena are common among children with major depressive disorder, in which both hallucinations and, less commonly, delusions may occur. The congruence of mood with psychotic features is most pronounced in depressed children, although children with schizophrenia may also seem sad. The hallucinations and delusions of schizophrenia are more likely to have a bizarre quality than those of children with depressive disorders. In children and adolescents with bipolar I disorder, it often is difficult to distinguish a first episode of mania with psychotic features from schizophrenia if the child has no history of previous depressions. Grandiose delusions and hallucinations are typical of manic episodes, but clinicians often must follow the natural history of the disorder to confirm the presence of a mood disorder. Pervasive developmental disorders, including autistic disorder with normal intelligence, may share some features with schizophrenia. Most notably, difficulty with social relationships, an early history of delayed language acquisition, and ongoing communication deviance occur in both disorders; however, hallucinations, delusions, and formal thought disorder are core features of schizophrenia and are not expected features of pervasive developmental disorders. Pervasive developmental disorders usually are diagnosed by 3 years of age, but schizophrenia with childhood onset can rarely be diagnosed before 5 years of age.

The abuse of alcohol and other substances sometimes can result in a deterioration of function, psychotic symptoms, and paranoid delusions. Amphetamines, lysergic acid diethylamide (LSD), and phencyclidine (PCP) may lead to a psychotic state. A sudden, flagrant onset of paranoid psychosis is more suggestive of substance-induced psychotic disorder than an insidious onset. Medical conditions that may induce psychotic features include thyroid disease, systemic lupus erythematosus, and temporal lobe disease.

COURSE AND PROGNOSIS

Important predictors of the course and outcome of early-onset schizophrenia include the child's level of functioning before the onset of schizophrenia, the age of onset, how much functioning the child regained after the first episode, and the amount of support available from the family. Children with developmental delays, learning disorders, and premorbid behavioral disorders, such as attention-deficit/hyperactivity disorder and conduct disorder, seem to respond poorly to medication treatment of schizophrenia and are likely to have the most guarded prognoses. In a long-term outcome study of patients with schizophrenia with onset before 14 years of age, the worst prognoses

occurred in children with schizophrenia that was diagnosed before they were 10 years of age and who had preexisting personality disorders.

An additional issue in outcome studies is the stability of the diagnosis of schizophrenia. As many as one third of children who receive a diagnosis of schizophrenia may end up with a diagnosis of a mood disorder (instead of schizophrenia) in adolescence. Children and adolescents with bipolar I disorder may have a better long-term prognosis than children and adolescents with schizophrenia. In adult-onset schizophrenia, family interactions, such as high expressed emotion, may be associated with increased relapse rates. No clear-cut data are available regarding childhood schizophrenia, but the degree of supportiveness, as opposed to critical and overinvolved family responses, probably influences the prognosis.

In general, schizophrenia with childhood onset seems to respond less to medication than schizophrenia with adult onset or adolescent onset, and the prognosis may be poorer. Positive symptoms—that is, hallucinations and delusions—are likely to be more responsive to medication than negative symptoms such as withdrawal. In a recent report of 38 children with schizophrenia who had been hospitalized, two thirds required placement in residential facilities, and only one third improved enough to return home.

TREATMENT

The treatment of schizophrenia with childhood onset includes a multimodality approach. Antipsychotic medications are indicated, given the degree of impairment in both social relationships and academic function exhibited by children with schizophrenia. Children with schizophrenia seem to have less robust responses to antipsychotic medications than adolescents and adults with the same disorder. Family education and ongoing family interventions are critical to maximize the level of support that the family can give the patient. The proper educational setting for the child is also important, because social skills deficits, attention deficits, and academic difficulties often accompany childhood schizophrenia.

Pharmacotherapy

Dopamine receptor antagonists have been largely replaced by the newer atypical antipsychotics as first-line treatment for children and adolescents with schizophrenia, because of their more favorable adverse-effect profiles. These serotonin-dopamine agonists, including risperidone, olanzapine, and clozapine (Clozaril) differ from the conventional antipsychotics in that they are serotonin receptor antagonists with some dopamine (D_2) activity, but without a predominance of D_2 receptor antagonism. They are believed to be more effective in reducing positive and negative symptoms of schizophrenia, and have some, but less, risk of causing extrapyramidal adverse effects. Additional atypical antipsychotics such as quetiapine (Seroquel) and ziprasidone (Geodon) are also serotonin-dopamine antagonists and are being used in clinical practice for children and adolescents with psychotic disorders who do not respond to other atypical antipsychotics.

Several recent studies have suggested that risperidone, a benzisoxazole derivative, is as effective as, and has less troublesome adverse effects than, high-potency conventional antipsychotics such as haloperidol (Haldol) in the treatment of schizophrenia in older adolescents and adults. Published case reports, and limited larger controlled studies have suggested the efficacy of risperidone in the treatment of psychosis in children and adolescents. Risperidone has been reported to cause weight gain and dystonic reactions and other extrapyramidal adverse effects in children and adolescents. Olanzapine is generally well tolerated with respect to extrapyramidal adverse effects compared to conventional antipsychotics and risperidone but is associated with moderate sedation and weight gain.

High-potency conventional antipsychotics, such as haloperidol and trifluoperazine (Stelazine), may be chosen over lower-potency antipsychotics as second-line treatments because of their minimal sedative effects. The dosage for haloperidol ranges from about 1 to 10 mg a day in divided doses. Acute dystonic reactions do occur in children, and 1 to 2 mg a day of benztropine usually is enough to treat the extrapyramidal adverse effects.

Children and adolescents who are treated with antipsychotic medications are at risk for withdrawal dyskinesis when the medication is withdrawn. The long-term adverse effects, including tardive dyskinesia, are perpetual risks for any patients treated with an antipsychotic medication.

Psychotherapy

Psychotherapists who work with children with schizophrenia must take into account a child's developmental level. They must continually support the child's good reality testing and be sensitive to the child's sense of self. Long-term intensive and supportive psychotherapy combined with pharmacotherapy is the most effective approach to this disorder.

References

Adams M, Kutcher S, Antonis E, Bird D. Diagnostic utility of endocrine and neuroimaging screening tests in first-onset adolescent psychosis. *J Am Acad Child Adolesc Psychiatry.* 1996;35:67.

Calderoni D, Wudarsky M, Bhangoo R, et al. Differentiating childhood-onset schizophrenia from psychotic mood disorders. *J Am Acad Child Adolesc Psychiatry.* 2001;40:1190.

Caplan R, Guthrie D, Foy JG. Communication deficits and formal thought disorder in schizophrenic children. *J Am Acad Child Adolesc Psychiatry.* 1992;31:151.

Caplan R, Guthrie D, Komo S. Conversational repair in schizophrenic and normal children. *J Am Acad Child Adolesc Psychiatry.* 1996;35:950.

Cohen D, Lazar G, Couvert P, et al. MECP2 mutation in a boy with a language disorder and schizophrenia. *Am J Psychiatry.* 2002;159:148.

Johns LC, Nazroo JY, Bebbingyon P, Kuipers E. Occurrence of hallucinatory experiences in a community sample and ethnic variations. *Br J Psychiatry.* 2002;180:174.

Kumra S, Shaw M, Merka P, Nakayama E, Augustin R. Childhood-onset schizophrenia: research update. *Can J Psychiatry.* 2001;46:965.

Lykes WC, Cuerva JE. Risperidone in children with schizophrenia. *J Am Acad Child Adolesc Psychiatry.* 1996;35:405.

McClennan JM. Early-onset schizophrenia. In: Sadock BJ, Sadock VA, eds. *Kaplan & Sadock's Comprehensive Textbook of Psychiatry.* 7th ed. Vol 2. Baltimore: Lippincott Williams & Wilkins; 2000:2782.

Miller PM, Byrne M, Hodges A, Lawrie SM, Johnstone EC. Childhood behavior, psychotic symptoms and psychosis onset in young people at high risk of schizophrenia: early findings from the Edinburgh High Risk Study. *Psycho Med.* 2002;32:173.

Quintana H, Ketapang M. Case study: risperidone in children and adolescents with schizophrenia. *J Am Acad Adolesc Psychiatry.* 1995;34:292.

Volkmar FR. Childhood and adolescent psychosis: a review of the past 10 years. *J Am Acad Child Adolesc Psychiatry.* 1996;35:843.

Volva J, Cobol P, Sheinmann B, et al. Clozapine, olanzapine, risperidone, and haloperidol in the treatment of patients with chronic schizophrenia and schizoaffective disorder. *Am J Psychiatry.* 2002;159:255.

51 Adolescent Substance Abuse

Adolescent substance use and abuse remain serious concerns regarding today's youth. Estimates of nearly 25 percent have been made of illicit drug use among adolescents from 12 to 17 years of age. Approximately one of five adolescents has used marijuana or hashish. Approximately one third of adolescents have used cigarettes by age 17 years. Studies of alcohol use among adolescents in the United States have shown that by 13 years of age, one third of boys and almost one fourth of girls have tried alcohol. By 18 years of age, 92 percent of males and 73 percent of females reported trying alcohol, and 4 percent reported using alcohol daily. Of high school seniors, 41 percent reported using marijuana; 2 percent reported using the drug daily. Emergency room visits for heroin use among 18- to 25-year-olds increased over 50 percent from 1997 to 2000.

Drinking among adolescents follows adult demographic drinking patterns: The highest proportion of alcohol use occurs among adolescents in the Northeast; whites are more likely to drink than are other groups; among whites, Roman Catholics are the least likely nondrinkers. The four most common causes of death in persons between the ages of 10 and 24 years are motor vehicle accidents (37 percent), homicide (14 percent), suicide (12 percent), and other injuries or accidents (12 percent). Of adolescents treated in pediatric trauma centers, more than one third are treated for alcohol or drug use.

Studies considering alcohol and illicit drug use by adolescents as psychiatric disorders have demonstrated a greater prevalence of substance use, particularly alcoholism, among biological children of alcoholics than among adopted youngsters. This finding is supported by family studies of genetic contributions, by adoption studies, and by observing children of substance users reared outside the biological home.

During the past decade, several risk factors have been identified for adolescent substance abuse. These include high levels of family conflict, academic difficulties, comorbid psychiatric disorders such as conduct disorder and depression, parental and peer substance use, impulsivity, and early onset of cigarette smoking. The greater the number of risk factors, the more likely it is that an adolescent will be a substance user.

EPIDEMIOLOGY

Alcohol

A recent survey showed that drinking was a significant problem for 10 to 20 percent of adolescents. In the age range of 13 to 17 years, in the United States, there are 3 million problem drinkers and 300,000 adolescents with alcohol dependence. The gap between male and female alcohol consumers is narrowing. Drinking was reported by 70 percent of 8th-grade students: 54 percent reported drinking within the past year, 27 percent reported having gotten drunk at least once, and 13 percent reported binge drinking in the 2 weeks before the survey. By the 12th grade, 88 percent of high school students reported drinking, and 77 percent drank within the past year; 5 percent of 8th-grade students, 1.3 percent of 10th-grade students, and 3.6 percent of 12th-grade students reported daily alcohol use.

Marijuana

Marijuana is the most widely used illicit drug among high school students. It has been termed a "gateway drug," because the strongest predictor of future cocaine use is frequent marijuana use during adolescence. Of 8th-grade, 10th-grade, and 12th-grade students, 10, 23, and 36 percent, respectively, report using marijuana, a slight decrease from the year preceding the survey. Of 8th-grade, 10th-grade, and 12th-grade students, 0.2, 0.8, and 2 percent, respectively, report daily marijuana use. Prevalence rates for marijuana are highest among Native American males and females; these rates are nearly as high in white males and females and Mexican American males. The lowest annual rates are reported by Latin American females, African American females, and Asian American males and females. Among juvenile arrests for illicit drug use in 2000, marijuana was the most commonly used drug by both males (55 percent) and females (60 percent).

Cocaine

The annual cocaine use reported by high school seniors decreased more than 30 percent between 1990 and 2000. Currently about 0.5 percent of 8th-grade students, 1 percent of 10th-grade students, and 2 percent of 12th-grade students are estimated to have used cocaine. The prevalence rates for crack cocaine use, however, is increasing and is most common among those between the ages of 18 and 25.

Lysergic Acid Diethylamide (LSD)

Lysergic acid diethylamide (LSD) is reportedly used by 2.7 percent of 8th-grade students, 5.6 percent of 10th-grade students, and 8.8 percent of 12th-grade students. Of 12th-grade students, 0.1 percent report daily use. The current LSD rates are lower than rates of LSD use during the past 2 decades.

Inhalants

The use of inhalants in the form of glue, aerosols, and gasoline is relatively more common among younger than older adolescents. Among 8th-grade, 10th-grade, and 12th-grade students, 17.6, 15.7, and 17.6

percent, respectively, report using inhalants; 0.2 percent of 8th-grade students, 0.1 percent of 10th-grade students, and 0.2 percent of 12th-grade students report daily use of inhalants.

Multiple Substance Use

Among adolescents enrolled in substance abuse treatment programs, 96 percent are polydrug users; 97 percent of adolescents who abuse drugs also use alcohol.

The reader is referred to Chapter 12, Substance-Related Disorders, for a thorough overview of illicit drug use epidemiologic data.

ETIOLOGY

Genetic Factors

The concordance for alcoholism is reportedly higher among monozygotic than dizygotic twins. Considerably fewer studies have been conducted of families of drug abusers. One twin study of drug users showed that the drug-abuse concordance for male monozygotic twins was twice that for dizygotic twins. Studies of children of alcoholics reared away from their biological homes have shown that these children have about a 25 percent chance of becoming alcoholics.

Psychosocial Factors

A recent study concluded that children in families with the lowest measures of parental supervision and monitoring initiated alcohol, tobacco, and other drug use earlier than children from families with more supervision. The risk was greatest for children below 11 years of age. With more rigorous parental monitoring, young adolescents might be delayed in, or prevented from, initiating drug and alcohol use. Furthermore, increased supervision during middle childhood years may diminish drug and alcohol sampling and ultimately diminish the risk of using marijuana, cocaine, or inhalants in the future.

Comorbidity

Rates of alcohol and drug use are reportedly higher in relatives of children with depression and bipolar disorders. On the other hand, mood disorders are common among those with alcoholism. There is evidence of a strong link between early antisocial behavior, conduct disorder, and substance abuse. Substance abuse may be viewed as one form of behavioral deviance that, unsurprisingly, is associated with other forms of social and behavioral deviance. Early intervention with children who show early signs of social deviance and antisocial behavior may conceivably impede the processes that contribute to later substance abuse.

Comorbidity, the occurrence of more than one substance use disorder or the combination of a substance use disorder and another psychiatric disorder, is common. It is important to know about all comorbid disorders, which may show differential responses to treatment. Surveys of adolescents with alcoholism show rates of 50 percent or higher for additional psychiatric disorders, especially mood disorders. A recent survey of adolescents who used alcohol found that more than 80 percent met criteria for another disorder. The disorders most frequently present were depressive disorders, disruptive behavior disorders, and drug use disorders. These rates of comorbidity are even higher than those for adults. The diagnosis of alcohol abuse or dependence was likely to follow, rather than precede, other disorders; the fact that a large proportion of adolescents with alcoholism have a previous childhood disorder may have both etiological and treatment implications. In this survey, the onset of alcohol disorders did not systematically precede drug abuse or dependence. In 50 percent of cases, alcohol use followed drug use. Alcohol use may be a gateway to drug use but is not in most cases. The presence of other psychiatric disorders was associated with an earlier onset of alcohol disorder, but it did not seem to indicate a more protracted course of alcoholism.

DIAGNOSIS AND CLINICAL FEATURES

According to the text revision of the fourth edition of *Diagnostic and Statistical Manual of Mental Disorders* (DSM-IV-TR), substance-related disorders include substance dependence, substance abuse, substance intoxication, substance withdrawal, and various substance-induced disorders (e.g., alcohol-induced anxiety disorder). *Substance dependence* refers to a cluster of cognitive, behavioral, and physiological symptoms indicating that a person continues the use of a substance despite significant substance-related problems. A pattern of repeated self-administration may result in tolerance, withdrawal, and compulsive drug-taking behavior. Dependence can be applied to every substance, with the exception of caffeine. It requires the presence of at least three symptoms of the maladaptive pattern, which can occur at any time during the same 12-month period. Symptoms of dependence can include tolerance, withdrawal, heavier use of the substance than was intended, an unsuccessful desire to cut down or control use, and reduction of social or occupational activities because of substance use. In addition, the user knows that the substance causes significant impairment but does not give it up. Physiological dependence (evidence of tolerance or withdrawal) may or may not be present.

Substance abuse refers to a maladaptive pattern of substance use leading to clinically significant impairment or distress, manifest by one or more of the following symptoms within a 12-month period: recurrent substance use in situations that cause physical danger to the user, recurrent substance use in the face of obvious impairment in school or work situations, recurrent substance use despite resulting legal problems, or recurrent substance use despite social or interpersonal problems. To meet the criteria for substance abuse, the symptoms must never have met the criteria for substance dependence for this class of substance.

Substance intoxication refers to the development of a reversible, substance-specific syndrome caused by use of a substance. Clinically significant maladaptive behavioral or psychological changes must be present.

Substance withdrawal refers to a substance-specific syndrome caused by the cessation of, or reduction in, prolonged substance use. The substance-specific syndrome causes clinically significant distress or impairs social or occupational functioning.

The diagnosis of alcohol or drug use in adolescents is made through careful interview, observations, laboratory findings, and history provided by reliable sources. Many nonspecific signs may point to alcohol or drug use, and clinicians must be careful to corroborate hunches before jumping to conclusions. Substance use may be viewed on a continuum with experimentation (the mildest use), regular use without obvious impairment, abuse, and finally, dependence. Changes in academic performance, nonspecific physical ailments, changes in relationships with family members,

changes in peer group, unexplained phone calls, or changes in personal hygiene may indicate substance use in an adolescent. Many of these indicators, however, also can be consistent with the onset of depression, adjustment to school, or the prodrome of a psychotic illness. Therefore, it is important to keep the channels of communication with an adolescent open when substance use is suspected.

Substance use is related to a variety of high-risk behaviors, including the use of a weapon, suicidal behavior, early sexual experimentation, risky driving, "heavy metal" or alternative music, and, occasionally, preoccupation with cults or Satanism. Although none of these behaviors necessarily predicts substance use, suspicion may be raised. Adolescents with inadequate social skills may use a substance as a way to try to fit in with a peer group. In some cases, adolescents begin their substance use at home with their parents, who also use substances to enhance their social interactions. Although there is no evidence of a typical adolescent user of alcohol or drugs, many substance users seem to have underlying social skills deficits, academic difficulties, and less than optimal peer relationships.

TREATMENT

Treatment settings that serve adolescents with alcohol or drug use disorders include inpatient units, residential treatment facilities, halfway houses, group homes, partial hospital programs, and outpatient settings. Basic components of adolescent alcohol or drug use treatment include individual psychotherapy, drug-specific counseling, self-help groups (Alcoholics Anonymous [AA], Narcotics Anonymous [NA], Alateen, Al-Anon), substance abuse education and relapse prevention programs, and random urine drug testing. Family therapy and psychopharmacological intervention may be added.

Before deciding on the most appropriate treatment setting for a particular adolescent, a screening process must take place in which structured and unstructured interviews help to determine the types of substances being used and their quantities and frequencies. Determining coexisting psychiatric disorders is also critical. Rating scales are typically used to document pretreatment and posttreatment severity of abuse. The Teen Addiction Severity Index (T-ASI), the Adolescent Drug and Alcohol Diagnostic Assessment (ADAD), and the Adolescent Problem Severity Index (APSI) are several severity-oriented rating scales. The T-ASI is broken down into dimensions that include a family function, school or employment status, psychiatric status, peer social relationships, and legal status.

After most of the information about substance use and the patient's overall psychiatric status has been obtained, a treatment strategy must be chosen and an appropriate setting must be decided on. Two very different approaches to the treatment of substance abuse are embodied in the Minnesota model and the multidisciplinary professional model. The Minnesota model is based on the premise of AA; it is an intensive 12-step program with a counselor who functions as the primary therapist. The program uses self-help participation and group processes. Inherent in this treatment strategy is the need for adolescents to admit that substance use is problematic and that help is necessary. Furthermore, they must be willing to work toward altering their lifestyle to eradicate substance use. The multidisciplinary professional model consists of a team of mental health professionals that usually is led by a physician. Following a case-management model, each member of the team has specific areas of treatment for which he or she is responsible. Interventions may include cognitive-behavioral therapy, family therapy, and pharmacological intervention. This approach usually is suited for adolescents with comorbid psychiatric diagnoses.

Cognitive-behavioral approaches to psychotherapy for adolescents with substance use generally require that adolescents be motivated to participate in treatment and refrain from further substance use. The therapy focuses on relapse prevention and maintaining abstinence.

Psychopharmacological interventions for adolescent alcohol and drug users are still in their early stages. When mood disorders are present, there are clear indications for antidepressants, and generally, the selective serotonin reuptake inhibitors are the first line of treatment. In the past, some pharmacological interventions have been aimed at aiding the abstinence process. For example, disulfiram (Antabuse) has been used in alcoholism to cause an aversive reaction if alcohol is ingested. In certain instances, administration of a medication has been used to block the reinforcing effect of the illicit drug, for instance, giving naltrexone (ReVia) for opioid or alcohol abuse. Some medications mitigate the craving or withdrawal symptoms for a drug that is no longer being used. Clonidine (Catapres) has been used transiently during heroin withdrawal. Occasionally, an intervention is made to substitute the illicit drug with another drug that is more amenable to the treatment situation, for example, using methadone instead of heroin. Adolescents are required to have two documented attempts at detoxification and consent from an adult before they can enter such a treatment program.

Fred is a 16-year-old male admitted to substance abuse treatment for the second time, following a relapse and threats of suicide. He was initially admitted to an inpatient program following a serious suicide attempt. He reported a long history of disruptive behavior and academic failure since childhood. He was increasingly truant and difficult for his family to control. During his first treatment episode, he reported an onset of substance use at age 11 years, rapid progression in substance involvement since age 13 years, then current use of marijuana on a daily basis, drinking alcohol up to several times a week, frequent trips on LSD, and experimentation with a variety of substances. Fred attended group sessions focusing on his initial denial of a substance use problem and then learned the process of recovery while attending other groups and AA and NA meetings. Family group sessions showed him and his parents the need for better communication and more adaptive interactions. Fred gradually responded to the structure of the treatment program, although he had frequent problems with anger control when confronted by peers or staff or when frustrated. Depressive symptoms failed to remit following 2 weeks of abstinence, and Fred was given fluoxetine (Prozac). He showed rapid improvement in mood and treatment compliance. Upon discharge, he was attending NA meetings and outpatient therapy. However, family conflict soon recurred, and Fred became noncompliant with outpatient treatment, medication, and meetings. He resumed old relationships with deviant peers and relapsed into daily marijuana use and occasional alcohol use. (Courtesy of Oscar G. Bukstein, M.D.)

Efficacious treatments for cigarette smoking cessation include nicotine-containing gum, patches, or nasal spray or inhaler. Bupropion (Zyban) aids in diminishing cravings for nicotine and is beneficial in the treatment of smoking cessation.

Because comorbidity influences treatment outcome, it is important to pay attention to other disorders such as mood disorders, anxiety disorders, conduct disorder, or attention-deficit/hyperactivity disorder during the treatment of substance use disorders.

References

Adalbjarnardottir S, Rafnsson FD. Adolescent antisocial behavior and substance use: longitudinal analyses. *Addict Behav.* 2002;27:227.

Arria AM, Yacoubian GS Jr, Fost E, Wish ED. The pediatric forum: ecstasy use among club rave attendees. *Arch Pediatr Adolesc Med.* 2002;156:295.

Bernard RM, Lockhart IA, Boermeester F, Tredoux C. Cigarette smoking in an adolescent population. *S Afr Med J.* 2002;92:58.

Botvin GJ, Griffin KW, Diaz T, Scheier LM, Williams C, Epstein JA. Preventing illicit drug use in adolescents: long-term follow-up data from a randomized control trial of a school population. *Addict Behav.* 2000;25:769.

Bukstein OG. Adolescent substance abuse. In: Sadock BJ, Sadock VA, eds. *Kaplan & Sadock's Comprehensive Textbook of Psychiatry.* 7th ed. Vol 2. Baltimore: Lippincott Williams & Wilkins; 2000:2932.

Chilcoat HD, Anthony J. Impact of parent monitoring on initiation of drug use through late childhood. *J Am Acad Child Adolesc Psychiatry.* 1996;35:91.

Copans SA, Kinney J. Adolescents. In: Kinney J, ed. *Clinical Manual of Substance Abuse.* St. Louis: Mosby-Year Book; 1996:288.

Degenhardt L, Hall W, Linskey M. Alcohol, cannabis and tobacco use among Australians: a comparison of the associations with other drug use and use disorders, affective and anxiety disorders, and psychosis. *Addiction.* 2001;96:1603.

De Micheli D, Formigoni ML. Are reasons for the first use of drugs and family circumstances predictors of future use patterns? *Addict Behav.* 2002;1:87.

Duffy A, Milin R. Case study: withdrawal syndrome in adolescent chronic cannabis users. *J Am Acad Child Adolesc Psychiatry.* 1996;35:1618.

Kaminer Y. *Adolescent Substance Abuse: A Comprehensive Guide to Theory and Practice.* New York: Plenum, 1994.

King CA, Ghaziuddin N, McGovern L, Brand E, Hill E, Naylor M. Predictors of comorbid alcohol and substance abuse in depressed adolescents. *J Am Acad Child Adolesc Psychiatry.* 1996;35:743.

Robbins MS, Kumar S, Walker-Barnes C, Feaster DJ, Briones E, Szapocznik J. Ethnic differences in comorbidity among substance-abusing adolescents referred to outpatient therapy. *J Am Acad Child Adolesc Psychiatry.* 2002;4:394.

Van Kampen J, Katz M. Persistent psychosis after a single ingestion of "ecstasy." *Psychosomatics.* 2001;42:525.

Weinberg NZ. Risk factors for adolescent substance abuse. *J Learn Disabil.* 2001;34:343.

Wills TA, Sandy JM, Yaeger AM, Cleary SD, Shinar O. Coping dimensions, life stress, and adolescent substance use: a latent growth analysis. *J Abnorm Psychol.* 2001;110:309.

52

Child Psychiatry: Additional Conditions That May Be a Focus of Clinical Attention

BORDERLINE INTELLECTUAL FUNCTIONING

The intellectual functioning of children plays a major role in their adjustment to school, social relationships, and family function. Children who cannot quite understand class work and may also be slow in understanding rules of games and the "social" rules of their peer group are often bitterly rejected. Some children with borderline intellectual functioning can mingle socially better than they can keep up academically in class. In these cases, the strengths of these children may be peer relationships, especially if they excel at sports, but eventually, their academic struggles will take a toll on self-esteem, if they are not appropriately remediated.

According to the text revision of the fourth edition of *Diagnostic and Statistical Manual of Mental Disorders* (DSM-IV-TR), a child with borderline intellectual functioning has an intelligence quotient (IQ) in the range of 71 to 84. Impaired adaptive functioning accompanies the disorder, which is diagnosed when difficulties in academic, social, or vocational areas pertaining to borderline intellectual functioning become the focus of clinical attention.

Clinicians must assess a patient's intellectual level and current and past levels of adaptive functioning to diagnose borderline intellectual functioning. In patients with major mental disorders whose current level of adaptive functioning has deteriorated, the diagnosis of borderline intellectual functioning may not be clearly evident. In such situations, clinicians must evaluate the patient's history to determine whether the level of adaptive functioning was compromised even before the onset of the mental disorder.

Only about 6 to 7 percent of the population has a borderline IQ as determined by the Stanford-Binet test or the Wechsler scales. The premise behind the inclusion of borderline intellectual functioning in DSM-IV-TR is that persons may experience difficulties in their adaptive capacities as a result of the intellectual deficits and thus may require attention. In the absence of specific intrapsychic conflicts, developmental traumas, biochemical abnormalities, and other factors linked to any other mental disorder, such persons may experience severe emotional distress. Frustration and embarrassment over their difficulties may shape their life choices and lead to circumstances warranting psychiatric intervention.

Etiology

Genetic factors are increasingly found to play a role in intellectual deficits. Environmental deprivation and infectious and toxic exposures can also contribute to cognitive impairment. Twin and adoption studies support hypotheses that many genes contribute to the development of a particular IQ. Specific infectious processes (e.g., congenital rubella), prenatal exposures (e.g., fetal alcohol syndrome), and specific chromosomal abnormalities (e.g., fragile X syndrome) result in mental retardation.

Diagnosis

DSM-IV-TR contains the following statement about borderline intellectual functioning:

> This category can be used when the focus of clinical attention is associated with borderline intellectual functioning, that is, an IQ in the 71 to 84 range. Differential diagnosis between Borderline Intellectual Functioning and Mental Retardation (an IQ of 70 or below) is especially difficult when the coexistence of certain mental disorders (e.g., Schizophrenia) is involved. Coding note: This is coded on Axis II.

Treatment

The main focus of treatment is to improve practical adaptive skills, social skills, and self-esteem. The goal is to improve the match between the person's capabilities and lifestyle. After the underlying problem becomes known to the therapist, psychiatric treatment can be useful. Many persons with borderline intellectual functioning can function at a superior level in some areas while being markedly deficient in others. By directing such persons to appropriate areas of endeavor, by pointing out socially acceptable behavior, and by teaching them living skills, the therapist can help improve their self-esteem.

ACADEMIC PROBLEM

The editors of DSM-IV-TR refer to *academic problem* as a problem that is not caused by a mental disorder or, if caused by a mental disorder, is severe enough to warrant clinical attention.

This diagnostic category is used when a child or adolescent is having significant academic difficulties that are not deemed to be due to a specific learning disorder or communication disorder or directly related to a psychiatric disorder. Nevertheless, intervention is necessary because the child's achievement in school is significantly impaired. Therefore, a child or adolescent who is of normal intelligence and is free of a learning disorder or a communication disorder but is failing in school or doing poorly falls into this category.

Etiology

Many emotional factors contribute to a child's confidence, competence, and academic success. Children who are troubled by family conflict, social isolation, or shyness may not fulfill their potential. Academic problems have many contributing factors and may arise at any time during the school years. School is the major occupation of children and adolescents and is their main social and educational instrument. Adjustment and success in the school setting depend on children's physical, cognitive, social, and emotional adjustment. Children's general coping mechanisms in many developmental tasks usually are reflected in their academic and social success in school. Boys and girls must cope with the process of separation from parents, adjustment to new environments, adaptation to social contacts, competition, assertion, intimacy, and exposure to unfamiliar attitudes. A corresponding relation often exists between school performance and how well these tasks are mastered.

Anxiety may play a major role in interfering with children's academic performances. Anxiety may hamper their abilities to perform well on tests, to speak in public, and to ask questions when they do not understand something. Some children are so concerned about the way others view them that they cannot attend to their academic tasks. For some children, conflicts about success and fears of the consequences imagined to accompany the attainment of success may hamper academic success. Sigmund Freud described persons with such conflicts as "those wrecked by success." For example, an adolescent girl may be unable to succeed in school because she fears social rejection or the loss of femininity, or both, and she perceives success as being involved with aggression and competition with boys.

Depressed children also may withdraw from academic pursuits; they require specific interventions to improve their academic performances and to treat their depression. Children who do not have major depressive disorder but who are consumed by family problems such as financial troubles, marital discord in their parents, and mental illness in family members may be distracted and unable to attend to academic tasks. Children who receive mixed messages from their parents about accepting criticism and redirection from their teachers may become confused and unable to perform well in school. The loss of the parents as the primary and predominant teachers in a child's life may result in identity conflicts for some children. Some students lack a stable sense of self and cannot identify goals for themselves, a situation that leads to a sense of boredom or futility.

Cultural and economic background can play a role in how well accepted a child feels in school and can affect the child's academic achievement. Familial socioeconomic level, parental education, race, religion, and family functioning can influence a child's sense of fitting in and can affect preparation to meet school demands.

Schools, teachers, and clinicians can share insights about how to foster productive and cooperative environments for all students in a classroom. Teachers' expectations about their students' performance influence these performances. Teachers serve as agents whose varying expectations can shape the differential development of students' skills and abilities. Such conditioning early in school, especially when negative, can disturb academic performance. Therefore, a teacher's affective response to a child can prompt the appearance of an academic problem. Most important is the teachers' humane approach to students at all levels of education, including medical school.

Diagnosis

DSM-IV-TR contains the following statement about academic problem:

> This category can be used when the focus of clinical attention is an academic problem that is not due to a mental disorder or, if due to a mental disorder, is sufficiently severe to warrant independent clinical attention. An example is a pattern of failing grades or of significant underachievement in a person with adequate intellectual capacity in the absence of a Learning or Communication Disorder or any other mental disorder that would account for the problem.

A 17-year-old student who had been getting As and Bs was active on the school football team and had a steady girlfriend. His parents were pleased when he obtained a part-time job, but after 3 months he was failing math. Psychiatric evaluation uncovered no evidence of depression, adjustment disorder, or other psychiatric condition. Family assessment revealed a history of financial difficulties and strong imperatives to earn money. The student modified his work schedule and repeated math in summer school; he went on to attend college without difficulty. (Courtesy of James J. McGough, M.D.)

Treatment

The initial step in determining a useful intervention for an academic problem is a comprehensive diagnostic evaluation. After it is known that another disorder is not directly influencing academic performance, an appropriate intervention can be developed. Although not considered a mental disorder, an academic problem often can be alleviated by psychological means. Psychotherapeutic techniques can be used successfully for scholastic difficulties related to poor motivation, poor self-concept, and underachievement. Early efforts to relieve the problem are critical: Sustained problems in learning and school performance frequently are compounded and precipitate severe difficulties. Feelings of anger, frustration, shame, loss of self-respect, and helplessness—emotions that most often accompany school failures—damage self-esteem emotionally and cognitively, disabling future performance and clouding expectations for success. Generally, children with academic problems require either school-based intervention or individual attention.

Tutoring is an effective technique for dealing with academic problems and should be considered in most cases. Tutoring has proved of value in preparing for objective multiple choice examinations, such as the Scholastic Aptitude Test (SAT) and

Medical College Aptitude Test (MCAT). Taking such examinations repetitively and using relaxation skills are two behavioral techniques of great value in diminishing anxiety.

CHILDHOOD OR ADOLESCENT ANTISOCIAL BEHAVIOR

According to DSM-IV-TR, *child or adolescent antisocial behavior* refers to behavior that is not caused by a mental disorder and includes isolated antisocial acts, not a pattern of behavior. This category covers many acts by children and adolescents that violate the rights of others, such as overt acts of aggression and violence and covert acts of lying, stealing, truancy, and running away from home. Certain antisocial acts, such as fire setting, possession of a weapon, or a severe act of aggression toward another child, require intervention for even a single occurrence. Sometimes, children without a pattern of recurrent aggression or antisocial behavior become involved in occasional less severe behaviors that nevertheless require some intervention. The DSM-IV-TR definition of conduct disorder requires a repetitive pattern of at least three antisocial behaviors for at least 6 months, but childhood or adolescent antisocial behavior may consist of isolated events that do not constitute a mental disorder but do become the focus of clinical attention. The emergence of occasional antisocial symptoms is common among children who have a variety of mental disorders, including psychotic disorders, depressive disorders, impulse-control disorders, and disruptive behavior and attention-deficit disorders, such as attention-deficit/hyperactivity disorder and oppositional defiant disorder.

A child's age and developmental level affect the manifestations of disturbed conduct and influence the child's likelihood to meet the diagnostic criteria for a conduct disorder, as opposed to childhood antisocial behavior. Therefore, a child of 5 or 6 years of age is not likely to meet the criteria for three antisocial symptoms—for example, physical confrontations, the use of weapons, and forcing someone into sexual activity—but a single symptom, such as initiating fights, is common in the 5- to 6-year-old age group. The term *juvenile delinquent* is defined by the legal system as a youth who has violated the law in some way, but the term does not imply that the youth meets the criteria for a mental disorder.

Epidemiology

Estimates of antisocial behavior range from 5 to 15 percent of the general population and somewhat less among children and adolescents. Reports have documented a higher frequency of antisocial behaviors in urban settings than in rural areas. In one report, the risk of coming into contact with the police for antisocial behavior was estimated to be 20 percent for teenage boys and 4 percent for teenage girls.

Etiology

Antisocial behaviors may occur in the context of a mental disorder or in its absence. Antisocial behavior is multidetermined and occurs most frequently in children or adolescents with many risk factors. Among the most common risk factors are harsh and physically abusive parenting, parental criminality, and a child's tendency toward impulsive and hyperactive behavior. Additional associated features of children and adolescents with antisocial behavior are low IQ, academic failure, and low levels of adult supervision. (See Chapter 33 for a discussion of genetic and social factors as causes of adult antisocial behavior.)

Psychological Factors. If their parenting is poor, children experience emotional deprivation, which leads to low self-esteem and unconscious anger. When children are not given any limits, their consciences are deficient because they have not internalized parental prohibitions that account for superego formation. Therefore, they have so-called superego lacunae, which allow them to commit antisocial acts without guilt. At times, such children's antisocial behavior is a vicarious source of pleasure and gratification for parents who act out their own forbidden wishes and impulses through their children. A consistent finding in persons who perform repeated acts of violent behavior is a history of physical abuse.

Diagnosis and Clinical Features

DSM-IV-TR contains the following statement about childhood or adolescent antisocial behavior:

> This category can be used when the focus of clinical attention is antisocial behavior in a child or adolescent that is not due to a mental disorder (e.g., Conduct Disorder or an Impulse-Control Disorder). Examples include isolated antisocial acts of children or adolescents (not a pattern of antisocial behavior).

The childhood behaviors most associated with antisocial behavior are theft, incorrigibility, arrests, school problems, impulsiveness, promiscuity, oppositional behavior, lying, suicide attempts, substance abuse, truancy, running away, associating with undesirable persons, and staying out late at night. The more symptoms present in childhood, the greater the probability of adult antisocial behavior; however, the presence of many symptoms also indicates the development of other mental disorders in adult life.

Differential Diagnosis

Substance-related disorders (including alcohol, cannabis, and cocaine use disorders), bipolar I disorder, and schizophrenia in childhood often manifest themselves as antisocial behavior.

Treatment

Disturbances of conduct frequently accompany the onset of various other psychiatric disorders. The first step in determining the appropriate treatment for a child or an adolescent who is manifesting antisocial behavior is to evaluate the need to treat any coexisting mental disorder, such as bipolar I disorder, a psychotic disorder, or a depressive disorder that may be contributing to the antisocial behavior. The treatment of antisocial behavior usually involves behavioral management, which is most effective when the patient is in a controlled environment or when the child's family members cooperate in maintaining the behavioral program. Schools can help modify antisocial behavior in classrooms. Rewards for prosocial behaviors and positive reinforcement for the control of unwanted behaviors have merit.

Medications generally are not used in patients with rare or occasional antisocial behaviors. Medications have been used

with some success when repetitive episodes of explosive behavior, aggression, or violent outbursts ensue. Lithium (Eskalith) and haloperidol (Haldol) may reduce explosive behavior and rage outbursts. When hyperactivity and impulsivity are contributing factors, methylphenidate (Ritalin) may help to reduce impulsivity and decrease aggression.

It is more difficult to treat children and adolescents who exhibit long-term patterns of antisocial behavior, particularly covert behaviors such as stealing and lying. Group therapy has been used to treat these behaviors, and cognitive problem-solving approaches are potentially helpful.

IDENTITY PROBLEM

According to DSM-IV-TR, *identity problem* refers to uncertainty about issues relating to identity, such as goals, career choice, friendships, sexual behavior, moral values, and group loyalties. An identity problem can cause severe distress for a young person and can lead a person to seek psychotherapy or guidance. Identity problem is, however, not recognized as a mental disorder in DSM-IV-TR. It sometimes manifests in the context of such mental disorders as mood disorders, psychotic disorders, and borderline personality disorder.

Epidemiology

No reliable information is available regarding predisposing factors, familial pattern, sex ratio, or prevalence, but problems with identity formation seem to be a result of life in modern society. Today, children and adolescents often experience great instability in family life, problems with identity formation, conflicts between adolescent peer values and the values of parents and society, and exposure through the media and education to various moral, behavioral, and lifestyle possibilities.

Etiology

The causes of identity problems often are multifactorial and include the pressures of a highly dysfunctional family and the influences of coexisting mental disorders. In general, adolescents who suffer from major depressive disorder, psychotic disorders, and other mental disorders report feeling alienated from family members and experience some turmoil. Children who have had difficulty mastering expected developmental tasks all along are likely to have difficulty with the pressure to establish a well-defined identity during adolescence. Erik Erikson used the term *identity versus role diffusion* to describe the developmental and psychosocial tasks challenging adolescents to incorporate past experiences and present goals into a coherent sense of self.

Diagnosis and Clinical Features

DSM-IV-TR contains the following statement about identity problem:

> This category can be used when the focus of clinical attention is uncertainty about multiple issues relating to identity such as long-term goals, career choice, friendship patterns, sexual orientation and behavior, moral values, and group loyalties.

The essential features of identity problem seem to revolve around the question "Who am I?" Conflicts are experienced as irreconcilable aspects of the self that the adolescent cannot integrate into a coherent identity. If the symptoms are not recognized and resolved, a full-blown identity crisis may develop. As Erikson described, youth manifests severe doubting and an inability to make decisions (abulia), a sense of isolation and inner emptiness, a growing inability to relate to others, disturbed sexual functioning, a distorted time perspective, a sense of urgency, and the assumption of a negative identity. The associated features frequently include marked discrepancy between the adolescent's self-perception and the views that others have of the adolescent; moderate anxiety and depression that are usually related to inner preoccupation, rather than external realities; and self-doubt and uncertainty about the future, with either difficulty making choices or impulsive experiments in an attempt to establish an independent identity. Some persons with identity problem join cultlike groups.

Differential Diagnosis

Identity problem must be differentiated from a mental disorder (such as borderline personality disorder, schizophreniform disorder, schizophrenia, or a mood disorder). At times, what initially seems to be an identity problem may be the prodromal manifestations of one of these disorders. Intense but normal conflicts associated with maturing, such as adolescent turmoil and midlife crisis, may be confusing, but they usually are not associated with marked deterioration in school, vocational, or social functioning or with severe subjective distress. Considerable evidence indicates that adolescent turmoil often is not a phase that is outgrown but an indication of true psychopathology.

Course and Prognosis

The onset of identity problem is most frequently in late adolescence, as teenagers separate from the nuclear family and attempt to establish an independent identity and value system. The onset usually is characterized by a gradual increase in anxiety, depression, regressive phenomena (e.g., loss of interest in friends, school, and activities), irritability, sleep difficulties, and changes in eating habits. The course usually is relatively brief, as developmental lags respond to support, acceptance, and the provision of a psychosocial moratorium.

Extensive prolongation of adolescence with continued identity problem may lead to the chronic state of role diffusion that may indicate a disturbance of early developmental stages and the presence of borderline personality disorder, a mood disorder, or schizophrenia. An identity problem usually resolves by the mid-20s. If it persists, the person with the identity problem may be unable to make career commitments or lasting attachments.

Treatment

Individual psychotherapy directed toward encouraging growth and development usually is considered the therapy of choice. Adolescents with identity problems often feel developmentally unprepared to deal with the increasing demands for social, emotional, and sexual independence. Issues of separation and individuation from their families can be challenging and overwhelming. Treatment is aimed at helping these adolescents develop a sense of competence and mastery about necessary social and voca-

tional choices. A therapist's empathic acknowledgment of an adolescent's struggle can be helpful in the process.

References

Lenzenweger MF, Clarkin JF, Kernberg OF, Foelsch PA. The inventory of personality organization: psychometric properties, factorial composition, and criterion relations with affect, aggressive dyscontrol, psychosis proneness, and self-domains in a nonclinical sample. *Psychol Assess.* 2001;13:577.

Lewis DO, Yeager CA, Lovely R, Stein A, Coham-Portorreal CS. A clinical follow-up of delinquent males: ignored vulnerabilities, unmet needs, and the perpetuation of violence. *J Am Acad Child Adolesc Psychiatry.* 1994;33:518.

Lundy MS, Pfohl B, Kuperman S. Adult criminality among formerly hospitalized child psychiatric patients. *J Am Acad Child Adolesc Psychiatry.* 1993;32:568.

McGough JJ. Border intellectual functioning and academic problem. In: Sadock BJ, Sadock VA, eds. *Kaplan & Sadock's Comprehensive Textbook of Psychiatry.* 7th ed. Vol 2. Baltimore: Lippincott Williams & Wilkins; 2000:1916.

Newcorn JH, Halpern JM. Comorbidity among disruptive behavior. *Child Adolesc Clin North Am.* 1994;3:227.

Rapoport JL, Castellanos FX, Gogate N, Janson K, Kohler S, Nelson P. Imaging normal and abnormal brain development: new perspectives for child psychiatry. *Aust N Z J Psychiatry.* 2001;35:272.

Steiner H, Feldman SS. Childhood or adolescent antisocial behavior. In: Sadock BJ, Sadock VA, eds. *Kaplan & Sadock's Comprehensive Textbook of Psychiatry.* 7th ed. Vol 2. Baltimore: Lippincott Williams & Wilkins; 2000:2903.

Verhulst IC, Eussen MLJM, Berden GFMG, Sanders-Woodstra J, van der Ende J. Pathways of problem behaviors from childhood to adolescence. *J Am Acad Child Adolesc Psychiatry.* 1993;32:388.

53

Psychiatric Treatment of Children and Adolescents

▲ 53.1 Individual Psychotherapy

To approach a child therapeutically, one must have a sense of normal development for a child of a given age as well as an understanding of the life story of the particular child. Wide normal variation exists with respect to how facile children are at describing their emotions in words and the level of motivation they engage in this process. Individual psychotherapy with children focuses on improving children's adaptive skills in and outside the family setting. Treatment reflects an understanding of children's developmental levels and shows sensitivity toward families and environments in which children live. Most children do not seek psychiatric treatment; they are taken to a psychotherapist because of a disturbance noted by a family member, a schoolteacher, or a pediatrician. Children often believe that they are being taken for treatment because of their misbehavior or as a punishment for wrongdoing.

Children can disclose their own thoughts, feelings, moods, and perceptual experiences better than others; however, even when external behavior problems have been identified by others, children's internal experiences may be largely unknown. Children often can describe their feelings in a particular situation but cannot make changes without an advocate's help. Thus, child psychotherapists function as advocates for their child patients in interactions with schools, legal agencies, and community organizations. Child psychotherapists may be called on to make recommendations that affect various aspects of children's lives.

THEORIES AND TECHNIQUES

To best address the emotional, social, and academic issues of children of varying ages and developmental levels, clinicians must have a working knowledge of several psychotherapeutic techniques and their applications in childhood. Psychodynamic approaches are generally mixed with supportive components and behavioral management techniques to build a comprehensive treatment plan for children. Individual psychotherapy with children frequently takes place in conjunction with family therapy, group therapy, and, when indicated, psychopharmacology. Several theoretical systems underlie psychotherapeutic approaches with children, including psychoanalytic theories, behavioral theories, family systems theories, and developmental theories.

Psychoanalytic Theories

In classic psychoanalytic theory, exploratory psychotherapy applies to patients of all ages by reversing the evolution of psychopathological processes. A principal difference noted with advancing age is a sharpening distinction between psychogenetic and psychodynamic factors. The younger the child, the more the genetic and dynamic forces are intertwined. The development of these pathological processes generally is believed to begin with experiences that have proved to be particularly significant to children and have affected them adversely. Although in one sense the experiences were real, in another sense, they may have been misinterpreted or imagined. In any event, to children, these were traumatic experiences that caused unconscious complexes. Being inaccessible to conscious awareness, the unconscious elements readily escape rational adaptive maneuvers and are subject to pathological misuse of adaptive and defensive mechanisms. The result is the development of conflicts leading to distressing symptoms, character attitudes, or patterns of behavior that constitute the emotional disturbance.

The psychoanalytic view of emotional disturbances in children has increasingly assumed a developmental orientation. Thus, the maladaptive defensive functioning is directed against conflicts between impulses that characterize a specific developmental phase and environmental influences or a child's internalized representations of environment. In this framework, disorders result from environmental interference with maturational timetables or conflicts with the environment engendered by developmental progress. The result is difficulty achieving or resolving developmental tasks and fulfilling capacities that are specific to later phases of development. These developmental stages can be expressed in various ways, from Anna Freud's lines of development to Erik Erikson's concept of sequential psychosocial capacities.

The goal of therapy is to help develop good conflict-resolution skills in children so they can function at their appropriate developmental levels. Therapy may again be necessary as children face the challenges of subsequent developmental periods.

Psychoanalytic psychotherapy is a modified form of psychotherapy that is expressive and exploratory and that endeav-

ors to reverse the evolution of emotional disturbance through reenacting and desensitizing traumatic events by freely expressing thoughts and feelings in an interview-play situation. Ultimately, therapists help patients understand the warded-off feelings, fears, and wishes that have beset them.

Whereas the psychoanalytic psychotherapeutic approach seeks improvement by exposure and resolution of buried conflicts, suppressive-supportive-educative psychotherapy works in the opposite fashion by aiming to facilitate repression. Therapists, capitalizing on patients' desire to please, encourage patients to substitute new adaptive and defensive mechanisms. In this therapy, clinicians use interpretations minimally; instead, they emphasize suggestion, persuasion, exhortation, operant reinforcement, counseling, education, direction, advice, abreaction, environmental manipulation, intellectual review, gratification of the patient's current dependent needs, and similar techniques.

Behavioral Theories

All behavior, whether adaptive or maladaptive, is a consequence of the same basic principles of behavior acquisition and maintenance. Behavior is either learned or unlearned. What renders behavior abnormal or disturbed is its social significance. Although theories and their derivative therapeutic intervention techniques have become increasingly complex over the years, all learning can be subsumed in two global basic mechanisms. One is classic respondent conditioning, akin to Ivan Pavlov's famous experiments, and the second is operant instrumental learning, which is associated with B. F. Skinner, although it is basic to both Edward Thorndike's law of effect, which is about the influence of reinforcing consequences of behavior, and to Sigmund Freud's pain-pleasure principle. Both of these basic mechanisms assign the highest priority to the immediate precipitants of behavior and deemphasize remote underlying causal determinants that are important in the psychoanalytic tradition.

The respondent conditioning theory asserts that there are only two types of abnormal behavior: behavioral deficits that result from a failure to learn and deviant maladaptive behavior that is a consequence of learning inappropriate things. Such concepts have always been an implicit part of the rationale underlying all child psychotherapy. Intervention strategies derive much of their success, particularly with children, from rewarding previously unnoticed good behavior, thereby highlighting it, and making it occur more frequently than in the past.

Family Systems Theories

Although families have long been an interest of child psychotherapists, the understanding of transactional family processes has been greatly enhanced by conceptual contributions from cybernetics, systems theory, communications theory, object relations theory, social role theory, ethology, and ecology. The bedrock premise entails the idea of a family functioning as a self-regulating open system that possesses its own unique history and structure. This structure is constantly evolving as a consequence of dynamic interaction between the family's mutually interdependent systems and persons who share a complementarity of needs. From this conceptual foundation, a wealth of ideas has emerged under rubrics such as family development, life cycle, homeostasis, functions, identity, values, goals, congruence, symmetry, myths, rules, roles (spokesperson, symptoms bearer, scapegoat, affect barometer, pet, persecutor, victim, arbitrator, distractor, saboteur, rescuer, breadwinner, disciplinarian, nurturer), structure (boundaries, splits, pairings, alliances, coalitions, enmeshed, disengaged), double bind, scapegoating, pseudomutuality, and mystification. Increasingly, appreciation of the family system sometimes explains why a minute therapeutic input at a critical junction may result in far-reaching changes, whereas in other situations, huge amounts of therapeutic effort seem to be absorbed with minimal evidence of change.

Developmental Theories

Underlying child psychotherapy is the assumption that in the absence of unusual interference, children mature in basically orderly, predictable ways that can be codified in a variety of interrelated psychosociobiological sequential systematizations. The central, overriding role of a developmental frame of reference in child psychotherapy distinguishes it from adult psychotherapy. A therapist's orientation should entail more than a knowledge of age-appropriate behavior derived from such studies as Arnold Gesell's description of the morphology of behavior. It should encompass more than psychosexual development with ego psychological and sociocultural amendments, exemplified by Erikson's epigenetic schema. It extends beyond familiarity with Jean Piaget's sequence of intellectual evolution as a basis for knowing the level of abstraction at which children of various ages may be expected to function or for assessing their capacities for moral orientation.

TYPES OF PSYCHOTHERAPIES

Developing a psychotherapeutic intervention for a particular child includes evaluation of the child's age, developmental level, type of problem, and communication style. Whichever style or combination of techniques a therapist chooses to use in psychotherapy, the relationship between child and therapist is a critical element. The relationship itself often is the primary, if not the sole, ingredient in psychotherapy. The therapist provides a safe space in which to listen, empathize, and solve problems with the child.

Cognitive-behavioral therapy is an amalgam of behavioral therapy and cognitive psychology. It emphasizes how children may use thinking processes and cognitive modalities to reframe, restructure, and solve problems. A child's distortions are addressed by generating alternative ways of dealing with problematic situations. Cognitive-behavioral strategies have been useful in the treatment of mood disorders and anxiety disorders.

Remedial, educational, and patterning psychotherapy is focused on teaching new attitudes and patterns of behavior to children who persist in using immature and inefficient patterns that are often presumed to be due to a maturational lag. Supportive psychotherapy is particularly helpful in enabling a well-adjusted youngster to cope with emotional turmoil engendered by a crisis. It also is used with disturbed youngsters whose less-than-adequate ego functioning may be seriously disrupted by an expressive-exploratory mode or by other forms of therapeutic intervention.

At the beginning of most psychotherapy, regardless of a patient's age and the nature of the therapeutic interventions, the principal therapeutic elements perceived by patients tend to be supportive as a consequence of therapists' universal efforts to be reliably and sensitively responsive. In fact, some therapy may never proceed beyond the supportive level, whereas other therapy develops an expressive-exploratory or behavioral modification flavor on top of the supportive foundation.

Release therapy, described initially by David Levy, facilitates the abreaction of pent-up emotions. Although abreaction is an aspect of many therapeutic undertakings, in release therapy, the treatment situation is structured to encourage only this factor. It is indicated primarily for preschool-age children who have a distorted emotional reaction to an isolated trauma.

Preschool-age children are sometimes treated through the parents, a process called *filial therapy.* Therapists using the strategy should be alert to the possibility that apparently successful filial treatment can obscure a significant diagnosis because patients are not treated directly. The first case of filial therapy was that of Little Hans, reported by Freud in 1905. Hans was a 5-year-old phobic child who was treated by his father under Freud's supervision.

Psychotherapy with children often is psychoanalytically oriented. Through the vehicle of self-understanding, it is focused on enabling children to develop their potential. This development is accomplished by liberating for constructive use psychic energy presumed to be expended in defenses against fantasied dangers. Children generally are unaware of these unreal dangers, their fear of them, and the psychological defenses they use to avoid both the danger and the fear. With the awareness that is facilitated, patients can evaluate the usefulness of their defensive maneuvers and can relinquish unnecessary maneuvers that constitute the symptoms of their emotional disturbance.

Child psychoanalysis, an intensive, uncommon form of psychoanalytic psychotherapy, works on unconscious resistance and defenses during three to four sessions a week. Under these circumstances, therapists anticipate unconscious resistance and allow transference manifestations to mature to a full transference neurosis, through which neurotic conflicts are resolved. Interpretations of dynamically relevant conflicts are emphasized in psychoanalytic descriptions, and elements that are predominant in other types of psychotherapies are not overlooked. Indeed, in all psychotherapy, children should derive support from the consistently understanding and accepting relationship with their therapists. Remedial educational guidance is provided when necessary.

Probably the most vivid examples of the integration of psychodynamic and behavioral approaches, although they are not always explicitly conceptualized as such, appear in the milieu of child and adolescent psychiatric therapy in inpatient, residential, and day treatment facilities. Behavioral change is initiated in these settings, and its repercussions are explored concurrently in individual psychotherapeutic sessions, so that the action in one arena and the information stemming from it augment and illuminate what transpires in the other arena.

Cognitive therapy has been used with children, adolescents, and adults. The approach attempts to correct cognitive distortions, particularly negative conceptions of self, and is used mainly in depressive disorders.

DIFFERENCES BETWEEN CHILDREN AND ADULTS

Logic suggests that psychotherapy with children, who generally are more flexible than adults and who have simpler defenses and other mental mechanisms, should consume less time than comparable treatment of adults. Experience usually does not confirm this expectation, because children usually lack some elements that contribute to successful treatment. A child, for example, typically does not seek help. As a consequence, one of a therapist's first tasks is to stimulate a child's motivation for treatment. Children commonly begin therapy involuntarily, often without the benefit of true parental support. Although parents may want their children to be helped or changed, the desire often is generated by frustrated anger toward the children. Typically, the anger is accompanied by relative insensitivity to what therapists perceive as the children's need and the basis for a therapeutic alliance. Therefore, whereas adult patients frequently perceive advantages in getting well, children may envision therapeutic change as nothing more than conforming to a disagreeable reality, an attitude that heightens the likelihood of their perceiving a therapist as the parent's punitive agent. This is hardly the most fertile soil in which to nurture a therapeutic alliance.

Children tend to externalize internal conflicts in search of alloplastic adaptations, and they find it difficult to conceive of problem resolution except by altering an obstructing environment. A passive, masochistic boy who is the constant butt of his schoolmates' teasing finds it inconceivable that the situation can be rectified by altering his mode of handling his aggressive impulses rather than by someone's controlling his tormentors, a view that may be reinforced by significant adults in his environment. The tendency of children to reenact their feelings in new situations facilitates the early appearance of spontaneous and global transference reactions that may be troublesome. Concurrently, children's eagerness for new experiences, coupled with their natural developmental fluidity, tends to limit the intensity and therapeutic usefulness of subsequent transference developments.

Children have a limited capacity for self-observation, with the notable exception of some obsessive children who resemble adults in this ability. Such obsessive children, however, usually isolate the vital emotional components. In exploratory-interpretative psychotherapies, the development of a capacity for ego splitting—that is, simultaneous emotional involvement and self-observation—is most helpful. Only by identifying with a trusted adult and in alliance with this adult can children approach such an ideal. A therapist's gender and the relatively superficial aspects of the therapist's demeanor may be important elements in the development of a trusting relationship with a child.

Regressive behavioral and communicative modes can be wearing on child therapists. Typically motor-minded, even when they do not require external controls, children may demand a physical stamina that is not a significant factor in therapy with adults. The age appropriateness of such primitive mechanisms as denial, projection, and isolation hinders the process of working through, which relies on a patient's synthesizing and integrating capacities, both of which are immature in children. Environmental pressures on therapists are also generally greater in psychotherapeutic work with children than in work with adults.

Although children compare unfavorably with adults in many qualities that are generally considered desirable in therapy, children have the advantage of their active maturational and developmental forces. The history of psychotherapy for children is punctuated by efforts to harness these assets and to overcome the liabilities. Recognition of the importance of play constituted a major forward stride in these efforts.

PLAYROOM

The structure, design, and furnishing of the playroom are important. Some therapists maintain that the toys should be few, simple, and carefully selected to facilitate the communication of fantasy. Other therapists suggest that a wide variety of playthings should be available to increase the range of feelings that children can express. These contrasting recommendations have been attributed to differences in therapeutic methods. Some therapists tend to avoid interpretation, even of conscious ideas, whereas others recommend the interpretation of unconscious content directly and quickly.

Therapists tend to change their preferences in equipment as they accumulate experience and develop confidence in their abilities. Although special equipment—such as genital dolls, amputation dolls, and see-through anatomically complete (except for genitalia) models—has been used in therapy, many therapists have observed that the unusual nature of such items risks making children wary and suspicious of a therapist's motives. Until dolls available to children in their own homes include genitalia, the psychological content that special dolls are designed to elicit may be more available at the appropriate time with conventional dolls.

Although the choices of play materials vary among therapists, the following equipment can constitute a well-balanced playroom or play area: multigenerational families of flexible but sturdy dolls of various races; additional dolls representing special roles and feelings, such as police officer, doctor, and soldier; dollhouse furnishings with or without a dollhouse; toy animals; puppets; paper, crayons, paint, and blunt-ended scissors; a spongelike ball; clay or something comparable; tools such as rubber hammers, rubber knives, and guns; building blocks, cars, trucks, and airplanes; and eating utensils. The toys should enable children to communicate through play. Therapists should avoid toys and materials that are fragile or break easily, that can result in physical injury to a child, or that can increase a child's guilt.

Each child should have a special drawer or box, if space is available, in which to store items the child brings to the therapy session or to store projects, such as drawings and stories, for future retrieval. Limits must be set so that the private storage area is not used to hoard communal play equipment and thus deprive the other patients. Some therapists assert that absence of such arrangements evokes material about sibling rivalry; others believe that this assertion is a rationalization for not respecting children's privacy, since sibling feelings can be expressed in other ways.

INITIAL APPROACH

Various approaches are associated with each therapist's individual style and perception of children's needs, from approaches in which a therapist endeavors to direct children's thought content and activity (release therapy, some behavior therapy, and certain educational patterning techniques) to exploratory methods in which a therapist endeavors to follow children's leads. Even though children determine the focus, therapists structure the situation. Encouraging children to say whatever they wish and to play freely, as in exploratory psychotherapy, establishes a definite structure. Therapists create an atmosphere in which they get to know all about a child—the good side as well as the bad side, as children would put it. A therapist may communicate to a child that the child's response elicits neither anger or pleasure but only understanding from the therapist. Such an assertion does not imply that therapists have no emotions, but it assures the young patient that the therapist's personal feelings and standards are subordinate to understanding the youngster.

THERAPEUTIC INTERVENTIONS

Psychotherapy with children and adolescents generally is more directed and active than it often is with adults. Children usually cannot synthesize histories of their own lives, but they are excellent reporters of their current internal states. Even with adolescents, a therapist often takes an active role, is somewhat less open-ended than with adults, and offers more direction and advocacy than with adults. A child or adolescent therapist often makes exclamations and expresses confrontations in which the therapist directs attention to data of which patients are cognizant. A therapist may use interpretations, designed to expand patients' conscious awareness of themselves, by making explicit the elements that have previously been expressed implicitly in the patients' thoughts, feelings, and behavior. Beyond interpretation, therapists may educatively offer new information to which patients have not been exposed previously. At the most active end of the continuum are advising, counseling, and directing, which are designed to help patients adopt a course of action or a conscious attitude.

Nurturing and maintaining a therapeutic alliance may require educating children about the process of therapy. Another educational intervention may entail assigning labels to affects that have not been part of a youngster's past experience. Rarely does therapy have to compensate for a real absence of education about acceptable decorum and playing games. Children usually are not in therapy because they have never been exposed to educational efforts but because repeated educational efforts have failed. Therefore, therapy generally need not include additional teaching efforts, despite the frequent temptation to offer them.

Adults' natural educational fervor with children often is accompanied by a paradoxical tendency to protect children from learning about some of life's realities. In the past, this tendency contributed to the stork's role in childbirth, the story that persons who have died are taking a long trip, and similar fairy-tale explanations about natural phenomena that adults are uncomfortable communicating to children. Although adults are more honest with children today, therapists can find themselves in situations in which their overwhelming urge to protect a hurt child may be as disadvantageous to the child as the stork myth. Alternatively, information given to the child must account for individual problems and developmental levels.

The temptation for therapists to offer themselves as a model for identification may also stem from helpful educational attitudes toward children. Although this may sometimes be an appropriate therapeutic

strategy, therapists should not lose sight of the pitfalls of this apparently innocuous maneuver.

PARENTS

Psychotherapy with children requires parental involvement, which does not necessarily reflect parental culpability for a youngster's emotional difficulties but is a reality of a child's dependent state. This fact cannot be stressed too much because of an occupational hazard shared by many who work with children—the urge to rescue children from their parents' negative influences, a desire that sometimes is related to an unconscious competitive desire to be a better parent than the child's or the therapist's own parents.

Parents are involved in child psychotherapy to varying degrees. For preschool-age children, the entire therapeutic effort may be directed toward the parents, without any direct treatment of the child. At the other extreme, children can be treated in psychotherapy without any parental involvement beyond the payment of fees and perhaps transporting the child to the therapy sessions. Most practitioners, however, prefer to maintain an informative alliance with parents for the purpose of obtaining additional information about the child.

Probably the most frequent parental arrangements are those developed in child guidance clinics—that is, parent guidance focused on the child or the parent–child interaction and therapy for the parents' own individual needs concurrent with the child's therapy. Parents may be seen by their child's therapist or by someone else. Recently, there have been increasing efforts to shift the focus from the child as the primary patient to the child as the family's emissary to the clinic. In such family therapy, all or selected members of the family are treated simultaneously as a family group. Although the preferences of specific clinics and practitioners for either an individual or a family therapeutic approach may be unavoidable, the final decision regarding which therapeutic strategy or combination to use should be derived from the clinical assessment.

CONFIDENTIALITY

The issue of confidentiality takes on greater meaning as children grow older. Very young children are unlikely to be as concerned about this issue as adolescents are. Confidentiality usually is preserved unless a child is believed to be in danger or to be a danger to someone else. In other situations, a child's permission usually is sought before a specific issue is raised with parents. There are advantages to creating an atmosphere in which children can feel that all words and actions are viewed by therapists as simultaneously both serious and tentative. In other words, children's communications do not bind therapists to a commitment; nevertheless, they are too important to be communicated to a third party without a patient's permission. Although such an attitude may be implied, sometimes therapists should explicitly discuss confidentiality with children. The bulk of what children do and say in psychotherapy is common knowledge to the parents.

The therapist should try to enlist parents' cooperation in respecting the privacy of children's therapeutic sessions. The respect is not always readily honored, because parents are naturally curious about what transpires, and they may be threatened by a therapist's apparently privileged position.

Routinely reporting to a child the essence of communications with third parties about the child underscores the therapist's reliability and respect for the child's autonomy. In certain treatments, the report may be combined with soliciting the child's guesses about these transactions. A therapist also may find it fruitful to invite children, particularly older children, to participate in discussions about them with third parties.

INDICATIONS

Psychotherapy usually is indicated for children with emotional disorders that seem to be permanent enough to impede maturational and developmental forces. Psychotherapy also may be indicated when a child's development is not impeded but is inducing reactions in the environment that are considered pathogenic. Such disharmonies ordinarily are dealt with by the child with parental assistance; however, when these efforts are persistently inadequate, psychotherapeutic interventions may be indicated.

Psychotherapy should be limited to instances in which positive indicators point to its potential usefulness. For a child to benefit from psychotherapy, the home situation must provide a certain amount of nurturance, stability, and motivation for therapy. A child must have adequate cognitive resources to participate in the process and profit from it. Psychotherapy must be judged with common sense. If a psychotherapy situation is not effective, one must determine whether the therapist and patient are poorly matched, whether the type of psychotherapy is inappropriate to the nature of the problems, and whether the child is cognitively inappropriate for the treatment.

REFERENCES

Braun-Scharm H. Diagnosis of schizophrenia. Puberty-related crisis or psychosis? *MMW Fortsch Med.* 2001;143:44.

Caplan R, Guthrie D, Tang B, Komo S, Asarnow RF. Thought disorder in childhood schizophrenia: replication and update of concept. *J Am Acad Child Adolesc Psychiatry.* 2000;39:771.

Cohen JA, Mannarino AP. A treatment model for sexually abused preschoolers. *J Interpers Violence.* 1993;8:115.

Eyberg SM. Assessing therapy outcome with preschool children: progress and problems. *J Clin Child Psychol.* 1992;21:306.

Fonagy P, Target M. The efficacy of psychoanalysis for children with disruptive behavior disorders. *J Am Acad Child Adolesc Psychiatry.* 1994;33:45.

Forehand R, Wierson M. The role of developmental factors in planning behavioral interventions for children: disruptive behavior as an example. *Behav Ther.* 1993;24:117.

Gabel S, Bemporad JR. Variations in countertransference reactions in psychotherapy with children. *Am J Psychother.* 1994;48:11.

Hibbs ED. Child psychiatry: short-term psychotherapy. In: Sadock BJ, Sadock VA, eds. *Kaplan & Sadock's Comprehensive Textbook of Psychiatry.* 7th ed. Vol 2. Baltimore: Lippincott Williams & Wilkins; 2000:2797.

Kazdin AE. Psychotherapy for children and adolescents: current progress and future research directions. *Am Psychol.* 1993;48:644.

Kernberg PF. A reevaluation of estimates of child therapy effectiveness: discussion. *J Am Acad Child Adolesc Psychiatry.* 1992;31:710.

Kumra S. The diagnosis and treatment of children and adolescents with schizophrenia; "My mind is playing tricks on me." *Child Adolesc Psychiatr Clin North Am.* 2000;9:183.

Leichtman M. Psychotherapeutic interventions with brain-injured children and their families: II. Psychotherapy. *Bull Menninger Clin.* 1992;56:338.

Lewis O. Child psychiatry: individual psychodynamic psychotherapy. In: Sadock BJ, Sadock VA, eds. *Kaplan & Sadock's Comprehensive Textbook of Psychiatry.* 7th ed. Vol 2. Baltimore: Lippincott Williams & Wilkins; 2000:2790.

Mullins LL, Olson RA, Chaney JM. A social learning/family systems approach to the treatment of somatoform disorders in children and adolescents. *Fam Syst Med.* 1992;10:201.

Racusin RJ. Brief psychodynamic therapy with young children. *J Am Acad Child Adolesc Psychiatry.* 2000;39:791.

Ronen T. Cognitive therapy with young children. *Child Psychiatry Hum Dev.* 1992;23:19.

Shapiro T, Esman A. Psychoanalysis and child and adolescent psychiatry. *J Am Acad Child Adolesc Psychiatry.* 1992;31:6.

Shirk SR, Russell RL. A reevaluation of estimates of child therapy effectiveness. *J Am Acad Child Adolesc Psychiatry.* 1992;31:703.

Target M, Fanagy P. The efficacy of psychoanalysis for children with emotional disorders. *J Am Child Adolesc Psychiatry.* 1994;33:361.

Weisz JR, Weiss B, Donenberg GR. The lab versus the clinic: effects of child and adolescent psychotherapy. *Am Psychol.* 1992;47:1578.

▲ 53.2 Group Psychotherapy

Group therapy is an effective modality that can be structured in a variety of ways to address issues of interpersonal competence, peer relationships, and social skill. Group psychotherapy can be modified to suit groups of children in various age groups and can focus on behavioral, educational, and social skills and psychodynamic issues. The mode in which the group functions depends on children's developmental levels, intelligence, and problems to be addressed. In behaviorally oriented groups, the group leader is a directive, active participant who facilitates prosocial interactions and desired behaviors. In groups using psychodynamic approaches, the leader may monitor interpersonal interactions less actively than in behavior therapy groups.

Groups are highly effective in providing peer feedback and support to children who are either socially isolated or unaware of their effects on their peers. Groups with very young children generally are highly structured by the leader and use imagination and play to foster socially acceptable peer relationships and positive behavior. Therapists must be keenly aware of the level of children's attention span and the need for consistency and limit setting. Leaders of preschool-age groups can model supportive adult behavior in meaningful ways for children who have been deprived or neglected. School-age children's groups may be single sex or may include both boys and girls. School-age children are more sophisticated in verbalizing their feelings than preschoolers, but they also benefit from structured therapeutic games. Children of school age need frequent reminders about rules, and they are quick to point out infractions of the rules to each other. Interpersonal skills can be addressed nicely in group settings with school-age children.

Same-sex groups are often used among early adolescents. Physiological changes in early adolescence and the new demands of high school lead to stress that may be ameliorated when groups of same-age peers compare and share. In older adolescence, groups more often include both boys and girls. Even with older adolescents, the leader often uses structure and direct intervention to maximize the therapeutic value of the group. Adolescents who are feeling dejected or alienated may find a special sense of belonging in a therapy group.

Johnny was a high-functioning, 14-year-old boy diagnosed with autistic disorder. He had been in individual and family therapy for several months before he was considered ready for group therapy. Johnny was an awkward-looking adolescent who looked and acted younger than his chronological age. His academic level was above average, but his social development was very limited. A supercilious, hypermoralistic attitude of more recent development contributed considerably to his social isolation, particularly after starting seventh grade. He was assigned to an established group of early adolescents with a mixture of clinical conditions, meeting once weekly for 75 minutes. Initially Johnny limited his participation to monosyllabic answers to direct questions, then he would go back to reading a book on the history of Napoleon, his favorite subject and object of fascination. Group members chose to ignore him after a while. Over a period of several weeks his interest in the book seemed to abate. Johnny brought it, but it remained unopened on his lap. He would make an occasional remark, mostly to criticize another group member for his "vulgarity." The group laughed at his remarks but scapegoating could be avoided. They seemed to respect his "differentness." Two months later, Peter, a very shy schizoid 13-year-old boy joined the group. After a few sessions Johnny developed an unexpected interest in Peter and sat by him and encouraged him to interact with the group. Soon Johnny was not bringing a book any longer and was more actively involved with group members. He responded to social cues in a more age-typical and appropriate manner, and though he continued having morbid preoccupations with power and a fascination with Napoleon, the intensity was considerably diminished. Johnny's growing interest in people was clinically evident. Group therapy was used in combination with individual and family therapy and psychotropic medication over 18 months. Although the group experience was only one component of the treatment plan, it became a most significant tool to help Johnny with his interpersonal deficits. (Courtesy of Alberto C. Serrano, M.D.)

PRESCHOOL-AGE AND EARLY SCHOOL-AGE GROUPS

Work with a preschool-age group usually is structured by a therapist through the use of a particular technique such as puppets or artwork or is couched in terms of a permissive play atmosphere. In therapy with puppets, children project their fantasies onto the puppets in a way not unlike ordinary play. The main value lies in the cathexis afforded children, especially if they show difficulty expressing their feelings. Here, the group aids the child less by interaction with other members than by action with the puppets.

In play group therapy, the emphasis rests on children's interactional qualities with each other and with the therapist in the permissive playroom setting. A therapist should be a person who can allow children to produce fantasies verbally and in play but who can also use active restraint when children undergo excessive tension. The toys are the traditional ones used in individual play therapy. The children use the toys to act out aggressive impulses and to relive their home difficulties with group members and with the therapist. The children selected for group treatment have a common social hunger and need to be like their peers and be accepted by them. Selected children usually include those with phobias, effeminate boys, shy and withdrawn children, and children with disruptive behavior disorders.

Modifications of these criteria have been used in group psychotherapy for autistic children, parent group therapy, and art

therapy. A modification of group psychotherapy has been used for toddlers with physical disabilities who show speech and language delays. The experience of twice-weekly group activities involves mothers and children in a mutual teaching–learning setting. This experience has proved effective for mothers who received supportive psychotherapy in the group experience; their formerly hidden fantasies about their children emerged and were dealt with therapeutically.

SCHOOL-AGE GROUPS

Activity group psychotherapy is based on the idea that poor, divergent experiences have led to deficits in children's appropriate personality development; therefore, corrective experiences in a therapeutically conditioned environment modify them. Because some latency-age children have deep disturbances involving fears, high anxiety levels, and guilt, a modification of activity-interview group psychotherapy has evolved. The format uses interview techniques, verbal explanations of fantasies, group play, work, and other communications. In this type of group psychotherapy, children verbalize in a problem-oriented manner, with the awareness that problems brought them together and that the group aims to change them. They report dreams, fantasies, daydreams, and traumatic and unpleasant experiences. Open discussion includes both the experiences and the group behavior.

Therapists vary in their use of time, cotherapists, food, and materials. Most groups meet after school for at least 1 hour, although other group leaders prefer a 90-minute session. Some therapists serve food during the last 10 minutes; others prefer serving times when the children are together for talking. Food, however, does not become a major feature and is never central to the group's activities.

PUBERTAL AND ADOLESCENT GROUPS

Group therapy methods similar to those used in younger-age groups can be modified to apply to pubertal children, who are often grouped monosexually. Their problems resemble those of late latency-age children, but they (especially the girls) are also beginning to feel the effects and pressures of early adolescence. Groups offer help during a transitional period; they seem to satisfy the social appetite of preadolescents, who compensate for feelings of inferiority and self-doubt by forming groups. This therapy takes advantage of the influence of the socialization process during these years. Because pubertal children experience difficulties in conceptualizing, pubertal therapy groups tend to use play, drawing, psychodrama, and other nonverbal modes of expression. The therapist's role is active and directive.

Activity group psychotherapy has been the recommended group therapy for pubertal children who do not have significantly disturbed personality patterns. The children, usually of the same sex and in groups of not more than eight, freely engage in activities in a setting especially designed and planned for its physical and environmental characteristics. Samuel Slavson, a pioneer in group psychotherapy, pictured the group as a substitute family in which the passive, neutral therapist becomes the surrogate for parents. The therapist assumes various roles, mostly in a nonverbal manner, as each child interacts with the therapist and other group members. Currently, however, therapists tend to see the group as a form of peer group, with its attendant socializing processes, rather than a reenactment of the family.

Late adolescents, 16 years of age and older, often may be included in groups of adults. Group therapy has been useful in the treatment of substance-related disorders. Combined therapy (the use of group and individual therapy) also has been used successfully with adolescents.

OTHER GROUP SITUATIONS

Groups are also helpful in more focused treatments, such as specific social skills training for children with attention-deficit/hyperactivity disorder, cognitive-behavioral group interventions for depressed children and children with bereavement problems or eating disorders. In these more specialized groups, the issues are more specific, and actual tasks (as in social skills groups) may be practiced within the group. Some residential and day treatment units use group psychotherapy techniques. Group psychotherapy in schools for underachievers and children from low socioeconomic levels has relied on reinforcement and on modeling theory, in addition to traditional techniques, and has been supplemented by parent groups.

In controlled conditions, residential treatment units have been used for specific studies in group psychotherapy, such as behavioral contracting. Behavioral contracting with reward-punishment reinforcement provides positive reinforcements among preadolescent boys with severe concerns in basic trust, low self-esteem, and dependence conflicts. Somewhat akin to formal residential treatment units are social group work homes. For children who undergo many psychological assaults before placement, supportive group psychotherapy offers ventilation and catharsis, but more often it succeeds in letting children become aware of the enjoyment of sharing activities and developing skills.

Public schools—also a structured environment, although not usually considered the best site for group psychotherapy—have been used by several workers. Group psychotherapy as group counseling readily lends itself to school settings. One such group used gender- and problem-homogeneous selection for groups of six to eight students, who met once a week during school hours over 2 to 3 years.

INDICATIONS

Many indications exist for the use of group psychotherapy as a treatment modality. Some indications are situational; a therapist may work in a reformatory setting, in which group psychotherapy seems to reach adolescents better than individual treatment does. Another indication is time economics; more patients can be reached in a given time by the use of groups than by individual therapy. Group therapy best helps a child at a given age and developmental stage and with a given type of problem. In young age groups, children's social hunger and their potential need for peer acceptance help determine their suitability for group therapy. Criteria for unsuitability are controversial and have been loosened progressively.

PARENT GROUPS

In group psychotherapy, as in most treatment procedures for children, parental difficulties present obstacles. Sometimes,

uncooperative parents refuse to bring a child or to participate in their own therapy. The extreme of this situation reveals itself when severely disturbed parents use a child as their channel of communication to work out their own needs. In such circumstances, a child is in the intolerable position of receiving positive group experiences that seem to create havoc at home.

Parent groups, therefore, can be a valuable aid to group psychotherapy for their children. Parents of children in therapy often have difficulty understanding their children's ailments, discerning the line of demarcation between normal and pathological behavior, relating to the medical establishment, and coping with feelings of guilt. Parent groups assist in these areas and help members formulate guidelines for action.

References

Cerda RA, Nemiroff HW, Richmond AH. Therapeutic group approaches in an inpatient facility for children and adolescents: a 15-year perspective. *Group.* 1991;15:71.

Chase JL. Inpatient adolescent and latency-age children's perspectives on the curative factors in group psychotherapy. *Group.* 1991;15:95.

Clifford MW. A model for group therapy with latency-age boys. *Group.* 1991;15:116.

Garland JA. The establishment of individual and collective competency in children's groups as a prelude to entry into intimacy, disclosure, and bonding. *Int J Group Psychother.* 1992;42:395.

Kymissis P, Licamele WL, Boots S, Kessler E. Training in child and adolescent group therapy: two surveys and a model. *Group.* 1991;15:163.

Schamess G. Reflections on a developing body of group-as-a-whole theory for children's therapy groups: an introduction. *Int J Group Psychother.* 1992;42:351.

Scheidlinger S. Short-term group psychotherapy for children: an overview. *Int J Group Psychother.* 1984;34:573.

Scheidlinger S. Group treatment of adolescents. *Am J Orthopsychiatry.* 1985;55:102.

Scheidlinger S. An overview of nine decades of group psychotherapy. *Hosp Community Psychiatry.* 1994;45:217.

Serrano AC. Child psychiatry: group psychotherapy. In: Sadock BJ, Sadock VA, eds. *Kaplan & Sadock's Comprehensive Textbook of Psychiatry.* 7th ed. Vol 2. Baltimore: Lippincott Williams & Wilkins; 2000:2813.

Shechtman Z, Ben-David M. Individual and group psychotherapy of childhood aggression: a comparison of outcomes and processes. *Group Dynamics.* 1999;3:263.

Suger M. Research in child and adolescent group psychotherapy. *J Child Adolesc Group Ther.* 1993;3:207.

Trad PV. Diagnostic peer group assessments in preschoolers with anxiety disorders. *J Child Adolesc Group Ther.* 1992;3:207.

Yalom ID. *Inpatient Group Psychotherapy.* New York: Basic Books; 1983.

Zimpfer DG. Group work with juvenile delinquents. *J Spec Group Work.* 1992;17:116.

▲ 53.3 Residential, Day, and Hospital Treatment

Residential treatment centers and facilities are appropriate settings for children and adolescents with mental disorders who require a highly structured and supervised setting for a substantial time. Such settings have the advantage of providing a stable, consistent environment with a high level of psychiatric monitoring but less intensive than in a hospital. Children and adolescents with serious psychiatric disturbances often end up in residential facilities because of difficulties managing their own psychiatric problems and because of family situations in which appropriate supervision and parenting are impossible. Residential settings offer many treatments, including behavioral management, psychotherapy, medication, special education, and the therapeutic milieu itself. Children and adolescents who benefit from residential settings have a wide variety of psychiatric problems and commonly have difficulty with impulse control and structuring their own time. Many residents of such programs also have families with serious psychiatric, financial, and parenting difficulties.

Day treatment programs are excellent alternatives for children and adolescents who require more intensive support, monitoring, and supervision than is available in the community but who can to live successfully at home if they receive the proper level of intervention. In most cases, children and adolescents who attend day hospital programs have serious mental disorders and might warrant psychiatric hospitalization without the program's support. Family therapy, group and individual psychotherapy, psychopharmacology, behavioral management programs, and special education are integral parts of these programs.

Psychiatric hospitalization is needed when a child or adolescent exhibits dangerous behavior, is contemplating suicide, or is experiencing an exacerbation of a psychotic disorder or another serious mental disorder. Safety, stabilization, and effective treatment are the goals of hospitalization. Recently, the length of stay for child and adolescent psychiatric patients has decreased because of financial pressures and increased availability of day treatment programs. Psychiatric hospitalization may be some children's first opportunity to experience a stable, safe environment. Hospitals often are the most appropriate places to start use of new medications, and they provide an around-the-clock setting in which to observe a child's behavior. Children may show remission of some symptoms by virtue of their removal from a stressful or abusive environment. After a child has been observed for several weeks, the best treatment and disposition may become clear.

RESIDENTIAL TREATMENT

More than 20,000 emotionally disturbed children are in residential treatment centers in the United States, and this number is increasing. Deteriorating social conditions, particularly in cities, often make it impossible for a child with a serious mental disorder to live at home. In these cases, residential treatment centers serve a real need. They provide a structured living environment in which children may form strong attachments to, and receive commitments from, staff members. The purpose of the center is to provide treatment and special education for children and their families.

Staff and Setting

Staffing patterns include various combinations of child-care workers, teachers, social workers, psychiatrists, pediatricians, nurses, and psychologists; therefore, residential treatment can be very expensive. The Joint Commission on the Mental Health of Children made the following structural and setting recommendations: In addition to space for therapy programs, there should be facilities for a first-rate school and a rich evening activity program, and there should be ample space for play, both indoors and out. Facilities should be small, seldom exceeding 60 patients in capacity with a limit of 100 patients, and they should make provisions for children to live in small groups. The centers should be located near the families they serve and should be readily accessible by public transportation. They should be located for ready access to

special medical and educational services and to various community resources, including consultants. The centers should be open institutions whenever possible; locked buildings, wards, or rooms should be required only rarely. In designing residential programs, the guiding principle should be that children should be removed from their normal life settings the least possible distance in space, in time, and in the psychological texture of the experience.

Indications

Most children who are referred for residential treatment have had multiple evaluations by professionals such as school psychologists, outpatient psychotherapists, juvenile court officials, or state welfare agency staff. Attempts at outpatient treatment and foster home placement usually precede residential treatment. Sometimes, the severity of a child's problems or the inability of a family to provide for the child's needs prohibits sending a child home. Many children sent to residential treatment centers have disruptive behavior problems in addition to other problems, including mood disorders and psychotic disorders. In some cases, serious psychosocial problems such as physical or sexual abuse, neglect, indigence, or homelessness necessitate out-of-home placement. The age range of the children varies among institutions, but most children are between 5 and 15 years of age. Boys are referred more frequently than girls.

An initial review of data enables the intake staff to determine whether a particular child is likely to benefit from the treatment program; often, for every child accepted for admission, three are rejected. The next step usually is interviews with the child and the parents by various staff members, such as a therapist, a group-living worker, and a teacher. Psychological testing and neurological examinations are given, when indicated, if they have not already been performed. The child and parents should be prepared for these interviews.

Group Living

Most of a child's time in a residential treatment setting is spent in group living. The group-living staff consists of child-care workers who offer a structured environment that forms a therapeutic milieu; the environment places boundaries and limitations on the children. Tasks are defined within the limits of children's abilities; incentives, such as additional privileges, encourage them to progress rather than regress. In milieu therapy, the environment is structured, limits are set, and a therapeutic atmosphere is maintained.

The children often select one or more staff members with whom to form a relationship; through this relationship, they express, consciously and unconsciously, many of their feelings about their parents. The child-care staff should be trained to recognize such transference reactions and to respond to them in a way that differs from the children's expectations, which are based on their previous or even current relationships with their parents.

To maintain consistency and balance, the group-living staff members must communicate freely and regularly with each other and with the other professional and administrative staff members of the residential setting, particularly the children's teachers and therapists. The child-care staff members must recognize any tendencies toward becoming the good (or bad) parent in response to a child's splitting behavior. This tendency may be manifest as a pattern of blaming other staff members for a child's disruptive behavior. Similarly, the child-care staff must recognize and avoid such individual and group countertransference reactions as sadomasochistic and punitive behavior toward a child.

The structured setting should offer a corrective emotional experience and opportunities for facilitating and improving children's adaptive behavior, particularly when such problems as speech and language deficits, intellectual retardation, inadequate peer relationships, bedwetting, poor feeding habits, and attention deficits are present. Some attention deficits are the basis of a child's poor academic performance and unsocialized behavior, including temper tantrums, fighting, and withdrawal.

Behavior modification principles also have been used, particularly in group work with children. Behavior therapy is part of a residential center's total therapeutic effort.

Education

Children in residential treatment frequently have severe learning disorders, disruptive behavior, and attention-deficit disorders. Usually, the children cannot function in a regular community school and consequently need a special on-grounds school. A major goal of the on-grounds school is to motivate children to learn. The educational process in residential treatment is complex; Table 53.3–1 shows some of its components.

Therapy

Most residential facilities use a basic behavior modification program to set guidelines and to give the residents a concrete sense of how to earn privileges. These behavioral programs range in detail and intensity. Some programs operate with level systems that are associated with privileges and responsibilities. Some programs use a token economy system in which residents earn points for appropriate behavior and for meeting specific goals. Most programs include basic tasks of living as well as specific therapeutic goals for the residents.

Psychotherapy offered in the program generally is supportive and oriented toward reunion with the family when possible. Insight-oriented psychotherapy is included when it can be used by a resident.

Parents

Concomitant work with parents is essential. Children usually have a strong tie to at least one parent, no matter how disturbed the parent may be. Sometimes, a child idealizes the parent, who repeatedly fails the child. Other times, the parent has an ambivalent or unrealistic expectation that the child will return home. In some instances, the parent must be helped to enable the child to live in another setting when it is in the child's best interest. Most residential treatment centers offer individual or group therapy for parents, couples or marital therapy, and in some cases, conjoint family therapy.

DAY TREATMENT

The concept of daily comprehensive therapeutic experiences that do not require removing children from their homes or families is derived partly from experiences with a therapeutic nurs-

Table 53.3–1
Education Process in Residential Treatment

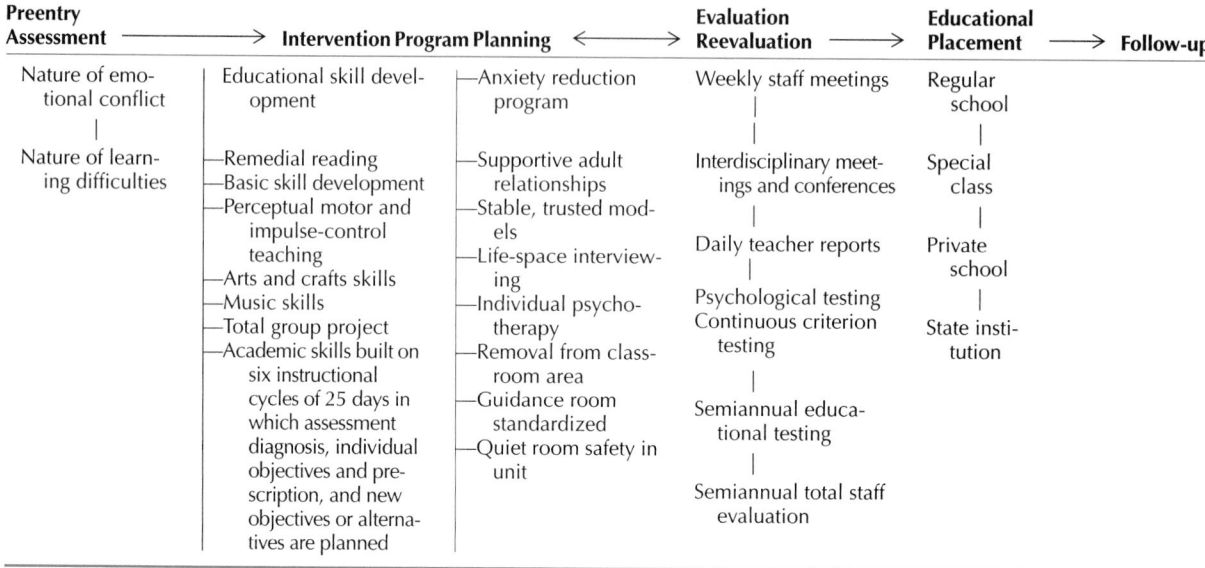

Preentry Assessment →	Intervention Program Planning ↔		Evaluation Reevaluation →	Educational Placement →	Follow-up
Nature of emotional conflict	Educational skill development	—Anxiety reduction program	Weekly staff meetings	Regular school	
Nature of learning difficulties	—Remedial reading	—Supportive adult relationships	Interdisciplinary meetings and conferences	Special class	
	—Basic skill development	—Stable, trusted models	Daily teacher reports	Private school	
	—Perceptual motor and impulse-control teaching	—Life-space interviewing	Psychological testing	State institution	
	—Arts and crafts skills	—Individual psychotherapy	Continuous criterion testing		
	—Music skills	—Removal from classroom area	Semiannual educational testing		
	—Total group project	—Guidance room standardized	Semiannual total staff evaluation		
	—Academic skills built on six instructional cycles of 25 days in which assessment diagnosis, individual objectives and prescription, and new objectives or alternatives are planned	—Quiet room safety in unit			

Courtesy of Melvin Lewis, M.B., B.S. (London), F.R.C.Psych., D.C.H.

ery school. Day hospital programs for children were then developed, and the number of programs continues to grow. The main advantages of day treatment are that children remain with their families and the families can be more involved in day treatment than they are in residential or hospital treatment. Day treatment also is much less expensive than residential treatment. At the same time, the risks of day treatment are a child's social isolation and confinement to a narrow band of social contacts in the program's disturbed peer population.

Indications

The primary indication for day treatment is the need for a more structured, intensive, and specialized treatment program than can be provided on an outpatient basis. At the same time, the home in which the child is living should be able to provide an environment that is at least not destructive to the child's development. Children who are likely to benefit from day treatment may have a wide range of diagnoses, including autistic disorder, conduct disorder, attention-deficit/hyperactivity disorder, and mental retardation. Exclusion symptoms include behavior that is likely to be destructive to the children themselves or to others under the treatment conditions. Therefore, some children who threaten to run away, set fires, attempt suicide, hurt others, or significantly disrupt the lives of their families while they are at home may not be suitable for day treatment.

Programs

The same ingredients that lead to a successful residential treatment program apply to day treatment. These ingredients include clear administrative leadership, team collaboration, open communication, and an understanding of children's behavior. Indeed, having a single agency offer both residential and day treatment has advantages.

A major function of child-care staff in day treatment for psychiatrically disturbed children is to provide positive experiences and a structure that enables the children and their families to internalize controls and to function better than in the past regarding themselves and the outside world. Again, the methods used are essentially similar to those in full residential treatment programs.

Because the ages, needs, and range of diagnoses of children who may benefit from some form of day treatment vary, many day treatment programs have been developed. Some programs specialize in special educational and structured environmental needs of mentally retarded children. Others offer special therapeutic efforts required to treat children with autism and schizophrenia. Still other programs provide the total spectrum of treatment usually found in full residential treatment, of which they may be a part. Children may move from one part of the program to another and may be in residential treatment or day treatment according to their needs. The school program always is a major component of day treatment, and psychiatric treatment varies according to a child's needs and diagnosis.

Results

Recently, attempts have been made to analyze the treatment outcome of day treatment and partial hospitalization. There are many different dimensions to analyzing overall benefits of such programs. Assessment of level of improvement in clinical status, academic progress, peer relationships, community interactions (legal difficulties), and family relationships are some pertinent areas to measure. In a recent follow-up 1 year after discharge from a partial hospital program, comparison of patients at admission and 1 year postdischarge showed statisti-

cally significant improvement in clinical symptoms on each subscale of the Child Behavior Checklist except for sex problems. These improvements included mood symptoms, somatic complaints, attention problems, thought problems, delinquent behavior, and aggressive behavior. The assessment of long-term effectiveness of day treatment is fraught with difficulties, from the point of view of a child's maintenance of gains, a therapist's view of psychological gains, or cost-benefit ratios.

At the same time, the advantage of day treatment has encouraged further development of programs. Moreover, the lessons learned from day treatment programs have moved mental health disciplines toward having services follow children, rather than perpetuating discontinuities of care. The experiences of day treatment for psychiatric conditions of children and adolescents have also encouraged pediatric hospitals and departments to adopt a model that promotes continuity of care for the medical treatment of children with chronic physical illnesses.

HOSPITAL TREATMENT

Beginning in the 1920s, inpatient psychiatric treatment of children includes two types of units: acute-care hospital units and long-term hospital units. Acute-care units generally accept children who exhibit dangerous (suicidal, assaultive, or psychotically disorganized) behavior. Diagnosis, stabilization, and formulation and initiation of a treatment plan are the goals of acute-care units. Disposition usually is to home, to residential treatment centers, or to long-term (usually state) hospitals for continued care. Acute-care hospitalization generally lasts from 6 to 12 weeks and often is extended because of the wait for beds in residential treatment centers and state hospitals.

Long-term hospitalization generally lasts many months to years. The staffs of inpatient units are interdisciplinary and include psychiatrists, psychologists, social workers, nurses, activity therapists, and teachers.

REFERENCES

Angold A, Costello EJ, Burns BJ, Erkanli A, Farmer EMZ. Effectiveness of nonresidential specialty mental health services for children and adolescents in the "real world." *J Am Acad Child Adolesc Psychiatry.* 2000;39:154.

Ascherman LI. The impact of unstructured games of fantasy and role playing on an inpatient unit for adolescents. *Int J Group Psychother.* 1993;43:335.

Bishop EG, McNally G. An in-home crisis intervention program for children and their families. *Hosp Community Psychiatry.* 1993;44:182.

DeAntonio M. Child psychiatry: residential and inpatient treatment. In: Sadock BJ, Sadock VA, eds. *Kaplan & Sadock's Comprehensive Textbook of Psychiatry.* 7th ed. Vol 2. Baltimore: Lippincott Williams & Wilkins; 2000:2846.

Gold J, Shera D, Clarkson B. Private psychiatric hospitalization of children: predictors of length of stay. *J Am Acad Child Adolesc Psychiatry.* 1993;32:135.

Grizenko N, Papineau D, Sayegh L. Effectiveness of a multimodal day treatment program for children with disruptive behavior problems. *J Am Acad Child Adolesc Psychiatry.* 1993;32:127.

Kayser JA, Teitelman M. Design and implementation of a continuum of care for children and youth in private mental health settings. *Continuum.* 1994;1:15.

Kiser LJ, Heston JD, Millsap PA, Pruitt DB. Testing the limits: special treatment procedures for child and adolescent partial hospitalization. *Int J Partial Hosp.* 1991;7:37.

Kiser LJ, Millsap PA, Hickerson S, et al. Results of treatment one year later: child and adolescent partial hospitalization. *J Am Acad Child Adolesc Psychiatry.* 1996;35:81.

Lundy M, Pumariega AJ. Psychiatric hospitalization of children and adolescents: treatment in search of a rationale. *J Child Fam Stud.* 1993;2:1.

Lyman RD, Prentice-Dunn S, Gabel S, eds. *Residential and Inpatient Treatment of Children and Adolescents.* New York: Plenum; 1989.

Lyons JS, Uziel-Miller ND, Reyes F, Sokol PT. Strengths of children and adolescents in residential settings: prevalence and associations with psychopathology and discharge placement. *J Am Acad Child Adolesc Psychiatry.* 2000;39:176.

Mikkelsen EJ, Bereika GM, McKenzie JC. Short-term family-based residential treatment: an alternative to psychiatric hospitalization for children. *Am J Orthopsychiatry.* 1993;63:28.

Pedersen J, Aakrog B. A 10-year follow-up of an adolescent psychiatric clientele and early predictors of readmission. *Nord J Psychiatry.* 2001;55:11.

Perrin EC. Children in hospitals. *J Dev Behav Pediatr.* 1993;14:50.

Pfeiffer SI, Strzelecki SC. Inpatient psychiatric treatment of children and adolescents: a review of outcome studies. *J Am Acad Child Adolesc Psychiatry.* 1990;29:847.

Zimet SG, Farley GK. Academic achievement of children with emotional disorders treated in a day hospital program: an outcome study. *Child Psychiatry Hum Dev.* 1993;23:183.

▲ 53.4 Biological Therapies

PHARMACOTHERAPY

Over the last decade, there have been many advances in the pharmacotherapy of psychiatric disorders in childhood, including data supporting the efficacy of selective serotonin reuptake inhibitors (SSRIs) in the treatment of depressive disorders, obsessive-compulsive disorders, and anxiety disorders. Double-blind, placebo-controlled studies have provided evidence for the efficacy of fluoxetine (Prozac) and paroxetine (Paxil) in the treatment of child and adolescent depression. The tricyclic drugs have rarely been recommended since SSRIs appeared on the market, because the SSRIs have more favorable adverse-effect profiles than the tricyclics. Fluoxetine, sertraline (Zoloft), paroxetine, fluvoxamine (Luvox), and nefazodone (Serzone) are relatively frequently used with children and adolescents. Concern about tricyclic drugs centers on their potential cardiotoxicity, which may have contributed to the sudden deaths of four children being treated with desipramine (Norpramin, Pertofrane) for attention-deficit/hyperactivity disorder (ADHD). Additional antidepressants, including bupropion (Wellbutrin) and venlafaxine (Effexor), are commonly used second-line antidepressants when SSRI agents are not efficacious.

The management of severe aggression, disruptive behavior, and ADHD remains a challenge. Combinations of antipsychotics with mood-stabilizing agents or stimulants are sometimes used in treatment-resistant cases, although few studies attest to the efficacy or safety of drug combinations. Newer "atypical" antipsychotic medications—serotonergic-dopamine antagonists (SDAs)—such as risperidone (Risperdal), olanzapine (Zyprexa), clozapine (Clozaril), and ziprasidone (Geodon) have enabled a wider range of treatment-resistant patients to benefit from neuroleptic treatment. The SDAs are believed to relieve both the positive and negative symptoms of schizophrenia and to produce less risk of extrapyramidal adverse effects and less potential for the development of tardive dyskinesia. Nevertheless, all antipsychotics pose some risk of extrapyramidal adverse effects and tardive dyskinesia. One challenge in obtaining optimal pharmacological treatment for children is to decrease maladaptive behaviors and promote productive academic functioning. To this end, clinicians must consider medication adverse effects that result in cognitive "dulling." Certain pharmacological agents used in pediatric populations are associated with a specific disorder or with target symptoms that appear in several disorders. For example, haloperidol (Haldol) was shown in past studies to be effective in the treatment of Tourette's disorder,

Table 53.4–1
Diagnostic Processes of Biological Therapy

1. Diagnostic evaluation
2. Symptom measurement
3. Risk-benefit ratio analysis
4. Establishment of a contract for therapy
5. Periodic reevaluation
6. Termination and tapered drug withdrawal

but it has also been used to control severe aggression, a symptom that emerges in the context of a variety of disorders. Currently, the SDAs have generally replaced the conventional antipsychotics (dopamine receptor antagonists) in the treatment of psychotic disorders and aggressive behavior management.

Therapeutic Considerations

An evaluation for psychopharmacotherapy must first include an assessment of a child's psychopathology and physical condition to rule out any predisposition for side effects (Table 53.4–1). An assessment of the child's caregivers focuses on their ability to provide a safe, consistent environment in which a clinician can conduct a drug trial. The physician must consider the benefit-risk ratio and must explain it to the patient, if he or she is old enough, and to the child's caregivers and others (e.g., child welfare workers) who may be involved in the decision to medicate.

The clinician must obtain baseline ratings before medicating. Behavioral rating scales help objectify the child's response to medication. The physician generally starts at a low dose and titrates upward on the basis of the child's response and the appearance of adverse effects. Optimal drug trials cannot be rushed (e.g., by insurance-imposed inadequately short hospital stays or by infrequent outpatient visits), nor can drug trials be prolonged by the physician's insufficient contact with the patient and the caregivers. The success of drug trials often hinges on the physician's daily accessibility.

Childhood Pharmacokinetics

Compared with adults, children have greater hepatic capacity, more glomerular filtration, and less fatty tissue. Thus, stimulants, antipsychotics, and tricyclic drugs are eliminated more rapidly by children than by adults; lithium (Eskalith) may be eliminated more rapidly, and children may be less able to store drugs in their fat. Because of children's quick elimination, the half-lives of many medications may be shorter in children than in adults.

Little evidence indicates that clinicians can predict a child's blood level from the dosage or a treatment response from the plasma level. Relatively low serum levels of haloperidol seem to be adequate to treat Tourette's disorder in children. No correlation is seen between the methylphenidate (Ritalin) serum level and a child's response. The data are incomplete and conflicting about major depressive disorder and serum levels of tricyclic drugs. Serum level is related to response for tricyclic drugs in the treatment of enuresis.

With lithium therapy, a ratio of lithium concentration in saliva to that in serum can be established for a child by averaging three to four individual ratios. The average ratio can then be used to convert subsequent saliva levels to serum levels and thus avoid some venipunctures in children who are stressed by blood tests. As with serum levels, regular clinical monitoring for adverse effects is necessary. Table 53.4–2 lists representative drugs and their indications, dosages, adverse reactions, and monitoring requirements.

Indications

Mental Retardation. The psychopharmacotherapy for mental retardation most often addresses behavioral problems, especially aggression, and the coexistence of other mental disorders. Medications are overused to control the behavior of institutionalized children who are retarded because other therapies and services are not available. For severe aggression, antipsychotics are most commonly used, and cognitive dulling can best be avoided with high-potency drugs. β-Adrenergic receptor antagonists have reduced aggression in uncontrolled studies of adults and children with mental retardation. Lithium and anticonvulsants such as carbamazepine (Tegretol) may also be tried. Antipsychotics have the advantage of a fast onset of action and little need for laboratory monitoring of their adverse effects, but the use of other drugs eliminates the risk for tardive dyskinesia.

The endogenous opioid antagonists, such as naltrexone (ReVia), and the SSRIs, such as fluoxetine, have been prescribed in an attempt to diminish self-injurious behavior in patients with mental retardation. When ADHD coexists with mental retardation, methylphenidate often is effective.

Recently, attempts have been made to treat the behavioral problems associated with fragile X syndrome with folic acid supplements. Some prepubescent children experienced less active or less aggressive behavior and concentrated better when they took folic acid than they did before treatment.

Learning Disorders. No pharmacological agent significantly improves any learning disorder, but many children with other mental disorders also have learning disorders, and many who have learning disorders also have behavioral problems. These associations and the importance of school and learning in children's lives raise questions about the cognitive effects of psychotropics. Table 53.4–3 summarizes the effects of drugs on cognitive tests of learning functions. In children with learning disorders but no other mental disorder, methylphenidate facilitates performance on several standard cognitive, psycholinguistic, memory, and vigilance tests but does not improve children's academic achievement ratings or teacher ratings. Cognitive impairment from psychotropic drugs, especially antipsychotics, may be an even greater problem for persons who are mentally retarded than for those with learning disorders.

Autistic Disorder. The behavioral problems of children with autistic disorder can be extreme. In short-term and long-term studies, haloperidol, often in nonsedating dosages, has proved efficacious in reducing temper tantrums, aggression, stereotypies, self-injurious behavior, hyperactivity, and withdrawal, but dyskinesia is a risk. Recently, the SSRIs have been studied in autistic disorder, as researchers posited an association between the compulsive behaviors in obsessive-compulsive disorder and stereotypic behaviors common in children with autism. To date, clomipramine (Anafranil) and fluoxetine have

Table 53.4–2
Common Psychoactive Drugs in Childhood and Adolescence

Drug	Indications	Dosage	Adverse Reactions and Monitoring
Antipsychotics—also known as *major tranquilizers, neuroleptics* Divided into (1) high-potency, low-dosage (e.g., haloperidol (Haldol), pimozide (Orap), trifluoperazine (Stelazine), thiothixene (Navane); (2) low-potency high-dosage (more sedating) (e.g., chlorpromazine (Thorazine); and (3) atypicals (e.g., risperidone (Risperdal), olanzapine (Zyprexa), quetiapine (Seroquel), and clozapine (Clozaril)	Psychoses; agitated self-injurious behaviors in MR, PDDs, CD, and Tourette's disorder—haloperidol and pimozide Clozapine—refractory schizophrenia in adolescence	All can be given in two to four divided doses or combined into one dose after gradual buildup Haloperidol—child 0.5–6 mg/d, adolescent 0.5–16 mg/d Clozapine—dosage not determined in children; <600 mg/d in adolescents Risperidone—1–3 mg/d Olanzapine—2.5–10 mg/d Quetiapine—25–500 mg/d	Sedation, weight gain, hypotension, lowered seizure threshold, constipation, extrapyramidal symptoms, jaundice, agranulocytosis, dystonic reaction, tardive dyskinesia Hyperprolactinemia with atypicals except quetiapine Monitor blood pressure, CBC count, LFTs and prolactin if indicated; with thioridazine, pigmentary retinopathy is rare but dictates ceiling of 800 mg in adults and proportionally lower in children; with clozapine, weekly WBC counts for development of agranulocytosis and EEG monitoring because of lowering of seizure threshold
Stimulants			
Dextroamphetamine (Dexedrine) and amphetamine-dextroamphetamine (Adderall) FDA-approved for children 3 years and older Methylphenidate (Ritalin, Concerta) and pemoline (Cylert)—FDA-approved for children 6 years and older	In ADHD for hyperactivity, impulsivity, and inattentiveness Narcolepsy	Dextroamphetamine and methylphenidate are generally given at 8 AM and noon Dextroamphetamine—about half the dosage of methylphenidate Methylphenidate—10–60 mg/d or up to about 0.5 mg/kg per dose Adderall—about half the dosage of methylphenidate	Insomnia, anorexia, weight loss (possibly growth delay), rebound hyperactivity, headache, tachycardia, precipitation or exacerbation of tic disorders With pemoline, monitor LFTs, as hepatotoxicity and liver failure are possible
Mood stabilizers			
Lithium—considered an antimanic drug; also has antiaggression properties	Studies support use in MR and CD for aggressive and self-injurious behaviors; can be used for same in PDD; also indicated for early-onset bipolar disorder	600–2,100 mg in two or three divided doses; keep blood levels to 0.4–1.2 mEq/L	Nausea, vomiting, polyuria, headache, tremor, weight gain, hypothyroidism Experience with adults suggests renal function monitoring
Divalproex (Depakote)	Bipolar disorder, aggression	Up to about 20 mg/kg per day; therapeutic blood level range appears to be 50–100 μg/mL	Monitor CBC count and LFTs for possible blood dyscrasias and hepatotoxicity Nausea, vomiting, sedation, hair loss, weight gain, possibly polycystic ovaries
Carbamazepine (Tegretol)—an anticonvulsant	Aggression or dyscontrol in MR or CD Bipolar disorder	Start with 10 mg/kg per day, can build to 20–30 mg/kg per day; therapeutic blood-level range appears to be 4–12 mg per day	Drowsiness, nausea, rash, vertigo, irritability Monitor CBC count and LFTs for possible blood dyscrasias and hepatotoxicity; must obtain blood concentrations
Antidepressants			
Tricyclic antidepressants—imipramine (Tofranil), nortriptyline (Pamelor), clomipramine (Anafranil)	Major depressive disorder, separation anxiety disorder, bulimia nervosa, enuresis; sometimes used in ADHD, sleepwalking disorder, and sleep terror disorder Clomipramine is effective in childhood OCD and sometimes in PDD	Imipramine—start with divided doses totaling about 1.5 mg/kg per day; can build up to not more than 5 mg/kg per day and eventually combine in one dose, which is usually 50–100 mg before sleep Clomipramine—start at 50 mg/d; can raise to not more than 3 mg/kg per day or 200 mg/d	Dry mouth, constipation, tachycardia, arrhythmia
Selective serotonin reuptake inhibitors—fluoxetine (Prozac), sertraline (Zoloft), fluvoxamine (Luvox), paroxetine (Paxil), citalopram (Celexa)	OCD; may be useful in major depressive disorder, anorexia nervosa, bulimia nervosa, repetitive behaviors in MR or PDD	Less than adult dosages	Nausea, headache, nervousness, insomnia, dry mouth, diarrhea, drowsiness, disinhibition

(continued)

Table 53.4–2 (*continued*)

Drug	Indications	Dosage	Adverse Reactions and Monitoring
Bupropion (Wellbutrin)	ADHD	Start low and titrate up to between 100 and 250 mg/d	Disinhibition, insomnia, dry mouth, gastrointestinal problems, tremor, seizures
Anxiolytics			
Benzodiazepines			
Clonazepam (Klonopin)	Panic disorder, generalized anxiety disorder	0.5–2.0 mg/d	Drowsiness, disinhibition
Alprazolam (Xanax)	Separation anxiety disorder	Up to 1.5 mg/d	Drowsiness, disinhibition
Buspirone (BuSpar)	Various anxiety disorders	15–90 mg/d	Dizziness, upset stomach
α_2-Adrenergic receptor agonists			
Clonidine (Catapres)	ADHD, Tourette's disorder, aggression	Up to 0.4 mg/d	Bradycardia, arrhythmia, hypertension, withdrawal hypotension
Guanfacine (Tenex)	ADHD	0.5–3.0 mg/d	Same as with clonidine plus headache, stomachache
β-Adrenergic receptor antagonist (beta blocker)			
Propranolol (Inderal)	Explosive aggression	Start at 20–30 mg/d and titrate	Monitor for bradycardia, hypotension, bronchoconstriction Contraindicated in asthma and diabetes
Other agents			
Naltrexone (ReVia)	Hyperactivity or self-injurious behavior in autism or MR	0.5–1.0 mg/kg per day	Drowsiness, vomiting, anorexia, headache, nasal congestion, hyponatremic seizures
Desmopressin (DDAVP)	Nocturnal enuresis	20–40 μg intranasally	Headache, nasal congestion, hyponatremic seizures (rare)

MR, mental retardation; PDD, pervasive development disorder; CD, conduct disorder; CBC, complete blood count; LFT, liver function test; WBC, white blood cell; ADHD, attention-deficit/hyperactivity disorder; OCD, obsessive-compulsive disorder.

shown promise in ending stereotypies and other behaviors in autistic children and adults.

The opioid antagonists naloxone (Narcan) and naltrexone have not been proved effective in diminishing self-injurious behavior in children with autistic disorder. The behavioral difficulties of children with autism can be difficult to manage. Much effort, firmness, and consistency are required from caregivers, and a variety of medications may need to be tried to determine which ones are beneficial. β-Adrenergic receptor antagonists (beta blockers), lithium, or anticonvulsants may be helpful. Polypharmacy is not unusual but has not been studied formally. Stimulants can be tried to reduce hyperactivity and inattentiveness in relatively manageable children with autism.

Attention-Deficit/Hyperactivity Disorder. Studies continue to support the use of stimulants in treating ADHD. The most frequently researched and used stimulant is methylphenidate. Dextroamphetamine (Dexedrine) has comparable efficacy and, unlike methylphenidate, is approved by the Food and Drug Administration (FDA) for children 3 years of age and older; the starting age for methylphenidate is 6 years. Another stimulant preparation, Adderall combines dextroamphetamine

Table 53.4–3
Effects of Psychotropic Drugs on Cognitive Tests of Learning Functions[a]

			Test Function			
Drug Class	Continuous Performance Test (Attention)	Matching Familiar Figures (Impulsivity)	Paired Associates (Verbal Learning)	Porteus Maze (Planning Capacity)	Short-Term Memory[a]	WISC (Intelligence)
Stimulant	↑	↑	↑	↑	↑	↑
Antidepressant	↑	0		0	0	0
Antipsychotic	↑↓		↓	↓	↓	0

↑, Improved; ↑↓, inconsistent; ↓, worse; 0, no effect.
[a]Various tests; digit span, word recall, etc.
Adapted from Amar MG. Drugs, learning and the psychotherapies. In: Werry JS, ed. *Pediatric Psychopharmacology: The Use of Behavior Modifying Drugs in Children.* New York: Brunner/Mazel; 1978:356.

Table 53.4–4
Common Dose-Related Side Effects of Stimulants

Insomnia
Decreased appetite
Irritability or nervousness
Weight loss

and amphetamine salts. Several extended-release preparations such as Concerta (extended-release methylphenidate) and Adderall XR (extended-release Adderall) have come on to the market, allowing children who use them to continue to benefit from the medication without needing to take a dose during the school day. Pemoline (Cylert) is no longer recommended because of the risk for hepatotoxicity. Stimulants reduce hyperactivity, inattentiveness, and impulsivity in about 75 percent of children with ADHD. The effects are not paradoxical, as normal children respond similarly. The dose-related adverse effects of stimulants are listed in Table 53.4–4.

ADHD often coexists with oppositional defiant disorder or conduct disorder. With these added disorders comes aggression. In some cases, stimulants seem to reduce aggression, but a common mistake is prolonging stimulant trials when the aggression is not subsiding and a switch to, or the addition of, a more specifically antiaggression drug is indicated.

Antidepressants can be tried for children with ADHD who are resistant to stimulants and children with preexisting tic disorders. Bupropion is commonly tried when stimulants are ineffective in treating ADHD. Desipramine has been somewhat effective in the treatment of ADHD, but its use is limited because of the associated risks. Since the sudden death of four children being treated with desipramine for ADHD, extra caution must be recommended. Other tricyclic drugs, currently rarely recommended, including nortriptyline (Pamelor) and clomipramine, have been tried with some success. Children with ADHD can respond to antidepressants within days of the beginning of treatment.

A few studies have shown that clonidine (Catapres), an α-adrenergic agonist agent, has some success in ADHD. Guanfacine (Tenex), another α-adrenergic agonist has also been used in clinical practice for children and adolescents with ADHD who do not respond to the stimulants. Antipsychotics are not indicated in the treatment of ADHD, unless there is accompanying psychosis, given the risks of sedation and tardive dyskinesia. ADHD often precedes and then coexists with tic disorders. (Chapter 46 discusses pharmacotherapy for children with both conditions.)

The dietary management of hyperactivity has received much public attention, but controlled studies have not substantiated its benefit. Similarly, in most controlled studies, caffeine was not superior to placebo for alleviating ADHD.

Conduct Disorder. The assaultiveness frequently associated with conduct disorder may be reduced with pharmacotherapy. Antipsychotics such as risperidone, olanzapine or haloperidol may quell aggression, but sedation and the risk of tardive dyskinesia are major drawbacks. With newer antipsychotics such as risperidone on the market, the hope of fewer long-term adverse effects supports its use. Lithium has reduced aggression in conduct disorder, and propranolol (Inderal) has been effective in open studies. Carbamazepine has not been shown to be effective in controlling aggression.

When conduct disorder is associated with ADHD and when the aggression is mild, a trial of a stimulant may be indicated; stimulants are faster acting and easier to monitor than the previously noted drugs. Clonidine may be effective and deserves further study.

Aggressive behavior can occur in the context of a variety of psychiatric disorders including comorbid ADHD and conduct disorder. Some evidence indicates that stimulant medications may also have some efficacy in controlling aggressive behavior in children with these disorders.

Tourette's Disorder. The high-potency antipsychotics haloperidol and pimozide (Orap) are the most effective medications for Tourette's disorder. Pimozide prolongs the QT interval and thus requires electrocardiographic (ECG) monitoring. Clonidine, a presynaptic α-adrenergic blocking agent, is less effective than the two antipsychotics but avoids the risk for tardive dyskinesia; sedation is a frequent side effect of clonidine.

Tic disorders often coexist with ADHD in children and adolescents. Stimulant use, which can precipitate tics, should be avoided in these patients, although recent studies indicate that the prohibition may not be totally warranted. Clonidine reduces tics in both ADHD and the comorbid cases. A small study supports the use of nortriptyline.

Enuresis. Before initiating psychopharmacotherapy for treating enuresis, clinicians must consider the merits of waiting for a possible spontaneous remission and of using behavioral techniques; bell-and-pad conditioning (a bell awakens the child when the mattress becomes wet), perhaps the most elaborate behavioral treatment, seems to be more successful than medication.

Tricyclic drugs are effective in reducing enuresis in about 60 percent of patients, and desmopressin (DDAVP) is effective in about 50 percent of patients. Improvement ranges from complete cessation of wetting to continued wetting but with less urine volume. Tricyclic drugs are given about 1 hour before bedtime. The starting dosage usually is 25 mg a day, a lower dosage than is used in trials for depression. The dosage can be increased to 75 mg a day for an adolescent but should not exceed 2 mg/kg a day. Children usually respond within days. Desmopressin is taken intranasally in dosages of 10 to 40 mg a day. When used over months, nasal discomfort can occur, and water retention is potentially a problem. Patients who respond with full dryness should continue to take the medication for several months to prevent relapses.

Separation Anxiety Disorder. SSRIs are currently recommended as first-line medications in the treatment of a variety of anxiety disorders in children and adolescents. Few studies support the use of anxiolytics in pediatric psychopharmacology. A recent double-blind, placebo-controlled study did not replicate a similar study performed by the same workers 20 years before, when imipramine (Tofranil) was shown to be effective for school refusal. Alprazolam (Xanax) may be helpful in separation anxiety disorder, but the data are conflicting.

Schizophrenia. SDAs are generally recommended currently as first-line agents in the treatment of psychotic disorders

55 Geriatric Psychiatry

Geriatric psychiatry is concerned with preventing, diagnosing, and treating psychological disorders in older adults. It is also concerned with promoting longevity; persons with a healthy mental adaptation to life are likely to live longer than those stressed with emotional problems. Mental disorders in the elderly often differ in clinical manifestations, pathogenesis, and pathophysiology from disorders of younger adults and do not always match the categories in the text revision of the fourth edition of *Diagnostic and Statistical Manual of Mental Disorders* (DSM-IV-TR). Diagnosing and treating older adults can present more difficulties than treating younger persons because older persons may have coexisting chronic medical diseases and disabilities, may take many medications, and may show cognitive impairments.

Prevalence data for mental disorders in elderly persons vary widely, but a conservatively estimated 25 percent have significant psychiatric symptoms. The number of mentally ill elderly persons was estimated to be about 9 million in the year 2000. That figure is expected to rise to 20 million by the middle of the century. The American Board of Psychiatry and Neurology established geropsychiatry (from the Greek *geros* ["old age"] and *iatros* ["physical"]) as a subspecialty in 1991, and today geriatric psychiatry is one of the fastest growing fields in psychiatry.

PSYCHIATRIC EXAMINATION OF THE OLDER PATIENT

Psychiatric history-taking and the mental status examination of older adults follow the same format as those of younger adults, but because of the high prevalence of cognitive disorders in older persons, psychiatrists must determine whether a patient understands the nature and purpose of the examination. When a patient is cognitively impaired an independent history should be obtained from a family member or caretaker. The patient still should be seen alone—even if there is clear evidence of impairment—to preserve the privacy of the doctor–patient relationship and to elicit any suicidal thoughts or paranoid ideation, which may not be voiced in the presence of a relative or nurse.

When approaching the examination of the older patient, one must remember that older adults differ markedly from one another. The approach to examining the older patient must take into account whether the person is a healthy 75-year-old who recently retired from a second career or a frail 96-year-old who just lost the only surviving relative with the death of the 75-year-old caregiving daughter.

Psychiatric History

A complete psychiatric history includes preliminary identification (name, age, sex, marital status), chief complaint, history of the present illness, history of previous illnesses, personal history, and family history. A review of medications (including over-the-counter medications) that the patient is currently using or has used in the recent past is also important.

Patients older than age 65 often have subjective complaints of minor memory impairments, such as forgetting persons' names and misplacing objects. Minor cognitive problems also may occur because of anxiety in the interview situation. These age-associated memory impairments are of no significance; the term *benign senescent forgetfulness* has been used to describe them.

A patient's childhood and adolescent history can provide information about personality organization and give important clues about coping strategies and defense mechanisms used under stress. A history of learning disability or minimal cerebral dysfunction is significant. The psychiatrist should inquire about friends, sports, hobbies, social activity, and work. The occupational history should include the patient's feeling about work, relationships with peers, problems with authority, and attitudes toward retirement. The patient also should be questioned about plans for the future. What are the patient's hopes and fears?

The family history should include a patient's description of parents' attitudes and adaptation to their old age and, if applicable, information about the causes of their deaths. Alzheimer's disease is transmitted as an autosomal-dominant trait in 10 to 30 percent of the offspring of parents with Alzheimer's disease; depression and alcohol dependence also run in families. The patient's current social situation should be evaluated. Who cares for the patient? Does the patient have children? What are the characteristics of patient–child relationships? A financial history helps the psychiatrist evaluate the role of economic hardship in the patient's illness and to make realistic treatment recommendations.

The marital history includes a description of the spouse and the characteristics of the relationship. If the patient is a widow or a widower, the psychiatrist should explore how grieving was handled. If the loss of the spouse occurred within the past year, the patient is at high risk for an adverse physical or psychological event.

The patient's sexual history includes sexual activity, orientation, libido, masturbation, extramarital affairs, and sexual symptoms (such as impotence and anorgasmia). Young clini-

The court-appointed child psychiatrist recorded the father's complaints but also failed to confirm abuse. In the joint interview with father and child, the boy was playing at the dollhouse. His father picked up a miniature bathtub and told him, "Billy, show the doctor how Mommy pushes your head underwater and tries to scare you. Go on, Billy, show the doctor." The child refused and became quite anxious. He moved away from the dollhouse.

The child psychiatrist concluded that the father suffered from delusions about abuse and that these delusions were harmful to the child, because he acted upon them and caused the child to undergo many unnecessary examinations and tests. He recommended that for these and other reasons, custody be awarded to the mother. He also recommended supervised visitation for the father. The judge granted custody to the mother but initially did not order that the father have supervised visitation. When he was with the child, the father continued to take him to emergency rooms. After another year, the judge stopped the visits altogether. (Courtesy of Stephen P. Herman, M.D.)

JUVENILE OFFENDERS

The creation of a separate juvenile court system in the United States occurred by statute in the state of Illinois in the late 1800s. Its mandate was to rehabilitate rather than to punish. The omission of various constitutional safeguards, such as the rights to counsel, confrontation, and cross-examination of an accuser, eventually led to criticism and disillusionment with this system. Juvenile offenders of small and significant crimes often were sent to state-run residential programs that were criticized for being overcrowded, neglectful, and frankly abusive. Despite the strong sentiment to increase due process protection for juveniles rather than pretrial, trial, and sentencing, the juvenile court system includes intake, adjudication, and disposition. The intake is a determination of whether there is probable cause that the youth committed a crime. If they confess, juveniles can be diverted from the court system altogether at this time, and appropriate plans for rehabilitation can be made in a community setting. For more serious crimes or when juveniles deny perpetrating a crime, the process continues. Juveniles must be represented by counsel, and an attorney is provided if the family cannot afford to provide its own.

Unlike adult court, in juvenile court guilt or innocence is determined by a judge, not a jury. The case is argued by a prosecuting attorney and a defense attorney, and the judge is bound by the same standards as in adult court; that is, a judgment of delinquency requires proof beyond a reasonable doubt. When the charge is substantiated and the judgment is for delinquency, the juvenile is an "adjudicated delinquent." Disposition must next be determined. Dispositions include a wide range of options, from placement in youth correctional facilities, to residential treatment settings, to psychiatric hospitalizations for further evaluation. *Delinquent acts* refer to ordinary crimes committed by juveniles; *status offenses* refer to behaviors that would not be criminal if perpetrated by adults, such as truancy, running away, or drinking alcohol. Sometimes, youths who are believed to have committed a serious crime are turned over (receive a waiver) to adult criminal court.

Psychiatrists are not infrequently consulted to provide recommendations at any phase of the juvenile justice process. A psychiatrist may be asked to evaluate a juvenile to make recommendations about appropriate diversion plans. Psychiatric evaluation may be sought for adjudicated delinquents to determine whether treatment for a psychiatric illness would work in favor of preventing future delinquent acts and, if so, in what setting. Psychiatric evaluations also may be requested when the court is considering a waiver to adult court. In some states, such decisions are based, in part, on the juvenile's psychiatric history and current mental status.

ADVERSE LIFE EVENTS AND PSYCHIATRIC SYMPTOMS

Child and adolescent psychiatrists are frequently sought out to evaluate children or adolescents who have been exposed to a traumatic or adverse life event and are exhibiting a variety of psychiatric symptoms. The child and adolescent psychiatrist may be asked to determine whether a child or adolescent is experiencing posttraumatic stress disorder or whether a given set of symptoms is likely to have been caused by exposure to the adverse life event. Another common request to a child and adolescent psychiatrist is to render an expert opinion regarding whether, for example, a child diagnosed with autistic disorder is likely to have been at greater risk for the disorder because of a particular treatment given to the mother during pregnancy. It is much easier for a child and adolescent psychiatrist to verify the presence of a psychiatric disorder in a child than to determine its exact cause. Evaluations requiring a psychiatrist to make a judgment identifying a single cause of a complex psychiatric disorder are generally difficult or impossible because of the lack of data linking psychiatric disorders to single causes.

References

Alessi N. Information technology and child and adolescent psychiatry: ethical issues. *Drug Benefit Trends.* 2001;13:24.

American Academy of Child and Adolescent Psychiatry. *Code of Ethics.* Washington, DC: American Academy of Child and Adolescent Psychiatry; 1980.

Barnum R. Clinical evaluation of juvenile delinquents facing transfer to adult court. *J Am Acad Child Adolesc Psychiatry.* 1987;26:922.

Berlin FS, Malin MH, Dean S. Effects of statutes requiring psychiatrists to report suspected sexual abuse of children. *Am J Psychiatry.* 1991;148:449.

Billick SB, Perry CD. Role of the psychiatric evaluator in child custody disputes. In: Rosner R, ed. *Principles and Practice of Forensic Psychiatry.* New York: Chapman & Hall; 1994:271.

Girouard C, Medaris M. Protecting children in cyberspace: the ICAC task force program. *Juvenile Justice Bull.* 2002;8:213.

Grisso T, Miller MO, Sabos B. Competency to stand trial in juvenile court. *Int J Law Psychiatry.* 1987;10:1.

Gunn J. Future directions for treatment in forensic psychiatry. *Br J Psychiatry.* 2000;176;332.

Herman SP. Forensic child and adolescent psychiatry. In: Sadock BJ, Sadock VA, eds. *Kaplan & Sadock's Comprehensive Textbook of Psychiatry.* 7th ed. Vol 2. Baltimore: Lippincott Williams & Wilkins; 2000:2938.

Kalogerakis M. Juvenile delinquency. In: Schetky DH, Benedek EP, eds. *Clinical Handbook of Child Psychiatry and the Law.* New York: Brunner/Mazel; 1992:97.

Lewis DO, Lovely R, Yeager G. Toward a theory of the genesis of violence: a follow-up study of delinquents. *J Am Acad Child Adolesc Psychiatry.* 1989;28:744.

Ratner RA. Juvenile delinquency. In: Rosner R, ed. *Principles and Practice of Forensic Psychiatry.* New York: Chapman & Hall; 1994:36.

Rosenberg JE. Forensic aspects of PTSD in children and adolescents. In: Eth S, ed. PTSD in children and adolescents. *Review of Psychiatry.* Vol 20, no. 1. Washington, DC: American Psychiatric Association; 2001:33.

Shields JM, Johnson A. Collision between law and ethics: consent for treatment with adolescents. *Bull Am Acad Psychiatry Law.* 1992;20:309.

Weintrob A. Confidentiality and its dilemmas in child and adolescent psychiatry. In: Rosner R, ed. *Principles and Practice of Forensic Psychiatry.* New York: Chapman & Hall; 1994:197.

55 Geriatric Psychiatry

Geriatric psychiatry is concerned with preventing, diagnosing, and treating psychological disorders in older adults. It is also concerned with promoting longevity; persons with a healthy mental adaptation to life are likely to live longer than those stressed with emotional problems. Mental disorders in the elderly often differ in clinical manifestations, pathogenesis, and pathophysiology from disorders of younger adults and do not always match the categories in the text revision of the fourth edition of *Diagnostic and Statistical Manual of Mental Disorders* (DSM-IV-TR). Diagnosing and treating older adults can present more difficulties than treating younger persons because older persons may have coexisting chronic medical diseases and disabilities, may take many medications, and may show cognitive impairments.

Prevalence data for mental disorders in elderly persons vary widely, but a conservatively estimated 25 percent have significant psychiatric symptoms. The number of mentally ill elderly persons was estimated to be about 9 million in the year 2000. That figure is expected to rise to 20 million by the middle of the century. The American Board of Psychiatry and Neurology established geropsychiatry (from the Greek *geros* ["old age"] and *iatros* ["physical"]) as a subspecialty in 1991, and today geriatric psychiatry is one of the fastest growing fields in psychiatry.

PSYCHIATRIC EXAMINATION OF THE OLDER PATIENT

Psychiatric history-taking and the mental status examination of older adults follow the same format as those of younger adults, but because of the high prevalence of cognitive disorders in older persons, psychiatrists must determine whether a patient understands the nature and purpose of the examination. When a patient is cognitively impaired an independent history should be obtained from a family member or caretaker. The patient still should be seen alone—even if there is clear evidence of impairment—to preserve the privacy of the doctor–patient relationship and to elicit any suicidal thoughts or paranoid ideation, which may not be voiced in the presence of a relative or nurse.

When approaching the examination of the older patient, one must remember that older adults differ markedly from one another. The approach to examining the older patient must take into account whether the person is a healthy 75-year-old who recently retired from a second career or a frail 96-year-old who just lost the only surviving relative with the death of the 75-year-old caregiving daughter.

Psychiatric History

A complete psychiatric history includes preliminary identification (name, age, sex, marital status), chief complaint, history of the present illness, history of previous illnesses, personal history, and family history. A review of medications (including over-the-counter medications) that the patient is currently using or has used in the recent past is also important.

Patients older than age 65 often have subjective complaints of minor memory impairments, such as forgetting persons' names and misplacing objects. Minor cognitive problems also may occur because of anxiety in the interview situation. These age-associated memory impairments are of no significance; the term *benign senescent forgetfulness* has been used to describe them.

A patient's childhood and adolescent history can provide information about personality organization and give important clues about coping strategies and defense mechanisms used under stress. A history of learning disability or minimal cerebral dysfunction is significant. The psychiatrist should inquire about friends, sports, hobbies, social activity, and work. The occupational history should include the patient's feeling about work, relationships with peers, problems with authority, and attitudes toward retirement. The patient also should be questioned about plans for the future. What are the patient's hopes and fears?

The family history should include a patient's description of parents' attitudes and adaptation to their old age and, if applicable, information about the causes of their deaths. Alzheimer's disease is transmitted as an autosomal-dominant trait in 10 to 30 percent of the offspring of parents with Alzheimer's disease; depression and alcohol dependence also run in families. The patient's current social situation should be evaluated. Who cares for the patient? Does the patient have children? What are the characteristics of patient–child relationships? A financial history helps the psychiatrist evaluate the role of economic hardship in the patient's illness and to make realistic treatment recommendations.

The marital history includes a description of the spouse and the characteristics of the relationship. If the patient is a widow or a widower, the psychiatrist should explore how grieving was handled. If the loss of the spouse occurred within the past year, the patient is at high risk for an adverse physical or psychological event.

The patient's sexual history includes sexual activity, orientation, libido, masturbation, extramarital affairs, and sexual symptoms (such as impotence and anorgasmia). Young clini-

fathers' property. At the beginning of this century, the "tender years" doctrine became the standard for determining child custody. According to this doctrine, the relationship between mother and infant, later generalized to mother and child, is responsible for the optimal emotional development of the child; the doctrine thus supported custody decisions in the mother's favor in most cases. With this doctrine as its guide, psychological issues in developing children became an acceptable dimension to consider in the determination of custody. In controversial and unclear cases, psychological expert testimony began to be accepted as a valuable part of child custody decision making.

The "best interest of the child" standard replaced the "tender years" doctrine and expanded considerations of the optimal parent to include assessing issues of emotional climate, safety, and educational and social opportunities for the children. The "best interest of the child" grew from the movement to support legislation about the rights of children in the areas of compulsory education, child labor laws, and child abuse and neglect protection laws. Therefore, although "best interest" standards have broadened the dimensions considered in evaluating which parent is best able to serve the best interest of the child, there is vagueness about how to measure these qualities in a parent. In view of the lack of clarity regarding what specific parameters in a parent best correspond to the interest of the child, child and adolescent psychiatrists have increasingly been asked to help make decisions by defining relevant psychological conditions in parents and in the relationships between parents and children.

Psychiatric evaluators may be asked to give an opinion about child custody at various points during the separation and divorce process. Sometimes, a psychiatric evaluation is requested by the parents before any legal action occurs. When the parents and an evaluator can agree on custody decisions before the legal process, a court is likely to go along with these decisions rather than launch an additional investigation. A psychiatric evaluation may be ordered by the court or by the attorneys representing feuding parents. In such cases, an evaluator is faced with two disgruntled parents who often are consumed by their mutual conflict to the point that neither is willing to compromise, even in the child's interest. The advantage in such cases, however, is that evaluators represent the court and can act as advocate for the child without the same pressures that an evaluator hired by only one parent faces. A psychiatric evaluation also may be initiated by a *guardian ad litem*, an attorney who is appointed by the court to represent the child. Psychiatric evaluators also may be requested to give an opinion about custody during a mediation process. Mediation is a legal process that usually involves one attorney and one evaluator. Because mediation can occur outside the judicial system, some families may prefer it to going through a trial. In addition to custody, psychiatric evaluators often are asked to give opinions about visitation.

In undertaking a custody evaluation, an evaluator is expected to determine the best interests of the child while keeping in mind the standard elements that the court considers. These considerations include the wishes of the parents and the child; relationships with significant others in the child's life; the child's adjustment to the current home, school, and community; the psychiatric and physical health of all parties; and the level of conflict and potential danger to the child under the care of either parent. A psychiatric evaluator must maintain his or her role as an advocate for the best interest of the child and does not consider the fairest outcome for parents. The psychiatric evaluator conducts a series of interviews, often including at least one separate interview with each parent and the child alone and one interview with the child and both parents. The evaluator may obtain a written waiver of confidentiality from all parties because he or she may have made disclosures to opposing attorneys and in court before the judge. The evaluator uses direct questioning as well as observations of the relationships between the child and each parent. The age and developmental needs of the child are considered in making a judgment regarding which parent may better serve the child's interests. As part of the psychiatric assessment of the child custody evaluation, the evaluator determines the need for psychiatric treatment of any of the parties involved.

The child custody evaluation generally is provided in a written report. This document is not confidential and may be used in court. The report contains a description of the relationship between the child and parents, the capabilities of the parents, and finally, the custody recommendations. In view of data supporting the importance of continuing a relationship with both parents in most cases, it is recommended that joint custody be considered before other options. When there is enough cooperation to negotiate for joint custody, the best interests of the child often are served. Joint custody may not be the best option for a child when the relationship of the child with either parent is jeopardized and undermined by the other. The next most frequent choice when joint custody is not advisable is full custody by one parent with visitation rights for the other parent. The parent awarded full custody should be able to support the visitations and relationship with the noncustodial parent. In custody disputes involving a biological parent and a nonbiological parent, the biological parent generally has the right to custody unless he or she is shown to be unable to provide for the child. After the custody evaluation has been submitted in writing, the results must be communicated to the parents, the child, and possibly their respective attorneys. The evaluator may be called on to testify in court, and the parties may use the custody evaluation to mediate other areas of their dispute.

Many complications can occur in an ongoing bitter dispute between divorcing or divorced parents. Both true and false allegations of psychiatric illness, drug or alcohol abuse, or sexual or physical abuse are not uncommon during custody battles. The evaluator must be prepared to verify any allegations and to carefully discuss their effects on custody and visitation. Evidence suggests that markedly elevated numbers of unfounded allegations of child sexual abuse occur during the course of custody disputes.

Two parents were locked in a bitter custody dispute over their 4-year-old son. Throughout the litigation, the father made numerous allegations that his wife was physically abusing the boy, burning him with cigarettes, sticking him with pins, poisoning his milk, and terrifying him by holding his head under water while giving him a bath. The father had called Child Protective Services numerous times, had taken his son to every emergency room in the city, and had sent out milk samples for toxicological analysis. Results of all physical examinations and laboratory tests were normal, and no doctor or city social worker had ever confirmed signs or symptoms of abuse. Yet the father persisted in his accusations.

54

Forensic Issues in Child Psychiatry

Child and adolescent psychiatrists are increasingly being sought out by patients and attorneys for evaluations and expert opinions related to child custody and criminal behaviors perpetrated by minors and to evaluate the relations between traumatic life events and the emergence of psychiatric symptoms in children and adolescents. In medicine, ethics historically has alluded to moral obligations as well as to the accepted behavior that physicians follow; on the broadest scale, the Hippocratic oath summarizes ethical values in medicine. During the past few decades, however, new ethical and moral dilemmas have arisen with the growth of medical knowledge and technology. The traditional ethical tenet that physicians must consider each patient above all else has often been challenged. For example, a patient may be kept alive for long periods while in a coma or a pregnant woman's life may be saved by aborting her fetus.

Society's view of children and their rights has evolved dramatically in the 20th century. The institution of a juvenile court system about 100 years ago was an acknowledgment that children must be protected and provided for differently than adults. In 1980, the American Academy of Child and Adolescent Psychiatry published a code of ethics that was developed to publicly endorse the ethical standards of this discipline. The code is based on the assumption that children are vulnerable and unable to take adequate care of themselves, but as they mature, their capacity to make judgments of, and choices about, their well-being develop as well. The code has several caveats: From the standpoint of child and adolescent psychiatrists, issues of consent, confidentiality, and professional responsibility must be seen in the context of overlapping and potentially conflicting rights of children, parents, and society.

Confidentiality, or intensive trust, refers to the relationship between two persons with respect to the "entrustment of secrets." Until the 1970s, little attention was paid to issues of confidentiality pertaining to minors. In 1980, among the items in the American Academy of Child and Adolescent Psychiatry's Code of Ethics, six principles were related to confidentiality. Breaches and limits of confidentiality can obtain in cases of child abuse or maltreatment or for purposes of appropriate education. Although unnecessary with a child or adolescent, consent for disclosure should be obtained when possible. In 1979, the American Psychiatric Association (APA) stated that a child 12 years of age could give consent for disclosure of confidential information, and that with the exception of safety issues, a minor's consent is required for disclosure of information to others, including the child's parents. According to the Academy of Child Psychiatry's Code of Ethics, the consent of a minor is not required for disclosure of confidential information. Specific ages for consent are not addressed in the code. Child and adolescent psychiatrists often face the dilemma of weighing the potential benefits and possible harm in sharing information obtained confidentially from a child with the child's parents. Although the smoothest transition occurs when the child and the physician agree that certain information can be shared, in many situations that border on "dangerousness to the child or others," the child or adolescent does not agree to share the information with a parent or another responsible adult. Among adolescents, these secrets that are sometimes shared with a psychiatrist may involve drug or alcohol use, unsafe sex practices, or a thrill-seeking act that places the adolescent in danger. A psychiatrist may choose to work with the child or adolescent toward agreeing to share confidential information when it is determined by the treating psychiatrist that the probable outcome would be beneficial. The initial treatment contract, however, limits confidentiality to situations of "danger" to the child or others.

Other arenas that can pose confidentiality dilemmas include educational and scientific settings, research activities, and third-party agencies. Professional settings such as annual psychiatric conventions often include individual case presentations. In the context of a clinical symposium, doctors should realize that confidentiality means more than changing or dropping a patient's name; other information in a case study may pose a threat to a patient's privacy. Research projects sometimes are impeded by laws designed to protect the privacy of children and their families. In some cases, long-term follow-up studies may no longer be "legal" because of a time limitation on a written consent for study. Third-party payers are requiring more and more confidential information before they consider reimbursement of psychiatric services. Information disclosed to insurance companies often is shared with many reviewers in the company; it also is in danger of being merged into a database in a computer system that is neither highly restricted nor confidential.

In general, there is no way to simplify the many difficult, complex confidentiality issues that may emerge in treating children and adolescents. Child and adolescent psychiatrists function as advocates for their patients and must always remain aware of minors' vulnerabilities and of the importance of maintaining trust in the treatment relationship.

CHILD CUSTODY

The evolution of child custody decision making has been influenced by increasing awareness and recognition of the rights of children and women, as well as by a broadening perspective on the developmental and psychological needs of the children involved. Historically, children were considered to be their

even if based on examination and testing to rule out pathophysiology, may not suffice. An adolescent's distress may show as sexual or delinquent acting out, withdrawal, or problems at school that are serious enough to warrant therapeutic intervention. Therapy also may be prompted by similar disturbances in some adolescents who fail to achieve peer-valued stereotypes of physical development despite normal pubertal physiology.

Substance-Related Disorders

Some experimentation with psychoactive substances is almost ubiquitous among adolescents, especially if this category of behavior includes alcohol use. However, most adolescents do not become abusers, particularly of prescription drugs and illegal substances. Any regular substance abuse represents disturbance. Substance abuse sometimes is self-medication against depression or schizophrenic deterioration and sometimes signals a character disorder in teenagers whose ego deficits render them unequal to the stresses of puberty and the tasks of adolescence. But, many substances, especially cocaine, have a physiologically reinforcing action that acts independently of preexisting psychopathology. Regardless of why the abuse developed, it becomes a problem in itself. Ego development depends on confronting and learning to cope adaptively with reality. The substances become both a substitute for reality and an avoidance of it and thus impair ego development and perpetuate the abuse to conceal poor coping skills.

When substance abuse covers an underlying illness or is a maladaptive response to current stresses or disturbed family dynamics, treatment of the underlying cause may take care of the substance abuse. Outpatient psychotherapy, however, generally is useless with long-term abusers, who require a structured setting in which the substances are not available.

Suicide

Suicide currently is the second leading cause of death among adolescents. Many hospital admissions of adolescents result from suicidal ideation or behavior. Suicide is the final common pathway for a number of disorders, and its high incidence reflects grave psychopathology. Some authorities believe that in adolescence, in contrast to adulthood, schizophrenia more often underlies suicide than major mood disorders do. Among adolescents who are not psychotic, the highest suicidal risks occur in those who have a history of parental suicide, who are unable to form stable attachments, who display impulsive behavior or episodic dyscontrol, and who abuse alcohol or other substances. Many adolescent suicides show a common pattern of long-standing family and social problems throughout childhood and the escalation of subjective distress under the pressure and stresses of puberty and adolescence, followed by a suicide attempt precipitated by the sudden real or perceived loss of a person or social support believed to be the one source of meaning or closeness.

Normal developmental losses of childhood dependence, of parents, of childhood—also can cause psychogenic depression in adolescents. The rapid and extreme mood swings in adolescence, coupled with adolescents' difficulties in seeing beyond the intensity of the moment, contribute to catastrophic despair and impulsive suicide attempts over losses that adults could withstand. Moreover, alcohol and other substances can decrease the resistance to suicidal impulses. Normally persistent magical thinking may impair the sense of permanence of death and may allow adolescents to contemplate suicide more lightly than adults do.

During both evaluation and treatment, suicidal thoughts, plans, and past attempts must be discussed directly when the concern arises and information is not volunteered. Long-term or recurring thoughts should be taken seriously, and an agreement or contract should be negotiated with adolescents not to attempt suicide without first calling and talking about it with the psychiatrist. Adolescents usually are honest about making and keeping, or refusing, such agreements; if they refuse, closed hospitalization is indicated. Hospitalization is a sign of serious, protective concern and may be as therapeutic as the opportunity to conduct or plan further treatment in a safe environment. See Chapter 49 for a more complete discussion of suicide in adolescents.

References

Blos P. *On Adolescence.* New York: Free Press; 1962.

Davis M, Raffe IH. The holding environment in the inpatient treatment of adolescents. *Adolesc Psychiatry.* 1985;12:434.

Erikson EH. The problem of ego identity. *J Am Psychoanal Assoc.* 1966;4:56.

Etain B, Le Heuzey MF, Mouren-Simeoni MC. Electroconvulsive therapy in the adolescent: clinical considerations apropos of a series of cases. *Can J Psychiatry.* 2001;46:976.

Feldman LB. Integrating individual and family therapy in the treatment of symptomatic children and adolescents. *Am J Psychother.* 1988;42:272.

Hendren RL, De Backer I, Pandina GJ. Review of neuroimaging studies of child and adolescent psychiatric disorders from the past 10 years. *J Am Acad Child Adolesc Psychiatry.* 2000;39:815.

March JS, Mulle K, Herbel B. Behavioral psychotherapy for children and adolescents with obsessive-compulsive disorder: an open trial of a new protocol-driven package. *J Am Acad Child Adolesc Psychiatry.* 1994;33:333.

Moreau D, Mufson L, Weissman MM, Klerman GL. Interpersonal psychotherapy for adolescent depression: description of modification and preliminary application. *J Am Acad Child Adolesc Psychiatry.* 1991;30:642.

Mufson L, Moreau D, Weissman MM, Wickramaratne P, Martin J, Samoilov A. Modification of interpersonal psychotherapy with depressed adolescents (IPT-A): phase I and II studies. *J Am Acad Child Adolesc Psychiatry.* 1994;33:695.

O'Brien JD. Current prevention concepts in child and adolescent psychiatry. *Am J Psychother.* 1991;45:261.

Pedersen J, Aakrog T. A 10-year follow-up study of an adolescent psychiatric clientele and early predictors of readmission. *Nord J Psychiatry.* 2000;55:11.

Pedersen J, Aakrog T. A 20-year study of an adolescent psychiatric clientele with special reference to the age of onset. *Nord J Psychiatry.* 2001;55:5.

Pfeffer CR. Psychiatric treatment of adolescents. In: Sadock BJ, Sadock VA, eds. *Kaplan & Sadock's Comprehensive Textbook of Psychiatry.* 7th ed. Vol 2. Baltimore: Lippincott Williams & Wilkins; 2000:2859.

Shaffer D, Garland A, Vieland V, Underwood M, Busner C. The impact of curriculum-based suicide prevention programs for teenagers. *J Am Acad Child Adolesc Psychiatry.* 1991;30:588.

Sholevar GP, Burland A, Frank JL, Etezady MH, Goldstein J. Psychoanalytic treatment of children and adolescents. *J Am Acad Child Adolesc Psychiatry.* 1989;28:685.

Wichstrøm L. Predictors of adolescent suicide attempts: a nationally representative longitudinal study of Norwegian adolescents. *J Am Acad Child Adolesc Psychiatry.* 2002;39:603.

reuptake inhibitors [SSRIs]) and schizophrenia (e.g., serotonin-dopamine antagonists [SDAs] including risperidone [Risperdal], olanzapine [Zyprexa], and clozapine [Clozaril]). While these medications have been used to treat adolescent disorders, systematic research is required to determine the efficacy and safety profiles of these medications for treatment of adolescent psychopathology.

A comprehensive workup is needed before starting psychopharmacotherapy with adolescents, including a physical examination; blood tests to evaluate hematological, kidney, liver, thyroid and other physiological functions; and an electrocardiogram (ECG) to measure cardiac function. Neurological assessment with an electroencephalogram (EEG) is necessary if seizure disorder is suspected or if the medication is likely to lower the seizure threshold.

A 17-year-old girl complained of episodes of rapid heartbeat, sweating, trembling, and fears of going out alone to the shopping mall. She had entered her senior year in high school, was considering her choice of colleges, and was planning to take her college entrance examination. Her parents wanted her to maintain the family tradition and go to the college from which her mother graduated. Psychoanalytically oriented outpatient treatment and treatment with an SSRI were instituted to alleviate the panic disorder symptoms. The psychotherapy focused on the patient's conflicts with her parents, highlighting her chronic concern that she could not meet parental expectations and fears of her independence. Medication appeared to reduce symptoms of tachycardia, tremulousness, and preoccupation with lack of competence. Psychotherapy was maintained for 8 months during her last year in high school. (Courtesy of Cynthia R. Pfeffer, M.D.)

Group Psychotherapy

In many ways group psychotherapy is a natural setting for adolescents. Most teenagers are more comfortable with peers than with adults. A group diminishes the sense of unequal power between the adult therapist and the adolescent patient. Participation varies, depending on an adolescent's readiness. Not all interpretations and confrontations should come from the parent-figure therapist; group members often are adept at noticing symptomatic behavior in each other, and adolescents may find it easier to hear and consider critical or challenging comments from their peers.

Group psychotherapy usually addresses interpersonal and current life issues. However, some adolescents are too fragile for group psychotherapy or have symptoms or social traits that are too likely to elicit peer group ridicule; they need individual therapy to attain enough ego strength to struggle with peer relationships. Conversely, other adolescents must resolve interpersonal issues in a group before they can tackle intrapsychic issues in the intensity of one-on-one therapy.

Family Therapy

Family therapy is the primary modality when adolescents' difficulties mainly reflect a dysfunctional family (e.g., teenagers with school refusal, runaways). The same may be true when developmental issues, such as adolescent sexuality and striving for autonomy, trigger family conflicts or when family pathology is severe, as in cases of incest and child abuse. In these instances, adolescents usually need individual therapy as well, but family therapy is mandatory if an adolescent is to remain in the home or return to it. Serious character pathology, such as that underlying antisocial and borderline personality disorders, often develops from highly pathogenic early parenting. Family therapy is strongly indicated whenever possible for such disorders, but most authorities consider it adjunctive to intensive individual psychotherapy when individual psychopathology has become so internalized that it persists regardless of the current family status.

Inpatient Treatment

Residential treatment schools often are preferable for long-term therapy, but hospitals are more suitable for emergencies, although some adolescent inpatient hospital units also provide educational, recreational, and occupational facilities for long-term patients. Adolescents whose families are too disturbed or incompetent, who are dangerous to themselves or others, who are out of control in ways that preclude further healthy development, or who are seriously disorganized require, at least temporarily, the external controls of structured environment.

Long-term inpatient therapy is the treatment of choice for severe disorders that are considered wholly or largely psychogenic in origin, such as major ego deficits that are caused by early massive deprivation and that respond poorly or not at all to medication. Severe borderline personality disorder, for example, regardless of the behavioral symptoms, requires a full-time corrective environment in which regression is possible and safe and in which ego development can take place. Psychotic disorders in adolescence often require hospitalization, but psychotic adolescents often respond to appropriate medication so that therapy usually is feasible in an outpatient setting, except during exacerbation. Adolescent schizophrenia patients who exhibit a long-term deteriorating course may require hospitalization periodically.

Day Hospitals

In day hospitals, which have become increasingly popular, adolescents spend the day in class, individual and group psychotherapy, and other programs, but they go home in the evenings. Day hospitals are less expensive than full hospitalization and usually are preferred by patients.

CLINICAL PROBLEMS

Atypical Puberty

Pubertal changes that occur $2\frac{1}{2}$ years earlier or later than the average age are within the normal range. However, body image is so important to adolescents that extremes of the norm may be distressing to some, either because markedly early maturation subjects them to social and sexual pressures for which they are unready or because late maturation makes them feel inferior and excludes them from some peer activities. Medical reassurance,

Respect and knowledgeable concern are human qualities and are not group restricted.

INTERVIEWS

Whenever circumstances permit, both an adolescent patient and his or her parents should be interviewed. Other family members also may be included, depending on their involvement in the teenager's life and difficulties. Clinicians should see the adolescent first, however; preferential treatment helps avoid the appearance of being the parents' agent. In psychotherapy with an older adolescent, the therapist and the parents usually have little contact after the initial part of the therapy, because ongoing contact inhibits the adolescent's desire to open up.

Interview Techniques

All patients test and mistrust therapists, but adolescents often manifest these reactions crudely, intensely, provocatively, and for prolonged periods. Clinicians must establish themselves as trustworthy and helpful adults to promote a therapeutic alliance. They should encourage adolescents to tell their own stories, without interrupting to check discrepancies; such a tactic seems like correcting and expressing disbelief. Clinicians should ask patients for explanations and theories about what happened. Why did these behaviors or feelings occur? When did things change? What caused the identified problems to begin when they did?

Sessions with adolescents generally follow the adult model; the therapist sits across from the patient. In early adolescence, however, board games (such as checkers) may help to stimulate conversation in an otherwise quiet, anxious patient.

Language is crucial. Even when a teenager and a clinician come from the same socioeconomic group, their languages are seldom the same. Psychiatrists should use their own language, explain any specialized terms or concepts, and ask for an explanation of unfamiliar in-group jargon or slang. Many adolescents do not talk spontaneously about illicit substances and suicidal tendencies but do respond honestly to a therapist's questions. A therapist may need to ask specifically about each substance and the amount and frequency of its use.

The sexual histories and current sexual activities of adolescents are increasingly important pieces of information for adequate evaluation. The nature of adolescents' sexual behaviors often is a vignette of their whole personality structures and ego development, but a long time may elapse in therapy before adolescents begin to talk about their sexual behavior.

TREATMENT

The best choices for treatment of psychiatric disorders in adolescents must take into account the characteristics of the individual adolescent and the family or social milieu. Adolescents' striving for autonomy may complicate problems of compliance with therapy and may result in the need for stabilization in inpatient settings whereas this level of care may not be necessary at a different stage of life. Therefore, the following discussion is less a set of guidelines than a brief summary of what each treatment modality can or should offer.

Individual Psychotherapy

Few adolescent patients are trusting or open without considerable time and testing, and it is helpful to anticipate the testing period by letting patients know that it is to be expected and is natural and healthy. Pointing out the likelihood of therapeutic problems—for instance, impatience and disappointment with the psychiatrist, with the therapy, with the time required, and with the often-intangible results—may help keep problems under control. Therapeutic goals should be stated in terms that adolescents understand and value. Although they may not see the point in exercising self-control, enduring dysphoric emotions, or forgoing impulsive gratification, they may value feeling more confident than in the past and gaining more control over their lives and the events that affect them.

Typical adolescent patients need a real relationship with a therapist they can perceive as a real person. The therapist becomes another parent, because adolescents still need appropriate parenting or reparenting. Thus, a professional who is impersonal and anonymous is a less useful model than one who can accept and respond rationally to an angry challenge or confrontation without fear or false conciliation, can impose limits and controls when adolescents cannot, can admit mistakes and ignorance, and can openly express the gamut of human emotions. Adolescents perceive the failure to take a stand about self-damaging and self-destructive behavior or to respond actively to manipulative and dishonest behavior as indifference or collusion.

Countertransference reactions can be intense in psychotherapeutic work with adolescents, and therapists must be aware of them. An adolescent often expresses hostile feelings toward adults, such as parents and teachers. A therapist may react with overidentification with the adolescent or with the parents. Such reactions are determined, at least in part, by a therapist's own experiences during adolescence or, when applicable, the therapist's own experiences as a parent.

Individual outpatient therapy is appropriate for adolescents whose problems are manifest in conflicted emotions and nondangerous behavior, who are not too disorganized to be maintained outside a structured setting, and whose families or other living environments are not disturbed enough to negate the influence of therapy. Such therapy characteristically focuses on intrapsychic conflicts and inhibitions; on the meanings of emotions, attitudes, and behavior; and on the influence of the past and the present. Antianxiety agents can be considered in adolescents whose anxiety may be high at certain times during psychotherapy, but adolescents' potential for abusing these drugs must be weighed carefully.

Psychopharmacotherapy and Combined Therapy

Attention-deficit/hyperactivity disorder has been studied most systematically with regard to combinations of psychotherapy and medications. Psychostimulants such as methylphenidate (Ritalin) and dextroamphetamine (Dexedrine) when combined with behavior therapy or cognitive behavioral therapy are most effective in improving social behavior and academic performance. No empirical studies of combined psychotherapeutic and medication treatment of mood disorders, anxiety disorders, or schizophrenia in adolescents have been published, but studies of adult patients, such as those with major depressive disorder, obsessive-compulsive disorder, and schizophrenia suggest that psychotherapy plus medication is most effective in reducing symptoms.

Advances in drug development have widened the choice of medications to treat mood disorders (e.g., selective serotonin

known treatment is effective. Tardive dyskinesia has not been reported in patients taking less than 375 to 400 g of chlorpromazine equivalents. Because nonpersistent choreiform movements of the extremities and trunk are common after abrupt discontinuation of antipsychotics, clinicians must distinguish these symptoms from persistent dyskinesias.

Whenever clinically feasible, children receiving antipsychotics should be periodically withdrawn from the medication, so that clinicians can assess the patient's current clinical needs and the possible development of tardive dyskinesia.

Stimulants. The current belief is that any growth suppression is temporary and that children taking stimulants eventually reach their normal height.

OTHER BIOLOGICAL THERAPIES

Electroconvulsive therapy (ECT) is rarely, if ever, indicated in childhood or adolescence. Psychosurgery for severe and intransigent obsessive-compulsive disorder should probably be delayed until adulthood, after all attempts at less drastic treatment have failed and when the patient can participate fully in the process of informed consent.

Little evidence indicates that food allergies or sensitivities play a role in childhood mental disorders. Diets that eliminate food additives, colorings, and sugar are difficult to maintain and usually have no effect. Megavitamin therapy usually is ineffective (unless the child has a frank vitamin deficiency) and can cause serious adverse effects.

References

Chalasani L, Kant R, Chengappa KN. Clozapine impact on clinical outcomes and aggression in severely ill adolescents with childhood-onset schizophrenia. *Can J Psychiatry.* 2001;46:965.

Clein PD, Riddle MA. Pharmacokinetics in children and adolescents. *Child Adolesc Psychiatr Clin North Am.* 1995;4:59.

Coffey BJ. Pediatric psychopharmacology. In: Sadock BJ, Sadock VA, eds. *Kaplan & Sadock's Comprehensive Textbook of Psychiatry.* 7th ed. Vol 2. Baltimore: Lippincott Williams & Wilkins; 2000:2831.

Colle LM, Belair JF, DiFeo M, Weiss J, LaRoache C. Extended open-label fluoxetine treatment of adolescents with major depression. *J Child Adolesc Psychopharmacol.* 1994;4:225.

Geller B. Psychopharmacology of children and adolescents: pharmacokinetics and relationships of plasma/serum levels to response. *Psychopharmacol Bull.* 1991;27:401.

Greenhill L. Pharmacotherapy: stimulants. *Child Adolesc Psychiatr Clin North Am.* 1992;1:411.

Hardan A, Johnson K, Johnson C, Kreczny B. Case study: risperidone treatment of children and adolescents with developmental disorders. *J Am Acad Child Adolesc Psychiatry.* 1996;35:1551.

Kowatch RA, Suppes T, Carmody TJ, et al. Effect size of lithium, divalproex sodium, and carbamazepine in children and adolescents with bipolar disorder. *J Am Acad Child Adolesc Psychiatry.* 2000;39:713.

Lamps CA. Citalopram and psychotic symptoms. *J Am Acad Child Adolesc Psychiatry.* 2002;1:6.

Miller PM, Byrne M, Hodges A, Lawrie SM, Johnstone EC. Childhood behavior, psychotic symptoms and psychosis onset in young people at high risk of schizophrenia: early findings from the Edinburgh Study. *Psychol Med.* 2002;32:173.

Ratey JJ, Gordon A. The psychopharmacology of aggression: toward a new day. *Psychopharmacol Bull.* 1993;29:65.

Remschmidt H, Fleischaker C, Hennighausen K, Schulz E. Management of schizophrenia in children and adolescents. The role of clozapine. *Paediatr Drugs.* 2000;2:253.

Riddle MA, Geller B, Ryan N. Another sudden death in a child treated with desipramine. *J Am Acad Child Adolesc Psychiatry.* 1993;32:792.

Spencer T, Biederman J, Wilens T, Steingard R, Geist D. Nortriptyline treatment of children with attention-deficit/hyperactivity disorder and tic disorder or Tourette's syndrome. *J Am Acad Child Adolesc Psychiatry.* 1993;32:205.

Steingard R, Biederman J, Spencer T, Wilens T, Gonzalez A. Comparison of clonidine response in the treatment of attention-deficit/hyperactivity disorder with and without comorbid tic disorders. *J Am Acad Child Adolesc Psychiatry.* 1993;32:350.

Volavka J, Czobor P, Sheitman B, et al. Clozapine, olanzapine, risperidone and Haldol in the treatment of patients with chronic schizophrenia and schizoaffective disorder. *Am J Psychiatry.* 2002;159:255.

▲ 53.5 Psychiatric Treatment of Adolescents

A variety of serious psychiatric disorders including schizophrenia and bipolar disorder have their onset during adolescence. In addition, the risk for completed suicide drastically increases in adolescence. Although some stress is virtually universal in adolescence, most teenagers without mental disorders can cope well with the environmental demands. Teenagers with preexisting mental disorders may experience exacerbations during adolescence and may become frustrated, alienated, and demoralized.

Clinicians and parents must be sensitive to adolescents' perceptions of themselves. In a group of teenagers of the same age, there is a range of emotional maturity. Issues that are specific to adolescents are related to their new evolving identities, the development of sexual activity, and their plans to meet future life goals.

DIAGNOSIS

Adolescents can be assessed in both their specific stage-appropriate functions and their general progress in accomplishing the tasks of adolescence. For almost all adolescents in today's culture, at least until their late teens, school performance is the prime barometer of healthy functioning. Intellectually normal adolescents who are not functioning satisfactorily in some form of schooling have significant psychological problems whose nature and causes should be identified.

Questions to be asked regarding adolescents' stage-specific tasks are the following: What degree of separation from their parents have they achieved? What sort of identities are evolving? How do they perceive their past? Do they perceive themselves as responsible for their own development or only the passive recipients of their parents' influences? How do they perceive themselves with regard to the future, and how do they anticipate their future responsibilities for themselves and others? Can they think about the varying consequences of different ways of living? How do they express their sexual and affectionate interests? These tasks occupy all adolescents and normally are performed at varying times.

Adolescents' object relations must be evaluated. Do they perceive and accept both good and bad qualities in their parents? Do they see their peers and boyfriends or girlfriends as separate persons with needs and identities of their own, or do others exist only for the adolescents' own needs?

A respect for, and (if possible) some actual understanding of, an adolescent's subcultural and ethnic background are essential. For example, in some groups, depression is acceptable; in other groups, overt depression is a sign of weakness and is masked by antisocial acts, substance misuse, and self-destructive risks. A psychiatrist need not be of the same race or group identity as an adolescent to treat him or her effectively.

Table 53.4–4
Common Dose-Related Side Effects of Stimulants

Insomnia
Decreased appetite
Irritability or nervousness
Weight loss

and amphetamine salts. Several extended-release preparations such as Concerta (extended-release methylphenidate) and Adderall XR (extended-release Adderall) have come on to the market, allowing children who use them to continue to benefit from the medication without needing to take a dose during the school day. Pemoline (Cylert) is no longer recommended because of the risk for hepatotoxicity. Stimulants reduce hyperactivity, inattentiveness, and impulsivity in about 75 percent of children with ADHD. The effects are not paradoxical, as normal children respond similarly. The dose-related adverse effects of stimulants are listed in Table 53.4–4.

ADHD often coexists with oppositional defiant disorder or conduct disorder. With these added disorders comes aggression. In some cases, stimulants seem to reduce aggression, but a common mistake is prolonging stimulant trials when the aggression is not subsiding and a switch to, or the addition of, a more specifically antiaggression drug is indicated.

Antidepressants can be tried for children with ADHD who are resistant to stimulants and children with preexisting tic disorders. Bupropion is commonly tried when stimulants are ineffective in treating ADHD. Desipramine has been somewhat effective in the treatment of ADHD, but its use is limited because of the associated risks. Since the sudden death of four children being treated with desipramine for ADHD, extra caution must be recommended. Other tricyclic drugs, currently rarely recommended, including nortriptyline (Pamelor) and clomipramine, have been tried with some success. Children with ADHD can respond to antidepressants within days of the beginning of treatment.

A few studies have shown that clonidine (Catapres), an α-adrenergic agonist agent, has some success in ADHD. Guanfacine (Tenex), another α-adrenergic agonist has also been used in clinical practice for children and adolescents with ADHD who do not respond to the stimulants. Antipsychotics are not indicated in the treatment of ADHD, unless there is accompanying psychosis, given the risks of sedation and tardive dyskinesia. ADHD often precedes and then coexists with tic disorders. (Chapter 46 discusses pharmacotherapy for children with both conditions.)

The dietary management of hyperactivity has received much public attention, but controlled studies have not substantiated its benefit. Similarly, in most controlled studies, caffeine was not superior to placebo for alleviating ADHD.

Conduct Disorder. The assaultiveness frequently associated with conduct disorder may be reduced with pharmacotherapy. Antipsychotics such as risperidone, olanzapine or haloperidol may quell aggression, but sedation and the risk of tardive dyskinesia are major drawbacks. With newer antipsychotics such as risperidone on the market, the hope of fewer long-term adverse effects supports its use. Lithium has reduced aggression in conduct disorder, and propranolol (Inderal) has been effective in open studies. Carbamazepine has not been shown to be effective in controlling aggression.

When conduct disorder is associated with ADHD and when the aggression is mild, a trial of a stimulant may be indicated; stimulants are faster acting and easier to monitor than the previously noted drugs. Clonidine may be effective and deserves further study.

Aggressive behavior can occur in the context of a variety of psychiatric disorders including comorbid ADHD and conduct disorder. Some evidence indicates that stimulant medications may also have some efficacy in controlling aggressive behavior in children with these disorders.

Tourette's Disorder. The high-potency antipsychotics haloperidol and pimozide (Orap) are the most effective medications for Tourette's disorder. Pimozide prolongs the QT interval and thus requires electrocardiographic (ECG) monitoring. Clonidine, a presynaptic α-adrenergic blocking agent, is less effective than the two antipsychotics but avoids the risk for tardive dyskinesia; sedation is a frequent side effect of clonidine.

Tic disorders often coexist with ADHD in children and adolescents. Stimulant use, which can precipitate tics, should be avoided in these patients, although recent studies indicate that the prohibition may not be totally warranted. Clonidine reduces tics in both ADHD and the comorbid cases. A small study supports the use of nortriptyline.

Enuresis. Before initiating psychopharmacotherapy for treating enuresis, clinicians must consider the merits of waiting for a possible spontaneous remission and of using behavioral techniques; bell-and-pad conditioning (a bell awakens the child when the mattress becomes wet), perhaps the most elaborate behavioral treatment, seems to be more successful than medication.

Tricyclic drugs are effective in reducing enuresis in about 60 percent of patients, and desmopressin (DDAVP) is effective in about 50 percent of patients. Improvement ranges from complete cessation of wetting to continued wetting but with less urine volume. Tricyclic drugs are given about 1 hour before bedtime. The starting dosage usually is 25 mg a day, a lower dosage than is used in trials for depression. The dosage can be increased to 75 mg a day for an adolescent but should not exceed 2 mg/kg a day. Children usually respond within days. Desmopressin is taken intranasally in dosages of 10 to 40 mg a day. When used over months, nasal discomfort can occur, and water retention is potentially a problem. Patients who respond with full dryness should continue to take the medication for several months to prevent relapses.

Separation Anxiety Disorder. SSRIs are currently recommended as first-line medications in the treatment of a variety of anxiety disorders in children and adolescents. Few studies support the use of anxiolytics in pediatric psychopharmacology. A recent double-blind, placebo-controlled study did not replicate a similar study performed by the same workers 20 years before, when imipramine (Tofranil) was shown to be effective for school refusal. Alprazolam (Xanax) may be helpful in separation anxiety disorder, but the data are conflicting.

Schizophrenia. SDAs are generally recommended currently as first-line agents in the treatment of psychotic disorders

in children and adolescents. A few double-blind studies showed modest effectiveness of conventional antipsychotics in adolescent schizophrenia, and only one of these studies was placebo controlled. In the only double-blind placebo-controlled study of childhood schizophrenia, haloperidol was significantly superior to placebo. Schizophrenia with onset in late adolescence is treated like adult-onset schizophrenia.

Mood Disorders. The SSRIs currently are the drugs of choice in the pharmacological treatment of depressive disorders in children and adolescents. One controlled study supports the efficacy of fluoxetine in this population. Tricyclic drugs have not been shown to be superior to placebo in double-blind, placebo-controlled studies of children and adolescents with major depressive disorder. In children, developmental differences in neurotransmitters and neuroendocrine systems may be associated with responses to antidepressants.

Most clinicians advocate a trial of antidepressant medication in severe, prolonged major depressive disorder. The SSRIs are favored because of their apparent efficacy, mild adverse-effect profile, and lower risk in overdose. When treating a child or an adolescent at risk for suicide, one should always use the safest medication.

Manic episodes in childhood and adolescence are treated as they are in adulthood. No double-blind, placebo-controlled studies have demonstrated the effectiveness of lithium in treating adolescent mania, but many open trials support its use. Divalproex (Depakote) is currently used frequently to treat bipolar disorder in children and adolescents.

Obsessive-Compulsive Disorder. Current literature supports the use of SSRIs as first-line agents for children and adolescents with obsessive-compulsive disorder. Previously, clomipramine was proved effective in diminishing obsessions and compulsions in children and adolescents, but although clomipramine is often well tolerated, the SSRIs have a more favorable adverse-effect profile and appear to be as effective as clomipramine.

Eating Disorders. The treatment of anorexia nervosa does not focus primarily on pharmacological interventions, but drugs can be important adjuncts in many cases. The SSRIs are not used uncommonly in this population; the target symptoms are obsessions and compulsions and high levels of anxiety and depressive symptoms. Cyproheptadine (Periactin) was used historically and reported to benefit some patients with anorexia, and antidepressants may benefit those with comorbid depressive disorders. However, the compromised metabolism of many patients with anorexia can put them at high risk for cardiac arrhythmias if tricyclic drugs are administered.

There is evidence from controlled studies that high-dosage SSRI treatment (fluoxetine at doses of approximately 60 mg per day) can reduce binge eating and purging in bulimia nervosa. Bupropion must be used with care in patients with bulimia nervosa because of the risk of seizures.

Sleep Terror Disorder and Sleepwalking Disorder. Sleep terror disorder and sleepwalking disorder occur in the transition from deep delta-wave sleep (stages 3 and 4) to light sleep. Benzodiazepines and tricyclics are effective in these disorders. They work by reducing both delta-wave sleep and arousals between sleep stages. The medications should be used temporarily and only in severe cases, because tolerance to the medications develops. Cessation of these medications can lead to severe rebound worsening of the disorders, and reducing delta sleep in children may have deleterious effects; thus, behavioral approaches are preferred for these disorders.

Other Disorders. Buspirone (BuSpar) has been effective in an open trial of adolescents with generalized anxiety disorder. Patients with early-onset panic disorder and panic attacks have benefited from clonazepam (Klonopin) in several open trials.

Adverse Effects and Complications

Antidepressants. Adverse effects related to antidepressants have been diminished significantly since SSRI antidepressants have been widely accepted as first-line treatments for depressive disorders in children and adolescents. Tricyclics are rarely recommended due to the significant risks of dangerous adverse effects. The adverse effects of tricyclics for children usually are similar to those for adults and result from the drugs' anticholinergic properties. The adverse effects include dry mouth, constipation, palpitations, tachycardia, loss of accommodation, and sweating. The most serious adverse effects are cardiovascular; in children, diastolic hypertension is more common and postural hypotension occurs more rarely than in adults. ECG changes are most apt to be seen in children receiving high dosages. Slowed cardiac conduction (PR interval > 0.20 seconds or QRS interval > 0.12) may necessitate lowering the dosage. FDA guidelines limit dosages to a maximum of 5 mg/kg a day. The drugs can be toxic in an overdose, and in small children, ingestion of 200 to 400 mg can be fatal. When the dosage is lowered too rapidly, withdrawal effects occur, mainly gastrointestinal symptoms—cramping, nausea, and vomiting—and sometimes apathy and weakness. Treatment is tapering the dosage more slowly.

Antipsychotics. The SDAs have generally replaced the conventional antipsychotics as first-line agents in the treatment of all psychotic disorders in children and adolescents. Historically, the best-studied antipsychotics given to pediatric age groups are chlorpromazine (Thorazine) and haloperidol. High-potency and low-potency antipsychotics are believed to differ in their adverse-effect profiles. The phenothiazine derivatives (chlorpromazine and thioridazine) have the most pronounced sedative and atropinic actions, whereas the high-potency antipsychotics are commonly believed to be associated with extrapyramidal reactions, such as parkinsonian symptoms, akathisia, and acute dystonias. Caution is warranted in assuming that these reactions are also true for children. In particular, when comparisons are made at low-dosage levels of equivalent potency, differences may not be detected.

Even if the frequency of the adverse effects differs among medications, the effects are always caused by the antipsychotics. Evidence in children of impaired cognitive function and, most importantly, tardive dyskinesia calls for great caution in the use of drugs. Tardive dyskinesia—which is characterized by persistent abnormal involuntary movements of the tongue, face, mouth, or jaw and sometimes the extremities—is a known hazard when giving antipsychotics to patients of all age groups. No

cians may have to overcome their own biases about taking a sexual history: Sexuality is an area of concern for many geriatric patients, who welcome the chance to talk about their sexual feelings and attitudes.

Mental Status Examination

The mental status examination offers a cross-sectional view of how a patient thinks, feels, and behaves during the examination. With older adults, a psychiatrist may not be able to rely on a single examination to answer all of the diagnostic questions. Repeat mental status examinations may be needed because of fluctuating changes in the patient's family.

General Description. A general description of the patient includes appearance, psychomotor activity, attitude toward the examiner, and speech activity.

Motor disturbances (e.g., shuffling gait, stooped posture, "pill rolling" movements of the fingers, tremors, and body asymmetry) should be noted. Involuntary movements of the mouth or tongue may be adverse effects of phenothiazine medication. Many depressed patients seem to be slow in speech and movement. A masklike facies occurs in Parkinson's disease.

The patient's speech may be pressured in agitated, manic, and anxious states. Tearfulness and overt crying occur in depressive and cognitive disorders, especially if the patient feels frustrated about being unable to answer one of the examiner's questions. The presence of a hearing aid or another indication that the patient has a hearing problem (e.g., requesting repetition of questions) should be noted.

The patient's attitude toward the examiner—cooperative, suspicious, guarded, ingratiating—can give clues about possible transference reactions. Because of transference, older adults can react to younger physicians as if the physicians were parent figures, despite the age difference.

Functional Assessment. Patients older than 65 years of age should be evaluated for their capacity to maintain independence and to perform the activities of daily life, which include toileting, preparing meals, dressing, grooming, and eating. The degree of functional competence in their everyday behaviors is an important consideration in formulating a plan of treatment for these patients.

Mood, Feelings, and Affect. Suicide is a leading cause of death of older persons, and an evaluation of a patient's suicidal ideation is essential. Loneliness is the most common reason cited by older adults who consider suicide. Feelings of loneliness, worthlessness, helplessness, and hopelessness are symptoms of depression, which carries a high risk for suicide. Nearly 75 percent of all suicide victims suffer from depression, alcohol abuse, or both. The examiner should specifically ask the patient about any thoughts of suicide, whether the patient feels life is no longer worth living, and whether a person is better off dead or, when dead, is no longer a burden to others. Such thoughts—especially when associated with alcohol abuse, living alone, recent death of a spouse, physical illness, and somatic pain—indicate a high suicidal risk.

Disturbances in mood states, most notably depression and anxiety, may interfere with memory functioning. An expansive or euphoric mood may indicate a manic episode or may signal a dementing disorder. Frontal lobe dysfunction often produces *witzelsucht*, which is the tendency to make puns and jokes and then laugh aloud at them.

The patient's affect may be flat, blunted, constricted, shallow, or inappropriate, all of which can indicate a depressive disorder, schizophrenia, or brain dysfunction. Such affects are important abnormal findings, even though they are not pathognomonic of a specific disorder. Dominant lobe dysfunction causes dysprosody, an inability to express emotional feelings through speech intonation.

Perceptual Disturbances. Hallucinations and illusions by older adults may be transitory phenomena resulting from decreased sensory acuity. The examiner should note whether the patient is confused about time or place during the hallucinatory episode; confusion points to an organic condition. It is particularly important to ask the patient about distorted body perceptions. Because hallucinations may be caused by brain tumors and other focal pathology, a diagnostic workup may be indicated. Brain diseases cause perceptive impairments; agnosia, the inability to recognize and interpret the significance of sensory impressions, is associated with organic brain diseases. The examiner should note the type of agnosia—the denial of illness (anosognosia), the denial of a body part (atopognosia), or the inability to recognize objects (visual agnosia) or faces (prosopagnosia).

Language Output. This category of the geriatric mental status examination covers the aphasias, which are disorders of language output related to organic lesions of the brain. The best described are nonfluent or Broca's aphasia, fluent or Wernicke's aphasia, and global aphasia, a combination of fluent and nonfluent aphasias. In nonfluent or Broca's aphasia, the patient's understanding remains intact, but the ability to speak is impaired. The patient cannot pronounce "Methodist Episcopalian." Speech generally is mispronounced and may be telegraphic. A simple test for Wernicke's aphasia is to point to some common objects—such as a pen or a pencil, a doorknob, and a light switch—and ask the patient to name them. The patient also may be unable to demonstrate the use of simple objects, such as a key and a match (ideomotor apraxia).

Visuospatial Functioning. Some decline in visuospatial capability is normal with aging. Asking a patient to copy figures or a drawing may be helpful in assessing the function. A neuropsychological assessment should be performed when visuospatial functioning is obviously impaired.

Thought. Disturbances in thinking include neologisms, word salad, circumstantiality, tangentiality, loosening of associations, flight of ideas, clang associations, and blocking. The loss of the ability to appreciate nuances of meaning (abstract thinking) may be an early sign of dementia. Thinking is then described as concrete or literal.

Thought content should be examined for phobias, obsessions, somatic preoccupations, and compulsions. Ideas about suicide or homicide should be discussed. The examiner should determine whether delusions are present and how such delusions affect the patient's life. Delusions may be present in nurs-

ing home patients and may have been a reason for admission. Ideas of reference or of influence should be described. Patients who are hard of hearing may be classified mistakenly as paranoid or suspicious.

Sensorium and Cognition. *Sensorium* concerns the functioning of the special senses; *cognition* concerns information processing and intellect. The survey of both areas, known as the neuropsychiatric examination, consists of the clinician's assessment and a comprehensive battery of psychological tests.

CONSCIOUSNESS. A sensitive indicator of brain dysfunction is an altered state of consciousness in which the patient does not seem to be alert, shows fluctuations in levels of awareness, or seems to be lethargic. In severe cases, the patient is somnolescent or stuporous.

ORIENTATION. Impairment in orientation to time, place, and person is associated with cognitive disorders. Cognitive impairment often is observed in mood disorders, anxiety disorders, factitious disorders, conversion disorder, and personality disorders, especially during periods of severe physical or environmental stress. The examiner should test for orientation to place by asking the patient to describe his or her present location. Orientation to person may be approached in two ways: Does the patient know his or her own name, and are nurses and doctors identified as such? Time is tested by asking the patient the date, the year, the month, and the day of the week. The patient also should be asked about the length of time spent in a hospital, during what season of the year, and how the patient knows these facts. Greater significance is given to difficulties concerning person than to difficulties of time and place, and more significance is given to orientation to place than to orientation to time.

MEMORY. Memory usually is evaluated in terms of immediate, recent, and remote memory. Immediate retention and recall are tested by giving the patient six digits to repeat forward and backward. The examiner should record the result of the patient's capacity to remember. Persons with unimpaired memory usually can recall six digits forward and five or six digits backward. The clinician should be aware that the ability to do well on digit-span tests is impaired in extremely anxious patients. Remote memory can be tested by asking for the patient's place and date of birth, the patient's mother's name before she was married, and names and birthdays of the patient's children.

In cognitive disorders, recent memory deteriorates first. Recent memory assessment can be approached in several ways. Some examiners give the patient the names of three items early in the interview and ask for recall later. Others prefer to tell a brief story and ask the patient to repeat it verbatim. Memory of the recent past also can be tested by asking for the patient's place of residence, including the street number; the method of transportation to the hospital; and some current events. If the patient has a memory deficit such as amnesia, careful testing should be performed to determine whether it is retrograde amnesia (loss of memory before an event) or anterograde amnesia (loss of memory after the event). Retention and recall also can be tested by having the patient retell a simple story. Patients who confabulate make up new material in retelling the story.

INTELLECTUAL TASKS, INFORMATION, AND INTELLIGENCE. Various intellectual tasks may be presented to estimate the patient's fund of general knowledge and intellectual functioning. Counting and calculation can be tested by asking the patient to subtract 7 from 100 and to continue subtracting 7 from the result until the number 2 is reached. The examiner records the responses as a baseline for future testing. The examiner can also ask the patient to count backward from 20 to 1, and can record the time necessary to complete the exercise. The patient also can be asked to do simple arithmetic—for example, to state the number of nickels in $1.35.

The patient's fund of general knowledge is related to intelligence. The patient can be asked to name the president of the United States, to name the three largest cities in the United States, to give the population of the United States, and to give the distance from New York to Paris. The examiner must take into account the patient's educational level, socioeconomic status, and general life experience in assessing the results of some of these tests.

READING AND WRITING. It may be important for the clinician to examine the patient's reading and writing and to determine whether the patient has a specific speech deficit. The examiner may have the patient read a simple story aloud or write a short sentence to test for a reading or writing disorder. Whether the patient is right-handed or left-handed should be noted.

Judgment. Judgment is the capacity to act appropriately in various situations. Does the patient show impaired judgment? What would the patient do on finding a stamped, sealed, addressed envelope in the street? What would the patient do if he or she smelled smoke in a theater? Can the patient discriminate? What is the difference between a dwarf and a boy? Why are couples required to get a marriage license?

Neuropsychological Evaluation

A thorough neuropsychological examination includes a comprehensive battery of tests that can be replicated by various examiners and can be repeated over time to assess the course of a specific illness. The most widely used test of current cognitive functioning is the Mini-Mental State Examination (MMSE), which assesses orientation, attention, calculation, immediate and short-term recall, language, and the ability to follow simple commands (see Table 10.1–4 in Section 10.1). The MMSE is used to detect impairments, follow the course of an illness, and monitor the patient's treatment responses. It is not used to make a formal diagnosis. The maximum MMSE score is 30. Age and educational level influence cognitive performance as measured by the MMSE.

The assessment of intellectual abilities is performed with the Wechsler Adult Intelligence Scale-Revised (WAIS-R), which gives verbal, performance, and full-scale intelligence quotient (IQ) scores. Some test results, such as those of vocabulary tests, hold up as aging progresses; results of other tests, such as tests of similarities and digit-symbol substitution, do not. The performance part of the WAIS-R is a more sensitive indicator of brain damage than the verbal part.

Visuospatial functions are sensitive to the normal aging process. The Bender Gestalt test is one of a large number of instruments used to test visuospatial functions; another is the Halstead-Reitan battery, which is the most complex battery of tests covering the entire spectrum of information processing and cognition. Depression, even in the absence of dementia, often impairs psychomotor performance, especially visuospatial functioning and timed motor performance. The Geriatric Depression Scale is a useful screening instrument that excludes somatic complaints from its list of items. The presence of

somatic complaints on a rating scale tends to confound the diagnosis of a depressive disorder.

Medical History. Elderly patients have more concomitant, chronic, and multiple medical problems and take more medications than younger adults; many of these medications can influence their mental status. The past medical history includes all major illnesses, traumata, hospitalizations, and treatment interventions. The psychiatrist should also be alert to underlying medical illness. Infections, metabolic and electrolyte disturbances, and myocardial infarction and stroke may first be manifested by psychiatric symptoms. Depressed mood, delusions, and hallucinations may precede other symptoms of Parkinson's disease by many months. On the other hand, a psychiatric disorder can also cause such somatic symptoms as weight loss, malnutrition, and inanition of severe depression.

Careful review of medications (including over-the-counter medications, laxatives, vitamins, tonics, and lotions) and even substances recently discontinued is extremely important. Drug effects may be long lasting and may induce depression (e.g., antihypertensives), cognitive impairment (e.g., sedatives), delirium (e.g., anticholinergics), seizures (e.g., neuroleptics). The review of medications must include sufficient detail to identify misuse (overuse, underuse) and relate medication use to special diets. A dietary history is also important; deficiencies and excesses (e.g., protein, vitamins) may influence physiological function and mental status.

MENTAL DISORDERS OF OLD AGE

The National Institute of Mental Health's Epidemiologic Catchment Area (ECA) program has found that the most common mental disorders of old age are depressive disorders, cognitive disorders, phobias, and alcohol use disorders. Older adults also have a high risk for suicide and drug-induced psychiatric symptoms. Many metal disorders of old age can be prevented, ameliorated, or even reversed. Of special importance are the reversible causes of delirium and dementia; but if not diagnosed accurately and treated in a timely fashion, these conditions can progress to an irreversible state requiring a patient's institutionalization. Table 55–1 lists the general cognitive domains assessed in a neuropsychological evaluation, with the tests used to measure that skill and a description of the specific behaviors measured by each test. The tests listed in the table constitute a comprehensive test battery generally appropriate for use with a geriatric population. Use of a comprehensive battery is preferable for confident determination of presence and type of dementia or other cognitive disorder in elderly persons, but in some circumstances, administering a several-hour battery is not possible. Tests marked with an asterisk are the core tests that are most sensitive for detection of a dementia.

Table 55–1
Cognitive Domains

Gross cognitive functioning
- Mini-Mental State Examination: *orientation, repetition, following commands, naming, constructional skill, written expression, memory, mental flexibility, and calculations*

Intelligence
- Wechsler Adult Intelligence Scale-Revised (WAIS-R) or Wechsler Intelligence Scale-III (WAIS-III): *verbal and nonverbal intelligence*

Basic attention
- WAIS-R or WAIS-III Digit Span: *repetition of digits forward and backward*

Information-processing speed
- WAIS-R or WAIS-III Digit Symbol: *rapid graphomotor tracking*
- Trailmaking Part A: *rapid graphomotor tracking*
- Stroop A and B: *rapid word reading and color naming*

Motor dexterity
- Finger tapping: *right and left index finger dexterity*

Language
- Boston Naming Test: *word retrieval*
- WAIS-R or WAIS-III Vocabulary: *vocabulary range*

Visual perceptual/spatial
- WAIS-R or WAIS-III Picture Completion: *visual perception*
- WAIS-R or WAIS-III Block Design: *constructional ability*
- Rey-Osterrieth Complex Figure: *paper-and-pencil copy of complex design*
- Beery Developmental Test of Visual Motor Integration: *paper-and-pencil copy of simple-to-complex designs*

Learning and memory
- 8- to 10-item word list learning task: *learning and recall of rote verbal information*
- Wechsler Memory Scale-Revised (WMS-R) or Wechsler Memory Scale-III (WMS-III)
  - Logical Memory subtest: *immediate and delayed recall of paragraph information*
  - Visual Reproduction subtest: *immediate and delayed recall of visual designs*
- Rey-Osterrieth Complex Figure 3-minute delayed recall: *delayed recall of complex design*

Executive functions
- Trailmaking Part B: *rapid alternation between tasks*
- Stroop C: *inhibition of an overlearned response*
- Wisconsin Card Sorting Test: *categorization and mental flexibility*
- Verbal fluency (FAS and category): *rapid word generation*
- Design fluency: *rapid generation of novel designs*

Courtesy of Kyle Brauer Boone, Ph.D.

Several psychosocial risk factors also predispose older persons to mental disorders. These risk factors include loss of social roles, loss of autonomy, the deaths of friends and relatives, declining health, increased isolation, financial constraints, and decreased cognitive functioning.

Many drugs can cause psychiatric symptoms in older adults. These symptoms can result from age-related alterations in drug absorption, a prescribed dosage that is too large, not following instructions and taking too large a dose, sensitivity to the medication, and conflicting regimens presented by several physicians. Almost the entire spectrum of mental disorders can be caused by drugs.

Dementing Disorders

Only arthritis is a more common cause of disability among adults age 65 and older than dementia, a generally progressive and irreversible impairment of the intellect, the prevalence of which increases with age. About 5 percent of persons in the United States older than age 65 have severe dementia, and 15

Table 55–2
Summary of Cognitive Deficits for Various Clinical Disorders

			Early Dementia		
	Medical Illness	Depression	Alzheimer's Disease	Vascular	Frontotemporal
Intelligence					
Verbal IQ			Mild to moderate	Mild to moderate	Mild to moderate
Performance IQ		Mild	Mild to moderate	Mild to moderate	Mild to moderate
Attention	Mild				
Mental speed	Mild	Mild	Mild to moderate	Mild to moderate	Mild to moderate
Motor speed	Mild			Mild to moderate	
Language			Mild to moderate	Mild to moderate	Mild to moderate
Visual spatial		Mild	Mild to moderate	Mild to moderate	Mild to moderate
Memory					
Verbal	Mild		Marked	Marked	Mild to moderate
Nonverbal	Mild	Mild	Marked	Marked	Mild to moderate
Executive	Mild	Mild	Mild to moderate	Mild to moderate	Marked

Courtesy of Kyle Brauer Boone, Ph.D.

percent have mild dementia. Of persons older than age 80, about 20 percent have severe dementia. Known risk factors for dementia are age, family history, and female sex.

In contrast to mental retardation, the intellectual impairment of dementia develops over time—that is, previously achieved mental functions are lost gradually. The characteristic changes of dementia involve cognition, memory, language, and visuospatial functions, but behavioral disturbances are common as well and include agitation, restlessness, wandering, rage, violence, shouting, social and sexual disinhibition, impulsiveness, sleep disturbances, and delusions. Delusions and hallucinations occur during the course of the dementias in nearly 75 percent of patients.

Cognition is impaired by many conditions, including brain injuries, cerebral tumors, acquired immune deficiency syndrome (AIDS), alcohol, medications, infections, chronic pulmonary diseases, and inflammatory diseases. Although dementias associated with advanced age typically are caused by primary degenerative central nervous system (CNS) disease and vascular disease, many factors contribute to cognitive impairment; in older persons, mixed causes of dementia are common. Table 55–2 provides a summary of cognitive deficits for various clinical disorders.

About 10 to 15 percent of all patients who exhibit symptoms of dementia have potentially treatable conditions. The treatable conditions include systemic disorders, such as heart disease, renal disease, and congestive heart failure; endocrine disorders, such as hypothyroidism; vitamin deficiency; medication misuse; and primary mental disorders, most notably depressive disorders.

Depending on the site of the cerebral lesion, dementias are classified as cortical and subcortical. A subcortical dementia occurs in Huntington's disease, Parkinson's disease, normal pressure hydrocephalus, vascular dementia, and Wilson's disease. The subcortical dementias are associated with movement disorders, gait apraxia, psychomotor retardation, apathy, and akinetic mutism, which can be confused with catatonia. Table 55–3 lists some potentially reversible conditions that may resemble dementia. The cortical dementias occur in dementias

Table 55–3
Some Potentially Reversible Conditions That May Resemble Dementia

Substances
- Anticholinergic agents
- Antihypertensives
- Antipsychotics
- Corticosteroids
- Digitalis
- Narcotics
- Nonsteroidal antiinflammatory agents
- Phenytoin
- Polypharmacotherapy
- Sedative hypnotics

Psychiatric disorders
- Anxiety
- Depression
- Mania
- Delusional (paranoid) disorders

Metabolic and endocrine disorders
- Addison's disease
- Cushing's syndrome
- Hepatic failure
- Hypercarbia (chronic obstructive pulmonary disease)
- Hypernatremia
- Hyperparathyroidism
- Hyperthyroidism
- Hypoglycemia
- Hyponatremia
- Hypothyroidism
- Renal failure
- Volume depletion

Miscellaneous conditions
- Fecal impaction
- Hospitalization
- Impaired hearing or vision

Courtesy of Gary W. Small, M.D.

of the Alzheimer's type, Creutzfeldt-Jakob disease (CJD), and Pick's disease, which frequently manifest aphasia, agnosia, and apraxia. In clinical practice, the two types of dementias overlap, and in most cases, an accurate diagnosis can be made only by autopsy. Human prion diseases result from coding mutations in the prion protein gene (PRNP) and may be inherited, acquired, or sporadic. They include familial CJD, Gerstmann-Sträussler-Scheinker syndrome, and fatal familial insomnia. These are inherited as autosomal-dominant mutations. The acquired diseases include kuru and iatrogenic CJD. Kuru was an epidemic prion disease of the Fore people of Papua, New Guinea, caused by cannibalistic funeral rituals, which peaked in incidence in the 1950s. Iatrogenic disease is rare and is caused, for example, by the use of contaminated dura mater and corneal grafts and treatment with human cadaveric pituitary-derived growth hormone and gonadotropin. Sporadic CJD accounts for 85% of the human prion diseases and occurs worldwide, with a uniform distribution and an incidence of about 1 in 1 million per annum, with a mean age at onset of 65 years. It is exceedingly rare in individuals under 30 years of age. (Additional information on dementia and prion disease is contained in Chapter 10, Section 10.3.)

Dementia of the Alzheimer's Type. Of all patients with dementia, 50 to 60 percent have dementia of the Alzheimer's type, which is the most common type of dementia. About 5 percent of all persons who reach age 65 have dementia of the Alzheimer's type, compared with 15 to 25 percent of those aged 85 or older. The prevalence of dementia of the Alzheimer's type is higher in women than in men. Patients with dementia of the Alzheimer's type occupy more than 50 percent of all nursing home beds.

This dementia has an insidious onset and is progressive. The mean survival for persons with dementia of the Alzheimer's type is approximately 8 years (range, 1 to 20 years). The diagnosis is made on the basis of the patient's history and a mental status examination. Brain-imaging techniques may also be useful.

Dementia of the Alzheimer's type is characterized by the gradual onset and progressive decline of cognitive functions. Memory is impaired, and at least one of the following is seen: aphasia, apraxia, agnosia, and disturbances in executive functioning. The general sequence of deficits is memory, language, and visuospatial functions. Initially, a patient may have an inability to learn and recall new information; then, he or she develops impaired naming, followed by an inability to copy figures. Early dementia of the Alzheimer's type may be difficult to diagnose because a patient's IQ may be normal.

Personality changes (e.g., depression, obsessiveness, and suspiciousness) occur. Outbursts of anger are common, and there is a risk of violent acts. Disorientation leads to wandering; a patient may be discovered far from home in a dazed condition. Loss of initiative is common. Neurological defects (e.g., gait disturbances, aphasia, apraxia, and agnosia) eventually appear.

ETIOLOGY. The cause of Alzheimer's disease is unknown, although postmortem neuropathological and biochemical studies have shown a selective loss of cholinergic neurons. Structural and functional changes occur. Gross anatomical findings include reduced gyral volume in the frontal and temporal lobes, with relative sparing of the primary motor and sensory cortex. Typical microscopic alterations include senile plaques and neurofibrillary tangles, which are derived from tau proteins. Blocking the aberrant phosphorylation of tau proteins is being explored as a possible therapeutic intervention in dementia of the Alzheimer's type.

TREATMENT. Dementia of the Alzheimer's type has no known prevention or cure. Treatment is palliative and consists of proper nutrition, exercise, and supervision of daily activity. Medication may be helpful in managing agitation and behavioral disturbances. Propranolol (Inderal), pindolol (Visken), buspirone (BuSpar), and valproate (Depakene) all have been reported to help reduce agitation and aggression. Haloperidol (Haldol) and other high-potency dopamine-blocking agents may be used to control acute behavior disturbances. Some patients with dementia of the Alzheimer's type show improvement in cognitive and functional measures when treated with tacrine (Cognex) or donepezil (Aricept). Reports of vitamin E supplementation (400 to 600 mg a day) retarding the progress of dementia are encouraging. Drugs such as memantine that protect neurons from excessive glutamate stimulation are under investigation.

Vascular Dementia. The second most common type of dementia is vascular dementia. It is characterized by the same cognitive deficits as dementia of the Alzheimer's type, but vascular dementia has focal neurological signs and symptoms, such as exaggerated deep tendon reflexes, extensor plantar response, pseudobulbar palsy, gait abnormalities, and weakness of an extremity. Compared with dementia of the Alzheimer's type, vascular dementia has an abrupt onset and a stepwise, deteriorating course. Vascular dementia may be prevented by reducing known risk factors such as hypertension, diabetes, cigarette smoking, and arrhythmias. Diagnosis can be confirmed with magnetic resonance imaging (MRI) and cerebral blood flow studies.

Dementia Due to Pick's Disease. Pick's disease causes a slowly progressing dementia and is associated with focal cortical lesions, primarily on the frontal lobe, that produce aphasia, apraxia, and agnosia. The disease lasts from 2 to 10 years; the average duration is 5 years. Clinically, Pick's disease is difficult to distinguish from Alzheimer's disease. On autopsy, however, the brain reveals intraneuronal inclusions called *Pick bodies,* which differ from the neurofibrillary tangles of Alzheimer's dementia. Pick's disease is much rarer than Alzheimer's dementia, and no treatment is available. It is also called *frontotemporal dementia.*

Other Dementias. Dementia due to Huntington's disease, dementia due to normal pressure hydrocephalus, Parkinson's disease, and other causes are covered in Chapter 10.

Depressive Disorders

Depressive symptoms are present in about 15 percent of all older adult community residents and nursing home patients. Age itself is not a risk factor for the development of depression, but being widowed and having a chronic medical illness are associated with vulnerability to depressive disorders. Late-onset depression is characterized by high rates of recurrence.

The common signs and symptoms of depressive disorders include reduced energy and concentration, sleep problems (especially early morning awakening and multiple awakenings), decreased appetite, weight loss, and somatic complaints.

Table 55–4
Geriatric Depression Scale (Short Version)

Answers indicating depression are boldfaced. Each answer counts one point; scores greater than 5 indicate probable depression.

1. Are you basically satisfied with your life?	Yes/**No**
2. Have you dropped many of your activities and interests?	**Yes**/No
3. Do you feel that your life is empty?	**Yes**/No
4. Do you often get bored?	**Yes**/No
5. Are you in good spirits most of the time?	Yes/**No**
6. Are you afraid that something bad is going to happen to you?	**Yes**/No
7. Do you feel happy most of the time?	Yes/**No**
8. Do you often feel helpless?	**Yes**/No
9. Do you prefer to stay at home, rather than going out and doing new things?	**Yes**/No
10. Do you feel you have more problems with memory than most?	**Yes**/No
11. Do you think it is wonderful to be alive now?	Yes/**No**
12. Do you feel pretty worthless the way you are now?	**Yes**/No
13. Do you feel full of energy?	Yes/**No**
14. Do you feel that your situation is hopeless?	**Yes**/No
15. Do you think that most people are better off than you are?	**Yes**/No

Special Instructions. The scale can be used as a self-rating or observer-rated metric. It has also been used as an observer-rated scale in mildly demented subjects.

Reprinted with permission from Yesavage JA. Geriatric Depression Scale. *Psychopharmacol Bull.* 1988;24:709.

The presenting symptoms may be different in older depressed patients from those seen in younger adults because of an increased emphasis on somatic complaints in older persons. They are particularly vulnerable to major depressive episodes with melancholic features, characterized by depression, hypochondriasis, low self-esteem, feelings of worthlessness, and self-accusatory trends (especially about sex and sinfulness) with paranoid and suicidal ideation. A geriatric depression scale is shown in Table 55–4.

Cognitive impairment in depressed geriatric patients is referred to as the *dementia syndrome of depression* (*pseudodementia*), which can be confused easily with true dementia. In true dementia, intellectual performance usually is global, and impairment is consistently poor; in pseudodementia, deficits in attention and concentration are variable. Compared with patients who have true dementia, patients with pseudodementia are less likely to have language impairment and to confabulate; when uncertain, they are more likely to say "I don't know"; and their memory difficulties are more limited to free recall than to recognition on cued recall tests. Pseudodementia occurs in about 15 percent of depressed older patients, and 25 to 50 percent of patients with dementia are depressed.

Bipolar I Disorder

Bipolar I disorder usually begins in middle adulthood, although the lifetime prevalence of 1 percent remains steady throughout life. A vulnerability to recurrence remains, so patients with a history of bipolar I disorder may display a manic episode late in life. In most instances, a first episode of manic behavior after age 65 should alert clinicians to search for an associated physiological or organic cause, such as an adverse effect of medication or early dementia. The signs and symptoms of mania in older persons are similar to those in younger adults and include an elevated, expansive, or irritable mood; a decreased need to sleep; distractibility; impulsivity; and, often, excessive alcohol intake. Hostile or paranoid behavior is usually present. Cognitive impairment, disorientation, or fluctuating levels of awareness should make clinicians suspect an organic cause.

Lithium (Eskalith) remains a treatment of choice for mania, but its use by older patients must be monitored carefully, because their reduced renal clearance makes lithium toxicity a significant risk. Neurotoxic effects are also more common in older persons than in younger adults.

Schizophrenia

Schizophrenia usually begins in late adolescence or young adulthood and persists throughout life. Although first episodes diagnosed after age 65 are rare, a late-onset type beginning after age 45 has been described. Women are more likely to have a late onset of schizophrenia than men. Another difference between early-onset and late-onset schizophrenia is the greater prevalence of paranoid schizophrenia in the late-onset type. About 20 percent of persons with schizophrenia show no active symptoms by age 65; 80 percent show varying degrees of impairment. Psychopathology becomes less marked as patients age.

The residual type of schizophrenia occurs in about 30 percent of persons with schizophrenia. Its signs and symptoms include emotional blunting, social withdrawal, eccentric behavior, and illogical thinking. Delusions and hallucinations are uncommon. Because most persons with residual schizophrenia cannot care for themselves, long-term hospitalization is required.

Older persons with schizophrenic symptoms respond well to antipsychotic drugs. Medication must be administered judiciously, and lower-than-usual dosages often are effective for older adults.

The patient was a 57-year-old divorced white man who required psychiatric hospitalization for the first time at the age of 49, after presenting with a 6-month history of being under surveillance by the police, Central Intelligence Agency (CIA), and detectives who were following him and monitoring his actions. He became very distraught and claimed to have gotten "tired of dodging them" and turned himself in to the police. He was taken by the police to the hospital for admission. He denied hearing voices but reported a ringing in his ears warning him that something harmful would soon happen. The patient admitted seeing faces in pictures that changed from time to time while he looked at them. At the time of admission the patient was working full-time as a painter and lived with his elderly father as he had since his divorce 19 years earlier. He frequently saw his three sons who lived in the area. The family reported no previous history of mental illness in the patient.

The patient's hobby was collecting model trains. His medical history was unremarkable, but the family history was significant for a maternal aunt who spent many years in a psychiatric hospital and his mother who required state hospitalization for 7 years for a "nervous breakdown." Results of the neurological and other physical examination were within normal limits as were routine laboratory tests and MRI of the brain. The patient was treated with haloperidol up to 4 mg a day with resolution of his delusional system except for episodic paranoid ideation and hearing voices. The patient was no longer employed but helped care for his 90-year-old father. (Courtesy of M. Jackuelyn Harris, M.D., and Dilip V. Jeste, M.D.)

Delusional Disorder

The age of onset of delusional disorder usually is between ages 40 and 55, but it can occur at any time during the geriatric period. Delusions can take many forms; the most common are persecutory—patients believe that they are being spied on, followed, poisoned, or harassed in some way. Persons with delusional disorder may become violent toward their supposed persecutors. Some persons lock themselves in their rooms and live reclusive lives. Somatic delusions, in which persons believe they have a fatal illness, also may occur in older persons. In one study of persons older than 65 years of age, pervasive persecutory ideation was present in 4 percent of persons sampled.

Among those who are vulnerable, delusional disorder can occur under physical or psychological stress and may be precipitated by the death of a spouse, loss of a job, retirement, social isolation, adverse financial circumstances, debilitating medical illness or surgery, visual impairment, and deafness. Delusions also may accompany other disorders—such as dementia of the Alzheimer's type, alcohol use disorders, schizophrenia, depressive disorders, and bipolar I disorder—which need to be ruled out. Delusional syndromes also may result from prescribed medications or be early signs of a brain tumor. The prognosis is fair to good in most cases; best results are achieved through a combination of psychotherapy and pharmacotherapy.

A late-onset delusional disorder called *paraphrenia* is characterized by persecutory delusions. It develops over several years and is not associated with dementia. Some workers believe that the disorder is a variant of schizophrenia that first becomes manifest after age 60. Patients with a family history of schizophrenia show an increased rate of paraphrenia.

The patient was a 74-year-old divorced white man referred by his primary care physician for paranoid delusions. The patient reported that a black gang was after him, especially "Mad Dog," the leader of the 5,000-member gang. The patient and his son said that the onset of the patient's concerns began 4 years earlier, and this resulted in the patient's changing residences four times during this period and retiring from his job as a sales clerk in a clothing store 2 years ago. He called the police several times to show them the gang's footprints in the grass and to report noise outside his window. The patient denied depressed mood, change in sleep or appetite, memory impairment, or problems with concentration. He denied auditory or visual hallucinations or any past psychiatric history. The patient lived alone in his apartment and took care of his finances and other activities of daily living. He had a high school diploma, was divorced, and had worked as a sales clerk "all his life." Medical problems were significant for hypercholesterolemia treated with medication. His MMSE score was 30/30. His physical (including neurological) examination and routine laboratory test results were unremarkable. The patient refused to take the prescribed antipsychotic drug but did come to the clinic to discuss his concerns. (Courtesy of M. Jackuelyn Harris, M.D., and Dilip V. Jeste, M.D.)

Anxiety Disorders

The anxiety disorders include panic disorder, phobias, obsessive-compulsive disorder, generalized anxiety disorder, acute stress disorder, and posttraumatic stress disorder. Anxiety disorders begin in early or middle adulthood, but some appear for the first time after age 60. An initial onset of panic disorder in older persons is rare but can occur. The ECA study determined that the 1-month prevalence of anxiety disorders in persons age 65 and older is 5.5 percent. By far the most common disorders are phobias (4 to 8 percent). The rate for panic disorder is 1 percent.

The signs and symptoms of phobia in older adults are less severe than those that occur in younger persons, but the effects are equally, if not more, debilitating for older patients. Existential theories help explain anxiety when there is no specifically identifiable stimulus for a chronically anxious feeling. Older persons must come to grips with death. The person may deal with the thought of death with a sense of despair and anxiety, rather than with equanimity and Erik Erikson's "sense of integrity." The fragility of the autonomic nervous system in older persons may account for the development of anxiety after a major stressor. Because of concurrent physically disability, older persons react more severely to posttraumatic stress disorder than younger persons.

Obsessions and compulsions may appear for the first time in older adults, although older adults with obsessive-compulsive disorder usually had demonstrated evidence of the disorder (e.g., being orderly, perfectionistic, punctual, and parsimonious) when they were younger. When symptomatic, patients become excessive in their desire for orderliness, rituals, and sameness. They may become generally inflexible and rigid and have compulsions to check things again and again. Obsessive-compulsive disorder (in contrast to obsessive-compulsive personality disorder) is characterized by ego-dystonic rituals and obsessions and may begin late in life.

Treatment of anxiety disorders must be tailored to individual patients and must take into account the biopsychosocial interplay producing the disorder. Both pharmacotherapy and psychotherapy are required.

Somatoform Disorders

Somatoform disorders, characterized by physical symptoms resembling medical diseases, are relevant to geriatric psychiatry

because somatic complaints are common among older adults. More than 80 percent of persons over 65 years of age have at least one chronic disease—usually arthritis or cardiovascular problems. After age 75, 20 percent have diabetes and an average of four diagnosable chronic illnesses that require medical attention.

Hypochondriasis is common in persons over 60 years of age, although the peak incidence is in the 40- to 50-year-old age group. The disorder usually is chronic, and the prognosis guarded. Repeated physical examinations help reassure patients that they do not have a fatal illness, but invasive and high-risk diagnostic procedures should be avoided unless medically indicated.

Telling patients that their symptoms are imaginary is counterproductive and usually engenders resentment. Clinicians should acknowledge that the complaint is real, that the pain is really there and perceived as such by the patient, and that a psychological or pharmacological approach to the problem is indicated.

Alcohol and Other Substance Use Disorder

Older adults with alcohol dependence usually give a history of excessive drinking that began in young or middle adulthood. They usually are medically ill, primarily with liver disease, and are either divorced, widowers, or men who never married. Many have arrest records and are numbered among homeless persons. A large number have chronic dementing illness such as Wernicke's encephalopathy and Korsakoff's syndrome. Twenty percent of nursing home patients have alcohol dependence.

Over all, alcohol and other substance use disorders account for 10 percent of all emotional problems in older persons, and dependence on such substances as hypnotics, anxiolytics, and narcotics is more common in old age than is generally recognized. Substance-seeking behavior characterized by crime, manipulativeness, and antisocial behavior is rarer in older than in younger adults. Older patients may abuse anxiolytics to allay chronic anxiety or to ensure sleep. The maintenance of chronically ill cancer patients with narcotics prescribed by a physician produces dependence, but the need to provide pain relief takes precedence over the possibility of narcotic dependence and is entirely justified.

The clinical presentation of older patients with alcohol and other substance use disorders varies and includes confusion, poor personal hygiene, depression, malnutrition, and the effects of exposure and falls. The sudden onset of delirium in older persons hospitalized for medical illness is most often caused by alcohol withdrawal. Alcohol abuse also should be considered in older adults with chronic gastrointestinal problems.

Older persons may misuse over-the-counter substances, including nicotine and caffeine. Thirty-five percent use over-the-counter analgesics, and thirty percent use laxatives. Unexplained gastrointestinal, psychological, and metabolic problems should alert clinicians to over-the-counter substance abuse.

Sleep Disorders

Advanced age is the single most important factor associated with the increased prevalence of sleep disorders. Sleep-related phenomena reported more frequently by older than by younger adults are sleeping problems, daytime sleepiness, daytime napping, and the use of hypnotic drugs. Clinically, older persons experience higher rates of breathing-related sleep disorder and medication-induced movement disorders than younger adults.

In addition to altered regulatory and physiological systems, the causes of sleep disturbances in older persons include primary sleep disorders, other mental disorders, general medical disorders, and social and environmental factors. Among the primary sleep disorders, dyssomnias are the most frequent, especially primary insomnia, nocturnal myoclonus, restless legs syndrome, and sleep apnea. Of the parasomnias, rapid eye movement (REM) sleep behavior disorder occurs almost exclusively among elderly men. The conditions that commonly interfere with sleep in older adults also include pain, nocturia, dyspnea, and heartburn. The lack of a daily structure and of social or vocational responsibilities contributes to poor sleep.

As a result of the decreased length of their daily sleep–wake cycle, older persons without daily routines, especially patients in nursing homes, may experience an advanced sleep phase, in which they go to sleep early and awaken during the night.

Even modest amounts of alcohol can interfere with the quality of sleep and can cause sleep fragmentation and early morning awakening. Alcohol may also precipitate or aggravate obstructive sleep apnea. Many older persons use alcohol, hypnotics, and other CNS depressants to help them fall asleep, but data show that these persons experience more early morning awakening than trouble falling asleep. When prescribing sedative-hypnotic drugs for older persons, clinicians must monitor the patients for unwanted cognitive, behavioral, and psychomotor effects, including memory impairment (anterograde amnesia), residual sedation, rebound insomnia, daytime withdrawal, and unsteady gait.

Changes in sleep structure among persons over 65 years of age involve both REM sleep and non–rapid eye movement (NREM) sleep. The REM changes include the redistribution of REM sleep throughout the night, more REM episodes, shorter REM episodes, and less total REM sleep. The NREM changes include the decreased amplitude of delta waves, a lower percentage of stages 3 and 4 sleep, and a higher percentage of stages 1 and 2 sleep. In addition, older persons experience increased awakening after sleep onset.

Much of the observed deterioration in the quality of sleep in older persons is due to the altered timing and consolidation of sleep. For example, with advanced age, persons have a lower amplitude of circadian rhythms, a 12-hour sleep-propensity rhythm, and shorter circadian cycles.

SUICIDE RISK

Elderly persons have a higher risk for suicide than any other population. The suicide rate for white men over the age of 65 is five times higher than that of the general population. One third of elderly persons report loneliness as the principal reason for considering suicide. Approximately 10 percent of elderly individuals with suicidal ideation report financial problems, poor medical health, or depression as reasons for suicidal thoughts. Suicide victims differ demographically from individuals who attempt suicide. About 60 percent of those who commit suicide are men; 75 percent of those who attempt suicide are women. Suicide victims as a rule use guns or hang themselves, whereas 70 percent of suicide attempters take a drug overdose, and 20 percent cut or slash themselves. Psychological autopsy studies suggest that most elderly persons who commit suicide have had a psychiatric disorder, most commonly depression. However,

psychiatric disorders of suicide victims often do not receive medical or psychiatric attention. More elderly suicide victims are widowed and fewer are single, separated, or divorced than is true of younger adults. Violent methods of suicide are more common in the elderly, and alcohol use and psychiatric histories appear to be less frequent. The most common precipitants of suicide in older individuals are physical illness and loss, whereas problems with employment, finances, and family relationships are more frequent precipitants in younger adults. Most elderly persons who commit suicide communicate their suicidal thoughts to family or friends prior to the act of suicide.

Older patients with major medical illnesses or a recent loss should be evaluated for depressive symptomatology and suicidal ideation or plans. Thoughts and fantasies about the meaning of suicide and life after death may reveal information that the patient cannot share directly. There should be no reluctance to question patients about suicide, since there is no evidence that such questions increase the likelihood of suicidal behavior.

OTHER CONDITIONS OF OLD AGE

Vertigo

Feelings of vertigo or dizziness, a common complaint of older adults, cause many older adults to become inactive because they fear falling. The causes of vertigo vary and include anemia, hypotension, cardiac arrhythmia, cerebrovascular disease, basilar artery insufficiency, middle ear disease, acoustic neuroma, and Ménière's disease. Most cases of vertigo have a strong psychological component, and clinicians should ascertain any secondary gain from the symptom. The overuse of anxiolytics can cause dizziness and daytime somnolence. Treatment with meclizine (Antivert), 25 to 100 mg daily, has been successful in many patients with vertigo.

Syncope

The sudden loss of consciousness associated with syncope results from a reduction of cerebral blood flow and brain hypoxia. A thorough medical workup is required to rule out the various causes listed in Table 55–5.

Table 55–5
Causes of Syncope

Cardiac disorders
Anatomical/valvular
Aortic stenosis
Mitral prolapse and regurgitation
Hypertrophic cardiomyopathy
Myxoma
Electrical
Tachyarrhythmia
Bradyarrhythmia
Heart block
Sick sinus syndrome
Functional
Ischemia and infarct
Situational hypotension
Dehydration (diarrhea, fasting)
Orthostatic hypotension
Postprandial hypotension
Micturition, defecation, coughing, swallowing
Abnormal cardiovascular reflexes
Carotid sinus syndrome
Vasovagal syncope
Drugs
Vasodilators
Calcium channel blockers
Diuretics
Beta blockers
Central nervous system abnormalities
Cerebrovascular insufficiency
Seizures
Metabolic abnormalities
Hypoxemia
Hypoglycemia or hyperglycemia
Anemia
Pulmonary disorders
Chronic obstructive pulmonary disease
Pneumonia
Pulmonary embolus

Hearing Loss

About 30 percent of persons over age 65 have significant hearing loss (presbycusis). After age 75, that figure rises to 50 percent. Causes vary. Clinicians should be sensitive to hearing loss in patients who complain they can hear but can't understand what is being said or who ask that questions be repeated. Most elderly persons with hearing loss can be treated with hearing aids.

ELDER ABUSE

An estimated 10 percent of persons above 65 years of age are abused. *Elder abuse* is defined by the American Medical Association as "an act or omission which results in harm or threatened harm to the health or welfare of an elderly person." Mistreatment includes abuse and neglect—physically, psychologically, financially, and materially. Sexual abuse does occur. Acts of omission include withholding food, medicine, clothing, and other necessities. The types of elder abuse are listed in Table 55–6.

Family conflicts and other problems often underlie elder abuse. The victims tend to be very old and frail. They often live with their assailants, who may be financially dependent on the victims. Both the victim and the perpetrator tend to deny or minimize the presence of abuse. Interventions include providing legal services, housing, and medical, psychiatric, and social services.

SPOUSAL BEREAVEMENT

Demographic data suggest that 51 percent of women and 14 percent of men over the age of 65 will be widowed at least once. Spousal loss is among the most stressful of all life experiences. As a group, older adults appear to have a more favorable outcome than expected following the death of a spouse. Depressive symptoms peak within the first few months after a death but decline significantly within a year. There is a relationship between spousal loss and subsequent mortality. Elderly survivors of spouses who committed suicide are especially vulnerable, as are those with psychiatric illness.

Table 55–6
Types of Elder Abuse

Physical or sexual abuse
- Bruises (bilateral and at various stages of healing)
- Welts
- Lacerations
- Punctures
- Fractures
- Evidence of excessive drugging
- Burns
- Physical restraints (tying to beds, etc.)
- Malnutrition and dehydration
- Lack of personal care
- Inadequate heating
- Lack of food and water
- Unclean clothes or bedding
- Lack of needed medication
- Lack of eyeglasses, hearing aids, false teeth
- Difficulty walking or sitting
- Venereal disease
- Pain or itching, bruises, or bleeding of external genitalia, vaginal area, or anal area

Psychological abuse (vulnerable adults react by exhibiting resignation, fear, depression, mental confusion, anger, ambivalence, insomnia)
- Threats
- Insults
- Harassment
- Withholding of security and affection
- Harsh orders
- Refusal on the part of the family or those caring for the adult to allow travel, visits by friends or other family members, attendance at church

Exploitation
- Misuse of vulnerable adult's income or other financial resources (victim is best source of information but in most cases has turned management of financial affairs over to another person; as a result, there may be some confusion about finances)

Medical abuse
- Withholding or improper administration of medications or necessary medical treatments for a condition or the withholding of aids the person would medically require, such as false teeth, glasses, hearing aids
- May be a cause of
  - Confusion
  - Disorientation
  - Memory impairment
  - Agitation
  - Lethargy
  - Self-neglect

Neglect
- Conduct of vulnerable adult or others that results in deprivation of care necessary to maintain physical and mental health
- May be manifest by
  - Malnutrition
  - Poor personal hygiene
  - Any of the indicators for medical abuse

Reprinted with permission from Washington State Medical Association. *Elder Abuse: Guidelines for Intervention by Physicians and Other Service Providers.* Seattle: Washington State Medical Association; 1985.

PSYCHOPHARMACOLOGICAL TREATMENT OF GERIATRIC DISORDERS

Certain guidelines should be followed regarding the use of all drugs in older adults. A pretreatment medical evaluation is essential, including an electrocardiogram (ECG). It is especially useful to have the patient or a family member bring in all currently used medications, because multiple drug use may be contributing to the symptoms.

Most psychotropic drugs should be given in equally divided doses three or four times over a 24-hour period. Older patients may not be able to tolerate a sudden rise in drug blood level resulting from one large daily dose. Any changes in blood pressure and pulse rate and other side effects should be watched. For patients with insomnia, however, giving the major portion of an antipsychotic or antidepressant at bedtime takes advantage of its sedating and soporific effects. Liquid preparations are useful for older patients who cannot or will not swallow tablets. Clinicians should frequently reassess all patients to determine the need for maintenance medication, changes in dosage, and development of adverse effects. If a patient is taking psychotropic drugs at the time of the evaluation, the clinician should, if possible, discontinue these medications and, after a washout period, reevaluate the patient during a drug-free baseline state.

Adults over 65 years of age use the greatest number of medications of any age group; 25 percent of all prescriptions are written for them. Adverse drug reactions caused by medications result in the hospitalization of nearly 250,000 persons in the United States each year. Psychotropic drugs are among the most commonly prescribed, along with cardiovascular and diuretic medications; 40 percent of all hypnotics dispensed in the United States each year are to those older than 75 years of age, and 70 percent of older persons use over-the-counter medications, compared with only 10 percent of young adults. (Chapter 36 presents a comprehensive survey of the psychopharmacological agents.)

Principles

The major goals of the pharmacological treatment of older persons are to improve the quality of life, maintain persons in the community, and delay or avoid their placement in nursing homes. Individualization of dosage is the basic tenet of geriatric psychopharmacology.

Alterations in drug dosages are required because of the physiological changes that occur as persons age. Renal disease is associated with decreased renal clearance of drugs; liver disease results in a decreased ability to metabolize drugs; cardiovascular disease and reduced cardiac output can affect both renal and hepatic drug clearance; and gastrointestinal disease and decreased gastric acid secretion influence drug absorption. As a person ages, the ratio of lean to fat body mass also changes. With normal aging, lean body mass decreases and body fat increases. Changes in the ratio of lean to fat body mass that accompany aging affect the distribution of drugs. Many lipid-soluble psychotropic drugs are distributed more widely in fat than in lean tissue, so a drug's action can be unexpectedly prolonged in older persons. Similarly, changes in end-organ or receptor-site sensitivity must be taken into account. In older

persons, the increased risk of orthostatic hypotension from psychotropic drugs is related to reduced functioning of blood pressure–regulating mechanisms.

As a general rule, the lowest possible dose should be used to achieve the desired therapeutic response. Clinicians must know the pharmacodynamics, pharmacokinetics, and biotransformation of each drug prescribed and the effects of the interaction of the drug with other drugs that a patient is taking.

Tricyclic Antidepressants

The secondary amines nortriptyline (Aventyl, Pamelor) and desipramine (Norpramin) are the most frequently used tricyclic antidepressant drugs in geriatric depression. They have lower anticholinergic and sedative effects than the tertiary amines amitriptyline (Elavil), doxepin (Adapin), and imipramine (Tofranil). Nortriptyline appears to have a lower potential for orthostatic hypotension than other tricyclic antidepressant agents. The plasma concentrations of antidepressant medications required for the treatment of depressed elderly patients are similar to those needed by young adults (nortriptyline plasma concentrations of 60 to 150 ng/mL and desipramine above 115 ng/mL). Elderly patients often develop therapeutic blood concentrations of nortriptyline or desipramine while on low daily doses. Most elderly patients develop therapeutic plasma concentrations with daily doses of nortriptyline of 1 to 1.2 mg/kg of body weight and of desipramine, 1.5 to 2 mg/kg. Elderly patients on nortriptyline often develop higher plasma levels of the nortriptyline metabolite 10-hydroxynortriptyline than do young adults, even when the plasma levels of the parent compound are similar. The increased levels of hydroxynortriptyline may in part be due to the lower renal clearance in elderly than in younger subjects. High 10-hydroxynortriptyline levels may contribute to cardiac conduction defects in elderly patients.

High intellectual functions, orthostatic blood pressure, the ECG, and the ability to urinate should be monitored frequently in depressed elderly patients receiving nortriptyline or desipramine. Pretreatment systolic orthostatic hypotension has been found to correlate with antidepressant response to nortriptyline in some elderly patients. Therefore, nortriptyline rather than desipramine use should be considered for such patients, and orthostatic blood pressure and subjective symptoms of orthostasis (feeling lightheaded upon standing) should be monitored carefully.

Tricyclic medications have anticholinergic properties, so these drugs should be avoided for patients with prosthetic hypertrophy or patients with narrow-angle glaucoma. Nortriptyline and desipramine have properties similar to those of type 1_A antiarrhythmic drugs (quinidinelike drugs). When administered to patients with right or left bundle branch block, tricyclic agents may cause second-degree block in approximately 10 percent of cases. For this reason, an ECG should always precede the use of tricyclic drugs in the elderly. The type 1_A properties of tricyclic medications necessitate cautious use of these drugs in patients with ischemic heart disease. A multicenter study demonstrated that type 1_A antiarrhythmics increase cardiac mortality in post–myocardial infarction patients. Although tricyclic medications were not used in this study, the type 1_A antiarrhythmic properties of tricyclic drugs suggest cautious use in patients with depression and ischemic heart disease.

Selective Serotonin Reuptake Inhibitors

Studies of elderly outpatients observed that selective serotonin reuptake inhibitors (SSRIs) are equally effective as tertiary amine tricyclic agents in the short-term treatment of depressive disorder. It is unclear whether SSRIs can help hospitalized elderly depression patients with severe, melancholic depression. A study that did not use random assignment suggested that cardiac inpatients with severe, melancholic depression have a poor response to fluoxetine (Prozac) but have a robust response to nortriptyline at therapeutic plasma concentrations. Although research inpatient studies of SSRI use are lacking, clinical experience suggests that these agents are effective in inpatients with a broad spectrum of depressive syndromes.

The dosages of SSRIs should be increased gradually. The starting daily doses may be fluoxetine 5 to 10 mg, paroxetine (Paxil) 5 to 10 mg, sertraline (Zoloft) 25 mg, and citalopram (Celexa) 10 mg. For most patients, daily doses of fluoxetine 20 mg, paroxetine 20 mg, sertraline 75 mg, and citalopram 20 to 30 mg suffice, although some require higher doses. The SSRI fluvoxamine (Luvox) may be effective in the treatment of geriatric depression, although research data are still sparse. The SSRIs have fewer cardiac adverse effects than tricyclic antidepressant agents and often are used as drugs of first choice, especially in patients with mild, nonmelancholic depression or in patients with cardiac disease. The most frequent adverse effects of SSRIs are insomnia, akathisia, nausea, anorexia, pseudoparkinsonism, and inappropriate secretion of antidiuretic hormone leading to hyponatremia.

Drug interactions should be considered in elderly patients receiving SSRIs. Fluoxetine and paroxetine inhibit the liver cytochrome P450 isoenzyme 2D6 (CYP 2D6). Sertraline is a weaker inhibitor of CYP 2D6, and citalopram has an insignificant inhibiting effect. CYP 2D6 is essential for the hydroxylation of nortriptyline and desipramine and the metabolism of antipsychotic agents and type 1_A antiarrhythmic drugs (encainide, flecainide [Tambocor]), β-adrenergic receptor antagonists (beta-blockers), and verapamil (Calan), whose plasma concentrations may be raised in SSRI-treated patients. Thus, dosage reduction and monitoring of plasma levels of tricyclic antidepressant, antipsychotic, and antiarrhythmic drugs are required in patients treated with fluoxetine or paroxetine. An exception is the SSRI fluvoxamine, which inhibits CYP 3A4 and CYP 1A2 but does not significantly inhibit the CYP 2D6. CYP 3A4 is responsible for the metabolism of alprazolam (Xanax), triazolam (Halcion), carbamazepine (Tegretol), quinidine (Cardioquin), erythromycin, terfenadine (Seldane), and astemizole (Hismanal) and may lead to an increase in the plasma concentration of these agents. These drugs should be avoided in patients receiving fluvoxamine. Similarly, theophylline (Aerolate) should be prescribed cautiously for fluvoxamine-treated patients because fluvoxamine may produce a threefold decrease in theophylline clearance by inhibiting the CYP 1D12 isoenzyme.

MAO Inhibitors

Monoamine oxidase inhibitors (MAOIs) are effective in patients with major depressive disorder; they are also effec-

tive in depressed patients with panic attacks. Low dosages of MAOIs—for example, phenelzine (Nardil) 30 to 45 mg daily or tranylcypromine (Parnate) 20 to 30 mg daily—should be used in the elderly. Orthostatic hypotension is the most frequent adverse effect of MAOIs. This adverse effect is of concern in the elderly because it may lead to falls and fractures, especially of the hip or the humerus. Other adverse effects include weight gain, lack of energy, and insomnia; lack of energy and daytime somnolence in phenelzine-treated patients; and nervousness, insomnia, and excessive perspiration in tranylcypromine-treated patients. Peripheral neuropathy occurs in a small percentage of patients taking MAOIs and often responds to pyridoxine. Sympathomimetic amines, monoamine precursors, tricyclic drugs, SSRIs, venlafaxine (Effexor), concomitant administration of two MAOIs, and tyramine-rich food may cause a hypertensive crisis and should be avoided in patients taking MAOIs. Drug interactions and dietary restrictions often prevent the use of MAOIs in the elderly.

Other Antidepressant Agents

Venlafaxine was found effective in hospitalized depressed patients as well as in drug-resistant depressed patients and in depressed patients with chronic pain. For this reason, venlafaxine should be considered in severe depression and in depression unresponsive to other agents.

Bupropion (Wellbutrin) has efficacy comparable to that of other antidepressant agents. Bupropion has fewer adverse effects than tricyclic drugs, including lack of cognitive impairment or sedation, safety in overdose, and lack of cardiotoxicity. Bupropion was found safe in patients with heart disease, and it should be considered in elderly cardiac patients. Bupropion has few drug interactions, but it should not be prescribed for patients receiving MAOIs. Bupropion may exacerbate preexisting hypertension. For this reason, blood pressure monitoring is required.

Nefazodone (Serzone) promotes sleep, has anxiolytic effects, is well tolerated, and is safe in overdose. Nefazodone does not influence the sleep architecture and does not cause sexual dysfunction. However, sedation and the need for two daily doses may be a problem for some elderly patients. A total daily dose of 300 to 500 mg may be required.

Augmentation of antidepressant drugs may improve the response of partially remitted geriatric depression. Lithium may augment tricyclic antidepressant response in elderly patients. The lithium dosage required by depressed elderly patients receiving tricyclics may be one third to one half that of younger adults. In younger patients, combinations of tricyclics with SSRIs have yielded an antidepressant response faster than tricyclics alone. Other augmentation techniques include combinations of tricyclics or SSRIs with thyroid hormones, psychostimulants, bupropion, pindolol, and other agents. Clinical experience suggests that augmentation techniques can be effective in some depressed geriatric patients with an incomplete response to a single antidepressant agent. However, the role of augmentation techniques is limited in geriatric depression because elderly patients often cannot tolerate combination therapies.

Table 55–7
Geriatric Dosages of Psychostimulants

Generic Name	Trade Name	Geriatric Dosage Range (mg a day)
Dextroamphetamine	Dexedrine	2.5–10
Pemoline	Cylert	18.75–37
Methylphenidate	Ritalin	2.5–20

Psychostimulants

The psychostimulants, also called *sympathomimetics* and *analeptics,* include amphetamines (e.g., dextroamphetamine [Dexedrine]), methylphenidate (Ritalin), and pemoline (Cylert). In selected patients, they can improve the mood, apathy, and anhedonia of depressed older persons, especially when these symptoms are caused by an associated chronic medical illness such as rheumatoid arthritis or multiple sclerosis. Amphetamines also may augment analgesia for patients who require pain medication. The use of psychostimulants is controversial because of the risk of abuse, but when prescribed judiciously in small dosages, they are of value. The geriatric dosages of the psychostimulants are listed in Table 55–7.

Antimanics

The use of lithium in elderly patients is more hazardous than its use in young patients because of the common occurrence of age-related morbidity and physiological changes of the heart, the thyroid, and the kidneys. Lithium is excreted by the kidneys, and decreased renal clearance and renal disease can increase the risk of toxicity. Thiazide diuretics decrease the renal clearance of lithium; consequently, the concomitant use of these medications can necessitate adjustments in lithium dosage. Other medications also may interfere with lithium clearance. Lithium may cause CNS effects, to which older persons often are especially sensitive. Because of these factors, frequent serum monitoring of lithium levels is recommended. In addition, cardiac, kidney, and thyroid workups are essential before initiating therapy. The geriatric dosages of drugs used in bipolar I disorder are listed in Table 55–8.

Table 55–8
Drugs Used to Treat Bipolar Disorder

Generic Name	Trade Name	Geriatric Dosage Range (mg a day)
Lithium carbonate	Eskalith, Lithane, Lithotabs	75–900
Carbamazepine	Tegretol	200–1,200
Valproate, divalproex	Depakene, Depakote	250–1,000
Clonazepam	Klonopin	0.5–1.5

A 78-year-old man with bipolar I disorder since age 40 became manic while residing in a nursing home. His mental illness had been complicated by chronic dependence, and he was now mildly demented. He had no history of renal disease, and his serum creatinine level was normal. After an initial period of typical manic grandiosity, when he was often seen near a local tavern, he soon deteriorated to crawling on his hands and knees, growling and barking like a dog, and striking out at all who approached. His lithium concentration was 1.2 mEq/L, with a maintenance dosage of 750 mg a day. After reducing the lithium dosage to achieve a concentration of 0.6 mEq/L, temporary addition of low-dose haloperidol and close attention to adequate fluid intake and preventing access to alcohol, both the manic episode and the superimposed delirium cleared within 3 weeks without need for another psychiatric hospitalization. (Courtesy of Soo Borson, M.D., and Jurgen Unützer, M.D.)

Antipsychotics

In addition to treating overt signs of psychosis such as hallucinations and delusions, antipsychotics have been used to deal effectively with violent, agitated, and abusive geriatric patients. In general, psychosis in older persons frequently responds to much lower dosages of medication than those used for younger patients. Older adults also are much more sensitive to many of the adverse effects of antipsychotic medications than young patients, specifically the extrapyramidal (parkinsonian) effects. Older patients have been known to stop speaking, ambulating, and swallowing as a result of these adverse effects. The same dosages of medication are not likely to produce significant problems for young patients.

Neurological Adverse Effects. The most common adverse effects of antipsychotic drugs are extrapyramidal signs, such as akathisia and acute dystonia. Akathisia may be misinterpreted as psychotic agitation, and the acute dyskinesias (especially of the face, tongue, and neck) may simulate the bizarre movements of schizophrenia. Parkinsonian symptoms are a late complication of drug therapy. The dyskinesias—manifest mainly by buccolingual movements—are noted late in the course of high-dosage antipsychotic therapy, especially in older persons. Autonomic adverse effects are particularly troublesome because they may upset the homeostasis of organs innervated by the autonomic nervous system, such as the bladder, the gastrointestinal tract, and the cardiovascular system. Alterations in sleep (e.g., insomnia, bizarre dreams, and sleepwalking) can occur. All drugs with anticholinergic properties may produce a toxic confusional state, which may also cause mydriasis and blurring of vision. Other drugs have adrenergic properties causing miosis.

Hip fracture resulting from falls, partly associated with medication use, is a major cause of morbidity in older persons and can be a proximal or distal factor associated with demise. Consequently, to minimize the potentially deleterious and even life-threatening adverse effects, clinicians should monitor drug use. Hip fractures are least often associated with short half-life anxiolytics and most often associated with antipsychotics.

An 83-year-old woman with long-standing diabetes and ischemic and hypertensive cardiovascular disease had gradually become bedfast over several years in a nursing home. Two months before psychiatric consultation was requested, she developed a psychotic illness characterized by delusions of being beaten during the night, aggressive outbursts, and pervasive despondency, which led to frequent and disruptive nocturnal phone calls to her daughter and to the local fire station. Initial clinical assessment disclosed moderately severe dementia in a personable but angry, frightened, and desperate woman eager for relief. Collateral history confirmed progressive cognitive deterioration over the course of her chronic medical illness, on a background of dysthymia of many years' duration. Trials of several antipsychotics and antidepressant medications had exacerbated both her symptoms and the problems of nursing staff in managing her care. A review of her medications showed that 4 of the 12 drugs she was taking on a regular basis were not essential for her medical management. (Courtesy of Soo Borson, M.D., and Jurgen Unützer, M.D.)

Clinical experience indicates that the therapeutic effects of antipsychotic medications in older persons may not become evident on a given dosage of medication for 4 weeks or longer. Because of the therapeutic factors and risks, the dictum in treating psychosis in persons over 65 years of age is to "start low and go slow." As in younger patients, adverse effect profiles should help determine the choice of medication, but no consensus exists about the choice or the dosage level of antipsychotics for older adults. There is no need to administer prophylactic antiparkinsonian agents on a regular basis when prescribing antipsychotics. The anticholinergic aspects of these drugs can create unwanted side effects, especially memory impairment. The geriatric dosages for commonly used antipsychotic agents are listed in Table 55–9.

Anxiolytics and Sedative-Hypnotics

The population older than 65 years of age constitutes less than 12 percent of the total population but includes 15 percent of long-term anxiolytic drug users. Their rate of regular use is five times that of the general population. Furthermore, among men with equivalent degrees of high emotional distress, those over 60 years of age are four times more likely to use an antianxiety drug than men between the ages of 18 and 29.

Geriatric patients with mild or moderate anxiety can benefit from anxiolytics, among which the benzodiazepines are the most widely used. Most patients are treated for brief periods, although some may have to be maintained on small dosages for long periods. The long-term use of benzodiazepines is controversial, because they are controlled substances with a potential for abuse; therefore, benzodiazepines with short or intermediate half-lives are preferable for use as hypnotics. Benzodiazepines may cause short periods of memory impairment, such as anterograde amnesia, which may aggravate an existing cognitive disorder in an older patient. Elderly patients accumulate the long-acting benzodiazepines (e.g., diazepam [Valium]) in adipose tissue,

Table 55–9
Geriatric Dosages of Commonly Used Antipsychotics

Generic Name	Trade Name	Geriatric Dosage Range (mg a day)
Phenothiazines		
Aliphatic		
Chlorpromazine	Thorazine	30–300
Triflupromazine	Vesprin	1–15
Piperazine		
Perphenazine	Trilafon	8–32
Trifluoperazine	Stelazine	1–15
Fluphenazine	Prolixin, Permitil	1–10
Piperidine		
Mesoridazine	Serentil	50–400
Thioxanthenes		
Chlorprothixene	Taractan	30–300
Thiothixene	Navane	2–20
Dibenzoxazepine		
Loxapine	Loxitane	50–250
Dihydroindole		
Molindone	Moban	50–225
Butyrophenone		
Haloperidol	Haldol	2–20
Benzisoxazole		
Risperidone	Risperdal	2–4

Table 55–10
Geriatric Dosages of Drugs Used to Treat Anxiety and Insomnia

Generic Name	Trade Name	Geriatric Dosage Range (mg a day)
Benzodiazepines		
Alprazolam	Xanax	0.5–6
Chlordiazepoxide	Librium	15–100
Clorazepate	Tranxene	7.5–60
Diazepam	Valium	2–60
Flurazepam	Dalmane	15–30
Halazepam	Paxipam	60–160
Lorazepam	Ativan	2–6
Oxazepam	Serax	30–120
Prazepam	Centrax	20–60
Temazepam	Restoril	15–30
Triazolam	Halcion	0.125–0.25
Nonbenzodiazepines		
Buspirone	BuSpar	5–60
Secobarbital	Seconal	50–300
Meprobamate	Miltown	400–800
Chloral hydrate	Noctec	500–1,000
Zolpidem	Ambien	2.5–5
β-Adrenergic receptor antagonists		
Propranolol	Inderal	40–160
Atenolol	Tenormin	25–100

and this process increases such adverse effects as ataxia, insomnia, and confusion (sundowner syndrome). These effects can be avoided if the lowest possible dosage is prescribed and intake is monitored until a therapeutic response is achieved.

Barbiturates may be substituted for the benzodiazepines in the few patients who do not respond to benzodiazepines. Geriatric patients are particularly prone to paradoxical dysphoria and cognitive disorganization, which can result from barbiturates. The barbiturates have a higher abuse potential than the benzodiazepines. Barbiturates are controlled substances, and the Drug Enforcement Agency (DEA) imposes constraints on their use.

Buspirone is an anxiolytic drug without sedative properties. It has a longer onset of action—up to 3 weeks—than either the benzodiazepines or the barbiturates and does not cause cognitive impairment. Moreover, it does not have any potential for abuse. A summary of the geriatric dosages of drugs used to treat anxiety and insomnia is presented in Table 55–10.

Estrogens

Estrogens may improve cognitive function through cholinergic neuroprotective and neurotropic effects. Furthermore, estrogen replacement therapy might augment the response to cholinesterase inhibitors such as tacrine. Adverse effects of estrogen replacement therapy are generally dose dependent and include endometrial hyperplasia and cancer, uterine bleeding (when taken with a progestin), breast tenderness, and nausea, among others. Because of the enhanced relative risk for endometrial cancer, periodic administration of progestins is recommended for women with intact uteri. The evidence for estrogen replacement therapy is stronger for a protective effect than for a symptomatic one. Ongoing clinical trials are assessing the effect of conjugated equine estrogens (Premarin) on cognition in women with Alzheimer's disease. Another ongoing trial is assessing whether hormone replacement therapy delays onset of Alzheimer's disease (National Institutes of Health Women's Health Initiative). In summary, a possible role for estrogen replacement therapy appears promising but is not substantiated.

Pharmacological Management of Agitation and Aggression in Dementia

A common issue in the treatment of older patients with dementia is the management of agitation and aggression. The use of antipsychotics is generally unsatisfactory because of their limited efficacy and their parkinsonian adverse effects. Benzodiazepines, although frequently used to treat behavior disturbances, may produce cognitive impairment, sedation, and paradoxical worsening of the patient's behavior. Buspirone, trazodone (Desyrel), and some β-adrenergic receptor antagonists, such as propranolol and pindolol, have been reported to reduce agitation, aggression, and impulsivity in patients with dementia and other cognitive disorders.

ELECTROCONVULSIVE THERAPY

Electroconvulsive therapy (ECT) has been controversial in the United States. It can be the most effective treatment option,

however, with the lowest risk of complications for older individuals with comorbid medical conditions likely to produce drug–disease and drug–drug interactions. ECT can provide a rapid response, which is vitally important in seriously ill patients, those at risk due to malnutrition or agitation related to psychiatric illness, and those at high risk for suicide. The current use of general anesthesia and medications to prevent musculoskeletal seizures has changed the procedure so that ECT is now generally considered as safe as, if not safer than, medication for use in frail elderly patients.

PSYCHOTHERAPY FOR GERIATRIC PATIENTS

The standard psychotherapeutic interventions—such as insight-oriented psychotherapy, supportive psychotherapy, cognitive therapy, group therapy, and family therapy—should be available to geriatric patients. According to Sigmund Freud, persons older than 50 years of age are not suited for psychoanalysis because their mental processes lack elasticity. In the view of many who followed Freud, however, psychoanalysis is possible after 50. Advanced age certainly limits plasticity of the personality, but as Otto Fenichel stated, "It does so in varying degrees and at very different ages so that no general rule can be given." Insight-oriented psychotherapy may help remove a specific symptom, even in older persons. It is of most benefit when patients have possibilities for libidinal and narcissistic gratification, but it is contraindicated if it would bring only the insight that life has been a failure and that the patient has no opportunity to make up for it.

Common age-related issues in therapy involve the need to adapt to recurrent and diverse losses (e.g., the deaths of friends and loved ones), the need to assume new roles (e.g., the adjustment to retirement and the disengagement from previously defined roles), and the need to accept mortality. Psychotherapy helps older persons to deal with these issues and the emotional problems surrounding them and to understand their behavior and the effects of their behavior on others. In addition to improving interpersonal relationships, psychotherapy increases self-esteem and self-confidence, decreases feelings of helplessness and anger, and improves the quality of life. As described by Alvin Goldfarb, geriatric psychotherapy has the general aim of assisting older adults to have minimal complaints, to help them make and keep friends of both sexes, and to have sexual relations when they have interest and capacity.

Psychotherapy helps relieve tensions of biological and cultural origins and helps older persons work and play within the limits of their functional status and as determined by their past training, activities, and self-concept in society. In patients with impaired cognition, psychotherapy can produce remarkable gains in both physical and mental symptoms. In one study conducted in an old-age home, 43 percent of the patients receiving psychotherapy showed less urinary incontinence, improved gait, greater mental alertness, improved memory, and better hearing than before psychotherapy.

Therapists must be more active, supportive, and flexible in conducting therapy with older than with younger adults, and they must be prepared to act decisively at the first sign of an incapacity that requires the active involvement of another physician such as an internist or that requires consulting with, or enlisting the aid of, a family member.

Older persons usually seek therapy for a therapist's unqualified and unlimited support, reassurance, and approval. Patients often expect a therapist to be all powerful, all knowing, and able to effect a magical cure. Most patients eventually recognize that the therapist is human and that they are engaged in a collaborative effort. In some cases, however, the therapist may have to assume the idealized role, especially when the patient is unable or unwilling to test reality effectively. With the help of the therapist, the patient deals with problems that had been avoided previously. As the therapist offers direct encouragement, reassurance, and advice, the patient's self-confidence increases as conflicts are resolved.

Supportive Psychotherapy

Frail, institutionalized, cognitively impaired, or chronically ill elderly patients require such psychotherapeutic techniques as support of healthier defense mechanisms, ventilation, and advice and help with acceptance of diminished capacities and increased dependency needs. In addition, they need caring, nurturing environments and assistance of families with their care giving. The patient's life history and psychodynamics (obtained from the patient or family members) enable the therapist to institute specific supportive therapeutic strategies.

An elderly woman with progressive cognitive impairment and lifelong personality traits of dependency and passivity is anxious and depressed about entering a nursing home. She may adapt well to the home if assigned to a roommate who is nurturing and protective.

Goldfarb has described a brief, supportive therapy technique for institutionalized, cognitively impaired patients. The therapist promotes patients' foundering self-esteem, sense of control, and safety by permitting them to develop an apparent special relationship with the therapist, who is perceived as a benevolent and powerful figure. The patients believe they have some control over the benevolent physician. This is accomplished in small, subtle ways. For example, the physician elicits the patient's preferences for the frequency of sessions, daily timetables, diet, or socializing and then acquiesces to the patient's wishes, while maintaining a quiet caution about being unduly manipulative. The technique includes weekly, short (15 minutes) visits and gratifying the patient's realistic requests when possible.

Life Review or Reminiscence Therapy

Robert Butler and others have noted the universal tendency of the aging person to reflect on, and reminisce about, the past. Reminiscence is characterized by the progressive return of memories of past experiences, especially those that were meaningful and conflictual. To varying degrees, elderly patients in therapy reminisce about the past, search for meaning in their lives, and strive for some resolution of past interpersonal and intrapsychic conflicts. Life review therapy systematically enhances this reminiscing process and makes it more conscious and deliberate. The therapist may guide the process by encouraging the patient to write or tape a biography with review of special events and turning points. Techniques include reunions with family and good friends and looking through memorabilia such as scrapbooks or picture albums. This technique has been

reported to resolve old problems, increase tolerance of conflict, relieve guilt and fears, and enhance self-esteem, creativity, generosity, and acceptance of the present.

Cognitive-Behavioral Therapy

In adapting cognitive-behavioral therapy to elderly patients, the therapist is often more active, redirecting the patient from reminiscence to here-and-now issues. The pace of therapy is sometimes slower than with younger adults, and when appropriate, the therapeutic alliance may be enhanced by permitting the patient to adopt a senior, teaching role with the younger therapist. To compensate for specific deficits such as hearing loss or cognitive slowing, information may be presented in different modalities, such as written material or taped sessions for the patient to take home. With older patients, termination is managed gradually rather than abruptly.

Brief (Time-Limited) Psychodynamic Psychotherapy

Brief, or time-limited, psychodynamic therapy can be considered for elderly patients with clearly defined, age-related problems that can be expected to resolve within a brief period of psychotherapy, such as an adjustment disorder, unresolved grief reaction, or new-onset anxiety disorder. Setting a time limit at the beginning of therapy reinforces the patients' confidence in their ability to resolve problems within a circumscribed period of time, focuses and accelerates the therapeutic process, diminishes their fear of dependency, and accommodates limited financial resources. Brief therapy uses the therapist's psychodynamic understanding of the patient and the patient's transference to the therapist to clarify and help resolve the patient's emotional reactions to a current life stress. During brief dynamic psychotherapy, the patient often uses the therapist to validate competency and normalcy, which helps to support and restore feelings of mastery and self-esteem. Symptomatic improvement often exceeds the achievement of insight or self-understanding.

Insight-Oriented Psychotherapy

The basic approach to insight-oriented therapy for older patients who are physically and cognitively intact is largely the same as that for younger patients. However, most clinicians agree that the themes introduced in therapy by elderly patients are more focused on issues of loss, sexual and physical decline, cumulative trauma, fear of pain and disability, decline in self-esteem, and increasing dependency. During longer-term psychotherapy, the condition and circumstances of the older patient evolve and change. The development of physical illness may require medical referral, collaboration with family members, or advocacy on behalf of the patient for community and other support services. Such active intrusions of the patient's real-life problems into the therapeutic process are not commonly dealt with by psychodynamic therapists, but when treating elderly patients, techniques must be adapted. Therapists are most effective when they learn to integrate different therapeutic modalities while maintaining a psychodynamic focus on the therapeutic relationship, the transference, and the goal of inner conflict resolution. Indeed, the necessity to integrate modalities of treatment is one of the hallmarks of the flexibility necessary to treat and manage the evolving therapeutic issues of elderly patients effectively.

Integrated Therapy

Integration of psychotherapies often is the most effective way to proceed.

At the age of 70, Mrs. S. was referred for psychiatric assessment because of her distress over her husband's declining physical state secondary to advanced Parkinson's disease. In the initial interview the therapist tried to determine three separate but interrelated factors: the patient's surface conflicts; the aspects of the conflicts that might be amenable to practical, environmental intervention; and the deeper psychological conflicts that were coloring the patient's ability to deal with the situation.

The manifest problems were loss of her husband's companionship and feeling helpless to cope with his illness. For example, he could not lie comfortably in bed and spent most nights sleeping in a living room chair, a situation that she could not tolerate. Mrs. S. feared her own growing incapacity from many years of arthritis and worried about the fate of her husband should she become immobilized.

In approaching the manifest difficulties, the therapist helped Mrs. S. define the specific areas of emotional conflict (especially her grief at the loss of the husband she once knew) and express and ventilate feelings of fearful anticipation, helplessness, and vulnerability. A cognitive therapy approach was used to help her recognize which parts of her feelings were based on unrealistic thoughts. Focusing on her feelings of failure and aloneness, the therapist helped her understand that others had struggled as she was struggling and that her sense of failure was not her fault but an inevitability of the illness. Concurrently, she was encouraged to distinguish her ideas of what was best for her husband from his actual needs.

At the same time, Mrs. S. examined the practical realities posed by her husband's illness and experimented with alternative methods of coping. For example, she gradually came to accept that there was no harm to her husband if he slept in a chair, as long as he felt comfortable. This simple change in perspective, arising from direct explanation and advice from the therapist, relieved much of her tension and guilt and allowed her to sleep more restfully.

The third concurrent component of therapy was an exploration of deeper sources of feeling. This part of therapy revealed the patient's rage at her husband. She had been unaware of how his illness had reactivated her long-standing belief that she had never been understood or cared for as she had wanted. She spoke of her conflicted feelings about her childhood and her lonely, restricted life with which she appeared to cope on the surface, while actually experiencing abandonment and fear. The therapist actively encouraged her reminiscence in the early phases of therapy, attempting to evoke the emotions that accompanied the memories. Gradually, she moved into a phase of meaningful exploration

of her inner state. The resulting improved comfort helped her carry on in her caregiving role but also freed her to begin to seek sources of essential nurturance and gratification for herself.

The successful outcome of this treatment probably delayed Mrs. S.'s own decline and enabled her husband to remain safely at home for a much longer time. This case illustrates both the efficacy of psychotherapy and its potential cost-effective and humanitarian outcome. (Courtesy of Joel Sadavoy, M.D., and Lawrence W. Lazarus, M.D.)

NEUROIMAGING STUDIES IN DEMENTIA

Dementia of the Alzheimer's type has been studied quite extensively by both computed tomography (CT) and MRI. The findings from neuroimaging studies in dementia closely parallel the more established pathological hallmarks of the disorder. Cross-sectional neuroimaging studies demonstrate smaller brain volumes and larger cerebrospinal fluid (CSF) volumes in these patients than in age-matched controls without dementia. Longitudinal studies using CT demonstrate progressive ventricular enlargement in patients with dementia, significantly greater than the minimal progressive dilation seen in controls without dementia. Also, while ventricular enlargement was noted relatively early in the course of the illness (when memory impairment dominates the clinical picture), the rate of enlargement appears to increase substantially when nonmemory cognitive aspects of the dementia become clinically apparent. In addition to the more global measures of atrophy, investigators have demonstrated focal volumetric reductions in both medial and lateral temporal lobe structures in patients with dementia (compared with controls). Even in patients with mild dementia, hippocampal volume reductions between patients and controls were striking. Other reports indicate that volumes of the left amygdala and the entorhinal cortex best discriminate patients with dementia of the Alzheimer's type from controls. In an effort to examine the neuroanatomical correlates of patients in the predementia stage, one study found that patients with minimal cognitive impairment and CT evidence of hippocampal atrophy progressed to clinical dementia on follow-up. Thus, focal hippocampal atrophy may serve as a marker for dementia of the Alzheimer's type. Focal neuroanatomical perturbations captured by CT and MRI early in the course of the disease may reflect the early pathological changes that occur in circumscribed brain regions in the limbic/mesial temporal areas. Progression of Alzheimer's disease is clearly associated with progressive neuronal loss, and the neuroimaging evidence clearly corroborates these changes.

In spite of the fact that structural and functional brain-imaging studies find statistical differences between groups of patients with psychiatric disorders other than dementia (e.g., depression, schizophrenia) and normal controls, these techniques are not yet indicated in the clinical diagnosis of these disorders. It remains to be established how well these techniques distinguish the psychiatric disorder of interest from other disorders (e.g., distinguish depressive pseudodementia from other forms of dementia), predict clinical course, correspond to postmortem histopathology, or influence decisions about treatment.

NURSING HOMES

Problems and Reforms

Nursing homes account for approximately 4.1 percent of elderly Americans, with 1.55 million older persons living in nursing homes at any time. This figure, however, greatly underestimates the number of individuals who use nursing home services. In 1995, 1.7 million persons were admitted to nursing homes; two thirds to three fourths of them were discharged after several months. It has been estimated that the number of nursing home residents will double by the year 2020 and triple by 2040 and that the probability that any person will require nursing home care at some point in his or her life exceeds 40 percent. The total costs of institutional care for elderly patients in the United States were estimated for 1993 at $74.9 million, with $36.9 million coming from Medicaid and $4.8 million from Medicare.

Nursing home care represents approximately 8 percent of the nation's total health care costs, but the burden of payment is markedly different from that of other aspects of health care, with approximately 50 percent of costs borne directly by residents and their families and most of the remainder shared equally by the federal and state governments through Medicaid programs. Medicare payments are limited to subacute care. In spite of recent trends toward a leveling of growth, the number of nursing homes and nursing home beds has increased dramatically since the mid-1960s when Medicaid programs were first developed. In parallel, there has been increasing recognition of the problems with nursing home care and the need for reform. As stated in a 1986 Institute of Medicine report, "Improving the Quality of Care in Nursing Homes," many nursing homes provide good care.

> But in many other government certified nursing homes, individuals who are admitted receive very inadequate—sometimes shockingly deficient—care that is likely to hasten the deterioration of their physical, mental, and emotional health. They also are likely to have their rights violated and may even be subject to physical abuse.

Several major issues raised about the quality of nursing home care were related to its psychiatric aspects; they included concerns that physical and chemical restraints were inappropriately being used to control residents' behavior and that psychiatric disorders (primarily depression) were being undertreated. Estimates of the prevalence of the use of physical restraints, such as wrist or ankle cuffs, belts, vest restraints, or geriatric chairs designed to restrict mobility, ranged from 25 to 85 percent. Use of these devices was endemic despite evidence from observational studies that they do not safely control agitated behavior and suggestions from cross-national studies that similar patient populations can be managed without their use. Surveys of medication use in long-term care facilities found prevalence rates of up to 74 percent for medications that act on the CNS.

Antipsychotic agents have been the most frequently prescribed psychotropic medications, with most reports of prevalence in the range of 20 to 50 percent. Evidence suggesting the misuse of those drugs came from findings that variables unrelated to patient characteristics (e.g., facility size, ratio of patients to staff, and the

size of the physician's nursing home practice) were directly associated with use of drugs. Substantial numbers of patients received psychotropic drugs without any diagnosis of mental disorder and without any chart note indicating the presence of relevant target symptoms. The importance of this issue for patients, families, and advocacy groups was poignantly captured by the newspaper headline "America's Other Drug Problem."

In 1987 the federal government, the largest single source of payment for nursing home care, used Medicaid and Medicare legislation to mandate nursing home reform that was enacted in the Omnibus Budget Reconciliation Act (OBRA) of 1987. OBRA 1987 (with modification in 1990) required preadmission screening and annual resident review (PASARR) to ensure that patients who belong in psychiatric hospitals were not inappropriately admitted to nursing homes. Other regulations stated that "the resident has a right to be free from any physical and chemical restraints imposed for purposes of discipline or convenience and not required to treat the resident's medical symptoms." OBRA 1987 requires that "residents who have not used antipsychotic drugs are not given these drugs unless antipsychotic drug therapy is necessary to treat a specific condition as diagnosed and documented in the clinical record," and "residents who use antipsychotic drugs receive gradual dose reductions and behavioral interventions, unless clinically contraindicated, in an effort to discontinue these drugs." Regulations also state that each resident must be free from unnecessary drugs, which are defined as any drug used without appropriate indications, in excessive dosage, for excessive duration, without adequate monitoring, or in the presence of adverse consequences that indicate that the medication should be reduced or discontinued. Although the definition of unnecessary drugs is rather general, guidelines used by surveyors to monitor facilities' compliance with OBRA regulations focus on antipsychotic, anxiolytic, and sedative-hypnotic drugs. The primary goal in the implementation of the antipsychotic drug and unnecessary drug regulations is to decrease the use of medications as chemical restraints.

Quality of Life

Nursing homes are communities consisting of residents, families, staff, and health care providers in which many patients with chronic disease and disability live out their lives. Accordingly, regulations developed to implement OBRA 1987 include the requirement that "a facility must care for its residents in a manner and in an environment that promotes maintenance or enhancement of each resident's quality of life." Specific provisions require attention to issues of dignity; individuality; self-determination; participation in resident and family groups; participation in social, religious, and community activities; availability of ongoing activity programs designed in accordance with the resident's interests and well-being; and delivery of all services in a manner that reasonably accommodates the individual needs and preferences of the resident. The high prevalence of psychiatric disorders, primarily dementia and depressive disorders, implies that expertise regarding the psychiatric disorders of late life is essential to meet quality-of-life and quality-of-care requirements.

A generation of research has established the general principle that both quality of life and health outcomes for nursing home residents are improved when the care environment is designed to foster the resident's sense of autonomy and control. M. Powell Lawton and his colleagues have emphasized that optimizing the resident's quality of life requires attention to the fit between individuals and their care environment. According to his ecological theory of aging and adaptation, the demands from the environment must match the resident's competencies and capabilities. Maximal performance can be elicited when the demands and challenges from the environment slightly exceed the level that would match the resident's current abilities; this may be most appropriate in a rehabilitation program. Alternatively, maximal comfort can be elicited when the environmental pressure is slightly below the resident's current abilities; this may be most appropriate during convalescence from acute illness or injury. According to Lawton, affective or behavioral pathology can occur when environmental demands exceed the zone of maximal performance and become overwhelming or when they fall below the zone of maximal comfort and represent a form of deprivation.

It is an ongoing challenge for nursing home staff to modify demands on the resident appropriately and to determine whether a change in activity level is a matter of changing physical ability or personal preference and when it is a symptom of psychopathology. Nursing homes each day must struggle with the way psychiatric disorders affect medical decision making. Development of institutional policies, procedures, and programs requires that psychiatric consultation be available to nursing home administrators and staff. Nursing homes are in fact neuropsychiatric institutions, and input from mental health professionals is necessary if the homes are to fulfill their missions.

PSYCHIATRIC SYMPTOMS ASSOCIATED WITH SPECIFIC MEDICAL DISORDERS

Cerebrovascular Disease

Significant depressions are common, occurring in up to 50 percent of all patients following an acute cerebrovascular accident. Depressive disorders after neocortical strokes resemble primary depressions in both clinical presentation and response to antidepressant pharmacotherapy. Manic episodes (which may respond to lithium or antimanic anticonvulsants) and apathetic behavioral states without depressive affect or mood appear especially likely after right hemisphere strokes. *Subcortical dementia* is a clinically useful concept designating a syndrome of psychomotor slowing, depressed mood, inattentiveness, forgetfulness, motor impairment, and seemingly disproportionate functional dependency occurring in patients with diseases of the thalamus, basal ganglia, and upper brainstem. This syndrome commonly results from subcortical ischemic disease (vascular depression) as well as from classic neurological diseases such as parkinsonism.

Acute confusional states frequently occur after stroke and may be the only presenting sign in a small minority of patients, particularly those with basal ganglia and other subcortical infarcts.

Psychotic symptoms with delusions, hallucinations, or a full schizophrenialike syndrome may result from focal brain injury, particularly after lesions of limbic cortical and subcortical structures. Paranoid and persecutory delusions and ideas of reference are common and may be circumscribed or highly elaborate and pervasive. Personality changes, particularly those

producing inappropriate aggressive or sexual behaviors, are encountered with regularity in patients with strokes, especially men with frank dementia, and frequently lead to psychiatric consultation and psychotropic drug treatment and sometimes to permanent psychiatric hospitalization.

Cardiovascular Disease

Acute myocardial infarction and chronic congestive heart failure may both be accompanied by psychiatric disturbances. Confusional states due to cerebral hypoperfusion or complications of treatment (e.g., cardiovascular drugs, electrolyte imbalances due to diuretics, or repeated resuscitations for ventricular arrhythmias) are best managed by primary efforts to improve compromised cardiac function and metabolic status. About 10 percent of patients who undergo open-heart surgery suffer mild but lasting neuropsychological impairment as a result. Barring major intraoperative complications, most of these impairments are mild; most affected patients are elderly.

Depression and anxiety disorders following myocardial infarction or heart failure require attention to both possible medical causes and psychological factors, especially patients' concerns about risk of death and disability and the adequacy of supportive care. Untreated or inadequately treated major depression worsens the prognosis in heart disease.

Chronic Diseases of the Lung, Kidneys, and Liver

Obstructive lung disease, caused in large part by cigarette smoking, is the most prevalent of the chronic respiratory diseases of the second half of life. Psychiatric complications include acute and chronic encephalopathies related to acute infarction or respiratory failure, to sustained hypoxemia and hypercapnia, or to the CNS effects of drugs used in management (oral or inhaled bronchodilators, high-dose prednisone, cough suppressants, or benzodiazepines). Depressions are common, as in other chronic medical illnesses, but tend to be characterized by prominent anxiety and paniclike episodes, accounting for frequent prescription of anxiolytics. Psychotic states may occur and are usually related to acute impairment of brain function.

Chronic renal and hepatic diseases produce encephalopathic states through their effects on nutrition, metabolism, excretory clearance, and drug disposition. The prevalence of other psychiatric disorders in these conditions approximates those for chronic disease in general; treatment considerations include evaluating the effects of disease on effective plasma drug levels and half-lives. Chronic hemodialysis has been associated with dementia due to brain accumulation of aluminum present in dialysis solutions, a discovery that has led to its exclusion from the formula.

Arthritis

The two major forms of arthritis in the elderly, osteoarthritis and rheumatoid arthritis, are important to the psychiatrist chiefly because together they constitute the leading cause of chronic disability in old age, affecting one of every two persons over 65. Mood disorders, the most prevalent psychiatric complications of degenerative arthritis, occur in up to 25 percent of patients and are primary determinants of the severity of functional disability. Because of the widespread comorbidity of arthritis and depression, recognition and treatment of mood disorder can contribute significantly to improving the functional health of the elderly population. Occasionally, psychiatric symptoms arise as a complication of treatment with nonsteroidal antiinflammatory drugs (NSAIDs) or prednisone.

Thyroid Disease, Malnutrition, and Anemia

Thyroid disease, malnutrition, and anemia are relatively common, particularly in older adults with significant comorbid medical illness. They may be responsible for such psychiatric symptoms as lethargy, weakness, confusion, and behavioral changes and should be actively sought and treated.

References

Coyne AC, Reichman WE, Berbig LJ. The relationship between dementia and elder abuse. *Am J Psychiatry.* 1993;150:643.

Crome IB, Day E. Substance misuse and dependence: older people deserve better services. *Rev Clin Gerontol.* 1999;9:327.

Dada F, Sethi S, Grossberg GT. Generalized anxiety disorder in the elderly. *Psychiatr Clin North Am.* 2001;24:155.

Draper B. The effectiveness of old age psychiatry services. *Int J Geriatr Psychiatry.* 2000;15:687.

Finnema E, Droees RM, Ribbe M, van-Tilburg W. A review of psychosocial models in psychogeriatrics: implications for care and research. *Alzheimer Dis Assoc Disord.* 2000;14:68.

Freudenstein U, Jagger C, Arthur A, Donner-Banzhoff N. Treatments for late life depression in primary care—a systematic review. *Fam Pract.* 2001; 18:321.

Harvey PD. Cognitive and functional impairments in elderly patients with schizophrenia: a review of the recent literature. *Harv Rev Psychiatry.* 2001;9:59.

Hsich G, Kenney K, Gibbs CJ Jr, Lee KH, Harrington MG. The 14-3-3 brain protein in cerebrospinal fluid as a marker for transmissible spongiform encephalopathies. *N Engl J Med.* 1996;335:921.

Jarvik LF, contributing ed. Geriatric psychiatry. In: Sadock BJ, Sadock VA, eds. *Kaplan & Sadock's Comprehensive Textbook of Psychiatry.* 7th ed. Vol 2. Baltimore: Lippincott Williams & Wilkins; 2000:2980.

Mallucci GR, Collinge J. Neuropsychiatric presentations of prion disease. *Curr Opin Psychiatry.* 1997;10:59.

Phelan EA, Larson B. Successful aging. *J Am Geriatr Soc.* 2002;50:1306.

Salzman C, Tune L. Neuroleptic treatment of late-life schizophrenia. *Harv Rev Psychiatry.* 2001;9:77.

Schachter AS, Davis KL. Guidelines for the appropriate use of cholinesterase inhibitors in patients with Alzheimer's disease. *CNS Drugs.* 1999;11:281.

Solomon K, Manepalli J, Ireland GA, Mahon GM. Alcoholism and prescription drug abuse in the elderly: St. Louis University grand rounds. *J Am Geriatr Soc.* 1993;41:57.

Sultzer DL. Selective serotonin reuptake inhibitors and trazodone for treatment of depression, psychosis and behavioral symptoms in patients with dementia. *Int Psychogeriatr.* 2000;12(suppl 1):245.

Thomas C, Kelman HR, Kennedy GJ, Ahn C. Depressive symptoms and mortality in elderly persons. *J Gerontol.* 1992;47:S80.

Umapathy C, Mulsant BH, Pollack BG. Bipolar disorder in the elderly. *Psychiatr Ann.* 2000;30:473.

Van-Gerpen MW, Johnson JE, Wionstead DK. Mania in the geriatric patient population: a review of the literature. *Am J Geriatr Psychiatry.* 1999;7:188.

Will RG, Ironside JW, Zeidler M, et al. A new variant of Creutzfeldt-Jakob disease in the UK. *Lancet.* 1996;347:921.

Woodward M. Hypnosedatives in the elderly: a guide to appropriate use. *CNS Drugs.* 1999;11:263.

56 End-of-Life Care and Palliative Medicine

Regardless of their specialty, at some point in their careers almost all practicing physicians have to deal with dying patients. Most medical training programs, however, address this reality inadequately, so that doctors and other professionals often must learn on their own to contend with problems of death. A recent review of 50 major nursing and medical textbooks found little or no mention of end-of-life care and a lack of helpful information on caring for patients dying from fatal disease. As a result of this neglect, treatment of terminal patients can be needlessly painful for patients as well as for family, friends, physicians, nurses, and other personnel who care for them. (In addition to this chapter, the reader is referred to Section 2.6, Death, Dying, and Bereavement.)

End-of-Life Care Defined

End of life refers to all those issues involved in caring for the terminally ill. It begins when curative therapy ceases and encompasses the following areas: (1) communication of prognosis to family and patient, and defining the patient's understanding of his or her illness; (2) advance directives about life-sustaining treatment; (3) the need for hospitalization and hospice care; (4) legal and ethical matters; (5) bereavement support and psychiatric care; and finally (6) palliative care to relieve pain and suffering. Each of these issues is discussed below.

GENERAL APPROACHES TO CARING FOR THE DYING PATIENT

The most important task for physicians caring for dying patients is to provide compassionate concern and continuing support. The hallmarks of appropriate care are predicated on a good doctor–patient relationship and include visiting patients regularly, maintaining eye contact, listening and touching appropriately, and being willing to answer questions respectfully and honestly.

Problems Facing the Physician

Physicians' abilities to care compassionately and effectively for patients who are dying depend largely on their own beliefs about death and dying. Indeed, some physicians are so upset by death that they are reluctant to discuss end-of-life issues with their patients; others may steadfastly refuse to use palliative care services for the terminally ill. Such terminally ill patients may be subject to unnecessary worry and discomfort if their doctors are unwilling to confront death with them.

Ideally, physicians should strive to extend life and decrease suffering, but at the same time, they should also accept that death is a defining characteristic of life. This ideal may be unattainable, but as long as physicians are aware their own beliefs and motivations, these factors will be less likely to hamper life-and-death decisions. Unfortunately, some physicians have developed dysfunctional attitudes about death, which have been reinforced throughout their lives by their experiences and training. It has been postulated that doctors are more frightened of death than members of other professional groups and that many enter the study of medicine so that they may gain control of their own mortality. In this way, these physicians are dealing with their underlying fear of death through extensive intellectualization.

Even if they themselves do not fear death, many physicians have been led by modern medicine and their training to unconsciously assume that they can prevent death. This false feeling of omnipotence is challenged by encounters with dying patients, because these doctors equate these patients with failure. It is no surprise, then, that these physicians may avoid their dying patients when their condition elicits fear or calls into question their own competence. Ultimately, their failure to accept their own inadequacies and limitations in treating disease often comes at the expense of patient care and comfort.

COMMUNICATION AND ITS IMPORTANCE

After a diagnosis and prognosis have been made, physicians need to talk to the patient and the patient's family. Formerly, doctors subscribed to a conspiracy of silence, believing that their patient's chances for recovery would improve if they knew less, because news of impending death might bring despair. The current practice is now one of honesty and openness toward patients; in fact, the question is not whether or not to tell the patient, but when and how. The American Hospital Association in 1972 drafted the Patient's Bill of Rights, declaring that patients have the "right to obtain complete, current information regarding diagnosis, treatment and prognosis in terms the patient can be reasonably expected to understand."

When breaking news of impending death to the patient, as when relating any bad news, diplomacy and compassion should be guiding principles. Often, bad news is not completely related

during one meeting but rather is absorbed gradually over a series of separate conversations. Advance preparations, including scheduling enough time for the visit, researching pertinent information such as test results and facts about the case, and even arranging furniture appropriately can only make the patient feel more comfortable.

If possible, these conversations should take place in a private, suitable space with the patient on equal terms with the physician (i.e., the patient dressed and the physician seated). If it is possible and desired by the patient, the patient's spouse or partner should be present. The treating physician should explain the current situation to the patient in clear, simple language, even when speaking to highly educated patients. Information may need to be repeated or additional meetings may be necessary to communicate all of the information. A gentle, sensible approach will help modulate the patient's own denial and acceptance. At no time should physicians take their patient's angry comments personally, and they should never criticize the patient's response to the bad news.

Physicians can signal their availability for honest communication by encouraging and answering questions from patients. Estimates as to how long a patient has to live are usually inaccurate and thus should not be given. Also, physicians should make it clear to their patients that they are willing to see them through until death occurs. Ultimately, physicians must choose how much information to give and when on the basis of each patient's needs and capacities.

The same general approaches apply as physicians seek to comfort members of the patient's family. Helping family members deal with feelings about the patient's illness can be just as important as comforting the patient, because family members are often the main source of emotional support for patients. Table 56–1 lists seven promises that physicians may make to dying patients.

TELLING THE TRUTH

Tactful honesty is the doctor's most important aid. Honesty, however, need not preclude hope or guarded optimism. One should always be aware that if 85 percent of patients with a particular disease die in 5 years, 15 percent are still alive after that time. The principles of doing good and not doing harm inform the decision of whether or not to tell the patient the truth. In general, most patients want to know the truth about their condition. Various studies of patients with malignancies show that 80 to 90 percent want to know their diagnosis.

However, doctors should ask patients how much they want to know about the illness because some persons do not want to know the facts about their illness. Such patients, if told the truth, deny that they ever were told, and they cannot participate in end-of-life decisions such as the use of life-sustaining equipment. The patients who openly request that they not be given "bad news" are often those who most fear death. Physicians should deal with these fears directly, but if the patient still cannot bear to hear the truth, someone closely related to the patient must be informed.

Ned Cassem suggests seven essential features in the management of the dying patient, which are listed in Table 56–2.

Table 56–1
The Seven Promises a Physician Should Make to a Dying Patient

- You will have the best of medical treatment, aiming to prevent exacerbation, improve function and survival, and ensure comfort.
- You will never have to endure overwhelming pain, shortness of breath, or other symptoms.
- Your care will be continuous, comprehensive, and coordinated.
- You and your family will be prepared for everything that is likely to happen in the course of your illness.
- Your wishes will be sought and respected, and followed whenever possible.
- We will help you consider your personal and financial resources and we will respect your choices about their use.
- We will do all we can to see that you and your family will have the opportunity to make the best of every day.

From Mitka M. Suggestions for help when the end is near. *JAMA*. 2000; 284:2441.
Adapted from National Coalition on Health Care (NCHC) and the Institute for Health-care Improvement (IHI). *Promises to Keep: Changing the Way We Provide Care at the End of Life,* released October 12, 2000, with permission.

Table 56–2
Seven Essential Features in the Management of the Dying Patient

1. Concern: Empathy, compassion, and involvement are essential; concern is ranked as the quality most appreciated by patients.
2. Competence: Skills and knowledge can be as reassuring as warmth and concern. In particular, health care providers must adeptly manage the main medical and psychiatric complications of terminal illness: pain, nausea, shortness of breath, and hopelessness. Patients benefit immeasurably from the reassurance that their providers will not allow them to live or die in pain.
3. Communication: Open lines of communication are essential in every stage of illness and dying, without exception.
4. Children: Allowing children or family members who want to visit the dying patient to do so is generally advisable; family provides consolation to dying patients.
5. Cohesion: Cohesion between the patient, family members, and caretakers maximizes patient support and helps the family through bereavement.
6. Cheerfulness: A gentle, appropriate sense of humor can be palliative; a somber or anxious demeanor should be avoided.
7. Consistency: Continuing, persistent attention is highly valued by patients, who often fear that they are a burden and will be abandoned; consistent physician involvement mitigates these fears.

Data from Ned Cassem, M.D.

Informed Consent

In the United States, informed consent is legally required for both conventional and experimental treatment. Patients must be given enough information about their diagnosis, prognosis, and treatment options to make a knowledgeable decision. This includes discussion of potential risks and benefits, available alternative treatments, and the results of not receiving treatment. This approach may come at some psychological cost; severe anxiety and occasional psychiatric decompensation can occur when patients feel overburdened by demands to make decisions. Nevertheless, patients respond best to doctors who explain the various options in detail. Some patients ask, "What

Table 56–3
Some Difficult Questions from Patients

"Why me?"
"Why didn't you catch this earlier? Did you make a mistake?"
"How long do I have?"
"What would you do in my shoes?"
"Should I try long-shot or experimental therapy?"
"Should I go to a 'medical mecca' for treatment or a second opinion?"
"If my suffering gets really bad, will you help me die?"
"Will you work with me all the way through to my death, no matter what?"

From Quill TF. Initiating end-of-life discussions with seriously ill patients. *JAMA.* 2000;284:2502, with permission.

would you do, doctor, if you were in my shoes? Or, if it were your wife, your husband, your child?" Physicians must be prepared to deal with these and other difficult questions posed by patients. Some of them are listed in Table 56–3.

End-of-life discussions are challenging, especially since they can influence how patients make informed choices. Table 56–4 lists representative questions that doctors can ask their patients to initiate the discussion of such end-of-life issues as do not resuscitate (DNR) orders, pain management, and advance directives.

TERMINAL CARE DECISIONS

Modern society is poorly equipped to cope with the life-and-death decisions spawned by technology. When it first emerged, cardiopulmonary resuscitation was enthusiastically supported by the medical profession. It was endowed with magical power and eventually became a ritualized rite rather than an optional medical treatment. That practice played into the therapeutic activism characteristic of many physicians. By the end of the 20th century, however, a countermovement began. First, the right to refuse treatment was established, thanks in large part to synergy between the consumer movement and the bioethics movement with its emphasis on patient autonomy. Next, the legality of DNR orders and the moral equivalence of stopping and not starting treatment were established. The medical profession was less enthusiastic than the public about these changes, perhaps because practitioners know too well the emotional ambiguities that surround death and must repeatedly experience them.

Advance Directives. Advance directives are wishes and choices about medical intervention when the patient's condition is considered terminal. Advance directives are legally binding in all 50 states and there are 3 types: living will, health care proxy, and DNR and do not intubate (DNI) orders.

LIVING WILL. In a living will, a patient who is mentally competent gives specific instructions that doctors must follow when the patient cannot communicate them because of illness. These instructions may include rejection of feeding tubes, artificial airways, or any other measures to prolong life.

HEALTH CARE PROXY. Also known as *durable power of attorney,* the health care proxy gives another person the power to make medical decisions if the patient cannot do so. That person, also known as the *surrogate,* is empowered to make all decisions about terminal care on the basis of what he or she thinks the patient would want.

DO NOT RESUSCITATE AND DO NOT INTUBATE ORDERS. These orders prohibit doctors from attempting to resuscitate (DNR) or intubate (DNI) the patient who is in extremis. DNR and DNI orders are

Table 56–4
Representative Questions for Initiating the Discussion about End-of-Life Issues

Domain	Representative Questions[a]
Goals	Given the severity of your illness, what is most important for you to achieve? What do you think about balancing quality of life with length of life in terms of your treatment? What are your most important hopes? What are your biggest fears?
Values	What makes life most worth living for you? Would there be any circumstances under which you would find life not worth living? What do you consider your quality of life to be like now? Have you seen or been with someone who had a particularly good death or particularly difficult death?
Advance directives	If with future progression of your illness you are not able to speak for yourself, who would be best able to represent your views and values? (health care proxy) Have you given any thought to what kind of treatment you would want (and not want) if you become unable to speak for yourself in the future? (living will)
Do-not-resuscitate order	If you were to die suddenly, that is, you stopped breathing or your heart stopped, we could try to revive you by using cardiopulmonary resuscitation (CPR). Are you familiar with CPR? Have you given thought as to whether you would want it? Given the severity of your illness, CPR would in all likelihood be ineffective. I would recommend that you choose not to have it, but that we continue all potentially effective treatments. What do you think?
Palliative care (pain and other symptoms)	Have you ever heard of hospice (palliative care)? What has been your experience with it? Tell me about your pain. Can you rate it on a 10-point scale? What is your breathing like when you feel at your best? How about when you are having trouble?
Palliative care ("unfinished business")	If you were to die sooner rather than later, what would be left undone? How is your family handling your illness? What are their reactions? Has religion been an important part of your life? Are there any spiritual issues you are concerned about at this point?

[a]Physicians should give the patient an opportunity to respond to each question. Base follow-up questions and responses on careful listening to the patient, using his or her own words whenever possible.
From Quill TE. Initiating end-of-life discussions with seriously ill patients. *JAMA.* 2000;284:2502.

Table 56–5
Advance Directive Living Will and Health Care Proxy

Death is a part of life. It is a reality like birth, growth, and aging. I am using this advance directive to convey my wishes about medical care to my doctors and other people looking after me at the end of my life. It is called an advance directive because it gives instructions in advance about what I want to happen to me in the future. It expresses my wishes about medical treatment that might keep me alive. I want this to be legally binding.

If I cannot make or communicate decisions about my medical care, those around me should rely on this document for instructions about measures that could keep me alive.

I do not want medical treatment (including feeding and water by tube) that will keep me alive if:

- I am unconscious and there is no reasonable prospect that I will ever be conscious again (even if I am not going to die soon in my medical condition), or
- I am near death from an illness or injury with no reasonable prospect of recovery.

I do want medicine and other care to make me more comfortable and to take care of pain and suffering. I want this even if the pain medicine makes me die sooner.

I want to give some extra instructions: *[Here list any special instructions, e.g., some people fear being kept alive after a debilitating stroke. If you have wishes about this, or any other condition, please write them here.]*

The legal language in the box that follows is a health care proxy. It gives another person the power to make medical decisions for me.

I name ______________________________,
who lives at ______________________________,
phone number ____________________, to make medical decisions for me if I cannot make them myself. This person is called a health care "surrogate," "agent," "proxy," or "attorney in fact." This power of attorney shall become effective when I become incapable of making or communicating decisions about my medical care. This means that this document stays legal when and if I lose the power to speak for myself, for instance, if I am in a coma or have Alzheimer's disease.

My health care proxy has power to tell others what my advance directive means. This person also has power to make decisions for me based either on what I would have wanted, or, if this is not known, on what he or she thinks is best for me.

If my first choice health care proxy cannot or decides not to act for me, I name ______________________________,
address ______________________________,
phone number ____________________, as my second choice.

I have discussed my wishes with my health care proxy, and with my second choice if I have chosen to appoint a second person. My proxy(ies) has(have) agreed to act for me.

I have thought about this advance directive carefully. I know what it means and want to sign it. I have chosen two witnesses, neither of whom is a member of my family, nor will inherit from me when I die. My witnesses are not the same people as those I named as my health care proxies. I understand that this form should be notarized if I use the box to name (a) health care proxy(ies).

Signature ______________________________
Date ______________________________
Address ______________________________
Witness's signature ______________________________
Witness's printed name ______________________________
Address ______________________________
Witness's signature ______________________________
Witness's printed name ______________________________
Address ______________________________
Notary [to be used if proxy is appointed] ____________________

Reprinted with permission from Choice in Dying, Inc.—the National Council for the Right to Die. (Choice in Dying is a national not-for-profit organization that works for the rights of patients at the end of life. In addition to this generic advance directive, Choice in Dying distributes advance directives that conform to each state's specific legal requirements and maintains a national Living Will Registry for completed documents.)

made by the patient who is competent to do so. They can be made part of the living will or expressed by the health care proxy. A sample advance directive that incorporates both a living will and a health care proxy is given in Table 56–5.

The *Uniform Rights of the Terminally Ill Act*, drafted by the National Conference on Uniform State Laws, was approved and recommended for enactment in all states. This act authorizes an adult to control the decisions regarding the administration of life-sustaining treatment by executing a declaration instructing a physician to withhold or to withdraw life-sustaining treatment if the person is in a terminal condition and cannot participate in medical treatment decisions. In 1991 the *Federal Patients Self-Determination Act* became law in the United States and required that all health care facilities (1) provide each patient admitted to a hospital with written information about the right to refuse treatment, (2) ask about advance directives, and (3) keep written records of whether the patient has an advance directive or has designated a health care proxy.

Today patients who have left no advance directives or who are legally incompetent to do so have access to hospital ethics committees that hold active legal and ethical debates about these issues. These ethics committees are also of help to doctors, who can gain both legal and moral support when recommending that no further treatment occur. It is much easier for all parties, however, if the patient has advance directives or a

Table 56–6
Tasks of Family Members

1. Administering medications
2. Dealing with adverse effects of medications
3. Providing help with, or actually performing, activities of daily living (ADLs)
4. Changing wound dressing
5. Managing ambulatory infusion pumps or other equipment
6. Providing symptom management (e.g., for pain, nausea and vomiting, shortness of breath, seizures, and terminal agitation)
7. Notifying the nurse or doctor when they are needed
8. Shopping for needed items and picking up prescriptions
9. Providing a presence and companionship
10. Attending to spiritual and religious needs
11. Carrying out advance directives
12. Managing financial matters

proxy. Ideally, physicians should initiate discussions with patients about advance directives and proxies early, even while the patient is healthy. The patient should be reminded that these early formulations can be modified but that even having preliminary advance directives will ensure that treating physicians observe the patient's wishes in the event of an emergency.

CARING FOR THE FAMILY

Family members play an important role as caregivers to the terminally ill and have needs of their own that often go unrecognized. Their responsibilities can be overwhelming, especially if only one family member is available or if family members themselves are infirm or elderly. Table 56–6 lists some family caregiving tasks. Many of these tasks require long hours of work or supervision that can lead to physical and emotional fatigue. One study of caregivers reports that 25 to 30 percent lost their jobs and more than half moved to lower-paying jobs to accommodate the need for flexibility. The highest stress level was found in families who cared for a terminally ill patient at home, especially when death occurs in the home, and realize in retrospect that they would have preferred an environment in which death occurs in the presence of skilled caretakers.

Family therapy sessions allow family members to explore feelings about death and dying. They serve as a forum in which anticipatory grief and mourning can take place. The ability to share feelings can be cathartic, especially if guilt is involved. Family members often have to deal with feelings of guilt about past interactions with the dying patient. Family sessions also help to achieve consensus about the patient's advance directives. If family members disagree about the patient's wishes, the medical staff may be unable to act. In such cases, legal action may be needed to resolve family disputes about what course of action to pursue.

PALLIATIVE CARE

Palliative care is the most important part of end-of-life care. It refers to providing relief from the suffering caused by pain or other symptoms of terminal disease. While this is most commonly associated with analgesic drug administration, many other medical interventions and surgical procedures fall under the umbrella of palliative care because they can make the patient more comfortable. Monitors and their alarms, peripheral and central lines, phlebotomy, measurement of signs, and even supplemental oxygen are usually discontinued to allow the patient to die peacefully. Relocating the patient to a quiet, private room (as opposed to an intensive care unit) and allowing family members to be present is another very important palliative care modality.

The shift from active treatment to palliative care is sometimes the first tangible sign that the patient will die, a transition that is emotionally difficult for everyone concerned about the patient to accept. The discontinuation of machines and measurements, which up until this point have been an integral part of the hospital experience, can be extremely disconcerting to the patient, family members, and even other physicians. Indeed, if these parties are not active in planning this transition it can easily seem that persons have given up on the patient.

Because of this difficulty, palliative care is sometimes avoided altogether (i.e., curative treatment is continued until the patient dies). This approach is likely to cause problems if it is adopted merely to avoid the reality of impending death. A well-negotiated transition to palliative care often decreases anxiety after the patient and family go through an appropriate anticipatory grief reaction. Furthermore, a positive emotional outcome is much more likely if the physician and staff project a conviction that palliative care will be an active, involved process, without hint of withdrawal or abandonment. When this does not occur or when the family cannot tolerate the transition, the ensuing stress frequently results in a need for psychiatric consultation.

A 36-year-old physician with end-stage leukemia was seen in psychiatric consultation because he reported seeing the "angel of death" at the foot of his hospital bed. He described the experience as frightening and inexplicable. The consultant asked the patient, "Are you afraid that you are going to die?" That was the first time anyone had mentioned death or dying in any context to the patient. He welcomed the opportunity to talk openly about his fears to the medical staff and to his family and eventually died a peaceful death.

Psychiatric consultation is indicated for patients who become severely anxious, suicidal, depressed, or overtly psychotic. In each instance, appropriate psychiatric medication can be prescribed to provide relief. Patients who are suicidal do not always have to be transferred to a psychiatric service. An attendant or nurse can be assigned to the patient on a 24-hour basis (one-on-one coverage). In such instances, the relationship that develops between the observer and the patient may have therapeutic overtones, especially with patients whose depression is related to a sense of abandonment. Terminal patients who are at high risk for suicide are usually in pain. When pain is relieved, suicidal ideation is likely to diminish. A careful evaluation of suicide potential is required for all patients. A premorbid history of past suicide attempts is a high risk factor for suicide in terminally ill patients. In patients who become psychotic, impaired cognitive function secondary to metastatic lesions to the brain must always be considered. Such patients respond to antipsychotic medications, and psychotherapy may also be of use.

Table 56–7
Types of Pain

Nociceptive pain	
Somatic pain	Usually but not always constant, aching, gnawing, and well localized; e.g., bone metastases
Visceral pain	Usually but not always constant, deep, squeezing, poorly localized, with possible cutaneous referral; e.g., pleural effusion leading to (1) deep chest pain, (2) diaphragmatic irritation referred to shoulder
Neuropathic pain	Burning dysesthetic pain with shocklike paroxysms associated with direct damage to peripheral receptors, afferent fibers, or CNS, leading to loss of central inhibitory modulation and spontaneous firing; e.g., phantom limb pain; can involve sympathetic somatic afferents
Psychogenic pain	Variable characteristics, secondary to psychological factors in the absence of medical factors; vanishingly rare as a pure phenomenon in cancer patients but often an additional factor in the presence of organic pain

Courtesy of Marguerite S. Lederberg, M.D., and Jimmie C. Holland, M.D.

PAIN MANAGEMENT

Types of Pain

Dying patients are subject to several different kinds of pain, summarized in Table 56–7. The distinctions are important because they call for different treatment strategies; somatic and visceral pain are more responsive to opiates, while neuropathic and sympathetically maintained pain respond better to adjuvant medications. Most advanced cancer patients, for example, have more than one kind of pain and require complex treatment regimens. Tables 56–8 and 56–9 outline the neurophysiology of pain and pain-suppression pathways.

A highly mobile and independent man with a malignant illness developed brain metastases that resulted in paralysis of his legs. His motility became markedly impaired and he was confined to a wheelchair. Having always been in control of his life circumstances, he now perceived others as "controlling his life." Subsequently he began to accuse his wife of trying to kill him by giving him too much medicine and became highly suspicious of all persons in his household, feeling that they were plotting ways to harm him or force him into total submission. He developed outbursts of intense anger, which occurred without provocation. As his disease progressed, he became increasingly confused and disoriented and began to hear persons "talking about him" when no one was present. The patient was treated with small dosages of antipsychotic medications in order to control the psychotic symptoms. The family was encouraged to include him in planning activities of the household so as to increase his sense of control and participation. His wife received counseling to assist her in coping with the behavior. (From Barton D. Approaches to the clinical care of the dying person. In: Barton D, ed. *Dying and Death: A Clinical Guide for Caregivers*. Baltimore: Williams & Wilkins; 1977:87.)

Table 56–8
Neurophysiology of Nociceptive Pain

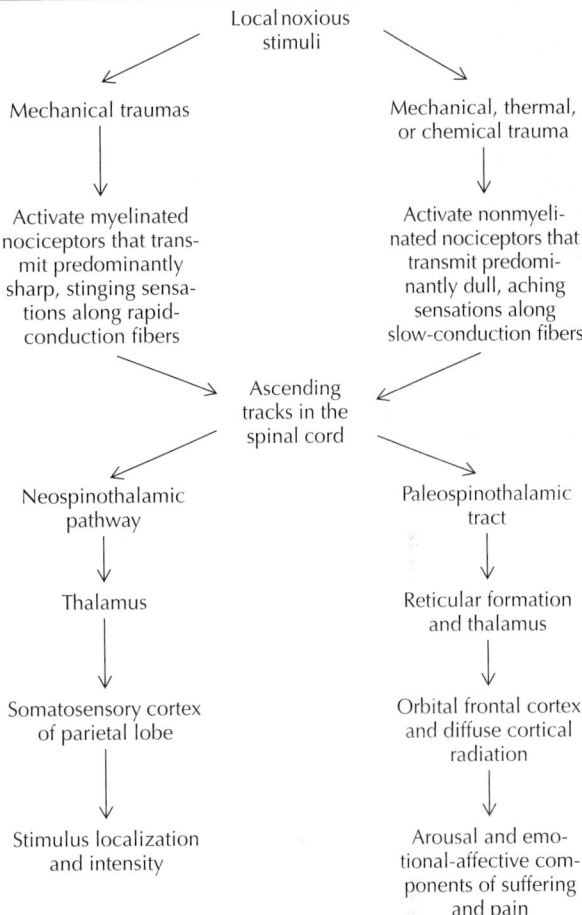

Local noxious stimuli

Mechanical traumas	Mechanical, thermal, or chemical trauma
↓	↓
Activate myelinated nociceptors that transmit predominantly sharp, stinging sensations along rapid-conduction fibers	Activate nonmyelinated nociceptors that transmit predominantly dull, aching sensations along slow-conduction fibers

→ Ascending tracks in the spinal cord ←

Neospinothalamic pathway	Paleospinothalamic tract
↓	↓
Thalamus	Reticular formation and thalamus
↓	↓
Somatosensory cortex of parietal lobe	Orbital frontal cortex and diffuse cortical radiation
↓	↓
Stimulus localization and intensity	Arousal and emotional-affective components of suffering and pain

Courtesy of Marguerite S. Lederberg, M.D., and Jimmie C. Holland, M.D.

Treatment of Pain

It cannot be overemphasized that pain management should be aggressive, and treatment should be multimodal. In fact, a good

Table 56–9
Endogenous Pain Suppression Pathways

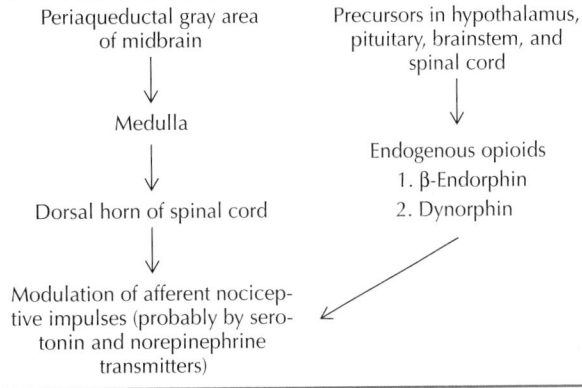

Periaqueductal gray area of midbrain	Precursors in hypothalamus, pituitary, brainstem, and spinal cord
↓	↓
Medulla	Endogenous opioids 1. β-Endorphin 2. Dynorphin
↓	↙
Dorsal horn of spinal cord	
↓	
Modulation of afferent nociceptive impulses (probably by serotonin and norepinephrine transmitters)	

Courtesy of Marguerite S. Lederberg, M.D., and Jimmie C. Holland, M.D.

Table 56–10
Opioid Analgesics for Management of Pain

Drug and Equianalgesic Dose Relative Potency	Dose (mg IM or oral)	Plasma Half-Life (hr)[a]	Starting Oral Dose[b] (mg)	Available Commercial Preparations
Morphine	10 IM 60 oral	3–4	30–60	Oral: tablet, liquid, slow-release tablet Rectal: 5–30 mg Injectable: sc, IM, IV, epidural, intrathecal
Hydromorphone	1.5 IM 7.5 oral	2–3	2–18	Oral: tablets: 1, 2, 4 mg Injectable: sc, IM, IV 2 mg/mL, 3 mg/mL, and 10 mg/mL
Methadone	10 IM 20 oral	12–24	5–10	Oral: tablets, liquid Injectable: sc, IM, IV
Levorphanol	2 IM 4 oral	12–16	2–4	Oral: tablets Injectable: sc, IM, IV
Oxymorphone	1	2–3	NA	Rectal: 10 mg Injectable: sc, IM, IV
Heroin	5 IM 60 oral	3–4	NA	NA
Meperidine	75 IM 300 oral	3–4 (normeperidine 12–16)	75	Oral: tablets Injectable: sc, IM, IV
Codeine	130 oral 200 oral	3–4	60	Oral: tablets and combination with acetylsalicylic acid, acetaminophen, liquid
Oxycodone[c]	15 oral 30 oral	—	5	Oral: tablets, liquid, oral formulation in combination with acetaminophen (tablet and liquid) and aspirin (tablet)

[a]The time of peak analgesia in nontolerant patients ranges from 1/2 hour to 1 hour, and the duration from 4 to 6 hours. The peak analgesic effect is delayed, and the duration is prolonged after oral administration.
[b]Recommended starting IM doses; the optimal dose for each patient is determined by titration, and the maximal dose is limited by adverse effects.
[c]A long-acting sustained-release form of oxycodone (Oxycontin) has been abused by drug addicts and its use has been criticized because of this; however, it is a very useful preparation available in 10-, 20-, 40-, and 160-mg doses that need to be taken once every 12 hours. It is used as a maintenance therapy for severe persistent pain.
Adapted from Foley K. Management of cancer pain. In: DeVita VT, Hellman S, Rosenberg SA, eds. *Cancer: Principles and Practice of Oncology.* 4th ed. Philadelphia: JB Lippincott; 1993:936.

pain regimen may require several drugs or the same drug used in different ways and administered via different routes. For example, intravenous morphine may be supplemented by self-administered oral "rescue" doses, or a continuous epidural drip may be supplemented by bolus intravenous doses. Transdermal patches may provide baseline concentrations in patients for whom intravenous or oral intake is difficult. Patient-controlled analgesia systems for intravenous opiate administration result in better pain relief with lower amounts dispensed than in staff-administered dosing.

Opioids commonly cause delirium and hallucinations. A frequent mechanism of psychotoxicity is the accumulation of drugs or metabolites whose duration of analgesia is shorter than their plasma half-life (morphine, levorphanol [Levo-Dromoran], and methadone [Dolophine]). Use of drugs like hydromorphone (Dilaudid), which have half-lives closer to their analgesic duration, can relieve the problem without loss of pain control. Cross-tolerance is incomplete between opiates; hence, several should be tried in any patient with the dosage lowered when switching drugs. Table 56–10 lists opioid analgesics.

The benefits of maintenance analgesia administration in terminally ill patients compared with as-needed administration cannot be overemphasized. Maintenance dosing improves pain control, increases drug efficiency, and relieves patient anxiety, whereas as-needed orders allow pain to increase while waiting for the drug to be given. Moreover, as-needed analgesia administration perversely sets up the patient for staff complaints about drug-seeking behavior. Even when maintenance treatment is used, extra doses of medication should be available for breakthrough pain, and repeated use of these medications should signal the need to raise the maintenance dose. Depending on their previous experiences with opioid analgesics and their weight, it is not unusual for some patients to require 2 g or more of morphine per day for relief of symptoms.

Knowing doses of different drugs and different routes of administration is important to avoid accidental undermedication. For example, when changing a patient from intramuscular to oral morphine use, one must multiply the intramuscular dose by 6 to avoid causing the patient pain and provoking drug-seeking behavior. Many adjuvant drugs used for pain are psychotropics with which psychiatrists are familiar, but in some cases, their analgesic effect is separate from their primary psychotropic effect. Commonly used adjuvants include antidepressants, phenothiazines, butyrophenones, antihistamines, amphetamines, and steroids (Table 56–11). They are particularly important in neuropathic and sympathetically maintained pain, for which they can be the mainstay of treatment.

Other developments in pain management include more intrusive procedures such as nerve blocks or the use of continuous epidural infusions. Additionally, radiation therapy, chemotherapy, and even surgical resection should always be considered as pain management modalities in palliative care. Short courses of radiotherapy or chemotherapy can be used to shrink tumors or manage metastatic lesions that cause pain or impairment. In patients with end-stage Hodgkin's disease, for example, systemic chemotherapy can improve the patient's quality of life by

Table 56–11
Nonopioid and Adjuvant Analgesic Drugs in the Management of Pain

Class or Drug	Indications	Starting Oral Dose (mg range, 24 hr)	Comments
Nonsteroidal antiinflammatory drugs			
Aspirin	Soft tissue and metastatic bone	650 650–1,000	Used in combination with opioids, GI and hematological effects; avoid combination with steroids
Acetaminophen	Like aspirin	650 650–1,000	Fewer GI effects, no effects on platelet function, no significant antiinflammatory effects
Ibuprofen		400 200–800	Higher analgesic potential than aspirin, fewer GI and hematological effects than aspirin
Choline magnesium trisalicylate	Like aspirin	1,500	Antiinflammatory and analgesic effects; similar to aspirin without hematological effects
Fenoprofen	Like aspirin	200 200–100	Higher analgesic potential than aspirin, fewer GI and hematological effects than aspirin
Diflunisal	Like aspirin	500 500–1,000	Longer duration of action than ibuprofen, higher analgesic potential than aspirin
Naproxen	Like aspirin	250 250–500	Longer duration of action than ibuprofen, higher analgesic potential than aspirin
Anticonvulsants			
Phenytoin	Neuropathic pain, acute lancinating type (tic)	100 200–800	Useful in paroxysmal nerve pain
Antidepressants			
Amitriptyline	Neuropathic pain; e.g., postherpetic neuralgia	10 10–150	Start at low dose and titrate slowly; has analgesic properties
Imipramine		50–100	
Antihistamines			
Hydroxyzine	Somatic and visceral pain	25 25–100	Additive analgesia in combination with opioids, antiemetic, antianxiety properties
Phenothiazines			
Methotrimeprazine	Somatic and visceral pain; useful in opioid-tolerant patients with GI obstruction and pain	5–16 IM	Has anxiolytic and antiemetic effects, available only in IM preparation
Steroids			
Prednisone	Somatic and neuropathic pain; e.g., inflammatory bone pain	5 5–60	Antiinflammatory, antiemetic, analgesic effects
Dexamethasone	Reflex sympathetic dystrophy; brachial, lumbar plexopathy	0.5–16	
Neurostimulants			
Dextroamphetamine	Somatic and visceral pain; e.g., postoperative pain	2.5 2.5–10	Additive analgesia in combination with opioids; reduces sedative effects
Methylphenidate	Opioid-induced sedation	5 5–15	Additive analgesia in combination with opioids; reduces sedative effects
Caffeine		300 300–600	Additive analgesia in combination with opioids; reduces sedative effects

Adapted from Foley K. Management of cancer pain. In: DeVita VT, Hellman S, Rosenberg SA, eds. *Cancer: Principles and Practice of Oncology.* 4th ed. Philadelphia: JB Lippincott; 1993.

decreasing tumor burden. Surgical resection of invasive tumors, most notably breast carcinomas, can be useful for the same reason.

PALLIATION OF OTHER SYMPTOMS

Symptom management is a high priority in palliative care. Patients are often more concerned about the day-to-day distress of their symptoms than they are about their impending death, which may not be as real to them. Table 56–12 lists common end-of-life symptoms. A comprehensive approach to palliation involves attending to these end-of-life symptoms as well as pain. Sources of distress include psychiatric symptoms such as anxiety and physical symptoms. Foremost among physical symptoms are those involving the gastrointestinal system,

Table 56–12
Common End-of-Life Symptoms/Signs

Symptom/Sign	Comments
Delusions	Occur in 90% of all terminal patients; can be reversed if cause is treatable, e.g., pain, medication; respond to antipsychotic medication
Fatigue or weakness	Most common occurrence in terminal illness; psychostimulants can be used for short-term relief
Dysphagia	Common in neurological disease end states, e.g., multiple sclerosis, amyotrophic lateral sclerosis
Incontinence	May follow pelvic radiation, which can produce fistulas; use indwelling or condom catheter
Dyspnea or cough	Produces severe anxiety with fear of suffocation; occurs in 80% of terminal lung cancer patients; opioids, bronchodilators of use
Nausea or vomiting	Adverse effect of radiation and chemotherapy; antiemetics, e.g., metoclopramide, prochlorperazine, of use; marijuana cigarettes of use in selected patients
Anorexia	All terminal disease states are associated with cachexia secondary to anorexia and dehydration; feeding tubes do not prevent aspiration
Loss of skin integrity	Decubiti most common on weight-bearing areas, e.g., hips, sacrum, outer ankle; important to turn body frequently; elbow and hip pads of use
Anxiety or depression	Psychological factors, e.g., fear of death, abandonment; physiological factors, e.g., pain, hypoxia; antianxiety and antidepressant medication of use; opioids have strong antianxiety effects

From Mitka M. Suggestions for help when the end is near. *JAMA* 2000; 284:2441; adapted from National Coalition on Health Care (NCHC) and the Institute for Health Care Improvement (IHI). *Promises to Keep: Changing the Way We Provide Care at the End of Life*, release, October 12, 2000. With permission.

including diarrhea, constipation, anorexia, nausea, vomiting, and bowel obstruction. Other important symptoms include insomnia, confusion, mouth sores, dyspnea, cough, pruritus, decubitus ulcers, and urinary frequency or incontinence. Caretakers should follow these symptoms closely and establish appropriate early and aggressive care for these symptoms before they become burdensome.

An effective treatment for nausea and vomiting associated with chemotherapy is the use of Δ-tetrahydrocannabinol (THC), the active ingredient of marijuana. Oral synthetic cannabinoid, dronabinol (Marinol) is used in 1- to 2-mg doses every 8 hours. The use of marijuana cigarettes to deliver THC is believed to be more effective than pills. Proponents say that its absorption is faster and antiemetic properties are more potent via the pulmonary system. Repeated attempts to legalize marijuana cigarettes for medical use have met with only limited success in this country.

A 47-year-old man with incurable lung cancer who had been treated unsuccessfully with chemotherapy and radiotherapy had been suffering from intractable dyspnea for 1 week. His family, nursing, and other staff were increasingly upset by his difficulty breathing and his pleas for relief. The attending physician refused to prescribe anything stronger than codeine. The palliative care team at the hospital intervened at the family's request. Relief was obtained with the use of 5 to 10 mg of intravenous bolus of morphine every 15 minutes. When the patient became comfortable, a continuous drip of intravenous morphine was instituted, complemented by subcutaneous morphine as needed.

The American Medical Association supports the position that terminal patients require substantial doses of opioids on a regular basis and should not be denied drugs for fear of producing physical dependence. A similar view is endorsed in *Goodman and Gilman's the Pharmacological Basis of Therapeutics* as follows:

> The physician should not wait until the pain becomes agonizing; no patient should ever wish for death because of a physician's reluctance to use adequate amounts of effective opioids. Accordingly, physicians who treat the terminally ill should not be intimidated by legal oversight.

DYING AT HOME

Depending on the patient's wishes and the nature of his or her disease, the choice to die at home is one that should be explored. While it is more burdensome on a family than dying in a hospital or hospice, death at home can be a welcome alternative for the patient and family seeking to spend quality time together. A home care team can assess a home for its suitability and suggest ways to facilitate activities of daily living, including modifications to furniture, hospital bed leasing, and installation of assistive devices such as handrails and commodes. The family's care can be supplemented with house calls by physicians, nurses, therapists, and chaplains. In any case, the family must know what their responsibilities are and must be well prepared to take care of the patient.

HOSPICE CARE

In 1967 the founding of St. Christopher's Hospice in England by Cicely Saunders launched the modern hospice movement. Several factors in the 1960s propelled the development of hospices, including concerns about inadequately trained physicians, inept terminal care, gross inequities in health care, and neglect of the elderly. Life expectancy had increased, and heart disease and cancer were becoming more common. Saunders emphasized an interdisciplinary approach to symptom control, care of the patient and family as a unit, the use of volunteers, continuity of care including home care, and follow-up with family members after a patient's death. The first hospice in the United States, Connecticut Hospice, opened in 1974. By 2000, there were over 3,000 hospices in the United States. Round-the-clock pain control with opioids is an essential component of hospice management. In 1983 Medicare began reimbursing hospice care. Medicare hospice guidelines emphasize home care, with benefits provided for a broad spectrum of physician, nursing, psychosocial, and spiritual services at home or, if necessary, in a hospital or nursing home. To be eligible, the patient

must be physician certified as having 6 months or less to live. By electing hospice care, patients agree to receive palliative rather than curative treatment. Many hospice programs are hospital-based, sometimes in separate units and sometimes in the form of hospice beds interspersed throughout the facility. Other program models include free-standing hospices and programs, hospital-affiliated hospices, nursing home hospice care, and home care programs. Nursing homes are the site of death for many elderly patients with incurable chronic illness, yet dying nursing home residents have limited access to palliative and hospice care. For example, in 1997, 3 percent of hospice enrollees were in nursing homes, while 87 percent were in private homes. Families generally express satisfaction with their personal involvement in hospice care. Savings with hospice care vary, but home care programs generally cost less than conventional institutional care, particularly in the final months of life. Hospice patients are less likely to receive diagnostic studies or such intensive therapy as surgery or chemotherapy. Hospice care is a proved, viable alternative for patients who elect a palliative approach to terminal care. In addition, hospice goals of dignified, comfortable death for the terminally ill and care for patient and family together have been increasingly adopted into mainstream medicine.

NEONATAL AND INFANT END-OF-LIFE CARE

Advances in reproductive medicine have increased the number of infants born prematurely as well as the number of multiple births. These advances have increased the need for life-sustaining methods of care and made decisions about when to use palliative care more complex. Some bioethicists believe that withholding life-sustaining interventions is appropriate under certain circumstances; others maintain that life-sustaining methods should not be used at all. An extensive study of attitudes among neonatologists about end-of-life decisions found no consensus about if and when to terminate life.

Most decisions to forego life-sustaining procedures for newborns concern those whose death is imminent. Even if their future quality of life is determined to be bleak, most physicians feel that some life is better than no life at all. Those physicians who support withholding intensive care consider the following quality-of-life issues: (1) extent of bodily damage (e.g., severe neurological impairment), (2) the burden that a disabled child will place on the family, and (3) the ability of the child to derive some pleasure from existence (e.g., having an awareness of being alive and being able to form relationships).

The American Academy of Pediatrics permits nontreatment decisions for newborns when the infant is irreversibly comatose or when treatment would be futile and only prolong the process of dying. These standards do not permit the parents to have any input into the decision-making process. In a well-publicized case in England in 2000, it was decided to surgically separate conjoined twins knowing that one would die as a result of the procedure and despite the objections of the parents, who believed that nature should take its course even if that led to the death of both infants. Neonatal end-of-life decisions remain in a state of limbo. There are no clear-cut criteria about which patients should receive intensive care and which should receive palliative care.

CHILD END-OF-LIFE CARE

After accidents, cancer is the second most common cause of death in children. While many childhood cancers are treatable, palliative care is necessary for children with cancers that are not. Children require more support than adults in coping with death. On average, a child does not view death as permanent until the age of about 10; prior to that, death is viewed as a sleep or separation. Therefore, children should be told only what they can understand; if they are capable, they should be involved in the decision-making process about treatment plans. Assurances that patients are pain-free and physically comfortable are just as important for children as they are for adults.

A unique aspect of end-of-life care in children involves addressing their fear of being separated from their parents. It is helpful to have parents participate in end-of-life care tasks within their capacities. Family sessions with the child in attendance allow feelings to emerge and questions to be answered.

SPIRITUAL ISSUES

The inclusion of a section on religious or spiritual problems in the text revision of the fourth edition of *Diagnostic and Statistical Manual of Mental Disorders* (DSM-IV-TR) is but one sign of increasing awareness of the importance of this area to patients, families, and many staff members as well. Several studies have shown that religious beliefs are often associated with mature and active coping methods, and the field of psychological and spiritual interfaces in terminally ill patients is spawning a whole new area of psychological research within the traditional medical establishment. The psychiatric consultant should inquire about faith, its meaning, associated religious practices, and impact on the coping response. It can be a source of strength or guilt at all stages of the disease, ranging from the earliest "What did I do to cause this?" through "Will God give me only what I can carry?" to the poignant life review of the late stage. It is often a primary factor in the reactions to suicidality and in attitudes toward terminal care decisions. Mental health professionals should deal with these areas in an unself-conscious and noncondescending manner and work to help patients fully integrate this aspect of their personality into their current crisis. The professional should also work in harmony with the patient's spiritual guide, if one is available. Sometimes an experienced, effective chaplain working with the appropriate patient can achieve positive results more directly than any psychotherapy. The following case exemplifies how creative pastoral care can relieve suffering.

A young woman was admitted to a hospice in a terminal state. She was experiencing a severe depression, which she attributed to not being able to see her oldest daughter receive her first communion. Arrangements were made for a ceremonial communion for her daughter to take place at the hospice. After the ceremony, the patient's mood improved markedly as one of her fears was alleviated and a religious need was satisfied. As her mood improved, she was able to address other unresolved issues and have quality visits with her children in her remaining days. (From O'Neil MT. Pastoral care. In: Cimino JE, Brescia MJ, eds. *Calvary Hospital Model for Palliative Care in Advanced Cancer.* Bronx: Palliative Care Institute; 1998, with permission.)

ALTERNATIVE AND COMPLEMENTARY MEDICINE

Many patients, once they are told they are terminally ill, seek alternative treatments, ranging from innocuous programs aimed at enhancing general health to more aggressive, harmful, or fraudulent regimens. Although most patients combine the alternative and the traditional, a substantial number favor complementary medicine as the only treatment for their disease.

Complementary methods to cure terminal illness, especially cancer, emphasize a holistic approach, involving purification of the body, detoxification through internal cleansing, and attention to nutritional and emotional well-being. Despite their widespread appeal, none of these methods has been demonstrated to cure cancer or prolong life, yet all have strong followings bolstered by anecdotal accounts of their efficacy. The popular *metabolic therapy* attributes cancer and other potentially fatal illnesses to toxins and waste materials accumulating in the body; treatment is based on reversing this process by diet, vitamins, minerals, enzymes, and colonic irrigations. Another approach includes macrobiotic diets or megavitamins to enhance the body's capacity to destroy malignancy. In 1987 the National Research Council recommended minimizing carcinogenic substances and fat in the diet and increasing whole-grain, fruit, and vegetable consumption as preventive guidelines. *Psychological approaches* cite maladaptive personality and coping styles as contributors to fatal diseases; treatment consists of shaping a positive attitude. *Spiritual approaches* aim at achieving harmony between the patient and nature. Some groups use spirituality as a way to ward off illness, which is sometimes seen as an external evil to be exorcised. *Immunotherapies* have gained popularity in recent years; cancer is attributed to a defective immune system, and restoration of immunocompetency is seen as the cure.

Society's present emphasis on health consciousness, mind-body relationships, and individual responsibility is reflected in the current popularity of alternative treatments. Staff working with terminally ill patients, especially those with cancer, must be informed of these approaches and be prepared to discuss them with patients. They must assess the patient's wish for these therapies, especially because such a wish often reflects emotional needs unmet by conventional treatment. A most important consideration is that many patients find increased strength to endure the suffering of terminal illness with the help of alternative medicine, even though the course of the disease may not be affected. (For a further discussion of alternative medicine, see Chapter 29.)

EUTHANASIA AND PHYSICIAN-ASSISTED SUICIDE

In the Hippocratic oath, physicians swear not to prescribe a deadly drug or to give a patient advice that may cause death. As a result, physicians must walk a fine line between their responsibility to relieve pain and suffering and their obligation to preserve life. With developments in technology and life-support systems and the increase in longevity, various groups are trying to develop a comprehensive policy regarding euthanasia that is acceptable to patients, physicians, lawyers, and theologians. Euthanasia and physician-assisted suicide have become sources of continuing controversy and are likely to be so for the foreseeable future.

Euthanasia

Euthanasia is defined as a physician's deliberate act to cause a patient's death by directly administering a lethal dose of medication or other agent. Because such patients are thought of as hopelessly ill or injured, euthanasia has been called "mercy killing." On the basis of the doctor's action and the patient's condition, several types of euthanasia have been described: *active euthanasia*, in which a physician deliberately intends to kill a patient to alleviate or prevent uncontrollable suffering; *passive euthanasia*, in which a physician withholds artificial life-sustaining measures; *voluntary euthanasia*, in which the person who is to die is competent to give consent and does so; and *involuntary euthanasia*, in which the person who is to die is incompetent or incapable of giving consent. Euthanasia assumes that the intent of the physician is to aid and abet the patient's wish to die.

Physician-Assisted Suicide

Suicide is a deliberate taking of one's own life. *Assisted suicide* is the imparting of information or means to enable such an act to take place. When the assistance is provided by a physician, the suicide is *physician assisted*. Assisted suicide and euthanasia should not be confused with palliative care designed to alleviate the suffering of dying patients. Palliative care includes giving pain relief and emotional, social, and spiritual support, as well as psychiatric care if indicated. The intent of palliative care is to relieve pain and suffering, not to end a patient's life, even though death may result from palliative care.

The issue of physician-assisted suicide came to national attention in 1990 when Jack Kevorkian, a physician in Michigan, connected Janet Adkins, a victim of dementia of the Alzheimer's type, to a so-called suicide machine that enabled her to give herself an infusion of potassium chloride (KCl) that ended her life. After that, Kevorkian helped over 100 persons take their own lives. In Michigan, where Kevorkian practiced, he was indicted for manslaughter and, in 1999, was sentenced to prison.

At one time, suicide was considered a type of murder, although no one was or is prosecuted for the crime. Assisted suicide, however, is a crime, and in some states (e.g., California) can be prosecuted as murder. Over 40 states in the United States, however, currently consider aiding and abetting suicide a crime without defining it as murder. In 1996, in both New York and California, state courts upheld the right to bring about one's own death through assisted suicide. In a 1994 landmark decision the people of Oregon approved a referendum permitting physicians to prescribe lethal medication for terminally ill patients (the Oregon Death with Dignity Act).

In a survey of physicians in Oregon (the only U.S. state where assisted suicide is legal), 5 percent of 2,649 physicians reported that they had received one or more requests for lethal prescriptions between late 1997 and early 1999. Most patients in question had cancer and a life expectancy of less than 6 months. In 30 percent of the cases, interventions such as pain control and hospice referral changed the patient's mind about assisted suicide. Of 165 patients for whom respondents reported the outcome of a request, 29 received prescriptions, and 17 died after taking the medication. Finally, Oregon physicians are required to notify the Oregon Health Division when they have pre-

scribed lethal medication. The division was notified of 33 such cases in 1999; 27 patients died after taking the medication, up from 16 in 1998. The data indicate that assisted suicide is not increasing dramatically in Oregon. In June 1997 the U.S. Supreme Court ruled that there is no constitutional right to assisted suicide; however, they did not overturn the Oregon law.

In the United States, physician-assisted suicide and euthanasia have been consistently opposed by the American Psychiatric Association, the American Medical Association, the American Nurses Association, the National Legal Center for the Disabled, and the Roman Catholic Church. The World Medical Association issued the following declaration on euthanasia in October 1987:

> Euthanasia, that is the act of deliberately ending the life of a patient, even at his own request or at the request of his close relatives, is unethical. This does not prevent the physician from respecting the will of a patient to allow the natural process of death to follow its course in the terminal phase of sickness.

The New York State Committee of Bioethical Issues is also opposed to euthanasia but has stated that physicians have an obligation to provide effective treatment to relieve pain and suffering, even though the treatment may on occasion hasten death. The committee stated the following:

> The principle of patient autonomy requires that physicians respect the decision of a patient who possesses decision-making capacity to forgo life-sustaining treatment. Life-sustaining treatment is defined as any medical treatment that serves to prolong life without reversing the underlying medical condition. Life-sustaining treatment includes, but is not limited to, mechanical ventilation, renal dialysis, blood transfusions, chemotherapy, antibiotics, and artificial nutrition and hydration.

Physicians are obligated to relieve pain and suffering and to promote the dignity and autonomy of dying patients in their care. This obligation includes providing effective palliative treatment even though such treatment may occasionally hasten death. But physicians should not perform euthanasia or participate in assisted suicide. Support, comfort, respect for patient autonomy, good communication, and adequate pain control may dramatically decrease the demand for euthanasia and assisted suicide. In certain carefully defined circumstances, it is humane to recognize that death is certain and suffering is great.

In the Netherlands, physicians are allowed to participate in active euthanasia provided certain conditions are met. The patient must make repeated requests that are well informed and enduring. The patient's mental or physical condition must be considered incurable. All other options for care must have been exhausted. The assisting physician must have the agreement of another physician. About 3 percent of all deaths in Holland result from euthanasia.

In the United States, a group called the Hemlock Society actively promotes the practice of euthanasia. Its founder, Derek Humphry, in his book *Final Exit*, gave explicit directions on suicide techniques. The book has been a bestseller in this country and abroad and attests to the interest and controversy surrounding the issue. Similar right-to-die societies include Choice in Dying and Americans for Death with Dignity.

The American Association of Suicidology in its 1996 *Report of the Committee on Physician-Assisted Suicide and Euthanasia* concluded that involuntary euthanasia can never be condoned; the report also stated, however, that "intolerable, prolonged suffering of persons in extremis should never be insisted upon, against their wishes, in single-minded efforts to preserve life at all cost." This position acknowledges that patients may die as a result of treatment given to them for the explicit purpose of relieving suffering; but death associated with palliative care differs greatly from physician-assisted suicide in that death is not the goal of treatment and is not intentional.

Requests for Suicide

To help guide clinicians facing requests for physician-assisted suicide, the AMA's Institute for Ethics has proposed the following 8-step clinical protocol:

1. Evaluation of the patient for depression or other psychiatric conditions that could cause disordered thought
2. Evaluation of the patient's "decision-making competence"
3. Discussion with the patient about his or her goals for care
4. Evaluation and response to the patient's "physical, mental, social, and spiritual suffering"
5. Discussion with the patient about the full range of treatment and care options
6. Consultation by the attending physician with other professional colleagues
7. Assurance that care plans chosen by the patient are being followed, including removal of unwanted treatment and the provision of adequate pain and symptom relief
8. Discussion with the patient explaining why physician-assisted suicide is to be avoided and why it is not compatible with the principled nature of the care protocol

Most psychiatrists view suicide as an irrational act that is the product of mental illness, usually depression. In almost every case in which a patient asks to be put to death, there is depression associated with an incurable medical condition that causes the patient intolerable pain. In these instances, every effort should be made to alleviate both conditions: antidepressants or psychostimulants for depression and opioids for pain. Psychotherapy, spiritual counseling, or both may be needed. In addition, family therapy to help with the stress of dealing with a dying patient may be necessary. It is also useful because some patients may ask to be put to death because they do not wish to be a burden to their families; others may feel coerced by their families into believing that they are or will be a burden and may choose death as a result. Currently, no professional codes countenance euthanasia or assisted suicide in the United States. Therefore, psychiatrists must stand on the side of responsible rescue and treatment.

A distinction also is needed between major depression and suffering. The nature of suffering has not been sufficiently studied by psychiatrists. It remains the province of theologians and philosophers. Suffering is a complex mix of spiritual, emotional, and physical factors that transcends pain and other symptoms of terminal illness. Physicians are more skilled at dealing with depression than with suffering. Anatole Broyard,

who chronicled his own death in his book *Intoxicated by My Illness,* wrote the following:

> I see no reason or need for my doctor to love me nor would I expect him to suffer with me. I wouldn't demand a lot of my doctor's time; I just wish he would brood on my situation for perhaps five minutes, that he would give me his whole mind just once, be bonded with me for a brief space, survey my soul as well as my flesh, to get at my illness, for each man is ill in his own way.

FUTURE DIRECTIONS

Advances in technology bring more complex medical, legal, moral, and ethical controversies regarding life, death, euthanasia, and physician-assisted suicide. Some forms of euthanasia have found a place in modern medicine, and expansion of the boundaries of patients' rights and their ability to choose the way they live and die are inevitable. Both patients and physicians need to be better educated about depression, pain management, palliative care, and quality of life. Medical schools and residency training programs need to give the topics of death, dying, and palliative care the attention they deserve. Society must ensure that economics, ageism, and racism do not get in the way of adequate and humane management of patients with a chronic terminal illness. Finally, national health care policy must provide adequate insurance coverage, home care, and hospice services to all appropriate patients. If these mandates are followed, the argument for physician assistance in dying will lose much of its impact.

References

Ganzini L. Physicians' experiences with the Oregon Death with Dignity Act. *N Engl J Med.* 2000;342:557.

Ganzini L, Fenn DS, Lee MA, Heintz RT, Bloom JD. Attitudes of Oregon psychiatrists towards physician-assisted suicide. *Am J Psychiatry.* 1996;153:11.

Gronenewoud JH. Clinical problems with the performance of euthanasia and physician-assisted suicide in the Netherlands. *N Engl J Med.* 2000;342:551.

Hendin H. *Seduced by Death: Doctors, Patients, and the Dutch Cure.* New York: WW Norton; 1997.

Hendin H, Klerman G. Physician-assisted suicide: the dangers of legalization. *Am J Psychiatry.* 1993;150:143.

Humphry D. *Final Exit: The Practicalities of Self-Deliverance and Assisted Suicide for the Dying.* Eugene, OR: Hemlock Society; 1991.

Jeret JS. Discussing dying: changing attitudes among patients, physicians, and medical students. *Pharos.* 1996;52:15.

Kastenbaum RJ. *Death, Society and Human Experience.* 2nd ed. New York: Macmillan; 1991.

Lazar TS. Physician-assisted suicide and the state of the law in California. *Action Rep Med Board Calif.* 1996;59:5.

Lee MA, Nelson HD, Tilden VP, Ganzini L, Schmidt TA, Tolle SW. Legalizing assisted suicide—views of physicians in Oregon. *N Engl J Med.* 1994; 334:310.

Lo B, Ruston D, Kates LW, et al. Discussing religious and spiritual issues at the end of life. A practical guide for physicians. *JAMA.* 2002;287:7490.

McCorkle R, Pasacreta JV. Enhancing caregiver outcomes in palliative care. *Cancer Control.* 2001;8:36.

Quill TE, Cassel CK, Meier DE. Care of the hopelessly ill: proposed clinical criteria for physician-assisted suicide. *N Engl J Med.* 1992;327:1380.

Rabow MW, Hardie GE, Fair JM, McPhee SJ. End-of-life-care content in 50 textbooks from multiple specialties. *JAMA.* 2000;283:771.

Robert G, Owens J. The near-death experience. *Br J Psychiatry.* 1988;153:607.

Rosner F, Rogatz P. Physicians-assisted suicide: Committee of Bioethical Issues of the Medical Society of the State of New York. *N Y State J Med* 1992;92:388.

Snyder L, Caplan AL, eds. *Assisted Suicide.* Bloomington, IN: Indiana University Press; 2002.

Yates P, Stetz KM. Families' awareness of and response to dying. *Oncol Nurs Forum.* 1999;26:113.

Zisook S, Downs NS. Death, dying, and bereavement. In: Sadock BJ, Sadock, VA, eds. *Kaplan & Sadock's Comprehensive Textbook of Psychiatry.* 7th ed. Vol 2. Baltimore: Lippincott Williams & Wilkins; 2000:1963

57 Forensic Psychiatry

Forensic psychiatry is the branch of medicine that deals with disorders of the mind and their relation to legal principles. The word *forensic* means belonging to the courts of law. At various stages in their historical development, psychiatry and the law have converged. Today, the two disciplines often intersect, especially when dealing with the criminal who, by violating the rules of society secondary to mental disorder, adversely affects the functioning of the community. Traditionally, the psychiatrist's efforts help explain the causes and, through prevention and treatment, reduce the self-destructive elements of harmful behavior. The lawyer, as the agent of society, is concerned that the social deviant is a potential threat to the safety and security of other persons. Both psychiatry and the law seek to implement their respective goals through the application of pragmatic techniques based on empirical observations.

Thomas Gutheil, an influential forensic psychiatrist, points out that the interface between psychiatry and the law contains much complexity and potential for gross misunderstanding, as illustrated in the following example.

During a routine outpatient psychotherapy appointment, a male middle-level manager began to complain to his therapist about his boss. Feeling the freedom of expression that the therapeutic situation is intended to foster, the man worked himself up to a higher pitch than usual, and in the emotional intensity of the moment, he stated that he would like to kill his boss. He then calmed down, somewhat relieved by having let off steam, went on to discuss other subjects, and departed at the end of the session.

The therapist did not believe that the patient was anywhere near the point of seriously acting on the feelings that were expressed. However, the therapist had heard of a case in which a therapist got into trouble for not warning third parties, so he decided to take action.

On a sheet with his letterhead, he typed a warning to the employer that his patient, John Jones, had expressed the desire to kill him. He sent the letter by first-class mail—not express or registered—and he addressed it not to the employer but to the personnel department of the company.

The resulting uproar, although perhaps predictable, surprised the therapist. During the subsequent liability suit for breach of confidentiality, he was heard to sputter, "But I was only doing what the law requires of me!"

In this case the therapist was not required to inform because he did not believe that his patient was going to act on his impulses; if he did believe so, his letter should have been addressed to the potential victim (return receipt requested) and not to the personnel department.

MEDICAL MALPRACTICE

Medical malpractice is a tort, or civil wrong. It is a noncriminal, noncontract wrong resulting from a physician's negligence. Simply put, negligence means doing something that a physician with a duty to care for the patient should not have done or failing to do something that should have been done as defined by current medical practice. Usually, the standard of care in malpractice cases is established by expert witnesses. The standard of care is also determined by reference to journal articles, professional textbooks and treatises, professional practice guidelines, and ethical practices promulgated by professional organizations.

To prove malpractice, the plaintiff (e.g., patient, family, or estate) must establish by a preponderance of the evidence that (1) a doctor–patient relationship existed that created a *duty* of care, (2) there was a *deviation* from the standard of care, (3) the patient was *damaged,* and (4) the deviation *directly* caused the damage.

These elements of a malpractice claim are sometimes referred to as the 4 Ds (duty, deviation, damage, direct causation). Proof by a preponderance of the evidence as required in a malpractice suit means simply more likely than not. Although the law does not assign a percentage, a preponderance of the evidence is akin to 51 to 49 percent, or just enough evidence to tip the scale one way or the other.

Each of the four elements of a malpractice claim must be present or there can be no finding of liability. For example, a psychiatrist whose negligence is the direct cause of harm to an individual (physical, psychological, or both) is not liable for malpractice if no doctor–patient relationship existed to create a duty of care. Psychiatrists are not likely to be sued successfully if they give negligent advice on a radio program that is harmful to a caller, particularly if a caveat was given to the caller that no doctor–patient relationship was being created. No malpractice claim will be sustained against a psychiatrist if a patient's worsening condition is unrelated to negligent care. Finally, if a psychiatrist treats a patient who is then harmed, no malpractice exists if the psychiatrist did not deviate from the standard of care.

Not every bad outcome is the result of negligence. Psychiatrists cannot guarantee correct diagnoses and treatments. When the psychia-

trist provides due care, mistakes may be made without necessarily incurring liability. Most psychiatric cases are complicated. Psychiatrists make judgment calls when selecting a particular treatment course among the many options that may exist. In hindsight, the decision may prove wrong but not be a deviation in the standard of care.

In addition to negligence suits, psychiatrists can be sued for the intentional torts of assault, battery, false imprisonment, defamation, fraud or misrepresentation, invasion of privacy, and intentional infliction of emotional distress. In an intentional tort, wrongdoers are motivated by the intent to harm another person or realize or should have realized that such harm is likely to result from their actions. For example, telling a patient that sex with the therapist is therapeutic perpetrates a fraud. Most malpractice policies do not provide coverage for intentional torts. Other legal theories of liability include breach of contract and civil rights violations of the U.S. Constitution, state constitutions, or federal civil right statutes.

Table 57–1
Informed Consent: Reasonable Information to Be Disclosed

Although there exists no consistently accepted standard for information disclosure for any given medical or psychiatric situation, as a rule of thumb, five areas of information are generally provided:

1. Diagnosis—description of the condition or problem
2. Treatment—nature and purpose of proposed treatment
3. Consequences—risks and benefits of the proposed treatment
4. Alternatives—viable alternatives to the proposed treatment including risks and benefits
5. Prognosis—projected outcome with and without treatment

Reprinted with permission from Simon RI. *Clinical Psychiatry and the Law.* 2nd ed. Washington, DC: American Psychiatric Press; 1992.

MANAGED CARE

National Practitioner Data Bank

On September 1, 1990, the Health Care Quality Improvement Act of 1986 established the National Practitioner Data Bank. The data bank tracks disciplinary actions, malpractice judgments, and settlements against physicians, dentists, and other health care professionals.

Hospitals, health maintenance organizations, professional societies, state medical boards, and other health care organizations are required to report any disciplinary action taken against providers that lasts more than 30 days. Disciplinary actions include limitation, suspension, or revocation of privileges or professional society membership. Under the Health Care Quality Improvement Act, health care entities and providers are granted immunity from liability when making good-faith peer review reports. This information about physicians is available online.

Negligent Prescription Practices

Negligent prescription practices usually include exceeding recommended dosages and then failing to adjust the medication level to therapeutic levels, unreasonable mixing of drugs, prescribing medication that is not indicated, prescribing too many drugs at one time, and failing to disclose medication effects. Elderly patients frequently take a variety of drugs prescribed by different physicians. Multiple psychotropic medications must be prescribed with special care because of possible harmful interactions and adverse effects.

Psychiatrists who prescribe medications must explain the diagnosis, risks, and benefits of the drug within reason and as circumstances permit (Table 57–1). Obtaining competent informed consent may be problematic if a psychiatric patient has diminished cognitive capacity because of mental illness or chronic brain impairment; a substitute health care decision maker may need to provide consent.

Informed consent should be obtained each time a medication is changed and a new drug is introduced. If patients are injured because they were not properly informed of the risks and consequences of taking a medication, sufficient grounds may exist for a malpractice action.

The question is often asked: How frequently should patients be seen for medication follow-up? The answer is that patients should be seen according to their clinical needs. No stock answer about the frequency of visits can be given. The longer the time interval between visits, however, the greater the likelihood of adverse drug reactions and clinical developments. Patients taking medications should probably not go beyond 6 months for follow-up visits. Managed care policies that do not reimburse for frequent follow-up appointments may result in a psychiatrist prescribing large amounts of medications. The psychiatrist is duty bound to provide appropriate treatment to the patient, quite apart from managed care or other payment policies.

Other areas of negligence involving medication that have resulted in malpractice actions include failure to treat adverse effects that have or should have been recognized; failure to monitor a patient's compliance with prescription limits; failure to prescribe medication or appropriate levels of medication according to the treatment needs of the patient; prescribing addictive drugs to vulnerable patients; failure to refer a patient for consultation or treatment by a specialist; and negligent withdrawal of medication treatment.

Split Treatment

In split treatment the psychiatrist provides medication and a nonmedical therapist conducts the psychotherapy. The following vignette illustrates a possible complication.

A psychiatrist provided medications for a depressed 43-year-old woman. A master's level counselor saw the patient for outpatient psychotherapy. The psychiatrist saw the patient for 20 minutes during the initial evaluation and prescribed a tricyclic drug, and the patient was prescribed enough drugs for follow-up in 3 months. The psychiatrist's initial diagnosis was recurrent major depression. The patient denied suicidal ideation. Appetite and sleep were markedly diminished. The patient had a long history of recurrent depression with suicide attempts. No further discussions were held between the psychiatrist and the counselor, who saw the patient once a week for 30 minutes in psychotherapy. Within 3 weeks, after a failed romantic relationship, the patient stopped taking her antidepressant medication, started to drink heavily, and committed suicide with an overdose of alcohol and antidepressant drugs. The counselor and psychiatrist were sued for negligent diagnosis and treatment.

Psychiatrists must do an adequate evaluation, obtain prior medical records, and understand that there is no such thing as a partial patient. Split treatments are potential malpractice traps because patients can "fall between the cracks" of fragmented care. The psychiatrist retains full responsibility for the patient's care in a split treatment situation. This does not preempt the responsibility of the other mental health professionals involved in the patient's treatment. Section V, annotation 3 of the *Principles of Medical Ethics with Annotations Especially Applicable to Psychiatry* states: "When the psychiatrist assumes a collaborative or supervisory role with another mental health worker, he/she must expend sufficient time to assure that proper care is given."

In managed care or other settings, a marginalized role of merely prescribing medication apart from a working doctor–patient relationship does not meet generally accepted standards of good clinical care. The psychiatrist must be more than just a medication technician. Fragmented care in which the psychiatrist only dispenses medication while remaining uninformed about the patient's overall clinical status constitutes substandard treatment that may lead to a malpractice action. At a minimum, such a practice diminishes the efficacy of the drug treatment itself or may even lead to the patient's failure to take the prescribed medication.

Split-treatment situations require that the psychiatrist remain fully informed of the patient's clinical status as well as the nature and quality of treatment the patient is receiving from the nonmedical therapist. In a collaborative relationship, the responsibility for the patient's care is shared according to the qualifications and limitations of each discipline. The responsibilities of each discipline do not diminish those of the other disciplines. Patients should be informed of the separate responsibilities of each discipline. The psychiatrist and the nonmedical therapist must periodically evaluate the patient's clinical condition and requirements to determine whether the collaboration should continue. Upon termination of the collaborative relationship, both treaters should inform the patient either separately or jointly. In split treatments, if the nonmedical therapist is sued, the collaborating psychiatrist will likely be sued, and vice versa.

Psychiatrists who prescribe medications in a split-treatment arrangement should be able to hospitalize a patient, if that should become necessary. If the psychiatrist does not have admitting privileges, prearrangements should be made with other psychiatrists who can hospitalize patients if emergencies arise. Split treatment is increasingly used by managed care companies and is a potential malpractice minefield.

PRIVILEGE AND CONFIDENTIALITY

Privilege

Privilege is the right to maintain secrecy or confidentiality in the face of a subpoena. Privileged communications are statements made by certain persons within a relationship—such as husband–wife, priest–penitent, or doctor–patient—that the law protects from forced disclosure on the witness stand. The right of privilege belongs to the patient, not to the physician, and so the patient can waive the right.

Psychiatrists, who are licensed to practice medicine, may claim medical privilege, but the privilege is so riddled with qualifications that it is practically meaningless. Purely federal cases have no psychotherapist–patient privilege. Moreover, the privilege does not exist at all in military courts, regardless of whether the physician is military or civilian and whether the privilege is recognized in the state in which the court martial takes place. The privilege has numerous exceptions, which often are viewed as implied waivers. In the most common exception, patients are said to waive the privilege by injecting their mental condition into the litigation, thereby making their condition an element of their claim or defense. Another exception involves proceedings for hospitalization, in which the interests of both the patient and the public are said to call for a departure from confidentiality. In several contests, clinicians may be ordered to give the court information that is ordinarily considered privileged. Yet another exception is made in child-custody and child-protection proceedings in regard to the best interest of the child. Furthermore, the privilege does not apply to *actions* between a therapist and a patient. Therefore, in a fee dispute or a malpractice claim, the complainant's lawyer can obtain the necessary therapy records to resolve the dispute.

Under medical privilege, psychiatrists and other physicians do not legally enjoy the same privilege that exists between client and attorney, priest and churchgoer, and husband and wife. Most physicians are not aware of this fact.

Confidentiality

A long-held premise of medical ethics binds physicians to hold secret all information given by patients. This professional obligation is called *confidentiality*. Confidentiality applies to certain populations and not to others; a group that is within the circle of confidentiality shares information without receiving specific permission from a patient. Such groups include, in addition to the physician, other staff members treating the patient, clinical supervisors, and consultants. Parties outside the circle include the patient's family, attorney, and previous therapist; sharing information with such persons requires the patient's permission. Nevertheless, in numerous instances, a psychiatrist may be asked to divulge information imparted by a patient. Although a court demand for information is most worrisome to psychiatrists, demands most frequently come from sources such as insurers, who cannot compel disclosure but can withhold a benefit without it. A patient generally makes a disclosure or authorizes the psychiatrist to make disclosures to receive a benefit, such as employment, welfare benefits, or insurance.

A subpoena can force a psychiatrist to breach confidentiality, and courts must be able to compel witnesses to testify for the law to function adequately. A subpoena ("under penalty") is an order to appear as a witness in court or at a deposition. Physicians usually are served with a *subpoena duces tecum,* which requires that they also produce their relevant records and documents. Although the power to issue subpoenas belongs to a judge, they are routinely issued at the request of an attorney representing a party to an action.

In bona fide emergencies, information may be released in as limited a way as feasible to carry out necessary interventions. Sound clinical practice holds that a psychiatrist should make the effort, time allowing, to obtain the patient's permission anyway and should debrief the patient after the emergency.

As a rule, clinical information may be shared with the patient's permission—preferably written permission, although oral permission suffices with proper documentation. Each release is good for only one piece of information, and permis-

sion should be reobtained for each subsequent release, even to the same party. Permission overcomes only the legal barrier, not the clinical one; the release is permission, not obligation. If a clinician believes that the information may be destructive, the matter should be discussed, and the release may be refused, with some exceptions.

Third-Party Payers and Supervision. Increased insurance coverage for health care is precipitating a concern about confidentiality and the conceptual model of psychiatric practice. Today, insurance covers about 70 percent of all health care bills; to provide coverage, an insurance carrier must be able to obtain information with which it can assess the administration and costs of various programs.

Quality control of care necessitates that confidentiality not be absolute; it also requires a review of individual patients and therapists. The therapist in training must breach a patient's confidence by discussing the case with a supervisor. Institutionalized patients who have been ordered by a court to get treatment must have their individualized treatment programs submitted to a mental health board.

Discussions about Patients. In general, psychiatrists have multiple loyalties: to patients, to society, and to the profession. Through their writings, teaching, and seminars, they can share their acquired knowledge and experience and provide information that may be valuable to other professionals and to the public. However, it is not easy to write or talk about a psychiatric patient without breaching the confidentiality of the relationship. Unlike physical ailments, which can be discussed without anyone's recognizing the patient, a psychiatric history usually entails a discussion of distinguishing characteristics. Psychiatrists have an obligation not to disclose identifiable patient information (and, perhaps, any descriptive patient information) without appropriate informed consent. Failure to obtain informed consent may result in a claim based on breach of privacy, defamation, or both.

Child Abuse. In many states, all physicians are legally required to take a course on child abuse for medical licensure. All states now legally require that psychiatrists, among others, who have reason to believe that a child has been the victim of physical or sexual abuse, make an immediate report to an appropriate agency. In this situation, confidentiality is decisively limited by legal statute on the ground that potential or actual harm to vulnerable children outweighs the value of confidentiality in a psychiatric setting. Although many complex psychodynamic nuances accompany the required reporting of suspected child abuse, such reports generally are considered ethically justified.

HIGH-RISK CLINICAL SITUATIONS

Tardive Dyskinesia

It is estimated that at least 10 to 20 percent of patients and perhaps as high as 50 percent of patients treated with neuroleptic drugs for more than 1 year exhibit some probable tardive dyskinesia. These figures are even higher for elderly patients. Despite the possibility for a large number of tardive dyskinesia–related suits, relatively few psychiatrists have been sued. In addition, patients who develop tardive dyskinesia may not have the physical energy and psychological motivation to pursue litigation. Allegations of negligence involving tardive dyskinesia are based on a failure to evaluate a patient properly, a failure to obtain informed consent, a negligent diagnosis of a patient's condition, and a failure to monitor.

Most of the above-noted allegations of negligence were claimed in the landmark case *Clites v. State*. The plaintiff was a mentally retarded man who was institutionalized from age 11 and treated with major tranquilizers from age 18 to 23. After tardive dyskinesia was diagnosed at age 23, the plaintiff's family sued. The family claimed that the defendants negligently prescribed medication, did not inform the patient of the possibility of developing tardive dyskinesia, and failed to monitor and subsequently treat the patient for the adverse effects of the drugs. The jury found for the plaintiff and awarded damages in the amount of $760,165. This award was affirmed on appeal.

The appellate court ruled that the defendants were negligent and deviated from the standards of the "industry." Among the "deviations" the court noted were the failure to conduct regular physical examinations and laboratory tests, the failure to intervene at the first signs of tardive dyskinesia, the inappropriate use of multiple medications at the same time, the use of drugs for convenience (e.g., "behavior management") rather than for therapy, and the failure to obtain the plaintiff's informed consent.

Suicidal Patients

Psychiatrists are more likely to be sued when their patients commit suicide, particularly when psychiatric inpatients kill themselves. Psychiatrists are assumed to have more control over inpatients, making the suicide preventable.

The evaluation of suicide risk is one of the most complex, dauntingly difficult clinical tasks in psychiatry. Suicide is a rare event. In our current state of knowledge, clinicians cannot accurately predict when or if a patient will commit suicide. No professional standards exist for predicting who will or will not commit suicide. Professional standards do exist for assessing suicide risk, but at best, only the degree of suicide risk can be judged clinically following a comprehensive psychiatric assessment.

A review of the case law on suicide reveals that certain affirmative precautions should be taken with a suspected or confirmed suicidal patient. For example, failing to perform a reasonable assessment of a suicidal patient's risk for suicide or implement an appropriate precautionary plan will likely render a practitioner liable. The law tends to assume that suicide is preventable if it is foreseeable. Courts closely scrutinize suicide cases to determine if a patient's suicide was foreseeable. *Foreseeability* is a deliberately vague legal term that has no comparable clinical counterpart, a common-sense rather than a scientific construct. It does not (and should not) imply that clinicians can predict suicide. Foreseeability should not be confused with preventability, however. In hindsight, many suicides seem preventable that were clearly not foreseeable.

Violent Patients

Psychiatrists who treat violent or potentially violent patients may be sued for failure to control aggressive outpatients and for the discharge of violent inpatients. Psychiatrists may be sued for failing to protect society from the violent acts of their

patients if it was reasonable for the psychiatrist to have known about the patient's violent tendencies and if the psychiatrist could have done something that could have safeguarded the public. In the landmark case *Tarasoff v. Regents of the University of California,* the California Supreme Court ruled that mental health professionals have a duty to protect identifiable, endangered third parties from imminent threats of serious harm made by their outpatients. Since then, courts and state legislatures have increasingly held psychiatrists to a fictional standard of having to predict the future behavior (dangerousness) of their potentially violent patients. Research has consistently demonstrated that psychiatrists cannot predict future violence with any dependable accuracy.

The duty to protect patients and endangered third parties should be considered primarily a professional and moral obligation and, only secondarily, a legal duty. Most psychiatrists acted to protect both their patients and threatened others from violence long before *Tarasoff.*

If a patient threatens harm to another person, most states require that the psychiatrist perform some intervention that might prevent the harm from occurring. In states with duty-to-warn statutes, the options available to psychiatrists and psychotherapists are defined by law. In states offering no such guidance, health care providers are required to use the clinical judgment that will protect endangered third persons. Typically, a variety of options to warn and protect are clinically and legally available, including voluntary hospitalization, involuntary hospitalization (if civil commitment requirements are met), warning the intended victim of the threat, notifying the police, adjusting medication, and seeing the patient more frequently. The duty to protect allows the psychiatrist to consider a number of clinical options. Warning others of danger, by itself, is usually insufficient. Psychiatrists should consider the *Tarasoff* duty to be a national standard of care, even if they practice in states that do not have a duty to warn and protect.

TARASOFF I. This issue was raised in 1976 in the case of *Tarasoff v. Regents of University of California* (now known as *Tarasoff I*). In this case, Prosenjiit Poddar, a student and a voluntary outpatient at the mental health clinic of the University of California, told his therapist that he intended to kill a student readily identified as Tatiana Tarasoff. Realizing the seriousness of the intention, the therapist, with the concurrence of a colleague, concluded that Poddar should be committed for observation under a 72-hour emergency psychiatric detention provision of the California commitment law. The therapist notified the campus police both orally and in writing that Poddar was dangerous and should be committed.

Concerned about the breach of confidentiality, the therapist's supervisor vetoed the recommendation and ordered all records relating to Poddar's treatment destroyed. At the same time, the campus police temporarily detained Poddar but released him on his assurance that he would "stay away from that girl." Poddar stopped going to the clinic when he learned from the police about his therapist's recommendation to commit him. Two months later, he carried out his previously announced threat to kill Tatiana. The young woman's parents thereupon sued the university for negligence.

As a consequence, the California Supreme Court, which deliberated the case for the unprecedented time of about 14 months, ruled that a physician or a psychotherapist who has reason to believe that a patient may injure or kill someone must notify the potential victim, the victim's relatives or friends, or the authorities.

The discharge of the duty imposed on the therapist to warn intended victims against danger may take one or more various steps, depending on the case. Therefore, stated the court, it may call for the therapist to notify the intended victim or others likely to notify the victim of the danger, to notify the police, or to take whatever other steps are reasonably necessary under the circumstances.

The *Tarasoff I* decision has not drastically affected psychiatrists; it has long been their practice to warn the appropriate persons or law enforcement authorities when a patient presents a distinct and immediate threat to someone. According to the American Psychiatric Association, confidentiality may, with careful judgment, be broken in the following ways. A patient probably will commit murder, and the act can be stopped only by the psychiatrist notifying the police. A patient probably will commit suicide, and the act can be stopped only by the psychiatrist notifying the police. A patient, such as a bus driver or an airline pilot, who has potentially life-threatening responsibilities, shows marked impairment of judgment.

The *Tarasoff I* ruling does not require therapists to report a patient's fantasies; instead, it requires them to report an intended homicide, and it is the therapist's duty to exercise good judgment.

TARASOFF II. In 1982, the California Supreme Court issued a second ruling in the case of *Tarasoff v. Regents of University of California* (now known as *Tarasoff II*), which broadened its earlier ruling, the duty to *warn*, to include the duty to *protect* (Fig. 57–1).

The *Tarasoff II* ruling has stimulated intense debates in the medicolegal field. Lawyers, judges, and expert witnesses argue the definition of protection, the nature of the relationship between the therapist and the patient, and the balance between public safety and individual privacy.

Clinicians argue that the duty to protect hinders treatment because a patient may not trust a doctor if confidentiality is not maintained. Furthermore, because it is not easy to determine whether a patient is dangerous enough to justify long-term incarceration, unnecessary involuntary hospitalization may occur because of a therapist's defensive practices.

As a result of such debates in the medicolegal field, since 1976, the state courts have not made a uniform interpretation of the *Tarasoff II* ruling (the duty to protect). Generally, clinicians should note whether a specific identifiable victim seems to be in imminent and probable danger from the threat of an action contemplated by a mentally ill patient; the harm, in addition to being imminent, should be potentially serious or severe. Usually, the patient must be a danger to another person and not to property; the therapist should take clinically reasonable action.

In a few cases (none successful so far), claims have already been advanced that a *Tarasoff*-like duty applies to the infection of partners with human immunodeficiency virus (HIV) by patients under mental health treatment. The breach of confidentiality in *Tarasoff* cases is justified only by the threat of violence. Laws vary confusingly by jurisdiction. The ideal solution is to persuade the patient to make the disclosure and report the matter to the public health authorities.

HOSPITALIZATION

All states provide for some form of involuntary hospitalization. Such action usually is taken when psychiatric patients present a danger to themselves or others in their environment to the extent that their urgent need for treatment in a closed institution is evident. Certain states allow involuntary hospitalization when patients are unable to care for themselves adequately.

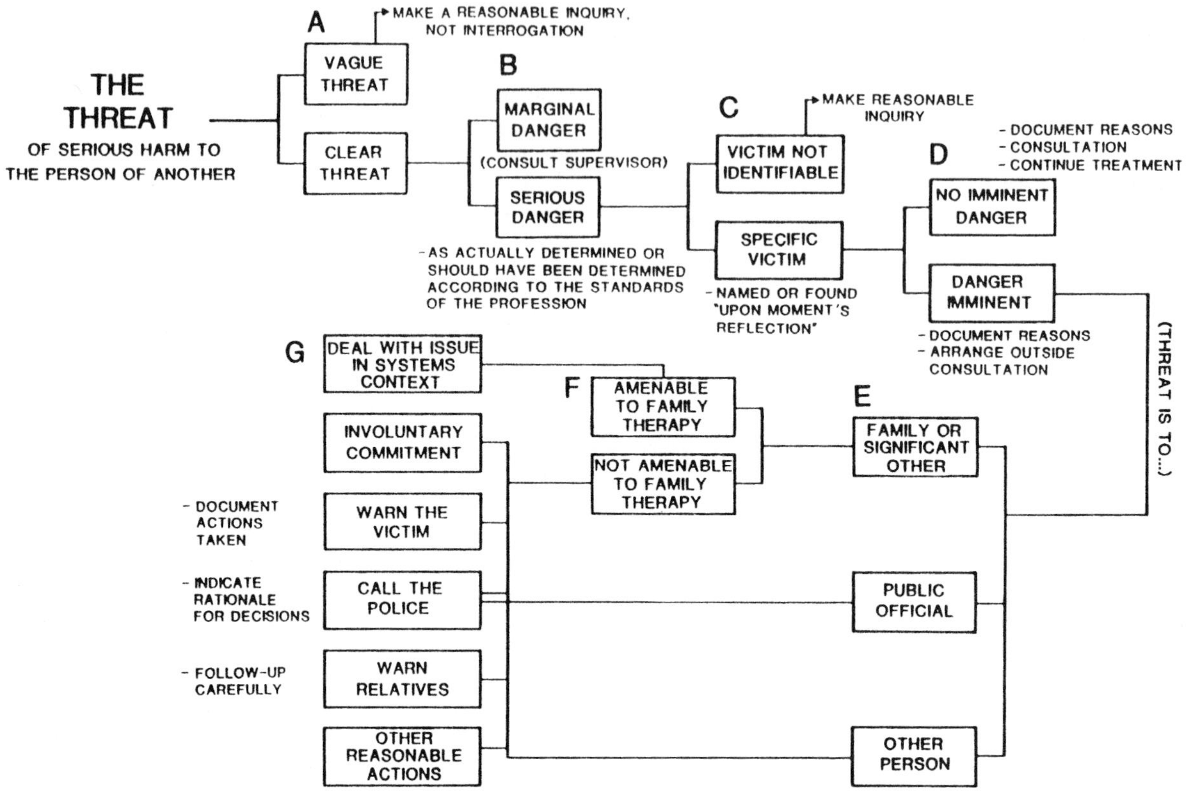

FIGURE 57–1
Tarasoff II decision chart. (Reprinted with permission from Gross BH, Weiberjer LE, ed. *The Mental Health Professional and the Legal System.* San Francisco: Jossey-Bass; 1998.)

The doctrine of *parens patriae* allows the state to intervene and to act as a surrogate parent for those who are unable to care for themselves or who may harm themselves. In English common law, *parens patriae* ("father of his country") dates to the time of King Edward I and originally referred to a monarch's duty to protect the people. In U.S. common law, the doctrine has been transformed into a paternalism in which the state acts for persons who are mentally ill and for minors.

The statutes governing hospitalization of persons who are mentally ill generally have been designated *commitment laws,* but psychiatrists have long considered the term to be undesirable. *Commitment* legally means a warrant for imprisonment. The American Bar Association and the American Psychiatric Association have recommended that the term *commitment* be replaced by the less offensive and more accurate term *hospitalization,* which most states have adopted. Although this change in terminology does not correct the punitive attitudes of the past, the emphasis on hospitalization is in keeping with psychiatrists' views of treatment rather than punishment.

False imprisonment is the legal action arising from the claim that a patient has been hospitalized negligently. It is an uncommon basis for malpractice litigation and is rarely successful when invoked. For instances in which hospitalization is necessary, a clinician's guidelines are to obtain an emergency or involuntary hospitalization in good faith, for reasonable cause, with data obtained from personal examination or a reliable report of danger; to seclude the patient for proper indications according to local regulations; and to obtain consultation in ambiguous cases.

Procedures of Admission

Four procedures of admission to psychiatric facilities have been endorsed by the American Bar Association to safeguard civil liberties and to make sure that no person is railroaded into a mental hospital. Although each of the 50 states has the power to enact its own laws on psychiatric hospitalization, the procedures outlined here are gaining much acceptance.

Informal Admission. Informal admission operates on the general hospital model, in which a patient is admitted to a psychiatric unit of a general hospital in the same way that a medical or surgical patient is admitted. Under such circumstances, the ordinary doctor–patient relationship applies, with the patient free to enter and to leave, even against medical advice.

Voluntary Admission. In cases of voluntary admission, patients apply in writing for admission to a psychiatric hospital. They may come to the hospital on the advice of a personal physician, or they may seek help on their own. In either case, patients are admitted if an examination reveals the need for hospital treatment.

Temporary Admission. Temporary admission is used for patients who are so senile or so confused that they require hospitaliza-

tion and are not able to make decisions of their own and for patients who are so acutely disturbed that they must be admitted immediately to a psychiatric hospital on an emergency basis. Under the procedure, a person is admitted to the hospital on the written recommendation of one physician. Once the patient has been admitted, the need for hospitalization must be confirmed by a psychiatrist on the hospital staff. The procedure is temporary because patients cannot be hospitalized against their will for more than 15 days.

Involuntary Admission. Involuntary admission involves the question of whether patients are suicidal and thus a danger to themselves or homicidal and thus a danger to others. Because these persons do not recognize their need for hospital care, the application for admission to a hospital may be made by a relative or a friend. Once the application is made, the patient must be examined by two physicians, and if both physicians confirm the need for hospitalization, the patient can then be admitted.

Involuntary hospitalization involves an established procedure for written notification of the next of kin. Furthermore, the patients have access at any time to legal counsel, who can bring the case before a judge. If the judge does not think that hospitalization is indicated, the patient's release can be ordered.

Involuntary admission allows a patient to be hospitalized for 60 days. After this time, if the patient is to remain hospitalized, the case must be reviewed periodically by a board consisting of psychiatrists, nonpsychiatric physicians, lawyers, and other citizens not connected with the institution. In New York State, the board is called the Mental Health Information Service.

Persons who have been hospitalized involuntarily and who believe that they should be released have the right to file a petition for a writ of habeas corpus. Under law, a writ of habeas corpus may be proclaimed by those who believe that they have been illegally deprived of liberty. The legal procedure asks a court to decide whether a patient has been hospitalized without due process of law. The case must be heard by a court at once, regardless of the manner or the form in which the motion is filed. Hospitals are obligated to submit the petitions to the court immediately.

RIGHT TO TREATMENT

Among the rights of patients, the right to the standard quality of care is fundamental. This right has been litigated in much publicized cases in recent years under the slogan of "right to treatment."

In 1966, Judge David Bazelon, speaking for the District of Columbia Court of Appeals in *Rouse v. Cameron,* noted that the purpose of involuntary hospitalization is treatment and concluded that the absence of treatment draws into question the constitutionality of the confinement. Treatment in exchange for liberty is the logic of the ruling. In this case, the patient was discharged on a writ of habeas corpus, the basic legal remedy to ensure liberty. Judge Bazelon further held that, if alternative treatments that infringe less on personal liberty are available, involuntary hospitalization cannot take place.

Alabama Federal Court Judge Frank Johnson was more venturesome in the decree he rendered in 1971 in *Wyatt v. Stickney.* The *Wyatt* case was a class-action proceeding brought under newly developed rules that sought not release but treatment. Judge Johnson ruled that persons civilly committed to a mental institution have a constitutional right to receive such individual treatment as will give them a reasonable opportunity to be cured or to have their mental condition improved. Judge Johnson set out minimum requirements for staffing, specified physical facilities, and nutritional standards, and required individualized treatment plans.

The new codes, more detailed than the old ones, include the right to be free from excessive or unnecessary medication; the right to privacy and dignity; the right to the least restrictive environment; the unrestricted right to be visited by attorneys, clergy, and private physicians; and the right not to be subjected to lobotomies, electroconvulsive treatments, and other procedures without fully informed consent. Patients can be required to perform therapeutic tasks but not hospital chores, unless they volunteer for them and are paid the federal minimum wage. This requirement is an attempt to eliminate the practice of peonage, in which psychiatric patients were forced to work at menial tasks, without payment, for the benefit of the state.

In a number of states today, medication or electroconvulsive therapy cannot be forcibly administered to a patient without first obtaining court approval, which may take as long as 10 days. The right to refuse treatment is a legal doctrine that holds that except in emergencies, persons cannot be forced to accept treatment against their will. An *emergency* is defined as a condition in clinical practice that requires immediate intervention to prevent death or serious harm to the patient or other or to prevent deterioration of the patient's clinical state.

In the 1976 case of *O'Connor v. Donaldson*, the Supreme Court of the United States ruled that harmless mentally ill patients cannot be confined against their will without treatment if they can survive outside. According to the Court, a finding of mental illness alone cannot justify a state's confining persons in a hospital against their will. Instead, involuntarily confined patients must be considered dangerous to themselves or others or possibly so unable to care for themselves that they cannot survive outside. As a result of the 1979 case of *Rennie v. Klein,* patients have the right to refuse treatment and to use an appeal process. As a result of the 1981 case of *Roger v. Oken,* patients have an absolute right to refuse treatment, but a guardian may authorize treatment. Questions have been raised about psychiatrists' ability to accurately predict dangerousness and about the risk to psychiatrists, who may be sued for monetary damages if persons are thereby deprived of their civil rights.

The ethical controversy concerning applications of the law to psychiatric patients came to the fore through Thomas Szasz, a professor of psychiatry at the State University of New York. In his book *The Myth of Mental Illness*, Szasz argued that the various psychiatric diagnoses are totally devoid of significance and contended that psychiatrists have no place in the courts of law and that all forced confinements because of mental illness are unjust. Szasz's opposition to suicide prevention and the imposition of treatment, with or without confinement, is interesting but is viewed by the psychiatric community with strong misgivings.

CIVIL RIGHTS OF PATIENTS

Thanks to several clinical, public, and legal movements, criteria for the civil rights of persons who are mentally ill, apart from their rights as patients, have been both established and affirmed.

Least Restrictive Alternative

Clinicians often are puzzled by the right of least restrictive alternative, which is perhaps the most legalistic civil right;

nothing in clinical work or training prepares psychiatrists to think in terms of restrictiveness. Instead, clinical interventions are undertaken according to their effectiveness, positive benefit-to-risk ratio, and other operational certainties. A series of legal decisions on state intervention in organizations maneuvered the concept of the least restrictive alternative into mental health law, where it has taken solid root.

The principle holds that patients have the right to receive the least restrictive means of treatment for the requisite clinical effect. Therefore, if a patient can be treated as an outpatient, commitment should not be used; if a patient can be treated on an open ward, seclusion should not be used.

Although apparently fairly straightforward on first reading, difficulty arises when clinicians attempt to apply the concept to choose among involuntary medication, seclusion, and restraint as the intervention of choice. Distinguishing among these interventions on the basis of restrictiveness proves to be a purely subjective exercise fraught with personal bias. Moreover, each of these three interventions is both more and less restrictive than each of the other two. Nevertheless, the effort should be made to think in terms of restrictiveness when deciding how to treat patients.

Visitation Rights

Patients have the right to receive visitors and to do so at reasonable hours (customary hospital visiting hours). Allowance must be made for the possibility that at certain times, a patient's clinical condition may not permit visits. This fact should be clearly documented, however, because such rights must not be suspended without good reason.

Certain categories of visitors are not limited to the regular visiting hours; these include a patient's attorney, private physician, and members of the clergy—all of whom have, broadly speaking, unrestricted access to the patient, including the right to privacy in their discussions. Even here, a bona fide emergency may delay such visits. Again, the patient's needs come first. Under similar reasoning, certain noxious visits may be curtailed (e.g., a patient's relative bringing drugs into the ward).

Communication Rights

Patients should, in general, have free and open communication with the outside world by telephone or mail, but this right varies regionally to some degree. Some jurisdictions charge the hospital administration with a responsibility for monitoring the communications of patients. In some areas, hospitals are expected to make available reasonable supplies of paper, envelopes, and stamps for patients' use.

Specific circumstances affect communication rights. A patient who is hospitalized in relation to a criminal charge of making harassing or threatening phone calls should not be given unrestricted access to the telephone, and similar considerations apply to mail. As a rule, however, patients should be allowed private telephone calls, and their incoming and outgoing mail should not be opened by hospital staff members.

Private Rights

Patients have several rights to privacy. In addition to confidentiality, they are allowed private bathroom and shower space, secure storage space for clothing and other belongings, and adequate floor space per person. They also have the right to wear their own clothes and to carry their own money.

Table 57–2
Indications for Seclusion and Restraint

1. Prevent clear, imminent harm to the patient or others
2. Prevent significant disruption to treatment program or physical surroundings
3. Assist in treatment as part of ongoing behavior therapy
4. Decrease sensory overstimulation[a]
5. At patient's voluntary reasonable request

[a]Seclusion only.
Reprinted with permission from Simon RI: *Concise Guide to Psychiatry and the Law for Clinicians.* 2nd ed. Washington, DC: American Psychiatric Press; 1998.

Economic Rights

Apart from special considerations related to incompetence, psychiatric patients generally are permitted to manage their own financial affairs. One feature of this fiscal right is the requirement that patients be paid if they work in the institution (e.g., gardening or preparing food). This right often creates tension between the valid therapeutic need for activity, including jobs, and exploitative labor. A consequence of this tension is that valuable occupational, vocational, and rehabilitative therapeutic programs may have to be eliminated because of the failure of legislatures to supply the funding to pay wages to patients who participate in these programs.

SECLUSION AND RESTRAINT

Seclusion and restraint raise complex psychiatric legal issues. Seclusion and restraint have both indications and contraindications (Tables 57–2 and 57–3). Seclusion and restraint have become increasingly regulated over the past decade.

Legal challenges to the use of restraints and seclusion have been brought on behalf of institutionalized mentally ill and mentally retarded persons. Typically, these lawsuits do not stand alone but are part of a challenge to a wide range of alleged abuses.

Generally, courts hold, or consent decrees provide, that restraints and seclusion be implemented only when a patient creates a risk of harm to self or others and no less restrictive alternative is available. Additional restrictions include the following:

Table 57–3
Contraindications to Seclusion and Restraint

1. Extremely unstable medical and psychiatric conditions
2. Delirious or demented patients unable to tolerate decreased stimulation
3. Overtly suicidal patients
4. Patients with severe drug reactions, overdoses or requiring close monitoring of drug dosages
5. For punishment or convenience of staff

1. Restraint and seclusion can only be implemented by a written order from an appropriate medical official
2. Orders are to be confined to specific, time-limited periods
3. A patient's condition must be regularly reviewed and documented
4. Any extension of an original order must be reviewed and reauthorized

The acceptability of restraint or seclusion for the purposes of training was recognized by the Supreme Court in *Youngberg v. Romeo,* which challenged the "treatment" practices at the Pennhurst State School and Hospital in Pennsylvania. The Court held that patients could not be restrained except to ensure their safety or, in certain undefined circumstances, "to provide needed training." Although recognizing that the defendant had a liberty interest in safety and freedom from bodily restraint, the Court noted that these interests were not absolute or in conflict with the need to provide training. The Court also held that decisions made by appropriate professionals regarding restraining the patient would be presumed correct. Psychiatrists and other mental health professionals have lauded the decision because the Court recognized that professionals are better able than the courts to determine the needs of patients, including deciding when restraint is appropriate.

The APA Task Force on the Psychiatric Uses of Seclusion and Restraint has developed guidelines for the appropriate use of seclusion and restraints, and the Joint Committee on Accreditation of Healthcare Organizations has promulgated guidelines for hospitals regarding seclusion and restraint requirements. Professional opinion concerning the clinical uses of physical restraints and seclusion varies considerably among psychiatrists. Seclusion can be justified on both clinical and legal grounds for a variety of uses, unless precluded by state freedom from restraint and seclusion statutes.

INFORMED CONSENT

Lawyers representing an injured claimant now invariably add to a claim of negligent performance of procedures (malpractice) an informed consent claim as another possible area of liability. Ironically, this is one claim under which the requirement of expert testimony may be avoided. The usual claim of medical malpractice requires the litigant to produce an expert to establish that the defendant physician departed from accepted medical practice. But in a case in which the physician did not obtain informed consent, the fact that the treatment was technically well performed, was in accord with the generally accepted standard of care, and effected a complete cure is immaterial. As a practical matter, however, unless the treatment had adverse consequences, a complainant will not get far with a jury in an action based solely on an allegation that the treatment was performed without consent.

In classic tort theory—a *tort* is a civil wrongful act other than a breach of contract—intentional touching to which a person has not given consent is *battery.* Therefore, the administration of electroconvulsive therapy or chemotherapy, although therapeutic, is a battery when performed without consent. Indeed, any unauthorized touching outside conventional social intercourse constitutes a battery and is an offense to the dignity of the person and an invasion of the person's right of self-determination, for which punitive and actual damages may be imposed. Justice Benjamin Cardozo wrote: "Every human being of adult years and sound mind has a right to determine what shall be done with his own body; and a surgeon who performs an operation without his patient's consent commits [a battery] for which he is liable in damages." Because informed consent has become a broadly recognized part of the standard of care, a procedure performed without informed consent may be malpractice as well as battery.

According to Justice Cardozo, the patient's consent to the treatment, not the effectiveness or the timeliness of the treatment, allows a physician to take care of a patient. Therefore, a mentally competent adult may refuse treatment, even though it is effective and involves little risk. But, for example, when gangrene sets in and the patient is psychotic, treatment—even of such momentous proportions as amputation—may be ordered to save the patient's life. The state also is said to have a compelling interest in preventing its citizens from committing suicide, and such interest allows treatment without consent in this situation as well.

In the case of minors, the parent or guardian is legally empowered to give consent to medical treatment. By statute, most states, however, list specific diseases and conditions that a minor can consent to have treated—including venereal disease, pregnancy, substance dependence, alcohol abuse, and contagious diseases. In an emergency, a physician can treat a minor without parental consent. The trend is to adopt the so-called mature minor rule, which allows minors to consent to treatment under ordinary circumstances. As a result of the Supreme Court's 1967 *Gault* decision, all juveniles must now be represented by counsel, must be able to confront witnesses, and must be given proper notice of any charges. Emancipated minors have the rights of an adult when it can be shown that they are living as adults with control over their own lives.

In the past, to obviate a claim of battery, physicians needed only to relate what they proposed to do and then to obtain the patient's consent thereto. Simultaneously with the growth of product liability and consumer law, however, the courts began to require that physicians also relate sufficient information to allow patients to decide whether such a procedure is acceptable in the light of the risks, the benefits, and the available alternatives, including no treatment at all. In general, informed consent requires that there be an understanding of the nature and the foreseeable risks and benefits of a procedure; a knowledge of alternative procedures; an awareness of the consequences of withholding consent; and the recognition that the consent is voluntary. Physicians must convey to patients a readiness to listen and to discuss anything a patient may fear as a risk, a side effect, or a concern about the proposed treatment.

Consent Form

The introduction of consent forms followed revelations of harm done to patients during clinical experimentation. Consent forms are written documents outlining a patient's informed consent to a proposed procedure. These forms usually are designed by attorneys, whose aim is to protect an institution from liability; therefore, the forms often are exhaustive and require a level of reading comprehension that is beyond many patients. Paradoxically, if such a form truly covered all possible eventualities, it probably would be too long to be comprehensible, and it if were

short enough to be comprehensible, it might be incomplete; some theorists have therefore recommended that the form be replaced by a standardized discussion and a progress note.

The basic elements of a consent form should include a fair explanation of the procedures to be followed and their purposes, including identification of any procedures that are experimental; a description of any attendant discomforts and risks reasonably to be expected; a description of any benefits reasonably to be expected; a disclosure of any appropriate alternative procedures that may be advantageous to the patient; an offer to answer any inquiries concerning the procedures; and an instruction that the patient is free to withdraw patient consent and to discontinue participation in the project or activity at any time without prejudice. The patient has the right to refuse treatment.

CHILD CUSTODY

The action of a court in a child-custody dispute is now predicated on the child's best interests. The maxim reflects the idea that a natural parent does not have an inherent right to be named a custodial parent, but the presumption, although a bit eroded, remains in favor of the mother in the case of young children. As a rule, the courts presume that the welfare of a child of tender years generally is best served by maternal custody when the mother is a good and fit parent. The best interest of the mother may be served by naming her as the custodial parent, because a mother may never resolve the effects of the loss of a child, but her best interest is not to be equated ipso facto with the best interest of the child. Care and protection proceedings are the court's interventions in the welfare of a child when the parents are unable to care for the child.

More fathers are asserting custodial claims. In about 5 percent of all cases, fathers are named custodians. The movement supporting women's rights also is enhancing the chances of paternal custody. With more women going to work outside the home, the traditional rationale for maternal custody has less force today than it did in the past.

Currently, every state has a statute allowing a court, usually a juvenile court, to assume jurisdiction over a neglected or abused child and to remove the child from parental custody. It usually orders that the care and custody of the child be supervised by the welfare or probation department.

TESTAMENTARY AND CONTRACTUAL CAPACITY AND COMPETENCE

Psychiatrists may be asked to evaluate patients' testamentary capacities and their competence to make a will. Three psychological abilities are necessary to prove this competence. Patients must know the nature and the extent of their bounty (property), the fact that they are making a bequest, and the identities of their natural beneficiaries (spouse, children, and other relatives).

When a will is being probated, one of the heirs or another person often challenges its validity. A judgment in such cases must be based on a reconstruction, using data from documents and from expert psychiatric testimony, of the testator's mental state at the time the will was written. When a person is unable to, or does not exercise the right to, make a will, the law in all states provides for the distribution of property to the heirs. If there are no heirs, the estate goes to the public treasury.

Witnesses at the signing of a will, who might include a psychiatrist, may attest that the testator was rational at the time the will was executed. In unusual cases, a lawyer may videotape the signing to safeguard the will from attack. Ideally, persons who are thinking of making a will and believe that questions might be raised about their testamentary competence hire a forensic psychiatrist to perform a dispassionate examination antemortem to validate and record their capacity.

An incompetence proceeding and the appointment of a guardian may be considered necessary when a family member spending the family's assets and property is in danger of dissipation as in the case of aged, retarded, alcohol-dependent, and psychotic persons. At issue is whether such persons are capable of managing their own affairs. A guardian appointed to take control of the property of one deemed incompetent, however, cannot make a will for the ward (the incompetent person).

Competence is determined on the basis of a person's ability to make a sound judgment—to weigh, to reason, and to make reasonable decisions. Competence is task specific, not general; the capacity to weigh decision-making factors (competence) often is best demonstrated by a person's ability to ask pertinent and knowledgeable questions after the risks and the benefits have been explained. Although physicians (especially psychiatrists) often give opinions on competence, only a judge's ruling converts the opinion into a finding; a patient is not competent or incompetent until the court so rules. The diagnosis of a mental disorder is not, in itself, sufficient to warrant a finding of incompetence. Instead, the mental disorder must cause an impairment in judgment for the specific issues involved. After they have been declared incompetent, persons are deprived of certain rights: they cannot make contracts, marry, start a divorce action, drive a vehicle, handle their own property, or practice their professions. Incompetence is decided at a formal courtroom proceeding, and the court usually appoints a guardian who will best serve a patient's interests. Another hearing is necessary to declare a patient competent. Admission to a mental hospital does not automatically mean that a person is incompetent.

Competence also is essential in contracts, because a contract is an agreement between parties to do a specific act. A contract is declared invalid, if, when it was signed, one of the parties was unable to comprehend the nature and effect of his or her act. The marriage contract is subject to the same standard and, thus, can be voided if either party did not understand the nature, duties, obligations, and other characteristics entailed at the time of the marriage. In general, however, the courts are unwilling to declare a marriage void on the basis of incompetence.

Whether competence is related to wills, contracts, or the making or breaking of marriages, the fundamental concern is a person's state of awareness and capacity to comprehend the significance of the particular commitment made.

Durable Power of Attorney

A modern development that permits persons to make provisions for their own anticipated loss of decision-making capacity is called a *durable power of attorney.* The document permits the advance selection of a substitute decision maker who can act without the necessity of court proceedings when the signatory

becomes incompetent through illness, progressive dementia, or perhaps a relapse of bipolar I disorder.

CRIMINAL LAW

Competence to Stand Trial

The Supreme Court of the United States stated that the prohibition against trying someone who is mentally incompetent is fundamental to the U.S. system of justice. Accordingly, the Court, in *Dusky v. United States*, approved a test of competence that seeks to ascertain whether a criminal defendant "has sufficient present ability to consult with his lawyer with a reasonable degree of rational understanding—and whether he has a rational as well as factual understanding of the proceedings against him."

One of the most useful clinical guides for determining a patient's competence to stand trial is the McGarry instrument, which identifies 13 areas of functioning:

1. Ability to appraise the legal defenses available
2. Level of unmanageable behavior
3. Quality of relating to the attorney
4. Ability to plan legal strategy
5. Ability to appraise the roles of various participants in the courtroom procedures
6. Understanding of court procedure
7. Appreciation of the charges
8. Appreciation of the range and the nature of the possible penalties
9. Ability to appraise the likely outcome
10. Capacity to disclose to the attorney available pertinent facts surrounding the offense
11. Capacity to challenge prosecution witnesses realistically
12. Capacity to testify relevantly
13. Manifestation of self-serving versus self-defeating motivation

One strength of such a guide is that it helps clinicians, even those without courtroom experience, picture the effects of the familiar forms of psychopathology on these parameters.

Clinicians merely offer opinions about competence. The judge is free to honor, modify, or disregard these opinions, and a patient is not competent or incompetent until the judge so rules. Psychiatrists would do well to refrain from protesting a competence judgment that contradicts clinical opinion. Disagreeing with a judgment is a matter for appeals courts, not for clinical objections.

Competence to Be Executed

One of the new areas of competence to emerge in the interface between psychiatry and the law is the question of a person's competence to be executed. The requirement for competence in this area is believed to rest on three general principles. First, a person's awareness of what is happening is supposed to heighten the retributive element of the punishment. Punishment is meaningless unless the person is aware of it and knows the punishment's purpose. Second, a competent person who is about to be executed is believed to be in the best position to make whatever peace is appropriate with religious beliefs, including confession and absolution. Third, a competent person who is about to be executed preserves, until the end, the possibility (admittedly slight) of recalling a forgotten detail of the events or the crime that may prove exonerating.

The need to preserve competence was supported recently in the Supreme Court case of *Ford v. Wainwright*. But no matter the outcome of legal struggles with this question, most medical bodies have gravitated toward the position that it is unethical for any clinician to participate, no matter how remotely, in state-mandated executions; a physician's duty to preserve life transcends all other competing requirements. Major medical societies, such as the American Medical Association (AMA) believe that doctors should not participate in the death penalty. A psychiatrist who agrees to examine a patient slated for execution may find the person incompetent on the basis of a mental disorder and may recommend a treatment plan, which, if implemented, would ensure the person's fitness to be executed. While there is room for a difference of opinion regarding whether or not a psychiatrist should become involved, the authors of *Synopsis* believe such involvement to be inhumane.

Criminal Responsibility

According to criminal law, committing an act that is socially harmful is not the sole criterion of whether a crime has been committed. Instead, the objectionable act must have two components: voluntary conduct (*actus reus*) and evil intent (*mens rea*). There cannot be an evil intent when an offender's mental status is so deficient, so abnormal, or so diseased as to have deprived the offender of the capacity for rational intent. The law can be invoked only when an illegal intent is implemented. Neither behavior, however harmful, nor the intent to do harm is, in itself, a ground for criminal action.

Until recently, in most U.S. jurisdictions, persons could be found not guilty by reason of insanity if they had a mental illness, did not know the difference between right and wrong, and did not know the nature and consequences of their acts. The persistence of the insanity defense seems to derive from two profound medicolegal forces. One is the moral imperative. The insanity defense is perhaps more nearly a moral than either a clinical or a legal issue. The moral dimension speaks to the reluctance to hold blameworthy or culpable those in society who do not seem to merit such labels because of their psychological or neurological conditions—a state the law calls *mental disease or defect*. Children and persons who are severely retarded have traditionally occupied this moral niche; persons who are mentally ill have always been in an ambiguous position. The second force sustaining the insanity defense is the perception of fairness. Society's sense of the fairness of its courts is undermined when, as one judge stated, "drooling idiots are treated as if they were responsible defendants." Ultimately, the legal system requires a class of nonculpable persons and a system and standards for defining this class—in short, the theory and practice of an insanity defense.

From a societal viewpoint, the insanity defense generates two common misconceptions that make it unpopular. First, many hardened criminals are believed to use the legal loophole to escape conviction. In reality, the insanity defense is used in only a tiny fraction of cases, and it prevails in a tiny fraction of this fraction—precisely because of its unpopularity. Second, the insanity defense is believed to allow psychiatrists to get

criminals off by acting as apologists for their evil actions. This view fails because the adversarial system requires two psychiatric opinions and because no psychiatrist ever decides a case.

M'Naghten Rule. The precedent for determining legal responsibility was established in 1843 in the British courts. The so-called M'Naghten rule, which has, until recently, determined criminal responsibility in most of the United States, holds that persons are not guilty by reason of insanity if they labored under a mental disease such that they were unaware of the nature, the quality, and the consequences of their acts or if they were incapable of realizing that their acts were wrong. Moreover, to absolve persons from punishment, a delusion used as evidence must be one that, if true, would be an adequate defense. If the delusional idea does not justify the crime, such persons are presumably held responsible, guilty, and punishable. The M'Naghten rule is known commonly as the right-wrong test.

The M'Naghten rule derives from the famous M'Naghten case of 1843 (Fig. 57–2). When Daniel M'Naghten murdered Edward Drummond, the private secretary of Robert Peel, M'Naghten had been suffering from delusions of persecution for several years, had complained to many persons about his "persecutors," and finally had decided to correct the situation by murdering Robert Peel. When Drummond came out of Peel's home, M'Naghten shot Drummond, whom he mistook for Peel. The jury, as instructed under the prevailing law, found M'Naghten not guilty by reason of insanity. In response to questions about what guidelines could be used to determine whether a person could plead insanity as a defense against criminal responsibility, the English chief judge wrote:

1. To establish a defense on the ground of insanity, it must be clearly proved that, at the time of committing the act, the party accused was laboring under such a defect of reason, from disease of the mind, as not to know the nature and quality of the act he was doing, or if he did know it, he did not know he was doing what was wrong.
2. Where a person labors under partial delusions only and is not in other respects insane and as a result commits an offense, he must be considered in the same situation regarding responsibility as if the facts with respect to which the delusion exists were real.

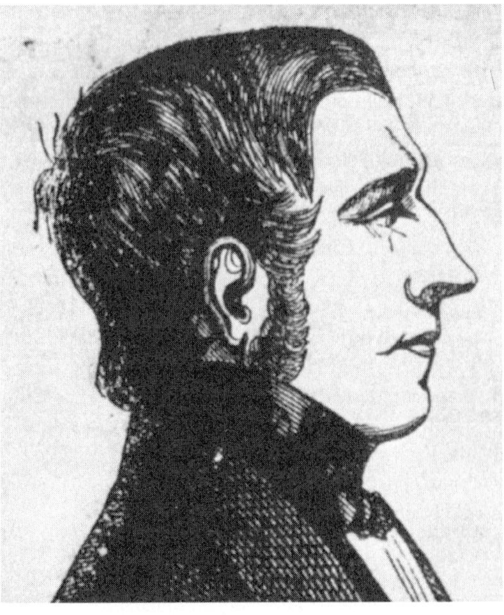

FIGURE 57–2
Daniel M'Naghten. His 1843 murder trial led to the establishment of rules still generally observed in legal insanity pleas. (Courtesy of Culver Pictures.)

According to the M'Naghten rule, the question is not whether the accused knows the difference between right and wrong in general, it is whether the defendant understood the nature and the quality of the act and whether the defendant knew the difference between right and wrong with respect to the act—that is, specifically whether the defendant knew the act was wrong or perhaps thought the act was correct, a delusion causing the defendant to act in legitimate self-defense.

Irresistible Impulse. In 1922, a committee of jurists in England reexamined the M'Naghten rule. The committee suggested broadening the concept of insanity in criminal cases to include the irresistible impulse tests, which rules that a person charged with a criminal offense is not responsible for an act if the act was committed under an impulse that the person was unable to resist because of mental disease. The courts have chosen to interpret this concept in such a way that it has been called the policeman-at-the-elbow law. In other words, the court grants an impulse to be irresistible only when it can be determined that the accused would have committed the act even if a policeman had been at the accused's elbow. To most psychiatrists, this interpretation is unsatisfactory because it covers only a small, special group of those who are mentally ill.

Durham Rule. In the case of *Durham v. United States*, Judge Bazelon handed down a decision in 1954 in the District of Columbia Court of Appeals. The decision resulted in the product rule of criminal responsibility, namely that an accused is not criminally responsible if his or her unlawful act was the product of mental disease or mental defect. In the Durham case, Judge Bazelon expressly stated that the purpose of the rule was to get good and complete psychiatric testimony. He sought to release the criminal law from the theoretical straitjacket of the M'Naghten rule, but judges and juries in cases using the *Durham* rule became mired in confusion over the terms "product," "disease," and "defect." In 1972, some 18 years after the rule's adoption, the Court of Appeals for the District of Columbia, in *United States v. Brawner*, discarded the rule. The court—all nine members, including Judge Bazelon—decided in a 143-page opinion to throw out its *Durham* rule and to adopt in its place the test recommended in 1962 by the American Law Institute in its mode penal code, which is the law in the federal courts today.

Model Penal Code. In its model penal code, the American Law Institute recommended the following test of criminal responsibility: Persons are not responsible for criminal conduct if, at the time of such conduct, as a result of mental disease or defect, they lacked substantial capacity either to appreciate the criminality (wrongfulness) of their conduct or to conform their

conduct to the requirement of the law. The term *mental disease or defect* does not include an abnormality manifest only by repeated criminal or otherwise antisocial conduct.

Subsection 1 of the American Law Institute rule contains five operative concepts: mental disease or defect, lack of substantial capacity, appreciation, wrongfulness, and conformity of conduct to the requirements of law. The rule's second subsection, stating that repeated criminal or antisocial conduct is not, of itself, to be taken as mental disease or defect, aims to keep the sociopath or psychopath within the scope of criminal responsibility.

Other Tests. The test of criminal responsibility and other tests of criminal liability refer to the time of the offense's commission, whereas the test of competence to stand trial refers to the time of the trial.

The 1982 verdict of a District of Columbia jury, which found John W. Hinckley, Jr., the would-be assassin of President Ronald Reagan, not guilty by reason of insanity, ignited moves to limit or abolish the special plea. Hinckley's trial by jury also turned out to be a trial of law and psychiatry. The psychiatrists and the law that allows their testimony were made the culprit for the unpopular verdict. "The psychiatrists spun sticky webs of pseudoscientific jargon," wrote a prominent columnist, "and in these webs the concept of justice, like a moth, fluttered feebly and was trapped." The American Bar Association and the American Psychiatric Association quickly issued statements calling for a change in the law. More than 40 bills were introduced in Congress to amend the law; none was passed, but the bills helped defuse the public criticism. At present, Hinckley is hospitalized indefinitely at the federal St. Elizabeth's Hospital in Washington, DC.

Attempts at legal reform have included the plea of guilty but mentally ill, which is already used in some jurisdictions. This standard has the advantage of identifying guilt while allowing some adaptation to psychiatric conditions; for example, it allows for treatment in restricted settings while permitting the courts to maintain an active role. "Guilty but insane" is a contradiction in terms; insanity has no legal meaning except as exculpation. The defense of diminished capacity is based on the claim that the defendant suffered an impairment (usually but not always because of mental illness) sufficient to interfere with the ability to formulate a specific element (such as forethought) of the particular crime charged. Therefore, the defense finds its most common use with so-called specific-intent crimes, such as first-degree murder.

Under this concept, the crime of Dan White, who killed two city officials of San Francisco, was reduced from murder to manslaughter. White's "Twinkie defense" involved psychiatrists who testified that he was depressed and that his compulsive eating of junk foods was a symptom of depression. His depression led to a manslaughter conviction, rather than a first-degree murder conviction. After he was released from prison, White committed suicide.

The AMA has proposed yet another reform—limiting the insanity exculpation to cases in which the person is so ill as to lack the necessary criminal intent (*mens rea*). This approach would all but eliminate the insanity defense and place a burden on the prisons to accept large numbers of persons who are mentally ill.

The American Bar Association and the American Psychiatric Association, in their 1982 statements, recommended a defense of nonresponsibility, which focuses solely on whether defendants, as a result of mental disease or defect, are unable to appreciate the wrongfulness of their conduct. These proposals would limit the evidence of mental illness to cognition and would exclude control, but apparently a defense would still be available under a not-guilty plea—such as extreme emotional disturbance, automatism, provocation, or self-defense—that would be established without psychiatric testimony about mental illness. The American Psychiatric Association also urged that "mental illness" be limited to severely abnormal mental conditions. These proposals still are controversial, and the issue probably will arise again with each sensational case in which the insanity defense is used.

OTHER AREAS OF FORENSIC PSYCHIATRY

Emotional Damage and Distress

There has been a rapidly rising trend to sue for psychological and emotional damage in recent years, both secondary to physical injury or as a consequence of witnessing a stressful act and from the suffering endured under the stress of such circumstances as concentration camp experiences. The West German government heard many of these claims from persons detained in Nazi camps during World War II. In the United States, the courts have moved from a conservative to a liberal position in awarding damages for such claims. Psychiatric examinations and testimony are sought in these cases, often by both the plaintiffs and the defendants.

Worker's Compensation

The stresses of employment may cause or accentuate mental illness. Patients are entitled to be compensated for their job-related disabilities or to receive disability retirement benefits. A psychiatrist is often called upon to evaluate such situations.

Civil Liability

Psychiatrists who sexually exploit their patients are subject to civil and criminal actions in addition to ethical and professional licensure revocation proceedings. Malpractice is the most common legal action (Table 57–4).

Table 57–4
Sexual Exploitation: Legal and Ethical Consequences

Civil lawsuit
Negligence
Loss of consortium
Breach-of-contract action
Criminal sanctions (e.g., statutory, adultery, sexual assault, rape)
Civil action for intentional tort (e.g., battery, fraud)
License revocation
Ethical sanctions
Dismissal from professional organizations

Reprinted with permission from Simon RI. *Clinical Psychiatry and the Law.* 2nd ed. Washington, DC: American Psychiatric Press; 1992.

RECOVERED MEMORIES

The current clamorous controversy concerning recovered memories of sexual abuse as described by Robert Simon threatens to undermine the credibility of the mental health professions. The debate has generated intense passions that have driven an increasing number of recovered memory cases into the courts. Patients alleging recovered memories of abuse have sued parents and other alleged perpetrators. In a number of instances, the alleged victimizers have sued therapists who, they claim, negligently induced false memories of sexual abuse. In an about face, some patients have recanted and joined forces with others (usually their parents) to sue therapists.

The memory debate has polarized a number of therapists into believers and disbelievers. Most therapists hold personal beliefs about the validity of recovered memories of sexual abuse that are somewhere between the extremes. Strongly held personal biases about recovered memories represent a new occupational hazard for clinicians. Such feelings can undermine the therapists' duty of neutrality to their patients, creating deviant treatment boundaries and the provision of substandard care.

Litigation in recovered memory cases is expected to soar in the coming years. A fundamental allegation in these cases is that the therapist abandoned a position of neutrality to suggest, persuade, coerce, and implant false memories of childhood sexual abuse. The guiding principle of clinical risk management in recovered memory cases is maintenance of therapist neutrality and establishment of sound treatment boundaries (Table 57–5).

Further complicating the matter is the empirical evidence about memory mechanisms, which (as is typical for any emerging science) reveals contradictory findings about how and what persons retain in memory and forget in various settings. Empirical studies often fail to distinguish whether allegedly repressed memories are not retrieved or simply not reported to researchers.

Table 57–5
Some Risk Factors in Treatment

1. Maintain therapist neutrality—do not suggest abuse
2. Stay clinically focused—provide adequate evaluation and treatment for patients presenting problems and symptoms
3. Carefully document the memory recovery process
4. Manage personal bias and countertransference
5. Avoid mixing treater and expert witness roles
6. Closely monitor supervisory and collaborative therapy relationships
7. Clarify nontreatment roles with family members
8. Avoid special techniques (e.g., hypnosis or sodium amytal) unless they are clearly indicated; obtain consultation first
9. Stay within professional competence—do not take cases you cannot handle

Data from Robert Simon, M.D.

References

Farber NJ, Aboff BM, Weiner J, Davis LR, Boyer EG, Ubel PA. Physicians' willingness to participate in the process of lethal injection for capital punishment. *Ann Intern Med.* 2001;135:884.

Goldstein RL. Paranoids in the legal system: the litigious paranoid and the paranoid criminal. *Psychiatr Clin North Am.* 1995;18:303.

Gunn J. Future directions for treatment in forensic psychiatry. *Br J Psychiatry.* 2000;176:332.

Gutheil TG. Approaches to forensic assessment of false claims of sexual misconduct by therapists. *Bull Am Acad Psychiatry Law.* 1992;20:289.

Jaworoski S, Zabow A. Involuntary psychiatric hospitalization of minors. *Med Law.* 1995;14:635.

Kantor JE. *Medical Ethics for Physicians-in-Training.* New York: Plenum; 1989.

Miller RD. Need-for-treatment criteria for involuntary civil commitment: impact in practice. *Am J Psychiatry.* 1992;149:1380.

Noonan JR, Johnson RK. The misuse of the diagnosis of bipolar disorder in the forensic context. *Am J Forensic Psychol.* 2002;20:5.

Palermo GB, Perracuti S, Palermo MT. Malingering a challenge for the forensic examiner. *Med Law.* 1996;15:143.

Roback HB, Moore RF, Bloch FS, Shelton M. Confidentiality in group psychotherapy: empirical findings and the law. *Int J Group Psychother.* 1996;46:117.

Saks E. The criminal responsibility of people with multiple personality disorder. *Psychiatr Q.* 1995;66:119.

Simon RI. Legal issues in psychiatry. In: Sadock BJ, Sadock VA, eds. *Kaplan & Sadock's Comprehensive Textbook of Psychiatry.* 7th ed. Vol 2. Baltimore: Lippincott Williams & Wilkins; 2000:3272.

Stone A. *Law Psychiatry and Morality.* Washington, DC: American Psychiatric Press; 1984.

Thomson L. Clinical management in forensic psychiatry. *J Forensic Psychiatry.* 1999;10:367.

58 Ethics in Psychiatry

Ethics in psychiatry refers to the principles of conduct that govern the behavior of psychiatrists as well as other mental health professionals. Ethics as a discipline deals with what is good and what is bad, what is right and what is wrong, and moral duties, obligations, and responsibilities.

PROFESSIONAL CODES

Most professional organizations and many business groups have codes of ethics. Such codes reflect a consensus about the general standards of appropriate professional conduct. The American Medical Association's *Principles of Medical Ethics,* the American Psychiatric Association's *Principles of Medical Ethics with Annotations Especially Applicable to Psychiatry,* and the *American College of Physicians Ethics Manual* articulate ideal standards of practice and professional virtues of practitioners. These codes include exhortations to use skillful and scientific techniques, to self-regulate misconduct within the profession, and to respect the rights and needs of patients, families, colleagues, and society. Such exhortations are reinforced by core ethical principles such as beneficence, autonomy, nonmaleficence, and justice (discussed below).

In recent years, interest has increased in the use of professional codes of ethics as a standard of criticism and a means of regulating professional misconduct. For ethical violations, the American Psychiatric Association (APA) may expel members from its organization or, for less severe violations, suspend membership for a time. During this period, a member may be required to undergo supervision or extra training. For still less severe violations, a member may be reprimanded or admonished, with no effect on membership status. Expulsion from the APA is reported publicly, but whether less severe violations are reported is left to the discretion of the local APA branch. Some hospitals withdraw privileges from a psychiatrist who has been expelled for ethical reasons, and malpractice coverage may be denied.

The Principles of Medical Ethics with Annotations Especially Applicable to Psychiatry (hereafter, *The Principles*) provides a useful and comprehensive example of a professional code geared to the psychiatric profession. The manual covers a broad array of psychiatric ethical issues, from fee splitting and sex with former patients to psychiatrists' participation in executions, all of which are unethical. Developed by the APA Ethics Committee members and consultants, it provides answers to commonly asked ethical questions. A summary of these principles is provided in Table 58–1.

CORE ETHICAL PRINCIPLES

Ethicists base their decisions on fewer core principles: autonomy, nonmaleficence, beneficence, and justice. On one hand, respect for patient autonomy is salient when psychosurgery is proposed, but the principle of social justice may be in force in deciding who receives a new medication that is scarce and expensive. The most pervasive ethical conflict in psychiatry and in medicine as a whole is that between *autonomy,* the right of patients to self-determination, and *beneficence,* the duty of physicians to act in the best interest of their patients.

Autonomy

The principle of *patient autonomy* has central importance and, conceptually, is in many ways coextensive with the legal concept of competence. A patient makes an autonomous choice by giving informed consent when that choice is (1) intentional, (2) free of undue outside influence, and (3) made with rational understanding. Usually, when patients respond to a choice by saying "yes," the desire to comply is assumed. However, that assumption may not be valid with a highly confused patient.

Nonmaleficence

Nonmaleficence is the duty of the psychiatrist to avoid either inflicting physical and emotional harm on the patient or increasing the risk of such harm. That principle is captured by *primum non nocere,* "first, do no harm."

Beneficence

The principle of *beneficence*—to prevent or remove harm and promote well-being—was the primary driving principle of medical and psychiatric practice throughout history until the rise of consumerism and other factors in the late 1960s. The expression of the principle is paternalism, the use of the psychiatrist's judgment about the best course of action for the patient or research subject.

Psychiatrists have historically justified beneficent paternalism on the basis of their superior knowledge, greater objectivity, and powerful desire to help their patients. A common example of the primacy of beneficence is the decision to hospitalize a suicidal patient involuntarily. That unilateral act implies either that the patient's autonomy is intact but must be overridden by the potential for dangerous behavior or that the patient's capacity for autonomous choice is impaired by the mental illness and must be ignored. Here is an example of the distinction between *weak paternalism* (acting beneficently when the patient's

Table 58–1
The Principles of Medical Ethics with Annotations Especially Applicable to Psychiatry

Each of the AMA principles of medical ethics printed separately (in italics) along with annotations especially applicable to psychiatry.

Preamble

The medical profession has long subscribed to a body of ethical statements developed primarily for the benefit of the patient. As a member of this profession, a physician must recognize responsibility not only to patients but also to society, to other health professionals, and to self. The following Principles, adopted by the American Medical Association, are not laws but standards of conduct, which define the essentials of honorable behavior for the physician.

Section 1

A physician shall be dedicated to providing competent medical service with compassion and respect for human dignity.[a]

1. A psychiatrist shall not gratify his/her own needs by exploiting a patient. The psychiatrist shall be ever vigilant about the impact that his/her conduct has upon the boundaries of the doctor–patient relationship and thus upon the well-being of the patient. These requirements become particularly important because of the essentially private, highly personal, and sometimes intensely emotional nature of the relationship with the psychiatrist.
2. A psychiatrist should not be a party to any type of policy that excludes, segregates, or demeans the dignity of any patient because of ethnic origin, race, sex, creed, age, socioeconomic status, or sexual orientation.
3. In accord with the requirements of law and accepted medical practice, it is ethical for a physician to submit his/her work to peer review and to the ultimate authority of the medical staff executive body and the hospital administration and its governing body.
4. A psychiatrist should not be a participant in a legally authorized execution.

Section 2

A physician shall deal honestly with patients and colleagues, and strive to expose those physicians deficient in character or competence, or who engage in fraud or deception.

1. The requirement that the physician conduct himself/herself with propriety in his/her profession and in all the actions of his/her life is especially important for the psychiatrist because the patient tends to model his/her behavior on that of his/her psychiatrist by identification. Further, the necessary intensity of the treatment relationship may tend to activate sexual and other needs and fantasies of both patient and psychiatrist, while weakening the objectivity necessary for control. Additionally, the inherent inequality in the doctor–patient relationship may lead to exploitation of the patient. Sexual activity with a current or former patient is unethical.
2. The psychiatrist should diligently guard against exploiting information furnished by the patient and should not use the unique position of power afforded by the psychotherapeutic situation to influence patients in any way not directly relevant to the treatment goals.
3. A psychiatrist who regularly practices outside his/her area of professional competence should be considered unethical. Determination of professional competence should be made by peer review boards or other appropriate bodies.
4. Special consideration should be given to psychiatrists who, due to illness, jeopardize the welfare of their patients and their own reputations and practices. It is ethical, even encouraged, for another psychiatrist to intercede in such situations.
5. Psychiatric services, like all medical services, are dispensed in the context of a contractual arrangement between the patient and the treating physician. The provisions of the contractual arrangement, which are binding on both the physician and the patient, should be explicitly established.
6. It is ethical for a psychiatrist to make a charge for a missed appointment when it falls within the terms of the specific contractual agreement with the patient. Charging for a missed appointment or for one not canceled 24 hours in advance need not, in itself, be considered unethical if a patient is fully advised that the physician will make such a charge. The practice, however, should be resorted to infrequently and always with the utmost consideration for the patient and his/her circumstances.
7. An arrangement in which a psychiatrist provides supervision or administration to other physicians or nonmedical persons for a percentage of their fees or gross income is not acceptable; this would constitute fee splitting.

Section 3

A physician shall respect the law and also recognize a responsibility to seek changes in those requirements which are contrary to the best interests of the patient.

1. It would seem self-evident that a psychiatrist who is a lawbreaker might be ethically unsuited to practice his/her profession. When such illegal activities bear directly upon his/her practice, this would obviously be the case. However, in other instances, illegal activities such as those concerning the right to protest social injustices might not bear on either the image of the psychiatrist or the ability of the specific psychiatrist to treat his/her patient ethically and well.

Section 4

A physician shall respect the rights of patients, of colleagues, and of other health professionals, and shall safeguard patient confidences within the constraints of the law.

1. Psychiatric records, including even the identification of a person as a patient, must be protected with extreme care. Confidentiality is essential to psychiatric treatment. This is based in part on the special nature of psychiatric therapy as well as on the traditional ethical relationship between physician and patient. Growing concern regarding the civil rights of patients and the possible adverse effects of computerization, duplication equipment, and data banks make the dissemination of confidential information an increasing hazard. Because of the sensitive and private nature of the information with which the psychiatrist deals, he/she must be circumspect in the information that he/she chooses to disclose to others about a patient. The welfare of the patient must be a continuing consideration.
2. A psychiatrist may release confidential information only with the authorization of the patient or under proper legal compulsion. The continuing duty of the psychiatrist to protect patients includes fully apprising him/her of the connotations of waiving the privilege of privacy. This may become an issue when the patient is being investigated by a government agency, is applying for a position, or is involved in legal action. The same principles apply to the release of information concerning treatment to medical departments of government agencies, business organizations, labor unions, and insurance companies. Information gained in confidence about patients seen in student health services should not be released without the students' explicit permission.
3. Clinical and other materials used in teaching and writing must be adequately disguised to preserve the anonymity of the individuals involved.
4. The ethical responsibility of maintaining confidentiality holds equally for consultations in which the patient may not have been present and in which the consultee was not a physician. In such instances, the physician consultant should alert the consultee to his/her duty of confidentiality.
5. Ethically, the psychiatrist may disclose only the information that is relevant to a given situation. He/she should avoid offering speculation as fact. Sensitive information such as an individual's sexual orientation or fantasy material is usually unnecessary.

(*continued*)

Table 58–1 (*continued*)

6. Psychiatrists are often asked to examine individuals for security purposes, to determine suitability for various jobs, and to determine legal competence. The psychiatrist must fully describe the nature, purpose, and lack of confidentiality of the examination to the examinee at the beginning of the examination.
7. Careful judgment must be exercised by the psychiatrist to include, when appropriate, the parents or guardian in the treatment of a minor. At the same time, the psychiatrist must assure the minor proper confidentiality.
8. When in the clinical judgment of the treating psychiatrist the risk of danger is deemed to be significant, the psychiatrist may reveal confidential information disclosed by the patient.
9. When the psychiatrist is ordered by the court to reveal the confidences entrusted to him/her by patients, he/she may comply or he/she may ethically hold the right to dissent within the framework of the law. When a psychiatrist is in doubt, the right of the patient to confidentiality and, by extension, to unimpaired treatment, should be given priority. The psychiatrist should reserve the right to raise the question of adequate need for disclosure. In the event the necessity for legal disclosure is demonstrated by the court, the psychiatrist may request the right to disclose only that information which is relevant to the legal question at hand.
10. With regard for the person's dignity and privacy and with truly informed consent, it is ethical to present a patient to a scientific gathering if the confidentiality of the presentation is understood and accepted by the audience.
11. When involved in funded research, the ethical psychiatrist advises human subjects of the funding source, retains his/her freedom to reveal data and results, and follows all appropriate and current guidelines relative to human subject protection.
12. Ethical considerations in medical practice preclude the psychiatric evaluation of any person charged with criminal acts prior to access to, or availability of, legal council. The only exception is rendering care to the person for the sole purpose of medical treatment.
13. Sexual involvement between a faculty member or supervisor and a trainee or student, in situations in which an abuse of power can occur, often takes advantage of inequalities in the working relationship and may be unethical because (a) any treatment of a patient being supervised may be deleteriously affected; (b) it may damage the trust relationship between teacher and student; and (c) teachers are important professional role models for their trainees and affect their trainees' future professional behavior.

Section 5

A physician shall continue to study, apply, and advance scientific knowledge, make relevant information available to patients, colleagues, and the public, obtain consultation, and use the talents of other health professionals when indicated.

1. Psychiatrists are responsible for their own continuing education and should remember that theirs must be a lifetime of learning.
2. In the practice of their specialty, the psychiatrists consult, associate, collaborate, or integrate their work with that of many professionals, including psychologists, psychometricians, social workers, alcoholism counselors, marriage counselors, and public health nurses. Furthermore, the nature of modern psychiatric practice extends the psychiatrist's contacts to such people as teachers, juvenile and adult probation officers, attorneys, welfare workers, agency volunteers, and neighborhood aides. Psychiatrists should ensure that the allied professionals or paraprofessionals with whom they are dealing and who refer patients for treatment, counseling, or rehabilitation are recognized members of their own discipline and are competent to carry out the therapeutic task required. Psychiatrists should have the same attitude toward members of the medical profession to whom they refer patients. Psychiatrists should not refer patients whenever they have reason to doubt the training, skill, or ethical qualifications of the allied professional.
3. When psychiatrists assume a collaborative or supervisory role with another mental health worker, they must expend sufficient time to ensure that proper care is given. It is contrary to the interests of the patient and to patient care if they allow themselves to be used as a figurehead.
4. In relationships between psychiatrists and practicing licensed psychologists, physicians should not delegate to the psychologist or, in fact, to any nonmedical person any matter requiring the exercise of professional medical judgment.
5. Psychiatrists should agree to the request of a patient for consultation or to such a request from the family of an incompetent or minor patient. Psychiatrists may suggest possible consultants, but the patient or family should be given free choice of the consultant. If psychiatrists disapprove of the professional qualifications of the consultant or if they cannot resolve difference of opinion they may, after suitable notice, withdraw from the case. If this disagreement occurs within an institution or agency framework, the differences should be resolved by mediation or arbitration by higher professional authority within the institution or agency.

Section 6

A physician shall, in the provision of appropriate patient care, except in emergencies, be free to choose whom to serve, with whom to associate, and the environment in which to provide medical services.

1. Physicians generally agree that the doctor–patient relationship is such a vital factor in effective treatment of the patient that preservation of optimal conditions for development of a sound working relationship between the doctors and their patient should take precedence over all other considerations.

Section 7

A physician shall recognize a responsibility to participate in activities contributing to an improved community.

1. Psychiatrists should foster the cooperation of those legitimately concerned with the medical, psychological, social, and legal aspects of mental health and illness. Psychiatrists are encouraged to serve society by advising and consulting with the executive, legislative, and judiciary branches of the government. Psychiatrists should clarify whether they speak as an individual or as a representative of an organization. Furthermore, psychiatrists should avoid cloaking their public statements with the authority of the profession (e.g., "Psychiatrists know that. . . .")
2. Psychiatrists may interpret and share with the public their expertise in the various psychosocial issues that may affect mental health and illness. Psychiatrists should always be mindful of their separate roles as dedicated citizens and as experts in psychological medicine.
3. On occasion psychiatrists are asked for an opinion about individuals who are in the light of public attention or who have disclosed information about themselves through public media. In such circumstance, psychiatrists may share their expertise about psychiatric issues in general with the public. However, it is unethical for psychiatrists to offer a professional opinion about a specific individual unless they have conducted an examination and have been granted proper authorization for such a statement.
4. Psychiatrists may permit their certification to be used for the involuntary treatment of any person only after their personal examination of that person. To do so, they must find that the person, because of mental illness, cannot form a judgment about what is in his/her own best interests and that without such treatment, substantial impairment is likely to occur to that person or others.

[a]Statements in italics are taken directly from the American Medical Association's Principles of Medical Ethics. Reprinted with permission from American Psychiatric Association. *The Principles of Medical Ethics with Annotations Especially Applicable to Psychiatry.* Washington, DC: American Psychiatric Association; 1995.

impaired faculties prevent an autonomous choice) and *strong paternalism* (acting beneficently despite the patient's intact autonomy).

Guidelines have been proposed for permitting beneficence to overrule patient autonomy; when the patient faces substantial harm or risk of harm, the paternalistic act is chosen that ensures the optimal combination of maximal harm reduction, low added risk, and minimum necessary infringement on patient autonomy. For example, convincing an acutely suicidal patient to enter the hospital voluntarily confers the environment necessary to contain the suicidal behavior, poses little added risk for most patients, and preserves more patient autonomy than involuntary hospitalization or a breach of confidentiality to an intervening third party on an outpatient basis.

Justice

Like the principles of autonomy, nonmaleficence, and beneficence, the principle of justice in psychiatry does not operate in a vacuum but responds to the ever-changing social, political, religious, and legal mores of the moment.

SPECIFIC ISSUES

From a practical point of view, several specific issues most frequently involve psychiatrists. These include (1) sexual boundary violations, (2) nonsexual boundary violations, (3) violations of confidentiality, (4) mistreatment of the patient (incompetence, double agentry), and (5) illegal activities (insurance, billing, insider stock trading).

Sexual Boundary Violations

For a psychiatrist to engage a patient in a sexual relationship is clearly unethical. Furthermore, legal sanctions against such behavior make the ethical question moot. Various criminal law statutes have been used against psychiatrists who violate this ethical principle. Rape charges may be, and have been, brought against such psychiatrists; sexual assault and battery charges also have been used to convict psychiatrists.

In addition, patients who have been victimized sexually by psychiatrists and other physicians have won damages in malpractice suits. Insurance carriers for the APA and the American Medical Association (AMA) no longer insure against patient–therapist sexual relations, and the carriers exclude liability for any such sexual activity.

The issue of whether sexual relations between an ex-patient and a therapist violate an ethical principle, however, remains controversial. Proponents of the view "Once a patient always a patient" insist that any involvement with an ex-patient—even one that leads to marriage—should be prohibited. They maintain that a transferential reaction that always exists between the patient and the therapist prevents a rational decision about their emotional or sexual union. Others insist that, if a transferential reaction still exists, the therapy is incomplete and that as autonomous human beings, ex-patients should not be subjected to paternalistic moralizing by physicians. Accordingly, they believe that no sanctions should prohibit emotional or sexual involvements by ex-patients and their psychiatrists. Some psychiatrists maintain that a reasonable time should elapse before such a liaison. The length of the "reasonable" period remains controversial: Some have suggested 2 years. Other psychiatrists maintain that any period of prohibited involvement with an ex-patient is an unnecessary restriction. *The Principles,* however, states: "Sexual activity with a current or *former* patient is unethical."

A male therapist is treating a female patient who may have some borderline personality traits. During a particularly emotional session, the doctor holds the patient's hand or puts his arm around her shoulder to comfort her. Perhaps there is even a hug; later, another emotional session and another hug, this time a bit longer. Soon each session ends with a hug, maybe a hug and a kiss on the cheek. Later the patient calls the doctor in the evening, sobbing. The doctor makes a house call; more hugs, more kisses. A suicide gesture is often catalytic. This scenario can get quite complicated and involved, but it is not uncommon. At this point the situation is, without question, a psychiatric emergency. The doctor must obtain an immediate consultation from an experienced colleague. Unfortunately, this option is rarely taken. Whether due to embarrassment, fear of criticism from the community, denial, or unwarranted omnipotence, the scenario usually progresses down the slippery slope, and sexual activity replaces treatment. (Courtesy of Peter Gruenberg, M.D.)

An argument occasionally put forward is that the sexual activity is consensual; that is, it takes place between two autonomous adults, and consequently, they should be able to do as they please. Yet even a rudimentary knowledge of dynamic psychiatry reveals that the two adults are rarely autonomous. Powerful, unconscious forces are at work in all doctor–patient relationships. The patient does not have to lie on a couch five times a week to develop transference. Transference occurs in every encounter with a patient. Even the brief medication-management visit produces transference (and countertransference). *The Principles* is quite clear in Section 2.1.

Although not spelled out in *The Principles*, sexual activity with a patient's family member is also unethical. This is most important when the psychiatrist is treating a child or adolescent. Most training programs in child and adolescent psychiatry emphasize that the parents are patients too and that the ethical and legal proscriptions apply to parents (or parent surrogates) as well as to the child. Nevertheless, some psychiatrists misunderstand this concept. Sexual activity between a doctor and a patient's family member is also unethical.

Nonsexual Boundary Violations

The relationship between a doctor and a patient for the purposes of providing and obtaining treatment is what is usually called the *doctor–patient relationship.* That relationship has both boundaries around it and boundaries within it. Either person may cross the boundary.

Not all boundary crossings are boundary violations. For example, a patient may say to a doctor at the end of an hour "I have left my money at home and I need a dollar to get my car out of the garage. Will you lend me a dollar until next time?" The patient has invited the doctor to cross the doctor–patient boundary and set up a lender–borrower relationship as well.

Depending upon the doctor's theoretical orientation, the clinical situation with the patient, and other factors, the doctor may elect to cross the boundary. One can then debate whether the boundary crossing is also a boundary violation. A *boundary violation* is a boundary crossing that is exploitative. It gratifies the doctor's needs at the expense of the patient. The doctor is responsible for preserving the boundary and for ensuring that boundary crossings are held to a minimum and that exploitation does not occur.

A resident in psychiatry was admonished by her psychotherapy supervisor to never, under any circumstances, accept a gift from a patient. In the course of treating a young girl with schizophrenia, she was offered a Christmas gift (a cotton scarf), which she refused to accept, explaining as gently as possible that it was not permitted by the "rules of the hospital." The next day the patient attempted suicide. She experienced the resident's refusal to accept the gift as a profound rejection (to which schizophrenia patients are exquisitely sensitive), which she could not tolerate. The case illustrates the need to understand the dynamics of gift giving and the transferential meaning to the patients of rejecting (or accepting) the gift.

The story (possibly apocryphal) is told of how Freud, who was an inveterate cigar smoker, was offered a box of difficult-to-find Havana cigars by a patient during the course of his analysis. Freud accepted the gift and then proceeded to ask his patient to explore his motivations in offering the gift. His reasons for accepting the cigars were more obvious than the patient's unconscious reason for giving them, about which there is no information.

Harm to the patient is not a component of a boundary violation. For example, using information supplied by the patient (e.g., a stock tip) is an unethical boundary violation, although no obvious harm may come to the patient. For purposes of discussion, nonsexual boundary violations may be grouped into several arbitrary (overlapping and not mutually exclusive) categories.

Business. Almost any business relationship with a former patient is problematic, and almost any business relationship with a current patient is unethical. Naturally, the circumstance and location may play a significant role in this admonition. In a rural area or a small community, one might be treating the only pharmacist (or plumber or couch upholsterer) in town; then one does business with the pharmacist/patient and tries to keep boundaries in check. Ethical psychiatrists try to avoid doing business with a patient or a patient's family member or asking a patient to hire one of their family members. Ethical psychiatrists avoid investing in a patient's business or collaborating with a patient in a business deal.

Ideological Issues. Ideological issues can cloud one's judgment and may lead to ethical lapses. Any clinical decision should be based on what is best for the patient; the psychiatrist's ideology should play as little a part as possible in such a decision. The ethical psychiatrist, then, must attend to current research, new approaches, and the results of such approaches. An obvious example of this problem is the psychiatrist who is convinced that an analytic approach is the only way to treat such conditions as major depression, bipolar disorder, and schizophrenia. Current research suggests that other approaches are as useful or more useful in many cases. The patient's welfare and the patient's wishes must be considered in such a situation. A psychiatrist who is consulted by a patient with an illness such as this should tell the patient what forms of treatment are available to treat the illness and allow the patient to decide upon a course of treatment. Naturally, psychiatrists should recommend the treatment that they feel is in the best interest of the patient, but ultimately, the patient should be free to choose.

Social. The particular locale and circumstances must be considered in any discussion of the behavior of an ethical psychiatrist in social situations. The overarching principle is that the boundaries of the psychiatrist–patient relationship should be respected. Further, if options exist, they should be exercised in favor of the patient. Problems often arise in treatment situations when friendships develop between the psychiatrist and the patient. Objectivity is compromised, therapeutic neutrality is impaired, and factors outside the consciousness of either party may play a destructive role. Such friendship should be avoided during treatment. Similarly, psychiatrists should not treat their social friends for the same set of reasons. Obviously, in an emergency, one does what one must.

Financial. For psychiatrists who practice in the private sector, dealing with the patient about money is a part of treatment. Issues surrounding setting the fee, collecting the fee, and other financial matters are grist for the mill. Even so, ethical concerns must be observed. *The Principles* advises the doctor on such matters as charging for missed appointments and other contractual problems. Ethics complaints against doctors are frequently precipitated by financial issues; thus the doctor must recognize the power that these issues have in the therapeutic relationship. Since the psychotherapeutic relationship is so much like a social relationship—the office looks like a living room, the doctor wears regular clothes, some patients might, without recognizing it, assume that a friendship exists that forgives payment of a fee. When the bill is presented, feelings, even though they are unconscious, are ruffled. The idea that psychiatric services are dispensed in a contractual context cannot be emphasized enough. Early in their careers psychiatrists are often reluctant to discuss fees openly out of a sense of embarrassment over discussing money or a sense of protecting the patient.

How an ethical psychiatrist handles the situation when a patient temporarily or permanently runs out of money is important. There are many options—some more problematic than others. The psychiatrist can certainly lower the fee, but caution is needed because a fee lowered to the point where the treatment is not somehow being compensated may evoke countertransference resentment. The number of patients being seen at a reduced fee is a similar consideration. Running up a bill can also be a problem. Is there an expectation of eventually being paid? Is the hypertrophic bill a sham? The frequency of sessions may have to be altered. Any psychiatrist who sees private patients will definitely face these problems.

Confidentiality

> All that may come to my knowledge in the exercise of my profession or outside of my profession or in the daily

commerce with men, which ought not to be spread abroad, I will keep secret and will never reveal.

Hippocrates

No provider of health care shall disclose medical information regarding a patient of the provider without first obtaining an authorization.

California Civil Code 56.10(a)

The identification of a person as a patient must be protected with extreme care. A psychiatrist may release confidential information only with the authorization of the patient or under proper legal compulsion.

The Principles

Although the medical profession overall is bound by rules of confidentiality—from Hippocrates to current state law—such rules seem to apply especially to the field of psychiatry. Psychiatrists are generally not troubled by hearing an internist ask a patient at a cocktail party how the new antihypertensive medicine is working out. However, psychiatrists are quite concerned if a psychiatrist in a similar situation asks a patient how he or she is doing with the new antipsychotic medicine. Psychiatrists take in stride the orthopedist who comments on an athlete's rotator cuff injury (his or her patient or not) but are outraged if a psychiatrist comments on a celebrity's substance abuse problem (his or her patient or not). Both psychiatrists and the public have every right to be outraged, and one can only wonder why the outrage does not apply to the internist and the orthopedist.

Patients expect confidentiality from psychiatrists, and patients own the confidentiality. That confidentiality survives even the death of the patient and is subsequently owned by the executor, not by the psychiatrist. A confidence cannot be broken just because the patient died. Psychiatrists must guard diligently against breaking confidences even with a release if that release was not signed by someone in an informed state of mind. A blanket release of information, often signed upon applying for insurance, submitting a claim, entering a hospital, and similar circumstances, is not an informed consent. The psychiatrist must ensure that release of information applies to the situation at hand. It is often suggested that whenever a request for information about a patient appears, the doctor should call the patient to verify consent to the disclosure.

Frequently psychiatrists get official-looking documents with the words "Subpoena Duces Tecum" on top and a signature at the bottom directing them to allow certain records to be copied or commanding them to produce the records somewhere. Most such documents do not come from a court, but from a lawyer's office. If there is any question that the patient has not consented to such disclosures and has not signed an informed consent to release such records, the ethical psychiatrist should contact the patient and come to some understanding. Patients who do not wish such records released may wish to have their lawyer attempt to quash the subpoena. Failing that, the psychiatrist may wish to ask the court to uphold the patient's right to privacy or at least determine what must (and what must not) be released. In certain jurisdictions patients may waive their right to privacy and confidentiality under certain circumstances (e.g., bringing their own mental state into a lawsuit). It is not within the psychiatrist's field of expertise to determine if the patient has waived that right. It is the job of the patient's lawyer, a judge, or both.

Overall, psychiatrists should never discuss their patients outside the office. Some psychiatrists feel that it is all right to discuss cases at the dinner table with their spouse and family. "After all," they say, "I trust my spouse and kids." However, trust is beside the point. Patients assume that what they tell the psychiatrist stays inside the consulting room. Merely informing a spouse of the identity of one's patient violates the ethical principles.

Dealing with the Press

Section 7.3 of *The Principles* is quite specific about doctors talking about mental illness. Psychiatrists may comment on mental illness generally but may not offer opinions about either their patient(s) or a person who is not their patient.

In 1964, Barry Goldwater, an outspoken, conservative man, ran for president of the United States. A magazine sent a questionnaire to nearly all the psychiatrists in the United States asking, "Do you believe Goldwater is psychologically fit to serve as President of the United States?" The magazine sent out 12,356 questionnaires and received 2,417 responses. Of these, 1,189 psychiatrists said the candidate was not psychologically fit to serve as president. The cover of the magazine ran its main story with the title "1,189 Psychiatrists Say Goldwater is Psychologically Unfit to be President!" How many of these psychiatrists actually examined the candidate? How many of them obtained permission to reveal the results of their examination? On what basis, then, did so many outstanding psychiatrists lose their moral bearings and offer a psychiatric or medical opinion on this man's mental state? By reading about him in the newspaper? By watching him on TV? The authors of *The Principles,* which was written 9 years later in 1973, considered this event when they wrote Section 7.3.

Ethics in Managed Care

Recent changes in how psychiatrists are compensated for their services have stimulated much criticism of both the managed care industry and the doctors who work in and for it. Some claim that the inner conflicts caused by working in a managed care environment are insurmountable. Some have declared that participating in a managed care scheme is per se unethical. Others, while lamenting the existence of managed care, have said that one can function ethically in such an environment. A significant number of psychiatrists believe that managed care provides the answer to overuse of limited services, contains costs, and offers the opportunity for outcome studies. There may be some truth to each point of view.

The ethical principles provide a clear course for the psychiatrist to follow regarding managed care. *The Principles,* Section 1, annotation 1, states, "A psychiatrist shall not gratify his or her own needs by exploiting a patient." This clearly applies in both the fee-for-service environment and the managed care environment. Thus, it would be unethical for psychiatrists working as managed care reviewers to deny needed care to patients on the basis of their employer's cost-containment policy rather than on the honest belief that they did not require the service. On the same principle, it would be unethical for a treating psychiatrist to dishonestly claim that a patient was suicidal (if that were not the case) to obtain payment for services that the treating psychiatrist believes is necessary.

Impaired Physicians

A physician may become impaired as the result of psychiatric or medical disorders or the use of mind-altering and habit-forming substances (e.g., alcohol and drugs). Many organic illnesses can interfere with the cognitive and motor skills required to provide competent medical care. Although the legal responsibility to report an impaired physician varies, depending on the state, the ethical responsibility remains universal. An incapacitated physician should be reported to an appropriate authority, and the reporting physician is required to follow specific hospital, state, and legal procedures. A physician who treats an impaired physician should not be required to monitor the impaired physician's progress or fitness to return to work. This monitoring should be performed by an independent physician or group of physicians who have no conflicts of interest.

The Office of Professional Medical Conduct (OPMC) in New York State regulates the practice of medicine by investigating illegal or unethical practice by physicians and other health professionals, such as physician assistants. Similar regulatory agencies exist in other states. Professional misconduct in New York State is defined as one of the following:

1. Practicing fraudulently and with gross negligence or incompetence.
2. Practicing while the ability to practice is impaired.
3. Being habitually drunk or being dependent on, or a habitual user of, narcotics or a habitual user of other drugs having similar effects.
4. Immoral conduct in the practice of the profession.
5. Permitting, aiding, or abetting an unlicensed person to perform activities requiring a license.
6. Refusing a client or patient service because of creed, color, or national origin.
7. Practicing beyond the scope of practice permitted by law.
8. Being convicted of a crime or being the subject of disciplinary action in another jurisdiction.

Professional misconduct complaints derive mainly from the public in addition to insurance companies, law enforcement agencies, and doctors, among others.

Physicians in Training

It is unethical to delegate authority for patient care to anyone who is not appropriately qualified and experienced, such as a medical student or a resident, without adequate supervision from an attending physician. Residents are physicians in training and, as such, must provide a good deal of patient care. Within a healthy, ethical teaching environment, residents and medical students may be involved with, and responsible for, the day-to-day care of many ill patients, but they are supervised, supported, and directed by highly trained and experienced physicians. Patients have the right to know the level of training of their care providers and should be informed about the resident's or medical student's level of training. Residents and medical students should know and acknowledge their limitations and should ask for supervision from experienced colleagues as necessary.

Table 58–2
Physician Charter of Professionalism

Fundamental principles

- **Primacy of patient welfare.** Altruism contributes to the trust central to doctor–patient relationships. Market forces, societal pressures, and administrative exigencies must not compromise this principle.
- **Patient autonomy.** Physicians must be honest with patients and empower them to make informed decisions about treatment.
- **Social justice.** Physicians should work actively to eliminate discrimination in health care whether based on race, gender, socioeconomic status, ethnicity, religion, or any other social category.

A set of commitments

- **Professional competence.** Physicians must be committed to lifelong learning. The profession, as a whole, must strive to see that all of its members are competent.
- **Honesty with patients.** Physicians must ensure that patients are completely and honestly informed before consenting to a treatment; they must be empowered to decide about the course of therapy. Physicians should also acknowledge that medical errors that injure patients sometimes occur. If a patient is injured through error, he or she should be informed promptly, since failure to do so seriously compromises patient and societal trust.
- **Patient confidentiality.** Fulfilling the commitment to confidentiality is more pressing now than ever before, given the widespread use of electronic information systems for compiling patient data.
- **Maintaining appropriate relations with patients.** Physicians should never exploit patients for any sexual advantage, personal financial gain, or other private purpose.
- **Improving quality of care.** This commitment entails not only maintaining clinical competence, but working collaboratively with other professionals to reduce medical error, increase patient safety, minimize overuse of health care resources, and optimize the outcomes of care.
- **Improving access to care.** Physicians must individually and collectively strive to reduce barriers to equitable health care.
- **Just distribution of finite resources.** Physicians should be committed to working with other physicians, hospitals, and payers to develop guidelines for cost-effective care. The physician's professional responsibility for appropriate allocation of resources requires scrupulous avoidance of superfluous tests and procedures.
- **Scientific knowledge.** Physicians have a duty to uphold scientific standards, to promote research, and to create new knowledge and ensure its appropriate use.
- **Maintaining trust by managing conflicts of interest.** Physicians have an obligation to recognize, disclose to the general public, and address conflicts of interest. Relationships between industry and opinion leaders should be disclosed.
- **Professional responsibilities.** Physicians are expected to participate in the process of self-regulation, including remediation and discipline of members who have failed to meet professional standards.

Physician Charter of Professionalism

In 2001, a movement to clarify the concept of "professionalism" was begun by the American Board of Internal Medicine. A set of principles called the *Physician Charter of Professionalism* was developed, which describes what it means for physicians to perform at their highest and most ethical level. Table 58–2 lists the principles and commitments of professional behaviors in the *Physician Charter of Professionalism* to which all physicians (including psychiatrists) are expected to adhere.

A summary of ethical issues discussed in this section is presented in a question-and-answer format in Table 58–3.

Table 58–3
Ethical Questions and Answers

Topic	Question	Answer
Abandonment	How can psychiatrists avoid being charged with patient abandonment upon retirement?	Retiring psychiatrists are not abandoning patients if they provide their patients with sufficient notice and make every reasonable effort to find follow-up care for the patients.
	Is it ethical to provide only outpatient care to a seriously ill patient, who may require hospitalization?	This could constitute abandonment unless the outpatient practitioner or agency arranges for their patients to receive inpatient care from another provider.
Bequests	A dying patient bequeaths his or her estate to his or her treating psychiatrist. Is this ethical?	No. Accepting the bequest seems improper and exploitational of the therapeutic relationship. However, it may be ethical to accept a token bequest from a deceased patient who named his or her psychiatrist in the will without that psychiatrist's knowledge.
Competency	Is it ethical for psychiatrists to perform vaginal exams? Hospital physicals?	Psychiatrists may provide nonpsychiatric medical procedures if they are competent to do so and if the procedures do not preclude effective psychiatric treatment by distorting the transference. Pelvic exams carry a high risk of distorting the transference and would be better performed by another clinician.
	Can ethics committees review issues of physician competency?	Yes. Incompetency is an ethical issue.
Confidentiality	Must confidentiality be maintained after the death of a patient?	Yes. Ethically, confidences survive a patient's death. Exceptions include protecting others from imminent harm or proper legal compulsions.
	Is it ethical to release information about a patient to an insurance company?	Yes, if the information provided is limited to that which is needed to process the insurance claim.
	Can a videotaped segment of a therapy session be used at a workshop for professionals?	Yes, if informed, uncoerced consent has been obtained, anonymity is maintained, the audience is advised that editing makes this an incomplete session, and the patient knows the purpose of the videotape.
	Should a physician report mere suspicion of child abuse in a state requiring reporting of child abuse?	No. A physician must make several assessments before deciding whether to report suspected abuse. One must consider whether abuse is ongoing, whether abuse is responsive to treatment, and whether reporting will cause potential harm. Check specific statutes. Make safety for potential victims the top priority.
Conflict of interest	Is there a potential ethical conflict if a psychiatrist has both psychotherapeutic and administrative duties in dealing with students or trainees?	Yes. You must define your role in advance to the trainees or students. Administrative opinions should be obtained from a psychiatrist who is not involved in a treatment relationship with the trainee or student.
Diagnosis without examination	Is it ethical to offer a diagnosis based only upon review of records to determine, for insurance purposes, if suicide was the result of illness?	Yes.
	Is it ethical for a supervising psychiatrist to sign a diagnosis on an insurance form for services provided by a supervisee when the psychiatrist has not examined the patient?	Yes, if the psychiatrist ensures that proper care is given and the insurance form clearly indicates the role of supervisor and supervisee.
Exploitation (also see Bequests)	What constitutes exploitation of the therapeutic relationship?	Exploitation occurs when the psychiatrist uses the therapeutic relationship for personal gain. This includes adopting or hiring a patient as well as sexual or financial relationships.
Fee splitting	What is fee splitting?	Fee splitting occurs when one physician pays another for a patient referral. This would also apply to lawyers giving a forensic psychiatrist referrals in exchange for a percentage of the fee. Fee splitting may occur in an office setting if the psychiatrist takes a percentage of his or her office-mates' fees for supervision or expenses. Costs for such items or services must be arranged separately. Otherwise, it would appear that the office owner could benefit from referring patients to a colleague in the office. Fee splitting is illegal.
Informed consent	Is it ethical to refuse to divulge information about a patient who has agreed to give this information to those requesting it?	No. It is the patient's decision, not the therapist's.
	Is informed consent needed when presenting or writing about case material?	Not if the patient is aware of the supervisory/teaching process and confidentiality is preserved.
Moonlighting	Can psychiatric residents ethically "moonlight"?	They can if their duties are not beyond their ability, if they are properly supervised, and if the moonlighting does not interfere with their residency training.

(*continued*)

Table 58–3 (*continued*)

Topic	Question	Answer
Reporting	Should psychiatrists expose or report unethical behavior of a colleague or colleagues? Can a spouse bring an ethical complaint?	Psychiatrists are obligated to report colleagues' unethical behavior. A spouse with knowledge of unethical behavior can bring an ethical complaint as well.
Research	How can ethical research be performed with subjects who cannot give informed consent?	Consent can be given by a legal guardian or via a living will. Incompetent persons have the right to withdraw from the research project at any time.
Retirement	See Abandonment.	
Supervision	What are the ethical requirements when a psychiatrist supervises other mental health professionals?	The psychiatrist must spend sufficient time to ensure that proper care is given and that the supervisee is not providing services that are outside the scope of his or her training. It is ethical to charge a fee for supervision.
Taping and recording	Can videotapes of patient interviews be used for training purposes on a national level (e.g., workshops, board exam preparation)?	Appropriate and explicit informed consent must be obtained. The purpose and scope of exposure of the tape must be emphasized in addition to the resulting loss of confidentiality.

Table by Eugene Rubin, M.D. (Data derived from American Psychiatric Association. *Opinions of the Ethics Committee on the Principles of Medical Ethics with Annotations Especially Applicable to Psychiatry.* Washington, DC: American Psychiatric Association; 1995.)

References

American Psychiatric Association. *Opinions of the Ethics Committee on the Principles of Medical Ethics with Annotations Especially for Psychiatry.* Washington, DC: American Psychiatric Association; 1993.

American Psychiatric Association. *The Principles of Medical Ethics with Annotations Especially for Psychiatry.* Washington, DC: American Psychiatric Association; 1995.

Block S, Chodoff P, eds. *Psychiatric Ethics.* New York: Oxford University Press; 1993.

Dunn LB, Jeste DV. Enhancing informed consent for research and treatment. *Neuropsychopharmacology.* 2001;24:595.

Epstein RS. *Keeping Boundaries: Maintaining Safety and Integrity in the Psychotherapeutic Process.* Washington, DC: American Psychiatric Press; 1994.

Epstein RS, Simon RI, Kay GG. Assessing boundary violations in psychotherapy: survey results with the Exploitation Index. *Bull Menninger Clin.* 1992;56:150.

Farber S, Green M. *Hollywood on the Couch.* New York: William Morrow; 1993.

Gabbard GO. *Sexual Exploitation in Professional Relationships.* Washington, DC: American Psychiatric Press; 1989.

Gabbard GO, Lester EP. *Boundaries and Boundary Violations in Psychoanalysis.* New York: Basic Books; 1996.

Gruenberg PB. Nonsexual exploitation of patients—an ethical perspective. *J Am Acad Psychoanal.* 1995;23:425.

Gruenberg PB. Ethics in psychiatry In: Sadock BJ, Sadock VA, eds. *Kaplan & Sadock's Comprehensive Textbook of Psychiatry.* 7th ed. Vol 2. Baltimore: Lippincott Williams & Wilkins; 2000:3290.

Gutheil TG, Gabbard GO. The concept of boundaries in clinical practice: theoretical and risk management dimensions. *Am J Psychiatry.* 1993;150:188.

Kupfer DJ, Frank E. Placebo in clinical trials for depression: complexity and necessity. *JAMA.* 2002;287:1853.

Lindsay G, Clarkson P. Ethical dilemmas of psychotherapists. *Psychologist.* 1999;12:182.

Mender D. Moral dilemmas faced by psychiatrists. *Am J Psychiatry.* 2002; 159:1443.

Schoener GR, Milgrom JH, Gonsiorek JC, Luepker ET, Conroe RM. *Psychotherapists' Sexual Involvement with Clients: Intervention and Prevention.* Minneapolis: Walk-in Counseling Center; 1989.

Vestig B. Annals of Internal Medicine's Harold Sax, M.D. describes Physician Charter of Professionalism. *JAMA.* 2001;266:3096.

Waldinger RJ. Boundary crossings and boundary violations: thoughts on navigating a slippery slope. *Harv Rev Psychiatry.* 1994;2:225.

59

Public and Hospital Psychiatry

PUBLIC PSYCHIATRY

Public psychiatry encompasses all mental health service systems that are primarily sponsored and funded by governments—federal, state, and local. It is no longer appropriate to conceptualize hospital and community services as separate treatment systems; they are integral components of the spectrum of services essential to any public mental health treatment system. All aspects of care from hospitalization, case management, and crisis intervention to day treatment and supportive living arrangements are the province of public psychiatry. Services may be provided directly by civil servants or contracted by government to either nonprofit or for-profit agencies. The essential feature is that all services are the responsibility of government and are offered to those who do not have the means to provide for their own care.

The present idea of public psychiatry was largely shaped by federal regulations passed in the 1960s to offer persons who were mentally ill financial support in their communities and to establish community mental health centers. Rather than isolating persons with mental disorders for long periods in state hospitals (Fig. 59–1), legislators thought it preferable to treat these persons in the community and to hospitalize them only briefly and under certain restrictions.

One unfortunate result of this approach is the numerous homeless, mentally ill persons who would once have lived in state institutions but are now left to the understaffed, financially limited, often grossly inadequate public health services. Public psychiatry must grapple with the almost unsolvable problem of providing these persons with continuous, comprehensive integrated care at a time when federal, state, and local budgets are sharply curtailed.

COMMUNITY MENTAL HEALTH

In 1963, under the leadership of President John F. Kennedy, Congress passed the Community Mental Health Centers Act, which provided funds for the construction of community mental health centers with specified catchment areas (geographical regions with a population of 75,000 to 200,000). Each community health center must provide five basic psychiatric services: inpatient care, emergency services (on a 24-hour basis), community consultation, day care (including partial hospitalization programs, halfway houses, aftercare services, and a broad range of outpatient services), and research and education. In 1975, Congress added the requirements of services for children and older persons, prehospitalization, screening, follow-up services for those who have been hospitalized, transitional housing, and alcoholism and drug-abuse services to the community centers' responsibilities. By the early 1980s, the community mental health center movement had strongly influenced mental health services, the practice of psychiatry, and the other mental health professions.

Eventually, a block grant program was created to provide federal funds to states for drug abuse, alcohol abuse, and other mental health programs. Several states established community support systems to help furnish needed mental health services; these programs are currently available nationwide. In spite of such efforts, state mental hospitals still receive most state-allocated mental health dollars, and financial limitations have interfered with the block grant and state programs.

BASIC CONCEPTS IN COMMUNITY MENTAL HEALTH

Commitment

Commitment to a population's health care implies a responsibility for planning. Commitment suggests that the plan should identify all the mental health needs of the population, inventory the resources available to meet these needs, and organize a system of care; that citizens and political figures should be involved in the planning process; that prevention is at least as important as direct treatment; and that all the population, including children, older persons, minorities, persons who are chronically and acutely ill, and those who live in geographically remote areas, should receive care. The federal requirement that mental health services be located close to persons' residences or workplaces is meant to make it easy for persons to get treatment and to identify illness early so that hospitalization, when required, is likely brief.

Services

Public mental health is a total system, not a single service. To be effective, services must be integrated and balanced, so that appropriate treatment modalities are available to fit patients' needs. A lack of services in one area (e.g., community placements) can delay other services (e.g., hospital discharges) and can lead to lack of services for some patients (e.g., those who cannot gain admission to overcrowded hospitals). A central authority must provide the needed integration.

The public mental health team includes psychiatrists (including child psychiatrists), clinical psychologists, psychiatric social workers, psychiatric nurses, administrative and clerical staff members, and occupational and recreational therapists for inpatient and partial hospitalization programs. Links to welfare workers, the clergy, family agencies, schools, and other human services groups are also maintained.

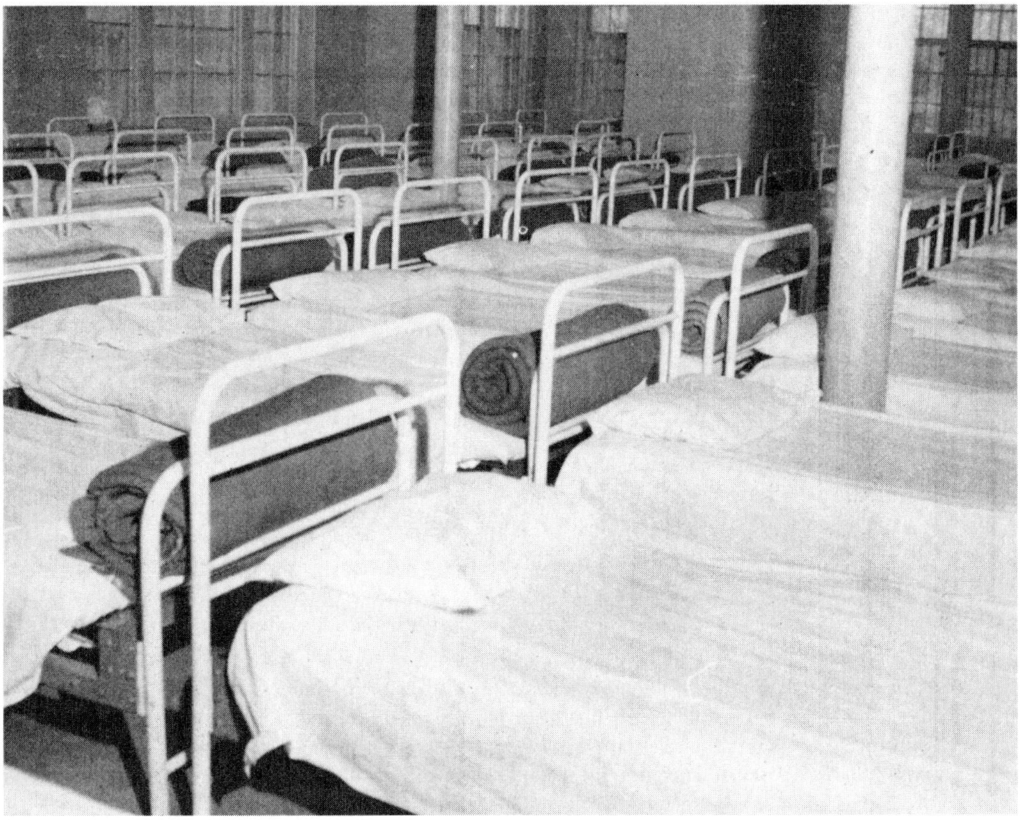

FIGURE 59–1
The crowded sleeping area in this illustration of a state hospital ward in the 1960s was antitherapeutic and exerted an unfavorable influence on both patients and staff. (National Association of Mental Health, New York.)

Long-Term Care. Because of concerns about the fragmentation of care and the tendency to keep patients hospitalized or unnecessarily restricted to one type of service, public mental health programs must encourage continuity of care. Continuity of care enables a single clinician to follow a patient through emergency services, hospitalization, partial hospitalization as a transition to the community, and outpatient treatment as follow-up. Continuity also provides an exchange of information and team responsibility for the patient when various therapists, for reasons of convenience or economy, treat the patient in several settings. A free exchange of clinical information between centers and a liaison between agencies are also part of the total system of care.

Case Management. Intensive case managers are clinicians who can provide continuity of care by following patients through all the phases of treatment while helping them negotiate a complex and fragmented system. Intensive case managers provide support, advocacy, and systems management. They engage patients in treatment through outreach in single-room-occupancy residences and shelters; they ensure continuing treatment by initiating contact during hospitalization and continuing support through aftercare; and they serve as liaisons between patients and other mental health providers and between the providers themselves. Ideally, intensive care managers should have small caseloads that allow intensive contact with their patients.

Community Participation. Communities should participate in decisions about their mental health care needs and programs instead of having them defined solely by professionals. Mental health services are sensitive to the needs of those served when the public is actively involved. The National Mental Health Association (NMHA) and the National Alliance for the Mentally Ill (NAMI) are two lay advocacy groups working at local, state, and national levels to improve care for persons who are mentally ill. Liaisons with these groups can provide links to the general public and facilitate outreach and educational efforts.

Consultation. Consultations range from attention to, or treatment of, a person's emotional problems to using knowledge about human behavior to help organizations achieve their professional goals with their programs and patients. Consultants offer assistance to mental health professionals who work in outpatient centers or agencies and also provide direct educational activities, liaison with consumer and advocacy groups, and administrative services.

Evaluation and Research. *Evaluation* is the process of obtaining information about a total community mental health program and its effects on people, institutions, and communities. Program evaluation should also provide feedback to planners and decision makers, so that operating programs can be modified and new ones planned. Evaluation is required for federally funded centers, which must spend at least 2 percent of their budgets on it. Research may focus specifically on key issues rather than on a total program and may address a particular disorder or a treatment method.

Least Restrictive Alternatives. The well-accepted concept of *least restrictive alternatives* means that mentally ill persons should be treated in settings that interfere least with their civil rights and freedom to participate in society. Patients should not be hospitalized (especially against their will in locked facilities) if their illness can be treated in a more open setting. Most states now have legislation protecting the rights of patients, and treatment in the least restrictive setting is usually one of those rights.

How far the concept of least restrictive care should be carried remains controversial. Patient rights advocates argue that this is the overriding principle, even if the therapeutic potential of the least restrictive facility is seriously compromised. Clinicians argue that therapeutic efficacy is the greatest concern and that the least restrictive principle can be compromised in the interest of better treatment. One must consider carefully whether any restriction on a patient is for the convenience of the psychiatrist and staff or for the protection of the patient.

PREVENTION

The disabilities associated with chronic mental illness are major social, economic, and public health problems. In the United States, these disabilities afflict more than 3 million persons; they are costly and create suffering for those affected, their families, and society. Although the term *chronic mental illness* has traditionally been associated with older patients who have a long history of mental hospitalization, it has been broadened to include young adults with repeated episodes of mental disorders. Many of these persons have never been hospitalized, but their ability to lead productive lives in the community is severely impaired. Psychiatric rehabilitation addresses the medical, psychiatric, and social needs of persons who are persistently mentally ill.

Preventive psychiatry is part of public psychiatry. The goal of prevention is to decrease the onset (incidence), duration (prevalence), and residual disability of mental disorders. The prevention of mental disorders is based on public health principles and is divided into primary, secondary, and tertiary prevention.

Primary Prevention

The goal of *primary prevention* is to prevent the onset of a disease or disorder and thereby reduce its incidence (the ratio of new cases to the population in a specific period). This goal is reached by eliminating causative agents, reducing risk factors, enhancing host resistance, and interfering with disease transmission. For some physical disorders, the identification and modification of one or more of these factors revolutionized health care, exemplified by the virtual elimination of many infectious diseases and vitamin deficiency states and by the reduction of some forms of cancer, heart disease, and lung disease.

Examples of primary prevention to help persons cope with life include mental health education programs (e.g., parent training in child development and alcohol and drug education programs); efforts at competence building (e.g., Outward Bound, Head Start, and other enriched day-care programs for disadvantaged children); the development and use of social support systems to reduce the effects of stress on those at high risk (e.g., widow-to-widow programs); anticipatory guidance programs to assist persons to prepare for expected stressful situations (e.g., counseling Peace Corps volunteers); and crisis intervention after stressful life events, such as bereavement, marital separation, divorce, traumas, and group disasters. The hostage-release program, in which U.S. hostages released from captivity are prepared for reentry into society, is an example of primary prevention. The "debriefing" group programs for victims of the World Trade Center and Pentagon terrorist attacks that occurred on September 11, 2001, are examples of specific techniques used to prevent posttraumatic stress disorder.

Primary prevention programs also aim at eradicating stressful agents and reducing stress. Such programs include prenatal and perinatal care to decrease the incidence of mental retardation and cognitive disorders in children (e.g., advice about improved nutrition and abstinence from alcohol and other substances during pregnancy, improved obstetrical services, specific dietary modification for neonates vulnerable to phenylketonuria); strict lead-elimination laws to reduce the incidence of lead encephalopathy; modification of divorce, adoption, and child abuse laws to provide a healthy environment for child development; enrichment or replacement of institutional settings for infants, children, and older persons; modification of certain risk factors for mental disorders that appear to be associated with low socioeconomic status; genetic counseling for parents at high risk for chromosomal abnormalities to prevent the unwitting conception of compromised infants; and efforts to reduce the spread of certain sexually transmitted diseases (e.g., acquired immune deficiency syndrome [AIDS] and syphilis) that can lead to mental disorders.

Secondary Prevention

Secondary prevention is defined as the early identification and prompt treatment of an illness or disorder, with the goal of reducing the prevalence (the proportion of existing cases in the population at risk at a specified time) of the condition by shortening its duration. Crisis intervention and public education are components of secondary prevention. In psychiatry, secondary prevention targets children who are emotionally ill for early intervention. The National Institute of Mental Health's (NIMH) Child and Adolescent Services System identifies and treats these children to support their family structures and prevent or reduce later disability.

On a broader scale, secondary prevention is embodied in the work of most psychiatrists and other mental health professionals. All try to initiate treatment and alleviate suffering at the earliest possible moment. Crisis intervention theories and services are important attempts at secondary prevention. Efforts to educate the public and reduce stigma to allow persons to seek treatment earlier is also secondary prevention.

Tertiary Prevention

The goal of *tertiary prevention* is to reduce the prevalence of residual defects and disabilities caused by an illness or a disorder. In the case of mental disorders, tertiary prevention enables those with chronic mental illness to reach the highest feasible level of functioning. Tertiary prevention, or rehabilitation, in psychiatry nearly always addresses patients suffering from the most severe and debilitating illnesses—schizophrenia, the most severe affective disorders, and the most disabling personality disorders. All of these illnesses, especially schizophrenia, tend to strike in late adolescence and young adulthood. These individuals are effectively removed from society during those years when most persons complete their education, learn trades, establish careers, begin families, and develop social support systems in the community. Consequently, even if the illness were completely cured without any residual functional deficits, these persons would still need extensive social rehabilitation.

Unfortunately the illness leaves residuals in many cases. These persons can have a wide range of psychological deficits that impair their ability to interact with others, handle the usual stresses of daily life, and achieve their potential. Therefore, psychiatric rehabilitation involves a complex process in which the professional attempts to address the psychological, social, and often the medical needs of the patient simultaneously. Obviously, the better the patient's functioning in society can be maintained during the acute exacerbations of illness, the less psychosocial rehabilitation will be necessary. This is why modern public psychiatry attempts to limit the lengths of hospitalizations by rapid intervention and to maintain social support systems even when patients are acutely ill. Rehabilitation is often an ongoing dynamic process carried out for the patient's lifetime because of the chronic relapsing nature of many types of mental illness, especially schizophrenia.

DEINSTITUTIONALIZATION

Deinstitutionalization is the process by which large numbers of patients are discharged from public psychiatric hospitals back into the community to receive outpatient care. This policy, which began in the late 1950s, decreased the state psychiatric hospital population from more than 560,000 beds at that time to roughly 100,000 beds today. Many patients were released into various aftercare clinics, where they continued to receive psychiatric treatment and rehabilitative services. Others were placed in new types of institutions, such as halfway houses, board and care facilities, and public housing units. Many had to be rehospitalized, and a revolving-door policy developed, with up to 80 percent of patients being readmitted within 2 years of discharge.

Deinstitutionalized patients need extensive social support, such as vocational and recreational counseling, comprehensive psychiatric treatment, paying jobs, and affordable housing. This support has not been given to the extent that planners and supporters of deinstitutionalization think necessary, primarily because of the lack of adequate funding on federal, state, and local levels. It is scandalous that funding for aftercare community services for those who are mentally ill continues to decline; unless this trend is reversed, deinstitutionalization will remain a failed public policy. Some have suggested that the limited funds available be channeled into improving existing state hospitals, so that chronically mentally ill patients and homeless mentally ill persons can be referred to the system and receive appropriate care.

Transinstitutionalization

The transfer of state hospital patients to other facilities is known as *transinstitutionalization*. Many workers believe that one set of problem has been exchanged for another without solving the problems of persons who are chronically mentally ill. As the number of state hospital beds has been reduced, the number of general hospital psychiatric beds has increased to over 50,000, the number of private psychiatric beds has increased to 80,000, and the number of Department of Veterans Affairs (VA) beds has increased to 25,000.

A significant percentage of persons who are mentally ill receive psychiatric services as prison inmates, and incarceration remains a significant component of transinstitutionalization. One study estimated that 31 percent of mentally ill persons in an urban jail were homeless before arrest. Severe mental illness is two to three times more prevalent in prison populations than among the general public. Many of the incarcerated homeless mentally ill persons are arrested for minor crimes that are survival strategies (e.g., trespassing in buildings or cars as a means of obtaining shelter) or for behavior directly produced by psychosis.

Several studies have found that without an active, multifaceted treatment system that assumes ongoing responsibility for all facets of patients' care, mentally ill patients regress in the community as they did in state hospitals. A major problem faced by chronically ill patients is that their illnesses interfere with their coping skills and render them particularly likely to drift downward into even more stressful, impoverished environments. The end result is an increase in homeless persons in urban areas.

HOMELESS MENTALLY ILL PERSONS

The homeless mentally ill population continues to grow; one major survey found a 7 percent rise in urban homeless persons who are mentally ill over a 19-month period, with a concurrent decline in the number of shelter beds. An average of 33 percent of homeless persons are mentally ill. The percentage ranges from 15 percent of homeless persons in Kansas City, Missouri, to 70 percent of homeless single adults in Boston. On average, 45 percent of homeless mentally ill persons are also dependent on alcohol or other substances. The estimated percentage of these persons with dual diagnoses ranges from 23 percent in Philadelphia to more than 60 percent in several major cities. There was a 9 percent rise in the number of dually diagnosed homeless persons during a recent 19-month period, with a concurrent increase in the average length of time of homelessness for those who are homeless and mentally ill.

Qualities of the Homeless

Like those who are chronically mentally ill, homeless mentally ill persons are a heterogeneous population, with no uniformity in diagnosis, demographics, functional performance, or residential history. One categorization divides them into street people, episodically homeless persons, and situationally homeless persons. Street people usually have schizophrenia or substance dependence or both, a history of psychiatric hospitalization, and a variety of health problems. Episodically homeless persons are usually younger than street people and are likely to be regarded as difficult patients with personality disorders, substance abuse, and mood disorders; they sporadically use a wide variety of mental health services. Situationally homeless persons have problems of situational stress more than of psychopathology.

Homeless mentally ill persons are not simply undomiciled. They are often totally disaffiliated, with few, if any, links to the community. They are unemployed, socially isolated, and out of contact with their families. Homeless women may be more likely than men to have intact social skills and social networks. In general, homeless mentally ill persons are difficult to treat because of their high levels of withdrawal and suspicion, psychopathology, homeless lifestyle, or negative past experiences with the mental health system.

In one group of homeless mentally ill patients studied, most suffered from schizophrenia and schizoaffective disorder. Many had histories of alcohol and other substance abuse. Close to one

third had concomitant physical illnesses that were secondary to alcohol dependence. The patients also suffered from significant medical problems, including anemia, lice infestation, nutritional deficiencies (B_{12}, folate, and iron deficiencies), cellulitis, and evidence of exposure to, and an increased incidence of, tuberculosis.

A 35-year-old man with a 10-year history of paranoid schizophrenia complicated by alcohol abuse resided in a city-run shelter, where he was identified as psychotic on the basis of his bizarre behavior related to hallucinations. He was enrolled in an intensive case management program. Through repeated outreach efforts, his intensive case manager helped him obtain benefits and begin treatment with fluphenazine (Prolixin), as prescribed by a visiting psychiatrist.

After the patient stabilized, his intensive case manager placed him in a supportive residence with on-site social workers and psychiatric staff members. The residence acted as the representative payee of the patient's entitlement check. At the same time, the patient attended an intensive program for mentally ill substance abusers at a nearby city hospital. He remained in the program and continued taking his medication for 2 years before leaving the program because of his desire for more control over his finances.

One year later, an outreach team found him posturing bizarrely and talking to himself in a city train terminal. He accepted a sandwich and voluntary transport to a specialized ward for the treatment of homeless mentally ill persons. After stabilization, he was transferred to a state hospital for intermediate care. As his insight into the interplay of his psychiatric illness and his alcohol abuse improved, community placement was sought.

Treatment

Some persons who are homeless and mentally ill remain within geographical limits; others travel from one part of the country to another. Because demography, epidemiology, history, and treatment needs vary, no single treatment method is recommended. In addition to the full range of traditional services—evaluation, crisis intervention, medication review, psychosocial skills training, and housing—homeless mentally ill patients may require less traditional services, such as a mailbox where welfare checks can be delivered, bathing facilities, and delousing services.

Traditional mental health service systems may present barriers to access for homeless mentally ill persons. Sometimes the barriers are simply the result of a lack of services to meet patients' special needs or of geographical or functional limitations. Housing programs for chronically mentally ill persons are often limited to high-functioning patients and screen out poorly functioning street people. Effective service programs include provisions for shelter and food, drop-in centers, outreach contact, and a cooperative endeavor between mental health agencies and other agencies in the community (e.g., the Salvation Army and church-affiliated organizations).

Homeless mentally ill persons can be treated through outreach programs and treatment geared to their specific needs. Effective treatment can be achieved with appropriate community placements and mentally ill substance abuser programs. Many patients cannot function in the community, even with significant support, and long-term state hospitalization may be the only way to safeguard their well-being. Governments must accept this reality if the patients' needs are to be met.

Outreach Programs

Street outreach programs are crucial components in addressing the problems of homeless mentally ill persons, as many persons do not use shelters. Those who do use shelters require shelter-based outreach programs, because they rarely seek treatment by traditional routes.

Street outreach programs have succeeded by using a multidisciplinary team of psychiatrists, social workers, and nurses. They approach homeless mentally ill persons by making repeated brief contacts while offering food and concrete services as a means of engagement. Street people do not tolerate a standard psychiatric interview; therefore, assessment must be made by observation, with particular attention to self-care, bizarre behavior, possible physical problems, and changing trends in appearance or behavior over time. Collateral histories from the police and workers in the community are often valuable.

PSYCHOGERIATRIC LONG-TERM CARE

The elderly population will increase an estimated 125 percent by the year 2030 and will need 3 times the nursing home care now available. The cost of such care will grow from $44 billion in 1990 to an estimated $187 billion in 2030. The growing need for professional care results from the increasing proportion of older persons who will lack family supports. As a result, future long-term care financing is a major problem.

Some have suggested private-sector solutions, which include making long-term-care insurance affordable through tax incentives, insurance regulations, and an increased emphasis on the provision of home care as a substitute for nursing home care, to decrease insurance payments and premiums. Others have called for a national long-term-care program as part of a national health plan. At present, much of the burden of elderly long-term care falls on families: More than 70 percent of the persons receiving long-term care rely on unpaid caretakers. It is clear that sweeping changes in the financing and delivery of long-term care will be needed to meet the increasing needs of this growing portion of the population.

OUTPATIENT COMMITMENT PROGRAM (OCP)

Mental patients discharged from public hospitals are often noncompliant with attending outpatient clinics for continued psychosocial or psychopharmacological treatment. In 1993, a program was begun at Bellevue Hospital Center to provide involuntary outpatient treatment of mentally ill persons, the goals of which are to help patients live and function in the community and to avoid relapse resulting in rehospitalization. Involuntary outpatient treatment is mandated by a judge, and patients report to the clinic for medication, individual or group therapy, psychosocial therapy, and vocational training. In addition, living arrangements are made for the patient and a case

manager is assigned. The court may order medication if the patient cannot make a treatment decision. All court-mandated outpatient commitment procedures are made after the patient is evaluated by a psychiatrist. Noncompliance is minimal because of close supervision and the patient's preference for OCP over involuntary hospitalization.

An alternative to outpatient commitment, conservatorship, is used in many states. Conservators—usually not part of the treatment system and often family members—are given responsibility for the patients' well-being and varying amounts of authority over their life, up to and including the ability to place them in a locked facility if their condition demands such placement. Of course, treatment staff must agree that the patient needs to be admitted. Thus these patients are being admitted because of their condition, not as punishment for not complying with treatment.

HOSPITAL PSYCHIATRY

Hospital treatment characteristically involves a multidisciplinary group of mental health professionals. Each team member addresses different elements of the patient's difficulty: psychiatrist (medical or psychiatric, medication, psychotherapy), nurse and mental health technician (personal care and interaction), psychologist (diagnostic assessment of cognitive strengths and weaknesses, psychotherapy), social worker (relations with family), and activity therapist—occupational, recreational, music, (avocational and vocational skills). The diagnostic assessment and treatment of the patient are enhanced by the collaboration and integration of these multidisciplinary perspectives.

The phases of hospital treatment include (1) admission, (2) immediate assessment and intervention, (3) continued diagnostic evaluation and refinement, (4) clarification of treatment goals and discharge criteria, (5) progress toward and achievement of goals, (6) discharge, and (7) appropriate aftercare or follow-up. The impact of managed care review has shortened the time allotted for these phases. When the hospital has a full continuum of care, ranging from intensive inpatient treatment to partial hospital programs for aftercare, the phase will continue into the partial hospital period.

Each patient should have a well-defined master treatment plan that addresses the reason for admission and the need for hospitalization, an assessment of patient problems, patient's strengths and assets, formal diagnoses, discharge criteria, and anticipated placement and posthospital treatment. Further, the treatment plan should identify problems to be focused on by the members of the treatment team, particularly problems that reflect the primary reason for hospitalization. Generally, the problems will be evident in one or more of the following areas: self-concept, interpersonal relationships, thinking and cognition, emotional functioning, impulse regulations or addiction, adaptive skills, or family. Goals should be articulated in measurable terms so that the patient's progress can be readily observed by all members of the treatment team. Prescribed diagnostic and treatment modalities should be recorded, as well as which staff members are responsible for carrying out these tasks (Table 59–1).

Hospital treatment programs may be characterized by their length of stay, primary treatment modality, and treatment goals. Inpatient programs are generally categorized as (1) short-term crisis intervention (1 to 4 weeks) or (2) extended treatment (longer than 4 weeks). Partial hospitalization programs are gener-

Table 59–1
Indications for Brief Hospitalization and Extended Hospitalization

Brief Hospitalization	Extended Hospitalization
Severity of illness factors	
Danger to self or others, or	
Symptoms that are of sufficient severity to interfere with functioning in work or family life and that are unresponsive to outpatient treatment, or	Impulsive or psychotic symptomatology that is extraordinarily severe and unremitting, including severely impaired schizophrenia patients who do not respond to psychiatric drugs, patients with impulse-ridden personality disorders, and those with severe eating disorders.
Impulsive behavior uncontrolled by outpatient treatment, or	Pervasive and continual suicidal, self-destructive, or violent behavior that does not respond to less intensive treatments.
Noncompliance with outpatient treatment with a deteriorating clinical picture, or	Axis I disorders complicated by severe Axis II pathology, including treatment-refractory addictions.
Complex psychopathology in association with family dynamics that require comprehensive inpatient evaluation, or	
Dual-diagnosis patients who have substance abuse complicated by another psychiatric disorder or disorders, or	Patients with long-term schizophrenia who cannot function outside the hospital without extensive vocational and social rehabilitation efforts.
Life-threatening withdrawal syndromes, or	
Transference crisis interfering with continuity of outpatient treatment.	Treatment-defeating patients with borderline personality disorder, including those who passively refuse to cooperate with treatment, those who make unrelenting hateful attacks on treaters, and those who evoke countertransference reactions that are destructive to treatment.
Treatment factors	
History of good response to previous hospitalization, or	Failure of previous treatment efforts, including pharmacotherapy, psychotherapy, and brief hospitalization.
No previous hospitalization.	
No major treatment complications.	Major treatment complications.
Limited treatment goals.	Treatment goals involving intrapsychic change or significant vocational and social rehabilitation.
Environmental factors	
Supportive family systems, or	Family system that is chaotic, unsupportive, absent, or undermining treatment, or
Other posthospitalization support system that is in place or can be made readily available.	Lack of a viable posthospital support system.
Clear precipitating stressor.	

Adapted from Gabbard GO. Comparative indications for brief and extended hospitalization. In: Tasman A, Riba MB, eds. *Review of Psychiatry.* Vol 11. Washington, DC: American Psychiatric Press; 1992.

ally open-ended and may serve as a transition from inpatient to outpatient care or they may be entered directly. These programs include various combinations of day hospital supervision and activities and night accommodations—night hospital, halfway house, family care, cooperative housing, and independent living.

Short-Term Inpatient Programs. Short-term or brief hospitalization seeks to arrest and reverse emotional decompensation, alleviate acute mental illness, reduce symptoms, restore defenses, and facilitate readjustment of the patient to the prior environment. These goals are achieved by separating the patient from the environment with admission to the hospital, administering appropriate psychiatric medication, exploring and negotiating with significant others in the patient's life, and supportive and exploratory psychotherapy with the patient. Sometimes specialized treatment procedures such as electroconvulsive therapy (ECT) may be indicated. Short-term hospitalization may also be used for in-depth diagnostic patient evaluation. Short-term stays are possible when no untoward treatment complications arise and when posthospital resources or support systems are available, accessible, or rapidly developed.

Specialized or focused programs have been developed for a wide range of mental illnesses, such as alcohol or other substance abuse, eating disorders, and dissociative disorders. In the 1970s, the prototype of these programs was developed for the treatment of alcohol use disorders, including a time-limited treatment program consisting of patient education about all facets of the condition, group confession and confrontation, self-help groups (Alcoholics Anonymous), and social work with the family. Now, these programs may use the controlled environment of the hospital to curb the patient's impulse to pursue symptomatic behavior while providing psychotherapeutic, educational, social work, and rehabilitative support.

Extended-Treatment Programs. Extended-treatment programs remain necessary for difficult-to-treat illnesses that do not respond to brief intervention or short-term treatment. Longer-term treatment may be indicated when briefer treatments have failed, treatment complications are severe, a treatment alliance is absent or resisted, life stressors are so profound or persistent that they impair recompensation, or an extended period of treatment is needed to achieve any beneficial effect. Extended-treatment programs may be modeled after a psychoanalytic psychotherapeutic model, a therapeutic community model, a token economy behavioral treatment model, or a moral treatment custodial care model.

The psychoanalytic perspective views symptoms as a product of unconscious psychic conflict within the patient, a compromise formation that expresses both the unconscious drive derivative and the ego's defense against the impulse. The assumption is that all behavior is determined and has meaning. The psychoanalytic model of hospital treatment seeks to identify and resolve the conflicts and symptomatic ego defenses of the individual as they are played out in the interactions with other staff and patients in the hospital. As articulated by William Menninger:

> It is our hates and our mismanaged loves that account for most if not all of our emotional sickness. In other words, our reactions to the people about us and their reactions to us result in adjustment or in varying degrees of maladjustment. Similarly, within the hospital, it is the relationships with other human beings—with other patients and with the hospital personnel—and the understanding of these relationships which lead the patient back to emotional health. The hospital must provide a variety of opportunities for resolution of the patient's conflicts through his expressing his hate in appropriate or constructive ways, in his learning to find new or renewed satisfactions in his activities, in his learning to love and be loved.

The therapeutic community was originally introduced in England, conceived by T. F. Main, and popularized by Maxwell Jones. This model looks at the hospital unit as a social system. It seeks to optimize the patient's healthy functioning in a setting that levels the hierarchy of the hospital and involves patients in decision making on the unit. It places responsibility on the patients to serve as agents of change, with a significant role in the rehabilitation of other patients on the unit. This model depends upon older patients transmitting to newer patients the norms, skills, and values essential for meaningful participation in the therapeutic community. Jones' treatment program was primarily designed for patients with personality disorders. Therapeutic community approaches are more difficult to implement in units that treat a large number of psychotically disturbed patients, because groups may be overstimulating to them.

The token economy model applies principles derived from experimental psychology and operant conditioning, with token rewards used as positive reinforcement for desired behaviors. These programs are used with more regressed, lower-functioning, chronically ill patients. As the patients receive rewards for preferred, adaptive behavior, they can exchange the tokens for desired privileges and activities.

In all models of inpatient hospital treatment, psychiatric nursing plays an essential role. Nursing personnel provide the direct supervision of the patients and administer prescribed medication. They also provide for basic needs of the patients, offer organization and structure, give support and aid intrapsychic growth, assist patients with interpersonal and interactional skills, and promote coping skills in a teaching and learning environment.

Partial Hospitalization. Partial hospitalization offers an alternative to 24-hour hospitalization, with some structured treatment programs that represent a transitional care setting between hospital and community. For some chronically ill patients the partial hospitalization may continue for an extended period. Most programs provide an informal, clublike setting that facilitates social interaction, features therapeutic activities, and diminishes dependency and isolation. Patients have a case manager or treatment coordinator who functions as their advocate and facilitator. Rehabilitation and vocational programs include assistance with daily living skills, recreational activity, and job training. Other services provided are medication review, group therapy, family treatment, and crisis treatment.

CLINICAL ISSUES

Indications for Hospitalization. Indications for hospital treatment are determined by factors within the individual patient—severity of the illness, level of awareness or insight regarding the illness, and the capacity to contain impulsive,

destructive behavior—and factors in the environment such as presence or absence of support and intensity of ongoing stressors. In general, hospital treatment is indicated when patients are so severely disturbed that someone else must step in and protect them from harming self or others, and their environment cannot provide this protection. In recent years, various checklists of admission criteria have been published; essentially, a patient merits hospitalization when there are serious problems in three parameters: the degree of dangerousness, the adequacy of the support system, and the ability to cooperate with care.

Glen Gabbard has outlined comparative indications for brief and extended hospitalization according to a grid of (1) severity of illness factors, (2) treatment factors, and (3) environmental factors. Illness factors include the danger to self or others, the interference of symptoms with functioning in work or family and their responsiveness to outpatient treatment, impulsive or noncompliant behavior, and dual diagnosis, with substance abuse complicated by another psychiatric disorder. Relevant treatment factors are the history of any previous hospitalization and the response to any prior treatment, the presence of any treatment complications, and the goals of treatment. Environmental factors are the family system, the posthospital support system, and the existence of clear precipitating stressors.

With regard to criteria for hospitalization for children, a review of 375 children seen at the Western Psychiatric Institute and Clinic at the University of Pittsburgh identified six items that distinguished children who were hospitalized from those who were not:

1. Aggressive outbursts toward other persons
2. Aggressive outbursts toward animals or objects
3. Patient's condition was deteriorating rapidly or failing to improve despite adequate outpatient treatment
4. Physical or neurological conditions or a psychotic, disorganized state that requires hospitalization to initiate treatment or to establish a diagnosis
5. A pathological or noxious situation that exists among the patient's family or associates and makes treatment without hospitalization impossible, or the patient's disordered state creates such difficulties for the family that the patient has to be hospitalized
6. Evaluation of the patient's condition requires 24-hour observation and evaluation that only a hospital can provide, including stabilization or reevaluation of medication or treatment of drug or alcohol dependence

Patient's Family. The family both influences and is influenced by hospitalization of a family member. Rather than focus on a pathological interaction between patient and family, modern hospital treatment attempts to engage the family as a caring and concerned resource in the treatment process. Models have been developed for inpatient family intervention, initiating family therapy with the patient's hospitalization. This approach does not assume that the cause of major psychotic disorders lies in family functioning or communication, but rather that the present-day functioning of a family with which the patient is living or is in frequent contact can be a major source of stress or support. The intervention seeks to help the family understand, live with, and deal with the patient and the patient's illness. Psychoeducational workshops and multiple family group meetings are especially helpful to families of patients who are chronically mentally ill.

References

Bachrach LL. What we know about homelessness among mentally ill persons: an analytical review and commentary. *Hosp Community Psychiatry.* 1992;43:453.

Blumenthal D. Controlling health care expenditures. *N Engl J Med.* 2001;344:766.

Breakey WR, ed. *Integrated Mental Health Services: Modern Community Psychiatry.* New York: Oxford University Press; 1996.

Burns BJ, Taube JE, Permutt T, et al. Evaluation of a Maryland fiscal incentive plan for placing state hospital patients in nursing homes. *Hosp Community Psychiatry.* 1991;42:1228.

Cohen CI. Poverty, social problems, and serious mental illness. *Psychiatr Serv.* 2002;53:899.

Cummins RA. The subjective well-being of people caring for a family member with a severe disability at home: a review. *J Intellect Dev Disabil.* 2001;26:83.

Dencker K, Gottfries C-G. The closure of a major psychiatric hospital: can psychiatric patients in long-term care be integrated into existing nursing homes? *J Geriatr Psychiatry Neurol.* 1991;4:149.

Draper B. The effectiveness of old age psychiatry services. *Int J Geriatr Psychiatry.* 2000;15:687.

Elpers JR. Public psychiatry. In: Sadock BJ, Sadock VA, eds. *Kaplan & Sadock's Comprehensive Textbook of Psychiatry.* 7th ed. Vol 2. Baltimore: Lippincott Williams & Wilkins; 2000:3185.

Epstein AM. Health policy 2001—a new series. *N Engl J Med.* 2001;344:673.

Goering P, Wasylenski D, St. Onge M, Paduchak D, Lancee W. Gender differences among clients of a case management program for the homeless. *Hosp Community Psychiatry.* 1992;43:160.

Hess R, Morgan J, eds. *Prevention in Community Mental Health Centers.* New York: Haworth; 1990.

Kahn JG. Prospects for expanding health insurance coverage. *N Engl J Med.* 2001;344:1948.

Katz SE, Nardacci D, Sabatini A, eds. *Intensive Treatment of the Homeless Mentally Ill.* Washington, DC: American Psychiatric Press; 1993.

Kawas JCH, Brookmeyer R. Aging and the public health effects of dementia. *N Engl J Med.* 2001;344:1098.

Marshall EJ, Reed JL. Psychiatric morbidity in homeless women. *Br J Psychiatry.* 1992;160:761.

Moak GS, Fisher WH. Geriatric patients and services in state hospitals: data from a national survey. *Hosp Community Psychiatry.* 1992;42:273.

Moffic HS. Cultural issues in community psychiatry. In: Vaccaro JV, Clark GH Jr, eds. *Practicing Psychiatry in the Community: A Manual.* Washington, DC: American Psychiatric Press; 1996.

Moon M. Medicare. *N Engl J Med.* 2001;344:928.

Saathoff GB, Cortina JA, Jacobson R, Aldrich CK. Mortality among elderly patients discharged from a state hospital. *Hosp Community Psychiatry.* 1992;43:280.

Solomon PL, Drain JN, Marcenko MO, Meyerson AT. Homelessness in a mentally ill jail population. *Hosp Community Psychiatry.* 1992;43:169.

Stein REK. Home-based comprehensive care services for children with chronic conditions. *Child Serv Soc Policy Res Pract.* 2001;4:189.

60

Health Care Delivery in Psychiatry and Medicine

An ideal health care delivery system in the United States would provide high-quality, affordable medical care for all citizens while promoting medical research and new technology. Social and economic factors, however, significantly affect a nation's health status and the delivery of health services. *Health*, according to the World Health Organization (WHO), is not merely the absence of disease but a state of complete physical, mental, and social well-being. To affect the factors that shape a population's health, illness, and death rate, the population must be studied to ascertain health care needs, use, accessibility, and optimal financial allocations for delivery.

Currently, workers in health care emphasize prevention and promoting good health as well as diagnosing and treating medical disorders. Escalating health care costs, however, have become a significant obstacle to fulfilling the requirements of an ideal health care system. The need to focus on cost control affects distribution of funds, delivery of services, and mechanisms for reimbursing medical personnel for these services.

HEALTH CARE PROVIDERS

Health care providers include a broad array of persons from a variety of professions who care for the sick. In addition to physicians, health care personnel include nurses, dentists, psychologists, social workers, podiatrists, speech therapists, and occupational therapists. More than 11 million persons were employed in health-related occupations in 2001.

Physician Supply

In 2000, there were about 772,000 physicians, 155,000 dentists, and 2.1 million nurses practicing in the United States. The number of allopathic physicians in graduate medical education has been steady at 98,000 since the mid-1990s.

Primary care physicians are usually defined as general practitioners, family practitioners, internists, and pediatricians. *Primary care* is defined as a type of medical care delivery that emphasizes first-contact care and assumes ongoing responsibility for patients in both health maintenance and therapy. Gynecologists serve as the sole health care provider for many women. In 1998, there were 59 primary care physicians per 100,000 population. According to *JAMA,* the number of medical doctors in primary care training programs has increased about 25 percent from 1995 to 2000; however, their distribution remains a problem. High physician–patient ratios exist in the Northeast and in California; low concentrations of physicians are the norm in the South and in the mountain states. Many rural areas are without a primary care provider, and the government has made an attempt to staff underserved areas through loan reimbursements for medical personnel.

Female Physicians

The proportion of female physicians nearly tripled between 1970 and 1994, and by 2010, women will represent 30 percent of the physician workforce. Women accounted for 6,825 of the 15,000 allopathic medical school graduates in 2001 and represent 66 percent of pediatric and obstetrics-gynecology residents. Though 84 percent report they are at least "satisfied" with their career choice, 38 percent of women doctors reported to *JAMA* that they would reconsider their specialty choice if given the opportunity, particularly older physicians who may have had fewer opportunities to enter traditionally male-dominated fields during their training. Physicians practicing in a medical school environment were much more likely to be satisfied with their career choice; however, women have not been promoted as far as or paid as much as their male counterparts in medical academia.

Some 33 percent of female physicians report that they are the primary caretaker for their children under age 12, and women physicians are often penalized for having children, either during residency or by group practices without adequate maternity benefits. Some residency programs are more flexible than others, offering half-time status to new mothers and prorated pay; others allow vacation planning to coordinate with public schools to accommodate families, and allow women to spread training over 6 years rather than 3 or 4, depending on the specialty. These types of arrangements result in greater productivity for physicians and easier debt management and child rearing; they should be encouraged in graduate medical education nationwide.

Medical Education

About 26 percent of medical doctors were educated outside the United States or Canada, a figure that has risen over the past 15 years, particularly in specialties such as pathology and rehabilitation. The number of international medical graduates (IMGs) entering residency in 2000 increased by 6.5 percent over 1999. IMGs are significantly more likely to have had previous graduate medical training before starting their residencies in the United States. Allopathic medical school applications dropped nearly 25 percent from 1990 to 2000. The number of appli-

cants to osteopathic medical schools has been holding steady, and more than 50 percent of DOs are entering family practice or other primary care fields.

Some states have given prescription privileges to physician assistants and nurse practitioners, who work under the supervision of a physician. Other groups, such as nurse midwives, nurse anesthetists, and optometrists, have skills and practices that overlap with their allopathic equivalents—obstetricians, gynecologists, anesthesiologists, and ophthalmologists. There is a trend toward an increased number of health care providers who are not trained as medical doctors.

U.S. Physician Needs

About 40 percent of U.S. physicians are primary care generalists; but the American Medical Association is predicting a shortage of physicians overall in the United States by 2010. The distribution of physicians shows that rural areas and inner cities have a shortage of all types of physicians, both generalists and specialists. Like most persons in the United States, doctors prefer metropolitan areas; there is no incentive for them to practice in rural areas where they are generally in solo practice without other professionals with whom they can interact. Solo practitioners face difficulties with burdensome billing and increased practice costs for contracting with private insurance companies; larger practices can share high administrative costs. There were 4,500 psychiatry residents in training in 1999, or 4.6 percent of MDs. There are 11.1 psychiatrists per 100,000 persons; however, they tend to be concentrated in urban areas, and that ratio is greatly increased, for example, in New York, where there are 24 psychiatrists per 100,000 persons. In 2002, only about 3 percent of medical students decided to enter psychiatry, a decrease that began in the 1980s and continues.

Physician Earnings

The median physician net income in 1999 was $163,170 per year, a 9 percent increase overall since 1994. Neurosurgery, orthopedic surgery, and cardiothoracic surgery are the highest paid specialties; pediatrics, general practice, and psychiatry are the lowest paid specialties (Table 60–1). Of the medical subspecialties, invasive cardiologists and gastroenterologists had the highest incomes, likely because of the large number of reimbursable procedures performed by both. The median gross income of office-based general internists fell nearly 11 percent in 2000 according to *Medical Economics*. Women net nearly $90,000 less per year than their male counterparts in internal medicine, and the discrepancy is present but narrower in other fields. Doctors in the Midwest and Southern states tend to make a bit more money, most likely because there are fewer physicians concentrated in those areas.

Physician Earnings in Context. In assessing the level of physician income relative to that of the typical worker, one must bear in mind several factors. Physicians work long hours, often under stress, and must continually keep up with new medical developments. The average primary care doctor sees 110 patients per week and works 55 to 60 hours. Physicians do not begin their careers until later in life. In 2001, the average age of a medical school graduate was 28. Counting postgraduate education, many physicians are in their early 30s before beginning to practice. In addition, most physicians incur high educational debt before they begin to practice. In 1999, 81 percent of graduates reported some debt, with the average debt amounting to $90,745.

Table 60–1
Average Physician Net Income by Specialty

Specialty	Yearly Income (thousands of $)
Pediatrics	139.3
General/family practice	141.5
Internal medicine	142.9
Psychiatry	171.5
Obstetrics/gynecology	223.6
Anesthesiology	233.8
General surgery	243.4
Radiology	250.7
Neurosurgery	492.6

Data are from the American Medical Group Association and surveys of MDs in group practice; these are pretax dollars for the year 1999, when the latest figures were available.

Physician income also varies greatly on the basis of years of postgraduate training required, number of patients with private insurance versus number on Medicare, practice size, and overhead costs of office equipment, all of which influence overall income. The proportion of Medicare patients treated by a physician affects income, as the payment rates for services are determined by the "sustainable growth rate" which factors in not only overall Medicare enrollment, but also changes in gross domestic product and inflation, to determine physicians' fees. The fee schedule for 2002 decreased physician payments by 5.4 percent, even as practice expenses rise.

Liability Insurance

One of the most expensive components of physician practices is liability insurance. From 1990 to 1996, premiums were lower than they had been for some time; however, by the end of 2002 they increased from 8 to 18 percent in various states. The high premiums result from the increased incidence of malpractice claims and high jury awards. Median jury awards in malpractice cases rose to $800,000 in 1999. More than one third of all physicians have been sued at least once during their medical careers; however, over 70 percent of cases are won by physicians, settled, or dismissed. Obstetricians and surgeons have the highest liability risk; at low risk are pathologists and psychiatrists. Internists have been hit with higher insurance premium increases in the last few years than specialists, possibly because of more lawsuits for medication errors or failure to diagnose problems at an early stage. Physicians who have a positive relationship with their patients have fewer liability suits than those who do not establish good rapport with their patients.

Working Hours of Interns and Residents

Teaching hospitals often rely on interns and residents to perform services such as phlebotomies and intravenous therapy and to serve as messengers and transporters, tasks that are more appropriately performed by ancillary personnel. In addition, house staff are often required to work long hours, and sleep deprivation can impair their judgment and clinical skills. The average resident works more than 80 hours per week, with a shift of 30 hours every third or fourth night. Because of this, in 1988, a limit on the number of hours interns and residents may work was set forth by the

U.S. Health Care Financing Administration (HCFA), now officially known as the Center for Medicare and Medicaid Services (CMS). Their work rules are (1) residents are limited to no more than 12 consecutive hours per assignment in emergency services; (2) residents may not work more than 80 hours per week over a 4-week period and cannot be scheduled to work more than 24 consecutive hours; and (3) scheduled rotations must be separated by not less than 8 nonworking hours, with at least one 24-hour period of nonworking time provided for each week. Nonworking time is time away from training and patient care activities. In 2000, 8 percent of residency training programs nationwide were cited by the Accreditation Council for Graduate Medical Education for violating the CMS work hour requirements.

In response to the death of a patient at a New York hospital in 1989, the NY State Legislature enacted the Bell Commission Report, which implied that resident work hours contributed in part to that accidental death. The state responded by establishing rules for resident work hours including 80-hour work week limits and 24-hour consecutive call limits. The impact of these limits on the continuity of care remains to be seen.

The CMS defined medical student responsibilities as follows: (1) students can take histories and perform physical examinations with the approval of the patient's attending physician, (2) they may write in the patient's chart, but all entries must be countersigned by the attending physicians, and (3) medical or surgical procedures may be performed if they are under direct in-person supervision.

Many medical educators believe that the current CMS rules do not go far enough and that interns and residents are not used properly by many teaching hospitals. It is not uncommon for a resident in cardiac surgery to be assisting at an operation for 14 hours and then stay on duty an additional 10 hours. Similarly, a pediatric resident may be in the emergency room for 24 hours without sleep. Even though their hours fall within the CMS guidelines, they are not conducive to a high level of functioning in either situation; nor do they contribute to the resident's education in view of the inevitable fatigue when a person is without sleep for 24 hours. For residents with families, especially those who are mothers, current work schedules disrupt both marital harmony and child rearing. This added stress interferes with optimal functioning. It has been suggested that chronic sleep deprivation may put residents at increased risk for motor vehicle crashes, medication errors, and decreased mental clarity. There are no easy answers to these problems, but the current situation clearly requires resolution.

HEALTH CARE COSTS

The provision of adequate cost-effective services to the U.S. public is a critical concern. Spending for all types of health care, including the care of persons who are mentally ill, continues to escalate. The growth of health care expenditures continues to outdistance the growth of the economy. Health care has become increasingly expensive as a result of inflation, population growth, and advanced technology.

The CMS predicts that by 2008 national health expenditures will reach \$2.6 trillion, or 16 percent of the U.S. gross domestic product. In 2001, the United States spent \$1.4 trillion on health care—\$484 billion from private insurance and \$631 billion from federal and state funds. The federal government's monetary contribution to health care has grown steadily over the years. Medicare now accounts for 17.6 percent of the public national health expenditure, and Medicaid represents 15.5 percent. Forty million persons over 65 were enrolled in Medicare in 1999 and 33 million were enrolled in Medicaid, most of whom are children under 18.

Some 84 percent of persons in the United States under age 65 had some form of health insurance in 1999; 12 percent of children under 18 years old have no insurance at all. In 2000, private health insurance premiums totaled \$438 billion, up 9.3 percent from 1999. In general, the scope of insurance coverage has widened as more persons enroll in managed care plans that more fully cover preventive services. In 1999, 29 percent of the population with private insurance—78 million persons—were enrolled in a health maintenance organization (HMO) in 1999, up from 18 percent in 1989. About 60 percent of Americans working for medium-sized and large companies are enrolled in managed care plans. Employer-based insurance is by far the largest provider in this country for persons under 65, followed by independent purchasing of plans (7 percent of the population can afford this option), Medicaid, and the Department of Veterans Affairs (VA).

HOSPITALS

Hospitals are the institutional providers of general medical and surgical services in the U.S. health care system. There were 5,810 hospitals in the United States in 2000, with about 983,000 beds. About 66 percent of all beds are occupied at any one time. According to the WHO, hospitals must have physician staff, offer continuous medical and nursing care to patients, and maintain inpatient facilities. Because hospitals consume the biggest percentage of health dollars, their use is the focus of current cost-containment strategies. The United States spent \$395 billion on hospital expenses in 2000; clearly, some of those strategies are not containing costs.

The number of yearly hospital admissions had been falling steadily since 1981. There were 34.8 million hospital admissions in 2000. A slight future increase may be expected as the number of persons aged 65 and older, with their greater needs for health services, continues to grow. Technological advances and the growth of managed care, however, have prompted the shift of care to less costly outpatient settings.

The length of stay for inpatients in community hospitals has been falling for the last decade. The average length of stay in 1999 was 5 days. Possible explanations for this drop include the expansion of managed care among the Medicare and Medicaid populations, as well as improved integration of services through networking, which may allow hospitals to discharge patients to more appropriate settings for their continued recovery.

Mental disorders account for a large proportion of health care expenditures, \$67 billion in 1990, including specialty hospitals and institutions. Most persons with health insurance have more restrictive coverage for mental illness than for other types of illnesses. The average length of stay in psychiatric hospitals is 10 days, a decrease of 57 percent over the previous decade, when inpatients enjoyed stays of 23 days. Psychiatric hospitals have moved from a curative to a stabilization goal, with more focus on continuing outpatient treatment after discharge, using partial hospitalization programs to achieve this goal. The United States has approximately 600 psychiatric hospitals today, with a total of 78,000 inpatient psychiatric beds in general, city, state, VA, and private hospitals.

Hospitals may be classified on the basis of ownership, length of stay, or the nature of the service offered. Table 60–2 presents an overview of important aspects of hospital organization.

Table 60–2
Aspects of Hospital Organization

Criteria	Voluntary Hospital	Investor-Owned Hospital	State Mental Hospital System	Municipal Hospital System	Federal Hospital System	Special Hospital
Patient population	All illnesses	All illnesses, although hospital may specialize	Mental illness	All illnesses	All illnesses	70% of facility must be for single diagnosis
Profit orientation	Nonprofit	For profit	Nonprofit	Nonprofit	Nonprofit	For profit or nonprofit
Ownership	Private management board	Private corporation; may be owned by medical doctors	State	City government	Federal government	Private or public
Affiliation	Church-affiliated, privately owned, or university-sponsored	May be owned by large chains such as Humana Corporation, Columbia/HCA	Free standing or affiliated with various medical schools	Voluntary teaching hospitals and medical schools	Department of Defense, Public Health Service, Coast Guard, prison, Merchant Marine, Indian Health Service, VA	Optional affiliation with medical schools
Other	Provide bulk of care in U.S.	Increasing in importance nationally	Deinstitutionalization—number of patients has been reduced	Most physicians at municipal hospitals are employed by their affiliated medical school	VA hospitals usually have affiliations with medical schools	Less regulated than other types of hospitals

Notes: (1) To be designated a teaching hospital, a hospital must offer at least four types of approved residencies, clinical experiences for medical students, and an affiliation with a medical school. (2) Short-term hospitals have an average patient stay of less than 30 days; long-term hospitals, an average of longer duration. (3) Special hospitals include obstetrics and gynecology; eye, ear, nose, and throat. They do not include psychiatric hospitals or substance abuse hospitals.

REGULATION OF HEALTH CARE

Hospital Standards and Performance

A group of agencies, such as the Joint Commission on Accreditation of Healthcare Organizations (JCAHO) and the Liaison Committee on Medical Education (LCME), influence the standards of hospital care and performance. In addition, hospitals must comply with government regulations (city and state health rules). The JCAHO inspects hospitals every 2 years and is also responsible for determining the requirements for hospital accreditation. Hospital reimbursements from Medicare and Medicaid are contingent on meeting these standards, but the accreditation is done on a voluntary basis. The LCME and the Liaison Committee on Graduate Medical Education are charged with accrediting medical schools and residency training programs, respectively. The two accrediting committees review education and training programs every 4 years; the procedure is voluntary.

Currently, all the hospitals in a community tend to be monitored as a single health entity and community resource. Thus no one unit has the prerogative to develop new facilities without concern for the services offered by the other hospitals in the area.

Hospital Utilization Review. This in-house evaluation process was created to make sure that institutions provide efficient, high-quality health care that meets patients' needs. The utilization review committee, consisting of hospital administrators, physicians, and nurses, reviews each patient's chart within a specified number of days of admission. The appropriateness of the admission, treatment strategies, and the length of the hospital stay are reviewed to facilitate the patient's discharge. Through this process the utilization review committee determines whether a particular admission was really indicated and whether the hospital stay was longer than necessary. A hospital must conduct utilization reviews to be eligible for JCAHO accreditation.

Professional Standards Review Organization. The Professional Standards Review Organization (PSRO) was set up by the federal government to review and monitor care received by patients whose care is paid for with government funds (including Medicare, Medicaid, as well as the VA). Local medical associations have elected physicians to make up PSROs, which serve several functions: They attempt to ensure high-quality care, control costs, determine maximum lengths of stay by patients in hospitals, conduct utilization reviews, and censure physicians who do not adhere to established guidelines. A PSRO may conduct a medical audit to evaluate the quality of care retrospectively by carefully examining charts, and it also reviews providers randomly to deter abuse.

Peer Review Organization. In the early 1980s, Peer Review Organizations (PROs) replaced PSROs as the federal review organizations for hospitals receiving Medicare funds. To promote compliance with federal guidelines for health and hospital care, PROs conduct independent utilization reviews and quality-of-care studies, validate diagnosis-related group (DRG) assignments, and review hospital admissions and readmissions.

Federally mandated and funded, the PROs have greater authority than the PSROs. PROs can impose sanctions on hospitals for inadequate care; they can even recommend terminating federal funding to hospitals that consistently violate federal standards. In addition, PROs can adjust or refuse payment for health services that they consider unnecessary.

PROs operate on a statewide level and can be either nonprofit or for profit. To reduce costs, a PRO is chosen through a competitive bidding process from among qualified physician-sponsored organizations.

Health Systems Agency. Health systems agencies (HSAs) are nonprofit organizations mandated by the federal government and set up on a statewide basis. HSAs promote or limit the development of health services and facilities, depending on the needs of a particular locality or state. They are made up of consumers and have considerable power in medicine. For example, before a new hospital can be built or an existing hospital can be extensively renovated, the HSA must approve a certificate of need (CON). Before a CON is issued, the necessity for a new facility in a specified locale must be established. HSAs control capital expenditures and, therefore, the availability of health resources. In each state, HSAs develop both long-term and short-term goals and plans, approve health care proposals requesting federal funding, review existing facilities and services, and suggest future construction and renovation projects on the basis of their findings.

HEALTH CARE INSURANCE

Government Reimbursement Programs

Medicare (Title 18). Set up by the Federal Social Security Act of 1965, Medicare is a federally funded health insurance program. It provides both hospital and medical insurance for persons 65 years of age and older and for persons with certain disabilities (e.g., blindness and renal disease). Medicare consists of two parts: Part A covers inpatient hospital care, dialysis, and skilled nursing facilities, hospice care, and some home health care. Funding is derived from a federal trust fund, which, in turn, receives its funds from Social Security contributions. $129 billion was spent from this fund in 1999 on Part A. Part B is optional medical insurance that can be purchased to cover such services as physicians' fees, medical supplies, some diagnostic tests, outpatient hospital care, and therapy services. Medicare benefits and eligibility standards are uniform throughout the United States, and more than 40 million persons are enrolled. The benefits available to Medicare members are listed in Table 60–3. Medicare does not cover hearing aids, dental care, dentures, or prescription drugs. This has been the impetus behind the creation of the Medicare/managed care program, through which senior citizens can choose to participate in managed care plans as part of their Medicare plan; 18 percent of seniors do so. However, recent reports indicate that these plans are resulting in huge out-of-pocket costs to the sickest patients, who require the most expensive drugs and quickly reach their small annual plan limit.

Table 60–3
Medicare Benefits

Benefits—Part A	Current Provisions[a]
Hospital	The beneficiary is responsible for a Part A deductible ($792 in 2002). Medicare covers all costs for the first 60 days; $198 per day for days 61–90 and $396 per day for days 91–150. Medicare pays nothing after day 150.
Skilled nursing facility (SNF)	Medicare pays all costs for the first 20 days if a patient has been released from the hospital prior to SNF care. From days 21–100, the patient pays $99 per day. After 100 days, Medicare pays nothing.
Home health care	Medicare covers all home health services and 80% of home medical equipment if patients meet the restrictive eligibility requirements.
Hospice care	Patients pay a $5 copay for prescription drugs in hospice care and 5% of the cost of inpatient care.
Benefits—Part B	**Current Provisions[b]**
Medical services	Beneficiaries pay an annual $100 deductible, after which Medicare pays 80% of the government fee schedule for outpatient care, lab fees, radiology, outpatient occupational and physical therapy. The beneficiary pays the remaining 20% and anything left above Medicare's approved fee schedule. This part includes 50% coverage (NOT 80%) of outpatient mental health treatment.
Clinical laboratory services	100% covered.
Home health care services	Part-time skilled nursing care while receiving Medicare-approved home care is covered.

[a]There are gaps in Medicare. The following are not covered by Parts A or B:
Physician charges above the Medicare-approved amount
Routine physical exams
Eye exams or eyeglasses, dental care or dentures, hearing aids, or foot care
Prescription drugs
[b]Major Medicare benefits provided under Part A (hospital insurance benefits) and Part B (medical insurance) as of March 2002.

Medicaid (Title 19). Mandated by the federal government in 1965, Medicaid is an assistance program for certain needy and low-income persons. It is financed by both federal and state governments, but each state defines its requirements for eligibility and is responsible for its administration. Although benefits vary from state to state, federal provisions require that Medicaid cover inpatient and outpatient hospital care (including psychiatric care), physicians' services, laboratory tests, diagnostic imaging, home health care services, and nursing home care. Medicaid also covers family planning and prenatal care, and states can choose to extend coverage to optometrists, glasses, and dental services. Medicaid, unlike Medicare, does cover prescription medications. Private psychiatric hospitals are not covered under Medicaid. Increasingly tight eligibility requirements have left many low-income persons without coverage and unable to pay. Currently, about 37 million persons are covered by Medicaid, and the number rises annually.

Risk Pools. In a disturbing trend, some insurance companies are raising the premiums of patients who develop an illness and wish to maintain their coverage to levels that are no longer affordable. Many states offer temporary high-risk health insurance plans ("risk pools") for persons who, because of their current physical condition, cannot purchase insurance at any price or have insurance that excludes treatment of their current health condition. These plans often have limited maximum benefits, limits on the number of persons who can enroll at any one time, and specific exclusions for certain diseases and health problems.

Self-Pay and "Fee-for-Service"

Patients contract with commercial insurance companies to cover both inpatient and outpatient costs, including physicians' fees, diagnostic procedures, and laboratory tests. For this type of insurance, self-pay patients pay a premium that may be based on an experience rating determined by the risk or previous record for reimbursement on insur-

ance claims or a community rating system in which each participant pays the same premium because the plan's cost is divided equally among group members. Before the rise of managed care, most health insurance was "fee-for-service." In this model, persons pay a predetermined percentage (e.g., 20 percent) of the cost of health care services. Patients are free to choose their doctors, who determine fees.

Managed Care

Managed care is a system by which a health care insurer and providers work together to ensure cost containment. The goal of managed care is to eliminate unnecessary medical procedures and obtain discounted services from physicians and hospitals. Business and insurance companies have advocated managed care in an effort to cut their medical costs for employees and insurance beneficiaries. The number of doctors participating in managed care has increased rapidly. According to one survey, 87 percent of primary care doctors have at least some managed care contracts, and 22 percent report more than half of their patients are insured through managed care.

The cost-cutting procedures used by managed care companies involve payment arrangements for hospitals, physicians, and pharmaceutical services. Cost-control procedures are put in place to evaluate doctors' decisions, to restrict coverage of certain kinds of care deemed experimental or cosmetic, and to limit the range of medications available to patients for various illnesses. HMOs and other managed care companies also lower health care costs by limiting the number of new hospitalizations and by discharging patients from hospitals earlier than usual. The emphasis on prevention and health promotion and on performing as much diagnosis and therapy as possible on an outpatient basis further helps control expenses. Managed care is beneficial in covering outpatient tests and surgery, and their prescription drug coverage is usually comprehensive. Employees' continuity of care is often disrupted by finding a new primary care physician every year whose services are covered by the new plan, however, because some employers switch health insurance plans frequently to lower rates.

Most HMOs are for-profit corporations, and their motivation to cut costs and increase earnings is strong. They have a large number of nonmedical employees, many of whom receive large salaries, far in excess of what physicians earn.

According to Families USA, a consumer health care advocacy organization, the CEO of United HealthGroup was the highest paid health plan executive in the year 2000—$54 million in compensation annually with an additional $357 million in stock options. Aetna/US Healthcare Corporation, the largest for-profit health care organization in the United States, reported revenues of $26.5 billion in 2000 (*Wall Street Journal,* February 16, 2000). An increased number of patients enrolled in HMOs, coupled with decreased medical costs in the form of lower fees to doctors and hospitals, contributed to HMOs' revenue growth. In addition to executive compensation, HMOs spend over $40 million annually on advertising and marketing their product. They have introduced a level of bureaucracy consisting of care managers and utilization review personnel, who not only must be paid but who also serve as intermediaries between doctor and patient. Obviously, health care has become a lucrative business in the United States; but the profits often come from denying medical, surgical, and drug reimbursement services; reducing payments to doctors and hospitals; and introducing complex procedures that serve to discourage patients and providers from pursuing denied claims.

Health Maintenance Organizations

An HMO is an organized system providing comprehensive (both inpatient and outpatient) health care in all specialties, including psychiatry. Members voluntarily enroll in the plan and pay a prepayment or capitation fee to cover all health care services for a fixed period (a month or a year). There are more than 500 HMOs in the United States, with an enrollment of about 79 million persons.

There are three types of HMOs: the *staff model,* in which physicians receive a salary to provide services in the HMO's own facility; the *group model,* in which health care is furnished by one or more groups of doctors and payment is received on a contractual basis at a predetermined rate; and the *individual practice association* (IPA) *network model,* in which the HMO negotiates with individual physicians to receive a capitation fee for providing services to each IPA member seen in their private offices. Physicians retain their office-based private practices when they join an IPA. Physicians in staff and group models often own stock in their HMOs.

An egregious cost cutting by HMOs was the provision that allowed only 24 hours of hospitalization for newborn deliveries. In 1996, the U.S. Congress agreed to legislation that prohibits the insurance company practice known as drive-through deliveries. Under the law, the decision about how long a mother and her newborn child remain in the hospital is now made by the mother and her physician. This new law represents a strong first step by the federal government toward ensuring that cost containment will not be allowed to be the primary or sole consideration in determining how, and which, health care services will be paid for in the new era of managed care. Also in response to this, a national Consumers for Quality Care group was established to advocate greater accountability for HMOs and cost-cutting practices. As of 2001, health insurers have been held liable for their practices in 10 states, including Texas, and 40 states guaranteed an independent appeals process for consumers denied care by their HMO or health insurer. A national patient's bill of rights, including the right to appeal a decision to deny health care made by a health insurance plan, has been tentatively passed in Congress, but a decision on whether to limit damage awards to avoid frivolous lawsuits has prevented a final bill from coming through. The insurance industry has lobbied powerfully against a patient's bill of rights, claiming that an increase in litigation will drive up premiums.

Relation of Medicare and Medicaid to HMOs. It is now possible for those eligible for fee-for-service Medicare and Medicaid benefits to become members of HMOs. Nationwide, Medicare HMO enrollment is about 6.8 million or about 18 percent of the elderly population, but persons over 65 who switch to HMOs can no longer visit the doctors of their choice, and access to specialists is also restricted. Furthermore, most HMOs do not cover members who live outside the HMO area. Disputes arise about unapproved emergency room visits, specialist referrals, and nursing home stays. The advantages claimed for HMO membership are that persons with Medicare HMO coverage do not have to pay a deductible of 20 percent of doctor bills but only a small copayment of $5 to $15. Some persons with chronic illness may find the annual cost of medication lower in HMOs. HMOs were anxious to enroll Medi-

caid beneficiaries at the program's inception, because they received over $4,000 annually for each enrollee. However, in an attempt to control costs, HMOs have been cutting ties with Medicare because its patients are often sicker and cost more to treat than younger patients and are thus less cost effective for managed care companies.

Primary Care Physicians. In most HMOs, every patient must choose a primary care physician, who has usually received training in internal medicine, family medicine, or pediatrics. Primary care physicians are fast becoming the foundation on which the current system of health delivery in the United States is based. These physicians deal not only with the physical complaints of their patients but also with their mental, emotional, and social concerns—a field called *primary care psychiatry*. Unfortunately, most primary care physicians have limited knowledge of the full range of psychiatric disorders and therapeutic options. Psychiatric educators face the challenge of upgrading the skills of primary care physicians in managing mental illness, particularly in prescribing psychotropic medications, more of which are dispensed by primary care physicians in the United States than by psychiatrists. Psychiatrists use potent pharmacology agents with a wide range of adverse effects, some of which may be fatal. Nonpsychiatric physicians must have an in-depth knowledge of these agents to practice psychopharmacological therapy effectively and safely.

Gatekeeper. The term *gatekeeper* has been applied to primary care physicians who, as part of providing total care for patients, must decide when to refer a patient to a specialist. Most HMOs require "preapproval" for a specialist referral; primary care physicians must request permission from the HMO to refer the patient. Some plans have utilization committees (which may or may not include physicians) whose goal is to review physician referrals to see whether they are indicated; these committees developed as protection against soaring health care expenditures. Most physicians acknowledge the need for accountability but view the procedures as cumbersome and inequitable. A nationwide survey of primary care physicians found that 38 percent believed their ability to make the right decisions for their patients had been declining, and 10 percent reported they had financial incentives not to refer patients to specialists if they had any doubt about the necessity of the referral.

One troubling aspect of review organizations is the denial of payment that occurs for some treatments labeled experimental but that actually are considered advisable treatment by medical experts. Payment denials of this sort are increasing and threaten to interfere with both innovative medical treatment and traditional medical care. Another particularly troubling issue resulting from these oversight activities is the breaching of confidentiality in doctor–patient relationships. Moreover, denials of payment, demands to justify clinical decisions, and requirements for preapproval of procedures undermine professional decision making and contribute to a growing sense of frustration among physicians in all specialties. Most complaints by patients about HMOs involve decisions by utilization review committees not to approve certain treatments; thus HMOs force patients to forgo the therapy or pay for it out of pocket, neither of which is satisfactory.

Preferred Provider Organizations

Like HMOs, preferred provider organizations (PPOs) use a prospective payment system. In a PPO, however, a corporation or an insurance company makes an agreement with a particular group of community hospital, doctors, and other health care providers to supply health services to PPO members at a previously determined discounted rate. PPOs have become the most common type of managed care, representing 38 percent of the market in 2000.

QUALITY OF CARE

Quality of care has several definitions, ranging from patient satisfaction with health care to the rate of death associated with a particular procedure, such as coronary bypass grafting. A database currently exists to record individual physicians' performance, but physicians are concerned that the data are flawed because the severity of illness, other concurrent illness, or case mix may not be taken into account. It is unfair to attempt to rate the competence of a psychiatrist on the basis of the number of suicide attempts in his or her practice if one psychiatrist's caseload is composed mainly of patients with severe mood disorders and another's is composed mainly of anxiety disorders. Similarly, rating cardiovascular surgeons on the basis of the mortality rate of their patients without considering the severity of illnesses and coexisting illness is illusory. One result of the release of these data to the public is that some cardiovascular surgeons have refused to operate on patients who are considered at high risk because of the chance of adversely affecting their standing. At present, no valid, reliable, or useful techniques exist to assess the quality of care. Some hospitals are being ranked by the number of procedures performed, to assure patients that their facility is experienced at performing certain operations.

The American Psychiatric Association (APA) has attempted to outline guidelines for the treatment of psychiatric disorders, but the APA is careful to point out that their guidelines are not "official" and are not meant to be followed slavishly. Thus psychiatrists have the latitude to individualize treatment plans for patients. When physicians deviate from published guidelines, however, they should document their reasons for the alternative method of care. By doing so, the physician can justify and maintain his or her autonomy.

In a 2001 study by the Harvard School of Public Health and the Kaiser Family Foundation of patients enrolled in private insurance plans, about 50 percent of patients voiced some type of problem with their health plan during the previous year. The most common problems involved denial of coverage or care or delays in seeing physicians. Managed care organizations typically restrict payments to specialists unless care is approved in advance by a designated primary care doctor. This practice contributed to patient dissatisfaction, because patients cannot seek a specialist of their own choosing.

In an attempt to deal with patients' desires to have a free choice of physician, most choose the type of payment method (e.g., PPO, HMO, traditional) at the time of service. Such plans offer a point-of-service (POS); patients may see any doctor they choose without a referral. POS plans are more expensive for patients and do not reimburse doctors at the same rate as doctors who belong to the HMO system. The U.S. government, in an effort to cut Medicare and Medicaid costs, is encouraging beneficiaries to enroll in managed care plans; however, those over 75 and those who are sick are unlikely to do so. Also, plans to reduce Medicare HMO-reimbursement dollars will decrease the managed care for-profit motive to continue to enroll the sick elderly.

Patients enrolled in HMO plans typically have a harder time getting access to care, suffer the longest waits for appointments, and have more complaints about choice of physician than those in PPOs; however,

their premiums are generally the lowest. PPO plans offer more choice and give consumers the freedom to see specialists without a referral, but PPOs may cause sicker patients greater problems with reimbursement and paperwork. The more health problems persons have, the less satisfied they are with their health care in general.

Americans without insurance have more severe problems. Lengthy delays in treatment can cost patients valuable time in diagnosis; once patients *are* diagnosed, often in emergency rooms, there are 3- to 4-month waits at the few thousand federally funded clinics where specialists often see patients for free. These are persons whose jobs may be part time and do not offer insurance or whose income is just far enough above the poverty level to make them ineligible for Medicaid. For patients with chronic disease and no insurance, the costs of medication and treatment can result in bankruptcy. In 2002, 39 million Americans were without health insurance.

PSYCHIATRIC CARE DELIVERY

Psychiatric care is provided by a variety of mental health organizations in addition to private practitioners. The organizations include psychiatric hospitals, including VA psychiatric hospitals, state and county mental hospitals, and private mental hospitals; psychiatric units of general hospitals; residential treatment centers for emotionally disturbed children; federally funded community mental health centers; and independent psychiatric outpatient clinics, where a psychiatrist has medical responsibility for all patients in the program. Most psychiatric patients are seen in one of these organizations; fewer than 5 percent of all psychiatric patients are seen by psychiatrists in private practice. There are approximately 600 free-standing psychiatric hospitals in the United States.

Recent studies indicate that over 30 million persons in the United States have anxiety disorders, and 19 million have a mood (affective) disorder. There are 2.2 million patients with schizophrenia and 5 million with severe cognitive impairment, such as Alzheimer's disease. HMOs clearly cannot handle such a large, serious caseload.

Mental health care is usually provided as part of the health benefit package offered by employers to their employees. It is also offered as a Medicare and Medicaid service. In almost all instances, however, mental health benefits are reviewed by so-called managed behavioral health care companies in an effort to reduce the costs of care and to provide some type of quality control over service. In doing their job, however, managed care programs seriously interfere with the practice of psychiatry as it is known today.

Many programs limit the number of psychotherapy visits to 5 to 20 sessions a year, and although some types of psychotherapies can be conducted within this framework, other types, such as insight-oriented or psychodynamic therapies, require frequent visits over an extended period. In addition, patients must be referred to a psychiatrist by their primary care physician, who is encouraged to try to deal with the patients' problems before making a referral. During this time pharmacotherapy rather than psychotherapy is most likely to be prescribed, and most primary care physicians have neither the training nor the time to provide therapy. When a referral to a psychiatrist is made, the psychiatrist must provide an initial report to the managed care company about the patient's condition and must submit periodic reports thereafter, a process that violates a basic tenet of successful psychotherapy, confidentiality. Finally, managed care companies encourage primary care physicians to refer patients to nonpsychiatrists, such as psychologists and social workers, for psychotherapy because they accept lower fees than do psychiatrists. Psychiatrists are used primarily to prescribe medication or to treat patients who require hospitalization. Managed behavioral health care companies receive a predetermined annual fee or, more often, a percentage of the amount of money saved as payment for their services, practices that have led to charges of conflict of interest.

In 2001, the New Mexico state legislature and governor extended the first prescription privileges in the United States to psychologists. Their decision was based, they said, on arguments that there are too few psychiatrists to staff rural areas in their state; thus they are trying to supply a demand. However, psychologists are no more likely to settle in rural areas than psychiatrists are, and they still require the supervision of a physician to prescribe under the new rules. Under capitation, psychologists are often reimbursed less for their services than psychiatrists, which makes their services even more attractive in times of severe cost cutting if they can prescribe medicine as well. Similar bills have been proposed in 13 other states and were all rejected; the American Medical Association (AMA) and the APA have successfully lobbied against allowing persons without a background in medicine to dispense potentially dangerous or fatal medications.

Claims Review

When psychiatric (or other medical) benefits are denied or curtailed, a claims review may be initiated by a patient or doctor. The first level of claims review generally consists of a clerical examination to determine whether the bill shows the necessary administrative information and whether the claimant is covered for the prescribed treatment. There is no determination of the appropriateness of the care given. The second level of claims review is generally done by trained personnel, often nurses. Here the claims reviewer compares the treatment rendered with previously established treatment criteria considered appropriate for the condition.

The second-level reviewer may approve payment for the claim. If the second-level reviewer has questions or if the treatment is considered inappropriate according to the criteria, the claim is reviewed by a third-level group or a true peer review committee. Here a professional determination is made concerning the appropriateness of the care rendered. The peer review committee (e.g., one or more psychiatrists) reviews each claim and may approve or disapprove. Levels of appeal exist for the practitioner who is dissatisfied with the committee determination. The appeals process often goes to a special committee of the county or state medical society.

Parity of Mental Health Services

Most employer health benefits set annual and lifetime payment caps for mental illness that are below that for physical illness. In 1996, Congress passed a bill (sponsored by Senators Peter Domenici and Paul Wellstone) that sought to achieve total equality or parity for benefits for mental and physical illness. Some disparity remains; not all mental disorders are included, and substance abuse and alcoholism are excluded from the mental illness

parity requirement. The bill also prohibits health plans from imposing lower lifetime financial limits on mental health benefits than on physical health benefits. The bill has come up for vote again to widen benefits, but despite a WHO report focusing on the worldwide morbidity of mental health in 2001, the bill has not passed nationwide, and mental health benefit limits continue to be lower than those of other types of illnesses. Most states have passed some form of limited parity legislation.

Gag Rule

Managed care plans prohibit doctors enrolled in their plans from advising patients about treatments not covered by the HMO, such as specialized or experimental procedures; doctors are also forbidden to refer patients to physicians who are experts in certain rare diseases but who are not members of an HMO. These and other prohibitions (including criticizing HMOs) are collectively known as the gag rule. Many states have passed laws prohibiting gag rules in contracts between HMOs and physicians, and the issue is currently under legislative review by the U.S. Congress. Several major HMOs have eliminated gag clauses as a result of public and professional pressure. The AMA has launched a major effort to achieve bipartisan elimination of health plan gag clauses. According to the AMA, there is intense lobbying by the insurance industry against implementation of gag clause legislation.

In an effort to regain control of the medical decision process, some states prohibit nonphysicians from making clinical decisions. The Texas State Board of Medical Examiners adopted a position statement (October 5, 1996) on what constitutes the practice of medicine in that state. According to the statement, "the determination of medical necessity appropriateness of proposed care so as to effect the diagnosis or treatment of a patient is the practice of medicine." The board warned that individuals or entities who make determinations of medical necessity or appropriateness who do not have a Texas medical license may be subject to investigation, criminal prosecution, injunctive action, and possibly monetary penalties. In concluding its statement, the board further warned, "To avoid a violation of the law regarding unlicensed practice, reviewers, insurers, medical directors, and managed care gatekeepers should be particularly conscientious in allowing physician providers to exercise independent medical judgment to the greatest extent possible." Sadly, 41 percent of physicians surveyed by the Commonwealth Fund reported having less time to spend with individual patients over the previous 3 years, and 35 percent were "unhappy" with the practice of medicine in general. Many reported having to spend extra time keeping up-to-date with utilization rules and managed care practice guidelines, rather than with colleagues and reading medical literature.

Some experts believe that the future of managed care is bleak over the long term. Managed care firms lack a social conscience, in that they do not contribute to teaching, research, or care of the poor. As governmental regulation of managed care policies and practices increases to ensure the social good, the profit-making goals of managed care companies and big business become more difficult to achieve. If they are to have a stronger presence in the future, as Jerome P. Kassner pointed out in the *New England Journal of Medicine* (April 8, 1997), "managed care plans will have to show that they have become better citizens: that they care about more than profits, that they do not skimp on care, that they support their just share of teaching, research, and the care of the poor, that they no longer muzzle physicians, and that they offer something special (including control of costs) by managing care."

FUTURE TRENDS

A new concept of medical services as *market driven* has emerged. This concept now dominates the health care industry and will do so for the foreseeable future. Paradoxically, the role of government must increase as legislation is required to regulate this new industry, whose preoccupation is the cost of health. There is growing conflict between medicine, whose expertise is in the quality of health, and industry, whose expertise is in business and profit.

Unfortunately an adversarial and litigious atmosphere has developed. Physicians are suing HMOs to gain autonomy among other issues; HMOs are suing physicians for alleged breaches of contract; patient are suing HMOs for denial of payment to themselves or their doctors; and various federal agencies are investigating HMOs' physicians, hospitals, and patients for purported infractions of a variety of complex rules and regulations. Only a small proportion of the health care dollar is earmarked for that purpose; the remainder supports the health care industry. The United States is far from achieving affordable medical care for all citizens, mentioned as an ideal health care delivery system in the opening of this section. Ultimately the U.S. Congress will become the arbiters between the consumers of health care (patients), the providers (physicians and other health professionals), and the payers (insurance companies, HMOs, and the federal government).

References

Embry RA, Buddenhagen P, Bolles S. Managed care and child welfare: challengers to implementation. *Child Youth Serv Rev.* 2000;22:93.

Galanter M, Keller DS, Dermatis H, Egelko S. The impact of managed care on substance abuse treatment: a report of the American Society of Addiction Medicine. *J Addict Dis.* 2000;19:13.

Gonzales ML, ed. *Socioeconomic Characteristics of Medical Practice, 1995.* Chicago: American Medical Association; 1995.

Himmelstein DU, Woolhandler S. A national health program for the United States: a physician's proposal. *N Engl J Med.* 1989;320:102.

Kassirer JD. Is managed care here to stay? *N Engl J Med.* 1997;336:1013.

McCormick D, Himmelstein DU, Woolhandler S, et al. Relationship between low quality-of-care scores and HMOs' subsequent disclosure of quality-of-care scores. *JAMA.* 2002;12:1484.

National Center for Health Statistics. *Health, United States, 1995.* Hyattsville, MD: Public Health Services; 1995.

Rice AH. Interdisciplinary collaboration in health care: education, practice and research. *Natl Acad Pract Forum.* 2000;2:59.

Rosenberg S. Health maintenance organization penetration and general hospital psychiatric services: expenditure and utilization trends. *Prof Psychol Res Pract.* 1996;27:345.

Vaccaro JV. Managed care. In: Sadock BJ, Sadock VA, eds. *Kaplan & Sadock's Comprehensive Textbook of Psychiatry.* 7th ed. Vol 2. Baltimore: Lippincott Williams & Wilkins; 2000:3136.

Weissman E, Pettigrew K, Sotsky S, Regier DA. The cost of access to mental health services in managed care. *Psychiatr Serv.* 2000;51:664.

Index

Page numbers followed by *t* and *f* indicate tables and figures, respectively. Page numbers in **boldface** indicate main discussions.

A

AA, 388, 402
AAMR, 1161
Abandonment, ethics concerning, 1372*t*
Abnormal Involuntary Movement Scale (AIMS), 996*t*, 1059, 1060*t*
Abnormal swallowing syndrome, sleep-related, **779**
Abortion
  by adolescent girls, 39
  induced, **874–875**
    in adolescence, 39
  spontaneous, 874
  techniques, 876*t*
Abraham, Karl, **217,** 785
  on depression, 541
  on grief, 64
Abreaction, 194, 689
  definition of, 281
  in group psychotherapy, 938*t*
Absences, **357,** 358*f*
Absorption, of psychotherapeutic drugs, **975**
Abstract thinking
  in adolescents, 138, 139
  assessment of, in mental status examination, 242
  definition of, 287
Abulia
  definition of, 282
  pharmacotherapy for, 1119
Abuse
  and attachment, 142
  child. *See* Child abuse and neglect
  elder, 879, **1327,** 1328*t*
  physical, of adults, **890**
  problems related to, **883–893,** 884*t*
    DSM-IV-TR classification of, 883
  sexual. *See* Sexual abuse
  of spouse, 151, **890,** 891*t*
  substance. *See* Substance abuse
Academic problem, 142, **1290–1292**
  diagnosis of, 1291
  DSM-IV-TR classification of, 1290
  etiology of, 1291
  treatment of, 1291–1292
Acalculia, definition of, 287. *See also* Mathematics disorder
Acamprosate, in alcohol use disorders, 389, 412–413
Acathexis, definition of, 281
Acceptance
  in dying patient, 60
  in group psychotherapy, 938*t*
Accident-prone personality, 157
Accident(s), **156–158**
  motivations in, 157–158
  psychophysiological considerations with, 157
Acculturation problem, **899–900**
ACE. *See* Angiotensin converting enzyme (ACE) inhibitors
Acebutolol, 999*t*, 1009*t*. *See also* β-Adrenergic receptor antagonist(s)
  chemistry of, 1008*f*
  pharmacological actions of, 1009
Acetaldehyde, 399
Acetaminophen
  blood level data for clinical assessment, 268*t*
  for pain management, 1345*t*
Acetazolamide, and lithium, 1072*t*
Acetic acid, 399
Acetophenazine, 999*t*
  preparations, 1064*t*
  structure of, 1052*f*
Acetylation status of patients, 533
Acetylcholine, **105–107**
  in Alzheimer's disease, 332
  and drugs, 105–106
  life cycle, 105
  metabolism, 105
  neurotransmitter function, 90*t*, 91*f*, 93*t*
  and psychopathology, 106
  receptors, 93*t*
  and sleep, 758
  synthesis of, 105
Acetylcholinesterase, 93, 105
Acetylcholinesterase inhibitors, 126
Acetylsalicylic acid, blood level data for clinical assessment, 268*t*
Acid phosphatase test, 269*t*
Ackerman, Nathan, on goals of couples (marital) therapy, 947
ACL, 181*t*
Acquired aphasia with convulsion, 1213
Acquired immune deficiency syndrome (AIDS), 371. *See also* Human immunodeficiency virus, infection (HIV)
  course of, 372
  dementia in, 256
  diagnosis of, 372–374
    counseling about, 373
  emergency manifestations of, 907*t*
  emergency treatment of, 907*t*
  fetal transmission, 455
  history of, 371
  medical considerations with, 845*t*
  neuropsychiatric aspects of, **371–379**
  pediatric, 1168
  personality change due to, 819, 819*t*
  psychiatric considerations with, 845*t*
  serum, testing for, 372–373
  stress and progression of, 132–133
  and suicide, 915
  and worried well, 376
Acromegaly, 257
Acrophobia, definition of, 284
ACT, 501
ACTH. *See* Adrenocorticotropic hormone (corticotropin) (ACTH)
Acting out, 207*t*
  definition of, 282
  in personality disorders, 802
Action potentials, **89–90,** 90*f*
  all-or-none phenomenon, 91
  translation into chemical neurotransmission, 89–90
Active therapy, 220
Actual self, 221
Actus reus, 1361
Aculalia, definition of, 285
Acupressure, **852**
Acupuncture, **852, 1145**
Acute intermittent porphyria, 366
  medical considerations with, 846*t*
  psychiatric considerations with, 846*t*
Acute stress disorder. *See also* Posttraumatic stress disorder
  diagnostic criteria for, 626–627, 626*t*
  differential diagnosis of, 679, 797
Acute stress reaction
  ICD-10 classification of, 797
  ICD-10 diagnostic criteria for, 595–598, 598*t*
ADAD, 1288
Adalat. *See* Nifedipine
Adam (drug). *See* Methylenedioxyamphetamine
Adapin. *See* Doxepin
Adaptational dynamics, 226
Adaptive mental mechanisms, **20–21**

Adderall, 1116. *See also* Sympathomimetics (and related drugs)
with dextroamphetamine, for attention-deficit/hyperactivity disorder, 1227, 1227*t*
pharmacological action of, 1117
Addict, 381
Addiction, 381. *See also specific substance*
Addison's disease
medical considerations with, 845*t*
neuropsychiatric manifestations of, 366
psychiatric considerations with, 845*t*
Additional conditions that may be a focus of clinical attention, **894–900**
in child psychiatry, **1290–1294**
Adenine, 123
Adenosine triphosphate, in protein phosphorylation, 95*f,* 96
Adenylyl cyclase, 94
ADH, 399
ADHD. *See* Attention-deficit/hyperactivity disorder (ADHD)
Adiadochokinesia, definition of, 286
Adiposogenital dystrophy, 752
Adjective Checklist (ACL), 181*t*
Adjustment disorder(s), **795–799**
with anxiety, **796**
clinical features of, 796
course of, 798
crisis intervention for, 798–799
with depressed mood, **796**
diagnosis of, 796
diagnostic criteria for, 796*t*
differential diagnosis of, 797–798
with disturbance of conduct, **797**
DSM-IV-TR classification of, 795
epidemiology of, 795
etiology of, 795–796
family factors in, 796
genetic factors in, 796
in ICD-10, 797, 798*t*
with mixed anxiety and depressed mood, **797**
with mixed disturbance of emotions and conduct, **797**
pharmacotherapy for, 799
prognosis for, 798
psychodynamic factors in, 795–796
psychotherapy for, 798–799
treatment of, 798–799
unspecified, **797**
Adler, Alfred, **217–218,** 218*f*
Admission, for hospitalization
informal, 1356
involuntary, 1357
procedures of, 1356–1357
temporary, 1356–1357
voluntary, 1356
Adolescence, **35–41**
abortions during, 39
asceticism in, 36–37, 208*t*
cognitive development in, 37
disorders of, 1259–1273
early, 35
end of, 35, 40
hormonal changes in, 36
and identity problems, **1293–1294**
late, 35
legal issues, 40*t*
middle, 35
mood disorders during, **1274–1279**
moral development in, 38
negativism in, 37
neurological changes in, 37
normality in, 18
occupational choice in, 38
onset of, 36
peer groups in, 37–38
personality development in, 37
pregnancy in, **39,** 40*t*
prostitution in, 39
psychosexual development in, 36–37
pyromania in, 787
violence in, 39–40
Adolescent antisocial behavior, **1292–1293**
clinical features of, 1292
diagnosis of, 1292
differential diagnosis of, 1292
epidemiology of, 1292
etiology of, 1292
psychological factors in, 1292
treatment of, 1292–1293
Adolescent crises
emergency manifestations of, 907*t*
emergency treatment of, 907*t*
Adolescent Drug and Alcohol Diagnostic Assessment (ADAD), 1288
Adolescent Problem Severity Index (APSI), 1288
Adolescent(s)
abstract thinking in, 138, 139
anabolic (androgenic) steroid use, 466
attitudes toward death, 61
biological therapies for, **1305–1311**
clinical interviews with, 1152–1153
clinical problems in, 1313–1314
day treatment with, **1303–1305,** 1313
deductive reasoning in, 138
depression in, clinical features of, 552–553
developmental tasks of, 215, 228
normative description of, 18
drug use, 38–39
dying, 61
gender identity disorders in, **732**
group psychotherapy with, **1301,** 1313
hallucinogen use, 437
hospital treatment of, **1305**
hypotheticodeductive thinking in, 138
identity confusion in, 215
identity diffusion in, 37
individual psychotherapy with, **1295–1300,** 1312
psychoanalytic theories in, 1295–1296
theories and techniques of, 1295–1296
inhalant use, 440–441, 443
inpatient treatment with, 1313
intelligence tests for, **1159**
lithium and, 1071
major depressive disorder in, 1277
mania in, 553, 1277
mental disorders in, 38
with opioid dependence, 450–451
parenting of, 38
posttraumatic stress disorder in, 627–628
psychiatric treatment of, **1295–1314, 1311–1314**
in residential treatment, **1302–1303**
risk-taking behavior in, 38
role diffusion in, 213–214, 215
and substance abuse, **1286–1289**
and substance-related disorders, **1314**
and suicide, 34, **1279–1281, 1314**
turmoil, 37, 139, 166–167
Adoption, 34, 45–46
availability, 46
biological parents in, 34
informing children of, 34
parental concerns in, 45
Adoption studies, 167
of mood disorders, 540
Adrenal axis, and major depressive disorder, 538
Adrenal disorder(s)
neuropsychiatric manifestations of, 366
psychological correlates of, **832–833**
Adrenal hormones, 129–130
Adrenal hyperplasia, virilizing, 693*t*
α-Adrenergic receptor agonist(s), 102
α-Adrenergic receptor antagonist(s)
implicated in sexual dysfunction, 711
α_2-Adrenergic receptor antagonist(s), **1005–1007**. *See also* Clonidine; Guanfacine
adverse reactions to, 1006
clinical features of, 1007
dosage of, 1007, 1007*t*
drug interactions, 1007
effects on specific organs and systems, 1005
indications for, 1005–1006
laboratory interferences, 1007
overdose of, 1006
precautions with, 1006
withdrawal, 1007
β-Adrenergic receptor antagonist(s), 102, 405, **1008–1011**. *See also* Atenolol; Metoprolol; Nadolol; Propranolol
adverse effects of, 1010, 1010*t*
for aggression, 1009–1010
for alcohol withdrawal, 1010
antidepressant augmentation with, 1010
chemistry of, 1008, 1008*f*
dosage and administration, 1011
drug interactions, 1010, 1035, 1062*t*
drugs used in psychiatry, 1009*t*
effects on specific organs and systems, 1009
geriatric dosage, 1332*t*
implicated in sexual dysfunction, 711
indications for, 1008*t,* 1009–1010
for intermittent explosive disorder, 785
intoxication/overdose, 984*t*
for lithium-induced postural tremor, 1009
for neuroleptic-induced acute akathisia, 1009
pharmacological actions, 1009
precautions with, 1010
for separation anxiety disorder, 1263
toxicity of, 1010*t*
for violent behavior, 1009–1010
β-Adrenergic receptor kinase, 93
β-Adrenergic receptor(s), 93, 94, 101–102
Adrenocortical insufficiency
medical considerations with, 845*t*
psychiatric considerations with, 845*t*
Adrenocorticotropic hormone (corticotropin) (ACTH)
synthesis of, 104
test for, 269*t*
Adrenogenital syndrome, 693*t,* **733–735,** 734*f*
Adrenoleukodystrophy, 1166
Adult antisocial behavior, **896–897**
clinical features of, 896, 897*t*
diagnosis of, 896
DSM-IV-TR classification of, 896
epidemiology of, 896
etiology of, 896
genetic factors in, 896
prevention of, 897

social factors in, 896
treatment of, 897
Adultery, 50
Adulthood, **41–50**
developmental tasks of, 214–215
early, **41–46**
developmental tasks of, 41–43
marriage in, 43–45, 44*t*
occupation in, 43
parenthood in, 45–46
unemployment in, 43
women and work, 43
evolution of, 40–41
history-taking about, 236–237
late, 41, **50–58**
attitudes toward death in, 61
maturity, 50
middle, 41, **46–48**
developmental tasks of, 46
divorce in, 48–50
empty-nest syndrome in, 48
features of, 45, 46*t*
gender changes in, 46
sexuality in, 47
midlife crisis, **47–48**
Adult(s)
and attention-deficit/hyperactivity disorder, 1229
gender identity disorders in, **732–733**
neuropsychological assessment of, **185–190**
physical abuse of, **890**
in psychotherapy, differences from children, 1297–1298
sexual abuse of, **890–892**
Advance directives, **1340–1342**
Advanced sleep phase syndrome, 772
Advice
in interview, 10
in psychotherapy, definition of, 927*t*
Adynamia, definition of, 281
Affect
appropriate
definition of, 280
in mental status examination, 238–239
blunted, definition of, 238, 280
constricted, definition of, 238, 280
definition of, 238, 280
in delusional disorder, 514
in elderly patients, 1319
evaluation of, in child psychiatric evaluation, 1156
flat, definition of, 238, 280
inappropriate, definition of, 280
instability, in autistic disorder, 1211
labile, definition of, 280
in mental status examination, 238
restricted, definition of, 280
Affective disorder(s). *See* Mood disorder(s)
Affirmation, in psychotherapy, definition of, 927*t*
Afterlife phenomena, 59
Age
and amphetamine (or amphetaminelike substance)-use disorders, 414
and anabolic (androgenic) steroid abuse, 466
and benzodiazepine abuse, 461
and hallucinogen-use disorders, 437
and inhalant-related disorders, 440–441
posttraumatic stress disorder and, 630
and schizoaffective disorder, 508–509
and suicide, 914, 914*f*
Ageism, 56
Age-related cognitive decline, **900**
Age 30 transition, 41–42
Aggression, **150–158**. *See also* Intermittent explosive disorder
β-adrenergic receptor antagonists for, 1009–1010
and air pollution, 153
and alcohol, 151
buspirone for, 1032
causes of, 153–154
environmental, 153–154
genetic, 154–155
situational, 154
social, 153
in children, pharmacotherapy for, 1006
chromosomal influences on, 154–155
and conduct disorder, 1235–1237
control of, 155–156
and crowding, 154
definition of, 282
in dementia, pharmacological management of, 1332
and direct provocation, 153
drive theory of, 153, 153*t*
and drugs, 154
DSM-IV disorders associated with, 150, 151*t*
fantasies versus acts, 150
Freud's theory of, 151, 200
and frustration, 153
and hormones, 154
as instinctive behavior, 151
instinct theory of, 151, 153*t*
interviewing agitated/violent patients, 249
as learned social behavior, 151–153
limbic system and, 84
Lorenz's theory of, 151, 158–159
in mental retardation, pharmacological intervention for, 1177–1178
as neuroanatomical damage, 154
and noise, 153
and pain, 154
pedigree studies of, 154
pharmacotherapy for, 156, 356, **1068,** 1132
and physiological arousal, 154
predictors of, 150–151
prevention of, 153*t,* 155–156
psychopharmacological interventions for, 157*t*
sex differences in, 151
and sexual arousal, 154
in sociobiology, 164
and substance abuse, 154
and televised violence, 32, 153
theories of, 151–154, 153*t*
twin studies of, 154
victims of, 156, 157*t*
Aging. *See also* Elderly; Geriatric psychiatry
biology of, 51–55, 52*t*
normal
versus amnestic disorder, 349
versus dementia, 339
memory problems in, 339, 349, 1318
psychosocial aspects of, 55–58
robust, 56
Aging parents, care of, **879**
Agitation, 103. *See also* Intermittent explosive disorder
acupuncture for, 1145
benzodiazepines for, 1022
definition of, 281
in dementia, pharmacological management of, 1332
pharmacotherapy for, **1055**
and psychotherapeutic drugs, **981**
Agnosia
definition of, 286
in elderly patients, 1319
visual, definition of, 286
Agoraphobia. *See also* Panic disorder, with agoraphobia
and alcohol use disorders, 397
associated symptoms, 605
behavior therapy for, 954*t*
clinical features of, 605
comorbidity with, 599–600
course of, 606
definition of, 284, 599
diagnosis of, 603
diagnostic criteria for, 603, 603*t*
emergency manifestations of, 907*t*
emergency treatment of, 907*t*
epidemiology of, 599
genetic factors in, 600–601
ICD-10 diagnostic criteria for, 596*t*
and pathological gambling, 788
prognosis for, 606
psychoanalytic theory of, 611
psychosocial factors in, 601
treatment of, 606–609
without history of panic disorder
diagnostic criteria for, 603, 603*t*
differential diagnosis of, 606
Agranulocytosis, 498
with antipsychotic drug therapy, 265, 266*t*
emergency manifestations of, 907*t,* 910*t*
emergency treatment of, 907*t,* 910*t*
Agraphia, definition of, 287
AIDS, 371. *See also* Human immunodeficiency virus (HIV), infection
Ailurophobia, definition of, 284
AIMS, 996*t*, 1059, 1060*t*
Ainsworth, Mary, 28, 140–141
Air pollution, and aggression, 153
Akathisia, 497. *See also* Medication-induced movement disorders; Neuroleptic-induced acute akathisia
anticholinergics for, 1013
definition of, 282
emergency manifestations of, 907*t*
emergency treatment of, 907*t*
pharmacotherapy for, 1013, **1026**
and psychotherapeutic drugs, **981**
Akinesia, definition of, 281
Akineton. *See* Biperiden hydrochloride
Akiskal, Hagop, 817
Alanine aminotransferase (ALT)
effects of alcohol on, 401
test for, 269*t*
Albumin, test for, 269*t*
Alcohol
absorption, 399
abuse/dependence, 395, **401–403**
acupuncture for, 1145
behavior therapy for, 954*t*
clinical features of, 401–402
delta, 402–403
diagnosis of, 401–402
differential diagnosis of, 575
in elderly, 1326
gamma, 402
mood disorder and, 351*t*, 553
pharmacotherapy for, 1046–1047, 1069
and schizophrenia, 476
subtypes of, 402–403
and suicide, **916**
type A, 402

Alcohol—*continued*
type B, 402
type I, male limited, 403
type II, male limited, 403
and aggression, 151
biochemistry of, 399
characteristics of, 398
with chloral hydrate, 1041
and disulfiram, adverse effects of, 1047
drug interactions, 401, 462, 464, 1007, 1021, 1022, 1028
effects, **398–401**
behavioral, 399, 400*t*
on brain, 399
on cardiovascular system, 400
on gastrointestinal system, 400
impairment charts, 400*t*
in laboratory tests, 401
on liver, 399
physiological, 398–401
on sleep, 399
fetal alcohol syndrome, 24, 24*f*, **409–410,** 1168–1169, 1172*t*
hallucinosis, 404*f*
intoxication, **403**
acute, diagnostic criteria for, 390*t*
clinical features of, 403
diagnosis of, 403
diagnostic criteria for, 401, 402*t*
emergency manifestations of, 908*t*
emergency treatment of, 908*t*
idiosyncratic, 408
emergency manifestations of, 908*t*
emergency treatment of, 908*t*
treatment of, 408
pathological, diagnostic criteria for, 390*t*
treatment of, 403, 404*t*
and lithium, 1072*t*
metabolism, 399, 533
ethnic differences in, 399
sex differences in, 399
and mirtazapine, 1075
tolerance, 399
in urinalysis, 268*t*
use
among adolescents, 1286
and educational status, 396
and ethnicity, 396
and geographic region, 396
medical complications of, 409, 409*t*
neurological complications of, 409, 409*t*
patterns of, 396*t*
prevalence of, 396
and race, 396
sex distribution of, 396
and urbanicity, 396
withdrawal, **403–405**
α_2-adrenergic receptor antagonists for, 1005
β-adrenergic receptor antagonists for, 1010
brain imaging in, 403, 404*f*
buspirone for, 1032
clinical features of, 403
diagnosis of, 403
diagnostic criteria for, 393*t*, 401, 402*t*
emergency manifestations of, 405, 908*t*
emergency treatment of, 908*t*
hallucinations and, 403, 406
mild or moderate, 411
mood disorder and, 351*t*
with perceptual disturbances, 403
pharmacotherapy for, 1005, 1010, 1026, **1037,** 1132
seizures in, 404, 404*t*
severe, 411
treatment of, 404–405, 404*t*
Alcohol dehydrogenase (ADH), 399
Alcoholic blackouts, 347, 396, 401, **407**
Alcoholic encephalopathy, 406
Alcoholic hepatitis, 399
Alcoholic pellagra encephalopathy, 409
Alcoholics Anonymous (AA), 388, 402
Alcoholism, 395. *See also* Drinker(s)
antisocial, 403
developmentally cumulative, 403
developmentally limited, 403
and jealous delusions, 515
negative-affect, 403
Alcohol-related disorder(s), 382*t*, **395–413**
amnestic disorder, persisting, 406–407
clinical features of, 406
diagnosis of, 406
emergency manifestations of, 908*t*
emergency treatment of, 908*t*
treatment of, 406
and antisocial personality disorder, 397
and anxiety disorders, 397, 408
and attention-deficit/hyperactivity disorder, 397
childhood history and, 397
comorbidity with, 397
counseling, 412
delirium, **405–406**
clinical features of, 405
diagnosis of, 405
emergency manifestations of, 405, 908*t*
emergency treatment of, 908*t*
treatment, 406
psychotherapy in, 406
dementia, persisting, 406
emergency manifestations of, 908*t*
emergency treatment of, 908*t*
and depression, 397
DSM-IV-TR classification of, 401, 401*t*
epidemiology of, 395–396
etiology of, 397–398
behavioral factors in, 398
biological factors in, 398
cultural factors in, 398
genetic influences, 398, 398*t*
learning factors in, 398
psychodynamic factors in, 397–398
social factors in, 398
family involvement, 411
hospitalization in, 405
intervention, 410–411
medications, 412–413
and mood disorders, 351*t*, 397, 407–408, 553
not otherwise specified, 408, 408*t*
and obsessive-compulsive disorder, 617
and opioid dependence, 450
pharmacotherapy for, 389, 399, 412–413, 1002*t*–1003*t*
prognosis, 410
psychodynamic theories, 397–398
psychotherapy for, 388
psychotic disorder and, 407
clinical features of, 407
diagnosis of, 407
with hallucinations
emergency manifestations of, 908*t*
emergency treatment of, 908*t*
and pyromania, 786
rehabilitation, 411–412
self-help groups, 413
sexual dysfunction, 408, 711
sleep disorders, 408
sociocultural theories, 398
socioeconomic class and, 396–397
statistical factors in, 396
and suicide, 397
treatment, 410–413
trends in, 395–396
Alcohol seizures
emergency manifestations of, 908*t*
emergency treatment of, 908*t*
Aldehyde dehydrogenase, 399
Aldolase, test for, 269*t*
Aldomet. *See* Methyldopa
Alexander, Franz, **218,** 218*f*, 852, 928
and brief psychotherapy, 930
Alexander technique, **852,** 853*f*, 866, 867
Alexia. *See also* Reading disorder
definition of, 287
Alexithymia, definition of, 280
Algophobia, definition of, 284
Alkaline phosphatase, test for, 269*t*
Alkaloid, 104
Allopathic medicine, 851
Allopathy, definition of, 851
All-or-none phenomenon, in action potentials, 91
Allport, Gordon, **218**
Alogia, definition of, 285
Alopecia areata, 791*f*
Alprazolam, 267, 999*t*. *See also* Benzodiazepine(s)
adverse effects of, 981*t*
adverse reactions to, 1027–1028
dosage of, 1025*t*
drug interactions, 378, 1081
CYP-induced, 976
geriatric dosage, 1332*t*
half-life of, 1025*t*
indications for, 500, 1024
pharmacokinetics of, 1022
precautions with, 1027–1028
for separation anxiety disorder, 1263
structure of, 1023*f*
Alprostadil, for sexual dysfunction, 715, 980
ALT. *See* Alanine aminotransferase (ALT)
Alter ego, 223
Alternative lifestyle
parenting, 45
pregnancy, 869
Alternative medicine, **851–867**
and end-of-life care, 1348
Altruism, 208*t*
in group psychotherapy, 938*t*
in sociobiology, 164
Aluminum toxicity, 332
Alurate. *See* Aprobarbital
Alzheimer's disease, 82, 331–333. *See also* Dementia, of Alzheimer's type
biochemical markers, 274*t*
cholinesterase inhibitors for. *See* Cholinesterase inhibitors
diagnosis of, 126
and estrogen replacement therapy, 1332
genetics of, 126, 127*f*, 331
glucose metabolism, in temporoparietal region of brain, 118*f*
infectious agents and, 133
insulin and, 129
neuroimaging in, 108, 111*f*, 117*f*, 118*f*
neuropathology of, 126, 331–332, 331*f*
neurotransmitters in, 332

senile plaques in brain, 332*f*
treatment of, 106
Amantadine, 999*t*, **1011–1012**
adverse effects of, 1012
for autistic disorder, 1215
chemistry of, 1011, 1011*f*
clinical guidelines for, 1012
for cocaine users, 435
dosage of, 1012
drug interactions, 1012, 1031
effects on specific organs and systems, 1011
for extrapyramidal disorders, 1059*t*
indications for, 1011–1012
intoxication/overdose, 984*t*
pharmacological actions of, 1011
precautions with, 1012
for sexual dysfunction, 980–981
structure of, 1011*f*
Ambien. *See* Zolpidem
Ambivalence
definition of, 281
in obsessive-compulsive disorder, 619
Amenorrhea, 256
American Academy of Child and Adolescent Psychiatry, code of ethics, 1315
American Association for Mental Retardation (AAMR), 1161
American Board of Psychiatry and Neurology, 246
American Dance Therapy Association, 854
American Herbal Association, 856
American Psychiatric Association (APA)
on confidentiality in child psychiatry, 1315
Practice Guideline for Psychiatric Evaluation of Adults, 6*t*
American School of Naturopathy, 864
American School of Osteopathy, 864
Amiloride, and lithium, 1072*t*
Amimia, definition of, 281
Amino acid(s), 123, **1146**. *See also* Dietary supplements
neurotransmitter function, 88, 91*f*, **96–97, 105–107**
in schizophrenia, 478
γ-Aminobutyric acid (GABA). *See* GABA
Aminoketones, adverse effects of, 981*t*
Aminophylline, blood level data for clinical assessment, 268*t*
Amitriptyline, 999*t*. *See also* Tricyclic drugs (tricyclic antidepressants)
adverse effects of, 567*t*, 981*t*, 1127*t*
for anorexia nervosa, 745
blood level data for clinical assessment, 268*t*
clinical information, 1130*t*
dosage and administration, 569*t*
drug interactions, 1134
mechanism of action, 567*t*
neurotransmitter effects of, 1126*t*
for pain management, 1345*t*
plasma levels, monitoring, 265
preparations of, 1130*t*
structure of, 1125*f*
Amlodipine, 999*t*, 1034*t*
dosage and administration, 1035
Ammonia, serum, test for, 269*t*
Ammonium chloride, indications for, 459
Amnesia. *See also* Dissociative amnesia
anterograde, definition of, 286
and benzodiazepine(s), 345, 463
definition of, 286
generalized, in dissociative amnesia, 677
localized, in dissociative amnesia, 677
medical causes of, 82
retrograde, definition of, 286
selective, in dissociative amnesia, 677
systematized, in dissociative amnesia, 677
transient global, 348, 349*f*
differential diagnosis of, 678
Amnestic disorder(s), **345–349**
alcohol-induced persisting, 406–407, 908*t*
with cerebrovascular disease, 347
clinical features of, 346–348
cognition in, 320–321
cognitive rehabilitation, centers for, 349–350
computed tomography, 323, 348–349
course of, 349
definition of, 319, 345
versus delirium, 349
versus dementia, 349
diagnosis of, 346
diagnostic criteria for, 350*t*
differential diagnosis of, 349
versus dissociative disorders, 349
DSM-IV classification of, 320*t*
due to a general medical condition, diagnostic criteria for, 345, 346*t*
with electroconvulsive therapy, 347–348
electroencephalography, 322
epidemiology of, 345
etiology of, 345, 345*t*, 346*t*
versus factitious disorder, 349
with head injury, 348
ICD-10, 350, 350*t*
with Korsakoff's syndrome, 347
laboratory evaluation of patient, 322, 322*t*, 348–349
magnetic resonance imaging, 323, 348–349
functional, 323
mental status examination, 320, 321*t*
with multiple sclerosis, 347
neuropsychological testing, 323
versus normal aging, 349
not otherwise specified, diagnostic criteria for, 346*t*
physical examination of patient, 321, 322*t*
positron emission tomography, 323
prognosis for, 349
psychiatric history, 320
psychotherapy for, 349
sedative-, hypnotic-, or anxiolytic-related, persisting, 463
signs and symptoms of, 319, 346
single photon emission computed tomography, 323
substance-induced
diagnostic criteria for, 394*t*
persisting, 381*t*, 382*t*. *See also specific substance*
diagnostic criteria for, 345, 346*t*
subtypes of, 319, 346–348
treatment of, 349
Amniocentesis, 23–24, 24
Amobarbital, 460, 999*t*. *See also* Amytal (amobarbital) interview; Barbiturate(s)
dosage of, 1020*t*
indications for, 1018
structure of, 1018*f*
Amok, 530*t*, 784
Amotivational syndrome, 427
Amoxapine, 999*t*
adverse effects of, 567*t*, 981*t*, 1127*t*
clinical information, 1130*t*
dosage and administration, 569*t*
mechanism of action, 567*t*
neurotransmitter effects of, 1126*t*
preparations of, 1130*t*
structure of, 1125*f*
Amphetamine salt preparations, for attention-deficit/hyperactivity disorder, 1227, 1227*t*
Amphetamine(s) (or amphetaminelike substance)-related disorder(s), 382*t*, **413–419,** 1116
clinical features of, 417
diagnosis of, 414
DSM-IV classification of, 415*t*
DSM-IV-TR classification of, 414
epidemiology of, 414
not otherwise specified, 417
diagnostic criteria for, 414, 416*t*
rehabilitation, 418–419
treatment, 418–419
Amphetamine(s) (or amphetaminelike substances), 100, 414, 999*t*. *See also* Sympathomimetics
abuse, 256, **414–415**
addiction potential, 100
adverse effects of, 417
physical, 417
psychological, 417
and age, 414
anxiety disorder, 417
blood level data for clinical assessment, 268*t*
classic, 414–418
dependence, **414–415**
designer, 414–418, 436
adverse effects of, 417, 418*f*
drug interactions, 1062*t*
effects of, 414
indications for, 413
intoxication delirium, 416
diagnosis of, 416
intoxication/overdose, **415,** 984*t*
diagnostic criteria for, 414, 415*t*
emergency manifestations of, 908*t*
emergency treatment of, 908*t*
with perceptual disturbances, 415
khat, 418
mood disorder, 417
for narcolepsy, 769
neuropharmacology of, 414
pharmacological action of, 1117
preparations, 413–414
psychotic behavior and, 163
psychotic disorder, 416
diagnosis of, 416
paranoia in, 416
versus paranoid schizophrenia, 416
treatment of, 416
sexual dysfunction, 417
sleep disorder, 417
substituted, 414, 417, 436
adverse effects of, 417, 418*f*
mechanisms of action, 417
subjective effects, 417–418
toxicity, 418
tolerance, 414
in urinalysis, 268*t*
for weight reduction, 755*t*
withdrawal, **416**
depression in, 416
diagnostic criteria for, 414–415, 415*t*
Amphetamine sulfate, 413
Amygdala, 78, 83–84
in memory formation, 80

Amylase, serum, test for, 270*t*
Amyl nitrite, 468
Amyloid plaque, of Alzheimer's disease, 331, 332*f*
Amyloid precursor protein, in Alzheimer's disease, 331
Amyotrophic lateral sclerosis, neuropsychiatric manifestations of, 363
Amytal. *See* Amobarbital
Amytal (amobarbital) interview, 267, 1148
"Amytal interview," 1018
ANA, 270*t*
Anabolic (androgenic) steroid(s)
abuse, **466–468**
in athletics, 467
clinical features of, 467
diagnosis of, 467
epidemiology of, 466
etiology of, 467
addiction, 467
adverse effects of, 467
commonly used, 466*t*
neuropharmacology of, 467
personality change due to, 467, **819**
synthetic, 467
use
and age, 466
prevalence of, 466
sex distribution of, 466
Anaclitic depression, 142
Anafranil. *See* Clomipramine
Analgesic(s)
abuse, 395*t*
end-of-life care, 1343–1345
indications for, 423
Anal personality, 215
Anal stage, 19, 200, 201*t*
Analysis of variance, 174
Analytically oriented group therapy, features of, 936*t*
Analytic psychology, 222
Anamnesis, 234
Anandamides, neurotransmitter function, 107
Androgen insensitivity syndrome, 693*t,* 735
Androgen(s)
and aggression, 154
for sex drive, 715
Androstenedione, 467
Anectine. *See* Succinylcholine
Anemia, with antipsychotic drug therapy, 266*t*
Anergia
definition of, 282
pharmacotherapy for, 1119
Anesthesia, for electroconvulsive therapy, 1140–1141
Angelica, 854*t*
Angelman syndrome, 1171*t*
Anger, in dying person, 60
Angiography, postprocedure complications, 1249*t*
Angiotensin converting enzyme (ACE) inhibitors
drug interactions, 1062*t*
and lithium, 1072*t*
Angst, 591
Anhedonia, 491
definition of, 280
orgasmic, 712
Anilingus, 723
Anima, 222
Animal models, **126–127,** 161–163
pharmacological syndromes, 163
stress syndrome, 161
Animistic thinking, 60–61, 137
Animus, 222
Anna O., 194
Anorexia, definition of, 281
Anorexia nervosa, 256, **739–746**. *See also* Eating disorder(s)
amenorrhea in, 256
behavior therapy for, 954*t*
binge eating-purging type, 741–742
biological factors in, 739–740
biological therapy for, 745
clinical features of, 741–742, 742*f*
cognitive-behavioral therapy, 745
cognitive profile of, 957*t*
comorbidity with, 739
course of, 744
diagnosis of, 741–742
diagnostic criteria for, 741*t*
differential diagnosis of, 743–744
ECG findings in, 741
emergency manifestations of, 908*t*
emergency treatment of, 908*t*
epidemiology of, 739
etiology of, 739–740
family therapy, 745
hospitalization for, 744–745
ICD-10 research criteria for, 745–746, 746*t*
laboratory examination, 743
laboratory findings in, 743
medical complications of, 741, 742*t*
neuroendocrine changes in, 740*t*
pathology of, 743
pharmacotherapy for, 745
prognosis for, 744
psychodynamic factors in, 740
psychological factors in, 740
and psychotherapeutic drugs, **982**
psychotherapy for, 745
restricting type, 741–743
social factors in, 740
treatment of, 744–745
Anorexiants, drug interactions, 1062*t*
Anorgasmia, **704–705,** 704*t*
Anosognosia, 83
definition of, 286
ANOVA. *See* Analysis of variance
Antabuse. *See* Disulfiram
Antacid(s)
abuse, 395*t*
drug interactions, 1061, 1062*t*
Anthropology
and psychiatry, **166–168**
psychoanalytical, **166**
Anthroposophically extended medicine, **852–853**
Anthroposophy, **852–853**
Antiandrogen agent(s), in aggressive sex offenders, 156
Antiandrogens, 715–716
Anti-anxiety agents. *See* Anxiolytic(s)
Antiarrhythmic drugs, drug interactions, 1035
CYP-induced, 976
Antibiotics, and lithium, 1072*t*
Anticholinergic(s), **1012–1015**. *See also* Benztropine; Trihexyphenidyl
adverse effects of, 1014
chemistry of, 1012, 1013*f*
clinical guidelines for, 1014–1015
dosage of, 1014–1015
drug interactions, 1014, 1061, 1062*t*
effects on specific organs and systems, 1013
herbal, 533
implicated in sexual dysfunction, 711
indications for, 1013
intoxication/overdose of, 984*t,* 1014
emergency manifestations of, 908*t*
emergency treatment of, 908*t*
mechanism of action, 105
pharmacological actions of, 1013
precautions with, 1014
Anticholinergic side effects, 256, 567*t*
Anticipation, 208*t*
Anticipatory grief, 63
Anticipatory response, 146
Anticoagulants, drug interactions, 1047
Anticonvulsant(s), 360, 360*t*
for aggressive/violent behavior, 156
for bipolar I disorder, 571
for cocaine users, 435
drug interactions, 1061
Gabapentin. *See* Gabapentin
indications for, 500
intoxication
emergency manifestations of, 908*t*
emergency treatment of, 908*t*
Lamotrigine. *See* Lamotrigine
Topiramate. *See* Topiramate
Antidepressant(s), 565–572. *See also* Monoamine oxidase inhibitors; Selective serotonin reuptake inhibitors
abuse, 395*t*
adverse effects of, 566, 567*t,* 981*t*
for aggressive/violent behavior, 156
alternatives to, 566
for anxiety disorders, 353
for attention-deficit/hyperactivity disorder, 1228
augmentation of, **989–990**
with β-Adrenergic receptor antagonist(s), 1010
for geriatric depression, 1330
available drugs, 566
children, adverse effects of use with, 1310
in combination with benzodiazepines, 1029
cyclic, laboratory testing with, 265
dosage and administration, guidelines for, 568, 569*t*
drug interactions, 566–568, 568*t,* 1061, 1062*t*
duration of treatment with, 568–569
for elderly, 1329, 1330
failure of drug trial with, 569
implicated in sexual dysfunction, 711
indications for, 427
mechanism of action, 92, 96, 103–104, 566, 567*t*
patient education about, 566
for postpartum psychosis, 527
prophylaxis with, 568–569
selection of, 567*t*
and sleep, 759
tetracyclic. *See* Tetracyclic drugs
thyroid hormones as adjuvants to, 1122
tricyclic. *See* Tricyclic drugs (tricyclic antidepressants)
type-specific treatments with, 568
Antiepileptics, drug interactions, 1010
Antiestrogens, 715–716
Antihistamine(s), **1015–1017**
adverse effects, 1016
chemistry of, 1015, 1015*f*
clinical guidelines for, 1016
dosage of, 1016, 1017*t*

drug interactions, 1016, 1028
effects on specific organs and systems, 1016
implicated in sexual dysfunction, 711
indications for, 1016
intoxication/overdose of, 984*t*
laboratory interferences, 1016
for nonpsychiatric disorders, 1015*t*
pharmacological actions of, 1016
precautions with, 1016
Antihypertensives, drug interactions, 1007, 1062, 1129
Antimanic agents, for elderly, 1330, 1330*t*
Antinuclear antibody (ANA) test, 270*t*
Antipsychotic(s), 85
adverse effects of, 497–499
for aggressive/violent behavior, 156
for alcoholism, 413
for attention-deficit/hyperactivity disorder, 1228
atypical, 471, 497–499
with benzodiazepines, 1029
children, use with, 1307*t*
adverse effects of, 1310–1311
classes of, 497
classic, 497
for cocaine users, 435
development of, 1051
drug interactions, 1028, 1129, 1133
for elderly, 1331, 1332*t*
neurological adverse effects of, 1331
implicated in sexual dysfunction, 711
indications for, 409, 419
for intermittent explosive disorder, 785
laboratory testing with, 265, 266*t*
and lithium, 1072*t*
mechanism of action, 100, 102
for schizophrenia, 471, 497–499
Serotonin-dopamine antagonists. *See* Serotonin-dopamine antagonist(s) (atypical antipsychotics)
standard, 497
Antiretroviral drugs, 376–377, 376*t*
psychotropic drug interactions, 377–378
Antisocial behavior
adult, **896–897**
in childhood/adolescence, **1292–1293**
Antisocial personality disorder, **807–808**. *See also* Personality disorder(s), cluster B
and alcohol use disorders, 397
clinical features of, 807–808
course of, 808
diagnosis of, 807
diagnostic criteria for, 807, 807*t*
differential diagnosis of, 784, 808
epidemiology of, 807
and opioid dependence, 450
and pathological gambling, 788
pharmacotherapy for, 808
prognosis for, 808
psychotherapy for, 808
and substance-related disorders, 387–388
treatment of, 808
Anton's syndrome, 70
Anxiety. *See also* Anxiety disorder(s); *specific anxiety disorder*
and academic problems, 1291
actual neuroses, 209
acupuncture for, 1145
adaptive functions of, 592
with adjustment disorder, **796**
animal model of, 161
and attachment, 141–142
and attention-deficit/hyperactivity disorder, 1226
basic, 221
benzodiazepines for, 1022
Bowlby's theory of, 141–142
buspirone for, 1032
castration, 593
cholecystokinin and, 105
cognitive symptoms of, 592–593
conflict and, 592
definition of, 281
with dementia, 108
differential diagnosis of, 902–904, 903*t*
disintegration, 593
fear and, 591–592
free-floating, definition of, 281
Freud's theory of, **206–209,** 591, 593
generalized. *See also* Generalized anxiety disorder
due to a general medical condition, 636
genetics of, 126
hierarchy of, 148
and insomnia, 760
mood disorder and, 553
normal, **591–593**
versus pathological, 591
paranoid, 593
pathological, **593–595**
peripheral manifestations of, 591, 592*t*
persecutory, 222, 593
pharmacotherapy for, 1003*t*, **1024,** 1032, 1075
psychological symptoms of, 592–593
and psychotherapeutic drugs, **981**
serotonin and, 103, 104
signal, 209
as signal, 593
stress and, 592
and stuttering, 1203
superego, 209, 592
Anxiety-blissfulness psychosis, **484,** 584
Anxiety disorder(s), **591–632**. *See also* Generalized anxiety disorder; Mixed anxiety-depressive disorder; *specific disorder*
β-adrenergic receptor antagonists for, 1009
alcohol-induced, 397, 408
amphetamine-induced, 417
Aplysia californica model for, 595
autonomic nervous system and, 594
behavioral theories of, 593–594
biological theories of, 594–595
brain imaging in, 595
caffeine-induced, 422–423
cannabis-induced, 426–427
cerebral cortex in, 595
cocaine-related, 433
cognitive profile of, 957*t*
and conversion disorder, 648
DSM-IV-TR classification of, 591, 595
due to a general medical condition, 636–638
clinical features of, 636–637
course of, 638
diagnosis of, 636
diagnostic criteria for, 636, 637*t*
differential diagnosis of, 638
epidemiology of, 636
etiology of, 636, 637*t*
prognosis for, 638
treatment of, 638
in elderly, 1325
epidemiology of, 593
existential theories of, 594
and expressive language disorder, 1195
GABAergic system in, 104
generalized. *See* Generalized anxiety disorder
due to a general medical condition, **353**
genetic studies of, 595
hallucinogen-related, 439
ICD-10 classification of, 595–598, 596*t*–597*t*
inhalant-related, 442–443
and intermittent explosive disorder, 783
and kleptomania, 785
limbic system in, 595
meprobamate for, 1021
neuroanatomical considerations in, 595
neuroimaging in, 109
neurotransmitters in, 594–595
not otherwise specified, **640–642**
diagnostic criteria for, 640, 640*t*
and opioid dependence, 450
other, ICD-10 diagnostic criteria for, 597*t*
PCP-induced, 458
pharmacotherapy for, 1006, 1009, 1021, 1081
phobic. *See also* Phobia(s); *specific phobia*
ICD-10 diagnostic criteria for, 596*t*
and posttraumatic stress disorder, 624
psychoanalytic theories of, 593
psychological theories of, 593–594
sedative-, hypnotic-, or anxiolytic-related, 463
substance-induced, 381*t*, 382*t*, **638–640**. *See also specific substance*
clinical features of, 638
course of, 640
diagnosis of, 638
diagnostic criteria for, 638, 639*t*
differential diagnosis of, 639
epidemiology of, 638
etiology of, 638
prognosis for, 640
treatment of, 640
and suicide, **917**
and transcranial magnetic stimulation, 1144–1145
and trichotillomania, 790
valvular heart disease and, 830
Anxiety dreams, 198
Anxiety hysteria, 610
Anxiolytic(s). *See also* Benzodiazepine(s); Sedative-, hypnotic-, or anxiolytic-related disorder(s)
for aggressive/violent behavior, 156
definition of, 460
for elderly, 1331–1332
implicated in sexual dysfunction, 711
indications for, 419, 427
Anxious-ambivalent attachment, 143
APA. *See* American Psychiatric Association (APA)
Apathy
definition of, 281
treatment of, 356
Aphasia(s), 78, 82, 189, 903, 904*t*
acquired, with convulsion, differential diagnosis of, 1213
anomic, 79*t*
Broca's, 79*t*, 82, 1319
conduction, 79*t*

Aphasia(s)—*continued*
differential diagnosis of, 1197
in elderly patients, 1319
fluent, 1319
global, 79*t*
definition of, 285
jargon, definition of, 285
localization of syndromes, 78, 79*t*
motor, definition of, 285
nominal, definition of, 285
nonfluent, 83, 1319
and phonological disorders, 1203*t*
in schizophrenia, 495
sensory, definition of, 285
syntactical, definition of, 285
transcortical
mixed, 79*t*
motor, 79*t*
sensory, 79*t*
types of, 79*t*
Wernicke's, 79*t,* 82, 1319
Aphasia Screening Test, 191*t*
Aphasic disturbances, definition of, 285
Aphonia, 255
Aphrodisiacs, 715
Aplysia californica, 147–148
model for anxiety disorders, 595
Apomorphine, 448, 715, 999*t*
for erectile dysfunction, 1050
Appearance
in medical assessment, 256–257
in mental status examination, 238
of schizophrenic patient, 487*f,* 490–491, 492*f*
Apperceptive visual agnosia, 70
Applied relaxation, for panic disorder, 608
Applied tension technique, **949–950**
Appointment(s)
missed, **12**
patient management of time, 246–247
Apraxia(s), **75, 77**
definition of, 286
ideational, 77
ideomotor, 75, 77, 1319
limb-kinetic, 75
oculomotor, 71
in schizophrenia, 495
Aprobarbital, 999*t*. *See also* Barbiturate(s)
dosage of, 1020*t*
indications for, 1018
structure of, 1018*f*
APSI, 1288
ARAS, 80, 119, 163
Archetypes, 222
Arginine vasopressin, 129*t*
Aricept. *See* Donepezil
Arieti, Silvano, on depression, 541
Aripiprazole, 999*t*
Aromatherapy, **853,** 854*t*
Arousal
brain function and, 80
physiological arousal, and aggression, 154
sexual
and aggression, 154
disorders. *See* Sexual arousal disorder(s)
β-Arrestin, 93
Arrhythmia(s), cardiac, biofeedback for, 949*t*
Arsenic, **367**
blood level data for clinical assessment, 268*t*
Arson, distinguished from pyromania, 786
Artane. *See* Trihexyphenidyl
Artificial insemination, 873*t*
Arylcyclohexylamine(s), 456
Ascending reticular activating system (ARAS), 80, 119, 163
Asceticism, in adolescence, 36–37, 208*t*
Ascorbic acid, indications for, 459
Asendin. *See* Amoxapine
Asher, Irvin, 365
Asia, nutrition in, 855
As-if personality, 809
Aspartate aminotransferase (AST)
effects of alcohol on, 401
test for, 270*t*
Asperger, Hans, 1218
Asperger's disorder, 1219
Asperger's syndrome, **1218–1219**
clinical features of, 1218
course of, 1218–1219
definition of, 1218
diagnosis of, 1218
diagnostic criteria for, 1218, 1218*t*
differential diagnosis of, 1218
etiology of, 1218
ICD-10 diagnostic criteria for, 1219, 1221*t*
prognosis for, 1218–1219
treatment of, 1219
Aspirin, for pain management, 1345*t*
Assaultive behavior, **904**
emergency manifestations of, 909*t*
emergency treatment of, 909*t*
Assertive Community Treatment (ACT) program, for schizophrenia, 501
Assertiveness training, in behavior therapy, **953**
Assessment instruments
for epidemiologic studies, 173–174, 174*t*
predictive value of, 175*t*
sensitivity of, 175*t*
specificity of, 175*t*
Association systems, **78–85**
Associative play, 31
Associative visual agnosia, 70
AST. *See* Aspartate aminotransferase (AST)
Astasia abasia, definition of, 282
Astereognosis, 67
definition of, 286
Asthma, 255, 831
biofeedback for, 949*t*
psychological correlates of, 826*t,* **831**
sleep-related, **779**
Astrocytoma, 108
Ataque de nervios, 530*t*
Atarax. *See* Hydroxyzine
Ataxia, 256
and benzodiazepine(s), 1028
definition of, 282
Atenolol, 999*t,* 1009*t*. *See also* β-Adrenergic receptor antagonist(s)
chemistry of, 1008*f*
geriatric dosage, 1332*t*
pharmacological actions of, 1009
Ativan. *See* Lorazepam
Atopic dermatitis, 833, 833*f*
psychological correlates of, **833**
Attachment, **28, 28–30**
abuse and, 142
animal model of, 159–160
and anxiety, 141–142
versus bonding, 140
clear-cut, 140
definition of, 140
disorders, **142–143**
ethological studies of, 140
fathers and, 29
mother–child, 28–29
normal, **139–140,** 141*t*
phases of, 140, 141*t*
relationship disorders, 143
severing, 142
Attachment behavior, 28–30
Attachment in the making, 140
Attachment theory, **139–142**
application of, 142
Attention
assessment of, in mental status examination, 241–242
brain function and, 80
disturbances of, definition of, 280
impairment, assessment for, 189–190
and phonological disorder, 1200
Attention cathexis, 199
Attention-deficit/hyperactivity disorder (ADHD), 80, **1223–1229**
in adults, manifestations of, 1229
and alcohol use disorders, 397
and brain damage, 1224
bupropion for, 1030
in children, 1225–1226
clinical features of, 1225–1226
combined psychotherapy and pharmacotherapy for, 970, 1312
and conduct disorder, 1226–1227, 1233
course of, 1227
definition of, 1223
and depression, 1226
and developmental coordination disorder, 1190
developmental factors in, 1223–1224
diagnosis of, 1224–1225
diagnostic criteria for, 1223, 1225*t,* 1229–1230, 1229*t,* 1230*t*
differential diagnosis of, 1187, 1226–1227, 1237
drug augmentation therapy for, **992**
epidemiology of, 1223
etiology of, 1223–1224
evaluation of therapeutic progress, 1229
and expressive language disorder, 1195
genetic factors in, 1223
in infants, 1225–1226
laboratory examination of, 1226
and mental retardation, 1163
pharmacological intervention for, 1177–1178
neurochemical factors in, 1224
neuroimaging in, 109
neurophysiological factors in, 1224
nonstimulant medications for, 1228, 1228*t*
not otherwise specified, **1229**
diagnostic criteria for, 1229*t*
and pathological gambling, 788
pathology of, 1226
pharmacotherapy for, 970, 992, 1003*t,* 1030, 1116, **1118,** 1227–1228, **1308–1309**
drug augmentation therapy, **992**
prognosis for, 1227
psychosocial factors in, 1224
psychosocial interventions for, 1229
psychotherapy for, 1229
and pyromania, 787
Rating Scale, 1158*t*
and reading disorder, 1181
and stuttering, 1203
subtypes of, 1223
sympathomimetics for, 1116

Tourette's disorder and, 1246
treatment of, 1227–1229
and written expression disorder, 1186
Attributable risk, definition of, 176
Attribution theory, **147**
Atypical puberty, **1313–1314**
Auditory Analysis Test, 191*t*
Auditory hallucinations, with schizophrenia with childhood onset, 1283
Auditory processing defect, 86–87
Auditory sound agnosia, 71
Auditory system, **71,** 73
disorders in, 71
language, auditory processing and, 86–87
Aura, definition of, 286
Aurorix. *See* Moclobemide
Austen Riggs Center, 217
Authority anxiety, and group psychotherapy, **935**
Autism
atypical, ICD-10 diagnostic criteria for, 1219, 1220*t*
childhood, ICD-10 diagnostic criteria for, 1219, 1220*t*
infantile. *See* Infantile autism
normal, 29*t*
Autistic disorder, **1208–1215**. *See also* Pervasive developmental disorder(s)
versus acquired aphasia with convulsion, 1213
behavioral characteristics in, 1210–1211
biochemical factors in, 1210
biological factors in, 1209
characteristics of, 1219
in children, pharmacotherapy for, **1306–1308**
clinical features of, 1210–1212
versus congenital deafness, 1213–1214
course of, 1214
diagnosis of, 1210–1212
diagnostic criteria for, 1210, 1210*t*
differential diagnosis of, 1212–1214, 1213*t,* 1269
epidemiology of, 1208
etiology of, 1208–1210
family factors in, 1209
genetic factors in, 1209
historical perspective on, 1208
immunological factors in, 1209
infantile
and language disorders, 1200*t*
and phonological disorders, 1203*t*
and mental retardation, 1163
versus mental retardation with behavioral symptoms, 1213
versus mixed receptive-expressive language disorder, 1213, 1214*t*
neuroanatomical factors in, 1209–1210
neurological factors in, 1209
pathogenesis of, 1208–1210
perinatal factors in, 1209
physical characteristics and, 1210
physical illness, associated, 1211–1212
prevalence of, 1208
prognosis for, 1214
versus psychosocial deprivation, 1214
psychosocial factors in, 1209
and schizophrenia with childhood onset, 1282
versus schizophrenia with childhood onset, 1213, 1213*t*
sex distribution of, 1208
and socioeconomic status, 1208
treatment of, 1214–1215
Autistic psychopathy, 1218
Autistic thinking, definition of, 283
Autoerotic asphyxiation, 712, 724
Autogenic training, **949,** 950*t*
Automatic hyperreflexia, 998*t*
Automatic Language Sequences, 191*t*
Automatic obedience, definition of, 282
Automatism, definition of, 281
Autonomic motor system, 77–78
parasympathetic, 77
sympathetic, 77
Autonomic nervous system, and anxiety disorder, 594
Autonomic sensory system, 72
Autonomy
Erikson's concept of, 19, **215**
patient autonomy, 1365
versus shame and doubt, 19, 212–213
Autopsy, psychological, 60
Autoscopic psychosis, **525–526**
Autosomal dominant transmission, 125
Autosomal recessive transmission, 125
Autotopagnosia, definition of, 286
Aventyl. *See* Nortriptyline
Aversion therapy, in behavior therapy, **953,** 954*f*
Aversive control, 146
Avoidance learning, 146
Avoidant attachment, 143
Avoidant personality disorder, 142, **812–813**. *See also* Personality disorder(s), cluster C
clinical features of, 812–813
course of, 813
diagnosis of, 812
diagnostic criteria for, 812, 813*t*
differential diagnosis of, 813
epidemiology of, 812
pharmacotherapy for, 813
prognosis for, 813
psychotherapy for, 813
treatment of, 813
Awareness, changes in, with brain tumor, 361
Axonal varicosities, 91
Axon hillock, 91
Ayahuasca, 436*t*
Ayurveda, **853**

B

Babinski reflex, 25
Back pain
acupuncture for, 1145
lower. *See* Low back pain
Bad trips, in hallucinogen use disorders, 438
Balint, Michael, 205, **218–219**
and brief focal psychotherapy, 931
Balint's syndrome, 70–71
Bandura, Albert, 147, 151
Barbital, 460
Barbituratelike substance(s), 460
intoxication/overdose, 462, 464
neuropharmacology of, 461
withdrawal, 462–463
Barbiturate(s), 460, **460, 1017–1022**. *See also specific drug*
abuse, 460–461
intravenous, 463–464
adverse effects of, 464, 1019
blood level data for clinical assessment, 268*t*
chemistry of, 1017, 1018*f*
clinical guidelines, 1019
in combination products, 1019, 1020*t*
dosage of, 1019, 1020*t*
drug interactions, 1007, 1019, 1019*t,* 1021, 1022, 1028, 1031, 1047, 1062*t*
effects on specific organs and systems, 1018
for elderly, 1332
indications for, 1018
intoxication/overdose, 462, 464, 984*t*
treatment of, 465
neuropharmacology of, 461
pharmacological actions of, 1018
precautions with, 1019
and sexual dysfunction, 711–712
similarly acting drugs, 1019–1022
in urinalysis, 268*t*
withdrawal, 462–463
pentobarbital test dose procedure for, 464, 465*t*
treatment of, 464–465
Bargaining, in dying person, 60
Basal ganglia, **75,** 76*f*
anatomy of, 75
disorders of, 75
neuroimaging in, 108
in schizophrenia, 477, **479**
BASC, 1158*t*
Basic fault, 219
Basic mistrust, 211–212, 215
Basic trust, **211–212, 215,** 221
versus basic mistrust, 19, 211–212
Basil, 854*t*
Bates, William H., 853
Bates method, **853**
Bateson, Gregory, 484
Battered wives, **890**
physician reference card, 891*t*
Battery, 1359
Bayley Scales of Infant Development, 1159
Bayley Scales of Infant Development-Second Edition, 1158*t*
Bazelon, David, 1357, 1362
Beard, George, 427, 664*f,* 665–665, 667
Beaumont, William, 822
Beck, Aaron, 139, 147, 564, 918
and cognitive therapy, 956
Bed-wetting. *See* Enuresis
Beery-Buktenika Developmental Test of Visual-Motor Integration, 1158*t*
Befloxatone, 999*t,* 1076
Behavior
change, mechanism of, 147
cross-cultural universals of, 168
operant, 144–145
overt, in mental status examination, 238
respondent, 144–145
shaping, 146
stereotyped, in autistic disorder, 1211
tension-reduction theory of, 148–150
Behavioral development, landmarks of, 22*t*
Behavioral disorder(s)
animal model of, 161–163
due to brain disease, damage and dysfunction, ICD-10 classification of, 382*t*
Behavioral genetics, **122–128**
Behavioral group therapy
classification of, 935
features of, 936*t*
Behavioral inhibition, and separation anxiety disorder, 1259
Behavioral management, for childhood/adolescent antisocial behavior, 1292

Behavioral psychology, versus psychoanalytic model, 149*t*, 150
Behavioral skills therapy. *See* Social skills training
Behavior Assessment System for Children (BASC), 1158*t*
Behaviorism, 227
Behavior modification, 109, 227
Behavior problems, symptoms of, history of, 235
Behavior therapy, **950–956**
for anorexia nervosa, 745, 954*t*
for anxiety disorders, 353
assertiveness training in, **953**
aversion therapy in, **953,** 954*f*
for bulimia nervosa, 750, 954*t*
with children, 1296
clinical applications of, 954*t*
and cognitive therapy, 957–959
for depression, 565
dialectical, **954–955**
for borderline personality disorder, 810, 954
for dysthymic disorder, 575
for elderly, 1334
for enuresis, 1257
and eye movement desensitization and reprocessing, **953–954**
flooding in, **952–953**
graded exposure in, **952**
history of, 951
immunological function, 132
implosion in, 952
in mental retardation, 1176
for obsessive-compulsive disorder, 623
for pain disorder, 658
for panic disorder, 601, 608
for paraphilias, 724–725
participant modeling in, **953**
for phobias, 615
positive reinforcement in, **954**
for posttraumatic stress disorder, 625
for psychosomatic illness, 842
questions in, 950–951, 951*t*
results of, 955
for sexual dysfunction, 714, 954*t*
social skills training in, **953**
and systematic desensitization, **951**
therapist role in, 955*t*
virtual stimuli, exposure to, **953**
Being, existential, 227
Benadryl. *See* Diphenhydramine
Bender, Lauretta, 187
Bender Visual-Motor Gestalt Test, 187–188, 188*f*–189*f*, 1159, 1191
for developmental coordination disorder, 1191
Benedict, Ruth, 166
Beneficence, 1365, 1368
Benign senescent forgetfulness, 1318
Bennett, Abram E., 1138
Benson, Herbert, 864
Benton Visual-Motor Gestalt test, 1158*t*
Benton Visual Retention Test, 186, 187*f*, 1158*t*
Benzamide
chemistry of, 1053
structure of, 1052*f*
Benzedrine. *See* Amphetamine(s) (or amphetaminelike substances); Amphetamine sulfate
Benzodiazepine(s), **460, 1022–1029**. *See also specific agent*
abuse, 460–461
and age, 461
and race, 461
sex distribution of, 461
adverse effects of, 464, 1026–1028
amnesia with, 345
and amnestic episodes, 463
for anxiety disorder due to a general medical condition, 353
augmentation of, **991**
buspirone, switching to, 1033
chemistry of, 1022, 1023*f*, 1024*f*
children, use with, 1308*t*
choice of drug, 1028–1029
comparison with buspirone, 1032*t*
dependence, 460, 1027–1028
pharmacotherapy for, 1003*t*
discontinuation of therapy, 1028
dosage and administration of, 1025*t*, 1028–1029
in drug combinations, 1029
drug interactions, 401, 462, 464, 1021, 1022, 1028, 1049, 1062*t*
duration of treatment, 1028
effects on specific organs and systems, 1024
for elderly, 1331–1332, 1332*t*
equivalent doses of, 464*t*
for generalized anxiety disorder, 635
half-lives of, 1025*t*
indications for, 404–405, 404*t*, 406, 423, 459, 500, 1024–1026
for insomnia, in delirium, 328
interviews, 267
intoxication/overdose, 462, 464, 985*t*
emergency manifestations of, 908*t*
emergency treatment of, 908*t*
flumazenil for, 1026
treatment of, 464–465
laboratory testing with, 265
mechanism of action, 106
and mirtazapine, 1075
for neuroleptic-induced acute dystonia, 1014
neuropharmacology of, 461
for nicotine addiction, 448
for panic disorder, 607
pharmacokinetics of, 1022–1023
pharmacological actions of, 1022–1024
potency of, 1028–1029
precautions with, 1026–1028
preparation of, 1025*t*
prescriptions, numbers of, 460, 465
for primary insomnia, 765
for psychotic disorders, 527
for separation anxiety disorder, 1263
tolerance to, 1027–1028
in urinalysis, 268*t*
withdrawal, 462, 982, 1027–1028, 1027*t*
buspirone for, 1032
pharmacotherapy for, 1003*t*, 1005, **1037**
treatment of, 464, 465*t*
Benzphetamine, 999*t*, 1116. *See also* Sympathomimetics (and related drugs)
for weight reduction, 755*t*
Benztropine, 999*t*
for extrapyramidal disorders, 1059*t*
mechanism of action, 100
for neuroleptic-induced acute dystonia, 1014
for neuroleptic-induced parkinsonism, 1014
Benztropine mesylate, 1014*t*. *See also* Anticholinergic(s)
structure of, 1013*f*
Bequests, ethics concerning, 1372*t*
Bereavement, **61–65, 894**
in childhood, 64, **1277**
definition of, 61
emergency manifestations of, 908*t*
emergency treatment of, 908*t*
major depressive disorder, differentiated, 63*t*
spousal, 1327
stages of, 62
uncomplicated, 557
Bergamot, 854*t*
Berne, Eric, **219,** 219*f*
and transactional group therapy, 935
Bernheim, Hippolyte-Marie, 194
and hypnosis, 961
Best interest standard, 1316
Beta blockers. *See* β-Adrenergic receptor antagonist(s)
Betel nuts, 470
Bethanechol
with cholinesterase inhibitors, 1044
for sexual dysfunction, 980
Bhakti yoga, 866
Bibring, Edward, on depression, 541
Bicarbonate, serum, test for, 270*t*
Bilirubin
serum, 264
test for, 270*t*
Bilis and colera, 530*t*
Binet, Alfred, 178
Binge drinking, 396
and educational status, 396
and ethnicity, 396
and geographic region, 396
and race, 396
and urbanicity, 396
Binge eating disorder, 295, 750–751, 750*t*, 753
Bini, Lucio, 1138
Binswanger's disease, 333
Bioavailability, of psychotherapeutic drugs, 975
Biochemical markers, **269,** 274*t*
Bioenergetics, **853**
Biofeedback, 843, **948–950**
applications of, 949*t*
applied tension technique, **949–950**
autogenic training, **949,** 950*t*
instrumentation methods of, 948
methods of, 948–950
for pain disorder, 658
progressive muscular relaxation therapy, **949,** 950*t*
relaxation therapy, **948–949**
results of, 950
theory of, 948
Biogenic amine(s)
in major depressive disorder, 536–537, 536*t*, 537*t*
and mood disorders, 102, 104
neuromodulatory systems, 96, 98*f*
neurotransmitter function, 88, 91*f*, 93*t*, **97–104**
receptors, 93*t*
Biological determinism, 167
Biological rhythms, **134–135**
Biological therapy
for children, **1305–1311**
therapeutic considerations with, 1306, 1306*t*
for sexual dysfunction, 714–715
Bion, Wilfred, **219**
Biopsychosocial model, of disease, 1–2

Biostatistic(s), **174–177**
  definition of, 174
  glossary of terms, 174–177
Biotransformation, of psychotherapeutic drugs, 975–976
Biperiden hydrochloride, 999*t*, 1014*t*. *See also* Anticholinergic(s)
  for extrapyramidal disorders, 1059*t*
  structure of, 1013*f*
Bipolar disorder(s), **534–572, 583**. *See also* Mood disorder(s)
  bipolar I, 535
    age distribution of, 536
    and alcohol use disorders, 397
    in children, 558–559, **1277**
    chromosome 11 and, 540
    and combined psychotherapy and pharmacotherapy, **968–969**
    comparison of treatments for, 1134*t*
    course of, 558–559, 560*f*
    definition of, 544
    diagnosis of, 544–545
    differential diagnosis of, 557, 1292
    in elderly, 558–559, 1324
    epidemiology of, 535
    family studies of, 539–540
    genetics of, 123, 125
    lifetime prevalence, 535*t*
    maintenance drug therapy for, 571–572
    marital status and, 536
    versus medical conditions, 557
    most recent episode depressed, diagnostic criteria for, 547*t*
    most recent episode hypomanic, diagnostic criteria for, 546*t*
    most recent episode manic, diagnostic criteria for, 546*t*
    most recent episode mixed, diagnostic criteria for, 547*t*
    most recent episode unspecified, diagnostic criteria for, 547*t*
    pharmacotherapy for, 570–572, **1026, 1035, 1037, 1054, 1068–1069, 1132,** 1134*t*
    prognosis for, 559–560
    rapid cycling, 571
      pharmacotherapy for, 1131
    recurrent, 545, 546*t*–547*t*
    single manic episode, 545, 546*t*
    twin studies of, 540
    X chromosome and, 540
  bipolar II, 535
    clinical features of, 553
    course of, 560
    diagnosis of, 545, 548*t*
    diagnostic criteria for, 548*t*
    differential diagnosis of, 557–558
    epidemiology of, 535
    lifetime prevalence, 535*t*
    pharmacotherapy for, 572
    prognosis for, 560
  bupropion for, 1030
  calcium channels inhibitors for, 1035
  carbamazepine for, 1037
  drug augmentation therapy for, **991**
  DSM-IV-TR classification of, 535
  genetics of, 123. 125
  ICD-10 diagnostic criteria, 587*t*–588*t*
  lifetime prevalence, 535*t*
  not otherwise specified, 583
    diagnostic criteria for, 583, 583*t*
  pharmacotherapy for, 96, 1003*t*
    bipolar I, 570–572, **1026, 1035, 1037, 1054, 1068–1069, 1132,** 1134*t*
    bipolar II, 572
    drug augmentation therapy, **991**
  and posttraumatic stress disorder, 624
Birth order, 218
  effects of, 33–34
Birth trauma, 226
Bisexual, definition of, 694
Black-out, 530*t*
Blackout(s)
  alcoholic, 347, 396, 401, **407**
  definition of, 286
Bladder control disorder(s), **1254–1258**. *See also* Enuresis
Bleuler, Eugen, **471–472,** 472*f*, 508, 681
Bleuler, Mandred, 502
Blink rate, in schizophrenia, 495
Blocking, 207*t*, 239
  definition of, 283
Blood alcohol levels, 398
Blood dyscrasias, and carbamazepine, **1037**
Blood flow
  in functional magnetic resonance imaging, 113
  in single photon emission computed tomography, 113
Blood level(s)
  data for clinical assessment, 268*t*
  procedure for taking, 265
Blood urea nitrogen (BUN), 263, 264*f*
  test for, 270*t*
Blurred vision, and psychotherapeutic drugs, **982**
Body anxiety, 1225
Body dysmorphic disorder, **653–655,** 753
  clinical features of, 644*t*, 654, 654*t*
  course of, 655
  diagnosis of, 654
  diagnostic criteria for, 654*t*
  differential diagnosis of, 655
  epidemiology of, 653–654
  etiology of, 654
  plastic surgery, relation to, 655
  prognosis for, 655
  treatment of, 655
Body image problems, 726
Body language, 82
  nonverbal skills, normal development of, 1195*t*
Bohannan, Paul, 49
Bonding, 28
  versus attachment, 140
  definition of, 140
  skin-to-skin contact in, 140
Borderline intellectual functioning, 142, **1290**
  diagnosis of, 1290
  etiology of, 1290
  treatment of, 1290
Borderline personality disorder, 222, **808–810**. *See also* Personality disorder(s), cluster B
  clinical features of, 809
  and combined psychotherapy and pharmacotherapy, **970–971**
  course of, 810
  diagnosis of, 809, 809*t*
  diagnostic criteria for, 809, 809*t*
  dialectical behavior therapy for, 810, 954
  differential diagnosis of, 784, 809–810
  emergency manifestations of, 908*t*
  emergency treatment of, 908*t*
  epidemiology of, 809
  and pathological gambling, 788
  pharmacotherapy for, 810, 1054, 1068–1069, 1132
  prognosis for, 810
  psychotherapy for, 810
  treatment of, 810, 810*t*
  and trichotillomania, 790
Borderline personality organization, 222
Boston Diagnostic Aphasia Examination, 189
Boston Naming Test, 191*t*
Bouffée délirante, 488–489, 522, 530*t*
Bowel control disorder(s), **1254–1258**. *See also* Encopresis
Bowen, Murray, and family therapy, 942–943
Bowen model, of family therapy, **942–943**
Bowlby, John, 28, 140*f*, **219**
  anxiety theory, 141–142
  attachment theory, 139–140, 167
  on bereavement, 62
  on depression, 541
Bradykinesia, 75
  definition of, 282
Bradylalia, definition of, 285
Bradyphrenia, in Parkinson's disease, 334
Braid, James, and hypnosis, 961
Brain. *See also* Neuroanatomy
  atrophy, in Alzheimer's disease, 331, 331*f*
  basal ganglia. *See* Basal ganglia
  damage
    in adults, assessment for, 185–191
    and attention-deficit/hyperactivity disorder, 1224
    catastrophic reaction to, 221
    hemispheric deficits, 187, 188*t*
    and mental retardation, 1169
    and obesity, 752
  disease, in elderly patients, 1319
  dorsal surface, 74*f*
  electric potential of, 119
  fontal lobes. *See* Frontal lobe(s)
  functional units of, 66
  hemispheric deficits/dominance, 187–189, 188*t*
  imaging, **108–122**. *See also* Computed tomography; Magnetic resonance imaging; Neuroimaging; Positron emission tomography
    in alcohol use disorders, 403, 404*f*
    in anxiety disorders, 595
    in cocaine use disorders, 430
    in depressive disorders, 111*f*
    electrophysiological techniques, 119–121. *See also* Electroencephalography; Event-related potentials; Evoked potentials
    functional techniques, 108, 112–119
    in generalized anxiety disorder, 633, 633*f*
    in major depressive disorder, 539, 540*f*
    in MPTP ingestion, 454
    in obsessive-compulsive disorder, 617, 617*f*
    in opioid use disorders, 449
    in panic disorder, 600
    in schizophrenia, 471, 479–481, 480*f*, 481*f*
    in schizophreniform disorder, 505, 506*f*
    structural techniques, 110–111
    in suicidal patients, 111, 111*f*
  injury, pathophysiology of, 361–362
  localization, mental status cognitive tests for, 190
  myelination of, 86
  organization of, 78–80

Brain—*continued*
precentral gyrus, 69*f*
regional functions of, 78–80, 80–83, 80*t*
reward systems, in substance-related disorders, 387, 388*f*, 414, 425
Brain death, 59, 59*t*
Brain-derived neurotropic factor, 93
Brain fag, 530*t*
Brainstem auditory evoked potentials, 119
Brain stimulation, and reinforcement, 150, 162–163
Brain tumor(s), 108, **360–361**
and headaches, 254
medical considerations with, 844*t*
mental disorder due to
clinical features of, 361
course of, 361
prognosis for, 361
and mental retardation, 1169
neuroimaging of, 110, 111*f*, 117*f*
personality change due to, 819, 819*t*
psychiatric considerations with, 844*t*
Brainwashing, 163, **629**
as dissociative disorder, 689
Breast feeding. *See* Lactation
Breathing-related sleep disorder, **769–770**
diagnostic criteria for, 769–770, 770*t*
Breathlessness, in depression, 255
Breuer, Joseph, 194, 197*f*
Brevital. *See* Methohexital
Bridge Reading Program, 1183
Brief focal psychotherapy, **931**
exclusion criteria for, 931*t*
interpersonal psychotherapy. *See* Interpersonal psychotherapy
requirements for, 931
techniques of, 931, 931*t*
Brief Psychiatric Rating Scale, 299*t*
Brief psychotherapy, **930–933**
for elderly, 1334
history of, 930–931
outcome of, 933
types of, 931–932
Brief psychotic disorder, 496, **520–529**
clinical features of, 522–524
comorbidity with, 521
course of, 524
definition of, 529
diagnosis of, 521, 521*t*
diagnostic criteria for, 521, 521*t*, 522*t*
differential diagnosis of, 524
emergency manifestations of, 908*t*
emergency treatment of, 908*t*
epidemiology of, 521
etiology of, 521
historical perspective on, 520–521
hospitalization for, 524
pharmacotherapy for, 524–525
precipitating stressors in, 523–524
prognosis for, 524, 524*t*
psychotherapy for, 525
treatment of, 524–525
Briquet, Paul, 643
Briquet's syndrome, 643
differential diagnosis of, 674
Broca, Pierre, 147
Broca's aphasia, 79*t*, 82
Brodmann's areas, 75
Brofaromine. *See also* Monoamine oxidase inhibitors
chemistry of, 1076*f*
for social phobia, 616
Bromide
blood level data for clinical assessment, 268*t*
intoxication
emergency manifestations of, 908*t*
emergency treatment of, 908*t*
serum, test for, 270*t*
Bromocriptine, 999*t*, **1047–1050**. *See also* Dopamine receptor antagonist(s), and precursors
for cocaine users, 435
drug interactions, 1031, 1062*t*
for hyperprolactinemia, 715
intoxication/overdose of, 985*t*
Bruininks-Oseretsky Test of Motor Development, for developmental coordination disorder, 1191
Bruxism, sleep-related, **776–777**
Buffalo adiposity, 752
Bufotenin, 436*t*
Bulimia
definition of, 281, 746
pharmacotherapy for, 1030, 1132
Bulimia nervosa, 256, **746–751**. *See also* Eating disorder(s)
behavior therapy for, 954*t*
binge eating/nonpurging type, 748
binge eating/purging type, 748–749, 749*f*
biological factors in, 747
clinical features of, 747–749
cognitive-behavioral therapy, 750
course of, 749
definition of, 746–747
diagnosis of, 747–749
diagnostic criteria for, 747–749, 747*t*
differential diagnosis of, 749
dynamic psychotherapy, 750
epidemiology of, 747
etiology of, 747
ICD-10 research criteria for, 745–746, 746*t*, 751
and kleptomania, 785
laboratory findings in, 749
nonpurging type, 746–747
pathology of, 749
pharmacotherapy for, 750, 1069
prognosis for, 749
psychological factors in, 747
psychotherapy for, 750
purging type, 746–747
social factors in, 747
treatment of, 749–750
BUN. *See* Blood urea nitrogen (BUN)
Buprenex. *See* Buprenorphine
Buprenorphine, 448, 999*t*, **1082–1085**
adverse reactions to, 1084
chemistry of, 1083, 1083*f*
dosage of, 1085
drug interactions, 1084
effects on organs and systems, 1082
for heroin addiction, 389
indications for, 455, 1083–1084
laboratory interferences, 1084
overdose of, 1084
pharmacological actions of, 1082
precautions with, 1084
withdrawal symptoms, 1084
Bupropion, 377, 1000*t*, **1029–1031**
adverse effects of, 567*t*, 981*t*, 1030–1031
for attention-deficit/hyperactivity disorder, 1228, 1228*t*
chemistry of, 1029–1030, 1029*f*
clinical guidelines for, 1031
for cocaine users, 435
dosage of, 569*t*, 1031
drug interactions, 378, 982, 1031
effects on specific organs and systems, 1030
for elderly patients, 1329, 1330
implicated in sexual dysfunction, 711
indications for, 1030
intoxication/overdose of, 985*t*
laboratory interferences, 711, 1031
mechanism of action, 100, 567*t*
for nicotine addiction, 447
precautions with, 1030–1031
for tobacco dependence, 389
BuSpar. *See* Buspirone
Buspirone, 1000*t*, **1031–1033**
adverse effects of, 1032
for alcoholism, 413
augmentation of, **991**
benzodiazepine, switching from, 1033
chemistry of, 1031, 1031*f*
children, use with, 1308*t*
comparison with benzodiazepines, 1032*t*
dosage and administration, 1033
drug interactions, 1032
effects on specific organs and systems, 1032
for generalized anxiety disorder, 635, 1032
geriatric dosage, 1332*t*
indications for, 1032
for intermittent explosive disorder, 785
intoxication/overdose of, 985*t*
laboratory interferences, 1033
mechanism of action, 104
for mood disorders, 1278–1279
for obsessive-compulsive disorder, 623
pharmacological actions of, 1032
for posttraumatic stress disorder, 630
precautions with, 1032
for separation anxiety disorder, 1263
Butabarbital, 1000*t*. *See also* Barbiturate(s)
dosage of, 1020*t*
indications for, 1018
structure of, 1018*f*
Butalbital, structure of, 1018*f*
Butaperazine, 1000*t*
Butisol. *See* Butabarbital
Butler, Robert, 46
Butorphanol, 448
Butyl nitrite, 468
Butyrophenones, 1051*t*
chemistry of, 1053
structure of, 1052*f*

C

Cabaj, Robert, 699
Cade, John F. J., 1067
Caffeine
adverse effects of, 419, 423
cerebral blood flow, effects on, 421
consumption, by age, 419, 420*t*
drug interactions, 1047, 1062*t*
epidemiology of, 419
genetics and use, 420–421
intoxication, 419
acute, diagnostic criteria for, 391*t*
diagnosis of, 421–423
diagnostic criteria for, 421*t*, 422
emergency manifestations of, 908*t*
emergency treatment of, 908*t*
and lithium, 1072*t*
neuropharmacology of, 420
for pain management, 1345*t*
serum level, test for, 270*t*
sources of, 419, 420*t*
as substance of abuse, 421

use
genetics and, 420–421
prevalence of, 419
signs and symptoms of, 423
withdrawal, 419
diagnosis of, 421–423
diagnostic criteria for, 394*t*
research criteria for, 422, 422*t*
Caffeine-related disorder(s), 382*t*, **419–424**
anxiety disorder, 419, 422–423
clinical features of, 423
comorbidity with, 420
diagnosis of, 421–423
DSM-IV-TR classification of, 421, 421*t*
epidemiology of, 419
not otherwise specified, 423
diagnostic criteria for, 421*t*
sleep disorder, 419, 423
and substance-related disorders, 420
treatment, 423
Calan. *See* Verapamil
Calcium
as second messenger, 86, 95
serum, test for, 270*t*
Calcium-calmodulin kinase II (CaMKII), 81, 127
Calcium channel inhibitors
adverse effects, 1035
chemistry of, 1033, 1034*f*
clinical guidelines for, 1035
dosage of, 1034*t*, 1035
drug interactions, 1035
effects on specific organs and systems, 1034
half-lives of, 1034*t*
for HIV infection, 377
for intermittent explosive disorder, 785
intoxication/overdose of, 985*t*
pharmacological actions of, 1033–1034
precautions with, 1035
use of, 1033
California Personality Inventory (CPI), 181*t*
Cameron, Norman, 513
CaMKII, 81, 127
cAMP. *See* Cyclic adenosine monophosphate (cAMP)
Campbell, Robert, 18
Canalization, 225
Cancellation Tests, 191*t*
Cancer
psycho-oncology, **838–839**
and suicide, 839*t*, 915
Cannabinoid receptors, 425, 426*t*
Cannabinoid(s)
intoxication, acute, diagnostic criteria for, 391*t*
withdrawal, 393*t*
Cannabis, 424
abuse, 426
and schizophrenia, 476
adolescent use, 1286
adverse effects of, 425
amotivational syndrome, 427
dependence, 425, 426
physiological, 425, 426
psychological, 425, 426
flashbacks, 427
intoxication, **426**
diagnostic criteria for, 426, 426*t*
effects of, 425, 426
emergency manifestations of, 908*t*
emergency treatment of, 908*t*
with perceptual disturbances, 426
intoxication delirium, 426
diagnosis of, 426
medical use of, 427
neuropharmacology of, 425, 425*f*
therapeutic uses of, 427
tolerance, 425
transient paranoid ideation, 426
in urinalysis, 268*t*
use
demographic correlates, 424
frequent, 425
history of, 425
medical, 427
prevalence, 424
recent trends, 424
withdrawal, 425
Cannabis-related disorder(s), 382*t*, **424–428**
anxiety disorder, 426–427
clinical features of, 425–427
diagnosis of, 425–427
DSM-IV classification of, 426, 426*t*
epidemiology of, 424
mood disorder, 427
not otherwise specified, 427
diagnostic criteria for, 427*t*
psychotic disorder, 426
rehabilitation, 427
sexual dysfunction, 427, 711
treatment, 427
Cannabis sativa, 424
Cannon, Walter, 822
CAP, 1158*t*
CAPA, 1153
Carbamazepine, 1000*t*, **1036–1040**
adverse effects of, 1037–1038, 1037*t*
for affective lability and impulsivity, 356
for bipolar disorder, 570, 571, 1037, 1134*t*
blood levels, 1040
data for clinical assessment, 268*t*
for bulimia nervosa, 750
with bupropion, 1031
chemistry of, 1036, 1036*f*
for cocaine users, 435
for conduct disorder, 1238
with donepezil, 1044
dosage and administration, 1038–1039
drug interactions, 378, 1028, 1031, 1035, 1038, 1039*t*, 1062*t*
CYP-induced, 976
effects on specific organs and systems, 1036
geriatric dosage, 1330*t*
indications for, 360, 404*t*, 405, 464, 500, 1037
initiation of treatment, 1039
intoxication/overdose of, 985*t*
laboratory interferences, 1038
laboratory monitoring with, 264, 267, 267*t*, 1040, 1040*t*
and lithium, 1072*t*
pharmacological actions of, 1036
precautions with, 1037–1038
pretreatment medical evaluation, 1039
for schizoaffective disorder, 511
and weight gain, 752
Carbidopa, 1000*t*
Carbon dioxide inhalation, 267, 270*t*
Carbonic anhydrase inhibitors, and lithium, 1072*t*
Carbon monoxide poisoning, 75, 1249*t*
Cardiovascular disease, and suicide, 915
Cardiovascular disorder(s), psychological correlates of, **829–831**
Cardiovascular drugs, and lithium, 1072*t*
Cardiovascular symptoms, sleep-related, **779**
Cardiovascular system, medical assessment of, 255–256
Cardizem. *See* Diltiazem
Cardozo, Benjamin, 1359
Career choice, 895
Carisoprodol, intoxication/overdose of, 985*t*
Carphenazine, 1000*t*
Case-control studies, 171
Case-history studies, 171
Case management, 501
Castration, preoccupation with, **735–736**
Castration anxiety, 593
CAT, 1159
Catalepsy, definition of, 281
Cataplexy
definition of, 281
with narcolepsy, 769
Catapres. *See* Clonidine
Catastrophic reaction, 221
in dementia, 337
Catastrophizing, 958*f*
Catatonia. *See also* Schizophrenia, catatonic type
definition of, 281
electroconvulsive therapy for, 1140
lethal, 998*t*
pharmacotherapy for, 1026
in schizophrenia, 490
Catatonic disorder due to a general medical condition, 350, 355*t*, 495
Catatonic excitement, definition of, 281
Catatonic posturing, definition of, 281
Catatonic rigidity, definition of, 281
Catatonic stupor
definition of, 281
in schizophrenia, 490
Catecholamines. *See also* Dopamine; Epinephrine; Norepinephrine
amphetamines and amphetaminelike substances and, 414
effects of cocaine on, 430
laboratory testing for, 263
plasma, test for, 270*t*
in substance-related disorders, 387, 388*f*
synthesis of, 98
urinary, test for, 270*t*
Catechol-*O*-methyltransferase, 101
Catha edulis, 418
Catharsis
Freud's use of, 194–196
in group psychotherapy, 938*t*
and prevention of aggression, 155
Cathinone, 418
Catnip, 469–470
Cat's cry syndrome, 1165
Cattell, Raymond, **219**–220
Cattell Infant Intelligence Scale, 1159
Causality, assuming, 958*f*
CBF. *See* Cerebral blood flow (CBF)
CCK. *See* Cholecystokinin (CCK)
CEC, 1161
Cellular phone compulsion, **793**
Center-surround response, 69
Central achromatopsia, 70
Central alveolar hypoventilation, **770**
Central nervous system (CNS), **85–88**
cholinergic tracts of, 105
depressants, drug interactions, 401, 1021, 1028, 1062, 1129
development, 85–88
experience and, 87
disorders
focal, with behavioral features, 903, 904*t*
neuroimaging and, 108
that require immediate treatment, 903, 904*t*

Central nervous system (CNS)—*continued*
  dopaminergic tracts of, 97–98, 99*f*
  and mirtazapine, 1075
  noradrenergic tracts of, 101, 101*f*
  psychoneuroendocrinology, **128–132**
  serotonergic tracts of, 102, 103*f*
  and sympathomimetics, 1117
Centrax. *See* Prazepam
Cerea flexibilitas, definition of, 281
Cerebellar tumor
  medical considerations with, 844*t*
  psychiatric considerations with, 844*t*
Cerebellum, **75**
  in schizophrenia, **479**
Cerebral blood flow (CBF)
  in alcohol intoxication, 403
  caffeine and, 421
  cocaine and, 430
  nicotine and, 446
  opioids and, 449
  regional, in schizophrenia, 481
  in schizophrenia, 481
Cerebral cortex
  in anxiety disorders, 595
  areas, classification of, 78
  association areas, 69–70, 70*f,* 78*f*
  in auditory system, 71, 73
  cytoarchitectonics of, 68*f*
  and emotion, 83
  and language, 82–83
  language areas of, 78*f*
  mapping, 73
  motor, 75, 77
  in olfaction, 71–72, 74
  rhythmical activity in, 122
  in somatosensory system, 66–68, 67*f,* 72–73
  in taste, 72
  in visual system, 69, 70*f,* 73
Cerebral infarctions, in cocaine use disorders, 434
Cerebrospinal fluid (CSF), testing, 270*t*
Cerebrovascular disease, 347
  amnestic disorder with, 347
  personality change due to, 819, 819*t*
Cerletti, Ugo, 1138
Ceruloplasmin, serum, testing, 270*t*
Cervical caps, 875*t*
cGMP, as second messenger, 95
Chace, Marian, 854
Character. *See also* Personality
  compulsive, 226
  formation of, 209
    Freud's concept of, 209
  hysterical, 226
  masochistic, 226
  narcissistic, 226
  types, 220, 226
Character armor, 226, 801
Character traits, 209
Charcoal, drug interactions, 1062*t*
Charcot, Jean-Martin, 194, 681
  and hypnosis, 961
Chelation therapy, **853**
Chemical convulsive therapies, **1149**
Chess, Stella, 26, 817
Chicago Study, 171–172
Chief complaint, **233**
Child abuse and neglect, **883–890**
  and attachment, 142
  and childhood/adolescent antisocial behavior, 1292
  clinical features of, 884–888
  and conduct disorder, 1235
  confidentiality and, 1354
  course of, 889
  diagnosis of, 884–888
  differential diagnosis of, 888–889
  emergency manifestations of, 907*t*
  emergency treatment of, 907*t*
  epidemiology of, 883
  etiology of, 883–884
  laboratory examinations for, 888, 888*f*
  pathology of, 888
  physical, **884–885,** 885*f*
  prevention of, 889–890
  prognosis for, 889
  reporting of, 889
  sexual, **885–887,** 886*t*
  treatment of child, 889–890
  treatment of parents, 889
Child and Adolescent Psychiatric Assessment (CAPA), 1153
Child Attention Profile (CAP), 1158*t*
Child Behavior Checklist, **1154**
Child custody, 49, **1315–1316, 1360**
Child development, stages of, 211–215
Childhood, 21
  bereavement in, 64, **1277**
  disorders of, 1259–1273
  early, history of, 235
  eating disorders of, **1241–1245**
  feeding disorders of, **1244**
  late, history of, 235
  middle, history of, 235
  mood disorders during, **1274–1279**
  normal development, 20–21
  psychoneurotic reactions to, 209–210, 210*t*
  pyromania in, 787
  sexual learning in, 692
Childhood antisocial behavior, **1292–1293**
  clinical features of, 1292
  diagnosis of, 1292
  differential diagnosis of, 1292
  epidemiology of, 1292
  etiology of, 1292
  psychological factors in, 1292
  treatment of, 1292–1293
Childhood disintegrative disorder, **1216–1218,** 1219
  course of, 1217–1218
  definition of, 1216–1217
  diagnosis of, 1217
  diagnostic criteria for, 1217, 1217*t*
  differential diagnosis of, 1217
  epidemiology of, 1217
  etiology of, 1217
  other, ICD-10 diagnostic criteria for, 1219, 1221*t*
  prognosis for, 1217–1218
  treatment of, 1218
Childhood onset schizophrenia. *See* Schizophrenia
Childhood psychosis, definition of, 1282
Child psychiatric evaluation, **1155–1160**
  history taking in, 1155
  identifying data in, 1155
  mental status examination in, 1155–1156, 1155*t*
  diagnosis in, 1160
  forensic issues in, **1315–1317**
  interviews in
    clinical interviews, 1151–1153
    "interviewer-based" interviews, 1153
    "respondent-based" interviews, 1153–1154
  neuropsychiatric assessment in, 1156–1157
  pictorial diagnostic instruments, 1154
  questionnaires in, 1154–1155
  rating scales in, 1154–1155
  recommendations in, 1160
  treatment plans in, 1160
Child psychiatry
  additional conditions that may be a focus of clinical attention, **1290–1294**
  adverse events, exposure to, **1317**
  assessment, examination, and psychological testing, **1151–1160**
  developmental, psychological, and educational testing in, 1157*t*–1158*t*, **1158–1160**
Child psychoanalysis, 1297
Child(ren)
  with AIDS, 1168
  and attention-deficit/hyperactivity disorder, 1225–1226
  attitudes toward death, 60–61
  with autistic disorder, pharmacotherapy for, **1306–1308**
  behavior therapy for, 1296
  biological therapies for, **1305–1311**
  bipolar I disorder in, 558–559, **1277**
  and conduct disorder, **1309**
  day care centers for, **880**
  day care for, 35
  day treatment with, **1303–1305**
  depression in
    clinical features of, 552–553
    separation anxiety and, 1260
  difficult versus easy, 29
  divorce and, 34
  dreams in, 33
  dying, 60–61
  early school-age, group psychotherapy with, **1300–1301**
  end-of-life care, 1347
  gender identity disorders in, **731–732**
  grief in, 64
  group psychotherapy with, **1300–1302**
  hospitalized, 61, 139
  hospital treatment of, **1305**
  and identity problem, **1293–1294**
  individual psychotherapy with, **1295–1300**
    psychoanalytic theories in, 1295–1296
    theories and techniques of, 1295–1296
  latency-age groups, group psychotherapy with, **1301**
  parent–child relational problems, **880**
  and pharmacotherapy, **979**
  posttraumatic stress disorder in, 627–628
  preschool-age
    clinical interviews with, 1152
    group psychotherapy with, **1300–1301**
  psychiatric treatment of, **1295–1314**
  psychotherapy with
    confidentiality in, 1299
    differences from adults, 1297–1298
    Erikson's technique, 216–217
    indications for, 1299
    initial approach to, 1298
    parental involvement in, 1299
    in playroom, 1298
    therapeutic interventions, 1298–1299
  in residential treatment, **1302–1303**
  rights of, 1315
  school-age
    clinical interviews with, 1152
    intelligence tests for, **1159**
  sleep in, 33
  spacing of, 33
  of working mothers, 35

Children's Apperception Test (CAT), 1159
Children's Personality Questionnaire, 1158*t*
Chinese medicine, 864
 and acupuncture/acupressure, **852**
Chiropractic, **853–854**
Chi-square test, 174
Chloral hydrate, 1000*t*, **1040–1041**
 adverse effects of, 1041
 blood level data for clinical assessment, 268*t*
 chemistry of, 1040, 1040*f*
 clinical guidelines for, 1041
 dosage of, 1041
 drug interactions, 401, 1041
 effects on specific organs and systems, 1041
 geriatric dosage, 1332*t*
 indications for, 1041
 intoxication/overdose of, 985*t*
 laboratory interferences, 1041
 pharmacological actions of, 1040–1041
 precautions with, 1041
 for primary insomnia, 765
Chlordiazepoxide, 460. *See also* Benzodiazepine(s)
 blood level data for clinical assessment, 268*t*
 dosage of, 1025*t*
 drug interactions, 1047
 geriatric dosage, 1332*t*
 half-life of, 1025*t*
 indications for, 404*t*, 405, 406
 pharmacological actions for, 1023
 structure of, 1023*f*
Chloride, serum, testing, 270*t*
Chlorpromazine, 497, 1000*t*. *See also* Dopamine receptor antagonist(s)
 for anorexia nervosa, 745
 blood level data for clinical assessment, 268*t*
 children, use with, 1307*t*
 geriatric dosage, 1332*t*
 and lithium, 1072*t*
 preparations, 1064*t*
 structure of, 1052*f*
Chlorprothixene, 1000*t*
 geriatric dosage, 1332*t*
 structure of, 1052*f*
Chlorthalidone, and lithium, 1072*t*
Chocolate, 470
Cholecystokinin (CCK)
 neurotransmitter function, 105
 octapeptide, 91*f*
 testing, 270*t*
Choline acetyltransferase, 332
Choline magnesium trisalicylate, for pain management, 1345*t*
Cholinergic receptors, 93*t*, 105
 muscarinic, 105
 nicotinic, 105
Cholinergic tracts, of central nervous system, 105
Cholinesterase inhibitors, **1041–1045**
 adverse effects of, 1043–1044
 chemistry of, 1042, 1042*f*
 clinical guidelines for, 1044
 dosage of, 1044
 drug interactions, 1044
 effects on specific organs and systems, 1043
 indications for, 1043
 laboratory interferences, 1044
 memantine. *See* Memantine
 neurotransmission, potentiation of, 1041, 1042*f*
 pharmacological actions of, 1042–1043
 precautions with, 1043–1044
Choo-choo phenomenon, 160*f*
Chorea, definition of, 282
Chorionic villus sampling, 23
Chromosomal aberrations, and mental retardation, 1165
Chromosome(s), 123
 definition of, 123
Chronic emotional illness, and relational problems, 879–880
Chronic fatigue syndrome, 133, **661–664**
 CDC criteria for, 661, 662*t*
 clinical features of, 661–662, 662*t*
 course of, 663
 diagnosis of, 661–662
 differential diagnosis of, 662–663, 663*t*
 epidemiology of, 661
 etiology of, 661
 ICD-10 classification of, 661
 pharmacotherapy for, 663, 664*t*, 1119
 prognosis for, 663
 self-help groups, 664
 sex distribution of, 661
 treatment of, 663–664
 virus and, 661
 workup for, 662, 663*t*
Chronic illness, and relational problems, 879
Chronic motor or vocal tic disorder, **1250–1251**
 clinical features of, 1251
 course of, 1251
 definition of, 1250
 diagnosis of, 1251
 diagnostic criteria for, 1251, 1251*t*
 differential diagnosis of, 1251
 epidemiology of, 1251
 etiology of, 1251
 prognosis for, 1251
 treatment of, 1251
Chronic paroxysmal hemicrania, sleep-related, **779**
Chronobiology, **134–135**
Chum period, 32, 228
Cigarettes
 drug interactions, 1062
 smoking. *See* Smoking
Cimetidine
 drug interactions, 1028, 1031, 1035, 1049, 1062*t*, 1079
 indications for, 1015
 and pramipexole, 1049
 psychotic disorder
  emergency manifestations of, 908*t*
  emergency treatment of, 908*t*
Ciprofloxacin and ropinirole, 1049
Circadian rhythms, in depression, 539
Circadian rhythm sleep disorder, **771–773**
 delayed sleep phase type, **771**
 diagnostic criteria for, 771*t*
 jet lag type, **771**
 shift work type, **772**
 unspecified, **772–773**
Circumcision, **888**
Circumstantiality, 239
 definition of, 283
Cisapride, drug interactions, 1029
Citalopram, 103, 1000*t*
 for elderly patients, 1329
 for separation anxiety disorder, 1263
Citric acid cycle, 96
Claims review, **1389**
Clang association(s), 239
 definition of, 283
Clarification
 in interview, 9
 in psychotherapy, definition of, 927*t*
Classification, in psychiatry, 288
Claustrophobia, definition of, 284
Clérambault-Kandinsky complex, 284
Client-centered group psychotherapy, classification of, 935
Client-centered psychotherapy, 226–227
Climacterium, 47
Clinical trials, 171
Clomipramine, 1000*t*
 adverse effects of, 567*t*, 981*t*
 for anorexia nervosa, 745
 for autistic disorder, 1215
 children, use with, 1307*t*
 clinical information, 1130*t*
 dosage and administration, 569*t*
 mechanism of action, 109, 567*t*
 neurotransmitter effects of, 1126*t*
 for obsessive-compulsive disorder, 622
 preparations of, 1130*t*
 structure of, 1125*f*
Clonazepam, 1000*t*. *See also* Benzodiazepine(s)
 for bipolar I disorder, 570
 chemistry of, 1022
 dosage of, 1025*t*
 drug interactions, 1028
 for extrapyramidal disorders, 1059*t*
 geriatric dosage, 1330*t*, 1332*t*
 half-life of, 1025*t*
 metabolism of, 533
 for obsessive-compulsive disorder, 623
 pharmacological actions for, 1023
 for separation anxiety disorder, 1263
 structure of, 1023*f*
Clonidine, 1000*t*, **1005–1007**
 adverse reactions to, 1006
 for attention-deficit/hyperactivity disorder, 1224, 1228
 children, use with, 1308*t*
 clinical features of, 1007
 for conduct disorder, 1238
 dosage of, 1007, 1007*t*
 drug interactions, 1007, 1062*t*
 effects on specific organs and systems, 1005
 for extrapyramidal disorders, 1059*t*
 indications for, 405, 450, 1005–1006
 intoxication/overdose of, 985*t*
 laboratory interferences, 1007
 mechanism of action, 102
 for nicotine addiction, 447
 overdose of, 1006
 precautions with, 1006
 withdrawal, 1007
  emergency manifestations of, 909*t*
  emergency treatment of, 909*t*
Cloning, molecular, 88
Cloning, positional, 125–126
Clorazepate. *See also* Benzodiazepine(s)
 dosage of, 1025*t*
 geriatric dose, 1332*t*
 half-life of, 1025*t*
 pharmacokinetics of, 1022–1023
 pharmacological actions for, 1023
 structure of, 1023*f*
Closed-circuit television, in electroencephalographic monitoring, 120
Closing-in error, 188*f*
Clouding of consciousness, 240
Clozapine, 497–499, 1000*t*. *See also* Serotonin-dopamine antagonist(s) (atypical antipsychotics)
 adverse effects of, 498
  laboratory monitoring for, 498
 agranulocytosis caused by, 498, 907*t*

Clozapine—*continued*
for autistic disorder, 1215
children, use with, 1307*t*
drug interactions, 976, 1028, 1134
for early-onset schizophrenia, 1285
indications for, 471, 497–499
intoxication/overdose of, 985*t*
laboratory monitoring of, 265, 266*t*
mechanism of action, 102, 478
for schizophrenia, 498
and weight gain, 752
Clozaril. *See* Clozapine
Clozaril National Registry, 265
Clumsiness. *See* Developmental coordination disorder
Clumsy child syndrome. *See* Developmental coordination disorder
Cluster headaches
pharmacotherapy for, 1069
sleep-related, **779**
Cluttering, **1205**
definition of, 285
differential diagnosis of, 1204
CMV, testing for, 270*t*
CNS. *See* Central nervous system (CNS)
Cobalamin deficiency, neuropsychiatric manifestations of, 367
Cocaine, 92, 100, 428, 428*f*
abuse, 431–433, 460
defined, 428–429
diagnosis of, 431
pharmacotherapy for, 1030
and schizophrenia, 476
addiction, 430
brain imaging in, 430
addiction potential, 100
adverse effects of, 255, 434
in animal models, 125
blood level data for clinical assessment, 268*t*
death caused by, 434
dependence, 430, 431–433
acupuncture for, 1145
defined, 428
diagnosis of, 431
pharmacotherapy for, 1003*t*
physiological, 430
psychological, 430
detoxification, 435
pharmacology for, 1030, 1131
effects
behavioral, 430
cardiac, 434
on cerebral blood flow, 430
cerebrovascular, 434
nasal congestion, 431
intoxication, 433
acute, diagnostic criteria for, 391*t*
diagnostic criteria for, 431, 431*t*, 433
emergency manifestations of, 909*t*
emergency treatment of, 909*t*
hallucinations in, 433
intoxication delirium, 433
diagnosis of, 433
neuropharmacology of, 429–430
pharmacological agents, 435
seizures, 434
sensitivity, 430
tolerance, 430
in urinalysis, 268*t*
use, 428
among adolescents, 1286
frequent, 430
history of, 430
methods of, 428, **430**
personality changes in, 431
rate of initiation, 430
withdrawal, 433
diagnostic criteria for, 394*t*, 431, 431*t*
emergency manifestations of, 909*t*
emergency treatment of, 909*t*
pharmacotherapy for, 1003*t*
self-medication in, 433
symptoms of, 433
Cocaine-related disorder(s), 382*t*, **428–435**
anxiety disorder, 433
brain imaging in, 430
clinical features of, 430–434
comorbidity with, 429
conditioning influences, 429
diagnosis of, 430–434
DSM-IV-TR classification of, 430–431, 430*t*
epidemiology of, 428, 429
etiology of, 429
genetic factors, 429
learning influences, 429
mood disorder, 433
New Haven Study, 172, 172*t*, 429
not otherwise specified, 433–434, 434*t*
pharmacological factors, 429
psychotic disorder, 433
hallucinations in, 433
paranoid delusions in, 433
rehabilitation, 434
sexual dysfunction, 433
sleep disorder, 433
sociocultural factors, 429
treatment, 434
Codeine. *See also* Opioid(s)
blood level data for clinical assessment, 268*t*
for pain management, 1344*t*
in urinalysis, 268*t*
Codependence, 381, 383
Codons, 123
Cogentin. *See* Benztropine
Cognex. *See* Tacrine
Cognition
in amnestic disorder(s), 320–321
contributing to noncompliance, 959, 959*t*
definition of, 147
in delirium, 320–321
in dementia, 320–321, 337
in elderly, 1320, 1321, 1321*t*, 1322*t*
evaluation of, in child psychiatric evaluation, 1156
impairment, with brain tumor, 361
in mania, 556
in mental status examination, 240–242
in schizophrenia, 495
Cognition-affect flow chart, 958*f*
Cognitive development
in adolescence, 37
history-taking about, 235
in infancy, 25–26
in middle (childhood) years, 32
Piaget's theory of, 19–20, 28*t*, 136–138
in preschool period, 31
in toddler period, 30
Cognitive disorder(s)
DSM-IV classification of, 320*t*
not otherwise specified, 320, 320*t*
Cognitive dissonance, **147**
Cognitive errors, derived from assumptions, 958*f*
Cognitive learning theory, **147**
Cognitive map, 81
Cognitive profile, of psychiatric disorders, 957*t*
Cognitive strategies, 147
Cognitive therapy, 139, **956–960**
for anorexia nervosa, 745
approach to depression, 960*t*
automatic thoughts in
elicitation of, 957
testing of, 957
behavioral techniques in, 957–959
for bulimia nervosa, 750
with children, 1296, 1297
cognitive techniques of, 957
for depression, 564–565, **956**
didactic aspects of, 957
for dysthymic disorder, 575
efficacy of, 959–960
for elderly, 1334
general assumptions of, 956, 956*t*
identification of maladaptive assumptions in, 957
imagery in, 958–959
indications for, 959*t*
in mental retardation, 1176
for panic disorder, 601, 608
for paraphilias, 724–725
for posttraumatic stress disorder, 625
for schizophrenia, 501
strategies and techniques of, 956–957, 957*t*
Cohesion, in group psychotherapy, 938*t*
Cohoba, 436*t*
Cohort studies, 171
Coitus interruptus, 875*t*
Colarusso, Calvin, 42
Colitis, psychological correlates of, 826*t*
Collective unconscious, 222
Colloid cysts, 361
Color agnosia, 70
Color anomia, 70
Color therapy, **854**
Coma, definition of, 280
Coma-inducing therapies, **1149**
Coma vigil, definition of, 280
Combat neurosis, 624
Combination drugs, 1002
Combination drug therapy, **989–992**
Combined individual and group psychotherapy, **940**
results of, 940
techniques of, 940
Command automatism, definition of, 281
Commitment
definition of, 1356
versus hospitalization, 1355–1356
Common sense psychiatry, 224
Communication, disturbances of, in autistic disorder, 1211
Communication, human characteristics of, 159
Communication disorder(s), **1194–1207**
comorbidity with, 1194–1196
differential diagnosis of, 1200*t*
in ICD-10, 1205–1206, 1206*t*
laboratory examination, 1197
not otherwise specified, **1205,** 1205*t*
pathology of, 1197
Communication rights, of patients, 1358
Community mental health, **1374–1376**. *See also* Public psychiatry
case management, 1375
commitment and, 1374
community participation, 1375
consultation and, 1375
evaluation, 1375
least-restrictive alternatives, 1375
long-term care, 1375
research, 1375
services, 1374

Compazine. *See* Prochlorperazine
Competence
  to be executed, 1361
  contractual, 1360–1361
  to stand trial, 1361
  testamentary, 1360–1361
Competency, ethics concerning, 1372*t*
Competition, in sociobiology, 164
Complementary medicine, **851–867**
  and end-of-life care, 1348
Complexes, Jung's concept of, 222
Compliance, **10–12**
  definition, 10
  factors affecting, 11
  strategies for improving, 11–12
Comprehensive Evaluation of Language Functions-Revised, 191*t*
Compulsion(s), 621*t*
  definition of, 282, 284, 616
Compulsive buying, 792–793
Compulsive character, 226
Compulsive gamblers. *See* Pathological gambling
Computed tomography (CT), **110**. *See also* Neuroimaging
  for amnestic disorder(s), 323, 348–349
  in attention-deficit/hyperactivity disorder, 1224
  of brain, 108, 110
    versus magnetic resonance imaging, 110, 110*f*, 111
  for cognitive disorders, 323
  for Creutzfeldt-Jakob disease, 364
  in delirium, 323
  in dementia, 323, 1335
  in obsessive-compulsive disorder, 109
  in schizophrenia, 109, 479–480
  SPECT. *See* Single photon emission computed tomography (SPECT)
Comrey Personality Scales (CPS), 181*t*
Conation, definition of, 281
Concentration
  ability, assessment for, 189–190
  assessment of, in mental status examination, 241–242
Concept formation, assessment of, 186
Concrete operations stage, 19, 28*t*
  Piaget's theory of, 137–138
Concrete thinking, definition of, 287
Condensation
  definition of, 283
  in dreams, 198
Conditioned insomnia, **765–767**
Conditioned response, 143
Conditioning
  applications of, 148
  avoidance, 145*t*
  classical, **143–144**
  escape, 145*t*
  instrumental, 144, 145*t*
  operant, 143, **144–146,** 145*t*
  primary reward, 145*t*
  respondent, 143
  secondary reward, 145*t*
Condoms, 875*t*, 876*f*
Conduct disorder(s), **1234–1238**
  and attention-deficit/hyperactivity disorder, 1226–1227, 1233
  and child abuse and maltreatment, 1235
  in children, pharmacotherapy for, **1309**
  clinical features of, 1235–1237
  course of, 1237
  diagnosis of, 1235–1237, 1236*t*
  differential diagnosis of, 1237
  epidemiology of, 1234
  etiology of, 1235
  and expressive language disorder, 1195
  in ICD-10, 1238, 1238*t*–1239*t*
  laboratory examination of, 1237
  and mental retardation, 1163
  mixed with emotional disorders, in ICD-10, 1240*t*
  neurobiological factors in, 1235
  parental factors in, 1235
  pathology of, 1237
  prognosis of, 1237
  psychological factors in, 1235
  and reading disorder, 1181
  sociocultural factors in, 1235
  treatment of, 1237–1238
Confabulation, 241
  definition of, 286
Confidence interval(s), 174–175
Confidentiality, **12, 1353–1355, 1369–1370**
  and child abuse, 1354
  in child psychiatry, 1152, 1315
  and discussions about patients, 1354
  ethics concerning, 1372*t*
  and HIV testing for, 374
  in psychotherapy with children, 1299
  and supervision, 1354
  and third-party payers, 1354
Conflict, and anxiety, 592
Conflict of interest, ethics concerning, 1372*t*
Confrontation
  in interview, 9
  in psychotherapy, definition of, 927*t*
Confusion
  acute, causes of, 81*t*
  definition of, 280
Confusional psychosis, **484,** 584
Congenital adrenal hyperplasia, 734*f*
Congenital arithmetic disorder. *See* Mathematics disorder
Congenital virilizing adrenal hyperplasia, **733–735,** 734*f*
Conjoint therapy, **946**
Conjugal paranoia, 515
Connors Abbreviated Parent-Teacher Rating Scale for ADHD, 1154–1155
Conscious mind, **199**
Consciousness
  clouding of, definition of, 240, 280
  definition of, 280
  dialectic with Being, 227
  disturbances of, definition of, 280
  in elderly, 1320
  level of, in mental status examination, 240–241
Consensual validation, in group psychotherapy, 938*t*
Consent form, 1359–1360
Conservation, 137, 138*f*
Consonar. *See* Brofaromine
Constipation
  definition of, 281
  and psychotherapeutic drugs, **982**
Consultation-liaison psychiatry, **843–850**
  diagnosis in, 843, 844*t*–847*t*
  in hemodialysis unit, 848–849
  problems seen in, 822, 823*t*, 843, 848*t*
  in surgical unit, 849, 849*t*
  transplantation issues, 849–850
  treatment in, 843–848
Contagion, in group psychotherapy, 938*t*
Containment, in object relations theory, 924
Continuous Performance Test, 191*t*
Continuous sleep therapy, 1149
Contraception, **874–877**
  methods of, 875*t*, 876*f*
  misuse of, 39, 39*t*
  oral. *See* Oral contraceptives
Contraceptive sponges, 875*t*
Contractual capacity, 1360–1361
Control group, 175
Controlling, 208*t*
Conversion disorder, **647–651**
  biological factors in, 648
  clinical features of, 644*t*, 648–649
  cognitive profile of, 957*t*
  comorbidity with, 647–648
  course of, 650
  diagnosis of, 648
  diagnostic criteria for, 648, 648*t*
  differential diagnosis of, 649–650
  epidemiology of, 647
  etiology of, 648
  identification in, 649
  la belle indifférence in, 649, 653
  learning theory and, 648
  motor symptoms in, 649
  physical examination findings in, 650*t*
  primary gain in, 649
  prognosis for, 650
  psychoanalytic factors in, 648
  secondary gain in, 649
  seizure symptoms in, 649
  sensory symptoms in, 649
  symptoms of, 647, 647*t*, 649
  treatment of, 650–651
Convulsion. *See also* Seizure(s)
  clonic, definition of, 282
  definition of, 282
  tonic, definition of, 282
Coombs' test, 270*t*
Cooper, John, 508
Copper
  serum, testing, 270*t*
  urine, testing, 270*t*
Coprolalia, 1246
  definition of, 284
Coprophagia, definition of, 282
Coprophilia, 724
Coprophrasia, definition of, 285
Copropraxia, 1246
Corgard. *See* Nadolol
Cornelia de Lange syndrome, 1171*t*
Coronary artery bypass surgery, 830
Coronary artery disease, psychological correlates of, **829–830**
Corrective emotional experience, 87, 218
  in psychoanalytic psychotherapy, **928**
Corrective familial experience, in group psychotherapy, 938*t*
Correlation coefficient, 175
Cortical columns
  in somatosensory system, 73
  in visual system, 73
Cortical rhythms, 121
Corticotropin-releasing hormone, 128, 129*t*
Cortisol, 262–263
  and major depressive disorder, 538
  testing, 270*t*
Council for Exceptional Children (CEC), 1161
Council for Responsible Nutrition, 856
Counterphobic attitude, 611
Countertransference, **4,** 193, 210
  and aging, 56
  HIV therapists, 378
  in psychoanalysis, **926**
Couple problems, **725**

Couples (marital) therapy, 45, **946–947**
  approaches to, 944*t*–945*t*
  combined therapy for, 946
  and conjoint therapy, **946**
  contraindications for, 947
  four-way session, **946**
  goals of, 947
  and group psychotherapy, **946**
  indications for, 946–947
  and individual therapy, **946**
  types of, 946
CPS, 181*t*
Crack (drug), 414, 428, **430**
  use, methods of, 430
Crank (drug), 414
Creatine phosphokinase, testing, 270*t*
Creatinine
  serum, testing, 270*t*
  urinary, testing for, 273*t*
Creatinine clearance, 263, 264*f*
Creativity, in adolescence, 37
Creutzfeldt-Jakob disease, **364,** 1322–1323
  dementia in, ICD-10 diagnostic criteria for, 344*t*
  familial, 1322–1323
  iatrogenic, 1322–1323
  sporadic, 1322–1323
  variant, **364–365**
Cri du chat syndrome, 1165, 1171*t*
Crime, emotional effects of, 157*t*
Criminal law, 1361–1363
Criminal responsibility, 1362–1363
Crisis, Erikson's concept of, 19
Crohn's disease, psychological correlates of, **827–828**
Cross-cultural psychiatry, **168–170**
Cross-cultural universals, 168
Cross-dressing, **735**
  in children, 731–732
  treatment of, 738
Crossover studies, 171
Cross-sectional studies, 171
Crowding, and aggression, 154
Crying, in infants, 141–142
Cryptococcosis, 108
Crystal (drug), 413–414
Crystal meth, 413
CSF, testing, 270*t*
CT. *See* Computed tomography (CT)
Cults, **899**
Cultural determinism, 167
Cultural identity, 169–170
Culturally diverse patients, 14
Culture
  and behavior, 166
  and bipolar I disorder, 536
  definition of, 166, 168–169
  ethnicity, 169
  and major depressive disorder, 536
  personality and, 166
  and psychopathology, 169
  and psychopharmacology, 532–533
  race, 169
  scope of, 169
  universal features of, 168
Culture-bound syndromes, 170, 295, **529–533**
  course of, 532
  indigenous healers, 532
  prognosis, 532
  representative syndromes, 529, 530*t*–531*t*, 531–532
  treatment of, 532
Cunnilingus, 723
Cushing's disease, obesity in, 752, 753*f*
Cushing's syndrome, 257, 832, 832*f*
  differential diagnosis of, 526
  medical considerations with, 845*t*
  neuropsychiatric manifestations of, 366
  psychiatric considerations with, 845*t*
  psychological correlates of, **832–833**
  and suicide, 915
Custody, child, 49, **1315–1317**
Cyclic adenosine monophosphate (cAMP), 101
  response element, 95
  as second messenger, 92, 95
Cyclic antidepressants. *See also* Tetracyclic drugs; Tricyclic drugs (tricyclic antidepressants)
  laboratory testing with, 265
  therapy with, 263
Cyclic guanosine monophosphate (cGMP), as second messenger, 95
Cyclic nucleotides, as second messenger, 95
Cyclothymia, ICD-10 diagnostic criteria, 589*t*
Cyclothymic disorder, 535, **576–578**. *See also* Bipolar disorder(s)
  biological factors in, 577
  biological therapy for, 578
  in childhood, **1277**
  clinical features of, 577–578
  course of, 578
  definition of, 576
  diagnosis of, 577–578
  diagnostic criteria for, 577, 577*t*
  differential diagnosis of, 578
  epidemiology of, 576
  etiology of, 576–577
  lifetime prevalence, 535*t*
  prognosis for, 578
  psychosocial factors in, 577
  psychosocial therapy for, 578
  signs and symptoms of, 577–578
  and substance abuse, 578
  treatment of, 578
Cylert. *See* Pemoline
Cyproheptadine, 1000*t*, **1015–1017**. *See also* Antihistamine(s)
  for anorexia nervosa, 745
  dosage and administration, 1017*t*
  implicated in sexual dysfunction, 711
  indications for, 1016
  pharmacological actions of, 1016
  for sexual dysfunction, 981
  structure of, 1015*f*
Cytoarchitectonics, cortical, 68*f*
Cytochrome P450 isoenzymes, 533, 976
  drug interactions, 566–568, 568*t*, 976, 977*t*, 1121
Cytomegalic inclusion disease, 1168
Cytomegalovirus (CMV), testing for, 270*t*
Cytomel. *See* Liothyronine
Cytosine, 123

D

DaCosta, Jacob Mendes, 599, 624
DaCosta's syndrome, 599, 624
Dalmane. *See* Flurazepam
Dance therapy, **854–855**
Dantrium. *See* Dantrolene
Dantrolene, 1000*t*, **1045–1046**
  adverse effects of, 1045–1046
  chemistry of, 1045, 1045*f*
  dosage and administration, 1046
  drug interactions, 1046
  effects on specific organs and systems, 1045
  indications for, 1045
  intoxication/overdose of, 985*t*
  laboratory interferences, 1046
  pharmacological actions of, 1045
  precautions with, 1045–1046
DAP, 1158*t*
Darvon. *See* Propoxyphene
Darwin, Charles, on fear, 591–592
Data
  definition of, 174
  interval ratios, definition of, 174
  nominal, definition of, 174
  ordinal, definition of, 174
Date rape, **892**
Davanloo, Habib, and short-term dynamic psychotherapy, 931–932, 932*t*
Davy, Humphry, 1067
Day care, for children, 35
Day care centers, **880**
Day residue, in dreams, 198
Day treatment
  with adolescents, 1313
  with children, **1303–1305**
    indications for, 1304
    programs in, 1304
    results of, 1304–1305
DBT. *See* Dialectical behavior therapy (DBT)
DDAVP. *See* Desmopressin (DDAVP)
Deafness
  congenital, differential diagnosis of, 1213–1214
  and phonological disorders, 1203*t*
Death
  attitudes toward, across life cycle, 60–61
  bereavement. *See* Bereavement
  causes of, 52–53
  of child, parent's response to, 64
  criteria for, 59, 59*t*
  definition of, 58–59
  impending, reactions to, 59–60
  intentional, 59
  legal aspects of, 59–60
  meaning of, 58
  near-death experience, 59
  psychogenic, 59
  reactions to, 59
  subintentional, 59
  sudden. *See* Sudden death
  timely, 59
  Uniform Determination of Death Act, 59
  unintentional, 59
  untimely, 59
  voodoo, 59
Death instinct, 151, 222, 917
  Freud's concept of, 200
Decathexis, definition of, 281
Decision trees, DSM-IV-TR and, 296, 297*f*
de Clerambault syndrome, 516
Deductive reasoning, 138
Defense mechanisms, **205–206**, 207*t*–208*t*
  in adolescence, 36–37
  classification of, 206, 207*t*–208*t*
  in delusional disorder, 513
  immature, 206, 207*t*
  mature, 208*t*
    adaptive, **20–21**
  narcissistic, 206, 207*t*
  neurotic, 206, 208*t*
  in obsessive-compulsive disorder, 618
  in personality disorders, 802–803
Defensive Functioning Scale, 296, 306*t*
Dehydroepiandrosterone (DHEA), 467–468, **1147**
  adverse effects of, 467

Deinstitutionalization, **1377**
Déja entendu, definition of, 286
Déja pensé, definition of, 286
Déja vu, 81
definition of, 286
Delinquency, 142
Delinquent acts, definition of, 1317
Delirium, **323–324**
in cancer patients, 839*t*
causes of, 323–324, **324–325,** 324*t*
characteristics of, 319, 323
cognition in, 320–321
computed tomography, 323
course of, 328
definition of, 280, 319, 323
versus dementia, **327,** 328*t,* 339
versus depression, 328
diagnosis of, 325–326
diagnostic criteria for, ICD-10, 329, 329*t*
differential diagnosis of, 327–328
DSM-IV classification of, 320*t*
due to a general medical condition, diagnostic criteria for, 325*t*
due to multiple etiologies, diagnostic criteria for, 326*t*
electroconvulsive therapy, 329
electroencephalography, 322
emergency manifestations of, 909*t*
emergency treatment of, 909*t*
epidemiology of, 324
functional magnetic resonance imaging, 323
laboratory evaluation of patient, 322, 322*t*
laboratory examinations in, 327, 327*t*
magnetic resonance imaging, 323
mental status examination, 320, 321*t*
neurological symptoms in, 327*t*
neuropsychological testing, 323
not otherwise specified, diagnostic criteria for, 326*t,* 329
opioid-induced, 1344
pharmacotherapy for, 328–329
physical examination of patient, 321, 322*t*
physical findings in, 327, 327*t*
positron emission tomography, 323
prognosis for, 328
prognostic significance of, 324
psychiatric history, 320
risk factors for, 324
versus schizophrenia, 328
single photon emission computed tomography, 323
sleep–wake disturbances in, 328
substance-induced, 324–325, 325*t,* 329, 381*t,* 382*t,* 458, 463. *See also specific substance*
substance intoxication, 381*t,* 382*t*
diagnostic criteria for, 325*t,* 329
substance withdrawal, 381*t,* 382*t,* 393*t*
diagnostic criteria for, 326*t,* 329
treatment of, 328–329
types of, 319
Delirium tremens (DTs), 403, 404*t,* 406
definition of, 285
Delusional disorder, 496, **511–520**. *See also* Schizophrenia
affect in, 514
biological factors in, 512–513
clinical features of, 513–517
cognition in, 514
course of, 518–519
defense mechanisms in, 513
definition of "delusion," 511, 512*t*
versus delirium, 518
versus dementia, 518
denial in, 513
diagnosis of, 511
diagnostic criteria for, 513, 514*t*
differential diagnosis of, 518
in elderly, 1325
emergency manifestations of, 909*t*
emergency treatment of, 909*t*
epidemiology of, 511
erotomanic type, 516
etiology of, 512–513
feelings in, 514
grandiose type, 517
in hearing-impaired, 255
hospitalization for, 519–520
impulse control in, 515
insight in, 515
jealous type, 515–516
judgment in, 515
mental status in, 513–515
mixed type, 517
mood in, 514
orientation in, 514
patient characteristics in, 513
perceptual disturbances in, 514
persecutory type, 515
pharmacotherapy for, 520, 1054
prognosis for, 518–519
psychodynamic factors in, 513
Freud's contributions on, 513
psychotherapy for, 519
reliability in, 515
risk factors associated with, 513, 513*t*
sensorium in, 514
somatic type, 516
versus substance-related disorders, 518
thought in, 514
treatment of, 519–520, 519*t*
types of, 515–517
unspecified type, 517
Delusional jealousy, 515
definition of, 284
Freud's contributions on, 513
Delusion(s)
with alcohol withdrawal, 403
bizarre, definition of, 283
of control, definition of, 284
definition of, 240, 283
in dementia, 336–337
of grandeur, definition of, 284
of infidelity, definition of, 284
mood-congruent, 240
definition of, 283
mood-incongruent, 240
definition of, 283
nihilistic, definition of, 283
paranoid, definition of, 284
of persecution, definition of, 284
of poverty, definition of, 283
of reference, definition of, 284
in schizophrenia, 471–472, 492–493
with childhood onset, 1283
of self-accusation, definition of, 284
somatic, definition of, 284
in substance-induced psychotic disorders, 528
systematized, definition of, 283
De Materia Medica, 856
Démence précoce, 471
Dementia, **108–109,** 254, **329–344,** 1321–1323
aggression in, pharmacological management of, 1332
agitation in, pharmacological management of, 1332
in AIDS patients, 256
alcohol-induced persisting, 406, 908*t*
of Alzheimer's type, 108, 331–333, 337–338, 1323
clinical features of, 1323
course of, 1323
DSM-IV diagnostic criteria for, 335*t,* 337
epidemiology of, 330, 1323
etiology of, 1323
genetic factors in, 331
neuroimaging in, 110
neuropathology of, 331–332, 331*f*
neurotransmitters in, 332
pathophysiology of, 106
pharmacotherapy for, 1003*t*
and sleep patterns, 759
treatment of, 340–341, 1323
versus vascular dementia, 339
versus amnestic disorder, 339
with anxiety, 108
with atherosclerosis, 108
catastrophic reaction in, 337
causes of, 330–334, 330*t,* 1322
cognition in, 320–321, 337
computed tomography, 323, 1335
cortical, 333, 334*t,* 1322–1323
course, 339–340, 1322
psychosocial determinants and, 340
in Creutzfeldt-Jakob disease, 1323
ICD-10 diagnostic criteria for, 344*t*
definition of, 287, 319, 329
versus delirium, **327,** 328*t,* 339
delusions in, 336–337
versus depression, 339, 340*t*
with depression, 108
diagnosis of, 334–338
differential diagnosis of, 339
DSM-IV classification of, 320*t*
DSM-IV diagnostic criteria for, 334, 335*t*–337*t*
due to multiple etiologies, DSM-IV-TR diagnostic criteria for, 336*t*
due to other general medical condition, 1322
DSM-IV diagnostic criteria for, 336*t,* 338
early-onset, 329
electroencephalography in, 120, 322
emergency manifestations of, 909*t*
emergency treatment of, 909*t*
epidemiology of, 329–330, 1321–1322
estrogen replacement therapy, 341
versus factitious disorder, 339
functional magnetic resonance imaging, 323
hallucinations in, 336–337
head trauma–related, 108, 334
HIV-related, 109, 334, 374–375
ICD-10 diagnostic criteria for, 344*t*
in Huntington's disease, 333–334, 334*t,* 1323
ICD-10 diagnostic criteria for, 344*t*
ICD-10, 341, 342*t*–344*t*
infectious, 334
inhalant-related persisting, 442, 443
laboratory evaluation of patient, 322, 322*t,* 338
magnetic resonance imaging, 108, 323, 1335
versus malingering, 339
versus mental retardation, 339
mental status examination, 320, 321*t*
mood changes in, 337
multi-infarct, 108
neuroimaging in, 111*f,* 117*f*
and neuroimaging, 108–109, 1335
neuropsychological testing, 323

Dementia—*continued*
versus normal aging, 339
not otherwise specified, DSM-IV-TR diagnostic criteria for, 337*t*
in Parkinson's disease, 334
ICD-10 diagnostic criteria for, 344*t*
pathophysiology of, 106, 1322–1323
personality changes in, 336
pharmacotherapy for, 341, 1003*t*
physical examination of patient, 321, 322*t,* 339–340
in Pick's disease, 333, **1323**
ICD-10 diagnostic criteria for, 344*t*
versus pituitary disorder, 339
positron emission tomography, 323
presenile, in familial multiple system taupathy, 332–333
prognosis for, 339–340
pseudodementia. *See* Pseudodementia
psychiatric history, 320
with psychosis, 108
psychosocial therapies, 341
versus schizophrenia, 339
sedative-, hypnotic-, or anxiolytic-related, persisting, 463
signs and symptoms, 319
single photon emission computed tomography, 323
subcortical, 333, 334*t,* 1322–1323
substance-induced. *See specific substance*
substance-induced persisting, 381*t,* 382*t*
alcohol-induced persisting, 406
DSM-IV-TR diagnostic criteria for, 336*t,* 338
inhalant-related persisting, 442
sedative-, hypnotic-, or anxiolytic-related, persisting, 463
and suicide, 915
treatment of, 340–341
experimental approaches, 341
types of, 319
vascular, **333,** 333*f,* 1323
DSM-IV diagnostic criteria for, 335*t*
DSM-IV-TR diagnostic criteria for, 338
epidemiology of, 330
ICD-10 diagnostic criteria for, 343*t*
versus transient ischemic attacks, 339
Dementia precox, 471–472
Demerol. *See* Meperidine
Demethylphenidate
for attention-deficit/hyperactivity disorder, 1227, 1227*t*
pharmacological action of, 1117
Demyelinating disorder(s), 109, 119
mental disorder due to, 362
mood disorder and, 351*t*
Denial, 207*t*
in delusional disorder, 513
in dying person, 60
Denver Developmental Screening Test, 1159
Deoxyribonucleic acid (DNA), 104, **123**
chemical structure of DNA molecule, 124*f*
definition of, 123
microassay analyses, 125
sequencing, 127
Depakene. *See* Valproate
Depakote. *See* Divalproex; Valproic acid
Dependence, substance. *See* Substance dependence
Dependence syndrome, 392*t*–393*t*
Dependent personality disorder, **814**. *See also* Personality disorder(s), cluster C
clinical features of, 813–814
course of, 814
diagnosis of, 813
diagnostic criteria for, 813, 814*t*
differential diagnosis of, 814
epidemiology of, 813
pharmacotherapy for, 814
prognosis for, 814
psychotherapy for, 814
treatment of, 814
Dependent variables, definition of, 177
Depersonalization
causes of, 687, 687*t*
definition of, 286, 685–686
Depersonalization disorder, 676, **685–687**
clinical features of, 686–687
course of, 687
definition of, 685–686
diagnosis of, 686–687
diagnostic criteria for, 686, 686*t*
differential diagnosis of, 687
epidemiology of, 686
etiology of, 686
prognosis for, 687
treatment of, 687
Depletion hypothesis, of neurasthenia, 665
Deprenyl. *See* Selegiline
Depression. *See also* Major depressive disorder; Mood disorder(s)
and academic problems, 1291
acupuncture for, 1145
with adjustment disorder, **796**
in adolescents, clinical features of, 552–553
and alcohol use disorders, 397
with amphetamine (or amphetaminelike substance) withdrawal, 416
anaclitic, 142
animal model of, 160, 161–162
anorexia nervosa and, 739
and attention-deficit/hyperactivity disorder, 1226
atypical, **583**
behavior therapy for, 565
brain magnetic resonance imaging, 111*f*
breathlessness in, 255
in children
clinical features of, 552–553
and separation anxiety disorder, 1260
cognitive theory of, 541, **956,** 956*t*
cognitive therapy for, 147
definition of, 280
versus delirium, 328
versus dementia, 339, 340*t*
with dementia, 108
dexamethasone-suppression test in, 262–263
double, 552, 575, 1276
drug augmentation therapy for, 989–991
in dying person, 60
in elderly, 58, 1323–1324, 1324*t*
clinical features of, 553
exercise as treatment for, 856
versus grief, 63–64
in hypothyroidism, 260–261
immune response and, 133
insight in, 555
insulin and, 129
interpersonal psychotherapy for, 565, 933–934, 960*t*
interviews, 249
judgment in, 556
learned helplessness theory of, 150, 161, 542
in middle age, 216
objective rating scales for, 555
panic disorder and, 606
Parkinsonism and, 75
pathophysiology of, 102, 104
pharmacotherapy for, 561, 564*t,* **565–572, 1026,** 1030, 1055, 1075, 1081
drug augmentation therapy, 989–991
postpartum. *See* Postpartum depression and psychoses
postpsychotic, 496
schizophrenia, postpsychotic depressive disorder of, **582–583**
postschizophrenic, 503*t*
with pseudodementia, 108
psychodynamic factors in, 541
psychotherapeutic approaches to, 960*t*
psychotherapy for, 561, 561*t*–564*t*
psychotic, 555
reserpine and, 163
and sleep, 134*f,* 135, 759
with strokes, 108
substance-induced, etiology of, 584, 585*t*
and substance-related disorders, 388
suicide in, 916, 918, 921
transcranial magnetic stimulation and, 121
and written expression disorder, 1186
Depression-related cognitive dysfunction, 339
Depressive disorder(s), 142
bupropion for, 1030
buspirone for, 1032
cognitive profile of, 957*t*
and conversion disorder, 648
drug augmentation therapy for, **990–991**
emergency manifestations of, 909*t*
emergency treatment of, 909*t*
and generalized anxiety disorder, 632
in mental retardation, 1178
mixed anxiety-depressive disorder, **583**
not otherwise specified, diagnostic criteria for, 578, 579*t*
pharmacotherapy for, 1003*t,* 1030, 1032, 1116, **1118, 1124**
and posttraumatic stress disorder, 624
and reading disorder, 1181
sleep stage histograms of patients with, 777*f*
suicide risk in, 916, **916**
Depressive episode(s)
clinical features of, 552
differential diagnosis of, 902, 903*t*
ICD-10 diagnostic criteria, 588*t*
mental status examination in, 553–555, 554*f*
mild, ICD-10 diagnostic criteria, 588*t*
moderate, ICD-10 diagnostic criteria, 588*t*
other, ICD-10 diagnostic criteria, 589*t*
pharmacotherapy for, **1068**
severe
with psychotic symptoms, ICD-10 diagnostic criteria, 588*t*
without psychotic symptoms, ICD-10 diagnostic criteria, 588*t*
Depressive equivalent, 552
Depressive personality disorder, 295, **817–818**
clinical features of, 817–818
course of, 818
diagnosis of, 817–818
differential diagnosis of, 818
epidemiology of, 817
etiology of, 817
pharmacotherapy for, 1119
prognosis for, 818
research criteria for, 818*t*
treatment of, 818
Depressive position, 222

Derailment, definition of, 283
Derealization, definition of, 286, 685–686
Dereism, definition of, 283
Dermatitis factitia, 257
Dermatological disorder(s), psychological correlates of, **833–834**
Descriptive statistics, 174, 175
Desipramine, 1000*t*
  adverse effects of, 567*t*, 981*t*, 1127*t*
  for attention-deficit/hyperactivity disorder, 1224, 1228
  blood level data for clinical assessment, 268*t*
  for bulimia nervosa, 750
  clinical information, 1130*t*
  for cocaine users, 435
  dosage and administration, 569*t*
  drug interactions, 378, 1134
  for elderly patients, 1329
  mechanism of action, 102, 567*t*
  neurotransmitter effects of, 1126*t*
  plasma levels, monitoring, 265
  preparations of, 1130*t*
  structure of, 1125*f*
Desmopressin (DDAVP)
  children, use with, 1308*t*
  for enuresis, 1258
Desoxyn. *See* Methamphetamine
Despair
  in children separated from mothers, 142
  Erikson's concept of, 214–215
Desyrel. *See* Trazodone
Detachment, in children separated from mothers, 142
Determinism
  biological, 167
  cultural, 167
  reciprocal, 147
Deutsch, Helene, 809
Development, **16–58,** 205, 206*f*, 228
  Adler's theory of, 217
  early, history of, 235
  epigenetic principle of, 87–88, **211–215**
    relation to Freudian theory, 211
  Erikson's theory of, **211–215**
  Kohut's theory of, 223
Developmental arithmetic disorder. *See* Mathematics disorder
Developmental coordination disorder, **1190–1193**
  clinical features of, 1191
  comorbidity with, 1190
  course of, 1192
  diagnosis of, **1191**
  diagnostic criteria for, 1191*t*
  differential diagnosis of, 1192
  epidemiology of, **1190**
  etiology of, **1191**
  and expressive language disorder, 1195
  and mathematics disorder, 1184
  and phonological disorder, 1200
  prognosis for, 1192
  treatment of, 1192–1193
Developmental disorder(s), versus tic disorder, 1249*t*
Developmentally based psychotherapy, 139
Developmental testing
  in child psychiatry, 1157*t*–1158*t*, **1158–1160**
  for infants and preschoolers, **1159**
Developmental theories, with children, 1296
Developmental word blindness. *See* Reading disorder
Devereux, George, 166
DEWS, 1187
Dexamethasone, 261
  with donepezil, 1044
  for pain management, 1345*t*
Dexamethasone suppression test (DST), **262–263,** 264*f*, **538**
  false-negative results, 262–263, 263*t*
  false-positive results, 262–263, 263*t*
  and mood disorders, 1278
  procedure of, 261
  reliability of, 262–263
  in schizophrenia, 482
  sensitivity of, 262–263, 263*t*
  specificity of, 262–263, 263*t*
Dexedrine. *See* Dextroamphetamine
Dexfenfluramine, for weight reduction, 755*t*
Dexmethylphenidate, 1000*t*, 1116
Dextroamphetamine, 413, 1000*t*, 1116. *See also* Sympathomimetics; Sympathomimetics (and related drugs)
  for attention-deficit/hyperactivity disorder, 1227, 1227*t*
  children, use with, 1307*t*
  geriatric dosage, 1330*t*
  intoxication/overdose of, 986*t*
  for pain management, 1345*t*
  pharmacological action of, 1116–1117, 1117
  for weight reduction, 755*t*
Dhat, 530*t*
DHEA. *See* Dehydroepiandrosterone (DHEA)
Diabetes mellitus, 256
  psychological correlates of, **832**
Diabetic ketoacidosis, 366
Diacetylmorphine. *See* Heroin
Diagnosis, **229**
Diagnosis without examination, ethics concerning, 1372*t*
Diagnostic Evaluation of Writing Skills (DEWS), 1187
Diagnostic and Statistical Manual of Mental Disorders (DSM), 125
  first edition, 288
  second edition, 288
  third edition, 288
  fourth edition. *See Diagnostic and Statistical Manual of Mental Disorders,* fourth edition (text revision)
  history of, 288
Diagnostic and Statistical Manual of Mental Disorders, fourth edition (text revision) (DSM-IV-TR), 150, **288–289**. *See also specific disorder*
  Axis I, 289, 289t
  Axis II, 289, 289*t*
  Axis III, 289, 289*t*
  Axis IV, 289–290, 290*t*
  Axis V, 290–291
  basic features, 288–289
  cautionary statement for, 295
  caveats, 295–296
  classes or groups of conditions in, 289
  classification of mental disorders, 293–294
    limitations of, 295–296
    updated to include ICD-9-CM numerical codes, 307*t*–313*t*
  clinical judgment, use of, 296
  criteria for mental disorder due to a general medical condition, 293
  criteria for substance-induced disorders, 293
  criteria used to exclude other diagnoses and to suggest differential diagnoses, 292–293
  and decision trees, 296, 297*f*
  definition of mental disorder, 293–294
  descriptive approach, 288
  diagnostic criteria, 288
  diagnostic uncertainties, 289
  in forensic psychiatry, 296
  frequently used criteria, 292–293
  guidelines, 295–296
  multiaxial evaluation, 289–291
    report form, 291, 291*t*
  multiple diagnoses, 292
  new and controversial categories, 294–295
  nonaxial format, 291, 292*t*
  not otherwise specified categories, 292
  organizational plan of, 294
  prior history in, 292
  provisional diagnosis, 292
  rating scales used in, 296
  severity of disorder, 291–292
  signs and symptoms, 275
  systematic description, 288
Diagnostic Interview for Children and Adolescents (DICA), 1154
Diagnostic test(s)
  interpreting performance of, 175*t*
  predictive value of, 175*t*
  sensitivity of, 175*t*
  specificity of, 175*t*
Dialectical behavior therapy (DBT), **954–955**
  for borderline personality disorder, 810, 954
Diarrhea, and psychotherapeutic drugs, **981**
Diazepam, 460, 1000*t*. *See also* Benzodiazepine(s)
  for adjustment disorders, 799
  blood level data for clinical assessment, 268*t*
  dosage of, 1025*t*
  drug interactions, 1047, 1134
  geriatric dosage, 1332*t*
  half-life of, 1025*t*
  indications for, 404*t*, 405, 419, 438, 459, 500
  pharmacokinetics of, 1022–1023
  pharmacological actions for, 1023
  structure of, 1023*f*
  for systematic desensitization, 951
  withdrawal, 462
Dibenzoxazepine
  adverse effects of, 981*t*
  chemistry of, 1053
  structure of, 1052*f*
DICA, 1154
Dichotomous thinking, 958*f*
Diencephalon, in memory formation, 80
Diet, **855**
  and aging, 53
  biological effects of, 53, 55*t*
Dietary supplements, **856**
  list of, 857*t*–858*t*
  Web sites, 859*t*
Diethylpropion, 1000*t*, 1116. *See also* Sympathomimetics (and related drugs)
  for weight reduction, 755*t*
Differentiation, stage of, 29*t*, 224
Diflunisal, for pain management, 1345*t*
Digoxin
  blood level data for clinical assessment, 268*t*
  drug interactions, 1081, 1124
  and lithium, 1072*t*
Dihydroepiandrosterone, 130
Dihydroindole
  chemistry of, 1053
  structure of, 1052*f*
Dilantin. *See* Phenytoin
Dilaudid. *See* Hydromorphone

Diltiazem. *See also* Calcium channel inhibitors
 dosage and administration, 1035
 and lithium, 1072*t*
 structure of, 1034*f*
2,5-Dimethoxy-4-methylamphetamine (DOM), 414
Dimethyltryptamine (DMT), 435, 436*t*
Dioscorides, 856
Diphenhydramine, 1000*t*, **1015–1017**. *See also* Antihistamine(s)
 blood level data for clinical assessment, 268*t*
 clinical guidelines for, 1016
 dosage and administration, 1016, 1017*t*
 for extrapyramidal disorders, 1059*t*
 indications for, 1015
 laboratory interferences, 1016
 pharmacological actions of, 1016
 for separation anxiety disorder, 1263
 structure of, 1015*f*
Diphenylbutylpiperidine, 1051*t*
 chemistry of, 1053
 structure of, 1052*f*
Diplopia, 255
Dipsomania, definition of, 282
Disabilities Act, 1161
Discriminant analysis, 175
Discrimination, **144**
Disinhibited attachment disorder of infancy or early childhood, 1270*t*
Disinhibition, definition of, 280
Disintegration anxiety, 593
Disorder of infancy, childhood, or adolescence not otherwise specified, **1273**, 1273*t*
Disorder of written expression. *See* Written expression disorder
Disorientation, definition of, 280
Dispal. *See* Orphenadrine
Displacement, 208*t*
 in dreams, 198
Displacement activity, with stress, 159
Disruptive behavior disorder, not otherwise specified, **1238**
 diagnostic criteria for, 1238*t*
Disruptive behavior disorders, **1232–1240**
Dissociation
 as defense, 208*t*
 definition of, 286
 in personality disorders, 802
 and splitting, 676
Dissociative amnesia, 676, **676–679**
 clinical features of, 677
 course of, 679
 diagnosis of, 677
  questions used to reveal symptoms in, 677, 678*t*
 diagnostic criteria for, 677, 677*t*
 differential diagnosis of, 677–678, 678*t*
 epidemiology of, 676
 etiology of, 676–677
 ICD-10 diagnostic criteria for, 690*t*
 prognosis for, 679
 treatment of, 679
Dissociative anesthesia and sensory loss, ICD-10 diagnostic criteria for, 690*t*
Dissociative convulsions, ICD-10 diagnostic criteria for, 690*t*
Dissociative disorder(s), **676–691**
 brainwashing, 689
 definition of, 676
 DSM-IV-TR classification of, 676
 ICD-10 classification of, 689
 ICD-10 diagnostic criteria for, 689, 690*t*
 not otherwise specified, 676, **687**, 688*t*
Dissociative fugue, 676, **679–680**
 clinical features of, 679–680
 course of, 680
 definition of, 679
 diagnosis of, 679–680
 diagnostic criteria for, 679–680, 679*t*
 differential diagnosis of, 680
 epidemiology of, 679
 etiology of, 679
 ICD-10 diagnostic criteria for, 690*t*
 prognosis for, 680
 treatment of, 680
Dissociative identity disorder, 471, 676, **680–685**
 clinical features of, 681–683, 682*t*
 course of, 684
 definition of, 286, 680–681
 diagnosis of, 681–683
 diagnostic criteria for, 681–682, 681*t*
 differential diagnosis of, 683
 epidemiology of, 681
 etiology of, 681
 forensic issues, 685
 historical perspective on, 681
 prognosis for, 684
 treatment of, 684–685, 684*t*–685*t*
Dissociative motor disorders, ICD-10 diagnostic criteria for, 690*t*
Dissociative phenomena, normal, 676
Dissociative stupor, ICD-10 diagnostic criteria for, 690*t*
Dissociative trance disorder, 295, 676, **688**, 688*t*
Distal tubule diuretics, and lithium, 1072*t*
DISTAR, 1183
Distortion, 207*t*
Distortions, in phonological disorders, 1201
Distractibility, definition of, 280
Distribution, 175
 definition of, 175
 frequency, 175
 normal, 175
 of psychotherapeutic drugs, 975
Disulfiram, 388, 1000*t*, **1046–1047**
 adverse effects, 1047
 for alcoholism, 412
 in alcohol use disorders, 389, 399
 chemistry, 1046, 1046*f*
 dosage and administration, 1047
 drug interactions, 1020, 1028, 1047, 1062*t*
 indications for, 1046–1047
 intoxication/overdose of, 986*t*
 laboratory interferences, 1047
 pharmacological actions of, 1046
 precautions with, 1047
Diuretics
 drug interactions, 1072
 and lithium, 1072*t*
Divalproex, 267, 1000*t*
 for bipolar I disorder, 570
 children, use with, 1307*t*
 geriatric dosage, 1330*t*
Divorce, **48–50**
 among physicians, **881**
 child custody and, 49
 community, 49
 coparental, 49
 economic, 49
 effects on children, 34
 legal, 49
 psychic, 49
 reasons for, 49–50
Dizziness, 254–255, 255*t*
DMT, 435, 436*t*
DNA. *See* Deoxyribonucleic acid (DNA)
DNI orders, **1340–1341**
DNR orders, **1340–1341**
Doctor–patient relationship, **1–15**
 and compliance, 10–12
 confidence, 1
 continuity of, **12–13**
 countertransference in, 4
 defensiveness, 1
 deliberative model, 3
 development of, 1
  with psychosomatic illness, 840
 empathy, 1
 informative model, 3
 interpretive model, 3
 models of, 2–3
 paternalistic model, 3
 rapport in, 1, 6–7
 transference in, **4**
 trust, 1
Dogmatil. *See* Sulpiride
Dollard, John, 143, 148
 frustration-aggression hypothesis, 153
Dolophine. *See* Methadone
DOM, 414
Domestic violence, 151. *See also* Battered wives; Child abuse and neglect
Dominance hierarchy, 162
Dominic-R, 1154
Donepezil, 106, 126, 341, 1000*t*
 adverse effects of, 1043
 for Alzheimer's disease and similar disorders, 1041
 dosage of, 1044
 drug interactions, 1044
 pharmacological action of, 1042
Don Juanism, 728
Do not intubate (DNI) orders, **1340–1341**
Do not resuscitate (DNR) orders, **1340–1341**
L-Dopa, 1000*t*, **1047–1050**. *See also* Dopamine receptor antagonist(s), and precursors
 adverse effects of, 100
 for cocaine users, 435
 drug interactions, 1031
 intoxication
  emergency manifestations of, 909*t*
  emergency treatment of, 909*t*
 intoxication/overdose of, 986*t*
Dopamine, 85, **97–100**
 and aggression, 154
 antagonists, 98, 100
 antidepressant effects on, 567*t*
 and drugs, 92, 100
 life cycle, 98, 100
 in major depressive disorder, 537
 metabolism, 98, 100
 neurotransmitter function, 90*t*, 91*f*, 93*t*
 and psychopathology, 100
 receptors, 93*t*, **100**
  effects of cocaine on, 430
  type 1 (D1), 100
  type 2 (D2), 100
   in addiction, 430
   in schizophrenia, 479, 481
  type 3 (D3), 100
  type 4 (D4), 100
  type 5 (D5), 100
 reuptake, effects of cocaine on, 430
 reuptake mechanism, 98
 and sleep, 759
 and stereotypic movements, 1271
 in substance-related disorders, 387, 388*f*

synthesis of, 98
testing, 270*t*
Dopamine agonists, for stereotypic movement disorder, 1272
Dopamine hypothesis, of schizophrenia, 100, 477–478
Dopamine receptor antagonist(s), 98, 100 **1050–1067**. *See also specific drug*
adverse effects, 1055–1061, 1055*t*
nonneurological, 1056–1057
alternative maintenance regimens, 1065
augmentation of, **991**
cardiac effects of, 1056
central anticholinergic effects, 1061
chemistry of, 1051–1053
choice of drug, 1063
classification of, 1051*f*, 1053
in combination therapy, 1054
dermatological effects, 1057
dosage and administration, 1063–1066
drug interactions, 1014, 1028, 1061–1063, 1062*t*
CYP-induced, 976
early treatment with, 1065
effects on specific organs and systems, 1054
endocrine effects, 1056
epileptogenic effects of, 1060
given as needed medications, 1065
hematological effects of, 1056
history of, 1050–1051
indications for, 416, 442, 459, 1054–1055
intoxication/overdose of, 986*t*, 1057
and jaundice, 1057
laboratory interferences, 1063
and lactation, 1061
list of, 1051*t*
long-acting depot medications, 1065–1066, 1065*t*
maintenance treatment with, 1065
and neuroleptic-induced acute akathisia, 1058–1059
and neuroleptic-induced acute dystonia, 1058
and neuroleptic-induced movement disorders, prevention of, 1061
and neuroleptic-induced parkinsonism, 1058
and neuroleptic-induced tardive dyskinesia, 1059–1060
and neuroleptic malignant syndrome, 1060
ophthalmological effects, 1057
and orthostatic hypertension, 1056
peripheral anticholinergic effects, 1056
pharmacological actions of, 1053–1054
plasma concentrations, 1066
precautions with, 1055–1061
and precursors, **1047–1050**
adverse reactions to, 1049
chemistry of, 1048, 1048*f*
clinical guidelines, 1049–1050
dosage of, 1049–1050, 1050*t*
drug interactions, 1049
effects on specific organs and systems, 1049
indications for, 1049
laboratory interferences, 1049
pharmacological actions of, 1048
precautions with, 1049
and pregnancy, 1061
rapid neuroleptization of, 1064
schedule of, 1064–1066
for schizophrenia, 477–478, 497, 1068
and sedation, 1060
serotonin-dopamine antagonists. *See* Serotonin-dopamine antagonist(s) (atypical antipsychotics)
for sexual dysfunction, 980
sexual side effects, 1057
short-term treatment with, 1064
side effects, neurological, 1057–1061
sudden death with, 1056
for Tourette's disorder, 1250
and treatment-resistant patients, 1066
and weight gain, 1057
withdrawal from, 982
Dopaminergic agonists, for cocaine users, 435
Dopaminergic tracts, of central nervous system, 97–98, 99*f*
Dopar. *See* L-Dopa
Doppler ultrasound, 270*t*
Doral. *See* Quazepam
Doriden. *See* Glutethimide
Dorsolateral region, 85
Dose-response curves, 975*f*
Double-bind concept, 484
Double-blind studies, 171
Double depression, 552, 1276
differential diagnosis of, 575
Double insanity, 517–518, 517*t*, 518*t*
Double simultaneous stimulation, 187
Down syndrome, 105, 1164, 1171*t*
chromosomal aberrations in, 1165
course of, 1165
diagnosis of, 1165
epidemiology of, 1165
mental retardation in, 1165, 1171*t*
Doxepin, 1000*t*
adverse effects of, 567*t*, 981*t*, 1127*t*
blood level data for clinical assessment, 268*t*
clinical information, 1130*t*
dosage and administration, 569*t*
mechanism of action, 567*t*
neurotransmitter effects of, 1126*t*
preparations of, 1130*t*
structure of, 1125*f*
Draw-a-Person (DAP) test, 178, 183*t*, 185
Drawings, children's, 31–32
Dreaming, during sleep, 756*f*, 758
Dreamlike state, definition of, 280
Dream(s)
affects in, 198
anxiety, 198
cerebral damage and, 83
in children, 33
condensation in, 198
day residue in, 198
displacement in, 198
Erikson's approach to, 216
Freud's theory of, **197–198**
history-taking about, 237–238
interpretation of, **197–198,** 756*f*, **926**
in group therapy, 936*t*
latent content, 198
manifest content, 197
and nocturnal sensory stimuli, 198
punishment, 198
secondary revision, 198
symbolic representation in, 198
Dream work, 197–198
Dress, physician's, 247
Drinker(s)
affiliative, 402
early-stage problem, 402
schizoid-isolated, 402
Drinking, binge. *See* Binge drinking
Drives, 199
control and regulation by ego, 205
Drive theory, Freud's, **199–204**
Dronabinol, 427
Droperidol, 1000*t*
chemistry of, 1053
for delirium, 328
preparations, 1064*t*
structure of, 1052*f*
Drowsiness, definition of, 280
Drug-assisted interviews, 1026, **1148**
Drug augmentation therapy, **989–992**
Drug Enforcement Agency (DEA), control levels of, 978*t*
Drug-induced extrapyramidal reactions, 992
Drug-induced movement disorders, 997*t*
Drug(s)
abuse. *See* Substance abuse
in adolescence, 38–39
and aggression, 154
delirium caused by, 324–325
dependence. *See* Substance dependence
depression caused by, 584, 585*t*
female sexual dysfunction caused by, 710–712, 710*t*
implicated in sexual dysfunction, 708*t*–709*t*, 710–712, **710–712,** 710*t*
male sexual dysfunction caused by, 708*t*, 710–712
pregnancy, use during, 24
and suicide, 915
teratogenicity, 24
Drummond, Edward, 1362
Dry mouth, and psychotherapeutic drugs, **982**
DSM. *See Diagnostic and Statistical Manual of Mental Disorders*
DST. *See* Dexamethasone suppression test (DST)
DTs. *See* Delirium tremens (DTs)
Dual-instinct theory, 199
Dual-sex therapy, 712–713
Duchenne's muscular dystrophy, 1249*t*
Duloxetine, 1000*t*, **1136–1137**
Durable power of attorney, 1360–1361
Durham v. United States, 1362
Durkheim, Emile, 917
Dusky v. United States, 1361
Dwarfism, psychosocial, 1269
differential diagnosis of, 1269
Dying patients
acceptance in, 60
alternative and complementary medicine, 1348
caring for, 1338
child care, 1347
communicating with, 1338–1339
definition of "dying," 58–59
denial in, 60
depression in, 60
dying at home, 1346
euthanasia, 1348
family care, 1342
hospice care, 1346–1347
infant care, 1347
informed consent, 1339–1340
management of, essential features, 1339*t*
neonatal care, 1347
pain management, 1343–1345
palliative care, 1342–1346
physician-assisted suicide, 1348–1349
promises physicians should make to, 1339*t*
questions from, 1340*t*
reactions to impending death, 59–60
spiritual issues, 1347
suicide requests, 1349–1350

Dying patients—*continued*
telling the truth, 1339
terminal care decisions, 1340–1342
Dynamic structures, 220
Dynorphins, synthesis of, 104
Dysarthria
and benzodiazepine(s), 1028
definition of, 285
differential diagnosis of, 1202
and phonological disorders, 1203*t*
Dyscalculia, definition of, 287. *See also* Mathematics disorder
Dysgraphia, 189
definition of, 287
and written expression disorder, 1186
Dyskinesia, definition of, 282
Dyskinetic movements, differential diagnosis of, 1272
Dyslexia, 113, 189. *See also* Reading disorder
developmental, 82–83
definition of, 82
Dysmorphophobia, 653, 753
Dyspareunia, **706,** 706*t*
due to a general medical condition, 707
nonorganic, ICD-10 diagnostic criteria for, 717*t*–718*t*
Dysphasia
differential diagnosis of, 1197
pharmacotherapy for, 1006
and phonological disorders, 1203*t*
Dysphonia, definition of, 285
Dyspnea, 255
Dysprosody, definition of, 285
Dyssomnia(s), **763–774**
in ICSD, 764*t*
not otherwise specified, 772*t*, **773–774**
Dysthymia
ICD-10 diagnostic criteria, 589*t*–590*t*
pharmacotherapy for, 1119
Dysthymic disorder, 535, **572–578**. *See also* Depressive disorder(s)
biological factors in, 573
in childhood, **1276–1277**
epidemiology of, 1274–1275
clinical features of, 573–574, 574*t*
cognitive theory of, 573
course of, 575
definition of, 572
diagnosis of, 573–574
diagnostic criteria for, 573–574, 573*t*, 574*t*
differential diagnosis of, 575
DSM-IV-TR classification of, 572
epidemiology of, 572
etiology of, 573
Freud's contributions on, 573
hospitalization for, 576
major depressive disorder, distinguished, 572
neuroendocrine studies in, 573
pharmacotherapy for, 576
prognosis for, 575
psychosocial factors in, 573
sleep studies in, 573
treatment of, 575–576
variants of, 574
Dystonia. *See also* Medication-induced movement disorders
acute
emergency manifestations of, 909*t*
emergency treatment of, 909*t*
definition of, 282
neuroleptic-induced acute. *See* Neuroleptic-induced acute dystonia
Dystonia musculorum deformans, 1249*t*

E

Ear, medical assessment of, 255
Early Intervention programs, 88
Early morning awakening, polysomnogram measures of, 760*t*
Eating disorder(s), **739–755**. *See also* Anorexia nervosa; Bulimia nervosa; Obesity
in children, pharmacotherapy for, **1310**
combined psychotherapy and pharmacotherapy for, 970
cyproheptadine for, 1017
epidemiology of, 739
in ICD-10, 1245
ICD-10 criteria for, 745–746, 746*t*, 751
of infancy or early childhood, **1241–1245**
and intermittent explosive disorder, 783
medical complications of, 741, 742*t*
not otherwise specified, 750–751, 750*t*
and obsessive-compulsive disorder, 617
pathophysiology of, 105
pharmacotherapy for, 1003*t*, 1017, **1127**
and trichotillomania, 790
EBV. *See* Epstein-Barr virus (EBV)
Echocardiography, 271*t*
Echolalia, 1246
definition of, 283
Echopraxia, 491, 1246
definition of, 281
Economic rights, of patients, 1358
Ecstasy, definition of, 280
Ecstasy (drug), 104, 414. *See* Methylenedioxyamphetamine
ECT. *See* Electroconvulsive therapy (ECT)
EDTA, 853
Educational psychotherapy, with children, 1296–1297
Educational status, and alcohol-related disorders, 396
Educational testing, in child psychiatry, 1157*t*–1158*t*, **1158–1160**
Education for all Handicapped Children Act, 1161, 1180
Education history, 236
Edwards Personal Preference Schedule (EPPS), 181*t*
EEG. *See* Electromyography (EMG)/electromyogram(s) (EEG)
Effexor. *See* Venlafaxine
Ego, **204–205,** 223
autonomous functions
primary, 205
secondary, 205
in character formation, 209
functions of, 197, 204, **205**
in neurotogenesis, 209
superego. *See* Superego
synthetic function of, 205
Ego boundaries, loss of, in schizophrenia, 492
Egocentrism, in children, 137
Ego defect, in schizophrenia, 483
Ego defenses, 197
Ego instincts, 199–200
Ego libido, 204
Egomania, definition of, 284
Ego psychology, 197, **204–209**
Ego states, Berne's concept of, 219
Ehrhardt, Anke, 693
Eicosanoid(s)
neurotransmitter function, 95, 107
as second messengers, 95
Eidetic image, definition of, 286
Ejaculation
premature. *See* Premature ejaculation
retarded, 256
retrograde, 256
Elation, definition of, 280
Elavil. *See* Amitriptyline
Eldepryl. *See* Selegiline
Elder abuse, 879, **1327,** 1328*t*
Elderly, **50–58,** 214–215. *See also* Geriatric psychiatry
accidents among, 157
alcohol abuse/dependence in, 1326
anemia, psychiatric symptoms with, 1337
antidepressant therapy for, 1329, 1330
antimanic agents for, 1330–1331, 1330*t*
antipsychotics for, 1331, 1332*t*
neurological adverse effects of, 1331
anxiety disorders in, 1325
anxiolytics for, 1331–1332
arthritis, psychiatric symptoms with, 1337
attitudes toward death in, 60
bipolar I disorder in, 1324
brief psychodynamic psychotherapy for, 1334
calcium channels inhibitors for, 1035
cardiovascular disease, psychiatric symptoms with, 1337
cerebrovascular disease, psychiatric symptoms with, 1336–1337
cognition in, 1320, 1321, 1321*t*, 1322*t*
cognitive-behavioral therapy for, 1334
delusional disorder in, 1325
dementing disorders in, 1321–1323
conditions resembling, 1322*t*
demographics of, **50,** 51*t*
depression in, 58, 1323–1324, 1324*t*
clinical features of, 552–553
developmental theorists, 55*t*
drug-related psychiatric symptoms in, 1321
electroconvulsive therapy for, 1332–1333
Erikson's view of, 214–215
functional assessment of, 1319
general description of patient, 1319
geographic distribution of, 53
health status of, 56, 56*t*
hearing loss in, 1327
insight-oriented therapy for, 1334
integrated therapy for, 1334–1335
judgment in, 1320
kidney disease (chronic), psychiatric symptoms with, 1337
language output in, 1319
life review therapy for, 1333–1334
and lithium, 1071–1072
liver disease (chronic), psychiatric symptoms with, 1337
long-term care of, 57–58, 57*f*
lung disease (chronic), psychiatric symptoms with, 1337
malnutrition, psychiatric symptoms with, 1337
medical history in, 1321
memory in, 1320
mental disorders in, 1321–1326
mental status examination, 1319–1320
monoamine oxidase inhibitors for, 1329–1330
neuropsychological assessment of, 1320–1321
normality among, 20
obsessive-compulsive disorder in, 1325
perceptual disturbances in, 1319
personality development, 53–55
pharmacotherapy for, **979,** 979*t*, 1328–1333
principles of, 1328–1329

phobias in, 1325
psychiatric assessment of, 1318–1321
family history in, 1318
marital history in, 1318
medical history in, 1321
psychiatric examination of, 1318–1319
sexual history in, 1318–1319
psychiatric problems of, 58
psychogeriatric long-term care, 1378
psychosocial risk factors in, 1321
psychostimulants for, 1330, 1330*t*
psychotherapy for, 1333–1335
reminiscence therapy for, 1333–1334
schizophrenia in, 1324–1325
sedative-hypnotics for, 1331–1332
selective serotonin reuptake inhibitors for, 1329
sensorium in, 1320
and sexuality, 57
sleep disorders in, 1326
socioeconomic status of, 56–57
somatoform disorders in, 1325–1326
spousal bereavement, 1327
substance abuse in, 1326
suicide in, 58, 1319, 1326–1327
supportive psychotherapy for, 1333
syncope in, 1327, 1327*t*
thyroid disease, psychiatric symptoms with, 1337
thyroid hormones for, 1122
tricyclic antidepressants for, 1329
vertigo in, 1327
visuospatial functioning in, 1319
Elders, Joycelyn, 380
Elective mutism, 1266, 1270*t*
Electrocardiography, with cyclic antidepressant therapy, 265
Electroconvulsive therapy (ECT), 263, **1138–1144**
adverse effects of, 1143–1144
for aggression, 156
amnestic disorder with, 347–348
and anesthetics, 1140–1141
barbiturates for, 1018
central nervous system effects, 1143–1144
children, use with, 1311
clinical guidelines for, 1140–1143
and concomitant medications, 1140
contraindications with, 1143
for delirium, 329
drug interactions, 1124
for elderly, 1332–1333
electrical stimulus in, 1142
electrode placement in, 1141–1142, 1142*f*
electrophysiological principles of, 1138–1139
failure of, 1143
fractures from, 1144
and general anesthetics, 1140–1141
headaches from, 1144
history of, 1138
indications for, 1139–1140
maintenance treatment, 1143
mechanism of action, 1139
and memory, 1143–1144
for mood disorder due to a general medical condition, 352
for mood disorders, 352
in childhood, 1279
and mortality, 1143
multiple monitored, 1143
and muscarinic anticholinergic drugs, 1140
and muscle relaxants, 1141, 1141*t*
muscle soreness from, 1144
number of, 1143
for obsessive-compulsive disorder, 623
and Ohm's law, 1139
and premedications, 1140–1141
pretreatment evaluation for, 1140
for schizophrenia, 500
seizures induced by, 1142–1143
monitoring of, 1142
prolonged, 1142–1143
tardive, 1142–1143
spacing of, 1143
Electroencephalography, 108, **119–121,** 271*t*
for attention-deficit/hyperactivity disorder, 1224
for biofeedback, 948
bipolar montages, 120
for cognitive disorders, 322
in dementia, 120, 322
of epileptic focus, 120
24-hour CCTV monitoring, 120
phase reversal, 120
referential montage, 120
in schizophrenia, 481
in seizures, 120, 357*f,* 358*f,* 359*f*
in sleep, 121, 756
in thought, 121
Electromyography (EMG)/electromyogram(s) (EEG)
for biofeedback, 948
in sleep, 756
Electrophysiology, **89–90**
in personality disorders, 801
Electroshock therapy (EST), 1138. *See also* Electroconvulsive therapy
Elimination disorder(s), **1254–1258**. *See also* Encopresis; Enuresis
E-mail
interviews, 248
medical record, 252
Embryo, 21
EMDR, **953–954**
Emergency psychiatric interview, 901, 902*t*
Emergency psychiatric medicine. *See* Psychiatric emergencies
EMG. *See* Electromyography (EMG)/electromyogram(s) (EEG)
Emotional damage and distress, damages awarded for, 1363
Emotional development
Freud's concept of, 167
in infancy, 26, 28*t*
in preschool period, 31–32
in toddler period, 30
Emotional disturbances, in children, psychoanalytic view of, 1295
Emotional insight, definition of, 283
Emotional problems, history-taking about, 235
Emotion(s), **83**
basic drives and, 83
childhood experience and, 87
definition of, 280
expressed, in families, 484
limbic system and, 83–84
and memory, 80
nature and nurture, 87
neuroanatomy and, 83
in psychoanalytic psychotherapy, **928**
Empathic validation, in psychotherapy, definition of, 927*t*
Empathy
development of, 32
in group psychotherapy, 938*t*
during interviews, 250
and prevention of aggression, 156
Empty-nest syndrome, 48
Encephalitis, and mental retardation, 1169
Encephalitis lethargica, 1249*t*
Encephalopathy
alcoholic, 406
alcoholic pellagra, 409
hepatic, 366
medical considerations with, 846*t*
psychiatric considerations with, 846*t*
HIV, 375
hypoglycemic, 366
pharmacology for, 1118
uremic, 366
Wernicke's, 406
emergency manifestations of, 908*t*
emergency treatment of, 908*t*
Encopresis, **1254–1256**
clinical features of, 1254–1255
course of, 1256
diagnosis of, 1254–1255
diagnostic criteria for, 1254–1255, 1255*t*
differential diagnosis of, 1256
epidemiology of, 1254
etiology of, 1254
laboratory findings in, 1255
nonorganic, ICD-10 diagnostic criteria for, 1258*t*
pathologic testing in, 1255
prognosis for, 1256
treatment of, 1256
Encouragement to elaborate, in psychotherapy, definition of, 927*t*
Endep. *See* Amitriptyline
Endocrine assessment, 132
Endocrine disorder(s)
mood disorder and, 351*t*
neuropsychiatric manifestations of, 365–366
personality change due to, 819, 819*t*
psychological correlates of, **831–832**
and suicide, 915
Endocrine therapies, **1147**
End-of-life care
alternative and complementary medicine, 1348
approaches to, 1338
child care, 1347
communication and its importance, 1338–1339
definition of, 1338
dying at home, 1346
euthanasia, 1348
family care, 1342
future directions in, 1350
hospice care, 1346–1347
infant care, 1347
informed consent, 1339–1340
neonatal care, 1347
pain management, 1343–1345
palliative care, 1342–1346
physician-assisted suicide, 1348–1349
problems facing the physician, 1338
reactions to impending death, 59–60
spiritual issues, 1347
suicide requests, 1349–1350
symptom management, 1345–1346, 1346*t*
telling the truth, 1339
terminal care decisions, 1340–1342
Endomorphins, 104
β-Endorphin, synthesis of, 104
Endorphins, 104, 449
Engel, George, 1–2
English language, neural activity and, 86

Enkephalins, 104, 449
Enuresis, **1256–1258**
  behavioral therapy for, 1257
  biofeedback for, 949*t*
  in children, pharmacotherapy for, **1309**
  clinical features of, 1257
  course of, 1257
  diagnosis of, 1257
  diagnostic criteria for, 1257, 1257*t*
  differential diagnosis of, 1257
  diurnal, 1257, 1257*t*
  epidemiology of, 1256
  etiology of, 1256–1257
  and expressive language disorder, 1196
  in ICD-10, 1258, 1258*t*
  nocturnal, 1257, 1257*t*
  nocturnal and diurnal, 1257, 1257*t*
  nonorganic, ICD-10 diagnostic criteria for, 1258*t*
  pathology and laboratory testing in, 1257
  pharmacotherapy for, 1127, 1258
  and phonological disorder, 1200
  prognosis for, 1257
  psychotherapy for, 1258
  and pyromania, 786–787
  treatment of, 1258
Environmental medicine, **856**
Enzyme deficiency disorder(s), 1167, 1167*t*–1168*t*
Eosinophilia-myalgia syndrome, 103–104
Ephedra, 470
Ephedrine, 414
Epidemiology, **170–174**
Epigenetic principle, 18, 88, **211–215**
Epilepsy, **356–360**. *See also* Seizure disorder
  brain function and, 79
  complex partial, and schizophrenia, 481
  definition of, 356
  diagnosis of, 359–360
  and dissociative amnesia, 677–678
  electroencephalography in, 120
    electroencephalographs of seizures, 357*f*, 358*f*, 359*f*
  epidemiology of, 356
  ICD-10, 358*t*
  mental disorders related to, 356–360
  and mental retardation, 1163
  mood disorder symptoms in, 359
  personality change due to, 819, 819*t*
  personality disturbances in, 358–359
  petit mal, **357,** 358*f*
  psychotic symptoms in, 359
  and suicide, 915
  symptoms
    ictal, 357–358
    interictal, 358–359, 359*f*
    preictal, 357
  temporal lobe, 83
  treatment of, 360
  vagal nerve stimulation for, 1145
  violence and, 359
Epileptic seizures, sleep-related, **779**
Epileptoid personality, 783
Epinephrine, **100–102**
  drug interactions, 1062–1063, 1062*t*
  laboratory testing for, 263
  life cycle, 101
  neurotransmitter function, 91*f*, 93*t*
  receptors, 93*t*
  synthesis of, 101
EPPS, 181*t*
EPQ, 181*t*
EPs. *See* Evoked potentials (EPs)
Epstein-Barr virus (EBV)
  and chronic fatigue syndrome, 661
  testing for, 271*t*
Eptastigmine, for Alzheimer's disease and similar disorders, 1042
Equanil. *See* Meprobamate
Erectile dysfunction, 701*t*, **703–704,** 703*t*
  dopamine receptor antagonists for, 1049
  due to a general medical condition, 707, 708*t*
  sublingual apomorphine for, 1050
  treatment of, 712–716, 1137
Ergasia, 224
Ergot alkaloids and bromocriptine, 1049
Erikson, Erik, **211–217,** 211*f*, 1293
  Childhood and Society, 166, 211
  on early adulthood, 43
  epigenetic principle, 88, **211–215**
    relation to Freudian theory, 211
  on old age, 55*t*
  on personality development, 53–54
  theory
    of development, 211
    of life cycle, 19, 46, 60, **211–215**
    of personality, 211
    of psychopathology, **215–216**
    of treatment, 216–217
EROS, 716
Eros, 151, 200
Eroticized child, 719
Erotic stimuli, 696
Erotomania, 516
  definition of, 284
ERPs. *See* Event-related potentials (ERPs)
Error
  type I, definition of, 177
  type II, definition of, 177
Erythrocyte sedimentation rate (ESR), testing for, 271*t*
Erythromycin
  with buspirone, 1033
  with paroxetine, 1044
Erythrophobia, definition of, 284
Erythroxylon coca, 428
Escape learning, 146
Escitalopram, 1000*t*
Esimil. *See* Guanethidine
Eskalith. *See* Lithium
ESR, testing for, 271*t*
Essential tremor, 256
EST, 1138
Estazolam, 1000*t*. *See also* Benzodiazepine(s)
  dosage of, 1025*t*
  half-life of, 1025*t*
  pharmacokinetics of, 1022
  pharmacological actions for, 1023
  structure of, 1023*f*
Estrogen(s), 130, 263, **1147**
  for dementia, 341
  drug interactions, 1028, 1046
  for elderly women, 1332
  for sex drive, 715
  testing for, 271*t*
Ethacrynic acid, and lithium, 1072*t*
Ethanol, 398. *See also* Alcohol
  blood level data for clinical assessment, 268*t*
  drug interactions, 1062*t*
Ethchlorvynol, 1000*t*, 1019, **1021–1022**
  intoxication/overdose of, 986*t*
Ethics, **1365–1373**
  beneficence, 1365, 1368
  business issues, 1369
  in child psychiatry, **1315–1317**
  confidentiality, 1369–1370
  financial issues, 1369
  ideological issues, 1369
  impaired physicians, 1371
  and integrative psychiatry, 867
  intersex surgery, 737
  justice, 1368
  managed care issues, 1370
  media relations, 1370
  medical record issues, 252–254
  military psychiatry, 252
  nonmaleficence, 1365
  nonsexual boundary violations, 1368–1369
  patient autonomy, 1365
  Physician Charter of Professionalism, 1371, 1371*t*
  physicians in training, 1371
  principles of, 1365, 1366*t*–1367*t,* 1368
  questions and answers, 1372*t*–1373*t*
  sexual boundary violations, 1368
  social issues, 1369
  suicide requests, 1349
Ethnicity, 169
  and alcohol use disorders, 396
Ethological studies, of attachment, 140
Ethological terminology, 165*t*
Ethology, **158–166**
Ethopropazine, 1000*t*
Ethopropazine hydrochloride, structure of, 1013*f*
Ethyl alcohol, 398. *See also* Alcohol
Ethylenediaminetetraacetic acid (EDTA), 853
N-Ethyl-3,4-methylenedioxyamphetamine, 414
Euphoria, definition of, 280
Euthanasia, **1348**
Eve (drug), 414
Event-related potentials (ERPs), 121–122
  in language tasks, 122
Evoked potentials (EPs), 121–122
  higher cognitive processing in, 122
  negative waves, 122
  positive waves, 122
  in schizophrenia, 481–482
Evolution, in sociobiology, 163
Evolutionary psychology, **163–164**
Excessive daytime sleepiness. *See* Hypersomnia
Excitation-contraction coupling, 90
Excretion, of psychotherapeutic drugs, 975–976
Exercise, 856
  and aging, 53
  biological effects of, 53, 55*t*
Exfoliative dermatitis, and carbamazepine, **1038**
Exhibitionism. *See also* Paraphilias
  clinical features of, 720
  diagnosis of, 720
  diagnostic criteria for, 720, 720*t*
  ICD-10 diagnostic criteria for, 726*t*
Existentialism, 227
Existential psychoanalysis, 227
Exocytosis, 92
Exons, 123
Experimental disorders, 149
Experimental models, 161–163
  pharmacological syndromes, 163
  stress syndrome, 161
Exploitation, ethics concerning, 1372*t*
Exploitative personality, 220
Exploratory psychotherapy, with children, 1295–1296
Expressive language development, in DSM-IV-TR, 1194
Expressive language disorder, **1194–1198**
  clinical features of, 1196

course of, 1197
diagnosis of, 1196, 1196*t*
differential diagnosis of, 1197
epidemiology of, 1194
etiology of, 1196
and language disorders, 1200*t*
and mathematics disorder, 1184
and phonological disorder, 1200
prognosis for, 1197
and stuttering, 1203
treatment of, 1197–1198
and written expression disorder, 1186
External genitalia, 693, 693*f*
Externalization, 208*t*
Extinction, **144**
Extrapyramidal disorders, pharmacotherapy for, 1059*t*
Extrapyramidal reactions, drug-induced, 992
Extroverts, 222
Eye, medical assessment of, 255
Eye movement desensitization and reprocessing (EMDR), **953–954**
Eye movement dysfunction, in schizophrenia, 482
Eye-roll sign for hypnotizability, 960, 961*f*
Eysenck Personality Questionnaire (EPQ), 181*t*

F

Fabry's disease, 1167*t*
Face, visual assessment of, 257
Facial Recognition Test, 189
Facilitation, in interview, 9
Factitious disorder(s), **668–675**
biological factors of, 669
clinical features of, 669
with combined psychological and physical signs and symptoms, **672**
comorbidity with, 668
course of, 674–675
versus dementia, 339
diagnosis of, 669, 669*t*
differential diagnosis of, 673–674
epidemiology of, 668
etiology of, 668–669
feigned syndromes, 670*t*
in ICD-10, 673, 673*t*
laboratory examination of, 673
not otherwise specified, **672–673**
diagnostic criteria for, 672*t*
pathology, 673
pharmacotherapy for, 675
with predominantly physical signs and symptoms, **670–672**
with predominantly psychological signs and symptoms, **669–670**
prognosis for, 674–675
by proxy, 295, 672, 673*t*
psychosocial factors of, 668–669
versus schizophrenia, 495–496
treatment of, 675
Factor analysis, 219
Failure to thrive, 142
and reactive attachment disorder of infancy or early childhood, 1267–1269, 1268*f*
Fairbairn, Ronald, 205, **220**
Faith healing, **865**
Falling-out, 530*t*
Fallopian tubal ligation, **877**
Falret, Jules, 534
False memory, definition of, 286
False memory syndrome, 689
Familial multiple system taupathy, 332–333
Family
birth order in, 33–34, 218
and child development, 34–35
clinical interviews with, in child psychiatry, 1153
dysfunction, and conduct disorder, 1235
expressed emotion in, 484
and mood disorder, 539–540
and personality, 167–168
pseudohostile, 484
pseudomutual, 484
relational problems in, 879–882
schisms in, 484
and schizophrenia, theories about, 483–484
single-parent, 45
skewed, 484
stability, and child development, 34
Family group therapy, **944**
Family history, **234**
Family-life chronology, 942*f*
rationale for, 943*t*
Family planning, **874–877**
Family studies, 167–168
Family systems therapy, with children, 1296
Family therapy, **941–948**
with adolescents, 1313
for anorexia nervosa, 745
approaches to, 944*t*–945*t*
Bowen model of, **942–943**
for cocaine use disorders, 434
in depression, 565
for dysthymic disorder, 576
family group therapy, **944**
frequency of treatment, 942
general systems model of, **943–944**
goals of, 946
initial consultation, 941–942
interview technique, 942
length of treatment, 942
models of, 942–944, 944*t*–945*t*
with obsessive-compulsive disorder, 623
in panic disorder, 608
paradoxical therapy, **945**
for phobias, 615
positive connotation in, **946**
psychodynamic-experiential model of, **942**
for psychosomatic illness, 842
reframing, **946**
for schizophrenia, 500–501
social network therapy, **944–945**
structural, **943**
techniques of, 944–946
initial consultation, 941–942
interview technique, 942
termination of treatment, 944*t*
theory of, 941
Fantasy
history-taking about, 237–238
in personality disorders, 802
Farber's lipogranulomatosis, 1167*t*
Fatal familial insomnia, **365,** 1323
Fathers
attachment and, 29
effect of pregnancy on, 869
Fatigue
definition of, 281
persistent. *See* Chronic fatigue syndrome
Fausse reconnaissance, definition of, 286
FDA. *See* Food and Drug Administration (FDA)
FDC, 977
Fear
and anxiety, 591–592
Darwin's contributions on, 591–592
definition of, 281, 591
limbic system and, 84
Fear response, 87
Feature extraction, in sensory systems, 66, 68–69, 78
Fecal incontinence, biofeedback for, 949*t*
Federn, Paul, theory of schizophrenia, 483
Feeding, limbic system and, 84
Feeding disorder of infancy or early childhood, **1244,** 1244*t*
course of, 1244–1245
differential diagnosis of, 1244
DSM-IV-TR diagnostic criteria, 1244*t*
epidemiology of, 1244
in ICD-10, 1244*t,* 1245, 1245*t*
prognosis for, 1244–1245
treatment of, 1245
Feeding habits, in early childhood, history of, 235
Feelings, in elderly patients, 1319
Fees, **12**
Fee splitting, ethics concerning, 1372*t*
Feldenkrais, Moshe, 856
Feldenkrais method, **856,** 858*f*
Fellatio, 723
Female genital mutilation, **887–888**
Female orgasmic disorder, **704–705,** 704*t*
premature orgasm, 712
Female pseudohermaphroditism, 734*f*
Fenfluramine
for autistic disorder, 1215
intoxication/overdose of, 986*t*
for obsessive-compulsive disorder, 622
for weight reduction, 755*t*
Fenichel, Otto, 611, 925
Fenoprofen, for pain management, 1345*t*
Ferenczi, Sándor, **220**
Fernald Method, 1183
Ferritin, serum, testing for, 271*t*
Fertility awareness method, 875*t*
Fetal alcohol syndrome, 24, 24*f,* **409–410,** 1168–1169, 1172*t*
Fetal blood sampling, 23
Fetal demise, 874
Fetal genetic disorders, 23–24
Fetal life, 21–23
α-Fetoprotein screening, 23
Fetishism. *See also* Paraphilias
clinical features of, 720, 720*t*
diagnosis of, 720, 720*t*
diagnostic criteria for, 720, 720*t*
ICD-10 diagnostic criteria for, 726*t*
Fetoscopy, 23–24, 24
Fetus, 21
behavior of, 21
small, 25
vulnerability to maternal stress, 23
Fibromyalgia, 837
diagnostic criteria for, 837*t*
pharmacotherapy for, 1119
psychological correlates of, **837**
Field, definition of, 223
Field theory, 223
Fight or flight response, 77
Filial therapy, with children, 1297
First-generation antihistamines, 1015
Fixation(s), 221
Flashbacks
after cannabis use, 427
complications of, 438

Flashbacks—*continued*
definition of, 438
in hallucinogen use disorders, 437, 437*t*, 438
triggers of, 438
Flight of ideas, 239
definition of, 283
Floccillation, definition of, 281
Flooding, in behavior therapy, **952**
Flumazenil, 1000*t*
for benzodiazepine overdose, 1026
dosage of, 1025*t*
half-life of, 1025*t*
indications for, 464
molecular structure of, 1024*f*
Flunitrazepam, 460
abuse, 460
Fluorescent treponemal antibody-absorption (FTA-ABS) test, 264
Fluorodeoxyglucose, in neuroimaging, 111*f*, 114, 117*f*
Fluoxetine, 93, 102, 981*t*, 1000*t*. *See also* Selective serotonin reuptake inhibitors
adverse effects of, 567*t*, 981*t*
for anorexia nervosa, 745
for bulimia nervosa, 750
with bupropion, 1031
for cataplexy, 769
children, use with, 1307*t*
for cocaine users, 435
for conduct disorder, 1238
detection of, by magnetic resonance spectroscopy, 112
dosage and administration, 569*t*
drug interactions, 378, 1031, 1079, 1124, 1134
CYP-induced, 976
for elderly patients, 1329
intoxication/overdose of, 986*t*
mechanism of action, 102, 109
for postpsychotic depressive disorder of schizophrenia, 583
for schizoaffective disorder, 511
for selective mutism, 1266
for separation anxiety disorder, 1263
and weight loss, 752
Fluoxymesterone, 467
Flupenthixol, for cocaine users, 435
Fluphenazine, 1000*t*. *See also* Dopamine receptor antagonist(s)
geriatric dosage, 1332*t*
indications for, 498
and lithium, 1072*t*
preparations, 1064*t*
structure of, 1052*f*
Fluphenazine decanoate, preparations, 1064*t*
Fluphenazine enanthate, preparations, 1064*t*
Flurazepam, 460, 1000*t*
dosage of, 1025*t*
geriatric dosage, 1332*t*
half-life of, 1025*t*
pharmacological actions for, 1023
for primary insomnia, 765
Fluvoxamine, 1000*t*. *See also* Selective serotonin reuptake inhibitors
adverse effects of, 567*t*, 981*t*
children, use with, 1307*t*
dosage and administration, 569*t*
drug interactions, 1016, 1028, 1062*t*, 1329
CYP-induced, 976
for elderly patients, 1329
intoxication/overdose of, 986*t*
mechanism of action, 103
for separation anxiety disorder, 1263
withdrawal from, 982
fMRI. *See* Magnetic resonance imaging, functional (fMRI)
Focal brain disease, 256
Folate, **1146**
serum, testing for, 271*t*
Folie à deux, 814
definition of, 280
Folie à trois, definition of, 280
Folie impose, 517–518, 517*t*, 518*t*
Folie simultanée, 518
Folk remedies, abuse of, 395*t*
Follicle-stimulating hormone (FSH), 263
in schizophrenia, 482
testing for, 271*t*
Follow-up interviews, 248
Food, Drug, and Cosmetic (FDC) Act, 977
Food allergies, 855
Food and Drug Administration (FDA)
approval process of, 977
and herbal medicine, 856
Food guide pyramid, 855, 855*f*
Ford v. Wainwright, 1361
Forensic psychiatry, **1351–1364**
child psychiatry, **1315–1317**
definition of, 1351
DSM-IV-TR and, 296
Formal operations stage, 19, 28*t*
Piaget's theory of, 138
Formal thought disorders, 239*t*. *See also* Thought disorder(s)
definition of, 283
Formication
in cocaine use disorders, 433
definition of, 285
fosB transcription factor, 127
Four-way session, in couples (marital) therapy, **946**
Fragile X syndrome, 1163–1164, 1171*t*, 1209, 1249*t*
mental retardation in, 1165, 1171*t*
Frankincense, 854*t*
Free association, 182, 193, 196, 210, 216
in psychoanalysis, **925**
Freebase, 428, 430
Free-floating attention, in psychoanalysis, **925**
Freeman, Walter, 1148
French, Thomas, and brief psychotherapy, 930
Frequency distribution, 175
Freud, Anna, **220–221**, 220*f*, 785
on child development, 21
developmental theory of, 36–37
Freud, Sigmund, **193–210**, 194*f*–197*f*
on accident-prone personality, 157
on adjustment disorders, 795
Beyond the Pleasure Principle, 200
on body dysmorphic disorder, 653
on child development, 20–21
on delusional disorder, 513
on depression, 541
developmental theory, 19, 167, 200
on dissociative identity disorder, 681
and dream interpretation, 197–198, 756*f*, 926
The Ego and the Id, 204
on emotion, 87
on gender identity disorders, 731
on homosexuality, 698
and hypnosis, 961
on impotence, 704
on incest, 196–197
The Interpretation of Dreams, 197–198
life of, 193–194
on love and intimacy, 699
Mourning and Melancholia, 64, 573
On Narcissism, 200
on narcissism, 204
on neurasthenia, 665
on normality, 17
on obsessive-compulsive symptoms, 618
on old age, 55*t*
on personality traits, 801
on phobic neurosis, 610–611
on pleasure principle, 150, **200**, 692
psychoanalytic method, 87
psychoanalytic theories of, 925–926
reality principle, **200**
on sensory deprivation, 163
on sexual desire disorder, 702
structural theory of mind, **204–205**, 204*f*
theory
of aggression, 151, 200
of anxiety neurosis, **206–209**, 591, 593, 599
of character, 209
of dreams, **197–198**
of homosexuality, 204
of infantile sexuality, **200**
of instincts, **199–204**
of neurosis, 196–197, **209**
of psychosexual development, 19
of schizophrenia, 483
of suicide, 917
Three Essays on the Theory of Sexuality, 19, 200
topographical model of mind, **198–199**
Totem and Taboo, 166
Freudian slip, definition of, 282
Frölich's syndrome, 752
Fromm, Erich, **220**, 220*f*
Frontal cortex, in schizophrenia, 477
Frontal lobe(s)
and antipsychotics, 85
and attention, 80
dysfunction, 80, 85
and emotion, 84
functions, 80*t*, 84–85
injury, 85
and language, 82
in memory impairment, 82
in mood and affect disorders, 109
in schizophrenia, 84, 109, 479, 482
subdivisions of, 85
testing, 85
Frontal lobe syndrome(s), 85, 903, 904*t*
Frontal lobe tumor(s)
medical considerations with, 844*t*
psychiatric considerations with, 844*t*
Frosch, John, 809
Frostig Movement Skills Test Battery, for developmental coordination disorder, 1191
Frotteurism. *See also* Paraphilias
clinical features of, 721
diagnosis of, 721
diagnostic criteria for, 721, 721*t*
FSH. *See* Follicle-stimulating hormone (FSH)
FTA-ABS test, 264
Fucosidosis, 1167*t*
Fugue, definition of, 286
Fulton, John F., 1147
Functional magnetic resonance imaging. *See* Magnetic resonance imaging, functional (fMRI)
Furosemide
drug interactions, 1041
and lithium, 1072*t*

G

GA, 789
GABA
  and aggression, 154
  in alcohol use disorders, 397
  in anxiety disorders, 595
  and drugs, 104, 106
  neurotransmitter function, 90*t*, 91*f*, 106
  in panic disorder, 600
  and psychopathology, 106
  receptors, GABAA
    barbiturate binding to, 461
    barbituratelike substance binding to, 461
    benzodiazepine binding to, 461
  in schizophrenia, 478
  in substance-related disorder(s), 387, 388*f*
Gabapentin, 1000*t*, **1089–1093**
  adverse reactions to, 1090–1091
  for bipolar I disorder, 570, 571
  chemistry of, 1089, 1089*f*
  dosage of, 1091
  drug interactions, 378, 1091
  indications for, 1090
  laboratory interferences, 1091
  pharmacological actions of, 1089
  precautions with, 1090–1091
Gabbard, Glen O., 608–609
GAF, 290, 290*t*, 296
Gag rule, 1390
Gait
  assessment of, 256
  disorders, 108
Galactosemia, 1168*t*, 1172*t*
Galantamine, 1000*t*
  adverse effects of, 1044
  for Alzheimer's disease and similar disorders, 1041
  dosage of, 1044
  drug interactions, 1044
  pharmacological action of, 1042–1043
Galvanic skin response (GSR) gauge, 948
Gamblers Anonymous (GA), 789
Gambling, pathological. *See* Pathological gambling
Games, psychological, definition of, 219
Gamete donors, 873*t*
Gamete intrafallopian transfer (GIFT), 873*t*
Gamma hydroxybutyrate (GBH) (GHB), **468**
Gampo, Songsten, 866
Gangliosidosis, generalized, 1167*t*
Gangs, and conduct disorder, 1236–1237
Ganser's syndrome, **689**
Gantt, W. Horsley, 161
Gap junctions, 91
Gardner Expressive One Word Picture Vocabulary Test-Revised, 191*t*
Gardner Receptive One Word Picture Vocabulary Test-Revised, 191*t*
GARF, 296, 305*t*–306*t*
Garrod, Alfred, 1067
Gas(es)
  neurotransmitter function, 88, 95
  as second messenger, 95
Gasner's syndrome, differential diagnosis of, 674
Gasoline inhalation, 1249*t*
Gastroesophageal reflux
  psychological correlates of disease, **827**
  sleep-related, **779–780**
Gastrointestinal disorder(s), 828*t*
  drugs for, 828, 829*t*
  psychological correlates of, **826–829**
Gastrointestinal system, medical assessment of, 256
Gastrointestinal upset, and psychotherapeutic drugs, **981**
Gatekeepers, HMOs, 1388
Gattefosse, René-Maurice, 853
Gault decision, 1359
Gay men, 697. *See also* Homosexuality
GBH, **468**
Gender identity, 32–33, **692–693,** 693*f*
  definition of, 730
  in toddler period, 30
Gender identity disorders, **730–738**
  in adolescents, **732**
  in adults, **732–733**
  biological factors, 730
  in children, **731–732**
  clinical features of, 731–735
  course of, 736
  definition of, 730
  diagnosis of, 731, 731*t*
  DSM-IV-TR classification of, 730
  etiology of, 730–731
  and homosexuality, 736
  in ICD-10, 738, 738*t*
  not otherwise specified, **733–735**
    diagnostic criteria for, 733*t*
  prognosis for, 736
  psychosocial factors, 730–731
  treatment of, 736–738
Gender issues, in psychotherapy, **929–930**
Gender role, 693–694
  in toddler period, 30
General adaptation syndrome, 822–823
Generalized anxiety disorder
  and alcohol use disorders, 397
  biological factors in, 632–633
  brain imaging in, 633, 633*f*
  buspirone for, 635, 1032
  characteristics of, 1262*t*
  of childhood, 1264*t*
  in children, pharmacotherapy for, 1310
  clinical features of, 633–634
  comorbidity with, 632
  course of, 634
  definition of, 632
  diagnosis of, 633
  diagnostic criteria for, 633, 634*t*
  differential diagnosis of, 634
  epidemiology of, 632
  etiology of, 632–633
  ICD-10 diagnostic criteria for, 597*t*
  and obsessive-compulsive disorder, 617
  pharmacotherapy for, 635, 1003*t*, 1006, 1009, **1024**, 1032, **1127**
  prognosis for, 634
  propranolol for, 1009
  psychosocial factors in, 633
  psychotherapy for, 634–635
  sex distribution of, 632
  treatment of, 634–635
  and trichotillomania, 790
Generalized gangliosidosis, 1167*t*
General systems model, of family therapy, **943–944**
Generation gap, 38
Generativity
  Erikson's concept of, 19, 46, **216**
  versus stagnation, 19, 46, 214
Gene(s), 123
  E4, multiple, in Alzheimer's disease, 331
  modifier, 124
Gene targeting, 127
Gene therapy, 128
Genetic epistemology, 133
Genetics
  animal models in, 126–127
  behavioral, **122–128**
  clinical research in, 128
  and drugs, 128
  fetal disorders, 23–24
  inheritance patterns, 125
  mapping, 125
  and mental illness, 125–126
  molecular biology, neurogenetics and, **122–128**
  and personality, 167–168
  traits, 124–125
Genital mutilation, **887–888**
Genital response, failure of, ICD-10 diagnostic criteria for, 717*t*
Genital stage, 203*t*
Genitourinary system, medical assessment of, 256
Genogram, in family therapy, 943
Geographic relocation anxiety, 1261
Gepirone, 1000*t*, **1033**
Geranium, 854*t*
Geriatric depression scale, 1324*t*
Geriatric psychiatry, **1318–1337**. *See also* Elderly
  definition of, 1318
  psychogeriatric long-term care, 1378
  psychopharmacological treatment in, 1328–1333
German measles. *See* Rubella
Gerontology, 50
Gerstmann-Sträussler-Scheinker syndrome, 1323
Gerstmann-Straussler syndrome, **365**
Gerstmann syndrome, 71. *See also* Mathematics disorder
Gesell, Arnold, 21
Gessell Infant Scale, 1159
Gestalt, definition of, 225
Gestalt group therapy, classification of, 935
Gestalt theory, 225
Gestalt therapy, 225
GH. *See* Growth hormone (GH)
GHB, **468**
Ghost sickness, 530*t*
GIFT, 873*t*
Gill, Merton M., **221**
Gilles de la Tourette syndrome. *See* Tourette's disorder
Ginkgo, 1146
Ginseng root, 715
Glioblastoma multiforme, 108
Global Assessment of Functioning (GAF) Scale, 290, 290*t*, 296
Global Assessment of Relational Functioning (GARF), 296, 305*t*–306*t*
Glomerulus/glomeruli, 71, 74
Glossolalia, definition of, 283
Glucose
  Alzheimer's patients, metabolism in temporoparietal region of brain of, 118*f*
  cerebral metabolism of, 114
  fasting blood level, testing for, 271*t*
  metabolism, 96, 117*f*
Glutamate
  and drugs, 106–107
  neurotransmitter function, 90*t*, 91*f*, 106
  and psychopathology, 107
  receptors, 81, 86, 90*t*
  in schizophrenia, 478
Glutamyl transaminase, serum, testing for, 271*t*

γ-Glutamyl transpeptidase, effects of alcohol on, 399
Glutethimide, 460, 1000*t*, 1019, **1022**
blood level data for clinical assessment, 268*t*
intoxication/overdose of, 986*t*
Glycine, 91*f*, 105
GnRH. *See* Gonadotropin-releasing hormone (GnRH)
Goldstein, Kurt, **221**
Gonadal hormones, 129–130
Gonadotropin-releasing hormone (GnRH), 128, 129*t*, 263
in schizophrenia, 482
testing for, 271*t*
Good-enough mother, 228, 796
Good-enough mothering, 29–30
Goodness of fit, 29
GORT-R, 1160
Gould, Roger, developmental theory of, 42–43
G protein(s), **94**
subunits, 94
Graded exposure, in behavior therapy, **952**
Grammar, 1194
Grandiose self, 223
Grand mal epilepsy, biofeedback for, 949*t*
Grandma's rule, 146
Grandmother cell, 69
Grapefruit juice, and buspirone, 1032, 1033
Graves' disease, 831, 831*f*
psychological correlates of, 831
Gray matter. *See also* Cerebral cortex
Gray Oral Reading Test-Revised (GORT-R), 1160
Green, Richard, 736–737
Greenspan, Stanley, 139
Grief, **61–65**
anniversary reactions, 63
anticipatory, 63
biology of, 64
in children, 64
complicated, 63
definition of, 61, 280
versus depression, 63–64
with divorce, 49
normal, 61–62
in parents, 64
pathological (abnormal), 63
period of, 62–63
phases of, 62, 62*f*, 65*t*
in children, 64
phenomenology of, 64, 64*t*
physician's role in, 64–65
psychodynamics of, 64
psychosis in, 63
Grief therapy, 64–65
"Grievance collectors," 13–14
Grooming, assessment of, 256
Group dynamics, 223
Group hysteria
emergency manifestations of, 909*t*
emergency treatment of, 909*t*
Group psychotherapy, **935–940**
with adolescents, **1301,** 1313
and attention-deficit/hyperactivity disorder, 1229
and authority anxiety, 935
behavioral patterns in, 939*t*
with children, **1300–1302**
indications for, 1301
latency-age groups, 1301
parental involvement in, 1301–1302
preschool/early school-age, 1300–1301
pubertal and adolescent groups, 1301
in residential settings, 1301
school-age groups, 1301
specialized groups, 1301
classification of, 935
for cocaine use disorders, 434
combined with individual psychotherapy, **940**
and couples (marital) therapy, **946**
diagnosis in, 936–937
for dysthymic disorder, 576
with families, **944**
features of, 935*t*
frequency of sessions in, 937
group formation, 937
homogenous versus heterogenous groups, 937
inpatient, **938–939**
inpatient versus outpatient, 939, 940*t*
length of sessions in, 937
mechanisms in, 937
membership criteria for, 936*t*
for obsessive-compulsive disorder, 623
open versus closed groups, 937
patient selection in, 935, 936*t*
and peer anxiety, **935–936**
preparation for, 937
for psychosomatic illness, 842
role of therapist in, 937–938
for schizophrenia, 501
self-help groups. *See* Self-help groups
for sexual dysfunction, 714
size of group in, 937
structural organization of, **937**
therapeutic factors in, 937, 938*t*
therapist's tasks in, 937*t*
types of, 936*t*
Groups, Bion's concept of, 219
Growth hormone (GH), 131, 263
and major depressive disorder, 538
testing, 271*t*
Growth-hormone-releasing hormone, 128, 129*t*
G-spot, 713
GSR, 948
Guanethidine, 256
drug interactions, 1062*t*, 1120
Guanfacine, 1000*t*, **1005–1007**
adverse reactions to, 1006
for attention-deficit/hyperactivity disorder, 1228
children, use with, 1308*t*
clinical features of, 1007
dosage of, 1007, 1007*t*
drug interactions, 1007
effects on specific organs and systems, 1005
indications for, 1005–1006
laboratory interferences, 1007
overdose of, 1006
precautions with, 1006
withdrawal, 1007
Guanine, 123
Guilt
definition of, 281
Erikson's concept of, 215
Gulf War syndrome, 628–629
Gulf war syndrome, 134
Gutheil, Thomas E., 689, 1351

H

HAAg, testing for, 271*t*
Habit and impulse disorders, ICD-10 classification of, 793–794, 793*t*
Habituation, 147–148, 381
Hacker, Ewold, 471
Hahnemann, Samuel, 851, 859, 863, 863*f*
Halazepam, 1000*t*. *See also* Benzodiazepine(s)
dosage of, 1025*t*
geriatric dosage, 1332*t*
half-life of, 1025*t*
pharmacological actions for, 1023
structure of, 1023*f*
Halcion. *See* Triazolam
Haldol. *See* Haloperidol
Hallervorden-Spatz disease, 1249*t*
Hallucination(s)
with alcohol withdrawal, 403, 406
auditory, definition of, 285
in autoscopic psychosis, 525
cenesthesic, definition of, 285
cenesthetic, in schizophrenia, 492
in cocaine intoxication, 433
command, definition of, 285
definition of, 285
in dementia, 336–337
in elderly patient, 1319
eliciting experience of, in mental status examination, 239
gustatory, definition of, 285
hallucinogen psychotic disorder with
emergency manifestations of, 909*t*
emergency treatment of, 909*t*
in hallucinogen use disorders, 439
haptic, definition of, 285
hypnagogic, 239
definition of, 285
hypnopompic, 239
definition of, 285
lilliputian, definition of, 285
mood-congruent, definition of, 285
mood-incongruent, definition of, 285
olfactory, definition of, 285
opioid-induced, 1344
in schizophrenia, 84, 471–472, 491–492
with childhood onset, 1283
symbolic meaning, 483
sleep–wake cycle and, 134
somatic, definition of, 285
in substance-induced psychotic disorders, 528
tactile, definition of, 285
visual, definition of, 285
Hallucinogen-related disorder(s), 382*t*, **435–440**
anxiety disorder, 439
clinical features of, 439
diagnosis of, 437–439
DSM-IV-TR classification of, 437, 437*t*
epidemiology of, 436–437
mood disorder, 438–439
not otherwise specified, 439
diagnostic criteria for, 439, 439*t*
persisting perception disorder (flashback), 438
diagnosis of, 438
diagnostic criteria for, 437, 437*t*
treatment of, 440
psychotic disorder, 438
diagnosis of, 438
emergency manifestations of, 909*t*
emergency treatment of, 909*t*
treatment of, 440, 909*t*
rehabilitation, 439–440
sexual dysfunction, 711
treatment, 439–440
Hallucinogen(s), 435–436, 436*t*
abuse, 438, 461

dependence, 438
psychological, 438
effects of, 439
and hallucinations, 439
intoxication, 438
acute, diagnostic criteria for, 391*t*–392*t*
diagnostic criteria for, 437, 437*t*, 438
treatment of, 438, 439–440
intoxication delirium, 438
diagnosis of, 438
neuropharmacology of, 437
tolerance, 437
use, 436–437
and age, 437
and geographic regions, 436
morbidity in, 436–437
mortality in, 436–437
prevalence of, 436–437
and race, 436
sex distribution of, 436
trends in, 436–437
Hallucinogen therapy, **1149**
Hallucinosis, 404*t*
definition of, 285
Haloperidol, 497, 1000*t*. *See also* Dopamine receptor antagonist(s)
adverse effects of, 106
for autistic disorder, 1215
blood level data for clinical assessment, 268*t*
with buspirone, 1032
chemistry of, 1053
for childhood/adolescent antisocial behavior, 1293
children, use with, 1307*t*
for conduct disorder, 1238
for delirium, 328
drug interactions, 1032, 1081
geriatric dosage, 1332*t*
indications for, 409, 416, 419, 438, 442, 459, 498
for inhalant-induced psychotic disorder, 443
and lithium, 1072*t*
and neuroleptic-induced parkinsonism, 1014
preparations, 1064*t*
for psychotic disorders, 527
structure of, 1052*f*
for Tourette's disorder, 1250
Haloperidol decanoate, preparations, 1064*t*
Halstead, Ward, 190
Halstead-Reitan Battery, **190**
Hamilton Anxiety Rating Scale, 181, 300*t*
Hamilton Rating Scale for Depression, 181, 300*t*–301*t*, 555
Hammond, William, 1067
Handedness, cerebral dominance for, 82, 84
Hard signs, 1156
Harlow, Harry, 28, 160, 692
Harmaline, 435
Harmine, 435
Hartmann, Heinz, 17
Hartnup disease, 1168*t*
Hathaway, Starke, 180
Hatha yoga, 866
Hawkins, David, 697
Hb. *See* Hemoglobin (Hb)
HBcAg, testing for, 271*t*
HBsAg, testing for, 271*t*
Hct, 271*t*
Head
medical assessment of, 254
visual assessment of, 257
Headache(s). *See also* Migraine
acupuncture for, 1145
cluster
pharmacotherapy for, 1069
sleep-related, **779**
from electroconvulsive therapy, 1144
medical assessment of, 254
postcoital, 712
psychological correlates of, **837–838**
and psychotherapeutic drugs, **981–982**
tension, 838, 838*t*
biofeedback for, 949*t*
Head banging, **1271–1272**
Head injury, 254. *See also* Head trauma
amnestic disorder with, 348
and suicide, 915
Head Start, 88
Head trauma, blunt, 361–362. *See also* Head injury
dementia related to, 108, 334
medical considerations with, 845*t*
mental disorder due to
symptoms of, 362
treatment of, 362
and mental retardation, 1169
pathophysiology of, 361–362
penetrating, 361–362
personality change due to, 819, 819*t*
psychiatric considerations with, 845*t*
Healing
attempts at, 168
cultural considerations, 168*f*
Health and aging, 53
Health care
costs of, **1384**
and cigarette smoking, 444
future trends in, 1390
insurance, **1386–1388**
providers. *See* Physician(s)
quality of care, 1388–1389
regulation of, 1385–1386
Health care proxies, **1340,** 1341*t*
Health maintenance organization(s) (HMOs), **1387–1388**
and alternative medicine, 851
Health systems agencies (HSAs), **1386**
Hearing, medical assessment of, 257
Hearing impairment
in elderly, 1327
and language disorders, 1200*t*
and phonological disorders, 1203*t*
severe, differential diagnosis of, 1213–1214
"Heavy metal" music, and substance abuse, 1288
Heavy metal poisoning, personality change due to, 819, 819*t*
Hebb, D.O., 163
Heidegger, Martin, 227
"Help-rejecting complainers," 14
Hematocrit (Hct), 271*t*
Hemisphere(s), cerebral, 78
and emotion, 83
functions of, 78
and language, 78, 78*f*, 82
lateralization, 78, 82
and memory, 80–82
transcranial magnetic stimulation and, 121
Hemodialysis unit, consultation-liaison psychiatry in, 848–849
Hemoglobin (Hb), 271*t*
oxygenated, 113
Hemoglobin SC disease, 124
Hemolysis, sleep-related, **780**
Hemp insanity, 426
Hepatic cirrhosis, 399
Hepatic encephalopathy, 366
medical considerations with, 846*t*
psychiatric considerations with, 846*t*
Hepatitis
alcoholic, 399
and carbamazepine, 1038, **1038**
transmission of, 454
Hepatitis A viral antigen (HAAg), testing for, 271*t*
Hepatitis B virus
c antigen (HBcAg), testing for, 271*t*
surface antigen (HBsAg), testing for, 271*t*
Hepatocellular injury, 263
Hepatolenticular degeneration. *See* Wilson's disease
Herbal medicines/remedies, 533, **856, 1146–1147**
abuse of, 395*t*
psychoactive herbs, 859, 860*t*–862*t*
Web sites for, 859*t*
Hermaphroditism, 693*t*, 736*f*
Heroin. *See also* Opioid(s)
neuropharmacology of, 449
for pain management, 1344*t*
in urinalysis, 268*t*
withdrawal, 452–453
Heroin behavior syndrome, 450–451
Herpes simplex encephalitis, 363
Herpes simplex virus, 1168
Heterocyclics, adverse effects of, 981*t*
Heterosexism, 697
Heterosexual, definition of, 694
Heterotopia, 86
5-HIAA. *See* 5-Hydroxyindoleacetic acid (5-HIAA)
Hinckley, John W., Jr., 1363
Hippocampus. *See also* Limbic system
and cognitive map, 81
and memory, 114, 148
in memory formation, 80
in neuroimaging, 114
place code, 127
and place code, 80
Histamine, 105, 1015
neurotransmitter function, 91*f*, 93*t*
receptors, 93*t*
Histamine receptor antagonists, 1015
Historical treatments, **1149**
History. *See also* Psychiatric history
of cognitive development, 235
current living situation, 237
early childhood, 235
education, 236
of emotional problems, 235
family, 234
late childhood, 235
legal, 237
marital, 236
medical, 233, 254
menstrual, 256
middle childhood, 235
military, 236
of motor development, 235
occupational, 235–236, 254
of past illness, 233
perinatal, 234–235
personal, **234–238,** 234*t*
of physical problems, 235
prenatal, 234–235
of present illness, 233
relationship, 235
religion, 236
school, 235

History—*continued*
sexual, 237, 237*t*, 699, 699*t*–700*t*
social activity, 236
values, 238
Histrionic personality disorder, **810–811**. *See also* Personality disorder(s), cluster B
clinical features of, 811
course of, 811
diagnosis of, 810–811
diagnostic criteria for, 811, 811*t*
differential diagnosis of, 811
epidemiology of, 810
pharmacotherapy for, 811
prognosis for, 811
psychotherapy for, 811
treatment of, 811
HIT, 183*t*
HIV. *See* Human immunodeficiency virus (HIV)
HMOs. *See* Health maintenance organization(s) (HMOs)
Hoarding personality, 220
Hoch, August, 508
Hoch, Paul, 809
Hoffman, Albert, 436
Holding environment, 228
Holistic medicine, 851
Holistic psychology, **221**
Holocoenosis, 221
Holter monitor, 271*t*
Holtzmann Inkblot Technique (HIT), 183*t*
Homeless mentally ill, **1377–1378**
outreach programs for, 1378
qualities of, 1377–1378
schizophrenic, 477
treatment of, 1378
Homeopathy, 851, **859–863**. *See also* Herbal medicines/remedies
Home Solutions Questionnaire-Revised (HSQ-R), 1158*t*
Homicidal behavior
emergency manifestations of, 909*t*
emergency treatment of, 909*t*
Homicide
incidence of, 155
risk of committing, assessing, 151*t*
in schizophrenia, 493–494
Homocystinuria, 1167*t*
Homophobia, 697
Homosexual, definition of, 694
Homosexual experience, in adolescence, 37
Homosexuality, **697–699**
biological factors in, 698
definition of, 697
in Freud's concept of narcissism, 204
Freud's contributions on, 513
and gender identity disorders, 736
neuroanatomy and, 78
parenting by, 45
prevalence of, 697*t*, 698–698
psychoanalytic factors in, 698
psychological factors in, 698
and psychopathology, 698
sexual behavior patterns in, 698
Homosexual panic
emergency manifestations of, 909*t*
emergency treatment of, 909*t*
Homovanillic acid, 100
in alcohol use disorders, 397
in schizophrenia, 478
Homunculus, 67, 73, 75
Hormonal replacement therapy, **877**
Hormonal treatment, for gender identity disorders, **737**
Hormone(s), 154. *See also specific hormone*
adolescence, changes in, 36
and aggression, 154
classification of, 129*t*
psychoneuroendocrinology, **128–132**
secretion of, 128
and sexual behavior, 696
for sexual dysfunction, 715
in substance abuse, 395*t*
Horney, Karen, **221,** 221*f*
Hospital addiction. *See* Munchausen syndrome
Hospitalism, 142
admission for. *See* Admission, for hospitalization
of adolescents, **1305**
for brief psychotic disorder, 524
of children, 60, 139, **1305**
Hospitalization, **1379–1381**
and adjustment disorders, 795
and alcohol use disorders, 405
for anorexia nervosa, 744–745
for delusional disorder, 519–520
extended-treatment programs, 1380
family issues, 1381
indications for, 1380–1381
legal considerations with, 1355–1357
for mood disorder, 560–561
partial hospitalization, 1380
for schizophrenia, 477, 497
for shared psychiatric disorder, 519
short-term inpatient programs, 1380
Hospitals, **1384,** 1385*t*
standards and performance, 1385
utilization review, 1385
HSAs, 1386
5-HT (5-hydroxytryptamine). *See* Serotonin
Hufeland, Christoph W., 863
Hull, Clark L., 147
Human constancy, 235
Human immunodeficiency virus (HIV), 371–372
antiretroviral drugs, 376–377, 376*t*
psychotropic drug interactions, 377–378
dementia related to, 109, 334, 374–375
ICD-10 diagnostic criteria for, 344*t*
encephalopathy, 375
history of, 371
infection, 133
adjustment disorder in, 375
antiretroviral/psychotropic drug interactions, 377–378
anxiety disorders in, 375
associated conditions, 374, 375*t*
clinical features of, 374–376
course of, 372
delirium in, 375
dementia in, 334, 374–375
ICD-10 diagnostic criteria for, 344*t*
dementia with, 109
depressive disorder in, 375
history-taking with, 376
mania in, 375
mood disorder in, 375
neurocognitive disorder in, 375
neurological features of, 374, 375*t*
neuropsychiatric aspects of, **371–379**
nonneurological features of, 374
pharmacotherapy for, 376–377
prevention of, 376
psychiatric syndromes in, 374–376
psychotherapy with, 378
psychotic disorder in, 376
stress and progression of, 132–133
substance abuse in, 375
and suicide, 375–376
treatment, involvement of significant others in, 378
treatment of, 376–378
and worried well, 376
psychotropic/antiretroviral drug interactions, 377–378
testing for, 264–265, 271*t*
confidentiality and, 374
counseling about, 373
indications for, 372–373, 373*t*
methods for, 372–373
posttest counseling about, 373, 374*t*
pretest counseling about, 373, 373*t*
transmission, 371–372
to fetus, **455**
intravenous drug abuse and, 454, 464
prevention, CDC guidelines for, 372, 372*t*
prevention of
education and, 456
needle exchange and, 456
Humanistic school, 218
Humor
as defense, 208*t*
and prevention of aggression, 156
Hunter syndrome, 1172*t*, 1175*f*
Huntington's disease, 51, 75, 109*f*, 333–334, 334*t*, 1249*t*
dementia in, 333–334, 334*t*, 1323
ICD-10 diagnostic criteria for, 344*t*
medical considerations with, 847*t*
mood disorder and, 351*t*
neuroimaging in, 108, 111*f*, 117*f*
pathophysiology of, 104
personality change due to, 819, 819*t*
psychiatric considerations with, 847*t*
psychosis in, 75
and suicide, 75, 915
Hurler's syndrome, 1167*t*, 1172*t*, 1175*f*
Husserl, Edmund, 275
Hwa-byung, 530*t*
Hydrocephalus, normal pressure, dementia in, 108
Hydromorphone, 448
for pain management, 1344*t*
17-Hydroxycorticosteroid, testing for, 271*t*
5-Hydroxyindoleacetic acid (5-HIAA), 97*f*, 102
testing for, 271*t*
5-Hydroxytryptamine. *See* Serotonin
Hydroxyzine, 1000*t*, **1015–1017**. *See also* Antihistamine(s)
dosage and administration, 1017*t*
for insomnia, in delirium, 328
laboratory interferences, 1016
for pain management, 1345*t*
structure of, 1015*f*
Hydroxyzine hydrochloride, indications for, 1015
Hydroxyzine pamoate, indications for, 1015
Hyperactive syndrome, 1223
Hyperactivity
biofeedback for, 949*t*
in children, pharmacotherapy for, 1006
definition of, 282
Hyperemesis gravidarum, in pregnancy, **872**
Hyperglycemia
medical considerations in, 844*t*
psychiatric considerations in, 844*t*
Hyperhidrosis, psychological correlates of, 834
Hyperkinesis
in autism, 1211
definition of, 281

Hyperkinetic disorders
diagnostic criteria for, 1230*t*
ICD-10 classification of, 1229–1230
Hypermnesia, definition of, 286
Hyperparathyroidism
medical considerations with, 846*t*
psychiatric considerations with, 846*t*
Hyperphagia, definition of, 281
Hyperprolactinemia, 833
psychological correlates of, **833**
Hypersalivation, pharmacotherapy for, 1006
Hypersexuality, in epilepsy, 359
Hypersomnia, **760–761**
causes of, 761*t*
definition of, 281
in ICD-10, 766*t*
primary, **767–768**
diagnostic criteria for, 767*t,* 768
treatment of, 768
related to another mental disorder
diagnostic criteria for, 779*t*
related to Axis I or Axis II disorder, 778–779
Hypertension
and dopamine activity, 1049
psychological correlates of, 826*t,* **830**
Hypertensive crisis
emergency manifestations of, 909*t*
emergency treatment of, 909*t*
from monoamine oxidase inhibitors, 1078
tyramine-induced, 1078
Hyperthermia, 998*t*
emergency manifestations of, 909*t*
emergency treatment of, 909*t*
malignant, 998*t*
Hyperthermic syndromes, 998, 998*t*
Hyperthyroidism, 260, 831
medical considerations in, 844*t*
neuropsychiatric manifestations of, 365
psychiatric considerations in, 844*t*
psychological correlates of, **831**
Hyperventilation, 255
behavior therapy for, 954*t*
emergency manifestations of, 909*t*
emergency treatment of, 909*t*
and panic attacks, 267
Hyperventilation syndrome, 831
psychological correlates of, **831**
Hypervigilance, definition of, 280
Hypnagogic hallucinations, 239
definition of, 285
Hypnopompic hallucinations, 239
definition of, 285
Hypnosis, 74, **960–964**
definition of, 74, 280, 960
for dietary change, 843
eye-roll sign for hypnotizability, 960, 961*f*
Freud's use of, 194
history of, 961
neurophysiological correlates of, 961
for pain disorder, 658
for phobias, 615
and sensory perception, 74
for smoking cessation, 843
for stuttering, 1205
trance state, 964
for weight loss, 843
Hypnotherapy, **964**
contraindications to, 964
indications for, 964
for sexual dysfunction, 713–714
Hypnotic capacity, **961–962**
Hypnotic induction, **961–962**
instructions for profile, 963*t*
Hypnoticlike experiences, 961, 962*t*
Hypnotic(s). *See also* Sedative-, hypnotic-, or anxiolytic-related disorder(s); Sedative, hypnotic, or anxiolytic substance(s)
definition of, 460
intoxication, acute, diagnostic criteria for, 391*t*
for primary insomnia, 765
withdrawal from
barbiturates for, 1018
diagnostic criteria for, 393*t*
Hypnotizability, 961–962
Hypoactive sexual desire disorder, 701*t,* 702–703, 702*t*
due to a general medical condition, 709, 710*t*
Hypoactivity, definition of, 282
Hypochondria, definition of, 284
Hypochondriacal disorder, ICD-10 diagnostic criteria, 659*t*
Hypochondriasis, 207*t,* **651–653**
clinical features of, 644*t,* 652
cognitive profile of, 957*t*
course of, 653
definition of, 651
diagnosis of, 651, 651*t*
diagnostic criteria for, 651, 651*t*
differential diagnosis of, 653, 673–674
epidemiology of, 651
etiology of, 651
prognosis for, 653
treatment of, 653
Hypoglycemia
in alcohol use disorders, 401
medical considerations in, 844*t*
psychiatric considerations in, 844*t*
Hypoglycemic encephalopathy, 366
Hypokinesis, definition of, 282
Hypomagnesemia, in alcohol use disorders, 404
Hypomania, 427
definition of, 280
ICD-10 diagnostic criteria, 586*t*–587*t*
Hypomanic episode
cognitive profile of, 957*t*
diagnostic criteria for, 543*t*
Hyponatremia, 495
in alcohol use disorders, 404
medical considerations with, 845*t*
psychiatric considerations with, 845*t*
Hypoparathyroidism
medical considerations with, 846*t*
psychiatric considerations with, 846*t*
Hyposexuality, in epilepsy, 359
Hypotension, and dopamine activity, 1049
Hypotensives, drug interactions, 1035
Hypothalamic-pituitary-adrenal axis, 129–130
Hypothalamic-pituitary-gonadal axis, 129
Hypothalamic-pituitary-thyroid axis, 130–131
Hypothalamus, 78
and appetite, 78
and rage, 78
and sexual orientation, 78
Hypothermia
emergency manifestations of, 909*t*
emergency treatment of, 909*t*
Hypotheticodeductive thinking, 138
Hypothyroidism, 131, 131*f,* 260
differential diagnosis of, 526
laboratory diagnosis of, 260, 262*t*
lithium and, 260
medical considerations in, 844*t*
neuropsychiatric manifestations of, 365–366
psychiatric considerations in, 844*t*
psychiatric symptoms in, 260–261
psychological correlates of, **832**
Hypoxyphilia, 724
Hysteria [term], 643
Hysterical anesthesia, definition of, 286
Hysterical character, 226
Hysteroid dysphoria, **583**

I

Ibogaine, 435, 436*t*
Ibuprofen
and lithium, 1072*t*
for pain management, 1345*t*
ICD-9. *See International Classification of Diseases,* ninth revision (ICD-9)
ICD-10. *See International Classification of Diseases,* tenth revision (ICD-10)
Ice (drug), 413–414
I-cell disease, 1167*t*
ICSD, 744, 764*t*
ICSI, 873*t*
Id, **204,** 222
Idealized parental image, 223
Idealized self, 221
Idealizing transference, 223
Ideas of influence, 240
Ideas of reference, 240, 492
Ideational apraxia, 77
Identical twins reared apart, studies of, 164–165
Identification
in conversion disorder, 649
in group psychotherapy, 938*t*
Identification phenomena, 62
Identifying data, for patient, 230–233
Identity
cultural, 169–170
dissociative disorder. *See* Dissociative identity disorder
Erikson's concept of, 19, **215**
establishing, 213–214
gender. *See* Gender identity
versus role confusion, 19
versus role diffusion, 213–214
Identity diffusion, definition of, 37
Identity problem, **1293–1294**
clinical features of, 1293
course of, 1293
diagnosis of, 1293
differential diagnosis of, 1293
epidemiology of, 1293
etiology of, 1293
prognosis for, 1293
treatment of, 1293–1294
Identity versus role diffusion, 1293
Ideomotor apraxia, 75, 77
Idiopathic hypertension, biofeedback for, 949*t*
Idiopathic insomnia, 767
Idiopathic psychoses, pharmacotherapy for, **1054**
Illness behavior, 2, 2*t*
assessment of, 2, 2*t*
Illness(es)
intercurrent, in patient in psychiatric treatment, **259**
medical, 260, 261*t*
importance of, 259–260
past, history of, 233
present, history of, 233
reactions to, 5*t*
Illogical thinking, definition of, 283

Illusion(s)
  definition of, 285
  in elderly patient, 1319
  versus hallucinations, 492
  in schizophrenia, 492
Imagery, in cognitive therapy, 958–959
Imaginary companions, 32
Imipramine, 1000*t*
  adverse effects of, 567*t*, 981*t*, 1127*t*
  blood level data for clinical assessment, 268*t*
  for bulimia nervosa, 750
  for cataplexy, 769
  children, use with, 1307*t*
  clinical information, 1130*t*
  for cocaine users, 435
  dosage and administration, 569*t*
  mechanism of action, 567*t*
  neurotransmitter effects of, 1126*t*
  for pain management, 1345*t*
  plasma levels, monitoring, 265
  preparations of, 1130*t*
  structure of, 1125*f*
Imitation, in group psychotherapy, 938*t*
Immanent justice, 137
Immune system
  disorder(s)
    acquired immune deficiency syndrome. *See* Acquired immune deficiency syndrome
    human immunodeficiency virus. *See* Human immunodeficiency virus
    neuropsychiatric manifestations of, 365
  psychoneuroimmunology, **132–134**
    in schizophrenia, 482
Impairment, of physician, ethics concerning, **1371**
Implosion, in behavior therapy, 952
Imposture, 670
Impotence. *See* Erectile dysfunction
Imprinting, 140, 158, 158*f*
Impulse control
  definition of, 281
  in delusional disorder, 515
  in depression, 555
  in mania, 556
Impulse-control disorder(s)
  and kleptomania, 785
  not elsewhere classified, **782–794**
    biological factors in, 782–783
    etiology of, 782
    ICD-10 classification of, 793–794, 793*t*
    psychodynamic factors in, 782
    psychosocial factors in, 782
  not otherwise specified, **792–793**
    diagnostic criteria for, 792, 792*t*
  and pathological gambling, 788
  pharmacotherapy for, **1037**
Impulsiveness, in schizophrenia, 493–494
Impulsivity, assessment of, in mental status examination, 242
Inappropriateness of affect, 238–239
Inapsine. *See* Droperidol
Inborn errors of metabolism, 1167*t*–1168*t*
Incest, 721, **886–887**
  emergency manifestations of, 909*t*
  emergency treatment of, 909*t*
  treatment for, 889
Incidence, 175–176
Incoherence, definition of, 283
Incompetence, ethics concerning, 1371
Independent variables, definition of, 177
Inderal. *See* Propranolol
Individual couples therapy, **946**
Individual psychology, 217
Individual psychotherapy
  with children and adolescents, **1295–1300,** 1312
    psychoanalytic theories in, 1295–1296
    theories and techniques of, 1295–1296
  combined with group psychotherapy, **940**
  and couples (marital) therapy, **946**
Individuation, 222
Indomethacin, and lithium, 1072*t*
Induced psychotic disorder, 517–518, 517*t*, 518*t*
Inductive reasoning, 138
Industrial psychiatry, 894–896
Industry
  Erikson's concept of, 19, **215**
  versus inferiority, 19, 213
Ineffability, definition of, 281
Inertia, treatment of, 356
Infancy, **25–30**
  developmental landmarks in, 22*t*, 25–26
  disorders of, 1259–1273
  eating disorders of, **1241–1245**
  feeding disorders of, **1244**
Infant end-of-life care, 1347
Infantile autism, 1208
  and language disorders, 1200*t*
  Tinbergen's study of, 159
Infantile Gaucher's disease, 1167*t*
Infantile sexuality, Freud's theory of, **200**
Infant(s)
  and attention-deficit/hyperactivity disorder, 1225–1226
  clinical interviews with, 1152
  crying in, 141–142
  developmental tasks of, 211–212
  postmature, 25
  premature, 25
    contrast with full-term infant, 25*f*
  temperamental differences in, 26
  terrifying experiences and, 87
Infection, and mental retardation, 1169
Infectious dementia, 334
Infectious disease
  mood disorder and, 351*t*
  neuropsychiatric manifestations of, 363–365
  psychiatric disorders, manifestations of, 133–134
Inferential statistics, 174
Inferiority, Erikson's concept of, 213, 215
Inferiority complex, 217
Infertility, **872–874**
Infiltrative glial cell tumors, 108
Information, fund of
  assessment of, in mental status examination, 242
  in elderly patient, 1320
Information processing, 147
Informed consent, **1359–1360**
  ethics concerning, 1372*t*
  prescription practices, 1352, 1352*t*
Inhalant-related disorder(s), 382*t*, **440–444**
  anxiety disorder, 442–443
    diagnosis of, 442–443
    treatment of, 443
  clinical features of, 443
  dementia, persisting, 442
    treatment of, 443
  diagnosis of, 442
  DSM-IV classification of, 441*t*, 442
  epidemiology of, 440–441
  mood disorder, 442–443
    diagnosis of, 442–443
    treatment of, 443
  not otherwise specified, 443
    diagnostic criteria for, 443, 443*t*
  psychotic disorder, 442
    diagnosis of, 442
    treatment of, 443
  rehabilitation, 443
  suburban/urban distribution of, 441
  treatment, 443
Inhalant(s)
  abuse, 442
  adverse effects of, 443
  death caused by, 443
  dependence, 442
  effects of, 443
  intoxication, 442
    diagnostic criteria for, 441*t*, 442
    treatment of, 443
  intoxication delirium, 442
  neuropharmacology of, 441
  nitrite, **468**
  tolerance, 441, 443
  use, 440–441
    and age, 440–441
    among adolescents, 1286–1287
    methods of, 440
    prevalence of, 440–441
    and race, 441
    trends in, 440–441
  withdrawal, 441, 443
Inhibition, 208*t*
Initiative
  Erikson's concept of, 19, **215**
  versus guilt, 19, 213
Injury/injuries, **156–158**
  psychophysiological considerations with, 157
  requiring ambulatory surgical evaluation and treatment
    medical considerations with, 845*t*
    psychiatric considerations with, 845*t*
  requiring inpatient surgical evaluation and treatment
    medical considerations with, 846*t*
    psychiatric considerations with, 846*t*
Innate releasing mechanisms, 159
Inositol phosphate, metabolism of, 1068
Inpatient group psychotherapy, **938–939**
  composition of group in, 939
  goals for, 939*t*
  short-term, 939*t*
  techniques for, 939*t*
Inpatient treatment, with adolescents, 1313
Insanity defense, 1362
Insight
  assessment of, in mental status examination, 242
  definition of, 242, 287
  in delusional disorder, 515
  in depression, 555
  evaluation of, in child psychiatric evaluation, 1156
  in group psychotherapy, 938*t*
  impaired, definition of, 287
  intellectual, 242
    definition of, 287
  levels of, 242
  in mania, 556
  in schizophrenia, 495
  true, definition of, 287
  true emotional, 242
Insight-oriented psychotherapy
  for dysthymic disorder, 575
  for elderly, 1334
  in panic disorder, 608
  for phobias, 615
  for schizophrenia, 501–502

Insomnia, **760**
acupuncture for, 1145
causes of, 761*t*
definition of, 281
in delirium, 328
diphenhydramine for, 1016
emergency manifestations of, 910*t*
emergency treatment of, 910*t*
ethchlorvynol for, 1021
fatal familial, **365**
glutethimide for, 1022
in ICD-10, 766*t*
idiopathic, 767
initial, definition of, 281
middle, definition of, 281
pharmacotherapy for, 1016, 1021, 1022, **1024–1025,** 1041, **1124**
primary, **763–767**
diagnostic criteria for, 763, 767*t*
treatment of, 765–767
psychophysiological, **765–767**
and psychotherapeutic drugs, **981**
related to another mental disorder
diagnostic criteria for, 777*t*
related to Axis I or Axis II disorder, **777–778**
secondary
to environmental conditions, 761*t*
to medical conditions, 761*t*
to psychiatric conditions, 761*t*
terminal, definition of, 281
Inspiration, in group psychotherapy, 938*t*
Instinct(s), 199–200
aim, 199
characteristics of, 199
death instinct, 151, 200, 222, 917
impetus, 199
life instinct, 151, 200
object, 199
source, 199
Instinct theory
of aggression, 151, 153*t*
Freud's, **199–204**
object relationships in, 200
Instinctual attachment system, 140
Insufficient sleep, **773**
Insulin
learning and, 129
memory and, 129
Insurance
health care, **1386–1388**
health maintenance organizations, 1387
managed care. *See* Managed care
Medicaid, 1386
Medicare, 1386
physicians' liability insurance, 1383
preferred provider organizations, 1388
risk pools, 1386
self-pay and "fee-for-service," 1386–1387
Integration, stage of, 224
Integrative psychiatry, **866–867**
Integrity
versus despair, 214–215
versus despair and isolation, 19
Erikson's concept of, 19, **216**
Intellectual functioning, in autism, 1212
Intellectual insight, 242, 287
Intellectualism, in adolescence, 37
Intellectualization, 208*t*
Intellectual tasks, in elderly patient, 1320
Intelligence
assessment of, in mental status examination, 242
borderline, 142, **1290**
classification of, by IQ range, 178–179, 180*t*
definition of, 178, 287
in elderly patient, 1320
long-term stability of, 1159
Intelligence quotient (IQ), 85, 178–179, 180*t*
and aggression, 154
with borderline intellectual functioning, 1290
interpretation of, 180
normal, 179–180
Intelligence test(s), **178–179**. *See also specific test*
for adolescents, **1159**
for children, 179
in schizophrenia, 490
for school age-children, **1159**
Interaction, in group psychotherapy, 938*t*
Intermittent explosive disorder, **783–785**
biological factors, 783
clinical features of, 783–784
course of, 784
diagnosis of, 783–784
diagnostic criteria for, 784
differential diagnosis of, 784
emergency manifestations of, 910*t*
emergency treatment of, 910*t*
epidemiology of, 783
etiology of, 783
familial factors, 783
genetic factors, 783
laboratory examinations, 784
pharmacotherapy for, 1003*t*
physical findings, 784
prognosis for, 784
psychosocial factors, 783
treatment of, 785
International Classification of Diseases, ninth revision (ICD-9), 288
International Classification of Diseases, tenth revision (ICD-10). *See also specific disorder*
classification of mental disorders, 294, 314*t*–318*t*
DSM-IV-TR, relation to, 288
epileptic seizures, 358*t*
on hyperkinetic disorders, 1229–1230
mental disorders related to medical conditions in, 390*t*–394*t*
organic mental disorders in, 323
signs and symptoms, 275
International Classification of Sleep Disorders (ICSD), 744, 764*t*
Internet compulsion, **793**
Interpersonal psychotherapy (ITP), **933–935,** 933*t*
for depression, 565, 933–934, 960*t*
for dysthymic disorder, 576
requirements and techniques, 933–934
results of, 934
Interpretation
of dreams, 197–198, 756*f,* 926
in group therapy, 936*t*
in group therapy, 936*t,* 938*t*
in interview, 9
of play, 222
in psychoanalysis, **925–926**
with psychosomatic illness, 840–841
in psychotherapy, definition of, 927*t*
Intersex conditions, **733**
treatment of, 737
Intersexual disorder(s), 693*t*
Interview(s), **4–12**
with adolescents, 1152–1153, 1312
advice in, 10
agitated/violent patients, 249
"Amytal interview," 1018
beginning, 7–8
with children, 1151–1154
clarification in, 9
common techniques, 8*t*
concluding, 10
confrontation in, 9
content, 8
factors affecting, 4–5
culturally diverse patients, 14
depressed patients, 249
drug-assisted, 267, 267*t,* **1148**
emergency, 901, 902*t*
empathy during, 250
ending, 248
explanation of treatment in, 9
facilitation in, 9
with family, in child psychiatry, 1153
family/friend present during, 7
functions of, 4, 5*t*
"help-rejecting complainers," 14
with infants and young children, 1152
insight-oriented, 5
interpretation in, 9
length of, 246–247
lying patients, 249–250
manipulative patients, 14
medical-surgical, 5
for mentally retarded patient, 1170
obstructive interventions, 247–248, 247*t*
office arrangement, 247
with parents, in child psychiatry, 1153
positive reinforcement in, 10
problem patients, 13–14
process, 8–10
factors affecting, 4
psychiatric, **5–6, 246–248**
follow-up, 248
goals of, 5
insight-oriented, 5
versus medical-surgical, 5–6
note taking in, 248
seating arrangements for, 247
symptom-oriented, 5
time management in, 246–247
psychodynamic, 5
psychotic patients, 248–249
questions in, 8
rapport in, 6, 7*t*
reassurance in, 10
reflection in, 9
with school-age children, 1152
seating in, 247
self-revelation in, 10
semistructured, 1153
silence in, 9
stress, 248
structured "respondent-based," 1153–1154
suicidal patients, 249
summation in, 9
supportive interventions, 247–248, 247*t*
suspicious patients, 13–14
symptom-oriented, 5
transition in, 9
Intimacy, **699**
Erikson's concept of, 19, **215–216**
versus isolation, 19, 214
Intoxication. *See specific substance*
Intracytoplasmic sperm injection (ICSI), 873*t*
Intrahepatic bile stasis, 264
Intrauterine devices (IUDs), 875*t*
Intravaginal foams, 875*t*
Introjection, 207*t,* 222

Introns, 123
Introverts, 222
In vitro fertilization and embryo transfer (IVF-ET), 873*t*
In vivo exposure, for panic disorder, 608
Iodides, and lithium, 1072*t*
Ion channel(s), **89**
effects of alcohol on, 399
gating, 89, 90*t*
Iproniazid, 1000*t*
history of, 1076
IQ. *See* Intelligence quotient (IQ)
Iron, testing for, 272*t*
Irrelevant answer, definition of, 283
Irresistible impulse, 1362
Irritable heart. *See* DaCosta's syndrome
Isay, Richard, 698
Islets of precocity, in autism, 1212
Ismelin. *See* Guanethidine
Isobutyl nitrite, 468
Isocarboxazid, 1000*t*, 1076. *See also* Monoamine oxidase inhibitors
adverse effects of, 981*t*
pharmacological action of, 1072–1073
Isolation
as defense mechanism, 208*t*
Erikson's concept of, 214
versus integrity, 19
versus intimacy, 19, 214
in personality disorders, 802
studies with monkeys, 159–160, 159*f*, 160*t*
Isoniazid, drug interactions, 1028, 1047
Isoptin. *See* Verapamil
Isradipine, 1000*t*, 1034*t*
dosage and administration, 1035
ITP. *See* Interpersonal psychotherapy; Interpersonal therapy (ITP)
Itraconazole, and buspirone, 1033
IUDs, 875*t*
IVF-ET, 873*t*

J

Jackson Personality Inventory (JPI), 181*t*
Jacobsen, C.F., 1147
Jacobson, Edith, **221**
on depression, 541
Jacobson, Edmund, on relaxation, 948
Jactatio capitis nocturna, **777**
Jak-STAT system, 95
Jamais vu, definition of, 286
Jamison, Kay Redfield, 913
Janet, Pierre, 653, 681
Janus kinase, 95
Japanese language, neural activity and, 86
Jasmine, 854*t*
Jaspers, Karl, 17, 472
phenomenology, school of, 275
Jaundice
emergency manifestations of, 910*t*
emergency treatment of, 910*t*
JC virus, 109
Jealousy, delusional, 515–516
definition of, 284
Freud's contributions on, 513
Johnson, Frank, 1357
Johnson, Virginia, 36, 47, 57, 703, 713
and four-way session therapy, 946
and sex therapy, 954*t*
Joint Commission on the Mental Health of Children, 1301
Joint custody, 1316
JPI, 181*t*
Judgment, 205
assessment of, in mental status examination, 242
automatic, definition of, 287
critical, definition of, 287
definition of, 287
in delusional disorder, 515
in depression, 555
in elderly patient, 1320
evaluation of, in child psychiatric evaluation, 1156
impaired, definition of, 287
in mania, 556
in schizophrenia, 495
Judgment of Line Orientation Test, 189, 189*f*
Jung, Carl Gustav, 19, **222,** 222*f*
Symbols and Transformations, 166
word-association technique, 185
Justice, 1368
Juvenile delinquency, and conduct disorder, 1236–1237
Juvenile delinquent, definition of, 1292
Juvenile offenders, rights of, **1317**

K

K-ABC, 1157*t*, 1159
Kahlbaum, Karl, 471, 534
KAIT, 1157*t*
Kandel, Eric, 147
Kanner, Leo, 1208
Kaplan, Harold, and structured interactional group psychotherapy, 940
Karasu, Toksoz Byram, 842
Kardiner, Abraham, 166
Karma yoga, 866
Karyotype, human, 118*f*
Kasanin, Jacob, 508
Kaufman Adolescent and Adult Intelligence Test (KAIT), 1157*t*
Kaufman Assessment Battery for Children (K-ABC), 1157*t*, 1159
Kaufman Test of Educational Achievement (K-TEA), 1157*t*, 1160
Kava, 470
drug interactions, 1028
Kemadrin. *See* Procyclidine
Kernberg, Otto, **222**
Ketalar. *See* Ketamine
Ketamine, 456, **459**
Kevorkian, Jack, 1348
Key-math Diagnostic Arithmetic Test, 1185
KFD, 1158*t*
Khat, 418
Kiddie Schedule for Affective Disorders and Schizophrenia (K-SADS), **1153**
Kidney function tests, 263–264
Kindling, 539
Kinetic Family Drawing (KFD), 1158*t*
Kinsey, Alfred, 47, 696–698, 724
Kirby, George H., 508
Klein, Donald, 818
Klein, Melanie, 222, **222,** 223*f*
on depression, 541
Kleine-Levin syndrome, **773**
Kleptomania, **785–786**
biological factors in, 785
clinical features of, 785–786
course of, 786
definition of, 282
diagnosis of, 785–786
diagnostic criteria for, 785, 786*t*
differential diagnosis of, 786
epidemiology of, 785
etiology of, 785
family factors in, 785
genetic factors in, 785
ICD-10 classification of, 793–794, 793*t*
pharmacotherapy for, 1132
prognosis for, 786
psychosocial factors in, 785
treatment of, 786
Klerman, Gerald, 565
Klinefelter's syndrome, 257, 693*t*, **733**
and suicide, 915
Klinger, Richelle, 699
Klismaphilia, 724
Klonopin. *See* Clonazepam
Klüver-Bucy syndrome, 83, 333
Knockout technology, 127
Knowledge-participation, 217
Kohlberg, Lawrence, 38
Köhler, Wolfgang, 225
Kohut, Heinz, **223**
on depression, 541
on old age, 55*t*
Kolb, Laurence, 817
Koro, 530*t*
Korsakoff's syndrome, 82, 186, 406, 1146
amnestic disorder with, 347
course of, 347
emergency manifestations of, 908*t*
emergency treatment of, 908*t*
Krabbe's disease, 1167*t*
Kraepelin, Emil, **471,** 472*f*, 508, 534, 556, 653
Kraft, Thomas, and hierarchy construction, 951
Kretschmer, Ernst, 472, 817
Krieger, Dolores, 866
K-SADS, **1153**
K-TEA, 1157*t*, 1160
Kübler-Ross, Elisabeth, 60
Kuru, 1323
neuropsychiatric manifestations of, 365

L

LA, testing for, 272*t*
La belle indifférence, 281, 649, 653
Labetalol, 1000*t*, 1009*t*. *See also* β-Adrenergic receptor antagonist(s)
chemistry of, 1008*f*
pharmacological actions of, 1009
Laboratory test(ing), in psychiatry, **260–269,** 269*t*–273*t*
neuroendocrine, 260–264
Lacan, Jacques, **223**
Lactate dehydrogenase (LDH), testing for, 272*t*
Lactate provocation, 267
Lactation, **871**
and dopamine receptor antagonists, 1061
pharmacotherapy during, **979**
Lamaze method, 870
Lamivudine, 376
LAMM, 455
Lamotrigine, 1000*t*, **1089–1093**
adverse reactions to, 1091
for bipolar I disorder, 570, 571
chemistry of, 1089, 1089*f*
dosage of, 1091–1092, 1092*t*
drug interactions, 1091
indications for, 1090

laboratory interferences, 1091
pharmacological actions of, 1090
precautions with, 1091
Lange, Carl, 1067
Lange, Fritz, 1067
Langfeldt, Gabriel, 472
Language
acquisition of, 73, 86–87
assessment of, 189
in adults, 189
auditory processing and, 86–87
cerebral dominance for, 82
changes, with brain tumor, 361
disturbances of, in autism, 1211
elderly language output, 1319
English, neural activity and, 86
evaluation of, in child psychiatric evaluation, 1156
event-related potentials and, 122
grammar, 1194
Japanese, neural activity and, 86
lexical categories, neural circuit for, 113
neuroanatomy and, 78, 78*f*, 82
and neuroimaging, 113
normal development of skills, 1195*t*
output, in elderly patient, 1319
phonology, 1194
pragmatics, 1194
processing, 82
production, 82
rhyming, 113, 116*f*
semantics, 1194
Language development
in infancy, 25–26, 27*f*, 27*t*
in middle (childhood) years, 32
in preschool period, 31
in toddler period, 30
windows for, 86
Language disorder(s), 82–83
and developmental coordination disorder, 1190
expressive. *See* Expressive language disorder
hearing impairment and, 1200*t*
infantile autism and, 1200*t*
mixed receptive-expressive. *See* Mixed receptive-expressive language disorder
receptive-expressive. *See* Receptive-expressive language disorder
written expression. *See* Written expression disorder
Language therapy, for mixed receptive-expressive language disorder, 1199
Larodopa. *See* L-Dopa
Latah, 530*t*
Latency stage, 19, 203*t*
Laughing gas, **468–469**
Laughter, common variants of, 87*f*
Lavender, 854*t*
Law of coercion to the biosocial mean, 220
Laxatives, abuse of, 395*t*
LDH, testing for, 272*t*
LE, test, 272*t*
Lead
blood level data for clinical assessment, 268*t*
poisoning, neuropsychiatric symptoms caused by, 367
Learned helplessness, 150, **161,** 542
Learning
of aggression, 151–153
avoidance, 143, 146
definition of, 143
escape, 146
in group psychotherapy, 938*t*
history of, 235
insulin and, 129
neurochemistry of, 143
neurophysiology of, 147–148, 148
operant, 227
and performance, 143
psychotropic(s) effect on, 1308*t*
sexual, in childhood, 692
state-dependent, 143
and stress, 148
trial-and-error, 144
types of, 143–147
Learning disability. *See* Learning disorder(s); Reading disorder
Learning disorder(s), **1180–1189**
and attention-deficit/hyperactivity disorder, 1226
auditory processing defect, 86–87
in children, pharmacotherapy for, **1306,** 1308*t*
definition of, 1180
developmental nonverbal, 83
differential diagnosis of, 1237
DSM-IV-TR classification of, 1180
history of, 235
in ICD-10, 1188, 1188*t*–1189*t*
and mixed receptive-expressive language disorder, 1198
not otherwise specified, **1188**
diagnostic criteria for, 1188*t*
and phonological disorder, 1200
Learning functions, effects of psychotropic drugs on, 1308*t*
Learning theory, **143–148**
and conversion disorder, 648
of phobias, 610
and psychoanalytic theory, 143
of schizophrenia, 483
terminology used in, 149*t*
Least restrictive alternative, 1357–1358
Legal history, 237
Leptin, 126
Lesbian(s), 697
Lesch-Nyhan syndrome, 1166, 1168*t*, 1172*t*
and stereotypic movements, 1271
Lethologica, definition of, 286
Leuenkephalin, 104
Leukocytosis, with antipsychotic drug therapy, 266*t*
Leukoencephalopathy, 109
Leukopenia
with antipsychotic drug therapy, 266*t*
emergency manifestations of, 910*t*
emergency treatment of, 910*t*
Levallorphan, 448, 455
Levinson, Daniel J., 20
developmental theory of, 41–42, 42*f*, 48
on old age, 55*t*
Levo-α-acetylmethadol (LAMM), 455
Levodopa. *See* L-Dopa
Levomethadyl, 1000*t*, **1082–1085**
adverse reactions to, 1084
chemistry of, 1082, 1083*f*
dosage of, 1085
drug interactions, 1084
effects on organs and systems, 1082
indications for, 1083
laboratory interferences, 1084
overdose of, 1084
pharmacological actions of, 1082
precautions with, 1084
withdrawal symptoms, 1084
Levomethadyl acetate, for heroin addiction, 389
Levorphanol, for pain management, 1344*t*
Levothroid. *See* Levothyroxine; Thyroxine
Levothyroxine, 1001*t*, 1122. *See also* Thyroid hormone(s)
Levoxyl. *See* Levothyroxine; Thyroxine
Lewin, Kurt, **223,** 225
Lewis, Dorothy, 154
Lewis, Melvin, 20
Lewy body disease, 333
Lexical processing, 71, 82
LFTs. *See* Liver function tests
LH. *See* Luteinizing hormone
Libido. *See* Sex drive
Librium. *See* Chlordiazepoxide
Liddell, Howard Scott, 161
Lidone. *See* Molindone
Lidz, Theodore, 18, 484
Liebault, Ambroise-August, 194
Life cycle, **16–58**
stages of, 19
Erikson's concept of, 19, 211–215
theories of, 19
Life events, and mood disorders, 540–541, 559*t*
Life expectancy, **51–53,** 53*t*
and ethnicity, 53
and race, 53
and sex, 53, 54*f*
Life instinct, 151
Freud's concept of, 200
Life space, 223
Lifetime expectancy, 176
Lifetime prevalence, 176
Light therapy, **863, 1145**
for primary insomnia, 765
Limbic system, 72, 78
in anxiety disorders, 595
behavioral aspects of, 83–84
and emotion, 72, 78, 83–84
and memory, 72, 78
and schizophrenia, 84
in schizophrenia, 471, 477, **478–479,** 479*f*, 480
Limb-kinetic apraxia, 75
Lindemann, Eric, and brief psychotherapy, 930
Linkage analysis, 128
Liothyronine, 1001*t*, 1122. *See also* Thyroid hormone(s)
dosage and administration, 569–570
and tricyclic/tetracyclic drugs, 1131
Lipkin, Mack, Jr., 5
Liquid ecstasy. *See* Gamma hydroxybutyrate
Lisuride, for cocaine users, 435
Lithium, 1001*t*, **1067–1074**
and adolescent patients, 1071
adverse effects of, 260, 567*t*, 1069–1073, 1069*t*
for affective lability and impulsivity, 356
for aggressive/violent behavior, 156, 356
for alcoholism, 413
augmentation of, **990**
for autistic disorder, 1215
Bear Lithia Water advertisement, 1067*f*
and bipolar disorder, 96
for bipolar I disorder, 570, 571, 1134*t*
blood level data for clinical assessment, 268*t*
for bulimia nervosa, 750
with carbamazepine, 1038–1039
cardiac effects, 1070–1071
chemistry of, 1067
for childhood/adolescent antisocial behavior, 1293

Lithium—*continued*
children, use with, 1307*t*
for cocaine users, 435
cognitive effects, 1070
for conduct disorder, 1238
dermatological effects, 1071
detection of, by magnetic resonance spectroscopy, 112
discontinuation of, 1074
dosage recommendations, 569, 1073
drug interactions, 378, 1028, 1031, 1062*t*, 1072–1073, 1072*t*, 1081, 1133
effects on specific organs and systems, 1068
and elderly patients, 1071–1072
factors predicting response to, 1068, 1068*t*
failure of treatment, 1074
gastrointestinal effects, 1069–1070
geriatric dosage, 1330*t*
history of, 1067
and hypothyroidism, 260
implicated in sexual dysfunction, 711
indications for, 500, 1068–1069
initial medical workup, 1073
intoxication/overdose of, 986*t*, 1071
laboratory interferences, 1073, 1073*t*
laboratory testing with, 264*f*, 266–267
maintenance treatment with, 1069
mechanism of action, 567*t*
neurological effects, 1070, 1072
for obsessive-compulsive disorder, 622
overdose of, 1071
and patient education, 1074
pharmacological actions of, 1067–1068
plasma concentrations, 1073–1074
for postpartum psychosis, 527
precautions with, 1069–1073
and pregnancy, 1072
renal effects, 1070
renal function monitoring in, 263–264, 264*f*
for schizoaffective disorder, 511
and schizophrenia, 500
serum concentrations, 1073–1074
thyroid effects, 1070
thyroid function monitoring in, 260, 262*t*
toxicity, 256, 1071
emergency manifestations of, 910*t*
emergency treatment of, 910*t*
signs and symptoms of, 1071*t*
tremors and, 100, 1070
and tricyclic/tetracyclic drugs, 1131
and weight gain, 752
withdrawal from, 982
Lithium-induced postural tremor, β-adrenergic receptor antagonists for, 1009
Lithobid. *See also* Lithium
Lithonate. *See* Lithium
Little Albert, 610
Little Hans, 610
Livedo reticularis, 1012
Liver function tests, 264, 267
Living situation, current, in history-taking, 237
Living wills, **1340,** 1341*t*
Llinas, Rudolfo, 134
LNNB, 190
LNNB-C, 1158*t*
Locura, 530*t*
Locus, genetic, 123
Logorrhea, definition of, 284
Longevity, 51
Long-term care
community mental health, 1375
for elderly, 57–58, 57*f*, 1378
Loop diuretics, and lithium, 1072*t*
Loose associations, 239
Loosening of associations, definition of, 283
Lopressor. *See* Metoprolol
Loratadine, indications for, 1015
Lorazepam, 1001*t*. *See also* Benzodiazepine(s)
for bipolar I disorder, 570
dosage of, 1025*t*
for extrapyramidal disorders, 1059*t*
geriatric dosage, 1332*t*
half-life of, 1025*t*
indications for, 404*t*, 406, 493, 500
pharmacokinetics of, 1022
pharmacological actions for, 1023
structure of, 1023*f*
Lorenz, Konrad, **158–159**
theory of aggression, 151, 158–159
Loss, in old age, 58
Love, **699**
maternal, 218–219
productive, 220
Love object, choice of, Freud's view of, 200, 204
Low back pain, 837
psychological correlates of, **837**
treatment of, 837
Loxapine, 1001*t*
chemistry of, 1053
geriatric dosage, 1332*t*
preparations, 1064*t*
structure of, 1052*f*
Loxitane. *See* Loxapine
LSD. *See* Lysergic acid diethylamide (LSD)
Lu, Frances G., 169
Ludiomil. *See* Maprotiline
Lumbar puncture, 268
Luminal. *See* Phenobarbital
Lupus anticoagulant (LA), testing for, 272*t*
Lupus erythematosus (LE) test, 272*t*
Luria, Alexander, 190
Luria-Nebraska Neuropsychological Battery (LNNB), 190
Luria-Nebraska Neuropsychological Battery: Children's Revision (LNNB-C), 1158*t*
Luscher, Max, 854
Lust Angst, 785
Lusz, Benedict, 864
Luteinizing hormone, 263
in schizophrenia, 482
testing for, 272*t*
Luvox. *See* Fluvoxamine
Lying patients, interviewing, 249–250
Lyme disease, 108, 133–134, **363–364**
bull's eye rash, 363, 364*f*
Lysergic acid diethylamide (LSD), 435, 436*t*
blood level data for clinical assessment, 268*t*
effects of, 439
mechanism of action, 104
neuropharmacology of, 437
psychotic disorder, 438
use among adolescents, 1286

M

Mace, 436*t*
Machover Draw-A-Person Test (DAP), 1158*t*
Macrobiotics, **863**
Macropsia, definition of, 286
Magical thinking
definition of, 283
in obsessive-compulsive disorder, 619
Magnesium, testing for, 272*t*
Magnetic resonance imaging (MRI), **110–111**. *See also* Neuroimaging
for amnestic disorder(s), 323, 348–349
in basal ganglia disorders, 108
of brain, 108, 110–111. *See also* Brain, imaging
versus computed tomography, 110, 110*f*, 111
for cognitive disorders, 323
for Creutzfeldt-Jakob disease, 364
in delirium, 323
in dementia, 108, 323, 1335
functional (fMRI), 108, 112–113
amnestic disorders, 323
blood flow, 113
of brain, 112–113
for cognitive disorders, 323
delirium, 323
dementia, 323
language in, 113
in rhyming, 113, 116*f*
in schizophrenia, 480
in sensory functions, 113
for intermittent explosive disorder, 784
in multiple sclerosis, 109
in obsessive-compulsive disorder, 109
in psychiatric diagnosis, 108
in schizophrenia, 109, 471, 480, 480*f*, 481*f*
in strokes, 108
terminology, 112–113
Magnetic resonance spectroscopy (MRS), **111–112,** 112*t*
of brain, 111–112
Magnetoencephalography (MEG), **121**
Maharishi Majesh Yogi, 864
Mahler, Margaret
on child development, 21
developmental theory of, 29, 29*t*
theory, of schizophrenia, 483
Major depressive disorder, **534–572**. *See also* Mood disorder(s)
in adolescents, 1277
adoption studies of, 540
adrenal axis and, 538
age distribution of, 536
bereavement, differentiated, 63*t*
biogenic amines in, 536–537, 536*t*, 537*t*
brain imaging in, 539, 540*f*
buspirone for, 1032
in childhood, **1275–1276**
epidemiology of, 1274–1275
and combined psychotherapy and pharmacotherapy, **969**
and cortisol, 538
course of, 558
criteria for severity/psychotic/remission specifiers for current (most recent) episode, 543*t*
and culture, 536
development of manic episodes in, 558
diagnosis of, 542–544
differential diagnosis of, 556–557, 1284
and dopamine, 537
DSM-IV-TR classification of, 534–535
duration of, 558
dysthymic disorder, distinguished, 572
electroconvulsive therapy for, 1139
epidemiology of, 535
etiology of, 536–542
family studies of, 539–540
and generalized anxiety disorder, 632
genetics of, 123, 539–540

growth hormone and, 538
infectious agents and, 133
lifetime prevalence, 535*t*
linkage studies of, 540
marital status and, 536
versus medical disorders, 556
neuroanatomical considerations in, 539
neurochemistry of, 536–539
neuroendocrine system and, 538
neuroimmune regulation and, 539
versus neurological conditions, 556
and norepinephrine, 536
and obsessive-compulsive disorder, 617
onset, 558
and opioid dependence, 450
versus other mental disorders, 556–557
pharmacotherapy for, 565–570, 1032, **1068, 1126,** 1132. *See also* Antidepressant(s)
prognosis for, 558
prognostic indicators in, 558
and prolactin, 539
psychosocial factors in, 540–542
recurrent
diagnosis of, 544, 545*t*
diagnostic criteria for, 545*t*
and serotonin, 536–537
sex distribution of, 535–536
single episode
diagnosis of, 543–544, 545*t*
diagnostic criteria for, 545*t*
and sleep, 539, 759
and socioeconomic status, 536
and somatostatin, 538–539
thyroid axis and, 538
and trichotillomania, 790
twin studies of, 540
vagal nerve stimulation for, 1145
Major depressive episode
diagnostic criteria for, 542*t*
with psychotic features
emergency manifestations of, 910*t*
emergency treatment of, 910*t*
Make-a-Picture Story (MAPS), 183*t*
Malan, Daniel
and brief focal psychotherapy, 931
on outcome of brief therapy, 933
Mal de ojo, 530*t*
Male erectile disorder. *See* Erectile dysfunction
Male genital mutilation, **888**
Male orgasmic disorder, **705,** 705*t*
Malformations, in first year of life, 24*t*
Malignant hyperthermia, 998*t*
Malingering, **897–898**
clinical features of, 897–898
versus dementia, 339
diagnosis of, 897–898
differential diagnosis of, 674, 898, 898*t*
epidemiology of, 897
versus schizophrenia, 495–496
treatment of, 898
Malinowski, Bronislaw, 166
Malnutrition
in elderly, psychiatric symptoms, 1337
and reading disorder, 1181
Malpractice, **1351–1352**
sexual exploitation of patient, 1363
Managed care, **1352–1353, 1387–1388**
ethical issues, 1370
gag rule, 1390
medical records and, 253–254
National Practitioner Data Bank, 1352
negligent prescription practices, 1352
psychiatric care delivery, 1389–1390
split treatment, 1352–1353
and substance-related disorders, 389–390
Mandarin, 854*t*
Mandrakes (drug). *See* Methaqualone
Mandrax. *See* Methaqualone
Manganese poisoning, neuropsychiatric symptoms caused by, 367
Mania. *See also* Mood disorder(s)
in adolescents, 553, 1277
and attention-deficit/hyperactivity disorder, 1226
cognition in, 556
definition of, 281
differential diagnosis of, 784
due to a general medical condition, etiology of, 585*t*
with HIV infection, 375
impulse control in, 556
insight in, 556
judgment in, 556
and nefazodone, 1081
nefazodone and activation of, 1081
perceptual disturbances in, 556
pharmacotherapy for, **1054**
psychodynamic factors in, 541
with psychotic symptoms, ICD-10 diagnostic criteria, 587*t*
rebound, 982
reliability in, 556
sensorium in, 556
thought in, 556
without psychotic symptoms, ICD-10 diagnostic criteria, 587*t*
Manic episode(s)
clinical features of, 553
criteria for severity/psychotic/remission specifiers for current (most recent) episode, 544*t*
diagnostic criteria for, 542*t*
differential diagnosis of, 902, 903*t*
electroconvulsive therapy for, 1139–1140
emergency manifestations of, 910*t*
emergency treatment of, 910*t*
mental status examination in, 555–556
pharmacotherapy for, 266, **1068**
signs and symptoms of, 553
Manipulative patients, 14
Mann, James, and time-limited psychotherapy, 931
Mannerism, definition of, 281
Mannitol, and lithium, 1072*t*
Mannosidosis, 1167*t*
MAO. *See* Monoamine oxidase (MAO)
MAO_B, 127
MAOIs. *See* Monoamine oxidase inhibitors (MAOIs)
Maple syrup urine disease, 1166–1167, 1167*t*
Maprotiline
adverse effects of, 567*t,* 981*t,* 1127*t*
clinical information, 1130*t*
dosage and administration, 569*t*
mechanism of action, 567*t*
neurotransmitter effects of, 1126*t*
preparations of, 1130*t*
structure of, 1125*f*
MAPS, 183*t*
Marijuana. *See* Cannabis
Marital adjustment, 44
Marital crises
emergency manifestations of, 910*t*
emergency treatment of, 910*t*
Marital history, 236
Marital problems, 44–45, **880–881**
Marital status
and bipolar I disorder, 536
and major depressive disorder, 536
and suicide, 914
Marital therapy. *See* Couples (marital) therapy
Marjoram, 854*t*
Marketing personality, 220
Maroteaux-Lamy syndrome, 1167*t*
Marplan. *See* Isocarboxazid
Marriage
demographics, 44*t*
in early adulthood, 43–45
interracial, 44
to physician, **881**
and relational problems, 880–881
unconsummated, 725
Marriage counseling/therapy, 45. *See also* Couples (marital) therapy
Marsilid. *See* Iproniazid
Masculine protest, 217
Maslow, Abraham, **223,** 224*f*
Masochism
and factitious disorders, 668
sadomasochism, ICD-10 diagnostic criteria for, 726*t*
sexual, 721, 722*t*
Masochistic character, 226
Massage, **863,** 866
Masters, William, 36, 47, 57, 703, 713
and four-way session therapy, 946
and sex therapy, 954*t*
Masturbation, **696–697,** 724
in adolescence, 37
Masturbatory pain, 712
Maternal drug use, 24
Mathematics, and music, 87
Mathematics disorder, **1183–1185**
clinical features of, 1184–1185
comorbidity with, 1184
course of, 1185
definition of, 1183
diagnosis of, 1184, 1184*t*
differential diagnosis of, 1185
epidemiology of, 1184
etiology of, 1184
laboratory examination of, 1184
pathology of, 1184
prognosis for, 1185
treatment of, 1185
and written expression disorder, 1186
Mature defense mechanisms, **20–21**
Mature thinking, versus primitive thinking, 956*t*
Maturity
adulthood, 49
Allport's concept of, 218
Maudsley, Henry, 1208
May, Rollo, on love and intimacy, 699
Mazes, 191*t*
Mazicon. *See* Flumazenil
Mazindol, 1001*t,* 1116. *See also* Sympathomimetics (and related drugs)
for cocaine users, 435
for weight reduction, 755*t*
McCarthy Scales of Children's Abilities (MSCA), 1159
McGarry instrument, 1361
McKinley, J. Charnley, 180
MCMI-II, 181*t*
MCV. *See* Mean corpuscular volume (MCV)
MDEA, 414
MDMA. *See* Methylenedioxymethamphetamine
Mead, Margaret, 166–167, 167*f*
Mean, definition of, 176

Mean corpuscular volume (MCV)
  effects of alcohol on, 401
  testing, 272*t*
Measure of central tendency, 176
Mebaral. *See* Mephobarbital
Medial region, of prefrontal cortex, 85
Medial temporal lobe, in memory formation, 80
Media relations, 1370
Medicaid, **1386**
  and HMOs, 1387–1388
Medical assessment, 254–260
Medical illness(es)
  history of, 254
  importance of, 259–260
  mood disorder and, 553
  with neuropsychiatric symptoms, 261*t*
  pharmacotherapy during, **979**
  with psychiatric symptoms, **844*t*–847*t***
  screening tests for, 261*t*
Medical malpractice, **1351–1352**
  sexual exploitation of patient, 1363
Medical record(s), **250–254,** 250*t*
  E-mail, 252
  ethical issues, 252–254
  managed care issues, 253–254
  military psychiatry, 252
  patient access to, 251
  personal note/observations, 251
  problem-oriented, 251–252
  psychiatric report, **243,** 243*t*–246*t*
  third parties
    payer documentation issues, 251*t*
    requests by, 251
  use of, 250–251
Medicare, 57, **1386**
  benefits, 1386*t*
  and HMOs, 1387–1388
Medication, adverse effects of, not otherwise specified, 998, 998*t*
Medication, common reasons for noncompliance with, 10–11, 11*t*
Medication-induced acute akathisia, 997*t*
Medication-induced acute dystonia, 997*t*
Medication-induced movement disorders, 295, **992–999,** 997*t*, 1058. *See also* Neuroleptic malignant syndrome
  dopamine receptor antagonists for, 1049
  not otherwise specified, **996–997**
    diagnostic criteria for, 996*t*
  pharmacotherapy for, 1003*t*
Medication-induced parkinsonism, 997*t*
Medication-induced postural tremor, **996,** 997*t*
  research criteria for, 996*t*
Meditation, **863–864,** 866
MEG, **121**
Megacolon, psychogenic, 1254
Megaloblastic anemia, 367
Megalomania, 517
Megavitamin therapy for children, 1311
Melancholia, definition of, 281
Melatonin, 131–132, 263, **1147**
  for primary insomnia, 765
  and sleep, 759
  testing for, 272*t*
Melissa, 854*t*
Mellanby effects, 399
Mellaril. *See* Thioridazine
Memantine, 377, 1001*t*, **1044–1045**
  for Alzheimer's disease and similar disorders, 1042
Memory, **80–82**
  Alzheimer's disease. *See* Alzheimer's disease
  assessment of, **186**
    in child psychiatric evaluation, 1156
    in elderly, 1320
    in mental status examination, 241, 241*t*
  brain function and, 80–82
  buffer, 148
  changes in, with brain tumor, 361
  definition of, 286
  dementia. *See* Dementia
  in depression, 555
  disturbances of, definition of, 286
  in elderly, 339, 349, 1318, 1320
  and electroconvulsive therapy, 1143–1144
  and emotion, 80, 148
  episodic, 186
  factual, 81
  false memory, definition of, 286
  false memory syndrome, 689
  formation of, 148
  immediate, 80, 148, 186
    definition of, 80, 286
    phonological, 80
    visuospatial, 80
  immediate retention and recall, assessment of, 241, 241*t*
  impairment, 81–82
  implicit, 186
  insulin and, 129
  levels of, 286
  limbic system and, 72, 78
  long-term, 148
  in mental status examination, 241
  and motor acts, 80–81
  primary, 148
  problems, in normal aging, 339, 349, 1318
  procedural, 81
  recent, 80, 148, 186
    assessment of, 241, 241*t*
    definition of, 80, 286
  recent past, 148, 186
    assessment of, 241, 241*t*
    definition of, 286
  recovered memory syndrome, **689**
  remote, 80, 148, 186
    assessment of, 241, 241*t*
    definition of, 80, 286
  retrospective falsification, definition of, 286
  in schizophrenia, 495
  screen memory, definition of, 286
  secondary, 148
  semantic, 186
  short-term, 148, 186
  and smell, 72, 148
  storage of, 148
  and stress, 148
  study of, with human subject, 81
  types of, 186
  visual system and, 69
  working, 80, 148
    definition of, 80
    emotional value and, 80
Memory quotient (M.Q.), 186
Men. *See also specific concern or disorder*
  climacterium, 47
  elderly, socioeconomic status of, 56–57
  in middle adulthood, 46
  rape of, **892**
  REM sleep in, 757
  sexual functioning, in midlife, 47
Menarche, 37
Meningiomas, skull-based, 108
Meningitis
  chronic, neuropsychiatric manifestations of, 363
  and mental retardation, 1169
Menkes' kinky-hair disease, 1168*t*
Menninger, Karl A., **224,** 917
  The Crime of Punishment, 224
  The Human Mind, 224
  Man Against Himself, 224
  Theory of Psychoanalytic Technique, 224
  The Vital Balance, 224
Menopause, 47, **877**
Mens rea, 1361, 1363
Menstrual-associated syndrome, **773**
Menstrual history, 256
Mental age, 178
Mental disorder(s)
  in adolescence, 38
  definition of, 282
  from demyelinating disorder, 362
  with depressive features, 556, 557*t*
  DSM-IV-TR classification of, 293–294, 307*t*–313*t*
  DSM-IV-TR definition of, 293–294
  due to brain disease, damage and dysfunction, ICD-10 classification of, 390*t*–394*t*
  in elderly, 1321–1326
  in full remission, 292
  due to a general medical condition, **350–370,** 351*t*
    anxiety disorders, **353**
    brain tumors, **360–361**
    catatonia, **355**
    demyelinating disorders, **362–363**
    endocrine disorders, **365–366**
    epilepsy, **356–360,** 357*f*, 358*f*, 358*t*, 359*f*, 360*t*
    head trauma, **361–362,** 361*t*
    ICD-10, **367,** 368*t*–370*t*
    immune disorders, **365**
    infectious diseases, **363–365**
    metabolic disorders, **366**
    mood disorders, **350–352,** 351*t*
    nutritional disorders, **366–367**
    personality change, **355–356,** 356*t*, 367, 368*t*
    psychotic disorders, **352–353,** 353*t*
    sexual dysfunctions, **354–355,** 354*t*
    sleep disorders, **353–354,** 354*t*
    toxins, **367**
  medical causes of, indicators of, 903, 904*t*
  mild, 291
  moderate, 291
  not otherwise specified, due to a general medical condition, 350, 355*t*
  of old age, 1321–1326
  versus panic disorder, 606
  in partial remission, 292
  severe, 292
  severity of, 291–292
  and sleep disorders, **353–354,** 354*t*, 764*t*, 777
Mental health, and suicide, 915
Mental retardation, **1161–1179**
  acquired childhood disorders and, 1169
  aggression in, pharmacological intervention for, 1177–1178
  and attention-deficit/hyperactivity disorder, 1163
    pharmacological intervention for, 1177–1178
  and autistic disorder, 1163, 1213
  with behavioral symptoms, differential diagnosis of, 1213
  behavior therapy in, 1176
  blood analysis, 1174
  brain damage and, 1169

in children, pharmacotherapy for, **1306**
chromosomal aberrations and, 1165
chromosome studies, 1174
classification of, 1161–1162, 1178*t*
clinical features of, 1173–1174
cognitive therapy in, 1176
comorbid psychopathology in, 1163–1164
genetic syndromes and, 1163–1164
neurological impairment and, 1163
prevalence of, 1163
psychosocial factors and, 1164
risk factors for, 1163–1164
complications of pregnancy and, 1169
conduct disorders and, 1163
course of, 1175
definition of, 287, 1178
degrees of severity, 1162–1163
versus dementia, 339
and depressive disorders, 1178
developmental characteristics in, 1162*t*
diagnosis of, 1170–1175
differential diagnosis of, 1175–1176, 1192, 1269
in Down's syndrome, 1165, 1171*t*
DSM-IV-TR diagnostic criteria for, 1170*t*
education for child with, 1176
electroencephalography, 1174
encephalitis and, 1169
environmental factors in, 1169–1170
epidemiology of, 1163
epilepsy and, 1163
etiology of, 1164–1170
explosive rage behavior in, pharmacological intervention for, 1178
family education about, 1177
family resources, 1177*t*
fetal alcohol syndrome and, 409–410, 1172*t*
in fragile X syndrome, 1165, 1171*t*
genetic factors in, 1165–1167
genetic syndromes and, 1163–1164
head trauma and, 1169
hearing evaluation in, 1174–1175
history-taking with, 1170
ICD-10 classification of, 1178
ICD-10 diagnostic criteria for, 1178*t*
infection and, 1169
laboratory tests in, 1174
and language disorders, 1200*t*
meningitis and, 1169
mild, 1162
clinical features of, 1173–1174
moderate, 1162–1163
clinical features of, 1173–1174
mood disorders, 1163
neuroimaging, 1174
neurological examination in, 1172–1173
neurological impairment in, 1163
nomenclature, 1161
perinatal factors and, 1169
and pervasive developmental disorder, 1176
pharmacological intervention for, 1177–1178
and phonological disorders, 1203*t*
physical findings in, 1170–1172
pregnancy complications and, 1163
prenatal factors and, 1168–1169
prenatal substance exposure and, 1169
prevention
primary, 1176
secondary, 1176–1178
tertiary, 1176–1178
profound, 1163
clinical features of, 1173–1174
prognosis for, 1175
psychiatric interview in, 1170
psychodynamic therapy in, 1176
psychological assessment in, 1175
psychosocial factors in, 1164
psychotic disorders and, 1163
and pyromania, 786
schizophrenia and, 1163
self-injury in, 1163
pharmacological intervention for, 1177–1178
severe, 1163
clinical features of, 1173–1174
social intervention for, 1177
sociocultural factors in, 1169–1170
speech evaluation in, 1174–1175
stereotypical motor movements in, 1271
pharmacological intervention for, 1178
syndromes associated with, 1171*t*–1172*t*
tardive dyskinesia and, 1177–1178
treatment of, 1176–1178, 1177*t*
and trichotillomania, 790
urine analysis, 1174
Mental status examination, 108, **238–243**
amnestic disorder(s), 320, 321*t*
for attention-deficit/hyperactivity disorder, 1225
attitude toward examiner in, 238
in child psychiatric evaluation, 1155–1156, 1155*t*
for delirium, 320, 321*t*
in delusional disorder, 513–515
for dementia, 320, 321*t*
in depressive episode, 553–555, 554*f*
in elderly, 1319–1321
format for, 238
in manic episode, 555–556
in mood disorder, 553–556
for obsessive compulsive disorder, 621
outline for, 238*t*
in schizophrenia, **490–494**
sensorium section questions testing cognitive functions, 320, 321*t*
Meperidine, 377, 448
blood level data for clinical assessment, 268*t*
drug interactions, 378, 454, 1062*t*
overdose, 455
for pain management, 1344*t*
withdrawal, 453
Mephobarbital, 1001*t*. *See also* Barbiturate(s)
dosage of, 1020*t*
indications for, 1018
structure of, 1018*f*
Meprobamate, 460, 1001*t*, 1017, 1019, **1021**
blood level data for clinical assessment, 268*t*
geriatric dosage, 1332*t*
intoxication/overdose of, 987*t*
Mercury
blood level data for clinical assessment, 269*t*
poisoning, neuropsychiatric symptoms caused by, 367
Mescaline, 435, 436*t*
Mesmer, Friedrich Anton, and hypnosis, 961
Mesolimbic dopamine system, in addiction, 430
Mesolimbic mesocortical tract, 98, 99*f*
Mesoridazine, 1001*t*
geriatric dosage, 1332*t*
preparations, 1064*t*
structure of, 1052*f*
Metabolic disorder(s)
differential diagnosis of, 1269
neuropsychiatric manifestations of, 366
Metabolism
of acetylcholine, 105
alcohol, 399, 533
of clonazepam, 533
of dopamine, 98, 100
of glucose, 96, 117*f*
Alzheimer's patients, metabolism in temporoparietal region of brain of, 118*f*
cerebral metabolism of, 114
of phenelzine, 533
of psychotherapeutic drugs, 975–976
of psychotropic drugs, 533
of serotonin, 97*f*
Metachromatic leukodystrophy, 1167*t*
Metal intoxication, testing for, 272*t*
Metanephrine, 264
Metenkephalin, 104
Methadone, 388, 448, **455,** 1001*t*, **1082–1085**
adverse reactions to, 1084
blood level data for clinical assessment, 269*t*
chemistry of, 1082, 1083*f*
dosage of, 1085
drug interactions, 378, 1084
effects on organs and systems, 1082
for heroin addiction, 389
indications for, 1083
intoxication/overdose of, 987*t*
laboratory interferences, 1084
overdose of, 1084
for pain management, 1344*t*
pharmacological actions of, 1082
precautions with, 1084
in urinalysis, 268*t*
withdrawal, 453, 455
symptoms, 1084
Methamphetamine, 414, 1001*t*, 1116. *See also* Sympathomimetics; Sympathomimetics (and related drugs)
blood level data for clinical assessment, 269*t*
use, prevalence of, 414
for weight reduction, 755*t*
Methanol, blood level data for clinical assessment, 269*t*
Methaqualone, 460
abuse, 460
blood level data for clinical assessment, 269*t*
overdose, 464
and sexual dysfunction, 712
in urinalysis, 268*t*
Methcathinone, 418
Methohexital, 1001*t*. *See also* Barbiturate(s)
as anesthetic for electroconvulsive therapy, 1018
dosage of, 1020*t*
indications for, 1018
structure of, 1018*f*
Methohexital sodium, intravenous
for sexual dysfunction, 715
Methotrimeprazine, for pain management, 1345*t*
3-Methoxy-4-hydroxyphenylglycol (MHPG)
in depression, 263
testing for, 272*t*
5-Methoxy-3,4-methylenedioxyamphetamine (MMDA), 414
3-Methoxymorphine. *See* Codeine
N-Methyl-D-aspartate receptor, 81, 85
phencyclidine (or phencyclidinelike substance) and, 457
Methyldopa
drug interactions, 1062*t*
and lithium, 1072*t*
mechanism of action, 102

Methylenedioxyamphetamine, 414, 436, 436*t*
effects of, 419
neurotoxic, 418*f*
pharmacology of, 414
Methylenedioxymethamphetamine, 104, 436*t*. *See also* Ecstasy
drug interactions, 378
Methylmalonic acidemia, 1168*t*
Methylphenidate, 413, 1001*t*, 1116. *See also* Sympathomimetics; Sympathomimetics (and related drugs)
for attention-deficit/hyperactivity disorder, 1227, 1227*t*, 1228
blood level data for clinical assessment, 269*t*
for childhood/adolescent antisocial behavior, 1293
children, use with, 1307*t*
for cocaine users, 435
drug interactions, 1007
geriatric dosage, 1330*t*
implicated in sexual dysfunction, 711
for narcolepsy, 769
for pain management, 1345*t*
pharmacological action of, 1117
Methylphenidate hydrochloride, intoxication/overdose of, 987*t*
Methylphenyltetrahydropyridine, 100
N-Methyl-4-phenyl-1,2,3,6-tetrahydropyridin (MPTP), parkinsonism induced by, 454
Methyltestosterone, 467
Methylxanthines, 419
Methyprylon intoxication/overdose, 987*t*
Metoclopramide, and lithium, 1072*t*
Metolazone, and lithium, 1072*t*
Metoprolol, 1001*t*, 1009*t*. *See also* β-Adrenergic receptor antagonist(s)
chemistry of, 1008*f*
pharmacological actions of, 1009
Metrifonate, for Alzheimer's disease and similar disorders, 1042
Metronidazole, and lithium, 1072*t*
Meyer, Adolf, **224,** 224*f*, 472
MHPG. *See* 3-Methoxy-4-hydroxyphenylglycol (MHPG)
"Mickey Finns," and chloral hydrate, 1041
Micronase. *See* Guanethidine
Midazolam, 1001*t*. *See also* Benzodiazepine(s)
dosage of, 1025*t*
drug interactions, 378
half-life of, 1025*t*
structure of, 1023*f*
Middle (childhood) years, 21, **32**
developmental landmarks of, 32
Midlife crisis, **47–48**
Midtown Manhattan Study, 172
Migraine, 254
biofeedback for, 949*t*
clinical features, 838*t*
cluster, 838
emergency manifestations of, 910*t*
emergency treatment of, 910*t*
psychological correlates of, 826*t*, **838**
vascular, 838
Mild cognitive disorder, 370*t*
Milieu therapy, **966**
Military history, 236
Miller, Neal, 143, 148
and biofeedback, 843, 948
Million Clinical Multiaxial Inventory (MCMI), 181*t*.
Million Clinical Multiaxial Inventory-II (MCMI-II), 181*t*
Millon Adolescent Personality Inventory (MAPI), 1158*t*
Mills, Gregory, 818
Miltown. *See* Meprobamate
Mimicry, definition of, 282
Mind
Freud's structural theory of, **204–205,** 204*f*
Freud's topographical model of, **198–199**
Mini-Mental State Examination (MMSE), 321*t*
in geriatric psychiatry, 1320
score
age and, 1320
educational level and, 1320
Minnesota model, of substance abuse treatment, 1288
Minnesota Multiphasic Personality Inventory (MMPI), 17, 178, **180,** 181*t*, 182*t*, 490, 1158*t*
Minnesota Multiphasic Personality Inventory-2 (MMPI-2), 180, 181*t*
Minor depressive disorder, 295, **579**
clinical features of, 579
course of, 579
diagnosis of, 579, 580*t*
diagnostic criteria for, 579
differential diagnosis of, 575, 579
epidemiology of, 579
etiology of, 579
prognosis for, 579
research criteria for, 579, 580*t*
treatment of, 579
Mirror stage, 223
Mirror transference, 223
Mirtazapine, 1001*t*, **1074–1076**
adverse effects of, 981*t*, 1075, 1075*t*
central nervous system effects, 1075
chemistry of, 1074, 1074*f*
dosage and administration, 1075–1076
drug interactions, 982, 1075
effects on specific organs and systems, 1075
gastrointestinal effects, 1075
indications for, 1075
intoxication/overdose of, 987*t*
mechanism of action, 102
for mood disorders, 1279
pharmacological actions of, 1075
precautions with, 1075
Misarticulations, in phonological disorders, 1201
Mitral valve prolapse
emergency manifestations of, 910*t*
emergency treatment of, 910*t*
and panic disorder, 600
Mixed affective episode, ICD-10 diagnostic criteria, 590*t*
Mixed anxiety-depressive disorder, 295, 583, **641**
with adjustment disorder, **797**
clinical features of, 642
course of, 642
diagnosis of, 641–642, 642*t*
differential diagnosis of, 642
epidemiology of, 641
etiology of, 641
ICD-10 diagnostic criteria for, 597*t*
pharmacotherapy for, **1024**
prognosis for, 642
research criteria for, 641, 642*t*
treatment of, 642
Mixed receptive-expressive language disorder, **1198–1199**
clinical features of, 1198–1199
comorbidity with, 1198
course of, 1199
diagnosis of, 1198, 1198*t*
differential diagnosis of, 1199, 1200*t*, 1213, 1214*t*
in DSM-IV-TR, 1194
epidemiology of, 1198
etiology of, 1198
laboratory examination of, 1199
and language disorders, 1200*t*
and mathematics disorder, 1184
pathology of, 1199
and phonological disorder, 1200
prognosis for, 1199
and stuttering, 1203
treatment of, 1199
MMDA, 414
MMECT, 1143
MMPI, 17, 178, **180**, 181*t*, 182*t*, 490, 1158*t*
MMPI-2. *See* Minnesota Multiphasic Personality Inventory-2 (MMPI-2)
MMSE. *See* Mini-Mental State Examination (MMSE)
M'Naghten, Daniel, 1362, 1362*f*
M'Naghten rule, 1362
Moban. *See* Molindone
Mobile phone compulsion, **793**
Moclobemide, 1001*t*, 1076. *See also* Monoamine oxidase inhibitors
adverse effects, of, 567*t*
chemistry of, 1076*f*
mechanism of, action, 567*t*
Moclobemide, for social phobia, 616
Modafinil, 1001*t*, **1120–1121**. *See also* Sympathomimetics (and related drugs)
abuse of, 1121
adverse effects of, 1121
for attention-deficit/hyperactivity disorder, 1228
cardiovascular effects, 1121
chemistry of, 1117*f*, 1121
dosage and administration, 1121
drug interactions, 1121
effects on specific organs and systems, 1121
indications for, 1121
laboratory interferences, 1121
for narcolepsy, 769
pharmacological actions of, 1121
precautions with, 1121
for pregnant patients, 1121
Modeling, 147
in behavior therapy, **953**
Model penal code, 1362–1363
Molecular biology, **122–128**
Molindone, 1001*t*
chemistry of, 1053
geriatric dosage, 1332*t*
preparations, 1064*t*
structure of, 1052*f*
Money, John, 693
Moniz, Antonio Egas, 1148
Monkey(s), 159*f*–162*f*
behavior, individual differences in, 161
catecholamine depletion, and social interaction, 163
developmental processes in, 159–161
isolate-reared, rehabilitation of, 160–161
social isolation studies with, 159–160, 159*f*, 160*t*
Monoamine oxidase (MAO), 92–93, 97*f*, 102, 103
antidepressant effects on, 567*t*
platelet
in personality disorders, 801
testing for, 272*t*
type B (MAO_B), 127

Monoamine oxidase inhibitors (MAOIs), 256, **1076–1080**
adverse effects of, 981*t,* 1077–1079
for attention-deficit/hyperactivity disorder, 1224
for bulimia nervosa, 750
with buspirone, 1032–1033
chemistry of, 1076, 1076*f*
clinical guidelines, 1079–1080
for cocaine users, 435
with dopamine receptor antagonists, 1049
dosage, 1079–1080, 1080*t,* 1082
drug interactions, 454, 982, 1012, 1014, 1031, 1032–1033, 1079, 1079*t,* 1081, 1124
effects on specific organs and systems, 1077
for elderly, 1329–1330
history of, 1076
implicated in sexual dysfunction, 711
indications for, 1077
intoxication/overdose of, 987*t,* 1078–1079
laboratory interferences, 1079
laboratory testing with, 265–266
mechanism of action, 92, 102
and mirtazapine, 1075
for mood disorder due to a general medical condition, 352
for mood disorders, 352
for obsessive-compulsive disorder, 622
for panic disorder, 607
pharmacological actions of, 1076–1077
precautions with, 1077–1079
and tricyclic/tetracyclic drugs, 1131
types of, 1077*t*
and tyramine-induced hypertensive crisis, 1078
tyramine-rich foods to be avoided, 1078*t*
withdrawal from, 1078
Monoamines, 274*t*
Monomania, definition of, 284
Montagu, Ashley, 169
Montessori technique, for developmental coordination disorder, 1193
Mood
changes in, in dementia, 337
definition of, 238, 280
in delusional disorder, 514
diurnal variation, definition of, 281
dysphoric, definition of, 280
in elderly patient, 1319
elevated, 92
definition of, 280
euthymic, definition of, 280
evaluation of, in child psychiatric evaluation, 1156
expansive, definition of, 280
instability, in autism, 1211
irritable, definition of, 280
labile, definition of, 280
in mental status examination, 238
neuroanatomy and, 83
physiological disturbances associated with, definition of, 281
Mood disorder(s), **534–590**
acetylcholine in, 106
adoption studies of, 540
alcohol-induced, 351*t,* 397, 407–408, 553
amphetamine-induced, 417
anxiety-blissful psychosis, **484**
with atypical features, 548–549, 549*t*
biogenic amine hypothesis of, 102, 104
bipolar. *See* Bipolar disorder(s)
in cancer patient, 839*t*
cannabis-induced, 427
with catatonic features, 549–550, 549*t*
in childhood and adolescence, **1274–1279**
biological factors, 1275
clinical features of, 1275–1278
course of, 1278
diagnosis of, 1275–1278
differential diagnosis of, 1237, 1278
DSM-IV-TR classification of, 1274
electroconvulsive therapy for, 1279
epidemiology of, 1274–1275
etiology of, 1275
genetic factors, 1275
laboratory examination of, 1277–1278
pathology of, 1277–1278
pharmacotherapy for, 1278–1279, **1310**
prognosis for, 1278
psychotherapy for, 1278
social factors, 1275
treatment of, 1278–1279
chronic, 550, 550*t*
clinical features of, 552–553
cocaine-related, 433
coexisting disorders in, 553
cognitive theory of, 542
combined psychotherapy and pharmacotherapy for, 1312
confusional psychosis, **484**
course of, 558–560
cyclothymic. *See* Cyclothymic disorder
in demyelinating disorders, 351*t*
dexamethasone suppression test and, 1278
diagnosis of, 542–552
DSM-IV-TR classification of, 534–535
due to a general medical condition, 584
diagnostic criteria for, 584, 584*t*
etiology of, 585*t*
due to medical condition with depressive features, pharmacotherapy for, **1126**
dysthymic. *See* Dysthymic disorder
electroconvulsive therapy for, 352
in childhood, 1279
in endocrine disorders, 351*t*
in epilepsy, 359
and factitious disorders, 668
and family, 539–540
frontal lobes and, 109
due to a general medical condition, **350–352,** 351*t,* 584, 584*t*
genetics of, 539–540
hallucinogen-related, 438–439
history of, 534
with HIV infection, 375
hospitalization for, 560–561
in Huntington's disease, 351*t*
hysteroid dysphoria, **583**
ICD-10 classification of, 586
ICD-10 diagnostic criteria, 586*t*–590*t*
infectious disease and, 351*t*
inhalant-related, 442–443
and intermittent explosive disorder, 783
and kleptomania, 785
life events and, 540–541, 559*t*
linkage studies of, 540
longitudinal course specifiers, 551*t,* 552
major depressive. *See* Major depressive disorder
medical illness and, 553
with melancholic features, 547–548, 548*t*
mental disorder, due to a general medical condition and, **350–352**
and mental retardation, 1163
mental status examination in, 553–556
mixed episode
criteria for severity/psychotic/remission specifiers for current (most recent) episode, 544*t*
diagnostic criteria for, 543*t*
motility psychosis, **483–484**
in multiple sclerosis, 351*t*
non-DSM-IV-TR types, 552
not otherwise specified, 585
diagnostic criteria for, 585, 586*t*
in nutritional disorders, 351*t*
opioid-induced, 453
and Parkinson's disease, 351*t*
and pathological gambling, 788
pathophysiology of, 102, 103, 109
PCP-induced, 458
persistent, ICD-10 diagnostic criteria, 589*t*–590*t*
personality and, 541
pharmacotherapy for, 352, 561, 564*t,* **565–572,** 1279
Phencyclidine (or phencyclidinelike substance)-induced, 458
with postpartum onset, 550, 550*t*
postpsychotic depressive disorder of schizophrenia, **582–583**
prognosis for, 558–560
psychosocial factors in, 540–542
psychosocial therapy for, 561
with psychotic features, 546
with rapid cycling, 550–552, 550*t*
recurrent, describing course of, 550–552, 550*t*
with seasonal pattern, 263, 550*t,* 552
sedative-, hypnotic-, or anxiolytic-related, 463
specifiers describing most recent episode, 546–550
and stress, 540–541
substance-induced, 381*t,* 382*t,* 553, **584–585**. *See also specific substance*
clinical features of, 585
course of, 585
diagnosis of, 584–585
diagnostic criteria for, 584, 586*t*
differential diagnosis of, 585
epidemiology of, 584
etiology of, 584, 585*t*
prognosis for, 585
treatment of, 585
suicidal behavior in, 917, 917*f*
treatment of, 560–572
and trichotillomania, 790
twin studies of, 540
Mood swings, definition of, 280
Moonlighting, ethics concerning, 1372*t*
Mora, George, 16
Moral development, 32, 138
in adolescence, 38
Morality, 38. *See also* Ethics
of conventional-role conformity, 38
preconventional, 38
of self-accepted moral principles, 38
Morel, Benedict, 471
Moreno, Jacob, and psychodrama, 940
Morgan, Christiana, 184
Morning glory seeds, 436*t,* 469
use disorders, 390
Moro reflex, 25, 26*f*
Morphine, 104
blood level data for clinical assessment, 269*t*
for pain management, 1344*t*
in urinalysis, 268*t*
withdrawal, 452–453

Morquio's disease, 1167*t*
Mother
good-enough, 29–30, 228
working, children of, 34
Mother–child relationship, and gender identity disorders, 731
Mother–infant attachment, 28–29
Mother–infant bonding, 140
Motility psychosis, **483–484,** 583
Motion therapy, 854–855
Motivation, Murray's concept of, 225
Motivation(s), 148
Motor area, supplementary, 75
Motor behavior
definition of, 281
evaluation of, in child psychiatric evaluation, 1156
Motor commands, corticalization of, 81
Motor cortex, 75, 77
Motor development, history-taking about, 235
Motor skills disorder, **1190–1193**
in ICD-10, 1193, 1193*t*
Motor strip, cerebral, 75
Motor system(s), **74–78**
autonomic, 77–78
parasympathetic, 77
sympathetic, 77–78
Motrin. *See* Ibuprofen
Mourning, **61–65**
definition of, 61, 280
Freud's concept of, 64
Movement, patient's, medical assessment of, 256
Movement disorder(s)
medication-induced, 295, 1058
pathophysiology of, 105
Moxibustion, **864**
MPTP, parkinsonism induced by, 454
M.Q., 186
MRI. *See* Magnetic resonance imaging (MRI)
mRNA. *See* Ribonucleic acid, messenger (mRNA)
MRS. *See* Magnetic resonance spectroscopy (MRS)
MSCA, 1159
Mucopolysaccharidoses
type I, 1167*t*
type II, 1167*t*
type III, 1167*t*
type IV, 1167*t*
type VI, 1167*t*
Mugwort leaves, 864
Mullen Scales of Early Learning, 1158*t*
Multidisciplinary professional model, of substance abuse treatment, 1288
Multigenic trait, 125
Multi-infarct dementia. *See* Dementia, vascular
Multiple monitored electroconvulsive therapy (MMECT), 1143
Multiple personality. *See also* Dissociative identity disorder
definition of, 286
Multiple sclerosis, 133
amnestic disorder with, 347
evoked potential protocols, 122
medical considerations with, 846*t*
mood disorder and, 351*t*
in neuroimaging, 109
neuropsychiatric manifestations of, 362–363, 363*f*
personality change due to, 819, 819*t*
psychiatric considerations with, 846*t*
and suicide, 915
Multiple self-organizations, 228
Multivariate analysis, 176, 219
Munchausen syndrome, 668, 670. *See also* Factitious disorder(s)
by proxy, 884
Murdock, George P., 169
Murphy, Gardner, **224–225**
Murray, Henry, 184, **225**
Muscarinic anticholinergic drugs, and electroconvulsive therapy, 1140
Muscarinic receptors, 93*t*, 105
Muscle relaxants, and electroconvulsive therapy, 1141
Muscle rigidity, definition of, 282
Musculoskeletal disorder(s)
from monoamine oxidase inhibitors, 1078
psychological correlates of, **834–837**
Music
brain function and, 83, 87
"heavy metal" music, and substance abuse, 1288
and mathematics, 87
Music therapy, **865**
Mutilation
female genital, **887–888**
male genital, **888**
repetitive self-mutilation, **793**
Mutism
definition of, 282
in schizophrenia, 487
selective, **1265–1266**
Mutual analysis, 220
Mutuality, Erikson's concept of, 216
Mu waves, 121
Myelin, 90
Myoclonic disorders, 1249*t*
Myoclonic dystonia, 1249*t*
Myofascial joint pain, biofeedback for, 949*t*
Myoglobin, urine, testing for, 272*t*
Myrrh, 854*t*
Mysoline. *See* Primidone
Myxedema, 752
medical considerations in, 844*t*
psychiatric considerations in, 844*t*
Myxedema madness, 365

N

Nadelson, Carol, 929
Nadolol, 1001*t*, 1009*t*. *See also* β-Adrenergic receptor antagonist(s)
chemistry of, 1008*f*
pharmacological actions of, 1009
Nail biting, 1271, **1272**
Nalmefene, 1001*t*, **1085–1089**
adverse reactions to, 1087–1088
chemistry of, 1086, 1086*f*
clinical guidelines for, 1088–1089
dosage of, 1088–1089
drug interactions, 1088
indications for, 1086–1087
laboratory interferences, 1088
precautions with, 1087–1088
Nalorphine, 448
indications for, 455
Naloxone, 448
challenge, 1087
test, 1088, 1088*t*
indications for, 455
stressors, reversal of, 131
Naltrexone, 131, 448, 1001*t*, **1085–1089**
adverse reactions to, 1087–1088
for alcoholism, 412
in alcohol use disorders, 389
for autistic disorder, 1215
chemistry of, 1086, 1086*f*
children, use with, 1308*t*
clinical guidelines for, 1088–1089
dosage of, 1088–1089
drug interactions, 1088
indications for, 455, 1086–1087
intoxication/overdose of, 987*t*
laboratory interferences, 1088
precautions with, 1087–1088
NAMI, 501
Naproxen
and lithium, 1072*t*
for pain management, 1345*t*
NARC, 1161
Narcan. *See* Naloxone
Narcissism, 223
Freud's concept of, 199–200, **204**
and intermittent explosive disorder, 783
secondary, 204
Narcissistic character, 226
Narcissistic defense mechanisms, 206, 207*t*
Narcissistic patients, 13
Narcissistic personality disorder, **811–812**. *See also* Personality disorder(s), cluster B
clinical features of, 811–812
course of, 812
diagnosis of, 811
diagnostic criteria for, 811, 812*t*
differential diagnosis of, 812
epidemiology of, 811
and pathological gambling, 788
pharmacotherapy for, 812
prognosis for, 812
psychotherapy for, 812
treatment of, 812
Narcoanalysis, 1148
Narcoanalysis, barbiturates for, 1018
Narcolepsy, **768–769**
diagnostic criteria for, 768, 769*t*
pharmacotherapy for, 1116, **1118,** 1127
polysomnographic recording of, 769, 769*f*
treatment of, 769
Narcotherapy, 1148
Narcotics. *See also* Opioid(s)
drug interactions, 401
Narcotics Anonymous, 434
Nardil. *See* Phenelzine
National Alliance for the Mentally Ill (NAMI), 501
National Association for Retarded Citizens (NARC), 1161
National Association of Black Social Workers, 46
National character, 166
National Institute of Mental Health Interview Schedule for Children Version IV (NIMH DISC-IV), 1153–1154
National Institutes of Health (NIH), Office of Alternative Medicine of, 851–852, 852*t*
National Practitioner Data Bank, 1352
National Strategy for Suicide Prevention, **921–922**
Naturopathy, **864**
Navane. *See* Thiothixene
NDA, 977
Near-death experience, 59
Necrophilia, 723
NE:E, 263
Needle phobia, definition of, 284

Needs
  hierarchy of, 223
  inborn, 225
Nefazodone, 1001*t*, **1080–1082**
  and activation of mania, 1081
  adverse effects of, 567*t*, 981*t*, 1081
  and buspirone, 1032, 1033
  cardiovascular effects, 1081
  chemistry of, 1080, 1080*f*
  clinical guidelines, 1082
  dosage, 569*t*, 1082
  drug interactions, 378, 982, 1028
  drug interactions, CYP-induced, 976
  effects on specific organs and systems, 1081
  for elderly depression, 1330
  for elderly patients, 1329
  indications for, 1081
  intoxication/overdose of, 987*t*
  mania, activation of, 1081
  mechanism of action, 103, 567*t*
  pharmacological actions of, 1080
  precautions with, 1081
Negative skewness in distributions, 172*f*
Negativism
  in adolescence, 37
  definition of, 281
Neglect
  of children, **887**. *See also* Child abuse and neglect
  maternal, 28
  problems related to, **883–893,** 884*t*
    DSM-IV-TR classification of, 883
Nembutal. *See* Pentobarbital
β-Neoendorphin, synthesis of, 104
Neologism, 240
  definition of, 283
Neonatal death, 874
Neonatal end-of-life care, 1347
Neonatal hypothyroidism, 261
Neonatal opioid withdrawal, 455
Neostigmine, for sexual dysfunction, 980
Neroli, 854*t*
Nervios, 530*t*
Nervous system, **85–88**
  development, 85–88
    experience and, 87
  fetal development, 21, 23*f*
  fetal development of, 21–23
Neugarten, Bernice, 47
  on old age, 20, 55*t*
Neuralgia, acupuncture for, 1145
Neurasthenia, **664–667,** 724
  Beard's contributions on, 665–666, 665*f*, 667
  clinical features of, 665–666
  course of, 667
  cultural classification as disease, 664
  definition of, 664
  depletion hypothesis of, 665
  diagnosis of, 665–666
  diagnostic criteria for, 665–666, 665*f*
  differential diagnosis of, 666–667
  epidemiology of, 664–665
  etiology of, 665
  experimental, in animals, 161
  ICD-10 classification of, 664
  pharmacotherapy for, 1119
  prognosis for, 667
  signs and symptoms reported by patients with, 665–666, 665*f*
  treatment of, 667
Neuroacanthocytosis, 1249*t*
Neuroanatomy, **66–88**
Neurochemistry, **88–107**
Neurocirculatory asthenia. *See* DaCosta's syndrome
Neurodermatitis, psychological correlates of, 826*t*
Neuroendocrine tests, **260–264**
Neurofibrillary tangles, 331
  in Alzheimer's disease, 126
  in Down's syndrome, 1165
Neurofibromatosis, **1166**
  type 1, 1172*t*
Neurogenetics and molecular biology, **122–128**
Neurohormones, **96,** 128, 129*t*
Neuroimaging, **108–122**. *See also* Computed tomography; Magnetic resonance imaging
  functional, 70, 80, 108, 109, 112–119
  indications for ordering in clinical practice, 108
  indications for ordering in clinical research, 109
  and neurological deficits, 108
  and psychiatry, 108
  techniques, 110–122
  uses, 109
Neuroleptic-induced acute akathisia, **994–995,** 1015
  β-adrenergic receptor antagonists for, 1009
  anticholinergics for, 1015
  antihistamines for, 1015
  dopamine receptor antagonists and, 1058–1059
  research criteria for, 995*t*
  treatment of, 995
Neuroleptic-induced acute dystonia, **994,** 1014
  amantadine for, dosage and administration of, 1018
  anticholinergics for, 1013, 1018
  antihistamines for, 1013
  benzodiazepine for, 1014
  benztropine for, 1014
  diphenhydramine for, 1016
  dopamine receptor antagonists for, 1058
  research criteria for, 994*t*
  treatment of, 994
Neuroleptic-induced movement disorders, **993–996**
  dopamine receptor antagonists for, 1061
Neuroleptic-induced parkinsonism, **993**
  anticholinergics for, 1014
  antihistamines for, 1015
  benztropine for, 1014
  diagnostic and research criteria for, 993*t*
  dopamine receptor antagonists and, 1058
  haloperidol for, 1014
  treatment of, 993
Neuroleptic-induced tardive dyskinesia, **995–996**
  Abnormal Involuntary Movement Scale, 995, 996*t*
  dopamine receptor antagonists and, 1059–1060
  research criteria for, 995*t*
Neuroleptic malignant syndrome, 497, **993–994,** 998*t*
  dopamine receptor antagonists and, 1060
  emergency manifestations of, 910*t*
  emergency treatment of, 910*t*
  pharmacotherapy for, 1004*t*, 1045
  research criteria for, 994*t*
Neuroleptic(s), 497. *See also* Antipsychotic(s)
Neurological abnormalities, differential diagnosis of, 1269
Neurological examination, 108, **258**
Neurological findings
  localizing, 495
  nonlocalizing, 495
  in schizophrenia, 495
Neurological hard signs, 1156
Neurological soft signs, 1156
Neuromodulator(s), **96**
Neuromuscular blocking agents, and lithium, 1072*t*
Neuromuscular rehabilitation, biofeedback for, 949*t*
Neuronal heterotopia, 86
Neuronal migration, during development, 85–86
Neuron(s)
  action potentials, **89–90,** 90*f*
  activity, in neuroimaging, 112–113
  charge, 89
  electrophysiology of, 89–90
  information processing, 88
  life cycle of, 85–86
  membrane, 89
  motor, 74
Neurontin. *See* Gabapentin
Neuropathies, acupuncture for, 1145
Neuropeptides, 104–105
  coexistence with other neurotransmitters, 104
  receptors, 104
  in schizophrenia, 478
  synthesis of, 104
Neuropeptide Y, 105
Neurophysiology, **88–107**
Neuropsychiatric assessment, in child psychiatry, **1156–1157**
Neuropsychological assessment, 178
  of adults, **185–191**
    aim of, 185–186
    purposes of, 185–186
  reliability of, 190
  validity of, 190
Neurosis, 196–197, 200
  and anxiety, 209
  classic psychoanalytic theory of, 209
  definition of, 275–276
  DSM-IV-TR classification of, 591
  experimental, in dogs, 161
  Sartre's concept of, 227
Neurosyphilis, 108, 264
  neuropsychiatric manifestations of, 363
  personality change due to, 819, 819*t*
Neurotensin, neurotransmitter function, 91*f*, 105
Neurotic symptoms, 209
Neurotransmission, chemical, 88, **96–97**
  translation of action potentials, 90
Neurotransmitter receptors, **93–94**
  postsynaptic, 93–94
  presynaptic, 92–93
  subsensitivity, 93
  in substance-related disorders, 387
  supersensitivity, 93
  types of, 90*t*, 93–94, 94*t*
Neurotransmitter(s), 88, **96–97,** 96*t*
  action of, 90
  and aggression, 154
  in Alzheimer's disease, 332
  amino acid, **105–107**
  antidepressant effects on, 567*t*
  in anxiety disorders, 594–595
  classification of, 91*f*, 92, 96–97
  excitability, 88
  excitatory, 89

Neurotransmitter(s)—*continued*
gene regulation, 123
inhibitory, 89
in obsessive-compulsive disorder, 617
in panic disorder, 600
in personality disorders, 801
putative, 96
in schizophrenia, 478
in substance-related disorders, 387
Neurotransmitter transporters, 93
New Drug Application (NDA), 977
New Haven Study, 172, 172*t*, 429
News media relations, 1370
Niacin deficiency, 409
neuropsychiatric manifestations of, 367
Nicardipine, 1001*t*
Nicotinamide deficiency
medical considerations with, 847*t*
psychiatric considerations with, 847*t*
Nicotine. *See also* Smoking
addiction, 444
pharmacotherapy for, 447, 448
adverse effects of, 446
dependence, 445
diagnosis of, 445
pharmacotherapy for, 1004*t*
effects, 446
on cerebral blood flow, 446
on sleep, 446
intoxication, acute, diagnostic criteria for, 392*t*
neuropharmacology of, 445
and sleep, 781
stimulation, 100, 106
testing for, 272*t*
use
death caused by, 444–445
and educational status, 444
prevalence of, 444
withdrawal, 445
diagnostic criteria for, 394*t*, 445, 445*t*
pharmacotherapy for, 1004*t*, 1005
Nicotine gum, 447
Nicotine inhalers, 447
Nicotine patches, 447
Nicotine-related disorder(s), 382*t*, **444–448**
clinical features of, 446
diagnosis of, 445
DSM-IV-TR classification of, 445, 445*t*
epidemiology of, 444
nicotine replacement therapies, 447
nonnicotine medications, 447–448
not otherwise specified, 445
diagnostic criteria for, 445, 446*t*
psychopharmacological therapies, 447–488
psychosocial therapies, 447
sleep disorders, 781
treatment, 446–448
Nicotine sprays, 447
Nicotine vaccine, 448
Nicotinic receptors, 93*t*, 105
Niemann-Pick disease, 1167*t*
Nifedipine, 1001*t*. *See also* Calcium channel inhibitors
dosage and administration, 1035
structure of, 1034*f*
Night-eating syndrome, 753
Nightmare disorder, **774–775**
pharmacotherapy for, 1127
Nightmares, in ICD-10, 766*t*
Night terrors. *See* Sleep terrors
Nigrostriatal tract, 97, 99*f*
NIH, 851–852, 852*t*
NIMH DISC-IV, 1153–1154
NIMH Epidemiologic Catchment Area Survey, 172–173, 173*t*
Nimodipine, 1001*t*, 1034*t*. *See also* Calcium channel inhibitors
dosage and administration, 1035
structure of, 1034*f*
Nimotop. *See* Nimodipine
Nisoldipine, 1001*t*
Nitrendipine, 1001*t*
Nitrite inhalants, **468**
Nitrous oxide, **468–469**
toxicity, emergency manifestations and treatment of, 910*t*
NMDA. *See N*-Methyl-D-aspartate
Noctec. *See* Chloral hydrate
Nocturnal myoclonus, **773**
Nocturnal myoclonus index, polysomnogram measures of, 760*t*
Nocturnal penile tumescence, 272*t*, 757
Nocturnal sensory stimuli, in dreams, 198
Nodes of Ranvier, 90
Noesis, definition of, 284
Noise, and aggression, 153
Noludar. *See* Methyprylon
Noncompliance, **899,** 968
Nonketotic hyperglycinemia, 1168*t*
Nonmaleficence, 1365
Nonnucleoside reverse transcriptase inhibitors, 376–377, 376*t*
Nonsteroidal antiinflammatory drugs (NSAIDs)
drug interactions, 1072
and lithium, 1072*t*
Nonverbal skills, normal development of, 1195*t*
Noradrenergic receptors, 101–102
Noradrenergic tracts, of central nervous system, 101, 101*f*
Norepinephrine, **100–102**
and aggression, 154
in Alzheimer's disease, 332
antidepressants and, 567*t*
in anxiety disorders, 594
drug interactions, 1062*t*
and drugs, 92, 102
laboratory testing for, 263
life cycle, 101
in major depressive disorder, 536
neurotransmitter function, 90*t*, 91*f*, 93*t*
in panic disorder, 600
and psychopathology, 102
receptors, 93*t*
in schizophrenia, 478
synthesis of, 101
Norepinephrine to epinephrine ratio (NE:E), 263
Normal autism, 29*t*
Normal distribution, 175, 172*f*
Normality, **16–17, 16–21**
adaptive mental mechanisms, 20–21
in adolescence, 18
as average, 17
child development, 20–21
functional perspectives of, 16–17
as health, 16–17
life cycle theory, 18–19
in old age, 20
as process, 17
psychoanalytic theories of, 17, 18*t*
as utopia, 17
Normal pressure hydrocephalus, 108, 254
Normetanephrine, 263
Norpramin. *See* Desipramine
Nortriptyline, 1001*t*
adverse effects of, 567*t*, 981*t*, 1127*t*
blood level data for clinical assessment, 269*t*
children, use with, 1307*t*
clinical information, 1130*t*
dosage and administration, 569*t*
drug interactions, 1134
for elderly patients, 1329
mechanism of action, 567*t*
neurotransmitter effects of, 1126*t*
for nicotine addiction, 447
plasma levels, monitoring, 265
preparations of, 1130*t*
structure of, 1125*f*
Nose, medical assessment of, 255
Noyes, Arthur, 817
NSAIDs. *See* Nonsteroidal antiinflammatory drugs (NSAIDs)
Nuclear magnetic resonance, 110
Nucleoside reverse transcriptase inhibitors, 376–377, 376*t*
Nucleotide(s), neurotransmitter function, 88, 96, 105
Null hypothesis, definition of, 176
Nursing homes, **1335–1336**
Nutmeg, 436*t*, 469
intoxication, emergency manifestations and treatment of, 910*t*
Nutrition, **855**
malnutrition. *See* Malnutrition
Nutritional disorder(s)
eating disorders. *See* Eating disorder(s)
mood disorder and, 351*t*
neuropsychiatric manifestations of, 366–367
Nutritional status, assessment of, 257
Nymphomania, 728
definition of, 282

O

Obesity, 105, **751–755**
brain damage and, 752
clinical features of, 753
comprehensive management approach to, 755
in Cushing's disease, 752
definition of, 751
developmental factors in, 752
dietary therapy for, 754
differential diagnosis of, 753
effects
on health, 753, 754*t*
on life expectancy, 754
etiology of, 751–753
exercise therapy for, 754
genetic factors in, 752
index measures of, 751
medical disorders associated with, 752, 753*f*
olanzapine for, 752
pharmacotherapy for, 754–755, 755*t*, **1118**
physical activity and, 752
prevalence of, 751
psychological factors in, 752–753
psychotherapy for, 755
psychotropic drugs for, 752
surgery for, 755
treatment of, 754–755
Object constancy, 29*t*
in schizophrenia, 483
Objectivity-participation, 216
Object libido, 204
Object permanence, 136
Object relations, 205, 220, 222, 228
in Freud's instinct theory, 200

Object relations theory, 924
Klein's theory, 222
therapeutic action in, 923–924
Obsession de la honte du corps, 653
Obsession(s), 621*t*
definition of, 284, 616
Obsessive-compulsive disorder (OCD), **616–623**
anorexia nervosa and, 739
behavioral factors in, 618
behavior therapy for, 623
biological factors in, 75, 617–618
brain imaging in, 617, 617*f*
buspirone for, 1032
in children, pharmacotherapy for, **1310**
clinical features of, 619–621
cognitive profile of, 957*t*
and combined psychotherapy and pharmacotherapy, **970**
comorbidity with, 617
course of, 622
defense mechanisms in, 618
definition of, 616
diagnosis of, 619
diagnostic criteria for, 619, 619*t*
differential diagnosis of, 621–622, 1272
drug augmentation therapy for, **991**
in elderly, 1325
electroconvulsive therapy for, 623
electrophysiologic abnormalities in, 617–618
epidemiology of, 616–617
etiology of, 617–619
family therapy with, 623
genetics of, 617
group therapy for, 623
ICD-10 diagnostic criteria for, 595–598, 598*t*
intrusive thoughts in, 620
versus medical conditions, 621
mental status examination in, 621
need for symmetry in, 621
neuroimaging in, 109
neuroimmunology and, 617
neurotransmitters in, 617
nonpsychiatric clinical specialists likelihood of seeing patients with, 612, 612*t,* 619, 620*t*
noradrenergic system and, 617
obsession of contamination in, 620
pathological doubt in, 620
and pathological gambling, 788
personality factors in, 618
pharmacotherapy for, 622–623, 1004*t,* **1024,** 1069, **1127,** 1132
drug augmentation therapy for, **991**
phototherapy for, 1145
prognosis for, 622
psychodynamic factors in, 618–619
psychosocial factors in, 618–619
psychotherapy for, 623
serotonergic system and, 617
symptom patterns, 620–621
in adults, 620, 620*t*
in children and adolescents, 620, 621*t*
Tourette's disorder and, 617, 618, 621, 1246
treatment of, 622–623
and trichotillomania, 790
Obsessive-compulsive personality disorder, **814–816**. *See also* Personality disorder(s), cluster C
clinical features of, 815–816
course of, 816
diagnosis of, 815
diagnostic criteria for, 815, 815*t*
differential diagnosis of, 816
epidemiology of, 814–815
pharmacotherapy for, 816
prognosis for, 816
psychotherapy for, 816
treatment of, 816
and trichotillomania, 790
Obsessive-compulsive symptoms, in a general medical condition, 637–638
Obstructive interventions, 247–248, 247*t*
Obstructive sleep apnea syndrome, **770**
Occipital lobe(s), functions of, 80*t*
Occipital lobe syndrome(s), 903, 904*t*
Occipital lobe tumor(s)
medical considerations with, 844*t*
psychiatric considerations with, 844*t*
Occupation
in early adulthood, 43
and suicide, 914–915
Occupational choice, 38
Occupational history, 235–236, 254
Occupational problems, **894–896**
OCD. *See* Obsessive-compulsive disorder (OCD)
O'Connor v. Donaldson, 1357
OCPs, **1378–1379**
Ocular dominance columns, 69, 70*f,* 73
Oculomotor apraxia, 71
Odorant binding, 71
Oedipus complex, 166, 221
Offer, Daniel, 16
Office, psychiatrist's, 247
Office of Alternative Medicine (OAM), of National Institutes of Health, 851–852
classification of alternative medicines, 854*t*
Office of Professional Medical Conduct (OPMC), 1371
Ohm's law, 89, **1139**
Olanzapine, 498, 1001*t*. *See* Serotonin-dopamine antagonist(s) (atypical antipsychotics)
adverse effects of, 498
for autistic disorder, 1215
for bipolar I disorder, 570
for early-onset schizophrenia, 1285
indications for, 498
intoxication/overdose of, 987*t*
for obesity, 752
for psychotic disorders, 527
for schizophrenia, 498
for Tourette's disorder, 1250
Old age. *See* Elderly
Olfaction, **71–72,** 74
and memory, 72, 148
and sexual responses, 71
Olfactory bulb, 71
Olivopontocerebellar atrophy, neuroimaging in, 111*f,* 117*f*
Omissions, in phonological disorders, 1201
Oneiroid state, 489
Oniomania, 792
Operant learning, 227
Operational fatigue, 624
Operational thought, 137
Opiate antagonists, for stereotypic movement disorder, 1272–1273
Opiate(s)
definition of, 448
neurotransmitter function, 90*t*
in substance-related disorders, 387, 388*f*
Opioid antagonist(s), 448, 452, **455**
Opioid receptor agonists, **1085–1089**
adverse reactions to, 1087–1088
buprenorphine. *See* Buprenorphine
chemistry of, 1086, 1086*f*
clinical guidelines for, 1088–1089
dosage of, 1088–1089
drug interactions, 1088
indications for, 1086–1087
laboratory interferences, 1088
levomethadyl. *See* Levomethadyl
methadone. *See* Methadone
nalmefene. *See* Nalmefene
naltrexone. *See* Naltrexone
pharmacological actions of, 1086
precautions with, 1087–1088
Opioid receptor(s), 449
Opioid-related disorder(s), 382*t,* **448–456**
biological factors in, 451
brain imaging in, 449
clinical features of, 453–454
comorbidity with, 450, 450*t*
definition of, 449
diagnosis of, 451
DSM-IV-TR classification of, 449, 451, 451*t*
epidemiology of, 449
etiology of, 450–451
genetic factors in, 451
mood disorder, 453
not otherwise specified, 453
diagnostic criteria for, 453, 453*t*
pharmacotherapy for, 1004*t*
psychodynamic theory of, 451
psychosocial factors in, 450–451
psychotherapy for, 455
psychotic disorder, 453
rehabilitation, 454–456
self-help, 456
sexual dysfunction, 453, 711
sleep disorder, 453
therapeutic communities for, 455–456
treatment, 454–456
Opioid(s), 448
abuse, 452, 460
definition of, 449
diagnosis of, 452
adverse effects of, 454
definition of, 448
dependence, 387, 448–456
acupuncture for, 1145
in adolescents, 450–451
brain imaging in, 449
definition of, 448–449
diagnosis of, 452
in pregnant women, 455
self-help, 456
social factors in, 450–451
and suicide attempts, 450
drug interactions, 454, 1028
effects, 453–454
on cerebral blood flow, 449
endogenous, 104, 131
intoxication
acute, diagnostic criteria for, 391*t*
diagnosis of, 452
diagnostic criteria for, 451, 451*t*
emergency manifestations of, 910*t*
emergency treatment of, 910*t*
intoxication delirium, 453, 1344
naturally occurring, 448
neuropharmacology of, 449, 450*f*
overdose, 454–455
treatment of, 454–455
for pain management, 1344, 1344*t*
receptors, 104
substitutes, for treatment of opioid use disorders, 455
synthetic, 448

Opioid(s)—*continued*
tolerance, 449–450
use
epidemiology of, 449
and hepatitis transmission, 454
and HIV transmission, 454
prevention, 456
methods of, 453, 454f
withdrawal, 449–450, 452–453, 453
diagnosis of, 452
diagnostic criteria for, 451, 452t
emergency manifestations of, 910t
emergency treatment of, 910t
neonatal, 455
pharmacotherapy for, 104, 1005
Oppositional defiant disorder, **1232–1233**
clinical features of, 1233
course of, 1234
diagnosis of, 1233, 1233t
differential diagnosis of, 1233–1234, 1237
epidemiology of, 1232
etiology of, 1232
and expressive language disorder, 1195
in ICD-10, 1238, 1238t–1239t
laboratory examinations for, 1233
pathology of, 1233
prognosis of, 1234
treatment for, 1234
Optical illusions, 71f
Optic ataxia, 71
Oral contraceptives, 875t
and bromocriptine, 1049
drug interactions, 1028, 1129
Oral stage, 19, 200, 201t
Oralstat, for weight reduction, 755, 982
Orap. *See* Pimozide
Orbitofrontal region, 85
Organic mental disorders, ICD-10 classification of, 323
Organic personality disorder, 382t
Organ inferiority, 218
Organ transplantation, consultation-liaison psychiatry and, 849–850
Orgasm, 694t–695t, 695–696
Orgasm disorders, 701t, **704–706**
female orgasmic disorder, **704–705,** 704t
premature orgasm, 712
premature ejaculation, **705–706,** 705t
ICD-10 diagnostic criteria for, 717t
treatment of, 713
retarded ejaculation, 256
retrograde ejaculation, 256
Orgasmic anhedonia, 712
Orgasmic dysfunction, ICD-10 diagnostic criteria for, 717t
Oriental medicine, **864**
Orientation
assessment of, 186–187
in delusional disorder, 514
in depression, 555
in elderly, 1320
evaluation of, in child psychiatric evaluation, 1155
in mental status examination, 241
in schizophrenia, 495
temporal, assessment of, 186–187, 187t
Orne, Martin, definition of hypnosis, 960
Ornish, Dean, 855
Ornish diet, 855
Orphenadrine, 1001t
for extrapyramidal disorders, 1059t
Orphenadrine citrate, 1014t. *See also* Anticholinergic(s)
structure of, 1013f
Orthostatic hypotension
biofeedback for, 949t
and psychotherapeutic drugs, **982**
Orton Gillingham reading program, 1183
Osler, William, 15
Osmotic diuretics, and lithium, 1072t
Osteopathic medicine, **864**
Othello syndrome, 515
Other mental disorders due to brain disease, damage and dysfunction, ICD-10 classification of, 370t
Other psychotic disorders, **505–533**
Othmer, Ekkehard and Sieglinde, 6
Out-of-body experiences, 59
Outpatient commitment programs (OCPs), **1378–1379**
Overactive disorder associated with mental retardation and stereotyped movements, ICD-10 diagnostic criteria for, 1219, 1221t
Overactivity, definition of, 282
Overdose. *See specific substance*
Overgeneralizing, 958f
Overvalued idea, definition of, 283
Overweight, 751. *See also* Obesity
Ovulation augmentation or induction, 873t
Oxazepam, 460, 1001t. *See also* Benzodiazepine(s)
dosage of, 1025t
geriatric dosage, 1332t
half-life of, 1025t
pharmacological actions for, 1023
structure of, 1023f
Oxcarbazepine, 1001t
Oxycodone
blood level data for clinical assessment, 269t
for pain management, 1344t
Oxymorphone, for pain management, 1344t
Oxytocin, 129t, 132
levels after orgasm, 696
neurotransmitter function, 105
Ozone therapy, **864**

P

Paced Auditory Serial Addition Test, 191t
Pain, 66–68
and aggression, 154
back pain
acupuncture for, 1145
lower. *See* Low back pain
management of, **1342–1346**
palliative care, **1342–1346**
perception of, 66, 104
types of, 1343
Pain control programs, for pain disorder, 658
Pain disorder, **655–658**
behavioral factors in, 656
behavioral therapy for, 658
biofeedback for, 658
biological factors in, 656
clinical features of, 644t, 656–657
course of, 657
definition of, 655
diagnosis of, 656
diagnostic criteria for, 656, 656t
differential diagnosis of, 657
epidemiology of, 655
etiology of, 655–656
hypnosis for, 658
interpersonal factors in, 656
nerve blocks for, 658
nerve stimulation for, 658
pain control programs for, 658
pharmacotherapy for, 657–658, **1127**
prognosis for, 657
psychodynamic factors in, 655
psychotherapy for, 658
surgical ablative procedures for, 658
treatment of, 657–658
Palilalia, 1246
Palliative care, **1342–1346**
Palmer, David Daniel, 853, 855f
Pamelor. *See* Nortriptyline
Pancreatic carcinoma
medical considerations with, 845t
psychiatric considerations with, 845t
Pancuronium bromide, and lithium, 1072t
Panic, definition of, 281
Panic attack(s)
carbon dioxide inhalation and, 267
in children, pharmacotherapy for, 1310
clinical features of, 603–605
definition of, 599
diagnosis of, 601–602
diagnostic criteria for, 601–602, 602t
due to a general medical condition, 637
hyperventilation and, 267
provocation of, with sodium lactate, 267
Panic disorder
with agoraphobia, 599
diagnosis of, 602
diagnostic criteria for, 602, 602t
pharmacotherapy for, **1126–1127**
and alcohol use disorders, 397
associated symptoms, 605
behavior therapy for, 601, 608
biological factors in, 107, 600
brain imaging in, 600
buspirone for, 1032
characteristics of, 599
in children, pharmacotherapy for, 1310
clinical features of, 603
cognitive-behavioral theories of, 601
cognitive profile of, 957t
cognitive therapy for, 601, 608
combined psychotherapy and pharmacotherapy for, 608–609, **969–970**
comorbidity with, 599–600
course of, 606
definition of, 599
and depression, 606
diagnosis of, 602
differential diagnosis of, 605–606, 605t
emergency manifestations of, 910t
emergency treatment of, 910t
epidemiology of, 599
etiology of, 600–601
family therapy in, 608
and generalized anxiety disorder, 632
genetic factors in, 600–601
historical perspective on, 599
ICD-10 diagnostic criteria for, 597t
insight-oriented psychotherapy in, 608
versus medical disorders, 605t, 606
versus mental disorders, 606
mitral valve prolapse and, 600
neuroimaging in, 112
neurotransmitters in, 600
and obsessive-compulsive disorder, 617
and pathological gambling, 788
pathophysiology of, 105
pharmacotherapy for, 606–608, 607t, 1004t, **1024,** 1032, 1132
duration of, 608
prognosis for, 606
propranolol for, 1009

psychoanalytic theories of, 601
psychodynamic themes of, 601*t*
psychosocial factors in, 601
relaxation training for, 608
respiratory training for, 608
sex distribution of, 599
versus social phobia, 606
versus specific phobia, 606
and suicide, 606
treatment failures, 607–608
treatment of, 606–609
in vivo exposure for, 608
without agoraphobia
diagnosis of, 602
diagnostic criteria for, 602, 602*t*
Panic-inducing substances, 600
Panicogens, 600
Panphobia, definition of, 284
Papaver somniferum, 448
Papez circuit, 83
Pappenheim, Bertha. *See* Anna O.
Paradoxical sleep, 756
Paradoxical therapy, **945**
Paral. *See* Paraldehyde
Paraldehyde, 1001*t,* 1019, **1020–1021**
blood level data for clinical assessment, 269*t*
drug interactions, 1020–1021, 1047
Parallel play, 31
Paramnesia, definition of, 286
Paranoid anxiety, 593
Paranoid personality disorder, **803–804**. *See also* Personality disorder(s), cluster A; Schizophrenia, paranoid type
clinical features of, 803
cognitive profile of, 957*t*
course of, 804
diagnosis of, 803
diagnostic criteria for, 803, 803*t*
differential diagnosis of, 803
epidemiology of, 803
pharmacotherapy for, 804
prognosis for, 804
psychotherapy for, 804
treatment of, 804
Paranoid pseudocommunity, 513
Paranoid-schizoid position, 222
Paraphasia, 257
Paraphilias, **718–729**
behavior therapy for, 954*t*
biological factors in, 719–720
classification of, 725, 726*t*
clinical features of, 720–724
cognitive-behavioral therapy for, 724–725
course of, 724
diagnosis of, 720–724
differential diagnosis of, 724
epidemiology of, 718–719, 719*t*
etiology of, 719–720
harmful nature of, 718
imprisonment for, 724
not otherwise specified, 723–724, 723*t*
prognosis for, 724
psychosocial factors in, 719
treatment of, 724–725
Paraphrenia, **489,** 1325
Parapraxis, 193
definition of, 282
Parapsychology, 225
Parasomnia(s), **761, 774–777**
in ICSD, 764*t*
not otherwise specified, **776–777**
diagnostic criteria for, 776*t*
Parasuicidal behavior, 919
dialectical behavior therapy for, 954
Parataxic mode, 228
Parathyroid disorder(s), neuropsychiatric manifestations of, 366
Parathyroid hormone, testing for, 272*t*
Parens patriae, 1356
Parental fit, 29
Parent–child interaction, evaluation of, in child psychiatric evaluation, 1155
Parent–child relational problems, **880**
Parenthood, in early adulthood, 45–46
Parenting
of adolescents, 38
alternative lifestyle, 45
of infants, 29
of toddlers, 30–31
Parenting styles, 34–35
Parent(s)
death of, effects on children, 34
grief in, 64
in group psychotherapy, with children, 1301–1302
interviews with, in child psychiatry, 1153
involvement in child psychotherapy, 1299
involvement in residential treatment of children, 1303
Parietal lobe(s)
functions of, 80*t*
and intelligence quotient, 85
in memory impairment, 81, 82
Parietal lobe tumor(s)
medical considerations with, 844*t*
psychiatric considerations with, 844*t*
Parkinsonianlike symptoms, 497
Parkinsonism, 97. *See also* Medication-induced movement disorders; Neuroleptic-induced movement disorders
characteristics of, 75
and depression, 75
emergency manifestations of, 910*t*
emergency treatment of, 910*t*
MPTP-induced, **454**
pharmacology for, 1014, 1076
Parkinson's disease, 75, 97
dementia in, 334
ICD-10 diagnostic criteria for, 344*t*
and memory, 81
mood disorder and, 351*t*
neuroimaging in, 119
pharmacotherapy for, 1026
transcranial magnetic stimulation and, 121
Parlodel. *See* Bromocriptine
Parnate. *See* Tranylcypromine
Paroxetine, 1001*t*. *See also* Selective serotonin reuptake inhibitors
adverse effects of, 567*t,* 981*t*
for conduct disorder, 1238
dosage and administration, 569*t*
for elderly patients, 1329
with erythromycin, 1044
intoxication/overdose of, 987*t*
mechanism of action, 103
for posttraumatic stress disorder, 630
for separation anxiety disorder, 1263
withdrawal from, 982
Paroxysmal myoclonic dystonia with vocalization, 1249*t*
Paroxysmal nocturnal hemoglobinuria, **780**
Partial complex status epilepticus, 434
Partialism, 723–724
Partial recovery, in conditioning, 144
Participant modeling, in behavior therapy, **953**
Participant observer, 228
Partner relational problems, **880–881**
Passion flower, 1146
Passive aggression, in personality disorders, 802
Passive-aggressive behavior, 207*t*
Passive-aggressive personality disorder, 295, **816–817**
clinical features of, 816–817
course of, 816–817
diagnosis of, 816
diagnostic criteria for, 816, 817*t*
differential diagnosis of, 817
epidemiology of, 816
pharmacotherapy for, 817
prognosis for, 817
psychotherapy for, 817
treatment of, 817
Past life medicine, **864–865**
Pastoral counseling, **899**
Pathological fire setting, ICD-10 classification of, 793–794, 793*t*
Pathological gambling, **788–789**
biological factors in, 788
clinical features of, 788–789
comorbidity with, 788
course of, 789
definition of, 788
diagnosis of, 788–789
diagnostic criteria for, 788, 788*t*
differential diagnosis of, 789
epidemiology of, 788
etiology of, 788
ICD-10 classification of, 793–794, 793*t*
laboratory examinations, 789
prognosis for, 789
psychological testing, 789
psychosocial factors in, 788
treatment of, 789
Pathological stealing, ICD-10 classification of, 793–794, 793*t*
Patient autonomy, 1365
Patient referral, guidelines for, 929, 929*t*
Patient(s). *See also* Doctor–patient relationship
acetylation status of, 533
auditory evaluation of, 257
civil rights of, **1357–1358**
clinically defined groups, analysis of, 109
demanding, 13
dependent, 13
expectations of and responses to physician. *See* Transference
general observation of, in medical assessment, 256–257
histrionic, 13
interviewing. *See* Interview(s)
introduction to, 6–7
isolated, 14
narcissistic, 13
obsessive, 14
olfactory evaluation of, 257
physical examination of, **257–258**
physician's expectations of and responses to. *See* Countertransference
problem, 13–14
psychiatric, diagnosis of intercurrent illness in, **259**
visual evaluation of, 256–257
Patient's Bill of Rights, 1338
Patient-therapist sexual relations, **1368**
Patterning psychotherapy, with children, 1296–1297
Pauling, Linus, 1146
Pavlov, Ivan Petrovich, 143–144, 144*f,* 161
Paxil. *See* Paroxetine
Paxipam. *See* Halazepam
PBG, testing for, 272*t*

PCP. *See* Phencyclidine (PCP) (or phencyclidinelike substance)
Peabody, Francis, 1
Peabody Individual Achievement Test (PIAT), 1159
Peabody Individual Achievement Test-Revised, 1182
Peabody Picture Vocabulary Test-III, 191*t*
Peabody Picture Vocabulary Test-Revised (PPVT-R), 1157*t*
Peak experience, 223
Pedigree study, of aggression, 154
Pedophilia
  clinical features of, 721
  diagnosis of, 721
  diagnostic criteria for, 721, 721*t*
  ICD-10 diagnostic criteria for, 726*t*
Peer anxiety, and group psychotherapy, **935–936**
Peer groups, in adolescence, 37–38
Peer Review Organizations (PROs), **1385–1386**
Pelvic pain, **878**
Pemoline, 1001*t*, 1116. *See also* Sympathomimetics; Sympathomimetics (and related drugs)
  for attention-deficit/hyperactivity disorder, 1228
  for cocaine users, 435
  geriatric dosage, 1330*t*
  intoxication/overdose of, 987*t*
  pharmacological action of, 1117
Penfield, Wilder, 73
Pentazocine, 448
  blood level data for clinical assessment, 269*t*
Pentobarbital, 460, 1001*t*. *See also* Barbiturate(s)
  dosage of, 1020*t*
  indications for, 1018
  structure of, 1018*f*
Pentobarbital challenge test, 1018, 1019*t*
Peonage, 1357
People orientation, evaluation of, in child psychiatric evaluation, 1155
Peptic ulcer disease
  pharmacotherapy for, 1127
  psychological correlates of, 826*t*, **827**
Peptidase, 104
Peptide(s), neurotransmitter function, 88, 91*f*, 104–105
Percentile rank, definition of, 176
Perception
  changes in, with brain tumor, 361
  definition of, 285
  in mental status examination, 239
Perceptual disturbances. *See also* Flashbacks
  in alcohol withdrawal, 403
  associated with cognitive disorder and medical condition, definition of, 286
  associated with conversion and dissociative phenomena, definition of, 286
  definition of, 285
  in delusional disorder, 514
  in elderly patient, 1319
  hallucinogen-related. *See* Hallucinogen-related disorder(s), persisting perception disorder (flashback)
  in mania, 556
  on mental status examination, 239
  in schizophrenia, 491–492
  substance-induced. *See specific substance*
Perceptual motor tests, 1159
Perceptual performance, assessment of, 187–189, 188*f*–189*f*
Perceptual tests, 1159
Perceptuomotor performance, assessment of, 187–189, 188*f*–189*f*
Percodan. *See* Oxycodone
Pergolide, 1001*t*, **1047–1050**. *See also* Dopamine receptor antagonist(s), and precursors
  for cocaine users, 435
Periactin. *See* Cyproheptadine
Perimenstrual mood changes, 256
Perinatal death, 874
Perinatal disorder(s), versus tic disorder, 1249*t*
Perinatal history, 234–235
Period prevalence, 176
Perioral tremor
  emergency manifestations of, 910*t*
  emergency treatment of, 910*t*
Peripheral nervous system, 85
  development of, 85
Perls, Frederick, **225**, 225*f*
  and gestalt group therapy, 935
Permissive hypothesis, 104
Permitil. *See* Fluphenazine
Perphenazine, 1001*t*
  blood level data for clinical assessment, 269*t*
  geriatric dosage, 1332*t*
  and lithium, 1072*t*
  preparations, 1064*t*
  structure of, 1052*f*
Persecutory anxiety, 222, 593
Perseveration, definition of, 283
Persistent somatoform pain disorder, ICD-10 diagnostic criteria, 660*t*
Persona, Jung's concept of, 222
Personal dispositions, 218
Personal history, **234–238**
Personality, 209
  accident prone, 157
  adult, assessment, **180–185**
  anal, 215
  assessment
    objective, 180–181, 181*t*
    projective, 182–185, 183*t*
  Cattell's study of, 219–220
  childhood, 235
  and child-rearing, 167–168
  and culture, 166
  definition of, 800
  disturbances, in epilepsy, 358–359
  epileptoid, 783
  Erikson's theory of, 211
  exploitative, 220
  family and, 167–168
  genetics and, 167–168
  hoarding, 220
  marketing, 220
  and mood disorder, 541
  productive, 220
  receptive, 220
  Roger's view of, 226
  serotonin and, 801
  Skinner's view of, 227
  traits, 218
  twin studies. *See* Twin studies
  variance in, 167–168
  viscosity of, in epilepsy, 358–359
Personality Assessment Inventory (PAI), 181*t*
Personality change
  in AIDS patients, 819, 819*t*
  with anabolic steroid use, 467, **819**
  from cocaine use, 431
  in dementia, 336
  due to a general medical condition, 350, 356*t*, 818–819
    clinical features of, 819
    course of, 819
    diagnosis of, 819
    differential diagnosis of, 819
    etiology of, 819, 819*t*
    prognosis for, 819
    treatment of, 819
Personality development
  in adolescence, 37
  in elderly, 54
  Murphy's theory of, 225
Personality disorder(s), **800–821**. *See also specific disorder*
  and alcohol use disorders, 397
  biological factors in, 801
  and brief psychiatric disorder, 521
  classification of, 800
  cluster A, 800
    genetic factors in, 800
  cluster B, 800
    genetic factors in, 800–801
  cluster C, 800
    genetic factors in, 800
  and conversion disorder, 648
  defense mechanisms in, 802–803
  diagnostic criteria for, 801*t*
  differential diagnosis of, 674, 784
  DSM-IV-TR classification of, 800, 801*t*
  due to brain disease, damage and dysfunction, ICD-10 classification of, 382*t*
  electrophysiology in, 801
  etiology of, 800–803
  and factitious disorders, 668
  genetic factors in, 800–801
  harm avoidance, psychobiology of, 820–821
  hormones in, 801
  ICD-10 classification of, 821
  and kleptomania, 785
  neurotransmitters in, 801
  not otherwise specified, **816**, 816*t*
  novelty seeking, psychobiology of, 821
  and obsessive-compulsive disorder, 617
  passive aggression in, 802
  persistence, psychobiology of, 821
  pharmacotherapy for, 820*t*
  platelet monoamine oxidase in, 801
  psychoanalytic factors in, 801–803
  reward dependence, psychobiology of, 821
  sadistic, 818
  sadomasochistic, 818
  signs and symptoms of, 800
  smooth pursuit eye movements in, 801
  and suicide, **917**
  temperament dimensions, 820–821, 821*t*
  treatment, psychobiological model of, 819–821
  and trichotillomania, 790
16 Personality Factor Questionnaire (16 PF), 181*t*
Personality test(s)
  for children, **1159**
  in schizophrenia, 490
Person-centered theory, 226
Personology, 225
Perspective, 71*f*
Pertofrane. *See* Desipramine
Pervasive developmental disorder(s), **1208–1222**
  characteristics of, 1219
  differential diagnosis of, 1192, 1197, 1269, 1284
  ICD-10 classification of, 1219, 1220*t*–1221*t*

not otherwise specified, 1219, 1219*t*
other, ICD-10 diagnostic criteria for, 1219, 1221*t*
types of, 1219
unspecified, ICD-10 diagnostic criteria for, 1219, 1221*t*
PET. *See* Positron emission tomography (PET)
Petit mal epilepsy, **357,** 358*f*
Pfizer. *See* Ziprasidone
Phallic stage, 19, 200, 202*t*
Phantom limb, definition of, 285
Pharmacogenetics, 533
Pharmacological syndromes, in experimental models, 163
Pharmacotherapy. *See also specific agent; specific disorder*
adverse effects of, **979–982,** 980*t*
for children, **979, 1305–1311**
adverse effects of, 1310–1311
indications for, 1306–1310
pharmacokinetics of, 1306, 1307*t*–1308*t*
therapeutic considerations with, 1306, 1306*t*
drug augmentation therapy, **989—992**
with geriatric patients, **979,** 979*t,* 1328–1333
with hepatic insufficiency, **979**
during lactation, **979**
with medical illness, **979**
during pregnancy, **979**
with psychosocial treatment, 967
with psychotherapy, **967–973**
clinical considerations, 971–972
cost effectiveness of, 972
one-person model of, 971
specific disorders treated with, 968–971
two-person model of, 971–972
with renal insufficiency, **979**
withdrawal syndromes, 982–983
Phase of life problem, 898–899
Phencyclidine (PCP) (or phencyclidinelike substance)
abuse, 461
diagnosis of, 457
blood level data for clinical assessment, 269*t*
contaminants, 457
dependence
diagnosis of, 457
physical, 457
psychological, 457
intoxication, 457–458
behavioral disturbances in, 457–458
diagnostic criteria for, 457, 457*t*
emergency manifestations of, 911*t*
emergency treatment of, 911*t*
perceptual disturbances in, 457–458
intoxication delirium, 458
ketamine, 459
neuropharmacology of, 456–457
tolerance, 457
in urinalysis, 268*t*
use, 456, 527
and geographic region, 456
history of, 456
methods of, 456
variability of dose, 459
users, crystallized, 456
withdrawal, 457
Phencyclidine (or phencyclidinelike substance)-related disorder(s), 382*t,* **456–460**
anxiety disorder, 458
clinical features of, 459
diagnosis of, 457–458
differential diagnosis of, 459
DSM-IV-TR classification of, 457, 457*t*
epidemiology of, 456
mood disorder, 458
not otherwise specified, diagnostic criteria for, 458, 458*t*
psychotic disorder, 458
rehabilitation, 459
treatment, 459
Phendimetrazine, 1001*t,* 1116. *See also* Sympathomimetics (and related drugs)
for weight reduction, 755*t*
Phenelzine, 1001*t,* 1076. *See also* Monoamine oxidase inhibitors
adverse effects of, 981*t*
chemistry of, 1076*f*
dosage and administration, 569*t*
drug interactions, 1012
for elderly patients, 1329
mechanism of action, 567*t*
metabolism of, 533
for obsessive-compulsive disorder, 622
pharmacological action of, 1072–1073
psychotic disorder induced by
emergency manifestations of, 911*t*
emergency treatment of, 911*t*
for selective mutism, 1266
for social phobia, 616
Phenmetrazine, 1001*t,* 1116. *See also* Sympathomimetics (and related drugs)
Phenobarbital, 460, 1001*t*. *See also* Barbiturate(s)
with donepezil, 1044
dosage of, 1020*t*
drug interactions, 378, 401, 1028, 1119, 1133–1134
hepatic effects, 264
indications for, 464–465, 1018
structure of, 1018*f*
withdrawal, 463
Phenomenalistic causality, 137
Phenomenology, **275**
Phenothiazine(s), 1051*t*
chemistry of, 1053
geriatric dosage, 1332*t*
indications for, 419
for intermittent explosive disorder, 785
laboratory testing with, 263
structure of, 1052*f*
Phentermine, 1001*t,* 1116. *See also* Sympathomimetics (and related drugs)
for weight reduction, 755*t*
Phentermine resin, for weight reduction, 755*t*
Phentolamine
indications for, 459
oral, 715
Phenylalanine, 1146
Phenylbutazone
drug interactions, 1119
and lithium, 1072*t*
Phenylethanolamine-*N*-methyltransferase (PNMT), 101
Phenylethylamine, adverse effects of, 981*t*
Phenylketonuria (PKU), **1166,** 1167*t,* 1172*t*
Phenylpiperazines, adverse effects of, 981*t*
Phenylpropanolamine (PPA), 414
toxicity of
emergency manifestations of, 911*t*
emergency treatment of, 911*t*
for weight reduction, 755*t*
Phenytoin
blood level data for clinical assessment, 269*t*
for cocaine users, 435
with donepezil, 1044
drug interactions, 1028, 1031, 1047, 1049, 1062*t,* 1119, 1124, 1133
and lithium, 1072*t*
for pain management, 1345*t*
Pheochromocytoma, 255–256, 263
medical considerations with, 847*t*
psychiatric considerations with, 847*t*
Pheromones, 71–72
Phobia(s). *See also* Panic disorder
and alcohol use disorders, 397
behavioral factors in, 610
behavior therapy for, 615, 954*t*
childhood, development of, 144
clinical features of, 614
cognitive profile of, 957*t*
course of, 614–615
definition of, 284, 609
differential diagnosis of, 614
in elderly, 1325
emergency manifestations of, 911*t*
emergency treatment of, 911*t*
epidemiology of, 609–610
family therapy for, 615
Freud's contributions on, 610–611
in a general medical condition, 638
insight-oriented psychotherapy for, 615
learning theory of, 610
pharmacotherapy for, 1004*t*
prognosis for, 614–615
psychoanalytic factors in, 610–611
psychodynamic themes in, 611*t*
social, 102, **609–616**
and alcohol use disorders, 397
anorexia nervosa and, 739
buspirone for, 1032
characteristics of, 1262*t*
comorbidity with, 610
course of, 615
definition of, 284, 609
diagnosis of, 613–614
diagnostic criteria for, 613, 613*t*
differential diagnosis of, 614
epidemiology of, 609–610, 610*t*
etiology of, 610–612
and generalized anxiety disorder, 632
genetic factors in, 612
ICD-10 diagnostic criteria for, 596*t*
lifetime prevalence, 610, 610*t*
neurochemical factors in, 611–612
and obsessive-compulsive disorder, 617
versus panic disorder, 606
pharmacotherapy for, **1024**
prognosis, 615
propranolol for, 1009
treatment of, 616
and trichotillomania, 790
specific, **609–616**
classification of phobias, 612
comorbidity with, 610
course of, 614
definition of, 284, 609
diagnosis of, 612–613
diagnostic criteria for, 612, 612*t*
differential diagnosis of, 614
epidemiology of, 609–610
etiology of, 610–612
and generalized anxiety disorder, 632
genetic factors in, 611
ICD-10 diagnostic criteria for, 596*t*
and obsessive-compulsive disorder, 617
versus panic disorder, 606
prognosis, 614
treatment of, 615

Phobia(s)—*continued*
treatment of, 615–616
Phobic anxiety, 1260
Phobic anxiety disorder. *See also* Phobia(s); *specific phobia*
of childhood, 1264*t*
ICD-10 diagnostic criteria for, 596*t*
Phoenix House, 456
Phonemes, 86
Phonological disorder, **1199–1202**
clinical features of, 1201–1202
comorbidity with, 1200
course of, 1202
diagnosis of, 1201, 1201*t*
differential diagnosis of, 1202, 1203*t*
DSM-IV-TR diagnostic criteria for, 1201, 1201*t*
environmental factors, 1201
epidemiology of, 1200
etiology of, 1200–1201
and expressive language disorder, 1196
and language disorders, 1200*t*
prognosis for, 1202
spontaneous remission of, 1202
and stuttering, 1203
treatment of, 1202
Phonological memory, immediate, 80
Phonological processing, 82
Phonology, 1194
Phosphoinositol metabolites, as second messenger, 95
Phosphorus, serum, testing for, 272*t*
Photosensitivity
emergency manifestations of, 911*t*
emergency treatment of, 911*t*
Photo therapy, **1145**
Physical abuse
of adults, **890**. *See also* Elder abuse
of children, **884–885,** 885*f*. *See also* Child abuse and neglect
of spouse, **890,** 891*t*
Physical appearance, evaluation of, in child psychiatric evaluation, 1155
Physical examination of patient, **257–258**
deferring, 258
incidental findings in, 258–259
psychological factors in, 258
selection for, 257–258
timing of, 258
Physical exercise, 856
Physical health, and suicide risk, 915
Physical problems, history-taking about, 235
Physician-assisted suicide, **1348–1349**
Physician Charter of Professionalism, 1371, 1371*t*
Physician marriages, **881**
Physician(s). *See also* Doctor–patient relationship
availability to patients, **12–13**
character and qualities, 14–15, 15*t*
earnings, 1383
expectations of and responses to patient. *See* Countertransference
female, 1382
impaired, ethical considerations with, **1371**
interns' working hours, 1383–1384
introduction to patient, 6–7
liability insurance, 1383
medical education, 1382–1383
patient's expectations of and responses to. *See* Transference
primary care, 1388
residents' working hours, 1383–1384
stresses on, 14–15, 15
suicide risk among, 914–915
supply of, 1382
U.S. needs, 1383
Physicians in training, ethics concerning, **1371**
Physostigmine
for Alzheimer's disease and similar disorders, 1041–1042
for anticholinergic intoxication, 1014
Piaget, Jean, **136–139,** 137*f*
theory, of cognitive (intellectual) development, 19, 24–26, 28*t,* 38, 60, **136–138**
applications to psychiatry, 139
PIAT, 1159
Piblokto, 531*t*
Pica
definition of, 281
in infancy or early childhood, **1241–1242**
clinical features of, 1241–1242
course of, 1242
diagnosis of, 1241–1242
diagnostic criteria for, 1242*t*
differential diagnosis of, 1242
epidemiology of, 1241
etiology of, 1241
in ICD-10, 1245*t*
laboratory examination of, 1242
pathology of, 1242
prognosis for, 1242
treatment of, 1242
in pregnant women, **872**
PICA-III-R, 1154
Pick bodies, 1323
Pick's disease, 83
dementia in, 333, **1323**
ICD-10 diagnostic criteria for, 344*t*
Pickwickian syndrome, 257, 753
Pictorial Instrument for Children and Adolescents (PICA-III-R), 1154
Pigmentary retinopathy
emergency manifestations of, 911*t*
emergency treatment of, 911*t*
Pimozide, 1001*t*
for anorexia nervosa, 745
chemistry of, 1053
preparations, 1064*t*
structure of, 1052*f*
for Tourette's disorder, 1250
Pindolol, 1001*t,* 1009*t*. *See also* β-Adrenergic receptor antagonist(s)
augmentation of, **990**
chemistry of, 1008*f*
pharmacological actions of, 1009
Piperacetazine, 1001*t*
Piperazine, structure of, 1052*f*
Piperazinoazepines, adverse effects of, 981*t*
1-Piperidenocyclohexane carbonitrite, 457
Piperidine, 457
Pituitary disorder(s), neuropsychiatric manifestations of, 366
PKU, **1166,** 1167*t,* 1172*t*
Placebos, **1148–1149**
Place orientation, evaluation of, in child psychiatric evaluation, 1155
Placidyl. *See* Ethchlorvynol
Platelet count, 272*t*
Play
analytic interpretation of, 222
in preschool years, 31–32
sex differences in, 32
as treatment modality, 216
Play group therapy, 1300
Playroom, psychotherapy in, 1298
Play therapy, 216
Pleasure principle, 150, **200**
PNI. *See* Psychoneuroimmunology (PNI)
PNMT, 101
Poikilothermia, 757
Point prevalence, 176
Point-to-point pattern, in sensory systems, 66, 68, 69
Politan, Phillip, 809
Polyphagia, definition of, 282
Polysomnogram, 120
Polysubstance related disorder, 470
Polysubstance use disorder, 382*t*
Polysurgical addiction. *See* Munchausen syndrome
Pondimin. *See* Fenfluramine
Population, statistical, 176
definition of, 174
Porphobilinogen (PBG), testing for, 272*t*
Positional cloning, 125–126
Positive connotation, in family therapy, **946**
Positive reinforcement, 145
in behavior therapy, **954**
in interview, 10
Positive skewness in distributions, 172*f*
Positron emission tomography (PET), 84, 108, **113–119**
in alcohol withdrawal, 403, 404*f*
in Alzheimer's disease, 111*f,* 118*f*
in attention-deficit/hyperactivity disorder, 1224
of brain, 113–119, 122
function, 113–119
neurologic disorders and, 117*f*
in brain tumor, 111*f,* 117*f*
in cocaine addiction, 430
for cognitive disorders, 323, 404*f*
for Creutzfeldt-Jakob disease, 364
in Huntington's disease, 111*f,* 117*f*
in language tasks, 120
in MPTP ingestion, 454
in multi-infarct dementia, 111*f,* 117*f*
in obsessive-compulsive disorder, 109
in olivopontocerebellar atrophy, 111*f,* 117*f*
in opioid use disorders, 449
pharmacological and neuropsychological probes, 119
reading disorder studies, 1181
in schizophrenia, 481
in temporal lobe epilepsy, 111*f,* 117*f*
Postangiographic complications, 1249*t*
Postcoital dysphoria, **725**
Postcoital headache, 712
Postconcussional disorder, 294, 361, 361*t*
Postconcussional syndrome, 368*t*
Postencephalitic syndrome, 368*t*
Postinfectious syndromes, 1249*t*
Postpartum blues, 526–527
Postpartum depression and psychoses, **526–527**
antidepressants for, 527
emergency manifestations of, 870, 870*t,* 911*t*
emergency treatment of, 911*t*
Postpsychotic depressive disorder of schizophrenia, **582–583**
Postsynaptic components, 93–94
Postsynaptic potentials, 89
Posttraumatic stress disorder, 87, **623–632**
and age, 630
biological factors in, 87, 625–626
brainwashing and, 629
buspirone for, 1032
in children and adolescents, 627–628
clinical features of, 627–629
cognitive-behavioral factors in, 625

comorbidity with, 624
course of, 630
diagnosis of, 626–627
diagnostic criteria for, 626–627, 626*t*
differential diagnosis of, 629, 679, 797
emergency manifestations of, 911*t*
emergency treatment of, 911*t*
epidemiology of, 624
eponyms for, 628, 628*t*
etiology of, 624–625
eye movement desensitization and reprocessing therapy, 631
Gulf War syndrome, 628–629
historical perspective on, 624
HPA axis, corticotropin-releasing factor and, 625–626
ICD-10 diagnostic criteria for, 595–598, 598*t*
noradrenergic system and, 625
opioid system and, 625
pharmacotherapy for, 630, 1004*t*, 1006, **1024,** 1032, **1037,** 1069, 1127, 1132
prognosis for, 630
propranolol for, 1009
psychodynamic factors in, 625, 625*t*
psychotherapy for, 630–631
risk factors, 624, 624*t*
September 11, 2001, 631
stressor in, 624
symptoms in, 628, 628*t*
torture and, 629
treatment of, 630–631
Posttraumatic syndromes, 1249*t*
Postural abnormalities, definition of, 281
Postural hypotension, 102
Posture
and Alexander technique, **852,** 853*f*
assessment of, 256
and Feldenkrais method, **856,** 858*f*
Potassium-sparing diuretics, and lithium, 1072*t*
Power analysis, 176
POWs, **900**
PPA. *See* Phenylpropanolamine (PPA)
PPOs, **1388**
PPVT-R, 1157*t*
Practicing, in development, 29*t*
Prader-Willi syndrome, 1163, 1164, 1165, 1171*t*
Pragmatics, 1194
Praise, in psychotherapy, definition of, 927*t*
Pramipexole, 1001*t*, **1047–1050**. *See also* Dopamine receptor antagonist(s), and precursors
Praxis, 75
Prayer, **865**
Prazepam, 1001*t*. *See also* Benzodiazepine(s)
dosage of, 1025*t*
geriatric dosage, 1332*t*
half-life of, 1025*t*
pharmacokinetics of, 1022–1023
pharmacological actions for, 1023
structure of, 1023*f*
Preattachment stage, 140
Precentral gyrus, 69*f*
Preconscious mind, **199**
Precox feeling, 491
Predictive value, of assessment instruments, 175*t*
Prednisone, for pain management, 1345*t*
Preferred provider organizations, **1388**
Prefrontal cortex, 85
regions of, 85
syndromes of, 85
Pregnancy, **868–874**
in adolescence, 38–39
and alcohol use disorders, 409–410
alternative lifestyle, 869
attitudes toward, 869
biology of, 868
bupropion and, 1030
carbamazepine and, 1038
coitus during, 869–870
complications of
and mental retardation, 1169
and reading disorder, 1181
and dopamine receptor antagonists, 1061
drug safety in, 871, 871*t*
drug use during, 24
false, 256, 281, 871–872
first trimester, 868
hyperemesis gravidarum in, 872
infertility and, 872–874
lactation. *See* Lactation
Lamaze method, 870
lithium and, 1072
marriage and, 869
modafinil in, 1121
opioid dependence in, 455
parturition and, 870
perinatal death, 874
pharmacotherapy during, **979**
pica in, **872**
postpartum blues, 526–527
postpartum depression and psychoses. *See* Postpartum depression and psychoses
prenatal screening, 871
psychology of, 868–869
psychotropics in, 871
radiation exposure during, 24
second trimester, 868
and sexual behavior, 869–870
sleep disturbance in, 773
smoking during, 24, 446
stages of, 868
teratogens in, 871
and tetracyclic drugs, 1129
third trimester, 868
and tricyclic drugs, 1129
Pregnancy tests, and dopamine receptor antagonists, 1063
Prejudice, and relational problems, 881
Premack, David, 146
Premack's principle, 146
Premature birth(s), 25, 25*f*
Premature ejaculation, **705–706,** 705*t*
ICD-10 diagnostic criteria for, 717*t*
treatment of, 713
Premature female orgasm, 712
Premenstrual dysphoric disorder, 295, **581, 878,** 878*f*
buspirone for, 1032
clinical features of, 581
course of, 581
diagnosis of, 581
differential diagnosis of, 581
epidemiology of, 581
etiology of, 581
pharmacotherapy for, 1004*t*, 1032, 1068
prognosis for, 581
research criteria for, 581, 582*t*
treatment of, 581
Premenstrual syndrome, pharmacotherapy for, 1004*t*
Prenatal disorders, 23–24
Prenatal history, 234–235
Prenatal period, **21–24**
Prenatal screening/testing, 23–24, 871
Prenatal substance exposure, 1169
Preoccupation with castration, **735–736**
Preoperational stage, 19, 28*t*
Piaget's theory of, 136–137
Preschool period, 21, **31–32**
developmental landmarks of, 22*t*, 31–32
Prescription, triplicate. *See* Triplicate prescription(s)
Prescription practices, negligent, 1352
Present State Examination, 475*t*, 489
Pressure, somatosensory, 66–68
Presynaptic components, 92–93
Prevalence, 176
definition of, 176
lifetime, 176
period, 176
point, 176
treated, 176
Preventive psychiatry, **1376–1377**
primary prevention, 1376
secondary prevention, 1376
tertiary prevention, 1376–1377
Priapism, trazodone-induced
emergency manifestations of, 911*t*
emergency treatment of, 911*t*
Pride system, 221
Primary care physicians, 1388
Primary gain, in conversion disorder, 649
Primary process thinking, 223
definition of, 283
Primate development, subhuman, **159–163**
Primatene. *See* Theophylline
Primidone
blood level data for clinical assessment, 269*t*
drug interactions, 1119
Primitive reflex circuit, 78
Primitive thinking, versus mature thinking, 956*t*
Prion disease, **364–365,** 1323
Prisoners of war (POWs), **900**
Pritikin, Nathan, 855
Pritikin diet, 855
Privacy, patients' right to, 1358
Privilege, **1353**
Probability, definition of, 176
Problem solving, assessment of, 186
Procardia. *See* Nifedipine
Process notes, 248
Prochlorperazine, 1001*t*
preparations, 1064*t*
structure of, 1052*f*
Procyclidine, 1001*t*
for extrapyramidal disorders, 1059*t*
Procyclidine hydrochloride, 1014*t*. *See also* Anticholinergic(s)
structure of, 1013*f*
Productive love, 220
Productive personality, 220
Prodynorphin, 104
Proenkephalin, 104
Professional codes, **1365**
Professional misconduct, **1371**
Professional patient syndrome. *See* Munchausen syndrome
Professional Standards Review Organization (PSRO), **1385**
Progesterone, 130
Progestins and bromocriptine, 1049
Progressive muscular relaxation therapy, **949,** 950*t*
Projection, 207*t*, 215, 222
in delusional disorder, 513
in personality disorders, 802
Projective identification, 219
in personality disorders, 803
Projective test(s), in schizophrenia, 490
Proketazine. *See* Carphenazine

Prolactin, 130, 263
hyperprolactinemia, psychological correlates of, **833**
and major depressive disorder, 539
serum, testing for, 273*t*
Prolixin. *See* Fluphenazine
Promazine, 1001*t*
preparations, 1064*t*
structure of, 1052*f*
Promethazine, 1001*t*, **1015–1017**. *See also* Antihistamine(s)
dosage and administration, 1017*t*
laboratory interferences, 1016
structure of, 1015*f*
Proopiomelanocortin, 104
Propionicacidemia, 1168*t*
Propoxyphene, 448
blood level data for clinical assessment, 269*t*
in urinalysis, 268*t*
Propranolamine, 414
Propranolol, 1002*t*, **1008–1011,** 1009*t*. *See also* β-Adrenergic receptor antagonist(s)
for aggression, 356
blood level data for clinical assessment, 269*t*
chemistry of, 1008*f*
children, use with, 1308*t*
drug interactions, 1010, 1081
for extrapyramidal disorders, 1059*t*
geriatric dosage, 1332*t*
for intermittent explosive disorder, 785
pharmacological actions of, 1009
for separation anxiety disorder, 1263
toxicity
emergency manifestations of, 911*t*
emergency treatment of, 911*t*
Proprioception, 66–68
PROs, **1385–1386**
Prosody, 78, 82, 495
definition of, 285
ProSom. *See* Estazolam
Prosopagnosia, 70
definition of, 286
Prospective studies, 171
Prostaglandin(s), neurotransmitter function, 88
Prosthetic devices, for erectile dysfunction, 716
Prostitution, in adolescence, 39
Protease inhibitors, 376–377, 376*t*
Protein kinase(s), 95*f*, 96
Protein(s)
phosphorylation, 95*f*, 96
synthesis of, 123
total serum, testing for, 273*t*
Protest stage, in children separated from mothers, 142
Prothrombin time (PT), testing for, 273*t*
Prototaxic mode, 228
Protriptyline, 1002*t*
adverse effects of, 567*t*, 981*t*, 1127*t*
for cataplexy, 769
clinical information, 1130*t*
dosage and administration, 569*t*
mechanism of action, 567*t*
for narcolepsy, 769
neurotransmitter effects of, 1126*t*
preparations of, 1130*t*
structure of, 1125*f*
Prozac. *See* Fluoxetine
Pruritus, localized, psychological correlates of, 833–834
Pruritus ani, psychological correlates of, 833–834
Pruritus vulvae, psychological correlates of, 834
Pseudocyesis, 256, **871–872**
definition of, 281
Pseudodementia, 108, 556
definition of, 287
versus dementia, 339, 340*t*
Pseudohermaphroditism, 693*t*, **735,** 735*f*
female, 734*f*
Pseudologia phantastica, 670
definition of, 284
Pseudoneurotic schizophrenia, 809
Pseudoseizures
in conversion disorder, 649
versus seizures, 359, 360*t*
PSI, 181*t*
Psilocybin, 435, 436*t*
Psoriasis, 833
psychological correlates of, **833**
PSRO, 1385
Psychedelics, 435. *See also* Hallucinogen(s)
Psychiatric care delivery, **1389–1390**
Psychiatric case register, 171
Psychiatric disorder(s)
and mixed receptive-expressive language disorder, 1198
not otherwise specified, **525–527**
opioid-induced, 453
PCP-induced, 458
postpartum psychosis, **525–526**
sedative-, hypnotic-, or anxiolytic-related, 463
shared psychotic disorder, **517–518**
substance-induced, 381*t*, 382*t*, 390, 495, **527–529**. *See also specific substance*
diagnostic criteria for, 394*t*
late-onset, 394*t*
residual, 394*t*
Psychiatric disorders, cognitive profile of, 957*t*
Psychiatric emergencies, **901–922**. *See also* Suicide
diagnosis of, 901–902, 902*f*
differential diagnosis of, 902–904
disposition of, 906–907
documentation of, 907
epidemiology of, 901
pharmacotherapy for, 906
psychotherapy for, 905–906
specific emergencies, 907*t*–912*t*
treatment of, 905
Psychiatric evaluation, of children, **1155–1160,** 1155*t*
Psychiatric history, **229–238**
format for, 229–230, 230*t*
identifying data in, 230–233
questions for, 230*t*–231*t*
Psychiatric rating scales, **296,** 298*t*
characteristics of, 296
used in DSM-IV-TR, 296
Psychiatric report, **243,** 243*t*–246*t*
Psychiatric research, categorization of patients, 109
Psychiatric treatment
of adolescents, **1295–1314, 1311–1314**
combined psychotherapy and pharmacotherapy for, 1312–1313
diagnosis in, 1311–1312
interviews in, 1312
treatment of, 1312–1313
of children, **1295–1314**
Psychiatry
and alternative medicine, 851–867
ethics in, **1365–1373**
Psychoactive substance(s). *See also* Substance abuse; Substance-related disorder(s)
definition of, 390
use, mental and behavioral disorders due to, 390, ***390t–394t***
Psychoanalysis, **923–930**
analytic process in, 925–926
analytic setting of, 925
beginnings of, 193–197
contraindications for treatment, 926
controlled clinical trials in, 929
countertransference in, **926**
dream interpretation in, 756*f*, **926**
duration of treatment, 925
free association in, 193, **925**
free-floating attention in, **925**
fundamental rule of, 925
future directions, 930
goals of, 923–925
of group, features of, 936*t*
indications for treatment, 926
interpretation in, **925–926**
meanings in, 193
principles of, 193
resistance in, **926**
schools derived from, **217–228**
scope of, 924*t*
social constructivist view of, 221
technique, 193, **210**
therapeutic action in, 923–925
therapeutic alliance in, 926
transference in, **925**
treatment by, **210**
treatment methods in, 925
use of couch in, 925
Psychoanalytic psychotherapy, **926–928**
controlled clinical trials in, 929
corrective emotional experience in, **928**
for depression, 565
expressive subtype, 923, 924*t*, **927–928**
indications for, 928*t*
expressive-supportive continuum of, 927, 927*t*
future directions, 930
goals and therapeutic action, 923–925
interventions in, definitions of, 927*t*
scope of, 924*t*
supportive subtype, 923, 924*t*, **928,** 929*t*
indications for, 928*t*
types of, 927–928
Psychoanalytic theory
versus behavioral psychology, 149*t*, 150
classic, of neurosis, **209**
and learning theory, 143
of schizophrenia, 483
tenets of, 200
Psychobiology, 224
Psychodrama, **940–941**
auxiliary ego in, 941
director in, 940–941
group in, 941
protagonist in, 941
roles in, 940–941
techniques of, 941
Psychodynamic-experiential model, of family therapy, **943**
Psychodynamic therapy
approach to depression, 960*t*
of opioid use disorders, 451
Psychogenic cardiac nondisease. *See also* DaCosta's syndrome
Psychogenic excoriation, 833, 834*f*
psychological correlates of, **833**

Psychological and behavioral factors associated with disorders or diseases classified elsewhere, ICD-10 classification of, 823*t*
Psychological factors affecting medical condition, **822–850**
  classification of, 822
  definition of, 822
  diagnostic criteria for, 823*t*
  stress theory, 822–823, 825
Psychological Screening Inventory (PSI), 181*t*
Psychological testing
  in child psychiatry, 1157*t*–1158*t*, **1158–1160**
  for children, **1151–1160**
Psychology, schools derived from, **217–228**
Psychomotor activity, in mental status examination, 238
Psychomotor agitation, definition of, 282
Psychoneuroendocrinology, **128–132**
Psychoneuroimmunology (PNI), **132–134**
  in schizophrenia, 482
Psycho-oncology, **838–839**
Psychopathology, Erikson's theory of, **215–216**
Psychopharmacology
  choice of drug in, 976–979
  classification of drugs, **974**
  clinical guidelines for, 976–979
  general principles of, **974–989**
  and neurotransmission, 88
  nonapproved dosages and uses, 977
  off-label use, 977
  pharmacodynamics of, 974–975
  pharmacokinetics of, 975–976
  pharmacological actions of, 974–976
  therapeutic failures in, 978–979, 978*t*
  therapeutic trials in, 977–978
Psychophysiological disorders, psychological correlates of, 826*t*
Psychophysiological insomnia, 765–767
Psychose passionelle, 516
Psychosexual [term], 692
Psychosexual development
  in adolescence, 36–37
  Freud's theory of, 19
  stages of, 200, 201*t*–203*t,* 217
Psychosexual development disorder(s), ICD-10 diagnostic criteria for, 727*t*
Psychosexual factors, 692–697
Psychosexuality, **692**
Psychosis. *See also* Schizophrenia
  acute delusional, **488–489**
  anxiety-blissfulness, **484,** 584
  childhood, 1282
  confusional, **484,** 584
  definition of, 276, 282
  with dementia, 108
  electroconvulsive therapy for, 1140
  in grief, 63
  hallucinogen-induced, 440
  in Huntington's disease, 75
  interviewing psychotic patients, 248–249
  motility, 583
  pharmacotherapy for, **1054–1055**
  postpartum. *See* Postpartum depression and psychoses
  risk for, with psychosomatic illness, 841
Psychosocial deprivation, differential diagnosis of, 1214
Psychosocial dwarfism, 142, 1269
  differential diagnosis of, 1269
Psychosocial growth
  universals in, 167
  variations in, 167–168
Psychosocial rehabilitation. *See* Psychosocial treatment and rehabilitation
Psychosocial therapy
  for dementia, 341
  for nicotine-related disorders, 447
  for schizophrenia, 500–502
Psychosocial treatment and rehabilitation, **966–967**
  clubhouses, **966**
  drug therapy with, 967
  milieu therapy, **966**
  results of, 967
  self-help programs, **966**
  social skills training, **964–965**
  token economy, **966,** 966*t*
  and vocational training, 966–967
Psychosomatic [term], 822
Psychosomatic illness, 215–216, 825*t*
  behavioral change, 841–842
  combined treatment of, 840
  family therapy for, 842
  group psychotherapy for, 842
  relapsing patients, 842, 842*t*
  treatment of, 840–843
    medical aspects, 841
    psychiatric aspects, 840–841
Psychosomatic medicine, 822
  historical perspective on, 822, 824*t*
  stress theory, 822–823, 825
Psychostimulant(s), 414
  for elderly, 1330, 1330*t*
Psychosurgery, **1147–1148**
  children, use with, 1311
  history of, 1147–1148
Psychotherapeutic drugs, **999–1138**
  absorption of, 975
  bioavailability of, 975
  development of new drugs, **983**
  distribution of, 975
  drug interactions, **983**
  intoxication/overdose of, **983–984,** 984*t*–988*t*
  in treatment of substance-related disorders, 388
Psychotherapeutic management, **968**
Psychotherapy, **923–973**
  for adjustment disorder, 798–799
  for alcohol use disorders, 388, 406
  for amnestic disorder, 349
  for anorexia nervosa, 745
  for antisocial personality disorder, 808
  and attachment theory, 142
  for attention-deficit/hyperactivity disorder, 1229
  for avoidant personality disorder, 813
  for borderline personality disorder, 810
  brief. *See* Brief psychotherapy
  for brief psychotic disorder, 525
  for bulimia nervosa, 750
  with children. *See also* Group psychotherapy; Individual psychotherapy
    confidentiality in, 1299
    differences from adults, 1297–1298
    Erikson's technique, 216–217
    indications for, 1299
    initial approach, 1298
    parental involvement in, 1299
    in playroom, 1298
    therapeutic interventions, 1298–1299
  current problems in, 929
  for delusional disorder, 519
  for dependent personality disorder, 814
  for depression, 561, 561*t*–564*t*
  developmentally based, 139
  for enuresis, 1258
  Erikson's view of, 216–217
  gender issues in, **929–930**
  for generalized anxiety disorder, 634–635
  for geriatric patients, 1333–1335
  for histrionic personality disorder, 811
  for HIV-infected (AIDS) patients, 378
  for identity problem, 1293–1294
  individual, for schizophrenia, 501–502
  insight-oriented. *See* Insight-oriented psychotherapy
  interpersonal. *See* Interpersonal psychotherapy
  interruption for medical emergency, with psychosomatic illness, 841
  for narcissistic personality disorder, 812
  for obsessive-compulsive disorder, 623
  for obsessive-compulsive personality disorder, 816
  for opioid use disorders, 455
  for pain disorder, 658
  for paranoid personality disorder, 804
  for passive-aggressive personality disorder, 817
  with pharmacotherapy, **967–973**
    clinical considerations, 971–972
    cost effectiveness of, 972
    one-person model of, 971
    specific disorders treated with, 968–971
    two-person model of, 971–972
  for posttraumatic stress disorder, 630–631
  referral for, by nonpsychiatric physician, 929, 929*t*
  resistance during, with psychosomatic illness, 841
  resistance to, with psychosomatic illness, 841
  for schizoid personality disorder, 805–806
  for schizotypal personality disorder, 807
  for sex addiction, 728
  for substance-related disorders, 388
  supportive. *See* Supportive psychotherapy
  types of, with children, 1296–1297
Psychotic agitation, pharmacotherapy for, 1026
Psychotic character disorder, 809
Psychotic depression, 555
Psychotic depressive disorder of schizophrenia, 294
Psychotic disorder(s). *See also* Schizophrenia
  alcohol-induced, 407, 908*t*
  amphetamine-induced, 416
  autoscopic psychosis, **525–526**
  cannabis-induced, 426
  cocaine-related, 433
  differential diagnosis of, 297*f*
  due to a general medical condition, 495
  due to a general medical condition, **352–353, 527–529**
  hallucinogen-induced, 440
  hallucinogen-related, 439, 909*t*
  with HIV infection, 376
  inhalant-related, 442, 443
  and mental retardation, 1163
  postpartum. *See* Postpartum depression and psychoses
Psychotic symptoms, pathophysiology of, 105
Psychotomimetics, 435. *See also* Hallucinogen(s)
Psychotropic(s)
  abuse, 395*t*
  antiretroviral drug interactions, 376–377
  drug interactions, 401
  effects on learning functions, 1308*t*
  laboratory tests related to, 265
  metabolism of, 533

Psychotropic(s)—*continued*
for obesity, 752
in pregnancy, 871
PT, testing for, 273*t*
Puberty, **35–36**
age of onset, 36
atypical, **1313–1314**
stages of, 35, 36*t*
Public psychiatry, **1374–1381**
community mental health, 1374–1376, **1374–1376**
deinstitutionalization, 1377
homeless mentally ill, 1377–1378
outpatient commitment programs, 1378–1379
preventive psychiatry, 1376–1377
psychogeriatric long-term care, 1378
Puerperal psychosis, **526–527**
Punishment
versus negative reinforcement, 146
and prevention of aggression, 155
Punishment dreams, 198
Punning, 239
p value, definition of, 176
Pylorospasm, 399
Pyridoxine
deficiency
medical considerations with, 847*t*
psychiatric considerations with, 847*t*
drug interactions, 1049
Pyromania, **786–787**
biological factors in, 787
clinical features of, 787
comorbidity with, 786–787
course of, 787
definition of, 786
diagnosis of, 787
diagnostic criteria for, 787, 787*t*
differential diagnosis of, 787
epidemiology of, 786
etiology of, 787
ICD-10 classification of, 793–794, 793*t*
and intermittent explosive disorder, 783
prognosis for, 787
psychosocial factors in, 787
treatment of, 787

Q

Qi-gong psychotic reactions, 531*t*
Quaalude. *See* Methaqualone
Quality of life, **1388–1389**. *See also* End-of-life care
Quantity, understanding of, 137–138, 138*f*
Quazepam, 1002*t*. *See also* Benzodiazepine(s)
chemistry of, 1022
dosage of, 1025*t*
half-life of, 1025*t*
pharmacological actions for, 1023
for primary insomnia, 765
structure of, 1023*f*
Question(s)
open-ended versus closed-ended, 8, 9*t*
opening, in interview, 8
Quetiapine, 498. *See* Serotonin-dopamine antagonist(s) (atypical antipsychotics)
adverse effects of, 498
for autistic disorder, 1215
for early-onset schizophrenia, 1285
indications for, 471, 498
mechanism of action, 478
for schizophrenia, 498
and weight gain, 752
Quinidine, blood level data for clinical assessment, 269*t*
Quinine, blood level data for clinical assessment, 269*t*

R

Rabbit syndrome, 1014. *See also* Medication-induced movement disorders
medication-induced, 997*t*
Rabbit tremor. *See* Perioral tremor
Rabies, encephalitis, 363
Race, 169
and alcohol use disorders, 396
and benzodiazepine abuse, 461
and hallucinogen use disorders, 436
and inhalant-related disorders, 441
and life expectancy, 53
and sedative, hypnotic or anxiolytic substance use disorders, 460
Racial distribution, of suicide, 914
Radiation exposure during pregnancy, 24
Rado, Sandor, **225–226,** 225*f*
Ramon y Cajal, Santiago, 88
Randolf, Theron, 856
Randomization, definition of, 176
Rank, Otto, **226,** 226*f*
The Trauma of the Birth, 226
Rape, **890–892**
date, **892**
emergency manifestations of, 911*t*
emergency psychiatric medicine, **904–905**
emergency treatment of, 911*t*
of men, **892**
statutory, **887**
of women, **890–892**
Rapid tranquilization, **906**
Rappaport, David, 221
Rapport, in interview, **6,** 7*t*
Rapprochement, 29*t*
Raskin Depression Scale, 555
Rating instruments. *See* Psychiatric rating scales
Rating scales, in child psychiatry, **1154–1155**
Rationalization, 208*t*
Rauwolfia alkaloid, structure of, 1052*f*
Raven's Progressive Matrices Test, 191*t*
Raynaud's syndrome, biofeedback for, 949*t*
Reaction formation, 205–206, 208*t*
in delusional disorder, 513
Reaction time, to stimulus, 190
Reactive attachment disorder of infancy or early childhood, **1266–1271**
clinical features of, 1267–1269
course of, 1269
diagnosis of, 1267–1269, 1267*t*
differential diagnosis of, 1269
disinhibited type, 1267–1269, 1270*t*
DSM-IV classification of, 1266–1267
epidemiology of, 1267
etiology of, 1267
and failure to thrive, 1267–1269, 1268*f*
in ICD-10, 1270, 1270*t*
inhibited type, 1267–1269
laboratory examination of, 1269
pathology of, 1269
prognosis of, 1269
subtypes of, 1267–1269
treatment of, 1270
Reactive psychosis, 520
Reading backward. *See* Reading disorder
Reading disorder, 82–83, **1180–1183**
clinical features of, 1182–1183
comorbidity with, 1181
course of, 1183
diagnosis of, 1181–1182, 1182*t*
differential diagnosis of, 1183
epidemiology of, 1180–1181
etiology of, 1181
and expressive language disorder, 1195
laboratory examination of, 1182–1183
and mathematics disorder, 1184
pathology of, 1182–1183
and phonological disorder, 1200
prognosis for, 1183
treatment of, 1183
and written expression disorder, 1186
Reading skills
assessment of, in mental status examination, 242
brain function and, 82–83
Reality
adaptation to, 205
ego relation to, 205
Gill's concept of, 221
sense of, 205
Reality principle, **200**
Reality testing, 205
definition of, 283
in group psychotherapy, 938*t*
Real self, 221
Reasoning, assessment of, 186
Rebound mania, 982
Reboxetine, 1002*t*, **1092–1093**
drug interactions, 982
Receptive-expressive language disorder, 1194
and written expression disorder, 1186
Receptive personality, 220
Reciprocal determinism, 147
Reciprocal inhibition, 148
Recommended daily allowances (RDA), 855
Recording, ethics concerning, 1373*t*
Recovered memory syndrome, **689**
Recurrent brief depressive disorder, 295, **579–581**
calcium channels inhibitors for, 1035
clinical features of, 580
course of, 580
diagnosis of, 580
diagnostic criteria for, 579
differential diagnosis of, 575, 580
epidemiology of, 580
etiology of, 580
ICD-10 diagnostic criteria, 590*t*
prognosis for, 580
research criteria for, 579, 581*t*
treatment of, 581
Recurrent depressive disorder
current episode mild, ICD-10 diagnostic criteria, 589*t*
current episode moderate, ICD-10 diagnostic criteria, 589*t*
current episode severe with psychotic symptoms, ICD-10 diagnostic criteria, 589*t*
current episode without psychotic symptoms, ICD-10 diagnostic criteria, 589*t*
currently in remission, ICD-10 diagnostic criteria, 589*t*
ICD-10 diagnostic criteria, 589*t*
Redux. *See* Dexfenfluramine
Reed, David, 44
Reflection, in interview, 9
Reflective self, 227

Reflex(es)
Babinski, 25
Moro, 25, 26*f*
newborn, 25
prenatal development of, 21
Reflexology, **865**
Reframing, in family therapy, 946
Regional cerebral blood flow (rCBF), in schizophreniform disorder, 505, 506*f*
Regitine. *See* Phentolamine
Regression, 207*t*
stress and, 139
Regression analysis, definition of, 176
Reich, Wilhelm, **226,** 226*f,* 801, 853
Reiki, **865,** 866
Reinforcement
adventitious, 146
brain stimulation and, 150, 162–163
negative, 146
partial, 145
positive, 145–146
in behavior therapy, **954**
in interview, 10
Reinforcement schedule, in operant conditioning, 145–146, 142*f*
continuous, 145
fixed-interval, 145, 142*f*
fixed ratio, 142*f*
variable-interval, 145, 142*f*
variable-ratio, 142*f*
Reinforcer(s), 145
primary, 145
secondary, 145
Reitan, Ralph, 190
Reitan-Indiana Neuropsychological Test Battery for Older Children, 1158*t*
Relapse prevention therapy (RPT), 434
Relational problems, **879–882**
definition of, 879
epidemiology of, 879
not otherwise specified, **881**
parent–child, **880**
partner, **880–881**
related to mental disorder or medical condition, **879–880**
sibling, **881**
Relationship disorders, 143
Relationship history, 235
Relative risk, definition of, 176
Relaxation response, 864
Relaxation training, 842, **948–949**
and integrative psychiatry, 866
for panic disorder, 608
progressive muscular relaxation therapy, **949,** 950*t*
for stuttering, 1205
for systematic desensitization, 951
Release therapy, with children, 1297
Reliability
in depression, 555
in mania, 556
patient's, assessment of, in mental status examination, 242–243
of schizophrenic patient, 495
in tests, 178
Religion, 2
and end-of-life care, 1347
faith healing, **865**
history-taking about, 236
and suicide, 914
Religiosity, in epilepsy, 358
Religious problem, **899**
Remedial psychotherapy, with children, 1296–1297
Remeron. *See* Mirtazapine
Renal function tests, 263–264, 264*f*
Rennie v. Klein, 1357
Reno, Janet, 427
Repetition compulsion, 200
Repetitive self-mutilation, **793**
Report, psychiatric, **243,** 243*t*–246*t*
Reporting, ethics concerning, 1373*t*
Repression, 196, 199, 208*t*
definition of, 286
and dreams, 197
Reproduction, **868–878**
assisted techniques, 873, 873*t*
rates of, in schizophrenia, 476
senescence, **877**
in sociobiology, 164
Research, ethics concerning, 1373*t*
Reserpine, 1002*t*
animal model of depression using, 163
intoxication
emergency manifestations of, 911*t*
emergency treatment of, 911*t*
mechanism of action, 100
and sleep, 759
structure of, 1052*f*
Residential treatment
with children, **1302–1303**
education in, 1303, 1304*t*
group living in, 1303
indications for, 1303
parental involvement in, 1303
setting of, 1302–1303
staff of, 1302–1303
therapy during, 1303
group psychotherapy in, 1301
Resistance, 193, 196, 210
in psychoanalysis, **926**
during psychotherapy, with psychosomatic illness, 841
to psychotherapy, with psychosomatic illness, 841
Respiratory disorder(s), psychological correlates of, **831**
Respiratory system, medical assessment of, 255
Respiratory training, for panic disorder, 608
Responsibility, excessive, 958*f*
Restless leg syndrome, **773,** 773*f*
Restoril. *See* Temazepam
Restraint(s), **1358–1359,** 1358*t*
use of, 406, 409, 493, **906,** 907*t*
Restriction fragment length polymorphism (RFLP), in substance abuse studies, 387
Reticulocyte count, 273*t*
Retina, 69
center-surround response in, 69
Retirement, 57
ethics concerning, 1373*t*
Ritonavir, drug interactions, 378
Retrospective falsification, definition of, 286
Retrospective studies, 171
Rett's disorder, 1166, **1215–1216,** 1219
clinical features of, 1216
course of, 1216
diagnosis of, 1216
diagnostic criteria for, 1216, 1216*t*
differential diagnosis of, 1216
etiology of, 1216
prognosis for, 1216
treatment of, 1216
Rett's syndrome, ICD-10 diagnostic criteria for, 1219, 1220*t*–1221*t*
Reunion, evaluation of, in child psychiatric evaluation, 1155
Reverse transcriptase inhibitors, 376–377, 376*t*
Reversibility, 138
ReVia. *See* Naltrexone
Review of systems, **254–256**
Revised Behavior Problem Checklist, **1154**
Rewards, versus reinforcers, 145
RFLP, in substance abuse studies, 387
Rhabdomyolysis, in phencyclidine (or phencyclidinelike substance) use disorder, 459
Rheumatoid arthritis, 834
psychological correlates of, **834**
Rhyming
dyslexia and, 113
gender differences in, 113
neuroimaging in, 113, 116*f*
Wernicke's area in, 113
Rhythm method, 875*t*
Ribonucleic acid (RNA), 104, **123**
Ribonucleic acid, messenger (mRNA), 104, 123
transcription, 123
Rifampin, drug interactions, 1028, 1044
Right-hand movement, brain activity and, 115*f*
Right to refuse treatment, 1357
Right to treatment, **1357**
Risk
attributable, definition of, 176
factor-related, definition of, 176
factor-specific, definition of, 176
relative, definition of, 176
Risk factor, definition of, 176
Risk-taking behavior, in adolescence, 38
Risperdal. *See* Risperidone
Risperidone, 497–499, 1002*t*. *See* Serotonin-dopamine antagonist(s) (atypical antipsychotics)
for autism, 1215
for bipolar I disorder, 570
children, use with, 1307*t*
for early-onset schizophrenia, 1285
geriatric dosage, 1332*t*
indications for, 471, 497–499
intoxication/overdose of, 988*t*
for schizophrenia, 498
for suicidal patients, 921
for Tourette's disorder, 1250
Ritalin. *See* Methylphenidate
Ritual, definition of, 282
Rivastigmine, 1002*t*
adverse effects of, 1044
for Alzheimer's disease and similar disorders, 1041
dosage of, 1044
pharmacological action of, 1042
RNA, 104, **123**
Robust aging, 56
Rocking, as stereotypic movement disorder, 1271
Rogers, Carl, **226–227,** 227*f*
and client-centered group psychotherapy, 935
Roger v. Oken, 1357
Rohypnol. *See* Flunitrazepam
Roid rage, 467
Role diffusion, Erikson's concept of, 213–214, 215
Role playing, 139
Rolf, Ida, 865
Rolfing, **865**
Romazicon. *See* Flumazenil
Roofies (drug). *See* Flunitrazepam
Rootwork, 531*t*
Ropinirole, 1002*t,* **1047–1050**. *See also* Dopamine receptor antagonist(s), and precursors

Rorschach, Hermann, 182, 183*f*
Rorschach Inkblots, 1158*t*
Rorschach test, 178, **182–183,** 183*f,* 183*t,* 490, 1159
Rotter Incomplete Sentences Blank, 1158*t*
Rouse v. Cameron, 1357
RPT, 434
Rubella, 1168
Rubinstein-Taybi syndrome, 1172*t*
Rumination disorder, in infancy or early childhood, **1242–1244**
  clinical features of, 1243
  course of, 1244
  diagnosis of, 1243
  diagnostic criteria of, 1243*t*
  differential diagnosis of, 1243–1244
  epidemiology of, 1243
  etiology of, 1243
  laboratory examination of, 1243
  pathology of, 1243
  prognosis for, 1244
  treatment of, 1244
Rush, Benjamin, 681
Rutter, Michael, 34

S

Sabshin, Melvin, 16
Sacher-Masoch, Leopold von, 721
Sadism
  Freud's concept of, 200
  sexual, 722, 722*t*
Sadistic personality disorder, 818
Sadock, Benjamin, and structured interactional group psychotherapy, 940
Sadomasochism, ICD-10 diagnostic criteria for, 726*t*
Sadomasochistic personality disorder, 818
Safe-sex guidelines, 371, 372*t*
St. John's Wort, 533, 1147
Sakel, Manfred, 1149
Salicylate
  blood level data for clinical assessment, 269*t*
  serum, testing for, 273*t*
Sample, definition of, 174
Sample from population, 177
Sanfilippo's syndrome, 1167*t*
Sangue dormido, 531*t*
SANS, 303*t*
SAPS, 304*t*
Sarno, John, 837
Sartre, Jean-Paul, **227**
Satanism, and substance abuse, 1288
Satiety, **751–752**
Satir, Virginia, and family therapy, 942
Satyriasis, definition of, 282
Saunders, Cicely, 1346
Scale for the Assessment of Negative Symptoms (SANS), 303*t*
Scale for the Assessment of Positive Symptoms (SAPS), 304*t*
Scales of Independent Behavior, 1157*t*
Scapegoating, in families, 944
Scatologia, telephone and computer, 723
Schemas, of permanent object, 136
Schilder, Paul, and imagery, 866, 958
Schizoaffective disorder, 496, **508–511**. *See also* Bipolar disorder(s); Depressive disorder(s); Schizophrenia
  age differences in, 508–509
  carbamazepine for, 1037
  in childhood, **1277**
  clinical features of, 509–510
  course of, 510–511
  definition of, 508
  diagnosis of, 509, 509*t*
  diagnostic criteria for, 509, 509*t,* 510*t*
  differential diagnosis of, 510
  emergency manifestations of, 911*t*
  emergency treatment of, 911*t*
  epidemiology of, 508–509
  etiology of, 509
  gender differences in, 508–509
  historical perspective on, 508
  outcome for, 510–511
  pharmacotherapy for, **1037,** 1054, **1068, 1132**
  prognosis for, 510–511
  psychosocial treatment of, 511
  treatment of, 511
Schizoid fantasy, 207*t*
Schizoid personality disorder, **804–806**. *See also* Personality disorder(s), cluster A
  clinical features of, 804–805
  course of, 805
  diagnosis of, 804
  diagnostic criteria for, 804, 804*t*
  differential diagnosis of, 805
  epidemiology of, 804
  pharmacotherapy for, 806
  prognosis for, 805
  psychotherapy for, 805–806
  treatment of, 805–806
Schizophrenia, **471–504**. *See also* Postpsychotic depressive disorder of schizophrenia
  affect in, 238–239, 491
  aftercare in, 497
  ambulatory, 809
  amino acids in, 478
  among immigrants, 477
  animal model of, 163
  anticonvulsant therapy for, 500
  antipsychotics for, 471, 497–499
    choice of drug, 497–499
    combined with other drugs, 500
    decisions on use, 499*f*
    in emergency, 498
    failure of drug trial, 498
    initial workup, 498
    megadose, 499
    noncompliance with, 498
    therapeutic principles, 498
    in treatment of refractory illness, 498–499
  aphasia in, 495
  appearance of patient in, 487*f,* 490–491, 492*f*
  apraxia in, 495
  Assertive Community Treatment program, 501
  auditory processing in, 126
  behavior therapy for, 954*t*
  benzodiazepines for, 500
  biological factors in, 477–482
  biological therapies for, **497–500**
  blink rate in, 495
  borderline, 489
  brain imaging in, 471, 479–481, 480*f,* 481*f*
  carbamazepine for, 500, 1037
  case management in, 501
  catatonic type, 487–488
    diagnostic criteria for, 485*t*
    differential diagnosis of, 784
    emergency manifestations of, 908*t*
    emergency treatment of, 908*t*
  with childhood onset, 490, **1282–1285**
    clinical features of, 1283–1284
    course of, 1284–1285
    diagnosis of, 1283–1284
    differential diagnosis of, 1213, 1213*t,* 1284
    DSM-IV-TR classification of, 1282
    epidemiology of, 1282
    etiology of, 1282–1283
    laboratory examinations for, 1284
    pathology of, 1284
    pharmacotherapy for, 1285, **1309–1310**
    prognosis for, 1284–1285
    psychotherapy for, 1285
    stability of diagnosis, 1285
    treatment of, 1285
  chromosomal markers in, 482
  and cigarette smoking, 444, 476
  clinical features of, **490–495**
  cognition in, 495
  cognitive behavioral therapy for, 501
  and combined psychotherapy and pharmacotherapy, **968–969**
  and complex partial epilepsy, 481
  and conversion disorder, 648
  course of, **496–497**
  cultural considerations in, 476–477
  versus delirium, 328
  delusions in, 471–472, 492–493
  versus dementia, 339
  description of, 471
  dexamethasone suppression test and, 482
  diagnosis of, **484–489**
  diagnostic criteria for, 473*t*–475*t,* 489
    DSM-IV-TR, 484–485, 484*t*
    flexible system, 474*t*
    ICD-10, 502, 502*t*–503*t*
    Langfeldt, 473*t*
    New Haven Schizophrenia Index, 473*t*
    Present State Examination, 475*t,* 489
    Research Diagnostic Criteria, 474*t*
    Schneider, 473*t*
    St. Louis Criteria, 474*t*
    Taylor and Abrams, 475*t*
    Tsuang and Winokur, 475*t*
  differential diagnosis of, **495–496,** 496*t,* 557, 674, 784, 1292
  disorganized type, 486–487
    diagnostic criteria for, 485*t*
  dopamine hypothesis of, 100, 477–478
  downward drift hypothesis of, 477
  drug augmentation therapy for, **991–992**
  DSM-IV-TR subtypes of, 485–488
    diagnostic criteria for, 484*t*
  early-onset, 489
  in elderly, 1324–1325
  electroconvulsive therapy for, 500, 1140
  electroencephalography in, 481
  electrophysiology in, 481
  emergency manifestations of, 911*t*
  emergency treatment of, 911*t*
  epidemiology of, 472–477
  etiology of, 477–484
  evoked potentials in, 481–482
  in exacerbation
    emergency manifestations of, 912*t*
    emergency treatment of, 912*t*
  eye movement dysfunction in, 482
  and family, theories about, 483–484
  family-oriented therapies for, 500–501
  feelings in, 491
  financial impact of, 477
  four As of, 85, 471–472
  GABA in, 478
  genetic factors in, 482, 482*t*
  genetics of, 123. 125–126
  geographical distribution of, 476

group therapy for, 501
hallucinations in, 84, 471–472, 491–492
cenesthetic, 492
childhood onset schizophrenia, 1283
symbolic meaning of, 483
hebephrenic, 486
historical perspective on, 471–472
and homelessness, 477
homicide in, 493–494
hospitalization for, 497
patterns in, 477
ICD-10 classification of, 485
ICD-10 diagnostic criteria, 502, 502*f*–503*f*
illusions in, 492
impulsiveness in, 493–494
infectious agents and, 133
insight in, 495
judgment in, 495
latent, 489
late-onset, 489
learning theories of, 483
lifetime prevalence of, 472
lithium therapy for, 500
and medical illness, 476
memory in, 495
and mental retardation, 1163
mental status examination in, **490–494**
mood in, 491
motor function in, 487, 491
neuroanatomy and, 84, 85
neurochemical hypotheses of, 100, 104
neuroimaging in, 109, 119
neurological findings in, 495
neuropathology of, 478–479
neurotransmitters in, 478
nonremitting, 472
norepinephrine in, 478
nuclear, 472
oneiroid, 489
onset
ages of, 475
sex differences in, 472–475
orientation in, 495
other (cenesthopathic), 489
paranoid type, 485–486
diagnostic criteria for, 485*t*
differential diagnosis of, 784
emergency manifestations of, 910*t*
emergency treatment of, 910*t*
pathophysiology of, 105, 107, 471, 477–482
perceptual disturbances in, 491–492
personal therapy for, 502
pharmacotherapy for, 497, 1004*t*, 1006, 1026, **1037, 1054, 1068**
children, **1309–1310**
decisions in, 499*f*
drug augmentation therapy, **991–992**
physical anomalies in, 495
pictures by schizophrenics, 493*f*, 494*f*
and population density, 476
postpsychotic depressive disorder of, 489, **582–583**
precox feeling with, 491
process, 472
prognosis for, **497**
factors affecting, 485*t*
pseudoneurotic, **489,** 809
psychoanalytic theories of, 483, 483*f*
psychological testing, 489–490
psychoneuroendocrinology in, 482
psychoneuroimmunology in, 482
psychosocial factors in, 471, **483–484**
psychosocial therapies for, 500–502
psychotherapy for
individual, 501–502
insight-oriented, 501–502
supportive, 501–502
recovery rates in, 496–497
reliability of patient with, 495
and reproduction rates, 476
residual type, 488
diagnostic criteria for, 485*t*
and seasonality of birth, 475–476
sensorium in, 495
serotonin in, 478
sex distribution of, 472–475
signs and symptoms of, 484*t*
accessory (secondary), 471
disorganized, 490
first-rank, 472
fundamental (primary), 471
negative, 490, 491*t*
neurological, 495
positive, 490, 491*t*
premorbid, 490
prodromal, 490
symbolic meaning of, 483
simple, 489. *See* Simple deteriorative disorder
social causation hypothesis of, 476–477
social skills training in, 500, 500*t*, 965*t*
social theories of, 484
socioeconomic considerations in, 477
speech in, 495
stress-diathesis model in, 477, 482
and substance use and abuse, 476
suicide in, 476, 493–494, **916**
tests in
intelligence, 490
personality, 490
projective, 490
psychological, 490
thought disorders in, 486, 492–493
thought in, 492–493
content of, 492–493
form of, 493
process of, 493
treatment, **497–502**
of refractory illness, 498–499
true, 472
twin studies of, 477, 480, 480*f*, 482, 482*t*
types I and II, 490, 491*t*
types of, 1283
undifferentiated type, 488
diagnostic criteria for, 485*t*
valproate for, 500
violence in, 493–494, 493*f*
vocational therapy for, 502
writing style, 493*f*
Schizophreniform disorder, 496, **505–508**
biological factors in, 505–506
brain imaging in, 505, 506*f*
clinical features, 506–507
course of, 508
diagnosis of, 506
diagnostic criteria for, 506, 507*t*
differential diagnosis of, 507–508
epidemiology of, 505
etiology of, 505–506
prognosis for, 508
treatment of, 508
Schizotypal personality disorder, **806–807,** 1282. *See also* Personality disorder(s), cluster A
clinical features of, 806
course of, 806
diagnosis of, 806
diagnostic criteria for, 806, 806*t*
differential diagnosis of, 806, 1284
epidemiology of, 806
pharmacotherapy for, 807
prognosis for, 806
psychotherapy for, 807
treatment of, 807
Schneider, Kurt, 472
School history, 235
School phobia, 1262
School refusal, 32
Schools, group psychotherapy in, 1301
School Situations Questionnaire (SSQ-R), 1158*t*
Schou, Mogens, 1067
Schreber, Daniel Paul, 513
SCID-D, 181
Scotopic sensitivity syndrome, 1181
Screen memory, definition of, 286
SDAs. *See* Serotonin-dopamine antagonist(s) (SDAs) (atypical antipsychotics)
Season, and suicide risk, 915
Seasonal affective disorder, 263
light therapy for, 1145
Seclusion, **1358–1359,** 1358*t*
Secobarbital, 460, 1002*t*. *See also* Barbiturate(s)
dosage of, 1020*t*
geriatric dosage, 1332*t*
indications for, 1018
structure of, 1018*f*
Secobarbital and amobarbital, 460
Seconal. *See* Secobarbital
Secondary gain, 233
in conversion disorder, 649
Secondary mood disorders
mood disorders due to a general medical condition. *See* Mood disorder(s), due to a general medical condition
mood disorders not otherwise specified, 585, 586*t*
substance-induced mood disorders. *See* Mood disorder(s), substance-induced
Secondary psychoses, pharmacotherapy for, **1054–1055**
Second-generation antihistamines, 1015
Secondhand smoke, 448
Second messenger(s), 94–95
Secure attachment style, 143
Secured base effect, 28
Security, versus anxiety, 28, 142
Sedation, mechanism of action, 102
Sedative-, hypnotic-, or anxiolytic-related disorder(s), 382*t*, **460–466**
buspirone for, 1032
clinical features of, 463–464
diagnosis of, 461–463
DSM-IV-TR classification of, 461–462, 461*t*
emergency manifestations of, 912*t*
emergency treatment of, 912*t*
epidemiology of, 460–461
legal issues, 465
not otherwise specified, diagnostic criteria for, 463, 463*t*
pharmacotherapy for, 1004*t*, 1032
rehabilitation, 464–465
substances, 460
treatment, 464–465
Sedative, hypnotic, or anxiolytic substance(s), 1019–1022. *See also* Barbiturate(s); Benzodiazepine(s)
abuse, 462
patterns of, 463–464
anxiety disorders, 463
delirium, 463
dependence, 462
drug interactions, 401, 1007

Sedative, hypnotic, or anxiolytic substance(s)—*continued*
for elderly, 1331–1332
intoxication, 462
diagnostic criteria for, 461–462, 461*t*
mood disorders, 463
neuropharmacology of, 461
overdose, 464
treatment of, 465
persisting amnestic disorder, 463
persisting dementia, 463
psychotic disorders, 463
sexual dysfunction, 463
sleep disorders, 463
use
intravenous, 464
oral, 463
and race, 460
sex distribution of, 460
withdrawal, 462–463
diagnostic criteria for, 461–462, 462*t*
pharmacotherapy for, 1018, 1132
Sedative(s). *See also* Sedative-, hypnotic-, or anxiolytic-related disorder(s)
definition of, 460
herbal, 533
intoxication, acute, diagnostic criteria for, 391*t*
use disorders, 382*t*
withdrawal, diagnostic criteria for, 393*t*
Seizure disorder. *See also* Epilepsy
emergency manifestations of, 912*t*
emergency treatment of, 912*t*
medical considerations with, 846*t*
psychiatric considerations with, 846*t*
Seizure(s)
absence, **357,** 358*f*
alcohol
emergency manifestations of, 908*t*
emergency treatment of, 908*t*
with alcohol withdrawal, 404, 404*t*
barbiturates for, 1018
classification of, 356–357, 358*t*
cocaine-related, 434
complex partial, definition of, 282
definition of, 282, 356
and electroconvulsive therapy, 1142–1143
electroencephalography in, 120, 357*f*, 358*f*, 359*f*
focus, 120
generalized, 120, **356–357**
generalized tonic-clonic, definition of, 282
international classification of, 358*t*
partial, **357,** 358*f*
versus pseudoseizures, 359, 360*t*
simple partial, definition of, 282
treatment of, 360
Selective abstraction, 958*f*
Selective inattention, definition of, 280
Selective mutism, **1265–1266**
clinical features of, 1265–1266
course of, 1266
diagnosis of, 1265–1266, 1265*t*
differential diagnosis of, 1197, 1266
epidemiology of, 1265
etiology of, 1265
in ICD-10, 1266
and language disorders, 1200*t*
prognosis of, 1266
treatment of, 1266
Selective serotonin reuptake inhibitors (SSRIs), 92, 103, **1093–1104**. *See also specific agent*
for adjustment disorders, 799
adverse reactions to, 981*t*, 1098–1100
for alcoholism, 413
for anxiety disorders, 353
for autistic disorder, 1215
chemistry of, 1093, 1093*f*
children, use with, 1307*t*
clinical guidelines for, 1102–1104
for cocaine users, 435
dosage of, 1102–1104
drug interactions, 982, 1028, 1062*t*, 1100–1102
CYP-induced, 976
for elderly, 1329
for generalized anxiety disorder, 636
implicated in sexual dysfunction, 711
indications for, 496, 1095–1098
for intermittent explosive disorder, 785
laboratory interferences, 1102
mechanism of action, 567*t*
for mood disorder due to a general medical condition, 352
for mood disorders, 352
for obsessive-compulsive disorder, 622
for panic disorder, 607
pharmacological actions of, 1093–1095
precautions with, 1098–1100
for separation anxiety disorder, 1263
withdrawal from, 982
Selegiline, 1002*t*, 1076. *See also* Monoamine oxidase inhibitors
chemistry of, 1076*f*
for cocaine users, 435
Self
actual, 221
grandiose, 223
Horney's concept of, 221
idealized, 221
real, 221
reflective, 227
true, 228
Self-actualization, 221, 223, 226
Self-determination, and oppositional defiant disorder, 1232
Self-direction, 226225
Self-efficacy, 147
Self-esteem
in Freud's concept of narcissism, 204
and written expression disorder, 1186
Self-help groups, **939–940**
alcohol-related disorders, 413
in grief, 65
Self-injury, 1271
in mental retardation, 1163
pharmacological intervention for, 1177–1178
repetitive self-mutilation, **793**
Self-object transferences, 223
Self psychology, goal of, 925
Self-realization, 221
Self-references, 958*f*
Self-regulation, 226
Self-reliance, growth of, 141
Self-revelation, 10
Self-stimulation, limbic system and, 84
Self-system, 228
Self-therapy, for stuttering, 1205
Seligman, Martin, 161
Selye, Hans, 822–823
Semans, James H., 713
Semantic processing, 82
Semantics, 1194
Semiotic function, 137
Semiotics, 223
Senescence, 51
reproduction, **877**
Senile plaque, in Alzheimer's disease, 126, 332
Senses, primary, **66–72**
Sensitivity
of assessment instruments, 175*t*
definition of, 177
Sensitization, 147–148
Sensorimotor period, 19, 28*t*
Piaget's theory of, 136, 134*t*
Sensorium
in elderly, 1320
in mania, 556
in mental status examination, 240–242
in schizophrenia, 495
Sensory deprivation, **163**
characteristic symptoms of, 163
theories of
cognitive, 163
physiological, 163
psychological, 163
Sensory perception, conscious, alteration of, through hypnosis, 74
Sensory stimuli, response to, in autism, 1211
Sensory system(s), **66–74**
activity-dependent mechanisms in, 68
association areas in, 70, 70*f*, 77–78
auditory, **71,** 73
autonomic, 72
cell specialization in, 69
disorders of, 66–67, 70–71
and evoked potentials, 121–122
feature extraction in, 66, 68–69, 78
genetic mechanisms in, 68
nature and nurture in, 69
neuroimaging in, 113
olfaction, **71–72,** 74
paradigms for, 68–69
role of, 66–67
somatosensory, **66–68,** 67*f*, 72–73
taste, **72**
visual, **68–71,** 70*f*, 73
Sentence Completion Test, 178, 183*t*, **185**
Separation, 142
animal studies of, 159–160
evaluation of, in child psychiatric evaluation, 1155
Separation anxiety, 29, 32, 142
Separation anxiety disorder, 142, **1259–1265**
biopsychosocial factors in, 1259
characteristics of, 1262*t*
in children, pharmacotherapy for, **1309**
clinical features of, 1260–1262
course of, 1262–1263
diagnosis of, 1260–1262, 1260*t*
differential diagnosis of, 1262, 1262*t*
DSM-IV-TR classification of, 1259
epidemiology of, 1259
etiology of, 1259–1260
genetic factors in, 1260
in ICD-10, 1263, 1263*t*–1264*t*
learning factors in, 1260
pharmacotherapy for, 1263
prognosis for, 1262–1263
treatment of, 1263
Separation-individuation, 29, 29*t*
September 11, 2001, 631
Sequential Tests of Educational Progress (STEP), 1160
Serax. *See* Oxazepam
Serentil. *See* Mesoridazine
Serlect. *See* Sertindole
Serological studies, 109
Seroquel. *See* Quetiapine

Serotonergic agents. *See also specific agent*
for generalized anxiety disorder, 636
Serotonergic receptors, 102–103
effector mechanisms, 93*t*
effects of, 102–103
Serotonergic tracts, of central nervous system, 102, 103*f*
Serotonin, 73, 88, **102–104**
and aggression, 154
in animal models, 127
antidepressant effects on, 567*t*
in anxiety disorders, 594–595
and drugs, 92, 102
laboratory testing for, 263
life cycle, 102
in major depressive disorder, 536–537
metabolism, 97*f*
neurotransmitter function, 90*t*, 91*f*, 93*t*
in panic disorder, 600
and personality, 801
and psychopathology, 104
receptors, 93*t*, 102–103
in schizophrenia, 478
synthesis of, 97*f*, 102
type 2 blockade, antidepressants and, 567*t*
Serotonin discontinuation syndrome, 982–983
Serotonin-dopamine antagonist(s) (SDAs) (atypical antipsychotics), 100, 1050, **1104–1113**
augmentation of, **991**
for autistic disorder, 1215
chemistry of, 1105, 1105*f*
clinical guidelines, 1111–1113
dosage of, 1111–1113
drug interactions, 1110–1111
for early-onset schizophrenia, 1285
indications for, 1106–1110
for intermittent explosive disorder, 785
pharmacological actions of, 1105–1106
for schizophrenia, 497–499
early-onset, 1285
Serotonin-specific reuptake inhibitors. *See* Selective serotonin reuptake inhibitors; *specific agent*
Serpasil. *See* Reserpine
Sertindole, 498. *See* Serotonin-dopamine antagonist(s) (atypical antipsychotics)
adverse effects of, 498
indications for, 471, 498
for schizophrenia, 498
Serotonergic pathways, 79*f*
Sertraline, 1002*t*. *See also* Selective serotonin reuptake inhibitors
adverse effects of, 567*t*, 981*t*
children, use with, 1307*t*
for conduct disorder, 1238
dosage and administration, 569*t*
for elderly patients, 1329
intoxication/overdose of, 988*t*
mechanism of action, 103
for posttraumatic stress disorder, 630
for schizoaffective disorder, 511
for separation anxiety disorder, 1263
withdrawal from, 982
Serum glutamic pyruvic transaminase. *See* Alanine aminotransferase
Serzone. *See* Nefazodone
SES. *See* Socioeconomic status (SES)
Session length, **12**
Sex, limbic system and, 84
Sex addiction, **726–729, 793**
behavioral patterns of, 727–728
comorbidity with, 728
diagnosis of, 727
pharmacotherapy for, 728–729
psychotherapy for, 728
signs of, 727*t*
treatment of, 728
Sex compulsivity, **726–729**
Sex distribution
of alcohol use disorders, 396
of anabolic (androgenic) steroid abuse, 466
of benzodiazepine abuse, 461
of hallucinogen use, 436
of schizoaffective disorder, 508–509
of schizophrenia, 472–475
of sedative, hypnotic or anxiolytic substance use disorders, 460
of suicide, 913
Sex drive
in adolescence, 36
androgens for, 715
estrogen for, 715
gender differences in, 696
libido, 692
Freud's concept of, **199,** 204
Jung's concept of, 19
in pregnancy, 869
Sex hormones, effects of, in adolescence, 36
Sex-reassignment surgery, **737**
Sex role behavior, and gender, 166
Sex roles, development of, **32–33**
Sex therapy, 954*t*
analytically oriented, 714
specific techniques, 713
Sexual abuse
of adults, **890–892**
of children, **885–887,** 886*t*
emergency manifestations of, 909*t*
emergency psychiatric medicine, **904–905,** 909*t*
recovered memories of, **1364**
Sexual activity, in old age, 57
Sexual arousal, and aggression, 154
Sexual arousal disorder(s), 701*t*, **703–704,** 703*t*
female, 703, 703*t*
male. *See* Erectile dysfunction
Sexual assault. *See* Rape
Sexual aversion, ICD-10 diagnostic criteria for, 717*t*
Sexual aversion disorder, 701*t*, 702–703, 702*t*
Sexual behavior, 694–697
changes in, in epilepsy, 359
changes in, in pregnancy, 869–870
Sexual coercion, **892**
Sexual desire
androgens to increase, 715
antiandrogens to decrease, 715–716
antiestrogens to decrease, 715–716
disorders, 701*t*, **702–703,** 702*t*
lack or loss of, ICD-10 diagnostic criteria for, 717*t*
Sexual development, in toddler period, 30
Sexual dimorphism, 164
Sexual disorder(s), not otherwise specified, 725–729, 727*t*
Sexual dysfunction(s), **701–718**
alcohol-induced, 408, 711
amphetamine-induced, 417
behavior therapy for, 714, 954*t*
biological treatments for, 714–715
cannabis-induced, 427, 711
cocaine-related, 433
defined, 701
definition of, 701
dopamine receptor antagonists for, 1049
dual-sex therapy for, 712–713
female, due to a general medical condition, 709, 710*t*
due to a general medical condition, **354–355,** 354*t*, **707–709,** 707*t*
group therapy for, 714
hallucinogen-related, 711
hormone therapy, 715
hypnotherapy for, 713–714
ICD-10 classification of, 716
ICD-10 diagnostic criteria for, 716, 717*t*
male, due to a general medical condition, **707–709,** 707*t*
mechanical treatments, 715, 716
neurophysiology of, 709, 709*t*
not otherwise specified, 712, 712*t*
opioid-induced, 453, 711
pharmacological agents implicated in, 708*t*–709*t*, 710–712, **710–712,** 710*t*, 715–716
pharmacotherapy for, 714–716, 1004*t*, 1137
and psychotherapeutic drugs, **980–981**
sedative-, hypnotic-, or anxiolytic-related, 463
sexual response cycle, dysfunctions not associated with, 701, 702*t*
substance-induced, 381*t*, 382*t*, 709*t*–710*t*, 710. *See also specific substance*
surgical treatments, 716
treatment of, 712–716
Sexual enjoyment, lack of, ICD-10 diagnostic criteria for, 717*t*
Sexual exploitation of patient, 1363, 1363*t*
Sexual harassment in the workplace, 881, **893**
educational material to reduce, 893*t*
Sexual history, **237,** 237*t*, 699, 699*t*–700*t*
in elderly, 1318–1319
Sexual identity. *See* Gender identity
Sexual instinct, Freud's concept of, 199
Sexual intercourse
in adolescence, 37
outside marriage, and divorce, 50
during pregnancy, 869–870
withdrawal method of contraception, 875*t*
Sexuality
laws and, 699
in midlife, 47
normal, **692–701**
Sexualization, 208*t*
Sexual learning in childhood, 692
Sexually transmitted diseases (STDs), **877–878**
AIDS. *See* Acquired immune deficiency syndrome
blood test for, 264–265
syphilis. *See* Syphilis
Sexual masochism. *See also* Paraphilias
clinical features of, 721
diagnosis of, 721
diagnostic criteria for, 721, 722*t*
Sexual maturation disorder, ICD-10 diagnostic criteria for, 727*t*
Sexual orientation, 694
ego-dystonic, 698
ICD-10 diagnostic criteria for, 727*t*
neuroanatomy and, 78
persistent and marked distress about, **729**
Sexual pain disorders, **706–707**
Sexual preference
disorders of, ICD-10 diagnostic criteria for, 726*t*
multiple disorders of, ICD-10 diagnostic criteria for, 726*t*
other disorders of, ICD-10 diagnostic criteria for, 726*t*

Sexual relations, between patient and therapist, **1368**
Sexual relationship disorder, ICD-10 diagnostic criteria for, 727*t*
Sexual response cycle, **694–696**
female, 695*t*, 696*f*
male, 694*t*, 696*f*
phase 1: desire, 695
sexual dysfunctions related to, 701*t*
phase 2: excitement, 694*t*, 695, 695*t*
sexual dysfunctions related to, 701*t*
phase 3: orgasm, 694*t*–695*t*, 695–696
sexual dysfunctions related to, 701*t*
phase 4: resolution, 694*t*–695*t*, 696
sexual dysfunctions related to, 701*t*
and sexual dysfunctions, 701*t*
not associated with sexual response cycle, 701, 702*t*
Sexual sadism. *See also* Paraphilias
clinical features of, 722
diagnosis of, 722
diagnostic criteria for, 722, 722*t*
Sexual seduction, childhood, and Freud's concept of neuroses, 196–197
SGOT. *See* Aspartate aminotransferase
SGPT (serum glutamic pyruvic transaminase). *See* Alanine aminotransferase
Shalala, Donna, 427
Shamanism, **865**
Shame
definition of, 281
Erikson's concept of, 215
Shaping behavior, 146
Shared psychotic disorder, **517–518,** 814
diagnostic criteria for, 517, 517*t*, 518*t*
Shell shock, 624
Shenjing shuariuo, 531*t*
Shen-k'uei, 531*t*
Shin-byung, 531*t*
Shneidman, Edwin, 921
on suicide, 913
Shock, in dying person, 60
Short stature, psychosocially determined, 1269
Short-term anxiety-provoking psychotherapy, **932,** 933*t*
requirements for, 932
techniques of, 932
Short-term dynamic psychotherapy, **931–932**
requirements for, 932
techniques of, 932
Shy bladder, 609
behavior therapy for, 954*t*
Shyness
and separation anxiety disorder, 1259
transient adaptational, 1266
and transient mutism, 1266
Sibling relational problems, **881**
Sibling rivalry, 31, **881**
Sibling rivalry disorder, 1264*t*
Sibutramine, 1002*t*, **1113–1114**
drug interactions, 982
for weight reduction, 755, 982
Sickle cell anemia, genetics of, 123
Sickle-thalassemia, 124
Sick-old, 50
Sifneos, Peter, and short-term anxiety-provoking psychotherapy, 932
Sigma (Σ) receptors, neurotransmitter function, 96, 107
Signal anxiety, 209
Signal indicators, 142
Signs and symptoms, **275–287, 280–287**
index to, 276*t*–279*t*
on rating instruments, 296
Sildenafil, 355, 714–715, 980, 1002*t*, **1114–1116**
adverse reactions to, 1115
chemistry of, 1114, 1114*f*
clinical guidelines for, 1116
dosage of, 1116
drug interactions, 1116
indications for, 1115
laboratory interferences, 1116
pharmacological actions of, 1114–1115
precautions with, 1115
Sill, Andrew Taylor, 864
Simple deteriorative disorder, 295, 489
Simple schizophrenia. *See* Simple deteriorative disorder
Simultagnosia, 71
definition of, 286
Sinequan. *See* Doxepin
Single photon emission computed tomography (SPECT), 108, **113**
of brain, 113
for cognitive disorders, **113,** 323
for Creutzfeldt-Jakob disease, 364
in obsessive-compulsive disorder, 109
pharmacological and neuropsychological probes, 119
in schizophrenia, 481
superimposition with other neuroimages, 113, 116*f*
Skin, visual assessment of, 257
Skin disorder(s), psychological correlates of, **833–834**
Skinner, B.F., 143–145, **227,** 227*f*
Skinner box, 145
Skin sampling, fetal, 23
Skin-to-skin contact, in bonding, 140
SLE. *See* Systemic lupus erythematosus (SLE)
Sleep, 756
abnormalities, and major depressive disorder, 539
alcohol effects on, 399, 781
in children, 33
definition of, 756
and depression, 134*f*, 135, 759
dreaming during, 756*f*, 758
in dysthymic disorder, 573
electrophysiology of, 756–757
functions of, 759
inadequate sleep hygiene, 765
induction of, 767*t*
insufficient, **773**
nicotine effects on, 781
non-rapid eye movement, 756–758
normal, **756–760**
paradoxical, 756
pattern of, 758*f*
patterns, 757*f*
rapid eye movement, 119
behavior disorder of, **777**
polysomnogram findings in, 756–758
polysomnogram measures of, 760*t*
regulation of, 758–759
requirements for, 759
in toddler period, 30
Sleep apnea
obstructive syndrome, **770**
laboratory recordings of, 770, 771*f*
nasal continuous positive airway pressure of, 770, 771*f*
polysomnogram measures of, 760*t*
Sleep attacks, 769
Sleep deprivation, 759, **1145**
Sleep disorder(s), **760–781.** *See also specific disorder*
alcohol-induced, 408
amphetamine-induced, 417
associated with medical-psychiatric disorders, in ICSD, 764*t*
associated with mental disorders, in ICSD, 764*t*
associated with neurological disorders, in ICSD, 764*t*
barbiturates for, 1018
breathing-related, **769–770**
caffeine-induced, 419, 423
cannabis-induced, 427
circadian rhythm, **771–773**
classification of, 761–763
cocaine-related, 433
in DSM-IV-TR, 761–762
due to general medical condition, **779–780**
diagnostic criteria for, 779*t*
in elderly, 1326
due to a general medical condition, **353–354,** 354*t*
in ICD-10, 763, 766*t*
in ICSD, 763, 764*t*
inadequate sleep hygiene, 765
major symptoms of, 760–761
and mental disorders, **353–354,** 354*t*, 764*t*, 777
nicotine-related, 781
opioid-induced, 453
pharmacotherapy for, 1004*t*, 1075
phototherapy for, 1145
polysomnogram measures of, 760*t*
in pregnancy, 773
primary, **763–777**
proposed, in ICSD, 764*t*
related to another mental disorder, **777**
sedative-, hypnotic-, or anxiolytic-related, 463
sleep state misperception, 767
substance-induced, 381*t*, 382*t*, **780–781,** 780*t*. *See also specific substance*
Sleep drunkenness, **774**
Sleep efficiency, polysomnogram measures of, 760*t*
Sleep history questionnaire, 761, 762*t*
Sleep hygiene, 765, 767*t*
Sleep latency, polysomnogram measures of, 760*t*
Sleep-onset REM period, polysomnogram measures of, 760*t*
Sleep paralysis, 769, **777**
Sleep-related abnormal swallowing syndrome, **779**
Sleep-related asthma, **779**
Sleep-related bruxism, **776–777**
Sleep-related cardiovascular symptoms, **779**
Sleep-related chronic paroxysmal hemicrania, **779**
Sleep-related cluster headaches, **779**
Sleep-related epileptic seizures, **779**
Sleep-related gastroesophageal reflux, **779–780**
Sleep-related head banging, **777**
Sleep-related hemolysis, **780**
Sleep schedule, alteration of, **1145**
Sleep state misperception, 767
Sleeptalking, **777**
Sleep terror disorder, **775**
in children, pharmacotherapy for, **1310**
diagnostic criteria for, 775*t*
polysomnogram of, 775
Sleep terrors, in ICD-10, 766*t*

Sleep–wake cycle, 134
Sleep–wake pattern, disorganized, 772–773
Sleep–wake rhythm, **759**
Sleep–wake schedule disturbance, **761**
in ICD-10, 766*t*
Sleepwalking, 33
definition of, 282
in ICD-10, 766*t*
Sleepwalking disorder, **775–776**
case example of, 776
in children, pharmacotherapy for, **1310**
diagnostic criteria for, 776*t*
differential diagnosis of, 678–679
Smell. *See also* Olfaction
patient's, assessment of, 257
Smith-Magenis syndrome, 1171*t*
Smoke-free environments, 448
Smoking. *See also* Nicotine
among psychiatric patients, 444
cessation of
bupropion for, 1030, 1031
health benefits of, 446
hypnosis for, 843
treatments for, 446–448
death caused by, 444–445
drug interactions, 1028, 1062*t*
epidemiology, 444
and health care costs, 444
during pregnancy, 24, 446
prevalence of, 444
rate of quitting, 444
in schizophrenia, 444, 476
treatment, 446–448
trends in, 444
Smooth pursuit eye movements, in personality disorders, 801
Soapers (drug). *See* Methaqualone
Social activity, history of, 236
Social and Occupational Functioning Assessment Scale (SOFAS), 296, 305*t*
Social anxiety disorder of childhood, 1264*t*
Social constructivist view, of psychoanalysis, 221
Social deprivation syndromes, 28
Social development
in infancy, 22*t*, 26
in preschool period, 22*t*, 31–32
in toddler period, 22*t*, 30
Social interaction, qualitative impairments, in autism, 1210–1211
Social isolation, studies with monkeys, 159–160, 159*f*, 160*t*
rehabilitation of abnormal behavior in, 160–161
Sociality, 167
Social learning theory, 143, **146–147**
Social network therapy, **944–945**
Social Readjustment Rating Scale, 825*t*
Social relatedness, evaluation of, in child psychiatric evaluation, 1156
Social relationship history, 235
Social Security, 57
Social skills training, **964–965**
in behavior therapy, **953**
goals of, 965–966
information-processing, 965–966
and mathematics disorder, 1184
methods of, 965
perception skills, 965
and prevention of aggression, 156
results of, 965
for schizophrenia, 965*t*
in schizophrenia, 500, 500*t*
Sociobiology, **163–164**
Socioeconomic status (SES)
and alcohol-related disorder(s), 396–397
and autistic disorder, 1208
and bipolar I disorder, 536
and elderly, 56–57
and major depressive disorder, 536
and schizophrenia, 477
and women, 57
Sodium, serum, testing for, 273*t*
Sodium bicarbonate, and lithium, 1072*t*
Sodium bicarbonate infusion, 271*t*
Sodium chloride, and lithium, 1072*t*
Sodium lactate, provocation of panic attacks with, **267**
Sodium methohexital, for systematic desensitization, 951
SOFAS, 296, 305*t*
Soft signs, 1156
Soldier's heart, 624
Solitary confinement, 163
Soma. *See* Carisoprodol
Somatic syndrome, ICD-10 diagnostic criteria, 588*t*
Somatization, 207*t*
Somatization disorder, **643–647**
biological factors in, 645
clinical features of, 644*t*, 645–646
and conversion disorder, 648
course of, 646
diagnosis, 645, 645*t*
diagnostic criteria for, 645, 645*t*
differential diagnosis of, 646
epidemiology of, 643–645
etiology of, 645
historical perspective on, 643
ICD-10 diagnostic criteria, 659*t*
prognosis for, 646
psychosocial factors in, 645
treatment of, 647
Somatoform autonomic dysfunction, ICD-10 diagnostic criteria, 659*t*–660*t*
Somatoform disorder(s)
clinical features of, 644*t*
definition of, 643
differential diagnosis of, 673–674, 679
DSM-IV-TR classification of, 643, 644*t*
in elderly, 1325–1326
ICD-10 diagnostic criteria, 659, 659*t*–660*t*
not otherwise specified, 658*t*, **659**
other, ICD-10 diagnostic criteria, 660*t*
undifferentiated, **658–659,** 658*t*. *See also* Neurasthenia
ICD-10 diagnostic criteria, 659*t*
unspecified, ICD-10 diagnostic criteria, 660*t*
Somatopagnosia, definition of, 286
Somatosensory evoked potentials, 122
Somatosensory system, **66–68,** 72–73
modalities of, 66–68, 67*f*
organization of, 66–68, 67*f*
prenatal development of, 67–68
Somatostatin, 105, 263
and major depressive disorder, 538–539
Somatotopic organization, 66, 67*f*
Somatotropin release-inhibiting factor, 128, 129*t*
Somnambulism, 33. *See also* Sleepwalking
definition of, 282
Somniloquy, **777**
Somnolence, 760
definition of, 280
and psychotherapeutic drugs, **982**
Sontag, Susan, 59
Sopor. *See* Methaqualone
Sound therapy, **865**
Sparine. *See* Promazine
Spastic dysphonia, differential diagnosis of, 1204
Special K (drug). *See* Ketamine
Specificity
of assessment instruments, 175*t*
definition of, 177
Specificity hypothesis, 218
Speck, Richard, 155*f*
SPECT. *See* Single photon emission computed tomography (SPECT)
Spectinomycin, and lithium, 1072*t*
Speech
assessment of, 257
brain function and, 82
definition of, 284
disturbances in, definition of, 284–285
evaluation of, in child psychiatric evaluation, 1156
evolution of, 72*f*
excessively loud or soft, definition of, 285
impaired, 73
in manic episode, 555–556
in mental status examination, 239
nonspontaneous, definition of, 284
normal development of skills, 1195*t*
poverty of, definition of, 284
poverty of content of, definition of, 285
pressure of, definition of, 284
prosody, 78, 82, 495
recognition, 71, 73
in schizophrenia, 495
Speech disorders
and developmental coordination disorder, 1190
and expressive language disorder, 1195
and mixed receptive-expressive language disorder, 1198
phonological disorder. *See* Phonological disorder
stuttering disorder. *See* Stuttering
Speech Foundation of America, 1205
Speech therapy
for mixed receptive-expressive language disorder, 1199
for phonological disorder, 1202
for stuttering, 1205
Speedballs (drug), 434
Speed (drug), 414
Spell, 531*t*
Spelling disorder. *See also* Written expression disorder
Spelling dyslexia. *See also* Written expression disorder
Spermatogenesis, induction of, 873*t*
Sphincter control, in toddler period, 30
Spiegel, David, 838
Spiegel, Herbert, on hypnosis, 960
Spikenard, 854*t*
Spike threshold, 88
Spirituality, 2
Spiritual problem, **899**
Spironolactone, and lithium, 1072*t*
Spitz, René, 28, 142
Splinter functions, in autism, 1212
Split personality. *See* Dissociative identity disorder
Splitting
dissociation and, 676
in personality disorders, 802
Split treatment, **1352–1353**
Spontaneous abortion, 874
Spousal bereavement, 1327
Spousal relational problems, **880–881**

Spouse abuse, **890**
  physician reference card, 891*t*
Squeeze technique, 713
SRA Basic Reading Program, 1183
SSQ-R, 1158*t*
SSRIs. *See* Selective serotonin reuptake inhibitors (SSRIs)
Stadol. *See* Butorphanol
Stagnation, Erikson's concept of, 46, 214
Stalking, **893**
Stammering. *See* Stuttering
Standard deviation, definition of, 177
Standardization, in testing, 178
Standardized score, 177
Stanford-Binet Intelligence Scale, 4th edition, 1157*t*, 1159
State-dependent learning, 143
Statistic(s)
  descriptive, 174
  glossary of terms, 174–177
  inferential, 174
Status epilepticus, 404, 434
Status offenses, definition of, 1317
Statutory rape, **887**
STDs. *See* Sexually transmitted diseases (STDs)
Steiner, Rudolf, 852–853
Stelazine. *See* Trifluoperazine
STEP, 1160
Stepparents, 34
Stereotypic movement disorder, **1271–1273**
  clinical features of, 1271–1272
  concurrent disorders, 1272
  course of, 1272
  diagnosis of, 1271–1272, 1272*t*
  differential diagnosis of, 1272
  DSM-IV-TR classification of, 1271
  epidemiology of, 1271
  etiology of, 1271
  in ICD-10, 1273*t*
  pharmacotherapy for, 1272–1273
  prognosis of, 1272
  treatment of, 1272–1273
Stereotypy, definition of, 281
Sterilization, 875*t*, **876–877**
Steroid(s)
  abuse, 395*t*
    anabolic (androgenic), **466–468**
  anabolic (androgenic). *See also* Anabolic (androgenic) steroid(s)
Stevens-Johnson syndrome, 571
Stillbirths, 874
Stimulant(s), 413–414
  abuse, 461
  adverse effects of, 1309*t*
  for children and adolescents, 156, 1307*t*
    adverse effects of, 1311
  herbal, 533
  intoxication, acute, diagnostic criteria for, 391*t*
  for mood disorder due to a general medical condition, 352
  withdrawal, diagnostic criteria for, 394*t*
Stimulus
  in classical conditioning, 143
  conditioned, 144
  generalization, 144
  unconditioned, 143
Stirling County Study, 172
Stop-start technique, 713
STP. *See* 2,5-dimethoxy-4-methylamphetamine
Stranger anxiety, 29, 142, 1259
Strange situation, 141, 141*t*
Stress
  adjustment disorders. *See* Adjustment disorder(s)
  and anxiety, 592
  and coronary artery disease, **829–830**
  endocrine responses to, 823
  factors, specific versus nonspecific, 826
  general adaptation syndrome, 822–823
  immune response to, 132–133, 825
  interviews, 248
  maternal, transmission to fetus, 23
  and mood disorder, 540–541
  neurotransmitter responses to, 823
  nonspecific stress theory, 826
  on physician, 14–15
  psychological, and illness or death, 1
  and regression, 139
  severe, reactions to
    ICD-10 classification of, 595–598
    ICD-10 diagnostic criteria for, 595–598, 598*t*
  specific stress theory, 826
  syndromes, animal models of, 161, 162*f*
  theory of, 822–823, 825
  unpredictable, in animal model, 162
  vicissitudes of life and, 825–826
  and weight gain, 256
  workplace and, **895**
Stress-diathesis model, 477, 482
Stressors, and adjustment disorders, 795–799
Stroke
  and depression, 108
  neuroimaging and, 108
Strokes, psychological, Berne's concept of, 219
Stroop Color Word Test, 191*t*
Structural model, of family therapy, **943**
Structured clinical diagnostic assessments, 181
Structured Clinical Interview for DSM-IV Dissociative Disorders (SCID-D), 181
Structured interactional group psychotherapy, 940
Stupor, definition of, 280
Stuttering, **1202–1205**
  clinical features of, 1204
  comorbidity with, 1203
  course of, 1204–1205
  definition of, 285, 1202
  diagnosis of, 1204, 1204*t*
  differential diagnosis of, 1204
  epidemiology of, 1203
  etiology of, 1203–1204
  phases of, 1204
  prognosis for, 1204–1205
  treatment of, 1205
Subacute sclerosing panencephalitis, neuropsychiatric manifestations of, 363
Subarachnoid hemorrhage, 254
Subdural hematoma, 254
Subhuman primate development, **159–163**
Sublimation, 208*t*
Subpoena duces tecum, 1353
Substance abuse. *See also* Substance-related disorder(s); *specific substance*
  among adolescents, **1286–1289**
    clinical features of, 1287–1288
    and comorbidity, 1287
    diagnosis of, 1287–1288
    DSM-IV-TR classification of, 1287
    epidemiology of, 1286–1287
    etiology of, 1287
    genetic factors in, 1287
    multiple substance abuse, 1287
    pharmacotherapy for, 1288
    psychosocial factors in, 1287
    treatment of, 1288–1289
  and attention-deficit/hyperactivity disorder, 1227
  current trends, 385–386
  definition of, 1287
  differential diagnosis of, 575, 674, 1237
  in elderly, 1326
  epidemiology of, 383–386
  and intermittent explosive disorder, 783
  during pregnancy, 24
  in schizophrenia, 476
Substance dependence, 381, 382*t*. *See also* Substance-related disorder(s); *specific substance*
  and aggression, 154
  behavioral, 381
  codependence, 381, 383
  and combined psychotherapy and pharmacotherapy, **970**
  course modifiers, 381, 384*t*
  current trends, 385–386
  definition of, 381, 1287
  diagnostic criteria for, 381, 383*t*, 392*t*–393*t*
  epidemiology of, 383–386
  etiology of, 386–387, 386*f*
    behavioral theories of, 386*f*, 387
    genetic factors in, 387
    neurochemical factors in, 387, 388*f*
    psychodynamic factors in, 386–387
  mood disorder and, 351*t*
  of non-dependence-producing substances, diagnostic criteria for, 395*t*
  physical, 381
  psychological, 381
  and suicide, **917**
Substance exposure, prenatal, 1169
Substance-induced
  agitation, pharmacotherapy for, 1026
  amnestic disorders. *See* Amnestic disorder(s)
  anxiety disorders. *See* Anxiety disorder(s)
  delirium, 324–325, 325*t*, 329, 381*t*, 382*t*, 458, 463. *See also specific substance*
  delusions, in substance-induced psychotic disorders, 528
  dementia. *See* Dementia
  depression, etiology of, 584, 585*t*
  disorders, in DSM-IV, 293, 381*t*, 382*t*
  hallucinations, in substance-induced psychotic disorders, 528
  mood disorders. *See* Mood disorder(s)
  perceptual disturbances. *See specific substance*
  psychiatric disorders. *See* Psychiatric disorder(s)
  sexual dysfunctions, 381*t*, 382*t*, 709*t*–710*t*, 710. *See also specific substance*
  sleep disorders, 381*t*, 382*t*, **780–781,** 780*t*. *See also specific substance*
Substance intoxication, 382*t*. *See also specific substance*
  acute, diagnostic criteria for, 390*t*
  definition of, 1287
  delirium, 381*t*, 382*t*
  diagnostic criteria for, 381, 383*t*
Substance P, 132
  neurotransmitter function, 90*t*, 104
Substance-related disorder(s), **380–470**. *See also* Substance abuse; Substance dependence; *specific substance*
  in adolescence, **1314**
  and antisocial personality disorder, 387–388
  brain reward systems in, 387, 388*f*

comorbidity with, 387–388, 389
comparative nosology of, 380
and depression, 388
differential diagnosis of, 1292
epidemiology of, 383
etiology of, 386–387
and factitious disorders, 668
and generalized anxiety disorder, 632
managed care and, 389–390
other (or unknown), 468–470
overview of, 380–395
and pathological gambling, 788
polysubstance related disorder, 470
and posttraumatic stress disorder, 624
psychotherapy for, 388
rehabilitation, **388–390**
substances associated with, 380, 382*t*
and suicide, 388
terminology, 380–381, 383
treatment, **388–390**
approaches in, 388
drug therapy in, 388
goals of, 388
for other or unknown substances, 470
and trichotillomania, 790
Substance-seeking behavior, 386*f*, 387, 387*f*
Substance withdrawal, 382*t*. *See also specific substance*
definition of, 1287
delirium, 381*t*, 382*t*, 393*t*
diagnostic criteria for, 381, 383*t*, 393*t*
emergency manifestations of, 912*t*
emergency treatment of, 912*t*
Substitutions, in phonological disorders, 1201
Successive approximation, 146
Succinylcholine, 1138
drug interactions, 1044
and lithium, 1072*t*
Sucking reflex, 136
Sudden death, 59
ADHD patients on desipramine, 1228
associated with antipsychotic medication
emergency manifestations of, 912*t*
emergency treatment of, 912*t*
of psychogenic origin
emergency manifestations of, 912*t*
emergency treatment of, 912*t*
Suggestibility, disturbances of, definition of, 280
Suggestion techniques, for stuttering, 1205
Suicidal behavior, cognitive profile of, 957*t*
Suicidal ideation, 1279
definition of, 280
Suicidal patients
brain MRI, 111*f*
as high-risk clinical situation, **1354**
interviewing, 249
Suicide, **913–922**
by adolescents, 34, **1279–1281, 1314**
biological factors in, 1280
clinical features of, 1280
diagnosis of, 1280
epidemiology of, 1279
etiology of, 1280
genetic factors in, 1280
social factors in, 1280
treatment of, 1280–1281
age distribution of, 914, 914*f*
and alcohol abuse/dependence, **916**
and alcohol use disorders, 397, **397**
from amantadine overdoses, 1012
anxiety disorder and, **917**
associated factors, 913–917
biological factors, 918, 918*f*
Cushing's syndrome and, 915
Danish-American adoption studies, 918–919
and dementia, 915
in depression, **916,** 918, 921
Durkheim's theory of, 917
dying patients' requests for, 1349–1350
in elderly, 58, 1319, 1326–1327
emergency manifestations of, 912*t*
emergency treatment of, 912*t*
endocrine disorders and, 915
epidemiology of, 913–917
ethical considerations, 921
etiology of, 917–918
Freud's theory of, 917
genetic factors, 918
and HIV-infected (AIDS) patients, 375–376
Huntington's disease and, 75
incidence of, 913
legal considerations, 921
marital status and, 914
Menninger's theory of, 917
mental health and, 915
methods, 915
molecular genetic studies, 919, 919*f*
National Strategy for Suicide Prevention, 921–922
occupation and, 914–915
panic disorder and, 606
parasuicidal behavior, 919
dialectical behavior therapy for, 954
personality disorders and, **917**
physical health and, 915
physician-assisted, **1348–1349**
potential, treatment of, 920–921
inpatient versus outpatient, 920–921
prediction, 919
prevalence of, 913
prevention, 920–921
National Strategy for Suicide Prevention, 921–922
previous suicidal behavior and, 917, 917*f*
in psychiatric patients, 915–917
psychological factors in, 917–918
racial distribution of, 914
rates
by age group and sex, 914*f*
by state, 913
in young people, 914
recent theories of, 917–918
religion and, 914
risk
evaluation of, 920, 920*t*
factors, 913, 913*t*
in schizophrenia, 476, 493–494, **916**
seasonality, 915
sex distribution of, 913
sociological factors in, 917
substance dependence and, **917**
and substance-related disorders, 388
twin studies, 918
Sullivan, Harry Stack, 32, **227–228,** 228*f*
life-cycle theory of, 19
theory of schizophrenia, 472, 483
Sulloway, Frank, 33–34
Sulpiride, 497
chemistry of, 1053
structure of, 1052*f*
Summation, in interview, 9
Sundowner syndrome, **337**
Sundowning, definition of, 280
Suomi, Stephen, 160
Superconducting quantum interference devices, 121
Superego, 204–205, 222
in character formation, 209
Superego anxiety, 209, 593
Superego lacunae, and childhood/adolescent antisocial behavior, 1292
Supervision, ethics concerning, 1373*t*
Supervisors, use of, **12**
Supportive group therapy, features of, 936*t*
Supportive interventions, 247–248, 247*t*
Supportive psychotherapy
for anxiety disorder due to a general medical condition, 353
for phobias, 615
for schizophrenia, 501–502
Suppression, 208*t*
Surgeon General's Report on the Health Consequences of Smoking: Nicotine Addiction, The, 444
Surgical unit, consultation-liaison psychiatry in, 849, 849*t*
Surmontil. *See* Trimipramine
Suronacrine, for Alzheimer's disease and similar disorders, 1042
Surrogate mothers, 873*t*
Survival analysis, 177
Survival systems, newborn, 25
Survivor guilt, 61
Suspicious patients, 13–14
Susto, 531*t*
Sydenham, Thomas, 643
Sydenham's chorea, 1249*t*
Syllogistic reasoning, 137
Symadine. *See* Amantadine
Symbiosis (symbiotic phase), 29*t*
Symbol Digit Modalities Test, 191*t*
Symbolic representation, in dreams, 198
Symbolization, 136
Symmetrel. *See* Amantadine
Sympathomimetics (and related drugs), 414, **1116–1122**
adverse effects, 1119, 1119*t*
augmentation of, **990**
cardiovascular effects, 1117
central nervous system effects, 1117
chemistry of, 1116, 1117*f*
dosage and administration, 1120, 1120*t*
drug interactions, 1119–1120, 1123, 1129
effects on specific organs and systems, 1117
endocrine effects, 1117
implicated in sexual dysfunction, 711
indications for, 1118–1119
laboratory interferences, 1120
pharmacological actions of, 1116–1117
precautions with, 1119
withdrawal
emergency manifestations of, 912*t*
emergency treatment of, 912*t*
Synapse(s), **91–96,** 92*f*
axoaxonic, 91
axodendritic, 91
axosomatic, 91
chemical, 91
components of, 92–94
conjoint, 91
electrical, 90, 91
Synaptic cleft, 91
Synaptic compartment, 93
Synaptic pruning, 86
in schizophrenia, 478
Synaptic transmission, process of, 975
Synaptogenesis, 86
Syncope, in elderly, 1327, 1327*t*
Synesthesia
definition of, 285
in hallucinogen use disorders, 439
Syntaxic mode, 227

Synthroid. *See* Levothyroxine; Thyroxine
Syphilis, 1168
tertiary
medical considerations with, 847*t*
psychiatric considerations with, 847*t*
tests for, 264–265
Systematic desensitization, 148, **951**
adjunctive use of drugs in, 951
and desensitization of stimulus, 951
hierarchy construction in, 951, 952*t*
indications for, 951
Systemic lupus erythematosus (SLE), 834, 835*f*
medical considerations with, 846*t*
neuropsychiatric manifestations of, 365
psychiatric considerations with, 846*t*
psychological correlates of, **834**
Szasz, Thomas, 16, 1357

T

T4. *See* Thyroxine (T4)
Tacrine, 341, 1002*t*
adverse effects of, 1044
for Alzheimer's disease and similar disorders, 1041
dosage of, 1044
drug interactions, 1044
intoxication/overdose of, 988*t*
pharmacological action of, 1042
serum transaminase levels, monitoring, 267
Tactile agnosia, 67
Tai chi chuan, **865–866**
Taijin kyofu sho, 531*t*
Talking down, in phencyclidine (or phencyclidinelike substance) use disorders, 459
Talwin. *See* Pentazocine
Tangentiality, 239
definition of, 283
Taping, ethics concerning, 1373*t*
Taractan. *See* Chlorprothixene
Tarasoff v. Regents of University of California, 1355, 1356*f*
Tardive dyskinesia, 100, 255, 497–499, 982
as high-risk clinical situation, 1354
differential diagnosis for, 1059, 1060*t*
emergency manifestations of, 912*t*
emergency treatment of, 912*t*
neuroleptic-induced, dopamine receptor antagonists and, 1059–1060
and mental retardation, 1177–1178
pharmacotherapy for, 1006
Tardive seizures, and electroconvulsive therapy, 1142–1143
Tardive Tourette's disorder syndromes, 1249*t*
T-ASI, 1288
Task assignments, graded, 958, 958*f*
Taste, **72**
TAT, 1158*t*, 1159
Tau protein, 126
in Alzheimer's disease, 331
in familial multiple system taupathy, 332–333
Tay-Sachs disease, 1167*t*
Teen Addiction Severity Index (T-ASI), 1288
Tegretol. *See* Carbamazepine
Television violence, aggression and, 32, 153, 153*t*
Temazepam, 1002*t*. *See also* Benzodiazepine(s)
dosage of, 1025*t*
geriatric dosage, 1332*t*
half-life of, 1025*t*
pharmacological actions for, 1023
structure of, 1023*f*
Temperament
genetics and, 162
inborn differences in, 26
Temperature, somatosensory, 66–68
Temporal arteritis, 254
Temporality, 176
Temporal lobe epilepsy (TLE), 83
emotional intensity in, 83
hyposexuality in, 83
neuroimaging in, 111*f*, 117*f*
and schizophrenia, 83
viscosity in, 83
Temporal lobe(s)
and emotion, 84
functions of, 80*t*
injury, 83
and language, 82
in memory impairment, 82
and schizophrenia, 84, 109
Temporal lobe syndrome(s), 903, 904*t*
Temporal lobe tumor(s)
medical considerations with, 844*t*
psychiatric considerations with, 844*t*
Temporomandibular joint (TMJ) pain, 949*t*
Tender years doctrine, 1315–1316
Tennessee Self-Concept Scale (TSCS), 181*t*
Tenormin. *See* Atenolol
Tension, definition of, 281
Tension headache
biofeedback for, 949*t*
psychological correlates of, **838**
Tension myositis syndrome, 837
Tension reduction theory, 148–150
Teratogen(s), 24
in pregnancy, 871
Terminal care decisions, **1340–1342**
Terrible 2s, 215
Terrorism, 631
Testamentary capacity, 1360–1361
Testicular feminization syndrome, 693*t*
Test of Early Written Language (TEWL), 1187
Test of Language Development-2, 191*t*
Test of Written Language (TOWL), 1187
Testosterone, 130, 263, 466, **1147**
serum, testing for, 273*t*
Test(s). *See also* Neuropsychological assessment; Personality, assessment; *specific test*
integration of findings, 185
objective, 178
projective, 178
reliability in, 178
in schizophrenia, 490
types of, 178
validity in, 178
Tetrabenazine, mechanism of action, 100
Tetracyclic drugs, **1125–1131**
adverse effects, 1127–1129, 1127*t*
allergic effects, 1128
anticholinergic effects, 1127–1128
autonomic effects, 1128
cardiac effects, 1128
chemistry of, 1125, 1125*f*
clinical guidelines, 1129–1130
dosage, 1129–1130
drug interactions, 982, 1014, 1028, 1119, 1129
CYP-induced, 976
effects on specific organs and systems, 1126
failure of drug trial, 1131
hematological effects, 1128
indications for, 1126–1127
intoxication/overdose of, 988*t*, 1130
laboratory testing with, 265
and MAOI, combination therapy with, 570
neurological effects, 1128
neurotransmitter effects of, 1126*t*
for panic disorder, 607
pharmacodynamics of, 1128*f*
pharmacological actions of, 1126
plasma concentrations, 1130
precautions with, 1127–1129
preparations of, 1130*t*
psychiatric effects, 1127
and sedation, 1128
termination of short-term treatment, 1131
therapeutic drug monitoring, 1130
and treatment-resistant depression, 1131
withdrawal from, 982
Tetracycline, and lithium, 1072*t*
Tetrahydrocannabinol (THC), 425, 427
drug interactions, 1047
TEWL, 1187
Thalamus
and arousal, 80
and rhythmical cortical activity, 120
and seizures, 120
somatosensory fibers in, 66–67
Thanatology, **58–65**
Thanatos, 151, 200, 917
THC. *See* Tetrahydrocannabinol (THC)
Thematic Apperception Test, 178, 183*t*, **184–185,** 184*f*, 225, 490
Thematic Apperception Test (TAT), 1158*t*, 1159
Theophylline, 419
blood level data for clinical assessment, 269*t*
drug interactions, 976, 1046, 1047
and lithium, 1072*t*
Therapeutic alliance, in psychoanalysis, 926
Therapeutic communities, for opioid use disorders, 455–456
Therapeutic touch, **866**
Thiamine deficiency, 82, 406, **1146**
medical considerations with, 847*t*
neuropsychiatric manifestations of, 367
psychiatric considerations with, 847*t*
Thiamylal. *See also* Barbiturate(s)
structure of, 1018*f*
Thiazides, and lithium, 1072*t*
Thinking
abstract, 138, 139
assessment of, in mental status examination, 242
definition of, 287
animistic, 60, 137
definition of, 282
form of, **239–240**
generalized disturbances in form or process of, definition of, 283
hypotheticodeductive, 138
parataxic mode, 227
primary process, 199, 223
primitive versus mature, 956*t*
prototaxic mode, 227–228
secondary process, 205
syntaxic mode, 227226
Thiopental, 1002*t*. *See also* Barbiturate(s)
structure of, 1018*f*
Thioridazine, 1002*t*. *See also* Dopamine receptor antagonist(s)
blood level data for clinical assessment, 269*t*
children, use with, 1307*t*
geriatric dosage, 1332*t*
indications for, 498
and lithium, 1072*t*

preparations, 1064*t*
structure of, 1052*f*
Thiothixene, 1002*t*
children, use with, 1307*t*
geriatric dosage, 1332*t*
preparations, 1064*t*
structure of, 1052*f*
Thioxanthenes, 1051*t*
chemistry of, 1053
Thomas, Alexander, 26
Thorazine. *See* Chlorpromazine
Thorndike, Edward L., 144
Thought
cognitive therapy, automatic thoughts in, 957
content, **240**
definition of, 239
in delusional disorder, 514
evaluation of, in child psychiatric evaluation, 1156
poverty of, definition of, 283
in schizophrenia, 492–493
specific disturbances in, definition of, 284
in delusional disorder, 514
in depression, 555
disturbances, in elderly, 1319–1320
electroencephalography of, 121
form of
in schizophrenia, 493
specific disturbances in, definition of, 283
in mania, 556
in mental status examination, 239–240, 240*t*
in obsessive-compulsive disorder, 620
operational, 137
process, **239–240**
definition of, 239
in schizophrenia, 493
trend or preoccupation of, definition of, 284
Thought broadcasting, definition of, 284
Thought control, definition of, 284
Thought disorder(s), 239, 239*t*
differential diagnosis of, 902, 904*t*
in schizophrenia, 486, 492–493
Thought insertion, definition of, 284
Thought process, evaluation of, in child psychiatric evaluation, 1156
Thought stoppage, 958–959
Thought withdrawal, definition of, 284
Three-dimensional constructional praxis test, 188*f*
Throat, medical assessment of, 255
Thumb sucking, 1271
Thymine, 123
Thyroid axis, and major depressive disorder, 538
Thyroid disorder(s), neuropsychiatric manifestations of, 365–366
Thyroid function tests, 260–261, 262*t*, 273*t*
Thyroid hormone(s), 130, **1122–1123**. *See also* Thyroxine
adverse effects, 1122–1123
augmentation of, **990**
chemistry of, 1122, 1122*f*
dosage and administration, 1123
drug interactions, 1123
effects on specific organs and systems, 1122
indications for, 1122
intoxication/overdose of, 988*t*
laboratory interferences, 1123
pharmacological actions of, 1122
precautions with, 1122–1123
Thyroid scan, 262*t*
Thyrotoxicosis
emergency manifestations of, 912*t*
emergency treatment of, 912*t*
Thyrotropin-releasing hormone (TRH), 91*f*, 128, 129*t*, 130
in schizophrenia, 482
stimulating test, 260–261, 263*t*
Thyroxine (T4)
serum, laboratory evaluation of, 260, 262*t*
structure of, 1122*f*
Tibetan medicine, **866**
Tic disorder(s), **1246–1253**. *See also* Chronic motor or vocal tic disorder; Transient tic disorder
differential diagnosis of, 1248, 1249*t*, 1272
ICD-10 classification of, 1252
ICD-10 diagnostic criteria for, 1252*t*
not otherwise specified, 1252, 1252*t*
pharmacotherapy for, 1004*t*, 1005
Tic(s). *See also* Chronic motor or vocal tic disorder
complex, 1246
definition of, 282, 1246
motor, 1246
simple, 1246
in Tourette's disorder, 1247
vocal, 1246
Time-limited psychotherapy, **931**. *See also* Brief psychotherapy
interpersonal. *See* Interpersonal psychotherapy
requirements for, 931
techniques of, 931, 932*t*
Time orientation, evaluation of, in child psychiatric evaluation, 1155
Tinbergen, Nicholaas, **159**
Tindal. *See* Acetophenazine
Tinea capitus, 791*f*
Title 18. *See* Medicare
Title 19. *See* Medicaid
TLE. *See* Temporal lobe epilepsy (TLE)
TM, **864**
TMJ, 949*t*
TMS. *See* Transcranial magnetic stimulation (TMS)
Tobacco. *See also* Nicotine; Smoking
intoxication, acute, diagnostic criteria for, 392*t*
smokeless
adverse effects of, 444
use, 444
prevalence of, 444
withdrawal, diagnostic criteria for, 394*t*
Toddler period, 21, **30–31**
developmental landmarks of, 22*t*, 30
Toddler(s), developmental tasks of, 212–213, 215
Tofranil. *See* Imipramine
Toilet training, 30, 215
history-taking about, 235
Token economy, **966,** 966*t*
Token Test, 191*t*
Tolerance-indignation, 217
Toluene abuse
emergency manifestations of, 912*t*
emergency treatment of, 912*t*
Topamax. *See* Topiramate
Topiramate, 1002*t*, **1089–1093**
adverse reactions to, 1091
for bipolar I disorder, 570, 571
chemistry of, 1089, 1089*f*
dosage of, 1092
drug interactions, 1091
indications for, 1090
laboratory interferences, 1091
pharmacological actions of, 1090
precautions with, 1091
and weight gain, 752
Tort, 1359
Torture victims, **900**
posttraumatic stress syndrome among, **629**
Touch, light, 66–68
Tourette, Georges Gilles de la, 1246
Tourette's disorder, **1246–1250**. *See also* Tic disorder(s)
and attention-deficit/hyperactivity disorder, 1246
in children, pharmacotherapy for, **1309**
clinical features of, 1247–1248
course of, 1248
definition of, 1246
diagnosis of, 1247–1248
diagnostic criteria for, 1247*t*
differential diagnosis of, 1248, 1249*t*
epidemiology of, 1246
etiology of, 1246–1247
genetics of, 123, 125, 1246
immunological factors in, 1247
as multigenic trait, 125
neuroanatomical factors in, 1246–1247
neurochemical factors in, 1246–1247
and obsessive-compulsive disorder, 617, 618, 621, 1246
and pathological gambling, 788
pathology and laboratory examination in, 1248
pharmacotherapy for, 1004*t*, 1005, **1055,** 1250
postinfection, 1247
prognosis for, 1248
and stereotypic movements, 1271
tics in, 1247
treatment of, 1250
Tower of Hanoi, 191*t*
Toxin(s)
exposure to, syndromes associated with, 628, 628*t*
neuropsychiatric symptoms caused by, 367
Toxoplasmosis, 1168
Trager, Milton, 866
Trager method, **866**
Trailing phenomenon, definition of, 285
Trail Making Test, 191*t*, 1158*t*
Trait(s)
biological, 219–220
environmentally learned, 219–220
genetic, 124–125
personality, 218
Trance, definition of, 280
Trance and possession disorders, ICD-10 diagnostic criteria for, 690*t*
Trance state, **964**
indicators of, 962*t*
Transaction, definition of, 219
Transactional group therapy
classification of, 935
features of, 936*t*
Transcendental meditation (TM), **864**
Transcranial magnetic stimulation (TMS), **121, 1144–1145**
techniques of, 1144
Transcription factors, 123
Transference, **4,** 193, 210
definition of, 193
and gender issues, 929–930
in group psychotherapy, 938*t*
in group therapy, 936*t*
idealizing, 223
mirror, 223
outside of psychotherapy, 968
in psychoanalysis, **925**

Transference—*continued*
with psychosomatic illness, 840
self-object, 223
in social constructivist view, 221
twinship, 223
Transference neurosis, 925
Transient adaptational shyness, 1266
Transient ischemic attacks
in cocaine use disorders, 434
differential diagnosis of, 339
Transient tic disorder, **1251–1252**
clinical features of, 1251–1252
course of, 1252
definition of, 1251
diagnosis of, 1251–1252
diagnostic criteria for, 1252, 1252*t*
epidemiology of, 1251
etiology of, 1251
prognosis for, 1252
treatment of, 1252
Transitional object, 28, 141, 205, 228
Transplantation issues, in consultation-liaison psychiatry, 849–850
Transinstitutionalization, **1377**
Transvestic fetishism, 735. *See also* Paraphilias
clinical features of, 722–723
diagnosis of, 722–723
diagnostic criteria for, 722–723, 723*t*
ICD-10 diagnostic criteria for, 726*t*
Tranxene. *See* Clorazepate
Tranylcypromine, 1002*t*, 1076. *See also* Monoamine oxidase inhibitors
adverse effects of, 981*t*
chemistry of, 1076*f*
dosage and administration, 569*t*
drug interactions, 1047
for elderly patients, 1329
mechanism of action, 567*t*
pharmacological action of, 1072–1073
Traumatic mutism, 1265
Trazodone, 1002*t*, **1123–1125**
adverse effects of, 567*t*, 981*t*, 1124
for bulimia nervosa, 750
chemistry of, 1123, 1123*f*
dosage and administration, 569*t*, 1124
drug interactions, 982, 1007, 1124
effects on specific organs and systems, 1123–1124
implicated in sexual dysfunction, 711
indications for, 1124
for intermittent explosive disorder, 785
intoxication/overdose of, 988*t*
mechanism of action, 103, 567*t*
precautions with, 1124
Treated prevalence, 176
Tremor(s)
with alcohol withdrawal, 403, 404*t*
definition of, 282
essential, 256
lithium-induced, 102, 1070
patient's, in medical assessment, 256
Treponema pallidum, 264
TRH. *See* Thyrotropin-releasing hormone (TRH)
Trial-and-error learning, 144
Triamterene, and lithium, 1072*t*
Triangulation, in Bowen model of family therapy, 943
Triazolam, 463, 1002*t*. *See also* Benzodiazepine(s)
dosage of, 1025*t*
drug interactions, 378, 1081
CYP-induced, 976
geriatric dosage, 1332*t*
half-life of, 1025*t*
pharmacokinetics of, 1022
for primary insomnia, 765
structure of, 1023*f*
Triazolobenzodiazepines, adverse effects of, 981*t*
Triazolopyridines, adverse effects of, 981*t*
Trichotillomania, **790–792,** 791*f*
clinical features of, 790
comorbidity with, 790
course of, 792
definition of, 282, 790
diagnosis of, 790
diagnostic criteria for, 790, 790*t*
differential diagnosis of, 791, 791*f*
epidemiology of, 790
etiology of, 790
ICD-10 classification of, 793–794, 793*t*
laboratory examination, 791
pathology of, 791
pharmacotherapy for, 1069
prognosis for, 792
treatment of, 792
Tricyclic drugs (tricyclic antidepressants), **1125–1131**
adverse effects, 1127–1129, 1127*t*
allergic effects, 1128
for anorexia nervosa, 745
anticholinergic effects, 1127–1128
for attention-deficit/hyperactivity disorder, 1224, 1228
autonomic effects of, 1128
cardiac effects, 1128
children, use with, 1307*t*
with cholinesterase inhibitors, 1044
clinical guidelines, 1129–1130
in combination with benzodiazepines, 1029
with dopamine receptor antagonists, 1049
dosage, 1129–1130
drug interactions, 982, 1007, 1014, 1028, 1047, 1119, 1129
CYP-induced, 976
effects on specific organs and systems, 1126
for elderly, 1329
failure of drug trial, 1131
hematological effects, 1128
implicated in sexual dysfunction, 711
indications for, 496, 1126–1127
for intermittent explosive disorder, 785
intoxication/overdose of, 988*t*, 1130
laboratory testing with, 263, 265
and lithium, 1072*t*
and MAOI, combination therapy with, 570
mechanism of action, 92, 102
for mood disorder due to a general medical condition, 352
neurological effects, 1128
neurotransmitter effects of, 1126*t*
overdose, 998*t*
for panic disorder, 607
pharmacodynamics of, 1128*f*
pharmacological actions of, 1126
plasma concentrations, 1130
precautions with, 1127–1129
preparations of, 1130*t*
psychiatric effects, 1127
and sedation, 1128
for separation anxiety disorder, 1263
termination of short-term treatment, 1131
therapeutic drug monitoring, 1130
and treatment-resistant depression, 1131
withdrawal from, 982
Trifluoperazine, 1002*t*
blood level data for clinical assessment, 269*t*
children, use with, 1307*t*
detection of, by magnetic resonance spectroscopy, 112
geriatric dosage, 1332*t*
preparations, 1064*t*
structure of, 1052*f*
for Tourette's disorder, 1250
Triflupromazine, 1002*t*
geriatric dosage, 1332*t*
preparations, 1064*t*
structure of, 1052*f*
Trigeminal neuralgia, acupuncture for, 1145
Triglycerides, effects of alcohol on, 400
Trihexyphenidyl, 1002*t*
for extrapyramidal disorders, 1059*t*
Trihexyphenidyl hydrochloride, 1014*t*. *See also* Anticholinergic(s)
structure of, 1013*f*
Triiodothyronine, laboratory evaluation of, 260, 262*t*
Trilafon. *See* Perphenazine
Trimipramine, 1002*t*
adverse effects of, 567*t*, 981*t*, 1127*t*
clinical information, 1130*t*
dosage and administration, 569*t*
mechanism of action, 567*t*
neurotransmitter effects of, 1126*t*
preparations of, 1130*t*
structure of, 1125*f*
Triplicate prescription(s), 465
disadvantages of, 466*t*
True self, 228
Trust
basic, 221
Erikson's concept of, 19, 215
L-Tryptophan
deficiency, and poor sleep patterns, 758, 1146
dosage and administration, 570
mechanism of action, 103–104
for obsessive-compulsive disorder, 623
for primary insomnia, 765
Tryptophan hydroxylase, 97*f*, 102
TSCS, 181*t*
Tsuang, Ming T., 484
T-Test, 177
Tubal ligation, **877**
Tuberculosis, 108
Tuberculosis sclerosis complex 1 and 2, 1172*t*
Tuberoinfundibular tract, 97, 98, 99*f*,
Tuberose, 854*t*
Tuberous sclerosis, **1166**
Turner's syndrome, 693*t*, **733,** 733*f*
Twilight state, definition of, 280
Twinship transference, 223
Twin studies
of aggression, 154
on alcohol abuse, 1287
of bipolar I disorder, 540
identical twins reared apart, 164–165
of major depressive disorder, 540
of mood disorders, 540
of personality, 167
of schizophrenia, 477, 480, 480*f*, 482, 482*t*
of suicide, 918
Twirling, definition of, 282
Type A behavior, behavior therapy for, 954*t*
Type I error, definition of, 177
Type II error, definition of, 177
Tyramine-induced hypertensive crisis, and monoamine oxidase inhibitors, 1078
Tyrosine, 1146
Tyrosine hydroxylase, 98
Tyrosine kinase receptor, 93

Tyrosine kinase(s), 96
Tyrosinosis, 1167*t*

U

Ulcerative colitis, psychological correlates of, **827**
Ultrasound, carotid, 270*t*
Ultrasound examinations, 23
Unconditional positive regard, 226
Unconditioned response, 143
Unconscious mind, 193, **199,** 222
  and dreams, 197
Unconsummated marriage, 726
Undifferentiated somatoform disorder, **658–659,** 658*t*
Undifferentiated wholeness stage, 224
Unemployment, in early adulthood, 43
Uniform Determination of Death Act, 58
Uniform Rights of the Terminally Ill Act, 1341
Unio mystica, definition of, 284
United States v. Brawner, 1362
Universalization, in group psychotherapy, 938*t*
Ure, Alexander, 1067
Urea, and lithium, 1072*t*
Urea cycle disorders, 1168*t*
Uremic encephalopathy, 366
Urethral stage, 202*t*
Uric acid, effects of alcohol on, 401
Urinalysis, 273*t*
  for mental retardation, 1174
  for substance abuse, 268, 268*t*
Urinary retention, and psychotherapeutic drugs, **982**
Urophilia, 724

V

Vacuum pumps, for sexual dysfunction, 716
Vagal nerve stimulation (VNS), **1145**
Vagina dentata, 702
Vaginismus, **706–707,** 706*t*
  nonorganic, ICD-10 diagnostic criteria for, 717*t*
  treatment of, 713
Vaillant, George, 20
  developmental theory of, 46–47, 56
Valences, 223
Validity, in tests, 178
Valium. *See* Diazepam
Valproate, 1002*t,* **1131–1135**
  adverse effects, 1132–1133, 1133*t*
  for bipolar I disorder, 570, 571, 1134*t*
  with carbamazepine, 1039
  chemistry of, 1131, 1132*f*
  dosage and administration, 1135
  drug interactions, 378, 1133–1134, 1134*t*
  effects on specific organs and systems, 1133
  geriatric dosage, 1330*t*
  indications for, 500, 1132
  laboratory interferences, 1135
  laboratory testing with, 264
  pharmacokinetics of, 1135*t*
  pharmacological actions of, 1131–1132
  precautions with, 1132–1133
  preparations, 1135*t*
  serum levels, monitoring, 267
  and weight gain, 752
Valproic acid, 1002*t,* 1131
  for affective lability and impulsivity, 356
  for bipolar I disorder, 570
  with bupropion, 1031
  with carbamazepine, 1039
  chemistry of, 1131, 1132*f*
  for cocaine users, 435
  drug interactions, 1031, 1062*t*
  indications for, 360
  intoxication/overdose of, 988*t*
Values, history-taking about, 238
Vanillylmandelic acid (VMA), 263
Variable(s)
  definition of, 177
  dependent, 175
  dependent, definition of, 177
  independent, definition of, 177
Variant Creutzfeldt-Jakob disease, 364–365
Vascular dementia. *See* Dementia, vascular
Vasectomy, 875*t,* **877**
Vasopressin, neurotransmitter function, 105
Vasovagal syncope, 830
VDRL test, 264, 273*t*
Vegetative signs, definition of, 281
Vegetative state, persistent, 80
Venereal Disease Research Laboratory (VDRL) test, 264, 273*t*
Venlafaxine, 1002*t,* **1135–1137**
  adverse reactions to, 567*t,* 981*t,* 1136
  for attention-deficit/hyperactivity disorder, 1228
  chemistry of, 1135, 1135*f*
  dosage and administration, 569*t,* 1136
  drug interactions, 982, 1136
  for elderly depression, 1330
  for elderly patients, 1329
  for generalized anxiety disorder, 636
  implicated in sexual dysfunction, 711
  indications for, 1136
  intoxication/overdose of, 988*t*
  laboratory interferences, 1136
  mechanism of action, 102, 103, 567*t*
  for mood disorders, 1279
  for obsessive-compulsive disorder, 622
  pharmacological actions of, 1135–1136
  precautions with, 1136
  withdrawal from, 982
Ventilation, in group psychotherapy, 938*t*
Ventral tegmental area, 98, 99*f*
Veraguth's fold, in depression, 554*f*
Verapamil, 1002*t,* 1034*t*. *See also* Calcium channel inhibitors
  dosage and administration, 1035
  and lithium, 1072*t*
  structure of, 1034*f*
Verbal fluency test, 191*t*
Verbigeration, definition of, 283
Veronal. *See* Barbital
Versed. *See* Midazolam
Vertigo, in elderly, 1327
Vesprin. *See* Triflupromazine
Viagra. *See* Sildenafil
Vibration, 66–68
Vicissitudes of life and stress, 825–826
Vineland Adaptive Behavior Scales, 1157*t*
Violence, **904**. *See also* Intermittent explosive disorder
  in adolescence, 39–40
  β-adrenergic receptor antagonists for, 1009–1010
  and alcohol, 151
  assessing, 905*t*
  control of, 155–156
  differential diagnosis of, 157*t*
  domestic, 151. *See also* Battered wives; Child abuse and neglect
  DSM-IV disorders associated with, 150, 151*t*
  and epilepsy, 359
  high-risk clinical situations, 1354–1355
  incidence of, 155
  mechanisms of, 155, 156*f*
  pharmacotherapy for, 906, **1055**
  predicting, 150–151, 151*t*–152*t,* 905*t*
  prevention of, 155–156
  and previous abuse, 151
  psychopharmacological interventions for, 156, 157*t*
  in schizophrenia, 493–494
  televised, 32, 153, 153*t*
  victims of, 156, 157*t*
Virilizing adrenal hyperplasia, 693*t*
Viscosity, of personality, in epilepsy, 358–359
Vision, medical assessment of, 256
Visitation rights, of patients, 1358
Visken. *See* Pindolol
Vistaril. *See* Hydroxyzine
Visual discrimination, complex, assessment of, 189
Visual evoked potentials, 122
Visual hallucinations, with schizophrenia with childhood onset, 1283
Visual system, **68–71,** 73
  activity-dependent mechanisms in, 68
  association areas in, 69–70, 70*f*
  cell specialization in, 69
  center-surround response in, 69
  cortical columns in, 69
  development of, 73
  disorders in, 70–71
  feature extraction in, 68–69
  genetic mechanisms in, 68
  memory and, 69
  nature and nurture in, 68–69
  optical illusions, 71*f*
  paradigms for, 68–69
Visuoconstructive capacity, assessment of, 187
Visuoperceptive capacity, assessment of, 187
Visuospatial ability, assessment of, in mental status examination, 242
Visuospatial functioning, in elderly, 1319
Vitamin A, serum, testing for, 273*t*
Vitamin B_{12}
  deficiency, **1146**
    emergency manifestations of, 912*t*
    emergency treatment of, 912*t*
    medical considerations with, 847*t*
    psychiatric considerations with, 847*t*
  serum, testing for, 273*t*
Vitamin(s). *See also* Dietary supplements
  A, serum, testing for, 273*t*
  abuse, 395*t*
  B_{12}. *See* Vitamin B_{12}
  deficiencies, **1145–1146**
  megavitamin therapy for children, 1311
Vivactil. *See* Protriptyline
VMA, 263
VNS, **1145**
Vocalization innervation, evolution of, 72*f*
Vocational rehabilitation, 896
Vocational training, **966–967**
  for schizophrenics, 502
Volatile nitrate use
  emergency manifestations of, 912*t*
  emergency treatment of, 912*t*
Volatile solvent(s), intoxication, acute, diagnostic criteria for, 392*t*
Volubility, definition of, 284
Vomeronasal organ, 71
von Frisch, Karl, 159

von Meduna, Ladislas J., 1138
Von Munchausen, Baron, 668, 669*f*
Voodoo, 59
Voyeurism. *See also* Paraphilias
  clinical features of, 722
  diagnosis of, 722, 723*t*
  diagnostic criteria for, 722, 723*t*
  ICD-10 diagnostic criteria for, 726*t*

W

WAIS, **179–180**, 179*f*
WAIS-R, 85, 1157*t*
Warfarin
  with chloral hydrate, 1041
  drug interactions, 1063, 1119, 1123
  and ethchlorvynol, 1021
  and glutethimide, 1022
Watson, John B., 144, 610
Watts, Alan, 867
Watts, James, 1148
Waxy flexibility, definition of, 281
WBC. *See* White blood cell count (WBC)
WCST, 191*t*
Wechsler, David, 179
Wechsler Adult Intelligence Scale (WAIS), **179–180,** 179*f*
Wechsler Adult Intelligence Scale-Revised (WAIS-R), 85, 1157*t*
  in geriatric psychiatry, 1319
Wechsler Individual Achievement Test (WIAT), 1157*t*
Wechsler Intelligence Scale for Children, 3rd edition (WISC-III), 179, 1157*t,* 1159
Wechsler Memory Scale-Revised (WMS-R), 186
Wechsler Preschool and Primary Scale of Intelligence (WPPSI), 179, 1157*t*
Weight gain, 751
  and psychotherapeutic drugs, **982**
  stress and, 256
Weight loss
  in depression, 256
  hypnosis for, 843
Weiss, Brian, and integrative psychiatry, 866
Wellbutrin. *See* Bupropion
Well-old, 50
Wernicke, Karl, 147
Wernicke-Korsakoff syndrome, 406
Wernicke's aphasia, 79*t,* 82
Wernicke's area, 113
Wernicke's encephalopathy, 406, 1146
  emergency manifestations of, 908*t*
  emergency treatment of, 908*t*
Wertheimer, Max, 225
White, Dan, 1363
White blood cell count (WBC), 273*t*
  with antipsychotic drug therapy, 266*t*
White matter. *See also* Cerebral cortex
WIAT, 1157*t*
Wide-Range Achievement Test-Revised (WRAT-R), 1157*t,* 1159
Wife abuse, **890**
  physician reference card, 891*t*
Will development, 226
Williams syndrome, 1171*t*
Will therapy, 226
Wilson's disease, 75, 1168*t,* 1249*t*
  medical considerations with, 847*t*
  psychiatric considerations with, 847*t*
Winnicott, Donald W., 28, 141, 205, **228,** 795–796
Winokur, George, 484
WISC-III, 179, 1157t, 1159
WISC-III Symbol Search, 191*t*
Wisconsin Card Scoring Test (WCST), 191*t*
Wisconsin Card Sorting Test, **186,** 1158*t*
Wish fulfillment, 197, 199
Withdrawal, substance. *See* Substance withdrawal
Withdrawal state, 393*t*
Witzelsucht, 83, 1319
WMS-R, 186
Wolff, Harold, 822
Wolf-Man, 653
Wolman's disease, 1167*t*
Wolpe, Joseph, 148
  and progressive muscular relaxation, 949
  and systematic desensitization, 951
Women. *See also specific concern or disorder*
  career problems of, 895–896
  climacterium, 47
  economic status of, 43
  elderly, socioeconomic status of, 57
  in middle adulthood, 46, 48
  rape of, **890–892**
  sexual functioning, in midlife, 47
  sexual harassment, 881, **893,** 893*t*
  unemployment, in early adulthood, 43
  work, in early adulthood, 43
Woodcock-Johnson Psycho-Educational Battery, 1157*t*
Woodcock-Johnson Psycho-Educational Battery-Revised, 1182
Word-association technique, 185
Word deafness, 71
Word production, assessment of, 257
Word salad, 82, 239
  definition of, 283
Workmen's compensation, 1363
Workplace
  circadian rhythm sleep disorder, shift work type, **772**
  sexual harassment, 881, **893**
    educational material to reduce, 893*t*
  stress and, **895**
  women, in early adulthood, 43
Worried well, 376
WPPSI, 179, 1157*t*
WRAT-R, 1157*t,* 1159
Writing skills, assessment of, in mental status examination, 242
Written expression disorder, **1185–1188**
  clinical features, 1186–1187
  comorbidity with, 1186
  definition of, 1185–1186
  diagnosis of, 1186
  differential diagnosis of, 1187
  epidemiology of, 1186
  etiology of, 1186
  laboratory examination of, 1187
  and mathematics disorder, 1184
  pathology of, 1187
  treatment of, 1188
Wyatt v. Stickney, 1357
Wynne, Lyman, 484

X

Xanax. *See* Alprazolam
Xanthines, and lithium, 1072*t*
Xenical. *See* Oralstat
Xenophobia, definition of, 284
X-linked disorders, 23
X-linked recessive transmission, 125
X-rays, 23
XTC. *See* Methylenedioxyamphetamine
XXY and 9p mosaicism, 1249*t*
XY genotype, enzymatic defects in, 693*t*
XYY genetic disorder, 154–155, 1249*t*

Y

Yale-Brown Obsessive Compulsive Scale (YBOCS), 181, 302*t*
Yocon. *See* Yohimbine
Yoga, **866**
Yohimbine, 715, 1002*t,* **1137–1138**
  adverse effects of, 1137
  chemistry of, 1137, 1137*f*
  dosage and administration, 1138
  drug interactions, 1007, 1138
  effects on specific organs and systems, 1137
  indications for, 1137
  mechanism of action, 1137
  pharmacological actions of, 1137
  precautions with, 1137
  for sexual dysfunction, 981
Yopo, 436*t*
Young-old, 50

Z

Zaleplon, 1002*t,* **1028**
  adverse reactions to, 1027
  dosage of, 1025*t*
  drug interactions, 1028
  half-life of, 1025*t*
  indications for, 1024–1025
  molecular structure of, 1024*f*
  pharmacological actions for, 1023–1024
  precautions with, 1027, 1028
  for primary insomnia, 765
Zar, 531*t*
Zeitgebers, 539
Zeldox. *See* Ziprasidone
Zen Buddhism, and integrative psychiatry, 867
Zidovudine, 376, 377
Ziprasidone, 498
  adverse effects of, 498
  for autistic disorder, 1215
  for early-onset schizophrenia, 1285
  indications for, 498
  for schizophrenia, 498
  and weight gain, 752
Zoloft. *See* Sertraline
Zolpidem, 1002*t,* **1028**
  adverse reactions to, 1027
  dosage of, 1025*t*
  drug interactions, 378, 1028
  geriatric dosage, 1332*t*
  half-life of, 1025*t*
  indications for, 1024–1025
  pharmacological actions for, 1023–1024
  precautions with, 1027, 1028
  for primary insomnia, 765
Zoophilia, 724. *See also* Paraphilias
Zoophobia, definition of, 284
Z-score, 177
Zung Self-Rating Depression Scale, 555
Zyban. *See* Bupropion
Zyprexa. *See* Olanzapine